CONTENTS

MEDICAL-SURGICAL NURSING

Patient-Centered Collaborative Care

MEDICAL-SURGICAL NURSING

Patient-Centered Collaborative Care

EIGHTH EDITION

Donna D. Ignatavicius, MS, RN, ANEF
Speaker and Curriculum Consultant for Academic Nursing Programs
Founder, Boot Camp for Nurse Educators®
President, DI Associates, Inc.
Placitas, New Mexico

M. Linda Workman, PhD, RN, FAAN
Senior Volunteer Faculty
College of Nursing
University of Cincinnati
Cincinnati, Ohio;
Formerly Gertrude Perkins Oliva Professor of Oncology
Frances Payne Bolton School of Nursing
Case Western Reserve University
Cleveland, Ohio

Section Editors:

Meg Blair, PhD, MSN, RN, CEN
Professor
Nebraska Methodist College
Omaha, Nebraska

Cherie Rebar, PhD, MBA, RN, FNP, COI
Director, Division of Nursing
Chair, Prelicensure Nursing Programs
Kettering College
Kettering, Ohio

Chris Winkelman, RN, PhD, CCRN, ACNP, CNE, FCCM, FANP
Associate Professor
Frances Payne Bolton School of Nursing
Case Western Reserve University
Cleveland, Ohio

ELSEVIER

ELSEVIER

3251 Riverport Lane
St. Louis, Missouri 63043

MEDICAL-SURGICAL NURSING:
PATIENT-CENTERED COLLABORATIVE CARE,
EIGHTH EDITION

ISBN (single volume): 978-1-4557-7255-1
ISBN (2-volume set): 978-1-4557-7258-2

This book and the individual contributions contained in it are protected under copyright by the Publisher (other than as may be noted herein).

Notices

Knowledge and best practice in this field are constantly changing. As new research and experience broaden our understanding, changes in research methods, professional practices, or medical treatment may become necessary.

Practitioners and researchers must always rely on their own experience and knowledge in evaluating and using any information, methods, compounds, or experiments described herein. In using such information or methods they should be mindful of their own safety and the safety of others, including parties for whom they have a professional responsibility.

With respect to any drug or pharmaceutical products identified, readers are advised to check the most current information provided (i) on procedures featured or (ii) by the manufacturer of each product to be administered, to verify the recommended dose or formula, the method and duration of administration, and contraindications. It is the responsibility of practitioners, relying on their own experience and knowledge of their patients, to make diagnoses, to determine dosages and the best treatment for each individual patient, and to take all appropriate safety precautions.

To the fullest extent of the law, neither the Publisher nor the authors, contributors, or editors, assume any liability for any injury and/or damage to persons or property as a matter of products liability, negligence or otherwise, or from any use or operation of any methods, products, instructions, or ideas contained in the material herein.

Previous editions copyrighted 2013, 2010, 2006, 2002, 1999, 1995, 1991

International Standard Book Number (single volume): 978-1-4557-7255-1
International Standard Book Number (2-volume set): 978-1-4557-7258-2

Executive Content Strategist: Lee Henderson
Traditional Content Development Manager: Billie C. Sharp
Senior Content Development Specialist: Rae L. Robertson
Publishing Services Manager: Deborah L. Vogel
Senior Project Manager: Jodi M. Willard
Design Direction: Margaret Reid

Printed in Canada

Last digit is the print number: 9 8 7 6 5 4 3 2 1

CONSULTANTS AND CONTRIBUTORS

CONSULTANTS

Richard Lintner, RT(R), (CV), (CT), (MR)
Clinical Instructor
Interventional Radiology
Kansas University Hospital
Kansas City, Kansas

Deanne Blach, MSN, RN
President, Nursing Education
DB Productions of NW AR, Inc.
Green Forest, Arkansas

Stephanie Ignatavicius, MA
Phoenix, Arizona

CONTRIBUTORS

Katherine L. Byar, MSN, APN, BC
Hematological Nurse Practitioner
Department of Internal Medicine/Oncology-Hematology
University of Nebraska Medical Center
Omaha, Nebraska

Lara L. Carver, PhD, RN, CNE
Associate Professor
Department of Nursing
National University
Las Vegas, Nevada

Robin Chard, PhD, RN, CNOR
Associate Professor
College of Nursing
Nova Southeastern University
Fort Lauderdale, Florida

Tammy Coffee, MSN, RN, ACNP
Preceptor
Department of Nursing
Case Western Reserve University;
Nurse Practitioner
Department of Surgery
MetroHealth Medical Center
Cleveland, Ohio

Janice Zeigler Cuzzell, RN, MA, CWS
Senior Rheumatology Clinical Coordinator
Immunology and Ophthalmology
Genentech, Inc.
San Francisco, California

Barbara J. Daly, PhD, RN, FAAN
Professor
School of Nursing
Case Western Reserve University;
Director
Clinical Ethics
University Hospitals Case Medical Center
Cleveland, Ohio

Laura M. Dechant, APN, MSN, CCRN, CCNS
Clinical Nurse Specialist
Heart, Vascular, and Interventional Services
Christiana Care Health System
Newark, Delaware

Cheryl Dumont, PhD, RN, CRNI
Director, Nursing Research and Vascular Access Team
Nursing Administration
Winchester Medical Center
Winchester, Virginia

June Eilers, PhD, APRN-CNS, BC
Research Associate Professor
College of Nursing
University of Nebraska
Omaha, Nebraska

Rachel L. Gallagher, MS, ANP-BC
Staff Officer
Physical Disability Board of Review
Diversified Technical Services, Inc.
El Paso, Texas

Nicole M. Heimgartner, RN, MSN
Assistant Professor
Division of Nursing
Kettering College
Kettering, Ohio

Stephanie Ignatavicius, MA
Phoenix, Arizona

Mary F. Justice, MSN, RN, CNE
Associate Professor
Department of Nursing
University of Cincinnati Blue Ash College
Cincinnati, Ohio

Mary Kazanowski, PhD, APRN, ACHPN
Palliative and Hospice Nurse Practitioner
VNA Hospice of Manchester and Southern New Hampshire
Manchester, New Hampshire;
Palliative Care Nurse Practitioner
Palliative Care Team
Concord Hospital
Concord, New Hampshire

Linda A. LaCharity, PhD, RN
Assistant Professor (Retired)
Adult Health
University of Cincinnati
Cincinnati, Ohio

Linda Laskowski-Jones, MS, RN, ACNS-BC, CEN, FAWM
Vice President
Emergency & Trauma Services
Christiana Care Health System
Wilmington, Delaware

Rona F. Levin, PhD, RN
Clinical Professor and Director, Doctor of Nursing Practice Program
College of Nursing
New York University;
Visiting Faculty
Quality Management Services
Visiting Nurse Service of New York
New York, New York;
Professor Emeritus
Felician College
Lodi, New Jersey

Margaret Elaine McLeod, MSN, APN, BC-ADM, ACNS-BC, CDE
Clinical Nurse Specialist
Department of Nursing
Tennessee Valley Health Care System
Nashville, Tennessee

Chris Pasero, MS, RN-BC, FAAN
Pain Management Educator and Clinical Consultant
El Dorado Hills, California

Jennifer Powers, MSN, FNP-BC
Clinical Assistant Professor
School of Health and Human Services
National University
San Diego, California;
Family Nurse Practitioner
Health Care Partners
Las Vegas, Nevada

Cherie Rebar, PhD, MBA, RN, FNP, COI
Director, Division of Nursing;
Chair, Prelicensure Nursing Programs
Division of Nursing
Kettering College
Kettering, Ohio

Harry C. Rees, III, MSN, ACNP-BC
Acute Care Nurse Practitioner
Cleveland Clinic Health System;
Metro Life Flight
MetroHealth Medical Center
Cleveland, Ohio

James G. Sampson, DNP, NP-C
Adjunct Assistant Professor
College of Nursing
University of Colorado
Aurora, Colorado;
Clinical Supervisor, Adult Nurse Practitioner
Department of Internal Medicine
Denver Health Medical Center
Denver, Colorado

Karen Toulson, RN, MSN, MBA, CEN, NE-BC
Nurse Manager
Emergency Department, Christiana Hospital
Christiana Care Health Services
Newark, Delaware

Shirley E. Van Zandt, MS, MPH, CRNP
Assistant Professor
School of Nursing
Boise State University
Boise, Idaho

Laura M. Willis, MSN, RN
Assistant Professor, Service Learning Coordinator
Department of Nursing, Service Learning
Kettering College
Kettering, Ohio

Chris Winkelman, RN, PhD, CCRN, ACNP, CNE, FCCM, FANP
Associate Professor
Frances Payne Bolton School of Nursing
Case Western Reserve University;
Clinical Nurse
Trauma/Critical Care
MetroHealth Medical Center
Cleveland, Ohio

Fay Wright, MS, RN, APRN-BC
Doctoral Student
The Florence S. Downs PhD Program in Nursing Research and Theory Development
New York University College of Nursing
New York, New York

CONTRIBUTORS TO TEACHING/LEARNING RESOURCES

PowerPoint® Slides

Nicole Heimgartner, RN, MSN, COI
Associate Professor of Nursing
Kettering College
Kettering, Ohio

Cherie Rebar, PhD, MBA, RN, FNP, COI
Director, Division of Nursing;
Chair, Prelicensure Nursing Programs
Division of Nursing
Kettering College
Kettering, Ohio

Laura M. Willis, MSN, APRN, FNP-C
Adjunct Professor
Kettering College
Kettering, Ohio;
Family Nurse Practitioner
The Little Clinic;
President, Connect RN2ED
Englewood, Ohio

TEACH® for Nurses Lesson Plans

Carolyn Gersch, PhDc, MSN, RN, CNE
Associate Director, Division of Nursing
Kettering College
Kettering, Ohio

Cherie Rebar, PhD, MBA, RN, FNP, COI
Director, Division of Nursing;
Chair, Prelicensure Nursing Programs
Division of Nursing
Kettering College
Kettering, Ohio

Test Bank

Meg Blair, PhD, MSN, RN, CEN
Professor
Nursing Division
Nebraska Methodist College
Omaha, Nebraska

Linda Hughes, PhD, RN, BSN, MS
Dean of Nursing
Nebraska Methodist College
Omaha, Nebraska

Tami Kathleen Little, RN, DNP, CNE
Dean of Nursing
Brookline College
Albuquerque, New Mexico

Case Studies

Candice Kumagai, RN, MSN
Formerly Clinical Instructor
University of Texas at Austin
Austin, Texas

Linda A. LaCharity, PhD, RN, MN, BSN
Adjunct Faculty
Formerly Accelerated Program Director and Assistant Professor
College of Nursing
University of Cincinnati
Cincinnati, Ohio

Concept Maps

Deanne A. Blach, MSN, RN
President, Nursing Education
DB Productions of NW AR, Inc.
Green Forest, Arkansas

Review Questions for the NCLEX® Examination

Lisa A. Hollett, RN, BSN, MA, MICN, Certified Forensic Nurse
Stroke Coordinator
Hillcrest Medical Center
Tulsa, Oklahoma

Mary Beth Flynn Makic, PhD, RN, CNS, CCNS, FAAN
Research Nurse Scientist
University of Colorado Hospital;
Critical Care and Associate Professor
College of Nursing
University of Colorado
Aurora, Colorado

Andrea R. Mann, MSN, RN, CNE
Interim Dean, Third Level Chair
Aria Health School of Nursing
Trevose, Pennsylvania

Denise Robinson, RN, MS, CNE
Assistant Professor of Nursing
Monroe County Community College
Monroe, Michigan

Kathryn Schartz, RN, MSN, PPCPNP-BC
Assistant Professor of Nursing
School of Nursing
Baker University
Topeka, Kansas

Mitch Seal, RN, EdD, Med-IT, BSN
Director of Strategic Planning & Partnerships
Medical Education and Training Campus Joint Base
San Antonio, Texas

Peggy Slota, DNP, RN, FAAN
Associate Professor of Nursing
Carlow University
Pittsburgh, Pennsylvania

REVIEWERS

CONTENT REVIEW PANEL

Diane K. Daddario, MSN, ACNS-BC, RN, BC, CMSRN
Adjunct Faculty, School of Nursing
Pennsylvania State University
University Park, Pennsylvania

Denise A. Foster, MSN, RN, CNE
Associate Professor
Sentara College of Health Sciences
Chesapeake, Virginia

Bradley Harrell, DNP, APRN, ACNP-BC, CCRN
Chair and Associate Professor
Germantown Undergraduate Nursing
Union University School of Nursing
Jackson, Tennessee

LaWanda Herron, PhD, MSA, MSN, FNP-BC
Director of Nursing
Holmes Community College
Grenada, Mississippi

Jamie Lynn Jones, MSN, RN, CNE
Assistant Professor
University of Arkansas at Little Rock
Little Rock, Arkansas

Tamara Kear, PhD, RN, CNS, CNN
Assistant Professor of Nursing
College of Nursing
Villanova University
Villanova, Pennsylvania

Melissa S. McNulty, PhD, ARNP
Professor
Pasco-Hernando State College
Wesley Chapel, Florida

Jason Mott, PhD, RN
Instructor of Nursing
Bellin College
Green Bay, Wisconsin

CLINICAL CHAPTER REVIEWERS

Sameeya N. Ahmed-Winston, RN, MSN, CPNP, CPHON
Pediatric Nurse Practitioner
Children's National Medical Center
Washington, D.C.

Margaret-Ann Carno, PhD, RN, MBA, CPNP, FAAN
Associate Professor of Clinical Nursing and Pediatrics
University of Rochester, School of Nursing
Rochester, New York

Laura M. Dechant, APN, MSN, CCRN, CCNS
Clinical Nursing Specialist
Christiana Care Health System
Newark, Delaware

Kathleen Sanders Jordan, DNP, MS, RN, FNP-BC, ENP-BC, SANE-P
Clinical Assistant Professor
School of Nursing
University of North Carolina Charlotte;
Nurse Practitioner
Mid-Atlantic Emergency Medicine Association
Charlotte, North Carolina

Kari Jean Ksar, RN, MS, CPNP
Pediatric Nurse Practitioner
Pediatric Gastroenterology, Hepatology, and Nutrition
Lucile Packard Children's Hospital at Stanford
Palo Alto, California

Martha E. Langhorne, MSN, RN, FNP, AOCN
Nurse Practitioner
Binghamton Gastroenterology
Binghamton, New York

Casey Norris, MSN, BSN, APRN, BC
Nursing Instructor
ITT Technical Institute
Madison, Alabama

Charles D. Rogers, MSN, RN
Assistant Professor of Nursing
Morehead State University
Morehead, Kentucky

Mark Stevens, MSN, RN, CNS, CEN, MICN
Professor of Nursing
National University
Fresno, California

Laura C. Williams, MSN, CNS, ONC, CCNS
Orthopedic Clinical Nurse Specialist
Orlando Regional Medical Center
Orlando, Florida

PREFACE

The first edition of this textbook, entitled *Medical-Surgical Nursing: A Nursing Process Approach,* was in many ways a groundbreaking work. The following six editions built on that achievement and further solidified the book's position as a major trendsetter for the practice of adult health nursing. Now in its eighth edition, "Iggy" charts an essential course for the future of adult nursing practice—a course reflected in its current title: *Medical-Surgical Nursing: Patient-Centered Collaborative Care.* The focus of this new edition continues to be to help students learn how to provide safe, quality care that is patient-centered, evidence-based, and collaborative. In addition to print formats as single- and two-volume texts, this edition is now available in a variety of electronic formats, including Pageburst on VST, Pageburst on Kno, and e-book formats for Kindle, Nook, and other e-readers.

The book's subtitle was carefully chosen to emphasize the nurse's role in providing care in collaboration with the patient, family, and members of the interdisciplinary team in both acute care and community-based settings. The Institute of Medicine (IOM), The Joint Commission, the Quality and Safety Education for Nurses (QSEN) Institute, and the 2010 IOM *Future of Nursing* report have called for all health professionals to coordinate and deliver evidence-based patient care as a collaborative care team.

KEY THEMES FOR THE 8TH EDITION

The key themes for this edition strengthen the book's focus on safety, quality care, and clinical judgment to best prepare the student for collaborative patient-centered practice in medical-surgical health settings. Each theme is outlined and described below.

- **New Focus on Concepts.** Enhanced compatibility with the concept-based nursing curriculum in pre-licensure programs and a conceptual approach to teaching and learning is the key feature that sets this edition apart. To help students connect previously-learned concepts with new information in the text, six Concept Overviews introduce groups of content units. These unique features review basic concepts learned in nursing fundamentals courses—such as oxygenation and protection—to help students make connections between foundational concepts and patient care for medical-surgical conditions. The Concept Overviews are now even more accessible with color sidebars to identify these pages. For continuity and reinforcement, a list of more specific Priority Nursing Concepts has been added at the beginning of each chapter. This placement is designed to help students better understand the role of the nurse when caring for patients with selected health problems. When these concepts are explicated in the body of each chapter, they are presented in small capital letters (e.g., OXYGENATION) to help students relate and apply essential concepts to provide more focused nursing care. Nursing Concepts and Clinical Judgment Reviews at the end of most chapters apply these same concepts to the health problems presented in the chapter.
- **Improved Focus on the Core Body of Knowledge and QSEN Competencies.** This edition not only continues to emphasize need-to-know content for the RN level of practice, but also includes an increased emphasis on Quality and Safety Education for Nurses (QSEN) Institute core competencies. Clinical practice settings emphasize the essential need for safe practices and quality improvement to provide collaborative patient-centered care that is evidence-based. Many hospitals and other health care agencies have formally adopted these QSEN competencies as core values and goals for patient care. To help prepare students for the work environment as new graduates, as well as to highlight the integration of safety and quality into all nursing actions, this edition incorporates an enhanced focus on these competencies.
- **Emphasis on Patient Safety.** Patient safety is emphasized throughout this edition, not only in the narrative but also in **Nursing Safety Priority boxes** that enable students to immediately identify the most important care needed for patients with specific health problems. These highlighted features are further classified as Action Alerts, Drug Alerts, or Critical Rescue. We also continue to include our leading-edge Best Practice for Patient Safety & Quality Care charts to emphasize the most important nursing care. Highlighted yellow text also demonstrates the application of The Joint Commission's National Patient Safety Goals initiative (http://www.jointcommission.org/standards_information/npsgs.aspx) and Core Measures content into every day nursing practice.
- **Focus on Patient-Centered Care.** Patient-centered care is enhanced in the eighth edition in several ways. The eighth edition continues to use the term "patient" instead of "client" throughout. Although the use of these terms remains a subject of discussion among nursing educators, we have not defined the patient as a dependent person. Rather, the patient can be an individual, a family, or a group—all of whom have rights that are respected in a mutually trusting nurse-patient relationship. Most health care agencies and professional organizations use "patient" in their practice and publications. In addition, most nursing organizations support the term.
- **New Focus on Gender Considerations.** To increase our emphasis on patient-centered care, we delineated **Gender Health Considerations** rather than restricting our emphasis on Women's Health Considerations as we did in previous editions. To further expand that focus on differences in patient values, preferences, and beliefs, we have added new, cutting-edge **Chapter 73, Care of Transgender Patients,** dedicated to transgender patient care. Along with other individuals in the lesbian, gay, bisexual, and questioning population, the health needs of transgender patients have gained national attention through their inclusion in *Healthy People 2020* and The Joint Commission's standards. This new chapter provides tools to help prepare students and faculty to care for transgender patients who are considering or who have undergone the gender transition process.
- **Emphasis on Evidence-Based Practice.** The updated **Chapter 5, Evidence-Based Practice in Medical-Surgical Nursing** (written by evidence-based practice (EBP) experts Dr. Rona F. Levin and Fay Wright), discusses the importance of *using best current evidence in nursing practice* and how to locate and use this evidence to improve patient care. This chapter, along with the **Evidence-Based Practice boxes** throughout the book, offers a solid foundation in this

essential aspect of nursing practice. Each box summarizes a useful research article and explains the implications of its findings for practice and further research, as well as a rating of the level of evidence based on a well-respected scale.

- **New Focus on Quality Improvement.** The QSEN Institute and clinical practice agencies require that all nurses have *quality improvement* knowledge and skills. To help prepare students for that role, this edition includes new and unique **Quality Improvement boxes.** Each box summarizes a quality improvement project published in the health care literature and the implications of the project's success in improving nursing care. The inclusion of these boxes, in addition to disseminating information and research, helps students understand that quality improvement has its underpinnings in practice change at the "grass roots" level. It also emphasizes the role of the bedside nurse in identifying potential solutions to practice problems.
- **Refocused Emphasis on Clinical Judgment.** Stressing the importance of clinical judgment skills, including an enhanced emphasis on prioritization and delegation, helps to best prepare students for practice and the NCLEX® Examination. As in the seventh edition, the eighth edition emphasizes the importance of nursing judgment to make timely and appropriate clinical decisions and prioritize care. To help achieve that focus, all-new case based **Clinical Judgment Challenges** (formerly called "Decision-Making Challenges"), based primarily on the QSEN core competencies, have been integrated throughout the text. Selected Clinical Judgment Challenges highlight ethical dilemmas and delegation and supervision issues. These exercises provide clinical situations in which students can use on-the-spot nursing judgment to help prepare them for the fast-paced world of medical-surgical nursing and become competent nurses. Suggested answer guidelines for these Clinical Judgment Challenges are provided on the book's Evolve website (http://evolve.elsevier.com/Iggy/). In addition, Dr. Christine Tanner's clinical judgment framework (Tanner, 2006) is used to help students apply selected concepts in the **Nursing Concepts and Clinical Judgment Reviews** at the end of most chapters. The components of this model include that clinical nurses use nursing judgment to provide safe, quality care by:
  - Noticing
  - Interpreting
  - Responding
  - Reflecting
- **Emphasis on Preparation for the NCLEX® Examination.** An enhanced emphasis on the NCLEX Examination and consistency with the 2013 NCLEX-RN® test plan has been refined in this edition. Like the seventh edition, the eighth edition also emphasizes "readiness"—readiness for the NCLEX® Examination, readiness for major emergencies such as those we see with all-too-frequent mass casualty events, readiness for safe drug administration, and readiness for the new and continually unfolding world of genetics and genomics. An increased number of new **NCLEX® Examination Challenges** are interspersed throughout the text to allow students the opportunity for practice in test-taking and decision-making. Answers to these Challenges are provided in the back of the book, and their rationales are provided on the Evolve website (http://evolve.elsevier.com/Iggy). As the NCLEX® Examination becomes more challenging, it is more critical than ever that students be ready to pass the licensure exam on the first try. To help both students and faculty achieve that outcome, chapter-opening **Learning Outcomes** are now more consistent with the competencies outlined in the detailed 2013 NCLEX-RN Test Plan. The eighth edition also continues to include an innovative end-of-chapter feature called **Get Ready for the NCLEX® Examination!** This unique and effective learning aid consists of a list of **Key Points** *organized by Client Needs Category* as found in the NCLEX-RN® Test Plan. Relevant QSEN competency categories are identified for selected Key Points.
- **Expanded Content on Community-Based Care.** Expanded coverage on this important nursing area, including long-term care, is included in this edition. A recent editorial article in the journal *Medical-Surgical Nursing* stated that the future of medical-surgical nurses will change to an increased role in care coordination and transition management between acute care and community-based care (Lattavo, 2014). To help students prepare for this new role, the eighth edition of our text expands coverage of community-based care, including essential collaborative management that is needed in home, long-term, rehabilitation, and ambulatory settings.
- **Collaborative Problems and NANDA-I Nursing Diagnoses.** This edition also features an improved delineation of **NANDA-I nursing diagnoses and collaborative patient problems.** As health care becomes increasingly more collaborative, nurses need to be able to communicate with other members of the health care team, including the patient and family. To help students learn how to facilitate that communication, the eighth edition identifies patient problems and specifies which actual and potential problems are NANDA-I nursing diagnoses and which are collaborative health problems.

CLINICAL CURRENCY AND ACCURACY

To ensure the book's currency and accuracy, we listened to students and faculty who have used the previous editions, focusing on their impressions of and experiences with the book. We reviewed documents crafted by a variety of health care organizations, including the Institute of Medicine (IOM), The Joint Commission (TJC), and the Institute for Healthcare Improvement (IHI). Recent nursing education publications were also examined, such as those authored by the National League for Nursing (NLN), the American Association of Colleges of Nursing (AACN), and Dr. Patricia Benner and her colleagues in their book *Educating Nurses: A Call for Radical Transformation* (2010). A thorough nursing education literature search of best current evidence helped us validate best practices and national health care trends to help shape the focus of the eighth edition.

We also commissioned in-depth reviews of every chapter by a dedicated panel of instructors and clinicians across the United States, and we used their reviews to guide us in revising the chapters into their final form. A well-respected interventional radiologist ensured the accuracy of selected diagnostic testing procedures and associated patient care.

The results of these efforts are reflected in the eighth edition's:

- Strong, consistent focus on NCLEX-RN® Examination preparation, clinical judgment, patient-centered collaborative care, pathophysiology, drug therapy, evidence-based clinical practice, and community-based care

- Foundation of relevant research and best practice guidelines
- Emphasis on the critical "need to know" information that beginning nurses must master to provide safe patient care

With today's knowledge explosion, it is easy for a book to become larger with each new edition. However, today's nursing students have a limited time to absorb and begin to apply the information essential for medical-surgical nursing care. Therefore in this eighth edition we eliminated some of the content found in previous foundation courses or other specialty textbooks. We limited our discussions to how this content is *used* in adult nursing and focused on content that was "need to know" for safe, patient-centered, quality nursing practice.

OUTSTANDING READABILITY

Today's students need to be able to read information once and understand it; they do not have time to repeatedly read the same information. To achieve this level of readability, the text employs a direct-address style (wherever appropriate) that speaks directly to the reader, and sentences are as short as possible without sacrificing essential content. In addition, we ensured that this new edition has improved consistency of difficulty level from chapter to chapter.

Reading level is highly influenced by the length of sentences and the length of words. Although we can control the length of the sentences, medical terms are often 4 to 5 syllables long and tend to skew a chapter's reading level. Nevertheless, the result of our efforts is a med-surg text of consistently outstanding readability. The average reading level is 10th to 11th grade. It is important to note that reducing the reading level of this edition did not reduce the quality or depth of content that students need to know. Instead, the content is clear, focused, and accessible.

EASE OF ACCESS

To make the text as easy to use as possible, we have maintained the previous editions' approach of smaller chapters of more uniform length. Consistent with our focus on the "need to know," we eliminated some of the less foundational content in the first unit of the last edition and added one new chapter. The more focused eighth edition contains 74 chapters.

The overall presentation of the eighth edition has been updated, including more recent and high-quality photographs for realism, and design change features to improve content access. The design of the eighth edition includes better placement of display elements (e.g., figures, tables, boxes, and charts) for a chapter flow that enhances text reading without splintering content or confusing the reader. Additional ease-of-access features for this edition include tabbed markings for the glossary, index, illustration credits, and bibliography for quick reference. To increase the smoothness of flow and reader concentration, side-turned tables and charts have been reduced throughout the text, as have tables and charts covering multiple pages. Tables and charts now feature an alternating pattern of light and dark shading to ensure essential content for a specific topic or characteristic is not confused with another topic or characteristic.

We also have maintained the unit structure of previous editions, with vital body systems (cardiovascular, respiratory, and neurologic) appearing earlier in the book. In these three units we continue to provide complex care content in separate chapters that discuss managing critically ill patients with coronary artery disease, respiratory health problems, and neurologic health problems.

To help break up long blocks of text and also to highlight key information, we continue to include streamlined yet eye-catching headings, bulleted lists, tables, charts, and in-text highlights. Key Terms are in boldface color type and are defined in the text to foster the learning of need-to-know vocabulary. A glossary is located in the back of the book. Chapter bibliographies have been moved to the back of the book to save space in chapters for need-to-know content. These current bibliographic resources include research articles, nationally accepted clinical guidelines, and other sources of evidence when available for each chapter. Classic sources from before 2011 are noted with an asterisk (*).

A PATIENT-CENTERED COLLABORATIVE CARE APPROACH

As in all previous editions, we take a collaborative care approach to patient care. We believe that in the real world of health care, nurses, patients, and other health care providers (including physicians, advanced-practice nurses, and physician's assistants) *share* responsibility for the management of patient problems. Thus we present patient care in a collaborative care framework. In this framework we make no *artificial* distinctions between medical treatment and nursing care. Instead, under each Patient-Centered Collaborative Care heading we discuss how the nurse coordinates care and interacts with members of the health care team as appropriate for the patient's health problems, including health promotion and illness prevention.

This edition includes newly redesigned patient-centered Concept Maps that underscore this collaborative care approach. Each Concept Map contains a case scenario. It then shows how a selected complex health problem is addressed. Each Concept Map spells out the steps of the nursing process and related concepts to illustrate the relationships among disease processes, priority patient problems, collaborative management, and more.

Although our approach is collaborative, the text is first and foremost a *nursing* text. We therefore use a nursing process approach as a tool to organize discussions of patient health problems and their management. Discussions of *major* health problems follow a full nursing process format using this structure:

[Health problem]
Pathophysiology
- Etiology (and Genetic Risk when appropriate)
- Incidence and Prevalence

Health Promotion and Maintenance (when appropriate)
Patient-Centered Collaborative Care
- Assessment
- Analysis
- Planning and Implementation
  - [Collaborative Intervention Statement (based on priority patient problems)]
  - Planning: Expected Outcomes
  - Interventions
- Community-Based Care
  - Home Care Management
  - Self-Management Education
  - Health Care Resources
- Evaluation: Outcomes

The Analysis sections list the priority patient problems (collaborative problems and nursing diagnoses) associated with major health problems and disorders. This eighth edition uses official NANDA-I nursing diagnosis language where it applies; however, most health care agencies prefer to identify collaborative patient problems or needs as the basis for the interdisciplinary plan of care rather than being restricted to NANDA-I language, which addresses primarily nursing-oriented patient problems. With its more flexible interweaving of NANDA-I diagnoses and collaborative patient problems or needs, the eighth edition more closely aligns with the language of clinical practice. The nursing diagnoses used in this edition are the 2012-2014 NANDA-I diagnoses—the most recently approved diagnoses at the time of publication of this edition. Health Promotion and Maintenance sections are found in selected discussions.

Discussions of less common or less complex disorders, although not given this complete subhead structure, nonetheless follow the same basic format: a discussion of the problem itself (including pertinent information on pathophysiology) followed by a section on patient-centered collaborative care of patients with the disorder. To demonstrate our commitment to providing the content foundational to nursing education and consistent with the recommendations of Benner and colleagues through the Carnegie Foundation for the Future of Nursing Education, we highlight throughout this edition essential pathophysiologic concepts that are key to understanding the basis for collaborative management.

Integral to this collaborative care approach is a clear delineation of just who is responsible for what. When a responsibility is primarily the nurse's, the text says so. When a decision must be made jointly by the patient, nurse, physician, and physical therapist, for example, this is clearly stated. When different health care practitioners in different care settings might be involved in the patient's care, this is stated.

ORGANIZATION

The 74 chapters of *Medical-Surgical Nursing: Patient-Centered Collaborative Care* are grouped into 16 units. Unit 1, Foundations for Medical-Surgical Nursing, lays the foundation for the health care concepts incorporated throughout the text. Unit 2 consists of three chapters on concepts of emergency and trauma care and disaster preparedness.

Unit 3 consists of three chapters on the management of patients with fluid, electrolyte, and acid-base imbalances. Chapters 11 and 12 review key assessments and related patient care in a clear, concise discussion. The chapter on infusion therapy (Chapter 13) is supplemented with an online Fluids & Electrolytes Tutorial on the companion Evolve website.

Unit 4 presents the perioperative nursing content that medical-surgical nurses need to know. This content provides a solid foundation to help the student better understand the collaborative care required for the surgical patient regardless of surgical setting. Even more emphasis is placed on continuous assessment during the perioperative period to prevent complications and improve outcomes in this era of increased ambulatory care.

Unit 5 provides core content on health problems related to immune system function. This content includes normal inflammation and the immune response, altered cell growth and cancer development, and interventions for patients with connective tissue disease, HIV infection, and other immunologic disorders, cancers, and infections.

The remaining 11 units, subdivided and introduced by the six Concept Overviews, cover medical-surgical content by body system. Each of these units begins with an Assessment chapter and continues with one or more Nursing Care chapters for patients with selected health problems in that body system. This framework is familiar to students who learn the body systems in preclinical foundational science courses such as anatomy and physiology.

MULTINATIONAL, MULTICULTURAL, MULTIGENERATIONAL FOCUS

To reflect the increasing diversity of our society, *Medical-Surgical Nursing: Patient-Centered Collaborative Care* takes a multinational, multicultural, and multigenerational focus. Addressing the needs of both U.S. and Canadian readers, we have included examples of trade names of drugs available in the United States and in Canada. Drugs that are available only in Canada are designated with a 🍁 symbol. When appropriate, we identify specific Canadian health care resources, including their websites. In many areas, Canadian health statistics are combined with those of the United States for provide an accurate "North American" picture.

To help nurses provide quality care for patients whose preferences, beliefs, and values may differ from their own, numerous **Cultural Considerations** and **Gender Health Considerations boxes** highlight important aspects of culturally competent care throughout the text. In addition, a new chapter (Chapter 73) is dedicated to the special health care needs of transgender patients.

Increases in life expectancy and the "graying" of the baby-boom generation add up to a steadily increasing older adult population. To help equip nurses for this challenge, the eighth edition continues to provide thorough coverage of the care of older adults. Chapter 2 offers content on the role of the nurse and health care team in promoting health for older adults in the community. It also provides coverage of common health problems that older adults may have in the health care setting, such as falls and inadequate nutrition. The text includes many **Nursing Focus on the Older Adult charts.** Laboratory values and drug dosages typical for older patients are also included throughout the book. Charts specifying normal physiologic changes to expect in the older population are found in each Assessment chapter. In addition, **Considerations for Older Adults boxes** are included throughout the text to emphasize key points to consider when caring for these patients.

ADDITIONAL LEARNING AIDS

As in previous editions, the eighth edition continues to include a rich array of learning aids geared toward adult learners to help students quickly identify and understand key information and to serve as study aids.

- Written in "patient-friendly" language, **Patient and Family Education: Preparing for Self-Management charts** provide the types of instructions that nurses must learn to provide to patients and their families to help them cope with life changes caused by illness.
- **Laboratory Profile charts** summarize important information on laboratory tests commonly used to evaluate

health problems. Information typically includes normal ranges of laboratory values (including differences for older adults, when appropriate) and the possible significance of abnormal findings.

- **Common Examples of Drug Therapy charts** summarize important information about commonly used drugs. Most charts include both U.S. and Canadian trade names for typically used drugs, usual dosages (including dosages for older patients, as appropriate), and nursing interventions with rationales.
- **Key Features charts** highlight the clinical manifestations of important health problems based on pathophysiologic concepts.
- **Evidence-Based Practice boxes**, provided in many chapters, give synopses of recent nursing research articles and other scientific articles applicable to nursing. Each box provides a brief summary of the research, its level of evidence (LOE), and a brief commentary with implications for nursing practice and future research. The purpose of this feature is to help students identify the strengths and weaknesses of the research and to see how research guides nursing practice.
- New to this edition, **Quality Improvement boxes** offer anecdotes of recent nursing articles that focus on this important QSEN competency. These features, similar to the Evidence-Based Practice boxes, provide a brief summary of the research with commentary on the implications for nursing practice and research.
- As in the previous editions, **Home Care Assessment charts** serve as a convenient summary of essential assessment points for patients who need follow-up home health nursing care.
- Subtypes of **Clinical Judgment Challenges** (CJCs) emphasize the six QSEN core competencies: Patient-Centered Care, Teamwork and Collaboration, Evidence-Based Practice, Quality Improvement, Safety, and Informatics.

AN INTEGRATED MULTIMEDIA RESOURCE BASED ON PROVEN STRATEGIES FOR STUDENT ENGAGEMENT AND LEARNING

Medical-Surgical Nursing: Patient-Centered Collaborative Care, 8th edition, is the centerpiece of a comprehensive package of electronic and print learning resources that break new ground in the application of proven strategies for student engagement, learning, and evidence-based educational practice. This integrated multimedia resource actively engages the student in problem solving and practicing clinical decision-making skills.

Resources for Instructors

For the convenience of faculty, all Instructor Resources are available on a streamlined, secure instructor area of the Evolve website (http://evolve.elsevier.com/Iggy/). Included among these Instructor Resources are the reorganized ***TEACH for Nurses*** **Lesson Plans.** These Lesson Plans focus on the most important content from each chapter and provide innovative strategies for student engagement and learning. Lesson Plans are provided for each chapter and are categorized into several parts:

Learning Outcomes
Teaching Focus
Key Terms
Nursing Curriculum Standards
  QSEN
  Concepts
  BSN Essentials
Student Chapter Resources
Instructor Chapter Resources
Teaching Strategies

Additional Instructor Resources provided on the Evolve website include:

- A completely revised, updated, high-quality **Test Bank** consisting of more than 1750 items, both traditional multiple-choice and NCLEX-RN® "alternate" item types. Each question is coded for correct answer, rationale, cognitive level, NCLEX Integrated Process, NCLEX Client Needs Category, and new Keywords to facilitate question searches. Page references are provided for Remembering (Knowledge)- and Understanding (Comprehension)-level questions. (Questions at the Applying [Application] and above cognitive level require the student to draw on understanding of multiple or broader concepts not limited to a single textbook page, so page cross references are not provided for these higher-level critical thinking questions.) The Test Bank is provided in the Evolve Assessment Manager and in ExamView and ParTest formats.
- An electronic **Image Collection** containing all images from the book (approximately 550 images), delivered in a format that makes incorporation into lectures, presentations, and online courses easier than ever.
- **PowerPoint Presentations**—a revised collection of more than 2000 slides corresponding to each chapter in the text and highlighting key content with integrated images and Unfolding Case Studies. Audience Response System Questions (three discussion-oriented questions per chapter for use with iClicker and other audience response systems) are included in these slide presentations. Answers and rationales to the Audience Response System Questions and Unfolding Case Studies are found in the "Notes" section of each slide.

Also available for adoption and separate purchase:

- Corresponding chapter-by-chapter to the textbook, ***Elsevier Adaptive Quizzing (EAQ)*** integrates seamlessly into your course to help students of all skill levels focus their study time and effectively prepare for class, course exams, and the NCLEX® certification exam. ***EAQ*** is comprised of a bank of high-quality practice questions that allows students to advance at their own pace—based on their performance—through multiple mastery levels for each chapter. A comprehensive dashboard allows students to view their progress and stay motivated. The educator dashboard, grade book, and reporting capabilities enable faculty to monitor the activity of individual students, assess overall class performance, and identify areas of strength and weakness, ultimately helping to achieve improved learning outcomes.
- *Simulation Learning System (SLS) for Medical-Surgical Nursing* is an online toolkit designed to help you effectively incorporate simulation into your nursing curriculum, with scenarios that promote and enhance the clinical decision-making skills of students at all levels. It offers detailed instructions for preparation and implementation

of the simulation experience, debriefing questions that encourage critical thinking, and learning resources to reinforce student comprehension. Modularized simulation scenarios correspond to Elsevier's leading medical-surgical nursing texts, reinforcing students' classroom knowledge base, synthesizing lecture and clinicals, and offering remediation content that's critical to debriefing.

Resources for Students

Resources for students include a revised, updated, and retitled Clinical Nursing Judgment Study Guide, a Clinical Companion, Elsevier Adaptive Learning (EAL), Virtual Clinical Excursions (VCE), and Evolve Learning Resources.

The ***Clinical Nursing Judgment Study Guide*** has been completely revised and updated and features a fresh emphasis on clinical decision making, priorities of delegation, management of care, and pharmacology.

The pocket-sized ***Clinical Companion*** is a handy clinical resource that retains its easy-to-use alphabetical organization and streamlined format. It includes "Critical Rescue," "Drug Alert," and "Action Alert" highlights throughout based on the Nursing Safety Priority features in the textbook. National Patient Safety Goals highlights have been expanded as a QSEN feature, focusing on one of six QSEN core competencies, while still underscoring the importance of observing vital patient safety standards. This "pocket-sized Iggy" has been tailored to the special needs of students preparing for clinicals and clinical practice.

Corresponding chapter-by-chapter to the textbook, ***Elsevier Adaptive Learning (EAL)*** combines the power of brain science with sophisticated, patented Cerego algorithms to help students to learn faster and remember longer. It's fun, it's engaging, and it's constantly tracking student performance and adapting to deliver content precisely when it's needed to ensure core information is transformed into lasting knowledge.

Virtual Clinical Excursions, featuring an updated and easy-to-navigate "virtual" clinical setting, is once again available for the eighth edition. This unique learning tool guides students through a virtual clinical environment and helps them "learn by doing" in the safety of a "virtual" hospital.

Also available for students is a dynamic collection of Evolve Student Resources, available at http://evolve.elsevier.com/Iggy/. The Evolve Student Resources include the following:

- Review Questions for the NCLEX® Examination
- Answer Guidelines for NCLEX® Examination and Clinical Judgment Challenges
- Interactive Case Studies
- Concept Maps (digital versions of the 12 Concept Maps from the text)
- Concept Map Creator (a handy tool for creating customized Concept Maps)
- Fluid & Electrolyte Tutorial (a complete self-paced tutorial on this perennially difficult content)
- Key Points (downloadable expanded chapter reviews for each chapter)
- Audio Glossary
- Audio Clips and Video Clips
- Content Updates

In summary, *Medical-Surgical Nursing: Patient-Centered Collaborative Care*, 8th edition, together with its fully integrated multimedia ancillary package, provides the tools you will need to equip nursing students to meet the challenges of nursing practice both now and in an emerging healthcare environment that may look very different from today's. The only elements that remain to be added to this package are those that you alone can provide—your diligence, your commitment, your innovation, *your nursing expertise.*

Donna D. Ignatavicius
M. Linda Workman

To all the nursing educators who are passionate about teaching and all the nursing students who are passionate about learning.

Also, to my husband, Charles, who has endured countless hours of loneliness while I've worked on this project and to Stephanie, my daughter, who has educated me about the LGBTQ community's special needs. Thank you!

Donna

To students everywhere.
To John, still my one.

Linda

ABOUT THE AUTHORS

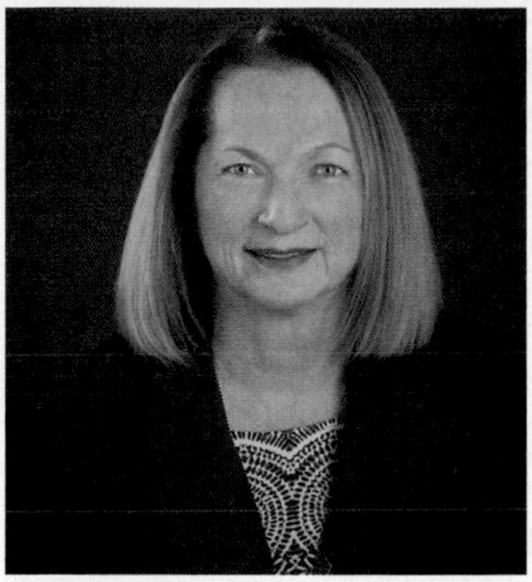

Donna D. Ignatavicius received her diploma in nursing from the Peninsula General School of Nursing in Salisbury, Maryland. After working as a charge nurse in medical-surgical nursing, she became an instructor in staff development at the University of Maryland Medical Center. She then received her BSN from the University of Maryland School of Nursing. For 5 years she taught in several schools of nursing while working toward her MS in Nursing, which she received in 1981. Donna then taught in the BSN program at the University of Maryland, after which she continued to pursue her interest in gerontology and accepted the position of Director of Nursing of a major skilled-nursing facility in her home state of Maryland. Since that time, she has served as an instructor in several associate degree nursing programs. Through her consulting activities and faculty development workshops, Donna has gained national recognition in nursing education. She is currently the President of DI Associates, Inc. (http://www.diassociates.com/), a company dedicated to improving health care through education and consultation for faculty. In recognition of her contributions to the field, she was inducted as a charter Fellow of the prestigious Academy of Nursing Education in 2007.

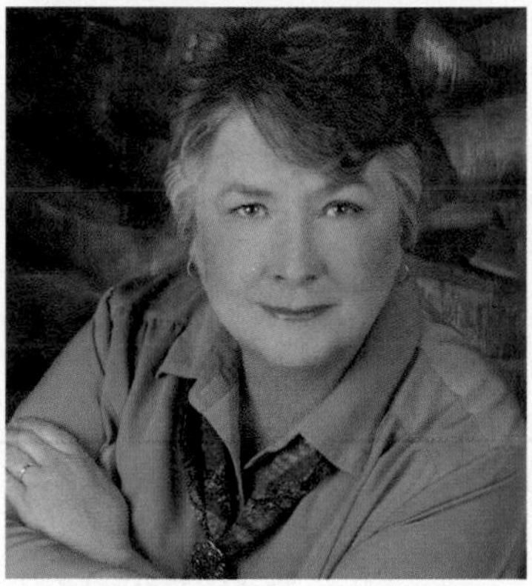

M. Linda Workman, a native of Canada, received her BSN from the University of Cincinnati College of Nursing and Health. After serving in the U.S. Army Nurse Corps and working as an Assistant Head Nurse and Head Nurse in civilian hospitals, Linda earned her MSN from the University of Cincinnati College of Nursing and a PhD in Developmental Biology from the University of Cincinnati College of Arts and Sciences. Linda's 30-plus years of academic experience include teaching at the diploma, associate degree, baccalaureate, and master's levels. Her areas of teaching expertise include medical-surgical nursing, physiology, pathophysiology, genetics, oncology, and immunology. Linda has been recognized nationally for her teaching expertise and was inducted as a Fellow into the American Academy of Nursing in 1992. She received Excellence in Teaching awards at the University of Cincinnati and at Case Western Reserve University. She is a former American Cancer Society Professor of Oncology Nursing and held an endowed chair in oncology for 5 years. In addition to authoring several textbooks and serving as a consult for major universities, she is Senior Volunteer Faculty at the College of Nursing, University of Cincinnati.

ACKNOWLEDGMENTS

Publishing a textbook and ancillary package of this depth and breadth would not be possible without the combined efforts of many people. Stephanie M. Ignatavicius assisted with literature searches. For this eighth edition, we welcomed three section editors to assist in our revision process: Meg Blair, Cherie Rebar, and Chris Winkelman. Each of these nursing educators worked with us on our seventh edition as contributors and/or ancillary material authors. For this eighth edition they updated and reviewed selected units of the text to provide their expertise.

Our contributing authors once again provided consistently excellent manuscripts in a timely fashion. Special thanks to Deanne Blach, who revised our Concept Maps, and Dr. Richard Lintner, who again provided expertise in interventional radiologic procedures and associated care. Our reviewers—expert clinicians and instructors from around the United States and Canada—provided invaluable suggestions and encouragement throughout the book's development.

The staff of Elsevier/Saunders once again provided us with crucial guidance and support throughout the planning, writing, revision, and production of the eighth edition. In particular, Executive Content Strategist Lee Henderson worked closely with us from the early stages of this edition to help us hone and focus our revision plan, and Lee coordinated the project from start to finish. Senior Content Development Specialist Rae Robertson then worked with us step-by-step to bring the eighth edition from vision to publication. Rae, Julia Curcio, and Kelly McGowan held the reins of our complex ancillary package and worked with a gifted group of writers and content experts to provide an outstanding library of resources to complement and enhance the text. Special thanks to Content Coordinators/Content Development Specialists Courtney Daniels and Samantha Taylor, who not only managed the *Clinical Companion* but also handled the countless administrative details associated with a project of this size.

Senior Project Manager Jodi Willard was once again a joy to work with. If, as is said, the mark of a good editor is that her work is invisible to the reader, then Jodi is the consummate editor. Her unwavering attention to detail, flexibility, and conscientiousness not only helped to make this edition the most consistently readable ever, but also made the entire production process incredibly smooth.

Special thanks also to Publishing Services Manager Debbie Vogel. For four editions now, Debbie has worked quietly behind the scenes to help bring the book to publication precisely on schedule and with a very high level of quality.

Designer Margaret Reid is responsible for the beautiful cover and the new interior design of the eighth edition. The praise of a book designer's work is often unsung, but Margaret's work on this edition has cast important features in exactly the right light, with neither too much nor too little emphasis, making this edition not only practical and easy to read, but also beautiful.

Our acknowledgments would not be complete without recognizing our dedicated team of Educational Solutions Consultants and other key members of the Sales and Marketing staff who helped to put this book into your hands.

Finally, we wish to thank John Danaher (President, Education) and Loren Wilson (Senior Vice President and General Manager, Content) for their ongoing vision, direction, and support for state-of-the-art educational resources for nurses.

Donna D. Ignatavicius
M. Linda Workman

CONTENTS

CONCEPT OVERVIEW: Metabolism, 1082

Unit XIII Problems of Digestion, Nutrition, and Elimination: Management of Patients with Problems of the Gastrointestinal System

Unit XIV Problems of Regulation and Metabolism: Management of Patients with Problems of the Endocrine System

GUIDE TO SPECIAL FEATURES

BEST PRACTICE FOR PATIENT SAFETY & QUALITY CARE

COMMON EXAMPLES OF DRUG THERAPY

CONCEPT MAP

EVIDENCE-BASED PRACTICE

FOCUSED ASSESSMENT

HOME CARE ASSESSMENT

KEY FEATURES

LABORATORY PROFILE

NURSING FOCUS ON THE OLDER ADULT

PATIENT AND FAMILY EDUCATION: PREPARING FOR SELF-MANAGEMENT

QUALITY IMPROVEMENT

CHAPTER 1

Introduction to Medical-Surgical Nursing Practice

Donna D. Ignatavicius

http//evolve.elsevier.com/Iggy/

PRIORITY CONCEPTS

- Safety
- Patient-Centered Care
- Teamwork and Collaboration
- Evidence-Based Practice
- Quality Improvement
- Informatics

LEARNING OUTCOMES

Safe and Effective Care Environment

1. Briefly describe the scope of medical-surgical nursing.
2. Explain the current priority focus on patient SAFETY and quality of care.
3. Identify the purpose and function of the Rapid Response Team (RRT).
4. Differentiate the six core Quality and Safety Education for Nurses (QSEN) competencies that health care professionals need to provide safe, PATIENT-CENTERED health care.
5. Identify six major ethical principles that help guide decision making and clinical judgment.
6. Communicate patient values, preferences, and expressed needs to other members of the health care team for effective COLLABORATION.
7. Outline the five rights of the delegation and supervision process.
8. Describe the SBAR procedure for successful hand-off communication in health care agencies.
9. Describe the nurse's role in the systematic QUALITY IMPROVEMENT process.
10. Identify three ways that INFORMATICS and technology are used in health care.

Medical-surgical nursing, sometimes called *adult health nursing,* is a specialty practice area in which nurses promote, restore, or maintain optimal health for patients from 18 to older than 100 years of age (Academy of Medical-Surgical Nurses [AMSN], 2012). A separate chapter on care of older adults is part of this textbook because the majority of medical-surgical patients are older than 65 years (see Chapter 2). To be consistent with the most recent health care literature, the authors use the term *patient* rather than *client* (except in NCLEX Examination Challenge questions). The *family* refers to the patient's relatives and significant others in the patient's life.

SCOPE OF MEDICAL-SURGICAL NURSING PRACTICE

The practice of medical-surgical nursing requires "specialized knowledge and clinical skills to manage actual or potential health problems that affect individuals, their significant others, and the community" (AMSN, 2012, p. 4). Therefore medical-surgical nursing is practiced in many types of health care settings, such as acute care facilities, skilled nursing facilities, home care agencies, and ambulatory care clinics. The role of the nurse in these settings includes care coordinator, caregiver, patient educator, and patient and family advocate (Fig. 1-1).

The nursing process and critical thinking are tools that help the medical-surgical nurse make decisions using clinical judgment while being respectful of the patient's and family's cultural diversity, age, gender, and lifestyle choices (AMSN, 2012). Most fundamentals textbooks have information on cultural diversity and competence. This textbook presents many *Clinical Judgment Challenges* and *NCLEX Examination Challenges* to help you practice how to use clinical judgment to make appropriate decisions for diverse patients.

Medical-surgical health problems occur when a patient's basic needs are not met. These needs, also called *concepts,* were introduced in your fundamentals of nursing course. This

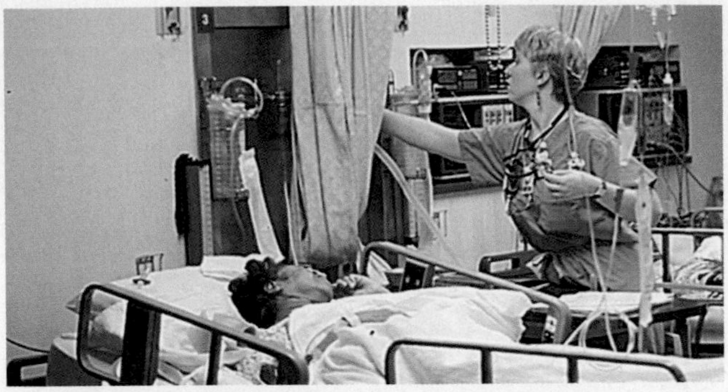

FIG. 1-1 A medical-surgical nurse providing care in an acute care hospital.

textbook builds on those concepts but focuses most on the role of nurses in safely meeting biologic (physiologic) needs for patients with selected medical-surgical health problems. Discussions of psychosocial (emotional), cultural, and spiritual needs are presented when appropriate to describe a holistic approach to patient care. For example, *Cultural Considerations* features highlight important content related to culture.

To further build a bridge between your basic fundamentals course and medical-surgical nursing care, several special features at the beginning of each textbook section review these selected concepts:

- Protection
- Oxygenation and Tissue Perfusion
- Mobility, Sensory Perception, and Cognition
- Nutrition, Metabolism, and Bowel Elimination
- Urinary Elimination
- Sexuality

Then, at the beginning of each chapter, a priority list highlights additional nursing concepts that apply to specific content in the chapter. These concepts are also emphasized in the concept maps for selected health problems. In addition to specified nursing concepts for each chapter, the QSEN core competency areas (professional nursing concepts) are integrated throughout the text.

PRIORITY FOCUS ON SAFETY AND QUALITY OF CARE

Nurses who practice medical-surgical nursing must have a broad knowledge base to meet the needs of patients. Rapid advances in technology, massive increases in available knowledge, and dramatic changes in the health care delivery system require that medical-surgical nurses use expert clinical judgment *to ensure patient safety as the priority in practice.*

Health care errors by physicians, nurses, and other health care professionals have been widely publicized for the past 20 years. Many of these errors have resulted in patient deaths and injuries and increased health care costs. As a result of these errors, a number of national and international organizations have implemented new programs and standards to combat this growing problem.

In 2000, the Institute of Medicine (IOM) stated in its *To Err Is Human: Building a Safer Health Care System* publication that between 44,000 and 98,000 patient *deaths* result each year from preventable errors in acute care hospitals. The report identified several factors that contributed to these findings and motivated other national bodies to examine ways they could improve patient safety and quality care. One of these groups, The Joint Commission (TJC), requires that health care organizations create a culture of SAFETY and encourage patients and families to become safety partners in protecting patients from harm.

The Joint Commission is one of several national organizations that offer peer evaluation for accreditation every 3 years for all types of U.S. health care agencies that meet their standards. Although acute care hospitals are accredited more often than other types of settings, many home care agencies, nursing homes, and ambulatory care centers are also TJC-accredited. Some agencies chose accreditation by organizations other than TJC (e.g., DNV Healthcare), but SAFETY is a major focus for all of them.

In 2002, TJC published its first annual **National Patient Safety Goals (NPSGs)**. These goals require health care organizations to focus on specific priority safety practices, many of which involve establishing nursing and health system approaches to care. Since that time, TJC continues to add new goals each year. NPSGs address high-risk issues such as safe drug administration, health care–associated infections, and communication effectiveness among health care team members. When appropriate, this textbook highlights related NPSGs. A complete list of these 2015 goals can be found on the TJC website at www.jointcommission.org.

TABLE 1-1 IHI Interventions to Save Patient Lives and Prevent Patient Harm

INTERVENTIONS TO SAVE PATIENT LIVES	INTERVENTIONS TO PREVENT PATIENT HARM
Deploy Rapid Response Teams.	Prevent harm from High-Alert Drugs (e.g., anticoagulants, insulin, opioids).
Provide reliable, evidence-based care for acute myocardial infarction.	Reduce surgical complications.
Prevent central line infections.	Prevent pressure ulcers.
Prevent adverse drug events (ADEs).	Reduce methicillin-resistant *Staphylococcus aureus* (MRSA) infections.
Prevent surgical site infections (SSIs).	Provide reliable, evidence-based care for congestive heart failure.
Prevent ventilator-associated pneumonia (VAP).	Get boards of health care organizations to support measures to promote safe patient care.

IHI, Institute for Healthcare Improvement.

Protecting Five Million Lives from Harm

As a result of the IOM report and other data from national studies, the Institute for Healthcare Improvement (IHI) concluded that there are millions of health care errors in U.S. hospitals each year. In 2004, the IHI and its partner health care organizations launched the *100,000 Lives Campaign*—an effort to save patient lives over an 18-month targeted time frame. Six interventions for QUALITY IMPROVEMENT changes in care were implemented by partnering health care agencies (Table 1-1). As a result of this project, an estimated 122,000 patient lives were saved!

The next IHI objective was to *protect patients from five million incidents of medical harm* over a 2-year period (December 2006 to December 2008) (Institute for Healthcare Improvement [IHI], 2005). **Medical harm** refers not only to physician incidents but also to errors caused by *all* members of the health care team or system that lead to patient injury or death. To meet this IHI objective, six interventions for changes in care were added to the original list. As seen in Table 1-1, many of these interventions are within the scope of nursing practice and are therefore emphasized throughout this textbook. Some interventions, such as pressure ulcer prevention and adverse drug event reduction, are also part of TJC's NPSGs.

One of the most successful IHI initiatives was the creation of the Rapid Response Team (RRT), also called the *Medical Emergency Team (MET)*. **Rapid Response Teams** save lives and decrease the risk for harm by providing care to patients *before* a respiratory or cardiac arrest occurs. Although the RRT does not replace the Code Team who responds to patient arrests, it intervenes rapidly when needed for those who are *beginning* to clinically decline.

! NURSING SAFETY PRIORITY (QSEN)

Critical Rescue

Early clinical changes in condition occur in most patients for up to 48 hours before a "Code Blue." Therefore observe for, document, and report early indicators of patient decline, including decreasing blood pressure, increasing heart rate, increasing pain, and changes in mental status.

Members of an RRT are critical care experts who are on-site and available at any time. Although membership varies among facilities, the team may consist of an intensive care unit (ICU) nurse, respiratory therapist, **intensivist** (physician who specializes in critical care), and/or **hospitalist** (family practice physician or internist employed by the hospital). In other hospitals, acute care nurse practitioners or medical residents may be part of the team. The team responds to emergency calls, usually from nurses, according to established agency protocols and policies. Patient families may also activate the RRT. Outcome data demonstrate that the RRT approach to emergency care reduces medical complications and decreases the number of cardiac and respiratory arrests (Bogert et al., 2010).

TJC's NPSGs also include the need for early intervention for patients who are clinically changing. They require each health care organization to establish criteria for patients, families, or staff to call for additional assistance in response to an actual or perceived change in the patient's condition. NPSGs are highlighted in yellow throughout this text as they apply to the content.

Quality and Safety Education for Nurses Core Competencies

The IOM published many reports during the past 15 years suggesting ways to improve patient safety and quality care. One of its reports, *Health Professions Education: A Bridge to Quality*, identified five broad core competencies for health care professionals to ensure patient safety and quality care (Institute of Medicine [IOM], 2003). All of these competencies are interrelated and include:

- Provide patient-centered care.
- Collaborate with the interdisciplinary health care team.
- Implement evidence-based practice.
- Use quality improvement in patient care.
- Use informatics in patient care.

Several years later, the QSEN initiative, now called the *QSEN Institute*, validated the IOM competencies for nursing practice and added SAFETY as a separate competency to emphasize its importance. In addition, the QSEN project team created specific knowledge, skills, and attitudes (KSAs) needed to develop each core competency, using a Delphi research approach. More information about the QSEN Institute can be found on its website at www.qsen.org. QSEN core competency areas are identified in the Key Points at the end of each chapter of this text as appropriate.

This text also highlights the QSEN competencies in its *Clinical Judgment Challenges*. Teaching/learning activities to help students develop specific KSAs can be found in the *Instructor Resources* on the Evolve website and accompanying *Clinical Nursing Judgment Study Guide*. Each QSEN competency is briefly described in the following six sections.

Patient-Centered Care

To be competent in PATIENT-CENTERED CARE, the medical-surgical nurse recognizes "the patient or designee as the source of control and full partner in providing compassionate and coordinated care based on respect for [the] patient's preferences, values, and needs" (Quality and Safety Education for Nurses [QSEN], 2011). The KSAs for competence in patient-centered care focus on communication, compassion, culture, patient education and empowerment, and respect for patients and their families (Table 1-2).

TABLE 1-2 Examples of Knowledge, Skills, and Attitudes (KSAs) Needed to Develop the IOM/QSEN Patient-Centered Care Competency

KNOWLEDGE	SKILLS	ATTITUDES
Describe how diverse cultural, ethnic, and social backgrounds function as sources of patient, family, and community values.	Provide patient-centered care with sensitivity and respect for the diversity of human experience.	Recognize personally held attitudes about working with different ethnic, cultural, and social backgrounds.
Demonstrate comprehensive understanding of the concepts of pain and suffering, including physiologic models of pain and comfort.	Assess presence and extent of pain and suffering.	Recognize personally held values and beliefs about the management of pain and suffering.
Examine how the safety, quality, and cost-effectiveness of health care can be improved through the active involvement of patients and families.	Engage patients or designated surrogates in active partnerships that promote health, safety and well-being, and self-care management.	Respect patient preferences for degree of active engagement in care processes.
Explore ethical and legal implications of patient-centered care.	Facilitate informed patient consent for care.	Respect and encourage individual expression of patient values, preferences, and expressed needs.

Data from Quality and Safety Education for Nurses, 2011 (www.qsen.org).
IOM, Institute of Medicine; *QSEN*, Quality and Safety Education for Nurses.

Nurses also provide family-centered care. As an advocate for the patient and family, teach them how to be empowered and have more control over their care. To assist in this process, TJC recommends a Speak Up™ campaign to provide information to patients and families to increase their empowerment (TJC, 2011). The basic framework of the campaign urges patients and their families to:

- Speak up if you have questions or concerns, and if you don't understand, ask again. It's your body and you have a right to know.
- Pay attention to the care you are receiving. Make sure you're getting the right treatments and medications by the right health care professionals. Don't assume anything.
- Educate yourself about your diagnosis, the medical tests you are undergoing, and your treatment plan.
- Ask a trusted family member or friend to be your advocate.
- Know what medications you take and why you take them. Medication errors are the most common health care errors.
- Use a hospital, clinic, surgery center, or other type of health care organization that has undergone a rigorous on-site evaluation against established state-of-the-art quality and safety standards, such as that provided by TJC.
- Participate in all decisions about your treatment. You are the center of the health care team.

Patient and family empowerment is one way to demonstrate respect for patients in their ability to be care partners.

Ethical Principles. Respect for people is the basis for six essential *ethical principles* that nurses and other health care professionals should use as a guide for clinical decision making. Respect implies that patients are treated as autonomous individuals capable of making informed decisions about their care. This patient **autonomy** is also referred to as *self-determination* or *self-management.* When the patient is not capable of self-determination, you are ethically obligated to protect him or her as an advocate within the professional scope of practice, according to the American Nurses Association (ANA) Code of Ethics for Nurses (ANA, 2010).

The second ethical principle is **beneficence,** which promotes positive actions to help others. In other words, it encourages the nurse to do good for the patient. **Nonmaleficence** emphasizes the importance of preventing harm and ensuring the patient's well-being. Harm can be avoided only if its causes or possible causes are identified. As described earlier in this chapter, patient safety is currently a major national focus to prevent deaths and injuries.

Fidelity refers to the agreement that nurses will keep their obligations or promises to patients to follow through with care. **Veracity** is a related principle in which the nurse is obligated to tell the truth to the best of his or her knowledge. If you are not truthful with a patient, his or her respect for you will diminish and your credibility as a health care professional will be damaged.

Social justice, the last principle, refers to equality and fairness; that is, all patients should be treated equally and fairly, regardless of age, gender identity, sexual orientation, religion, race, ethnicity, or education. For example, a patient who cannot afford health care receives the same quality and level of care as one who has extensive insurance coverage. An older patient with dementia is shown the same respect as a younger patient who can communicate. A Hispanic patient who can communicate only in Spanish receives the same level of care as a Euro-American patient whose primary language is English. More information on ethics and ethical principles can be found in your fundamentals textbook.

The ANA recognizes the need for nurses to provide culturally competent care, emphasizing that nurses should practice with respect and compassion to ensure the dignity and uniqueness of every person (ANA, 2010). The individual's unique values, preferences, and needs must be communicated to each member of the health care team. Some of the *Clinical Judgment Challenges* in this textbook focus on ethical issues.

Special Needs of the LGBTQ Population. Nurses today have been made aware of cultural variations and learned how to incorporate those differences to individualize patient care. However, one group that is rarely addressed in the nursing literature is the lesbian, gay, bisexual, transgender, and queer and/or questioning (LGBTQ) population (Pettinato, 2012). This terminology is widely accepted by the LGBTQ community and is commonly used, although *LGBT* may be seen more often in health care literature. Queer and/or questioning individuals prefer not having strict labels on their sexualities or genders. Another term that may also be used is *LGBTQI* to include intersex individuals. Intersex individuals have sexual or reproductive organs that are not clearly male or female or may have a combination of both male and female organs.

Many studies provide evidence that LGBTQ individuals do not feel comfortable with or trust health care professionals because of previous discrimination (IOM, 2011). The *Healthy People 2020* initiative added a category for these individuals because of health disparities in this population and the need in the United States to improve LGBTQ health. The complete document can be found on www.healthypeople.gov/2020. This textbook includes special health needs of this population as part of its *Gender Health Considerations* features. A new chapter on transgender health has also been added to this edition of the text to help students learn about the special needs of transgender patients.

The health care system, like other facets of society, often overlooks sexualities and genders that are alternative to the standard of heterosexuality and clearly delineated maleness or femaleness. As a health care professional, it is essential to not be restricted by rigid standards of identity. A good way of rethinking concepts of sexuality and gender is to think of each as existing along a spectrum as opposed to the confinement of heterosexual/homosexual and male/female.

To begin to gain trust and show respect for the LGBTQ patient, health care professionals need to know their patient's sexual orientation and gender identity. Do not assume that every patient is heterosexual or clearly gendered. *Include questions about gender identity and sexual activity as part of your patient's health assessment.* Table 1-3 lists recommended patient interview questions about sexual orientation, gender identity, and health care.

Teamwork and Collaboration

To provide patient- and family-centered care, the nurse "functions effectively within nursing and inter-professional teams, fostering open communication, mutual respect, and shared decision-making to achieve quality patient care" (QSEN, 2011). Therefore the KSAs for this competency emphasize the importance of communication and team functioning. Communication is an essential process for successful collaboration. **Collaboration** entails planning, implementing, and evaluating patient care together using an interdisciplinary (ID) plan of care. To help meet this purpose, health care agencies have frequent and regular ID meetings and conduct ID patient care rounds.

Electronic mail (e-mail) allows for quick communication among health care professionals to enhance collaboration and coordination of care. *However, it should not replace face-to-face and phone communication.*

Although there are many health care team members, some caregivers work more closely with nurses than others. For example, the physician or other health care provider and medical-surgical nurse collaborate frequently in a given day regarding patient care. The occupational therapist may not work as closely with the nurse unless the patient is receiving rehabilitation services. Collaboration with the rehabilitation team is discussed in Chapter 6.

One of the most important members of the ID team is the case manager (CM) or discharge planner, who is typically a nurse or social worker in health care agencies. The purpose of the **case management** process is to provide quality and cost-effective services and resources to achieve positive patient outcomes. In collaboration with the nurse, the CM coordinates inpatient and community-based care before discharge from a hospital or other facility. Part of that process may involve communicating with other CMs who are employed by third-party health care payers (e.g., Medicare) to keep patients from being readmitted to the hospital.

Communication. Poor communication between professional caregivers and health care agencies causes many medical errors and patient safety risks. In 2006, The Joint Commission began to require systematic strategies for improving communication. Two years later, another National Patient Safety Goal mandated that nurses communicate continuing patient care needs, such as pain management or respiratory support, to post-discharge caregivers.

To improve communication between staff members and health care agencies, procedures for hand-off communication were established. An effective procedure used in many agencies today is called *SBAR* (pronounced S-Bar). **SBAR** is a formal method of communication between two or more members of the health care team. The SBAR process includes these four steps:

- **S**ituation: Describe what is happening at the time to require this communication.
- **B**ackground: Explain any relevant background information that relates to the situation.
- **A**ssessment: Provide an analysis of the problem or patient need based on assessment data.
- **R**ecommendation: State what is needed or what the desired outcome is.

Several modifications of SBAR include I-SBAR and I-SBAR-R. In these procedures, the "I" reminds the individual to *identify* himself or herself. The last "R" stands for the *response* that the receiver provides based on the information given. Be sure to follow the established documentation and reporting protocols in your agency.

One of the most recent projects to improve communication was provided in 2010 by the Center for Transforming Health Care (www.centerfortransforminghealthcare.org). Every transition of care is potentially risky for patients because vital information needs to be communicated among caregivers and from one health care agency to another to keep patients safe. This QUALITY IMPROVEMENT (QI) project recommends these targeted solutions to ensure successful communication using the acronym ***SHARE*** as outlined in Table 1-4.

TABLE 1-3 Recommended Patient Interview Questions about Sexual Orientation, Gender Identity, and Health Care

- Do you have sex with men, women, both, or neither?
- Does anyone live with you in your household?
- Are you in a relationship with someone who does not live with you?
- If you have a sexual partner, have you or your partner been evaluated about the possibility of transmitting infections to each other?
- If you have more than one sexual partner, how are you protecting both of you from infections, such as hepatitis B or hepatitis C or HIV?
- Have you disclosed your gender identity and sexual orientation to your health care provider?
- If you have not, may I have your permission to provide that information to members of the health care team who are involved in your care?
- Who do you consider as your closest family members?

HIV, Human immune deficiency virus.

TABLE 1-4 Center for Transforming Health Care Targeted Solutions to Enhance Successful Hand-Off Communication and Collaboration: SHARE

TARGETED SOLUTION	DESCRIPTION OF SOLUTION
Standardize critical content.	Providing details of the patient's history to the receiver, emphasizing key information about the patient, and synthesizing information from various sources before passing it on.
Hardwire within your system.	Developing standardized forms, tools, and methods, such as checklists; identifying new and existing technologies to assist in successful hand-off; and stating expectations about how to conduct a successful hand-off.
Allow opportunity to ask questions.	Using critical-thinking skills when discussing a patient's case as well as sharing and receiving Information as an interdisciplinary team ("pit crew"). Receivers should expect to receive all key information about the patient, scrutinize and question the data, and exchange contact information with the sender for additional questions.
Reinforce quality and measurement.	Demonstrating leadership commitment to successful hand-offs, such as holding staff accountable, monitoring compliance with use of standardized forms, and using data to determine a systematic approach for improvement.
Educate and coach.	Teaching staff throughout the organization about what constitutes a successful hand-off, standardizing training on how to conduct a hand-off, providing performance feedback at the time of the hand-off, and making successful hand-offs an organizational priority.

Data from the Joint Commission Center for Transforming Healthcare. (2010). *Joint Commission Center for Transforming Healthcare tackles miscommunication among caregivers.* Retrieved January 15, 2013, from www.centerfortransforminghealthcare.org.

Specific examples of ways to improve communication among nurses and other health care professionals using the SHARE principles have been cited in recent nursing literature. For instance, Maxson et al. (2012) reported a process for shift reporting from one nurse to another in which both shift nurses made bedside rounds during each patient's report. In this way, the patient and family were included in the communication process and patient safety was improved (see Evidence-Based Practice box). Burns (2011) reported a pilot study on a medical unit in which the unit's nurse, hospitalist physician, and physician's nurse made patient rounds as a team to improve health team communication and increase the patient's perception of and satisfaction with his or her care.

Delegation and Supervision. As a nursing leader, you will delegate certain nursing tasks and activities to unlicensed assistive personnel (UAP), such as patient care technicians (PCTs) or patient care assistants (PCAs). **Delegation** is the process of transferring to a competent person the authority to perform a selected nursing task or activity in a selected patient care situation. This process requires precise and accurate communication. *The nurse is always accountable for the task or activity that is delegated!*

An important process that is sometimes not consistently performed by busy medical-surgical nurses is supervision of the UAP to whom the task or activity has been delegated. **Supervision** is guidance or direction, evaluation, and follow-up by the nurse to ensure that the task or activity is performed appropriately. Examples of delegated tasks are turning and positioning, vital signs, and intake and output measurements.

Be sure to follow these five rights when you delegate and supervise a nursing task or activity to a UAP:

- *Right task:* The task is within the UAP's scope of practice and competence.
- *Right circumstances:* The patient care setting and resources are appropriate for the delegation.
- *Right person:* The UAP is competent to perform the delegated task or activity.
- *Right communication:* The nurse provides a clear and concise explanation of the task or activity, including limits and expectations.
- *Right supervision:* The nurse appropriately monitors, evaluates, intervenes, and provides feedback on the delegation process as needed.

Other activities or patient care responsibilities may be assigned by a registered nurse (RN) to another RN or to a licensed practical or vocational nurse (LPN/LVN). Each state designates which tasks may be safely delegated and assigned to nursing team members. Interventions that you can typically delegate or assign in any state are indicated throughout this text. Some of the *Clinical Judgment and NCLEX Examination Challenges* throughout this book will test your understanding of the delegation and supervision process.

EVIDENCE-BASED PRACTICE QSEN

Does a Bedside Nurse Reporting Process Promote Patient Safety?

Maxson, P.M., Derby, K.M., Wrobleski, D.M., & Foss, D.M. (2012). Bedside nurse-to-nurse handoff promotes patient safety. *MEDSURG Nursing, 21*, 140-144.

Patient handoff at shift change in most hospitals has typically included a verbal or taped report, allowing nurses to communicate necessary patient information for continuity of care. Bedside handoff between shifts allows the patient and family to have an opportunity for input into the plan of care. This process helps meet the Joint Commission's National Patient Safety Goals and encourages patients to be an active part of their own care.

A convenience sample of 60 patients was used in a small study to examine the effects of bedside nurse-to-nurse handoff on a hospital unit. Thirty (30) patients were enrolled before the change in shift reporting, and 30 were enrolled after the change to bedside handoff. All nursing staff were invited to participate. Patients and staff completed surveys before and after the practice change. Fifteen nurses completed the pre- and post-survey indicating that they were more satisfied with the bedside handoff method when compared with the previous method of reporting. Patient satisfaction also increased as a result of the bedside nurse-to-nurse handoff process.

Level of Evidence: 4

This research was a small descriptive study that used a convenience sample.

Commentary: Implications for Practice and Research

Use of bedside nursing handoff increases patient and staff satisfaction and standardizes the shift report. This process also improves patient safety because both nurses see the patient during the change-of-shift period. Patients feel they are more active partners in their care and have the opportunity to ask questions and provide information during the handoff time. Additional studies using larger samples are needed to demonstrate the advantages and possible disadvantages of the shift change nurse-to-nurse handoff.

Evidence-Based Practice

Evidence-based practice (EBP) is the integration of the best current evidence to make decisions about patient care. It considers the patient's preferences and values as well as one's own clinical expertise for the delivery of optimal health care (Melnyk & Fineout-Overholt, 2011; QSEN, 2011). Health care agencies follow the Core Measures developed by the Centers for Medicare & Medicaid (CMS) in collaboration with TJC to ensure that best practices are followed. Examples of Core Measures are highlighted throughout this textbook, such as those related to heart failure, stroke, and acute myocardial infarction.

The best source of evidence is research. However, available nursing research is limited and in some areas may not reflect the highest or best level of evidence. Some nursing research is designed as small, descriptive studies to explore new concepts. The findings of these studies cannot be generalized, but they provide a basis for future larger and better-controlled research.

As we did in the last edition of our text, this edition devotes a chapter to EBP (Chapter 5). In addition, *Evidence-Based Practice* boxes are found throughout the text to provide the most current research that serves as a basis for nursing practice. Each of these features presents a brief summary of the research, identifies the level (strength) of evidence using the scale in Chapter 5, and concludes with a "Commentary: Implications for Practice and Research" discussion to help you apply the findings of the study to your daily practice.

Quality Improvement

Ensuring patient and staff safety requires individual and systematic evaluation and change. To meet the **quality improvement** competency, nurses are expected to "use data to monitor the outcomes of care processes and use improvement methods to design and test changes to continuously improve the quality and safety of health care systems" (QSEN, 2011). The KSAs stress the importance of learning how to use specific QI tools, participating in root cause analyses, and impacting changes in care processes.

As a medical-surgical nurse, you will be expected to:

- Identify indicators to monitor quality and effectiveness of health care.
- Access and evaluate data to monitor the quality and effectiveness of health care.
- Recommend ways to improve care processes.
- Implement activities to improve care processes.

A new feature for this edition of our textbook is *Quality Improvement* boxes that summarize articles on QI projects and end with a "Commentary: Implications for Practice and Research" discussion. Additional information about the QI process can be found in nursing leadership and management resources.

Informatics

Informatics involves using information and technology to communicate, manage knowledge, mitigate error, and support decision making (QSEN, 2011; Yoder-Wise, 2011). The emphasis of the KSAs for informatics is documentation, electronic data access, and data utilization.

Although most health care settings have information technology (IT) departments, nurses retrieve and use valuable information for patient care. The largest application of health care informatics is use of the electronic health record (EHR) (also called *electronic patient record [EPR]* or *electronic medical record [EMR]*) for documenting nursing and interdisciplinary care. Computers may be located at the nurses' work station or at the patient's bedside (point of care [POC]) (Fig. 1-2) or near the nurses' station. Handheld mobile devices are also popular because of their ease of use and portability.

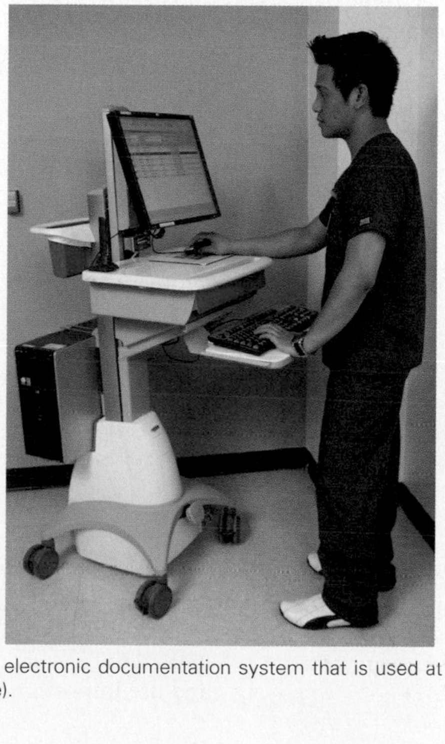

FIG. 1-2 An electronic documentation system that is used at the bedside (point of care).

Another major purpose of informatics is for retrieval of data for the evidence-based practice process described in Chapter 5. The Internet provides ways to search for multiple sources of information very efficiently. However, all data sources must be evaluated for their credibility and reliability. Some health care agencies provide handheld mobile devices, such as the iPod Touch™, to health care professionals for data access and team communication via text or e-mail.

New technologies for patient, staff, and resource (inventory) management are emerging in health care agencies to promote patient safety and improve efficiency. An example of these technologies is radio frequency identification (RFID). RFID allows any person or object to be tracked electronically. For example, patients wear electronic identification wristbands.

Nurses need to be involved in decisions about introducing new or advanced health care technologies into the health care agency. They should also be included in designing technology that improves the effectiveness and efficiency of health care while providing for patient and staff privacy.

Safety

As discussed earlier in this chapter, nurses play a key role in promoting safety and preventing errors, including "missed nursing care," the necessary care that should have been provided by one or more nurses. The nurse "minimizes risk of harm to patients and providers through both system effectiveness and individual performance" (QSEN, 2011). The KSAs for safety stress the importance of examining care processes (QI), integrating national patient resources, and using appropriate tools to reduce reliance on memory, such as checklists.

The National Council of State Boards of Nursing (NCSBN) published findings of an extensive study of nursing practice breakdowns (Benner et al., 2010). These results identified nine key areas where nursing practice should be improved, including:

- Medication administration
- Clearly communicating patient data and clinical assessments
- Attentiveness/surveillance of patients
- Clinical reasoning or judgment
- Prevention of errors or complications
- Intervention (carrying out nursing actions in an appropriate and timely manner)
- Interpretation of authorized provider orders
- Professional responsibility and patient advocacy
- Mandatory reporting

The research report also provided case examples and analyses to assist in the development of quality improvement processes.

Three types of *Nursing Safety Priority* boxes are found throughout this text to emphasize the importance of safety when in daily practice. These features delineate safety based on patient need. For example, *Nursing Safety Priority: Critical Rescue* emphasizes the need for action for potential or actual life-threatening problems. *Nursing Safety Priority: Action Alert* boxes focus on the need for action but not necessarily for life-threatening situations. These safety alerts are essential, though, to ensure optimal patient outcomes. As the name implies, *Nursing Safety Priority: Drug Alert* boxes specify actions needed to ensure safety related to drug administration, monitoring, or related patient and family education.

GET READY FOR THE NCLEX® EXAMINATION!

KEY POINTS

Review these Key Points for each NCLEX Examination Client Needs Category.

Safe and Effective Care Environment

- Medical-surgical nursing is a specialty practice that requires a broad knowledge base and clinical skills to meet the needs of adult patients in a variety of settings.
- Medical-surgical nurses help meet human needs of adult patients, such as mobility and oxygenation, in a caring, respectful relationship.
- The Joint Commission requires that health care organizations create a culture of SAFETY by following the National Patient Safety Goals (NPSGs). **Safety** QSEN
- The Institute for Healthcare Improvement (IHI) interventions to save lives and prevent patient harm are listed in Table 1-1. **Safety** QSEN
- Rapid Response Teams (RRTs) save lives and decrease the risk for patient harm before a respiratory or cardiac arrest occurs. **Safety** QSEN
- Remember to always observe for slow and sudden changes in patient condition, especially changes in vital signs and mental status. **Safety** QSEN
- A vital role of the nurse is as an advocate to empower patients and their families to have control over their health care and function as safety partners.
- The six core competencies for health care professionals based on research by the Institute of Medicine (IOM) and Quality and Safety Education for Nurses (QSEN) are PATIENT-CENTERED CARE, TEAMWORK AND COLLABORATION, EVIDENCE-BASED PRACTICE, QUALITY IMPROVEMENT, INFORMATICS, and SAFETY.
- Examples of the knowledge, skills, and attitudes needed for patient-centered care are found in Table 1-2. **Patient-Centered Care** QSEN
- Six essential ethical principles to consider when making clinical decisions are autonomy, beneficence, nonmaleficence, fidelity, veracity, and social justice.
- Nurses must show respect and compassion for the uniqueness of every individual to ensure PATIENT-CENTERED CARE.
- The lesbian, gay, bisexual, transgender, queer and/or questioning (LGBTQ) population typically does not trust health care professionals; use sensitive questioning about sexual orientation and gender identity as part of your interview with patients in this group (see Table 1-3). **Patient-Centered Care** QSEN
- Nurses COLLABORATE by communicating patient's needs and preferences with members of the health care team to establish an individualized approach to care. **Teamwork and Collaboration** QSEN
- The SBAR procedure or similar established protocol is used for successful hand-off communication between caregivers and between health care agencies as part of the SHARE collaborative process (see Table 1-4).
- When delegating a nursing task to unlicensed assistive personnel (UAP), the nurse is always accountable to ensure that the task was performed safely and accurately. **Safety** QSEN
- EVIDENCE-BASED PRACTICE (EBP) is the integration of best current evidence to make decisions about patient care. It considers the patient's preferences and values, as well as one's own clinical expertise. **Evidence-Based Practice** QSEN
- Nurses are active participants in the systematic QUALITY IMPROVEMENT process in their health care agency. **Quality Improvement** QSEN
- INFORMATICS and technology are used for patient documentation, electronic data access, and health care resource tracking. **Informatics** QSEN

CHAPTER 2

Common Health Problems of Older Adults

Donna D. Ignatavicius

http//evolve.elsevier.com/Iggy/

PRIORITY CONCEPTS

- Nutrition
- Mobility
- Sensory Perception
- Cognition
- Elimination
- Tissue Integrity

LEARNING OUTCOMES

Safe and Effective Care Environment

1. Explain the need to collaborate with members of the health care team to help the patient/family achieve health goals.
2. Identify risk factors for falls and impaired driving ability, including problems with mobility, in older adults who live in the community or are hospitalized.
3. Explain evidence-based falls risk and prevention interventions for older adults in the hospital and community.
4. Describe best practices to promote patient safety when using restraints.

Health Promotion and Maintenance

5. Teach selected evidence-based lifestyle practices to promote healthy activities in older adults.
6. Conduct a medication assessment for potential risks for adverse drug events in older adults.

Psychosocial Integrity

7. Assess the older patient's risk for and signs of neglect and abuse.
8. Use valid and reliable assessment tools to document mental/behavioral health problems in the older adult.
9. Compare characteristics of common problems of cognition: depression, delirium, and dementia.
10. Develop a plan of care to assist the older adult to cope with relocation stress syndrome.

Physiological Integrity

11. Identify four subgroups of older adults.
12. Explain factors that contribute to nutrition-related problems among older adults in the community and inpatient facilities.
13. Describe the effects of drugs on the older adult.
14. Identify key interventions to prevent problems related to tissue integrity in older adults.

About 13% of the people in the United States are older than 65 years, but this number is expected to grow to 25% by 2050 (U.S. Census Bureau, 2013). In general, women live longer than men, although the exact reason for this difference is not known. Most patients on adult acute care and nursing home units are older than 65 years; many of these patients are discharged for home health services. Therefore nurses and other health care professionals need to know about the special needs of older adults to care for them in a variety of settings.

This chapter describes the major health issues, sometimes referred to as **geriatric syndromes**, associated with late adulthood in community and inpatient settings (Brown-O'Hara, 2013). The care of older adults (sometimes referred to as *elders*) with specific acute and chronic health problems is discussed as appropriate throughout this text. *Nursing Focus on the Older Adult* charts and *Considerations for Older Adults* boxes highlight the most important information. A brief review of major physiologic changes of aging are listed in the Assessment chapter of each body system unit. A number of gerontologic nursing textbooks and journals are available for additional information about older adult care.

OVERVIEW

Late adulthood can be divided into four subgroups:

- 65 to 74 years of age: the young old
- 75 to 84 years of age: the middle old
- 85 to 99 years of age: the old old
- 100 years of age or older: the elite old

The fastest growing subgroup is the old old, sometimes referred to as the advanced older adult population. Members of this subgroup are sometimes referred to as the "frail elderly," although a number of 85- to 95-year-olds are very healthy and do not meet the criteria for being frail. *Frailty* is a geriatric syndrome in which the older adult has unintentional weight loss, weakness and exhaustion, and slowed physical activity, including walking. Frail older adults are also at high risk for adverse outcomes (Brown-O'Hara, 2013; Rocchiccioli & Sanford, 2009).

The vast majority of older adults live in the community at home, in assisted-living facilities, or in retirement or independent living complexes. Of all older adults, only about 5% live in long-term care (LTC) facilities (mostly nursing homes) and another 10% to 15% are ill but are cared for at home. Older adults from any setting usually experience one or more hospitalizations in their lifetime. About half of all older adults will likely be admitted at some time during their life for short-term stays in a skilled unit of a LTC facility, usually for rehabilitation or complex medical-surgical follow-up care.

Other institutions also have an increase in aging adults. For example, men older than 50 years are the fastest growing group of prisoners today. Like the rest of the older population, older prisoners have multiple chronic health problems. However, these problems are often complicated by a history of alcohol and substance abuse and poor NUTRITION that require deliberate management strategies. Nurses who work in these settings must have expertise in care of older adults.

The number of homeless people older than 60 years is also growing. The inability to pay for housing and family/partner relationship problems are primary factors that contribute to this trend. Most homeless adults have one or more chronic health problems, including mental/behavioral health disorders (Gerber, 2013). A growing number are veterans of war.

HEALTH ISSUES FOR OLDER ADULTS IN COMMUNITY-BASED SETTINGS

Health is a major concern for many older adults. Health status can affect the ability to perform ADLs and to participate in social roles. A failure to perform these activities may increase dependence on others and may have a negative effect on morale and life satisfaction. When older adults lose the ability to function independently, they often feel empty and worthless. Loss of autonomy is a painful event related to the physical and mental changes of aging.

Older adults may also experience a number of losses that can affect a sense of control over their lives, such as the death of a spouse and friends or the loss of social and work roles. Nurses need to support older adults' self-esteem and feelings of independence by encouraging them to maintain as much control as possible over their lives, to participate in decision making, and to perform as many tasks as possible.

Like younger and middle-aged adults, older adults need to practice health promotion and illness prevention to maintain or achieve a high level of wellness. Teach them the importance of promoting wellness and strategies for meeting this outcome (Chart 2-1).

Common health issues and geriatric syndromes that often affect older adults in the community include:

- Decreased NUTRITION and hydration
- Decreased MOBILITY
- Stress and loss
- Accidents
- Drug use and misuse
- Mental health/COGNITION problems (including substance abuse)
- Elder neglect and abuse

CHART 2-1 Patient and Family Education: Preparing for Self-Management

Lifestyles and Practices to Promote Wellness

Health-Protecting Behaviors

- Have yearly influenza vaccinations (after October 1).
- Obtain a pneumococcal vaccination.
- Obtain a shingles vaccination.
- Have a tetanus immunization, and get a booster every 10 years.
- Wear seat belts when you are in an automobile.
- Use alcohol in moderation or not at all.
- Avoid smoking; if you do smoke, do not smoke in bed.
- Install and maintain working smoke detectors and/or sprinklers.
- Create a hazard-free environment to prevent falls; eliminate hazards such as scatter rugs and waxed floors.
- Use medications, herbs, and nutritional supplements according to your health care provider's prescription.
- Avoid over-the-counter medications unless your physician directs you to use them.

Health-Enhancing Behaviors

- Have a yearly physical examination; see your health care provider more often if health problems occur.
- Reduce dietary fat to not more than 30% of calories; saturated fat should provide less than 10% of your calories.
- Increase your daily dietary intake of complex carbohydrate– and fiber-containing food to five or more servings of fruits and vegetables and six or more servings of grain products.
- Increase calcium intake to between 1000 and 1500 mg daily; take a vitamin D supplement every day if not exposed daily to sunlight.
- Allow at least 10 to 15 minutes of sun exposure two or three times weekly for vitamin D intake; avoid prolonged sun exposure.
- Exercise regularly three to five times a week.
- Manage stress through coping mechanisms that have been successful in the past.
- Get together with people in different settings to socialize.
- Reminisce about your life through reflective discussions or journaling.

Decreased Nutrition and Hydration

The minimum nutritional requirements of the human body remain consistent from youth through old age, with a few exceptions. Older adults need an increased dietary intake of calcium, vitamin D, vitamin C, and vitamin A because aging changes disrupt the ability to store, use, and absorb these substances. For older adults who have a sedentary lifestyle and reduced metabolic rate, a reduction in total caloric intake to maintain an ideal body weight is needed. NUTRITION-related problems can occur in older adults when these needs are not met.

Many physical aging changes influence nutritional status or the ability to consume needed nutrients. Diminished senses of taste and smell often result in a loss of desire for food. Older adults have less ability to taste sweet and salt than to taste bitter and sour. This aging change may result in an overuse of table sugar and salt to compensate. Some older adults consume numerous desserts and other sweet foods, which can cause them to become overweight or obese. Teach older adults how to balance their diets with healthy food selections. Remind them to substitute herbs and spices to season food and vary the textures of food substances to feel satisfied.

Tooth loss and poorly fitting dentures from inadequate dental care or calcium loss can also cause the older adult to avoid important nutritious foods. Unlike today, dental preventive programs were not readily available or stressed as being important when today's older adults were younger. Older people with dentition problems may eat soft, high-calorie foods such as ice cream and mashed potatoes, which lack roughage and fiber. Unless the person carefully chooses more nutritious soft foods, vitamin deficiencies, constipation, and other problems can result. The extensive use of prescribed and over-the-counter (OTC) drugs, including herbal supplements, may decrease appetite, affect food tolerances and food absorption, and cause constipation.

Constipation can reduce quality of life for older adults and cause pain, depression, anxiety, and decreased social activities (Toner & Claros, 2012). In some cases, it leads to a small or large bowel obstruction, potentially life-threatening events. Constipation is common among older adults and can be caused by multiple risk factors, including foods, drugs, and diseases.

! NURSING SAFETY PRIORITY QSEN

Action Alert

Teach older adults to increase fiber and fluid intake, exercise regularly, and avoid risk factors that contribute to constipation. Older adults should consume 35 to 50 g of fiber each day and drink at least 2 L a day unless medically contraindicated. Some people may also add a "colon cocktail" of equal portions of prune juice, applesauce, and psyllium (e.g., Metamucil) to their daily diet. Remind older adults to take 1 to 2 tablespoons of the mixture daily. If these measures do not prevent constipation, teach them to take a stool softener. For opioid-induced constipation (OIC), methylnaltrexone (Relistor) may be prescribed. This drug is given subcutaneously once every other day as needed and tends to have quick results (Toner & Claros, 2012).

Reduced income, chronic disease, fatigue, and decreased ability to perform ADLs are other factors that contribute to inadequate NUTRITION and constipation among older adults. "Fast food" is often inexpensive and requires no preparation. However, it is usually high in fat, carbohydrates, and calories but lacking in healthy nutrients. Older adults can become overweight or obese when they consume a diet high in fast food.

Other older adults may reduce their intake of food to near-starvation levels, even with the availability of programs such as food stamps (Supplemental Nutritional Assistance Program [SNAP]), community food banks, and Meals on Wheels. Many senior centers and homeless shelters offer meals, as well as group social activities. The lack of transportation, the necessity of traveling to obtain such services, and the inability to carry large or heavy groceries prevent some older adults from taking advantage of food programs. Others are too proud to accept free services.

Inadequate NUTRITION may also be related to loneliness. Older adults may respond to loneliness, depression, and boredom by not eating, which can lead to weight loss. Many who live alone lose the incentive to prepare or eat balanced diets, especially if they do not "feel well." Men who live at home alone are especially at risk for not eating enough calories to maintain their weight.

Some older adults are at risk for **geriatric failure to thrive (GFTT)**—a complex syndrome including under-nutrition, impaired physical functioning, depression, and cognitive impairment (Rocchiccioli & Sanford, 2009). However, drug therapy, chronic diseases, major losses, and poor socioeconomic status can cause these same health problems. Be sure to consider these factors when screening for GFTT. For those at risk for or who have GFTT, collaborate with the older adult and family to plan referral to his or her primary care provider for extensive evaluation. Early supportive intervention can help prevent advanced levels of deterioration.

! NURSING SAFETY PRIORITY QSEN

Action Alert

Perform nutritional screening for older adults in the community who are at risk for inadequate NUTRITION—either weight loss or obesity. Ask the person about unintentional weight loss or gain, eating habits, appetite, prescribed and over-the-counter drugs, and current health problems. Determine contributing factors for older adults who have or are at risk for poor NUTRITION, such as transportation issues or loneliness. Based on these data, develop and implement a plan of care in collaboration with the registered dietitian, pharmacist, and/or case manager to manage these problems. Chapter 60 describes nutritional assessment and management of NUTRITION problems in detail.

People older than 65 years are also at risk for dehydration because they have less body water content than younger adults. In severe cases, they require emergency department visits or hospital stays.

! NURSING SAFETY PRIORITY QSEN

Action Alert

Older adults sometimes limit their fluid intake, especially in the evening, because of problems associated with MOBILITY, prescribed diuretics, and urinary incontinence. *Teach older adults that fluid restrictions make them susceptible to dehydration and electrolyte imbalances (especially sodium and potassium) that can cause serious illness or death.*

Incontinence may actually increase because the urine becomes more concentrated and irritating to the bladder and urinary sphincter. Teach older adults the importance of drinking 2 liters of water a day plus other fluids as desired. Remind them to avoid excessive caffeine and alcohol because they can cause dehydration. Chapter 11 discusses fluid and electrolyte imbalances in detail.

Decreased Mobility

Exercise and activity are important for older adults as a means of promoting and maintaining MOBILITY and overall health (Fig. 2-1). Physical activity can help keep the body in shape and maintain an optimal level of functioning. Regular exercise has many benefits for older adults in community-based settings. The advantages of maintaining appropriate levels of physical activity include:

- Decreased risk for falls
- Increased muscle strength and balance
- Increased MOBILITY
- Increased sleep
- Reduced or maintained weight
- Improved sense of well-being and self-esteem
- Decreased depression symptoms
- Improved longevity
- Reduced risks for diabetes, coronary artery disease, and dementia

Assess older adults in any setting regarding their history of exercise and any health concerns they may have. For independent older adults, remind them to check with their health care provider to implement a supervised plan for regular

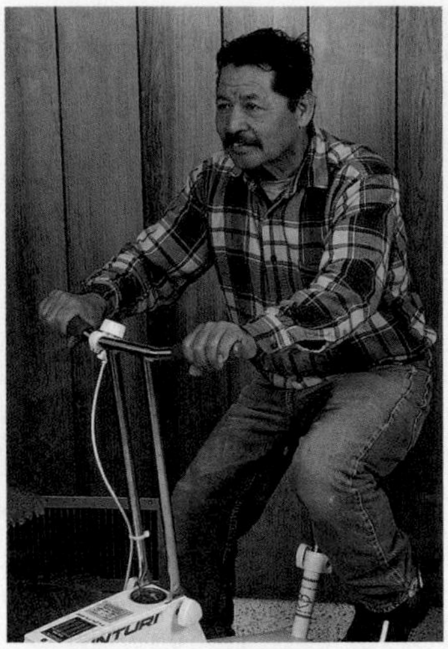

FIG. 2-1 Exercise is important to older adults for health promotion and maintenance.

physical activity. Teach all older adults about the value of physical activity.

For people who are homebound, focus on functional fitness, such as performing ADLs. For those who are not homebound, teach the importance of other types of exercise. Resistance exercise, for example, maintains muscle mass. Aerobic exercise, like walking, improves strength and endurance. One of the best exercises is walking at least 30 minutes, 3 to 5 times a week. During the winter, indoor shopping centers and other public places can be used. In addition, many senior centers and community centers offer exercise programs for older adults. For those who have limited MOBILITY, chair exercises are provided.

Swimming is also recommended but does not offer the weight-bearing advantage of walking. Weight bearing helps build bone, an especially important advantage for older women to prevent osteoporosis (see Chapter 50). Teach older adults who have been sedentary to start their exercise programs slowly and gradually increase the frequency and duration of activity over time, under the direction of their health care provider.

NCLEX EXAMINATION CHALLENGE

Health Promotion and Maintenance

Which statement by an older adult regarding diet and exercise indicates a need for further teaching by the nurse?

A. "I need to include more fiber in my diet like whole grains, raw vegetables, and fruits."
B. "I just joined our local fitness center and plan to go there three times a week"
C. "I will stop drinking fluids after 4 PM to prevent getting up during the night."
D. "I drink prune juice every day and that keeps my bowels very regular."

Stress and Loss

Stress can speed up the aging process over time, or it can lead to diseases that increase the rate of degeneration. It can also impair the reserve capacity of older adults and lessen their ability to respond and adapt to changes in their environment.

Although no period of the life cycle is free from stress, the later years can be a time of especially high risk. Frequent sources of stress and anxiety for the older population include:

- Rapid environmental changes that require immediate reaction
- Changes in lifestyle resulting from retirement or physical incapacity
- Acute or chronic illness
- Loss of significant others
- Financial hardships
- Relocation

How people react to these stresses depends on their personal coping skills and support networks. For instance, losses leave many older adults without friends for support and help. As a result, many must rely solely on their personal resources to maintain their mental health/behavioral health. A combination of poor physical health and social problems leaves older adults susceptible to stress overload, which can result in illness and premature death.

The ways in which people adapt to old age depend largely on the personality traits and coping strategies that have characterized them throughout their lives. Establishing and maintaining relationships with others throughout life are especially important to the older person's happiness. Even more important than having friends is the nature of the friendships. People who have close, intimate, stable relationships with others in whom they confide are more likely to cope with crisis.

Some older adults have chosen to return to work at least on a part-time basis to increase their income and socialize with other people. If a person retired between the ages of 55 and 65 years and lives into his or her 80s, funds can deplete; additional income is needed to meet basic needs, including money for prescription drugs. Although U.S. government Medicare Part A pays for inpatient hospital care, older adults pay for Medicare Part B to reimburse for 80% of most ambulatory care services, Medicare Part D for prescription drugs, and often a private Medi-Gap insurance (e.g., United or Blue Cross/Blue Shield) to cover the costs not paid for by Medicare. The premiums for these insurances are very expensive and may still require that older adults pay out-of-pocket copayments for health care services and prescription drugs.

Fortunately, most older adults are relatively healthy and live in and own their own homes. Physical and/or mental health problems may force some to relocate to a retirement center or an assisted-living facility, although these facilities can be very expensive. Others move in with family members or to apartment buildings funded and designated for seniors. Older adults usually have more difficulty adjusting to major change when compared with younger and middle-aged adults. Being admitted to a hospital or nursing home is a particularly traumatic experience. Older adults often suffer from relocation stress syndrome, also known as *relocation trauma.* **Relocation stress syndrome** is the physical and emotional distress that occurs after the person moves from one setting to another. Examples of physiologic behaviors are sleep disturbance and increased physical symptoms, such as GI distress. Examples of emotional manifestations are withdrawal, anxiety, anger, and depression. Chart 2-2 lists nursing interventions that may help decrease the effects of relocation.

Family members and facility staff need to be aware that older adults need personal space in their new surroundings. Older adults need to participate in deciding how the space will be arranged and what they can keep in their new home to help offset potential feelings of powerlessness. Suggest that the patient or family bring in personal items, such as pictures of

CHART 2-2 **Best Practice for Patient Safety & Quality Care** QSEN

Minimizing the Effects of Relocation Stress in Older Adults

- Provide opportunities for the patient to assist in decision making.
- Carefully explain all procedures and routines to the patient before they occur.
- Ask the family or significant other to provide familiar or special keepsakes to keep at the patient's bedside (e.g., family picture, favorite hairbrush).
- Reorient the patient frequently to his or her location.
- Ask the patient about his or her expectations during hospitalization or assisted-living or nursing home stay.
- Encourage the patient's family and friends to visit often.
- Establish a trusting relationship with the patient as early as possible.
- Assess the patient's usual lifestyle and daily activities, including food likes and dislikes and preferred time for bathing.
- Avoid unnecessary room changes.
- If possible, have a family member, significant other, staff member, or volunteer accompany the patient when leaving the unit for special procedures or therapies.

relatives and friends, favorite clothing, and valued knickknacks, to assist in making the new setting seem more familiar and comfortable. This same intervention can be carried out in a hospital setting.

Accidents

Accidents are very common among older adults; falls are the most common. Motor vehicle crashes increase as well because of physiologic changes of aging or chronic diseases like Alzheimer's or peripheral neuropathy.

Fall Prevention

Most accidents occur at home. Teach older adults about the need to be aware of safety precautions to prevent accidents, such as falls. Incapacitating accidents are a primary cause of decreased MOBILITY and chronic pain in old age. Some people develop **fallophobia** (fear of falling) and avoid leaving their homes.

Home modifications may help prevent falls. Collaborate with family and significant others when recommending useful changes to prevent older adult injury. Safeguards such as handrails, slip-proof pads for rugs, and adequate lighting are essential in the home. Avoiding scatter rugs, slippery floors, and clutter is also important to prevent falls. Installing grab bars and using non-slip bathmats can help prevent falls in the bathroom. Raised toilet seats are also important. Remind older adults to avoid going out on days when steps are wet or icy and to ask for help when ambulating. To minimize sensory overload, advise the older adult to concentrate on one activity at a time.

Changes in SENSORY PERCEPTION and MOBILITY can create challenges for older adults in any environment. For example, **presbyopia** (farsightedness that worsens with aging) may make walking more difficult; the person is less aware of the location of each step. In addition, the older adult may have disorders that affect visual acuity, such as macular degeneration, cataracts, glaucoma, or diabetic retinopathy. Teach the person to look down at where he or she is walking and have frequent eye examinations to update glasses or contact lenses to improve vision. Drug therapy or surgery may be needed to correct glaucoma or cataracts.

A reduced sense of touch decreases the awareness of body orientation (e.g., whether the foot is squarely on the step). The decreased reaction time that commonly results from age-related changes in the neurologic system may also impair the ability to recognize or move from a dangerous setting. Chronic diseases such as peripheral neuropathy and arthritis can affect MOBILITY and SENSORY PERCEPTION in the older adult as well. If needed, encourage the use of visual, hearing, or ambulatory assistive devices. High costs and a fear of appearing old sometimes prevent older adults from obtaining or using hearing aids, eyeglasses, walkers, or canes.

Once an older person has been identified as being at high risk for falls, choose interventions that help prevent falls and possible serious injury. For example, for those in the community, tai chi exercise is very helpful to improve balance and functional MOBILITY, as well as to decrease the fear of falling, especially among older women (Wooten, 2010).

Driving Safety

Motor vehicle crashes are the most common cause of injury-related death in the young-old population—those between 65 and 74 years of age. Increased national concerns about this growing problem have prompted many states to require more frequent testing for older drivers. As one ages, reaction time and the ability to multitask decrease. Sleep disturbances, especially insomnia, are also common in older adults but are *not* part of normal aging. Some crashes occur because the person falls asleep while driving.

The older the person, the more likely he or she will have chronic diseases and the drugs needed to manage them. These health problems and treatments can contribute to motor vehicle crashes. For instance, drugs used for hypertension can cause orthostatic hypotension (low blood pressure when changing body position from a supine to sitting or standing position).

Physicians and other health care professionals play a major role in identifying driver safety issues. Yet, many are reluctant to intervene because older patients feel they will lose their independence if they cannot drive. They may also be angry and resistant to the idea of giving up perhaps their only means of transportation. As an alternative, health care professionals can recommend driving refresher courses and suggest that high-risk driving conditions, like wet roads, be avoided. Newer vehicles have some safety features to help older adults, such as large-print digital readouts for speed and other data. Chart 2-3 lists additional ways to improve older adult driver safety.

Drug Use and Misuse

Drug therapy for the older population is another major health issue. Because of the multiple chronic and acute health problems that occur in this age-group, drugs for older adults account for about one third of all prescription drug costs. The term **polymedicine** has been used to describe the use of many drugs to treat multiple health problems for older adults. **Polypharmacy** is the use of multiple drugs, duplicative drug therapy, high-dosage medications, and drugs prescribed for too long a period of time (Planton & Edlund, 2010). Another term, hyperpharmacy, has also been used to describe the excessive use of drugs to treat disease (Messina & Escallier, 2011).

Older adults commonly take multiple nonprescription (OTC) drugs, such as analgesics, antacids, cold and cough preparations, laxatives, and herbal/nutritional supplements, often without consulting a health care provider. Therefore this

CHART 2-3 Best Practice for Patient Safety & Quality Care QSEN

Recommendations for Improving Older Adult Driver Safety

- Discuss driving ability with the patient to assess his or her perception.
- Assess physical and mental deficits that could affect driving ability.
- Consult with appropriate health care providers to treat health problems that could interfere with driving.
- Suggest community-based transportation options, if available, instead of driving.
- Discuss driving concerns with patients and their families.
- Remind the patient to wear glasses and hearing aids, if prescribed.
- Encourage driver refresher classes, often offered by AARP (formerly the American Association of Retired Persons).
- Consult a certified driving specialist for an on-road driving assessment.
- Encourage avoiding high-risk driving locations or conditions, such as busy urban interstates and wet or icy weather conditions.
- Report unsafe drivers to the state department of motor vehicles if they continue to drive.

population is at high risk for adverse drug events (ADEs) directly related to the number of drugs taken and the frequency with which they are taken. Drug-drug, food-drug, drug-herb, and drug-disease interactions are common ADEs that often lead to hospital admission.

Effects of Drugs on Older Adults

Older adults often do not tolerate the standard dosage of drugs traditionally prescribed for younger adults. The physiologic changes related to aging make drug therapy more complex and challenging. These changes affect the absorption, distribution, metabolism, and excretion of drugs from the body. Even common antibiotics can lead to temporary memory loss or acute confusion. More commonly, antibiotic therapy can cause a *Clostridium difficile* infection, as discussed in Chapter 23.

Age-related changes that can potentially affect drug *absorption* from an oral route include an increase in gastric pH, a decrease in gastric blood flow, and a decrease in GI motility. Despite these changes, older adults do not have major absorption difficulties because of age-related changes alone.

Age-related changes that affect drug *distribution* include smaller amounts of total body water, an increased ratio of adipose tissue to lean body mass, a decreased albumin level, and a decreased cardiac output. Increased adipose tissue in proportion to lean body mass can cause increased storage of lipid-soluble drugs. This leads to a decreased concentration of the drug in plasma but an increased concentration in tissue.

Drug *metabolism* often occurs in the liver. Age-related changes affecting metabolism include a decrease in liver size, a decrease in liver blood flow, and a decrease in serum liver enzyme activity. These changes can result in increased plasma concentrations of a drug (Lilley, Collins, & Snyder, 2014). Monitor liver function studies, and teach older adults to have regular physical examinations.

Changes in the kidneys can also result in high plasma concentrations of drugs. The *excretion* of drugs usually involves the renal system. Age-related changes of the renal system include decreased renal blood flow and reduced glomerular filtration rate. These changes result in a decreased creatinine clearance and thus a slower excretion time for medications. Consequently,

TABLE 2-1 Common Adverse Drug Events (ADEs) in Older Adults

• Edema	• Dizziness
• Severe nausea and vomiting	• Syncope
• Anorexia	• Urinary retention
• Dehydration	• Diarrhea
• Dysrhythmias	• Constipation/impaction
• Fatigue	• Hypotension
• Weakness	• Acute confusion

Data from Berryman, S.N., Jennings, J., Ragsdale, S., Lofton, T., Huff, D.C., & Rooker, J.S. (2012). Beers criteria for potentially inappropriate medication use in older adults. *MEDSURG Nursing, 21,* 129-133.

serum drug levels can become toxic and the patient can become extremely ill or die. *Monitor renal studies, especially serum creatinine and creatinine clearance, when giving drugs to older adults!*

A creatinine clearance test measures the glomerular filtration rate of the kidneys. A commonly used formula for calculating creatinine clearance for men rather than directly measuring it is:

$$\frac{(140 - \text{Age in years}) \times \text{Lean body weight in kg}}{\text{Serum creatinine in mg/dL} \times 72}$$

For women, use this formula and multiply the answer by 0.85. A normal creatinine clearance for men is 107 to 139 mL/min and for women is 87 to 107 mL/min. Values decrease by 6.5 mL/min for each decade of life after 20 years of age (Pagana & Pagana, 2014).

When chronic disease is added to the physiologic changes of aging, drug reactions have a more dramatic effect and take longer to correct. Often a lower dose of a drug is necessary to prevent ADEs. The policy of "start low, go slow" is essential when health care providers prescribe drugs for older adults. The physiologic changes of aging are highly individual. Alterations in drug therapy should always be individualized according to the actual physiologic changes present and the occurrence and severity of chronic disease. Common ADEs are listed in Table 2-1.

Self-Administration of Drugs

Most people older than 65 years take their own medications. Because the risk for drug toxicity is considerably increased in the older population, assist patients in assuming this task responsibly. Teach patients and their caregivers, providing clear and concise directions and developing ways to assist them in overcoming difficulties with self-administration.

Older adults may make errors in self-administration or do not adhere to the drug regimen for several reasons. First, they may simply forget. In the rush of daily activities, they may not take their drugs or may take them too often because they cannot remember when or whether they have taken the medications. It is often helpful if they associate pill taking with daily events (e.g., meals) or keep a simple chart or calendar. Pill boxes are available for a daily, weekly, or monthly supply of medicine that can be placed in small compartments (Fig. 2-2). Egg cartons can be very cost-effective pill boxes. Large print on the drug label assists patients who have poor vision. Writing the drug regimen on the top of the bottle with large letters and numbers is helpful for some older adults. Colored labels or dots can also be applied. Easy-open bottle caps help older adults with limited hand mobility or strength.

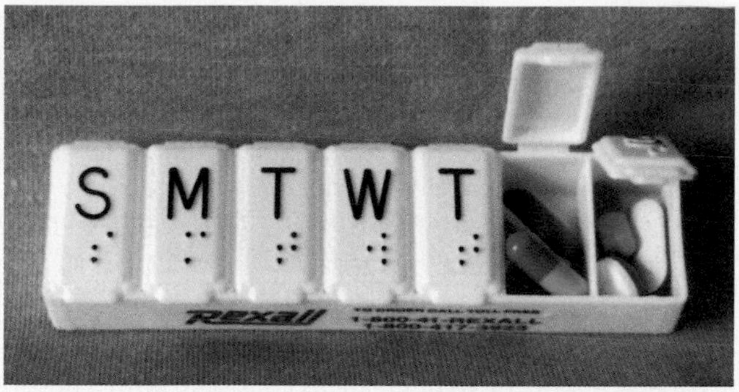

FIG. 2-2 A medication system for safe self-administration.

A second reason for drug errors is poor communication with health care professionals. These problems result from poor explanations that are not understood because of educational limitations, language barriers, or difficulty with hearing and vision. Health care professionals often presume that their patients have learned the information if they have taught them about the drugs. Assist older adults in planning their drug therapy schedules as needed.

Complementary and Alternative Therapies. A third reason for errors is the varying ways that older adults take their medications. Many people older than 65 years use a multitude of complementary and alternative therapies. Some add to their drug regimen by taking OTC drugs, which can interact with prescription drugs and cause serious problems (Vitale, 2012). For example, a patient receiving warfarin (Coumadin, Warfilone ✤) for anticoagulation may take ibuprofen (Motrin) regularly for arthritis or garlic for hypertension. Because ibuprofen and garlic can inhibit clotting, this combination can cause serious bleeding. When obtaining a drug history, ask patients about all OTC drugs, including herbal and food supplements.

Some other older adults avoid taking their prescribed drugs. The fear of dependency or the cost of the drugs may cause many to discontinue their drug therapy too soon or not begin taking the drug. In addition, the actions or side effects of some drugs may not be desirable. For example, diuretics may cause incontinence when patients cannot get to the bathroom quickly enough. Others may think that two pills are twice as effective and, therefore, better than taking just one. Some older adults take drugs that are leftover from a previous illness or one that is borrowed from someone else. Teach patients to take their medications exactly as prescribed by their health care providers.

Medication Assessment and Health Teaching

The *Healthy People 2020* initiative recommends that older adults be interviewed regarding their medication use and include these questions:

- Do you take five or more prescription medications?
- Do you take herbs, vitamins, or other dietary supplements, or OTC medications?
- Do you have your prescriptions filled at more than one pharmacy?
- Is more than one health care practitioner prescribing your medications?
- Do you take your medications more than once a day?
- Do you have trouble opening your medication bottles?
- Do you have poor eyesight or hearing?
- Do you live alone?

TABLE 2-2 Examples of Beers Criteria for Potentially Inappropriate Medication Use in Older Adults

• meperidine (Demerol) • cyclobenzaprine (Flexeril) • digoxin (Lanoxin) (Should not exceed 0.125 mg daily except for atrial fibrillation) • ticlopidine (Ticlid) • fluoxetine (Prozac) • amitriptyline (Elavil) • diazepam (Valium)	• promethazine (Phenergan) • ketorolac (Toradol) • short-acting nifedipine (e.g., Procardia) • ferrous sulfate (Iron) (Should not exceed 325 mg daily) • chlorpropamide (Diabinese) • diphenhydramine (Benadryl)

Data from Berryman, S.N., Jennings, J., Ragsdale, S., Lofton, T., Huff, D.C., & Rooker, J.S. (2012). Beers criteria for potentially inappropriate medication use in older adults. *MEDSURG Nursing, 21,* 129-133.

- Do you have a hard time remembering to take your medications?

The Beers Criteria for Potentially Inappropriate Medication Use in Older Adults assessment tool, simply known as the *Beers criteria,* is also very useful in screening for medication-related risks in older adults who have chronic health problems (Berryman et al., 2012). The tool lists multiple medications and related concerns. Examples of these "at-risk" drugs are listed in Table 2-2.

To reduce drug-related risks in older adults, perform a medication assessment every 6 months or more often if an acute illness or exacerbation of a chronic disease occurs. Be sure to:

- Obtain a list of all medications taken on a regular and as-needed basis; include OTC and prescribed drugs, herbs, and nutritional supplements. If a list is not available, ask the older adult or family to gather all ointments, pills, lotions, eyedrops, inhalers, injectable solutions, vitamins, minerals, herbs, and other OTC medications and place into a bag for review.
- Highlight all medications that are part of the Beers criteria; highlight any medication for which the indication for its use is not clear, inappropriate, or could be discontinued (e.g., duplicative drug).
- Collaborate with the older adult, family, pharmacist, and primary health care provider if appropriate to determine the need for medication changes. Suggest once-a-day dosing if possible.
- Give older adults verbal and written information (at the appropriate reading level) regarding any change or new medication prescribed.
- Promote adherence to the drug therapy regimen exactly as prescribed; remind older adults to check with their primary care provider if they want to change their regimen or add an OTC medication or natural product (nutritional or herbal supplement, or probiotic).

NCLEX EXAMINATION CHALLENGE

Physiological Integrity

A home care nurse conducts an assessment of an older woman's medications and herbal/nutritional supplements. Which supplement is most likely to cause an interaction with prescribed medications?

A. Calcium
B. Vitamin C
C. St. John's wort
D. Vitamin B complex

- Encourage lifestyle changes and other nonpharmacologic interventions to help manage or prevent health problems.
- Remind older adults not to share or borrow medications.

Mental Health/Behavioral Health Problems

Older adults are usually mentally sound and competent. Some changes in COGNITION have been identified as age related and are linked to specific cognitive functions rather than intellectual capacity. These changes include a decreased reaction time to stimuli and an impaired memory for recent events. *However, severe cognitive impairment, depression, hallucinations, and delusions are not common.*

Two forms of competence exist: legal competence and clinical competence. A person is **legally competent** if he or she is:

- 18 years of age or older
- Pregnant or a married minor
- A legally emancipated (free) minor who is self-supporting
- Not declared incompetent by a court of law

If a court determines that an older adult is not legally competent, a **guardian** is appointed to make health care decisions. Guardians may be family members or a person who is not related to the patient. When no one is available, a guardian may be appointed from a local Area Agency on Aging, an organization with comprehensive services and resources for older adults.

A person is **clinically competent** if he or she is legally competent and can make clinical decisions. Decisional capacity is determined by a person's ability to identify problems, recognize options, make decisions, and provide the rationale supporting the decisions. Selected behavioral/mental illnesses often affect both legal and clinical competence.

Nurses are in a unique position to teach older adults about ways to promote cognitive health. In a recent systematic literature review, Williams and Kemper (2010) found that collaborative interventions targeting cognitive training (e.g., learning a new skill), physical activity, social engagement, and NUTRITION were the most helpful in optimizing cognitive aging.

As older adults age, they are at increasing risk for severe mental health problems—depression, delirium, and dementia, often referred to as the *3Ds.* Many older veterans of the Korean and Vietnam wars also suffer from chronic pain, depression, post-traumatic stress disorder (PTSD), and severe anxiety. Substance abuse, especially alcoholism, is common among veterans and older adults in general. Alcoholism can contribute to cognitive decline and may be used as a coping mechanism for loss. Several mental health problems are discussed briefly here; more comprehensive discussions can be found in mental health/behavioral health textbooks.

Depression

Depression is the most common mental health/behavioral health problem among older adults in the community, affecting 15 of every 100 older adults (National Institute of Mental Health [NIMH], 2011). It increases in incidence when older adults are admitted to the hospital or nursing home. **Depression** is broadly defined as a mood disorder that can have cognitive, affective, and physical manifestations. It can be primary or secondary and can range from mild to severe, or major. As a *primary* problem, depression is thought to result from a lack of the neurotransmitters *norepinephrine* and *serotonin* in the brain. *Secondary* depression, sometimes called *situational* depression, can result when there is a sudden change in the person's life, such as an illness or loss. Common illnesses that can cause secondary depression include stroke, arthritis, and cardiac disease. It is often underdiagnosed by physicians and is therefore undertreated.

Families and nurses are in the best position to suspect depression in an older adult. Several screening tools are available to help determine if the patient has clinical depression. The **Geriatric Depression Scale—Short Form (GDS-SF)** is a valid and reliable screening tool and is available in multiple languages. The patient selects "yes" or "no" to 15 questions, or a nurse or other health care professional can ask the questions to the patient. A score of 10 or greater is consistent with a possible diagnosis of clinical depression (Fig. 2-3). These patients are then evaluated more thoroughly by the health care provider for treatment. Without diagnosis and treatment, depression can result in:

- Worsening of medical conditions
- Risk for physical illness
- Alcoholism and drug abuse
- Increased pain and disability
- Delayed recovery from illness
- Suicide

Older adults with depression may have early morning insomnia, excessive daytime sleeping, poor appetite, a lack of energy, and an unwillingness to participate in social and recreational activities. The primary treatment for depression usually includes drug therapy and psychotherapy. Selective serotonin reuptake inhibitors (SSRIs) are the first choice for drug therapy but take 2 to 3 weeks to work. They act by increasing the amount of serotonin and norepinephrine at nerve synapses in the brain.

! NURSING SAFETY PRIORITY QSEN

Drug Alert

Tricyclic antidepressants should not be used because they have anticholinergic properties that can cause acute confusion, severe constipation, and urinary incontinence. For older adults who may be prescribed this group of drugs, question the health care provider and request an SSRI or other treatment.

Recent research has demonstrated that reminiscence or reflective therapies also help older adults overcome feelings of depression and despair. A study by McCaffrey et al. (2010) determined that frequent walking through a large garden and reflective journaling decreased depression as measured by the Geriatric Depression Scale (see the Evidence-Based Practice box). More information about depression, including strategies for preventing depression, is available in mental health/behavioral health nursing textbooks.

Dementia

Dementia is a broad term used for a syndrome that involves a slowly progressive cognitive decline, sometimes referred to as *chronic confusion.* This syndrome represents a global impairment of intellectual function and is generally chronic and progressive. There are many types of dementia, the most common being Alzheimer's disease. Multi-infarct dementia, the second most common dementia, results from a vascular disorder. Chapter 42 discusses dementias in detail, with a focus on Alzheimer's disease.

Geriatric Depression Scale—Short Form

Choose the best answer for how you have felt over the past week:

1. Are you basically satisfied with your life? YES / **NO**
2. Have you dropped many of your activities and interests? **YES** / NO
3. Do you feel that your life is empty? **YES** / NO
4. Do you often get bored? **YES** / NO
5. Are you in good spirits most of the time? YES / **NO**
6. Are you afraid that something bad is going to happen to you? **YES** / NO
7. Do you feel happy most of the time? YES / **NO**
8. Do you often feel helpless? **YES** / NO
9. Do you prefer to stay at home, rather than going out and doing new things? **YES** / NO
10. Do you feel you have more problems with memory than most? **YES** / NO
11. Do you think it is wonderful to be alive now? YES / **NO**
12. Do you feel pretty worthless the way you are now? **YES** / NO
13. Do you feel full of energy? YES / **NO**
14. Do you feel that your situation is hopeless? **YES** / NO
15. Do you think that most people are better off than you are? **YES** / NO

Answers in bold indicate depression. Score 1 point for each bolded answer.

A score > 5 points is suggestive of depression.
A score ≥ 10 points is almost always indicative of depression.
A score > 5 points should warrant a follow-up comprehensive assessment.

FIG. 2-3 The Geriatric Depression Scale—Short Form.

EVIDENCE-BASED PRACTICE QSEN

Do Reflective Activities Improve Symptoms of Depression and Despair in Older Adults?

McCaffrey, R., Hanson, C., & McCaffrey, W. (2010). Garden walking for depression: A research report. *Holistic Nursing Practice, 24*(5), 252-259.

Depression affects 15 of every 100 older adults at some point in their later years, which leads to physical, mental, and social dysfunction. In this mixed-method design study, the researchers created a walking guide and reflective journal entitled *Stroll for Well-Being: Garden Walks at the Morikami Museum* (Stroll) to be used by 40 community-dwelling older adults at their convenience for 12 visits over a period of 6 months. The participants were either self-diagnosed or were being treated by a health care provider for depression. The sample was 62.5% white and 12.5% African American. The remaining group was a mix of ethnic backgrounds. Most participants were educated at a high school level or higher.

The *Stroll* was structured so that they would spend about 2 hours each at 6 stops in the Morikami Museum and Japanese Gardens. At each stop, the participants made entries into a reflective journal to share their lived experience.

Using the short-form Geriatric Depression Scale (GDS) as a quantitative measure before and after the intervention, the researchers found a statistically significant change in depression scores, with lower scores indicating less depression. For the qualitative aspect of the study, a 4-step thematic analysis of the journal entries included:

- Being forced to spend time away from pressures of the day
- A sense of the beauty of nature
- Using the gardens to provide insight and depth to the experience
- Gratitude for the beauty of nature and the "life I have led"

Level of Evidence: 4

This study is a small descriptive study but includes both quantitative and qualitative methods to study the effect of the intervention for a selected convenience sample.

Commentary: Implications for Practice and Research

Depression is usually treated with psychotherapy and drugs, which often cause adverse drug effects in older adults. When nurses care for older adults with depression, they need to recommend alternative and complementary interventions that may help relieve depressive symptoms and possibly decrease dependence on drug therapy. Using the findings of this study, it is clear that enjoying the beauty of nature and reflecting on life experiences can benefit patients who have been diagnosed with or suspect that they have depression.

Delirium

Whereas dementia is a chronic, progressive disorder, **delirium** is an *acute* state of confusion. Delirium also differs from dementia in that it is often short-term and reversible within a month or less. It is often seen among older adults in a setting with which they are unfamiliar. It occurs in up to 50% of older adults who are hospitalized (Sendelbach & Guthrie, 2009). In addition to cognitive changes, some patients have physical and emotional manifestations. The types of delirium are *hyperactive, hypoactive, mixed,* and *unclassifiable. Hyperactive* patients may try to climb out of bed or become agitated, restless, and aggressive. *Hypoactive* patients are quiet, apathetic, and withdrawn. *Mixed* delirium patients have a combination of hyperactive and hypoactive manifestations. Others cannot be classified in one of these categories.

Some of the multiple factors that can cause delirium are:
- Drug therapy (especially anticholinergic and psychoactive drugs)
- Electrolyte imbalances
- Infections, especially urinary tract, pneumonia, and sepsis
- Fecal impaction or severe diarrhea
- Surgery
- Metabolic problems, such as hypoglycemia
- Neurologic disorders, such as tumors
- Circulatory, renal, and pulmonary disorders
- Nutritional deficiencies
- Hypoxemia (decreased arterial oxygen level)
- Relocation
- Major loss

! NURSING SAFETY PRIORITY QSEN

Action Alert

Acutely confused patients who are discharged from the hospital are at an increased risk for functional decline, falls, and incontinence at home. Therefore carefully assess older patients in any setting for acute confusion so that it can be managed.

A number of tools have been developed for point-of-care screening for delirium, including the Confusion Assessment Method (CAM), Delirium Index (DI), NEECHAM Confusion Scale, and Mini-Cog (Sendelbach & Guthrie, 2009). The CAM consists of nine open-ended questions and a diagnostic algorithm for determining delirium (Table 2-3). This screening tool is easily adaptable for computerized point-of-care charting (Swan et al., 2011).

TABLE 2-3 The Confusion Assessment Method (CAM)

1. Acute onset and fluctuating course (e.g., Is there evidence of an acute change in mental status from the patient's baseline?)
2. Inattention (e.g., Does the patient have difficulty focusing attention or keeping track of what is being said?)
3. Disorganized thinking (e.g., Is the patient's thinking and conversation disorganized or incoherent?)
4. Altered level of consciousness (e.g., Is the patient lethargic, hyperalert, or difficult to arouse?)

The diagnosis of delirium by the CAM is the presence of features 1 and 2 *and* either 3 *or* 4.

Data from Sendelbach, S., & Guthrie, P.F. (2009). Evidence-based guideline—Acute confusion/delirium: Identification, assessment, treatment, and prevention. *Journal of Gerontological Nursing, 35*(11), 11-17.

Collaborate with the health care team to remove or treat risk or causative factors for acute confusion. For example, if the patient has a low oxygen saturation level, provide supplemental oxygen therapy to increase oxygen to the brain. If the patient has a urinary tract infection (UTI), it is treated. The primary clinical manifestation of UTIs in older adults is acute confusion.

To help prevent and manage delirium, use a calm voice to frequently reorient the patient. For example, playing tapes of soothing music may have a calming effect. Providing a doll or stuffed animal to "fidget" with may prevent the patient from removing important medical tubes or equipment. Some nurses believe that providing dolls and stuffed animals is treating the adult like a child, but this intervention can sometimes be very effective when used for therapeutic purposes. If the patient has a favorite item, such as an afghan blanket or a picture, ask the family or significant others to provide it for the same purpose.

Table 2-4 highlights the major differences between delirium and dementia and lists the major nursing considerations for each. The most difficult challenge is caring for a patient who is experiencing both problems at the same time.

Alcohol Use and Abuse

Excessive alcohol consumption increases the risk for falls and other accidents, affects mood and COGNITION, and leads to complications of chronic diseases like diabetes mellitus, hypertension, and gastroesophageal reflux disease (GERD). Isolation, depression, and delirium can result from alcohol abuse. The National Institute on Alcohol Abuse and Alcoholism (NIAAA) recommends that people older than 65 years have no more than one alcoholic drink a day or seven drinks in a week (NIAAA, 2011).

The Short Michigan Alcoholism Screening Test—Geriatric Version (SMAST-G) is often used by nurses and other health care professionals in ambulatory care settings to detect alcohol abuse or alcoholism. The 10 yes/no question test is available in English and Spanish and can be either self-administered

TABLE 2-4 Differences in the Characteristics of Delirium and Dementia

VARIABLE	DEMENTIA	DELIRIUM
Description	A chronic, progressive cognitive decline	An acute confusional state
Onset	Slow	Fast
Duration	Months to years	Hours to less than 1 month
Cause	Unknown, possibly familial, chemical	Multiple, such as surgery, infection, drugs
Reversibility	None	Usually
Management	Treat signs and symptoms	Remove or treat the cause
Nursing interventions	Reorientation not effective in the late stages; use validation therapy (acknowledge the patient's feelings, and do not argue); provide a safe environment; observe for associated behaviors, such as delusions and hallucinations	Reorient the patient to reality; provide a safe environment

or administered by a clinician. Examples of questions on the tool are:

- Do you drink to take your mind off your problems?
- When you feel lonely, does having a drink help?

A "yes" answer is worth one point. A total score of two or more points indicates that the person has a problem with alcohol.

Other screening tools for alcohol misuse in older adults include the CAGE questionnaire and the Alcohol-Related Problems Survey (ARPS) and the Short ARPS (shARPS). The acronym *CAGE* comes from four questions:

- Have you ever tried to cut down on your drinking?
- Have people annoyed you by criticizing your drinking?
- Have you ever felt bad or guilty about your drinking?
- Have you ever had a drink first thing in the morning to settle your nerves to get rid of a hangover (eye-opener)?

The ARPS and shARPS were created specifically for use with older adults. In a classic study by Fink et al. (2002), these tools were shown to be more sensitive than the SMAST-G and CAGE screening tests in identifying older adults at risk for alcohol abuse. Those who were identified as non-hazardous and harmful drinkers by the ARPS tool were not identified by other tools. These groups were not diagnosed as having alcoholism but were at risk for this problem.

CLINICAL JUDGMENT CHALLENGE

Patient-Centered Care; Safety QSEN

A 67-year-old man recently lost his wife after being married for 42 years. He met his wife shortly after he returned from Vietnam as a combat soldier. He visits his physician and reports decreased appetite, moodiness, and extreme fatigue, even though he sleeps 10 to 12 hours a night. When giving his medical history, he admits that he drinks 4 or 5 beers and smokes marijuana almost every day.

1. What do you think caused this man's new symptoms and why?
2. As this man's office nurse, what other assessment data do you need to collect? What screening tools might you use?
3. For what safety issues is this older adult at risk and why?
4. With whom might you collaborate to develop his plan of care?

Elder Neglect and Abuse

Another problem for some older adults is neglect and abuse, both verbal and physical. Some older adults are more vulnerable to these problems than others, especially widows who may have difficulty being assertive. Elder abuse and neglect is a serious problem that affects an estimated 2 million older adults each year (U.S. Census Bureau, 2013). Older persons who are neglected or abused are often physically dependent. The abuser is often a family member who becomes frustrated or distraught over the burden of caring for the older adult. Unfortunately, only a few cases of elder abuse are reported (Stark, 2012).

Prolonged caregiving by a family member is a new and unexpected role for adult children, usually women. This new role may result in role fatigue, conflict, and strain. As a result, **neglect** can occur when a caregiver fails to provide for an older adult's basic needs, such as food, clothing, medications, or assistance with ADLs. The caregiver refuses to let other people, like nursing assistants or home care nurses, into the home. Whether intentional or unintentional, neglect accounts for almost half of all cases of actual elder abuse.

Physical abuse is the use of physical force that results in bodily injury, especially in the "bathing suit" zone (abdomen, buttocks, genital area, upper thighs). Examples of physical abuse are hitting, burning, pushing, and molesting the patient. Sedating the older adult is also abusive. **Financial abuse** occurs when the older adult's property or resources are mismanaged or misused; this is more common than physical abuse. **Emotional abuse** is the intentional use of threats, humiliation, intimidation, and isolation toward older adults.

Carefully assess the patient for signs of abuse, such as bruises in clusters or regular patterns; burns, commonly to the buttocks or the soles of the feet; unusual hair loss; or multiple injuries, especially fractures. If the older adult is too weak or has no other resources or support systems, he or she may not admit that abuse is occurring. Neglect may be manifested by pressure ulcers, contractures, dehydration or malnutrition, urine burns, excessive body odor, and listlessness. Depression and dementia are common in community older adults who are abused or neglected.

Be sure to screen for abuse and neglect of older adults using an appropriate assessment tool. Table 2-5 lists tools that can be used by nurses and other health care professionals to screen for elder abuse and neglect (Stark, 2012). The older adult should be referred to the appropriate service when there is:

- Evidence of mistreatment without sufficient clinical explanation
- Report by an older adult of being abused or neglected
- A belief by the health care professional that there is a high risk for or probable abuse, neglect, abandonment, or exploitation

All states in the United States and other Western countries have laws requiring health care professionals to report suspected elder abuse. In the community, if physical abuse or neglect is suspected, notify the local Adult Protective Services agency. In a hospital or nursing home, notify the social worker or case manager, who then will report the problem to the appropriate agency.

HEALTH CARE ISSUES FOR OLDER ADULTS IN HOSPITALS AND LONG-TERM CARE SETTINGS

Older adults who are admitted to hospitals and long-term care settings such as nursing homes have special needs and potential health problems. Many of these problems are similar to those seen among community older adults as discussed in this chapter. The Joint Commission and other agencies have addressed some of the most common problems seen in older adults. In addition, since 1996, the Hartford Institute for Gerontological Nursing has worked to ensure that all hospitalized patients 65 years of age and older be given quality care.

Nurses may not be aware that the needs of older adults differ from those of younger adults. Some health care systems have designated Acute Care of the Elderly (ACE) units with geriatric

TABLE 2-5 Examples of Elder Abuse Screening Tools

- Elder Abuse Suspicion Index
- Elder Assessment Instrument
- Indicators of Abuse Screen
- Questions to Elicit Elder Abuse
- Hwalek-Sengstock Elder Abuse Screening Tool
- Caregiver Abuse Screen
- Brief Abuse Screen for the Elderly
- Vulnerability to Abuse Screening Scale

CULTURAL CONSIDERATIONS

Patient-Centered Care QSEN

The health of Hispanic older adults continues to lag behind that for non-Hispanic whites due to a number of factors, such as language barriers, inadequate health insurance, and lack of health care access. To add to this health disparity, most nurses and other health care professionals are not trained in the language or culture of Hispanic older adults. Some older Hispanic patients may have beliefs and values that conflict with traditional Western health care views. Be respectful of these differences and incorporate them into your patient's plan of care. Become educated about the Hispanic culture and learn to speak basic medical Spanish to foster communication and trust (Strunk et al., 2013).

GENDER HEALTH CONSIDERATIONS

Patient-Centered Care QSEN

Significant health disparities are also associated with the lesbian, gay, bisexual, transgender, and questioning (LGBTQ) older adult population. Compared with heterosexual adults, LGBTQ older adults are at an elevated risk for disability from chronic disease and mental distress (Fredriksen-Goldsen, 2011). When admitted to the hospital or nursing home, they may hide their gender identity and sexual orientation from the nurse and other health care providers because of fear of rejection, discrimination, or lack of adequate health care.

Do not assume that your older patients or visitors are heterosexual. Establish a safe and trusting relationship with the patient and discuss sexual orientation and gender issues in a private setting to emphasize confidentiality. Do not force patients to answer any questions with which they feel uncomfortable. Teach direct caregivers, such as nursing assistants, that they may observe patients with sexual organs that conflict with the patient's gender identity. If this situation occurs, remind them not to be offensive or judgmental but, rather, carry out the task as planned. Chapter 73 in this text describes care of transgender patients in detail.

resources nurses and geriatric clinical nurse specialists. The patients are cared for by geriatricians who specialize in the care of older adults.

Other hospitals have developed interdisciplinary programs system-wide to meet the special needs of older patients. The incentive for these new programs is the Nurses Improving Care for Healthsystem Elders (NICHE) project, which continues to generate evidence-based practice guidelines for older adult care.

The purpose of all of these programs and units is to focus on the special health care issues or geriatric syndromes seen in the older population (Brown-O'Hara, 2013). The **Fulmer SPICES** framework was developed as part of the NICHE project and identifies six serious "marker conditions" that can lead to longer hospital stays, higher medical costs, and even deaths. These conditions are:

- Sleep disorders
- Problems with eating or feeding
- Incontinence
- Confusion
- Evidence of falls
- Skin breakdown

Each of these problems is briefly described here and also is discussed in more detail in other parts of this chapter and the textbook. Other problems, such as depression and constipation, are also common in older hospitalized patients. Rather than being fully comprehensive, the SPICES framework is intended to be an easy tool that has been called "geriatric vital signs" (Fulmer, 2007).

Problems of Sleep, Nutrition, and Continence

Sleep disorders are common in hospitalized patients, especially older adults. Adequate rest is important for healing, as well as for physical and mental functioning. Pain, chronic disease, environmental noise and lighting, and staff conversations are a few of the many contributing factors to insomnia in the acute and long-term care setting. Assess the patient, and ask how he or she is sleeping. If the patient is not able to answer, observe for restlessness and other behaviors that could indicate lack of adequate rest. Manage the patient's pain by giving pain medication before bedtime. Attempt to keep patients awake during the day to prevent insomnia. Keep staff conversations as quiet as possible and away from patients' rooms. Dim the lights to make the patient area as dark as possible. Avoid making loud noises such as slamming doors. Postpone treatments until waking hours or early morning if they can be delayed safely. If possible, place a "Do not Disturb" sign on the patient's door to avoid unnecessary interruptions in sleep.

Problems with eating and feeding prevent the older patient from receiving adequate NUTRITION. Malnutrition is common among older adults and is associated with poor clinical outcomes, including death. In a study by Volkert et al. (2010), NUTRITION-related problems were present in half of 205 older patients admitted to a community hospital, but only 8.3% of them received enteral nutrition supplements. The researchers concluded that nutritional screenings and standard protocols should be implemented for older patients in all hospitals. Nurses need to perform nutritional screenings on the first day of patient admission, including a thorough nutritional history, weight, height, and body mass index (BMI) calculation. Chapter 60 describes nutritional screening in more detail.

Collaborate with the registered dietitian (RD) about the patient's nutritional status as needed to achieve health goals. Consider cultural preferences, and determine what foods the patient likes. Manage symptoms such as pain, nausea, and vomiting. If the patient has difficulty chewing or swallowing, coordinate a plan of care with the speech-language pathologist and dietitian. If there are no dietary restrictions, encourage family members or friends to bring in food that the patient might enjoy. Additional interventions to prevent nutrition-related problems are discussed in Chapter 60.

Urinary and bowel ELIMINATION *issues* vary in type and severity and may be caused by many factors, including acute or chronic disease, ADL ability, and available staff. Assess the patient to identify causes for incontinence or retention. *These problems are not physiologic changes of aging but are very common in both the hospital and long-term care setting.* Place the patient on a toileting schedule or a bowel or bladder training program, if appropriate. Delegate and supervise this activity to unlicensed assistive personnel. Chapters 6 and 66 discuss bladder training in detail; Chapter 6 describes bowel training as well. Constipation was described earlier in this chapter.

Confusion, Falls, and Skin Breakdown

Acute and chronic confusion affect many older patients in both the hospital and nursing home. Whereas chronic confusion states such as dementia are not reversible, acute confusion, or delirium, may be avoidable and is often reversible when the cause is resolved or removed (see Table 2-4). For example, avoiding multiple drugs and promoting adequate sleep can help prevent acute confusion. Help the patient by reorienting him or her to reality as much as needed. Keep the patient as

NCLEX EXAMINATION CHALLENGE

Physiological Integrity

An older adult returns to the orthopedic unit after an open reduction, internal fixation surgery for a fractured hip. Upon admission, she is combative and screaming profane language. What is the nurse's first action?

A. Increase the client's rate of intravenous fluids.
B. Give the client IV morphine stat.
C. Start oxygen via mask at 6 L/min.
D. Assess for risk factors that could cause her behaviors.

comfortable as possible; for example, provide interventions to control pain. Delirium is discussed earlier in this chapter. Chapter 42 describes dementia in detail.

The most common accident among older patients in a hospital or nursing home setting is falling. A **fall** is an unintentional change in body position that results in the patient's body coming to rest on the floor or ground. Some falls result in serious injuries such as fractures and head trauma. The Joint Commission's **National Patient Safety Goals (NPSGs)** require that all inpatient health care settings have admission and daily fall risk assessment tools and a fall reduction program for patients who are at high risk.

Assess all older patients for risk for falls. Many evidence-based assessment tools, such as the Morse Fall Scale, STRATIFY, and the Hendrich II Fall Risk Model (HIIFRM), have been developed to help the nurse focus on factors that increase an older person's risk for falling. Some of these tools also recommend selected interventions depending on the patient's fall risk score (Swartzell et al., 2013). Chart 2-4 lists some of the common risk factors that should be assessed and evidence-based, collaborative interventions for preventing falls in high-risk patients. *A recent history of falling is the single most important predictor for falls.*

Toileting-related falls are very common, especially at night (Tzeng & Yin, 2012). Older patients often have **nocturia** (urination at night) and get out of bed to go to the bathroom. They may forget to ask for assistance and may subsequently fall as a result of disorientation in the darkness in an unfamiliar environment. In some cases, they may crawl over the siderail, which can make the fall more serious. Because of this, full or split siderails are used far less often in both hospitals and nursing homes. In both settings, siderails are classified as restraints unless the use of rails helps patients increase mobility.

A **restraint** is any device or drug that prevents the patient from moving freely and must be prescribed by a health care provider. In 1990, the federal government enforced a law that gives nursing home residents the right to be restraint free. Removing physical restraints from nursing home residents has reduced serious injuries, although falls and minor injuries have increased in some cases. Mattresses placed on floors next to patient beds or "low beds" have helped reduce injury.

Hospitals have also reduced the use of physical restraints. The Joint Commission has specific standards that limit the use of physical restraints in hospitals and nursing homes. Chemical restraints (psychoactive drugs) such as haloperidol (Haldol) have sometimes been used in place of physical restraints.

Experts agree that older adults should not be placed in a physical restraint or sedated just because they are old. Use alternatives before applying any type of restraint (Chart 2-5). However, if all other interventions (e.g., reminding patients to call for assistance when needed; asking a family member to stay with patients) are not effective in fall prevention, a physical restraint may be required for a limited period. Applying a restraint is a serious intervention and should be analyzed for its risk versus its benefit. Check the patient in a restraint every 30 to 60 minutes, and release the restraint at least every 2 hours for turning, repositioning, and toileting. Physical restraints such

CHART 2-4 Best Practice for Patient Safety & Quality Care QSEN

Assessing Risk Factors and Preventing Falls in Older Adults

Assess for the presence of these risk factors:

- History of falls
- Advanced age (>80 years)
- Multiple illnesses
- Generalized weakness or decreased mobility
- Gait and postural instability
- Disorientation or confusion
- Use of drugs that can cause increased confusion, mobility limitations, or orthostatic hypotension
- Urinary incontinence
- Communication impairments
- Major visual impairment or visual impairment without correction
- Alcohol or other substance abuse
- Location of patient's room away from the nurses' station (in the hospital or nursing home)
- Change of shift or mealtime (in the hospital or nursing home)

Implement these nursing interventions for all patients, regardless of risk:

- Monitor the patient's activities and behavior as often as possible, preferably every 30 to 60 minutes.
- Teach the patient and family about the fall prevention program to become safety partners.
- Remind the patient to call for help before getting out of bed or a chair.
- Help the patient to get out of bed or a chair if needed; lock all equipment, such as beds and wheelchairs, before transferring patients.
- Teach patients to use the grab bars when walking in the hall without assistive devices or when using the bathroom.
- Provide or remind the patient to use a walker or cane for ambulating if needed; educate him or her on how to use these devices.
- Remind the patient to wear eyeglasses or a hearing aid if needed.
- Help the incontinent patient to toilet every 1 to 2 hours.
- Clean up spills immediately.
- Arrange the furniture in the patient's room or hallway to eliminate clutter or obstacles that could contribute to a fall.
- Provide adequate lighting at all times, especially at night.
- Observe for side effects and toxic effects of drug therapy.
- Orient the patient to the environment.
- Keep the call light and patient care articles within reach; ensure that the patient can use the call light.
- Place the bed in the lowest position with the brakes locked.
- Place objects that the patient needs within reach.
- Ensure that adequate handrails are present in the patient's room, bathroom, and hall.
- Have the physical therapist assess the patient for mobility and safety.

For patients at a high risk for falls:

- Implement all assessments and interventions listed above.
- Relocate the patient for best visibility and supervision.
- Encourage family members or significant other to stay with the patient.
- Collaborate with other members of the health care team, especially the rehabilitative services.
- Use technologic devices to alert staff to patients getting out of bed, such as mattress sensor pads and chair alarms.
- Use low beds or futon-type beds to prevent injury if the patient falls out of bed.

CHART 2-5 Best Practice for Patient Safety & Quality Care QSEN

Using Restraint Alternatives

- If the patient is acutely confused, reorient him or her to reality as often as possible.
- If the patient has dementia, use validation to reaffirm his or her feelings and concerns.
- Check the patient often, at least every hour.
- If the patient pulls tubes and lines, cover them with roller gauze or another protective device; be sure that IV insertion sites are visible for assessment.
- Keep the patient busy, with an activity, pillow or apron, puzzle, or art project.
- Provide soft, calming music.
- Place the patient in an area where he or she can be supervised. (If the patient is agitated, do not place him or her in a noisy area.)
- Turn off the television if the patient is agitated.
- Ask a family member or friend to stay with the patient at night.
- Help the patient to toilet every 2 to 3 hours, including during the night.
- Be sure that the patient's needs for food, fluids, and comfort are met.
- If agency policy allows, provide the patient with a pet visit.
- Provide familiar objects or cherished items that the patient can touch.
- Document the use of all alternative interventions.
- If a restraint is applied, use the least restrictive device (e.g., mitts rather than wrist restraints, a roller belt rather than a vest).

as vests have caused serious injury and even death. *If restraint is needed, use the least restrictive device first. Be sure to follow your facility's policy and procedure for using restraints.*

Chemical restraints are often overused in hospital settings. Examples include:

- Antipsychotic drugs
- Antianxiety drugs
- Antidepressant drugs
- Sedative-hypnotic drugs

The most potent group of psychoactive drugs is the antipsychotics. These drugs are appropriate only for the control of certain behavioral problems, such as delusions, acute psychosis, and schizophrenia. Typical antipsychotic drugs include haloperidol (Haldol, Peridol ♣) and thiothixene (Navane). These drugs should not be used to treat anxiety or induce sedation.

! NURSING SAFETY PRIORITY QSEN

Drug Alert

Closely monitor older adults receiving antipsychotics for adverse drug events (ADEs). Assess patients for:

- Anticholinergic effects, the most common problem, causing constipation, dry mouth, and urinary retention
- Orthostatic hypotension, which increases the patient's risk for falls and fractures
- Parkinsonism, including tremors, bradycardia, and a shuffling gait
- Restlessness and the inability to stay still in any one position
- Hyperglycemia and diabetes mellitus, which occur more with drugs like risperidone (Risperdal) and quetiapine (Seroquel)

If any of these ADEs occur, notify the health care provider immediately.

Skin breakdown, especially pressure ulcers, is a major TISSUE INTEGRITY problem among older adults in hospitals and nursing homes. In some cases, these wounds cause death from infection. Therefore prevention is the best approach. The Joint Commission's NPSGs require that all health care agencies have a program to prevent agency-associated pressure ulcers. The program should include these evidence-based interventions:

- Nutritional support
- Avoidance of skin injury from friction or shearing forces
- Repositioning and support surfaces
- A plan to increase MOBILITY and activity level, when appropriate
- Skin cleansing and use of moisture barriers

Assess older adults for their risk for pressure ulcers, using an assessment tool such as the Braden Scale for Predicting Pressure Sore Risk (see Chapter 25). Implement evidence-based interventions to prevent agency-acquired pressure ulcers and maintain TISSUE INTEGRITY. Coordinate these interventions with members of the health care team, including the dietitian and wound care specialist.

! NURSING SAFETY PRIORITY QSEN

Action Alert

Supervise unlicensed assistive personnel (UAP) for frequent turning and repositioning for the patient who is immobile. Assess the skin every 8 hours for reddened areas that do not blanch. Remind UAP to keep the skin clean and dry. Use pressure-relieving mattresses, and avoid briefs or absorbent pads that can cause skin irritation and excess moisture. Chapter 25 describes in detail additional interventions for prevention and management of pressure ulcers.

Skin tears are also common in older adults, especially the old-old group and those who are on chronic steroid therapy. Teach UAP to use extreme caution when handling these patients. Use a gentle touch, and report any open areas. Avoid bruising because older adults have increased capillary fragility.

Care Transition from the Hospital or Long-Term Care Setting to Home

Some older adults and their families experience a breakdown in communication and coordination of care when transitioning from the hospital or long-term care (LTC) setting (nursing home) to the home setting. If the transition is not optimal, older adults experience high readmission rates and an increase in visits to the emergency department or health care provider's office.

A qualitative study by Dossa et al. (2012) showed that health care professionals, especially nurses, did not communicate effectively as they prepared for the discharge of older adults. Care was not coordinated among health care professionals, which led to confusion for the older adult and family caregivers. To help prevent these problems, the authors recommended that a system needs to be in place to address patients' communication needs. The system should include follow-up phone calls after discharge to home and having one case manager to coordinate care during and after the transition from the inpatient agency to home. A home care nurse or other health care professional can serve as a "health coach" to ensure understanding of discharge instructions, consistent follow-up appointments, and a designated emergency contact for the patient and family. Discharge instructions should be easy to read, in large print, and accurate. Continuity of care for high quality transition between settings is essential to achieve positive outcomes for older adults.

GET READY FOR THE NCLEX® EXAMINATION!

KEY POINTS

Review these Key Points for each NCLEX Examination Client Needs Category.

Safe and Effective Care Environment

- Collaborate with members of the health care team when providing care to older adults in the community or inpatient setting. For example, consult with the registered dietitian for problems with NUTRITION; consult with the pharmacist to discuss the patient's drug regimen. **Teamwork and Collaboration** QSEN
- Assess all older adults for risk factors for impaired driving ability, such as decreased MOBILITY, SENSORY PERCEPTION, and COGNITION (see Chart 2-3).
- Assess older adults in the community and inpatient settings for falls risk factors (e.g., cognitive decline and vision impairment) and implement interventions as delineated in Chart 2-4. **Safety** QSEN
- Physical and chemical restraints should not be used for older adults until all other alternatives have been tried (see Chart 2-5).
- Follow The Joint Commission's National Patient Safety Goals and federal/state standards when using patient restraints to maintain patient safety. **Safety** QSEN

Health Promotion and Maintenance

- Teach older adults about the benefits of regular physical exercise.
- Provide information regarding community resources for older adults to help them meet their basic needs.
- Teach health promotion practices as listed in Chart 2-1.
- Conduct a medication assessment for potential risks in older adults using the Beers criteria.

Psychosocial Integrity

- Depression is the most common yet most underdiagnosed and undertreated mental health/behavioral health disorder among older adults.
- Delirium is acute confusion; dementia is chronic confusion (see Tables 2-3 and 2-4). Confusion is not part of the normal aging process.
- Screen older adults for alcohol abuse or alcoholism, and refer those with identified problems to appropriate resources. **Evidence-Based Practice** QSEN
- Screen older adults for neglect and abuse, which are serious problems; family caregivers are usually the abusers (see Table 2-5). **Safety** QSEN
- Relocation stress syndrome is the reaction of an older adult when transferred to a different environment; ways to minimize this problem are listed in Chart 2-2.

Physiological Integrity

- The four subgroups of the older adult population are the young old, middle old, old old, and elite old.
- The biggest concern regarding accidents among older adults in both the community and inpatient setting is falls. **Safety** QSEN
- Physiologic changes of aging predispose older adults to toxic effects of medication; drugs are absorbed, metabolized, and distributed more slowly than in younger people. They are also excreted more slowly by the kidneys.
- Medication use in older adults is often a problem when they commit errors when self-medicating, avoid needed medications, or have problems understanding their medication regimen. **Evidence-Based Practice** QSEN
- Follow The Joint Commission's National Patient Safety Goals and best practice guidelines to prevent agency-acquired pressure ulcers.
- Promote sleep and rest for older adults to decrease the incidence of delirium and to prevent falls.
- Use the SPICES assessment tool for identifying serious health problems that can be prevented or managed early.

3 CHAPTER

Assessment and Care of Patients with Pain

Chris Pasero and Donna D. Ignatavicius

http//evolve.elsevier.com/Iggy/

PRIORITY CONCEPTS

- Pain
- Cognition
- Sensory Perception

LEARNING OUTCOMES

Safe and Effective Care Environment

1. Identify the role of the nurse as an advocate for patients with acute pain or chronic cancer or non-cancer pain.
2. Explain the importance of collaborating with the health care team in developing the pain management plan of care.

Health Promotion and Maintenance

3. Develop a teaching plan for patients to include complementary and alternative therapies for pain management.
4. Incorporate special considerations for older adults related to pain assessment and management.
5. Describe how to provide patient-centered care by respecting patients' preferences, values, and beliefs regarding pain and its management.

Psychosocial Integrity

6. Discuss the attitudes and knowledge of patients and their families regarding pain assessment and management.
7. Explain the importance of assessing expectations of patient and family for relief of pain, discomfort, or suffering.

Physiological Integrity

8. Demonstrate comprehensive understanding of the concepts of pain and suffering, including physiologic models of PAIN and comfort.
9. Perform a complete pain assessment, and document per agency policy.
10. Compare and contrast the characteristics of the major types of PAIN and examples of each.
11. Explain the role of the three analgesic groups in pain management.
12. Differentiate between addiction, pseudoaddiction, tolerance, and physical dependence.
13. Develop a plan of care to prevent common side effects of opioid analgesics.
14. Compare the advantages and disadvantages of drug administration routes.
15. Describe the benefits and limitations of selected safety-enhancing technologies used in pain management.
16. Prioritize care for the patient receiving patient-controlled analgesia.
17. Outline care for a patient receiving epidural analgesia.
18. Identify the importance of incorporating nonpharmacologic interventions into the patient's plan of care as needed to control pain.

OVERVIEW

PAIN is a universal, complex, and personal experience that everyone has at some point in life. It is the most common reason people seek medical care and the number-one reason people take medication. Unrelieved pain can alter or diminish quality of life more than any other single health-related problem. Despite more than 30 years of education and dissemination of guideline recommendations, the failure to adequately manage pain remains a major health problem worldwide.

In response to mandates by many professional organizations and The Joint Commission (TJC), many hospitals and other health care agencies in the United States have implemented interdisciplinary PAIN initiatives to help ensure patients receive the best possible treatment. Some hospitals address this by establishing pain resource nurse (PRN) programs. As the name implies, one or more nurses per clinical unit are trained to serve as a resource to other members of the health care team in managing pain. Other hospitals have a formal team or pain service consisting of one or more nurses, pharmacists, case managers, and/or physicians. In larger facilities, pain services may specialize by type of pain (e.g., acute pain service or pain and palliative care team). Although a large part of the team's plan may center on drug therapy, these groups also recommend nonpharmacologic measures when appropriate.

SCOPE OF THE PROBLEM

PAIN is a major economic problem and a leading cause of disability that hampers the lives of many people, especially older adults. Chronic non-cancer pain, such as osteoarthritis, rheumatoid arthritis, diabetic neuropathy, and post-stroke pain syndrome, is the most common cause of long-term disability, affecting millions of Americans and others throughout the world.

Pain is inadequately treated in all health care settings. Populations at the highest risk in medical-surgical nursing are older adults, substance abusers, and those whose primary language differs from that of the health care professional. Older adults in nursing homes are at especially high risk because many residents are unable to report their PAIN. In addition, there often is a lack of staff members who have been trained to manage pain in the older adult population.

Inadequate PAIN management can lead to many adverse consequences affecting the patient and family members (Table 3-1). Therefore nurses have a legal and ethical responsibility to ensure that patients receive adequate pain control. Many professional organizations, including the American Society for Pain Management Nursing (ASPMN), the American Pain Society (APS), and TJC state that patients in all health care settings, including home care, have a right to effective pain management.

Patients rely on nurses and other health care professionals to adequately assess and manage their PAIN. As the coordinator of patient care, be sure to accurately document your assessments and actions, including patient and caregiver teaching. Communication and collaboration among the patient and members of the interdisciplinary health care team about the patient's pain, expectations, and progress toward control are equally important.

DEFINITIONS OF PAIN

Pain is defined as an unpleasant sensory and emotional experience associated with actual or potential tissue damage. McCaffery (1968) offered a more personal definition when she stated that PAIN is whatever the experiencing person says it is and exists whenever he or she says it exists. This has become the clinical definition of PAIN worldwide and reflects an understanding that the patient is the authority on the PAIN and the *only* one who can describe the experience. *In other words, self-report is always the most reliable indication of pain.* Nurses who approach pain from this perspective can help the patient achieve effective management by advocating for proper control. If the patient cannot provide self-report, a variety of other methods, such as observation of behavioral indicators, are used to assess the PAIN (see later in this chapter).

TABLE 3-1 Impact of Unrelieved Pain

Physiologic Impact	Quality-of-Life Impact
• Prolongs stress response • Increases heart rate, blood pressure, and oxygen demand • Decreases GI motility • Causes immobility • Decreases immune response • Delays healing • Poorly managed acute pain increases risk for development of chronic pain	• Interferes with ADLs • Causes anxiety, depression, hopelessness, fear, anger, and sleeplessness • Impairs family, work, and social relationships **Financial Impact** • Costs Americans billions of dollars per year • Increases hospital length of stay • Leads to lost income and productivity

CATEGORIZATION OF PAIN BY DURATION

PAIN is often described as being acute or chronic based on its duration (Table 3-2). *Acute pain* is usually short-lived, whereas *chronic pain* can last a person's lifetime. *Acute pain* often results from sudden, accidental trauma (e.g., fractures, burns, lacerations) or from surgery, ischemia, or acute inflammation. *Chronic pain or persistent pain* is further divided into two subtypes. *Chronic cancer pain* is pain associated with cancer and is usually the result of tissue changes from tumor growth. *Chronic non-cancer pain* is associated with past or ongoing tissue damage, such as chronic back or neck pain or osteoarthritis pain. *Non-cancer pain is the most common type of chronic pain.*

Acute Pain

Almost everyone experiences acute PAIN at some time. Brief **acute pain** serves a biologic purpose in that it acts as a warning signal by activating the sympathetic nervous system and causing various physiologic responses. Although not consistent in all people, when acute PAIN is severe, you may see responses similar to those found in "fight-or-flight" reactions, such as increased vital signs, sweating, and dilated pupils. Most people protect themselves by drawing away from the painful stimulus. Behavioral signs may include restlessness (especially among cognitively impaired older adults who sometimes fidget and pick at clothing), an inability to concentrate, apprehension, and overall distress of varying degrees. These heightened physiologic and behavioral responses are often referred to as the *acute pain model.* It is important to remember that the response to pain is highly individual and that humans quickly adapt physiologically and behaviorally to pain. Be careful not to expect certain responses when assessing any type of pain. *The absence of the*

TABLE 3-2 Characteristics of Acute Pain and Chronic Pain

ACUTE	CHRONIC* (OR PERSISTENT)
• Has short duration • Usually has a well-defined cause • Decreases with healing • Is usually reversible • Initially serves a biologic purpose (warning sign to withdraw from painful stimuli or seek help) • When prolonged, serves no useful purpose • Ranges from mild to severe intensity • May be accompanied by anxiety and restlessness • When unrelieved, can increase morbidity and mortality and prolong hospital length of stay	• Usually lasts longer than 3 months • May or may not have well-defined cause • Usually begins gradually and persists • Serves no useful purpose • Ranges from mild to severe intensity • Often accompanied by multiple quality-of-life and functional adverse effects, including depression, fatigue, financial burden, and increased dependence on family, friends, and the health care system • Can impact the quality of life of family members and friends

*Includes chronic cancer pain and chronic non-cancer pain.

physiologic and behavioral responses does not mean the absence of pain.

Acute pain is usually temporary, has a sudden onset, and is easily localized. The PAIN is typically confined to the injured area and may subside with or without treatment. As the injured area heals, the SENSORY PERCEPTION of pain changes and, in most cases, diminishes and resolves. Both the caregiver and the patient can see an end to the pain, which usually makes coping somewhat easier.

PAIN that accompanies surgery is one of the most common examples of acute pain, but it is not always well managed. *The response to pain after surgery is highly individual and variable.* There is no evidence that shows one type of surgery is consistently more or less painful than another. Usually, poorly managed postoperative pain is a result of inadequate drug (analgesic) therapy. Poorly managed and prolonged acute pain serves no useful purpose and has many adverse effects including inability of the patient to participate in the recovery process with subsequent increased disability. The severity of early postoperative pain may be a predictor of long-term PAIN. Those who experience unrelieved severe postoperative pain are at high risk for the development of chronic persistent postsurgical PAIN (Pasero, 2011).

Chronic Pain

Chronic pain (also called *persistent pain*) is often defined as PAIN that lasts or recurs for an indefinite period, usually for more than 3 months. The onset is gradual, and the character and quality of the pain often change over time. *Chronic pain serves no biologic purpose.* Because it persists for an extended period, it can interfere with personal relationships and performance of ADLs. Chronic pain can also result in emotional and financial burdens, depression, and hopelessness for patients and their families. It is important to remember that the body adapts to persistent pain, and thus vital signs, such as pulse and blood pressure, may actually be lower than normal in people with chronic pain. *Although many characteristics of chronic pain are similar in different patients, be aware that each patient is unique and requires a highly individualized plan of care.*

Chronic Cancer Pain

Many patients with cancer report PAIN at the time of diagnosis, which increases in advanced stages of the disease. Most cancer pain can be successfully managed by giving adequate amounts of oral opioids around the clock, yet patients with cancer are often inadequately treated for what can be persistent, excruciating pain and suffering.

Most cancer PAIN is the result of tumor growth, including nerve compression, invasion of tissue, and/or bone metastasis, an extremely painful condition. Cancer treatments also can cause *acute pain* (e.g., from repetitive blood draws and other procedures, surgery, and toxicities from chemotherapy and radiation therapy).

Patients with cancer PAIN generally have pain in two or more areas of the body but usually talk about only the primary area. Be sure to perform a complete pain assessment to ensure an effective plan of care (see the Concept Map).

Chronic Non-Cancer Pain

Chronic non-cancer PAIN is a global health problem, occurring most often in people older than 65 years. This type of pain was formerly called *chronic nonmalignant* PAIN. However, most experts, and certainly patients who suffer daily, believe that all pain is malignant. There are many sources and types of chronic non-cancer PAIN. Among the most common are neck, shoulder, and low back pain following injury. Chronic conditions, such as diabetes, rheumatoid arthritis, Crohn's disease, and interstitial cystitis, often are associated with chronic pain. People who have had a stroke or are paralyzed may report persistent pain as a result of central nervous system (CNS) damage. Sometimes the exact cause of the pain is unclear as with fibromyalgia.

CATEGORIZATION OF PAIN BY UNDERLYING MECHANISMS

PAIN is more commonly categorized as either nociceptive (normal pain processing) or neuropathic (abnormal pain processing) (Table 3-3). The duration of nociceptive and neuropathic pain can be either acute (short-lived) or chronic (persistent), and a person can have both types.

Nociceptive Pain

The classic *gate control theory* is credited with stimulating intense research that led to discoveries that form the basis of what is known about PAIN transmission today. According to this theory, a gating mechanism exists in the spinal cord. It was proposed that when the gate is open, pain impulses ascend to the brain where the person perceives that PAIN is present (Pasero & McCaffery, 2011). When the gate is closed, the impulses are blocked and PAIN is not perceived. It is no longer necessary to discuss pain transmission in terms of theories because much is known today about this phenomenon, known as *nociception.*

Nociception is the term that is used to describe how PAIN becomes a conscious experience. It involves the *normal functioning of physiologic systems* that process noxious stimuli with the ultimate result being that the stimuli are perceived to be painful. In short, nociception means "normal" pain transmission and is generally discussed in terms of four processes: transduction, transmission, perception, and modulation (Fig. 3-1). Although it is helpful to consider nociception in the context of these four processes, it is important to understand that they do not occur as four separate and distinct entities. They are continuous, and the processes overlap as they flow from one to another.

Transduction is the first process of nociception and refers to the means by which noxious events activate neurons that exist throughout the body (skin, subcutaneous tissue, and visceral, or somatic, structures) and have the ability to respond selectively to specific noxious stimuli. These neurons are called *nociceptors.* When they are stimulated directly, a number of excitatory compounds (e.g., serotonin, bradykinin, histamine, substance P, and prostaglandins) are released that further activate more nociceptors (see Fig. 3-1) (Yaksh & Wallace, 2011).

Transmission is the second process involved in nociception. Nociceptors have small-diameter axons—either A-delta or C fibers (see Fig. 3-1). Effective transduction generates an electric signal (action potential) that is transmitted in these nerve fibers from the periphery toward the CNS. *A-delta fibers* are lightly myelinated and faster conducting than unmyelinated C fibers. The endings of A-delta fibers detect thermal and mechanical injury. The SENSORY PERCEPTION accompanying A-delta fiber activation is sharp and well-localized and leads to an appropriately rapid protective response, such as reflex withdrawal from

CONCEPT MAP

PAIN — SENSORY PERCEPTION — COGNITION

CHRONIC CANCER PAIN

HISTORY

62-year-old Jack Brown is receiving end-of-life PALLIATIVE care with metastasis of colon cancer. Palliative surgery removed an obstructive cancerous tumor but he continues to have persistent abdominal pain described as dull with an intensity of 7/10. He is receiving hydromorphone (Dilaudid) via PCA pump for pain control and Fentora lozenges are available for breakthrough pain.

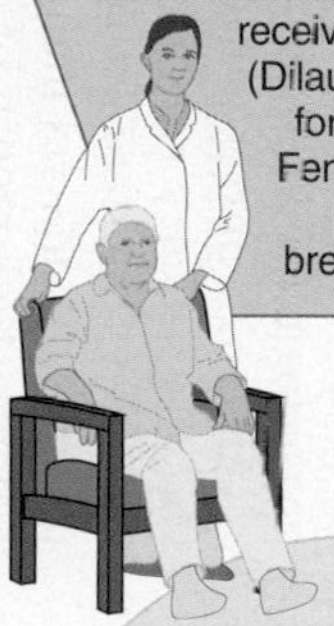

PAIN Assessment

- Grimacing, crying at times
- Verbalization of pain
- Restlessness
- Changes in interpersonal interaction–irritable with family interventions
- Changes in activity pattern/routine; hesitant to get out of bed

PAIN Management

- Hydromorphone-basal infusion 0.5 mg/hr, demand dose of 0.2 mg with lockout interval of 10 min and 4-hr limit of 6 mg
- Fentora: oral transmucosal lozenge, one lozenge as needed
- Massage therapy daily

Data Synthesis

PATIENT PROBLEMS

Pain – metastasis of colon cancer requiring palliation for end-of-life care

SENSORY PERCEPTION – pain interfering with clear thought, family relations, and ADLs

Planning

EXPECTED OUTCOMES

- Maintain level of pain control that allows patient to function and have acceptable quality of life
- Maximize independence and ability to perform ADLs
- Not experience unsafe effects from pharmacologic pain management
- Feel safe and well-cared for with physical/psychosocial needs met; provide closure with earthly life

INTERVENTIONS

1 Comprehensive Pain Assessment

- Perform complete pain assessment and document findings. Ask patient to point to **area(s)** of pain on the body; rank **severity** of pain using the NRS; document using patient's own description, what makes pain better/worse, and how it impacts daily life. *Assesses sensory perception of pain and determines effectiveness of pain management for palliative therapy.*
- **Assess** impact of pain on performing ADLs. *Determines whether chronic pain interferes with ADLs.*
- Collaborate with interdisciplinary team about patient's pain, expectations, and progress toward control. *Coordinated efforts achieve effective pain management and palliation.*

2 Pharmacologic Pain Management

- Develop treatment plan to clarify outcomes, discussing options with patient and family. *Individualizes safe and effective use of analgesics based on comprehensive assessment.*
- Monitor effectiveness of around-the-clock dosing of analgesics. Give Fentora lozenges for breakthrough pain. *Successfully manages cancer pain.*
- Prevent common side effects: give antiemetics and fluids for nausea/vomiting; give a daily stool softener plus a mild peristaltic stimulant for constipation. *Side effects are a primary reason people stop taking pain medication.*

3 Nursing Safety Priority: Action Alert!

Teach patient how to use the PCA device and to report side effects. Monitor sedation level and respiratory status at least every 2 hours. Promptly decrease dose if increased sedation is detected. *Ensures patient is able to understand relationships between pain, accepting an analgesic dose, and pain relief. Ensures patient is cognitively and physically able to use the equipment.*

4 Nonpharmacologic Pain Management

- Explore nonpharmacologic interventions to complement drug therapy. *Cognitive-behavioral therapy, distraction, and imagery may strongly influence pain perception.*
- Teach alternative methods: heat, cold, pressure; Therapeutic Touch; massage; vibration; TENS unit; distraction; imagery; relaxation; hypnosis. *Facilitates relaxation and reduces anxiety, stress, and depression.*

5 Psychosocial Assessment

- Assist patient to verbalize concerns about body image, self-concept, role performance, self-esteem, sexuality. *Sets realistic goals based on patient preferences and values of palliative care at end of life.*
- Have patient describe personal attitudes about pain. *Prevents worries about addiction, death, or body mutilation, and thoughts of being punished or a spiritual significance to lingering pain.*
- Respect patient's verbal and nonverbal expressions of pain. *Avoids depression and hopelessness arising from uncontrolled chronic pain.*
- Explore support systems and coping strategies. *Helps keep unpredictability and uncertainty of terminal disease from affecting the entire family.*

6 Self-Management Education

- Teach patient and family about drug therapy. *Maximizes relief and symptom control at home, and eliminates unnecessary hospital readmissions.*
- Help patient establish an analgesic regimen that helps with sleep, rest, appetite, and activity level. *Helps patient identify and plan important activities with adequate rest periods.*
- Evaluate family support systems to assist patient in adhering to proposed treatment and plan of care. *Includes family members in activities during and after hospitalization.*

Concept Map by Deanne A. Blach, MSN, RN

TABLE 3-3 Physiologic Sources of Nociceptive Pain and Neuropathic Pain

PHYSIOLOGIC STRUCTURE	CHARACTERISTICS OF PAIN	SOURCES OF ACUTE POSTOPERATIVE PAIN	SOURCES OF CHRONIC PAIN SYNDROMES
Nociceptive Pain (normal pain processing)			
Somatic Pain			
Cutaneous or superficial: skin and subcutaneous tissues	Sharp, burning	Incisional pain, pain at insertion sites of tubes and drains, wound complications, orthopedic procedures, skeletal muscle spasms	Bony metastases, osteoarthritis and rheumatoid arthritis, low back pain, peripheral vascular diseases
Deep somatic: bone, muscle, blood vessels, connective tissues	Dull, aching, cramping		
Visceral Pain			
Organs and the linings of the body cavities	Poorly localized Diffuse, deep cramping or splitting, sharp, stabbing	Chest tubes, abdominal tubes and drains, bladder distention or spasms, intestinal distention	Pancreatitis, liver metastases, colitis, appendicitis
Neuropathic Pain (abnormal pain processing)			
Peripheral or central nervous system: nerve fibers, spinal cord, and higher central nervous system	Poorly localized Shooting, burning, fiery, shocklike, sharp, painful numbness	Phantom limb pain, postmastectomy pain, nerve compression	HIV-related pain, diabetic neuropathy, postherpetic neuralgia, chemotherapy-induced neuropathies, cancer-related nerve injury, radiculopathies

HIV, Human immune deficiency virus.

the painful stimuli. *C fibers* are unmyelinated or poorly myelinated slow conductors and respond to mechanical, thermal, and chemical stimuli. Activation after acute injury yields a poorly localized (more widely distributed) typically aching or burning pain. In contrast to the intermittent nature of A-delta sensations, C fibers usually produce more continuous pain.

Perception is the third broad process involved in nociception. Perception, which may be viewed as the end result of the neural activity associated with transmission of information about noxious events, involves the conscious awareness of PAIN (see Fig. 3-1). It requires the activation of higher brain structures, including the cortex, and involves both awareness and the occurrence of emotions and drives associated with pain. The physiology of pain perception is very poorly understood but presumably can be targeted by therapies that activate higher cortical functions to achieve pain control or coping. Cognitive-behavioral therapy and specific approaches such as distraction and imagery (discussed later in the chapter) have been developed based on evidence that brain processes can strongly influence pain perception.

Modulation of afferent input generated in response to noxious stimuli happens at every level from the periphery to the cortex (see Fig. 3-1). The neurochemistry of modulation is complex and not yet fully understood, but it is known that multiple peripheral and central systems and dozens of neurochemicals are involved. For example, the endogenous opioids (endorphins) are found throughout the peripheral nervous system (PNS) and CNS and, like the exogenous opioids administered therapeutically, they inhibit neuronal activity by binding to opioid receptors. Other central inhibitory neurotransmitters important in the modulation of pain include serotonin and norepinephrine, which are released in the spinal cord and brainstem by the descending fibers of the modulatory system to inhibit pain.

Nociceptive pain is the result of actual or potential tissue damage or inflammation and is often categorized as being somatic or visceral. *Somatic pain* arises from the skin and musculoskeletal structures, and *visceral pain* arises from organs. Examples include PAIN-associated trauma, surgery, burns, and tumor growth.

Neuropathic Pain

Neuropathic pain is a descriptive term used to refer to PAIN that is believed to be sustained by a set of mechanisms that is driven by damage to or dysfunction of the PNS and/or CNS. In contrast to nociceptive pain, which is sustained by ongoing activation of essentially *normal* neural systems, neuropathic pain is sustained by the *abnormal* processing of stimuli. Whereas nociceptive pain involves tissue damage or inflammation, neuropathic pain may occur in the absence of either.

It is not clear why noxious stimuli result in neuropathic PAIN in some people and not in others and why some treatments work in some and not in others. Neuropathic pain is difficult to treat and often resistant to first-line analgesics. Asking patients to describe it is the best way to identify the presence of neuropathic pain. Common distinctive descriptors include "burning," "shooting," "stabbing," and feeling "pins and needles." Much is unknown about what causes and maintains neuropathic pain; it is the subject of intense ongoing research.

PATIENT-CENTERED COLLABORATIVE CARE

Pain Assessment

All accepted guidelines identify the patient's self-report as the gold standard for assessing the existence and intensity of PAIN (Pasero & McCaffery, 2011). Because pain is such a private and personal experience, it may be difficult for the person to describe or explain it to others. However, subjective descriptions of the experience and measurement of pain intensity are more reliable and accurate than observable qualities of pain. The amount of pain and responses to it vary from person to person; therefore interpreting it solely on actions or behaviors can be misleading and is not recommended. Patients may report pain in the absence of any observable or documented physiologic changes.

Although nurses are entitled to their doubts and opinions about a patient's PAIN, those doubts and opinions cannot be allowed to interfere with appropriate patient care. The nurse's primary role in PAIN management is to advocate for patients by *accepting* their reports of pain and acting promptly to relieve it,

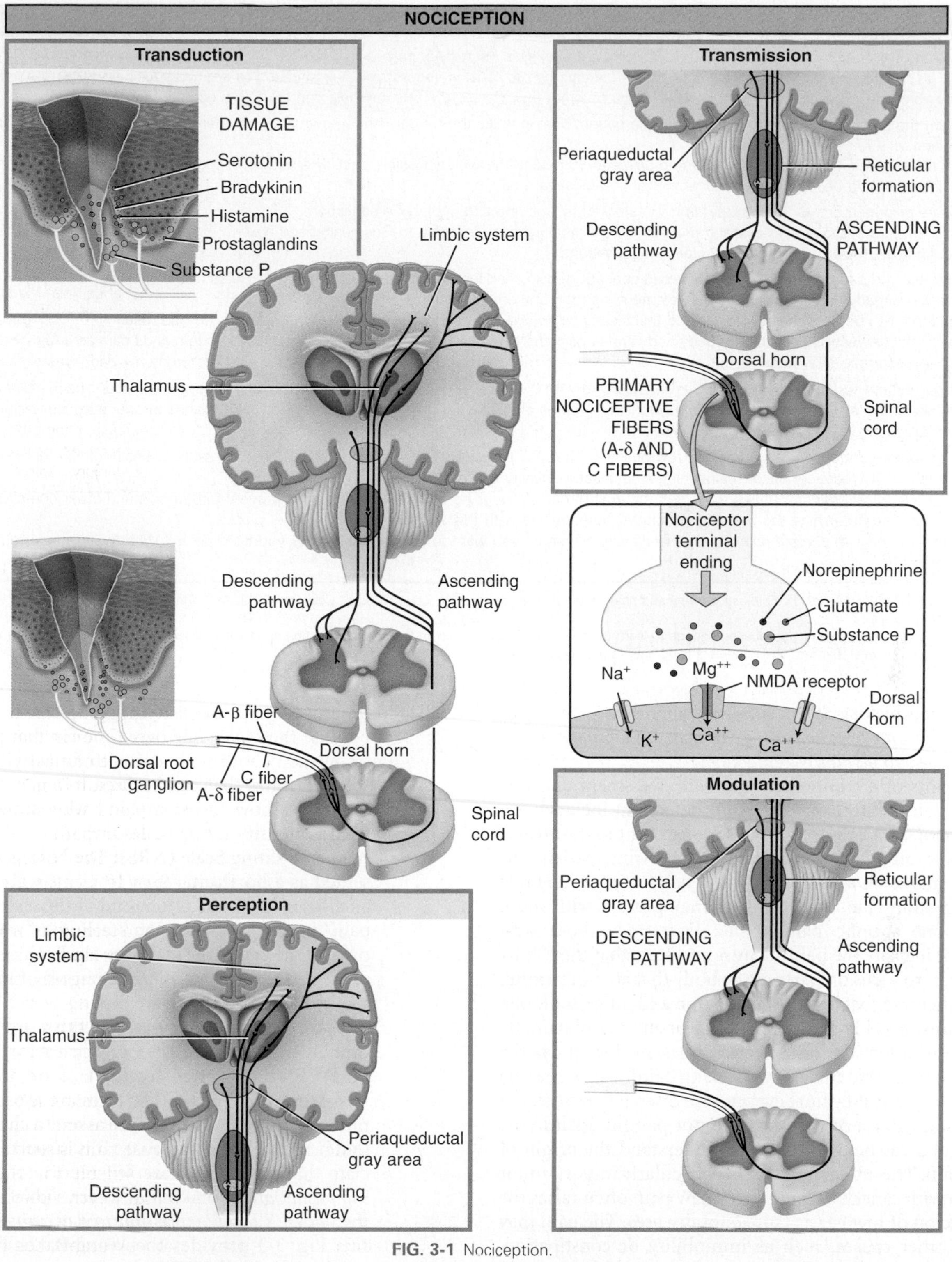

FIG. 3-1 Nociception.

while respecting patients' preferences and values (Quality and Safety Education for Nurses [QSEN], 2011).

To be patient-centered, always respect the patient's verbal and nonverbal expressions of PAIN without making judgments or inferences about the reality of it. If patients perceive that health care professionals doubt the existence of their pain, mistrust and other negative feelings can arise and interfere with a therapeutic nurse-patient relationship.

The Comprehensive Pain Assessment

A comprehensive pain assessment should be conducted during the initial interview with the patient, with each new report of pain, and whenever indicated by changes in the patient's condition or treatment plan during the course of care. PAIN assessment at these intervals serves as the foundation for developing and evaluating the effectiveness of the treatment plan. Remember that patients' personal preferences and values affect how

TABLE 3-4 Teaching Patients and Their Families How to Use A Pain Rating Scale*

Step 1. Show the pain rating scale to the patient and family, and explain its primary purpose. *Example:* "This is a pain rating scale that many of our patients use to help us understand their pain and to set goals for pain relief. We will ask you regularly about pain, but any time you have pain you must let us know so that we can help control it. We don't always know when you hurt."
Step 2. Explain the parts of the pain rating scale. If the patient does not like it or understand it, switch to another scale (e.g., vertical presentation, VDS, or faces). *Example:* "On this pain rating scale, 0 means no pain and 10 means the worst possible pain. The middle of the scale, around 5, means moderate pain. A 2 or 3 would be mild pain, but 7 or higher means severe pain."
Step 3. Discuss pain as a broad concept that is not restricted to a severe and intolerable sensation. *Example:* "Pain refers to any kind of discomfort anywhere in your body. Pain also means aching and hurting. Pain can include pulling, tightness, burning, knifelike feelings, and other unpleasant sensations."
Step 4. Verify that the patient understands the broad concept of pain. Ask the patient to mention two examples of pain he or she has experienced. If the patient is already in pain that requires treatment, use the present situation as the example. *Example:* "I want to be sure that I've explained this clearly, so would you give me two examples of pain you've had recently?" If the patient examples include various parts of the body and various pain characteristics, that indicates that he or she understands pain as a fairly broad concept. An example of what a patient might say is "I have a mild, sort of throbbing headache now, and yesterday my back was aching."
Step 5. Ask the patient to practice using the pain rating scale with the present pain or select one of the examples mentioned. *Example:* "Using the scale, what is your pain right now? What is it at its worst?" OR "Using the pain rating scale and one of your examples of pain, what is that pain usually? What is it at its worst?"
Step 6. Set goals for comfort and function/recovery/quality of life. Ask patients what pain rating would be acceptable or satisfactory, considering the activities required for recovery or for maintaining a satisfactory quality of life. *Example for a surgical patient:* "I have explained the importance of coughing and deep breathing to prevent pneumonia and other complications. Now we need to determine the pain rating that will not interfere with this so that you may recover quickly." *Example for patient with chronic pain or terminal illness:* "What do you want to do that pain keeps you from doing? What pain rating would allow you to do this?"

From Pasero, C., & McCaffery, M. (2011). *Pain assessment and pharmacologic management.* St. Louis: Mosby. Copyright 2011, McCaffery, M., & Pasero, C. Used with permission.
VDS, Verbal descriptor scale.
*When a patient is obviously in pain or not focused enough to learn to use a pain rating scale, pain treatment should proceed without pain ratings. Teaching can be undertaken when pain is reduced to a level that facilitates understanding how to use a pain scale.

they report their history. *When culturally appropriate, be sure to include families and significant others in this information-gathering process to be family-centered.*

Components of a comprehensive PAIN assessment and tips on how to elicit the information from the patient include:

- *Location(s):* Ask the patient to state or point to the area(s) of PAIN on the body. Sometimes allowing patients to make marks on a body diagram is helpful in gaining this information (Fig. 3-2). Patients may present with more than one specific painful site. Encourage those who cannot identify the painful areas and state that they "hurt all over" to focus on parts of the body that are not painful. Ask them to begin with the hand and fingers of one extremity and identify the presence or absence of pain. By focusing attention on selected areas of the body, the patient is assisted in better localizing painful areas. People who state that they hurt everywhere often begin to realize that some parts of the body are not painful. Identifying painful areas helps the patient understand the origin of the pain. This understanding is particularly important for those with cancer, because every new pain often raises the suspicion of metastasis (spread of disease). The pain may have other causes, such as immobility or constipation. Pain may be described as belonging to one of four categories related to its location:
  1. Localized pain is confined to the site of origin.
  2. Projected pain is diffuse around the site of origin and is not well localized.
  3. Referred pain is felt in an area distant from the site of painful stimuli.
  4. Radiating pain is felt along a specific nerve or nerves.
- *Intensity:* Ask the patient to rate the severity of the PAIN using a reliable and valid assessment tool. Various self-report scales have been developed to help patients communicate PAIN intensity. Once a scale is selected, be sure to use the *same* scale over time for that patient, and assess intensity both with and without activity. See Table 3-4 for strategies that can be used to teach patients and their families how to use a pain rating scale. The most common intensity rating scales are:
  - Numeric Rating Scale (NRS): The NRS is usually presented as a horizontal 0-to-10 point scale, with word anchors of "no pain" at one end of the scale, "moderate pain" in the middle of the scale, and "worst possible pain" at the end of the scale (see Fig. 3-3). Some patients relate better to a vertical presentation of the scale.
  - Wong-Baker FACES® Pain Rating Scale: The FACES scale consists of 6 cartoon faces with word descriptors, ranging from a smiling face on the left for "no pain (or hurt)" to a frowning, tearful face on the right for "worst pain (or hurt)." The faces are most commonly numbered 0 to 10. Patients are asked to choose the face that best describes their PAIN. It is important to appreciate that faces scales are self-report tools; *clinicians should not attempt to match a face shown on a scale to the patient's facial expression to determine pain intensity.* Fig. 3-3 provides the Wong-Baker FACES scale combined with the NRS.
  - Faces Pain Scale-Revised (FPS-R): The FPS-R has 7 faces to make it consistent with other scales using the 0 to 10 metric. The faces range from a neutral facial expression to one of intense pain. As with the Wong-Baker FACES® scale, patients are asked to choose the face that best reflects their PAIN. Some research shows that the FPS-R is preferred by both cognitively intact and impaired older adults.
  - Verbal Descriptor Scale (VDS): A VDS uses different words or phrases to describe the intensity of PAIN,

McGill-Melzack PAIN QUESTIONNAIRE

Patient's name ____________ Age ________

File No. ____________ Date ________

Clinical category (e.g., cardiac, neurologic)

Diagnosis: ________

____

____

Analgesic (if already administered):

1. Type ____________
2. Dosage ____________
3. Time given in relation to this test ______

Patient's intelligence: circle number that represents best estimate.

1 (low) 2 3 4 5 (high)

****

This questionnaire has been designed to tell us more about your pain. Four major questions we ask are

1. Where is your pain?
2. What does it feel like?
3. How does it change with time?
4. How strong is it?

It is important that you tell us how your pain feels now. Please follow the instructions at the beginning of each part.

Part 1. Where Is Your Pain?

Please mark, on the drawings below, the areas where you feel pain. Put E if external, or I if internal, near the areas you mark. Put EI if both external and internal.

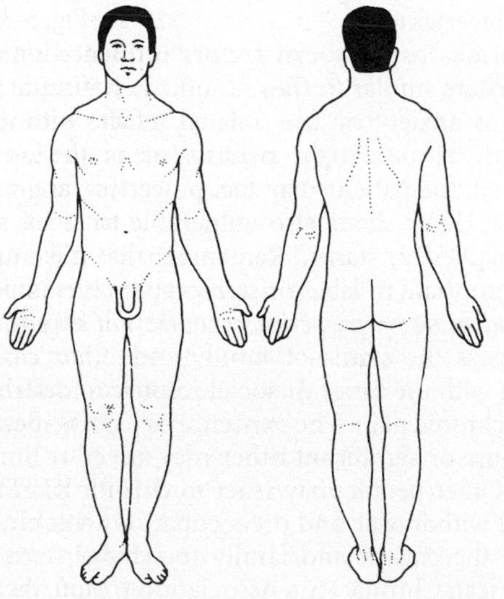

Part 2. What Does Your Pain Feel Like?

Some of the words below describe your *present* pain. Circle *ONLY* those words that best describe it. Leave out any category that is not suitable. Use only a single word in each appropriate category—the one that applies best.

1
Flickering
Quivering
Pulsing
Throbbing
Beating
Pounding

2
Jumping
Flashing
Shooting

3
Pricking
Boring
Drilling
Stabbing
Lancinating

4
Sharp
Cutting
Lacerating

5
Pinching
Pressing
Gnawing
Cramping
Crushing

6
Tugging
Pulling
Wrenching

7
Hot
Burning
Scalding
Searing

8
Tingling
Itchy
Smarting
Stinging

9
Dull
Sore
Hurting
Aching
Heavy

10
Tender
Taut
Rasping
Splitting

11
Tiring
Exhausting

12
Sickening
Suffocat-
ing

13
Fearful
Frightful
Terrifying

14
Punishing
Grueling
Cruel
Vicious
Killing

15
Wretched
Blinding

16
Annoying
Troublesome
Miserable
Intense
Unbearable

17
Spreading
Radiating
Penetrating
Piercing

18
Tight
Numb
Drawing
Squeezing
Tearing

19
Cool
Cold
Freezing

20
Nagging
Nauseating
Agonizing
Dreadful
Torturing

Part 3. How Does Your Pain Change With Time?

1. Which word or words would you use to describe the *pattern* of your pain?

1	2	3
Continuous	Rhythmic	Brief
Steady	Periodic	Momentary
Constant	Intermittent	Transient

2. What kind of things *relieve* your pain?
3. What kind of things *increase* your pain?

Part 4. How Strong Is Your Pain?

People agree that the following 5 words represent pain of increasing intensity. They are:

1	2	3	4	5
Mild	Discomforting	Distressing	Horrible	Excruciating

To answer each question below, write the number of the most appropriate word in the space beside the question.

1. Which word describes your pain right now? ____
2. Which word describes it at its worst? ____
3. Which word describes it when it is least? ____
4. Which word describes the worst toothache you ever had? ____
5. Which word describes the worst headache you ever had? ____
6. Which word describes the worst stomachache you ever had? ____

FIG. 3-2 The McGill-Melzack Pain Questionnaire.

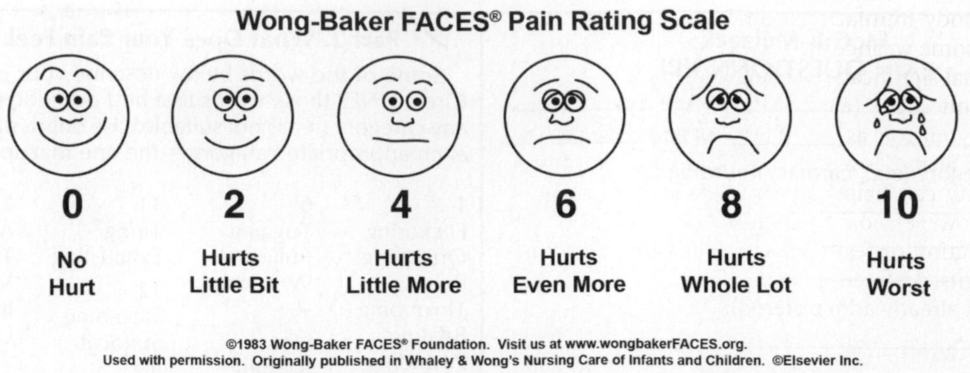

FIG. 3-3 Wong-Baker FACES® pain rating scale.

such as "*no pain, mild pain, moderate pain, severe pain very severe pain,* and *worst possible pain.*" The patient is asked to select the phrase that best describes the pain intensity.

- *Quality:* Ask the patient to describe how the PAIN feels. He or she may use one word or a group of words to convey the SENSORY PERCEPTION of the pain. *Avoid suggesting descriptive words for the pain; allow patients to use their own words to describe the pain.* Descriptors such as "sharp," "shooting," or "burning" may help identify the presence of neuropathic pain. Ask the patient whether the pain is superficial or deep. In general, those with pain involving superficial or cutaneous (skin) structures describe it as superficial and can often localize the pain to a specific area.
- *Onset and duration:* Ask the patient when the PAIN started and whether it is constant or intermittent.
- *Aggravating and relieving factors:* Ask the patient what makes the PAIN worse and what makes it better. Ask about strategies the patient has used before to manage pain.
- *Effect of pain on function and quality of life:* The effect of PAIN on the ability to perform recovery activities should be regularly evaluated. It is particularly important to ask patients with persistent pain about how it has affected their lives. Ask what they could do before the pain began that they can no longer do and what they want to do but cannot do.
- *Comfort-function (pain intensity) outcomes:* For patients with *acute pain,* identify expected short-term functional outcomes. Reinforce to the patient that adequate PAIN control will lead to more successful achievement of those outcomes. For example, tell surgical patients that they will be expected to ambulate or participate in physical therapy postoperatively. Ask patients to identify a level of pain that will allow accomplishment of the expected outcomes. A realistic outcome for most patients is 2 or 3 on a scale of 0 to 10. Pain intensity that is consistently above the desired level requires further evaluation and consideration of possible adjustment of the treatment plan.
- *Other information:* Consider the patient's culture, past PAIN experiences, and pertinent medical history such as comorbidities. Current treatments and diagnostic studies are considered when performing an assessment. For example, patients who are intubated may be awake and alert but unable to speak. Strategies to assess the presence and severity of PAIN in these patients include (Tate et al., 2012):

CONSIDERATIONS FOR OLDER ADULTS

Patient-Centered Care QSEN

PAIN is not an inevitable consequence of aging; however, the incidence is higher in older adults. Sensitivity to pain does not diminish with age. Many older adults, even those with mild to moderate dementia, are able to use a self-report assessment tool if nurses and other caregivers take the time to administer it. Many older adults are reluctant to report pain for a variety of reasons including the belief that it is normal and that they are bothering the nurse. It is essential that attempts be made to elicit the patient's self-report and pain be assessed frequently with a focus on functional and quality-of-life indicators in this vulnerable population.

Psychosocial Assessment

PAIN holds unique meaning for the person experiencing it. Patients having *acute pain* from surgery may interpret it as necessary and expected. It may be viewed with relief as a sign that some greater problem has been resolved or alleviated by the surgery. Knowing that the duration of the pain is limited may be reassuring for a patient. In contrast, acute chest pain associated with angina may mark the beginning of a life of fear and uncertainty.

Various psychosocial factors influence *chronic* PAIN. Some factors are similar to those found in the acute pain experience, such as anxiety or fear related to the meaning of the pain. Because chronic pain persists or is perhaps only partially relieved, the patient may feel powerless, angry, hostile, or desperate. He or she is also vulnerable to labels such as "chronic complainer" or "faker." Remember that it is unprofessional and inappropriate to label or stereotype patients. *Remain objective, and advocate for proper pain control for all patients.*

Assess the status of family and other close relationships, along with the range of social resources available to the patient with chronic pain. The existence of a pain-specific conflict with a spouse or significant other may affect or limit coping strategies. Other people may react to chronic pain with depression, social withdrawal, and preoccupation with physical symptoms. Refer the patient and family to self-help groups, such as the American Chronic Pain Association (http://theacpa.org), which provides the "10-Step Program from Patient to Person."

If the chronic PAIN is associated with a progressive disease such as cancer, rheumatoid arthritis, or peripheral vascular disease, the patient may have worries and concerns about the consequences of the illness. People with cancer-related pain may fear death or body mutilation. Some may think they are being punished for some wrongdoing in life. Others may attach a religious or spiritual significance to lingering pain.

Ask open-ended questions (e.g., "Tell me how your pain has affected your job or your role as a mother.") to allow the patient to describe personal attitudes about PAIN and its influence on life. This opportunity can help someone whose life has been changed by pain. However, some patients choose not to share their private information or fears. As a patient-centered nurse, always respect patients' preferences and values.

NCLEX EXAMINATION CHALLENGE

Physiological Integrity

A client who had a laminectomy reports new onset of severe back pain. What responses by the nurse are most appropriate for the client at this time? **Select all that apply.**

A. "How is your pain on a 0-10 scale with 10 being the worst possible pain you've had?"
B. "Could you describe the pain in your back?"
C. "When you had visitors, you seemed to be laughing and not in any pain."
D. "I'll get you some pain medication that the surgeon ordered."
E. "Can you tell me what positions make the pain feel worse and better?"

Assessment Challenges

Patients who are unable to report their PAIN using the customary self-report assessment tools are at higher risk for undertreated pain than those who can report. These include patients who are cognitively impaired, critically ill (intubated, unresponsive), comatose, or imminently dying. Patients who are receiving neuromuscular blocking agents or are sedated from general anesthetics and other drugs given during surgery are also among this at-risk population.

First suggested in 1999 by McCaffery and Pasero, the *Hierarchy of Pain Measures* is recommended by many professional organizations today as a framework for assessing PAIN in patients who cannot self-report. The key components of the Hierarchy require the nurse to (1) attempt to obtain self-report; (2) consider underlying pathology or conditions and procedures that might be painful (e.g., surgery); (3) observe behaviors; (4) evaluate physiologic indicators; and (5) conduct an analgesic trial. See Table 3-5 for detailed information on each component of the Hierarchy of Pain Measures.

Patients with problems of COGNITION are among those at highest risk for undertreated PAIN because they are unable or have difficulty reporting their pain. The Hierarchy of Pain Measures (Table 3-5) lists several strategies to use when obtaining self-report is a challenge. When these are ineffective, the Hierarchy suggests that a number of behaviors have been shown to be indicators of pain. Behavioral pain assessment tools are often used to systematically evaluate behaviors to help determine the presence of pain. Improvement in the behavioral pain score helps confirm suspicions that pain is present and provides a reference point for assessing the effectiveness of interventions.

It is important for nurses to remember that *a score obtained from the use of a behavioral tool is not the same as a self-reported pain intensity score.* Although it may seem logical to assume that the higher the behavioral score, the more intense the pain, this cannot be proven without the patient's report. Some patients remain nonverbal and lie completely still (which would yield a

TABLE 3-5 Hierarchy of Pain Measures

1. Attempt to obtain the patient's self-report, the single most reliable indicator of pain. Do not assume a patient cannot provide a report of pain; many cognitively impaired patients are able to use a self-report tool if simple actions are taken.
   - Try using a standard pain assessment tool (see Fig. 3-3).
   - Ensure eyeglasses and hearing aids are functioning.
   - Increase the size of the font and other features of the scale.
   - Present the tool in vertical format (rather than the frequently used horizontal).
   - Try using alternative words, such as "ache," "hurt," and "sore" when discussing pain.
   - Ask about pain in the present.
   - Repeat instructions and questions more than once.
   - Allow ample time to respond.
   - Remember that head nodding and eye blinking or squeezing the eyes tightly can also be used to signal presence of pain and sometimes used to rate intensity.
   - Ask awake and oriented ventilated patients to point to a number on the numeric scale if they are able.
   - Repeat instructions and show the scale each time pain is assessed.
2. Consider the patient's condition or exposure to a procedure that is thought to be painful. If appropriate, *assume pain is present* (APP) and document APP when approved by institution policy and procedure. As an example, pain should be assumed to be present in an unresponsive, mechanically ventilated, critically ill trauma patient. Nurses should assume that certain procedures are painful and premedicate based on that assumption.
3. Observe behavioral signs (e.g., facial expressions, crying, restlessness, and changes in activity). A pain behavior in one patient may not be in another. Try to identify pain behaviors that are unique to the patient ("pain signature"). Many behavioral pain assessment tools are available that will yield a pain behavior score and may help determine if pain is present. However, it is important to remember that a behavioral score is not the same as a pain intensity score. Behavioral tools are used to help identify the presence of pain and whether an intervention is effective, but the pain intensity is unknown if the patient is unable to provide it.
   - A surrogate who knows the patient well (e.g., parent, spouse, or caregiver) may be able to provide information about underlying painful pathology or behaviors that may indicate pain.
   - Although surrogates may be helpful in identifying behaviors that may indicate pain, research has shown that they commonly underestimate or overestimate the intensity of the pain. Therefore they should not be asked to rate the patient's pain intensity.
4. Evaluate physiologic indicators with the understanding that they are the *least* sensitive indicators of pain and may signal the existence of conditions other than pain or a lack of it (e.g., hypovolemia, blood loss). Patients quickly adapt physiologically despite pain and may have normal or below normal vital signs in the presence of severe pain. The overriding principle is that the absence of an elevated blood pressure or heart rate does not mean the absence of pain.
5. Conduct an analgesic trial to confirm the presence of pain and to establish a basis for developing a treatment plan if pain is thought to be present. An analgesic trial involves administering a low dose of analgesic and observing patient response. The initial low dose may not be enough to illicit a change in behavior and should be increased if the previous dose was tolerated, or another analgesic may be added. If behaviors continue despite optimal analgesic doses, other possible causes should be investigated.
   - In patients who are unresponsive, no change in behavior will be evident and the optimized analgesic dose should be continued.

From Pasero, C., & McCaffery, M. (2011). *Pain assessment and pharmacologic management.* St. Louis: Mosby.

low behavioral score) despite having severe PAIN. The reality is that if a patient cannot report the intensity of pain, the exact intensity is unknown. Two of the most commonly used behavioral assessment tools that are used for patients with problems of COGNITION such as delirium (acute confusion) or dementia (chronic confusion) are:

- Checklist of Nonverbal Pain Indicators (CNPI) has been tested in the acute care setting in patients with varying levels of cognitive impairment. The tool groups behavioral indicators of PAIN into six categories. Each category allows a score of 0 if the behavior is not observed and a 1 if the behavior occurred even briefly during activity or rest:
  - Facial expression (e.g., grimacing, crying)
  - Verbalizations or vocalizations (e.g., screaming)
  - Body movements (e.g., restlessness)
  - Changes in interpersonal interactions
  - Changes in activity patterns or routines
  - Mental status changes (e.g., confusion, increased confusion)
- Pain Assessment in Advanced Dementia (PAINAD) scale, which has been tested in patients with severe dementia (Herr et al., 2011). The tool groups behavioral indicators into five categories for scoring using a graduated scale of 0 (least intense behaviors) to 2 (most intense behaviors) per category for a maximum behavioral score of 10:
  - Breathing (independent of vocalization)
  - Negative vocalization
  - Facial expression
  - Body language
  - Consolability (ability to calm the patient)

NCLEX EXAMINATION CHALLENGE

Psychosocial Integrity

An older client who has advanced Alzheimer's disease is admitted to the clinical unit after abdominal surgery and is guarding her abdomen and moaning. What action will the nurse take?

A. Ask the client's family to rate the intensity of the client's pain using the 0-to-10 scale.
B. Use a behavioral pain assessment tool to determine the presence of pain.
C. Ask the client to rate the intensity of her pain using the 0-to-10 scale.
D. Contact the primary health care provider to request an order for an antianxiety drug.

For patients who are mechanically ventilated or may not be able to use other tools for communication, you can use these interventions:

- Establishing a reliable yes-no signal (e.g., thumbs up or down, head nods, or eye blinks) may be appropriate in some patients to establish the presence of pain.
- Use of communication boards, alphabet boards, computer, or picture boards with word labels may be helpful for patients with COGNITION problems.
- Correctly interpreting lip reading by maintaining eye contact, encouraging the patient to speak slowly, and using dentures if required are recommended.

Pharmacologic Management of Pain

Safe and effective use of analgesics requires the development of an individualized treatment plan based on a comprehensive assessment. This plan includes clarifying the desired outcomes of treatment and discussing options and preferences with the patient and family. Desired outcomes are periodically re-evaluated and changes made depending on patient response and, in some cases, disease progression.

Multimodal Analgesia

PAIN is complex, which explains why there is no single, universal treatment for it. Its complexity is also the basis for the widespread recommendation that a multimodal analgesic approach be used regardless of the type of pain (American Society of Anesthesiologists [ASA], 2012; Pasero & McCaffery, 2011; Portenoy, 2011; Turk et al., 2011; Wu & Raja, 2011). Multimodal treatment involves the use of two or more classes of analgesics to target different pain mechanisms in the PNS or CNS. It relies on the thoughtful and rational combination of analgesics to maximize relief and prevent analgesic gaps that may lead to worsening pain or unnecessary episodes of uncontrolled pain.

A multimodal approach may allow lower doses of each of the drugs in the treatment plan. Lower doses have the potential to produce fewer side effects. Further, multimodal analgesia can result in comparable or greater relief than can be achieved with any single analgesic. For postoperative PAIN, the use of combination therapy to prevent both inflammatory and neuropathic pain is likely to yield the best immediate results. It also offers the promise of reducing the incidence of prolonged or persistent postsurgical pain.

The multimodal strategy also has a role in the management of persistent PAIN. The complex nature of the many chronic conditions indicates the need for appropriate combinations of analgesics, such as anticonvulsants, antidepressants, and local anesthetics, to target differing underlying mechanisms.

Preemptive analgesia involves the administration of local anesthetics, opioids, and other drugs (multimodal analgesia) along the continuum of care, during the preoperative, intraoperative, and postoperative periods. This continuous approach is designed to decrease PAIN severity in the postoperative period, reduce analgesic dose requirements, prevent morbidity, shorten hospital stay, and avoid complications after discharge. Continuous multimodal analgesia may inhibit changes in the spinal cord that can lead to changes in the peripheral and central nervous systems that initiate and sustain chronic persistent postsurgical pain (see Nociception earlier in the chapter).

Routes of Administration

The oral route is the preferred route of analgesic administration and should be used whenever feasible because it is generally the least expensive, best tolerated, and easiest to administer. Other routes of administration are used when the oral route is not possible, such as in patients who are NPO, nauseated, or unable to swallow. For example, early postoperative pain and pain that is severe and escalating is managed with the IV route of administration. Then patients are transitioned to oral analgesics when they are able to tolerate oral intake.

Around-the-Clock Dosing

Two basic principles of providing effective management are (1) preventing PAIN and (2) maintaining a level of pain control that allows the patient to function and have an acceptable quality of life. Accomplishment of these desired outcomes may require the mainstay analgesic to be administered on a scheduled around-the-clock (ATC) basis, rather than PRN ("as needed"), to maintain stable analgesic levels. *ATC dosing regimens are designed to control pain for patients who report it being present 12 hours or more during a 24-hour period*, such as that associated with most chronic syndromes and pain during the first 24 to 48 hours after surgery or other tissue injury. PRN dosing of analgesics is appropriate for intermittent PAIN, such as before painful procedures and **breakthrough pain** (additional pain that "breaks through" the pain being managed by the mainstay analgesic), for which supplemental doses of analgesic are provided.

Patient-Controlled Analgesia

Patient-controlled analgesia (PCA) is an interactive method of management that allows patients to treat their pain by self-administering doses of analgesics. It is used to manage all types of PAIN and given by multiple routes of administration, including IV, subcutaneous, epidural, and perineural. A PCA infusion device ("pump") is used when PCA is delivered by invasive routes of administration and is programmed so that the patient can press a button ("pendant") to self-administer a set dose of analgesic ("PCA dose") at a set time interval ("demand" or "lockout") as needed. *Patients who use PCA must be able to understand the relationships between pain, pressing the PCA button and taking the analgesic, and pain relief. They must also be cognitively and physically able to use any equipment that is used to administer the therapy.*

PCA may be given with or without a basal rate (continuous infusion). The use of a basal rate is common when patient-controlled epidural analgesia (PCEA) is used. It is often added for opioid-tolerant patients and occasionally for opioid-naïve patients receiving IV PCA to allow them to achieve pain control. Remember that the patient has no control over the delivery of a continuous infusion. Essential to the safe use of a basal rate is prompt discontinuation of the basal rate if increased sedation or respiratory depression occurs.

! NURSING SAFETY PRIORITY QSEN

Action Alert

Teach patients how to use the PCA device and to report side effects, such as dizziness, nausea and vomiting, and excessive sedation. As with all opioids, monitor the patient's sedation level and respiratory status at least every 2 hours. Promptly decrease the opioid dose (i.e., discontinue basal rate) if increased sedation is detected.

The primary benefit of PCA is that it recognizes that only the patient can feel the PAIN and only the patient knows how much analgesic will relieve it. This fact reinforces that *PCA is for patient use only and that unauthorized activation of the PCA button (called "PCA by proxy") can be very dangerous.* Instruct staff, family, and other visitors to contact the nurse if they have concerns about pain control rather than pressing the PCA button for the patient.

The Three Analgesic Groups

Analgesics are categorized into three main groups: (1) non-opioid analgesics, which include acetaminophen and the NSAIDs; (2) opioid analgesics, such as morphine, hydromorphone, fentanyl, and oxycodone; and (3) adjuvant analgesics (sometimes referred to as *co-analgesics*), which make up the largest group and include a variety of agents with unique and widely differing mechanisms of action. Examples are local anesthetics and some anticonvulsants and antidepressants. Table 3-6 lists the three analgesic groups and examples of drugs in each group.

Non-opioid Analgesics. Acetaminophen and NSAIDs make up the non-opioid analgesic group. *Acetaminophen* is thought to relieve PAIN by underlying mechanisms in the CNS. It has analgesic and antipyretic properties but is not effective to treat inflammation. In contrast, *NSAIDs* have analgesic, antipyretic, and anti-inflammatory properties. These drugs produce pain relief by blocking prostaglandins through inhibition of the enzyme *cyclooxygenase (COX)* in the peripheral nervous system (see Nociception and Fig. 3-1 earlier in the chapter).

Non-opioids are available in a variety of formulations and given by multiple routes of administration. They are also flexible analgesics used for a wide range of conditions. Non-opioid drugs are appropriate alone for mild to moderate nociceptive pain (e.g., from surgery, trauma, or osteoarthritis) or are added to opioids, local anesthetics, and/or anticonvulsants as part of a multimodal analgesic regimen for more severe nociceptive pain. *However, they are not effective for neuropathic pain.*

Acetaminophen and an NSAID may be given together, and there is no need for staggered doses. Unless contraindicated, all surgical patients should routinely be given acetaminophen and an NSAID in scheduled doses as the foundation of the pain treatment plan throughout the postoperative course, preferably initiated preoperatively.

The non-opioids are often combined in a single tablet with opioids, such as oxycodone (Percocet) or hydrocodone (Vicodin, Lortab, Vicoprofen), and are very popular for the treatment of mild to moderate acute pain. Many people with persistent pain also take a combination non-opioid/opioid analgesic. However, it is important to remember that these combination drugs are not appropriate for severe pain of any type because the maximum daily dose of the non-opioid limits the escalation of the opioid dose.

Acetaminophen. Oral acetaminophen (Tylenol, Abenol ♣) has a long history of safety in recommended doses in all age-groups and most patient populations. It is recommended as first-line for musculoskeletal pain (e.g., osteoarthritis) in older adults but has no inflammatory properties so is less effective than NSAIDs for chronic inflammatory pain (e.g., rheumatoid arthritis). IV acetaminophen (Ofirmev) is approved for treatment of pain and fever in adults and children age 2 years and older and is given by a 15-minute infusion in single or repeated doses. It is given alone for mild to moderate pain or in combination with opioid analgesics for more severe pain and has been shown to be well tolerated and to produce a significant opioid dose-sparing effect and superior pain relief compared with placebo (Pasero & Stannard, 2012).

The most serious complication of acetaminophen is hepatotoxicity (liver damage) as a result of overdose. Patient's hepatic risk factors must always be considered before administration of acetaminophen. In the healthy adult, a maximum daily dose below 4000 mg is rarely associated with liver toxicity (Pasero & Stannard, 2012). Many experts recommend reducing the daily dose (e.g., 2500-3000 mg daily) when used for *long-term* treatment in older adults. Acetaminophen does not increase bleeding time and has a low incidence of GI adverse effects, making it the analgesic of choice in many people with comorbidities.

TABLE 3-6 The Three Analgesic Groups

Non-Opioid Analgesics

Advantages
- Versatile with multiple agents, formulations, and routes of administration available
- Flexible and useful for a wide variety of mild to moderate nociceptive-type pain conditions
- Identified as the foundation of a multimodal approach for nociceptive-type pain
- Can produce opioid dose-sparing effects
- Available in combination with opioids

Disadvantages
- Wide inter-individual differences in response
- Ineffective for neuropathic pain
- Acetaminophen adverse effects require careful consideration of patient's hepatic status before administration and care not to exceed recommended daily dose
- NSAID adverse effects prohibit use or suggest cautionary use in some patient populations, including older adults, patients with high CV and/or GI risk factors, and those with bleeding disorders
- All of the non-opioids and combination non-opioid/opioid formulations have a maximum daily dose that should not be exceeded

Examples
- Acetaminophen (Tylenol)
- Nonselective NSAIDs:
  - Aspirin
  - Diclofenac (Voltaren; Voltaren gel; Flector patch)
  - Ibuprofen (Motrin)
  - Ketoprofen (Orudis)
  - Ketorolac (Toradol)
  - Meloxicam (Mobic)
  - Naproxen (Naprosyn)
- COX-2-selective NSAIDs:
  - Celeçoxib (Celebrex)

Opioid Analgesics

Advantages
- Cornerstone of moderate to severe nociceptive-type pain
- Mu agonists have no ceiling on analgesia
- Opioid rotation can be initiated for development of tolerance
- With the exception of constipation, tolerance develops to side effects with regular daily doses over several days

Disadvantages
- Constipation is an almost universal opioid side effect and the number-one reason people stop taking pain medication
- Although most side effects are manageable, undetected excessive sedation and respiratory depression are life threatening
- Close monitoring of sedation and respiratory status is indicated during at least the first 24 hours of opioid therapy
- Screening for appropriateness and ongoing monitoring via a therapeutic relationship between the patient and prescriber are required for safe and effective long-term opioid therapy
- Some opioids produce metabolites that can accumulate and produce toxicity, for example, morphine (morphine 3-glucuronide [M3G])

Examples of Mu Opioid Agonists
- Morphine (MS Contin; Kadian; Avinza; Roxanol; Duramorph; Astramorph)
- Fentanyl (Sublimaze; Duragesic; Actiq; Fentora; Onsolis)
- Hydromorphone (Dilaudid; Hydromorph; Exalgo)
- Hydrocodone (Zogenix ER; Lortab; Vicodin [also contain acetaminophen]; Vicoprofen [also contains ibuprofen])
- Oxycodone (OxyIR; OxyContin; Percocet [also contains acetaminophen]; Percodan [also contains aspirin])
- Oxymorphone (Opana; Opana ER)
- Methadone (Dolophine; Methadose)

Adjuvant Analgesics

Advantages
- Largest and most diverse analgesic group; wide variety of agents, formulations, and routes of administration available depending on agent
- Side effects often are responsive to dose reduction
- Tolerance develops to most of the adverse effects

Disadvantages
- Contain the agents that are recommended for treatment of neuropathic pain
- Considerable variability among people in their response to agents used to treat chronic neuropathic pain, including to agents within the same class; a "trial and error" strategy must be used, and multiple analgesic trials are sometimes necessary
- Most require titration of dose over several weeks to evaluate effectiveness; patients must be forewarned of delayed onset of analgesia
- Most have a maximum daily dose
- Side effects can be significant and may limit dose escalation

Examples
- Anticonvulsants:
  - Gabapentin (Neurontin)
  - Pregabalin (Lyrica)
- Antidepressants:
  - Tricyclic antidepressants:
    - Nortriptyline (Aventyl; Pamelor)
    - Desipramine (Norpramin)
  - Serotonin-norepinephrine reuptake inhibitors (SNRIs):
    - Duloxetine (Cymbalta)
    - Venlafaxine (Effexor)
- Alpha$_2$-adrenergic agonists:
  - Clonidine (Catapres, Duraclon)
  - Tizanidine (Zanaflex)
- Local anesthetics:
  - Bupivacaine (Marcaine)
  - Ropivacaine (Naropin)
  - Lidocaine injectable
  - Lidocaine patch 5% (Lidoderm)
- Muscle relaxants/antispasmodics:
  - Baclofen (Lioresal)
  - Cyclobenzaprine (Flexeril)
- NMDA antagonists:
  - Ketamine (Ketalar)

CV, Cardiovascular; *NMDA*, *N*-methyl-D-aspartate.

! NURSING SAFETY PRIORITY QSEN

Drug Alert

Teach patients to tell their primary health care provider about the amounts of acetaminophen and NSAIDs they take each day. Remind patients of the importance of being alert to the adverse effects of the medications they take and to complete any prescribed laboratory tests (e.g., liver enzymes) to identify early indicators of adverse effects.

NSAIDs. A benefit of the NSAID group is the availability of a wide variety of agents for administration via noninvasive routes. Ibuprofen (Motrin, Novo-Profen♣), naproxen (Naprosyn, Nu-Naprox♣), and celecoxib (Celebrex) are the most widely used oral NSAIDs in the United States and Canada (see Table 3-6). Diclofenac (Voltaren) is prescribed in patch and gel form for topical administration. An intranasal patient-controlled formulation of ketorolac (Sprix) has been approved for short-term treatment of acute PAIN. IV formulations of ketorolac (Toradol) and ibuprofen (Caldolor) are also used to manage acute pain. Both have been shown to produce excellent analgesia alone for mild to moderate nociceptive pain and significant opioid dose-sparing effects when administered as part of a multimodal analgesic plan for more severe pain (Pasero & McCaffery, 2011).

NSAIDs have more adverse effects than acetaminophen, with gastric toxicity and ulceration being the most common of the adverse effects. Risk factors for NSAID adverse effects include being older than 60 years or having a history of peptic ulcer or cardiovascular (CV) disease. An important principle of NSAID use is to administer the lowest dose for the shortest time necessary.

All NSAIDs carry a risk for CV adverse effects through prostaglandin inhibition. The U.S. Food and Drug Administration (FDA) cautions against the use of any NSAIDs after high-risk open heart surgery because of an elevated CV risk with NSAIDs in this population. Prostaglandins also affect renal function. Be sure that the patient is adequately hydrated when administering NSAIDs to prevent acute renal failure.

! NURSING SAFETY PRIORITY QSEN

Drug Alert

NSAIDs can cause GI disturbances and decrease platelet aggregation (clotting), which can result in bleeding. Therefore observe the patient for gastric discomfort or vomiting and for bleeding or bruising. Tell the patient and family to stop taking these drugs and report these effects to the primary health care provider immediately if any of these problems occur. Celecoxib has no effect on bleeding time and produces less GI toxicity compared with other NSAIDs.

Health Teaching. When taking a patient history, ask about the use of non-opioids, keeping in mind that most people do not understand the difference between the generic and brand names of over-the-counter (OTC) drugs. Patients may be taking both a generic non-opioid (e.g., acetaminophen, naproxen, or ibuprofen) and a brand name of the same non-opioid (e.g., Tylenol, Naprosyn, or Advil) at the same time and exceeding the safe maximum daily dose. They also may not realize that many OTC medications, such as sleep and cold remedies, contain non-opioids. Ask the patient or patient's family to provide the name of each drug (prescription and OTC) that the patient is taking, as well as the daily dose. Teach patients to be aware of the amount of non-opioid in combination products such as hydrocodone (e.g., Vicodin, Vicoprofen) and oxycodone (e.g., Percocet). Stress to patients that exceeding the safe maximum daily non-opioid dose places the patient at a high risk for adverse effects, such as liver toxicity (acetaminophen) and GI bleeding and CV complications (NSAIDs).

CONSIDERATIONS FOR OLDER ADULTS

Patient-Centered Care QSEN

Older adults are at increased risk for NSAID-induced GI toxicity. Acetaminophen should be used for mild pain. If an NSAID is needed for inflammatory pain or additional analgesia, the least ulcerogenic NSAID is recommended. The addition of a proton pump inhibitor (e.g., lansoprazole, omeprazole) to NSAID therapy, or opioid analgesics rather than an NSAID, is recommended for high-risk patients.

? NCLEX EXAMINATION CHALLENGE

Physiological Integrity

An older client takes acetaminophen (Tylenol) 2000 mg daily for osteoarthritis. What health teaching will the nurse provide for the client related to this medication?

A. "Be sure and take your medication with food to prevent stomach ulcers."
B. "Take your medication only when you need it for chronic pain."
C. "Avoid any over-the-counter medications that may contain acetaminophen."
D. "Take your blood pressure often because acetaminophen can cause it to go up."

Opioid Analgesics. Opioid analgesics are the mainstay in the management of moderate to severe nociceptive types of PAIN, such as postoperative, surgical, trauma, and burn pain (see Table 3-6). Although it is often used, the term "narcotic" is considered obsolete and inaccurate when discussing the use of opioids for pain management. "Narcotic" is used loosely by law enforcement and the media to refer to a variety of substances of potential abuse. Legally, controlled substances classified as narcotics include opioids, cocaine, and others. *The preferred term is "opioid analgesics" when discussing these agents in the context of pain management.* Some patients prefer the term "pain medications" or "pain medicine."

GENETIC/GENOMIC CONSIDERATIONS

Patient-Centered Care QSEN

It has long been known that the cytochrome (CY) *P450* enzyme system is important to the metabolism of some opioids. Interethnic variations in phenotypes of the *CYP450* enzymes are common, causing decreased metabolism of selected analgesics in a small percentage of Caucasians and Asians. These variations have clinical implications when the opioid *codeine*, which is metabolized by the *CYP450* enzyme system, is administered. Slow metabolizers may not respond well to codeine, and ultra-rapid metabolizers may have an exaggerated response (Pasero & McCaffery, 2011).

Opioids produce their effects by interacting with opioid receptor sites located throughout the body, including in the peripheral tissues, in the GI system, and in the spinal cord and brain (Yaksh & Wallace, 2011). When an opioid binds to the opioid receptor sites, it produces analgesia as well as unwanted effects, such as constipation, nausea, sedation, and respiratory depression. There are three classifications of opioids:

- Full or *mu agonists* ("morphine-like") bind primarily to the mu type opioid receptors in the CNS and, among other actions, block the release of the neurotransmitter *substance P,* which prevents the opening of calcium channels and the transmission of PAIN (Yaksh & Wallace, 2011). A major benefit of the mu opioid agonists is that they have no ceiling on analgesia. This means that increases in dose produce increases in pain relief and that there is no maximum dose (see Physical Tolerance later in the chapter). This property makes the mu opioid agonists the first-line opioid analgesics for moderate to severe nociceptive pain. Examples are morphine, fentanyl, hydromorphone, oxycodone, and hydrocodone.
- *Mixed agonists antagonists* bind to more than one type of opioid receptor. They bind as agonists to the kappa opioid receptors to produce analgesia and other effects and to the mu opioid receptors as antagonists. This antagonistic property explains why these drugs can trigger severe PAIN and opioid withdrawal syndrome characterized by rhinitis, abdominal cramping, nausea, agitation, and restlessness in patients who have been taking regular daily doses of a mu agonist opioid for several days. Another undesirable effect of these drugs is that they produce a dose-ceiling effect, which means further increases in dose will not produce further relief. This latter property limits their usefulness in pain management. Occasionally, these drugs are used in very low doses to antagonize (in hopes of relieving) opioid-induced side effects, such as pruritus. However, this approach risks reversing analgesia, so patients must be assessed frequently to ensure adequate PAIN control is maintained. Examples are butorphanol (Stadol) and nalbuphine (Nubain).
- *Partial agonists* have some kappa and mu opioid receptor activity but produce an analgesia plateau and are not easily reversed by opioid antagonists, such as naloxone (Narcan). These properties limit their role in PAIN management. Buprenorphine is a partial agonist opioid, available in a transdermal patch (Butrans) for stable pain management. The drug has been formulated alone (Subutex) and with naloxone (Suboxone) for the treatment of the disease of addiction.

Opioid antagonists (e.g., naloxone [Narcan], naltrexone [Revia]) are drugs that also bind to opioid receptors but produce no analgesia (Yaksh & Wallace, 2011). If an antagonist is present, it competes with opioid molecules for binding sites on the opioid receptors and has the potential to block analgesia and other effects. They are used most often to reverse opioid effects, such as excessive sedation and respiratory depression.

Key Principles of Opioid Administration. Many factors are considered when determining the appropriate opioid analgesic for the patient with pain. These include the unique characteristics of the various opioids and patient factors, such as type of pain, pain intensity, age, gender, coexisting disease, current drug regimen and potential drug interactions, prior treatment outcomes, and patient preference.

Titration (dose increases or decreases) of the opioid dose is usually required at the start and throughout the course of treatment when opioids are administered. Whereas patients with cancer pain most often are titrated upward over time for progressive pain, patients with acute pain, particularly postoperative pain, are eventually titrated downward as pain resolves. Although the dose and analgesic effect of mu agonist opioids have no ceiling, the dose may be limited by side effects. The absolute dose administered is unimportant as long as a balance between pain relief and side effects is favorable. *The desired outcome of titration is to use the smallest dose that provides satisfactory pain relief with the fewest side effects.*

When an increase in the opioid dose is necessary and safe, the increase can be titrated by percentages. When a slight improvement in analgesia is needed, a 25% increase in the opioid dose may be sufficient; a 50% increase for moderate improvement; and a 100% increase may be indicated for strong improvement, such as when treating severe, escalating pain (Pasero & McCaffery, 2011). The time at which the dose can be increased is determined by the onset and peak effects of the opioid and its formulation. For example, the frequency of IV opioid doses during initial titration may be as often as every 5 to 15 minutes (see later discussion of specific opioids). In contrast, at least 24 hours should elapse before the dose of transdermal fentanyl is increased after the first patch application.

GENDER HEALTH CONSIDERATIONS

Patient-Centered Care QSEN

Research has identified differences between females and males in a number of factors that influence the pharmacokinetics (absorption, distribution, metabolism, and excretion) and pharmacodynamics (effects on the body) of drugs. Some of these factors are organ physiology, body composition, gastric emptying time, enzyme activity, and drug clearance (Snidvongs, 2008). Abundant research shows that women are at substantially greater risk for more pain conditions than men and that they may experience more postoperative and procedural pain than men (Fillingim et al., 2009). In the immediate postoperative period, women seem to have a higher opioid requirement but men demonstrate higher opioid consumption after the initial recovery period. This difference may be partly explained by the faster recovery after general anesthesia in women. Side effects and complications associated with opioid and non-opioid analgesics appear to be more prevalent in women than in men. Creatinine clearance (drug excretion) is generally higher in men than in women due to increased muscle mass, and clearance varies with the menstrual cycle in women.

CONSIDERATIONS FOR OLDER ADULTS

Patient-Centered Care QSEN

Although the patient's weight is not a good indicator of analgesic requirement, *age is considered an important factor to consider when selecting an opioid dose.* For older adults, the guideline is to "start low and go slow" with all drug dosing. For example, the starting opioid dose should be reduced by 25% to 50% in older adults because they are more sensitive to opioid side effects than are younger adults. The amount of subsequent doses is based on patient response, which should be evaluated frequently. Monitor sedation level and respiratory status, and promptly reduce the drug dose if sedation occurs or the respiratory rate is markedly decreased, depending on agency policy. Chart 3-1 describes best practices for pain assessment and management in the older adult.

Physical Dependence, Tolerance, and Addiction. The terms *physical dependence* and *tolerance* often are confused with *addiction,* so clarification of definitions is important. The most widely accepted definitions of these terms are:

- *Physical dependence is a normal response* that occurs with repeated administration of an opioid for several days. It

CHART 3-1 **Nursing Focus on the Older Adult**

Pain

Prevalence of Pain

- Recognize that older adults are at high risk for undertreated pain and those with cognitive impairment are at even higher risk.
- Common caregiver and health care team misconceptions, such as that pain sensitivity decreases with aging and older adults cannot tolerate analgesics without significant adverse effects, contribute to the under-treatment of pain in older adults.

Beliefs About Pain

- Older adults tend to report pain less often than younger adults, which frequently results in members of the health care team administering suboptimal analgesics and doses. The failure of older adults to report pain may be related to common beliefs and concerns they have about pain and the reporting of pain, such as:
  - Pain is an inevitable consequence of aging and little can be done to relieve it.
  - Expressing pain is unacceptable or is a sign of weakness.
  - Reporting pain will result in being labeled as a "bad" patient or a "complainer."
  - Nurses and physicians are too busy to listen to reports of pain.
  - Pain signifies a serious illness or impending death.
- Be aware of the common beliefs of older patients regarding pain and its management and correct misconceptions to help prevent barriers to achieving optimal pain relief.
- Nurses and other caregivers can overcome their reluctance to administer prescribed analgesics in adequate doses by following the principles of pain management in older persons (see *Management of Pain section*).

Assessment of Pain

- Ask the patient to provide his or her own report of pain; even mild to some moderate cognitively impaired older adults are able to provide self-report if nurses and caregivers take the time to obtain it.
  - Offer various self-report pain tools.
  - Always show tools in hard copy with large lettering, adequate space between lines, non-glossy paper, and color for increased visualization.
  - Be sure the patient is wearing glasses and hearing aids if needed and available.
  - Provide adequate lighting and privacy to avoid distracting background noise.
  - Repeat questions more than once, and allow adequate time for response.
  - Use verbal descriptions such as "ache," "sore," and "hurt" if the patient seems to have difficulty relating to the word "pain."
  - Ask about present pain only.
  - If the patient is able to use a self-report tool, use the same tool and reteach the tool each time pain is assessed.

Considerations for Cognitively Impaired Patients (also see Table 3-5)

- Remember to "assume pain is present" in patients with diseases and conditions or procedures commonly associated with pain (see discussion below on *analgesic trial*).
- If the patient is unable to provide self-report, look for behaviors that may indicate the presence of pain.
  - Someone who knows the patient well, such as a family member or caregiver, may be helpful in identifying behaviors that might indicate pain. Do not ask others to rate pain intensity, and do not attempt to rate it yourself. Only the patient knows how severe the pain is, and if he or she cannot rate or describe the intensity, the exact intensity is unknown.
- Assess using a reliable and valid behavioral pain assessment tool.
  - Remember that behavioral tools tell us that pain might be present and provide a reference point to help determine the effectiveness of interventions, but the scores on behavioral tools have not been correlated with the ratings on pain intensity scales. A behavioral score is not a pain intensity rating.
  - Use the same behavioral assessment tool each time pain is assessed.
- Consider an analgesic trial to help determine the presence of pain and to establish an ongoing treatment plan in patients who are thought to have pain. This involves the administration of a low-dose analgesic; changes or decreases in the intensity of behaviors indicate that pain may be the cause of the behaviors. Doses should be increased or additional analgesics added as appropriate.

Management of Pain

- Use a multimodal approach that combines analgesics with different underlying mechanisms with the desired outcome of achieving optimal pain relief with lower doses than would be possible with a single analgesic; lower doses result in fewer side effects.
- Consider the type of pain, and begin therapy with the first-line analgesics that are recommended for that type of pain.
  - Non-opioids (acetaminophen, NSAIDs), opioids, and local anesthetics are first-line analgesics for nociceptive-type pain (e.g., postoperative pain, osteoarthritis pain, cancer pain).
  - Antidepressants, anticonvulsants, and local anesthetics are first-line analgesics for neuropathic-type pain (e.g., postherpetic neuralgia, diabetic neuropathy, phantom limb pain, post-stroke pain).
- Do not give meperidine to older adults because most have decreased renal function and are unable to efficiently eliminate its CNS-toxic metabolite *normeperidine*.
- Use around-the-clock (ATC) dosing of analgesics for pain that is of a continuous nature (e.g., chronic osteoarthritis or cancer pain; chronic neuropathic pain, first 24 to 48 hours after surgery).
- Use as needed (PRN) dosing for intermittent pain and before painful activities, such as before ambulation and physical therapy.
- Be aware of the main side effects of the analgesics that are administered and that they may be more likely to occur or be more severe in older than in younger adults.
- *Start low and go slow* with drug dosing; increase doses to achieve adequate analgesia based on patient's response to the previous dose.
- Teach the patient and family or other caregiver about the pain management plan (analgesics and nonpharmacologic strategies) and when to notify the primary health care provider for unrelieved pain or unmanageable or intolerable drug side effects.
- To promote adherence to the pain management plan in the home setting, suggest using a pillbox to organize each day's medications and keeping a diary to identify times of the day or activities that increase pain. The diary can be presented to the primary health care provider who can use it to make necessary adjustments in the treatment plan.

is manifested by the occurrence of withdrawal symptoms when the opioid is suddenly stopped or rapidly reduced or an antagonist such as naloxone is given. Withdrawal symptoms may be suppressed by the natural, gradual reduction of the opioid as pain decreases or by gradual, systematic reduction, referred to as *tapering. Physical dependence is not the same as addictive disease.*

- *Tolerance is also a normal response* that occurs with regular administration of an opioid and consists of a decrease in one or more effects of the opioid (e.g., decreased analgesia, sedation, or respiratory depression). Like physical dependence, *tolerance is not the same as addictive disease.* Tolerance to analgesia usually occurs in the first days to 2 weeks of opioid therapy but is uncommon after that. It may be treated with increases in dose or rotation to a different opioid. However, disease progression, not tolerance to analgesia, appears to be the reason for most dose escalations. Stable pain usually results in stable opioid

TABLE 3-7 Equianalgesic Dose Chart for Common MU Opioid Analgesics

- *Equianalgesic* means approximately the same pain relief.
- The equianalgesic chart is a guideline for selecting doses for opioid-naïve patients. Doses and intervals between doses are titrated according to each person's responses.
- The equianalgesic chart is helpful when switching from one drug or route of administration to another.

OPIOID	ORAL	PARENTERAL	COMMENTS
Morphine	30 mg	10 mg	Standard for comparison; first-line opioid via multiple routes of administration; once-daily and twice-daily oral formulations; clinically significant metabolites.
Fentanyl	No formulation	100 mcg IV 100 mcg/hr of transdermal fentanyl is approximately equal to 4 mg/hr of IV morphine; 1 mcg/hr of transdermal fentanyl is approximately equal to 2 mg/24 hr of oral morphine	First-line opioid via IV, transdermal, and intraspinal routes; available in oral transmucosal and buccal formulations for breakthrough pain in opioid-tolerant patients; no clinically relevant metabolites.
Hydrocodone	30 mg (NR)	No formulation	Available only in combination with non-opioid and as such is appropriate only for mild to some moderate pain.
Hydromorphone (Dilaudid)	7.5 mg	1.5 mg	First-line opioid via multiple routes of administration; once-daily oral formulation; clinically significant metabolites noted with long-term, high-dose infusion.
Oxycodone	20 mg	No formulation in the United States	Short-acting and twice-daily oral formulations.
Oxymorphone	10 mg	1 mg	Parenteral and short-acting and twice-daily oral formulations.

Data from Pasero, C., & McCaffery, M. (2011). *Pain assessment and pharmacologic management.* St. Louis: Mosby.
NR, Not recommended.

doses. With the exception of constipation, tolerance to the opioid side effects develops with regular daily dosing of opioids over several days.

- *Opioid addiction is a chronic neurologic and biologic disease.* The development and characteristics of addiction are influenced by genetic, psychosocial, and environmental factors. No single cause of addiction, such as taking an opioid for pain relief, has been found. It is characterized by one or more of these behaviors: impaired control over drug use, compulsive use, continued use despite harm, and craving. *The disease of addiction is a treatable disease; as for any other suspected disease, refer the patient to an expert for diagnosis and treatment.*
- *Pseudoaddiction* is a mistaken diagnosis of addictive disease. When a patient's PAIN is not well controlled, the patient may begin to manifest symptoms suggestive of addictive disease. For example, in an effort to obtain adequate pain relief, the patient may respond with demanding behavior, escalating demands for more or different medications, and repeated requests for opioids on time or before the prescribed interval between doses has elapsed. PAIN relief typically eliminates these behaviors and is often accomplished by increasing opioid doses or decreasing intervals between doses.

Opioid Naïve versus Opioid Tolerant. Patients are often characterized as being either opioid naïve or opioid tolerant. An *opioid-naïve* person has not recently taken enough opioid on a regular basis to become tolerant to the effects of an opioid. An *opioid-tolerant* person has taken an opioid long enough at doses high enough to develop tolerance to many of the effects, including analgesia and the undesirable effects, such as nausea and sedation. There is no set time for the development of tolerance with wide individual variation among people. Some patients do not develop tolerance at all. Patients who have taken opioids regularly for about 7 days or longer are considered to be opioid tolerant.

Equianalgesia. The term *equianalgesia* means approximately "equal analgesia." An equianalgesic chart provides a list of analgesic doses, both oral and parenteral (IV, subcutaneous, and IM), that are approximately equal to each other in ability to provide pain relief (Table 3-7). Equianalgesic conversion of doses is used to help ensure patients receive approximately the same pain relief when they are switched from one opioid or route of administration to another. It requires a series of calculations based on the daily dose of the current opioid to determine the equianalgesic dose of the opioid to which the patient is to be switched. Consult and collaborate with the pharmacist whenever equianalgesic conversion is indicated.

Relative potency is the ratio of drug doses required to produce the same effect. For example, note in Table 3-7 that a single dose of 1.5 mg of parenteral hydromorphone produces approximately the same analgesia as 10 mg of parenteral morphine. This means that hydromorphone is more potent than morphine, but increased potency does not mean the drug is therapeutically superior or that it provides any advantage. Safe and effective pain management requires nurses to appreciate the differences in the potencies of the various opioids and apply the principles of equianalgesia when administering opioids.

Drug Formulation Terminology. The terms *short acting, fast acting, immediate release (IR),* and *normal release* have been used interchangeably to describe oral opioids that have an onset of action of about 30 minutes and a relatively short duration of 3 to 4 hours. The term *immediate release* is misleading because none of the oral analgesics have an immediate or even a fast onset of analgesia. The term *short acting* is preferred to reflect the short duration of oral opioids. Oral transmucosal and intranasal formulations are appropriately referred to as *ultra fast acting* because they have a peak effect of 5 to 15 minutes, depending on formulation.

The terms *modified-release, extended release (ER), sustained release (SR),* and *controlled release* are used to describe opioids that are formulated to release over a prolonged period of time.

For the purposes of this chapter, the term *modified-release* will be used when discussing these opioid formulations. *Long-acting* is applied to drugs with a long *half-life,* such as methadone. A drug's half-life provides an estimate of how fast the drug leaves the body. By definition, **half-life** is the time it takes for the amount of drug in the body to be reduced by 50%.

! NURSING SAFETY PRIORITY QSEN

Drug Alert

Modified-release opioids should never be crushed, broken, or chewed because doing so alters the formulation of the drug and can result in adverse events, including death from respiratory depression if consumed. Teach the patient to swallow the drug whole and allow the "time release" function of the drug to take effect. Intact modified-release tablets may be administered rectally in some patients who cannot swallow.

Selected Opioid Analgesics. *Morphine* is the standard against which all other opioid drugs are compared. It is the most widely used opioid throughout the world, particularly for cancer pain, and its use is established by extensive research and clinical experience. Morphine is a *hydrophilic* drug (readily absorbed in aqueous solution), which accounts for its slow onset and long duration of action when compared with other opioid analgesics (Table 3-8). It is available in a wide variety of short-acting and modified-release oral formulations and is given by multiple other routes of administration, including rectal, subcutaneous, and IV.

Fentanyl (Sublimaze) differs from morphine significantly in characteristics. It is a *lipophilic* (readily absorbed in fatty tissue) opioid and, as such, has a fast onset and short duration of action (see Table 3-8). These characteristics make it the most commonly used IV opioid when rapid analgesia is desired, such as for the treatment of severe, escalating acute PAIN and for procedural pain when a short duration of action is desirable. Fentanyl is the recommended opioid for patients with end-organ failure because it has no clinically relevant metabolites (Pasero & McCaffery, 2011). It also produces fewer hemodynamic adverse effects than other opioids so is often preferred in patients who are hemodynamically unstable, such as the critically ill.

Its lipophilicity makes fentanyl ideal for drug delivery by transdermal patch (Duragesic) for long-term opioid therapy and by the oral transmucosal (Actiq) and buccal (Fentora) routes for breakthrough PAIN treatment in opioid-tolerant patients. After application of the transdermal patch, a subcutaneous depot of fentanyl is established in the skin near the patch. After absorption from the depot into the systemic circulation, the drug distributes to fat and muscle. When the first patch is applied, 12 to 18 hours are required for clinically significant analgesia to be obtained. Be aware that the patient may need adequate supplemental analgesia during that time. Change the patch every 48 to 72 hours depending on patient response.

TABLE 3-8 Characteristics of Selected First-Line Opioid Analgesics*

OPIOID	ONSET (MINUTES)	PEAK (MINUTES)	DURATION (HOURS)
Morphine	30-45 (oral) 5-10 (IV)	60 90 (oral) 15-30 (IV)	3-4 (oral) 3-4 (IV)
Fentanyl	5 (OT) 3-5 (IV)	15 (OT) 10-20 (IV)	2 (OT) 2 (IV)
Hydromorphone	15-30 (oral) 5 (IV)	30-90 (oral) 10-30 (IV)	3-4 (oral) 3-4 (IV)

Data from Pasero, C., & McCaffery, M. (2011). *Pain assessment and pharmacologic management.* St. Louis: Mosby.
IV, Intravenous; *OT,* oral transmucosal.
*Characteristics do not apply to modified-release formulations.

! NURSING SAFETY PRIORITY QSEN

Drug Alert

Teach patients taking transdermal fentanyl not to apply heat (e.g., hot packs, heating pads) directly over the patch because heat increases absorption of the drug and can result in adverse events, including death from fentanyl-induced respiratory depression. Ask patients about the presence of patches on admission, and document and communicate this information to other members of the interdisciplinary health care team.

Hydromorphone (Dilaudid) is less hydrophilic than morphine but less lipophilic than fentanyl, which contributes to an onset and duration of action that is intermediate between morphine and fentanyl (see Table 3-8). The drug is often used as an alternative to morphine, especially for acute PAIN, most likely because the two drugs produce similar analgesia and have comparable side effects. It is a first- or second-choice opioid (after morphine) for postoperative management via IV PCA and is available in a once-daily modified-release oral formulation for long-term opioid treatment.

? NCLEX EXAMINATION CHALLENGE

Physiological Integrity

A client has a one-time order for morphine 2 mg IV push. The drug is available as 5 mg/mL. The nurse administers _____ mL of morphine for one dose.

Oxycodone is available in the United States for administration by the oral route only and is used to treat all types of PAIN. In combination with acetaminophen or ibuprofen, it is appropriate for mild to some moderate pain. Single-entity, short-acting (OxyIR) and modified-release (OxyContin) oxycodone formulations are used most often for moderate to severe cancer PAIN and in some patients with moderate to severe non-cancer pain. It has been used successfully as part of a multimodal treatment plan for postoperative pain as well. Like morphine, it is available in liquid form for patients who are unable to swallow tablets.

Hydrocodone in combination with non-opioids limits its use to the treatment of mild to some moderate PAIN. It is one of the most commonly prescribed analgesics in the United States, but its prescription for treatment of persistent pain (except for breakthrough dosing) should be carefully evaluated because of its ceiling on efficacy and safety related to the non-opioid constituent (ingredient).

Methadone (Dolophine) is a unique opioid analgesic that may have advantages over other opioids in carefully selected patients. In addition to being a mu opioid, it is an antagonist at the NMDA (*N*-methyl-D-aspartate) receptor site and thus has the potential to produce analgesic effects as a second- or third-line option for some neuropathic pain states (Dworkin et al., 2010). It may be given as an alternative when it is necessary to switch a patient to a new opioid because of inadequate analgesia or unacceptable side effects during long-term opioid therapy.

Although it has no active metabolites, methadone has a very long and highly variable half-life (5 to 100+ hours; average is 20 hours). Watch patients closely for excessive sedation—a sign of drug accumulation during the titration period. Other limitations are its tendency to interact with a large number of medications and prolong QTc interval.

Dual Mechanism Analgesics. The dual mechanism analgesics, *tramadol* (Ultram) and *tapentadol* (Nucynta), are relatively new to the PAIN management arena. These drugs bind weakly to the mu opioid receptor site and block the reuptake (resorption) of the inhibitory neurotransmitters *serotonin* and/or *norepinephrine* in the spinal cord and brainstem of the modulatory descending PAIN pathway (see Nociception earlier in this chapter). This makes these neurotransmitters more available to fight pain. Because they have the opioid receptor binding property, they are discussed in the Opioid Analgesics section of this chapter. However, they are usually referred to as dual mechanism rather than opioid analgesics.

Tramadol is used for both acute and chronic PAIN and is available in oral short-acting (Ultram) and modified-release (Ultram ER) formulations, including a short-acting tablet in combination with acetaminophen (Ultracet). It is appropriate for acute pain and has been designated as a second-line analgesic for the treatment of neuropathic pain (Dworkin et al., 2010). Side effects are similar to those of opioids. The drug can lower seizure threshold and interact with other drugs that block the reuptake of serotonin, such as the selective serotonin reuptake inhibitor (SSRI) antidepressants. Although rare, this combination can have an additive effect and result in serotonin syndrome, characterized by agitation, diarrhea, heart and blood pressure changes, and loss of coordination.

The newer dual mechanism analgesic *tapentadol* is also available in short-acting (Nucynta) and modified-release (Nucynta ER) formulations and is appropriate for both acute and chronic PAIN. Major benefits of tapentadol are that it has no active metabolites and a significantly more favorable side effect profile (particularly GI effects) compared with opioid analgesics.

Opioids to Avoid. *Meperidine* (Demerol) was once the most widely used opioid analgesic in the inpatient setting. In recent years, it has either been removed from or severely restricted on U.S. hospital formularies for the treatment of pain in an effort to improve patient safety. A major drawback to the use of meperidine is its active metabolite, *normeperidine*, a CNS stimulant that can cause delirium, irritability, tremors, myoclonus, and generalized seizures. It is a particularly poor choice in older adults because they have decreased renal function, which prevents the elimination of the toxic metabolite. Meperidine has no advantages over any other opioid, and it has no place in the treatment of persistent pain or in delivery systems, such as PCA. If prescribed, meperidine should not be used for more than 48 hours or at doses exceeding 600 mg/24 hours (Pasero & McCaffery, 2011).

Codeine in combination with non-opioids (e.g., with acetaminophen in Tylenol #3) has been used for many years for the management of mild to moderate pain; however, it has largely been replaced by analgesics that are more efficacious and better tolerated (e.g., Percocet, Vicodin). Research has shown that codeine/acetaminophen is less effective and associated with more adverse effects than NSAIDs, such as ibuprofen and naproxen, for acute pain.

Intraspinal Analgesia. Intraspinal analgesia involves the administration of analgesics via a needle or catheter placed in the epidural space or the intrathecal (subarachnoid) space by an anesthesia provider. The intraspinal routes of administration are used to manage both acute pain, such as postoperative pain, and some chronic cancer and non-cancer pain.

Epidural analgesia can be delivered by intermittent bolus technique, continuous infusion, or patient-controlled epidural analgesia (PCEA) with or without continuous infusion. The most commonly administered analgesics by the epidural route are the opioids *morphine, hydromorphone,* and *fentanyl* in combination with a long-acting local anesthetic, such as bupivacaine (Marcaine) or ropivacaine (Naropin). This multimodal approach allows lower doses of both the opioid and local anesthetic and produces fewer side effects. A single epidural injection of preservative-free morphine (Duramorph) is effective for about 24 hours. An extended-release formulation of preservative-free epidural morphine (DepoDur) is effective for 48 hours.

Intrathecal (spinal) analgesia is usually delivered via single bolus technique for patients with acute pain (e.g., hysterectomy) or continuous infusion via an implanted device for the treatment of chronic pain. Because the drug is delivered directly into the aqueous cerebral spinal fluid (CSF), morphine with its hydrophilic nature is used most often for intrathecal analgesia. Extremely small amounts of drug are administered by the intrathecal route (about 10 times less than by the epidural route) because the drug is so close to the spinal action site.

The side effects of intraspinal analgesia depend on the type of drug administered. In other words, if opioids are administered, the same opioid-induced side effects that occur with other routes of administration can occur with intraspinal administration. If local anesthetics are administered, common side effects are urinary retention, hypotension, and numbness and weakness of lower extremities. The latter can occur on a continuum (mild and localized) to a complete block (undesirable and requires prompt anesthesia evaluation). In most cases, the side effects that occur during continuous infusion or PCEA can be managed by decreasing the dose.

Complications of intraspinal analgesia are rare but can be life threatening. Perform frequent neurologic assessments and promptly report abnormal findings to the anesthesiologist or nurse anesthetist.

! NURSING SAFETY PRIORITY QSEN

Drug Alert

Assess patients receiving epidural local anesthetic for their ability to bend their knees and lift their buttocks off the mattress (if not prohibited by surgical procedure). Ask them to point to any areas of numbness and tingling. Mild, transient lower extremity motor weakness and orthostatic hypotension may be present, necessitating assistance with ambulation. Most undesirable effects can be managed with a reduction in local anesthetic dose. Promptly report areas of numbness outside of the surgical site, inability to bear weight, and severe hypotension to the anesthesia provider. *Do not delegate assessment of local anesthetic effects to unlicensed assistive personnel!*

SENSORY PERCEPTION manifestations (e.g., increasing numbness and tingling of extremities), decreasing ability to bear weight, and/or changes in bowel or bladder function can indicate the development of an epidural hematoma or abscess. If not detected, a hematoma or abscess can cause spinal cord compression and paralysis.

Nurses have an extensive role in the management and monitoring of intraspinal techniques, including infusion device operation, replacing empty drug reservoirs, checking and protecting infusion sites and systems, treating side effects, preventing complications, discontinuing therapy, and removing catheters.

Adverse Effects of Opioid Analgesics. The most common side effects of opioid analgesics are constipation, nausea, vomiting, pruritus, and sedation (Pasero & McCaffery, 2011). Respiratory depression is less common but the most feared of the opioid side effects. *Most of the opioid side effects are dose-related, so simply decreasing the opioid dose is sufficient to eliminate or make most of the side effects tolerable for most patients.* Table 3-9 lists interventions to prevent and manage opioid-induced side effects.

Opioids can result in delayed gastric emptying, slowed bowel motility, and decreased peristalsis, all of which can result in slow-moving, hard stool that is difficult to pass. Risk for *constipation* is elevated with opioid use, advanced age, and immobility, but it is an almost universal opioid side effect in all populations (i.e., tolerance rarely develops). Constipation is a primary reason people stop taking their pain medication. Therefore teach the importance of taking a preventive approach and aggressive management if symptoms occur. To prevent constipation, remind patients to take a daily stool softener plus a mild peristaltic stimulant, such as senna, for as long as they are taking an opioid.

Postoperative nausea and vomiting (PONV) are among the most unpleasant of the side effects associated with surgery. It is less common in older than younger adults. Evaluate patients for PONV risk, reduce risk factors if possible, and provide multimodal analgesia so that the lowest effective opioid dose can be given.

Pruritus (itching) is a side effect, not an allergic reaction to opioids. Although antihistamines such as diphenhydramine (Benadryl) are commonly used, there is no strong evidence that they relieve opioid-induced pruritus. Patients may report being less bothered by itching after taking an antihistamine, but this is likely the result of sedating effects. Sedation can be problematic in those already at risk for excessive sedation, such as postoperative patients. This problem can lead to life-threatening respiratory depression (Jarzyna et al., 2011; Pasero & McCaffery, 2011). *Remember that the single most effective, safest, and least expensive treatment for pruritus is opioid dose reduction.*

As patients become opioid tolerant, *tolerance to the opioid side effects (with the exception of constipation) develops.* It is reassuring for patients receiving long-term opioid therapy to know that most of the side effects will subside with regular daily doses of opioids over several days.

Most patients experience sedation at the beginning of opioid therapy and whenever the opioid dose is increased significantly. *If undetected or left untreated, excessive sedation can progress to clinically significant respiratory depression.* Like most of the other opioid side effects, sedation and respiratory depression are dose-related. Prevention of clinically significant opioid-induced respiratory depression begins with administration of the lowest effective opioid dose (multimodal analgesia with a non-opioid foundation), careful titration, and close monitoring of sedation and respiratory status throughout therapy. *Unless the patient is at*

TABLE 3-9 Nursing Interventions to Prevent and Treat Selected Opioid Side Effects*

Constipation

- Assess previous bowel habits.
- Keep a record of bowel movements.
- Remind patients that tolerance to this side effect does not develop, so *a preventive approach must be used;* administer a stool softener plus mild stimulant laxative for duration of opioid therapy; do not give bulk laxatives because these can result in obstruction in some patients.
- Provide privacy, encourage adequate fluids and activity, and give foods high in roughage.
- If ineffective, try suppository or Fleet's enema.

Nausea and Vomiting (N/V)

- Use a multimodal antiemetic preventive approach (e.g., dexamethasone plus ondansetron in moderate- to high-risk patients).
- Assess cause of nausea and eliminate contributing factors if possible.
- Reduce opioid dose if possible.
- Reassure patients taking long-term opioid therapy that tolerance to this side effect develops with regular daily opioid doses.
- Treat with antiemetic drug as prescribed.
- Consider switching to another opioid for unresolved N/V.

Sedation

- Remember that sedation precedes opioid-induced respiratory depression; identify patient and iatrogenic risk factors and monitor sedation level and respiratory status frequently during the first 24 hours of opioid therapy.
- Use a simple sedation scale to monitor for unwanted sedation (see Table 3-10).
- If excessive sedation is detected, reduce opioid dose to prevent respiratory depression.
- Eliminate unnecessary sedating drugs such as antihistamines, anxiolytics, muscle relaxants, and hypnotics. If it is necessary to administer these drugs during opioid therapy, monitor sedation and respiratory status closely.
- Reassure patients taking long-term opioid therapy that tolerance to this side effect develops with regular daily opioid doses.
- Be aware that stimulants such as caffeine may counteract opioid-induced sedation.
- Consider switching to another opioid for unresolved excessive sedation during long-term opioid therapy.

Respiratory Depression

- Be aware that counting respiratory rate alone does not constitute a comprehensive respiratory assessment. Proper assessment of respiratory status includes observation of the rise and fall of the patient's chest to determine depth and quality in addition to counting respiratory rate for 60 seconds.
- Recognize that *snoring is respiratory obstruction* and an ominous sign (see text).
- Remember that sedation precedes opioid-induced respiratory depression; identify patient and iatrogenic risk factors and monitor sedation level and respiratory status frequently during the first 24 hours of opioid therapy (see Sedation section).
- Stop opioid administration immediately for clinically significant respiratory depression, stay with patient, continue attempts to arouse patient, support respirations, call for help (consider Rapid Response Team or Code Blue), and consider giving naloxone.
- Reassure patients taking long-term opioid therapy that tolerance to this side effect develops with regular daily opioid doses.

*With the exception of constipation, opioid side effects are dose-related. This means that a multimodal analgesic approach that incorporates non-opioid analgesics as its foundation and administers the lowest effective opioid dose should be used. The simplest and most effective method for managing opioid side effects when they occur is to reduce the opioid dose.

the end of life, promptly reduce opioid dose or stop titration whenever increased sedation is detected to prevent respiratory depression. In some patients (e.g., those with obstructive sleep apnea, pulmonary dysfunction, multiple comorbidities), mechanical monitoring, such as capnography (to measure exhaled carbon dioxide) and pulse oximetry (to measure oxygen saturation), is needed (Jarzyna et al., 2011; Pasero & McCaffery, 2011).

Occasionally, drugs that produce significant sedation are used to treat side effects and other conditions that accompany the PAIN experience. For example, *antianxiety agents* (anxiolytics), such as alprazolam (Xanax) and lorazepam (Ativan), are prescribed to reduce anxiety. Many of the drugs used to treat opioid side effects are sedating, such as the antihistamines (diphenhydramine) for pruritus and the antiemetics *promethazine (Phenergan)* and *hydroxyzine (Vistaril)* for nausea. It is important to recognize that administration of these drugs together has an additive sedating effect. If administered, closely monitor for sedation and assess respiratory status frequently.

To assess sedation, use a simple, easy-to-understand sedation scale developed for assessment of *unwanted* sedation that includes what should be done at each level of sedation (Jarzyna et al., 2011; Pasero & McCaffery, 2011). Table 3-10 presents a widely used sedation scale. The key to assessing sedation is to determine how easy it is to arouse the patient. Assess each person's response to the first dose of an opioid. If opioids are administered by bolus technique, assess sedation level and respiratory status at the opioid's peak time after each bolus. *If a patient is difficult to arouse, always stop the opioid, stay with the patient, continue vigorous attempts to arouse, and call for help!*

Respiratory depression is assessed on the basis of what is normal for a particular person and is usually described as clinically significant when there is a decrease in the rate, depth, and regularity of respirations from baseline, rather than just by a specific number of respirations per minute. Risk factors for opioid-induced respiratory depression include age 55 years or older, obesity, obstructive sleep apnea, and pre-existing pulmonary dysfunction or other comorbidities.

TABLE 3-10 Pasero Opioid-Induced Sedation Scale (POSS) with Interventions*

S = Sleep, easy to arouse
Acceptable; no action necessary; may increase opioid dose if needed.

1 = Awake and alert
Acceptable; no action necessary; may increase opioid dose if needed.

2 = Slightly drowsy, easily aroused
Acceptable; no action necessary; may increase opioid dose if needed.

3 = Frequently drowsy, arousable, drifts off to sleep during conversation
Unacceptable; monitor respiratory status and sedation level closely until sedation level is stable at less than 3 and respiratory status is satisfactory; decrease opioid dose 25% to 50%[1] or notify primary[2] or anesthesia provider for orders; consider administering a non-sedating, opioid-sparing non-opioid, such as acetaminophen or a NSAID, if not contraindicated; ask patient to take deep breaths every 15-30 minutes.

4 = Somnolent, minimal or no response to verbal and physical stimulation
Unacceptable; stop opioid; consider administering naloxone[3,4]; call Rapid Response Team (Code Blue); stay with patient, stimulate, and support respiration as indicated by patient status; notify primary[2] or anesthesia provider; monitor respiratory status and sedation level closely until sedation level is stable at less than 3 and respiratory status is satisfactory.

From Pasero, C., & McCaffery, M. (2011). *Pain assessment and pharmacologic management.* St. Louis: Mosby. Copyright 1994. Used with permission.
*Appropriate action is given in italics at each level of sedation.
[1]Opioid analgesic orders or a hospital protocol should include the expectation that a nurse will decrease the opioid dose if a patient is excessively sedated.
[2]For example, the physician, nurse practitioner, advanced practice nurse, or physician assistant responsible for the pain management prescription.
[3]For adults experiencing respiratory depression, administer dilute solution (0.4 mg of naloxone in 10 mL of normal saline) very slowly (0.5 mL over 2 minutes) while observing the patient's response (titrate to effect).
[4]Hospital protocols should include the expectation that a nurse will administer naloxone to any patient suspected of having life-threatening opioid-induced sedation and respiratory depression.

! NURSING SAFETY PRIORITY QSEN

Critical Rescue

An accurate respiratory assessment requires watching the rise and fall of the patient's chest to determine depth and regularity of respirations in addition to counting the respiratory rate for 60 seconds. Listening to the sound of the patient's respiration is critical as well—*snoring indicates airway obstruction and must be attended to promptly* with repositioning and, depending on severity, a request for respiratory therapy consultation and further evaluation (Pasero & McCaffery, 2011). For accuracy, respiratory assessment is done before arousing the sleeping patient.

CONSIDERATIONS FOR OLDER ADULTS

Patient-Centered Care QSEN

The incidence of opioid side effects in the older adult population varies depending on the side effect. Older adults are sensitive to the sedating effects of opioids, making them higher risk for respiratory depression than younger adults.

? NCLEX EXAMINATION CHALLENGE

Physiological Integrity

A nursing technician reports that a postoperative client who is receiving IV PCA morphine is very drowsy, unable to complete a sentence without falling asleep, and has a respiratory rate of 12 breaths per minute. What is the nurse's first action at this time?

A. Arouse the client and raise the head of the bed to a 90-degree angle.
B. Promptly call the primary health care provider to request an order to reduce the opioid dose.
C. Take away the client's PCA button and tell the family to notify staff when pain returns.
D. Reduce environmental stimuli by darkening the room so that the client can sleep.

! NURSING SAFETY PRIORITY QSEN

Drug Alert

Unless the patient is at the end of life, promptly administer the opioid antagonist *naloxone (Narcan)* IV to reverse clinically significant opioid-induced respiratory depression. When giving the opioid antagonist *naloxone,* administer it slowly until the patient is more arousable and respirations increase to an acceptable rate. The desired outcome is to reverse just the sedative and respiratory depressant effects of the opioid but not the analgesic effects. Giving too much naloxone too fast not only can cause severe PAIN but also can lead to ventricular dysrhythmias, pulmonary edema, and even death. Continue to closely monitor the patient after giving naloxone because the duration of naloxone is shorter than the duration of most opioids and respiratory depression can recur. Sometimes more than one dose of naloxone is needed.

Adjuvant Analgesics. Adjuvant analgesics (sometimes called *co-analgesics*) are drugs that have a primary indication other than PAIN but are analgesic for some painful conditions (see Table 3-6). For example, the primary indication for antidepressants is depression, but some antidepressants help relieve some types of pain. The adjuvant analgesics are the largest and most diverse of the three analgesic groups. Drug selection and dosing are based on both experience and evidence-based practice guidelines (Dworkin et al., 2010).

Anticonvulsants and Antidepressants. *Anticonvulsants* (also called *antiepileptic drugs [AEDs]* when used for seizure management) produce analgesia by blocking sodium and calcium channels in the CNS, thereby diminishing the transmission of PAIN. The gabapentinoids *gabapentin (Neurontin)* and *pregabalin (Lyrica)* are recommended as first-line analgesics for persistent neuropathic pain (Dworkin et al., 2010). They are increasingly being added to postoperative treatment plans to address the neuropathic component of surgical pain. Primary side effects are sedation and dizziness, which are usually transient and most notable during the titration phase of treatment.

Antidepressants relieve PAIN on the descending modulatory pathway by blocking the body's reuptake of the inhibitory neurochemicals *norepinephrine* and *serotonin.* Antidepressant adjuvant analgesics are divided into two major groups: the *tricyclic antidepressants* (TCAs) and the newer *serotonin and norepinephrine reuptake inhibitors* (SNRIs). Evidence-based guidelines recommend the TCAs *desipramine (Norpramin)* and *nortriptyline (Aventyl, Pamelor)* and the SNRIs *duloxetine (Cymbalta)* and *venlafaxine (Effexor)* as first-line options for neuropathic pain treatment (Dworkin et al., 2010).

The most common side effects of the TCAs are dry mouth, sedation, dizziness, mental clouding, weight gain, and constipation. Orthostatic hypotension is a potentially serious TCA side effect making TCAs a poor choice for older adults. The most serious adverse effect is cardiotoxicity, especially for patients with existing significant heart disease. The SNRIs have a more favorable side effect profile and are better tolerated than the TCAs. The most common SNRI side effects are nausea, headache, sedation, insomnia, weight gain, impaired memory, sweating, and tremors.

CONSIDERATIONS FOR OLDER ADULTS

Patient-Centered Care QSEN

Older adults are often sensitive to the effects of the adjuvant analgesics that produce sedation and other CNS effects, such as anticonvulsants and antidepressants. Therapy should be initiated with low doses, and titration should proceed slowly with systematic assessment of patient response. Caregivers in the home setting must be taught to take preventive measures to reduce the likelihood of falls and other accidents. A home safety assessment is highly recommended and can be arranged by social services before discharge.

Local Anesthetics. Local anesthetics relieve PAIN by blocking the generation and conduction of the nerve impulses necessary to transmit pain (Catterall & Mackie, 2011). The local anesthetic effect is dose-related. A high enough dose of local anesthetic can produce complete anesthesia, and a low enough dose (subanesthetic) can produce analgesia.

Local anesthetics have a long history of safe and effective use for the treatment of all types of PAIN. Allergy to local anesthetics is rare, and side effects are dose-related. CNS signs of systemic toxicity include ringing in the ears, metallic taste, irritability, and seizures. Signs of cardiotoxicity include circumoral tingling and numbness, bradycardia, cardiac dysrhythmias, and CV collapse.

The *lidocaine patch 5%* (Lidoderm) is 10 cm by 14 cm and contains 700 mg of lidocaine. The patch is placed directly over or adjacent to the painful area for absorption into the tissues directly below. A major benefit of the drug is that it produces minimal systemic absorption and side effects. The patch is left in place for 12 hours and then removed for 12 hours (12-hours-on, 12-hours-off regimen). This application process is repeated as needed for continuous analgesia.

Topical local anesthetic creams for superficial procedures, such as IV insertion, include *EMLA* (eutectic mixture of local anesthetics*) and LMX-4. EMLA* contains a combination of lidocaine 2.5% and prilocaine 2.5% and is applied to intact skin for 60 to 120 minutes before the procedure. *LMX-4* contains 4% lidocaine and is applied 30 minutes before the procedure. EMLA has a longer duration of action (2 hours) than LMX-4 (30 minutes) after cream removal. Topical local anesthetic side effects are rare and usually transient, with local skin reactions being the most common.

For many years, *regional anesthesia* has been administered by single-injection peripheral nerve blocks using a long-acting local anesthetic, such as bupivacaine or ropivacaine, to target a specific nerve or nerve plexus. This technique is highly effective in producing PAIN relief, but the effect is temporary (4-12 hours). *Continuous peripheral nerve block* (also called *perineural regional analgesia*) offers an alternative with longer lasting analgesia. A continuous peripheral nerve block involves establishment by an anesthesia provider of an initial block followed by placement of a catheter through which an infusion of local anesthetic is administered continuously, with or without PCA capability. When PCA capability is added, this is referred to as *PCRA* (patient-controlled regional analgesia). Just as with epidural and intrathecal analgesia, nurses are responsible for monitoring and managing the therapy (Pasero & McCaffery, 2011).

Use of Placebos

A placebo is defined as any medication or procedure, including surgery, which produces an effect in a patient because of its implicit or explicit intent, not because of its specific physical or chemical properties. A saline injection is one example of a placebo. Administration of a medication at a known subtherapeutic dose (e.g., 0.05 mg of morphine in an adult) is also considered a placebo.

Placebos are appropriately used as controls in research evaluating the effects of a new medication. Patients or volunteers who participate in placebo-controlled research must be able to give informed consent or have a guardian who can provide informed consent. Unfortunately, occasionally placebos are used clinically in a deceitful manner and without informed consent. This is often done when the clinician does not accept the patient's report of pain. Pain relief resulting from a placebo, should it occur, is mistakenly believed to invalidate a patient's report of pain. This typically results in the patient being deprived of pain-relief measures despite research showing that many patients who have obvious physical stimuli for pain (e.g., abdominal surgery) report pain relief after placebo administration. The use of placebos has both ethical and legal implications, violates the nurse-patient relationship, and deprives patients of more appropriate methods of assessment or treatment.

! NURSING SAFETY PRIORITY QSEN

Drug Alert

Deceitful administration of a placebo violates informed consent law and jeopardizes the nurse-patient therapeutic relationship. Never administer a placebo to a patient. Promptly contact your nursing supervisor if you are given an order to do so.

Nonpharmacologic Management of Pain

Most people use self-management and nonpharmacologic strategies to deal with their health issues and promote well-being (Bruckenthal, 2010). Nonpharmacologic methods are appropriate alone for mild- and some moderate-intensity PAIN and should be used to complement, not replace, pharmacologic therapies for more severe pain. The effectiveness of nonpharmacologic methods can be unpredictable. Although not all have been shown to relieve pain, they offer many benefits to some patients of all ages (see Evidence-Based Practice box). For example, research has shown that nonpharmacologic methods can facilitate relaxation and reduce anxiety, stress, and depression, which often accompany the pain experience (Bruckenthal, 2010). Many patients find the use of nonpharmacologic methods helps them cope better and feel greater control over the pain experience. Nurses play an important role in providing and teaching their patients about nonpharmacologic strategies. Many of the methods are relatively easy for nurses to incorporate into daily clinical practice and may be used individually or in combination with other nonpharmacologic therapies.

Nonpharmacologic interventions are categorized as being body-based (physical) modalities; mind-body (cognitive-behavioral) methods; biologically based therapies; and energy therapies (Bruckenthal, 2010). Biologically based and energy therapies are used most often in the ambulatory care setting and are beyond the scope of this chapter.

Physical Modalities

The physical modalities have the best evidence for reducing pain. In the acute care setting, the physical modalities are used most often because of their ease in implementation and their role in postoperative recovery. In the ambulatory care setting, sustained physical regimens, such as regular low-impact exercise, in combination with analgesics improve outcomes for people with chronic pain. Many of the physical modalities require a prescription for use and reimbursement. Some require a trained expert to administer the technique (e.g., acupuncture). Among the most effective physical modalities used to manage or prevent pain are:

- Physical therapy
- Occupational therapy
- Aquatherapy
- Functional restoration (also has cognitive-behavioral components)
- Acupuncture
- Low-impact exercise programs, such as slow walking and yoga

The physical modalities are often administered using an interdisciplinary approach. The assistance of physical and occupational therapists to help design and implement an individualized plan with realistic goal setting promotes effectiveness of these methods. Coordinate with the therapist to implement strategies to decrease pain before therapy sessions with the purpose of increasing function and preventing further deterioration. Teach patients to adhere to their drug regimen to maximize effectiveness of the treatment plan. Expected patient outcomes include an increase in the range of motion, strength, and function of the affected area and an improved quality of life. The occupational therapist may also help decrease pain by making one or more splints to rest severely inflamed joints.

A number of *cutaneous (skin) stimulation* strategies, which apply mild stimulation to the skin and subcutaneous tissues, have been used for many years to relieve pain. Examples of cutaneous stimulation include:

- Application of heat, cold, or pressure
- Therapeutic massage
- Vibration
- Transcutaneous electrical nerve stimulation (TENS)

EVIDENCE-BASED PRACTICE QSEN

Does Education About the Use of Nonpharmacologic Methods Improve Pain Management in Rural Community-Dwelling Older Adults?

Fouladbakhsh, J.M., Szczesny, S., Jenuwine, E.S., & Vallerand, A.H. (2011). Nondrug therapies for pain management among rural older adults. *Pain Management Nursing, 12*(2), 70-81.

Researchers used a quasi-experimental two-group (experimental and control) design to test an educational intervention aimed at educating older adults in a rural community about the appropriate use of nonpharmacologic treatments for pain relief. The interventions were (1) the application of a moist hot pack and/or (2) cold pack to a part of the body for a specified period of time, and/or (3) the use of relaxation breathing exercises while experiencing pain. The sample consisted of 55 adult volunteers who were 60 years of age or older, English-speaking, and had experienced pain in the past 2 weeks. The subjects enrolled in an educational session by date and location that were convenient to them. Surveys to establish baseline pain, pain-related distress, and perception of control over pain were conducted before intervention to establish baseline levels. Participants were randomized to receive either a 30-minute (control) or 60-minute (experimental) education program and a follow-up evaluation session 2 weeks later. Both groups received an additional 30-minute session focused on safe use of over-the-counter (OTC) analgesics. The experimental group received an additional 30-minute session on the safe and appropriate use of the three nonpharmacologic treatments, and each participant in the experimental group was given one hot pack and one cold pack to take home after the education sessions.

At follow-up, there was a significant increase in the use of all three of the nonpharmacologic interventions in the experimental group with two to three times more participants reporting their use than those in the control group. The most frequently used nonpharmacologic therapy was topical application of heat and cold in both groups.

Level of Evidence: 3

The researchers used a quasi-experimental two-group (experimental and control) design to test the interventions.

Commentary: Implications for Practice and Research

This study suggests that older adults with pain may benefit from the use of simple nonpharmacologic interventions and that a structured educational program is helpful in increasing their use of these methods. However, further research and a larger sample size are needed to detect statistically significant changes over time.

Cold applications are especially helpful for inflamed areas, such as for patients with rheumatoid arthritis and those who have knee surgery. Heat is appropriate when an increased blood flow is desired, such as for patients with osteoarthritis pain. Paraffin dips for the hands can be helpful to increase movement for those patients as well. Warm showers and compresses that can be done at home are useful in reducing stiffness and promoting movement in patients with arthritis, especially after awakening. Local short-acting gels and creams may provide *cryotherapy (cold treatment)* to relieve muscle aches and pains. These products can often be bought over the counter (OTC) (e.g., Bengay, Icy Hot). The effects of this type of application can last up to 2 hours. Discuss this information with the patient before the use of a cutaneous method:

- The benefits of these techniques are highly unpredictable and may vary from application to application.
- PAIN relief is generally sustained only as long as the stimulation continues.
- Multiple trials may be necessary to establish the desired effects.
- Stimulation itself may aggravate pre-existing pain or may produce new pain.

Despite these potential drawbacks, cutaneous stimulation can be effective in the management of both acute and chronic PAIN in selected patients. A major benefit of these methods is that many are easy for patients to self-administer.

TENS is used occasionally as an adjunctive treatment for PAIN. Although there are several types of TENS units, each involves the use of a battery-operated device capable of delivering small electrical currents through electrodes applied to the painful area. The voltage or current is regulated by adjusting a dial to the point at which the patient perceives a prickly "pins-and-needles" SENSORY PERCEPTION rather than the pain. The current is adjusted based on the degree of desired relief. TENS requires the person to be skilled in the use of the necessary equipment and to be able to apply leads to the correct areas of the body. These factors are cited by patients as drawbacks and can be barriers to older adults who live alone and who may have difficulty with lead application.

Spinal cord stimulation is an *invasive* stimulation technique that provides PAIN control by applying an electrical field over the spinal cord. A trial with a percutaneous epidural stimulator is conducted to determine whether permanent placement of the device is appropriate. If the trial is successful, electrodes are surgically placed in the epidural space and connected to an external or implanted programmable generator. The patient is taught to program and adjust the device to maximize comfort. Spinal cord stimulation can be extremely effective in selected patients but is reserved for intractable neuropathic pain syndromes that have been unresponsive to less invasive methods.

Cognitive-Behavioral Strategies

Cognitive-behavioral strategies are less effective in relieving PAIN than physical modalities. However, they help patients feel more in control and cope better with pain and the conditions that often accompany it, such as depression, anxiety, and stress. Cognitive-behavioral strategies are useful in reducing the patient's focus on pain but do not physiologically block pain transmission. They are most appropriate as an adjunct to pharmacologic therapy for more severe pain. In addition to potential benefits, the limitations of cognitive-behavioral methods should be explained to patients to prevent unrealistic expectations.

Cognitive-behavioral methods range from simple (e.g., prayer, relaxation breathing, artwork, reading, and watching television) to more complex (e.g., meditation, guided imagery, hypnosis, biofeedback, and virtual reality). It is important to recognize that many of the methods require patient teaching and subsequent patient participation. Therefore it is inappropriate to attempt to teach the more complex cognitive-behavioral methods to patients who are unfamiliar with them and are experiencing severe pain, anxiety, or agitation. Not all patients are receptive to the use of these methods. To respect their wishes, values, and preferences as part of patient-centered care, do not insist that patients use any method.

Distraction is probably the most commonly used cognitive-behavioral method. All of us use simple distraction measures in our daily life when we watch television or read a book. Nurses often observe that patients request less PAIN medication when family members are present and when talking on the phone. After visiting hours, it is not unusual for patients to request pain medication because they are no longer distracted.

Visual distracters (e.g., looking at a picture, watching television, playing a video game) can divert the attention to something pleasant or interesting. Auditory distracters (e.g., listening to music or relaxation tapes) can have a calming effect. Changing the environment involves removing or reducing unpleasant stressors that can interfere with the patient's ability to cope with pain, such as loud noise and bright lights. Ask patients if they use any cognitive-behavioral techniques in their daily life. Encourage them to apply those methods to their current pain experience.

Imagery is a more complex form of distraction in which the patient is encouraged to visualize or think about a pleasant or desirable feeling, sensation, or event. The person is encouraged to sustain a sequence of thoughts aimed at diverting attention away from the pain. Patients who practice this technique can mentally and vividly experience sights, sounds, smells, events, or other sensations. Intense concentration is required to visualize images; therefore patients must have fairly well-controlled pain to participate.

Before suggesting imagery, assess the patient's level of concentration to determine whether he or she can sustain a particular thought or thoughts for a desired time. The time interval for mental imagery can vary from 5 to 60 minutes. Behaviors that may be helpful in assessing whether a patient is a candidate for teaching guided imagery include that the patient is able to:

- Read and comprehend a newspaper or magazine article
- Tap to a rhythm or sing while listening to music
- Follow the logic and participate in sustained conversation
- Have an interest in environmental surroundings

When the patient has demonstrated ability to concentrate, assist him or her in identifying a pleasant or favorable thought. Encourage the patient to focus on this thought to divert attention away from painful stimuli. CDs or other audio recordings, either commercial or created by the patient and family, may help form and maintain images. This is an example of guided imagery instructions:

> Imagine being on the beach of a deserted island. You can hear the sound of waves rushing onto the shore, the cry of seagulls flying high above, and the rustling of trees as they are brushed gently by the wind. You can feel the warmth of the sun over your body and the cooling breeze.

Patients may also use *relaxation techniques* to reduce anxiety, tension, and emotional stress, all of which can exacerbate pain. For example, before and during a painful procedure, patients can be reminded to breathe slowly, deeply, and rhythmically to divert attention and promote relaxation. Relaxation techniques can be both physical and psychological. Physical relaxation techniques include:

- Relaxation breathing
- Receiving a body massage, back rub, or warm bath
- Modifying the environment to reduce distractions
- Moving into a comfortable position

Psychological relaxation techniques include:

- Pleasant conversation
- Laughter and humor
- Music (provide a range of choices)
- Relaxation tapes

CLINICAL JUDGMENT CHALLENGE

Patient-Centered Care; Evidence-Based Practice QSEN

An older woman visits the neurologist for low back pain that she has had for several months. She has been taking high doses of ibuprofen and acetaminophen every day with some pain relief. After a thorough physical examination, the neurologist starts her on pregabalin (Lyrica) 75 mg twice daily for pain. As her office nurse, you are preparing for health teaching.

1. What questions will you ask the patient at this time in preparation for teaching?
2. How might you find the best evidence to help prepare her teaching plan?
3. What are the concerns about her current pain management regimen?
4. What nonpharmacologic methods might benefit her? How will you determine if they are appropriate for her values and beliefs?

Community-Based Care

Before patients are discharged from an acute care setting, collaborate with members of the health care team to optimize PAIN control. Before discharge or transfer from a hospital, ensure that the patient, especially one who will receive opioid analgesia, has appropriate prescriptions and enough doses to last at least until the first follow-up visit with the primary health care provider.

Home Care Management

Fatigue exacerbates PAIN. If physical modifications in the home (e.g., installing a downstairs bathroom) are unrealistic, suggest changes in schedules, role responsibilities, and daily routines to help prevent or reduce fatigue.

At home, patients may require a referral for physical therapy, especially to start or continue exercise regimens or treatment with cutaneous stimulation or heat or cold techniques. Patients may need a social worker to assist them develop coping strategies or maintain adequate family dynamics. A hospice or palliative care referral (hospital- or community-based) can help maintain continuity of care in the management of terminally ill patients and those who require treatment of some chronic conditions.

Home infusion therapy programs provide a wide variety of services to patients who require technology-supported PAIN care at home. Many of these services depend on approval by the insurance carrier, usually before analgesic options are considered and therapy is started. Case managers can be helpful in answering insurance and other payment questions. Well-defined home agency practices and professional support at home are required if patients leave the hospital with infusion therapy for pain management. Often, family members are taught to assume the responsibilities of home infusion therapy.

Self-Management Education

Teach the patient and family about analgesic regimens, including any technical skills needed to administer the analgesic; the purpose and action of various drugs, their side effects, and complications; and the importance of correct dosing and dosing intervals. Explain how to prevent or treat the constipation commonly associated with taking opioid analgesics and other medications. Inform the patient about what to do and who to contact if the prescribed management regimen is not controlling pain well or when side effects are intolerable or unmanageable.

Help the patient establish an analgesic regimen that does not interfere with sleep, rest, appetite, and level of physical mobility. Ensure that patients are aware of any dangers associated with driving or operating mechanical equipment. Tell patients to ask their primary health care provider when these activities are safe to perform. Older patients and others at risk for falls or accidents in the home setting may benefit from a home safety assessment.

In patients with PAIN from advanced cancer, all efforts are directed toward maximizing relief and symptom control at home and eliminating unnecessary hospital re-admissions. This may mean that the primary health care provider prescribes a flexible analgesic schedule that allows the patient to adjust analgesics according to the amount of pain. Teach the patient and family how to safely treat breakthrough pain and increase drug doses within the prescribed dosing guidelines. If painful ambulatory care treatments or procedures are expected, tell the patient how important it is to talk with his or her primary health care provider to determine available options for preventing procedural pain (e.g., premedicating).

Evaluate family support systems to assist the patient in adhering to and continuing the proposed medical treatment and nursing plan of care. Inform and include family members in activities during and after hospitalization. To achieve a reasonable level of involvement in life activities for the patient, suggest ways to continue participation in household, social, sexual, and work-oriented activities after discharge. Help the patient identify important activities and plan to do them with adequate rest periods.

The patient with chronic pain needs continued support to cope with the anxiety, fear, and powerlessness that often accompany this type of pain. Help the patient and family or significant others identify coping strategies that have worked in the past. Outside support systems are often extremely helpful, such as organizations like the *American Chronic Pain Association* (http://theacpa.org). This organization has the "10-Step Program from Patient to Person" and provides numerous educational materials and facilitates the establishment of local support groups for people with chronic PAIN.

Health Care Resources

Ask the prescriber for a home health care or hospice referral, as appropriate, for patients who require assistance or supervision with the PAIN management regimen at home. Important information to provide to the home health care nurse includes the patient's condition, level of sedation, weakness or fatigue, possible constipation or nutritional problem, sleep patterns, and functional status. Detailed information about the patient's current pain management regimen and how well it has been tolerated is essential. Use a structured procedure such as SBAR (situation, background, assessment, recommendations) to communicate this information.

In addition to explaining the patient's physical status to the home health care nurse, describe the patient's level of anxiety and general expectations about PAIN after discharge. Close relationships and available support networks are important factors in providing ongoing support for effective pain intervention strategies.

Referral to an advanced practice nurse pain specialist, social worker, or psychologist may be necessary for some patients and families to provide continued support, reinforce instructions for complex pharmacologic or nonpharmacologic strategies, or evaluate overall physical and emotional adaptation after discharge. When severe chronic or intractable pain exists, health care professionals should direct the patient and family to appropriate resources such as pain centers or health care providers who specialize in long-term PAIN management.

GET READY FOR THE NCLEX® EXAMINATION!

KEY POINTS

Review these Key Points for each NCLEX Examination Client Needs Category.

Safe and Effective Care Environment

- The nurse is legally and ethically responsible for acting as an advocate for patients experiencing PAIN.
- Coordinate the patient's plan of care as he or she transfers between health care agencies; be sure to clearly communicate the plan of care to the new agency. **Teamwork and Collaboration** QSEN

Health Promotion and Maintenance

- Provide information to the patient and family about nonpharmacologic therapies such as ice and heat; these modalities are additions to, not replacements for, the established plan of care.
- Consider the special needs of older adults when assessing and managing their PAIN (see Chart 3-1). **Patient-Centered Care** QSEN
- Assess and meet the patient's need for PAIN management promptly to promote relief; be sensitive to the cultural preferences and values of the patient and family. **Patient-Centered Care** QSEN

Psychosocial Integrity

- Be aware that some nurses and physicians may have biases about pain assessment and management; be objective when caring for patients with PAIN.
- Assess and document the patient's and family's expectations for management of PAIN. **Patient-Centered Care** QSEN
- Provide accurate information to patients who have misconceptions and misunderstandings about PAIN and pain management to prevent these from becoming barriers to effective pain management.

Physiological Integrity

- Remember that PAIN is what the patient says it is; self-report is always the most reliable indicator of pain. **Patient-Centered Care** QSEN
- Perform and document a complete PAIN assessment, including duration, location, intensity, and quality of pain. **Informatics** QSEN
- Never use placebos to assess the presence of PAIN; their deceitful use is prohibited by state boards of nursing and numerous professional organizations.
- Factors that affect PAIN and its management include age, gender, race, genetics, and culture. **Patient-Centered Care** QSEN
- The two major types of PAIN are nociceptive pain and neuropathic pain. Pain is also classified by its duration as acute or chronic. Chronic pain is further classified as cancer or non-cancer chronic pain.
- Examples of causes for acute PAIN include surgery and trauma; arthritis and cancer are common causes of chronic pain.
- Multimodal analgesia is the recommended approach for the management of all types of pain (see Table 3-6). Multimodal analgesia combines different drugs with different underlying mechanisms of action with the goal of producing better pain relief at lower analgesic doses than would be possible with any single analgesic alone. Lower doses result in fewer side effects. Non-opioid analgesics (acetaminophen, NSAIDs) are the first-line therapy for mild to moderate nociceptive pain and the foundation for a multimodal treatment plan for more severe nociceptive pain. **Evidence-Based Practice** QSEN
- Assess patients on acetaminophen for clinical manifestations of hepatotoxicity and nephrotoxicity; these adverse drug effects may occur when the medication is taken in higher than recommended daily doses. **Safety** QSEN
- Recall that NSAIDs should be used with caution in older adults because of adverse effects, such as GI toxicity, bleeding, and fluid retention, for which they are at higher risk than younger adults. **Safety** QSEN
- The mu opioid agonists are first-line therapy for moderate to severe nociceptive pain. Morphine, fentanyl, hydromorphone, and oxycodone are the most commonly used mu opioid agonists and are available in a wide variety of formulations for administration by a variety of routes of administration for both acute and chronic PAIN. **Evidence-Based Practice** QSEN
- Meperidine is not recommended for the treatment of any type of PAIN. Its toxic metabolite (normeperidine) can accumulate and cause confusion, seizures, and even death. It is a particularly poor choice in older adults and those with decreased renal clearance. **Evidence-Based Practice** QSEN
- Physical dependence is a normal response that occurs with repeated administration of an opioid for several days. It is manifested by the occurrence of withdrawal symptoms when

the opioid is suddenly stopped or rapidly reduced or an antagonist such as naloxone is given. It cannot be equated with addictive disease.

- Tolerance is a normal response that occurs with regular administration of an opioid and consists of a decrease in one or more effects of the opioid (e.g., decreased analgesia, sedation, or respiratory depression). It cannot be equated with addictive disease. With the exception of constipation, tolerance to the opioid side effects develops with regular daily dosing of opioids over several days.
- Opioid addiction is a chronic neurologic and biologic disease. The development and characteristics of addiction are influenced by genetic, psychosocial, and environmental factors. No single cause of addiction, such as taking an opioid for PAIN relief, has been found. It is characterized by one or more of these behaviors: impaired control over drug use, compulsive use, continued use despite harm, and craving.
- Use an equianalgesic chart (see Table 3-7 when changing from one opioid or route of administration to another to help ensure the patient receives about the same relief with the new opioid or route as with the previous. **Evidence-Based Practice** QSEN
- Be aware of the advantages and disadvantages of the various routes of analgesic administration.
- Observe for and prevent common side effects of analgesics (see Table 3-9). Remember that the single most effective treatment of most side effects is to decrease the dose of the drug causing the side effect.
- Remember that sedation precedes opioid-induced respiratory depression; assess sedation using a sedation scale, and decrease the opioid dose if excessive sedation is detected (see Table 3-10). **Safety** QSEN
- The intraspinal routes include the intrathecal (also called *spinal*) and epidural routes of administration. Intrathecal analgesia is given by single injection of opioid (most often) into the subarachnoid space for acute pain or implanted device for chronic pain; epidural analgesia is given by single injection or continuous infusion with or without PCA capability for all types of pain and usually combines an opioid with a local anesthetic.
- Adjuvant analgesics are drugs that have a primary indication other than pain but are analgesic for some painful conditions. The most commonly used are antidepressants, anticonvulsants, and local anesthetics. Examples are listed in Table 3-6.
- Nonpharmacologic therapies may be effective alone for mild pain and are used to complement, not replace, pharmacologic interventions for moderate to severe pain. **Evidence-Based Practice** QSEN
- PAIN can be managed in any setting, including the home. All patients require teaching with regard to their pain management regimen to ensure continuity of care. Patients or family members will require specialized training when infusion therapy is used in the home setting.
- Request referral or consultation with pain specialists and/or pain centers for patients with PAIN that cannot be managed with customary methods. **Teamwork and Collaboration** QSEN

CHAPTER 4

Genetic and Genomic Concepts for Medical-Surgical Nursing

M. Linda Workman

http://evolve.elsevier.com/Iggy/

PRIORITY CONCEPTS

- Ethics
- Collaboration

LEARNING OUTCOMES

Safe and Effective Care Environment

1. Ensure collaboration with health care team members and genetics professionals when providing genetic testing information to patients and families.

Health Promotion and Maintenance

2. Teach the patient and family who are at increased genetic risk for a disease or disorder to implement environmental modifications to reduce the risk when possible.

Psychosocial Integrity

3. Reduce the psychological impact for the patient and family regarding genetic assessment and genetic testing.

Physiological Integrity

4. Incorporate genetic and genomic principles into patient and family assessment techniques.
5. Ensure the use of professional ethics when integrating genomic health into medical-surgical nursing practice.

Genomic health is a growing part of today's comprehensive health care. Although the terms *genetics* and *genomics* often are used interchangeably, there are some differences. **Genetics** is concerned with the general mechanisms of heredity and the variation of inherited traits. Thus how genetic traits are transmitted from one generation to the next is part of genetics. The definition of **genomics** is both broader and more specific, focusing on the function of all of the human DNA, including genes and noncoding DNA regions. Thus how a gene is expressed within a person or family constitutes genomics. **Genomic health care** is the application of known genetic variation to enhance health care to individuals and their families.

Many adult-onset health problems have a genetic basis, meaning that variation of gene sequences and expression contributes to a person's risk for disease development. Some of these health problems also demonstrate **heritability**, meaning that the risk for developing the disorder can be transmitted to one's children in a recognizable pattern. Some adult-onset disorders, such as Huntington disease, are unavoidable when a person inherits a specific genetic mutation that causes the disorder. For other health problems, the risk is increased but is not absolute, indicating a *predisposition* or *susceptibility* toward the problem when a specific genetic mutation is inherited, but such a disorder may never occur. For example, certain gene variations increase the risk for type 2 diabetes; however, the disease is more likely to develop only when the person with the genetic variations has a sedentary lifestyle and is overweight. One outcome of genomic health care is to identify personal risk for disease development and assist the person to reduce the risk by modifying his or her environment (Manuck & McCaffery, 2014).

Specific discoveries regarding each person's genetic differences are being used to assess disease risk, enhance disease prevention strategies, and personalize disease management approaches (Bielinski et al., 2014). As a result, all health care professionals, including registered nurses, are expected to have at least a minimum knowledge of basic genetics to provide the best possible care for patients and families (Calzone et al., 2013). Table 4-1 lists selected genetic competencies important in medical-surgical nursing. Nurses are expected to know enough about basic genetics to recognize when a patient or family has a possible genetic risk for a health problem and to coordinate the attention of health care team members to ensure appropriate care.

GENETIC BIOLOGY REVIEW

Genes are the coded instructions for the making of all the different proteins the human body produces. For every hormone, enzyme, and other proteins the human body makes, it is the specific genes that tell each cell what protein to make, how to make it, when to make it, and how much to make. Think of each gene as a specific "recipe" for making a protein.

Every human somatic cell with a nucleus contains the entire set of human genes, known as the **genome**. The human genome contains between 20,000 and 25,000 genes. For example, all cells have the gene for insulin. However, the only cell type that allows the insulin gene to be **expressed** (turned on, activated) and

TABLE 4-1 Selected Essential Genetic Competencies for Medical-Surgical Nursing Practice

- Use appropriate genetic terminology.
- Recognize that a person/family with an identified genetic variation is a full member of society deserving of the same quality of health care as that provided to all others.
- Differentiate between genetic predisposition to a health problem and the actual expression or diagnosis of the health problem.
- Recognize the genetic and environmental influences on development of common adult-onset health problems.
- Be aware of genetic-based individual variation in responses to drug therapy.
- Consider genetic transmission patterns when performing a detailed patient and family history assessment.
- Ask appropriate questions during assessment to obtain information relevant to potential genetic risk or predisposition to a specific health problem(s).
- Construct a family pedigree, using standard symbols, that encompasses at least three generations.
- Identify patients/families at increased genetic risk for potential disease development.
- Ensure that patients/families identified to be at increased genetic risk for potential disease development are referred to the appropriate level of genetics professional.
- Individualize patient teaching about genetic issues using terminology and language the patient/family understands.
- Inform patients/families about potential risks and potential benefits of genetic testing.
- Advocate for patients with regard to their rights of accurate information, informed consent, competent counseling, refusal of genetic testing, freedom from coercion, and sharing of testing results.
- Assist patients/families to find credible resources regarding a specific genetic issue.
- Maintain patient/family confidentiality regarding any issue related to genetic testing, genetic predisposition, or genetic diagnosis, including whether genetic testing is even being considered.
- Support the patient's/family's decisions regarding any aspect of genetic testing or genetic diagnosis.

Data from competencies identified by American Association of Colleges of Nursing. (2008). *The essentials of baccalaureate education for nursing practice.* Washington, DC: Author; American Nurses Association. (2008). *Essentials of genetic and genomic nursing: Competencies, curricula guidelines, and outcome indicators* (2nd ed.). Silver Springs, MD: Author; Kirk, M., Calzone, K., Arimori, N., & Tonkin, E. (2011). Genetic-genomics competencies and nursing regulation. *Journal of Nursing Scholarship, 43*(2), 107-116.

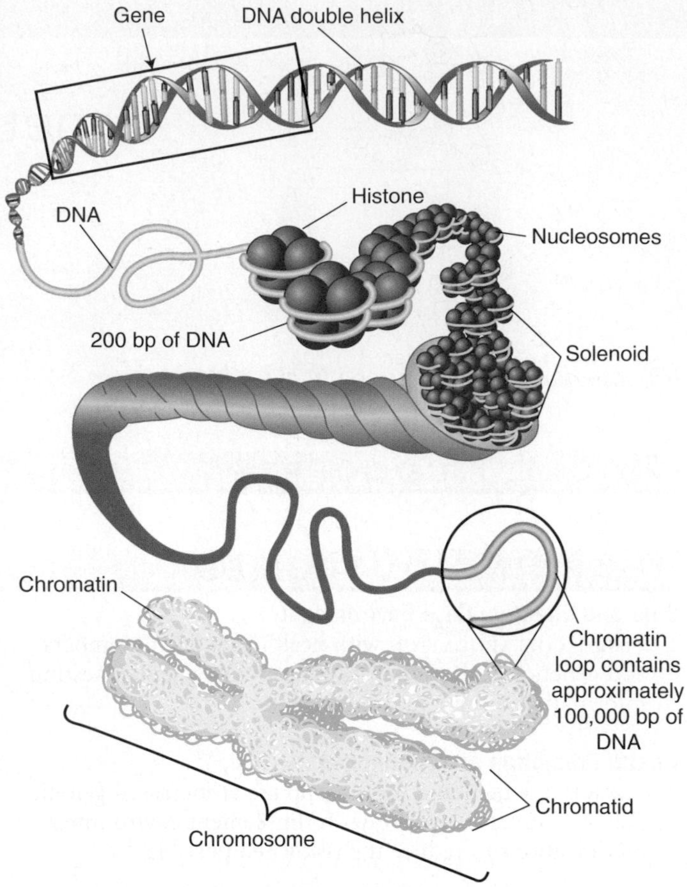

FIG. 4-1 The various forms of DNA from a loose double helix to coiled tightly into a chromosome. *bp,* Base pair.

make insulin is the beta cell of the pancreas. So, although the insulin gene is present in skin cells, heart cells, brain cells, and other cells, only in the beta cells is this gene selectively expressed when insulin is needed.

Genes are composed of DNA, which is present as 46 separate large chunks within the nucleus (Fig. 4-1). During cell division, each large chunk of DNA replicates and then organizes into a chromosome form to ensure precise delivery of the genetic information to each of the two new daughter cells. Thus DNA, chromosomes, and genes are all the same basic thing; only the structures differ.

Each chromosome has many genes within it. Humans have 23 pairs of chromosomes—46 individual chromosomes. The Y chromosome is small and has fewer than 100 genes. Larger chromosomes, such as the number 1 chromosome, contain thousands of genes.

One way to think of it is to consider all the DNA in any cell's nucleus (genome) to be a giant "cookbook" containing all the recipes needed to make all the proteins, hormones, enzymes, and other substances your body needs. The chromosome pairs are the different book chapters (so the human genome cookbook has 23 chapters), and the genes are the individual recipes contained within the chapters.

There is a specific chromosome location (**locus**) for every gene. For example, the locus of the gene for blood type is on chromosome 9. The location and the exact DNA sequence for many, but not all, genes is now known.

DNA

DNA Structure

In humans, DNA is a linear, double-stranded structure composed of multiple units of four different nitrogenous bases, each attached to a sugar molecule. The bases in each strand are linked together by phosphate groups. These two individual strands are held together loosely. This double-stranded DNA is arranged like a long set of railroad tracks. The "backbones" of the track are the two long steel rails. For DNA, these backbones are the phosphate groups that hold the bases in place. The bases are the individual railroad ties. Think of each tie as having two pieces—one piece attached to the right-hand rail and one piece attached to the left-hand rail.

Fig. 4-2 shows a very small piece of double-stranded DNA on the left (containing only four base pairs) taken from the larger piece of DNA on the right. The phosphate groups that hold the nucleotides together as a strand are in the red box. The green box in the lower left-hand section shows a whole nucleotide (a base with the sugar and the phosphate group) in place

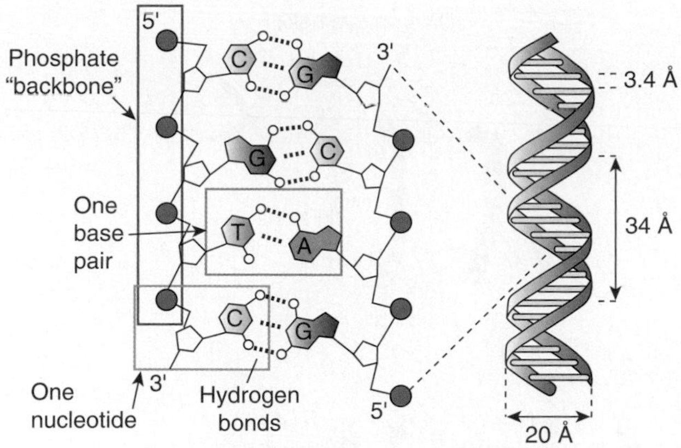

FIG. 4-2 The structure of DNA.

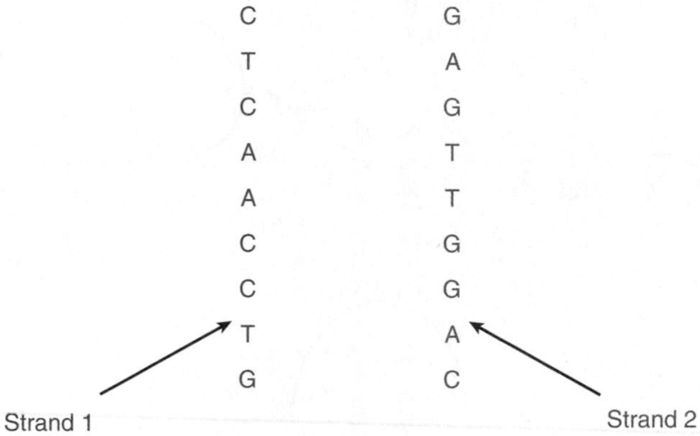

FIG. 4-3 Complementary strands of DNA.

in the left-hand DNA strand. The blue box in the middle of the two strands shows how the base from the left strand lines up with and pairs to a complementary base in the right strand.

Bases are the essential parts of DNA. Many trillions of bases in the DNA are found in the nucleus of just one cell. The four bases in DNA are adenine (A), guanine (G), cytosine (C), and thymine (T). Each base becomes a complete **nucleotide** when a five-sided sugar (known as a *deoxyribose sugar*) and a phosphate group are attached (see Fig. 4-2). Nucleotides form the DNA strands with the phosphate groups holding the bases in place.

Base pairs are the linked bases in the two opposite strands of DNA. The bases always link together across from each other in a very specific way. Thymine always forms a pair with adenine, and cytosine always forms a pair with guanine. Thus the bases of each pair are *complementary* to each other. Because these complementary base pairs in DNA are specific, if the base sequence of one strand of DNA is known, the opposite strand's sequence could be accurately predicted. For example, if the left-hand section of DNA (strand 1 in Fig. 4-3) had the sequence C-T-C-A-A-C-C-T-G, the corresponding (complementary) right-hand section (strand 2 in Fig. 4-3) of DNA would have the sequence G-A-G-T-T-G-G-A-C.

When the two strands of DNA are lined up properly, they twist into a loose helical shape (see Fig. 4-1). In this shape, the DNA is so fine that it can be seen only with electron microscopes. Only when a cell undergoes mitosis does the DNA super-coil tightly into dense pieces called *chromosomes* (Fig. 4-1), which can be seen with standard microscopes.

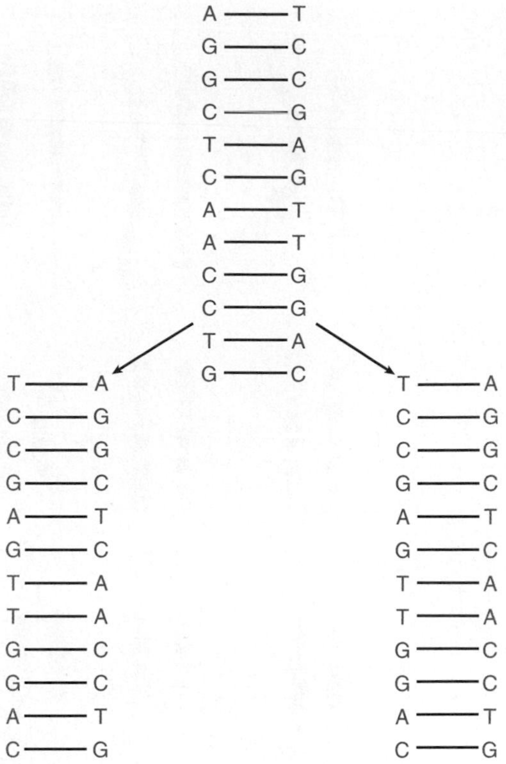

FIG. 4-4 DNA replication. *Blue type,* Original DNA; *red type,* newly replicated DNA.

DNA Replication

DNA must reproduce itself (**replicate**) every time a cell divides (undergoes mitosis). The purpose of mitosis is for one cell to reproduce into two new daughter cells, each of which is identical to the parent cell that started mitosis. For each new cell to have exactly the right amount of DNA and genes, the DNA in the dividing cell must exactly replicate. This process involves having the double strands of DNA separate and then build two new strands that are perfectly complementary to the original strands (Fig. 4-4). The result is two sets of double-stranded DNA. At the time of actual cell division with the separation into two new cells, one set of DNA will move into one of the two new cells made during mitosis and the second set will move into the other new cell. In this way, every new cell ends up with exactly the right amount of DNA with all the genes.

Chromosomes

As shown in Fig. 4-1, a chromosome is a specific large chunk of highly condensed double-stranded DNA, with each chunk containing billions of bases and hundreds (and sometimes thousands) of genes. Each chromosome forms and moves to the center of the cell that is about to divide. Just before the cell splits into two cells, each chromosome is pulled apart so that half of each chromosome goes into one new cell and the other half goes into the other new cell. Thus chromosomes are temporary structures to ensure the precise delivery of DNA to the two new cells. Humans have 46 chromosomes divided into 23 pairs.

Some things about a person can be known by examining his or her chromosomes, but limited information can be obtained by chromosomal analysis because each chromosome is composed of a large chunk of DNA. Only very large deletions, additions, or rearrangements of DNA show up at the level of the

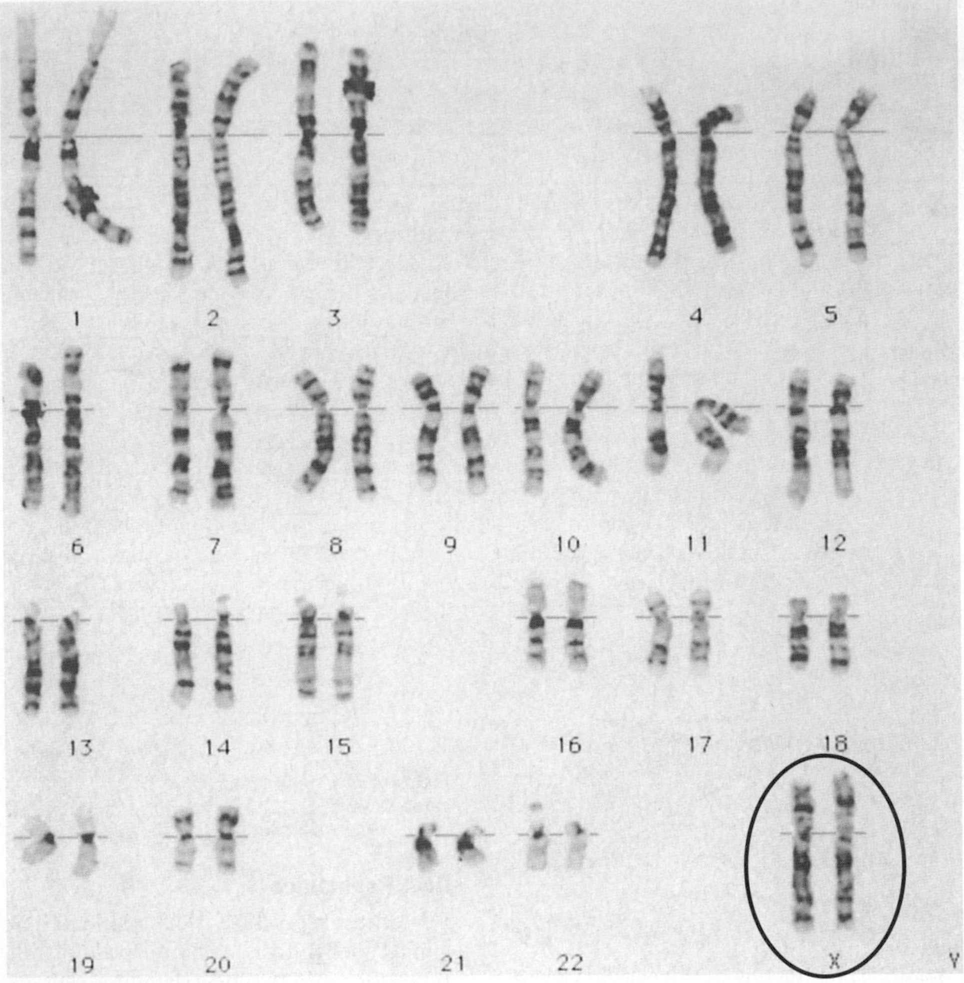

FIG. 4-5 A karyotype of a chromosomally normal female. (The sex chromosomes are *circled in red.*)

chromosome. Losses or gains of even tens of thousands of bases cannot be detected by chromosome analysis.

A **karyotype** is an organized arrangement of all of the chromosomes present in a cell during the metaphase section of mitosis (Fig. 4-5). A picture of the chromosomes is made. Chromosomes are first paired up and then arranged according to size (largest first) and centromere position. This gross organization of DNA can be used to determine missing or extra whole chromosomes and some large structural rearrangements. *A missing gene or a mutated gene would not show up at this level of analysis.* What can be learned about the person from whom the karyotype in Fig. 4-5 was made is that the person is human, female, and **euploid** (has the correct number of chromosome pairs for the species). This person is chromosomally "normal," although she probably has some genes that are different from (variant from or mutated from) the same genes in other people. If the karyotype is abnormal in any way (has more or less than the normal number or has broken chromosomes), the karyotype would be called **aneuploid**.

Autosomes are the 22 pairs of human chromosomes (numbered 1 through 22) that do not code for the sexual differentiation of a person. **Sex chromosomes** are the pair of chromosomes that include the genes for the sexual differentiation of the person. Chromosomally normal males have an X and a Y as the sex chromosomes. Chromosomally normal females have two Xs (XX) as the sex chromosomes (see Fig. 4-5).

Gene Structure and Function

A **gene** is a specific segment(s) of DNA that contains the code (recipe) for a specific protein (see Fig. 4-1). Thus genes are the smallest functional unit of the DNA. Each chromosome is a large segment of DNA that contains hundreds of genes.

For many human traits, one gene controls the expression of that trait in any person. Such traits are known as "single gene traits" *(monogenic traits)*. For each single gene, we have two alleles. An **allele** (pronounced "ah-**lee**-el") is an alternate form (or variation) of a gene. For example, there is one gene for blood type but there are three possible gene alleles (A, B, and O). Each person has only two of the three specific gene alleles for blood type. One of these alleles is on one chromosome 9 of the pair; the other allele is located on the other number 9 chromosome. Because each person only has two number 9 chromosomes, he or she can have only two of the three possible alleles for blood type. One gene allele was inherited from the person's mother, and the other gene allele was inherited from the person's father. *Some traits have even more than three possible alleles, but each person has only two.* Which blood type gene alleles are inherited from a person's parents determines which blood type he or she expresses.

If a person has inherited a blood type A allele from his or her mother and a blood type B allele from his or her father, he or she has the A and B alleles; the blood type expressed when

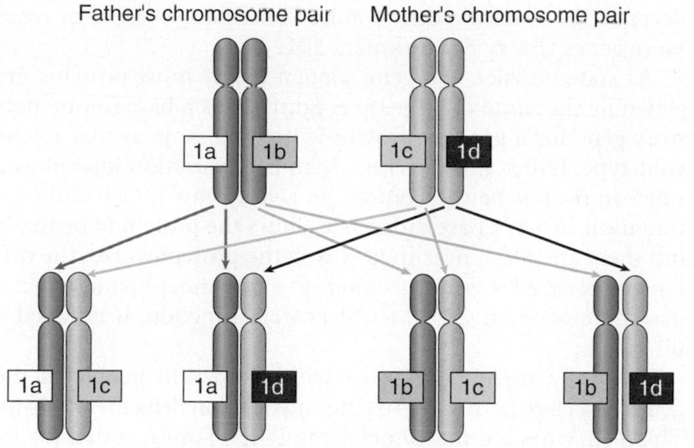

FIG. 4-6 Inheritance of four possible alleles for the single gene trait 1. (Any one person can have only two alleles for a single gene trait.)

the blood bank determines type is type AB. Fig. 4-6 shows this concept. In Fig. 4-6, two people are about to become pregnant. What are the possibilities for this baby to have a specific type of ear shape (pointy, rounded, square, triangular)? The gene for ear shape is trait 1, and it (for the purposes of this explanation) is on chromosome number 6.

Each of the father's sperm contains only one number 6 chromosome and each of the mother's eggs contains only one number 6 chromosome (so that when the sperm fertilizes the egg, the resulting person conceived will have only one pair of chromosome number 6 instead of two pairs of chromosome number 6).

Half the father's sperm have the 1a allele for ear shape, and the other half have allele 1b for ear shape. Half the mother's eggs have 1c for ear shape, and the other half have 1d. The resulting baby can inherit only either a 1a or a 1b from the father, not both; and this same baby can inherit only a 1c or a 1d from the mother—again, not both. The lower portion of Fig. 4-6 shows all the combinations possible for each ear shape gene alleles for any child these two people have.

If a person has two identical alleles for a single gene trait, that person is said to be *homozygous* for that trait. So if a person has an A blood-type gene allele on one number 9 chromosome and an A blood-type gene allele on the other number 9 chromosome, he or she is homozygous for that trait and will express the A blood type.

If a person has two different alleles for a single gene trait, he or she is *heterozygous* for that trait. So if a person has an A blood-type gene allele on one number 9 chromosome and a B blood-type gene allele on the other number 9 chromosome, that person is heterozygous for that trait and will express the AB blood type. Because the A and B alleles are equally dominant *(co-dominant),* they will both be expressed in the actual blood type.

There are differences in expression of the alleles for a trait depending on whether an allele is dominant or is recessive. If a person has an A blood-type gene allele on one number 9 chromosome and an O blood-type gene allele on the other number 9 chromosome, that person is heterozygous for that trait and expresses only the A blood type. Because the A allele is dominant and the O allele is recessive, they will not both be expressed in the actual blood type. Only the dominant allele is expressed, and the recessive allele is "silent." More information about dominant, recessive, and co-dominant expression is presented later in the Patterns of Inheritance section on p. 56.

Phenotype

The **phenotype** of any gene for a person is what characteristic can actually be observed or, in some cases, determined by a laboratory test. For example, the person who has the AO gene alleles for blood type has the phenotype of type A blood. A person with curly hair has a curly hair phenotype regardless of whether he or she has two alleles for curly hair or one allele for curly hair and one allele for straight hair.

Genotype

The **genotype** for a person's single gene trait is what the actual alleles are for that trait—not just what can be observed. A person with a phenotype of type A blood could have either an AA genotype or an AO genotype. The person who has type O blood would have an OO genotype. When a person has homozygous alleles for a trait, we would expect the genotype and phenotype to be the same. When a person has heterozygous alleles for a trait, the phenotype and the genotype are not always the same. *Recessive traits are expressed only when the person is homozygous for the alleles.* Thus for expressed recessive traits, phenotype and genotype are the same. Dominant traits are expressed whether the person is homozygous for the gene alleles or heterozygous for the gene alleles. Thus for dominant traits, phenotype and genotype can be the same but do not have to be the same.

Gene Expression

The purpose of a gene is to code for the making of a specific protein. For example, the hormone *insulin* is a protein. When a person's blood glucose level starts to rise, the beta cells of the pancreas rapidly make insulin to maintain the person's blood glucose homeostasis.

To continue the cookbook analogy, each gene is the recipe needed to make a specific protein. All the "stuff" that a human body makes—every hormone, every enzyme, every growth factor, every chemical needed to keep the person functioning—is a protein. These proteins are *gene products* because they are produced when the right gene is *expressed.* Just a few examples of gene products are insulin, hemoglobin, erythropoietin, angiotensin, and estrogen.

Protein Synthesis

Protein synthesis is the process by which genes are used to make the proteins needed for physiologic function. Proteins are made up of individual amino acids hooked together like beads on a string. There are 22 different amino acids. Every protein has a specific number of each of the amino acids and a specific order in which they are placed. *If even one amino acid is out of order or completely deleted from the sequence, the protein may be less functional or, perhaps, nonfunctional and unable to perform its job in the body.*

For example, the hormone *insulin* is a protein that contains 51 amino acids in a specific sequence. If some of the amino acids are missing or are in the wrong position, the protein made would be different from real insulin and could not reduce blood glucose levels. *Thus the actual order of the amino acids is critical for the final function of any protein.*

Within the DNA there is a three-nucleotide (base) code for each amino acid. A gene for a specific protein contains all the

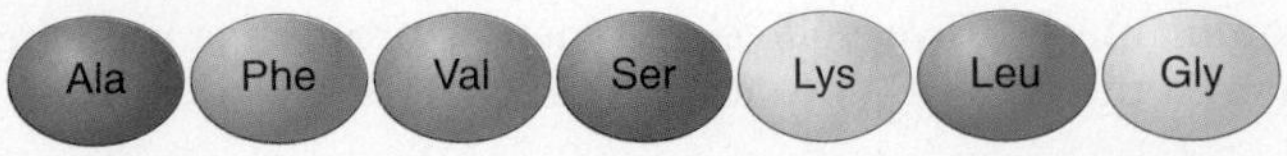

FIG. 4-7 A sample protein composed of seven amino acids.

amino acid codes in exactly the right order for that protein. For example, the final active form of the protein *insulin* has 51 amino acids. Thus the minimum number of bases needed in the gene for insulin would be 153 (3 bases per amino acid × 51 amino acids). Fig. 4-7 shows an example of a short protein made up of only 7 amino acids.

The key for making a functional protein is accurate placement of all the amino acids in the order specified by the gene. When problems exist in the base sequence of a gene, its expression may not result in a functional protein. In addition, the process of protein synthesis involves many complex steps and a problem at any step could result in the failure to produce a functional protein.

Mutations

Many human genes have been sequenced, meaning that their base sequence is known and so is the sequence of their amino acids in the expressed proteins. Most people have the same base sequence for a specific gene, like the gene for insulin. When this sequence is the most common one found in a large population of humans, it is referred to as the *wild-type* gene sequence. Think of the term *wild-type* as meaning "normal" or "expected." When a person has a different sequence for a gene compared with the known wild-type sequence, the gene has a variation or mutation. Mutations as small variations in gene sequences occur more often in very large genes, and the significance of some of these changes is not known. It is these differences or variations in the sequences of some genes from the wild-type that are now being examined more closely in health care. Some of these variations can reduce the function of the protein produced, some can eliminate the function of the protein produced, and a few variations have been found that enhance the function of the produced protein compared with the function of the wild-type protein.

Mutations are DNA changes that are passed from one generation to another and thus are *inherited.* An inherited mutation does not have to mean that the mutation is passed from one human generation to another. It can mean that the mutation is passed from one *cell* generation to another and may affect only certain tissues within a person rather than be a problem within a family. These mutations occur in general body cells (somatic cells) and are known as *somatic mutations.* Because these mutations occur in a person's cells after conception, the person cannot pass a somatic mutation on to his or her children. One possible outcome of somatic mutations is an increased risk for cancer in cells with such mutations.

When mutations occur in sex cells, they are called *germline mutations.* A germline mutation *can* be passed on to a person's children, and each of that child's cells, including his or her somatic cells and sex cells, will contain the mutated DNA.

When mutations resulting in sequence variation occur in a gene area of the DNA, the change can alter the expression of that gene and an incorrect gene product (protein) might result. Mutations can have serious results, although some mutations may be beneficial. Gene mutations that increase the risk for a disorder are known as *susceptibility* genes. Gene mutations that decrease the risk for a disorder are known as *protective* or *resistance* genes (Beery & Workman, 2012).

As stated earlier, the gene sequences for most proteins are generally the same in all people. Sometimes a base in one person's gene for a specific protein is not the same as that in the wild-type. Either this difference can be a variation known as a *single nucleotide polymorphism,* or *SNP* ("snip"), or it can be a mutation. When a base difference allows the protein to be made but there are differences in how well the protein works, the difference is called a *gene variation* or a **polymorphism**. When a base difference causes a loss of protein function, it is called a **mutation**.

Clinically, many SNPs exist within different people in the genes of a large family of enzymes involved in drug metabolism. These enzymes are the cytochrome P-450 family, coded for by at least ten separate extremely large genes, with as many as 100 subsets of genes. Cytochrome p is abbreviated as CYP (pronounced "sip"). SNPs in these genes can make the resulting enzyme less active than normal or more active than normal. Either way, a change in activity of any one of these enzymes can affect a person's response to drug therapy. For example, the drug *warfarin* (Coumadin) is metabolized for elimination primarily by two enzymes from this system, CYP2CP and CYP2C19. About 17% to 37% of white people have a SNP variation in CYP2CP that slows the metabolism of warfarin. This means that warfarin remains in the person's system longer, greatly increasing the risk for bleeding and other side effects. For people who have this gene mutation, warfarin doses need to be much lower than those for the general population (Cheek, 2013).

CULTURAL CONSIDERATIONS

Patient-Centered Care QSEN

Most people of Asian heritage have a SNP in the *CYP2C19* gene that results in low activity of the enzyme produced. This mutation greatly reduces the metabolism of warfarin, leading to a longer warfarin half-life and increased bleeding risks along with other serious side effects. Any person of Asian heritage who needs anticoagulation therapy should be started on very low dosages of warfarin and have his or her international normalized ratio (INR) monitored more frequently than people who do not have a variation of the *CYP2C19* gene.

The most devastating gene mutations are the ones that change the amino acid codes so that a proper protein is not made. Other changes may alter how often or how well a group of cells divides. Gene mutations or variations may cause one person to have a greater-than-normal risk for developing a disease. A different variation in the same gene may cause another person to have a smaller-than-normal risk for developing the same disease.

PATTERNS OF INHERITANCE

For every single gene trait, a person inherits one allele for that gene from his or her mother and one allele from his or her father. How these traits are expressed depends on whether one or both alleles are "dominant" or "recessive." Expression also depends on whether the gene for the trait is located on an autosome or on a sex chromosome.

It is possible to determine how the gene for a specific trait is passed from one human generation to the next *(transmitted)*. By looking at how that trait is expressed through several generations of a family, patterns emerge that indicate whether the gene for the trait is dominant or recessive and whether it is located on an autosomal chromosome or on one of the sex chromosomes. This information can be determined through *pedigree analysis*. Determining inheritance patterns for a specific trait makes it possible to predict the relative risk for any one person to have a trait or transmit that trait to his or her children.

Pedigree

A **pedigree** is a graph of a family history for a specific trait or health problem over several generations. Fig. 4-8 shows common symbols used when creating a pedigree. Fig. 4-9 shows a typical three-generation pedigree. Although the term *pedigree* is the correct genetic term, it can offend some patients. Use the term *family tree* in place of pedigree when talking with patients. Construct a pedigree that includes at least three generations when taking the family history. When analyzing a pedigree, note the answers to these:

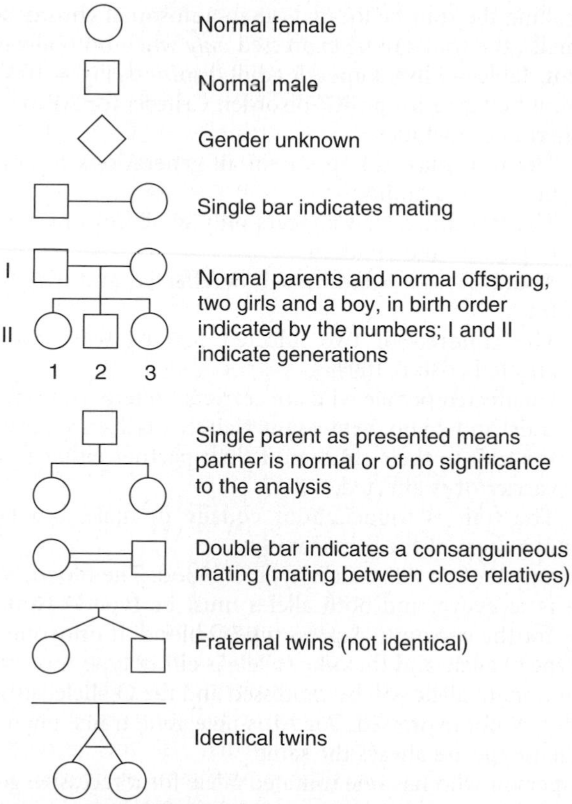

FIG. 4-8 Standard pedigree symbols.

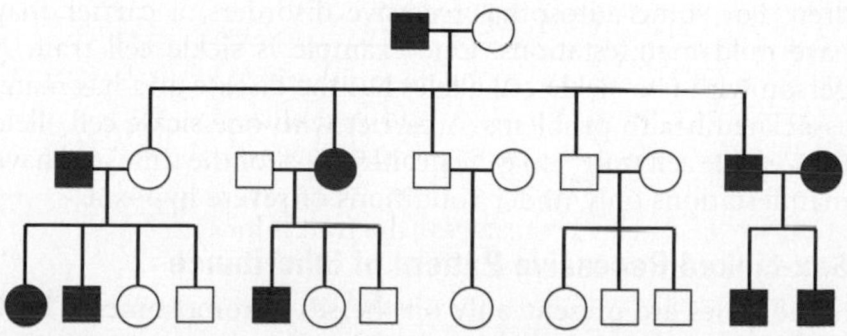

FIG. 4-9 A three-generation pedigree showing an autosomal dominant pattern of inheritance.

- Is any pattern of inheritance recognized, or does the trait appear sporadic?
- Is the trait expressed equally among male and female family members or unequally?
- Is the trait present in every generation, or does it skip one or more generations?
- Do only affected people have children who are affected with the trait, or do unaffected people also have children who express the trait?

The four types of inheritance patterns associated with single gene–controlled traits are autosomal dominant, autosomal recessive, sex-linked dominant, and sex-linked recessive. Each inheritance pattern has specific defining criteria. Table 4-2 lists the patterns of inheritance for some disorders that occur in adults or may be identified in children who live to adulthood.

Autosomal Dominant Pattern of Inheritance

Autosomal dominant (AD) single gene traits require that the gene alleles controlling the trait be located on an autosomal chromosome. A dominant gene allele is usually expressed even

TABLE 4-2 Patterns of Inheritance for Genetic Disorders Among Adults

PATTERN OF INHERITANCE	DISORDER
Autosomal dominant	Breast cancer* (mutation of *BRCA1* or *BRCA2* genes) Diabetes mellitus type 2* Familial adenomatous polyposis Familial melanoma Familial hypercholesterolemia Hereditary nonpolyposis colon cancer (HNPCC) Huntington disease Long QT syndrome and sudden cardiac death Malignant hyperthermia (MH) Marfan syndrome Myotonic dystrophy Neurofibromatosis (types 1 and 2) Ovarian cancer* (mutation of *BRCA1* genes) Polycystic kidney disease† (types 1 and 2) Retinitis pigmentosa† von Willebrand's disease
Autosomal recessive	Albinism Alpha$_1$-antitrypsin deficiency Beta thalassemia Bloom syndrome Cystic fibrosis Hereditary hemochromatosis Sickle cell disease Xeroderma pigmentosum
Sex-linked recessive	Glucose-6-phosphate dehydrogenase deficiency Hemophilia Red-green color blindness
Complex disorders/ Familial clustering	Alzheimer's disease Autoimmune disorders Bipolar disorder Parkinson disease Schizophrenia Hypertension Rheumatoid arthritis

*Some disorders have both a genetic and nongenetic form.
†Some disorders have more than one genetic form and can also be autosomal recessive.

when only one allele of the pair is dominant. Other criteria for AD inheritance include:

- The trait appears in every generation with no skipping.
- The risk for an affected person to pass the trait to a child is 50% with each pregnancy.
- Unaffected people do not have affected children; therefore their risk is essentially 0%.
- The trait is found about equally in males and females.

An example of an AD trait is blood type A. If a person is homozygous for the blood type A allele, he or she will express type A blood (with genotype being identical to the phenotype). If a person is heterozygous for the blood type A allele with the other allele being type O (which is a recessive trait), he or she will also express type A blood. In this case, however, the phenotype is not identical to the genotype. *When a dominant allele is paired with a recessive allele, only the dominant allele is expressed.* The blood type B allele is a dominant allele. When a B allele is paired with an O allele, B blood type is expressed. When a person has one blood type A allele and a blood type B allele, however, both alleles are expressed because they are equally dominant (co-dominant) and the person has type AB blood.

Some health problems inherited as autosomal dominant (AD) single gene traits are not apparent at birth but develop as the person ages (see Table 4-2). Two factors that affect the expression of some AD single gene traits are penetrance and expressivity.

Penetrance

Penetrance is how often or how well, within a population, a gene is expressed when it is present. Some genes are more penetrant than others. For example, the gene for Huntington disease (HD) has an autosomal dominant pattern of transmission. This gene is "highly penetrant" (sometimes called "fully penetrant"). This means that if a person has the HD gene allele, his or her risk for expressing the gene and developing the disease is about 99.99%. Therefore a person who has one HD allele is at high risk for developing HD.

Some dominant gene alleles have "reduced" penetrance. So a person who has the gene mutation has a lower risk for this gene being expressed and actually developing the disorder.

Penetrance has been calculated by examining a population of people known to have the gene mutation and assessing the percentage that go on to express the gene by developing the disorder. For example, the *BRCA2* gene mutation increases a person's risk for breast cancer. This gene is not fully penetrant, so some women (and men) who have the gene do not develop breast cancer. The penetrance rate for this gene mutation is calculated to be between 60% and 80%, meaning that a person who has the gene mutation has a 60% to 80% risk for developing breast cancer. Although this risk is far higher than among people who do not have the mutated gene, the risk is not 100%. Having the gene mutation does not absolutely predict that the person will develop breast cancer—just that the risk is high. However, the person with the mutation can pass on this genetic mutation to his or her children, who will then have an increased risk for breast cancer development.

Expressivity

Expressivity is the degree of expression a person has when a dominant gene is present. So it is a personal issue, not a population issue. The gene is *always* expressed, but some people have more severe problems than do other people. For example, the gene mutation for one form of neurofibromatosis *(NF1)* is dominant. Some people with this gene mutation have only a few light brown skin tone areas known as *café au lait spots*. Other people with the same gene mutation develop hundreds of tumors (neurofibromas) that protrude through the skin. Expressivity accounts for some variation in genetic disease severity.

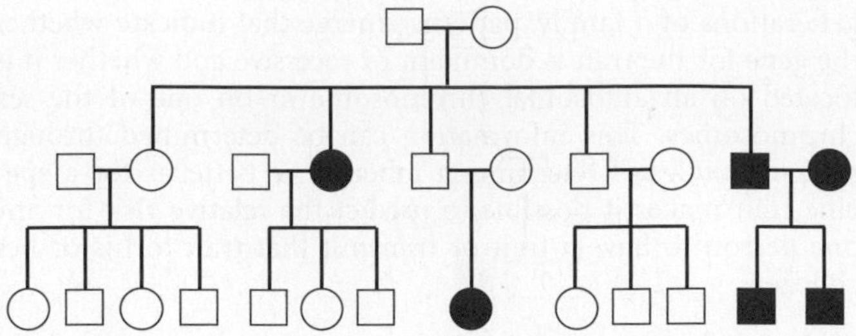

FIG. 4-10 A typical pedigree showing an autosomal recessive pattern of inheritance.

Autosomal Recessive Pattern of Inheritance

Autosomal recessive (AR) single gene traits require that the gene controlling the trait be located on an autosomal chromosome. Normally, the trait can be expressed *only* when both alleles are present. Table 4-2 lists some AR adult disorders. Fig. 4-10 shows a typical pedigree for an AR disorder. Criteria for AR patterns of inheritance include:

- The trait may not appear in all generations of any one branch of a family.
- The trait often first appears only in siblings rather than in parents and children.
- About 25% of a family will be affected and express the trait.
- The children of two affected parents will *always* be affected (risk is 100%).
- Unaffected people who are carriers (heterozygous for the trait) and do not express the trait themselves *can* transmit the trait to their children if their partner either is also a carrier or is affected.
- The trait is found about equally in male and female members of the same family.

An example of an AR trait is type O blood. The blood-type O allele is recessive, and both alleles must be type O (homozygous) for the person to express type O blood. If only one allele is a type O allele and the other allele is either type A or type B, the dominant allele will be expressed and the O allele, although present, is not expressed. For AR single gene traits, phenotype and genotype are always the same.

A person who has one mutated allele for a recessive genetic disorder is a **carrier**. A carrier, even though he or she may have one mutated allele, may not have any manifestations of the disorder but can pass this mutated allele on to his or her children. For some autosomal recessive disorders, a carrier may have mild manifestations. One example is sickle cell trait. A person with two sickle cell alleles has the disease and has many associated health problems. A carrier with one sickle cell allele (has "sickle cell trait") may be healthy most of the time and have manifestations only under conditions of severe hypoxia.

Sex-Linked Recessive Pattern of Inheritance

Some genes are present only on the sex chromosomes. The Y chromosome has only a few genes that are not also present on the X chromosome. These genes are important for male sexual

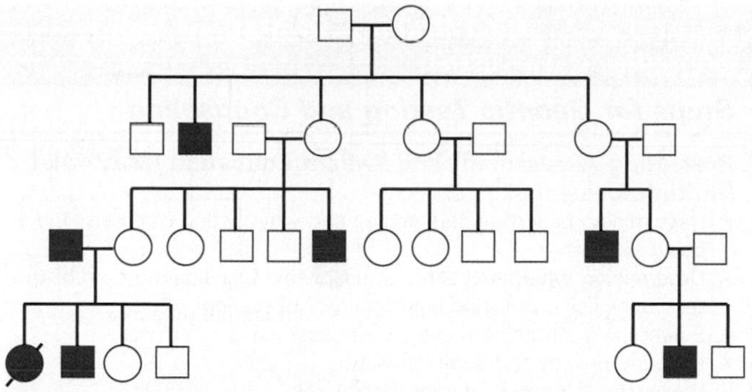

FIG. 4-11 A typical pedigree showing a sex-linked (X-linked) recessive pattern of inheritance.

development. The X chromosome has many single genes that are not present on the Y or elsewhere in the genome. Some of these genes are specific for female sexual development, but there are also several hundred genes on the X chromosome that code for other functions. Few disorders have X-linked dominant expression and are not discussed in this chapter.

Because the number of X chromosomes in males and females is not the same (1:2), the number of X-linked chromosome genes in the two genders is also unequal. Males have only one X chromosome. As a result, X-linked recessive genes have dominant expression in males and recessive expression in females. This difference in expression is because males do not have a second X chromosome to balance the presence of a recessive gene on the first X chromosome.

Sex-linked (X-linked) recessive single gene traits require that the gene allele be present on both of the X chromosomes for the trait to be expressed in females (homozygous) and on only one X chromosome for the trait to be expressed in males. Fig. 4-11 shows a typical pedigree for a sex-linked recessive disorder. Features of a sex-linked recessive pattern of inheritance are:

- The incidence of the trait is much higher among males in a family than among females.
- The trait cannot be passed down (transmitted) from father to son.
- Transmission of the trait is from father to all daughters (who will be carriers).
- Female carriers have a 50% risk (with each pregnancy) of passing the gene to their children.

Complex Inheritance and Familial Clustering

Some health problems appear in families at a rate higher than normal and greater than can be accounted for by chance alone; however, no specific pattern occurs within a family. Although clusters suggest a genetic influence, it is likely that additional factors, such as gender and the environment, also influence disease development or disease severity. Such disorders include Alzheimer's disease, type 1 diabetes, and many others. These disorders are often called *complex* and *multifactorial*, because although an increased genetic risk may be present, the risk is changed by diet, lifestyle, exposure to toxins, infectious agents, and other factors.

GENETIC TESTING

Purpose of Genetic Testing

Many people are eager to have genetic testing but also are fearful of genetic testing. The lay public often believe that a single genetic test can "tell everything about a person." Although genetic testing has the potential to be that informative, this is not currently the case. *It is important to remember that no single person is genetically perfect.*

TABLE 4-3 Purposes of Genetic Testing for Adults

PURPOSE/TYPE	DEFINITION
Carrier testing	Determining whether a patient without symptoms has an allele for a recessive disorder that could be transmitted to his or her children. Disorders for which carrier testing is common include sickle cell disease, hemophilia, hereditary hemochromatosis, cystic fibrosis, beta thalassemia, and Tay-Sachs disease.
Diagnostic testing	Determining whether a patient has or does not have a mutation that increases the risk for a specific disorder.
Symptomatic	Patient has clinical manifestations; test results confirm a diagnosis.
Presymptomatic	Patient has no clinical manifestations but is at high risk for inheriting a specific genetic disorder for which there is no known prevention or treatment. A disorder for which presymptomatic testing is commonly performed is Huntington disease.
Predisposition	Family history or genetic testing indicates risk is high for a known genetic disorder. The patient does not have any manifestations but wants to know whether he or she has the specific mutation and what the chances are that it will be expressed. Disorders for which predisposition testing is often performed include hereditary breast/ovarian cancer and hereditary colorectal cancers. The advantage of predisposition testing is that the patient can then engage in heightened screening activities or medical and surgical interventions that reduce risk.

Genetic testing can be performed with many different techniques. Some genetic tests are specific for a disorder. Others may show a gene variation but the significance of the variation may not be known. Unexpected information can be found during genetic testing. Some ordinary tests, such as blood typing and tissue typing, provide genetic information. Tests that measure the amount of an enzyme or protein also provide genetic information.

Testing for the purpose of assessing genetic information can be performed at many levels. Cellular or biochemical tests provide information about gene products made by a cell, tissue, or organ. Chromosomes and chromosome segments can be assessed for missing, extra, broken, or rearranged chromosomes. The sequence of a gene can be examined to determine variation or mutation. At present, not all genes can be analyzed and the analysis of even one gene is limited by expense and availability. Specific base pairs can be evaluated for mutations (Conley et al., 2013). Many tests are expensive, and the results may not be conclusive. Table 4-3 lists purposes of genetic testing for adults.

Benefits and Risks of Genetic Testing

Genetic testing is different from any other type of testing. Informed consent is required before genetic testing is performed. The person tested is the one who gives consent, even though genetic testing *always* gives information about family members—not just the patient (Badzek et al., 2013).

Benefits of genetic testing include the ability to confirm a diagnosis or to test people who are at risk for a health problem but do not as yet have any manifestations (presymptomatic testing). The information can help a person, family, and their health care provider develop a specific plan of care or early detection. For example, in the case of a strong genetic predisposition for colon cancer, identifying a patient before symptoms appear allows interventions to prevent the disease or to diagnosis it earlier, when cure is more likely.

Risks are associated with genetic testing that are not associated with other types of tests. Genetic testing results do not change. Thus a positive test result cannot be "taken back." Other risks may include psychological or social risks, as well as a risk for family disruption. Often genetic tests are expensive and may not be covered by insurance. Some genetic tests have limited value for predicting future risk. Testing may identify a patient at great risk for the future development of a serious health problem that cannot be prevented or managed. Such a disorder is Huntington disease (HD), which currently has no treatment. Knowing positive test results in this case can lead to depression, blame, and guilt.

Another risk of genetic testing is that positive results may be used to discriminate against a person or a family. Some protection is in place to prevent health insurance companies from failing to insure a person or dropping the coverage of a person who is at high risk for developing a serious illness (e.g., breast or ovarian cancer). However, there are no protections against rate hikes or exclusions of specific treatments. Patients often fear workplace discrimination and personal discrimination if positive test results become known.

Genetic Counseling

Genetic testing is not a standard test that any person should have performed without knowing the benefits and risks. Counseling patients before, during, and after testing is critical and is required by the professional ETHICS governing genetic medicine. Entire families may be a part of the genetic evaluation and follow-up. For example, a 45-year-old woman has breast cancer. In her family, her mother, grandmother, brother, and one sister have all had breast cancer. Genetic testing indicates that she has a *BRCA1* gene mutation. This woman's older daughter wonders whether she has a gene mutation for breast cancer and asks to be tested. When she and her younger sister are tested, the older daughter does not have the mutation but the younger sister does.

Genetic counseling is a process—not a single session or a single recommendation. This process should begin when the patient or family is first identified as potentially having a genetic problem. The process continues through actual testing if the decision to test is made, and it continues through interpretation of results and follow-up. Chart 4-1 lists the steps in the process.

As a nurse and patient advocate, it is your professional duty to determine whether the patient understands the consequences of testing. Often a patient may request genetic testing even when there is no indication of an increased risk for a genetic disorder. Counseling and evaluation can help patients understand whether any useful information could be obtained from testing.

CHART 4-1 Best Practice for Patient Safety & Quality Care QSEN

Steps for Genetic Testing and Counseling

Pretesting Assessment and Patient Education (May Take Multiple Sessions)

- Determining patient understanding and why testing or counseling is being sought
- Determining whether testing is reasonable (considering cost of the test, specificity, probable risk, accuracy of testing)
- Establishing a trusting professional relationship
- Ensuring privacy and confidentiality
- Reviewing informed consent procedures
- Assessing the patient's ability to communicate accurately (including language issues, cognitive function, sensory perception)
- Assessing the patient's psychosocial status and availability of social support
- Taking a detailed patient health history (including drugs, diet, exercise, hormonal history, lifestyle issues)
- Obtaining physical assessment data relevant to the at-risk disorder
- Taking a detailed family history and constructing a three-generation pedigree (minimum)
- Obtaining and verifying information obtained from:
  - Patient
  - Family members
  - Medical records
  - Pathology reports
  - Death certificates
- Interpreting the family history
- Discussing the consequences of testing
- Discussing patient rights and obligations regarding disclosure of information
- Discussing testing options
- Assessing to determine whether coercion is occurring
- Obtaining material to be tested (usually blood)

Test Result Presentation

- Re-assessing the patient's wish to know or not know the test results
- Respecting the patient's decision to not know the test results
- Ensuring privacy and confidentiality
- Presenting the test results
- Interpreting the test results
- Assessing the patient's perception of the test results

Follow-Up

- Supporting the patient's decision to disclose or not disclose the information to other family members
- Discussing the potential risks for other family members
- Ensuring privacy and confidentiality
- Addressing the patient's concerns
- Discussing prevention, early detection, and treatment options
- Discussing family concerns
- Addressing psychosocial issues
- Discussing available resources for information, support, and further counseling
- Providing summary of results and consultation to the patient

Adapted from Beery, T., & Workman, M.L. (2012). *Genetics and genomics in nursing and health care*. Philadelphia: F.A. Davis.

Counseling should be a COLLABORATION performed by a professional or a team who have defined expertise in interpretation of genetic testing results. Such professionals include advanced practice nurses with specialization in genetics, certified genetic counselors, clinical geneticists, and medical geneticists. Each profession has a different level of preparation in genetics and different skills or roles in the counseling process. For example, an advanced practice nurse may counsel a patient about the Huntington disease gene mutation because this test is not ambiguous and the gene is highly penetrant. When a genetic test shows a variation or mutation in an unusual gene region or when penetrance is reduced, the patient may best be served by counseling from a certified genetic counselor or a clinical or medical geneticist.

No matter which professional is involved in genetic counseling, a key feature of this counseling is to be "nondirective." When using a nondirective approach, the counselor provides as much information as possible about the risks and benefits but does not influence the patient's decision to test or not to test. Once the patient has made the decision, the counselor supports the patient and the decision.

Ethical Issues

ETHICS and ethical issues are involved at every level of genetic testing. Some of the most important issues focus on the patient's right to know versus the right not to know his or her gene status, confidentiality, coercion, and sharing of information.

The right to know genetic risk versus the right to not know is the individual patient's choice. Sometimes a patient's right to know has an impact on the right of another family member to not know.

Confidentiality is crucial to the genetic counseling process. *The results of a genetic test must remain confidential to the patient. The results cannot be given to a family member, other health care provider, or insurance carrier without the patient's permission.*

Coercion is possible by other family members and by health care professionals. *The final decision to have genetic testing or to not have testing rests with the patient.* Other people may believe it is important for the patient to have the test; however, the patient must make the decision without such pressures. As a patient advocate, professional ETHICS require you to assess whether the patient is freely making the decision to have genetic testing or whether someone else is urging the patient to test. This important issue can be difficult to assess. Ask the patient who else in his or her family wants to know the results of testing.

Sharing of test result information, negative or positive, can be stressful. The patient makes the final decision whether to share the information with family members. Some patients choose not to share this information even when other family members may also be at risk. This can be difficult for the health care provider who knows the patient has a positive test result for a serious inherited condition and the patient chooses not to tell other family members who may be at risk (Berkman & Hull, 2014). For example, hereditary nonpolyposis colon cancer (HNPCC) has an autosomal dominant inheritance pattern and each child of the patient has a 50% risk for having the gene. If the patient chooses not to tell his or her grown children, they then do not have the opportunity for increased screening to find the cancer at an early stage when cure is possible. An ethical dilemma arises when the health care provider wants to inform the children of their risk.

THE ROLE OF THE MEDICAL-SURGICAL NURSE IN GENETIC COUNSELING

Medical-surgical nurses help patients during the assessing, testing, and counseling processes, although they do not provide in-depth genetic counseling. Patients often feel most comfortable sharing information with nurses and asking nurses to clarify information.

? CLINICAL JUDGMENT CHALLENGE

Ethical/Legal

A 22-year-old man has a maternal grandfather with Huntington disease (HD). His father, mother, and paternal grandfather are all healthy and free of HD manifestations. He wants to know whether he also has the HD gene and arranges to be tested. His mother does not want to know whether she has the gene mutation. The man is tested and is found to be positive for the gene mutation that causes HD.

1. Why could a positive test affect this man's mother?
2. Does the mother's right to not know her HD status override the son's right to know his status? Explain your reasoning.
3. Review the ethical principles in Chapter 1. Which principle(s) would be violated if the son informs his mother of his positive test results?

Nurses may be the first health care professionals to identify a patient at specific genetic risk. Some of the "red flags" that a patient may have a genetic risk for a disease or disorder are:

- The disease or disorder occurs at a higher incidence within the family compared with the general population.
- The patient or close family members have another identified genetic problem.
- The incidence of a specific disease or disorder occurs in the patient or in family members at an unusually early age.
- A rare disease is present in two or more family members.
- More than one type of cancer is present in any one person.
- The specific manifestation is associated with one or more genetic disorders (e.g., unusual freckling or skin pigmentation, bicuspid aortic valve, deafness).

The nurse may be the health care professional who first verifies information to bring a genetic problem to light. For example, during an assessment, a patient reveals that her mother died of bone cancer when she was 40 years old. Bone cancer is quite rare among adults; thus the nurse might then ask, "Did your mother ever have any other type of cancer?" Often the patient may then reveal that her mother had breast cancer some years before ("bone cancer" was actually breast cancer that had spread to the bones). Breast cancer at an early age can indicate a genetic predisposition.

Patients may ask questions that indicate they have an interest in genetic testing. These are examples of questions that may be cues that the patient has genetic concerns:

- Will my children get this disease?
- Because my sister has this problem, what are the chances I might also develop it?
- Is there a way to test and see whether my chances of getting this disease or problem are high or low?

Areas of responsibility for any medical-surgical nurse in working with a patient who is considering or having genetic testing include communication, privacy and confidentiality, information accuracy, patient advocacy, and support.

Communication

In congruence with professional ETHICS, act as a patient advocate by ensuring that communication between the patient and whoever is providing the genetic information is clear. First, assess the patient's ability to receive and process information. Can the patient see and hear clearly, or are assistive devices needed? Does the patient understand English, or will an interpreter be needed? Does the patient have adequate cognition at the time of meeting with the genetics professional, or is it impaired by medication, disease, anxiety, or fear?

If the patient appears not to understand terms or jargon during a discussion between him or her and a genetics professional, ask the professional to use common terms and examples for the patient. Verify with the patient that he or she understands or does not understand.

After any discussion about genetic risk or genetic testing, assess the patient's understanding of what was said. Ask the patient to explain, in his or her own words, what the issue means and what his or her expectations are.

Privacy and Confidentiality

Professional ETHICS require that all conversations regarding potential diagnoses or genetic testing need to occur in a private environment. The patient has the right to determine who may be a part of the discussion and can decide to exclude the primary physician and any family member from the discussion with a genetics professional. It is important that health care professionals who may be present during such discussion do not disclose information, formally or informally, without the patient's permission. It is the nurse's ethical duty and responsibility to protect this information from improper disclosure to family members, other health care professionals, other patients, insurance providers, or anyone not specified by the patient.

Information Accuracy

Correct myths about genetic disorders, and teach patients about the nature of genetic testing. In addition, help patients find accurate and helpful resource materials or websites. Medical-surgical nurses are not genetics experts and would not be expected to be the final source of definitive information; however, with COLLABORATION they can help ensure that the patient is referred to the correct level of genetic counseling. If you are present during the patient's discussions with a genetics professional, assess whether the patient understands the issues regarding the health problem.

Patient Advocacy and Support

Ensure that the patient's rights are not neglected or ignored. Ask the patient privately what his or her wishes are regarding genetic testing. Ask whether another person or agency is insisting on the testing. Remind the patient that he or she does not have to agree to be tested. Verify that he or she has signed an informed consent statement for the test.

Considering or having genetic testing is a stressful experience. The patient and family require support and may need help with coping. Ethically, genetic testing should be performed only after genetic counseling has occurred and should be followed with more counseling.

Patients may feel anger, depression, guilt, or hopelessness. Patients who have positive results (results that indicate a specific mutation is present) from genetic testing may have issues of risk for early death or disability and the possibility of having passed the risk for a health problem on to their children. Patients who have an ambiguous test result or one of unknown significance may feel that they have agonized over a decision, spent money, and still have no clear answer. Even patients who have negative genetic test results (results that indicate a specific mutation is not present) need counseling and support. Some patients may have an unrealistic view of what a negative result means for their general health. Others may feel guilty that they were "spared" when other family members were not.

Assess the patient's response to genetic test results. Determine what coping methods were used successfully in the past. If the patient has disclosed information to family members, assess whether they can help provide support or need support themselves. Assess whether the information about positive test results has strained family relationships. Refer the patient to appropriate support groups and general counseling services.

For some positive genetic test results, such as having a *BRCA1* gene mutation, the risk for developing breast cancer is high but is not a certainty. With high risk, the patient needs a plan for prevention and risk reduction. One form of prevention is early detection. Thus a patient who tests positive for a *BRCA1* mutation should have at least yearly mammograms and ovarian ultrasounds to detect cancer at an early stage when it is more easily cured. Teach the patient who has positive test results that indicate an increased risk for a specific health problem about the types of screening procedures that are available and how often screening should occur. For example, some patients at known high genetic risk for breast cancer and ovarian cancer choose the primary prevention methods of bilateral prophylactic mastectomies (surgical removal of the breasts) and oophorectomies (surgical removal of the ovaries). Although these strategies are severe, they are effective and the patient should be informed about their availability.

Teach patients at known high risk for a specific disorder how to modify the environment to reduce risk. For example, a patient who has a specific mutation in the *a1AT* (alpha$_1$-antitrypsin) gene is at increased risk for early-onset emphysema. The onset of emphysema is even earlier when the patient smokes or is chronically exposed to inhalation irritants. By modifying his or her environment, the disease can be delayed or the manifestations reduced.

NCLEX EXAMINATION CHALLENGE

Psychosocial Integrity

The client who has been found to have a mutation in a gene allele that greatly increases her risk for chronic obstructive lung disease asks the staff nurse to be present when she discloses the test results to her family. What is the nurse's role in this situation?

A. Primary health care provider
B. Genetic counselor
C. Patient advocate
D. Patient support

GET READY FOR THE NCLEX® EXAMINATION!

KEY POINTS

Review these Key Points for each NCLEX Examination Client Needs Category.

Safe and Effective Care Environment

- Ensure that a person or family with indications of an increased genetic risk for a disease or disorder is referred to an appropriate genetics professional. **Teamwork and Collaboration** QSEN
- Advocate for the patient with regard to whether or not to have genetic testing, informed consent before testing, and sharing of test results. **Patient-Centered Care** QSEN
- Ensure that confidentiality of genetic test results is maintained by all health care team members. **Safety** QSEN
- Determine whether an informed consent statement was obtained before any genetic test is performed.
- Keep all patient and family information regarding genetic testing confidential.

Health Promotion and Maintenance

- Identify patients and families at increased genetic risk for disease or disorder.
- Teach patients and families at known increased genetic risk for disease or disorder what types of screening procedures and schedules are most appropriate (check specific disorder chapters for the appropriate screening guidelines). **Evidence-Based Practice** QSEN
- Teach patients and families at known increased genetic risk for disease or disorder what types of environmental modifications can reduce risk, delay disease onset, or reduce symptom severity (check specific disorder chapters for appropriate modifications). **Evidence-Based Practice** QSEN

Psychosocial Integrity

- Assess patients who have received results of genetic testing for responses such as anger, guilt, or depression.
- Allow the patient and family who have been identified as being at increased genetic risk for serious health problems to express concerns and feelings.
- Ensure that the patient who undergoes genetic testing is appropriately counseled before testing, while waiting for test results, and after test results are obtained. **Teamwork and Collaboration** QSEN
- Support the decision of the patient and family to have or not to have genetic counseling or testing.

Physiological Integrity

- Be aware that mutations or variations in gene sequences can change the activity of a protein and have adverse effects on health.
- Keep in mind that many common adult diseases or disorders have a genetic basis (hypertension, diabetes, cancer) although some of these diseases also may occur among people with no genetic risk.
- Remind the patient that having a gene variation that increases the risk for a disorder does not necessarily mean that the disorder will ever develop.
- Ensure that patients understand that genetic testing reveals information about their family members, as well as about themselves.
- Construct a three-generation pedigree from data obtained during the family history section of patient assessment.
- Remind patients that the results of genetic testing cannot be "taken back."
- Be prepared to assume the accepted roles of the medical-surgical nurse in genetic counseling, which include examining assessment data for indications of genetic risk, acting as a patient advocate, correcting myths about genetic disorders and genetic testing, protecting the patient's privacy and rights, and helping to ensure that the patient and/or family at increased genetic risk are referred to a genetics professional.

5 CHAPTER

Evidence-Based Practice in Medical-Surgical Nursing

Rona F. Levin and Fay Wright

http://evolve.elsevier.com/Iggy/

PRIORITY CONCEPTS

- Evidence-Based Practice
- Teamwork and Collaboration
- Safety
- Quality Improvement

LEARNING OUTCOMES

Safe and Effective Care Environment

1. Describe evidence-based practice (EBP) to include the components of research evidence, clinical expertise, and patient/family values.
2. Explain the role of evidence in making clinical decisions and determining best clinical practice.
3. Explain how to use an EBP approach to identifying a clinical problem, issue, or challenge.
4. Differentiate clinical opinion from research and evidence summaries.
5. Formulate a focused clinical question about clinical practice.
6. List the steps of how to perform a systematic literature review to answer clinical questions.
7. Briefly describe two models of EBP for changing processes of care.
8. Explain the steps of the evidence-based practice improvement (EBPI) model.
9. Discuss how the EBPI model can be used to guide a clinical practice improvement project.

OVERVIEW

All health care professionals need to understand and use an evidence-based practice (EBP) approach to practice. In 2003, the Institute of Medicine (IOM) published a report entitled *Health Professions Education: A Bridge to Quality*. That report contained this mandate: "All health professionals should be educated to deliver patient-centered care as members of an interdisciplinary team, emphasizing evidence-based practice, quality improvement approaches and informatics" (IOM, 2003, p. 3). Since that report was published, EBP to improve the quality of patient care has been a consistent theme in the IOM's publications, with more than 24 reports found on their website to guide implementation of EBP (http://www.iom.edu/Reports.aspx).

In 2010, the IOM in partnership with the Robert Wood Johnson Foundation published *The Future of Nursing: Leading Change, Advancing Health* (IOM, 2010). Key among the four major recommendations is: "Nurses should be full partners, with physicians and other health care professionals, in redesigning health care in the United States" (p. 3). The specifics of this recommendation include the need for nurses to be prepared to be collaborators in health care improvement efforts and sometimes lead those projects. Aspects of this role include "taking responsibility for identifying problems and areas of system waste, devising and developing improvement plans, [and] tracking improvement over time …" (p. 3). Thus all nurses need to be equipped with the knowledge and skill that are required to be a full partner in making positive change in health care. This chapter provides the foundation to begin that preparation.

Definitions of Evidence-Based Practice

According to several nursing experts and the Quality and Safety Education for Nurses (QSEN) movement, EBP incorporates the best current evidence with the expertise of the clinician and the patient's values and preferences to make a decision about health care (Cronenwett et al., 2007; Levin et al., 2013; Melnyk & Fineout-Overholt, 2011). This definition was based on the work of Sackett et al. (2000), who had proposed three components of EBP—best evidence, clinical expertise, and patient values and preferences—as part of the definition of evidence-based medicine.

Ervin (2002) proposed this definition of EBP for nursing: "Evidence-based nursing practice is practice in which nurses make clinical decisions using the best available research and other evidence that is reflected in approved policies, procedures, and clinical guidelines in a particular healthcare agency" (Ervin, 2002, p. 12). DiCenso et al. (2005) further extended this definition to include information about the patient's clinical state and the setting or circumstances in which health care is being provided.

The EBP process is COLLABORATIVE and involves all members of the health care team, including the patient and family. This model is shared by many health care professions and is not unique to nursing. Therefore, although other professions might refer to the model as evidence-based medicine (EBM) or evidence-based social work similar to how DiCenso et al. (2005) specified the practice of nursing, the authors of this text refer to the model as EBP.

Steps of the Evidence-Based Practice Process

The process of EBP is systematic and includes several steps as presented by Sackett et al. (2000) in the context of practicing and teaching medicine.

1. Asking "burning" clinical questions
2. Finding the very best evidence to try to answer those questions
3. Critically appraising and synthesizing the relevant evidence
4. Making recommendations for practice improvement
5. Implementing accepted recommendations
6. Evaluating outcomes

Important to note is that the original approach to EBP developed in the medical community was intended to be used by physicians to solve individual patient problems for which physicians did not have ready answers. The adoption of EBP by nursing and other health care disciplines, however, required a different perspective that incorporated organizational data, goals, and priorities. Most nurses work within a health care agency, not in an independent practice setting. Nurses must COLLABORATE with those in other disciplines who are involved in practice changes within a health care agency. An example of how EBP works within a hospital system is provided later in this chapter.

Asking "Burning" Clinical Questions

Clinical questions are derived when clinicians do not have all the information they need to make the best possible decisions about patient care. A "burning" clinical question is one that usually arises in daily practice or when attending a class or reading a professional journal on a specific topic. The question may arise in relation to an individual patient, a group or population of patients, or a patient care unit or larger organizational area. An example of an *individual* patient question that a nurse might ask is: "My older hospitalized patient who has been placed on fall precautions fell in the bathroom. What else could I have done to prevent this patient from falling, and what can I do to prevent her from falling in the future?" At a *group or population* level, the nurse might ask: "What are current best practices for assessing hospital patients' risk for falls, and/or what are best practices for fall prevention in patients who are at risk for falls? At a *unit or organizational* level, the question might be: "Is the current policy and procedure for assessing patients' risk for falls and for implementing preventive practices based on the best available evidence?"

Once you critically think about and pose a question about clinical practice, you will need to find out at what level the question needs to be answered (i.e., at the individual patient level, patient population level, or organizational level). If the latter two levels are where the problem exists, then begin to gather background information from the literature and internal evidence from your organization to describe the problem more fully (Levin et al., 2010).

One way you can begin to use EBP in your practice is to review the policy and procedure for a specific nursing practice in your clinical setting and determine what type of evidence was used as the basis for that policy and procedure. Does the protocol list references? What types of references are cited?

Once you have described the clinical practice problem and can focus on exactly what concerns you have, ask yourself whether the question is a *background* or a *foreground* question. A *background* question usually asks for a fact, a statement on which most authorities or experts would agree. For example: What is the etiology of congestive heart failure? What are the most frequently prescribed analgesics for the management of postoperative pain? The answers to these types of questions can usually be found in a textbook and are not controversial. A *foreground* question, on the other hand, usually asks a question of relationship and may be controversial. An example of this type of question is: What are the most effective interventions for treating venous leg ulcers?

Qualitative Versus Quantitative Questions. If you are asking a foreground question, develop a more specific, detailed clinical question to guide your search for evidence. Clinical questions may be qualitative or quantitative. A **qualitative question** focuses on the meanings and interpretations of human phenomena or experiences of people and usually analyzes the content of what a person says during an interview or what a researcher observes. Examples of qualitative questions are:

- What is the experience of having cancer like for young adults?
- How do older women respond to a residential move to assisted-living facilities?
- What are the differences in nurses' work culture between acute care and home care agencies?

A **quantitative question** asks about the relationship between or among defined, measurable phenomena and includes a more objective approach to both data collection and data analysis. Answers to quantitative questions necessitate statistical analysis of information that is collected to answer a question. Examples of quantitative questions are:

- What is the effect of using a new assessment tool to predict the likelihood of falling to frequency and severity of falls in patients undergoing hip replacement?
- What is the effect of hydrocolloid dressings compared with silver-impregnated dressings on the rate of wound healing in patients with postsurgical incision wounds?

PICO(T) Format. Nursing authors suggest framing clinical questions in a PICO (Fleming, 2008; Levin, 2013) or PICO(T) format (Fineout-Overholt & Stillwell, 2011). The PICO(T) format is outlined in Table 5-1. The major components of a focused clinical question are the **p**opulation, **i**ntervention, **c**omparison, and **o**utcome, with an added **t**ime component when appropriate.

The *population* indicates the specific group of patients to whom the question applies. This component is important because evidence that may support an intervention with one group of patients may not apply to another group of patients. For example, a fall prevention program for older adults who live at home may be very different from a fall prevention program for patients who attend a rehabilitation program. Be sure to think about the age, gender, ethnicity/race, and specific health problems to narrow your population of interest.

The *intervention* component may pertain to (1) a new therapy that has been supported by best evidence, (2) exposure to disease

TABLE 5-1 **Examples of Components of PICO(T) Questions in Relation to Type of Question**

	THERAPY	ETIOLOGY	DIAGNOSIS	PREVENTION	PROGNOSIS	MEANING
Population						
Intervention						
Comparison						
Outcome						
Time						

or harm, (3) a prognostic factor, or (4) a risk behavior or factor—for example, the need for toileting to help prevent falls (Melnyk & Fineout-Overholt, 2011). In terms of a new therapy, one might compare the use of guided imagery to decrease nausea and vomiting among patients receiving chemotherapy with similar patients who receive the current drug therapy for nausea and vomiting, and then evaluate patient outcomes.

The *comparison* component of the clinical question may be either the standard or current treatment as in the above example or may be another intervention with which the innovative practice is compared. In the case of prognostic questions, the comparison may consider another factor or potential influence that could affect the outcome of the patient's health. A preventive question might examine the absence of the risk factor as the comparison—for example, the need for toileting compared with no need for toileting to prevent falls.

The *outcome* component specifies the measurable and desired outcomes of your practice innovation, which may be focused on improving how you assess patients to make a nursing diagnosis or on a prevention or therapeutic intervention. Outcomes must include measures of the results of introducing an innovation to determine whether it was successful. For example, for an intervention outcome, measures might include patients' perception of pain, number of days spent in a hospital, or need for rehabilitative services. Or when testing a way to improve diagnostic accuracy, your outcome might focus on the sensitivity and specificity of a diagnostic test or nursing assessment tool (e.g., What is the best tool for assessing the risk for patient falls on an orthopedic unit?).

Fineout-Overholt and Stillwell (2011) advocated adding a *time* component or time frame to the focused clinical question. The question may include specifying within what time period one would expect the outcome(s) to occur. An example of a completed PICO(T) question is: What is the effect of adding hourly rounding to the standard falls protocol for the geriatric unit (patients 65 years or older) in hospital Y on the process of care provision (to be more specifically defined) and the outcomes of rate of falls, fall morbidity, and clinician satisfaction within a 3-month period?

Arriving at the focused clinical question is not an easy task, even for seasoned clinicians. Clearly identifying each component of the PICO(T) question focuses the clinical question for the next step in the EBP process: finding the best evidence to improve the practice problem.

Finding the Best Evidence

Finding the best available evidence to answer a focused clinical question has been a challenge for clinicians and health care agencies. The major barrier that prevents nurses from engaging in evidence-based practice is lack of time (Pravikoff et al., 2005). Other barriers include:

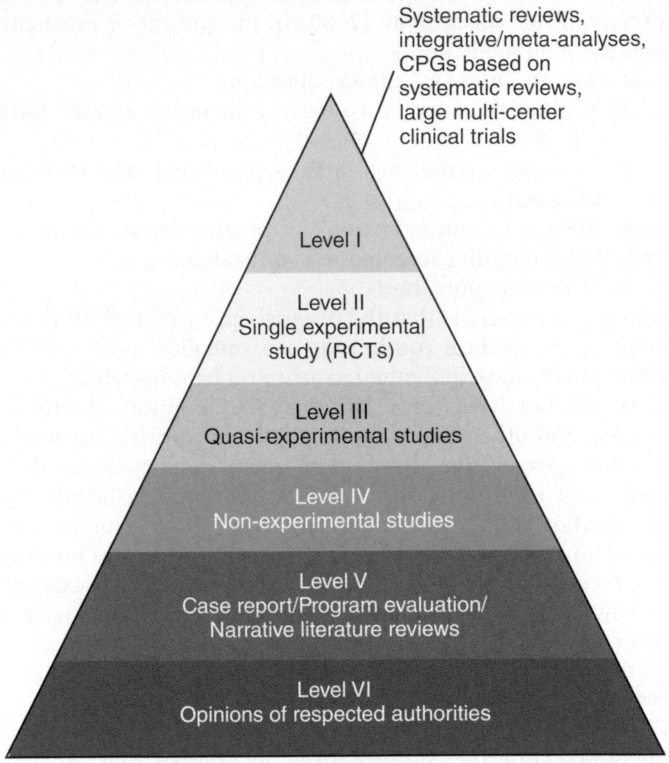

FIG. 5-1 Pyramid of evidence for questions of therapy. *CPGs,* Clinical practice guidelines; *RCTs,* randomized controlled trials.

- Lack of value for research in practice
- Lack of understanding of organization or structure of electronic databases
- Difficulty accessing research materials
- Lack of computer skills
- Difficulty understanding research articles

The health care system is addressing these challenges in many settings to improve the safety and quality of patient care. Many hospitals and community health care agencies are involved in promoting evidence-based practices and projects to reach national safety goals. An example of how staff nurses are essential contributors and collaborators on such projects is presented at the end of this chapter in the Application of the EBPI Model to Clinical Practice section.

Level of evidence (LOE) refers to the status or rank of evidence. Most evidence hierarchies are pyramids with the highest level of evidence at the top (Fig. 5-1). The type of evidence needed depends on the nature of the clinical question—is the question quantitative or qualitative? For example, if you are asking about the effectiveness of different types of compression bandages on healing of venous leg ulcers, you would want to *measure* the change in size of the ulcer as one indication of healing *(quantitative)*. On the other hand, you might be interested in what the experience of having a chronic venous ulcer is like for women *(qualitative)*. Each type of question requires different types and sources of evidence to find an answer. Table 5-2 provides an internationally accepted hierarchy for qualitative levels of evidence. The Evidence-Based Practice boxes in this text identify each study's LOE.

A preliminary evidence search entails identifying whether quality clinical practice guidelines (CPGs) exist to answer the clinical question. A **clinical practice guideline** is an "official recommendation" based on evidence to diagnose and/or manage a health problem (e.g., pain management). If these guidelines are of high quality and they contain the answer to your question, the search may be complete (Levin & Jacobs, 2012). The importance of CPGs is reinforced with the IOM's consensus report on the use and effectiveness of quality clinical practice guidelines for the implementation of EBP (IOM, 2011).

If the guidelines do not provide a sufficient answer to your question and/or they are not based on high-quality evidence, you need to search the "Fantastic Four" databases:

- Cochrane Library of Systematic Reviews
- Joanna Briggs Institute (JBI) systematic reviews
- Medline (or PubMed)
- Cumulative Index to Nursing and Allied Health Literature (CINAHL)

Other databases may also contain a wealth of information depending on the nature of the question. For example, if you are asking a psychological question about the best way to help patients deal with anxiety, then PsycINFO would be a good source. The instructional or health sciences librarian at the local college/university or clinical agency can assist in finding the best current evidence to answer your question. In some cases, you may need to revise the search if the original terms used did not access relevant citations. Table 5-3 provides a template that you can use for any evidence search that you undertake.

If a continued literature search is needed for *quantitative* clinical questions, start with looking for the top level of evidence (i.e., systematic reviews, which are meta-analyses, clinical practice guidelines based on top level evidence, and/or multisite randomized clinical trials) (see Fig. 5-1). If searching for answers to *qualitative* questions, look first for meta-syntheses. The major purpose of providing systematic reviews of evidence on a topic for both qualitative and quantitative questions is so that busy clinicians will not have to spend many hours finding original single studies and then reviewing, critiquing, and synthesizing each study's evidence. In some cases, evidence summaries are available (Table 5-4). Fig. 5-2 provides a guide for conducting a systematic evidence search.

Critically Appraising and Synthesizing Evidence

The key to this step is a collaborative team effort. One effective strategy is to have each member of an EBP team take responsibility for summarizing and critically appraising a select number of articles (depending, of course, on the number of relevant articles your search revealed) and then presenting a written summary and review to all team members. This allows collegial critique of the evidence, helps clarify areas of uncertainty, and facilitates team consensus on what the best evidence is to answer the clinical question. In addition, summarizing and critically appraising each piece of relevant evidence and entering the results of this activity into a table of evidence makes it easier to synthesize all the relevant evidence succinctly. This evidence synthesis will tell you if there is sufficient evidence to guide practice related to your clinical question.

Making Recommendations to Improve Practice

Once you have reviewed, critically appraised, and synthesized all the relevant evidence, you are ready to make practice recommendations in a written report to whoever needs to review them for potential approval. The clinical application at the end of the chapter illustrates this process.

Implementing Recommendations

This step is perhaps the most exciting and energizing component of an EBP project. After all the hard work of focusing the practice problem, developing a PICO question, retrieving and critically appraising the evidence, and getting practice recommendations approved, the protocol and implementation plan can be developed. This plan should improve practice, patient outcomes, and the desired outcomes of the system (e.g., cost savings). Approaches to implementation are varied. Examples of models to guide EBP projects from the beginning to the end are presented in the next section of this chapter.

TABLE 5-2 JBI Levels of Qualitative Evidence for Meaningfulness*

LEVEL OF EVIDENCE	MEANINGFULNESS M (1-4)
1	Meta-synthesis of research with unequivocal synthesized findings
2	Meta-synthesis of research with credible synthesized findings
3	a. Meta-synthesis of text/opinion with credible synthesized findings b. One or more single research studies of high quality
4	Expert opinion

*From Joanna Briggs Institute. (2008). *Reviewer's manual*. Adelaide, Australia: Author.
JBI, Joanna Briggs Institute.

TABLE 5-3 Example of a Search Strategy Table with Hypothetical Data

DATABASE	KEY WORDS	DATE RANGE	PEER REVIEWED	# OF CITATIONS	# RETRIEVED	# USED
Medline (PubMed)	Pain Postoperative Behavioral Assessment Scale	2002-2010	All	5	3	0
CINAHL	Pain Postoperative Behavioral Pain Scales	2000-2010	All	25	5	2

CINAHL, Cumulative Index to Nursing and Allied Health Literature.

Keep in mind that the process of implementation needs to be systematic, shared, and consistent. That is, the implementation protocol has to be followed strictly so that any outcomes that are achieved are actually based on the new EBP innovation being implemented. Therefore complete buy-in from the people who will be involved in implementing the new practice is essential.

Evaluating Outcomes

Evaluating outcomes requires valid and reliable measurement tools. For example, if the clinical question is evaluating the effect of music therapy on reducing postoperative abdominal pain, then a tool to measure pain intensity and quality would be used. Many of these tools are cited in the literature and can be used without permission. Others require that permission be obtained in writing. Be sure to determine whether permission is needed before you use any measurement tool.

TABLE 5-4 Sources for Pre-Appraised Evidence Guidelines/Summaries

PUBLISHER	WEBSITE
BMJ Clinical Evidence	www.clinicalevidence.com
DynaMed	www.ebscohost.com/dynamed
USPSTF Guidelines	www.ahrq.gov/clinic/prevenix.htm
AHRQ Evidence Reports	www.ahrq.gov/clinic/epcix.htm

AHRQ, Agency for Healthcare Research and Quality; *BMJ,* British Medical Journal; *USPSTF,* U.S. Preventive Services Task Force.

MODELS AND FRAMEWORKS FOR IMPLEMENTING EVIDENCE-BASED PRACTICE

Several authors have attempted to develop models or conceptual frameworks to facilitate an understanding of the complex process of introducing evidence-based improvement efforts (Rycroft-Malone & Bucknall, 2010). Each model highlights factors or processes that need to be considered when attempting to implement practice change.

Iowa Model

The major purpose of the Iowa model of EBP is to help health care professionals use evidence to improve patient outcomes. Originally developed as a model for research utilization, Titler revised and enhanced the model in 2010 to incorporate the elements of EBP. Important aspects of the current model include the (Titler, 2010):

- Triggers that lead to clinical questions
- Assessment of whether these questions are priorities for the health care organization
- Focus on forming a team to develop an EBP initiative
- General overview or steps for deciding about whether to implement and then adopt a change in practice

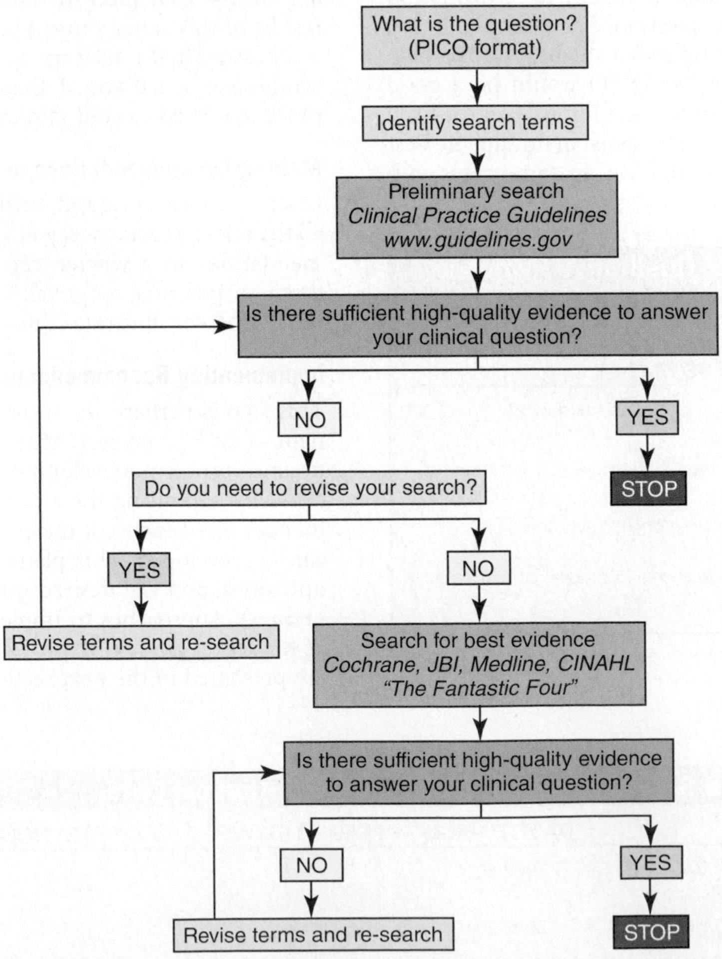

FIG. 5-2 Algorithm for systematic review of the published evidence. *CINAHL,* Cumulative Index to Nursing and Allied Health Literature.

CLINICAL JUDGMENT CHALLENGE

Evidence-Based Practice; Quality Improvement; Safety QSEN

An 82-year-old alert and oriented woman was admitted with a diagnosis of congestive heart failure. She also has urinary frequency. You notice on her chart that she is a "high falls risk." Over 70% of patients on your unit are also at high risk for falls. The written policy and procedure for fall prevention at your hospital states that patients at risk for falling should have:

- Their health care record flagged with a yellow flower
- A yellow flower placed on their room or bed
- A bed alarm installed
- Their siderails up at all times, except when a visitor, nurse, or nursing assistant is present

The patient felt the urge to urinate and pressed her call light. Someone on the intercom told her that she would assist her shortly. After 15 minutes, the patient had to make a decision to either urinate in bed or climb over the siderails to go to the bathroom. She decided to climb over the siderails and fell. The bed alarm went off after she left the bed.

1. Considering that over 70% of patients admitted to your unit are flagged as "at risk for falls," how do you think the nurses decide that a patient is at risk for falling? Are they using valid, reliable, sensitive, and specific assessment tools to make this determination?
2. In a population of inpatient older adults, what factors can predict patient falls with a high degree of accuracy?
3. Does the best available evidence support the use of bed alarms as an intervention that prevents falls in inpatient adults of any age?
4. In a population of adult inpatients, what are the factors that have been shown by research to be the most predictive of falls?
5. What interventions have been shown to decrease the fall rates in acute care institutions with this population? (Also see Chapter 3.)

Reavy and Tavernier Model

Reavy and Tavernier (2008) developed a model and process to implement EBP that uses concepts from previously developed models (e.g., Stetler model, Iowa model) and builds upon them. The emphasis of the Reavy and Tavernier model is on the crucial role of the direct caregiver (e.g., the staff nurse) in making changes to enhance clinical practice. The authors of the model view the staff nurse as the clinical expert. Given that the staff nurse may not have expertise in research and/or practice improvement, they believe that the expertise of a nurse researcher is needed to facilitate the EBP process. The nurse researcher serves as a role model and supports nursing staff in identifying areas for improvement, assists staff with literature reviews and synthesis of evidence, and helps with the implementation and evaluation of EBP projects. Reavy and Tavernier suggest that if a nurse researcher is not available in the practice setting, then a clinical nurse specialist, advanced practice nurse, or nurse manager might provide the needed support to staff nurses. Also included in this model is an emphasis on patient and family preferences and values; however, there is little explanation of the crucial role of patient as stakeholder in any practice improvement efforts. See Table 5-5 for a more detailed description of this model.

ARCC Model

The Advancing Research and Clinical Practice through Close Collaboration (ARCC) model of evidence-based practice was originally developed by Bernadette Melnyk in 1999 and was enhanced by Melnyk and Fineout-Overholt over a 10-year period (Melnyk & Fineout-Overholt, 2010). The current version of the model consists of several components and how they relate to each other. The major components of the model are:

TABLE 5-5 Processes Used for Implementation of the Reavy and Tavernier Evidence-Based Practice Model for Staff Nurses

	PATIENT VALUES AND PREFERENCES	STAFF NURSE/CLINICAL EXPERT	NURSE RESEARCHER/BEST AVAILABLE EVIDENCE
Assessment	Give verbal and nonverbal communication	Receive verbal and nonverbal messages (collect data)	
Identification and evaluation of problem		1. Identify problem(s) 2. Discuss potential interventions and outcome 3. Conduct literature search	Assist with literature search as needed
Analysis and synthesis of best available evidence		1. Analyze and critique best available evidence 2. Synthesize evidence	Assist with analysis, and critique as needed
Planning		1. Assess feasibility of change 2. Define proposed change 3. Identify resources 4. Define desired outcome	
Implementation and evaluation	Receive nursing care based on best evidence	1. Design and implement peer teaching strategies 2. Implement change 3. Conduct pilot study 4. Evaluate findings 5. Decide to adopt or reject change 6. Communicate findings	1. Provide assistance with pilot study 2. Receive communication related to ideas for research
Integration and maintenance	Receive nursing care based on best evidence	1. Integrate into policies 2. Monitor process 3. Monitor outcomes 4. Communicate updates	Receive communication related to ideas for research

- Organizational assessment and readiness to implement EBP
- Identification of strengths and barriers to EBP implementation
- Development and use of EBP mentors
- Implementation of EBP
- Measurement of nurse, system, and patient outcomes

Key to this model is the development and use of EBP mentors who teach, guide, and facilitate agency staff in the implementation and evaluation of evidence-based practices (Melnyk & Fineout-Overholt, 2010).

EVIDENCE-BASED PRACTICE IMPROVEMENT (EBPI) MODEL

The EBPI model developed by Levin et al. under the auspices of the Visiting Nurse Service of New York (Levin et al., 2010) combines the best of the EBP and PI/QI (process/QUALITY IMPROVEMENT) systems into one approach for implementing practice improvement.

Steps of the EBPI Model

The model is prescriptive and easy for guiding health care practitioners from any discipline and setting to achieve positive change. As depicted in Fig. 5-3, the model includes:

- Describing the practice problem
- Formulating a focused clinical question (in PICO format)
- Searching for evidence to answer the question

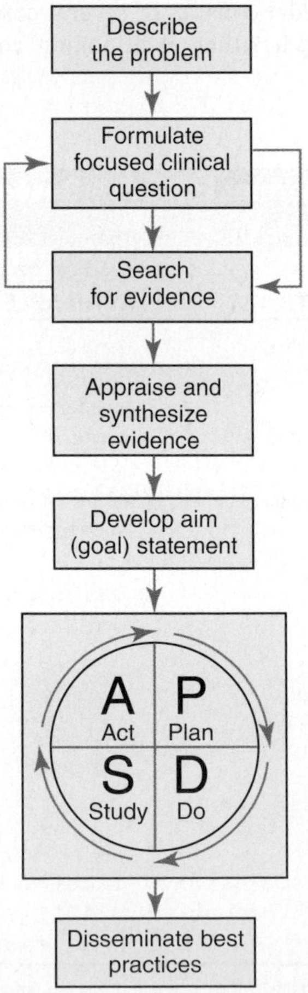

FIG. 5-3 The Evidence-Based Practice Improvement (EBPI) model.

- Appraising and synthesizing relevant evidence
- Developing an aim statement or project goal
- Developing, implementing, and evaluating the protocol for practice improvement
- Using small tests of change or **p**lan, **d**o, **s**tudy, **a**ct (PDSA) cycles to test methods
- Disseminating best practices

Adopted from the process improvement approach is the idea of PDSA cycles or small tests of change (Langley et al., 2009). Many professionals in health care, business, and other fields implement what they believe is a good idea for an improvement on too-large a scale before they have perfected the new practice or even assessed how successful it may or may not be in their setting with their populations (patients or consumers). One of the most important benefits of small tests of change is that you have a chance to perfect the process or practice that you want to implement before disseminating and using the practice on a wide scale. Small tests of change for EBPI projects in health care are conducted with a small group of people (e.g., patients or staff) for a short period and may be repeated several times until the implementation protocol is perfected (Levin, 2009).

During small tests of change, it is helpful to use the concept of PDSA cycles to guide the activities.

- "**P**" stands for "plan" and is the first step in introducing a practice change. During this phase, a project team develops a protocol for implementation, which includes not only the protocol or procedure for the practice innovation but also a total plan for the exact process that will be followed for implementing the project. It includes who will be administering the new practice, how it will be implemented, the time frame for implementation, and how the particular processes implemented for each small test of change will be evaluated.
- "**D**" stands for "do" and is the action-oriented phase of the process. The new innovation or a portion of it is tested according to the plan.
- "**S**" stands for "study" and refers to the review and analysis of data collected during the "do" phase of the cycle.
- "**A**" stands for "act" and is the evaluation of results from the small test to guide decisions about how to proceed with the EBP project.

Decisions then need to be made about how to revise or refine the practice protocol and institute another small test of change to try out the refined protocol and then decide whether the plan is worth continuing.

Application of the EBPI Model to Clinical Practice: A Case Study

Describe the Practice Problem

On an adult general surgical unit in a community hospital, the nursing staff identified that assessing patients' postoperative pain with the current practice of using a numeric 10-point rating scale did not seem to be an effective assessment tool when the patient was lying quietly or appeared to be asleep. The nurses thought that to ask the restful patient to scale his or her pain refocused the patient on the pain and was not supportive of patient relaxation and pain relief. When this type of clinical observational pain assessment was performed, the nurse often did not chart the assessment in the medical record—how could the nurse label the level of pain on the scale when patient behaviors were used to assess pain? To document pain assessment and management in the patient's health record, the nurse would make up a pain rating score. A nurse's note could have been added to the medical record to describe pain behaviors the nurse identified as indicators that pain appeared to be decreasing and pain medication was working. However, the nurses on the unit did not write notes until the end of the shift. Thus the health record appeared as if no re-assessment had taken place and that the nurses were not following hospital policy. Pain assessment and management is a key quality measure for hospital accreditation making EBP quality improvement not only a clinical priority but also an important hospital initiative (The Joint Commission, 2010).

The nurses on the unit identified that pain assessment needed to be improved for quality patient care. A small team of staff nurses who understand the EBP process was formed to lead the project to address the clinical concerns. The staff identified that the main focus of the problem was assessment of patients who were asleep or appeared asleep. Was there a reliable and valid method to assess pain by observing behaviors without disturbing the patient? The nurses identified that the numeric rating scale worked for most postoperative patients after the second postoperative day. The clinical concern was assessing and re-evaluating pain management within the first 24 hours after surgery when patients were tired and often asleep because of the remnants of anesthetic and being heavily medicated for pain.

A chart audit confirmed that the nursing staff consistently assessed and re-evaluated pain with the numeric rating scale on the second postoperative day. Pain was assessed according to standards 95% of the time. On the first day after surgery, the pain scale was documented only 12% of the time. Nurses' notes to describe the patients' pain were written only 60% of the time during the first postoperative day. Clearly, there was a problem documenting pain assessment on the first postoperative day.

No one doubted that the nurses assessed pain frequently and provided pain relief; however, only the administration of pain medication was documented. Pain assessments were not consistently charted and, from a legal standpoint, the pain assessment was not done. When the numeric pain scale was used, the nurses consistently met hospital standards for pain assessment and evaluation of pain relief. The chart audit showed that a new, easy-to-use tool that assessed pain behaviors was needed to improve the documentation of pain assessment.

Formulate a Focused Clinical Question

After conducting the chart audit, the EBP team defined the clinical problem and framed a PICO question to focus the literature search for evidence-based strategies to improve pain assessment. The PICO question developed was: In the adult hospitalized patient (**P**), does the implementation of a behavioral pain scale (**I**) compared with the use of a visual analog scale (**C**) improve the assessment and management of pain in patients on the first postoperative day (**O**)?

Search for Evidence

To start their search, the EBP team began at the Cochrane Library to try to find the highest level of evidence, a clinical practice guideline to answer their question. The Cochrane Library search revealed eight clinical practice guidelines related to pain assessment but none discussed nonverbal/behavioral assessment tools (www.thecochranelibrary.com). The EBP team then went to the hospital library and accessed the CINAHL database. The initial search term used was "Pain Assessment." This search provided 11,501 article results for the years 1966 to 2013 (www.EBSCOHOST.com). No matter how many nurses worked on the project, it would be impossible to read and evaluate over 11,000 articles. The team then remembered to use the PICO template as a guide to focus the search. Limits to narrow the search were added to the request, and only articles for pain assessment or measurement in adults ages 19 years and older were accessed. Just limiting the articles by the age of the patient reduced the number of articles to 4,836 (www.EBSCOHOST.com). This was a more manageable number of articles but still a huge number to review from a practical standpoint. So the search was further limited to the last 10 years, yielding, 3379 articles, still an insurmountable number of articles to read (www.EBSCOHOST.com). Further limiting the search using the term "inpatient" reduced the number of articles to 237—a much more manageable number, yet still overwhelming (www.EBSCOHOST.com)! Articles from 2013 appeared on the first page of the search screen. The titles revealed many interesting yet varied article topics. The search retrieved articles that addressed pain assessment with culture and pain assessment methods for specific medical diagnoses. Articles that specifically addressed behavioral pain assessment tools in the acute care setting were not immediately apparent in a list of articles.

The team realized that using the PICO question keywords might help narrow the search to the specific topic of interest and to a manageable number of articles to review. Using the search options of "postoperative pain" and "clinical assessment tools," the search engine revealed 89 articles for review (www.EBSCOHOST.com). The nurses then saved the complete search so that they could refer to the list and read other articles as they explored solutions to the PICO question.

The EBP team reviewed the search results and identified five articles that appeared to address the clinical question specifically. One article discussed the use of three evidence-based practices for postoperative pain assessment (Carlson, 2009). The nurses were intrigued by the title of this article—is it possible that the authors have already evaluated three different methods that address their specific clinical question and that it can be read in one article? Another article examined abdominal surgery patients' pain management from the postanesthesia care unit (PACU) to the surgical unit (Wilding et al., 2009). Because PACU-to-unit transition takes place during the early postoperative period, the time that pain assessment using current practice is a concern, this article seemed to address the PICO question. Two articles complemented each other with one reporting the feasibility of using a nonverbal pain assessment tool in the critical care unit (Gélinas, 2010) and another reporting the same tool's reliability (Keane, 2012).

The fifth article also focused on pain assessment tools in the critical care unit (Hall, 2007). This article evaluated three pain assessment tools. Thus the nurses chose to review these three articles in postoperative critical care patients to see if any of the tools discussed could be used on the general surgical floor.

Appraise and Synthesize the Evidence

The team read the articles and completed tables of evidence (TOEs) so the information from the articles could be organized and discussed. The TOEs also helped the nurses systematically organize what they read in a consistent format for group discussion and analysis (Table 5-6). These tables were used as the group discussed their individual review of the articles, which

TABLE 5-6 Sample Entry for a Table of Evidence

NURSING SERVICES TABLE OF EVIDENCE

PROJECT TITLE: PAIN ASSESSMENT
DATE OF REVIEW: FEBRUARY 2013

REVIEWER: F. WRIGHT

ARTICLE INFORMATION: AUTHORS, TITLE, DATE PUBLISHED, JOURNAL	SAMPLE CHARACTERISTICS AND SIZE	STUDY DESIGN, PATIENT SELECTION, EVIDENCE LEVEL/ QUALITY RATING	INTERVENTION	AUTHORS' CONCLUSIONS	REVIEWER'S COMMENTS (STRENGTHS, LIMITATIONS, POTENTIAL PRACTICE CHANGE?)
Keane, K.M. (2012). Validity and reliability of the critical care pain observation tool: a replication study. *Pain Management Nursing, 14*(4), e216-225.	21 postoperative patients assessed for pain at rest, and after repositioning 3 times on postoperative day 1. Mean age of 64 yrs. 67% male patients.	Prospective comparison to determine if there were differences in observed pain behaviors between 2 separate nurse observers and videotaped behaviors to test the reliability and validity of the CPOT instrument. **Level III: quasi-experimental design**	Patients' pain assessed using the CPOT. The CPOT was used to assess pain and compare the results with observations and self-reports of pain when the patient could report pain levels verbally.	Initial CPOT instrument testing: strong discriminant validity (t = 5.75, p >0.001). Good face validity; 93% inter-rater reliability; Kappa statistic was 0.36 to 0.72 (p = 05). The cognitively and non–cognitively impaired groups' CNPI scores did not differ significantly in total scores. The cognitively impaired group had more pain behaviors identified at rest than the non–cognitively impaired group.	This was a replication of the initial testing (Gélinas, 2010) of the CPOT to assess pain in nonverbal critically ill patients. It seems to be reliable and simple to use. The CPOT seems to be most effective in patients when not intubated and so may be useful on the acute care floor during immediate postoperative assessments.

CNPI, Checklist of nonverbal pain indicators; *CPOT,* Critical-Care Pain Observation Tool.

included a summary of the evidence contained in the article, the strengths and limitations of the evidence, and potential application to their specific PICO question. As the nurses critically appraised the evidence, the group referred to the quantitative evidence pyramid in Fig. 5-1 to identify the level of evidence of each article. The colorful pyramid was posted during the discussion for ease of reference. Through dialog about each article, the authors' methods, outcomes, and the limitations of the different tools to measure pain, the group rated the quality of the articles. This process was used to make an informed decision about the strength of the evidence before any practice recommendations could be made. The staff wanted to use the highest level of evidence possible to inform the practice change. One of the critical care articles was identified as a level III quasi-experimental study and presented a description of a tool that was reported as "easy to use" and reliable for nonverbal patients (Keane, 2012). The staff returned to the literature search to find more information on one of the behavioral pain tools discussed in the same article.

Develop the Aim Statement

After reviewing the evidence to answer the focused clinical question, the nurses developed this aim statement: Improve the frequency of nurses' assessment of first-day postoperative pain from 12% to 70% after 2 weeks of introducing a new behavioral pain assessment tool.

Implement the PDSA Cycles

After the second search for evidence to answer the clinical question and additional review of the new evidence, the team of nurses planned to make a practice change (**Plan**). A small test of the utility of the tool needed to be performed to see if the nurses could accurately assess pain using the behavioral assessment tool and to determine its practicality for use. To evaluate the inter-rater reliability of the tool to determine if the nurses could consistently assess a patient's pain in the same way with the same tool, three of the nurses used the tool simultaneously to assess pain in 10 postoperative patients (**Do**). The assessment results were compared and evaluated to identify whether the nurses were using the tool consistently (**Study**). This small test of change resulted in positive feedback from nurses as to the practicality of the tool, and inter-rater reliability was high (i.e., different nurses observing patients and assessing their pain at the same time using the new tool came up with consistently similar ratings of these patients' pain).

The next step was to perform another small test of change (**Act**) to evaluate if nurses on the EBP team could use the pain assessment tool effectively in the clinical unit to improve patient pain assessment. The team used the tool for 1 week on all first-day postoperative patients. Patient records were monitored daily by the nurse educator and unit manager to evaluate the frequency of pain assessment. Because the team had the initial chart audit data, collecting the same data with the new tool in use would help identify if the behavioral scale for assessment of pain was completed and documented more consistently than before the new scale was introduced. In addition, the EBP nurse team was able to develop a step-by-step process for use of the tool.

The next step in the EBPI implementation process was for the project team to educate the rest of the unit staff on all shifts about the evidence-based intervention—the behavioral pain assessment tool and the process for its use. The TOEs were summarized and discussed to provide the staff with concrete information about the new tool. The EBP nurse team demonstrated how the tool was used. A member of the project team pretended to be asleep in a bed as a patient so that the nurses could role-play how to perform the pain assessment with the proposed tool. Informational posters were placed on the unit and multiple copies were made of the tool for use during the small test of change. The unit secretaries were involved in the education since they were responsible for providing the tools and collecting them when they were completed.

For 2 weeks, the nursing staff used the new tool to assess the pain of first-day postoperative patients. The team reviewed patient charts daily and answered questions about the use of the tool and the documentation of the pain assessment. At the completion of this third small test of change, the team reviewed the chart audits and found that the unit nurses had appropriately documented pain assessment on the first postoperative day 85% of the time—a huge improvement! A short questionnaire was distributed to the nursing staff to determine their feedback about the use and effectiveness of the tool. All unit staff found the new tool easy to use and expressed positive beliefs in its value. They also were very proud to have achieved an outcome that exceeded their outcome in the aim statement.

Disseminate Best Practices

Given the success the nurses achieved on this one postoperative unit with their small tests of change using PDSA cycles, they recommended the introduction of the new behavioral pain assessment tool to the Hospital Standards of Practice Committee. The Committee, consisting of an interdisciplinary team of nurses, physicians, pharmacists, and other health care professionals, was excited about the evidence-based practice improvement effort. They decided to pilot the new tool on all surgical units for 1 month to see if the same results could be achieved with wider dissemination. If the initial benchmark of 70% was achieved in the pilot, then the new protocol for assessment of pain on the first postoperative day would be instituted hospital-wide as the standard of practice. At completion of the pilot, the benchmark of 70% was achieved and the Committee voted to incorporate the new policy and procedure as standard practice.

All nurses who worked on surgical units, the operating suites, and PACU were educated about the new hospital standards for pain assessment. The plan for evaluation of the new practice was to conduct random patient record audits each month for 6 months to determine whether the improvement effort continued after initial implementation. The nurse educator and the EBP mentor worked with the initial EBP nurse team (three staff nurses) to submit an abstract for presentation at an EBP conference. The Vice President of Patient Care Services agreed to pay all expenses for the five nurses who led the project to attend the conference if the abstract was accepted for presentation.

GET READY FOR THE NCLEX® EXAMINATION!

KEY POINTS

Review these Key Points for each NCLEX Examination Client Needs Category.

Safe and Effective Care Environment

- Describe EVIDENCE-BASED PRACTICE (EBP) to include the components of research evidence, clinical expertise, and patient/family values: EBP is a strategy for making clinical decisions about how we practice nursing and other health care professions.
- Describe EBP to include the components of research evidence, clinical expertise, and patient/family values: EBP incorporates the expertise of the clinician and the patient's values and preferences to make decisions about health care. **Evidence-Based Practice** QSEN
- Explain how to use an EBP approach to identifying a clinical problem, issue, or challenge, and formulate a focused clinical question about clinical practice: The first step of the EBP process is to ask a clinical "burning" question using the PICO(T) format (see Table 5-1).
- Recall that quantitative questions focus on the relationship among measurable phenomena and include statistical analysis of information.
- Remember that qualitative questions focus on the meanings and interpretations of human phenomena or experiences of people using interview or observation.
- Explain the roles of levels of evidence by reviewing Fig. 5-1 and Table 5-2, which refer to the status or rank of evidence.
- Briefly describe two models of EBP for changing processes of care: Examples of models of EBP include the Iowa model, the Reavy and Tavernier model (see Table 5-5), and the evidence-based practice improvement (EBPI) model. **Evidence-Based Practice** QSEN
- Differentiate clinical opinion from research and evidence summaries: When performing a literature search on current evidence to answer the clinical question, organize the data into a table of evidence like the one shown in Table 5-6.
- Discuss how the EBPI model can be used to guide a clinical practice QUALITY IMPROVEMENT project: When making changes based on findings from the literature, use PDSA cycles to test the changes on a small scale.
- Discuss how the EBPI model can be used to guide a clinical practice improvement project: Recall that PDSA stands for "Plan," "Do," "Study," and "Act." **Quality Improvement** QSEN
- List the steps of how to perform a systematic literature review to answer clinical questions using the steps in Table 5-5. Recall these steps include searching for clinical practice guidelines, summarizing and appraising research, making recommendations for change, implementing the change, and evaluating the outcomes.

6 CHAPTER

Rehabilitation Concepts for Chronic and Disabling Health Problems

Donna D. Ignatavicius

http://evolve.elsevier.com/Iggy/

PRIORITY CONCEPTS

- Nutrition
- Mobility
- Elimination
- Cognition
- Tissue Integrity

LEARNING OUTCOMES

Safe and Effective Care Environment

1. Identify the roles of each member of the interdisciplinary rehabilitation team.
2. Identify health care settings where rehabilitation care is provided.
3. Delegate and supervise selected nursing tasks as part of care for the rehabilitation patient.
4. Coordinate recommendations for home modifications with the patient, family, occupational therapist, and case manager.
5. Use safe patient handling practices based on current evidence to prevent self-injury.

Health Promotion and Maintenance

6. Develop a teaching plan to prevent complications for the rehabilitation patient who has impaired physical MOBILITY.

Psychosocial Integrity

7. Assess the patient's response to chronic or disabling health problems.
8. Identify special considerations for older adults undergoing rehabilitative care, including assessment of COGNITION.

Physiological Integrity

9. Interpret health assessment findings to plan appropriate collaborative care for the rehabilitation patient in the acute or long-term care setting.
10. Assess the ability of patients to use assistive/adaptive devices to promote MOBILITY.
11. Identify the role of NUTRITION in the care of the patient in a rehabilitation setting.
12. Plan interventions to prevent skin breakdown and impaired TISSUE INTEGRITY for rehabilitation patients.
13. Differentiate retraining methods for a patient with a spastic versus flaccid bladder and bowel to promote ELIMINATION.
14. Explain the primary concerns for patients being discharged to home after rehabilitation.

A **chronic health problem** is one that has existed for at least 3 months. A **disabling health problem** is any physical or mental health/behavioral health problem that can cause disability. This text focuses primarily on physical health problems; mental health/behavioral health problems are discussed in more detail in textbooks on mental health/behavioral health nursing.

Patients with chronic and disabling health problems often participate in rehabilitation programs to prevent further disability, maintain functional ability, and restore as much function as possible. The rehabilitation nurse collaborates with the nursing and health care team and coordinates the patient's interdisciplinary care.

OVERVIEW

Chronic and Disabling Health Problems

Chronic and disabling illnesses are a major health problem in the United States, with almost half of the population having one or more chronic health problems. Complications of chronic disease account for the majority of all deaths, and associated medical costs account for over two thirds of the nation's health care cost. The rate of chronic and disabling conditions is expected to increase as more "baby boomers" approach late adulthood. Some people with chronic and disabling problems are in inpatient settings like rehabilitation centers and skilled nursing facilities, whereas others are managed at home.

Stroke, coronary artery disease, cancer, chronic obstructive pulmonary disease (COPD), asthma, and arthritis are common chronic diseases that can result in varying degrees of disability. Most occur in people older than 65 years. Younger adults are also living longer with potentially disabling genetic disorders that, in the past, would have shortened life expectancy. These specific health problems are discussed throughout this text.

Chronic and disabling conditions are not always illnesses (e.g., heart disease); they may also result from accidents. Accidents are a leading cause of trauma and death among young and middle-aged adults. Increasing numbers of people survive accidents with severe injuries because of advances in medical technology and safety equipment such as motor vehicle airbags. As a result, they are often faced with chronic, disabling neurologic conditions, such as traumatic brain injuries (TBIs) and spinal cord injuries (SCIs).

These health problems are also common among military men and women survivors who served in Iraq and Afghanistan. The most common complications of these wars are TBI and single or multiple limb amputations. These disabilities require months to years of follow-up health care after returning to the community. Because of people living longer with chronic and disabling health problems, the need for rehabilitation is on the rise.

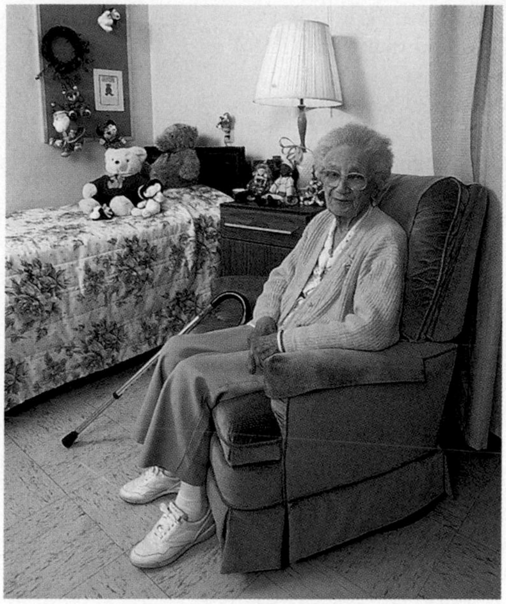

FIG. 6-1 Patient (resident) in a skilled nursing facility rehabilitation unit.

Rehabilitation Settings

Rehabilitation is the continuous process of learning to live with and manage chronic and disabling conditions. The desired outcome of rehabilitation is that the patient will return to the best possible physical, mental, social, vocational, and economic capacity. Rehabilitation is not limited to the return of function in post-traumatic situations. It also includes education and therapy for any chronic illness characterized by a change in a body system function or body structure. Rehabilitation programs related to respiratory, cardiac, and musculoskeletal health problems are common examples that do not involve trauma.

Rehabilitation ("rehab") can occur in a number of settings. This process starts in the acute care hospital (sometimes called *acute* or *short-term rehabilitation*) and continues after discharge from the hospital. The nurse coordinates care from acute care through community-based care to ensure successful rehabilitation.

For continuing rehabilitation services, the most common **inpatient rehabilitation facilities (IRFs)** are freestanding rehabilitation hospitals, rehabilitation or skilled units within hospitals (e.g., transitional care units [TCUs]), and skilled nursing facilities to which the patient is typically admitted for 1 to 3 weeks or longer. **Skilled nursing facilities (SNFs)** are part of either a hospital or long-term care (nursing home) setting (Fig. 6-1). Skilled rehabilitation and nursing services for older residents admitted to SNFs are reimbursed through Medicare A for the first 21 days after admission. After that time, reimbursement is a combination of Medicare and other payer sources for a specified number of days.

Patients in nursing homes or skilled nursing units in hospitals are called *residents*. The term **resident** implies that the person lives in the inpatient facility and has all the rights of anyone living in his or her home. Residents wear street clothes rather than hospital gowns and have choices in what they eat and how they plan each day.

Ambulatory care rehabilitation departments and home rehabilitation programs may be needed for continuing less-intensive services. Eighty percent (80%) of rehabilitation services are paid for by Medicare B for older adults for a specified period of time if they have this benefit. Some agencies have specialized clinics focused on rehabilitation of patients with specific health problems, such as those that care for patients with strokes; amputations; and large, chronic, and/or nonhealing wounds. After disabled patients become more confident and independent, they may choose to live at home or in a group home. Group homes are facilities in which patients live independently together with other disabled adults. Each patient or group of patients has a care provider, such as a personal care aide, to assist with ADLs and daily decisions requiring accurate judgments. The patients may or may not be actively employed. In some cases, the care home offers employment opportunities to the residents. The purpose of these homes is to provide independent living arrangements outside an institution, especially for younger patients with TBI or SCI.

The Rehabilitation Team

Successful rehabilitation depends on the coordinated effort of a group of the patient, family, and health care professionals in planning, implementing, and evaluating patient-centered care. The focus of the rehabilitation team is to restore and maintain the patient's function to the greatest extent possible.

In addition to the patient, family, and/or significant others, members of the interdisciplinary health care team in the rehabilitation setting may include:

- Physicians, nurse practitioners, and clinical nurse specialists
- Nurses and nursing assistants
- Physical therapists and assistants
- Occupational therapists and assistants
- Speech-language pathologists and assistants
- Rehabilitation assistants/restorative aides
- Recreational or activity therapists
- Cognitive therapists or neuropsychologists
- Social workers or case managers
- Clinical psychologists
- Vocational counselors

- Spiritual care counselors
- Registered dietitians (RDs)
- Pharmacists
- Biomedical technicians

Not all settings that offer rehabilitation services have all of these members on their team. Not all patients require the services of all health care team members.

A physician who specializes in rehabilitative medicine is called a **physiatrist**. Most inpatient rehabilitation settings employ physiatrists. A primary care physician or nurse practitioner may also oversee care for the patient's medical problems.

Rehabilitation nurses in the inpatient setting coordinate the efforts of health care team members and therefore function as the patient's case manager. Nurses also create a rehabilitation milieu, which includes (Pryor, 2010):

- Allowing time for patients to practice self-management skills
- Encouraging patients and providing emotional support
- Protecting patients from embarrassment (e.g., bowel training)
- Making the inpatient unit a more homelike environment

Table 6-1 summarizes the nurse's role as part of the rehabilitation team. Because of an increase in the need for older adult rehabilitation, some nurses specialize in gerontologic rehabilitation (Association of Rehabilitation Nurses [ARN], 2008b). Nurses and other health care professionals may be designated as **rehabilitation case managers** in the home or in acute care settings.

As their name implies, **nursing assistants** or **nursing technicians** assist in the care of patients. These members of the rehabilitation team are under the direct supervision of the registered nurse (RN) or licensed practical or vocational nurse (LPN or LVN).

Physical therapists (PTs), also called **physiotherapists**, intervene to help the patient achieve self-management by focusing on gross MOBILITY skills (e.g., by facilitating ambulation and teaching the patient to use a walker) (Fig. 6-2). They may also teach techniques for performing certain ADLs, such as transferring (e.g., moving into and out of bed), ambulating, and toileting, and can assist with cognitive retraining (often for patients with TBI). In some settings, PTs play a major role in providing wound care. Physical therapy assistants (PTAs) may be employed to help the PT.

Occupational therapists (OTs) work to develop the patient's fine motor skills used for ADL self-management, such as those required for eating, hygiene, and dressing. OTs also teach patients how to perform independent living skills, such as cooking and shopping. Many inpatient rehabilitation facilities have fully furnished and equipped apartments where patients can practice independent living skills in a mock setting under supervision. To accomplish these outcomes, OTs teach skills related to coordination (e.g., hand movements) and cognitive retraining (Fig. 6-3). Occupational therapy assistants (OTAs) may be available to help the OT.

TABLE 6-1 Nurse's Role in the Rehabilitation Team

- Advocates for the patient and family
- Creates a therapeutic rehabilitation milieu
- Provides and coordinates holistic patient care in a variety of health care settings, including the home
- Collaborates with the rehabilitation team to establish expected patient outcomes to develop a plan of care
- Coordinates rehabilitation team activities to ensure implementation of the plan of care
- Acts as a resource to the rehabilitation team having specialized knowledge and clinical skills needed to care for patient with chronic and disabling health problems
- Communicates effectively with all members of the rehabilitation team, including the patient and family
- Plans continuity of care when the patient is discharged from the health care facility
- Evaluates the effectiveness of the interdisciplinary plan of care for the patient and family

Adapted from Association of Rehabilitation Nurses. (2008). *Standards and scope of rehabilitation nursing practice*, Glenview, IL: Author.

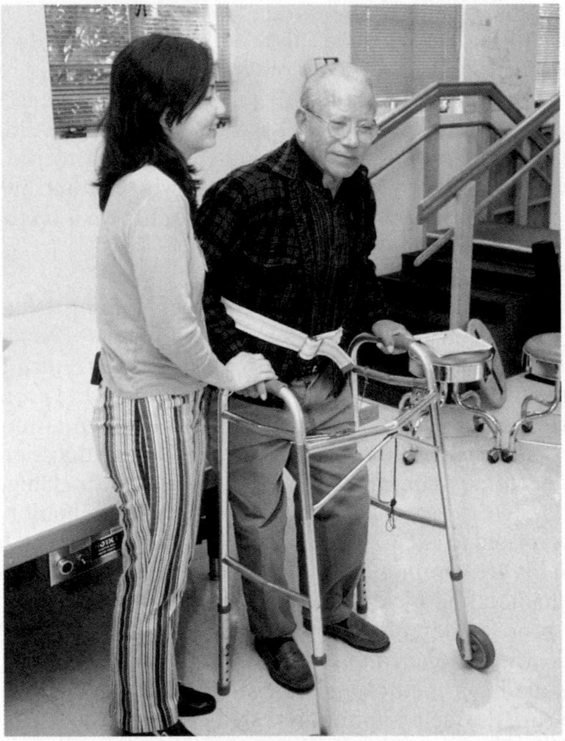

FIG. 6-2 A physical therapist helping a patient ambulate with a walker.

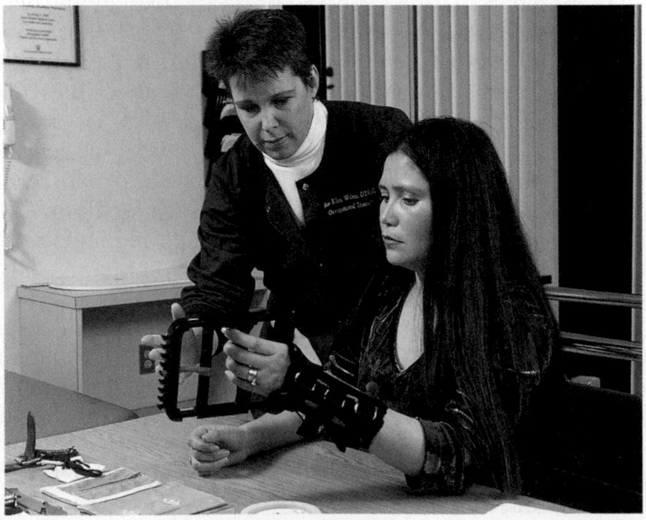

FIG. 6-3 A registered occupational therapist working with a patient on improving hand strength.

Speech-language pathologists (SLPs) evaluate and retrain patients with speech, language, or swallowing problems. *Speech* is the ability to say words, and *language* is the ability to understand and put words together in a meaningful way. Some patients, especially those who have experienced a head injury or stroke, have difficulty with both speech and language. Those who have had a stroke also may have dysphagia (difficulty with swallowing). SLPs provide screening and testing for dysphagia. If the patient has this problem, the SLP recommends appropriate foods and feeding techniques. Speech-language pathology assistants (SLPAs) may be employed to help the SLP.

PTs, OTs, and SLPs are collectively referred to as *rehabilitation therapists*. Assistants to PTs, OTs, and SLPs are called *rehabilitation assistants*. **Restorative aides**, usually in the nursing department, continue the rehabilitation therapy plan of care when therapists are not available. This model of care is common in long-term care settings, such as nursing homes.

Recreational or **activity therapists** work to help patients continue or develop hobbies or interests. These therapists often coordinate their efforts with those of the OT.

Cognitive therapists, usually neuropsychologists, work primarily with patients who have experienced head injuries with cognitive impairments. These therapists often use computers to assist with cognitive retraining.

Various counselors are helpful in promoting community reintegration of the patient and acceptance of the disability or chronic illness. **Social workers** help patients identify support services and resources, including financial assistance, and coordinate transfers to or discharges from the rehabilitation setting. **Clinical psychologists** also counsel patients and families on their psychological problems and on strategies to cope with disability. They may also perform a battery of assessments for COGNITION. **Spiritual counselors**, usually members of the clergy, specialize in spiritual assessments and care.

Vocational counselors assist with job placement, training, or further education. Work-related skills are taught if the patient needs to change careers because of the disability. If the patient has not yet completed high school, tutors may help with completion of the requirements for graduation.

Registered dietitians (RDs) may be needed to ensure that patients meet their needs for NUTRITION. For example, for patients who need weight reduction, a restricted calorie diet can be planned. For patients who need additional calories or other nutrients, including vitamins, dietitians can plan a patient-specific diet.

Pharmacists collaborate with the other members of the health care team to ensure that the patient receives the most appropriate drug therapy to meet the patient's needs. They oversee the prescription and preparation of medications and provide the health care team with essential information regarding drug safety.

Biomedical technicians maintain the safety of adaptive and electronic devices by monitoring their function and making repairs as needed.

Depending on the patient's health care needs, additional team members may be included in the rehabilitation program, such as the geriatrician, respiratory therapist, and prosthetist. Interdisciplinary team conferences for planning care and evaluating the patient's progress are held regularly with the patient, family members and significant others, and health care providers. The interdisciplinary patient record is shared and read by all team members.

❖ PATIENT-CENTERED COLLABORATIVE CARE

◆ Assessment

History. Collect the history of the patient's present condition, any current drug therapy, and any treatment programs in progress. Begin by obtaining general background data about the patient and family. This information includes cultural practices and the patient's home situation. In collaboration with the occupational therapist, the nurse or case manager addresses the layout of the home. Together they discuss whether the physical layout at home, such as stairs or the width of doorways, will present a problem to the patient after discharge.

Assess the patient's usual daily schedule and habits of everyday living. These include hygiene practices, NUTRITION, ELIMINATION, sexual activity, and sleep. Ask about the patient's preferred method and time of bathing and hygiene activity. In assessing dietary patterns, note food likes and dislikes. Also, obtain information about bowel and bladder function and the normal pattern of elimination.

In assessing sexuality patterns, ask about changes in sexual function since the onset of the disability. The patient's current and previous sleep habits, patterns, usual number of hours of sleep, and use of hypnotics are also assessed. Question whether the patient feels well rested after sleep. Sleep patterns have a significant impact on activity patterns. The assessment of activity patterns focuses on work, exercise, and recreational activities.

CONSIDERATIONS FOR OLDER ADULTS

Patient-Centered Care QSEN

Older adults who need rehabilitation often have other chronic diseases that need to be managed, including diabetes mellitus, coronary artery disease, osteoporosis, and arthritis. These health problems added to the normal physiologic changes associated with aging predispose the older adult to falls, pressure ulcers, and pneumonia. When discharged from a hospital setting, some older patients are undernourished, which causes weakness and fatigue. The longer the hospital stay, the more debilitated the older adult can become.

Health teaching may be challenging because some older patients may have beginning changes in cognition, including short-term memory loss. Sensory losses, like vision and hearing, may also affect their ability to give an accurate history or grasp new information.

Physical Assessment/Clinical Manifestations. Upon admission for baseline and at least daily (depending on agency policy and type of setting), collect physical assessment data systematically according to major body systems (Table 6-2). The primary focus of the assessment related to rehabilitation and chronic disease is the *functional* abilities of the patient.

Cardiovascular and Respiratory Assessment. An alteration in cardiac status may affect the patient's cardiac output or cause activity intolerance. Assess associated signs and symptoms of decreased cardiac output (e.g., chest pain, fatigue). If present, determine when the patient experiences these symptoms and what relieves them. The health care provider may prescribe a change in drug therapy or may prescribe a prophylactic dose of nitroglycerin to be taken before the patient resumes activities. Collaborate with the health care provider and appropriate therapists to determine whether activities need to be modified.

TABLE 6-2 Assessment of Patients in Rehabilitation Settings

BODY SYSTEM	RELEVANT DATA
Cardiovascular system	Chest pain Fatigue Fear of heart failure
Respiratory system	Shortness of breath or dyspnea Activity tolerance Fear of inability to breathe
Gastrointestinal system and nutrition	Oral intake, eating pattern Anorexia, nausea, and vomiting Dysphagia Laboratory data (e.g., serum prealbumin level) Weight loss or gain Bowel elimination pattern or habits Change in stool (constipation or diarrhea) Ability to get to toilet
Renal-urinary system	Urinary pattern Fluid intake Urinary incontinence or retention Urine culture and urinalysis
Neurologic system	Motor function Sensation Perceptual ability Cognitive abilities
Musculoskeletal system	Functional ability Range of motion Endurance Muscle strength
Integumentary system	Risk for skin breakdown Presence of skin lesions

For the patient showing fatigue, the nurse and patient plan methods for using limited energy resources. For instance, frequent rest periods can be taken throughout the day, especially before performing activities. Major tasks could be performed in the morning because most people have the most energy at that time.

A hindrance to rehabilitation for patients with cardiac disorders is fear, particularly for older adults. These patients may have survived a life-threatening experience (e.g., myocardial infarction) and may be so afraid of recurrence or death that they are unable or unwilling to resume any activity. They usually benefit from participation in a structured cardiac rehabilitation program. (See Chapter 38 for a complete description of cardiac rehabilitation.)

Ask the patient whether he or she has shortness of breath, chest pain, or severe weakness and fatigue during or after activity. *Determine the level of activity that can be accomplished without these symptoms.* For example, can the patient climb one flight of stairs without shortness of breath or does shortness of breath occur after climbing only two steps?

Gastrointestinal and Nutritional Assessment. Monitor the patient's oral intake and pattern of eating. Also, assess for the presence of anorexia, **dysphagia**, nausea, vomiting, or discomfort that may interfere with oral intake. Determine whether the patient wears dentures and, if so, whether they fit. Review the patient's height, weight, hemoglobin and hematocrit levels, serum prealbumin, and blood glucose levels. (See Chapter 60 for discussion of how to perform a screening for NUTRITION status.) Weight loss or weight gain is particularly significant and may be related to an associated disease or to the illness that caused the disability.

Bowel ELIMINATION habits vary from person to person. They are often related to daily job or activity schedules, dietary patterns, age, and family or cultural background. Elimination habits may be difficult to assess, because many nurses are hesitant to request (and many patients are afraid to volunteer) information pertaining to elimination. Ask about usual bowel patterns before the injury or the illness.

Note any changes in the patient's bowel routine or stool consistency. The most common problem for rehabilitation patients is constipation. In their classic best practice guidelines, the Association of Rehabilitation Nurses (ARN) (2002) defines **constipation** as the passage of hard, dry stool fewer than 3 times a week or significant change in the patient's usual habits for more than 3 months. Examples of significant changes include abdominal fullness and bloating and straining when having a bowel movement.

If the patient reports any alteration in ELIMINATION pattern, try to determine whether it is due to a change in diet, activity pattern, or medication use. Always assess bowel habits on what is normal for that person.

Ask whether the patient can manage bowel function independently. Independence in bowel elimination requires COGNITION, manual dexterity, sensation, muscle control, and MOBILITY. If the patient requires help, determine whether someone is available at home to provide the assistance. Also assess the patient's and family's ability to cope with any dependency in bowel elimination.

Renal and Urinary Assessment. Ask about the patient's baseline urinary ELIMINATION patterns, including the number of times he or she usually voids. Determine whether he or she routinely awakens during the night to empty the bladder (**nocturia**) or sleeps through the night. Record fluid intake patterns and volume, including the type of fluids ingested and the time they were consumed.

Question whether the patient has ever had any problems with urinary incontinence or retention. Also, monitor laboratory reports, especially the results of the urinalysis and culture and sensitivity, if needed. *Urinary tract infections (UTIs) among older adults are often missed because acute confusion may be the only indicator of the infection.* Many health care professionals expect older patients to be confused and may not detect this problem. If untreated, UTIs can lead to kidney infection and possible failure.

Neurologic and Musculoskeletal Assessment. The neurologic assessment includes motor function (MOBILITY), sensation, and COGNITION. Assess the patient's pre-existing problems, general physical condition, and communication abilities. Patients may have **dysphasia** (slurred speech) because of facial muscle weakness or may have **aphasia** (inability to speak or comprehend), usually the result of a cerebral stroke or traumatic brain injury (TBI). These communication problems are discussed in detail in the chapters on problems of the nervous system.

Determine if the patient has **paresis** (weakness) or **paralysis** (absence of movement). Observe the patient's gait. Identify sensory-perceptual changes, such as visual acuity, that could contribute to the patient's risk for injury. Assess his or her response to light touch, hot or cold temperature, and position change in each extremity and on the trunk. Identify levels of decreased sensation. For a perceptual assessment, the nurse evaluates the patient's ability to receive and understand what is heard and seen and the ability to express appropriate motor and verbal responses. During this portion of the assessment, begin to assess short-term and long-term memory.

Assess the patient's cognitive abilities, especially if there is a head injury or stroke. Several tools are available to evaluate COGNITION. One of the most commonly used tools in rehabilitation and long-term care settings is the Brief Interview for Mental Status (BIMS), which is described in detail in Chapter 41. The Confusion Assessment Method (CAM) is used to determine if the patient had delirium, an acute confusional state. (See Table 2-3 in Chapter 2 for description of the CAM tool.)

As with other body systems, nursing assessment of the musculoskeletal system focuses on function. Assess the patient's musculoskeletal status, response to the impairment, and demands of the home, work, or school environment. Determine the patient's endurance level, and measure active and passive joint range of motion (ROM). Review the results of manual muscle testing by physical therapy, which identifies the patient's ROM and resistance against gravity. In this procedure, the therapist determines the degree of muscle strength present in each body segment.

Skin Assessment. Identify actual or potential interruptions in skin and TISSUE INTEGRITY. To maintain healthy skin, the body must have adequate food, water, and oxygen intake; intact waste-removal mechanisms; sensation; and functional MOBILITY. Changes in any of these variables can lead to rapid and extensive skin breakdown. If the patient cannot protect or maintain the skin, assess and plan for his or her needs.

! NURSING SAFETY PRIORITY (QSEN)

Action Alert

Be sure to remind unlicensed assistive personnel to report changes in the patient's skin promptly, including any new onset of redness. Assess the patient frequently to determine the risk for skin breakdown before it occurs! Older adults are at a very high risk for heel and sacral pressure ulcers, which can occur within 24 hours after admission.

Most rehabilitation settings use special skin assessment tools to identify patients at risk for skin breakdown. For example, the classic Braden Scale for Predicting Pressure Ulcer Risk (see Chapter 25) assesses several areas: sensory perception, skin moisture, activity level, nutritional status, and potential for friction and shear.

Other skin risk assessment tools are available. Some tools also include additional indicators of nutritional status, such as the serum prealbumin. When these levels are low, the patient is at high risk for pressure ulcers. Some tools include incontinence and altered mental state as risk factors.

If a pressure ulcer or other change in skin integrity develops, accurately assess the problem and its possible causes. Inspect the skin every 2 hours until the patient learns to inspect his or her own skin several times a day. Measure the depth and diameter of any open skin areas in inches or centimeters, depending on the policy of the facility. Assess the area around the open lesion to determine the presence of cellulitis or other tissue damage. Chapter 25 includes several widely used classification systems for assessing skin breakdown. Determine the patient's knowledge about the cause and treatment of skin breakdown, as well as his or her ability to inspect the skin and participate in maintaining TISSUE INTEGRITY.

In most health care agencies, the skin assessment is documented on a special form or part of the electronic health record to keep track of each area of skin breakdown. A baseline assessment is conducted on admission to the agency and updated periodically depending on the agency's policy and the nurse's judgment. In most long-term care, acute care, and rehabilitation settings and with the patient's (or family's if the patient cannot communicate) permission, photographs of the skin are taken on admission and at various intervals for documentation.

? NCLEX EXAMINATION CHALLENGE

Physiological Integrity

An older adult is admitted for rehabilitation after a total hip replacement. Which statement by the nursing assistant will require follow-up by the nurse?

A. "The client has an abduction pillow between her legs."
B. "The client reports being tired after her physical therapy session."
C. "The client is resting in bed after she had her pain pill."
D. "The client's sacrum is reddened and uncomfortable."

Functional Assessment. *Functional ability* refers to the ability to perform **activities of daily living (ADLs)**, such as bathing, dressing, feeding, and ambulating, and **independent living skills**, including using the telephone, shopping, preparing food, and housekeeping. These latter skills are sometimes referred to as **instrumental activities of daily living (IADLs)**. Functional assessment tools are used to assess a patient's abilities. Rehabilitation nurses, physiatrists, or rehabilitation therapists complete one or more of these assessment tools based on the patient's abilities and the policy of the health care setting.

One classic uniform data system still used for outcome data collection across the United States is the Functional Independence Measure (FIM) developed by Granger and Gresham (1984). As a basic indicator of the severity of a disability, the FIM attempts to quantify what the person actually does, whatever the diagnosis or impairment. It does not measure what a person should do or how the person would perform under a different set of circumstances. To eliminate the bias of a particular discipline, the assessment may be performed by trained clinicians. The entire assessment may be performed by one person, or certain categories may be completed by various professionals.

Categories for assessment are self-care, sphincter control, MOBILITY and locomotion, communication, and COGNITION. Scoring is done with numbers that use predetermined criteria for measurement. The patient is evaluated when he or she is admitted to and discharged from a rehabilitation institution and at other specified times to determine progress. The FIM system has also been adapted for use in other health care settings, including acute care and home care, and is available in multiple languages.

In U.S. long-term care settings, the interdisciplinary **Minimum Data Set (MDS) 3.0** is required by the U.S. Centers for Medicare and Medicaid (CMS) to assess patients (residents) in nursing homes. The resident's MOBILITY, sensation, and COGNITION are evaluated, as well as the overall health status. A list

TABLE 6-3 Assessment Components of the Minimum Data Set (MDS) 3.0

• Hearing, Speech and Vision	• Swallowing and Nutritional Status
• Cognitive Patterns	• Oral/Dental Status
• Mood	• Skin Condition
• Behavior	• Medications
• Preferences for Customary Routines and Activities	• Special Treatments and Procedures
• Functional Status	• Restraints
• Bowel and Bladder	• Participation in Assessment and Goal Setting
• Active Disease Diagnoses	• Supplemental Therapies
• Health Conditions (e.g., pain, fall history)	

Data from Centers for Medicare and Medicaid Services (CMS). MDS 3.0 for nursing homes and swing bed providers, 2013. Retrieved September 2014 from http://www.cms.gov/Medicare/Quality-Initiatives-Patient-Assessment-Instruments/NursingHomeQualityInits/NHQIMDS30.html.

of assessment components for the MDS 3.0 is presented in Table 6-3. Similar to the FIM, all health care team members involved in the resident's care record their assessments on the MDS and the RN coordinates the comprehensive assessment.

Psychosocial Assessment. In addition to determining cognitive function, assess the patient's body image and self-esteem through verbal indicators and descriptions of self-care. Encourage the family to allow the patient to perform as many functions as possible independently to build feelings of self-worth.

Assess the patient's use of defense mechanisms and manifestations of anxiety. To assess the patient's response to loss, ask him or her to describe feelings concerning the loss of a body part or function. Assess for the presence of any stress-related physical problem. Some patients have symptoms of depression, such as fatigue, a change in appetite, or feelings of powerlessness. See Chapter 7 for a thorough discussion of loss and grieving and Chapter 2 for a brief description of depression among the older adult population.

Determine the availability of support systems for the patient. The major support system is typically the family or significant others. Patients who do not have these support systems are more likely to develop depression. Identify the patient's spiritual and/or religious needs, and refer to an appropriate health care team member as needed. Assess sexuality and intimacy needs, and document findings in the electronic health record (EHR).

Vocational Assessment. To assist patients in maximizing functional status, encourage them to resume usual activities. Vocational counselors can help patients find meaningful training, education, or employment after discharge from the rehabilitation setting, if needed.

Patients in the United States should be informed about the Americans with Disabilities Act, which was passed by Congress in 1991 to prevent employer discrimination against disabled people. The employer must offer *reasonable* assistance to a disabled employee to allow him or her to perform the job. For example, if an employee has a severe hearing loss, the employer may need to hire an interpreter for sign language. Workers have a right to ask for special adaptations based on their disabilities.

The rehabilitation team assesses the cognitive and physical demands of the patient's job to determine whether he or she can return to the former job or whether retraining in another field is necessary. The physical demands of jobs range from light in sedentary occupations (0 to 10 lbs often lifted) to heavy (more than 100 lbs often lifted). The nurse must also consider other aspects of the job, such as mobility or senses required (e.g., hearing).

Job analysis also involves assessing the work environment of the patient's former job. Collaborate with the vocational counselor to determine whether the environment is conducive to the patient's return. Job modifications may be needed to accommodate the patient at work. If an injured worker requires vocational rehabilitation, refer him or her to vocational rehabilitation personnel to evaluate present skills and learn new skills for employment if needed. In most states, Workers' Compensation insurance helps support vocational rehabilitation.

◆ Analysis

Regardless of age or specific disability, these priority patient problems are common. Additional problems depend on the patient's specific chronic illness or disability. The priority NANDA-I nursing diagnoses and collaborative problems for patients with chronic and disabling health problems include:

1. Impaired Physical Mobility related to neuromuscular impairment, sensory-perceptual impairment, and/or chronic pain (NANDA-I)
2. Decreased functional ability related to neuromuscular impairment and/or impairment in perception or cognition
3. Risk for Impaired Skin Integrity related to altered sensation and/or altered nutritional state (NANDA-I)
4. Urinary incontinence or Urinary Retention related to neurologic dysfunction and/or trauma or disease affecting spinal cord nerves (NANDA-I)
5. Constipation related to neurologic impairment, inadequate nutrition, or decreased mobility (NANDA-I)

◆ Planning and Implementation

Improving Physical Mobility

Planning: Expected Outcomes. The patient with chronic illness or disability is expected to reach a level of physical MOBILITY that allows him or her to function independently with or without assistive devices. In addition, the patient is expected to be free of complications of immobility.

Interventions. Most problems requiring rehabilitation relate to decreased physical MOBILITY. For example, patients with neurologic disease or injury, amputations, arthritis, and cardiopulmonary disease usually experience some degree of immobility. Coordinate care with physical and occupational therapists as the key rehabilitation team members in helping patients meet their mobility outcomes. Patients initially spend 5 to 6 hours a day for at least 5 days a week in rehabilitation therapy departments to regain MOBILITY and self-management skills.

Safe Patient Handling Practices. Before they learn to become independent, patients with decreased MOBILITY in any health care setting or at home often need assistance with positioning in bed and transfers, such as from a bed to a chair, commode, or wheelchair. Patients may not be able to bear full weight, may have inadequate balance, and/or may be very obese. For many years, nurses relied on "body mechanics" to prevent staff injury when moving patients or assisting them to move. This traditional, but outdated, approach was based on the belief that correct body positioning by staff members would protect them from the force of lifting and moving. For example, if the patient could not bear weight or did not have sufficient balance (e.g., quadriplegic spinal cord injury), nurses and therapists used a "bear hug" technique to lift the patient from bed to chair or back again. Obese patients were also lifted with multiple staff assistance.

Heavy lifting and dependent transfers by staff members have resulted in a very high incidence of **work-related musculoskeletal disorders (MSDs)**, most often chronic back injuries, which can be prevented. As a response to this costly problem, the National Institute for Occupational Safety and Health (NIOSH) established evidence-based guidelines for safe patient handling. Based on this document, the American Nurses Association, in partnership with NIOSH and the Veterans Health Administration, developed a curriculum for all nursing students and practicing nurses on how to safely handle and move patients in any health care setting or home environment (American Nurses Association, 2012). In collaboration with other health care team members, nurses assess patient MOBILITY and use best practices for safe patient handling (SPH).

Because each patient has unique needs and characteristics, assess the patient's MOBILITY level using a standardized tool to plan interventions for SPH. An example of an appropriate assessment tool for this purpose is shown in Fig. 6-4. Before moving the patient, assess his or her environment for potential hazards that could cause injury, such as a slippery or uneven floor.

Use these general SPH practices, and teach to staff members:

- Maintain a wide, stable base with your feet.
- Put the bed at the correct height—waist level while providing direct care and hip level when moving patients.
- Try to keep the patient or work directly in front of you to prevent your spine from rotating.
- Keep the patient as close to your body as possible to prevent reaching.

The Veterans Health Administration and many other health care systems follow a no-lift or limited-lift policy for all of their facilities due in large part to technology. That means that nurses and therapists either rely on the patient to independently move and transfer or use a powered, mechanical full-body lift that is either ceiling- or wall-mounted or portable (mobile) (Fig. 6-5). Most lifts use slings that are comfortable, safe, and easy to apply. Electric-powered, portable sit-to-stand devices are also available.

Instead of a no-lift policy, though, some long-term care facilities limit lifting to 35 pounds (15.9 kg). These changes involve intensive staff training and compliance to prevent staff injury. Mechanical lifts are also available for home use.

For patients who are learning to become independent in transfer or bed MOBILITY skills, the physical or occupational therapist usually specifies the procedure for these maneuvers. For example, a quadriplegic patient may use a sliding board for transfer, whereas a paraplegic patient may need a wheelchair with removable arms. A patient still in bed may be taught to turn independently using the siderails. In any case, for safety, always plan or teach the patient to plan the transfer technique before initiating it. The desired outcome is that the patient will eventually be able to transfer independently *and* safely.

If the patient has problems maintaining blood pressure while out of bed, the physical therapist may start him or her on a tilt table to gradually increase tolerance. A low blood pressure is a particularly common problem for patients who are quadriplegic because they have a delayed blood flow to the brain and upper part of the body.

! NURSING SAFETY PRIORITY (QSEN)

Critical Rescue

Before any transfer, carefully observe for potential problems. Orthostatic, or postural, hypotension is a common problem in rehabilitation settings and contributes to falls, which are common for any patient with impaired mobility. If the patient moves from a lying to a sitting or standing position too quickly, his or her blood pressure drops; as a result, he or she becomes dizzy or faints. This problem is worsened by antihypertensive drugs, especially in older adults. To prevent this situation, help the patient change positions slowly, with frequent rest periods to allow the blood pressure to stabilize. If needed, measure blood pressure with the patient in the lying, sitting, and standing positions to examine the differences. **Orthostatic hypotension** is indicated by a drop of more than 20 mm Hg in systolic pressure or 10 mm Hg in diastolic pressure between positions. Notify the health care provider and the therapists about this change.

Weight gain is another potential problem when rehabilitation patients have impaired MOBILITY. Excessive weight hinders transfers both for the nurse or the therapist who is assisting and for the patient who is learning to transfer independently. Weight is usually checked every week to monitor gains or losses. If needed, collaborate with the dietitian to plan a weight-reduction diet for the patient.

Gait Training. The physical therapist works with patients for gait training if they are able to ambulate. While regaining the ability to ambulate, patients may need to use assistive devices, such as a variety of canes or walkers (Fig. 6-6). The specific device selected for each patient depends on the amount of weight bearing that is allowed or tolerated. For example, a stroke patient who has problems with maintaining balance or a steady gait when walking might need a walker. Some patients use walkers with rollers made of tennis ball materials; others who fatigue easily may need a walker with a built-in seat to rest at intervals. A patient who had a total hip replacement 6 weeks ago may be able to use a straight (also called *single-point*) cane.

When working with patients who are using these devices, also known as **ambulatory aids**, the physical therapist ensures that there is a level surface on which to walk. The patient wears a transfer (gait) belt for safety so that the therapist or nurse can guide him or her during ambulation to help prevent falls. Use of transfer belts is recommended as one of the best practices for safe patient handling (Waters & Rockefeller, 2010).

Reinforce the physical therapist's instructions and encourage practice, with the outcome being to walk independently with or without an assistive device. Older patients typically use a walker, with or without rollers, for a broader base of support. Younger or minimally impaired patients often progress to the use of a hemi-cane or straight cane. Chart 6-1 outlines best practices for patient safety when teaching patients how to use ambulatory aids.

Some patients never regain the ability to walk because of their impairment, such as advanced multiple sclerosis or complete high spinal cord injury. They may become wheelchair dependent and need to learn wheelchair or motorized scooter mobility skills. With the help of physical and occupational therapy, most patients can learn to move anywhere in a wheelchair or scooter. For example, quadriplegic patients often use motorized wheelchairs that can be directed and propelled by moving their head or blowing into a device. Patients with multiple sclerosis often use scooters to get around.

Assessment Tool and Care Plan for Safe Patient Handling and Movement

I. Patient's Level of Assistance

____Independent—Patient performs task safely, with or without staff assistance, with or without assistive devices.
____Partial Assist—Patient requires no more help than standby, cueing, or coaxing, or caregiver is required to lift no more than 35 lbs of a patient's weight.
____Dependent—Patient requires nurse to lift more than 35 lbs of the patient's weight, or patient is unpredictable in the amount of assistance offered. In this case, assistive devices should be used.

An assessment should be made before each task if the patient has a varying level of ability to assist because of medical reasons, fatigue, medications, etc. When in doubt, assume the patient cannot assist with the transfer/repositioning.

II. Weight-Bearing Capability

____Full
____Partial
____None

III. Bilateral Upper-Extremity Strength

____Yes
____No

IV. Patient's Level of Cooperation and Comprehension

____Cooperative—May need prompting; able to follow simple commands.
____Unpredictable or variable (patient whose behavior changes frequently should be considered unpredictable)—Not cooperative or unable to follow simple commands.

V. Weight________ **Height** ________

Body Mass Index (BMI) (needed if patient's weight is over 300 lbs)*
If BMI exceeds 50, institute Bariatric Algorithms.

The presence of the following conditions is likely to affect the transfer/repositioning process and should be considered when identifying equipment and techniques needed to move the patient.

VI. Check Applicable Conditions Likely to Affect Transfer/Repositioning Techniques

____Hip/knee/shoulder replacements	____Respiratory/cardiac compromise	____Fractures
____History of falls	____Wounds affecting transfer/positioning	____Splints/traction
____Paralysis/paresis	____Amputation	____Severe osteoporosis
____Unstable spine	____Urinary/fecal stoma	____Severe pain/discomfort
____Severe edema	____Contractures/spasms	____Postural hypotension
____Very fragile skin	____Tubes (IV, chest, etc.)	

Comments: ____

____

____

____

____

____

VII. Appropriate Lift/Transfer Devices Needed

Vertical Lift:
Horizontal Lift:
Other Patient-Handling Devices Needed:

Sling Type

____Seated	____Seated (Amputee)	____Standing
____Supine	____Ambulation	____Limb Support

Sling Size ________

Signature ______________________ **Date** ______________________

*If patient weighs more than 300 lbs, the BMI is needed. For online BMI table and calculator, see http://www.nhlbi.nih.gov/guidelines/obesity/bmi_tbl.htm.

FIG. 6-4 Example of a tool to assess physical mobility.

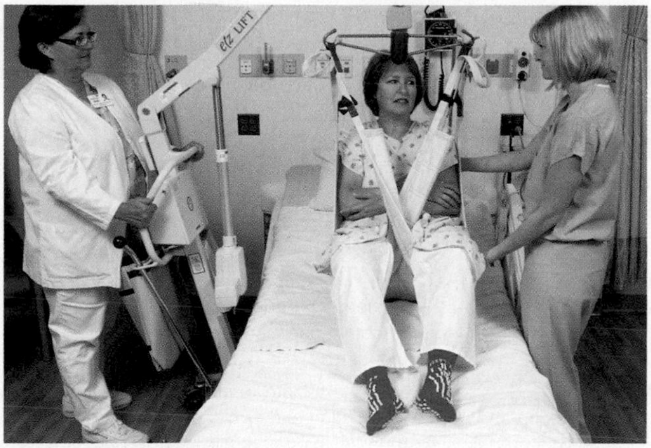

FIG. 6-5 Example of powered, mechanical full-body lift.

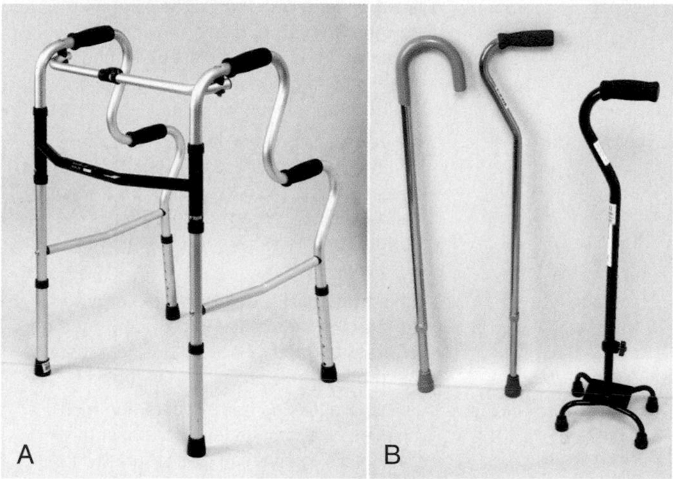

FIG. 6-6 Assistive devices for ambulation. Assistive devices vary in the amount of support they provide. A straight (single-point) cane provides less support than a walker **(A)** or quadripod cane **(B)**.

CHART 6-1 Best Practice for Patient Safety & Quality Care QSEN

Gait Training with Selected Ambulatory Aids

Walker Assisted

- Apply a transfer belt around the patient's waist.
- Guide the patient to a standing position.
- Remind the patient to place both hands on the walker.
- Ensure that the patient is well balanced.
- Teach the patient repeatedly to perform this sequence:
  - Lift the walker.
  - Move the walker about 2 feet forward, and set it down on all legs.
  - While resting on the walker, take small steps.
  - Check balance.
  - Repeat the sequence.

Cane Assisted

- Apply a transfer belt around the patient's waist.
- Guide the patient to a standing position.
- Be sure the cane is at the height of the patient's wrist when the arm is placed at his or her side. (Many canes can be adjusted to the required height.)
- Remind the patient to place his or her strong hand on the cane.
- Ensure that the patient is well balanced.
- Teach the patient to perform this sequence repeatedly:
  - Move the cane and weaker leg forward at the same time.
  - Move the stronger leg one step forward.
  - Check balance and repeat the sequence.

During the rehabilitation phase, patients are at risk for complications of immobility. Table 6-4 lists some of the common complications and strategies the nurse can use to help prevent each complication. Implementing range-of-motion (ROM) routines, adhering to schedules for turning and repositioning, and maintaining skin care are constant components of rehabilitation nursing care to prevent complications of immobility.

One way to increase MOBILITY, even with patients who are bedridden, is through ROM exercises. ROM techniques are beneficial for any patient with decreased mobility. Although simple ROM techniques are presented in basic nursing textbooks, a few key principles are pertinent to rehabilitation nursing care:

- The human body contains more joints than simply the knees, hips, elbows, and shoulders. For ROM techniques

TABLE 6-4 Prevention of the Common Complications of Immobility

BODY SYSTEM	COMPLICATIONS	PREVENTION
Musculoskeletal	Contractures Footdrop Osteoporosis Susceptibility to fractures Muscular atrophy	Foot support while in bed, range-of-motion exercises, high-top tennis shoes Ambulation if possible (walking) Other weight-bearing exercises
Gastrointestinal	Constipation	Sitting in an upright position Increased activity level Increased fluid and fiber intake
Cardiovascular	Decreased cardiac output Increased venous stasis Thrombus formation Embolism	Range-of-motion exercises Exercise Antiembolism stockings Avoidance of leg massage Low–molecular-weight heparin or other anticoagulant
Neurologic	Disorientation	Sleep-wake schedule in accord with light-dark pattern Reorientation (to person, place, time) Control of sensory stimulation
Renal/urinary	Calculi	Decreased dietary calcium level, if needed Increased fluid intake Ensuring low post-void residuals
	Infection	Intermittent catheterization instead of indwelling if possible
Respiratory	Pneumonia	Frequent oral hygiene Frequent repositioning in wheelchair or bed Breathing exercises
Integumentary (Skin)	Pressure ulcers	Frequent repositioning in wheelchair or bed Pressure reduction or relief devices (in bed and wheelchair) Meticulous skin care Adequate nutrition Frequent skin assessments

to be effective in preventing musculoskeletal contractures, the patient must exercise all joints, including each joint of the fingers, hands, toes, and so forth.
- In performing ROM activities, the nurse or patient performs full-range movement of each joint at least five times and completes the entire process at least three times daily.
- The nurse or PT does not move the joints beyond the point at which the patient expresses pain or beyond the point at which resistance occurs.

Patients with decreased MOBILITY who are able to follow directions are taught by the nurse and the physical therapist to perform active or active-assisted ROM exercises.

Increasing Functional Ability

Planning: Expected Outcomes. The patient with chronic illness or disability is expected to increase functional ability in self-care and other self-management skills with or without assistive/adaptive devices.

Interventions. ADLs, or self-care activities, include eating, bathing, dressing, grooming, and toileting. Encourage the patient to perform as much self-care as possible. Be patient because he or she often takes more time to complete a task than healthy adults do. Collaborate with the occupational therapist (OT) to identify ways in which self-care activities can be modified so the patient can perform them independently and with minimal frustration if possible. For example, the OT teaches a hemiplegic patient to put on a shirt by first placing the affected arm in the sleeve and then putting the unaffected arm in the appropriate sleeve. Slip-on shoes or shoes with Velcro straps may be recommended for some patients. Encourage patients to practice, and allow them time to try to be independent in ADLs.

In long-term care (LTC) settings, federal regulations require that residents not lose their functional skills while they are in the facility. Therefore most facilities have developed *restorative nursing* programs and have coordinated these programs with rehabilitation therapy and activity therapy. The focus of this coordinated effort includes:
- Bed mobility
- Walking
- Transfers
- Dressing
- Grooming
- Active range of motion
- Communication

A variety of devices are available for patients with chronic illness and disability for *assisting with self-care*. An **assistive/adaptive device**, or self-care support device, is any item that enables the patient to perform all or part of an activity independently and safely. Examples include long-handled shoehorns and reachers to prevent bending and losing one's balance. Table 6-5 identifies common devices and describes their use.

Many medical equipment stores and large pharmacies carry clothing and assistive/adaptive devices designed for patients with disabilities. The occupational therapist determines specific patient needs for this equipment. Collaborate with the occupational therapist to look for creative and inexpensive alternatives to meeting these needs. For example, barbecue tongs may be used as "reachers" for pulling up pants or obtaining items on high shelves. A foam curler with the plastic insert removed may be placed over a pencil or eating utensil to make a built-up device. The patient might use an extended shoehorn to operate light switches from wheelchair height. Hook-and-loop fasteners (Velcro) sewn on clothes can prevent the frustrations caused by buttons and zippers.

TABLE 6-5 Examples and Uses of Common Assistive/Adaptive Devices

DEVICE	USE
Buttonhook	Threaded through the buttonhole to enable patients with weak finger mobility to button shirts Alternative uses include serving as pencil holder or cigarette holder
Extended shoehorn	Assists in the application of shoes for patients with decreased mobility Alternative uses include turning light switches off or on while patient is in a wheelchair
Plate guard and spork (spoon and fork in one utensil)	Applied to a plate to assist patients with weak hand and arm mobility to feed themselves; spork allows one utensil to serve two purposes
Gel pad	Placed under a plate or a glass to prevent dishes from slipping and moving Alternative uses include placement under bathing and grooming items to prevent them from moving
Foam buildups	Applied to eating utensils to assist patients with weak hand grasps to feed themselves Alternative uses include application to pens and pencils to assist with writing or over a buttonhook to assist with grasping the device
Hook and loop fastener (Velcro) straps	Applied to utensils, a buttonhook, or a pencil to slip over the hand and provide a method of stabilizing the device when the patient's hand grasp is weak
Long-handled reacher	Assists in obtaining items located on high shelves or at ground level for patients who are unable to change positions easily
Elastic shoelaces or Velcro shoe closure	Eliminates the need for tying shoes

Assistive technology has further increased the ability for disabled patients to care for themselves using electronic equipment. For example, telephones and computer keyboards can be operated by voice-activation devices. **Robotic technology** provides mechanical parts for the extremities when they are not functional or have been amputated. The cost of these aids has prevented their widespread use (Stein, 2012).

Fatigue often occurs with chronic and disabling conditions. Therefore collaborate with the OT to assess the patient's self-care abilities and to determine possible ways of *conserving energy*. Coordinate with the therapist to develop strategies for energy conservation after evaluating the patient's self-care routines. Preparation for ADLs can help reduce effort and energy expenditure (e.g., gathering all necessary equipment before starting grooming routines). If a patient has high energy levels in the morning, he or she can be taught to schedule energy-intensive activities in the morning rather than later in the day or evening. Spacing activities is also helpful for conserving energy. In addition, allowing time to rest before and after eating and toileting decreases the strain on energy level.

CLINICAL JUDGMENT CHALLENGE

Evidence-Based Practice; Safety QSEN

A 61-year-old widower is admitted to an inpatient facility for rehabilitation after a right knee replacement for severe osteoarthritis that resulted from his carpentry job. He lives alone in a one-story house and has two daughters nearby who visit every week. After his wife died 10 years ago, the patient was diagnosed with diabetes mellitus type 2 and hypertension. His serum cholesterol is elevated, and he is overweight. His favorite foods are fried chicken, mashed potatoes and gravy, and homemade buttermilk biscuits, which his daughters frequently prepare for him. As his nurse, you complete his admission assessment.

1. What are this patient's priority problems?
2. With what health care team members will you need to collaborate?
3. What safe patient handling practices would you need to use?
4. What type of ambulatory assistive device would be most appropriate for him at this time?
5. What health teaching does the patient need regarding his mobility and nutrition?

Maintaining Skin Integrity

Planning: Expected Outcomes. The patient with chronic illness or disability is expected to have intact skin and TISSUE INTEGRITY.

Interventions. *The best intervention to prevent skin breakdown and maintain tissue integrity is frequent position changes in combination with adequate skin care and sufficient nutritional intake.* Teach staff to *turn and reposition all patients at least every 2 hours* if they are unable to perform this activity. This time frame may not be sufficient for people who are frail and have thin skin, especially older adults. To determine the best turning schedule, assess the patient's skin condition during each turning and repositioning. For example, if the patient has been sleeping for 2 hours and the nursing assistant decides to postpone turning for 1 hour, reddened areas over the bony prominences may be present. If reddened areas do not fade within 30 minutes after pressure relief or do not blanch, they may be classified as pre-ulcer areas, or stage I pressure areas (see Chapter 25).

Patients who sit for prolonged periods in a wheelchair need to be repositioned at least every 1 to 2 hours. Each patient is evaluated by the physical or occupational therapist for the best seating pad or cushion that is comfortable yet reduces pressure on bony prominences. Patients who are able are taught to perform "wheelchair push-ups" by using their arms to lift their buttocks off the wheelchair seat for 10 seconds or longer every hour, or more often if needed. The PT helps them strengthen their arm muscles in preparation for performing wheelchair push-ups.

If the patient wears high-top tennis shoes for foot positioning to prevent footdrop, remove the shoes and assess for pressure areas every 2 hours. Many patients with neurologic problems have decreased or absent sensation and may not be able to feel the discomfort of increased pressure. Also, check patients who are sitting in wheelchairs for signs of pressure, especially on the lower legs where the leg of the wheelchair could rub against the skin.

Adequate skin care is an essential component of prevention. Perform or assist patients in completing skin care each time they are turned, repositioned, or bathed. Delegate and supervise skin care to unlicensed assistive personnel (UAP), including cleaning soiled areas, drying carefully, and applying a moisturizer. If a patient is incontinent, use topical barrier creams or ointments to help protect the skin from moisture, which can contribute to skin breakdown. *To prevent damage to the already fragile capillary system, teach UAP to avoid rubbing reddened areas.* Instead, carefully observe the areas for further breakdown and relieve pressure on the areas as much as possible. Bed pillows are often good pressure-relieving devices. (See Chapter 25 for a complete discussion of skin care interventions.)

Sufficient NUTRITION is needed both to repair wounds and to prevent pressure ulcers. Collaborate with the dietitian to assess the patient's food selection and ensure that it contains adequate protein and carbohydrates. Both the nurse and the dietitian closely monitor the patient's weight and serum prealbumin levels. If either of these indices decreases significantly, the patient may need high-protein, high-carbohydrate food supplements (e.g., milkshakes) or commercial preparations. Chapter 60 describes nutritional supplementation in detail.

Pressure-relieving or pressure-reducing devices include waterbeds, gel mattresses or pads, air mattresses, low–air loss overlays or beds, and air-fluidized beds. Mattress overlays, such as air and gel types, and replacement mattresses are often effective in reducing pressure. *The use of any mechanical device (except air-fluidized beds) does not eliminate the need for turning and repositioning.*

Specialty beds are categorized as either "low air loss" or "air fluidized." Air-fluidized therapy (e.g., Clinitron Rite Hite® bed) provides the most effective pressure relief by distributing the patient's weight to prevent pressure in any one area. These beds are not often used to *prevent* skin breakdown because insurers may not reimburse the agency for the use of the bed. Therefore these special beds are reserved for *severe skin problems* that have not healed with the use of a conventional bed or other mechanical device. The primary disadvantage of this therapy is its expense, which may exceed several hundred dollars for each day of use. Patients also report discomfort from the heat generated by the bed. Although air-fluidized beds are heavy to move, lighter and more portable versions are available for home use. The cost of air-fluidized therapy is reimbursed by some health insurance providers if the bed is deemed medically necessary to treat the patient's skin problem.

Establishing Urinary Continence

Planning: Expected Outcomes. Most patients with chronic illness or disability are expected to have normal patterns of urinary ELIMINATION without retention, infection, or incontinence.

Interventions. Neurologic disabilities often interfere with successful bladder control in a patient undergoing rehabilitation. These disabilities result in two basic functional types of neurogenic bladder: overactive (e.g., reflex or spastic bladder) and underactive (e.g., hypotonic or flaccid bladder).

An overactive **spastic** (upper motor neuron) **bladder** causes incontinence with sudden, gushing voids. The bladder does not usually empty completely, and the patient is at risk for urinary tract infection. Neurologic problems affecting the upper motor neuron typically occur in patients with strokes or with high-level spinal cord injuries (cervical) or those above the mid-thoracic region. These injuries result in a failure of impulse transmission from the lower spinal cord areas to the cortex of the brain. Therefore when the bladder fills and transmits impulses to the spinal cord, the patient cannot perceive the sensation. Because there is no injury to the *lower* spinal cord and the voiding reflex arc is intact, the efferent (motor) impulse from a distended bladder is relayed and the bladder contracts.

Experimental technology using sacral neuromodulation is being tested with complete spinal cord–injury patients. The results have been positive in preventing urinary incontinence in patients with spastic bladders (Sievert et al., 2010).

Nonpharmacologic Management. An underactive **flaccid** or **areflexic** (lower motor neuron) **bladder** results in urinary retention and overflow (dribbling). Injuries that damage the lower motor neuron at the spinal cord level of S2-4 (e.g., multiple sclerosis, spinal cord injury or tumor below T12) may directly interfere with the reflex arc or may result in inaccurate interpretation of impulses to the brain. The bladder fills, and afferent (sensory) impulses conduct the message via the spinal cord to the brain cortex. Because of the injury, the impulse is not interpreted correctly by the brain's bladder center and there is a failure to respond with a message for the bladder to contract.

Patients who cannot completely empty their bladder are at risk for post-void residual urine and subsequent possible urinary tract infection. **Post-void residual (PVR)** is the amount of urine remaining in the bladder within 20 minutes after voiding. PVR assessments using a noninvasive ultrasound device called the *BladderScan* are performed by nurses at the bedside. The residual amount measured is accurate if the device is used correctly. It is not accurate when used for morbidly obese patients. The outcome of bladder ultrasonography is to prevent the use of an indwelling urinary catheter. Long-term urinary catheters cause urinary tract infections that are often chronic. A picture of the BladderScan device is in Chapter 65 (see Fig. 65-10).

The nurse can teach a variety of techniques to assist the patient in retraining or repatterning voiding, including (Table 6-6):

- Facilitating, or triggering, techniques
- Intermittent catheterization
- Consistent scheduling of toileting routines; "timed void"

These techniques may not be as effective in patients with physiologic changes associated with aging, including stress incontinence in women with weak pelvic floor muscles and overflow incontinence in men with enlarged prostate glands.

Facilitating (triggering) techniques are used to stimulate voiding. If there is an upper motor neuron problem but the reflex arc is intact (reflex bladder pattern), the voiding response can be initiated by any stimulus that sends the message to the spinal cord level S2-4 that the bladder might be full. Such techniques include stroking the medial aspect of the thigh, pinching the area above the groin, massaging the penoscrotal area, pinching the posterior aspect of the glans penis, and providing digital anal stimulation.

When the patient has a lower motor neuron problem, the voiding reflex arc is not intact (flaccid bladder pattern) and additional stimulation may be needed to initiate voiding. Two techniques used to facilitate voiding are the Valsalva maneuver and the Credé maneuver. For the Valsalva maneuver, teach the patient to hold his or her breath and bear down as if trying to defecate. This technique should not be used by spinal cord–injured patients who are at risk for bradycardia due to loss of vagus nerve control. Assist the patient in performing the **Credé maneuver** by placing the patient's hand in a cupped position directly over the bladder area and instructing him or her to push inward and downward gently as if massaging the bladder to empty.

Intermittent catheterization may be needed for a flaccid or spastic bladder. Initially, a urinary catheter is inserted to drain urine every few hours—after the patient has attempted voiding and has used the Valsalva and Credé maneuvers. If less than 100 to 150 mL of post-void residual is obtained, the nurse typically increases the interval between catheterizations. *The patient should not go beyond 8 hours between catheterizations.* If intermittent self-catheterization is needed at home after discharge from the rehabilitation facility, the patient may use a specialized appliance to help perform the procedure, especially if he or she has problems with manual dexterity. For patients who cannot catheterize themselves, a family member or significant other may need to be taught how to perform the procedure.

Most patients who need intermittent catheterization have chronic bacteriuria (bacteria in the urine with a positive culture), especially those with spinal cord injury (SCI). Unless the patient has symptoms of a urinary tract infection (UTI), such as fever or burning when voiding, the infection is not treated.

! NURSING SAFETY PRIORITY QSEN

Action Alert

To *prevent* UTI, teach patients and their caregivers to wash their hands thoroughly before and after catheterization and clean the genital area well. Remind the patient to drink at least 8 to 10 glasses of fluid (two quarts) every day by dinnertime and avoid carbonated beverages. If patients have indwelling urinary catheters, remind them to drink 15 glasses of fluid (three quarts) each day before dinner and avoid carbonated beverages.

TABLE 6-6 Management of Neurogenic Bladder

FUNCTIONAL TYPE	NEUROLOGIC DISABILITY	DYSFUNCTION	RE-ESTABLISHING VOIDING PATTERNS
Reflex (spastic)	Upper motor neuron spinal cord injury above T12	Urinary frequency, incontinence but may not empty completely	Triggering or facilitating techniques Drug therapy, as appropriate Bedside bladder ultrasound Intermittent catheterization Consistent toileting schedule Indwelling urinary catheter (as last resort) Increased fluids
Flaccid	Lower motor neuron spinal cord injury below T12 (affects S2-4 reflex arc)	Urinary retention, overflow	Valsalva and Credé maneuvers Increased fluids Intermittent or indwelling urinary catheterization

The Natural Medicines Comprehensive Database states that cranberry juice or extract may be effective to help *prevent* UTI (U.S. National Library of Medicine [NIH], 2011). It is not effective for *treating* urinary infection.

Consistent toileting routines may be the best way to re-establish voiding continence when the patient has an overactive bladder. Assess the patient's previous voiding pattern, and determine his or her daily routine. At a minimum, the nurse or nursing staff assists the patient with voiding after awakening in the morning, before and after meals, before and after physical activity, and at bedtime. *Remind the staff to toilet the patient every 2 hours during the day and every 3 to 4 hours at night.*

Consider the patient's bladder capacity, which may range from 100 to 500 mL, as well as MOBILITY limitations and restrictive clothing. Bladder capacity is determined by measuring urine output. Ensure that the patient is aware of nearby bathrooms at all times or has a call system to contact the nurse or unlicensed assistive personnel for assistance. Chapter 66 also describes methods of achieving bladder control.

Drug Therapy. Drugs are not commonly used for urinary ELIMINATION problems. Mild overactive bladder problems may be treated with antispasmodics, such as oxybutynin (Ditropan XL, Apo-Oxybutynin ♣), solifenacin (VESIcare), or tolterodine (Detrol LA), to prevent incontinence on a short-term basis.

CONSIDERATIONS FOR OLDER ADULTS

Patient-Centered Care QSEN

When urinary antispasmodic drugs are used in older adults, observe for, document, and report hallucinations, delirium, or other acute cognitive changes due to the anticholinergic effects of the drugs.

Patients with symptomatic UTIs are managed with short-term antibiotics, such as trimethoprim (Trimpex) or trimethoprim/sulfamethoxazole (Septra, Bactrim). Patients who have frequent UTIs may be placed on pulse antibiotic therapy in which they alternate one week of antibiotic therapy with 3 weeks without antibiotics. Report the patient's progress in bladder training to the rehabilitation team so that the best decision regarding drug therapy can be made.

Establishing Bowel Continence

Planning: Expected Outcomes. The patient with chronic illness or disability is expected to have regular evacuation of stool without constipation. If possible, patients will control their bowel ELIMINATION schedule.

Interventions. Neurologic problems often affect the patient's bowel pattern by causing a reflex (spastic) bowel, a flaccid bowel, or an uninhibited bowel. Bowel retraining programs are designed for each patient to best meet the expected outcomes (Table 6-7). Pardee et al. (2012) found that establishing a successful bowel program can also enhance the quality of life for patients, especially those who have a spinal cord injury (SCI).

Upper motor neuron diseases and injuries, such as a cervical or mid-level spinal cord injury, may result in a reflex (spastic) bowel pattern, with defecation occurring suddenly and without warning. With a reflex pattern, any facilitating or triggering mechanism may lead to defecation if the lower colon contains stool. An example of facilitating or triggering techniques is digital stimulation. For this technique, use a lubricated glove or finger cot and massage the anus in a circular motion for no less than 1 full minute.

! NURSING SAFETY PRIORITY QSEN

Critical Rescue

Do not use digital stimulation for patients with cardiac disease because of the risk for inducing a vagal nerve response. This response causes a rapid decrease in heart rate (bradycardia).

Lower motor neuron diseases and injuries interfere with transmission of the nervous impulse across the reflex arc and may result in a flaccid bowel pattern, with defecation occurring infrequently and in small amounts. The use of manual disimpaction may get the best results. Some patients also need oral laxatives and/or stool softeners (Coggrave & Norton, 2010) (see the Evidence-Based Practice box).

Neurologic injuries that affect the brain may cause an uninhibited bowel pattern, with frequent defecation, urgency, and reports of hard stool. Patients may manage uninhibited bowel patterns through a consistent toileting schedule, a high-fiber diet, and the use of stool softeners.

In some cases, patients are not able to regain their previous level of control over their bowel function. The rehabilitation team assists in designing a bowel ELIMINATION program that accommodates the disability.

TABLE 6-7 Management of Neurogenic Bowel

FUNCTIONAL TYPE	NEUROLOGIC DISABILITY	DYSFUNCTION	RE-ESTABLISHING DEFECATION PATTERNS
Reflex (spastic)	Upper motor neuron spinal cord injury above T12	Defecation without warning, but may not empty completely	Triggering mechanisms Facilitation techniques High-fiber diet Increased fluids Laxative use (for some patients) Consistent toileting schedule Manual disimpaction
Flaccid	Lower motor neuron spinal cord injury below T12 (affects S2-4 reflex arc)	Usually absent stools for patients with complete lesions	Triggering or facilitating techniques Increased fluids High-fiber diet Suppository use Consistent toileting schedule Manual disimpaction

EVIDENCE-BASED PRACTICE QSEN

Manual Bowel Disimpaction in Patients with Spinal Cord Injury

Coggrave, M.J., & Norton, C. (2010). The need for manual evacuation and oral laxatives in the management of neurogenic bowel dysfunction after spinal cord injury: A randomized controlled trial of a stepwise protocol. *Spinal Cord, 48*(6), 504-510.

The researchers used a randomized controlled design to test interventions needed to maintain bowel continence among patients who had spinal cord injuries for many years. The 68 volunteers were randomized into an intervention group of 35 and a control group of 33. The control group used their usual bowel management program. The intervention group used oral laxatives and manual disimpaction in a stepwise protocol and in combination. All study participants kept bowel diaries for 6 weeks.

Findings from the study showed that manual disimpaction significantly improved bowel continence more than oral laxatives or other bowel management programs. Some patients needed both laxatives and disimpaction to maintain bowel continence.

Level of Evidence: 1

This study used a randomized controlled design to compare bowel management interventions between a control group and an experimental group that used two specific bowel management interventions—manual disimpaction and oral laxatives.

Commentary: Implications for Practice and Research

This research added to the evidence for planning the best bowel management protocol for spinal cord–injured patients. Nurses can use this information to teach patients how to maintain bowel continence. Bowel control is a sensitive and embarrassing patient problem, and nurses can be instrumental in teaching patients about which methods achieve the best outcome.

Collaborate with patients to schedule bowel ELIMINATION as close as possible to their previous routine. For example, a patient who had stools at noon every other day before the illness or injury should have the bowel program scheduled in the same way. An exception is the patient who prefers another time that best fits into his or her daily routine. If the patient is employed during the day, a time-consuming bowel elimination program in the morning may not work. The bowel protocol can then be changed to the evening when there is more time.

Bowel retraining programs for patients with neurologic problems are often designed to include a combination of methods. Although drug therapy should not be a first choice when formulating a bowel training program, consider the need for a suppository if the patient does not re-establish defecation habits through a consistent toileting schedule, dietary modification, anal stimulation, and disimpaction.

Bisacodyl (Dulcolax), a commonly used laxative, may be prescribed either rectally or orally as part of a bowel training program. Suppositories must be placed against the bowel wall to stimulate the sacral reflex arc and promote rectal emptying. Results occur in 15 to 30 minutes. Administer the suppository when the patient expects to defecate, for example, after a meal to coincide with the gastrocolic reflex. Using the suppository every second or third day is usually effective in re-establishing defecation patterns.

Many rehabilitation patients are at high risk for constipation, especially older adults. Encourage fluids (at least 8 glasses a day) and 20 to 35 g of fiber in the diet. Teach patients to eat 2 to 3 daily servings of whole grains, legumes, and bran cereals and 5 daily servings of fruits and vegetables. Do not offer a bedpan when toileting. Instead, be sure that the patient sits upright on a bedside commode or bathroom toilet to facilitate defecation.

NCLEX EXAMINATION CHALLENGE

Physiological Integrity

Which statement by a quadriplegic client indicates a need for the nurse to provide further teaching about bowel retraining?

A. "I'll eat low-fiber foods each day to prevent diarrhea."
B. "I'll drink at least a quart of water or other liquids every day."
C. "I'll do my daily bowel training routine after I eat breakfast."
D. "I'll use a suppository to help empty my rectum."

Community-Based Care

Discharge planning begins at the time of the patient's admission. If the patient is transferred from a hospital to a rehabilitation unit or long-term care facility, orient him or her to the change in routine and emphasize the importance of self-care. When the patient is admitted, a nurse, case manager, and/or OT assess his or her current living situation at home. Together with the patient and family members or significant others, they determine the adequacy of the current situation and the potential needs after discharge to home. The patient with chronic illness and disability may require home care, assistance with ADLs, nursing care, or physical or occupational therapy after discharge.

Other health care professionals may be necessary to meet the unique needs of special populations. For example, patients with brain injury may benefit from life planning—a process that examines and plans to meet lifelong needs. External case managers specializing in life planning may be part of the interdisciplinary rehabilitation team.

Home Care Management. Before the patient returns home, the nurse assesses his or her readiness for discharge from the rehabilitation facility or hospital. The home may be assessed in multiple ways and points in time.

Predischarge Assessment. Before discharge, the case manager or OT may visit the home to assess its layout and accessibility. These professionals may be employed by the health care agency or by a third-party payer, such as a health maintenance organization. Because of the stress of hospitalization, a patient with a fractured hip who is ambulating well with a walker may neglect to explain to the nurse that the bathroom in the home is accessible by stairway only. The patient may not consider it important to mention that throw rugs, which can cause falls, are scattered throughout the apartment. Fall prevention strategies in the home environment for older adults are discussed in Chapter 2.

During a predischarge visit to the home, the accessibility of bathrooms, bedrooms, and kitchen is assessed. If the patient will be wheelchair dependent after discharge from the facility, home modifications may be needed, such as ramps to replace steps. Doorways should be checked for adequate width. A doorway width of 36 to 38 inches (slightly less than 1 meter [m]) is usually sufficient for a standard-size wheelchair. Obese patients require bariatric wheelchairs and furniture and therefore need a wider door opening. Any room that the patient needs to use is assessed. The bedroom should have sufficient space for the patient to maneuver transfers to and from the wheelchair and the bed, if needed. The bathroom may need a raised toilet seat to at least 17 inches (43 cm).

Space requirements depend on the patient's need to use a wheelchair, walker, or cane. In the bathroom, grab bars may need to be installed before the patient comes home. Bathtub benches can provide support for the patient who has difficulty with mobility and, when used in combination with a handheld showerhead, can provide easily accessible bathing facilities. Assessment of the kitchen may or may not be critical, depending on whether the patient has help with cooking and preparing meals. If the patient will be cooking after discharge, the kitchen may need to be assessed for wheelchair or walker accessibility, appliance accessibility, and the need for adaptive equipment.

Leave-of-Absence Visit. A second method of assessing the patient's home is through a brief home visit, also called a *leave-of-absence (LOA) visit*, before discharge. Explain the need for the trial home visit, and assess the patient's comfort level with this idea. The patient who has been hospitalized for a lengthy period may feel intense anxiety about returning home. The nurse may allay such anxieties with careful preparation. Before the visit, the rehabilitation nurse meets with the patient and family members or significant others to set goals for the visit and to identify specific tasks to be attempted while at home. After the home visit, interview the patient to determine the success of the visit and to assess additional education or training needs before final discharge.

Going home may not be an option for everyone. Some patients may not have a support network of family members or significant others. For example, many older adults have no spouse or close friends living nearby. Children may live far away, which can make home care difficult. If no caregiver is available, the family must decide whether care can be provided in the home by an outside resource. The patient may need to be admitted to a 24-hour supervised health care setting, such as a nursing home. Continued rehabilitation services are available in most long-term care settings (skilled nursing facilities) at least 5 days a week if it is medically necessary.

Self-Management Education. The OT and PT teach the patient to perform ADLs and IADLs independently. The patient's learning potential and cognitive capacity are assessed. The patient is asked to perform or direct each skill or technique independently to verify understanding. Written material explaining the steps in the procedure is provided to the patient and family members to reinforce learning and to provide support with the technique after discharge. Before distributing written material, the rehabilitation team assesses the reading level of the material and determines whether it is appropriate for the patient's reading ability and language skills.

Any chronic illness or disability necessitates changes in lifestyle and body image. Assist the patient in dealing with such changes by encouraging verbalization of feelings and emotions. A focus on existing capabilities instead of disabilities is emphasized.

The patient may fail to relate psychologically to the disability during hospitalization. For example, he or she may display anger or frustration in attempting to perform self-care routines before discharge from the rehabilitation facility. Encourage the patient to be open about such feelings and to talk about ways to prevent worries from becoming realities after discharge. If needed, refer the patient to a mental health care professional to help with adjustment and coping strategies.

The LOA home visit assists the patient and family members or significant others in psychosocial preparation for discharge. It allows the experience of the home situation while being able to return to the hospital environment after a few hours. Often the patient finds new problems in the home that must be addressed before discharge. Review this information with the patient in preparation for discharge to the home.

Health Care Resources. After discharge to the home, various health care resources (e.g., physical therapy, home care nursing, vocational counseling) are available to the patient with chronic illness and disability. Assess the need for additional care and support throughout the hospitalization, and coordinate with the case manager and physician in arranging for home services. A newer process using technology called *tele-health*, or *tele-rehabilitation* allows for care coordination in the home setting. Through the use of various electronic devices, phone, or computer software, a health care team member can monitor the patient's vital signs, weight, and other assessment data. Other programs, such as Rehab@Home, allow patients to perform therapeutic exercises at home using Wii, a webcam, and a computer.

◆ *Evaluation: Outcomes*

The patient and rehabilitation team evaluate the effectiveness of interdisciplinary interventions based on the common patient problems. Expected outcomes may include that the patient will:

- Reach a level of physical mobility that allows him or her to function independently with or without assistive devices
- Prevent complications of decreased physical mobility
- Perform self-care and other self-management skills independently or with minimal assistance, possibly using assistive/adaptive devices
- Have intact skin and underlying tissues
- Establish urinary continence without infection or retention
- Have regular evacuation of stool without constipation

GET READY FOR THE NCLEX® EXAMINATION!

KEY POINTS

Review these Key Points for each NCLEX Examination Client Needs Category.

Safe and Effective Care Environment

- Recall that rehabilitation is the process of learning to live with chronic and disabling conditions; the role of the rehabilitation nurse is outlined in Table 6-1.
- Collaborate with members of the interdisciplinary rehabilitation team, including physicians, nurse practitioners, physiotherapists, occupational therapists, dietitians, and speech/language pathologists; the patient and family are also members of the team. **Teamwork and Collaboration** QSEN
- Know that acute (short-term) rehabilitation care occurs in a variety of settings, including inpatient rehabilitation facilities (IRFs) and skilled nursing facilities (SNFs) in either a nursing home or hospital.
- Delegate and supervise selected nursing tasks, such as reporting reddened skin areas, as part of quality care for the rehabilitation patient.
- After assessing the home environment, the case manager, OT, and/or rehabilitation nurse make recommendations to the patient and family about home modifications.
- Use evidence-based safe patient handling practices, such as using mechanical lifts and working with other team members, when assessing and moving patients to prevent injury and improve MOBILITY. **Evidence-Based Practice** QSEN
- Recall that the rehabilitation therapists teach patients transfer, bed MOBILITY, and gait training techniques (see Chart 6-1).
- Encourage the patient to be as independent as possible when performing ADLs and safe MOBILITY skills.

Health Promotion and Maintenance

- In coordination with the PT and OT, assess the patient's ability to perform ADLs and MOBILITY skills using a functional assessment process. **Teamwork and Collaboration** QSEN
- Prevent complications of immobility for patients, and teach them how to prevent complications by using interventions listed in Table 6-4. Examples include pressure ulcers, urinary calculi, constipation, and venous thromboembolism. **Evidence-Based Practice** QSEN

Psychosocial Integrity

- Assess the patient's self-esteem and changes in body image caused by chronic or disabling health problems.
- Assess the patient's COGNITION to screen for depression, delirium, and dementia using tools such as the Confusion Assessment Method (CAM), especially for older adults.
- Assess the patient's and family's response to chronic and disabling conditions, including feelings of loss and grief.
- Assist patients in coping with their loss, and assess the availability of patient support systems, especially for older adults. **Patient-Centered Care** QSEN

Physiological Integrity

- Assess rehabilitation patients as outlined in Table 6-2 to help plan appropriate collaborative care.
- Review the Functional Independence Measure (FIM) system as one assessment tool used to assess functional ability of the patient in rehabilitation, including the need for assistive/adaptive devices.
- Recognize that the Minimum Data Set (MDS) 3.0 is the comprehensive assessment tool required by the Centers for Medicare and Medicaid Services that is used in long-term care/nursing home settings (see Table 6-3).
- Assess patients in rehabilitation for risk factors that make them likely to develop skin breakdown; interventions to prevent skin problems include repositioning and adequate NUTRITION. **Quality Improvement** QSEN
- Patients with neurogenic bladder and bowel problems are managed by training programs; overactive (spastic or reflex) and underactive (hypotonic or flaccid) elimination problems are managed differently (see Tables 6-6 and 6-7).
- In collaboration with the rehabilitation therapists, evaluate the ability of patients to use assistive/adaptive devices to promote independence. **Teamwork and Collaboration** QSEN
- Determine patient and family needs regarding discharge to home or other community-based setting.

End-of-Life Care

Mary K. Kazanowski

http://evolve.elsevier.com/Iggy/

PRIORTY CONCEPTS

- Palliation
- Pain
- Cognition
- Perfusion

LEARNING OUTCOMES

Safe and Effective Care Environment

1. Describe the importance of collaborating with members of the interdisciplinary team when caring for the dying patient and family or other caregivers.
2. Discuss the ethical and legal obligations of the nurse with regard to end-of-life care.

Health Promotion and Maintenance

3. Explain to patients and their families the purpose and procedure for advance directives.

Psychosocial Integrity

4. Assess the patient's and family's ability to cope with the dying process.
5. Assess and plan interventions to meet the dying patient's spiritual needs.
6. Incorporate the patient's cultural practices and beliefs when providing care during the dying process and death.
7. Identify the need for providing psychosocial support to the family or other caregivers during the patient's dying process.

Physiological Integrity

8. Describe the pathophysiology of death.
9. Compare the concepts of hospice and palliation.
10. Assess patients for signs and symptoms related to the end of life.
11. Explain how to provide evidence-based end-of-life care to the dying patient, including symptom management.
12. Explain best practice guidelines for performing postmortem care.

OVERVIEW OF DEATH AND DYING

Although dying is part of the normal life cycle, it is often feared as a time of pain and suffering. For the family, death of a member is a life-altering loss that can cause significant and prolonged suffering. As sad and difficult as the death may be, the experience of dying need not be physically painful for the patient or emotionally agonizing for the family. The dying process is an opportunity to change a potentially difficult situation into one that is tolerable, peaceful, and meaningful for the patient and the family left behind.

Because nurses spend more time with patients than do any other health care providers, it is the nurse who often has the greatest impact on a person's experience with death. A nurse can affect the dying process to prevent death without dignity (bad death) from occurring while striving to promote a peaceful and meaningful death (good death). To accomplish this desired outcome, nurses need to have knowledge of end-of-life care, compassion, advocacy, and therapeutic communication skills (Clabots, 2012).

A **good death** is one that is free from avoidable distress and suffering for patients, families, and caregivers; in agreement with patients' and families' wishes; and consistent with clinical practice standards. Persistent pain, not having one's wishes followed at the end of one's life, isolation, abandonment, and agonizing about losses associated with death are characteristics of a **bad death**.

Death in the United States

Table 7-1 lists the most common causes of death in the United States. Of all people who die, only a small percentage of them die suddenly and unexpectedly. Most people die after a long period of illness (e.g., cardiac, renal, respiratory disease), with gradual deterioration until an active dying phase before the death. Most people who die are older than 65 years.

The U.S. health care system is based on the acute care model, which is focused on prevention, early detection, and cure of disease. This focus and the advances in survival rates for once deadly diseases have made it difficult for many patients and

TABLE 7-1 Leading Causes of Death in the United States

1. Diseases of the heart
2. Malignant neoplasms (cancer)
3. Chronic lower respiratory diseases (e.g., chronic obstructive pulmonary disease [COPD])
4. Cerebrovascular diseases
5. Accidents (unintentional injuries)
6. Alzheimer's disease
7. Diabetes mellitus
8. Influenza and pneumonia
9. Nephritis, nephritic syndrome, and nephrosis
10. Intentional self-harm (suicide)
11. Septicemia
12. Chronic liver disease and cirrhosis
13. Essential hypertension and hypertensive renal disease
14. Parkinson disease
15. Pneumonitis caused by aspiration of solids and liquids

Data from Hoyert, D.L., & Xu, J. (2011). Deaths: Preliminary data for 2011. *National Vital Statistics Reports, 61*(6), 1-52. National Center for Health Statistics. Retrieved December 2013 from www.cdc.gov/nchs/data/nvsr/nvsr61/nvsr61_06.pdf.

CONSIDERATIONS FOR OLDER ADULTS

Patient-Centered Care QSEN

Older adults in the United States are estimated to account for 75% of deaths each year. Older adults are also more likely than younger adults to think about their needs and preferences related to end of life (EOL). Data suggest that older adults want early discussions with their health care provider in preparation for death (Gillick, 2010). Despite this desire, understanding of preferences and needs related to end of life is lacking.

health care providers to accept death as an outcome of disease. Many view death as a failure.

These negative views have led to a major deficiency in the quality of care provided to many people at the end of life. In 1995, a landmark study highlighted the poor quality of dying experienced by hospitalized patients. The Study to Understand Prognoses and Preferences for Outcomes and Risks of Treatment (SUPPORT) showed that more than 50% of a sample of 9105 hospitalized patients with a life-threatening disease had moderate to severe pain during the last days of their lives. In addition, they did not have their wishes met, even when their wishes were known.

Pathophysiology of Dying

Death is defined as the cessation of integrated tissue and organ function, manifested by lack of heartbeat, absence of spontaneous respirations, or irreversible brain dysfunction. It generally occurs as a result of an illness or trauma that overwhelms the compensatory mechanisms of the body, eventually leading to cardiopulmonary failure/arrest. Direct causes of death include:

- Heart failure secondary to cardiac dysrhythmias, myocardial infarction, or cardiogenic shock
- Respiratory failure secondary to pulmonary embolism, heart failure, pneumonia, lung disease, or respiratory arrest caused by increased intracranial pressure
- Shock secondary to infection, blood loss, or organ dysfunction, which leads to lack of blood flow (i.e., PERFUSION) to vital organs

Inadequate PERFUSION to body tissues deprives cells of their source of oxygen, which leads to anaerobic metabolism with acidosis, hyperkalemia, and tissue ischemia. Dramatic changes in vital organs lead to the release of toxic metabolites and destructive enzymes, referred to as *multiple organ dysfunction syndrome (MODS)*. As illness or organ damage progresses, the syndrome occurs with renal and liver failure. Renal or liver failure can also *start* the dying process.

When the body is hypoxic and acidotic, a lethal dysrhythmia such as ventricular fibrillation or asystole can occur, which ultimately leads to the lack of cardiac output and PERFUSION. Shortly after cardiac arrest, respiratory arrest occurs. When respiratory arrest occurs first, cardiac arrest follows within minutes.

Planning for End-of-Life and Advance Directives

In 1991, the U.S. Congress passed the Patient Self-determination Act (PSDA), which granted people the right to determine the medical care they wanted provided (or not provided) if they became incapacitated. Documentation of this self-determination is accomplished by completing an **advance directive (AD)**. The PSDA requires that a representative in every health care agency ask patients when admitted if they have written advance directives. Patients who do not have ADs should be provided with information on the value of having an AD in place and given the opportunity to complete the state-required forms. Ideally, advance directives should be completed long before a medical crisis.

Advance directives vary from state to state but are readily available through Caring Connections, an online program of the National Hospice and Palliative Care Organization (www.caringinfo.org). Anyone can complete the advance directive forms without legal consultation. Exact titles for each AD form vary from state to state. Generally speaking, most ADs have a section where one names a **durable power of attorney for health care (DPOAHC)**. The DPOAHC is not the same as DPOA for financial affairs. Most legal representatives recommend that the person who is the durable power of attorney be different from the person who is the durable power of attorney for one's finances.

The DPOAHC is the designation for the person or persons appointed to make one's decisions related to health care in the event the person loses decision-making capacity (Fig. 7-1). The DPOAHC, often referred to as a *health care proxy, health care agent,* or *surrogate decision maker,* does not make health care decisions until a physician states that the person loses or lacks the capacity to make his or her own health care decisions because of impairment in COGNITION.

To have decision-making ability, a person must be able to perform three tasks:

- Receive information (but not necessarily oriented × 4)
- Evaluate, deliberate, and mentally manipulate information
- Communicate a treatment preference

By definition, the comatose patient does not have decisional ability.

The second part of the Advance Directive is a **living will** (LW), which identifies what one would (or would not) want if he or she were near death. Treatments that are discussed include cardiopulmonary resuscitation (CPR), artificial ventilation, and artificial nutrition or hydration. The third type of advance directive is a do-not-resuscitate (DNR) form. A **DNR** is an actual order from a physician or other authorized health care provider who instructs that CPR not be attempted in the event

NEW HAMPSHIRE DURABLE POWER OF ATTORNEY FOR HEALTH CARE

INSTRUCTIONS

PRINT YOUR NAME

I,________________________________, hereby appoint ____________________________
(name) (name of agent)

PRINT THE NAME AND ADDRESS OF YOUR AGENT

of ____
(address)

as my agent to make any and all health care decisions for me, except to the extent I state otherwise in this document or as prohibited by law. This durable power of attorney for health care shall take effect in the event I become unable to make my own health care decisions.

INSTRUCTION STATEMENTS

STATEMENT OF DESIRES, SPECIAL PROVISIONS, AND LIMITATIONS REGARDING HEALTH CARE DECISIONS.

CIRCLE AND INITIAL THE RESPONSES THAT REFLECT YOUR WISHES

For your convenience in expressing your wishes, some general statements concerning the withholding or removal of life-sustaining treatment are set forth below. (Life-sustaining treatment is defined as procedures without which a person would die, such as but not limited to the following: cardiopulmonary resuscitation, mechanical respiration, kidney dialysis or the use of other external mechanical and technological devices, drugs to maintain blood pressure, blood transfusions, and antibiotics.) There is also a section that allows you to set forth specific directions for these or other matters. If you wish, you may indicate your agreement or disagreement with any of the following statements and give your agent power to act in those specific circumstances.

TERMINAL ILLNESS

1. If I become permanently incompetent to make health care decisions, and if I am also suffering from a terminal illness, I authorize my agent to direct that life-sustaining treatment be discontinued.
   YES NO (Circle your choice and initial beneath it.)

PERMANENTLY UNCONSCIOUS

2. Whether terminally ill or not, if I become permanently unconscious I authorize my agent to direct that life-sustaining treatment be discontinued.
   YES NO (Circle your choice and initial beneath it.)

ARTIFICIAL NUTRITION AND HYDRATION

3. I realize that situations could arise in which the only way to allow me to die would be to discontinue artificial feeding (artificial nutrition and hydration). In carrying out any instructions I have given above in #1 or #2 or any instructions I may write in #4 below, I authorize my agent to direct that (circle your choice of [a] or [b] and initial beside it):

   (a) artificial nutrition and hydration not be started or, if started, be discontinued,

   —OR—

   (b) although all other forms of life-sustaining treatment be withdrawn, artificial nutrition and hydration continue to be given to me.

If you do not complete item 3, your agent will <u>*not*</u> *have the power to direct the withdrawal of artificial nutrition and hydration.*

ADD PERSONAL INSTRUCTIONS (IF ANY)

4. Here you may include any specific desires or limitations you deem appropriate, such as when or what life-sustaining treatment you would want used or withheld, or instructions about refusing any specific types of treatment that are inconsistent with your religious beliefs or unacceptable to you for any other reason. You may leave this question blank if you desire.

(attach additional pages as necessary)

ALTERNATE AGENT

In the event the person I appoint above is unable, unwilling or unavailable, or ineligible to act as my health care agent, I hereby appoint

PRINT THE NAME AND ADDRESS OF YOUR ALTERNATE AGENT

______________________________ of ______________________________
(name of alternate agent) (address of alternate agent)

as alternate agent.

I hereby acknowledge that I have been provided with a disclosure statement explaining the effect of this document. I have read and understand the information contained in the disclosure statement.

LOCATION OF THE ORIGINAL AND COPIES

The original of this document will be kept at __________________ and the following persons and institutions will have signed copies:

DATE AND SIGN THE DOCUMENT HERE

In witness, whereof, I have hereunto signed my name this _________ day of ______________, 20 ______.
(day) (month) (year)

____
(signature)

WITNESSING PROCEDURE

WITNESSES MUST SIGN AND PRINT THEIR ADDRESSES

I declare that the principal appears to be of sound mind and free from duress at the time the durable power of attorney for health care is signed and that the principal has affirmed that he or she is aware of the nature of the document and is signing it freely and voluntarily.

Witness: __________________________ Address: _________________________________
Witness: __________________________ Address: _________________________________

AND A NOTARY PUBLIC OR JUSTICE OF THE PEACE MUST COMPLETE THIS SECTION

STATE OF NEW HAMPSHIRE, COUNTY OF ______________________________
The foregoing instrument was acknowledged before me this ______ day of _____, 20 ___, by ___________.

____
Notary Public/Justice of the Peace
My commission expires:

FIG. 7-1 An example of a durable power of attorney for health care (DPOAHC).

of cardiac or respiratory arrest. DNR directives are intended for people with known life-limiting conditions, such as terminal cancer. Depending on the state of residence, people who have made the decision not to be resuscitated may have portable DNR documents and or bracelets to identify themselves as having orders not to resuscitate. Some states also have directives referred to as *POLST* (physician orders for life-sustaining treatment), which document additional treatments in case of cardiac or pulmonary arrest. Like portable DNRs, POLST follow the patient across health care settings.

By law, all health care providers must initiate CPR for a person who is not breathing or is pulseless unless that person has a DNR order. The problem with performing CPR is that it can be a violent, likely painful intervention, which prevents a peaceful death. CPR is also likely to be unsuccessful when performed on a patient with advanced disease and comorbidities, especially when the patient is older than 65 years. Many patients and families, however, do not understand the limitations of CPR and do not realize it was never intended to be performed on patients with end-stage disease (Peberdy et al., 2008).

Hospice and Palliative Care

The concept of hospice in the United States came about from a grassroots effort in response to the unmet needs of terminally ill people. As both a philosophy and a system of care, **hospice** uses an interdisciplinary approach to assess and address the holistic needs of patients and families to facilitate quality of life and a peaceful death. This holistic approach neither hastens nor postpones death but provides relief of symptoms. Hospice systems of care are provided in a variety of settings. They are often affiliated with home care agencies, providing services to patients at home or in a long-term care or assisted-living facility. Some communities also have hospice houses, which provide care to patients in the terminal phase of their lives.

The *Medicare Hospice Benefit* serves as a guide for hospice care in the United States. This benefit pays for hospice services for Medicare recipients who have a prognosis of 6 months or less to live and who agree to forego curative treatment for their terminal illness. Historically, those with terminal cancer made up the majority of patients receiving hospice care. The proportion of patients with terminal cancer, however, has recently decreased, with increases in numbers of patients with other terminal illnesses, (e.g., dementia, end-stage chronic obstructive pulmonary disease [COPD], cardiac disease, or neurologic disease).

Guidelines are available to assist health care providers and families in identifying who is entitled to hospice care under Medicare. Patients who do not qualify for Medicare may have benefits through private insurance or government medical assistance programs (e.g., Medicaid).

CONSIDERATIONS FOR OLDER ADULTS

Patient-Centered Care QSEN

Although twice as many older adults died in hospice care as in a hospital or nursing home compared with a decade ago, hospice is often treated as a last resort after aggressive critical care (see the Evidence-Based Practice box). Earlier referrals to hospice care by physicians in collaboration with the health care team would increase its benefit for older adults and families.

EVIDENCE-BASED PRACTICE QSEN

When Do Medicare Patients Use Hospice Services?

Kelley, A.S., Deb, P., Du, Q., Aldridge Carlson, M.D., & Morrison, R.S. (2013). Hospice enrollment saves money for Medicare and improves care quality across a number of different lengths-of-stay. *Health Affairs, 32(3),* 552-561.

Despite the demonstrated potential to improve quality of care and lower costs, the Medicare Hospice Benefit has been found to produce savings only for patients enrolled 53 to 105 days before death. The researchers for this study reviewed data from the Health and Retirement Study data (2002-2008) for the most common hospice enrollment periods, which are: 1 to 7 days, 8 to 14 days, 15 to 30 days, and 53 to 105 days before death. Patients enrolling in these periods in hospice were compared with matched, non-hospice controls.

Within all enrollment periods, hospice patients had significantly lower rates of hospital and critical care use, hospital readmissions, and in-hospital death when compared with the matched non-hospice patients.

Level of Evidence: 1

This was a large systematic study that overcame limitations of previous research.

Commentary: Implications for Practice and Research

This study indicates that hospice is the best model of care for people near death, saves health care costs, and addresses quality of care at the end of life. Nurses should provide information to patients at end of life about the value of hospice to ensure a peaceful, dignified death.

Because benefits and care generally require a prognosis of 6 months or less, its use is limited. Many people with chronic, serious illness whose prognosis may be longer than 6 months often do not have access to the support services that work so well within the hospice model. In an effort to address this need, palliative care has evolved.

Palliative care is a philosophy of care for people with life-threatening disease that assists patients and families in identifying their goals of care, assists them with informed decision making, and facilitates quality symptom management. Unlike hospice, PALLIATION is provided by a physician, nurse practitioner, or team of providers, as a consultation visit, with one or more follow-up visits. Palliative care consults are provided in a large number of hospitals and on an ambulatory care basis in some communities. Table 7-2 compares palliative care to hospice care.

Because of their proximity to patients, nurses are often in the position of assisting patients in exploring their wishes for end-of-life care. To elicit this information, the nurse could ask these questions (Steed, 2012):

- Do you have advance directives?
- Have you thought who you would want to speak for you about your medical care, if you were not able to speak for yourself?
- What are your goals for end-of-life care?
- Have you discussed resuscitation with your health care provider?
- Do you want to be at home at the end of your life?
- Do you currently have any distressing symptoms that are not being controlled?
- Do you feel that your spiritual needs are being met? If not, how can we help meet them?

TABLE 7-2 Comparison of Hospice and Palliative Care

HOSPICE CARE	PALLIATIVE CARE
Patients have a prognosis of six (6) months or less to live.	Patients can be in any stage of serious illness.
Care is provided when curative treatment, such as chemotherapy, has been stopped.	A consult is provided that is concurrent with curative therapies or therapies that prolong life.
Care is provided in 60- and 90-day periods with an opportunity to continue if eligibility criteria are met.	Care is not limited by specific time periods.
Ongoing care is provided by RNs, social workers, chaplains, and volunteers.	Care is in the form of a consult visit by a physician or advanced practice nurse who makes recommendations; follow-up visits may be provided.

When developing a plan of care for people nearing the end of their lives, consideration should be given for where the person wants to die. A large percentage of Americans would like to die at home. If this is the patient's preference, work with the patient, family, and health care provider to determine if this goal is possible. Providers trained in end-of-life care are available through hospice agencies who can meet with the patient and family to evaluate their needs and assist them in the discharge plan.

CLINICAL JUDGMENT CHALLENGE

Patient-Centered Care QSEN

A 77-year-old female with stage IV heart failure has had two hospitalizations for congestive heart failure (CHF) exacerbations in the past month. The patient lives alone and has no durable power of attorney for health care or living will. She tells you she does not need an advance directive because she "can just come back to the hospital and they will take care of me."

1. How would you respond to the patient at this time?
2. What types of referral might you make for her? How would you do this?
3. Is the patient a candidate for hospice at this time? Why or why not?
4. What symptoms of distress do you anticipate?
5. How do you feel about the patient wanting re-hospitalization for heart failure?

PATIENT-CENTERED COLLABORATIVE CARE

Assessment

Obtain information about the patient's diagnosis, past medical history, and recent state of health to identify the risks for symptoms of distress at end of life. People with lung cancer, heart failure, or chronic respiratory disease are at high risk for respiratory distress and dyspnea as they decline. Those with brain tumors are at risk for seizure activity. Patients with tumors near major arteries (e.g., head and neck cancer) are at risk for hemorrhage. Those who have been experiencing PAIN often continue to have pain at the end of life, which may increase, decrease, or remain at the same level of intensity.

Physical Assessment/Clinical Manifestations. As death nears, patients often have signs and symptoms of decline in physical function, manifested as weakness, anorexia, and changes in cardiovascular function, breathing patterns, and GI and genitourinary function. As death nears, peripheral circulation decreases and the patient's skin is often cold, mottled, and cyanotic because of poor tissue PERFUSION. Blood pressure decreases and often is only palpable. The dying person's heart rate may increase, become irregular, and gradually decrease before stopping. Changes in breathing pattern are common, with breaths becoming very shallow and rapid. Periods of apnea and **Cheyne-Stokes respirations** (apnea alternating with periods of rapid breathing) are also common. Death occurs when respirations and heartbeat stop.

Although these signs and symptoms of physical decline are often disturbing to patients and families, they generally do not cause physical discomfort to the patient. However, symptoms that cause suffering can occur in patients with cancer and noncancer diagnoses.

Near the end of life, the patient often becomes weak and drowsy, often sleeping 23 or more hours of the day. Eventually he or she can become unresponsive. As the patient's ability to speak diminishes, it is difficult to assess his or her perception of symptoms. When caring for those who are unable to communicate their distress or needs, identify alternative ways to assess symptoms of distress. Teach family caregivers to watch closely for objective signs of discomfort (e.g., restlessness, grimacing, moaning) and identify when these symptoms occur in relation to positioning, movement, medication, or other external stimuli. Teach them how to perform interventions that can help relieve discomfort and stress as described in Chart 7-1.

Although the patient's point of view is the most valid indicator of comfort or distress, the family's perception of symptoms is also important. Family caregivers, health care providers, and dying patients may differ in their perceptions of symptoms in terms of intensity, significance, and meaning. Whereas health care providers are often able to identify symptoms of distress, families are often more knowledgeable about the patient's habits and preferences. Incorporate all pertinent information into the plan for symptom management, and work with patients and families toward a common outcome.

Assess any symptom of distress in terms of intensity, frequency, duration, quality, exacerbating (worsening) and relieving factors, and effect on the patient's comfort when awake or asleep. A method for rating the intensity of symptoms should be used to facilitate ongoing assessments and evaluate treatment response. A rating scale of 0 to 10 is commonly used, with 0 indicating no distress and 10 indicating the worst possible distress. The intensity of the symptom before and after an intervention (e.g., medication) is documented by the nurse or the family caregiver and is used daily to evaluate the patient's overall comfort.

Psychosocial Assessment. People facing death may have fear and/or anxiety about their impending death and experience

CULTURAL CONSIDERATIONS

Patient-Centered Care QSEN

Be aware that patients differ in their needs at end of life depending on their gender and ethnicity. For example, families may not want to know about the terminal conditions of their loved ones. In some cultures, this decision is based on respect for older family members. Ask the family what they want to know and if they desire the assistance of a language interpreter (Clabots, 2012).

CHART 7-1 Patient and Family Education: Preparing for Self-Management

Common Physical Signs and Symptoms of Approaching Death with Recommended Comfort Measures

Coolness of Extremities

Circulation to the extremities is decreased; the skin may become mottled or discolored.

- Cover the person with a blanket.
- Do not use an electric blanket, hot water bottle, electric heating pad, or hair dryer to warm the person.

Increased Sleeping

Metabolism is decreased.

- Spend time sitting quietly with the person.
- Do not force the person to stay awake.
- Talk to the person as you normally would, even if he or she does not respond.

Fluid and Food Decrease

Metabolic needs have decreased.

- Do not force the person to eat or drink.
- Offer small sips of liquids or ice chips at frequent intervals if the person is alert and able to swallow.
- Use moist swabs to keep the mouth and lips moist and comfortable.
- Coat the lips with lip balm.

Incontinence

The perineal muscles relax.

- Keep the perineal area clean and dry. Use disposable underpads (Chux) and disposable undergarments.
- If the person would be more comfortable, consider a Foley catheter.

Congestion and Gurgling

The person is unable to cough up secretions effectively.

- Position the patient on his or her side.
- Administer medications to decrease the production of secretions.

Breathing Pattern Change

Slowed circulation to the brain may cause the breathing pattern to become irregular, with brief periods of no breathing or shallow breathing.

- Elevate the person's head.
- Position the person on his or her side.

Disorientation

Decreased metabolism and slowed circulation to the brain may occur.

- Identify yourself whenever you communicate with the person.
- Reorient the patient as needed.
- Speak softly, clearly, and truthfully.

Restlessness

Decreased metabolism and slowed circulation to the brain may occur.

- Play soothing music, and use aromatherapy.
- Do not restrain the person.
- Massage the person's forehead.
- Reduce the number of people in the room.
- Talk quietly.
- Keep the room dimly lit.
- Keep the noise level to a minimum.
- Consider sedation if other methods do not work.

Adapted from the Hospice of North Central Florida, Inc.

CHART 7-2 Patient and Family Education: Preparing for Self-Management

Common Emotional Signs of Approaching Death

Withdrawal

The person is preparing to "let go" from surroundings and relationships.

Vision-like Experiences

The person may talk to people you cannot see or hear and see objects and places not visible to you. These are not hallucinations or drug reactions.

- Do not deny or argue with what the person claims.
- Affirm the experience.

Letting Go

The person may become agitated or continue to perform repetitive tasks. Often this indicates that something is unresolved or is preventing the person from letting go. As difficult as it may be to do or say, the dying person takes on a more peaceful demeanor when loved ones are able to say things such as, "It's okay to go. We'll be alright."

Saying Goodbye

When the person is ready to die and you are ready to let go, saying "goodbye" is important for both of you. Touching, hugging, crying, and saying "I love you," "Thank you," "I'm sorry," or "I'll miss you so much" are all natural expressions of sadness and loss. Verbalizing these sentiments can bring comfort both to the dying person and to those left behind.

Adapted from the Hospice of North Central Florida, Inc.

difficulty coping. Assess cultural considerations, values, and religious beliefs of the patient and family for their influence on the dying experience, control of symptoms, and family bereavement.

Families of people near death often manifest fear, anxiety, and knowledge deficits regarding the process of death and their role in providing care. Assess the patient and family for fear and anxiety and their expectations of the death experience. Ask them if they want to talk to a **bereavement** (grief) counselor or want guidance from clergy. Explain the common emotional signs of approaching death as described in Chart 7-2.

◆ *Interventions*

The desired outcomes for a patient near the end of life (EOL) are that the patient will have:

- Needs and preferences met
- Control of symptoms of distress
- Meaningful interactions with family
- A peaceful death

Interventions are planned to meet the physical, psychological, social, and spiritual needs of patients using an interdisciplinary approach. The coordinated, interdisciplinary care of hospice is the most successful approach to end-of-life care to date. *Although the perception of hospice is that it provides care for the dying, the major focus of hospice care is on quality of life.* Drug therapy is a major component of hospice care to provide symptom relief. Commonly used drugs are summarized in Chart 7-3.

Interventions to relieve symptoms of distress include positioning, administration of medications, and a variety of complementary and alternative therapies. When medications are used, they are often scheduled around the clock to maintain comfort and prevent reoccurrence of the symptom. The most

CHART 7-3 **Best Practice for Patient Safety & Quality Care** QSEN

Symptom Relief Kit for Patients in Home Hospice

- For unrelieved pain: Morphine solution (20 mg/1 mL solution) 0.25 to 0.5 mL orally or sublingually every 2 to 3 hours as needed.
- For unrelieved dyspnea: Morphine solution (20 mg/1 mL solution) 0.25 to 0.5 mL orally or sublingually every 2 hours as needed.
- For nausea or vomiting: Prochlorperazine 25-mg suppository rectally or 10-mg tablet orally every 6 hours as needed.
- For severe agitation and restlessness:
  - Determine if patient is in pain; treat accordingly.
  - Determine if patient is experiencing urinary retention; insert straight or Foley catheter.
  - Haloperidol 0.5 to 1 mg orally or sublingually every 6 hours.
  - Lorazepam 0.5 to 1 mg elixir or tablet dissolved in 0.5 mL water, administered against buccal mucosa every 4 hours to keep patient comfortable. If patient becomes more agitated after lorazepam, discontinue and contact hospice.
- For oral secretions or loud, wet respirations:
  - Atropine sulfate ophthalmic drops 1%, (2 drops orally or sublingually) every 4 hours as needed; or hyoscyamine drops (Levsin) (0.125-0.25 mg orally every 6 hours).
  - Scopolamine 1 to 3 transdermal patches every 72 hours.
- For unrelieved pain, dyspnea, nausea, vomiting, agitation, or secretions, call hospice.

common end-of-life symptoms that can cause the patient distress are:

- PAIN
- Weakness
- Breathlessness/dyspnea
- Nausea and vomiting
- Restlessness and agitation
- Seizures

Pain Management. *Pain is the most distressing symptom that dying patients fear the most.* Diseases such as cancer often cause tumor pain as a result of the infiltration of cancer cells into organs, nerves, and bones. Other causes of PAIN in dying patients include osteoarthritis, muscle spasms, and stiff joints secondary to immobility.

Patients who have had their PAIN controlled with either short-acting or long-acting opioids should continue their scheduled doses to prevent reoccurrence of the pain. As patients get closer to death, however, they often lose the ability to swallow. Long-acting oral opioids generally cannot be crushed, and rotation to rectal, transdermal, intravenous, or a subcutaneous route may be necessary. Short-acting opioids such as morphine sulfate, oxycodone, or hydromorphone elixir can be given sublingually, via the buccal mucosa, or rectally. They are quick-acting, effective, and safe to administer, even to comatose patients.

CONSIDERATIONS FOR OLDER ADULTS

Patient-Centered Care QSEN

Pain relief is often the priority need of older adults receiving PALLIATION. But PAIN is often underreported and undertreated. Do not withhold opioid drugs from older adults. Instead, reduce starting doses, make dose increases slowly, and monitor for changes in mental status or excessive sedation.

Some experts in symptom management at end of life (EOL) recommend discontinuing routine doses of opioids such as morphine when patients become oliguric or anuric. The rationale for this decision is to decrease the risk for delirium that may occur as the result of a failing kidney's inability to excrete morphine metabolites from the body. If delirium is interfering with the patient's ability to achieve a quality end of life, changing the opioid to fentanyl IV is an option. Fentanyl does not have active metabolites, and the delirium may improve. For patients with known renal failure, fentanyl should ideally be used from the start of opioid administration. In cases where it cannot be easily obtained (i.e., when not available by sublingual route or IV route), oxycodone is a better choice over morphine. Chapter 3 describes in detail the management of chronic PAIN.

Complementary and Alternative Therapies. Nonpharmacologic interventions are often integrated into the pain management plan. Some common approaches are presented here, as well as in Chapter 3.

Massage may decrease pain in people with cancer and is one of the most popular complementary interventions used for patients at EOL. This technique involves manipulating the patient's muscles and soft tissue, which improves circulation and promotes relaxation. Patients who are severely weak, are arthritic, or have advanced age may not tolerate extensive massage but may benefit from a short treatment to sites of their choice. In working with patients with cancer, use light pressure and avoid deep or intense pressure. Massage should not be done over the site of tissue damage (e.g., open wounds, tissue undergoing radiation therapy), in patients with bleeding disorders, and in those who are uncomfortable with touch.

Music therapy is another complementary therapy used by people near end of life that has been shown to decrease PAIN by promoting relaxation. Select music based on patient preferences and values.

Therapeutic Touch involves moving one's hands through the patient's energy field to relieve PAIN. Reiki therapy is another type of energy therapy being evaluated for its role in pain and symptom management. Use of Reiki requires a Reiki practitioner who is trained in the method.

Aromatherapy can be used in conjunction with other treatments to relieve pain near EOL. It is thought to decrease PAIN by promoting relaxation and reducing anxiety. Lavender, capsicum, bergamot, chamomile, rose, ginger, rosemary, lemongrass, sage, and camphor have been used in end-of-life care.

NCLEX EXAMINATION CHALLENGE

Physiological Integrity

A client with metastasis to the bone is receiving IV antibiotics for pneumonia but has declined further treatment for his disease. He is experiencing severe back pain rated as a 9 on a 0-to-10 scale. What interventions are the most appropriate for the nurse to implement for this client? **Select all that apply.**

A. Provide both non-opioid and opioid analgesics.
B. Offer music therapy to help the client relax and decrease anxiety.
C. Obtain an order for physical therapy to encourage ambulation.
D. Help the client assume the best position of comfort.
E. Offer Reiki therapy, if available.

Weakness Management. Patients commonly experience weakness and fatigue as death nears. Weakness combined with decreased neurologic function may impair the ability to swallow (dysphagia). Once the patient has difficulty swallowing, oral intake should be limited to soft foods and sips of liquids, only if the patient wants. Teach families about the risk for aspiration, and reassure them that anorexia is normal at this stage. Families often have difficulty accepting that their loved ones are not being fed and may request that IV fluids be started. With great sensitivity, reinforce that stopping food and liquid intake is a natural process. Inform families that giving fluids can actually increase discomfort in a person with multisystem slowdown (Buck, 2012). Discomfort from fluid replacement could lead to respiratory secretions (and distress), increased GI secretions, nausea, vomiting, edema, and ascites. Most experts believe that dehydration in the last hours of life (i.e., terminal dehydration) does not cause distress and may stimulate endorphin release that promotes the patient's sense of well-being. To avoid a dry mouth and lips, moisten them with soft applicators and apply an emollient to soften the lips.

! NURSING SAFETY PRIORITY (QSEN)

Action Alert

Dysphagia near death presents a problem for oral drug therapy. Although some tablets may be crushed, drugs such as sustained-release capsules should not be taken apart. Reassess the need for each medication. Collaborate with the prescriber about discontinuing drugs that are not needed to control PAIN, dyspnea, agitation, nausea, vomiting, cardiac workload, or seizures. In collaboration with a pharmacist experienced in PALLIATION, identify alternative routes and/or alternative drugs to maintain control of symptoms. Choose the least invasive route such as oral, buccal mucosa (inside cheek), transdermal (via the skin), or rectal. Some oral drugs can be given rectally. Depending on the patient needs, the subcutaneous or IV routes may be used if access is available. The IM route is almost never used at the end of life because it is considered painful and drug distribution varies among patients.

Breathlessness/Dyspnea Management. Dyspnea is a subjective experience in which the patient has an uncomfortable feeling of breathlessness, often described as terrifying. It is a common symptom of distress near the end of life, especially among older adults because of decreased oxygen reserves associated with aging. Patients, families, and health care providers often consider it the major cause of suffering at end of life. Dyspnea can be:

- Directly related to the primary diagnosis (e.g., lung cancer, breast cancer, coronary artery disease)
- Secondary to the primary diagnosis (e.g., pleural effusion)
- Related to treatment of the primary disease (e.g., heart failure caused by chemotherapy, pneumonitis or constrictive pericarditis caused by radiation therapy, anemia related to chemotherapy)
- Unrelated to the primary disease (e.g., pneumonia or congestive heart failure [CHF]).

Depending on the cause, the pathophysiology of dyspnea can involve:

- Obstructive, restrictive, or vascular disturbances in the airways with tumor or lymph node involvement
- Pulmonary congestion secondary to fluid overload and/or cardiac dysfunction
- Bronchoconstriction and bronchospasm as seen with respiratory infection, chronic obstructive pulmonary disease (COPD), or airway blockage by a tumor
- Decreased hemoglobin-carrying capacity as with anemia
- Hyperventilation secondary to neuromuscular disease with limited movement of the diaphragm

Perform a thorough assessment of the patient's dyspnea. Include onset, severity (e.g., 0-to-10 scale), and precipitating factors. Precipitating factors may include time of day, position, anxiety, PAIN, cough, or emotional distress.

Pharmacologic interventions should begin early in the course of dyspnea near death. Nonpharmacologic interventions can be used in conjunction with but not in place of drug therapy.

Opioids such as morphine sulfate are the standard treatment for dyspnea near death. They work by (1) altering the perception of air hunger, reducing anxiety and associated oxygen consumption and (2) reducing pulmonary congestion by dilating pulmonary blood vessels. Patients who have not been receiving opioids are given starting doses of morphine 5 to 6 mg (or less for patients of advanced age) orally every 4 hours during the day and 10 mg at bedtime. If dyspnea occurs only with activity, give morphine before the activity up to every 2 hours. Those who are taking morphine or other opioids for pain may need higher doses for breathlessness, at times up to 50% more than their usual dose.

If a patient is having severe respiratory distress and poor oxygenation, morphine by mouth may need to be repeated as often as every 30 minutes and an IV or subcutaneous route may need to be established. Subcutaneous or intravenous doses of 1 to 2 mg of morphine may be given every 5 to 10 minutes until dyspnea is relieved.

Oxygen therapy for dyspnea near death has not been established as a standard of care for all patients. However, those who do not respond promptly to morphine or other drugs should be tried on oxygen (2 to 6 L by nasal cannula) to assess its effect. Patients often feel more comfortable when the oxygen saturation is greater than 90%. If possible, provide oxygen by nasal cannula (NC) because masks can be frightening. If oxygen is not effective, discontinue it.

! NURSING SAFETY PRIORITY (QSEN)

Action Alert

Offer oxygen to any patient with dyspnea near death, regardless of his or her oxygen saturation, because comfort is the desired outcome. If the patient is feeling dyspneic even though the oxygen saturation is above 90%, be sure that he or she receives oxygen to relieve respiratory distress. In addition, offer a fan directed toward the patient's face. Some patients find the circulating air more comfortable than oxygen therapy.

Bronchodilators, such as albuterol (Proventil) or ipratropium bromide (Atrovent, Apo-Ipravent ♣) via a metered dose inhaler (MDI) or nebulizer, may be given for symptoms of bronchospasm (heard as wheezes). *Corticosteroids,* such as prednisone (Deltasone, Winpred ♣), may also be given for bronchospasm and inflammatory problems within and outside the lung. Superior vena cava syndrome and cancer-related lymphangitis causing dyspnea may also respond to corticosteroids (also see Chapter 22).

People who have fluid overload with dyspnea, crackles on auscultation, peripheral edema, and other signs of CHF may be given a *diuretic* such as furosemide (Lasix, Uritol ♣) to decrease blood volume, reduce vascular congestion, and reduce the workload of the heart. Furosemide can be administered by mouth, IV, or subcutaneously. IV push administration, which is effective within minutes, may be preferred for heart failure and pulmonary edema.

Antibiotics may be indicated for dyspnea from a respiratory infection. A thorough workup for a respiratory infection is not appropriate when death is imminent. However, if signs or symptoms of a respiratory infection occur with dyspnea, a trial of an appropriate antibiotic may be considered to make the patient comfortable.

Secretions in the respiratory tract and oral cavity may also contribute to dyspnea near death. Loud, wet respirations (referred to as **death rattle**) are disturbing to family and caregivers even when they do not seem to cause dyspnea or respiratory distress. Reposition the patient onto one side to reduce gurgling, and place a small towel under his or her mouth to collect secretions. *Anticholinergics,* such as atropine (ophthalmic) solution 1% given sublingually every 4 hours as needed or hyoscyamine (Levsin) every 6 hours, are commonly given to dry up secretions. Scopolamine may also be given transdermally to reduce secretion production. Oropharyngeal suctioning is not recommended for loud secretions in the bronchi or oropharynx because it is often not effective and may only agitate the patient.

Fear and anxiety may be components of respiratory distress at end of life. For this reason, benzodiazepines are commonly given when morphine does not fully control the person's dyspnea. Low-dose lorazepam (Ativan) is administered orally, sublingually, or IV every 4 hours as needed or around the clock.

Nonpharmacologic interventions include:

- Applying wet cloths on the patient's face
- Positioning the patient with the head of the bed up either in a hospital bed or a reclining chair to increase chest expansion
- Encouraging imagery and deep breathing

Insertion of a urinary (Foley) catheter to avoid the need for exertion with voiding may be a comfort measure if the patient or family agrees. Risk for infection should not be a consideration when a person is near death.

NCLEX EXAMINATION CHALLENGE

Physiological Integrity

The nurse is caring for a client who has severe dyspnea because of end-stage chronic obstructive pulmonary disease. Which interventions are the most appropriate to help improve his breathing? **Select all that apply.**

A. Administer morphine sulfate on an around-the-clock schedule.
B. Teach the client and family to keep him in a sitting position.
C. Use a large electric fan to circulate the air.
D. Keep the room temperature warm to prevent respiratory infection.
E. Teach the client and family that he should use bronchodilators as prescribed.

Nausea and Vomiting Management. Although not as common a problem as PAIN or dyspnea, nausea and vomiting occur frequently among terminally ill patients during the last week of life. It is particularly common in patients with acquired immune deficiency syndrome (AIDS) and with breast, stomach, or gynecologic cancers.

Other causes of nausea and vomiting at the end of life include:

- Uremia (increased serum urea nitrogen)
- Hypercalcemia
- Increased intracranial pressure
- Constipation or impaction
- Bowel obstruction

If constipation is identified as the cause of nausea and vomiting, give the patient a biphosphate enema (e.g., Fleet) to remove stool quickly. If stool in the rectum cannot be evacuated, a mineral oil enema followed by gentle disimpaction may relieve the patient's distress. Nausea and vomiting related to other causes can be controlled by one or more antiemetic agents such as prochlorperazine (Compazine), ondansetron (Zofran), dexamethasone (Decadron, Deronil♣, Dexasone♣), or metoclopramide (Reglan, Maxeran♣). Based on a patient's response, one or more of these drugs may be combined and compounded into rectal suppositories or oral troches. In addition to providing medications, be sure to remove sources of odors and keep the room temperature at a level that the patient desires.

Complementary and Alternative Therapies. Aromatherapy using chamomile, camphor, fennel, lavender, peppermint, and rose may reduce or relieve vomiting. Some patients, however, may have worse nausea with aroma. Ask the patient and family about their preferences, and respect culturally established practices.

Agitation and Delirium Management. Agitation at the end of life first requires assessing for PAIN or urinary retention, constipation, or another reversible cause. If constipation is ruled out as the cause and if analgesia and catheterization do not relieve restlessness, delirium (acute confusion) is suspected. ***Delirium*** *is a neuropsychiatric syndrome manifested by an acute change in the level of arousal. Clinical manifestations include altered sleep/wake cycle, mumbling speech, disturbance of memory and attention, and perceptual disturbances with delusions and hallucinations.* Delirium can be hyperactive or hypoactive. *Hypoactive (quiet)* delirium is probably not uncomfortable for patients. *Agitated (noisy)* delirium with emotional and behavioral symptoms (e.g., yelling, hallucinations) can be uncomfortable, especially for family. Chapter 2 discusses delirium in more detail.

When delirium occurs in the week or two before death, it is referred to as *terminal delirium.* Possible causes include the adverse effects of opioids, benzodiazepines, anticholinergics, or steroids. If drugs are suspected causes, they may be decreased or discontinued, particularly if recently started.

NURSING SAFETY PRIORITY QSEN

Drug Alert

Do not give the patient more than one antipsychotic drug at a time because of the risk for adverse drug events (ADEs). A neuroleptic such as a low dose of haloperidol (Haldol, Peridol ♣) 0.5-2 mg orally, IV, subcutaneously, or rectally is commonly used at end of life. Although haloperidol has the potential to cause extrapyramidal symptoms or adverse cardiovascular events and death in older adults with dementia, the benefits of treating delirium usually outweigh the risks.

Benzodiazepines are not generally used as a first choice for older adults with agitation because of their risk for causing delirium. Development of increased agitation after receiving a benzodiazepine could represent a paradoxical reaction—the opposite of what is expected.

Complementary and Alternative Therapies. Music therapy may produce relaxation by quieting the mind and promoting a restful state. Aromatherapy with chamomile may also help overcome anxiety, anger, tension, stress, and insomnia in dying patients.

Seizure Management. Seizures are not common at end of life but may occur in patients with brain tumors, advanced AIDS, and pre-existing seizure disorders. Around-the-clock drug therapy is needed to maintain a high seizure threshold for patients who can no longer swallow antiepileptic drugs (AEDs) and are at risk for seizures. Benzodiazepines, such as diazepam (Valium) and lorazepam (Ativan), are the drugs of choice. For home use, rectal diazepam gel or sublingual lorazepam oral solution (2 mg/mL) may be preferred. As a second choice, barbiturates such as phenobarbital may be given rectally or IV.

Management of the Refractory Symptoms of Distress. Patients receiving opioids for pain or dyspnea and other drugs such as antiemetics or antianxiety agents may experience mild sedation as a side effect to therapy. Depending on the patient and how soon death is expected, this side effect may decrease with time. What is important to understand is that drug therapy for symptoms of distress at end of life are guided by protocols, using medications believed to be safe, with the intent of alleviating suffering. *There is no evidence that administering medications for symptoms of distress using established protocols hastens deaths.* The ethical responsibility of the nurse in caring for patients near death is to follow guidelines for drug use to manage symptoms and to facilitate prompt and effective symptom management until death (Arnstein & Robinson, 2011).

A small percentage of patients have refractory symptoms of distress that do not respond to treatment near the end of life. These patients may be candidates for **proportionate palliative sedation**—a care management approach involving the administration of drugs such as benzodiazepines (e.g., midazolam [Versed]), neuroleptics, barbiturates, or anesthetic agents (e.g., propofol [Diprivan]) for the purpose of "lowering of patient consciousness." *The intent of palliative sedation to promote comfort and not hasten death distinguishes it from euthanasia (discussed later in this chapter).* The use of palliative sedation for refractory symptoms of distress is supported by a consensus of experts in palliative care as a comfort therapy of last resort (Arnstein & Robinson, 2011).

Psychosocial Management. The personal experience of dying or of losing a loved one through death is life altering. Unexpected deaths, particularly in young people, tend to be most traumatic. When a person has a chronic life-threatening disease, he or she and the family may have some knowledge of the expected outcome. Others, however, may have never considered their illness to be potentially terminal. It is important to first assess what patients and family understand about their illness and then help them identify the desired outcomes for care in the context of the illness.

Whereas death is the termination of life, dying is a process. People facing death may demonstrate emotional signs and symptoms of their response to the dying process through behaviors that equate to saying goodbye or through actual withdrawal. Some patients attempt to make families feel better by reassuring them that everything will be fine. Teach families that such behaviors are normal to the process of dying (see Chart 7-2).

Assisting Patients During the Grieving Process. **Grief** is the emotional feeling related to the perception of the loss. Patients who are dying suffer not only from the anticipated death but also from the loss of the ability to engage with others and in the world. **Mourning** is the outward social expression of the loss. Interventions to assist patients and families in grieving and mourning are based on cultural beliefs, values, and practices. Some patients and their families express their grief openly and loudly, whereas others are quiet and reserved. Table 7-3 lists basic beliefs regarding death, dying, and afterlife for some of the major religions.

Nursing interventions are aimed at providing appropriate emotional support to allow patients and their families to verbalize their fears and concerns. Support includes keeping the patient and family involved in health care decisions and emphasizing that the goal is to keep the patient as comfortable as possible until death. Interventions for providing psychosocial support are summarized in Chart 7-4.

Intervene with those grieving an impending death by "being with" as opposed to "being there." "Being with" implies that you are physically and psychologically with the grieving patient, empathizing to provide emotional support. Listening and acknowledging the legitimacy of the patient's and/or family's

TABLE 7-3 Basic Beliefs Regarding Care at End of Life and Death Rituals for Selected Religions

Christianity

- There are many Christian denominations, which have variations in beliefs regarding medical care near end of life.
- Roman Catholic tradition encourages people to receive Sacrament of the Sick, administered by a priest at any point during an illness. This sacrament may be administered more than once. Not receiving this sacrament will NOT prohibit them from entering heaven after death.
- People may be baptized as Roman Catholics in an emergency situation (e.g., person is dying) by a layperson. Otherwise, they are baptized by a priest.
- Christians believe in an afterlife of heaven or hell once the soul has left the body after death.

Judaism

- The dying person is encouraged to recite the confessional or the affirmation of faith, called the *Shema.*
- According to Jewish law, a person who is extremely ill and dying should not be left alone.
- The body, which was the vessel and vehicle to the soul, deserves reverence and respect.
- The body should not be left unattended until the funeral, which should take place as soon as possible (preferably within 24 hours).
- Autopsies are not allowed by Orthodox Jews, except under special circumstances.
- The body should not be embalmed, displayed, or cremated.

Islam

- Based on belief in one God Allah and his prophet Muhammad. Qur'an is the scripture of Islam, composed of Muhammad's revelations of the Word of God (Allah).
- Death is seen as the beginning of a new and better life.
- God has prescribed an appointed time of death for everyone.
- Qur'an encourages humans to seek treatment and not to refuse treatment. Belief is that only Allah cures but that Allah cures through the work of humans.
- Upon death, the eyelids are to be closed and the body should be covered. Before moving and handling the body, contact someone from the person's mosque to perform rituals of bathing and wrapping body in cloth.

Data from Giger, J.N. (2013). *Transcultural nursing: Assessment and intervention* (6th ed.). St. Louis: Mosby.

CHART 7-4 Best Practice for Patient Safety & Quality Care QSEN

Psychosocial Interventions for Care of the Dying Patient and the Family

- Offer physical and emotional support by "being with" the patient.
- Respect cultural preferences.
- Be realistic.
- Encourage reminiscence.
- Promote spirituality.
- Avoid explanations of the loss.
- Communicate with the patient.
- Provide referrals to bereavement specialists.
- Teach about the physical signs of death (see Chart 9-1).
- Ensure that the patient is receiving palliative care, with an emphasis on symptom management.

impending loss are often more therapeutic than speaking; this concept is often referred to as **presence**. Nurses facilitate the expression of grief by giving the person who is mourning permission to express himself or herself. Your manner and words show that these expressions of grief are acceptable and expected. An example of therapeutic communication might be "This must be very difficult for you" or "I'm sorry this is happening."

Do not minimize a patient's or family member's pain of loss. Avoid trite assurances such as "Things will be fine. Don't cry," "Don't be upset. She wouldn't want it that way," or "In a year you will have forgotten." Such comments can be barriers to demonstrating care and concern. Accept whatever the grieving person says about the situation. Remain present, be ready to listen attentively, and guide gently. In this way, you can help the bereaved family and significant others prepare for the necessary reminiscence and integration of the loss.

Storytelling through reminiscence and life review can be an important activity for patients who are dying. **Life review** is a structured process of reflecting on one's life, which is often facilitated by an interviewer. **Reminiscence** is the process of randomly reflecting on memories of events in one's life. The benefits of storytelling through either method provide the ability to attain perspective and enhance meaning. Suggest that the patient and family record autobiographic stories (print or video), write memories in a journal, or develop a scrapbook. Young dying parents often write letters for their children to read when they are older. If the patient does not have enough energy for these activities, familiar objects such as photographs and favorite jewelry can be used to spark ideas for stories.

Meeting Spiritual Needs. Spirituality is whatever or whoever gives ultimate meaning and purpose in one's life that invites particular ways of being in the world in relation to others, oneself, and the universe. A person's spirituality may or may not include belief in God. **Religions** are formal belief systems that provide a framework for making sense of life, death, and suffering and responding to universal spiritual questions. Religions often have beliefs, rituals, texts, and other practices that are shared by a community. For some patients, spirituality and religion can help them cope with the thought of death, contributing to quality of life during the dying process.

Perform a spiritual assessment to identify the patient's spiritual needs and to facilitate open expression of his or her beliefs and needs. A spiritual assessment could start with questions such as "What is important to you?" or "What gives you meaning or purpose in your life?"

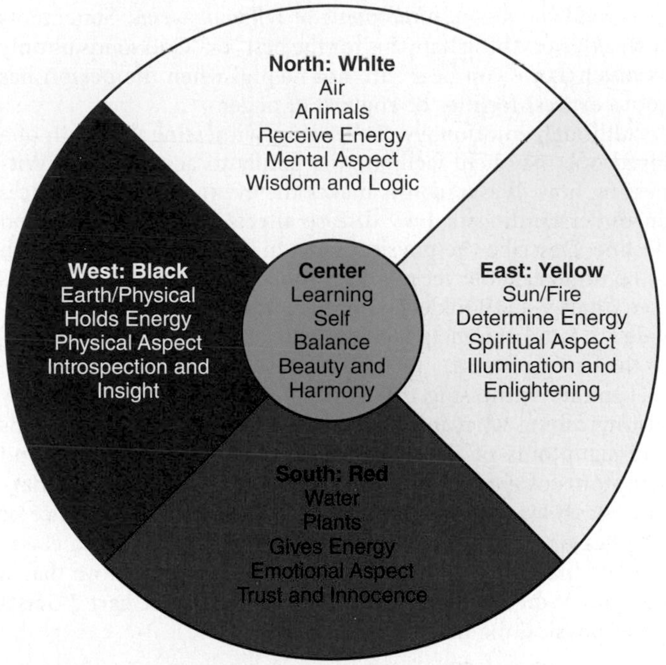

FIG. 7-2 An example of a medicine wheel used by indigenous people to provide harmony and balance in life and transition into the spirit worlds after death.

CULTURAL CONSIDERATIONS

Patient-Centered Care QSEN

When assessing the spiritual needs of the dying patient, consider end-of-life preferences based on ethnic beliefs and practices. For example, the medicine wheel represents the spiritual journey to find one's own path for indigenous people in many countries, including American Indians (e.g., Cherokee, Navajo, Lakota) and Aboriginal people (e.g., Inuit, First Nations) in Canada and Alaska (also known as *Alaska Natives*). The medicine wheel helps people in these groups maintain balance and harmony within four life dimensions (Clarke & Holtslander, 2010) (Fig. 7-2). Depending on specific tribal practices and beliefs, the dimensions may be represented by colors, seasons, or directions.

As part of the dying process, certain tribal ceremonies must take place for patients to have a peaceful transition into the Spirit World and experience a "good death." One special ceremony involves smudging: Selected tribal medicines are burned, and the smoke is passed over the patient's body to cleanse it.

Be aware that supporting patients and their families within their cultural framework is essential as part of the dying process for all patients. Respect all practices, and allow for privacy during ceremonies and ritual practices.

Regardless of whether a person has had an affiliation with a religion or a belief in God or other Supreme Being, he or she can experience what is referred to as *spiritual* or *existential distress.* Existential distress is brought about by the actual or perceived threat to one's continued existence. Terminal illness and facing death can pose a profound threat to one's personhood. The main task for a person at EOL is coming to terms with one's losses, which may include loss of meaning and loss of relationships and facing the unknown. Acknowledge the patient's spiritual pain, and encourage verbalization. Use a family tree to discuss relationships, fears, hopes, and unfinished business. If the patient or family prefers, arrange for counseling with chaplains or others trained in end-of-life care. *Do not try to explain the loss in philosophic or religious terms.* Statements such as "Everything happens for the best" or "God sends us only as much as we can bear" are not helpful when the person has yet to express feelings of anguish or anger.

Although emotionally challenging, witnessing the death of a loved one may help facilitate the family to accept death. Witnessing how ill a person is makes the event real and enhances an understanding of how disease affects bodily function and decline. Describe the physical signs in detail—realistic enough to be unmistakable yet not so graphic as to alarm the listeners (see Chart 7-1). Booklets with this information should be provided to families to help them see what is expected and "normal" to the dying process.

Families witnessing the dying process often have difficulty distinguishing what is a normal finding of decline from signs and symptoms of distress. Instructing families on signs and symptoms of PAIN (e.g., grimacing, moaning, guarding behaviors) or dyspnea is essential. Emphasize that in the absence of dyspnea or pain, patients often die very peacefully with cessation of breathing. Nurses and family members know that a person has died when he or she stops breathing. Chart 7-5 lists other physical manifestations of death.

POSTMORTEM CARE

If the death was in the home and expected, emergency assistance should not be notified. If the person was a patient in a hospice program, the family calls hospice. If a death is unexpected or suspicious, the medical examiner is notified. Otherwise, the nurse or physician performs the pronouncement and completes a death certificate (Chart 7-6). Most states allow nurses to pronounce death in nursing homes and other long-term care facilities, but only a few states permit nurses to pronounce in acute care facilities such as hospitals. Be sure to check your health care agency's policies for who can pronounce death and the specific procedure to follow.

After the patient dies, ask the family or other caregivers if they would like to spend time with the patient to assist them in coping with what has happened and say their good-byes. Even if the death has been anticipated, no one knows how he or she will feel until it occurs. It may take hours to days to weeks or months for each person to realize the full effect of the event. Some family members may find it therapeutic to bathe and prepare the person's body for transfer to the funeral home or the hospital morgue. Offer families this opportunity if it is culturally acceptable.

Before preparing the body for transfer, ask the physician whether an autopsy will be required. When the death is expected, an autopsy is not likely. An autopsy is generally performed only when the cause of death is not known. Some religions do not allow autopsies, such as Orthodox Jews.

After the family or significant others view the body, follow agency procedure for preparing the patient for transfer to either the morgue or a funeral home. In the hospital, a postmortem kit is generally used with a shroud and identification tags. Chart 7-7 describes best practice guidelines for postmortem care.

CHART 7-5 Patient and Family Education: Preparing for Self-Management

Signs That Death Has Occurred

- Breathing stops.
- Heart stops beating.
- Pupils become fixed and dilated.
- Body color becomes pale and waxen.
- Body temperature drops.
- Muscles and sphincters relax.
- Urine and stool may be released.
- Eyes may remain open, and there is no blinking.
- The jaw may fall open.
- Observers may hear trickling of fluids internally.

CHART 7-6 Best Practice for Patient Safety & Quality Care QSEN

Pronouncement of Death

- Note time of death that the family or staff reported the cessation of respirations.
- Identify the patient by the hospital identification (ID) tag; note the general appearance of the body.
- Ascertain that the patient does not rouse to verbal or tactile stimuli. Avoid overtly painful stimuli, especially if family members are present.
- Auscultate for the absence of heart sounds; palpate for the absence of carotid pulse.
- Look and listen for the absence of spontaneous respirations.
- Record the time at which your assessment was completed.
- Document the time of pronouncement and all notifications in the medical record (i.e., to attending physician). Document if the medical examiner needs to be notified (may be required for unexpected or suspicious death). Document if an autopsy is planned per the attending physician and family.
- If your state and agency policy allows an RN to pronounce death, document as indicated on the death certificate.

CHART 7-7 Best Practice for Patient Safety & Quality Care QSEN

Postmortem Care

- Provide all care with respect to communicate that the person was important and valued.
- Ask the family or significant others if they wish to help wash the patient or comb his or her hair; respect and follow their cultural practices for body preparation.
- If no autopsy is planned, remove or cut all tubes and lines according to agency policy.
- Close the patient's eyes unless the cultural/religious practice is for a family member or other person to close the eyes.
- Insert dentures if the patient wore them.
- Straighten the patient, and lower the bed to a flat position.
- Place a pillow under the patient's head.
- Wash the patient as needed, and comb and arrange the patient's hair unless the family desires to perform bathing and body preparation.
- Place waterproof pads under the patient's hips and around the perineum to absorb any excrement.
- Clean the patient's room or unit.
- Allow the family or significant others to see the patient in private and to perform any religious or cultural customs they wish (e.g., prayer).
- Assess that all who need to see the patient have done so, before transferring to the funeral home or morgue.
- Notify the hospital chaplain or appropriate religious leader if requested by the family or significant others.
- Ensure that the nurse or physician has completed and signed the death certificate.
- Prepare the patient for transfer to either a morgue or funeral home; wrap the patient in a shroud (unless the family has a special shroud to use), and attach identification tags per agency policy.

TABLE 7-4 Definitions of Ethical Concepts Related to Issues at End of Life

Withdrawing or withholding life-sustaining therapy (formerly called *passive euthanasia*) An act of omission (e.g., withholding or withdrawing treatment) that might prolong the life of a person who cannot be cured by the treatment. In this situation, the withdrawal of the intervention does not directly cause the patient's death.
Principle of double effect Involves taking an action intended to have a good effect, which also has a known harmful effect. This is not active euthanasia.
Voluntary active euthanasia An act by which the causative agent or treatment in the death of a patient is administered directly by another.
Involuntary active euthanasia The action to end the patient's life is taken without the patient's consent.
Physician-assisted suicide A practice whereby a physician provides a means (e.g., medication) to a patient with the knowledge that the patient will use the means to commit suicide.

THE CONCEPT OF EUTHANASIA

Nurses are usually in the best and most immediate position to discuss end-of-life issues. This includes assisting in the decision-making process regarding immediate or future needs. To do this, nurses must be knowledgeable about terminology and ethical issues related to death and dying (Table 7-4).

Much confusion exists regarding the concept of euthanasia. **Withdrawing or withholding life-sustaining therapy**, formerly called **passive euthanasia**, involves discontinuing one or more therapies that might prolong the life of a person who cannot be cured by the therapy. Another phrase sometimes used is "letting the person die naturally" or "allowing natural death (AND)," as discussed earlier in this chapter. *In this situation, the withdrawal of the intervention does not directly cause the patient's death.* The progression of the patient's disease or poor health status is the cause of death. Professional organizations (e.g., American Nurses Association, American Medical Association) and religious communities (e.g., the Catholic church) support the right of patients and their surrogate decision makers to refuse or stop treatment (e.g., mechanical ventilation, antibiotics, IV fluids) when patients are close to death and interventions are considered medically futile and/or capable of causing harm. The U.S. court system also supports withdrawal of aggressive treatment and the rights of surrogate decision makers to refuse or stop treatment.

By contrast, **active euthanasia** requires that health care providers take action (e.g., give medication or treatment) that purposefully and directly causes the patient's death. *Active euthanasia is not supported by most professional organizations, including the American Nurses Association.* In the states of Oregon, Washington, and Vermont, physician-assisted suicide is legal in certain situations. Nurses should not be involved in active euthanasia or physician-assisted euthanasia. They do, however, play a major role in end-of-life care by advocating for patients' wishes and ensuring quality symptom management and support at the end of life.

GET READY FOR THE NCLEX® EXAMINATION!

KEY POINTS

Review these Key Points for each NCLEX Examination Client Needs Category.

Safe and Effective Care Environment

- Hospice care uses an interdisciplinary approach to assess and address the holistic needs of patients who have a 6-month prognosis or less; examples of health care team members include the social worker, case manager, pharmacist, and physician. **Teamwork and Collaboration** QSEN
- Assess the patient and family to determine if they have written advance directives, such as a durable power of attorney for health care (DPOAHC), a living will, or portable DNR.
- The decision by DPOAHC to withdraw or withhold life-sustaining therapy is supported by the U.S. Supreme Court and other professional/religious organizations.
- Be aware that active euthanasia involves giving a patient a treatment or agent that causes death (see Table 7-4) and is legal only in Oregon, Washington State, and Vermont under certain circumstances.
- Be aware that nurses have an ethical obligation to provide timely information about expected care outcomes so that patients and families can make the best EOL decisions.

Health Promotion and Maintenance

- Stress the importance of having a DPOAHC to inform health care providers of your wishes if you lack capacity.
- Teach the patient and family that an advance directive is a written document that specifies what, if any, extraordinary actions the patient would want if he or she could no longer make decisions about care.

Psychosocial Integrity

- Assess the patient's emotional signs of impending death; assess coping ability of the patient and family or other caregiver (see Chart 7-2).
- Incorporate the patient's personal cultural practices and spiritual beliefs regarding death and dying (see Table 7-3). **Patient-Centered Care** QSEN
- Be aware that people facing death may experience fear and anxiety about their impending death and experience difficulty coping.
- Provide psychosocial interventions to support the patient and family during the dying process, as listed in Chart 7-4.

Physiological Integrity

- Death is defined as the cessation of integrated tissue and organ function, manifested by cessation of heartbeat, absence of spontaneous respirations, or irreversible brain dysfunction.
- Hospice and palliative care are different, as described in Table 7-2.

- Assess the patient for pain, dyspnea, agitation, nausea, and vomiting, which are common problems at the end of life. **Evidence-Based Practice** QSEN
- Recognize that older adults are often undertreated for pain or other symptoms at EOL.
- Assess for the common physical signs of approaching death, as listed in Chart 7-1.
- Medications are frequently given to control dyspnea, pain, nausea, vomiting, and agitation in patients near death (see Chart 7-3).
- Because of the risk for delirium, particularly in older adults, providers may avoid use of benzodiazepines for treatment of anxiety, even at end of life. Development of increased agitation after receiving benzodiazepine could represent a paradoxical reaction. **Safety** QSEN
- Terminal delirium may occur in a week or two before death. Haloperidol given orally or IV is the drug of choice.
- Assessment of oxygen saturation for patients at end of life is not necessary. Oxygen should be provided based on comfort. **Evidence-Based Practice** QSEN
- Common complementary and alternative therapies used for symptom management at end of life include aromatherapy, music therapy, and energy therapies, such as Therapeutic Touch.
- Follow Chart 7-7 for best practice guidelines for performing postmortem care; incorporate the patient's cultural and religious beliefs in body preparation and burial (see Table 7-3). **Patient-Centered Care** QSEN

CHAPTER 8

Concepts of Emergency and Trauma Nursing

Linda Laskowski-Jones and Karen L. Toulson

http://evolve.elsevier.com/Iggy/

PRIORITY CONCEPTS

- Safety
- Teamwork and Collaboration
- Communication

LEARNING OUTCOMES

Safe and Effective Care Environment

1. Describe the emergency department (ED) environment, including vulnerable populations and interdisciplinary team members.
2. Engage in collaboration with members of the interdisciplinary health care team members in the ED.
3. Plan and implement best practices to maintain staff and patient safety in the ED.
4. Explain selected core competencies that nurses need to function in the ED.
5. Triage patients in the ED to prioritize the order of care delivery.
6. Prioritize resuscitation interventions based on the primary survey of the injured patient.

Psychosocial Integrity

7. Describe the role of the ED nurse in providing support for families after the death of a loved one.

Physiological Integrity

8. Describe the general process of admission through disposition of a patient in the ED.
9. Prevent or reduce common risk factors in the ED that contribute to adverse events in older adults.

The demand for emergency care in the United States is growing rapidly. Emergency departments (EDs) function as safety nets for communities of all sizes by providing services to both insured and uninsured patients seeking medical care. They are also responsible for safety through public health surveillance and emergency disaster preparedness. Some hospital-based emergency departments also provide observation, procedural care, and employee or occupational health services. Other hospital-based emergency departments have interdisciplinary specialty teams who take part in collaboration to provide first-line care for patients with stroke and cardiac problems (Alberts et al., 2011). The role of the ED is so vital that the Centers for Medicare and Medicaid Services (2013) has a process for designating small rural facilities of 25 inpatient beds or fewer as **critical access hospitals** if they provide around-the-clock emergency care services 7 days a week. Critical access hospitals are considered *necessary providers of health care* to community residents that are not close to other hospitals in a given region.

Because of the multi-specialty nature of the environment, EDs play a unique role within the U.S. health care system. More than 119 million people visit the ED each year (Centers for Disease Control and Prevention [CDC], 2010). The demand for emergency care has greatly increased over the past 15 years, and the health care consumer has higher expectations. However, the capacity to provide necessary resources has not kept pace in most systems. Emergency department crowding occurs when the need for care exceeds available resources in the department, hospital, or both (Howard, 2009). The Joint Commission has established a set of metrics (Core Measure Sets) based on ED length of stay (LOS) that hospitals are required to submit. The longer the ED length of stay for admitted patients, the more overcrowded the ED becomes. That, in turn, limits access to other patients who are in need of ED beds for emergency care.

A prolonged LOS also indicates problems with inpatient bed availability and poor overall hospital throughput.

Health care reform initiatives stemming from the Affordable Care Act will certainly impact emergency services; the full spectrum of that impact is currently evolving. The widespread availability of health insurance may produce an increase in the number of patients who use the emergency department because they now have greater access to the necessary financial resources. Emergency department use may actually decrease for some types of patients as hospitals and providers partner in Accountable Care Organization models. This will better control costs by managing patient outcomes through primary care networks and disease management programs. Emergency departments may also experience a shift in focus from admitting the majority of acutely ill patients to the hospital for care to COLLABORATING more with home care services and establishing better access to resources in the community to enable patients to be safely discharged home from the ED when possible.

THE EMERGENCY DEPARTMENT ENVIRONMENT OF CARE

In the emergency care environment, rapid change is the rule. The typical ED is fast paced and, at the height of activity, might even appear chaotic. Patients seek treatment for a number of physical, psychological, spiritual, and social reasons. In general, nurses work in this environment because they dislike routines and thrive in challenging, stimulating work settings. Although most EDs have treatment areas that are designated for certain populations such as patients with trauma or cardiac, psychiatric, or gynecologic problems, care can actually take place almost anywhere. In a crowded ED, patients may receive initial treatment outside of the usual treatment rooms, including the waiting room and hallways.

The ED is typically alive with activity and noise, although the pace decreases at times because arrivals are random. Emergency nurses can expect background sounds that include ringing telephones, monitor alarms, vocal patients, crying children, and radio transmissions between staff and incoming ambulance or helicopter personnel. Interruptions and distractions are the norm, and the nurse must ensure these events do not impact patient SAFETY.

Demographic Data and Vulnerable Populations

Staff members in the ED provide care for people across the life span with a broad spectrum of issues, illnesses, and injuries—as well as various cultural and religious values. Especially vulnerable populations who visit the ED include the homeless, the poor, and older adults. During a given shift, for example, the emergency nurse may function as a cardiac nurse, a geriatric nurse, a psychiatric nurse, a pediatric nurse, and a trauma nurse. Patient acuity ranges from life-threatening emergencies to minor symptoms that could be addressed in a primary care office or community clinic. Some of the most common reasons that people seek ED care are:

- Abdominal pain
- Chest pain
- Breathing difficulties
- Injuries (especially falls in older adults)
- Headache
- Fever
- Pain (the most common symptom)

CONSIDERATIONS FOR OLDER ADULTS

Patient-Centered Care QSEN

Older adults usually visit the ED because of worsening of an existing chronic condition or because the condition affects their ability to perform ADLs. Older adults are also sometimes admitted from nursing homes or assisted-living facilities for procedures (e.g., insertion of a percutaneous endoscopic gastrostomy [PEG] tube or peripherally inserted central catheter [PICC]) or for treatments (e.g., blood transfusions). Some hospitals plan direct admission of the patient to same-day surgery or hold a bed for the procedure or treatment to bypass the ED. This arrangement decreases the patient's wait time and therefore decreases the risks for adverse events, such as pressure ulcer development or hospital-acquired infection. Incorporating family members of older adults into the ED care process can aid in overall patient evaluation, decision making, and satisfaction with the ED experience (Nikki et al., 2013).

Special Nursing Teams

Many EDs have specialized nursing teams that deal with high-risk populations of patients. One example is the forensic nurse examiner team. **Forensic nurse examiners (RN-FNEs)** are educated to obtain patient histories, collect forensic evidence, and offer counseling and follow-up care for victims of rape, child abuse, and domestic violence—also known as *intimate partner violence (IPV)* (Desy, 2010). They are trained to recognize evidence of abuse and to intervene on the patient's behalf. Forensic nurses who specialize in helping victims of sexual assault are called *sexual assault nurse examiners (SANEs)* or *sexual assault forensic examiners (SAFEs)*.

Interventions performed by forensic nurses may include providing information about developing a SAFETY plan or how to escape a violent relationship. Forensic nurse examiners document injuries and collect physical and photographic evidence. They may also provide testimony in court as to what was observed during the examination and information about the type of care provided.

The **psychiatric crisis nurse team** is another example of an ED specialty team. Many patients who visit the ED for their acute problems also have chronic mental health disorders. The availability of mental health nurses can improve the quality of care delivered to these patients who require specialized interventions in the ED and can offer valuable expertise to the emergency health care staff. For example, the team evaluates patients with emotional behaviors or mental illness and facilitates the follow-up treatment plan, including possible admission to an appropriate psychiatric facility. These nurses also interact with patients and families when sudden illness, serious injury, or death of a loved one may have caused a crisis. On-site interventions can help patients and families cope with these unexpected changes in their lives.

Interdisciplinary Team Collaboration

The emergency nurse is one member of the large interdisciplinary team who provides care for patients in the ED. A team approach to emergency care using COLLABORATION is considered a standard of practice (Fig. 8-1). In this setting, the nurse coordinates care with all levels of health care team providers, from prehospital emergency medical services (EMS) personnel to physicians, hospital technicians, and professional and ancillary support staff.

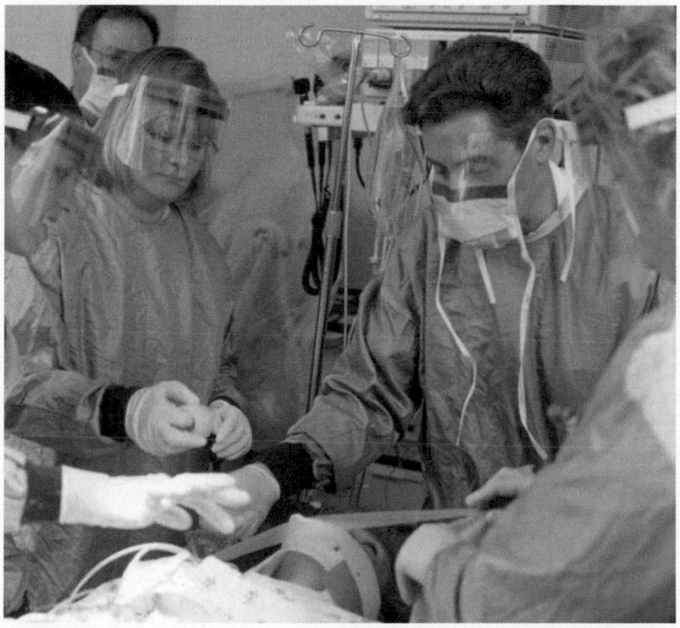

FIG. 8-1 The ability to work as part of an interdisciplinary team is crucial to positive outcomes for emergency department (ED) patients.

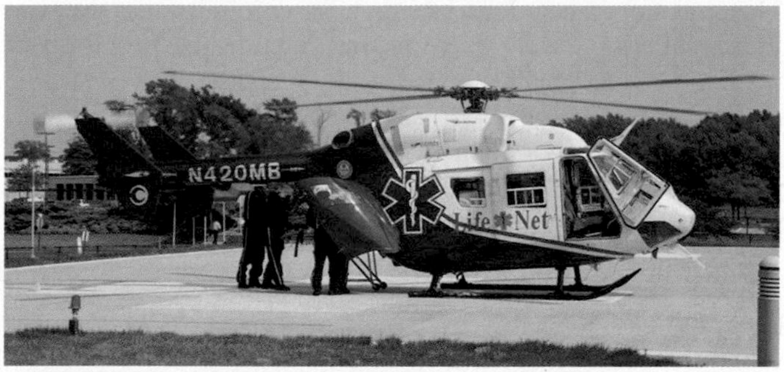

FIG. 8-2 Advanced life support helicopter arriving at emergency department landing zone. Helicopters are used to rapidly transport critically ill and injured patients to the hospital for emergent care.

Prehospital care providers are typically the first caregivers that patients see before transport to the ED by an ambulance or helicopter (Fig. 8-2). Local protocols define the skill level of the EMS responders dispatched to provide assistance. **Emergency medical technicians (EMTs)** offer basic life support (BLS) interventions such as oxygen, basic wound care, splinting, spinal immobilization, and monitoring of vital signs. Some units carry automatic external defibrillators (AEDs) and may be authorized to administer selected drugs such as an EpiPen or nitroglycerin based on established medical protocols. For patients who require care that exceeds BLS resources, paramedics are usually dispatched. **Paramedics** are advanced life support (ALS) providers who can perform advanced techniques, which may include cardiac monitoring, advanced airway management and intubation, establishing IV access, and administering drugs en route to the ED (Fig. 8-3).

The prehospital provider is a key source for valuable patient data. Emergency nurses rely on these providers to be the "eyes and ears" of the health care team in the prehospital setting and to ensure COMMUNICATION of this information to other staff members for continuity of care.

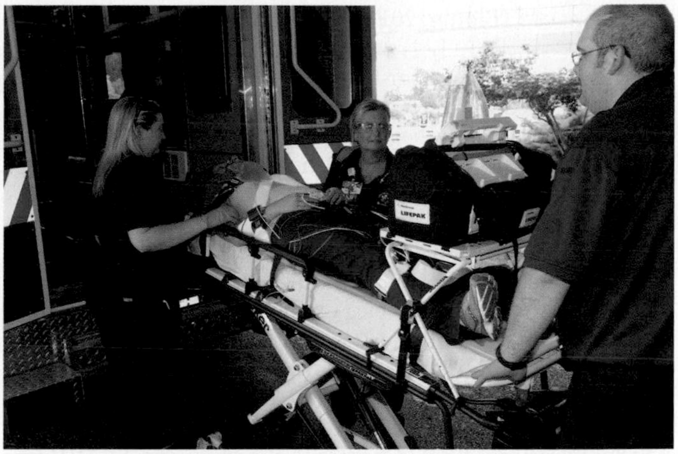

FIG. 8-3 Prehospital providers take a patient from the ambulance to be brought into the emergency department.

Another integral member of the emergency health care team is the **emergency medicine physician**. These medical professionals receive specialized education and training in emergency patient management. As emergency care has become increasingly complex and specialized, emergency medicine is a recognized physician specialty practice.

The emergency nurse interacts with a number of staff and community physicians involved in patient care but is involved in close COLLABORATION with emergency medicine physicians. Even though other physician specialists may be involved in ED patient treatment, the emergency medicine physician typically directs the overall care in the department. Many EDs also employ nurse practitioners (NPs) and physician assistants (PAs) to assume designated roles in patient assessment and treatment. Teaching hospitals also have resident physicians who train in the ED. They act in collaboration with or under the supervision of the emergency medicine physician to assist with emergency care delivery.

The emergency nurse interacts and regularly takes part in COLLABORATION with *professional and ancillary staff* who function in support roles. These personnel include radiology and ultrasound technicians, respiratory therapists, laboratory technicians, social workers, case managers, nursing assistants, and clerical staff. Each support staff member is essential to the success of the emergency health care team. The ED nurse is accountable for communicating pertinent staff considerations, patient needs, and restrictions to support staff (e.g., physical limitations, Transmission-Based Precautions) to ensure that ongoing patient and staff safety issues are addressed. For example, the respiratory therapist can assist the nurse to troubleshoot mechanical ventilator issues. Laboratory technicians can offer advice regarding best practice techniques for specimen collection. During the discharge planning process, social workers or case managers can be tremendous patient advocates in locating community resources, including temporary housing, durable medical equipment (DME), drug and alcohol counseling, health insurance information, and prescription services.

The emergency nurse's interactions extend beyond the walls of the ED. COMMUNICATION with nurses from the inpatient units is necessary to ensure continuity of patient care. Providing a concise but comprehensive report of the patient's ED experience is essential for the *hand-off communication* process and patient SAFETY (Blouin, 2011). Information should include the patient's:

- Situation (reason for being in the ED)
- Brief medical history
- Assessment and diagnostic findings
- Transmission-Based Precautions if needed
- Interventions
- Response to those interventions

The Joint Commission's National Patient Safety Goals (NPSGs) (The Joint Commission [TJC], 2013) advocate that hospitals and other health care agencies use a standardized approach to hand-off communications to prevent errors caused by poor or inadequate communication. Many agencies use the SBAR method (situation, background, assessment, response) or some variation of that method to ensure complete and clearly understood COMMUNICATION. Chapter 1 discusses the SBAR technique in more detail.

Both emergency nurses and nurses on inpatient units need to understand the unique aspects of their two practice environments to prevent conflicts. For example, nurses on inpatient units may be critical of the push to move patients out of the ED setting quickly, particularly when the unit activity is high. Similarly, the emergency nurse may be critical of the inpatient unit's lack of understanding or enthusiasm for accepting admissions rapidly. Effective interpersonal communication skills and respectful negotiation can optimize teamwork and COLLABORATION between the emergency nurse and the inpatient unit nurse. For instance, when ED patient volume or acuity is overwhelming, the unit nurse can volunteer to assist the ED nurse by moving a monitored patient to the hospital bed. Whenever possible, the emergency nurse may decide to delay sending admitted patients to inpatient units during change of shift or crisis periods such as a cardiac arrest on the unit.

STAFF AND PATIENT SAFETY CONSIDERATIONS

In the emergency department (ED) setting, staff and patient SAFETY are major concerns (Chart 8-1).

Staff Safety

Staff safety concerns center on the potential for transmission of disease and on personal safety when dealing with aggressive, agitated, or violent patients and visitors. The emergency nurse uses Standard Precautions at all times when a potential for contamination by blood or other body fluids exists. Patients with tuberculosis or other airborne pathogens are preferentially placed in a negative pressure room if available. The nurse wears a powered air-purifying respirator (PAPR) or a specially fitted facemask before engaging in any close interaction with these patients (see Chapter 23).

EDs employ several methods of ensuring SAFETY. Many EDs have at least one security guard present at all times for immediate assistance with these situations. Metal detectors may be used as a screening device for patients and visitors who are suspected of having weapons. Strategically located panic buttons and remote door access controls allow staff to get help and secure major ED or hospital entrances. The triage reception area—a particularly vulnerable access point into the ED—is often designed to serve as a security barrier with bullet-proof glass and staff-controlled door entry into the treatment area. Hospitals may even employ canine units made up of specially trained officers and dogs to patrol high-risk areas and respond to handle threatening situations (Johnson & Parker, 2009).

! NURSING SAFETY PRIORITY QSEN

Action Alert

Hostile patient and visitor behaviors also pose injury risks to staff members. Be alert for volatile situations or people who demonstrate aggressive or violent tendencies through verbal abuse or acting out. Be sure to follow the hospital's security plan, including looking for an escape route, attempting de-escalation strategies before harm can occur, and notifying security staff as well as supervisory staff of the situation. Emergency visits resulting from gang or domestic violence can produce particularly hazardous conditions. Report all episodes of assaultive or violent behaviors through the hospital's event documentation process so that hospital leaders and risk managers are aware of the scope of the problem and can plan safety strategies, including staff education, accordingly (Harding, 2011).

Patient Safety

In addition to concerns about staff safety, some of the most common *patient* SAFETY issues are:

- Patient identification
- Fall risk
- Skin breakdown in vulnerable populations
- High risk for medical errors or adverse events

Hospital emergency departments have unique factors that can affect patient SAFETY. These factors include the provision of

CHART 8-1 Best Practice for Patient Safety & Quality Care QSEN

Maintaining Patient and Staff Safety in the Emergency Department

SAFETY CONSIDERATION	INTERVENTIONS TO MINIMIZE RISK
Patient identification	Provide an identification (ID) bracelet for each patient. Use two unique identifiers (e.g., name, date of birth). If patient identity is unknown, use a special identification system.
Injury prevention for patients	Keep rails up on stretcher. Keep stretcher in lowest position. Remind the patient to use call light for assistance. Reorient confused patient frequently. If patient is confused, ask a family member or significant other to remain with him or her. Implement measures to protect skin integrity for patients at risk for skin breakdown.
Risk for errors and adverse events	Obtain a thorough patient and family history. Check the patient for a medical alert bracelet or necklace. Search the patient's belongings for weapons or other harmful devices when he or she has altered mental status.
Injury prevention for staff	Use Standard Precautions at all times. Anticipate hostile, violent patient, family, and/or visitor behavior. Plan options if violence occurs, including assistance from the security department.

complex emergency care, constant interruptions, and the need to interact with the many providers involved in caring for one patient.

Correct *patient identification* is critical in any health care setting. All patients are issued an identification bracelet at their point of entry in the ED—generally at the triage registration desk or at the bedside if emergent needs exist. For patients with an unknown identity and those with emergent conditions that prevent the proper identification process (e.g., unconscious patient without identification, emergent trauma patient), hospitals commonly use a "Jane/John Doe" or another identification system. Whatever method is used, always verify the patient's identity using two unique identifiers before each intervention and before medication administration per The Joint Commission's 2013 National Patient Safety Goals. Examples of appropriate identifiers include the patient's name, birth date, agency identification number, home telephone number or address, and/or Social Security number.

Fall prevention starts with identifying people at risk for falls and then applying appropriate fall precautions and SAFETY measures. Patients can enter the ED without apparent fall risk factors, but because of interventions such as pain medication, sedation, or lower extremity cast application, they can develop a risk for falls. Falls can also occur in patients with medical conditions or drugs that cause syncope ("blackouts"). Many older adults also experience orthostatic (postural) hypotension as a side effect of cardiovascular drugs. In this case, patients become dizzy when changing from a lying or sitting position (see Chapter 2).

! NURSING SAFETY PRIORITY QSEN

Action Alert

Help patients move slowly from a supine to an upright position and when ambulating, if needed. Also, confirm that siderails are up and locked on stretchers, that the call light is within reach, and that a patient's fall risk is communicated clearly to visitors and staff members who may assume responsibility for care.

Older adults who are on beds or stretchers should *always* have all siderails up and the bed or stretcher in the lowest position. Access to a call light is especially important; instruct the patient to call for the nurse if assistance is needed rather than attempt independent ambulation. Many older adults have difficulty adjusting to the noise and pace of the ED and/or have illnesses or injuries that cause delirium, an acute confusional state. Reorient the patient frequently, and re-assess mental status. Undiagnosed delirium increases the risk for mortality for older adults who are admitted to the hospital. Assess the need for a family member, significant other, or sitter to stay with the patient to prevent falls and assist with reorientation. Additional safety strategies are listed in Chart 8-1.

Some patients spend a lengthy time on stretchers while awaiting unit bed availability—possibly as long as 1 to 2 days in some hospitals, especially during high census periods as often occurs in flu season. During that time, basic health needs require attention, including providing nutrition, hygiene, SAFETY, and privacy for all ED patients. Waiting in the ED can cause increased pain in patients with back pain or arthritis.

Protecting skin integrity also begins in the ED. Emergency nurses need to assess the skin frequently and implement preventive interventions into the ED plan of care, especially when caring for older adults or those of any age who are immobilized. Interventions that promote clean, dry skin for incontinent patients, mobility techniques that decrease shearing forces when moving the immobile patient, and routine turning help prevent skin breakdown. Chapter 25 describes additional nursing interventions for preventing skin breakdown.

A significant SAFETY risk for all patients who enter the emergency care environment is the *potential for medical errors or adverse events,* especially those associated with medication administration. The episodic and often chaotic nature of emergency management in an environment with frequent interruptions can easily lead to errors.

To reduce error potential, the emergency nurse makes every attempt to obtain essential and accurate medical history information from the patient, family, or reliable significant others as necessary. When dealing with patients who arrive with an altered mental status, a quick survey to determine whether the person is wearing a medical alert bracelet or necklace is important to gain medical information. In addition, a two-person search of patient belongings may yield medication containers; the name of a physician, pharmacy, or family contact person; or a medication list. In this case, the nurse serves as a detective to find clues, which may not only promote SAFETY but also help determine the diagnosis and influence the overall emergency treatment plan. Automated electronic tracking systems are also available in some EDs to assist staff in identifying the location of patients at any given time and in monitoring the progress of care delivery during the visit. These valuable safety measures are especially important in large or busy EDs with a high population of older adults (Laskowski-Jones, 2008).

In addition to falls and pressure ulcer development, another adverse event that can result from a prolonged stay in the ED is a *hospital-acquired infection.* Older adults, in particular, are at risk for urinary tract or respiratory infections. Patients who are immune suppressed, especially those on chronic steroid therapy or immune modulators, are also at a high risk. Nurses and other ED personnel need to wash their hands frequently and thoroughly or use hand sanitizers to help prevent pathogen transmission.

? CLINICAL JUDGMENT CHALLENGE

Safety QSEN

The emergency department manager has created a task force to decrease the rate of adverse incidents in patients who have increased safety needs during their stay in the department. At their meeting, each person discussed a specific safety need and actions that can be taken to reduce that risk.

1. What populations are at highest risk for safety compromise while in the emergency department?
2. What specific procedures can the unit implement to decrease medication errors?
3. What actions can be delegated to unlicensed personnel in these areas: medication administration, skin protection, and fall risk?
4. How can the staff reduce hazard risk for patients who are confused (either as a chronic condition or as the result of medication side effects) or who have delirium?

SCOPE OF EMERGENCY NURSING PRACTICE

The scope of emergency nursing practice encompasses management of patients across the life span—from birth through death—and all health conditions that prompt a person of any age to seek emergency care.

Core Competencies

Emergency nursing practice requires that nurses be skilled in patient assessment, priority setting and clinical decision making, multitasking, and COMMUNICATION. A sound knowledge base is also essential. Flexibility and adaptability are vital traits because situations within the ED, as well as individual patients, can change rapidly.

Like that of any nurse in practice, the foundation of the emergency nurse's skill base is *assessment*. He or she must be able to rapidly and accurately interpret assessment findings according to acuity and age. For example, mottling of the extremities may be a normal finding in a newborn but it may indicate poor peripheral perfusion and a shock state in an adult.

CONSIDERATIONS FOR OLDER ADULTS

Patient-Centered Care QSEN

Some older adults may not be able to provide an accurate history because of memory loss or acute delirium. If possible, review their prior hospitalization records to obtain complete histories, or ask a family member or friend for pertinent information. Older adults usually have many pre-existing diseases (comorbidities) that must be considered as part of the assessment. *Knowing the history is vital because these conditions might adversely affect or complicate the cause for the ED visit.* For example, a patient who has rib fractures but has a history of chronic obstructive pulmonary disease (COPD) may not be able to maintain adequate oxygenation without endotracheal intubation and mechanical ventilatory support in the ED.

Another consideration for older adult assessment is that the presenting symptoms of older adults are often different or less specific than those of younger adults. For example, increasing weakness, fatigue, and confusion may be the only admission concerns. These vague symptoms can be caused by serious illnesses, such as an acute myocardial infarction (MI), urinary tract infection, or pneumonia. Diagnosing older adults often keeps them in the ED for extended periods, which can lead to patient safety concerns as discussed on p. 108.

Another skill for the emergency nurse is *priority setting*, which is essential in the triage process. Priority setting depends on accurate assessment, as well as good critical thinking and clinical decision-making skills. These skills are generally gained through hands-on clinical experience in the ED. However, discussion of case studies and the use of human patient simulation and simulation software and aids can help prepare nurses to acquire this skill base in a nonthreatening environment and then apply it in the actual clinical situation (Kisner & Johnson-Anderson, 2010).

The knowledge base for emergency nurses is broad and ranges from critical care emergencies to less common problems, such as snakebites and hazardous materials contamination (see Chapters 9 and 10). ED nurses also learn to recognize and manage the legal implications of societal problems such as domestic violence, elder abuse, and sexual assault.

Although most EDs have physicians available around the clock who are physically located within the ED, the nurse often initiates COLLABORATIVE interdisciplinary protocols for lifesaving interventions such as cardiac monitoring, oxygen therapy, insertion of IV catheters, and infusion of appropriate parenteral solutions. In many EDs, nurses function under clearly defined medical protocols that allow them to initiate drug therapy for emergent conditions such as anaphylactic shock and cardiac arrest. Emergency care principles extend to knowing what essential laboratory and diagnostic tests may be needed and, when necessary, obtaining them.

The emergency nurse must be proficient in performing a variety of technical skills (multitasking), sometimes in a stressful, high-pressure environment such as a cardiac or trauma resuscitation. In addition to basic skills, he or she may also need to be proficient with critical care equipment, such as invasive pressure monitoring devices and mechanical ventilators. This type of equipment is commonly found in EDs that are part of Level I and Level II trauma centers.

The nurse also COLLABORATES with and assists the physician with a number of procedures. Knowledge and skills related to procedural setup, patient preparation, teaching, and postprocedure care are key aspects of emergency nursing practice. Common ED procedures include:

- Simple and complex suturing for wound closure
- Foreign body removal
- Central line insertion
- Endotracheal intubation and initiation of mechanical ventilation
- Transvenous pacemaker insertion
- Lumbar puncture
- Pelvic examination
- Chest tube insertion
- Paracentesis
- Fracture management

More than one nurse may be necessary to assist with some procedures. For example, if moderate sedation is used to produce amnesia and relaxation during fracture reduction, one nurse assists the physician with the actual procedure while the other nurse monitors the patient before, during, and after the moderate sedation medications are administered.

Finally, an essential aspect of the emergency nurse's skill base is *COMMUNICATION*. The ED environment is complex; therefore multiple barriers to effective communication are likely. One common barrier is the patient's cultural beliefs and practices, especially if they differ from those of the health care team. Assess each patient as an individual, and be careful not to

CULTURAL CONSIDERATIONS

Patient-Centered Care QSEN

Be aware of the various cultural and religious values of patients that may influence care. Many people have distinct beliefs that must be respected in the health care setting. For example, some Mexican Americans are modest and do not like to have their bodies exposed. They often tend to be very family-oriented and affectionate toward each other.

Patients with language barriers can present a challenge. The population of non-English-speaking people is rapidly increasing in the United States. When a patient who is not proficient in English arrives to the ED seeking care, access available resources such as telephone language lines and dedicated interpreters contracted by the hospital to ensure an understanding of all aspects of care.

A religious belief system can also affect the delivery of care. For example, Jehovah's Witness patients do not accept blood transfusions and may not accept certain medications that are derived from human blood components.

Be aware that not all patients identify themselves as male or female. Some patients may be in the process of changing their gender identity from male to female or female to male (transgender people). Ask the patient what pronoun (he, she, or other term) that the person prefers to be called. Demonstrate professional behaviors that promote trust. Chapter 73 discusses the special care for this population in detail.

stereotype anyone based on his or her ethnicity, socioeconomic status, gender identity, or religion.

ED crowding and insufficient nursing personnel to meet the demand for services also create difficulties with COMMUNICATION of pertinent patient information and quality of written documentation. The high-stress ED environment can negatively affect effective interpersonal behaviors, particularly when nurses must deal with angry, violent, or demanding patients.

Training and Certification

Two general types of certification are referred to in emergency nursing practice: the "certification" that marks successful completion of a particular course of study; and emergency nursing specialty certification (Table 8-1). As part of the orientation and employment requirements for staff nurses in most U.S. EDs, successful completion of the Basic Life Support (BLS) for Healthcare Providers and Advanced Cardiac Life Support (ACLS) and Pediatric Advanced Life Support (PALS) provider courses through the American Heart Association is necessary. These courses provide instruction in fundamental, evidence-based management theory and techniques for cardiopulmonary resuscitation (CPR). Course participants include physicians, nurses, and prehospital personnel. The ACLS course builds on the BLS content to include:

- Advanced concepts in cardiac monitoring
- Invasive airway management skills
- Pharmacologic and electrical therapies
- Intravascular access techniques
- Special resuscitation situations
- Post-resuscitation management considerations

Additional certification may be required through successful completion of trauma continuing education courses.

EMERGENCY NURSING PRINCIPLES

Triage

ED **triage** is an organized system for sorting or classifying patients into priority levels depending on illness or injury severity. The organization of emergency care and the ED is structured through triage principles. The key concept is that patients who present to the ED with the highest acuity needs receive the quickest evaluation, treatment, and prioritized resource utilization such as x-rays, laboratory work, and computed tomography (CT) scans. These patients also have priority for hospital service areas, such as the operating room or cardiac catheterization laboratory. A person with a lower acuity problem may wait longer in the ED because the higher acuity patient is moved to the "head of the line." The staff may need to COMMUNICATE information about this system to the patient and family who may not understand why other patients are treated first.

TABLE 8-1 Descriptions of Training and Certifications for Emergency Nursing

CERTIFICATION	DESCRIPTION
Basic Life Support (BLS) (required)	Noninvasive assessment and management skills for airway maintenance and cardiopulmonary resuscitation (CPR)
Advanced Cardiac Life Support (ACLS) (usually required)	Invasive airway management skills, pharmacology, and electrical therapies, special resuscitation
Pediatric Advanced Life Support (PALS) (may be required)	Neonatal and pediatric resuscitation
Certified Emergency Nurse (CEN) (optional)	Validates core emergency nursing knowledge base

The triage nurse is the gatekeeper in the emergency care system. When patients present to the ED, regulatory standards dictate that a registered nurse (RN), physician, or physician assistant (PA) perform a rapid assessment to determine triage priority. However, the RN is typically the person assigned to perform the triage function in most hospitals. The triage nurse requires appropriate training and experience in both emergency nursing and triage decision-making concepts to develop an expert knowledge base, as well as ongoing mentoring and quality improvement feedback (Dateo, 2013). In some instances, the triage nurse may seek the input of an emergency physician, advanced practice nurse (e.g., nurse practitioner [NP]), or PA to help establish the acuity level if the patient's presentation is highly unusual.

Based on the triage priority, patients may be rushed into a treatment room, directed to a lower acuity area within the ED, or asked to sit in the waiting room. Variations on this theme include:

- Triage nurse–initiated protocols for laboratory work or diagnostic studies that may be performed before the patient is actually evaluated by a physician
- Initiation of care while the patient is on a stretcher in the hallway of a crowded ED

These protocols are especially beneficial for certain populations who require rapid diagnosis and COLLABORATIVE treatment within a defined time frame from ED arrival to meet established standards of care. Examples are patients with chest pain or those with a clinical presentation indicative of stroke, sepsis, or pneumonia.

Emergent, Urgent, and Nonurgent Categories

Many triage systems can be used by a hospital ED. Any system must be applied consistently by triage nursing staff and endorsed by the emergency medicine physician staff. Based on the severity of the patient's condition, a well-known triage scheme used in the United States is the three-tiered model of "emergent, urgent, and nonurgent" (Table 8-2). In this system, for example,

TABLE 8-2 Three-Tiered Triage System and Examples of Patients Triaged in Each Tier

TIER LEVEL	EXAMPLES OF PATIENTS TRIAGED IN EACH TIER
Emergent (life threatening)	Respiratory distress Chest pain with diaphoresis Stroke Active hemorrhage Unstable vital signs
Urgent (needs quick treatment, but not immediately life threatening)	Severe abdominal pain Renal colic Displaced or multiple fractures Complex or multiple soft tissue injuries New-onset respiratory infection, especially pneumonia in older adults
Nonurgent (could wait several hours if needed without fear of deterioration)	Skin rash Strains and sprains "Colds" Simple fracture

a patient experiencing crushing substernal chest pain, shortness of breath, and diaphoresis would be classified as emergent and triaged immediately to a treatment room within the ED. Similarly, a critically injured trauma patient or a person with an active hemorrhage would also be prioritized as emergent. The **emergent triage** category implies that a condition exists that poses an immediate threat to life or limb.

The **urgent triage** category indicates that the patient should be treated quickly but that an immediate threat to life does not exist at the moment. Reassessment is needed if a physician cannot evaluate the patient in a timely manner. In people with evidence of clinical deterioration, triage priority may be upgraded from urgent to emergent. Examples of patients who typically fall into the urgent category are those with a new onset of pneumonia (as long as respiratory failure does not appear imminent), renal colic, complex lacerations not associated with major hemorrhage, displaced fractures or dislocations, and temperature greater than 101° F (38.3° C). Those categorized as **nonurgent** can generally tolerate waiting several hours for health care services without a significant risk for clinical deterioration. Conditions within this classification include patients with sprains and strains, simple fractures, "cold" symptoms, and skin rashes.

Other Multi-Tiered Models

To further sort patient conditions within an acuity classification or triage priority system, four- and five-tier triage models also exist. Such models are based either on comprehensive lists of conditions that indicate the particular triage priority to which a patient should be assigned or on the nature of resources that a patient will use in the ED setting. A patient situation may generate various triage classifications in different hospitals depending on the triage priority system used at that particular institution. Some schemes may even take into account the presence of pre-existing conditions such as a history of anticoagulant use, diabetes, heart disease, and organ transplantation.

It is surprising that there is no universally accepted triage system recognized in the United States. Thus there is no standardization of triage acuity data to compare patient acuity among hospitals. Medical providers, health insurance companies, and patients often disagree on the definition of an emergent versus a nonurgent ED visit, making it essential to use a practical triage system to maintain department efficiency and allocation of resources (Aacharya et al., 2011). The Emergency Nurses Association in COLLABORATION with the American College of Emergency Physicians studied the available research literature on acuity scales and concluded that two standardized five-level systems, the **Emergency Severity Index (ESI)** and the **Canadian Triage Acuity Scale (CTAS)**, are the most reliable (Shelton, 2010). The ESI model uses an algorithm that fosters rapid, reliable, and clinically pertinent categorization of patients into five groups, from level 1 (emergent) to level 5 (nonurgent). The CTAS model differs from ESI in that lists of descriptors are used to establish the triage level.

Whatever triage model is used, triage nurses must employ a systematic approach, apply solid clinical decision-making skills, and maintain a caring ethic. Compassion fatigue, or burn-out, can hinder objectivity in dealing with patients who present to the ED. A biased approach threatens the ED nurse's ability to triage patients accurately. Mistriage is a patient SAFETY risk that can be the "root cause" of delayed or inadequate treatment with potentially deadly consequences.

NCLEX EXAMINATION CHALLENGE

Safe and Effective Care Environment

The emergency department nurse is assigned to five clients waiting for orders to be implemented. Which client does the nurse assess first?

A. 60-year-old waiting for transport to the operating room for an emergency appendectomy
B. 25-year-old with a closed femur fracture who received pain medication 10 minutes ago
C. 30-year-old with nausea and vomiting who has IV fluids infusing and is now sleeping
D. 28-year-old construction worker with a laceration to the arm that is waiting to be sutured

Disposition

At the conclusion of the assessment, the physician must make a decision regarding patient disposition (i.e., where the patient should go after being discharged from the ED). Should the patient be admitted to the hospital, transferred to a specialty care center, or be discharged to home with instructions for continued care and follow-up? Usually, the answer is straightforward. A patient who has an evolving myocardial infarction, stroke, or acute surgical need is admitted.

Sometimes, though, the ED disposition decision is less clear. Often the physician discusses this decision in COLLABORATION with the emergency nurse. The nurse may have a greater sense of how well a patient will manage in a home setting depending on whether other family members or friends are available to assist and are reliable. For example, in the event a patient with a minor head injury has suffered a loss of consciousness, someone is typically expected to remain with that person for

CONSIDERATIONS FOR OLDER ADULTS

Patient-Centered Care QSEN

If discharge from the ED to home is possible, ensure that safety issues are considered. For example, collaborate with the emergency department physician to evaluate the patient's prescription and over-the-counter medications to determine if the drug regimen should be continued. Involve the ED-based pharmacist if one is available for consultation when necessary. If the medication regimen needs to be changed, be sure that the patient and family member or significant other has the new information in writing and that it is explained verbally. If needed, assess whether the patient has someone who can dispense medications into a "medi-set" to ensure accuracy and prevent adverse drug events. Consider a social services or case management referral for those patients in need of financial resources to obtain prescribed medications.

To prevent future ED visits, screen older adults per agency policy for functional assessment, cognitive assessment, and risk for falls. Depression screening is also important because suicide rates are two times higher among older adults when compared with younger adults. White men older than 85 years are at the highest risk (Touhy & Jett, 2012).

More than half of all older patients are admitted to the hospital directly from the ED (Nolan, 2009). If hospitalization is needed, determine if the patient has advance directives or is able to make decisions about advance directives before admission. If the patient was admitted from a nursing home, contact the facility to let them know the patient's status. If the patient was receiving home health care services, notify the agency about the hospital admission. Contact the patient's primary physician and designated family member if he or she is not present with the patient.

the first 12 to 24 hours to be sure that he or she does not show any evidence of neurologic deterioration. Another common scenario involves the potential risk to the patient in cases of actual or suspected domestic violence. If discharge to home is not deemed safe, the patient may be admitted to the hospital in an observation status until resources can be organized to provide for a safe environment. Coordinate the discharge plan and continuing care with the social worker or case manager.

Case Management

Some EDs employ registered nurse case managers who screen ED patients and intervene when necessary to arrange appropriate referral and follow-up. This is an evolving role in the ED setting that can be beneficial in providing comprehensive care and as a strategy to avoid inappropriate use of resources.

ED case managers, supported by electronic information systems, can review the ED census on both a "real-time" and a retrospective basis to determine which patients have visited the ED frequently in a given period. The case manager can then determine the reasons they sought emergency services, such as lack of a primary health care provider, exacerbation ("flare-up") of a chronic condition, a lack of health education, or lack of the financial resources necessary to manage the health condition. COLLABORATIVE case management interventions include facilitating referrals to primary care providers or to subsidized community-based health clinics for patients or families in need of routine services.

For those with needs related to chronic conditions, the case manager can arrange referral into appropriate disease management programs in the community if available. Disease management programs are specific to a particular condition such as asthma, COPD, diabetes, hypertension, heart failure, and renal failure. They help patients learn how to manage their condition on a day-to-day basis to prevent exacerbations or clinical deterioration. The desired outcome is to keep the person out of the hospital as long as possible. Health teaching is a key component of these programs. For other health teaching needs, the ED case manager directs the patient to the appropriate educational resources such as a health educator, registered dietitian, or community organization (e.g., the American Cancer Society, the American Heart Association).

Other functions of the ED case manager might include working in COLLABORATION with staff to plan disposition for homeless people, locating a safe environment for victims of domestic violence or elder abuse, or providing information on resources for low-cost or free prescriptions. Homeless adults often have multiple chronic medical illnesses for which they visit emergency departments frequently. A large study of homeless adults with chronic medical illnesses demonstrated a decrease in ED visits and hospital admissions as a result of an organized follow-up system for housing and ongoing case management support. (See the Quality Improvement box.)

Patient and Family Education

A key role of the emergency nurse is health teaching. At the most basic level, nurses review discharge instructions with the patient and family before signing them out of the department.

In addition to discharge instructions, the ED environment and community-at-large present many opportunities for health education. Emergency nurses are in an ideal position to educate the public about wellness and injury-prevention strategies. If the patient presented after a motor vehicle crash, for instance, the nurse can reinforce the need to wear seat belts or use child safety seats correctly. ED visits that result from mishaps in the home provide an excellent opportunity to discuss home SAFETY issues (e.g., the need for smoke detectors and carbon monoxide

QUALITY IMPROVEMENT QSEN

Improving the Flow of Stable Patients Through an Emergency Department

Popovich, M.A., Boyd, C., Dachenhaus, T., & Kusler, D. (2012). Improving stable patient flow through the emergency department by utilizing evidence-based practice: One hospital's journey. *Journal of Emergency Nursing, 38*(5), 474-478.

Many nonemergent patients use emergency departments (EDs) for medical care, resulting in overcrowding, lengthy wait times, patient dissatisfaction, and increasing numbers of patients who leave without being seen (LWBS). Increased length of wait has been correlated with poorer outcomes. A project was designed in the country's fifth-largest pediatric emergency department to investigate whether an evidence-based, volume-driven protocol would increase rapid treatment of stable patients. The protocol included a volume-based driver, unlike other tools used in EDs to manage patient flow, staffing, and resource allocation, such as the Emergency Severity Index (ESI), which is a 5-level decision-making tool used in triage. The protocol was designed to determine when to open the satellite unit for stable patients.

A participating hospital contained a 68-bed Level I trauma center and a nearby 8-bed satellite unit. A benchmark of 120 minutes for total length of stay (TLOS) was established as the quality indicator. After reviewing ED statistics, a tool was developed that considered total patient census and the number of ESI 4 and 5 patients in the unit. The triggers were a total census of 55 and/or 11 to 16 ESI level 4 patients and/or 5 to 7 ESI level 5 patients in the department. Other considerations included more than two people in the triage line, more than three people in the lobby waiting to be seen, and whether the urgent care section was full. Training was conducted to ensure consistency among the nurses in categorizing level 4 and level 5 patients. Use of the tool increased the number of days the satellite was open and decreased the number of patients who LWBS by 29%. The 120-minute benchmark was not met, but only by 7.5 minutes.

Commentary: Implications for Practice and Research

This demonstrated that patient satisfaction and outcomes were diminished as waiting times for ED services increased. EDs using an evidence-based tool can eliminate personal opinions when considering whether to use additional resources to expedite the flow of stable patients through the department. Specifying triggers for activating these resources can allow for better use of ED services. Research should continue on fine-tuning the tool to meet the needs of individual EDs, correlating use of the tool and patient outcomes, and should investigate patient satisfaction with the resulting (it is hoped decreased) wait times.

CULTURAL CONSIDERATIONS

Patient-Centered Care QSEN

Most discharge instructions are either preprinted or computer generated and can be customized to address the patient's needs. Consider his or her reading level, primary language, and visual acuity. Educational materials and instructions should be available at no higher than the 6th-grade reading level. For patients who have English as a second language, many hospitals have educational materials available in Spanish and other regional languages. However, interpreters may be necessary to assist the health care provider customize the information appropriately. For older adults and others with vision deficits, large-print materials may be helpful.

detectors) and fall prevention tips (e.g., the need for proper lighting, removal of throw rugs). Injury is not the only topic that affords a teaching opportunity. A new onset or an exacerbation of a medical condition also allows for education, such as how to measure blood glucose and ways to control blood pressure or reduce the risk for heart disease.

Death in the Emergency Department

Not all critically ill or injured patients who come to the ED can be saved. Sometimes a patient's death is expected by family members, typically when they have dealt with a loved one's terminal condition or age-related decline. Usually, however, a death in the ED is a sudden and unexpected event that produces a state of crisis and chaos for family and significant others. Emergency department staff members need to address the needs of the family members in this overwhelming time.

If resuscitation efforts are still underway when the family arrives, one or two family members may be given the opportunity to be present during lifesaving procedures. Family presence during resuscitation is gaining wider acceptance in the health care community; however, a significant number of hospitals still have not devised clear policies or guidelines to facilitate family-witnessed resuscitation (Feagan & Fisher, 2011).

If the patient dies before family members arrive, ED staff members try to prepare the body and the room for viewing by the family. However, certain types of ED deaths may require forensic investigation or become medical examiner's cases. Therefore ED staff may not be able to remove IV lines and indwelling tubes or clean the patient's skin if these actions could potentially damage evidence. Trauma deaths, suspected homicide, or abuse cases always fall into this category. In these situations, cover the body with a sheet or blanket while leaving the patient's face exposed, and dim the lights before family viewing.

When dealing with family members in crisis, simple and concrete COMMUNICATION is best. Words such as *death* or *died*, although seemingly harsh, create less confusion than terms such as *expired* or *passed away*. Demonstrate caring, compassion, and empathy during all interactions, even in periods of heightened emotions. Intense grief can provoke a range of family reactions from silence to violence. If available, coordinate with crisis staff (social workers or psychiatric nurses) to assist families and maintain SAFETY during this time. Offer the family the option of speaking with clergy or calling someone of their choice for additional support. A family member may need to be admitted to the ED to be treated for anxiety or physical manifestations of stress such as chest pain, difficulty breathing, or severe headache.

Dealing with death is often difficult for ED personnel, especially during busy periods when the ability to console family members may be limited. In response, some emergency departments have developed bereavement committees that focus on meeting the needs of grieving families. Actions such as sending sympathy cards, attending funerals, making follow-up phone calls, and creating memory boxes are common. These actions help COMMUNICATE caring and compassion after the moment of crisis.

THE IMPACT OF HOMELESSNESS

Homelessness affected 636,000 people in 2011, an increase of 1% from the prior year (National Alliance to End Homelessness, 2012). The homeless population is made up of both adults and children who live from day to day in a state of fear, chaos, and confusion (Gerber, 2013). People become homeless as a result of a crisis or persistent poverty (Gerber, 2013). They have a high incidence of acute and chronic health conditions, psychiatric illnesses, physical disabilities or limitations, and problems with substance abuse (Gerber, 2013). They are vulnerable to physical trauma, weather exposure, sexually transmitted diseases, infestation, and infectious diseases such as tuberculosis and influenza.

Homeless patients often seek ED care for a variety of reasons. Because the ED is open 24 hours per day and is mandated by federal law to perform an emergency medical screening examination on all of their patients, patients who are homeless know that they will gain entry despite their inability to pay for services. The ED represents a safe place to go for shelter in poor weather and for food, medical care, pain relief, and human interaction. Some homeless patients simply seek a temporary respite from their current living conditions, which may be a park, homeless shelter, car, abandoned building, or cardboard box. Those people who have been persistently homeless may assimilate into the homeless culture, learn to take great pride in their survival skills, and fiercely protect their few belongings as well as their living space. They may develop a distrust of outsiders, including members of the health care profession, and are especially sensitive to any perceived bias or stereotyping (Gerber, 2013).

Patients who are homeless bring special challenges to their ED evaluation, treatment, and disposition. Some visit the ED frequently and do not adhere to treatment recommendations or follow-up with community referrals. Those with mental illness or substance abuse may act out or become disruptive, posing a SAFETY risk to staff and patients.

To best care for homeless patients in the ED setting, nurses must first maintain their situational awareness and attend to their own needs for personal safety. These include not only anticipating the potential for violent behavior but also using Standard Precautions and assessing the need to isolate the patient in a negative pressure room if airborne disease such as tuberculosis (TB) is a concern. The key nursing action is to demonstrate behaviors that promote trust. These include making eye contact (if culturally appropriate), speaking calmly, avoiding any prejudicial or stereotypical remarks, being patient, showing genuine care and concern by listening, following through on promises, and exercising caution when there is a need to enter into the patient's personal space (Gerber, 2013). Clear professional boundaries must be stated if the patient becomes disruptive, profane, or sexually inappropriate. While collaborating with the emergency care provider to ensure that the patient's emergency medical needs are identified and treated, consult a social worker or case manager to work with the patient in identifying safety needs, referral options, and community resources. It is also important to develop an individual care plan with the interdisciplinary health care team if the patient uses the ED frequently. This type of care plan is extremely beneficial in establishing a consistent approach to patient management, especially when the patient has complex conditions or exhibits drug-seeking and disruptive behavior.

TRAUMA NURSING PRINCIPLES

The general public tends to use the term *trauma* to mean any type of crisis ranging from a heart attack to psychological stress. Among health care professionals, though, **trauma** refers to bodily injury. More than 180,000 people in the United States die each year as a result of injuries, and nearly 2 million are hospitalized, often with permanent and disabling consequences (National Center for Injury Prevention and Control [NCIPC], 2012). Injuries can be categorized as either intentional (i.e., assault, homicide, suicide) or unintentional (i.e., accidents). *Unintentional injury,* such as a motor vehicle crash, is the leading cause of death for Americans younger than 35 years and is one of today's most significant public health problems (NCIPC, 2012).

Injury management is a key component of emergency department services. About 30 million people in the United States visit the ED each year to receive treatment for injuries (NCIPC, 2012). Therefore an important part of emergency nursing practice is a core competency in general trauma care. For emergency nurses who work in accredited trauma centers, opportunities typically exist to further develop expertise in trauma nursing through ongoing clinical practice, specialty training programs, and continuing education. Trauma nursing is a field that encompasses the continuum of care from injury prevention and prehospital services to acute care, rehabilitation, and, ultimately, community reintegration.

Trauma Centers and Trauma Systems

Trauma centers have their roots in military medicine. Injured soldiers who received rapid transport from the battlefield and treatment from skilled health care personnel had a survival advantage in the mobile army surgical hospital (MASH) units first deployed in the Korean and Vietnam wars. Consequently, the MASH unit became the original model for the development of civilian trauma centers. Today's **trauma center** in the United States is a specialty care facility that provides competent and timely trauma services to patients, depending on its designated level of capability.

Trauma Centers

Not all EDs that offer around-the-clock emergency services are trauma centers. The American College of Surgeons Committee on Trauma (2006) has set forth national standards for trauma center accreditation and categorizes the resource requirements necessary for the highest capability trauma center (Level I) to the lowest (Level IV) (Table 8-3).

A *Level I trauma center* is a regional resource facility that is capable of providing leadership and total COLLABORATIVE care for every aspect of injury, from prevention through rehabilitation. These centers also have a responsibility to offer professional and community education programs, conduct research, and participate in system planning. Because a significant resource and experience commitment is required to maintain strict accreditation standards, Level I trauma centers are usually located in large teaching hospitals and serve dense population areas (Fig. 8-4).

Level II trauma centers are usually located in community hospitals and are capable of providing care to the vast majority of injured patients. However, a Level II trauma center may not be able to meet the resource needs of patients who require very complex injury management, such as those in need of advanced surgical care. These people are generally transferred to a Level I trauma center for specialty care. In communities without a Level I trauma center, Level II centers play a significant leadership role in injury management, education, prevention, and emergency preparedness planning.

A *Level III trauma center* is a critical link to higher capability trauma centers in communities that do not have ready access to Level I or Level II centers. The primary focus is initial injury stabilization and patient transfer. Level III trauma centers are usually found in smaller, rural hospitals and serve areas with low population density. Because Level III trauma centers have general surgeons and orthopedic surgeons immediately available, patients with some major injuries may be admitted for care. However, if the injuries are severe or critical, transfer to a Level I or II trauma center occurs after ED assessment, resuscitation, and stabilization—sometimes after emergent, lifesaving surgery. Patients are typically transported out in either an advanced life support ambulance or helicopter with critical care transport personnel in attendance.

The function of a *Level IV trauma center* is to offer advanced life support care in rural or remote settings that do not have ready access to a higher-level trauma center, such as a ski area. Patients are stabilized to the best degree possible before transfer,

TABLE 8-3 Levels and Functions of Trauma Centers

LEVELS OF TRAUMA CENTER	FUNCTIONS OF TRAUMA CENTER
Level I	Usually located in large teaching hospital systems in densely populated areas Provides a full continuum of trauma services for all patients Conducting research is a requirement for designation
Level II and Level III	Both typically located in community hospitals **Level II** Provides care to most injured patients Transports patient if needs exceed resource capabilities **Level III** Stabilizes patients with major injuries Transports patient if needs exceed resource capabilities
Level IV	Usually located in rural and remote areas Provides basic trauma patient stabilization and advanced life support within resource capabilities Arranges transport to higher trauma center levels as necessary

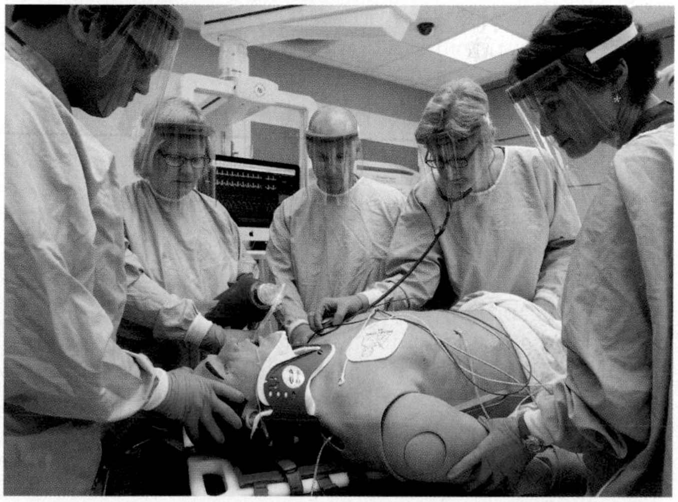

FIG. 8-4 A trauma team participates in a realistic trauma resuscitation simulation. This type of training ensures staff remain proficient in skills and able to care for any situation that might present to the emergency department (ED).

using available personnel such as advanced practice nurses, physician assistants, nurses, and paramedics. Resources, including the consistent availability of a physician, may be extremely limited. Transport time to the final care center can be prolonged because of both distance and bad weather conditions that may prevent transfer by air.

Level III and Level IV trauma centers establish close COLLABORATIVE relationships with Level I and Level II trauma centers. Based on accreditation standards, care providers at Levels I and II trauma centers have a responsibility to readily accept injured patients in transfer. They provide timely feedback to trauma personnel at referring hospitals and share expertise by offering educational opportunities to advance trauma care delivery in the region. In addition, personnel from all levels of trauma centers participate in focused system improvement and patient safety initiatives that enhance quality of care and solve identified problems.

Trauma Systems

Trauma centers save lives—but a trauma center is only as good as the overall trauma system that supports it. A **trauma system** is an organized and integrated approach to trauma care designed to ensure that all critical elements of trauma care delivery are aligned to meet the injured patient's needs. These elements include (Cooper & Laskowski-Jones, 2006):

- Access to care through COMMUNICATION technology (e.g., an enhanced 911 service)
- Timely availability of prehospital emergency medical care
- Rapid transport to a qualified trauma center
- Early provision of rehabilitation services
- System-wide injury prevention, research, and education initiatives

The overall desired outcome of an organized trauma system is to enable an injured patient not only to recover from trauma but also to return to a productive role in society.

A well-functioning trauma system is also essential to general public health and SAFETY. It provides the structure necessary for disaster readiness and community emergency preparedness (see Chapter 10). Although most states now have at least some basic elements of a trauma system in place, significant gaps still exist in many regions.

Mechanism of Injury

The **mechanism of injury (MOI)** describes how the patient's traumatic event occurred, such as a high-speed motor vehicle crash, a fall from a standing height, or a gunshot wound to the torso. Knowing key details about the MOI can provide insight into the energy forces involved and may help trauma care providers predict injury types and, in some cases, patient outcomes. Prehospital care providers report the MOI as a COMMUNICATION standard when handing off care to ED and trauma personnel. Similarly, patients who present to the ED for medical care will often relate the MOI by describing the particular chain of events that caused their injuries.

Two of the most common injury-producing mechanisms are blunt trauma and penetrating trauma. **Blunt trauma** results from impact forces like those sustained in a motor vehicle crash, a fall, and an assault with fists, kicks, or a baseball bat. **Blast effect** from an exploding bomb also causes blunt trauma. The energy transmitted from a blunt trauma mechanism, particularly the rapid **acceleration-deceleration** forces involved in high-speed crashes or falls from a great height, produces injury by tearing, shearing, and compressing anatomic structures. Trauma to bones, blood vessels, and soft tissues occurs.

Penetrating trauma is caused by injury from sharp objects and projectiles. Examples are wounds from knives, ice picks, and other comparable implements, as well as bullets (gunshot wounds [GSWs]) or pellets. Fragments of metal, glass, or other materials that become airborne in an explosion (shrapnel) can also produce penetrating trauma. Each mechanism has the risk for specific injury patterns and severity that the trauma team considers when planning diagnostic evaluation and management strategies. Certain injury mechanisms, such as a gunshot wound to the chest or abdomen or a stab wound to the neck, are so highly associated with life-threatening consequences that they automatically require trauma team intervention for a rapid and coordinated resuscitation response.

Primary Survey and Resuscitation Interventions

A basic tenet of emergency care in any environment is scene SAFETY. In the prehospital setting, emergency care providers must ensure that they are aware of any hazards that might pose a threat to rescuers and take actions to decrease or eliminate the risk. This same concept applies to the hospital ED setting. Before engaging in trauma resuscitation as a nurse member of the trauma team, keep in mind that there is a high risk for contamination with blood and body fluids. For this reason, use Standard Precautions in *all* resuscitation situations and at other times when exposure to blood and body fluids is likely. Proper attire consists of an impervious cover gown, gloves, eye protection, a facemask, and surgical cap, as well as shoe covers (if *significant* blood loss is anticipated, such as during an ED procedure).

The initial assessment of the trauma patient is called the **primary survey**, which is an organized system to rapidly identify and effectively manage immediate threats to life. The primary survey is based on a standard "ABC" mnemonic plus a "D" and "E" for trauma patients: airway/cervical spine (**A**); breathing (**B**); circulation (**C**); disability (**D**); and exposure (**E**). Resuscitation efforts occur simultaneously with each element of the primary survey (American College of Surgeons Committee on Trauma, 2008; Laskowski-Jones, 2009). Even though the resuscitation team may encounter multiple clinical problems or injuries, issues identified in the primary survey are managed before the team engages in interventions of lower priority, such as splinting fractures and dressing wounds.

A: Airway/Cervical Spine

Like for any patient, the highest priority intervention is to establish a patent airway. Even minutes without an adequate oxygen supply can lead to brain injury that can progress to anoxic brain death.

In general, a non-rebreather mask is best for the spontaneously breathing patient. Bag-valve-mask (BVM) ventilation with the appropriate airway adjunct and a 100% oxygen source is indicated for the person who needs ventilatory assistance during resuscitation. A patient with significantly impaired consciousness requires an endotracheal tube and mechanical ventilation (American College of Surgeons Committee on Trauma, 2008).

B: Breathing

After the airway is successfully secured, breathing becomes the next priority in the primary survey. *This assessment determines*

! NURSING SAFETY PRIORITY (QSEN)

Critical Rescue

Clear the airway of any secretions or debris either with a suction catheter or manually if necessary. Protect the cervical spine in any trauma patient with the potential for spinal injury by manually aligning the neck in a neutral, in-line position and using a jaw-thrust maneuver when establishing an airway. Provide supplemental oxygen for all patients who require resuscitation.

whether or not ventilatory efforts are effective—not only whether or not the patient is breathing. Listen to breath sounds and evaluate chest expansion, respiratory effort, and any evidence of chest wall trauma or physical abnormalities. Both apneic patients and those with poor ventilatory effort need BVM ventilation for support until endotracheal intubation is performed and a mechanical ventilator is used. If cardiopulmonary resuscitation (CPR) becomes necessary, the mechanical ventilator is disconnected and the patient is manually ventilated with a BVM device. Lung compliance can be assessed through sensing the degree of difficulty in ventilating the patient with the BVM.

C: Circulation

When effective ventilation is ensured, the priority shifts to circulation. The adequacy of heart rate, blood pressure, and overall perfusion becomes the focus of the assessment. Common threats to circulation include cardiac arrest, myocardial dysfunction, and hemorrhage leading to a shock state. Interventions are targeted at restoring effective circulation through cardiopulmonary resuscitation, hemorrhage control, IV vascular access with fluid and blood administration as necessary, and drug therapy. *External* hemorrhage is usually quite obvious and best controlled with firm, direct pressure on the bleeding site with thick, dry dressing material. This method is effective in decreasing blood flow for most wounds. *Tourniquets that occlude arterial blood flow distal to the injury may be considered to manage severe bleeding from extremity trauma when direct pressure fails to achieve hemorrhage control; hemostatic dressings (e.g., dressings impregnated with substances that speed the formation of a blood clot) are another essential tool to manage life-threatening hemorrhage (Strickler, 2010). Internal* hemorrhage is a more hidden complication that must be suspected in injured patients or those who present in a shock state.

In a resuscitation situation, blood pressure can be quickly and easily estimated before a manual cuff pressure can be obtained by palpating for the presence or absence of peripheral and central pulses:

- Presence of a radial pulse: BP at least 80 mm Hg systolic
- Presence of a femoral pulse: BP at least 70 mm Hg systolic
- Presence of a carotid pulse: BP at least 60 mm Hg systolic

By the time hypotension occurs, compensatory mechanisms used by the body in an attempt to maintain vital signs in a shock state have been exhausted. Timely, effective intervention is critical to preserve life and vital organ function.

IV access is best achieved initially with insertion of large-bore (16-gauge) peripheral IV lines in the antecubital area (inside bend of the elbow). Additional access can be obtained via central veins in the femoral, subclavian, or jugular sites using large-bore (8.5 Fr) central venous catheters. Intraosseous access is an excellent initial approach for critically ill patients when veins cannot be rapidly accessed by the resuscitation team (see Chapter 13 for discussion of intraosseous infusion therapy). Ringer's lactate and 0.9% normal saline (NS) are the crystalloid solutions of choice for resuscitation; hypertonic saline may also be prescribed in some situations, particularly in the case of head trauma. Fluids and blood products should be warmed before administration to prevent hypothermia. Anticipate the need for rapid blood component administration in a hemorrhagic shock state using packed red blood cells, fresh frozen plasma, and platelets to both replace blood loss and prevent coagulopathy when significant hypotension persists after infusion of 2 L of solution (Davis et al., 2012). However, the priority intervention is to stop the bleeding.

D: Disability

The disability examination provides a rapid baseline assessment of neurologic status. A simple method to evaluate level of consciousness is the "AVPU" mnemonic:

- A: <u>A</u>lert
- V: Responsive to <u>v</u>oice
- P: Responsive to <u>p</u>ain
- U: <u>U</u>nresponsive

Another common way of determining and documenting level of consciousness is the **Glasgow Coma Scale (GCS)**, an assessment that scores eye opening, verbal response, and motor response. The lowest score is 3, which indicates a totally unresponsive patient; a normal GCS score is 15. Metabolic abnormalities (e.g., severe hypoglycemia), hypoxia, neurologic injury, and illicit drugs or alcohol can impair level of consciousness. Frequent reassessment is needed for rapid intervention in the event of neurologic compromise or deterioration.

E: Exposure

The final component of the primary survey is **exposure.**

! NURSING SAFETY PRIORITY (QSEN)

Action Alert

Remove all clothing to allow for thorough assessment. Always *cut away* clothing with scissors:

- During resuscitation when rapid access to the patient's body is critical
- When manipulating a patient's limbs to remove clothing could cause further injury
- When thermal or chemical burns have caused fabrics to melt into the patient's skin

If evidence preservation is an issue, handle items per institutional policy. Evidence may include articles of clothing, impaled objects, weapons, drugs, and bullets. Emergency nurses are often called upon to provide testimony in court regarding their recall of the presentation and treatment of patients in the ED. Examples of types of cases in which evidence collection is vital are rape, elder abuse, domestic violence, homicide, suicide, drug overdose, and assault.

Once clothing is removed, hypothermia (body temperature less than or equal to 97° F [36° C]) poses a risk to injured patients, especially those with burns and traumatic shock states (Moore, 2011). Hypothermia is discussed in detail in Chapter 9.

Table 8-4 highlights the primary survey and associated resuscitation interventions.

TABLE 8-4 The Primary Survey and Resuscitation Interventions

PRIORITIES OF THE PRIMARY SURVEY	EXAMPLES OF SPECIFIC INTERVENTIONS
A: Airway/cervical spine	Establish a patent airway by positioning, suctioning, and oxygen as needed. Protect the cervical spine by maintaining alignment; use a jaw-thrust maneuver if there is a risk for spinal injury. If the Glasgow Coma Scale (GCS) score is 8 or less or the patient is at risk for airway compromise, prepare for endotracheal intubation and mechanical ventilation.
B: Breathing	Assess breath sounds and respiratory effort. Observe for chest wall trauma or other physical abnormality. Prepare for chest decompression if needed. Prepare to assist ventilations if needed.
C: Circulation	Monitor vital signs, especially blood pressure and pulse. Maintain vascular access using a large-bore catheter. Use direct pressure for external bleeding; anticipate need for a tourniquet for severe, uncontrollable extremity hemorrhage and use of a hemostatic dressing.
D: Disability	Evaluate the patient's level of consciousness (LOC) using the GCS. Re-evaluate the patient's LOC frequently.
E: Exposure	Remove all clothing for a complete physical assessment. Prevent hypothermia (e.g., cover the patient with blankets, use heating devices, infuse warm solutions).

NCLEX EXAMINATION CHALLENGE

Safe and Effective Care Environment

A trauma client has been brought to the emergency department after a motor vehicle crash. The client has severe injuries. What action does the nurse perform first?

A. Start 2 large-bore IVs and run normal saline.
B. Apply oxygen and an oximeter probe to the client.
C. Stabilize the cervical spine and assess the airway.
D. Place pressure on a large bleeding wound to the forehead.

The Secondary Survey and Resuscitation Interventions

After the ED resuscitation team addresses the immediate life threats, other activities that the emergency nurse can anticipate include insertion of a gastric tube for decompression of the GI tract to prevent vomiting and aspiration, insertion of a urinary catheter to allow careful measure of urine output, and preparation for diagnostic studies. The resuscitation team also performs a more comprehensive head-to-toe assessment, known as the **secondary survey**, to identify other injuries or medical issues that need to be managed or that might affect the course of treatment.

Disposition

The patient may be transported immediately to the operating room or interventional radiology suite directly from the ED, depending on the nature of the injury. When no immediate procedural intervention is indicated, patients are admitted to inpatient units for management and nursing care based on the nature and severity of their injuries, as well as any other pre-existing medical conditions that could complicate trauma care. However, if the facility does not have the resource capabilities to manage the injured patient, the physician arranges for transfer to a higher level of care.

Work in COLLABORATION with the interdisciplinary team to address the trauma patient's complex health care needs, including early consultation with social services and the rehabilitation team. Coordinate with other support services as necessary, such as pastoral care, nutrition support, psychiatry, behavioral health specialists, and substance abuse counselors. Trauma centers are required to incorporate systems to identify patients with high-risk alcohol use (American College of Surgeons Committee on Trauma, 2006). An effective strategy is to implement an SBIRT (screening, brief intervention, and referral to treatment) program in which interdisciplinary trauma team members, including emergency and trauma nurses, are educated to assess patients for problem drinking. The typical interaction involves a brief, respectful conversation that offers feedback, advice, and motivation to reduce alcohol consumption (Desy et al., 2010).

Consider the needs of family members in crisis and address them when planning nursing care. A trauma advanced practice nurse, if available, can help coordinate trauma care by offering clinical expertise, facilitating COMMUNICATION among caregivers, and serving as an educator for the patient, staff, and family (Mower-Wade & Pirrung, 2010). They can organize family meetings with the interdisciplinary team and arrange for necessary resources. If this resource is not available, a case manager or specially educated direct care nurse may perform these functions.

GET READY FOR THE NCLEX® EXAMINATION!

KEY POINTS

Review these Key Points for each NCLEX Examination Client Needs Category.

Safe and Effective Care Environment

- Understand that emergency departments (EDs) are fast-paced, often crowded environments where care occurs for patients across the life span with a variety of health problems.
- Recognize that some vulnerable populations who present to the ED include patients who are uninsured (poor), homeless, and older adults. **Patient-Centered Care** QSEN
- Anticipate that some of the most common reasons that patients seek ED care are chest pain, abdominal pain, difficulty breathing, injury, headache, fever, and pain.
- COLLABORATE with members of the interdisciplinary health care team in the ED, which includes prehospital providers,

physicians, nurses, specialty teams, and support staff. **Teamwork and Collaboration** QSEN

- Review Chart 8-1 to plan and implement best practices to maintain staff and patient SAFETY in the ED. **Safety** QSEN
- Explain the core competencies needed for nurses to function in the ED, including assessment, priority setting, knowledge, technical skills, and COMMUNICATION.
- Understand that the three-level triage model categorizes patients as emergent, urgent, and nonurgent (see Table 8-2). The Emergency Severity Index is a five-tier triage system that uses both acuity and the prediction of necessary resources to rapidly categorize the priority of patients.
- Recall that trauma centers are categorized as Levels I through IV, based on their resource capabilities as listed in Table 8-3.
- Remember that the mechanism of injury describes the manner in which the traumatic event occurred.
- Recall that the two most common injury-producing mechanisms are blunt trauma and penetrating trauma.
- Prioritize resuscitation interventions based on the primary survey of the injured patient by implementing the steps of the primary survey and trauma resuscitation as outlined in Table 8-4.
- Recall that patient education as part of the discharge plan is an important part of ED nursing practice.

Psychosocial Integrity

- Provide support by working in COLLABORATION with the psychiatric crisis team as needed.

Physiological Integrity

- Remember the general process of admission through discharge in the ED. Patients managed in the ED are treated and stabilized before discharge. Patients may be discharged to their homes or be admitted for observation or inpatient care.
- Recall that about half of all older adults who visit the ED are admitted to the hospital. **Patient-Centered Care** QSEN
- Understand that ED nurses are accountable for preventing or reducing risks such as falls, medication errors, pressure ulcers, and hospital-acquired infections. COMMUNICATION with the older adult may be challenging if he or she has memory loss or develops acute delirium while in the ED. **Safety** QSEN

9 CHAPTER

Care of Patients with Common Environmental Emergencies

Linda Laskowski-Jones

http://evolve.elsevier.com/Iggy/

PRIORITY CONCEPTS

- Pain
- Thermoregulation
- Tissue Integrity

LEARNING OUTCOMES

Safe and Effective Care Environment

1. Collaborate with the interdisciplinary health care team when providing care for patients with common environmental emergencies.

Health Promotion and Maintenance

2. Teach people at risk how to prevent heat-related and cold-related injuries, especially older adults.
3. Teach people at risk how to prevent arthropod bites and stings and snakebites.

Physiological Integrity

4. Assess patients at high risk for environmental emergencies.
5. Prioritize first aid/prehospital interventions for patients who have thermoregulation problems.
6. Prioritize first aid/prehospital interventions for patients who have arthropod bites affecting tissue integrity.
7. Prioritize first aid/emergency care interventions for patients who have venomous snakebites.
8. Apply knowledge of pathophysiology to identify best practices for care of patients with environmental emergencies.
9. Develop an evidence-based plan of care for a patient who is allergic to bees and is stung.
10. Prioritize care for patients who have been struck by lightning.
11. Prioritize care for patients who survive a drowning incident.
12. Explain best practices for patients who are at risk for or experience altitude-related illnesses.

Recreational activities, as well as home and work responsibilities, inspire people of all ages to leave their homes and go outdoors. However, seemingly harmless outside activities can have associated environmental risks, especially for older adults. Some risks, such as insect bites or stings, reptile bites, and environmental conditions, may also pose threats indoors. This chapter provides an overview of selected environmental emergencies, their initial emergency management (first aid), and acute care interventions. Illness and injury prevention strategies for nurses to incorporate into their own lifestyle and health teaching opportunities are also discussed.

HEAT-RELATED ILLNESSES

High environmental temperature (above 95° F [35° C]) and high humidity (above 80%) are the most common environmental factors causing heat-related illnesses. These thermoregulation-related illnesses include heat exhaustion and heat stroke. Some of the most vulnerable, at-risk populations for these problems are:

- Older adults
- People with mental health conditions
- People who work outside, such as construction and agricultural workers (more men than women)
- Homeless people
- Illicit drug users (especially cocaine users)
- Outdoor athletes (recreational and professional)
- Members of the military who are stationed in countries with hot climates (e.g., Iraq, Afghanistan)

Older adults have less body fluid volume and can easily become dehydrated when exposed to excessive heat and humidity. Wearing heavy clothing, inadequate acclimatization to hot weather, and social disadvantage (e.g., poor housing, lack of air-conditioning) are also significant contributing factors.

A patient's health status can also increase the risk for heat-related illness, especially obesity, heart disease, fever, infection, strenuous exercise, seizures, mental health disorders, and all degrees of burns (even sunburn). In addition, the use of certain prescribed drugs such as lithium, neuroleptics, beta-adrenergic blockers, anticholinergics, angiotensin-converting

CHART 9-1 Nursing Focus on the Older Adult

Heat-Related Illness Prevention

- Avoid alcohol and caffeine.
- Prevent overexposure to the sun; use a sunscreen with an SPF of at least 30 with UVA and UVB protection.
- Rest frequently, and take breaks from being in a hot environment. Plan to limit activity at the hottest time of day.
- Wear clothing suited to the environment. Lightweight, light-colored, and loose-fitting clothing is best.
- Pay attention to your personal physical limitations; modify activities accordingly.
- Take cool baths or showers to help reduce body temperature.
- Stay indoors in air-conditioned buildings, if possible.
- Ask a neighbor, friend, or family member to check on the older adult at least twice a day during a heat wave.

SPF, Sun protection factor; *UVA,* ultraviolet A; *UVB,* ultraviolet B.

enzyme (ACE) inhibitors, and diuretics increases the risk for heat-related illness (Cusack et al., 2011).

HEALTH PROMOTION AND MAINTENANCE

Teach older adults before participating in any hot weather activity how to consider their risks and to take steps to eliminate or minimize them whenever possible. Ask them to have a family member, friend, or neighbor check on them several times each day to ensure that there are no signs of heat-related illness. Chart 9-1 lists other essential heat-related illness prevention strategies for older adults, many of which apply to adults of any age.

HEAT EXHAUSTION

❖ PATHOPHYSIOLOGY

Heat exhaustion is a syndrome resulting primarily from dehydration. It is caused by heavy perspiration, as well as inadequate fluid and electrolyte intake during heat exposure over hours to days. Patients feel ill, and their clinical manifestations resemble the flu. Profuse diaphoresis can lead to profound, even fatal, dehydration and hyponatremia caused by excessive sodium lost in perspiration. *If untreated, heat exhaustion can lead to heat stroke, which is a true emergency condition that has a very high mortality rate.*

❖ PATIENT-CENTERED COLLABORATIVE CARE

In heat exhaustion, patients usually have flu-like symptoms with headache, weakness, nausea, and/or vomiting. Body temperature is not significantly elevated in this condition. The patient may continue to perspire despite dehydration.

! NURSING SAFETY PRIORITY (QSEN)

Action Alert

Assess the patient for orthostatic hypotension and tachycardia, especially the older adult who is predisposed to rapid dehydration. Older adults who are already dehydrated often experience acute confusion and are at risk for falls.

Ask the person experiencing heat exhaustion to immediately stop physical activity; move him or her to a cool place, and use cooling measures. Effective cooling measures include placing cold packs on the neck, chest, abdomen, and groin; soaking the person in cool water; or fanning him or her while spraying water on the skin. Remove any constrictive clothing. Provide an oral rehydrating solution such as a sports drink or an oral rehydration therapy solution. Mistakenly drinking plain water can worsen the sodium deficit. *Do not give salt tablets*—they can cause stomach irritation, nausea, and vomiting. If these signs and symptoms persist, call an ambulance to transport the patient to the hospital.

In the clinical setting, monitor vital signs. Rehydrate the patient with IV 0.9% saline solution if nausea or vomiting persists. Draw blood for serum electrolyte analysis. Hospital admission is indicated only for patients who have other health problems that are worsened by the heat-related illness or for those with severe dehydration. The management of hypovolemic dehydration is discussed in more detail in Chapter 11.

HEAT STROKE

❖ PATHOPHYSIOLOGY

Heat stroke is a *true medical emergency* in which body temperature may exceed 104° F (40° C). It has a high mortality rate if not treated in a timely manner. The victim's THERMOREGULATION mechanisms fail and cannot adjust for a critical elevation in body temperature (Laskowski-Jones, 2010). If the condition is not treated or the patient does not respond to treatment, organ dysfunction and death can result. In their cohort study of 16 emergency departments, Hausfater et al. (2010b) found that nine factors help predict mortality in patients admitted to emergency departments with non-exertional heat stroke (see the Evidence-Based Practice box).

The two major types of heat stroke are exertional and classic. **Exertional heat stroke** has a sudden onset and is often the result of strenuous physical activity in hot, humid conditions. Not being used to hot weather and wearing clothing too heavy for the environment are common contributing factors. **Classic heat stroke,** also referred to as *non-exertional heat stroke,* occurs over a period of time as a result of chronic exposure to a hot, humid environment, such as a home without air-conditioning in the high heat of the summer. It generally affects ill and older adults and causes several hundred deaths in the United States every year. The risk factors for heat stroke are similar to those for heat exhaustion.

❖ PATIENT-CENTERED COLLABORATIVE CARE

◆ Assessment

Victims of heat stroke have a profoundly elevated body temperature (above 104° F [40° C]). *Although the patient's skin is hot and dry, the presence of sweating does not rule out heat stroke—people with heat stroke may continue to perspire.*

Mental status changes occur as a result of thermal injury to the brain. Manifestations can include confusion, bizarre behavior, seizures, or even coma (Chart 9-2). Vital sign abnormalities may include hypotension, tachycardia, and tachypnea. Recent research demonstrates that cardiac troponin I (cTnI) is frequently elevated during non-exertional heat-related illnesses. A severe increase (>1.5 ng/mL) indicates severe myocardial damage and decreases the chance of patient survival 1 year after the event (Hausfater et al., 2010a).

Complications of THERMOREGULATION failure due to classic heat stroke include multiple organ dysfunction syndrome (MODS), renal impairment, electrolyte and acid-base

EVIDENCE-BASED PRACTICE QSEN

What Factors Predict Who Will Develop Non-exertional Heat Stroke?

Hausfater, P., Megarbane, B., Dautheville, S., Patzak, A., Andronikof, M., Andre, S., et al. (2010). Prognostic factors in non-exertional heatstroke. *Intensive Care Medicine, 36,* 272-280.

Heat-related illnesses are often medical emergencies that can lead to death. The authors presented findings of a large multi-center observational cohort study of 1456 patients who were admitted to 16 emergency departments (EDs) in teaching hospitals during heat waves. The mean age of the sample was 79 years, and 391 of them were critically ill on admission. All of the study patients had an elevated core body temperature. The survival rate for the study sample was only 57% at 1 year after diagnosis.

On retrospective review of the patients' charts, it was found that nine factors negatively influenced survival rates. They included an age older than 80 years, body temperature of over 104° F (40° C), systolic blood pressure less than 100 mm Hg, Glasgow Coma Scale score of less than 12, presence of cancer and/or cardiac disease, previous treatment with diuretics, living in an institution, and transported to the ED by ambulance.

Level of Evidence: 4

This study is a nonexperimental or descriptive cohort study, but it used a large sample size in multiple emergency departments. Random assignment or comparison of two groups was not appropriate for answering the research question.

Commentary: Implications for Practice and Research

The results of this study indicate that older, institutionalized patients with cardiac disease or cancer and heat stroke have a high risk for not surviving a year after the heat-related illness. The major nursing implication from this study is that more emphasis on preventing heat-related illnesses in institutionalized patients is needed, particularly if they are older than 80 years. Strengths of the study included the large sample size collected from multiple emergency departments. A weakness might be the level of evidence (Level 4: nonexperimental or descriptive cohort study), but this is probably outweighed by the sampling method and the fact that an experimental design was not appropriate to answer the research question. Nurses are in a key position to advocate for these patients and to implement interventions that can help prevent heat stroke. Early detection and treatment also are needed. Chart 9-1 lists best practices for decreasing the risk for heat-related illnesses in older adults.

disturbances, coagulopathy (abnormal clotting), pulmonary edema, and cerebral edema (O'Brien et al., 2012). Any of these problems can lead to death and are described in detail elsewhere in this book.

◆ *Interventions*

Coordinate care with the health care team to recognize and treat immediately and aggressively to achieve optimal patient outcomes. Chart 9-3 lists evidence-based emergency care of patients with heat stroke.

First Aid/Prehospital Care. Do not give food or liquid by mouth because vomiting and aspiration are risks in patients with neurologic impairment. Immediate medical care using advanced life support is essential.

Hospital Care. *The first priority for collaborative care is to monitor and support the patient's airway, breathing, and circulatory status.* Provide high-concentration oxygen therapy, start several IV lines with 0.9% saline solution, and insert an indwelling urinary catheter. Continue aggressive interventions to cool the patient until the rectal temperature is 102° F (38.9° C) (O'Brien et al., 2012). External continuous cooling methods include using cooling blankets and applying ice packs in the axillae and groin and on the neck and head. Internal cooling methods may include iced gastric and bladder lavage. Use a continuous core temperature–monitoring device (e.g., rectal or esophageal probe) or a temperature-monitoring urinary bladder catheter to prevent hypothermia.

If shivering occurs during the cooling process, give a parenteral benzodiazepine such as diazepam (Valium). Lorazepam (Ativan) is an alternative agent. Seizure activity can further elevate body temperature and is also treated with an IV benzodiazepine. Once the patient is stabilized, admission to a critical care unit is warranted to monitor for complications such as multi-system organ dysfunction syndrome and severe electrolyte imbalances; these problems increase mortality risk.

CHART 9-2 Key Features

Heat Stroke

- Body temperature more than 104° F (40° C)
- Hot and dry skin; may or may not perspire
- Mental status changes, such as:
  - Acute confusion
  - Bizarre behavior
  - Anxiety
  - Loss of coordination
  - Hallucinations
  - Agitation
  - Seizures
  - Coma
- Vital sign changes, including:
  - Hypotension
  - Tachycardia
  - Tachypnea (increased respiratory rate)
- Electrolyte imbalances, especially sodium and potassium
- Decreased renal function (oliguria)
- Coagulopathy (abnormal clotting)
- Pulmonary edema (crackles)

! NURSING SAFETY PRIORITY QSEN

Critical Rescue

After ensuring that the patient has a patent airway, effective breathing, and adequate circulation, use rapid cooling as the first priority for care. Methods for rapidly cooling include:

- Removing clothing
- Placing ice packs on the neck, axillae, chest, and groin
- Immersing the victim in cold water
- Wetting the patient's body with cold water and then fanning rapidly to aid in cooling by evaporation

Drenching the victim with large amounts of icy water may be the fastest, most effective means to reduce core body temperature (O'Brien et al., 2012).

? NCLEX EXAMINATION CHALLENGE

Physiological Integrity

An older client with heat exhaustion is being cooled with cool water spray and fanning. What assessment indicates to the nurse that the client needs hospitalization?

A. The client is alert and oriented.
B. The client's mucous membranes are dry and sticky.
C. The client reports weakness and nausea.
D. The client continues to sweat while being cooled.

CHART 9-3 **Best Practice for Patient Safety & Quality Care** QSEN

Emergency Care of the Patient with Heat Stroke: Restoring Thermoregulation

At the Scene

- Ensure a patent airway.
- Remove the patient from the hot environment (into air-conditioning or into the shade).
- Remove the patient's clothing.
- Pour or spray cold water on the patient's body and scalp.
- Fan the patient (not only the person providing care, but all surrounding people should fan the patient with newspapers or whatever is available).
- If ice is available, place ice in cloth or bags and position the packs on the patient's scalp, in the groin area, behind the neck, and in the armpits.
- Contact emergency medical services to transport the patient to the emergency department.

At the Hospital

- Give oxygen by mask or nasal cannula; be prepared for endotracheal intubation.
- Start at least one IV with a large-bore needle or cannula.
- Administer normal saline (0.9% sodium chloride) as prescribed, using cooled solutions if available.
- Use a cooling blanket.
- Do not give aspirin or any other antipyretics.
- Insert a rectal probe to measure core body temperature continuously, or use a rectal thermometer and assess temperature every 15 minutes.
- Insert an indwelling urinary drainage catheter.
- Monitor vital signs frequently as clinically indicated.
- Obtain baseline laboratory tests as quickly as possible: serum electrolytes, cardiac enzymes, liver enzymes, and complete blood count (CBC).
- Assess arterial blood gases.
- Administer muscle relaxants (benzodiazepines) if the patient begins to shiver.
- Measure urine output and specific gravity to determine fluid needs.
- Stop cooling interventions when core body temperature is reduced to 102° F (39° C).
- Obtain urinalysis, and monitor urine output.

SNAKEBITES

Although most snake species are nonvenomous (nonpoisonous) and harmless, there are two families of poisonous snakes in North America: pit vipers *(Crotalidae)* and coral snakes *(Elapidae)*.

Pit vipers are named for the characteristic depression between each eye and nostril that serves as a heat-sensitive organ for locating warm-blooded prey. They include various species of rattlesnakes, copperheads, and cottonmouths and account for the majority of the poisonous snakebites in the United States (Figs. 9-1 and 9-2).

Coral snakes are found from North Carolina to Florida and in the Gulf states through Texas and the southwestern United States. They have broad bands of red and black rings, separated by yellow or cream rings. These nonaggressive snakes have short, fixed fangs and inject highly neurotoxic venom into prey.

Most snakes fear humans and attempt to avoid contact with them. Sudden, unexpected confrontations at close range often lead to defensive strikes. Awareness is the key to snakebite prevention.

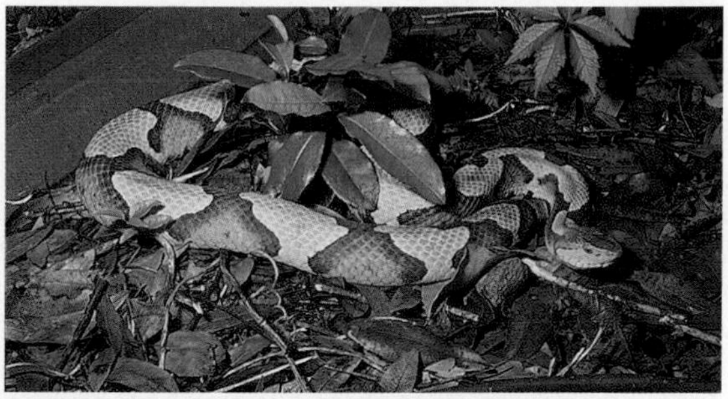

FIG. 9-1 Southern copperhead *(Agkistrodon contortrix)* has markings that make it almost invisible when lying in leaf litter.

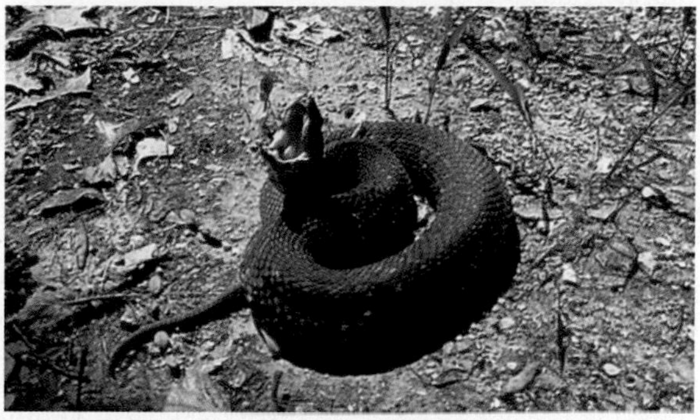

FIG. 9-2 Cottonmouth water moccasin *(Agkistrodon piscivorus)*. The open-mouthed threat gesture is characteristic of this semiaquatic pit viper.

CHART 9-4 **Patient and Family Education: Preparing for Self-Management**

Snakebite Prevention

- Do not keep venomous snakes as pets.
- Be extremely careful in locations where snakes may hide, such as tall grass, rock piles, ledges and crevices, woodpiles, brush, boxes, and cabinets. Snakes are most active on warm nights.
- Don protective attire such as boots, heavy pants, and leather gloves. When walking or hiking, use a walking stick or trekking poles.
- Inspect suspicious areas before placing hands and feet in them.
- Do not harass any snakes you may encounter. Striking distance can be up to two-thirds the length of the snake. Even young snakes pose a threat; they are capable of envenomation from birth.
- Be aware that newly dead or decapitated snakes can inflict a bite for up to an hour after death because of persistence of the bite reflex.
- Do not transport the snake with the victim to the medical facility for identification purposes; instead, take a digital photo of the snake at a safe distance if possible.

HEALTH PROMOTION AND MAINTENANCE

Chart 9-4 provides common-sense actions to avoid being bitten by a poisonous snake. Teach people who own snakes to follow these precautions. Remind them that snakebites can be life threatening.

NORTH AMERICAN PIT VIPERS

North American pit vipers can be differentiated from harmless snakes by these key anatomic features:

- A heat-sensing "pit"
- A triangular head that indicates the presence of venom glands and elliptical pupils

- Two retractable, curved fangs that have canals for venom flow
- Up to three sets of developing "replacement" fangs behind the primary fangs

Unlike copperheads and cottonmouths, rattlesnakes also have interlocking horny rings in their tails that vibrate and serve as a characteristic warning signal. Pit vipers can regulate the amount of venom flow through their fangs, depending, in part, on the size of the prey. The amount of venom injected in bites to humans varies. A bite might actually be "dry," meaning there is no **envenomation** (venom injection), yet there are distinctive fang marks on the patient. In contrast, "harmless" snakes do not have venom glands or fangs but can bite and leave skin marks.

❖ PATHOPHYSIOLOGY

When providing emergency care to a victim of snakebite, assess for evidence that venom has been injected into the body. The primary functions of venom are to immobilize, kill, and aid in digestion of prey. Therefore venom causes local and systemic toxic effects. The enzymes in venom break down human tissue proteins, alter membrane integrity, and impair blood clotting. The pathophysiologic effects of pit viper envenomation can lead to impaired TISSUE INTEGRITY from local tissue necrosis and massive tissue swelling, intravascular fluid shifts and hypovolemic shock, pulmonary edema, renal failure, hemorrhagic complications from disseminated intravascular coagulation (DIC), and death. These complications are discussed elsewhere in this book.

❖ PATIENT-CENTERED COLLABORATIVE CARE

◆ Assessment

The clinical manifestations of venom release are based on the type and amount of venom injected; the bite location; and the age, size, and health status of the victim. Puncture wounds in the skin are a key local sign of pit viper envenomation. One or more puncture wounds may be present, depending on how many fangs the snake has and how many times the snake struck the patient. Severe PAIN, swelling, and redness or **ecchymosis** (bruising) in the area around the bite are common. Hours later, vesicles or hemorrhagic bullae may form. Systemic responses to venom must be distinguished from the effects of anxiety and panic related to being bitten by a snake. Common reports by the victim include a minty, rubbery, or metallic taste in the mouth and tingling or paresthesias of the scalp, face, and lips. Other effects include muscle **fasciculations** (twitching) and weakness, nausea, vomiting, hypotension, seizures, and **coagulopathy** (clotting abnormalities) or DIC. If the bite site does not show evidence of local tissue swelling or redness within 8 hours, systemic effects are less likely to develop.

◆ Interventions

First Aid/Prehospital Care. First aid interventions for snakebite should begin in the field and can improve the victim's outcome.

Immobilizing the affected extremity in a position of function with a splint may help limit the spread of the venom. Maintain the extremity at the level of the heart. Keep the person warm, and provide calm reassurance. Do not offer any alcohol because it can cause the venom to spread through vasodilation (Bledsoe et al., 2009). *Do not incise or suck the wound, apply ice to it, or use a tourniquet—these actions are ineffective and can worsen the patient's outcome* (Norris et al., 2012).

> **! NURSING SAFETY PRIORITY (QSEN)**
>
> ***Critical Rescue***
>
> The first priority is to move the person to a safe area away from the snake and encourage rest to decrease venom circulation. Next, remove jewelry and constricting clothing before swelling worsens. Call for immediate emergency assistance. Do not attempt to capture or kill the snake, but do take digital photographs at a safe distance if possible to aid in snake identification.

Hospital Care. *Acute care in a hospital is required as soon as possible because envenomation is a medical emergency.* Supportive care includes supplemental oxygen, two large-bore IV lines, and infusion of crystalloid fluids such as normal saline solution or Ringer's lactate solution. Apply continuous cardiac and blood pressure monitoring equipment to quickly detect clinical deterioration. Because venom can cause severe PAIN at the bite site, opioids are indicated. Provide tetanus prophylaxis and wound care as part of the collaborative plan of care.

Severe pit viper bites cause coagulopathy and promote hemorrhage and tissue destruction. Along with typical baseline laboratory studies, anticipate obtaining specimens for a coagulation profile, complete blood count (CBC), creatine kinase (CK), type and crossmatch for possible blood transfusion, and urinalysis. An electrocardiogram (ECG) is necessary to detect evidence of myocardial ischemia or other cardiac abnormalities.

Obtain pertinent patient history related to the event, including a full description of the snake's appearance, the time the bite occurred, prehospital interventions, and any past incidence of snakebite or antivenom use. To accurately assess the development of tissue edema at the bite site, measure and record the circumference of the bitten extremity every 15 to 30 minutes. Delineate the border of skin discoloration or edema with a skin marker to better track the progression of venom effects.

Venom potency varies. Not all snakebite victims need antivenom administration. The decision whether or not to give antivenom is based on the severity of the snakebite. Table 9-1 classifies **envenomation** severity. *Contact the regional poison*

TABLE 9-1 Grades of Pit Viper Envenomation

ENVENOMATION	CHARACTERISTICS
None	Fang marks, but no local or systemic reactions
Minimal	Fang marks, local swelling and pain, but no systemic reactions
Moderate	Fang marks and swelling progressing beyond the site of the bite; systemic signs and symptoms, such as nausea, vomiting, paresthesias, and hypotension
Severe	Fang marks present with marked swelling of the extremity, subcutaneous ecchymosis, severe symptoms, including manifestations of coagulopathy

From Auerbach, P.S., Donner, H.J., & Weiss, E.A. (2013). *Field guide to wilderness medicine* (4th ed.). St. Louis: Mosby.

control center so that toxicologists can provide specific advice for antivenom dosing and medical management.

The newest and safest antivenom for pit viper bites is Crotalidae Polyvalent Immune Fab (CroFab), which is derived from sheep (ovine). This drug consists of specific antibody fragments of immunoglobulin G (IgG) that bind and neutralize toxins in pit viper venom to counteract its effects on the body (Norris et al., 2012). Unlike the older antivenoms that were derived from horse serum, serum sickness rarely occurs after IV CroFab administration. **Serum sickness** is a type III hypersensitivity reaction that develops within 3 to 21 days, first as a skin rash with progression to fever, joint PAIN, and **pruritus** (itching). Although mild to moderate allergic reactions such as pruritus and **urticaria** (hives) can occur, anaphylaxis is rare. If the patient has a known hypersensitivity to papain or papaya, which is used during the manufacturing process, CroFab is contraindicated unless the benefits are believed to outweigh the risks (Fougera Pharmaceuticals, Inc., 2008). Give CroFab cautiously to patients who have:

- A previous allergic reaction to antivenom therapy
- A hypersensitivity to bromelain (a pineapple-derived enzyme) or sheep protein
- Prior CroFab therapy for a past envenomation (patients can become sensitized to the foreign sheep protein)
- Pregnancy
- Sensitivity to mercury-containing products (the antivenom contains mercury)

CroFab should be given to patients as soon as possible, with the optimal timing within 6 hours of the bite (Fougera Pharmaceuticals, Inc., 2008). The recommended initial IV dose is 4 to 6 vials infused over 60 minutes. During the first 10 minutes, the infusion should be slow (25-50 mL/hr). Monitor the patient closely for an allergic reaction (e.g., hives, rash, difficulty breathing). If symptoms are not effectively controlled with the first dose, an additional 4 to 6 vials are recommended. Once the symptoms are under control, 2 more vials of CroFab are administered every 6 hours for a total of 18 hours of administration (Fougera Pharmaceuticals, Inc., 2008).

CORAL SNAKES

❖ PATHOPHYSIOLOGY

North American coral snakes are found in the southeastern and southwestern United States (Fig. 9-3). These snakes burrow into the ground and are nonaggressive. Coral snakes account for fewer than 1% of venomous snakebites in the United States (Norris, 2011). Their ability to inject venom is less efficient than that of the pit vipers. Their maxillary fangs are small and fixed in an upright position. Most bites occur when people attempt to handle the snake. Coral snake venom has two toxins: a nerve toxin and a muscle toxin. The amount of venom in an adult coral snake is enough to kill an adult.

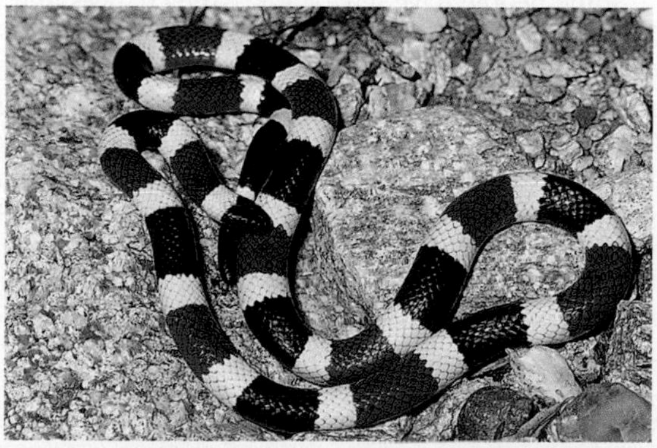

FIG. 9-3 Sonoran coral snake *(Micruroides euryxanthus)* is also known as the *Arizona coral snake.* No documented fatality has followed a bite by this species.

Coral snakes can be recognized by bands of black, red, and yellow that circle around the body of the snake. Several harmless snake species closely resemble the coral snake. If a black band lies between the red and yellow bands, the snake is usually nonvenomous. If the red band touches the yellow band, the snake is venomous. A helpful memory aid for identifying coral snakes is "red on yellow can kill a fellow" and "red on black, venom lack." *Be aware that this saying applies only to coral snakes found in the United States!*

❖ PATIENT-CENTERED COLLABORATIVE CARE

◆ Assessment

Manifestations of coral snake envenomation are the result of its neurotoxic properties. The physiologic effect is to block neurotransmission, which produces weakness, cranial nerve deficits (ptosis, diplopia, swallowing difficulty), an altered level of consciousness, and, ultimately, respiratory paralysis (Norris, 2011). Unlike the PAIN from pit viper bites, pain at the coral snakebite site may be only mild and transient. The venom is spread via the lymphatic system, but swelling, if present, is typically mild. Fang marks may be difficult to find because of the coral snake's small teeth. The toxic effects of coral snake venom also may be delayed up to 13 hours after a bite but then produce rapid clinical deterioration (Norris et al., 2012). Early signs and symptoms include nausea, vomiting, headache, pallor, and abdominal pain. Assess for neurologic manifestations, such as paresthesias (painful tingling), numbness, muscle fasciculations, and mental status changes, as well as cranial nerve and peripheral nerve deficits. Total flaccid paralysis may occur later, and the patient may have difficulty speaking, swallowing, and breathing. Clotting disorders do not occur.

Respiratory problems and cardiovascular collapse can occur in severe cases (Norris, 2011). Arterial blood gas analysis reveals respiratory insufficiency. The muscle toxin in the venom can cause an elevation in creatine kinase (CK) levels from muscle breakdown and produce **myoglobinuria** (release of muscle myoglobulin into the urine). Despite these clinical effects, death is rare if the patient receives timely management.

◆ Interventions

First Aid/Prehospital Care. Because several varieties of harmless snakes resemble the coral snake, the first priority, if possible, is to identify the snake as a coral snake. *However, if the snake cannot be positively identified, the victim should be treated as if venom has been injected.* Because coral snake venom does not destroy tissue, the field treatment to limit the spread of venom includes the use of pressure immobilization techniques (Norris et al., 2012). The affected extremity is encircled snugly with an elastic bandage or roller gauze dressing to impede lymphatic flow; it is then splinted. *This compression bandage must not be so tight that it impairs arterial flow. It should not be removed until the victim is managed at an acute care facility* (Norris et al., 2012).

Hospital Care. Once in an acute care setting, patients who have had an actual or potential coral snake envenomation will have continuous cardiac, blood pressure, and pulse oximetry monitoring and are admitted to a critical care unit. Prepare to provide aggressive airway management via endotracheal intubation if respiratory insufficiency or severe neurologic impairment occurs. Aspiration of secretions is a significant risk for this patient.

Coral snake antivenom is no longer manufactured in the United States. Until another drug manufacturer takes over production, supportive care is recommended as the primary patient management strategy (Norris, 2011). A patient can survive a coral snake bite without antivenom but may require prolonged mechanical ventilation; the effects of severe bites can persist for many days (Norris, 2011). *Contact the regional poison control center immediately for specific advice on patient management.*

! NURSING SAFETY PRIORITY QSEN

Critical Rescue

The most significant risk to the victim is airway compromise and respiratory failure. Therefore ensure that the patient's IV lines are patent and that resuscitation equipment is immediately available.

ARTHROPOD BITES AND STINGS

Arthropods include spiders, scorpions, bees, and wasps. Unlike snakes, almost all species of spiders are venomous to some degree—most are not harmful to humans either because their mouth is too small to pierce human skin or the quantity or quality of their venom is inadequate to produce major health problems. Brown recluse and black widow spiders, scorpions, bees, and wasps are examples of venomous arthropods that can cause toxic reactions in humans. Chart 9-5 lists actions that help prevent arthropod bites and stings.

CHART 9-5 Patient and Family Education: Preparing for Self-Management

Arthropod Bite/Sting Prevention

- Wear protective clothing, including gloves and shoes, when working in areas known to harbor venomous arthropods, such as spiders, scorpions, bees, and wasps.
- Cover garbage cans. Bees and wasps are attracted to uncovered garbage.
- Use screens in windows and doors to prevent flying insects from entering buildings.
- Inspect clothing, shoes, and gear for insects before putting on these items.
- Shake out clothing and gear that have been on the ground to prevent arthropod "stowaways" and inadvertent bites and stings.
- Consult an exterminator to control arthropod populations in and around the home. Eliminating insects that are part of the arthropod's food source may also limit their presence.
- Identify nesting areas such as yard debris and rock piles; remove them whenever possible.
- Do not place unprotected hands where the eyes cannot see.
- Avoid handling insects or keeping them as "pets."
- Do not swat insects, wasps, and Africanized bees because they can send chemical signals that alert others to attack.
- Carry a prescription epinephrine autoinjector and antihistamines if known to be allergic to bee and wasp stings. Ensure at least one family member is also able to use the autoinjector.

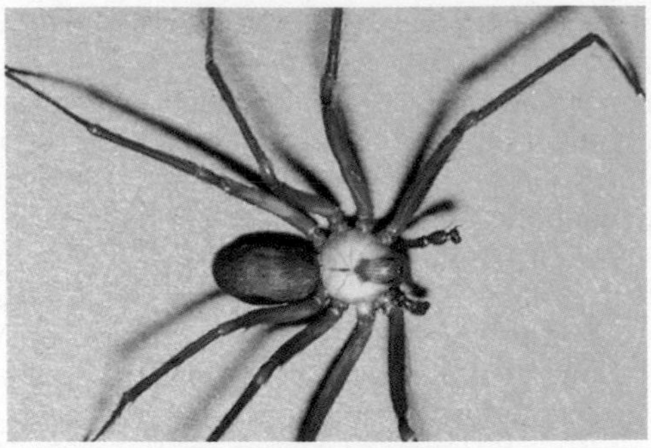

FIG. 9-4 Brown recluse spider *(Loxosceles reclusa).*

BROWN RECLUSE SPIDER

❖ PATHOPHYSIOLOGY

Brown recluse spiders are known for producing bites that result in skin ulcers. Also known as "fiddlebacks" or "violin spiders," they are medium-size spiders that are light brown and have a dark brown, fiddle-shaped mark that extends from their eyes down their back (Fig. 9-4). Like their name implies, brown recluse spiders are shy and hide in areas that are dark and secluded, such as boxes, closets, basements, sheds, and garages. Most indoor bites occur when people are sleeping, reaching into boxes or closets, or donning clothing that contains the spider. Few people ever see the spider that bit them. The only evidence may be impaired TISSUE INTEGRITY from a skin lesion or a necrotic wound or, less often, systemic effects from the injected toxin, commonly referred to as **loxoscelism**. Note that it is also common for patients to mistake a skin lesion for a spider bite; the lesion may actually be due to a skin infection, an insect bite, or even the manifestation of a health condition (Suchard, 2011).

❖ PATIENT-CENTERED COLLABORATIVE CARE

◆ Assessment

Brown recluse spider venom causes cell damage. The bite may be described as painless or stinging to sharp and painful. Some victims are unaware that they were bitten until intense local aching and pruritus develop over minutes to hours. The central bite site may demonstrate impaired TISSUE INTEGRITY appearing as a bleb or vesicle surrounded by edema and erythema, which may expand over the course of hours as the toxin spreads to surrounding tissues. The center of the bite becomes bluish purple. Some people have few or no tissue changes and therefore do not require medical attention.

For other people who are bitten, over the next 1 to 3 days the central part of the wound becomes dark and necrotic (Fig. 9-5). **Eschar** (a necrotic, leathery covering over the wound) eventually forms. The combination of these tissue changes is often referred to as the classic "red, white, and blue sign" that is associated with severe brown recluse spider bites.

When the eschar sloughs, TISSUE INTEGRITY is impaired by an open wound or ulcer that can remain for weeks to months. In rare cases, some patients may also have manifestations of systemic toxicity to brown recluse spider bites. These can include a rash, fever, chills, nausea, vomiting, malaise, and joint PAIN. In the worst cases, hemolytic reactions, renal failure, pulmonary edema, cardiovascular collapse, and death can occur.

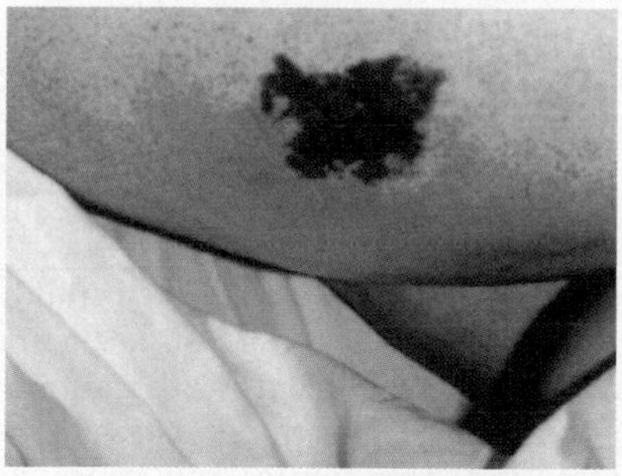

FIG. 9-5 Brown recluse spider bite after 24 hours, with central ischemia and rapidly advancing cellulitis.

◆ Interventions

First Aid/Prehospital Care. The basic first aid for a brown recluse spider bite is to apply cold compresses over the site intermittently until there is no further progression of the wound (Arnold, 2012). Cold helps decrease the enzyme activity of the venom and may limit tissue swelling and necrosis. *Do not use heat because it increases the enzyme activity and potentially worsens the wound.* Recommended actions include elevation of the affected extremity, local wound care, and rest.

Hospital Care. Supportive care and ongoing monitoring for complications meet the needs of most patients with a brown recluse spider bite. For patients with wounds that appear infected, topical antiseptic and sterile dressings are necessary. Wound cultures and antibiotics may also be indicated. Tetanus prophylaxis is recommended.

A surgeon evaluates patients whose wounds require interventions beyond conservative management. Débridement (removal of necrotic tissue) and skin grafting may be required to promote TISSUE INTEGRITY and healing in severe wounds. Where available, collaborate with a wound specialist nurse.

A small number of patients experience severe systemic complications (loxoscelism). Manifestations include:

- Fever and chills
- Nausea and vomiting
- Renal failure
- **Hemolytic anemia** (anemia caused by destruction of red blood cells)
- **Thrombocytopenia** (decreased platelets)
- Disseminated intravascular coagulation (DIC)
- Death

These problems are discussed elsewhere in this text. Critical care management, including aggressive hydration, blood transfusions, hemodialysis, and supportive therapies, is required to prevent further deterioration and promote recovery.

BLACK WIDOW SPIDER

❖ PATHOPHYSIOLOGY

Black widow spiders can be found in every state in the United States except Alaska. They can inflict deadly bites and are found in cool, damp environments like outdoor log piles, vegetation, and rocks. They also commonly inhabit barns, sheds, and garages. The female spider is best identified by her shiny black color and the red hourglass pattern on her abdomen. Male spiders are smaller in size and lighter in color with white and gray markings. The hourglass pattern is faint in males. Black widow spiders carry neurotoxic venom. Bites to humans are usually defensive when the spider is at risk for being crushed.

The initial bite of a black widow spider ranges from nearly painless to sharply painful. Typically, the person notices a tiny papule or small, red punctate mark. Some people have intense PAIN, which seems out of proportion to the lesion. In many cases, the symptoms do not progress beyond a local reaction in the area of the bite site. If systemic signs and symptoms do occur, they generally develop within 1 hour and involve the neuromuscular system.

❖ PATIENT-CENTERED COLLABORATIVE CARE

◆ Assessment

Black widow spider venom produces a syndrome known as **latrodectism**, in which the venom causes neurotransmitter release from nerve terminals. Severe abdominal PAIN, muscle rigidity and spasm, hypertension, and nausea and vomiting are common. The problem may be incorrectly diagnosed as an acute abdomen, and surgical consultation may be considered because of the clinical features similar to peritonitis (Boyer et al., 2012). Muscle spasms involve the large muscles of the abdomen, back, and limbs. Other problems include facial edema, **ptosis** (eyelid drooping), diaphoresis, weakness, increased salivation, respiratory difficulty from excessive secretions, fasciculations (twitching), and **paresthesias** (painful tingling or numbness). The effects of the bite are self-limited and generally resolve in a few days. *However, older adults with other health problems like cardiovascular disease are at much higher risk for complications.*

◆ Interventions

First Aid/Prehospital Care

! NURSING SAFETY PRIORITY QSEN

Action Alert

The priority intervention for a black widow spider bite in the prehospital setting is to apply an ice pack because cold application decreases the action of the neurotoxin.

Monitor the person for evidence of systemic toxicity as described in the previous Assessment section. If this problem occurs, support the patient's airway, breathing, and circulation. Patients should be transported to a medical facility as soon as possible for advanced life support care.

Hospital Care. In the emergency department, closely monitor vital signs, with special attention to blood pressure and respiratory function. Supportive therapy in the hospital includes administration of opioid pain medication and muscle relaxants such as diazepam (Valium) or other benzodiazepines. Provide tetanus prophylaxis as needed. Observe the patient for seizures related to a rapidly rising blood pressure (Boyer et al., 2012). For some patients, antihypertensive agents are needed. Although relapses may occur, the patient usually recovers within a week.

Less often, pulmonary edema, uncontrollable hypertension, seizures, respiratory arrest, and shock occur. These patients require critical care management. Antivenom is available for black widow spider bites. Although it can cause anaphylaxis and serum sickness, antivenom is considered effective in treating severe reactions (Boyer et al., 2012). The drug is also given to pregnant women because they may have uterine contractions from a black widow spider bite that can lead to a premature delivery (Boyer et al., 2012). The regional poison control center provides information about antivenom dosing and management for women who are pregnant.

SCORPIONS

❖ PATHOPHYSIOLOGY

Scorpions are found in many states within the United States although not typically in the Midwest or New England. However, stings are always possible when people keep scorpions as pets or when scorpions are accidentally transported in baggage and packaging. Unlike spiders that envenom their prey by inflicting a bite, scorpions inject venom through a stinging apparatus on their tail. Most scorpion stings produce a mild reaction characterized by local PAIN, inflammation, and mild systemic symptoms. These effects are usually self-limiting and best treated by analgesics, supportive management, and basic wound care.

One species of scorpion found in the southwestern United States that can inflict a sting associated with a potentially fatal systemic response is the bark scorpion (Fig. 9-6). It is often found in trees and woodpiles and around debris. Humans are usually stung when the scorpion gets into clothing, shoes, blankets, and personal items left on the ground.

❖ PATIENT-CENTERED COLLABORATIVE CARE

◆ Assessment

Because bark scorpion venom is neurotoxic, clinical manifestations result from cranial nerve and/or skeletal muscle involvement. The sting site may or may not show evidence of the venom release. There may be no redness or other obvious sign of inflammation. Gentle tapping at the potential sting site causing increased PAIN is associated with a bark scorpion sting (Suchard, 2012). The severity of the reaction varies from local pain to severe systemic manifestations, such as excessive salivation, hyperactivity, high fever, hypertension, GI disorders, tachycardia, cardiac dysfunction, pulmonary edema, and nervous system involvement. In rare cases, death can occur.

Symptoms usually begin immediately after the sting and can reach a crisis level within 12 hours. Recovery occurs gradually. PAIN and paresthesias can remain for up to 2 weeks (Suchard, 2012).

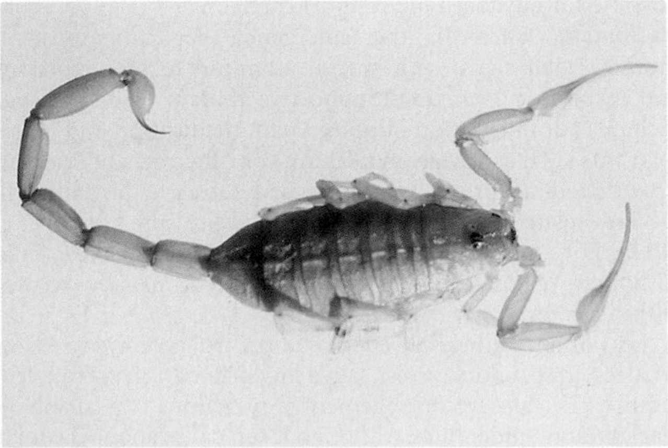

FIG. 9-6 The bark scorpion of Arizona *(Centruroides sculpturatus)*.

◆ Interventions

Hospital Care. *The first priority of patient management is vital sign assessment and continuous monitoring for several hours in a hospital emergency department or critical care unit.* As symptoms worsen, the patient may develop respiratory failure and need intubation and mechanical ventilation.

Provide supplemental oxygen and IV fluid replacement immediately. Apply an ice pack to the sting site to control pain. Give analgesic and sedative agents with caution in the non-intubated, spontaneously breathing patient. Potent opioids, benzodiazepines, and barbiturates can cause loss of airway reflexes and precipitate respiratory failure. Fever is treated with acetaminophen (Tylenol) and application of a cooling blanket as needed. Because scorpion stings produce a puncture wound impairing TISSUE INTEGRITY, provide tetanus prophylaxis and basic wound care with an antiseptic agent. *Contact the poison control center as soon as possible to assist with patient management, particularly in regard to use of pharmacologic agents for scorpion stings.*

BEES AND WASPS

❖ PATHOPHYSIOLOGY

Bees and wasps are also venomous arthropods. Stings can produce a wide range of reactions from discomfort at the sting site to severe PAIN, multi-system problems, and life-threatening anaphylaxis in allergic people. Bumblebees, hornets, and wasps are capable of stinging repeatedly when disturbed. They have a smooth stinger that may or may not become lodged in the victim. Only honeybees can sting just once. When a honeybee stings a person, the stinger and venom sac pull away from the bee. The bee dies, but venom injection continues because the stinger and sac remain in the victim.

"Africanized" bees, also called "killer bees," are a very aggressive species that are found in the southwestern states. They are known to attack in groups and can remain agitated for several hours. People under attack should attempt to outrun the bees, if possible, and keep their mouth and eyes protected from the swarm. A person should never go into a body of water because the bees will attack when he or she comes up for air. When a person sustains multiple stings, reactions are more severe and may be fatal because multiple venom doses have cumulative toxic effects.

Health Promotion and Maintenance

Chart 9-5 lists actions that may help prevent arthropod bites and stings.

❖ PATIENT-CENTERED COLLABORATIVE CARE

◆ Assessment

The person who is stung by a bee or wasp first has a local reaction of immediate PAIN and a wheal-and-flare skin reaction. For some people, swelling can be extensive and involve an entire limb or body area. Systemic effects can then develop based on the venom load and the person's sensitivity to the venom. These effects may include generalized edema, nausea, vomiting, and diarrhea and are reactions to the toxic effects of the venom itself, not necessarily an allergic reaction. Other toxic venom effects include destruction of red and white blood cells and platelets, damage to the blood vessel walls, acute kidney injury, renal failure, liver injury, and cardiac complications; multisystem organ failure can develop (Lin et al., 2011).

If the patient has an *allergy to the venom*, then **urticaria** (hives), pruritus (itching), and swelling of the lips and tongue may occur. An allergic response can rapidly progress to an anaphylactic reaction in highly sensitive patients. **Anaphylaxis** is a life-threatening allergic response and is evidenced by respiratory distress with bronchospasm and laryngeal edema, hypotension, deterioration in mental status, and cardiac dysrhythmias. *This type of reaction constitutes a true medical emergency that is imminently life threatening and may lead to cardiac arrest.* Initially it may be impossible to distinguish an allergic reaction from a toxic venom reaction because they both can cause the same types of early signs and symptoms.

◆ Interventions

First Aid/Prehospital Care. *Basic* emergency care for bee and wasp stings includes quick removal of the stinger (if present) and application of an ice pack (Laskowski-Jones, 2010). Tweezers formerly were avoided for stinger removal because it was believed that pinching the stinger would cause additional venom to be injected. However, this concern appears to be unfounded (Auerbach, 2009). The stinger is best removed with tweezers or by gently scraping or brushing it off with the edge of a knife blade, credit card, or needle. The method used to remove the stinger is not as important as the speed of removal (Auerbach, 2009).

Advanced prehospital emergency care interventions are prioritized to ensure that airway, breathing, and circulation are maintained. First, determine whether the patient has a history of allergic reactions to bee stings. If the patient has a severe allergic reaction with wheezing, facial swelling, and respiratory distress, epinephrine must be given immediately. Allergic adult patients typically carry an epinephrine autoinjector (e.g., EpiPen®, Auvi-Q™. This device administers a quick and simple single dose of epinephrine in an emergency with just a click of a button. The injection is given via the IM route, typically in the mid-portion of the outer thigh. (See Chapter 20 for further discussion of epinephrine administration for anaphylaxis management.)

After epinephrine administration, an antihistamine such as diphenhydramine (Benadryl, Allerdryl ♣) or chlorpheniramine (Chlor-Trimeton, Novo-Pheniram ♣) is also given. In the field setting, oral liquid diphenhydramine (available over the counter) may be easier for the victim to swallow than the tablet form if there is tongue or pharyngeal edema. *Call 911 to transport the patient to a medical facility as soon as possible, since epinephrine administration may need to be repeated in 15 minutes if symptoms persist.*

Hospital Care. Once in a clinical setting, patients who sustain serious reactions to bee or wasp stings need oxygen administration and continuous cardiac and blood pressure monitoring. Establish an IV infusion with normal saline solution to support blood pressure. Advanced life support drugs and resuscitation equipment should be made immediately available. If epinephrine IM fails to relieve the life-threatening reaction, a different epinephrine formulation may be requested as a very slow IV bolus.

Bronchospasm can be treated with albuterol (Proventil, Novo-Salmol ♣) via inhalation or a similar bronchodilating agent. Parenteral antihistamines, such as diphenhydramine (Benadryl, Allerdryl ♣), and corticosteroids are also commonly prescribed to decrease the immune response. The toxin in the bee and wasp venom may outlast the effects of the initial doses of epinephrine and antihistamines and cause a recurrence of the allergic reaction over time. Therefore doses may need to be repeated for hours or days. Corticosteroids in tapered doses are often given to manage or prevent delayed allergic effects, termed a *biphasic reaction,* which generally occurs within 4 to 6 hours of the sting; however, the evidence regarding the effectiveness of corticosteroid administration is unclear (Choo et al., 2013).

All patients who have sustained multiple stings (particularly more than 50) are observed in an emergency care setting for several hours to monitor for the development of toxic venom effects. A critical care admission may be needed.

> **! NURSING SAFETY PRIORITY (QSEN)**
> ***Drug Alert***
>
> IV epinephrine administration has much greater risk for adverse cardiovascular effects than IM epinephrine. Use the IV form of epinephrine with extreme caution, especially in older adults with cardiovascular disease, because it can dramatically increase pulse rate and blood pressure. Monitor the patient's vital signs frequently—at least every 10 to 15 minutes for 1 hour after IV administration.

> **! NURSING SAFETY PRIORITY (QSEN)**
> ***Action Alert***
>
> Teach anyone who develops an allergic reaction to bee or wasp stings to always carry a prescription epinephrine autoinjector and wear a medical alert tag or bracelet.

LIGHTNING INJURIES

❖ PATHOPHYSIOLOGY

Lightning is a year-round force of nature responsible for multiple injuries and deaths each year. It is caused by an electric charge generated within thunderclouds that may become cloud-to-ground lightning—the most dangerous form to people and structures. Young adult males account for the majority of lightning-related deaths. Most lightning-related injuries occur in the summer months during the afternoon and early evening because of increased thunderstorm activity and greater numbers of people spending time outside. Anyone without adequate shelter, including golfers, hikers, campers, beach-goers, and swimmers, is at risk.

Lightning has an enormous magnitude of energy and a different current flow than a typical high-voltage electric shock. The duration of contact is nearly instantaneous, resulting in a flashover phenomenon—an effect that may account for the relatively low overall mortality rate. Because water is a conductor of electricity and current takes the path of least resistance to the ground, any wetness on the body increases the flashover effect of a lightning strike. Lightning flashover produces an explosive force that can injure victims directly, as well as cause them to fall or to be thrown. The clothing and shoes of victims may be damaged or blown off in the process.

Lightning produces injury by directly striking a victim, by splashing off a nearby object, or by traveling through the ground. Although few people die after a lightning strike, many survivors are left with permanent disabilities.

Health Promotion and Maintenance

Injuries caused by lightning strike are highly preventable. Teach people to stay indoors during an electrical storm. Chart 9-6 lists common prevention strategies. For more information, the Wilderness Medical Society (http://wms.org) also offers evidence-based practice guidelines for the prevention and treatment of lightning injuries (Davis et al., 2012).

❖ PATIENT-CENTERED COLLABORATIVE CARE

◆ Assessment

Both the cardiopulmonary and the central nervous systems are profoundly affected by lightning injuries. *The most lethal initial effect of massive electrical current discharge on the cardiopulmonary system is cardiac arrest.* Because cardiac cells are autorhythmic, an effective cardiac rhythm may return spontaneously. However, prolonged respiratory arrest from impairment of the medullary respiratory center can produce hypoxia and, subsequently, a second cardiac arrest. Therefore, when attempting to manage multiple victims of a lightning strike, provide care to those who are in cardiopulmonary arrest first. Initiate resuscitation measures with immediate airway and ventilatory management, chest compressions, and other appropriate life-support interventions.

People who survive the immediate lightning strike may be treated in a less emergent fashion. However, these victims can have serious myocardial injury, which may be manifested by ECG and myocardial perfusion abnormalities, such as angina and dysrhythmias. The initial appearance of mottled skin and decreased to absent peripheral pulses usually arises from arterial vasospasm and typically resolves spontaneously in several hours.

Central nervous system (CNS) injury is common in lightning strike victims. A classic finding is an immediate but temporary paralysis that affects the lower limbs to a greater extent than the upper limbs. This condition usually resolves within hours, but the patient must be evaluated for spinal injury. Other clinical manifestations and complications resulting from lightning strikes include cataracts, tympanic membrane rupture, cerebral hemorrhage, depression, and post-traumatic stress disorder. Lightning strikes also cause skin burns. Most burns are superficial and heal without incident. Patients may have full-thickness burns, charring, and contact burns from overlying metal objects. An uncommon but characteristic skin manifestation of lightning is the appearance of branching or ferning marks on the skin called **Lichtenberg figures**.

CHART 9-6 Patient and Family Education: Preparing for Self-Management

Lightning Strike Prevention

- Observe weather forecasts when planning to be outside.
- Seek shelter when you hear thunder. Safe choices include going inside the nearest building or an enclosed vehicle. Isolated sheds and the entrances to caves are dangerous, however. Do not stand under an isolated tall tree or structure (e.g., ski lift, flagpole, boat mast, power line) in an open area such as a field, ridge, or hilltop; lightning seeks the highest point. A stand of dense trees offers better protection.
- Leave the water immediately (including an indoor shower or bathtub), and move away from any open bodies of water.
- Avoid metal objects like chairs or bleachers; put down tools, fishing rods, garden equipment, golf clubs, and umbrellas; stand clear of fences, exposed pipes, motorcycles, bicycles, tractors, and golf carts.
- If camping in a tent, stay away from the metal tent poles and wet walls.
- Once inside a building, stay away from open doors, windows, fireplaces, metal fixtures, and plumbing.
- Turn off electrical equipment including computers, televisions, and stereos.
- Stay off the telephone. Lightning can enter through the telephone line and produce head and neck trauma, including cataracts and tympanic membrane disruption. Death can result.
- If you are caught out in the open and cannot seek shelter, attempt to move to lower ground such as a ravine or valley; stay away from any tall trees or objects that could result in a lightning strike splashing over to you; place insulating material between you and the ground (e.g., sleeping pad, rain parka, life jacket). A lightning strike is imminent if your hair stands on end, you see blue halos around objects, and hear high-pitched or crackling noises. If you cannot move away from the area immediately, crouch on the balls of your feet and tuck your head down to minimize the target size; do not lie down on the ground or have hand contact with the ground.

Data from Auerbach, P.S., Donner, H.J., & Weiss, E.A. (2013). *Field guide to wilderness medicine* (4th ed.). St. Louis: Mosby.

◆ Interventions

First Aid/Prehospital Care. Because of lightning's powerful impact to the body, patients are at great risk for multi-system trauma. The full extent of injury may not be known until thorough monitoring and diagnostic evaluation can be performed in the hospital. Initial care includes spinal immobilization with priority attention to stabilization of airway, breathing, and circulation through standard basic and advanced life support measures. Cardiopulmonary resuscitation (CPR) is performed immediately when a person is in cardiac arrest. If cardiopulmonary or CNS injury is present, skin burns are *not* an initial priority. However, if time and resources permit, a sterile dressing may be applied to cover the sites. *Victims of lightning strike are not electrically charged; the rescuer is in no danger from physical contact.* Nonetheless, the storm can present a continued threat to everyone in the vicinity who lacks adequate shelter. Contrary to popular belief, lightning can and does strike in the same place more than once.

Hospital Care. Once in the acute care hospital setting, the focus of care is advanced life support management, including cardiac monitoring to detect cardiac dysrhythmias and a 12-lead ECG. The patient may require mechanical ventilation until spontaneous breathing returns. Collaborate with the health care team to perform a thorough physical and diagnostic evaluation

CLINICAL JUDGMENT CHALLENGE

Patient-Centered Care QSEN

A nurse is working at a day camp for church leaders when a sudden severe thunderstorm occurs. Several adults participating in outdoor activities appear to have been hit by lightning. The nurse arrives on scene and finds four injured people. One person appears to be unconscious, one has ferning marks and burns on his skin, and the other two are sitting up against the wall of a building and reporting severe weakness of their lower extremities.

1. What risk factors did these people have for lightning injury?
2. Which person should the nurse assess first and what is the priority of care of this patient?
3. What potential complication does the nurse plan to address in the immediate rescue period?
4. What direction should the nurse give the large crowd of campers and camp staff?

to identify obvious and occult (hidden) traumatic injuries because the patient may have suffered a fall or blast effect during the strike. A computed tomography (CT) scan of the head may be performed to identify intracranial hemorrhage. A creatine kinase (CK) measurement may be requested to detect skeletal muscle damage resulting from the lightning strike. In severe cases, **rhabdomyolysis** (circulation of by-products of skeletal muscle destruction) can lead to renal failure. Burn wounds are assessed and treated according to standard burn care protocols. Tetanus prophylaxis is necessary for burns or any break in skin integrity. Some institutions transfer these victims to a burn center for follow-up management.

COLD-RELATED INJURIES

Two common cold-related injuries are hypothermia and frostbite. Both types of injury can be prevented by implementing protection from the cold. Teach patients at risk ways to prevent these injuries through methods to maintain THERMOREGULATION, which can range from mild discomfort to major systemic complications.

HEALTH PROMOTION AND MAINTENANCE

When participating in cold weather activities, clothing choices are critical to the prevention of hypothermia and frostbite. Teach the importance of wearing synthetic clothing because it moves moisture away from the body and dries fast. Cotton clothing, especially as an undergarment, holds moisture, becomes wet, and contributes to the development of hypothermia. Cotton clothing should be strictly avoided in a cold outdoor environment; this rule applies to gloves and socks as well. Wet socks and gloves promote frostbite in the toes and fingers. Wearing too many pairs of socks can decrease circulation and lead to frostbite.

Clothing should be layered so that it can be easily added or removed as the temperature changes. The inner layers, such as polyester fleece, provide warmth and insulation. The outer layer's purpose is to block the wind and provide moisture protection. This layer is best made of a windproof, waterproof, breathable fabric. A hat is an essential clothing item that significantly decreases body heat loss through the head. Face protection with a facemask should be used on particularly cold days when wind chill poses a risk. Sunscreen (minimum sun protection factor [SPF] 30) and sunglasses are also important to protect skin and eyes from the sun's harmful rays.

Teach people to keep water, extra clothing, and food in their car when driving in winter in case the vehicle becomes stranded. Maintaining personal fitness and conditioning is also an important consideration to prevent hypothermia and frostbite. People should not diet or restrict food or fluid intake when participating in winter outdoor activities. Malnutrition and dehydration contribute to cold-related illnesses and injuries. Finally, it is important for people to know their physical limits and to come in out of the cold when these limits have been reached.

HYPOTHERMIA

❖ PATHOPHYSIOLOGY

Hypothermia is a core body temperature below 95° F (35° C). Common predisposing conditions that promote hypothermia include:

- Cold water immersion
- Acute illness (e.g., sepsis)
- Traumatic injury
- Shock states
- Immobilization
- Cold weather (especially for the homeless and people working outdoors)
- Advanced age
- Selected medications (e.g., phenothiazines, barbiturates)
- Alcohol intoxication and substance abuse
- Malnutrition
- Hypothyroidism
- Inadequate clothing or shelter (e.g., the homeless population)

An environmental temperature below 82° F (28° C) can produce impaired THERMOREGULATION and hypothermia in any susceptible person. *Therefore people, especially older adults, are actually at risk on a year-round basis in most areas of the world.* Wind chill is a significant factor: heat loss increases as wind speed rises. Wet conditions further increase heat loss through evaporation. Weather is the most common cause of hypothermia for outdoor sports enthusiasts and for those with inadequate clothing or shelter. It is also a problem for the older adult, the homeless, and the poor who cannot afford heating.

❖ PATIENT-CENTERED COLLABORATIVE CARE

◆ Assessment

Hypothermia is commonly divided into three categories by severity: *mild* (90° to 95° F [32° to 35° C]); *moderate* (82.4° to 90° F [28° to 32° C]); and *severe* (below 82.4° F [28° C]). Treatment decisions are based on the severity of hypothermia. Chart 9-7 summarizes by category the common key features for the patient who is hypothermic.

◆ Interventions

First Aid/Prehospital Care. For treatment of *mild hypothermia,* the person needs to be sheltered from the cold environment, have all wet clothing removed, and undergo passive or active external rewarming. Passive methods involve applying

CHART 9-7 Key Features

Hypothermia

Mild
- Shivering
- Dysarthria (slurred speech)
- Decreased muscle coordination
- Impaired cognition ("mental slowness")
- Diuresis (caused by shunting of blood to major organs)

Moderate
- Muscle weakness
- Increased loss of coordination
- Acute confusion
- Apathy
- Incoherence
- Possible stupor
- Decreased clotting (caused by impaired platelet aggregation and thrombocytopenia)

Severe
- Bradycardia
- Severe hypotension
- Decreased respiratory rate
- Cardiac dysrhythmias, including possible ventricular fibrillation or asystole
- Decreased neurologic reflexes
- Decreased pain responsiveness
- Acid-base imbalance

warm clothing or blankets. Active methods incorporate heating blankets, warm packs, and convective air heaters or warmers to speed rewarming. If a heating blanket is used, monitor the patient's skin at least every 15 to 30 minutes to reduce the risk for burn injury.

In the case of mild, uncomplicated hypothermia as the only health problem, having the victim drink warm high-carbohydrate liquids that do not contain alcohol or caffeine can aid in rewarming. Alcohol is a peripheral vasodilator; both alcohol and caffeine are diuretics. These effects can potentially worsen dehydration and hypothermia.

Hospital Care. General management principles apply to both *moderate* and *severe* hypothermia. Protect patients from further heat loss and handle them gently to prevent ventricular fibrillation. Positioning the patient in the supine position prevents orthostatic changes in blood pressure from cardiovascular instability. Follow standard resuscitation efforts with special attention to maintenance of airway, breathing, and circulation as recommended by the American Heart Association (2011):

- Administer drugs with caution and/or spaced at longer intervals because metabolism is unpredictable in hypothermic conditions.
- Remember that drugs can accumulate without obvious therapeutic effect while the patient is cold but may become active and potentially lead to drug toxicity as effective rewarming is underway.
- Consider withholding IV drugs, except vasopressors, until the core temperature is above 86° F (30° C).
- Initiate CPR for patients without spontaneous circulation.
- For a hypothermic patient in ventricular fibrillation or pulseless ventricular tachycardia, one defibrillation attempt is appropriate. Be aware that defibrillation attempts may be ineffective until the core temperature is above 86° F (30° C).

Treatment of *moderate* hypothermia may involve both active external and core (internal) rewarming methods. Applying external heat with heating blankets can promote core temperature "after-drop" by producing peripheral vasodilation. **"After-drop"** is the continued decrease in core body temperature after the victim is removed from the cold environment; it is caused by the return of cold blood from the periphery to the central circulation. Therefore the patient's trunk should be actively rewarmed before the extremities. Core rewarming methods for moderate hypothermia include administration of warm IV fluids, heated oxygen or inspired gas to prevent further heat loss via the respiratory tract, and heated peritoneal, pleural, gastric, or bladder lavage.

! NURSING SAFETY PRIORITY (QSEN)

Critical Rescue

Patients who are *severely* hypothermic are at high risk for cardiac arrest. Avoid using active *external* rewarming with heating devices because it is dangerous and contraindicated in this population due to rapid vasodilation.

The treatment of choice for *severe* hypothermia is to use *extracorporeal* rewarming methods such as cardiopulmonary bypass or hemodialysis (Leikin et al., 2012). Cardiopulmonary bypass is the fastest core rewarming technique. However, this device is not available in all hospitals. It also requires specialized personnel and resources to operate it properly. Monitor for early signs of complications that can occur after rewarming, such as fluid, electrolyte, and metabolic abnormalities; acute respiratory distress syndrome (ARDS); acute renal failure; and pneumonia.

A long-standing principle in the treatment of patients with hypothermic cardiac arrest is that "no one is dead until they are warm and dead." There is a factual basis to this statement when considering the number of survivors who have suffered a prolonged hypothermic cardiac arrest. Prolonged resuscitation efforts may not be reasonable in cases in which survival appears highly unlikely, such as in an anoxic event followed by a hypothermic cardiac arrest.

FROSTBITE

❖ PATHOPHYSIOLOGY

Another significant cold-related injury that may or may not be associated with hypothermia is frostbite. The main risk factor is inadequate insulation against cold weather; that is, either the skin is exposed to the cold or the person's clothing offers insufficient protection, leading to injury. Wet clothing, in particular, is a poor insulator and facilitates the development of frostbite. Fatigue, dehydration, and poor nutrition are other contributing factors. People who smoke, consume alcohol, or have impaired peripheral circulation have a higher incidence of frostbite. Any previous history of frostbite further increases a person's susceptibility.

? NCLEX EXAMINATION CHALLENGE

Health Promotion and Maintenance

An occupational health nurse is teaching a safety class to city employees who work outdoors year round. What does the nurse teach are risk factors for developing frostbite? **Select all that apply.**

A. Excessive fatigue
B. Prior episodes of frostbite
C. Diabetes or other peripheral vascular disease
D. Dehydration
E. Smoking
F. Wearing polyester socks

❖ PATIENT-CENTERED COLLABORATIVE CARE

◆ Assessment

Frostbite occurs when body tissue freezes and causes damage. Like burns, frostbite injuries can be superficial, partial, or full thickness. By contrast, **frostnip** is a type of superficial cold injury that may produce pain, numbness, and pallor of the affected area but is easily relieved by applying warmth; it does not cause tissue damage (impaired TISSUE INTEGRITY). Frostnip typically develops on skin areas such as the face, nose, finger, or toes. Untreated, it is a precursor to more severe forms of frostbite.

First-degree frostbite, the least severe type of frostbite, involves **hyperemia** (increased blood flow) of the involved area and edema formation. In *second-degree frostbite,* large fluid-filled blisters develop with partial-thickness skin necrosis (Fig. 9-7). *Third-degree frostbite* appears as small blisters that contain dark fluid and an affected body part that is cool, numb, blue, or red and does not blanch. Full-thickness and subcutaneous tissue

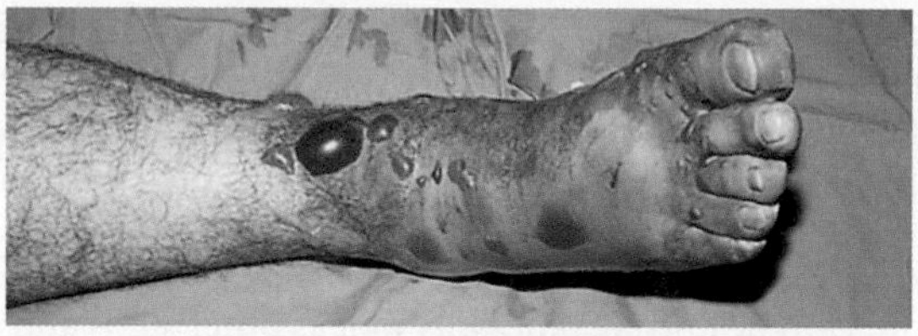

FIG. 9-7 Edema and blister formation 24 hours after frostbite injury occurring in an area covered by a tightly fitted boot.

necrosis occurs and requires débridement. In *fourth-degree frostbite,* the most severe form, there are no blisters or edema; the part is numb, cold, and bloodless. The full-thickness necrosis extends into the muscle and bone. At this stage, gangrene develops, which may require amputation of the affected part.

◆ Interventions

First Aid/Prehospital Care. *Recognition of frostbite is essential to early, effective intervention and prevention of further tissue damage.* Asking a partner to frequently observe for early signs of frostbite such as a white, waxy appearance to exposed skin, especially on the nose, cheeks, and ears, is an effective strategy to identify the problem before it worsens. In persons with dark skin, skin becomes paler, waxy, and somewhat gray. In this case, the best remedy is to have the person seek shelter from the wind and cold and to attend to the affected body part. Superficial frostbite is easily managed using body heat to warm the affected area. Teach patients to place their warm hands over the affected areas on their face or to place cold hands under the arms.

Hospital Care. Patients with more severe and deeper forms of frostbite need aggressive management. For all degrees of partial-thickness to full-thickness frostbite, rapid rewarming in a water bath at a temperature range of 104° to 108° F (40° to 42° C) is indicated to thaw the frozen part (Auerbach et al., 2010). Because patients experience severe PAIN during the rewarming process, this intervention is best accomplished in a medical facility; however, it may be done in another setting if no other options exist for prompt transport or rescue. Administer analgesics, especially IV opiates, and IV rehydration.

> **! NURSING SAFETY PRIORITY** QSEN
>
> **Critical Rescue**
>
> Do not apply dry heat or massage the frostbitten areas as part of the warming process. These actions can produce further tissue injury.

When the rewarming process is complete, handle the injured areas gently and elevate them above heart level if possible to decrease tissue edema. Sometimes splints are used to immobilize extremities during the healing process. Assess the person at least hourly for the development of compartment syndrome—a limb-threatening complication caused by severe neurovascular impairment. Observe for early manifestations, which include increasing pain (even after analgesics are given) and paresthesias (painful tingling and numbness). Compare the affected extremity with the unaffected one to assess for pallor. Assess for pulses and muscle weakness. Management of compartment syndrome is discussed in detail in Chapter 51.

Frostbite destroys tissue and produces a deep tetanus-prone wound; the patient should be immunized to prevent tetanus. Apply only loose, nonadherent sterile dressings to the damaged areas. Avoid compression of the injured tissues. Both topical and systemic antibiotics may be used. Once a patient's frozen part has thawed, do not allow it to refreeze, which worsens the injury. Antiprostaglandin therapy with ibuprofen may be used because it may decrease tissue damage for some patients (Auerbach et al., 2010).

In cases of severe, deep frostbite, débridement of necrotic tissue may be needed to evaluate tissue viability and provide wound management. Amputation may be indicated for patients with severe injuries or for those who develop gangrene or severe compartment syndrome.

ALTITUDE-RELATED ILLNESSES

❖ PATHOPHYSIOLOGY

High altitude illnesses, also known as **high altitude disease (HAD)** or *altitude sickness,* cause pathophysiologic responses in the body as a result of exposure to low partial pressure of oxygen at high elevations. Although most consider high altitude to be an elevation over 5000 feet, millions of people worldwide who ascend to or live at altitudes above 2500 feet are at risk for acute and chronic mountain sickness.

As altitude increases, atmospheric (barometric) pressure decreases. Oxygen makes up 21% of the pressure. Therefore, as this pressure falls, the partial pressure of oxygen in the air decreases, resulting in less available oxygen to humans. The pathophysiologic consequence is hypoxia. Hypoxia is more pronounced as elevation increases. Elevations higher than 18,000 feet are extreme altitudes. Supplemental oxygen is necessary at these levels in non-acclimatized people to prevent altitude-related illnesses, including death, from occurring during abrupt ascent.

The cause of HAD is an interaction of environmental and genetic factors (Guoen et al., 2009). Those who are obese or have chronic illnesses, especially cardiovascular problems, are more at risk than those who are thinner and healthier. Dehydration and central nervous system depressants, such as alcohol, also increase the risk. The age of the person does not seem to be a factor in altitude-related illnesses.

> **GENETIC/GENOMIC CONSIDERATIONS**
>
> **Patient-Centered Care** QSEN
>
> Genetic differences among certain ethnic groups who live in high altitude areas have been studied. For example, chronic mountain sickness is less common in Tibetans and Sherpas than in Andeans, Hans, or Peruvian Quechuas (Guoen et al., 2009).
>
> In addition, the pathogenesis of mountain sickness is associated with unidentified variations in hypoxia-related genes and the genes responsible for the human leukocyte antigen (HLA) system. Examples of genes with variants that may contribute to the development of HAD include:
>
> - *EPO* (erythropoietin), which regulates red blood cell production
> - *HIF1A* (hypoxia inducible factor), which mediates the effects of hypoxia on body cells
> - *EDN1* (endothelin), which causes vasoconstriction and thus increases blood pressure
> - *NOS3* (endothelial nitric oxide synthase), which makes nitric acid in vascular tissue to maintain vessel tone and altitude adaptation
>
> At this time, no clinical genetic testing to determine a person's risk for altitude sickness is available; however, further research is being conducted to identify specific gene variations that contribute to altitude-related illnesses.

The process of adapting to high altitude is called *acclimatization*. **Acclimatization** involves physiologic changes that help the body adapt to less available oxygen in the atmosphere. As the carotid bodies sense a decline in Pao_2 at about 5000 feet, they increase the respiratory rate to improve oxygen delivery. This mechanism is called the "hypoxic-ventilatory response." Increased respiratory rate causes **hypocapnia** (decreased carbon dioxide) and respiratory alkalosis, which limit further increases in respiratory rate. Rapid eye movement (REM) sleep is impaired. Hypoxia can occur from periods of apnea. Within 24 to 48 hours of being at high altitude, the kidneys excrete the excess bicarbonate, which helps the pH to return to normal and ventilatory rate to again increase.

Increased sympathetic nervous system activity increases heart rate, blood pressure, and cardiac output. Pulmonary artery pressure rises as an effect of generalized hypoxia-induced pulmonary vasoconstriction. Cerebral blood flow increases to maintain cerebral oxygen delivery. Hypoxia also induces red blood cell production by stimulating the release of erythropoietin. The result is an increase in red blood cells and hemoglobin concentration. Over time, polycythemia can develop in people who remain in a high altitude environment.

People who plan to climb to high altitudes are advised to ascend slowly, over the course of days or even weeks, depending on the degree of elevation. Ascending too rapidly is the primary cause of altitude-related illnesses. They are much more common in people who sleep at elevations above 8000 feet.

The three most common clinical conditions that are considered high altitude illnesses are acute mountain sickness (AMS), high altitude cerebral edema (HACE), and high altitude pulmonary edema (HAPE). AMS may occur with HACE and/or HAPE; the underlying pathophysiology is hypoxia. Chronic mountain sickness can occur in people who live at high elevations. Although each syndrome has several unique manifestations, the basic assessment and management approach are the same.

❖ PATIENT-CENTERED COLLABORATIVE CARE

◆ Assessment

Assessment findings for the typical patient with AMS include reports of throbbing headache, anorexia, nausea, and vomiting. Feeling chilled, irritable, and apathetic is also associated with AMS. The syndrome produces effects similar to an alcohol-induced hangover. The patient may relate a feeling of extreme illness. Vital signs are variable: the patient can be tachycardic or bradycardic, have normal blood pressure, or have postural hypotension. He or she may experience dyspnea both on exertion and at rest. Exertional dyspnea is expected as a person adjusts to high altitude. However, dyspnea at rest is abnormal and may signal the onset of HAPE.

If AMS progresses to *high altitude cerebral edema (HACE)*, the extreme form of this disorder, the patient cannot perform ADLs and has extreme apathy. A key sign of HACE is the development of ataxia (defective muscular coordination). The patient also has a change in mental status with confusion and impaired judgment. Cranial nerve dysfunction and seizures may occur. If untreated, a further decline in the patient's level of consciousness results. Stupor, coma, and death can result from brain swelling and the subsequent damage caused by increased intracranial pressure over the course of 1 to 3 days.

High altitude pulmonary edema (HAPE) often appears in conjunction with HACE but may occur during the progression of AMS within the first 2 to 4 days of a rapid ascent to high altitude, commonly on the second night. It is the most common cause of death associated with high altitude. Patients notice poor exercise tolerance and a prolonged recovery time after exertion. Fatigue and weakness, as well as other signs and symptoms of AMS, are present. Important clinical indicators of HAPE include a persistent dry cough and cyanosis of the lips and nail beds. Tachycardia and tachypnea occur at rest. Crackles may be auscultated in one or both lungs. Pink, frothy sputum is a late sign of HAPE. A chest x-ray demonstrates pulmonary infiltrates and pulmonary edema. Arterial blood gas analysis shows respiratory alkalosis and hypoxemia (decreased oxygen). Pneumonia also may be present. Pulmonary artery pressure is usually very elevated because of pulmonary edema.

◆ Interventions

First Aid/Prehospital Care. *The most important intervention to manage serious altitude-related illnesses is descent to a lower altitude.* Patients must be monitored carefully for any evidence of symptom progression. With mild AMS, the victim should be allowed to rest and acclimate at the current altitude. The person is instructed not to ascend to a higher altitude, especially for sleep, until symptoms lessen. If symptoms persist or worsen, he or she should be moved to a lower altitude as soon as possible. Even a descent of about 1600 feet may improve the patient's condition and reverse altitude-related pathologic effects. Oxygen should also be administered if available to effectively treat symptoms of AMS.

Prevention and Treatment. The oral drug *acetazolamide* (Diamox, Apo-Acetazolamide 🍁) is commonly used to both prevent and treat AMS (Hackett & Roach, 2012). Acetazolamide is a carbonic anhydrase inhibitor. It acts by causing a bicarbonate diuresis, which rids the body of excess fluid, and induces metabolic acidosis. The acidotic state increases respiratory rate and decreases the occurrence of periodic respiration during sleep at night. In this way, it helps patients acclimate faster to a high altitude. For best results, the drug should be taken 24 hours before ascent and be continued for the first 2 days of the trip.

! NURSING SAFETY PRIORITY (QSEN)

Drug Alert

Because acetazolamide is a sulfa drug, ask about an allergy to sulfa before the patient takes the drug because it may cause hypersensitivity reactions in those who are sulfa-sensitive.

Another drug that is indicated in the treatment of moderate to severe AMS is dexamethasone (Decadron, Deronil 🍁). This drug's mechanism of action is unclear for AMS treatment, but it reduces cerebral edema by acting as an anti-inflammatory in the central nervous system. It does not speed acclimatization like acetazolamide does, but it does relieve the symptoms of AMS. Symptoms may recur when the drug is stopped, an effect termed the "rebound phenomenon" (Hackett & Roach, 2012).

For the treatment of HACE, early recognition of ataxia or a change in level of consciousness should prompt a rapid descent by rescuers or companions to a lower altitude. While undergoing descent, the patient can be given supplemental oxygen and dexamethasone. If mental status is severely impaired and the patient's airway is at risk, all drugs should be given parenterally. Ultimately, the patient with HACE must be admitted to the hospital. Critical care management may be necessary.

Like HACE, early recognition of HAPE is essential to improve the patient's chance for survival. Phosphodiesterase inhibitors such as tadalafil (Cialis) and sildenafil (Viagra) may be used to prevent HAPE because of their pulmonary vasodilatory effects (Hackett & Roach, 2012). When it occurs, HAPE is a serious condition that requires quick evacuation to a lower altitude, oxygen administration, and bedrest to save the patient's life. If descent must be delayed because of weather conditions or other factors, oxygen administration is essential as soon as possible. Keep the patient warm at all times. Drugs are not substitutes for descent and oxygen. However, the treatment of HAPE may include the calcium channel blocker *nifedipine* (Procardia, Adalat PA ♣, Apo-Nifed ♣) to decrease pulmonary vascular resistance (Hackett & Roach, 2012). Hospital admission is required. In uncomplicated cases of HAPE, recovery occurs quickly but effects such as weakness and fatigue may persist for 2 weeks.

Chart 9-8 summarizes best practices for preventing, recognizing, and treating altitude-related illnesses.

NCLEX EXAMINATION CHALLENGE

Physiological Integrity

A client on a climbing expedition reports a headache and nausea. The client rests 1 day at the current altitude and then climbs further the following day. The third day, other members of the climbing team note that the client has developed gross motor coordination difficulties. What action by the team nurse takes priority?

A. Administering acetazolamide (Diamox)
B. Providing 100% oxygen by facemask
C. Having the client descend to a lower altitude
D. Ensuring that the client stays warm at all times

CHART 9-8 Best Practice for Patient Safety & Quality Care (QSEN)

Preventing, Recognizing, and Treating Altitude-Related Illnesses

- Plan a slow ascent to allow for acclimatization.
- Learn to recognize clinical manifestations of altitude-related illnesses.
- Avoid overexertion and overexposure to cold; rest at present altitude before ascending further.
- Ensure adequate hydration and nutrition.
- Avoid alcohol and sleeping pills when at high altitude.
- For progressive or advanced acute mountain sickness (AMS), recognize symptoms and implement an immediate descent; provide oxygen at high concentration.
- To prevent the occurrence of AMS, discuss the use of acetazolamide (Diamox) and other agents as indicated with your health care provider.
- Protect skin and eyes from the sun's harmful ultraviolet rays at high altitude. Wear sunscreen (at least SPF 30) and high-quality wrap-around sunglasses or goggles.

SPF, Sun protection factor.

DROWNING

❖ PATHOPHYSIOLOGY

Drowning is a leading cause of accidental death in the United States. It occurs when a person suffers primary respiratory impairment from submersion or immersion in a liquid medium (usually water) (Szpilman et al., 2012). **Near-drowning** was previously defined as recovery after submersion; however, this term is no longer used because language that describes drowning incidents has been standardized. Today the drowning process is considered a continuum with outcomes that range from survival to death.

Health Promotion and Maintenance

Prevention is the key to avoiding drowning incidents. When providing health teaching, include these points:

- Constantly observe people who cannot swim and are in or around water.
- Do not swim alone.
- Test the water depth before diving in head first; never dive into shallow water.
- Avoid alcoholic beverages when swimming and boating and while in proximity to water.
- Ensure that water rescue equipment, such as life jackets, flotation devices, and rope, is immediately available when around water.

❖ PATIENT-CENTERED COLLABORATIVE CARE

◆ Assessment

When water is aspirated into the lungs, the quantity and the makeup of the water are key factors in the pathophysiology of the drowning event. Aspiration of both fresh water and salt water causes surfactant to wash out of the lungs. Surfactant reduces surface tension within the alveoli, increases lung compliance and alveolar radius, and decreases the work of breathing. Loss of surfactant destabilizes the alveoli and leads to increased airway resistance. Salt water—a hypertonic fluid—also creates an osmotic gradient that draws protein-rich fluid from the vascular space into the alveoli. In both cases, pulmonary edema results. Salt water and fresh water aspiration cause similar degrees of lung injury (Szpilman et al., 2012). Another concern is water quality; the victim's outcome may be negatively affected by contaminants in the water such as chemicals, algae, microbes, sand, and mud. These substances can worsen lung injury and cause a lung infection.

The duration and severity of hypoxia are the two most important factors that determine outcomes for victims of drowning. Very cold water seems to have a protective effect. Successful resuscitations have been reported even after prolonged arrest intervals. Hypothermia might offer some protection to the hypoxic brain by reducing cerebral metabolic rate. The diving reflex is a physiologic response to asphyxia, which produces bradycardia, a reduction in cardiac output, and vasoconstriction of vessels in the intestine, skeletal muscles, and kidneys. These physiologic effects are thought to reduce myocardial oxygen use and enhance blood flow to the heart and cerebral tissues. Survival may be linked to some combination of the effects of hypothermia and the diving reflex.

The cause of the drowning should also be determined, if possible. The patient may have suffered a medical condition or injury that caused the drowning event such as a seizure, myocardial infarction, stroke, or spinal cord injury while in the water. Injuries sustained from diving into shallow water or body surfing, such as cervical spine trauma, can also increase the difficulty of rescue and resuscitation efforts.

◆ Interventions

First Aid/Emergency Care. *Immediate emergency care focuses on a safe rescue of the victim.* Potential rescuers must consider their own swimming abilities and limitations, as well as any natural or human-made hazards, before attempting to save the victim; failure to do so could place additional lives in jeopardy. *Once rescuers gain access to the victim, the priority is safe removal from the water.* Spine stabilization with a board or flotation device should be considered only for those victims who are at high risk for spine trauma (e.g., history of diving, use of a water slide, signs of injury or alcohol intoxication), as opposed to all drowning victims (Szpilman et al., 2012). Time is of the essence; efforts directed toward a rapid rescue have the most potential benefit. Initiate airway clearance and ventilatory support measures, including delivering rescue breaths while the patient is still in the water, as soon as possible (Szpilman et al., 2012). If hypothermia is a concern, handle the victim gently to prevent ventricular fibrillation.

! NURSING SAFETY PRIORITY QSEN

Critical Rescue

Do not attempt to get the water out of the victim's lungs; deliver abdominal or chest thrusts only if airway obstruction is suspected.

Hospital Care. Once the person is safely removed from the water, airway and cardiopulmonary support interventions begin, including oxygen administration, endotracheal intubation, CPR, and defibrillation, if necessary. In the clinical setting, gastric decompression with a nasogastric or orogastric tube is needed to prevent aspiration of gastric contents and improve ventilatory function. After a period of artificial ventilation by mask, the victim typically has a distended abdomen, which impairs movement of the diaphragm and decreases lung ventilation. Patients who experience drowning require complex care to support their major body systems. The full spectrum of critical care technology may be needed to manage the pathophysiologic complications of drowning, including pulmonary edema, infection, acute respiratory distress syndrome (ARDS), and CNS impairment. These complications are discussed elsewhere in this text.

? CLINICAL JUDGMENT CHALLENGE

Patient-Centered Care QSEN

Emergency Medical Services (EMS) brought a drowning victim to the emergency department (ED). The patient is mildly hypothermic, bradycardic, and hypotensive.

1. What further information will the nurse need to obtain from the paramedics?
2. How does the nurse explain the major pathophysiologic event of drowning to the nursing student observing in the ED?
3. The paramedics state that the patient was submerged in a polluted, fresh water pond. How does that environment affect the patient?
4. What action does the nurse take to prevent a complication from CPR in this patient and why?

NURSING CONCEPTS AND CLINICAL JUDGMENT REVIEW

What might you NOTICE if the patient has impaired THERMOREGULATION as a result of a cold-related injury?

- Body temperature below 95° F (35° C) (hypothermia)
- Shivering (hypothermia)
- Possible ventricular fibrillation (hypothermia)
- Cold, pale extremities (frostnip)
- Patient reports numbness or pain (frostnip)
- Hyperemia and edema (1st-degree frostbite)
- Fluid-filled blisters and deep skin necrosis (2nd-degree frostbite)
- Small blisters containing dark fluid, pale or red cool skin that does not blanch, patient reports numbness (3rd-degree frostbite)
- Numb, cold, bloodless body part that eventually develops necrosis (4th-degree frostbite)

What should you INTERPRET and how should you RESPOND to the patient with impaired THERMOREGULATION as a result of a cold-related injury?

Perform focused physical assessment findings and interpret their relationship to impaired thermoregulation, including:

- Temperature
- Skin integrity
- Reports of pain or numbness
- Other vital signs
- Cardiac assessment
- Neurologic assessment
- Fluid status

Respond by:

- *Providing rewarming measures:* Remove patient from the environment; remove wet, cold clothing; initiate passive external rewarming, active external rewarming, or internal rewarming measures as appropriate for hypothermia; thaw frozen body parts in a warm water bath and handle gently; handle hypothermic patients gently to prevent ventricular fibrillation
- Providing pain control measures
- Applying loose, dry dressings
- Administering tetanus prophylaxis and possible antibiotics for open wounds
- Preparing patient for possible débridement
- Using caution when administering drugs because of unpredictable metabolism; alternatively consider withholding drugs except vasopressors until core temperature is at least 86° F (30° C)

- Initiating CPR if needed; one defibrillation attempt is appropriate but may be ineffective if core temperature is lower than 86° F (30° C)
- Providing hydration

On what should you REFLECT?
- Monitor the patient's response to pain medication and rewarming techniques.
- Monitor for further injury from rewarming techniques.
- Evaluate the patient's and family's knowledge about the injury and treatment plans.
- Educate the patient and family on ways to prevent future cold-related injury.
- Monitor the patient's nutrition and hydration status.

GET READY FOR THE NCLEX® EXAMINATION!

KEY POINTS

Review these Key Points for each NCLEX Examination Client Needs Category.

Safe and Effective Care Environment
- Collaborate with the health care team to assess high-risk patients, especially older adults, for their knowledge of safety precautions to prevent THERMOREGULATION alterations such as heat-related and cold-related injuries. **Evidence-Based Practice** QSEN
- Assess high-risk patients, including those who do not know how to swim, for their knowledge of safety precautions to avoid drowning.

Health Promotion and Maintenance
- Teach people how to prevent heat-related illnesses as outlined in Chart 9-1.
- Educate people how to prepare for cold environments, including proper clothing (no cotton) and avoidance of wind and wet weather.
- Instruct people how to prevent arthropod bites and stings as described in Chart 9-5.
- Teach people how to avoid getting bitten by a snake as listed in Chart 9-4.

Physiological Integrity
- Recall that heat-related injuries can be mild (heat exhaustion) to severe (heat stroke).
- Recall that the priority for first aid for heat stroke, after a patent airway is established, is to cool the patient as quickly as possible (see Chart 9-3). **Patient-Centered Care** QSEN
- Remember that North American pit vipers can be identified by their triangular-shaped head and retractable fangs; nonpoisonous snakes do not have these features.
- Recall that the management of a patient who has a snakebite depends on the severity of envenomation (venom injection) (see Table 9-1); both local and systemic manifestations can occur.
- Remember that the priority for first aid/prehospital care when a patient has a snakebite is to decrease the venom circulation. **Patient-Centered Care** QSEN
- Administer antivenom drugs that are available for most types of poisonous snakebites; monitor for an allergic response when these medications are given.
- Recall that the bite of a brown recluse spider can cause tissue necrosis; in rare cases, systemic manifestations can occur, including death.
- Remember that cold applications, such as ice, should be used as first aid/prehospital care for poisonous spider bites.
- Understand that the effect of the bark scorpion venom is neurotoxic; monitor the patient for signs of respiratory failure that may require mechanical ventilation.
- Recall that single bee and wasp stings cause only local reactions unless the person is allergic to them.
- Remember that epinephrine is the drug of choice for bee and wasp sting allergic reactions, followed by an antihistamine drug. **Patient-Centered Care** QSEN
- Teach people that the best way to prevent lightning injury is to avoid places where lightning is likely to strike (see Chart 9-6).
- Recall that lightning causes central nervous system and cardiovascular complications, as well as skin burns.
- Instruct people that two common cold injuries are hypothermia and frostbite; both may be prevented by selecting appropriate layered clothing; cotton should not be worn.
- Teach patients that in moderate to severe cases of hypothermia, coagulopathy (abnormal clotting) or cardiac failure can occur.
- Remember that the priority for care of a patient with a cold injury is warming; alcohol should be avoided. **Patient-Centered Care** QSEN
- Recall that frostbite causes various degrees of impaired TISSUE INTEGRITY and is classified as mild (frostnip) to serious (fourth degree); severe frostbite can result in amputation due to compartment syndrome or gangrene.
- Know that high altitude can cause a range of physiologic consequences in the body, primarily due to hypoxia.
- Teach people that the priority for care of the patient with illness related to high altitude is descent to a lower altitude.
- Recall that acetazolamide (Diamox, Apo-Acetazolamide 🍁) is the drug of choice for prevention and treatment of mild altitude-related illness.
- Review Chart 9-8, which outlines best practice strategies for preventing, recognizing, and treating altitude-related illnesses.
- Remember that drowning victims often require cardiopulmonary support, including CPR.
- Recall that a drowning victim is at risk for pulmonary infection, ARDS, and central nervous system impairment.

10 CHAPTER

Concepts of Emergency and Disaster Preparedness

Linda Laskowski-Jones

http://evolve.elsevier.com/Iggy/

PRIORITY CONCEPTS

- Communication
- Safety
- Teamwork and Collaboration

LEARNING OUTCOMES

Safe and Effective Care Environment

1. Apply principles of triage to prioritize care delivery in a disaster situation.
2. Identify the roles of the nurse in emergency preparedness and response.
3. Compare the key personnel roles in an emergency preparedness and response plan.
4. Describe the components of an emergency preparedness and response plan.
5. Develop a personal emergency preparedness plan.
6. Identify which patients to recommend for hospital discharge in a disaster situation.

Psychosocial Integrity

7. Assess survivors for ability to adapt to the effects of disaster changes or traumatic events.
8. Provide support to the person and/or family in coping with life changes resulting from a disaster.

Physiological Integrity

9. Explain how to maintain physical safety when responding to disaster and mass casualty situations.

A **disaster** is commonly defined as an event in which illness or injuries exceed resource capabilities of a health care facility or community because of destruction and devastation. The disaster can be either *internal* to a health care facility or *external* from situations that create casualties in the community. Both internal and external disasters can occur simultaneously.

TYPES OF DISASTERS

An *internal* disaster is any event inside a health care facility or campus that could endanger the safety of patients or staff. The event creates a need for evacuation or relocation. It often requires extra personnel and the activation of the facility's emergency preparedness and response plan (also called an *emergency management plan*). Examples of potential internal disasters include fire, explosion, loss of critical utilities (e.g., electricity, water, and communications capabilities), and violence. Each health care organization develops policies and procedures for preventing these events through organized facility and security management plans. The most important outcome for any internal disaster is to maintain patient, staff, and visitor safety.

An *external* disaster is any event outside the health care facility or campus, somewhere in the community, which requires the activation of the facility's emergency management plan. The number of facility staff and resources may not be adequate for the incoming emergency department (ED) patients. External disasters can be either natural, such as a hurricane, earthquake or tornado, or technologic, such as an act of terrorism with explosive devices or a malfunction of a nuclear reactor with radiation exposure. Recent external disasters include the Boston Marathon bombing on April 15, 2013, and the West, Texas, fertilizer plant explosion 2 days later. St. John's Regional Medical Center in Joplin, Missouri, had an internal disaster compounding an external disaster on May 2011 when it was directly hit by an EF-5 tornado that destroyed a large part of the town. Of the 142 dead, only 6 people inside the hospital died (Letner, 2011) (Fig. 10-1).

Both internal and external disasters can result in many casualties, including death. Multi-casualty and mass casualty (disaster) events are not the same. The main difference is based on the scope and scale of the incident, considering the number and severity of victims or casualties involved. Both require specific response plans to activate necessary resources. In general, a **multi-casualty event** can be managed by a hospital using local resources; a **mass casualty event** overwhelms local medical capabilities and may require the collaboration of multiple agencies and health care facilities to handle the crisis (Smith,

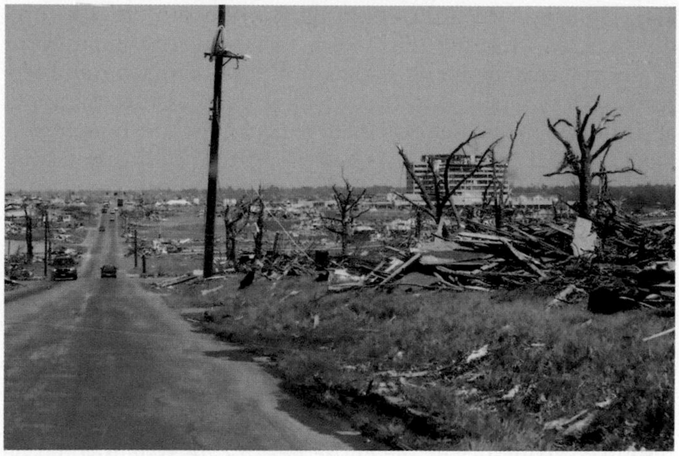

FIG. 10-1 St. John's Regional Medical Center in Joplin, Missouri, after a powerful tornado struck in May 2011.

2010). State, regional, and/or national resources may be needed to support the areas affected by the event. Trauma centers have a special role in all emergency preparedness activities because they provide a critical level of expertise and specialized resources for complex injury management.

To maintain ongoing disaster preparedness, hospital personnel participate in emergency training and drills regularly. In the United States, The Joint Commission (2008) mandates that hospitals have an emergency preparedness plan that is tested through drills or actual participation in a real event at least twice yearly. One of the drills or events must involve community-wide resources and an influx of actual or simulated patients to assess the ability of collaborative efforts and command structures. In addition, accredited health care organizations are required to take an "all-hazards approach" to disaster planning. Using this approach, preparedness activities must address *all credible threats* to the SAFETY of the community that could result in a disaster situation. Disaster drills, then, are ideally planned based on a risk assessment or vulnerability analysis that identifies the events most likely to occur in a particular community. For example, a flood is more likely in the Gulf of Mexico and an avalanche is more likely in ski areas of the Rocky Mountains. It is essential that staff actively participate in these drills and take them seriously to enable their ongoing competency. The importance of training was emphasized in all the recent disasters and is credited with saving lives (Caramenico, 2013).

Hospitals are not the only health care agencies that are required to practice disaster drills. Nursing homes and other long-term care (LTC) facilities are also mandated to have annual drills to prepare for mass casualty events. Part of the response plan must include a method for evacuation of residents from the facility in a timely and safe manner as was demonstrated in the West, Texas, nursing home evacuation.

An evacuation plan is also part of fire prevention and preparedness plans for health care facilities. The Life Safety Code® published by the National Fire Protection Association (2013) provides guidelines for building construction, design, maintenance, and evacuation. The Centers for Medicare and Medicaid Services (CMS) (2012) requires every health care facility to practice at least one fire drill or actual fire response once a year. Patient evacuation is not required if the event is a drill. All facility personnel are mandated to have training on fire prevention and responsiveness each year. Chart 10-1 lists general guidelines for fire responsiveness and building evacuation to ensure SAFETY.

CHART 10-1 Best Practice for Patient Safety & Quality Care QSEN

Nurse's Role in Responding to Health Care Facility Fires

- Remove any patient or staff from immediate danger of the fire or smoke.
- Discontinue oxygen for all patients who can breathe without it.
- For patients on life support, maintain their respiratory status manually until removed from the fire area.
- Direct ambulatory patients to walk to a safe location.
- If possible, ask ambulatory patients to help push wheelchair patients out of danger.
- Move bedridden patients from the fire area in bed, by stretcher, or in a wheelchair; if needed, have one or two staff members move patients on blankets or carry them.
- After everyone is out of danger, seek to contain the fire by closing doors and windows and using an ABC extinguisher (can put out any type of fire), if possible.
- Do not risk injury to you or staff members while moving patients or attempting to extinguish the fire.

IMPACT OF EXTERNAL DISASTERS

The events of September 11, 2001, substantially changed hospital and community disaster planning efforts (Wielawski, 2006). With the shocking terrorist attacks on the Twin Towers of the World Trade Center and the Pentagon and the actual and perceived threat of domestic terrorism, including the anthrax exposure that followed, hospital emergency preparedness concepts became much more fully integrated into the daily operations of emergency departments (EDs) by necessity. Weapons of mass destruction (WMD) rapidly became a focus of public health risk.

The term "NBC" was coined to describe **n**uclear, **b**iologic, and **c**hemical threats. In response, emergency medical services (EMS) agencies and hospitals improved SAFETY by upgrading their decontamination facilities, equipment, and all levels of personal protective equipment to better protect staff. ED physician and nursing staff now routinely undergo hazardous materials (HAZMAT) training and learn how to recognize patterns of illness in patients who present for treatment that potentially indicate biologic terrorism agents, such as anthrax or smallpox (Fig. 10-2). Protocols for the pharmacologic treatment of infectious disease agents, as well as stockpiles of antibiotics and nerve agent antidotes, are readily available.

The most immediate outcome of improving emergency preparedness after September 11 is that the ability to competently handle the more typical multi-casualty or mass casualty incident such as a bus crash, tornado, or building collapse has been greatly improved in many communities. However, disaster situations can still exceed the scope of usual day-to-day crisis operations, pointing to the necessity of well-defined regional and national emergency preparedness plans and the need for ongoing drills.

In 2005, Hurricane Katrina made landfall in Louisiana and other Gulf states as a category 4 storm and caused more than 1000 deaths and devastating environmental and property damage. Volunteers from all over the United States, as well as

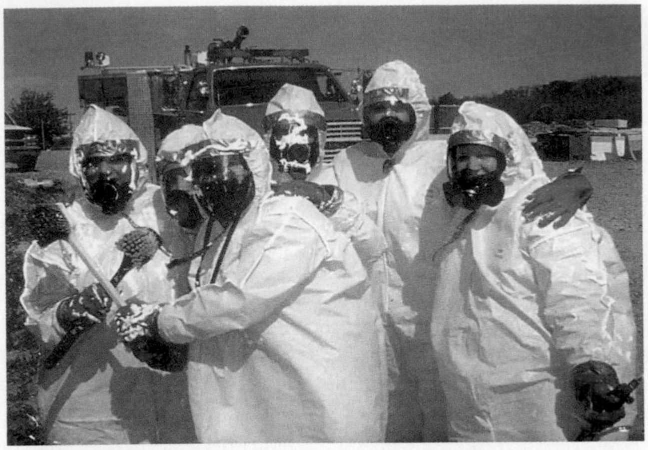

FIG. 10-2 Hazardous materials (HAZMAT) training to decontaminate people exposed to toxic agents in an outdoor decontamination area.

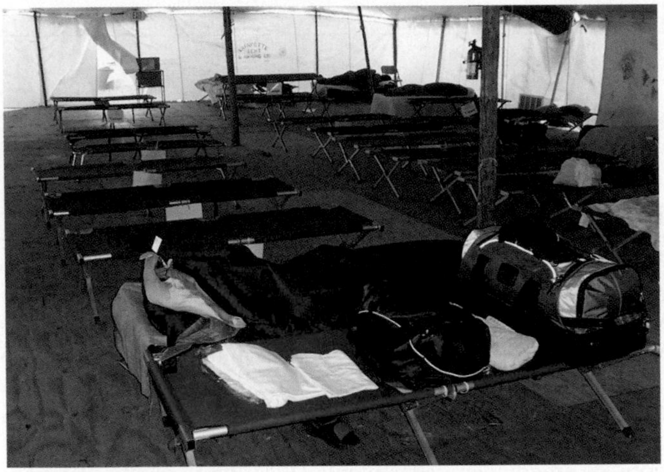

FIG. 10-3 Temporary shelter set up for homeless victims of Hurricane Katrina in New Orleans.

local, regional, and federal agencies, took part in the large-scale disaster evacuation, rescue, and relief effort that severely challenged available resources and established disaster plans. Critical systems failed and were eventually re-established through COLLABORATION with multiple agencies to ensure that the most basic human needs were met (Fig. 10-3). Hurricane Katrina overwhelmed the existing emergency care system and caused the mobilization of a national mutual aid response on a level that had not been experienced in recent U.S. history.

Many health care facilities still have not made structural changes that would offer SAFETY and protection from flooding and utilities failures. A case in point is the devastation brought by "Superstorm Sandy" that made landfall on New York City in October 2012. Though it was downgraded from a category 1 hurricane, the flooding that occurred destroyed critical equipment, including emergency power generators, in the lower levels of several health care facilities, causing the loss of utilities and crippling hospital operations. Hospitals that were severely impacted had to evacuate patients to other facilities, many of which were already overwhelmed by an influx of patients from the storm's damage in the community. Staff worked for several days in harsh conditions, evacuating critical patients via stairwells since elevators were nonfunctional, carrying glow sticks and flashlights and wearing headlamps (Evans, 2012).

Lessons learned from Hurricane Katrina and other natural disasters, as well as worldwide incidents such as Superstorm Sandy, the earthquakes in Japan and Haiti, tsunamis, and terrorist attacks, enable improved facility design, staff preparation, and coordination of efforts that are beneficial for future disasters. These insights also can be applied to health care facility and community agency plans for pandemic infections, including influenza.

A **pandemic** (an infection or disease that occurs throughout the population of a country or the world) leads a vast number of people to seek medical care, even the "worried well." Though not yet ill, the "worried well" want evaluation, preventive treatment, or reassurance from a health care provider. A pandemic influenza outbreak, such as the 2009-2010 swine flu outbreak caused by the H1N1 virus, raised significant concerns that the resource capabilities of the entire health care system could be overwhelmed and that community systems and critical supply chains could be severely damaged. Worker illness, absenteeism, and personal choices to remain quarantined to avoid being exposed to the illness negatively affect the number of health care staff available to care for patients. Fortunately, because of widespread vaccination programs and public information campaigns, the swine flu pandemic of 2009-2010 was well managed. Concern remains that avian influenza A strain (H5N1), also known as "bird flu," could pose a global pandemic threat if a gene mutation occurs to allow easy human-to-human spread. Because of the mass casualty nature of pandemic influenza, emergency preparedness planners must COLLABORATE to incorporate strategies for handling an influx of ill patients into the system as part of ongoing disaster readiness. Quarantine of selected nursing units or the entire hospital could become necessary, prompting closure until the risk has passed.

Common to all mass casualty events, the goal of **emergency preparedness** is to effectively meet the extraordinary need for resources such as hospital beds, staff, drugs, personal protective equipment (PPE), supplies, and medical devices, such as mechanical ventilators. The U.S. government stockpiles critical equipment and supplies in case they are needed for a pandemic influenza outbreak and organizes large-scale vaccination programs (see Chapter 23 for more information on emerging infections). Each state has its own specific emergency preparedness plan for pandemic influenza, including who would receive vaccines in a mass casualty event.

EMERGENCY PREPAREDNESS AND RESPONSE

Mass Casualty Triage

A key process in any multi-casualty or mass casualty response is effective **triage** to rapidly sort ill or injured patients into priority categories based on their acuity and survival potential.

Triage functions may be performed by EMS providers in the field, such as:

- Emergency medical technicians (EMTs) and paramedics
- Nurse and physician field teams who are called from the hospital to a disaster scene to assist EMS providers
- Nurse and physician hospital teams to assess and reassess incoming patients

Triage concepts in a mass casualty incident differ from the "civilian triage" methods discussed in Chapter 8 that are practiced during usual emergency department operations (Table 10-1). Although disaster triage practices can vary widely based

TABLE 10-1 Comparison of Triage Under Usual Versus Mass Casualty Conditions

TRIAGE UNDER USUAL CONDITIONS	TRIAGE UNDER MASS CASUALTY CONDITIONS
Emergent (immediate threat to life)	Emergent or class I (red tag) (immediate threat to life)
Urgent (major injuries that require immediate treatment)	Urgent or class II (yellow tag) (major injuries that require treatment)
Nonurgent (minor injuries that do not require immediate treatment)	Nonurgent or class III (green tag) (minor injuries that do not require immediate treatment)
Does not apply	Expectant or class IV (black tag) (expected and allowed to die)

on local EMS protocols, some concepts are fairly universal. Most mass casualty response teams both in the field (at the disaster site) and in the hospital setting use a **disaster triage tag system** that categorizes triage priority by color and number (Smith, 2010):

- Emergent (class I) patients are identified with a red tag.
- Patients who can wait a short time for care (class II) are marked with a yellow tag.
- Nonurgent or "walking wounded" (class III) patients are given a green tag.
- Patients who are expected to die or are dead are issued a black tag (class IV).

NURSING SAFETY PRIORITY (QSEN)

Action Alert

In mass casualty or disaster situations, implement a military form of triage with the overall desired outcome of doing the greatest good for the greatest number of people (Smith, 2010). This means that patients who are critically ill or injured and might otherwise receive attempted resuscitation during usual operations may be triaged into an "expectant" or "black-tagged" category and allowed to die or not be treated until others received care.

Typical examples of black-tagged patients are those with massive head trauma, extensive full-thickness body burns, and high cervical spinal cord injury requiring mechanical ventilation. The rationale for this seemingly heartless decision is that limited resources must be dedicated to saving the most lives rather than expending valuable resources to save one life at the possible expense of many others.

In general, *red-tagged* patients have immediate threats to life, such as airway obstruction or shock, and require immediate attention. *Yellow-tagged* patients have major injuries, such as open fractures with a distal pulse and large wounds that need treatment within 30 minutes to 2 hours. *Green-tagged* patients have minor injuries that can be managed in a delayed fashion, generally more than 2 hours. Examples of green-tag injuries include closed fractures, sprains, strains, abrasions, and contusions.

Green-tagged patients are often referred to as the "walking wounded" because they may actually evacuate themselves from the mass casualty scene and go to the hospital in a private vehicle. Green-tagged patients usually make up the greatest number in most large-scale multi-casualty situations. Therefore they can overwhelm the system if provisions are not made to handle them as part of the disaster plan. Also, because they often come to the hospital on their own, the hospital may not be able to determine how many actual casualties will arrive. A related concern is that green-tagged patients who self-transport may unknowingly carry contaminants from a nuclear, biologic, or chemical incident into the hospital environment with potentially disastrous consequences. ED staff must anticipate these issues and COLLABORATE to devise emergency response plans accordingly, including appropriate decontamination measures.

NCLEX EXAMINATION CHALLENGE

Physiological Integrity

The nurse is triaging clients arriving at the hospital after a large scale disaster. Which of these clients is correctly classified?

A. Young adult with closed fractures of her right leg and arm: Yellow tag
B. Older adult with severe abdominal pain who is dazed and confused: Black tag
C. Middle-aged adult with third-degree burns over 90% of his body: Red tag
D. Young adult with bruises and superficial lacerations: Green tag

Once patients are in the triage area of the hospital, they typically receive a special bracelet with a disaster number. Preprinted labels with this number can be applied to the patients' chart forms and personal belongings. Digital photos may be used as part of the identification process in some systems. The standard hospital registration process and identification band can be applied after the patient's identity is confirmed.

Automated tracking systems using infrared and radiofrequency technology (RFT) are available in some emergency departments to track a patient's triage priority upon arrival, location, and process of care. The interactions the patient has with caregivers can also be tracked, an important SAFETY strategy if the patient is later found to have contaminants or a disease that could pose a risk to staff members who had close contact and require decontamination or prophylaxis (Laskowski-Jones, 2008). These systems are valuable components of the hospital's emergency preparedness infrastructure because they can rapidly portray the overall census and acuity of patients. They also enable ED leaders to determine how many casualties of a particular acuity level a hospital can safely accept from the incident scene.

Notification and Activation of Emergency Preparedness/Management Plans

When the number of casualties exceeds the usual resource capabilities, a disaster situation exists. What may be a routine day in the emergency department of a large urban trauma center could be defined as a disaster for a small rural community hospital if the same number of patients were to arrive. Each facility, then, decides when criteria are met to declare a disaster. Flexibility is needed because resources may change by time of day and by day of the week. For instance, hospitals typically have the fewest staff available after midnight on the weekend. An incident that occurs in this time frame may require activation of the emergency preparedness plan to bring extra resources into the hospital. The same incident during weekday business hours might be handled with on-site personnel alone without the need for activation of the plan.

Notification that a multi-casualty or mass casualty situation exists usually occurs by radio, cellular, or electronic COMMUNICATION between the ED and EMS providers at the scene. A state or regional emergency management agency may also notify the ED of the event. Each hospital has its own policy that specifies *who* has the authority to activate and *how* to activate the disaster or emergency preparedness plan. Group paging systems, telephone trees, and instant computer-based alert messages are the most common means of notifying essential personnel of a mass casualty incident or disaster.

A catastrophic event, such as a major earthquake or tornado, or a terrorist incident involving weapons of mass destruction (WMD) also requires the COLLABORATION of volunteers from all levels of health care providers in the region. In this case, the media may be contacted to broadcast messages to the health care community-at-large via television, radio, and electronic announcements. For such incidents, the National Guard, the American Red Cross, the public health department, various military units, a Medical Reserve Corps (MRC), or a Disaster Medical Assistance Team (DMAT) can be activated by state and federal government authorities.

- An MRC is made up of a group of volunteer medical and public health care professionals, including physicians and nurses. They offer their services to health care facilities or to the community in a supportive or supplemental capacity during times of need such as a disaster or pandemic disease outbreak. This group may help staff hospitals or community health settings that face personnel shortages and establish first aid stations or special-needs shelters. As a means to alleviate emergency department and hospital overcrowding, the MRC may also set up an acute care center (ACC) in the community for patients who need acute care (but not intensive care) for days to weeks.
- A DMAT is a medical relief team made up of civilian medical, paraprofessional, and support personnel that is deployed to a disaster area with enough medical equipment and supplies to sustain operations for 72 hours (U.S. Department of Health & Human Services, 2013). DMATs are part of the National Disaster Medical System (NDMS) in the United States. They provide relief services ranging from primary health care and triage to evacuation and staffing to assist health care facilities that have become overwhelmed with casualties (Merchant et al., 2010). *Because licensed health care providers such as nurses act as federal employees when they are deployed, their professional licenses are recognized and valid in all states.* Additional examples of services provided by the NDMS include:
  - Disaster Mortuary Operational Response Teams (DMORTs) to manage mass fatalities
  - National Veterinary Response Teams (NVRTs) for emergency animal care
  - International Medical Surgical Response Teams (IMSuRTs) to establish fully functional field surgical facilities wherever they are needed in the world

Nurses can join these teams, complete the required training, and offer their expertise as part of a coordinated federal response team in times of critical need (U.S. Department of Health & Human Services, 2013).

Before going to the incident in the field, nurses, physicians, and support staff must have adequate training to prepare them to recognize the risks in an unstable environment (Laskowski-Jones, 2010; Olchin & Krutz, 2012; Yin et al., 2012). Such risks can include the potential for structural collapse, becoming the secondary target of a terrorist attack, interpersonal violence in unsecured locales, and working in an environment in which contagious diseases and natural hazards are common (e.g., poisonous snake bites and mosquito-borne illnesses). Disaster workers must take measures such as obtaining prophylactic medications and vaccinations, having a personal evacuation plan, and ensuring access to necessary supplies and protective equipment so that they do not become victims as well.

The National Disaster Life Support Foundation, Inc. (2013) offers Core, Basic, and Advanced Disaster Life Support training courses that include all essential aspects of disaster response and management. They include the core competencies of disaster management to all levels of health care professionals. In addition, the Federal Emergency Management Agency (FEMA) (2013) provides numerous online resources, including Community Emergency Response Team (CERT) training so that people are better prepared for disasters and are able to respond more self-sufficiently to incidents and hazard situations in their own communities. These courses include mass casualty triage education.

Hospital Emergency Preparedness: Personnel Roles and Responsibilities

Nurses play a major role in the emergency preparedness or emergency management plan. In the event of a disaster, the Hospital Incident Command System is established for organization and structure.

Hospital Incident Command System

The facility-level organizational model for disaster management is the **Hospital Incident Command System (HICS)**, which is a part of the National Incident Management System (NIMS) implemented by the Department of Homeland Security and FEMA to standardize disaster operations. In this system, roles are formally structured under the hospital or long-term care facility incident commander with clear lines of authority and accountability for specific resources (FEMA, 2013). Officers are named to oversee essential emergency preparedness functions such as public information, safety and security, and medical command. Chiefs are appointed to manage logistics, planning, finance, and operations as appropriate to the type and scale of the event. In turn, chiefs delegate specific duties to other departmental officers and unit leaders. The idea is to achieve a manageable span of control over the personnel or resources allocated to achieve efficiency. FEMA offers free courses on the NIMS model and HICS structure through their website (www.training.fema.gov/IS/).

Because mass casualty events typically involve large numbers of people and can create a chaotic work environment, many EMS agencies and health care facilities use brightly colored vests with large lettering to help identify key leadership positions. Specific job action sheets are distributed to all personnel with leadership roles in HICS that pre-define reporting relationships and list prioritized tasks and responsibilities. The HICS personnel also establish an **emergency operations center (EOC)** or **command center** in a designated location with accessible communication technology. They then use their collective expertise to manage the overall incident. All internal requests for additional personnel and resources, as well as COMMUNICATION with

TABLE 10-2 Summary of Key Personnel Roles and Functions for Emergency Preparedness and Response Plan

PERSONNEL ROLE	PERSONNEL FUNCTION
Hospital incident commander	Physician or administrator who assumes overall leadership for implementing the emergency plan
Medical command physician	Physician who decides the number, acuity, and resource needs of patients
Triage officer	Physician or nurse who rapidly evaluates each patient to determine priorities for treatment
Community relations or public information officer	Person who serves as a liaison between the health care facility and the media

field teams and external agencies, should be coordinated through the EOC to maintain unity of command.

The roles and responsibilities of health care personnel in a mass casualty event or disaster are defined within the institution's emergency response or preparedness plan (Table 10-2). Each plan can be as individual as the particular facility's operations. However, virtually all plans identify certain key functions. For example, one of the primary roles in a hospital to be established at the onset of an incident is that of a **hospital incident commander** who assumes overall leadership for implementing the institutional plan. This person is usually either a physician in the ED or a hospital administrator who has the authority to activate resources. The role can also be fulfilled by a nursing supervisor functioning as the on-site hospital administrator after usual business hours. The hospital incident commander's role is to take a global view of the entire situation and facilitate patient movement through the system. The commander brings in both personnel and supply resources to meet patient needs. For example, a hospital incident commander might dictate that all patients due to be discharged from an inpatient unit be moved to a lounge area immediately to free up hospital beds for mass casualty victims. He or she could also direct departments such as physical therapy or a surgical clinic to cancel their usual operations to convert the space into a minor treatment area. The incident commander assists in the organization of hospital-wide services to rapidly expand hospital capacity, recruit paid or volunteer staff, and ensure the availability of medical supplies.

Another typical role defined in hospital or other health care emergency preparedness plans is that of the **medical command physician**. He or she focuses on determining the number, acuity, and medical resource needs of victims arriving from the incident scene to the hospital and organizing the emergency health care team response to the injured or ill patients. Responsibilities include identifying the need for and calling in specialty-trained providers such as:

- Trauma surgeons
- Neurosurgeons
- Orthopedic surgeons
- Pulmonologists
- Plastic surgeons
- Burn surgeons
- Infectious disease physicians
- Industrial hygienists
- Radiation safety personnel

In smaller hospitals with limited specialty resources, the medical command physician might also help determine which patients should be transported out of the facility to a higher level of care or to a specialty hospital (e.g., burn center).

Closely affiliated with the medical command physician is the **triage officer**. This person is generally a physician in a large hospital who is assisted by triage nurses. When physician resources are limited, an experienced nurse may assume this role. The triage officer rapidly evaluates each person who presents to the hospital, even those who come in with triage tags in place. Patient acuity is re-evaluated for appropriate disposition to the area within the ED or hospital best suited to meet the patient's medical needs.

Many other roles and responsibilities can be defined within the institutional emergency response plan and may include the supply officer, the COMMUNICATIONS officer, the infection control officer, and the community relations/public information officer, to name a few. The community relations or public information officer is an especially important role to delineate in advance. Mass casualty incidents tend to attract a large amount of media attention. This staff member can draw media away from the clinical areas so that essential hospital operations are not hindered. He or she can also serve as the liaison between hospital administration and the media to release only appropriate and accurate information.

Role of Nursing in Health Care Facility Emergency Preparedness and Response

Nurses play key roles before, during, and after a disaster. Before an event, they contribute to developing internal and external emergency response plans, including defining specific nursing roles. Nurses take into account the security needs, COMMUNICATION methods, training, alternative treatment areas, staffing for high-demand or surge situations, and requirements for resources, equipment, and supplies. They then test the plans by actively participating in disaster drills and evaluating the outcomes.

During an actual disaster, the ED charge nurse, trauma program manager, and other ED nursing leadership personnel act in COLLABORATION with the medical command physician and triage officer to organize nursing and ancillary services to meet patient needs. Telephone trees may be activated to call in ED nurses who are not working or are not scheduled to work. ED areas are identified and prepared to stage, triage, resuscitate, and treat the disaster victims. Efforts are made to quickly discharge or admit other ED patients as appropriate to make room for the new arrivals. ED nurses apply principles of triage as disaster victims enter the system to prioritize care delivery and direct patients to the designated areas best suited to meet their needs.

Nursing roles in a disaster extend to all areas within a health care facility. The level of involvement is determined by the scope and scale of the disaster. In any mass casualty event, nurses from medical-surgical nursing units may be asked, in COLLABORATION with the health care provider, to recommend patients for discharge to free up inpatient beds for disaster victims. Patients who are the most medically stable may be discharged early, including those who:

- Were admitted for observation and are not bedridden
- Are having diagnostic evaluations and are not bedridden
- Are soon scheduled to be discharged or could be cared for at home with support from family or home health care services

- Have had no critical change in condition for the past 3 days
- Could be cared for in another health care facility, such as rehabilitation or long-term care

NCLEX EXAMINATION CHALLENGE

Safe and Effective Care Environment

The ED charge nurse is assigning duties to nurses who have been floated to the ED or who have volunteered to help staff the ED during a mass casualty situation. Which assignments are most appropriate? **Select all that apply.**

A. GI laboratory nurse assigned to orthopedic clients having sedation procedures
B. Critical care nurse assigned to client, not related to the mass casualty, having chest pain
C. Medical-surgical nurse assigned to accompany clients to radiology
D. Nursing manager from an inpatient unit assigned to monitor clients in the waiting room
E. Liaison nurse from the operating room assigned to work with families

General staff nurses also may be recruited to COLLABORATE in providing care for stable ED patients, thus allowing ED nurses to focus their efforts on aiding the mass casualty victims. Critical care unit nurses need to identify patients who can be transferred out of the unit to rapidly expand critical care bed capacity. In addition, they can supplement ED nurses in the resuscitation setting or assist in monitored care and transport to critical care units. Hospital and ED nurse leaders also typically direct the ancillary departments to deliver supplies, instrument trays, medications, food, and personnel to meet service demands.

Hospital staff of all levels may be required to alter their routine operations to accommodate a high volume of patients, including those with special needs such as decontamination, burn management, or quarantine. Emergency plans dictate specific actions by staff members, such as who should be called when the plan is activated, who should report, where to report, what supplies or equipment carts should be brought to a predesignated location, and what type of paperwork or system should be implemented for patient identification in a large-scale event. Some staff may even have their roles changed completely. For example, nurses from the performance improvement department or case management may be reassigned to fulfill a clinical responsibility for a nursing unit. The key concept is that staff members are expected to remain flexible in a mass casualty situation and perform at their highest level to address the needs of both the health care system and the patients. The greatest good for the greatest number of people is still the organizing principle when considering roles and responsibilities in mass casualty events—not necessarily individual staff preferences. However, the SAFETY of all patients is vital.

Creativity and flexibility of nursing leaders and nursing staff are essential to provide the staffing coverage necessary for a large-scale or extended incident. The willingness of staff to show up for work is directly impacted by their concerns for their home and family in a disaster; inadequate staffing can jeopardize a facility's ability to provide care. A **personal emergency preparedness plan** developed by each nurse can help in such situations. It should outline the preplanned specific arrangements that are to be made for childcare, pet care, and older adult care if the need arises, especially if the event prevents returning home for an extended period.

TABLE 10-3 Basic Supplies for Personal Preparedness (3-Day Supply)

- Backpack
- Clean clothing, sturdy footwear
- Potable water—at least 1 gallon per person per day for at least 3 days
- Food—non-perishable, no cooking required
- Headlamp or flashlight—battery powered; extra batteries and/or chemical light sticks (**NOTE**: a headlamp is superior because it allows hands-free operation)
- Pocket knife or multi-tool
- Personal identification (ID) with emergency contacts and phone numbers, allergies, and medical information; lists of credit card numbers and bank accounts (keep in watertight container)
- Towel and washcloth; towelettes, soap, hand sanitizer
- Paper, pens, and pencils; regional maps
- Cell phone and charger
- Sunglasses/protective and/or corrective eyewear
- Emergency blanket and/or sleeping bag and pillow
- Work gloves
- Personal first aid kit with over-the-counter (OTC) and prescription medications/vitamins
- Rain gear
- Roll of duct tape and plastic sheeting
- Radio—battery powered or hand-crank generator
- Toiletries (toothbrush and toothpaste, comb, brush, razor, shaving cream, mirror, feminine supplies, deodorant, shampoo, lip balm, sunscreen, insect repellent, toilet paper)
- Plastic garbage bags and ties, resealable plastic bags
- Matches in a waterproof container
- Whistle
- Household liquid bleach for disinfection

NURSING SAFETY PRIORITY QSEN

Action Alert

Include emergency contact names, addresses, and telephone numbers to use in a crisis as part of a personal emergency preparedness plan. In addition, pre-assemble **personal readiness supplies** or **"go bag"** (disaster supply kit) for the home and automobile with clothing and basic survival supplies, which allows for a rapid response for disaster staffing coverage (Table 10-3). "Go bags" are needed for all members of the family, including pets, in the event the disaster requires evacuation of the community or people to take shelter in their own homes.

When called to respond to work during a mass casualty event, some nurses may experience ethical and moral conflict between their family obligations and professional responsibilities (Chaffee, 2006). The American Nurses Association's (ANA's) *Code of Ethics for Nurses with Interpretive Statements* (2001) does not offer clear guidance in this situation. Each person has to make a choice about whether to be involved in helping during the emergency or when to become involved.

EVENT RESOLUTION AND DEBRIEFING

When the last major casualties have been treated and no more are expected to arrive in numbers that could overwhelm the health care system, the incident commander considers "standing down" or deactivating the emergency response plan.

However, although the casualties may have left the ED, other areas in the hospital may still be under stress and need the support of the supplemental resources provided by emergency plan activation. Before terminating the response, it is essential to ensure that the needs of the other hospital departments have been met and all are in agreement to resume normal operations.

A vital consideration in event resolution is staff and supply availability to meet ongoing operational needs. If nursing staff and other personnel were called in from home during their off hours or if they worked well beyond their scheduled shifts to meet patient and departmental needs, provision for adequate rest periods should be made. Exhaustion poses a risk not only to patient safety but also to the nurse when he or she must drive home. Sleeping quarters at the hospital might be necessary in this case, especially if the disaster event contributed to treacherous travel conditions.

Severe shortages of supplies also pose a threat to usual operations at the conclusion of a mass casualty incident. Taking inventory and restocking the ED are high priority assignments. COLLABORATION between the ED and the central supply department is essential to resolving stock availability problems. Instrument trays must be washed, packaged, and re-sterilized. Critical supplies that have been depleted from hospital stores must be reordered and delivered to the hospital quickly. Contracts with key vendors outlining emergency re-supply expectations and arrangements should be a part of the hospital's overall emergency preparedness plan.

Two general types of **debriefing**, or formal systematic review and analysis, occur after a mass casualty incident or disaster. The first type entails bringing in critical incident stress debriefing (CISD) teams to provide sessions for small groups of staff to promote effective coping strategies. The second type of debriefing involves an administrative review of staff and system performance during the event to determine whether opportunities for improvement in the emergency management plan exist.

Critical Incident Stress Debriefing

CISD is only one component of a much broader critical incident stress management (CISM) program. CISM programming addresses pre-crisis through post-crisis interventions for small to large groups, including communities. After working through the turmoil and the emotional impact of the incident as well as the aftermath, the staff may find it difficult to "get back to normal." Without intervention during *and* after the emergency, they may develop post-traumatic stress disorder (PTSD). PTSD can lead to multiple characteristic psychological and physical effects, including flashbacks, avoidance, less interest in previously enjoyable events, and detachment, as well as rapid heart rate and insomnia. People suffering from PTSD can have great difficulty relating in their usual way to family and friends. Ultimately, professional "burnout" can stem from the inability to cope with the stress effectively. A resource for CISM is the International Critical Incident Stress Foundation, Inc. (2013); their mission is "to provide leadership, education, training, consultation, and support services in comprehensive crisis intervention and disaster behavioral health services to the emergency response professions, other organizations, and communities worldwide" (www.icisf.org/who-we-are). Chart 10-2 lists recommendations proposed by several national organizations to help prevent PTSD during the emergency situation.

CHART 10-2 Best Practice for Patient Safety & Quality Care QSEN

Preventing Staff Post-Traumatic Stress Disorder (PTSD) During a Mass Casualty Event

- Use available counseling.
- Encourage and support co-workers.
- Monitor each other's stress level and performance.
- Take breaks when needed.
- Talk about feelings with staff and managers.
- Drink plenty of water, and eat healthy snacks for energy.
- Keep in touch with family, friends, and significant others.
- Do not work for more than 12 hours per day.

Adapted from Papp, E. (2005). Preparing for disasters: Helping yourself as you help others. *AJN, 105*(5), 112.

A CISD team comprises two or three specially trained people who come together quickly when called to deal with the emotional needs of health care team members after a particularly devastating or disturbing incident. The team leader typically has background in a mental health/behavioral health field. The co-leader is ideally a peer of the group being debriefed. Thus, if nurses are debriefed, then a nurse member of the CISD team is generally assigned to the session. CISD-trained physicians, police, firefighters, EMTs, and paramedics may also be used, depending on the needs of the group. The third member of the team is known as the "doorkeeper." This person is responsible for keeping inappropriate people out (e.g., media, spectators) and talking with anyone who leaves the session early in an effort to have him or her return or accept follow-up. Staff involved in the incident need protected time to undergo stress debriefing, which generally lasts from 1 to 3 hours per session.

Typical "ground rules" for stress debriefing include strict confidentiality of information shared during the session and unconditional acceptance of the thoughts and feelings expressed by people within the group. The usual arrangement for the most effective group interaction is a circular configuration of chairs in a private setting. Food should be available so that hunger is not a distraction. CISD group leaders encourage group discussion through asking a series of questions designed to get everyone involved to tell his or her own story about the incident and explain the personal impact. The group leaders enable participants to place the incident into perspective and dispel any feelings of blame or guilt. They also educate participants about self-care concepts and coping strategies to use immediately. People who require more than a CISD session may need referral for mental health/behavioral health counseling.

Administrative Review

The second type of debriefing is an administrative evaluation directed at analyzing the hospital or agency response to an event while it is still in the forefront of the minds of everyone who participated in it. The goal of this type of debriefing is to discern what went right and what went wrong during activation and implementation of the emergency preparedness plan so that needed changes can be made. Typically, representatives from all groups that were involved in the incident come together soon after plan activation has been discontinued. They each are given an opportunity to hear and express both positive and negative comments related to their experiences with the event. Then, in the days after the plan activation, written critique forms are also solicited to gain additional information after participants have had time to consider their overall impressions of the response as well as the impact it had on their respective departments or clinical areas.

Although drills are important, implementing the emergency preparedness plan during an actual mass casualty event is the most effective means of "reality testing" the plan's utility. Feedback provided by participants can be used to modify or revise the plan and create new processes in preparation for future events.

ROLE OF NURSING IN COMMUNITY EMERGENCY PREPAREDNESS AND RESPONSE

During a community disaster, nurses and other emergency personnel may be needed for triage, first aid/emergency care, and shelter assistance. The first action of first-responders in a disaster is to remove people from danger, both the injured and uninjured. This job is typically managed by firefighters and other disaster-trained emergency personnel; unless they have had specific search and rescue training, nurses are not usually involved in this process. In all cases, developing and maintaining accurate *situational awareness* is critical for appropriate priority setting and SAFETY in a rapidly changing environment (Busby & Witucki-Brown, 2011).

After removal from danger, victims are triaged by health care personnel as described earlier in this chapter. After triage, nurses often provide on-site first aid and emergency care. They may also be involved in teaching and supervising volunteers. The American Red Cross sets up shelters for people who have lost their homes or have been evacuated from their homes.

Nurses may also need to teach those living temporarily in shelters about procedures that will be needed for SAFETY when they return home. For example, clean drinking water may not be available for several days or longer. Community residents may need to boil their water before drinking. If electricity and gas are not available, an outdoor grill or camp stove can be used. As alternative procedures, commercial water purification filters, sterilizing ultraviolet pens, or tablets or 10 to 20 drops of chlorine bleach added to a gallon of water will make the water safe to drink.

Human waste management creates another challenge if toilets do not flush. If not managed safely, enteric pathogens spread disease. A toilet bowl or bucket lined with a plastic bag can be used for human waste. To sanitize it and provide odor control, chlorine bleach can be added and the bag tied and sealed. Portable toilet chemicals or chlorinated lime may be used as alternatives. To prevent a toxic gas reaction, remind residents not to mix any chemicals. Treated human waste bags can be buried in the ground. In an austere environment, a pit can be dug in the ground as an improvised toilet. In all cases, emphasize the importance of handwashing with soap and water or using a hand sanitizer to prevent disease transmission.

PSYCHOSOCIAL RESPONSE OF SURVIVORS TO MASS CASUALTY EVENTS

One of the most important roles of the nurse after a community disaster is health assessment, including psychosocial health. Experiencing a disaster can produce both immediate and long-lasting psychosocial effects in people personally affected by the event. Depending on the nature and magnitude of the incident, survivors experience the tragic loss of loved ones, property, and valued possessions. They and their family members may have suffered injuries or illnesses brought about by the catastrophe. Lifestyles, roles, and routines are drastically altered, preventing people from achieving any sense of normalcy in the hours, the days, and perhaps even the weeks and months that follow a disaster. Coping abilities in survivors are severely stressed, leading to many individual responses that can range from functional and adaptive behaviors to maladaptive coping.

Survivors have to confront feelings of vulnerability resulting from the devastating event, knowing that it could occur again—a particularly relevant issue for people who live in areas prone to acts of terrorism or to natural disasters. The decision—be it voluntary or involuntary—to abandon a family home or geographic region and then relocate to a "safe" area either temporarily or permanently results in a further sense of loss and grief. Some people may feel guilty about living through an event that caused so many others to die. The range of intense emotions can appear as physical illness, as well as psychological and social dysfunction.

When helping people in crisis after a mass casualty event, be calm and reassuring. Establish rapport through active listening and honest COMMUNICATION. Survivors benefit from talking about their experiences and being helped as they work to problem-solve. Offer choices whenever possible to help survivors gain a sense of personal control. Help survivors adapt to their new surroundings and routines through simple, concrete explanations. Convey caring behaviors, and provide a sense of safety and security to the best extent possible. If available, request that crisis counselors respond and assist in providing compassionate support to victims and their families (Kallman & Feury, 2011).

A disaster may cause some survivors to develop post-traumatic stress disorder (PTSD), which can potentially last for a lifetime. People who are unable to sleep, are easily startled, have "flashbacks" to relive the disaster, or report "feeling numb" 2 weeks or more after a disaster or traumatic event are at risk for PTSD (Hyer & Brown, 2008).

CLINICAL JUDGMENT CHALLENGE

Patient-Centered Care QSEN

An ED nurse has gone on an emergent medical mission trip to a Third World country after an earthquake with multiple building collapses in a remote rural area. Hundreds are reported missing, and even more are injured. Medical resources in this country are scarce.

1. What challenges does this nurse face in terms of his or her own safety and health?
2. How can the nurse manage basic hygiene and meet basic needs?
3. Some local residents are so distraught that they are unable to function and are not eating or sleeping. What assistance can the nurse provide?
4. After returning from the mission trip, the nurse feels apathetic, disengaged with regular employment, and is often short tempered with co-workers and staff. What resources exist for the nurse?

Nurses caring for survivors with these manifestations should perform further assessment. One tool that can be used to assess survivor response to a disaster is the Impact of Event Scale—

Revised (IES-R). The IES-R is a 22-item self-administered questionnaire including several subscales, such as avoidance. Before giving the tool, determine the patient's reading level because it is written at a 10th-grade reading level. The tool should not be used for patients with short-term memory loss. For that reason, many older survivors are often not adequately assessed for post-disaster PTSD (Hyer & Brown, 2008). However, assess all older survivors of a disaster for this complication when possible.

! NURSING SAFETY PRIORITY QSEN

Action Alert

A high score on any IES-R subscale indicates a need for further evaluation and counseling. Refer the patient to a social worker or qualified mental health counselor. A high score on all subscales requires referral to a psychiatrist or clinical psychologist to evaluate the possibility of current or past trauma, such as abuse or neglect.

GET READY FOR THE NCLEX® EXAMINATION!

KEY POINTS

Review these Key Points for each NCLEX Examination Client Needs Category.

Safe and Effective Care Environment

- Describe the hospital emergency preparedness and response team that all hospitals are required to have in case of mass casualty (disaster). **Teamwork and Collaboration** QSEN
- Use the guidelines in Chart 10-1 to respond to a fire in any facility. **Safety** QSEN
- Apply principles of triage by using the typical triage system for a mass casualty situation, which includes an additional category for those patients allowed to die (black-tagged) (see Table 10-1).
- Describe the special roles that are assigned in a mass casualty incident as identified in Table 10-2.
- Understand how to assist in determining the need for initiating the emergency preparedness plan based on available resources, including staffing. **Teamwork and Collaboration** QSEN
- Be prepared for an emergency by developing a personal emergency preparedness plan, including a plan for child, pet, and older adult care; have a "go bag," or disaster supply kit, packed for both the automobile and the home (see Table 10-3).
- Compare key personnel roles in an emergency preparedness and response plan, including those involved in the two types of debriefing that occur after a mass casualty event or period—critical incident stress debriefing and an administrative review or evaluation. **Teamwork and Collaboration** QSEN
- Identify the important roles of nurses in preparing for, managing, and debriefing after internal health care facility and community disasters.
- Recall that nurses play a major role in triage, first aid and emergency care, and shelter assistance in external community disasters.
- Understand how to identify which patients to recommend for hospital discharge in a disaster situation. **Patient-Centered Care** QSEN

Psychosocial Integrity

- Assess survivors and families for their ability to adapt to the effects of disaster changes or traumatic events, including post-traumatic stress disorder (PTSD). **Patient-Centered Care** QSEN
- Provide emotional support to the person and/or family in coping with life changes resulting from a disaster by encouraging relaxation, listening to survivor feelings, and referring for appropriate counseling. **Patient-Centered Care** QSEN
- Be honest with victims and their families, and help them adapt to their changed or new surroundings.
- Provide support by taking precautions to prevent staff from developing PTSD as outlined in Chart 10-2.

Physiological Integrity

- Take precautions for meeting basic needs in a mass casualty situation; know your own limitations, and develop situational awareness when responding. **Safety** QSEN

11 CHAPTER

Assessment and Care of Patients with Fluid and Electrolyte Imbalances

M. Linda Workman

http://evolve.elsevier.com/Iggy/

PRIORITY CONCEPTS

- Fluid and Electrolyte Imbalance

LEARNING OUTCOMES

Safe and Effective Care Environment

1. Protect the patient with a change in fluid and electrolyte balance.

Health Promotion and Maintenance

2. Teach people how to prevent, recognize, and manage a change in fluid and electrolyte balance.

Psychosocial Integrity

3. Reduce the psychological impact for the patient experiencing a change in fluid and electrolyte balance.

Physiological Integrity

4. Use knowledge from anatomy and physiology to assess the patient's fluid and electrolyte balance.
5. Use laboratory data and clinical manifestations to determine the effectiveness of interventions to restore fluid and electrolyte balance.
6. Prioritize interventions for a patient who has a change in fluid and electrolyte balance.

HOMEOSTASIS

The body works best when fluid and electrolyte balance is kept within a narrow range of normal. For example, no body system works well if 2 liters of blood volume are gained or lost. To keep conditions as close to normal as possible (known as **homeostasis**), the body has many control actions (known as **homeostatic mechanisms**) to prevent dangerous changes.

Homeostasis requires that the body's volume and composition of fluids remain within normal limits. Water (fluid) is the most common substance in the body, making up about 55% to 60% of total weight for healthy younger adults and 50% to 55% of total weight for healthy older adults. This water is divided into two main compartments (spaces)—the fluid outside the cells (**extracellular fluid [ECF]**); and the fluid inside the cells (**intracellular fluid [ICF]**). The ECF space is about one third (about 15 L) of the total body water. The ECF includes **interstitial fluid** (fluid between cells, sometimes called the "third space"); blood, lymph, bone, and connective tissue water; and the transcellular fluids. **Transcellular fluids** are in special body spaces and include cerebrospinal fluid, synovial fluid, peritoneal fluid, and pleural fluid. ICF is about two thirds (about 25 L) of total body water. Fig. 11-1 shows normal total body water distribution.

Water is needed to deliver dissolved nutrients, electrolytes, and other substances to all organs, tissues, and cells. In health, the volume of water in the fluid compartments remains within the normal range although the water moves constantly between compartments. Changes in either the amount of water or the amount of electrolytes in body fluids can affect the functioning of all cells, tissues, and organs. *For proper function, the volume of all body fluids and the types and amount of dissolved substances must be carefully balanced.*

PHYSIOLOGIC INFLUENCES ON FLUID AND ELECTROLYTE BALANCE

Body fluids are composed of water and particles dissolved or suspended in water. The **solvent** is the water portion of fluids. **Solutes** are the particles dissolved or suspended in the water.

Solutes vary in type and amount from one fluid space to another. When solutes express an overall electrical charge, they are known as *electrolytes*. Body function depends on keeping the correct FLUID AND ELECTROLYTE BALANCE within each body fluid space (compartment).

Three processes control FLUID AND ELECTROLYTE BALANCE so the internal environment remains stable even when the external environment changes. These processes—filtration, diffusion, and osmosis—determine how, when, and where fluids and particles move across cell membranes.

FILTRATION

Physiologic Action

Filtration is the movement of FLUID (water) through a cell or blood vessel membrane because of water pressure (**hydrostatic pressure**) differences on both sides of the membrane. Water pressure is related to water volume pressing against confining membranes.

Fluid weight in a space is related to the amount of FLUID present in that area. Water molecules in a confined space constantly press outward against the membranes, creating hydrostatic pressure. This is a "water-pushing" pressure, because it is the force that pushes water outward from a confined space through a membrane (Fig. 11-2).

The amount (volume) of water in any body fluid space determines the hydrostatic pressure of that space. Blood, which is "thicker" than water (more *viscous*), is confined within the blood vessels. Blood has hydrostatic pressure because of its weight and volume. Another factor that affects blood hydrostatic pressure in arteries is the pumping action of the heart.

The hydrostatic pressures of two fluid spaces can be compared whenever a porous (**permeable**) membrane separates the two spaces. If the hydrostatic pressure is the same in both fluid spaces, there is no pressure difference between the two spaces and the hydrostatic pressure is at *equilibrium*. If the hydrostatic pressure is not the same in both spaces, **disequilibrium** exists. This means that the two spaces have a graded difference *(gradient)* for hydrostatic pressure: one space has a higher hydrostatic pressure than the other. *The human body constantly seeks equilibrium.* When a gradient exists, water movement (filtration) occurs until the hydrostatic pressure is the same in both spaces (see Fig. 11-2).

Water moves through the membrane (**filters**) from the space with higher hydrostatic pressure to the space with lower pressure. Filtration continues only as long as the hydrostatic pressure gradient exists. Equilibrium is reached when enough fluid leaves one space and enters the other space to make the hydrostatic pressure in both spaces equal. In equilibrium, water molecules are evenly exchanged between the two spaces but no net further filtration of fluid occurs. Neither space gains or loses water molecules, and the hydrostatic pressure in both spaces remains the same.

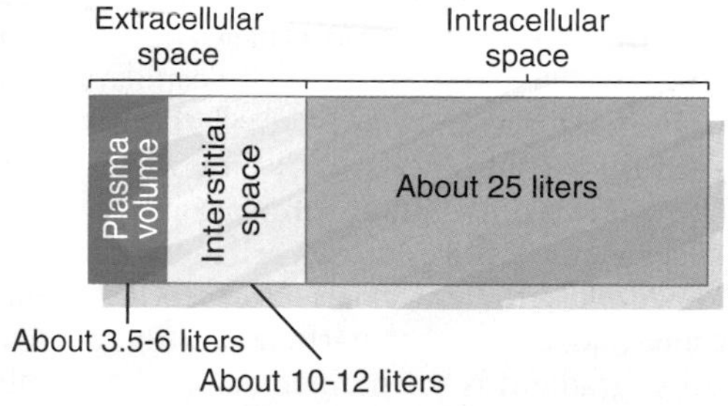

FIG. 11-1 Normal distribution of total body water in adults.

Clinical Significance

Blood pressure is an example of a hydrostatic filtering force. It moves whole blood from the heart to capillaries where filtration can occur to exchange water, nutrients, and waste products between the blood and the tissues. The hydrostatic pressure difference between the capillary blood and the interstitial fluid (fluid in the tissue spaces) determines whether water leaves the blood vessels and enters the tissue spaces.

Capillary membranes are only one cell layer thick, making a thin "wall" to hold blood in the capillaries. Large spaces (**pores**) in the capillary membrane help water filter freely when a hydrostatic pressure gradient is present (Fig. 11-3).

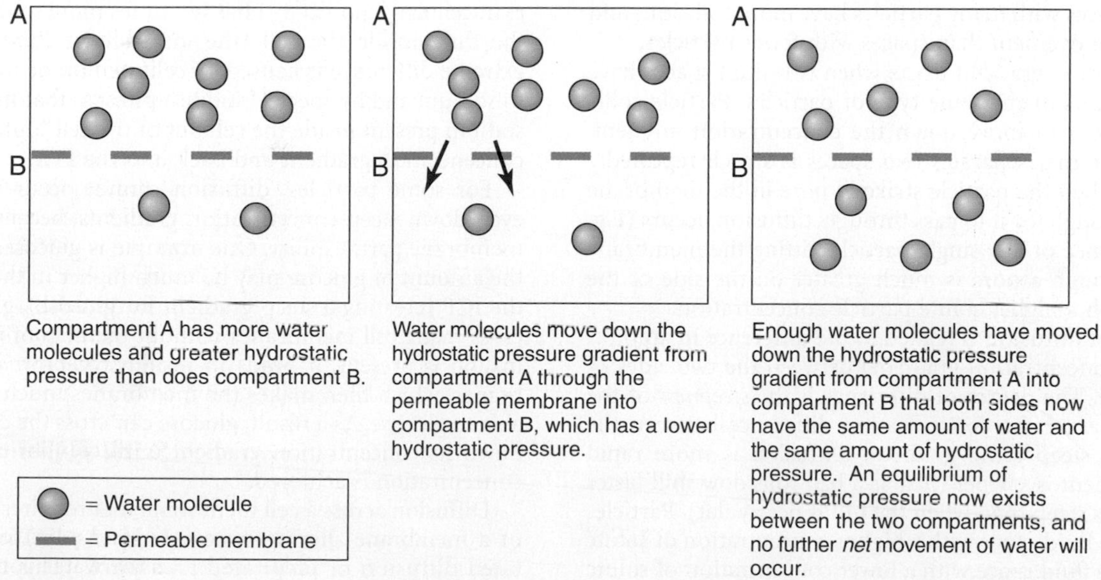

FIG. 11-2 The process of filtration.

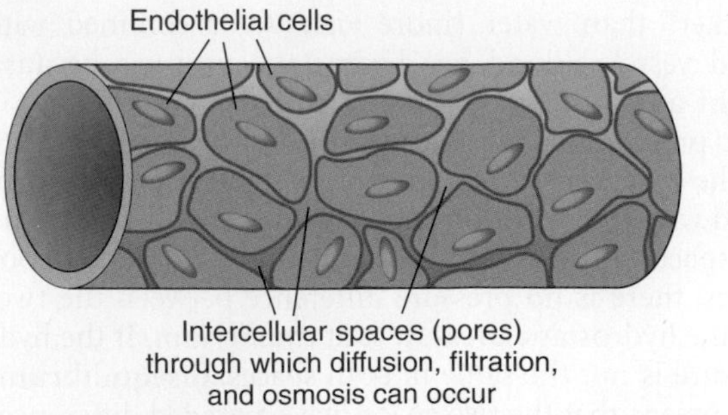

FIG. 11-3 The basic structure of a capillary.

Edema (tissue swelling from excess FLUID) forms with changes in hydrostatic pressure differences between the capillary blood and the interstitial fluid, such as in patients with right-sided heart failure. In this condition, the volume of blood in the right side of the heart increases because the right ventricle is too weak to pump blood efficiently into the lung blood vessels. As blood backs up into the venous and capillary systems, the capillary hydrostatic pressure rises until it is higher than the hydrostatic pressure in the interstitial space. Then, excess filtration of fluids from the capillaries into the interstitial tissue space occurs, forming visible edema.

DIFFUSION

Physiologic Action

Diffusion is the movement of particles (solute) across a permeable membrane from an area of higher particle concentration to an area of lower particle concentration (down a *concentration gradient*). Particles in a fluid have totally random movement from the vibration of atoms in the nucleus. This random movement allows molecules to bump into each other within a confined fluid space. Each collision increases the speed of particle movement. The more particles (higher concentration) present in the confined fluid space, the greater the number of collisions.

As a result of the collisions, molecules in a solution spread out evenly through the available space. They move from an area of higher amounts (higher concentration) of molecules to an area of lower amounts until an equal amount is present in all areas. Fluid spaces with many particles have more collisions and faster particle movement than spaces with fewer particles.

A concentration gradient exists when two fluid spaces have different amounts of the same type of particles. Particle collisions cause them to move down the concentration gradient. Any membrane that separates two spaces is struck repeatedly by particles. When the particle strikes a pore in the membrane that is large enough for it to pass through, diffusion occurs (Fig. 11-4). The chance of any single particle hitting the membrane and going through a pore is much greater on the side of the membrane with a higher solute particle concentration.

The speed of diffusion is related to the difference in amount of particles (concentration gradient) between the two sides of the membrane. The degree of difference is the *steepness* of the gradient: the larger the concentration difference between the two sides, the steeper the gradient. Diffusion is more rapid when the gradient is steeper (just as a ball rolls downhill faster when the hill is steep than when the hill is nearly flat). Particles move from the fluid space with a higher concentration of solute particles to the fluid space with a lower concentration of solute particles.

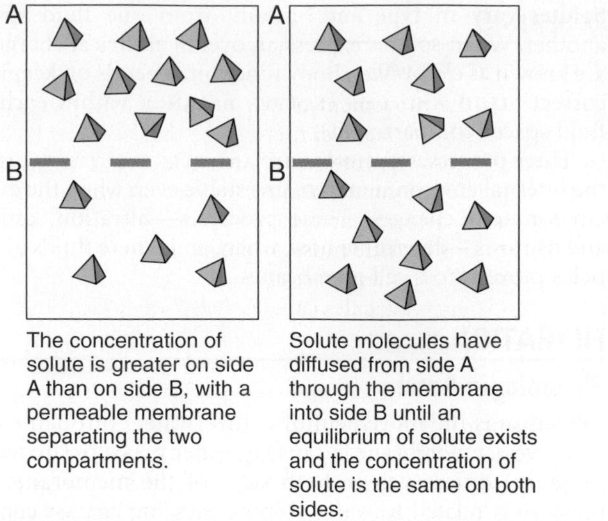

FIG. 11-4 Diffusion of solute particles through a permeable membrane from an area of higher solute concentration to an area of lower solute concentration until an equilibrium is reached.

Particle diffusion continues as long as a concentration gradient exists between the two sides of the membrane. When the concentration of particles is the same on both sides of the membrane, the particles are in equilibrium and only an equal exchange of particles continues.

Clinical Significance

Diffusion is what transports most ELECTROLYTES and other particles through cell membranes. Unlike capillary membranes, which permit the diffusion of most small-size particles down a gradient, cell membranes are *selective* for which particles can diffuse. They permit diffusion of some particles but not others. Some particles cannot move across a cell membrane, even when a steep "downhill" gradient exists, because the membrane is **impermeable** (closed) to that particle. For these particles, the concentration gradient is maintained across the membrane.

Impermeability and special transport systems cause differences in the amounts of specific particles from one fluid space to another. For example, usually the fluid outside the cell (the extracellular fluid [ECF]) has ten times more sodium ions than the fluid inside the cell (the intracellular fluid [ICF]). This extreme difference is caused by cell membrane impermeability to sodium and by special "sodium pumps" that move any extra sodium present inside the cell out of the cell "uphill" against its concentration gradient and back into the ECF.

For some particles, diffusion cannot occur without help, even down steep concentration gradients, because of selective membrane permeability. One example is glucose. Even though the amount of glucose may be much higher in the ECF than in the ICF (creating a steep gradient for glucose), glucose cannot cross many cell membranes without the help of insulin. When insulin is present, it binds to insulin receptors on cell membranes, which then makes the membranes much more permeable to glucose. As a result, glucose can cross the cell membrane down its concentration gradient until equilibrium of glucose concentration is achieved.

Diffusion across a cell membrane that requires the assistance of a membrane-altering system (e.g., insulin) is called **facilitated diffusion** or **facilitated transport**. This type of movement is still a form of diffusion.

OSMOSIS

Physiologic Action

Osmosis is the movement of water only through a selectively permeable *(semipermeable)* membrane. For osmosis to occur, a membrane must separate two fluid spaces and one space must have particles that cannot move through the membrane. (The membrane is impermeable to this particle.) A concentration gradient of this particle must also exist. Because the membrane is impermeable to these particles, they cannot cross the membrane but water molecules can. (Usually water can *always* move through a cell membrane.)

For the fluid spaces to have equal concentrations of the particle, the water molecules move down their concentration gradient from the side with the higher concentration of water molecules (and thus a lower concentration of particles along with a greater hydrostatic pressure) to the side with the lower concentration of water molecules (and a higher concentration of particles along with a lower hydrostatic pressure). This movement continues until both spaces contain the same proportions of particles to water. Dilute (less concentrated) FLUID has fewer particles and more water molecules than the more concentrated fluid. Thus water moves by osmosis down its hydrostatic pressure gradient from the dilute fluid to the more concentrated fluid until a concentration equilibrium occurs (Fig. 11-5).

At this point, the *concentrations* of particles in the fluid spaces on both sides of the membrane are equal even though the total amounts of particles and volumes of water are different. *The concentration equilibrium occurs by the movement of water molecules rather than the movement of solute particles.*

Particle concentration in body FLUID is the major factor that determines whether and how fast osmosis and diffusion occur. This concentration is expressed in milliequivalents per liter (mEq/L), millimoles per liter (mmol/L), and milliosmoles per liter (mOsm/L). **Osmolarity** is the number of milliosmoles in a *liter* of solution; **osmolality** is the number of milliosmoles in a *kilogram* of solution. The normal osmolarity value for plasma and other body fluids ranges from 270 to about 300 mOsm/L. The body functions best when the osmolarity of all body fluid spaces is close to 300 mOsm/L. When all fluids have this particle concentration, the fluids are **isosmotic** or **isotonic** (also called **normotonic**) to each other.

FLUIDS with osmolarities greater than 300 mOsm/L are **hyperosmotic**, or **hypertonic**, compared with isosmotic fluids. These fluids have a *greater* osmotic pressure than do isosmotic fluids and tend to pull water from the isosmotic fluid space into the hyperosmotic fluid space until an osmotic balance occurs. If a hyperosmotic IV solution (e.g., 3% or 5% saline) were infused into a patient with normal ECF osmolarity, the infusing fluid would make the person's blood hyperosmotic. To balance this situation, the interstitial fluid would be pulled into the circulation in an attempt to dilute the blood osmolarity back to normal. As a result, the interstitial volume would shrink and the plasma volume would expand.

FLUIDS with osmolarities of less than 270 mOsm/L are **hypo-osmotic**, or **hypotonic**, compared with isosmotic fluids. Hypo-osmolar fluids have a *lower* osmotic pressure than isosmotic fluids, and water is pulled from the hypo-osmotic fluid space into the isosmotic fluid space. An example of a hypotonic IV fluid is 0.45% saline.

Clinical Significance

Osmosis and filtration act together at the capillary membrane to maintain both extracellular fluid (ECF) and intracellular fluid (ICF) volumes within their normal ranges. The thirst mechanism is an example of how osmosis helps maintain homeostasis. The feeling of thirst is caused by the activation of cells in the brain that respond to changes in ECF osmolarity.

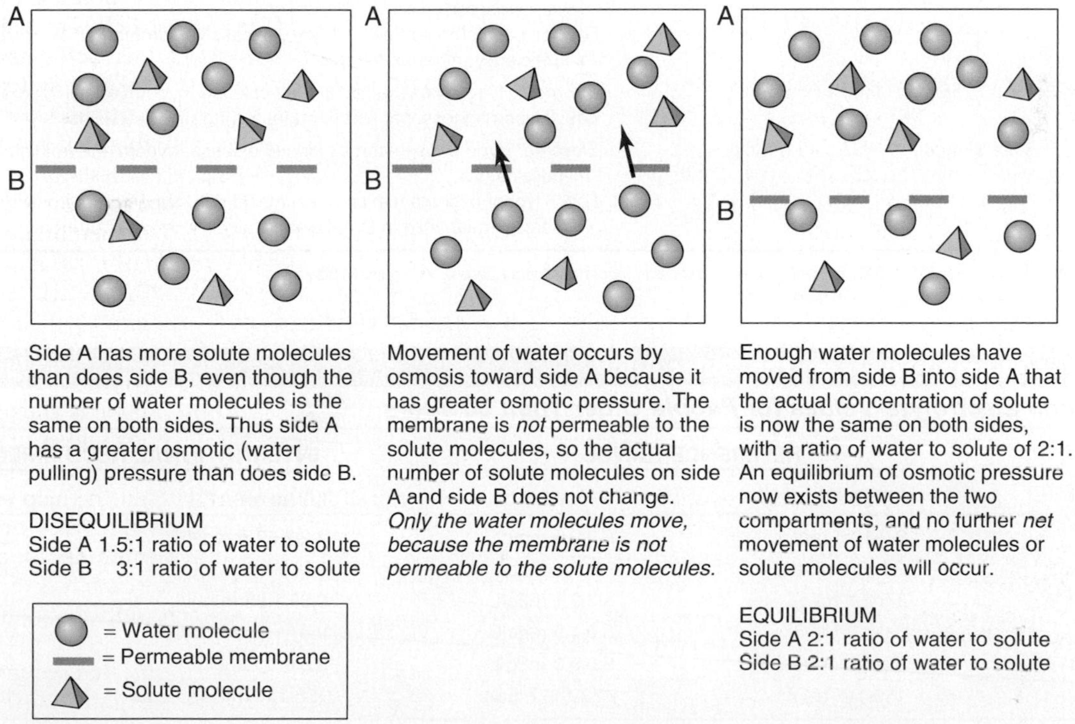

FIG. 11-5 The process of osmosis to generate a concentration equilibrium (but not a volume equilibrium) for a solute particle that cannot move through a cell membrane.

These cells, so very sensitive to changes in ECF osmolarity, are called *osmoreceptors.* When a person loses body water but most of the particles remain, such as through excessive sweating, ECF volume is decreased and osmolarity is increased (is hypertonic). The cells in the thirst center shrink as water moves from the cells into the hypertonic ECF. The shrinking of these cells triggers a person's awareness of thirst and increases the urge to drink. Drinking replaces the amount of water lost through sweating and dilutes the ECF osmolarity, restoring it to normal. The thirst mechanism is less sensitive in older adults, increasing their risk for dehydration.

FLUID BALANCE

BODY FLUIDS

FLUID BALANCE is closely linked to and affected by ELECTROLYTE concentrations. Table 11-1 lists the normal ranges of the major serum electrolytes. Chart 11-1 lists the normal electrolyte values for people older than 60 years.

A person's age, gender, and amount of fat affect the amount and distribution of body fluids. An older adult has less total body water than a younger adult. Chart 11-2 discusses age-related changes in FLUID BALANCE. An obese person has less total water than a lean person of the same weight because fat cells contain almost no water.

GENDER HEALTH CONSIDERATIONS

Patient-Centered Care QSEN

Women of any age have less total body water than men of similar sizes and ages. This difference is because men tend to have more muscle mass than women and because women have more body fat. (Muscle cells contain mostly water, and fat cells have little water.) This difference in water distribution may be responsible for differences seen in women's and men's responses to drugs.

Body fluids are constantly filtered and replaced as FLUID BALANCE is maintained through intake and output. The total amount of water within each fluid space is stable, but individual

TABLE 11-1 Major Serum Electrolyte Concentrations and Significance of Abnormal Values

ELECTROLYTE	REFERENCE RANGE	INTERNATIONAL RECOMMENDED UNITS	SIGNIFICANCE OF ABNORMAL VALUES
Sodium (Na^+)	136-145 mEq/L	136-145 mmol/L	*Elevated:* Hypernatremia; dehydration; kidney disease; hypercortisolism *Low:* Hyponatremia; fluid overload; liver disease; adrenal insufficiency
Potassium (K^+)	3.5-5.0 mEq/L	3.5-5.0 mmol/L	*Elevated:* Hyperkalemia; dehydration; kidney disease; acidosis; adrenal insufficiency; crush injuries *Low:* Hypokalemia; fluid overload; diuretic therapy; alkalosis; insulin administration; hyperaldosteronism
Calcium (Ca^{2+})	9.0-10.5 mg/dL	2.25-2.62 mmol/L	*Elevated:* Hypercalcemia; hyperthyroidism; hyperparathyroidism *Low:* Hypocalcemia; vitamin D deficiency; hypothyroidism; hypoparathyroidism; kidney disease; excessive intake of phosphorus-containing foods and drinks
Chloride (Cl^-)	98-106 mEq/L	98-106 mmol/L	*Elevated:* Hyperchloremia; metabolic acidosis; respiratory alkalosis; hypercortisolism *Low:* Hypochloremia; fluid overload; excessive vomiting or diarrhea; adrenal insufficiency; diuretic therapy
Magnesium (Mg^{2+})	1.3-2.1 mEq/L	0.65-1.05 mmol/L	*Elevated:* Hypermagnesemia; kidney disease; hypothyroidism; adrenal insufficiency *Low:* Hypomagnesemia; malnutrition; alcoholism; ketoacidosis
Phosphorus (P) (Phosphate [PO_4^{3+}]P)	3.0-4.5 mg/dL	0.97-1.45 mmol/L	*Elevated:* Hyperphosphatemia; kidney disease; hypoparathyroidism; acidosis; hypocalcemia *Low:* Hypophosphatemia; chronic antacid use; hyperparathyroidism; hypercalcemia; vitamin D deficiency; alcoholism; malnutrition

Data from Pagana, K., & Pagana, T. (2014). *Mosby's manual of diagnostic and laboratory tests* (5th ed). St. Louis: Mosby.

CHART 11-1 Nursing Focus on the Older Adult

Normal Plasma Electrolyte Values for People Older Than 60 Years

	REFERENCE RANGE		INTERNATIONAL RECOMMENDED UNITS	
ELECTROLYTE	60-90 YEARS	>90 YEARS	60-90 YEARS	>90 YEARS
Calcium (Ca^{2+})	9.0-10.5 mg/dL	8.2-9.6 mg/dL	2.2-2.62 mmol/L	2.05-2.40 mmol/L
Chloride (Cl^-)	98-106 mEq/L	98-111 mEq/L	98-106 mmol/L	98-111 mmol/L
Magnesium (Mg^{2+})	1.3-2.1 mEq/L	1.3-2.1 mEq/L	0.65-1.05 mmol/L	0.65-1.05 mmol/L
Phosphorus (P)	3.0-4.5 mg/dL	3.0-4.5 mg/dL	0.97-1.45 mmol/L	0.97-1.45 mmol/L
Potassium (K^+)	3.5-5.0 mEq/L	3.5-5.0 mEq/L	3.5-5.0 mmol/L	3.5-5.0 mmol/L
Sodium (Na^+)	136-145 mEq/L	132-146 mEq/L	136-145 mmol/L	132-146 mmol/L

Data for adults 60 to 90 years from Pagana, K., & Pagana, T. (2014). *Mosby's manual of diagnostic and laboratory tests* (5th ed). St. Louis: Mosby.
Data for adults >90 years from Tietz, N.W. (Ed.). (1995). *Clinical guide to laboratory tests* (3rd ed.). Philadelphia: Saunders.

water molecules move continually among all spaces. As a result, water in all spaces is exchanged continually while maintaining constant fluid volume.

Fluid intake is regulated through the thirst drive. FLUID enters the body as liquids and as solid foods, which contain up to 85% water (Table 11-2).

A rising blood osmolarity or a decreasing blood volume triggers the sensation of thirst. Sensations such as mouth dryness or the thought that a person has not had a drink recently also triggers the thirst drive. An adult takes in about 2300 mL of fluid daily from food and liquids.

Fluid loss occurs through several routes (see Table 11-2). The kidney is the most important and the most sensitive water loss route because it is regulated and is adjustable. The volume of urine excreted daily varies depending on the amount of FLUID taken in and the body's need to conserve fluids.

The minimum amount of urine per day needed to excrete toxic waste products is 400 to 600 mL. This minimum volume is called the **obligatory urine output**. If the 24-hour urine output falls below the obligatory output amount, wastes are retained and can cause lethal electrolyte imbalances, acidosis, and a toxic buildup of nitrogen.

CHART 11-2 Nursing Focus on the Older Adult

Impact of Age-Related Changes on Fluid Balance

SYSTEM	CHANGE	RESULT
Skin	Loss of elasticity Decreased turgor Decreased oil production	Skin becomes an unreliable indicator of fluid status, especially the back of the hand Dry, easily damaged skin
Kidney	Decreased glomerular filtration Decreased concentrating capacity	Poor excretion of waste products Increased water loss, increasing the risk for dehydration
Muscular	Decreased muscle mass	Decreased total body water Greater risk for dehydration
Neurologic	Diminished thirst reflex	Decreased fluid intake, increasing the risk for dehydration
Endocrine	Adrenal atrophy	Poor regulation of sodium and potassium, increasing the risk for hyponatremia and hyperkalemia

TABLE 11-2 Routes of Fluid Ingestion and Excretion

INTAKE	OUTPUT
Measurable	
Oral fluids	Urine
Parenteral fluids	Emesis
Enemas*	Feces
Irrigation fluids*	Drainage from body cavities
Not Measurable	
Solid foods	Perspiration
Metabolism	Vaporization through the lungs

*Measured by subtracting the amount returned from the amount instilled.

The ability of the kidneys to make either concentrated or very dilute urine helps maintain FLUID BALANCE. The kidney works with various hormones to maintain fluid balance when extracellular fluid concentrations, volumes, or pressures change.

Other normal water loss occurs through the skin, the lungs, and the intestinal tract. Water losses also can result from salivation, drainage from fistulas and drains, and GI suction.

Water loss from the skin, lungs, and stool is called **insensible water loss** because there are no mechanisms to control this loss. In a healthy adult, insensible water loss is about 500 to 1000 mL/day. This loss increases greatly during thyroid crisis, trauma, burns, states of extreme stress, and fever. Insensible water loss also increases when the environment is hot and dry. Patients at risk for increased insensible water loss include those being mechanically ventilated, those with rapid respirations *(tachypnea)*, and those undergoing continuous GI suctioning. Loss by sweating is variable and can reach a maximum rate of about 2 L/hr. Water loss through stool is normally minimal. However, this loss can increase greatly with severe diarrhea or excessive fistula drainage. If not balanced by intake, insensible loss can lead to severe dehydration and electrolyte imbalances.

HORMONAL REGULATION OF FLUID BALANCE

Three hormones help control FLUID AND ELECTROLYTE BALANCE. These are aldosterone, antidiuretic hormone (ADH), and natriuretic peptide (NP).

Aldosterone is a hormone secreted by the adrenal cortex whenever sodium levels in the extracellular fluid (ECF) are decreased. Aldosterone prevents both water and sodium loss. When aldosterone is secreted, it acts on the kidney nephrons, triggering them to reabsorb sodium and water from the urine back into the blood. This action increases blood osmolarity and blood volume. Aldosterone prevents excessive kidney excretion of sodium. It also helps prevent blood potassium levels from becoming too high.

Antidiuretic hormone (ADH), or vasopressin, is released from the posterior pituitary gland in response to changes in blood osmolarity. The hypothalamus contains the osmoreceptors that are sensitive to changes in blood osmolarity. Increased blood osmolarity, especially an increase in the level of plasma sodium, results in a slight shrinkage of these cells and triggers ADH release from the posterior pituitary gland. Because the action of ADH retains just water, it only indirectly regulates electrolyte retention or excretion.

ADH acts directly on kidney tubules and collecting ducts, making them more permeable to water only. As a result, more water is *reabsorbed* by these tubules and returned to the blood, decreasing blood osmolarity by making it more dilute. When blood osmolarity decreases with low plasma sodium levels, the osmoreceptors swell slightly and inhibit ADH release. Less water is then reabsorbed, and more is lost from the body in the urine. As a result, the amount of water in the extracellular fluid (ECF) decreases, bringing osmolarity up to normal.

Natriuretic peptides (NPs) are hormones secreted by special cells that line the atria of the heart (atrial natriuretic peptide [ANP]) and the ventricles of the heart. (The peptide secreted by the heart ventricular cells is known as *brain natriuretic peptide [BNP]* because it was first discovered in the brain.) These peptides are secreted in response to increased blood volume and blood pressure, which stretch the heart tissue. NP binds to receptors in the nephrons, creating effects that are opposite of aldosterone. Kidney reabsorption of sodium is inhibited at the same time that glomerular filtration is increased, causing increased urine output. The outcome is decreased circulating blood volume and decreased blood osmolarity.

SIGNIFICANCE OF FLUID BALANCE

The Renin-Angiotensin II Pathway

The human body requires FLUID AND ELECTROLYTE BALANCE, as well as a balance of acids and bases, for best function. The most important fluids to keep in balance are the blood volume (plasma volume) and the fluid inside the cells (intracellular fluid). Of these two, the most critical FLUID BALANCE to prevent death is maintaining blood volume at a sufficient level for blood pressure to remain high enough to ensure adequate perfusion and gas exchange of all organs and tissues. Balance of both water and electrolytes is needed for this very vital function.

Because low blood volume and low blood pressure can rapidly lead to death, the body has many specific actions (compensatory mechanisms) that guard against excessive fluid loss from the plasma volume. These actions involve specific hormone levels, kidney function, and blood vessel responses to change how water and sodium are handled to maintain blood pressure.

Because the kidney is a major regulator of water and sodium balance to maintain blood pressure and perfusion to all tissues and organs, the kidneys monitor blood pressure, blood volume, blood oxygen levels, and blood osmolarity (related to sodium concentration). When the kidneys sense that any one of these parameters is getting low, they begin to secrete a substance called *renin* that sets into motion a group of hormonal and blood vessel responses to ensure that blood pressure is raised back up to normal. Fig. 11-6 summarizes these responses.

So, the triggering event is any change in the blood that indicates to the kidney that tissue and organ perfusion are at risk. Low blood pressure is a triggering event because when it gets too low, blood cannot flow through vessels into tissues and organs. Anything that reduces blood volume (e.g., dehydration, hemorrhage) below a critical level *always* lowers blood pressure. Low blood oxygen levels also are triggering events because with too little oxygen in the blood, even if the blood reaches the tissues and organs, it cannot supply the needed oxygen and the tissues and organs could die. A low blood sodium level also is a triggering event because sodium and water are closely linked. Where sodium goes, water follows. So, anything that causes the blood to have too little sodium prevents water from staying in the blood. The result is low blood volume with low blood pressure and poor tissue perfusion.

Once the kidneys sense that tissue and organ perfusion are at risk, special cells in the kidney tubule begin to secrete renin into the blood. Renin then activates some blood proteins, one of which is *angiotensinogen.* Activated angiotensinogen is *angiotensin I,* which is relatively weak and has little action. It is then acted on by another enzyme known as *angiotensin-converting enzyme* or *ACE,* which converts angiotensin I into its most active form, angiotensin II.

Angiotensin II starts several different activities that all work to increase blood volume and blood pressure. First, because angiotensin II is a powerful vasoconstrictor, it causes constriction of small arteries and veins throughout the body. This action increases peripheral resistance and reduces the size of the vascular bed, which raises blood pressure as a compensatory

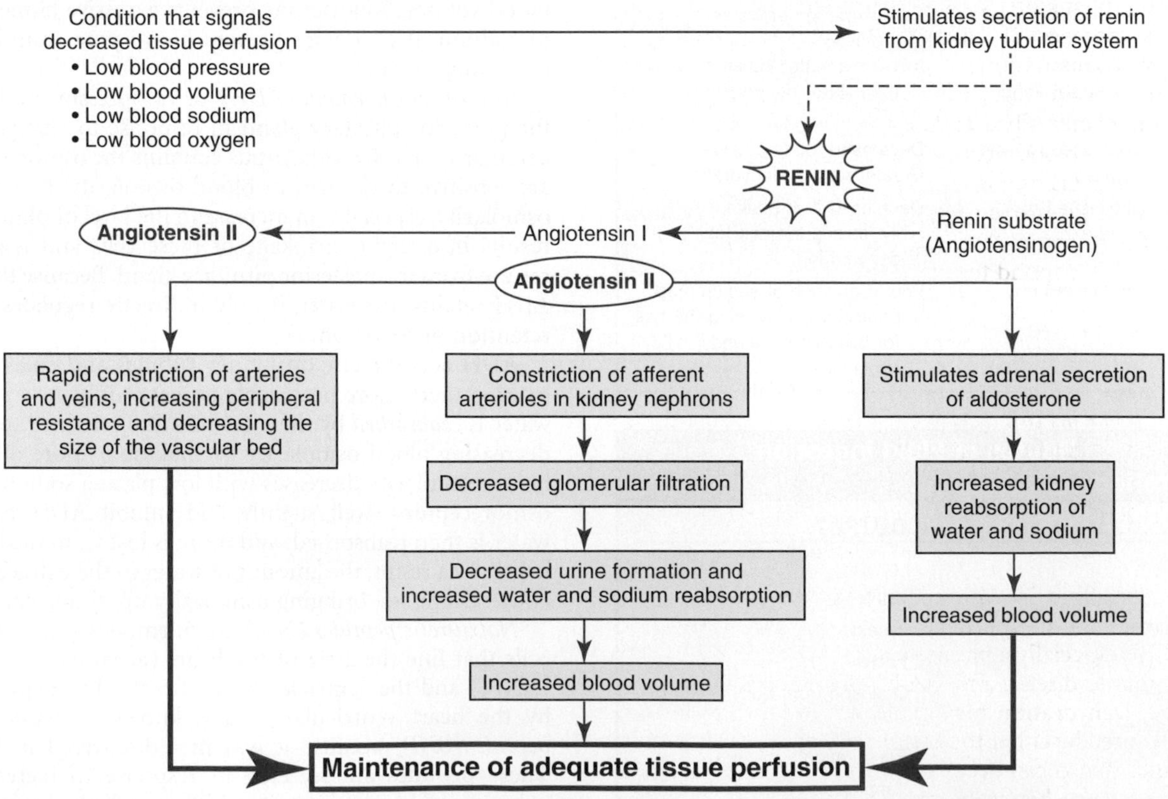

FIG. 11-6 The role of the renin-angiotensin II pathway in fluid and electrolyte balance and blood pressure regulation.

mechanism without adding more blood volume. At the same time, a second action of angiotensin II is that it constricts the size of the arterioles that feed the kidney nephrons. This action results in a lower glomerular filtration rate and a huge reduction of urine output. Decreasing urine output prevents further loss of water so that more is retained in the blood to help raise blood pressure. The last and slightly slower action of angiotensinogen II is to cause the adrenal glands to secrete the hormone *aldosterone.* Aldosterone is nicknamed the "water-and-sodium-saving hormone" because it causes the kidneys to reabsorb water and sodium, preventing them from being excreted into the urine. This response allows more water and sodium to be returned to the blood, increasing blood pressure and blood volume. All of these actions help maintain perfusion to vital organs.

Clinical Application

The renin-angiotensin II pathway is highly stimulated whenever the patient is in shock or when the stress response occurs. This is why urine output is used as an indicator of perfusion adequacy after surgery or any time the patient has undergone an invasive procedure and is at risk for hemorrhage.

An additional application of this pathway is related to management of *hypertension* (high blood pressure). Patients who have hypertension are often asked to limit their intake of sodium. The reason for this is that a high sodium intake raises the blood level of sodium, causing more water to be retained in the blood volume and raising blood pressure. Drug therapy for hypertension management may include diuretic drugs that increase the excretion of sodium so that less is present in the blood, resulting in a lower blood volume. Another class of drugs often used to manage blood pressure is the "ACE inhibitors." These drugs disrupt the renin-angiotensin II pathway by reducing the amount of angiotensin-converting enzyme (ACE) made so that less angiotensin II is present. With less angiotensin II, there is less vasoconstriction and reduced peripheral resistance, less aldosterone production, and greater excretion of water and sodium in the urine. All of these responses lead to decreased blood volume and blood pressure. Another class of drugs used to manage hypertension is the angiotensin receptor blockers (ARBs). These drugs disrupt the renin-angiotensin II pathway by blocking the receptors that bind with angiotensin II so that the tissues cannot respond to it and blood pressure is lowered.

FLUID IMBALANCES

All patients are at risk for some degree of fluid imbalance because many health problems can disrupt fluid intake or output. FLUID imbalances can occur in any setting.

DEHYDRATION

❖ PATHOPHYSIOLOGY

In dehydration, fluid intake or retention is less than what is needed to meet the body's fluid needs, resulting in a FLUID volume deficit, especially a plasma volume deficit. It is a condition rather than a disease and can be caused by many factors (Table 11-3). Dehydration may be an *actual* decrease in total body water caused by either too little intake of fluid or too great a loss of fluid. It also can occur without an actual loss of total body water, such as when water shifts from the plasma into the interstitial space. This condition is called *relative* dehydration.

Dehydration may occur with just water (fluid) loss or with water and electrolyte loss (isotonic dehydration). *Isotonic dehydration is the most common type of fluid loss problem.* FLUID is lost only from the extracellular fluid (ECF) space, including both the plasma and the interstitial spaces. There is no shift of fluids between spaces, so the intracellular fluid (ICF) volume remains normal (Fig. 11-7). Circulating blood volume is decreased (hypovolemia) and leads to inadequate tissue perfusion. The body's defenses adapt (compensate) during dehydration to maintain adequate blood flow to vital organs in spite of

CONSIDERATIONS FOR OLDER ADULTS

Patient-Centered Care QSEN

Older patients are at high risk for dehydration because they have less total body water than younger adults. In addition, many older adults have decreased thirst sensation and may have difficulty with walking or other motor skills needed for obtaining fluids. They also may take drugs such as diuretics, antihypertensives, and laxatives that increase fluid excretion.

TABLE 11-3 Common Causes of Fluid Imbalances

Dehydration	Fluid Overload
• Hemorrhage	• Excessive fluid replacement
• Vomiting	• Kidney failure (late phase)
• Diarrhea	• Heart failure
• Profuse salivation	• Long-term corticosteroid therapy
• Fistulas	• Syndrome of inappropriate antidiuretic hormone (SIADH)
• Ileostomy	• Psychiatric disorders with polydipsia
• Profuse diaphoresis	• Water intoxication
• Burns	
• Severe wounds	
• Long-term NPO status	
• Diuretic therapy	
• GI suction	
• Hyperventilation	
• Diabetes insipidus	
• Difficulty swallowing	
• Impaired thirst	
• Unconsciousness	
• Fever	
• Impaired motor function	

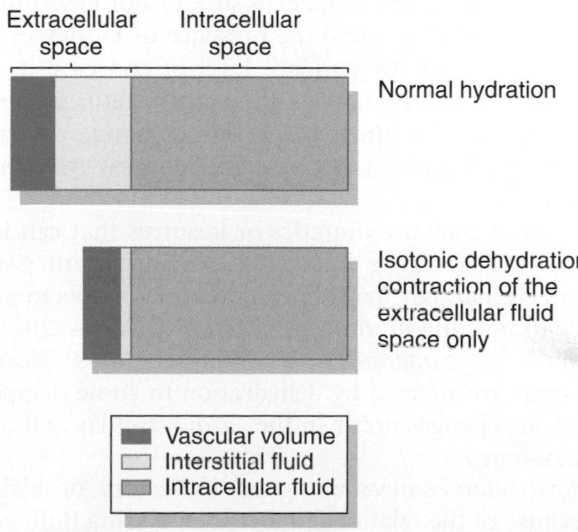

FIG. 11-7 Changes in fluid compartment volumes with dehydration.

hypovolemia. The main defense is increasing vasoconstriction and peripheral resistance to maintain blood pressure and circulation.

Health Promotion and Maintenance

Mild dehydration is very common among healthy adults and is corrected or prevented easily by matching fluid intake with fluid output. Teach all patients to drink more fluids, especially water, whenever they engage in heavy or prolonged physical activity or live in dry climates or at higher altitudes. Beverages with caffeine can increase fluid loss, as can drinks containing alcohol; thus these beverages should not be used to prevent or treat dehydration.

Moderate to severe dehydration is more likely to occur in people who are unable to obtain fluids without help, such as some older adults. Dehydration in older adults in long-term care facilities can be prevented with programs that include routinely offering residents fluids every hour or two during the day and when administering medications.

❖ PATIENT-CENTERED COLLABORATIVE CARE

◆ Assessment

History. The nutrition history can reveal problems that affect FLUID BALANCE. Ask specific questions about food and liquid intake. Also assess the types of fluids and foods ingested to determine amount and osmolarity. Many patients do not know that solid foods contain liquid. Other foods such as ice cream, gelatin, and ices are liquids at body temperature, and these must be included when calculating fluid intake.

Collect specific information about exact intake and output volumes, and obtain serial daily weight measurements. If possible, weigh the patient directly rather than asking what he or she weighs because weight loss is an indication of dehydration. *Because 1 L of water weighs 2.2 pounds (1 kg), changes in daily weights are the best indicators of fluid losses or gains. A weight change of 1 pound corresponds to a fluid volume change of about 500 mL.*

Output includes losses not only as urine but also as sweat, diarrhea, and insensible loss during fevers. Ask specific questions about prescribed and over-the-counter drugs, and check the dosage, the length of time taken, and the patient's adherence with the drug regimen.

Other important areas of the patient history include a sense of thirst or excessive drinking, exposure to hot environments, living at higher altitudes, and the presence of kidney or endocrine diseases. Assess the patient's level of consciousness and mental status, because changes in mental status occur with FLUID imbalance. Ask the patient about changes in ring or shoe tightness. A sudden decrease in tightness may indicate dehydration.

Older adults may use diuretics or laxatives that can lead to FLUID AND ELECTROLYTE imbalance. An important issue for older adults is that they may depend on other people to provide assistance in meeting fluid needs (Collins & Claros, 2011).

Physical Assessment/Clinical Manifestations. Nearly all body systems are affected by dehydration to some degree. The most obvious changes occur in the cardiovascular and integumentary systems.

Cardiovascular changes are good indicators of hydration status because of the relationship between plasma fluid volume and blood pressure. Heart rate increases in an attempt to maintain blood pressure with less blood volume. Peripheral pulses are weak, difficult to find, and easily blocked with light pressure. The blood pressure also decreases, as does the pulse pressure, with a greater decrease in the systolic blood pressure. Hypotension is more severe with the patient in the standing position than in the sitting or lying position (**orthostatic** or **postural hypotension**). Because the blood pressure with the patient standing may be much lower than in other positions, first measure blood pressure with the patient lying down, then sitting, and finally standing. (These measures are also called "ortho checks" or "ortho changes.") As the blood pressure decreases when changing position, the person may not have sufficient blood flow to the brain, causing the sensations of light-headedness and dizziness. This problem increases the risk for falling, especially among older adults.

Neck veins are normally distended when a patient is in the supine position, and hand veins are distended when lower than the level of the heart. Neck veins normally flatten when the patient moves to a sitting position. With dehydration, neck and hand veins are flat, even when the neck and hands are not raised above the level of the heart.

Respiratory changes include an increased rate because the decreased blood volume reduces perfusion and oxygenation. The increased respiratory rate is a compensatory mechanism that attempts to maintain oxygen delivery when perfusion is decreased.

Skin changes can indicate dehydration. Assess the skin and mucous membranes for color, moisture, and turgor. In older patients, this information is less reliable because of poor skin turgor resulting from the loss of elastic tissue and increased skin dryness from the loss of tissue FLUID with aging. Assess skin turgor by checking:

- How easily the skin over the back of the hand and arm can be gently pinched between the thumb and the forefinger to form a "tent"
- How soon the pinched skin resumes its normal position after release

In dehydration, skin turgor is poor, with the tent remaining for minutes after pinching the skin. The skin is dry and scaly.

CONSIDERATIONS FOR OLDER ADULTS

Patient-Centered Care QSEN

Assess skin turgor in an older adult by pinching the skin over the sternum or on the forehead, rather than the back of the hand (Fig. 11-8). With aging, the skin loses elasticity and tents on hands and arms even when the person is well hydrated.

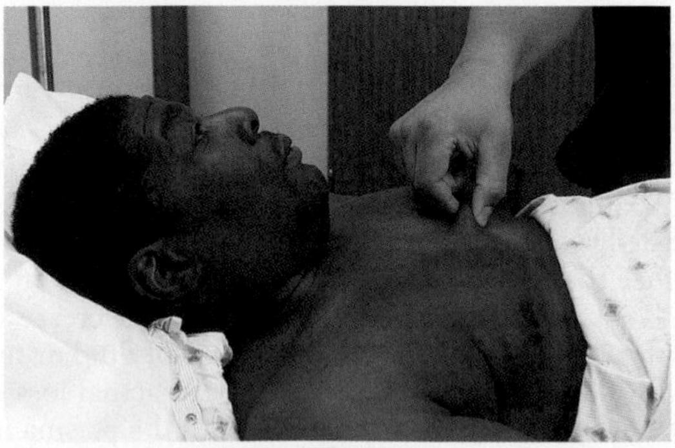

FIG. 11-8 Examining the skin turgor of an older patient.

In dehydration, oral mucous membranes are not moist. They may be covered with a thick, sticky coating and may have cracks and fissures. The surface of the tongue may have deep furrows. This manifestation may not be accurate for assessing dehydration in patients taking drugs that have the side effect of dry mouth.

Neurologic changes with dehydration include changes in mental status and temperature with reduced blood flow in the brain. Confusion is more common among older adults and may be the first indication of a FLUID imbalance. Check to determine whether the patient is alert and oriented. Chapter 41 provides more information about assessment of mental status.

The patient with dehydration often has a low-grade fever, and fever can also cause dehydration. A patient with a temperature higher than 102° F (39° C) for longer than 6 hours is especially at risk because the increased body temperature increases the rate at which FLUID is lost. For every degree (Celsius) increase in body temperature above normal, a minimum of an additional 500 mL of body fluid is lost.

Kidney changes in dehydration affect urine volume and concentration. Monitor urine output, comparing total output with total fluid intake and daily weights. The urine may be concentrated, with a specific gravity greater than 1.030. The color is dark amber and has a strong odor. *Urine output below 500 mL/day for any patient without kidney disease is cause for concern.* Use daily weights to assess fluid loss. Weight loss over a half pound per day is fluid loss.

Laboratory Assessment. No single laboratory test result confirms or rules out dehydration. Instead, dehydration is determined by laboratory findings along with clinical manifestations (see Table 11-1). Usually, laboratory findings with dehydration show elevated levels of hemoglobin, hematocrit, serum osmolarity, glucose, protein, blood urea nitrogen, and various ELECTROLYTES because more water is lost and other substances remain, increasing blood concentration (**hemoconcentration**). Hemoconcentration is not present when dehydration is caused by hemorrhage, because loss of all blood and plasma products occurs together.

◆ Interventions

The focus of management for the patient with dehydration is to prevent injury, prevent further fluid loss, and increase fluid volumes to normal. Nursing priorities include patient safety, fluid replacement, and drug therapy.

Patient safety issues and strategies are priorities of care before and during other therapies for dehydration. Monitor vital signs, especially heart rate and blood pressure. The patient with dehydration is at risk for falls because of orthostatic hypotension, dysrhythmia, muscle weakness, and possible confusion. Assess his or her muscle strength, gait stability, and level of alertness. Instruct the patient to get up slowly from a lying or sitting position and to immediately sit down if he or she feels light-headed. Implement the falls precautions listed in Chart 2-4 in Chapter 2.

Fluid replacement is key to correcting dehydration and preventing death from reduced perfusion. Best practices for nursing care of the patient with dehydration are listed in Chart 11-3. Mild to moderate dehydration is corrected with oral fluid replacement if the patient is alert enough to swallow and can tolerate oral fluids. Encourage fluid intake, and measure the amount ingested.

Determine whether the patient has any special fluid needs (e.g., sugar-free fluids, thickened fluids). Provide FLUID the patient enjoys, and time the intake schedule. Dividing the total amount of fluids needed by nursing shifts helps meet fluid needs more evenly over 24 hours with less danger of overload. Offer the conscious patient small volumes of fluids hourly.

Coordinate with unlicensed assistive personnel (UAP) to meet patients' specific fluid needs. Teach UAP to offer 2 to 4 ounces of fluid every hour to patients who are dehydrated or who are at risk for dehydration. If incontinence is a concern, ensure that UAP understand that withholding fluids is not appropriate to prevent the problem. Instruct them to take the time to stay with patients while they drink the fluid and to note the exact amount ingested. Direct UAP to report any difficulties patients may have in swallowing or managing fluids.

Oral rehydration solutions (ORS) for rehydration therapy are an effective way to replace fluids. Specifically formulated solutions containing glucose and ELECTROLYTES are absorbed even when the patient is vomiting or has diarrhea. These are more often used in the home setting, in long-term care, and for patients who have poor veins, making IV therapy difficult. A variety of commercial ORS are available over the counter.

Drug therapy for dehydration is directed at restoring FLUID BALANCE and controlling the causes of dehydration. Whenever possible, fluid is replaced orally. When dehydration is severe or the patient cannot tolerate oral fluids, IV fluid replacement is needed. Calculation of how much fluid to replace is based on the patient's weight loss and clinical manifestations. The rate of fluid replacement depends on the degree of dehydration and the patient's cardiac, pulmonary, or kidney status.

The type of fluid prescribed varies with the patient's cardiovascular status and the osmolarity of the blood. Table 11-4 lists

CHART 11-3 Best Practice for Patient Safety & Quality Care (QSEN)

The Patient with Dehydration

- When possible, provide oral fluids that meet the patient's dietary restrictions (e.g., sugar-free, low-sodium, thickened).
- Collaborate with other members of the health care team to determine the amount of fluids needed during a 24-hour period.
- Ensure the fluids are offered and ingested on an even schedule at least every 2 hours throughout 24 hours.
- Teach unlicensed assistive personnel to actively participate in the hydration therapy and not to withhold fluids to prevent incontinence.
- Administer prescribed IV fluids at a rate consistent with hydration needs and any known cardiac, pulmonary, or kidney problems.
- Monitor the patient's response to fluid therapy at least every 2 hours for indicators of adequate rehydration or the need for continuing therapy, especially:
  - Pulse quality
  - Urine output
  - Pulse pressure
  - Weight (every 8 hours)
- Monitor for and report indicators of fluid overload, including:
  - Bounding pulse
  - Difficulty breathing
  - Neck vein distention in the upright position
  - Presence of dependent edema
- Assess the IV and the infusion site at least hourly for indications of infiltration, extravasation, or phlebitis (e.g., swelling around the site, pain, cordlike veins, reduced drip rate).
- Administer drugs prescribed to correct the underlying cause of the dehydration (e.g., antiemetics, antidiarrheals, antibiotics, antipyretics).

TABLE 11-4 Characteristics of Common Intravenous Therapy Solutions

SOLUTION	OSMOLARITY (mOsm/L)	pH	CALORIES (KCAL) PER LITER	TONICITY
0.9% saline	308	5	0	Isotonic
0.45% saline	154	5	0	Hypotonic
5% dextrose in water (D_5W)	272	3.5-6.5	170	Isotonic*
10% dextrose in water ($D_{10}W$)	500	3.5-6.5	340	Hypertonic*
5% dextrose in 0.9% saline	560	3.5-6.5	170	Hypertonic*
5% dextrose in 0.45% saline	406	4	170	Hypertonic*
5% dextrose in 0.225% saline	321	4	170	Isotonic*
Ringer's lactate	273	6.5	9	Isotonic
5% dextrose in Ringer's lactate	525	4-6.5	179	Hypertonic*

Data from Trissel, L. (2013). *Handbook on injectable drugs* (17th ed.). Bethesda, MD: American Society of Hospital-System Pharmacists.
*Solution tonicity at the time of administration. Within a short time after administration, the dextrose is metabolized and the tonicity of the infused solution decreases in proportion to the osmolarity or tonicity of the non-dextrose components (electrolytes) within the water.

the composition of common IV fluids. The two most important areas to monitor during rehydration are pulse rate and quality and urine output.

Drug therapy may correct some causes of the dehydration. For example, antidiarrheal drugs are prescribed when diarrhea causes dehydration. Antimicrobial therapy may be used in patients with bacterial diarrhea. Antiemetics may be used when vomiting causes dehydration. Antipyretics to reduce fever are helpful when fever makes dehydration worse.

NCLEX EXAMINATION CHALLENGE

Safe and Effective Care Environment

Which assessment finding indicates to the nurse that fluid resuscitation therapy for the client with isotonic dehydration is effective?
A. Respiratory rate has changed from 16 to 18 breaths/min.
B. Urine specific gravity has increased from 1.040 to 1.050.
C. Neck veins are flat when the client moves to a sitting position.
D. Pulse pressure has changed from 22 mm Hg to 32 mm Hg.

FLUID OVERLOAD

❖ PATHOPHYSIOLOGY

Fluid overload, also called *overhydration,* is an excess of body FLUID. It is not a disease but, rather, a clinical indication of a problem in which fluid intake or retention is greater than the body's fluid needs. The most common type of fluid overload is hypervolemia (Fig. 11-9) because the problems result from excessive fluid in the extracellular fluid (ECF) space. Most problems caused by fluid overload are related to excessive fluid in the vascular space or to dilution of specific electrolytes and blood components. The conditions leading to fluid overload are related to excessive intake or inadequate excretion of fluids. See Table 11-3 for causes of fluid overload. Fig. 11-10 outlines the adaptive changes the body makes in response to mild or moderate fluid overload, especially increased urine output and edema formation. When overload is severe or occurs in a person with poor cardiac or kidney function, it can lead to heart failure and pulmonary edema. Dilution of electrolytes, especially sodium and potassium, can lead to seizures, coma, and death (McGraw, 2012).

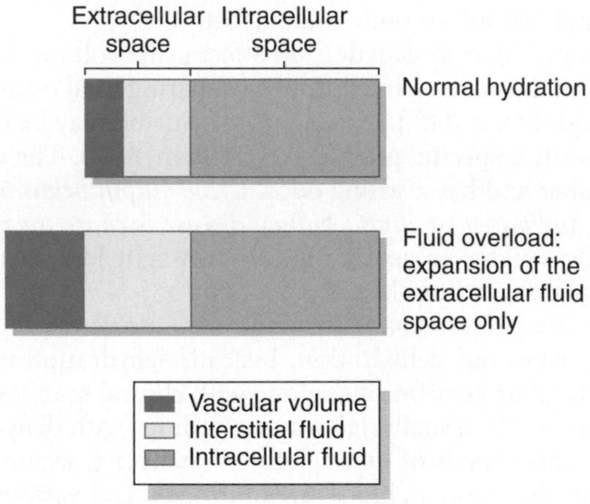

FIG. 11-9 Changes in fluid compartment volumes with fluid overload.

❖ PATIENT-CENTERED COLLABORATIVE CARE

◆ Assessment

Patients with fluid overload often have pitting edema (Fig. 11-11). Other manifestations are usually seen in the cardiovascular, respiratory, neuromuscular, integumentary, and GI systems (Chart 11-4).

Fluid overload is diagnosed based on assessment findings and the results of laboratory tests. Usually, serum electrolyte values are normal but decreased hemoglobin, hematocrit, and serum protein levels may result from excessive water in the vascular space (**hemodilution**).

◆ Interventions

The focus of priority nursing interventions for patients with fluid overload is to ensure patient safety, restore normal FLUID BALANCE, provide supportive care until the imbalance is resolved, and prevent future fluid overload. Drug therapy, nutrition therapy, and monitoring are the basis of intervention.

Patient safety is the first priority. Interventions are implemented to prevent fluid overload from becoming worse, leading to pulmonary edema, heart failure, and complications of electrolyte dilution. Any patient with fluid overload, regardless of age, is at risk for these complications. Older adults or those with cardiac problems, kidney problems, pulmonary problems, or liver problems are at greater risk.

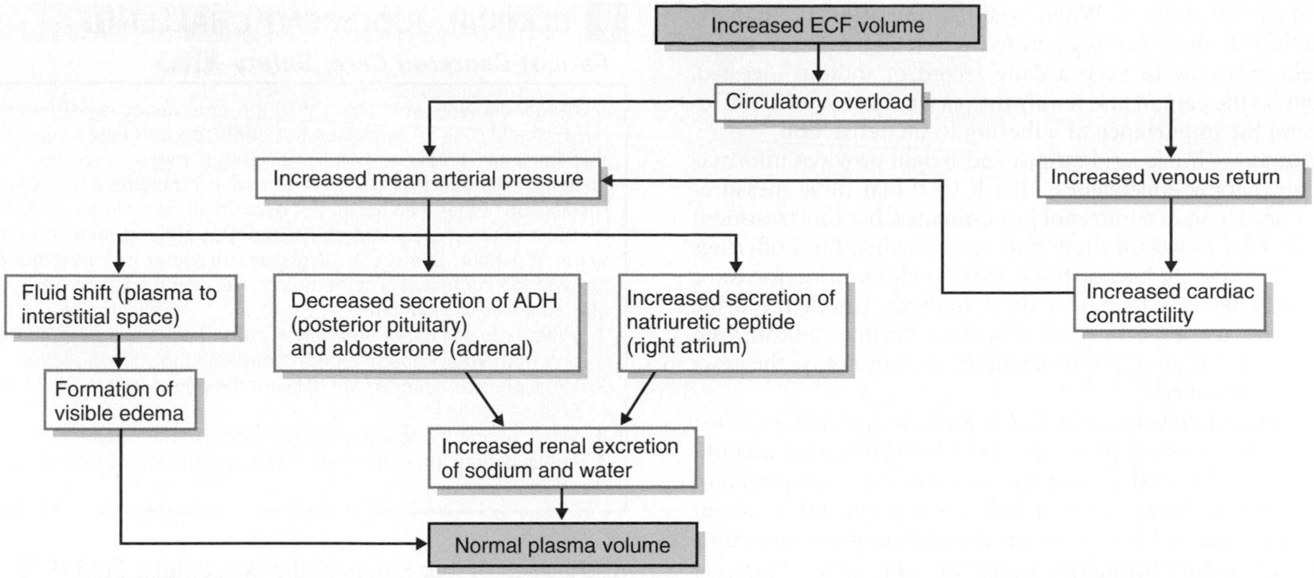

FIG. 11-10 Adaptive actions and mechanisms to prevent cardiac and pulmonary complications during fluid overload. (*ADH,* Antidiuretic hormone; *ECF,* extracellular fluid.)

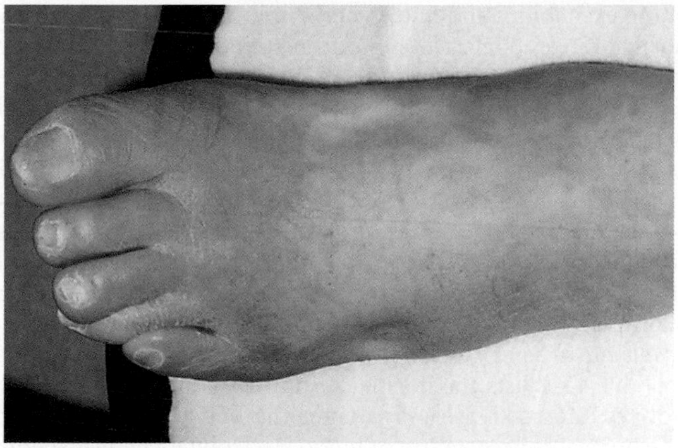

FIG. 11-11 Pitting edema of the left foot and ankle.

Monitor for indicators of increased fluid overload (bounding pulse, increasing neck vein distention, presence of crackles in lungs, increasing peripheral edema, reduced urine output) at least every 2 hours.

! NURSING SAFETY PRIORITY QSEN

Critical Rescue

Pulmonary edema can occur very quickly and can lead to death. Notify the health care provider of any change that indicates the fluid overload either is not responding to therapy or is becoming worse.

The patient with fluid overload and edema is at risk for skin breakdown. Use a pressure-reducing or pressure-relieving overlay on the mattress. Assess skin pressure areas daily for signs of redness or open area, especially the coccyx, elbows, hips, and heels. Because many patients with fluid overload may be receiving oxygen by mask or nasal cannula, check the skin integrity around the mask, nares, and ears and under the elastic band. Help the patient change positions every 2 hours, or ensure that unlicensed assistive personnel (UAP) perform this action.

CHART 11-4 Key Features

Fluid Overload

Cardiovascular Changes
- Increased pulse rate
- Bounding pulse quality
- Elevated blood pressure
- Decreased pulse pressure
- Elevated central venous pressure
- Distended neck and hand veins
- Engorged varicose veins
- Weight gain

Respiratory Changes
- Increased respiratory rate
- Shallow respirations
- Shortness of breath
- Moist crackles present on auscultation

Skin and Mucous Membrane Changes
- Pitting edema in dependent areas
- Skin pale and cool to touch

Neuromuscular Changes
- Altered level of consciousness
- Headache
- Visual disturbances
- Skeletal muscle weakness
- Paresthesias

Gastrointestinal Changes
- Increased motility
- Enlarged liver

Drug therapy focuses on removing the excess FLUID. Diuretics are prescribed for fluid overload if kidney failure is not the cause. Prescribed drugs may include high-ceiling (loop) diuretics, such as furosemide (Lasix, Furoside ♣). If there is concern that too much sodium and other ELECTROLYTES would be lost using loop diuretics or if the patient has syndrome of inappropriate antidiuretic hormone (SIADH), conivaptan (Vaprisol) or tolvaptan (Samsca) may be prescribed.

Monitor the patient for response to drug therapy, especially weight loss and increased urine output. Observe for manifestations of electrolyte imbalance, especially changes in electrocardiogram (ECG) patterns. Assess laboratory findings, especially sodium and potassium values, every 8 hours or whenever they are drawn.

Nutrition therapy for the patient with *chronic* fluid overload may involve restrictions of both FLUID and sodium intake. Often sodium restriction involves only "no added salt" to ordinary table foods when fluid overload is mild. For more severe fluid overload, the patient may be restricted to 2 g/day to 4 g/day of sodium. When sodium restriction is ongoing, teach the patient and family how to check food labels for sodium content and how to keep a daily record of sodium ingested. Explain to the patient and family the reason for any fluid restriction and the importance of adhering to the restriction.

Monitoring intake and output and weight provides information on therapy effectiveness. Teach UAP that these measurements need to be accurate, not just estimated, because treatment decisions are based on these findings. Schedule fluid offerings throughout the 24 hours. Teach UAP to check urine for color and character and to report these findings. Check the urine specific gravity (a specific gravity below 1.005 may indicate fluid overload). If the patient is receiving IV therapy, infuse the exact amount prescribed.

Fluid retention may not be visible. Rapid weight gain is the best indicator of fluid retention and overload. Metabolism can account for only a half pound of weight gain in one day. Each pound of weight gained (after the first half pound) equates to about 500 mL of retained FLUID. Weigh the patient at the same time every day (before breakfast), using the same scale. Whenever possible, have the patient wear the same type of clothing for each weigh-in. When in-bed weights are taken, lift tubing and equipment off the bed. Record the number of blankets and pillows on the bed at the initial weigh-in, and ensure ongoing weights always include the same number.

If the patient is discharged to home before the fluid overload has completely resolved or has continuing risk for fluid overload, teach him or her and the family to monitor weight at home. Suggest that a record of these daily weights be kept to show the health care provider at checkups. Patients may choose to use mobile "apps" to record and trend this information. Also, instruct the patient to call his or her health care provider for more than a 3-pound gain in a week or more than a 2-pound gain in 24 hours.

ELECTROLYTE BALANCE AND IMBALANCES

Electrolytes, or **ions**, are substances dissolved in body FLUID that carry an electrical charge. **Cations** have positive charges; **anions** have negative charges. Body fluids are electrically neutral, which means that the number of positive ions is balanced by an equal number of negative ions. However, the distribution of ions differs in the extracellular fluid (ECF) and the intracellular fluid (ICF) (Fig. 11-12).

CLINICAL JUDGMENT CHALLENGE

Patient-Centered Care; Safety QSEN

A 39-year-old woman is brought to the emergency department by her husband. She is conscious but confused and keeps repeating that her head hurts so much she feels it might "explode." The husband tells you that she has no health problems and takes no medications other than aspirin for occasional pain. He also tells you that she entered a contest earlier today to try and drink the most water in 1 hour. She drank 10 glasses of water in 1 hour but did not win the contest and came home. Her confusion and headache started about an hour later.

1. What type of fluid or electrolyte imbalance is she likely to have and from what cause? Explain your selection.
2. What physical assessment data are the priority to obtain? Explain your selection.
3. What laboratory data would you expect to be ordered?
4. Is this patient at risk for heart failure or pulmonary edema? Why or why not?

Most ELECTROLYTES have different concentrations in the ICF and ECF. This concentration difference helps maintain membrane excitability and allows nerve impulse transmission. The normal ranges of electrolyte concentration are very narrow. So, even small changes in these levels can cause major problems.

Electrolyte imbalances can occur in healthy people as a result of changes in fluid intake and output. These imbalances are usually mild and are easily corrected. Severe electrolyte imbalances with actual losses or retention of specific electrolytes are life threatening and can occur in any setting. People at greatest risk for severe imbalances are older patients, patients with chronic kidney or endocrine disorders, and those who are taking drugs that alter FLUID AND ELECTROLYTE BALANCE. *All ill people are at some risk for electrolyte imbalances.*

Table 11-1 lists the normal serum levels of the major electrolytes. Most ELECTROLYTES enter the body in ingested food. The normal concentration of blood electrolytes changes slightly with the aging process. Chart 11-1 lists the normal electrolyte values for people older than 60 years.

ELECTROLYTE BALANCE occurs by matching the dietary intake of electrolytes with the kidney excretion or reabsorption of

Plasma volume	Interstitial fluid	Intracellular fluid
Volume 3.5-5.5 L	Volume ~10 L	Volume 25-30 L
Osmolarity 270-300 mOsm	Osmolarity 270-300 mOsm	Osmolarity 270-300 mOsm
Sodium 136-145 mEq/L	Sodium 135-145 mEq/L	Sodium 14 mEq/L
Potassium 3.5-5.0 mEq/L	Potassium 3.5-5.0 mEq/L	Potassium 140 mEq/L
Chloride 96-109 mEq/L	Chloride ~118 mEq/L	Chloride ~4-6 mEq/L
Calcium 9.0-10.5 mg/dL	Calcium 7.0-9.0 mg/dL	Calcium 1.0-8.0 mg/dL
Magnesium 1.3-2.1 mEq/L	Magnesium ~1.3 mEq/L	Magnesium 6-30 mEq/L
Protein 7-8 g/L	Protein ~2 g/L	Protein 16 g/L

FIG. 11-12 The electrolyte composition of various body fluids.

electrolytes. For example, the plasma level of potassium is maintained between 3.5 and 5.0 mEq/L (mmol/L). The high potassium level in foods such as meat and citrus fruit could increase the ECF potassium level and lead to major problems. In health, this does not occur because kidney excretion of potassium keeps pace with potassium intake and prevents major changes in the blood potassium level.

CONSIDERATIONS FOR OLDER ADULTS

Patient-Centered Care QSEN

Older adults are at risk for electrolyte imbalances as a result of age-related organ changes, especially reduced kidney function. They are more likely to be taking drugs that affect fluid or electrolyte balance.

SODIUM

Sodium (Na^+), a mineral, is the major *cation* (positively charged particle) in the extracellular fluid (ECF) and maintains ECF osmolarity. Sodium levels of the ECF are high (136 to 145 mEq/L [mmol/L]), and the intracellular fluid (ICF) sodium levels are low (about 14 mEq/L [mmol/L]). Keeping this difference in sodium levels is vital for skeletal muscle contraction, cardiac contraction, and nerve impulse transmission. Sodium levels and movement influence water balance because "where sodium goes, water follows." The ECF sodium level determines whether water is retained, excreted, or moved from one fluid space to another.

To maintain electrical balance, the sodium (a cation) level within body FLUIDS must be matched by an equal number of anions (negatively charged substances). When this balance is present, the fluid is electrically neutral. Changes in plasma sodium levels seriously change fluid volume and the distribution of other ELECTROLYTES.

Sodium enters the body through the ingestion of many foods and fluids. Foods with the highest sodium levels are those that are processed or preserved, such as smoked or pickled foods, snack foods, and many condiments. Foods lowest in sodium include fresh fish and poultry and most fresh vegetables and fruit.

Despite variation in sodium intake from one day to the next, the blood sodium level usually remains within the normal range. Serum sodium balance is regulated by the kidney under the influences of aldosterone, antidiuretic hormone (ADH), and natriuretic peptide (NP), as described on p. 153.

Low serum sodium levels inhibit the secretion of ADH and NP and trigger aldosterone secretion. Together these compensatory actions increase serum sodium levels by increasing kidney reabsorption of sodium and enhancing kidney loss of water.

High serum sodium levels inhibit aldosterone secretion and directly stimulate secretion of ADH and NP. Together these hormones increase kidney excretion of sodium and kidney reabsorption of water.

HYPONATREMIA

❖ *PATHOPHYSIOLOGY*

Hyponatremia is an ELECTROLYTE imbalance in which the serum sodium (Na^+) level is below 136 mEq/L (mmol/L). Sodium imbalances often occur with a fluid imbalance because the same hormones regulate both sodium and water balance. The problems caused by hyponatremia occur from two changes—reduced excitable membrane depolarization and cellular swelling.

TABLE 11-5 Common Causes of Hyponatremia

Actual Sodium Deficits
- Excessive diaphoresis
- Diuretics (high-ceiling diuretics)
- Wound drainage (especially gastrointestinal)
- Decreased secretion of aldosterone
- Hyperlipidemia
- Kidney disease (scarred distal convoluted tubule)
- Nothing by mouth
- Low-salt diet
- Cerebral salt-wasting syndrome
- Hyperglycemia

Relative Sodium Deficits (Dilution)
- Excessive ingestion of hypotonic fluids
- Psychogenic polydipsia
- Freshwater submersion accident
- Kidney failure (nephrotic syndrome)
- Irrigation with hypotonic fluids
- Syndrome of inappropriate antidiuretic hormone secretion
- Heart failure

Excitable cell membrane depolarization depends on high extracellular fluid (ECF) levels of sodium being available to cross cell membranes and move into cells in response to a stimulus. Hyponatremia makes depolarization slower so that excitable membranes are less excitable.

With hyponatremia, the osmolarity of the ECF is lower than that of the intracellular fluid (ICF). As a result, water moves into the cell, causing swelling. Even a small amount of swelling can reduce cell function. Larger amounts of swelling can make the cell burst *(lysis)* and die.

Many conditions and drugs can lead to hyponatremia (Table 11-5). A common cause of low sodium levels is the prolonged use and overuse of diuretics, especially in older adults. When these drugs are used to manage FLUID overload, sodium is lost along with the extra water. Hyponatremia can result from the loss of total body sodium, the movement of sodium from the blood to other fluid spaces, or the dilution of serum sodium from excessive water in the plasma.

❖ *PATIENT-CENTERED COLLABORATIVE CARE*

◆ *Assessment*

The manifestations of hyponatremia are caused by its effects on excitable cellular activity. The cells especially affected are those involved in cerebral, neuromuscular, intestinal smooth muscle, and cardiovascular functions.

Cerebral changes are the most obvious problems of hyponatremia. Behavioral changes result from cerebral edema and increased intracranial pressure. Closely observe and document the patient's behavior, level of consciousness, and mental status. A sudden onset of acute confusion or increased confusion is often seen in older adults who have low serum sodium levels. When sodium levels become very low, seizures, coma, and death may occur (McGraw, 2012).

Neuromuscular changes are seen as general muscle weakness. Assess the patient's neuromuscular status during each nursing shift for changes from baseline. Deep tendon reflexes diminish, and muscle weakness is worse in the legs and arms. Test arm muscle strength by having the patient squeeze your hand.

Another way to test arm muscle strength is to have the patient flex his or her arms against the chest and keep them flexed while you attempt to pull them away from the chest. Test leg muscle strength by having the patient push both feet against a flat surface (like a box or a board) while you apply resistance to the opposite side of the flat surface.

! NURSING SAFETY PRIORITY QSEN

Action Alert

If muscle weakness is present, immediately check respiratory effectiveness because ventilation depends on adequate strength of respiratory muscles.

Intestinal changes include increased motility, causing nausea, diarrhea, and abdominal cramping. Assess the GI system by listening to bowel sounds and observing stools. Bowel sounds are hyperactive, with rushes and gurgles over the splenic flexure and in the lower left quadrant. Bowel movements are frequent and watery.

Cardiovascular changes are seen as changes in cardiac output. The cardiac responses to hyponatremia with **hypovolemia** (decreased plasma volume) include a rapid, weak, thready pulse. Peripheral pulses are difficult to palpate and are easily blocked with light pressure. Blood pressure is decreased, and the patient may have severe orthostatic hypotension, leading to lightheadedness or dizziness. The central venous pressure is low.

When hyponatremia occurs with **hypervolemia** (FLUID overload), cardiac changes include a full or bounding pulse with normal or high blood pressure. Peripheral pulses are full and difficult to block; however, they may not be palpable if edema is present.

◆ Interventions

The specific cause of the low sodium level is determined to plan the most appropriate management. Interventions with drug therapy and nutrition therapy are used to restore serum sodium levels to normal and prevent complications from FLUID overload or a too-rapid change in serum sodium level. *The priorities for nursing care of the patient with hyponatremia are monitoring the patient's response to therapy and preventing hypernatremia and fluid overload.*

Drug therapy involves reducing the doses of any drugs that increase sodium loss, such as most diuretics. Other regimens vary depending on whether a FLUID imbalance occurs with hyponatremia. When hyponatremia occurs with a fluid deficit, IV saline infusions are prescribed to restore both sodium and fluid volume. Severe hyponatremia may be treated with small-volume infusions of hypertonic saline, most often 3% saline (Schreiber, 2013b) although 5% saline can be used for extreme hyponatremia. These infusions are delivered using a controller to prevent accidental increases in infusion rate. Monitor the infusion rate and the patient's response.

When hyponatremia occurs with FLUID excess, drug therapy includes giving drugs that promote the excretion of water rather than sodium, such as conivaptan (Vaprisol) or tolvaptan (Samsca). Drug therapy for hyponatremia caused by inappropriate secretion of antidiuretic hormone (ADH) may include lithium and demeclocycline (Declomycin). Assess hourly for signs of excessive fluid loss, potassium loss, and increased sodium levels.

Nutrition therapy can help restore sodium balance in mild hyponatremia. Collaborate with the registered dietitian (RD) to teach the patient about which foods to increase in the diet. Therapy involves increasing oral sodium intake and restricting oral fluid intake. Fluid restriction may be needed long-term when FLUID overload is the cause of the hyponatremia or when kidney fluid excretion is impaired. Nursing actions for patient safety, skin protection, monitoring, and patient and family teaching are the same as those for fluid overload on pp. 161-162.

HYPERNATREMIA

❖ PATHOPHYSIOLOGY

Hypernatremia is an ELECTROLYTE imbalance in which the serum sodium level is over 145 mEq/L (mmol/L). It can be caused by or can cause changes in FLUID volume. Table 11-6 lists causes of hypernatremia.

As serum sodium level rises, a larger difference in sodium levels occurs between the extracellular fluid (ECF) and the intracellular fluid (ICF). More sodium is present to move rapidly across cell membranes during depolarization, making excitable tissues more easily excited. This condition is called **irritability**, and excitable tissues over-respond to stimuli. In addition, water moves from the cells into the ECF to dilute the hyperosmolar ECF. So, when serum sodium levels are high, severe cellular dehydration with cellular shrinkage occurs. Eventually the dehydrated excitable tissues may no longer be able to respond to stimuli.

❖ PATIENT-CENTERED COLLABORATIVE CARE

◆ Assessment

The manifestations of hypernatremia vary with the severity of sodium imbalance and whether a FLUID imbalance is also present. Changes are first seen in excitable membrane activity, especially nerve, skeletal muscle, and cardiac function.

Nervous system changes start with altered cerebral function. Assess the patient's mental status for attention span and cognitive function. In hypernatremia with normal or decreased FLUID volumes, the patient may have a short attention span and be agitated or confused. When hypernatremia occurs with fluid overload, the patient may be lethargic, drowsy, stuporous, and even comatose.

Skeletal muscle changes vary with the degree of sodium increases. Mild rises cause muscle twitching and irregular muscle contractions. As hypernatremia worsens, the muscles and nerves are less able to respond to a stimulus and muscles become progressively weaker. Late, the deep tendon reflexes are reduced or absent. Muscle weakness occurs bilaterally and has

TABLE 11-6 Common Causes of Hypernatremia

Actual Sodium Excesses	Relative Sodium Excesses
• Hyperaldosteronism	• Nothing by mouth
• Kidney failure	• Increased rate of metabolism
• Corticosteroids	• Fever
• Cushing's syndrome or disease	• Hyperventilation
• Excessive oral sodium ingestion	• Infection
• Excessive administration of sodium-containing IV fluids	• Excessive diaphoresis
	• Watery diarrhea
	• Dehydration

no specific pattern. Observe for twitching in muscle groups. Assess muscle strength by having the patient perform handgrip and arm flexion against resistance as described on pp. 161-162. Assess deep tendon reflexes by lightly tapping the patellar (knee) tendons and Achilles (heel) tendons with a reflex hammer and measuring the movement.

Cardiovascular changes include decreased contractility because high sodium levels slow the movement of calcium into the heart cells. Measure blood pressure and the rate and quality of the apical and peripheral pulses. Pulse rate and blood pressure may be normal, above normal, or below normal, depending on the FLUID volume and how rapidly the imbalance occurred.

Pulse rate is increased in patients with hypernatremia and hypovolemia. Peripheral pulses are difficult to palpate and are easily blocked. Hypotension and severe orthostatic (postural) hypotension are present, and pulse pressure is reduced.

Patients with hypernatremia and hypervolemia have slow to normal bounding pulses. Peripheral pulses are full and difficult to block. Neck veins are distended, even with the patient in the upright position. Blood pressure, especially diastolic blood pressure, is increased.

◆ Interventions

Drug and nutrition therapies are used to prevent further sodium increases and to decrease high serum sodium levels. Interventions used when sodium levels become life threatening include hemodialysis. *Priorities for nursing care of the patient with hypernatremia include monitoring his or her response to therapy and ensuring patient safety by preventing hyponatremia and dehydration.*

Drug therapy is used to restore FLUID balance when hypernatremia is caused by fluid loss. Isotonic saline (0.9%) and dextrose 5% in 0.45% sodium chloride are most often prescribed (Schreiber, 2013a). Although the dextrose 5% in 0.45% sodium chloride is hypertonic in the IV bag, once it is infused, the glucose is rapidly metabolized and the fluid is really hypotonic. Hypernatremia caused by poor kidney excretion of sodium requires drug therapy with diuretics that promote sodium loss, such as furosemide (Lasix, Furoside🍁) or bumetanide (Bumex). Assess the patient hourly for symptoms of excessive losses of fluid, sodium, or potassium.

Nutrition therapy to prevent or correct mild hypernatremia involves ensuring adequate water intake, especially among older adults. Dietary sodium restriction may be needed to prevent sodium excess when kidney problems are present. Collaborate with the dietitian to teach the patient how to determine the sodium content of foods, beverages, and drugs. Nursing actions for patient safety, skin protection, monitoring, and patient and family teaching are similar to those for fluid overload on pp. 158-160.

NCLEX EXAMINATION CHALLENGE

Physiological Integrity

Which condition or manifestation in the client with a serum sodium level of 149 mEq/L indicates to the nurse that this electrolyte imbalance may be caused by excessive fluid loss?

A. The client has twitching muscle contractions in the lower extremities.
B. The client's skin is cool and clammy.
C. The urine specific gravity is increased.
D. The hematocrit is 52%.

POTASSIUM

Potassium (K^+) is the major cation of the intracellular fluid (ICF). The normal plasma potassium level ranges from 3.5 to 5.0 mEq/L (mmol/L) (see Table 11-1). The normal ICF potassium level is about 140 mEq/L (mmol/L). Because of its high levels inside cells, potassium has some control over intracellular osmolarity and volume. Keeping this large difference in potassium concentration between the ICF and the extracellular fluid (ECF) is critical for excitable tissues to depolarize and generate action potentials.

Because potassium levels in the blood and interstitial fluid are so low, any change seriously affects physiologic activities. For example, a decrease in blood potassium of only 1 mEq/L (from 4 mEq/L to 3 mEq/L) is a 25% difference in total ECF potassium concentration. In contrast, a 1 mEq/L decrease in blood sodium level (from 130 mEq/L to 129 mEq/L) is, overall, a much smaller change (less than 1%) in total ECF sodium concentration.

Almost all foods contain potassium. It is highest in meat, fish, and many (but not all) vegetables and fruits. It is lowest in eggs, bread, and cereal grains. Typical potassium intake is about 2 to 20 g/day. Despite heavy potassium intake, the healthy adult keeps plasma potassium levels within the narrow range of normal values.

The main controller of ECF potassium level is the sodium-potassium pump within the membranes of all body cells. This pump moves extra sodium ions from the ICF and moves extra potassium ions from the ECF back into the cell. In this way, the serum potassium level remains low and the cellular potassium remains high. At the same time, this action also helps the serum sodium level remain high and the cellular sodium level remain low.

About 80% of potassium is removed from the body by the kidney. Kidney excretion of potassium is enhanced by aldosterone.

HYPOKALEMIA

❖ PATHOPHYSIOLOGY

Because 98% of total body potassium (K^+) is inside cells, minor changes in extracellular potassium levels cause major changes in cell membrane excitability. **Hypokalemia** is an ELECTROLYTE imbalance in which the serum potassium level is below 3.5 mEq/L (mmol/L). *It can be life threatening because every body system is affected.*

Low serum potassium levels increase the difference in the amount of potassium between the fluid inside the cells (ICF) and the fluid outside the cells (ECF). This increased difference reduces the excitability of cells. As a result, the cell membranes of all excitable tissues, such as nerve and muscle, are less responsive to normal stimuli. Gradual potassium loss may have no manifestations until the loss is extreme. Rapid reduction of serum potassium levels causes dramatic changes in function. Table 11-7 lists causes of hypokalemia.

Actual potassium depletion occurs when potassium loss is excessive or when potassium intake is not adequate to match normal potassium loss. Relative hypokalemia occurs when total body potassium levels are normal but the potassium distribution between fluid spaces is abnormal or it is diluted by excess water.

TABLE 11-7 Common Causes of Hypokalemia

Actual Potassium Deficits
- Inappropriate or excessive use of drugs:
  - Diuretics
  - Digitalis
  - Corticosteroids
- Increased secretion of aldosterone
- Cushing's syndrome
- Diarrhea
- Vomiting
- Wound drainage (especially gastrointestinal)
- Prolonged nasogastric suction
- Heat-induced excessive diaphoresis
- Kidney disease impairing reabsorption of potassium
- Nothing by mouth

Relative Potassium Deficits
- Alkalosis
- Hyperinsulinism
- Hyperalimentation
- Total parenteral nutrition
- Water intoxication
- IV therapy with potassium-poor solutions

❖ PATIENT-CENTERED COLLABORATIVE CARE

◆ Assessment

Age is important because urine concentrating ability decreases with aging, which increases potassium loss. Older adults are more likely to use drugs that lead to potassium loss.

Drugs, especially diuretics, corticosteroids, and beta-adrenergic agonists or antagonists, can increase potassium loss through the kidneys. Ask about prescription and over-the-counter drug use. In patients taking digoxin (Lanoxin, Novo-Digoxin 🍁), hypokalemia increases the sensitivity of the cardiac muscle to the drug and may result in digoxin toxicity, even when the digoxin level is within the therapeutic range. Ask whether the patient takes a potassium supplement, such as potassium chloride (KCl), or eats foods that have high concentrations of potassium, such as bananas, citrus juices, raisins, and meat. The patient may not be taking the supplement as prescribed because of its unpleasant taste.

Disease can lead to potassium loss. Ask about chronic disorders, recent illnesses, and medical or surgical interventions. A thorough nutrition history, including a typical day's food and beverage intake, helps identify patients at risk for hypokalemia.

Respiratory changes occur because of respiratory muscle weakness resulting in shallow respirations. *Thus respiratory status should be assessed first in any patient who might have hypokalemia.* Assess the patient's breath sounds, ease of respiratory effort, color of nail beds and mucous membranes, and rate and depth of respiration.

! NURSING SAFETY PRIORITY (QSEN)

Action Alert

Assess the respiratory status of a patient who has hypokalemia at least every 2 hours because respiratory insufficiency is a major cause of death for these patients.

Musculoskeletal changes include skeletal muscle weakness. A stronger stimulus is needed to begin muscle contraction. A patient may be too weak to stand. Hand grasps are weak, and deep tendon reflexes may be reduced (hyporeflexia). Severe hypokalemia causes flaccid paralysis. Assess for muscle weakness and the patient's ability to perform ADLs.

Cardiovascular changes are assessed by palpating the peripheral pulses. In hypokalemia, the pulse is usually thready and weak. Palpation is difficult, and the pulse is easily blocked with light pressure. The pulse rate can range from very slow to very rapid, and an irregular heartbeat (dysrhythmia) may be present. Measure blood pressure with the patient in the lying, sitting, and standing positions, because orthostatic (postural) hypotension occurs with hypokalemia.

Neurologic changes from hypokalemia include altered mental status. The patient may have short-term irritability and anxiety followed by lethargy that progresses to acute confusion and coma as hypokalemia worsens.

Behavioral changes caused by hypokalemia can occur quickly. The patient may be lethargic and unable to perform simple problem-solving tasks such as counting by threes. As hypokalemia progresses, confusion increases and coma may develop.

Intestinal changes occur with hypokalemia because GI smooth muscle contractions are decreased, which leads to decreased peristalsis. Bowel sounds are hypoactive, and nausea, vomiting, constipation, and abdominal distention are common. Measure abdominal girth, and auscultate for bowel sounds in all four abdominal quadrants. *Severe hypokalemia can cause the absence of peristalsis* ***(paralytic ileus)****.*

Laboratory data confirm hypokalemia (serum potassium value below 3.5 mEq/L [mmol/L]). Hypokalemia causes ECG changes in the heart, including ST-segment depression, flat or inverted T waves, and increased U waves. *Dysrhythmias can lead to death, particularly in older adults who are taking digoxin.*

◆ Interventions

Interventions for hypokalemia focus on preventing potassium loss, increasing serum potassium levels, and ensuring patient safety. Drug and nutrition therapies help restore normal serum potassium levels. *The priorities for nursing care of the patient with hypokalemia are (1) ensuring adequate oxygenation, patient safety for falls prevention, and prevention of injury from potassium administration and (2) monitoring the patient's response to therapy.* Chart 11-5 highlights best practice activities when caring for a patient with hypokalemia.

Drug therapy for management and prevention of hypokalemia includes additional potassium and drugs to prevent potassium loss (Scotto et al., 2014). Most potassium supplements are potassium chloride, potassium gluconate, or potassium citrate. The amount and the route of potassium replacement depend on the degree of loss.

Potassium is given IV for severe hypokalemia. The drug is available in different concentrations, and this drug carries a high alert warning as a concentrated electrolyte solution. The Joint Commission's National Patient Safety Goals has mandated that concentrated potassium be diluted and added to IV solutions only in the pharmacy by a registered pharmacist and that vials of concentrated potassium not be available in patient care areas. *Before infusing any IV solution containing potassium chloride (KCl), check and recheck the dilution of the drug in the IV solution container.*

CHART 11-5 Best Practice for Patient Safety & Quality Care QSEN

The Patient with Hypokalemia

- Question the continued use of drugs that increase excretion of potassium (e.g., thiazide and loop diuretics).
- Administer prescribed oral potassium supplement, well diluted and with a meal or just after a meal or snack to prevent nausea and vomiting.
- Prevent accidental overdose of IV potassium by checking and re-checking the concentration of potassium in the IV solution, ensuring that the maximum concentration is no greater than 1 mEq/10 mL of solution.
- Establish an IV access in a large vein with a high volume of flow, avoiding the hand.
- Assess the IV access for placement and an adequate blood return *before* administering potassium-containing solutions.
- Use a controller for solution delivery, maintaining an infusion rate not faster than 5 to 10 mEq of potassium per hour.
- Assess the IV site hourly.
- Stop the infusion immediately if the patient reports pain or burning or if any manifestation of infiltration occurs.
- If possible, monitor electrocardiography (ECG) continuously.
- Monitor patient responses every 1 to 2 hours to determine therapy effectiveness and the potential for hyperkalemia.
    - Indications of therapy effectiveness:
        - Respiratory rate is greater than 12 breaths per minute
        - Oxygen saturation is at least 95% (or has returned to the patient's normal baseline)
        - The patient can cough effectively
        - Hand grasp strength increases
        - Deep tendon reflexes are present
        - Bowel sounds are present and active
        - Pulse is easily palpated and regular
        - Systolic blood pressure when standing remains within 20 mm Hg of the systolic pressure obtained when the patient is sitting or lying down
        - ST segment returns to the isoelectric line
        - T waves increase in size and are positive
        - U waves decrease or disappear
        - Patient's cognition resembles his or her prehypokalemic state
        - Serum potassium level is between 3.5 and 5.0 mEq/L
    - Indications of hyperkalemia:
        - Heart rate is less than 60 beats per minute
        - P waves are absent
        - T waves are tall
        - PR intervals are prolonged
        - QRS complexes are wide
        - Deep tendon reflexes are hyperactive
        - Bowel sounds are hyperactive
        - Numbness or tingling is present in the hands and feet and around the mouth
        - The patient is anxious
        - Serum potassium level is above 5.0 mEq/L
- Keep patient on bedrest until hypokalemia resolves, or provide assistance when out of bed to prevent falls.

! NURSING SAFETY PRIORITY QSEN

Drug Alert

A dilution no greater than 1 mEq of potassium to 10 mL of solution is recommended for IV administration. The maximum recommended infusion rate is 5 to 10 mEq/hr; this rate is never to exceed 20 mEq/hr under any circumstances. In accordance with National Patient Safety Goals (NPSGs), potassium is not given by IV push to avoid causing cardiac arrest.

Potassium is a severe tissue irritant and is never given by IM or subcutaneous injection. Tissues damaged by potassium can become necrotic, causing loss of function and requiring surgery. IV potassium solutions irritate veins and cause phlebitis. Check the prescription carefully to ensure that the patient receives the correct amount of potassium. Assess the IV site hourly, and ask the patient whether he or she feels burning or pain at the site.

! NURSING SAFETY PRIORITY QSEN

Action Alert

If infiltration of solution containing potassium occurs, stop the IV solution immediately, remove the venous access, and notify the health care provider or Rapid Response Team. Document these actions along with a complete description of the IV site.

Oral potassium preparations may be taken as liquids or solids. Potassium has a strong, unpleasant taste that is difficult to mask, although it can be mixed with many liquids. Because potassium chloride can cause nausea and vomiting, give the drug during or after a meal and advise patients using the drug at home not to take it on an empty stomach.

Diuretics that increase the kidney excretion of potassium can cause hypokalemia, especially high-ceiling (loop) diuretics (e.g., furosemide [Lasix, Furoside 🍁] and bumetanide [Bumex]) and the thiazide diuretics. These drugs are avoided in patients with hypokalemia. A potassium-sparing diuretic may be prescribed to increase urine output without increasing potassium loss. Potassium-sparing diuretics include spironolactone (Aldactone, Novospiroton 🍁), triamterene (Dyrenium), and amiloride (Midamor).

Nutrition therapy involves collaboration with a dietitian to teach the patient how to increase dietary potassium intake. Eating foods that are naturally rich in potassium helps prevent further loss, but supplementation is needed to restore normal potassium levels.

Implement safety measures with a patient who has muscle weakness from hypokalemia, including the falls precautions listed in Chart 2-4 in Chapter 2. Be sure to have the patient wear a gait belt when ambulating with assistance.

Respiratory monitoring is performed at least hourly for severe hypokalemia, especially checking for increasing rate and decreasing depth. Also check oxygen saturation by pulse oximetry to determine breathing effectiveness. Assess respiratory muscle effectiveness by checking the patient's ability to cough. Examine the face, oral mucosa, and nail beds for pallor or cyanosis. Evaluate arterial blood gas values (when available) for decreased blood oxygen levels (**hypoxemia**) and increased arterial carbon dioxide levels (**hypercapnia**), which indicate inadequate breathing effectiveness.

? NCLEX EXAMINATION CHALLENGE

Physiological Integrity

Which question is most important for the nurse to ask the client who has a serum potassium level of 2.9 mEq/L?

A. "Do you use sugar substitutes?"
B. "Do you use diuretics or laxatives?"
C. "Have you had any muscle twitches or cramps, especially at night?
D. "Have you or any member of your family ever been diagnosed with lung disease?"

HYPERKALEMIA

❖ PATHOPHYSIOLOGY

Hyperkalemia is an ELECTROLYTE imbalance in which the serum potassium level is higher than 5.0 mEq/L (mmol/L). Even small increases above normal values can affect excitable tissues, especially the heart.

A high serum potassium increases cell excitability; as a result, most excitable tissues respond to less intense stimuli and may even discharge spontaneously. The heart is very sensitive to serum potassium increases, and hyperkalemia interferes with electrical conduction, leading to heart block and ventricular fibrillation.

The problems that occur with hyperkalemia are related to how rapidly ECF potassium levels increase. Sudden potassium rises cause severe problems at serum levels between 6 and 7 mEq/L. When serum potassium rises slowly, problems may not occur until potassium levels reach 8 mEq/L or higher.

Hyperkalemia is rare in people with normal kidney function. Most cases of hyperkalemia occur in hospitalized patients and in those undergoing medical treatment. Those at greatest risk are chronically ill patients, debilitated patients, and older adults (Table 11-8).

❖ PATIENT-CENTERED COLLABORATIVE CARE

◆ Assessment

Age is important because kidney function decreases with aging. Ask about kidney disease, diabetes mellitus, recent medical or surgical treatment, and urine output, including frequency and amount of voidings. Ask about drug use, particularly potassium-sparing diuretics and angiotensin-converting enzyme (ACE) inhibitors. Obtain a nutrition history to determine the intake of potassium-rich foods and the use of salt substitutes (which contain potassium).

Collect specific information about manifestations related to hyperkalemia. Ask whether the patient has had palpitations, skipped heartbeats, other cardiac irregularities, muscle twitching, leg weakness, or unusual tingling or numbness in the hands, feet, or face. Ask about recent changes in bowel habits, especially diarrhea.

Cardiovascular changes are the most severe problems from hyperkalemia and are the most common cause of death in patients with hyperkalemia. Cardiac manifestations include bradycardia, hypotension, and ECG changes of tall, peaked T waves, prolonged PR intervals, flat or absent P waves, and wide QRS complexes. As serum potassium levels rise, ectopic beats may appear. Complete heart block, asystole, and ventricular fibrillation are life-threatening complications of severe hyperkalemia.

Neuromuscular changes with hyperkalemia have two phases. Skeletal muscles twitch in the early stages of hyperkalemia, and the patient may be aware of tingling and burning sensations followed by numbness in the hands and feet and around the mouth (**paresthesia**). As hyperkalemia worsens, muscle weakness occurs followed by flaccid paralysis. The weakness moves up from the hands and feet and first affects the muscles of the arms and legs. Respiratory muscles are not affected until serum potassium levels reach lethal levels.

Intestinal changes include increased motility with diarrhea and hyperactive bowel sounds. Bowel movements are frequent and watery.

Laboratory data confirm hyperkalemia (potassium level over 5.0 mEq/L). If it is caused by dehydration, levels of other ELECTROLYTES, hematocrit, and hemoglobin also are elevated. Hyperkalemia caused by kidney failure occurs with elevated serum creatinine and blood urea nitrogen, decreased blood pH, and normal or low hematocrit and hemoglobin levels.

TABLE 11-8 Common Causes of Hyperkalemia

Actual Potassium Excesses
- Overingestion of potassium-containing foods or medications:
  - Salt substitutes
  - Potassium chloride
  - Rapid infusion of potassium-containing IV solution
  - Bolus IV potassium injections
- Transfusions of whole blood or packed cells
- Adrenal insufficiency
- Kidney failure
- Potassium-sparing diuretics
- Angiotensin-converting enzyme inhibitors (ACEIs)

Relative Potassium Excesses
- Tissue damage
- Acidosis
- Hyperuricemia
- Uncontrolled diabetes mellitus

◆ Interventions

Interventions for hyperkalemia focus on reducing the serum potassium level, preventing recurrences, and ensuring patient safety. Drug therapy is key. *The priorities for nursing care of the patient with hyperkalemia are assessing for cardiac complications, patient safety for falls prevention, monitoring the patient's response to therapy, and health teaching.*

Drug therapy can restore normal potassium balance by enhancing potassium excretion and promoting the movement of potassium from the extracellular fluid (ECF) into the cells.

Stop potassium-containing infusions, and keep the IV access open. Withhold oral potassium supplements, and provide a potassium-restricted diet.

Increasing potassium excretion helps reduce hyperkalemia if kidney function is normal. Potassium-excreting diuretics, such as furosemide, are prescribed. When kidney problems exist, drug therapy to increase potassium excretion includes cation exchange resins that promote intestinal sodium absorption and potassium excretion, such as sodium polystyrene sulfonate (Kayexalate). However, this therapy may take hours to reduce potassium levels. If potassium levels are dangerously high, additional measures, such as dialysis, are needed.

Movement of potassium from the extracellular fluid (ECF) to the intracellular fluid (ICF) can help reduce serum potassium levels temporarily. Potassium movement into the cells is enhanced by insulin. Insulin increases the activity of the sodium-potassium pumps, which move potassium from the ECF into the cell. IV fluids containing glucose and insulin are prescribed to help decrease serum potassium levels (usually 100 mL of 10% to 20% glucose with 10 to 20 units of regular insulin) (Cottrell, 2012). These IV solutions are hypertonic and are infused through a central line or in a vein with a high blood flow to avoid local vein inflammation. Observe the patient for manifestations of hypokalemia and hypoglycemia during this therapy.

CHART 11-6 Patient and Family Education: Preparing for Self-Management

Nutritional Management of Hyperkalemia

You Should Avoid	You May Eat
• Meats, especially organ meat and preserved meat • Dairy products • Dried fruit • Fruits high in potassium: ▪ Bananas ▪ Cantaloupe ▪ Kiwi ▪ Oranges • Vegetables high in potassium: ▪ Avocados ▪ Broccoli ▪ Dried beans or peas ▪ Lima beans ▪ Mushrooms ▪ Potatoes (white or sweet) ▪ Seaweed ▪ Soybeans ▪ Spinach	• Eggs • Breads • Butter • Cereals • Sugar • Fruits low in potassium (fresh, frozen, or canned): ▪ Apples ▪ Apricots ▪ Berries ▪ Cherries ▪ Cranberries ▪ Grapefruit ▪ Peaches ▪ Pineapple • Vegetables low in potassium: ▪ Alfalfa sprouts ▪ Cabbage ▪ Carrots ▪ Cauliflower ▪ Celery ▪ Eggplant ▪ Green beans ▪ Lettuce ▪ Onions ▪ Peas ▪ Peppers ▪ Squash

Data from Pennington, J.A., & Spungen, J.S. (2010). *Bowes and Church's food values of portions commonly used* (19th ed.). Philadelphia: Lippincott Williams & Wilkins.

Cardiac monitoring allows for the early recognition of dysrhythmias and other manifestations of hyperkalemia on cardiac muscle. Compare recent ECG tracings with the tracings obtained when the patient's serum potassium level was close to normal.

! NURSING SAFETY PRIORITY (QSEN)

Critical Rescue

Notify the health care provider or Rapid Response Team if the patient's heart rate falls below 60 beats per minute or if the T waves become spiked, both of which accompany hyperkalemia.

Health teaching is key to the prevention of hyperkalemia and the early detection of complications. The teaching plan includes diet, drugs, and recognition of the manifestations of hyperkalemia. Collaborate with the dietitian to teach the patient and family about which foods to avoid (those high in potassium). Foods that are low in potassium are listed in Chart 11-6. Instruct the patient and family to read the labels on drug and food packages to determine the potassium content. Warn them to avoid salt substitutes, which contain potassium.

CALCIUM

Calcium (Ca^{2+}) is a mineral with functions closely related to those of phosphorus and magnesium. It is an ion having two positive charges *(divalent cation)* that exists in the body in a bound form and an ionized (unbound or free) form.

Bound calcium is usually attached to serum proteins, especially albumin. Ionized calcium is present in the blood and other extracellular fluid (ECF) as free calcium. Free calcium is the active form and must be kept within a narrow range in the ECF. The body functions best when blood calcium levels are maintained between 9.0 and 10.5 mg/dL, or between 2.25 and 2.62 mmol/L (see Table 11-1). Calcium has a steep gradient between ECF and intracellular fluid (ICF) because the amount of calcium in the ICF is very low. This mineral is important for maintaining bone strength and density, activating enzymes, allowing skeletal and cardiac muscle contraction, controlling nerve impulse transmission, and allowing blood clotting.

Calcium enters the body by dietary intake and absorption through the intestinal tract. Dairy products are common foods high in calcium. Absorption of dietary calcium requires the active form of vitamin D. Calcium is stored in the bones. When more calcium is needed, parathyroid hormone (PTH) is released from the parathyroid glands. PTH increases serum calcium levels by:

- Releasing free calcium from bone storage sites (bone *resorption* of calcium)
- Stimulating vitamin D activation to help increase intestinal *absorption* of dietary calcium
- Inhibiting kidney calcium excretion
- Stimulating kidney calcium *reabsorption*

When excess calcium is present in plasma, PTH secretion is inhibited and the secretion of *thyrocalcitonin (TCT)*, a hormone secreted by the thyroid gland, is increased. TCT causes the plasma calcium level to decrease by inhibiting bone resorption of calcium, inhibiting vitamin D–associated intestinal uptake of calcium, and increasing kidney excretion of calcium in the urine.

HYPOCALCEMIA

❖ PATHOPHYSIOLOGY

Hypocalcemia is an ELECTROLYTE imbalance in which a total serum calcium (Ca^{2+}) level is below 9.0 mg/dL or 2.25 mmol/L. Calcium is stored in bone, with only a small amount of total body calcium present in extracellular fluid (ECF). Because the normal blood level of calcium is so low, any change in calcium levels has major effects on function.

Calcium is an excitable membrane stabilizer, regulating depolarization and the generation of action potentials. It decreases sodium movement across excitable membranes, slowing the rate of depolarization. Low serum calcium levels increase sodium movement across excitable membranes, allowing depolarization to occur more easily and at inappropriate times.

Hypocalcemia is caused by many chronic and acute conditions, as well as medical or surgical treatments. Table 11-9 lists causes of hypocalcemia. Acute hypocalcemia results in the rapid onset of life-threatening manifestations. Chronic hypocalcemia occurs slowly over time, and excitable membrane manifestations may not be severe because the body has adjusted to the gradual reduction of serum calcium levels.

Actual calcium loss (a reduction in total body calcium) occurs when the absorption of calcium from the GI tract slows or when calcium is lost from the body. Relative calcium loss causes total body calcium amounts to remain normal while serum calcium levels are low. This problem occurs when the

TABLE 11-9 Common Causes of Hypocalcemia

Actual Calcium Deficits
- Inadequate oral intake of calcium
- Lactose intolerance
- Malabsorption syndromes:
  - Celiac sprue
  - Crohn's disease
- Inadequate intake of vitamin D
- End-stage kidney disease
- Diarrhea
- Steatorrhea
- Wound drainage (especially gastrointestinal)

Relative Calcium Deficits
- Hyperproteinemia
- Alkalosis
- Calcium chelators or binders
  - Citrate
  - Mithramycin
  - Penicillamine
  - Sodium cellulose phosphate (Calcibind)
  - Aredia
- Acute pancreatitis
- Hyperphosphatemia
- Immobility
- Removal or destruction of parathyroid glands

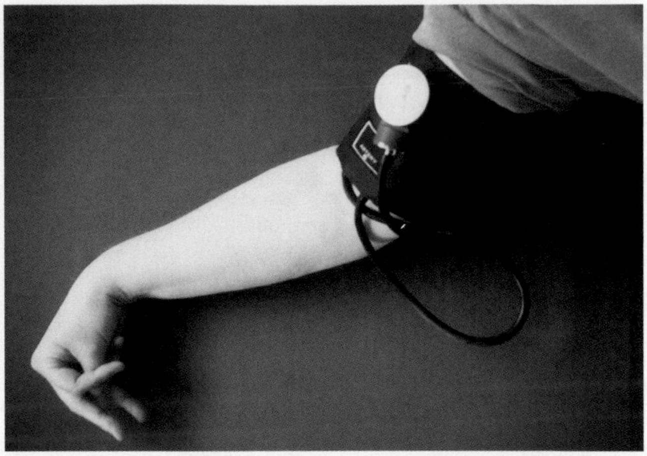

FIG. 11-13 Palmar flexion indicating a positive Trousseau's sign in hypocalcemia.

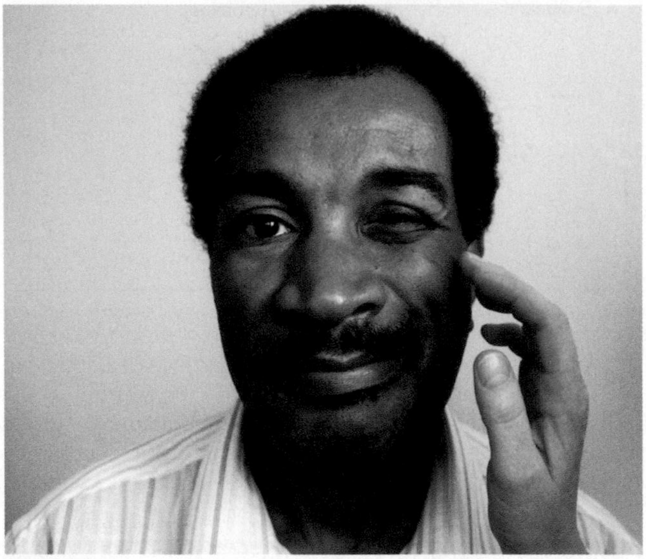

FIG. 11-14 Facial muscle response indicating a positive Chvostek's sign in hypocalcemia.

GENDER HEALTH CONSIDERATIONS

Patient-Centered Care QSEN

Postmenopausal women are at risk for chronic calcium loss. This problem is related to reduced weight-bearing activities and a decrease in estrogen levels. As they age, many women decrease weight-bearing activities such as running and walking, which allows osteoporosis to occur at a more rapid rate. Also, the estrogen secretion that protects against osteoporosis diminishes. (See Chapter 50 for a complete discussion of osteoporosis.)

unbound calcium in the body is reduced or when parathyroid gland function is decreased.

❖ PATIENT-CENTERED COLLABORATIVE CARE

◆ Assessment

Assess the nutrition history for the risk for hypocalcemia. Ask the patient about his or her intake of dairy products and whether he or she takes a calcium supplement regularly.

One indicator of hypocalcemia is a report of frequent, painful muscle spasms ("charley horses") in the calf or foot during rest or sleep. Ask about a history of recent orthopedic surgery or bone healing. Endocrine disturbances and treatments are risk factors for hypocalcemia. A history of thyroid surgery, therapeutic irradiation of the upper middle chest and neck area, or a recent anterior neck injury increases the risk for hypocalcemia. Most manifestations of acute hypocalcemia are caused by overstimulation of the nerves and muscles.

Neuromuscular changes often occur first in the hands and feet. Paresthesias occur at first, with sensations of tingling and numbness. If hypocalcemia continues or worsens, muscle twitching or painful cramps and spasms occur. Tingling may also affect the lips, nose, and ears. These problems may signal the onset of neuromuscular overstimulation and tetany (Crawford & Harris, 2012).

Assess for hypocalcemia by testing for Trousseau's and Chvostek's signs. To test for Trousseau's sign, place a blood pressure cuff around the upper arm, inflate the cuff to greater than the patient's systolic pressure, and keep the cuff inflated for 1 to 4 minutes. Under these hypoxic conditions, a positive Trousseau's sign occurs when the hand and fingers go into spasm in palmar flexion (Fig. 11-13). To test for Chvostek's sign, tap the face just below and in front of the ear (over the facial nerve) to trigger facial twitching of one side of the mouth, nose, and cheek (Fig. 11-14).

Cardiovascular changes involve heart rate and ECG changes. The heart rate may be slower or slightly faster than normal, with a weak, thready pulse. Severe hypocalcemia causes severe hypotension and ECG changes of a prolonged ST interval and a prolonged QT interval.

Intestinal changes include increased peristaltic activity. Auscultate the abdomen for hyperactive bowel sounds. The patient may report painful abdominal cramping and diarrhea.

Skeletal changes are common with chronic hypocalcemia. Calcium leaves bone storage sites, causing a loss of bone density (osteoporosis). The bones are less dense, more brittle, and fragile and may break easily with slight trauma. Vertebrae become more compact and may bend forward, leading to an overall loss of height. See Chapter 50 for discussion of osteoporosis.

Ask about changes in height and any unexplained bone pain. Observe for spinal curvatures and any unusual bumps or protrusions in bones that may indicate old fractures.

◆ Interventions

Interventions focus on restoring normal calcium levels and preventing complications. These include drug therapy, nutrition therapy, reducing environmental stimuli, and preventing injury. Patient safety during restoration of serum calcium levels is a nursing care priority.

Drug therapy for hypocalcemia includes direct calcium replacement (oral and IV) and drugs that enhance the absorption of calcium, such as vitamin D. When hypocalcemia is a result of hyperphosphatemia, aluminum hydroxide may help raise serum calcium levels. When neuromuscular manifestations are troublesome, drugs that decrease nerve and muscle responses also may be used.

Nutrition therapy involves a high-calcium diet for patients with mild hypocalcemia and for those who are at continuing risk for hypocalcemia. Collaborate with the dietitian to assist the patient in selecting calcium-rich foods.

Environmental management for safety is needed because the excitable membranes of the nervous system and the skeletal system are overstimulated in hypocalcemia. Reduce stimulation by keeping the room quiet, limiting visitors, adjusting the lighting, and using a soft voice.

Use seizure precautions for the patient with hypocalcemia (see Chapter 42). Keep emergency equipment (e.g., oxygen, suction) at the bedside.

Injury prevention strategies are needed because the patient with long-standing calcium loss may have brittle, fragile bones that fracture easily and cause little pain. When lifting or moving a patient with fragile bones, use a lift sheet rather than pulling the patient. Observe for normal range of joint motion and for any unusual surface bumps or depressions over bony areas that may indicate bone fracture.

HYPERCALCEMIA

❖ PATHOPHYSIOLOGY

Hypercalcemia is an ELECTROLYTE imbalance in which the total serum calcium level is above 10.5 mg/dL or 2.62 mmol/L. Even small increases above normal have severe effects. Although the effects of hypercalcemia occur first in excitable tissues, all systems are affected.

Hypercalcemia means either that the amount of serum calcium is so great that the normal calcium-controlling actions cannot keep pace or that a control action is not functioning properly (Table 11-10). Hypercalcemia causes excitable tissues to be less sensitive to normal stimuli, thus requiring a stronger stimulus to function. The excitable tissues affected most by hypercalcemia are the heart, skeletal muscles, nerves, and intestinal smooth muscles.

TABLE 11-10 Common Causes of Hypercalcemia

Actual Calcium Excesses	Relative Calcium Excesses
• Excessive oral intake of calcium	• Hyperparathyroidism
• Excessive oral intake of vitamin D	• Malignancy
• Kidney failure	• Hyperthyroidism
• Use of thiazide diuretics	• Immobility
	• Use of glucocorticoids
	• Dehydration

❖ PATIENT-CENTERED COLLABORATIVE CARE

◆ Assessment

The manifestations of hypercalcemia are related to its severity and how quickly the imbalance occurred. The patient with a mild but rapidly occurring calcium excess often has more severe problems than the patient whose imbalance is severe but has developed slowly.

Cardiovascular changes are the most serious and life-threatening problems of hypercalcemia. Mild hypercalcemia at first causes increased heart rate and blood pressure. Severe or prolonged calcium imbalance depresses electrical conduction, slowing heart rate.

Measure pulse rate and blood pressure, and observe for indications of poor tissue blood flow, such as cyanosis and pallor. Examine ECG tracings for dysrhythmias, especially a shortened QT interval.

Hypercalcemia allows blood clots to form more easily whenever blood flow is poor. Blood clotting is more likely in the lower legs, the pelvic region, areas where blood flow is blocked by internal or external constrictions, and areas where venous obstruction occurs.

Assess for slowed or impaired blood flow. Measure and record calf circumferences with a soft tape measure. Assess the feet for temperature, color, and capillary refill to determine the blood flow to and from the area.

Neuromuscular changes include severe muscle weakness and decreased deep tendon reflexes without paresthesia. The patient may be confused and lethargic.

Intestinal changes are first reflected as decreased peristalsis. Constipation, anorexia, nausea, vomiting, and abdominal distention and pain are common. Bowel sounds are hypoactive or absent. Assess abdominal size by measuring abdominal girth with a soft tape measure in a line circling the abdomen at the umbilicus.

◆ Interventions

Interventions for hypercalcemia focus on reducing serum calcium levels through drug therapy, rehydration, and, depending on the cause and severity, dialysis. Cardiac monitoring is also important.

Drug therapy involves preventing increases in calcium, as well as drugs to lower calcium levels. IV solutions containing calcium (e.g., Ringer's lactate) are stopped. Oral drugs containing calcium or vitamin D (e.g., calcium-based antacids) are discontinued.

FLUID volume replacement can help restore normal serum calcium levels. IV normal saline (0.9% sodium chloride) is usually given because sodium increases kidney excretion of calcium.

Thiazide diuretics are discontinued and are replaced with diuretics that enhance the excretion of calcium, such as furosemide (Lasix, Furoside ♣). Calcium chelators (calcium binders) help lower serum calcium levels. Such drugs include plicamycin (Mithracin) and penicillamine (Cuprimine, Pendramine ♣).

Drugs to prevent hypercalcemia include agents that inhibit calcium resorption from bone, such as phosphorus, calcitonin (Calcimar), bisphosphonates (etidronate), and prostaglandin synthesis inhibitors (aspirin, NSAIDs).

Cardiac monitoring of patients with hypercalcemia is needed to identify dysrhythmias and decreased cardiac output. Compare recent ECG tracings with the patient's baseline tracings. Especially look for changes in the T waves and the QT interval and changes in rate and rhythm.

NCLEX EXAMINATION CHALLENGE

Health Promotion and Maintenance

Which intervention is most important for the nurse to teach the client who is at continuing risk for hypercalcemia and has normal kidney function?

A. "Report a weight gain of 1 lb or more a day to your health care provider immediately."
B. "Keep track of the number of bowel movements you have each day."
C. "Avoid taking aspirin or any aspirin-containing products."
D. "Be sure to drink at least 2 liters of fluids each day."

PHOSPHORUS

Normal serum levels of phosphorus range from 3.0 to 4.5 mg/dL, or 0.97 to 1.45 mmol/L (see Table 11-1). Most phosphorus (80%) can be found in the bones. It is the major anion in the ICF, and its levels inside cells are much higher than in the ECF. Phosphorus is needed for activating vitamins and enzymes, forming energy supplies, and assisting in cell growth and metabolism. It also functions in acid-base balance and calcium homeostasis.

Phosphorus balance and calcium balance are intertwined. Plasma levels of calcium and phosphorus exist in a balanced, reciprocal relationship, which means that when you multiply the two values, the product remains constant. Therefore a change in the level of serum phosphorus results in an equal and opposite change in the level of serum calcium (and vice versa).

The regulation of ECF phosphorus occurs through the activity of parathyroid hormone (PTH). Increased PTH levels cause a net loss of phosphorus. Reduced PTH levels enhance kidney reabsorption of phosphorus, resulting in increased plasma levels of phosphorus.

HYPOPHOSPHATEMIA

❖ *PATHOPHYSIOLOGY*

Hypophosphatemia is an electrolyte imbalance in which the serum phosphorus level is below 3.0 mg/dL. Body functions are not usually impaired with rapid changes in serum phosphorus levels. Reduced function occurs more often with chronic hypophosphatemia. Table 11-11 lists causes of phosphorus imbalance.

Most effects of hypophosphatemia are related to decreased energy metabolism, as well as to other FLUID AND ELECTROLYTE imbalances. Because phosphorus and calcium are inter-related, *decreases* in serum phosphorus levels cause *increases* in serum calcium levels.

TABLE 11-11 Common Causes of Phosphorus Imbalance

Hypophosphatemia
- Malnutrition
- Starvation
- Use of aluminum hydroxide–based antacids
- Use of magnesium-based antacids
- Hyperparathyroidism
- Hypercalcemia
- Kidney failure
- Malignancy
- Hyperglycemia
- Hyperalimentation
- Respiratory alkalosis
- Uncontrolled diabetes mellitus
- Alcohol abuse

Hyperphosphatemia
- Decreased kidney excretion resulting from kidney disease
- Tumor lysis syndrome
- Increased intake of phosphorus
- Hypoparathyroidism

❖ *PATIENT-CENTERED COLLABORATIVE CARE*

◆ *Assessment*

Manifestations of hypophosphatemia are most apparent in the cardiac, musculoskeletal, hematologic, and central nervous systems. Cardiac changes include weak contractility, decreased stroke volume, and decreased cardiac output. Peripheral pulses are slow, difficult to find, and easy to block. Prolonged hypophosphatemia causes progressive but reversible cardiac muscle damage.

Musculoskeletal changes include weak skeletal muscles that may progress to acute muscle breakdown (**rhabdomyolysis**). With profound muscle weakness, respiratory efforts are ineffective, leading to respiratory failure. Assess for muscle strength, and observe respiratory effort.

The manifestations of *chronic* hypophosphatemia are most evident in the skeletal system. Bone density is decreased, which leads to fractures. Assess the patient for unusual lumps or depressions over bony areas that indicate bone fractures.

Central nervous system changes are not apparent until hypophosphatemia is severe. These first appear as irritability and may progress to seizure activity followed by coma.

◆ *Interventions*

Drugs that promote phosphorous loss (e.g., antacids, osmotic diuretics, calcium supplements) are discontinued. Oral replacement of phosphorus along with a vitamin D supplement may correct moderate hypophosphatemia. IV phosphorus is given only when serum phosphorus levels fall below 1 mg/dL and the patient has serious manifestations. Infuse IV phosphorus slowly because the problems caused by hyperphosphatemia are equally serious.

Nutrition therapy involves increasing the intake of phosphorus-rich foods while decreasing the intake of calcium-rich foods. Collaborate with the dietitian to teach the patient and family which foods to eat and which to avoid.

HYPERPHOSPHATEMIA

Hyperphosphatemia is an electrolyte imbalance in which the serum phosphorus level is above 4.5 mg/dL. High levels are well tolerated by most body systems. Causes of increased serum phosphorus levels include kidney disease, certain cancer treatments, increased phosphorus intake, and hypoparathyroidism. Table 11-11 lists common causes of hyperphosphatemia.

The problems caused by hyperphosphatemia center on the hypocalcemia that results when serum phosphorus levels increase. These problems include increased membrane excitability and can cause life-threatening side effects (see p. 168). Thus the management of hyperphosphatemia entails the management of hypocalcemia (see p. 169).

MAGNESIUM

Magnesium (Mg^{2+}) is a mineral that forms a cation when dissolved in water. Most magnesium is stored in bones and cartilage. Little magnesium is present in the extracellular fluid (ECF). Plasma levels of free magnesium range from 1.3 to 2.1 mEq/L, or 0.65 to 1.05 mmol/L (see Table 11-1). The intracellular fluid (ICF) has more magnesium and it has more functions inside the cells than in the blood. It is important for skeletal muscle contraction, carbohydrate metabolism, generation of energy stores, vitamin activation, blood coagulation, and cell growth. Magnesium regulation occurs through the kidney and the intestinal tract although the exact mechanisms are not known. When blood magnesium levels are low, ingested magnesium is rapidly absorbed and kidney excretion of magnesium stops. When blood magnesium levels are high, little magnesium is absorbed from food and kidney magnesium excretion increases.

HYPOMAGNESEMIA

Hypomagnesemia is an electrolyte imbalance in which the serum magnesium (Mg^{2+}) level is below 1.3 mEq/L. It is most often caused by decreased absorption of dietary magnesium or increased kidney magnesium excretion. Table 11-12 lists the specific causes of hypomagnesemia.

The effects of hypomagnesemia are caused by increased membrane excitability and the accompanying serum calcium and potassium imbalances. Excitable membranes, especially nerve cell membranes, may depolarize spontaneously.

Neuromuscular changes are caused by increased nerve impulse transmission. Normally, magnesium inhibits nerve impulse transmission at synapse areas. Decreased levels increase impulse transmission from nerve to nerve or from nerve to skeletal muscle. The patient has hyperactive deep tendon reflexes, numbness and tingling, and painful muscle contractions. Positive Chvostek's and Trousseau's signs may be present because hypomagnesemia may occur with hypocalcemia (see the earlier discussion of these assessment signs of neuromuscular changes on p. 168 in the Hypocalcemia section). The patient may have tetany and seizures as hypomagnesemia worsens.

Intestinal changes are from decreased intestinal smooth muscle contraction. Reduced motility, anorexia, nausea, constipation, and abdominal distention are common. A paralytic ileus may occur when hypomagnesemia is severe.

Interventions for hypomagnesemia aim to correct the imbalance and manage the specific problem that caused it. In addition, because hypocalcemia often occurs with hypomagnesemia, interventions also aim to restore normal serum calcium levels.

Drugs that promote magnesium loss, such as high-ceiling (loop) diuretics, osmotic diuretics, aminoglycoside antibiotics, and drugs containing phosphorus, are discontinued. Magnesium is replaced intravenously with magnesium sulfate ($MgSO_4$) when hypomagnesemia is severe. Assess deep tendon reflexes at least hourly in the patient receiving IV magnesium to monitor effectiveness and prevent hypermagnesemia. If hypocalcemia is also present, drug therapy to increase serum calcium levels is prescribed.

HYPERMAGNESEMIA

Hypermagnesemia is an ELECTROLYTE imbalance in which the serum magnesium level is above 2.1 mEq/L. Table 11-12 lists the specific causes of hypermagnesemia.

Magnesium is a membrane stabilizer. Most manifestations of hypermagnesemia occur as a result of reduced membrane excitability. They usually are not apparent until serum magnesium levels exceed 4 mEq/L.

Cardiac changes include bradycardia, peripheral vasodilation, and hypotension. These problems become more severe as serum magnesium levels increase. ECG changes show a prolonged PR interval with a widened QRS complex. Bradycardia can be severe, and cardiac arrest is possible. Hypotension is also severe, with a diastolic pressure lower than normal. *Patients with severe hypermagnesemia are in grave danger of cardiac arrest.*

Central nervous system changes result from depressed nerve impulse transmission. Patients may be drowsy or lethargic. Coma may occur if the imbalance is prolonged or severe.

Neuromuscular changes include reduced or absent deep tendon reflexes. Voluntary skeletal muscle contractions become progressively weaker and finally stop.

Hypermagnesemia has no direct effect on the lungs; however, when the respiratory muscles are weak, respiratory insufficiency can lead to respiratory failure and death.

Interventions for hypermagnesemia focus on reducing the serum level and correcting the underlying problem that caused the imbalance. All oral and parenteral magnesium is discontinued. When kidney failure is not present, giving magnesium-free IV fluids can reduce serum magnesium levels. High-ceiling (loop) diuretics such as furosemide (Lasix, Furoside 🍁) can

TABLE 11-12 Common Causes of Magnesium Imbalance

Hypomagnesemia

- Malnutrition
- Starvation
- Diarrhea
- Steatorrhea
- Celiac disease
- Crohn's disease
- Drugs (diuretics, aminoglycoside antibiotics, cisplatin, amphotericin B, cyclosporine)
- Citrate (blood products)
- Ethanol ingestion

Hypermagnesemia

- Increased magnesium intake:
  - Magnesium-containing antacids and laxatives
  - IV magnesium replacement
- Decreased kidney excretion of magnesium resulting from kidney disease

further reduce serum magnesium levels. When cardiac problems are severe, giving calcium may reverse the cardiac effects of hypermagnesemia.

CHLORIDE

Chloride (Cl^-) is the major anion of the extracellular fluid (ECF) and works with sodium to maintain ECF osmotic pressure. The normal plasma concentration of chloride ranges from 98 to 106 mEq/L or mmol/L (see Table 11-1). It enters the body through dietary intake and is important in the formation of hydrochloric acid in the stomach.

Only a small amount of chloride is present inside the cells because negative charges on the cell membrane repel chloride and prevent it from crossing the membrane. However, extracellular chloride can enter cells when exchanged for another anion that is leaving the cell. This situation, called a *chloride shift*, decreases plasma chloride without a net body loss of chloride. Bicarbonate (HCO_3^-) is the anion most commonly exchanged for chloride.

Imbalances of chloride usually occur as a result of other electrolyte imbalances. An exception is chloride loss from excessive vomiting or prolonged gastric suction. Imbalances of chloride are usually corrected by interventions for correcting other electrolyte or acid-base problems.

CLINICAL JUDGMENT CHALLENGE

Patient-Centered Care; Safety QSEN

The patient is a 29-year-old woman admitted 20 hours ago for an acute exacerbation of Crohn's disease with intense abdominal pain. She is NPO and receiving normal saline intravenously at 175 mL per minute. She was last given hydromorphone (Dilaudid) 4 mg IV 30 minutes ago. Because she did have an episode of hypotension earlier after Dilaudid, you now take her vital signs. On inflating the blood pressure cuff, she develops palmar flexion. The flexion remains after the cuff is deflated.

1. What is most likely the cause of this problem?
2. What electrolytes are most likely to be out of balance and why?
3. What is your best first action?
4. Should the Rapid Response Team be called? Why or why not?
5. What additional assessment data are most important to collect? Explain your selection.

NURSING CONCEPTS AND CLINICAL JUDGMENT REVIEW

What might you NOTICE in a patient who has adequate FLUID AND ELECTROLYTE BALANCE?

Vital signs:

- Heart rate and rhythm within usual range for the patient
- Respiratory rate and depth within usual range for the patient

Physical assessment:

- Skin turgor normal, no tenting, no edema
- Skin color normal (no cyanosis or pallor)
- Oral mucous membrane and nail beds pink with rapid capillary refill
- Strong and equal peripheral pulses
- Deep tendon reflexes present and normal
- Muscle strength consistent with what is normal for the patient
- Urine output about equal to fluid intake

Psychological assessment:

- Oriented and not confused
- Easily aroused from sleep

Laboratory assessment:

- Serum electrolyte values within normal limits
- Normal electrocardiogram

GET READY FOR THE NCLEX® EXAMINATION!

KEY POINTS

Review these Key Points for each NCLEX Examination Client Needs Category.

Safe and Effective Care Environment

- Assess any patient with a problem of FLUID AND ELECTROLYTE BALANCE for falls risk.
- Ensure access to adequate fluids for patients who cannot talk or who have limited mobility.
- Supervise the oral fluid therapy and intake and output measurement aspects of care delegated to unlicensed assistive personnel.
- Use a pump or controller to deliver IV fluids to patients with fluid overload. **Safety** QSEN
- Do not give IV potassium at a rate greater than 20 mEq/hr.
- Never give potassium supplements by the IM, subcutaneous, or IV push routes. **Safety** QSEN
- Use a pump or controller when giving IV potassium-containing solutions. **Safety** QSEN
- Use a gait belt when assisting a patient with muscle weakness to walk or transfer. **Safety** QSEN
- Collaborate with the dietitian to teach patients about diets that are restricted in potassium, sodium, or calcium.
- Use a lift sheet to move or reposition a patient with chronic hypocalcemia. **Safety** QSEN

Health Promotion and Maintenance

- Encourage all patients to maintain an adequate fluid intake (minimum of 2 L per day) unless another condition requires fluid restriction.
- Teach all people to increase fluid intake when exercising, when in hot or dry environments, or during conditions that increase metabolism (e.g., fever).

- Instruct patients at risk for FLUID imbalance to weigh themselves on the same scale daily, close to the same time each day, and with about the same amount of clothing on each time and to monitor these daily weights for changes or trends. **Patient-Centered Care** QSEN
- Instruct patients who exercise heavily (athletes) to take scheduled fluid replacement breaks.
- Instruct caregivers of older adults who have cognitive impairments or mobility problems to schedule offerings of fluids at regular intervals throughout the day. **Patient-Centered Care** QSEN
- Teach patients how to determine electrolyte content of processed foods by reading labels.
- Teach patients who are prescribed to take diuretics to take the drugs as prescribed.
- Teach patients who are taking digoxin to measure their pulse for rate, rhythm, and quality.
- Teach patients who are taking diuretics to measure their pulse for rate, rhythm, and quality.

Psychosocial Integrity

- Explain the purpose of fluid restriction to the patient and the family to ensure cooperation and prevent any misunderstandings.
- Assess patients who have a sudden change in cognition for a change in FLUID AND ELECTROLYTE BALANCE. **Safety** QSEN
- Determine the patient's food preferences and dislikes when planning an electrolyte-restricted diet.

Physiological Integrity

- Assess skin turgor on the forehead or the sternum of older patients.
- Use daily weights to determine fluid gains or losses. **Evidence-Based Practice** QSEN
- Ask patients about the use of drugs such as diuretics, laxatives, salt substitutes, and antihypertensives that may alter FLUID AND ELECTROLYTE BALANCE.
- Correctly interpret laboratory electrolyte values.
- Do not give oral fluids to an unconscious patient.
- Monitor the cardiac and pulmonary status at least every hour when patients with dehydration are receiving IV fluid replacement therapy.
- Offer or ensure that oral care is performed at least every 4 hours for patients with dehydration.
- Assess the IV site hourly of a person receiving IV solutions containing potassium, and document its condition. **Safety** QSEN
- Immediately stop the infusion of potassium-containing solutions if infiltration is suspected.
- Assess all patients with hyperkalemia for cardiac dysrhythmias and ECG abnormalities, especially tall T waves, conduction delays, and heart block.
- Assess the respiratory status of all patients with hypokalemia.
- Assess the bowel sounds; heart rate, rhythm and quality; and muscle strength to evaluate the patient's responses to therapy for an ELECTROLYTE imbalance.

12 CHAPTER

Assessment and Care of Patients with Acid-Base Imbalances

M. Linda Workman

http://evolve.elsevier.com/Iggy/

PRIORITY CONCEPTS

- Acid-Base Balance

LEARNING OUTCOMES

Safe and Effective Care Environment

1. Identify patients at risk for falls as a result of problems with ACID-BASE BALANCE, especially older adults.

Health Promotion and Maintenance

2. Teach patients measures to take to maintain ACID-BASE BALANCE and avoid imbalances.

Psychosocial Integrity

3. Reduce the psychological impact for the patient experiencing a problem with ACID-BASE BALANCE.

Physiological Integrity

4. Apply knowledge of anatomy and physiology to explain regulation of ACID-BASE BALANCE.
5. Assess the patient for ACID-BASE BALANCE status, using laboratory data and clinical manifestations.
6. Prioritize nursing care for the patient with a problem affecting ACID-BASE BALANCE.

ACID-BASE BALANCE occurs through control of hydrogen ion (H^+) production and elimination. Body fluid **pH** is a measure of the body fluid's free hydrogen ion level. *This value has the narrowest range of normal and the tightest control mechanisms of all the electrolytes.* The level of free hydrogen ions, formed from acids, must be rigidly controlled. Even small changes in the free hydrogen ion level (pH) of body fluids can cause major problems in function. Keeping the pH within the normal range involves balancing acids and bases in body fluids. Normal pH ranges from 7.35 to 7.45 for arterial blood and from 7.31 to 7.41 for venous blood.

The normal free hydrogen ion level of blood and other body fluids is quite low (less than 0.0001 mEq/L) compared with other electrolytes (see Chapter 11). Because it is so low, the hydrogen ion concentration is not measured directly but, instead, is calculated in negative logarithm units. The value of pH is *inversely* related (negatively related) to the level of free hydrogen ions. Thus the *lower* the pH value of a fluid, the *higher* the level of free hydrogen ions in that fluid. The pH of a solution may range from 1 (as acidic as possible) to 14 (as alkaline as possible), with 7 being neutral. *A change of 1 pH unit actually represents a tenfold change in free hydrogen ion level.* Therefore any pH unit change (e.g., a change from 7.4 to 7.3) represents a large increase in the free hydrogen ion level.

Keeping the pH of the blood within the normal range by regulating ACID-BASE BALANCE is important because changes from normal interfere with many functions. These include:

- Changing the shape and reducing the function of hormones and enzymes
- Changing the distribution of other electrolytes, causing fluid and electrolyte imbalances
- Changing excitable membranes, making the heart, nerves, muscles, and GI tract either less or more active than normal
- Decreasing the effectiveness of many drugs

ACID-BASE BALANCE

Most body fluids have a pH value between 7.35 and 7.45 even though they contain acidic substances and basic substances. This value is slightly alkaline rather than strictly neutral (7.0 is neutral). Normal body fluid pH remains at this near-neutral value when the acids and bases are nearly balanced, limiting the total number of free or unbalanced hydrogen ions. ACID-BASE BALANCE occurs by matching the rate of hydrogen ion production (which is a continuous normal process) with hydrogen ion loss.

Acid-Base Chemistry

Acids

Acids are substances that release hydrogen ions when dissolved in water (H_2O), *increasing* the amount of free hydrogen ions in that solution. The strength of an acid is measured by how easily it releases a hydrogen ion in solution. A strong acid, such as hydrochloric acid (HCl), separates completely in water and releases *all* of its hydrogen ions, as shown in Fig. 12-1.

A weak acid releases only *some,* not all, of its hydrogen ions. In the following example, each molecule of acetic acid (CH_3COOH), a weak acid, contains a total of four hydrogen molecules. When acetic acid combines with water, as shown in Fig. 12-2, it releases only one of its four hydrogen molecules, keeping the other three hydrogen molecules bound to the molecule (CH_3COO^-).

Bases

A **base** binds free hydrogen ions in solution and *lowers* the amount of free hydrogen ions in solution. Strong bases bind hydrogen ions easily. Examples are sodium hydroxide (NaOH) and ammonia (NH_3).

Weak bases bind hydrogen ions less readily. An example of a weak base is bicarbonate (HCO_3^-). Although a weak base, the many bicarbonate ions in the body are critical in preventing major changes in body fluid pH.

Buffers

Buffers are critical in keeping body fluid pH at normal levels because they can react either as an acid (releasing a hydrogen ion) or as a base (binding a hydrogen ion). How a buffer reacts depends on the existing ACID-BASE BALANCE of that fluid. Buffers always try to bring the fluid as close as possible to the normal body fluid pH of 7.35 to 7.45. If the fluid is basic (with few free hydrogen ions), the buffer *releases hydrogen ions* into the fluid (Fig. 12-3). If the fluid is acidic (with many free hydrogen ions), the buffer *binds some of the excess hydrogen ions.* In this way, buffers act like hydrogen ion "sponges," soaking up hydrogen ions when too many are present and squeezing out hydrogen ions when too few are present. This flexibility allows buffers to keep body fluid pH in the normal range.

Liquids with a pH of 7.0 are neutral by having a free hydrogen ion level in which the amount and strength of acids and bases are equal. Fig. 12-4 shows the concept of neutral pH in which the combined *strength* and *amount* of all acids are equal to the combined *strength* and *amount* of all bases in a given solution. With human acid-base homeostasis, the relative

$$HCl + H_2O \leftrightarrow H^+ + Cl^- + H_2O$$

Hydrochloric acid, Water, Hydrogen ion, Chloride ion, Water

FIG. 12-1 Release of hydrogen ions by a strong acid (hydrochloric acid) in which the strong acid completely dissociates in water.

$$CH_3COOH + H_2O \leftrightarrow H^+ + CH_3COO^- + H_2O$$

Acetic acid (not ionized), Water, Hydrogen ion, Acetic acid (ionized), Water

FIG. 12-2 Release of hydrogen ions by a weak acid (acetic acid) in which the weak acid only partially dissociates in water and most of its hydrogen ions remain bound.

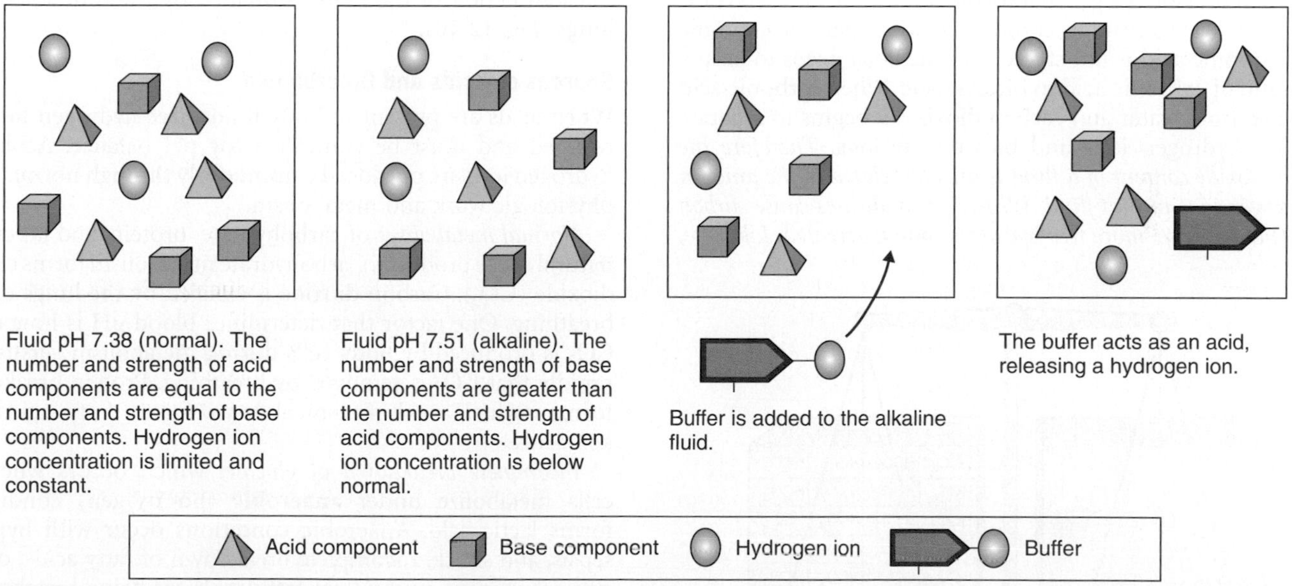

FIG. 12-3 Action of buffer in solution.

AAABBB AAABBB AAABBB	AAAABBB AAAABBB AAAABBB	AAABB AAABB AAABB
Neutral or acid-base balance	Acidic (acid excess) (actual acidosis)	Acidic (base deficit) (relative acidosis)

FIG. 12-4 Concept of acidic versus normal pH. (A = acid; B = base.)

AAABBB AAABBB AAABBB	AAABBBB AAABBBB AAABBBB	AABBB AABBB AABBB
Neutral	Alkaline (base excess)	Alkaline (acid deficit)

FIG. 12-5 Concept of alkaline versus normal pH. (A = acid; B = base.)

amounts and strengths of acids and bases are nearly equal and, normally, hydrogen ion production is balanced with hydrogen ion loss so that the overall free hydrogen ion levels remain constant.

Liquids with a pH ranging from 1.0 to 6.99 have more or stronger (or both) acids compared with bases. These liquids are *acidic* (see Fig. 12-4), with more free hydrogen ions released than bound, increasing the amount of free hydrogen ions in the liquid.

Liquids with a pH ranging from 7.01 to 14.0 have more or stronger (or both) bases compared with acids. These liquids are *basic,* in which more hydrogen ions are being bound than released, decreasing the amount of free hydrogen ions (Fig. 12-5).

Body Fluid Chemistry

Bicarbonate Ions

Body fluids contain different types of acids and bases. The most common base in human body fluid is bicarbonate (HCO_3^-); the most common acid is carbonic acid (H_2CO_3). In health, the body keeps these substances at a constant ratio of 1 molecule of carbonic acid to 20 free bicarbonate ions (1:20) (Fig. 12-6). To maintain this ratio, both carbonic acid and bicarbonate must be carefully controlled. This constant ratio is related to balancing the production and elimination of carbon dioxide (CO_2) and hydrogen ions (H^+).

Relationship Between Carbon Dioxide and Hydrogen Ions

A key process in understanding ACID-BASE BALANCE is the carbonic anhydrase equation. This equation, driven by the enzyme *carbonic anhydrase,* shows how hydrogen ion levels and carbon dioxide levels are directly related to one another, so that an increase in one causes an equal increase in the other (Fig. 12-7).

Carbon dioxide is a gas that forms carbonic acid when combined with water, making carbon dioxide a part of carbonic acid. Carbonic acid is not stable, and the body needs to keep a 1:20 ratio of carbonic acid to bicarbonate. When carbonic acid is formed from water and carbon dioxide, it begins to separate into free hydrogen ions and bicarbonate ions. *Therefore the carbon dioxide content of a fluid is directly related to the amount of hydrogen ions in that fluid. Whenever conditions cause carbon dioxide to increase, more free hydrogen ions are created. Likewise, whenever free hydrogen ion production increases, more carbon dioxide is produced.*

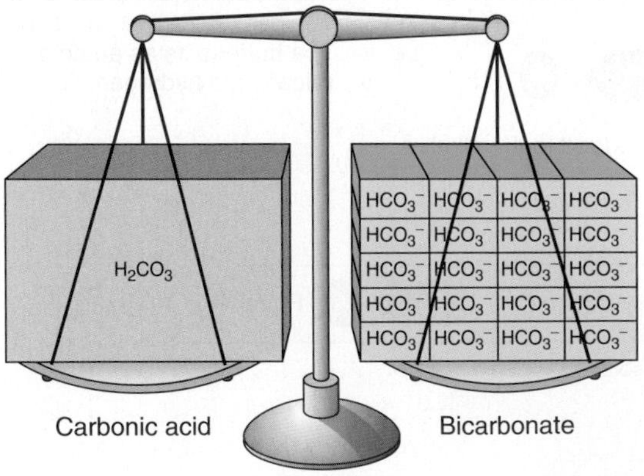

FIG. 12-6 Normal ratio of carbonic acid to bicarbonate is 1:20.

$$CO_2 + H_2O \leftrightarrow H_2CO_3 \leftrightarrow HCO_3^- + H^+$$

FIG. 12-7 The carbonic anhydrase equation showing that the concentration of carbon dioxide is directly related to the concentration of hydrogen ions.

When excess carbon dioxide is produced, the equation shifts to the *right,* causing an *increase* in hydrogen ions (and a *decrease* in pH), as shown in Fig. 12-8. When very little carbon dioxide is produced, no free hydrogen ions are created by this equation.

When excess hydrogen ions are present, the carbonic anhydrase equation shifts to the *left,* causing the creation of more carbon dioxide, as shown in Fig. 12-9. When the amount of free hydrogen ions in body fluids is low, no extra carbon dioxide is produced.

How is the relationship between free hydrogen ions and carbon dioxide helpful? Carbon dioxide is a gas that can be eliminated during exhalation, and this action is important for ACID-BASE BALANCE. When any condition causes the hydrogen ion concentration of body fluids to increase, extra CO_2 is produced in the same proportion. This extra CO_2 is eliminated during exhalation, helping to bring the hydrogen ion concentration down to normal. Whenever the CO_2 level changes, the pH changes to the same degree, in the opposite direction. Thus when the CO_2 level of a liquid increases, the pH drops, indicating more free hydrogen ions (more acidic). Likewise, when the CO_2 level of a liquid decreases, the pH rises, indicating fewer free hydrogen ions (more alkaline).

An increase in bicarbonate causes the amount of hydrogen ions to decrease and the pH to increase, or become more alkaline (basic). Likewise, a decrease in bicarbonate causes the free hydrogen ion level to increase and the pH to decrease, or become more acidic.

Because the kidneys control bicarbonate levels and the lungs control CO_2 levels in the healthy person, pH is also described as the function of the kidneys divided by the function of the lungs (Fig. 12-10).

Sources of Acids and Bicarbonate

When acids are present in body fluids, free hydrogen ions are released and must be controlled for pH balance. Acids and hydrogen ions are produced continuously through normal body physiologic work and metabolism.

Normal metabolism of carbohydrate, protein, and fat creates natural waste products. Carbohydrate metabolism forms carbon dioxide (CO_2). Carbon dioxide is exhaled by the lungs during breathing. One factor that determines blood pH is how much CO_2 is produced by body cells during metabolism versus how rapidly that CO_2 is removed by breathing. Protein breakdown forms sulfuric acid. Fat breakdown forms fatty acids and ketoacids.

Incomplete breakdown of glucose, which occurs whenever cells metabolize under **anaerobic** (no oxygen) conditions, forms lactic acid. Anaerobic conditions occur with hypoxia, sepsis, and shock. Incomplete breakdown of fatty acids, occurring when large amounts of fatty acids are being metabolized, forms ketoacids.

Cell destruction allows cell contents to be released, including the structures that contain acids. These released acids in the extracellular fluid (ECF) increase free hydrogen ion levels.

$$\mathbf{CO_2} + H_2O \rightarrow H_2CO_3 \rightarrow HCO_3^- + \mathbf{H^+}$$

FIG. 12-8 Increased carbon dioxide levels force the equation to the right and increase the concentration of hydrogen ions proportionately.

$$CO_2 + H_2O \leftarrow H_2CO_3 \leftarrow HCO_3^- + H^+$$

FIG. 12-9 Increased hydrogen ion levels force the equation to the left and increase the concentration of carbon dioxide levels proportionately.

$$pH = \frac{\overset{\text{(Slow but powerful response)}}{\text{Kidney function = Bicarbonate levels}}}{\underset{\text{(Rapid but limited response)}}{\text{Lung function = Carbon dioxide levels}}}$$

FIG. 12-10 Contribution of pH balance by kidney and lung function.

CHART 12-1 Laboratory Profile

Acid-Base Assessment

TEST	NORMAL RANGE FOR ADULTS: ARTERIAL	NORMAL RANGE FOR ADULTS: VENOUS	SIGNIFICANCE OF ABNORMAL FINDINGS
pH			
Adult <90 yr	7.35-7.45	7.31-7.41	Increased: metabolic alkalosis, loss of gastric fluids, decreased potassium intake, diuretic therapy, fever, salicylate toxicity, respiratory alkalosis, hyperventilation
>90 yr	7.25-7.45	7.31-7.41	Decreased: metabolic or respiratory acidosis, ketosis, renal failure, starvation, diarrhea, hyperthyroidism
Pao_2			
Adult <90 yr	80-100 mm Hg		Increased: increased ventilation, oxygen therapy, exercise
>90 yr	70-90 mm Hg		Decreased: respiratory depression, high altitude, carbon monoxide poisoning, decreased cardiac output
$Paco_2$	35-45 mm Hg	40-50 mm Hg	Increased: respiratory acidosis, emphysema, pneumonia, cardiac failure, respiratory depression Decreased: respiratory alkalosis, excessive ventilation, diarrhea
Bicarbonate	21-28 mEq/L	24-29 mEq/L	Increased: metabolic alkalosis, bicarbonate therapy Decreased: metabolic acidosis, diarrhea, pancreatitis
Lactate	3-7 mg/dL 0.3-0.8 mmol/L	5-20 mg/dL 0.6-2.2 mmol/L	Increased: hypoxia, exercise, insulin infusion, alcoholism, pregnancy Decreased: fluid overload

Data from Pagana, K., & Pagana, T. (2014). *Mosby's manual of diagnostic and laboratory tests* (5th ed). St. Louis: Mosby.

$Paco_2$, Partial pressure of arterial carbon dioxide; *Pao_2*, partial pressure of arterial oxygen.

Bicarbonate, a weak base, is the main buffer of the ECF. It comes from the GI absorption of ingested bicarbonate, pancreatic production of bicarbonate, movement of cellular bicarbonate into the ECF, kidney reabsorption of filtered bicarbonate, and the breakdown of carbonic acid. Once bicarbonate is in the ECF, it is kept at a level 20 times greater than that of carbonic acid.

Acid-Base Regulatory Actions and Mechanisms

As long as body cells are healthy, they continuously produce acids, carbon dioxide, and free hydrogen ions. Despite this production, hydrogen ion, bicarbonate, oxygen, and carbon dioxide levels are kept within normal limits when ACID-BASE BALANCE controlling actions are normal. Chart 12-1 lists their normal values in arterial and venous blood. This homeostasis depends on:

- Hydrogen ion production being consistent and not excessive
- CO_2 loss from the body through breathing keeping pace with all forms of hydrogen ion production

To keep the free hydrogen ion level (pH) of the ECF within the narrow normal range, the body has chemical, respiratory, and kidney actions (mechanisms) for acid-base balance (Table 12-1).

Chemical Acid-Base Control Actions and Mechanisms

Buffers are the first line of defense against changes in free hydrogen ion levels. These buffers are always present in body fluids and act fast to reduce or raise the amount of free hydrogen ions to normal. By acting as hydrogen ion "sponges," buffers can bind hydrogen ions when too many are present or release hydrogen ions when not enough are present.

Buffers are composed of chemicals or proteins. The two most common chemical buffers are bicarbonate (which is active in both the extracellular fluid [ECF] and intracellular fluid [ICF]) and phosphate (which is active in the ICF). Protein buffers are the most common buffers. Extracellular protein buffers are albumin and globulins. A major intracellular protein buffer is hemoglobin. When the amount of free hydrogen ions in the blood increases, some of the excess hydrogen ions cross the membranes of red blood cells and bind to the large numbers of hemoglobin molecules in each red blood cell. This binding of hydrogen ions to hemoglobin results in fewer hydrogen ions remaining in the blood, bringing blood pH back up toward normal.

Respiratory Acid-Base Control Actions and Mechanisms

When chemical buffers alone cannot prevent changes in blood pH, the respiratory system is the second line of defense against changes. Breathing controls the amount of free hydrogen ions by controlling the amount of carbon dioxide (CO_2) in arterial blood. Because CO_2 is converted into hydrogen ions with the carbonic anhydrase reaction, the CO_2 level is *directly* related to the hydrogen ion level. Breathing rids the body of any excess CO_2.

The CO_2 level in venous blood increases with metabolism. This CO_2 moves into lung capillary blood. Because the amount (pressure) of CO_2 is far higher in lung capillary blood than it is

TABLE 12-1 **Acid-Base Regulatory Mechanisms**

MECHANISM TYPE	KEY CHARACTERISTICS
Chemical	
Protein buffers (albumin, globulins, hemoglobin) Chemical buffers (bicarbonate, phosphate)	Very rapid response Provide immediate response to changing conditions Can handle relatively small fluctuations in hydrogen ion production during normal metabolic and health conditions
Respiratory	
Increased hydrogen ions or increased carbon dioxide: Triggers the brain to increase the rate and depth of breathing, causing more carbon dioxide to be lost and decreasing the hydrogen ion concentration Decreased hydrogen ions or decreased carbon dioxide: Inhibits brain stimulation, leading to decreased rate and depth of breathing, causing carbon dioxide to be retained and increasing the hydrogen ion concentration	Primarily assist buffering systems when the fluctuation of hydrogen ion concentration is acute
Kidney	
Actions to decrease pH: Increased kidney excretion of bicarbonate Increased kidney reabsorption of hydrogen ions Actions to increase pH: Decreased kidney excretion of bicarbonate Decreased kidney reabsorption of hydrogen ions	The most powerful regulator of acid-base balance Respond to large or chronic fluctuations in hydrogen ion production or elimination Slowest response (hours to days) Longest duration

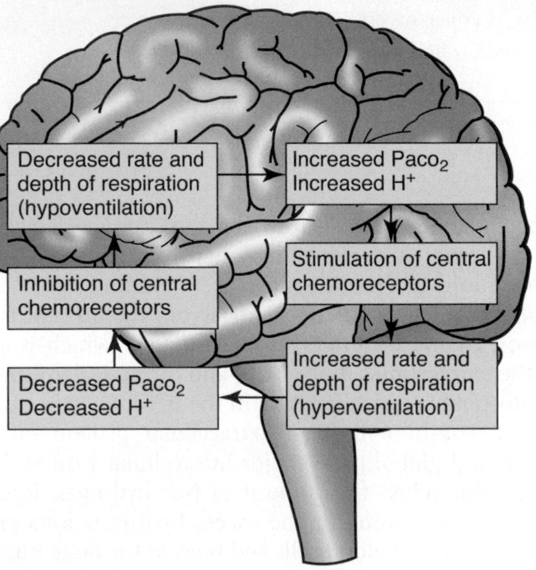

FIG. 12-11 Neural regulation of respiration and hydrogen ion concentration. (*H*+, Hydrogen ion, *Paco₂*, partial pressure of arterial carbon dioxide.)

in the air in the alveoli, CO_2 diffuses freely from the blood into the alveolar air. Once in the alveoli, CO_2 is exhaled during breathing and is lost from the body. Because the amount (pressure) of CO_2 in room air is nearly zero, CO_2 can continue to be exhaled even when breathing is impaired.

Respiratory regulation of ACID-BASE BALANCE is under the control of the central nervous system (Fig. 12-11). Special receptors in the respiratory areas of the brain are sensitive to changes in the amount of CO_2 in brain tissues. As the amount of CO_2 begins to rise above normal in brain blood and tissues, these central receptors trigger the neurons to increase the rate and depth of breathing (**hyperventilation**). As a result, more CO_2 is exhaled ("blown off") from the lungs and the CO_2 level in the ECF decreases. When the arterial CO_2 level returns back down to normal, the rate and depth of breathing return to levels that are normal for the person.

If the amount of ECF free hydrogen ions is too low, then the CO_2 level also is too low. Central receptors sense these low CO_2 levels and stop or slow the neuron activity in the respiratory centers of the brain, decreasing the rate and depth of breathing (**hypoventilation**). As a result, less CO_2 is lost through the lungs and more CO_2 is retained in arterial blood. This retention of already-formed CO_2, together with the normal production of CO_2 from metabolism, results in a rapid return of the arterial CO_2 levels (and hydrogen ion levels) back up to normal. When these levels are normal, the rate and depth of breathing also return to normal levels.

The respiratory system's response in acid-base balance is rapid. Changes in the rate and depth of breathing occur within minutes after changes in the hydrogen ion level or CO_2 level of the ECF occur.

Kidney Acid-Base Control Actions and Mechanisms

The kidneys are the third line of defense against wide changes in body fluid pH. Kidney actions are stronger for regulating ACID-BASE BALANCE but take 24 to 48 hours to completely respond. When blood pH changes are persistent, kidney actions to increase excretion and reabsorption rates of acids or bases (depending on which way pH changes) start. These actions are kidney movement of bicarbonate, formation of acids, and formation of ammonium.

Kidney movement of bicarbonate is the first kidney pH control action. It occurs in the kidney tubules in two ways: (1) kidney movement of bicarbonate produced elsewhere in the body and (2) kidney movement of bicarbonate produced in the kidneys. Much of the bicarbonate made in other body areas is excreted in the urine. When blood hydrogen ion levels are high, this bicarbonate is reabsorbed from the kidneys back into circulation, where it can help buffer excess hydrogen ions. The kidney tubules also can make additional bicarbonate and reabsorb it to increase the buffer effect. When blood hydrogen ion levels are low, the bicarbonate stays in the urine and is excreted.

Formation of acids occurs through the phosphate-buffering system inside the cells of the kidney tubules. When the newly created bicarbonate made in kidney cells is reabsorbed into the blood, the urine has an excess of anions, including phosphate (HPO_4^{2-}). This negatively charged fluid draws hydrogen ions (which have a positive charge) into the urine. Once in the urine, the hydrogen ion binds to phosphate ions, forming an acid (H_2PO_4) that is then excreted in the urine.

Formation of ammonium converts the ammonia (NH_3), which is formed during normal protein breakdown, into ammonium (NH_4^+) in the urine. The ammonium "traps" the hydrogen ions and then allows them to be excreted in the urine. The result is a loss of hydrogen ions and an increase in blood pH.

Compensation

In the process of *compensation,* the body adapts to attempt to correct changes in blood pH and maintain ACID-BASE BALANCE. A pH below 6.9 or above 7.8 is usually fatal. The normal pH range for human extracellular fluid (ECF) is 7.35 to 7.45. Both the kidneys and the lungs can compensate for acid-base imbalances, but they are not equal in their final responses. The respiratory system is much more sensitive to acid-base changes and can begin compensation efforts within seconds to minutes after a change in pH. However, these efforts are limited and can be overwhelmed easily. The kidney compensatory actions are much more powerful and result in rapid changes in ECF composition. However, these more powerful actions are not fully triggered unless the acid-base imbalance continues for several hours to several days.

Respiratory compensation occurs through the lungs, usually to correct for acid-base imbalances from metabolic problems. For example, when prolonged running causes buildup of lactic acid, hydrogen ion levels in the ECF increase and the pH drops. To bring the pH back to normal, breathing is triggered in response to increased carbon dioxide levels. Both the rate and depth of respiration increase. These respiratory efforts cause the blood to lose carbon dioxide with each exhalation, so ECF levels of carbon dioxide and free hydrogen ions gradually decrease. When the lungs can *fully compensate,* the pH returns to normal.

Kidney compensation results when a healthy kidney works to correct for changes in blood pH that occur when the respiratory system either is overwhelmed or is not healthy. For example, in a person with chronic obstructive pulmonary disease (COPD), the respiratory system cannot exchange gases adequately. Carbon dioxide is retained continuously, hydrogen ion levels increase, and the blood pH falls (becomes more acidic). To oppose this process, the kidney excretes more hydrogen ions and increases the reabsorption of bicarbonate back into the blood. As a result, the blood pH remains either within or closer to the normal range. When these backup actions are completely effective, acid-base problems are *fully compensated* and the pH of the blood returns to normal even though the levels of oxygen and bicarbonate may be abnormal (Blevins, 2014).

Sometimes, however, the respiratory problem causing the acid-base imbalance is so severe that kidney actions can only *partially compensate* and the pH is not quite normal. Partial compensation helps because it prevents the acid-base imbalance from becoming severe (Blevins, 2014).

ACID-BASE IMBALANCES

Acid-base imbalances are problems of ACID-BASE BALANCE resulting from changes in the blood hydrogen ion level or pH. These changes are caused by problems with the acid-base regulatory actions or by exposure to dangerous conditions. Imbalances in which blood pH is below normal reflect **acidosis**, and imbalances in which blood pH is above normal reflect **alkalosis**. Acid-base imbalances impair the function of many organs and can be life threatening.

ACIDOSIS

❖ PATHOPHYSIOLOGY

In acidosis, the acid-base balance of the blood and other extracellular fluid (ECF) is upset by an excess of hydrogen ions (H^+). This is seen as an arterial blood pH below 7.35. The amount of acids present is greater than normal compared with the amount or strength of bases.

Acidosis is not a disease; it is a condition caused by a disorder or pathologic process. It can be caused by metabolic problems, respiratory problems, or both. Patients at greatest risk for acute acidosis are those with problems that impair breathing. Older adults with chronic health problems are at greater risk for developing acidosis (Chart 12-2).

Acidosis can result from an actual or relative increase in the amount or strength of acids. An *actual acid excess* results in acidosis by either overproducing acids (and release of hydrogen ions) or undereliminating normally produced acids (retention of hydrogen ions). Either way, more hydrogen ions are present than should be. Problems that increase acid production include diabetic ketoacidosis and seizures. Problems that decrease acid

CHART 12-2 Nursing Focus on the Older Adult

The Older Patient Experiencing Acid-Base Imbalance

When Obtaining a Patient's History

- Assess risk factors for acid-base imbalance, including drugs, chronic health problems (especially kidney disease, pulmonary disease), and acute health problems.
- Ask the patient to list all prescribed and over-the-counter drugs (especially diuretics and antacids). If the patient is unable to provide this information, ask the family to bring the drugs in from home.
- Ask the patient to recall what liquids were taken in the past 24 hours and whether urination amounts have changed.

When Assessing the Patient

- Compare the patient's mental status with what the family, significant other, or health record states is the patient's baseline.
- Observe the rate and depth of respiration.
  - Determine whether the patient can complete a sentence without stopping for breath.
- Examine the color of nail beds and mucous membranes.
- Obtain a urine specimen, and observe for color and character. Test for specific gravity and pH.
- Examine skin turgor for dehydration. Attempt to pinch the skin to form a tent over the sternum and on the forehead. If a tent forms, record how long it remains.
- Measure the rate and quality of the pulse.
- Monitor clinical responses and laboratory values while the acid-base imbalance is being corrected.
- Administer IV therapy by pump or controller.

elimination include respiratory impairment and kidney impairment.

In *relative* acidosis, the amount of acids does not increase. Instead, the amount or strength of the bases decreases (to create a *base deficit*), which makes the fluid relatively more acidic than basic. A relative acidosis *(base deficit)* is caused by either overeliminating or underproducing bicarbonate ions (HCO_3^-) (see Fig. 12-4). Problems that underproduce bases include pancreatitis and dehydration. A condition that overeliminates bases is diarrhea.

Regardless of its cause, acidosis causes major changes in body function. The main problems occur because hydrogen ions are positively charged ions. An increase in hydrogen ions creates imbalances of other positively charged electrolytes, especially potassium. The changes in potassium levels because of excess hydrogen ions is described in the Laboratory Assessment section for acidosis. These electrolyte imbalances then disrupt the functions of nerves, cardiac muscle, and skeletal muscle. Manifestations of acidosis first appear in the musculoskeletal, cardiac, respiratory, and central nervous systems. Even slight increases in blood hydrogen ion levels reduce the activity of many hormones and enzymes, leading to death.

Acidosis can be caused by metabolic problems, respiratory problems, or combined metabolic and respiratory problems. Specific causes of acidosis are listed in Table 12-2.

Metabolic Acidosis

Four processes can result in metabolic acidosis: overproduction of hydrogen ions, underelimination of hydrogen ions, underproduction of bicarbonate ions, and overelimination of bicarbonate ions.

TABLE 12-2 Common Causes of Acidosis

PATHOLOGY	CONDITION
Metabolic Acidosis	
Overproduction of hydrogen ions	Excessive oxidation of fatty acids:
	Diabetic ketoacidosis
	Starvation
	Hypermetabolism:
	Heavy exercise
	Seizure activity
	Fever
	Hypoxia, ischemia
	Excessive ingestion of acids:
	Ethanol or methanol intoxication
	Salicylate intoxication
Underelimination of hydrogen ions	Kidney failure
Underproduction of bicarbonate	Kidney failure
	Pancreatitis
	Liver failure
	Dehydration
Overelimination of bicarbonate	Diarrhea
Respiratory Acidosis	
Underelimination of hydrogen ions	Respiratory depression:
	Anesthetics
	Drugs (especially opioids)
	Electrolyte imbalance
	Inadequate chest expansion:
	Muscle weakness
	Airway obstruction
	Alveolar-capillary block

Overproduction of hydrogen ions can occur with excessive breakdown of fatty acids, anaerobic glucose breakdown *(lactic acidosis)*, and excessive intake of acids. Excessive breakdown of fatty acids occurs with diabetic ketoacidosis or starvation. When insufficient glucose is available for fuel, the body breaks down fats (lipids). The products of excessive fatty acid breakdown are strong acids *(ketoacids)*, which release large amounts of hydrogen ions.

Lactic acidosis occurs when cells use glucose without adequate oxygen *(anaerobic metabolism)*; glucose then is incompletely broken down and forms lactic acid. This acid releases hydrogen ions, causing acidosis. Lactic acidosis occurs whenever the body has too little oxygen to meet metabolic oxygen demands (e.g., heavy exercise, seizure activity, reduced oxygen).

Excessive intake of acids floods the body with hydrogen ions. Agents that cause acidosis when ingested in excess include ethyl alcohol, methyl alcohol, and acetylsalicylic acid (aspirin).

Underelimination of hydrogen ions leads to acidosis when hydrogen ions are produced at the normal rate but are not removed at the same rate they are produced. Most hydrogen ion loss occurs through the lungs and the kidneys. Kidney failure causes acidosis when the kidney tubules cannot secrete hydrogen ions into the urine and they are retained. Severe lung problems also can result in retention of CO_2 with a corresponding retention of hydrogen ions.

Underproduction of bicarbonate ions (base deficit) leads to acidosis when hydrogen ion production and removal are normal but too few bicarbonate ions are present to balance the hydrogen ions. Because bicarbonate is made in the kidneys and in the pancreas, kidney failure and impaired liver or pancreatic function can cause a base-deficit acidosis.

Overelimination of bicarbonate ions (base deficit) leads to acidosis when hydrogen ion production and removal are normal but too many bicarbonate ions have been lost. One cause of base deficit acidosis is diarrhea.

Respiratory Acidosis

Respiratory acidosis results when respiratory function is impaired and the exchange of oxygen (O_2) and carbon dioxide (CO_2) is reduced. This problem causes CO_2 retention, which leads to the same increase in hydrogen ion levels and acidosis. (See the carbonic anhydrase equation in Fig. 12-7.)

Unlike metabolic acidosis, respiratory acidosis results from only one cause—retention of CO_2, causing increased production of free hydrogen ions. Table 12-2 lists the four types of respiratory problems and their possible causes.

Respiratory depression results from depressed function of the brainstem neurons that trigger breathing movements. This lowered rate and depth of breathing leads to poor gas exchange and retention of carbon dioxide. Common causes include anesthetic agents, opioids, and poisons. Physical respiratory depression occurs when respiratory neurons are damaged or destroyed by trauma or when problems in the brain increase the intracranial pressure. Problems causing cerebral edema and respiratory depression include brain tumors, cerebral aneurysm, stroke, and overhydration.

Inadequate chest expansion reduces gas exchange and leads to acidosis. Chest expansion can be restricted by skeletal trauma or deformities, respiratory muscle weakness, or external constriction. Respiratory muscle weakness, caused by electrolyte imbalances, fatigue, muscular dystrophy, muscle damage, or muscle breakdown, reduces chest movement. External conditions, such as casts, tight scar tissue around the chest, obesity, and ascites, can restrict chest movement.

Airway obstruction prevents air movement into and out from the lungs *(ventilation)* and leads to poor gas exchange, CO_2 retention, and acidosis. External obstruction can be caused by clothing, neck edema, and local lymph node enlargement. Internal obstruction can be caused by aspiration of foreign objects, bronchoconstriction, mucus, and edema.

Reduced alveolar-capillary diffusion causes poor gas exchange and leads to CO_2 retention and acidosis. Disorders that reduce diffusion include pneumonia, pneumonitis, tuberculosis, emphysema, acute respiratory distress syndrome, chest trauma, pulmonary emboli, pulmonary edema, and drowning.

Combined Metabolic and Respiratory Acidosis

Metabolic and respiratory acidosis can occur at the same time. Uncorrected acute respiratory acidosis always leads to poor oxygenation and lactic acidosis (McCance et al., 2014). For example, a person who has diabetic ketoacidosis and chronic obstructive pulmonary disease has a combined metabolic and respiratory acidosis. Combined acidosis is more severe than either metabolic acidosis or respiratory acidosis alone.

❖ PATIENT-CENTERED COLLABORATIVE CARE

◆ Assessment

History. Collect data about risk factors related to the development of acidosis. Information about age, nutrition, and current manifestations are especially important.

Older adults are more at risk for problems leading to acid-base imbalance, including cardiac, kidney, or pulmonary impairment. Also, older adults may be taking drugs that disrupt ACID-BASE BALANCE, especially diuretics and aspirin. Ask about specific risk factors, such as any type of breathing problem, kidney failure, diabetes mellitus, diarrhea, pancreatitis, and fever.

Obtain a detailed nutrition history to determine total caloric intake and the proportions of carbohydrates, fats, and proteins ingested. Ask whether the patient has fasted or followed a strict diet within the past week.

Ask about headaches, behavior changes, increased drowsiness, reduced alertness, reduced attention span, lethargy, anorexia, abdominal distention, nausea or vomiting, muscle weakness, or increased fatigue. Ask the patient to relate activities of the previous 24 hours to identify activity intolerance, behavior changes, and fatigue. Because the central nervous system is often depressed in acidosis, you may need to obtain this information from the patient's family.

Physical Assessment/Clinical Manifestations. Manifestations of acidosis are similar whether the cause is metabolic or respiratory (Chart 12-3). Acidosis reduces the ability of excitable membranes to respond appropriately, especially in cardiovascular tissue, neurons, skeletal muscle, and GI smooth muscle.

Cardiovascular changes are first seen with mild acidosis and are more severe as the condition worsens. Early changes include increased heart rate and cardiac output. With worsening acidosis or with acidosis and **hyperkalemia** (elevated blood potassium levels), heart rate decreases, T waves become tall and peaked, and QRS complexes are widened. Peripheral pulses may be hard to find and are easily blocked. Hypotension occurs with vasodilation.

CHART 12-3 Key Features

Acidosis

Cardiovascular Manifestations
- Delayed electrical conduction:
  - Ranges from bradycardia to heart block
  - Tall T waves
  - Widened QRS complex
  - Prolonged PR interval
- Hypotension
- Thready peripheral pulses

Central Nervous System Manifestations
- Depressed activity (lethargy, confusion, stupor, coma)

Neuromuscular Manifestations
- Hyporeflexia
- Skeletal muscle weakness
- Flaccid paralysis

Respiratory Manifestations
- Kussmaul respirations (in metabolic acidosis with respiratory compensation)
- Variable respirations (generally ineffective in respiratory acidosis)

Integumentary Manifestations
- Warm, flushed, dry skin in metabolic acidosis
- Pale to cyanotic and dry skin in respiratory acidosis

! NURSING SAFETY PRIORITY QSEN

Critical Rescue

Assess the cardiovascular system first in any patient at risk for acidosis, because acidosis can lead to cardiac arrest from the accompanying hyperkalemia.

Central nervous system (CNS) changes include depression of CNS function. Problems may range from lethargy to confusion, especially in older patients. As acidosis worsens, the patient may become unresponsive. Assess the patient's mental status (see Chapter 41).

Neuromuscular changes include reduced muscle tone and deep tendon reflexes as a result of the accompanying hyperkalemia. Assess arm muscle strength and leg muscle strength. Test arm muscle strength by having the patient squeeze your hand. Test leg muscle strength by having the patient push both feet against a flat surface (like a box or a board) while you apply resistance to the opposite side of the flat surface. Muscle weakness is bilateral and can progress to paralysis.

Respiratory changes may cause the acidosis and can be caused by the acidosis. Assess the patient's rate, depth, and ease of breathing. Use pulse oximetry to determine how well oxygen is delivered to the peripheral tissues.

If acidosis is metabolic in origin, the rate and depth of breathing increase as the hydrogen ion level rises. Breaths are deep and rapid and not under voluntary control, a pattern called **Kussmaul respiration.**

If acidosis is caused by respiratory problems, breathing efforts are reduced. Respirations are usually shallow and rapid. Muscle weakness makes this problem worse.

Skin changes occur with metabolic or respiratory acidosis. With metabolic acidosis, breathing is unimpaired and the rate is increased and CO_2 is lost. This causes vasodilation and makes the skin and mucous membranes warm, dry, and pink. With respiratory acidosis, breathing is ineffective and skin and mucous membranes are pale to cyanotic.

Psychosocial Assessment. *Behavioral changes may be the first manifestations of acidosis.* Observe and document the patient's behavior by description (objectively) rather than by interpretation (subjectively). Ask family members if the patient's behavior is typical for him or her, and establish a baseline for comparison with later assessment findings.

Laboratory Assessment. Arterial blood pH is the laboratory value used to confirm acidosis. Acidosis is present when arterial blood pH is less than 7.35. However, this test alone does not indicate what is causing the acidosis. Manifestations of metabolic acidosis and respiratory acidosis are similar, but their treatments are different. *Therefore it is critical to obtain and interpret other laboratory data, such as arterial blood gas (ABG) values and blood levels of electrolytes* (Chart 12-4).

Metabolic acidosis is reflected by several changes in ABG values. The pH is low (<7.35) because buffering and respiratory compensation are not adequate to keep the amount of free hydrogen ions at a normal level. The bicarbonate level is low (<21 mEq/L). It is low because (1) bicarbonate has been lost, causing a base-deficit acidosis; (2) bicarbonate production is inadequate, causing a base-deficit acidosis; or (3) bicarbonate may be bound to other substances. The partial pressure of arterial oxygen (Pao_2) is normal because gas exchange is not impaired. The partial pressure of arterial carbon dioxide ($Paco_2$) is normal or even slightly decreased because gas exchange is adequate and carbon dioxide retention is not a factor (Jones, 2010).

The serum potassium level is often high in acidosis as the body attempts to maintain electroneutrality during buffering. Fig. 12-12 shows the movement of potassium ions as serum pH changes. As the blood hydrogen ion level rises, some of the excess hydrogen ions enter red blood cells for intracellular buffering. The movement of hydrogen ions into the cells creates an excess of positive ions inside the cells. To balance these extra positive charges, an equal number of potassium ions (that also have a positive charge) move from the cells into the blood. This increases the blood potassium level, causing hyperkalemia.

Respiratory acidosis is reflected by several changes in ABG values. The pH is low (<7.35) because of the increased amount of free hydrogen ions in the blood. Buffering and kidney compensation are not adequate to keep the amount of free hydrogen ions at a normal level. If the kidneys partially compensate for this acidosis, pH is low but not as abnormal as could be expected with the degree of CO_2 retention.

CHART 12-4 Laboratory Profile

Acid-Base Imbalances (Uncompensated)

	LABORATORY VALUE CHANGES						
IMBALANCE	pH	HCO_3^-	Pao_2	$Paco_2$	K^+	Ca^{2+}	Cl^-
Metabolic acidosis	↓	↓	Ø	Ø and ↓	↑	Ø	Ø and ↑
Respiratory acidosis	↓	Ø	↓	↑	↑	Ø	↑↓
Combined acidosis	↓	↓↑	↓	↑	↑	Ø	↑
Metabolic alkalosis	↑	↑	Ø	Ø and ↑	↓	↓	↓
Respiratory alkalosis	↑	Ø	Ø	↓↓	↓	↓	↑
Combined alkalosis	↑	↑	Ø	↓	↓	↓	↓

↑, Above normal; ↓, below normal; ↑↓, value can increase or decrease depending on other factors; Ø, normal; Ca^{2+}, calcium ions; Cl^-, chloride ions; $Paco_2$, partial pressure of arterial carbon dioxide; Pao_2, partial pressure of arterial oxygen; HCO_3^-, bicarbonate ions; K^+, potassium ions.

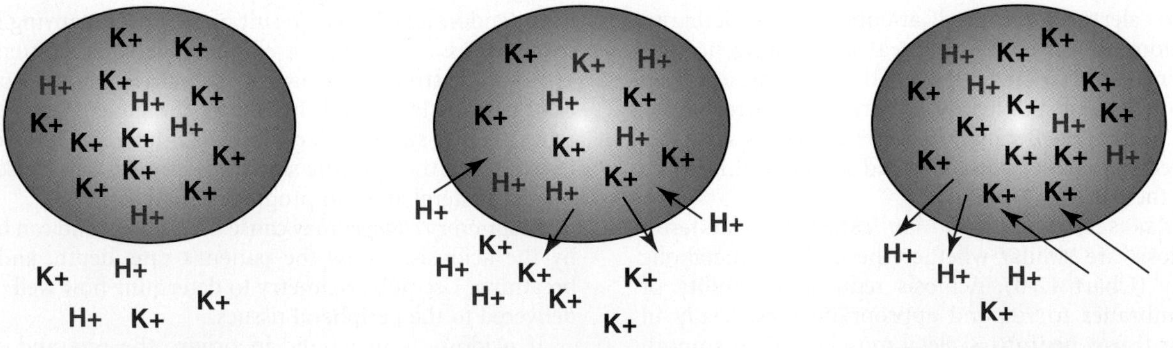

Under normal conditions, the intracellular potassium content is much greater than that of the extracellular fluid. The concentration of hydrogen ions is low in both compartments.

In acidosis, the extracellular hydrogen ion content increases and the hydrogen ions move into the intracellular fluid. To keep the intracellular fluid electrically neutral, an equal number of potassium ions leave the cell, creating a relative hyperkalemia.

In alkalosis, more hydrogen ions are present in the intracellular fluid than in the extracellular fluid. Hydrogen ions move from the intracellular fluid into the extracellular fluid. To keep the intracellular fluid electrically neutral, potassium ions move from the extracellular fluid into the intracellular fluid, creating a relative hypokalemia.

FIG. 12-12 Movement of potassium (K^+) in response to changes in the extracellular fluid hydrogen ion (H^+) concentration.

The partial pressure of arterial oxygen (Pa_{O_2}) is low and the partial pressure of arterial carbon dioxide (Pa_{CO_2}) is high because the pulmonary problem impairs gas exchange, causing poor oxygenation and CO_2 retention. *(The hallmarks of respiratory acidosis are a decreasing* Pa_{O_2} *coupled with a rising* Pa_{CO_2}*.)* Because carbon dioxide diffuses more easily across the alveolar membrane than oxygen, a decreased Pa_{O_2} usually occurs before an increased Pa_{CO_2}.

The serum bicarbonate level is variable. A patient with rapid onset of respiratory acidosis often has a normal bicarbonate level because kidney compensation has not started. When the acidosis persists for 24 hours or longer, kidney compensation increases the levels of bicarbonate. Chronic respiratory acidosis is indicated by an elevated bicarbonate level and increased Pa_{CO_2}.

Serum potassium levels are elevated in acute respiratory acidosis. They are normal or low in chronic respiratory acidosis when kidney compensation is present.

Priority Patient Problems. Priority problems for the patient experiencing acidosis are associated with the decreased function of excitable membranes. These problems include hypotension and decreased perfusion, impaired memory and cognition, and increased risk for falls.

◆ Interventions

Interventions for acidosis focus on correcting the underlying problem and monitoring for changes. To ensure appropriate interventions, first identify the specific type of acidosis present.

Metabolic Acidosis. Interventions for metabolic acidosis include hydration and drugs or treatments to control the problem causing the acidosis. For example, if the acidosis is a result of diabetic ketoacidosis, insulin is given to correct the hyperglycemia and halt the production of ketone bodies. Rehydration and antidiarrheal drugs are given if the acidosis is a result of prolonged diarrhea. *Bicarbonate is administered only if serum bicarbonate levels are low.*

Nursing priorities include continuously monitoring the patient for changes that indicate either he or she is responding to the treatment or the acidosis is becoming worse. The cardiovascular system and the skeletal muscle system are sensitive to acidosis and are the most important systems to monitor. Interpreting ABG results is an important part of monitoring.

Respiratory Acidosis. Priority interventions for respiratory acidosis are focused on improving ventilation and oxygenation and maintaining a patent airway. These include drug therapy, oxygen therapy, pulmonary hygiene (positioning and breathing techniques), ventilatory support, and prevention of complications. (See Chapter 30 for disorders causing respiratory acidosis.)

Drug therapy is focused on improving ventilation and oxygenation rather than directly on altering pH. Drug categories useful for respiratory acidosis include bronchodilators, anti-inflammatories, and mucolytics.

Oxygen therapy helps promote gas exchange for patients with respiratory acidosis. Carefully monitor oxygen saturation to ensure that the lowest flow of oxygen that prevents hypoxemia is used to avoid oxygen-induced tissue damage.

Ventilation support with mechanical ventilation may be needed for patients who cannot keep their oxygen saturation at 90% or who have respiratory muscle fatigue. Chapter 32 discusses the nursing care needs of patients who are being mechanically ventilated.

Preventing complications is a nursing priority when caring for a patient with respiratory acidosis. Monitoring breathing status hourly and intervening when changes occur are critical in preventing complications. Listen to breath sounds, and assess how easily air moves into and out of the lungs. Check for any muscle retractions, the use of accessory muscles (especially the neck muscles [sternocleidomastoids]), and whether breathing produces a grunt or wheeze that can be heard without a stethoscope. Assess nail beds and oral membranes for cyanosis (a late finding).

NCLEX EXAMINATION CHALLENGE
Physiological Integrity

What type of acid-base problem does the nurse expect in a client who is being insufficiently mechanically ventilated and whose most recent arterial blood gas results include a pH of 7.29?

A. Metabolic acidosis with an acid excess
B. Metabolic acidosis with a base deficit
C. Respiratory acidosis with an acid excess
D. Respiratory acidosis with a base deficit

ALKALOSIS

❖ PATHOPHYSIOLOGY

In patients with alkalosis, the ACID-BASE BALANCE of the blood is disturbed and has an excess of bases, especially bicarbonate (HCO_3^-). The amount or strength of the bases is greater than normal compared with the amount of the acids. Alkalosis is a *decrease* in the free hydrogen ion level of the blood and is reflected by an arterial blood pH *above* 7.45. Like acidosis, alkalosis is not a disease but, rather, is a manifestation of a problem. It can be caused by metabolic problems, respiratory problems, or both (Table 12-3).

Alkalosis can result from an actual or relative increase in the amount or strength (or both) of bases. In an actual base excess, alkalosis occurs when base (usually bicarbonate) is either overproduced or undereliminated.

TABLE 12-3 Common Causes of Alkalosis

PATHOLOGY	CONDITION
Metabolic Alkalosis	
Increase of base components	Oral ingestion of bases: Antacids Parenteral base administration: Blood transfusion Sodium bicarbonate Total parenteral nutrition
Decrease of acid components	Prolonged vomiting Nasogastric suctioning Hypercortisolism Hyperaldosteronism Thiazide diuretics
Respiratory Alkalosis	
Excessive loss of carbon dioxide	Hyperventilation, fear, anxiety Mechanical ventilation Salicylate toxicity High altitudes Shock Early-stage acute pulmonary problems

AAABBB AAABBB AAABBB	AAABBBB AAABBBB AAABBBB	AABBB AABBB AABBB
Acid-base balance	Actual alkalosis (base excess)	Relative alkalosis (acid deficit)

FIG. 12-13 Concepts of actual and relative alkalosis. (A = acid; B = base.)

In *relative* alkalosis, the actual amount or strength of bases does not increase but the amount of the acids decreases, creating an *acid deficit.* A relative base-excess alkalosis (actual acid deficit) results from an overelimination or underproduction of acids (Fig. 12-13).

The problems of alkalosis are serious and can be life threatening. Management focuses on correcting the cause after identifying whether the alkalosis origin is respiratory or metabolic.

Whether metabolic, respiratory, or both, alkalosis affects specific functions. The pathologic effects are caused by the electrolyte imbalances that occur in response to decreased blood cation (positively charged particles) levels. Most problems of alkalosis are related to increased stimulation of the nervous, neuromuscular, and cardiac systems.

Metabolic alkalosis is an acid-base imbalance caused by either an increase of bases (base excess) or a decrease of acids (acid deficit). Base excesses are caused by excessive intake of bicarbonates, carbonates, acetates, and citrates. Excessive use of bicarbonate-containing antacids can cause a metabolic alkalosis. Other base excesses can occur during medical treatments, such as citrate excesses during massive blood transfusions and IV sodium bicarbonate given to correct acidosis. The hallmark of a base-excess acidosis is an ABG result with an elevated pH and an elevated bicarbonate level along with normal oxygen and carbon dioxide levels.

Acid deficits can be caused by disease processes or medical treatment. Disorders causing acid deficits include prolonged vomiting, excess cortisol, and hyperaldosteronism. Treatments that promote acid loss causing metabolic alkalosis include thiazide diuretics and prolonged gastric suctioning.

Respiratory alkalosis is usually caused by an excessive loss of CO_2 through hyperventilation (rapid respirations). Patients may hyperventilate in response to anxiety, fear, or improper settings on mechanical ventilators. Hyperventilation can also result from direct stimulation of central respiratory centers because of fever, central nervous system lesions, and salicylates. The hallmark of respiratory alkalosis is an ABG result with an elevated pH coupled with a low carbon dioxide level. Usually, the oxygen and bicarbonate levels are normal.

❖ PATIENT-CENTERED COLLABORATIVE CARE

◆ Assessment

Manifestations of problems with ACID-BASE BALANCE are the same for metabolic and respiratory alkalosis. Many symptoms are the result of the low calcium levels (**hypocalcemia**) and low potassium levels (**hypokalemia**) that usually occur with alkalosis (see Fig. 12-12). These problems change the function of the nervous, neuromuscular, cardiac, and respiratory systems (Chart 12-5).

Central nervous system (CNS) changes are caused by overexcitement of the nervous systems. Patients have dizziness, agitation, confusion, and hyperreflexia, which may progress to seizures. Tingling or numbness may occur around the mouth and in the toes. Other indicators of alkalosis with hypocalcemia are positive Chvostek's and Trousseau's signs (see Chapter 11).

CHART 12-5 Key Features

Alkalosis

Central Nervous System Manifestations
- Increased activity
- Anxiety, irritability, tetany, seizures
- Positive Chvostek's sign
- Positive Trousseau's sign
- Paresthesias

Neuromuscular Manifestations
- Hyperreflexia
- Muscle cramping and twitching
- Skeletal muscle weakness

Cardiovascular Manifestations
- Increased heart rate
- Normal or low blood pressure
- Increased digitalis toxicity

Respiratory Manifestations
- Increased rate and depth of ventilation in respiratory alkalosis
- Decreased respiratory effort associated with skeletal muscle weakness in metabolic alkalosis

Neuromuscular changes are related to the hypocalcemia and hypokalemia that occur with alkalosis. Nervous system activity increases, causing muscle cramps, twitches, and "charley horses." Deep tendon reflexes are hyperactive. **Tetany** (continuous contractions) of muscle groups also may be present. Tetany is painful and indicates a rapidly worsening condition.

Skeletal muscles may contract as a result of nerve stimulation, but they become weaker because of the hypokalemia. Handgrip strength decreases, and the patient may be unable to stand or walk. Respiratory efforts become less effective as the respiratory muscles weaken.

Cardiovascular changes occur because alkalosis increases myocardial irritability, especially when accompanied by hypokalemia. Heart rate increases, and the pulse is thready. When decreased blood volume is also present, the patient may have severe hypotension. The hypokalemia increases heart sensitivity to digoxin, which increases the risk for digoxin toxicity.

Respiratory changes, especially increases in the rate of breathing, are the main causes of respiratory alkalosis. Although the volume of air inhaled and exhaled with each breath is nearly normal, the total volume of air inhaled and exhaled each minute rises with the increased respiratory rate. The increased minute volume may be caused by anxiety or physiologic changes.

Arterial blood pH greater than 7.45 confirms alkalosis, but this test alone does not identify its cause. Because the manifestations of metabolic alkalosis and respiratory alkalosis are similar, it is critical to obtain additional laboratory data, especially arterial blood gas (ABG) values and specific serum electrolyte levels (see Chart 12-4) (Blevins, 2014).

◆ Interventions

Interventions are planned to prevent further losses of hydrogen, potassium, calcium, and chloride ions; to restore fluid balance; to monitor changes; and to provide for *patient safety.* Treatments that may have caused alkalosis (e.g., prolonged gastric suctioning, excessive infusion of certain IV solutions, drugs that promote hydrogen ion excretion) are modified or stopped. Drug therapy is prescribed to resolve the causes of alkalosis and to restore normal fluid, electrolyte, and acid-base balance. For example, the patient with metabolic alkalosis caused by diuretic therapy receives fluid and electrolyte replacement, and the diuretic therapy is adjusted or stopped. Antiemetic drugs are prescribed for vomiting. Monitor the patient's progress, and adjust fluid and electrolyte therapy. Monitor electrolytes daily until they return to near normal.

During correction of alkalosis, a nursing care priority is prevention of injury from falls. The patient with alkalosis has hypotension and muscle weakness, which increase the risk for falls, especially among older adults. Implement the general falls prevention nursing interventions and the high-risk falls prevention nursing interventions outlined in Chart 2-4 in Chapter 2.

CLINICAL JUDGMENT CHALLENGE

Patient-Centered Care; Safety QSEN

The patient is a 21-year-old college student brought to the emergency department by his friends when he was found unconscious during a fraternity party. He was seen drinking heavily at the party and had not eaten for 2 days before the event. He takes no prescription drugs, and his current vital signs are: T = 97.8° F; P = 48, slightly irregular and thready; R = 28, deep and regular; BP = 88/50. His current arterial blood gas results are: pH = 7.31; HCO_3^- = 25 mEq/L; $PaCO_2$ = 28 mm Hg; PaO_2 = 99 mm Hg.

1. What specific type of acid-base problem does this patient have? Explain your choice.
2. What is the most probable origin of the acid-base imbalance?
3. Should oxygen be applied? Why or why not?
4. What nursing interventions for safety are most appropriate for this patient?
5. What additional laboratory and assessment data should be performed? Provide a rationale for your selections.

NURSING CONCEPTS AND CLINICAL JUDGMENT REVIEW

What might you NOTICE in a patient with appropriate ACID-BASE BALANCE?

Vital signs:
- Respiratory rate and depth within usual range for the patient
- Heart rate and rhythm within usual range for the patient
- Oxygen saturation of 95% or higher

Physical assessment:
- Able to speak a sentence of 12 words without stopping for breath
- Able to walk and talk without stopping for breath
- Skin color normal (no cyanosis or pallor)
- Oral mucous membrane and nail beds pink with rapid capillary refill
- Breathing quiet
- Muscle strength consistent with what is normal for the patient
- Urine output about equal to fluid intake

Psychological assessment:
- Oriented and not confused
- Energy level good; can engage in desired work, recreational, and personal activities

Laboratory assessment:
- Arterial blood gas values within normal limits
- Serum electrolyte values, especially potassium and calcium, within normal limits

GET READY FOR THE NCLEX® EXAMINATION!

KEY POINTS

Review these Key Points for each NCLEX Examination Client Needs Category.

Safe and Effective Care Environment
- Assess the ACID-BASE BALANCE of any patient with new-onset muscle weakness.
- Use fall precautions for any patient with a problem in ACID-BASE BALANCE. **Safety** QSEN

Health Promotion and Maintenance
- Teach patients to take drugs as prescribed, especially diuretics, antihypertensives, and cardiac drugs.
- Instruct patients at continuing risk for respiratory acidosis to stop smoking.

Psychosocial Integrity
- Assess the oxygenation status of any patient with acute confusion.
- Monitor the neurologic status at least every 2 hours in patients being treated for a problem with ACID-BASE BALANCE.
- Assist patients who have anxiety-induced respiratory alkalosis to identify causes of anxiety.

Physiological Integrity
- Be aware of how the following principles, processes, and mechanisms influence the regulation of ACID-BASE BALANCE:
  - The normal pH of the body's extracellular fluids (including blood) is 7.35 to 7.45.
  - The more hydrogen ions present, the more acidic the fluid; the fewer hydrogen ions present, the more alkaline the fluid.
  - pH values below 7.35 indicate acidosis; pH values above 7.45 indicate alkalosis.
  - Anything that increases the CO_2 level in the blood increases the hydrogen ion content and lowers the pH.

- Acids are normally formed in the body as a result of metabolism.
- Chemical blood buffers are the immediate way that acid-base imbalances are corrected.
- The lungs control the amount of CO_2 that is retained or exhaled.
- The kidneys regulate the amount of hydrogen and bicarbonate ions that are retained or excreted by the body.
- If a lung problem causes retention of carbon dioxide, the healthy kidney compensates by increasing the amount of bicarbonate that is produced and retained.
- Acidosis reduces the excitability of cardiovascular muscle, neurons, skeletal muscle, and GI smooth muscle.
- Alkalosis increases the sensitivity of excitable tissues, allowing them to over-respond to normal stimuli and respond even without stimulation.
- Check the serum potassium level for any patient who has acidosis. **Evidence-Based Practice** **QSEN**
- Assess the cardiovascular system first in any patient at risk for acidosis because acidosis can lead to cardiac arrest from the accompanying hyperkalemia. **Evidence-Based Practice** **QSEN**
- Assess the airway of any patient who has acute respiratory acidosis.
- Assess heart rate and rhythm at least every 2 hours for any patient with an acid-base imbalance.
- Monitor arterial blood gas (ABG) values to evaluate the effectiveness of therapy for acid-base imbalances. **Evidence-Based Practice** **QSEN**

CHAPTER 13

Infusion Therapy*

Cheryl J. Dumont

http://evolve.elsevier.com/Iggy/

PRIORITY CONCEPTS

- Fluid and Electrolyte Balance
- Tissue Integrity
- Infection
- Perfusion

LEARNING OUTCOMES

Safe and Effective Care Environment

1. Prevent IV administration errors by following best practices that ensure patient and staff safety.
2. Describe the benefits and limitations of selected safety-enhancing technologies used for infusion therapy.
3. Identify the evidence-based guidelines for prevention of intravenous (IV) catheter–related bloodstream INFECTION (CR-BSI).

Health Promotion and Maintenance

4. Describe the special needs and care for older adults receiving IV therapy.
5. Teach the patient and family about the type and care related to the patient's infusion therapy.

Physiological Integrity

6. Explain how to check the accuracy of prescriptions for IV fluids and drug therapy.
7. Identify the appropriate veins for peripheral IV catheter insertion.
8. Differentiate types of vascular access devices (VADs) used for peripheral and central IV therapy.
9. Outline best practice for inserting peripheral VADs.
10. Assess the patient's infusion site frequently for local complications, such as phlebitis and infiltration.
11. Prioritize nursing interventions for maintaining an infusion system.
12. Assess, prevent, and manage systemic complications related to infusion therapy and VADs.
13. Describe nursing care associated with intra-arterial, intraperitoneal, subcutaneous, intraosseous, and intraspinal infusion therapy.

Infusion therapy is the delivery of medications in solution and fluids by parenteral (piercing of skin or mucous membranes) route through a wide variety of catheter types and locations using multiple procedures. IV therapy is the most common route for infusion therapy. It delivers solutions directly into the veins of the vascular system. This chapter focuses on access for and administration of all types of infusion therapy.

OVERVIEW

Infusion therapy is delivered in all health care settings, including hospitals, home care, ambulatory care clinics, physicians' offices, and long-term care facilities. The most common reasons for using infusion therapy are to:

- Maintain FLUID BALANCE or correct fluid imbalance
- Maintain ELECTROLYTE or acid-base BALANCE or correct electrolyte or acid-base imbalance
- Administer medications
- Replace blood or blood products

IV therapy is the most common invasive therapy administered to hospitalized patients. Advances in medicine and technology have made it possible for people with chronic diseases such as diabetes mellitus, chronic kidney disease, and malabsorption syndromes to live long and productive lives. These patients often depend on long-term infusion therapy of some kind. They often have very poor vascular integrity and, therefore, accessing their peripheral veins takes a high level of skill.

Having a specialized team of infusion nurses to initiate and maintain infusion therapy has been recommended as best practice by the Centers for Disease Control and Prevention (CDC) to reduce complications of infusion therapy (O'Grady et al., 2011). These teams have demonstrated value in cost savings, patient satisfaction, and patient outcomes.

*With recognition given to the Winchester Medical Center Vascular Access Team: Meredith Baker, Tammy Brannon, Cathy Dalton, Ronee Fertig, Ozlem Getz, Debbie Knippenberg, Paula McCarren, Sheri Miller, and Nancy Stoop.

Infusion nurses may perform any or all of these activities:

- Develop evidence-based policies and procedures
- Insert and maintain various types of peripheral and central venous catheters
- Monitor patient outcomes of infusion therapy
- Educate staff, patients, and families regarding infusion therapy
- Consult on product selection and purchasing decisions
- Provide therapies such as blood withdrawal, therapeutic phlebotomy, hypodermoclysis, intraosseous infusions, and administration of medications including chemotherapy

The registered nurse (RN) generalist is taught to insert peripheral IVs; most institutions have a process for credentialing this skill. Depending on the state's nurse practice act, licensed practical/vocational nurses (LPNs/LVNs) and technicians may be trained and credentialed to perform the skill of peripheral IV insertion and assist with infusions. *The RN is ultimately accountable for all aspects of infusion therapy and delegation of associated tasks (Infusion Nurses Society [INS], 2011).* You have a strategic role in selection of the correct device and managing the patient requiring infusion therapy (Santolim et al., 2012).

The Infusion Nurses Society (INS) publishes guidelines and standards of practice for policy and procedure development in all health care settings. These standards establish the criteria for all nurses delivering infusion therapy. The Infusion Nurses Certification Corporation (INCC) offers a written certifying examination. Nurses who successfully complete this examination have mastered an advanced body of knowledge in this specialty and may use the initials *CRNI*, which stand for *certified registered nurse infusion.*

Types of Infusion Therapy Fluids

Many types of parenteral fluids are used for infusion therapy. These fluids are IV solutions, including parenteral nutrition, blood and blood components, and drug therapy.

Intravenous Solutions

More than 200 IV fluids (solutions) are available that meet the requirements established by the United States Pharmacopeia (USP). Each solution is classified by its tonicity (concentration) and pH. Tonicity is typically categorized by comparison with normal blood plasma as osmolarity (mOsm/L). As discussed in Chapter 11, normal serum osmolarity for adults is between 270 and 300 mOsm/L. Parenteral solutions within that normal range are **isotonic**; those fluids greater than 300 mOsm/L are **hypertonic**; and those fluids less than 270 mOsm/L are **hypotonic**.

When an *isotonic* **infusate** (solution that is infused into the body) is used, water does not move into or out of the body's cells. Therefore patients receiving isotonic solutions are at risk for fluid overload, especially older adults (see Chapter 11). *Hypertonic* solutions are used to correct FLUID AND ELECTROLYTE and acid-base imbalances by moving water out of the body's cells and into the bloodstream. Electrolytes and other particles also move across cell membranes across a concentration gradient (from higher concentration to lower concentration). Parenteral nutrition solutions are hypertonic (see Chapter 60). Instead of moving water out of cells, *hypotonic* infusates move water into cells to expand them. Patients receiving either hypertonic or hypotonic fluids are at risk for phlebitis and infiltration. **Phlebitis** is the inflammation of a vein caused by mechanical, chemical, or bacterial irritation. **Infiltration** occurs when IV solution leaks into the tissues around the vein.

The pH of IV solutions is a measure of the acidity or alkalinity and usually ranges from 3.5 to 6.2. Extremes of both osmolarity and pH can cause vein damage leading to phlebitis and **thrombosis** (blood clot in the vein). Thus FLUIDS and medications with a pH value less than 5 and more than 9 and with an osmolarity more than 600 mOsm/L are best infused in the central circulation where greater blood flow provides adequate hemodilution (Perucca, 2010). For example, total parenteral nutrition (TPN) solutions have an osmolarity greater than 1400 mOsm/L. TPN should not be infused in peripheral circulation because it can damage blood cells and the endothelial lining of the veins and decrease PERFUSION.

! NURSING SAFETY PRIORITY (QSEN)

Drug Alert

Drugs such as amiodarone (Cordarone), vancomycin (Vancocin), and ciprofloxacin (Cipro I.V.) are venous irritants that have a pH less than 5. Phlebitis occurs when patients require long-term infusion of these drugs in peripheral circulation. Drugs with vasoconstrictive action (e.g., dopamine or chemotherapeutic agents [e.g., vinblastine]) are **vesicants** (chemicals that damage body tissue on direct contact) that can cause extravasation. **Extravasation** results in severe TISSUE INTEGRITY impairment as manifested by blistering, tissue sloughing, or necrosis from infiltration into the surrounding tissues. (See Complications of Intravenous Therapy section on p. 204 for further explanation and Chapter 22 for more detail.) Monitor the IV insertion site carefully for early manifestations of infiltration, including swelling, coolness, or redness. If any of these symptoms are present, discontinue the drug immediately and notify the infusion therapy team, if available. If an infusion specialist is not available, plan to remove the IV catheter and consider central line placement.

Blood and Blood Components

Blood transfusion is given by using packed red blood cells, created by removing a large portion of the plasma from whole blood. Other available blood components include platelets, fresh frozen plasma, albumin, and several specific clotting factors. Each component has detailed requirements for blood-type compatibility and infusion techniques. For patient safety, The Joint Commission's (TJC) 2014 National Patient Safety Goals (NPSGs) require agencies to ensure that blood components are properly ordered, handled and dispensed, and administered and that patients are appropriately monitored. Positive patient identification using two patient identifiers and requiring two qualified health care professionals is essential before any blood or blood component is administered.

Most organizations use the International Society of Blood Transfusion (ISBT) universal bar-coding system to ensure the right blood for the right patient (Fig. 13-1). The ISBT system includes four components that must be present on the blood label both in bar code and in eye-readable format. These four components are (1) a unique facility identifier, (2) the lot number relating to the donor, (3) the product code, and (4) the ABO group and Rh type of the donor.

An acute hemolytic transfusion reaction caused by an incompatible blood transfusion is a "sentinel event." The Joint Commission defines a **sentinel event** as an unexpected occurrence involving serious physical or psychological injury or

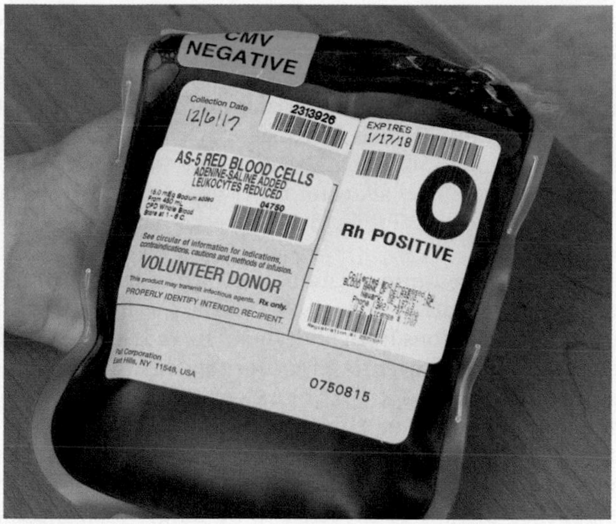

FIG. 13-1 Unit of blood showing the International Society of Blood Transfusion (ISBT) universal bar code for blood transfusions.

the risk thereof and requiring an intense analysis of the contributing factors and corrective action. As a measure to improve the quality of health care, The Joint Commission reviews organizations' activities in response to sentinel events. Established policies and procedures must be rigidly followed to ensure a safe transfusion and reduce the risk for complications. (See Chapter 40 for a complete discussion of blood transfusion administration.)

Drug Therapy

IV drugs provide a rapid therapeutic effect but can lead to immediate serious reactions, called **adverse drug events (ADEs)**. Hundreds of drugs are available for infusion by a variety of techniques. As with all drug administration, nurses must be knowledgeable about drug indications, proper dosage, contraindications, and precautions. IV administration also requires knowledge of appropriate dilution, rate of infusion, pH and osmolarity, compatibility with other IV medications, appropriate infusion site (peripheral versus central circulation), potential for vesicant/irritant effects, and specific aspects of patient monitoring because of its immediate effect. *Regardless of familiarity with the drug, never assume that IV administration is the same as giving that drug by other routes.* New information is continuously being published, and new drugs are rapidly being introduced.

Medication safety is extremely important in all health care settings today. The Joint Commission's 2014 NPSGs include as a major goal improving the safety of high-alert drugs. An example of these drugs is concentrated electrolyte solutions (e.g., potassium chloride), which require restricted access, prominent warnings about the concentration, and storage in a secured location.

Procedures must be established to prevent errors resulting from look-alike, sound-alike drugs such as Celebrex IV (celecoxib) and Cerebyx (fosphenytoin). Other strategies to reduce errors include limiting available concentrations of drugs and dispensing all drugs, including catheter flush solutions, in single-dose containers. Smart pumps with drug libraries (see Infusion Systems section), in combination with computer provider (physician, nurse practitioner, physician assistant) order entry (CPOE) and bar code medication administration (BCMA) systems, use recent technology to help reduce adverse drug events (ADEs). Electronic medication administration records (MARs) and multiple checks by pharmacists, as required by The Joint Commission's NPSGs, also help reduce errors.

Prescribing Infusion Therapy

A prescription for infusion therapy written by an authorized provider (physician, nurse practitioner, or physician assistant) is necessary before IV therapy begins. To be complete, the prescription for infusion fluids should include:

- Specific type of fluid
- Rate of administration written in milliliters per hour (mL/hr) or the total amount of fluid and the total number of hours for infusion (e.g., 125 mL/hr or 1000 mL/8 hr)
- Drugs and the specific dose to be added to the solution, such as electrolytes or vitamins

A drug prescription should include:

- Drug name, preferably by generic name
- Specific dose and route
- Frequency of administration
- Time of administration
- Length of time for infusion
- Purpose (required in some health care agencies, especially nursing homes)

Some continuously infused drugs, such as those for pain management, are prescribed as milligrams per hour. The type and volume of dilution for infusion medications may be included in the prescription or calculated by the infusion pharmacist.

! NURSING SAFETY PRIORITY (QSEN)

Action Alert

Determine that the IV prescription is appropriate for the patient and clarify any questions with the health care provider before administration. Be sure to check for the accuracy and completeness of the treatment prescription. An example of an incomplete one is "5% dextrose in water to keep the vein open" (TKO or KVO). This statement does not specify the rate of infusion and is not considered complete.

Vascular Access Devices

An infusion catheter, also known as a **vascular access device (VAD)**, is a plastic tube placed in a blood vessel to deliver fluids and medications. This catheter should not be confused with the ventricular assist device also called a VAD. In this chapter, VAD refers to vascular access devices. The specific type and purpose of the therapy determine whether the infusion can be given safely through peripheral veins or if the large central veins of the chest are needed. Advances in catheter materials and insertion techniques have radically expanded the types of VADs currently used. This discussion includes the description of each type of catheter used for peripheral and central IV therapy. Seven major types are described:

- Short peripheral catheters
- Midline catheters
- Peripherally inserted central catheters (PICC)
- Nontunneled percutaneous central venous catheters (CVCs)
- Tunneled catheters
- Implanted ports
- Hemodialysis catheters

Assess the patient's needs for vascular access, and choose the device that has the best chance of infusing the prescribed therapy for the required length of time. Depending on the patient and type of VAD to be inserted, a topical anesthetic agent or intradermal lidocaine HCl 1% may be helpful to decrease patient discomfort. Obtain a health care provider's order and check for patient allergies before administering any anesthetic.

NCLEX EXAMINATION CHALLENGE

Safe and Effective Care Environment

A client receiving ciprofloxacin intravenously reports that the peripheral IV insertion site has become painful and reddened. In what order will the nurse perform the needed actions to manage this problem?

A. Report the patient's problem to the health care provider.
B. Document findings and actions in the electronic health record.
C. Change the IV insertion site to a new location.
D. Stop the infusion of the drug immediately.

PERIPHERAL INTRAVENOUS THERAPY

Short infusion catheters are the most commonly used vascular access devices (VADs) for **peripheral IV therapy**. They are usually placed in the veins of the arm. Another catheter used for peripheral IV therapy is a midline catheter.

Short Peripheral Catheters

Short peripheral catheters are composed of a plastic cannula built around a sharp stylet extending slightly beyond the cannula (Fig. 13-2). The stylet (sharp) allows for the venipuncture, and the cannula is advanced into the vein. Once the cannula is advanced into the vein, the stylet is withdrawn. These catheters are designed with a safety mechanism to cover the sharp end of the stylet after it is removed from the patient. The stylet is a hollow-bore, blood-filled needle that carries a high risk for exposure to bloodborne pathogens if needle stick injury occurs. A federal law enacted in 2000 amended the Bloodborne Pathogen Standards from the Occupational Safety and Health Administration (OSHA) requiring the use of catheters with an engineered safety mechanism to prevent needle sticks.

Insertion and Placement Methods

Short peripheral catheters are most often inserted into superficial veins of the forearm using sterile technique. In emergent situations, these catheters can be used also in the external jugular vein of the neck. *Avoid the use of veins in the lower extremities of adults, if possible, because of an increased risk for deep vein thrombosis and infiltration.*

Short catheters range in length from $\frac{3}{4}$ inch to $1\frac{1}{4}$ inch with gauge sizes from 26 gauge (the smallest) to 14 gauge (large bore). *Choose the smallest gauge catheter capable of delivering the prescribed therapy.* Current design improves the fluid flow through the catheter while using a smaller gauge and thereby decreases the possibility of vein irritation from a large catheter. For example, a thin-walled 24-gauge Insyte catheter has about the same flow-rate ability as a 22-gauge non–thin-walled Angiocath. Larger gauge sizes allow for faster flow rates but also cause phlebitis more often. Table 13-1 lists each gauge size and its common uses.

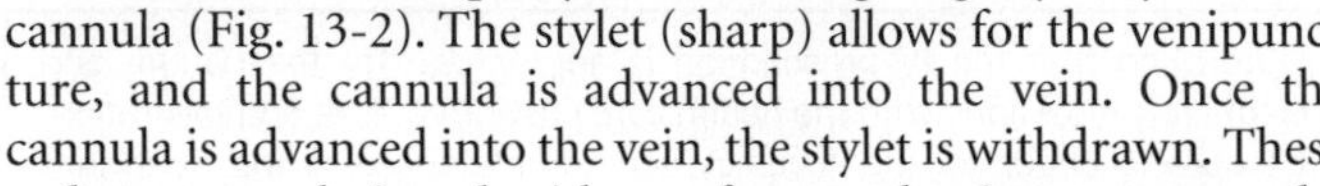

FIG. 13-2 BD Insyte Autoguard IV catheter. With the push of a button, the needle instantly retracts, reducing the risk for accidental needle stick injuries.

The current recommendations for dwell (stay in) time of short peripheral catheters do not include a specific time frame. The recommendations from both the CDC and the INS are that the catheter should be removed and/or rotated to a different site based on clinical indications (e.g., signs of phlebitis [warmth, tenderness, erythema or palpable venous cord], infection, or malfunction) (CDC, 2011; INS, 2011). This process requires conscientious and frequent assessment of the site. However, if the patient's therapy is expected to be longer than 6 days, a midline catheter or PICC should be chosen (O'Grady et al., 2011). When selecting the site for insertion of a peripheral catheter, consider the patient's age, history, and diagnosis; the type and duration of the prescribed therapy; and, whenever possible, the patient's preference. Chart 13-1 lists the major criteria for the placement of peripheral VADs.

Vein transilluminators and ultrasound devices are now available as tools to assist in IV line placement. Several different types of portable *vein transilluminators* are available, such as VeinViewer, Veinlite LED, and AccuVein AV 300 (Fig. 13-3). Although they may have different mechanisms of action (some use infrared light and some use laser), these devices penetrate only up to about 10 mm and are limited to finding superficial veins.

TABLE 13-1 Choosing the Gauge Size for Peripheral Catheters

CATHETER GAUGE	INDICATIONS	APPROXIMATE FLOW RATES
24-26 gauge Smallest, shortest ($\frac{3}{4}$-inch length)	Not ideal for viscous infusions Expect blood transfusion to take longer Preferred for infants and small children	24 mL/min (1440 mL/hr)
22 gauge	Adequate for most therapies; blood can infuse without damage	38 mL/min (2280 mL/hr)
20 gauge ($1\text{-}1\frac{1}{4}$-inch length)	Adequate for all therapies Most providers of anesthesia prefer not to use a smaller size than this for surgery cases	65 mL/min (3900 mL/hr)
18 gauge	Preferred size for surgery Vein needs to be large enough to accommodate the catheter	110 mL/min (6600 mL/hr)
14-16 gauge	For trauma and surgical patients requiring rapid fluid resuscitation Needs to be in a vein that can accommodate it	

Ultrasound-guided peripheral IV insertion can allow insertion into deeper veins (White et al., 2010). This technology has been shown to be very valuable in assisting with cannulation of peripheral veins that the nurse cannot access with sight and touch. However, there are risks the nurse must be aware of when using ultrasound guidance. This technology should be used only by nurses who have been trained and whose competencies are maintained. Arteries and nerves lie parallel to deep veins, and training is needed to learn to identify these structures and avoid damaging them. In addition, when deeper veins are accessed, infiltration may go undetected until a significant amount of fluid has collected in the tissues. This complication can be particularly devastating if the solution is an irritant or vesicant.

CHART 13-1 Best Practice for Patient Safety & Quality Care QSEN

Placement of Short Peripheral Venous Catheters

- Verify that the prescription for infusion therapy is complete and appropriate for infusion through a short peripheral catheter.
- For adults, choose a site for placement in the upper extremity. DO NOT USE THE WRIST.
- Choose the patient's nondominant arm when possible.
- Choose a distal site, and make all subsequent venipunctures proximal to previous sites.
- Do not use the arm on the side of a mastectomy, lymph node dissection, arteriovenous shunt or fistula, or paralysis.
- Avoid choosing a site in an area of joint flexion.
- Avoid choosing a site in a vein that feels hard or cordlike.
- Avoid choosing a site close to areas of cellulitis, dermatitis, or complications from previous catheter sites.
- Choose a vein of appropriate length and width to fit the size of the catheter required for infusion.

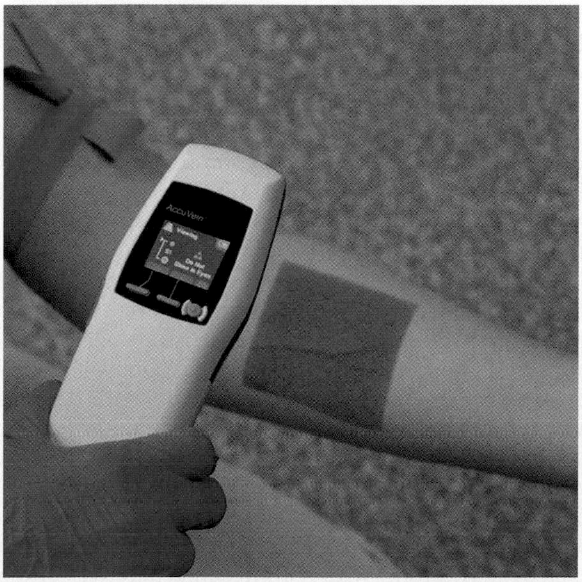

FIG. 13-3 The AccuVein AV300 is a vein illumination device that helps health care professionals locate veins for blood draw, IV infusion, and blood donation by projecting a pattern of light on the patient's skin to reveal the position of underlying veins on the skin's surface. The device uses red and infrared light, which the hemoglobin in blood absorbs to detect the position of the vein.

For patients who need IV access but are at risk for fluid overload or do not need extra IV fluids, the peripheral vascular access device (VAD) can be converted into an intermittent IV lock, also called a *saline lock.* This device allows administration of specific drugs given IV push (e.g., furosemide [Lasix, Furoside 🍁]) or on an intermittent basis using a medication administration set. IV antibiotics are frequently given this way. In some cases, the saline lock is placed in case there is a need for emergency drug administration via IV push. The intermittent device is flushed with saline before and after drug administration to ensure patency and prevent occlusion with a blood clot.

Site Selection and Skin Preparation

The most appropriate veins for peripheral catheter placement include the dorsal venous network, basilic, cephalic, and median veins, as well as their branches (Fig. 13-4). *However, cannulation of veins on the hand is not appropriate for older patients with a loss of skin turgor and poor vein condition and for active patients receiving infusion therapy in an ambulatory care clinic or home care. Use of veins on the dorsal surface of the hands should be reserved as a last resort for short-term infusion of non-vesicant and non-irritant solutions in young patients.*

Mastectomy, axillary lymph node dissection, lymphedema, paralysis of the upper extremity, and the presence of dialysis grafts or fistulas alter the normal pattern of blood flow through the arm. Using veins in the extremity affected by these conditions requires a physician's request. Short peripheral catheters are not recommended for obtaining routine blood samples.

! NURSING SAFETY PRIORITY QSEN

Critical Rescue

Avoid veins on the palmar side of the wrist because the median nerve is located close to veins in this area, making the venipuncture more painful and difficult to stabilize. The cephalic vein begins above the thumb and extends up the entire length of the arm. This vein is usually large and prominent, appearing as a prime site for catheter insertion. Damage to the nerve from any injury can result in permanent loss of function or complex regional pain syndrome, type 2 (CRPS) (Watts & Kremer, 2011). Reports of tingling, feeling "pins and needles" in the extremity, or numbness during the venipuncture procedure can indicate nerve puncture. If any of these symptoms occur, stop the IV insertion procedure immediately, remove the catheter, and choose a new site.

Winged needles ("butterfly needles") are easy to insert but are associated with a high frequency of infiltration. They are most commonly used for injection of single-dose drugs or for drawing blood samples. Like a short peripheral catheter, winged needles should also have an engineered safety mechanism to house the needle when removed.

Aseptic skin preparation and technique before IV insertion are crucial. Catheter-related bloodstream INFECTION (CR-BSI) can occur from a peripheral IV site. The CDC recommendations include:

- Perform evidence-based hand hygiene before palpating the insertion site.
- Clip hair—do not shave.
- Ensure that skin is clean. If visibly soiled, cleanse with soap and water.
- Wear clean gloves for peripheral IV insertion; do not touch the access site after application of antiseptics.

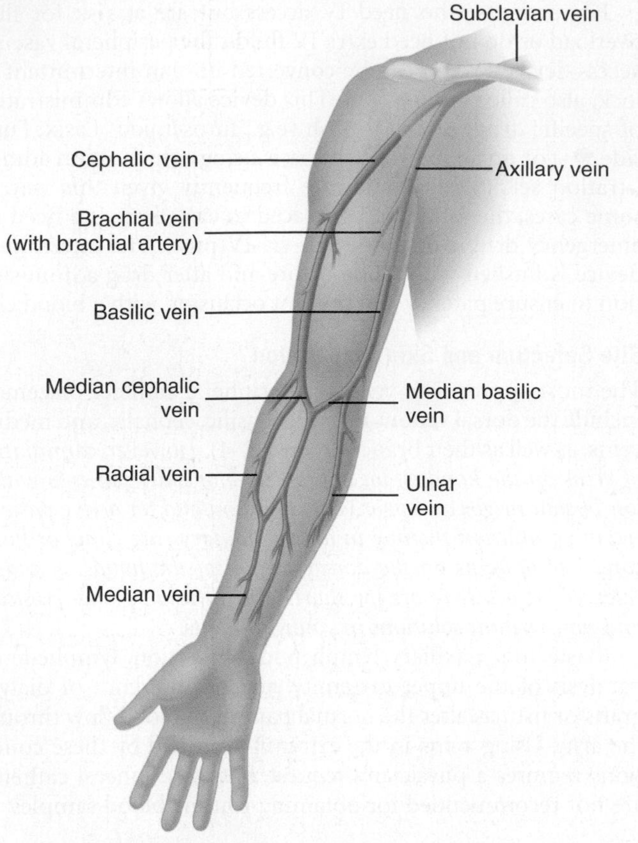

FIG. 13-4 Common IV sites in the inner arm.

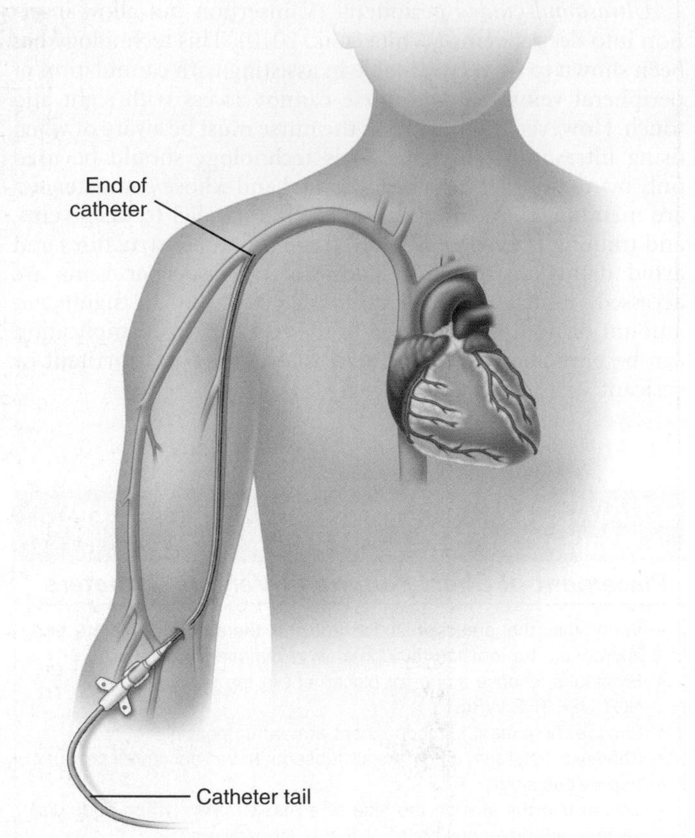

FIG. 13-5 Midline catheter; the tip of this catheter resides in a peripheral vein.

- Prepare clean skin with a skin antiseptic (chlorhexidine 2% with 70% alcohol, 70% isopropyl alcohol, or povidone-iodine) using a back-and-forth motion for 30 seconds, and allow the solution to dry before peripheral venous catheter insertion.

Midline Catheters

Midline catheters can be anywhere from 3 to 8 inches long, 3 to 5 Fr, and double or single lumen. They are inserted through the veins of the upper arm. The median antecubital vein is used most often if insertion is done without the aid of ultrasound guidance. With ultrasound guidance, deeper veins can be accessed and the insertion site can be further above the antecubital fossa. The basilic vein is preferred over the cephalic vein because of its larger diameter and straighter path. It also allows greater hemodilution of the fluids and medications being infused. The catheter tip is located in the upper arm with the tip residing no further into the venous network than the axillary vein (Fig. 13-5). These catheters are used for therapies lasting from 1 to 4 weeks; however, there are no recommendations for the optimal dwell time. In a 2014 study, the average dwell time for midlines was identified as 6.9 days (Dumont, Getz, & Miller, 2014). Because of the extended dwell time, strict sterile technique is used for insertion and dressing changes for a midline catheter. Additional education and skill assessment are required for the nurse to be qualified to insert midline catheters.

Midline catheters have been found to reduce the number of repeated IV cannulations, which reduces patient discomfort, increases patient satisfaction, and contributes to organizational efficiency (Alexandrou et al., 2011). A midline catheter can be used when skin integrity or limited peripheral veins make it difficult to maintain a short peripheral catheter. Indications for these catheters include fluids for hydration and drug therapy that is given longer than 6 days and up to 4 weeks, such as antibiotics, heparin, steroids, and bronchodilators.

Midline catheters are considered to dwell in the peripheral circulation; the recommendations for infusates (fluids or drugs) are the same as for short peripheral IVs. Fluids and medications infused through a midline catheter should have a pH between 5 and 9 and a final osmolarity of less than 600 mOsm/L (Perucca, 2010). The pH and osmolarity outside these parameters increase the risk for complications like phlebitis and thrombosis. Midline catheters should not be used for infusion of **vesicant medications**—drugs that cause severe tissue damage if they escape into the subcutaneous tissue (**extravasation**). There is concern that at a midline tip location, larger amounts of the drug may extravasate before the problem is detected.

All parenteral nutrition formulas, including those with low concentrations of dextrose, and solutions that have an osmolarity greater than 600 mOsm/L should not be infused through a midline catheter. Do not draw blood from these catheters routinely. Midline catheters should not be placed in extremities affected by mastectomy with lymphedema, paralysis, or dialysis grafts and fistulas. When using a double-lumen midline catheter, do not administer incompatible drugs simultaneously through both lumens because the blood flow rate in the axillary vein is not high enough to ensure adequate hemodilution and prevention of drug interaction in the vein.

A new midline, PowerGlide, has been developed by Bard Access Systems. This catheter is approved for power injection of 5 mL/sec for computed tomography (CT) scans (Bard, 2013). There is no evidence in the literature to date on the efficacy of this practice.

NCLEX EXAMINATION CHALLENGE

Physiological Integrity

The health care provider prescribes 1 L 5%D/0.9%NS to be infused over 10 hours. The nurse sets the rate at _______mL/hr of IV solution.

CENTRAL INTRAVENOUS THERAPY

In **central IV therapy**, the vascular access device (VAD) is placed in the central circulation, specifically within the superior vena cava (SVC) near its junction with the right atrium, also called the *caval-atrial junction (CAJ)*. Blood flow in the SVC is about 2 L/min compared with about 200 mL/min in the axillary vein. Most central vascular access devices require confirmation of tip location at the CAJ by chest radiograph before solutions are infused. However, newer technologies use either a magnet tip locator or identification of the CAJ by electrocardiogram rather than by x-ray. Both the Sherlock 3CG by Bard and the VasoNova/Teleflex systems have received Food and Drug Administration (FDA) approval as an alternative to chest x-ray or fluoroscopy to verify PICC tip location.

A number of types of central vascular access devices (CVADs) are available, depending on the purpose, duration, and insertion site availability. Several recent improvements in catheter materials allow antimicrobial and heparin coatings to reduce INFECTION risk and improve the longevity of the catheter. Not all central line catheters are approved for power injection used in radiologic tests. The catheter can rupture if it is not designed to handle the injection pressure necessary for some tests such as pulmonary CT angiography or CT angiography of the aorta (5 mL/sec and 300 per square inch [psi]). Check with the radiology department and read the indications on the packaging before using them for power injection (Macha et al., 2009).

Peripherally Inserted Central Catheters

A **peripherally inserted central catheter (PICC)** is a long catheter inserted through a vein of the antecubital fossa (inner aspect of the bend of the arm) or the middle of the upper arm. Nurses who insert these CVADs require special training and certification.

In adults, the PICC length ranges from 18 to 29 inches (45-74 cm) with the tip residing in the superior vena cava (SVC) ideally at the caval-atrial junction (CAJ) (Fig. 13-6). Placement of the catheter tip in veins distal to the SVC is avoided. This inappropriate tip location, often called a *mid-clavicular catheter*, is associated with much higher rates of thrombosis than when the tip is located in the SVC at the CAJ. Mid-clavicular tip locations are used only when anatomic or pathophysiologic changes prohibit placing the catheter into the SVC.

PICCs should be inserted early in the course of therapy before veins of the extremity have been damaged from multiple venipunctures and infusions. Insertion methods using guidewires and ultrasound systems greatly improve insertion success. The basilic vein is the preferred site for insertion; the cephalic vein can be used if necessary. Two brachial veins are not recommended because they are more difficult to access; they are deeper in the arm and run close to the brachial artery. *Sterile technique is used for insertion to reduce the risk for catheter-related bloodstream* INFECTION *(CR-BSI). Before the catheter can be used for infusion, a chest x-ray indicating that the tip resides in the lower SVC is required when the catheter is not placed under fluoroscopy or with the use of the electrocardiogram tip locator technique.*

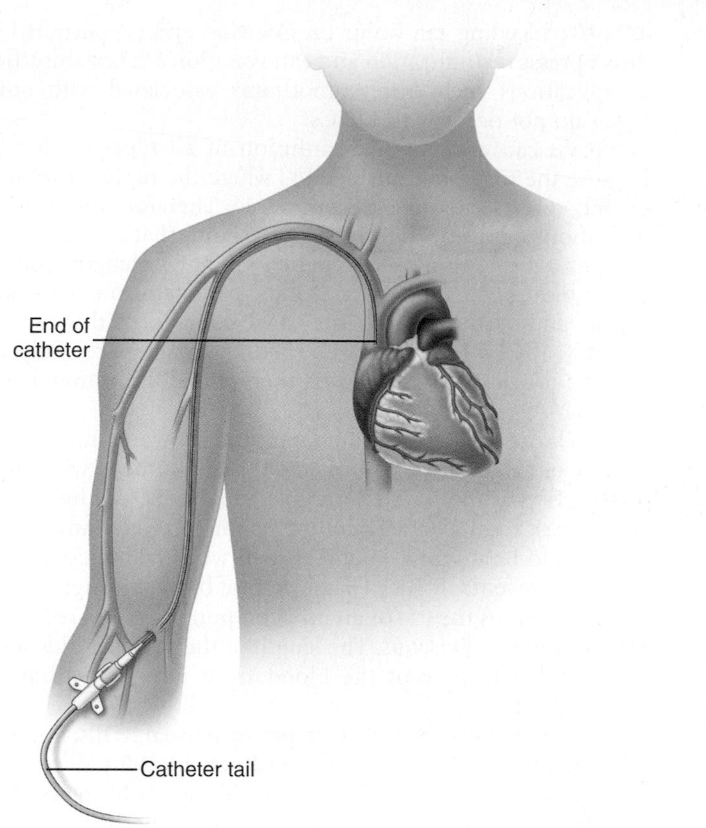

FIG. 13-6 Peripherally inserted central catheter (PICC) is placed peripherally in a vein of the upper arm with the tip resting in the superior vena cava.

PICCs are available in single-, dual-, or triple-lumen configurations and are available with both the Groshong valve and the pressure-activated safety valve (PASV). PICCs are also available as "Power PICCs" and can be used for contrast injection at a maximum of 5 mL/sec and a maximum pressure of 300 psi. They can also be connected to transducers and used to monitor central venous pressure (Bard Access Systems, 2011).

The most common complications from PICCs include phlebitis, thrombophlebitis, deep vein thrombosis (DVT), and CR-BSIs. Thrombophlebitis and DVT can be very serious, threaten the integrity of the vein, and decrease PERFUSION. The smallest possible French size should be used to decrease the rate of upper extremity DVT, a potentially life-threatening event.

CR-BSI has been noted to be less common in PICCs than in other central venous catheters (CVCs) because of the insertion site in the upper extremity. The cooler, drier skin of the upper arm has fewer types and numbers of microorganisms, leading to lower rates of INFECTION. Accidental arterial puncture or excessive bleeding can occur on insertion and is controlled by direct pressure. Infiltration and extravasation are rare. Insertion complications such as pneumothorax associated with other CVCs do not occur with PICCs.

PICCs can accommodate infusion of all types of therapy because the tip resides in the SVC where the rapid blood flow quickly dilutes the fluids being infused. Therefore there are no limitations on the pH or osmolality of fluids that can be infused through a PICC. For example, patients requiring lengthy courses of antibiotics, chemotherapy agents, parenteral nutrition formulas, and vasopressor agents can benefit from this type of catheter. PICCs have been reported to dwell successfully for months or even years; however, the optimal dwell time is not known.

PICCs can be used for blood sampling; however, lumen sizes of 4 Fr or larger are recommended. Using lumens with small diameters may not yield a sample capable of producing the needed test results. In addition, frequent entry into any central line should be minimized and treated with strict aseptic technique to prevent CR-BSI. Transfusion of blood through a PICC usually requires the use of an infusion pump. Packed red blood cells are cold and viscous. The length of the catheter adds resistance and may prevent the blood from infusing within the 4-hour limit.

Teach patients with a PICC to perform usual ADLs; however, they should avoid excessive physical activity. Muscle contractions in the arm from physical activity like heavy lifting can lead to catheter dislodgment and possible lumen occlusion. PICCs may be contraindicated in paraplegic patients who rely on their arms for mobility and in patients using crutches that provide support in the axilla.

PICC insertion is commonly performed in the patient's hospital room, an ambulatory care treatment facility, or the imaging department. Regardless of where they are inserted, the same precautions must be taken as with any other central line insertion using the catheter-related bloodstream INFECTION (CR-BSI) prevention bundle. Major components of this prevention bundle include:

- Hand hygiene
- Maximal barrier precautions upon insertion
- Chlorhexidine skin antisepsis
- Optimal catheter site selection and post-placement care with avoidance of the femoral vein for central venous access in adult patients
- Daily review of line necessity with prompt removal of unnecessary lines

Other helpful interventions include use of a check list for sterility during the procedure, a line cart with all equipment, and a stop sign on the door of the room to stop unnecessary traffic through the room during the procedure.

! NURSING SAFETY PRIORITY QSEN

Action Alert

The INS recommendation for flushing PICC lines not actively used is 5 mL of heparin (10 units/mL) in a 10-mL syringe at least daily when using a non-valved catheter and at least weekly with a valved catheter. Use 10 mL of sterile saline to flush before and after medication administration; 20 mL of sterile saline is flushed after drawing blood. *Always use 10-mL barrel syringes to flush any central line because the pressure exerted by a smaller barrel poses a risk for rupturing the catheter.*

Nontunneled Percutaneous Central Venous Catheters

Nontunneled percutaneous central venous catheters (CVCs) are inserted by a physician, trained physician assistant, or nurse practitioner through the subclavian vein in the upper chest or the internal jugular veins in the neck using sterile technique. Occasionally the patient's condition may require insertion of the CVC in a femoral vein, but the rate of infection is very high. If the femoral site must be used, it is removed as soon as possible.

CVCs are usually 7 to 10 inches (18 to 25 cm) long and have one to as many as five lumens (Fig. 13-7). These catheters are also available with antimicrobial coatings such as chlorhexidine and silver sulfadiazine. The tip resides in the superior vena cava (SVC) and is confirmed by a chest x-ray. Nontunneled percutaneous CVCs are most commonly used for emergent or trauma situations, critical care, and surgery. There is no recommendation for optimal dwell time. However, these catheters are commonly used for short-term situations and are *not* the catheter of choice for home care or ambulatory clinic settings.

Insertion of these central catheters requires the patient to be placed in the Trendelenburg position, usually with a rolled towel between the shoulder blades. This position may be difficult or contraindicated for patients with respiratory conditions, spinal curvatures, and increased intracranial pressure, especially for older adults. Trauma, surgery, or radiation in the neck or chest prohibits the use of these devices as well. Insertion with ultrasound guidance has been demonstrated to

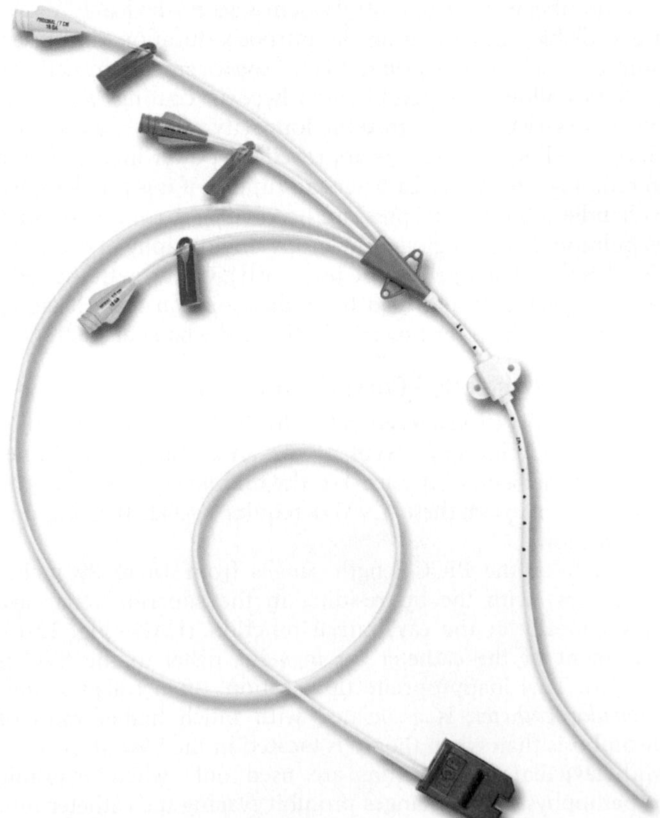

FIG. 13-7 The Edwards Lifesciences PreSep central venous catheter (CVC); often placed in the subclavian or internal jugular vein with the tip of the catheter resting in the superior vena cava.

improve the safety of insertion in the internal jugular site (Griswold-Theodorson et al., 2009). The presence of a tracheotomy increases the risk for cross-contamination of the insertion site. The warmer, moister skin of the neck and upper chest has more types and higher numbers of microorganisms, resulting in more CR-BSIs with this type of catheter.

Tunneled Central Venous Catheters

Tunneled central venous catheters are VADs that have a portion of the catheter lying in a subcutaneous tunnel, separating the points where the catheter enters the vein from where it exits the skin. This separation is intended to prevent the organisms on the skin from reaching the bloodstream (Fig. 13-8). Today these catheters are usually inserted by physicians in the radiology suite, rather than placed surgically. The catheter has a cuff made of a rough material that is positioned inside the subcutaneous tunnel. These cuffs commonly contain antibiotics, which also reduce the risk for INFECTION. The tissue granulates into the cuff, providing a mechanical barrier to microorganisms and anchoring the catheter in place.

The design of tunneled CVCs requires surgical techniques for insertion and removal. Single-, dual-, and triple-lumens are available. These catheters were originally named for the physicians who designed them, including Broviac, Hickman, and Leonard catheters.

Tunneled catheters are used primarily when the need for infusion therapy is frequent and long-term. Patients needing parenteral nutrition for months, years, or the remainder of their life commonly choose a tunneled catheter. Tunneled catheters are also chosen when several weeks or months of infusion therapy are needed and a PICC is not a good choice. For example, paraplegic patients needing 6 to 8 weeks of antibiotics are not good candidates for a PICC because of the excessive use of the upper extremities for mobility. Some oncology patients may prefer a tunneled catheter instead of an implanted port because they cannot tolerate the needle sticks required for accessing those devices.

Implanted Ports

Implanted ports are very different from other central vascular access devices (CVADs). This type of device is chosen for patients who are expected to require IV therapy for more than a year (Santolim et al., 2012). This device is typically inserted by a physician in the radiology department or by a surgeon in the operating suite. Implanted ports consist of a portal body, a dense septum over a reservoir, and a catheter. They can be single- or double-lumen and come in various sizes. A subcutaneous pocket is surgically created to house the port body. The catheter is inserted into the vein and attached to the portal body. The septum is made of self-sealing silicone and is located in the center of the port body over the reservoir; the catheter extends from the side of the port body. The incision is closed, and no part of the catheter is visible externally; therefore this device has the least impact on body image (Fig. 13-9).

Some implanted ports are power-injectable and can be used for obtaining contrast-enhanced computed tomography (CECT). These devices can withstand 5 mL/sec at up to 300 psi pressure. The BARD PowerPort can be identified by palpation of three bumps on the top of the septum and a triangular-shaped port. Be careful not to press firmly on the bumps because it can be painful to the patient. Be sure to use a power-injection–rated noncoring needle with this type of port when it is used for this purpose. These needles come with labeling identifying that they are power-injection rated (Fig. 13-10).

Venous ports may be placed on the upper chest or the upper extremity. The venous catheter may enter either the subclavian or internal jugular vein. Although an implanted port is most commonly used in the venous system, the catheter may be placed in arteries, the epidural space, or the peritoneal cavity, with the port pocket located over a bony prominence.

Implanted ports are accessed by using a noncoring needle (a common brand name is *Huber*) that is specially designed with a deflected tip. This design slices through the dense septum

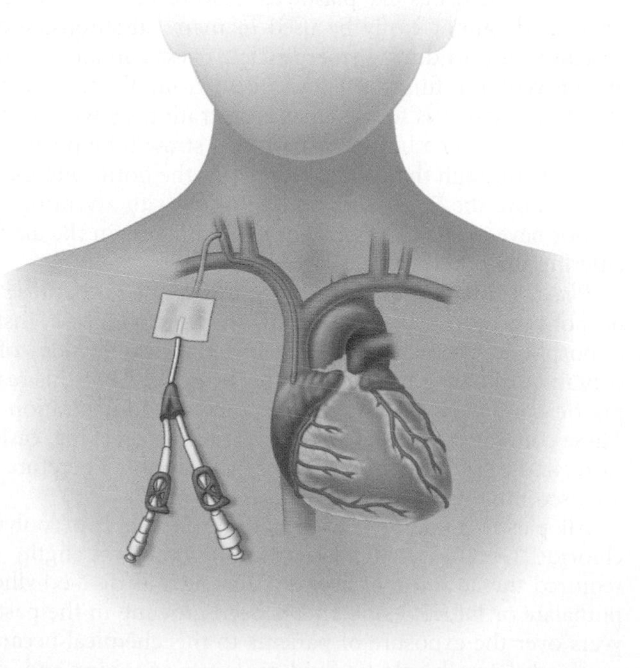

FIG. 13-8 Tunneled catheter. A portion of this catheter lies in a subcutaneous tunnel, separating the point where the catheter enters the vein from where it exits the skin.

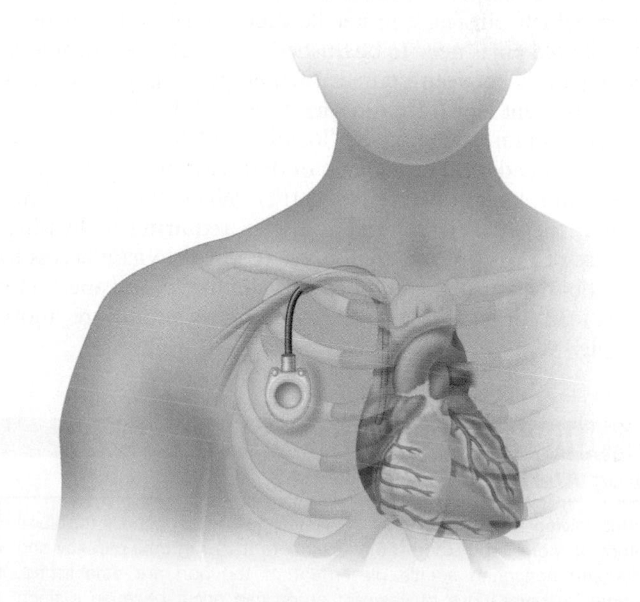

FIG. 13-9 Positioning of an implanted port.

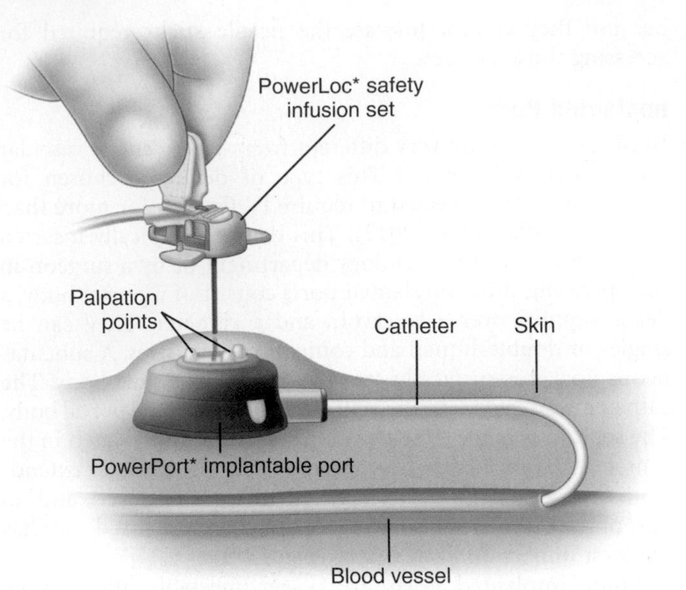

FIG. 13-10 A noncoring needle for accessing an implanted powerport.

without coring out a small piece of it, thus preserving the integrity of the septum. Port bodies placed in the chest have a larger septum and usually tolerate about 2000 punctures. Port bodies placed in the upper extremity are smaller and are rated to tolerate about 750 punctures.

Port access should be done only by formally trained health care professionals using a mask and aseptic technique. Implanted ports are used most often for patients receiving chemotherapy. These patients are immune-compromised making them highly susceptible to INFECTION. Before puncture, palpate the port to locate the septum. Carefully palpate to feel the shape and depth of the port body to ensure puncture of the septum, not the attached catheter. Some have attached extension sets and wings to stabilize the needle. One important feature is an engineered safety mechanism to contain the needle when it is removed from the septum. Because the dense septum holds tightly to the needle, there can be a rebound when it is pulled from the septum, which can result in needle stick injury to the nurse.

Implanted ports need to be flushed after each use and at least once a month between courses of therapy. This procedure is done to prevent clot formation in the internal chamber of the port and is often referred to as "locking" or "de-accessing." The INS recommendation for locking or de-accessing a port is 5 mL of 100 units heparin/mL (INS, 2011). When the port is not accessed, there is no external catheter requiring a dressing. Puncture of the skin over the port is required to gain access to the port body, causing pain for some patients. Topical anesthetic creams can be used to make the access procedure more tolerable.

! NURSING SAFETY PRIORITY QSEN

Drug Alert

Before giving a drug through an implanted port, always check for blood return. If there is no blood return, withhold the drug until patency and adequate noncoring needle placement of the port are established. Serious extravasations of vesicant drugs can occur because a fibrin sheath (flap or tail) may occur at the tip of the catheter, clot it, and cause retrograde subcutaneous leakage.

Hemodialysis Catheters

Hemodialysis catheters have very large lumens to accommodate the hemodialysis procedure or a pheresis procedure that harvests specific blood cells. They may be tunneled for long-term needs or nontunneled for short-term needs. A hemodialysis catheter is critical to the management of renal failure and must function well. CR-BSIs and vein thrombosis are common problems; therefore this catheter should not be used for administration of other fluids or drugs except in an emergency.

The concentration of heparin used to lock hemodialysis catheters ranges from 1,000 to 10,000 units/mL. Researchers have demonstrated that using 1,000 units/mL reduces the incidence of postinsertion bleeding but may be associated with an increased need for recombinant tissue plasminogen activator (tPA) to maintain patency. A flush of 1,000 units heparin/mL or a solution of 4% sodium citrate in the amount of the dwell volume of each lumen has been recommended (Moran & Ash, 2008). Heparin is most often used because sodium citrate has not been as commercially available in the preparation needed. To prevent systemic anticoagulation and subsequent bleeding, be sure to aspirate the heparin from the lumens before use.

INFUSION SYSTEMS

Nurses administering infusion therapies need to understand how infusion systems work. This knowledge ensures that the patient can benefit from a particular system's advantages while minimizing any potential complications.

Containers

Infusion containers are made of glass or plastic. *Glass* bottles were the original fluid container to be mass produced. They are easily sterilized, and it is easy to read the amount of fluid remaining in the bottle. Also, glass is inert and so cannot interact with some drugs like plastic can. However, glass bottles are heavy and cannot easily be used in many situations, such as patient transport during emergencies. These containers require an air vent for fluids to flow freely from them. The most common method is to use an administration set with a special filtered vent. Some bottles may have a straw tube open to the room air through the rubber stopper in the bottle and extending to above the level of the fluid. Bottles with a venting straw do not have a barrier to prevent contaminants in the air from entering the fluid.

Plastic containers are considered *closed systems* because they do not rely on outside air to allow the fluid to infuse. Instead, atmospheric pressure pushes against the flexible sides of the container, allowing the fluid to flow by gravity. For this reason, plastic containers do not require vented administration sets. These containers are lightweight, resistant to breaking, easier to store, and easy to use in emergency conditions. Therefore they are used more frequently than glass containers.

All plastic containers were commonly made of polyvinyl chloride (PVC). To increase flexibility and strength, PVC required the addition of a plasticizer, such as di-2-ethylhexylphthalate or DEHP. Concern has been growing in the past few years over the exposure of patients to this chemical because it can leach from the plastic fluid container or tubing and infuse into the patient with the IV fluid or medication. The FDA has determined that there is little to no risk posed to most patients by exposure to the amount of DEHP released from IV bags with infusion of crystalloids or drugs. However, there is concern about the buildup of chemical exposure from many sources over a lifetime and specifically the potential effects of DEHP on the development of the male reproductive system. Therefore many hospitals are using PVC-free and DEHP-free IV bags, especially for high-risk groups.

One disadvantage of removing DEHP from the plastic bags is that the bags are less pliable and more prone to rupture. Some institutions do not allow these bags to be sent through a pneumatic tube system because the pressure exerted has caused the bags to rupture during transport.

A problem with plastic containers is that they are not compatible with insulin, nitroglycerin, lorazepam (Ativan), fat emulsions, and lipid-based drugs. Nitroglycerin and insulin adhere to the walls of the PVC container, making it impossible to know exactly how much medication the patient is receiving. There is evidence that a priming volume of 20 mL of insulin solution is required to minimize the effect of insulin absorption losses to the plastics in IV lines (Thompson et al., 2012).

Another concern with plastic bags is the accuracy of reading the amount of fluid remaining in the container. The middle graduations have been shown to be 10% above or below the actual amount of fluid, but the first and last markings could be inaccurate by as much as 40% (Perucca, 2010).

! NURSING SAFETY PRIORITY (QSEN)

Action Alert

Regardless of the type of fluid container being used, check it for cracks or pinholes before use. Always observe the fluid for **turbidity** (cloudiness) or any unusual color that could indicate contamination.

Administration Sets

The administration set is the connection between the catheter and the fluid container. Numerous sets are available in many different configurations. The type and purpose of the infusion determine the type of administration set needed. Some sets are *generic*, meaning that they are appropriate for most infusions. Other sets are used for specific types of infusions, such as blood transfusion. Still others are *dedicated*, meaning that they must be used with a specific manufacturer's infusion controlling device. Information that describes their proper use is provided on the packaging of administration sets.

Secondary Administration Sets

A primary continuous administration set is used to infuse the primary IV fluid by either a gravity infusion or an electronic infusion pump. A short **secondary administration set**, also known as a **piggyback set**, is attached to the primary set at a Y–injection site and is used to deliver intermittent medications (Fig. 13-11). Directions and diagrams for use are typically on the packaging. Once attached, these sets should remain connected together as an infusion system. Primary and secondary continuous infusion administration sets used to infuse fluids other than parenteral nutrition, lipids, blood, or blood products should be changed no more frequently than every 96 hours (INS, 2011).

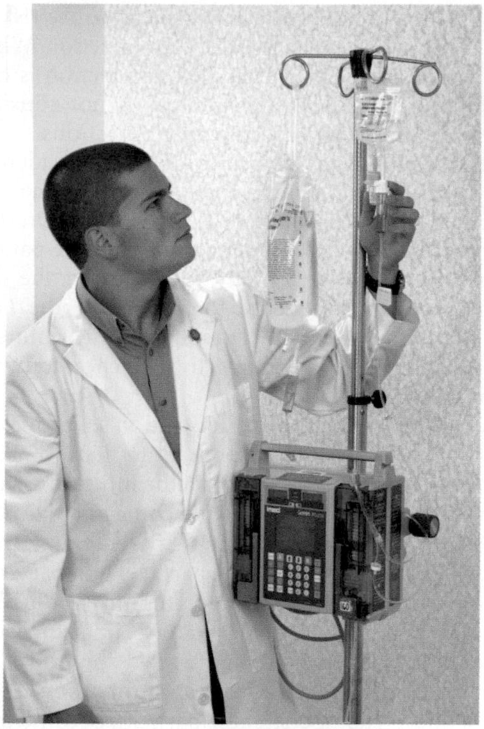

FIG. 13-11 Secondary IV administration set attached to the primary set at a Y-injection site.

Intermittent Administration Sets

When no primary continuous fluid is being infused, use an intermittent administration set to infuse multiple doses of medications through a catheter that has been capped with a needleless connection device. Remove the medication bag from the previous dose, and attach the new one. Remove the sterile cap covering the distal end of the set, and attach the set to the catheter. Because both ends of the set are being manipulated with each dose, the INS standards of practice state that this set should be changed every 24 hours. When the administration set is used for infusion of parenteral nutrition or lipid solution, change it every 24 hours. Change blood tubing within 4 hours; use new tubing to infuse propofol (Diprivan) every 6 to 12 hours (McGoldrick, 2010).

Administration sets are sterile in the fluid pathway and under the sterile caps on each end of the set. The set is not packaged as a completely sterile product and cannot be added to a sterile field. Careful attention is required to maintain the sterility of the spike and the connection end of the tubing to prevent introduction of microorganisms into the catheter and bloodstream.

Add-on Devices

Several other types of add-on devices include short extension sets, injection caps, and filters. Extension sets may be packaged as a sterile product for adding to a sterile field; however, always check the product label for this information.

Administration sets have two ways to connect to the catheter hub: a slip lock or a Luer-Lok. The *slip lock* is a male end that slips into the female catheter hub. A *Luer-Lok* connection has the same male end with a threaded collar that requires twisting onto the corresponding threads of the catheter hub. All connections, including *extension sets*, should have a Luer-Lok design to ensure that the set remains firmly connected. Loose connections lead to fluid leakage and increase the risk for contamination and subsequent bloodstream infection. When using a central venous catheter, a Luer-Lok connection is critical to reduce the risk for air embolism. Tape is not considered an adequate mechanism for securing set connections.

Luer-Lok devices may be purposefully or accidentally disconnected. Patients or visitors may disconnect the system to allow the patient to get out of bed or the chair. Or, the device may become accidentally disconnected when the patient turns or moves. In either case, be sure to reconnect the device by following the proper sequence to reassemble the IV system components. Fatalities have resulted when nurses have accidently reconnected IV tubing to a tracheostomy or other inappropriate port.

Filters may be part of the administration set or may be separate add-on pieces. Their purpose is to remove particulate matter, microorganisms, and air from the infusion system. Filter sizes depend on the pore size, with common sizes being 1.2 microns used to filter lipid-containing parenteral nutrition and 0.2 microns intended to remove all particles and bacteria. Filters should be placed as close to the catheter hub as possible.

Particulate matter in the IV fluid, a primary reason to use filters, comprises undissolved, unintended substances and may include rubber pieces, glass particles, cotton fibers, drug particles, paper, and metal fibers. These particles become trapped in the small circulation of the lungs. A red blood cell is about 5 microns in diameter and is the largest size that can pass through the pulmonary capillary bed; IV fluids may contain particles larger than 5 microns. For patients receiving infusion therapy for long periods, a significant number of particles could block the blood flow through the pulmonary circulation. Microcirculation in the spleen, kidneys, and liver could also be affected. Particulate matter has also been implicated in the development of phlebitis in peripheral veins.

Other concerns with using filters include the possibility for their rupture, their use with certain drugs that bind to the filter surface, using the incorrect size of filter for drugs with large molecules, and choosing a filter that will not tolerate the pressure exerted by infusion pumps. Rupture is most commonly associated with the exertion of high pressure exceeding the limit tolerated by the specific filter. Some drugs cannot be filtered because they are retained inside the filter because of their chemical nature or molecule size. For these reasons, medication filtration during the process of admixing is commonly used today as an alternative to final filtration at the bedside. Drugs of a very small quantity should be administered below the filter.

Filters used on blood administration sets have much larger pore size and are not interchangeable with filters used for fluids and medications. A standard blood filter ranges from 170 to 260 microns and removes microclots and other debris caused by blood collection and storage. Microaggregate filters have a pore size of 20, 40, or 80 microns and are used to remove degenerating platelets, white blood cells, and fibrin strands. Leukocyte-removal filters are used to remove white blood cells that cause febrile and allergic blood transfusion reactions.

Needleless Connection Devices

In July 1992, the Occupational Safety and Health Administration (OSHA) published guidelines entitled *Occupational Exposure to Bloodborne Pathogens, Final Rule.* This document requires health care organizations to initiate engineering controls "that isolate or remove the bloodborne pathogen hazard from the workplace." This standard was amended in 2001 with the passage of the Needlestick Safety and Prevention Act. This regulation requires the use of devices engineered with safety mechanisms and mandates that staff who perform these tasks be directly involved with selecting products. It also requires each employer to maintain a sharps injury log with details of each incident. Many products are designed to minimize health care workers' exposure to contaminated needles. Luer-activated devices are the most common design for needleless systems today.

Although these devices have reduced the incidence of accidental needle sticks for health care professionals, concern remains about a possible increase in the risk for catheter-related bloodstream infections (CR-BSIs) (Jarvis et al., 2009). This concern stems from the crevices created with the diaphragm and Luer-Lok design. Blood and bacteria can be trapped in the crevices, and meticulous cleaning is required with each use.

Various designs are available for connectors that provide positive or negative displacement of fluid when the needleless syringe is removed. Needleless positive-pressure valve (PPV) connectors were developed to prevent backflow of blood into the IV catheter, thereby decreasing chances of thrombus formation and CR-BSI. Several newer connectors are silver-impregnated to reduce bacterial growth (Fig. 13-12). Be sure to check which type of connector valve is used in your facility because the flushing technique differs depending on type. Researchers have found conflicting results about the relationships between these devices and CR-BSI and catheter occlusion (Khalidi et al., 2009; Mitchell et al., 2009; O'Grady et al., 2011).

Conclusive studies are needed to determine the best design for needleless systems. Until then, implement these interventions to reduce infection risk:

- Clean all needleless system connections vigorously with antimicrobial for 30 seconds (usually 70% alcohol or alcohol and 2% chlorhexidine swabs) before connecting infusion sets or syringes, paying special attention to the small ridges in the Luer-Lok device. There are newer caps that are impregnated with alcohol or chlorhexidine that may be used to keep the port aseptic; however, these will increase costs and research is needed to demonstrate the benefit.
- Do not tape connections between tubing sets.
- Use evidence-based hand hygiene guidelines from the CDC and OSHA

Rate-Controlling Infusion Devices

The ability to regulate the rate and volume of infusions is critical to the safe and accurate administration of medications and

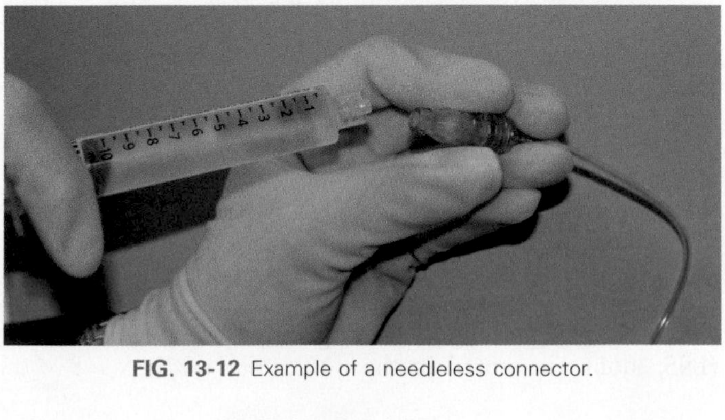

FIG. 13-12 Example of a needleless connector.

fluids to patients. Nurses have a choice of numerous devices that can be electronically or mechanically regulated.

Electronic infusion devices (IV pumps) are used universally in acute care institutions. They are also used in long-term care settings and at home. In addition, "smart pumps" provide the latest infusion computer technology to promote patient safety and save nursing time. *Remember that the use of pumps does not decrease your responsibility to carefully monitor the patient's infusion site and the infusion rate.*

In inpatient settings, IV pumps are pole-mounted. As their name implies, these electronic devices with battery backup pump drugs or fluids under pressure. They accurately measure the volume of fluid being infused by using one of three mechanisms:

- A syringe-type mechanism that fills and empties
- A wavelike, peristaltic action that pushes fluid along the tubing
- A series of microchambers that fill and empty

Regardless of the pumping mechanism, these devices require dedicated cassette tubing designed to match the pump.

Syringe pumps use an electronic or battery-powered piston to push the plunger continuously at a selected milliliter-per-hour rate. The use of syringe pumps is limited to small-volume continuous or intermittent infusions and depends on the syringe size. Antibiotics and patient-controlled analgesia are frequently delivered with syringe pumps. Patients requiring fluid restrictions can also benefit from using a syringe pump because smaller yet accurate volumes can be used to dilute medications.

Ambulatory pumps are generally used for home care patients and allow them to return to their usual activities while receiving infusion therapy. These pumps have a wide range of sizes, with some requiring a backpack, but they usually weigh less than 6 pounds. They are typically used to accurately deliver continuous infusions, such as parenteral nutrition, pain medication, and many programmable drug schedules. Frequent battery recharging or replacement is usually necessary.

Electronic infusion devices can be programmed in many different ways and require a thorough knowledge of the specific brand being used. Infusion rate and the volume to be infused are usually entered in single milliliter increments, but some can be programmed as fractions of a milliliter. Some pumps allow the rate to be programmed to taper or ramp up and down at the beginning and ending of the infusion. Secondary syringe infusion, secondary infusion rate, remote site programming, adjustable infusion pressure, and integration into the nurse call system also are possible.

Electronic infusion devices have a variety of alarms, such as air-in-line, upstream and downstream occlusion, infusion complete, and low-battery or power warnings. All devices must have some mechanism to prevent free flow of the infusing fluid or medication. When the cassette or tubing is removed from the pump, this mechanism automatically stops fluid flow until it is properly replaced in the pump. This safety measure prevents accidental rapid infusion of large amounts of fluid or medication, which could lead to serious clinical problems.

In the past few years, **smart pumps** (infusion pumps with dosage calculation software) have been promoted to reduce adverse drug events (ADEs). Incorrect programming of pumps without this feature is one of the most common types of drug errors, especially in hospitals. Multiple libraries of drug information are stored in the pump manufacturer's medical management system. This software allows the facility to preprogram dosing limits, especially for high-alert drugs. Examples of smart pumps are the B. Braun Outlook 400ES and the Baxter Sigma Spectrum infusion system.

The newest development in smart pumps is a wireless network connection. Drug libraries can be updated via a wireless connection, thus eliminating the necessity of manually updating each pump. In addition to preventing drug errors, smart pump systems record potential errors that would have occurred without these safety mechanisms (Breland, 2010).

Dose-track technology is intended to transmit the infusion data to the institution's pharmacy so that the correct patient receives the correct medication. Dose-guard technology alerts the nurse if institution-defined dose limits are exceeded. These newer technologies provide safeguards for patients to keep them safe. However, the "smarter" the pump, the more extensive the programming steps are and the more alarms that the nurse must respond to. In addition, technology and wireless connections can fail. The challenge for nurses is to maintain the skill of manual dose calculation and rate control, to acknowledge and validate all alarms, and to guard against becoming desensitized to alarms.

Mechanically regulated devices can be used to deliver intermittent medications such as antibiotics or continuous pain medications in community-based health or home care settings. In acute care settings, devices called "infusers" may be found in surgical services. They are powered by positive pressure from the collapsing balloon or roller returning to its coiled position.

The systems include elastomeric balloons, spring-coiled syringes and containers, and a multi-chambered fluid container placed in a mechanical roller (Accufuser or On-Q PainBuster) (Fig. 13-13). These small portable devices do not require power sources such as batteries or electricity. They deliver a preset

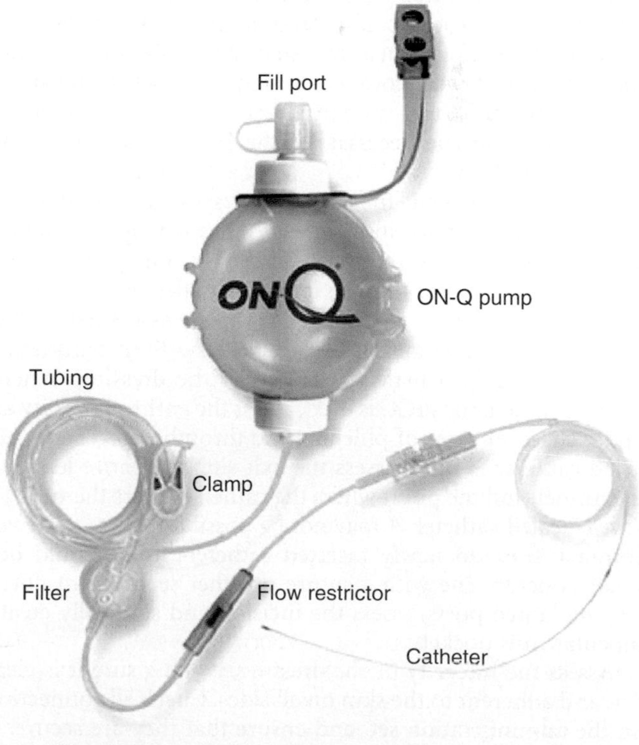

FIG. 13-13 On-Q PainBuster pump (mechanical infuser).

infusion rate, and fluid volume is determined by the size of the fluid container; however, most hold only 50 to 100 mL.

NURSING CARE FOR PATIENTS RECEIVING INTRAVENOUS THERAPY

Educating the Patient

The current trend in health care demands that we partner with our patients to provide the best patient-centered care. In 2010, The Joint Commission added the requirement that all patients who have central lines placed in the hospital must have education on prevention of catheter-related bloodstream infection (CR-BSI). Before catheter insertion, educate the patient and family about:

- The type of catheter to be used
- Hand hygiene and aseptic technique for care of the catheter
- The therapy required
- Alternatives to the catheter and therapy
- Activity limitations
- Any signs or symptoms of complications that should be reported to a health care professional

Provide written information before placement of a long-term catheter, and continue to assess the patient's knowledge level and provide more information or answers as needed. Most manufacturers of PICCs, tunneled catheters, and implanted ports provide patient information booklets. However, specific information about the chosen procedures and supplies may be required. Conversation and pictures will be helpful for patients who are *literacy challenged* (have a low reading level ability).

Performing the Nursing Assessment

All central VADs require documentation of tip location at the CAJ by either electrocardiogram technology, fluoroscopy, or chest x-ray. The initial verbal and subsequent written report should contain specific information about the catheter tip location in relation to anatomic structures. The nurse's knowledge of accurate tip location is required before beginning infusion through the catheter. Repeating the x-ray during catheter use may be necessary if the patient reports unusual pain or sensation.

Nursing assessment for all infusion systems should be systematic. Begin with the insertion site and work upward, following the tubing. Know the type of catheter your patient has in place. Be sure to find out the length of catheter, the insertion site, and tip location to perform a complete assessment. Assess the insertion site by looking for redness, swelling, hardness, or drainage. Lightly palpate the area over the dressing. When a midline catheter or PICC is used, assess the entire extremity and upper chest for signs of phlebitis and thrombosis. When a tunneled catheter is used, assess the exit site, the entire length of the tunnel, and the point where the catheter enters the vein. For a well-healed catheter, it may not be possible to detect the vein entrance site. On newly inserted catheters, there could be a small puncture site with a suture or other securement device. For implanted ports, assess the incision and surgically created subcutaneous pocket.

Assess the integrity of the dressing, making sure it is clean, dry, and adherent to the skin on all sides. Check all connections on the administration set, and ensure that they are secure. Be sure they are not taped. Check the rate of infusion for all fluids by either counting drops or checking the infusion pump. Assess the amount of fluid that has infused from the container. Is it accurate, or is it infusing too fast or too slow? Adjust the rate to the prescribed flow rate. Check all labels on containers for the patient's name and fluid or medication. *Be sure that the correct solution is being infused!*

! NURSING SAFETY PRIORITY (QSEN)

Action Alert

Remind unlicensed assistive personnel (UAP) to avoid taking blood pressures in an extremity with any type of catheter in place. If a short peripheral catheter is being used for continuous infusion, the compression while taking the blood pressure can increase venous pressure, causing fluid to overflow from the puncture site and infiltration. When a midline catheter or PICC is being used, compression from the blood pressure cuff could increase vein irritation and lead to phlebitis.

Draw blood samples in the extremity opposite from all catheters. Blood should not be drawn from a venipuncture site proximal to (above) an infusing peripheral catheter because the infusing fluid could alter the results of the test to be performed. Venipuncture at or near the insertion site of a midline catheter or PICC could damage the catheter, add to areas of venous inflammation, and decrease PERFUSION.

Securing and Dressing the Catheter

Adequate catheter securement is vital to prevent many complications. Tape, sutures, and specially designed securement devices can be used for this purpose. For a short peripheral catheter, tape strips are most common; however, the tape should be *clean*. Tape strips from a peripheral IV start kit are preferred. Strips of tape should not be taken from rolls of tape moved between patient's rooms, from other procedures, or from uniform pockets. Precutting tape and placing it on the patient's bedrails, your uniform or scrubs, or other object should also be avoided to prevent infection.

Newer *securement devices* are designed for all catheter types and provide an evidence-based method to prevent VAD movement (INS, 2011). Recent studies have shown that these devices, such as the StatLock IV stabilization device, prevent peripheral and central catheters from becoming dislodged (Fig. 13-14) (see the Evidence-Based Practice box). In addition, they prevent complications like phlebitis and infiltration. To prevent skin tears, remove the adhesive on a StatLock with 70% alcohol.

PICCs and nontunneled percutaneous central catheters may be sutured in place; however, this creates additional breaks in the skin that could become infected. If these sutures are loose or broken, notify the health care provider to replace them. IV catheter sutures are being replaced with securement devices and Dermabond glue in some facilities, which can decrease infection and avoid the need to remove sutures after infusion therapy is discontinued.

Tunneled catheters usually have sutures placed near the skin exit site, which are removed after the tunnel has healed. The incision over an implanted port pocket will have sutures until it has healed. After it is healed and when it is not accessed, no dressing is required. When an implanted port is accessed, the sterile occlusive dressing should cover the entire needle and site.

Sterile dressings used over the insertion site protect the skin and puncture site. For a short *peripheral* catheter, the transparent membrane dressings do not require routine changes. Short peripheral lines do not usually dwell longer than a few days, and as long as the dressing is dry, clean, and intact, it does not have

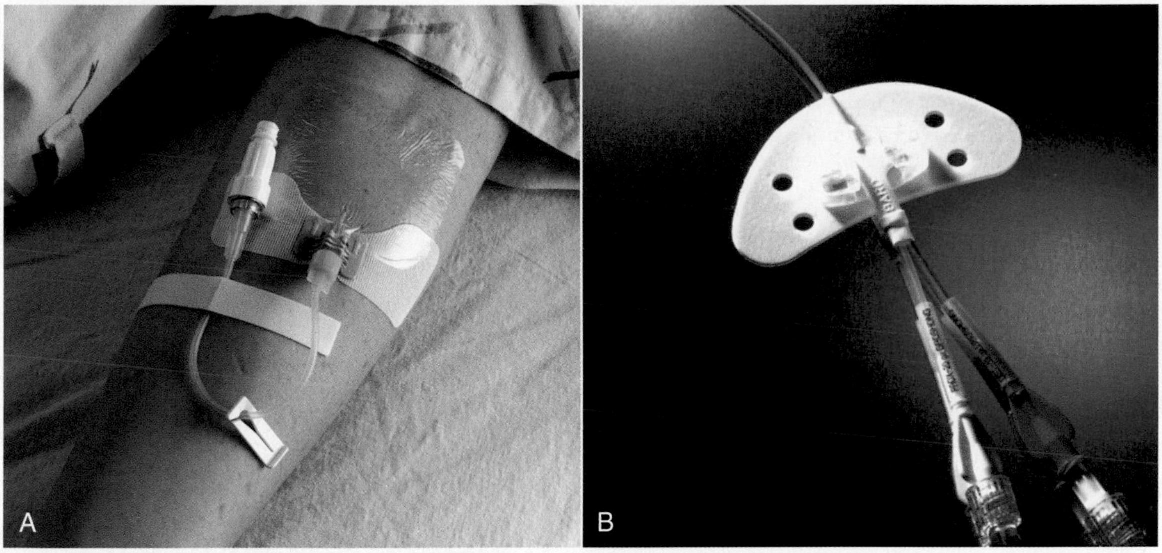

FIG. 13-14 The StatLock provides a standardized method to prevent catheter movement.

EVIDENCE-BASED PRACTICE QSEN

What is the Best Method for Securing a Patient's Peripheral IV Line?

Alekseyev, S., Byrne, M., Carpenter, A., Franker, C., Kidd, C., & Hulton, L. (2012). Prolonging the life of a patient's IV: An integrative review of intravenous securement devices. *MEDSURG Nursing, 21*(5), 285-292.

Intravenous catheter stabilization is recognized as an important intervention to maintain peripheral IV therapy. The researchers sought to answer this clinical question: What is the best device or method for securing a patient's IV to preserve its integrity and prevent migration and loss of access? A thorough literature search for available research was performed, and 13 articles were identified as usable for this review. Twelve of the reported studies found that manufactured catheter stabilization devices were preferred over traditional tape and surgical strips methods. Although most studies included use of the StatLock anchoring device, no one securement device was recommended. Studies of the StatLock device showed that it significantly improved peripheral IV survival rates and reduced complication rates. These findings reduced health care costs and staff time.

Level of Evidence: 1

This study used an integrative research review and analysis methodology to determine best practices for use of IV securement devices.

Commentary: Implications for Practice and Research

This research validated the effectiveness of manufactured IV catheter securement and stabilization devices for all patients receiving peripheral infusion therapy. These devices reduce the need for IV restarts, IV complications, and costs associated with IV therapy. Future studies are needed to determine which device(s) are the best to standardize care of patients receiving peripheral infusion therapy.

to be changed. Any VAD dressing should be changed when it is loose or soiled.

For central lines and midline catheters, tape and sterile gauze or a transparent membrane dressing may be used. Change tape and gauze dressings every 48 hours; change transparent membrane dressings, such as Tegaderm, every 5 to 7 days (INS, 2011). The initial dressing on a midline catheter or PICC is usually tape and gauze, changed within 24 hours after insertion because some bleeding is likely. Transparent membrane dressings can be used for subsequent dressing. For patients who develop erythema (redness) from Tegaderm, the IV3000 dressing from Smith and Nephew may be used. Document when you change the sterile dressing and your IV site assessments in the appropriate electronic health record according to agency policy.

! NURSING SAFETY PRIORITY QSEN

Action Alert

Site protection may be needed for short peripheral catheters or for port access needles. Plastic shields can be placed over the site to prevent accidental bumping or pressure from clothing. Make sure you can easily assess the site frequently. Never place a restraint or opaque dressing over a peripheral IV site, especially when infusing an irritant or vesicant.

When changing the dressing, remove it by pulling laterally from side to side. It can also be removed by holding the external catheter and pulling it off toward the insertion site. *Never pull it off by pulling away from the insertion site because this could dislodge the catheter!*

After removing the dressing from a midline catheter or any central venous catheter, note the external catheter length. Compare this length with the original length at insertion. If the length has changed, the catheter tip location has also changed and may no longer be in a vein appropriate for infusion. Follow agency policy or notify the health care provider about the length change. A chest x-ray may be needed, and careful assessment of the type of therapy and remaining length of therapy will likely be required.

Protect the external catheter, dressing, and all attached tubing from water because it is a source of contamination. *Remind unlicensed assistive personnel (UAP) to cover the extremity where the IV is located when giving the patient a bath.* A plastic bag or wrap can be taped over the extremity to keep the dressing and site dry.

CLINICAL JUDGMENT CHALLENGE

Evidence-Based Practice; Safety QSEN

A new graduate nurse is being oriented to your medical-surgical nursing unit. Today he is assigned to care for three patients. One patient is an older adult with an infiltrated peripheral IV in her forearm. The second patient has a PICC line for antibiotic therapy, and the third patient has an arterial implanted port for chemotherapy. As his preceptor, you are responsible for teaching him how to assess patients with these devices and prevent and/or monitor for complications. Your unit has several memory checklists for IV care that you plan to review with him.

1. What best clinical practices will you teach the new nurse about how to care for patients who have a PICC line?
2. For what life-threatening complication is the patient with the implanted port most at risk?
3. You observe the new nurse as he prepares to restart the IV for the older adult patient. He chooses a vein in the dorsum of the hand. What is your best response about his IV site selection?
4. What is the value of memory checklists to ensure consistency among nurses caring for patients receiving IV therapy?

Changing Administration Sets and Needleless Connectors

Plan the change of administration sets and fluid containers to occur at the same time, if possible, to minimize the number of times the system is opened. For short peripheral catheters, the administration set and catheter should also be changed at the same time to avoid excessive manipulation of the catheter. Document these changes per agency policy.

Needleless connector devices can be changed when the administration set is changed. If it is being used for intermittent infusions, the device should be changed at least once per week. Fluid leakage from the device indicates the integrity has been compromised, and it should be changed immediately.

Precautions to prevent *air emboli* are required when changing the set or connectors attached to any catheter; however, central venous catheters require special attention. Most catheters have a pinch clamp that can be closed during this procedure. Techniques used to increase the intrathoracic pressure and prevent air embolism during IV set change include:

- Placing the patient in a flat or Trendelenburg position to ensure that the catheter exit site is at or below the level of the heart
- Asking the patient to perform a Valsalva maneuver by holding his or her breath and bearing down
- Timing the IV set change to the expiratory cycle when the patient is spontaneously breathing
- Timing the IV set change to the inspiratory cycle when the patient is receiving positive-pressure mechanical ventilation

Controlling Infusion Pressure

Fluid flow through the infusion system requires that the pressure on the external side be greater than the pressure at the catheter tip. Fluid flow can be slowed or obstructed by many causes. Inside the catheter lumen, resistance is created by the catheter length and diameter or by deposits of fibrin, thrombus, or drug precipitate. Near the catheter tip, resistance to flow comes from the catheter tip impinging on the vein wall, thrombus, or venous spasm.

All catheter manufacturers have warnings about the use of excessive pressure. Gravity and infusion pumps do not exert pressure too high for the catheter to handle; however, excessive pressure from syringes can lead to catheter damage. For this reason, use 10-mL syringes for central venous catheters. Although these larger syringes generate less pressure, it is still possible to reach excessive pressure levels if great force is applied against a syringe attached to a catheter that is partially occluded.

Flushing the Catheter

Catheter flushing prevents contact between incompatible drugs and maintains patency of the lumens. Normal saline alone or normal saline followed by heparinized saline may be used. When using valved catheters and certain positive fluid-displacement needleless devices, normal saline alone is acceptable because these devices have mechanisms that prevent the backflow of blood into the catheter lumen.

NURSING SAFETY PRIORITY QSEN

Critical Rescue

Assess catheter patency carefully before each use. Use sterile technique to flush with normal saline while applying slow, gentle pressure to the syringe plunger. If you feel any resistance, stop the procedure immediately! If you continue, catheter rupture or forcing a blood clot into circulation could result. During the flushing procedure, always aspirate for a brisk blood return from the catheter lumen.

If the catheter will not yield a blood return, further diagnostic studies may be needed to determine the cause of the problems. Thrombolytic agents such as alteplase (Cathflo Activase) may be used to dissolve blood clots in venous catheters (Genentech, 2011).

For short peripheral catheters, usually 3 mL normal saline is adequate to flush the catheter. For all other catheters, 5 to 10 mL of preservative-free normal saline is needed. Bacteriostatic normal saline is limited to no more than 30 mL in a 24-hour period in adults. By using 10 mL before and after each dose of medication, it is easy to exceed this limitation. Check your agency's policy and procedure about specific flushing amounts.

Flush catheters immediately after each use. Delay in disconnecting the intermittent administration set and flushing the catheter could cause lumen occlusion from blood that backflows into the lumen when the infusion pressure is lower than venous pressure.

All fluids used to flush catheters should be obtained from single-dose containers or prefilled syringes. Vials used for multiple doses contribute to medication errors and increase the risk for contamination.

Obtaining Blood Samples from Central Venous Catheters

Short peripheral catheters should not be used routinely for obtaining blood samples. This additional manipulation could lead to vein irritation that requires removal of the catheter. Central venous catheters and midlines can be used for obtaining blood samples after a careful assessment of the risks versus the benefits. If your patient has no peripheral venipuncture sites or is fearful of needles, using the central venous catheter may be appropriate. The risks associated with obtaining blood samples from a central venous catheter are numerous. This procedure requires additional hub manipulation, which is a major cause of CR-BSI. Consider the laboratory tests needed and the types of fluids that have recently been infused. For

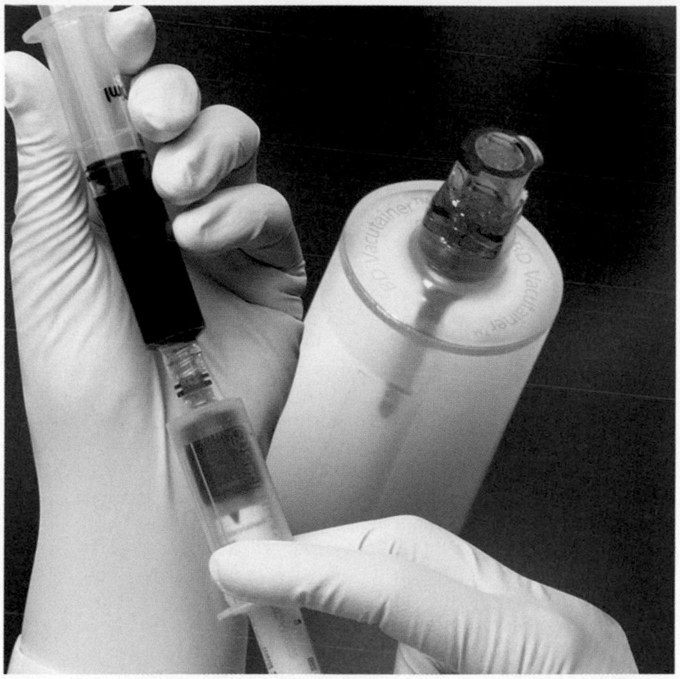

FIG. 13-15 Vacutainer needle holder prevents needle stick injuries when drawing blood.

example, heparin interferes with coagulation studies and electrolytes in the fluid may alter the results of serum electrolytes. Drawing blood from catheters for blood culture should not be done within an hour of completion of antimicrobial infusions (Garcia & Isenberg, 2010).

If blood sampling from a central venous catheter is the best alternative, vigorous cleaning of the connections with 70% alcohol is necessary. Use methods that do not require exposed needles. Vacuum tubes attached via a "vacutainer" to the catheter hub eliminate the need to transfer the blood from a syringe into the tubes. For small-diameter catheters, the vacuum in the tube may cause the catheter to temporarily collapse, preventing the backflow of blood into the tube. In this situation, small syringes should be used because they create less pressure on aspiration, the opposite of what small syringes do on injection. Transfer of the blood from the syringe to the vacuum tube requires the use of a "vacutainer needle holder." This device keeps the needle housed in a plastic case and covered, preventing needle stick injuries (Fig. 13-15). After blood draw from any catheter, a flush of 10 to 20 mL sterile normal saline is necessary to ensure a patent line. Be sure to clear the line and cap of blood to prevent a breeding ground for infection.

Removing the Vascular Access Device

To remove a short peripheral IV, lift opposite sides of the transparent dressing and pull laterally to remove the dressing from the site while stabilizing the catheter. Slowly withdraw the catheter from the skin, and immediately cover the puncture site with dry gauze. Hold pressure on the site until hemostasis is achieved. Assess the catheter tip to make sure it is intact and completely removed. Document the time of catheter removal and the appearance of the IV site.

Removal of midline catheters and PICCs must be performed with the same slow, gentle techniques used to insert the catheter. Veins can develop venospasms when rapid or forceful techniques are used. After explaining to the patient that this procedure will not be painful, remove the dressing and withdraw the catheter in short segments by pulling from the insertion site. *If you feel resistance, always stop and never apply force to the catheter. Extreme traction or force could cause the catheter to break and embolize (travel) to the heart or pulmonary circulation.*

Simple distraction techniques and deep breathing may be sufficient to relax the patient and remove the catheter. If these fail, replace the dressing and apply heat; allow time for the vein wall to relax. Keeping the extremity warm and dry and asking the patient to drink warm liquids could facilitate removal. Use of medications to relax the vein wall may be required if the catheter cannot be removed after several hours. Imaging studies may also be needed to determine whether the cause is a thrombosis instead of venospasm.

Nontunneled percutaneous central catheters are removed by clipping any sutures and withdrawing the catheter in short segments. Venospasm does not commonly occur when removing these catheters because the vein diameter is large.

To prevent venous air embolism when removing any central venous catheter (including PICCs), position the patient in a flat supine or Trendelenburg position according to agency policy. To ensure the intrathoracic pressure is higher than atmospheric pressure, have the patient hold his or her breath or perform a Valsalva maneuver during removal. If the patient is mechanically ventilated, time the removal to the delivery of an inhalation by the ventilator. Be sure to keep the catheter clamped during this procedure. When a central venous catheter is removed, a tract between the skin and vein may create a conduit that could allow air to be pulled into the vein.

After removal, measure the catheter length and compare it with the length documented on insertion. *If the entire catheter length was not removed, contact the health care provider immediately!* Removal of tunneled catheters and implanted ports is usually performed by nurse practitioners or physicians.

Documenting Intravenous Therapy

Intravenous therapy is risk prone. Nurses can protect themselves from malpractice claims with conscientious assessment, intervention, and documentation. Be sure you document after insertion of a vascular access device (VAD) and throughout the course of the therapy. When inserting a venous catheter, remember to document the:

- Date and time of the VAD insertion
- Name of the nurse (you) who inserted the VAD
- Vein that was used for insertion
- Type of VAD used
- Number of insertion attempts and locations of attempts before successful insertion
- Response of the patient to the VAD insertion process
- Type of dressing applied
- Type of securement device, if used
- Special barrier precautions used, if any
- Patient and family education provided related to IV therapy

During the course of the patient's infusion therapy, be sure to continue documenting in the electronic health record your assessments and any interventions needed as a result of complications. Follow your agency's policies and procedures for additional requirements.

COMPLICATIONS OF INTRAVENOUS THERAPY

Complications from IV therapy can be minor and limited or life threatening. Serious life-altering or life-threatening complications are dramatically increasing in frequency and severity and present a tremendous financial burden to the U.S. health care system. Catheter-related bloodstream INFECTION (CR-BSI) is one of the most serious problems, often resulting in patient death. They are more common in patients with central VADs but can also occur with peripheral catheters.

Catheter-Related Bloodstream Infection

The Institute for Healthcare Improvement identified catheter-related bloodstream INFECTION (CR-BSI) as one of several preventable hospital-acquired infections (HAIs). They report that CR-BSIs are responsible for up to 28,000 deaths per year. As part of their previous *100,000 Lives Campaign*, a number of evidence-based interventions were combined into the CR-BSI prevention bundle. As a nurse, your accountability is to ensure that these interventions are followed (Table 13-2).

Other Complications of Intravenous Therapy

Local complications of IV therapy occur at or near the catheter. A priority for care for patients with IV therapy is to prevent, assess, and detect these complications. In some cases, nurses also manage these problems. Definitions, causes, signs and symptoms, treatment, and prevention of local complications are summarized in Table 13-3. *Systemic complications* of IV therapy involve the entire vascular system or multiple systems.

TABLE 13-2 The Catheter-Related Bloodstream Infection (CR-BSI) Prevention Bundle

- Use a *checklist* during insertion to make sure everything is done correctly. Tell anyone who violates the correct steps to stop the procedure immediately.
- *Hand hygiene* before inserting a central line must be thorough (i.e., no quick scrub). Anyone who touches the central line must also perform thorough hand hygiene.
- *Maximal barrier precautions* during line insertion require that the patient be draped from head to toe with a sterile barrier.
- The health care provider who inserts the VAD wears sterile *gloves, gown, and mask.* Anyone in the room during the procedure must also wear a mask.
- *Traffic in and out of the room must be minimized.* Many institutions use a "stop" sign on the door of the room to prevent people from coming in and going out during the procedure and a special "central line cart" to ensure they have everything they need in the room.
- *Chlorhexidine is used for skin disinfection* because it has best outcomes for preventing infection.
- *Use preferred sites.* PICC in the upper arm and subclavian veins are the first choice. The next preference is the internal jugular vein, and the least preferred is the femoral vein.
- *Post-placement care* requires meticulous dressing changes and care of all parts of the IV system, such as keeping ports and stopcocks clean; hanging bags using sterile technique; vigorous scrub of catheter hub with alcohol when used.
- *Review daily the need* for the patient's VAD. The incidence of CR-BSI increases each day the device is in place. As soon as it is determined that the patient no longer needs the IV line, it should be removed.

PICC, Peripherally inserted central catheter; *VAD,* vascular access device.

TABLE 13-3 Local Complications of Intravenous Therapy

COMPLICATION	CAUSE	SIGNS AND SYMPTOMS	TREATMENT	PREVENTION
Infiltration Leakage of a non-vesicant IV solution or medication into the extravascular tissue	Peripheral catheter has punctured opposite vein wall Obstruction of blood flow causing backflow through original entrance site Inflammatory process causing fluid leakage at the capillary level Fibrin sheath fully encasing a central venous catheter leading to retrograde flow and leakage from venipuncture site Damaged septum of implanted port Dislodged port access needle	IV rate slows Increasing edema around site Patient report of skin tightness; blanching or coolness of skin; burning, tenderness, or general discomfort at the insertion site; fluid leaking from puncture site; absence of a blood return (though this may not be reliable with a short peripheral catheter)	Stop infusion and remove short peripheral catheter immediately after identification of problem. Apply sterile dressing if weeping from tissue occurs. Elevate extremity. Warm or cold compresses may be used according to the solution infiltrated and organizational policy. Warm compresses increase circulation to the area and speed healing. Cool compresses may be used to relieve discomfort and reduce swelling. Insert a new catheter in the opposite extremity. For all central venous catheters, obtain a study to determine the cause of the problem. For implanted port, remove and insert a new port access needle. Rate the infiltration using the INS Infiltration Scale and document (Table 13-7).	Catheter stabilization—use smallest catheter appropriate; avoid area of flexion, or use arm board. Avoid placing restraints at the IV site. Make successive venipunctures proximal to the previous site. Monitor site frequently; educate patient about activities and signs and symptoms. Central venous catheters—obtain a brisk blood return before using the catheter for infusion. Frequently assess proper positioning of port access needle. Stabilize it well, and protect from clothing.

TABLE 13-3 **Local Complications of Intravenous Therapy—cont'd**

COMPLICATION	CAUSE	SIGNS AND SYMPTOMS	TREATMENT	PREVENTION
Extravasation				
Leakage of a vesicant IV solution or medication into the extravascular tissue This can occur with both peripheral and central catheters	Same as for infiltration	Same as for infiltration Blistering and tissue sloughing may not appear for a few days and resolves over 1-4 wk with infiltration of some chemotherapeutic agents such as anthracycline and alkylating agents	Stop infusion, and disconnect administration set. Aspirate drug from short peripheral catheter or port access needle. Leave short peripheral catheter or port access needle in place to deliver antidote, if indicated by established policy. If possible, aspirate residual drug from the exit site of a central venous catheter. Administer antidote according to established policy. Apply cold compresses for all drugs EXCEPT vinca alkaloids and epipodophyllotoxins. Photograph site. Monitor at 24 hr, 1 wk, 2 wk, and as needed. Surgical interventions may be required. Provide written instructions to patient and family.	Same as for infiltration. Know the vesicant potential before giving any IV medication. Prevention is key.
Phlebitis				
Inflammation of the vein Post-infusion phlebitis presents within 48-96 hr after the catheter has been removed	Mechanical cause from insertion technique, catheter size, and lack of catheter securement Chemical cause from extremes of pH and/or osmolarity of the fluid or medication Bacterial cause from a break in aseptic technique, poor securement, and extended dwell time	Patient may report pain at the IV site; nurse may observe that vein appears red and inflamed along the length; vein may become hard and cordlike (Table 13-6)	Remove short peripheral catheter at the first sign of phlebitis; use warm compresses to relieve pain. Monitor frequently. Document using Phlebitis Scale. Insert a new catheter using the opposite extremity. Mechanical phlebitis occurring in the first week after PICC insertion may be treated without catheter removal. Apply continuous heat; rest and elevate the extremity. Significant improvement is seen in 24 hr, and complete resolution is seen within 72 hr. Remove catheter if treatment is unsuccessful.	Choose the smallest-gauge catheter for the required therapy. Avoid sites of joint flexion, or stabilize with an armboard. Avoid infusing fluids or medications with a pH below 5 or above 9 through a peripheral vein. Avoid infusing fluids or medications with a final osmolarity above 500 mOsm/L through a peripheral vein. Rotate sites every 72-96 hr according to established policy. Adequately secure the catheter. Use aseptic technique. For PICCs, teach patient to avoid excessive physical activity with the extremity.
Thrombosis				
Blood clot inside the vein	Anything that damages the endothelial lining of the intima can initiate clot formation Traumatic venipuncture Multiple venipuncture attempts Use of catheters too large for the chosen vein Hyper-coagulable state and venous stasis	Slowed or stopped infusion rate Swollen extremity Tenderness and redness Engorged peripheral veins of the ipsilateral chest and extremity	Stop infusion and remove short peripheral catheter immediately. Apply cold compresses to decrease blood flow and stabilize the clot. Elevate extremity. Surgical intervention may be required. For central venous catheters, notify the physician and obtain requests for a diagnostic study. Low-dose thrombolytic agents can be used to lyse the clot.	Use evidence-based venipuncture technique. Make only two attempts to perform venipuncture. Choose the smallest-gauge catheter in the largest vein possible. Secure catheter adequately. Use armboards if short peripheral catheters are placed in areas of joint flexion. Ensure adequate hydration to avoid changes in blood composition and flexion of the extremity. Prophylactic low-dose warfarin (Coumadin, Warfilone🍁) may be prescribed for patients with a central venous catheter.

Continued

TABLE 13-3 Local Complications of Intravenous Therapy—cont'd

COMPLICATION	CAUSE	SIGNS AND SYMPTOMS	TREATMENT	PREVENTION
Thrombophlebitis				
The presence of a blood clot and vein inflammation	Same as for phlebitis and thrombosis	Same as for phlebitis and thrombosis	Same as for phlebitis and thrombosis. Apply cold compresses initially, followed by warm.	Same as for phlebitis and thrombosis.
Ecchymosis and Hematoma				
Ecchymosis results from infiltration of blood into the surrounding tissue Hematoma results from uncontrolled bleeding	Unskilled or multiple IV insertion attempts Patients with coagulopathy or fragile veins (e.g., older adults and patients on steroids) Accidental laceration of a large vein or artery	Swelling Bruising Pain or tenderness	When removing device, apply light pressure; excessive pressure could cause other fragile veins in the area to rupture. For hematoma, apply direct pressure until bleeding has stopped. Elevate extremity, apply ice for first 24 hours, and then warm compress for comfort.	Avoid veins that cannot be easily seen or palpated. Use extra caution in patients with coagulopathies. Use evidence-based venipuncture technique.
Site Infection				
Invasion of microorganisms at the insertion site in the absence of simultaneous bloodstream infection Infection localized at the insertion site, the port pocket, or subcutaneous tunnel	Break in aseptic technique during insertion or the handling of sterile equipment Lack of proper hand hygiene and skin antisepsis	Site appears red, swollen, and warm; patient may report tenderness at the site; may observe purulent or malodorous exudates	Clean exit site with alcohol, expressing drainage if present. For short peripheral catheter, midline catheter, or PICC, remove using sterile technique and avoid contact between skin and catheter. Send catheter tip for culture, if requested. Clean site with alcohol, and cover with dry sterile dressing; physician to evaluate for septic phlebitis and need for antimicrobial therapy or surgical intervention.	Use strict aseptic technique when inserting, maintaining, or removing catheters. Practice evidence-based hand hygiene. Ensure dressing remains clean, dry, and adherent to skin at all times.
Venous Spasm				
A sudden contraction of the vein	A normal response to irritation or injury of the vein wall	Cramping or pain at or above the insertion site Numbness in the area Slowing of the infusion rate Inability to withdraw midline catheter or PICC	Temporarily slow infusion rate. Apply warm compress. Do not immediately remove short peripheral catheter. If occurring during midline catheter or PICC removal, do not apply tension or attempt forceful removal. Reapply a dressing, apply heat, encourage patient to drink warm liquids, and keep extremity covered and dry. 12-24 hr may be required before catheter can be removed.	Allow time for vein diameter to return to normal after tourniquet removal and before advancing catheter. Infuse fluids at room temperature, if possible. For a midline catheter or PICC, gently withdraw the catheter in short segments.
Nerve Damage				
Inadvertent piercing or complete transection of a nerve	Venipuncture near known nerve locations Unanticipated nerve locations	Reports of tingling or feeling "pins and needles" at or below the insertion site Numbness at or near the insertion site	Immediately stop the insertion procedure if the patient reports extreme pain. Remove the catheter if reports of discomfort do not improve when the catheter is secured.	Avoid using the cephalic vein near the wrist. Avoid using veins on the palm side of the wrist. Adequately secure the catheter, but avoid tape that is too tight. Support areas of joint flexion with an armboard.

INS, Infusion Nurses Society; *PICC*, peripherally inserted central catheter.

TABLE 13-4 **Systemic Complications of Intravenous Therapy**

COMPLICATION	CAUSE	SIGNS AND SYMPTOMS	TREATMENT	PREVENTION
Circulatory Overload				
Disruption of fluid homeostasis with excess fluid in the circulatory system	Infusion of fluids at a rate greater than the patient's system can accommodate	Patient may report shortness of breath and cough; patient's blood pressure is elevated, and there is puffiness around the eyes and edema in dependent areas; patient's neck veins may be engorged, and nurse may hear moist breath sounds.	Slow the IV rate, and notify physician; raise patient to an upright position; monitor vital signs, and administer oxygen as prescribed; administer diuretics as prescribed.	Monitor intake and output carefully, and notify physician as soon as an imbalance is noticed between the patient's intake and output.
Speed Shock				
Systemic reaction to the rapid infusion of a substance unfamiliar to the patient's circulatory system	Rapid infusion of drugs or bolus infusion, which causes the drug to reach toxic levels quickly	Patient may report lightheadedness or dizziness and chest tightness; nurse may note that patient has a flushed face and an irregular pulse; without intervention, patient may lose consciousness and go into shock and cardiac arrest.	Immediately discontinue the drug infusion and hang isotonic solution to keep the vein open; monitor vital signs carefully, and notify physician for further treatments.	Be aware of the appropriate infusion rate of medications and adhere to them; use of infusion control devices assists in prevention of speed shock.
Catheter Embolism				
A shaving or piece of catheter breaks off and floats freely in the vessel	Anything that damages the catheter—during insertion, dressing change, excessive force with flushing or medication administration	Depending on where the catheter embolizes, this could be life threatening. Cardiopulmonary arrest could occur.	Emergently notify the physician. Remove the catheter, and apply a tourniquet high on the limb of the catheter site; inspect catheter to determine how much may have embolized; an x-ray is taken to determine the presence of any catheter piece; surgical intervention may be necessary.	When inserting over-the-needle catheters, never reinsert the needle into the catheter; avoid pulling a through-the-needle catheter back through the needle during insertion. Avoid scissors near the catheter with dressing changes.

Information on common systemic complications can be found in Table 13-4. For central venous catheters (CVCs), complications can occur during the insertion procedure or during the dwell time (Table 13-5). Tables 13-6 and 13-7 are the INS criteria for grading phlebitis and infiltrations. Document all assessments and complications in the patient's electronic health record. Notify the infusion therapy team and/or health care provider per agency policy when complications occur.

IV THERAPY AND CARE OF THE OLDER ADULT

The aging process causes numerous changes in all body functions, and yet aging occurs differently in each person. Nutrition, environment, genetics, social factors, and education are just a few of the factors that influence the older adult's needs. Because all body functions are affected, IV therapy can be affected by these changes.

Skin Care

Aging skin becomes thinner and loses subcutaneous fat, decreasing the skin's ability for thermal regulation. Fewer nerve endings mean the decreased ability to feel pain. Older patients *may* not perceive acute pain from traumatic venipuncture requiring excessive probing or multiple attempts. However, this action increases the risk for fluid leakage and subsequent infiltration or extravasation injury. Inserting and removing a catheter and dressing could tear the skin layers.

Skin antisepsis is extremely important because of the decreased immunity seen as part of the aging process. Lipids are normally found in skin as a protective agent, and alcohol easily dissolves lipids. Although greater numbers of organisms may be killed, the skin can also become excessively dry and cracked. Current recommendations call for using friction when cleaning the skin to penetrate the layers of the epidermis. However, excessive friction may damage fragile skin and cause impaired TISSUE INTEGRITY. Chlorhexidine is the preferred agent, and the product currently available contains alcohol. Check for allergies to iodine before using iodine or iodophors. Iodophors such as povidone-iodine require contact with the skin for a minimum of 2 minutes to be effective. All antiseptic solutions must be thoroughly dry before applying the dressing or tape.

Skin should never be shaved before venipuncture, but excessive amounts of hair should be clipped. Shaving causes microabrasions that can lead to infection. The skin of an older adult may be more delicate and therefore more easily nicked while shaving.

Skin and TISSUE INTEGRITY can easily be compromised by the application of tape or dressings. Use of skin protectant solutions puts a protective barrier between the skin and dressing and improves the adherence of the dressing to the skin. Removal of tape and dressings may require adhesive remover solutions, or an alcohol pad may accomplish the same purpose. Securement devices like the StatLock require the use of a skin

TABLE 13-5 Complications During the Dwell of Central Venous Catheters

COMPLICATION	POSSIBLE CAUSES	SIGNS AND SYMPTOMS	TREATMENT	PREVENTION
Catheter Migration				
Movement of a properly placed catheter tip to another vein No change in the external catheter length	Changes in intrathoracic pressure caused by coughing, vomiting, sneezing, heavy lifting, and congestive heart failure	For migration to the jugular vein: reports of hearing a running stream or gurgling sound on the side of catheter insertion For migration to the azygos vein: back pain between the shoulder blades Neurologic complications if medications are infused	Stop all infusions, and flush catheter. Notify physician. Obtain a chest radiograph, if required, to assess tip location. Spontaneous repositioning back to the SVC is possible. Repositioning by radiology may be required.	Place catheter tip properly in the lower third of the SVC near the junction with the right atrium. Instruct patient to perform usual ADLs but to avoid excessive physical activity.
Catheter Dislodgment				
Movement of catheter into or out of the insertion site	Inadequate catheter securement Excessive physical activity with a PICC	External catheter length has changed, also changing the internal tip location No other signs or symptoms may be immediately noticed	Stop all infusions, and flush catheter. NEVER re-advance the catheter into the insertion site. Determine the amount of external catheter length, and compare with the length documented on insertion. Notify the physician or nurse inserting the catheter for further assessment.	Use proper catheter securement device. Instruct patient to perform normal ADLs but to avoid excessive physical activity.
Catheter Rupture				
Catheter is broken, damaged, or separated from hub or port body	Forcefully flushing a catheter with any size syringe against resistance Using scissors to remove a dressing Catheter compression of a subclavian inserted catheter between the clavicle and first rib (also known as *pinch-off syndrome*)	Fluid leaking from insertion site Pain or swelling during infusion Reflux of blood into the catheter extension Inability to aspirate blood from catheter	Repair the damaged segment; depends on the availability of a repair kit designed for the specific brand of catheter being used; repair may be considered a temporary measure instead of a permanent treatment. Remove catheter.	NEVER use excessive force when flushing a catheter, regardless of syringe size. On injection, small syringes generate more pressure than larger syringes. Use of a 10-mL syringe is generally recommended for flushing procedures. Insert catheter through jugular or upper extremity sites instead of subclavian site.
Lumen Occlusion				
Catheter lumen is partially or totally blocked	Drug or mineral precipitate (calcium, diazepam, and phenytoin are common) Lipid sludge from long-term infusion of fat emulsion Blood clots and fibrin sheath caused by blood reflux into lumen Allowing administration sets to remain connected for extended periods after medication has infused	Infusion stops, or pump alarm sounds Inability or difficulty administering fluids Inability or difficulty drawing blood Increased resistance to flushing of the catheter	Assess history of catheter use. A suddenly developing problem may indicate contact between incompatible medications. A problem that develops over an extended period may indicate a gradual clot formation. For drug precipitate, determine the pH of the precipitated drug. Use hydrochloric acid for acidic drug. Use sodium bicarbonate for alkaline drugs. For blood clot, use thrombolytic enzymes such as alteplase.	Always flush with normal saline between, before, and after each medication given through the catheter. Use positive-pressure flushing techniques when a negative fluid displacement needleless connector is being used. Use a positive fluid displacement needleless connector. Flush catheters immediately when medication infusion is complete.
Catheter-Related Bloodstream Infection (CR-BSI)				
Pathogenic organisms invade the patient's circulation The CDC has specific criteria to classify these infections	Lack of sterile field during insertion Inadequate skin antiseptic agents and application techniques Manipulation of the catheter hub leading to intraluminal contamination Inadequate hand hygiene Long dwell time	Early symptoms include fever, chills, headache, and general malaise	Change the entire infusion system from solution to IV device; notify physician, obtain cultures, and administer antibiotics as prescribed. If the infusate is the suspected cause, send a specimen to the laboratory for evaluation.	Maintain sterile technique. Use the recommended CR-BSI prevention bundle.

CDC, Centers for Disease Control and Prevention; *PICC,* peripherally inserted central catheter; *SVC,* superior vena cava.

TABLE 13-6 Phlebitis Scale from INS Standards of Practice

GRADE	CLINICAL CRITERIA
0	No symptoms
1	Erythema with or without pain
2	Pain at access site with erythema and/or edema
3	Pain at access site with erythema and/or edema Streak formation Palpable cord
4	Pain at access site with erythema and/or edema Streak formation Palpable venous cord more than 1 inch long Purulent drainage

Data from Infusion Nurses Society (INS). (2011). Infusion nursing standards of practice. *Journal of Infusion Nursing, 34(IS),* S8.

TABLE 13-7 Infiltration Scale from INS Standards of Practice

GRADE	CLINICAL CRITERIA
0	No symptoms
1	Skin blanched Edema <1 inch in any direction Cool to touch With or without pain
2	Skin blanched Edema 1-6 inches in any direction Cool to touch With or without pain
3	Skin blanched, translucent Gross edema >6 inches in any direction Cool to touch Mild to moderate pain Possible numbness
4	Skin blanched, translucent Skin tight, leaking Skin discolored, bruised, swollen Gross edema >6 inches in any direction Deep pitting tissue edema Circulatory impairment Moderate to severe pain Infiltration of any amount of blood product, irritant, or vesicant

Data from Infusion Nurses Society (INS). (2011). *Standards of Practice*, Norwood, MA.

protectant (e.g., Skin-Prep) before applying the device. The protectant prevents skin tearing when the device is removed.

Vein and Catheter Selection

Vein and catheter selection are of highest importance in older adults. Choose insertion sites carefully after considering the patient's skin integrity, vein condition, and functional ability. The general principle of starting with the most distal sites usually indicates use of hand veins. *However, avoid fragile skin and small, tortuous veins on the back of the hand (dorsum); select the initial IV site higher on the arm.*

Venous distention must be accomplished with a flat tourniquet; however, the veins may require longer to adequately distend. Allowing a tourniquet to remain in place for extended periods causes an overfilling of the vein and can result in a hematoma when the vein is punctured. On extremely fragile skin, the tourniquet application can lead to ecchymotic areas or skin tears. Protect the skin by placing a wash cloth or the patient's gown between the skin and tourniquet. A tourniquet may not be required in veins that are already distended; however, carefully palpate these veins to determine their condition. Avoid hard, cordlike veins. Blood pressure cuffs can also be used for venous distention. Inflate the cuff and release until the pressure is slightly less than diastolic pressure. Other methods to distend veins include:

- Tapping lightly, but avoiding forceful slapping
- Asking the patient to open and close the fist so the muscles can force blood into the veins, making sure the hand is relaxed when the venipuncture is attempted
- Placing the extremity lower than the heart
- Applying warm compresses or a heating pad (be careful not to make it too hot) to the entire extremity for 10 to 20 minutes and removing just before making the venipuncture

As with all patients, venipuncture technique requires adequate skin and vein stabilization during the puncture and complete catheter advancement. Veins of an older adult are more likely to roll away from the needle. Low angles of 10 to 15 degrees between the skin and catheter will improve your success with venipuncture.

As soon as the catheter enters the vein, it may be necessary to release the tourniquet. Release of venous pressure from the puncture can lead to ecchymosis. Allowing the tourniquet to remain in place during the complete catheter advancement could increase this problem.

! NURSING SAFETY PRIORITY QSEN

Action Alert

Catheter securement may mean that administration sets are placed out of easy reach of a confused patient. Use flexible netting over the extremity to help prevent the patient from pulling at the dressing or tubing, while allowing easy access to the site. A device such as the I.V. House UltraDressing shown in Fig. 13-16 can also protect the site. Do not use rolled bandages to cover the extremity because they prevent insertion site assessment. Complications may progress to an advanced state before they are noticed.

Choosing a midline catheter or PICC may be best in older patients with poor skin turgor, limited venous sites, or veins that are fragile, tortuous, or hard. These catheters are placed in the upper extremity where venous distention techniques can be used. Inserting nontunneled percutaneous central catheters in older adults can be much more challenging. Venous distention for insertion requires the Trendelenburg position and a well-hydrated patient. FLUID volume deficit prevents adequate distention of the subclavian or jugular veins. Patients with conditions like chronic obstructive pulmonary disease and kyphosis cannot tolerate the Trendelenburg position. Tunneled catheters and implanted ports may be appropriate after considering the surgical techniques required to insert these catheters.

Cardiac and Renal Changes

Because of changes in cardiac and renal status in older adults, the accuracy of infusion volume and flow rate measurements is

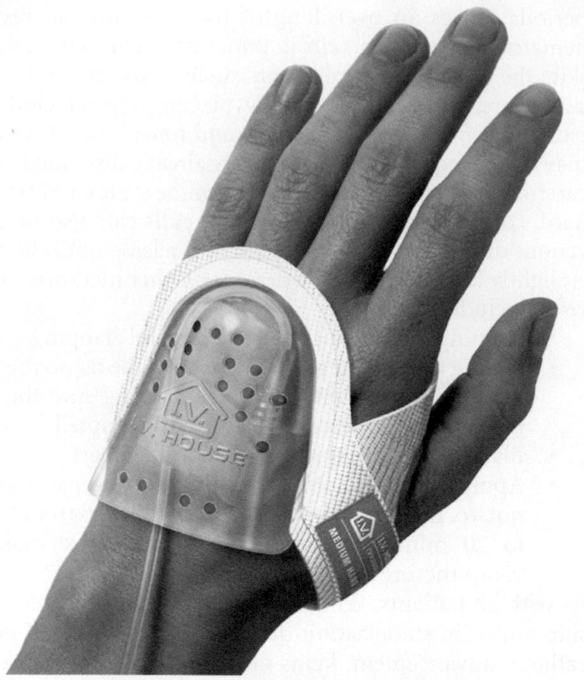

FIG. 13-16 I.V. House UltraDressing IV site protector, a safety device used for IV site protection, guards the integrity of the older adult's skin while helping secure the site.

CLINICAL JUDGMENT CHALLENGE

Patient-Centered Care; Teamwork and Collaboration; Informatics QSEN

A 63-year-old obese, diabetic woman is transferred from the hospital to the skilled nursing facility (SNF) where you work as a charge nurse. The resident is being managed with IV cefoxitin 2 g IV piggyback (IVPB) every 8 hours for osteomyelitis resulting from an arterial foot ulcer. On review of her admission orders, you note that she has a newly inserted intermittent saline lock in her right forearm and is prescribed to receive the antibiotic for 4 more weeks.

1. The SNF policy for administration of drugs prescribed every 8 hours is a 6 PM–2 AM–10 AM schedule. Would you schedule her antibiotic at these times? Why or why not?
2. Two days later as you are planning to end your shift, the resident reports that her IV site seems red and swollen. What action will you take at this time? What will you document on the resident's electronic health record?
3. Is a peripheral vascular access device (VAD) the best choice for this resident? Why or why not? With whom will you or the oncoming nurse collaborate to make this decision? What does the evidence say about the type of VAD that would be best to meet this resident's needs? Where would you go to find the answer to this clinical question?
4. Using the SBAR technique, what will you report to the oncoming nurse about the resident's IV complications?

very important in the older adult. The health care provider's prescription for infusion therapy should be assessed for appropriateness for the patient's condition. Older adults are very prone to FLUID overload and resulting congestive heart failure. Electronic controlling devices may be required to ensure the necessary accuracy. Clinical manifestations of fluid overload are described in Chapter 11.

When fluid restrictions are required, medications could be diluted in small quantities and delivered using a syringe pump or a manual IV push. Consult with a pharmacist to determine the smallest amount of diluent required. This alternative may allow the patient to have more fluid to drink. Serum sodium levels should be considered when normal saline is routinely used for dilution in patients with hypertension or cardiac problems.

An increasing number of patients with chronic illness require repeated and frequent IV therapies. Many of these patients are vein depleted and need vein preservation. Subcutaneous and intraosseous routes have demonstrated effectiveness in emergency resuscitation. These procedures may also be beneficial for routine infusion of isotonic, non-irritant, non-vesicant solutions in patients with chronic illness and vein depletion (Aguiar, 2010).

Specific therapies requiring infusion into arteries and peritoneal, epidural, and intrathecal space are also available. These therapies are most commonly used to administer chemotherapy, lytic therapy, or pain medication.

SUBCUTANEOUS INFUSION THERAPY

Subcutaneous infusion therapy has been used for a variety of drug infusions. Most commonly it is used for administration of pain medications and insulin therapy. It is beneficial for palliative care patients who cannot tolerate oral medications, when IM injections are too painful, or when vascular access is not available or is too difficult to obtain.

Hypodermoclysis or "clysis" involves the slow infusion of isotonic FLUIDS into the patient's subcutaneous tissue. Although common in the early twentieth to mid-twentieth century, this method had not been widely used again until the 1990s. The growth of geriatric and palliative health care has helped spur the use of this method of infusion therapy for selected patients (Scales, 2011).

Hypodermoclysis can be used for short-term FLUID volume replacement. The patient must have sufficient sites of intact skin without INFECTION, inflammation, bruising, scarring, or edema. The most common sites are the front and sides of the thighs and hips, the upper abdomen, and the area under the clavicle. Unlike IV therapy, the upper extremities should not be used because fluid is absorbed more readily from sites with larger stores of adipose tissue. Hypodermoclysis is not appropriate for emergency resuscitations and should not be used if the fluid replacement needs exceed 2000 to 3000 mL/day and should not exceed 1500 mL/day at any single infusion site (Scales, 2011).

Hyaluronidase may be ordered by the health care provider and is mixed with each liter of infusion fluid. This substance is an enzyme that improves the absorption of the infusion from the subcutaneous tissue (Connolly et al., 2011; INS, 2011).

A small-gauge (25 to 27) winged infusion or "butterfly" needle, a small-gauge short peripheral catheter, or an infusion set specially designed for subcutaneous infusion can be chosen. The subcutaneous infusion sets have a small needle extending at a right angle from a flat disk that helps stabilize the needle.

When choosing the infusion site, consider the patient's level of activity. The area under the clavicle or the abdomen prevents difficulty with ambulation. Clip excess hair in the area, and clean the chosen site with the antiseptic solution, preferably 2% chlorhexidine gluconate in 70% isopropyl alcohol to prevent infection (Candon et al., 2010). Prime the infusion tubing and the attached subcutaneous infusion set or winged needle. Gently pinch an area of about 2 inches (5 cm), and insert the needle using sterile technique. After securing the needle, cover the site with a transparent dressing. Flow rates for hydration fluids begin at 30 mL/hr. After 1 hour, the rate can be increased if the patient has experienced no discomfort. The maximum rate is usually 2 mL/min or 120 mL/hr. Assess the site every 4 hours while in a hospital setting and at least twice daily while at home. Redness, warmth, leakage, bruising, swelling, and reports of pain indicate tissue irritation and possible impaired tissue integrity. If these symptoms occur, remove the infusion needle. Rotate the site at least once a week. More frequent rotation may be needed depending on TISSUE INTEGRITY (INS, 2011).

Other complications include pooling of the fluid at the insertion site and an uneven fluid drip rate. Both of these problems may be resolved by restarting the infusion in another location. An infusion pump may also be used. Small ambulatory infusion pumps can be used to allow for greater mobility.

INTRAOSSEOUS INFUSION THERAPY

Intraosseous (IO) therapy allows access to the rich vascular network in the red marrow of bones. Although IO has previously been regarded as a pediatric procedure, it is now considered acceptable for use in adults. Victims of trauma, burns, cardiac arrest, diabetic ketoacidosis, and other life-threatening conditions benefit from this therapy because often clinicians cannot access these patients' vascular systems for traditional IV therapy (Aguiar, 2010). Intraosseous catheters may be established in the prehospital setting when IV access cannot be readily obtained in an emergency.

Absorption rates of large-volume parenteral (LVP) infusions and drugs administered via the IO route are similar to those achieved with peripheral or central venous administration. The IO route should be used only during the immediate period of resuscitation and should not be used longer than 24 hours (Aguiar, 2010). After establishing access, efforts should continue to obtain IV access as well.

There are few contraindications for intraosseous infusion. The only absolute contraindication is fracture in the bone to be used as a site. Conditions such as severe osteoporosis, osteogenesis imperfecta, or other conditions that increase the risk for fracture with insertion of the IO needle and skin infection over the site may also be contraindications for some patients. Repeated attempts to access the same site should be avoided (Madigan, 2008).

Any needle could be used to provide therapy and access the medullary space (marrow). However, 15- or 16-gauge needles specifically designed for IO are preferred. New technology using a battery-powered drill has improved the ease of IO insertion. A number of sites can be used, including the proximal tibia (tibial tuberosity), distal femur, medial malleolus (inner ankle), proximal humerus, and iliac crest. The proximal tibia is the most common site accessed for IO therapy (Fig. 13-17).

If IV access cannot be obtained within the first few minutes of resuscitation procedures, IO may be attempted. The leg is restrained, and the site is cleaned with an antiseptic agent such as chlorhexidine. After successful insertion, the needle must be secured to prevent movement out of the bone. The same doses of fluids and medications can be infused IO as IV. An infusion pump may be used for rapid flow rates.

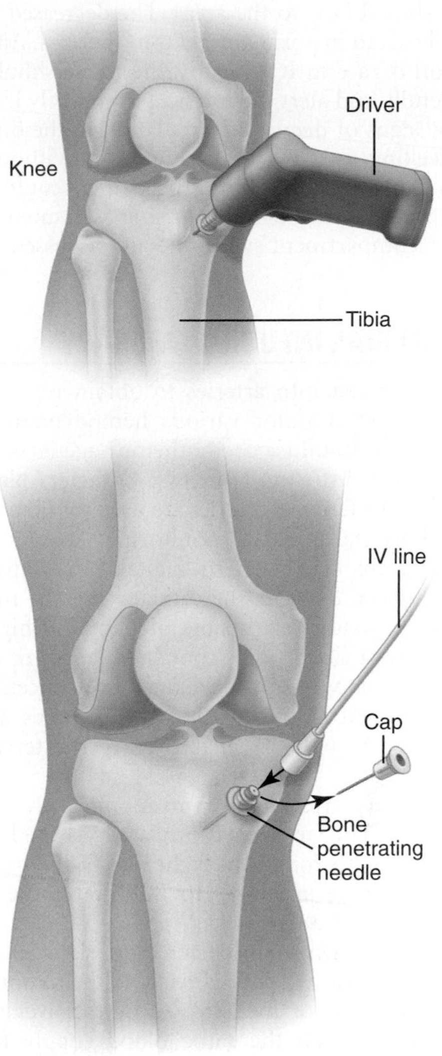

FIG. 13-17 Proximal tibial intraosseous (IO) access.

During the procedure, most patients rate the pain as a 2 or 3 on a scale of 0 to 10. Lidocaine 1% is used to anesthetize the skin, the subcutaneous tissue, and the periosteum to promote comfort (Madigan, 2008). Pain is also reported during the initial infusion. This may be reduced by injecting 0.5 mg/kg of preservative-free lidocaine through the intraosseous port before initiating the infusion (Phillips et al., 2010).

Improper needle placement with infiltration into the surrounding tissue is the most common complication of IO therapy. An accumulation of fluid under the skin at either the insertion site or on the other side of the limb indicates that the needle either is not far enough in to penetrate the bone marrow or is too far into the limb and has protruded through the other side of the shaft. Needle obstruction occurs when the puncture has been accomplished but flushing has been delayed. This delay may cause the needle to become clotted with bone marrow.

Osteomyelitis is an unusual but serious complication of IO therapy. You can help prevent this with meticulous aseptic technique, hand hygiene, and removal of the catheter as soon as it is no longer needed.

Compartment syndrome is a condition in which increased tissue pressure in a confined anatomic space causes decreased

PERFUSION (blood flow to the area). The decreased circulation to the area leads to hypoxia and pain in the area. Although the complication is rare in IO therapy, the nurse should monitor the site carefully and alert the physician promptly if the patient exhibits any signs of decreased circulation to the limb, such as coolness, swelling, mottling, or discoloration. Without improvement in PERFUSION to the limb, the patient could ultimately require amputation of the limb. Nursing assessment and interventions for compartment syndrome are discussed in detail in Chapter 51.

INTRA-ARTERIAL INFUSION THERAPY

Catheters are placed into arteries to obtain repeated arterial blood samples, to monitor various hemodynamic pressures continuously, and to infuse chemotherapy agents or fibrinolytics (**intra-arterial infusion therapy**). Catheters placed in the radial, brachial, or femoral arteries are used for obtaining blood samples and arterial pressure monitoring. Arterial waveforms and pressures are converted to digital values displayed on attached monitors. Between the catheter and the monitor is a special administration set capable of handling high infusion pressure, a pressurized fluid container, a continuous flush attachment, a three-way stopcock, and a transducer. The transducer is positioned at the level of the patient's atrium and secured to an IV pole to enable correct arterial pressure measurements.

The pulmonary artery is used to monitor pressures in the heart and lungs. This artery is cannulated via the large central venous system and through the right side of the heart. Hemodynamic monitoring and how to interpret these values are described in Chapter 38.

Chemotherapy agents administered arterially allow infusion of a high concentration of drug directly to the tumor site before it is diluted in blood or metabolized by the liver or kidneys. Drug infusion through the same blood supply feeding the tumor optimizes cell destruction at the tumor site while minimizing systemic side effects. The most common arterial sites include the hepatic and celiac arteries for liver tumors, although the carotid artery for tumors of the head, neck, or brain and pelvic arteries for cervical tumors have been used. Arterial catheter insertion can be performed through the skin via a surgical procedure or by an interventional radiologist. Implanted ports are commonly used for extended therapies. For short-term therapy, an external catheter may be used for 3 to 7 days, although the risks for complications increase during dwell time.

! NURSING SAFETY PRIORITY QSEN

Critical Rescue

Carefully secure all junctions on the administration sets with Luer-Lok devices. Life-threatening hemorrhage can occur if an accidental disconnection occurs! When an infusion pump is used, be sure that it has a pressure high enough to overcome arterial pressure. Closely monitor the arterial insertion site and affected extremity. Assess the extremity for warmth, sensation, capillary refill, and pulse.

When the carotid artery is involved, perform neurologic assessments. When a femoral catheter is used, apply antiembolic stockings or other measures to prevent deep vein thrombosis. Complications from arterial catheters are similar to those from venous catheters, including infection, bleeding from the insertion site, hemorrhage from a catheter disconnection, catheter migration, infiltration, and catheter lumen or arterial occlusion. Specialized training is required to manage patients with arterial catheters.

INTRAPERITONEAL INFUSION THERAPY

Intraperitoneal (IP) infusion therapy is the administration of chemotherapy agents into the peritoneal cavity. IP therapy is used to treat intra-abdominal malignancies such as ovarian and gastrointestinal tumors that have moved into the peritoneum after surgery.

Catheters used for IP therapy may be an implanted port for long-term treatment or an external catheter for temporary use. These catheters, including those attached to an implanted port, have large internal lumens with multiple side-holes along the catheter length to allow for delivery of large quantities of fluid. Administration of IP therapy includes three phases: the instillation phase; the dwell phase, usually 1 to 4 hours; and the drain phase. Because this treatment involves the delivery of biohazardous agents, additional competency is required to handle the infusion properly.

The patient should be in the semi-Fowler's position for the infusion. He or she may experience nausea and vomiting caused by increasing pressure on the internal organs from the infusing fluid. Pressure on the diaphragm may cause respiratory distress. Reducing the flow rate and treatment with antiemetic drugs may be needed. Severe pain may indicate that the catheter has migrated, and an abdominal x-ray is needed to determine its location.

During the dwell and drainage phases, the patient may need assistance in frequently moving from side to side to distribute the fluid evenly around the abdominal cavity. After the fluid has drained, the catheter is flushed with normal saline, although heparinized saline may be used in implanted ports. Catheter lumen occlusion is caused by the formation of fibrous sheaths or fibrin clots or plugs inside the catheter or around the tip.

Exit site INFECTION, indicated by redness, tenderness, and warmth of the tissue around the catheter, can occur. Microbial peritonitis and inflammation of the peritoneal membranes from the invasion of microorganisms are other complications. If peritonitis occurs, the patient may experience a fever and report abdominal pain. Abdominal rigidity and rebound tenderness may be present. This condition is preventable by using strict aseptic technique in the handling of all equipment and infusion supplies. Management includes antimicrobial therapy administered either IV or intraperitoneally.

INTRASPINAL INFUSION THERAPY

The spinal column is covered by three layers: the dura mater, or outermost covering; the arachnoid, or middle layer; and the pia mater, which is closest to the spinal cord. Two spaces used for infusion are the **epidural** space between the dura mater and vertebrae and the **subarachnoid** space. The epidural space consists of fat, connective tissue, and blood vessels that protect the spinal cord. Medications infused into the epidural space must diffuse through the dura mater, and there is the possibility that some drug will be absorbed systemically. **Intrathecal** medications are infused into the subarachnoid space and directly into the cerebral spinal fluid, allowing reduced doses (McHugh et al., 2012). Care of patients with these therapies requires competency training and validation.

Postoperative and chronic pain is the primary indication for epidural infusion (see Chapter 3). Opioids administered epidurally slowly diffuse across the dura mater to the dorsal horn of the spinal cord. They lock onto receptors and block pain impulses from ascending to the brain. The patient receives pain relief from the level of the injection caudally (toward the toes). Local anesthetics administered epidurally work on the sensory nerve roots in the epidural space to block pain impulses. The physician administers the first dose of medication; then, depending on state law, the type of medication, and facility policies, nurses trained in epidural therapy may administer subsequent doses.

Intrathecal infusion of chemotherapy has been used for treating central nervous system (CNS) cancers. The belief was that lower total body doses delivered directly to the tumor would help prevent side effects. However, more recent studies have linked intrathecal infusion of methotrexate with increased neuromuscular impairments in acute lymphoblastic leukemia (ALL) survivors (Ness et al., 2012). Intrathecal infusion has also been used to manage chronic pain and to treat spasticity of neurologic diseases such as cerebral palsy, multiple sclerosis, reflex sympathetic dystrophy, and traumatic and anoxic acquired brain injuries (Hayek et al., 2011; McHugh et al., 2012).

A temporary catheter used for epidural therapy can be a percutaneous catheter that is secured at the site and extends up the back toward the shoulder. These catheters are used for postoperative pain management and usually dwell for only several hours or a few days. Infection and subsequent meningitis and catheter migration are the possible complications.

Epidural catheters used for longer periods include a tunneled catheter and implanted port. Tunneled catheters are tunneled toward the abdomen and have a subcutaneous cuff to act as a barrier to infection. The external catheter exits the skin on the abdomen, so it can be easily reached for use by the patient or caregiver. An epidural implanted port is the same design as an IV implanted port and is accessed with the same noncoring needle. The catheter extends from the lumbar puncture site to the port pocket and is located over a bony prominence on the abdomen through a subcutaneous tunnel. Surgically implanted pumps can also be used to deliver epidural and intrathecal infusion.

Using sterile technique, an intraspinal catheter usually is inserted in the lumbar region. The external portion of a temporary epidural catheter is laid along the back toward the head and usually extends over the shoulder. The entire catheter length is taped for added security. Dressings are usually not routinely changed because they are used only for short periods. If bleeding or fluid leakage requires dressing removal, use extreme care to prevent dislodging the catheter.

For a tunneled catheter or implanted port, the entire subcutaneous tunnel and port pocket should be frequently assessed. Measurement of an external catheter segment could help identify catheter migration.

An in-line filter is used on all intraspinal infusions to block the infusion of particulate matter. Medications commonly contain preservatives such as alcohol, phenols, or sulfites; however, these are toxic to the CNS. All medications used for intraspinal infusion must be free of preservatives. Alcohol and products containing alcohol should not be applied to the insertion site because the solution could track along the catheter and cause nerve damage. Povidone-iodine solutions are preferred for skin antisepsis before insertion and during catheter dwell, including tunneled catheter exit sites and implanted port pockets.

Complications from epidural and intrathecal infusion can be caused by the type of medication being infused or can be related to the catheter. It is important to know the specific location of the intraspinal catheter because the doses of medications are quite different. When used for pain management, doses are usually 10 times greater for epidural than for intrathecal infusion. Assess the patient for response to the drugs being given, level of alertness, respiratory status, and itching.

Catheter-related complications include INFECTION, bleeding, leakage of cerebrospinal fluid (CSF), occlusion of the catheter lumen, and catheter migration. It is important to be aware of coagulopathy and timing of anticoagulant therapy when epidural catheters are inserted. Epidural hematoma can cause neurologic damage if not corrected promptly. Infection in the patient receiving either epidural or intrathecal therapy could be the result of a lack of asepsis when handling the medication or during the administration. Evidence of local infection, such as redness or swelling at the catheter exit site, may be present. The patient may also exhibit neurologic and systemic signs of infection (e.g., meningitis), such as headache, stiff neck, or temperature higher than 101° F (38.3° C). Report any neurologic change to the health care provider immediately!

GET READY FOR THE NCLEX® EXAMINATION!

KEY POINTS

Review these Key Points for each NCLEX Examination Client Needs Category.

Safe and Effective Care Environment

- Check IV administration orders for accuracy and completeness before implementing them. **Safety** QSEN
- Prevent IV administration errors by using smart pumps and other emerging technology-based safety infusion systems; these devices do not replace careful monitoring and assessment of the patient receiving infusion therapy. **Informatics** QSEN
- Devices engineered with safety mechanisms are required by the Occupational Safety and Health Administration (OSHA) to prevent staff injuries from needles, thus preventing bloodborne pathogen hazards. **Safety** QSEN
- Use the evidence-based catheter-related bloodstream infection (CR-BSI) prevention bundle during insertion and care of patients who have central lines, including using a checklist

during insertion, hand hygiene, maximal barrier precautions, and chlorhexidine for skin disinfection (see Table 13-2). **Evidence-Based Practice** QSEN

Health Promotion and Maintenance

- Older adults present special challenges when infusion therapy is used; physiologic changes of the skin and cardiac/renal systems must be considered.
- Use small IV catheters for older adults, and insert using a 10- to 15-degree angle to prevent rolling of the vein. **Patient-Centered Care** QSEN
- Teach patients and their families about the patient's infusion therapy, including purpose, type, and safety precautions.

Physiological Integrity

- Infusion therapy is the delivery of parenteral medications and fluids through a wide variety of catheters and locations.
- Infusion therapy is used for establishing FLUID AND ELECTROLYTE BALANCE, achieving optimum nutrition, maintaining hemostasis, and treating or preventing illnesses with medications.
- Vascular access devices (VADs) are catheters that are used to deliver fluids and electrolytes and medications into the intravascular space.
- Common types of VADs include short peripheral catheters, midline catheters, peripherally inserted central catheters (PICCs), nontunneled percutaneous and tunneled central catheters, implanted ports, and hemodialysis catheters.
- Use best practice for placement of short peripheral VADs, including avoiding the small veins of the hands (see Chart 13-1). **Evidence-Based Practice** QSEN
- Document care for the patient receiving IV therapy, including the type of VAD inserted. **Informatics** QSEN
- The type of VAD that is used depends on the reason for infusion therapy, the patient's condition, and the length of therapy.
- Choose the appropriate peripheral catheter gauge size of the VAD depending on its purpose (see Table 13-1).
- PICCs, tunneled central catheters, and implanted ports are commonly used for long-term infusion therapy.
- Infusion controllers and pumps are electronic devices used to regulate the flow of infusion fluids and medications, but be sure to monitor the infusion rate.
- Nursing care for patients receiving all types of infusion therapy includes using sterile technique when starting the therapy and when changing components of the infusion system, changing and securing the site dressing, and assessing the site for local complications (see Table 13-3). **Evidence-Based Practice** QSEN
- Assess and document the presence of phlebitis using the INS Phlebitis Scale (see Table 13-6). **Evidence-Based Practice** QSEN
- Use normal saline to flush IV catheters on a periodic basis per agency policy.
- Assess, prevent, and manage systemic complications related to IV therapy as outlined in Table 13-4.
- Assess, prevent, and manage complications during the course of central IV therapy as listed in Table 13-5.
- Subcutaneous therapy of fluids (hypodermoclysis) involves a slow infusion for a short time; the thighs, hips, and abdomen are commonly used.
- Intraosseous infusion therapy allows fluids and medications to be absorbed by the rich vascular network of the bones; it is used for both children and adults, particularly in emergency situations.
- Arterial therapy is used primarily for the administration of chemotherapy agents directly into a tumor site; the liver is the most common arterial site for this purpose.
- Intraperitoneal therapy is used for chemotherapy agent administration into the peritoneal cavity, especially for ovarian and gastrointestinal tumors that have metastasized into the peritoneum.
- Epidural and intrathecal administration of medications are the common uses for intraspinal infusion. Epidural infusions are usually for pain management; intrathecal infusions are usually chemotherapy agents used for cancers that cross the blood-brain barrier into the central nervous system.

CHAPTER 14

Care of Preoperative Patients

Robin Chard

http://evolve.elsevier.com/Iggy/

PRIORITY CONCEPTS

- INFECTION

LEARNING OUTCOMES

Safe and Effective Care Environment

1. Differentiate among the various types and purposes of surgery.
2. Examine personal factors for each patient for potential threats to safety, especially with older adults.
3. Protect the patient from injury and INFECTION during the perioperative period.

Health Promotion and Maintenance

4. Teach patients about dietary restrictions, preoperative preparations, and interventions to perform after surgery to prevent complications.

Psychosocial Integrity

5. Reduce the psychological impact for the patient and family regarding the preoperative experience.
6. Ensure patient concerns and needs are communicated to other members of the health care team.

Physiological Integrity

7. Use knowledge of physiology and behavioral principles to describe an accurate and complete preoperative assessment.
8. Implement interventions to reduce the risk for perioperative complications.
9. Use laboratory and clinical data to assess for changes that may affect the patient's response to drugs, anesthesia, and surgery.

Patients undergoing surgery have benefitted greatly from advances in surgical techniques, anesthesia, pharmacology, medical devices, and supportive interventions. Research defining best practices has resulted in improved outcomes in all areas of the perioperative experience. New interventions, such as robotics and other types of minimally invasive surgeries (MISs), are continually being developed. Advances in anesthetic agents and techniques have made surgery safer than ever before. Many surgical procedures have moved from the operating room to other departments such as interventional radiology, cardiac catheterization, and endoscopy. Ambulatory care facilities, known as ambulatory surgical centers (ASCs), are being used for many surgical procedures outside acute care hospitals and account for more than 23 million surgical procedures performed annually (Ambulatory Surgery Center Association, 2013). These changes affect the role of the perioperative nurse and have an impact on how patient teaching is performed.

Cost-reduction is a driving force for the management of the surgical patient. Shortened stays and ambulatory surgeries are common. Patient histories may be conducted by telephone or online before surgery rather than in person. Some patients may be observed only after surgery and not admitted as an inpatient. In response to the ongoing health care delivery changes and the use of multiple settings, nurses have modified their interventions, remaining focused on patient care before (**preoperative**), during (**intraoperative**), and after (**postoperative**) surgery. Together, these time periods are known as the **perioperative** experience.

Patient safety throughout the perioperative period is the number-one priority for all personnel. Fig. 14-1 shows an

Surgical Safety Checklist

World Health Organization | Patient Safety — A World Alliance for Safer Health Care

Before induction of anaesthesia → **Before skin incision** → **Before patient leaves operating room**

Before induction of anaesthesia

(with at least nurse and anaesthetist)

Has the patient confirmed his/her identity, site, procedure, and consent?
- ☐ Yes

Is the site marked?
- ☐ Yes
- ☐ Not applicable

Is the anaesthesia machine and medication check complete?
- ☐ Yes

Is the pulse oximeter on the patient and functioning?
- ☐ Yes

Does the patient have a:

Known allergy?
- ☐ No
- ☐ Yes

Difficult airway or aspiration risk?
- ☐ No
- ☐ Yes, and equipment/assistance available

Risk of >500ml blood loss (7ml/kg in children)?
- ☐ No
- ☐ Yes, and two IVs/central access and fluids planned

Before skin incision

(with nurse, anaesthetist and surgeon)

- ☐ **Confirm all team members have introduced themselves by name and role.**
- ☐ **Confirm the patient's name, procedure, and where the incision will be made.**

Has antibiotic prophylaxis been given within the last 60 minutes?
- ☐ Yes
- ☐ Not applicable

Anticipated Critical Events

To Surgeon:
- ☐ What are the critical or non-routine steps?
- ☐ How long will the case take?
- ☐ What is the anticipated blood loss?

To Anaesthetist:
- ☐ Are there any patient-specific concerns?

To Nursing Team:
- ☐ Has sterility (including indicator results) been confirmed?
- ☐ Are there equipment issues or any concerns?

Is essential imaging displayed?
- ☐ Yes
- ☐ Not applicable

Before patient leaves operating room

(with nurse, anaesthetist and surgeon)

Nurse Verbally Confirms:
- ☐ The name of the procedure
- ☐ Completion of instrument, sponge and needle counts
- ☐ Specimen labeling (read specimen labels aloud, including patient name)
- ☐ Whether there are any equipment problems to be addressed

To Surgeon, Anaesthetist and Nurse:
- ☐ What are the key concerns for recovery and management of this patient?

This checklist is not intended to be comprehensive. Additions and modifications to fit local practice are encouraged.

Revised 1 / 2009

FIG. 14-1 A surgical safety checklist.

overview of a surgical safety checklist as recommended by the World Health Organization (WHO). Quality measures such as wrong-site surgery, patient falls, hospital-acquired pressure ulcers, and vascular catheter–associated INFECTIONS must now be reported to the Centers for Medicare and Medicaid Services (CMS). These data are used for tracking patient outcomes and ensuring patient-centered care and accountability on the part of health care facilities.

Because surgery is invasive and involves exposure to various anesthetic agents and drugs, as well as positioning and other environmental hazards, complications are common. Some complications are predictable and are considered preventable or "never events." As a result, The Joint Commission (TJC) has partnered with other groups and agencies and developed a plan for the reduction and eventual elimination of preventable surgical complications known as the *Surgical Care Improvement Project (SCIP)*. Implementation of these core measures is now mandatory for patient safety. The current plan focuses on INFECTION prevention, prevention of serious cardiac events, and prevention of venous thromboembolism (VTE) (also known as *deep vein thrombosis [DVT]*). Ten specific core measures have been identified as actions required for prevention of these complications in patients identified as at risk. Table 14-1 provides an overview of these core measures areas. (The numbers associated with the core measures are not always chronologic, indicating that some areas are still in development.) The preoperative areas of responsibility for these core measures and their prevention strategies are highlighted in the appropriate areas of this chapter. In addition, some core measures also are discussed in patient care chapters most associated with the complication.

NCLEX EXAMINATION CHALLENGE

Safe and Effective Care Environment

Because of an unexpected emergency case, a client scheduled for colon surgery at 8 AM has been rescheduled for 11 AM. What is the nurse's best action related to preoperative prophylactic antibiotic administration according to the Surgical Care Improvement Project (SCIP) guidelines?

A. Administer the preoperative antibiotic at 7 AM as originally prescribed.
B. Administer the antibiotic at the same time as the other prescribed preoperative drugs.
C. Adjust the antibiotic administration time to be within 1 hour before the surgical incision.
D. Hold the preoperative antibiotic until the client is actually in the operating room and has been anesthetized.

OVERVIEW

The preoperative period begins when the patient is scheduled for surgery and ends at the time of transfer to the surgical suite. As a nurse, you will function as an educator, an advocate, and a promoter of health. The surgical environment demands the

TABLE 14-1 **Surgical Care Improvement Project (SCIP) Core Measure Overview**

CORE MEASURE IDENTIFICATION	MEASUREMENT NAME/DESCRIPTION
SCIP Infection-1 (SCIP Inf-1)	*Prophylactic Antibiotic Received Within One Hour Prior to Surgical Incision* The purpose is to use short-duration antibiotics to establish bactericidal blood and tissue levels by the time the surgical incision is made.
SCIP Infection-2 (SCIP Inf-2)	*Prophylactic Antibiotic Selection for Surgical Patients* The purpose is to ensure that prophylactic antibiotics are used for patients who are at increased risk for surgical site infections. The guidelines for risk and for the exact antibiotic to be used are specific to each type of surgical procedure and follow evidence-based published recommendations.
SCIP Infection-3 (SCIP Inf-3)	*Prophylactic Antibiotics Discontinued Within 24 Hours After Surgery End Time* The purpose is to ensure that prophylactic antibiotic therapy provides benefit without risk. Prolonged prophylactic antibiotic therapy has not been shown to increase benefit and is known to increase the risk for *C. difficile* infection and the development of microorganisms that are resistant to antimicrobial drugs.
SCIP Infection-4 (SCIP Inf-4)	*Cardiac Surgery Patients with Controlled 6 AM Postoperative Blood Glucose* (Applies to cardiac surgery patients only) The purpose is to avoid hyperglycemia (which is defined as blood glucose levels above 200 mg/dL and is associated with increased complications and mortality) in cardiac surgery patients, especially patients undergoing coronary artery bypass graft surgery and patients with diabetes who are having cardiac surgery.
SCIP Infection-6 (SCIP Inf-6)	*Surgery Patients with Appropriate Hair Removal* The purpose is to avoid hair removal procedures, specifically shaving, that cause skin abrasions and increase the risk for surgical site infections. If hair must be removed from the surgical site, removal is performed with electric clippers or chemical depilatories.
SCIP Infection-9 (SCIP Inf-9)	*Urinary Catheter Removed on Postoperative Day 1 (POD 1) or Postoperative Day 2 (POD 2) with Day of Surgery Being Day Zero* The purpose is to avoid urinary catheter–associated urinary tract infections, which increase with longer duration indwelling catheters. It is unacceptable to have an indwelling urinary catheter in place longer than 48 hours after surgery unless there is a documented specific and medically validated reason for it.
SCIP Infection-10 (SCIP Inf-10)	*Surgery Patients with Perioperative Temperature Management* The purpose is to prevent prolonged hypothermia, which is associated with impaired wound healing, serious cardiac complications, altered drug metabolism, coagulation problems, and a higher incidence of surgical site infections. Temperature must be measured within 15 minutes from the end of anesthesia administration. Intentional hypothermia must be documented.
SCIP CARD-2	*Surgery Patients on Beta-Blocker Therapy Prior to Arrival Who Received a Beta-Blocker During the Perioperative Period* The purpose is to ensure that patients with specific medical conditions receive beta-blocker therapy before surgery and continue the therapy in the immediate postoperative period. This evidence-based action has resulted in a significant reduction in coronary events, cardiovascular mortality, and overall mortality.
SCIP Venous thromboembolism-1 (SCIP VTE-1)	*Surgery Patients with Recommended Venous Thromboembolism Prophylaxis Ordered* The purpose is to reduce the complications from postoperative venous thromboembolism (VTE). Surgery is a major risk factor responsible for VTE formation and subsequent pulmonary embolism. Although VTE prophylaxis is effective, it is underused. Specific preoperative and postoperative VTE prophylaxis strategies are recommended on the basis of patient risk, type and duration of surgery, and extent of expected postoperative immobilization.
SCIP Venous thromboembolism-2 (SCIP VTE-2)	*Surgery Patients Who Received Appropriate Venous Thromboembolism Prophylaxis Within 24 Hours Prior to Surgery to 24 Hours After Surgery* The purpose is to reduce the complications from postoperative venous thromboembolism (VTE), particularly among patients undergoing the types of surgeries in which the risk is highest.

Data from The Joint Commission. (2014). *National Patient Safety Goals.* Retrieved April 2014, from www.jointcommission.org/surgical_care_improvement_project/.
C. difficile, Clostridium difficile.

use of knowledge, judgment, and skills based on the principles of nursing science. Perioperative nursing places special emphasis on safety, advocacy, and patient education, although ensuring a "culture of safety" is the responsibility of all health care team members.

The patient's readiness for surgery is critical to the outcome. Preoperative care focuses on preparing the patient for the surgery and ensuring patient safety. This care includes education and any intervention needed before surgery to reduce anxiety and complications and to promote patient cooperation in procedures after surgery. Use adult teaching and learning principles in teaching patients and families before surgery. Validate, clarify, and reinforce information the patient has received from the surgeon or other members of the surgical team. In addition, during the nursing assessment before surgery, problems may be identified that warrant further patient assessment or intervention before the procedure. As required by The Joint Commission's National Patient Safety Goals (NPSGs), communication and collaboration with the surgical team are essential so that correct actions are taken to achieve the desired outcome.

Categories and Purposes of Surgery

Surgical procedures are categorized by the purpose, body location, extent, and degree of urgency. Table 14-2 explains the categories and gives examples of surgical procedures.

TABLE 14-2 **Selected Categories of Surgical Procedures**

CATEGORY	DESCRIPTION	CONDITION OR SURGICAL PROCEDURE
Reasons for Surgery		
Diagnostic	Performed to determine the origin and cause of a disorder or the cell type for cancer	Breast biopsy Exploratory laparotomy Arthroscopy
Curative	Performed to resolve a health problem by repairing or removing the cause	Cholecystectomy Appendectomy Hysterectomy
Restorative	Performed to improve a patient's functional ability	Total knee replacement Finger reimplantation
Palliative	Performed to relieve symptoms of a disease process, but does not cure	Colostomy Nerve root resection Tumor debulking Ileostomy
Cosmetic	Performed primarily to alter or enhance personal appearance	Liposuction Revision of scars Rhinoplasty Blepharoplasty
Urgency of Surgery		
Elective	Planned for correction of a nonacute problem	Cataract removal Hernia repair Hemorrhoidectomy Total joint replacement
Urgent	Requires prompt intervention; may be life threatening if treatment is delayed more than 24 to 48 hr	Intestinal obstruction Bladder obstruction Kidney or ureteral stones Bone fracture Eye injury Acute cholecystitis
Emergent	Requires immediate intervention because of life-threatening consequences	Gunshot or stab wound Severe bleeding Abdominal aortic aneurysm Compound fracture Appendectomy
Degree of Risk of Surgery		
Minor	Procedure without significant risk; often done with local anesthesia	Incision and drainage (I&D) Implantation of a venous access device (VAD) Muscle biopsy
Major	Procedure of greater risk; usually longer and more extensive than a minor procedure	Mitral valve replacement Pancreas transplant Lymph node dissection
Extent of Surgery		
Simple	Only the most overtly affected areas involved in the surgery	Simple/partial mastectomy
Radical	Extensive surgery beyond the area obviously involved; is directed at finding a root cause	Radical prostatectomy Radical hysterectomy
Minimally invasive surgery (MIS)	Surgery performed in a body cavity or body area through one or more endoscopes; can correct problems, remove organs, take tissue for biopsy, re-route blood vessels and drainage systems; is a fast-growing and ever-changing type of surgery	Arthroscopy Tubal ligation Hysterectomy Lung lobectomy Coronary artery bypass Cholecystectomy

Surgical Settings

The term **inpatient** refers to a patient who is admitted to a hospital. The patient may be admitted the day before or, more often, the day of surgery (often termed *same-day admission [SDA]*), or the patient may already be an inpatient when surgery is needed. The terms **outpatient** and **ambulatory** refer to a patient who goes to the surgical area the day of the surgery and returns home on the same day (i.e., *same-day surgery [SDS]*). Hospital-based ambulatory surgical centers, freestanding surgical centers, physicians' offices, and ambulatory care centers are common. More than half of all surgical procedures in North America are performed in ambulatory centers (Ambulatory Surgery Center Association, 2013).

One advantage of outpatient surgery is that patients are not separated from the comfort and security of their home and family. Same-day surgery, however, places more responsibility on the patient and family, especially for care after surgery. Often a case manager is needed to coordinate post-discharge care for the patient.

❖ PATIENT-CENTERED COLLABORATIVE CARE

◆ Assessment

History. Data collection about the patient before surgery begins in various settings (e.g., the surgeon's office, the preadmission or admission office, the inpatient unit, the telephone, the Internet). Use privacy to increase the patient's comfort with the interview process. Anesthesia and surgery are both physical and emotional stressors. Collect these data:

- Age
- Use of tobacco, alcohol, or illicit substances, including marijuana
- Current drugs
- Use of complementary or alternative practices, such as herbal therapies, folk remedies, or acupuncture
- Medical history
- Prior surgical procedures and how these were tolerated
- Prior experience with anesthesia, pain control, and management of nausea or vomiting
- Autologous or directed blood donations
- Allergies, including sensitivity to latex products
- General health
- Family history
- Type of surgery planned
- Knowledge about and understanding of events during the perioperative period
- Adequacy of the patient's support system

When taking a history, screen the patient for problems that increase the risk for complications during and after surgery. Some problems that increase the surgical risk or increase the risk for complications after surgery are listed in Table 14-3.

Older patients are at increased risk for complications from both anesthesia and surgery (Doerflinger, 2009). The normal aging process decreases immune system functioning and delays wound healing. The frequency of chronic illness increases in older patients. Gas exchange is more profoundly affected by general anesthetic agents and by opioid analgesics. Age-related changes in kidney and liver function may delay the elimination of anesthetic and analgesic agents, increasing the risk for adverse reactions. See Chart 14-1 for other changes in older adults that may alter the operative response or risk.

Drugs and substance use may affect patient responses to surgery. Tobacco use increases the risk for pulmonary complications because of changes to the lungs, blood vessels, and chest cavity. Alcohol and illicit substance use can alter the patient's responses to anesthesia and pain medication. Withdrawal of alcohol before surgery may lead to delirium tremens. Prescription and over-the-counter drugs may also affect how the patient reacts to the operative experience. Adverse effects can occur with the use of some herbs. Thus asking about and documenting past and current use of herbs or botanicals are important.

Medical history is important to obtain because many chronic illnesses increase surgical risks and need to be considered when planning care. For example, a patient with systemic lupus erythematosus may need additional drugs to offset the stress of the surgery. A patient with diabetes may need a more extensive bowel preparation because of decreased intestinal motility. An INFECTION may need to be treated before surgery.

TABLE 14-3 Selected Factors That Increase the Risk for Surgical Complications

Age
• Older than 65 years
Medications
• Antihypertensives
• Tricyclic antidepressants
• Anticoagulants
• Nonsteroidal anti-inflammatory drugs (NSAIDs)
Medical History
• Decreased immunity
• Diabetes
• Pulmonary disease
• Cardiac disease
• Hemodynamic instability
• Multi-system disease
• Coagulation defect or disorder
• Anemia
• Dehydration
• Infection
• Hypertension
• Hypotension
• Any chronic disease
Prior Surgical Experiences
• Less-than-optimal emotional reaction
• Anesthesia reactions or complications
• Postoperative complications
Health History
• Malnutrition or obesity
• Drug, tobacco, alcohol, or illicit substance use or abuse
• Altered coping ability
Family History
• Malignant hyperthermia
• Cancer
• Bleeding disorder
Type of Surgical Procedure Planned
• Neck, oral, or facial procedures (airway complications)
• Chest or high abdominal procedures (pulmonary complications)
• Abdominal surgery (paralytic ileus, venous thromboembolism)

Ask the patient specifically about cardiac problems because complications from anesthesia occur more often in patients with cardiac problems (Johnson, 2011). A patient with a history of rheumatic heart disease may be prescribed antibiotics before surgery. Cardiac problems that increase surgical risks include coronary artery disease, angina, myocardial infarction (MI) within 6 months before surgery, heart failure, hypertension, and dysrhythmias. These problems impair the patient's ability to withstand hemodynamic changes and alter the response to anesthesia. The risk for an MI during surgery is higher in patients who have heart problems. Patients with cardiac disease may require perioperative therapy with beta-blocking drugs, as recommended by core measures for SCIP CARD-2 (see Table 14-1).

Pulmonary complications during or after surgery are more likely to occur in older patients, those with chronic respiratory

CHART 14-1 Nursing Focus on the Older Adult

Age-Related Changes as Surgical Risk Factors

PHYSIOLOGIC CHANGE	NURSING INTERVENTIONS	RATIONALES
Cardiovascular System		
Decreased cardiac output Increased blood pressure	Determine normal activity levels, and note when the patient tires.	Knowing limits helps prevent fatigue.
Decreased peripheral circulation	Monitor vital signs, peripheral pulses, and capillary refill.	Having baseline data helps detect deviations.
Respiratory System		
Reduced vital capacity Loss of lung elasticity	Teach coughing and deep-breathing exercises.	Pulmonary exercises help prevent pulmonary complications.
Decreased oxygenation of blood	Monitor respirations and breathing effort.	Having baseline data helps detect deviations.
Renal/Urinary System		
Decreased blood flow to kidneys Reduced ability to excrete waste Decline in glomerular filtration rate	Monitor intake and output. Assess overall hydration. Monitor electrolyte status.	Ongoing assessment helps detect fluid and electrolyte imbalances and decreased renal function.
Nocturia common	Assist frequently with toileting needs, especially at night.	Frequent toileting helps prevent incontinence and falls.
Neurologic System		
Sensory deficits Slower reaction time	Orient the patient to the surroundings. Allow extra time for teaching the patient.	An individualized preoperative teaching plan is developed based on the patient's orientation and any neurologic deficits.
Decreased ability to adjust to changes in the surroundings	Provide for the patient's safety.	Safety measures help prevent falls and injury.
Musculoskeletal System		
Increased incidence of deformities related to osteoporosis or arthritis	Assess the patient's mobility. Teach turning and positioning. Encourage ambulation.	Interventions help prevent complications of immobility.
	Place on falls precautions, if indicated.	Safety measures help prevent injury.
Skin		
Dry with less subcutaneous fat makes the skin at greater risk for damage; slower skin healing increases risk for infection	Assess the patient's skin before surgery for lesions, bruises, and areas of decreased circulation.	Having baseline data helps detect changes and evaluate interventions.
	Pad bony prominences.	Padding can protect at-risk areas.
	Use pressure-avoiding or pressure-reducing overlays.	Overlays can prevent pressure ulcer formation by redistributing body weight.
	Avoid applying tape to skin.	Tape removal damages thin skin.
	Teach the patient to change position at least every 2 hours.	Changing position frequently helps prevent reduced blood flow to an area and changes external pressure patterns.

problems, and smokers because of smoking- or age-related lung changes (Doerflinger, 2009). Increased chest rigidity and loss of lung elasticity reduce anesthetic excretion. Smoking increases the blood level of **carboxyhemoglobin** (carbon monoxide on oxygen-binding sites of the hemoglobin molecule), which decreases oxygen delivery to organs. Action of cilia in pulmonary mucous membranes decreases, which leads to retained secretions and predisposes the patient to INFECTION (pneumonia) and **atelectasis** (collapse of alveoli). Atelectasis reduces gas exchange and causes intolerance of anesthesia. It is also a common problem after general anesthesia.

Chronic lung problems such as asthma, emphysema, and chronic bronchitis also reduce the elasticity of the lungs, which reduces gas exchange. As a result, patients with these problems have reduced tissue oxygenation.

Previous surgical procedures and anesthesia affect the patient's readiness for surgery. Previous experiences, especially with complications, may increase anxiety about the scheduled surgery. Ask about the patient's experience with anesthesia and all allergies. These data provide information about tolerance of and possible fears about the use of anesthesia. The family medical history and problems with anesthetics may indicate possible reactions to anesthesia, such as malignant hyperthermia (see Chapter 15).

An allergy to certain substances alerts you to a possible reaction to anesthetic agents or to substances that are used before or during surgery. For example, povidone-iodine (e.g., Betadine) used for skin cleansing contains the same allergens found in shellfish. Patients who are allergic to shellfish may have an adverse reaction to povidone-iodine. The patient with an allergy to avocados, bananas, strawberries, and other fruits may also have a latex sensitivity or allergy. Patients who have an egg, peanut, or soy allergy may have a reaction to propofol (Diprivan), which is an anesthetic agent often used in the induction and maintenance of anesthesia (MDConsult, 2012).

Blood donation for surgery can be made by the patient (**autologous donations**) a few weeks just before the scheduled surgery date. Then, if blood is needed during or after surgery, an autologous blood transfusion can be given. This practice eliminates transfusion reactions and reduces the risk for acquiring bloodborne disease. Specific patient criteria, which may vary by surgical type and patient health problem, must be met to qualify for autologous transfusion.

A special tag is placed on the blood bag when an autologous blood donation has been made. The blood donor center gives the patient a matching tag that he or she wears or brings to the surgical area before surgery as required by The Joint Commission's National Patient Safety Goals (NPSGs). This procedure helps ensure that patients receive only their own donated blood. Patients may wish to have family and friends donate blood exclusively for their use, if needed. This practice (called *directed blood donation*) is possible only if the blood types are compatible and the donor's blood is acceptable. Directed donation is not practiced in all blood donation centers. When directed blood donations are used, a special tag is attached to the blood bag. This tag notes the names of the patient and the donor and bears the patient's signature.

Ask whether autologous or directed blood donations have been made, and document this information in the chart. It is important to know the specific blood collection center where the donation was made and whether the blood has arrived before the patient goes into surgery. The hospital receives and stores the blood units until they are used or are no longer needed. Unused blood is returned to the collection center.

Increased use of "bloodless surgery" and minimally invasive surgery (MIS) provides alternatives for patients with religious or medical restrictions to blood transfusions. These programs reduce the need for transfusion during and after surgery. Some techniques used are limiting blood samples (the number of samples, as well as the volume of blood drawn per sample) before surgery and stimulating the patient's own red blood cell production with epoetin alpha (e.g., Epogen, Procrit). Supplemental iron, folic acid, vitamin B_{12}, and vitamin C may be prescribed to help red blood cell formation. Newer equipment and surgical techniques cause less blood loss than older techniques. Such advances include recycling blood suctioned during surgery and immediately transfusing it back into the patient. Assess, monitor, teach, and support the patient during the bloodless surgery process.

Discharge planning is started before surgery. Assess the patient's home environment, self-care capabilities, and support systems and anticipate postoperative needs before surgery. *All patients, regardless of how minor the procedure or how often they have had surgery, should have discharge planning.* Older patients and dependent adults may need transportation referrals to and from the physician's office or the surgical setting. A home care nurse may be needed to monitor recovery and to provide instructions. Patients with few support systems may need follow-up care at home. Some patients need a planned direct admission to a rehabilitation facility or center for physical therapy after surgery, especially joint replacement surgery. Shortened hospital stays require adequate discharge planning to achieve the desired outcomes after surgery.

Physical Assessment/Clinical Manifestations. The preoperative patient may be any age, with a health status that varies from well to debilitated. Perform a complete assessment before surgery to obtain baseline data. Use this information to identify current health problems, potential complications related to anesthesia, and risk for complications that may occur after surgery.

Begin the assessment by obtaining a complete set of vital signs. You may need to obtain vital signs several times at different time intervals for accurate baseline values. Previous vital signs from another admission (if available) are helpful to compare with current vital signs. Abnormal vital signs may require postponement of surgery until the problem is treated and the patient's condition is stable. Also assess for anxiety, which could increase blood pressure, pulse, and respiratory rate. Document these findings as part of the overall assessment.

CHART 14-2 Nursing Focus on the Older Adult

Specific Considerations When Planning Care for the Older Preoperative Patient

- Greater incidence of chronic illness
- Greater incidence of malnutrition
- More allergies
- Increased incidence of impaired self-care abilities
- Inadequate support systems
- Decreased ability to withstand the stress of surgery and anesthesia
- Increased risk for cardiopulmonary complications after surgery
- Risk for a change in mental status when admitted (e.g., related to unfamiliar surroundings, change in routine, drugs)
- Increased risk for a fall and resultant injury

Throughout the assessment, focus on problem areas identified from the patient's history and on all body systems affected by the surgical procedure. The older adult (Chart 14-2; see also Chapter 2) or chronically ill patient is at increased risk for complications during and after surgery. The number of serious problems **(morbidity)** and death **(mortality)** during or after surgery is higher in older and chronically ill patients (Johnson, 2011).

Report any abnormal assessment findings to the surgeon and to anesthesia personnel, as required by The Joint Commission's NPSGs. In this way, you are a proactive patient advocate exercising professional legal responsibility. Often, established protocols or care maps identify what interventions are to be performed before surgery.

Cardiovascular status is critical to assess because cardiac problems are associated with many surgery-related deaths. Check the patient for hypertension, which is common, is often undiagnosed, and can affect the response to surgery. Cardiac assessment includes listening to heart sounds for rate, regularity, and abnormalities. Ask whether the patient has ever had a venous thromboembolism (VTE). Examine the patient's hands and feet for temperature, color, peripheral pulses, capillary refill, and edema. Report any problems (e.g., absent peripheral pulses, pitting edema, cardiac manifestations, chest pain, shortness of breath, and dyspnea) to the surgeon for further assessment and evaluation. (Cardiac assessment is discussed in Chapter 33.)

Respiratory status considers age, smoking history (including exposure to secondhand smoke), and any chronic illness (Doerflinger, 2009). Obese patients may have undiagnosed respiratory problems such as obstructive sleep apnea (OSA), which can lead to complications from anesthesia (Graham et al., 2011). Observe the patient's posture; respiratory rate, rhythm, and depth; overall respiratory effort; and lung expansion. Document any clubbing of the fingertips (swelling at the base of the nail beds caused by a chronic lack of oxygen) or cyanosis. Auscultate the lungs to assess for any abnormal breath sounds (crackles, wheezes, rubs). (More information on respiratory assessment is found in Chapter 27.)

Kidney function affects the excretion of drugs and waste products, including anesthetic and analgesic agents. If kidney function is reduced, fluid and electrolyte balance can be altered, especially in older patients. Ask about problems such as urinary frequency, **dysuria** (painful urination), **nocturia** (awakening during nighttime sleep because of a need to void), difficulty starting urine flow, and **oliguria** (scant amount of urine). Ask the patient about the appearance and odor of the urine. Assess the patient's usual fluid intake and degree of continence. If the patient has kidney or urinary problems, consult with the physician about further workup. (Kidney/urinary assessment is discussed further in Chapter 65.)

Kidney impairment decreases the excretion of drugs and anesthetic agents. As a result, drug responses may be prolonged. Scopolamine (Buscopan ♣), morphine, other opioids, benzodiazepines, and barbiturates often cause confusion, disorientation, apprehension, and restlessness when given to patients with decreased kidney function.

Neurologic status includes the patient's overall mental status, level of consciousness, orientation, and ability to follow commands. This information is needed before planning preoperative teaching and care after surgery. A problem in any of these areas affects the type of care needed during the surgical experience. Determine the patient's baseline neurologic status to be able to identify changes that may occur later. Also assess for any motor or sensory deficits. (See Chapter 41 for complete nervous system assessment.)

The usual neurologic status of a mentally impaired patient may be difficult to assess (Doerflinger, 2009). The patient who has been independent and oriented at home may become disoriented in the hospital setting. Family members can often provide information about what the patient was like at home.

The Joint Commission's NPSGs require that you ensure patient safety by assessing the patient's risk for falling, especially older patients. Evaluate factors such as mental status, muscle strength, steadiness of gait, and sense of independence to determine the patient's risk. Document the patient's ability to ambulate and the steadiness of gait as baseline data.

Musculoskeletal status problems may interfere with positioning during and after surgery. For example, patients with arthritis may be able to assume surgical positions but have discomfort after surgery from prolonged joint immobilization. Other anatomic features, such as the shape and length of the neck and the shape of the chest cavity, may interfere with respiratory and cardiac function or require special positioning during surgery.

! NURSING SAFETY PRIORITY (QSEN)

Action Alert

Ask about a history of joint replacement, and document the exact location of any prostheses. Communicate this information to operating room personnel to ensure that electrocautery pads, which could cause an electrical burn, are not placed on or near the area of the prosthesis. Other areas to avoid electrocautery pad placement include on or near bony prominences, scar tissue, hair, tattoos, weight-bearing surfaces, pressure points, and metal piercings (Spruce & Braswell, 2012).

Nutrition status, especially malnutrition and obesity, can increase surgical risk. Surgery increases metabolic rate and depletes potassium, vitamin C, and B vitamins, all of which are needed for wound healing and blood clotting. In poorly nourished patients, decreased serum protein levels slow recovery. Negative nitrogen balance may result from depleted protein stores. This problem increases the risk for skin breakdown, delayed wound healing, possible dehiscence or evisceration (see Chapter 16), dehydration, and sepsis.

Some older patients may have poor nutrition because of chronic illness, diuretic or laxative use, poor dietary planning or habits, anorexia, lack of motivation, or financial limitations (Touhy & Jett, 2014). Indications of poor fluid or nutrition status include:

- Brittle nails
- Muscle wasting
- Dry or flaky skin, decreased skin turgor, and hair changes (e.g., dull, sparse, dry)
- Orthostatic (postural) hypotension
- Decreased serum protein levels and abnormal serum electrolyte values

The obese patient is often malnourished because of an imbalanced diet. Obesity increases the risk for poor wound healing because of excessive ***adipose*** (fatty) tissue. Fatty tissue has few blood vessels, little collagen, and decreased nutrients, all of which are needed for wound healing. Obesity stresses the heart and reduces the lung volumes, which can affect the surgery and recovery. Obese patients may need larger drug doses and may retain them longer after surgery.

Skin assessment is important. Many insurers have denied coverage to hospitals for care provided to patients who develop skin breakdown or pressure ulcers during the perioperative period. Assess the patient's skin for signs of breakdown, open sores, or areas that may be exposed to excessive pressure during the surgical procedure, and document these findings. Communicate this information to the circulating nurse so that precautions can be taken to prevent injury.

? NCLEX EXAMINATION CHALLENGE

Safe and Effective Care Environment

An 81-year-old client, scheduled for a long orthopedic procedure, appears to have a low body mass index. In addition to the body mass index value, which additional client information is most important for the nurse to report to the surgeon and perioperative team as indicating an increased risk for skin breakdown?

A. Negative nitrogen balance
B. Previous abdominal surgery
C. Allergy to latex products
D. Change in mental status upon admission

Psychosocial Assessment. Perform a psychosocial assessment to determine the patient's level of anxiety, coping ability, and support systems. Provide information and offer support as needed.

Most patients have some degree of anxiety or fear before surgery. The extent of these reactions varies according to the type of surgery, the perceived effects of the surgery and its potential outcome, and the patient's personality. Surgery may be seen as a threat to life, body image, self-esteem, self-concept, or lifestyle. Patients may fear death, pain, helplessness, a change in role or work status, a diagnosis of life-threatening conditions, possible disabling or crippling effects, or the unknown.

Anxiety or fear affects the patient's ability to learn, cope, and cooperate with teaching and operative procedures. Anxiety may also influence the amount and type of anesthetic needed and may slow recovery. In some cases, severe preoperative anxiety can increase the degree of pain after surgery. Be aware of potential anxiety when interviewing the patient and planning teaching.

Assess coping mechanisms used by the patient under similar situations or in the past when confronted with a stressful situation. Ask open-ended questions about the patient's feelings about the entire surgical experience. Factors that influence coping include age, previous surgical or sick-role experiences, and physical discomfort. Manifestations of anxiety include anger, crying, restlessness, profuse sweating, increased pulse rate, palpitations, sleeplessness, diarrhea, and urinary frequency.

Laboratory Assessment. Laboratory tests before surgery provide baseline data about the patient's health and help predict potential complications. The patient scheduled for surgery in an ambulatory surgical center or admitted to the hospital on the morning of or day before surgery may have preadmission testing (PAT) performed from 24 hours to 28 days before the scheduled surgery. These test results are usually valid unless there has been a change in the patient's condition that warrants repeated testing or the patient is taking drugs that can alter laboratory values (e.g., warfarin [Coumadin], aspirin, diuretics). Some facilities have time limits for tests, especially pregnancy testing or any other test results that would require altering the surgical plan.

The choice of laboratory testing before surgery varies among facilities and depends on the patient's age, medical history, and type of anesthesia planned (Rothrock, 2011). The most common tests include:

- Urinalysis
- Blood type and screen
- Complete blood count or hemoglobin level and hematocrit
- Clotting studies (prothrombin time [PT], international normalized ratio [INR], activated partial thromboplastin time [aPTT], platelet count)
- Electrolyte levels
- Serum creatinine and blood urea nitrogen levels
- Depending on a female patient's age and the nature of the planned procedure, a pregnancy test may also be needed

Urinalysis is performed to assess for abnormal substances in the urine such as protein, glucose, blood, and bacteria. If kidney disease is suspected or if the patient is older, the physician may request other tests to determine the type and degree of disease present.

Report electrolyte imbalances or other abnormal results to the anesthesia team and the surgeon before surgery. **Hypokalemia** (decreased serum potassium level) increases the risk for toxicity if the patient is taking digoxin, slows recovery from anesthesia, and increases cardiac irritability. **Hyperkalemia** (increased serum potassium level) increases the risk for dysrhythmias, especially with the use of anesthesia.

! NURSING SAFETY PRIORITY QSEN

Critical Rescue

Any potassium imbalance—hypokalemia or hyperkalemia—must be corrected before surgery.

Other studies may be needed, depending on the patient's medical history. For example, baseline arterial blood gas (ABG) values are assessed before surgery for patients with chronic pulmonary problems. Chart 14-3 lists abnormal laboratory findings and their possible causes.

CHART 14-3 Laboratory Profile

Perioperative Assessment

TEST	NORMAL RANGE FOR ADULTS	SIGNIFICANCE OF ABNORMAL FINDINGS: INCREASED IN	SIGNIFICANCE OF ABNORMAL FINDINGS: DECREASED IN
Potassium (K^+)	3.5-5.0 mEq/L, or 3.5-5.0 mmol/L	Dehydration Kidney impairment Acidosis Cellular/tissue damage Hemolysis of the specimen	NPO status when potassium replacement is inadequate Excessive use of non–potassium-sparing diuretics Vomiting Malnutrition Diarrhea Alkalosis
Sodium (Na^+)	90 yr or younger: 136-145 mEq/L, or 136-145 mmol/L Older than 90 yr: 132-146 mEq/L, or 132-146 mmol/L	Cardiac failure or kidney impairment Hypertension Excessive amounts of IV fluids containing sodium chloride Edema Dehydration (hemoconcentration)	Nasogastric drainage Vomiting or diarrhea Excessive use of laxatives or diuretics Excessive amounts of IV fluids containing water Syndrome of inappropriate antidiuretic hormone (SIADH)
Chloride (Cl^-)	90 yr or younger: 98-106 mEq/L, or 98-106 mmol/l Older than 90 yr: 98-111 mEq/L, or 98-111 mmol/L	Respiratory alkalosis Dehydration Kidney impairment Excessive amounts of IV fluids containing sodium chloride (NaCl)	Excessive nasogastric drainage Vomiting Excessive use of diuretics Diarrhea
Carbon dioxide (CO_2)	60 yr or younger: 23-30 mEq/L, or 23-30 mmol/L 60-90 yr: 23-31 mEq/L, or 23-31 mmol/L Older than 90 yr: 20-29 mEq/L, or 20-29 mmol/L	Chronic pulmonary disease Intestinal obstruction Vomiting or nasogastric suctioning Metabolic alkalosis	Hyperventilation Diabetic ketoacidosis Diarrhea Lactic acidosis Renal failure Salicylate toxicity

Continued

CHART 14-3 **Laboratory Profile—cont'd**

Perioperative Assessment

TEST	NORMAL RANGE FOR ADULTS	SIGNIFICANCE OF ABNORMAL FINDINGS: INCREASED IN	SIGNIFICANCE OF ABNORMAL FINDINGS: DECREASED IN
Glucose (fasting)	60 yr or younger: 70-110 mg/dL, or 4.1-5.9 mmol/L 60-90 yr: 82-115 mg/dL, or 4.6-6.4 mmol/L Older than 90 yr: 75-121 mg/dL, or 4.2-6.7 mmol/L	Hyperglycemia Excessive amounts of IV fluids containing glucose Stress Steroid use Pancreatic or hepatic disease	Hypoglycemia Excess insulin
Creatinine	*Females:* 60 yr or younger: 0.5-1.1 mg/dL, or 44-97 µmol/L 60-90 yr: 0.6-1.2 mg/dL, or 53-106 µmol/L Older than 90 yr: 0.6-1.3 mg/dL, or 53-115 µmol/L *Males:* 60 yr or younger: 0.6-1.2 mg/dL, or 53-106 µmol/L 60-90 yr: 0.8-1.3 mg/dL, or 71-115 µmol/L Older than 90 yr: 1.0-1.7 mg/dL, or 88-150 µmol/L	Kidney damage with destruction of large number of nephrons Renal insufficiency Acute kidney injury Chronic kidney disease End-stage kidney disease (ESKD)	Atrophy of muscle tissue
Blood urea nitrogen (BUN)	Younger than 60 yr: 10-20 mg/dL, or 3.61-7.1 mmol/L 60-90 yr: 8-23 mg/dL, or 2.9-8.2 mmol/L Older than 90 yr: 10-31 mg/dL, or 3.6-11.1 mmol/L	Dehydration Kidney impairment Excessive protein in diet Liver failure	Overhydration Malnutrition
Prothrombin time (pro time, PT)	11-12.5 sec, 85%-100%, or 1 : 1.1 patient-control ratio	Coagulation defect (bleeding disorder) Vitamin K deficiency	Coagulation (clotting) disorder, such as thrombophlebitis or pulmonary embolus
International normalized ratio (INR)	0.7-1.8	Anticoagulant therapy (aspirin, warfarin)	Extensive cancer
Partial thromboplastin time, activated (aPTT)	30-40 sec	Coagulation defect (bleeding disorder) Anticoagulant therapy (heparin) Liver disease	Coagulation (clotting) disorder, such as thrombophlebitis or pulmonary embolus Extensive cancer
White blood cell (WBC) count (leukocyte count)	Total: 5,000-10,000/mm^3	Infection Inflammation Stress Tissue necrosis	Immune disorder Immunosuppressant therapy
Hemoglobin, total	*Females:* 18-44 yr: 12-16 g/dL, or 117-155 g/L 45-64 yr: 11.7-16.0 g/dL, or 117-160 g/L 65-74 yr: 11.7-16.1 g/dL, or 117-161 g/L *Males:* 18-44 yr: 14-18 g/dL, or 132-173 g/L 45-64 yr: 13.1-17.2 g/dL, or 131-172 g/L 65-74 yr: 12.6-17.4 g/dL, or 126-174 g/L	Dehydration Polycythemia Chronic pulmonary disease Congestive heart failure	Blood loss Anemia Renal failure
Hematocrit	*Females:* 18-44 yr: 35%-45% 45-74 yr: 37%-47% *Males:* 18-44 yr: 42%-52% 45-64 yr: 39%-50% 65-74 yr: 37%-51%	Dehydration Polycythemia High altitude	Blood loss Anemia Kidney failure

Source: Pagana, K., & Pagana, T. (2014). *Mosby's manual of diagnostic and laboratory tests* (5th ed). St. Louis: Mosby.

Imaging Assessment. A chest x-ray may be requested before surgery. Often, healthy adults are not required to have a chest x-ray. A chest x-ray determines the size and shape of the heart, lungs, and major vessels and provides evidence of the presence of pneumonia or tuberculosis. It also provides baseline data in case of complications. Abnormal x-ray findings alert the surgeon to potential cardiac or pulmonary complications. Heart failure, cardiomyopathy, pneumonia, or infiltrates may cause cancellation or delay of elective surgery. For emergency surgery, x-ray results assist the anesthesia provider in selecting anesthesia type.

Other imaging studies are based on patient need, medical history, and the nature of the surgical procedure. For example, a patient with back pain may have CT scans or MRI examinations before spinal surgery to identify the exact location of the problem.

Other Diagnostic Assessment. An electrocardiogram (ECG) may be required for patients older than a specific age who are to have general anesthesia. The age varies among facilities but is often 40 to 45 years. An ECG may also be required for patients with a history of cardiac disease or those at risk for cardiac complications. It provides baseline information on new or existing cardiac problems, such as an old myocardial infarction (MI). A patient with a known cardiac problem may need a cardiology consultation before surgery. Drugs for problem prevention, such as nitroglycerin, beta blockers, and antibiotics, may be needed throughout the surgical period to reduce or prevent stress on the heart. Abnormal or potentially life-threatening ECG results may cause the cancellation of surgery until the patient's cardiac status is stable.

A focused assessment of the preoperative patient is shown in Chart 14-4.

NCLEX EXAMINATION CHALLENGE

Physiological Integrity

The preoperative admitting nurse notices that the client scheduled for total joint replacement surgery in 2 hours has a smell of alcohol on his breath even though he has just stated that he has fasted completely for the past 10 hours. What is the nurse's best first action?

A. Accept the client's statement and continue the preoperative preparation.
B. Report the discrepancy to the surgeon and anesthesiologist immediately.
C. Tell the client the observation and provide the opportunity for him to explain.
D. Remind the client that alcohol consumption may require changes in anesthesia procedure.

◆ *Analysis*

The priority NANDA-I nursing diagnoses and collaborative problems for preoperative patients include:

1. Deficient Knowledge related to unfamiliarity with surgical procedures and preparation (NANDA-I)
2. Anxiety related to new or unknown experience, possibility of pain, and possible surgical outcomes (NANDA-I)

◆ *Planning and Implementation*

As the nurse, your role is to ensure coordination of care for the patient before surgery. This responsibility continues until the patient is transferred to the operating room (OR).

Providing Information

Planning: Expected Outcomes. The patient needs to know what to expect during and after surgery and participate in his or her recovery as indicated by consistently demonstrating these behaviors:

- Explaining in his or her own words the purpose and expected results of the planned surgery
- Asking questions when a term or procedure is not known
- Adhering to the NPO requirements
- Stating an understanding of preoperative preparations (e.g., skin preparation, bowel preparation)
- Demonstrating correct use of exercises and techniques to be used after surgery for the prevention of complications (e.g., splinting the incision, using an incentive spirometer, performing leg exercises, ambulating as early as permitted)

Interventions. Because the surgical experience is foreign to many people, focus on teaching the patient and family members. Teaching may begin in the surgeon's office for planned or elective surgery. Pamphlets, written instructions, approved websites, and video recordings or DVDs may be given or sent to the patient. More teaching may occur when the patient has preadmission testing. Some facilities hold classes before surgery for groups of patients or show videos for those who are having the same or similar surgical procedures. A tour of the operating suite and the postanesthesia care unit (PACU) may be included.

Explore the patient's level of knowledge and understanding. Increased access to information via the Internet may be helpful but is also a concern. Some Internet information may not be accurate or may not apply to a specific patient's plan of care.

The Joint Commission's NPSGs require that you provide information about informed consent, dietary restrictions, specific preparation for surgery (bowel and skin preparations), exercises after surgery, and plans for pain management to promote patients' participation and help achieve the expected outcome. A sample educational checklist is shown in Table 14-4. Because education occurs in a variety of settings, coordination of patient teaching efforts is challenging. When you care for the patient just before surgery (same-day, ambulatory surgery [outpatient] unit, inpatient hospital unit), assess the patient's

CHART 14-4 **Focused Assessment**

The Preoperative Patient

As part of the cardiopulmonary assessment, take and record vital signs; report:

- Hypotension or hypertension
- Heart rate less than 60 or more than 120 beats/min
- Irregular heart rate
- Chest pain
- Shortness of breath or dyspnea
- Tachypnea
- Pulse oximetry reading of less than 94%

Assess for and report any signs or symptoms of infection, including:

- Fever
- Purulent sputum
- Dysuria or cloudy, foul-smelling urine
- Any red, swollen, draining IV or wound site
- Increased white blood cell count

Assess for and report signs or symptoms that could contraindicate surgery, including:

- Increased prothrombin time (PT), international normalized ratio (INR), or activated partial thromboplastin time (aPTT)
- Hypokalemia or hyperkalemia
- Patient report of possible pregnancy or positive pregnancy test

Assess for and report other clinical conditions that may need to be evaluated by a physician or advanced practice nurse before proceeding with the surgical plans, including:

- Change in mental status
- Vomiting
- Rash
- Recent administration of an anticoagulant drug

TABLE 14-4 Preoperative Teaching Checklist

Consider these items when planning individualized preoperative teaching for patients and families:

- Fears and anxieties
- Surgical procedure
- Preoperative routines (e.g., NPO, blood samples, showering)
- Invasive procedures (e.g., lines, catheters)
- Coughing, turning, deep breathing
- Incentive spirometer
  - How to use
  - How to tell when used correctly
- Lower extremity exercises
- Stockings and pneumatic compression devices
- Early ambulation
- Splinting
- Pain management

and family members' knowledge and provide additional information as needed. If the patient is receiving sedation or general anesthesia, stress the importance of having another person drive the patient home after the procedure. Document in the patient record information about who was involved in teaching, what specifically was taught, and what education materials were given to the patient and family.

Ensuring Informed Consent. Surgery of any type involves invasion of the body and requires informed consent from the patient or legal guardian (Fig. 14-2). The Joint Commission's NPSGs state that patients deserve to be informed and involved in decisions affecting their health care. Consent implies that the patient has sufficient information to understand:

- The nature of and reason for surgery
- Who will be performing the surgery and whether others will be present during the procedure (e.g., students)
- All available options and the risks associated with each option
- The risks associated with the surgical procedure and its potential outcomes
- The risks associated with the use of anesthesia

Informed consent is one way to help ensure patient safety. It helps protect the patient from any unwanted procedures and protects the surgeon and the facility from lawsuit claims related to unauthorized surgery or uninformed patients. Written record of informed consent is documented on a "consent form" but can also be documented in the surgeon's notes. The consent form documents the patient's consent and signature for the procedure listed.

As a competent adult, it is the patient's right to refuse treatment for any reason, even when refusal might lead to death. For example, in the case of Jehovah's Witnesses, some patients will not accept blood transfusions because of their religious convictions.

The surgeon is responsible for having the consent form signed before sedation is given and before surgery is performed. *You, as a nurse, are not responsible for providing detailed information about the surgical procedure. Rather, your role is to clarify facts that have been presented by the surgeon and dispel myths that the patient or family may have about the surgical experience. You verify that the consent form is signed, and you serve as a witness to the signature, not to the fact that the patient is informed (Rock & Hoebeke, 2014).*

! NURSING SAFETY PRIORITY QSEN

Action Alert

If you believe that the patient has not been adequately informed, contact the surgeon and request that he or she see the patient for further clarification. Document this action in the medical record.

Patients who cannot write may sign with an X, which must be witnessed by two people. In an emergency, telephone or telegram authorization is acceptable and should be followed up with written consent as soon as possible. The number of witnesses (usually two) and the type of documentation vary according to the facility's policy. For a life-threatening situation in which every effort has been made to contact the person with medical power of attorney, consent is desired but not essential. In place of written or oral consent, written consultation by at least two physicians who are not associated with the case may be requested by the surgeon. This formal consultation legally supports the decision for surgery until the appropriate person can sign a consent form. If the patient is not capable of giving consent and has no family, the court can appoint a legal guardian to represent the patient's best interests.

A blind patient may sign his or her own consent form, which usually needs to be witnessed by two persons. Patients who do not speak the general language of the facility or who are hearing impaired may require a qualified translator and a second witness. Many facilities have consent forms written in more than one language and also have health care professionals who are proficient with American Sign Language. Qualified translators may be health care professionals, other types of hospital employee, or family members. They are required to keep patient information confidential.

Some surgical procedures, such as sterilization and experimental procedures, may require a special permit in addition to the standard consent. National and local governing bodies and the individual facility determine which procedures require a separate permit. Separate consents for anesthesia and blood products may be required.

Surgical procedures that are site-specific, such as left, right, or bilateral, require patient identification before surgery. As required by The Joint Commission's NPSGs, to ensure the correct site is selected and the wrong site is avoided, the site is marked by a licensed independent practitioner and, whenever possible, involves the patient. The surgeon is accountable and should be present during the procedure. The nurse is an important part of this safety measure. Before starting the operative procedure, facilities use a "time-out" procedure to verify the correct site, patient, and procedure. The perioperative nurse is in a position of ensuring these safety measures are implemented immediately before the procedure is started (Association of periOperative Registered Nurses [AORN], 2014c). The "time-out" involves the participation of all members of the procedure team including the surgeon, anesthesia provider, circulating nurse, scrub person, and any other active participants.

! NURSING SAFETY PRIORITY QSEN

Critical Rescue

At a minimum, the patient's identity, correct side and site, correct patient position, and agreement on the proposed procedure must be verified by all members of the surgical team.

GENERAL REQUEST AND CONSENT

FOR OFFICE USE ONLY:
Patient Name: ____________________
Date of Birth: ____________________
Date of Procedure: ____________________

I ______________________ request and give consent to ______________________
(Type or print patient name) (Type or print Doctor or Practitioner Name(s))

to perform the following procedure(s) ______________________
(Please list site and side if appropriate)

The benefits, risks, complications, and alternatives to the above procedure(s) have been explained to me.

I understand that the procedure(s) will be performed at Christiana Care by and under supervision of my doctor or practitioner. My doctor or practitioner may use the services of other doctors or practitioners, or members of the resident staff as he or she deems necessary or advisable.

I authorize my doctor or practitioner and his or her associates and assistants to perform such additional procedures, which in their judgment are necessary and appropriate to carry out my diagnosis or treatment.

I authorize the hospital to retain, preserve and use for scientific, teaching or transplant purposes, or to make other dispositions of, at their convenience, any specimens, tissues, or parts taken from my body during the course of this operation.

I consent to observers in the operating room in accordance with hospital policy. I consent to photography or video taping of my surgical procedure for educational purposes, provided my identity remains anonymous and confidential.

I agree to being given blood or blood products as deemed advisable during the course of my procedure. The risks, benefits, and alternatives to receiving blood or blood products have been explained to me.

I consent to the administration of sedation or analgesia during my procedure. The risks, benefits, and alternatives to receiving sedation or analgesia have been explained to me.

If anesthesia is required, I consent to the administration of anesthesia by members of the Department of Anesthesiology. I also consent to the use of non-invasive and invasive monitoring techniques as deemed necessary. I understand that anesthesia involves risks that are in addition to those resulting from the operation itself including, but not limited to, dental injury, hoarseness, vocal cord injury, infection, nerve injury, corneal abrasion, seizures, heart attack, stroke and even death.

Please initial one of the following statements (females only):

______ To the best of my knowledge I am not pregnant. ______ I believe I am pregnant.

I certify that I have read and understand the above consent statements. In addition, I have been offered the opportunity to ask my doctor or practitioner any questions I have regarding the procedure(s) to be performed and they have been answered to my satisfaction. I acknowledge that I have been given no guarantee or assurance as to the results that may be obtained from the procedure(s).

Signature of Patient or Decision Maker — Date and Time	Doctor or Practitioner Signature — Date and Time
Relationship to Patient if Decision Maker	Doctor ID # or Print Name
Witness Signature — Date and Time	Practitioner Print Name/Title
Witness Print Name	

Telephone Consent: ______________________
Name of person obtained from/Relationship to Patient

Witness's (es') Signature(s) — Date and Time	Witness's (es') Signature(s) — Date and Time
Witness's (es') Print Name(s)	Witness's (es') Print Name(s)

FIG. 14-2 A surgical consent form.

CLINICAL JUDGMENT CHALLENGE

Safety QSEN

The patient states the surgeon discussed the addition of a second procedure to the one indicated on the consent. The patient is visibly upset that the consent he is asked to sign with the surgical resident reflects only one procedure and cannot understand why the nurse and resident do not have the authority to "fix" the consent. In addition, he states he will not take his wedding ring off because it has never left his hand since his wife put it there 30 years ago.

1. How would you address the patient's immediate concern regarding the consent?
2. Under what conditions could the second procedure be performed?
3. What remedy would you propose to prevent such occurrences in the future?
4. How will you respond to the patient's unwillingness to remove his wedding ring?

Patient Self-Determination. Patients receiving medical care have the right to have or to initiate advance directives, such as a living will or durable power of attorney, as mandated by the Patient Self-Determination Act. Advance directives provide legal instructions to the health care providers about the patient's wishes and are to be followed. *Surgery does not provide an exception to a patient's advance directives or living will* (AORN, 2014b). Chapter 7 discusses advance directives in more detail.

Implementing Dietary Restrictions. Regardless of the type of surgery and anesthesia planned, the patient is restricted to NPO status before surgery. **NPO** means no eating, drinking (including water), or smoking (nicotine stimulates gastric secretions). The exact amount of time a patient must be NPO before surgery is controversial. Patients, especially older adults, who fast for 8 or more hours may have imbalances of fluids, electrolytes, and blood glucose levels. The American Society of Anesthesiologists (ASA) recommends a reduced NPO time—6 or more hours for easily digested solid food and 2 hours for clear liquids (Crenshaw, 2011; Sendelbach, 2010). A major problem is that these guidelines for duration of fasting have not been implemented universally.

NPO status ensures that the stomach contains a limited volume of gastric secretions, which decreases the risk for aspiration. Outpatients and patients who are scheduled for admission to the hospital on the same day that surgery is performed must receive written and oral instructions about when to begin NPO status.

NURSING SAFETY PRIORITY QSEN

Action Alert

Emphasize the importance of adhering to the prescribed NPO restriction. Failure to adhere can result in cancellation of surgery or increase the risk for aspiration during or after surgery.

Administering Regularly Scheduled Drugs. On the day of surgery, the patient's usual drug schedule may need to be altered. Consult the medical health care provider and the anesthesia provider for instructions about drugs such as those taken for diabetes, cardiac disease, or glaucoma, as well as regularly scheduled anticonvulsants, antihypertensives, anticoagulants, antidepressants, and corticosteroids. The surgeon may prescribe some drugs, including over-the-counter drugs such as aspirin, other NSAIDs, and herbal supplements, to be stopped until after surgery. Other drugs may be given IV to maintain the drug level in the blood. *Drugs for cardiac disease, respiratory disease, seizures, and hypertension are commonly allowed with a sip of water before surgery.* Some antihypertensive or antidepressant drugs are withheld on the day of surgery to reduce adverse effects on blood pressure during surgery. Even when beta blockers are not part of a patient's usual medications, they may be prescribed for some patients who are at risk for cardiac problems. Check with the health care provider, surgeon, or anesthesia provider to determine whether a specific patient requires perioperative therapy with beta-blocking drugs, as recommended by core measures for SCIP CARD-2 (see Table 14-1).

The patient who takes insulin for diabetes may be given a reduced dose of intermediate- or long-acting insulin based on the blood glucose level or may be given regular (fast-acting) insulin in divided doses on the day of surgery. As an alternative, an IV infusion of 5% dextrose in water may be given with the insulin to prevent low blood sugar during surgery. Because of the many treatment approaches to diabetes, clarify drug and IV prescriptions with the health care provider. (See Chapter 64 for more information about diabetes.)

Intestinal Preparation. Bowel or intestinal preparations are performed to prevent injury to the colon and to reduce the number of intestinal bacteria. Bowel evacuation is needed when a patient is having major abdominal, pelvic, perineal, or perianal surgery. In addition, colonoscopy procedures, routinely performed in outpatient ambulatory care facilities, require the patient to follow a strict preoperative protocol for bowel evacuation. The surgeon's preference and the type of surgical procedure determine the type of bowel preparation. Enemas ordered to be given until return flow is clear is a stressful procedure, especially for the older patient. Repeated enemas can cause electrolyte imbalance, fluid volume imbalances, vagal stimulation, and postural (orthostatic) hypotension. Enemas cause severe anal discomfort in patients with hemorrhoids. Some physicians prescribe potent laxatives instead of enemas, especially for older patients. Bowel preparations can exhaust the patient, and you must take safety precautions to prevent falls.

Skin Preparation. The skin is the body's first line of defense against INFECTION. A break in this barrier increases the risk for infection, especially for older patients. Skin preparation before surgery is the first step to reduce the risk for surgical site infection (AORN, 2014d).

One or two days before the scheduled surgery, the surgeon may ask the patient to shower using an antiseptic solution. Instruct the patient to be especially careful to clean well around the proposed surgical site. If the patient is hospitalized before surgery, showering and cleaning are repeated the night before surgery or in the morning before transfer to the surgical suite. This cleaning reduces contamination of the surgical field and reduces the number of organisms at the site. Remove any soil or debris from the surgical site and surrounding areas.

Factors that predispose to wound contamination and surgical site INFECTION (SSI) include bacteria found in hair follicles, disruption of the normal protective mechanisms of the skin, and nicks in the skin. Shaving of hair creates the potential for infection. Hair clipping with electrical clippers and depilatories are to be used for hair removal as required by The Joint Commission's NPSGs (Tanner et al., 2011). This type of skin preparation is part of the Surgical Care Improvement Project's (SCIP) core measures for SCIP Inf-6 (see Table 14-1).

The Centers for Disease Control and Prevention (CDC) recommends that if shaving is necessary, the hair should be removed using disposable sterile supplies and aseptic principles *immediately* before the start of the surgical procedure. If needed, shaving is performed in the treatment room, the holding area of the operating suite, or the operating room (OR). Fig. 14-3 shows areas of hair removal for various surgical procedures.

Preparing the Patient for Tubes, Drains, and Vascular Access. Prepare the patient for possible placement of tubes, drains, and vascular access devices. Preparation reduces the

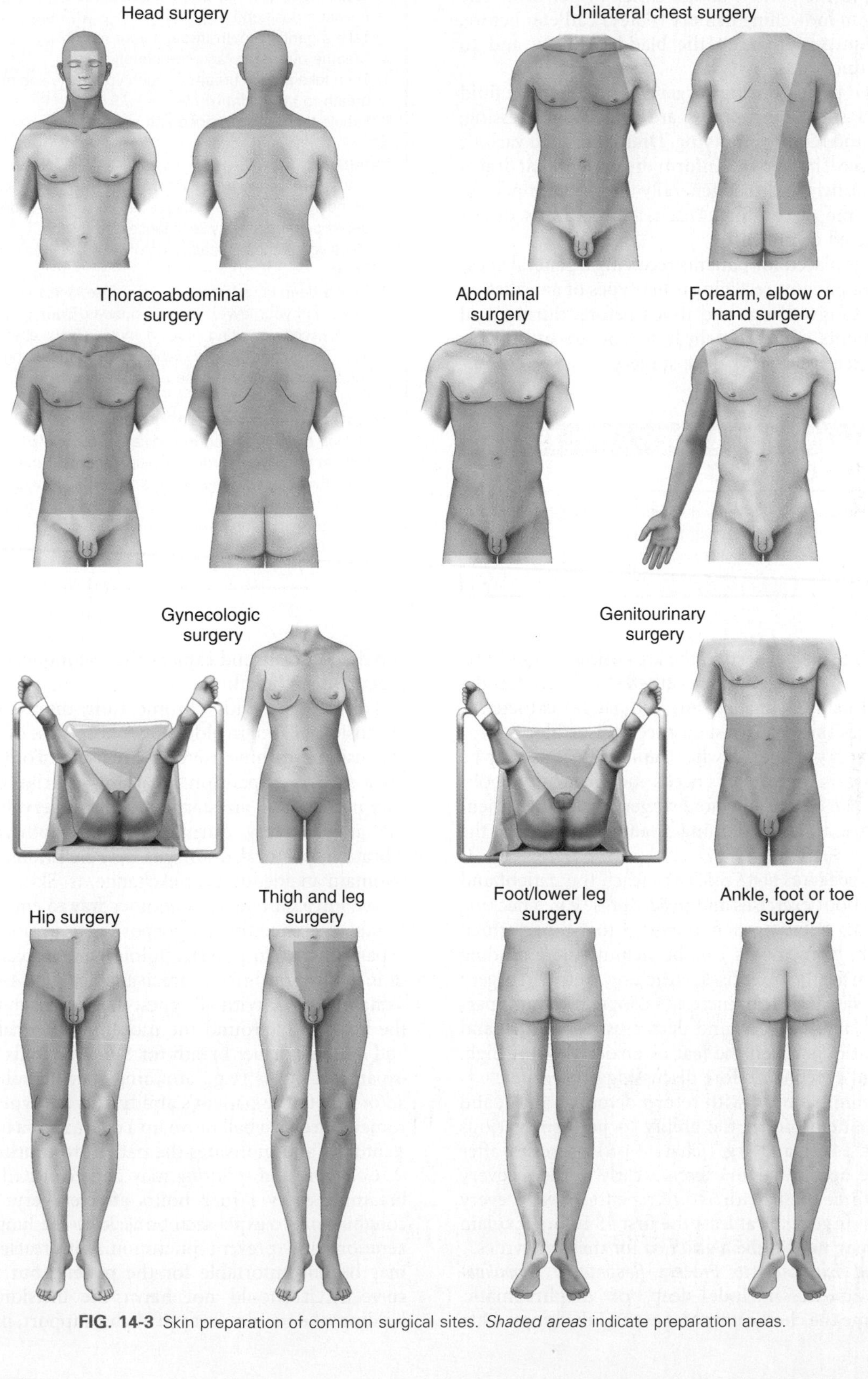

FIG. 14-3 Skin preparation of common surgical sites. *Shaded areas* indicate preparation areas.

patient's anxiety and fear and the family's negative reaction. Be careful not to scare the patient while providing information about the purpose of each tube.

Tubes of all sorts are common after surgery. A nasogastric (NG) tube may be inserted before abdominal surgery to decompress or empty the stomach and the upper bowel. Usually the tube is placed after the induction of anesthesia, when insertion is less disturbing to the patient and is easier to perform. The patient may need an indwelling urinary (Foley) catheter before, during, or after surgery to keep the bladder empty and to monitor kidney function.

Drains are often placed during surgery to help remove fluid from the surgical site. Some drains are under the dressing; others are visible and require emptying. Drains come in various shapes and sizes (see Chapter 16). Inform the patient that drains are often used routinely and that generally they are not painful but may cause some discomfort. Discuss the reasons drains should not be kinked or pulled.

Vascular access is placed for patients receiving a general anesthetic and for most patients receiving other types of anesthetics. Access is needed to give drugs and fluids before, during, and after surgery. Patients who are dehydrated or are at risk for dehydration may receive fluids before surgery.

CONSIDERATIONS FOR OLDER ADULTS

Patient-Centered Care QSEN

Older adult patients are at greater risk for dehydration because their fluid reserves are lower than those of young or middle-aged adults. Carefully monitor older adult patients and patients with cardiac disease receiving IV fluids. (See Chapter 13 for more information on IV therapy.)

CHART 14-5 Patient and Family Education: Preparing for Self-Management

Perioperative Respiratory Care

Deep (Diaphragmatic) Breathing

1. Sit upright on the edge of the bed or in a chair, being sure that your feet are placed firmly on the floor or a stool. (After surgery, deep breathing is done with the patient in Fowler's position or in semi-Fowler's position.)
2. Take a gentle breath through your mouth.
3. Breathe out gently and completely.
4. Then take a deep breath through your nose and mouth, and hold this breath to the count of five.
5. Exhale through your nose and mouth.

Expansion Breathing

1. Find a comfortable upright position, with your knees slightly bent. (Bending the knees decreases tension on the abdominal muscles and decreases respiratory resistance and discomfort.)
2. Place your hands on each side of your lower rib cage, just above your waist.
3. Take a deep breath through your nose, using your shoulder muscles to expand your lower rib cage outward during inhalation.
4. Exhale, concentrating first on moving your chest, then on moving your lower ribs inward, while gently squeezing the rib cage and forcing air out of the base of your lungs.

Splinting of the Surgical Incision

1. Unless coughing is contraindicated, place a pillow, towel, or folded blanket over your surgical incision and hold the item firmly in place.
2. Take three slow, deep breaths to stimulate your cough reflex.
3. Inhale through your nose, and then exhale through your mouth.
4. On your third deep breath, cough to clear secretions from your lungs while firmly holding the pillow, towel, or folded blanket against your incision.

The IV access is usually placed in the arm using a large-bore, short catheter (e.g., 18-gauge, 1-inch catheter) or placed in the back of the hand using a smaller-bore (20-gauge) catheter. A larger vein provides the least resistance to fluid or blood infusion, especially in an emergency when rapid infusions may be needed. Depending on the patient's needs and the facility's policies, the IV access can be placed before surgery when the patient is in the hospital room, in the holding or admission area of the surgical suite, or in the OR.

Postoperative Procedures and Exercises. Teach the patient and family members about exercises and procedures (e.g., checking dressings, obtaining vital signs frequently) to be performed after surgery. Family members can be helpful in reminding patients to perform the exercises. Teaching before surgery reduces apprehension and fear, increases cooperation and participation in care after surgery, and decreases respiratory and vascular complications. When the fear or anxiety level is high, explore the patient's feelings before discussing procedures.

Discussion, demonstration with return demonstration, and practice by the patient aid in the ability to perform various breathing (Chart 14-5) and leg (Chart 14-6) exercises after surgery. Stress the need to begin exercises early in the recovery phase and to continue them, with 5 to 10 repetitions each, every 1 to 2 hours after surgery for at least the first 48 hours. Explain that the patient may need to be awakened for these activities.

Procedures and Exercises to Prevent Respiratory Complications. Breathing exercises include deep, or diaphragmatic, breathing to enlarge the chest cavity and expand the lungs. After you demonstrate and explain the technique, urge the patient to practice deep breathing.

For patients with chronic lung disease or limited chest expansion, as seen in older patients because of the aging process, expansion breathing exercises are useful. For the patient having chest surgery, expansion breathing exercises strengthen accessory muscles and are started before surgery. Expansion breathing after surgery during chest physiotherapy (percussion, vibration, postural drainage) may help loosen secretions and maintain an adequate air exchange.

Incentive spirometry is another way to encourage the patient to take deep breaths. Its purpose is to promote complete lung expansion and to prevent pulmonary problems. Various types of incentive spirometers are available; Fig. 14-4 shows a patient using one type. With all types, the patient must be able to seal the lips tightly around the mouthpiece, inhale spontaneously, and hold his or her breath for 3 to 5 seconds for effective lung expansion. Goals (e.g., attaining specific volumes) can be set according to the patient's ability and the type of incentive spirometer. Seeing a ball move up a column or a bellows expanding reinforces and motivates the patient to continue performance.

Coughing and splinting may be performed along with deep breathing every 1 to 2 hours after surgery. The purposes of coughing are to expel secretions, keep the lungs clear, allow full aeration, and prevent pneumonia and atelectasis. Coughing may be uncomfortable for the patient, but when performed correctly, it should not harm the incision. Splinting (i.e., holding) the incision area provides support, promotes a feeling

CHART 14-6 **Patient and Family Education: Preparing for Self-Management**

Postoperative Leg Exercises

Exercise No. 1

1. Lie in bed with the head of your bed elevated to about 45 degrees.
2. Beginning with your right leg, bend your knee, raise your foot off the bed, and hold this position for a few seconds.
3. Extend your leg by unbending your knee, and lower the leg to the bed.
4. Repeat this sequence four more times with your right leg; then perform this same exercise five times with your left leg.

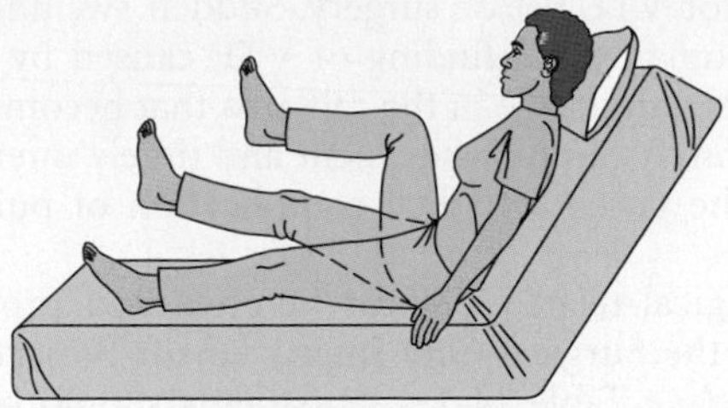

Exercise No. 2

1. Beginning with your right leg, point your toes toward the bottom of the bed.
2. With the same leg, point your toes up toward your face.
3. Repeat this exercise several times with your right leg; then perform this same exercise with your left leg.

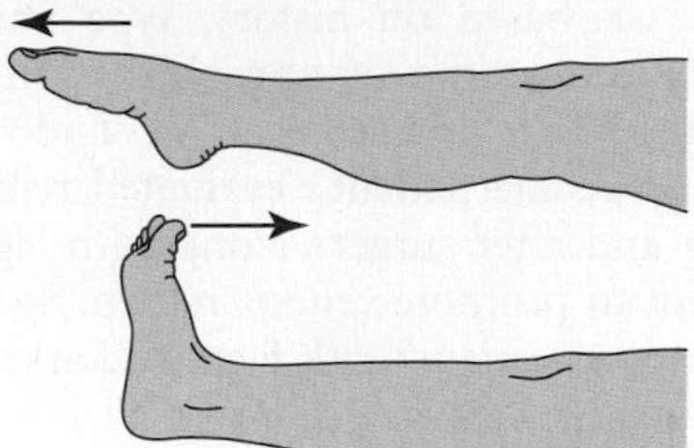

Exercise No. 3

1. Beginning with your right leg, make circles with your ankle, first to the left and then to the right.
2. Repeat this exercise several times with your right leg; then perform this same exercise with your left leg.

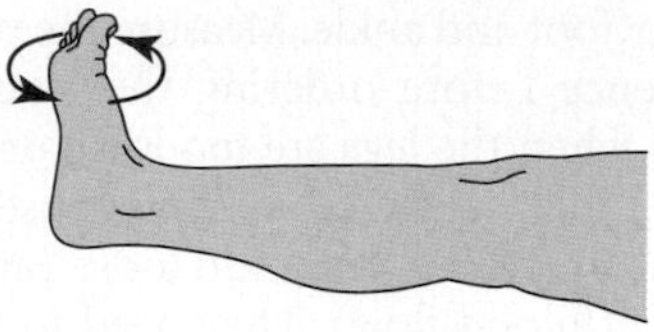

Exercise No. 4

1. Beginning with your right leg, bend your knee and *push* the ball of your foot into the bed or floor until you feel your calf and thigh muscles contracting.
2. Repeat this exercise several times with your right leg; then perform this same exercise with your left leg.

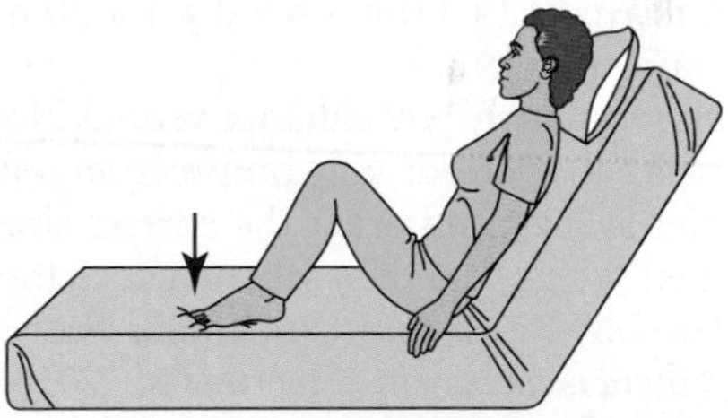

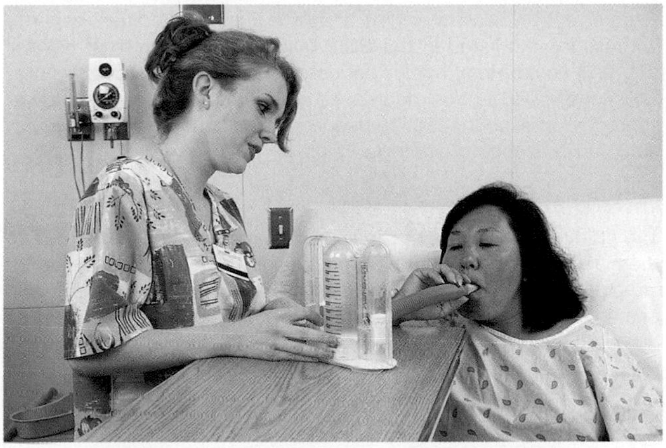

FIG. 14-4 A patient using an incentive spirometer.

of security, and reduces pain during coughing. The proper technique for splinting the incision site and coughing is described in Chart 14-5. A folded bath blanket or pillow is helpful to use as a splint. Cardiac surgery patients may receive their own heart-shaped pillow for splint use.

The use of routine coughing exercises after surgery is controversial. Some surgeons believe coughing may harm the surgical wound and that it would be better to use other, safer measures for lung hygiene, such as deep breathing and incentive spirometer exercises. When routine coughing exercises should be avoided for a specific patient, such as after a hernia repair or craniotomy, the surgeon usually writes a "do not cough" prescription.

Procedures and Exercises to Prevent Cardiovascular Complications. Venous stasis and venous thromboembolism (VTE) (a group of vascular disorders that includes deep vein thrombosis [DVT] and pulmonary embolism [PE]) are potential but often avoidable complications of surgery. VTE or DVT can lead to a PE if the blood clot breaks off and travels to the lungs. Patients at greater risk for VTE:

- Are obese
- Are older than 40 years
- Have cancer
- Have decreased mobility or are immobile
- Have a spinal cord injury
- Have a history of VTE, DVT, PE, varicose veins, or edema
- Are taking oral contraceptives

- Smoke
- Have decreased cardiac output
- Have hip fracture or total hip or total knee surgery

Always assess for VTE before surgery. Sudden swelling in one leg is a common physical finding of VTE caused by DVT. A patient may feel a dull ache in the calf area that becomes worse with ambulation. A careful assessment and timely intervention may prevent the potentially fatal complication of pulmonary embolism.

Because surgical-related VTE can be prevented, prophylaxis is required by the Surgical Care Improvement Project (SCIP) core measures (see Table 14-1). All patients should be evaluated for VTE risk based on history, type and duration of surgery, and expected time of immobilization after surgery. VTE prophylaxis may involve devices and drug therapy, depending on a specific patient's evaluated risk. Devices may be used during and after surgery along with leg exercises and early ambulation to promote venous return. Specific interventions depend on the patient's risk factors (Larkin et al., 2012). (See the Evidence-Based Practice box.)

Antiembolism stockings (TED or Jobst stockings) and elastic (Ace) wraps provide graduated compression of the legs, starting at the end of the foot and ankle. Measure the patient's leg length and circumference before ordering the stocking size. Elastic wraps are used when the legs are too large or too small for the stockings. Assist the patient in applying the stockings or wraps, and ensure that they are neither too loose (are ineffective) nor too tight (inhibit blood flow). They need to be worn properly and should be removed 1 to 3 times per day for 30 minutes for skin inspection and skin care.

Pneumatic compression devices enhance venous blood flow by providing intermittent periods of compression on the legs. Measure the patient's legs, and order the correct size. Place the boots on the patient's legs, and then set and check the compression pressures (usually 35-55 mm Hg). *Unless these devices are applied properly, there is no benefit (Elpern et al., 2013).* Fig. 14-5 shows various types of sequential compression devices. Antiembolism stockings may be worn in addition to the boots and may reduce some of the uncomfortable sensations of the boots (e.g., itching, sweating, heat).

Leg exercises also promote venous return. Teach the leg exercises outlined in Chart 14-6, and then urge the patient to practice these exercises before surgery. The exercises are important, even when other devices are used.

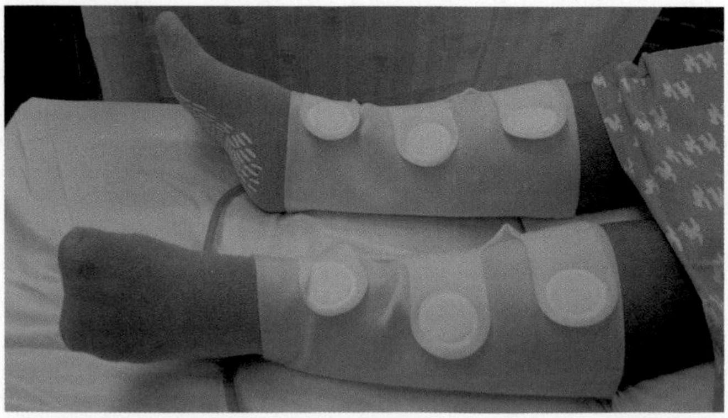

FIG. 14-5 An external pneumatic compression device used to promote venous return and prevent deep vein thrombosis (DVT).

Mobility soon after surgery (early ambulation) has many cardiovascular and other benefits. It stimulates intestinal motility, enhances lung expansion, mobilizes secretions, promotes venous return, prevents joint rigidity, and relieves pressure. For most types of surgery, teach the patient to turn at least every 2 hours after surgery while confined to bed. Teach patients how

EVIDENCE-BASED PRACTICE QSEN

VTE Prevention Beyond the Surgical Care Improvement Project (SCIP): What Works?

Larkin, B., Mitchell, K., & Petrie, K. (2012). Translating evidence to practice for mechanical venous thromboembolism prophylaxis. *AORN Journal, 96*(5), 513-527.

Both pharmacologic and mechanical prophylaxis for prevention of venous thromboembolism (VTE) are being used extensively to prevent VTE after surgery. Many health care professionals, including nurses, believe that pharmacologic prophylaxis is more effective and more important than mechanical prophylaxis. However, some patients cannot use pharmacologic prophylaxis. This integrative review of the literature sought to determine the evidence for best practices related to mechanical prophylaxis to prevent surgical-related venous thromboembolism (VTE) events. Variables compared included the types of mechanical prophylaxis, timing of application, the effects of combining prophylaxis methods, and the use of unilateral prophylaxis for some orthopedic procedures.

A variety of research reports and previous meta-analyses from appropriate sources were reviewed. The criteria and need for mechanical prophylaxis and its optimal initiation varied by institution and profession. Most surgeons followed the SCIP guidelines, whereas experienced perioperative nurses expanded the risk factors to include history of VTE events, level of general immobility, and presence of varicosities. Also examined were issues related to availability of prescribed devices and the timing of their application.

Results of the study indicated that use of mechanical prophylaxis for VTE is increasing, although the timing and duration of application is not consistent. Overall, the best outcomes were obtained when devices, whether they were graduated compression stockings or intermittent pneumatic compression devices, were applied correctly in the preoperative period rather than intraoperatively or postoperatively. No evidence supports the combination of devices to be more effective than either type of device alone. In addition, patients with issues not listed in the SCIP guidelines were also at risk for VTE and could benefit from perioperative mechanical prophylaxis. These include older age, decreased general mobility, irritable bowel syndrome, oral contraceptive use, malignant disease, severe infection, and presence of varicose veins.

Level of Evidence: 1

The study is an analysis of previous research studies on the use of mechanical prophylaxis for perioperative prevention of VTE, examining practices and specific devices. The methods used were appropriate to answer the question posed, and the large numbers of human subjects resulted in credible evidence to support the need for practice consistency.

Commentary: Implications for Practice and Research

The current SCIP criteria for VTE mechanical prophylaxis are beginning points, not end points, for this evolving prevention strategy. Nurses can contribute to the desired outcome of reducing surgical-related VTE events by identifying patients who have other risk factors for VTE that may be less obvious or are not included in the SCIP criteria. By partnering with surgeons to ensure that such patients are prescribed mechanical prophylaxis and that the devices are applied correctly during the preoperative period, the goal of VTE as a "never" event is closer to being achieved.

to use the bed siderails safely for turning and how to protect the surgical wound by splinting when turning. Assure patients that assistance and pain drugs will be given as needed to reduce any anxiety and pain they may have with this activity.

For certain surgical procedures, such as some brain, spinal, and orthopedic procedures, the surgeon may prescribe turning restrictions. Ask the surgeon about other interventions to prevent complications of immobility in patients with turning restrictions. During teaching before surgery, inform the patient of anticipated turning restrictions.

Most patients are allowed and encouraged to get out of bed the day of or the day after surgery. Assist the patient into a chair or with ambulation after the surgery, the next day, or when the surgeon specifies. If a patient must remain in bed, help him or her turn, deep breathe, and perform leg exercises at least every 2 hours to prevent complications from immobility.

Minimizing Anxiety

Planning: Expected Outcomes. Before surgery, the patient is expected to have manageable anxiety as indicated by consistently demonstrating these behaviors:

- Expressing a reduced level of anxiety
- Showing an absence of body language indicators of anxiety (e.g., hand wringing, facial tension, restlessness, dilated pupils, sweating, elevated blood pressure, elevated pulse rate)

Interventions. Anxiety often causes restlessness and sleeplessness. The patient may perceive the surgical experience as a threat to life and function. Assess the patient's level of anxiety, as discussed on p. 222 in the Psychosocial Assessment section. Interventions such as teaching and communicating with the patient before surgery, enabling the patient to use previously successful coping mechanisms, and giving antianxiety drugs help reduce the anxiety. Incorporate available support systems into the plan of care.

Preoperative teaching involves first assessing the patient's knowledge about the surgical experience (see p. 225 in the Providing Information section) and then providing factual information to promote his or her understanding. Allow ample time for questions. Respond to the questions accurately, and refer unanswered questions to the proper professional. During the discussion, continually assess the patient's responses and anxiety level. Be careful not to provide information that might increase anxiety. The informed, educated patient is better able to anticipate events and maintain self-control and is thus less anxious.

Encouraging communication by having the patient state feelings, fears, and concerns can help reduce anxiety. Use an honest and open approach so that the patient can express feelings freely without fear of ridicule or judgment. Keep the patient informed by clarifying information, answering questions, and allaying fears about the surgery.

Promoting rest is helpful because the stress and anxiety of impending surgery often interfere with the patient's ability to sleep and rest the night before surgery. The period before surgery is physically and emotionally stressful. To help the patient relax, determine what he or she usually does to relax and fall asleep. If the patient is able, urge him or her to continue these methods of relaxation. A back rub is relaxing and can be performed by a nurse, unlicensed assistive personnel (UAP), or family member. The surgeon may prescribe a sedative or hypnotic drug to help the patient be well rested for surgery.

Distraction may be used as an intervention for anxiety, especially in the 24 hours immediately before surgery. Listening to music may decrease anxiety, as may watching television, reading, or visiting with friends and family members.

Teaching family members helps reduce anxiety by increasing the likelihood of support and involvement in the patient's care. Assess the readiness and desire of the family to take an active part in the patient's care. A positive sign of family interest is that of members asking questions about the surgical experience. After family readiness is determined, keep family members informed and encourage their involvement in all aspects of education. Emphasize the important role of the family before surgery, but guide discussions and practice sessions so that the patient is the focus of the discussion. Family members can encourage and help the patient practice exercises to be performed after surgery.

Inform the family of the time for surgery, if known, and of any schedule changes. If the patient is an outpatient, provide clear directions to the patient and family regarding any specific night-before procedures, what time and where to report, and what to bring with them. Encourage the family to stay with the patient before surgery for support.

Most families are anxious about the surgery planned for their loved one. To reduce their anxiety, explain the routines expected before, during, and after surgery. Tell the family that after the patient leaves the hospital room or admission area, there is usually a 30- to 60-minute preparation period in the operating area (holding room, treatment area) before the surgery actually begins. After surgery, the patient is taken to the postanesthesia care unit (PACU) usually for 1 to 2 hours before returning to the hospital room or discharge area. The length of stay in the PACU depends on the type of surgery, the type of anesthesia, any complications, and the patient's responses. Tell the family about the best place to wait for the patient or surgeon according to the facility's policy and the surgeon's preference. Many hospitals and surgical centers have surgical waiting areas so that families can wait in comfortable surroundings and be easily located when the procedure is completed. Often families are provided with a beeper to let them know when to report to a specific area to receive updates about the patient's status, meet with the surgeon, or see the patient.

Preoperative Chart Review. Review the patient's chart to ensure that all documentation, preoperative procedures, and orders are completed. Check the surgical informed consent form and, if indicated, any other special consent forms to see that they are signed and dated and that they contain the witnesses' signatures. Confirm that the scheduled procedure, including the identification of left versus right when necessary, is what is listed on the consent form. Even though it might be obvious, inform the patient that the site for surgery will be marked before the procedure begins. If possible, encourage the patient to assist with the marking, as suggested by The Joint Commission's NPSGs. Document allergies according to facility policy. Accurate measuring and recording of height and weight are important for proper dosage of the anesthetic agents. Ensure that the results of all laboratory, radiographic, and diagnostic tests are on the chart. Document any abnormal results, and report them to the surgeon and the anesthesia provider. If the patient is an autologous blood donor or has had directed blood donations made, those special slips must be included in the chart. Record a current set of vital signs (within 1 to 2 hours of the scheduled surgery time), and document any significant physical or psychosocial observations.

Report special needs, concerns, and instructions (including advance directives) to the surgical team, as required by The Joint Commission's NPSGs. For example, advise the surgical team if the patient is a member of Jehovah's Witnesses and does not accept blood products or if the patient is hard of hearing and does not have his or her hearing aid. This information assists the surgical team in providing personalized care while the patient is in the surgical area.

Preoperative Patient Preparation. Facilities usually require the patient to remove most clothing and wear a hospital gown into the OR; however, underpants may be worn in above-the-waist surgery and socks may be worn, except in foot or leg surgery. If prescribed by the surgeon, apply antiembolism stockings or pneumatic compression devices before surgery. In some ambulatory settings, such as for cataract surgery, no or minimal clothes are removed.

Patients are advised to leave all valuables at home. If he or she has valuables, including jewelry, money, or clothes, they are given to a family member or locked in a safe place, according to the facility's policy. If rings cannot be removed, tape them in place. Depending on the type and location of surgery, pierced jewelry may need to be removed. Religious emblems may be pinned or fastened securely to the patient's gown. Some facilities have paper emblems from a religious leader.

The patient wears an identification band that clearly gives the first and last name, hospital number, surgeon, and birth date. An additional bracelet, usually red, identifies any allergies. A bracelet indicating that a blood sample for type and screen has been drawn may be worn, depending on the facility's policy.

If dentures are to be removed, including partial dental plates, place them in a labeled denture cup. Denture removal is a safety measure to prevent aspiration and obstruction of the airway. If a patient has any capped teeth, document this finding on the checklist.

All prosthetic devices, such as artificial eyes and limbs, are removed and given to a family member or safely stored, as are contact lenses, glasses, wigs, and toupees. Check and remove hairpins and clips, which can conduct electrical current used during surgery and cause scalp burns.

Some facilities allow hearing aids in the surgical suite to help communication before and after surgery. If the patient is sent to surgery with a hearing aid, communicate this to the surgical nurse to prevent accidental loss of or damage to the device. Some facilities allow dentures, wigs, and glasses to be worn into the operating suite to prevent embarrassment to the patient. These items are removed when absolutely necessary.

The removal of fingernail polish or artificial nails is controversial. Polish and artificial nails have been thought to affect the accuracy of pulse oximetry readings. Recent studies have indicated that pulse oximetry readings taken on fingers are affected by brown or blue polish but not by red or lighter color polish. In addition, pulse oximetry does not have to be measured on fingers only. Some facilities still require that at least one artificial nail must be removed to monitor oxygen saturation by pulse oximetry.

After the patient is prepared for surgery and the operating suite is ready to receive him or her, ask him or her to empty the bladder. This action prevents incontinence or overdistention and is a starting point for intake and output measurement. A full bladder may hinder access to the surgical site. Answer questions, offer reassurance as needed, and give prescribed drugs.

Preoperative Drugs. Preoperative drugs may be prescribed regardless of the type of planned anesthesia. Various drugs reduce anxiety, promote relaxation, prevent laryngospasm, reduce vagal-induced bradycardia, inhibit oral and gastric secretions, and decrease the amount of anesthetic needed for the induction and maintenance of anesthesia. Drug selection is based on the patient's age, physical and psychological condition, medical history, and height and weight; other drugs the patient takes routinely; test results; and the type and extent of the planned surgical procedure. If more than one response is required, combination therapy may be prescribed.

Drug types for preoperative purposes may include sedatives (e.g., hydroxyzine [Atarax, Vistaril]); hypnotics (e.g., lorazepam [Ativan]); anxiolytics (e.g., midazolam [Versed]); opioid analgesics (e.g., morphine, hydromorphone); and an anticholinergic agent (e.g., atropine). Other specific-purpose drugs also may be added. For example, if rapid emptying of the stomach is needed, metoclopramide (Reglan) may be prescribed. When procedures are long or stress ulcers are likely, an H_2 histamine blocker (e.g., cimetidine [Tagamet]; ranitidine [Zantac]) is used.

Preoperative drugs may be given when the patient is "on call" to the surgical suite. After positively identifying the patient as required by The Joint Commission's NPSGs (using the armband and asking the patient to state his or her name and birth date) and making sure the operative permit is signed, give the correct drugs in the correct doses. Then raise the siderails, place the call light within easy reach of the patient, and remind him or her not to try to get out of bed. Place the bed in a low position. Tell the patient that he or she may become drowsy and have a dry mouth as a result of the drugs.

A more common practice is for the preoperative drugs to be given *after* the patient is transferred to the preoperative area. This practice permits the surgical team and anesthesia personnel to make more accurate assessments and have last-minute discussions with a patient not yet affected by drugs. In addition, after the patient is in the preoperative area, drugs can be given by the IV route. Monitoring equipment such as continuous pulse oximetry and ECG are more readily available in this area. The oral or IM route is used less often because of variable absorption rates. The surgeon may order a prophylactic antibiotic to be given right before or during surgery to reduce the risk for a surgical site INFECTION (SSI), as suggested by The Joint Commission's NPSGs. When needed, the antibiotic is given within 60 minutes before the incision is made, as mandated by the Surgical Care Improvement Project (SCIP) core measures, SCIP Inf-1 (see Table 14-1).

Patient Transfer to the Surgical Suite. In the immediate preoperative period, review and update the patient's chart, reinforce teaching, ensure that the patient is correctly dressed for surgery, and give prescribed preoperative drugs. Use an electronic or hardcopy preoperative checklist for a smooth, efficient transfer to the surgical suite (Fig. 14-6). The patient, along with the signed consent form, the completed preoperative checklist, the chart, and the patient identification card, is transported to the surgical suite.

Most patients in the hospital setting are transferred to the surgical suite on a stretcher with the siderails up. In special circumstances (e.g., patients requiring traction, those having some types of orthopedic surgery, those who should be moved as little as possible), the patient is transferred in the hospital bed. Other factors that influence the decision to transfer in a

PREOPERATIVE CHECKLIST **PATIENT INFORMATION**

Date and Time of Arrival to Presurgical Holding Area:__________

INITIAL APPROPRIATELY

1. Hospital identification band intact and legible including patient name, date of birth, medical record number ____ Yes ____ No	
A. If yes, which arm? ________	
B. If no, make and apply arm band	
C. Is the extremity involved in the surgery? ____ Yes ____ No	
D. If yes, change to another extremity ____ Yes ____ No	

	IN PLACE	REMOVED
2. Glasses, contact lenses		
3. Hearing aid(s)		
4. Jewelry, piercings, religious medals, ring taped to finger		
5. Dentures (full, partial)		
6. Other prostheses (list)		
7. Hairpiece, wig, pins/combs		
8. Makeup, nail polish		
9. Clothing		
	YES	**NO**
10. Antiembolic stockings, compression devices		
11. Patient voided		
12. Advance directives on MR		
13. IV started by:		
14. Permission for surgeon to speak to family		
15. Family has pager #		
16. Informed consent signed, witnessed, on chart		

INITIAL APPROPRIATE COLUMN

	YES	NO
17. Site of site-specific surgery verified by patient and surgeon		
18. History and physical on chart		
19. Pregnancy test date within the past 10 days for females age 11–55 (unless documented hysterectomy)		
20. Type and screen verified with blood bank		
21. Test results (circle those on chart) CBC H&H UA EPI PT/PTT METAPNL ECG CXR		
22. OR notified of latex allergy		
23. ID plate on chart		
24. NPO with appropriate meds		

LIST KNOWN ALLERGIES

PRE-OP MEDS & DOSAGES	TIME
VITAL SIGNS	**TIME**
BP Pulse	
Resp O2 sat	
Temp Ht Wt	
MISCELLANEOUS	**YES/NO**
Risk for falls	
Communication barrier	

COMMENTS__________

RN________ **PHONE/PAGER**________ **DATE**________ **TIME**________

FIG. 14-6 A preoperative checklist.

bed are the patient's age, size, and physical condition. In ambulatory settings, patients either walk or are transferred to the surgical suite on a stretcher or in a wheelchair.

◆ *Evaluation: Outcomes*

Evaluate the care of the preoperative patient based on the identified patient problems. The expected outcomes include that the patient:

- States understanding of the informed consent and preoperative procedures
- Demonstrates postoperative exercises and techniques for prevention of complications
- Has reduced anxiety

Specific indicators for these outcomes are listed for each patient problem in the Planning and Implementation section (see earlier).

NURSING CONCEPTS AND CLINICAL JUDGMENT REVIEW

What might you NOTICE in a patient who is preparing for surgery and has adequate body defenses related to INFECTION?

Vital signs:
- Body temperature within normal range
- No sweating or chills

Physical assessment:
- Skin intact (no rashes, abnormal lesions, open areas, or drainage)
- Skin color normal for ethnicity
- Lymph nodes normal, no enlargement or pain
- Absence of sore throat, pain or burning on urination, productive cough
- Lung sounds clear to auscultation

Psychological assessment:
- Oriented, not confused

Laboratory assessment:
- White blood cell levels within normal limits for age and gender
- All cultures negative for pathogenic organisms
- Urinalysis result shows clear urine, no bacteria, white blood cells, or nitrates present
- Chest x-ray clear

GET READY FOR THE NCLEX® EXAMINATION!

KEY POINTS

Review these Key Points for each NCLEX Examination Client Needs Category.

Safe and Effective Care Environment
- Determine the purpose of surgery for each patient in your care.
- Assess each patient's personal factors for threats to safety.
- Ensure that the patient is wearing proper identification.
- Use at least two appropriate identifiers (e.g., hospital number, the identification band, asking the patient to state his or her name and birthdate) to identify the patient when providing instruction, administering drugs, marking surgical sites, and performing any procedure. *Do not use room number or bed number to identify the patient.* **Safety** QSEN
- Check that the informed consent has been properly signed by the patient and witness and that the presurgical checklist is complete and accurate. **Safety** QSEN
- Ask the patient to explain in his or her own words what surgical procedure is being done and why.
- Check that documentation for any procedure to be performed on one of a paired organ or extremity clearly indicates which organ or extremity is involved. **Safety** QSEN
- If the patient's explanation of the scheduled surgery is not consistent with the documentation, notify the surgeon and request that he or she speak to the patient. **Safety** QSEN
- Ensure that the patient is not asked to sign an operative permit or any other legal document after the preoperative drugs have been given.
- After the patient has received preoperative drugs, keep the siderails up and the bed in the low position.
- Communicate during hand-off to the operating room personnel all care that has been provided and what care may still be needed.

Health Promotion and Maintenance
- Teach patients about dietary restrictions, preoperative preparations, and specific interventions to perform after surgery to prevent complications (incision splinting, deep-breathing exercises, range-of-motion exercises—as described in Charts 14-5 and 14-6). **Patient-Centered Care** QSEN

Psychosocial Integrity
- Assess the extent of the patient's and family members' knowledge about the scheduled surgical procedure to identify learning needs. **Patient-Centered Care** QSEN
- Encourage the patient to express his or her feelings regarding the surgical procedure or its possible outcome.
- Explain and provide written information for all diagnostic procedures, restrictions, and follow-up care to the patient and his or her family.

- Communicate to the surgeon and anesthesia personnel any concerns, fears, or preferences the patient has. **Patient-Centered Care** QSEN
- Apply appropriate interventions to reduce patient anxiety.

Physiological Integrity

- Perform a complete and accurate preoperative assessment.
- If required, ensure that dentures and any other personal items are removed from the patient before he or she is transferred to the surgical suite.
- Apply prescribed antiembolic stockings, sequential compression boots, or other devices to reduce or prevent vascular complications. **Evidence-Based Practice** QSEN
- Communicate to the surgeon and anesthesia personnel any physical or laboratory change that may alter the patient's response to drugs, anesthesia, or surgery.

15 CHAPTER

Care of Intraoperative Patients

Robin Chard

http://evolve.elsevier.com/Iggy/

PRIORITY CONCEPTS

- Infection
- Gas Exchange
- Sensory Perception
- Clotting
- Thermoregulation

LEARNING OUTCOMES

Safe and Effective Care Environment

1. Differentiate the roles and responsibilities of various intraoperative personnel.
2. Use appropriate patient identifiers when administering drugs, ensuring informed consent, and verifying surgical sites during the intraoperative period.
3. Protect the patient from injury, poor thermoregulation, and infection during the intraoperative period.
4. Communicate care provided and needed at each transition in care during the intraoperative period.

Psychosocial Integrity

5. Reduce the psychological impact for the patient and family regarding the intraoperative experience.
6. Ensure patient concerns and needs are communicated to other members of the health care team during the intraoperative period.

Physiological Integrity

7. Use knowledge of anatomy, physiology, and principles of aging to modify and prioritize patient care during the intraoperative period to prevent skin breakdown and positioning injury.
8. Coordinate appropriate care for the patient with malignant hyperthermia.

The *intraoperative period* begins when the patient enters the surgical suite and ends at the time of transfer to the postanesthesia recovery area, same-day surgery unit, or the intensive care unit. The main concerns of perioperative nurses are safety and patient advocacy by preventing, reducing, controlling, and managing many hazards. In the operating room (OR) the patient is at risk for infection, impaired skin integrity, increased anxiety, poor thermoregulation and altered body temperature, and injury related to positioning and other hazards. The surgical phase is filled with unfamiliar experiences and uncertain outcomes. Nursing care during this period affects the patient's physical needs, spiritual needs, comfort, safety, dignity, and psychological status. Specific procedures and policies may differ among agencies but should all reflect the standards and recommended practices as published by the Association of periOperative Registered Nurses (AORN) (2014a). Perioperative nurses practice within a specific, patient-focused model that incorporates professional practice with attainable, measurable outcomes.

OVERVIEW

Members of the Surgical Team

The surgical team usually consists of the surgeon, one or more surgical assistants, the anesthesia provider, and the OR nursing staff. Perioperative, or OR, nurses include the holding area nurse, circulating nurse, scrub nurse or a non-nurse "scrub person," and specialty nurse. The number of assistants, circulating nurses, and scrub nurses depends on the complexity and length of the surgical procedure. For some minor procedures, only a circulating nurse and scrub person may be needed in addition to the surgeon. More complex procedures may require additional nursing staff to either circulate or scrub.

Surgeon and Surgical Assistant

The *surgeon* is a physician who is responsible for the surgical procedure and any surgical judgments about the patient. The *surgical assistant* might be another surgeon (or physician, such as a resident or intern) or an advanced practice nurse, physician assistant, certified registered nurse first assistant (CRNFA), or surgical technologist. Under the direction of the surgeon and within the legal scope of practice for each state, the assistant may hold retractors, suction the wound (to improve viewing of the operative site), cut tissue, suture, and dress wounds.

Anesthesia Providers

The *anesthesiologist* is a physician who specializes in giving anesthetic agents. A *certified registered nurse anesthetist (CRNA)* is an advanced practice registered nurse with additional education and credentials who delivers anesthetic agents under the supervision of an anesthesiologist, surgeon, dentist, or podiatrist. The anesthesia provider gives anesthetic drugs to induce and maintain anesthesia and delivers other drugs to support the patient during surgery.

The anesthesia provider monitors the patient during surgery by assessing and monitoring:

- The level of anesthesia (i.e., by using a peripheral nerve stimulator or electroencephalogram [EEG] bispectral analysis)
- Cardiopulmonary function (using electrocardiographic [ECG] monitoring, pulse oximetry, end-tidal carbon dioxide monitoring, arterial blood gases [ABGs], and hemodynamic monitoring via arterial lines and/or pulmonary artery catheters)
- Capnography (monitors ventilation for non-intubated patients)
- Vital signs
- Intake and output

Depending on the patient's needs, anesthesia personnel give IV fluids, including blood products.

Perioperative Nursing Staff

Perioperative nursing staff have several roles during surgery, depending on their education, experience, skill, and job responsibilities. Regardless of their role, the OR nurse uses clinical decision-making skills, develops a plan of nursing care, and coordinates care delivery to patients and their family members.

Holding area nurses work in those operating suites that have a presurgical holding area next to the main ORs. The holding area nurse coordinates and manages the care while the patient waits in this area until the OR is ready. Responsibilities include greeting the patient on arrival, reviewing the medical record and preoperative checklist, verifying that the operative consent forms are signed, and documenting the risk assessment (Fig. 15-1). This nurse also assesses the patient's physical and emotional status, gives emotional support, answers questions, and provides additional education as needed.

The holding area is busy, with many staff members performing different procedures before surgery (e.g., starting IV lines, inserting catheters). The nurse promotes comfort, privacy, and confidentiality. In some facilities, family members may wait here with the patient.

Circulating nurses, or "circulators," are registered nurses who coordinate, oversee, and are involved in the patient's nursing care in the OR. This nurse's actions are vital to the smooth flow of events before, during, and after surgery. He or she coordinates all activities within that particular OR. The circulator sets up the OR and ensures that needed supplies, including blood products and diagnostic support, are available. All anticipated equipment is gathered and inspected by the circulator to ensure safety and function before surgery. Depending on the procedure and position required, the circulator makes up the operating bed (OR table) with gel pads (to prevent pressure ulcers), safety straps and armboards, and either heating pads under the sheets or disposable warming blankets placed over the patient as needed to prevent hypothermia.

If there is no holding area nurse, the circulator also assumes the responsibilities of that role. Even when there is a holding area nurse, the circulator also greets the patient and reviews findings with the holding area nurse.

Once the patient is moved into the OR, the circulating nurse, along with the OR team, assists the patient in transferring to the OR table. The nurse positions the patient, protecting bony areas with padding while providing comfort and reassurance. While observing the patient, the circulating nurse also assists the anesthesia provider with the induction of anesthesia by positioning the patient and applying cricoid pressure, when requested. The circulator then may assist with additional positioning, insert a Foley catheter if needed, apply the grounding pad, test equipment, and "prep" (scrub) the surgical site before the patient is draped with sterile drapes.

Throughout the surgery, the circulating nurse:

- Protects the patient's privacy
- Ensures the patient's safety
- Monitors traffic in the room
- Assesses the amount of urine and blood loss
- Reports findings to the surgeon and anesthesia provider
- Ensures that the surgical team maintains sterile technique and a sterile field
- Anticipates the patient's and surgical team's needs, providing supplies and equipment
- Communicates information about the patient's status to family members during long or unique procedures
- Documents care, events, interventions, and findings

Depending on facility policy, the circulating nurse may record drugs, blood, and blood components given. (This also may be a function of the anesthesia provider.)

Before the procedure is over, the circulating nurse completes documentation in the OR and nursing records, including the presence of drains or catheters, the length of the surgery, and a count of all sponges, "sharps" (needles, blades), and instruments. He or she notifies the postanesthesia care unit (PACU) of the patient's estimated time of arrival and any special needs.

Scrub nurses or scrub persons set up the sterile table (Fig. 15-2), drape the patient, and hand sterile supplies, sterile equipment, and instruments to the surgeon and the assistant. Knowledge of the surgical procedure allows the scrub person to anticipate which instruments and types of sutures the surgeon will need, which reduces the duration of anesthesia. Collaboration and coordination of activities between the surgeon and the scrub person help promote the best surgical outcome for the patient. Throughout the procedure, the scrub person (with the circulating nurse) maintains an accurate count of sponges, sharps, and instruments and amounts of irrigation fluid and drugs used.

A specially trained person who is not a nurse may perform the scrub role. Such people are called *operating room technicians (ORTs)* or *surgical technologists.* Often certified surgical technologists (CSTs) are used in the OR.

Specialty nurses may be in charge during some types of specialty surgery (e.g., orthopedic, cardiac, ophthalmologic) and provide specific nursing care during surgery. This nurse assesses, maintains, and recommends equipment, instruments, and supplies used in that specialty.

Identification of Patient, Procedure, and Surgical Side/Sites, and Fire Risk Assessment

Procedure: ______________________ ____________ Date of Procedure

Preoperative verification process to be completed by assigned personnel in designated areas. Mark appropriate blocks. Side 1

PEP	Sending Unit	Prep & Holding/Admission Area
Posting Card	Patient verbalizes	Patient verbalizes
Patient verbalizes	ID Bracelet (e.g., Name & DOB)	ID Bracelet (e.g., Name & DOB)
Other	OR Schedule	OR Schedule
	Surgical Consent	Surgical Consent
	Site marked with "Yes" ☐ N/A	Site marked with "Yes" ☐ N/A
	H & P	H & P
	X-ray Report / X-ray	X-ray Report / X-ray
	Other studies	Other studies
Signature:	Signature:	Signature:
Print Name:	Print Name:	Print Name:
Date/Time:	Date/Time:	Date/Time:

Surgical Site Marking Verification

* Not applicable (N/A) meets exemption criteria (see instructions on side 2).
* After 2 methods of verification (patient verbalized, consent, H & P, other), the patient (in presence of RN) will write "Yes" with a permanent marker on or as near to surgical site:

☐ N/A ☐ RIGHT ☐ LEFT

Signature ____________ Print Name ____________ Date / Time

Side/Sites Marked by: ______________________

COMMENTS

Signature ____________ Date/Time

ANESTHESIA (Time-out) — **CONFIRMATION OF PATIENT IDENTIFICATION, PROCEDURE, & SURGICAL SITE PRIOR TO THE START OF ANESTHESIA BLOCK**

The anesthesiologist ______________________ (Provider Name(s)) and the identification assistant (perianesthesia nurse, operating room RN, another anesthesia provider, another physician or physician assistant) have verbally agreed that ______________________ (Patient Name) will have the following block performed: ______________________ Identification Assistant ______________________

Re-verification completed ____________ Re-verification completed ____________ Re-verification completed ____________

SURGICAL TEAM (Time-out) — **CONFIRMATION OF PATIENT IDENTIFICATION, PROCEDURE, SURGICAL SITE, AND AS APPLICABLE, IMPLANT WITH START OF PROCEDURE**

The surgical team (Surgeon/Resident, Anesthesia Provider, and Circulating RN) has verbally agreed that ______________________ (Patient Name) will have the above procedure performed.
Document procedure/site only if the procedure/site is different or left blank at top of form. ______________________

Circulating RN: ______________________ Signature / Print Name ____________ Date / Time

SURGICAL TEAM — **SURGICAL SITE FIRE RISK ASSESSMENT SCORE**

Alcohol based prep solution had sufficient time for fumes to dissipate. ☐ YES ☐ NO ☐ N/A

(Circle appropriate option)	Y	N
• Surgical site or incision above the xiphoid	1	0
• Open oxygen source (Patient receiving supplemental oxygen via any variety of face mask or nasal cannula)	1	0
• Available ignition source (i.e., electrosurgery unit, laser, fiberoptic light source)	1	0
Scoring 3 = High risk; 2 = Low risk w/potential to convert to high risk; 1 = Low risk — Total Score		

Verified by: ______________________ (Circulating RN Signature)
Print Name: ______________________
☐ High Risk Fire Protocol initiated

(Complete this section if Risk Score increases to "3" during procedure)
☐ High Risk Fire Protocol Initiated Signature/Title: ____________ Print Name: ____________ Time: ____________

FIG. 15-1 Identification of patient, procedure, and surgical side/sites, and fire risk assessment.

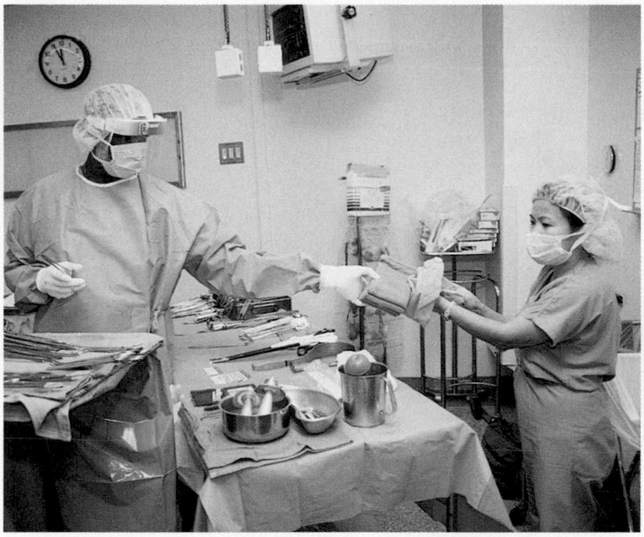

FIG. 15-2 Setting up the sterile table.

If the facility uses laser technology, a nurse specially trained in the use, care, and maintenance of the laser is needed (laser specialty nurse or a laser nurse coordinator). (**Laser** is an acronym for **l**ight **a**mplification by the **s**timulated **e**mission of **r**adiation.) A laser creates intense heat, rapidly clots blood vessels or tissue, and turns target tissue (e.g., a tumor) into vapor. All personnel must observe safety measures (e.g., wear eye shields, read door signs) during laser procedures to prevent injury to the patient and staff (AORN, 2014h).

Preparation of the Surgical Suite and Team Safety

The patient is unable to protect himself or herself during surgery; protection is provided by all members of the surgical team. The OR layout helps prevent INFECTION by reducing contaminants through air exchanges in the room, maintaining recommended temperature and humidity levels, and limiting the traffic and activities in the OR. Safety straps are used for the patient, and the OR bed is locked in place. Blankets or warming units are used to prevent hypothermia from poor THERMOREGULATION, and interventions are used to prevent skin breakdown.

The nurse ensures electrical safety through proper placement of grounding pads and use of electrical equipment that meets safety standards. All equipment used during surgery must be functional and in proper working condition as determined by the safety procedure of that facility. Equipment is cleaned and, when required, sterilized before use. The scrub and circulating nurses together ensure a correct count of surgical instruments, sharps, and sponges. Counts are performed before the procedure, during the procedure as items are added or when personnel are relieved from that assignment, at closure of the first layer of the surgical wound, and immediately before complete skin closure (AORN, 2014l).

All OR personnel work to prevent fire and complications from the use of hazardous or toxic substances. Ignition sources, oxidizers, and fuels are present in the OR and increase the risk for fires. Such events are rare but can occur during any procedure. A cool room temperature (between 68° and 73° F [20° and 23° C]) with low humidity (30% to 60%) is optimal. The nurse is aware of emergency measures to take in the event of a fire or spill.

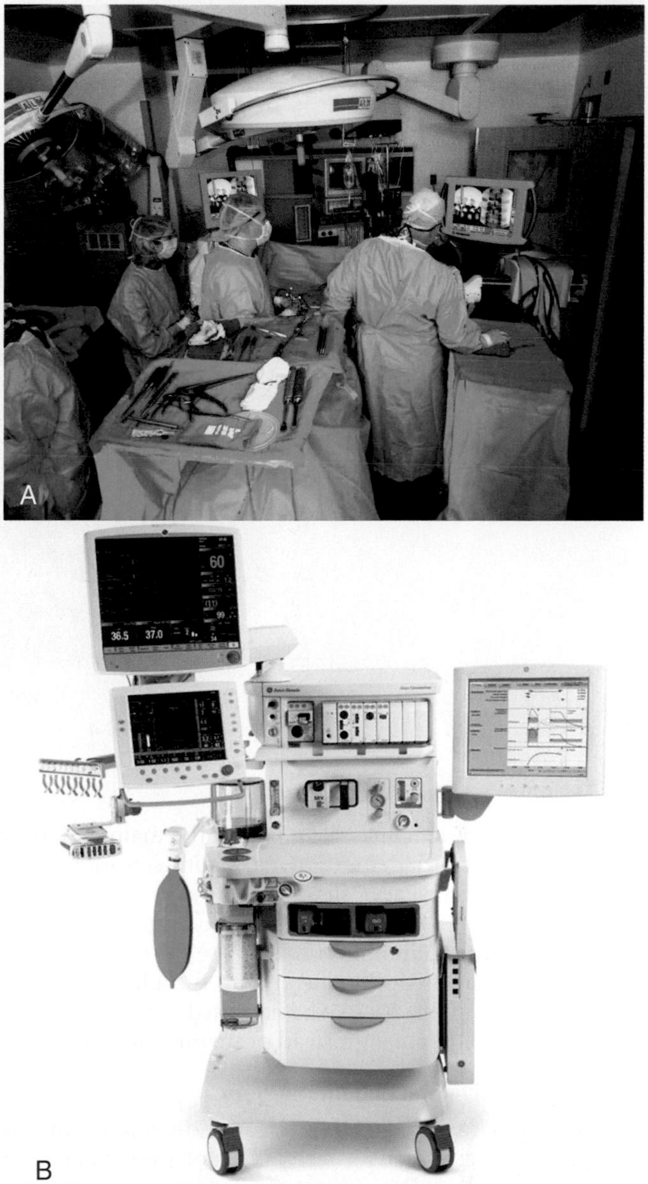

B

FIG. 15-3 A, A typical operating room. **B,** A typical anesthesia station with an anesthesia machine.

Layout

The surgical suite is located out of the mainstream of the hospital and near the PACU and support services (e.g., blood bank, pathology, and laboratory departments). Traffic flow is patterned to reduce contamination from outside the suite. Within the suite, clean and contaminated areas are separate. The surgical area is divided into three zones—unrestricted, semirestricted, and restricted—to ensure proper movement of patients and personnel.

Most suites contain staff areas as well as areas related to patient care, surgery, and surgical support. Staff areas include locker rooms and staff lounges. Patient care areas include an admission or holding area and operating rooms (ORs). Support areas include ORs, cabinets for sterile supplies, separate utility rooms for clean and soiled equipment, and a clean linen room.

Fig. 15-3 shows a typical OR. The number of tables and equipment in a room is based on the needs of each patient. A

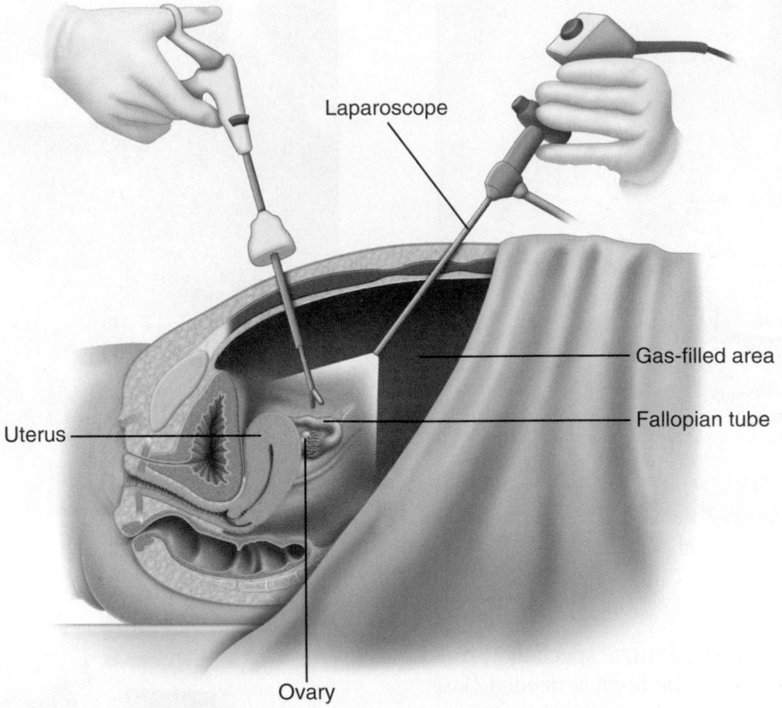

FIG. 15-4 How an operative laparoscope is used.

communication system links the OR with the main desk of the surgical suite and includes an intercom with separate systems for routine and emergency calls.

New OR designs use computers with the surgical equipment, lights, OR bed, and communications. These "hi-tech" rooms are similar to traditional ORs but larger with the addition of computer equipment. Many have voice-activated command systems to operate some equipment instead of manual operation.

Minimally Invasive and Robotic Surgery

Minimally invasive surgery (MIS) is a common practice and now is the preferred technique for many types of surgery, including cholecystectomy, cardiac surgery, splenectomy, and spinal surgery. It is even being used for cancer surgeries, such as the removal of a lung lobe (lobectomy) or even the entire lung (pneumonectomy) and colectomy. Benefits of MIS include reduced surgery time for some surgeries, smaller incisions, reduced blood loss, faster recovery time, and less pain after surgery.

During MIS, one or more small incisions is made in the surgical area and an **endoscope** (a tube that allows viewing and manipulation of internal body areas) is placed through the opening (Fig. 15-4). These instruments may be rigid, semirigid, or flexible and may have self-contained light sources. Endoscopes have different names and shapes for different surgical purposes. For example, laparoscopes are used for abdominal surgery, arthroscopes are used for joint surgery, and ureteroscopes are used for urinary tract surgery.

In addition to being used for examination and obtaining specimens for biopsy, endoscopes can be used for organ removal, reconstruction, blood vessel grafting, and many other procedures. Cutting, suturing, stapling, cautery, and laser surgery can all be performed through or with endoscopes. An important part of MIS for abdominal surgery, pelvic surgery, and surgery in some other body cavity areas is injecting gas or air into the cavity before the surgery to separate organs and improve visualization. This injection is known as **insufflation** and may contribute to complications and patient discomfort. This factor is considered when deciding whether to perform a procedure by traditional surgery or by endoscopy.

Patient preparation for endoscopic surgery is similar to the preparation for the same procedure when performed by open surgical methods. An endoscopic surgical procedure has a chance for becoming an open surgical procedure depending on what patient-related or procedure-related variables are discovered or develop during the surgery.

Robotic technology takes MIS to a new level and is changing how surgery is performed and how the OR is organized. Many gynecologic, urologic, and cardiovascular procedures are being performed by using robotics. The robotic system consists of a console, surgical arm cart, and video cart (Fig. 15-5). The surgeon first inserts the required instruments and positions the articulating arms; he or she then breaks scrub and performs the surgery while sitting at the console. A three-dimensional (3-D) view of the patient's anatomy allows precise control and dexterity. The vision cart holds the monitors, cameras, and recorder equipment. This new technology requires a perioperative robotics nurse specialist who teaches patients and family and trains members of the surgical team.

Mechanical trauma and thermal injury are two types of injury that a patient can incur during MIS and robotic surgery (Ulmer, 2010). Both MIS and robotic surgery are limited by the cost of special equipment, OR settings, and the lengthy training and practice periods for the surgeon to become proficient in even one procedure using these methods.

Health and Hygiene of the Surgical Team

People are a source of contamination in the surgical setting from the bacteria on the skin and the hair and in the airways.

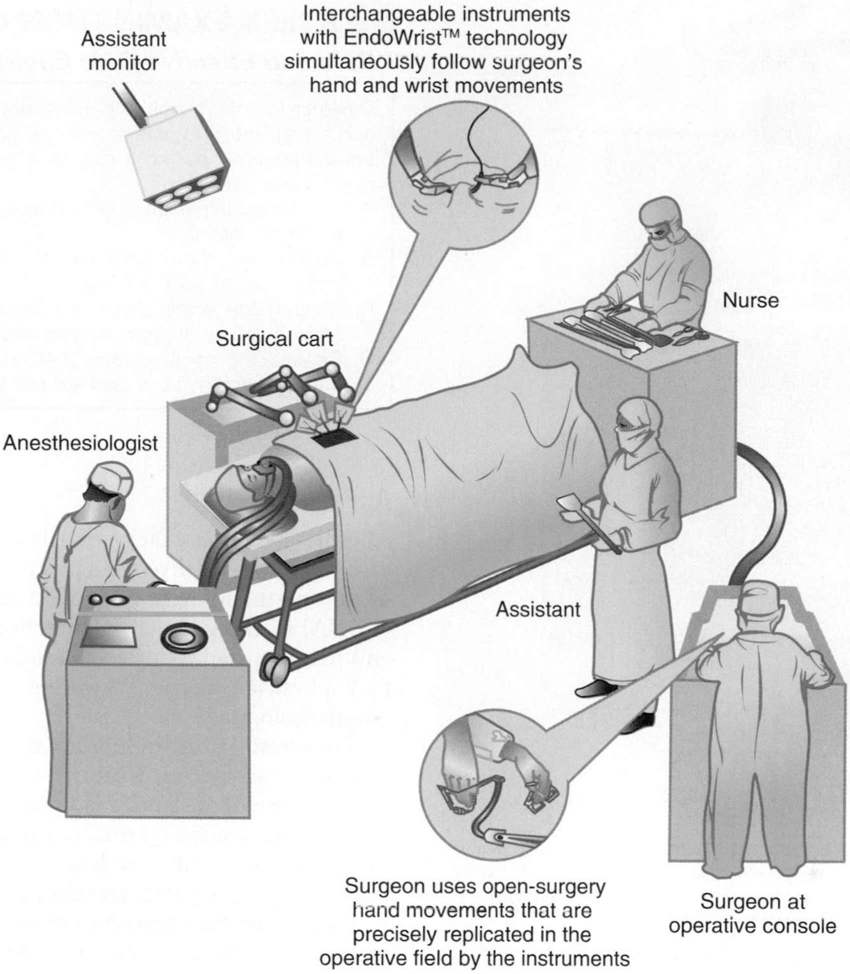

FIG. 15-5 The operating room layout for robotic surgery with the da Vinci Surgery System.

To avoid transmitting these organisms to the patient, policies and procedures for special health standards and dress must be followed. All members of the surgical team and support personnel in the surgical suite must be free of communicable diseases. No one who has an open wound, cold, or any INFECTION should participate in surgery.

Good personal hygiene and frequent handwashing help prevent and control INFECTION. Jewelry carries many organisms and should be minimal. All personnel must wash their hands between touching patients and performing procedures. Hands of surgical personnel may be cultured on a regular basis to assess for potential **nosocomial** (health care–acquired) infections and to identify sources of pathogens. Further interventions or cultures are needed if quality reports indicate a problem. Routine cultures are usually obtained every 3 to 6 months. Surgical attire and the surgical scrub help prevent contaminations.

Surgical Attire

All members of the surgical team and all OR personnel must wear scrub attire while in the surgical suite. Scrub attire, provided by the hospital, is clean (not sterile) and is worn to reduce contamination and risk for INFECTION from areas outside of the surgical setting. Basic surgical attire is a shirt and pants and a cap or hood (Fig. 15-6). Shoe coverings may be worn only to protect the shoes. *Staff change into clean surgical attire in the OR suite locker rooms, not at home* (AORN, 2014o). All members of the surgical team must cover their hair, including any facial hair.

In addition to basic attire, everyone must wear protective attire (mask, eyewear, gloves, and gown). Everyone who enters an OR where a sterile field is present must wear a mask. Surgical team members who are scrubbed and at the bedside during the surgery must also wear a sterile fluid-resistant gown, sterile gloves, and eye protectors or face shields. Team members who are *not* scrubbed (e.g., anesthesia provider, circulator) may wear cover scrub jackets that are snapped or buttoned closed and eyewear, as warranted. For some procedures, the surgical team wears what amounts to surgical "space suits" to prevent wound contamination.

Surgical Scrub

The surgeon, assistants, and the scrub nurse perform a surgical scrub after putting on a mask and before putting on a sterile gown and gloves (Fig. 15-7). *The scrub does not make the skin sterile.* Correctly performed, the scrub reduces the number of organisms from the hands, arms, and nails. Rings, watches, and bracelets are removed before scrubbing. Fingernails are kept short, clean, and healthy. Artificial nails, which have been proven to harbor organisms even after appropriate

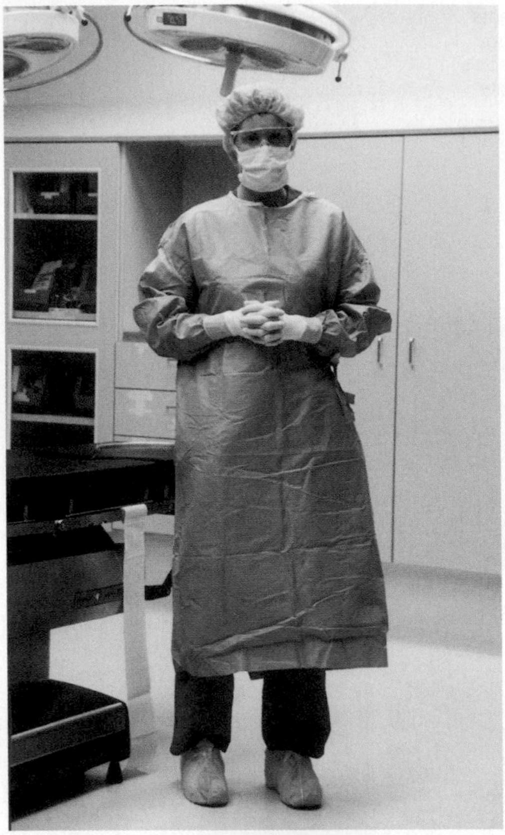

FIG. 15-6 Typical attire for all scrubbed personnel. Note complete hair covering, eye shields, mask, sterile gloves over the sleeves of the sterile gown, and shoe coverings. Note that when not in use, the hands are typically folded in front of the body, never below the waist.

scrub techniques are used, are not worn (World Health Organization, 2014).

A surgical antimicrobial solution is used for the surgical scrub. Plain or antimicrobial soap is used for washing hands immediately before the surgical scrub. Vigorous rubbing that creates friction is used from the fingertips to the elbow. The scrub continues for 3 to 5 minutes, followed by a rinse. For rinsing, hands and arms are positioned so that water runs off, rather than up or down, the arms (AORN, 2014p). After scrubbing, personnel enter the OR with their hands held higher than the elbows and thoroughly dry their hands and forearms with a sterile towel. This person is then assisted into a sterile gown *("gowning")* and puts on sterile gloves *("gloving")*. Newer, alcohol-based surgical scrub agents may or may not require the use of water. Operating room personnel wash and dry their hands with soap and water before applying the agent to their hands and forearms, rubbing thoroughly until dry.

Gowns, gloves, and materials used at the operative field must be sterile. These items are changed between procedures and as they become contaminated. The surgical gown is considered sterile only on the front from the chest to the level of the sterile field. The entire sleeves of the gown are considered sterile from 2 inches above the elbow to the cuff. The back of the gown is not considered sterile because it cannot be seen by the wearer. Only when they are properly scrubbed and attired do members of the surgical team handle sterile drapes and equipment.

NCLEX EXAMINATION CHALLENGE

Safe and Effective Care Environment

While at the scrub sink, the scrub person informs the circulating nurse that she now wears artificial nails because her own nails break frequently posing a risk for a glove puncture. What is the nurse's best response?

A. Ask the scrub person to wear double-gloves to prevent puncture or contamination.
B. Confirm with the scrub person that artificial nails are acceptable and do not affect hand hygiene.
C. Support the scrub person's rationale that broken nails are a serious source of cross-contamination.
D. Remind the scrub person that artificial nails alter skin flora, impede hand hygiene, and are not permitted.

Anesthesia

Anesthesia reduces or temporarily eliminates SENSORY PERCEPTION. Anesthesia delivery is a precise science. It requires the skill of an anesthesiologist, a certified registered nurse anesthetist (CRNA) working under the direction of an anesthesiologist or another physician, or an anesthesiologist assistant (AA—similar to a physician assistant working under the direction of an anesthesiologist).

Anesthesia is an induced state of partial or total loss of SENSORY PERCEPTION, with or without loss of consciousness. The purpose of anesthesia is to block nerve impulse transmission, suppress reflexes, promote muscle relaxation, and, in some cases, achieve a controlled level of unconsciousness. Anesthesia providers use a separate anesthesia record for documentation.

Usually the anesthesia provider selects the type of anesthesia to be used after consulting with the patient and surgeon and after considering specific patient factors. The nurse and patient communicate preferences and fears about anesthesia to the anesthesia provider. Patient health problems are factors in the selection and dose of anesthetic. Selection is also influenced by:

- Type and duration of the procedure
- Area of the body having surgery
- Safety issues to reduce injury, such as airway management
- Whether the procedure is an emergency
- Options for management of pain after surgery
- How long it has been since the patient ate, had any liquids, or had any drugs
- Patient position needed for the surgical procedure
- Whether the patient must be alert enough to follow instructions during surgery
- The patient's previous responses and reactions to anesthesia

The physical status of a patient is ranked according to a classification system developed by the American Society of Anesthesiologists (ASA). The anesthesiologist assesses the patient and assigns him or her to one of six categories based on current health and the presence of diseases and disorders. The categories rank patients in a range from a totally healthy patient (P1 ranking) to a patient who is brain dead (P6 ranking) (Johnson, 2011). This system is used to estimate potential risks during surgery and patient outcomes.

Anesthesia delivery begins with selecting and giving preoperative drugs (see Chapter 14). The nurse must know the actions of the drugs used and their effects during and after surgery.

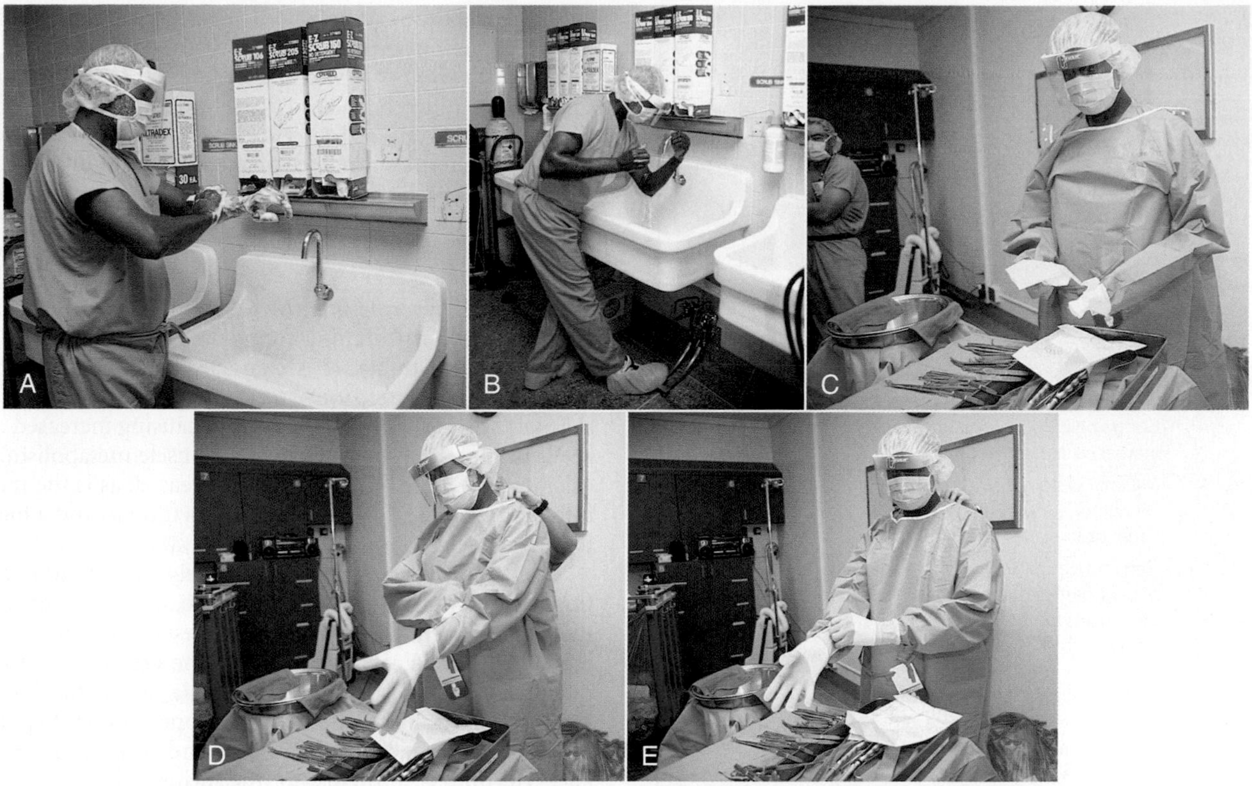

FIG. 15-7 The scrubbing, gowning, and gloving process. **A,** The surgical scrub. **B,** Rinsing. Note the water falling off the hands and arms. Also note the foot-operated handle that controls the water flow. (After scrubbing and rinsing, the scrub nurse dries his hands and arms with a sterile towel inside the operating room and then is assisted into a sterile gown.) **C,** The scrub nurse prepares sterile gloves. Note that the scrub nurse's hands are *inside* the sleeve of the gown and that he is touching the sterile gloves only with the sterile sleeve. **D,** The scrub nurse puts on his first sterile glove while the sterile gown is being tied in the back. Note again that his hand never emerges from under the sterile sleeve. **E,** The scrub nurse puts on his second sterile glove.

Anesthetic agents affect many systems and can worsen other health problems. For example, most anesthetics are metabolized by the liver and excreted by the kidneys. Liver or kidney impairment increases anesthetic effects and the risk for toxicity. In addition, interactions may occur between the anesthetics and other drugs the patient has received.

Anesthesia can be induced in many ways. The most common forms of anesthesia used in North America include general, regional, and local anesthesia (Table 15-1). Less commonly used forms include hypnosis, cryothermia (use of cold), and acupuncture.

General Anesthesia

General anesthesia is a reversible loss of consciousness induced by inhibiting neuronal impulses in several areas of the central nervous system (CNS). This state can be achieved with a single agent or a combination of agents. General anesthesia depresses the CNS, resulting in analgesia (pain relief or pain suppression), amnesia (memory loss of the surgery), and unconsciousness, with loss of muscle tone and reflexes. The patient is unconscious and has no SENSORY PERCEPTION. General anesthesia is used most often in surgery of the head, neck, upper torso, and abdomen.

Stages of General Anesthesia. Induction of general anesthesia involves four stages. Table 15-2 lists the expected patient responses and nursing care for each stage. The speed of emergence (recovery from the anesthesia) depends on the anesthetic agent, the duration of anesthesia administration, and whether a reversal agent is used. Retching, vomiting, and restlessness may occur during emergence, although not all patients have these responses. Suction equipment must be available to prevent aspiration. During recovery, shivering, rigidity, and slight cyanosis may occur. These responses are caused by a temporary change in the body's THERMOREGULATION. The nurse provides warm blankets, radiant heat, and oxygen to decrease the effects of emergence.

Administration of General Anesthesia. General anesthesia agents are administered by inhalation and IV injection. A combination of types of agents (balanced anesthesia) is used to provide hypnosis, amnesia, analgesia, muscle relaxation, and reduced reflexes with minimal disturbance of physiologic function. This method provides safe and controlled anesthetic delivery, especially for older and high-risk patients. An example of balanced anesthesia is the use of thiopental or propofol for induction, morphine for analgesia, and pancuronium for muscle relaxation. Agent selection is based on the individual patient and the specific surgical procedure.

Other drugs, such as hypnotics, opioid analgesics, and neuromuscular blocking agents, may be used as part of the anesthesia regimen. Hypnotics and opioid analgesics can be used for sedation before surgery, for IV moderate sedation for short procedures, and as an adjunct to general anesthesia during surgery. The neuromuscular blocking agents are used to relax the jaw and vocal cords immediately after induction so that the

TABLE 15-1 Features of Various Types of Anesthesia

TYPE	FEATURES
Inhalation	Most controllable method Induction and reversal accomplished with pulmonary ventilation Must be used in combination with other agents for painful or prolonged procedures Limited muscle relaxant effects Postoperative nausea and shivering common
Intravenous	Rapid and pleasant induction Low incidence of postoperative nausea and vomiting Must be metabolized and excreted from the body for complete reversal Contraindicated in presence of liver or kidney disease Increased cardiac and respiratory depression
Balanced	Minimal disturbance to physiologic function Can be used with older and high-risk patients Drug interactions can occur
Regional or Local	Gag and cough reflexes stay intact Allows participation and cooperation by the patient Less disruption of physical and emotional body functions No way to control agent after administration Increased nervous system stimulation (overdose) Not practical for extensive procedures because of the amount of drug that would be required to maintain anesthesia

endotracheal tube can be placed. These drugs also may be used during surgery to provide continued muscle relaxation.

Complications of General Anesthesia. Complications can range from minor (e.g., sore throat) to death. Improvement in anesthesia delivery and surgical techniques has resulted in a decline in anesthesia-related deaths, even among higher-risk patients. Although the anesthesia provider has the main responsibility for monitoring patient responses during surgery, the circulating nurse also remains alert for changes in the patient's condition.

Malignant hyperthermia (MH), an inherited muscle disorder, is an acute, life-threatening complication of certain drugs used for general anesthesia. It is characterized by many problems, including poor THERMOREGULATION. The reaction begins in skeletal muscle exposed to the drugs, causing increased calcium levels in muscle cells and increased muscle metabolism. Serum calcium and potassium levels are increased, as is the metabolic rate, leading to acidosis, cardiac dysrhythmias, and a high body temperature.

Onset of MH may occur immediately after anesthesia induction, several hours into the procedure, or even after the anesthetic has been terminated. Manifestations are caused by increased muscle calcium level and the greatly increased body metabolism. These include tachycardia, dysrhythmias, muscle rigidity (especially of the jaw and upper chest), hypotension, tachypnea, skin mottling, cyanosis, and **myoglobinuria** (presence of muscle proteins in the urine). *The most sensitive*

TABLE 15-2 The Four Stages of General Anesthesia and Related Nursing Interventions

DESCRIPTION	NURSING INTERVENTIONS	RATIONALES
Stage 1 (Analgesia and Sedation, Relaxation)		
Begins with induction and ends with loss of consciousness.	Close operating room doors, dim the lights, and control traffic in the operating room.	Avoiding external stimuli in the environment promotes relaxation.
Patient feels drowsy and dizzy, has a reduced sensation to pain, and is amnesic.	Position patient securely with safety belts.	Using safety measures in stage 1 prepares for stage 2.
Hearing is exaggerated.	Keep discussions about the patient to a minimum.	Being sensitive to the patient maintains his or her dignity.
Stage 2 (Excitement, Delirium)		
Begins with loss of consciousness and ends with relaxation, regular breathing, and loss of the eyelid reflex.	Avoid auditory and physical stimuli.	Sensory stimuli can contribute to the patient's response.
Patient may have irregular breathing, increased muscle tone, and involuntary movement of the extremities.	Protect the extremities.	Safety measures help prevent injury.
Laryngospasm or vomiting may occur.	Assist the anesthesiologist or CRNA with suctioning as needed.	Adequate suctioning of vomitus can prevent aspiration.
Patient is susceptible to external stimuli.	Stay with patient.	Staying with the patient is emotionally supportive.
Stage 3 (Operative Anesthesia, Surgical Anesthesia)		
Begins with generalized muscle relaxation and ends with loss of reflexes and depression of vital functions.	Assist the anesthesiologist or CRNA with intubation.	Providing assistance helps promote smooth intubation and prevent injury.
The jaw is relaxed, and breathing is quiet and regular. The patient cannot hear. Sensations (i.e., to pain) are lost.	Place patient into operative position. Prep (scrub) the patient's skin over the operative site as directed.	Performing procedures as soon as possible promotes time management to minimize total anesthesia time for the patient.
Stage 4 (Danger)		
Begins with depression of vital functions and ends with respiratory failure, cardiac arrest, and possible death. Respiratory muscles are paralyzed; apnea occurs. Pupils are fixed and dilated.	Prepare for and assist in treatment of cardiac and/or pulmonary arrest. Document occurrence in the patient's chart.	Teamwork and preparedness help decrease injuries and complications and promote the possibility of a desired outcome for the patient.

CRNA, Certified registered nurse anesthetist.

indication is an unexpected rise in the end-tidal carbon dioxide level with a decrease in oxygen saturation and tachycardia. Extremely elevated temperature, as high as 111.2° F (44° C), is a late sign of MH. Survival depends on early diagnosis and the immediate actions of the entire surgical team. Dantrolene sodium, a skeletal muscle relaxant, is the drug of choice along with other interventions (Mitchell-Brown, 2012).

NURSING SAFETY PRIORITY QSEN

Critical Rescue

Monitor patients for the cluster of elevated end-tidal carbon dioxide level, decreased oxygen saturation, and tachycardia related to malignant hyperthermia. If these changes begin, alert the surgeon and anesthesia provider immediately.

When the patient has a known history or risk for MH, treatment with dantrolene can begin before, during, and after surgery to prevent it. Chart 15-1 lists best practices for care of the patient with MH. The AORN recommends that all operating rooms have a dedicated MH cart containing drugs for management (normal saline, dantrolene, sodium bicarbonate, insulin, 50% dextrose, lidocaine, and calcium chloride), a protocol card listing interventions, and the MH hotline number. Additional nursing support is needed during this true perioperative emergency.

GENETIC/GENOMIC CONSIDERATIONS

Patient-Centered Care QSEN

MH is a genetic disorder with an autosomal dominant pattern of inheritance. The patient with a genetic predisposition for MH is at risk for this complication from halothane, enflurane, isoflurane, desflurane, sevoflurane, and succinylcholine. This rare problem is most common in young adults. Males are affected more often than females (despite the autosomal dominant pattern of inheritance) because of gender differences in muscle mass. The muscle biopsy tested with the caffeine halothane contracture test (CHCT) is still considered the most commonly used MH testing even though this disorder is inherited and only five centers are approved to perform the test (Online Mendelian Inheritance in Man [OMIM], 2013). There is also a genetic test that is performed on blood to assess whether a mutation in the *RYR1* gene is present. Usually, the cost of the genetic test is not covered by insurance. Always ask the patient about any previous problems or difficulties with anesthesia.

Overdose of anesthetic can occur if the patient's metabolism and drug elimination are slower than expected, such as with patients who are older or who have liver or kidney problems. Other drugs (e.g., antihypertensives) also alter metabolism, and interactions can occur between the anesthetic and the patient's regular drugs. Accurate information about the patient's height, weight, and medical history, especially liver and kidney function, is vital in determining the anesthetic type and dosage.

Unrecognized hypoventilation is an anesthesia-induced complication. Failure of adequate GAS EXCHANGE can lead to cardiac arrest, permanent brain damage, and death. Monitoring standards include the use of an end-tidal carbon dioxide monitor to confirm carbon dioxide levels in the patient's expired gas and a breathing system disconnect monitor to detect any break in the breathing circuit equipment.

Intubation complications can include many problems (e.g., broken teeth and caps, swollen lip, vocal cord trauma). Difficult intubation may be caused by anatomic issues or disease presence (e.g., small oral cavity, tight jaw joint, tumor). Improper neck extension during intubation may cause injury. The surgeon should be in the OR during the intubation process in case a

CHART 15-1 Best Practice for Patient Safety & Quality Care QSEN

Emergency Care of the Patient with Malignant Hyperthermia

- Stop all inhalation anesthetic agents and succinylcholine.
- If an endotracheal tube (ET) is not already in place, intubate immediately.
- Ventilate the patient with 100% oxygen, using the highest possible flow rate.
- Administer dantrolene sodium (Dantrium) IV at a dose of 2 to 3 mg/kg.
- If possible, terminate surgery. If termination is not possible, continue surgery using anesthetic agents that do not trigger malignant hyperthermia (MH).
- Assess arterial blood gases (ABGs) and serum chemistries for metabolic acidosis and hyperkalemia.
- If metabolic acidosis is evident by ABG analysis, administer sodium bicarbonate IV.
- If hyperkalemia is present, administer 10 units of regular insulin in 50 mL of 50% dextrose IV.
- Use active cooling techniques:
  - Administer iced saline (0.9% NaCl) IV at a rate of 15 mL/kg every 15 minutes as needed.
  - Apply a cooling blanket over the torso.
  - Pack bags of ice around the patient's axillae, groin, neck, and head.
  - Lavage the stomach, bladder, rectum, and open body cavities with sterile iced normal saline.
- Insert a nasogastric tube and a rectal tube.
- Monitor core body temperature to assess effectiveness of interventions and to avoid hypothermia.
- Monitor cardiac rhythm by electrocardiography (ECG) to assess for dysrhythmias.
- Insert a Foley catheter to monitor urine output.
- Treat any dysrhythmias that do not resolve on correction of hyperthermia and hyperkalemia with antidysrhythmic agents *other than calcium channel blockers.*
- Administer IV fluids at a rate and volume sufficient to maintain urine output above 2 mL/kg/hr.
- Monitor urine for presence of blood or myoglobin.
- If urine output falls below 2 mL/kg/hr, consider using osmotic or loop diuretics, depending on the patient's cardiac and kidney status.
- Contact the Malignant Hyperthermia Association of the United States (MHAUS) hotline for more information regarding treatment: (800) 644-9737.
- Transfer the patient to the intensive care unit (ICU) when stable.
- Continue to monitor the patient's temperature, ECG, ABGs, electrolytes, creatine kinase, coagulation studies, and serum and urine myoglobin levels until they have remained normal for 24 hours.
- Instruct the patient and family about testing for MH risk.
- Refer the patient and family to the Malignant Hyperthermia Association of the United States at (800) 986-4287 or www.mhaus.org.
- Report the incident to the North American Malignant Hyperthermia Registry at the Malignant Hyperthermia Association of the United States: (800) 644-9737.

Data from Malignant Hyperthermia Association of the United States. (2014). *Emergency therapy for MH acute phase treatment.* Retrieved April 2014, from www.mhaus.org/healthcare-professionals/#.UPGIEGeN58F

tracheotomy is needed when the endotracheal tube (ET) is placed. Intubation causes tracheal irritation and edema. Often the patient has a sore throat after surgery.

NCLEX EXAMINATION CHALLENGE

Safe and Effective Care Environment

Which change in the anesthetized client alerts the nurse to the possibility of malignant hyperthermia?

A. Widening pulse pressure
B. Increasing output of dilute urine
C. Increasing end-tidal carbon dioxide level
D. Ascending flaccid paralysis of skeletal muscles

Local or Regional Anesthesia

Local or regional anesthesia briefly disrupts sensory nerve impulse transmission from a specific body area or region, thus reducing SENSORY PERCEPTION in a limited area. Motor function may or may not be affected. The patient remains conscious and can follow instructions. The gag and cough reflexes remain intact, and the risk for aspiration is low. This type of anesthesia may be supplemented with sedatives, opioid analgesics, or hypnotics to reduce anxiety and increase comfort. The OR nurse provides the patient with information, directions, and emotional support before, during, and after the procedure.

Local Anesthesia. **Local anesthesia** is delivered topically (applied to the skin or mucous membranes of the area to be anesthetized) and by local infiltration (injected directly *into* the tissue around an incision, wound, or lesion). Sometimes when the term *local* is used, it means *any* form of anesthesia that is not general or monitored anesthesia.

Regional Anesthesia. **Regional anesthesia** is a type of local anesthesia that blocks multiple peripheral nerves and reduces SENSORY PERCEPTION in a specific body region. It can be used under a variety of conditions and surgeon and patient preferences. It is often used when pain management after surgery is enhanced by regional anesthesia, such as after a total knee replacement. If the patient has eaten and the surgery is an emergency, it may be possible to perform surgery with the patient under regional anesthesia to decrease the risk for aspiration. Regional anesthesia includes field block, nerve block, spinal, and epidural (Table 15-3). Figs. 15-8 and 15-9 show common sites of nerve blocks, spinal anesthesia, and epidural anesthesia.

The nurse's role in the delivery of regional anesthesia consists of:

- Assisting the anesthesia provider
- Observing for breaks in sterile technique
- Providing emotional support for the patient
- Staying with the patient
- Offering information and reassurance
- Positioning the patient comfortably and safely

TABLE 15-3 Types of Regional Anesthesia

ANESTHESIA TYPE	DEFINITION AND COMMON USE
Field block	A series of injections *around* the operative field Most commonly used for chest procedures, hernia repair, dental surgery, and some plastic surgeries
Nerve block	Injection of the local anesthetic agent *into or around* one nerve or group of nerves in the involved area Most commonly used for limb surgery or to relieve chronic pain
Spinal anesthesia	Injection of an anesthetic agent into the cerebrospinal fluid in the subarachnoid space (see Fig. 15-9) Most commonly used for lower abdominal, pelvic, hip, and knee surgery
Epidural anesthesia	Injection of an agent into the epidural space (see Fig. 15-9) Most commonly used for anorectal, vaginal, perineal, hip, and lower extremity surgeries

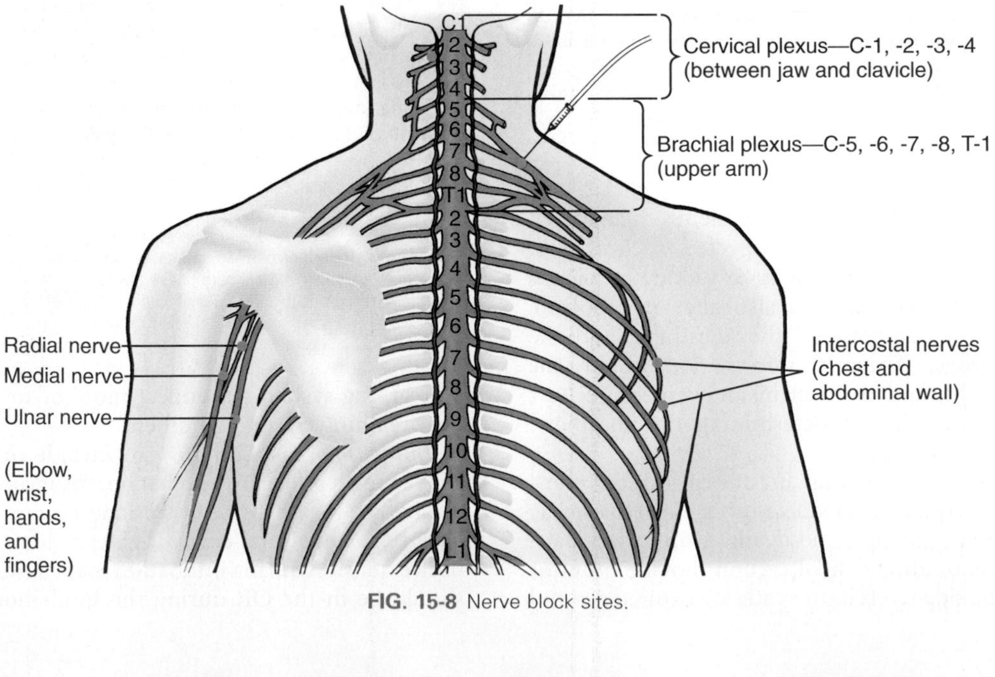

FIG. 15-8 Nerve block sites.

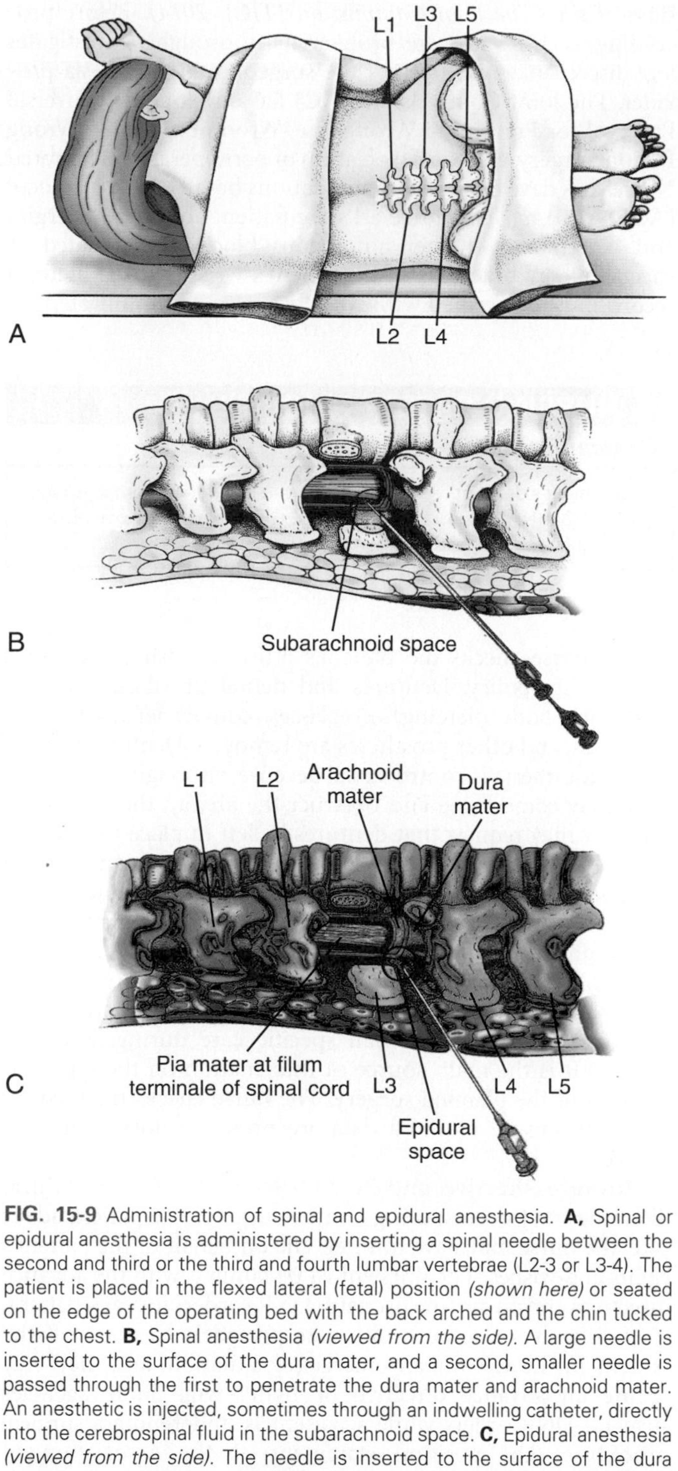

FIG. 15-9 Administration of spinal and epidural anesthesia. **A,** Spinal or epidural anesthesia is administered by inserting a spinal needle between the second and third or the third and fourth lumbar vertebrae (L2-3 or L3-4). The patient is placed in the flexed lateral (fetal) position *(shown here)* or seated on the edge of the operating bed with the back arched and the chin tucked to the chest. **B,** Spinal anesthesia *(viewed from the side).* A large needle is inserted to the surface of the dura mater, and a second, smaller needle is passed through the first to penetrate the dura mater and arachnoid mater. An anesthetic is injected, sometimes through an indwelling catheter, directly into the cerebrospinal fluid in the subarachnoid space. **C,** Epidural anesthesia *(viewed from the side).* The needle is inserted to the surface of the dura mater, and the anesthetic is injected, usually through an indwelling catheter, into the epidural space.

Complications of Local or Regional Anesthesia. Complications of local or regional anesthesia are related to patient sensitivity to the anesthetic agent (anaphylaxis), incorrect delivery technique, systemic absorption, and overdose. The nurse observes for central nervous system (CNS) stimulation followed by CNS and cardiac depression, which are indications of a systemic toxic reaction. The nurse also assesses for restlessness, excitement, incoherent speech, headache, blurred vision, metallic taste, nausea, tremors, seizures, and increased pulse, respiration, and blood pressure. Interventions include establishing an open airway, giving oxygen, and notifying the surgeon. Usually a fast-acting barbiturate is needed for treatment. If the toxic reaction is untreated, unconsciousness, hypotension, apnea, cardiac arrest, and death may result.

Cardiac arrest may occur as a rare complication of spinal anesthesia. Epinephrine is given to prevent cardiac arrest in patients who develop sudden, unexplained bradycardia.

Local early complications include edema and inflammation. Abscess formation, tissue necrosis, and/or gangrene may occur later. Abscesses result from contamination during injection of the agent. Necrosis and gangrene may occur as a result of prolonged blood vessel constriction in the injected area.

Moderate Sedation

Moderate sedation (conscious sedation) is the IV delivery of sedative, hypnotic, and opioid drugs to reduce SENSORY PERCEPTION but allow the patient to maintain a patent airway. The amnesia action is short, and the patient has a rapid return to ADLs. Etomidate (Amidate), diazepam (Valium, Vivol 🍁, Novo-Dipam 🍁), midazolam (Versed), fentanyl (Sublimaze), alfentanil (Alfenta), propofol (Diprivan), and morphine sulfate are the most commonly used drugs. Moderate sedation is used to reduce the level of consciousness during endoscopy, cardiac catheterization, closed fracture reduction, cardioversion, and other short procedures.

Selection of patients for moderate sedation is based on specific criteria. The physician determines whether the patient is a candidate. In most states, a credentialed registered nurse may deliver moderate sedation under physician supervision and within the state-defined scope of nursing practice. Credentialing includes advanced training in IV drug delivery, airway management, and advanced cardiac life support (ACLS).

The nurse monitors the patient during and after the procedure for response to the procedure and the drugs. The airway, level of consciousness, oxygen saturation, capnography (measure of carbon dioxide level), ECG status, and vital signs are monitored every 15 to 30 minutes until the patient is awake and oriented and vital signs have returned to baseline levels (AORN, 2014i).

Evaluation of consciousness for recovery sedation is performed using a sedation scale. The Ramsay Sedation Scale (RSS) lists specific patient responses or behaviors to a continuum of environmental stimulation demonstrating degree of arousal from sedation (Table 15-4).

The patient receiving IV moderate sedation can be discharged to go home with a responsible adult if capnography indicates GAS EXCHANGE is adequate and arousal from sedation is at an RSS 2 level. If the patient returns to the general medical-surgical nursing unit, the unit nurses continue monitoring. The patient is expected to be sleepy but arousable for several hours after the procedure. Oral intake is not permitted until 30 minutes after the patient has received the sedation or according to the physician's prescription. If the patient was intubated or had oral endoscopy, return of the gag reflex is required before oral intake. When fluids are permitted, the nurse makes sure that the patient is awake and positioned to avoid aspiration.

TABLE 15-4 Ramsay Sedation Scale for Assessing Post-Sedation Consciousness

RAMSAY SCORE	RESPONSE DESCRIPTORS
RSS 1	Patient is anxious and agitated or restless, or both.
RSS 2	Patient is cooperative, oriented, and tranquil (calm, not agitated).
RSS 3	Patient responds quickly, but only to commands.
RSS 4	Patient exhibits brisk response to stimulus.
RSS 5	Patient exhibits a sluggish response to stimulus.
RSS 6	Patient exhibits no response to stimulus. The RSS must be reapplied at intervals until full consciousness is achieved.

Data from Dawson, R., von Fintel, N., & Naim, S. (2010). Sedation assessment using the Ramsay scale. *Emergency Nurse, 18*(3), 18-20.
RSS, Ramsay Sedation Scale.

❖ PATIENT-CENTERED COLLABORATIVE CARE

◆ Assessment

History. On arrival in the surgical suite, the patient is taken to the holding area or directly into the operating suite. The holding area nurse or the circulating nurse greets the patient on arrival. As indicated in The Joint Commission's National Patient Safety Goals (NPSGs), *correct identification of the patient is the responsibility of every member of the health care team.* Check the patient's identification bracelet and ask, "What is your name and birth date?" This practice prevents errors by drowsy or confused patients. For example, if a patient is asked "Are you Mr. Gates?," he may respond inappropriately if he is anxious or sedated. The nurse always validates identification using the medical record and identification bracelet and by asking the patient or family.

! NURSING SAFETY PRIORITY (QSEN)

Critical Rescue

The Joint Commission's NPSGs require that you verify the patient's identity with two types of identifiers (name, medical record number, telephone number, or other person-specific identifier). Ask the patient to tell you his or her name.

After completing the identification process, the nurse validates that the surgical consent form has been signed and witnessed. The nurse asks "What kind of operation are you having today?" to ascertain that the patient's perception of the procedure, the surgical consent, the surgeon's order, and the operative schedule are the same. *When the procedure involves a specific site, validating the side on which a procedure is to be performed (e.g., for amputation, cataract removal, hernia repair) is the responsibility of each health care professional before and at the time of surgery. The Joint Commission now recommends that the patient and the licensed independent practitioner who is ultimately accountable for the procedure and will be present during the procedure (usually the surgeon performing the surgery) mark the surgical site (The Joint Commission [TJC], 2014).* Before proceeding, each health care professional thoroughly investigates *any* discrepancy and notifies the surgeon and anesthesia provider. The Joint Commission (TJC) has developed a Universal Protocol for Preventing Wrong Site, Wrong Procedure, Wrong Person Surgery, and the Association of periOperative Registered Nurses has developed recommendations based on this protocol (AORN, 2014r). The nurse asks the patient about any allergies and determines whether autologous blood was donated. A special allergy bracelet on the patient's wrist and the medical record must be verified with what has been communicated.

! NURSING SAFETY PRIORITY (QSEN)

Critical Rescue

If the patient's description of the surgical site is different from that listed on the informed consent, form a time-out with the patient, yourself, and the surgeon to ascertain and mark the correct site.

The nurse checks the patient's attire to ensure adherence with facility policy. Dentures and dental prostheses, jewelry (including body piercing), eyeglasses, contact lenses, hearing aids, wigs, and other prostheses are removed. Denture removal before anesthesia is controversial because, although the denture plate may come loose and obstruct the airway, the anesthesia provider may request that dentures be left in place to ensure a snug fit of the bag-mask. In some facilities, patients may wear eyeglasses and hearing aids until after anesthesia induction.

Medical Record Review. The circulating nurse and anesthesia provider review the patient's medical record in the holding area or the operating room (OR). This record provides information to identify patient needs during surgery and allows the nurse to assess and plan specific care during and after surgery. It is the main source of information on the type and location of the planned surgery. The nurse checks the medical record to ensure required data are present before surgery is started.

Advance Directives and Do-Not-Resuscitate Orders. Ethical dilemmas may occur during or after surgery. As a patient advocate, the nurse may have to intervene on behalf of the patient's rights and wishes. The nurse must be familiar with the advance directives and do-not-resuscitate (DNR) orders for each patient. It is difficult for some health care providers to not treat the patient in the OR for an emergency situation, and they may ignore an advance directive or living will. Some agencies suspend DNR orders while a patient is undergoing a surgical procedure. The position statement of the Association of periOperative Registered Nurses regarding the care of patients with DNR orders states that automatically suspending a DNR or allow-natural-death order during surgery undermines a patient's right to self-determination (AORN, 2014c).

! NURSING SAFETY PRIORITY (QSEN)

Action Alert

Advance directives are to be honored in the surgical environment regardless of the situation.

Allergies and Previous Reactions to Anesthesia or Transfusions. The nurse asks about allergies and previous reactions to anesthesia or blood transfusions. Allergies to iodine products or shellfish indicate a risk for a reaction to the agents used to clean the surgical area. Latex allergies are assessed with all patients because anaphylaxis can occur with latex contact during surgery. Latex-free equipment and supplies are used when there is a latex allergy. The nurse documents the allergy in the medical record and notifies the OR team.

The patient's previous experience with anesthesia helps the nurse and anesthesia provider anticipate needs and plan interventions. For example, if a patient is restless or agitated as a reaction to anesthesia, the nurse can have padding for the siderails and protective restraints available. The use of blood products during surgery may be influenced by the patient's history, religious beliefs, preferences, and past transfusion reactions.

Autologous Blood Transfusion. **Autologous blood transfusion** (reinfusing the patient's own blood) may be used for surgery. Chapters 14 and 40 discuss autologous transfusion in more detail. Chart 15-2 outlines best practices for autologous blood transfusion using blood salvage techniques during surgery.

Laboratory and Diagnostic Test Results. The OR nurse reviews the most recent laboratory findings and test results to inform the surgical team about the patient's health and to alert them for potential problems. These results are usually obtained within 24 to 48 hours before surgery for hospitalized patients and within 4 weeks for ambulatory surgery patients. The nurse reports all abnormal findings or results to the surgeon and anesthesia provider. Laboratory values greater than or less than the normal range are potentially life threatening during surgery (see Chapter 14). For example, if the hemoglobin level is less than 10 g/dL, oxygen transport and GAS EXCHANGE are reduced, affecting the amount and type of anesthesia used.

Medical History and Physical Examination Findings. The nurse performs a final assessment for threats to patient safety, starting with the patient's age and general physical condition. Older patients and those who are thin or overweight are at greater risk for skin injury. Assessing mental status is important because confused patients and those who are unable to either follow instructions or communicate may not be able to tell you when a problem exists. Patients who have impaired SENSORY PERCEPTION of any type are at increased risk for injury. Specific drugs, such as long-term steroid use (which increases capillary fragility and thins the skin), as well as limitations of range or motion, require modification during positioning and threaten patient safety.

CHART 15-2 Best Practice for Patient Safety & Quality Care QSEN

Intraoperative Autologous Blood Salvage and Transfusion

- Be aware of the cell-processing method to be used.
- Make sure that collection containers are labeled for the patient.
- Assist with sterile setup as necessary.
- Assist with processing and reinfusing procedures as needed.
- Document the transfusion process.
- Monitor the patient's vital signs during the transfusion procedure.

The OR nurse checks that the medical history and examination findings, including usual pulse and blood pressure, are recorded. This information provides baseline data to assess the patient's reaction to the surgery and anesthesia. Drugs taken before surgery may affect the patient's reaction to surgery and wound healing. For example, aspirin and other NSAIDs that can increase CLOTTING time and the risk for hemorrhage.

Knowing the patient's medical history and age allows the nurse to plan interventions for the care and safety of high-risk patients (Chart 15-3). The nurse carefully monitors older patients and those with cardiac disease for potential fluid overload.

After completing the medical record review, the nurse may insert an IV catheter and perform a surgical skin preparation. He or she provides emotional support and explains procedures to the patient. If the patient is in the holding area, he or she is moved to the OR after the preoperative routine is completed.

! NURSING SAFETY PRIORITY QSEN

Action Alert

Once the patient has been moved into the holding area or the OR, do not leave him or her alone.

? CLINICAL JUDGMENT CHALLENGE

Ethical/Legal; Safety; Teamwork and Collaboration; Quality Improvement QSEN

A patient scheduled for a palliative, pain-relieving procedure has a do-not-resuscitate (DNR) order confirmed in the medical record. However, after being premedicated, the patient requests the order be suspended during the procedure and that a family member be contacted.

1. Is the patient permitted to suspend the DNR order in light of the fact that he has already received premedication?
2. What principle of ethical behavior guides your response? (You may need to review the ethical principles in Chapter 1.)
3. How should the OR nurse proceed with the patient request?
4. What steps could be taken to ensure that patient requests and revisions of requests can be handled appropriately in the future?

CHART 15-3 Nursing Focus on the Older Adult

Intraoperative Nursing Interventions

- Allow patients to retain eyeglasses, dentures, and hearing aids until anesthesia has begun.
- Use a small pillow under the patient's head if his or her head and neck are normally bent slightly forward.
- Lift patients into position to prevent shearing forces on fragile skin.
- Position arthritic and artificial joints carefully to prevent postoperative pain and discomfort from strain on those joints.
- Pad bony prominences to prevent pressure sores.
- Provide extra padding for those patients with decreased peripheral circulation.
- Use warming devices to prevent hypothermia.
- Cover the patient's head and feet.
- Warm IV and irrigation fluids as indicated by agency policy and manufacturer's recommendations.
- Follow strict aseptic technique.
- Carefully monitor intake and output, including blood loss.

Data from Clayton, J. (2008). Special needs of older adults undergoing surgery. *AORN Journal, 88*(3), 557-570.

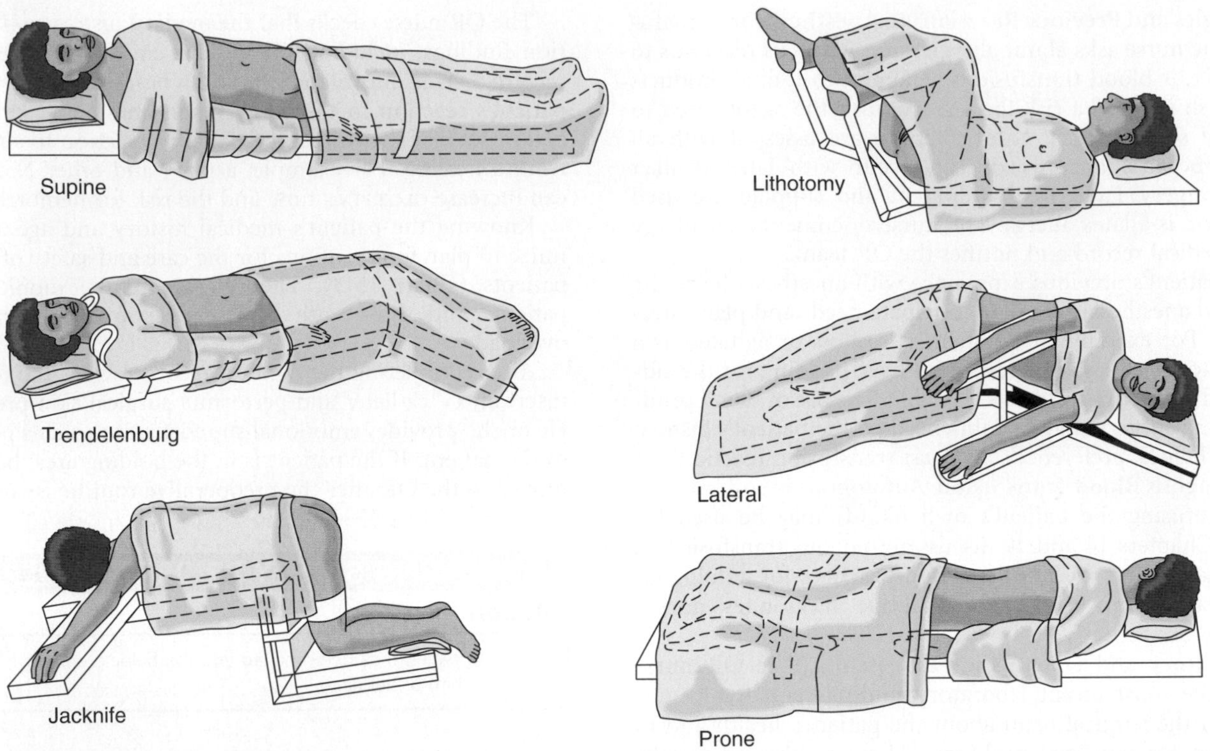

FIG. 15-10 Common surgical positions.

◆ *Analysis*

The priority NANDA-I nursing diagnoses and collaborative problems for patients during surgery include:

1. Risk for Perioperative Positioning Injury related to improper positioning (NANDA-I)
2. Risk for Infection related to invasive procedures (NANDA-I)
3. Impaired Gas Exchange related to anesthesia, pain, reduced respiratory effort (NANDA-I)

◆ *Planning and Implementation*

Preventing Injury

Planning: Expected Outcomes. The patient is expected to be free of injury as indicated by:

- Adequate capillary refill and peripheral pulses in all extremities
- Sensory perception and motor function after surgery at the same level as before surgery
- Absence of skin redness or open skin areas
- Absence of bruising

Interventions. Interventions are needed to prevent injury from positioning because of anesthesia and the narrow OR bed. The patient cannot guard against nerve or joint damage and muscle stretch or strain. In addition, pressure ulcers often start to develop during surgery. Thus proper positioning is important. The circulating nurse pads the operating bed with foam and/or silicone gel pads and properly places the grounding pads. He or she coordinates the transfer to the operating bed and helps the patient to a comfortable position. The skin is assessed, especially of older patients, for bruising or injury, and extra padding is placed as indicated.

The patient is usually in a supine position after transfer to the operating bed. Anesthesia may be initiated with the patient supine, and the patient then may be repositioned for surgery (Fig. 15-10).

The circulating nurse coordinates positioning of the patient for surgery and modifies the position according to the patient's safety and special needs. The OR nurse ensures that there is an adequate number of personnel to assist in positioning the patient.

Factors influencing the *timing* of repositioning include:

- The surgical site
- The age and size of the patient
- The anesthetic delivery technique
- Pain on movement (conscious patient)

Factors influencing the actual *position* include:

- The specific procedure being performed
- The surgeon's preference
- The patient's age, size, and weight
- Any pulmonary, skeletal, or muscular limitations, such as arthritis, joint replacements, emphysema, or implanted devices

Chart 15-4 lists best practices to prevent complications related to prolonged immobility during surgery.

The dorsal recumbent (supine), prone, lithotomy, and lateral positions are most often used for surgery. Fig. 15-10 shows many surgical positions and the use of protective padding. When general anesthesia is used, the nurse positions the patient slowly to prevent hypotension from blood vessel dilation. Proper positioning is ensured by assessing for:

- Anatomic alignment
- Interference with circulation and breathing
- Protection of skeletal and neuromuscular structures

CHART 15-4 Best Practice for Patient Safety & Quality Care QSEN

Prevention of Complications Related to Intraoperative Positioning

Prevention of Brachial Plexus Complications (Paralysis, Loss of Sensation in Arm and Shoulder)
- Pad the elbow if tucked at the side.
- Avoid excessive abduction.
- Secure the arm firmly on a padded armboard, positioned at shoulder level, and extended less than 90 degrees.

Prevention of Radial Nerve Complications (Wrist Drop)
- Support the wrist with padding.
- Be careful not to overtighten wrist straps.

Prevention of Medial or Ulnar Nerve Complications (Hand Weakness, Claw Hand)
- Place the safety strap above or below the nerve locations.

Prevention of Peroneal Nerve Complications (Foot Drop)
- Pad knees and ankles.
- Maintain minimal external rotation of the hips.
- Support the lower extremities.
- Be careful not to overtighten leg straps.

Prevention of Tibial Nerve Complications (Loss of Sensation on the Plantar Surface of the Foot)
- Place the safety strap above the ankle.
- Do not place equipment on lower extremities.
- Urge operating room (OR) personnel to avoid leaning on the patient's lower extremities.

Prevention of Joint Complications (Stiffness, Pain, Inflammation, Limited Motion)
- Place a pillow or foam padding under bony prominences.
- Maintain the patient's extremities in good anatomic alignment.
- Slightly flex joints and support with pillows, trochanter rolls, or pads.

Data from Association of periOperative Registered Nurses. (2010). Recommended practices for positioning the patient in the perioperative practice setting. In *Perioperative standards and recommended practices* (pp. 327-350). Denver: Author.

- Optimal exposure of the operative site and IV line
- Adequate access to the patient for the anesthesia provider
- The patient's comfort, safety, and dignity

Care is modified to reduce the potential complications from specific positions. For example, patients in the lithotomy position may develop leg swelling, pain in the legs or back, reduced foot pulses, or reduced SENSORY PERCEPTION from compression of the peroneal nerve. The nurse ensures proper padding and position changes at regular intervals. He or she continually assesses circulation adequacy by checking pulses and capillary refill below pressure points. Throughout surgery, the nurse prevents obstruction of circulation, respiration, or nerve conduction caused by tight straps, poorly placed pads and pillows, or the position of the bed.

Preventing Infection

Planning: Expected Outcomes. The patient is expected to have an uninfected surgical wound or wounds. Indicators include:
- Wound edges are closed and not excessively red or swollen
- Wound is free from purulent drainage
- White blood cell counts remain at expected levels after surgery
- Patient is afebrile

Interventions. Surgical wound INFECTIONS interfere with recovery, delay wound healing, contribute to rising health care costs, and are a source of nosocomial infections. The Centers for Disease Control and Prevention (CDC) defines surgical site infections as occurring 30 days post-surgery (CDC, 2014). Aseptic technique must be strictly practiced by all OR personnel to ensure that the patient is free from infection, as required by The Joint Commission's NPSGs. The Surgical Care Improvement Project (SCIP), as described in Table 14-1 of Chapter 14, has core measures related for the prevention of surgical site infections.

Assess the risk for INFECTION by identifying patients with health problems such as diabetes mellitus, immunodeficiency, obesity, and kidney disease. The nurse performs the prescribed skin preparation, protects against cross-contamination, keeps traffic to a minimum, and administers prescribed antimicrobial prophylaxis. Surgery increases risk for wound complications (e.g., incisional tears, lacerations), infection, and loss of body fluids. Sterile surgical technique and the use of protective drapes, skin closures, and dressings reduce complications and promote wound healing. When a wound is already infected or is at high risk for infection, antibiotics may be used directly in the wound before wound closure.

Skin and tissue closures include sutures, staples, special tape, and tissue adhesive (surgical "glue"). Fig. 15-11 shows commonly used wound closures. They are used to:
- Hold wound edges in place until wound healing is complete
- Occlude blood vessels, preventing poor CLOTTING and hemorrhage
- Prevent wound contamination and INFECTION

Sutures are absorbable or nonabsorbable. *Absorbable sutures* are digested over time by body enzymes. *Nonabsorbable sutures* become encapsulated in the tissue during the healing process and remain in the tissue unless they are removed. Body enzymes do not affect nonabsorbable sutures. Retention (stay) sutures (see Fig. 15-11) may be used in addition to standard sutures for patients at high risk for impaired wound healing (obese patients, patients with diabetes, and those taking steroids).

After the incision is closed, the surgeon may inject a local anesthetic or instill an antibiotic into the wound. A gauze or spray dressing may be applied to protect the incision from contamination. A variety of dressings are used to absorb drainage and support the incision. A pressure dressing may be applied to prevent poor CLOTTING and bleeding. One or more drains (see Chapter 16) may be inserted to remove secretions and fluids around the surgical area. These secretions, if not drained, slow healing and promote bacterial growth, which could result in wound INFECTION.

The nurse coordinates the surgical team in positioning and transferring the patient. When needed, a roller board or a lift sheet is used to move the patient from the operating bed to a stretcher or bed. The circulating nurse and anesthesia provider go with the patient to the PACU and report his or her surgical experience to the PACU nurse (see Chapter 16).

Preventing Hypoventilation

Planning: Expected Outcomes. The patient is expected to be free of damaging events related to impaired GAS EXCHANGE and hypoventilation as indicated by:
- Maintenance of Sao_2, Pao_2, and blood pH within normal limits

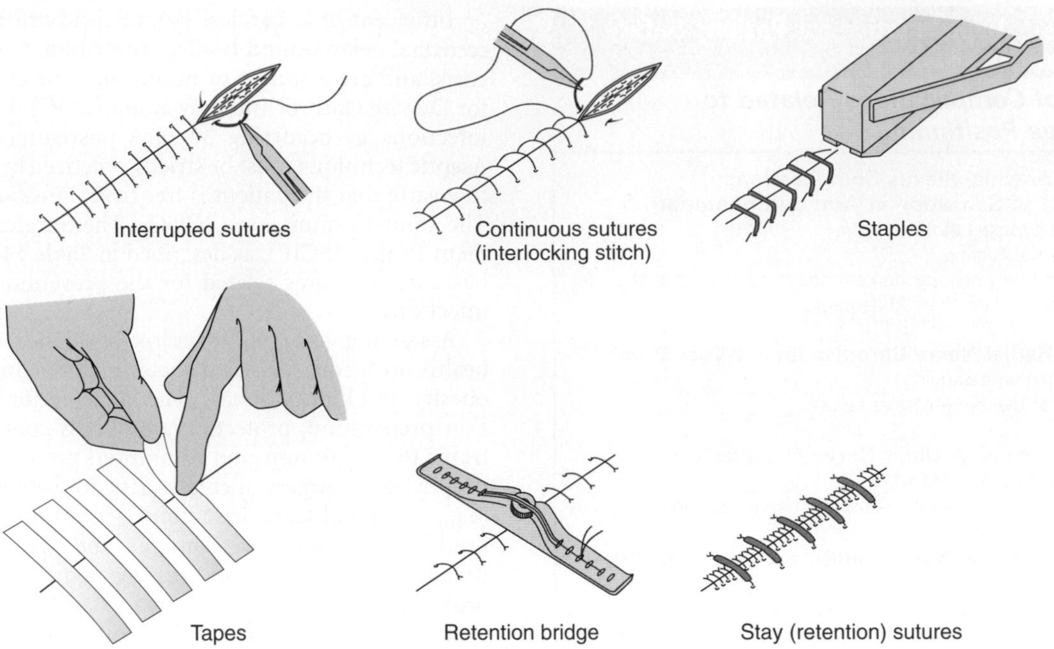

FIG. 15-11 Common skin closures.

- Vital signs within normal limits
- Return to presurgical level of cognitive function

Interventions. The purpose of interventions is to prevent injury resulting from the anesthesia effect on breathing and GAS EXCHANGE. The nurse, surgeon, and anesthesia provider monitor the patient according to official standards. These standards, adopted by both the American Society of Anesthesiologists and the American Association of Nurse Anesthetists, include continuous monitoring of breathing, circulation, and cardiac rhythms; blood pressure and heart rate recordings every 5 minutes; and the constant presence of an anesthesia provider during the case.

◆ *Evaluation: Outcomes*

The nurse evaluates the care of the patient during surgery based on the identified priority patient problems. The expected outcomes are that the patient:

- Is safely anesthetized without complications
- Does not experience any injury related to surgical positioning or equipment
- Is free of skin or tissue contamination and INFECTION during surgery
- Is free of skin tears, bruises, redness, or other injury over pressure points and elsewhere
- Maintains normal THERMOREGULATION and body temperature

Specific indicators for these outcomes are listed for each priority patient problem under the Planning and Implementation section (see earlier).

NURSING CONCEPTS AND CLINICAL JUDGMENT REVIEW

What might you NOTICE in a patient during surgery who has adequate body defenses related to INFECTION?

Vital signs:
- Body temperature within normal range
- No sweating or chills

Physical assessment:
- Skin color normal for ethnicity
- Any drainage is not purulent
- Urine is clear

GET READY FOR THE NCLEX® EXAMINATION!

KEY POINTS

Review these Key Points for each NCLEX Examination Client Needs Category.

Safe and Effective Care Environment

- Review preoperative checklist and informed consent forms, including any allergies.
- Highlight any known allergies. **Safety** QSEN
- Ensure that all personnel entering the OR are wearing proper OR attire for their role.
- Observe for and inform OR personnel of any break in sterile field or sterile technique. **Safety** QSEN
- Use appropriate patient identifiers when administering drugs or marking surgical sites. **Safety** QSEN
- Report to the surgeon any discrepancy between what type of surgery the patient says is going to be performed and what the informed consent form indicates. **Safety** QSEN
- Apply grounding pads as needed. **Safety** QSEN
- Complete any needed skin preparation.
- Perform an accurate "sharps," sponge, and instrument count with the scrub nurse or surgical technologist. **Safety** QSEN

Psychosocial Integrity

- Communicate patient preferences or fears about anesthesia to the anesthesia provider. **Patient-Centered Care** QSEN
- Preserve the patient's privacy and dignity by keeping body exposure to a minimum.
- Stay with the patient during induction of anesthesia.
- Communicate information about the patient's status to waiting family members.
- Ensure that the patient's wishes, as expressed in the advance directives statement, are honored in the surgical setting. **Patient-Centered Care** QSEN

Physiological Integrity

- Apply padding to the OR bed to maintain the patient's skin integrity. **Evidence-Based Practice** QSEN
- Position the patient comfortably and safely.
- Maintain the malignant hyperthermia cart.
- Monitor the patient's airway, level of consciousness, oxygen saturation, ECG, and vital signs during and immediately after moderate sedation.
- Assess the patient for tachycardia, increased end-tidal carbon dioxide level, and increased body temperature as indicators of malignant hyperthermia.
- Assess all skin areas and document findings before transferring the patient to the postanesthesia care unit.
- Communicate clearly and accurately information about the patient's surgical experience when handing off the patient to the postanesthesia care nurse. **Teamwork and Collaboration** QSEN

16 CHAPTER

Care of Postoperative Patients

Robin Chard

http://evolve.elsevier.com/Iggy/

PRIORITY CONCEPTS

- Gas Exchange
- Pain
- Clotting
- Infection
- Tissue Integrity

LEARNING OUTCOMES

Safe and Effective Care Environment

1. Protect the patient from injury and INFECTION during the postoperative period.
2. Communicate care provided and needed at each transition in care during the postoperative period.

Health Promotion and Maintenance

3. Evaluate patient risk for complications of wound healing, INFECTION, and development of venous thromboembolism.
4. Continue to provide perioperative education for patients and family members after surgery.

Psychosocial Integrity

5. Reduce the psychological impact for the patient and family regarding the postoperative experience.

Physiological Integrity

6. Perform an ongoing head-to-toe assessment of the postoperative patient.
7. Implement appropriate PAIN relief strategies for the postoperative patient.
8. Apply knowledge of anatomy, physiology, and pathophysiology to monitor the patient for the complications of shock, respiratory depression, and impaired wound healing.
9. Prioritize nursing interventions for the patient during the postoperative period.
10. Collaborate with health care team members to perform emergency procedures for surgical wound dehiscence or wound evisceration.

The **postoperative period** starts with completion of surgery and transfer of the patient to a specialized area for monitoring such as the postanesthesia care unit (PACU) and may continue after discharge from the hospital until all activity restrictions have been lifted. The period of postanesthesia care is divided into three phases that are based on the level of care needed, not the physical place of care. Not every patient will need all three phases.

Phase I care occurs immediately after surgery, most often in a PACU, although care in an ambulatory care unit is becoming common. For those patients who have very complicated procedures or many serious health problems, phase I care may occur in an intensive care unit (ICU). The length of time the patient remains at a phase I level of observation depends on his or her health status, the surgical procedure, anesthesia type, and rate of progression to complete alertness and hemodynamic stability. It can range from less than 1 hour to days. This level features very close monitoring of the airway, vital signs, and indicators of recovery that varies from every 5 to 15 minutes initially. The time between assessments gradually increases as the patient progresses toward recovery.

Phase II postoperative recovery focuses on preparing the patient for care in an extended care environment, such as a medical-surgical unit, step-down unit, skilled nursing facility, or home. This phase can occur in a PACU, on a medical-surgical unit, or in the same-day surgery (SDS) unit (ambulatory care unit) and may last only 15 to 30 minutes, although 1 to 2 hours is more typical. Patients are discharged from this phase when presurgery level of consciousness has returned, oxygen saturation is at baseline, and vital signs are stable. Some patients achieve this level of recovery in phase I and can be discharged directly to home. Others may require further observation.

The third phase of postoperative recovery, known as the *extended-care environment,* most often occurs on a hospital unit or in the home. For patients who have continuing care needs that cannot be met at home, discharge may be from the hospital unit to an extended-care facility. Although vital signs continue to be monitored in this type of environment, the frequency ranges from several times daily to just once daily.

The actual time spent away from home after surgery varies according to age, physical health, self-care ability, support systems, type and length of surgical procedure, anesthesia, any complications, home environmental conditions, and community resources. The core measures recommended by the Surgical Care Improvement Project (SCIP) that were initiated during the preoperative period to prevent certain surgical complications are continued or re-evaluated during the postoperative period. (See Chapter 14 and Table 14-1 for an explanation of these measures.)

OVERVIEW

The purpose of a **postanesthesia care unit (PACU)** (recovery room) is the ongoing evaluation and stabilization of patients to anticipate, prevent, and manage complications after surgery. The PACU is usually located close to the surgical suite for ease of access and patient transfer. The unit is usually a large and open room to provide direct observation of all patients and easy access to supplies and emergency equipment. The patient area may be divided into individual cubicles. So that each patient can be observed continuously, privacy curtains or screens are partially open and are fully closed only during bedside procedures. Each cubicle has equipment to monitor and care for the patient, such as oxygen, suction equipment, cardiac monitors, pulse oximetry, airway equipment, and emergency drugs.

After the surgery is completed, the circulating nurse and the anesthesia provider accompany the patient to the PACU. For patients in critical condition, transfer may be directly from the operating room (OR) to the ICU. On arrival, the anesthesia provider and the circulating nurse give the PACU nurse a verbal "hand-off" report to communicate the patient's condition and care needs.

A hand-off report that meets The Joint Commission's National Patient Safety Goals requires effective communication between health care professionals. It is at least a two-way verbal interaction between the health care professional giving the report and the nurse receiving it. The language used to give the report is clear and cannot be interpreted in more than one way. The nurse receiving the report focuses on the report and is not distracted by the environment or other responsibilities. Standardizing the information reported helps prevent omission of critical patient-centered information and helps avoid irrelevant details (Association of periOperative Registered Nurses [AORN], 2014). The receiving nurse takes the time to restate (report back) the information to verify what was said and to make certain he or she has the same understanding as the reporting person. The receiving nurse takes the time to ask questions and the reporting professional must respond to the questions until a common understanding is established. Chart 16-1 gives an example of critical information to include in a standard hand-off report.

The PACU nurse is skilled in the care of patients with multiple medical and surgical problems immediately after a surgical procedure. This area requires in-depth knowledge of anatomy and physiology, anesthetic agents, pharmacology, PAIN management, extubation, surgical procedures, and advanced cardiac life support (ACLS). The PACU nurse is skilled in assessment and can make knowledgeable, quick decisions if emergencies or complications occur. The patient is monitored closely. The anesthesia provider and surgeon are consulted as needed.

CHART 16-1 Best Practice for Patient Safety & Quality Care (QSEN)

Postoperative Hand-off Report

- Type and extent of the surgical procedure
- Type of anesthesia and length of time the patient was under anesthesia
- Allergies (especially to latex or drugs)
- Any health problems or pathologic conditions
- Status of vital signs, including temperature and oxygen saturation
- Type and amount of IV fluids and drugs administered
- Estimated blood loss (EBL)
- Any intraoperative complications, such as a traumatic intubation
- Primary language, any sensory impairments, any communication difficulties
- Special requests that were verbalized by the patient preoperatively
- Preoperative and intraoperative respiratory function and dysfunction
- Location and type of incisions, dressings, catheters, tubes, drains, or packing
- Intake and output, including current IV fluid administration and estimated blood loss
- Prosthetic devices
- Joint or limb immobility while in the operating room, especially in the older patient
- Other intraoperative positioning that may be relevant in the postoperative phase
- Intraoperative complications, how managed, patient responses (e.g., laboratory values)

❖ PATIENT-CENTERED COLLABORATIVE CARE

◆ Assessment

History. Use the surgical team's report to plan the care for an individual patient. After receiving the report and assessing the patient, review the medical record for information about the patient's history, physical condition, and emotional status. If the patient remains as an inpatient, the surgical and anesthesia information is incorporated into the postoperative plan of care. Chapter 14 identifies factors that increase the risk for the potential complications listed in Table 16-1.

Physical Assessment/Clinical Manifestations. Assess the patient, and record data on a PACU flow chart record (Fig. 16-1). Assessment data include level of consciousness, temperature, pulse, respiration, oxygen saturation, and blood pressure. Examine the surgical area for bleeding. Monitor vital signs as often as your facility's policy states, the patient's condition warrants, and the surgeon prescribes. Once the patient is discharged from the PACU, vital signs are measured as prescribed or as often as the patient's condition indicates.

! NURSING SAFETY PRIORITY (QSEN)

Action Alert

Respiratory assessment is the most critical assessment to perform after surgery for any patient who has undergone general anesthesia or moderate sedation or has received sedative or opioid drugs.

TABLE 16-1 General Potential Complications of Surgery

Respiratory System Complications
- Atelectasis
- Pneumonia
- Pulmonary embolism (PE)
- Laryngeal edema
- Ventilator dependence
- Pulmonary edema

Cardiovascular Complications
- Hypertension
- Hypotension
- Hypovolemic shock
- Dysrhythmias
- Venous thromboembolism (VTE), especially deep vein thrombosis (DVT)
- Heart failure
- Sepsis
- Disseminated intravascular coagulation (DIC)
- Anemia
- Anaphylaxis

Skin Complications
- Pressure ulcers
- Wound infection
- Wound dehiscence
- Wound evisceration
- Skin rashes or contact allergies

Gastrointestinal Complications
- Paralytic ileus
- Gastrointestinal ulcers and bleeding

Neuromuscular Complications
- Hypothermia
- Hyperthermia
- Nerve damage and paralysis
- Joint contractures

Kidney/Urinary Complications
- Urinary tract infection
- Acute urinary retention
- Electrolyte imbalances
- Acute kidney injury (AKI)
- Stone formation

CHART 16-2 Focused Assessment

The Patient on Arrival at the Medical-Surgical Unit After Discharge from the Postanesthesia Care Unit

Airway
- Is it patent?
- Is the neck in proper alignment?

Breathing
- What is the quality and pattern of the breathing?
- What is the respiratory rate and depth?
- Is the patient using accessory muscles to breathe?
- Is the patient receiving oxygen? At what setting? What is the pulse oximetry reading?

Mental Status
- Is the patient awake, able to be aroused, oriented, and aware?
- Does the patient respond to verbal stimuli?

Surgical Incision Site
- How is it dressed?
- Review the amount of drainage on the dressing immediately.
- Is there any bleeding or drainage under the patient?
- Are any drains present?
- Are the drains set properly (e.g., compressed if they should be compressed, not kinked, patient not lying on them)?
- How much drainage is present in the drainage container?

Temperature, Pulse, and Blood Pressure
- Are these values within the patient's baseline range?
- Are these values significantly different from when the patient was in the postanesthesia care unit (PACU)?

Intravenous Fluids
- What type of solution is infusing and with what additives?
- How much solution was remaining on arrival?
- How much solution infused in the transport time from PACU?
- At what rate is the infusion supposed to be set? Is it?

Other Tubes
- Is there a nasogastric or intestinal tube?
- What is the color, consistency, and amount of drainage?
- Is suction applied to the tube if ordered? Is the suction setting correct?
- Is there a Foley catheter?
- Is the Foley draining properly?
- What is the color, clarity, and volume of urine output?

The health care team determines the patient's readiness for discharge from the PACU by the presence of a recovery score rating of 9 to 10 on the recovery scale (see Fig. 16-1). Other criteria for discharge (e.g., stable vital signs; normal body temperature; no overt bleeding; return of gag, cough, and swallow reflexes; the ability to take liquids; and adequate urine output) may be specific to the facility. After you determine that all criteria have been met, the patient is discharged by the anesthesia provider to the hospital unit or to home. If an anesthesia provider has not been involved, which may be the case with local anesthesia or moderate sedation, the surgeon or nurse discharges the patient once the discharge criteria have been met.

Assessment continues from the PACU to the intensive care or medical-surgical nursing unit. If the patient is to be discharged from the PACU to home, assessment and any needed nursing care are continued by home care nurses or by the patient or family members after health teaching. When the patient is transferred to an inpatient unit, complete an initial assessment on arrival (Chart 16-2).

During the postoperative period, all patients remain at risk for pneumonia, shock, cardiac arrest, respiratory arrest, CLOTTING and venous thromboembolism (VTE), and GI bleeding. These serious complications can be prevented or the consequences reduced with collaborative care. Nursing observations and interventions are part of critical rescue management for patient safety and quality care.

Respiratory System. *When the patient is admitted to the PACU, immediately assess for a patent airway and adequate GAS EXCHANGE. Although some patients may be awake and able to speak, talking is not a good indicator of adequate gas exchange.* An artificial airway, such as an endotracheal tube

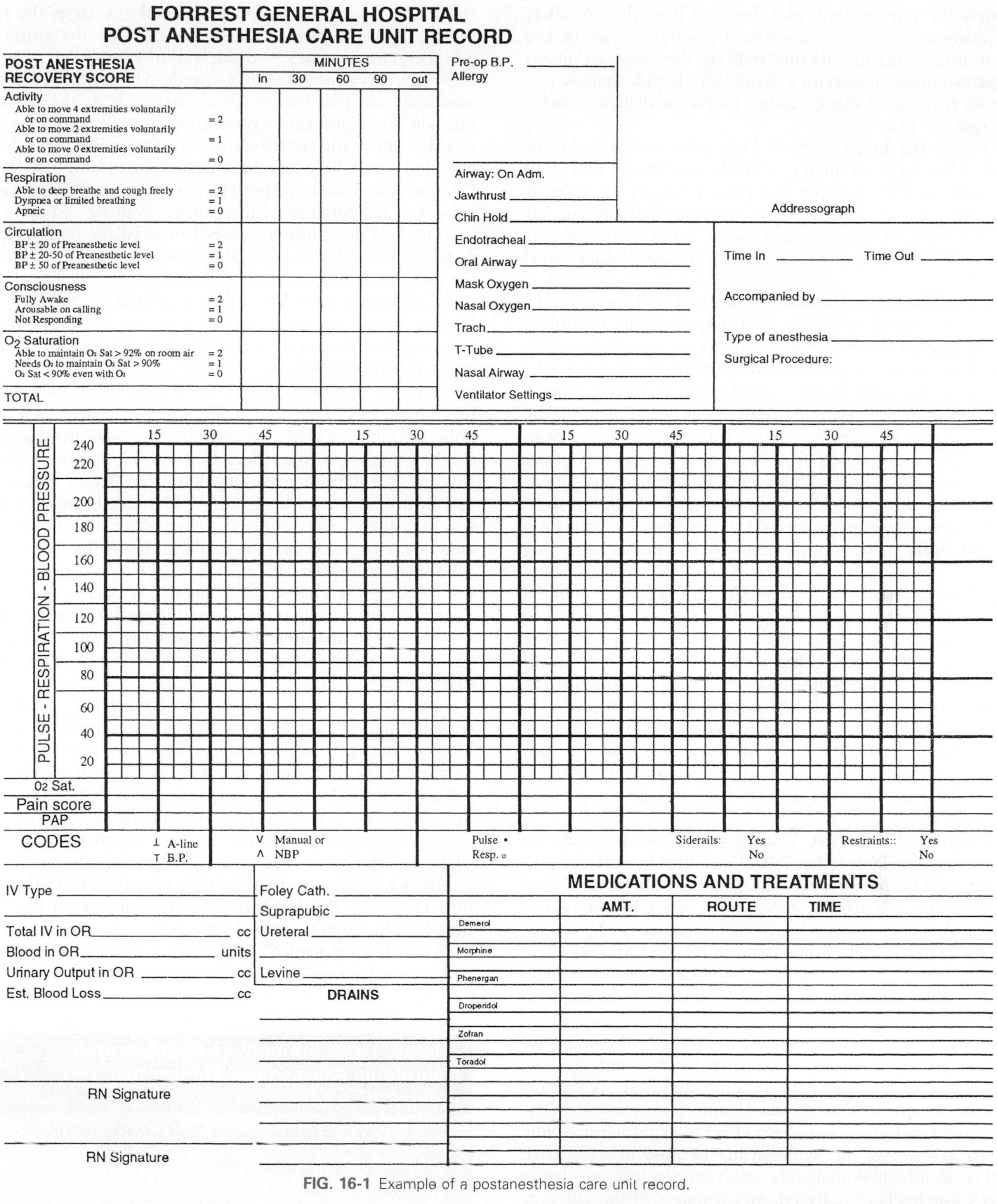
FORREST GENERAL HOSPITAL
POST ANESTHESIA CARE UNIT RECORD

POST ANESTHESIA RECOVERY SCORE		MINUTES in	30	60	90	out
Activity						
Able to move 4 extremities voluntarily or on command	= 2					
Able to move 2 extremities voluntarily or on command	= 1					
Able to move 0 extremities voluntarily or on command	= 0					
Respiration						
Able to deep breathe and cough freely	= 2					
Dyspnea or limited breathing	= 1					
Apneic	= 0					
Circulation						
BP ± 20 of Preanesthetic level	= 2					
BP ± 20-50 of Preanesthetic level	= 1					
BP ± 50 of Preanesthetic level	= 0					
Consciousness						
Fully Awake	= 2					
Arousable on calling	= 1					
Not Responding	= 0					
O_2 Saturation						
Able to maintain O_2 Sat > 92% on room air	= 2					
Needs O_2 to maintain O_2 Sat > 90%	= 1					
O_2 Sat < 90% even with O_2	= 0					
TOTAL						

Pre-op B.P. ______
Allergy

Airway: On Adm.
Jawthrust ______
Chin Hold ______
Endotracheal ______
Oral Airway ______
Mask Oxygen ______
Nasal Oxygen ______
Trach ______
T-Tube ______
Nasal Airway ______
Ventilator Settings ______

Addressograph

Time In ______ Time Out ______
Accompanied by ______
Type of anesthesia ______
Surgical Procedure:

PULSE - RESPIRATION - BLOOD PRESSURE
15 30 45 15 30 45 15 30 45 15 30 45
240
220
200
180
160
140
120
100
80
60
40
20
O_2 Sat.
Pain score
PAP

CODES ⊥ A-line T B.P. V Manual or ^ NBP Pulse • Resp. o Siderails: Yes No Restraints:: Yes No

IV Type ______
Total IV in OR ______ cc
Blood in OR ______ units
Urinary Output in OR ______ cc
Est. Blood Loss ______ cc

Foley Cath. ______
Suprapubic
Ureteral ______
Levine ______

DRAINS

MEDICATIONS AND TREATMENTS

	AMT.	ROUTE	TIME
Demerol			
Morphine			
Phenergan			
Droperidol			
Zofran			
Toradol			

RN Signature

RN Signature

FIG. 16-1 Example of a postanesthesia care unit record.

(ET), a nasal trumpet, or an oral airway, may be in place. If the patient is receiving oxygen, document the type of delivery device and the concentration or liter flow of the oxygen. Continuously monitor pulse oximetry for oxygen saturation (Spo_2) while the patient is in the PACU. The Spo_2 should be above 95% (or at the patient's presurgery baseline).

! NURSING SAFETY PRIORITY (QSEN)

Critical Rescue

If the oxygen saturation drops below 95% (or below the patient's presurgery baseline), notify the surgeon or anesthesia provider. If it drops by 10 percentage points and you are certain it is an accurate measure, call the Rapid Response Team.

Assess the rate, pattern, and depth of breathing to determine adequacy of GAS EXCHANGE. A respiratory rate of less than 10 breaths per minute may indicate anesthetic- or opioid analgesic–induced respiratory depression. Rapid, shallow respirations may signal shock, cardiac problems, increased metabolic rate, or PAIN.

Listen to the lungs over all lung fields to assess breath sounds. Also check symmetry of breath sounds and chest wall movement. If, for example, the patient has an ET tube, it could move down into the right bronchus and prevent left lung expansion. In this case, lung sounds on the left are absent or decreased and only the right chest wall rises and falls with breathing.

Perform ongoing inspection of the chest wall for accessory muscle use, sternal retraction, and diaphragmatic breathing. These manifestations may indicate an excessive anesthetic effect, airway obstruction, or paralysis, which could result in hypoxia. Listen for snoring and **stridor** (a high-pitched crowing sound). Snoring and stridor occur with airway obstruction resulting from tracheal or laryngeal spasm or edema, mucus in the airway, or blockage of the airway from edema or tongue relaxation. When neuromuscular blocking agents are retained, the patient has muscle weakness, which could impair GAS EXCHANGE. Indicators of muscle weakness include the inability to maintain a head lift, weak hand grasps, and an abdominal breathing pattern.

If the patient returns to an inpatient unit, complete an initial assessment on arrival (see Chart 16-2) and then continue to assess for respiratory depression or hypoxemia. Listen to the lungs to check for effective expansion and for abnormal breath sounds. Check the lungs at least every 4 hours during the first 24 hours after surgery and then every 8 hours, or more often, as indicated. Older patients, smokers, and patients with a history of lung disease are at greater risk for respiratory complications after surgery and need more frequent assessment (Sullivan, 2011). Obese patients are also at high risk for respiratory complications.

Cardiovascular System. *Vital signs* and heart sounds are assessed on admission to the PACU and then at least every 15 minutes until the patient's condition is stable. Automated blood pressure cuffs and cardiac monitoring assist in continuous assessment.

Review vital signs after surgery for trends, and compare them with those taken before surgery. Report blood pressure changes that are 25% higher or lower than values obtained before surgery (or a 15- to 20-point difference, systolic or diastolic) to the anesthesia provider or the surgeon. Decreased blood pressure and pulse pressure and abnormal heart sounds indicate possible cardiac depression, fluid volume deficit, shock, hemorrhage, or the effects of drugs (see Chapters 11 and 37). Bradycardia could indicate an anesthesia effect or hypothermia. Older patients are at risk for hypothermia because of age-related changes in the hypothalamus (the temperature regulation center), low levels of body fat, and coolness of the OR suite (Sullivan, 2011; Touhy & Jett, 2014). An increased pulse rate could indicate hemorrhage, shock, or PAIN.

Cardiac monitoring is maintained until the patient is discharged from the PACU. For patients at risk for dysrhythmias, monitoring may continue either on telemetry units or on general medical-surgical units. In assessing the vital signs of a patient who is not being monitored continuously, compare the rate, rhythm, and quality of the apical pulse with the rate, rhythm, and quality of a peripheral pulse, such as the radial pulse. A **pulse deficit** (a difference between the apical and peripheral pulses) could indicate a dysrhythmia.

Peripheral vascular assessment needs to be performed because anesthesia and positioning during surgery (e.g., the lithotomy position for genitourinary procedures) may impair the peripheral circulation and contribute to CLOTTING and venous thromboembolism (VTE), especially deep vein thrombosis (DVT). Compare distal pulses on both feet for pulse quality, observe the color and temperature of extremities, evaluate sensation and motion, and determine the speed of capillary refill. Palpable pedal pulses indicate adequate circulation and perfusion of the legs.

In adherence with The Joint Commission's Surgical Care Improvement Project (SCIP) core measures for prevention of inappropriate CLOTTING and VTE, continue the prophylactic measures initiated before surgery (Myles, 2012). Although these measures vary in type (e.g., drug therapy with anticoagulants or antiplatelet drugs, sequential compression devices, antiembolic stockings or elastic wraps, early ambulation) depending on the patient's specific risk factors and the type and extent of surgery, any preventive strategies started before surgery are usually needed for at least the first 24 hours after surgery. Reassess the patient's risk for CLOTTING and VTE and the effectiveness of the preventive strategies daily. Assess the feet and legs for redness, pain, warmth, and swelling, which may occur with DVT. Foot and leg assessment may be performed once during a nursing shift or once daily depending on the patient's risk for complications and the facility's or agency's policy. (See Chapters 14 and 36 for more information on prevention of inappropriate CLOTTING and VTE.)

Neurologic System. *Cerebral functioning* and the level of consciousness or awareness must be assessed in *all* patients who have received general anesthesia (Table 16-2) or any type of sedation. Observe for lethargy, restlessness, or irritability, and test coherence and orientation. Determine awareness by observing responses to calling the patient's name, touching the patient, and giving simple commands such as "Open your eyes" and "Take a deep breath." Eye opening in response to a command indicates wakefulness or arousability but not necessarily awareness. Determine the degree of orientation to person, place, and time by asking the conscious patient to answer questions such as "What is your name?" (person), "Where are you?" (place), and "What day is it?" (time).

TABLE 16-2 Immediate Postoperative Neurologic Assessment: Return to Preoperative Level

Order of Return to Consciousness After General Anesthesia

1. Muscular irritability
2. Restlessness and delirium
3. Recognition of pain
4. Ability to reason and control behavior

Order of Return of Motor and Sensory Functioning After Local or Regional Anesthesia

1. Sense of touch
2. Sense of pain
3. Sense of warmth
4. Sense of cold
5. Ability to move

CLINICAL JUDGMENT CHALLENGE

Patient-Centered Care QSEN

The patient is a 71-year-old woman who came from the operating room to the postanesthesia recovery unit about an hour ago after a short procedure (dilation and curettage) under general anesthesia for dysfunctional uterine bleeding. She awakens when her name is called, but she does not know where she is or why. In addition, she has pulled off her oxygen cannula and keeps trying to pull out her IV. Her last vital signs, taken 15 minutes ago, were BP, 140/92; pulse, 88; respirations, 18. When you check her vital signs now, they are BP, 128/102; pulse 110; respirations 24. She is saying she is thirsty and wants some water.

1. Are any of the changes in vital signs a cause for concern? If so which ones?
2. Given her surgery, where should you look for bleeding? (Check Chapter 71 for information about this procedure.)
3. Should you apply oxygen? Why or why not?
4. Should you give her sips of water? Why or why not?
5. Should you notify the surgeon or anesthesia provider? Why or why not?

CONSIDERATIONS FOR OLDER ADULTS

Patient-Centered Care QSEN

For an older adult, a rapid return to his or her level of orientation before surgery may not be realistic. Preoperative drugs and anesthetics may delay the older patient's return of orientation.

Reassure family members that most episodes of postoperative confusion or delirium resolve within a day or two (Brooks, 2012).

Compare the patient's baseline neurologic status (obtained before surgery) with the findings after surgery. Patients who had altered cerebral functioning before surgery because of another condition usually continue to have that alteration after surgery. After the patient is alert (and all other criteria have been met), he or she is discharged from the PACU. On the medical-surgical nursing unit, assess the level of consciousness every 4 to 8 hours or as indicated by the patient's condition and the facility's policy.

Motor function and sensory function after general anesthesia are altered and must be assessed. General anesthesia depresses all voluntary motor function. Regional anesthesia alters the motor and sensory function of only part of the body. (See Chapter 15 for more information on anesthesia.)

Motor and sensory function after spinal and epidural anesthesia are profoundly affected and critical to assess. Assess the level of sensation loss remaining by lightly pricking the patient's skin with a needle or pin and having the patient indicate when the sensation feels sharp rather than dull (just pressure). Evaluate motor function by asking the patient to move each extremity. The patient who had epidural or spinal anesthesia remains in the PACU until sensory function (feeling) and voluntary motor movement of the legs have returned (see Table 16-2). Also assess the strength of each limb, and compare the results on both sides. Test for the return of sympathetic nervous system tone by gradually elevating the patient's head and monitoring for hypotension. Begin this evaluation after the patient's sensation has returned to at least the spinal dermatome level of T10.

Specific assessment findings for complications of spinal and epidural anesthesia are listed in Chart 16-3. After the patient is transferred to the nursing unit, continue neurologic assessment as indicated.

CHART 16-3 Best Practice for Patient Safety & Quality Care QSEN

Recognizing Serious Complications of Spinal and Epidural Anesthesia

Respiratory Depression (can occur if the anesthetic agent moves higher in the epidural or subarachnoid space)

- What is the quality and pattern of the breathing?
- What is the respiratory rate and depth?
- Is the patient receiving oxygen? At what setting? What is the pulse oximetry result?
- Notify the anesthesia provider if pulse oximetry drops or if the patient is unable to increase the depth of respiration.

Hypotension (can occur when regional anesthesia causes widespread vasodilation)

- What is the patient's blood pressure?
- Is the blood pressure now lower than in the preoperative or operative period?
- Has the pulse pressure widened?
- Notify the anesthesia provider if systolic blood pressure remains more than 10 mm Hg below the patient's baseline or if other manifestations of shock are present.
- Notify the anesthesia provider if hypotension is accompanied by other manifestations of autonomic nervous system blockade (bradycardia, nausea, vomiting).

Epidural Hematoma

- Assess for delayed or regressing return of sensory and motor function.
- If return is delayed or is taking longer than usual, alert the anesthesia provider.
- Determine whether sensory or motor deficits are improving, remaining the same, or worsening.
- If motor deficits are worsening or decreasing after brief improvement, notify the anesthesia provider immediately.
- Assess for return of deep tendon reflexes of extremities on both sides.
- Compare reflexes from one side of the body with the other.
- If reflexes regress, notify the anesthesia provider immediately.
- Assess pain level in the back.
- If the patient feels pressure or increasing back pain while coughing or straining, notify the anesthesia provider immediately.

Infection (Meningitis)

- Assess for mental status changes.
- Assess for increasing temperature.
- Assess for ability to turn the neck.
- Notify the anesthesia provider immediately for temperature elevations above 101° F (38.3° C), inability to move the neck, acute confusion.

Postdural Puncture Headache

- Assess for report of headache in the occipital region, especially when the patient is permitted to sit upright.

NCLEX EXAMINATION CHALLENGE

Physiological Integrity

Which assessment parameter is most important for the nurse to employ for the client admitted to the postanesthesia care unit (PACU) for recovery after surgery under epidural anesthesia?

A. Determining the client's level of consciousness
B. Checking for pain on dorsi and plantar flexion of the foot
C. Assessing the response to pinprick stimulation from feet to mid-chest level
D. Comparing blood pressure taken in the right arm with blood pressure taken in the left arm

Fluid, Electrolyte, and Acid-Base Balance. Fasting before and during surgery, the loss of fluid during the procedure, and the type and amount of blood or fluid given affect the patient's fluid and electrolyte balance after surgery. Fluid volume deficit or fluid volume overload may occur after surgery. Sodium, potassium, chloride, and calcium imbalances also may result, as may changes in other electrolyte levels. Fluid and electrolyte imbalances occur more often in older or debilitated patients and in those with health problems such as diabetes mellitus, Crohn's disease, or heart failure.

Intake and output measurement is part of the operative record and is reported by the circulating nurse to the PACU nurse. Record any intake or output, including IV fluid intake, vomitus, urine, wound drainage, and nasogastric (NG) tube drainage. You must know the total intake and output from both the OR and the PACU to assess fluid balance accurately and to complete the 24-hour intake and output record.

Hydration status is assessed in the PACU and the medical-surgical unit. To determine hydration status, inspect the color and moisture of mucous membranes; the turgor, texture, and "tenting" of the skin (test over the sternum or forehead of an older patient); the amount of drainage on dressings; and the presence of axillary sweat. Measure and compare total output (e.g., NG tube drainage, urine output, wound drainage) with total intake to identify a possible fluid imbalance. Consider insensible fluid loss, such as sweat, when reviewing total output. Continue to assess intake and output as long as the patient is at risk for fluid imbalances. Some facilities require intake and output to be measured if the patient receives IV fluids or has a catheter, drains, or an NG tube. In addition, patients who have heart disease or kidney disease may need a longer period of intake and output measurement.

IV fluids are closely monitored to promote fluid and electrolyte balance. Isotonic solutions such as lactated Ringer's (LR), 0.9% sodium chloride (normal saline), and 5% dextrose with lactated Ringer's (D_5/LR) are used for IV fluid replacement in the PACU. After the patient returns to the medical-surgical unit, the type and rate of IV infusions are based on need.

Acid-base balance is affected by the patient's respiratory status; metabolic changes during surgery; and losses of acids or bases in drainage. For example, NG tube drainage or vomitus causes a loss of hydrochloric acid and leads to metabolic alkalosis. Examine arterial blood gas (ABG) values and other laboratory values. (See Chapter 12 for more detailed information on acid-base imbalances.)

Kidney/Urinary System. Control of urination may return immediately after surgery or may not return for hours after general or regional anesthesia. The effects of preoperative drugs (especially atropine), anesthetic agents, or manipulation during surgery can cause urine retention. Assess for urine retention by inspection, palpation, and percussion of the lower abdomen for bladder distention or by the use of a bladder scanner (see Chapter 65). Assessment may be difficult to perform after lower abdominal surgery. Urine retention is common early after surgery and requires intervention, such as intermittent (straight) catheterization, to empty the bladder.

When the patient has an indwelling urinary (Foley) catheter, assess the urine for color, clarity, and amount. If the patient is voiding, assess the frequency, amount per void, and any manifestations. Urine output should be close to the total intake for a 24-hour period. Consider sweat, vomitus, or diarrhea stools as sources of output. Report a urine output of less than 30 mL/hr (240 mL per 8-hour nursing shift) to the surgeon. Decreased urine output may indicate hypovolemia or renal complications. (See Chapter 65 for kidney/urinary assessment.)

Gastrointestinal System. *Postoperative nausea and vomiting (PONV)* are among the most common reactions after surgery. Many patients who receive general anesthesia have some form of GI upset within the first 24 hours after surgery; however, some patients are more at risk than others (Tinsley & Barone, 2013). Patients with a history of motion sickness are more likely to develop nausea and vomiting after surgery. Obese patients may be at risk because many anesthetics are retained by fat cells and remain in the body longer. Abdominal surgery and the use of opioid analgesics reduce intestinal peristalsis after surgery. These problems increase the risk for prolonged nausea and vomiting after surgery. Preventive drug therapy, often started in the preoperative period, is effective in reducing the incidence. Drugs often used are a serotonin antagonist such as ondansetron (Zofran), a sedating H_1 histamine antagonist such as dimenhydrinate (Dramamine), and an anticholinergic agent such as scopolamine.

PONV can stress and irritate abdominal and GI wounds, increase intracranial pressure in patients who had head and neck surgery, elevate intraocular pressure in patients who had eye surgery, and increase the risk for aspiration. Assess the patient continuously for PONV. Often patients have nausea as the head of the bed is raised early after surgery. Help reduce this distressing symptom by having the patient in a side-lying position before raising the head slowly.

Intestinal peristalsis may be delayed because of prolonged anesthesia time, the amount of bowel handling during surgery, and opioid analgesic use. In the PACU and later on the medical-surgical unit, assess for the return of peristalsis. *Patients who are recovering from abdominal surgery often have decreased or no peristalsis for at least 24 hours.* This problem may persist for several days for those who have GI surgery.

Listen for bowel sounds in all four abdominal quadrants and at the umbilicus. If NG suction is being used, turn off the suction before listening to prevent mistaking the sound of the suction for bowel sounds. *The presence of active bowel sounds usually indicates return of peristalsis; however, the absence of bowel sounds does not confirm a lack of peristalsis. The best indicator of intestinal activity is the passage of flatus or stool (Massey, 2012).* Abdominal cramping along with distention denotes trapped, nonmoving gas—not peristalsis.

Decreased peristalsis occurs in patients who have a paralytic ileus. The abdominal wall is distended with no visible intestinal movement. Assess for the manifestations of paralytic ileus (distended abdomen, abdominal discomfort, vomiting, no passage of flatus or stool). In some patients, bowels sounds can be heard even when a true paralytic ileus is present. The passage of flatus or stool is the best indicator of resolution of a paralytic ileus. See the Evidence-Based Practice box.

A nasogastric (NG) tube may be inserted during surgery to decompress and drain the stomach, to promote GI rest, and to allow the lower GI tract to heal. It may also be used to monitor any gastric bleeding and to prevent intestinal obstruction. Usually low suction is applied to promote drainage. Suction is either continuous or intermittent.

Record the color, consistency, and amount of the NG drainage every 8 hours (Table 16-3). In some instances, an occult blood test (Gastroccult) may be performed. Normal NG drainage fluid is greenish yellow. Red or pink drainage fluid

EVIDENCE-BASED PRACTICE QSEN

Evidence-Based Practice or Sacred Cow?

Massey, R. (2012). Return of bowel sounds indicating an end of postoperative ileus: Is it time to cease this long-standing nursing tradition? *MEDSURG Nursing, 21*(3), 146-150.

Abdominal surgery, especially surgery involving bowel anastomosis, is known to reduce or stop intestinal peristalsis and result in postoperative ileus (POI) with a duration of 3 to 5 days. POI causes a cluster of patient symptoms, which include abdominal pain, distention, nausea, and vomiting. In addition, POI delays nutrition and lengthens hospital stay. For more than a century, the classic indicator for return of bowel function after POI was the presence of bowel sounds. Recommended assessment is auscultation of the four abdominal quadrants for 5 minutes each, a total time task of 20 minutes. A variety of previous research suggests that assessment of bowel sounds for return of function after POI is an unreliable "tradition" that wastes nursing care time and may, in fact, cause harm.

Problems associated with assessment of bowel sounds as an indicator of bowel function return include the fact that the small intestine usually recovers bowel sounds ahead of the colon but that the sounds do not always correlate to peristaltic movement of retained gas and fluids. This means that positive bowel sounds in some quadrants may result in early enteral feeding of a patient before true peristalsis returns. Also, some patients have no loss of bowel sounds after abdominal surgery but do experience the symptom cluster associated with POI, again making the presence of bowel sounds an unreliable indicator of peristalsis. Moreover, studies indicate that most nurses auscultate the abdomen for only 30 to 60 seconds in each quadrant, not the recommended but unvalidated time of 5 minutes per quadrant. Even this smaller amount of time represents unproductive nursing activity.

The current study examined the return of bowel sounds and other manifestations as indicators for resolution of POI among 66 patients who all had intestinal surgery with anastomosis for cancer. The average return of bowel sounds among these 66 patients was 2.23 days and was not related to the average time to first passage of flatus.

Level of Evidence: 3

This quasi-experimental study with a two-group, post-test only design was randomized and had sufficient subjects to provide result validity. The use of objective measurements added to study strength.

Commentary: Implications for Practice and Research

This study provides evidence for the rational elimination of 20 minutes of nursing time spent in auscultation of bowel sounds several times daily after abdominal surgery. The findings of this study support other studies that recommend using the practice of using passage of flatus or stool as the marker for the end of POI rather than the time-honored but unsupported practice of auscultating bowel sounds for 20 minutes. Actual passage of flatus or stool demonstrates an end of POI and complete return of peristalsis with forward propulsion of intestinal contents for the entire GI tract. Additional positive indicators for evidence of an end to POI include elimination of abdominal distention, nausea, and vomiting and the tolerance of oral intake. Nurses need to understand the physiologic basis for why return of bowel sounds may be an unreliable indicator of an end to POI and may result in inappropriate initiation of dietary intake.

indicates active bleeding, and brown liquid or drainage with a "coffee-ground" appearance indicates old bleeding. Assess that the NG tube is securely taped to the nose, and note any skin irritation.

Assess the patient for complications related to NG tube use, such as fluid and electrolyte imbalances, aspiration, and nares discomfort. To prevent aspiration, check the tube placement every 4 to 8 hours and before instilling any liquid, including drugs, into the tube. (See Chapter 55 for information on tube placement and care.) Electrolyte imbalances can result from NG drainage and tube irrigation with water instead of saline. Imbalances include fluid volume deficit, hypokalemia and hyponatremia (see Chapter 11), hypochloremia, and metabolic alkalosis (see Chapter 12).

TABLE 16-3 Calculating Nasogastric Tube Drainage

Formula

Drainage in collection device − Amount of irrigant = True (actual) amount of drainage

Example

A patient's drainage container was marked at 150 mL at 7 AM. At 3 PM, there was 525 mL in the container. During the nursing shift, the nurse instilled 30 mL of saline as an irrigant into the tube four times, as prescribed by the physician.

525 mL − 150 mL = 375 mL of drainage
30 mL × 4 = 120 mL of irrigant
375 mL − 120 mL = 255 mL of actual drainage

! NURSING SAFETY PRIORITY QSEN

Action Alert

After gastric surgery, do not move or irrigate the NG tube unless prescribed by the surgeon.

Constipation may occur after surgery as a result of anesthesia, analgesia (especially opioids), decreased activity, and decreased oral intake. Assess the abdomen by inspection, auscultation, palpation, and percussion and record the elimination pattern to determine whether intervention is needed. *Auscultate before palpation or percussion because these two maneuvers can affect peristalsis.* Increased dietary fiber intake, the use of mild laxatives or bulk-forming agents, or the use of enemas may be needed.

? NCLEX EXAMINATION CHALLENGE

Safe and Effective Care Environment

The assessment findings for the nasogastric tube drainage of a client recently transferred from the PACU include the presence of 140 mL of greenish yellow drainage. What is the nurse's best action?

A. Instruct the client to drink water until the drainage is clear.
B. Reposition the tube to increase the drainage.
C. Call and report this finding to the surgeon.
D. Document the finding as the only action.

Skin Assessment. The clean surgical wound regains TISSUE INTEGRITY (heals) at skin level in about 2 weeks in the absence of trauma, connective tissue disease, malnutrition, or the use of some drugs, such as steroids. Smokers and patients who are older, obese, or have diabetes or whose immunity is reduced have delayed wound healing. Complete tissue integrity (healing) of all layers within the surgical wound may take 6 months to 2 years. The physical health and age of the patient, size and location of the wound, and stress on the wound all affect healing time. Head and facial wounds heal more quickly than abdominal and leg wounds because of the better blood flow to the head and neck.

Normal Wound Healing. During the first few days of normal wound healing, the incised tissue regains blood supply and begins to bind together. Fibrin and a thin layer of epithelial cells seal the incision. After 1 to 4 days, epithelial cells continue growing in the fibrin and strands of collagen begin to fill in the wound gaps. *This process continues for 2 to 3 weeks. At that time,* TISSUE INTEGRITY *appears regained; however, healing is not complete for up to 2 years, until the scar is strengthened.* (See Chapters 24 and 25 for discussion of wound healing and wound infection.)

When the patient is an inpatient, the surgeon usually removes the original dressing on the first or second day after surgery. Assess the TISSUE INTEGRITY of the incision on a regular basis, at least every 8 hours, for redness, increased warmth, swelling, tenderness or PAIN, and the type and amount of drainage. Some drainage, changing from **sanguineous** (bloody) to serosanguineous to **serous** (serum-like, or yellow), is normal during the first few days. Serosanguineous drainage continuing beyond the fifth day after surgery or increasing in amount instead of decreasing alerts you to the possibility of dehiscence (discussed below), and the surgeon should be notified. Crusting on the incision line is normal, as is a pink color to the line itself, which is caused by inflammation from the surgical procedure. Slight swelling under the sutures or staples is also normal. Redness or swelling of or around the incision line, excessive tenderness or pain on palpation, and purulent or odorous drainage indicate wound INFECTION and must be reported to the surgeon.

Impaired Wound Healing. Impaired wound healing with loss of TISSUE INTEGRITY may be caused by INFECTION, distention, stress at the surgical site, and health problems that cause delayed wound healing (e.g., diabetes). Wound **dehiscence** is a partial or complete separation of the outer wound layers, sometimes described as a "splitting open of the wound." **Evisceration** is the total separation of all wound layers and protrusion of internal organs through the open wound (Fig. 16-2). Both of these problems occur most often between the fifth and tenth days after surgery. Wound separation occurs more often in obese patients and those with diabetes, immune deficiency, or malnutrition or who are using steroids. Dehiscence or evisceration may follow forceful coughing, vomiting, or straining and when not splinting the surgical site during movement. The patient may state, "Something popped" or "I feel as if I just split open."

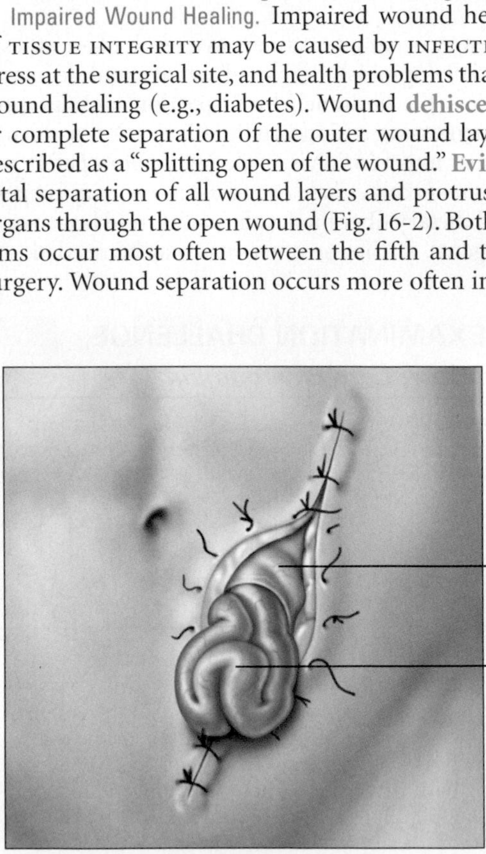

FIG. 16-2 Complications of surgical wound healing.

Dressings and Drains. Assess all dressings, including casts and elastic (Ace) bandages, for bleeding or other drainage on admission to the PACU and then hourly thereafter. When the patient is on the nursing unit, assess the dressing each time vital signs are taken (at least every 8 hours). During dressing inspection, check for drainage and record its amount, color, consistency, and odor. If drainage is present on a dressing or cast, monitor its progression by outlining it with a pencil and indicating the date and time. Check the area underneath the patient also, because drainage or blood may leak from the side of the dressing and not appear on the dressing itself.

Ensure that the dressing does not restrict circulation or sensation. This problem is most likely to occur when dressings are tight or completely encircle an arm or a leg. Chest dressings that are too tight or that encircle the chest can restrict breathing.

The surgeon inserts a drain into or close to the wound if more than a minimal amount of drainage is expected. A Penrose drain (a single-lumen, soft, open, latex tube) is a gravity-type drain under the dressing. Drainage on the dressing is expected with open tube drains but is not expected with closed drainage systems. Assess closed-suction drains, such as Hemovac, Vacu-Drain, and Jackson-Pratt drains, for maintenance of suction. Specialty drains, such as a T-tube, may be placed for specific drainage purposes. For example, a T-tube drains bile after a cholecystectomy. Chronic wounds or wounds that heal by delayed primary intention are drained with a negative pressure wound device. Fig. 16-3 shows commonly used drains.

Assess all drains for patency when the patient is admitted to the PACU and every time vital signs are taken. Monitor the amount, color, and type of drainage while the patient is in the PACU and at least every 8 hours after he or she is transferred to the medical-surgical nursing unit. Large amounts of sanguineous drainage may indicate poor CLOTTING and possible internal bleeding.

Discomfort/Pain Assessment. The patient almost always has PAIN or discomfort after surgery. Pain is a subjective experience and may be more intense than you can appreciate. Pain after surgery is related to the surgical wound, tissue manipulation, drains, positioning during surgery, presence of an endotracheal tube, and the patient's experience with pain (Ward, 2014). In accordance with The Joint Commission's National Patient Safety Goals, assess the patient's discomfort and need for medication by considering the type, extent, and length of the surgical procedure. Assess for physical and emotional signs of acute pain, such as increased pulse and blood pressure, increased respiratory rate, profuse sweating, restlessness, confusion (in the older adult), wincing, moaning, and crying. When possible, ask the patient to rate the pain before and after drugs are given (e.g., on a scale of 0 to 10, with 0 being no pain and 10 being extreme pain). Plan the patient's activities around the timing of analgesia to improve mobility. Observe for a return of baseline physical and emotional behaviors. (See Chapter 3 for further discussion of pain assessment.)

PAIN assessment is started by the PACU nurse. After the patient is transferred from the PACU, the medical-surgical nurse continues to assess the patient's comfort level. Pain usually reaches its peak on the second day after surgery, when the

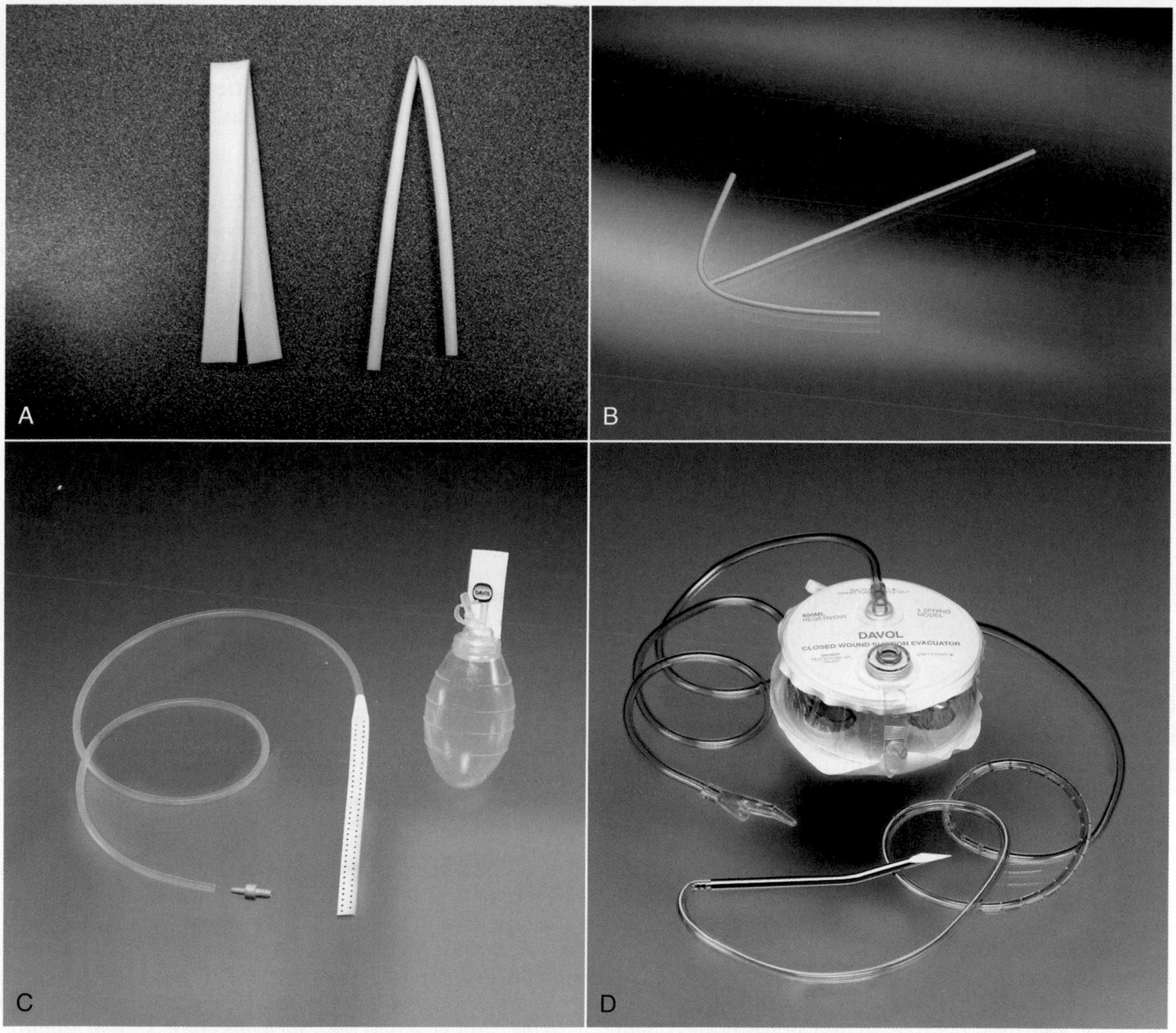

FIG. 16-3 Types of surgical drains. Gravity drains, such as the Penrose **(A)** and the T-tube **(B)** drain directly through a tube from the surgical area. In closed wound drainage systems, such as the Jackson-Pratt **(C)** and Hemovac **(D)**, drainage collects in a collecting vessel by means of compression and re-expansion of the system.

patient is more awake and more active and the anesthetic agents and drugs given during surgery have been excreted.

Psychosocial Assessment. Consider the psychological, social, and cultural issues of the patient after surgery as you provide physical care. This assessment may be delayed or difficult to perform in the PACU when the patient is drowsy or confused. Consider the patient's age and medical history, the surgical procedure, and the impact of surgery on recovery, body image, roles, and lifestyle.

Indications of anxiety include restlessness; increased pulse, blood pressure, and respiratory rate; and crying. The patient may be anxious and ask questions about the results or findings of the surgical procedure. Reassure the patient that the surgeon will speak with him or her after he or she is fully awake. If the surgeon has already spoken with the patient, reinforce what was said.

After the patient returns to the medical-surgical unit, continue the psychosocial assessment and also assess family members for psychological discomfort.

Laboratory Assessment. Laboratory tests are performed after surgery to monitor for complications. Tests are based on the surgical procedure, the patient's medical history, and clinical manifestations after surgery. Common tests include analysis of electrolytes and a complete blood count (see Chart 14-3 in Chapter 14). Changes in electrolyte, hematocrit, and hemoglobin levels often occur during the first 24 to 48 hours after surgery because of blood and fluid loss and the body's reaction to the surgical process. Fluid loss with minimal blood loss may cause elevated laboratory values. Such test results appear increased but actually are concentrated normal values.

An indication of INFECTION is an increase in the band cells (immature neutrophils) in the white blood cell differential count, known as a "left-shift" or *bandemia.* The source of infection may be the respiratory system, urinary tract, surgical wound, or IV site. Obtain specimens for culture and sensitivity testing, and monitor the culture reports at 24, 48, and 72 hours. Notify the surgeon of positive culture results. (See Chapters 17 and 23 for information on infection.)

Arterial blood gas (ABG) tests may be needed for patients who have respiratory or cardiac disease, those undergoing mechanical ventilation after surgery, and those who had chest surgery. Review ABG results, and notify the surgeon of any acid-base imbalance or hypoxemia that indicates poor GAS EXCHANGE. (For more discussion on arterial blood gases and acidosis, see Chapter 12.)

Urine and kidney laboratory tests also may be obtained (e.g., urinalysis, urine electrolyte levels, serum creatinine levels). Other laboratory tests depend on the diagnosis, type of surgical procedure, and other health problems. Examples are a serum amylase level for a patient who had pancreatic surgery and a blood glucose level for a patient with diabetes.

◆ Analysis

The priority NANDA-I nursing diagnoses and collaborative problems for patients after surgery include:

1. Potential for hypoxemia related to the effects of anesthesia, pain, opioid analgesics, and immobility
2. Potential for wound infection and delayed healing related to wound location, decreased mobility, drains and drainage, and tubes
3. Acute Pain related to the surgical incision, positioning during surgery, and endotracheal (ET) tube irritation (NANDA-I)

◆ Planning and Implementation

Preventing Hypoxemia

Planning: Expected Outcomes. The patient is expected to attain or maintain optimal lung expansion and breathing patterns after surgery as indicated by:

- Partial pressure of arterial oxygen (Pao_2) within normal range
- Partial pressure of arterial carbon dioxide ($Paco_2$) within normal range
- Oxygen saturation values within normal range

Interventions

Airway Maintenance. After assessing the airway and GAS EXCHANGE, you may need to insert an oral airway if the patient does not already have one. The oral airway pulls the tongue forward and holds it down to prevent obstruction. If the patient had oral surgery or has clenched teeth, a large tongue, or upper airway obstruction, insert a nasal airway (nasal trumpet) to keep the airway open. Keep the manual resuscitation bag and emergency equipment for intubation or tracheostomy nearby. For patients whose only airway is a tracheostomy or laryngectomy stoma, alert other staff members by posting signs in the room and notes on the chart.

Monitoring. Monitor the patient's oxygen saturation (Spo_2) for adequacy of GAS EXCHANGE with pulse oximetry at least every hour or more often, according to the patient's condition. Patients who normally have a low Pao_2, such as those with lung disease or older adults, are at higher risk for hypoxemia. An older adult is often prescribed low-dose oxygen therapy for the first 12 to 24 hours after surgery to reduce confusion from anesthesia and sedation (Sullivan, 2011). A patient who received moderate sedation with a benzodiazepine such as midazolam (Versed) or lorazepam (Ativan, Nu-Loraz ♣) may be overly sedated or have respiratory depression sufficient to need reversal with flumazenil (Romazicon) (Chart 16-4). Hypothermia after surgery causes shivering, which increases oxygen demand and can induce hypoxemia. Many rewarming methods can be used, although prevention is more important. The highest incidence of hypoxemia after surgery occurs on the second postoperative day.

CHART 16-4 Best Practice for Patient Safety & Quality Care QSEN

Emergency Care of the Patient Experiencing a Benzodiazepine Overdose

- Secure the airway and IV access before starting benzodiazepine antagonist therapy.
- Prepare to administer flumazenil (Romazicon)* in a dose of 0.2 mg to 1 mg IV.
- Repeat drug every 2 to 3 minutes up to 3 mg, as needed, depending on the patient's response.
- Give oxygen if hypoxia is present or if respirations are below 10 breaths per minute.
- Have suction equipment available because flumazenil can trigger vomiting and a drowsy patient is at risk for aspiration.
- Continuously monitor vital signs and level of consciousness for reversal of overdose.
- Do not leave the patient until he or she is fully responsive.
- Continue to monitor the patient's vital signs and level of consciousness every 10 to 15 minutes for the first 2 hours because flumazenil is eliminated from the body more quickly than is the benzodiazepine.
- Determine the need for additional flumazenil therapy 1 to 2 hours after the patient initially becomes fully responsive.
- Observe the patient for tremors or convulsions because flumazenil can lower the seizure threshold in patients who have seizure disorders.
- Assess the IV site every shift because flumazenil can cause thrombophlebitis at the injection site.
- Observe the patient for side effects of flumazenil, including skin rash, hot flushes, dizziness, headache, sweating, dry mouth, and blurred vision. The incidence of these side effects increases with higher total doses of flumazenil.

*There are other benzodiazepine antagonists; however, flumazenil is used most often to manage adult benzodiazepine overdose in the postoperative period.

Positioning. *In the PACU, immediately position the patient in a semi-Fowler's position unless contraindicated. If the patient cannot have the head of the bed raised, either place him or her in a side-lying position or turn the head to the side to prevent aspiration.*

Oxygen Therapy. Hypoxemia is prevented and managed with oxygen therapy. Apply oxygen by face tent, nasal cannula, or mask to eliminate inhaled anesthetic agents, increase oxygen levels, raise the level of consciousness, and reduce confusion. After the patient is fully reactive and stable, raise the head of the bed to promote respiratory function.

For some patients, oxygen therapy may continue through the second day after surgery. When hypoxemia occurs despite preventive care, interventions such as respiratory treatments and mechanical ventilation may be used to manage the cause of the hypoxemia.

Breathing Exercises. After the patient regains the gag and cough reflexes and meets the agency's criteria for extubation (if intubated), remove the airway or ET tube. Usual extubation criteria include the ability to raise and hold the head up and evidence of thoracic breathing. Help the patient splint the incision, cough, and deep breathe to promote GAS EXCHANGE and eliminate anesthetic agents. Chart 14-5 in Chapter 14 reviews breathing exercises and splinting of the surgical area. As soon as the patient is awake enough to follow commands, urge him or her to cough, use the incentive spirometer, and take deep breaths hourly while awake throughout the postoperative period. The patient who is unable to remove mucus or sputum requires oral or nasal suctioning. Perform mouth care after removing secretions.

Movement. Assist the patient out of bed and to ambulate as soon as possible to help remove secretions and promote ventilation. Even when the patient has had extensive surgery, the expectation may be to get out of bed the day of or the first day after surgery. If this is not possible, assist him or her to turn at least every 2 hours (side to side) and ensure that breathing exercises and leg exercises are performed (see Charts 14-5 and 14-6 in Chapter 14). Early ambulation reduces the risk for pulmonary complications, especially after abdominal, pelvic, or spinal surgery. It increases circulation to extremities and reduces the risk for CLOTTING and venous thromboembolism (VTE), especially deep vein thrombosis (DVT). The patient may resist getting up, but you must stress the importance of activity to prevent complications. When indicated, offer pain medication 30 to 45 minutes before he or she gets out of bed.

Preventing Wound Infection and Delayed Healing

Planning: Expected Outcomes. The patient is expected to have incision healing without wound complications as indicated by:

- Wound edges remaining together
- No purulent drainage, induration, or redness in, from, or around the incision

Interventions. Nursing assessment of the surgical area is critical (see the discussion of skin assessment on p. 263). Although most wound complications do not require additional surgical intervention, emergency surgical procedures may be needed.

Nonsurgical Management. Wound care includes reinforcing the dressing, changing the dressing, assessing the wound for healing and infection, and caring for drains, including emptying drainage containers/reservoirs, measuring drainage, and documenting drainage features. Emphasize the importance of early deep-breathing exercises to prevent forceful coughing. Urge the patient to bend the hips when in the supine position to reduce tension on a chest or abdominal wound. Remind him or her to always splint the chest or abdominal incision when coughing. Promote wound healing and protection of the skin, especially for the older patient (Sullivan, 2011). Chart 16-5 lists best practices for skin care of the older patient after surgery.

Dressings. The surgeon usually performs the first dressing change to assess the wound, remove any packing, and advance (pull partially out) or remove drains. Before the first dressing change, reinforce the dressing (add more dressing material to the existing dressing) if it becomes wet from drainage. Document the added material, as well as the color, type, amount, and odor of drainage fluid and time of observation. Assess the surgical site at least every shift, and report any unexpected findings to the surgeon.

After removal of the dressing, the surgeon may leave the suture or staple line open to the air, which allows easy assessment of the wound and early detection of poor wound edge adherence, drainage, swelling, or redness. Some surgeons believe that air-drying promotes healing. A draining wound, however, is always covered with a dressing.

Dressing changes are prescribed by the surgeon; however, the facility or unit may have standards or policies that dictate specific protocols for dressing changes and incision care. An unchanged wet or damp dressing is a source of INFECTION. Change dressings using aseptic technique until the sutures or staples are removed.

CHART 16-5 Nursing Focus on the Older Adult

Best Practice in Postoperative Skin Care

Improve perfusion to the wound to promote wound healing:
- Keep the patient adequately hydrated to maintain cardiac output.
- Keep the airway patent, and provide adequate oxygenation.
- Keep the patient's oxygen saturation on pulse oximetry at greater than 93%.

Conserve the patient's energy:
- Allow the patient to sleep in a darkened, quiet room.
- Administer drugs to combat pain and sleeplessness, as prescribed.
- Provide rest periods throughout the day.
- Control the patient's room temperature.
- Assist in ADLs.

Place the patient on a safety program to prevent falls, if indicated.

Use strict aseptic technique in caring for breaks in the integument (e.g., IV or other catheters, indwelling urethral catheter, wound).

Maintain the patient's psychosocial health:
- Prevent unnecessary stressors.
- Allow the patient liberal visitation of supportive others.
- Enable the patient to use individual successful coping mechanisms.
- Keep the patient well groomed and bathed.

Protect fragile skin:
- Minimize the use of tape on the skin.
- Use hypoallergenic tape or Montgomery straps.
- Change dressings as soon as they become wet.
- Lift the patient during transfer or repositioning.

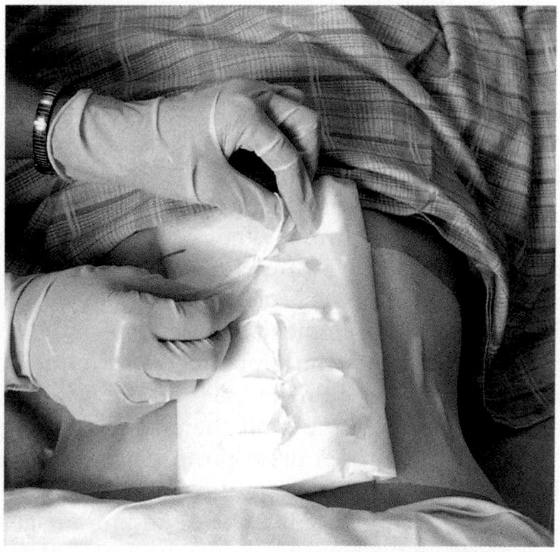

FIG. 16-4 Patient with a dressing held in place with Montgomery straps.

Dressings vary with the surgical procedure and the surgeon's preference. Common dressings for large incisions consist of gauze or nonadherent pads covered with a larger absorbent pad held in place by tape, a tubular stretchy net, or Montgomery straps (Fig. 16-4). Some incisions may be covered with a transparent plastic surgical dressing (e.g., OpSite) or a spray in the operating room. This type of dressing stays intact for 3 to 6 days, allows direct observation of the wound, prevents contamination, and eliminates the need for dressing changes.

Wound or suture line care consists of changing gauze dressings at least once during a nursing shift or daily and may include cleaning the area with sterile saline or some other solution. Some suture lines are left open to air without any dressing to cover the incision. The hospital's policy, the unit's standards, and the surgeon's preference determine what solution, if any, is used to clean the wound and how often dressings are changed. For large dressing changes or drain removal, offer the patient a prescribed analgesic before the procedure. Always assess the skin for redness, rash, or blisters in areas where tape has been used. Tape can cause a skin reaction after surgery even among patients who are not known to be tape sensitive.

Skin sutures or staples are usually removed 5 to 10 days after surgery, although this varies up to 30 days depending on the type of surgery and the patient's health. After sutures or staples are removed, the incision may then be secured with Steri-Strips, which stay in place until they fall off on their own. The surgeon or the nurse removes the sutures or staples, depending on the agency's policy. Clean the incision with the prescribed solution before removing sutures or staples. Before removing sutures, examine the condition and healing stage of the wound. First remove every other suture or staple and re-assess the wound for integrity. If wound healing is progressing normally, the rest of the sutures or staples may then be removed. If the wound does not appear to be healing well or if any manifestations of INFECTION are present, notify the surgeon before removing any sutures.

Drains. Drains (see Fig. 16-3) may be placed in the wound or through a separate small incision (known as a "stab" wound) close to the incision during surgery. Drains provide an exit route for air, blood, and bile. Drains also help prevent deep INFECTION and abscess formation during healing.

The Penrose drain is placed into the external aspect of the incision and drains directly onto the dressing and skin around the incision. Change a damp or soiled dressing, and carefully clean under and around the Penrose drain. Then place absorbent pads under and around the exposed drain to prevent skin irritation, wound contamination, and INFECTION. Whether sutured in place or not, the drain can be dislodged or pulled out accidentally during a dressing change. It is also possible for the drain to slip back through the wound into the patient. Usually this complication is prevented when the drain is first placed in the OR. The surgeon pins a sterile safety pin through the drain at an angle perpendicular to the drain and the wound, which prevents the drain from slipping. As the wound heals, the surgeon or nurse shortens (advances) the drain by pulling it out a short distance and trimming off the excess external portion so that only 2 to 3 inches of drain protrudes through the incision. The safety pin must be repositioned each time the drain is advanced. The drain remains in place until drainage stops.

Jackson-Pratt and Hemovac drains are two self-contained drainage systems that drain wounds directly through a tube via gravity and vacuum. These drains are sutured in place with a suture that seals the area when the drain is removed. Use sterile technique to empty the reservoir. Record the amount and color of drainage during every nursing shift or more often if prescribed. After emptying and compressing the reservoir to restore suction, secure the drain to the patient's gown (never to the sheet or mattress) to prevent pulling and stress on the surgical wound.

Drug Therapy. Wound INFECTION is a major complication after surgery. It usually results from contamination during surgery, preoperative infection, debilitation, or immunosuppression. In accordance with the Surgical Care Improvement Project (SCIP) core measures for prevention of surgical site infection, a patient at risk for wound infection may have received antibiotic therapy with drugs that are effective against organisms common to the specific surgical site both before and during surgery. The need for these antibiotics is re-evaluated at 24 hours after surgery. If manifestations of infection are not present, the antibiotic is discontinued at that time (SCIP Infection-3, see Table 14-1 in Chapter 14). If manifestations of wound infection are present, they are documented to justify continuation of antibiotic therapy.

Wounds that become infected and open are treated with dressing changes and systemic antibiotic therapy. Depending on the surgeon's prescription, irrigate the wound (e.g., with sterile saline, hydrogen peroxide, povidone-iodine, or acetic acid), loosely pack it with solution-soaked gauze (e.g., neomycin, gentamicin, iodoform, povidone-iodine, saline, or acetic acid), and cover the wound with dry, sterile dressings. These wet-to-damp dressing changes, done 1 to 3 times daily, promote healing from within the wound and **débridement** (removal of the infected or dead tissue) as the wound heals. Negative pressure wound care systems such as Wound VAC may be prescribed to help close the wound. Chapter 25 discusses these systems.

Surgical Management. Poorly healing wounds, infected wounds, or complicated wounds may require surgical intervention.

Management of Dehiscence. If dehiscence (wound opening) occurs, apply a sterile nonadherent (e.g., Telfa) or saline dressing to the wound and notify the surgeon. Instruct the patient to bend the knees and to avoid coughing. A wound that becomes infected dehisces by itself, or it may be opened by the surgeon through an incision and drainage (I&D) procedure. In either case, the wound is left open and is treated as described previously.

Management of Evisceration. An ***evisceration*** *(a wound opening with protrusion of internal organs) is a surgical emergency.* Chart 16-6 lists best practices for emergency care of the patient with surgical wound evisceration. Provide support by explaining what happened and reassuring the patient that the emergency will be handled competently.

! NURSING SAFETY PRIORITY QSEN

Critical Rescue

When a surgical wound evisceration occurs, one nurse tends to the patient while another nurse immediately notifies the surgeon.

The surgeon may prescribe a nasogastric (NG) tube to decompress the stomach and relieve internal pressure or to remove the stomach's contents if the patient has been eating and general anesthesia is needed. Prepare the patient for surgery (see Chapter 14) to close the wound. Regional or local anesthesia may be used, depending on the location and type of wound. Nausea and vomiting, which stress the already fragile incision, are reduced when regional or local anesthesia is used. To increase the incision's integrity, stay or retention sutures of wire or nylon are used along with standard sutures or staples (see Fig. 15-11 in Chapter 15).

Prevention. Patients also are at risk for developing pressure ulcers from positioning during surgery, from contact with damp surgical linens, and from unpadded surfaces. Pressure ulcers acquired during the surgical period prolong stays and increase the risk for complications. Early intervention of pressure ulcers can prevent progression and complications.

Examine the patient's skin for areas of redness or open areas. Document and report any abnormalities. Use padding and

CHART 16-6 Best Practice for Patient Safety & Quality Care QSEN

Emergency Care of the Patient with Surgical Wound Evisceration

1. Call for help! Instruct the person who responds to notify the surgeon or Rapid Response Team immediately and to bring any needed supplies into the patient's room.
2. Stay with the patient.
3. Cover the wound with a nonadherent dressing premoistened with warmed sterile normal saline. **NOTE:** The supplies needed for this emergency should be in the patient's room, especially if the patient is at high risk for dehiscence or evisceration.
4. If premoistened dressings are not available, moisten sterile gauze or sterile towels in a sterile irrigation tray with sterile saline and then cover the wound.
5. If saline is not immediately available, cover the wound with gauze and then moisten with sterile saline using a sterile irrigation tray as soon as someone brings saline.
6. Do not attempt to reinsert the protruding organ or viscera.
7. While covering the wound, note the patient's response and assess for manifestations of shock.
8. Place the patient in a supine position with the hips and knees bent.
9. Raise the head of the bed 15 to 20 degrees.
10. Take vital signs, and document them. **NOTE:** If the person who answered the call for help is back in the room before this, instruct him or her to take vital signs while you focus on covering the wound and repositioning the patient.
11. Provide support and reassurance to the patient.
12. Continue assessing the patient, including vital signs assessment, every 5 to 10 minutes until the surgeon arrives.
13. Keep dressings continuously moist by adding warmed sterile saline to the dressing as often as necessary. Do not let the dressing become dry.
14. When the surgeon arrives, report your finding and your interventions. Then follow the surgeon's directions.
15. Document the incident, the activity the patient was engaged in at the time of the incident, your actions, and your assessments.

positioning to relieve pressure. Treat any open areas according to facility guidelines and the surgeon's prescription. Ensure that information about the patient's skin condition in the PACU is communicated to the medical-surgical nurse. For patients at high risk, collaborate with a certified Wound, Ostomy, and Continence registered nurse (WOCRN) to plan preventive or interventional skin care.

Managing Pain

Planning: Expected Outcomes. The postoperative patient is expected to attain or maintain optimal comfort levels. Indicators include:

- Reporting that pain is controlled
- Absence of physiologic indicators of acute pain (increased heart rate and blood pressure)
- Absence of facial grimacing, teeth clenching
- Willingness to move and participate in self-care

Interventions. PAIN management after surgery includes drug therapy and other methods of management, such as positioning, massage, relaxation techniques, and diversion. Often the patient has better pain relief from a combination of approaches. Assess the patient's comfort level and the effectiveness of the therapies. See Chapter 3 for discussion of pain assessment and management. The patient who has optimal pain control is better able to cooperate with the therapies and exercises to prevent complications and promote rehabilitation.

Drug Therapy. *The use of opioids or other analgesics for pain management may mask or increase the severity of symptoms of an anesthesia reaction. Therefore give these drugs with caution, especially in the PACU when the patient's condition is not stable.* When pain drugs are used in the PACU, they are usually given IV in small doses. After receiving any drug for PAIN, the patient remains in the PACU for a defined period (often 45 to 60 minutes). Assess for hypotension, respiratory depression, and other side effects. Within 5 to 10 minutes after an IV injection, assess the effectiveness of the drug (i.e., on a rating scale) in relieving pain.

Opioid analgesics are given during the first 24 to 48 hours after surgery to control acute PAIN. Around-the-clock scheduling or the use of patient-controlled analgesia (PCA) systems is more effective than "on demand" scheduling because more constant blood levels are achieved. Drugs commonly used include morphine (Statex ♣), hydromorphone (Dilaudid), ketorolac (Toradol), codeine, butorphanol (Stadol), and oxycodone with aspirin (Percodan) or oxycodone with acetaminophen (Tylox, Percocet).

! NURSING SAFETY PRIORITY QSEN

Drug Alert

The usual dosage for hydromorphone is much smaller (about one-fifth to one-tenth) that of morphine.

Assess the type, location, and intensity of the pain before and after giving medication (see also Discomfort/Pain Assessment, p. 264). Monitor the patient's vital signs for hypotension and hypoventilation after giving opioid drugs. Chart 16-7 lists more information about analgesics used after surgery.

Patient-controlled analgesia (PCA) by IV infusion or internal pump (the catheter is sutured into or near the surgical area) and epidural analgesia are often used for better pain control. In PCA, the patient adjusts the dosage of the analgesic based on the pain level and response to the drug. This method allows more consistent pain relief and more control by the patient. The maximum dose per hour is "locked in" to the pump so that the patient cannot accidentally overdose. Common drugs used in PCA include morphine and hydromorphone.

Epidural analgesia can be given intermittently by the anesthesia provider or by continuous infusion through an epidural catheter left in place after epidural anesthesia. Drugs given by epidural catheter include the opioids *fentanyl (Sublimaze), preservative-free morphine (Duramorph),* and *bupivacaine (Marcaine).*

Take care not to overmedicate or undermedicate, especially with older patients. In assessing for overmedication, monitor vital signs, especially blood pressure and respiratory rate, and level of consciousness. Complications from the use of opioid analgesics include respiratory depression, hypotension, nausea, vomiting, and constipation. An opioid antagonist, such as naloxone (Narcan), may be needed to reverse the acute effects of opioid depression. Because of the short effect of the opioid antagonist, monitor the patient's blood pressure and respirations every 15 to 30 minutes until the full effect of the opioid analgesic has passed. You may need to give more doses of the antagonist during this time because it is eliminated from the body more quickly than is the opioid. (See Chart 16-8 for more information on using opioid antagonists to reverse opioid

CHART 16-7 Common Examples of Drug Therapy

Management of Postoperative Pain

DRUG	USUAL DOSAGE	NURSING INTERVENTIONS	RATIONALES
Morphine sulfate (Epimorph 🍁, Statex 🍁)	2-15 mg IM or IV incrementally 10-30 mg orally every 4 hr	Monitor respiratory status. Monitor blood pressure. Assess for GI motility and urine output.	Respiratory depression can be severe and require medical intervention. Hypotension, constipation, and urinary retention can occur.
Hydromorphone hydrochloride (Dilaudid)	1-4 mg IV or IM every 3-4 hr 2-4 mg orally every 3-4 hr	Monitor respirations. Monitor blood pressure. Monitor for food intolerance. Monitor fluid and electrolyte balance. Assess GI motility.	Respiratory depression, hypotension, anorexia, nausea, vomiting, and constipation can occur.
Codeine sulfate, codeine phosphate (Paveral 🍁)	15-60 mg IM or orally every 4 hr	Monitor respiratory status. Monitor for food intolerance. Monitor fluid and electrolyte balance. Assess GI motility.	Respiratory depression, nausea, and vomiting can occur. Constipation is common; prophylactic interventions may be indicated.
Butorphanol tartrate (Stadol)	1-4 mg IM every 3-4 hr 0.5-2 mg IV	Monitor neurologic status and changes in level of consciousness. Monitor respiratory status.	Butorphanol can cause increased intracranial pressure and respiratory depression.
Oxycodone hydrochloride and aspirin (Percodan, Endodan 🍁, Oxycodan 🍁)	1-2 tablets (5-10 mg) orally every 3-4 hr	Assess GI tolerance of medication. Assess for GI bleeding. Monitor GI motility. Monitor coagulation studies (PT, aPTT). Monitor respiratory status.	The aspirin component can irritate the stomach and could cause GI bleeding. Bleeding times and other coagulation study results may be increased because of the aspirin component. Respiratory depression and constipation can be caused by the oxycodone component.
Oxycodone hydrochloride and acetaminophen (Tylox, Percocet, Endocet 🍁, Oxycocet 🍁)	1-2 tablets (5-10 mg) orally every 3-4 hr	Monitor blood pressure and respiratory status. Assess for GI motility.	Respiratory depression, hypotension, and constipation can occur.
Ketorolac tromethamine (Toradol)	15-60 mg IM or IV every 6 hr	Monitor for GI bleeding. Monitor for kidney effects, especially in older adults.	GI bleeding, ulceration, and perforation can occur. Decreased urine output, increased serum creatinine, hematuria, and proteinuria can occur. Ketorolac is cleared more slowly in older adults. Older persons are more sensitive to the kidney effects of NSAIDs.
Ibuprofen (Motrin, Amersol 🍁, Novoprofen 🍁)	300-800 mg orally every 4-6 hr	Monitor upper GI tolerance of medication. Give with food or milk. Monitor coagulation studies (PT, aPTT). Assess for signs of bleeding or delayed clotting.	Food or milk helps decrease irritation of the stomach. Bleeding times and other coagulation study results may be increased. Monitoring leads to early detection of complications.

aPTT, Activated partial thromboplastin time; *GI,* gastrointestinal; *NSAID,* nonsteroidal anti-inflammatory drug; *PT,* prothrombin time.

overdose.) In addition, the patient has breakthrough PAIN after the opioid antagonist is given, so other interventions to promote comfort are needed.

Assess for undermedication by asking the patient about degree of PAIN relief and observing for other cues of discomfort (e.g., restlessness, increased confusion, "picking" at bedcovers). Offer prescribed drug(s) after checking for hypotension and respiratory depression.

As recovery progresses, reduce the doses and frequency of drugs for PAIN control. Drugs are changed from injectable or PCA to oral as soon as the patient can tolerate oral agents. Nonopioid analgesics, such as acetaminophen (Tylenol, Atasol 🍁), and NSAIDs, such as ibuprofen (Motrin, Novo-Profen 🍁) and ketorolac (Toradol), are used alone or with an opioid analgesic. Antianxiety drugs may be given with an opioid analgesic to decrease pain-related anxiety, reduce muscle tension, and control nausea.

! NURSING SAFETY PRIORITY QSEN

Drug Alert

Do not confuse Toradol with Tramadol (a drug used for central analgesia).

CHART 16-8 **Best Practice for Patient Safety & Quality Care** QSEN

Emergency Care of the Patient Experiencing an Opioid Overdose

- Prepare to administer naloxone hydrochloride (Narcan)* in a dose of 1 to 2 mg IV.
- Repeat naloxone every 2 to 3 minutes up to 10 mg, as needed, depending on the patient's response.
- Maintain an open airway.
- Give oxygen if hypoxia is present or if respirations are below 10 breaths per minute.
- Have suction equipment available because naloxone can trigger vomiting and a drowsy patient is at risk for aspiration.
- Continuously monitor vital signs and level of consciousness for reversal of overdose.
- Do not leave the patient until he or she is fully responsive.
- Assess the patient for pain because reversal of the opioid overdose also reverses the analgesic effects.
- Continue to monitor the patient's vital signs and level of consciousness every 10 to 15 minutes for the first hour. Naloxone is eliminated from the body more quickly than is the opioid, and it may induce side effects, including blood pressure changes, tachycardia, and dysrhythmias.
- Determine the need for additional antagonist therapy 1 hour after the patient initially becomes fully responsive.

*There are other opioid antagonists; however, naloxone hydrochloride is used most often to manage adult opioid overdose in the postoperative period.

Complementary and Alternative Therapies. Provide other comfort measures that may lower the amount of drugs needed to control PAIN. These measures, such as positioning, massage, relaxation, and diversion, reduce anxiety and allow the patient to relax and rest.

In positioning the patient, consider the position during surgery, the location of the surgical incision and drains, and problems such as arthritis and chronic lung disease. Assist the patient to a position of comfort. Support the extremities with pillows. Turn or help the patient turn at least every 2 hours while he or she is bedridden to prevent complications of immobility.

! NURSING SAFETY PRIORITY QSEN

Action Alert

Unless the surgeon prescribes pillow support, place no pillows under the knees, and do not raise the knee gatch, because this position could restrict circulation and increase the risk for venous thromboembolism.

Based on the surgeon's prescription and your assessment of the patient's tolerance, urge the patient to increase activity progressively to prevent complications. When he or she is first allowed out of bed, assist the patient to the side of the bed and into a chair. Teach him or her to splint the surgical wound for support and comfort during the transfer.

Use gentle massage on stiff joints or a sore back to decrease discomfort. Assist the patient to a side-lying position, and apply lotion with smooth, gentle strokes to increase blood flow to the area and promote relaxation. *Do not massage the calves because of the risk for loosening a clot and causing a life-threatening pulmonary embolus.*

CHART 16-9 **Best Practice for Patient Safety & Quality Care** QSEN

Nonpharmacologic Interventions to Reduce Postoperative Pain and Promote Comfort

- Control or remove noxious stimuli.
- Cushion and elevate painful areas; avoid tension or pressure on those areas.
- Provide adequate rest to increase pain tolerance.
- Encourage the patient's participation in diversional activities.
- Instruct the patient in relaxation techniques; use audio recordings or CDs and breathing exercises.
- Provide opportunities for meditation.
- Help the patient stimulate sensory nerve endings near the painful areas to inhibit ascending pain impulses.
- Use ice to reduce and prevent swelling, as indicated.
- Find a general position of comfort for the patient.
- Help the patient stimulate the area contralateral (opposite) to the painful area.

Relaxation and diversion are also used to control acute episodes of PAIN during dressing changes and injections. (See Chapter 3 for how to instruct and guide the patient through these pain control methods.) Music and noise reduction may help decrease awareness of discomfort. Chart 16-9 lists other interventions that may help reduce pain and promote comfort.

NCLEX EXAMINATION CHALLENGE

Psychosocial Integrity

The nurse is about to give the prescribed pain medication to a client 30 minutes before a scheduled dressing change. The client states that the drug makes him feel sick and he would rather "tough it out." What is the nurse's best first response?

A. "Tell me more about the sick feeling."
B. "That's fine. You have the right to refuse any drug."
C. "Your surgeon would not have prescribed the drug if it wasn't needed."
D. "Remember that the pain of the dressing change would be worse than feeling sick."

Community-Based Care

Many patients are discharged after a brief hospital stay or directly from the PACU to home. Because of the shortened length of hospital stays, discharge planning, teaching, and referral begin before surgery and continue after surgery.

Home Care Management. If the patient is discharged directly to home, assess information about the home environment for safety, patient accessibility, cleanliness, and availability of caregivers. Use the data obtained on admission before surgery to determine the patient's needs. For example, if the patient is unable or not allowed to climb stairs and lives in a two-story house with only one bathroom, advise the patient to rent a bedside commode. Collaborate with the social worker or discharge planner to identify needs related to care after surgery, including meal preparation, dressing changes, drain management, drug administration, equipment rental, physical therapy, and personal hygiene. A referral to a home care nursing agency may be indicated.

The patient is usually concerned about complications, PAIN, changes in the usual activity level, or payment of the hospital bill. The more extensive the surgical procedure is, the more fearful the patient is of assuming self-care. Support the patient and family members as they make discharge plans. The patient with visible scars after surgery may need more emotional support from and acceptance by his or her family. The patient may be angry about the surgical outcome or about role changes. He or she may be concerned about financial matters and work. The surgical outcome may not have met the patient's expectations, and further interventions may be needed to assist in resolving his or her feelings. Ensure that referrals are made for additional counseling as indicated.

Self-Management Education. The teaching plan for the patient and family after surgery includes:

- Prevention of infection
- Care and assessment of the surgical wound
- Management of drains or catheters
- Nutrition therapy
- Pain management
- Drug therapy
- Progressive increase in activity

If dressing changes and drain or catheter care are needed, instruct the patient and family members on the importance of proper handwashing to prevent infection. Explain and demonstrate wound care to the patient and family, who then perform a return demonstration. During teaching sessions, evaluate learning and promote adherence after discharge. At the same time, teach about the manifestations of complications such as wound INFECTION. Also instruct the patient and family about what to do if complications occur.

A diet high in protein, calories, and vitamin C promotes wound healing. Supplemental vitamin C, iron, zinc, and other vitamins are often prescribed after surgery to aid in wound healing and red blood cell formation. Instruct the patient who needs dietary restrictions about the importance of following the prescribed diet while recovering from surgery. Encourage the older adult or debilitated patient to continue using dietary supplements, if prescribed, between meals until the wound is completely healed and the energy levels are restored.

Teach the patient about drugs for PAIN, especially about the proper dosage and frequency. Instruct the patient to notify the surgeon if pain is not controlled or if the pain suddenly increases. If antibiotics or other drugs are prescribed, stress the importance of completing the entire prescription.

Surgery stresses the body, and time and rest are needed for healing. Teach the patient to increase activity level slowly, rest often, and avoid straining the wound or the surrounding area. The surgeon decides when the patient may climb stairs, return to work, drive, and resume other usual activities, such as sexual intercourse. The amount of weight that the patient can lift safely after surgery is specifically defined by the surgeon (i.e., in pounds or kilograms). Remind patients of the weights of grocery bags, women's handbags, and common items in the home.

Instruct the patient in the use of proper body mechanics. A patient whose work involves a moderate amount of physical labor may return to work about 6 weeks after abdominal surgery. Stress the importance of adherence to prevent complications or disability. A referral for a home care nurse may be needed for follow-up.

! NURSING SAFETY PRIORITY (QSEN)

Action Alert

Always ensure that the patient and family receive written discharge instructions to follow at home. Assess the patient's and family's understanding of the instructions by having them explain the instructions in their own words.

Health Care Resources. After returning home, the patient may need supplies or equipment and assistance with dressing changes, ADLs, and meal preparation. Referral to a home care agency is made if needed. Home care may be paid for by third-party insurance payers, including Medicare, if the patient is homebound and requires skilled care such as dressing changes or physical therapy. The home care nurse provides skilled nursing assessments, dressing supplies, education in self-care, and referrals for services as needed. Such referrals include Meals on Wheels, support groups, and homemaker services (e.g., for housekeeping, food shopping).

◆ Evaluation: Outcomes

Evaluate the care of the patient after surgery based on the identified priority patient problems. The expected outcomes include that the patient:

- Attains and maintains adequate lung expansion and respiratory function
- Has complete wound healing without complications
- Has acceptable comfort levels after surgery

Specific indicators for these outcomes are listed for each priority patient problem in the Planning and Implementation section (see earlier).

NURSING CONCEPTS AND CLINICAL JUDGMENT REVIEW

What might you NOTICE in a patient after surgery who has a surgical wound INFECTION?

- Elevated body temperature
- Heart rate elevated above the patient's baseline
- Sweating and chills present
- Wound edges are red for 1 cm or more on each side of the wound
- Incision line is swollen, and skin adjacent to the incision is warmer to the touch than is the skin further away from the incision
- Purulent drainage is present
- An odor may emanate from the incision
- An open area or areas may be present within the incision

What should you INTERPRET and how should you RESPOND to a patient who has a wound INFECTION after surgery?

Perform and interpret physical assessment, including:

- Assessing vital signs with temperature at least every 4 hours
- Assessing for increase in pain perception
- Assessing cognition
- Assessing the wound for pain, size, open areas, and drainage

- Assessing the skin immediately surrounding the wound for redness and swelling
- Assessing serial white blood cell counts with differential for changes, including elevations above normal, decreases below normal, and presence of a "left shift"

Respond by:
- Documenting wound features
- Notifying the surgeon or health care provider
- Cleansing the wound (obtaining cultures, if within agency policy)
- Maintaining or starting IV line
- Administering prescribed drug therapy
- Monitoring laboratory test results to determine therapy effectiveness
- Continuing to assess for changes in the patient's condition, especially indications of infection in any other body area.

On what should you REFLECT?
- Identify the patient's personal factors that could have contributed to the wound infection.
- Think about what steps could be taken to identify the problem earlier.

GET READY FOR THE NCLEX® EXAMINATION!

KEY POINTS

Review these Key Points for each NCLEX Examination Client Needs Category.

Safe and Effective Care Environment
- Examine individual patient factors for potential threats to safety, especially risk for surgical site INFECTION, hypoventilation, and venous thromboembolism. **Safety** QSEN
- Use aseptic technique during all dressing changes. **Safety** QSEN
- Use established criteria to determine when a patient is ready to leave the postanesthesia care unit (PACU) for discharge to home or a medical-surgical nursing unit.
- Keep suction equipment, oxygen, and artificial breathing equipment near the patient in the PACU. **Safety** QSEN

Health Promotion and Maintenance
- Reinforce to the patient and family after surgery the specific interventions to use to prevent complications (incision splinting, deep-breathing exercises, range-of-motion exercises—as described in Charts 14-5 and 14-6 in Chapter 14).
- Encourage early ambulation.
- Stress the need for following the activity restrictions prescribed by the surgeon.
- Teach the patient and family about any drugs to be continued after discharge from the facility. **Patient-Centered Care** QSEN
- Instruct the patient and family about the clinical manifestations of complications and when to seek assistance. **Patient-Centered Care** QSEN

Psychosocial Integrity
- Keep family members informed of the patient's progress during the time that he or she is in the postanesthesia recovery area.
- Reassure patients and family members that taking pain medication when needed, even opioids, does not make them drug abusers. **Patient-Centered Care** QSEN

Physiological Integrity
- Begin every assessment of the patient after surgery by checking the airway and breathing effectiveness. **Safety** QSEN
- Assess the incision site each shift (on the medical-surgical nursing unit).
- Offer alternative therapies for relaxation, pain reduction, and distraction, such as massage, music therapy, and guided imagery.
- In the event of wound dehiscence or evisceration, have the patient lie flat (supine) with knees bent to reduce intra-abdominal pressure; apply sterile, nonadherent dressing materials to the wound; and follow the steps outlined in Chart 16-6. **Evidence-Based Practice** QSEN

CONCEPT OVERVIEW

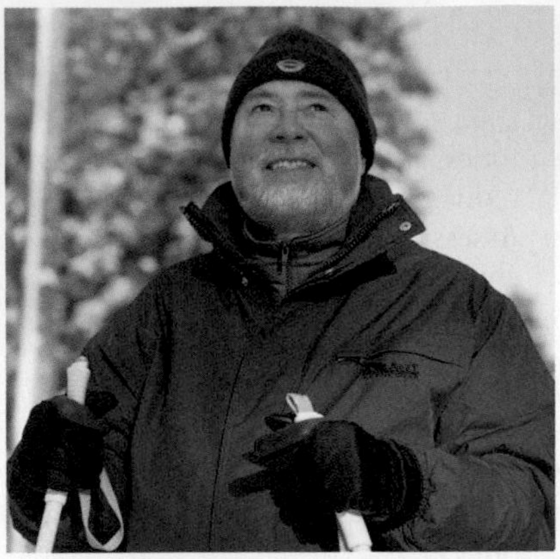

Protection

The human need for protection is provided through the actions of the concepts of INFLAMMATION and IMMUNITY (Giddens, 2013). The body works best when the internal environment is kept separate from the external environment. This is especially important for substances and organisms that could harm body cells, tissues, and organs. Normal protection is provided by three types of defenses—similar to how people living in a castle are protected against invaders (Fig. 1).

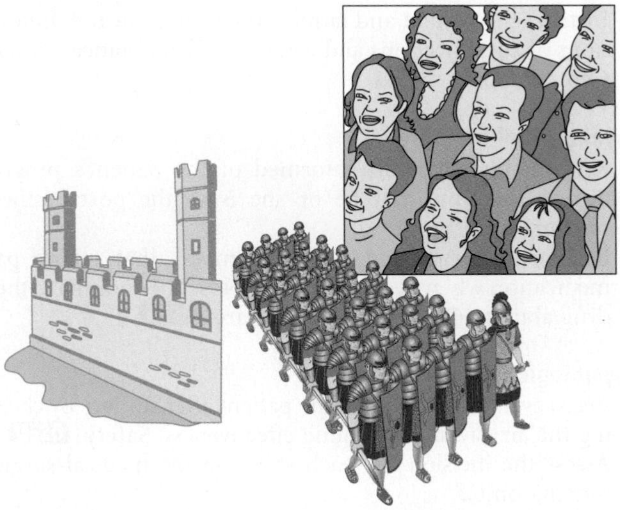

FIG. 1 Three levels of protection (moat, castle wall, knights and soldiers) for people.

The first defense is the moat surrounding the castle walls. Although the moat seldom kills invaders directly, it at least slows them down and sometimes repels them. The human "moat" is the normal flora on the surface of the skin and mucous membranes, sometimes referred to as types of general or innate IMMUNITY. This normal flora is made up of bacteria and other organisms that belong on the skin, live peacefully with the human host, and help repel more harmful microorganisms. When the normal flora is changed as a result of some types of drug therapy, procedures, diseases, excessive dryness, and normal aging, this small protection is damaged or lost.

The second defense is the castle wall and the "watchers" and alarm systems embedded within it. When it is tall, thick, and intact and when the watchers and alarms are working, penetration of the castle by invaders is greatly reduced. In humans, this type of protection is provided by intact skin and mucous membranes, which are also part of innate IMMUNITY. These structures are a formidable barrier to invaders and help prevent dangerous changes in the internal environment. However, the castle walls do suffer some damage over time and must be repaired and maintained to provide continuing protection.

The last and strongest defense consists of the knights and soldiers within the castle. These individuals have the skills to capture or kill invaders. Some of these skills are common to all the knights and soldiers, and others are unique to different groups. In humans, the white blood cells (leukocytes) and the substances they produce serve as knights and soldiers, which provide the responses of INFLAMMATION and IMMUNITY. In addition to the work related directly to the invaders, this defense helps repair and maintain the castle walls. It is important to remember that this level of protection relies on the alarms of the castle wall and its physical barrier to recognize invaders and trigger the protective responses of the knights and soldiers.

Protection occurs best when all three defenses are intact and are working at their highest functional levels. These defenses of INFLAMMATION and IMMUNITY begin at birth and are at the maximum function in early to middle adulthood. The defenses decline slowly over time, making an older adult at greater risk for illnesses related to invasion and a decreased ability to repair damage. External factors and health status can reduce the ability of INFLAMMATION and IMMUNITY to provide complete protection. Specific nursing strategies can help reduce risk and protect the person whose defenses are less than perfect.

CHAPTER 17

Inflammation and Immunity

M. Linda Workman

http://evolve.elsevier.com/Iggy/

PRIORITY CONCEPTS

- INFLAMMATION
- IMMUNITY

LEARNING OUTCOMES

Physiological Integrity

1. Describe the concept of self-tolerance.
2. Explain the differences between INFLAMMATION and IMMUNITY in terms of cells, functions, and features.
3. Discuss the influences of the aging process on INFLAMMATION and IMMUNITY and how these changes increase health risks for older adults.
4. Interpret laboratory data to assess a patient's immune status and risk for infection.
5. Differentiate the protection provided by active IMMUNITY, passive IMMUNITY, and cell-mediated IMMUNITY.
6. Describe the expected immune system responses to the presence of transplanted organs and the need for drug therapy to prevent transplant rejection.

The immune system involves the concepts of both INFLAMMATION and IMMUNITY to work with other defenses in providing *protection* from harmful microorganisms and cells. As indicated in the Concept Overview defining the issue of *protection* using the concepts of inflammation and immunity, the cells and cell products of inflammation and immunity are represented mostly by the knights and soldiers behind the castle walls. The products made by cells (e.g., cytokines, growth factors, antibodies) are the weapons of the knights and soldiers. Some of these cells serve as watchers and alarm systems within the castle walls (skin and mucous membranes) and help repair these walls when damage occurs.

Although infectious diseases are common, most people are healthy more often than they are ill. INFLAMMATION and IMMUNITY are the major defenses that protect against disease when the body is invaded by organisms. These same defenses also help the body recover after tissue damage. Thus inflammation and immunity are critical to maintaining health and preventing disease. When all the different parts and functions of inflammation and immunity are working well, the person is **immunocompetent** and has maximum protection against infection.

IMMUNITY is reduced by many diseases, injuries, and medical therapies. *Whether immunity is reduced temporarily or permanently, it always endangers the patient's health.* Chapter 19 discusses inadequate immunity and inflammatory responses. Other problems occur when immunity and inflammation are excessive or occur at inappropriate times. Chapters 18 and 20 discuss issues related to excess or inappropriate inflammatory or immune responses.

OVERVIEW

IMMUNITY is composed of many cell functions that protect against the effects of injury or invasion. People interact with many other large and small living organisms (bacteria, viruses, molds, spores, pollens, protozoa, and cells from other people or animals). As long as organisms do not enter the body, they pose no health threat. Body defenses to prevent organisms from entering include intact skin and mucous membranes, skin surface normal flora, and natural chemicals that inhibit bacterial growth. These defenses are not perfect, and invasion can occur. However, most invasions do not result in disease or illness because of proper immunity.

The purpose of INFLAMMATION and IMMUNITY is to provide *protection* by neutralizing, eliminating, or destroying organisms that invade the body. To protect without harming the body,

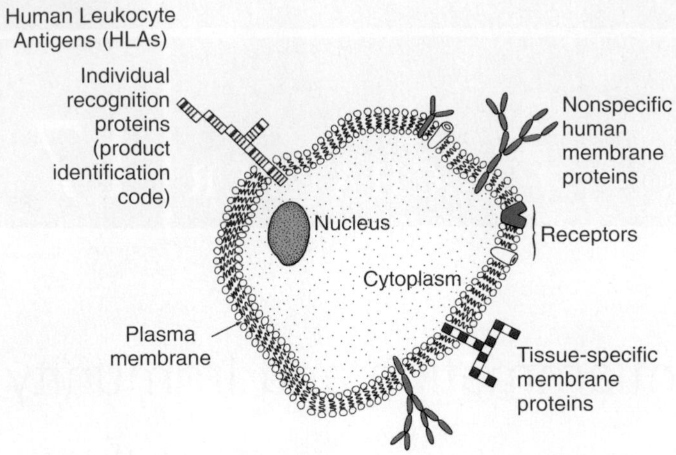

FIG. 17-1 Proteins on human cell plasma membranes.

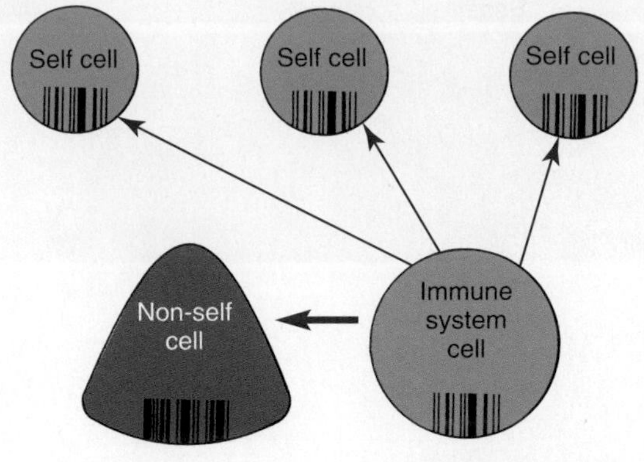

FIG. 17-2 Determination by immune system cell of self versus non-self cells.

immune system cells exert these actions only against non-self proteins and cells. Immune system cells can distinguish between the body's own healthy self cells and non-self proteins and cells.

Self Versus Non-Self

Non-self proteins and cells include infected body cells, cancer cells, cells from other people, and invading organisms. Recognizing self versus non-self, which is necessary to prevent healthy body cells from being destroyed along with the invaders, is called **self-tolerance**. The immune system cells are the only cells capable of determining self from non-self. Self-tolerance is possible because of the different proteins present on cell membranes.

Each cell is surrounded by a plasma membrane with different proteins protruding through the surface (Fig. 17-1). For example, in liver cells, many different protein types are present on the liver cell membranes. The amino acid sequence of each protein type differs from that of all other protein types. Some of these protein types are found only on human cells, because these protein types are specific markers for human tissues. Also, each person's cells have surface proteins that are specific to that person. These unique proteins would be identical only to the proteins of an identical sibling. These unique proteins, known as **human leukocyte antigens (HLAs)**, are found on the surface of all body cells of that person and serve as a "universal product code" for that person. One person's HLAs are recognized as "foreign," or non-self, by the immune system of another person. Because the cell-surface proteins are non-self to another person's immune system, they are **antigens**, which are proteins capable of stimulating an immune response.

Human leukocyte antigens are on the surfaces of most body cells—not just leukocytes. They are a normal part of the person and determine the *tissue type* of a person. Other names for these HLAs are *human histocompatibility antigens* and *class I antigens.*

There are many different human major HLAs that are determined by a set of genes called the *major histocompatibility complex (MHC)*. However, each human expresses only six of the major HLAs. The specific antigens that any person has (of a large number of possible antigens) are determined by which MHC gene alleles were inherited from his or her parents.

The HLAs are key for recognition and self-tolerance. The immune system cells constantly come into contact with other body cells and with any invader that enters the body. At each encounter, the immune system cells compare the surface protein HLAs to determine whether the encountered cell belongs in the body (Fig. 17-2). If the encountered cell's HLAs perfectly match the HLAs of the immune system cell, the encountered cell is "self" and is not attacked. If the encountered cell's HLAs do not perfectly match the HLAs of the immune system cell, the encountered cell is non-self, or foreign. The immune system cell then takes action to neutralize, destroy, or eliminate this foreign invader.

IMMUNITY changes during a person's life as a result of nutrition status, environmental conditions, drugs, disease, and age. Immunity is most efficient when people are in their 20s and 30s and slowly declines with increasing age (Touhy & Jett, 2014). Older adults have decreased immune function, increasing their risk for many health problems (Chart 17-1).

Organization of the Immune System

The immune system is present throughout the body and is influenced by the nervous system, the endocrine system, and the GI system. Most immune system cells come from the bone marrow. Some cells mature in the bone marrow; others leave the bone marrow and mature in different body sites. When mature, many immune system cells are released into the blood, where they circulate to most body areas and have specific effects.

The bone marrow is the source of all blood cells, including most immune system cells. The bone marrow produces immature, undifferentiated cells called **stem cells**. Stem cells are **pluripotent**, meaning that each cell has more than one potential outcome. When the stem cell is first generated in the bone marrow, it is undifferentiated, not yet committed to maturing into a specific blood cell type. This stem cell is flexible (pluripotent) and could become any one of many mature blood cells. Fig. 17-3 shows the possible outcomes for maturation of stem cells. The type of mature cell that the stem cell becomes depends on which pathway it follows.

The maturational pathway of any stem cell depends on body needs and on the presence of specific growth factors that direct the cell to a pathway. For example, erythropoietin is a growth factor for red blood cells (**erythrocytes [RBCs]**). When immature stem cells are exposed to erythropoietin, they commit to the erythrocyte pathway and eventually become mature RBCs.

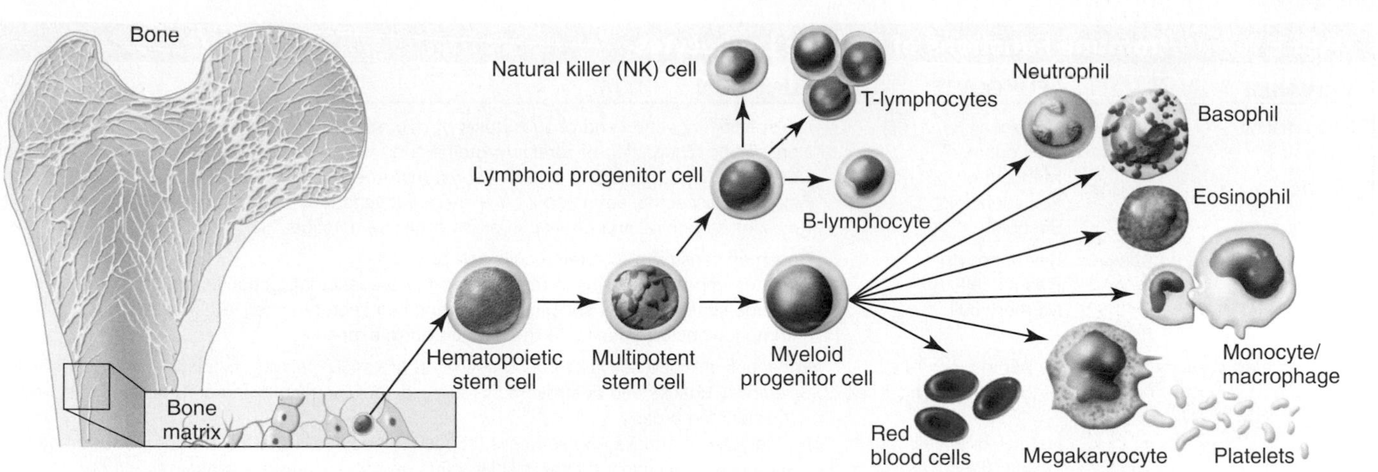

FIG. 17-3 Stem cell differentiation and maturation.

CHART 17-1 **Nursing Focus on the Older Adult**

Changes in Immune Function Related to Aging

IMMUNE COMPONENT	FUNCTIONAL CHANGE	NURSING IMPLICATIONS
Inflammation	Reduced neutrophil function.	Neutrophil counts may be normal, but activity is reduced, increasing the risk for infection.
	Leukocytosis does not occur during acute infection.	Patients may have an infection but not show expected changes in white blood cell counts.
	Older adults may not have a fever during inflammatory or infectious episodes.	Not only is there potential loss of protection through inflammation, but also minor infections may be overlooked until the patient becomes severely infected or septic.
Antibody-mediated immunity	The total number of colony-forming B-lymphocytes and the ability of these cells to mature into antibody-secreting cells are diminished.	Older adults are less able to make new antibodies in response to the presence of new antigens. Thus they should receive immunizations, such as "flu shots," the pneumococcal vaccination, and the shingles vaccination.
	There is a decline in natural antibodies, decreased response to antigens, and reduction in the amount of time the antibody response is maintained.	Older adults may not have sufficient antibodies present to provide protection when they are re-exposed to microorganisms against which they have already generated antibodies. Thus older patients need to avoid people with viral infections and need to receive "booster" shots for old vaccinations and immunizations, especially tetanus and pertussis (whooping cough).
Cell-mediated immunity	The number of circulating T-lymphocytes decreases.	Skin tests for tuberculosis may be falsely negative.
		Older patients are more at risk for bacterial and fungal infections, especially on the skin and mucous membranes, in the respiratory tract, and in the genitourinary tract.

White blood cells (**leukocytes** [**WBCs**]) protect the body from the effects of invasion by organisms. These cells are the immune system cells, the knights and soldiers protecting the castle inhabitants after invaders get through the castle wall. Table 17-1 lists the functions of different immune system cells. The leukocytes provide protection through these defensive actions:

- Recognition of self versus non-self
- Destruction of foreign invaders, cellular debris, and unhealthy or abnormal self cells
- Production of antibodies directed against invaders
- Complement activation
- Production of cytokines that stimulate increased formation of leukocytes in bone marrow and increase specific leukocyte activity

The three processes needed for human protection through IMMUNITY are (1) INFLAMMATION, (2) antibody-mediated immunity (AMI), and (3) cell-mediated immunity (CMI). Each process uses different defensive actions, and each influences or requires assistance from the other two processes (Fig. 17-4). *Therefore full immunity (immunocompetence) requires the function and interaction of all three processes.*

INFLAMMATION

INFLAMMATION, also called *innate-native immunity* or *natural immunity,* provides immediate protection against the effects of tissue injury and invading foreign proteins. Innate-native immunity is any natural protective feature of a person. It can be a barrier to prevent organisms from entering the body or can be an attacking force that eliminates organisms that have already entered the body. This type of IMMUNITY cannot be transferred from one person to another and is not an adaptive response to exposure or invasion by foreign proteins.

TABLE 17-1 Immune Functions of Specific Leukocytes

VARIABLE	LEUKOCYTE	FUNCTION
Inflammation	Neutrophil	Nonspecific ingestion and phagocytosis of microorganisms and foreign protein
	Macrophage	Nonspecific recognition of foreign proteins and microorganisms; ingestion and phagocytosis
	Monocyte	Destruction of bacteria and cellular debris; matures into macrophage
	Eosinophil	Releases vasoactive amines during allergic reactions to limit these reactions
	Basophil	Releases histamine and heparin in areas of tissue damage
Antibody-mediated immunity	B-lymphocyte	Becomes sensitized to foreign cells and proteins
	Plasma cell	Secretes immunoglobulins in response to the presence of a specific antigen
	Memory cell	Remains sensitized to a specific antigen and can secrete increased amounts of immunoglobulins specific to the antigen on re-exposure
Cell-mediated immunity	Helper/inducer T-cell	Enhances immune activity through secretion of various factors, cytokines, and lymphokines
	Cytotoxic/cytolytic T-cell	Selectively attacks and destroys non-self cells, including virally infected cells, grafts, and transplanted organs
	Natural killer cell	Nonselectively attacks non-self cells, especially body cells that have undergone mutation and become malignant; also attacks grafts and transplanted organs

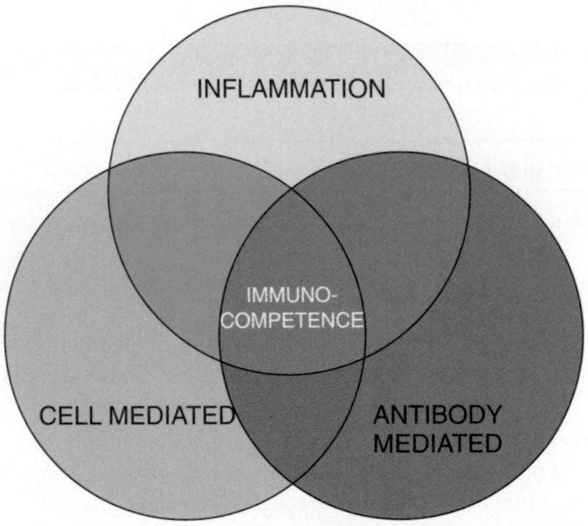

FIG. 17-4 The three divisions of immunity: inflammation, antibody-mediated immunity, and cell-mediated immunity. Optimal function of all three divisions is necessary for complete immunity.

The inflammatory responses are part of innate IMMUNITY. Other parts of innate immunity include skin, mucosa, antimicrobial chemicals on the skin, complement, and natural killer cells.

The ability to respond with inflammation is critical to health and well-being. INFLAMMATION differs from AMI and CMI in two important ways:

- Inflammatory protection is immediate but short-term. It does not provide true immunity on repeated exposure to the same organisms.
- Inflammation is a *nonspecific* body defense to invasion or injury and can be started quickly by almost any event, regardless of where it occurs or what causes it.

So, inflammation triggered by a scald burn to the hand is the same as inflammation triggered by bacteria in the middle ear. How widespread the manifestations of INFLAMMATION are depends on the intensity, severity, and duration of exposure to the initiating event. For example, a splinter in the finger triggers inflammation only at the splinter site, whereas a burn injuring 50% of the skin leads to an inflammatory response involving the entire body.

INFLAMMATION starts tissue actions that cause visible and uncomfortable manifestations that are important in ridding the body of harmful organisms. However, if the inflammatory response is excessive, tissue damage may result. Inflammation also helps start both antibody-mediated and cell-mediated actions to activate full IMMUNITY.

Infection

A confusing issue about INFLAMMATION is that this process occurs in response to tissue injury, as well as to infection by organisms. *Infection is usually accompanied by inflammation; however, inflammation can occur without infection.* Examples of inflammation without infection include joint sprain injuries, myocardial infarction, and blister formation. Examples of inflammation caused by noninfectious invasion include allergic rhinitis, contact dermatitis, and other allergic reactions. Inflammations from infection include otitis media, appendicitis, and viral hepatitis, among many others. *Inflammation does not always mean that an infection is present.*

Cell Types Involved in Inflammation

The leukocytes (white blood cells [WBCs]) involved in INFLAMMATION are neutrophils, macrophages, eosinophils, and basophils. An additional cell type important in inflammation is the tissue mast cell. Neutrophils and macrophages destroy and eliminate foreign invaders. Basophils, eosinophils, and mast cells release chemicals that act on blood vessels to cause tissue-level responses that help neutrophil and macrophage actions.

Neutrophils

Mature neutrophils make up between 55% and 70% of the normal total WBC count. Neutrophils come from the stem cells and complete the maturation process in the bone marrow (Fig. 17-5). They are also called *granulocytes* because of the large number of granules present inside each cell. Other names for neutrophils are based on their appearance and maturity. Mature neutrophils are also called *segmented neutrophils* ("segs") or *polymorphonuclear cells* ("polys," PMNs) because of their segmented nucleus. Less mature neutrophils are called *band neutrophils* ("bands" or "stabs") because of their nuclear shape.

Usually, growth of a stem cell into a mature neutrophil requires 12 to 14 days. This time is shortened by the presence of specific growth factors (cytokines), such as granulocyte-macrophage colony-stimulating factor (GM-CSF) and granulocyte colony-stimulating factor (G-CSF). The purpose and action of cytokines are described on p. 286 in the Cytokines section.

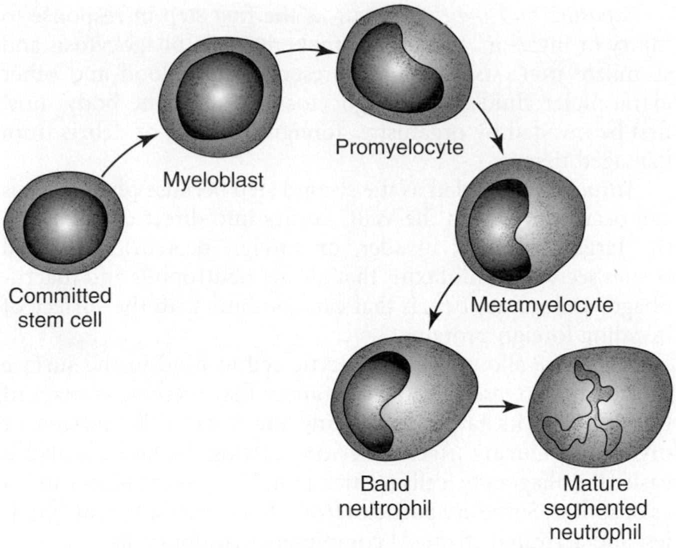

FIG. 17-5 Stem cell maturation into fully functional segmented neutrophils.

TABLE 17-2 Values of a White Blood Cell Differential for Peripheral Blood Representing a Normal Count

WBC TYPE	%	/MM³
Total WBC	**100**	**10,000**
Segs	62	6200
Bands	5	500
Monos	3	300
Lymphs	28	2800
Eosins	1.5	150
Basos	0.5	50

WBC, White blood cell.

In the healthy person with full IMMUNITY, more than 100 billion fresh, mature neutrophils are released from the bone marrow into the circulation daily. This huge production is needed because the life span of each neutrophil is short—about 12 to 18 hours.

Neutrophil function provides protection after invaders, especially bacteria, enter the body. This powerful army of small cells destroys invaders by phagocytosis and enzymatic digestion, although each cell is small and can take part in only one episode of phagocytosis.

Mature neutrophils are the only stage of this cell capable of phagocytosis. Because this cell type is responsible for continuous, instant, nonspecific protection against organisms, the percentage and actual number of mature circulating neutrophils are used to measure a patient's risk for infection: the higher the numbers, the greater the resistance to infection. This measurement is the **absolute neutrophil count (ANC)**, also called the *absolute granulocyte count* or *total granulocyte count.*

The differential of a normal white blood cell count shows the number and percent of the different types of circulating leukocytes (Table 17-2). Usually, most neutrophils released into the blood from the bone marrow are segmented neutrophils; only a small percentage are band neutrophils or other less mature forms. Some problems, such as sepsis, cause the neutrophils in the blood to change from being mostly segmented neutrophils to being less mature forms. This situation is termed a **left shift** or *bandemia* because the segmented neutrophil (at the far right of the neutrophil pathway in Fig. 17-5) is no longer the most numerous type of circulating neutrophils. Instead, more of the circulating cells are bands—the less mature cell type found farther left on the neutrophil pathway.

A left shift indicates that the patient's bone marrow cannot produce enough mature neutrophils to keep pace with the continuing infection and is releasing immature neutrophils into the blood. These immature cells are of no benefit because they are not capable of phagocytosis.

TABLE 17-3 Tissue Macrophages

TISSUE	MACROPHAGE
Lung	Alveolar macrophage
Connective tissue	Histiocyte
Brain	Microglial cell
Liver	Kupffer cell
Peritoneum	Peritoneal macrophage
Bone	Osteoclast
Joint	Synovial type A cell
Kidney	Mesangial cell

Macrophages

Macrophages come from the committed myeloid stem cells in the bone marrow and form the mononuclear-phagocyte system. The stem cells first form monocytes, which are released into the blood at this stage. Until they mature, monocytes have limited activity. Most monocytes move from the blood into body tissues, where they mature into macrophages. Some macrophages become "fixed" in position within the tissues, whereas others can move within and between tissues. Macrophages in various tissues have slightly different appearances and names (Table 17-3). The liver, spleen, and intestinal tract contain large numbers of these cells.

Macrophage function protects the body in several ways. These cells are important in immediate inflammatory responses and also stimulate the longer-lasting immune responses of antibody-mediated IMMUNITY (AMI) and cell-mediated IMMUNITY (CMI). Macrophage functions include phagocytosis, repair, antigen presenting/processing, and secretion of cytokines for immune system control.

The inflammatory function of macrophages is phagocytosis. Macrophages can easily distinguish between self and non-self, and their large size makes them very effective at trapping invading cells. They have long life spans and can take part in many phagocytic events.

Basophils

Basophils come from myeloid stem cells and make up only about 1% of the total circulating WBC count. These cells cause the manifestations of INFLAMMATION.

Basophil function acts on blood vessels with basophil chemicals (vasoactive amines), which include heparin, histamine, serotonin, kinins, and leukotrienes. Basophils have sites that bind the base portion of immunoglobulin E (IgE) molecules, which binds to and is activated by allergens. When allergens bind to the IgE on the basophil, the basophil membrane opens and releases the vasoactive amines into the blood, where most of them act on smooth muscle and blood vessel walls. Heparin inhibits blood and protein clotting. Histamine constricts small veins, inhibiting blood flow and decreasing venous return. This effect causes blood to collect in capillaries and arterioles. Kinins dilate arterioles and increase capillary permeability. These actions cause blood plasma to leak into the interstitial space *(vascular leak syndrome)*. Thus basophils stimulate both general INFLAMMATION and the inflammation of allergy and hypersensitivity reactions.

Eosinophils

Eosinophils come from the myeloid line and contain many vasoactive chemicals. Only 1% to 2% of the total WBC count normally is composed of eosinophils.

Eosinophil function is very active against infestations of parasitic larvae and also limits inflammatory reactions. The eosinophil granules contain many different substances. Some are enzymes that degrade the vasoactive chemicals released by other leukocytes. This is why the number of circulating eosinophils increases during an allergic response.

Tissue Mast Cells

Tissue mast cells look like and have functions very similar to basophils and eosinophils. Although mast cells do originate in the bone marrow, they come from a different parent cell than leukocytes and do not circulate as mature cells (Abbas et al., 2012). Instead, they differentiate and mature in tissues, especially those near blood vessels, nerves, lung tissue, skin, and mucous membranes. Like basophils, mast cells have binding sites for the base of IgE molecules and are involved in hypersensitivity reactions. Some mast cells also respond to the inflammatory products made and released by T-lymphocytes. The tissue mast cells have important roles in maintaining and prolonging inflammatory and hypersensitivity reactions.

Phagocytosis

A key process of INFLAMMATION is **phagocytosis**, the engulfing and destruction of invaders, which also rids the body of debris after tissue injury. Neutrophils and macrophages are most efficient at phagocytosis. Phagocytosis involves the seven steps shown in Fig. 17-6.

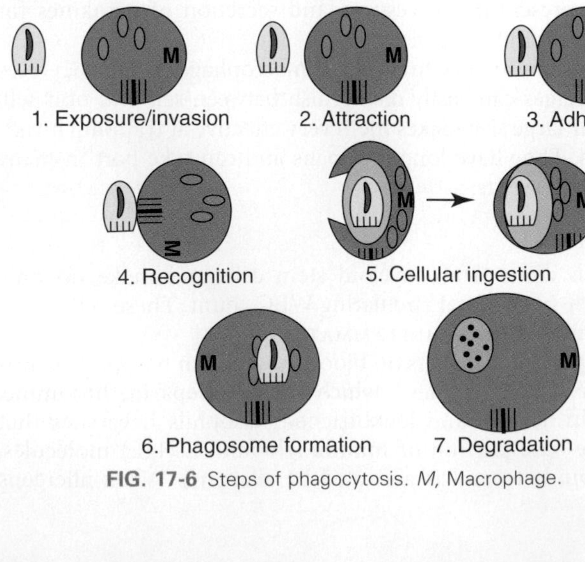

FIG. 17-6 Steps of phagocytosis. *M*, Macrophage.

Exposure and invasion occur as the first step in response to injury or invasion. Leukocytes that engage in phagocytosis and stimulate INFLAMMATION are present in the blood and other extracellular fluids. For phagocytosis to start, the body must first be invaded by organisms, foreign proteins, or debris from damaged tissues.

Attraction is needed as the second step because phagocytosis can occur only when the WBC comes into direct contact with the target (antigen, invader, or foreign protein). Damaged tissues secrete chemotaxins that attract neutrophils and macrophages and release debris that can combine with the surface of invading foreign proteins.

Adherence allows the phagocytic cell to bind to the surface of the target. *Opsonins* are substances that increase contact of the cell with its target by coating the target cell (antigen or organism). During INFLAMMATION, coating the target makes it easier for phagocytic cells to stick to it. Many substances can act as opsonins. Some are particles from dead neutrophils, antibodies, and activated (fixated) complement components.

Complement activation and fixation are part of opsonization and help with adherence. Twenty different inactive complement proteins are present in the blood. When stimulated, each complement protein is activated, joins other activated complement proteins, surrounds an antigen, and "fixes" or sticks to the antigen. Complement fixation occurs quickly as a cascade.

Recognition occurs when the phagocytic cell sticks to the target cell and "recognizes" it as non-self. The phagocytic cells examine the universal product codes (human leukocyte antigens [HLAs]) of whatever they encounter. Recognition of non-self is made easier by opsonins on the target cell surface. Phagocytic cells start phagocytosis only when the target cell is recognized as non-self or debris.

Cellular ingestion is needed because phagocytic destruction occurs inside the cell. The target cell is brought inside the phagocytic cell by phagocytosis (engulfment).

Phagosome formation occurs when the phagocyte's granules break and release enzymes that attack the ingested target.

Degradation is the final step. The enzymes in the phagosome digest the engulfed target.

Sequence of Inflammation

INFLAMMATION (inflammatory responses) occurs in a predictable three-stage sequence. The sequence is the same regardless of the triggering event. Responses at the tissue level cause the **five cardinal manifestations of inflammation**: warmth, redness, swelling, pain, and decreased function. The timing of the stages may overlap.

Stage I is the vascular part of the inflammatory response that first involves changes in blood vessels. Injured tissues and the leukocytes and tissue mast cells in this area secrete histamine, serotonin, and kinins that constrict the small veins and dilate the arterioles in the area of injury. These blood vessel changes cause redness and warmth of the tissues. This increased blood flow increases delivery of nutrients to injured tissues.

Blood flow to the area increases **(hyperemia)**, and swelling **(edema)** forms at the site of injury or invasion. Capillary leak also occurs, allowing blood plasma to leak into the tissues. This response causes swelling and pain. Edema at the site of injury or invasion protects the area from further injury by creating a cushion of fluid. The duration of these responses depends on the severity of the initiating event, but usually they subside within 24 to 72 hours.

The macrophage is the major cell involved in stage I of INFLAMMATION. The action is rapid because macrophages are already in place at the site of injury or invasion. This action is limited because the number of macrophages is so small. To enhance the inflammatory response, the tissue macrophages secrete several cytokines. One cytokine is colony-stimulating factor (CSF), which triggers the bone marrow to shorten the time needed to produce white blood cells (WBCs) from 14 days to a matter of hours. Some cytokines cause neutrophils from the bone marrow to move to the site of injury or invasion, which leads to the next stage of inflammation.

Stage II is the cellular exudate part of the response. In this stage, **neutrophilia** (an increased number of circulating neutrophils) occurs. Exudate in the form of pus occurs, containing dead WBCs, necrotic tissue, and fluids that escape from damaged cells.

The most active cells in stage II are the neutrophils, basophils, and tissue mast cells. Under the influence of cytokines, the neutrophil count can increase hugely within 12 hours after inflammation starts. Neutrophils attack and destroy organisms and remove dead tissue through phagocytosis. Basophils and tissue mast cells continue or sustain the initial responses.

In acute INFLAMMATION, the healthy person produces enough mature neutrophils to keep pace with invasion and prevent the organisms from growing. At the same time, the WBCs and inflamed tissues secrete cytokines, which allow tissue macrophages to increase and trigger bone marrow production of monocytes. This reaction begins slowly, but its effects are long lasting.

During this phase, the arachidonic acid cascade starts to increase the inflammatory response. This action begins by the conversion of fatty acids in plasma membranes into arachidonic acid (AA). The enzyme *cyclooxygenase* (COX) converts AA into many chemicals that are further processed into the substances (mediators) that promote the continued inflammatory response in the tissues. These mediators include histamine, leukotrienes, prostaglandins, serotonin, and kinins. Many anti-inflammatory drugs, including NSAIDs, stop this cascade by preventing cyclooxygenase from converting AA into inflammatory mediators.

When an infection stimulating INFLAMMATION lasts longer than just a few days, the bone marrow begins to release immature neutrophils, reducing the number of circulating mature neutrophils. This reduction of mature neutrophils limits the helpful effects of inflammation and increases the risk for sepsis.

Stage III features tissue repair and replacement. Although this stage is completed last, it begins at the time of injury and is critical to the final function of the inflamed area.

Some of the WBCs involved in INFLAMMATION start the replacement of lost tissues or repair of damaged tissues by inducing the remaining healthy cells to divide. In tissues that cannot divide, WBCs trigger new blood vessel growth and scar tissue formation. Because scar tissue does not act like the tissue it replaces, function is lost wherever scar tissue forms. The degree of function lost depends on how much normal tissue is replaced by scar tissue. For example, when heart muscles are destroyed because of a myocardial infarction (heart attack), scar tissue forms in the area to prevent a hole from forming in the muscle wall as the ischemic cells die. (Remember that heart muscle is non-dividing tissue and the heart cannot replace these muscle cells.) The scar tissue serves only as a patch; it does not contract or act in any way like heart muscle. So, if 20% of the left ventricle is replaced with scar tissue, the effectiveness of left ventricular contraction is reduced by at least 20%.

INFLAMMATION alone cannot provide IMMUNITY. Inflammatory cells must interact with lymphocytes to provide long-lasting immunity. Long lasting immune actions develop through antibody-mediated immunity (AMI) and cell-mediated immunity (CMI).

NCLEX EXAMINATION CHALLENGE

Safe and Effective Care Environment

The white blood cell count with differential of a client undergoing preadmission testing before surgery indicates a total count of 10,000 cells per cubic millimeter (mm^3) of blood. Which differential counts or percentages does the nurse report to the physician?

A. Eosinophils 200/mm^3
B. Monocytes 2000/mm^3
C. Segmented neutrophils 5700/mm^3
D. Lymphocytes 2100/mm^3

IMMUNITY

IMMUNITY is an *adaptive* internal protection that results in long-term resistance to the effects of invading microorganisms. This means that the responses are not automatic. The body has to learn to generate specific immune responses when it is infected by or exposed to specific organisms. Lymphocytes develop actions and products that provide the protection of true immunity. These cells develop specific actions in response to specific invasion (Fig. 17-7).

Antibody-Mediated Immunity

Antibody-mediated immunity (**AMI**), also known as *humoral immunity*, involves antigen-antibody interactions to neutralize, eliminate, or destroy foreign proteins. Antibodies are produced by sensitized B-lymphocytes (B-cells).

B-cells become sensitized to a specific foreign protein (antigen) and produce antibodies directed specifically against that protein. The antibody, rather than the actual B-cell, then causes one of several actions to neutralize, eliminate, or destroy that antigen.

B-cells have the most direct role in AMI. Macrophages and T-lymphocytes (discussed on p. 285 in the Cell-Mediated Immunity section) work with B-cells to start and complete antigen-antibody interactions. *For optimal AMI, the entire immune system must function adequately.*

B-cells start as stem cells in the bone marrow, the primary lymphoid tissue, that commit to the lymphocyte pathway (see Fig. 17-3) and are then restricted in development. The lymphocyte stem cells are released from the bone marrow into the blood. They then migrate into many secondary lymphoid tissues to mature. The secondary lymphoid tissues for B-cell maturation are the spleen, parts of lymph nodes, tonsils, and the mucosa of the intestinal tract.

Antigen-Antibody Interactions

The body learns to make enough of any specific antibody to provide long-lasting immunity against specific organisms or toxins. The seven steps needed to produce a specific antibody directed against a specific antigen whenever the person is

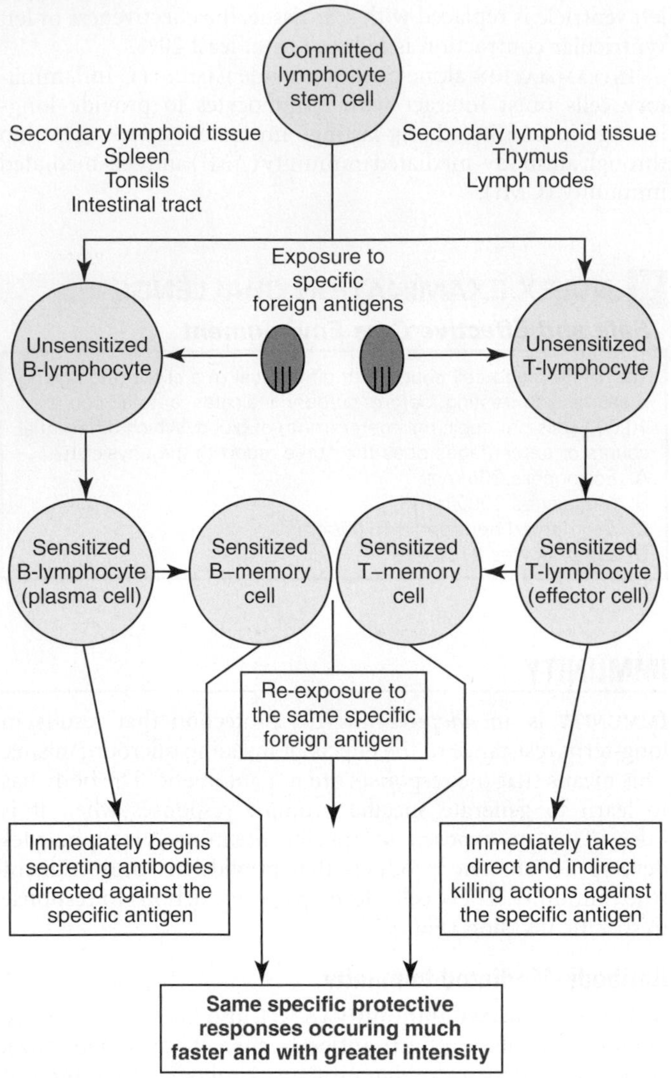

FIG. 17-7 B-lymphocyte and T-lymphocyte differentiation, maturation, and function.

exposed to that antigen are shown in Fig. 17-8 and described below.

Exposure or invasion is needed because antibody actions occur inside the body or on a few body surfaces. Thus the antigen must first enter the person to generate an antibody, although not all exposures result in antibody production. Invasion by the antigen must occur in such large numbers that some of the antigen evades detection by the body's natural nonspecific defenses or overwhelms the ability of the inflammatory response to get rid of the invader.

For example, a person who has never been exposed to the viral disease *influenza A* now baby-sits for three children who develop influenza symptoms within the next 10 hours. These children, in the pre-symptomatic stage, shed many millions of live influenza A virus particles by droplets from the upper respiratory tract. They expose the baby-sitter by drinking out of the baby-sitter's cup, kissing him or her directly on the lips, and sneezing and coughing directly into his or her face. During the 5 hours spent with the children, the baby-sitter is heavily invaded by the influenza A virus and will become sick with this disease within 2 to 4 days. While the virus is growing and the disease is developing, the baby-sitter's white blood cells are taking part in antibody-antigen actions to prevent him or her from having influenza A more than once.

Antigen recognition is the next step to begin making antibodies against an antigen. The unsensitized B-cell must first recognize the antigen as non-self. B-cells need the help of macrophages and helper/inducer T-cells to recognize an antigen.

Recognition is started by the macrophages. After the antigen surface has been altered by opsonization (see discussion of "adherence" on p. 280), the macrophage recognizes the invading antigen as non-self and attaches itself to the antigen. This attachment allows the macrophage to "present" the attached antigen to the helper/inducer T-cell. Then the helper/inducer T-cell and the macrophage together process the antigen to expose the antigen's recognition sites (universal product code). After processing the antigen, the helper/inducer T-cell brings the antigen into contact with the B-cell so that the B-cell can recognize the antigen as non-self.

Sensitization occurs when the B-cell recognizes the antigen as non-self and is now "sensitized" to this antigen. A single unsensitized B-cell can become sensitized only once. *So, each B-cell can be sensitized to only one type of antigen.*

Sensitizing allows this B-cell to respond to any substance that carries the same antigens (codes) as the original antigen. The sensitized B-cell always remains sensitized to that specific antigen. In addition, all cells produced by that sensitized B-cell also are already pre-sensitized to that same specific antigen.

Immediately after it is sensitized, the B-cell divides and forms two types of B-lymphocytes, each one remaining sensitized to that specific antigen (see Fig. 17-7). One new cell becomes a **plasma cell**, which starts immediately to produce antibodies against the sensitizing antigen. The other new cell becomes a memory cell. The **memory cell** is a sensitized B-cell but does not produce antibodies until the next exposure to the same antigen (see discussion of sustained immunity (memory) on p. 284).

Antibody production and release allow the antibodies to search out specific antigens. Antibodies are produced by plasma cells, and each plasma cell can make as many as 300 molecules of antibody per second. Each plasma cell produces antibody specific only to the antigen that originally sensitized the parent B-cell. For example, in the case of the baby-sitter who was invaded by the influenza A virus, the plasma cells from those B-cells sensitized to the influenza A virus can make only anti–influenza A antibodies. The antibody class (e.g., immunoglobulin G [IgG] or immunoglobulin M [IgM]) that the plasma cell produces may vary, but the antibody can be forever directed only against the influenza A virus.

Antibody molecules made by plasma cells are released into the blood and other body fluids as free antibody. Because the antibody is in body fluids (or body "humors") and is separate from the B-cells, this type of IMMUNITY is sometimes called **humoral immunity**. *Circulating antibodies can be transferred from one person to another to provide the receiving person with immediate immunity of short duration.*

Antibody-antigen binding is needed for anti-antigen actions. Antibodies are Y-shaped molecules (Fig. 17-9). The tips of the short arms of the Y recognize the specific antigen and bind to it. Because each antibody molecule has two tips (Fab fragments, or arms), each antibody can bind either to two separate antigens or to two areas of the same antigen.

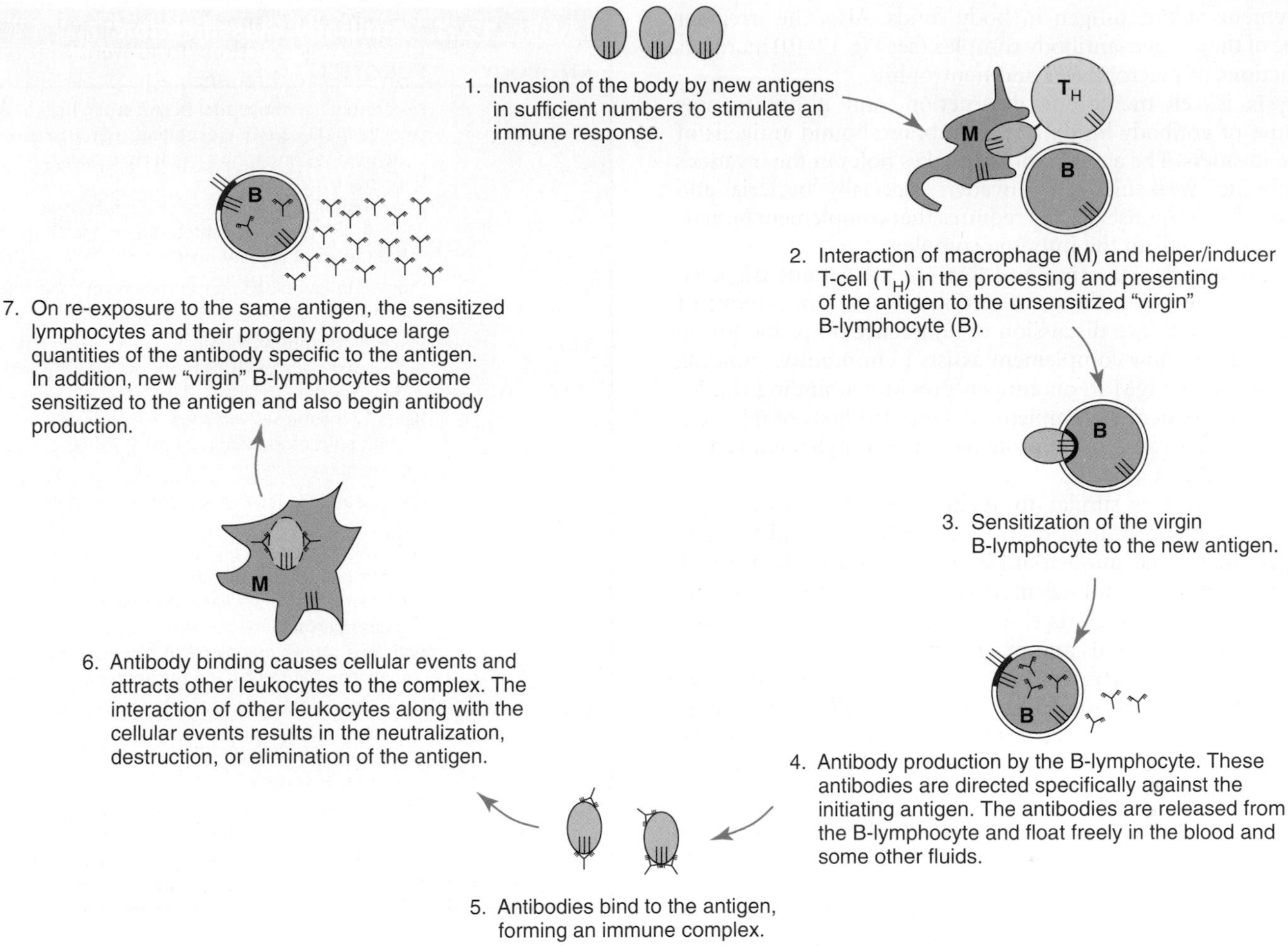

FIG. 17-8 Sequence of the seven steps required to stimulate antibody-mediated immunity.

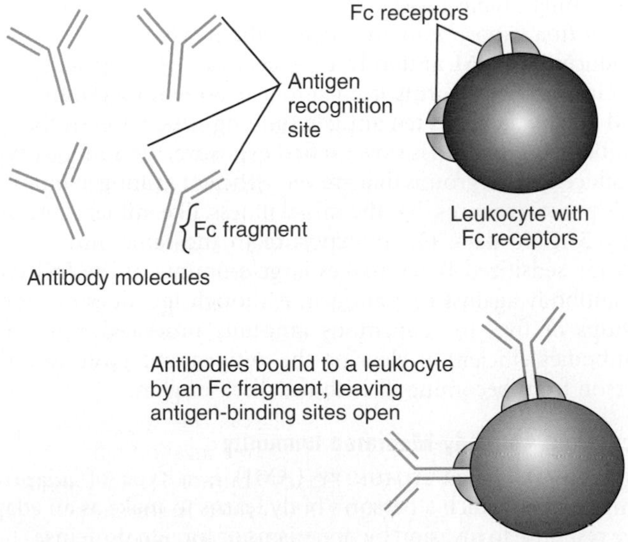

FIG. 17-9 Antibody structure and the Fc receptors on leukocytes.

The stem of the Y is the "Fc fragment." This area can bind to Fc receptor sites on white blood cells (WBCs). The WBC then not only has its own means of attacking antigens but also has the added power of having surface antibodies that can stick to antigens (see Fig. 17-9).

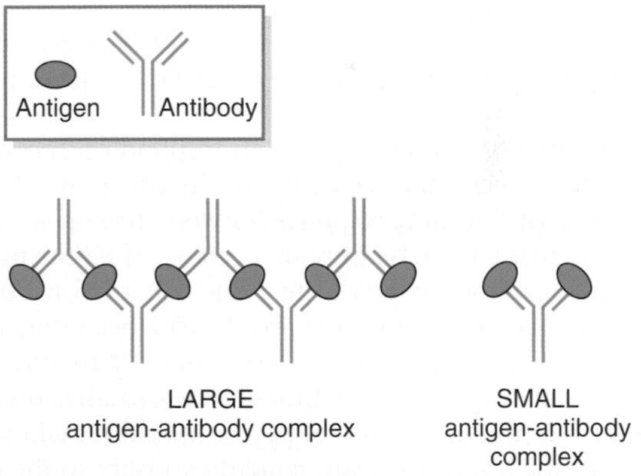

FIG. 17-10 Formation of large and small antigen-antibody complexes (immune complexes).

The binding of antibody to antigen may not be lethal to the antigen. Instead, antibody-antigen binding starts other actions that neutralize, eliminate, or destroy the antigen.

Antibody-binding actions are triggered by binding of antibody to antigen. The resulting reactions of agglutination, lysis, complement fixation, precipitation, and inactivation can then neutralize, eliminate, or destroy the bound antigen.

Agglutination is a clumping action that results from the antibody linking antigens together, forming large and small immune complexes (Fig. 17-10). Agglutination slows the movement of the antigen in body fluids. Also, the irregular shape of the antigen-antibody complex (see Fig. 17-10) increases the actions of macrophages and neutrophils.

Lysis is cell membrane destruction, and it occurs now because of antibody binding to membrane-bound antigens of some invaders. The actual binding makes holes in the invader's membrane, weakening the invader, especially bacteria and viruses. This response usually requires that complement be activated and "fixed" to the immune complex.

Complement activation and fixation are actions triggered by the IgG and IgM classes of antibodies that can remove or destroy antigen. (See discussion of adherence on p. 280 for an explanation of how complement assists in immunity.) Binding of either IgG or IgM to an antigen provides a binding site for the first component of complement. Once the first complement molecule is activated, other proteins of the complement system are activated in a cascade.

Precipitation is similar to agglutination but has a larger response. With precipitation, antibody molecules bind so much antigen that large antigen-antibody complexes are formed. These complexes cannot stay in suspension in the blood. Instead, they form a large precipitate, which then can be acted on and removed by neutrophils and macrophages.

Inactivation (neutralization) is the process of making an antigen harmless without destroying it. Usually only a small area of the antigen, the active site, causes the harmful effects. When an antibody binds to an antigen's active site, covering it up, the antigen is made harmless without destroying it.

Sustained immunity (memory) provides us with long-lasting IMMUNITY to a specific antigen. Sustained immunity results from memory B-cells made during the lymphocyte sensitization stage. These memory cells remain sensitized to the specific antigen to which they were originally exposed. On re-exposure to the same antigen, the memory cells rapidly respond by first dividing and forming new sensitized blast cells and plasma cells. The blast cells continue to divide, producing many more sensitized plasma cells. These new sensitized plasma cells rapidly make large amounts of the antibody specific for the sensitizing antigen.

This ability of the memory cells to respond on re-exposure to the same antigen that originally sensitized the B-cell allows a rapid and large immune response *(anamnestic response)* to the antigen. Because so much antibody is made, often the invading organisms are removed completely and the person does not become ill. This process prevents people from becoming ill with chickenpox or any infectious disease more than once, even though they are exposed many times to the causative organism. Without immunologic memory, people would remain susceptible to specific diseases on subsequent exposure to the organisms and no long-term IMMUNITY would be generated (Abbas et al., 2012; McCance et al., 2014).

Antibody Classification

All antibodies are immunoglobulins, also called *gamma globulins.* These names are based on the structure and function of antibodies. A globulin is a protein that is globular rather than straight. Because antibodies are globular proteins, they are "globulins." The term **immunoglobulin** is used for antibodies because they are globular proteins that provide IMMUNITY. Antibodies also are called **gamma globulins** because all free antibodies in the plasma separate out in the gamma fraction of plasma proteins during electrophoresis. The five antibody types are classified by differences in size, location, amount, function, and timing (Table 17-4).

TABLE 17-4 Antibody Classification

ANTIBODY	FUNCTION
IgA	"Secretory" antibody that is present in high concentrations in the secretions of mucous membranes and in the intestinal mucosa Very low circulating levels Most responsible for preventing infection in the upper and lower respiratory tracts, the GI tract, and the genitourinary tract
IgD	Present in low blood concentrations in conjunction with IgM
IgE	Variable concentration in blood Associated with antibody-mediated hypersensitivity reactions Binds to mast cells and causes their degranulation when an allergen (antigen) binds to IgE antigen recognition sites
IgG	Composes at least 75% of circulating antibody population Is heavily expressed on second and subsequent exposures to antigens to provide sustained, long-term immunity against invading microorganisms Activates classic complement pathway, and enhances neutrophil and macrophage actions
IgM	First antibody formed by a newly sensitized B-lymphocyte plasma cell Composes about 10% to 15% of circulating antibody population Especially effective at the antibody actions of agglutination and precipitation because of having 10 potential binding sites per molecule Activates complement pathway

On first exposure to an antigen, the newly sensitized B-cell produces the IgM antibody type against the antigen. IgM is special because it forms itself into a five-member group. Each IgM group, then, has ten antigen binding sites. So, even though antibody production is slow on first exposure, the antibody type produced forms groups that are very efficient at antigen binding. This process ensures that the initial illness, like influenza A, lasts only 5 to 10 days. On re-exposure to the same antigen, the already sensitized B-cell makes large amounts of the IgG type of antibody against that antigen. Although IgG does not form groups of five, the enormous amounts produced make IgG antibodies efficient at clearing the antigen and protecting the person from becoming ill with the disease again.

Acquiring Antibody-Mediated Immunity

Antibody-mediated IMMUNITY (AMI) is a type of **adaptive immunity** in which a person's body learns to make as an adaptive response to invasion by organisms or foreign proteins. Thus antibody-mediated immunity is an *acquired immunity.* Adaptive immunity occurs either naturally or artificially through lymphocyte responses and can be either active or passive.

Active immunity occurs when antigens enter a person's body and it responds by making specific antibodies against the antigen. This type of IMMUNITY is *active* because the body takes an active part in making antibodies. Active immunity occurs under natural or artificial conditions.

Natural active IMMUNITY occurs when an antigen enters the body naturally without human assistance and the body responds by actively making antibodies against that antigen (e.g., influenza A virus). Usually, the invasion that triggers antibody production also causes the disease. However, processes occurring in the body at the same time as infection create immunity to that antigen. Thus the person will not become ill after a second exposure to the same antigen. *Natural active immunity is the most effective and the longest lasting.*

Artificial active IMMUNITY is the protection developed by vaccination or immunization. This type of immunity is used to prevent serious and potentially deadly illnesses (e.g., tetanus, diphtheria, polio). Small amounts of specific antigens are placed as a vaccination into a person. The person's immune system responds by actively making antibodies against the antigen. Because antigens used for this procedure have been specially processed to make them less likely to grow in the body (**attenuated**), this exposure usually does not cause the disease. Artificial active immunity lasts many years, although repeated but smaller doses of the original antigen are required as a "booster" to retain the protection.

Passive IMMUNITY occurs when the antibodies against an antigen are transferred to a person's body after first being made in the body of another person or animal. Because these antibodies are foreign to the receiving person, they are recognized as non-self and eliminated quickly. For this reason, passive immunity provides only immediate, short-term protection against a specific antigen. It is used when a person is exposed to a serious disease for which he or she has little or no actively acquired immunity. Instead, the injected antibodies are expected to inactivate the antigen. Artificial passive immunity may be used to prevent disease or death for patients exposed to rabies, tetanus, and poisonous snake bites.

Natural passive IMMUNITY occurs when antibodies are passed from the mother to the fetus via the placenta or to the infant through colostrum and breast milk.

AMI works with INFLAMMATION to protect against infection. However, AMI can provide the most effective long-lasting IMMUNITY only when its actions are combined with those of cell-mediated immunity.

Cell-Mediated Immunity

Cell-mediated IMMUNITY (CMI), or cellular immunity, involves many white blood cell (WBC) actions and interactions. CMI is another type of adaptive or acquired true immunity that is provided by lymphocyte stem cells that mature in the secondary lymphoid tissues of the thymus and pericortical areas of lymph nodes (see Fig. 17-7). Certain CMI responses influence and regulate the activities of antibody-mediated immunity (AMI) and INFLAMMATION by producing and releasing cytokines. For total or full immunity, CMI must function optimally.

Cell Types Involved in Cell-Mediated Immunity

The WBCs with the most important roles in CMI include several specific T-lymphocytes (T-cells) along with a special population of cells known as *natural killer (NK) cells.* T-cells have a variety of subsets, each of which has a specific function.

Different T-cell subsets can be identified by the presence of "marker proteins" (antigens) on the cell membrane's surface. More than 200 different T-cell proteins have been identified on the cell membrane, and some of these are commonly used clinically to identify specific cells (Abbas et al., 2012). Most T-cells have more than one antigen on their cell membrane. For example, all mature T-cells contain T1, T3, T10, and T11 proteins.

The names used to identify specific T-cell subsets include the specific membrane antigen and the overall actions of the cells in a subset. The three T-lymphocyte subsets that are critically important for the development and continuation of CMI are helper/inducer T-cells, suppressor T-cells, and cytotoxic/cytolytic T-cells. An additional cell, the natural killer cell, although not a true T-cell, also contributes to CMI.

Helper/inducer T-cells have the T4 protein on their membranes. These cells are usually called *T4+ cells* or T_H *cells.* The most correct name for helper/inducer T-cells is *CD4+* (cluster of differentiation 4).

Helper/inducer T-cells easily recognize self cells versus non-self cells. When they recognize non-self (antigen), helper/inducer T-cells secrete cytokines that can enhance the activity of other WBCs and increase overall immune function. These cytokines increase bone marrow production of stem cells and speed up their maturation. Thus helper/inducer T-cells act as organizers in "calling to arms" various squads of WBCs involved in inflammatory, antibody, and cellular protective actions.

Suppressor T-cells have the T8-lymphocyte antigen on membrane surfaces. These cells are commonly called *T8+ cells, CD8+ cells,* or T_S*-cells.* Suppressor T-cells help regulate CMI.

Suppressor T-cells prevent **hypersensitivity** (immune overreactions) on exposure to non-self cells or proteins. This function is important in preventing the formation of antibodies directed against normal, healthy self cells, which is the basis for many autoimmune diseases. The suppressor T-cells secrete cytokines that have an overall *inhibitory* action on most cells of the immune system.

Suppressor T-cells have the opposite action of helper/inducer T-cells. For optimal function of CMI, then, a balance between helper/inducer T-cell activity and suppressor T-cell activity must be maintained. This balance occurs when the helper/inducer T-cells outnumber the suppressor T-cells by a ratio of 2:1. When this ratio increases, indicating that helper/inducer T-cells vastly outnumber the suppressor cells, overreactions can occur, some of which are tissue damaging as well as unpleasant. When the helper/suppressor ratio decreases, indicating fewer-than-normal helper/inducer T-cells, IMMUNITY is suppressed and the person's risk for infections increases.

Cytotoxic/cytolytic T-cells are also called T_C*-cells.* Because they have the T8 protein present on their surfaces, they are a subset of suppressor cells. Cytotoxic/cytolytic T-cells destroy cells that contain a processed antigen's human leukocyte antigens (HLAs). This activity is most effective against self cells infected by parasites, such as viruses or protozoa.

Parasite-infected self cells have both self HLA proteins (universal product code) and the parasite's antigens on the cell surface. This allows the person's immune system cells to recognize the infected self cell as abnormal, and the cytotoxic/cytolytic T-cell can bind to it, punch a hole, and deliver a "lethal hit" of enzymes to the infected cell, causing it to lyse and die.

Natural killer (NK) cells are also known as *CD16+ cells* and are very important in providing CMI. The actual site of NK cell differentiation and maturation is unknown, and it is not a true T-cell subset (Abbas et al., 2012).

NK cells have direct cytotoxic effects on some non-self cells without first being sensitized. They conduct "seek and destroy" missions in the body to eliminate non-self cells.

NK cells are most effective in destroying unhealthy or abnormal self cells. The non-self cells most often harmed by NK cells are cancer cells and virally infected body cells.

Cytokines

Cell-mediated IMMUNITY (CMI) regulates the immune system by the production and activity of cytokines. **Cytokines** are small protein hormones produced by the many WBCs (and some other tissues). Cytokines made by the macrophages, neutrophils, eosinophils, and monocytes are called **monokines.** Those produced by T-cells are called **lymphokines.** In addition, we now know that many other body cell types can produce and respond to cytokines.

Cytokines work like hormones: one cell produces a cytokine, which in turn exerts its effects on other cells of the immune system and on other body cells. The cells responding to the cytokine may be located close to or remote from the cytokine-secreting cell. Thus cytokines act like "messengers" that tell specific cells how and when to respond. The cells that change their activity when a cytokine is present are "responder" cells. For a responder cell to respond to the presence of a cytokine, the responder cell must have a specific receptor to which the cytokine can bind. Once the cytokine binds to its receptor, the responder cell changes its activity.

Cytokines control many inflammatory and immune responses and are controlled by interactions with other systems, especially the nervous system. Cytokines include the interleukins (ILs), interferons (IFNs), colony-stimulating factors, tumor necrosis factors (TNFs), and transforming growth factors (TGFs). The interleukins are the largest group of cytokines, with interleukin-33 (IL-33) being the most recently defined. There are many cytokines, and cytokine classification is undergoing changes. Some are considered "proinflammatory" and increase the actions of natural immunity (INFLAMMATION). These currently include TNF-α, IL-1, IL-10, IL-12, and interferons (α [alpha], β [beta], and γ [gamma]). Other cytokines have a major influence on AMI and CMI activities. These include IL-2, IL-4, IL-5, IL-10, TGF-β, and IFN-γ. Although there are many cytokines, not all their functions are known or clinically useful at this time; however, this is an area of continuing research and discovery. Table 17-5 lists the cytokines that have current clinical importance. Chapters discussing specific diseases (e.g., lymphoma, rheumatoid arthritis) caused by or treated with certain cytokines have more information about the role of specific cytokines in the disease and its treatment.

TABLE 17-5 Activity of Selected Cytokines

CYTOKINE	ACTIONS
Pro-inflammatory Cytokines	
Interleukin-1 (IL-1)	Induces fever Stimulates production of prostaglandins Increases growth of CD4+ T-cells
Interleukin-2 (IL-2)	Increases growth and differentiation of T-lymphocytes Enhances natural killer cell activity against cancer cells
Interleukin-6 (IL-6)	Stimulates liver to produce fibrinogen and protein C Increases rate of bone marrow production of stem cells Increases numbers of sensitized B-lymphocytes
Tumor Necrosis Factor (TNF)	Induces fever Major cytokine involved in rheumatoid arthritis damage Major cytokine involved in the acute inflammatory response to infectious bacteria and starts many of the systemic complications of severe infection or sepsis Participates in graft rejection Induces cell death Stimulates delayed hypersensitivity reactions and allergy
Growth Factors	
Granulocyte Colony-Stimulating Factor (G-CSF)	Increases numbers and maturity of neutrophils
Granulocyte-Macrophage Colony-Stimulating Factor (GM-CSF)	Increases growth and maturation of myeloid stem cells
Erythropoietin	Increases growth and differentiation of erythrocytes
Thrombopoietin	Increases growth and differentiation of platelets

Protection Provided by Cell-Mediated Immunity

Cell-mediated IMMUNITY (CMI) helps protect the body through the ability to differentiate self from non-self. The non-self cells most easily recognized by CMI are cancer cells and those self cells infected by organisms that live within host cells, especially viruses. CMI watches for and rids the body of self cells that might potentially harm the body. *CMI is important in preventing the development of cancer and metastasis after exposure to carcinogens.*

Transplant Rejection

Natural killer (NK) cells and cytotoxic/cytolytic T-cells also destroy cells from other people or animals. Although this action is normal and is usually helpful, it is also responsible for rejection of tissue grafts and transplanted organs (also termed *grafts*). Because the solid organ transplanted into the recipient is seldom a perfectly identical match of human leukocyte antigens (unless the organ is obtained from an identical sibling) between the donated organ and the recipient host, the patient's immune system cells recognize a newly transplanted organ as non-self. Without intervention, the recipient's immune system starts inflammatory and immunologic actions to destroy or eliminate these non-self cells. This activity causes rejection of the transplanted organ. Rejection of transplanted solid organs and other grafts is a result of a complex series of responses that change over time and involve different components of the immune system. Rejection can be hyperacute, acute, or chronic.

Hyperacute Rejection

Hyperacute rejection begins immediately on transplantation and is an antibody-mediated response. Antigen-antibody complexes form in the blood vessels of the transplanted organ. The recipient's (host's) blood has pre-existing antibodies to one or more of the antigens (including blood group antigens) present in the donated organ. The antigen-antibody complexes adhere to the lining of blood vessels and activate complement. The activated complement in the blood vessel linings triggers the blood clotting cascade, causing small clots to form throughout the new organ. Widespread clotting occludes blood vessels and leads to ischemic necrosis, INFLAMMATION with phagocytosis of the necrotic blood vessels, and release of lytic enzymes into the new organ. These enzymes cause massive cellular destruction within the transplanted organ and graft loss.

Hyperacute rejection occurs mostly in transplanted kidneys but is less common now as a result of greater efforts in HLA matching. The patients at greatest risk for hyperacute rejection are those who have received donated organs of an ABO blood type different from their own, have received multiple blood transfusions at any time in life before transplantation, have a history of multiple pregnancies, or have received a previous transplant.

The manifestations of hyperacute rejection are apparent within minutes of attachment of the donated organ to the recipient's blood supply. The process cannot be stopped once it has started, and the rejected organ is removed as soon as hyperacute rejection is diagnosed.

Acute Rejection

Acute rejection first occurs within 1 week to 3 months after transplantation and may occur sporadically after that. Two mechanisms are responsible. The first mechanism is antibody mediated and results in vasculitis within the transplanted organ. This reaction differs from hyperacute rejection in that blood vessel necrosis (not occlusion) leads to organ destruction.

The second mechanism is cellular. The recipient's cytotoxic/cytolytic T-cells and NK cells enter the transplanted organ through the blood, penetrate the organ cells, start an inflammatory response, and cause lysis of the organ cells.

Diagnosis of acute rejection is made by laboratory tests that show impaired function of the donated organ and by biopsy of the donated organ. Manifestations of acute rejection vary with each patient and with the specific organ transplanted. For example, when acute rejection occurs in a transplanted kidney, the patient usually has some tenderness in the kidney area and may have other general manifestations of INFLAMMATION.

An episode of acute rejection after solid organ transplantation does not automatically mean that the patient will lose the new organ. Drug management of the recipient's immune responses at this time may limit the damage to the organ and allow the graft to be maintained.

Chronic Rejection

The origin of *chronic rejection* is similar to chronic INFLAMMATION and scarring. The smooth muscles of blood vessels overgrow and occlude the vessels. The donated organ tissues are replaced with fibrotic, scarlike tissue. Because this fibrotic tissue is not organ tissue, the transplanted organ's function is reduced in proportion to the amount of normal tissue that is replaced by fibrotic tissue. This type of reaction is long-standing and occurs continuously as a response to chronic ischemia caused by blood vessel injury. The results of chronic rejection are unique to different transplanted organs. For example, in transplanted lungs, chronic rejection thickens small airways. In transplanted livers, chronic rejection destroys bile ducts. In transplanted hearts, this process is called *accelerated graft atherosclerosis (AGA)* and is the major cause of death in patients who have survived 1 or more years after heart transplantation.

Although good control over the recipient's immune function can delay this type of rejection, the process probably occurs to some degree with all transplanted solid organs obtained from donors who are not identical siblings of the recipients. Because the fibrotic changes are permanent, there is no cure for chronic graft rejection. When the fibrosis increases to the extent that the transplanted organ can no longer function, the only recourse is retransplantation.

Management of Transplant Rejection

Rejection of transplanted solid organs involves all three components of IMMUNITY, although cell-mediated immune (CMI) responses contribute the most to the rejection process. Approved drugs used to manage transplant rejection are listed in Chart 17-2.

Maintenance therapy is the continuous immunosuppression used after a solid organ transplant. The drugs used for routine therapy after solid organ transplantation are combinations of a calcineurin inhibitor, a corticosteroid, and an antiproliferative agent (Alexander & Susla, 2013). Which drugs are used depends on the transplant type and other patient-specific conditions. These are all oral agents and must be taken for the life of the transplanted organ. All are immunosuppressive to some degree, and the dosage is adjusted to the immune response of each patient. Treatment with these agents increases the risk for bacterial and fungal infections and for cancer development.

Rescue therapy is used to treat acute rejection episodes. The drug categories for this purpose are the monoclonal and polyclonal antibodies (see Chart 17-2). The drugs used for maintenance are often also used during rejection episodes at much higher dosages than for maintenance.

CHART 17-2 Common Examples of Drug Therapy

Transplant Rejection

DRUG/CLASS	ROUTE OF ADMINISTRATION	SIDE EFFECTS
Corticosteroids		
Broadly inhibit cytokine production in most leukocytes, resulting in generalized immunosuppression		
Prednisone (Deltasone)	Oral	Hypertension Hyperlipidemia Osteoporosis Weight gain Cushingoid appearance Opportunistic infection Glaucoma GI ulcer formation Hyperglycemia
Prednisolone (Millipred, Orapred, Veripred)	Oral	Same as for prednisone

Continued

CHART 17-2 Common Examples of Drug Therapy—cont'd

Transplant Rejection

DRUG/CLASS	ROUTE OF ADMINISTRATION	SIDE EFFECTS
Calcineurin Inhibitors		
The inhibition of calcineurin stops the production and secretion of IL-2, which then prevents the activation of lymphocytes involved in transplant rejection.		
Cyclosporine (Sandimmune, Neoral, Gengraf)	Oral	Nephrotoxic Hypertension Tremor Coronary artery disease Hirsutism Gingival hyperplasia Opportunistic infections Malignancies Hyperuricemia Hepatoxicity
Tacrolimus (Prograf)	Oral	Nephrotoxic Hypertension Hyperkalemia Hypomagnesemia Hyperglycemia Opportunistic infections Malignancies
Antiproliferatives		
The main action of all antiproliferatives is to inhibit something essential to DNA synthesis, which prevents cell division in activated lymphocytes. Some have additional immune suppressive actions.		
Azathioprine (Imuran)	Oral	Bone marrow suppression Thrombocytopenia Anemia Pancreatitis Hepatotoxicity Malignancies
Mycophenolate (CellCept, Myfortic)	Oral	Leucopenia Thrombocytopenia Nausea Opportunistic infection Malignancies
Sirolimus (Rapamune)	Oral	Leucopenia Thrombocytopenia Hypercholesterolemia Hypertriglyceridemia
Everolimus (Afinitor, Zortress)	Oral	Acne GI upsets Hepatoxicity Cushingoid appearance Gingival hyperplasia Hyperglycemia Hyperlipidemia Hypertension Leucopenia
Monoclonal Antibodies		
Specifically target the activation sites of T-lymphocytes, increasing their elimination from circulation		
Muromonab-CD3 (Orthoclone OKT3)	IV	Systemic inflammatory responses Aseptic meningitis Opportunistic infections Malignancies Hypersensitivity reactions
Basiliximab (Simulect)	IV	GI disturbances
Daclizumab (Zenapax)	IV	GI disturbances
Polyclonal Antibodies		
Antibodies derived from other animals (horses or rabbits) that bind to and eliminate most T-lymphocytes, thus stopping a transplant rejection episode.		
Antithymocyte globulin–equine (Atgam)	IV	Leukopenia Serum sickness Thrombocytopenia Pruritus Fever Arthralgias Opportunistic infections Malignancies
Antithymocyte globulin–rabbit (RATG, Thymoglobulin)	IV	Same as for antithymocyte globulin–equine

CLINICAL JUDGMENT CHALLENGE

Patient-Centered Care; Safety QSEN

A patient comes to the emergency room after stepping on a rusty nail while fixing a fence on his horse farm. He tells you that his last tetanus toxoid booster vaccination was about 12 years ago. The health care provider prescribes an injection of HyperTET, which contains concentrated pre-formed antibodies to the tetanus bacterium. The patient is instructed to return to his health care provider in 10 days to receive a tetanus "booster" vaccination.

1. What type of immunity is provided by the booster vaccination the patient received 12 years ago? Explain your choice.
2. Why does this patient need HyperTET now, and what type of immunity does it provide?
3. Why does the patient have to wait 10 days to receive the next tetanus booster?

NURSING CONCEPTS AND CLINICAL JUDGMENT REVIEW

What might you NOTICE in a patient with adequate protection as a result of appropriate responses for INFLAMMATION and IMMUNITY?

Vital signs:
- Body temperature within normal range

Physical assessment:
- Skin intact (no rashes, abnormal lesions)
- Skin color normal (no redness)
- No edema or excessively warm body areas
- All body areas fully functional with no pain
- No indicators of infection or illness

Laboratory assessment:
- White blood cell count and differential within the normal range
- No positive cultures of skin, blood, urine, sputum
- No evidence of allergic reactions

GET READY FOR THE NCLEX® EXAMINATION!

KEY POINTS

Review these Key Points for each NCLEX Examination Client Needs Category.

Physiological Integrity

- INFLAMMATION and IMMUNITY are provided through the actions and products of white blood cells (WBCs), also called *leukocytes.*
- Different types of WBCs provide different types of immune or inflammatory protection.
- The differential of the WBC count can be used to determine the patient's risk for infection, the presence or absence of infection, the presence or absence of an allergic reaction, and whether an infection is bacterial or viral.
- WBCs are the only body cells able to recognize non-self cells and to attack them.
- Self-tolerance is the special ability of WBCs to recognize healthy self cells and not attempt to attack or destroy them.
- Human leukocyte antigens (HLAs) are a person's tissue type and are inherited from parents.
- Immunocompetence requires that all three parts of INFLAMMATION and IMMUNITY have optimal functioning.
- INFLAMMATION is a general, nonspecific protective response also known as *innate immunity.*
- The five cardinal manifestations of INFLAMMATION are redness, warmth, swelling, pain, and loss of function.
- INFLAMMATION and infection are not the same thing. Infection almost always is accompanied by inflammation, but inflammation often occurs without infection.
- The tissue responses to INFLAMMATION are helpful if confined to the area of invasion or infection and do not extend beyond the acute phase.
- Chronic INFLAMMATION can damage tissues and reduce function.
- The cells and actions of cell-mediated IMMUNITY control and coordinate the entire inflammatory and immune responses.
- Inflammatory protection cannot be transferred from one person to another.
- Immune function declines with age, making the older adult at increased risk for infection and cancer development.
- Antibody-mediated IMMUNITY (also known as *humoral immunity*) can be transferred from one person or animal to another.
- Antibodies transferred from one person into another person have a short-term effect.
- Natural, active IMMUNITY is the most beneficial and long-lasting type of immunity.
- Vaccinations cause artificial active IMMUNITY and require "boosting" for best long-term effects.
- A person's normal membrane proteins would be antigens in another person.
- Transplant rejection is a normal response of the immune system that can damage or destroy the transplanted organ.
- Patients who receive transplanted organs (unless from an identical sibling) need to take immunosuppressive drugs daily to prevent transplant rejection.
- Patients who take immunosuppressive drugs have an increased risk for infection and cancer development.

18 CHAPTER

Care of Patients with Arthritis and Other Connective Tissue Diseases

Donna D. Ignatavicius

http://evolve.elsevier.com/Iggy/

PRIORITY CONCEPTS

- Pain
- Mobility
- Infection
- Immunity
- Inflammation

LEARNING OUTCOMES

Safe and Effective Care Environment

1. Identify interdisciplinary team members who collaborate to ensure quality care for patients with connective tissue diseases (CTDs).
2. Prioritize collaborative evidence-based interventions for patients with osteoarthritis (OA) and rheumatoid arthritis (RA).

Health Promotion and Maintenance

3. Identify community resources to help patients achieve or maintain independence in ADLs.
4. Describe risk factors for the development of arthritis and other CTDs.
5. Teach patients how to protect and exercise their joints to prevent injury.
6. Teach patients evidence-based strategies for how to prevent osteoarthritis.
7. Teach patients how to prevent Lyme disease and detect it early if it occurs.

Psychosocial Integrity

8. Assess the patient's and family's response to arthritis or other CTD, their support systems, and available resources.
9. Assess the patient's and family's sources of stress and coping mechanisms when living with arthritis or other CTD.

Physiological Integrity

10. Compare and contrast the pathophysiology and clinical manifestations of OA and RA, including those caused by joint inflammation and degenerative changes.
11. Interpret laboratory findings for patients with RA and other CTDs that affect immunity.
12. Assess presence and extent of pain and suffering in patients with arthritis.
13. Apply knowledge of pathophysiology to monitor for and prevent complications of total hip and knee arthroplasty.
14. Teach patients and their families about the postoperative care required after a total joint arthroplasty.
15. Provide information for patients and families about the use and side effects of drug therapy for arthritis or other CTD.
16. Identify the nursing implications associated with drug therapy for patients with rheumatoid arthritis and other CTDs.
17. Document and plan patient care in the electronic health care record for the patient with arthritis.
18. Differentiate between discoid lupus erythematosus and systemic lupus erythematosus.
19. Prioritize nursing interventions for patients who have systemic sclerosis.
20. Describe the patient-centered collaborative care of gout based on knowledge of pathophysiology.
21. Explain the differences between polymyositis, systemic necrotizing vasculitis, polymyalgia rheumatica, ankylosing spondylitis, Reiter's syndrome, and Sjögren's syndrome.
22. Describe current treatment strategies for patients with fibromyalgia syndrome and psoriatic arthritis.

Connective tissue disease (CTD) is the major focus of *rheumatology,* the study of rheumatic disease. A **rheumatic disease** is any disease or condition involving the musculoskeletal system. In this text, CTDs are discussed separately from other musculoskeletal conditions because most CTDs are classified as autoimmune disorders. In autoimmune disease, antibodies attack healthy normal cells and tissues. For reasons that are unclear, the immune system does not recognize body cells as self and therefore triggers an immune response. The usual *protective* nature of the immune system does not function properly in patients with autoimmune CTDs.

Most common CTDs are characterized by chronic pain and progressive joint deterioration, which results in decreased function and impaired mobility. Some of these disorders have additional localized clinical manifestations, whereas others are systemic. The economic and social costs of these diseases are staggering and will increase steadily as "baby boomers" continue to age. Patient care usually requires an interdisciplinary approach, including medicine, surgery, nursing, rehabilitation therapy, pharmacy, and/or case management.

Arthritis means INFLAMMATION of one or more joints. In clinical practice, however, arthritis is categorized as either noninflammatory or inflammatory. Noninflammatory, localized arthritis such as osteoarthritis (OA) is not systemic; OA is not an autoimmune disease. Systemic autoimmune diseases such as rheumatoid arthritis (RA) and systemic lupus erythematosus (SLE) are inflammatory disorders.

OSTEOARTHRITIS

❖ PATHOPHYSIOLOGY

Osteoarthritis is the most common arthritis and a major cause of disability among adults in the United States and the world. It is sometimes called *osteoarthrosis* or *degenerative joint disease (DJD)*.

Osteoarthritis is the progressive deterioration and loss of cartilage and bone in one or more joints. Articular cartilage, also known as *hyaline cartilage,* contains water and a matrix of:

- Proteoglycans (glycoproteins containing chondroitin, keratin sulfate, and other substances)
- Collagen (elastic substance)
- Chondrocytes (cartilage-forming cells)

As people age or experience joint injury, proteoglycans and water decrease in the joint. The production of synovial fluid, which provides joint lubrication and nutrition, also declines because of the decreased synthesis of hyaluronic acid and less body fluid in the older adult (Antonelli & Starz, 2012).

In patients of any age with OA, enzymes, such as stromelysin, break down the articular matrix. In early disease, the cartilage changes from its normal bluish white, translucent color to an opaque and yellowish brown appearance. As cartilage and the bone beneath the cartilage begin to erode, the joint space narrows and **osteophytes** (bone spurs) form (Fig. 18-1). As the disease progresses, fissures, calcifications, and ulcerations develop and the cartilage thins. Inflammatory cytokines (enzymes) such as interleukin-1 (IL-1) enhance this deterioration. The body's normal repair process cannot overcome the rapid process of degeneration (McCance et al., 2014). Secondary joint INFLAMMATION can occur when joint involvement is severe.

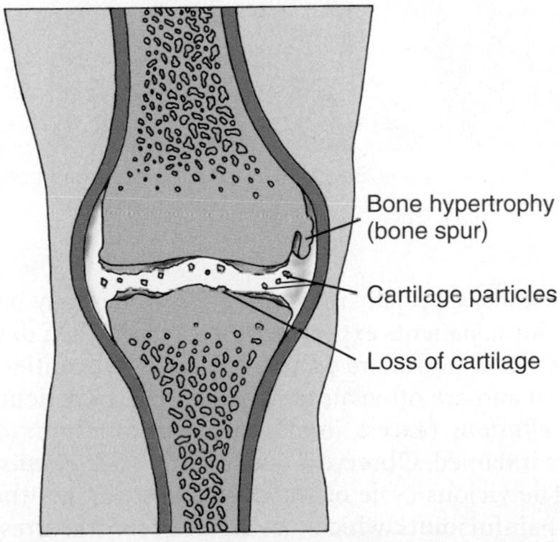

FIG. 18-1 Joint changes in degenerative joint disease.

Eventually the cartilage disintegrates and pieces of bone and cartilage "float" in the diseased joint causing **crepitus,** a grating sound caused by the loosened bone and cartilage. The resulting joint pain and stiffness can lead to decreased mobility and muscle atrophy. Muscle tissue helps support joints, particularly those that bear weight (e.g., hips, knees).

Etiology and Genetic Risk

The cause of OA is a combination of many factors. For patients with *primary* OA, the disease is caused by aging and genetic factors. Weight-bearing joints (hips and knees), the vertebral column, and the hands are most commonly affected, probably because they are used most often or bear the mechanical stress of body weight and many years of use.

Secondary OA occurs less often than primary disease and results from joint injury and obesity (Antonelli & Starz, 2012). Injury to the joints from excessive use, trauma, or other joint disease (e.g., rheumatoid arthritis) predisposes a person to OA. Heavy manual occupations (e.g., carpet laying, construction, farming) cause high-intensity or repetitive stress to the joints. The risk for hip and knee OA is increased in professional athletes, especially football players, runners, and gymnasts. Fractures or other joint tissue injuries can lead to OA years after the trauma. Certain metabolic diseases (e.g., diabetes mellitus, Paget's disease of the bone) and blood disorders (e.g., hemophilia, sickle cell disease) can also cause joint degeneration.

Obesity is a common contributing factor to osteoarthritis. Weight-bearing joints, such as hips and knees, are most often affected in obese people.

Incidence and Prevalence

The prevalence of OA varies among different populations but is a universal problem. Most people older than 60 years have joint changes that can be seen on x-ray examination, although not all of those people actually develop the disease. According to Arthritis Foundation (2013b) estimates, 27 million people in the United States have symptomatic osteoarthritis.

GENDER HEALTH CONSIDERATIONS

Patient-Centered Care QSEN

More men than women younger than 55 years have AO, but after 55, women have it more often than men (Antonelli & Starz, 2012). Although the cause for this difference is not known, contributing factors may include increased obesity in women after having children, broader hips in women than men, and more athletic injuries in young men as compared with young women (Arthritis Foundation, 2013b).

Lesbian women and bisexuals are more likely to be overweight or obese when compared with other populations. Although the reason for this difference is not known, it is possible that lesbian women and bisexual people use food as a coping strategy because many have fears and concerns about "coming out" about their sexual orientation, especially to health care professionals and family members (Pettinato, 2012). Be sure to assess all patients in the hospital or community-based setting, particularly those who are older and obese, for clinical manifestations of osteoarthritis.

Health Promotion and Maintenance

The Arthritis Foundation's Osteoarthritis Intervention Working Group produced an evidence-based document that proposed the Public Health Agenda needed to prevent and manage osteoarthritis.

❖ PATIENT-CENTERED COLLABORATIVE CARE

◆ Assessment

History. Patients with OA usually seek medical attention in ambulatory care settings for their joint pain. However, you will also care for those who have OA as a secondary diagnosis in acute and chronic care facilities. Ask the patient about the course of the disease. Collect information specifically related to OA, such as the nature and location of joint PAIN and how much pain and suffering he or she is experiencing. *Remember that older patients may underreport pain, resulting in inadequate management.* Use a 0-to-10 scale or other assessment tool to assess PAIN intensity. Chapter 3 discusses pain assessment in detail.

Other questions to ask include:

- If joint stiffness has occurred, where and for how long?
- When and where has any joint swelling occurred?
- What do you do to control the PAIN or stiffness?
- Do you have any loss of MOBILITY or difficulty in performing ADLs?

Because this disease occurs more often in older women, age and gender are important factors for the nursing history. Ask patients about their occupation, nature of work, history of injury (including falls), weight history, and current or previous involvement in sports. A history of obesity is significant, even for those currently within the ideal range for body weight. Document any family history of arthritis. Determine whether the patient has a current or previous medical condition that may cause joint symptoms.

Physical Assessment/Clinical Manifestations. In the early stage of the disease, the clinical manifestations of OA may appear similar to those of rheumatoid arthritis (RA). The distinction between OA and RA becomes more evident as the disease progresses. Table 18-1 compares the major characteristics of both diseases and their common drug therapy.

The typical patient with OA is a middle-aged or older woman who reports *chronic joint pain and stiffness.* Early in the course of the disease, the PAIN diminishes after rest and worsens after activity. Later the pain occurs with slight motion or even when at rest. Because cartilage has no nerve supply, the pain is caused by joint and soft-tissue involvement and by spasms of the surrounding muscles. During the joint examination, the patient may have tenderness on palpation or when putting the joint through range of motion. **Crepitus** may be felt or heard as the joint goes through range of motion. One or more joints may be affected. The patient may also report joint stiffness that usually lasts less than 30 minutes after a period of inactivity.

On inspection, the joint is often enlarged because of bony hypertrophy. The joint feels hard on palpation. The presence of INFLAMMATION in patients with OA indicates a secondary synovitis. About half of patients with hand involvement have **Heberden's nodes** (bony nodules at the distal interphalangeal [DIP] joints) and **Bouchard's nodes** (bony nodules at the proximal interphalangeal [PIP] joints) (Fig. 18-2). Although OA is *not* a bilateral, symmetric disease, these large bony nodes appear on both hands, especially in women. The nodes may be painful and red. Some patients experience discomfort when developing nodes or when nodes are palpated. These deformities tend to be familial and are often a cosmetic concern to patients.

Joint effusions (excess joint fluid) are common when the knees are inflamed. Observe any *atrophy of skeletal muscle* from disuse. The vicious cycle of the disease discourages the movement of painful joints, which may result in contractures, muscle atrophy, and further PAIN. *Loss of function* or MOBILITY may

TABLE 18-1 Differential Features of Rheumatoid Arthritis and Osteoarthritis

CHARACTERISTIC	RHEUMATOID ARTHRITIS	OSTEOARTHRITIS
Typical onset (age)	35-45 yr	Older than 60 yr
Gender affected	Female (3:1)	Female (2:1)
Risk factors or cause	Autoimmune (genetic basis) Emotional stress (triggers exacerbation) Environmental factors	Aging Genetic factor (possible) Obesity Trauma Occupation
Disease process	Inflammatory	Degenerative
Disease pattern	Bilateral, symmetric, multiple joints Usually affects upper extremities first Distal interphalangeal joints of hands spared Systemic	May be unilateral, single joint Affects weight-bearing joints and hands, spine Metacarpophalangeal joints spared Nonsystemic
Laboratory findings	Elevated rheumatoid factor, antinuclear antibody, ESR	Normal or slightly elevated ESR
Common drug therapy	NSAIDs (short-term use) Methotrexate Leflunomide (Arava) Corticosteroids Biological response modifiers Other immunosuppressive agents	NSAIDs (short-term use) Acetaminophen Other analgesics

ESR, Erythrocyte sedimentation rate; *NSAIDs*, nonsteroidal anti-inflammatory drugs.

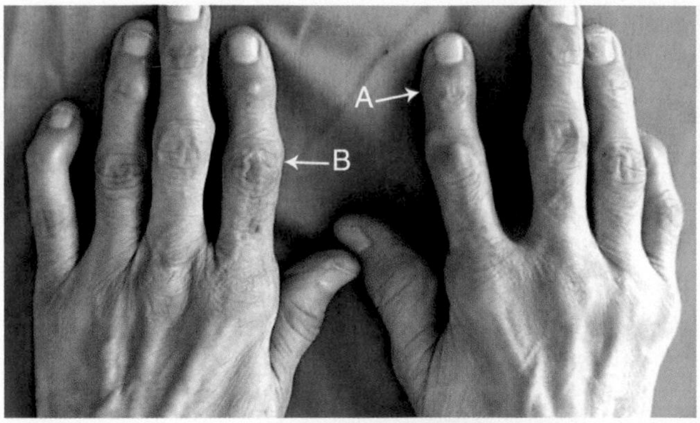

FIG. 18-2 Heberden's and Bouchard's nodes are enlarged bony nodules affecting the joints of the hand.

result, depending on which joints are involved. Hip or knee pain may cause the patient to limp and restrict walking distance.

Osteoarthritis (OA) can affect the spine, especially the lumbar region at the L3-4 level or the cervical region at C4-6 (neck). Compression of spinal nerve roots may occur as a result of vertebral facet bone spurs. The patient typically reports radiating PAIN, stiffness, and muscle spasms in one or both extremities.

Severe pain and deformity interfere with ambulation and self-care. In addition to performing a musculoskeletal assessment, collaborate with the physical and occupational therapists to conduct a functional assessment. Assess the patient's MOBILITY and ability to perform ADLs. Chapter 6 describes functional assessment.

Psychosocial Assessment. OA is a chronic condition that may cause permanent changes in lifestyle. An inability to care for oneself in advanced disease can result in role changes and other losses. Constant PAIN interferes with quality of life. Chronic pain can also affect sexuality. Patients may not have the energy for sexual intercourse or may find positioning uncomfortable.

Patients with continuous PAIN from arthritis may develop depression or anxiety. The patient may also have a role change in the family, workplace, or both. To identify changes that have been or need to be made, ask his or her roles before the disease developed. Identify coping strategies to help live with the disease. Ask the patient about his or her expectations regarding treatment for OA.

In addition to role changes, joint deformities and bony nodules often alter body image and self-esteem. Observe the patient's response to body changes. Does he or she ignore them or seem overly occupied with them? Ask patients directly how they perceive their body image. Document your assessment findings in the interdisciplinary electronic health record per agency policy.

Laboratory Assessment. The health care provider uses the history and physical examination to make the diagnosis of OA. The results of routine laboratory tests are usually normal but can be helpful in screening for associated conditions. The erythrocyte sedimentation rate (ESR) and high-sensitivity C-reactive protein (hsCRP) may be slightly elevated when secondary synovitis (synovial INFLAMMATION) occurs. The ESR also tends to rise with age, infection, and other inflammatory disorders.

Imaging Assessment. Routine x-rays are useful in determining structural joint changes. Specialized views are obtained when the disease cannot be visualized on standard x-ray film but is suspected. Magnetic resonance imaging (MRI) and computed tomography (CT) may be used to determine vertebral or knee involvement.

◆ Analysis

The priority NANDA-I nursing diagnoses and collaborative problems for patients with osteoarthritis (OA) include:

1. Chronic Pain related to cartilage deterioration (NANDA-I)
2. Impaired Mobility related to joint pain and muscle atrophy (NANDA-I)

◆ Planning and Implementation

In 2010, the Osteoarthritis Research Society International (OARSI) committee updated its evidence-based expert consensus guidelines for patients with knee, hand, and hip OA (Zhang et al., 2010). These interdisciplinary best practice guidelines were also supported by the Arthritis Foundation and have major implications for nursing care.

Managing Chronic Pain

Planning: Expected Outcomes. The patient with OA is expected to have PAIN control that is acceptable to the patient (e.g., at a 3 on a pain intensity scale of 0 to 10).

Interventions. No drug therapy can influence the course of OA. Optimal management of patients with OA requires a multimodal approach (combination of therapies) to manage PAIN. If these measures are ineffective, surgery may be performed to reduce pain (Zhang et al., 2010). Perform a pain assessment before and after implementing interventions.

Nonsurgical Management. Management of chronic joint PAIN can be challenging for both the patient and the health care professional. Drug therapy and a variety of nonpharmacologic therapies are used to manage the patient with OA. Chapter 3 elaborates on interventions for chronic non-cancer pain.

Drug Therapy. The purpose of drug therapy is to reduce PAIN caused by cartilage destruction, muscle spasm, and/or secondary joint INFLAMMATION. The American Pain Society, American Geriatrics Society, and OARSI committee recommend regular *acetaminophen* (Tylenol, Atasol♣) as the primary drug of choice because OA is not a primary anti-inflammatory disorder (Davies, 2011).

! NURSING SAFETY PRIORITY (QSEN)

Drug Alert

Patients are at risk for liver damage if they take more than 3000 mg daily of acetaminophen, have alcoholism, or have liver disease. *Older adults are particularly at risk because of normal changes of aging, such as slowed excretion of drug metabolites.* Remind patients to read the labels of over-the-counter (OTC) or prescription drugs that could contain acetaminophen before taking them. Teach them that their liver enzyme levels will be monitored while taking this drug.

Topical drug applications may help with temporary relief of PAIN. Prescription lidocaine 5% patches (Lidoderm) have been approved by the Federal Drug Administration (FDA) for postherpetic neuralgia (nerve pain) but may also relieve joint PAIN (especially the knee) for some patients. Teach the patient to apply the patch on clean, intact skin for 12 hours each day. Up to three patches may be applied to painful joints at one time. Remind him or her that Lidoderm can cause skin irritation. Teach the patient that the lidocaine patch is contraindicated in those patients taking class I antidysrhythmics. Topical salicylates, such as OTC Aspercreme patch, gel, or cream, are also useful for some patients as a temporary pain reliever, especially for knee pain. Buspirone HCl (Buspar) topical cream may also relieve local joint pain for some patients.

If acetaminophen or topical agents do not relieve PAIN, the analgesic drug class of choice is *nonsteroidal anti-inflammatory drugs (NSAIDs)* if the patient can tolerate them. These traditional drugs supported by OARSI guidelines include oral COX-2 nonselective and selective NSAIDs and topical NSAIDs.

Before beginning oral NSAID therapy, baseline laboratory information is obtained, including a complete blood count (CBC) and kidney and liver function tests. Celecoxib (Celebrex), a COX-2 inhibitor, is usually the first choice unless the patient has hypertension, kidney disease, or cardiovascular disease.

NURSING SAFETY PRIORITY (QSEN)

Drug Alert

All of the COX-2 inhibiting drugs are thought to cause cardiovascular disease, such as myocardial infarction, and kidney problems. Older NSAIDs, such as ibuprofen, can cause severe GI side effects, bleeding, and acute kidney failure. Therefore they are prescribed at the lowest effective dose for a short period of time (Davies, 2011). Teach your patient about adverse effects from NSAIDs and the need to report them to his or her health care provider. Examples include having dark, tarry stools; shortness of breath; edema; frequent dyspepsia (indigestion); **hematemesis** (bloody vomitus); and changes in urinary output.

Topical NSAIDs are considered to be safe and effective nonsystemic drugs for pain relief. For example, the diclofenac-epolamine patch and diclofenac solution are used for patients with signs and symptoms associated with knee OA.

When topical or systemic drugs are not effective and for temporary relief of PAIN in a single joint, the health care provider may inject an individual joint with cortisone, a commonly used steroid. Patients may have the same joint injected up to 4 times a year, or once every 3 months. Frequently injected joints include the knee, base of the thumb, shoulder, and trochanteric bursa, which people often call the *hip*.

Other agents, such as hyaluronate (Hyalgan) and hylan G-F 20 (Synvisc), are specific injections for knee and hip PAIN associated with OA. These synthetic joint fluid implants replace or supplement the body's natural hyaluronic acid, which is broken down by inflammation and aging.

Other oral drugs that can be given to patients with OA include muscle relaxants and opioids. Muscle relaxants, such as cyclobenzaprine hydrochloride (Flexeril), are sometimes given for painful muscle spasms, especially those occurring in the back from OA of the vertebral column. *These drugs should be used with caution in older adults because they can cause acute confusion. Remind any patient not to drive or operate dangerous machinery when taking muscle relaxants.* Weak opioid drugs such as tramadol (Ultram or Ultram ER) may also be given for patients with OA. Chapter 3 discusses drug therapy for pain relief in more detail.

NCLEX EXAMINATION CHALLENGE

Physiological Integrity

The health care provider prescribes celecoxib (Celebrex) for a client with osteoarthritis. What health teaching will the nurse provide for this client regarding this drug? **Select all that apply.**

A. "Take the drug on an empty stomach before breakfast."
B. "Stop taking the drug if unusual bleeding occurs and call your health care provider."
C. "Report frequent episodes of indigestion to your health care provider."
D. "Expect fluid accumulation in your legs and feet that usually gets worse during the day."
E. "Call 911 immediately if chest pain occurs."

Nonpharmacologic Interventions. In addition to analgesics, many nonpharmacologic measures can be used for patients with OA, such as rest balanced with exercise, joint positioning, heat or cold applications, weight control, and a variety of complementary and alternative therapies.

Teach the patient to *position joints in their functional position.* For example, when in a supine position (recumbent), he or she should use a small pillow under the head or neck but avoid the use of other pillows. The use of large pillows under the knees or head may result in flexion contractures. If needed, the legs may be elevated 8 to 12 inches (20 to 30 cm) to reduce back discomfort. Remind him or her to use proper posture when standing and sitting to reduce undue strain on the vertebral column. Teach the patient to wear supportive shoes; foot insoles may help relieve pressure on painful metatarsal joints. Collaborate with the physical therapist (PT) to plan a program for muscle-strengthening exercises to better support the joints.

Most patients apply *heat* or *cold* for temporary relief of PAIN, but not all patients find these modalities effective. Heat may help decrease the muscle tension around the tender joint and thereby decrease pain. Suggest hot showers and baths, hot packs or compresses, and moist heating pads. *Regardless of treatment, teach him or her to check that the heat source is not too heavy or so hot that it causes burns.* A temperature just above body temperature is adequate to promote comfort.

If needed, collaborate with the PT to provide special heat treatments, such as paraffin dips, diathermy (using electrical current), and ultrasonography (using sound waves). A 15- to 20-minute application usually is sufficient to temporarily reduce PAIN, spasm, and stiffness. Cold packs or gels that feel hot and cold at the same time may also be used.

Cold therapy has limited use for most patients in controlling PAIN. Cold works by numbing nerve endings and decreasing secondary joint inflammation, if present.

NURSING SAFETY PRIORITY (QSEN)

Action Alert

Teach the patient to use ice packs that are not too heavy. Do not place them directly on skin; instead, wrap them in a towel or soft cloth.

There is no one food that causes or cures arthritis. Instead, a well-balanced diet is recommended. Gradual *weight loss* for obese patients may lessen the stress on weight-bearing joints, decrease pain, and perhaps slow joint degeneration. If needed, collaborate with the registered dietitian to provide more in-depth teaching and meal planning or make referrals to community resources.

Complementary and Alternative Therapies. Some patients with OA have reported that a variety of complementary and alternative medicine (CAM) therapies are useful. However, the evidence supporting their effectiveness is often inconsistent and inconclusive (see the Evidence-Based Practice box).

Topical *capsaicin* products are safe over-the-counter (OTC) drugs. They work by blocking or modifying substance P and other neurotransmitters for PAIN. Tell the patient using capsaicin to expect a burning sensation for a short time after applying it. Recommend the use of plastic gloves for application. To prevent burning of eyes or other body areas, wash hands immediately after applying the substance.

Dietary supplements may complement traditional drug therapies. Glucosamine and chondroitin are widely used and are the most effective nonprescription supplements taken to decrease PAIN and improve functional ability. However, the evidence to support their use is inconsistent (Fouladbakhsh, 2012).

EVIDENCE-BASED PRACTICE QSEN

Which Complementary and Alternative Methods Best Relieve Osteoarthritis Symptoms?

Fouladbakhsh, J. (2012). Complementary and alternative modalities to relieve osteoarthritis symptoms. *Orthopaedic Nursing, 31*(2), 115-121.

The author conducted a systematic review of current literature to determine the effectiveness and safety of commonly used complementary and alternative medicine (CAM) therapies in patients with osteoarthritis (OA), including mind-body therapies, supplements, and body-based treatments.

Research findings related to mind-body therapies revealed limited evidence for the use of yoga and a moderate level of evidence supporting the use of tai chi for patients with OA. According to the literature review, the only energy therapy that is moderately effective for OA is acupuncture for pain relief. Evidence for the use of glucosamine and chondroitin sulfate supplement is inconsistent. No evidence exists to support the use of most other supplements except for pycnogenol (pine bark extract). Research shows that massage therapy, a body-based treatment, for patients with OA is moderately effective for the relief of back pain.

Level of Evidence: 1

The author conducted a systematic literature review (previous 10 years) to draw conclusions about the effectiveness of selected CAM therapies for patients who have OA.

Commentary: Implications for Practice and Research

Further study is needed to examine the effectiveness of commonly used CAM therapies by patients with OA. Consistency in studies is needed to provide clearer answers and explore the complexity of these therapies. Nurses caring for patients with OA need to provide information about the evidence or lack of evidence for CAM therapies. Before patients take supplements such as glucosamine, remind them to check with their health care provider about their safety.

CHART 18-1 Patient and Family Education: Preparing for Self-Management

Considerations for Taking Glucosamine Supplements

- Tell your health care provider if you decide to take glucosamine.
- Do not take glucosamine if you have hypertension.
- Do not take glucosamine if you are pregnant or breast-feeding.
- Monitor for bleeding if you take chondroitin with glucosamine or chondroitin alone if you are on anticoagulant therapy.
- If diabetic, monitor your blood glucose levels carefully because taking glucosamine for a prolonged time can increase them.
- Be aware that glucosamine can cause adverse effects such as a rash; GI disturbances, especially diarrhea; drowsiness; and headache.
- Be sure to take the recommended dosage based on your weight.
- Read drug labels to ensure that you do not take too much glucosamine for your weight; some drug names may not indicate they contain glucosamine (e.g., Bioflex, Arth-X Plus, Nutri-Joint).

These natural products are found in and around bone cartilage for repair and maintenance. **Glucosamine** may decrease inflammation, and **chondroitin** may play a role in strengthening cartilage. These supplements are used topically or taken in oral form. Chart 18-1 summarizes what you should teach your patients about glucosamine, with or without chondroitin.

CLINICAL JUDGMENT CHALLENGE

Patient-Centered Care; Evidence-Based Practice QSEN

A 66-year-old woman visits a new health care provider for a physical examination. She tells you that she works in a school cafeteria and has to stand most of the day. When you take an admission history, she tells you that she has pain and stiffness in her knees, feet, hands, and cervical spine. She takes ibuprofen when needed with some pain relief but has frequent indigestion for which she takes OTC Zantac. The patient is 5′4″ tall and weighs 183 pounds today.

During her physical assessment, you note that the patient has multiple Heberden's and Bouchard's nodes on both hands and a swollen right knee. She has a joint effusion in her right third PIP, and she is right-handed. The health care provider diagnoses her joint involvement as osteoarthritis (OA).

1. What additional physical assessment do you need to perform to determine the patient's level of functioning?
2. What risk factors contribute to her diagnosis of OA?
3. What OTC, nonpharmacologic, or CAM therapies for joint pain and stiffness might you recommend? What evidence supports those recommendations?
4. How might this patient's OA affect her ability to continue working in her current job?
5. What health teaching is needed for this patient to help manage her OA?

Surgical Management. Surgery may be indicated when conservative measures or drug therapy no longer provides PAIN control, when MOBILITY becomes so restricted that the patient cannot participate in activities he or she enjoys, and when he or she cannot maintain the desired quality of life. The most common surgical procedure performed for *older adults* with OA is **total joint arthroplasty (TJA)** (surgical creation of a joint), also known as **total joint replacement (TJR)**. Almost any synovial joint of the body can be replaced with a prosthetic system that consists of at least two parts—one for each joint surface. TJAs are expected to increase exponentially as baby boomers age over the next 20 years.

Total joint arthroplasty is a procedure used most often to manage the PAIN of OA and to improve MOBILITY, although other conditions causing cartilage destruction may require the surgery. These disorders include RA, congenital anomalies, trauma, and osteonecrosis. **Osteonecrosis** is bony necrosis secondary to lack of blood flow, usually from trauma or chronic steroid therapy. Hip and knee joints are most commonly replaced, but finger and wrist joint, elbow, shoulder, toe joint, and ankle replacements have been improved in the past 15 years.

The *contraindications* for TJA are active infection anywhere in the body, advanced osteoporosis, and rapidly progressive inflammation. An infection elsewhere in the body or from the joint being replaced can result in an infected TJA and subsequent prosthetic failure. Therefore if a patient has a urinary tract infection, for example, the physician treats the infection before surgery. Advanced osteoporosis can cause bone shattering during insertion of the prosthetic device. Severe medical problems, such as uncontrolled diabetes or hypertension, put the patient at risk for major postoperative complications and possible death.

Total Hip Arthroplasty. The number of total hip arthroplasty (THA) procedures (also known as *total hip replacement [THR]*) has steadily increased over the past 35 years. The first time a patient receives any total joint arthroplasty, it is referred to as **primary arthroplasty**. If the implant loosens, **revision arthroplasty** may be performed. Availability of improved joint implant materials and better custom design features allow longer life of a replaced hip. Although patients of any age can undergo THR, the procedure is performed most often in those older than 60 years. *The special needs and normal physiologic changes of older adults often complicate the perioperative period and may result in additional postoperative complications.*

Preoperative Care. As with any surgery, preoperative care begins with assessing the patient's level of understanding about the surgery and his or her ability to participate in the postoperative plan of care. The surgeon explains the procedure and postoperative expectations (including possible complications) during the office visit, but this patient education may have occurred weeks or months before the scheduled surgery. Some patients may not know what questions to ask or may forget the important information that was taught. Information may be provided in a notebook or DVD format that the patient can take home to review and share with family. This is particularly useful to patients with poor reading skills or poor memory. Written materials or other media provided in the patient's language appropriate for the patient's educational level are essential.

In some hospitals or orthopedic office practices, the physical therapist (PT) may have the patient practice transfers, positioning, and ambulation. An occupational therapist (OT) may partner with the PT to assist in exercises or learning to ambulate with an assistive device, such as crutches or a walker. The OT may also help obtain assistive/adaptive equipment that will be needed after surgery. The cost of some items, such as an elevated toilet seat, is covered by Medicare and other insurers because they are essential to prevent hip dislocation. Other helpful equipment, such as grab bars and shower chairs, may not be paid for by third-party payers and can be purchased at local pharmacies or medical supply stores, based on the patient's specific needs.

All patients are also told to visit a dentist and have any necessary dental procedures done before surgery. After surgery, he or she must take extreme care not to acquire an infection that could migrate to the surgical area and cause prosthetic failure. *Remind the patient to tell any future health care provider that he or she has had any total joint arthroplasty.*

In addition to usual preoperative laboratory tests, the surgeon may ask the patient with RA to have a cervical spine x-ray if he or she is having general anesthesia. Those with RA often have cervical spine disease that can lead to subluxation during intubation. Hip x-rays, CT scan, and/or MRI may be done to assess the operative joint and surrounding soft tissues.

Because venous thromboembolism (VTE) is a serious postoperative complication, especially for hip surgery, assess the patient's risk factors for clotting problems, including history of previous clotting, obesity, smoking, and advanced age. *Teach patients that drugs that increase the risks for clotting and bleeding, such as NSAIDs, vitamins C and E, and hormone replacement therapy (HRT) or oral contraceptive drugs, must be discontinued about a week before surgery.*

Patients are also assessed for the need for possible blood transfusion after surgery. For patients who are at risk for postoperative anemia, one or more blood transfusions may be needed. Autologous (patient's own) or banked blood can be used. If desired, the patient may donate blood several weeks before surgery to be used after surgery. This pre-deposit autologous blood donation is a safe and cost-effective blood replacement alternative for those who are undergoing elective surgeries. It also decreases the risk for blood transfusion reactions.

For some patients, the surgeon may prescribe several weeks of epoetin alfa (Epogen, Procrit, Eprex ♣) with or without iron to prevent anemia that can occur after hip or knee replacement. Epoetin alfa is recombinant human erythropoietin, a substance that is essential for developing red blood cells. This drug is particularly useful for older adults, who frequently have mild anemia before surgery.

Remind patients that they will likely be asked to take a shower with special antiseptic soap the night before surgery to decrease bacteria that could cause infection after surgery. Tell them to wear clean nightwear after their shower and sleep on clean linen. Review which drugs are safe to take or necessary the morning of the operation, such as antihypertensives, and which ones should be avoided. Medication should be taken with a very small amount of water to prevent vomiting and aspiration during surgery. See Chapter 14 for additional preoperative care for any type of surgery.

Operative Procedures. Similar to other orthopedic surgeries, the patient receives an IV antibiotic, usually a cephalosporin such as cefazolin (Ancef), within an hour before the initial surgical incision to help prevent INFECTION.

The anesthesiologist or nurse anesthetist places the patient under general or **neuraxial** (epidural/spinal) anesthesia for lower extremity surgery. Neuraxial induction reduces blood loss and the incidence of deep vein thrombosis. Intraoperative blood loss with hypotensive neuraxial anesthesia is usually less than that with general anesthesia, thereby decreasing the need for postoperative blood transfusions. Patients receiving general anesthesia may have a regional nerve block, which lasts up to 24 hours after surgery.

Some patients are candidates for *minimally invasive surgery* (MIS) using a smaller incision with special instruments to reduce muscle cutting. This newer technique cannot be used for patients who are obese or those with osteoporosis. It is done only for primary THAs, not for revision surgeries. Like those of any MIS, the benefits of minimally invasive THA are decreased soft tissue damage and postoperative PAIN. Patients often have a shorter hospital stay and quicker recovery. They are generally satisfied with the cosmetic appearance of the incision because there is less scarring. Postoperative complications are not as common in patients having minimally invasive ("mini") hip replacements when compared with those having the traditional technique.

Regardless of procedure type, two components are used in the THA—the acetabular component and the femoral component (Fig. 18-3). A non-cemented prosthesis is most often used. Bone surfaces are smoothed as they are prepared to receive the artificial components. The non-cemented components are press-fitted into the prepared bone. The acetabular cup may be placed using computer or robotic assistance. If the prosthesis is cemented, polymethyl methacrylate (an acrylic fixating substance) is used. A closed wound drainage system may be placed in the wound before the surgeon closes the incision.

Considerations of a non-cemented prosthesis include protection of weight-bearing status to allow bone to grow into the prosthesis and decreased problems with loosening of the prosthesis. With a cemented prosthesis, cement can fracture or deteriorate over time, leading to loosening of the prosthesis, which causes pain and can lead to the need for a revision arthroplasty.

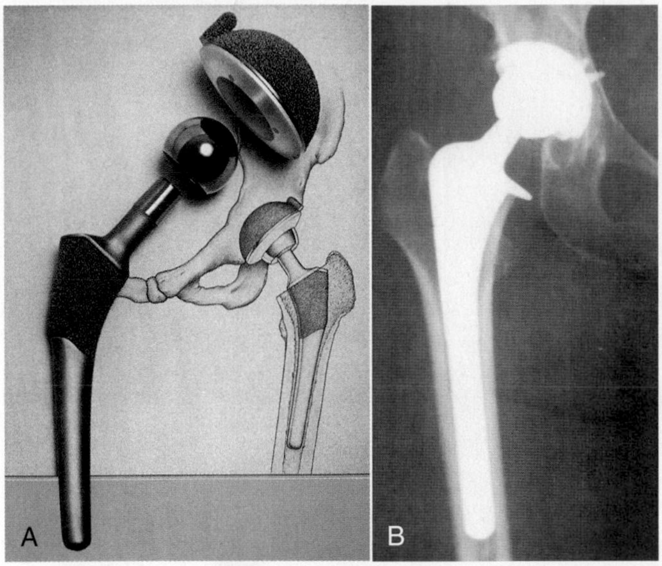

FIG. 18-3 **A,** Two major components of total hip arthroplasty. **B,** X-ray showing the components in place.

In revision arthroplasty, the old prosthesis is removed and new components are replaced. Bone graft may be placed if bone loss is significant. Outcomes from revision arthroplasty may not be as positive as with primary arthroplasty.

Postoperative Care. In addition to providing the routine postoperative care discussed in Chapter 16, assess for and help prevent possible postoperative complications. Table 18-2 summarizes these complications, including nursing measures for prevention, assessment, and intervention. Chart 18-2 highlights special concerns for the care of older adults in the postoperative period. Collaborate with your patient and his or her family to become safety partners to keep the patient free from harm, including complications, such as:

- Hip dislocation
- Venous thromboembolism (VTE)
- Infection
- Anemia
- Neurovascular compromise

Preventing Hip Dislocation. A major complication of THA is **subluxation** (partial dislocation) or total dislocation.

! NURSING SAFETY PRIORITY (QSEN)

Action Alert

Teach patients to maintain correct positioning at all times. When the patient returns from the postanesthesia care unit (PACU), place him or her in a supine position with the head slightly elevated. Place a regular or abduction pillow between the patient's legs to prevent adduction beyond the midline of the body according to agency policy or surgeon preference.

In some hospitals, abduction devices with straps are placed on patients who are restless or cannot follow instructions, especially older adults with delirium or dementia. One or two regular bed pillows are used in most cases to remind patients to keep their legs abducted. For devices with straps, be sure to loosen the straps every 2 hours and check the patient's skin for irritation or breakdown.

TABLE 18-2 Nursing Interventions to Prevent Complications of Lower Extremity Total Joint Arthroplasty

COMPLICATION	PREVENTION/INTERVENTION
Dislocation	Position correctly. For hip, keep leg slightly abducted. For hip, prevent hip flexion beyond 90 degrees. Assess for acute PAIN, rotation, and extremity shortening. Report immediately to physician.
Infection	Use aseptic technique for wound care and emptying of drains. Wash hands thoroughly when caring for patient. Culture drainage fluid, if change. Monitor temperature. Report excessive inflammation or drainage to physician.
Venous thromboembolism	Have patient wear elastic stockings and/or sequential compression device per agency policy. Teach leg exercises to patient. Encourage fluid intake. Observe for signs of thrombosis (redness, swelling, or pain). Observe patient for changes in mental status. Administer anticoagulant as prescribed. Do not massage legs. Do not flex knees for a prolonged period of time.
Hypotension, bleeding, or infection	Take vital signs at least every 4 hours. Observe patient for bleeding. Report excessively low blood pressure or bleeding to physician.

CHART 18-2 Nursing Focus on the Older Adult

Postoperative Care of the Older Adult with a Total Hip Arthroplasty

- Use an abduction pillow or splint to prevent adduction after surgery if the patient is very restless or has an altered mental state.
- Keep the patient's heels off the bed to prevent pressure ulcers.
- Do not rely on fever as a sign of infection; older patients often have infection without fever. Decreasing mental status typically occurs when the patient has an infection.
- When assisting the patient out of bed, move him or her slowly to prevent orthostatic (postural) hypotension.
- Encourage the patient to deep breathe and cough and to use the incentive spirometer every 2 hours to prevent atelectasis and pneumonia.
- As soon as permitted, get the patient out of bed to prevent complications of immobility.
- Anticipate the patient's need for pain medication, especially if he or she cannot verbalize the need for pain control.
- Expect a temporary change in mental state immediately after surgery as a result of the anesthetic and unfamiliar sensory stimuli. Reorient the patient frequently.

Place and support the affected leg in neutral rotation. *Keep the patient's heels off the bed to prevent skin breakdown, particularly older adults.* The procedure for postoperative turning is controversial and specified by agency policy or surgeon preference. In most cases, you are safe to turn the patient if the pillow

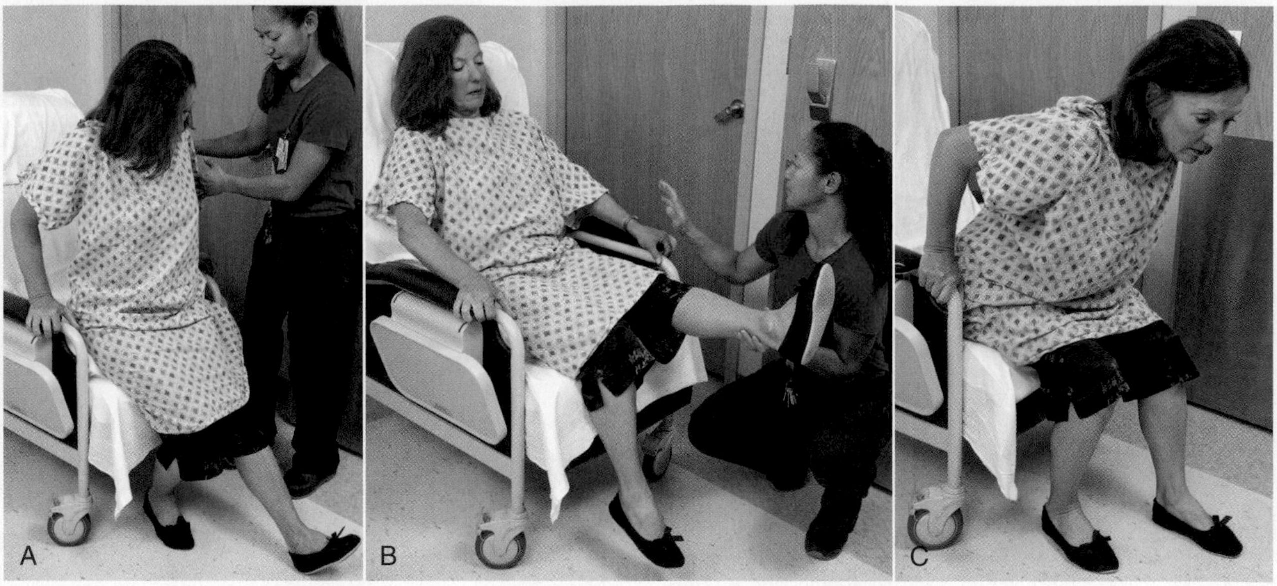

FIG. 18-4 Correct **(A, B)** and incorrect **(C)** hip flexion after a total hip replacement.

is in place. Some surgeons allow only turning directly onto one side or the other, depending on the surgical approach.

Teach the patient and family about other precautions to prevent dislocation as outlined in Chart 18-3. In addition to preventing adduction, remind them that the patient should avoid flexing the hips more than 90 degrees at all times. Use diagrams or demonstrate correct positioning to help reinforce this information before the patient gets out of bed (Fig. 18-4).

! NURSING SAFETY PRIORITY QSEN

Critical Rescue

Observe for possible signs of hip dislocation, which include severe hip PAIN, shortening of the affected leg, and leg rotation. If any of these clinical manifestations occur, keep the patient in bed and notify the surgeon immediately!

If the hip is dislocated, the surgeon manipulates and relocates the affected hip after the patient receives moderate sedation. The hip is then immobilized by an abduction splint or other device until healing occurs—usually in about 6 weeks.

Preventing Venous Thromboembolism. The most potentially life-threatening complication after THA is venous thromboembolism (VTE), which includes deep venous thrombosis (DVT) and pulmonary embolism (PE). *Older patients are especially at increased risk for VTE because of age and decreased circulation before surgery. Obese patients and those with a history of VTE are also at high risk for thrombi.* Apply sequential compression devices (SCDs) and/or antiembolism stockings according to agency policy.

Anticoagulants, such as warfarin (Coumadin, Warfilone 🍁), subcutaneous low-molecular-weight heparin (LMWH), or factor Xa inhibitors, help prevent VTE. Patients are usually on anticoagulants for 3 to 6 weeks after surgery, depending on the patient's response and risk factors. The use of subcutaneous LMWHs has markedly increased for patients with total hip and

CHART 18-3 Patient and Family Education: Preparing for Self-Management

Care of Patients with Total Hip Arthroplasty After Hospital Discharge

Hip Precautions
- Do not sit or stand for prolonged periods.
- Do not cross your legs beyond the midline of your body.
- Do not bend your hips more than 90 degrees.
- Do not twist your body when standing.
- Use an ambulatory aid, such as a walker, when walking.
- Use assistive/adaptive devices for dressing, such as for putting on shoes and socks.
- Do not put more weight on your affected leg than allowed.
- Resume sexual intercourse as usual on the advice of your surgeon.

Pain Management
- Report increased hip pain to the surgeon immediately.
- Take oral analgesics as prescribed and only as needed.
- Do not overexert yourself; take frequent rests.

Incisional Care
- Inspect your hip incision every day for redness, heat, or drainage; if any of these are present, call your physician immediately.
- Cleanse your hip incision with a mild soap and water every day; be sure to dry it thoroughly.

Other Care
- Continue walking and performing the leg exercises as you learned in the hospital.
- Do not cross your legs to help prevent blood clots.
- Report pain, redness, or swelling in your legs to your physician immediately.
- Call 911 for acute chest pain or shortness of breath.
- If you are taking an anticoagulant, follow the precautions learned in the hospital to prevent bleeding; avoid using a straight razor, avoid injuries, and report bleeding or excessive bruising to your surgeon immediately.
- Perform postoperative exercises as instructed, including straight leg raises, gluteal sets, ankle pumps, and "ham" sets.

knee replacements. Examples include enoxaparin (Lovenox), dalteparin (Fragmin), and tinzaparin (Innohep).

As an alternative to LMWHs, subcutaneous fondaparinux (Arixtra), a factor Xa inhibiting agent, may be prescribed for some patients undergoing hip and knee arthroplasty. A newer Xa inhibitor, rivaroxaban (Xarelto), is given orally once a day. You do not need to monitor the international normalized ratio (INR), prothrombin time (PT), or activated partial thromboplastin time (aPTT) for patients receiving these drugs because they do not affect coagulation values. Like other anticoagulants, however, patients are at risk for bleeding. A complete discussion of nursing care associated with patients taking anticoagulants and VTE is found in Chapter 36. The Joint Commission's *VTE Core Measures* are also discussed in that chapter.

Early ambulation and exercise help prevent VTE. Teach the patient about leg exercises, which should begin in the immediate postoperative period and continue through the rehabilitation period. These exercises include plantar flexion and dorsiflexion (heel pumping), circumduction (circles) of the feet, gluteal and quadriceps muscle setting, and straight-leg raises (SLRs). Teach the patient to perform gluteal exercises by pushing the heels into the bed and achieve **quadriceps-setting exercises** ("quad sets") by straightening the legs and pushing the back of the knees into the bed. In addition to preventing clots, these exercises improve muscle tone, which helps restore the function of the extremity.

Preventing Infection. INFECTION can occur during hospitalization or months or years later after a hip replacement. Most infections are caused by contamination during surgery and are considered "deep" infections.

Monitor the surgical incision and vital signs carefully—every 4 hours for the first 24 hours and every 8 to 12 hours thereafter. Observe for signs of INFECTION, such as an elevated temperature and excessive or foul-smelling drainage from the incision. *An older patient may not have a fever with infection but, instead, may experience an altered mental state.* If you suspect this problem, obtain a sample of any drainage for culture and sensitivity to determine the offending organisms and the antibiotics that may be needed for treatment.

Assessing for Bleeding and Managing Anemia. Observe the surgical hip dressing for bleeding or other type of drainage at least every 4 hours or when vital signs are taken. Empty and measure the bloody fluid in the surgical drain(s) every shift. The total amount of drainage is usually less than 50 mL/8 hr. Patients who have the minimally invasive procedure may not have a drain. The surgeon usually removes the drains and operative dressing 24 to 48 hours after surgery. *Take special care when removing tape from the skin to prevent tape burns and skin tears as the surgical dressing is changed, especially for older adults.*

The surgeon also requests periodic hemoglobin and hematocrit (H&H) tests to assess for anemia. Although some patients receive several units of blood during surgery, the H&H levels may continue to fall; in this case, additional blood is given 1 to 2 days after surgery. Blood pressure may be lower than usual because of blood loss during surgery.

Assessing for Neurovascular Compromise. As with other musculoskeletal surgery, monitor neurovascular assessments frequently for a possible compromise in circulation to the affected distal extremity.

In addition to implementing interventions to prevent potential postoperative complications and monitoring for early signs of complications, the interdisciplinary team plans care to manage PAIN, improve MOBILITY and activity, and promote self-management.

! NURSING SAFETY PRIORITY (QSEN)

Action Alert

Check and document color, temperature, distal pulses, capillary refill, movement, and sensation. Remember to compare the operative leg with the nonoperative leg. These assessments are performed at the same time the vital signs are checked. Report any changes in neurovascular assessment to the surgeon, and carefully monitor for changes. Early detection of changes in neurovascular status can prevent permanent tissue damage.

Managing Pain. Although hip arthroplasty is performed to relieve joint PAIN, patients experience pain related to the surgical procedure. Many state that their pain is different and less severe than before surgery. Immediate pain control is typically achieved by extended-release epidural morphine (EREM) or patient-controlled analgesia (PCA) with morphine or another opioid. An NSAID should be taken with the opioid to decrease INFLAMMATION. Chapter 3 contains information on the nursing care associated with these acute pain modalities. *Keep in mind that the patient may also receive additional analgesic drugs for chronic arthritic pain in other joints.*

Regardless of the PAIN management method used, most patients do not require parenteral analgesics after the first day. Oral opioids, such as oxycodone plus acetaminophen (Percocet, Tylox), are then commonly prescribed until the pain can be controlled by NSAIDs such as ketorolac (Toradol, Acular) or ibuprofen (Motrin, Apo-Ibuprofen 🍁).

Nonpharmacologic methods for acute and chronic PAIN control can also be used to decrease the amount of drug therapy used (see Chapter 3). A study by Thomas and Sethares (2010) found that guided imagery can be helpful in controlling pain in patients with total joint arthroplasty.

Promoting Mobility and Activity. Depending on the time of day that the surgery is performed, the patient with a THA gets out of bed with assistance the night of surgery to prevent problems related to impaired MOBILITY (e.g., atelectasis, pneumonia), especially in older adults.

! NURSING SAFETY PRIORITY (QSEN)

Action Alert

Be sure to assist the patient the first time he or she gets out of bed to prevent falls and observe for dizziness. When getting the patient out of bed, stand on the same side of the bed as the affected leg. After the patient sits on the side of the bed, remind him or her to stand on the unaffected leg and pivot to the chair with guidance. *To avoid injury, do not lift the patient!*

Remind the patient to avoid flexing the hips beyond 90 degrees as discussed earlier (see Fig. 18-4). Raised toilet seats and reclining chairs help prevent hyperflexion of the replaced hip joint. Be sure to teach the patient to also *avoid* twisting the body or crossing his or her legs to prevent hip dislocation.

The surgeon, type of prosthesis, and surgical procedure determine the amount of weight bearing that can be applied to the affected leg. A patient with a cemented implant is usually allowed immediate partial weight bearing (PWB) and progresses to full weight bearing (FWB). Typically, only "toe-touch" or minimal weight bearing is permitted for patients with uncemented prostheses. When x-ray evidence of bony ingrowth can be seen, the patient can progress to PWB and then to FWB.

In collaboration with the physical therapist (PT), teach the patient how to follow weight-bearing restrictions. Most patients use a walker (may be a rolling walker), but younger adults may use crutches. They are usually advanced to a single cane or crutch if they can walk without a severe limp 4 to 6 weeks after surgery. When the limp disappears, they no longer need an ambulatory/assistive device and may be permitted to sit in chairs of normal height, use regular toilets, and drive a car.

NCLEX EXAMINATION CHALLENGE

Physiological Integrity

A client had a right total hip arthroplasty 2 days ago. Which precautions will the nurse teach the client to prevent surgical complications? **Select all that apply.**

A. "Stand on your right leg and pivot to the chair."
B. "Do not bend your hips more than 90 degrees."
C. "Cross your legs to be most comfortable."
D. "Avoid twisting your body when moving."
E. "Use a long-handled shoe horn to put on your shoes."

Promoting Self-Management. The hospital's occupational therapy department may supply assistive/adaptive devices to help with ADLs, especially for those having traditional surgery. Particularly important are devices designed for reaching to prevent patients from bending or stooping and flexing the hips more than 90 degrees. Extended handles on shoehorns and dressing sticks may be very useful to achieve ADL independence. Third-party payers may or may not pay for these devices, depending on the patient's status.

For those who have *traditional surgery,* the length of stay in the acute care hospital is typically 2 to 3 days, but older adults or those experiencing postoperative complications may stay longer. Those who have the *minimally invasive THA* are discharged on the second postoperative day or the day of surgery (23-hour stay). Those patients are discharged to home on crutches to practice their own rehabilitative exercises. Most of them are able to return to work in 2 weeks. For that reason, some hospitals have started Rapid Recovery Hip Replacement programs for patients who are candidates for MIS.

Discharge for patients having *traditional surgery* may be to the home, a rehabilitation unit, a transitional care unit, or a skilled unit or long-term care facility for continued rehabilitation before discharge to home. The interdisciplinary team provides written instructions for posthospital care and reviews them with patients and their family members (see Chart 18-3). Be sure to provide a copy of these instructions for the patient.

In some acute care settings, postoperative classes are provided to the caregivers of patients who have joint replacements to improve the quality of the postoperative experience (Mazaleski, 2011). These classes are provided by the interdisciplinary team and include pain management, new medications, activity level, discharge instructions, and home preparation (see the Quality Improvement box).

Acute rehabilitation usually takes 1 to 2 weeks or longer, depending on the patient's age and tolerance and the type of prosthesis used. However, it often takes 6 weeks or longer for complete recovery. Some patients who are discharged to their home are able to attend physical therapy sessions in an office or ambulatory care setting. Others have no means or cannot use community resources and need physical therapy in the home, depending on their health insurance coverage. *Collaborate with the case manager to determine which option is best for your patient.*

QUALITY IMPROVEMENT (QSEN)

Improving Postoperative Total Joint Replacement Education for Caregivers

Mazaleski, A. (2011). Postoperative total joint replacement class for support persons: Enhancing patient and family centered care using a quality improvement model. *Orthopaedic Nursing, 30*(6), 361-364.

Postoperative education is essential to ensure positive patient outcomes and increase patient satisfaction. The orthopedic clinical nurse specialist for an active orthopedic unit suggested a postoperative class on the unit for caregivers of patients who had total joint replacements. The ultimate goal of the education was to promote patient- and family-centered care.

The Plan, Do, Study, Act (PDSA) quality improvement (QI) model was used to guide the planning and implementation of the project. A review of patient and family satisfaction scores revealed poor understanding of drug therapy and its side effects. The class included information on new medications, pain management, activity level, and home preparation. A post-class survey was given to class attendees and used to improve future classes. For example, specific discharge instruction sheets were developed for oxycodone and Warfarin. Since the classes were started, patient and family satisfaction scores increased and over 90% of the class attendees strongly agreed that the information was helpful.

Readmission rates will be monitored for patients whose caregivers attended the class. In addition, questions and concerns related to office staff during follow-up visits will be tracked.

Commentary: Implications for Practice and Research

Research indicates that discharge teaching after surgery improves quality of care and improves patient and family satisfaction. This QI project planned and implemented a class for caregivers of patients who had total joint replacements to educate them on postoperative care at home. The attendees for each class were surveyed to determine their satisfaction with the class. The staff made changes to subsequent classes based on those findings.

Other outcome data are needed to evaluate the effectiveness of the classes. The authors plan to collect these data, including hospital readmission rate and postoperative complications.

Total Knee Arthroplasty. Although many adults require total knee arthroplasty (TKA, also known as *total knee replacement [TKR]*), those who have a knee replaced are often younger than those who have a hip replaced. Continued improvements in total knee implants have increased the expected life of a TKA to 20 years or more, depending on the age and activity level of the patient. An increasing number of patients who have TKAs are overweight or obese. Obesity increases wear and tear on weight-bearing joints, which can lead to revision surgeries. Unilateral (one joint) or bilateral joint replacements done at the same time may be performed, depending on the patient.

Preoperative Care. TKA, like hip replacement, is performed when joint PAIN cannot be managed by conservative measures. When limited MOBILITY severely prevents patients from participating in work or activities they enjoy, this procedure can restore a high quality of life. The preoperative care and teaching for patients undergoing a TKA are similar to that for total hip replacement. However, precautions for positioning are not the same. Differences in patient and family teaching depend on the procedure used by the orthopedic surgeon.

Like the minimally invasive surgery (MIS) for the hip, the knee can also be replaced using MIS. Candidates for mini–knee replacement cannot have severe bone loss, obesity, or previous knee surgery. They should be in good general health. Patients having MIS usually have less blood loss during surgery, less pain, more joint range of motion (less stiffness from scarring), and a faster recovery, leading to a shorter hospital stay. Rapid Recovery Knee Replacement programs for patients having minimally invasive TKA are becoming popular in a number of hospitals.

All patients are given verbal and either written or video preoperative instructions, which include the activity protocol to follow after surgery. The PT and OT provide information about transfers, ambulation, postoperative exercises, and ADL assistance. Patients may practice walking with walkers or crutches to prepare them for ambulation after TKA. Teach patients about the possible need for assistive-adaptive devices to assist with ADLs, including an elevated toilet seat, safety handrails, and dressing devices like a long-handled shoehorn. Some third-party payers cover these devices, depending on the patient's condition and age; however, other insurers may not pay for them. Teach the patient and family how and where this equipment can be obtained to have it available after surgery.

Some surgeons prescribe a continuous passive motion (CPM) machine after knee surgery to increase joint MOBILITY. Others have found that the range of motion for the surgical knee is not improved by using this device. If the patient will have a CPM machine after surgery, be sure to explain what it is and how it is used.

Routine diagnostic testing is requested, as well as any additional tests, such as cervical spine x-rays for patients with rheumatoid arthritis (RA) to determine if the patient can be intubated for anesthesia. Cervical spine involvement occurs in about half of all patients with RA. Changes in the cricoarytenoid joint of the larynx can also make intubation difficult (Nelson, 2011). Knee x-rays, CT scan, and/or MRI may be done to assess the joint and surrounding soft tissues. Rheumatoid arthritis is discussed later in this chapter.

Teach patients that they will need to shower with a special antiseptic soap the night before surgery to decrease bacteria on the skin that could cause INFECTION after surgery. Remind them to wear clean nightwear and sleep on clean linen. Ask them to check with their surgeon about what medications they can take the morning of surgery, including antihypertensives and corticosteroids (taken by many patients with RA). Take these drugs with a small amount of water to prevent vomiting and aspiration during surgery. See Chapter 14 for additional preoperative care for any type of surgery.

Operative Procedures. As with the hip, the knee can be replaced with the patient under general or neuraxial (epidural or spinal) anesthesia. An antibiotic, usually an IV cephalosporin, is given shortly before surgical opening to help prevent INFECTION. In the *traditional surgery,* the surgeon makes a central longitudinal incision about 8 inches (20 cm) long. Osteotomies of the femoral and tibial condyles and of the posterior patella are performed, and the surfaces are prepared for the prosthesis. The femoral component is often non-cemented (using a press-fit) with the tibial component being cemented. The surgeon typically inserts a surgical drain and applies a pressure dressing to decrease edema and bleeding.

Minimally invasive TKA may be performed using a shorter incision and special instruments to spare muscle and other soft tissue. Computer-guided or robotic equipment may be used to ensure accurate positioning of the knee implants. This procedure is referred to as a *computer-assisted TKA.*

Complementary and Alternative Therapies. A newer intervention to reduce the severe PAIN that occurs after knee arthroplasty is the intraoperative insertion of Adlea, a refined capsaicin product, directly into the surgical joint. Most patients who were given Adlea during knee surgery have less acute postoperative pain when compared with others who did not receive the treatment.

Postoperative Care. Postoperative nursing care of the patient with a TKA is similar to that for the patient with a total hip arthroplasty; however, maintaining hip abduction is not necessary. The surgeon may prescribe a CPM machine, which can be applied in the postanesthesia care unit (PACU) or soon after the patient is admitted to the postoperative unit (Fig. 18-5). The CPM machine keeps the prosthetic knee in motion and may prevent the formation of scar tissue, which could decrease knee mobility and increase postoperative pain. In the immediate postoperative period, the surgeon may also prescribe ice packs or an ice machine to decrease swelling at the surgical site. Swelling and bruising are more common with this type of surgery than with hip surgery.

The surgeon, PT, or technician presets the CPM machine for the appropriate range of motion and cycles per minute. A typical initial setting is 20 to 30 degrees of flexion and full extension (0 degrees) at two cycles per minute, but this setting varies according to surgeon preference. The machine is generally used on an intermittent schedule of a designated number of hours several times a day, with the range of motion increased gradually. Observe and document the patient's response to the device, and follow the surgeon's protocol for settings. Chart 18-4 outlines your responsibility when caring for a patient using the CPM machine.

In general, pain control measures for patients with TKA are similar to those with total hip arthroplasty. Many patients report high ratings on the PAIN intensity scale and require IV opioid medications longer than patients with THA, particularly if they have had bilateral surgery. *Be sure to manage your patient's pain to provide comfort, increase his or her participation in physical therapy, and improve joint mobility.*

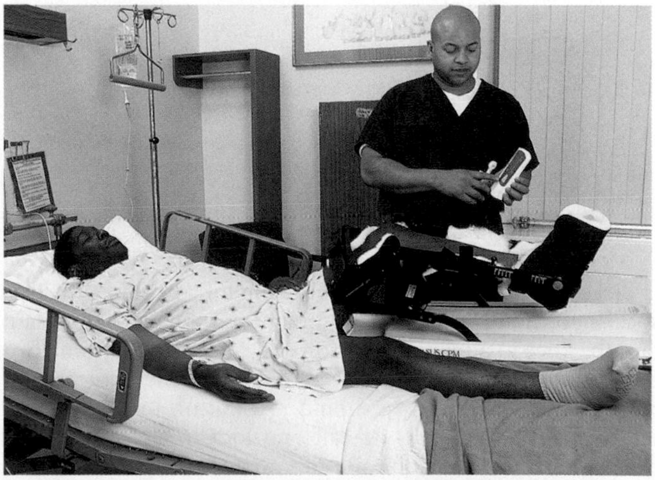

FIG. 18-5 A continuous passive motion (CPM) machine in use.

CHART 18-4 **Best Practice for Patient Safety & Quality Care** QSEN

The Patient Using a Continuous Passive Motion (CPM) Machine

- Ensure that the machine is well padded.
- Check the cycle and range-of-motion settings at least once every 8 hours.
- Ensure that the joint being moved is properly positioned on the machine.
- If the patient is confused, place the controls to the machine out of his or her reach.
- Assess the patient's response to the machine.
- Turn off the machine while the patient is having a meal in bed.
- When the machine is not in use, do not store it on the floor.

One of the most recent advances in postoperative PAIN management for lower extremity total joint arthroplasty is *peripheral nerve blockade (PNB)*. In this procedure, the anesthesiologist injects the femoral or sciatic nerve with local anesthetic; the patient may receive a continuous infusion of the anesthetic by portable pump. This method not only decreases pain but also allows patients to participate in rehabilitation earlier than when using opioid analgesia alone. Patients having continuous femoral nerve blockade (CFNB) after TKA require less opioids and antiemetics when compared with patients receiving no CFNB and those who had a single-shot femoral nerve blockade (FNB).

When caring for a patient receiving a CPNB, perform neurovascular assessments every 2 to 4 hours or according to hospital protocol. The patient should be able to plantarflex and dorsiflex the affected foot but not feel PAIN in the lower leg. Check for movement, sensation, warmth, color, pulses, and capillary refill.

! NURSING SAFETY PRIORITY QSEN

Critical Rescue

Monitor the patient for signs and symptoms that could indicate that the local anesthetic is getting into the patient's system, such as:

- Metallic taste
- Tinnitus
- Nervousness
- Slurred speech
- Bradycardia
- Hypotension
- Decreased respirations
- Seizures

Report any of these new signs and symptoms to the surgeon or anesthesiologist immediately, and carefully continue monitoring the patient for changes.

Because dislocation is a rare problem for a patient with TKA, special positioning to prevent adduction is not required. Maintain the knee in a neutral position and not rotated internally or externally. If a CPM machine is not used, the surgeon may recommend that the knee should rest flat on the bed or with one pillow under the lower calf and foot to encourage slight extension of the knee joint. Be sure that the surgical knee does not hyperextend.

Some complications that affect patients with total hip arthroplasty may also affect those having TKA, such as venous thromboembolism, infection, anemia, and neurovascular compromise. Assessments and interventions associated with these complications are described in the Postoperative Care section of the discussion of Total Hip Arthroplasty on pp. 297-300.

The desired outcome for discharge from the acute hospital unit is that the patient can walk independently with crutches, walker, or cane and has adequate flexion in the operative knee for ambulation. Patients who had minimally invasive TKA are discharged to home in 1 to 2 days with instructions for postoperative exercises, weight bearing, and activity progression. Many of these instructions (except for preventing hip dislocation) are similar to those provided for teaching patients after a total hip arthroplasty (see Chart 18-3).

Patients are able to partially weight bear unless the prosthesis is not cemented. During the home rehabilitation phase, the use of a stationary bicycle or CPM machine may help gain flexion. These patients can return to work and other usual activities in 2 to 3 weeks, depending on their age and other health status factors.

Acute rehabilitation for *traditional* TKA usually takes about 1 to 2 weeks longer, depending on the age and tolerance of the patient. These patients may be discharged to their home or to an acute rehabilitation unit, transitional care unit, skilled unit, or long-term care facility for therapy. They may also be instructed to use a continuous passive motion (CPM) machine at home. If able, they may attend physical therapy sessions in an office or ambulatory care setting. If not, home care services can provide physical therapy and nursing care in their home, depending on the insurance available. *Collaborate with the case manager to determine which option is best for your patient.* Total recovery from traditional TKA takes 6 weeks or longer, especially for those older than 75 years.

NCLEX EXAMINATION CHALLENGE

Safe and Effective Care Environment

A nursing technician is assigned to care for a client who has a CPM machine in place after a total knee arthroplasty. Which statement by the "tech" indicates a need for further teaching and supervision by the nurse?

A. "I will turn off the machine if the client has any pain."
B. "I will turn off the machine when the client eats."
C. "I will store the machine on a chair when not used."
D. "I will check to make sure the client's leg is correctly placed."

Other Joint Arthroplasties. After the hip and knee, the shoulder and hand are the most common joints replaced for severe OA, RA, or trauma. Elbow, wrist, ankle, and foot replacements are not performed as often as other types of arthroplasties. The shoulder and other upper extremity joints do not bear weight and therefore tend to have less degeneration and subsequent PAIN. Preoperative teaching for patients having any of these surgeries depends on the surgeon's technique and postoperative protocols. For example, the continuous passive motion (CPM) machine may be prescribed postoperatively in the hospital and in the posthospital setting (home or other facility). These devices are available for almost any joint surgery in the body. Some surgeons find that the CPM machine is not helpful in promoting joint mobility and may be uncomfortable for patients.

Total shoulder arthroplasty (TSA) has gained popularity as newer prostheses and technology have been developed. This procedure usually decreases arthritic PAIN and increases the patient's ability to perform ADLs. Because the shoulder joint is complex and has many **articulations** (joint surfaces), **subluxation** (partial dislocation) or complete dislocation is a major potential complication. Usually the glenohumeral joint, created by the glenoid cavity of the shoulder blade (scapula) and the head of the humerus, is replaced because it moves the most and is therefore most affected by arthritis. A **hemiarthroplasty** (replacement of part of the joint), typically the humeral component, may be performed as an alternative to TSA.

The surgeon makes an incision to replace the joint while the patient is under general anesthesia. The implant may be cemented or press-fitted without cement. Some surgeons perform *minimally invasive TSA,* which decreases postoperative complications like infection and nerve damage. A sling is applied to immobilize the joint until therapy begins.

In addition to dislocation, postoperative complications are similar to those for other total joint replacements and include infection and neurovascular compromise. Active and passive exercises are needed to begin shoulder movement. *As for any other total joint arthroplasty, perform frequent neurovascular assessments, at least every 4 to 8 hours.* The hospital stay for TSA is shorter than for a total hip or knee replacement. Rehabilitation with an occupational therapist generally takes several months.

Total elbow arthroplasty (TEA) is performed most often for patients with rheumatoid arthritis (RA), but it is done for anyone whose severe arthritis limits MOBILITY and causes uncontrolled PAIN. TEA may be successful in increasing range of motion, but infection and loosening may occur because of extensive tissue cutting during surgery. Active and passive exercises are used postoperatively. In general, elbow motion is allowed as tolerated. Occupational therapy may not be necessary, but the need depends on the individual patient. Lifting is usually restricted on a long-term basis after TEA. Generalized swelling usually resolves in 3 to 6 months.

Any joint of the hand or foot can be replaced *(phalangeal joint, metacarpal or metatarsal arthroplasties),* often for patients with RA. Hand prostheses are implanted without the use of cement because they stay in place and do not bear weight.

For the hand, a bulky dressing is used temporarily after surgery and is then replaced with a dynamic splint. Edema is controlled by having the patient elevate the arm as much as possible. The rehabilitation program for phalangeal joint arthroplasties may last for many weeks until normal function and strength return. These procedures are typically performed in specialized hand centers. Joint replacements in the toe usually require less rehabilitation.

Any bone of the *wrist* can also be replaced, including the heads of the radius and ulna. The postoperative pressure dressing is removed in 1 to 2 days, and a splint is applied. The patient usually regains full function within 6 to 12 weeks, but lifting may be restricted for a longer period. Special hand therapists work with these patients for the extensive rehabilitation that is required for phalangeal and wrist replacements.

Because the ankles support about 25% of the body's weight and are complex joints, developing an implant that is both small enough and strong enough has been difficult. Although total ankle arthroplasties (TAAs) have been problematic for more than three decades, newer non-cemented prosthetic systems have renewed interest in ankle replacements. Surgeons who specialize in foot and ankle surgeries are available in some parts of the country.

Postoperative complications include infection, delayed wound healing, nerve injuries, and loosening. Therefore TAA is not as successful as total hip or knee replacements. Noncemented prostheses seem to be preferred over cemented ones to prevent loosening. The patient is allowed to begin weight bearing at about 6 weeks, and rehabilitation continues for about 3 months.

Improving Mobility

Planning: Expected Outcomes. The patient with osteoarthritis (OA) is expected to maintain or improve a level of MOBILITY and activity that allows him or her to function independently with or without an assistive ambulatory device.

Interventions. Management of the patient with OA is an interdisciplinary effort. If needed, collaborate with the physical therapist (PT) and occupational therapist (OT) to meet the outcome of independent function and MOBILITY. Major interventions include therapeutic exercise and the promotion of ADLs and ambulation by teaching about health and the use of assistive devices.

Certain recreational activities may also be therapeutic, such as swimming to enhance chest and arm muscles. Aerobic exercises (e.g., walking, biking, swimming, aerobic dance) are also recommended. Kim et al. (2012) reported the effectiveness of an aquarobic (water exercise) program for patients with osteoarthritis in increasing MOBILITY and reducing PAIN. Exercises may be prescribed by rehabilitation therapists for the patient with OA, but you will need to reinforce their techniques and principles. The ideal time for exercise is immediately after the application of heat. To prevent further joint damage, teach patients to carefully follow the instructions for exercise outlined in Chart 18-5.

Collaborate with the PT to evaluate the patient's need for ambulatory aids such as canes, walkers, or platform crutches. Although some patients do not like to use these aids or may forget how to use them, they can help prevent further joint deterioration and PAIN. Collaborate with the OT, if needed, to provide suggestions and devices for assistance for ADLs.

CHART 18-5 Patient and Family Education: Preparing for Self-Management

Exercises for Patients with Osteoarthritis or Rheumatoid Arthritis

- Follow the exercise instructions that have been prescribed specifically for you. There are no universal exercises; your exercises have been specifically tailored to your needs.
- Do your exercises on both "good" and "bad" days. Consistency is important.
- Respect pain. Reduce the number of repetitions when the inflammation is severe and you have more pain.
- Use active rather than active-assist or passive exercise whenever possible.
- Do not substitute your normal activities or household tasks for the prescribed exercises.
- Avoid resistive exercises when your joints are severely inflamed.

Community-Based Care

The patient with OA is not usually hospitalized for the disease itself but is admitted for surgical management. Expect that any patient older than 60 years will have some degree of arthritis and possibly chronic pain that needs to be managed.

Home Care Management. If weight-bearing joints are severely involved, the patient may have difficulty going up or down stairs. Making arrangements to live on one floor with accessibility to all rooms is often the best solution. A home care nurse or case manager may collaborate with a rehabilitation therapist to assess the need for structural alterations to the home to accommodate ambulatory aids and enable the patient to perform ADLs. For example, a kitchen counter may need to be lowered or a seat and handrails may need to be installed in the shower. If the patient has undergone a total hip replacement, an elevated toilet seat is necessary for several weeks postoperatively to prevent excessive hip flexion. Patients who have TKAs may also find elevated toilet seats easier to use.

Self-Management Education. Self-management education (SME) is an effective psychosocially focused nonpharmacologic intervention (Shin & Kolanowski, 2010). Learning how to protect joints is the most important part of patient and family education. Preventing further damage to joints slows the progression of OA and minimizes PAIN. Explain the general principles of joint protection, and give practical examples (Chart 18-6).

As with other diseases in which drugs and nutritional therapy are used, teach the patient and family the drug therapy protocol, desired effects and potential side effects, and toxic effects. Emphasize the importance of reducing weight and eating a well-balanced diet to promote tissue healing.

Many patients with arthritis look for a cure after becoming frustrated and desperate about the course of the disease and treatment. Better control of arthritis is possible, but cure is not yet available. Unfortunately, tabloids, books, media, and the Internet often report "curative" remedies. People spend billions of dollars each year on quackery, including liniments, special diets, and copper bracelets. More hazardous substances, such as snake venom and industrial cleaners, are also advertised as remedies. Refer the patient to the Arthritis Foundation for up-to-date information about these "cures." The practice of wearing a copper bracelet will not cure arthritis, but it will not cause harm. If the patient is using a potentially harmful substance or method, however, reinforce the need to avoid the unproven remedy and explain why it should not be used. Respect the patient's preferences, values, and beliefs for using benign remedies that do not cause harm.

With most types of arthritis and connective tissue disease (CTD), patients must live with a chronic, unpredictable, and painful disorder. Their roles, self-esteem, and body image may be affected by these diseases. Body image is often not as devastating in OA as in the inflammatory arthritic diseases, such as RA. The psychosocial component associated with having arthritis is discussed in more detail later in this chapter in the Rheumatoid Arthritis section.

Health Care Resources. The patient who has undergone surgery may need help from community resources. After an arthroplasty, he or she may need assistance with MOBILITY. The patient may be discharged to home or an inpatient unit. Collaborate with the case manager and surgeon to determine the best placement. If the patient is discharged to home, home care nurses may be approved for third-party payment for several visits, depending on the presence of any existing systemic diseases. A home care aide may visit the home to help with hygiene-related needs, and a physical therapist may work with ambulatory and mobility skills. For older patients, a family member, significant other, or other caregiver should be in the home for at least the first few weeks when the patient needs the most assistance. Emphasize the need for patient safety, especially interventions to prevent falls as described in Chapter 2.

Provide written instructions about the required care, regardless of whether the patient goes home or to another inpatient facility. As required by The Joint Commission's National Patient Safety Goals (NPSGs) and other health care accrediting organizations, hand-off communication with the new care provider is essential for seamless continuity of care.

The Arthritis Foundation (www.arthritis.org) is an important community resource for all patients with arthritis and other CTDs. This organization provides information to lay people and health care professionals and refers patients and their families to other resources as needed. Local support groups can help them cope with these diseases.

CHART 18-6 Patient and Family Education: Preparing for Self-Management

Evidence-Based Instructions for Joint Protection

- Use large joints instead of small ones; for example, place your purse strap over your shoulder instead of grasping the purse with your hand.
- Do not turn a doorknob clockwise. Turn it counterclockwise to avoid twisting your arm and promoting ulnar deviation.
- Use two hands instead of one to hold objects.
- Sit in a chair that has a high, straight back.
- When getting out of bed, do not push off with your fingers; use the entire palm of both hands.
- Do not bend at your waist; instead, bend your knees while keeping your back straight.
- Use long-handled devices, such as a hairbrush with an extended handle.
- Use assistive/adaptive devices, such as Velcro closures and built-up utensil handles, to protect your joints.
- Do not use pillows in bed except a small one under your head.
- Avoid twisting or wringing your hands.

◆ *Evaluation: Outcomes*

Evaluate the care of the patient with OA on the basis of the identified priority problems. The expected outcomes are that he or she:

- Achieves PAIN control to a pain intensity level of 3 to 4 on a scale of 0 to 10 or at a level that is acceptable to the patient
- Moves and functions in his or her own environment independently with or without assistive devices

RHEUMATOID ARTHRITIS

❖ *PATHOPHYSIOLOGY*

Rheumatoid arthritis (RA) is a chronic, progressive, systemic inflammatory autoimmune disease process that affects primarily the synovial joints. **Systemic** means this disease affects the body system, affecting many joints and other tissues. RA affects over 1.3 million people, and Euro-Americans have the disease more often than other groups (Arthritis Foundation, 2013c). The cause for this trend is not known.

In RA, transformed autoantibodies (rheumatoid factors [RFs]) are formed that attack healthy tissue, especially synovium, causing inflammation. The disease then begins to involve the articular cartilage, joint capsule, and surrounding ligaments and tendons. IMMUNITY and INFLAMMATION factors cause cartilage damage in patients with RA (McCance et al., 2014):

- CD4 T–helper cells and other immune cells in synovial fluid promote cytokine release, especially interleukin-1 (IL-1) and tumor necrosis factor–alpha (TNFA), which attack cartilage.
- Neutrophils and other inflammatory cells in the joint are activated and break down the cartilage.
- Immune complexes deposit in synovium, and osteoclasts are activated.
- B- and T-lymphocytes of the immune system are stimulated and increase the inflammatory response. (Also see Chapter 17 for a complete discussion of the inflammatory response.)

The synovium then thickens and becomes hyperemic, fluid accumulates in the joint space, and a pannus forms. The **pannus** is vascular granulation tissue composed of inflammatory cells; it erodes articular cartilage and eventually destroys bone. As a result, in late disease, fibrous adhesions, bony ankylosis, and calcifications occur; bone loses density, and secondary osteoporosis occurs.

Permanent joint changes may be avoided if RA is diagnosed early. Early and aggressive treatment to suppress synovitis may lead to a remission. RA is a disease characterized by natural remissions and exacerbations. Interdisciplinary health care team management helps control the disease to decrease the intensity and number of exacerbations. Preventing flares helps prevent joint erosion and permanent joint damage.

Because rheumatoid arthritis is a systemic disease, areas of the body besides the synovial joints can be affected. Inflammatory responses similar to those occurring in synovial tissue may occur in any organ or body system in which connective tissue is prevalent. If blood vessel involvement (**vasculitis**) occurs, the organ supplied by that vessel can be affected, leading to eventual failure of the organ or system in late disease.

The etiology of RA remains unclear, but research suggests a *combination of environmental and genetic factors.* Some researchers also suspect that female reproductive hormones influence the development of RA because it affects women more often than men—usually young to middle-aged women. Others suspect that infectious organisms may play a role, particularly the Epstein-Barr virus (McCance et al., 2014). Physical and emotional stresses have been linked to exacerbations of the disorder and may be contributing factors or "triggers" to its development.

GENETIC/GENOMIC CONSIDERATIONS

Patient-Centered Care QSEN

Research has shown that there is a strong association between RA and several human leukocyte antigen (HLA)-*DR* alleles. The cause of this association is not clear, but most HLA diseases are autoimmune (Nussbaum et al., 2007). *DR* alleles, especially *DR4* and *DRB1*, are the primary genetic factors contributing to the development of RA. *DR4* is associated with more severe forms of the disease. Other contributing factors are being researched.

CHART 18-7 Key Features

The Patient with Rheumatoid Arthritis

Early Manifestations

Joint
- Inflammation

Systemic
- Low-grade fever
- Fatigue
- Weakness
- Anorexia
- Paresthesias

Late Manifestations

Joint
- Deformities (e.g., swan neck or ulnar deviation)
- Moderate to severe pain and morning stiffness

Systemic
- Osteoporosis
- Severe fatigue
- Anemia
- Weight loss
- Subcutaneous nodules
- Peripheral neuropathy
- Vasculitis
- Pericarditis
- Fibrotic lung disease
- Sjögren's syndrome
- Kidney disease
- Felty's syndrome

PATIENT-CENTERED COLLABORATIVE CARE

Assessment

The onset of rheumatoid arthritis (RA) may be acute and severe or slow and progressive; patients may have vague symptoms that last for several months before diagnosis. The onset of the disease is more common in the winter months than in the warmer months. The manifestations of RA can be categorized as early or late disease and as articular (joint) or extra-articular (Chart 18-7).

Physical Assessment/Clinical Manifestations

Early Disease Manifestations. The patient with RA typically reports joint signs and symptoms of joint INFLAMMATION, generalized weakness, and fatigue. Anorexia and a weight loss of about 2 to 3 pounds (1 kg) usually occur early in the disease process. Persistent low-grade fever may accompany these manifestations. In patients with early disease, the upper-extremity joints are involved initially—often the proximal interphalangeal (PIP) and metacarpophalangeal (MCP) joints of the hands. These joints may be slightly reddened, warm, stiff, swollen, and tender or painful, particularly on palpation (caused by synovitis). The typical pattern of joint involvement in RA is bilateral and symmetric (e.g., both wrists). The number of joints involved usually increases as the disease progresses. In early disease, the patient may report migrating symptoms known as **migratory arthritis.**

The presence of only *one* hot, swollen, painful joint (out of proportion to the other joints) may mean the joint is infected. *Refer the patient to the health care provider (generally the rheumatologist) immediately if this is the case.* Single hot, swollen joints are considered infected until proven otherwise and require immediate long-term antibiotic treatment.

Late Disease Manifestations. As the disease worsens, the joints become progressively inflamed and very painful. The patient usually has frequent morning stiffness (also called the **gel phenomenon**), which lasts for 45 minutes to several hours after awakening. On palpation, the joints feel soft and look puffy because of synovitis and **effusions** (joint swelling with fluid, especially the knees). The fingers often appear spindle-like. Note any muscle atrophy (which can result from disuse secondary to joint pain) and a decreased range of motion in the affected joints.

Most or all synovial joints are eventually affected. The temporomandibular joint (TMJ) may be involved in severe disease, but such involvement is uncommon. When the TMJ is affected, the patient may have PAIN when chewing or opening the mouth.

When the spinal column is involved, the cervical joints are most likely to be affected. During clinical examination, gently palpate the posterior cervical spine and identify it as cervical pain, tenderness, or loss of motion.

! NURSING SAFETY PRIORITY QSEN

Critical Rescue

Cervical disease may result in subluxation, especially of the first and second vertebrae. This complication may be life threatening because branches of the phrenic nerve that supply the diaphragm are restricted and respiratory function may be compromised. The patient is also in danger of becoming quadriparetic (weak in all extremities) or quadriplegic (paralyzed in all extremities). If a person with RA reports cervical PAIN (may radiate down one arm) or loss of range of motion in the cervical spine, notify the health care provider immediately.

Joint Involvement. *Joint deformity* occurs as a late, articular manifestation, and secondary osteoporosis can cause bone fractures. Observe common deformities, especially in the hands and feet (Fig. 18-6). Extensive wrist involvement can result in carpal tunnel syndrome (see Chapter 51 for assessment and management of carpal tunnel syndrome).

Gently palpate the tissues around the joints to elicit PAIN or tenderness associated with other rheumatoid complications, unless the patient is having severe joint pain. For example, **Baker's cysts** (enlarged popliteal bursae behind the knee) may occur and cause tissue compression and pain. Tendon rupture is also possible, particularly rupture of the Achilles tendon.

Systemic Complications and Associated Syndromes. Numerous extra-articular clinical manifestations are associated with advanced disease. Assess the patient to ascertain systemic involvement. In addition to increased joint swelling and tenderness, *moderate to severe weight loss, fever, and extreme fatigue* are common in late disease **exacerbations**, often called "flare-ups." Some patients have the characteristic round, movable, nontender **subcutaneous nodules**, which usually appear on the ulnar surface of the arm, on the fingers, or along the Achilles tendon. These nodules can disappear and reappear at any time and are associated with severe, destructive disease. Rheumatoid nodules usually are not a problem themselves; however, they occasionally open and become infected and may interfere with ADLs. Accidentally bumping the nodules may cause discomfort. Occasionally, nodules occur in the lungs.

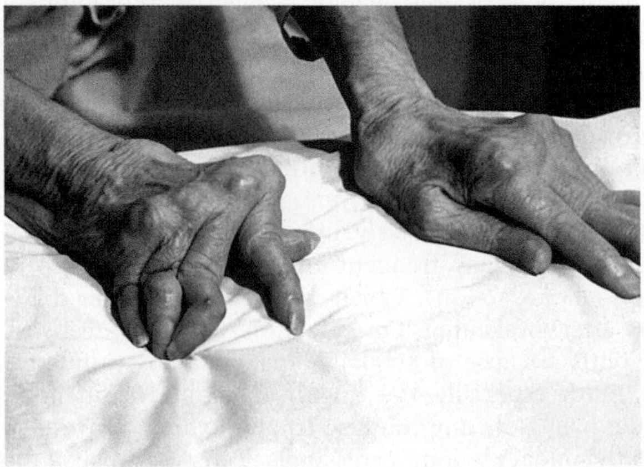

FIG. 18-6 Common joint deformities seen in rheumatoid arthritis.

Inflammation of the blood vessels results in *vasculitis*, particularly of small to medium-size vessels. When arterial involvement occurs, major organs can become ischemic and malfunction. Assess for ischemic skin lesions that appear in groups as small, brownish spots, most commonly around the nail bed (**periungual lesions**). Monitor the number of lesions, note their location each day, and report vascular changes to the health care provider. Increased lesions indicate increased vasculitis, and a decreased number indicates decreased vasculitis. Also carefully assess any larger lesions that appear on the lower extremities. These lesions can lead to ulcerations, which heal slowly as a result of decreased circulation. Peripheral neuropathy associated with decreased circulation can cause footdrop and **paresthesias** (burning and tingling sensations), usually in older adults.

Respiratory complications may manifest as *pleurisy, pneumonitis, diffuse interstitial fibrosis, and pulmonary hypertension.* Cardiac complications include *pericarditis and myocarditis.* These health problems are discussed elsewhere in this text. Assess for eye involvement, which typically manifests as *iritis and scleritis.* If either of these complications is present, the sclera of one or both eyes is reddened and the pupils have an irregular shape. Visual disturbances may occur.

Several syndromes are seen in patients with advanced RA. The most common is **Sjögren's syndrome**, which includes a triad of:

- Dry eyes (keratoconjunctivitis sicca [KCS], or the sicca syndrome)
- Dry mouth (**xerostomia**)
- Dry vagina (in some cases)

Note the patient's report of dry mouth or dry eyes. Some patients state that their eyes feel "gritty," as if sand is in their eyes. Inspect the mouth for dry, sticky membranes and the eyes for redness and lack of tearing.

Less commonly observed is **Felty's syndrome**, which is characterized by RA, hepatosplenomegaly (enlarged liver and spleen), and leukopenia. **Caplan's syndrome** is characterized by the presence of rheumatoid nodules in the lungs.

Psychosocial Assessment. Rheumatoid arthritis (RA) and other inflammatory types of arthritis are chronic diseases that can be crippling if not well controlled. Fear of becoming disabled and dependent, uncertainty about the disease process, altered body image, devaluation of self, frustration, and depression are common psychosocial problems. Physical limitations and PAIN caused by disease may limit MOBILITY and ADLs. These limitations can result in role changes in the family and society. For example, the person may not be able to cook for the family or be an active sexual partner. In addition, extreme fatigue often causes patients to desire an early bedtime and may result in a reluctance to socialize.

Body changes caused by joint changes and steroid therapy (if used) may also cause poor self-esteem and body image. Because many societies value people with physically fit, attractive bodies, the patient with RA may be embarrassed to be seen in public places. The patient may grieve or experience degrees of depression. He or she may have feelings of helplessness caused by a loss of control over a disease that can "consume" the body. Fortunately, newer drugs have improved the treatment of RA and provide the patient with hope and better disease control. Only a small percentage of patients with RA become wheelchair dependent.

Living with a chronic disease and its PAIN is difficult for the patient and family. Chronic suffering and pain affect quality of life. Assess the patient's emotional and mental status in relation to the disease and its problems. Evaluate his or her support systems and resources. Patients who are knowledgeable about their disease and treatment options feel emotionally stronger to cope with their disease and better able to discuss treatment options with their health care provider.

Laboratory Assessment. Laboratory tests help support a diagnosis of RA, but no single test or group of tests can confirm it. Chart 18-8 summarizes the most common laboratory tests that the health care provider may use for diagnosing connective tissue diseases.

The test for *rheumatoid factor (RF)* measures the presence of unusual antibodies of the immunoglobulins G (IgG) and M (IgM) types that develop in a number of connective tissue diseases. Many patients with RA have a positive titer (greater than 1:80), but not all positive results indicate the disease, *especially in older adults* (Pagana & Pagana, 2014).

The *antinuclear antibody (ANA)* test measures the titer of a group of antibodies that destroy the nuclei of cells and cause tissue death in patients with autoimmune disease. The fluorescent method is sometimes referred to as *FANA.* If this test result is positive (a value higher than 1:40), various subtypes of this antibody are identified and measured.

When RA patients also have Sjögren's syndrome (SS) or if the syndrome occurs as a separate disease, several unusual anti–SS antibody types may be present. In particular, *anti–SS-A (Ro)* and *anti–SS-B (La)* antibodies are present in about 60% to 70% of those with Sjögren's syndrome or those with secondary Sjögren's and RA (Pagana & Pagana, 2014).

Serum *complement proteins,* especially C3 and C4, are usually decreased in autoimmune diseases, including RA and lupus. An elevated *erythrocyte sedimentation rate (ESR),* or "sed rate," can confirm INFLAMMATION or INFECTION anywhere in the body. An elevated ESR helps support a diagnosis of an unspecified inflammatory disease. The test is most useful to monitor the course of a disease, especially for inflammatory autoimmune diseases. In general, the more severe the disease gets, the higher the ESR rises; as the disease improves or goes into remission, the ESR level decreases.

The *high-sensitivity C-reactive protein,* or *hsCRP,* is another useful test to measure INFLAMMATION and may be done with or instead of the ESR. As the name implies, it is more sensitive to inflammatory changes than the ESR. It is also very useful for detecting infection anywhere in the body.

The presence of most chronic diseases usually causes mild to moderate anemia, which contributes to the patient's fatigue. Therefore monitor the patient's complete blood count (CBC) for a low hemoglobin, hematocrit, and red blood cell (RBC) count. An increase in white blood cell (WBC) count is consistent with an inflammatory response. A decrease in the WBC count may indicate Felty's syndrome, a complication associated with late RA. Thrombocytosis (increased platelets) can also occur in patients with late RA. Additional laboratory tests may be performed depending on the body systems and organs that may be affected by the disease. For example, if heart involvement is suspected, the health care provider may request cardiac enzymes.

Other Diagnostic Assessment. A standard x-ray is used to visualize the joint changes and deformities typical of RA. A CT scan may help determine the presence and degree of cervical spine involvement.

CHART 18-8 Laboratory Profile

Connective Tissue Disease

TEST	NORMAL RANGE FOR ADULTS	SIGNIFICANCE OF ABNORMAL FINDINGS
Rheumatoid factor	Negative	Positive or increase indicative of possible RA or other CTD; may also be elevated in leukemia, liver disease, and kidney disease
ANA (total)	Negative (if positive, types of ANA identified [e.g., anti-ENA, anti-Smith, anti–ss-A (Ro)] to indicate what part of cells are involved)	Elevations common in SLE, SSc, RA, and other inflammatory CTDs (5% of healthy adults have positive ANA results)
Serum complement	*Total:* 30-75 units/mL (*C3:* 75-175 mg/dL; *C4:* 22-45 mg/dL)	Decreased values indicative of active autoimmune disease, such as SLE, and other problems like anemia, infection, and malnutrition
Erythrocyte sedimentation rate (ESR)	*Male:* up to 15 mm/hr *Female:* up to 20 mm/hr	Increased in inflammatory diseases, like RA, SLE, PMR, temporal arteritis; also elevated in patients with bacterial infections or severe anemias
SPEP	*Total:* 6.4-8.3 g/dL	
Albumin	3.5-5.0 g/dL	Decreased level occurs with chronic inflammation or infection; also decreased in malnutrition and advanced cirrhosis
Globulin	2.3-3.4 g/dL	
Alpha$_1$ globulin	0.1-0.3 g/dL	Increased level possible in RA
Alpha$_2$ globulin	0.6-1.0 g/dL	
Beta globulin	0.7-1.1 g/dL	
Gamma globulin	0.8-1.6 g/dL	Increased levels indicative of CTD (inflammatory type)
HLA testing *(HLA-B27)*	None	Presence of *HLA B27* indicative of Reiter's syndrome or ankylosing spondylitis

ANA, Antinuclear antibody; *CTD,* connective tissue disease; *ENA,* extractable nuclear antigens; *HLA,* human leukocyte antigen; *PMR,* polymyalgia rheumatica; *RA,* rheumatoid arthritis; *SLE,* systemic lupus erythematosus; *SPEP,* serum protein electrophoresis; *SSc,* systemic sclerosis.

An *arthrocentesis* is an invasive procedure that may be used for patients with joint swelling caused by excess synovial fluid (effusion). It may be performed at the bedside or in a health care provider's office or clinic. After administering a local anesthetic, the provider inserts a large-gauge needle into the joint (usually the knee) to aspirate a sample of synovial fluid to relieve pressure. The fluid is analyzed for inflammatory cells and immune complexes, including RF. Fluid from patients with RA typically reveals increased WBCs, cloudiness, and volume.

Teach the patient to use ice and rest the affected joint for 24 hours after arthrocentesis. Often the health care provider will recommend acetaminophen as needed for PAIN. If increased pain or swelling occurs, teach the patient or family to notify the health care provider immediately.

! NURSING SAFETY PRIORITY (QSEN)

Action Alert

After an arthrocentesis, monitor the insertion site for bleeding or leakage of synovial fluid. Notify the health care provider if either of these problems occurs.

A bone scan or joint scan can also assess the extent of joint involvement. MRI may be performed to assess spinal column disease or other joint involvement.

Because RA can affect multiple body systems, tests to diagnose specific systemic manifestations are performed as necessary. For example, electromyography helps confirm peripheral neuropathy. Pulmonary function tests help determine the presence of lung involvement.

? NCLEX EXAMINATION CHALLENGE

Physiological Integrity

Which assessment findings will the nurse expect for the client with early-stage rheumatoid arthritis? **Select all that apply.**

A. Heberden's nodes
B. Elevated erythrocyte sedimentation rate (ESR)
C. Positive antinuclear antibody (ANA) titer
D. Severe weight loss
E. Joint inflammation
F. Red, swollen joints

◆ *Interventions*

As in other types of arthritis, the interdisciplinary health care team manages PAIN by using a combination of pharmacologic and nonpharmacologic measures. A **synovectomy** to remove inflamed synovium may be needed for joints like the knee or elbow. Total joint arthroplasty (TJA) may be indicated when other measures fail to relieve PAIN. TJA is discussed in the Osteoarthritis section of this chapter.

Managing Inflammation and Pain. The expected outcome is that the disease goes into remission and its progression slows to decrease PAIN, prevent joint destruction, and increase MOBILITY. Drug therapy and nonpharmacologic interventions are used to help meet this outcome.

Drug Therapy. Some drugs prescribed for RA have anti-inflammatory and/or analgesic actions. Other drugs are immunosuppressive and disease modifying, which may cause remission of the illness and prevent erosive joint changes. Biological response modifiers make up the newest class of disease-modifying drugs that help reduce signals for the immune system to cause INFLAMMATION (Chart 18-9). Patients with inflammatory diseases other than RA are also using various biological response modifying drugs successfully. Although RA is a chronic disease and no cure is yet available, drugs now used can better control the disease and prevent further deterioration.

The health care provider, often a rheumatologist, makes decisions about appropriate drug therapy for patients with rheumatoid disease based on the severity of the disease. Initially, most patients are managed with **disease-modifying antirheumatic drugs (DMARDs)**. As the name implies, these drugs are given to slow the progression of the disease.

First-Line Disease-Modifying Antirheumatic Drugs. Methotrexate (MTX) (Rheumatrex), an immunosuppressive medication, in a low, once-a-week dose (generally 25 mg or less per week orally) is the mainstay of therapy for RA because it is effective and relatively inexpensive. It is a slow-acting drug, taking 4 to 6 weeks to begin to control joint INFLAMMATION. Observe for desired therapeutic drug effects, such as a decrease in joint PAIN and swelling.

Monitor patients for potential adverse effects, such as decreasing WBCs and platelets (as a result of bone marrow suppression) or elevations in liver enzymes or serum creatinine.

! NURSING SAFETY PRIORITY (QSEN)

Drug Alert

Patients taking MTX are at risk for INFECTION. Teach them to avoid crowds and people who are ill. Remind patients to avoid alcoholic beverages while taking MTX to prevent liver toxicity. Teach them to observe and report other side and toxic effects, which include mouth sores and acute dyspnea from pneumonitis. Rarely, lymph node tumor (lymphoma) has been associated in those who have RA and are taking MTX. Folic acid, one of the B vitamins, is often given to those who are taking MTX to help decrease some of the drug's side effects.

Pregnancy is not recommended while taking methotrexate because birth defects are possible. *Strict birth control is recommended for childbearing women who are in need of MTX to control their RA.* If pregnancy is ever desired, instruct the patient to consult the rheumatologist as well as an obstetric/gynecologic (OB/GYN) health care provider. Generally, the health care provider will discontinue the drug at least 3 months before planned pregnancy. MTX may be restarted after birth if the patient does not breast-feed (Lilley et al., 2014).

Leflunomide (Arava) may be prescribed for some patients. It is a slow-acting immune-modulating medication that helps diminish inflammatory symptoms of joint swelling and stiffness and improves MOBILITY. The drug is generally prescribed as a loading dose of 100 mg orally daily for 3 days followed by 20 mg orally daily thereafter. Inform the patient that Arava takes 4 to 6 weeks and sometimes up to 3 months before maximum benefit is realized.

Arava is a potent medication that is generally tolerated, but side effects of hair loss, diarrhea, decreased WBCs and platelets, or increased liver enzymes have been reported. *Teach patients to report these changes, and monitor laboratory results carefully. Remind them to avoid alcohol. Inform them that Arava can cause birth defects, and therefore recommend strict birth control to*

CHART 18-9 Common Examples of Drug Therapy

*Biological Response Modifiers Used for Rheumatoid Arthritis and Other Connective Tissue Diseases**

DRUG AND USUAL DOSAGE	PURPOSE OF DRUG	NURSING INTERVENTIONS	RATIONALES
For *all* biological response modifiers (BRMs) (also called *biologics*)	Neutralize biologic activity of tumor necrosis factor–alpha (TNFA), interleukins (IL), T-lymphocytes, or tyrosine kinase (TK) to decrease immune response and inflammation	Do not give BRMs if patient has a serious infection, TB, or MS. Teach patients taking BRMs to avoid getting live vaccines.	Drugs may exacerbate infections, MS, or lupus.
		Teach patient to avoid crowds and people with infections.	Serious infections, especially respiratory infections, can lead to hospitalization or cause death.
Etanercept (Enbrel): Usually 25 mg subcutaneously twice weekly	TNFA inhibitor	Teach patient to report site reaction. Teach patient how to self-administer drug.	Site reactions can be painful. Patients need to self-administer the drug at home or have another person learn how to give the injections.
Infliximab (Remicade): 3 mg/kg of body weight as IV infusion, followed by the same dose at Weeks 2 and 6. If patient responds, maintenance infusions are given at the same dose every 8 weeks.	TNFA inhibitor	Refrigerate all BRMs except Remicade. Teach patient to report chest pain or difficulty breathing during infusion; monitor blood pressure and infusion site.	Refrigeration prevents drug decomposition. Severe allergic reaction is potentially life threatening; infusion reactions usually subside.
Adalimumab (Humira): 40 mg subcutaneously every 2 weeks	TNFA inhibitor	Teach patient to report site reaction.	Site reactions may occur to indicate local allergic response.
Anakinra (Kineret): Typically 100 mg subcutaneously daily	IL-1 receptor antagonist	Teach patient to monitor site for reaction (occurs more commonly when compared with other BRMs).	Site reactions may occur.
		Monitor WBC count.	Drug can cause a severe decrease in WBC count and make patient very susceptible to infection.
		Teach patient to report respiratory symptoms, such as cough and fever. Teach patient that malignancies can result from taking this drug.	Drug can cause serious respiratory infections and various types of cancers.
Abatacept (Orencia): Based on body weight from 500 to 1000 mg IV each week for 2 wks, and then may be given at longer intervals for maintenance	Selective T-lymphocyte co-stimulator modulator (T-cell inhibitor)	Report cough, dizziness, and sore throat; do not receive live vaccines while taking the drug.	Serious respiratory infections can occur.
		Monitor for dyspnea, wheezing, flushing, itching.	This drug can cause a mild to moderate allergic reaction.
Rituximab (Rituxan): Two 1000-mg IV doses given 2 weeks apart initially, followed by the same dosing every 4-6 months depending on the patient's response	Monoclonal antibody	Observe for infusion reaction as above.	Drug can cause a local allergic response.
Golimumab (Simponi): 50 mg subcutaneously once a month	TNFA inhibitor	Teach patient to report signs and symptoms of infection, including fever and malaise; teach patient to avoid live vaccines while taking drug.	Drug has a black box warning about serious infections from opportunistic pathogens that can lead to hospitalizations or death.
		Teach patient about adverse drug effects including hypertension, GI distress, and infection from opportunistic pathogens; report signs and symptoms of these problems to the health care provider.	These adverse drug effects can lead to serious illness.
Tocilizumab (Actemra): Dose varies based on weight; given IV initially at 4 mg/kg and then increased to 8 mg/kg of body weight; drug may also be self-administered as a subcutaneous prefilled injection; dosing intervals depend on the patient's response and route of administration	IL-6 inhibitor	Teach patient the importance of having frequent WBC, platelet, and liver enzyme testing.	Drug can cause decreased WBCs and platelets, and liver dysfunction.

MS, Multiple sclerosis; *TB,* tuberculosis; *TNF,* tumor necrosis factor; *WBC,* white blood cell.

*This is not a comprehensive list; this chart lists only the common biological response modifiers (BRMs) used for rheumatoid arthritis and other connective tissue diseases.

women of childbearing age. Tell patients to contact the health care provider immediately if pregnancy occurs while taking the drug. Cholestyramine (Questran) is available to help block the drug's action.

Another DMARD sometimes used for RA is hydroxychloroquine (Plaquenil). This drug slows the progression of mild rheumatoid disease before it worsens (see Chart 18-9). It is an antimalarial drug that helps decrease joint and muscle PAIN. Patients generally tolerate Plaquenil quite well. In a few cases, mild stomach discomfort, light-headedness, or headache has been reported.

! NURSING SAFETY PRIORITY (QSEN)

Drug Alert

The most serious adverse effect of Plaquenil is retinal damage. Teach patients to report blurred vision or headache. Remind them to have an eye examination before taking the drug and every 6 months to detect changes in the cornea, lens, or retina. If this rare complication occurs, the health care provider discontinues the drug (Lilley et al., 2014).

Nonsteroidal Anti-inflammatory Drugs. *NSAIDs are sometimes used for RA to relieve PAIN and INFLAMMATION.* The choice of which one to prescribe depends on the patient's needs and tolerance, as well as the scientific evidence supporting the drug therapy. To decrease GI problems, the NSAID may be given with an H2-blocking agent, such as ranitidine (Zantac) or misoprostol (Cytotec). If there is no clinical change after 6 to 8 weeks, the health care provider may discontinue the current NSAID and try another one or change to a different drug class.

It was once thought that celecoxib (Celebrex), a COX-2 inhibiting NSAID, should be given rather than the older NSAIDs like ibuprofen. However, all COX-2 inhibiting drugs have recently been associated with cardiovascular disease, such as myocardial infarction, and some have been taken off the market. The risk for GI bleeding is also high in patients taking Celebrex, and the drug cannot be given to those who have had recent open heart surgery.

Biological Response Modifiers. As a group, **biological response modifiers (BRMs)**, sometimes called **biologics**, are one of the newest classes of DMARDs. Most BRMs neutralize the biologic activity of tumor necrosis factor–alpha (TNFA) by inhibiting its binding with TNF receptors. Any one of the BRMs may be tried. If one drug is not effective, the health care provider prescribes another drug in the same class. All these drugs are extremely expensive at this time, and insurance companies may not completely pay for their use. Some patients receive one of these drugs in addition to the drugs in this Drug Therapy section.

Teach patients receiving any one of the BRMs that they are at a high risk for developing INFECTION. Instruct them to stay away from people with infections and to avoid large crowds if possible. Remind patients with multiple sclerosis (MS), tuberculosis (TB), or a positive TB test that they should not receive TNF inhibitors because they make patients susceptible to flare-ups of these diseases. Determine whether the patient has had a recent negative purified protein derivative (PPD) test for TB. If not, a PPD skin test is typically administered and the selected BRM is not started until a negative test result is confirmed. Collaborate with the health care provider to ensure that this process is complete.

Etanercept (Enbrel) is given subcutaneously as 25 mg twice weekly for most patients. Immunosuppression with medications such as methotrexate is generally tried before using Enbrel or other biological response modifiers. Methotrexate is often given in combination with biologic therapies because the combination may be more effective than either drug alone (Cranwell-Bruce, 2011). Most patients tolerate Enbrel or Enbrel and methotrexate together; however, laboratory monitoring is important. Combination therapy requires CBC, serum creatinine, and a liver panel to be drawn regularly, generally every 4 to 8 weeks. In general, clinical outcomes with Enbrel have been excellent.

Teach the patient or family member how to self-administer Enbrel injections. Injection site reaction and systemic INFECTION (especially respiratory) are possible adverse effects. Ice and hydrocortisone 1% cream can be used if a red, itchy rash at the injection site develops. Teach the patient to notify the health care provider if infection or a delay in wound healing occurs.

Infliximab (Remicade), first approved to treat Crohn's disease, is given in a single IV infusion over several hours. The initial dose generally used for RA is 3 mg/kg of body weight. The drug dosage is repeated at weeks 2 and 6. After these first three infusions, a maintenance dose of 3 mg/kg of body weight is given every 8 weeks, depending on the response of the patient. For patients who do not respond to the first three infusions, the drug dosage may be increased up to 10 mg/kg of body weight given at 4-week intervals. The risk of side effects and adverse effects increases at higher doses. Patients typically take methotrexate before starting Remicade and continue on combination therapy.

! NURSING SAFETY PRIORITY (QSEN)

Drug Alert

Teach the patient to report and observe for symptoms of Remicade infusion reaction: chest discomfort, tachycardia, shortness of breath, or light-headedness. If any of these symptoms are reported, decrease the IV rate or discontinue it!

The symptoms of infusion reaction generally subside, but the health care provider must be notified in case medical assistance is needed. Dose, rate, and interval changes may be needed. Acetaminophen and Benadryl are medications often given before the start of Remicade and are often used at the time of reported infusion reaction. Those who experience serious adverse effects, such as hypertension or anaphylaxis, require permanent discontinuation of the drug.

Adalimumab (Humira) is the first fully human TNFA inhibitor and is given by subcutaneous injection. Symptoms of inflammatory arthritis tend to decrease with the use of Humira, including less joint swelling, less stiffness, and better MOBILITY. Injection site reactions and adverse effects similar to the other TNFA inhibitors have been reported. Careful monitoring, especially with combination therapy of Humira and methotrexate or other drug that affects the body's IMMUNITY, is important and similar to combination therapy with other BRMs.

Anakinra (Kineret) is another biological response modifier. Instead of affecting tumor necrosis factor–alpha (TNFA), however, it works to inhibit a different protein signal of the immune system called *interleukin-1 (IL-1).* IL-1 is also a pro-inflammatory protein that signals the immune system to increase INFLAMMATION (Cranwell-Bruce, 2011). It is thought that IL-1 is a weaker protein than TNF, but having an alternative drug that targets a different receptor site is helpful when a patient cannot take other biologics. Those who have multiple sclerosis or tuberculosis cannot take TNF inhibitors, but Kineret can be used with this population.

Injection site reactions occur more often with Kineret compared with other BRMs. Ice and hydrocortisone 1% cream are recommended. Remind patients to rotate injection sites. Kineret is administered with a simple jet for self-administration. The patient has the option to use the simple jet or administer the subcutaneous injection traditionally.

Abatacept (Orencia) and *rituximab (Rituxan, MabThera)* require IV infusions every 2 weeks to start and then may be more spread out, depending on the drug. Like the results of the other BRMs, patients usually report feeling a benefit from these drugs in 2 weeks, but it may take months for the maximum benefit to be seen. *Golimumab (Simponi)* is the first biologic that is administered only once each month for both RA and psoriatic arthritis. Teach patients that this drug has a black box warning for serious INFECTIONS that may lead to hospitalization or death from opportunistic pathogens (Cranwell-Bruce, 2011).

Tocilizumab (Actemra) is given when the patient cannot tolerate other drugs. Tocilizumab is different from other biologics because it is the first humanized interleukin-6 (IL-6) receptor-inhibiting monoclonal antibody that is available for patients with RA. It can be used alone or in combination with other DMARDs. Teach patients about adverse drug effects, including hypertension, GI distress, infection, and an increase in low-density lipoproteins (LDLs) and liver enzymes. Like for other biologics, teach the patient about the high risk of infection (e.g., tuberculosis) when taking Actemra.

One of the newest biologics is *tofacitinib (Xeljanz)*, which has been approved for moderate to severe RA as monotherapy or in combination with methotrexate. This drug is a tyrosine kinase inhibitor (TKI). Tyrosine kinases usually facilitate cytokine-mediated (e.g., interleukin) signals that promote the inflammatory process. Teach patients that tofacitinib carries a black box warning alerting patients about its potential for serious opportunistic INFECTIONS, tuberculosis, lymphoma, and other cancers.

Other Drugs. A few drugs may be given as adjuncts to or instead of the previously described drugs. It is not unusual for a patient to be taking several disease-modifying drugs, such as methotrexate, a BRM, and an adjunct medication. Each drug works differently to relieve symptoms and slow the progression of the disease.

Glucocorticoids (steroids)—usually prednisone (Deltasone)—are given for their fast-acting anti-inflammatory and immunosuppressive effects. Prednisone may be given in high dose for short duration (**pulse therapy**) or as a low chronic dose. Moderate-dose short-term tapering bridge therapy may be used when inflammation is symptomatic and other RA medications are insufficient or have not yet had an effect.

Chronic steroid therapy can result in numerous complications, such as:

- Diabetes mellitus
- INFECTION
- Fluid and electrolyte imbalances
- Hypertension
- Osteoporosis
- Glaucoma

Some drug effects are dose related, whereas others are not. Observe the patient for complications associated with chronic steroid therapy, and report them to the health care provider. For example, if blood pressure becomes elevated or significant laboratory values change, notify the health care provider.

Instruct patients taking chronic steroids to take calcium 1200 to 1500 mg daily plus vitamin D 400 mg daily to help prevent osteoporosis. Bisphosphonate drugs may also be prescribed. Bone density measurements (DEXA [dual-energy x-ray absorptiometry] scans) are done every 2 to 3 years to monitor for bone loss.

Patients with RA may experience one or a few joints that have more PAIN and INFLAMMATION than the others. Cortisone injections in single joints may be used to relieve local pain and inflammation. Have the patient ice and rest the joint for 24 hours after the procedure. Oral analgesics also are sometimes needed during that time.

Other immunosuppressive agents that may be used as a last resort are *azathioprine (Imuran)* and *cyclophosphamide (Cytoxan)*. Cyclophosphamide is sometimes given specifically to control RA vasculitis. Such immunosuppressive drugs may cause bone marrow suppression and occasionally leukemia or lymphoma. White blood cell counts are expected to decrease 7 to 14 days after the administration of IV cyclophosphamide; therefore monitor laboratory results closely to ensure safe limits. Hemorrhagic cystitis is a concern more with oral cyclophosphamide. Instruct the patient to drink water and void frequently (about every 2 hours while awake), which dilutes the urine and empties the bladder, thus decreasing opportunity for bladder irritation from residual drug. Hair thinning or loss can be seen with immunosuppressive medications. Cyclophosphamide may also cause sterility; strict birth control is recommended.

Nonpharmacologic Interventions. Adequate rest, proper positioning, and ice and heat applications are important in pain management. If acute INFLAMMATION is present, ice packs may be applied to "hot" joints for PAIN relief until the inflammation lessens. The ice pack should not be too heavy. At home, the patient can use a small bag of frozen peas or corn as an ice pack.

Heated paraffin (wax) dips may help increase comfort of arthritic hands. Finger and hand exercises are often done more easily after paraffin treatment. To relieve morning stiffness or the pain of late-stage disease, recommend a hot shower rather than a sponge bath or a tub bath. It is often difficult for the patient with RA to get into and out of a bathtub, although special hydraulic lifts and tub chairs are available to allow the patient to bathe. Safety (grab) bars and nonskid tread in the tub or shower floor are important safety features to discuss with all patients. Some older adults prefer using shower chairs and a walk-in shower that does not have a ledge that could cause falls.

Hot packs applied directly to involved joints may be beneficial. Most physical therapy departments have machines that keep hot packs ready anytime they are needed. Teach patients to use the microwave or stovetop heating instructions to warm heat packs at home. Remind them to follow the instructions given with each heating device used.

Plasmapheresis (sometimes called *plasma exchange*) is an in-hospital procedure prescribed by a health care provider in which the patient's plasma is treated to remove the antibodies causing the disease. Although not commonly done, this procedure may be combined with steroid pulse therapy for patients with severe, life-threatening disease.

Complementary and Alternative Therapies. Some patients may have pain relief from hypnosis, acupuncture, imagery, music therapy, or other technique. Stress management is also popular as a PAIN relief intervention. Chapter 3 discusses these therapies in more detail.

Adequate nutrition is an important part of the management of RA. Obesity should be avoided or treated if present. The inflammatory state may place a greater burden on the metabolism of some essential nutrients. This catabolic state may be related to increased cytokine production, specifically tumor necrosis factor.

According to the National Center for Complementary and Alternative Medicine, some supplements have been found to help decrease INFLAMMATION and include:

- Cold water fish or fish oil capsules containing omega-3 fatty acids at 2.5 to 5 g daily (should not be taken if the patient is taking anticoagulant therapy)
- Gamma-linolenic acid (GLA), an omega-6 fatty acid found in the oils of certain plant seeds, such as primrose and black currant

According to the Arthritis Foundation, no one food causes or cures RA; however, healthy nutrition in general is important. Refer the patient to the Arthritis Foundation's pamphlet regarding diet and arthritis. Refer him or her to the dietitian for vitamin- and nutrition-specific questions or recommendations. Teach patients to take any herbal or nutrition supplement under the supervision of a qualified health care provider to prevent adverse events and drug-food or drug-drug interactions.

Other complementary and alternative medicine (CAM) therapies are safe and have been scientifically proven to be effective to help control RA PAIN for most people. Examples include mind-body therapies, such as relaxation techniques, imagery, and spiritual practices. For information about these techniques, see Chapter 3.

Promoting Self-Management. Although the physical appearance of a patient with severe RA may create the image that ADL independence is not possible, a number of alternative and creative methods can be used to perform these activities. *Do not perform these activities for the patient unless asked. Those with RA do not want to be dependent.* For example, hand deformities often prevent a patient from opening packages of food, such as a box of crackers; however, he or she may prefer to use the teeth to open the crackers rather than depend on someone else.

In the hospital or long-term care facility, a patient may not eat because of the barriers of heavy plate covers, milk cartons, small packages of condiments, and heavy containers. Styrofoam or paper cups may bend and collapse as he or she attempts to hold them. A china or heavy plastic cup with handles may be easier to manipulate. Collaborate with the dietitian to assist with access to food and total independence in eating.

When fine motor activities (e.g., squeezing a tube of toothpaste) become impossible, larger joints or body surfaces can substitute for smaller ones. For example, teach how to use the palm of the hand to press the paste onto the brush. Devices such as long-handled brushes can help patients brush their hair; dressing sticks can assist with putting on pants. These examples illustrate the need to assess the problem area, suggest alternative methods, and refer the patient to an occupational or physical therapist for special assistive and adaptive devices if necessary.

Managing Fatigue. Nursing interventions depend in part on identifying the factors contributing to fatigue. For example, increases in PAIN, sleep disturbances, and weakness are positively associated with increased fatigue. Anemia may also be a contributing factor and may be treated with iron (if an iron deficiency anemia is present), folic acid, or vitamin supplements prescribed by the health care provider. Chronic normochromic or chronic hypochromic anemia often occurs in most chronic systemic diseases. Assess for drug-related blood loss, such as that caused by NSAIDs, by checking the stool for gross or occult blood. *Older white women are the most likely to experience GI bleeding as a result of taking these medications. The reason for this trend is not known.*

When fatigue results from muscle atrophy, the health care provider prescribes an aggressive physical therapy program to strengthen muscles and prevent further atrophy. Patients experience increased fatigue when pain prevents them from getting adequate rest and sleep. Measures to facilitate sleep include promoting a quiet environment, giving warm beverages, and administering hypnotics or relaxants as prescribed, if necessary.

In addition to identifying and managing specific reasons for fatigue, determine the patient's usual daily activities and teach principles of **energy conservation**, including:

- Pacing activities
- Allowing rest periods
- Setting priorities
- Obtaining assistance when needed

Chart 18-10 lists specific suggestions for conserving energy and thus increasing activity tolerance and MOBILITY.

Enhancing Body Image. Body image may be affected by both the disease process and drug therapy. Steroids can cause a moonfaced appearance, acne, striae, "buffalo humps," and weight gain. Determine the patient's perception of these changes and the impact of the reactions of family and significant others. The most important intervention is communicating acceptance of the patient. When a trusting relationship is established, encourage him or her to express personal feelings.

As a reaction to body image disturbance and the presence of a chronic, painful disease, some patients display behaviors indicative of loss. They may use coping strategies that range from denial or fear to anger or depression. In an attempt to regain control over the effects of the disease process, they may appear to be "manipulative and demanding" and sometimes may be referred to as having an "arthritis personality." *This personality, which represents a negative label, is a myth; using these terms should be avoided.* Patients are trying to cope with the effects of their illness and should be treated with patience and understanding. Continually assess and accept these behaviors, but remain realistic in discussing goals to improve self-esteem. Emphasize their strengths, and help them identify previously successful coping strategies.

CHART 18-10 Patient and Family Education: Preparing for Self-Management

Energy Conservation for the Patient with Arthritis

- Balance activity with rest. Take one or two naps each day.
- Pace yourself; do not plan too much for one day.
- Set priorities. Determine which activities are most important, and do them first.
- Delegate responsibilities and tasks to your family and friends.
- Plan ahead to prevent last-minute rushing and stress.
- Learn your own activity tolerance, and do not exceed it.

Community-Based Care

Patients with rheumatoid arthritis (RA) are usually managed at home but, in a few cases, may be institutionalized in a long-term care facility if they become restricted to bed or a wheelchair. Some patients may be transferred to a rehabilitation facility for several weeks to aid in developing strategies, techniques, and skills for independent living at home.

Home Care Management. The amount of home care preparation depends on the severity of the disease. Structural changes may be necessary if there are deficits in ADLs or MOBILITY. Doors must be wide enough to accommodate a wheelchair or walker if one is used. Ramps are needed to prevent the patient in a wheelchair from becoming homebound. If the person cannot use stairs, he or she must have access to facilities for all ADLs on one floor. Handrails should be available in the bathroom and halls.

To promote continued homemaking functions, countertops and appliances may require structural changes. The patient may also require handrails and elevated chairs and toilet seats, which facilitate transfers (Fig. 18-7). *These devices are especially important for older adults with arthritis.*

Self-Management Education. Self-management education (SME) is a vital role for nurses in collaborative management of arthritis. Many people have signs and symptoms of joint INFLAMMATION but do not seek medical attention. Teach them to seek professional health care to reduce PAIN and disability.

Teach patients to discuss any questions with their health care provider before trying any over-the-counter or home remedies. Some remedies may be harmful. Check with the Arthritis Foundation for the latest information on arthritis myths and quackery (www.arthritis.org).

Provide information to the patient and family about drug therapy, as well as joint protection, energy conservation, rest, and exercise. This SME is summarized in Charts 18-5, 18-6, and 18-10.

Assess the patient's coping strategies. The patient with RA often reports being on an "emotional roller coaster" from coping with a chronic illness every day. Control over one's life is an important human need. The patient with an unpredictable chronic disease may lose this control, and this lowers self-esteem. Health care providers must allow the patient to make decisions about care. Families and significant others must also include him or her in decision making. Although the patient's behavior may be perceived as demanding or manipulative, his or her self-esteem cannot be improved without this important aspect of interpersonal relationships.

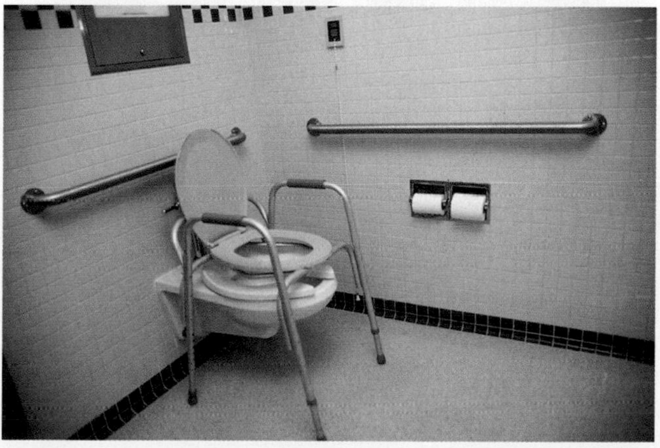

FIG. 18-7 Handrails and an elevated toilet seat make transfers easier for the patient.

Increased dependency also affects a sense of control and self-esteem. Some people ignore their health needs and portray a tough image for others by insisting that they need no assistance. Emphasize to the patient and family that asking for help may be the best decision at times to prevent further joint damage and disease progression.

RA may also affect work and social roles. The patient may have physical difficulty doing tasks that require lifting, climbing, grasp, or gross or fine motor activities. The severity of RA disease may cause difficulty with total number of hours worked. Some people with RA can do their jobs well without problem; others may have varying degrees of difficulty. Those who can no longer do their job at work may need to discuss with their employer having a lighter workload, but some may need to file for disability with their company and Social Security office.

Health Care Resources. The need for health care resources for the patient with RA is similar to that for the patient with osteoarthritis. A home care nurse or aide, physical therapist, or occupational therapist may be needed during severe exacerbations or as the disease progresses. In collaboration with the case manager, identify these resources and make sure they are available as needed. The Arthritis Foundation is an excellent source of information and support.

Arthritis support groups and self-help courses provide the education and the support that patients, families, and friends need. Refer the patient to a psychological counselor or religious or spiritual leader for emotional support and guidance during times of crisis or as needed. Identify and recommend other support systems within the family and community when necessary.

CLINICAL JUDGMENT CHALLENGE

Teamwork and Collaboration; Safety QSEN

An 81-year-old woman with RA has been controlled with methotrexate for 18 years. Recently she experienced increased joint pain and swelling in her right knee that have affected her mobility and activity level. She walks with a cane in the community but uses a walker at home. Earlier in the week, she almost fell while walking to her car after she left the bank. The rheumatologist plans to add etanercept (Enbrel) to her drug regimen.

1. With what members of the health care team might you collaborate as part of her plan of care?
2. What safety measures are needed before she begins taking Enbrel?
3. What self-management education will she need before starting Enbrel?
4. What home and community assessment might be needed to ensure her safety?

LUPUS ERYTHEMATOSUS

❖ PATHOPHYSIOLOGY

The two main classifications of lupus are discoid lupus erythematosus (DLE) and systemic lupus erythematosus (SLE). A small percentage of patients with lupus have the DLE type, which affects only the skin.

Unlike DLE, **systemic lupus erythematosus** is a chronic, progressive, inflammatory connective tissue disorder that can cause major body organs and systems to fail. It is characterized by spontaneous remissions and **exacerbations** ("flare-ups"), and the onset may be acute or insidious (slow). The condition is potentially fatal, but most patients with SLE live many years after diagnosis and lead productive lives. Improvements in determining the cause, diagnosis, and treatment of lupus account for the prolonged survival.

Lupus is thought to be an autoimmune process. Antinuclear antibodies (ANAs) primarily affect the DNA, ribonucleic acid (RNA), and other components within the cell nuclei. As a result, immune complexes form in the serum and organ tissues, which cause INFLAMMATION, damage, and destruction (McCance et al., 2014). These complexes invade organs directly or cause **vasculitis** (vessel inflammation), which deprives the organs of arterial blood and oxygen.

Autoimmune complexes in SLE tend to be most attracted to the glomeruli of the kidneys. Therefore many of these patients have some degree of kidney involvement, called *lupus nephritis*—the leading cause of death from the disease. Other causes of death are cardiac and central nervous system involvement.

CULTURAL CONSIDERATIONS

Patient-Centered Care QSEN

Lupus affects women 10 times more often than men; women of color are affected far more often than Euro-Americans. The reason for this difference is unknown (McCance et al., 2014). The disease also occurs among American Indians, Asian Americans, and Hispanics (Lupus Foundation of America, 2014).

The onset of the disease occurs most often during the child-bearing years (ages 20 to 40 years), but it has been reported in young children and older adults. A genetic predisposition is based on the trend to develop the disease in some twins and the occurrence of autoimmune disease in some families of patients who have lupus. However, it is not the only basis of the disease. Like RA, lupus is probably caused by a complex *combination of genetic and environmental factors.*

A transient lupus-like syndrome can occur in some patients taking select medications, especially procainamide (Pronestyl) and hydralazine (McCance et al., 2014). When these drugs are discontinued, the syndrome usually resolves. Neither of these drugs is commonly used.

❖ PATIENT-CENTERED COLLABORATIVE CARE

◆ Assessment

It is impossible to describe a typical textbook picture of a patient with lupus because of the extreme range of symptoms. There is no classic presentation of this disease. When lupus is in remission, the patient may appear healthy and have few or no activity limitations. When the disease flares, some patients may be so ill that admission to a critical care unit is needed. Chart 18-11 highlights the clinical manifestations that can occur with systemic lupus.

Physical Assessment/Clinical Manifestations

Skin Involvement. *The major skin manifestation of DLE and SLE is a dry, scaly, raised rash on the face* (**"butterfly" rash**) (Fig. 18-8). This rash may also appear on other sun-exposed areas. The rash is initially nonscarring and may increase in a lupus flare and disappear when the disease is in remission.

CHART 18-11 Key Features

Systemic Lupus Erythematosus (SLE) and Systemic Sclerosis (SSc)

SYSTEMIC LUPUS ERYTHEMATOSUS	SYSTEMIC SCLEROSIS
Skin Manifestations	
Inflamed, red rash	Inflamed
Discoid lesions	Fibrotic
	Sclerotic
	Edematous
Renal Manifestations	
Nephritis	Kidney failure
Cardiovascular Manifestations	
Pericarditis	Myocardial fibrosis
Raynaud's phenomenon	Raynaud's phenomenon
Pulmonary Manifestations	
Pleural effusions	Interstitial fibrosis
	Pulmonary hypertension
Neurologic Manifestations	
CNS lupus	Not common
Gastrointestinal Manifestations	
Abdominal pain	Esophagitis
	Ulcers
Musculoskeletal Manifestations	
Joint inflammation	Joint inflammation
Myositis	Myositis
Other Manifestations	
Fever	Fever
Fatigue	Fatigue
Anorexia	Anorexia
Vasculitis	Vasculitis

CNS, Central nervous system.

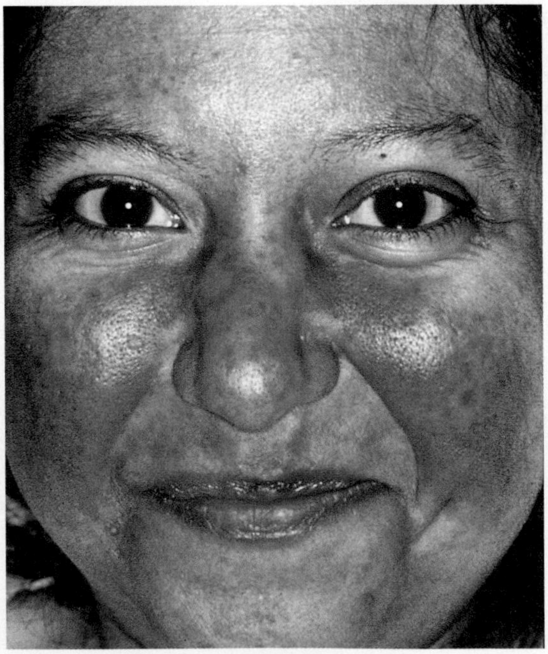

FIG. 18-8 The characteristic "butterfly" rash of systemic lupus erythematosus.

Individual round **discoid** (coinlike) **lesions** are the scarring lesions of discoid lupus. The lesions are especially evident when the patient is exposed to sunlight or ultraviolet light. Alopecia is also common in lupus. Observe and document all skin changes, and monitor them daily while the patient is in an acute care setting or during an ambulatory care or home visit. Mouth ulcers are not uncommon.

Other Manifestations. In addition to skin changes, *polyarthritis* occurs in most patients with SLE. The early joint changes are similar to those seen in rheumatoid arthritis (RA), but severe deformities are not common even in late disease. Small joints and the knees are most commonly inflamed. **Osteonecrosis** (bone necrosis from lack of oxygen) is often seen in those who have been treated for at least 5 years with steroids like prednisone. Chronic steroid therapy may cause the constriction of small blood vessels supplying the joint, which causes the tissue to die. The hip is most commonly affected, and reports of PAIN and decreased MOBILITY result. As a result, a total hip arthroplasty may be done.

Observe for *muscle atrophy,* which can result from disuse, from skeletal muscle invasion by the immune complexes (**myositis**), or from chronic steroid therapy. Myalgia (muscle pain) may also occur. Inspect and palpate the major muscles, especially those in the extremities.

Because SLE is an inflammatory condition, *fever* and *fatigue* are common findings. *Fever is the classic sign of a flare, or exacerbation.* Various degrees of generalized weakness, fatigue, anorexia, and weight loss may occur. These signs may be the only evidence of disease, which makes diagnosis by the health care provider difficult. Therefore some patients have a diagnosis of "probable SLE."

Any or all body systems may be affected by SLE. Because lupus nephritis is the leading cause of death, carefully assess for signs of renal involvement (e.g., changes in urine output, proteinuria, hematuria, fluid retention).

Pleural effusions or *pneumonia* is found in almost half of all cases of SLE, but this complication is usually not life threatening. Pulmonary restrictive or obstructive changes may not result in overt clinical signs; however, progressive involvement can lead to dyspnea and arterial blood gas abnormalities. Perform a complete respiratory assessment to determine any abnormalities in respiratory pattern or breath sounds.

Pericarditis is the most common cardiovascular manifestation and causes tachycardia, chest pain, and myocardial ischemia. Monitor the vital signs at least every 4 hours while the patient is in the hospital, and report chest pain immediately to the physician. *Anemia, leukopenia, and thrombocytopenia* are also common in patients with SLE.

Raynaud's phenomenon occurs in a small portion of lupus patients. On exposure to cold or extreme stress, the patient reports the characteristic red, white, and blue color changes and severe pain in the digits; these changes are caused by arteriolar vasospasm. Ask patients whether color changes occur when their hands or feet are exposed to cold or when they are extremely stressed.

Neurologic manifestations are varied. Central nervous system effects include psychoses, paresis, seizures, migraine headaches, and cranial nerve palsies. Peripheral neuropathies are also common. Perform a neurologic assessment as described in Chapter 41.

Monitor *abdominal* PAIN, which usually results from **serositis** (peritoneal involvement). Mesenteric arteritis, pancreatitis from arteritis of the pancreatic artery, and colonic ulcers also can cause abdominal pain with lupus. Jaundice is rare. Many patients have lymph enlargement, and a few have splenomegaly (enlarged spleen). Palpate the lymph nodes, and document findings. Vasculitis affecting any major or small vessels can lead to organ failure.

Psychosocial Assessment. The psychosocial results of lupus can be devastating. With either DLE or SLE, the rash can be disfiguring and embarrassing. Young adult women who never had a blemish are confronted with a rash that cannot be completely covered with makeup. If chronic steroid therapy is used, side effects such as acne, striae, fat pads, and weight gain intensify the problem of an already altered body image.

Chronic fatigue and generalized weakness may prevent the patient from being as active as in the past. He or she may avoid social gatherings and may withdraw from family activities. The unpredictability and chronicity of SLE can cause fear and anxiety. Fear may increase if the patient knows another person with the disease, particularly if the other person has more advanced severe disease. Unfortunately, the myth that lupus is fatal is still common. Inform the patient and family that control of lupus is generally possible with regular medical monitoring, medications, and healthy practices, such as limiting sun exposure to prevent exacerbation of the disease.

Assess the patient's and family's feelings about the illness to identify areas requiring intervention. Determine their usual coping mechanisms and support systems before developing a plan of care. See p. 293 in the Psychosocial Assessment section of the Rheumatoid Arthritis section for additional information.

Laboratory Assessment. Because discoid lupus erythematosus (DLE) is not a systemic condition, the only significant test is a *skin biopsy.* The physician gently scrapes skin cells from the rash for microscopic evaluation. The characteristic lupus cell and a number of inflammatory cells confirm the diagnosis.

Some of the immunologic-based laboratory tests used to diagnose SLE are the same as those performed for rheumatoid arthritis (RA): rheumatoid factor, antinuclear antibody, erythrocyte sedimentation rate, serum protein electrophoresis, serum complement (especially C3 and C4), and immunoglobulins (see Chart 18-8). A false-positive Venereal Disease Research Laboratory (VDRL) syphilis test is common with lupus (Pagana & Pagana, 2014).

More specific immunologic tests, such as anti–SS-a (Ro), anti–SS-b (La), anti-Smith (anti-Sm), anti-DNA, and extractable nuclear antigens (ENAs), are also performed (Pagana & Pagana, 2014). High titers of some of these antibodies are associated with lupus.

A CBC commonly shows **pancytopenia** (a decrease of all cell types), probably caused by direct attack of the blood cells or bone marrow by immune complexes. Serum electrolyte levels, kidney function, cardiac and liver enzymes, and clotting factors are also routinely assessed to determine other body system functioning.

◆ *Interventions*

The health care provider often prescribes potent drugs that are used topically and systemically. In addition, precautions are taken to prevent further skin impairment and exacerbations. Many of the skin lesions do not disappear, even with treatment, but they usually fade when the disease is in remission.

Managing Lupus with Drug Therapy. With DLE, the patient's major concern is the rash or discoid lesions. Patients with SLE are also concerned about skin changes. Topical cortisone preparations help reduce inflammation and promote fading of the skin lesions. Acetaminophen (Tylenol) or NSAIDs may be used to treat joint and muscle PAIN and INFLAMMATION.

In addition, the health care provider may prescribe the anti-malarial agent *hydroxychloroquine* (Plaquenil) for some patients. Plaquenil decreases the absorption of ultraviolet light by the skin and therefore decreases the risk for skin lesions. *Teach patients to have frequent eye examinations (before starting the drug and every 6 months thereafter) if they are receiving Plaquenil.*

The health care provider often prescribes chronic steroid therapy to treat the systemic disease process. For renal or central nervous system lupus, he or she may also prescribe immunosuppressive agents, such as methotrexate (Rheumatrex) or azathioprine (Imuran). Although clinical manifestations improve during remission, maintenance doses of these drugs are usually continued to prevent further exacerbations of the disease. These drugs make patients susceptible to INFECTION.

! NURSING SAFETY PRIORITY (QSEN)

Drug Alert

When patients are taking steroids and/or immunosuppressants, stress the importance of avoiding large crowds and people who are ill. Teach patients to report any early sign of INFECTION to their health care provider. Observe for side effects and toxic effects of these drugs, and report their occurrence immediately. Remind patients to take their medication early in the morning before breakfast because that is the time when the body's natural corticosteroid level is the lowest.

For severe renal involvement, immunosuppressants may be given in combination with steroids. For patients who do not respond to this regimen, a high-dose IV bolus of glucocorticoids, cyclophosphamide, and plasmapheresis may be tried for 3 consecutive days. Kidney transplantation has been successful for some patients.

The first drug approved for SLE in 60 years is *belimumab (Benlysta)*. In SLE, abnormal B-cells contribute to autoantibodies. Belimumab is an IV human monoclonal antibody (mAb) that prevents B-lymphocyte stimulator protein from binding to B-cell receptor sites, thus decreasing B-cell survival. It is given with other drugs to treat SLE. Like for other biologics, teach patients that the drug increases their risk for serious INFECTIONS. Teach patients not to receive live vaccines for 30 days before treatment.

Protecting the Skin. Teach patients to protect their skin to prevent an exacerbation of the disease.

! NURSING SAFETY PRIORITY (QSEN)

Action Alert

Instruct patients to avoid prolonged exposure to sunlight and other forms of ultraviolet lighting, including certain types of fluorescent light. Remind them to wear long sleeves and a large-brimmed hat when outdoors. Patients should use sun-blocking agents with a sun protection factor (SPF) of 30 or higher on exposed skin surfaces.

In addition, teach patients to clean the skin with mild soap (e.g., Ivory) and to avoid harsh, perfumed substances. The skin should be rinsed and dried well and lotion applied. Excess powder and other drying substances should be avoided. Cosmetics must be carefully selected and should include moisturizers and sun protectors. If desired, refer the patient to a medical cosmetologist who specializes in applying makeup for skin lesions of all types.

Patients' hair should receive special attention because alopecia (hair loss) is common. Recommend the use of mild protein shampoos and the avoidance of harsh treatments (e.g., permanents or highlights) until the hair regrows during remission.

Community-Based Care

Community-based care for the patient with lupus is similar to that for RA. In general, the patient is home but may need repeated hospitalizations during exacerbations of disease. He or she usually does not need rehabilitation unless having surgery, because severe joint deformity and prolonged immobility are not common in lupus.

Two major differences exist between SLE and RA in terms of education of the patient and family or significant others. First, instruct patients with SLE how to protect the skin (Chart 18-12). Second, teach them to monitor body temperature. Fever is the major sign of an exacerbation, during which they can become seriously ill. Teach the importance of reporting any other unusual or new clinical manifestations to the health care provider immediately.

Many patients become frustrated that family members, significant others, and lay people do not have a thorough understanding of lupus. When lupus is in complete remission, patients appear to be healthy; however, an exacerbation can lead to a critical care admission. This unpredictability disrupts the patient's life and can cause fear and anxiety. Help him or her identify coping strategies and support systems that can help with functioning in the community.

Teach the possible effects of the disease on lifestyle, including fatigue. Women of childbearing age need to know that pregnancy can be a stressor and can cause an exacerbation of the disease, either during pregnancy or after delivery. The pregnant woman also has an increased risk for miscarriage, stillbirth, or premature birth. Pregnancy is not recommended for those with cardiac, renal, or central nervous system involvement. Sexual counseling regarding contraception options may be necessary.

The Arthritis Foundation is a general resource for all patients with connective tissue disease. The Lupus Foundation

CHART 18-12 Patient and Family Education: Preparing for Self-Management

Evidence-Based Practice for Skin Protection in Patients with Lupus Erythematosus

- Cleanse your skin with a mild soap, such as Ivory.
- Dry your skin thoroughly by patting rather than rubbing.
- Apply lotion liberally to dry skin areas.
- Avoid powder and other drying agents, such as rubbing alcohol.
- Use cosmetics that contain moisturizers.
- Avoid direct sunlight and any other type of ultraviolet lighting, including tanning beds.
- Wear a large-brimmed hat, long sleeves, and long pants when in the sun.
- Use a sun-blocking agent with a sun protection factor (SPF) of at least 30.
- Inspect your skin daily for open areas and rashes.

(www.lupus.org) is a resource specific for patients with lupus. It is a national organization and has chapters in every state to provide information and assistance for patients with lupus and their families. Local support groups and services are offered free of charge.

NCLEX EXAMINATION CHALLENGE

Health Promotion and Maintenance

What self-management education by the nurse is important for clients diagnosed with systemic lupus erythematosus who are taking prednisone? **Select all that apply.**

A. "Take calcium supplements to prevent osteoporosis from the steroid."
B. "Stay away from crowds and people with infections."
C. "Avoid being in the sun to prevent disease flare-ups."
D. "Get up slowly to prevent dizziness from orthostatic hypotension."
E. "Take your prednisone early in the morning before breakfast."

SYSTEMIC SCLEROSIS

PATHOPHYSIOLOGY

Systemic sclerosis (SSc), also called *scleroderma,* is an uncommon chronic, inflammatory, autoimmune connective tissue disease. Formerly called *progressive systemic disease,* or *PSS,* this illness is not always progressive. **Scleroderma** means hardening of the skin, which is only one clinical manifestation of the problem. Some patients, often children, have only skin involvement, or localized scleroderma (also called *linear scleroderma*). However, adults usually have skin and other body system involvement. SSc is less common than systemic lupus erythematosus (SLE) but is associated with a higher mortality rate. See Chart 18-11 for a comparison of the clinical manifestations of these two diseases. The manifestations for both diseases vary widely from person to person.

The early inflammatory process of SSc is so similar to that of lupus that patients may first be diagnosed as having probable SLE until the disease progresses or until antibody testing supports the diagnosis. The inflamed tissue in patients with SSc becomes fibrotic and then **sclerotic** (hard). Renal involvement is the leading cause of death. Respiratory involvement and hypertension are also common. Patients with SSc do not respond well to the steroids and immunosuppressants used for lupus, and therefore the mortality rate is higher.

The classification for systemic sclerosis is:

- **Diffuse cutaneous SSc**—skin thickening on the trunk, face, and proximal and distal extremities (over most of the body)
- **Limited cutaneous SSc**—thickened skin limited to sites distal to the face, neck, and distal extremities

Patients with the *limited* form of the disease often have the **CREST syndrome**:

- Calcinosis (calcium deposits)
- Raynaud's phenomenon (first symptom that occurs)
- Esophageal dysmotility
- Sclerodactyly (scleroderma of the digits)
- Telangiectasia (spider-like hemangiomas)

The first symptom that usually occurs in patients with the *diffuse* form of the disease is hand and forearm edema, which may exist with bilateral carpal tunnel syndrome. Gastroesophageal reflux disease (GERD) is commonly present in patients with either type of the disease.

Little is known about the cause of SSc, but autoimmunity is suspected. The occurrence of more than one case per family is uncommon, but other connective tissue diseases may be noted in the family history. At this time, specific genetic causes have not been confirmed.

Systemic sclerosis has been described in people of all races and in all geographic areas and affects over 300,000 people. Women are affected more often than men. The onset of the disease is usually between 25 and 55 years of age, with most women getting it in their 40s (Scleroderma Foundation, 2013).

PATIENT-CENTERED COLLABORATIVE CARE

Assessment

Physical Assessment/Clinical Manifestations. **Arthralgia** (joint PAIN) and stiffness are common manifestations that you can assess during the musculoskeletal examination. The acute joint INFLAMMATION that occurs with rheumatoid arthritis (RA) is not common, and deformities are rare.

Findings on inspection of the skin depend on the stage of the scleroderma. Typically, a painless, symmetric, pitting edema of the hands and fingers is present, especially in patients with the diffuse form of the disease. The edema may progress to include the entire upper and lower extremities and face. In this phase, the fingers are described as *sausage-like.* The skin is taut, shiny, and free of wrinkles. If diffuse scleroderma occurs, swelling is replaced by tightening, hardening, and thickening of skin tissue; this phase is sometimes called the *indurative phase* (Fig. 18-9). The skin loses its elasticity, and range of motion is markedly decreased; ulcerations may occur. Joint contractures may develop, and the patient may be unable to perform ADLs independently.

Major organ damage is likely to develop with diffuse scleroderma, specifically affecting the renal and cardiopulmonary systems. The initial GERD symptoms progress into other problems, especially affecting the esophagus. The esophagus loses its motility, resulting in *dysphagia (difficulty swallowing).* Assess for the ability of the patient to swallow before allowing him or her to drink or eat food. A small, sliding hiatal hernia may be present, and swallowing may be difficult. Reflux of the gastric contents can cause esophagitis and subsequent ulceration, particularly in the lower two thirds of the esophagus. Intestinal changes are similar to those of the esophagus. Peristalsis is diminished, which causes clinical manifestations similar to a partial bowel obstruction. Malabsorption is a common complication, causing malodorous *diarrheal stools.*

In addition to assessing problems of the digestive tract, observe for *cardiovascular manifestations. Raynaud's phenomenon* occurs in various degrees in most patients with SSc. On exposure to cold or emotional stress, the small arterioles in the digits of both hands and feet rapidly constrict, which causes decreased blood flow. In severe cases, the patient experiences digit necrosis, excruciating pain, and **autoamputation of the distal digits** (the tips of the digits fall off spontaneously). In many patients, vasculitic lesions, often around the nail beds (**periungual lesions**), are evident. *Myocardial fibrosis,* another common problem, is evidenced by electrocardiographic (ECG) changes, cardiac dysrhythmias, and chest pain.

Lung involvement in the patient with SSc may go undetected until late in the disease or sometimes until autopsy. *Fibrosis of*

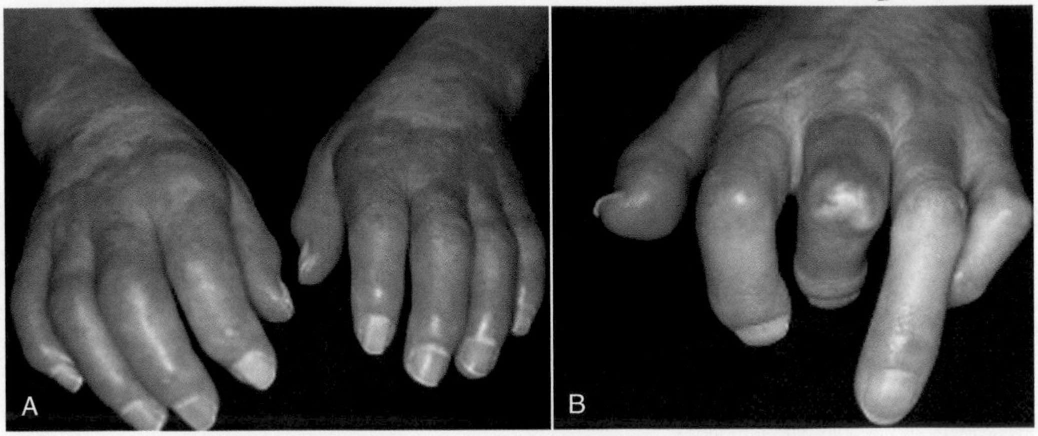

FIG. 18-9 Late-stage skin changes seen in patients with systemic sclerosis.

the alveoli and interstitial tissues is present in almost all cases of the disease, but clinical manifestations may not be present. Patients with scleroderma and *pulmonary arterial hypertension* have a more serious prognosis. *Renal involvement* is an important aspect of the overall disease process and often causes malignant hypertension and death. Assess for signs of impending organ failure, such as changes in urine output and increased blood pressure.

Laboratory Assessment. The laboratory findings for SSc are similar to those for SLE. Clinical findings and the patient's response to drug therapy help the health care provider differentiate between the two diseases. Additional tests depend on which organs seem to be affected. Upper and lower GI series are commonly performed because of the frequency of GI clinical manifestations.

◆ *Interventions*

The medical management of SSc aims to force the disease into remission and thus slow disease progression. The health care provider uses drug therapy primarily for this purpose, but it is often unsuccessful. Systemic steroids and immunosuppressants are used in large doses and often in combination. Another desired outcome of disease management is to identify early organ involvement and treat it before it becomes severe and irreversible. For example, a patient who has lung involvement receives aggressive respiratory therapy and other treatments as the condition requires.

Recently, bosentan (Tracleer), the first of a new class of drugs called *endothelin receptor antagonists,* demonstrated improved walk tests for patients with class III or class IV pulmonary arterial hypertension. Various doses improved patients' breathing during exercise, but the potential for liver injury at the highest dose caused recommended doses to be lowered. Teach the patient the desired and potential adverse effects, including liver toxicity and birth defects. Remind him or her of the importance of follow-up testing for liver enzyme levels.

New oral tyrosine kinase inhibitors (TKIs), including nilotinib (Tasigna) and imatinib mesylate (Gleevec), are being tested for use for patients with systemic sclerosis. These drugs work to decrease INFLAMMATION and slow the progression of the disease. They are currently approved in the United States for use in certain types of cancer.

Local skin protective measures can help maintain skin integrity. Teach the patient to use mild soap and lotions and gentle cleaning techniques. Inspect the skin for further changes or open lesions. Skin ulcers are treated according to their type and location.

In addition to drug therapy to control the overall disease process, specific measures can provide comfort. The patient with SSc not only experiences chronic joint PAIN but also has severe, acute pain during episodes of Raynaud's phenomenon. Remind unlicensed nursing personnel to use a bed cradle and foot board to keep bed covers away from the skin in severe cases. Adjust the room temperature to prevent chilling, which can precipitate digit vasospasm. The patient who can tolerate touching of the affected areas can wear gloves and socks to increase warmth. Because cigarette smoking and extreme emotional stress can also cause symptoms to recur, teach the patient to avoid or minimize these factors as much as possible.

If the patient has esophageal involvement, collaborate with the speech and language pathologist to schedule a swallowing study. The patient may need small, frequent meals rather than the traditional three meals daily. He or she should minimize the intake of foods and liquids that stimulate gastric secretion (e.g., spicy foods, caffeine, alcohol). Teach the patient to keep his or her head elevated for 1 to 2 hours after meals. He or she may need to be in this position continuously. Histamine antagonists and antacids help reduce and neutralize gastric acid. To help prevent choking, collaborate with the dietitian for dietary changes (Chart 18-13).

CHART 18-13 Best Practice for Patient Safety & Quality Care QSEN

The Patient with Systemic Sclerosis and Esophagitis

- Keep the patient's head elevated at least 60 degrees during meals and for at least 1 hour after each meal.
- Provide small, frequent meals rather than three large meals each day.
- Give the patient small amounts of food for each bite, and explain the importance of chewing each bite carefully before swallowing.
- Provide semisoft foods, such as mashed potatoes and pudding or custard; liquids are most likely to cause choking.
- Collaborate with the dietitian about the patient's diet.
- Teach the patient to avoid foods that increase gastric secretion, such as caffeine, pepper, and other spices.
- Give antacids or histamine antagonists as needed.

Nursing care for the patient with joint PAIN and decreased MOBILITY is very similar to that for rheumatoid arthritis (see the Interventions section of the Rheumatoid Arthritis section on p. 293). NSAIDs are given for INFLAMMATION and pain. Joint protection and energy conservation are also important for these patients.

Community-Based Care

Community-based care for the person with SSc is similar to that for lupus. The patient is treated at home but may need frequent hospitalizations if major organ involvement occurs during exacerbations. The Arthritis Foundation (www.arthritis.org) and Scleroderma Foundation (www.scleroderma.org) are excellent resources for more information about the disease and how to manage it.

GOUT

❖ PATHOPHYSIOLOGY

Gout, or gouty arthritis, is a systemic disease in which urate crystals deposit in the joints and other body tissues, causing inflammation. It is the most common inflammatory arthritis in older adults, affecting an estimated 6.1 million people (Arthritis Foundation, 2013a). The cause and treatment of gout have been firmly established. The classic case of well-advanced disease is seldom seen today unless the patient does not adhere to the therapeutic regimen. The two major types of gout are primary and secondary.

Primary gout is the most common type and results from one of several inborn errors of purine metabolism. An end product of purine metabolism is uric acid, which is usually excreted by the kidneys. In primary gout, the production of uric acid exceeds the excretion capability of the kidneys. Sodium urate is deposited in synovium and other tissues, resulting in inflammation. For some patients, primary gout is inherited as an X-linked trait; males are affected through female carriers. A number of patients have a family history of gout. Primary gout affects middle-aged and older men and postmenopausal women. The peak time of onset in men is between 40 and 50 years of age (McCance et al., 2014).

Secondary gout involves **hyperuricemia** (excessive uric acid in the blood) caused by another disease or factor. Secondary gout affects people of all ages. Renal insufficiency, diuretic therapy, "crash" diets, and certain chemotherapeutic agents decrease the normal excretion of uric acid and other waste products. Disorders such as multiple myeloma and certain carcinomas result in increased production of uric acid because of a greater turnover of cellular nucleic acids. Treatment involves management of the underlying disorder.

Hyperuricemia and gout are often seen in older patients with cardiovascular health problems, obese people, and postmenopausal women. The incidence of gout is increasing as the baby boomer generation reaches 65 years of age.

The three clinical stages of the primary disease process are asymptomatic hyperuricemia, acute gouty arthritis, and chronic or tophaceous gout (McCance et al., 2014). The patient is usually unaware of the *asymptomatic hyperuricemic stage* unless he or she has had a serum uric acid level determination. The serum level is elevated, but no obvious signs of the disease are present. No treatment is needed in this stage.

The first "attack" of gouty arthritis begins the *acute stage.* The patient experiences excruciating PAIN and INFLAMMATION in one or more small joints, usually the metatarsophalangeal joint of the great toe, called **podagra**. The erythrocyte sedimentation rate (ESR) is usually increased as a result of the inflammatory process. Months or years may pass before additional attacks occur. The patient is asymptomatic, and no abnormalities are found during examination of the joints.

After repeated episodes of acute gout, deposits of urate crystals develop under the skin and within the major organs, particularly in the renal system. The patient is then classified as having *chronic tophaceous gout.* In chronic gout, urate kidney stone formation is more common than renal insufficiency. Chronic gout can begin anywhere between 3 and 40 years after the initial gout symptoms occur (McCance et al., 2014).

❖ PATIENT-CENTERED COLLABORATIVE CARE

◆ Assessment

Note the patient's age, gender, and family history of gout. A complete history is needed to determine whether gout has been caused by another problem. Some women overuse diuretics, which can lead to secondary gout.

Overt manifestations are present in the acute and chronic phases of gout. You will likely encounter a patient with acute gout, but chronic gout is not as common in the United States today. *Joint INFLAMMATION is the most common finding of acute gout. The joint is usually so painful that the patient seeks medical care immediately.* Inspect the inflamed area. It is usually too painful and swollen to be touched or moved.

The health care provider requests a serum uric acid level to check for hyperuricemia. Because the level can be altered by food intake, several measurements may be obtained. A consistent level of more than 6.5 mg/dL is generally considered abnormal, depending on the laboratory test used. Urinary uric acid levels are also measured; an overproduction of uric acid is confirmed by an excretion of more than 750 mg/24 hr (Pagana & Pagana, 2014).

The health care provider may request kidney function tests, such as blood urea nitrogen (BUN) and serum creatinine levels, to monitor possible kidney involvement. A definitive diagnostic test for the disease is synovial fluid aspiration (arthrocentesis) to detect the needle-like crystals in the affected joint that are characteristic of the disorder.

With *chronic* gout, inspect the skin for **tophi**, or deposits of sodium urate crystals (Fig. 18-10). Although tophi are rarely

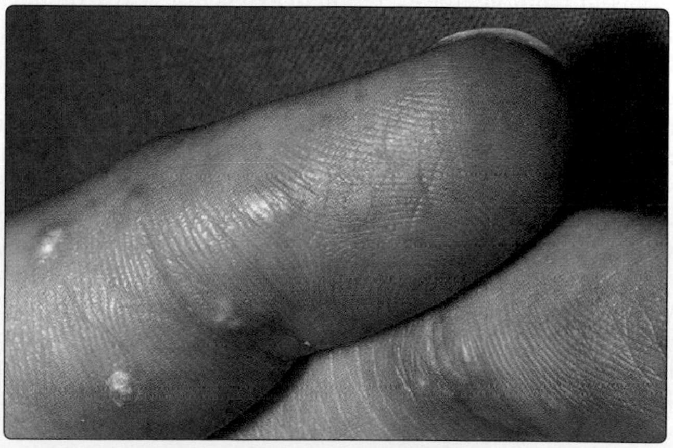

FIG. 18-10 Typical appearance of tophi, which may occur in chronic gout, on an index finger.

seen today, they may appear on the outer ear, arms, and fingers near the joints. The tophi are hard on palpation and are irregular in shape. When the skin over the tophi is irritated, it may break open and a yellow, gritty substance is discharged. Infection may result.

Other manifestations of chronic gout include signs of renal calculi (stones) or renal dysfunction, such as severe PAIN or changes in urinary output. In some cases, urate kidney stones occur before the arthritis is present.

◆ Interventions

Gout is one of the easiest diseases for the health care provider to diagnose and treat in its early phases. If the patient receives treatment and adheres to drug therapy, he or she should experience no further symptoms and no change in body image or lifestyle. The patient with gout is treated on an ambulatory basis, but hospitalized patients may have a secondary diagnosis of the disease.

Drug Therapy. Drug therapy is the key to managing patients with gout. In acute gouty "attacks," the inflammation subsides spontaneously within 3 to 5 days; however, most patients cannot tolerate the pain for that long. The drugs used for acute gout are different from those used for chronic gout. The health care provider typically prescribes a combination of colchicine (Colcrys) and an NSAID, such as indomethacin (Indocin, Novomethacin 🍁) or ibuprofen (Motrin, Amersol 🍁) for acute gout. IV colchicine works within 12 hours. The patient takes oral medications until the INFLAMMATION subsides, usually for 4 to 7 days.

For patients with repeated acute episodes or with chronic gout, the health care provider prescribes drugs on a continuous, maintenance basis to promote uric acid excretion or to reduce its production. Allopurinol (Zyloprim, Purinol 🍁) or febuxostat (Uloric) is the drug of choice. Febuxostat may cause a greater risk to cardiovascular health than allopurinol (Lilley et al., 2014). As xanthine oxidase inhibitors, these drugs prevent the conversion of xanthine to uric acid. Teach patients to take them after meals and drink a glass of water with each dose to prevent GI distress. Drinking at least 8 glasses of water each day helps prevent renal dysfunction. Remind patients that periodic follow-up laboratory tests, including liver enzymes, kidney function studies, and complete blood count, are important because xanthine oxidase inhibitors cause liver dysfunction and bone marrow suppression.

Probenecid can also be effective as a uricosuric drug in gout because it promotes the excretion of excess uric acid. Combination drugs that contain probenecid and colchicine (e.g., Col-BENEMID) are also available. The health care provider and nurse monitor serum uric acid levels to determine the effectiveness of these medications. Aspirin should be avoided because it inactivates the effects of the drug.

For patients with severe gout who do not respond to other drugs (refractory gout), pegloticase (Krystexxa) can be prescribed as an IV dose every 2 weeks. This drug is an enzyme that works directly on uric acid and converts it to allantoin, which can be excreted by the kidneys. Monitor patients carefully for allergic reactions, including anaphylaxis, during and immediately after drug administration because pegloticase is a protein that is foreign to the body.

Nutrition Therapy and Lifestyle Recommendations. The American College of Rheumatology best practice guidelines recommend a strict low-purine diet and suggest that patients avoid foods such as organ meats, shellfish, and oily fish with bones (e.g., sardines). Some health care providers and dietitians believe that limiting protein foods, especially red and organ meats, is sufficient. It is well known, however, that excessive alcohol intake and fad "starvation" diets can cause a gouty attack. *Teach patients to determine which foods precipitate acute attacks and try to avoid them.*

In addition to food and beverage restrictions, patients with gout should avoid all forms of aspirin and diuretics because they may precipitate an attack. Likewise, excessive physical or emotional stress can exacerbate the disease. Surgery or acute illness, like a myocardial infarction, can also trigger an attack. Stress-management techniques may be helpful for the patient with gout.

Teach the patient to drink plenty of fluids to prevent the formation of urinary stones. Increasing fluid intake helps dilute urine and prevent sediment formation. Uric acid is more soluble in urine with a high pH and therefore is less likely to form urinary stones in that environment. The patient's urinary pH can be increased with an intake of alkaline ash foods, such as citrus fruits and juices, milk, and certain other dairy products. The value of adhering to a strict diet rich in these foods is questionable, however. If the patient is overweight, recommend community resources for losing weight, including increasing exercise.

NCLEX EXAMINATION CHALLENGE

Physiological Integrity

The nurse is preparing to give medications to a group of clients. Which drug is not appropriate to treat the disease with which it is matched?

A. Rheumatoid arthritis—methotrexate (MTX)
B. Osteoarthritis—acetaminophen (Tylenol)
C. Acute gout—allopurinol (Zyloprim)
D. Systemic lupus erythematosus—prednisone (Deltasone)

INFECTIOUS ARTHRITIS

Any infectious agent can invade the joint space and cause PAIN, INFLAMMATION, and tissue destruction. Certain pathogens, such as *Staphylococcus aureus,* destroy tissue rapidly; others, especially viruses, do not cause irreversible damage. The cornerstone of management is local or systemic antibiotic therapy for 6 to 8 weeks.

LYME DISEASE

Lyme disease is a reportable systemic infectious disease caused by the spirochete *Borrelia burgdorferi* and results from the bite of an infected deer tick, also known as the *black-legged tick.* It is the most common vector-borne disease in the United States and Europe. Most cases of the disease in the United States are seen in New England; the mid-Atlantic states, including Maryland and Virginia; the upper Midwest, including Wisconsin and Minnesota; and northern California, especially during the summer months.

In the early and *localized stage I,* the patient appears with *flu-like symptoms,* **erythema migrans** (round or oval, flat or slightly raised rash), and *PAIN and stiffness in the muscles and joints.* Most patients in the United States tend to have only one

CHART 18-14 Patient and Family Education: Preparing for Self-Management

Prevention and Early Detection of Lyme Disease

- Avoid heavily wooded areas or areas with thick underbrush, especially in the spring and summer months.
- Walk in the center of the trail.
- Avoid dark clothing. Lighter-colored clothing makes spotting ticks easier.
- Use an insect repellent (DEET) on your skin and clothes when in an area where ticks are likely to be found.
- Wear long-sleeved tops and long pants; tuck your shirt into your pants and your pants into your socks or boots.
- Wear closed shoes or boots and a hat or cap.
- Bathe immediately after being in an infested area, and inspect your body for ticks (about the size of a pinhead); pay special attention to your arms, legs, and scalp.
- Check your pets for ticks.
- Gently remove with tweezers or fingers covered with tissue or gloves any tick that you find (do not squeeze). Dispose of the tick by flushing it down the toilet (burning a tick could spread infection).
- After removal, clean the tick area with an antiseptic such as rubbing alcohol.
- Wait 4 to 6 weeks after being bitten by a tick before being tested for Lyme disease (testing before this time is not reliable).
- Report symptoms, such as a rash or influenza-like illness, to your physician immediately.

lesion, sometimes referred to as a *"bull's-eye lesion."* Symptoms begin within 3 to 30 days of the tick bite, but most present in 7 to 14 days. Antibiotic therapy, such as doxycycline or amoxicillin, is prescribed during this uncomplicated stage for 14 to 21 days. Erythromycin can be used for patients who are allergic to penicillin. Without treatment, these symptoms may disappear in about 4 to 5 weeks.

If not treated or if treatment is not successful, the patient may progress to the more serious complications of Lyme disease. *Stage II (early disseminated stage)* occurs 2 to 12 weeks after the tick bite. The patient may develop *carditis* with *dysrhythmias, dyspnea, dizziness, or palpitations,* as well as central nervous system disorders such as *meningitis, facial paralysis* (often misdiagnosed as Bell's palsy), and *peripheral neuritis.* For severe disease, IV antibiotics (e.g., ceftriaxone or cefotaxime) are given for at least 30 days.

If Lyme disease is not diagnosed and treated in the earlier stages, later chronic complications (e.g., *arthritis, chronic fatigue, memory/thinking problems*) can result. This *late stage III (chronic persistent stage)* occurs months to years after the tick bite. *For some patients, the first and only sign of Lyme disease is arthritis.* In some cases, the disease may not respond to antibiotics in any stage and the patient develops permanent damage to joints and the nervous system. *Prevention is the best strategy for Lyme disease.* Teach patients to follow the measures outlined in Chart 18-14 to prevent Lyme and other tick-borne diseases. Tell them about community resources such as the Lyme Disease Foundation (www.lyme.org) for more information.

PSORIATIC ARTHRITIS

Psoriatic arthritis (PsA) affects some people who have psoriasis—a skin condition characterized by a scaly, itchy rash, usually on the elbows, knees, and scalp. Fingernail and toenail lifting and pitting may also occur (see Chapter 25 for discussion of this disease). The joint PAIN associated with psoriasis is often associated with stiffness, especially in the morning. Neck and back pain are particularly common, but various forms of the disease can cause small joint arthritis or involvement of the sacroiliac joints of the spine.

PsA occurs most often in people between 30 and 50 years of age in men and women of all races. Nail symptoms are common in patients who have the associated arthritis. Causes may include genetic and environmental factors, infectious agents, and immune system dysfunction.

Most patients do not experience destructive and deforming arthritis affecting more than three joints, but for those who do, the experience has a major impact on their quality of life. Treatment is focused on managing joint PAIN and INFLAMMATION, controlling skin lesions, and slowing the progression of the disease. Health teaching for skin care is similar to that for lupus. Management of joint inflammation is similar to that for rheumatoid arthritis as described earlier in this chapter. Methotrexate (Rheumatrex), sulfasalazine (Azulfidine), and biological response modifiers (also called *biologics*), such as etanercept (Enbrel) and golimumab (Simponi), are being used with success.

Teach the patient or family member how to self-administer Enbrel injections. Injection site reactions and infections (especially respiratory) are possible adverse effects. Ice and hydrocortisone 1% cream can be used if a red, itchy rash at the injection site develops.

Golimumab (Simponi) is the first biologic that is administered only once each month for psoriatic arthritis. Teach patients that this drug has a black box warning for serious infections that may lead to hospitalization or death from opportunistic pathogens (Cranwell-Bruce, 2011).

Several newer types of biologics have also been approved for psoriatic arthritis. Ustekinumab (Stelara) targets the cytokines *interleukin (IL)-12* and *IL-23* to decrease INFLAMMATION. Alefacept (Amevive) is an IV immunosuppressive drug (T-cell blocker) that is reserved for moderate to severe disease. Teach patients taking these drugs about their risk for INFECTION. Remind them to avoid crowds and anyone with an INFECTION.

Acitretin (Soriatane) is an oral retinoid given for patients with severe disease. Teach patients to take the drug once a day with a meal and follow up with laboratory testing for liver enzymes.

The National Psoriasis Foundation (www.psoriasis.org) is an excellent community resource for patients and their families. Further discussion regarding management of psoriasis can be found in Chapter 25.

FIBROMYALGIA SYNDROME

Fibromyalgia syndrome (FMS), also referred to as simply *fibromyalgia,* is a chronic PAIN syndrome, not an inflammatory disease. However, arthritis and other comorbidities are commonly present in patients diagnosed with FMS. Pain, stiffness, and tenderness are located at specific sites in the back of the neck, upper chest, trunk, low back, and extremities. These tender points are also known as **trigger points** and can typically be palpated to elicit pain in a predictable, reproducible pattern. The pain is typically described as burning and gnawing. Increased muscle tenderness may be caused by the inability to tolerate pain, possibly related to dysfunction in the brain, especially the thalamus and hypothalamus (McCance et al., 2014).

The PAIN and tenderness tend to come and go but typically worsen in response to stress, increased activity, and weather conditions. The patient reports mild to severe fatigue, and sleep disturbances are common. Some people report numbness or tingling in their extremities, and others are sensitive to noxious odors, loud noises, and bright lights. Headaches and jaw pain are also common. Secondary FMS can accompany any connective tissue disease (CTD), particularly lupus and rheumatoid disease, and may not necessarily be related to sleep patterns.

Other symptoms include:

- Gastrointestinal (GI), including abdominal PAIN, diarrhea and constipation, and heartburn
- Genitourinary, including dysuria, urinary frequency, urgency, and pelvic pain
- Cardiovascular, including dyspnea, chest pain, and dysrhythmias
- Visual, including blurred vision and dry eyes
- Neurologic, including forgetfulness and concentration problems

Many with these symptoms become frustrated because they are not properly diagnosed and are in constant pain and discomfort.

Some patients are diagnosed as having chronic fatigue syndrome (CFS). CFS, migraine headache, irritable bowel syndrome (IBS), and myofascial PAIN are often present in those with FMS. As a result, patients can become depressed and anxious.

Most patients are women between 30 and 50 years of age. It is unlikely that the disease is caused by one factor. Possible precipitating factors include CFS, Lyme disease, trauma, and flu-like illness (McCance et al., 2014). FMS may also be aggravated by deep-sleep deprivation. Teach patients to limit caffeine, alcohol, or other unnecessary substances that could interfere with deep sleep. Establish a regular sleep pattern.

Pregabalin (Lyrica) and duloxetine HCl (Cymbalta), which are antidepressant drugs, are approved for fibromyalgia nerve PAIN. These drugs work to increase the release of serotonin and norepinephrine, neurotransmitters in the brain (Lilley et al., 2014). Teach the patient that these drugs can cause drowsiness and sleepiness and that alcohol should be avoided while taking them.

Tricyclic antidepressive agents, such as amitriptyline (Elavil, Apo-Amitriptyline ♣) or nortriptyline (Pamelor), may promote sleep and reduce pain or muscle spasm. These drugs should be used with caution in older adults because they can cause confusion and orthostatic hypotension. Trazodone (Desyrel) may be preferred for this population because of its minimal side effects. Tramadol (Ultram) is also effective for managing fibromyalgia. This drug has tricyclic effects and opioid properties to help relieve PAIN (see Chapter 3).

Physical therapy along with NSAIDs and possibly muscle relaxants may also be prescribed to help decrease fibromyalgia PAIN. Instruct the patient to exercise regularly. Home exercise should include stretching, strengthening, and low-impact aerobic exercise. Walking, swimming, rowing, biking, and water exercise are good examples of low-impact exercise. Complementary and alternative therapies, such as tai chi, acupuncture, hypnosis, and stress management, may help some patients with symptom relief. Refer patients to the land, water, and walking exercise pamphlets produced by the Arthritis Foundation (www.arthritis.org). Inform them about the National Fibromyalgia Association for additional information and patient and family support (www.fmaware.org).

CHRONIC FATIGUE SYNDROME

Chronic fatigue syndrome (CFS), also known as *chronic fatigue and immune dysfunction syndrome (CFIDS)*, is a chronic illness in which patients have severe fatigue for 6 months or longer, usually following flu-like symptoms. In addition, four or more of these criteria must be met for a diagnosis of CFS:

- Sore throat
- Substantial impairment in short-term memory or concentration
- Tender lymph nodes
- Muscle PAIN
- Multiple joint PAIN with redness or swelling
- Headaches of a new type, pattern, or severity (not familiar to the patient)
- Unrefreshing sleep
- Postexertional malaise lasting more than 24 hours

Chronic fatigue syndrome is most common in women and is not limited to any socioeconomic group or age. There is no laboratory test to confirm the diagnosis, and therefore many people with the disease probably have not been diagnosed. The cause is unknown, although immune, endocrine, neurologic, and environmental factors are being studied.

Management of the patient is challenging in that there is no cure for CFS. Treatment is supportive and focuses on alleviation or reduction of symptoms. For example, NSAIDs may help with body aches and PAIN. Low-dose antidepressants, such as pregabalin (Lyrica), may also be effective in promoting sleep and preventing or treating depression. Teach the patient to follow healthy practices, such as adequate sleep, proper nutrition, regular exercise (but not excessive to increase fatigue), stress management, and energy conservation. Complementary and alternative therapies, such as acupuncture, tai chi, massage, and herbal supplements, may be helpful for some patients.

Refer the patient to the National Chronic Fatigue Syndrome and Fibromyalgia Association for information and support groups.

OTHER CONNECTIVE TISSUE DISEASES

Many other connective tissues diseases (CTDs) may be seen, but they are not as common as those health problems previously described. Table 18-3 describes some of these CTDs, their key assessments, and primary collaborative interventions.

OTHER DISEASE-ASSOCIATED ARTHRITIS

A number of other diseases can cause secondary arthritis. Tuberculosis, Crohn's disease, ulcerative colitis, hemophilia, and sickle cell anemia are typical examples. To manage joint involvement, the primary disease is treated. For example, when a patient with Crohn's disease is in remission, joint manifestations also subside. Conditions in which joint involvement can occur are presented in Table 18-4.

MIXED CONNECTIVE TISSUE DISEASE

A diagnosis of mixed CTD is made when a patient presents with clinical manifestations that are not typical of any one CTD.

TABLE 18-3 Other Connective Tissue Diseases That Affect Joints

DISEASE	DESCRIPTION/ PATHOPHYSIOLOGY	ASSESSMENT/CLINICAL MANIFESTATIONS	COLLABORATIVE INTERVENTIONS
Polymyositis/ dermatomyositis	Autoimmune, inflammatory disease that causes symmetric muscle atrophy; when skin rash is also present, disease is called *dermatomyositis (DM);* women between 30 and 60 years affected most often.	Severe muscle weakness Dysphagia (difficulty swallowing) Periorbital edema and lilac eyelid rash (DM) Malignant neoplasms in older patients	Comfort measures Swallowing precautions Nutritional support PT/OT support Immunosuppressant agents and/ or chronic steroid therapy (Teach about risk for infection.) Health teaching about progression of disease, comfort measures, and dietary needs
Systemic necrotizing vasculitis	A group of autoimmune diseases that result in arteritis (inflammation of arterial walls) causing ischemia in the tissues or organs that are supplied by the arteries.	Peripheral arterial disease causing severe pain and necrosis of toes or fingers Signs and symptoms of organ dysfunction or failure, such as kidney or heart failure; also can cause stroke-like symptoms	Chronic steroid therapy and other immunosuppressants Vasodilators, depending on type of vasculitis Management of organ dysfunction or failure
Polymyalgia rheumatica (PMR) and temporal arteritis (TA)	Autoimmune, genetic-based disease affecting middle-aged and older women most often that causes proximal muscle weakness (shoulder and pelvic girdles) (PMR). TA (also known as *giant cell arteritis*) may occur as a separate disease or with PMR.	Shoulder, neck, pelvic, and hip weakness, stiffness, joint aches, low-grade fever, fatigue, and weight loss caused by inflammation (PMR) Headache and visual disturbances (TA)	Responds well to high-dose steroid therapy to cause remission of disease Symptom management Short-term PT/OT as needed Health teaching about medication and pain modalities, such as heat application for joints
Ankylosing spondylitis	Autoimmune, inflammatory disease affecting the spine that is thought to be genetic (strongly associated with specific variations in the *HLA-27* allele on chromosome 6). Can occur in both men and women, but white men younger than 40 years most commonly affected.	Chronic back pain Compromised respiratory function due to rigid chest wall Visual disturbances caused by iritis (inflammation of the iris) Joint pain and aching Malaise Weight loss	Chronic pain management modalities NSAIDs DMARDs, such as methotrexate and biologic response modifiers Symptom management
Reiter's syndrome	Complex syndrome associated with the *HLA-27* allele causing a triad of arthritis, conjunctivitis, and urethritis (inflammation of the urethra). Triggered by exposure to infection, especially sexually transmitted disease or intestinal infection.	Joint pain Eye infection causing redness, pain, and drainage Pain or burning on urination and changes in urinary pattern	Antibiotic therapy to manage infection Pain management NSAIDs Other symptom management
Marfan syndrome	Autosomal dominant disorder resulting from mutations in the *fibrillin I* gene (FBNI). Fibrillin important in limiting the stretch of elastic connective tissues and allowing them to return to their original resting shape. Disease shortens life expectancy, often with death in the 30s.	Excessive height Elongated hands and feet Joint discomfort or pain Scoliosis Visual problems, such as decreased visual acuity or glaucoma Cardiovascular problems, such as mitral valve prolapse and aortic aneurysm, leading to heart failure or death	Symptom management Frequent echocardiography monitoring and physical examinations to detect heart problems Genetic counseling

DMARDs, Disease-modifying antirheumatic drugs; *OT,* occupational therapy; *PT,* physical therapy.

TABLE 18-4 Common Disorders Associated with Arthritis

- Crohn's disease
- Ulcerative colitis
- Tuberculosis
- Hemophilia
- Whipple's disease
- Intestinal bypass surgery
- Hyperparathyroidism
- Hyperthyroidism
- Diabetes mellitus
- Sickle cell anemia crisis
- Psoriasis
- Infection

About 10% of patients with CTDs are classified as having mixed disease. Some of these are overlap syndromes, in which two or more diseases occur at the same time. Common examples are (1) systemic lupus erythematosus (SLE) plus systemic sclerosis (SSc) and (2) rheumatoid arthritis (RA) plus SLE. Management depends on the clinical manifestations, but often the patient is treated as having SLE.

NURSING CONCEPTS AND CLINICAL JUDGMENT REVIEW

What might you NOTICE if the patient has impaired IMMUNITY as a result of arthritis or other connective tissue disease (CTD)?

- Joint inflammation (redness, swelling, pain)
- Impaired joint mobility and stiffness
- Joint deformity
- Difficulty ambulating
- Fever
- Rash
- Report of weight loss and fatigue
- Other manifestations that indicate organ involvement, such as dysrhythmias (heart) and decreased urinary output (kidneys)

What should you INTERPRET and how should you RESPOND to a patient with impaired IMMUNITY as a result of arthritis or other CTD?

Perform and interpret focused physical assessment findings, including:

- Joint assessment, including range of motion
- ADL ability
- Pain intensity and quality
- Body weight
- Ability to cope with disease
- Vital signs
- Other assessments related to specific organ involvement (e.g., cardiac assessment)

Respond:

- Provide pain control interventions, including drug therapy and nonpharmacologic measures (e.g., heat and cold application).
- Collaborate with members of the health care team to improve mobility and ambulation, if needed.
- Teach about drug therapy, including the expected and adverse effects.
- Teach about nonpharmacologic measures to control pain, including ice and heat, and CAM therapies, such as glucosamine.
- Report manifestations of organ involvement to the health care provider for possible immediate intervention (e.g., drug therapy for severe dysrhythmias).
- Monitor laboratory test results to determine progress of treatment.
- Continue to assess for changes in the patient's condition, including new or additional manifestations of organ involvement.
- Encourage patients and their families to discuss their feelings about chronic illness and possible body image changes.
- Help identify coping strategies, and provide information about community and professional resources and support groups.

On what should you REFLECT?

- Monitor the patient's response to pain control interventions.
- Evaluate the patient's and family's knowledge of the disease and its management.
- Evaluate the patient's and family's stress levels and coping strategies.
- Think about what else you might do to promote mobility.
- Decide whether you need to provide alternative interventions or additional health teaching.

GET READY FOR THE NCLEX® EXAMINATION!

KEY POINTS

Review these Key Points for each NCLEX Examination Client Needs Category.

Safe and Effective Care Environment

- Collaborate with the health care team to manage chronic PAIN and increase MOBILITY for patients with arthritis and other CTDs. **Teamwork and Collaboration** QSEN
- Prioritize care for patients with systemic lupus erythematosus (SLE) and systemic sclerosis (SSc) by monitoring for life-threatening complications, such as kidney failure.

Health Promotion and Maintenance

- Provide information about community resources for patients, especially professional organizations such as the Arthritis Foundation and Lupus Foundation.
- Teach patients to prevent joint trauma and reduce weight as needed to help prevent osteoarthritis. **Evidence-Based Practice** QSEN
- Recall that a combination of environmental, genetic, and immune risk factors can cause arthritis and other connective tissue diseases.
- Reinforce the importance of good health practices, such as adequate sleep, proper nutrition, regular exercise, and stress-management techniques for patients with arthritis and other CTDs.
- Teach patients with arthritis what exercises to do (Chart 18-5), joint protection techniques (Chart 18-6), and energy conservation guidelines (Chart 18-10). **Evidence-Based Practice** QSEN
- Teach patients with SLE to avoid sunlight; exacerbations of the disease may be triggered.
- Remind patients with gout to avoid factors that trigger an attack, such as aspirin, organ meats, and alcohol. **Evidence-Based Practice** QSEN
- Teach people ways to prevent or detect early Lyme disease as listed in Chart 18-14.

Psychosocial Integrity

- Recognize that patients with rheumatoid arthritis (RA) may have body image disturbance as a result of potentially deforming joint involvement and nodules.
- Encourage patients with arthritis and connective tissue diseases to discuss their chronic illness and identify coping strategies that have previously been successful. **Patient-Centered Care** QSEN
- Be aware that chronic, painful diseases affect the patient's quality of life and role performance.
- Recognize that patients with fibromyalgia syndrome (FMS) and chronic fatigue syndrome (CFS) are often frustrated because they have not been diagnosed or have been misdiagnosed.
- Teach patients with FMS and CFS that antidepressant drugs can promote sleep and decrease PAIN, as well as prevent or treat the depression that is common with these illnesses.

Physiological Integrity

- Be aware that most of the connective tissue diseases and arthritic disorders have a genetic basis as part of their etiology; most are also classified as autoimmune diseases and have remissions and exacerbations.
- Differentiate OA as primarily a degenerative joint problem that can affect one or more joints, and RA as a systemic disease that presents as a bilateral symmetric joint INFLAMMATION.
- Realize that older patients have OA more than younger patients; younger patients have RA more than older adults; other differences between the two diseases are summarized in Table 18-1.
- Teach patients who have osteoarthritis (OA) or are prone to the disease to lose weight (if obese), avoid trauma, and limit strenuous weight-bearing activities.
- Instruct patients with arthritic pain to use multiple modalities for pain relief, including ice/heat, rest, positioning, complementary and alternative therapies, and medications as prescribed.
- Teach patients to monitor and report side and adverse effects of drugs used to treat OA and other connective tissue diseases.
- Assess patients with rheumatoid arthritis for early or late clinical manifestations as listed in Chart 18-7.
- Teach patients who are taking hydroxychloroquine (Plaquenil) to have frequent (every 6 months) eye examinations to monitor for retinal changes. **Safety** QSEN
- Remind patients to avoid crowds and other possible sources of INFECTION when they are taking immunosuppressant drugs. **Safety** QSEN
- Implement interventions for patients having total joint arthroplasty (TJA) to prevent venous thromboembolitic complications (e.g., anticoagulants, exercises, sequential compression devices); observe the patient for bleeding when he or she is taking anticoagulants.
- Be careful when positioning a patient after a total hip arthroplasty (THA) to prevent dislocation; do not hyperflex the hips or adduct the legs (see Chart 18-3). **Safety** QSEN
- Be aware that disease-modifying antirheumatic drugs (DMARDs) and biological response modifiers (BRMs) slow the progression of connective tissue diseases, especially RA and SLE.
- Remind patients taking methotrexate (Rheumatrex) to avoid people with INFECTIONS; check the patient's PPD test or history of tuberculosis before starting the drug. **Safety** QSEN
- Teach patients receiving BRMs and other disease-modifying agents to avoid crowds and people with INFECTIONS; opportunistic pathogens may cause serious infections or death (see Chart 18-9).
- Monitor and interpret laboratory test results for patients with autoimmune connective tissue diseases as highlighted in Chart 18-8.
- Differentiate clinical manifestations and prognosis for patients with systemic lupus erythematosus (SLE) versus systemic sclerosis (SSc) as listed in Chart 18-11.
- Prioritize care by assessing for swallowing ability in patients who have SSc; collaborate with the dietitian for food modifications if needed. **Teamwork and Collaboration** QSEN
- Monitor for acute joint INFLAMMATION in patients with a history of gout; the great toe and other small joints are most typically affected.
- Keep in mind that patients with psoriatic arthritis have skin and joint involvement that require collaborative management (also see Chapter 25 for discussion of psoriasis).
- Assess for visual symptoms (indicating possible giant cell arteritis) in patients with polymyalgia rheumatica; report changes immediately to the health care provider.
- Be aware that arthritis often accompanies other diseases, such as Crohn's disease and hemophilia.

19 CHAPTER

Care of Patients with HIV Disease and Other Immune Deficiencies

James Sampson and M. Linda Workman

http://evolve.elsevier.com/Iggy/

PRIORITY CONCEPTS

- Immunity
- Infection
- Nutrition
- Tissue Integrity
- Pain

LEARNING OUTCOMES

Safe and Effective Care Environment

1. Use appropriate techniques to reduce the risk for infection in an immunosuppressed patient.
2. Prevent human immune deficiency virus (HIV) transmission to yourself and others.

Health Promotion and Maintenance

3. Assess all patients for high-risk behaviors related to HIV infection.

Psychosocial Integrity

4. Reduce the psychological impact of HIV disease or other immune deficiencies for the patient and family.
5. Work with other members of the health care team to ensure that the values, preferences, and expressed needs of patients with HIV disease or other immune deficiencies are respected.

Physiological Integrity

6. Use clinical manifestations and laboratory data to assess for immune deficiencies and their complications.
7. Integrate the contributions of others who play a role in helping the patient/family experiencing HIV disease achieve health goals.
8. Prioritize nursing care for the patient with AIDS.

Immunity is complex and functions to help the body stay healthy by preventing the growth of infectious organisms and abnormal cells, such as cancer cells. Infectious organisms and cancer cells are considered "non-self," as described in Chapter 17. The immune system monitors all cells and substances, maintaining those that are considered "self" (belonging to the body) and attacking and destroying "non-self" (foreign) substances. Infection from different organisms is a major threat, and exposure occurs daily. The efficiency of the immune system prevents disease despite this exposure. As discussed in Chapter 17, an important function of the immune system is detecting body cells that undergo changes to cancer cells. When detected early enough, the immune system destroys these precancerous cells before a tumor forms.

When the immune system fails to recognize infectious agents, severe local and systemic infections are not suppressed or controlled. Immune system failure can be the result of a primary (congenital) immune deficiency in which one or more parts of the system are not functioning properly from birth. It can also be secondary (acquired after birth) as the result of viral infection, contact with a toxin, or medical therapy that can cause a normal immune system to function less efficiently. Then the immune system can no longer recognize foreign invaders (non-self). The consequences can range from mild, localized health problems to total immunity failure, leaving the body open to attack from any foreign pathogen.

ACQUIRED (SECONDARY) IMMUNE DEFICIENCIES

HIV INFECTION AND AIDS

❖ *PATHOPHYSIOLOGY*

Human immune deficiency virus (HIV) infection and disease can progress to acquired immune deficiency syndrome (AIDS), which is the most common immune deficiency disease and is now a serious worldwide epidemic (World Health Organization [WHO], 2013).

Etiology and Genetic Risk

The cause of HIV infection is a virus—the human immune deficiency virus. HIV is a parasite looking for a way into a cell, to take over the cell, and to force the cell into making more copies of the virus (viral particles). These new viral particles then look for additional cells to infect, repeating the cycle as long as there are new host cells to infect.

The HIV Infectious Process. *Viral particle features* include an outer envelope with special "docking proteins," known as *gp41* and *gp120,* that assist in finding a host (Fig. 19-1). Inside, the virus has genetic material along with the enzymes *reverse transcriptase (RT)* and *integrase.* The HIV must get inside a host cell. It does this by first entering the host's bloodstream and then "hijacking" certain cells, especially the *CD4+ T-cell,* also known as the *CD4+ cell, helper/inducer T-cell,* or *T4-cell* (see Chapter 17). This cell directs immune system defenses and regulates the activity of all immune system cells. When HIV enters a CD4+ T-cell, it can then create more virus particles.

Virus-host interactions are needed after INFECTION for disease development. When a person is infected with HIV, the virus randomly "bumps" into many cells. The docking proteins on the outside of the virus must find special receptors on a host cell for the virus to bind and then enter the cell. The CD4+ T-cell has surface receptors known as *CD4, CCR5,* and *CXCR4* (Fig. 19-2). Proteins on the HIV particle surface, known as *gp120* and *gp41,* recognize these receptors on the CD4+ T-cell. For the virus to enter this cell, *both* the *gp120* and the *gp41* must bind to the receptors. The *gp120* first binds to the primary CD4 receptor, which changes its shape and allows the *gp120* to bind to either the *CCR5* co-receptor or the *CXCR4* co-receptor. Once co-receptor binding occurs, *gp41* inserts a fusion peptide into the T-cell membrane, boring a hole to allow insertion of viral genetic material and enzymes into the host cell. This attachment allows the virus to then enter the CD4+ T-cell (see Fig. 19-2). *Viral binding to the CD4 receptor and to either of the co-receptors is needed to enter the cell.* (The drug class known as *entry inhibitors* works here to prevent the interaction needed for entry of HIV into the CD4+ T-cell.)

After entering a host cell, HIV must get its genetic material into the host cell's DNA. HIV is a **retrovirus,** which is able to insert its single-stranded ribonucleic acid (ss-RNA) genetic material into the host's DNA. The genetic material of the human cell is double-stranded DNA (ds-DNA). To infect and take over a human cell, the genetic material must be the same. The HIV enzyme *reverse transcriptase (RT)* converts HIV's ss-RNA into ds-DNA, which makes the viral genetic material the same as human DNA. (The drug classes known as *nucleoside reverse transcriptase inhibitors [NRTIs]* and *non-nucleoside reverse transcriptase inhibitors [NNRTIs]* work here to prevent viral replication [Fig. 19-3] by reducing how well reverse transcriptase can convert HIV genetic material into human genetic material.) HIV then uses its enzyme *integrase* to get its DNA into the nucleus of the host's CD4+ T-cell and insert it into the host's ds-DNA. This action completes the infection of the CD4+ T-cell. (The drug class known as *integrase inhibitors* works here to prevent viral DNA from integrating into the host's DNA.)

HIV particles are made within the infected CD4+ T-cell, using all the metabolic machinery of the host. The new virus particle is made in the form of one long protein strand. The strand is clipped by the enzyme *HIV protease* into smaller functional pieces. These pieces are formed into a new finished viral particle. (The drug class known as *protease inhibitors* works here to inhibit HIV protease.) Once the new virus particle is finished, it fuses with the infected cell's membrane and then buds off in search of another CD4+ T-cell to infect (see Fig. 19-3).

Effects of HIV infection are related to the new genetic instructions that now direct CD4+ T-cells to change their role in immune system defenses. The new role is to be an "HIV factory," making up to 10 billion new viral particles daily. In addition, the immune system is made weaker by removing some CD4+ T-cells from circulation. In early HIV infection before HIV disease is evident, the immune system can still attack and destroy most of the newly created virus particles. With time, however, the number of HIV particles overwhelms the immune system. Gradually, CD4+ T-cell counts fall, viral numbers *(viral load)* rise, and without treatment, the patient eventually dies of opportunistic INFECTION or cancer.

Everyone who has AIDS has HIV infection; however, not everyone who has HIV infection has AIDS. The distinction is the number of CD4+ T-cells and whether any opportunistic infections have occurred. A healthy adult usually has at least 800 to 1000 CD4+ T-cells per cubic millimeter (mm^3) of blood. This number is reduced in the person with HIV disease.

Some people develop an acute INFECTION within 4 weeks of first being infected. Manifestations of this acute HIV infection can be fever, night sweats, chills, headache, and muscle aches, which are similar to those of any viral infection—not just HIV. A sore throat and rash also may accompany this acute HIV infection. With time, these symptoms cease and the person feels well again, although a "war is going on" between HIV and the immune system.

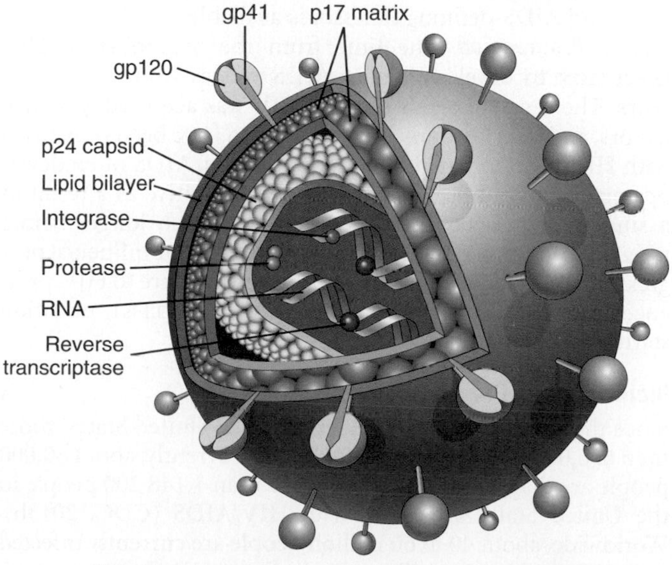

FIG. 19-1 The human immune deficiency virus (HIV).

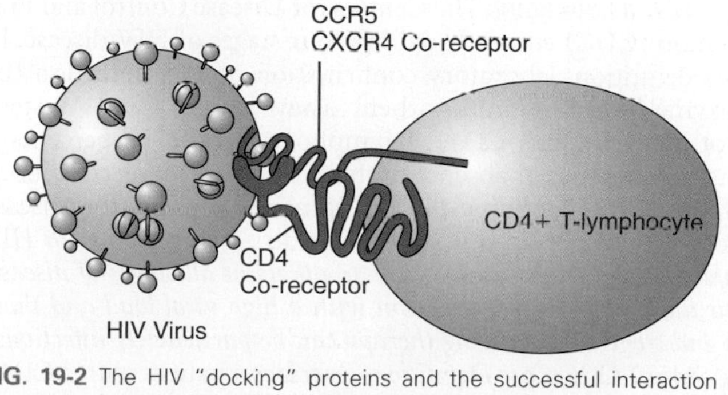

FIG. 19-2 The HIV "docking" proteins and the successful interaction of these proteins with the CD4+ T-lymphocyte receptors.

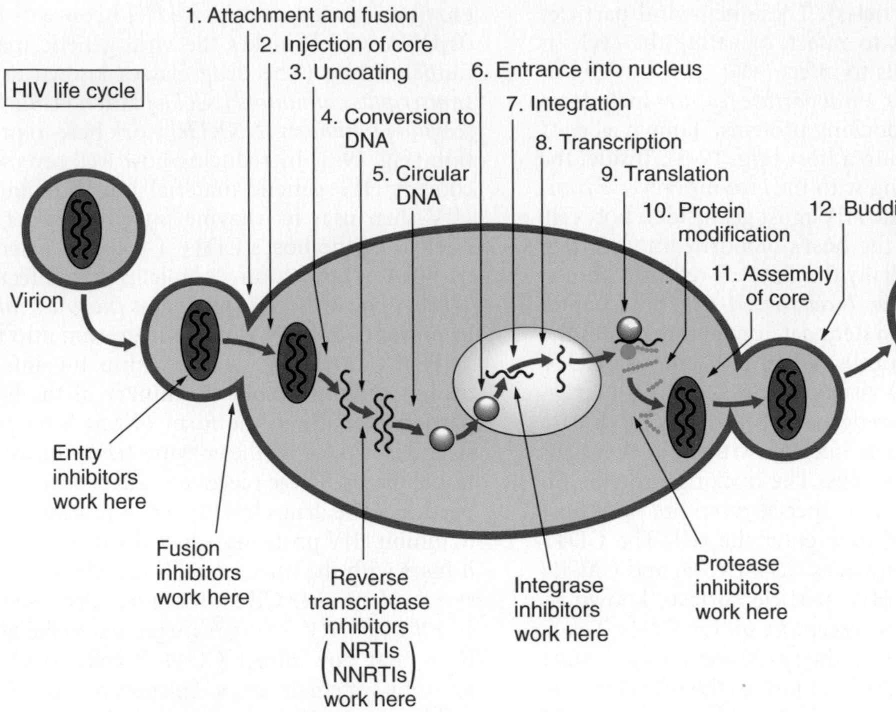

FIG. 19-3 The life cycle of the HIV and sites of action for anti-HIV therapy.

As time passes, more CD4+ T-cells are infected and taken out of service. The count decreases, and those that remain function poorly. Poor CD4+ T-cell function leads to these immune system abnormalities:

- Lymphocytopenia (decreased numbers of lymphocytes)
- Increased production of incomplete and nonfunctional antibodies
- Abnormally functioning macrophages

As the CD4+ T-cell level drops, the patient is at risk for bacterial, fungal, and viral INFECTIONS, as well as opportunistic cancers. **Opportunistic infections** are those caused by organisms that are present as part of the body's normal environment and are kept in check by normal immune function. They occur because of the profound immunosuppression in the person with AIDS.

A diagnosis of AIDS requires that the person be HIV positive and have either a CD4+ T-cell count of less than 200 cells/mm^3 or less than 14% (even if the total CD4+ count is above 200 cells/mm^3) or an opportunistic infection. Once AIDS is diagnosed, even if the patient's T-cell count goes higher than 200 cells/mm^3 or if the percentage rises above 14%, or the infection is successfully treated, the AIDS diagnosis remains and the patient does not revert to being just HIV positive.

HIV Classification. The Centers for Disease Control and Prevention (CDC) currently defines four stages of HIV disease. In this definition, laboratory confirmation of HIV infection (by enzyme-linked immunosorbent assay [ELISA] and Western blot analysis) plus CD4+ T-lymphocyte count or percentage and the presence or absence of the 27 AIDS-defining conditions (Table 19-1) determine the classification (Centers for Disease Control and Prevention [CDC], 2013b). *The person with HIV infection can transmit the virus to others at all stages of disease, but the recently infected person with a high viral load and those at end stage without drug therapy can be particularly infectious.*

Stage 1 CDC Case Definition describes a patient with a CD4+ T-cell count of greater than 500 cells/mm^3 or a percentage of 29% or greater. A person at this stage has no AIDS-defining illnesses.

Stage 2 CDC Case Definition describes a patient with a CD4+ T-cell count between 200 and 499 cells/mm^3 or a percentage between 14% and 28%. A person at this stage has no AIDS-defining illnesses.

Stage 3 CDC Case Definition describes any patient with a CD4+ T-cell count of less than 200 cells/mm^3 or a percentage of less than 14%. A person who has higher CD4+ T-cell counts or percentages but who also has an AIDS-defining illness meets the Stage 3 CDC Case Definition.

Stage 4 CDC Case Definition is used to describe any patient with a confirmed HIV infection but no information regarding CD4+ T-cell counts, CD4+ T-cell percentages, and AIDS-defining illnesses is available.

HIV Progression. The time from the beginning of HIV INFECTION to development of AIDS ranges from months to years. The range depends on how HIV was acquired, personal factors, and interventions. For people who have been transfused with HIV-contaminated blood, for example, AIDS often develops quickly. For those who become HIV positive as a result of a single sexual encounter, the period is much longer before progression to AIDS. Other personal factors that influence progression to AIDS include frequency of re-exposure to HIV, presence of other sexually transmitted diseases (STDs), nutrition status, and stress.

Incidence and Prevalence

Since the beginning of the epidemic in the United States, more than 636,000 people have died of AIDS. Currently, about 50,000 people are diagnosed yearly and more than 1,148,200 people in the United States are living with HIV/AIDS (CDC, 2013b). Worldwide, about 40 to 60 million people are currently infected with HIV, at least 30 million deaths from AIDs have occurred, and 33 million people are living with AIDS (WHO, 2013).

TABLE 19-1 Centers for Disease Control and Prevention Classification of Aids-Defining Conditions in Adults

- Bacterial infections, multiple or recurrent
- Candidiasis of bronchi, trachea, or lungs
- Candidiasis of esophagus
- Cervical cancer, invasive
- Coccidioidomycosis, disseminated or extrapulmonary
- Cryptococcosis, extrapulmonary
- Cryptosporidiosis, chronic intestinal (>1-month's duration)
- Cytomegalovirus disease (other than liver, spleen, or nodes)
- Cytomegalovirus retinitis (with loss of vision)
- Encephalopathy, HIV-related
- Herpes simplex: chronic ulcers (>1-month's duration) or bronchitis, pneumonitis, or esophagitis
- Histoplasmosis, disseminated or extrapulmonary
- Isosporiasis, chronic intestinal (>1-month's duration)
- Kaposi's sarcoma
- Lymphoid interstitial pneumonia or pulmonary lymphoid hyperplasia complex
- Lymphoma, Burkitt's (or equivalent term)
- Lymphoma, immunoblastic (or equivalent term)
- Lymphoma, primary, of brain
- *Mycobacterium avium* complex or *Mycobacterium kansasii*, disseminated or extrapulmonary
- *Mycobacterium tuberculosis* of any site, pulmonary, disseminated, or extrapulmonary
- *Mycobacterium*, other species or unidentified species, disseminated or extrapulmonary
- *Pneumocystis jiroveci* pneumonia
- Pneumonia, recurrent (two instances within 12 months)
- Progressive multifocal leukoencephalopathy
- *Salmonella* septicemia, recurrent
- Toxoplasmosis of brain
- Wasting syndrome attributed to HIV

From Schneider, E., Whitmore, S., Glynn, K.M., Dominguez, K., Mitsch, A., McKenna, M.T.; Centers for Disease Control and Prevention. (2008). Revised surveillance case definitions for HIV infection among adults, adolescents, and children aged <18 months and for HIV infection and AIDS among children aged 18 months to <13 years—United States, 2008. *Morbidity and Mortality Weekly Report: Recommendations and Reports, 57*(RR-10), 9. Retrieved December 2013 from www.cdc.gov/mmwr/preview/mmwrhtml/rr5710a2.htm

GENETIC/GENOMIC CONSIDERATIONS

Patient-Centered Care QSEN

About 1% of people with HIV infection are long-term nonprogressors (LTNPs). These people have been infected with HIV for at least 10 years and have remained asymptomatic, with CD4+ T-cell counts within the normal range and a viral load that is either undetectable or very low.

A genetic difference for this population is that their *CCR5/CXCR4* co-receptors on the CD4+ T-cells are abnormal and nonfunctional as a result of gene mutations for these co-receptors. The mutation creates defective co-receptors that do not bind to the HIV docking proteins. Cells with this defective co-receptor successfully resist the entrance of HIV. People who have only one mutated co-receptor gene allele have fewer normal co-receptors and can be infected with HIV, although disease progression is relatively slow.

Most AIDS cases in North America occur among men who have sex with men (MSM) (59%-69%) or people of either gender who have used injection drugs (16%) (CDC, 2013b). *The changing demographics of the infection indicate that the perception that HIV/AIDS is only a problem for homosexual white men is false (Kirton, 2011).*

CULTURAL CONSIDERATIONS

Patient-Centered Care QSEN

Most new HIV infections reported in the United States occur in racial and ethnic minority groups, particularly among African Americans and Hispanics (CDC, 2013b). These two groups show an increasing trend in HIV infection and disease compared with a leveling off among white people.

GENDER HEALTH CONSIDERATIONS

Patient-Centered Care QSEN

About 25% of newly diagnosed cases are women. In less affluent countries, 50% of cases occur in women (WHO, 2013). The largest risk factor is sexual exposure. Strategies specifically targeted to reducing sexual exposures of HIV to women may help prevent an increase in HIV infection in that group. Women with HIV disease have a poorer outcome with shorter mean survival time than that of men. This outcome may be the result of late diagnosis and social or economic factors that reduce access to medical care.

Gynecologic problems, especially persistent or recurrent vaginal candidiasis, may be the first signs of HIV disease in women. Other problems include pelvic inflammatory disease, genital herpes, other sexually transmitted diseases (STDs), and cervical dysplasia or cancer.

The effect of HIV on pregnancy outcomes includes higher incidence of premature delivery, low-birth-weight infants, and transmission of the disease to the infant. Appropriate antiretroviral drug therapy during pregnancy reduces the risk for transmitting the infection to the infant. (See the discussion on p. 332 in the Perinatal Transmission section.)

CONSIDERATIONS FOR OLDER ADULTS

Patient-Centered Care QSEN

Infection with HIV can occur at any age. Assess the older patient for risk behaviors, including a sexual and drug use history (Foster et al., 2012). (See the Evidence-Based Practice box for specific risky behaviors often practiced by older adults.) Age-related decline in immunity increases the likelihood that the older adult will develop the infection after an HIV exposure.

Health Promotion and Maintenance

AIDS is a disease with a mortality rate of at least 60% for adults. Although a very few people who have been given high doses of antiretroviral drugs immediately upon diagnosis have subsequently shown no detectable virus, there are too few cases to indicate whether such therapy can result in an enduring cure. Thus, at this time, there is no available cure for AIDS and a major focus for health care worldwide is prevention of HIV INFECTION.

HIV has been found in blood, semen, vaginal secretions, breast milk, amniotic fluid, urine, feces, saliva, tears, cerebrospinal fluid, lymph nodes, cervical cells, corneal tissue, and brain tissue of infected patients. The fluids with the highest concentrations of HIV are semen and blood. HIV is transmitted most often in these three ways:

- Sexual: genital, anal, or oral sexual contact with exposure of mucous membranes to infected semen or vaginal secretions
- Parenteral: sharing of needles or equipment contaminated with infected blood or receiving contaminated blood products

EVIDENCE-BASED PRACTICE QSEN

How Are Older Adults at Risk for HIV Infection?

Foster, V., Clark, P., Holstad, M., & Burgess, E. (2012). Factors associated with risky sexual behaviors in older adults. *Journal of the Association of Nurses in AIDS Care, 23*(6), 487-499.

The incidence of human immune deficiency virus (HIV) infection is significant among adults over 50 years of age in North America and contributes to earlier mortality and morbidity in this age-group. Many programs for HIV risk reduction focus on younger adults, teenagers, and racial/ethic minorities. However, the older adult age-group continues to develop HIV infection. This correlational study sought to (1) determine whether higher levels of HIV knowledge and higher levels of motivation to practice safer sex were associated with lower levels of risky sexual behaviors and (2) identify what factors were associated with continued practice of risky sexual behaviors among adults ages 50 years and older.

A convenience sample of 106 sexually active, community-dwelling, single men and women ranging in age from 50 to 74 years were recruited into the study. (Some participants planned to be sexually active, whereas others were sexually active during the study period.)

Level of Evidence: 4

The study method was prospective, cross-sectional, and correlational. Statistical evaluation methods were appropriate for the design.

Commentary: Implications for Practice and Research

The study is important for many reasons. First, it established the incidence of sexual behaviors in a relatively large group of older adult participants. It also highlighted the fact that many health care professionals, as well as older adult patients, are reluctant to discuss sexual behaviors and risk for HIV infection in the defined age-group. In addition, the knowledge of correct condom use, a well-established deterrent to HIV transmission, is lacking among many older adults.

The study defined important areas for future nursing research. Among these are the need for nurses and other health care professionals to understand that aging does not limit the risks for HIV transmission and the absolute need for consistently addressing sexuality in older adults. Strategies to increase correct condom use among sexually active older adults (who may only see the use as a no-longer-needed form of birth control) need to be developed and tested.

- Perinatal: from the placenta, from contact with maternal blood and body fluids during birth, or from breast milk from an infected mother to child

Teach everyone about the transmission routes and ways to reduce their exposure (discussed next). Also stress that HIV is not transmitted by casual contact in the home, school, or workplace. Sharing household utensils, towels and linens, and toilet facilities does not transmit HIV. In addition, HIV is not spread by mosquitoes or other insects.

! NURSING SAFETY PRIORITY QSEN

Action Alert

Teach all people, regardless of age, gender, ethnicity, or sexual orientation, that they are susceptible to HIV infection.

Sexual Transmission

Safer sex methods of *A, abstinence; B, be faithful;* and *C, condom use* can reduce HIV transmission. *Abstinence and mutually monogamous sex with a noninfected partner are the only absolutely safe methods of preventing HIV INFECTION from sexual contact.* Many forms of sexual expression can spread HIV infection if one partner is infected. *The risk for becoming infected from a partner who is HIV positive is always present,* although some sexual practices are more risky than others. Because the virus concentrates in blood and seminal fluid and is also present in vaginal secretions, risk differs by gender, sexual act, and the viral load of the infected partner.

Gender affects HIV transmission, like all other sexually transmitted diseases (STDs), and it is more easily transmitted from infected male to uninfected female than vice versa. This is because HIV is most easily transmitted when infected body fluids come into contact with mucous membranes or nonintact skin. The vagina has more surface area of mucous membrane than does the penis. Teach women the importance of always either using a vaginal or dental dam or female condom or having their male partners use a condom.

Sexual acts or practices that permit infected seminal fluid to come into contact with mucous membranes or nonintact skin are the most risky for sexual transmission of HIV. The practice with the highest risk is anal intercourse with the penis and seminal fluid of an infected person coming into contact with the mucous membranes of the uninfected partner's rectum. *Anal intercourse in which the semen depositor (inserting or active partner) is infected is a very risky sexual practice regardless of whether the semen receiver (receiving partner) is male or female.* Anal intercourse not only allows seminal fluid to make contact with the mucous membranes of the rectum but also tears the mucous membranes, making INFECTION more likely. Teach patients who engage in anal intercourse that the semen depositor needs to wear a condom during this act.

Viral load, or the amount of virus present in blood and other body fluids, affects transmission. The higher the blood level of HIV (**viremia**), the greater the risk for sexual and perinatal transmission. Current highly active antiretroviral therapy (HAART) has caused the viral load of some infected patients to drop below detectable levels. *Although there is less virus in seminal or vaginal fluids of people receiving HAART, the risk for transmission still exists.*

Safer sex practices are those that reduce the risk for nonintact skin or mucous membranes coming in contact with infected body fluids and blood. Teach everyone the importance of consistently using these safer sex practices:

- A latex or polyurethane condom for genital and anal intercourse
- A condom or latex barrier (dental dam) over the genitals or anus during oral-genital or oral-anal sexual contact
- Latex gloves for finger or hand contact with the vagina or rectum

New research for prevention of sexual transmission has resulted in the use of drug therapy for *pre-exposure prophylaxis* (Aschenbrenner, 2012). The use of the combination drug *Truvada* (emtricitabine and tenofovir) by HIV-1–negative sexual partners of known HIV-1–positive people appears to reduce HIV transmission.

For those who believe they have been exposed to HIV as a result of sexual relations or other types of non-occupational

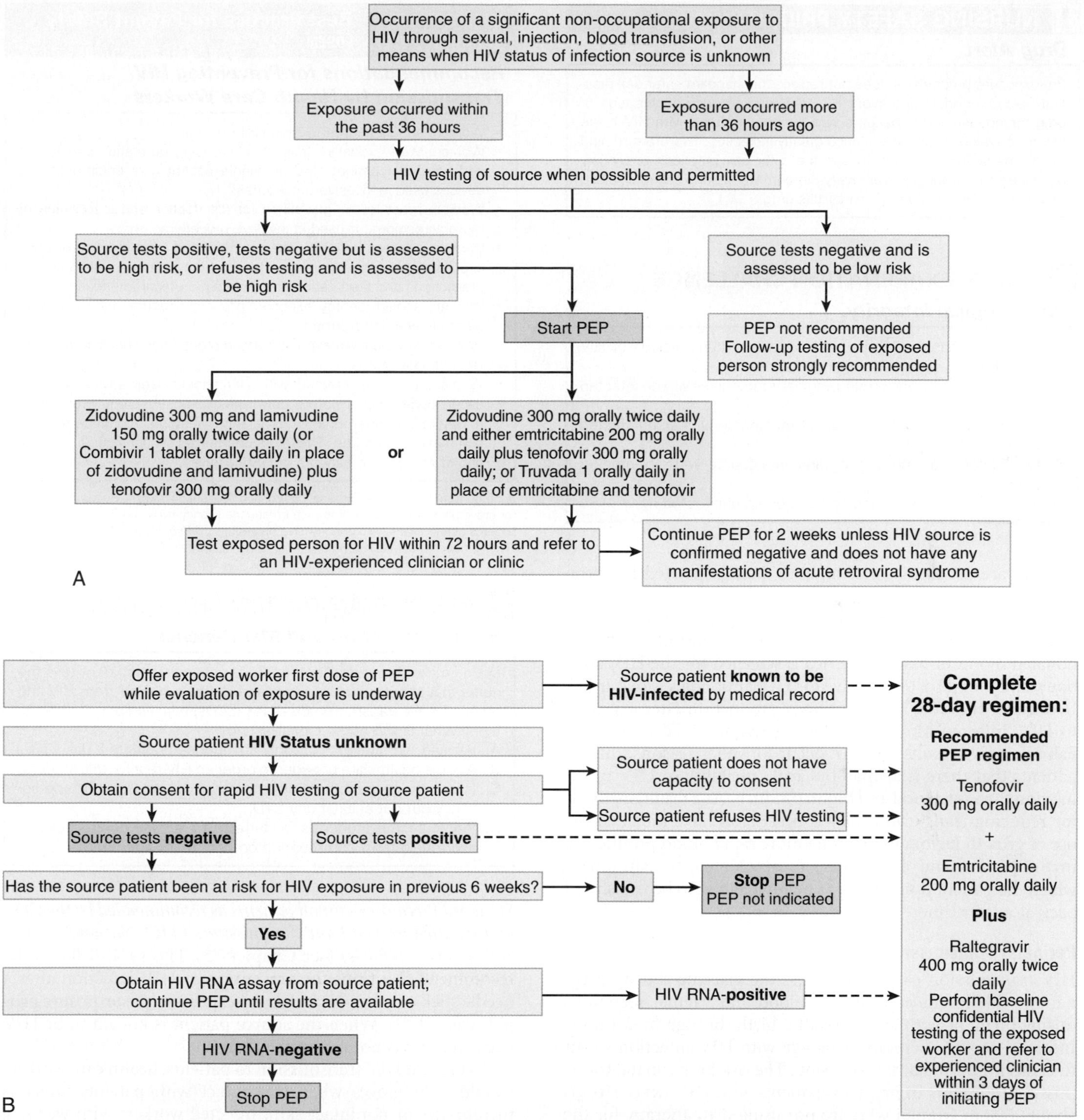

FIG. 19-4 New York State Health Department HIV guidelines. **A,** Recommendations for non occupational postexposure prophylaxis for HIV infection. **B,** Recommendations for occupational postexposure prophylaxis for HIV infection.

exposure, the CDC has guidelines for *postexposure prophylaxis*. The length and type of prophylaxis therapy depend on the nature of the exposure (Fig. 19-4, *A*).

Parenteral Transmission

Preventive practices to reduce transmission among injection drug users (IDUs) include the use of proper cleaning of "works" (needles, syringes, other drug paraphernalia). Instruct IDUs to clean a used needle and syringe by first filling and flushing them with clear water. Next, the syringe should be filled with ordinary household bleach. The bleach-filled syringe should be shaken for 30 to 60 seconds. Advise IDUs to carry a small container with this solution whenever sharing needles. Some communities have a needle exchange program in which needles and

NURSING SAFETY PRIORITY QSEN

Drug Alert

Pre-exposure prophylaxis does not replace the standard safer sex practices recommended to prevent HIV transmission. Also, if this type of drug therapy is used in patients who become infected with HIV-1, the risk for developing drug resistance greatly increases. Therefore remind people prescribed Truvada to use the safer sex practices previously described and to adhere to an every-3-month HIV testing schedule along with monitoring for side effects of this drug.

NCLEX EXAMINATION CHALLENGE

Physiological Integrity

Which couple has the highest risk for sexual transmission of HIV without the use of a condom or dental dam?

A. Uninfected male performing vaginal intercourse with an infected female
B. Infected male performing vaginal intercourse with an uninfected female
C. Uninfected male performing anal intercourse with an infected male
D. Infected male performing oral sex on an uninfected male

syringes are used only once and are then exchanged for clean ones.

The risk for AIDS transmission through blood and blood products has been reduced to a national average of 0.02%. All donated blood in North America is screened for the HIV antibody, and blood that is positive for HIV antibodies is discarded. Because of the time lag in antibody production after exposure to HIV, infected blood can test negative for HIV antibodies. False-negative results also can occur for other reasons. Inform patients that there is a small but real possibility of HIV transmission through blood and blood products. As a result, methods for reducing transfusion-related INFECTION have included the use of growth factors to promote more rapid blood production in the patient and an increase in autologous transfusion in which the patient donates his or her own blood to be transfused back at a later time.

Perinatal Transmission

HIV transmission can occur across the placenta during pregnancy, with infant exposure to blood and vaginal secretions during birth, or with exposure after birth through breast milk. Inform women of childbearing age with HIV infection about the risks for perinatal transmission. The risk for perinatal transmission to infants in pregnant patients with HIV INFECTION is about 25% in woman who are not using drug therapy for the disease compared with about 8% for women who are using drug therapy for HIV. Therefore encourage HIV-positive women who are pregnant to continue the therapy or, if they are not on antiviral therapy, to start the therapy as soon as possible.

Transmission and Health Care Workers

Needle stick or "sharps" injuries are the main means of occupation-related HIV infection for health care workers. In addition, health care workers can be infected through exposure of nonintact skin and mucous membranes to blood and body fluids. *The best prevention for health care providers is the consistent use of*

CHART 19-1 Best Practice for Patient Safety & Quality Care QSEN

Recommendations for Preventing HIV Transmission by Health Care Workers

- Workers should adhere to Standard Precautions.
- Workers with exudative lesions or weeping dermatitis should not perform direct patient care or handle patient care equipment and devices used in invasive procedures.
- Workers must follow guidelines for disinfection and sterilization of reusable equipment used in invasive procedures.
- Workers infected with HIV are not restricted from practice of non–exposure-prone procedures, as long as they comply with Standard Precautions and sterilization and disinfection recommendations.
- Workers should identify exposure-prone procedures by institutions where they are performed.
- Workers who perform exposure-prone procedures should know their HIV antibody status.
- Workers who are infected with HIV should seek advice from an expert review panel before performing exposure-prone procedures to determine under what circumstances they may continue to practice these procedures. These circumstances would include notification of prospective patients of HIV positivity.

Adapted from Centers for Disease Control and Prevention. (1991). Recommendations for preventing transmission of human immunodeficiency virus and hepatitis B virus to patients during exposure-prone invasive procedures. *Morbidity and Mortality Weekly Report: Recommendations and Reports, 40*(RR-8), 1-9.

NCLEX EXAMINATION CHALLENGE

Health Promotion and Maintenance

During a health assessment, a 22-year-old college student tells the nurse that she is sexually active and protects herself from HIV and other sexually transmitted diseases (STDs) by using oral contraceptives. What is the nurse's best action?

A. Remind the student that only abstinence prevents STDs.
B. Ask the health care provider to order an HIV test for this student.
C. Inform the student that oral contraceptives protect against pregnancy but not against any STD.
D. Reinforce the student's preferred use of oral contraceptives, and refrain from commenting on her sexual activity.

Standard Precautions for all patients as recommended by the CDC and required by The Joint Commission's (TJC) National Patient Safety Goals (NPSGs) (see Chapter 23). Fig. 19-4, *B* shows the recommended actions for prevention of HIV infection after a needle stick or other occupational exposure (postexposure prophylaxis [PEP]). When the source patient is known to be HIV negative, PEP is not recommended.

To prevent HIV transmission to patients, health care workers should wear gloves when in contact with patients' mucous membranes or nonintact skin. Infected workers with weeping dermatitis or open lesions should not perform direct care. The CDC guidelines for preventing HIV transmission by health care workers during exposure-prone invasive procedures are listed in Chart 19-1. These include any procedure in which there is a risk for broken skin injury to the health care worker and the worker's blood is likely to make contact with the patient's body cavity, subcutaneous tissues, or mucous membranes.

Testing

Testing for HIV antibodies or other features of the virus is complex, requiring interpretation, counseling, and confidentiality. Testing plays a role in prevention because tests are a way

CHART 19-2 **Patient and Family Education: Preparing for Self-Management**

CDC Recommendations for HIV Testing

You should be tested for HIV if you fall within one or more of these groups:
- People with sexually transmitted disease
- Injection drug users
- People who consider themselves at risk
- Women of childbearing age with identifiable risks, including:
  - Used injection drugs
  - Engaged in prostitution
  - Had sexual partners who were infected or at risk
  - Had sexual contact with men from countries with high HIV prevalence
- People who received a transfusion between 1978 and 1985
- People planning to get married
- People undergoing medical evaluation or treatment for manifestations that may be HIV related
- People admitted to hospitals
- People in correctional institutions such as jails and prisons
- Prostitutes and their customers

Adapted from Centers for Disease Control and Prevention. (1987). Public Health Service guidelines for counseling and antibody testing to prevent HIV infection and AIDS. *Morbidity and Mortality Weekly Report, 36*(31), 509-515.
CDC, Centers for Disease Control and Prevention.

of diagnosing HIV INFECTION before immune changes or disease manifestations develop. A primary health care focus for testing is to teach those who test positive to modify their behaviors to prevent transmission to others. *Therefore all sexually active people should know their HIV status.* Chart 19-2 lists additional conditions for which HIV antibody testing is advised.

Pretest and post-test counseling must be performed by personnel trained in HIV issues. These counselors may be nurses, physicians, social workers, health educators, or even lay educators who have specialized training. Counseling helps the patient make an informed decision about testing and provides an opportunity to teach risk-reduction behaviors. Post-test counseling is needed to interpret the results, discuss risk reduction, and provide psychological support and health promotion information for the patient with a positive test result. People who test positive should also be counseled on how to inform sexual partners and those with whom they have shared needles. Testing methods, their accuracy, and indications are presented on p. 336 in the Laboratory Assessment section.

❖ PATIENT-CENTERED COLLABORATIVE CARE

◆ Assessment

The person who has HIV disease is monitored on a regular basis for changes in immune function or health status that indicate disease progression and the need for intervention. The frequency of monitoring varies from every 2 to 6 months based on disease progression and responses to treatment. This continuing assessment of the patient with HIV disease is crucial, because he or she may have problems related to disease in many organ systems and to ensure that the drug continues to work optimally. Assess subtle changes so that INFECTIONS and other problems can be found early and treated.

History. Ask about age, gender, occupation, and where the person lives. Thoroughly assess the current illness, including when it started, the severity of symptoms, associated problems, and any interventions to date. Ask the patient about when the HIV INFECTION was diagnosed and what manifestations led to that diagnosis. Ask him or her to give a chronologic history of infections and problems since the diagnosis. Assess the patient's health history, including whether he or she received a blood transfusion between 1978 and 1985 in the United States (before routine blood testing for HIV contamination). Because blood testing for HIV contamination is not consistently performed in all parts of the world, ask the immigrant patient about his or her history of transfusion therapy before coming to the United States.

Ask the patient about sexual practices, sexually transmitted diseases (STDs), and major infectious diseases, including tuberculosis and hepatitis. If the patient has hemophilia, ask about treatment with clotting factors. Determine whether the patient has engaged in past or present injection drug use, including needle sharing. Assess the patient's level of knowledge regarding the diagnosis, symptom management, diagnostic tests, treatments, community resources, and modes of HIV transmission. Also assess his or her understanding and use of safer sex practices. If knowledge deficits are found, provide the appropriate patient teaching.

Physical Assessment/Clinical Manifestations. HIV disease and AIDS are a progression continuum. The patient with HIV disease may either have few manifestations and problems or may have problems that are acute rather than chronically present. As the disease progresses, however, more severe health problems occur and the patient may not realize that the disease is progressing. Assess for clusters of symptoms that may indicate disease progression (Chart 19-3).

Opportunistic Infections. The patient with HIV/AIDS often develops pathogenic INFECTIONS and opportunistic infections. *Pathogenic infections* are caused by virulent organisms and occur even among people with normal IMMUNITY. *Opportunistic infections* are those caused by organisms that are present as part of the body's normal environment and are kept in check by normal immune function. Only when immunity is depressed are such organisms capable of causing infection.

Opportunistic INFECTIONS occur because of the profound immunosuppression of the person with HIV disease. They may result from primary infection or reactivation of a latent infection. Opportunistic infections account for many of the clinical manifestations observed in HIV infection and can be protozoan, fungal, bacterial, or viral. More than one infection may be present at the same time. The presence of opportunistic infections may represent disease progression or a temporary further reduction of immune status. *In either case, these infections can result in death if appropriate treatment is not started quickly.* Priority nursing actions when caring for a patient who is HIV positive are continually assessing for and documenting the presence of an opportunistic infection and monitoring the patient's response to therapy. Report to the health care provider those manifestations that may indicate an infection.

Opportunistic infections do not pose a threat to the immunocompetent health care worker caring for a patient with HIV disease or AIDS. When the patient with HIV disease or AIDS has a pathogenic infection, however, health care personnel must use precautions appropriate to the specific disease to prevent disease spread. For example, when the person with HIV/AIDS also has tuberculosis at a transmissible stage, Airborne Precautions are needed in addition to Standard Precautions. See Chapter 23 for a more complete discussion on Transmission-Based Precautions for specific infectious diseases.

CHART 19-3 Key Features

AIDS

Immunologic Manifestations
- Low white blood cell counts:
  - CD4+/CD8+ ratio <2
  - CD4+ count <200/mm³
- Hypergammaglobulinemia
- Opportunistic infections
- Lymphadenopathy
- Fatigue

Integumentary Manifestations
- Dry skin
- Poor wound healing
- Skin lesions
- Night sweats

Respiratory Manifestations
- Cough
- Shortness of breath

Gastrointestinal Manifestations
- Diarrhea
- Weight loss
- Nausea and vomiting

Central Nervous System Manifestations
- Confusion
- Dementia
- Headache
- Fever
- Visual changes
- Memory loss
- Personality changes
- Pain
- Seizures

Opportunistic Infections
- Protozoal infections:
  - Toxoplasmosis
  - Cryptosporidiosis
  - Isosporiasis
  - Microsporidiosis
  - Strongyloidiasis
  - Giardiasis
- Fungal infections:
  - Candidiasis
  - *Pneumocystis jiroveci* pneumonia
  - Cryptococcosis
  - Histoplasmosis
  - Coccidioidomycosis
- Bacterial infections:
  - *Mycobacterium avium* complex infection
  - Tuberculosis
  - Nocardiosis
- Viral infections:
  - Cytomegalovirus infection
  - Herpes simplex virus infection
  - Varicella-zoster virus infection

Malignancies
- Kaposi's sarcoma
- Non-Hodgkin's lymphoma
- Hodgkin's lymphoma
- Invasive cervical carcinoma

Protozoal and fungal infections are common among patients with AIDS. *Pneumocystis jiroveci* pneumonia (PCP) is the most common opportunistic INFECTION in persons infected with HIV. This organism is now considered a fungus. Assess for dyspnea on exertion, tachypnea, a persistent dry cough, and a persistent low-grade fever. The patient may report fatigue and weight loss. Auscultate breath sounds for crackles.

Toxoplasmosis encephalitis, caused by *Toxoplasma gondii,* is acquired through contact with contaminated cat feces or by ingesting infected undercooked meat. Assess the patient for subtle changes in mental status, neurologic deficits, headaches, and fever. Additional changes may include difficulties with speech, gait, and vision; seizures; lethargy; and confusion. Perform a comprehensive mental status examination and monitor the patient to detect subtle changes.

Cryptosporidiosis is an intestinal INFECTION caused by *Cryptosporidium* organisms. In AIDS, this illness ranges from a mild diarrhea to a severe wasting with electrolyte imbalance. Diarrhea may result in fluid loss of up to 15 to 20 L/day. Ask the patient about the presence of diarrhea and whether he or she has had an unplanned weight loss of 5 pounds or more.

Fungal INFECTION occurs by overgrowth of normal body flora. *Candida albicans* is part of the intestinal tract's natural flora. In the person with AIDS, candidiasis (overgrowth of the

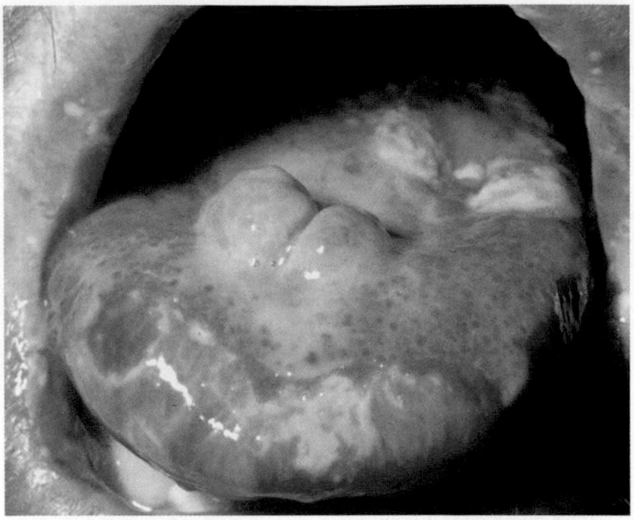

FIG. 19-5 Oral candidiasis (thrush).

Candida fungus) occurs because the immune system can no longer control fungal growth. *Candida* stomatitis or esophagitis occurs often in AIDS. Patients may report food tasting "funny," mouth pain, difficulty in swallowing, and pain behind the sternum. On examination of the mouth and throat, you may see cottage cheese–like, yellowish white plaques and inflammation (Fig. 19-5). Esophagitis is diagnosed by endoscopic examination with biopsy and culture. Women with HIV disease or AIDS may have persistent vaginal candidiasis with severe pruritus (itching), perineal irritation, and a thick, white vaginal discharge.

Cryptococcosis, caused by *Cryptococcus neoformans,* is a debilitating meningitis and can be a widely spread infection in AIDS. Ask about fever, headache, blurred vision, nausea and vomiting, neck stiffness, confusion, and other mental status changes. Patients may have seizures and other neurologic problems, or they may have mild malaise, fever, and headaches.

Histoplasmosis, caused by *Histoplasma capsulatum,* begins as a respiratory INFECTION and progresses to widespread infection in the person with AIDS. Assess for dyspnea, fever, cough, and weight loss. Check for enlargement of lymph nodes, the spleen, or the liver.

Bacterial infections are acquired from other people or sources and as overgrowth of skin flora. *Mycobacterium avium* complex (MAC) is the most common bacterial INFECTION associated with AIDS. This problem is caused by *M. intracellulare* or *M. avium,* which infects the respiratory or GI tract. MAC is a systemic infection. Assess for fever, debility, weight loss, malaise, and sometimes swollen lymph glands or organ disease.

Tuberculosis (TB), caused by *Mycobacterium tuberculosis,* occurs in 2% to 10% of persons with AIDS (CDC, 2009). More than 50% of all patients with AIDS and TB have extrapulmonary disease sites, including the central nervous system, bones, liver, spleen, skin, and intestinal tract. Ask about cough, dyspnea, chest pain, fever, chills, night sweats, weight loss, and anorexia. Manifestations of extrapulmonary infection vary with the site. *The person with TB and a CD4+ T-cell count below 200/mm³ may not have a positive TB skin test (purified protein derivative [PPD]) because of an inability to mount an immune response to the antigen, a condition known as **anergy**.* Blood analysis by the fully automated nucleic acid amplification test (NAAT) for tuberculosis with results available in less than 2 hours is the most sensitive and rapid test for the presence of *M. tuberculosis*. It is very useful in the acute care setting to determine whether a symptomatic patient actually has TB. Other diagnostic tests include a chest x-ray, acid-fast sputum smear, and sputum culture.

! NURSING SAFETY PRIORITY (QSEN)

Action Alert

Until parameters other than a skin test come back negative for TB in a patient with AIDS who also has TB manifestations, maintain Airborne Precautions along with Standard Precautions.

The tuberculosis bacillus is spread by airborne routes. When particles from the patient's respiratory tract are aerosolized, anyone near him or her is at risk for inhaling the particles and the bacillus. Therefore the nurse or respiratory therapist who gives cough-inducing aerosol treatments, such as pentamidine isethionate, to patients with AIDS should be screened with a PPD skin test or QuantiFERON blood test every 6 months to determine whether he or she has been infected with TB.

Pneumonia from bacterial INFECTION recurs often among patients with AIDS, and two or more episodes of any type of bacterial pneumonia in a 12-month period are an AIDS case definition. Assess for chest pain, productive cough, fever, and dyspnea.

Viral infection from a virus other than HIV is common among people with HIV disease that has progressed to AIDS. Cytomegalovirus (CMV) can infect many sites in persons with AIDS, including the eye (CMV retinitis), respiratory and GI tracts, and the central nervous system. CMV INFECTION can also cause many nonspecific problems such as fever, malaise, weight loss, fatigue, and swollen lymph nodes. CMV retinitis impairs vision, ranging from slight impairment to total blindness. CMV can also cause diarrhea, abdominal bloating and discomfort, and weight loss. Ask the patient whether he or she has any of these manifestations. In addition, CMV can cause encephalitis, pneumonitis, adrenalitis, hepatitis, and disseminated infection.

Herpes simplex virus (HSV) INFECTION in people with HIV disease or AIDS occurs in the perirectal, oral, and genital areas. The manifestations are more widespread and of longer duration among patients with HIV/AIDS than among those who are immunocompetent. Numbness or tingling at the site of infection occurs up to 24 hours before blisters form. Lesions are painful, with chronic open areas after blisters rupture. Assess for fever, pain, bleeding, and enlarged lymph nodes in the affected area. Also assess for headache, myalgia, and malaise.

Varicella-zoster virus (VZV) infection (*shingles*) is not a new INFECTION for people with AIDS. This virus causes chickenpox and then remains present in the nerve ganglia. When people who have had chickenpox previously are immunocompromised, VZV leaves the nerve ganglia and enters other tissue areas, causing shingles. Ask whether the patient has pain and burning along sensory nerve tracts (see Chapter 41 for the dermatomes of sensory nerve locations), headache, and low-grade fever. Examine the skin for fluid-filled blisters with or without crusts.

Malignancies. Weakened IMMUNITY increases the risk for some cancers. These include Kaposi's sarcoma, lymphomas, invasive cervical cancer, lung cancer, GI cancer, and anal cancer (Kirton, 2011).

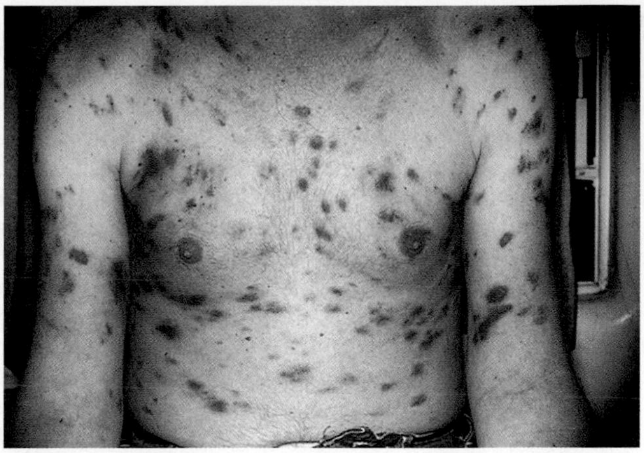

FIG. 19-6 Kaposi's sarcoma lesions.

Kaposi's sarcoma (KS) is the most common AIDS-related malignancy. The risk for KS appears to be related to co-infection with human herpes virus-8.

KS develops as small, purplish brown, raised lesions that are usually not painful or itchy. The skin and mucous membrane lesions can occur anywhere on the body (Fig. 19-6). In some patients, lesions develop in the lymph nodes, mouth and throat, intestinal tract, or lungs. KS is diagnosed by biopsy and histologic examination of the lesion. Assess KS lesions for number, size, location, and whether they are intact, and monitor their progression.

Malignant lymphomas occurring with AIDS are Hodgkin's lymphoma, non-Hodgkin's B-cell lymphomas (such as Burkitt's lymphoma), immunoblastic lymphoma, and primary brain lymphoma. Manifestations include swollen lymph nodes, weight loss, fever, and night sweats.

Human papilloma virus (HPV) INFECTION results in multiple types of malignancies and manifestations, but the most common in HIV infection are cervical and anal cancers. Cervical Papanicolaou (Pap) testing every 6 months is the standard of care for HIV-positive patients. In MSM patients, performing an anal Pap test, using the same medium as for a cervical Pap test, is now becoming standard of care and is being extended to both male and female patients for the early detection and treatment of cervical and anal cancers.

Endocrine Complications. Patients with HIV disease may have disease-related and treatment-related endocrine problems, such as gonadal dysfunction, body shape changes, adrenal insufficiency, diabetes mellitus, and elevated triglycerides and cholesterol (which increase the risk for cardiovascular problems).

Many HIV-positive men have low testosterone levels, and HIV-positive women often have irregular menstrual cycles. With this gonadal dysfunction comes a decrease in body muscle mass for both genders, with a decrease in weight, and a change in libido, accompanied by a decrease in energy and an increase in fatigue.

Body shape changes from fat redistribution or fat disposition (known as *lipodystrophy*) are common in patients receiving antiretroviral therapies, especially protease inhibitors and nucleoside reverse transcriptase inhibitors. Manifestations include "buffalo humps" or cervical (neck) fat development and large abdominal fat accumulations. Other body areas, such as the face, arms, and legs, have a wasted appearance and show prominent vein patterns or sunken facial cheeks from loss of subcutaneous fat, known as *lipoatrophy.*

Adrenal dysfunction can result from the glands being infected by opportunistic infections, resulting in adrenal insufficiency. This problem manifests as fatigue, weight loss, nausea, vomiting, low blood pressure, and electrolyte disturbances and can be life threatening.

Patients taking protease inhibitors have a higher-than-expected incidence of type 1 diabetes and hyperlipidemia. These problems are seen even among patients who have no other risks for these problems or the associated heart disease.

Other Clinical Manifestations. All body systems are affected in AIDS. *AIDS dementia complex (ADC)*, also called *HIV-associated dementia complex*, refers to the manifestations of central nervous system involvement. ADC occurs in about 70% of people with AIDS and is a result of infection of cells within the central nervous system by HIV. ADC causes cognitive, motor, and behavioral impairments. Manifestations range from barely noticeable to severe dementia. (See Chapter 42 for more discussion on dementia.)

Some neurologic problems may be a result of HIV INFECTION or drug side effects, including peripheral neuropathies and myopathies. Assess for manifestations of peripheral neuropathies, which include paresthesias and burning sensations, reduced sensory perception, pain, and gait changes. Myopathies are accompanied by leg weakness, ataxia, and muscle pain.

AIDS wasting syndrome is not due to any single factor. It may be a result of altered metabolism from cancer or INFECTION. Diarrhea, malabsorption, anorexia, and oral and esophageal lesions can all contribute to persistent weight loss, and the patient may appear quite emaciated.

Skin changes include dry, itchy, irritated skin and many types of rashes. Folliculitis, eczema, or psoriasis may occur. Ask the patient about skin sensation changes, and examine any rash or irritation. When the platelet count is low, petechiae or bleeding gums may be present.

Kidney problems, including HIV-associated nephropathy (HIVAN) are common. These problems range from discrete glomerular injury to acute and chronic kidney diseases. Compared with the general population, patients with HIV have a sixteenfold higher risk for requiring a renal replacement intervention.

Psychosocial Assessment. Psychosocial data collection for a patient with AIDS is very important. Ask about the patient's social support system, including family, significant others, and friends. To protect confidentiality, learn who in this support system is aware of the diagnosis so that it is not inadvertently mentioned. Health care professionals must respect the patient's choices as much as possible without compromising care. Offer resources to help with disclosure to sexual partners or significant others.

The patient may be closest to a lover or a friend who is not legally recognized as next of kin. Obtain the name and telephone number of that person, and learn whether a health care proxy or durable power-of-attorney document has been signed.

Ask about the patient's ADLs and any changes that may have occurred since the diagnosis. Assess his or her employment status and occupation, immigration status, social activities and hobbies, living arrangements, and financial resources, including health insurance. Ask whether he or she uses drugs, including tobacco, alcohol, supplements, opioids, benzodiazepines, cocaine, crystal methamphetamine, or injection drugs.

To plan care and monitor changes, assess the patient's anxiety level, mood, cognitive ability, and energy level. Ask about any experiences with discrimination and how they were handled. After assessing the patient's level of self-esteem and changes in body image, work with him or her to identify strengths and coping strategies. Gather information about any suicidal ideation, depression, or other psychological problems. Also ask about the use of support groups or other community resources.

The patient with HIV disease has less energy as the disease progresses, and there are many causes. Pace interviews, assessments, and interventions to match his or her energy level. When the patient is greatly fatigued, postpone or eliminate nonurgent tests or care activities.

Laboratory Assessment

Lymphocyte Counts. Lymphocyte counts are performed as part of a complete blood count (CBC) with differential (see Chapter 17). The normal white blood cell (WBC) count is between 5000 and 10,000 cells/mm^3, with a differential of about 30% to 40% lymphocytes (an absolute number of 1500 to 4500). Patients with AIDS are often leukopenic, with a WBC count of less than 3500 cells/mm^3, and lymphopenic (<1500 lymphocytes/mm^3).

CD4+ T-cell and CD8+ T-cell counts and percentages are part of an immune profile. People with HIV disease and AIDS usually have a lower-than-normal number of CD4+ T-cells, whereas the number of CD8+ T-cells remains normal. The normal ratio of CD4+ to CD8+ T-cells is 2 : 1. In HIV disease and AIDS, because of the low number of CD4+ T-cells, this ratio is low. Low CD4+ T-cell counts and a low ratio are associated with more disease manifestations.

Antibody Tests. Antibody tests are used to measure the patient's response to the virus (the antigen) rather than to measure parts of the virus. When the body is infected with HIV, the body makes an antibody to the virus, usually within 3 weeks to 3 months after the INFECTION first occurs. In some people, antibodies are not made until 36 months after initial infection.

HIV antibodies can be measured by enzyme-linked immunosorbent assay (ELISA) and Western blot analysis. False-negative results (incorrectly indicating the absence of HIV infection) have been reported early in the infection, in people with cancer, and in people receiving long-term immunosuppressive therapy.

ELISA is an inexpensive and accurate test. The patient's serum is mixed with HIV grown in culture. If the patient has antibodies to HIV, they bind to the HIV antigens and can be detected (a positive test). However, this test can be negative even when the person has HIV INFECTION if the test is performed before antibodies are made in sufficient amounts. The time between when a person is first infected with the virus and when viral replication is occurring but the immune system has not yet started making antibodies is called the "window period." *So, if the patient has unprotected sex with an HIV-positive person one night and comes in for testing a week later, the ELISA will be negative even though the patient may have active HIV. Thus testing during the window does not provide useful information.*

False-positive test results (incorrectly indicating HIV infection) occur in about 0.1% (1 of 1000) of those tested with ELISA. False-positive results sometimes occur in pregnant women and women who have had children, injection drug users, people who have had malaria, patients with lymphomas, and other conditions. Therefore anyone who has a positive ELISA needs to have additional testing to confirm or rule out INFECTION.

Western blot is used to confirm the diagnosis when the results of an ELISA are positive. This test is more sophisticated and expensive than the ELISA. The Western blot detects serum antibodies to four specific major HIV antigens. A positive Western blot result is based on the presence of antibodies to at least two of the major HIV antigens.

The result is inconclusive if two of the major antibodies are not detected but other antibodies to HIV are. The person should then be retested. *If a person has a positive test result for HIV antibodies, it does not mean that he or she has HIV disease or AIDS—only that he or she has been infected with the virus.*

Both the ELISA and Western blot are blood-based tests. This requires special equipment and trained personnel to test for HIV infection. Some HIV testing is simpler, using techniques that are not blood-based so that testing can be done anywhere, even at home. One test involves oral testing for HIV antibody. This test uses a device that is placed against the gum and cheek for 2 minutes. Fluid (called *transmucosal exudate,* not saliva) is drawn into an absorbable pad, which, in an HIV-positive person, contains HIV-specific antibodies. The pad is placed in a solution; a positive result shows a change similar to a positive result in a urine pregnancy test. Total testing time is about 20 minutes. This test has the same accuracy as blood testing and can provide results quickly. If results are positive for HIV, a blood test is needed to confirm the result.

Home test kits require that a drop of blood be placed on a test card with a special code number. The card is mailed to a laboratory where the blood is tested for HIV antibodies. A special telephone number is called and the code entered. Test results are then given.

A newly approved HIV home test kit is the OraQuick In-Home HIV Test. This test uses oral transmucosal exudate and results are ready in 20 to 40 minutes. The manufacturer recommends that the test be performed at least 3 months after a risk event has occurred. A positive result indicates the need for additional testing. The manufacturer provides a 24-hour telephone support service for correct use of the product and general counseling.

Viral Load Testing. Viral load testing (also called *viral burden testing*) measures the presence of HIV viral genetic material (RNA) or other viral proteins in the patient's blood rather than the body's response to the virus. These tests are quantitative and indicate the level of viral burden or viral load, which is useful to monitor disease progression and treatment effectiveness.

Quantitative RNA assays quantify viral load. These assays are the reverse transcriptase-polymerase chain reaction (RT-PCR), the branched DNA (bDNA) method, and the nucleic acid sequence–based assay (NASBA). All three assays use gene amplification to determine the amount of HIV RNA present in a patient's serum, and all have a specificity of 100%. Even if only a few infected cells are present in a serum sample, tiny amounts of the HIV RNA are amplified to allow detection and diagnosis of people who have no indication of INFECTION. These tests are used to monitor therapy effectiveness and the need to change drug regimens.

Other Laboratory Assessment. Other laboratory tests monitor the patient's overall health and detect or diagnose any infections or other problems related to HIV disease. These tests include blood chemistries, a CBC with differential and platelets, toxoplasmosis antibody titer, liver function tests, a serologic test for syphilis (STS), antigens and antibodies to hepatitis viruses A, B, and C, lipid profile, QuantiFERON TB testing or PPD, and cervical and anal Pap testing. Other tests to evaluate the immune profile may include bone marrow aspiration with biopsy and cultures. Other tests may be performed to monitor toxicities from antiretroviral drugs.

GENETIC/GENOMIC CONSIDERATIONS

Patient-Centered Care QSEN

The HIV genotype test is used to determine whether any mutations exist in the strain of HIV that has infected the patient. This test is useful before starting antiretroviral therapy to learn whether the patient is infected with a resistant strain of HIV. The test helps the clinician choose which antiretroviral drugs are most likely to be effective against viral replication. It is also useful in patients who demonstrate initial success in antiretroviral therapy and then have rapid disease progression. The human leukocyte antigen (HLA) *B5701* allele test is a genetic test to determine how a person will respond to a drug. Patients with a variant of this gene allele have a hypersensitivity reaction to abacavir (Ziagen) that ranges from mild fever, rash, nausea, and vomiting to fatal anaphylaxis. Abacavir should not be used without first testing for *B5701,* and if positive, abacavir is never used either as an individual drug or in combined drug preparations.

Other Diagnostic Assessment. Other diagnostic tests are performed on the basis of the patient's manifestations. These may include testing stool for ova and parasites; biopsies of the skin, lymph nodes, lungs, liver, GI tract, or brain; a chest x-ray; gallium scans; bronchoscopy, endoscopy, or colonoscopy; liver and spleen scans; CT scans; pulmonary function tests; and arterial blood gas (ABG) analysis.

◆ *Analysis*

The priority NANDA-I nursing diagnoses and collaborative problems for patients with AIDS include:

1. Risk for Infection related to immune deficiency (NANDA-I)
2. Inadequate oxygenation related to anemia, respiratory infection (*P. jiroveci* pneumonia [PCP], cytomegalovirus [CMV] pneumonitis), pulmonary Kaposi's sarcoma (KS), or anemia
3. Chronic Pain related to neuropathy, myelopathy, cancer, or infection (NANDA-I)
4. Imbalanced Nutrition: Less Than Body Requirements related to high metabolic need, nausea and vomiting, diarrhea, difficulty chewing or swallowing, or anorexia (NANDA-I)
5. Diarrhea related to infection, food intolerance, or drugs (NANDA-I)
6. Impaired Skin Integrity related to KS, infection, altered nutritional state, incontinence, immobility, hyperthermia, or cancer (NANDA-I)
7. Confusion (Acute and Chronic) related to AIDS dementia complex (ADC), central nervous system infection, or cancer (NANDA-I)
8. Reduced self-esteem related to changes in body image, role, or independence

◆ *Planning and Implementation*

Preventing Infection. The patient with AIDS is susceptible to opportunistic other INFECTIONS because of immune

CHART 19-4 Patient and Family Education: Preparing for Self-Management

Prevention of Infection

During the times when your white blood cell counts are low:

- Avoid crowds and other large gatherings of people who might be ill.
- Do not share personal toilet articles, such as toothbrushes, toothpaste, washcloths, or deodorant sticks, with others.
- If possible, bathe daily, using an antimicrobial soap. If total bathing is not possible, wash the armpits, groin, genitals, and anal area twice a day with an antimicrobial soap.
- Clean your toothbrush at least weekly by either running it through the dishwasher or rinsing it in liquid laundry bleach (and then rinsing out the bleach with hot running water).
- Wash your hands thoroughly with an antimicrobial soap before you eat or drink, after touching a pet, after shaking hands with anyone, as soon as you come home from any outing, and after using the toilet.
- Avoid eating salads; raw fruits and vegetables; undercooked meat, fish, and eggs; and pepper and paprika.
- Wash dishes between use with hot, sudsy water, or use a dishwasher.
- Do not drink water, milk, juice, or other cold liquids that have been standing for longer than an hour.
- Do not reuse cups and glasses without washing.
- Do not change pet litter boxes. If unavoidable, use gloves and wash hands immediately.
- Avoid turtles and reptiles as pets.
- Do not feed pets raw or undercooked meat.
- Take your temperature at least once a day and whenever you do not feel well.
- Report any of these manifestations of infection to your physician immediately:
  - Temperature greater than 100° F (37.8° C)
  - Persistent cough (with or without sputum)
  - Pus or foul-smelling drainage from any open skin area or normal body opening
  - Presence of a boil or abscess
  - Urine that is cloudy or foul smelling or that causes burning on urination
- Take all prescribed drugs.
- Do not dig in the garden or work with houseplants.
- Wear a condom (if you are a man) when having sex. If you are a woman having sex with a male partner, ensure that he wears a condom or use a female vaginal polyurethane condom.
- Avoid travel to areas of the world with poor sanitation or less-than-adequate health care facilities.

CHART 19-5 Best Practice for Patient Safety & Quality Care QSEN

Care of the Hospitalized Immunosuppressed Patient

- Place the patient in a private room whenever possible.
- Use good handwashing technique or use alcohol-based hand rubs before touching the patient or any of his or her belongings.
- Ensure that the patient's room and bathroom are cleaned at least once each day.
- Do not use supplies from common areas for neutropenic patients. For example, keep a dedicated box of disposable gloves in his or her room and do not share this box with any other patient. Provide single-use food products, individually wrapped gauze, and other individually wrapped items.
- Limit the number of health care personnel entering the patient's room.
- Monitor vital signs, including temperature, every 4 hours.
- Inspect the patient's mouth at least every 8 hours.
- Inspect the patient's skin and mucous membranes (especially the anal area) for the presence of fissures and abscesses at least every 8 hours.
- Inspect open areas, such as IV sites, every 4 hours for manifestations of infection.
- Change gauze-containing wound dressings daily.
- Obtain specimens of all suspicious areas for culture (as specified by the agency), and promptly notify the physician.
- Assist the patient in performing coughing and deep-breathing exercises.
- Encourage activity at a level appropriate for the patient's current health status.
- Keep frequently used equipment in the room for use with this patient only (e.g., blood pressure cuff, stethoscope, thermometer).
- Limit visitors to healthy adults.
- Use strict aseptic technique for all invasive procedures.
- Avoid the use of indwelling urinary catheters.
- Keep fresh flowers and potted plants out of the patient's room.
- Teach the patient to eat a low-bacteria diet (e.g., avoiding raw fruits and vegetables; undercooked meat, eggs, and fish; pepper and paprika as seasonings sprinkled on food right before eating).

deficiency. Initial management focuses on supporting the patient's IMMUNITY by controlling the HIV infection with antiretroviral therapy. When the patient's immunity declines, management includes both prophylaxis and treatment of opportunistic infections.

Planning: Expected Outcomes. The patient is expected to remain free of opportunistic diseases and other INFECTION. Indicators include:

- Absence of chills, fever, or temperature instability
- Absence of purulent drainage or sputum
- Absence of diarrhea
- Absence of chest x-ray infiltration
- Maintenance of white blood cell (WBC) count within the patient's normal range

Interventions. The person who has HIV infection and is immunosuppressed is at greater risk for any type of INFECTION. Teach him or her to avoid exposure to infection (Chart 19-4). Chart 19-5 outlines best practices for prevention of infection in a hospitalized patient with decreased immune function.

Drug Therapy. All currently licensed antiretroviral drugs have excellent activity against HIV; however, *it is important to remember that antiretroviral therapy only inhibits viral replication and does not kill the virus.* Treatment with only one antiretroviral agent (i.e., *monotherapy*) promotes drug resistance and does not improve the patient's life span. Instead, multiple drugs are used together in combinations from different classes of antiretroviral agents. This approach is termed *highly active antiretroviral therapy (HAART)* and has reduced viral load, improved CD4+ T-cell counts, and slowed disease progression. As a general rule, patients are told they must take the drugs correctly 90% of the time, making sure that out of 10 doses, 9 are taken on time and correctly. This is a tall order when considering that this drug therapy is for the rest of one's life.

An important issue with HAART is the development of drug-resistant mutations in the HIV organism. When resistance develops, viral replication is no longer suppressed by the drugs. Testing is now possible to determine whether a strain of HIV has developed resistance to specific drugs (see the Genetic/Genomic Considerations box on p. 337). Several factors contribute to the development of drug resistance to HAART, with the most important being missed doses of drugs. When doses are missed, the blood drug concentrations become lower than what are needed for inhibition of viral replication (often called the *minimum inhibitory concentration*). When this concentration is too low, the HIV can replicate and produce new viral particles that are resistant to the drugs being used.

An important understanding about HIV resistance to one or more drugs is that once a patient has HIV with resistant mutations, the resistant virus is stored in the body indefinitely, a process known as *archiving*. The drugs to which the virus is resistant are no longer used for that patient. Even years later, if the drug to which the HIV demonstrated resistance is tried again, the viruses with the resistant mutation come out of archival storage to defeat the drug.

! NURSING SAFETY PRIORITY QSEN

Drug Alert

Ensure that HAART drugs are not missed, delayed, or administered in lower-than-prescribed doses in the inpatient setting. Teach patients the importance of taking their drugs exactly as prescribed to maintain the effectiveness of HAART drugs. Even a few missed doses per month can promote drug resistance (remember the 90% rule).

The main actions of each drug category and representative drugs in each category are presented in Chart 19-6. These categories are nucleoside reverse transcriptase inhibitors (NRTIs), non-nucleoside reverse transcriptase inhibitors (NNRTIs), protease inhibitors (PIs), integrase inhibitors, fusion inhibitors, and entry inhibitors. Drawbacks to HAART include the expense of the drugs, food and timing requirements, and the number of daily drugs. Newer combination drug formulations have reduced the number of tablets and capsules that need to be taken daily; however, the daily regimen is lifelong and burdensome.

Most antiretroviral drugs have significant side effects and many possible drug interactions. Be sure to consult a drug reference book for usual dosages, side effects, and nursing interventions.

An interesting complication of effective HAART in some patients whose CD4+ T-cell counts rise and immune responses return to normal is the development of immune reconstitution inflammatory syndrome (IRIS) (Carr & Traufler, 2011). As the drugs begin to suppress HIV replication and the T-cells slowly

CHART 19-6 Common Examples of Drug Therapy

HIV Infection

DRUG CATEGORY	MECHANISM OF ACTION	REPRESENTATIVE DRUGS
Nucleoside Reverse Transcriptase Inhibitors (NRTIs)	Drugs have a similar structure to the four nucleoside bases of DNA, making them "counterfeit" bases. Fools the HIV enzyme *reverse transcriptase* into using these counterfeit bases so that viral DNA synthesis and replication are suppressed.	Abacavir (Ziagen) Didanosine (Videx EC) Emtricitabine (Emtriva) Lamivudine (Epivir) Stavudine (Zerit) Tenofovir (Viread) Zidovudine (Retrovir)
Non-Nucleoside Reverse Transcriptase Inhibitors (NNRTIs)	Drugs bind directly to the HIV-1 enzyme *reverse transcriptase,* preventing viral cell DNA replication, RNA replication, and protein synthesis. This action suppresses viral replication of the HIV-1 virus but does not affect HIV-2 viral replication.	Delavirdine (Rescriptor) Efavirenz (Sustiva) Etravirine (INTELENCE) Nevirapine (Viramune, Viramune XR) Rilpivirine (EDURANT)
Protease Inhibitors (PIs)	Drugs competitively block the HIV protease enzyme, preventing viral replication and release of viral particles. The HIV initially produces all of its proteins in one long strand, which must be broken down into separate smaller proteins by HIV protease to be active. Thus, when inhibited, viral proteins are not functional and viral particles cannot leave the cell to infect other cells.	Atazanavir (Reyataz) Darunavir (Prezista) Fosamprenavir (Lexiva) Indinavir (Crixivan) Lopinavir/ritonavir (Kaletra) Nelfinavir (Viracept) Saquinavir (Invirase) Tipranavir (Aptivus)
Integrase Inhibitors	Drugs inhibit the HIV enzyme *integrase,* which the virus uses to insert the viral DNA into the host cell's human DNA. Without this action, viral proteins are not made and viral replication is inhibited.	Dolutegravir (TIVICAY) Elvitegravir (EVG) Raltegravir (Isentress)
Fusion Inhibitors	Drugs block the fusion of HIV with a host cell by blocking the ability of *gp41* to fuse with the host cell's CD4 receptor. Without fusion, infection of new cells does not occur.	Enfuvirtide (Fuzeon)
Entry Inhibitors/*CCR5* Antagonists	Drug works to prevent infection by blocking the *CCR5* receptor on CD4+ T-cells. (The virus's *gp120* must bind to the CD4 receptor and its *gp41* must bind to the *CCR5* receptor or to the *CXCR4* receptor for entry into host cells. This class of drug prevents cellular infection with HIV.	Maraviroc (Selzentry)
Combination Products	Each ingredient has the same mechanism of action as the parent drug class.	Atripla (emtricitabine, tenofovir, & efavirenz) Combivir (lamivudine & zidovudine) Complera (emtricitabine, rilpivirine, & tenofovir) Epzicom (lamivudine & abacavir) Stribild (elvitegravir, cobicistat, emtricitabine, & tenofovir) Truvada (emtricitabine & tenofovir) Trizivir (lamivudine, zidovudine, & abacavir)

begin to rebound, the T4-cells "recognize" several opportunistic INFECTIONS (e.g., tuberculosis, cryptococcosis, *Mycobacterium avium* complex, pneumocystis pneumonia, cytomegalovirus, hepatitis, and others) that were present before but not recognized because of severe immunosuppression. With the T-cells now in sufficient numbers and active, they begin to sound the alarm about the presence of these opportunistic infections. The T4-cells generate an inflammatory reaction, high fever, chills and, depending on which opportunistic infection the immune system is reacting against, worsening disease. For example, IRIS is common with those co-infected with HIV and TB. TB manifestations initially become much worse after starting HAART. Because some of these manifestations are similar to those of drug therapy side effects and other problems, IRIS may go undiagnosed and untreated, increasing the risk for death. When IRIS is recognized, short-term therapy with corticosteroids can reduce the inflammatory responses.

CLINICAL JUDGMENT CHALLENGE

Safety; Evidence-Based Practice; Patient-Centered Care QSEN

J.L. and C.R. are two men in a 2-year monogamous relationship, who were recently married in Washington state. J.L. has been HIV-positive for 4 years. C.R. is HIV-negative and in good health. J.L. is currently an inpatient for an elective cholecystectomy this afternoon. His HIV infection is well controlled on a three-drug cocktail, which he is tolerating well. During the assessment, you ask J.L. how they keep C.R. HIV-negative. A sheepish grin follows. J.L. is generally the insertive (active) partner and C.R. and J.L. have mutually agreed to not use condoms for either oral or rectal sex, as that affects the quality of their sexual pleasure. They continue to make sure that J.L.'s viral load is kept undetectable and he always "pulls out" prior to ejaculation.

1. How safe are their sexual practices for C.R. if he chooses to remain HIV-negative?
2. What should you tell them about condom use?
3. Is C.R. an appropriate candidate for pre-exposure prophylaxis (Pr-EP)?
4. After checking out the information about Pr-EP, what can you tell them about the pros and cons of this therapy?

Immune Enhancement. Research is being conducted to evaluate treatments that may enhance or replenish the immune system of patients with AIDS. Some of these methods include bone marrow transplantation, lymphocyte transfusion, and infusions of lymphokines, white blood cell colony-stimulating factors, and red blood cell growth factors.

Complementary and Alternative Therapies. Complementary therapies are often used by people with HIV/AIDS. Such therapies include vitamins, shark cartilage, and botanical products available at health food stores. The usefulness of these products has yet to be established through well-controlled clinical trials. In addition, some botanicals alter the effects of prescription drugs. Ask the patient which botanicals or homeopathic agents he or she is using, and check with the pharmacist to determine known drug interactions with HAART therapy.

Enhancing Oxygenation

Planning: Expected Outcomes. The patient is expected to maintain adequate gas exchange with oxygenation and perfusion and to have minimal dyspnea. Indicators include:

- Rate and depth of respiration within the normal range
- Pulse oximetry within the normal range

NCLEX EXAMINATION CHALLENGE

Safe and Effective Care Environment

What is the most important question the nurse asks the client prescribed to begin highly active antiretroviral therapy?

A. Do you have any symptoms now of active infection?
B. Is there any possibility that you are pregnant?
C. Are you currently sexually active?
D. What other medications do you take?

- Absence of cyanosis or pallor and abnormal breath sounds

Interventions. The nurse or respiratory therapist uses drug therapy, respiratory support and maintenance, comfort, and rest to enhance oxygenation.

Drug therapy is a mainstay for gas exchange problems resulting from INFECTION. Drug therapy is started after an infectious cause for respiratory difficulty is identified. A common respiratory infection among people with HIV disease is *P. jiroveci* pneumonia (PCP). The treatment of choice for PCP is trimethoprim with sulfamethoxazole (Apo-Sulfatrim ♣, Bactrim, Cotrim, Septra). Many patients have adverse reactions to this drug, including nausea, vomiting, hyponatremia, rashes, fever, leukopenia, thrombocytopenia, and hepatitis.

Pentamidine isethionate (Pentacarinat ♣, Pentam), usually given IV or IM, is also used to treat PCP. Aerosolized pentamidine isethionate is used as prophylaxis for patients with CD4+ T-cell counts below 200 (or 14%), as well as for those who have already had PCP.

Other drug therapies include bronchodilators to improve airflow, as well as dapsone (Avlosulfon) and atovaquone (Mepron), which can be used as alternative therapies to trimethoprim-sulfamethoxazole for existing PCP or as prophylaxis. For moderate to severe PCP, steroids may be used to reduce the inflammation.

Respiratory support and maintenance help maintain respiratory function and avoid complications. Assess the respiratory rate, rhythm, and depth, breath sounds, and vital signs and monitor for cyanosis at least every 8 hours. Apply oxygen and humidify the room as prescribed. Also monitor mechanical ventilation, perform suctioning and chest physical therapy as needed, and evaluate blood gas results.

Comfort can help improve gas exchange. Assess the patient's comfort. The patient with difficulty breathing is often more comfortable with the head of the bed elevated. Pace activities to reduce shortness of breath and fatigue.

Rest and activity changes are needed when gas exchange is impaired. Most patients with HIV/AIDS have fatigue, especially when respiratory problems also are present. Some treatments worsen fatigue. Consult with the patient to pace activities to conserve energy. Guide the patient in active and passive range-of-motion (ROM) exercises. Schedule non–time-critical activities, such as bathing, so that he or she is not fatigued at mealtime.

Managing Pain. The patient with severe HIV disease or AIDS often has PAIN from many causes. Pain can result from enlarged organs stretching the viscera or compressing nerves. Tumor invasion of bone and other tissues can cause pain, as can compression of nerves from swollen lymph nodes. Many patients with AIDS have peripheral neuropathy–induced pain from the disease or drug therapies (Anastasi et al., 2013). Many have generalized joint and muscle pain.

Planning: Expected Outcomes. The patient is expected to achieve an acceptable level of comfort and PAIN reduction. Indicators include:

- Reporting that pain is controlled to a level that is acceptable to him or her
- Absence of indicators of acute pain (increased heart rate and blood pressure)
- Absence of facial grimacing, teeth clenching
- Willingness to move and participate in self-care

Interventions. Drug therapy and other approaches are used together to manage PAIN in the patient with HIV/AIDS, depending on the cause of the pain.

Comfort measures include the use of pressure-relieving mattress pads, warm baths or other forms of hydrotherapy, massage, and applying heat or cold to painful areas to reduce PAIN levels, with or without drug therapy. Take care when moving or assisting the patient. Use lift sheets to avoid pulling or grasping the patient with joint pain. The patient may be thin and have poor circulation, contributing to pain and discomfort. Help him or her change positions often.

Drug therapy with different drug classes is used to manage different types of PAIN. For arthralgia and myalgia, NSAIDs may reduce inflammation and increase comfort. Pregabalin (Lyrica) may provide some relief from muscle and joint pain. Neuropathic pain may respond to tricyclic antidepressants such as amitriptyline (Elavil) or to anticonvulsant drugs such as gabapentin (Neurontin), phenytoin (Dilantin), or carbamazepine (Tegretol), although these drugs often interact with antiretroviral drugs. These drugs may take days to weeks before a full effect is seen. During this time, opioids may be needed to control pain.

When opioids are used, assess the patient for PAIN intensity and quality. Mild to moderate pain is treated with weaker opioids such as hydrocodone, tramadol, or codeine. More intense pain is treated with stronger opioids such as oxycodone, morphine, hydromorphone (Dilaudid), or fentanyl transdermal (Duragesic). Combinations of weak and strong opioids along with non-opioid drugs may be used to provide the best sustained pain relief and allow the patient to participate in activities to the extent that he or she wishes.

Complementary and alternative therapies are used by many patients with PAIN from HIV/AIDS. These include acupuncture, massage, guided imagery, distraction, progressive relaxation, body-talk, and biofeedback and can be used with traditional and pharmacologic measures to improve comfort.

Enhancing Nutrition. Many patients with AIDS have difficulty maintaining their weight and NUTRITION status. This problem may be caused by fatigue, anorexia, nausea and vomiting, difficult or painful swallowing, diarrhea, intestinal malabsorption, or wasting syndrome.

Planning: Expected Outcomes. The patient is expected to maintain optimal weight through adequate NUTRITION and hydration. Indicators include:

- Selecting foods high in calories and protein
- Maintaining current weight or gaining weight
- Drinking at least 2 to 3 L of fluids per day
- Maintaining normal blood levels of ferritin, albumin, prealbumin, and hemoglobin

Interventions. Because there are many factors for poor NUTRITION in AIDS, diagnostic procedures are needed to determine the cause. Once the cause is determined, appropriate therapy is initiated. For example, in candidal esophagitis, nutrition is affected by swallowing difficulties.

Drug therapy can include ketoconazole (Nizoral) or fluconazole (Diflucan) orally, or IV amphotericin B (Fungizone). Administer the drug as prescribed, and monitor for side effects such as nausea and vomiting, which also affect NUTRITION. Provide mouth care and ice chips, and keep unpleasant odors out of the patient's environment. Antiemetics are used as needed.

Nutrition therapy includes monitoring weight, intake and output, and calorie count. Assess food preferences and dietary cultural or religious practices. Teach the patient about the need for a high-calorie and high-protein diet. Encourage him or her to avoid dietary fat, because fat intolerance often occurs as a result of the disease and as a side effect of some antiretroviral drugs. Collaborate with the registered dietitian to provide an appropriate diet, including small, frequent meals (better tolerated than large meals). Supplemental vitamins and fluids are indicated in some cases. For the patient who cannot achieve adequate NUTRITION through food, tube feedings or total parenteral nutrition may be needed.

Mouth care can improve appetite. When this nursing action is delegated to unlicensed assistive personnel (UAP), instruct them to offer the patient rinses of sodium bicarbonate with sterile water or normal saline several times a day. Explain to UAP why the patient should use a soft toothbrush and the need to drink plenty of fluids. For oral pain, general analgesics or oral anesthetic gels and solutions may be needed. Avoid the use of alcohol-based mouthwashes.

Complementary and alternative therapies to promote healing of mouth sores can help improve food intake. Some patients have found relief from oral thrush with the use of lemon juice and lemongrass infusions.

Minimizing Diarrhea. Patients with AIDS often suffer from diarrhea. Sometimes an infectious cause (e.g., *Giardia*, *Cryptosporidium*, or amoeba) can be determined and treated, or the cause is determined but no effective therapy is available. Many patients are lactose intolerant, and HIV disease worsens the condition. Diarrhea may occur as a side effect of drug therapy. In some cases, no cause can be identified.

Planning: Expected Outcomes. The patient is expected to have decreased diarrhea; to maintain fluid, electrolyte, and NUTRITION status; and to reduce incontinence. Indicators include:

- Has a stool amount and character that are appropriate for the diet
- Recognizes urge to defecate
- Maintains control of stool passage

Interventions. For most patients with AIDS and diarrhea, symptom management is all that is available. Antidiarrheals, such as diphenoxylate hydrochloride (Diarsed 🍁, Lomotil) or loperamide (Imodium), given on a regular schedule, provide some relief. Consult with the dietitian, and teach about appropriate foods. Recommended dietary changes include less roughage; less fatty, spicy, and sweet food; and no alcohol or caffeine. Some patients obtain relief when they eliminate dairy products or eat smaller amounts of food more often and drink plenty of fluids, especially between meals.

Assess the perineal skin every 8 to 12 hours for a change in skin TISSUE INTEGRITY. Provide the patient with a bedside commode or a bedpan if needed because some patients cannot reach the bathroom in time. Teach UAP performing this care to provide the patient with privacy, support, and understanding. Explain the need to keep the patient's perineal area clean and dry. Instruct UAP to report any skin changes in the perineal area, including persistent redness, rashes, blisters, or open areas. Collaborate with a wound care specialist for more interventions to manage anal excoriation and discomfort.

NCLEX EXAMINATION CHALLENGE

Health Promotion and Maintenance

Which dietary change does the nurse suggest for the client who has diarrhea associated with HIV disease?

A. "Avoid fatty foods."
B. "Increase your intake of fiber."
C. "Take an antacid 30 minutes before each meal."
D. "Restrict your intake of fluids to 1 liter per day."

Restoring Skin Integrity. Impaired TISSUE INTEGRITY in AIDS may be related to Kaposi's sarcoma (KS) of the skin, mucous membranes, and internal organs. Lesions may be localized or widespread. Large lesions can cause pain, restrict movement, and impede circulation, causing open, weeping, painful lesions. Another cause of impaired tissue integrity may be skin INFECTION with herpes simplex virus (HSV) or varicella zoster virus (VZV) (shingles).

Planning: Expected Outcomes. The patient is expected to have healing of any existing lesions and avoid increased skin breakdown or secondary INFECTION. Indicators include:

- Absence of new lesions or open skin areas
- Existing lesions become smaller in diameter
- Absence of pus, induration, or redness in, from, or around skin lesions

Interventions. Often, KS responds well to effective antiretroviral drug therapy. With time and HAART, many lesions disappear and do not reappear as long as the patient remains on HAART. For lesions that do not respond to HAART, KS can be treated with local radiation, intralesional or systemic chemotherapy, cryotherapy, or topical retinoids. Systemic therapy with chemotherapy or interferon is used in patients with rapidly progressive disease or with major involvement of the intestinal tract, lungs, or other organs.

Treatment of painful KS lesions includes analgesics and comfort measures. Keep open, weeping KS lesions clean and dressed to prevent infection. Many patients with KS are concerned about their appearance and the risk for being identified as HIV positive. Makeup (if lesions are closed), long-sleeved shirts, and hats may help maintain a normal appearance.

For the patient with a herpes simplex virus (HSV) outbreak, provide good skin care directly or delegate this care to UAP. Stress the importance of keeping the area clean and dry. Teach UAP to clean abscesses at least once per shift with normal saline and allow them to air-dry. This infection is painful and requires analgesics, assistance with position, and other comfort measures. Modified Burow's solution (Domeboro) soaks promote healing for some patients. HSV infection is treated with acyclovir (Zovirax) or valacyclovir (Valtrex).

Minimizing Confusion. Neurologic changes and confusion are major areas of concern for patients with HIV disease or AIDS. These changes may be due to psychological stressors accompanying the disease or to organic disorders caused by opportunistic INFECTIONS, cancer, or HIV encephalitis.

Planning: Expected Outcomes. The patient is expected to show improved mental status. Indicators include that the patient demonstrates these behaviors:

- Identifies self and significant others
- Identifies correct month and year
- Recalls immediate, recent, and remote information accurately

Interventions. Patients with AIDS suffer from enormous loss and psychological stress, which complicates the assessment of changes in behavior or affect. Assess baseline neurologic and mental status by using neurologic assessment tools (see Chapter 41) to compare any changes. Evaluate the patient for subtle changes in memory, ability to concentrate, affect, and behavior. It is important to determine whether the cause of the neurologic changes is treatable.

Reorient the confused patient to person, time, and place as needed. Coordinate with all members of the health care team to ensure that reorientation methods are performed by everyone who interacts with the patient. Remind the patient of your identity and explain what is to be done at any given time. Give simple directions; use short, uncomplicated sentences; explain activities in simple language; and involve him or her in daily planning. Ask significant others to bring in familiar items from home. When possible, arrange all items in the patient's environment in the same location as at home. Calendars, clocks, radios, and putting the bed close to a window may help keep the patient oriented.

Drug therapy is used for different conditions that can cause confusion in the person with AIDS. Psychotropic drugs are used to manage ongoing behavioral problems or emotional disorders. Antidepressants and anxiolytics may be prescribed.

Safety measures are crucial to the well-being of the confused patient. He or she may not be aware of activities or surroundings and may need help with bathing, dressing, eating, ambulating, and other ADLs. Make the environment, whether a hospital room or long-term care facility, safe and comfortable.

Some patients with AIDS have seizures. Institute seizure precautions, including keeping siderails in the up position and having oxygen and suctioning equipment available. Anticonvulsants may be added to the drug therapy.

Assess the patient with neurologic manifestations for increased intracranial pressure (ICP). If not recognized and managed early, ICP can lead to permanent brain damage and death. Increased ICP in patients with HIV disease is most commonly managed with corticosteroids.

NURSING SAFETY PRIORITY QSEN

Critical Rescue

Document and report immediately any changes in level of consciousness (one of the earliest signs of increased ICP), vital signs, pupil size or reactivity, or limb strength to the health care provider for appropriate intervention.

Support the family and friends of the patient who has neurologic impairment. There is great trauma in seeing a loved one unable to care for himself or herself or showing childlike behavior. Answer questions honestly and sensitively. Teach UAP, the family, and significant others how to reorient the patient. Encourage them to continue to provide the patient with news of family happenings or current events. Coordinate with the social worker to identify community resources for the patient and family.

Supporting Self-Esteem. The patient with AIDS may have changes in self-esteem resulting from dramatic changes in appearance. Many patients also have significant changes in their relationships and in day-to-day activities, including a job. All changes can reduce self-esteem.

Planning: Expected Outcomes. The patient is expected to identify his or her positive aspects and accept himself or herself. Indicators include that he or she often or consistently demonstrates these behaviors:

- Maintains eye contact
- Accepts compliments from others
- Expresses feelings of self-worth

Interventions. Provide a climate of acceptance for patients with AIDS by promoting a trusting relationship. Help them express feelings, and identify positive aspects of themselves. Allow for privacy, but do not avoid or isolate the patient. Encourage self-care, independence, control, and decision making by helping him or her set short-term, attainable goals and offering praise when goals are achieved.

Guided imagery is used by many patients to increase their sense of control and enhance self-esteem. Imagery can focus on helping them cope with distressing side effects or painful procedures. Some patients picture battle scenes in which HIV is killed by immune system cells.

Community-Based Care

HIV disease is manageable and chronic (Starr & Bradley-Springer, 2014). The usual course of illness is one of intermittent acute INFECTIONS and periods of relative wellness over years. This period is often followed by chronic, progressive debilitation. Because of the cyclic nature of HIV disease and AIDS, the patient often spends long periods at home between hospital admissions. In some instances, especially as the illness becomes more severe, he or she may need referral to a long-term care facility, home care agency, or hospice. In collaboration with the social worker, dietitian, and others, work with patients to plan what will be needed and how they will manage at home with self-care and ADLs.

Home Care Management. Before the patient is discharged to home, assess his or her status, ability to perform self-care activities, and plans to maintain communication with primary care providers. Home care can range from help with ADLs for those with weakness, debility, or limited function to around-the-clock nursing care, drugs, and nutrition support for severely or terminally ill patients. Assess available resources, including family members and significant others willing and able to be caregivers. Help the family make arrangements for outside caregivers or respite care, if needed. Patients may need referrals or help in planning housing, finances, insurance, legal services, and spiritual counseling. Coordinate with the case manager to ensure these issues are addressed.

Usually a home care nurse makes an initial visit to the patient with AIDS for assessment purposes, and care is followed up by home care aides. If the patient becomes more debilitated, a nurse re-assesses his or her status. Chart 19-7 lists focused assessment areas for the patient with AIDS at home.

Self-Management Education. *Teaching the patient, family, and friends is a high priority when preparing for discharge.* Instruct about modes of transmission and preventive behaviors (e.g., guidelines for safer sex; not sharing toothbrushes, razors, and other potentially blood-contaminated articles). Caregivers also need instruction about best practices for Infection Control Precautions to prevent transmission while caring for the patient in the home (Chart 19-8), nursing techniques to use in the home, and coping or support strategies.

CHART 19-7 Focused Assessment

The Person with AIDS

Assess cardiovascular and respiratory status:
- Vital signs
- Presence of acute chest pain or dyspnea
- Presence of cough
- Presence of fever
- Activity tolerance

Assess nutritional status:
- Food intake
- Weight loss or gain
- General condition of skin
- Financial resources

Assess neurologic status:
- Cognitive changes
- Motor changes
- Sensory disturbances

Assess gastrointestinal status:
- Mouth and oropharynx
- Presence of dysphagia
- Presence of abdominal pain
- Presence of nausea, vomiting, diarrhea, constipation

Assess psychological status:
- Presence of anxiety
- Presence of depression

Assess activity and rest:
- Activities of daily living (ADLs)
- Mobility and ambulation
- Fatigue
- Sleep pattern
- Presence of pain

Assess home environment:
- Safety hazards
- Structural barriers affecting functional ability

Assess patient's and caregiver's adherence and understanding of illness and treatment, including:
- Manifestations to report to nurse
- Medication schedule and side or toxic effects

Assess patient's and caregiver's coping skills.

Teach the patient, family, and friends how to protect the patient from INFECTION, how to identify the presence of infections, and what to do if these appear. Teach about the use of self-care strategies, such as good hygiene, balanced rest and exercise, skin care, mouth care, and safe administration and potential side effects of all prescribed drugs. During diet teaching, stress good NUTRITION; the need to avoid raw or rare fish, fowl, or meat; thorough washing of fruits and vegetables; and proper food refrigeration.

Teach the patient to avoid large crowds, especially in enclosed areas, not to travel to countries with poor sanitation, and to avoid cleaning pet litter boxes. Chart 19-4 lists more strategies to teach the patient and family how to avoid INFECTION.

Psychosocial Preparation. Patients with AIDS often fear social stigma and rejection. Be aware that this fear is realistic, and help identify ways to avoid problems, as well as identify coping strategies for difficult situations. Support family members and friends in efforts to help the patient and provide protection from discrimination.

Encourage patients to continue as many usual activities as possible. Except when too ill or too weak, they can continue to work and participate in most social activities. Support them in their selection of friends and relatives with whom to discuss the diagnosis. Stress that sexual partners and care providers should be informed; beyond that, it is up to the patient. Some patients have depression or anxiety about the future. Almost all feel the burden of having a fatal disease widely considered unacceptable and feel compelled to maintain some secrecy about the illness. Referrals to community resources, mental health/behavioral health professionals, and support groups can help the patient verbalize fears and frustrations and cope with the illness.

CHART 19-8 Best Practice for Patient Safety & Quality Care QSEN

Infection Control for Home Care of the Person with AIDS

Direct Care
- Follow Standard Precautions and good handwashing techniques.
- Do not share razors or toothbrushes.

Housekeeping
- Wipe up feces, vomitus, sputum, urine, or blood or other body fluids and the area with soap and water. Dispose of solid wastes and solutions used for cleaning by flushing them down the toilet. Disinfect the area by wiping with a 1:10 solution of household bleach (1 part bleach to 10 parts water). Wear gloves during cleaning.
- Soak rags, mops, and sponges used for cleaning in a 1:10 bleach solution for 5 minutes to disinfect them.
- Wash dishes and eating utensils in hot water and dishwashing soap or detergent.
- Clean bathroom surfaces with regular household cleaners, and then disinfect them with a 1:10 solution of household bleach.

Laundry
- Rinse clothes, towels, and bedclothes if they become soiled with feces, vomitus, sputum, urine, or blood. Then dispose of the soiled water by flushing it down the toilet. Launder these clothes with hot water and detergent with 1 cup of bleach added per load of laundry.
- Keep soiled clothes in a plastic bag.

Waste Disposal
- Dispose of needles and other "sharps" in a labeled puncture-proof container such as a coffee can with a lid or empty liquid bleach bottle, using Standard Precautions, to avoid needle stick injuries. Decontaminate full containers by adding a 1:10 bleach solution. Then seal the container with tape and place it in a paper bag. Dispose of the container in the regular trash.
- Remove solid waste from contaminated trash (e.g., paper towels or tissues, dressings, disposable incontinence pads, disposable gloves); then flush the solid waste down the toilet. Place the contaminated trash items in tied plastic bags, and dispose of them in the regular trash.

Health Care Resources. In many cities, community groups and volunteers assist people with AIDS. The types and number of services vary by agency and city, but many include HIV testing and counseling, clinic services, buddy systems, support groups, respite care, education and outreach, referral services, and housing. Patients may need referrals to other local resources, such as home care agencies, companies that provide home IV therapy, community mental health/behavioral health agencies, Meals on Wheels, transportation services, and others. In addition, educational materials and support groups are available through Internet access.

◆ *Evaluation: Outcomes*

The overall outcomes for care of patients with AIDS are to maintain the highest possible level of function for as long as possible, reduce INFECTIONS, and maintain quality of life and dignity during the course of progressive illness. Evaluate the care of the patient with AIDS on the basis of the identified priority problems. Expected outcomes include that he or she should:

- Adhere to the prescribed drug therapy regimen at least 90% of the time
- Practice safer sex techniques all of the time
- Remain free from opportunistic INFECTIONS
- Have adequate respiratory function
- Achieve an acceptable level of physical comfort
- Attain adequate weight and NUTRITION and fluid status
- Maintain TISSUE INTEGRITY
- Remain oriented
- Maintain self-esteem
- Maintain a support system and involvement with others

Specific indicators for these outcomes are listed for each patient problem in the Planning and Implementation section (see earlier).

CLINICAL JUDGMENT CHALLENGE

Ethical/Legal

Mark S. is a 24-year-old man who was diagnosed with HIV 3 years ago. He has been followed in the HIV clinic and has not been adherent to his medication regimen. In addition, he has struggled off and on with substance abuse. He currently lives with his mother and came to the emergency department today with severe pneumocystis pneumonia. He required intubation and admission to the ICU. On his first day in the unit, his mother asked about his condition. She was told that he had a severe pneumonia, but that it was likely he would recover. The staff ask the nurse manager whether Mark's mother has a right to know his HIV status since he lives with her and might be at risk for exposure to the virus.

1. What is the nurse manager's responsibility in this situation?
2. Is Mark's mother likely to be at risk for exposure to HIV? Why or why not?
3. Should the staff inform Mark's mother about his HIV status? Why or why not?
4. If his mother is informed about Mark's HIV status, what, if any, ethical issues/principles would be violated?

THERAPY-INDUCED IMMUNE DEFICIENCIES

Some acquired secondary immune deficiencies may be related to other conditions that cause the loss of immunoglobulins or destruction of lymphocytes. The most common cause of secondary immune deficiency is the use of drugs and other treatment modalities for various diseases. Sometimes immunosuppression is a desired effect, as in organ transplantation or for the treatment of autoimmune disorders. Often immunosuppression is an undesirable, complicating side effect of therapy that is used for another intent, such as cancer chemotherapy, and may even require changing the therapeutic regimen. Various therapies cause different types and degrees of immunosuppression. The challenge is to have maximum therapeutic effect without leaving the patient overly susceptible to serious complications.

Drug-Induced Immune Deficiencies

Several drug classes have major immunosuppressive effects. Some induce general immunosuppression; others are more specific and target one part of the immune system more than another.

Cytotoxic drugs are mostly those used in the treatment of cancer and autoimmune disorders. These drugs interfere with all rapidly dividing cells, especially the white blood cells (WBCs), which are responsible for providing IMMUNITY and protection against INFECTION. The result is a decrease in the number of these important cells, especially the neutrophils, greatly increasing the patient's risk for infection. Cytotoxic drugs also interfere with the ability of lymphocytes to produce and release products such as lymphokines and antibodies, causing general immunosuppression.

Corticosteroids are hormones that have both anti-inflammatory and immunosuppressive effects that are used to treat many autoimmune diseases, neoplasms, and endocrine disorders. They inhibit inflammation by blocking the movement of many WBCs. These drugs disrupt the synthesis of arachidonic acid, the main precursor for a variety of inflammatory chemicals.

Corticosteroids reduce the number of circulating T-cells and result in suppressed cell-mediated immunity. They also interfere with immunoglobulin G (IgG) production and reduce antibody-antigen binding. These drugs have many effects that alter disease activity, as well as numerous side effects, including:

- Central nervous system changes, such as euphoria, insomnia, or psychosis
- Cardiovascular changes, such as edema and hypertension
- GI effects, such as gastric irritation, ulcers, and increased appetite (with weight gain)
- Other changes (e.g., hyperglycemia, muscle weakness, delayed wound healing, bone density loss, body fat redistribution, adrenal suppression)

Cyclosporine (Sandimmune, Neoral) is a drug that selectively suppresses the CD4+ T-cells by blocking their growth and development. It is used to prevent organ transplant rejection and graft-versus-host disease and occasionally is used for autoimmune disorders.

Disease-modifying immunosuppressive drugs represent a large group of newer agents that specifically slow the damage caused by a variety of autoimmune diseases. Examples include alefacept (Amevive), etanercept (Enbrel), infliximab (Remicade), and many others. Regardless of their specific action in reducing cell damage, they always decrease the general immune responses to some degree and increase the risk for INFECTION, both newly acquired infections and dormant pre-existing infections. The health problems for which these drugs are most commonly prescribed are rheumatoid arthritis and psoriasis. Specific disease-modifying drugs are discussed in the chapters presenting the health problems for which they are prescribed.

Radiation-Induced Immune Deficiencies

Although chemotherapy suppresses IMMUNITY and inflammation more than radiotherapy does, radiation also is toxic to white blood cells (WBCs), especially lymphocytes and neutrophils. Some radiation exposures can induce profound general immunosuppression. Whether immune deficiency occurs after radiation therapy depends on the location and dose of radiation. Exposure to the ilium and femur in adults can cause generalized immunosuppression because these bone areas are the primary blood cell–producing sites.

Management of the patient with treatment-induced immune deficiency aims to improve immune function and prevent INFECTION. The most severe immunosuppression occurs while he or she is receiving the immunosuppressive drugs or during radiation treatment. The severity and duration of the immunosuppression are related to the dosage of specific drugs. Although this impairment is usually temporary, with good recovery of IMMUNITY and inflammation within weeks or months of therapy completion, the potential for severe infections makes this problem a major treatment concern. Common infections occurring during this period include those of fungal origin, especially yeast, residual viral breakthrough, and a variety of bacteria.

Coordinate with other health care professionals to provide safe care to patients at risk for INFECTION. Chart 19-5 lists specific actions to prevent infection among patients with any type of immunosuppression. Good handwashing by all health care personnel before contact with the patient is essential for infection prevention. Aseptic technique must be used with any invasive procedure as required by The Joint Commission's National Patient Safety Goals (NPSGs).

In some instances, drug-induced immunosuppression can be reduced or avoided by giving hematopoietic growth factors to stimulate bone marrow production of immune system cells. Although not appropriate for all types of disorders, this treatment can reduce the patient's risk for INFECTION during drug therapy. See Chapters 22 and 40 for discussion about this therapy.

Many patients remain at home during periods of immunosuppression. Teach the patient and family best practices to reduce the patient's risk for INFECTION (see Chart 19-4).

For patients receiving long-term therapy with immunosuppressive drugs, drug dosages are altered according to their responses. The lowest dose that achieves the desired effect is given.

CONGENITAL (PRIMARY) IMMUNE DEFICIENCIES

Congenital, or primary, immune deficiencies are rare disorders in which the person is born with a defect in the development or function of one or more immune components. Thus IMMUNITY does not adequately protect him or her from INFECTION or cancer.

Some congenital immune deficiencies are inherited as an X-linked trait (e.g., Bruton's agammaglobulinemia or Wiskott-Aldrich syndrome), and some are recessive (e.g., ataxia-telangiectasia). For many congenital immune deficiencies there is no identified genetic defect.

Congenital immune deficiencies are classified according to the type of immune function that is impaired: antibody-mediated, cell-mediated, or combined. Because cell-mediated and combined immune deficiencies are so severe and rare that the affected person is usually managed in a pediatric setting, only antibody-mediated problems (seen in adults) are discussed in this chapter.

SELECTIVE IMMUNOGLOBULIN A DEFICIENCY

Selective immunoglobulin A (IgA) deficiency is the most common congenital immune deficiency seen in adults, occurring in 1 per 600 to 800 people (McCance et al., 2014). The patient may be asymptomatic or have chronic recurrent INFECTIONS of the upper respiratory tract, skin, urinary tract, vaginal tract, and GI tract. Selective IgA deficiency does not reduce life span. Because IgA is the major antibody in secretions, bacterial infections are seen mostly in the respiratory, GI, and urogenital tracts.

Treatment for IgA deficiency is limited to vigorous treatment of INFECTIONS. Unlike other immunoglobulin deficiencies, IgA deficiency is not managed with exogenous immunoglobulin for two reasons. First, exogenous immunoglobulin contains little IgA and would not help boost IgA levels. Second, because patients with IgA deficiency make normal amounts of all other antibodies, they are at high risk for severe allergic reactions to exogenous immunoglobulin.

! NURSING SAFETY PRIORITY QSEN

Drug Alert

Never administer intravenous immunoglobulin (IVIG) to a patient who has selective immunoglobulin A deficiency.

BRUTON'S AGAMMAGLOBULINEMIA

A classic congenital antibody-mediated immune deficiency is Bruton's disease or Bruton's agammaglobulinemia. Boys born with this disease start to have recurrent INFECTIONS at about 6 months of age, after maternal antibodies, transferred through the placenta, have been lost. These infections include otitis, sinusitis, pneumonia, furunculosis, meningitis, and septicemia. Laboratory assessment shows an absence of circulating immunoglobulin (antibodies).

The prognosis for many patients with Bruton's disease is good if antibody replacement with immune serum globulin is started early. The globulin is regularly given to these patients, usually about 100 to 400 mg/kg IV every 3 to 4 weeks. The dosage and schedule are individualized. Antibiotics are used for specific infections. Long-term prophylactic antibiotic therapy may be used.

COMMON VARIABLE IMMUNE DEFICIENCY

The patient with common variable immune deficiency, or hypogammaglobulinemia, has recurrent bacterial INFECTIONS similar to those seen with Bruton's disease. The patient has low levels of circulating antibodies (immunoglobulins) of all classes.

Hypogammaglobulinemia differs from Bruton's disease in that it usually first appears later (in adolescence or young adulthood), it occurs almost equally in men and women, and the infections are less severe. Common problems include giardiasis (intestinal infection with *Giardia lamblia*), pneumonia, sinusitis, gastric cancer, bronchiectasis, and gallstones.

Treatment is similar to that for Bruton's disease. Regular infusions of immune serum globulin and regular or intermittent use of antibiotics protect the affected person against infection.

NURSING CONCEPTS AND CLINICAL JUDGMENT REVIEW

What might you NOTICE if the patient has impaired protection and increased INFECTION risk as a result of HIV disease and AIDS?

- Chronic or recurrent infections
- History or presence of opportunistic infections
- Decreasing CD4+ T-cell count
- Decreasing CD4+ T-cell to CD8+ T-cell ratio
- Diarrhea
- Report of weight loss and fatigue
- Swollen lymph nodes
- Poor wound healing
- Skin lesions
- Headache
- Fever
- Memory loss

What should you INTERPRET and how should you RESPOND to a patient who has impaired protection and increased INFECTION risk as a result of HIV disease and AIDS?

Perform and interpret focused physical assessment findings including:

- Assess cardiovascular and respiratory status:
  Vital signs
  Presence of acute chest pain or dyspnea
  Presence of cough
  Presence of fever
  Activity tolerance
- Assess nutrition status:
  Food intake
  Weight loss or gain
  General condition of skin
- Assess neurologic status:
  Cognitive changes
  Sensory disturbances
- Assess gastrointestinal status:
  Mouth and oropharynx
  Presence of dysphagia
  Presence of nausea, vomiting, diarrhea
- Assess psychological status:
  Presence of anxiety
  Presence of depression
- Assess activity and rest:
  Activities of daily living (ADLs)
  Fatigue
  Sleep pattern
  Presence of pain

Respond:

- Collaborate with members of the health care team to protect the patient from infection.
- Monitor laboratory test results to determine therapy effectiveness, progression of disease, indications of opportunistic infection.
- Teach the patient and significant other about highly active antiretroviral therapy (HAART) including dosages, schedule, side effects, and the need to take all drugs exactly as prescribed.
- Teach the patient and significant other how to avoid infection in the home environment.
- Teach the patient how to avoid transmission of the HIV.
- Continue to assess for changes in the patient's condition, especially indications of infection in any body area.

On what should you REFLECT?

- Consider your personal views on sexuality, lifestyle choices, what constitutes family membership, gender identification, and fear of HIV transmission.
- Evaluate the patient's, family's, and significant other's knowledge of the disease and its management.
- Evaluate the patient's, family's, and significant other's stress levels, use of coping strategies, and knowledge of community resources.
- Assess the knowledge and proficiency of unlicensed assistive personnel (UAP) in carrying out infection control measures.
- Evaluate the degree of compassion and interaction that UAP display toward patients with HIV infection and AIDS.

GET READY FOR THE NCLEX® EXAMINATION!

KEY POINTS

Review these Key Points for each NCLEX Examination Client Needs Category.

Safe and Effective Care Environment

- Use Standard Precautions for all patients regardless of age, gender, race or ethnicity, sexual orientation, education level, and profession. **Safety** QSEN
- Follow the best practices outlined in Chart 19-5 to protect the hospitalized immunosuppressed patient from INFECTION. **Evidence-Based Practice** QSEN
- Use good handwashing techniques before providing any care to a patient who is immune deficient.
- Ensure the confidentiality of the patient's HIV status. **Patient-Centered Care** QSEN
- Teach unlicensed assistive personnel (UAP) to use Standard Precautions. **Teamwork and Collaboration** QSEN
- Teach unlicensed assistive personnel (UAP) the differences in care required for a patient with a pathogenic infection versus a patient with an opportunistic INFECTION. **Teamwork and Collaboration** QSEN

Health Promotion and Maintenance

- Identify patients at high risk for INFECTION because of work environment or leisure activities.
- Urge all patients who are HIV positive to use condoms and other precautions during sexual intimacy even if the partner is also HIV positive.
- Teach patients with protein-calorie malnutrition what foods to include in the diet to promote better NUTRITION.
- Teach the patient and family to protect against INFECTION by following the recommendations in Chart 19-4.
- Teach the patient and family about the manifestations of INFECTION and when to seek medical advice.
- Urge patients to adhere to their antiviral drug regimen.

Psychosocial Integrity

- Treat all patients, regardless of diagnosis, with dignity.
- Do not assume that any visitor or family member knows the patient's diagnosis.
- Urge all patients who are HIV positive to inform their sexual partners of their HIV status.
- Respect the patient's right to inform or not to inform family members about his or her HIV status. **Patient-Centered Care** QSEN
- Use a nonjudgmental approach when discussing sexual practices, sexual behaviors, and recreational drug use.
- Pace your interview to match the learning needs and energy level of each patient.
- Encourage the patient to express his or her feelings about a change in health status or the diagnosis of an "incurable" disease.
- Refer patients newly diagnosed with HIV INFECTION to local resources and support groups.
- Teach family members reorientation techniques to use when the patient is confused.
- Explain all diagnostic procedures, restrictions, and follow-up care to the patient scheduled for tests.
- Allow patients who have a change in physical appearance to mourn this change.

Physiological Integrity

- Use prescribed oxygen therapy, drug therapy, and respiratory support to improve gas exchange and oxygenation for the patient with respiratory problems related to reduced IMMUNITY.
- Use pharmacologic and nonpharmacologic therapies to reduce pain for the patient with HIV disease and AIDS. **Patient-Centered Care** QSEN
- Pace nonurgent health care activities to reduce the risk for fatigue for patients with AIDS.
- Assess the immune-deficient patient every shift for manifestations of INFECTION. Document the assessment findings, and report any manifestation of infection immediately to the health care provider. **Safety** QSEN
- Assess the TISSUE INTEGRITY of the perianal region of a patient with AIDS-related diarrhea after every bowel movement.
- Collaborate with the health care provider, registered dietitian, respiratory therapist, pharmacist, social worker, and case manager to individualize patient care for the person with HIV disease and AIDS in any care setting. **Teamwork and Collaboration** QSEN

20 CHAPTER

Care of Patients with Immune Function Excess: Hypersensitivity (Allergy) and Autoimmunity

M. Linda Workman

http://www.elsevier.com/Iggy/

PRIORITY CONCEPTS

- Inflammation
- Immunity

LEARNING OUTCOMES

Safe and Effective Care Environment

1. Protect the patient who has hypersensitivities from injury related to inflammation.
2. Coordinate with other members of the health care team to ensure a safe environment for the patient with a latex allergy.

Health Promotion and Maintenance

3. Teach patients with allergies how to protect themselves against harm from a hypersensitivity reaction.

Psychosocial Integrity

4. Reduce the psychological impact for patients and families of patients who have immunity or inflammation excess.

Physiological Integrity

5. Assess all patients for the potential to have a severe hypersensitivity reaction.
6. Prioritize care for the patient experiencing anaphylaxis.

Usually, inflammation and immunity are protective and helpful responses. However, when inflammation or immunity is prolonged or excessive or occurs at an inappropriate time, normal tissues are damaged. These responses are "overreactions" to invaders and foreign antigens and are known as *hypersensitivity* or *allergic responses.* When these responses fail to recognize and protect self cells, normal body tissues are attacked and harmed. This type of reaction is known as an *autoimmune response.* Hypersensitivity and autoimmune responses can severely damage cells, tissues, and organs (Abbas et al., 2012).

HYPERSENSITIVITIES/ALLERGIES

Hypersensitivity or **allergy** is excessive inflammation occurring in response to the presence of an **antigen** (foreign protein or allergen) to which the patient usually has been previously exposed. It can cause problems that range from uncomfortable (e.g., itchy, watery eyes or sneezing) to life threatening (e.g., allergic asthma, anaphylaxis, bronchoconstriction, or circulatory collapse). The terms *hypersensitivity* and *allergy* are used interchangeably. Hypersensitivity reactions are classified into four basic types, determined by differences in timing, pathophysiology, and manifestations (Table 20-1). Each type may occur alone or along with one or more other types (McCance et al., 2014).

TYPE I: RAPID HYPERSENSITIVITY REACTIONS

Type I, or rapid hypersensitivity, also called *atopic allergy,* is the most common type of hypersensitivity from excess immunity. This type results from the increased production of the immunoglobulin E (IgE) antibody class. Acute inflammation occurs when IgE responds to an antigen, such as pollen, and causes the release of histamine and other vasoactive amines from basophils, eosinophils, and mast cells. Examples of type I reactions include anaphylaxis and allergic asthma (discussed in Chapter 30); atopic allergies such as hay fever and allergic rhinitis; and allergies to substances such as latex, bee venom, peanuts, iodine, shellfish, drugs, and thousands of other environmental allergens. Allergens can be contacted in these ways:

- Inhaled (plant pollens, fungal spores, animal dander, house dust, grass, ragweed)
- Ingested (foods, food additives, drugs)
- Injected (bee venom, drugs, biologic substances such as contrast dyes)
- Contacted (latex, pollens, foods, environmental proteins)

Some reactions occur just in the areas exposed to the antigen, such as the mucous membranes of the nose and eyes, causing symptoms of rhinorrhea, sneezing, and itchy, red, watery eyes. Other reactions may involve all blood vessels and bronchiolar smooth muscle causing widespread blood vessel dilation,

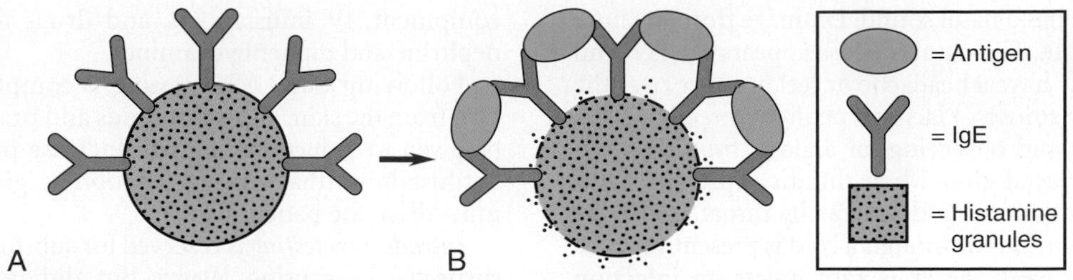

FIG. 20-1 Degranulation and histamine release. **A,** Mast cell with IgE. **B,** Mast cell degranulation and histamine release when allergen binds to IgE.

TABLE 20-1 Mechanisms and Examples of Types of Hypersensitivities

MECHANISM	CLINICAL EXAMPLES
Type I: Immediate	
Reaction of IgE antibody on mast cells with antigen, which results in release of mediators, especially histamine	Hay fever Allergic asthma Anaphylaxis
Type II: Cytotoxic	
Reaction of IgG with host cell membrane or antigen adsorbed by host cell membrane	Autoimmune hemolytic anemia Goodpasture's syndrome Myasthenia gravis
Type III: Immune Complex–Mediated	
Formation of immune complex of antigen and antibody, which deposits in walls of blood vessels and results in complement release and inflammation	Serum sickness Vasculitis Systemic lupus erythematosus Rheumatoid arthritis
Type IV: Delayed	
Reaction of sensitized T-cells with antigen and release of lymphokines, which activates macrophages and induces inflammation	Poison ivy Graft rejection Positive TB skin tests Sarcoidosis

IgE, Immunoglobulin E; *IgG,* immunoglobulin G; *TB,* tuberculosis.

decreased cardiac output, and bronchoconstriction. This condition is known as **anaphylaxis**, which is a medical emergency and must be treated immediately (see the Anaphylaxis section on p. 351).

ALLERGIC RHINITIS

❖ *PATHOPHYSIOLOGY*

Allergic rhinitis, or *hay fever,* is triggered by IMMUNITY and INFLAMMATION reactions to airborne allergens, especially plant pollens, molds, dust, animal dander, wool, food, and air pollutants. Some acute episodes are "seasonal," recurring at the same time each year and lasting only a few weeks. Chronic rhinitis, or perennial rhinitis, occurs intermittently (with no predictable seasonal pattern) or continuously when a person is exposed to certain allergens. In "nonallergic rhinitis," the same manifestations are present although no allergic cause is identified and the immune system does not appear to be involved.

On first exposure to an **allergen** (an antigen that causes allergic sensitization), the person responds by making antigen-specific IgE. This IgE binds to the surface of basophils and mast cells (see Fig. 17-9 on p. 283 in Chapter 17). These cells have many granules containing vasoactive amines (including histamine) that are released when stimulated. Once the antigen-specific IgE is formed, the person is sensitized to that allergen.

In a type I allergic reaction, the already sensitized person is re-exposed to the allergen. The resulting response has a primary phase and a secondary phase. In the primary phase, the allergen binds to two adjacent IgE molecules on the surface of a basophil or mast cell, which breaks the cell membrane. The membrane opens and releases the vasoactive amines into tissue fluids (Fig. 20-1).

The most common vasoactive amine is *histamine,* a short-acting biochemical. Histamine causes capillary leak, nasal and conjunctival mucus secretion, and itching (pruritus), often occurring with erythema (redness). These manifestations of INFLAMMATION last for about 10 minutes after histamine is first released. When the allergen is continuously present, mast cells continuously release histamine and other proteins, prolonging the response.

The secondary phase results from the release of other cellular proteins. These other proteins draw more white blood cells to the area and stimulate a more general inflammatory reaction through actions of leukotriene and prostaglandins (other mediators of INFLAMMATION; see Chapter 17). This reaction occurs in addition to the allergic reaction stimulated in the primary phase. The resulting inflammation increases the clinical manifestations and continues the response.

The production of high IgE levels in response to antigen exposure is genetically based on the inheritance of many genes. Although allergic tendencies are inherited, specific allergies are *not* inherited. For example, a mother who has an allergy to penicillin but not to peanuts may have a child with an allergy to peanuts but not to penicillin. Atopic allergies affect about 10% of the population in North America (McCance et al., 2014).

❖ *PATIENT-CENTERED COLLABORATIVE CARE*

◆ *Assessment*

History. An accurate and detailed history helps identify possible allergic rhinitis (Holmes & Scullion, 2012). Ask the patient to describe the onset and duration of problems in relation to possible allergen exposure. Ask about work, school, and home environments and about possible exposures through hobbies, leisure time, or sports activities. Because a tendency toward type I allergic responses can be inherited, ask about the presence of allergies among parents and siblings.

Physical Assessment/Clinical Manifestations. The patient with allergic rhinitis has **rhinorrhea** (a "runny" nose), a "stuffy" nose, and itchy, watery eyes. He or she may breathe through the mouth, and the voice has a nasal sound. Drainage from the nose is usually clear or white. The nasal mucosa appears swollen and pink. The patient may have a headache or feel pressure over the frontal and maxillary sinuses. Placing a penlight directly on the skin over the sinuses and observing for a glow *(transillumination)* often shows reduced glow when rhinitis is present. With postnasal drip, the patient has a dry, scratchy throat and pharyngitis. He or she often feels as though a cold is present that has lasted longer than a week. Fever is rare unless an infection occurs with the rhinitis.

Laboratory Assessment. A white blood cell (WBC) count and differential indicate the presence of excess IMMUNITY with an allergic response by an increase in eosinophils. A patient with severe seasonal allergic rhinitis may have an eosinophil count as high as 12% (normal being 1% to 2%). Some patients have an increased total WBC count, but the percentage of neutrophils remains normal (55% to 70%). If an acute infection occurs with allergic rhinitis, both the total WBC count and the neutrophils increase.

Other laboratory tests indicating an allergic reaction include serum immunoglobulin E (IgE) levels measured by enzyme-linked immunosorbent assay (ELISA) and the radioallergosorbent test (RAST) (Pagana & Pagana, 2014). A normal level of IgE for adults is about 39 IU/ mL (or less than 100 IU/mL). This level increases greatly with allergies. The usual IgE test does not indicate the specific allergen—only the tendency to have allergic responses. The radioimmunosorbent test (RIST) shows the blood level of IgE directed against a specific antigen and can determine specific allergies. The expense of this study limits its use in allergy testing.

Allergy Testing. *Skin testing* can show which specific allergens are the cause of a type I reaction. Skin testing is performed as scratch testing or intradermal testing. Patch testing is often reserved for contact dermatitis.

A scratch or prick test can show an *immediate* hypersensitivity reaction to an allergen and is used in routine allergy testing for type I reactions. Allergens introduced through a scratch or prick cause a localized reaction (wheal) when the test result is positive. Results are usually determined after 15 to 20 minutes.

Patient Preparation. Systemic glucocorticoids and antihistamines are discontinued 2 weeks before the test to avoid suppressing the test response. Nasal sprays to reduce mucous membrane swelling are permitted, except for sprays that contain an antihistamine.

Procedure. The best site for scratch testing is the inside of the forearm or on the back. Other sites are used if a rash or skin problem is present on the arms or back. Gently clean the skin with soap and water, and remove surface oils with alcohol.

Small drops of sera containing different known allergens are placed on the skin. The skin is scratched or pricked through the drop with a skin testing needle. Control drops are also applied to determine how a person reacts to substances that do not normally stimulate a reaction (negative control) and to substances that normally should stimulate an excess IMMUNITY reaction (positive control). The allergen-tested areas are examined for the presence and size of reactions. These areas are then compared with the control areas. Areas with erythema and wheal formation are positive for that antigen. Degree of sensitivity is estimated by the size of the response.

Although serious reactions in response to scratch testing are rare, ensure that emergency equipment is available during testing. This includes manual resuscitation bag, oxygen, suction equipment, IV infusion set, and drugs for anaphylaxis (epinephrine and diphenhydramine).

Follow-up Care. After testing is completed, wash the solution from the skin. Topical steroids and oral antihistamines may be given to reduce itching and increase patient comfort. If an antihistamine that causes sedation is given, another person must drive the patient home.

Intradermal testing is reserved for substances that are strongly suspected of causing allergy but did not test positive with scratch testing. Intradermal testing increases the risk for an adverse reaction, including anaphylaxis. Ensure that emergency equipment is in the room with the patient. Small amounts of testing sera (0.1 mL) are injected intradermally on the upper arm, and the area is observed for erythema and wheal formation. The degree of allergy is estimated by the size of the response. Preparation and follow-up care are the same as for scratch testing.

Oral food challenges are used for patients who have allergic rhinitis when the allergen is eaten rather than inhaled. This type of testing is used to identify specific allergens if skin testing is not conclusive and if keeping a food diary has failed to determine the offending food items. The test requires the patient to eliminate suspected foods for 7 to 14 days before testing. After this time, the patient is directed to eat a specific suspected food for at least 1 day and to monitor for manifestations of allergy. When many food allergies are present, the patient may have to eat only one food type per day of testing. *Oral food challenges are not performed using foods that have previously caused a serious or anaphylactic reaction in the patient being tested.*

◆ Interventions

Interventions for allergy management include avoidance therapy, drug therapy, complementary therapies, and desensitization therapy. Many patients use a combination of these therapies for management of allergic rhinitis and other manifestations of type I allergy.

Avoidance Therapy. Avoidance therapy can be successful when specific allergens have been identified. Teach the patient to avoid direct or close contact with these agents. Some allergens, such as foods or drugs, may be easy to avoid. Other allergens, such as pollen, mold, or dust mites, may require environmental changes.

Teach patients that airborne allergens can be reduced by air-conditioning and air-cleaning units. Removing cloth drapes, upholstered furniture, and carpeting also reduces airborne allergens. Covering mattresses and pillows with plastic or an ultra-mesh cover reduces exposure to dust mites and mold, as does laundering bed linens weekly in hot water and detergent.

Pet-induced allergies pose special challenges. Simple interventions, such as keeping pets out of the bedroom and thorough cleaning of the room to remove animal hair and dander, may reduce symptoms. Frequent bathing of the pet or keeping the pet outdoors can decrease allergen exposure. Depending on the severity of the allergy and how well other methods provide relief, pets with fur, feathers, or dander may need to be removed from the household.

Drug Therapy. Drug therapy for symptom relief can be effective in reducing the allergic response and making the patient more comfortable. This therapy involves the use of steroidal and nonsteroidal agents (to reduce inflammation), vasoconstrictors, antihistamines, mast cell stabilizers, and drugs that inhibit the release or action of leukotrienes.

Decongestants are available as systemic oral drugs or nasal sprays. These drugs do not clear the allergen or prevent the release of mediators such as histamine. They work by causing vasoconstriction in the inflamed tissue, thereby reducing the edema. Decongestants often contain ephedrine, phenylephrine, or pseudoephedrine. Secretions are reduced when vasoconstricting drugs are combined with an anticholinergic drug, such as scopolamine or atropine. Many decongestants are available by prescription and as over-the-counter cold and allergy drugs. Side effects include dry mouth, increased blood pressure, and sleep difficulties.

! NURSING SAFETY PRIORITY QSEN

Drug Alert

Because effects are systemic, teach patients with high blood pressure, glaucoma, or urinary retention to consult with a health care professional before taking any decongestant.

Antihistamines block histamine from binding to the receptor. This action prevents vasodilation and capillary leak. Many antihistamines also decrease secretions. Some antihistamines, such as diphenhydramine (Benadryl, Allerdryl ♣) and chlorpheniramine (Allergy, Aller-Chlor, Chlor-Trimeton), often induce sedation. Others, such as desloratadine (Clarinex), cetirizine (Zyrtec), and fexofenadine (Allegra), are less sedating.

Corticosteroids decrease INFLAMMATION and excess IMMUNITY in many ways, one of which is by preventing the synthesis of mediators. Corticosteroid nasal sprays (topical intranasal steroids) can prevent the symptoms of rhinitis. Systemic corticosteroids can produce severe side effects and are used only on a short-term basis for serious problems associated with type I reactions, rarely for rhinitis.

Mast cell stabilizing drugs include nasal sprays, such as cromolyn sodium (Nasalcrom), that prevent mast cell membranes from opening when an allergen binds to IgE. Thus these drugs prevent the symptoms of allergic rhinitis but are not useful during an acute episode.

Leukotriene antagonists may be used to manage and prevent allergic rhinitis. Zileuton (Zyflo) prevents leukotriene synthesis. (See Chapter 17 for a discussion of the role of leukotriene in INFLAMMATION and allergy.) Zafirlukast (Accolate) blocks the leukotriene receptor.

Complementary and Alternative Therapies. Complementary and alternative therapies have helped some patients with rhinitis obtain relief, especially through the use of aromatherapy. Possible mechanisms of action include competition and desensitization. Some patients with pollen allergies report decreased problems after eating unprocessed honey.

Desensitization Therapy. Desensitization therapy, commonly called "allergy shots," may be needed when allergens are identified and cannot be avoided easily. It involves subcutaneous injections of very dilute solutions of the identified allergen or allergens. A 0.05-mL dose of this solution is injected subcutaneously. Usually an increasing dose is given weekly until the patient is receiving a 0.5-mL dose. The patient is then started on the lowest dose of the next higher concentration of allergen solution. The process is repeated with increasing concentrations of allergen solutions until the patient is receiving the maximum dose of the greatest concentration (usually 1:100), depending on his or her response. The recommended full course of treatment is about 5 years.

Desensitization appears to reduce allergic responses by competition. In theory, the very small amounts of allergen first injected are too low to bind to the IgE already present but are enough to induce immunoglobulin G (IgG) production against that allergen. IgG is not attached to either mast cells or basal cells, and allergens that bind to IgG do not trigger allergic responses. IgG then clears the allergen from the body (see Chapter 17). By gradually increasing the allergen injection, large amounts of IgG are produced against the allergen. When the patient is then exposed to the allergen in the environment, the IgG binds to it and clears it from the body before IgE can bind to it and trigger an allergic reaction. Because so much more IgG can be produced compared with IgE, IgG is successful in the competition to bind the allergen (Abbas et al., 2012).

ANAPHYLAXIS

❖ PATHOPHYSIOLOGY

Anaphylaxis, the most life-threatening example of a type I hypersensitivity reaction, occurs rapidly and systemically. It affects many organs within seconds to minutes after allergen exposure. Anaphylaxis is not common, episodes can vary in severity, and *it can be fatal. The major factor in fatal outcomes for anaphylaxis is a delay in the administration of epinephrine* (Simons et al., 2011). Many substances can trigger anaphylaxis in a susceptible person (Table 20-2). Drugs and dyes are more

TABLE 20-2 Common Agents That Cause Anaphylaxis

Drugs/Foreign Proteins
- Antibiotics (penicillin, cephalosporins, tetracycline, sulfonamides [especially Bactrim and Septra]), streptomycin, vancomycin, chloramphenicol, amphotericin B, others)
- Adrenocorticotropic hormone, insulin, vasopressin, protamine*
- Allergen extracts, muscle relaxants, hydrocortisone, vaccines, local anesthetics (lidocaine, procaine)*
- Angiotensin-converting enzyme (ACE) inhibitors
- Angiotensin receptor blockers (ARBs)
- Chemotherapy agents (antineoplastic drugs)
- Monoclonal antibodies
- Whole blood, cryoprecipitate, immune serum globulin*
- Radiocontrast media*
- Opiates

Foods
- Peanuts
- Shellfish
- Eggs
- Legumes, nuts
- Grains
- Berries
- Preservatives
- Bananas

Other Agents
- Pollens
- Molds
- Latex
- Other

Insects/Animals
- Hymenoptera: bees, wasps, hornets
- Fire ants
- Snake venom

*Anaphylaxis caused by these substances is probably a result of direct mast cell degranulation rather than an immunoglobulin E (IgE)-mediated hypersensitivity event.

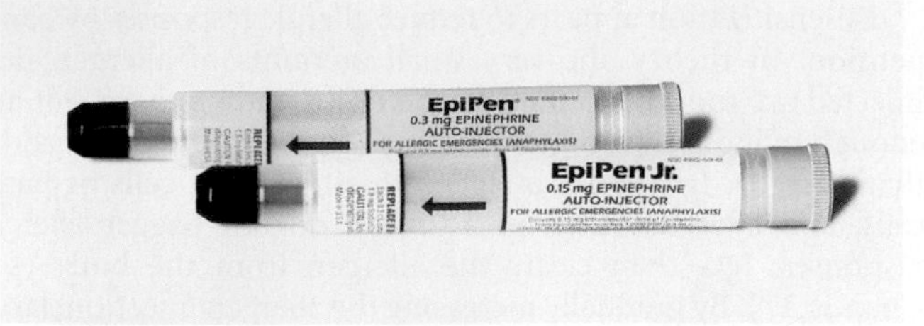

FIG. 20-2 EpiPen and EpiPen Jr. self-injectors for epinephrine.

CHART 20-1 Patient and Family Education: Preparing for Self-Management

Care and Use of Automatic Epinephrine Injectors

- Practice assembly of injection device with a non–drug-containing training device provided through the injection device manufacturer.
- Keep the device with you at all times.
- When needed, inject the drug into the top of your thigh, slightly to the outside, holding the device so that the needle enters straight down.
- You can inject the drug right through your pants; just avoid seams and pockets where the fabric is thicker.
- Use the device when *any* symptom of anaphylaxis is present and call 911. It is better to use the drug when it is not needed than to not use it when it is needed!!!
- Whenever you need to use the device, get to the nearest hospital for monitoring for at least the next 4 to 6 hours.
- Have at least two drug-filled devices on hand in case more than one dose is needed.
- Protect the device from light and avoid temperature extremes.
- Carry the device in the case provided by the manufacturer.
- Keep safety cap in place until you are ready to use the device.
- Check the device for:
  - Expiration date—If the date is close to expiring or has expired, obtain a replacement device.*
  - Drug clarity—If the drug is discolored, obtain a replacement device.
  - Security of cap—If the cap is loose or comes off accidently, obtain a replacement device.

*Some manufacturers have an automatic notification service to let you know your device is about to expire.

common causes of anaphylaxis in acute care settings; food and insect stings/bites are common causes in community settings.

Health Promotion and Maintenance

Anaphylaxis has a rapid onset and a potentially fatal outcome (even with appropriate medical intervention); thus prevention and early intervention are critical. *Teach the patient with a history of allergic reactions to avoid allergens whenever possible, to wear a medical alert bracelet, and to alert health care personnel about specific allergies.* Some patients must carry an emergency anaphylaxis kit (e.g., a kit with injectable epinephrine, sometimes called a "bee sting kit") or an epinephrine injector, such as the EpiPen or Twinject automatic injector. The EpiPen device is a spring-loaded injector that delivers 0.3 mg of epinephrine per 2-mL dose directly into the subcutaneous tissue or intramuscularly (Fig. 20-2). Teach patients prescribed the device how to care for and use it (Chart 20-1).

The medical records of patients with a history of anaphylaxis should prominently display the list of specific allergens. Ask the patient about drug allergies before giving any drug or agent. If he or she has a known allergy, be sure to document in the medical record the allergen and the typical response produced and communicate the allergy and its response to other members of the health care team. Skin tests should be performed before giving any substance that has a high incidence of causing anaphylactic reactions, such as iodine-containing dyes. Be aware of common cross-reacting agents. For example, a patient who is allergic to penicillin is also likely to react to cephalosporins because both have a similar chemical structure. People who have an allergy to bananas, avocados, and some nuts are more likely to have a latex allergy, although this is not universal.

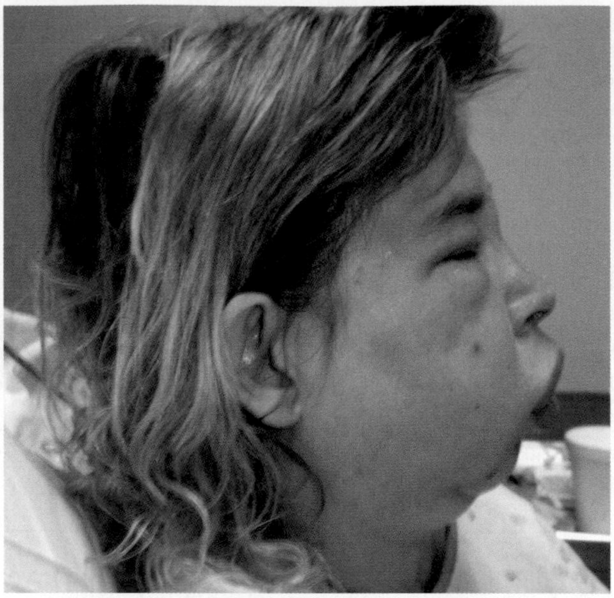

FIG. 20-3 Angioedema of the face, lips, and mouth.

Take precautionary measures if a drug or agent must be used despite a history of allergic reactions. Start an IV, and place intubation equipment and a tracheostomy set at the bedside. The patient is often premedicated with diphenhydramine (Benadryl, Allerdryl 🍁) or a corticosteroid. The allergy-causing substance is given first intradermally, then subcutaneously, and then intramuscularly in increasing doses at 20- to 30-minute intervals so the initial dose by the next route does not exceed the final dose by the previous route.

❖ PATIENT-CENTERED COLLABORATIVE CARE

◆ Assessment

A major problem with anaphylaxis management is that initial manifestations may be subtle, such as sudden severe abdominal cramping and diarrhea. A set of three criteria, listed in Chart 20-2, is used for diagnosis of anaphylaxis. A patient is considered to have anaphylaxis whenever any *one* of these three criteria is met.

A patient having an anaphylactic reaction first has feelings of uneasiness, apprehension, weakness, and impending doom. Often he or she is anxious and frightened. These feelings are followed, often quickly, by generalized itching and urticaria (hives). Erythema and sometimes **angioedema** (diffuse swelling) of the eyes, lips, or tongue occur next (Fig. 20-3). Intensely itchy skin wheals or hives may appear and sometimes merge to form large, red blotches.

Histamine and other mediators cause INFLAMMATION, bronchoconstriction, mucosal edema, and excess mucus production.

CHART 20-2 Key Features

Anaphylaxis

Clinical Criteria 1

Onset within minutes to hours of skin or mucous membrane problems involving swollen lips, tongue, soft palate, uvula; widespread hives; pruritus; or flushing along with any *one* of these new onset symptoms:

- Respiratory distress or ineffectiveness:
  - Dyspnea
  - Bronchospasms
  - Wheezes
  - Stridor
  - Hypoxia
  - Cyanosis
  - Peak expiratory rate flow lower than the patient's usual
- Hypotension or any indication of reduced perfusion resulting in organ dysfunction:
  - Loss of consciousness
  - Incontinence
  - Hypotonia
  - Absent deep tendon reflexes

Clinical Criteria 2

Onset within minutes to hours of *two* or more of these symptoms after a patient has been exposed to a potential allergen:

- Skin or mucous membrane problems involving swollen lips, tongue, soft palate, uvula; widespread hives; pruritus; or flushing
- Respiratory distress or ineffectiveness as evidenced by any dyspnea, bronchospasms, wheezes, stridor, hypoxia, cyanosis, or peak expiratory rate flow lower than the patient's usual
- Hypotension or any indication of reduced perfusion resulting in organ dysfunction, such as loss of consciousness, incontinence, hypotonia, or absent deep tendon reflexes
- Persistent GI problems such as nausea or vomiting, cramping, abdominal pain

Clinical Criteria 3

Onset within minutes to hours of hypotension with systolic blood pressure lower than 90 mm Hg or 30% lower than the patient's baseline systolic pressure.

Adapted from Simons, E., Ardusso, L., Bilo, M.B., El-Gamal, Y., Ledford, D., Ring, J., et al. (2011). World Allergy Organization guidelines for the assessment and management of anaphylaxis. *WAO Journal, 4*(2), 13-37.

Respiratory symptoms include congestion, rhinorrhea, dyspnea, and increasing respiratory distress with audible wheezing.

On auscultation, crackles, wheezing, and reduced breath sounds are heard. Patients may have laryngeal edema as a "lump in the throat," hoarseness, and stridor (a crowing sound). Distress increases as the tongue and larynx swell and more mucus is produced. Stridor increases as the airway begins to close. Increasing bronchoconstriction can lead to reduced chest movement and impaired airflow. Respiratory failure may follow from laryngeal edema, suffocation, or lower airway constriction causing hypoxemia (poor blood oxygenation).

The patient is usually hypotensive and has a rapid, weak, irregular pulse from extensive capillary leak and vasodilation. He or she is faint and diaphoretic with increasing anxiety and confusion.

◆ *Interventions*

Assess respiratory function first. Emergency respiratory management is critical during an anaphylactic reaction, because the severity of the reaction increases with time. The upper airways and lower airways are affected by bronchoconstriction that quickly impairs airflow and leads to hypoxemic arrest. Immediately establish or stabilize the airway. If an IV drug is suspected to be causing the anaphylaxis, stop the drug immediately but do not remove the venous access because restarting an IV may be very difficult when the patient becomes severely hypotensive. Change the IV tubing and hang normal saline. Additional emergency interventions for patients with anaphylaxis are listed in Chart 20-3.

The patient with anaphylaxis is usually anxious or frightened and often expresses a sense of impending doom. Stay with the patient and reassure him or her that the appropriate interventions are being instituted.

Epinephrine (1:1000) 0.3 to 0.5 mL is the first-line drug for anaphylaxis. It is given IM or IV when manifestations appear (see Chart 20-3). This drug constricts blood vessels, improves cardiac contraction, and dilates the bronchioles. The same dose may be repeated every 5 to 15 minutes if needed (Vacca & McMahon-Bowen, 2013). Other drugs used to treat anaphylaxis are listed in Chart 20-4.

CHART 20-3 Best Practice for Patient Safety & Quality Care QSEN

Emergency Care of the Patient with Anaphylaxis

- Immediately assess the respiratory status, airway, and oxygen saturation of patients who show any symptom of an allergic reaction.
- Call the Rapid Response Team.
- Ensure that intubation and tracheotomy equipment is ready.
- Apply oxygen using a high-flow, non-rebreather mask at 90% to 100%.
- Immediately discontinue the IV drug or infusing solution of a patient having an anaphylactic reaction to that drug or solution. **Do not** discontinue the IV, but change the IV tubing and hang normal saline.
- If the patient does not have an IV, start one immediately and run normal saline.
- Be prepared to administer epinephrine IV (preferred) or IM.
  - Epinephrine 1:1000 concentration, 0.3 to 0.5 mL IV push or IM
  - Repeat drug administration as needed every 5 to 15 minutes until the patient responds
- Keep the head of the bed elevated about 10 degrees if hypotension is present; if blood pressure is normal, elevate the head of the bed to 45 degrees or higher to improve ventilation.
- Raise the feet and legs.
- Stay with the patient.
- Reassure the patient that the appropriate interventions are being instituted.

! NURSING SAFETY PRIORITY QSEN

Critical Rescue

Immediately call the Rapid Response Team if you suspect anaphylaxis, because most anaphylactic deaths are related to treatment delay. If the patient is not treated immediately, he or she may lose consciousness. Dysrhythmias, shock, and cardiopulmonary arrest may occur within minutes as intravascular volume is lost and the heart becomes hypoxic.

! NURSING SAFETY PRIORITY QSEN

Critical Rescue

Administer epinephrine as quickly as possible. Most deaths from anaphylaxis are related to delay in epinephrine administration.

CHART 20-4 Common Examples of Drug Therapy

Anaphylaxis

DRUG	MECHANISM	SIDE EFFECTS
Sympathomimetics (First-Line Drugs)		
Epinephrine (Adrenalin)	Rapidly stimulates alpha- and beta-adrenergic receptors of autonomic nervous system (alpha: vasoconstriction; beta: bronchodilation).	Pallor, tachycardia and palpitations, nervousness, muscle twitching, sweating, anxiety, insomnia, hypertension, headache, hyperglycemia.
Isoproterenol (Isuprel)	Stimulates beta-adrenergic receptors, relaxing bronchial smooth muscles and dilating vessels.	Same as for epinephrine.
Ephedrine sulfate (Vatronol)	Similar to isoproterenol but with longer duration of action.	Same as for epinephrine.
Antihistamines (Second-Line Drugs)		
Diphenhydramine HCl (Allerdryl 🍁, Benadryl)	Competes with histamine for H_1 receptors on effector cells, thus blocking effects of histamine on bronchioles, gastrointestinal tract, and blood vessels.	Drowsiness, confusion, insomnia, headache, vertigo, photosensitivity, diplopia, nausea, vomiting, dry mouth.
Corticosteroids (Second-Line Drugs)		
Hydrocortisone sodium succinate (Solu-Cortef) (IV/IM) Dexamethasone (Decadron) (IV/IM) Methylprednisolone sodium succinate (Solu-Medrol) (IV/IM) Prednisone (orally)	Anti-inflammatory—inhibits production of many inflammatory mediators; inhibits mast cell degranulation.	Fluid and sodium retention, hypertension, cushingoid state, gastric distress, adrenal suppression, psychosis, osteoporosis, susceptibility to infection.
Vasopressors (Support Drugs)		
Norepinephrine (Levophed)	Raises blood pressure and cardiac output in severely decompensated states.	Headache, tachycardia, fibrillation, decreased urine output, hypertension, metabolic acidosis.
Dopamine (Intropin)	Raises blood pressure and cardiac output in severely decompensated states.	Dysrhythmias, tachycardia, hypertension, dyspnea, nausea and vomiting, azotemia, headache.

Antihistamines such as diphenhydramine (Benadryl, Allerdryl 🍁) 25 to 100 mg are second-line drugs and are given IV or IM for angioedema and urticaria. If needed, an endotracheal tube may be inserted or an emergency tracheostomy may be performed.

If the patient can breathe independently, give oxygen to reduce hypoxemia. Start oxygen therapy via a high-flow nonrebreather facemask at 90% to 100% before arterial blood gas results are obtained. Monitor pulse oximetry to determine oxygenation adequacy. Arterial blood gases may be drawn to determine therapy effectiveness. Use suction to remove excess mucus and other secretions, if indicated. Continually assess the respiratory rate and depth, and assess breath sounds continually for bronchospasm, wheezing, crackles, and stridor. Elevate the bed to 45 degrees unless severe hypotension is present.

For bronchospasms, the patient may be given an inhaled beta-adrenergic agonist such as metaproterenol (Alupent) or albuterol (Proventil) via high-flow nebulizer every 2 to 4 hours. Corticosteroids are added to emergency interventions, but they are not effective immediately. Oral steroids are continued (at lower doses) after the anaphylaxis is under control to prevent the late recurrence of manifestations.

Continually assess for changes in any body system or for adverse effects of drug therapy. For severe anaphylaxis, the patient is admitted to a critical care unit for cardiac, pulmonary arterial, and capillary wedge pressure monitoring. Observe the patient for fluid overload from the rapid drug and IV fluid infusions, and report changes to the health care provider immediately. The patient is discharged from the hospital when respiratory and cardiovascular systems have returned to baseline.

NCLEX EXAMINATION CHALLENGE

Safe and Effective Care Environment

The client having an intravenous injection of radiocontrast material (dye) for an angiogram starts to have skin wheals at the injection site and difficulty breathing. What is the nurse's best first action?

A. Administer oxygen by mask or nasal cannula.
B. Stop the infusion of the contrast material.
C. Prepare an injection of epinephrine.
D. Notify the Rapid Response Team.

LATEX ALLERGY

Latex allergy is a type I hypersensitivity reaction in which the specific allergen is a processed natural latex rubber protein. When the allergen enters the body through inhalation or direct contact with blood vessels (e.g., as might occur during surgery), interaction with IgE occurs, leading to a type I reaction and INFLAMMATION. For some people, latex allergen contact is limited to the skin or mucous membranes, causing contact dermatitis, a type IV hypersensitivity reaction (see p. 355). Others may have a "mixed" allergic response to latex, with symptoms of both type I and type IV hypersensitivities.

The incidence of latex hypersensitivity in the general population is increasing. People at greatest risk are those with a high exposure to natural latex products, such as patients with spina bifida, people who routinely use latex condoms, and health care workers who use latex gloves, especially gloves that are powdered (Wade, 2012).

Ask all patients about their use of and known reactions to natural latex products. Document all food allergies because some have cross-reactivity for latex allergy. In addition, consider your own exposure and risk for reactions to natural latex products.

Avoiding products that contain natural latex proteins can prevent reactions and initial sensitivity. Most surgical gloves, tubing, and vial closures are now being made from synthetic substances that do not contain latex proteins. Interventions for the patient who has a type I or a type IV reaction to latex are the same as for reactions caused by other allergens.

! NURSING SAFETY PRIORITY QSEN

Action Alert

Use only latex-free products in the care of a patient with a known latex allergy.

? NCLEX EXAMINATION CHALLENGE

Safe and Effective Care Environment

With which client is it most important for the nurse to use latex-free gloves?

A. 38-year-old woman taking oral contraceptives
B. 68-year-old man with total hip replacement
C. 38-year-old man allergic to shellfish and nuts
D. 28-year-old woman with spina bifida

TYPE II: CYTOTOXIC REACTIONS

In a type II (cytotoxic) reaction, the body makes autoantibodies directed against self cells that have some form of foreign protein attached to them. The autoantibody binds to the self cell and forms an immune complex (see Fig. 17-10 on p. 283 in Chapter 17). The self cell is then destroyed along with the attached protein. Clinical examples of type II reactions include immune hemolytic anemias, immune thrombocytopenic purpura, hemolytic transfusion reactions (when a patient receives the wrong blood type during a transfusion), Goodpasture's syndrome, and drug-induced hemolytic anemia.

Management of type II reactions begins with discontinuing the offending drug or blood product. Plasmapheresis (filtration of the plasma to remove specific substances) to remove autoantibodies may be beneficial. Otherwise, treatment is symptomatic. Complications such as hemolytic crisis and kidney failure can be life threatening.

TYPE III: IMMUNE COMPLEX REACTIONS

In a type III reaction, excess antigens cause immune complexes to form in the blood (Fig. 20-4). These circulating complexes usually lodge in small blood vessel walls of the kidneys, skin, and joints. The complexes trigger INFLAMMATION, and tissue or vessel damage results.

Many immune complex disorders (mostly connective tissue disorders) are caused by type III reactions. For example, the manifestations of rheumatoid arthritis are caused by immune complexes that lodge in joint spaces followed by tissue destruction, scarring, and fibrotic changes. Systemic lupus erythematosus (SLE) has immune complexes lodged in the vessels (vasculitis), the glomeruli (glomerulonephritis), the joints (arthralgia, arthritis), and other organs and tissues. (See Chapter 18 for a discussion of SLE.)

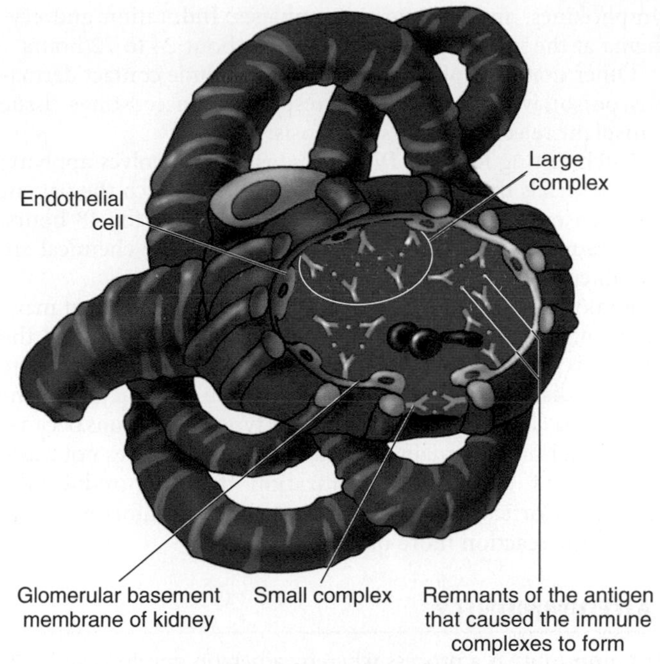

FIG. 20-4 An immune complex in a type III hypersensitivity reaction.

Serum sickness is a group of manifestations that occurs after receiving serum or certain drugs. Immune complexes are deposited in blood vessel walls of the skin, joints, and kidneys. Common causes of serum sickness are penicillin, other antibiotics, and some animal serum–based drugs. Other agents known to cause serum sickness include antilymphocyte globulin and antithymocyte globulin, used to treat organ transplant rejection.

The patient with serum sickness has fever, arthralgia (achy joints), rash, malaise, lymphadenopathy (enlarged lymph nodes), and possibly polyarthritis and nephritis about 7 to 12 days after receiving the causative agent. Teach him or her about the possibility of serum sickness and what manifestations to look for whenever you give a foreign serum. Also keep emergency equipment and drugs close at hand in case he or she has an anaphylactic reaction.

Serum sickness is usually self-limiting, and manifestations subside after several days. Management is symptomatic; antihistamines are given for itching and aspirin for arthralgias. Prednisone is given if manifestations are severe.

TYPE IV: DELAYED HYPERSENSITIVITY REACTIONS

In a type IV reaction, the reactive cell is the T-lymphocyte (T-cell). Antibodies and complement are not involved. Sensitized T-cells (from a previous exposure) respond to an antigen by releasing chemical mediators and triggering macrophages to destroy the antigen. A type IV response typically occurs hours to days after exposure. It consists of edema, induration, ischemia, and tissue damage at the site.

An example of a small type IV reaction is a positive purified protein derivative (PPD) test for tuberculosis (TB). In a patient previously exposed to TB, an intradermal injection of this agent causes sensitized T-cells to clump at the injection site, release lymphokines, and activate macrophages. Induration and erythema at the injection site appear after about 24 to 72 hours.

Other examples of type IV reactions include contact dermatitis, poison ivy skin rashes, local response to insect stings, tissue transplant rejections, and sarcoidosis.

Patch testing for type IV hypersensitivity involves applying test chemicals that contain the allergen(s) to which the patient has been exposed. The patches remain in place for 48 hours. After removal, the skin areas in contact with the chemical are examined for localized redness, swelling, and blisters.

Removal of the offending antigen is the major focus of management. The reaction is self-limiting in 5 to 7 days, and the patient is treated symptomatically. Monitor the reaction site and sites distal to the reaction for circulation adequacy. Diphenhydramine (Benadryl) is not useful for type IV reactions because histamine is not the main mediator. Because IgE does not cause this type of reaction, desensitization does not reduce the response. Corticosteroids can reduce the discomfort and help resolve the reaction more quickly.

AUTOIMMUNITY

Autoimmunity is a process whereby a person develops an inappropriate IMMUNITY. In this response, antibodies or lymphocytes are directed against healthy normal cells and tissues. (Antibodies directed against self tissues or cells are known as **autoantibodies**.) For unknown reasons, the immune system fails to recognize certain body cells or tissues as self and thus triggers immune reactions. The responses, both antibody- and cell-mediated responses, are directed against normal body cells (McCance et al., 2014).

Examples of diseases that have an autoimmune cause include systemic lupus erythematosus (SLE), polyarteritis nodosa, scleroderma, rheumatoid arthritis, autoimmune hemolytic anemia, rheumatic fever, and Hashimoto's thyroiditis (Table 20-3). Other diseases, such as type 1 diabetes mellitus, may have multiple causes, one of which is autoimmune.

Management of autoimmunities depends on the organ or organs affected. *There is no cure.* Anti-inflammatory drugs and immunosuppressive drugs are commonly used along with symptomatic treatment to suppress the excess IMMUNITY.

TABLE 20-3 Known or Probable Autoimmune Disorders

DISORDER	AUTOANTIGEN
Systemic or Non–Organ Specific	
Systemic lupus erythematosus	DNA, DNA proteins
Rheumatoid arthritis	IgG, possibly cartilage
Progressive systemic sclerosis	DNA proteins
Mixed connective tissue disorder	DNA proteins
Scleroderma	Endothelial cells; epithelial cells
Organ Specific	
Autoimmune hemolytic anemia	Erythrocytes
Autoimmune thrombocytopenic purpura	Platelets
Crohn's disease	Crypt epithelial cells
Diabetes mellitus, type I	Islet cells, insulin, insulin receptor
Dermatomyositis	Unknown
Glomerulonephritis	Glomerular basement membranes
Goodpasture's syndrome	Glomerular basement membranes, pulmonary basement membranes
Graves' disease	Thyroid-stimulating hormone receptor
Hashimoto's thyroiditis	Thyroid cell surface
Idiopathic Addison's disease	Adrenal cell
Myasthenia gravis	Acetylcholine receptor, acetylcholine
Pernicious anemia	Intrinsic factor, parietal cell, B_{12} complexes
Psoriasis	Stratum corneum
Reiter's syndrome	Possibly collagen, conjunctival cells
Sjögren's syndrome	Salivary gland cells, vaginal mucous cells, lacrimal gland cells
Uveitis	Uveal tract cells (eye)
Vasculitis	Unknown, possibly collagen or endothelial cells

IgG, Immunoglobulin G.

GENDER HEALTH CONSIDERATIONS

Patient-Centered Care QSEN

Virtually all autoimmune disorders, especially rheumatic disorders, occur much more commonly among women than men (McCance et al., 2014). The risk for autoimmune disease among women compared with men ranges from 5:1 to 20:1.

SJÖGREN'S SYNDROME

PATHOPHYSIOLOGY

Sjögren's syndrome (SS) is a group of problems that often appear with other autoimmune disorders. Problems include dry eyes, dry mucous membranes of the nose and mouth (xerostomia), and vaginal dryness. These problems are caused by autoimmune destruction (excess IMMUNITY) of the lacrimal, salivary, and vaginal mucus-producing glands. Often, the patient with SS also has rheumatoid arthritis or fibromyalgia.

Most patients with SS are women 35 to 45 years old. SS occurs more frequently among patients with certain tissue types, specifically HLA-DRW52, HLA-DR3, and HLA-B8. Although an exact triggering agent has not been identified, viral infection is strongly suspected, especially human immunodeficiency virus type 1 (HIV-1), human T-cell lymphotrophic virus type 1 (HTLV-1), and Epstein-Barr virus (EBV).

Insufficient tears cause INFLAMMATION and ulceration of the cornea. Insufficient saliva decreases digestion of carbohydrates, promotes tooth decay, and increases the risk for oral and nasal infections. Vaginal dryness increases the risk for infection and causes painful sexual intercourse.

PATIENT-CENTERED COLLABORATIVE CARE

The patient with Sjögren's syndrome (SS) usually has blurred vision, burning and itching of the eyes, and thick mattering in the conjunctiva. Difficulty swallowing food is common, as are changes in taste. Ask about nosebleeds (**epistaxis**) and frequent upper respiratory infections (Catanzaro & Dinkel, 2014).

Examination reveals enlarged lymph nodes. If rheumatoid arthritis (RA) accompanies SS, the patient has swollen, painful joints and limited joint mobility (see Chapter 18 for a discussion of RA). Laboratory assessment may show increased amounts of general antinuclear antibodies, anti–SS-A or anti–SS-B antibodies, and elevated levels of IgM rheumatoid factor.

There is no cure for SS. The intensity and the progression of the disorder can be slowed by suppressing IMMUNITY and INFLAMMATION. Drugs used to modulate the immune system in patients with SS include low-dose chemotherapy with methotrexate (Rheumatrex) or cyclophosphamide (Cytoxan). Both drugs have serious long-term side effects, especially on liver and bone marrow function. Other immunosuppressive drugs used to manage SS are corticosteroids, cyclosporine (Gengraf, Neoral, Sandimmune), and hydroxychloroquine (Plaquenil). The monoclonal antibody *rituximab* (Rituxan) has been beneficial for patients with severe inflammatory manifestations of SS (Poetzsch, 2012).

A variety of artificial tears and artificial saliva can help reduce the dry eye and dry mouth manifestations. Teach patients to use humidifiers in the home to increase environmental moisture. Use of water-soluble vaginal lubricants and moisturizers can increase patient comfort and reduce vaginitis. Some patients relieve dry mouth with drugs that increase salivation, such as systemic pilocarpine (Salagen). A drug that increase tears production is cyclosporine (Restasis) eyedrops.

Another intervention for dry eyes is to block the tear outflow channel with small plugs or close it surgically. Then, tears produced remain in contact with the eye longer.

CLINICAL JUDGMENT CHALLENGE

Patient-Centered Care; Evidence-Based Practice QSEN

The patient is a 49-year-old secretary who has just been diagnosed with Sjögren's syndrome (SS) when her health care provider investigated possible causes for her sudden increase in dental caries (15 in 1 year). Upon hearing about the possible dry eyes and vaginal dryness that often accompany SS, she tells you that she has noticed the dry eyes and thought it was just "old age" catching up with her. She also says that she has noticed some vaginal dryness but is not concerned about it because she is not sexually active. She then tells you that she feels bad about this diagnosis because it means that she probably has a poor immune system and is at a greater risk for infections and cancer.

1. Is she correct about her assessment of her immune function? Why or why not?
2. What should you tell her about the vaginal dryness even though she is not concerned?
3. In addition to follow-up by her primary health care provider for the SS, what other health promotion activities would be important for her?

GOODPASTURE'S SYNDROME

❖ *PATHOPHYSIOLOGY*

Goodpasture's syndrome is an autoimmune disorder in which autoantibodies attack the glomerular basement membrane and neutrophils. The two organs with the most damage are the lungs and the kidneys. A person with the disorder may have lung and/or kidney problems. Lung damage is manifested as pulmonary hemorrhage. Kidney damage shows as glomerulonephritis that may rapidly progress to complete kidney failure (see Chapters 67 and 68). Goodpasture's syndrome is most common in adolescent males or young men (McCance et al., 2014).

❖ *PATIENT-CENTERED COLLABORATIVE CARE*

Goodpasture's syndrome often is not diagnosed until serious lung or kidney problems are present. Manifestations include shortness of breath, hemoptysis (bloody sputum), decreased urine output, weight gain, generalized edema, hypertension, and tachycardia. Chest x-rays show areas of consolidation. The most common cause of death is uremia as a result of kidney failure.

Spontaneous resolution of Goodpasture's syndrome has occurred but is rare. Interventions focus on reducing damage from excess IMMUNITY and performing some type of renal replacement therapy.

Drug therapy is the mainstay of treatment for Goodpasture's syndrome. High-dose corticosteroids are most often used. Other drug therapy to suppress the autoimmune response is the same as that for Sjögren's syndrome (SS).

Additional therapy to reduce the excessive IMMUNITY involves plasmapheresis (filtration of the plasma to remove some proteins) to remove the autoantibodies. If the lungs and kidneys do not have permanent damage, patients undergoing plasmapheresis have shown clinical improvement. Some patients using plasmapheresis need infusions of intravenous immunoglobulin (IVIG) to maintain antibody protection against infection.

Depending on the level of kidney function remaining, the patient may need ongoing renal replacement therapy. Peritoneal dialysis or hemodialysis may be used, depending on the patient's health status, ability to self-manage the therapy, and lifestyle (see Chapter 68).

Kidney transplantation is an option for some patients with Goodpasture's syndrome. After transplantation, kidney function is normal and a few patients have been completely disease-free. In others, the kidney problems are improved but the lung destruction continues. Some of the drugs used to prevent kidney rejection also suppress the autoimmune response.

NURSING CONCEPTS AND CLINICAL JUDGMENT REVIEW

What might you NOTICE if the patient is experiencing excess IMMUNITY and loss of protective response in the form of a severe allergic reaction?

- Possible skin rash, blisters, wheals, especially on the skin at the IV site
- Swelling of the face, lips, tongue (angioedema)
- Difficulty breathing, hoarseness, stridor, wheezing
- Cyanosis
- Increasing anxiety

What should you INTERPRET and how should you RESPOND to a patient experiencing excess IMMUNITY and loss of protection as a result of a severe allergic reaction?

Perform and interpret physical assessment, including:
- Taking vital signs, especially respiratory rate and depth and blood pressure
- Auscultating all lung fields
- Monitoring oxygen saturation by pulse oximetry
- Assessing cognition
- Assessing for the use of accessory muscles
- Assessing for the presence of thick or excessive secretions
- Assessing the patient's ability to cough and clear the airway

Respond by:
- Removing or discontinuing the offending agent
- Ensuring a patent airway
- Notifying the Rapid Response Team
- Applying oxygen, and assessing the patient's responses to this intervention
- Maintaining IV access, changing IV tubing, hanging normal saline
- Keeping the patient's head elevated between 10 and 45 degrees
- Preparing to administer IV diphenhydramine and epinephrine
- Staying with the patient

On what should you REFLECT?
- Observe patient for evidence of drug therapy and oxygen therapy effectiveness (adequate tissue perfusion and oxygenation [see Chapter 27]).
- Think about what may have precipitated this episode and what steps could be taken to either prevent a similar episode or identify it earlier.
- Think about what additional resources could improve the nursing response to this situation.

GET READY FOR THE NCLEX® EXAMINATION!

KEY POINTS

Review these Key Points for each NCLEX Examination Client Needs Category.

Safe and Effective Care Environment
- Ensure that only latex-free products are used for a patient who has a known latex allergy. **Safety** QSEN
- Verify that all allergies are documented in a prominent place in the patient's medical record.
- Keep emergency equipment and drugs (epinephrine, Benadryl, cortisol) in or near the room of a patient with known severe allergies or a history of anaphylaxis. **Safety** QSEN

Health Promotion and Maintenance
- Urge all patients with severe allergies or those who have a history of anaphylaxis to wear a medical alert bracelet.
- Teach the patient and family about the manifestations of allergic reactions and when to seek medical help. **Patient-Centered Care** QSEN
- Teach the patient who has a known drug allergy about which other drugs are likely to stimulate the same reactions. **Patient-Centered Care** QSEN
- Teach the patient who carries an automatic epinephrine injector how to care for, assemble, and use the device. Obtain a return demonstration. **Patient-Centered Care** QSEN

Psychosocial Integrity
- Explain all diagnostic procedures, restrictions, and follow-up care to the patient scheduled for tests related to hypersensitivities.
- Stay with the patient in anaphylaxis.
- Reassure patients who are in anaphylaxis that the appropriate interventions are being instituted.

Physiological Integrity
- Identify patients at risk for hypersensitivity reactions, especially anaphylaxis. **Safety** QSEN
- Communicate a patient's allergies to all members of the health care team.
- Immediately assess the respiratory status and airway of patients who show any manifestations of an allergic reaction. **Evidence-Based Practice** QSEN
- Immediately discontinue the IV drug or solution of a patient having an anaphylactic reaction to that drug or solution. **Do not** discontinue the IV, but change the IV tubing and hang normal saline. **Evidence-Based Practice** QSEN
- Hold the dose of any prescribed drug when a patient develops angioedema. **Safety** QSEN
- Give oxygen to any patient in anaphylaxis.

CHAPTER 21

Cancer Development

M. Linda Workman

http://evolve.elsevier.com/Iggy/

PRIORITY CONCEPTS

- Cellular Regulation

LEARNING OUTCOMES

Health Promotion and Maintenance

1. Help people identify behaviors that reduce the risk for cancer development and cancer death.
2. Teach the recommended screening practices and schedules for specific cancer types.

Physiological Integrity

3. Explain why causes of specific cancers can be hard to establish.
4. Use knowledge of basic biology to understand how normal cells can lose cellular regulation and become malignant.
5. Distinguish the features of normal cells from those of benign tumors and cancer cells.
6. Discuss the roles of oncogenes and suppressor genes in cancer development.
7. Compare the cancer development processes of initiation and promotion.
8. Interpret cancer grading, ploidy, and staging reports.
9. Explain how cancer metastasis occurs and the expected sites of distant metastasis for common cancers.
10. Discuss the role of immunity in protection against cancer.
11. Assess the individual patient's need for genetic testing for cancer predisposition based on family history.

Abnormal cell growth includes moles or skin tags, which are **benign** (harmless) and do not require intervention, as well as **malignant cell growth** (cancer). Cancer is serious and without intervention leads to death. It is a common health problem in the United States and Canada. Over 1.8 million people are newly diagnosed with cancer each year (American Cancer Society [ACS], 2014; Canadian Cancer Society, 2014). Some types of cancer can be prevented; others have better cure rates if diagnosed early. As a nurse, you can have a vital impact in educating the public about cancer prevention and early detection methods.

Although cancer is common today, it is not a new disorder. Some types of cancer are more common today, especially among more affluent societies, than in centuries past. Two reasons for this increase are the longer life expectancy of people in more affluent countries and increased exposure to substances that cause cancer.

Cancer will occur in about 1 of every 3 people currently living in North America (ACS, 2014; Canadian Cancer Society, 2014), although cancer risk differs for each person. More than 13 million Americans with a history of cancer are alive today (ACS, 2014).

PATHOPHYSIOLOGY

During infancy and childhood, growth of cells and tissues is normal, and many body cells continue to "grow" by **mitosis** (cell division) long after maturation is complete. Such cells are located in tissues in which constant damage or wear is likely and continued cell growth is needed to replace dead tissues. Cells of the skin, hair, mucous membranes, bone marrow, and linings of organs such as the lungs, stomach, intestines, bladder, and uterus, among others have the ability to divide throughout a person's life span. The growth is well controlled through cellular regulation, ensuring that the right number of cells is always present in any tissue or organ.

Some tissues and organs stop growing by cell division after development is complete. For example, heart muscle cells no longer divide after fetal life; the number of heart muscle cells is fixed at birth. The size of the heart increases as the person grows because each cell gets larger, but the number of heart muscle cells does not increase. Growth that causes tissue to increase in size by enlarging each cell is **hypertrophy**. Growth that causes tissue to increase in size by increasing the number of cells is **hyperplasia** (Fig. 21-1).

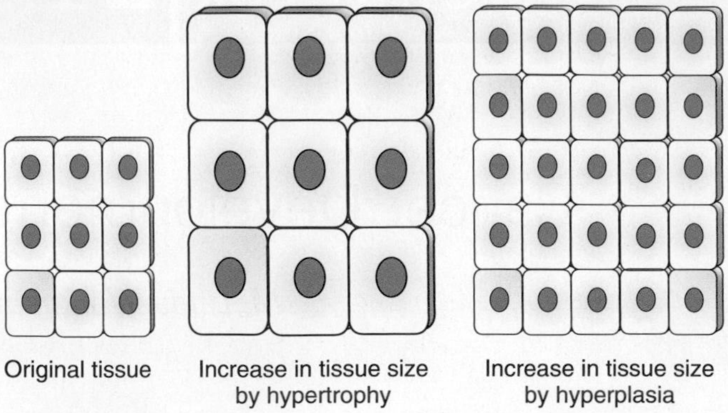

FIG. 21-1 Tissue growth by hypertrophy and hyperplasia.

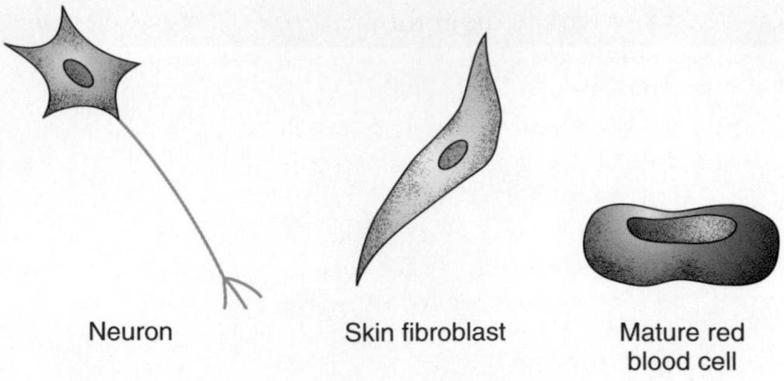

FIG. 21-2 Distinctive morphology of some normal cells.

Any new or continued cell growth not needed for normal development or replacement of dead and damaged tissues is called **neoplasia**. This cell growth is always abnormal even if it causes no harm. Whether the new cells are benign or cancerous, neoplastic cells develop from normal cells *(parent cells)*. Thus cancer cells were once normal cells but underwent genetic mutations to no longer look, grow, or function normally. The strict processes controlling normal growth and function, CELLULAR REGULATION, have been lost (Beery & Workman, 2012). To understand how cancer cells grow, it is helpful to first understand the regulation and function of normal cells.

Biology of Normal Cells

Many different normal cells work together to make the whole person function at an optimal level. For optimal function, each cell must perform in a predictable manner.

Specific morphology is the feature in which each normal cell type has a distinct and recognizable appearance, size, and shape, as shown in Fig. 21-2.

A smaller nuclear-to-cytoplasmic ratio means that the nucleus of a normal cell does not take up much space inside the cell. As shown in Fig. 21-2, the size of the normal cell nucleus is relatively small compared with the size of the rest of the cell, including the cytoplasm.

Differentiated function means that every normal cell has at least one function it performs to contribute to whole-body function. For example, skin cells make keratin, liver cells make bile, cardiac muscle cells contract, and red blood cells make hemoglobin.

Tight adherence occurs because normal cells make proteins that protrude from the membranes, allowing cells to bind closely and tightly together. One such protein is fibronectin, which keeps most normal tissues bound tightly to each other. Exceptions are blood cells. Red blood cells and white blood cells produce no fibronectin and do not usually adhere together.

Nonmigratory means that normal cells do not wander throughout the body (except for blood cells). This occurs in normal cells because they are tightly bound together, which prevents cell wandering from one tissue into the next.

Orderly and well-regulated growth or CELLULAR REGULATION is a very important feature of normal cells. They divide (undergo mitosis) for only two reasons: (1) to develop normal tissue or (2) to replace lost or damaged normal tissue. Even when they are capable of mitosis, normal cells divide only when body conditions are just right. Cell division (**mitosis**), occurring in a well-recognized pattern, is described by the cell cycle. Fig. 21-3 shows the phases of the cell cycle. Living cells not actively reproducing are in a reproductive resting state termed G_0. During the G_0 period, cells actively carry out their functions but do not divide. Normal cells spend most of their lives in the G_0 state rather than in a reproductive state.

Mitosis makes one cell divide into two new cells that are identical to each other and to the cell that began mitosis. The steps of entering and completing the cell cycle are tightly controlled. This CELLULAR REGULATION occurs through proteins produced by "suppressor genes."

Whether a cell enters and completes the cell cycle to form two new cells depends on the presence and absence of specific CELLULAR REGULATION proteins. Proteins that promote cells to enter and complete cell division are produced by oncogenes and are known as *cyclins.* When cyclins are activated, they allow a cell to leave G_0 and enter the cycle. These activated cyclins then drive the cell to progress through the different phases of the cell cycle and divide. Proteins produced by suppressor genes control the amount of cyclins present and ensure that cell division occurs only when it is needed. *Thus CELLULAR REGULATION of division is a balance between the proteins that promote cell division (cyclins) and the proteins that limit cell division (suppressor gene products).*

Fig. 21-4 shows the activities of the phases of the cell cycle (described below):

- **G_1.** In this phase, the cell is getting ready for division by taking on extra nutrients, making more energy, and growing extra membrane. The amount of cytoplasm also increases.
- **S.** Because making one cell into two cells requires twice as much of everything, including DNA, the cell must double its DNA content through DNA synthesis. This process occurs in S phase.
- **G_2.** In this phase, the cell makes important proteins that will be used in actual cell division and in normal physiologic function after cell division is complete.
- **M.** The single cell splits apart into two cells (actual mitosis) during M phase.

Contact inhibition is CELLULAR REGULATION that stops further rounds of cell division when the dividing cell is completely surrounded and touched (contacted) by other cells. Of the normal cells that can divide, each cell divides only when some of its surface is not in direct contact with another cell. Once a normal cell is in direct contact on all surface areas with other cells, it no longer undergoes mitosis. Thus normal cell division is contact inhibited.

Apoptosis is programmed cell death. Not only do normal cells have to divide only when needed and perform their specific differentiated functions, to ensure optimum body function, some cells also have to die at the appropriate time. Thus normal cells have a finite life span. With each cell division, the telomeric DNA at the ends of the cell's chromosomes shortens (see Chapter 4). When this DNA is gone, the cell responds to CELLULAR REGULATION signals for apoptosis. This ensures that each organ has an adequate number of cells at their functional peak.

Normal chromosomes (known as **euploidy**) is a feature of most normal human cells. These cells have 23 pairs of chromosomes, the correct number for humans.

Biology of Abnormal Cells

Body cells are exposed to a variety of conditions that can alter how the cells grow or function. When either cell growth or cell function is changed, the cells are considered abnormal. Table 21-1 compares features of normal, benign tumor, and cancer (malignant) cells.

Features of Benign Tumor Cells

Benign tumor cells are normal cells growing in the wrong place or at the wrong time as a result of a small problem with CELLULAR REGULATION. Examples include moles, uterine fibroid tumors, skin tags, endometriosis, and nasal polyps. Benign tumor cells have these characteristics:

- *Specific morphology* occurs with benign tumors. They look like the tissues they come from, retaining the specific morphology of parent cells.
- *A smaller nuclear-to-cytoplasmic ratio* is a feature of benign tumors just like completely normal cells.
- *Specific differentiated functions* continue to be performed by benign tumors. For example, in endometriosis, a type of benign tumor, the normal lining of the uterus (endometrium) grows in an abnormal place (e.g., on an ovary or in the chest cavity). This displaced endometrium acts just like normal endometrium by changing each month under the influence of estrogen. When the hormone level drops and the normal endometrium sheds from the uterus, the displaced endometrium, wherever it is, also sheds.
- *Tight adherence* of benign tumor cells to each other occurs because they continue to make fibronectin.
- *No migration* or wandering of benign tissues occurs because they remain tightly bound and do not invade other body tissues.
- *Orderly growth* with normal growth patterns occurs in benign tumor cells even though their growth is not needed. The fact that growth continues beyond an appropriate time or occurs in the wrong place indicates some problem with CELLULAR REGULATION, but the rate of growth is normal. The benign tumor grows by hyperplastic expansion. *It does not invade.*
- *Normal chromosomes* are usually found in benign tumor cells, with a few exceptions. Most of these cells have 23 pairs of chromosomes, the correct number for humans.

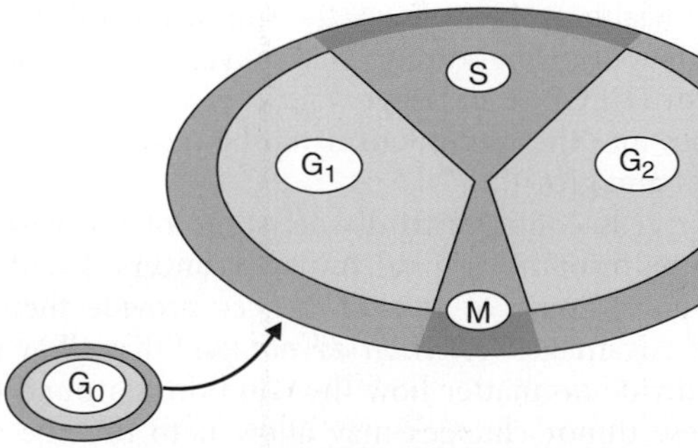

FIG. 21-3 The cell cycle.

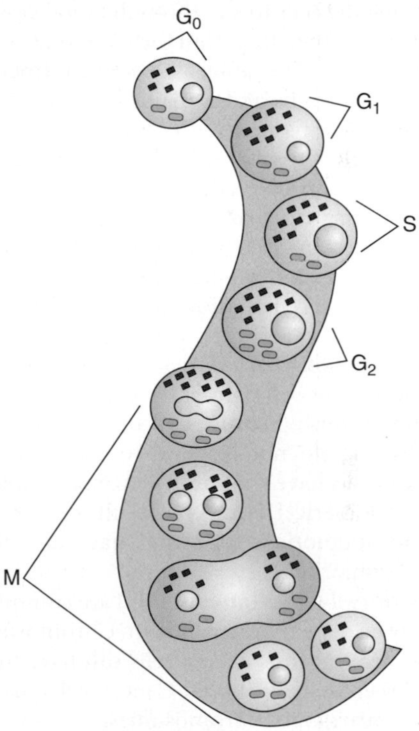

FIG. 21-4 Cellular events during mitotic cell division.

TABLE 21-1 Characteristics of Normal and Abnormal Cells

CHARACTERISTIC	NORMAL CELL	BENIGN TUMOR CELL	MALIGNANT CELL
Cell division	None or slow	Continuous or inappropriate	Rapid or continuous
Appearance	Specific morphologic features	Specific morphologic features	Anaplastic
Nuclear-to-cytoplasmic ratio	Smaller	Smaller	Larger
Differentiated functions	Many	Many	Some or none
Adherence	Tight	Tight	Loose
Migratory	No	No	Yes
Growth	Well regulated	Expansion	Invasion
Chromosomes	Diploid (euploid)	Diploid (euploid)	Aneuploid*
Mitotic index	Low	Low	High*

*Depends on the degree of malignant transformation.

Features of Cancer Cells

Cancer (**malignant**) cells are abnormal, serve no useful function, and are harmful to normal body tissues. Cancers commonly have these features:

- *Anaplasia* is the cancer cells' loss of the specific appearance of their parent cells. As a cancer cell becomes more malignant, it becomes smaller and rounded. Thus many different types of cancer cells look alike under the microscope.
- *A larger nuclear-cytoplasmic ratio* occurs because the cancer cell nucleus is larger than that of a normal cell and the cancer cell is smaller than a normal cell. The nucleus occupies much of the space within the cancer cell, creating a larger nuclear-to-cytoplasmic ratio.
- *Specific functions are lost* partially or completely in cancer cells. *Cancer cells serve no useful purpose.*
- *Loose adherence* is typical for cancer cells because they do not make fibronectin. As a result, cancer cells easily break off from the main tumor.
- *Migration* occurs because cancer cells do not bind tightly together and have many enzymes on their cell surfaces. These features allow the cells to slip through blood vessel walls and between tissues, spreading from the main tumor site to many other body sites. The ability to spread (**metastasize**) is unique to cancer cells and a major cause of death. Cancer cells invade other tissues, both close by and more remote from the original tumor. Invasion and persistent growth make untreated cancer deadly.
- *Contact inhibition does not occur* in cancer cells because of lost CELLULAR REGULATION, even when all sides of these cells are in continuous contact with the surfaces of other cells. This persistence of cell division makes the disease difficult to control.
- *Rapid or continuous cell division* occurs in many types of cancer cells because they re-enter the cell cycle for mitosis almost continuously because CELLULAR REGULATION is lost. These cells also do not respond to signals for apoptosis. Most cancer cells have a lot of the enzyme *telomerase,* which maintains telomeric DNA. As a result, cancer cells do not respond to apoptotic signals and have an unlimited life span (are "immortal").
- *Abnormal chromosomes* (**aneuploidy**) are common in cancer cells as they become more malignant. Chromosomes are lost, gained, or broken; thus cancer cells can have more than 23 pairs or fewer than 23 pairs. Cancer cells also may have broken and rearranged chromosomes.

CANCER DEVELOPMENT

Carcinogenesis/Oncogenesis

Carcinogenesis and **oncogenesis** are other names for cancer development. The process of changing a normal cell into a cancer cell is called **malignant transformation**, occurring through loss of CELLULAR REGULATION leading to the steps of initiation, promotion, progression, and metastasis (Beery & Workman, 2012).

Initiation is the first step in carcinogenesis. Normal cells can become cancer cells if they lose CELLULAR REGULATION by having their genes promoting cell division, **oncogenes**, turn on excessively (overexpressed). Initiation is a change in gene expression caused by anything that can penetrate a cell, get into the nucleus, and mutate the DNA, leading to loss of cellular regulation. Such changes can activate oncogenes that should have only limited expression and can damage suppressor genes, which normally limit oncogene activity. Thus initiation leads to excessive cell division through DNA damage that results in loss of cellular regulation by either loss of suppressor gene function or enhancement of oncogene function.

Initiation is an irreversible event that can lead to cancer development. After initiation, a cell can become a cancer cell if the CELLULAR REGULATION loss that occurred during initiation continues. *If growth conditions are right, widespread metastatic disease can develop from just one cancer cell.*

Substances that change the activity of a cell's genes so that the cell becomes a cancer cell are **carcinogens**. Carcinogens may be chemicals, physical agents, or viruses. More than 100 agents, substances, mixtures, and exposures are known or reasonably anticipated to cause cancer in humans, and about another 200 are suspected to be carcinogens. The National Toxicology Program's website (http://ntp.niehs.nih.gov/) lists these substances (U.S. Department of Health and Human Services [USDHHS], 2011). Chapters presenting the care of patients with specific cancers discuss specific known carcinogens within the Etiology sections.

Promotion is the enhanced growth of an initiated cell by substances known as **promoters**. Once a normal cell has been initiated by a carcinogen and is a cancer cell, it can become a tumor if its growth is enhanced. Many normal hormones and body proteins, like insulin and estrogen, can act as promoters and make cells divide more frequently. The time between a cell's initiation and the development of an overt tumor is called the **latency period**, which can range from months to years. Exposure to promoters can shorten the latency period.

Progression is the continued change of a cancer, making it more malignant over time. After cancer cells have grown to the point that a detectable tumor is formed (a 1-cm tumor has at least 1 billion cells in it), other events must occur for this tumor to become a health problem. First, the tumor must develop its own blood supply. The tumor makes vascular endothelial growth factor (VEGF) that triggers nearby capillaries to grow new branches into the tumor, ensuring the tumor's continued nourishment and growth.

As tumor cells continue to divide, some of the new cells change features from the original, initiated cancer cell and form different groups. Some of the differences provide these cell groups with advantages *(selection advantages)* that allow them to live and divide no matter how the conditions around them change. These tumor changes may allow it to become more malignant. Over time, the tumor cells have fewer and fewer normal cell features.

The original tumor is called the **primary tumor**. It is usually identified by the tissue from which it arose *(parent tissue),* such as in breast cancer or lung cancer. When primary tumors are located in vital organs, such as the brain or lungs, they can grow and either lethally damage the vital organ or interfere with that organ's ability to perform its vital function. At other times, the primary tumor is located in soft tissue that can expand without damage as the tumor grows. One such site is the breast. The breast is not a vital organ, and even with a large tumor, the primary tumor alone would not cause the patient's death. When the tumor spreads from the original site into vital areas, life functions can be disrupted and death may follow.

Metastasis occurs when cancer cells move from the primary location by breaking off from the original group and establishing remote colonies. These additional tumors are called

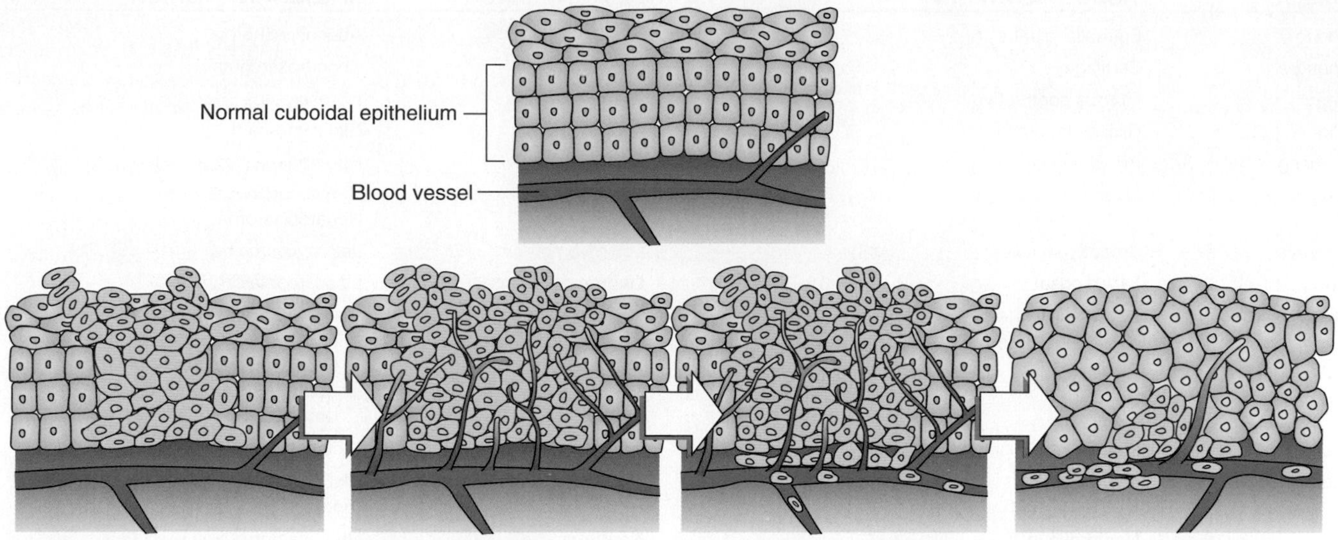

Malignant transformation
Some normal cuboidal cells have undergone malignant transformation and have divided enough times to form a tumorous area within the cuboidal epithelium.

Tumor vascularization
Cancer cells secrete vascular endothelial growth factor (VEGF), stimulating the blood vessels to bud and form new channels that grow into the tumor.

Blood vessel penetration
Cancer cells have broken off from the main tumor. Enzymes on the surface of the tumor cells make holes in the blood vessels, allowing cancer cells to enter blood vessels and travel around the body.

Arrest and invasion
Cancer cells clump up in blood vessel walls and invade new tissue areas. If the new tissue areas have the right conditions to support continued growth of cancer cells, new tumors (metastatic tumors) will form at this site.

FIG. 21-5 The steps of metastasis.

metastatic or **secondary tumors**. *Even though the tumor is now in another organ, it is still a cancer from the original altered tissue. For example, when breast cancer spreads to the lung and the bone, it is still breast cancer in the lung and bone—not lung cancer and not bone cancer.* Metastasis occurs through many steps, as shown in Fig. 21-5.

Tumors first extend into surrounding tissues by secreting enzymes that open up areas of surrounding tissue. Pressure, created as the tumor increases in size, forces tumor cells to invade new territory.

Spread to distant organs and tissues requires cancer cells to penetrate blood vessels. **Bloodborne metastasis** (tumor cell release into the blood) is the most common cause of cancer spread. Enzymes secreted by tumor cells also make large pores in the patient's blood vessels, allowing tumor cells to enter the blood and circulate. Because tumor cells are loosely held together, clumps of cells break off of the primary tumor into blood vessels for transport.

Tumor cells circulate through the blood and enter tissues at remote sites. Clumps of cancer cells can become trapped in capillaries. These clumps damage the capillary wall and allow cancer cells to leave the capillary and enter the surrounding tissue.

When conditions in the remote site can support tumor cell growth, the cells stop circulating (arrest) and invade the surrounding tissues, creating secondary tumors. Table 21-2 lists the common sites of metastasis for specific tumor types.

Another way cancers metastasize is by *lymphatic spread.* Lymphatic spread is related to the number, structure, and location of lymph nodes and vessels. Primary sites that are rich in lymphatics have more early metastatic spread than areas with few lymphatics.

TABLE 21-2 Common Sites of Metastasis for Different Cancer Types

Breast Cancer	**Prostate Cancer**
Bone*	Bone (especially spine and legs)*
Lung*	Pelvic nodes
Liver	
Brain	**Melanoma**
	GI tract
Lung Cancer	Lymph nodes
Brain*	Lung
Bone	Brain
Liver	
Lymph nodes	**Primary Brain Cancer**
Pancreas	Central nervous system
Colorectal Cancer	
Liver*	
Lymph nodes	
Adjacent structures	

*Most common site of metastasis for the specific malignant neoplasm.

Cancer Classification

Cancers are classified by the type of tissue from which they arise (e.g., glandular, connective) (McCance et al., 2014), as described in Table 21-3. Other ways to classify cancer include biologic behavior, anatomic site, and degree of differentiation.

About 100 different types of cancer arise from various tissues or organs. Fig. 21-6 compares cancer distribution by site and gender. Cancers are either solid or hematologic. Solid tumors develop from specific tissues (e.g., breast cancer and lung cancer). Hematologic cancers arise from blood cell–forming tissues (e.g., leukemias and lymphomas).

TABLE 21-3 Classification of Tumors By Tissue of Origin

PREFIX	TISSUE OF ORIGIN	BENIGN TUMOR	MALIGNANT TUMOR*
Adeno	Epithelial glands	Adenoma	Adenocarcinoma
Chondro	Cartilage	Chondroma	Chondrosarcoma
Fibro	Fibrous connective	Fibroma	Fibrosarcoma
Glio	Glial cells (brain)	Glioma	Glioblastoma
Hemangio	Blood vessel	Hemangioma	Hemangiosarcoma
Hepato	Liver	Hepatoma	Hepatocarcinoma Hepatoblastoma
Leiomyo	Smooth muscle	Leiomyoma	Leiomyosarcoma
Lipo	Fat/adipose	Lipoma	Liposarcoma
Lympho	Lymphoid tissues		Malignant lymphomas Hodgkin's lymphoma Non-Hodgkin's lymphoma Burkitt's lymphoma Cutaneous T-cell
Melano	Pigment-producing skin		Melanoma
Meningioma	Meninges	Meningioma	Malignant meningioma Meningioblastoma
Neuro	Nerve tissue	Neuroma Neurofibroma	Neurosarcoma Neuroblastoma
Osteo	Bone	Osteoma	Osteosarcoma
Renal	Kidney		Renal cell carcinoma
Rhabdo	Skeletal muscle	Rhabdomyoma	Rhabdomyosarcoma
Squamous	Epithelial layer of skin, mucous membranes, and organ linings	Papilloma	Squamous cell carcinoma of skin, bladder, lungs, cervix

*Carcinomas are tumors of glandular tissue; sarcomas are tumors of connective tissue; blastomas are tumors of less differentiated, embryonal tissues.

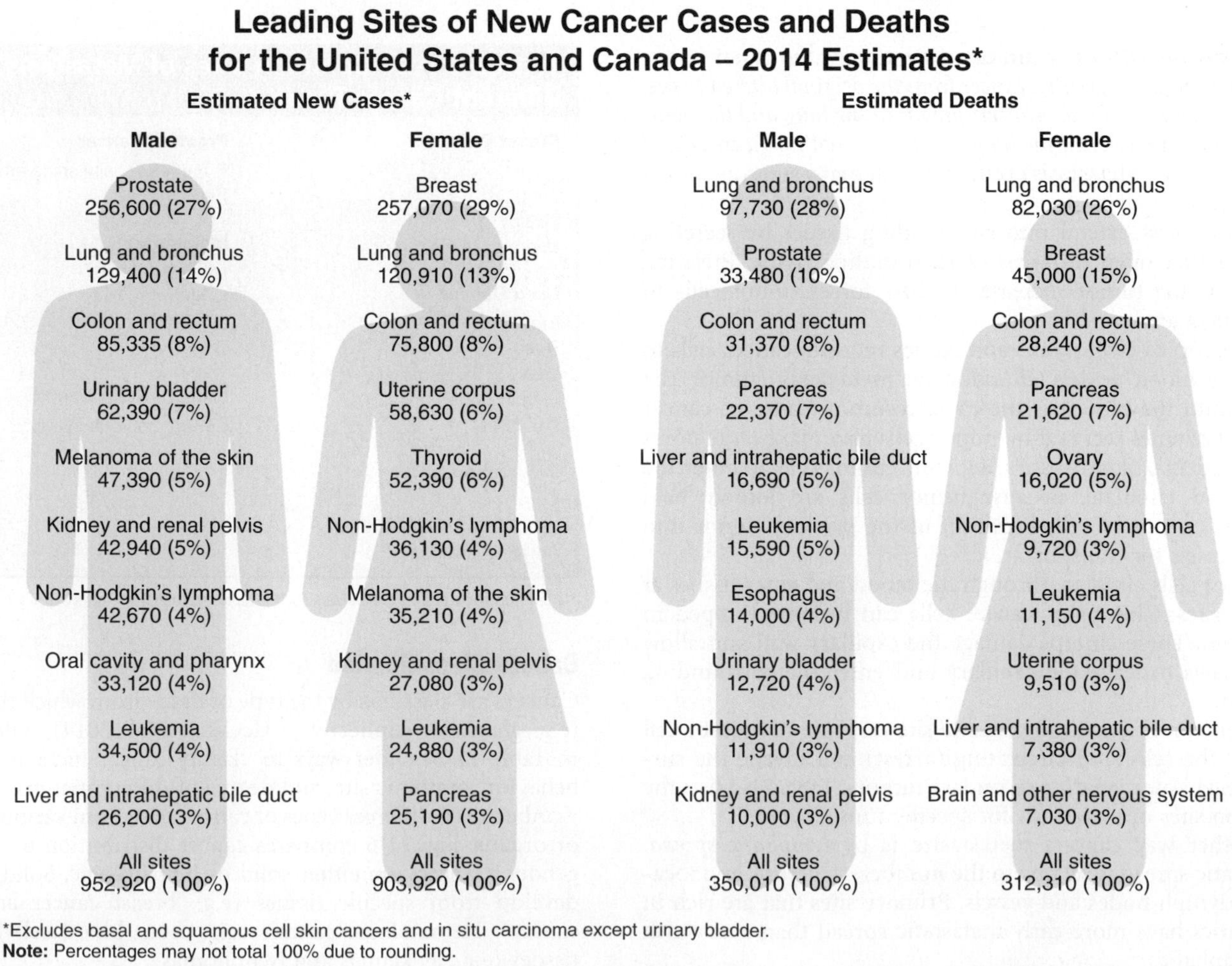

FIG. 21-6 Cancer incidence and death by site and gender. (Data from American Cancer Society, 2014 and Canadian Cancer Statistics, 2014.)

TABLE 21-4 Grading of Malignant Tumors

GRADE	CELLULAR CHARACTERISTICS
G_x	Grade cannot be determined.
G_1	Tumor cells are well differentiated and closely resemble the normal cells from which they arose. This grade is considered a low grade of malignant change. These tumors are malignant but are relatively slow growing.
G_2	Tumor cells are moderately differentiated; they still retain some of the characteristics of normal cells but also have more malignant characteristics than do G_1 tumor cells.
G_3	Tumor cells are poorly differentiated, but the tissue of origin can usually be established. The cells have few normal cell characteristics.
G_4	Tumor cells are poorly differentiated and retain no normal cell characteristics. Determination of the tissue of origin is difficult and perhaps impossible.

TABLE 21-5 Staging of Cancer—TNM Classification

Primary Tumor (T)	
T_x	Primary tumor cannot be assessed
T_0	No evidence of primary tumor
T_{is}	Carcinoma in situ
T_1, T_2, T_3, T_4	Increasing size and/or local extent of the primary tumor
Regional Lymph Nodes (N)	
N_x	Regional lymph nodes cannot be assessed
N_0	No regional lymph node metastasis
N_1, N_2, N_3	Increasing involvement of regional lymph nodes
Distant Metastasis (M)	
M_x	Presence of distant metastasis cannot be assessed
M_0	No distant metastasis
M_1	Distant metastasis

Cancer Grading, Ploidy, and Staging

Systems of grading and staging have been developed to help standardize cancer diagnosis, prognosis, and treatment. **Grading** of a tumor classifies cellular aspects of the cancer. **Ploidy** classifies tumor chromosomes as normal or abnormal. **Staging** classifies clinical aspects of the cancer.

Grading is needed because some cancer cells are "more malignant" than others, varying in their aggressiveness and sensitivity to treatment. Some cancer cells barely resemble the tissue from which they arose, are aggressive, and spread rapidly. These cells are a "high-grade" cancer. On the basis of cell appearance and activity, grading compares the cancer cell with the normal parent tissue from which it arose. It is a means of evaluating the patient with cancer for prognosis and appropriate therapy. Grading also allows health care professionals to evaluate the results of management.

Different clinical groups have established different grading systems for different types of cancer cells, but overall, they resemble the standard system listed in Table 21-4. This system rates cancer cells with the lowest rating given to those cells that closely resemble normal cells and the highest rating given to cancer cells that barely resemble normal cells. Grading systems for different cancers are presented in the clinical chapters in which care is discussed.

Ploidy is the description of cancer cells by chromosome number and appearance. Normal human cells have 46 chromosomes (23 pairs), the normal diploid number (**euploidy**). When malignant transformation occurs, changes in the genes and chromosomes also occur. Some cancer cells gain or lose whole chromosomes and may have structural abnormalities of the remaining chromosomes, a condition called **aneuploidy**. The degree of aneuploidy usually increases with the degree of malignancy. Some specific chromosome changes are associated with specific cancers, and their presence is used for diagnosis and prognosis. One example is the "Philadelphia" chromosome abnormality often present in chronic myelogenous leukemia cells (see Chapter 40).

Staging determines the exact location of the cancer and its degree of metastasis at diagnosis. Cancer stage influences selection of therapy. Staging is done by clinical staging, surgical staging, and pathologic staging. *Clinical staging* assesses the patient's clinical manifestations and evaluates them for tumor size and possible spread. *Surgical staging* assesses the tumor size, number, sites, and spread by inspection at surgery. *Pathologic staging* is the most definitive type, determining the tumor size, number, sites, and spread by pathologic examination of tissues obtained at surgery.

The **tumor, node, metastasis (TNM)** system is used to describe the anatomic extent of cancers. The TNM staging systems have specific prognostic value for each solid tumor type. Table 21-5 shows a basic TNM staging system. TNM staging is not useful for leukemia or lymphomas (see Chapter 40). Additional specific staging systems include Dukes' staging of colon and rectal cancer and Clark's levels method of staging skin cancer.

Tumor growth is assessed in terms of **doubling time** (the amount of time it takes for a tumor to double in size) and **mitotic index** (the percentage of actively dividing cells within a tumor). The smallest detectable tumor is about 1 cm in diameter and contains 1 billion cells. To reach this size, it must undergo at least 30 doublings. A tumor with a mitotic index of less than 10% is a slow-growing tumor; a tumor with an index of 85% is fast growing. Tumors have a wide range of growth rates.

NCLEX EXAMINATION CHALLENGE

Physiological Integrity

Which pathologic description of a client's tumor does the nurse interpret as being the "most malignant" or "high grade" cancer?

A. Poorly differentiated; mitotic index = 20%, euploid
B. Moderately differentiated; mitotic index = 50%, euploid
C. Undifferentiated; mitotic index = 50%, aneuploid
D. Highly differentiated; mitotic index = 10%, aneuploid

Cancer Etiology and Genetic Risk

Carcinogenesis takes years and depends on several tumor and patient factors (Santos et al., 2013). Three interacting factors influence cancer development: exposure to carcinogens, genetic predisposition, and immune function. These factors account for variation in cancer development from one person to another, even when each person is exposed to the same hazards.

Oncogene activation is the main mechanism of carcinogenesis regardless of the specific cause. These oncogenes are turned on (expressed) under controlled conditions for CELLULAR REGULATION when cells divide for normal growth and replacement of dead or damaged tissues. At other times they are turned off, controlled, or suppressed by products of "suppressor genes."

When a normal cell is exposed to any carcinogen (initiator), the normal cell's DNA can be damaged and mutated. The mutations damage suppressor genes, preventing them from producing proteins that control CELLULAR REGULATION for the expression of oncogenes. As a result, the oncogenes are overexpressed and can cause the cells to change from normal cells to cancer cells. When oncogenes are overexpressed in a cell, excessive amounts of cyclins are produced and upset the balance between cell growth enhancement and cell growth limitation. The effect of these excessive cyclins is greater than the effect of the suppressor gene products, thus losing cellular regulation and allowing uncontrolled cell division.

Oncogenes are not abnormal genes but are part of every cell's normal makeup. Oncogenes become a problem only if they are overexpressed as a result of exposure to carcinogenic agents or events with loss of CELLULAR REGULATION. Both external and personal factors can activate oncogenes.

External Factors Causing Cancer

External factors, including environmental exposure, are responsible for about 80% of cancer in North America (ACS, 2014). Environmental carcinogens are chemical, physical, or viral agents that cause cancer (USDHHS, 2011).

Chemical carcinogenesis can occur from exposures to many known chemicals, drugs, and other products used in everyday life. Chemicals vary in how carcinogenic they are. For example, tobacco and alcohol appear to be only mildly carcinogenic. For these substances, chronic, long-term exposure to large amounts is required before CELLULAR REGULATION is lost and a cancer develops. However, these two substances can act as *co-carcinogens,* meaning that when they are taken together, they enhance each other's carcinogenic activity.

Not all cells are susceptible to carcinogenesis to the same degree. Normal cells that have the ability to divide are at greater risk for cancer development than are normal cells that are not capable of cell division. For example, cancers commonly arise in bone marrow, skin, lining of the GI tract, ductal cells of the breast, and lining of the lungs. All of these cells normally undergo cell division. Cancers of nerve tissue, cardiac muscle, and skeletal muscle are rare. These cells do not normally undergo cell division.

About 30% of cancers diagnosed in North America are related to tobacco use (ACS, 2014; Canadian Cancer Society, 2014). Tobacco is the single most preventable source of carcinogenesis. It contains many different carcinogens and co-carcinogens. Long-term tobacco use first initiates and then promotes cancer. The risk for cancer development from tobacco use depends on a person's immune function, genetic susceptibility, and amount and types of tobacco exposure.

Tissues with the greatest risk for tobacco-induced cancer are those that have direct contact with tobacco or tobacco smoke. Cigarette smoking and tobacco use also promote the development of other cancers. Table 21-6 lists the specific cancers that are associated with tobacco use.

Physical carcinogenesis from physical agents or events also causes cancer by DNA damage. Two physical agents that are known to cause cancer are radiation and chronic irritation.

TABLE 21-6 Cancer Types Associated with Tobacco Use

• Lung	• Uterine cervix
• Oral cavity	• Kidney
• Pharynx	• Bladder
• Larynx	• Liver
• Esophagus	• Stomach
• Pancreas	• Myeloid leukemia

Data from American Cancer Society. (2014). *Cancer facts and figures—2014.* Report No. 00-300M–No. 500814. Atlanta: Author.

TABLE 21-7 Cancers Associated with a Known Viral Origin

VIRUS	MALIGNANCIES
Epstein-Barr virus	Burkitt's lymphoma, B-cell lymphoma, nasopharyngeal carcinoma
Hepatitis B virus	Primary liver carcinoma
Hepatitis C virus	Primary liver carcinoma, possibly B-cell lymphomas
Human papilloma virus	Cervical carcinoma, vulvar carcinoma, penile carcinoma, and other anogenital carcinomas
Human lymphotrophic virus type I	Adult T-cell leukemia
Human lymphotrophic virus type II	Hairy cell leukemia

From U.S. Department of Health and Human Services, Public Health Service, National Toxicology Program. (2011). *Report on carcinogens* (12th ed.). Retrieved January 2014, from http://ntp.niehs.nih.gov/go.roc12.

Even small doses of radiation affect cells to some degree. Some effects are temporary and are self-repaired. Other effects cannot be repaired and may induce cancer in the damaged cell. The two types of radiation that cause cancer are ionizing and ultraviolet (UV). Some ionizing radiation is found naturally in such elements as radon, uranium, and radium found in rocks and soil. Other sources of ionizing radiation include x-rays for diagnosis and treatment of disease, as well as cosmic radiation. UV radiation is a type of solar radiation, coming from the sun. Other sources of UV radiation include tanning beds and germicidal lights. UV rays do not penetrate deeply, and the most common cancer type caused by UV exposure is skin cancer.

Both ionizing and UV radiation mutate genes. Although radiation exposure induces cancers more often among cells that can divide, it can cause cancer also among nondividing cells.

Chronic irritation and tissue trauma are suspected to cause cancer. The incidence of skin cancer is higher in the scars of people with burn scars or other types of severe skin injury. Chronically irritated tissues undergo frequent cell division and thus are at an increased risk for DNA mutation.

Viral carcinogenesis occurs when viruses infect body cells and break DNA strands. Viruses then insert their own genetic material into the human DNA. Breaking the DNA, along with viral gene insertion, mutates the cell's DNA and can either activate an oncogene or damage suppressor genes. Viruses that cause cancer are **oncoviruses**. Table 21-7 lists cancers of known viral origin.

Dietary factors related to cancer development are poorly understood although dietary practices are suspected to alter cancer risk. Suspected dietary factors include low fiber intake and a high intake of red meat or animal fat. Preservatives,

CHART 21-1 Patient and Family Education: Preparing for Self-Management

Dietary Habits to Reduce Cancer Risk

- Avoid excessive intake of animal fat.
- Avoid nitrites (prepared lunch meats, sausage, bacon).
- Minimize your intake of red meat.
- Keep your alcohol consumption to no more than one or two drinks per day.
- Eat more bran.
- Eat more cruciferous vegetables, such as broccoli, cauliflower, Brussels sprouts, and cabbage.
- Eat foods high in vitamin A (e.g., apricots, carrots, leafy green and yellow vegetables) and vitamin C (e.g., fresh fruits and vegetables, especially citrus fruits).

preparation methods, and additives (dyes, flavorings, sweeteners) may have cancer-promoting effects. Chart 21-1 lists dietary habits that may reduce cancer risk.

Personal Factors and Cancer Development

Personal factors, including immune function, age, and genetic risk, also affect whether a person is likely to develop cancer.

Immune function protects the body from foreign invaders and non-self cells (see Chapter 17). Non-self cells include cells that are no longer normal, such as cancer cells. Cell-mediated immunity, especially natural killer (NK) cells and helper T-cells, provides immune surveillance.

Cancer incidence increases among immunosuppressed people. Adults older than 60 years have immune systems with reduced function and a higher incidence of cancer compared with that of the general population. Organ transplant recipients taking immunosuppressive drugs to prevent organ rejection also have a higher incidence of cancer. In patients with acquired immune deficiency syndrome (AIDS), cancer incidence may be as high as 70%.

Advancing age is the single most important risk factor for cancer (ACS, 2013b). As a person ages, immune protection decreases and external exposures to carcinogens accumulate. Teach older adults to be aware of and report manifestations such as the seven warning signs of cancer (Table 21-8) to health care providers. Health care providers should investigate all manifestations suggestive of disease. Cancer assessment considerations for the older adult are listed in Chart 21-2.

GENETIC/GENOMIC CONSIDERATIONS

Patient-Centered Care QSEN

Genetic risk for cancer occurs only in a small percent of the population; however, people who have a genetic predisposition are at very high risk for cancer development (Beery & Workman, 2012). Mutations in suppressor genes or oncogenes can be inherited when they occur in germline cells (sperm and ova) and are then passed on to one's children, in whom all cells contain the inherited mutations. Thus for some people, tight CELLULAR REGULATION is compromised by a mutation in a suppressor gene, which reduces or halts its function and allows oncogene overexpression. In other people, the suppressor genes are normal and the oncogene is mutated and does not respond to suppressor gene signals, thus reducing cellular regulation and increasing the risk for cancer development. Table 21-9 lists conditions associated with an increased genetic risk for cancer development. Be sure to include questions about these conditions when performing a family history.

TABLE 21-8 The Seven Warning Signs of Cancer

C	**C**hanges in bowel or bladder habits
A	**A** sore that does not heal
U	**U**nusual bleeding or discharge
T	**T**hickening or lump in the breast or elsewhere
I	**I**ndigestion or difficulty swallowing
O	**O**bvious change in a wart or mole
N	**N**agging cough or hoarseness

CHART 21-2 Nursing Focus on the Older Adult

Cancer Assessment

CANCER TYPE	ASSESSMENT CONSIDERATION
Colorectal cancer	Ask the patient whether bowel habits have changed over the past year (e.g., in consistency, frequency, color). Is there any obvious blood in the stool? Test at least one stool specimen for occult blood during the patient's hospitalization. Encourage the patient to have a baseline colonoscopy. Encourage the patient to reduce dietary intake of animal fats, red meat, and smoked meats. Encourage the patient to increase dietary intake of bran, vegetables, and fruit.
Bladder cancer	Ask the patient about the presence of: Pain on urination Blood in the urine Cloudy urine Increased frequency or urgency
Prostate cancer	Ask the patient about: Hesitancy Change in the size of the urine stream Pain in the back or legs History of urinary tract infections
Skin cancer	Examine skin areas for moles or warts. Ask the patient about changes in moles (e.g., color, edges, sensation).
Leukemia	Observe the skin for color, petechiae, or ecchymosis. Ask the patient about: Fatigue Bruising Bleeding tendency History of infections and illnesses Night sweats Unexplained fevers
Lung cancer	Observe the skin and mucous membranes for color. How many words can the patient say between breaths? Ask the patient about: Cough Hoarseness Smoking history Exposure to inhalation irritants Exposure to asbestos Shortness of breath Activity tolerance Frothy or bloody sputum Pain in the arms or chest Difficulty swallowing

TABLE 21-9 Conditions Associated with a Genetic Predisposition for Cancer

CONDITION	SPECIFIC CANCER TYPE
Inherited cancers*	Breast cancer Prostate cancer Ovarian cancer
Familial clustering	Breast cancer Melanoma
Bloom syndrome	Leukemia
Familial polyposis	Colorectal cancer
Chromosomal aberrations	
Down syndrome (47 chromosomes)	Leukemia
Klinefelter syndrome (47,XXY)	Breast cancer
Turner's syndrome (45,XO)	Leukemia Gonadal carcinoma Meningioma Colorectal cancer

*Not all breast, prostate, or ovarian cancers are inherited.

Genetic testing for cancer predisposition is available to confirm or rule out a person's genetic risk for some specific cancer types. These tests are performed on blood and are expensive, and the cost often is not covered by insurance. Genetic testing should not be performed unless a family history clearly indicates the possibility of increased genetic risk and the patient wants to have the test results. *These tests do not diagnose the presence of cancer; they only provide risk information.*

A variety of issues and potential problems exist with genetic testing for cancer risk. Correct interpretation of the results is critical. Ideally, a genetic counselor is involved in giving the patient information before, as well as after, testing is performed. *When a patient tests positive for a known cancer-causing gene mutation, his or her risk for cancer development is greatly increased; however, the cancer still may never develop.*

Other issues regarding genetic testing include who will have access to the information and whether to share the test results with family members. Genetic testing has implications for the entire family, not just the patient being tested. For more information on genetic testing, see Chapter 4.

CULTURAL CONSIDERATIONS

Patient-Centered Care QSEN

The incidence of cancer varies among races. American Cancer Society (ACS) data (2012; 2013) show that African Americans have a higher incidence of cancer than white people do and the death rate is higher for African Americans. Since 1960, the overall incidence among African Americans has increased 27% whereas for white people it has increased only 12%. Cancer sites and cancer-related mortality vary along racial lines as well. One explanation for this difference is that more African Americans have less access to health care. Thus they are more often diagnosed with later-stage cancer that is more difficult to cure or control. However, this disparity in health care access does not explain all differences.

When risks for cancer development are assessed, behavior and socioeconomic factors are assessed along with ethnicity and genetic predisposition. The American Cancer Society (2013) reports that cancer incidence and survival are often related to socioeconomic factors. These factors include the availability of health care services or the belief that seeking early health care has a positive effect on the outcome of cancer diagnosis.

CANCER PREVENTION

Cancer prevention activities focus on primary prevention and secondary prevention. **Primary prevention** is the use of strategies to prevent the actual occurrence of cancer. This type of cancer prevention is most effective when there is a known cause for a cancer type. **Secondary prevention** is the use of screening strategies to detect cancer early, at a time when cure or control is more likely.

Primary Prevention

Avoidance of known or potential carcinogens is an effective prevention strategy when a cause of cancer is known and avoidance is easily accomplished. For example, teach people to use skin protection during sun exposure to avoid skin cancer. Much lung cancer can be avoided by not using tobacco and by eliminating environmental asbestos exposure. Teach everyone about the dangers of cigarette smoking and other forms of tobacco use (see the *Health Promotion and Maintenance* feature in Chapter 27). Teach people who are exposed to carcinogens in the workplace to use personal protective equipment that reduces direct contact with this substance. As more cancer causes are identified, avoidance may become even more effective.

Modifying associated factors appears to have a positive influence in reducing cancer risk. Absolute causes are not known for many cancers, but some conditions appear to increase risk. Examples are the increased incidence of cancer among people who consume alcohol; the association of a diet high in fat and low in fiber with colon cancer, breast cancer, and ovarian cancer; and a greater incidence of cervical cancer among women who have multiple sexual partners. Modifying behavior to reduce the associated factor may decrease the risk for cancer development. Therefore teach all people to limit their intake of alcohol to no more than one ounce per day and to include more fruits, vegetables, and whole grains in their diets. Instruct women about the importance of limiting the number of sexual partners and to use safer sex practices to avoid exposure to viruses that can increase the risk for cervical cancer (see Table 21-7 for a listing of cancer-causing viruses).

Removal of "at risk" tissues reduces cancer risk for a person who has a known high risk for developing a specific type of cancer. Examples include removing moles to prevent conversion to skin cancer, removing colon polyps to prevent colon cancer, and removing breasts to prevent breast cancer. Not all "at risk" tissues can be removed (e.g., those that are part of essential organs).

Chemoprevention is a strategy that uses drugs, chemicals, natural nutrients, or other substances to disrupt one or more steps important to cancer development. These agents may be able to reverse existing gene damage or halt the progression of the transformation process. Currently, hundreds of agents are under investigation for chemoprevention. At this time, only a few agents have been found effective and are commonly prescribed. These include the use of aspirin and celecoxib (Celebrex) to reduce the risk for colon cancer, the use of vitamin D and tamoxifen to reduce the risk for breast cancer, and the use of lycopene to reduce the risk for prostate cancer (ACS, 2014).

Vaccination is a new method of primary cancer prevention. Although vaccines against colon cancer and others are being explored, currently the only vaccine approved for cancer prevention prevents infection from several forms of the human papilloma virus (HPV). These vaccines are Gardasil and Cervarix. As more viruses are identified as being cancer causing, it is hoped that vaccines will be developed to prevent those viral infections.

Secondary Prevention

Regular screening for cancer does not reduce cancer incidence but can greatly reduce some types of cancer deaths. Teach all adults the benefits of participating in specific routine screening techniques annually as part of health maintenance. General screening recommendations are listed in chapters discussing cancers by organ system. The age and type of participation in specific screening tests are different for people who have an identified increased risk for a specific cancer type. In addition, there is some controversy about when the age and frequency for screening has the greatest benefit. Examples of recommended screenings include (ACS, 2014):

- Yearly mammography for women older than 40 years
- Yearly clinical breast examination for women older than 40 years; every 3 years for women ages 20 to 39 years
- Colonoscopy at age 50 years and then every 10 years
- Yearly fecal occult blood for adults of all ages
- Digital rectal examination (DRE) for men older than 50 years

Because cancer development clearly involves gene changes (either inherited gene mutations or acquired damage-induced gene mutations), people can be screened for some gene mutations that increase the risk for cancer. A few examples of these known gene mutations are mutations in the *BRCA1* gene, which increases the risk for both breast and ovarian cancer; mutations in the *BRCA2* gene, which increases the risk for breast cancer; and mutations in the *APC*, *MLH1*, and *MSH2* genes, which increase the risk for colon cancer.

When taking a patient history and the person appears to have a strong family history of either breast cancer or colon cancer, create a three-generation pedigree to more fully explore the possibility of genetic risk. If a pattern of risk emerges, inform the person about the possible benefits of genetic screening and advise him or her to talk with an oncologist or genetics professional for more information. Screening can help a person at increased genetic risk for cancer to alter lifestyle factors, participate in early detection methods, or even have at-risk tissue removed. Genetic screening has some personal risks as well as potential benefits (see Chapter 4).

NCLEX EXAMINATION CHALLENGE

Health Promotion and Maintenance

A 65-year-old client tells the nurse she does not have mammograms because there is no history of breast cancer in her family. What is the nurse's best response?

A. "You are correct. Breast cancer is an inherited type of malignancy and your family history indicates a low risk for you."
B. "Performing breast self-examination monthly at home is sufficient screening for someone with your family history."
C. "Because your breasts are no longer as dense as they were when you were younger, your risk for breast cancer is now decreased."
D. "Breast cancer can be found more frequently in families; however, the risk for general, nonfamilial breast cancer increases with age."

GET READY FOR THE NCLEX® EXAMINATION!

KEY POINTS

Review these Key Points for each NCLEX Examination Client Needs Category.

Health Promotion and Maintenance

- Teach all people to avoid tanning beds and to use sunscreen and to wear protective clothing during sun exposure. **Patient-Centered Care** QSEN
- Encourage patients to participate in the recommended cancer-screening activities for their age-group and cancer risk category. **Patient-Centered Care** QSEN
- Inform all patients who smoke that smoking increases the risk for development of many cancer types.
- Assist anyone interested in smoking cessation to find an appropriate smoking cessation program (see Chapter 27). **Patient-Centered Care** QSEN
- Assess the patient's knowledge about causes of cancer and his or her screening/prevention practices. **Patient-Centered Care** QSEN
- Assist patients who fear a cancer diagnosis to understand that finding cancer at an early stage increases the chances for cure.
- Ask all patients about their exposures to environmental agents that are known or suspected to impair CELLULAR REGULATION and increase the risk for cancer.
- Obtain a detailed family history (at least three generations), and use this information to create a pedigree to assess the patient's risk for familial or inherited cancer. **Patient-Centered Care** QSEN
- Teach anyone, especially older adults, the "seven warning signs of cancer" (see Table 21-8).

Physiological Integrity

- Be aware of these facts regarding cancer risk and cancer development:
  - Cancer cells originate from normal body cells.
  - Transformation of a normal cell into a cancer cell involves mutation of the genes (DNA) of the normal cell and results in the loss of CELLULAR REGULATION.
  - Oncogenes that are overexpressed can cause a cell to develop into a tumor.
  - Only one cell has to undergo malignant transformation for cancer to begin.

- Benign tumors grow by expansion, whereas malignant tumors grow by invasion.
- Most tumors arise from cells that are capable of cell division.
- A key feature of cancer cells is the loss of CELLULAR REGULATION and apoptosis. These cells have an "infinite" life span.
- Primary prevention of cancer involves avoiding exposure to known causes of cancer.
- Secondary prevention of cancer involves screening for early detection.
- Tobacco use is a causative factor in 30% of all cancers.
- Tumors that metastasize from the primary site into another organ are still designated as tumors of the originating tissue.

Care of Patients with Cancer

June Eilers

http://evolve.elsevier.com/Iggy/

PRIORITY CONCEPTS

- INFECTION
- PAIN
- CLOTTING

LEARNING OUTCOMES

Safe and Effective Care Environment

1. Modify the environment to protect patients who have neutropenia, thrombocytopenia, or peripheral neuropathy from INFECTION and injury.
2. Protect yourself and others from cytotoxic agents and radiation.

Health Promotion and Maintenance

3. Teach patients and family members how to avoid injury and INFECTION when blood counts are low.
4. Teach patients and family members how to manage side effects of cancer treatment.

Psychosocial Integrity

5. Reduce the psychological impact of cancer treatment for the patient and family.
6. Work with other members of the health care team to ensure that patient values, preferences, and expressed needs related to cancer and its treatment are respected.

Physiological Integrity

7. Interpret laboratory data and clinical manifestations to determine the presence of cancer treatment side effects and oncologic emergencies.
8. Ensure that the patient with cancer has his or her PAIN effectively managed.
9. Prioritize nursing interventions for the patient with neutropenia or thrombocytopenia.
10. Prioritize nursing care for the patient receiving radiation therapy.
11. Prioritize nursing care for the patient receiving hormonal manipulation therapy.
12. Prioritize nursing care for the patient receiving biological response modifiers and growth factors as supportive therapy in the treatment of cancer.
13. Prioritize nursing care for the patient receiving targeted therapy for cancer.
14. Prioritize care for patients who experience an oncologic emergency.

Cancer is a serious common problem in all parts of the world. Most people fear cancer and associate a cancer diagnosis with PAIN, suffering, and death. In affluent countries, more than 68% of people diagnosed with cancer are cured and thousands of others live 5 years or longer (American Cancer Society, 2014; Canadian Cancer Society, 2014). *Regardless of treatment type, cancer always affects a person's physical and psychological functioning and stresses the family.*

Providing care to patients experiencing cancer and their families is complex and challenging. This chapter describes the general interventions for cancer and the problems associated with cancer treatment. For treatments and patient problems that occur with specific cancer types, consult the chapters in which the cancer is described. Table 22-1 lists common cancer types and the specific locations within this text where the interventions are presented.

GENERAL DISEASE-RELATED CONSEQUENCES OF CANCER

Cancer can develop in any organ or tissue and destroys normal tissue, which decreases function of that tissue or organ. Even when cancers occur in nonvital tissues or organs, they can cause death by **metastasizing** (spreading) into vital organs and disrupting critical physiologic processes (see Chapter 21). Advanced cancers often cause:

- Reduced immunity and blood-producing functions
- Altered GI structure and function

TABLE 22-1 Text Location of Specific Cancer Content

CANCER TYPE	CHAPTER
Bladder (urothelial)	66
Brain	45
Breast	70
Cervical	71
Colorectal	56
Esophageal	54
Head and Neck	29
Leukemia	40
Lung	30
Lymphoma	40
Ovarian	71
Prostate	72
Renal cell carcinoma	67
Skin	25
Stomach (gastric)	55

- Motor and sensory deficits
- Decreased respiratory function

REDUCED IMMUNITY AND BLOOD-PRODUCING FUNCTIONS

Impaired immune and blood-producing functions occur most often in patients with leukemia and lymphoma but can also occur with any cancer that invades the bone marrow. Tumor cells enter the bone marrow and reduce the production of healthy white blood cells (WBCs), which are needed for normal immune function. Thus patients who have cancer, especially leukemia, are at an increased risk for INFECTION (McCance et al., 2014).

When cancer invades the bone marrow, it also causes anemia by decreasing the number of red blood cells (RBCs) and causes thrombocytopenia by decreasing the number of platelets. These changes may be caused by the cancer itself or by cancer treatment, especially chemotherapy. The patient feels weak and fatigued and is at risk for impaired CLOTTING with bleeding. In addition, patients with anemia may be short of breath, especially if they also have respiratory involvement related to cancer.

ALTERED GI STRUCTURE AND FUNCTION

Abdominal tumors may obstruct or compress structures anywhere in the GI tract, reducing the ability to absorb nutrients and eliminate wastes. Tumors often also increase metabolic rate and the need for nutrients at a time when the patient has less energy for meal preparation or eating.

Tumors that invade the liver profoundly damage this organ, which has many important metabolic functions. This damage leads to malnutrition and death.

Many patients with cancer have anorexia that often interferes with their ability to meet energy needs. **Cachexia** (extreme body wasting and malnutrition) develops from an imbalance between food intake and energy use (increased catabolism). This problem may occur even when nutritional intake appears adequate. Changes in taste resulting from the cancer or the treatment can reduce appetite and cause food aversions. Some patients experience early satiety or a sense of fullness and inability to eat even though they have eaten only a small volume of food.

Nutrition support for the patient with cancer, especially one undergoing cancer therapy, is complex. A diet high in protein and carbohydrates is often prescribed to help him or her maintain weight and to provide the nutrients needed for energy and cellular repair. Patients and families often believe cancer can be cured more easily if weight is gained or maintained. Currently no one nutrition plan meets the needs of all patients with cancer. Challenges related to food intake often become an emotional problem for family members who struggle with watching nutrition changes in their loved ones.

MOTOR AND SENSORY DEFICITS

Motor and sensory deficits occur when cancers invade bone or the brain or compress nerves. In patients with bone metastasis, the primary cancer started in another organ (e.g., lung, prostate, breast). Bones become thinner with an increased risk for *pathologic fractures* that can occur with minimal trauma. Bone metastasis causes PAIN, fractures, spinal cord compression, and hypercalcemia, each of which reduces mobility.

Patients have sensory changes if the spinal cord is damaged or if nerves are compressed. Sensory, motor, and cognitive functions are impaired when cancer spreads to the brain. Any tumor, cancer or benign, growing in the brain can destroy healthy brain tissue and cause death.

Cancer treatments also contribute to sensory and motor deficits. Certain chemotherapy agents cause peripheral neuropathy that leads to altered sensation, PAIN, and modified gait. "Chemo brain" is an alteration of cognitive function experienced by some patients.

The patient with cancer may also have PAIN, especially chronic pain. Pain does not always accompany cancer, but it can be a major problem for those with terminal cancer. Chapter 3 provides an in-depth discussion of the causes and management of cancer pain. The concept map in Chapter 3 (p. 27) presents nursing care issues related to chronic cancer pain.

REDUCED GAS EXCHANGE

Cancer can disrupt oxygenation in several ways and often results in death. Tumors in the airways cause airway obstruction. If lung tissue is involved, lung capacity is decreased, leading to hypoxemia. Tumors can also press on blood and lymph vessels in the chest, which results in pulmonary edema and dyspnea. Tumors can thicken the alveolar membrane and damage pulmonary blood vessels, reducing gas exchange. With any lung tumor (primary or metastatic), patients are at risk for hypoxia, poor gas exchange, and poor tissue oxygenation.

CANCER MANAGEMENT

The purpose of cancer management is to prolong survival time and improve quality of life. Without cancer therapy, many patients with cancer would die within months of diagnosis. Cancer therapy includes surgery, radiation, chemotherapy, immunotherapy (biological response modifiers), molecularly targeted therapy, photodynamic therapy, and hormonal therapy. These therapies may be used separately or in combination to kill cancer cells. The types of therapy used depend on the specific type of cancer, whether the cancer has spread, and the health of the patient. Treatment regimens *(protocols)* have been established for most types of cancer.

SURGERY

Surgery is the earliest known treatment for cancer and continues to be a cornerstone of therapy. Most cancers are diagnosed with the assistance of surgery, and it is used as part of therapy in many cancers. For cancer, surgery involves the removal of diseased or suspicious tissue. If cancer is confined to the removed tissue, surgery alone can result in a "cure" for that cancer. Even when surgery cannot result in a cancer cure, it is often a useful part of diagnosis, treatment, follow-up, and rehabilitation. Current types of cancer surgery are used for prophylaxis, diagnosis, cure, control, palliation, assessing therapy effectiveness, and reconstruction.

Prophylactic surgery removes "at-risk" tissue to prevent cancer development. It is performed when a patient has either an existing premalignant condition or a strong predisposition for development of a specific cancer. For example, removing a benign polyp from the colon before it can develop into colon cancer is a prophylactic action.

Diagnostic surgery (biopsy) is the removal of all or part of a suspected lesion for examination and testing. It provides evidence for the presence of cancer. Other forms of therapy are seldom initiated without this confirmation of cancer. The extent of a biopsy varies from a fine needle aspiration to an open incision exploratory surgery.

Curative surgery removes all cancer tissue. Surgery alone can result in a cure rate of about 30% when all visible and microscopic tumor is removed or destroyed. This number could increase with screening and early detection efforts.

Cancer control, or *cytoreductive surgery*, removes part of but not the entire tumor. It is also known as "debulking" surgery and decreases the number of cancer cells, which increases the chances that other therapies can be successful.

Palliative surgery focuses on improving the quality of life during the survival time, not on cure. Examples include removal of tumor tissue that is causing PAIN, obstruction, or difficulty swallowing.

Second-look surgery is a repeat examination after treatment to assess the disease status in patients who have been treated and have no symptoms of remaining tumor. The results of this surgery are used to determine whether a specific therapy should be continued or discontinued.

Reconstructive or *rehabilitative surgery* increases function, enhances appearance, or both. Examples include breast reconstruction after mastectomy, replacement of the esophagus, bowel reconstruction, revision of scars, and cosmetic reconstruction in head and neck cancer.

Side Effects of Surgical Therapy

Unlike surgery performed for many other reasons, cancer surgery often involves the loss of a body part or its function. Sometimes whole organs are removed, such as the kidney, lung, breast, testis, leg, or tongue. *Any organ loss reduces function.* Some cancer surgery results in scarring or disfigurement. Patients are anxious about surviving the cancer and want to be "rid" of it. However, they also may be grieving a change in appearance or lifestyle.

❖ PATIENT-CENTERED COLLABORATIVE CARE

The care needs of the patient having surgery for cancer are similar to those related to surgery for other reasons (see Chapters 14, 15, and 16). For cancer surgery, additional priority care needs are psychosocial support and assisting the patient to achieve maximum function.

Often cancer surgery occurs within days of the diagnosis, before the patient and family have time to adjust. Be aware that the stress of the diagnosis can significantly impact the patient's and family's ability to understand any teaching provided at this time. Assess the patient's and family's ability to cope with the uncertainty of cancer and its treatment and with the changes in body image and role. For example, surgery involving the genitals, urinary tract, colon, or rectum may permanently damage these organs, resulting in changes in the patient's means of sexual expression or control of elimination. Procedures to create a urinary or fecal diversion may damage nerves, causing erectile dysfunction in men and painful intercourse in women.

Coordinate with the health care team to support the patient. Encourage the patient and family to express their concerns. Help the patient accept changes in appearance or function by encouraging him or her to look at the surgical site, touch it, and participate in dressing changes. Provide information about support groups such as those sponsored by the American Cancer Society (www.cancer.org) or Canadian Cancer Society (www.cancer.ca). Some cancer organizations have support groups for patients and separate support groups for patients' spouses and children. Discuss having a person who has coped with the same issues come for a visit. Such visits can help show the patient that many aspects of life can be the same after cancer treatment. For patients who have persistent depression as a result of the cancer diagnosis or appearance changes, a referral to a mental health counselor and drug therapy may be indicated.

Physical rehabilitation is often indicated after surgery. Reduced function may be an outcome for some types of cancer surgery. For example, a modified radical mastectomy for breast cancer can lead to muscle weakness and reduced arm function on that side. Performing specific exercises after surgery can reduce functional loss. Head and neck cancer surgery often requires therapy to improve swallowing and speech. Therapy can be painful and challenging. The patient needs encouragement to perform the expected activities. Teach patients about the importance of performing the exercises to regain as much function as possible and prevent complications. Coordinate with the physical therapist, occupational therapist, and family members to plan strategies individualized to each patient to regain or maintain optimal function.

The role of surgery in cancer care continues to change. Laparoscopic and other minimally invasive approaches with smaller incisions and robotic access to internal body cavities have reduced some risks (Yu et al., 2013) (see Chapters 14 and 15). Regardless of the surgical approach, nurses have a critical role in the patient's recovery after surgery. This includes reinforcing the importance of early mobility, PAIN management, and prevention of INFECTION.

The use of surgery in combination with other therapies has increased. Such combinations may include intraoperative radiation therapy, the placement of a radioactive source, or the administration of chemotherapy into a body cavity. Other uses include surgical placement of internal catheters into a specific vessel and placement of electronic pumps for chemotherapy or pain drugs.

CLINICAL JUDGMENT CHALLENGE

Ethical/Legal

Mrs. W. is an 80-year-old woman who has undergone exploratory surgery for an acute bowel obstruction. She had been relatively healthy, although growing more frail in recent years, and recently began to need home oxygen intermittently for chronic lung disease. Persistent abdominal pain and vomiting brought her to the emergency department. She lives alone in an assisted-living apartment near her daughter Joan, who provides some additional assistance with grocery shopping, bill paying, etc. Mrs. W. has just been admitted to the ICU after surgery, where she is expected to remain intubated and mechanically ventilated overnight. The surgeon and Mrs. W.'s daughter are talking outside of her room. You join the conversation in time to hear the surgeon explain that a large, disseminated cancer was found as the cause of the obstruction; he removed as much as he could but was not able to resect all of the cancer. Joan responds, "I was afraid of this. Whatever you do, don't tell my mother it was cancer—she'll never be able to cope with that. Please, just tell her that it was a benign tumor and you took it out." The surgeon looks uncertain but nods and then leaves the bedside. Joan turns to you and says, "Tell the other nurses—nobody can say it was cancer."

1. What, if anything, should you say to Joan at this point?

   It is now the next day. As expected, Mrs. W. has remained stable through the night and has been successfully extubated. She is still somewhat sleepy and has not asked any questions about her surgery. When Joan comes in to visit, she pulls you aside and says, "No one told her about the cancer, right?"

2. How should you respond to Joan now?
3. Review the ethical principles in Chapter 1. What ethical principle(s) are at risk or in play with this situation?

RADIATION THERAPY

Radiation therapy (radiotherapy) involves the use of radionuclides, ionizing radiation beams, or discrete gamma ray sources to treat cancer. The purpose of radiation therapy for cancer is to destroy cancer cells, have minimal damaging effects on the surrounding normal cells, and maintain a safe environment. Radiation may be used to cure, control, or palliate the disease.

The effects of radiation are seen only on tissues within the radiation path; thus this type of therapy usually is a *local* treatment. For example, radiation to the chest for lung cancer causes skin changes and hair loss only on the chest area actually being irradiated. The person does *not* lose his or her scalp hair. When total body irradiation (TBI) is used, all body areas are affected. Some effects are apparent within days or weeks, whereas other effects on deeper tissues may not be apparent for months to years after radiation therapy is completed.

Most radiation therapy for cancer is ionizing radiation. When cells are exposed to it, particles within the cell's nucleus are rearranged, resulting in a tremendous release of intracellular energy. Ionizing radiation is given off by many elements, including radium, and radioactive isotopes of specific elements.

As a radioactive element breaks down (decays), radiation energy is released as high energy particles (alpha particles and beta particles) and high energy photons (gamma rays). **X-rays** are radiation that is generated by machine. All types of radiation are identical in their effects on cells.

The energy produced by radioactive elements (gamma rays, alpha particles, beta particles) varies in its ability to penetrate tissues and damage cells (Fig. 22-1). *Gamma rays* are used most commonly for radiation therapy because of their ability to deeply penetrate tissues. *Beta particles* are weaker and must be placed within or very close to the cancer cells for cancer therapy (see discussion of brachytherapy on p. 375). *Alpha particles* are not used as cancer therapy.

The amount of radiation delivered to a tissue is the **exposure**; the amount of radiation absorbed by the tissue is the **radiation dose**. The dose is always less than the exposure because some energy is lost on the way to the tissue. The three factors determining the absorbed dose are the *intensity* of exposure, the *duration* of exposure, and the *closeness* (distance) of the radiation source to the cells. Absorbed radiation doses are described in units called **gray (gy)**. One gy is equal to one joule of energy absorbed by one kg of a material. The total dose of radiation used depends on tumor size and location and on the radiation sensitivity of the tumor and nearby tissues. Some normal tissues are more sensitive than others to radiation. For example, breast tissue tolerates much higher doses of radiation than the liver does. A total dose of 50 to 60 gy might be prescribed for a breast cancer. However, only 12 gy might be prescribed for a liver tumor because a higher dose would destroy healthy liver cells as well as the tumor.

Radiation therapy usually is given as a series of divided doses because of the varying responses of all cancer cells within one tumor. Most often, small doses of radiation are given on a daily basis for a set time period to allow greater destruction of cancer cells while reducing the damage to normal tissues.

The intensity of the radiation decreases with the distance from the radiation emitting source. This factor is known as the *inverse square law*. For example, the radiation dose received at

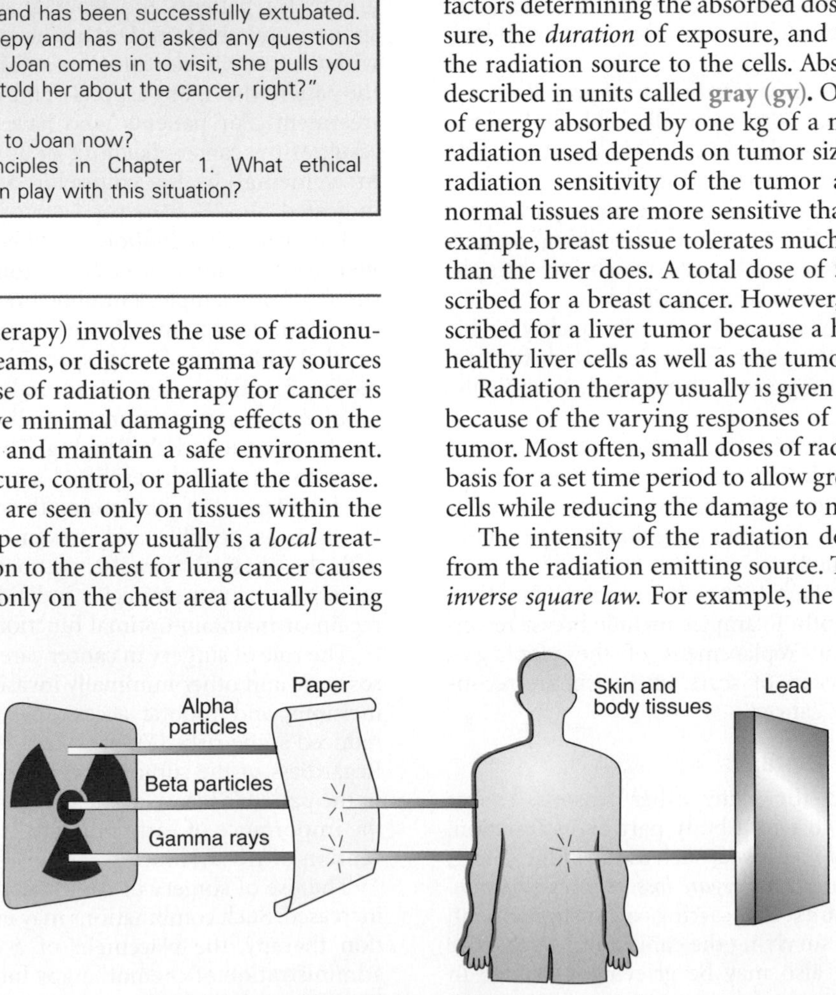

FIG. 22-1 Penetrating capacity of different types of radiation.

a distance of 2 meters from the radiation source is only one fourth of the dose received at a distance of 1 meter from the radiation source; the dose of radiation received at 3 meters is only one ninth of the dose received at 1 meter.

Cells damaged by radiation either die outright or become unable to divide. Radiation damage occurs anytime a cell is exposed to radiation, not just when it is dividing. However, the damage is greater to dividing cells than to non-dividing cells when exposed to radiation. Cancer radiation therapy does not immediately kill all cells within a tumor because these cells absorb the radiation dose slightly differently and their overall response to the radiation is slightly different. A few cells die immediately, and more die within the next few days. Some cells are unable to divide as a result of a single treatment. Still other cells repair the radiation-induced damage and recover.

Radiation may be used as a stand-alone treatment or may be combined with other cancer therapies. Combining therapies requires careful planning of sequencing, timing, and dose of each therapy to maximize tumor kill and limit damage to normal cells. Often, combining radiation with chemotherapy involves first giving agents that radiosensitize and actually enhance the radiation damage and result in a greater cell kill than either therapy used alone.

Radiation Delivery Methods and Devices

Radiation delivery types for cancer therapy are teletherapy and brachytherapy. The type used depends on the patient's general health and on the shape, size, and location of the tumor. The ideal radiation dose is one that kills the cancer cells with an acceptable level of damage to normal tissues (damage to normal tissues cannot be avoided).

Teletherapy is radiation delivered from a source outside of the patient. *Because the source is external, the patient is not radioactive and is not hazardous to others.* Newer teletherapy delivery methods improve the accuracy of the dose delivered. Intensity modulated radiation therapy (IMRT) breaks the single beam into thousands of smaller beams that better focus on the tumor. Stereotactic body radiotherapy (SBRT) uses three-dimensional tumor imaging to identify the exact tumor location, which allows precise delivery of higher radiation doses and spares more of the surrounding tissue. Usually, the total dosage is delivered in one to five separate treatment sessions.

Regardless of the delivery method, the exact tumor location is first determined for therapy accuracy. Once the pattern of radiation delivery is decided, the patient must always be in exactly the same position for all treatments. Ensure that the patient can get into and maintain this position. Position-fixing devices and markings, either on the patient's body or on the devices, ensure the proper position each day of treatment. The markings may be small permanent "tattoos," ink outlines on the skin, or a marked mask laid over the skin. Position-fixing devices include customized external body molds, foam-based body molds, and fiberglass splints.

Brachytherapy means "short" (close) therapy. The radiation source comes into direct, continuous contact with the tumor for a specific time period. This method provides a high dose of radiation in the tumor and a very limited dose in surrounding normal tissues.

Brachytherapy uses radioactive isotopes either in solid form or within body fluids. Isotopes can be delivered to the tumor in several ways. *With all types of brachytherapy, the radiation source is within the patient. Therefore the patient emits radiation for a period of time and is a potential hazard to others.* When the isotopes used are unsealed and suspended in a fluid, they are given by the oral or IV routes or instilled within body cavities. An example of brachytherapy with soluble isotopes is the ingestion or injection of the radionuclide *iodine-131* (^{131}I) (an iodine base with a half-life of 8.05 days) to treat some thyroid cancers. The iodine concentrates in the thyroid gland and destroys the thyroid cancer cells. *When isotopes are unsealed, they enter body fluids and eventually are eliminated in waste products. These wastes are radioactive and should not be directly touched by anyone. They must be handled according to guidelines established by the institution. After the isotope is completely eliminated from the body, neither the patient nor the body wastes are radioactive.*

Solid or sealed radiation sources are implanted within or near the tumor. These sources can be temporary or permanent. Most implants emit continuous, low-energy radiation to tumors. Some devices (e.g., seeds or needles) can be placed into the tumor and stay in place by themselves. Seeds are so small and the half-life of the isotope so short that this device is permanently left in place (often for prostate cancer) and, over time, completely loses its radioactivity. Other devices are removed and reused in other patients. Some sources must be held in place during therapy using special applicators. While the solid implants are in place, the patient emits radiation but excreta are not radioactive. Thus, at this time, the patient poses a hazard to others but the excreta do not.

Traditional implants deliver "low-dose rates" (LDRs) of radiation continuously, and patients are hospitalized for several days. "High-dose rate" (HDR) implant radiation is another delivery type. The patient comes into the radiation therapy department several times a week, and a stronger radiation implant is placed for only an hour or so each time. The patient is radioactive only when the implant is in place (Rupert, 2011). Chart 22-1 lists the best practices for the safety of the personnel providing care to the patient with a sealed radiation implant.

A newer approach of targeted therapy for liver cancers involves interventional radiology to place a catheter in the femoral artery and then position it into the liver. Yttrium-90 radioactive beads are injected into the blood vessels supplying liver tumors. These beads lodge in the tumor vessels and deliver a calculated dose of beta particles directly into the tumor(s). This dose travels only 1 to 2 centimeters, and the beads decay to near zero after about 96 hours. This method can deliver an effective therapy dose to the liver without damaging the healthy liver tissue.

Side Effects of Radiation Therapy

Side effects of radiation therapy include both acute and long-term site-specific changes (Table 22-2). These effects are limited to the tissues exposed to the radiation. Therefore the side effects vary according to the site (Ruppert, 2011). Skin changes and hair loss are local but are often permanent depending on the total absorbed dose.

Altered taste sensations and fatigue are two common systemic side effects noted by patients during radiation, regardless of the radiation site. Taste changes are thought to be caused by metabolites released from dead cells. Many patients develop an aversion to the taste of red meats. Fatigue may be related to the increased energy demands needed to repair damaged cells. Regardless of the cause, radiation-induced fatigue can be debilitating and may last for months (Poirier, 2011). Some degree of bone marrow suppression occurs regardless of the treatment

CHART 22-1 Best Practice for Patient Safety & Quality Care QSEN

Care of the Patient with Sealed Implants of Radioactive Sources

- Assign the patient to a private room with a private bath.
- Place a "Caution: Radioactive Material" sign on the door of the patient's room.
- If portable lead shields are used, place them between the patient and the door.
- Keep the door to the patient's room closed as much as possible.
- Wear a dosimeter film badge at all times while caring for patients with radioactive implants. The badge offers no protection but measures a person's exposure to radiation. Each person caring for the patient should have a separate dosimeter to calculate his or her specific radiation exposure.
- Wear a lead apron while providing care. Always keep the front of the apron facing the source of radiation (do not turn your back toward the patient).
- If you are attempting to conceive, do not perform direct patient care regardless of whether you are male or female.
- Pregnant nurses should not care for these patients; do not allow pregnant women or children younger than 16 years to visit.
- Limit each visitor to one-half hour per day. Be sure visitors stay at least 6 feet from the source.
- Never touch the radioactive source with bare hands. In the rare instance that it is dislodged, use a long-handled forceps to retrieve it. Deposit the radioactive source in the lead container kept in the patient's room.
- Save all dressings and bed linens in the patient's room until after the radioactive source is removed. After the source is removed, dispose of dressings and linens in the usual manner. Other equipment can be removed from the room at any time without special precautions and does not pose a hazard to other people.

site. The intensity of the suppression is related to the dose, site, and size of the area irradiated.

Radiation damage to normal tissues during therapy can start inflammatory responses that lead to tissue fibrosis and scarring. These effects may appear years after radiation treatment. For example, women who receive HDR therapy for uterine cancer may develop radiation-induced colon changes (which also was irradiated) years later, resulting in constipation and even obstruction. Because any form of radiation can damage and mutate normal cell DNA, radiation therapy increases the risk for development of second malignancies. This risk is lower when delivery methods involve less exposure to normal tissues.

Not all patients experience the same degree of side effects to normal tissues even when receiving the same dose of radiation therapy. Genetic differences appear to influence how sensitive a person's normal tissues are to radiation damage (Proud, 2014).

❖ PATIENT-CENTERED COLLABORATIVE CARE

Most patients and family members are anxious about radiation and look to the nurse to explain the purpose and side effects of radiation therapy. Accurate information about radiation therapy helps patients cope with the treatment (Ruppert, 2011).

Skin in the radiation path becomes dry and may break down. Teaching patients about skin care needs during radiation therapy is a priority intervention. Instruct the patient to not remove temporary ink markings when cleaning the skin until radiation therapy is completed. There are no universal evidence-based interventions for skin care during radiation therapy. It is important to teach patients to avoid skin irritation from

TABLE 22-2 Acute and Late Site-Specific Effects of Radiation Therapy

ACUTE EFFECTS	LATE EFFECTS
Brain	**Subcutaneous and Soft Tissue**
Alopecia and radiodermatitis of the scalp	Radiation-induced fibrosis
Ear and external auditory canal irritation	**Central Nervous System**
Cerebral edema	Brain necrosis
Nausea and vomiting	Leukoencephalopathy
Somnolence syndrome	Cognitive and emotional dysfunction
	Pituitary and hypothalamic dysfunction
Head and Neck	Spinal cord myelopathies
Oral mucositis	
Taste changes	**Head and Neck**
Oral candidiasis	Xerostomia and dental caries
Oral herpes	Trismus
Acute xerostomia	Osteoradionecrosis
Dental caries	Hypothyroidism
Esophagitis and pharyngitis	
Breast and Chest Wall	**Lung**
Skin reactions	Pulmonary fibrosis
Esophagitis	
	Heart
Chest and Lung	Pericarditis
Esophagitis and pharyngitis	Cardiomyopathy
Taste changes	Coronary artery disease
Pneumonia	
	Breast/Chest Wall
Abdomen and Pelvis	Atrophy, fibrosis of breast tissue
Anorexia	Lymphedema
Nausea and vomiting	
Diarrhea and proctitis	**Abdomen and Pelvis**
Cystitis	Small and large bowel injury
Vaginal dryness/vaginitis	
Eye	
Conjunctival edema and tearing	

clothing and to follow the radiation-oncology department's policy regarding the use and timing of skin care products. Use of skin care products designed to manage or protect the skin from radiation damage does reduce the degree of skin problems that develop during a full course of radiation therapy (Bergstrom, 2011). Chart 22-2 is an example of an established skin care protocol during external radiation therapy.

! NURSING SAFETY PRIORITY QSEN

Action Alert

Skin in the radiation path is more sensitive to sunburn and sun damage. Advise against direct skin exposure to the sun during treatment and for at least 1 year after completing radiation therapy.

The normal tissues most sensitive to external radiation are bone marrow cells, skin, mucous membranes, hair follicles, and germ cells (ova and sperm). When possible, these tissues are shielded from radiation during therapy. At times, they cannot be protected from exposure. Some changes caused by radiation are permanent. The long-term problems vary with the location and dose of radiation received (see Table 22-2). For example,

CHART 22-2 Patient and Family Education: Preparing for Self-Management

Skin Protection During Radiation Therapy

- Wash the irradiated area gently each day with either water or a mild soap and water as prescribed by your radiation therapy team.
- Use your hand rather than a washcloth when cleansing the therapy site to be gentler.
- Rinse soap thoroughly from your skin.
- If ink or dye markings are present to identify exactly where the beam of radiation is to be focused, take care not to remove them.
- Dry the irradiated area with patting motions rather than rubbing motions; use a clean, soft towel or cloth.
- Use only powders, ointments, lotions, or creams on your skin at the radiation site that are prescribed by the radiation oncology department.
- Wear soft clothing over the skin at the radiation site.
- Avoid wearing belts, buckles, straps, or any type of clothing that binds or rubs the skin at the radiation site.
- Avoid exposure of the irradiated area to the sun:
  - Protect this area by wearing clothing over it.
  - Try to go outdoors in the early morning or evening to avoid the more intense sun rays.
  - When outdoors, stay under awnings, umbrellas, and other forms of shade during the times when the sun's rays are most intense (10 AM to 7 PM).
- Avoid heat exposure.

radiation to the throat and upper chest can cause difficulty in swallowing and can lead to reduced nutrition. A registered dietitian is part of the radiation oncology team. Head and neck radiation may damage the salivary glands and cause dry mouth (**xerostomia**), which affects quality of life and increases the patient's lifelong risk for tooth decay. Thus teach patients that regular dental visits are essential. Bone exposed to radiation therapy is less dense and breaks more easily (the cause of pathologic fractures). Fatigue remains a common problem during and for some time after radiation therapy. Exercise and sleep interventions may be somewhat beneficial for fatigue. Teach about the symptoms that might be expected from the specific location and dose of radiation (see Table 22-1 for the location of this information for different cancer types).

NCLEX EXAMINATION CHALLENGE

Psychosocial Integrity

The client receiving brachytherapy with implanted radioactive "seeds" for prostate cancer asks the nurse when these seeds will be removed. What is the nurse's best response?

A. "The half-life of radiation in these seeds is so short that it is not necessary to remove them."
B. "They will be removed only if their presence is painful or leads to an enlarged prostate gland."
C. "When we know for certain that all cancerous cells have been killed, the seeds will be removed."
D. "The seeds are small enough to be absorbed by your body and excreted in the urine or stool."

CYTOTOXIC SYSTEMIC AGENT THERAPY

When cancer has spread beyond a localized area that can be removed with surgery or safely treated with radiation therapy, systemic therapy is indicated for optimal results. Systemic therapy has many effects on normal tissues as well as on cancerous tissue.

GENETIC/GENOMIC CONSIDERATIONS

Patient-Centered Care QSEN

A newer approach to selection of cancer treatment agents to be used is checking the patient's genetic profile to determine the likelihood of experiencing dangerous side effects. This process, known as *pharmacogenomics,* allows a more individualized approach to chemotherapy selection and side effect management. In addition, checking the genetic profile of the tumor can determine its sensitivity to various chemotherapy and targeted therapy agents (Boucher et al., 2014; Santos et al., 2013). This increasingly common practice individualizes cancer therapy and improves therapy outcomes. Expected future outcomes include an economic advantage for cancer care as decisions for treatment can be based on likelihood of effectiveness for an individual rather than on a tumor type or stage of disease. Remind patients that assessing genetic sensitivity can result in a selection of therapy that differs from that of other people with the same cancer type.

Systemic therapy with the use of antineoplastic agents is cytotoxic therapy in that the agents induce cell damaging/cell killing (cytotoxic) actions on cells, including cancer cells. Selection of agents to use as cytotoxic treatment of cancer is based on cellular kinetic concepts that include cell cycle, growth factors, and tumor burden. Most of the cytotoxic agents are not cancer cell specific and thus potentially affect all cells in the body. This effect is especially seen on rapidly dividing cells such as those in the bone marrow. The time when bone marrow activity and white blood cell counts are at their lowest levels after cytotoxic therapy is the **nadir**. It occurs at different times for different drugs. To reduce immunosuppression, combination cytotoxic therapy avoids using drugs with nadirs that occur at or near the same time.

CHEMOTHERAPY

Chemotherapy, the treatment of cancer with chemical agents, is used to cure and to increase survival time. It has some selectivity for killing cancer cells over normal cells. This killing effect on cancer cells is related to the ability of chemotherapy to damage DNA and interfere with cell division. Tumors with rapid growth are often more sensitive to chemotherapy.

As described in Chapter 21, cancer cells can separate from the original tumor, spread to new areas, and establish new cancers at distant sites (**metastasize**). Patients with metastatic cancer will die unless treatment eliminates the metastatic cancer cells along with the original cancer cells. Chemotherapy is useful in treating cancer because its effects are systemic, providing the opportunity to kill metastatic cancer cells that may have escaped local treatment. Chemotherapy used along with surgery or radiation is termed **adjuvant** therapy.

Drugs used for chemotherapy usually are given systemically and exert their cell-damaging (**cytotoxic**) effects against healthy cells as well as cancer cells. The normal cells most affected by chemotherapy are those that divide rapidly, including skin, hair, intestinal tissues, spermatocytes, and blood-forming cells. These drugs are classified by the specific types of action they exert in the cancer cell (Table 22-3).

Chemotherapy Drug Categories

Alkylating agents cross-link DNA, making the DNA strands bind tightly together. This action prevents proper DNA and ribonucleic acid (RNA) synthesis, which inhibits cell division.

TABLE 22-3 Categories of Chemotherapeutic Drugs

Antimetabolites
Azacitidine (Vidaza)
Capecitabine (Xeloda)
Cladribine (Leustatin)
Clofarabine (Clolar)
Cytarabine (Cytosar, ara-C)
Decitabine (Dacogen)
Floxuridine (FUDR)
5-Fluorouracil (Adrucil, Efudex, Fluoroplex)
Fludarabine (Fludara, FLAMP)
Gemcitabine (Gemzar)
6-Mercaptopurine (Purinethol)
Methotrexate (MTX, Mexate)
Nelarabine (Arranon)
Pemetrexed (Alimta)
Pentostatin (Nipent)
6-Thioguanine (Tabloid)

Antitumor Antibiotics
Bleomycin (Blenoxane)
Dactinomycin (Cosmegen)
Daunorubicin (Cerubidine, Daunomycin)
Doxorubicin (Adriamycin, Rubex)
Doxorubicin liposomal (Doxil)
Epirubicin (Ellence)
Idarubicin (Idamycin)
Mitomycin C (Mutamycin)
Mitoxantrone (Novantrone)
Valrubicin (Valstar)

Antimitotics
Cabazitaxel (Jevtana)
Docetaxel (Taxotere)
Etoposide (VP-16, VePesid)
Eribulin mesylate (Halaven)
Paclitaxel (Taxol)
Teniposide (Vumon)
Vinblastine (Velban, Velbe, Velsar)
Vincristine (Oncovin)
Vinorelbine (Navelbine)

Alkylating Agents
Altretamine (Hexalen)
Bendamustine (Treanda)
Busulfan (Busulfex)
Carboplatin (Paraplatin)
Carmustine (BiCNU, Gliadel)
Chlorambucil (Leukeran)
Cisplatin (Platinol)
Cyclophosphamide (Cytoxan, Procytox)
Dacarbazine (DTIC)
Estramustine (Emcyt, Estracyte)
Ifosfamide (Ifex)
Lomustine (CCNU, CeeNU)
Mechlorethamine (Mustargen)
Melphalan (Alkeran) (available in oral or IV form)
Oxaliplatin (Eloxatin)
Streptozocin (Zanosar)
Temozolomide (Temodar)
Thiotepa (Thioplex)

Topoisomerase Inhibitors
Irinotecan (Camptosar)
Topotecan (Hycamtin)

Miscellaneous Agents
Arsenic trioxide (Trisenox)
Asparaginase (Elspar)
Hydroxyurea (Droxia, Hydrea)
Ixabepilone (Ixempra)
Pegaspargase (Oncaspar)
Procarbazine (Matulane, Natulan 🍁)
Vorinostat (Zolinza)

Data from the U.S. Food and Drug Administration website at www.fda.gov/cder/index.html; and MD Consult at www.mdconsult.com/php/82925233-2/homepage.

Antimetabolites are similar to normal metabolites needed for vital cell processes. Most cell reactions require metabolites in order to begin or continue the reaction. Antimetabolites closely resemble normal metabolites and are "counterfeit" metabolites that fool cancer cells into using the antimetabolites in cellular reactions. Because antimetabolites cannot function as proper metabolites, their presence impairs cell division.

Antimitotic agents interfere with the formation and actions of microtubules so cells cannot complete mitosis during cell division. As a result, the cancer cell either does not divide at all or divides only once.

Antitumor antibiotics damage the cell's DNA and interrupt DNA or RNA synthesis. Exactly how the interruptions occur varies with each agent.

Topoisomerase inhibitors disrupt an enzyme (topoisomerase) essential for DNA synthesis and cell division. When drugs disrupt the enzyme, proper DNA maintenance is prevented, leading to DNA breakage and cell death.

Miscellaneous chemotherapy drugs are those with mechanisms of action that are either unknown or do not fit those of other drug categories.

Combination Chemotherapy

Successful cancer chemotherapy often involves giving more than one specific anticancer drug in a timed manner *(combination chemotherapy)*. Using more than one drug can be more effective in killing cancer cells than using just one drug. However, the side effects and damage caused to normal tissues also increase with combination chemotherapy.

Treatment Issues

Drugs selected for use with a given patient are based on the sensitivity of cancer cells to the drug and the stage or extent of disease. Dosages for most chemotherapy drugs are calculated according to the patient's size. Often, calculations are based on milligrams per square meter of total body surface area (TBSA), which considers the patient's height as well as weight.

Chemotherapy drugs are given on a regular basis and are timed to maximize cancer cell kill and minimize damage to normal cells. The intent is to allow normal cells time to recover from any injury but not allow adequate time for the cancer cells to recover. The schedule may vary slightly to accommodate a patient's response to therapy, but chemotherapy is usually scheduled every 3 to 4 weeks for a specified number of times. Maintaining the intended dosage and timing schedule to ensure the patient receives what was planned is a critical factor in the successful response to chemotherapy. Newer protocols of giving higher doses of chemotherapy more often, called **dose-dense chemotherapy**, may be used for aggressive cancer treatment, especially for breast cancer. This dose-dense therapy also results in more intense side effects.

Patient and family education are critical in helping patients maintain an optimal dosing schedule for best outcomes, reducing side effects, and preventing therapy complications. Many patient problems are managed in the home. Therefore comprehensive and consistent patient education efforts by knowledgeable nurses are key to patient safety (see the Quality Improvement box).

Many chemotherapy drugs are given IV, although other routes may be used. For specific cancer types, the chemotherapy may be infused or instilled into a body cavity. The *intrathecal* route delivers drugs into the spinal canal, and the *intraventricular* route delivers drugs directly into the ventricles of the brain. *Intraperitoneal* instillations place the drugs within the abdominal cavity, most often for ovarian cancer. Drugs for bladder cancer can be instilled directly into the bladder *(intravesicular route)*. In some instances, drugs may be applied as a *topical* preparation for skin lesions. *Intra-arterial* infusions may be used to deliver a higher dose locally. For examples, with liver tumors, an interventional radiologist places a catheter into the artery supplying the liver tumor. The concentrated chemotherapy drug, delivered in sponge-like beads, is infused, and the beads become trapped in the small arteries feeding the tumor. The techniques and care needs for different routes are described with the specific cancer type most commonly associated with the specific administration route.

The IV route is the most common for chemotherapy. The standard of care designated by the Oncology Nursing Society (ONS) and supported by the American Society of Clinical Oncologists (ASCO) for safe administration of IV

QUALITY IMPROVEMENT QSEN

Use of Checklists Can Help Ensure Important Information is Included in Patient Education

Dalby, C., Nesbitt, M., Frechette, C., Kennerley, K., Lacoursiere, L., & Buswell, L. (2013). Standardization of initial chemotherapy teaching to improve care. *Clinical Journal of Oncology Nursing, 17*(5), 472-475.

Chemotherapy for cancer treatment uses toxic drugs with many side effects and complications, and regimens often last for many months. Patients and families require much education and support to manage side effects and reduce the ongoing risks to patient safety. The oncology nurses at a large, well-known comprehensive cancer center that has multiple satellite ambulatory care sites noted that patients continued to have concerns for how to manage problems at home and when to seek professional help even after completing an initial chemotherapy teaching session. Closer examination of teaching techniques revealed that different satellites employed different resources and that individual oncology nurses used different approaches to patient teaching. To comply with the recently updated standards put forth by the American Society of Clinical Oncology and the Oncology Nursing Society to strengthen patient education, the nurses formed an improvement team consisting of nurse representatives from each treatment satellite, an oncology clinical nurse specialist, and a quality improvement expert. This team first agreed on what categories of patient education were critical and then reached consensus for developing category-specific appropriate checklists for teaching content to cover in each category.

Checklists were developed for content in the categories of (1) patient-specific information, (2) treatment regimen, (3) how and what to communicate (to health care providers), and (4) patient resources. Inclusion of content was determined by vote from experienced oncology nurses. In addition, a treatment-specific calendar for patient/family use was developed, as was a patient education assessment survey. The checklists and other resources were used at the initial chemotherapy visit. The survey was implemented at the third chemotherapy visit to determine checklist effectiveness, reassess patient educational needs, and reinforce key content from earlier teaching sessions.

Survey results at 4 months indicated a high degree of patient satisfaction (97%) with initial chemotherapy teaching. Patients indicated that they were confident in what to expect during chemotherapy and when to contact their providers. The nurses at the satellites involved in this project believed that the checklists helped them provide more consistent and comprehensive education.

Commentary: Implications for Practice and Research

Accurate patient and family education are critical in helping patients maintain an optimal dosing schedule for best outcomes, reducing side effects, and preventing serious therapy complications. This project demonstrated the checklists could help standardize the information and resources presented to patients at initial chemotherapy to ensure adequate patient preparation. Having input from experienced nurses at multiple sites helped ensure no critical information was omitted from teaching plans and helped obtain "buy-in" from all nurses working in these areas. This plan is now being expanded to all satellite clinics of the cancer center.

chemotherapy is that administration of these drugs requires special education and handling (Neuss et al., 2013; Polovich & Martin, 2011). Special education for competency does not mean that only an advanced practice nurse can perform this function; however, it does mean that the person should be a registered nurse who has completed an approved chemotherapy course. Responsibility for monitoring the patient during chemotherapy administration, however, rests with all nurses providing patient care.

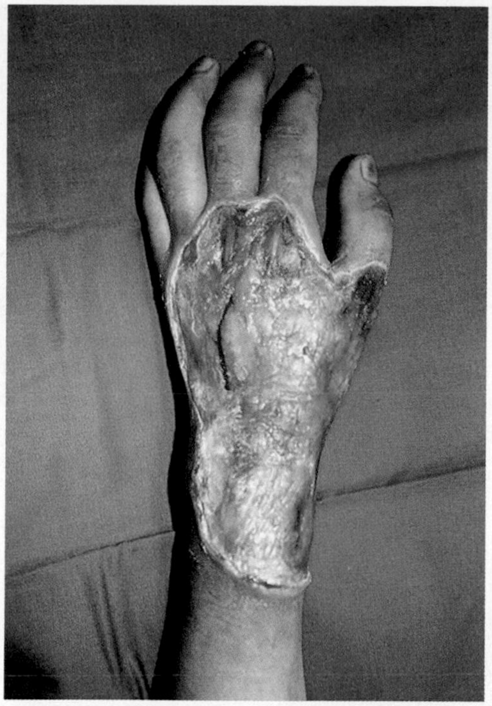

FIG. 22-2 Appearance of tissue damage and loss after chemotherapy extravasation.

A serious complication of IV infusion is **extravasation**, which occurs when drug leaks into the surrounding tissues (also called *infiltration*). When the drugs given are **vesicants** (chemicals that damage tissue on direct contact), the results of extravasation can include PAIN, INFECTION, and tissue loss (Fig. 22-2). Surgery is sometimes needed for severe tissue damage.

The most important nursing intervention for extravasation is prevention (Gonzales, 2013; Schulmeister, 2014). Small extravasations resolve without extensive treatment if less than 0.5 mL of the drug has leaked into the tissues. If a larger amount has leaked, extensive tissue damage occurs and surgery may be needed. Careful monitoring of the access site is critical during chemotherapy administration to prevent leakage of larger volumes. Institutions should have established evidenced-based policies and procedures that are drug specific to guide extravasation management. With some drugs, cold compresses to the area are prescribed; for other agents, warm compresses are used. Antidotes may be injected into the site of extravasation. Coordinate with the oncologist and pharmacist to determine the specific antidote needed for the extravasated drug. Increasingly, when vesicants are part of therapy, the use of an implanted port or central line to decrease the risk for extravasation is recommended. Even with these devices, the nurse must observe closely for any indication of leakage and initiate management guidelines immediately.

Most chemotherapy drugs, even oral drugs, are absorbed through the skin and mucous membranes. As a result, the health care workers who prepare or give these drugs (especially nurses and pharmacists) are at risk for absorbing them. Anyone preparing, giving, or disposing of chemotherapy drugs or handling excreta from patients within 48 hours of receiving IV chemotherapy must use extreme caution and wear personal protective equipment (PPE). Such equipment includes eye protection, masks, double gloves or "chemo" gloves, and gown. The Occupational Safety and Health Administration (OSHA)

TABLE 22-4 **Current Oral Chemotherapeutic Drugs**

AGENT	DRUG CATEGORY	CANCER TYPE
Altretamine (Hexalen)	Alkylating agent	Ovarian cancer
Capecitabine (Xeloda)	Antimetabolite	Breast cancer Colorectal cancer
Chlorambucil (Leukeran)	Alkylating agent	Chronic lymphocytic leukemia; Hodgkin's lymphoma Non-Hodgkin's lymphoma
Dasatinib (Sprycel)	Tyrosine kinase inhibitor	Chronic myelogenous leukemia; acute myelogenous leukemia that is Philadelphia chromosome positive
Erlotinib (Tarceva)	Epidermal growth factor receptor inhibitor	Non–small cell lung cancer Pancreatic cancer
Everolimus (Afinitor)	Angiogenesis inhibitor	Advanced renal cell carcinoma
Gefitinib (Iressa)	Epidermal growth factor receptor inhibitor	Non–small cell lung cancer
Hydroxyurea (Droxia, Hydrea)	Miscellaneous agent	Chronic myelogenous leukemia Head and neck cancer Melanoma Ovarian cancer Sickle cell disease
Imatinib (Gleevec)	Tyrosine kinase inhibitor	Chronic myelogenous leukemia that is Philadelphia chromosome positive Gastrointestinal stromal tumors Myelodysplastic syndrome
Lapatinib (Tykerb)	Tyrosine kinase inhibitor	Breast cancer
Lenalidomide (Revlimid)	Angiogenesis inhibitor	Multiple myeloma; myelodysplastic syndrome
Lomustine (CCNU, CeeNU)	Alkylating agent	Hodgkin's lymphoma Malignant glioma
Melphalan (Alkeran)	Alkylating agent	Multiple myeloma Ovarian cancer
Mercaptopurine (Purinethol)	Antimetabolite	Acute lymphocytic leukemia
Nilotinib (Tasigna)	Tyrosine kinase inhibitor	Chronic myelogenous leukemia that is Philadelphia chromosome positive
Pazopanib (Votrient)	Multikinase inhibitor	Advanced renal cell carcinoma
Procarbazine (Matulane, Natulan 🍁)	Miscellaneous agent	Hodgkin's lymphoma
Sorafenib (Nexavar)	Multikinase inhibitor	Advanced renal cell carcinoma; hepatocellular carcinoma
Sunitinib (Sutent)	Multikinase inhibitor	Advanced renal cell carcinoma; gastrointestinal stromal tumor
Temozolomide (Temodar)	Alkylating agent	Brain tumors (primary)
Thioguanine (Tabloid)	Antimetabolite	Acute myelogenous leukemia
Topotecan (Hycamtin)	Topoisomerase inhibitor	Small cell lung cancer
Vorinostat (Zolinza)	Histone inhibitor	Cutaneous T-cell lymphoma

and the Oncology Nursing Society (ONS) have established these practice guidelines and protective standards (Walton et al., 2012).

About two dozen anticancer drugs are available currently as oral agents (Table 22-4). This number is expected to double within the next 10 years. Only a few are actually oral formulations of classic cytotoxic chemotherapy agents; more are classified as specific types of targeted therapy agents (discussed later). Oral drugs are more convenient for the patient, and they can be taken at home. However, there are many problems with oral anticancer drugs. One of the biggest problems is the perception by patients and non-oncology nurses that these drugs are less toxic than those given intravenously (Davey, 2013; Neuss et al., 2013), which is **not** true. *Oral anticancer drugs are just as toxic to the person taking the drug and the person handling the drug as are standard chemotherapy drugs.* The responsibility for administration of these drugs often shifts from the oncology clinic to the home or to non-oncology acute care settings, and issues of protection, correct administration, adherence, and recognition and management of side effects are major concerns. Patients need education and support to self-manage this therapy, including the accidental ingestion by another person. Not all patients are willing or able to accept the responsibility of self-management, and this must be considered during patient selection for oral chemotherapy.

Because these oral agents can be absorbed through skin and mucous membranes and exert toxic effects, the person who handles and administers them needs to use PPE in the same way as during IV chemotherapy administration. This becomes a more critical issue when non-oncology nurses are administering the drugs. The ONS practice guidelines stress nurse education for competence to administer these drugs. All nurses administering these drugs must know the indications for drug use, dosage ranges, side effects and adverse effects, schedules, and specific precautions (Yagasaki & Komatsu, 2013). In addition, these oral agents must not be crushed, split, broken, or chewed. These drugs are biohazardous and must be discarded in accordance with agency policy.

Adherence to defined oral chemotherapy schedules and dosages is more of a problem than with IV administration (Davey, 2013). Studies have shown that even highly motivated patients with cancer consider that skipping doses or reducing doses of oral drugs has only a minor impact. As with teaching other aspects of self-care, nurses have to be certain that patients and caregivers understand the implications of the decisions they make. Disrupting the schedule or reducing dosages has a negative impact on therapy outcomes and leads to drug resistance among cancer cells, disease progression, and reduced survival.

Side Effects of Chemotherapy

Temporary and permanent damage can occur to normal tissues from chemotherapy because it is systemic and exerts its effects on all cells. Problems include hemorrhagic cystitis, cardiac muscle damage, and loss of bone density. For some cancer drugs, agents that protect specific healthy cells (cytoprotectants or chemoprotectants) are given ahead of or with chemotherapy drugs to decrease the impact of these drugs on normal tissues. For example, amifostine (Ethyol) reduces DNA damage and is used to prevent kidney damage in patients receiving cisplatin; to reduce neutropenia; and to reduce radiation-induced xerostomia for patients receiving radiation therapy for head and neck cancer. Mesna (Mesnex) binds toxic metabolites to decrease bladder toxicity from ifosfamide and high-dose cyclophosphamide use.

Serious short-term side effects occur with cytotoxic chemotherapy. The side effects on the hematopoietic (blood-producing) system can be life threatening and are the most common reason for changing the dosage or the treatment plan. The suppressive effects on the bone marrow blood-forming cells cause **anemia** (decreased numbers of red blood cells and hemoglobin), **neutropenia** (decreased numbers of white blood cells leading to immunosuppression), and **thrombocytopenia** (decreased numbers of platelets). Common distressing side effects include nausea and vomiting, **alopecia** (hair loss), **mucositis** (open sores on mucous membranes), many skin changes, anxiety, sleep disturbance, altered bowel elimination, and changes in cognitive function. The emotional impact of these side effects is referred to as *cancer therapy symptom distress,* which can vary from patient to patient.

Drug therapy is used to reduce symptom distress from some of these side effects. For other problems, such as alopecia, no evidence-based prevention strategies exist but the patient can be helped to reduce his or her distress from its presence. Nonpharmacologic nursing interventions for many types of symptom distress experienced include distraction, massage, guided imagery, and other forms of complementary therapy (Serra et al., 2012).

Psychosocial issues can occur during chemotherapy. For many chemotherapy regimens, drugs are given over a period ranging from 2 hours to as long as 8 hours. During this time, the patient may be confined to a treatment area and constantly reminded of the disease and its treatment. Distraction methods such as virtual reality, guided imagery, reading, watching television, and talking with visitors may help reduce the sense of unpleasantness.

❖ PATIENT-CENTERED COLLABORATIVE CARE

The priority care issues during chemotherapy are protecting the patient from the life-threatening side effects and managing the associated distressing symptoms. For some patients, the symptoms are so unpleasant that they want to stop treatment.

Bone Marrow Suppression

In addition to killing cancer cells, chemotherapy also destroys circulating blood cells and reduces replacement of these cells by suppressing bone marrow function, also known as *myelosuppression.* The numbers of all circulating leukocytes, erythrocytes, and platelets are decreased. Reduced leukocyte numbers, especially **neutropenia**, greatly increase the risk for INFECTION. Decreased erythrocytes and platelets cause hypoxia, fatigue, and impaired CLOTTING leading to an increased tendency to bleed.

INFECTION risk results from neutropenia, placing the patient at extreme risk for sepsis. This critical problem is the major dose-limiting side effect of cancer chemotherapy and can lead to death during treatment. Many chemotherapy drugs cause myelosuppression to some degree and decrease the patient's protective responses to infection. The severity of the risk is related to drug dosage. Impairment is temporary, and protection recovers within weeks after therapy completion. However, the seriousness of potential infections makes this problem a major treatment concern (Held-Warmkessel, 2011). The most common infections are fungal, bacterial, and viral breakthrough. Most infections during neutropenia result from overgrowth of the patient's own normal flora and entrance of these organisms into the bloodstream.

INFECTION risk can be managed with the use of biological response modifiers (BRMs) and growth factors to stimulate bone marrow production of immune system cells. Although not appropriate for all types of cancer, this supportive treatment can reduce the risk for infection during chemotherapy. This treatment is discussed in the Immunotherapy section on p. 387. Actual infections are treated with anti-infective drugs, such as antibiotic, antifungal, and antiviral drugs. Just like for any other infection, anti-infective therapy is specific for the organism(s) causing the infection.

CONSIDERATIONS FOR OLDER ADULTS

Patient-Centered Care QSEN

Older adults are at even greater risk for chemotherapy-induced neutropenia because of age-related changes in bone marrow function. Using growth factors, such as filgrastim (Neupogen) and pegfilgrastim (Neulasta), before neutropenia occurs rather than later can reduce the severity of neutropenia and the risk for infectious complications. Be extra vigilant in assessing older adults for early manifestations of infection.

! NURSING SAFETY PRIORITY QSEN

Action Alert

The priority nursing interventions for the patient with neutropenia are protecting him or her from INFECTION within the health care system and teaching the patient and family how to reduce infection risk in the home. Total patient assessment, including skin and mucous membrane inspection, lung sounds, mouth assessment, and inspection of venous access device insertion sites, must be performed every 8 hours by a registered nurse for hospitalized patients.

Explain to the patient the importance of reporting any change in skin and mucous membranes or other health status. Instruct him or her to report any pimple, sore, rash, or open skin area. Also teach him or her to report a cough, burning on urination, PAIN around the venous access site, or new drainage from any body area. Good handwashing before contact with the patient is essential for INFECTION prevention. Use aseptic technique with any invasive procedure. Chart 22-3 lists the best practices to prevent infection in patients with neutropenia.

When delegating any nursing care activity to unlicensed assistive personnel (UAP), teach them the importance of protecting the neutropenic patient from INFECTION. Stress the ways that cross-contamination can occur and how to avoid this source of infection. Also ensure that UAP understand that even when the neutropenic patient is very tired and does not feel well, certain aspects of personal hygiene cannot be deferred. *Teach the importance of mouth care and washing of the axillary and perianal regions at least every 12 hours.*

Monitoring for manifestations of INFECTION is critical for the hospitalized patient with neutropenia. The reduced numbers of neutrophils can limit the presence of common infection manifestations. Often the patient with neutropenia does not develop a high fever or have purulent drainage even when a severe infection is present. Hospital units specializing in care of neutropenic patients often have standard protocols that nurses initiate as soon as infection is suspected, *before* a physician examines the patient, because treatment delay can result in sepsis and death. These protocols specify what types of cultures to obtain (e.g., blood, urine, sputum, central line, wound), what diagnostic tests to obtain (e.g., chest x-ray), and what antibiotics to start immediately.

CHART 22-3 Best Practice for Patient Safety & Quality Care QSEN

Care of the Patient with Myelosuppression and Neutropenia

- Place the patient in a private room whenever possible.
- Use good handwashing technique or use alcohol-based hand rubs before touching the patient or any of the patient's belongings.
- Ensure that the patient's room and bathroom are cleaned at least once each day.
- Do not use supplies from common areas for patients with myelosuppression and neutropenia. For example, keep a dedicated box of disposable gloves in his or her room and do not share this box with any other patient. Provide single-use food products, individually wrapped gauze, and other individually wrapped items.
- Limit the number of health care personnel entering the patient's room.
- Monitor vital signs every 4 hours, including temperature.
- Inspect the patient's mouth at least every 8 hours.
- Inspect the patient's skin and mucous membranes (especially the anal area) for the presence of fissures and abscesses at least every 8 hours.
- Inspect open areas, such as IV sites, every 4 hours for manifestations of infection.
- Change wound dressings daily.
- Obtain specimens of all suspicious areas for culture (as specified by the agency), and promptly notify the physician.
- Assist the patient in coughing and deep-breathing exercises.
- Encourage activity at a level appropriate for the patient's current health status.
- Change IV tubing daily or according to unit protocol.
- Keep frequently used equipment in the room for use with this patient only (e.g., blood pressure cuff, stethoscope, thermometer).
- Limit visitors to healthy adults.
- Use strict aseptic technique for all invasive procedures.
- Monitor the white blood cell count daily.
- Avoid the use of indwelling urinary catheters.
- Follow agency policy for restriction of fresh flowers and potted plants in the patient's room.

! NURSING SAFETY PRIORITY QSEN

Critical Rescue

Consider any temperature elevation in a patient with neutropenia an indication of INFECTION. Report it to the health care provider immediately, and implement standard infection protocols.

Many patients remain at home during periods of neutropenia and are at continuing risk for INFECTION. The focus remains on keeping the patient's own normal flora under control and preventing transmission of organisms from other people to him or her. *The patient with neutropenia but no other manifestations of communicable disease is NOT an infection hazard to other people; however, other people can be an infection hazard to the patient.* Teach patients and families self-care actions to reduce the risk for infection (Chart 22-4), especially handwashing.

Anemia and *thrombocytopenia* also result from the bone marrow suppression caused by some chemotherapy drugs.

CHART 22-4 Patient and Family Education: Preparing for Self-Management

Prevention of Infection

During the times your white blood cell counts are low:

- Avoid crowds and other large gatherings of people who might be ill.
- Do not share personal toilet articles, such as toothbrushes, toothpaste, washcloths, or deodorant sticks, with others.
- If possible, bathe daily, using an antimicrobial soap. If total bathing is not possible, wash the armpits, groin, genitals, and anal area twice a day with an antimicrobial soap.
- Clean your toothbrush at least weekly by either running it through the dishwasher or rinsing it in liquid laundry bleach (and then rinsing the bleach out with hot running water).
- Wash your hands thoroughly with an antimicrobial soap before you eat and drink, after touching a pet, after shaking hands with anyone, as soon as you come home from any outing, and after using the toilet.
- Follow the cancer center's instructions for eating fresh salads; raw fruits and vegetables; meat, fish and eggs; and pepper and paprika.
- Wash dishes between use with hot, sudsy water, or use a dishwasher.
- Do not drink water, milk, juice, or other cold liquids that have been standing at room temperature for longer than an hour.
- Do not reuse cups and glasses without washing.
- Do not change pet litter boxes.
- Take your temperature at least once a day and whenever you do not feel well.
- Report any of these indications of infection to your physician immediately:
  - Temperature greater than 100°F (37.8°C)
  - Persistent cough (with or without sputum)
  - Pus or foul-smelling drainage from any open skin area or normal body opening
  - Presence of a boil or abscess
  - Urine that is cloudy or foul smelling or that causes burning on urination
- Take all prescribed drugs.
- Wear clean disposable gloves underneath gardening gloves when working in the garden or with houseplants.
- Wear a condom (if you are a man) when having sex. If you are a woman having sex with a male partner, ensure that he wears a condom.

Anemia causes patients to feel fatigued from a lack of adequate red blood cells to transport oxygen, and some tissues are hypoxic. Thrombocytopenia increases the risk for excessive bleeding from impaired CLOTTING. When the platelet count is less than 50,000/mm³, small trauma can lead to prolonged bleeding. With a count lower than 20,000 platelets/mm³, spontaneous and uncontrollable bleeding may occur. Both anemia and thrombocytopenia may require transfusion therapy.

The use of growth factors to stimulate production of red blood cells and platelets to improve CLOTTING is common. Erythropoiesis-stimulating agents (ESAs) such as darbepoetin alfa (Aranesp) and epoetin alfa (Epogen and Procrit) can prevent or improve anemia associated with chemotherapy and can reduce the need for transfusions. These drugs increase the production of many blood cell types, not just erythrocytes, increasing the patient's risk for hypertension, blood clots, strokes, and heart attacks, especially among older adults. Also, certain types of cancer cells grow faster in the presence of these ESAs, such as head and neck cancer cells, leukemias, and some lymphomas, and their use may be restricted. Dosing is based on each patient's hemoglobin levels to ensure that just enough red blood cells are produced to avoid the need for transfusion but not necessarily to bring hemoglobin or hematocrit levels up to normal.

An example of growth factor therapy for thrombocytopenia is the use of oprelvekin (Neumega). This drug increases the production of platelets. The drug may cause fluid retention and increase the risk for heart failure and pulmonary edema. Other side effects include conjunctival bleeding, hypotension, and tachycardia. Check whether patients have a working scale, and teach them to weigh themselves daily and keep a record. Remind them to immediately report sudden weight gain or dyspnea to the health care provider.

The priority for nursing care for the patient with thrombocytopenia is to provide a safe environment. Chart 22-5 lists the best practices for Bleeding Precautions for impaired CLOTTING. Teach UAP the importance of using Bleeding Precautions and the need to report any evidence of bleeding immediately. Caregivers at home also need to know these practices.

Teach patients with thrombocytopenia and their families to avoid injury and excessive bleeding when discharge occurs before the platelet count has returned to normal. Chart 22-6 reviews precautions to teach patients to prevent bleeding and what to do if bleeding occurs.

NCLEX EXAMINATION CHALLENGE

Physiological Integrity

The client receiving high-dose chemotherapy who has neutropenia asks the nurse whether he and his wife can have sexual intercourse while he is receiving chemotherapy. What is the nurse's best response?

A. "No, this activity will increase the side effects of the chemotherapy."
B. "No, the danger of impregnating your wife is too great."
C. "Yes, as long as you feel like it and use a condom."
D. "Yes, if you do not have an infection."

Chemotherapy-Induced Nausea and Vomiting

Chemotherapy-induced nausea and vomiting (CINV) arises from a variety of GI and neural mechanisms. It may manifest as *anticipatory* (before receiving the chemotherapy, often triggered by thoughts, sights, and sounds related to the anticipated chemotherapy), *acute* (within the first 24 hours after chemotherapy), *delayed* (occurring after the first 24 hours), *breakthrough* (occurring intermittently during therapy for CINV), or a combination of these. Many cancer drugs are **emetogenic** (vomiting inducing) to some degree, depending on the dose. Although evidence-based advances in prevention and control of CINV are helpful, it remains a common and distressing issue (Cherwin, 2012). Nausea often persists even when vomiting is controlled.

Acute CINV is more common than other types. It may persist for 1 to 2 days after chemotherapy is given. A few drugs, such as dacarbazine (DTIC), may trigger CINV almost as soon as the drug is started. Other drugs, such as cisplatin (Platinol), induce delayed nausea and vomiting that can continue as long as 5 to 7 days after receiving it. Patients who have CINV during one round of chemotherapy may begin to have the same manifestations before the next round as a result of sheer anticipation. Once considered the single most distressing side effect of chemotherapy, CINV often can be well controlled with appropriate evidence-based antiemetic therapy, especially with serotonin (5-HT3) antagonist drugs and the use of standardized protocols for its prevention and management.

Drug Therapy. Many antiemetics are available to relieve nausea and vomiting. These drugs vary in the side effects they

CHART 22-5 Best Practice for Patient Safety & Quality Care QSEN

Prevention of Injury for the Patient with Thrombocytopenia

- Handle the patient gently.
- Use and teach unlicensed assistive personnel (UAP) to use a lift sheet when moving and positioning the patient in bed.
- Avoid IM injections and venipunctures.
- When injections or venipunctures are necessary, use the smallest-gauge needle for the task.
- Apply firm pressure to the needle stick site for 10 minutes or until the site no longer oozes blood.
- Apply ice to areas of trauma.
- Test all urine and stool for the presence of occult blood.
- Observe IV sites every 4 hours for bleeding.
- Instruct patients to notify nursing personnel immediately if any trauma occurs and if bleeding or bruising is noticed.
- Avoid trauma to rectal tissues:
  - Do not administer enemas.
  - If suppositories are prescribed, lubricate liberally and administer with caution.
- Instruct the patient and UAP that the patient should use an electric shaver rather than a razor.
- When providing mouth care or supervising others in providing mouth care:
  - Use a soft-bristled toothbrush or tooth sponges.
  - Do not use water pressure gum cleaners.
  - Make certain that dentures and other dental devices fit and do not irritate.
- Instruct the patient not to blow the nose or insert objects into the nose.
- Instruct UAP and the patient that the patient should wear shoes with firm soles whenever ambulating.
- Practice fall prevention strategies according to the agency's policies.
- Keep pathways and walkways clear and uncluttered.

CHART 22-6 Patient and Family Education: Preparing for Self-Management

Preventing Injury or Bleeding

During the time your platelet count is low:
- Use an electric shaver.
- Use a soft-bristled toothbrush.
- Do not have dental work performed without consulting your cancer health care provider.
- Do not take aspirin or any aspirin-containing products. Read the label to be sure that the product does not contain aspirin or salicylates.
- Do not participate in contact sports or any activity likely to result in your being bumped, scratched, or scraped.
- If you are bumped, apply ice to the site for at least 1 hour.
- Avoid hard foods that would scrape the inside of your mouth.
- Eat only warm, cool, or cold foods to avoid burning your mouth. Be especially cautious with cheese topping on pizza.
- Check your skin and mouth daily for bruises, swelling, or areas with small reddish purple marks that may indicate bleeding.
- Notify your cancer health care provider if you:
  - Are injured and persistent bleeding results
  - Have excessive menstrual bleeding
  - See blood in your vomit, urine, or bowel movement
- Avoid trauma with intercourse.
- Avoid anal intercourse.
- Take a stool softener to prevent straining during a bowel movement.
- Do not use enemas or rectal suppositories.
- Avoid bending over at the waist, which increases pressure in the brain.
- Do not wear clothing or shoes that are tight or that rub.
- Avoid blowing your nose or placing objects in your nose. If you must blow your nose, do so gently without blocking either nasal passage.
- Avoid playing musical instruments that raise the pressure inside your head, such as brass wind instruments and woodwinds or reed instruments.

produce and how well they control CINV. One or more antiemetics are usually given before, during, and after chemotherapy. Drugs commonly used short-term to control CINV are listed in Chart 22-7. *Patient response to antiemetic therapy is variable, and the drug combinations are individualized for best effect (Barak et al., 2013).*

! NURSING SAFETY PRIORITY QSEN

Drug Alert

Do not confuse the antiemetic drug *Anzemet* (dolasetron) with the diabetes drug *Avandamet* (a combination of metformin and rosiglitazone). The drugs have similar sounding names but totally different actions.

Regardless of which drugs are being used to prevent or reduce CINV, they are most effective when used in an evidence-based approach for prevention and management on a scheduled basis (Davidson et al., 2012). Drug therapy for CINV works best when given before the nausea and vomiting are out of control. *The nursing priority is to coordinate with the patient and health care provider to ensure adequate control of CINV. Ensure that antiemetics are given before chemotherapy and are repeated based on the response and duration of CINV.* When patients are receiving dose-dense chemotherapy, the intensity of CINV also increases and more aggressive antiemetic therapy is needed. Teach patients to continue the therapy, even when CINV appears controlled. *When the patient stops taking the drug(s), teach him or her to start retaking the drug at the first sign of nausea to prevent it from becoming uncontrollable.*

CONSIDERATIONS FOR OLDER ADULTS

Patient-Centered Care **QSEN**

The older adult can become dehydrated more quickly than a younger adult if CINV is not controlled. Teach older adults to be proactive with taking their prescribed antiemetics and to contact their health care provider if the CINV either does not resolve within 12 hours or becomes worse.

Mucositis

Mucositis (sores in mucous membranes) often develops in the entire GI tract, especially in the mouth (**stomatitis** refers to reactions that involve the other tissues and structures in the oral cavity). Mucositis is believed to be a complex, multiphase process at the cellular level started in response to cytotoxic chemotherapy. Mouth sores cause PAIN and interfere with eating and quality of life. Chart 22-8 lists the patient education for self-management of mucositis.

Frequent mouth assessment and oral hygiene are key in managing mucositis. Stress the importance of good and frequent oral hygiene, including teeth cleaning and mouth rinsing. Because most patients with mucositis also have bone marrow suppression and are at risk for impaired CLOTTING with bleeding, they must take care to avoid traumatizing the oral mucosa. Instruct them to use a soft-bristled toothbrush or disposable mouth sponges. Recommendations include *gentle* flossing once daily. Encourage them to rinse the mouth with plain water or saline at frequent intervals during the day and night when awake. Frequency is guided by the intensity of the mucositis. Initially, the rinses start after meals and at bedtime, then every 2 hours, and then progressing to hourly if needed for comfort. Teach patients to avoid mouthwashes that contain alcohol or other drying agents that may further irritate the mucosa.

Oral hygiene equipment must be kept clean. Remind patients not to share toothbrushes. Toothbrushes can be cleaned weekly by using a home dishwasher or by rinsing them with a solution of liquid bleach or hydrogen peroxide and then rinsing with hot water.

Many compounds are available for PAIN relief from mucositis as "swish and spit" mixtures that contain a local anesthetic combined with anti-inflammatory agents, although their use is not evidence-based. Remind the patient that these mixtures are not to be swallowed. For multiple mouth lesions, most patients require systemic pain medications.

Alopecia

Alopecia, hair loss, may occur as whole-body hair loss or may be as mild as only a thinning of the scalp hair. When body hair loss includes pubic hair, patients may struggle with their sexual identity and may not discuss this problem. Reassure patients that hair loss is temporary. Regrowth usually begins about 1 month after completion of chemotherapy; however, the new hair may differ from the original hair in color, texture, and

CHART 22-7 **Common Examples of Drug Therapy**

Chemotherapy-Induced Nausea and Vomiting

DRUG/USUAL DOSAGE	PHYSIOLOGIC PURPOSE	NURSING INTERVENTIONS	RATIONALE
Serotonin Antagonists			
Ondansetron (Zofran) 8 mg IV or orally every 8 hr Granisetron (Kytril) 1 mg IV or orally every 12 hr Granisetron transdermal (Sancuso) 1 patch per day starting 24 to 48 hrs before chemotherapy administration and continuing for up to 7 days after chemotherapy administration Dolasetron (Anzemet) 100 mg IV or orally 30 minutes before chemotherapy administration Palonosetron (Aloxi) 0.25 mg IV as a single dose 30 minutes before chemotherapy administration	Prevent CINV by blocking the 5-HT3 receptors in the brain (chemotrigger zone) and in the intestines. This action prevents serotonin from binding to the receptors and activating the nausea and vomiting centers.	Teach patient to change positions slowly to avoid falls. Assess the patient for headache.	These drugs may induce bradycardia, hypotension, and vertigo. Headache is a common side effect of drugs from this class.
Neurokinin Receptor Antagonists			
Aprepitant (Emend) *3-day oral regimen:* Day 1, 125 mg 1 hour before chemotherapy administration Days 2 and 3, 80 mg in the morning (no chemotherapy these days) *IV regimen:* Day 1, 115 mg 30 minutes before chemotherapy, followed by oral regimen on Days 2 and 3	Reduce CINV by blocking the substance P neurokinin receptor. When used together with a serotonin antagonist and a corticosteroid, both acute and delayed nausea and vomiting are controlled.	Teach patients who are also taking warfarin (Coumadin) to have their INRs checked before and after the 3 days of this therapy. Teach women who are using oral contraceptives to use an additional form of birth control while on this drug.	This drug interferes with the effectiveness of warfarin. The drug reduces the effectiveness of oral contraceptives, increasing the risk for an unplanned pregnancy.
Corticosteroids			
Dexamethasone (Decadron) 5-10 mg IV or orally daily	Reduce CINV by decreasing swelling in the brain's chemotrigger zone.	Teach patients to reduce salt intake to about 4 g daily.	Drug causes fluid retention and hypertension.
Prokinetic Agents			
Metoclopramide (Reglan) 20-40 mg IM or IV twice or three times daily	Reduce CINV by blocking dopamine receptors in the brain's chemotrigger zone.	Teach the patient to avoid driving or operating heavy machinery.	Increased drowsiness is common.
Benzodiazepines			
Lorazepam (Ativan) 1-3 mg orally or IV twice or three times daily	Reduce CINV by enhancing cholinergic effects and by decreasing the person's awareness.	Teach the patient and family that the patient should avoid driving, operating heavy machinery, making legal decisions, and going up and down staircases unassisted.	The drug induces amnesia and profound drowsiness.

CINV, Chemotherapy-induced nausea and vomiting; *INR,* international normalized ratio.

thickness. No known evidence-based treatment safely prevents alopecia. *The priority nursing actions are to teach patients how to avoid scalp injury and to assist them in coping with this body image change.*

The hairless scalp is at risk for injury. Teach the patient to avoid direct sunlight on the scalp by wearing a hat or other head covering. Sunscreen use is essential to prevent sunburn because many drugs increase sun sensitivity, regardless of skin darkness. This skin can be damaged by helmets, headphones, headsets, wigs, and other items that rub the head. Teach the patient to wear some head covering underneath these items. Head coverings also are needed during cold weather and in cool environments to reduce body heat loss and prevent hypothermia.

Assist patients in selecting a type of head covering that suits their income and lifestyle. One recommendation is to coordinate wig purchases with the patient's hairdresser or barber. Having very short hair or a shaved head now is common and socially acceptable for men, and many men choose not to wear a wig during chemotherapy. Cutting the hair very short before chemotherapy begins allows a better wig fit.

Suggest that patients purchase a wig before therapy begins and have their hairdresser shape it to mimic their usual hairstyle to reduce appearance changes. High-quality wigs are expensive but can look very much like the patient's own hair. Many local units of the American Cancer Society (ACS) offer the loan of wigs that other patients have donated to be lent to others with cancer. Patients also can disguise hair loss with caps, scarves, and turbans. The ACS also provides instruction (Look Good-Feel Better) regarding makeup and the use of scarves, for example, to improve appearance and how patients feel about themselves. Patients in control of their appearance may improve their quality of life during therapy (Borsellino & Young, 2011).

Changes in Cognitive Function

Some patients receiving chemotherapy have reported changes in cognitive function—most commonly reduced ability to concentrate, memory loss, and difficulty learning new information during treatment and for months to years after treatment. Although most types of chemotherapy drugs do not cross the blood-brain barrier and were thought not to affect any part of

CHART 22-8 Patient and Family Education: Preparing for Self-Management

Mouth Care for Patients with Mucositis

- Examine your mouth (including the roof, under the tongue, and between the teeth and cheek) every 4 hours for fissures, blisters, sores, or drainage.
- If sores or drainage is present, contact your health care provider to determine whether these areas need to be cultured.
- Brush the teeth and tongue with a soft-bristled brush or sponges every 8 hours and after meals.
- Avoid the use of mouthwashes that contain alcohol or glycerin.
- "Swish and spit" room-temperature tap water, normal saline, or salt and soda water on a regular basis (at least 4 times a day) and as needed according to changes in the oral cavity.
- Drink 2 or more liters of water per day if another health problem does not require limiting fluid intake.
- Take antimicrobial drugs as prescribed.
- Use topical analgesic drugs as prescribed.
- Take pain medications on schedule as needed.
- Apply a water-based moisturizer to your lips after each episode of mouth care and as needed.
- Use prescribed "artificial saliva" or mouth moisturizers as needed.
- Avoid using tobacco or drinking alcoholic beverages.
- Avoid spicy, salty, acidic, dry, rough, or hard food.
- Cool liquids to prevent burns or irritation.
- If you wear dentures, use them only during meals. When not in place, soak dentures in an antimicrobial solution. Rinse thoroughly before placing them in your mouth.

brain function, the drugs can induce inflammation and general biochemical changes that could reduce cognitive function, at least temporarily (Kanaskie, 2012; Myers, 2012).

This problem, termed "chemo brain," is reported most often in women undergoing chemotherapy for breast cancer, although it is not limited either to women or to breast cancer treatment. The fact that it is reported more in this population reflects that breast cancer is very common, it is often treated with high-dose chemotherapy, and most patients with breast cancer survive a long time after therapy.

Comparisons of brain structure and cognitive function before, during, and after high-dose chemotherapy show some anatomic changes in brain white matter and gray matter. These changes are not usually present at 3 years after completion of therapy. It is not known why all patients receiving high-dose chemotherapy do not develop the problem; however, genetic differences may be partly responsible. Not only is the exact cause of this side effect unclear, so are the personal risk factors.

The priority for nursing care is to support the patient who reports this side effect. Listen to the patient's concerns, and tell him or her that other patients have also reported such problems. Providing absolute reassurance is difficult, but the results of early studies indicate that recovery is likely with time. A common sense approach includes that patients should be warned against participating in other behaviors that could alter cognitive functioning, such as excessive alcohol intake, recreational drug use, and activities that increase the risk for head injury. Research about reducing the effects of chemo brain is ongoing.

Chemotherapy-Induced Peripheral Neuropathy

Chemotherapy-induced peripheral neuropathy (CIPN) is the loss of sensory or motor function of peripheral nerves associated with exposure to certain anticancer drugs (Binner et al., 2011; Tofthagen et al., 2011). Some patients undergoing chemotherapy with nerve-damaging drugs (e.g., antimitotics and platinum-based drugs) have rapid onset of severe CIPN. The degree of CIPN is related to the dosage of the nerve-damaging drugs; higher doses lead to greater neuropathy. The results of CIPN on function are widespread, with the most common problems including loss of sensation in the hands and feet, orthostatic hypotension, erectile dysfunction, neuropathic PAIN, loss of taste discrimination, and severe constipation. CIPN is a long-term consequence and may be permanent in some people. No known interventions prevent CIPN.

The priority for nursing care of patients experiencing CIPN is teaching them to prevent injury. Loss of sensation increases the patient's risk for injury because he or she may not be aware of excessive heat, cold, or pressure. The risk for injury to the feet is very high. Falls are more likely because the patient cannot feel changes in terrain and because of orthostatic hypotension. Chart 22-9 lists teaching priorities for the patient with CIPN.

CHART 22-9 Patient and Family Education: Preparing for Self-Management

Chemotherapy-Induced Peripheral Neuropathy

- Protect feet and other body areas where sensation is reduced (e.g., do not walk around in bare feet or stocking feet; always wear shoes with a protective sole).
- Be sure shoes are long enough and wide enough to prevent creating sores or blisters.
- Buy shoes in the afternoon or evening to accommodate any size change needed for foot swelling.
- Provide a long break-in period for new shoes; do not wear new shoes for longer than 2 hours at a time.
- Avoid pointed-toe shoes and shoes with heels higher than 2 inches.
- Inspect your feet daily (with a mirror) for open areas or redness.
- Avoid extremes of temperature; wear warm clothing in the winter, especially over hands, feet, and ears.
- Test water temperature with a thermometer when washing dishes or bathing. Use warm water rather than hot water (less than 105° F or 40.6° C).
- Use potholders when cooking.
- Use gloves when washing dishes or gardening.
- Do not eat foods that are "steaming hot"; allow them to cool before placing them in your mouth.
- Eat foods that are high in fiber (e.g., fruit, whole grain cereals, vegetables).
- Drink 2 to 3 liters of fluid (nonalcoholic) daily unless your health care provider has told you to restrict fluid intake.
- Use the actions for "Falls Prevention" supplied by the cancer center during all activities.
- Get up slowly from a lying or sitting position. If you feel dizzy, sit back down until the dizziness fades before standing; then stand in place for a few seconds before walking or using the stairs.
- To prevent tripping or falling, look at your feet and the floor or ground where you are walking to assess how the ground, floor, or step changes.
- Avoid using area rugs, especially those that slide easily.
- Keep floors free of clutter that could lead to a fall.
- Use handrails when going up or down steps.

Some issues, such as erectile dysfunction, may be helped with devices or drug therapy (see Chapter 72 for options for erectile dysfunction). Other issues are not correctable and affect many aspects of quality of life. The loss of hand sensation may make some activities that require very fine motor skills difficult or impossible. Assess the patient's ability to cope with these changes. Coordinate with an occupational therapist to help the patient adjust for sensory deficits in performing activities. Patients who have an altered gait are at increased risk for falls and injury.

NCLEX EXAMINATION CHALLENGE

Health Promotion and Maintenance

Which precaution is most important for the nurse to teach the client who has chemotherapy-induced peripheral neuropathy?
A. Avoid taking aspirin or any aspirin-containing products.
B. Use a bath thermometer to check bath water temperature.
C. Do not use mouthwashes that contain alcohol or glycerin.
D. Bathe daily using an antimicrobial soap or gel.

IMMUNOTHERAPY: BIOLOGICAL RESPONSE MODIFIERS

Biological response modifiers (BRMs) modify the patient's biologic responses to tumor cells. BRMs can influence cancer cells in a variety of ways. Some have direct antitumor activity, helping the body recognize cancer cells as foreign so that the immune system destroys them. BRMs also can improve immune function and enhance the body's ability to repair or replace cells damaged by cancer treatment.

As discussed in Chapter 17, cytokines released from immune system cells are not usually cytotoxic alone but influence how immune system cells function. The cytokines include the interferons, interleukins, tumor necrosis factors, and colony-stimulating factors. Some cytokines enhance immune function, which plays an important role in cancer prevention (see Chapters 17 and 21). Cytokines and other BRMs work by stimulating the immune system to recognize cancer cells and take actions to eliminate or destroy them. Some BRMs stimulate faster recovery of bone marrow function after treatment-induced suppression. Additional BRMs include the monoclonal antibodies and vaccines.

BRMs as Cancer Therapy

Two common types of BRMs used as cancer therapy are the interleukins and interferons. Some agents can stimulate specific immune system cells to attack and destroy cancer cells; other agents block cancer cell access to an essential function or nutrient.

Interleukins (ILs) are a large group of substances the body makes to help regulate inflammation and immunity. Some are now synthesized as anticancer drugs. In particular, ILs have been useful for renal cell carcinoma and melanoma. ILs help different immune system cells recognize and destroy abnormal body cells. In particular, IL-1, IL-2, and IL-6 appear to "charge up" the immune system and enhance attacks on cancer cells by macrophages, natural killer (NK) cells, and tumor-infiltrating lymphocytes (Abbas et al., 2012).

Interferons (IFNs) are cell-produced proteins that have been effective to some degree in the treatment of melanoma, hairy cell leukemia, renal cell carcinoma, ovarian cancer, and cutaneous T-cell lymphoma. They assist in cancer therapy by:

- Slowing tumor cell division
- Stimulating the growth and activation of NK cells
- Inducing cancer cells to resume a more normal appearance and function
- Inhibiting the expression of oncogenes

TABLE 22-5 Common Biological Response Modifiers Used As Supportive Cancer Therapy

AGENT	CELL TYPE AFFECTED	INDICATIONS
Sargramostim (Leukine, Prokine)	All granulocytes Neutrophils Eosinophils Monocytes Macrophages	Chemotherapy-induced leukopenia
Filgrastim (Neupogen) Pegfilgrastim (Neulasta)	Neutrophils	Chemotherapy-induced neutropenia
Epoetin alfa (Epogen, Procrit) Darbepoetin alfa (Aranesp)	Erythrocytes	Chemotherapy-induced anemia Chemotherapy-induced fatigue Anemia induced by renal failure
Oprelvekin (Neumega)	Platelets	Chemotherapy-induced thrombocytopenia
Sipuleucel-T (Provenge) (product is a vaccine)	T-cells; antigen-processing cells (macrophages)	Hormone-refractory prostate cancer

One drug classified as a BRM that has a different action is thalidomide (Thalomid), which reduces the level of tumor-secreted vascular endothelial growth factor (VEGF). VEGF is needed to maintain blood supply to the tumor. When VEGF is reduced, the tumor is poorly nourished and cancer cells die. This drug is approved for treatment of multiple myeloma.

BRMs as Supportive Therapy

BRMs used for supportive therapy during cancer treatment are the colony-stimulating factors or "growth factors" (Table 22-5). These factors induce more rapid recovery of the bone marrow after suppression by chemotherapy. This effect has two benefits. First, when bone marrow suppression is shortened or less severe, patients are less at risk for life-threatening INFECTIONS, anemia, and impaired CLOTTING with bleeding. Second, because the growth factors allow more rapid bone marrow recovery, patients can receive their chemotherapy as scheduled and may even be able to tolerate higher doses, potentially increasing the chance for cure.

Side Effects of BRM Therapy

Patients receiving interleukins have generalized and often severe inflammatory reactions. Fluid shifts and capillary leak syndrome (CLS) are widespread with edema formation. Tissue swelling affects the function of all organs and can be life threatening. Patients receiving high-dose BRM therapy should receive care in an intensive care or monitoring unit. These effects occur during the period of acute drug infusion and resolve after therapy completion.

Many BRMs and growth factors induce manifestations of inflammation during and just after receiving the drug, including fever, chills, rigors, and flu-like symptoms (general malaise). Problems are worse when higher doses are given, but they seem to become less severe over time. The nursing priorities for patients receiving BRMs include assessing for complications of systemic inflammation and making patients as comfortable as possible. Fever is treated with acetaminophen. Patients with severe rigors are managed with meperidine (Demerol). Patients may also experience nausea, vomiting, diarrhea, and anorexia. Antiemetics are helpful in the management of nausea and vomiting.

Neurologic manifestations associated with BRM use can be significant. These include confusion, fatigue, somnolence, irritation or agitation, hallucinations, vivid dreams, anxiety, and sleep disturbances. Some patients have psychosocial issues of fear, tearfulness, depression, and mood swings. Early identification of these manifestations is an important nursing care activity.

Interferon therapy causes peripheral neuropathy. It is not known whether the neuropathy is temporary or permanent. (See the Chemotherapy-Induced Peripheral Neuropathy section on p. 386.)

Skin dryness, itching, and peeling occur with many types of BRM therapy. The skin problems are more severe with higher doses and when more than one type of BRM is used at the same time. Reactions are temporary but cause much discomfort and distress. Advise patients to apply moisturizers (unscented) to the skin and to use mild soap to clean the skin. Involved areas should be protected from the sun with clothing or the use of sunscreen agents. Teach patients to avoid swimming and to not use topical steroid creams on affected areas.

Monoclonal Antibodies

Monoclonal antibody therapy combines actions from immunotherapy and targeted therapy to help treat specific cancers. The body normally responds to foreign substances with the production of antibodies. These proteins are then able to target the antigen when present in the body, attacking and destroying the foreign antigen (nonself cells). In cancer therapy, human, mouse, and rabbit hybrid cells can produce antibodies against given targets known to be present in or on certain types of cancer cells.

Monoclonal antibodies bind to their target antigens, which are often specific cell surface membrane proteins. Binding prevents the protein from performing its functions. Some cancer cells express cell membrane surface proteins that are unique to cancer cells and have a role in cancer cell division. So, by binding these proteins, monoclonal antibodies prevent cell division. Some monoclonal antibodies actually make tumor cells more sensitive to chemotherapy and increase the effectiveness of immune system attacks on the cancer cells. The most well known monoclonal antibody for targeted therapy is rituximab (Rituxan). It binds to the protein *CD20,* which is often overexpressed on the surface of non-Hodgkin's lymphoma cell membranes. This protein activates an early step of the cell cycle division process. Binding *CD20* with rituximab prevents it from stimulating cell division in the non-Hodgkin's lymphoma cells.

Allergic reactions can be an issue in patients receiving monoclonal antibodies because of the incorporation of non-human proteins. Most of these antibodies initially were developed in mice and express some mouse proteins. Now many of these antibodies have been "humanized," reducing the risk for allergic reactions. Nursing assessment is key for early recognition of a potentially life-threatening allergic reaction.

The monoclonal antibodies to the epidermal growth factor receptor (EGFR) bind to those specific receptors on normal and cancerous cells. Thus side effects also occur in the skin, mucous membranes, and lining of the GI tract.

MOLECULARLY TARGETED THERAPY

Molecularly targeted therapies are technically biologic agents. However, their unique actions and roles in cancer therapy warrant separate discussion. These agents use molecular flaws in some cancer cells to specifically target cancer cells and have less of an impact on normal cells. Generally, molecularly targeted therapies block the growth and spread of cancer by interfering with the specific signals or molecules involved in the growth and progression of cancer cells (Beatty et al., 2011). These agents are providing patients with cancer a new sense of hope against a challenging disease.

As discussed in Chapter 21, normal cells have tightly controlled regulation over when and to what extent a cell divides; cancer cells have escaped this tight control. External events can indicate to a cell that cell division is needed. However, these external events must be communicated to the cell's nucleus to activate the genes that promote cell division (oncogenes) and turn off the genes that normally suppress cell division (suppressor genes). The key to communicating the need for cell division is the presence and activation of signal transduction pathways. Fig. 22-3 shows a segment of a cell with one signal transduction pathway. When this pathway is activated at the cell surface by binding growth factors to their receptors, having certain drugs interact with the cell's plasma membrane, binding of certain adhesion molecules (CAMs), changing movement of calcium and sodium across the membrane, or other cell-to-cell interactions, the first result is an increase in the cell's production of a family of enzymes known as *tyrosine kinases (TKs).* With increased TKs present, the pro–cell division signal activates many substances, known as *transcription factors,* within the pathway. When the pro–cell division transcription factors reach the cell's nucleus, oncogenes are activated, suppressor genes are inactivated, and a variety of proteins are produced to make cell division occur.

When cell division is not needed, external signals, such as growth factor inhibitors and the surrounding of a cell's plasma membrane with other cells, send signals that inhibit activation of TKs and the signal transduction pathway. As a result, fewer transcription factors are produced, suppressor genes are expressed, and oncogenes are suppressed. The proteins needed for cell division are not produced, and cell division does not occur.

Overall, cancer cells have more active signal transduction pathways and transcription factors that ultimately lead to excessive division of the cancer cells. Targeted therapies take advantage of differences in one or more parts of the signal transduction pathway to block it. Often these parts are overexpressed in cancer cells. Agents used as targeted therapies can disrupt the pathway and slow or stop cell division. They may work by blocking a growth factor receptor, by preventing the activation of tyrosine kinases, by limiting the production of transcription factors, and by other mechanisms that are not yet fully understood. Regardless of how a targeted therapy works, it will work only with those cancer cells that have the actual target. The result is that the signal for turning on cell division genes (oncogenes) does not get through to the cell's nucleus (Fig. 22-4) (Byar & Workman, 2012; Santos et al., 2013).

Drugs for targeted therapy have been approved as treatment for certain cancers. These drugs are classified based on the mechanism of action, and some have more than one action (Table 22-6). Because of the varying mechanisms of action and

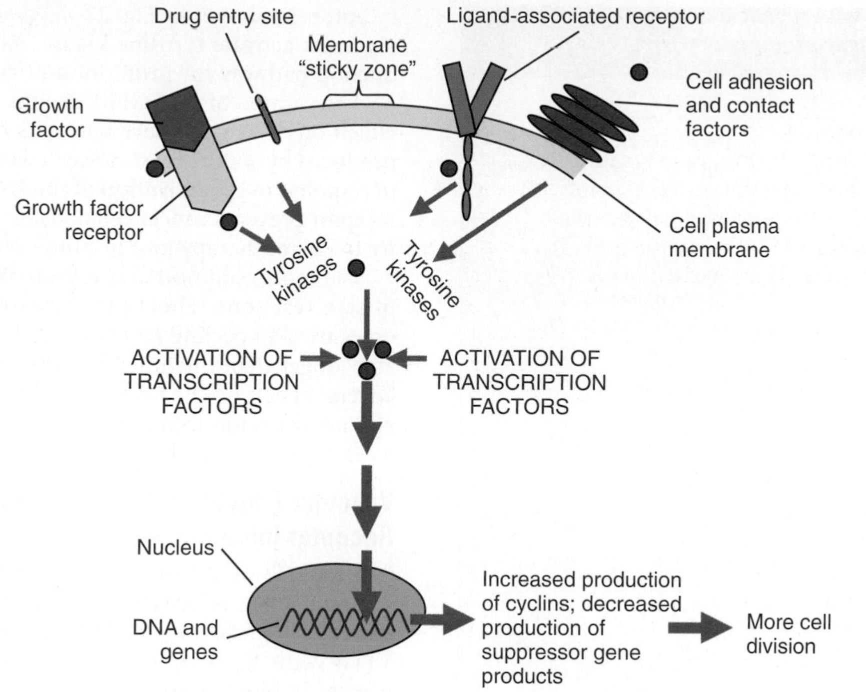

FIG. 22-3 Pro–cell division signal transduction pathway.

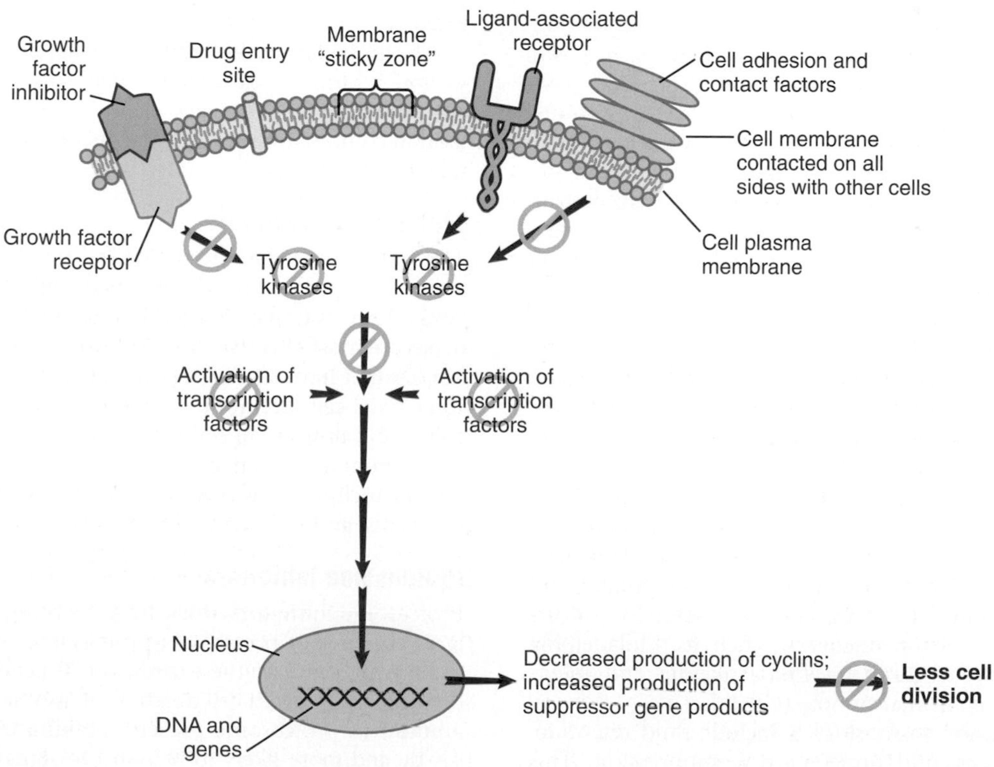

FIG. 22-4 Sites of action for targeted therapies that inhibit a signal transduction pathway and greatly reduce cell division.

the relative newness of these therapies, the priority nursing action is careful assessment for adverse reactions to therapy.

It is important to remember that these drugs will not work unless the cancer cell overexpresses the actual target substance. Thus not all patients with the same cancer type would benefit from the use of targeted therapy. Each person's cancer cells are evaluated to determine whether the cells have enough of a target to be affected by targeted therapy.

The targeted therapy agents are classified based on their action. The first application of these agents was against estrogen

TABLE 22-6 Common Targeted Therapy Agents

CLASSIFICATION	AGENT
Tyrosine kinase inhibitors	Dasatinib (Sprycel) Imatinib mesylate (Gleevec) Lapatinib (Tykerb) Nilotinib (Tasigna)
Epidermal growth factor receptor inhibitors (EGFRIs)	Cetuximab (Erbitux) Erlotinib (Tarceva) Gefitinib (Iressa) Panitumumab (Vectibix) Trastuzumab (Herceptin)
Vascular endothelial growth factor receptor inhibitors (VEGFRIs)	Bevacizumab (Avastin)
Multikinase inhibitors	Sorafenib (Nexavar) Sunitinib (Sutent) Pazopanib (Votrient)
Proteasome inhibitors	Bortezomib (Velcade)
Angiogenesis inhibitors	Everolimus (Afinitor) Lenalidomide (Revlimid) Temsirolimus (Torisel)
Monoclonal antibodies	Alemtuzumab (Campath) Ibritumomab (Zevalin) Rituximab (Rituxan) ^{131}I tositumomab (Bexxar)

in breast cancer (discussed in the Hormonal Manipulation section on p. 391). There now are a group of selective estrogen receptor modulators (SERMs). Aromatase inhibitors (AIs) have been developed to interfere with estrogen's ability to promote the growth of estrogen receptor positive breast cancers. Discussion in this section will focus on the tyrosine kinase inhibitors (TKIs), epidermal growth factor/receptor inhibitors (EGFRIs), vascular endothelial growth factor/receptor inhibitors (VEGFRIs), multikinase inhibitors (MKIs), proteasome inhibitors, and angiogenesis inhibitors.

Tyrosine Kinase Inhibitors

Drugs with the main action of inhibiting activation of tyrosine kinases (TKs) are **tyrosine kinase inhibitors (TKIs)**. There are many different TKs. Some are unique to the cell type; others may be present only in cancer cells that express a specific gene mutation. As a result, the different TKI drugs are effective in disrupting the growth of some cancer cell types and not others. An example of a TKI is imatinib mesylate (Gleevec). This drug binds to the energy site of the enzyme *tyrosine kinase* and prevents its activation. The drug is most useful in cancers that overexpress the *ABL1* oncogene, such as Philadelphia chromosome–positive chronic myeloid leukemia and metastatic gastrointestinal stromal tumors (GISTs).

Side effects common to most TKIs include fluid retention, electrolyte imbalances, and bone marrow suppression. This suppression can be severe enough to cause neutropenia, anemia, and thrombocytopenia. The problems associated with bone marrow suppression are increased when the patient also receives traditional chemotherapy with drugs that suppress bone marrow.

Epidermal Growth Factor/Receptor Inhibitors

The epidermal growth factor/receptor inhibitors (EGFRIs) block epidermal growth factor from binding to its cell surface receptor. As shown in Fig. 22-4, when this receptor is blocked, it cannot activate tyrosine kinase. As a result, the signal transduction pathway for promotion of cell division is inhibited.

An example of an EGFRI drug is trastuzumab (Herceptin), which binds the excessive amounts of a certain type of EGFR produced by some breast cancer, ovarian, and colon cancer cells in response to the activation of the *HER2/neu* gene. Binding this receptor prevents cancer cell division and increases the sensitivity to chemotherapy and immune system actions.

The most common side effects of EGFRIs include a variety of skin reactions. These may be as mild as a rash or result in excessive skin peeling and fissures. Trastuzumab has been available longer than the other EGFRIs and has been found to have adverse effects on the heart. It is not known if the cardiac effects also are common to other EGFRIs.

Vascular Endothelial Growth Factor/Receptor Inhibitors

An example of a vascular endothelial growth factor/receptor inhibitor drug is bevacizumab (Avastin). It binds to vascular endothelial growth factor (VEGF) and prevents the binding of VEGF with its receptors on the surfaces of endothelial cells present in blood vessels. This inhibits formation of new blood vessels within a tumor. As a result, tumor cells are poorly nourished and metastasis is inhibited. This drug is used with standard chemotherapy for many cancers that overexpress the receptor.

The most common side effects are hypertension and impaired wound healing. Bone marrow suppression with neutropenia and thrombocytopenia also occur, especially when the drug is used in combination with chemotherapy drugs that cause bone marrow suppression.

Multikinase Inhibitors

The multikinase inhibitors (MKIs) are drugs that inhibit the activity of specific kinases in cancer cells and in tumor blood vessels. An example of an MKI is sunitinib (Sutent). These drugs are most effective in preventing the activation of tyrosine kinases that have a specific gene mutation found most often in some renal cell carcinomas, GI stromal tumors, and pancreatic, colon, and non–small cell lung cancer cells.

A common side effect of this class of drugs is hypertension. Others include nausea and vomiting, diarrhea, constipation, mucositis, and mild neutropenia and thrombocytopenia.

Proteasome Inhibitors

Proteasome inhibitors work by preventing the formation of a large complex of proteins (a proteasome) in cells. The proteasome helps regulate the expression of genes that promote cell division and prevent cell death. Proteasome inhibitors limit the amount of proteasome present, making the cell less likely to divide and more likely to respond to signals for cell death. An example of a proteasome inhibitor is bortezomib (Velcade). Proteasomes are present in normal and cancer cells, but cancer cells are much more sensitive to the effects of proteasome inhibition than are normal cells.

The most common side effects of bortezomib are nausea, vomiting, anorexia, abdominal PAIN, bowel changes, and decreased taste sensation. Peripheral neuropathy is also common. Other side effects include headache, rash, pruritus, back and bone pain, and muscle aches.

Angiogenesis Inhibitors

Angiogenesis inhibitors target a specific protein kinase known as the *mammalian target of rapamycin (mTOR)*. An example of an angiogenesis inhibitor is temsirolimus (Torisel). When the drug binds to an intracellular protein, a protein-drug complex forms that inhibits the activity of mTOR. When mTOR is inhibited, the concentrations of vascular endothelial growth factor (VEGF) are greatly reduced and many pro–cell division signal transduction pathways are disrupted. This drug is especially useful in suppressing the growth of renal cell carcinomas.

Hypersensitivity reactions to these drugs are common and so is hyperglycemia. Bone marrow suppression is moderate to severe with anemia, neutropenia, and thrombocytopenia. Other general side effects include headache, nausea and vomiting, back PAIN, muscle and joint PAIN, mucositis, diarrhea, and skin problems.

PHOTODYNAMIC THERAPY

Photodynamic therapy (PDT) is the selective destruction of cancer cells through a chemical reaction triggered by types of laser light. It can be used to destroy some cancers, reduce the size of tumors and then allow more complete tumor removal by surgery, and shrink tumors in airways or the esophagus to relieve obstruction. PDT is used most often for non-melanoma skin cancers, ocular tumors, GI tumors, and lung cancers located in the upper airways.

An agent that sensitizes cells to light is injected IV along with a dye. The intent is to sensitize cancer cells to destruction by specific wavelengths of laser light administered later. These agents enter all cells but leave normal cells more rapidly than cancer cells. Usually, within 48 to 72 hours, most of the drug has collected in high concentrations in cancer cells. At this time, a laser light is focused on the tumor. The light activates a chemical reaction in those cells retaining the sensitizing drug that induces irreversible cell damage. Some cells die and slough immediately; others continue to slough for several days. Some lesions require only one exposure to the laser, and others must be re-exposed several days after the first treatment (Agostinis et al., 2011).

❖ *PATIENT-CENTERED COLLABORATIVE CARE*

Use of first-generation photosensitizers in PDT was limited by an intense general sensitivity to light for up to 12 weeks. This light sensitivity required strict protection from all light sources for weeks. Newer photosensitizers and laser technologies have less general sensitivity, allowing greater use of this therapy with less need for intense protection.

HORMONAL MANIPULATION

Hormonal manipulation involves changing usual hormone responses. Hormones are natural chemicals secreted by endocrine glands and picked up by capillaries where they circulate to all body areas. Hormones exert their effects only on their specific target tissues. Some hormones make hormone-sensitive tumors grow more rapidly. Thus decreasing the amount of these hormones available to hormone-sensitive tumors can slow the cancer growth rate.

Hormonal manipulation includes steroids, steroid analogues, and enzyme inhibitors (aromatase inhibitors, gonadotropin-releasing hormone analogues, antiandrogens, and antiestrogens). Many of these agents are used to block receptors and thus prevent the cancer cells from receiving normal hormonal growth stimulation.

TABLE 22-7 Common Agents Used for Hormonal Manipulation of Cancer

TYPE OF AGENT	EXAMPLE
Hormone Agonists	
Androgen	Fluoxymesterone (Halotestin) Testolactone (Teslac)
Estrogen	Chlorotrianisene (Tace) Conjugated equine estrogen (Premarin) Diethylstilbestrol (DES, Stilphostrol) Ethinyl estradiol (Estinyl)
Progestin	Medroxyprogesterone (Amen, Provera) Megestrol (Megace)
Luteinizing hormone–releasing hormone (LHRH)	Leuprolide (Eligard, Lupron, Viadur) Goserelin (Zoladex)
Hormone Antagonists	
Antiandrogens	Bicalutamide (Casodex) Flutamide (Eulexin)
Antiestrogens	Fulvestrant (Faslodex) Tamoxifen (Nolvadex) Toremifene (Fareston)
Hormone Inhibitors	Aminoglutethimide (Cytadren, Elipten) Anastrozole (Arimidex) Exemestane (Aromasin) Letrozole (Femara)

Hormonal manipulation can help control some types of cancer for many years but does not cure the disease. If a tumor depends on hormone A for growth and a large quantity of hormone B (similar to A) is given to the patient, hormone B will interfere with the tumor's uptake of hormone A or will limit the amount produced. As a result, tumor growth is slowed and survival time increases. Table 22-7 lists drugs used in hormonal manipulation for cancer therapy.

Some drugs are *hormone antagonists* that compete with natural hormones at the receptors. When hormone antagonists are given, they bind to the specific hormone receptor on or in the tumor cell and prevent the needed hormone from binding to the receptor. If a tumor needs a certain hormone to grow and the hormone can enter or activate the cell only through a receptor, hormone antagonists can slow tumor growth.

The hormone inhibitors also are used for hormonal therapy. These drugs inhibit the normal organ production of some specific hormones. For example, the aromatase inhibitor *anastrozole* (Arimidex) prevents the production of estrogen in the adrenal gland and reduces the blood level of estrogen, which results in slower growth of some breast cancers.

Side effects of hormonal manipulation are different from those of other types of chemotherapy. Androgens and the antiestrogen receptor drugs cause masculinizing effects in women. Chest and facial hair may develop, menstrual periods stop, and breast tissue shrinks. Patients may have some fluid retention. For men and women receiving androgens, acne may develop, hypercalcemia is common, and liver dysfunction may occur with prolonged therapy. Women receiving estrogens or progestins have irregular menses, fluid retention, and breast tenderness. All patients who take estrogen or progestins are at increased risk for venous thromboembolism.

Feminine manifestations appear in men who take estrogens, progestins, or antiandrogen receptor drugs. Facial hair thins, facial skin is smoother, body fat is redistributed, and breast development (**gynecomastia**) can occur. Bone loss is common, which increases the risk for osteoporosis and pathologic bone fractures (Limburg et al., 2014). Testicular and penile atrophy also occur to some degree. Teach patients and families about expected side effects. Encourage them to express their feelings about body changes. Refer them for counseling if needed.

ONCOLOGIC EMERGENCIES

Cancer is a chronic disease. However, a number of acute complications from the cancer and its treatment can occur. There is some controversy regarding which complications are considered oncologic emergencies (Denshar et al., 2011). This chapter includes sepsis and disseminated intravascular coagulation, syndrome of inappropriate antidiuretic hormone, spinal cord compression, hypercalcemia, superior vena cava syndrome, and tumor lysis syndrome as emergencies. Early diagnosis and immediate intervention of these emergency conditions are essential to avoid life-threatening situations. The role of the nurse is to implement interventions to prevent and detect these complications early for immediate treatment.

SEPSIS AND DISSEMINATED INTRAVASCULAR COAGULATION

Sepsis, or *septicemia,* is a condition in which organisms enter the bloodstream (bloodstream infection [BSI]) and can result in septic shock, a life-threatening condition. Patients with cancer are at risk for INFECTION and sepsis because their white blood cell counts are often low and immune function is impaired. Chapter 37 describes the pathophysiology of sepsis and septic shock.

Disseminated intravascular coagulation (DIC) is a problem with the blood-CLOTTING process. DIC is triggered by many severe illnesses, including cancer. In patients with cancer, DIC often is caused by gram-negative sepsis, although viral and other bacterial INFECTIONS can trigger it. A patient's normal flora can enter the bloodstream through any site of skin breakdown and cause a severe infection, especially when neutropenia is present. Additional causes of sepsis include liver disease, intravascular hemolysis, prosthetic devices, or metabolic acidosis.

Extensive, abnormal CLOTTING occurs throughout the small blood vessels of patients with DIC. This widespread clotting depletes the existing clotting factors and platelets. As this happens, extensive bleeding occurs. Bleeding from many sites is the most common problem and ranges from minimal to fatal hemorrhage. Clots block blood vessels and decrease blood flow to major body organs and result in PAIN, strokelike manifestations, dyspnea, tachycardia, reduced kidney function, and bowel necrosis.

DIC is a life-threatening problem with a high mortality rate even when proper therapies are instituted. *Thus the best management of sepsis and DIC is prevention. Identify patients at greatest risk for sepsis and DIC. Practice strict adherence to aseptic technique during invasive procedures and during contact with nonintact skin and mucous membranes. Teach patients and families the early manifestations of* INFECTION *and when to seek assistance.*

When sepsis is present and DIC is likely, management focuses on reducing the INFECTION and halting the DIC process. IV antibiotic therapy is initiated. During the early phase of DIC, anticoagulants (especially heparin) are given to limit CLOTTING and prevent the rapid consumption of circulating clotting factors. When DIC has progressed and hemorrhage is the primary problem, clotting factors are given. See Chapter 37 for a more detailed discussion of the management of DIC.

SYNDROME OF INAPPROPRIATE ANTIDIURETIC HORMONE

In healthy people, antidiuretic hormone (ADH) is secreted by the posterior pituitary gland only when more fluid (water) is needed in the body, such as when plasma volume is decreased. Certain conditions induce ADH secretion when not needed by the body, which leads to syndrome of inappropriate antidiuretic hormone (SIADH).

Cancer is a common cause of SIADH, especially small cell lung cancer. SIADH also may occur with other cancers, including head and neck, melanoma, gastrointestinal, prostate, and hematologic malignancies, especially when tumors are present in the brain. Some tumors make and secrete ADH, whereas others stimulate the posterior pituitary to secrete ADH. Drugs often used in patients with cancer also can cause SIADH (e.g., morphine sulfate, cyclophosphamide).

In SIADH, water is reabsorbed in excess by the kidney and put into systemic circulation. The retained water dilutes blood sodium levels. Mild manifestations include weakness, muscle cramps, loss of appetite, and fatigue. Serum sodium levels range from 115 to 120 mEq/L or lower (normal range is 135 to 145 mEq/L). With greater fluid retention, weight gain, nervous system changes, personality changes, confusion, and extreme muscle weakness occur. As the sodium level drops toward 110 mEq/L, seizures, coma, and death may follow depending on how rapidly the sodium value is lowered.

SIADH is managed by treating the condition and the cause. Nursing priorities focus on patient safety, restoring normal fluid balance, and providing supportive care. Management includes fluid restriction, increased sodium intake, and drug therapy. One drug, demeclocycline (Declomycin), works in opposition to ADH. Immediate cancer therapy with radiation or chemotherapy may cause enough tumor regression that ADH production returns to normal. Effective treatment of the cancer triggering the syndrome is the only cure for SIADH.

Patient safety includes preventing fluid overload from becoming worse, leading to pulmonary edema and heart failure. The older adult and those with coexisting cardiac problems,

! NURSING SAFETY PRIORITY QSEN

Action Alert

Monitor for increasing fluid overload (bounding pulse, increasing neck vein distention (jugular venous distention [JVD]), presence of crackles in lungs, increasing peripheral edema, reduced urine output) at least every 2 hours. *Pulmonary edema can occur very quickly and can lead to death.* Notify the health care provider of any change that indicates the fluid overload from SIADH either is not responding to therapy or is becoming worse.

kidney problems, lung problems, or liver problems are at greater risk for complications with SIADH. See Chapter 62 for a detailed discussion of SIADH management.

SPINAL CORD COMPRESSION

Spinal cord compression (SCC) and damage occur either when a tumor directly enters the spinal cord or the spinal column or when the vertebrae collapse from tumor degradation of the bone. It is a common cause of neurologic complications of cancer. Tumors may begin in the spinal cord but more often spread from the lung, prostate, breast, and colon. SCC may cause back PAIN or other problems before nerve deficits occur. Neurologic problems are specific to the level of spinal compression and can lead to paralysis, which is usually permanent if the compression is not alleviated promptly. Loss of neurologic function has a tremendous negative impact on quality of life for the patient and family.

Early recognition and treatment of spinal cord compression are key to a positive outcome. Assess for neurologic changes, including back PAIN, muscle weakness or a sensation of heaviness in the arms or legs, numbness or tingling in the hands or feet, inability to distinguish hot and cold, and an unsteady gait. Depending on how low the compression occurs, constipation, incontinence, and difficulty starting or stopping urination also may be present. Consider the possibility of SCC with new onset of any of these problems. Teach patients and families the manifestations of early SCC, and instruct them to seek help as soon as problems occur.

Treatment is often palliative with high-dose corticosteroids given first to reduce swelling around the spinal cord and relieve manifestations. High-dose radiation may be used to reduce the size of the tumor in the area and relieve compression. Surgery may be performed to remove the tumor and rearrange the bony tissue so less pressure is placed on the spinal cord. External back or neck braces may be used to reduce the weight borne by the spinal column and to reduce pressure on the spinal cord or spinal nerves.

HYPERCALCEMIA

Hypercalcemia (increased serum calcium level) occurs in up to a third of patients with cancer. At high levels it is regarded an emergency and can lead to death. Breast, lung, and renal cell carcinomas; multiple myeloma; and adult T-cell leukemia and lymphoma are the most common causes among cancer patients. These cancers can secrete parathyroid hormone, causing bone to release calcium. In addition, systemic secretion of vitamin D analogues by the tumor can also cause elevated calcium levels in the bloodstream. Decreased mobility and dehydration worsen hypercalcemia.

Early manifestations of hypercalcemia are nonspecific and lead to delayed recognition, thus worsening the impact of the problem. Common manifestations include skeletal PAIN, kidney stones, abdominal discomfort, and altered cognition. Additional manifestations include fatigue, loss of appetite, nausea, vomiting, constipation, and increased urine output. More serious problems include severe muscle weakness, loss of deep tendon reflexes, paralytic ileus, dehydration, and electrocardiographic (ECG) changes. Severity of manifestations depends on how high the calcium level is and how quickly it rose (see Chapter 11).

Cancer-induced hypercalcemia often develops slowly for many patients, which allows the body time to adapt to this electrolyte change. As a result, manifestations of hypercalcemia may not be evident until the serum calcium level is greatly elevated. Serum ionized calcium levels are the most reliable laboratory test for this complication.

Oral hydration may be enough to reduce calcium levels and relieve manifestations. Normal saline is used when IV hydration is needed. Loop diuretics can promote calcium loss in urine. Many drugs such as bisphosphonates, which block bone resorption of calcium, calcitonin, and oral glucocorticoids, can temporarily lower serum calcium levels. Treatment of the cancer is needed for long-term calcium control. When cancer-induced hypercalcemia is life threatening or occurs with kidney disease, dialysis can temporarily reduce serum calcium levels.

SUPERIOR VENA CAVA SYNDROME

The superior vena cava (SVC), which returns all blood from the cranial, neck, and upper extremity vasculature to the heart, has thin walls, and compression or obstruction by tumor growth or by clots in the vessel leads to congestion of the blood (Fig. 22-5). This is known as *superior vena cava (SVC) syndrome* and can occur quickly or develop gradually over time. With gradual development, increased collateral circulation to handle the blood flow can occur. SVC compression causes PAIN and is life threatening. It occurs most often in patients with lymphomas (especially with tumors in the mediastinum), thymoma, lung cancer, and breast cancer.

The manifestations result from the blockage of venous return from the head, neck, and upper trunk. Early manifestations occur when the patient arises after a night's sleep and include edema of the face, especially around the eyes, and tightness of the shirt or blouse collar. As the compression worsens, the patient develops engorged blood vessels and erythema of the upper body (Fig. 22-6), edema in the arms and hands, dyspnea, and epistaxis. Late manifestations include hemorrhage, cyanosis, mental status changes, decreased cardiac output, and hypotension. Radiographic imaging is essential for diagnosis and treatment planning. Death results if compression is not relieved.

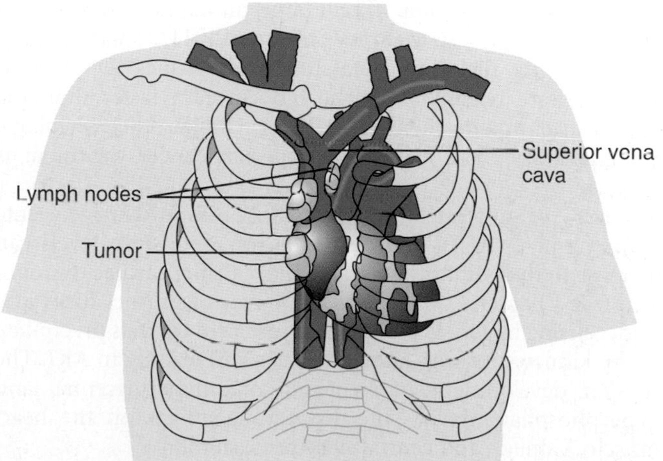

FIG. 22-5 Compression of the superior vena cava by lymph nodes and tumors in superior vena cava syndrome.

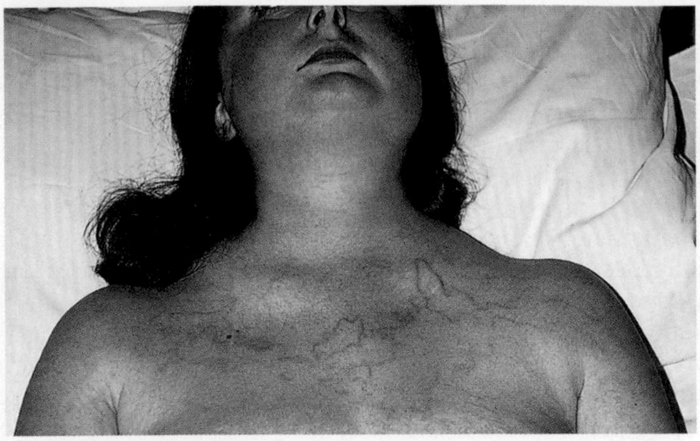

FIG. 22-6 Appearance of the face, neck, upper arms, and chest in a patient with superior vena cava syndrome.

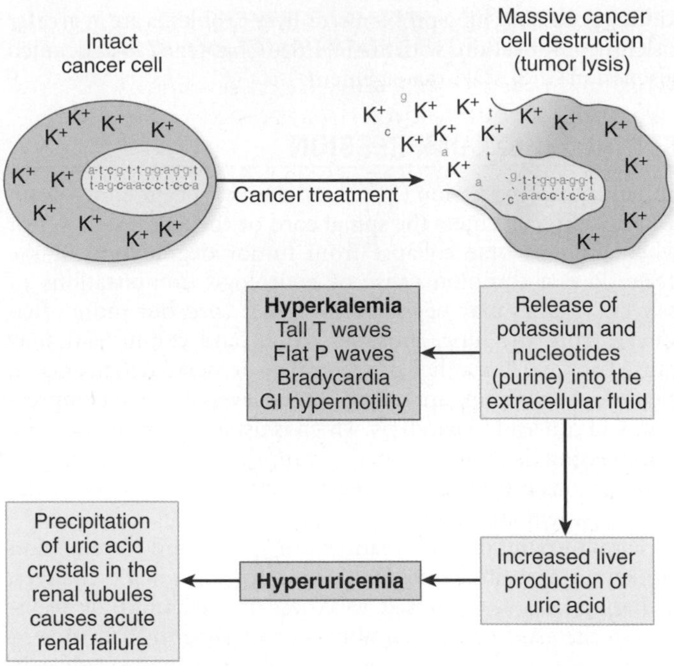

FIG. 22-7 Pathology of tumor lysis syndrome. *K*, Potassium.

SVC syndrome is often a late-stage manifestation; the tumor is usually widespread. High-dose radiation therapy to the upper chest area may be used to provide temporary relief. Chemotherapy may be the only option for long-term control of the cancer causing the compression. Surgery is rarely performed for this condition. A metal stent can be placed in the vena cava in an interventional radiology department to relieve swelling. Follow-up angioplasty can keep this stent open for a longer period.

NCLEX EXAMINATION CHALLENGE

Safe and Effective Care Environment

Which change in health status indicates to the nurse that the client's superior vena cava syndrome is worsening?

A. The client's systolic blood pressure is rising, and the diastolic pressure is decreasing.
B. The client's severe nausea and vomiting no longer respond to antiemetics.
C. The client has experienced four nosebleeds in the past 2 days.
D. Pedal edema is now present.

TUMOR LYSIS SYNDROME

In tumor lysis syndrome (TLS), large numbers of tumor cells are destroyed rapidly (Maloney & Denno, 2011). Their intracellular contents, including potassium and purines (DNA components), are released into the bloodstream faster than the body can eliminate them (Fig. 22-7). Unlike other oncologic emergencies, TLS is a positive sign that cancer treatment is effective.

Severe or untreated TLS can cause tissue damage, acute kidney injury (AKI), and death. Serum potassium levels can increase to the point of hyperkalemia, causing cardiac dysfunction (see Chapter 11). The large amounts of purines form uric acid, causing hyperuricemia. These uric acid crystals precipitate in the kidney, blocking kidney tubules and leading to AKI. The sudden development of hyperkalemia, hyperuricemia, and hyperphosphatemia has life-threatening effects on the heart muscle, kidneys, and central nervous system.

TLS is usually seen in patients receiving radiation or chemotherapy for cancers that are very sensitive to these therapies, including leukemia, lymphoma, small cell lung cancer, germ cell tumors, inflammatory breast cancer, melanoma, and multiple myeloma. Early manifestations include lethargy, nausea, vomiting, anorexia, diarrhea, cloudy urine, flank PAIN, muscle weakness, and cramps.

Hydration prevents and manages TLS by diluting the serum potassium level and increasing the kidney flow rates. These actions prevent the precipitation of uric acid crystals, increase the excretion of potassium, and flush any kidney precipitate.

With tumors known to be very sensitive to cancer therapy, instruct patients to drink at least 3000 mL (5000 mL is more desirable) of fluid the day before, the day of, and for 3 days after treatment. Some fluids should be alkaline (sodium bicarbonate) to help prevent uric acid precipitation. Stress the importance of keeping fluid intake consistent throughout the 24-hour day, and help patients draw up a schedule of fluid intake.

Because some patients have nausea and vomiting after cancer therapy and may not feel like drinking fluids, stress the importance of following the antiemetic regimen. Instruct patients to contact the cancer care provider immediately if nausea prevents adequate fluid intake so parenteral fluids can be started.

Prophylaxis is essential for high-risk patients receiving treatment that is expected to reduce tumor burden quickly. Management becomes more aggressive for patients who become hyperkalemic or hyperuricemic. In addition to fluids, diuretics (especially osmotic types) are given to increase urine flow through the kidney. These agents are used cautiously to avoid dehydration. Drugs that promote purine excretion, such as allopurinol (Aloprim, Zyloprim), rasburicase (Elitek), or febuxostat (Uloric), are given (Mackiewicz, 2012). To reduce serum potassium levels for mild to moderate hyperkalemia, sodium polystyrene sulfonate can be given orally or as a retention enema. For more severe hyperkalemia, IV infusions containing glucose and insulin may be given. Patients who have severe hyperkalemia and hyperuricemia may need dialysis.

NURSING CONCEPTS AND CLINICAL JUDGMENT REVIEW

What might you NOTICE if the patient has impaired protection and increased INFECTION risk as a result of cancer therapy?
- Recurring infections
- Presence of opportunistic infections
- Diarrhea
- Skin lesions
- Headache
- Fever

What should you INTERPRET and how should you RESPOND to a patient who has impaired protection and increased INFECTION risk as a result cancer therapy?

Perform and interpret focused physical assessment findings including:
- Assess cardiovascular and respiratory status:
  - Vital signs
  - Presence of acute chest pain or dyspnea
  - Presence of cough
  - Presence of fever above 100° F (37.8° C)
  - Activity tolerance
- Assess urinary status:
  - Color and clarity of urine
  - Pain or burning on urination
- Assess gastrointestinal status:
  - Mouth, oropharynx, and perineal area for manifestations of infection
  - Presence of dysphagia
  - Presence of nausea, vomiting, diarrhea

Respond by:
- Collaborating with members of the health care team to protect the patient from infection
- Monitoring laboratory test results to determine indications of infection
- Teaching the patient and family about reporting changes indicating infection immediately
- Teaching the patient and family how to avoid infection in the home environment
- Continuing to assess for changes in the patient's condition, especially indications of infection in any body area

On what should you REFLECT?
- Evaluate the patient's and family's knowledge of neutropenia and its management.
- Evaluate the patient's and family's stress levels, use of coping strategies, and knowledge about community resources.
- Assess the knowledge and proficiency of unlicensed assistive personnel (UAP) in carrying out infection control measures.

GET READY FOR THE NCLEX® EXAMINATION!

KEY POINTS

Review these Key Points for each NCLEX Examination Client Needs Category.

Safe and Effective Care Environment
- Use aseptic technique during care for open skin areas or any invasive procedure to prevent INFECTION. **Safety** QSEN
- Perform good handwashing before providing any care to patients with neutropenia.
- Use Bleeding Precautions for any patient with thrombocytopenia and impaired CLOTTING (see Chart 22-5). **Safety** QSEN
- Use appropriate personal protective equipment (gowns, gloves, masks, eye protection) when mixing or administering IV or oral chemotherapeutic drugs and when handling the excreta of a patient receiving chemotherapy and for 48 hours afterward. **Safety** QSEN
- Position shields properly when patients in inpatient settings are receiving brachytherapy. **Safety** QSEN

Health Promotion and Maintenance
- Teach patients receiving radiation therapy how to care for the skin in the radiation path (see Chart 22-2). **Patient-Centered Care** QSEN
- Teach the patient and family about the manifestations of INFECTION and when to seek medical advice. **Patient-Centered Care** QSEN
- Teach patients at risk for bleeding from impaired CLOTTING the precautions to avoid injury (see Chart 22-6). **Patient-Centered Care** QSEN
- Instruct patients to use prescribed antiemetic drugs on a schedule for maximum relief of nausea and vomiting. **Patient-Centered Care** QSEN

Psychosocial Integrity
- Allow the patient and family the opportunity to express concerns regarding the diagnosis of cancer or the treatment regimen. **Patient-Centered Care** QSEN
- Encourage the patient to verbalize feelings about changes in appearance resulting from cancer therapy. **Patient-Centered Care** QSEN
- Explain all procedures, restrictions, drugs, and follow-up care to the patient and family.
- Encourage patients to use strategies to improve their appearance when alopecia occurs. **Patient-Centered Care** QSEN
- Refer patients and family members to local cancer resources and support groups.
- Ensure that patient preferences are honored whenever possible. **Patient-Centered Care** QSEN

Physiological Integrity
- Perform a total assessment each time the patient with cancer is seen to determine the level of cancer treatment side effects

and whether an oncologic emergency exists. **Patient-Centered Care** QSEN

- Assess the patient's PAIN level on a regular basis. **Patient-Centered Care** QSEN
- Use pharmacologic and nonpharmacologic therapies to reduce PAIN for the patient with cancer. **Patient-Centered Care** QSEN
- Work with other members of the health care team to ensure the implementation of a personalized PAIN management regimen. **Teamwork and Collaboration** QSEN
- Assess the venous access device at least every 30 to 60 minutes during chemotherapy administration. **Safety** QSEN
- Assess the patient receiving chemotherapy for INFECTION at least every 8 hours. **Safety** QSEN
- Inspect the oral mucosa of patients with neutropenia at least every 8 hours. **Evidence-Based Practice** QSEN
- Report any temperature over 100° F (37.8° C) in a patient with neutropenia. **Evidence-Based Practice** QSEN
- Assess the patient with thrombocytopenia and impaired CLOTTING for bleeding. **Safety** QSEN
- Instruct the patient and family caring for skin in the path of radiation therapy.
- Assess the patient receiving hormonal therapy for evidence of blood clot formation. **Safety** QSEN
- Closely monitor patients receiving any type of targeted therapy for manifestations of severe side effects or adverse drug reactions. **Safety** QSEN
- Teach patients and families the manifestations of oncologic emergencies and when to notify the health care provider. **Patient-Centered Care** QSEN
- Assist patients and families experiencing cancer to find appropriate community resources for support, supplies, care, and other assistance.

CHAPTER 23

Care of Patients with Infection

Donna D. Ignatavicius

http://evolve.elsevier.com/Iggy/

PRIORITY CONCEPTS

- INFECTION
- IMMUNITY

LEARNING OUTCOMES

Safe and Effective Care Environment

1. Describe INFECTION control methods, such as hand hygiene and Transmission-Based Precautions.
2. Apply current principles of INFECTION prevention and control.

Health Promotion and Maintenance

3. Specify health teaching for patients, families, and staff about INFECTION control measures.

Psychosocial Integrity

4. Plan ways to help patients cope with Transmission-Based Precautions.

Physiological Integrity

5. Identify patients most at risk for INFECTION, including older adults.
6. Provide information to patient and family about drug therapy for infections.
7. Identify common clinical manifestations of infections and infectious diseases.
8. Interpret laboratory test findings related to infections and infectious diseases.
9. Evaluate nursing interventions for management of the patient with an INFECTION.
10. Explain why multidrug-resistant organisms are increasing.
11. Identify basic clinical management for common emerging diseases.

The human body has many *protective* systems that promote homeostasis. Physiologic mechanisms are the structural and functional defenses that protect people from stressors such as infection. When these mechanisms fail to work properly or are overcome with microbes, INFECTION can result.

INFECTIONS and infectious diseases have been the major cause of millions of deaths worldwide for centuries. Threats of bioterrorism have been added to the concerns about multidrug-resistant and emerging infections. Global travel and migration have increased exposure to a wider variety of infectious agents than in the past.

Advancing technology and invasive procedures also introduce microorganisms into the body, often resulting in INFECTION. In other environments these microorganisms are harmless. This chapter provides an overview of infection and general principles for prevention and management. Specific infections and their management are described elsewhere in this text.

OVERVIEW OF THE INFECTIOUS PROCESS

A **pathogen** is any microorganism (also called an *agent*) capable of producing disease. Infections can be **communicable** (transmitted from person to person [e.g., influenza]) or not communicable (e.g., peritonitis). Microorganisms with differing levels of **pathogenicity** (ability to cause disease) surround everyone. **Virulence** is a term for pathogenicity. However, virulence is related more to the frequency with which a pathogen causes disease (degree of communicability) and its ability to invade and damage a host. It can also indicate the severity of the disease.

Many microorganisms live in or on the human host without causing disease. Some microbes are beneficial. Each body location harbors its own characteristic bacteria, or **normal flora**. Normal flora often functions to compete with and prevent INFECTION from unfamiliar agents attempting to invade a body site. In some instances, microorganisms that are often pathogenic may be present in the tissues of the host and yet not cause symptomatic disease because of normal flora; this process is called *colonization*.

In the United States, the Centers for Disease Control and Prevention (CDC) collects information about the occurrence and nature of infections and infectious diseases. It then recommends guidelines to health care agencies for infection control and prevention. Certain diseases, such as tuberculosis, must be reported to health departments and the CDC. The infection control practitioner (ICP) for each health care agency is responsible for tracking infections (**surveillance**) and ensuring compliance with federal and local requirements and accreditation standards.

Transmission of Infectious Agents

Transmission of INFECTION requires three factors:

- Reservoir (or source) of infectious agents
- Susceptible host with a portal of entry
- Mode of transmission

Reservoirs (sources of infectious agents) are numerous. Animate reservoirs include people, animals, and insects. Inanimate reservoirs include soil, water, other environmental sources, and medical equipment (e.g., IV solutions, urine collection devices). Stethoscopes used for auscultation by many health care providers carry *Staphylococcus aureus* from the skin of one patient to another. These devices should be cleaned with an antibacterial solution between patients (Alspach, 2014). The host's body can be a reservoir; pathogens colonize skin and body substances (e.g., feces, sputum, saliva, wound drainage). A person with an active INFECTION or an asymptomatic **carrier** (one who harbors an infectious agent without active disease) is a reservoir. Examples of *community* reservoirs include sewage, stagnant or contaminated water, and improperly handled foods.

Bacteria like *Neisseria meningitidis* can exist in the respiratory tract while causing no illness. If the bacteria invade the bloodstream or cerebrospinal fluid, they become extremely pathogenic. Another example is *Enterococcus,* which lives as normal flora in the GI system, where it is nonpathogenic and assists in the digestive process. If it enters the bloodstream, *Enterococcus* can cause disease.

Continued multiplication of a pathogen is sometimes accompanied by toxin production. **Toxins** are protein molecules released by bacteria to affect host cells at a distant site. *Exotoxins* are produced and released by certain bacteria into the surrounding environment. Botulism, tetanus, diphtheria, and *Escherichia coli* 0157:H7–related systemic diseases are attributed to exotoxins. *Endotoxins* are produced in the cell walls of certain bacteria and released only with cell lysis. For example, typhoid and meningococcal diseases are caused by endotoxins.

Host factors influence the development of INFECTION (Table 23-1). Host defenses provide the body with an efficient system for *protection* against pathogens. Breakdown of these defense mechanisms may increase the **susceptibility** (risk) of the host for infection.

The patient's *immune status* plays a large role in determining risk for infection. Congenital abnormalities, as well as acquired health problems (e.g., renal failure, steroid dependence, cancer, acquired immune deficiency syndrome [AIDS]), can result in numerous immunologic deficiencies. Depression of IMMUNITY may make the host more susceptible to infection or impair the ability to combat organisms that have gained entry.

Immunity is resistance to INFECTION; it is usually associated with the presence of antibodies or cells that act on specific microorganisms. **Passive immunity** is of short duration (days or months) and either natural by transplacental transfer from the mother or artificial by injection of antibodies (e.g., immunoglobulin). **Active immunity** lasts for years and is natural by infection or artificial by stimulation of the body's immune defenses (e.g., vaccination). Chapter 17 discusses the immune system and IMMUNITY in detail.

Environmental factors can also influence patients' immune status and thus their susceptibility to or ability to fight INFECTION. Examples include alcohol consumption, nicotine use, inhalation of bone marrow–suppressing toxic chemicals, and certain vitamin deficiencies. Malnutrition, especially protein-calorie malnutrition, places patients at increased risk for infection. Diseases such as diabetes mellitus also predispose a patient to infection. Older adults have decreased immunity, as well as other physiologic changes that make them very susceptible to infection (Chart 23-1).

TABLE 23-1 Host Factors That Influence the Development of Infection

HOST FACTOR	INCREASED RISK FOR INFECTION
Natural immunity	Congenital or acquired immune deficiencies
Normal flora	Alteration of normal flora by antibiotic therapy
Age	Infants and older adults
Hormonal factors	Diabetes mellitus, corticosteroid therapy, and adrenal insufficiency
Phagocytosis	Defective phagocytic function, circulatory disturbances, and neutropenia
Skin/mucous membranes/ normal excretory secretions	Break in skin or mucous membrane integrity; interference with flow of urine, tears, or saliva; interference with cough reflex or ciliary action; changes in gastric secretions
Nutrition	Malnutrition or dehydration
Environmental factors	Tobacco and alcohol consumption and inhalation of toxic chemicals
Medical interventions	Invasive therapy such as endoscopy, urinary catheters, IVs; chemotherapy, radiation therapy, and steroid therapy (suppress immune system); surgery

CHART 23-1 Nursing Focus on the Older Adult

Factors That May Increase Risk for Infection in the Older Patient

FACTOR	AGING-ASSOCIATED CHANGES OR CONDITIONS
• Immune system	• Decreased antibody production, lymphocytes, and fever response
• Integumentary system	• Thinning skin, decreased subcutaneous tissue, decreased vascularity, slower wound healing
• Respiratory system	• Decreased cough and gag reflexes
• Gastrointestinal system	• Decreased gastric acid and intestinal motility
• Chronic illness	• Diabetes mellitus, chronic obstructive pulmonary disease, neurologic impairments
• Functional/cognitive impairments	• Immobility, incontinence, dementia
• Invasive devices	• Urinary catheters, feeding tubes, IV devices, tracheostomy tubes
• Institutionalization	• Increased person-to-person contact and transmission

Medical and surgical interventions may impair normal immune response. Steroid therapy, chemotherapy, and antirejection drugs increase the risk for INFECTION. Medical devices (e.g., intravascular or urinary catheters, endotracheal tubes, synthetic implants) may also interfere with normal host defense mechanisms. Surgery, trauma, radiation therapy, and burns result in nonintact skin. *The body's skin is one of the best barriers or defenses against infection.* When this barrier is broken, infection often results. Microorganisms may enter the body in a variety of ways, including the respiratory tract, GI tract, genitourinary tract, skin and mucous membranes, and bloodstream.

Routes of Transmission

Pathogens may enter the body through the *respiratory tract.* Microbes in droplets are sprayed into the air when people with infected oral or nasal tissues talk, cough, or sneeze. A susceptible host then inhales droplets, and pathogens localize in the lungs or are distributed via the lymphatic system or bloodstream to other areas of the body. Microorganisms that enter the body by the respiratory tract and produce distant infection include influenza virus, *Mycobacterium tuberculosis,* and *Streptococcus pneumoniae.*

Other pathogens enter the body through the *GI tract.* Some stay there and produce disease (e.g., *Shigella* causing self-limited disease). Others invade the GI tract to produce local and distant infection (e.g., *Salmonella enteritidis*). Some produce limited GI symptoms, causing systemic infection (e.g., *Salmonella typhi*) or profound involvement of other organs (e.g., hepatitis A virus). Millions of foodborne illness cases occur each year in the United States. This type of illness results in many hospitalizations and deaths.

Microorganisms also enter through the *genitourinary tract. Urinary tract infection (UTI) is one of the most common health care–associated infections (HAIs).* More than half of patients in adult intensive care units (ICUs) have urinary catheters in place. Indwelling urinary catheters are a primary cause of *catheter-associated urinary tract infections (CAUTIs),* especially in older adults. CAUTIs can increase hospital costs by prolonging the patient's length of stay and complicating the patient's recovery. In many settings, nurse-driven protocols have helped decrease the use of urinary catheters and associated infections (see the Quality Improvement box).

Although intact skin is the best barrier to prevent most infections, some pathogens such as *Treponema pallidum* can enter the body through intact *skin* or *mucous membranes.* Most enter through breaks in these normally effective surface barriers. Sometimes a medical procedure creates a break in cutaneous or mucocutaneous barriers, as in catheter-acquired **bacteremia** (bacteria in the bloodstream) and surgical-site infections (SSIs). *Fragile skin of older patients and of those receiving prolonged steroid therapy increases infection risk.*

Microorganisms can gain direct access to the *bloodstream,* especially when invasive devices or tubes are used. The incidence of bloodstream infections (BSIs) continues to increase in hospitals throughout the United States. Central venous catheters (CVCs) are a primary cause of these infections (see Chapter 13 for more discussion of CVC-related BSIs). In the community setting, biting insects can inject organisms into the bloodstream, causing infection (e.g., Lyme disease, West Nile viral encephalitis).

QUALITY IMPROVEMENT (QSEN)

Reducing Catheter-Associated Urinary Tract Infections

Mori, C. (2014). A-voiding catastrophe: Implementing a nurse-driven protocol. *MEDSURG Nursing, 23*(1), 15-21, 28.

In spite of the move to decrease the use of indwelling urinary catheters (e.g., Foley catheters), catheter-associated urinary tract infections (CAUTIs) remain a major cause of sepsis and increased hospital costs. The Centers for Medicare and Medicaid Services (CMS) recently began to link health care reimbursement to quality improvement efforts to prevent CAUTIs.

An interdisciplinary team led by a clinical nurse specialist in a Midwestern community hospital implemented a protocol that decreased the use of urinary catheters and ensured best practices for patients for whom the catheters were indicated. Using a screening checklist, each patient was assessed to determine the need for a Foley catheter. If certain criteria were not met, the catheter was removed by a nurse using a specific protocol during and after removal. For patients who had to have a Foley catheter, the nurse provided care to minimize the chance for urinary infection, including checking that the:

- Catheter was secure
- Tamper-evident seal was intact
- Catheter tubing was not twisted or had a dependent loop
- Catheter bag was positioned lower than the bladder level
- Drainage bag did not touch the floor or was overfilled.

Commentary: Implications for Practice and Research

Research demonstrates that decreasing the use of indwelling urinary catheters is the most important intervention to prevent hospital-acquired CAUTIs. This project used this research and showed how an interdisciplinary team led by a CNS in a community hospital could improve the quality of care by decreasing urinary tract infections. In addition, nurses provided evidence-based care for patients who needed urinary catheters to ensure adequate urinary flow.

A limitation of the project was that incremental changes or strategies to maintain the positive changes were not discussed. More quality improvement activities at a unit or health care agency are needed to use current research, sustain a change in nursing practice, and achieve positive patient outcomes.

Methods of Transmission

For INFECTION to be transmitted from an infected source to a susceptible host, a transport mechanism is required. Microorganisms are transmitted by several routes:

- Contact transmission (indirect and direct)
- Droplet transmission
- Airborne transmission

Contact transmission is the usual mode of transmission of most infections. Many INFECTIONS are spread by direct or indirect contact. With *direct contact,* the source and host have physical contact. Microorganisms are transferred directly from skin to skin or from mucous membrane to mucous membrane. Often called *person-to-person transmission,* direct contact is best illustrated by the spread of the "common cold."

Indirect contact transmission involves the transfer of microorganisms from a source to a host by passive transfer from a contaminated object. Contaminated articles or hands may be sources of infection. For example, patient-care devices like glucometers and electronic thermometers may transmit pathogens if they are contaminated with blood or body fluids. Uniforms, laboratory coats, and isolation gowns used as part of personal protective equipment (PPE) may be contaminated as well.

Indirect transmission may involve contact with infected secretions or *droplets.* Droplets are produced when a person talks or sneezes; the droplets travel short distances. Susceptible hosts may acquire infection by contact with droplets deposited on the nasal, oral, or conjunctival membranes. Therefore the CDC recommends that staff stay at least 3 feet (1 m) away from a patient with droplet infection. An example of droplet-spread INFECTION is influenza.

Airborne transmission occurs when small airborne particles containing pathogens leave the infected source and enter a susceptible host. These pathogens can be suspended in the air for a prolonged time. The particles carrying pathogens are usually contained in droplet nuclei or dust; they are usually propelled from the respiratory tract by coughing or sneezing. A susceptible person then inhales the particles directly into the respiratory tract. For example, tuberculosis is spread via airborne transmission.

Preventing the spread of microbes that are transmitted by the airborne route requires the use of special air handling and ventilation systems in an airborne infection isolation room (AIIR). *M. tuberculosis* and the varicella-zoster virus (chickenpox) are examples of airborne agents that require one of these systems. In addition to the AIIR, respiratory protection using a certified **powered air purifying respirator (PAPR)** is recommended for health care personnel entering the patient's room. This device has a high efficiency particulate air (HEPA) filter and battery to promote positive-pressure airflow and is more effective than N95 respirators.

Other sources of infectious agents include the environment, such as contaminated food, water, or vectors. Vectors are insects that carry pathogens between two or more hosts, such as the deer tick that causes Lyme disease.

The *portal of exit* completes the chain of INFECTION. Exit of the microbe from the host often occurs through the portal of entry. An organism, such as *M. tuberculosis,* enters the respiratory tract and then exits the same tract as the infected host coughs. Some organisms can exit from the infected host by several routes. For example, varicella-zoster virus can spread through direct contact with infective fluid in vesicles and by airborne transmission.

Physiologic Defenses for Infection

Strong and intact host defenses can prevent microbes from entering the body or can destroy a pathogen that has entered. Impaired host defenses may be unable to defend against microbial invasion, allowing entry of organisms that can destroy cells and cause INFECTION. Common defense mechanisms include:

- Body tissues
- Phagocytosis
- Inflammation
- Immune systems

Intact skin forms the first and most important physical barrier to the entry of microorganisms. In addition to providing a mechanical barrier, the skin's slightly acidic pH (resulting from breakdown of lipids into fatty acids), together with normal skin flora, creates an unfriendly environment for many bacteria.

Mucous membranes' mucociliary action provides some mechanical protection against pathogenic invasion. More important, however, mucous membranes are bathed in secretions that inactivate many microorganisms. Lysozymes, which dissolve the cell walls of some bacteria, are present in large quantities in many body secretions, particularly in tears and nasal mucus.

Other body systems provide natural barriers to INFECTION. For instance, the healthy respiratory tract clears most of all inhaled material by upper airway filtration, humidification, mucociliary transport, and coughing. Peristaltic action mechanically empties the GI tract of pathogenic organisms. Stomach acid, intestinal secretions, pancreatic enzymes, and bile, together with the competition from normal bowel flora, provide an environment that protects the GI tract from invasion by harmful organisms. In the genitourinary tract, the flushing action of urine eliminates pathogenic organisms. The low pH of urine also maintains a sterile environment, although some microorganisms, such as *E. coli,* can thrive in an acid medium.

Phagocytosis occurs when a foreign substance evades the first-line mechanical barriers and enters the body. Various leukocyte types function differently in the immune reaction, but neutrophils bear primary responsibility for phagocytosis. This process of engulfing, ingesting, killing, and disposing of an invading organism is an essential mechanism in host defense. Phagocytic dysfunction dramatically increases a patient's risk for INFECTION.

Inflammation is another important nonspecific defense mechanism for preventing the spread of INFECTION. It occurs when tissue becomes damaged. Damaged cells release enzymes, and polymorphonuclear (PMN) leukocytes (neutrophils) are attracted to the infected site from the bloodstream. One important substance, histamine, increases the permeability of the capillaries in inflamed tissues, thus allowing fluid, proteins, and white blood cells to enter an inflamed area. Other enzymes activate fibrinogen, which causes leaked fluid to clot and prevents its flow away from the damaged site into unaffected tissue, essentially "walling off" the inflamed tissue. The process of phagocytosis disposes of the invading microorganism and often dead tissue. If inflammation is caused by infection, the end products of inflammation form pus, which is then absorbed or exits the body through a break in the skin. Chapter 17 discusses the process of inflammation in more detail.

Specific defense responses to specific microorganisms are provided by the antibody- and cell-mediated immune systems. The **antibody-mediated immune system** produces antibodies directed against certain pathogens. These antibodies inactivate or destroy invading microorganisms as well as protect against future infection from that microorganism. Resistance to other microorganisms is mediated by the action of specifically sensitized T-lymphocytes and is called **cell-mediated immunity**. The components of the immune system work both independently and together to protect against infection. Chapter 17 describes the function of the immune system in detail.

HEALTH PROMOTION AND MAINTENANCE

Infections occur most often in high-risk patients, such as older adults and those who have inadequate immune systems (immunocompromised). Implement interventions to prevent infection and detect signs and symptoms as early as possible. Chart 23-2 summarizes nursing interventions for INFECTION prevention and control.

Infection Control in Health Care Settings

INFECTION acquired in the inpatient health care setting (not present or incubating at admission) is termed a **health**

CHART 23-2 Best Practices for Patient Safety & Quality Care QSEN

Nursing Interventions for the Patient at Risk for Infection

- Assess patients for risk for infections.
- Monitor for signs and symptoms of infection.
- Monitor laboratory tests results, such as cultures and white blood cell (WBC) count and differential.
- Screen all visitors for infections or infectious disease.
- Inspect skin and mucous membranes for redness, heat, pain, swelling, and drainage.
- Promote sufficient nutritional intake, especially protein for healing.
- Encourage fluid intake to treat fever.
- Teach the patient and family the signs and symptoms of infections and when to report them to the health care provider.
- Teach the patient and family how to avoid infections in health care agencies and the community.

CHART 23-3 Best Practice for Patient Safety & Quality Care QSEN

Hand Hygiene

- When hands are visibly soiled or contaminated with proteinaceous material or are visibly soiled with blood or other body fluids, wash hands with soap and water.
- If hands are not visibly soiled, use an alcohol-based hand rub (ABHR) for decontaminating hands or wash hands with soap and water.
- Use either ABHR or wash with soap and water (decontaminate hands) before having direct contact with patients.
- Decontaminate hands before donning sterile gloves to perform a procedure, such as inserting an invasive device (e.g., indwelling urinary catheter).
- Decontaminate hands after contact with a patient's intact skin (e.g., taking a pulse) or with body fluids or excretions/secretions.
- Decontaminate hands after removing gloves.
- Decontaminate hands after contact with inanimate objects (including medical equipment) in the immediate vicinity of the patient.

care–associated infection (HAI). When occurring in a hospital setting, they are sometimes referred to as *hospital-acquired infections,* but the former term is more accurate. HAIs can be *endogenous* (from a patient's flora) or *exogenous* (from outside the patient, often from the hands of health care workers, tubes, or implants). HAIs, including surgical site infections (SSIs), cause increased health care costs and many deaths (see discussion in Chapter 16). These infections tend to occur most often because health care workers do not follow basic infection control principles.

Infection control within a health care facility is designed to reduce the risk for HAIs and thus reduce morbidity and mortality, as recommended in The Joint Commission's National Patient Safety Goals (NPSGs). This expected outcome is consistent with the desire for health care facilities to create a *culture of safety* within their environments (see Chapter 1). INFECTION control and prevention is an interdisciplinary effort and includes:

- Facility- and department-specific infection control policies and procedures
- Surveillance and analysis
- Patient and staff education
- Community and interdisciplinary collaboration
- Product evaluation with an emphasis on quality and cost savings
- Bioengineering for designing health care facilities that help control the spread of infections

The INFECTION control program of a hospital is coordinated and implemented by a health care professional certified in infection control (CIC) who has clinical and administrative experience. The Centers for Disease Control and Prevention (CDC) recommends one person with CIC credentials for every 100 occupied acute care beds. Long-term care facilities may not have a practitioner who specializes in infection control. However, every facility must designate a health care professional to be responsible for coordinating and implementing an infection prevention and control program.

Long-term care facilities are unique in that they have a large group of older adults who are together in one setting for weeks to years. Nursing homes, in particular, are required to provide a homelike environment in which residents can move and interact freely. Therefore INFECTION control in these settings can be challenging. As a result, many infectious outbreaks may occur, such as pneumonia, *Clostridium difficile,* and multidrug-resistant organisms (discussed in the Multidrug-Resistant Organism Infections and Colonizations section on p. 405).

Ambulatory and home health care are the fastest growing segments of the health care system. INFECTION remains a common cause of death for dialysis patients. Little information is available about acquired infections in home health settings because data are not systematically collected, surveillance programs are not established, and best practices for infection prevention and control do not yet exist.

Methods of Infection Control and Prevention

All health care workers who come in contact with patients or care areas are involved in some aspect of the infection control program of the agency. According to the CDC, infections can be prevented or controlled in several ways:

- Hand hygiene
- Disinfection/sterilization
- Standard Precautions
- Transmission-Based Precautions
- Staff and patient placement and cohorting

Hand Hygiene

Health care workers' hands are the primary way in which infection is transmitted from patient to patient or staff to patient. **Hand hygiene** refers to both handwashing and alcohol-based hand rubs (ABHRs) ("hand sanitizers").

In 2002, the U.S. CDC released a document entitled "CDC Hand Hygiene Recommendations." These recommendations are summarized in Chart 23-3. *Handwashing is still an important part of hand hygiene, but it is recognized that in some health care settings, sinks may not be readily available.* Despite years of education, health care workers do not wash their hands or perform hand hygiene on a consistent basis (Upshaw-Owens & Bailey, 2012). The Quality Improvement box describes one hospital unit's project to improve the percentage of health care workers who perform hand hygiene.

Effective handwashing includes wetting, soaping, lathering, applying friction under running water for at least 15 seconds, rinsing, and adequate drying. Friction is essential to remove skin oils and to disperse transient bacteria and soil from hand surfaces. Performing adequate handwashing takes time that health care workers (HCWs) may not feel they have. Handwashing can

QUALITY IMPROVEMENT (QSEN)

Improving Nursing Staff Compliance with Proper Hand Hygiene

Foulk, K.C., Tocydlowski, P., Snow, T.M., McCloud, K., Cuevas, M., Bishop, D., et al. (2012). Infusing fun into quality and safety initiatives. *Nursing2012, 42*(11), 14-16.

Proper hand hygiene is essential for patient safety to prevent the spread of infection. Nurses on a medical-surgical unit in a large mid-Atlantic hospital recognized that their unit's compliance with using proper hand hygiene was only 71%, lower than the rate for the rest of the hospital. As a result, the unit had a total of 12 *Clostridium difficile* infections over a one-year period. The quality and safety (QI) council of the unit set a goal of achieving 90% compliance with proper hand hygiene and implemented a project to change practice over the next year.

Interventions used to increase compliance included reminders in monthly staff meetings and newsletters, e-mails, and bulletin board postings. A hand hygiene game and music video (entitled "Get Your Clean On") were developed and used by the nursing staff. Each shift's charge nurse gave red laminated hands to any staff member who was not performing proper hand hygiene. The member who collected the most "hot hands" at the end of the shift was considered the most noncompliant. As a result of these interventions, the data for the following year revealed a 98% compliance with proper hand hygiene and a total of only 6 *C. difficile* infections. These data suggest that increased compliance with hand hygiene resulted in a decrease in hospital-acquired infections.

Commentary: Implications for Practice and Research

Research demonstrates that proper hand hygiene is the most important intervention to prevent hospital-acquired infections. This project utilized this research and showed how one group of nurses on a hospital unit could improve the quality of care by decreasing unit infections. The staff took a unit view to develop a variety of approaches to change behaviors. They reported that the project was fun as well as informative.

A limitation of the project was that incremental changes or strategies to maintain the positive changes were not discussed. More quality improvement activities at a unit or health care agency are needed to utilize current research, sustain a change in nursing practice, and achieve positive patient outcomes.

also cause dry skin, and therefore hand moisturizers are essential to maintain good hand health and hygiene.

Alcohol-based hand rubs (ABHRs) allow care providers to spend less time seeking out sinks and more time delivering care. However, these hand rubs have their limitations.

! NURSING SAFETY PRIORITY (QSEN)

Action Alert

If your hands are visibly dirty or soiled or feel sticky or if you have just toileted, *wash your hands instead of using ABHRs.* Keep in mind that ABHRs are also ineffective against spore-forming organisms such as *Clostridium difficile,* a common cause of health care–associated diarrhea, especially in older adults. Do not use an ABHR before inserting eye drops, ointments, or contact lenses because alcohol can irritate the patient's eyes, causing burning and redness. The Joint Commission's National Patient Safety Goals require that health care agencies monitor handwashing practices and the use of ABHRs to make sure that HCWs are performing hand hygiene on a regular basis.

The CDC recommends using antiseptic solutions such as chlorhexidine for handwashing in caring for patients who are at high risk for infection (e.g., those who are immunocompromised).

The classic CDC guidelines (Centers for Disease Control and Prevention [CDC], 2002) also address the issue of artificial fingernails, which have been linked to a number of outbreaks due to poor fingernail health and hygiene. The guidelines recommend that artificial fingernails and extenders not be worn while caring for patients at high risk for infections, such as those in ICUs or operating suites. Most health care agencies have banned artificial nails for all health care workers providing direct patient care and require that natural nails be short. Some agencies also ban the use of nail polish.

Sterilization and Disinfection

Sterilization and disinfection have helped invasive procedures become much more common and safe. **Sterilization** means destroying all living organisms and bacterial spores. Many invasive procedures, such as inserting vascular access devices (VADs) and urinary catheters, require sterile technique. Sterile technique in the operating suite is discussed in detail in Chapter 15.

All items that invade human tissue where bacteria are not commonly found should be sterilized. **Disinfection** does not kill spores and only ensures a reduction in the level of disease-causing organisms. High-level disinfection is adequate when an item is going inside the body where the patient has resident bacteria or normal flora (e.g., GI and respiratory tracts). As with sterilization, no high-level disinfection can occur without first cleaning the item. This can be especially difficult with items that have narrow lumens in which organic debris can become trapped and is not easily visible. For example, endoscopes have been especially challenging to clean and have been linked to a number of infectious outbreaks.

Standard Precautions

The 2007 guidelines from the CDC focus on transmission mechanisms and the precautions needed to prevent the spread of infection. Included in these guidelines are Standard Precautions and Transmission-Based Precautions, including Airborne, Droplet, and Contact Precautions (Tables 23-2 and 23-3).

Standard Precautions are based on the belief that all body excretions, secretions, and moist membranes and tissues, excluding perspiration, are potentially infectious. As barriers to potential or actual infections, **personal protective equipment (PPE)** is used. PPE refers to gloves, isolation gowns, face protection (masks, goggles, face shields), and powered air purifying respirators (PAPRs) or N95 respirators (Fig. 23-1).

! NURSING SAFETY PRIORITY (QSEN)

Action Alert

Remember that gloves are an essential part of INFECTION control and should always be worn as part of Standard Precautions. Either handwashing or use of alcohol-based hand rubs should be done before donning and after removing gloves. The combination of hand hygiene and wearing gloves is the most effective strategy for preventing infection transmission!

Health care settings in the United States and Canada have switched from latex to non-latex gloves. The U.S. National Institute for Occupational Safety and Health (NIOSH) issued a public warning about potential allergic reactions to those exposed to latex in gloves and other medical products. Reactions include rashes, nasal or eye symptoms, asthma, and (rarely) shock. People with **latex allergy** usually have an allergy to foods such as bananas, kiwis, and avocados. Health care

TABLE 23-2 **Recommendations for Application of Standard Precautions for the Care of All Patients in All Health Care Settings**

COMPONENT	RECOMMENDATIONS
Hand hygiene	Perform hand hygiene after touching blood, body fluids, secretions, excretions, contaminated items; immediately after removing gloves; between patient contacts
Personal protective equipment (PPE)	Use appropriate PPE, including:
• Gloves	For touching blood, body fluids, secretions, excretions, contaminated items; for touching mucous membranes and nonintact skin
• Gown	During procedures and patient-care activities when contact of clothing/exposed skin with blood/body fluids, secretions, and excretions is anticipated
• Mask, eye protection (goggles), face shield*	During procedures and patient-care activities likely to generate splashes or sprays of blood, body fluids, secretions, especially suctioning, endotracheal intubation
Soiled patient-care equipment	Handle in a manner that prevents transfer of microorganisms to others and to the environment; wear gloves if visibly contaminated; perform hand hygiene
Environmental control	Develop procedures for routine care, cleaning, and disinfection of environmental surfaces, especially frequently touched surfaces in patient-care areas
Textiles and laundry	Handle in a manner that prevents transfer of microorganisms to others and to the environment
Needles and other sharps	Do not recap, bend, break, or hand-manipulate used needles; use safety features such as needleless systems when available; place used sharps in puncture-resistant container
Patient resuscitation	Use mouthpiece, resuscitation bag, other ventilation devices to prevent contact with mouth and oral secretions
Patient placement	Prioritize for single-patient room if patient is at increased risk for transmission, is likely to contaminate the environment, does not maintain appropriate hygiene, or is at increased risk for acquiring infection or developing adverse outcome following infection
Respiratory hygiene/cough etiquette (source containment of infectious respiratory secretions in symptomatic patients, beginning at initial point of encounter [e.g., triage and reception areas in emergency departments and physician offices])	Instruct symptomatic persons to cover mouth/nose when sneezing/coughing; use tissues and dispose in no-touch receptacle; observe hand hygiene after soiling of hands with respiratory secretions; wear surgical mask if tolerated or maintain spatial separation, >3 feet if possible

*During aerosol-generating procedures on patients with suspected or proven infections transmitted by respiratory aerosols, wear a powered air purifying respirator (PAPR) (most effective) or N95 mask in addition to gloves, gown, and face/eye protection.

workers (HCWs) have not been as strict with wearing gloves as they should because of poor fit or skin dryness, irritation, and dermatitis. One possible solution to dry skin is the use of aloe vera–coated gloves or moisturizers such as Eucerin or AmLactin products.

The respiratory hygiene/cough etiquette (RH/CE) requirement is directed at patients and visitors with signs of respiratory illness, such as sinus or chest congestion, cough, or rhinorrhea ("runny nose"). The elements for RH/CE include:

- Patient, staff, and visitor education
- Posted signs
- Hand hygiene
- Covering the nose and mouth with a tissue and prompt tissue disposal or using surgical masks (or sneezing/coughing into a shirt sleeve rather than the hand)
- Separation from the person with respiratory INFECTION by more than 3 feet (1 m)

Transmission-Based Precautions

Transmission-Based Precautions may also be referred to as *Isolation Precautions.* But, the word *isolation* implies that the patient is physically separated from everyone, which is not always the case.

Airborne Precautions are used for patients known or suspected to have INFECTIONS transmitted by the airborne transmission route. These infections are caused by organisms that can be suspended in air for prolonged periods. Negative airflow rooms are required to prevent airborne spread of microbes. Enclosed booths with high-efficiency particulate air (HEPA) filtration or ultraviolet light may be used for sputum induction procedures. Tuberculosis, measles (rubeola), and chickenpox (varicella) are examples of airborne diseases.

Droplet Precautions are used for patients known or suspected to have INFECTIONS transmitted by the droplet transmission route. Such infections are caused by organisms in droplets that may travel 3 feet but are not suspended for long periods. Examples of infectious conditions requiring Droplet Precautions include influenza, mumps, pertussis, and meningitis caused by either *N. meningitidis* or *Haemophilus influenzae* type B.

Contact Precautions are used for patients known or suspected to have INFECTIONS transmitted by direct contact or contact with items in the environment. Patients with significant multidrug-resistant organism (MDRO) infection or colonization, such as methicillin-resistant *Staphylococcus aureus* (MRSA) or vancomycin-resistant *Enterococcus* (VRE), are placed on Contact Precautions. Other infections requiring Contact Precautions include pediculosis (lice), scabies, respiratory syncytial virus (RSV), and *C. difficile.*

Staff and Patient Placement and Cohorting

Adequate staffing of nurses is an essential method for preventing INFECTION. In addition to a ratio of one infection control practitioner to 100 occupied acute care beds, nurse staffing is critical. When possible, bedside nurse staffing should consist of full-time nurses assigned regularly to the unit to ensure consistent practices (Upshaw-Owens & Bailey, 2012).

TABLE 23-3 **Transmission-Based Infection Control Precautions**

PRECAUTIONS (IN ADDITION TO STANDARD PRECAUTIONS)	EXAMPLES OF DISEASES IN CATEGORY
Airborne Precautions	
1. Private room required with monitored negative airflow (with appropriate number of air exchanges and air discharge to outside or through HEPA filter); keep door(s) closed 2. Special respiratory protection: • Wear PAPR for known or suspected TB • Susceptible persons not to enter room of patient with known or suspected measles or varicella unless immune caregivers are not available • Susceptible persons who must enter room must wear PAPR or N95 HEPA filter* 3. Transport: patient to leave room only for essential clinical reasons, wearing surgical mask	Diseases that are known or suspected to be transmitted by air: Measles (rubeola) *Mycobacterium tuberculosis,* including multidrug-resistant TB (MDRTB) Varicella (chickenpox)†; disseminated zoster (shingles)†
Droplet Precautions	
1. Private room preferred: if not available, may cohort with patient with same active infection with same microorganisms if no other infection present; maintain distance of at least 3 feet from other patients if private room not available 2. Mask: required when working within 3 feet of patient 3. Transport: as above	Diseases that are known or suspected to be transmitted by droplets: Diphtheria (pharyngeal) Streptococcal pharyngitis Pneumonia Influenza Rubella Invasive disease (meningitis, pneumonia, sepsis) caused by *Haemophilus influenzae* type B or *Neisseria meningitidis* Mumps Pertussis
Contact Precautions	
1. Private room preferred: if not available, may cohort with patient with same active infection with same microorganisms if no other infection present 2. Wear gloves when entering room 3. Wash hands with antimicrobial soap before leaving patient's room 4. Wear gown to prevent contact with patient or contaminated items or if patient has uncontrolled body fluids; remove gown before leaving room 5. Transport: patient to leave room only for essential clinical reasons; during transport, use needed precautions to prevent disease transmission 6. Dedicated equipment for this patient only (or disinfect after use before taking from room)	Diseases that are known or suspected to be transmitted by direct contact: *Clostridium difficile* Colonization or infection caused by multidrug-resistant organisms (e.g., MRSA, VRE) Pediculosis Respiratory syncytial virus Scabies

HEPA, High-efficiency particulate air; *MRSA,* methicillin-resistant *Staphylococcus aureus; PAPR,* powered air purifying respirator; *TB,* tuberculosis; *VRE,* vancomycin-resistant *Enterococcus.*
*Before use: training and fit testing required for personnel.
†Add Contact Precautions for draining lesions.

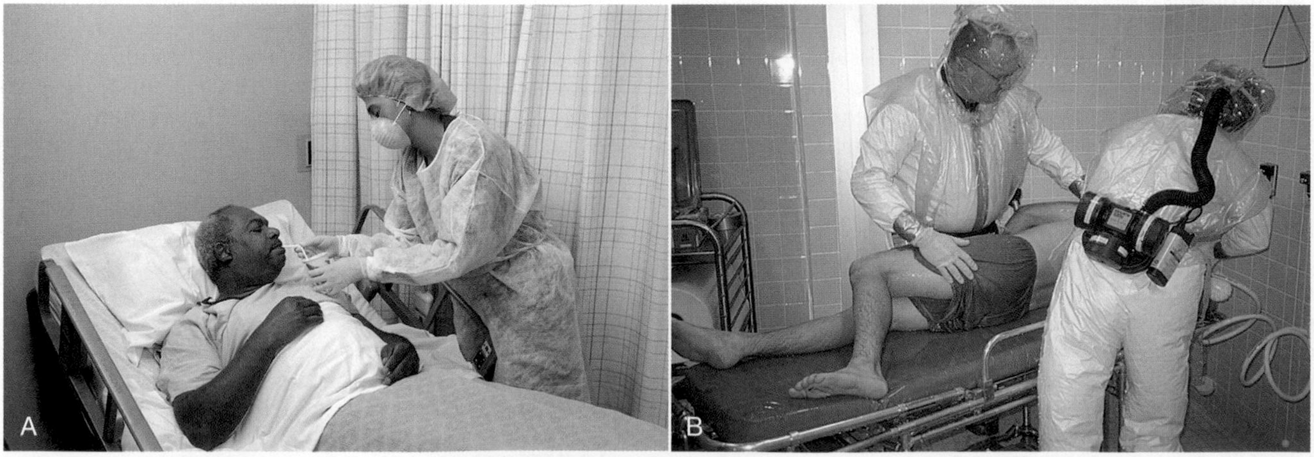

FIG. 23-1 A, Nurse in personal protective equipment (PPE) caring for a patient in a private room. **B,** Powered air purifying respirator (PAPR).

Patient placement has been used as a way to reduce the spread of INFECTION. The CDC does not mandate that all patients with infections have a private room. It does recommend that private rooms always be used for patients on Airborne Precautions and those in a protective environment (PE). A PE is architecturally designed and structured to prevent INFECTION from occurring in patients who are at extremely high risk, such as those having stem cell therapy. The CDC also prefers private rooms for patients who are on Contact and Droplet Precautions. If private rooms are not available, keep these patients at least 3 feet apart. Many hospitals are becoming totally private-room facilities. Large health care systems have biomedical engineers to assist in designing the best environment to reduce the spread of infection, including ventilation systems and physical layout.

Cohorting is another method of patient placement. **Cohorting** is the practice of grouping patients who are colonized or infected with the same pathogen. This method has been used the most with patients who have an outbreak of a multidrug-resistant organism like methicillin-resistant *Staphylococcus aureus* (MRSA). It is particularly effective in long-term care settings.

INFECTION control principles for *patient transport* include limiting movement to other areas of the facility, using appropriate barriers like covering infected wounds, and notifying other departments or agencies who are receiving the patient about the necessary precautions. Accurate hand-off communication between agencies is also very important to prevent the spread of infection, according to The Joint Commission's NPSGs.

NCLEX EXAMINATION CHALLENGE

Safe and Effective Care Environment

Which statement by a nursing student indicates a need for further teaching by the nurse regarding infection control for a client who has an open, draining wound?

A. "I will wear an isolation gown when providing direct care."
B. "I will wear gloves when changing the client's dressing."
C. "I will wear a mask each time I enter the client's room."
D. "I will use a hand sanitizer when I can't wash my hands."

MULTIDRUG-RESISTANT ORGANISM INFECTIONS AND COLONIZATIONS

Antibiotics have been available for many years. Unfortunately, these drugs were commonly prescribed for conditions that did not need them or were given at higher doses and for longer periods of time than were necessary. As a result, a number of microorganisms have become resistant to certain antibiotics; that is, drugs that were once useful no longer control these infectious agents (multidrug-resistant organisms [MDROs]). For this reason, a culture of safety related to INFECTION control has been mandated by the CDC, the Institute for Healthcare Improvement (IHI), and The Joint Commission: Standard Precautions must be strictly followed today in all health care settings to prevent more of these difficult and deadly infections.

One of the newest discoveries to explain the increase in health care–acquired infections (HCAIs), especially the rise in drug-resistant infections, is the formation of biofilms. A **biofilm**, also called *glycocalyx*, is a complex group of microorganisms that functions within a "slimy" gel coating on medical devices such as urinary catheters, orthopedic implants, and enteral feeding tubes; on parts of the body like the teeth (plaque) and tonsils; and in chronic wounds. These reservoirs become sources of INFECTION for which antibiotics and disinfection are not effective. Antibiotic therapy may increase the growth of microbes within biofilms.

Biofilms are extremely difficult to treat, and mechanical disruption strategies are the mainstay of management and research (Ramage et al., 2010). Studies on biofilms that cause the most common HCAIs, such as catheter-associated urinary tract infections (CAUTIs) and wound infections, continue to be conducted. Many specific biofilms have been identified, and methods to remove or disrupt them are being researched.

Patients with *indwelling urinary catheters* are at high risk for pyelonephritis (kidney infection) and septicemia. Current evidence shows that urease-producing bacteria, especially *Proteus mirabilis,* cause crystalline biofilms that create a crust that can block the catheter (Stickler & Feneley, 2010). Therefore indwelling urinary catheters are used only when absolutely necessary. Antimicrobial catheters, either silver-alloy or antimicrobial-coated, are recommended for short-term urinary catheter use to decrease encrustation (Parker et al., 2009). Little evidence is available to demonstrate methods to reduce CAUTIs in long-term indwelling catheters except for frequent catheter changes. In postoperative patients, Palese et al. (2010) found that the regular use of ultrasound bladder scanners reduces urinary tract infections by preventing the inappropriate use of urinary catheters. Nurses can use this information to provide the most current assessment interventions for reducing CAUTIs. Chapter 66 describes evidence-based interventions to prevent urinary tract infections.

Traditional débridement alone is not successful to prevent or manage *chronic wound* infections, often caused by *S. aureus.* A systematic review by Lo et al. (2008) found that silver-releasing dressings were very effective. Biofilms can be disrupted by using dry gauze to mechanically disrupt them after débridement. Antibacterial enzymes may also be used.

The most common MDROs are methicillin-resistant *Staphylococcus aureus,* vancomycin-resistant *Enterococcus,* and carbapenem-resistant *Enterococcus.* Other infections, such as vancomycin-intermediate *S. aureus* (VISA) and vancomycin-resistant *S. aureus* (VRSA), may also occur, which may be effectively treated with antibiotics such as linezolid (Zyvox) and quinupristin-dalfopristin (Synercid).

Methicillin-Resistant *Staphylococcus aureus* (MRSA)

Staphylococcus aureus (S. aureus) is a common bacterium found *on* the skin and perineum and in the nose of many people. It is usually not infectious when in these areas because the number of bacteria is controlled by good hygiene measures. However, when skin or mucous membranes are not intact, minor INFECTIONS, like boils or conjunctivitis, may occur. If the organism enters into deep wounds, surgical incisions, the lungs, or bloodstream, more serious infections occur that require strong antibiotics like methicillin.

Within the past 40 years, more and more *S. aureus* infections have not responded to methicillin or other penicillin-based drugs. Known as *MRSA,* these infections are one of the fastest growing and most common in health care today. In its *5 Million Lives Campaign,* the IHI included reducing MRSA infections as one of its six new goals (see Chapter 1). This type of INFECTION is called *health care–associated MRSA,* or *HA-MRSA.* Patients who have HA-MRSA have increased hospital stays at a very high cost. To add to this problem, about 25% of patients may be colonized with the organism. Health care staff members may also colonize. Patients who develop HA-MRSA pneumonia, abscesses, or bacteremia (bloodstream infection [BSI]) can quickly progress to sepsis and death.

MRSA is spread by direct contact and invades hospitalized patients through indwelling urinary catheters, vascular access devices, and endotracheal tubes. It is susceptible to only a few antibiotics, such as vancomycin (Lyphocin, Vancocin) and linezolid (Zyvox). A newer IV antibiotic, ceftaroline fosamil (Teflaro), is the first cephalosporin approved to treat MRSA.

Current evidence shows that bathing hospitalized patients with pre-moistened cloths or warm water containing chlorhexidine gluconate (CHG) solution can significantly reduce MRSA infection by 23% to 32% (Kassakian, et al., 2011; Powers, et al., 2012). In 2013, the American Association of Critical Care published a recommendation that nurses use CHG to bathe patients in critical care settings as a way to reduce MRSA and other multi-drug–resistant organisms.

! NURSING SAFETY PRIORITY QSEN

Action Alert

Patients most at risk for HA-MRSA are older adults and those who have suppressed IMMUNITY, have a long history of antibiotic therapy, or have invasive tubes or lines. ICU patients are especially at risk. Check with your agency policy regarding specific MRSA preventive measures. Examples include bathing patients with chlorhexidine wipes and administering nasal mupirocin ointment.

Although controversial, some health care facilities have a MRSA-surveillance program in which each patient's nose is swabbed and cultured for MRSA. Staff may also be cultured. All patients with HA-MRSA infection or colonization should be placed on Contact Precautions.

Community-associated MRSA, or CA-MRSA, causes infections in healthy, nonhospitalized people, especially those living in college housing and prisons. It is easily transmitted among family members and can cause serious skin and soft-tissue infections, including abscesses, boils, and blisters. The best way to decrease the incidence of this growing problem is health teaching, including:

- Performing frequent hand hygiene, including using hand sanitizers
- Avoiding close contact with people who have infectious wounds
- Avoiding large crowds
- Avoiding contaminated surfaces
- Using good overall hygiene

Minocycline (Minocin, Apo-Minocycline 🍁) and doxycycline (Doryx, Apo-Doxy 🍁) are usually effective in treating CA-MRSA.

? NCLEX EXAMINATION CHALLENGE

Safe and Effective Care Environment

A client is admitted with a catheter-associated methicillin-resistant *Staphylococcus aureus* (MRSA) infection. Which personal protective equipment is appropriate when providing client care? **Select all that apply.**

A. Mask
B. Gloves
C. Shoe covers
D. Goggles
E. Gown

Vancomycin-Resistant *Enterococcus* (VRE)

Enterococci are bacteria that live in the intestinal tract and are important for digestion. When they move to another area of the body, such as during surgery, they can cause an infection, usually treatable with vancomycin. However, in recent years, many of these infections have become resistant to the drug, and VRE results. Risk factors for this infection include prolonged hospital stays, severe illness, abdominal surgery, enteral nutrition, and immunosuppression. Place patients with VRE infections on Contact Precautions to prevent contamination from body fluids.

Unfortunately, VRE can live on almost any surface for days or weeks and still be able to cause an infection. Contamination of toilet seats, door handles, and other objects is very likely for a lengthy period.

Carbapenem-Resistant *Enterobacteriaceae* (CRE)

Carbapenem antibiotics, most often given for abdominal infections such as peritonitis, have been used extensively for the past 15 years. Examples of this class of antibiotics include imipenem (Cilastin) and meropenem (Merrum IV).

Klebsiella and *Escherichia coli* (*E. coli*) are types of *Enterobacteriaceae* that are located within the intestinal tract. Carbapenem-resistant *Enterobacteriaceae* (CRE) is a family of pathogens that are difficult to treat because they have a high level of resistance to carbapenems due to enzymes that break down the antibiotics. *Klebsiella pneumoniae* (KPC) and New Delhi mettalo-beta-lactamase are examples of these enzymes. Patients who are high risk for CRE include those in intensive care units or nursing homes and patients who are immunosuppressed, including older adults.

To prevent the transmission of this infection, place patients that are high-risk on Contact Precautions. The CDC (2013) also recommends chlorhexidine (2% dilution) bathing to prevent CRE or decrease colonization and other types of infections from MDROs.

OCCUPATIONAL AND ENVIRONMENTAL EXPOSURE TO SOURCES OF INFECTION

The U.S. Occupational Safety and Health Administration (OSHA) is a federal agency that protects workers from injury or illness at their place of employment. Unlike the voluntary guidelines developed by the CDC, OSHA regulations are law. Employers can be fined or disciplined for noncompliance with OSHA regulations. The regulation for prevention of exposure to bloodborne pathogens, such as hepatitis B and hepatitis C or the human immune deficiency virus (HIV), is one example of an OSHA regulation.

Reduction of skin and soft-tissue injuries (e.g., needle sticks) is essential to reduce bloodborne pathogen transmission to health care personnel. *OSHA mandates that sharp objects ("sharps") and needles be handled with care.* Many contaminated sharp-object exposures involve nurses. Needleless devices have helped decrease these exposures, especially when caring for patients receiving infusion therapy (see Chapter 13).

Other INFECTION control concerns that nurses and other HCWs have are the possibilities of pandemic influenza or biologic agent exposure. A large outbreak of one of the MDROs is also worrisome, especially if no drug is sensitive enough for successful management. Nurses may fear that they will accidentally bring the infectious agent to their homes and families.

! NURSING SAFETY PRIORITY QSEN

Action Alert

To help prevent the transmission of an MDRO, wear scrubs and change clothes before leaving work. Keep work clothes separate from personal clothes. Take a shower when you get home, if possible, to rid your body of any unwanted pathogens. Be careful not to contaminate equipment that is commonly used, such as your stethoscope.

Another environmental source for infection is animals or insects. For example, *hantaviruses* are caused by exposure to rodent-infected areas such as old sheds or cabins. Lyme disease can be caused by deer ticks (see Chapter 18).

Saliva and excrement from deer mice and rats living in the southwestern part of the United States are the primary sources of hantaviruses. While not a common infection, patients can die from complications such as *hantavirus pulmonary syndrome,* a severe and potentially lethal respiratory disease. Teach patients to avoid exposure to potential hantaviruses by avoiding rodent-infested areas. If infested areas need to be cleaned, teach patients to wear rubber or latex gloves and either a tight-seal negative-pressure respirator or a positive pressure powered air purifying respirator equipped with N100 or P100 filters (Ly, 2013).

PROBLEMS FROM INADEQUATE ANTIMICROBIAL THERAPY

Inadequate antimicrobial therapy may range from an incorrect choice of drug to poor patient adherence. Drug regimen **noncompliance** (deliberate failure to take the drug) or **nonadherence** (accidental failure to take the drug) also contributes to resistant-organism development.

Some diseases such as tuberculosis (TB) have legal sanctions that require that a patient complete treatment. Patients who are at risk for noncompliance or nonadherence with an anti-TB drug regimen may be placed on *directly observed therapy (DOT).* This means that a health care worker must observe and validate patient compliance with the drug regimen. DOT has been very effective at reducing the spread of multidrug-resistant TB.

Serious complications of INFECTION may also result from incomplete or inadequate antibiotic therapy. Local infections that could be cured without complications, such as cellulitis and pneumonia, may progress to abscess formation if appropriate drug therapy is not continued. Although drug therapy does not always prevent abscess, early therapy may prevent or limit the size of an abscess.

In addition to abscess formation, inadequate therapy may lead to systemic spread. If the infection is not resolved or if it is treated with drugs that are ineffective for the offending microorganism, the pathogen may enter the bloodstream (septicemia or bloodstream infection [BSI]). Inadequately treated local infections may also lead to BSI with leukocytosis (increased white blood cell count). In severe or advanced cases, leukopenia (decreased white blood cell count) and life-threatening disseminated intravascular coagulation (DIC) may occur. After pathogens invade the bloodstream, no site is protected from invasion.

BSI may progress to **septic shock,** more accurately called *sepsis-induced distributive shock.* In septic shock, insufficient cardiac output is compounded by hypovolemia. Inadequate blood supply to vital organs leads to hypoxia (lack of oxygen) and organ failure. Chapter 37 describes this type of shock and its management in detail.

❖ *PATIENT-CENTERED COLLABORATIVE CARE*

◆ *Assessment*

History. The patient's age, history of tobacco or alcohol use, current illness or disease (e.g., diabetes), past and current drug use (e.g., steroids), and poor nutritional status may place him or her at increased risk for INFECTION. Patients who are immunocompromised as a result of disease or therapies such as chemotherapy and radiation are also at a high risk for infection. Ask the patient about previous vaccinations or immunizations, including the dates of administration.

Ask the patient if he or she has recently been in a hospital or nursing home as a patient or visitor. Inquire about having invasive testing, such as a colonoscopy, or recent surgery. Ask if the patient had an indwelling urinary catheter or IV line. These invasive treatments often are the source of infections.

Determine whether the patient has been exposed to infectious agents. A history of recent exposure to someone with similar clinical symptoms or to contaminated food or water, as well as the time of exposure, assists in identifying a possible source of INFECTION. This information helps determine the incubation period for the disease and thus provides a clue to its cause.

Contact with animals, including pets, may increase exposure to infection. Question the patient about recent animal contact at home or work or in leisure activities (e.g., hiking). Insect bites should be documented.

Obtain a travel history. Travel to areas both within and outside the patient's home country may expose a susceptible person to infectious organisms not encountered in the local community.

A thorough sexual history may reveal behavior associated with an increased risk for sexually transmitted diseases. Obtain a history of IV drug use and a transfusion history to assess the patient's risk for hepatitis B, hepatitis C, and HIV infections.

Identifying the type and location of symptoms may point to affected organ systems. The onset order of symptoms gives clues to the specific problem. Gathering a history of past INFECTION or colonization with multidrug-resistant organisms will help determine which type of Transmission-Based Precautions is needed.

Physical Assessment/Clinical Manifestations. Disorders caused by pathogens vary depending on the INFECTION cause and site. Common clinical manifestations are associated with specific sites of infection. Carefully inspect the skin for symptoms of *local* infection at any site *(pain, swelling, heat, redness, pus).* Wounds can easily become infected because the integrity of the skin is broken.

CONSIDERATIONS FOR OLDER ADULTS

Patient-Centered Care QSEN

Fever (generally a temperature above 101° F [38.3° C]), chills, and malaise are primary indicators of a systemic infection. Fever may accompany other noninfectious disorders, and infection can be present without fever, especially in patients who have impaired immunity. The older adult, whose normal temperature may be 1° to 2° lower than the normal temperature in younger adults, may have a fever at 99° F (37.2° C). In most patients with an infection, fever (**hyperthermia**) is a normal immune response that can help destroy the pathogen. Assess the patient for these signs and symptoms, and carefully ask about their history and pattern.

Lymphadenopathy (enlarged lymph nodes), pharyngitis, and GI disturbance (usually diarrhea or vomiting) are often associated with infection. To detect enlargement, palpate the cervical, axillary, and other lymph nodes; examine the throat for redness. Ask about changes in stool and if the patient has had any nausea or vomiting.

Psychosocial Assessment. The patient with an infectious disease often has psychosocial concerns. Delay in diagnosis because of the need to await clinical test results produces anxiety. Assess the patient's and family's level of understanding about various diagnostic procedures and the time required to obtain test results. Plan education on infection risk reduction at a time when they are ready to learn.

Feelings of malaise and fatigue often accompany infection. Assess the patient's current level of activity and the impact of these symptoms on family, occupational, and recreational activities.

The potential spread of INFECTION to others is an additional stress associated with the diagnosis of infection. The patient may curtail family and social interactions for fear of spreading the illness. Determine the patient's and family's understanding of the infection, the mode of transmission, and mechanisms that may limit or prevent transmission. Special precautions, although sometimes necessary for preventing transmission of the organism, can be emotionally difficult for the patient and family.

A number of transmissible infectious diseases, especially those identified with social stigmas (e.g., IV drug abuse), are associated with labeling. The patient may feel socially isolated or have guilt related to behavior that increased the risk for infection. Observe carefully for the patient's reaction to labels and how these feelings further affect socialization.

Laboratory Assessment. The definitive diagnosis of an infectious disease requires identification of a microorganism in the tissues of an infected patient. Direct examination of blood, body fluids, and tissues under a microscope may not yield a definitive identification. However, laboratory assessment usually provides helpful information about organisms, such as shape, motility, and reaction to staining agents. Even when direct microscopy does not provide a conclusive specific diagnosis, often enough information is obtained for starting appropriate antimicrobial therapy.

The best procedure for identifying a microorganism is ***culture***, or isolation of the pathogen by cultivation in tissue cultures or artificial media. Specimens for culture can be obtained from almost any body fluid or tissue. The health care provider usually decides when and where the specimen for culture is taken.

Proper collection and handling of specimens for culture, using Standard Precautions, are essential for obtaining accurate results. Specimens collected must be appropriate for the suspected infection. Be sure that the specimen is of adequate quantity and is freshly obtained and placed in a sterile container to preserve the specimen and microorganism. Label the specimen properly including the date and time it was collected. Follow your agency's policy if you have any questions about how to perform a culture.

After isolation of a microorganism in culture, antimicrobial **sensitivity** testing is performed to determine the effects of various drugs on that particular microorganism. An agent that is killed by acceptable levels of an antibiotic, for example, is considered sensitive to that drug. An organism that is not killed by tolerable levels of an antibiotic is considered resistant to that drug. Preliminary results are usually available in 24 to 48 hours, but the final results generally take 72 hours. *Antimicrobial therapy should not begin until after the culture specimen is obtained.*

Rapid cultures or assays are used in ambulatory care settings to provide quicker assessments of infections. The most popular is the rapid antigen detection test for group A streptococci to rule out "strep throat" in patients who present with pharyngitis (sore, inflamed throat). Other examples of newer tests are those for tuberculosis (TB) and influenza ("flu"), discussed in Chapter 31.

A *white blood cell (WBC) count with differential* is often done for the patient with a suspected infection. Five types of leukocytes (white blood cells) are measured as part of the results:

- Neutrophils
- Lymphocytes
- Monocytes
- Eosinophils
- Basophils

In most active infections, especially those caused by bacteria, the total leukocyte count is elevated. Various infections are characterized by changes in the percentages of the different types of leukocytes. The differential count usually shows an increased number of immature neutrophils, or a **shift to the left** ("left shift"). A few infectious diseases, however, such as malaria and infectious mononucleosis, are associated with neutropenia (decreased neutrophils). See Chapter 17 for further discussion.

The *erythrocyte sedimentation rate (ESR)* measures the rate at which red blood cells fall through plasma. This rate is most significantly affected by an increased number of acute-phase reactants, which occurs with inflammation. Thus an elevated ESR (>20 mm/hr) indicates inflammation or infection somewhere in the body. Chronic INFECTION, especially osteomyelitis and chronic abscesses, is commonly associated with an elevated ESR. The ESR is chronically elevated with inflammatory arthritis and other connective tissue diseases as well (see Chapter 18). The effectiveness of therapy is often determined by a decrease in this value.

Serologic testing is performed to identify pathogens by detecting antibodies to the organism. The antibody titer tends to *increase* during the acute phase of infectious diseases such as hepatitis B. The titer *decreases* as the patient improves.

Imaging Assessment. X-ray films may be obtained to determine activity or destruction by an infectious microorganism. Radiologic studies (e.g., chest films, sinus films, joint films, GI studies) are available for diagnosis of infection in a specific body site.

More sophisticated techniques for INFECTION diagnosis include computed tomography (CT) scans and magnetic resonance imaging (MRI). CT and ultrasonography are helpful in assessing for abscesses. CT scans help identify suspected osteomyelitis and fluid collections that point to possible infection. MRI scans provide a cross-sectional assessment for infection.

Another diagnostic tool for the evaluation of a patient with an infectious disease is ultrasonography. This noninvasive procedure is particularly helpful in detecting infection involving the heart valves.

Scanning techniques using radioactive substances such as gallium can determine the presence of inflammation caused by INFECTION. Inflammatory tissue is identified by its increased uptake of the injected radioactive material.

◆ Analysis

The priority NANDA-I nursing diagnoses and collaborative problems for patients with an infection or infectious disease include:

1. Hyperthermia related to the immune response triggered by pathogenic invasion (NANDA-I)
2. Social Isolation related to being placed on Transmission-Based Precautions (NANDA-I)

◆ Planning and Implementation

Managing Hyperthermia

Planning: Expected Outcomes. Patients with an INFECTION or infectious disease are expected to have a body temperature within normal limits as a result of effective interdisciplinary management.

Interventions. The primary concern is to provide measures to eliminate the underlying cause of fever (also known as *hyperthermia*) and to destroy the causative microorganism. In collaboration with the health care team, nurses use a variety of methods to manage fever.

Drug therapy plays a major role in patient-centered collaborative care of patients with INFECTION. Antimicrobials, also called *anti-infective agents,* are the cornerstone of drug therapy. Antipyretics are used to decrease patient discomfort and reduce fever.

Antibiotics, antiviral agents, and antifungals are common types of antimicrobial drugs that are given for INFECTION, depending on its type. Effective antibiotics are available to treat nearly all bacterial infections, but misuse of antibiotics has contributed to the development of multidrug-resistant organisms (MDROs) discussed earlier in this chapter. A few effective antifungal agents have been developed, but these drugs generally cause more toxicity than antibacterial agents.

Effective antimicrobial therapy requires delivery of an appropriate drug, sufficient dosage, proper administration route, and sufficient therapy duration. These four requirements ensure delivery of a concentration of drug sufficient to inhibit or kill infecting microorganisms. To ensure effectiveness of antibiotic therapy such as vancomycin, health care providers may require serum trough and peak levels be drawn. Specimens for trough levels are drawn about 30 minutes prior to the next scheduled vancomycin dose. Specimens for peak levels are drawn 30 to 60 minutes after medication administration (Rosini & Srivastava, 2013).

Health care providers collaborate on selecting drugs and dosing. Antimicrobials act on susceptible pathogens by:

- Inhibiting cell wall synthesis (e.g., penicillins and cephalosporins)
- Injuring the cytoplasmic membrane (e.g., antifungal agents)
- Inhibiting biosynthesis, or reproduction (e.g., erythromycin and gentamicin)
- Inhibiting nucleic acid synthesis (e.g., actinomycin)

Teach the drug's actions, side effects, and toxic effects to patients and their families. Observe and report side effects and adverse events. These reactions vary according to the specific classification of the drug. Most antibiotics can cause nausea, vomiting, and rashes. Stress the importance of completing the entire course of drug therapy, even if symptoms have improved or disappeared.

Antipyretic drugs, such as acetaminophen (Tylenol, Ace-Tabs 🍁), are often given to reduce fever. Because these drugs mask fever, monitoring the course of the disease may be difficult. Therefore, unless the patient is very uncomfortable or if fever presents a significant risk (e.g., in the patient with heart failure, febrile seizures, or head injury), antipyretics are not always prescribed.

Teach patients that they may have waves of sweating after each dose. Sweating may be accompanied by a fall in blood pressure followed by return of fever. These unpleasant side effects of antipyretic therapy can often be alleviated by increasing fluid intake and by regular scheduling of drug administration.

Other interventions to reduce fever may include external cooling and fluid administration. Perform a thorough assessment before and after interventions are implemented.

External cooling by hypothermia blankets or ice bags or packs can be effective mechanisms for reducing a high fever. Alternative cooling methods may be used. Sponging the patient's body with tepid water or applying cool compresses to the skin and pulse points to reduce body temperature is sometimes helpful. *Teach unlicensed assistive personnel (UAP) to observe for and report shivering during any form of external cooling. Shivering may indicate that the patient is being cooled too quickly.*

The use of fans is discouraged because they can disperse airborne- or droplet-transmitted pathogens. Fans can also disturb air balance in negative pressure rooms, making them positive pressure rooms and allowing possible transmission of the agent to those outside the room.

In patients with fever, fluid volume loss is increased from rapid evaporation of body fluids and increased perspiration. As body temperature increases, fluid volume loss increases.

TABLE 23-4 Possible Allergic Reactions to Antibiotic Therapy

• Nausea and/or vomiting	• Erythema multiforme (Stevens-Johnson syndrome)
• Flushing	• Angioneurotic edema
• Wheezing	• Serum sickness (headache, fever, chills, hives, malaise, conjunctivitis)
• Sneezing	• Anaphylaxis (laryngeal edema, bronchospasm, hypotension, vascular collapse, cardiac arrest)
• Pruritus	• Death
• Urticaria	
• Rashes	
• Maculopapular to exfoliative dermatitis	
• Vascular eruptions	

! NURSING SAFETY PRIORITY QSEN

Drug Alert

Before administering an antimicrobial agent, check to see that the patient is not allergic to it (Table 23-4). Be sure to take an accurate allergy history before drug therapy begins to prevent possible life-threatening reactions, such as anaphylaxis!

! NURSING SAFETY PRIORITY QSEN

Action Alert

If fluid volume loss increases, patients may be at risk for dehydration and require additional fluids either orally or IV. Monitor carefully for signs of dehydration, such as increased thirst, decreased skin turgor, dry mucous membranes, and acute confusion, especially in older adults. Increase oral fluid intake and provide IV fluids as prescribed. Chapter 11 discusses interventions for dehydration in detail.

Responding to Feelings of Social Isolation

Planning: Expected Outcomes. The patient with an INFECTION or infectious disease who is placed on Transmission-Based Precautions is expected to cope with feelings of isolation and interact with others.

Interventions. Education is the major intervention for meeting this outcome. Teach the patient and family about the mode of transmission of infection and mechanisms that prevent spread to others. Assess coping mechanisms that the patient has used in the past. If he or she is in the hospital, collaborate with the certified hospital chaplain or social worker to help alleviate the patient's stress, anxiety, or depression.

As part of the health care team, ensure that the patient and family understand the disease process and its cause. If necessary, ensure that the patient and family can state specific ways in which precautions will be used in the home after discharge from the hospital.

Because the patient requiring precautions may feel secluded, encourage staff and family members to maintain contact with the patient. Remind them that the pathogen, not the patient, requires special precautions. Encourage family members and friends to visit and to use appropriate infection control measures. Communication by telephone or e-mail is often effective for continuing contact with loved ones. Television, Internet, and handheld mobile devices help bring the outside world into the life of the patient confined to the room.

In the long-term care setting, an outbreak of respiratory or GI INFECTION usually requires limiting visitors, activities, and admissions to the facility. Nurses working in these settings need to be familiar with federal and state regulations regarding managing infections.

Community-Based Care

Patients with infections may be cared for in the home, hospital, nursing home, or ambulatory care setting, depending on the type and severity of the INFECTION. Infections among older adults in nursing homes are common. Residents often have meals together in a communal dining room and participate in group activities. Confused residents may not wash their hands or may enter other resident rooms. Immunizing them against respiratory infections is highly recommended because these illnesses can cause severe complications or death in older adults.

Home Care Management. The patient with an infectious disease such as osteomyelitis may require continued, long-term antibiotic therapy at home or in a long-term care facility. Emphasize the importance of a clean home environment, especially for the patient who continues to have compromised IMMUNITY or who is uniquely susceptible to **superinfection** (i.e., reinfection or a second infection of the same kind) to reduce the chance of infection. Drugs often need to be refrigerated. Ensure that the patient has access to proper storage facilities, and teach him or her to check for signs of improper storage, such as discoloration of the drug.

Ask about the availability of handwashing facilities in the home, and check that supplies and instructions are provided as needed. Most people do not know how to wash hands correctly. Demonstrate the procedure with the patient and family, and request a repeat demonstration.

Self-Management Education. Explaining the disease and making certain that the patient understands what is causing the illness are the primary purposes of health teaching. Discuss whether the pathogen causing the INFECTION can be spread to others and the modes of transmission.

If the patient has an infectious disease that is potentially transmissible, teach the patient, family, and other home caregivers about precautions. Explain whether any special household cleaning is necessary and, if so, what those special steps include. If syringes with needles are used to administer drug therapy, explain how to dispose safely and legally of needles in the community. Clothing soiled with blood or other body fluids can be washed with bleach or disinfectant (e.g., Lysol). Recommended cleaning measures should be based on actual available equipment and facilities.

For the patient who is discharged to the home setting to complete a course of antimicrobial therapy, the importance of adherence to the planned drug regimen needs to be stressed. Explain the importance of both the timing of doses and the completion of the planned number of days of therapy. Teach the patient (and family as appropriate) how the agents need to be taken (e.g., before meals, with meals, without other agents) and the possible side effects. Side effects include those that are expected (e.g., gastric distress), as well as more severe adverse reactions (e.g., rash, fever, other systemic signs and symptoms). Teach the patient about allergic manifestations and the need to notify a health care provider if an adverse reaction occurs (see Table 23-4). Also discuss what to do if a drug dose is missed (e.g., doubling the dosage, waiting until the next dose time).

Many patients are discharged with an infusion device to continue drug therapy at home or in other inpatient facilities. The patient, family member, or home care nurse administers the drugs. Home care services are often used to teach appropriate administration of drug therapy in the patient's home. Health teaching and wound care may also be needed. These services have proved efficient, effective, psychologically supportive, and less expensive than hospitalization or skilled nursing facilities (SNFs).

The patient is often anxious and fearful that the INFECTION will be transmitted to family members or friends. Teaching the patient and the family ways of preventing the spread of disease allays these fears. Pay careful attention to the patient's and family's concerns. Making concrete suggestions (e.g., "Your wife can wear gloves when changing your dressing") to address specific concerns may reduce these fears.

The patient with an infectious disease associated with lifestyle behaviors, such as sexual activity or IV drug abuse, may have guilt related to the disease. Encourage discussion of feelings associated with the illness, and assist in locating support systems that may help alleviate these feelings, such as clergy or other spiritual or cultural leaders.

Health Care Resources. At times, a patient who has been hospitalized for an infectious disease may not be able to return to the home setting due to lack of caregiver support. In such cases, temporary placement in a SNF may be needed. Document care requirements, patient history of infection or colonization with multidrug-resistant organisms, medication schedules, and personal needs and preferences on transfer forms. Hand-off communication, such as the SBAR, between the two facilities is required to facilitate a smooth transition from the hospital to the intermediate care setting, according to The Joint Commission's National Patient Safety Goals.

TABLE 23-5 Centers for Disease Control and Prevention* Examples of Bioterrorism Agents and General Clinical Management

PATHOGEN OR AGENT AND DISEASE INFORMATION	CLINICAL MANAGEMENT
Anthrax (*Bacillus anthracis*)	
Cutaneous: 1-7 days after contact, exposed skin itching, progressing to papular and vesicular lesions, eschar, edema, ulceration, and sloughing. If untreated, may spread to lymph nodes and bloodstream. Fatality 5%-20%. **Inhalation:** 48 hr after organism or spore inhalation, flu-like illness with possible brief improvement. 2-4 days from initial symptoms, abrupt onset of severe cardiopulmonary illness (dyspnea, tachycardia, fever, diaphoresis, thoracic edema, shock, and respiratory failure). If antibiotics delayed until onset of cardiopulmonary symptoms, mortality high. May be confused with common upper respiratory infection (URI). **Other forms:** Gastrointestinal (GI), meningeal, and sepsis.	**For cutaneous and inhaled anthrax:** No person-to-person spread. Contact Precautions are not needed unless patient presents directly from exposure. Standard Precautions for: Prescribed wound cleansing and management of lesions Ventilator support for respiratory failure Postmortem care
Botulism (*Clostridium botulinum* and Neurotoxin)	
Toxin ingestion results in dysphasia, dry mouth, drooping eyelids, and blurred or double vision. Vomiting and constipation or diarrhea may be present initially, extending to symmetric flaccid paralysis in an alert person. Acute bilateral cranial nerve impairment and descending weakness or paralysis follow. Neurologic symptoms after 12-36 hr for foodborne botulism and in 24-72 hr after aerosol exposure. Case fatality up to 10%. Recovery may take months.	Standard Precautions: decontamination of patient is not required. No person-to-person spread. Consider outbreak with suspicion of a single case. Consult with CDC and health departments. Advise careful cleanup and disposal of suspected contaminated food source *after* consultation with health department about any needed laboratory sampling. Interdisciplinary planning for nutrition and rehabilitation support during lengthy neuromuscular and respiratory recovery.
Plague (*Yersinia pestis*)	
Lymphatic infection: 2-8 days after bites from fleas of an infected rodent (rarely after infected tissue or body fluid contact), onset of fever and chills, painful lymphadenopathy (or bubo—usually inguinal, axillary, or cervical lymph nodes), headache, GI symptoms, and rapidly progressive weakness. 50%-60% fatality if untreated. **Pneumonic:** 1-3 days after aerosolized organism inhalation, fever and chills, productive cough, hemoptysis, rapidly progressive weakness, GI symptoms, and bronchopneumonia. Survival unlikely if not treated within 18 hr of symptom onset. **Other forms:** Sepsis with coagulopathy, rarely meningitis.	Droplet Precautions: required for pneumonic plague (until 72 hr of antibiotic therapy). Contact Precautions until decontamination is complete: For any suspected gross contamination. See documentation information listed under Anthrax—above. For prescribed management of bubo(s) if incised to drain. Community and other environmental modifications: Apply insecticide to infested environment and pets (to kill fleas). Reduce food and water supply for rodents. Avoid sick or dead animals.
Smallpox (Variola Virus) (Variola Major and Minor)	
10-17 days after droplet or airborne virus inhalation or contact with bleeding lesions, onset of severe myalgias, headache, and high fever. 2-3 days later, a papular rash appears on face and spreads to extremities (and palms and soles). The rash quickly (simultaneously) becomes vesicular and then painful and pustular (contrasted to varicella rash that crops and concentrates more on trunk with various stages of macules to vesicles seen at one time). Patients are infectious at onset of rash until scabs separate (3 wk). Historically, variola major kills 20%. May be confused with varicella.	Standard, Contact, and Airborne Precautions for patients with vesicular rash pending diagnosis. Same for varicella and variola. Also, avoid contact with organism while handling contaminated clothes and bedding. Wear protective attire (gloves, gown, and N95 respirator). One case is a public health emergency—highly communicable. Consult CDC and health departments at earliest suspicion. Vaccine does not give reliable lifelong immunity. Previously vaccinated persons are considered susceptible. *Following exposure:* Initiate Airborne Precautions, and observe for unprotected contacts (from days 10-17). Vaccinate within 2-3 days of exposure.

Other Key Points

Assessment: Include account of symptoms, patient's incident (what, where, when, how, others exposed or ill, and officials aware).

Treatment: Antibiotic-resistance possible. Vaccine and postexposure prophylaxis are subject to change. If any of the above diseases are suspected, consult infection control practitioner for coordination with community health officials and CDC about current recommendations and specimen collection. *If bioterrorism suspected,* Federal Bureau of Investigation (FBI) will coordinate evidence collection and delivery.

Multiple exposures planning: Emergency and critical care managers must address availability and acquisition of stocks of medications, vaccines, equipment (e.g., ventilators), and communications with officials, as well as public information needs.

◆ Evaluation: Outcomes

Evaluating the care of the patient with an INFECTION or infectious disease on the basis of the identified priority problems is important. The expected outcomes include that the patient:

- Has body temperature and other vital signs within baseline
- Adheres to drug therapy regimen
- Copes with feelings of social isolation

Specific indicators for these outcomes are listed for each priority problem under the Planning and Implementation section (see earlier).

CRITICAL ISSUES: EMERGING INFECTIONS AND GLOBAL BIOTERRORISM

Current concerns related to INFECTION and infection control are the risk for global bioterrorism (Table 23-5), emerging

CLINICAL JUDGMENT CHALLENGE

Evidence-Based Practice; Quality Improvement; Informatics QSEN

The hospital quality improvement (QI) department reports a 25% increase in CRE infections on your surgical intensive care unit during the past month. A unit-based QI team is created to identify possible causes of this increase and strategies for decreasing these infections.

1. What are some possible causes of CRE infections?
2. Using the PICOT format in Chapter 5, develop a clinical question to address the problem.
3. How will your unit QI team begin to answer the clinical question?
4. What data sources might you use?
5. What will you do with the retrieved data?
6. How will you present your findings?

infectious diseases, and multidrug-resistant organisms (MDROs). As for any pathogen, strict infection control measures can prevent transmission of these microbes to you and your patients. Some of the most serious infections are briefly described here. Table 23-6 lists more emerging infections that may present as problems in the United States and other parts of the world.

The 2014 Ebola epidemic was labeled as the largest in history, with many West African countries affected (CDC, 2014). An epidemic occurs when new cases of a certain disease substantially exceed expectation during a given period. The ongoing struggle with the Ebola virus outbreak in West Africa became a concern within the United States when an individual who flew back from Liberia was diagnosed, although after initial discharge, at a Dallas hospital. That individual later died. Symptoms of Ebola, which can present from 2 to 21 days after exposure (with an average of 8 to 10 days), include fever greater than 101.5° F, severe headache, muscle pain, weakness, diarrhea, vomiting, abdominal pain, and unexplained hemorrhage (bleeding or bruising) (CDC, 2014). The virus is most commonly spread through exposure to bodily fluids of the infected individual and through needle sticks in which the needle has been contaminated with the virus (CDC, 2014). Recovery from this virus is contingent on appropriate clinical care and the immune response of the patient. Patients who recover from Ebola infection develop antibodies that can last for 10 years (CDC, 2014) (Table 23-7).

With the Dallas Ebola incident, there was reported to be a communication concern within the electronic medical record

TABLE 23-6 Examples of Global Emerging Infections

Recently Emerging Infections	Older Rapidly Growing Infections
• H1N1 influenza • West Nile virus • Avian influenza • Hemorrhagic fevers (e.g., Ebola, Marburg) • Monkeypox • Bovine spongiform encephalopathy • Vancomycin-intermediate *Staphylococcus aureus* (VISA) • Vancomycin-resistant *Staphylococcus aureus* (VRSA) • *Clostridium difficile* (new strain)	• Methicillin-resistant *Staphylococcus aureus* (MRSA) • Vancomycin-resistant *Enterococcus* (VRE) • Carbapenem-resistant *Enterobacteriaceae* (CRE) • Multidrug-resistant tuberculosis • *Clostridium difficile*

TABLE 23-7 Care for Patients with Ebola Virus Disease

TRANSMISSION OF DISEASE	PREVENTION OF DISEASE	ASSESSMENT	PATIENT-CENTERED COLLABORATIVE CARE
The primary source of the Ebola virus is most likely contaminated bats or primates (apes and monkeys) in West Africa. Information that is known about transmission includes: • The Ebola virus cannot be transmitted unless a person is sick and has clinical manifestations of the disease. • The Ebola virus is not spread via air, water, or food. • Nurses can help identify people at high risk for having or transmitting the disease by taking a complete history, including asking about travel to West Africa, or exposure to family and friends who have Ebola. • The disease can be transmitted by unprotected contact with people infected with the Ebola virus or with people who have died from Ebola. • Teach patients who recover from Ebola and their partners that the virus is present in semen for up to 3 months. Using a condom may prevent transmission.	Take special training *before* caring for patients with the Ebola virus. Use these precautions: • Avoid direct contact with body fluids (blood, feces, saliva, urine, vomit, and semen). • Use Standard, Contact, and Droplet Precautions, including appropriate PPE. • Isolate patient with Ebola in a single room. • Use dedicated or disposable medical equipment and supplies. • Practice proper sterilization measures.	Clinical manifestations occur 2-21 days after exposure to the Ebola virus. Assess for: • Fever • Severe headache • Muscle pain • Weakness • Fatigue • Diarrhea • Vomiting • Abdominal pain • Unexplained hemorrhage (bleeding and bruising)	No drug therapy or vaccine is yet FDA approved for Ebola. Remember that the virus can enter the body through broken skin or unprotected mucous membranes such as the eyes, nose, and mouth. Supportive care includes: • Intravenous fluid and electrolyte replacement • Oxygen and ventilation support • Blood pressure support • Treatment of other infections • Care and comfort measures • Symptomatic care • Emotional support • Possible end-of-life care

Data from CDC. (2014). *Ebola (Ebola virus disease)*. Accessed in November 2014 from www.cdc.gov/vhf/ebola/index/html.

(EMR) in which the physician was unable to view the nurse's notes and see that the nurse had recorded the patient's recent returne from West Africa. It is of vital importance that the nurse and provider of care be sure to communicate pertinent historical information both verbally and in the EMR so that appropriate interventions for both the individual and the general public can be undertaken immediately.

Pandemic infections, such as influenza, are another threat to the population. As recently as the early 1900s, the "Spanish flu" killed millions of people throughout the world. Health care workers are encouraged to have yearly influenza vaccines to prevent infection with common strains of the virus. The federal government and health care agencies around the United States include the risk for pandemic disease in their disaster planning (see Chapter 10).

Contaminated food is another source of INFECTION. The incidence of foodborne infections has risen in the United States as contaminated fresh spinach, ground beef, and other foods were found to contain *E. coli* 0157:H7. Many illnesses and thousands of recent deaths in the United States have been caused by this infection. Safer food preparation practices and increased monitoring by federal agencies have resulted from demand for public safety.

Another pathogen, *Clostridium difficile (C. difficile),* is associated with antibiotic therapy use, especially in older adults. Associated problems have led to the development of the diagnosis of **C. difficile–associated disease (CDAD)** (Grossman & Mager, 2010). A new more virulent strain of this pathogen has developed in the past decade due to the use of fluoroquinolone antibiotics, such as ciprofloxacin (Cipro).

C. difficile is spread by indirect contact with inanimate objects like medical equipment and commodes, and its toxins cause colon dysfunction and cell death from sepsis. CDAD is confirmed by stool culture. Patients who have three or more liquid stools per day for two or more days are suspected of having the infection. Fever and abdominal pain and cramping commonly occur with diarrheal stools. Oral metronidazole (Flagyl) and vancomycin have been the drugs of choice to treat CDAD. However, some patients experience recurrence of infection after treatment with these drugs. A new oral antibacterial drug available for specifically managing *C. difficile* is fidaxomicin (Dificid).

A new controversial treatment for CDAD is fecal bacteriotherapy to transplant stool with normal healthy flora into the infected patient. The donor stool is liquefied with saline, filtered, and administered to the patient with CDAD by nasogastric tube, fecal enema, or colonoscopy. Results of this treatment have been very positive (Meyers, 2011).

In addition to concerns about emerging infections, preparation for and education about *bioterrorism* have been major focuses of the U.S. government since September 11, 2001. In some cases, vaccines are no longer given for biologic agents like smallpox. Many people in the United States have never been vaccinated, and those who had vaccinations many years ago are not guaranteed to have lifelong immunity. Anthrax, usually seen in animals, may be spread to the skin or inhaled. These infections have a high fatality rate in humans. Plague, once seen centuries ago, is one of the biggest threats because the survival rate is low. Vaccines are being researched and stockpiled by the U.S. government for some of the common biologic agents.

NURSING CONCEPTS AND CLINICAL JUDGMENT REVIEW

What might you NOTICE if the patient has INADEQUATE PROTECTION as a result of infection or infectious disease?

- Flushing and sweating
- Localized skin inflammation (redness, warmth, swelling, pain)
- Open wound (draining or non-draining)
- Report of diarrhea or vomiting
- Report of sore throat
- Fatigue
- Rash
- Acute confusion (in older adults)

What should you INTERPRET and how should you RESPOND to a patient with INADEQUATE PROTECTION as a result of infection or infectious disease?

Perform and interpret focused physical assessment findings, including:

- Vital signs
- Skin and/or wound assessment
- Lymph palpation
- Throat inspection

Respond:

- Manage fever if present.
- Take culture of drainage and send to laboratory for analysis.
- Monitor laboratory findings, including complete blood count (CBC) with white blood cell (WBC) differential.
- Place on appropriate Transmission-Based Precautions.
- Teach patients and families about Transmission-Based Precautions and hand hygiene.
- Administer antimicrobial therapy as prescribed.
- Collaborate with the facility's infection control practitioner.
- Teach patients and families about the need to adhere to the drug therapy regimen.
- Follow CDC guidelines and The Joint Commission's National Patient Safety Goals (NPSGs).

On what should you REFLECT?

- Monitor the patient's response to drug therapy.
- Monitor the patient's vital signs for return to baseline.
- Evaluate the patient's and family's knowledge of infection, Transmission-Based Precautions, and drug therapy.
- Monitor the staff's compliance with hand hygiene and personal protective equipment (PPE).
- Evaluate the patient's and family's coping ability.
- Think about what else you might do to make the patient more comfortable.
- Decide whether you need to provide alternative or additional interventions or health teaching.

GET READY FOR THE NCLEX® EXAMINATION!

KEY POINTS

Review these Key Points for each NCLEX Examination Client Needs Category.

Safe and Effective Care Environment

- Handwashing and alcohol-based hand rubs are two methods of hand hygiene (see Chart 23-3).
- The Centers for Disease Control and Prevention (CDC) recommends a ban on artificial fingernails for health care professionals when they are caring for patients at high risk for infection. **Evidence-Based Practice** QSEN
- Infections can be prevented or controlled through hand hygiene, disinfection/sterilization, personal protective equipment (PPE), patient placement, and adequate staffing; proper hand hygiene and gloves are the most important interventions because health care workers' hands are the primary way in which disease is transmitted from patient to patient. **Evidence-Based Practice** QSEN
- Standard Precautions are used with all patients in health care settings, assuming that all body excretions and secretions are potentially infectious (see Table 23-2). **Safety** QSEN
- Airborne Precautions are used for patients who have infections transmitted through the air, such as tuberculosis.
- Droplet Precautions are used for patients who have infections transmitted by droplets, such as influenza and certain types of meningitis.
- Contact Precautions are used for patients who have infections transmitted by direct contact or contact with items in the patient's environment.

Health Promotion and Maintenance

- Health teaching about clinical manifestations of infection and drug therapy is important for the patient with an infection being managed at home; some patients may need health care nursing services for IV antimicrobial therapy.
- Teach patients about antimicrobial therapy and protective measures to prevent infection transmission.
- Teach patients how to avoid community-acquired MRSA by performing frequent hand hygiene and by avoiding crowds and direct contact with others who have infections. **Safety** QSEN

Psychosocial Integrity

- Patients who have Transmission-Based Precautions may feel isolated, anxious, or depressed; they may feel neglected and dissatisfied with their care. Help patients cope with these feelings through verbalization and collaboration with the health care team. **Teamwork and Collaboration** QSEN

Physiological Integrity

- Patients at the highest risk for infection include older adults, health care professionals at risk for needle sticks, and patients who have diabetes or are immunocompromised. Patients who take long-term steroid therapy or have had invasive procedures or therapies are also at a high risk for infection.
- Multidrug-resistant organisms (MDROs) are the result of the overuse of antibiotic therapy and include methicillin-resistant *Staphylococcus aureus* (MRSA), vancomycin-resistant *Enterococcus* (VRE), and carbapenem-resistant *Enterobacteriaceae* (CRE).
- A biofilm, also called *glycocalyx,* is a complex group of microorganisms that function within a "slimy" gel coating on medical devices, such as urinary catheters, orthopedic implants, and enteral feeding tubes; on parts of the body like the teeth (plaque) and tonsils; and in chronic wounds. Biofilms are difficult to treat, and research is examining methods to manage them to better treat.
- Common clinical manifestations of infections and infectious diseases include fever and lymphadenopathy. If infections are not treated or are inadequately treated, systemic sepsis (septicemia), septic shock, and disseminated intravascular coagulation (DIC) may result.
- A culture is the most definitive way to confirm and identify microorganisms; sensitivity testing determines which antibiotics will destroy the identified microbes.
- The white blood cell differential count usually shows a shift to the left (increased number of immature neutrophils) during active infections.
- Antimicrobials and antipyretics are the most common types of drugs used when infection is accompanied by fever.
- Antipyretics are used only when the fever presents a significant risk or the patient is very uncomfortable, because antipyretics may mask the disease. **Evidence-Based Practice** QSEN
- Critical issues for the next decade include bioterrorism, emerging infectious diseases, and multidrug-resistant organisms (MDROs).

CHAPTER 24

Assessment of the Skin, Hair, and Nails

Janice Cuzzell and M. Linda Workman

http://evolve.elsevier.com/Iggy/

PRIORITY CONCEPTS

- TISSUE INTEGRITY

LEARNING OUTCOMES

Safe and Effective Care Environment

1. Protect hospitalized patients from skin injury and loss of TISSUE INTEGRITY.

Health Promotion and Maintenance

2. Teach all people how to protect the skin from damage and cancer development.

Psychosocial Integrity

3. Reduce the psychological impact for the patient and family regarding the assessment and testing of the integumentary system.

Physiological Integrity

4. Use knowledge of anatomy and physiology to perform a focused assessment of the skin, hair, and nails, incorporating information about genetic risk and age-related changes affecting these structures.

The skin, hair, and nails are the tissues making up the integumentary system. Skin TISSUE INTEGRITY plays a major role in protection. Intact skin has barrier functions, alarm functions, and even combat functions. As shown in Fig. 24-1, the skin protects the body against invasion of pathogenic organisms by providing a first line of defense (the moat), a second line of defense (the castle wall), and even a third line of defense (the knights and soldiers). The normal flora on the surfaces of skin and mucous membranes repels some of the more harmful microorganisms. Specialized cells in the skin engulf foreign substances (antigens) that invade the body when skin TISSUE INTEGRITY is lost and then alert the immune system to the presence of the invader. Localized tissue inflammation and swelling work to contain the invading pathogen until white blood cells can respond and remove this threat.

The skin is the largest organ of the body and, when intact, helps regulate body temperature and maintains fluid and electrolyte balance. Skin changes can provide important information about a person's health and well-being. Emotional stress, systemic disease, some drugs, and skin injury or disease can alter skin function, appearance, and texture.

The skin's sensory function allows the use of touch as an intervention to provide comfort, relieve pain, and communicate caring. Because the skin has many sensory receptors, the patient can report subjective skin sensations that might indicate specific health problems.

ANATOMY AND PHYSIOLOGY REVIEW

Structure of the Skin

The skin has three layers: subcutaneous tissue (fat), dermis, and epidermis (Fig. 24-2). Each layer has unique properties that help the skin maintain its complex functions.

Subcutaneous fat (adipose tissue [fat]) is the innermost layer of the skin, lying over muscle and bone. Fat distribution varies with body area, age, and gender. Fat cells insulate the body and absorb shock, padding internal structures. Blood vessels go through the fatty layer and extend into the dermis, forming capillary networks that supply nutrients and remove wastes.

The dermis (corium) is the layer above the fat layer and contains no skin cells but does contain some protective mast cells and macrophages (see Chapter 17). The dermis is composed of interwoven collagen and elastic fibers that give the skin flexibility and strength.

Collagen, the main component of dermal tissue, is a protein produced by fibroblast cells. Its production increases in areas of tissue injury and helps form scar tissue. Fibroblasts also produce **ground substance**, a lubricant that contributes to skin suppleness and turgor.

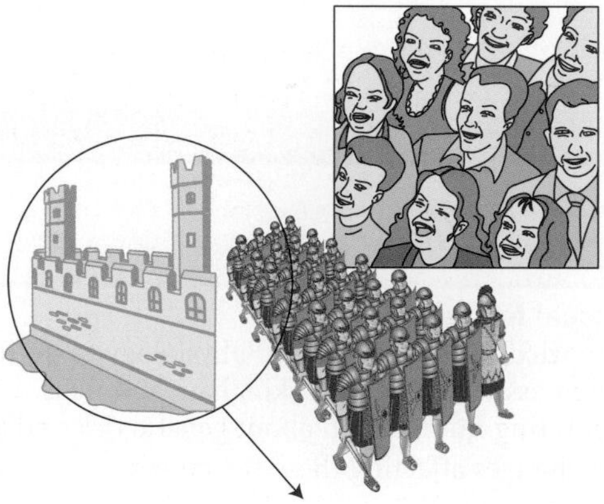

FIG. 24-1 Role of the skin in the concept of body protection.

Skin elasticity depends on the amount and quality of the dermal elastic fibers. The major component of the elastic fiber is elastin.

The dermis has capillaries and lymph vessels for the exchange of oxygen and heat. It is rich in sensory nerves that transmit the sensations of touch, pressure, temperature, pain, and itch.

The epidermis is the outermost skin layer. It is anchored to the dermis by fingerlike projections (**rete pegs**) that interlock with dermal structures called **dermal papillae.** Less than 1 mm thick, the epidermal layer is the first line of defense between the body and the environment.

The epidermis does not have its own blood supply. Instead it receives nutrients by diffusion from the blood vessels in the dermal layer. Attached to the basement membrane of the epidermis are the basal **keratinocytes**—skin cells that undergo cell division and differentiation to continuously renew skin TISSUE INTEGRITY and maintain optimal barrier function. As basal cells divide, keratinocytes are pushed upward and form the *spinous layer (stratum spinosum).* Together the basal layer and the spinous layer are referred to as the *germinative layer (stratum germinativum),* because these layers are responsible for new skin growth (McCance et al., 2014). The keratinocytes continue to enlarge and flatten as they move upward to form the outermost horny skin layer (**stratum corneum**)**.** When these cells reach the stratum corneum (in 28 to 45 days), they are no longer living cells and are shed from the skin surface. **Keratin**, a protein produced by keratinocytes, makes the horny layer waterproof.

On the palms of the hands and soles of the feet an additional thick layer of epidermis forms known as the *stratum lucidum.* This clear layer of nonliving cells pads and protects the underlying dermal and epidermal structures in these vulnerable areas.

Vitamin D is activated in the epidermis by ultraviolet (UV) light, such as sunlight. Once activated, it is distributed by the blood to the GI tract to promote uptake of dietary calcium.

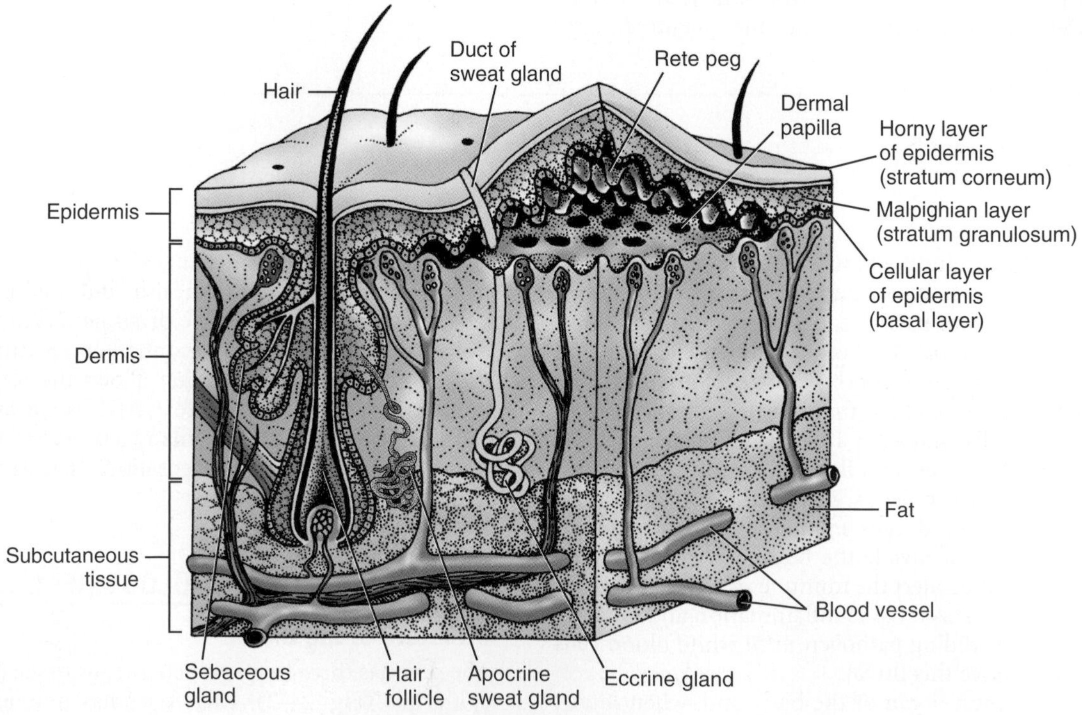

FIG. 24-2 Anatomy of the skin.

Melanocytes are pigment-producing cells found at the basement membrane. These cells give color to the skin and account for the ethnic differences in skin tone. Darker skin tones are not caused by increased numbers of melanocytes; rather, the size of the pigment granules *(melanin)* contained in each cell determines the color. Melanin protects the skin from damage by UV light, which stimulates melanin production. For this reason, people with dark skin are less likely to develop sunburn than lighter-skinned people. Freckles, birthmarks, and age spots are lesions caused by patches of increased melanin production. Melanin production also increases in areas that have endocrine changes or inflammation.

Structure of the Skin Appendages

Hair differs in type and function in various body areas. Hair growth varies with race, gender, age, and genetic predisposition. Individual hairs can differ in both structure and rate of growth, depending on body location.

Hair follicles are located in the dermal layer of the skin but are actually extensions of the epidermal layer (see Fig. 24-2). Within each hair follicle, a round column of keratin forms the hair shaft. Hair color is genetically determined by a person's rate of melanin production.

Hair growth occurs in cycles of a growth phase followed by a resting phase. Growth is dependent on a good blood supply and adequate nutrition. Stressors can alter the growth cycle and result in temporary hair loss. Permanent baldness, such as male pattern baldness, is inherited.

Nails on fingers and toes have cosmetic value and are useful for grasping and scraping. Like hair follicles, the nails are extensions of the keratin-producing epidermal layers of the skin.

The white, crescent-shaped portion of the nail at the lower end of the nail plate is the **lunula** and is where nail keratin is formed and nail growth begins (Fig. 24-3). Nail growth is a continuous but slow process. Fingernail replacement requires 3 to 4 months. Toenail replacement may take up to 12 months.

The cuticle attaches the nail plate to the soft tissue of the nail fold. The nail body is translucent, and the pinkish hue reflects a rich blood supply beneath the nail surface. Nail growth and appearance are often altered during systemic disease or serious illness.

Sebaceous glands are distributed over the entire skin surface except for the palms of the hands and soles of the feet. Most of these glands are connected directly to the hair follicles (see Fig. 24-2).

Sebaceous glands produce **sebum**, a mildly bacteriostatic, fat-containing substance. Sebum lubricates the skin and reduces water loss from the skin surface.

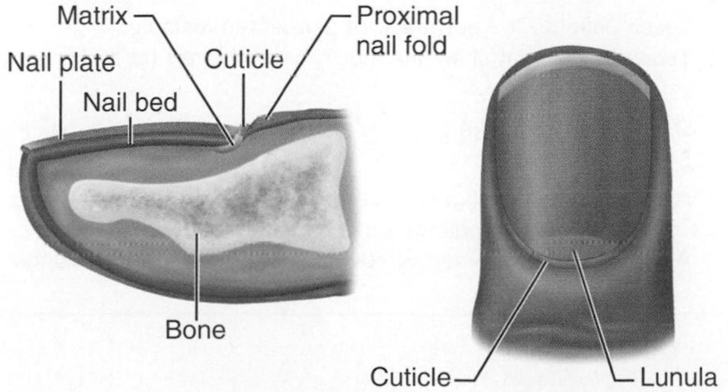

FIG. 24-3 Anatomy of the nail.

Sweat glands of the skin are of two types: eccrine and apocrine. Eccrine sweat glands arise from the epithelial cells. They are found over the entire skin surface and are not associated with the hair follicle. The odorless, colorless secretions of these glands are important in body temperature regulation. This sweat and the resultant water evaporation can cause the body to lose up to 10 to 12 L of fluid in a single day.

Apocrine sweat glands are in direct contact with the hair follicle and are found mostly in the axillae, nipple, umbilical, and perineal body areas. The interaction of skin bacteria with the secretions of these glands causes body odor.

Functions of the Skin

The skin is a complex organ responsible for the regulation of many body functions throughout the life span (Table 24-1) (McCance et al., 2014). In addition to the skin's protective and regulatory functions, its location on the outside of the body makes it an important way to communicate a patient's state of health and body image.

Skin Changes Associated with Aging

The process of aging begins at birth (Touhy & Jett, 2014). As changes in physiology progress with aging, the skin also undergoes age-related changes in structure and function (Chart 24-1). Figs. 24-4 through 24-8 show age-related skin changes.

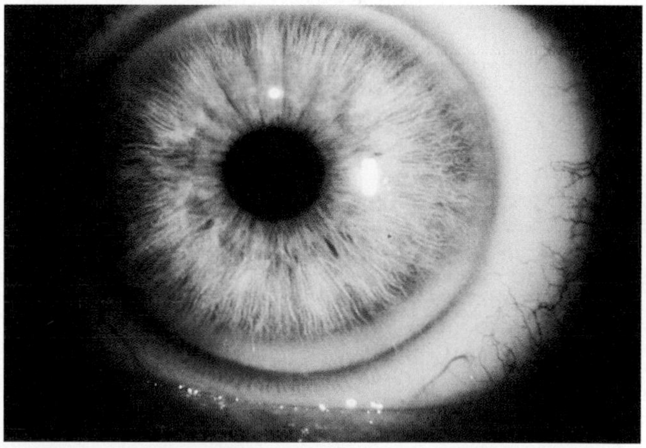

FIG. 24-4 Arcus senilis of the iris.

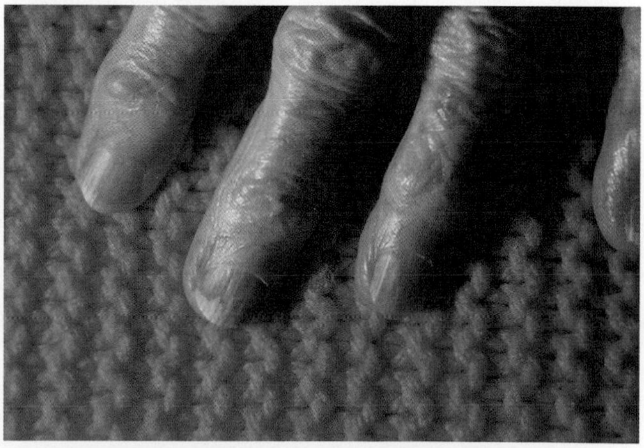

FIG. 24-5 Nail changes: longitudinal ridges and thickening.

TABLE 24-1 **Functions of the Skin**

EPIDERMIS	DERMIS	SUBCUTANEOUS TISSUE
Protection		
Keratin provides protection from injury by corrosive materials Inhibits proliferation of microorganisms because of dry external surface Mechanical strength through intercellular bonds	Provides cells for wound healing Provides mechanical strength: Collagen fibers Elastic fibers Ground substance Sensory nerve receptors signal skin injury and inflammation	Mechanical shock absorber Energy reserve Insulation
Homeostasis (Water Balance)		
Low permeability to water and electrolytes prevents systemic dehydration and electrolyte loss	Lymphatic and vascular tissues respond to inflammation, injury, and infection	No real function in water balance
Temperature Regulation		
Eccrine sweat glands allow dissipation of heat through evaporation of sweat secreted onto the skin surface	Cutaneous vasculature promotes or inhibits heat loss from the skin surface	Fat cells insulate and assist in retention of body heat
Sensory Organ		
Transmits a variety of sensations through the neuroreceptor system	Has many nerve receptors for relaying sensations to the brain	Contains large pressure receptors
Vitamin Synthesis		
Allows photoconversion of 7-dehydrocholesterol to active vitamin D	No function	No function
Psychosocial		
Body image alterations occur with many epidermal diseases	Body image alterations occur with many dermal diseases	Body image alterations may result from changes in body fat stores

CHART 24-1 **Nursing Focus on the Older Adult**

Changes in the Integumentary System Related to Aging

PHYSICAL CHANGES	CLINICAL FINDINGS	NURSING ACTIONS
Epidermis		
Decreased epidermal thickness	Skin transparency and fragility	Handle patients carefully to reduce skin friction and shear. Assess for excessive dryness or moisture. Avoid taping the skin.
Decreased cell division	Delayed wound healing	Avoid skin trauma, and protect open areas.
Decreased epidermal mitotic homeostasis	Skin hyperplasia and skin cancers (especially in sun-exposed areas)	Assess non–sun-exposed areas for baseline skin features. Assess exposed skin areas for sun-induced changes.
Increased epidermal permeability	Increased risk for irritation	Teach patients how to avoid exposure to skin irritants.
Decreased immune system cells	Decreased skin inflammatory response	Do not rely on degree of redness and swelling to correlate with the severity of skin injury or localized infection.
Decreased melanocyte activity	Increased risk for sunburn	Teach patients to wear hats, sunscreen, and protective clothing. Teach patients to avoid sun exposure from 10 AM to 4 PM.
Hyperplasia of melanocyte activity (especially in sun-exposed areas)	Changes in pigmentation (e.g., liver spots, age spots)	Teach patients to keep track of pigmented lesions. Teach them what changes should be evaluated for malignancy.
Decreased vitamin D production	Increased risk for osteomalacia	Urge patients to take a multiple vitamin or a calcium supplement with vitamin D.
Flattening of the dermal-epidermal junction	Increased risk for shearing forces, resulting in blisters, purpura, skin tears, and pressure-related problems	Avoid pulling or dragging patients. Assist patients confined to bed or chairs to change positions at least every 2 hours. Avoid or use care when removing adhesive wound dressings.

CHART 24-1 Nursing Focus on the Older Adult—cont'd

Changes in the Integumentary System Related to Aging

PHYSICAL CHANGES	CLINICAL FINDINGS	NURSING ACTIONS
Dermis		
Decreased dermal blood flow	Increased susceptibility to dry skin	Teach patients to apply moisturizers when the skin is still moist and to avoid agents that promote skin dryness.
Decreased vasomotor responsiveness	Increased risk for heat stroke and hypothermia	Teach patients to dress for the environmental temperatures.
Decreased dermal thickness	Paper-thin, transparent skin with an increased susceptibility to trauma	Handle patients gently, and avoid the use of tape or tight dressings. Use lift sheets when positioning patients.
Degeneration of elastic fibers	Decreased tone and elasticity	Check skin turgor on the forehead or chest.
Benign proliferation of capillaries	Cherry hemangiomas	Teach patients that these are benign.
Reduced number and function of nerve endings	Reduced sensory perception	Tell patients to use bath thermometer and to lower the water heater temperature to prevent scalds.
Subcutaneous Layer		
Thinning subcutaneous layer	Increased risk for hypothermia	Teach patients to dress warmly in cold weather.
	Increased risk for pressure injury	Assist patients confined to bed or chairs to change positions at least every 2 hours.
Hair		
Decreased number of hair follicles and rate of growth	Increased hair thinning	Suggest wearing hats to prevent heat loss in cold weather and to prevent sunburn.
Decreased number of active melanocytes in follicle	Gradual loss of hair color (graying)	Inform patients that hair color loss can occur at any age.
Nails		
Decreased rate of growth	Increased risk for fungal infections	Inspect the nails of all older adults. Teach patients to keep feet clean and dry.
Decreased nail bed blood flow	Longitudinal nail ridges	Use the oral mucosa to assess for cyanosis.
Thickening of the nail	Toenails thicken and may overhang the toes	Use fingernails to assess capillary refill. Cut toenails straight across. Do not use nail appearance alone to assess for a fungal infection. Assess skin next to the nail to determine whether the thick nail is irritating it.
Glands		
Decreased sebum production	Increased size of nasal pores; large comedones	Teach patients not to squeeze the pores or comedones to prevent skin trauma.
Decreased eccrine and apocrine gland activity	Increased susceptibility to dry skin	Urge patients to use soaps with a high fat content. Teach patients to avoid frequent bathing with hot water. Teach patients to apply moisturizers after bathing while skin is moist.
	Decreased perspiration with decreased cooling effect	Do not use sweat production as an indicator of hyperthermia.

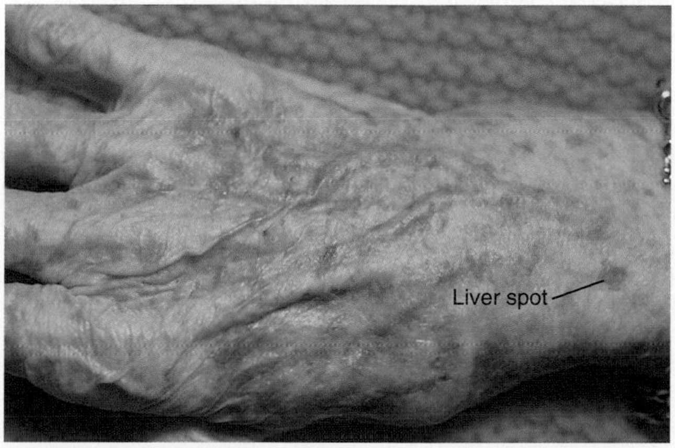

FIG. 24-6 Paper-thin, transparent skin with actinic lentigo (liver spots).

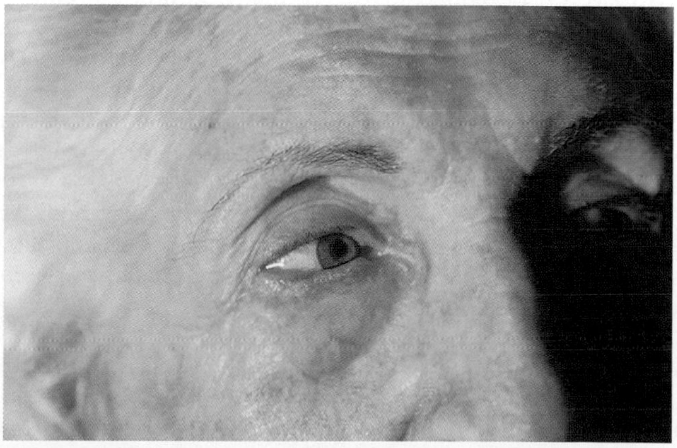

FIG. 24-7 Eyelid eversion, deepening of the eye orbit, and "bags" under the eye.

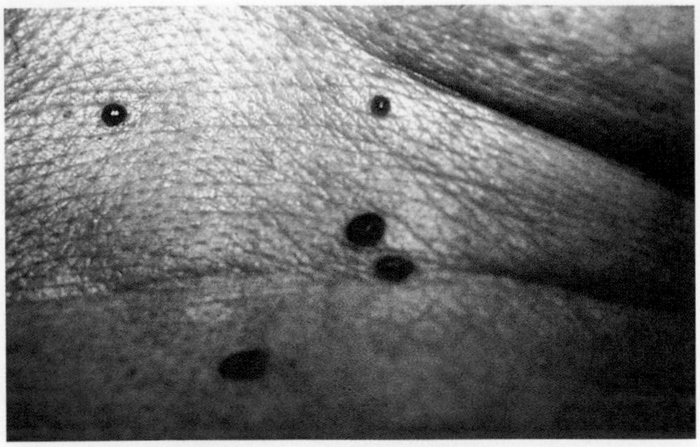

FIG. 24-8 Senile (cherry) angiomas.

Individual differences exist in how quickly and to what degree the skin ages. Although genetic factors, hormonal changes, and disease may change skin appearance over time, chronic sun exposure is the single most important factor leading to degeneration of the skin components.

ASSESSMENT METHODS

Patient History

Take an accurate history from the patient so that skin problems can be readily identified. Chart 24-2 highlights specific questions to ask during a skin assessment.

Demographic data include age, race, occupation, and hobbies or recreational activities. This information can help identify causative or aggravating factors for skin problems. Age is important because many changes in the skin, hair, and nails are normal for the aging process.

Ethnicity can also be important. Some variations in skin appearance are normal for patients of some ethnicities but are abnormal for those of other races or ethnicities.

Information about occupation and hobbies can provide clues to chronic skin exposure to chemicals, irritants, and other substances that can contribute to skin problems.

Socioeconomic status data can help identify environmental factors that might contribute to skin disease. Unhealthy or crowded living conditions promote the spread of contagious skin pathogens. Recent or frequent travel to tropical climates may be a source of unusual skin infections or infestations.

Regardless of skin color or ethnicity, always ask patients about the amount of time spent in the sun and tanning booths and identify skin problems related to sun overexposure. Use this time to teach the patient about the harmful aspects of sun exposure and how to reduce risk. Also determine whether he or she regularly assesses the skin for lesion development or changes.

Skin problems related to poor hygiene are common. Ask about living conditions and bathing practices. Teach people that keeping the skin and hair clean by bathing and shampooing regularly helps maintain the skin's health.

Information about drug use is important because prescribed drugs, over-the-counter (OTC) drugs, herbal preparations or remedies, and tobacco use can cause skin reactions or affect skin function. Ask about any recent use of prescription drugs, OTC drugs (e.g., laxatives, antacids, cold remedies), and herbal preparations or remedies. Determine when each drug was started, the dose and frequency of the drug, and the time the last dose was taken. Ask the patient whether skin changes began after starting a new drug. A drug history also helps identify skin changes that result from management of other health problems, such as the changes that occur with long-term steroid or anticoagulant therapy.

Allergies to environmental substances often have skin manifestations. The allergies may be well documented or have a new onset. Ask about the use of any new personal care product (e.g., shaving products, perfumes, soap, shampoo, lotion, makeup, hair gel), laundry detergents and softeners, and home cleaning products. Ask whether the patient wears gloves to avoid direct contact with cleaning solutions. New clothing may contain chemicals that irritate the skin. Noting the body location(s) of the skin problem can help determine its cause.

Nutrition Status

Document the patient's weight, height, body build and fat distribution, and food preferences. Protein deficiencies, vitamin deficiencies, and obesity can increase the risk for skin lesions and delay wound healing. Fat-free diets and chronic alcoholism

CHART 24-2 Best Practice for Patient Safety & Quality Care (QSEN)

Questions to Obtain an Accurate Nursing History of the Patient with a Skin Problem

Medical-Surgical History
- Do you have any current or previous medical problems?
- Have you undergone any recent or previous surgical procedures?

Family History
- Is there any family tendency toward chronic skin problems?
- Do any members of your immediate family have recent skin problems?

Medication History
- Are you allergic to any drugs? If so, describe the reaction.
- What prescription drugs have you taken recently? When was the drug started? What is the dose or frequency of administration? When was the last dose taken?
- What over-the-counter drugs have you taken recently? When was the drug started? What is the dose or frequency of administration? When was the last dose taken?

Social History
- What is your occupation?
- What recreational activities do you enjoy?
- Have you traveled recently?
- What is your nutrition status?
- Do you use tobacco or recreational drugs or drink alcohol?

Current Health Problem
- When did you first notice the skin problem?
- Where on the body did the problem begin?
- Has the problem gotten better or worse?
- Has a similar skin condition ever occurred before? If so, what was the course and how was it treated?
- Is the problem associated with any itching, burning, stinging, numbness, pain, fever, nausea and vomiting, diarrhea, sore throat, cold, stiff neck, new foods, new soaps or cosmetics, new clothing or bed linens, or stressful situations?
- What seems to make the problem worse?
- What seems to make the problem better?

can lead to vitamin deficiencies and related skin changes. Skin problems such as chronic urticaria and acne may be worsened by certain foods or food additives.

Hydration influences overall skin health, and the skin reflects hydration status. Reduced fluid intake can lead to dry skin. Skin manifestations of severe fluid losses are seen as loose skin that tents when pinched together. Fluid overload with edema can stretch the skin, masking wrinkles and allowing the formation of skin "pits" (i.e., pitting edema) when pressure is applied to it.

Family History and Genetic Risk

Many skin problems (e.g., psoriasis, keloid formation, eczema) have a familial predisposition. Explore any family tendency of chronic skin problems. Ask about immediate family members' current health to identify a transmittable disorder (e.g., ringworm, scabies).

Current Health Problems

Begin by gathering information about skin changes and skin care practices (see Chart 24-2).

If a skin problem is identified, obtain more information about the specific problem, such as:

- When did the patient first notice the rash or skin change?
- Where on the body did the rash begin?
- Has the problem improved or become worse?

If the problem has occurred before, ask the patient to describe the course of the skin lesion and how it was treated. Try to link the problem with manifestations, such as itching, burning, numbness, pain, fever, sore throat, stiff neck, or nausea and vomiting. Ask him or her to identify anything that seems to make the problem better or worse.

Skin Assessment

Inspection

Skin changes may be related to a specific skin disease or reflect a systemic disorder. Use a thorough skin assessment to identify clues about a patient's overall state of health.

A thorough assessment of the skin is best performed with the patient undressed. (Always provide privacy to maintain the patient's dignity.) Incorporate skin examination as a routine part of daily care during the bath or when assisting with hygiene.

Inspect the patient's skin surfaces in a well-lighted room; natural or bright fluorescent lighting makes subtle skin changes more visible. Use a penlight to closely inspect lesions and to illuminate the mouth.

Assess each skin surface systematically, including the scalp, hair, nails, and mucous membranes. Give particular attention to the skinfold areas. The moist, warm environment of skinfolds can harbor organisms, such as yeast or bacteria. Observe and document these features:

- Obvious changes in color and vascularity
- Presence or absence of moisture
- Edema
- Skin lesions
- Skin integrity

Check the cleanliness of the various body areas to determine whether the patient's self-care activities need to be evaluated.

Skin color is affected by blood flow, oxygenation, body temperature, and pigmentation. The wide variation in skin tones requires different techniques for patients who have darker skin. (See the Cultural Considerations box for tips for assessing patients with darker skin.)

Describe and document changes in skin color by their appearance (Table 24-2). Include in your description whether the changes are general or confined to one body region. Color changes are more visible in the areas of least pigmentation, such as the oral mucosa, sclera, nail beds, and palms and soles. Inspect these areas to help confirm more subtle color changes of general body areas.

Lesions in skin disease are clinically described in terms of primary and secondary lesions (Fig. 24-9). **Primary lesions** are an initial reaction to a problem that alters skin components. **Secondary lesions** are changes in the appearance of the primary lesion. These changes occur with progression of an underlying disease or in response to a topical or systemic therapeutic intervention. For example, acute dermatitis often occurs as primary vesicles with associated **pruritus** (itching). Secondary lesions in the form of crusts occur as the patient scratches, the vesicles are opened, and the exudate dries. With chronic dermatitis, the skin often becomes **lichenified** (thickened) because of the patient's continual rubbing of the area to relieve itching.

Describe lesions by color, size, location, and shape. Note whether they are isolated or are grouped and form a distinct pattern. Table 24-3 defines terms used to describe lesions.

Assess each lesion for these ABCDE features that are associated with skin cancer (The Skin Cancer Foundation, 2014):

- **A**symmetry of shape
- **B**order irregularity
- **C**olor variation within one lesion
- **D**iameter greater than 6 mm
- **E**volving or changing in any feature (shape, size, color, elevation, itching, bleeding, or crusting)

Teach patients these signs, and encourage them to perform skin self-examination on a monthly basis (American Cancer Society, 2014). *A patient who has a lesion with one or more of the ABCDE features should be evaluated by a dermatologist or surgeon.*

In describing location, determine whether lesions are generalized or localized. If the lesions are localized, identify the specific body areas involved. This information is important because some diseases have a specific pattern of skin lesions. For example, involvement of only the sun-exposed areas of the body is important when considering possible causes. Rashes limited to the skinfold areas (e.g., on the axillae, beneath the breasts, in the groin) may reflect problems related to friction, heat, and excessive moisture.

Edema causes the skin to appear shiny, **taut** (tightly stretched), and paler than uninvolved skin. During skin inspection, document the location, distribution, and color of areas of edema.

Skin elasticity is affected by edema. Using moderate pressure, place the tip of a finger against edematous tissue to determine the degree of indentation, or pitting (see Chapter 11).

Moisture content is assessed by noting the thickness and consistency of secretions. Normally, increased moisture in the form of sweat occurs with increased activity or elevated environmental temperatures. Dampness of skinfold areas occurs with reduced air circulation where the skin surfaces touch. Excess moisture can cause impaired TISSUE INTEGRITY with skin breakdown in bedridden and debilitated patients.

Overly dry skin is caused by a dry environment, poor skin lubrication, inadequate fluid intake, and the normal aging process. Dry skin usually has scaling and flaking and may be

TABLE 24-2 Common Alterations in Skin Color

ALTERATION	UNDERLYING CAUSE	LOCATION	SIGNIFICANCE
White (pallor)	Decreased hemoglobin level	Conjunctivae	Anemia
	Decreased blood flow to the skin (vasoconstriction)	Mucous membranes	Shock or blood loss
		Nail beds	Chronic vascular compromise
		Palms and soles	Sudden emotional upset
		Lips	Edema
	Genetically determined defect of the melanocyte (decreased pigmentation)	Generalized	Albinism
	Acquired patchy loss of pigmentation	Localized	Vitiligo, tinea versicolor
Yellow-orange	Increased total serum bilirubin level (jaundice)	Generalized	Hemolysis of red blood cells
		Mucous membranes	Liver disorders
		Sclera	
	Increased serum carotene level (carotenemia)	Perioral	Increased ingestion of carotene-containing foods (carrots)
		Palms and soles	Pregnancy
		Ears and nose	Thyroid deficiency
		Absent in sclera and mucous membranes	Diabetes
	Increased urochrome level	Generalized	Chronic kidney disease (uremia)
		Absent in sclera and mucous membranes	
Red (erythema)	Increased blood flow to the skin (vasodilation)	Generalized	Generalized inflammation (e.g., erythroderma)
		Localized (to area of involvement)	Localized inflammation (e.g., sunburn, cellulitis, trauma, rashes)
		Face, cheeks, nose, upper chest	Fever, increased alcohol intake
		Area of exposure	Exposure to cold
Blue	Increase in deoxygenated blood (cyanosis)	Nail beds	Cardiopulmonary disease
		Mucous membranes	Methemoglobinemia
		Generalized	
	Bleeding from vessels into tissue:		
	Petechiae (1-3 mm)	Localized	Thrombocytopenia
	Ecchymosis (>3 mm)	Localized	Increased blood vessel fragility
Reddish blue	Increased overall amount of hemoglobin	Generalized	Polycythemia vera
	Decreased peripheral circulation	Distal extremities, nose	Inadequate tissue perfusion
Brown	Increased melanin production	Localized (to area of involvement)	Chronic inflammation
		Pressure points, areolae, palmar creases, and genitalia	Exposure to sunlight
			Addison's disease
		Face, areolae, vulva, linea nigra	Pregnancy; oral contraceptives (melasma)
	Café au lait spots (tan-brown patches):		
	<6 spots	Localized	Nonpathogenic
	>6 spots	Generalized	Possible neurofibromatosis
	Melanin and hemosiderin deposits (bronze or grayish tan color)	Distal lower extremities	Chronic venous stasis
		Exposed areas or generalized	Hemochromatosis

TABLE 24-3 Terms Commonly Used to Describe Skin Lesion Configurations

annular Ringlike with raised borders around flat, clear centers of normal skin
circinate Circular
circumscribed Well-defined with sharp borders
clustered Several lesions grouped together
coalesced Lesions that merge with one another and appear confluent
diffuse Widespread, involving most of the body with intervening areas of normal skin; generalized
linear Occurring in a straight line
serpiginous With wavy borders, resembling a snake
universal All areas of the body involved, with no areas of normal-appearing skin

especially marked in areas of limited circulation, such as the feet and lower legs. It is a common problem during the winter months when the air contains less moisture, living in geographic areas with little humidity, and in the hospital environment where humidity is often low.

Vascular changes or markings may be normal or abnormal, depending on the cause. Normal vascular markings include birthmarks, cherry angiomas (see Fig. 24-8), spider angiomas, and venous stars. Bleeding into the skin is abnormal and results in **purpura** (bleeding under the skin that may progress from red to purple to brownish yellow), petechiae, and ecchymosis.

Petechiae are small, reddish purple lesions (<0.5 mm in diameter) that do not fade or blanch when pressure is applied (Fig. 24-10). They often indicate increased capillary fragility. Petechiae of the lower extremities often occur with stasis

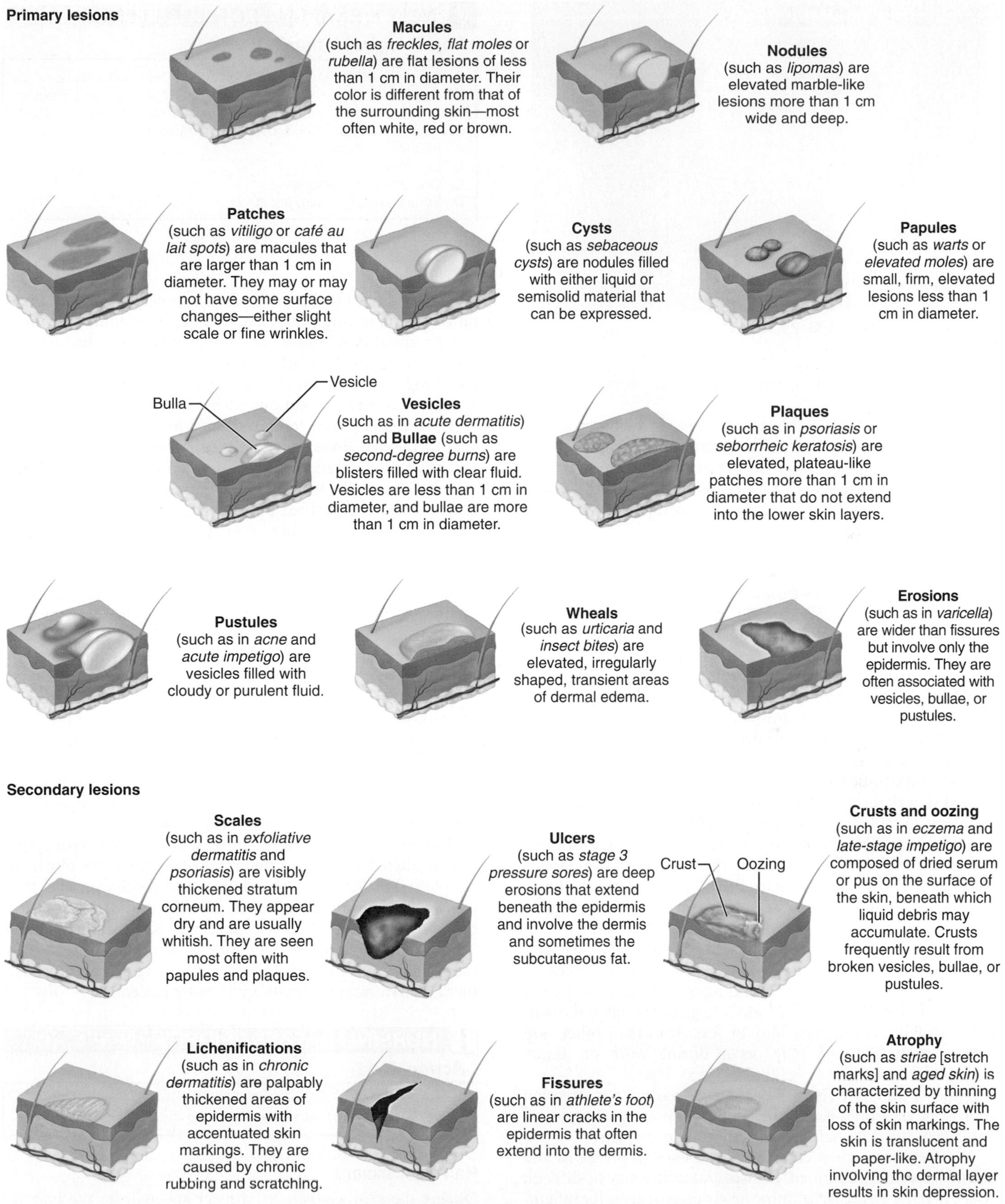

FIG. 24-9 Classification of skin lesions.

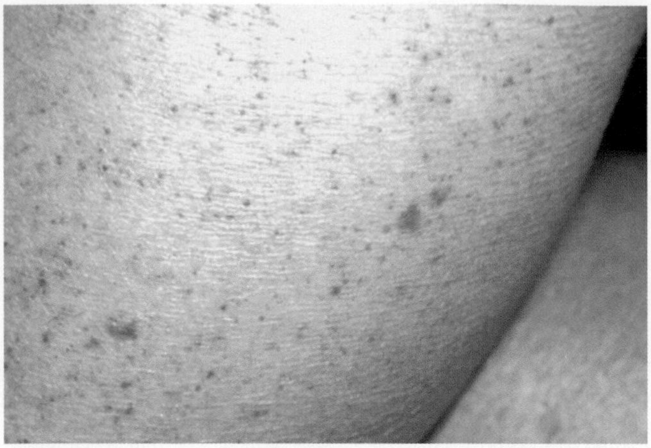

FIG. 24-10 Petechiae.

dermatitis, a condition usually seen with chronic venous insufficiency.

Ecchymoses (bruises) are larger areas of hemorrhage. In older adults, bruising is common after minor trauma to the skin. Certain drugs (e.g., aspirin, warfarin, corticosteroids) and low platelet counts lead to easy or excessive bruising. Anticoagulants and decreased numbers of platelets disrupt clotting action, resulting in ecchymosis.

Skin TISSUE INTEGRITY is assessed by first examining areas with actual breaks or open areas. For example, skin tears are a common finding in older people as a result of aging. The thin, fragile skin is easily damaged by friction or shearing forces, especially if bruising is already present. Look for skin tears in these areas:

- Where constricting clothing rubs against the skin
- On the upper extremities, where the skin is grasped when assisting a patient to ambulate or change position
- Where adhesive tapes or dressings have been applied and removed

Check for the presence of multiple abrasions or early pressure-related skin changes. These changes may indicate unrecognized problems in mobility or sensory perception.

Describe breaks in skin TISSUE INTEGRITY by their location, size, color, and distribution and by the presence of drainage or infection. The evaluation of partial-thickness and full-thickness wounds, including objective criteria that describe progress toward healing, is discussed in Chapter 25.

Cleanliness of the skin is evaluated to learn about self-care needs. Inspect the hair, nails, and skin closely for excessive soiling and offensive odor. Depending on a patient's degree of self-care deficit, hard-to-reach areas (e.g., perirectal and inguinal skinfolds, axillae, feet) may be less clean than other skin surface areas. Staining may occur during work or leisure activities.

Patients who have cognitive problems may not pay attention to hygiene measures. Assess the cognition of any patient whose hygiene of the skin, hair, or nails appears inadequate.

Tattoos and piercings can cause or mask skin problems and must be carefully examined. Bruises and rashes may be difficult to see in tattooed areas. Examine newly pierced areas for inflammation or infection. Scars may be present in old tattoos or pierced areas and should be documented. Closely examine any areas where tattoos have been removed. Skin cancer is more likely to occur in these areas.

NCLEX EXAMINATION CHALLENGE

Physiological Integrity

During skin inspection the nurse observes two brown lesions on the older client's upper back. The lesions are large and irregular with a consistently rough texture and a raised border. Which descriptors does the nurse use to document these observations?

A. Annular, macular
B. Confluent, fissured
C. Circumscribed, plaquelike
D. Serpiginous, pustular, linear

Palpation

Skin inspection can be misleading in areas of color changes, tattoos, and piercings. Use palpation to gather additional information about skin lesions, moisture, temperature, texture, and turgor (Table 24-4). Wash hands thoroughly before and after palpating a patient's skin. Use gloves to examine nonintact skin, and use Standard Precautions when skin areas are draining.

Palpation confirms lesion size and whether they are flat or slightly raised. Consistency of larger lesions can vary from soft and pliable to firm and solid. Subtle changes, such as the difference between a fine **macular** (flat) rash and a **papular** (raised) rash, are best determined by palpating with your eyes closed. Ask the patient whether skin palpation causes pain or tenderness.

In areas of excess dryness, rub your finger against the skin surface to determine the degree of flaking or scaling. Changes in skin temperature are detected by placing the back of your hand on the skin surface. First, make certain to have warm hands. Cold hands interfere with accurate assessment and are uncomfortable for the patient.

Palpate skin surfaces to assess texture, which differs according to body area and exposure to irritants. For example, areas of long-term sun exposure have a rougher texture than protected skin surfaces. The patient who has repeated exposure to harsh soaps or chemicals may show skin changes related to this exposure. Increased skin thickness from scarring, lichenification, or edema usually decreases elasticity.

Turgor indicates the amount of skin elasticity. Skin turgor can be altered by water content and aging. Gently pinch the patient's skin between your thumb and forefinger, and then release. If skin turgor is normal, the skin immediately returns to its original state when released. Poor skin turgor is seen as "tenting" of the skin, with a gradual return to the original state (see Chapter 11). Loss of elasticity with aging makes the assessment of skin turgor difficult in an older patient.

NURSING SAFETY PRIORITY QSEN

Action Alert

To avoid mistaking dehydration for dry skin in an older adult, always assess skin turgor on the forehead or chest.

Hair Assessment

During the skin assessment, inspect and palpate the hair for general appearance, cleanliness, distribution, quantity, and quality. Hair is normally found in an even distribution over most of the body surfaces, with the hair on the scalp, in the pubic region, and in the axillary folds thicker and coarser than

TABLE 24-4 **Common Clinical Findings In Skin Palpation**

CLINICAL FINDINGS	CAUSE	LOCATION	EXAMPLES OF PREDISPOSING CONDITIONS
Edema			
Localized	Inflammatory response	Area of involvement	Trauma
Dependent or pitting	Fluid and electrolyte imbalance Venous and cardiac insufficiency	Ambulatory: dorsum of foot and medial ankle Bedridden: buttocks, sacrum, and lower back	Congestive heart failure Kidney disease Liver cirrhosis Venous thrombosis or stasis
Nonpitting	Endocrine imbalance	Generalized, but more easily seen over the tibia	Hypothyroidism (myxedema)
Moisture			
Increased	Autonomic nervous system stimulation	Face, axillae, skinfolds, palms, and soles	Fever, anxiety, activity Hyperthyroidism
Decreased	Dehydration Endocrine imbalance	Buccal mucous membranes with progressive involvement of other skin surfaces	Fluid loss Postmenopausal status Hypothyroidism Normal aging
Temperature			
Increased	Increased blood flow to the skin	Generalized	Fever, hypermetabolic states Neurotrauma
		Localized	Inflammation
Decreased	Decreased blood flow to the skin	Generalized	Impending shock, sepsis, anxiety Hypothyroidism
		Localized	Interference with vascular flow
Turgor			
Decreased	Decreased elasticity of the dermis (tenting when pinched)	Abdomen, forehead, or radial aspect of the wrist	Severe dehydration Sudden, severe weight loss Normal aging
Texture			
Roughness or thickness	Irritation, friction	Pressure points (e.g., soles, palms, elbows) Localized areas of pruritus	Calluses Chronic eczema Atopic skin diseases
	Sun damage	Areas of sun exposure	Normal aging
	Excessive collagen production	Localized or generalized	Scleroderma Scars and keloids
Softness or smoothness	Endocrine disturbances	Generalized	Hyperthyroidism

hair on the trunk, arms, and legs. Although color and growth patterns vary, sudden changes in hair characteristics may reflect an underlying disease. Check any abnormal findings by obtaining a detailed history of the change.

How well the hair is groomed, including the cleanliness of areas of thicker hair growth, can confirm information about a patient's social history and health care needs. If the patient has intense itching or scratches continually, examine the scalp and pubis for lice and **nits** (lice eggs). Inspect the scalp for scaling, redness, open areas, crusting, and tenderness.

Dandruff, a collection of patchy or diffuse white or gray scales on the surface of the scalp, is common. The flaking that occurs with dandruff causes many people to mistakenly think the scalp is too dry; however, it is a problem of excessive oil production. Dandruff is a cosmetic problem, but a very oily scalp can induce inflammatory changes with redness and itching. Severe inflammatory dandruff can extend to the eyebrows and the skin of the face and neck. *If severe dandruff is not treated, hair loss can occur.* Teach the patient that dandruff is not caused by dryness and should be treated to prevent hair loss.

Although gradual hair loss occurs with aging, sudden asymmetric or patchy hair loss at any age is of concern. Assess the scalp for hair distribution and thickness, and document variations. Body hair loss, especially on the feet or lower legs, may occur with decreased blood flow to the area and also is a part of aging.

Hirsutism is excessive growth of body hair or hair growth in abnormal body areas. Increased hair growth across the face and chest in women is a sign of hirsutism. It may occur on the face of a woman as part of aging, is one manifestation of hormonal imbalance, and can also occur as a side effect of drug therapy. If hirsutism is present, look for changes in fat distribution and capillary fragility, which can occur in Cushing's disease, and for clitoral enlargement and deepening of the voice, which may indicate ovarian dysfunction.

Nail Assessment

Dystrophic (abnormal-appearing) nails may occur with a serious systemic illness or local skin disease involving the epidermal keratinocytes. Assess the fingernails and toenails for color, shape, thickness, texture, and the presence of lesions.

Many variations in color, texture, and grooming of the nails are influenced by factors unrelated to disease, such as occupation. When assessing the older adult, observe for minor variations associated with the aging process (see Fig. 24-5), such as a gradual thickening of the nail plate, the presence of longitudinal ridges, or a yellowish gray discoloration.

Color of the nail plate depends on nail thickness and transparency, amount of red blood cells, arterial blood flow, and pigment deposits (Table 24-5). Fig. 24-11 shows normal variations in nail color. Changes in color can be caused by chemical damage that occurs with some occupations and with the long-term use of nail polish. Regardless of skin color, the healthy nail blanches (lightens) with pressure.

During examination, the patient's fingers and toes should be free of any surface pressure that interferes with local blood flow or alters the appearance of the digits. To differentiate between color changes from the underlying blood supply and those from pigment deposits, blanch the nail bed to see whether the color changes with pressure. Gently squeeze the end of the finger or toe, exerting downward pressure on the nail bed, and then release the pressure. Color caused by blood flow changes as pressure is applied and returns to the original state when pressure is released. Color caused by pigment deposits remains unchanged.

Nail shape changes may be related to systemic disease. For example, fingernail clubbing occurs with impaired gas exchange. (See Fig. 30-10 in Chapter 30.)

Assess nail shape by examining the curve of the nail plate and surrounding tissue from all angles. Palpate the fingertips to

TABLE 24-5 Common Alterations in Nail Color

ALTERATION	CLINICAL FINDINGS	SIGNIFICANCE
White	Horizontal white banding or areas of opacity	Chronic liver or kidney disease (hypoalbuminemia)
	Generalized pallor of nail beds	Shock Anemia Early arteriosclerotic changes (toenails) Myocardial infarction
Yellow-brown	Diffuse yellow to brown discoloration	Jaundice Peripheral lymphedema Bacterial or fungal infections of the nail Psoriasis Diabetes Cardiac failure Staining from tobacco, nail polish, or dyes Long-term tetracycline therapy Normal aging (yellow-gray color)
	Vertical brown banding extending from the proximal nail fold distally	Normal finding in dark-skinned patients Nevus or melanoma of nail matrix in light-skinned patients
Red	Thin, dark red vertical lines 1-3 mm long (splinter hemorrhages)	Bacterial endocarditis Trichinosis Trauma to the nail bed Normal finding in some patients
	Red discoloration of the lunula	Cardiac insufficiency
	Dark red nail beds	Polycythemia vera
Blue	Diffuse blue discoloration that blanches with pressure	Respiratory failure Methemoglobinuria Venous stasis disease (toenails)

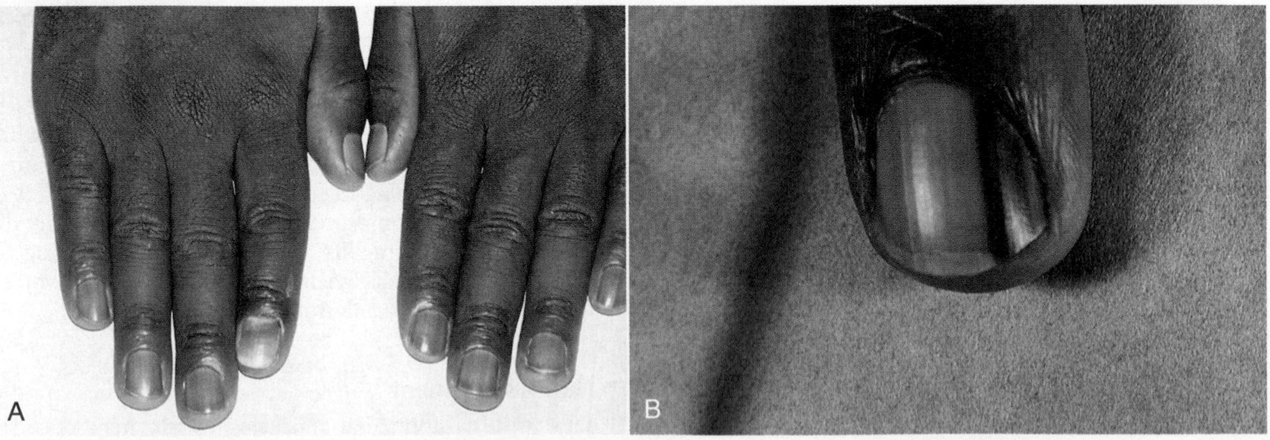

FIG. 24-11 **A,** Diffuse nail pigmentation. **B,** Linear nail pigmentation.

assess for sponginess, tenderness, or edema. Table 24-6 describes common variations in nail shape.

Thickness of the nail plate varies with age, trauma, dermatologic disease, or decreased arterial blood flow. In older patients, look for a "heaped-up" appearance of the toenails, which occurs with fungal infection *(onychomycosis)*.

Consistency of the nail is described as hard, soft, or brittle. Nail plates become hard, with thickening. A warm-water soak or lubrication with petroleum jelly is required to soften the nail plates before they can be trimmed. Soft nail plates, which are thin and bend easily with pressure, are associated with malnutrition, chronic arthritis, myxedema, and peripheral neuritis.

Brittle nails can split, as with onychomycosis or advanced psoriasis involving the fingers or toes. Splitting of the nail plate is caused by repeated exposure to water and detergents, which damage the plate over time.

Lesions can occur around, on, within, or under the nail. Separation of the nail plate from the nail bed *(onycholysis)* creates an air pocket beneath the plate. The pocket first appears as a grayish white opacity. The color changes as dirt and keratin collect in the pocket, and the area begins to have a bad odor. This problem occurs with fungal infections and after trauma. Separation of the nail plate may also occur with psoriasis or with prolonged chemical contact.

Inspect the tissue folds around the nail plate for redness, heat, swelling, and tenderness. **Acute paronychia** (inflammation of the skin around the nail) often occurs with a torn cuticle or an ingrown toenail.

Chronic paronychia is common and is an inflammation that persists for months. People at risk for chronic paronychia are those with frequent exposure to water, such as homemakers, bartenders, laundry workers, and nurses.

CULTURAL CONSIDERATIONS

Patient-Centered Care QSEN

Pallor, erythema, cyanosis, and other skin color changes are less visible in patients with naturally dark skin tones. Although physiologic processes are the same for both light-skinned and dark-skinned patients, the amount of skin pigmentation alters how the skin appears in response to physiologic alterations. Different assessment skills are needed to detect the more subtle color changes. Become familiar with the normal appearance of a dark-skinned patient's mucous membranes, nail beds, and skin tone so that variations from baseline can be identified. Chart 24-3 lists assessment techniques to assess skin manifestations in people with dark skin.

TABLE 24-6 Common Variations In Nail Shape

NAIL SHAPE	CLINICAL FINDINGS		SIGNIFICANCE
Normal	Angle of 160 degrees between the nail plate and the proximal nail fold Nail surface slightly convex Nail base firm when palpated	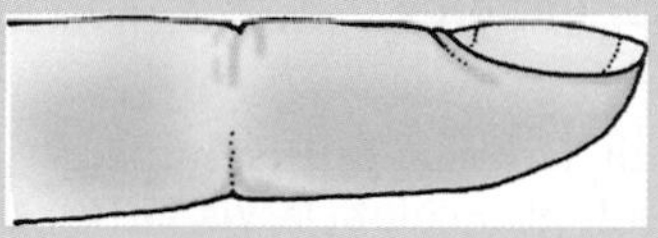	Normal finding
Clubbing:			
Early clubbing	Straightening of angle between the nail plate and the proximal nail fold to 180 degrees Nail base spongy when palpated	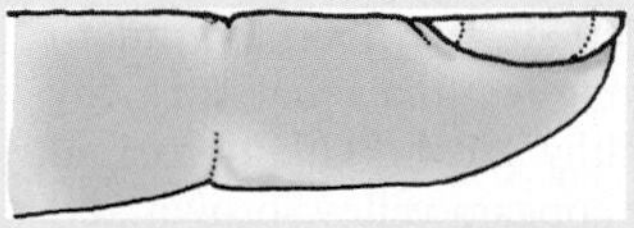	Hypoxia Lung cancer
Late clubbing	Angle between the nail plate and the proximal nail fold exceeds 180 degrees Nail base visibly edematous and spongy when palpated Enlargement of the soft tissue of the fingertips gives a "drumstick" appearance when viewed from above	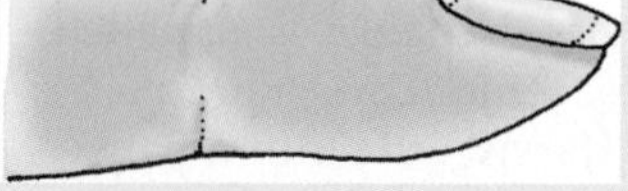	Prolonged hypoxia Emphysema Chronic obstructive pulmonary disease Advanced lung cancer Cystic fibrosis Chronic heart disease
Spoon nails (koilonychia):			
Early koilonychias	Flattening of the nail plate with an increased smoothness of the nail surface	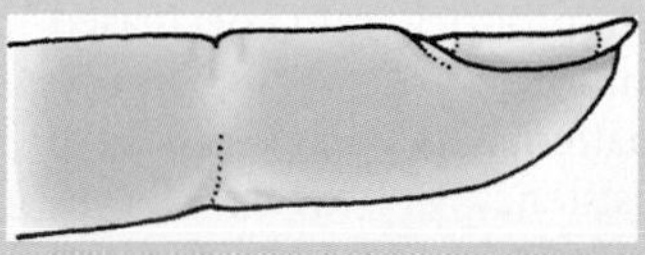	Iron deficiency (with or without anemia) Poorly controlled diabetes >15 yr in duration Local injury
Late koilonychias	Concave curvature of the nail plate		Psoriasis Chemical irritants Developmental abnormality
Beau's grooves	1-mm–wide horizontal depressions in the nail plates caused by growth arrest (involves all nails)	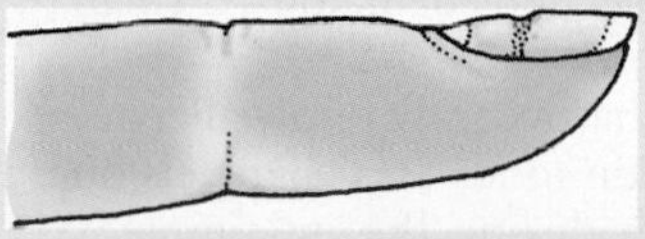	Acute, severe illness Prolonged febrile state Isolated periods of severe malnutrition
Pitting	Small, multiple pits in the nail plate May be associated with plate thickening and onycholysis Most often involves the fingernails (several or all)	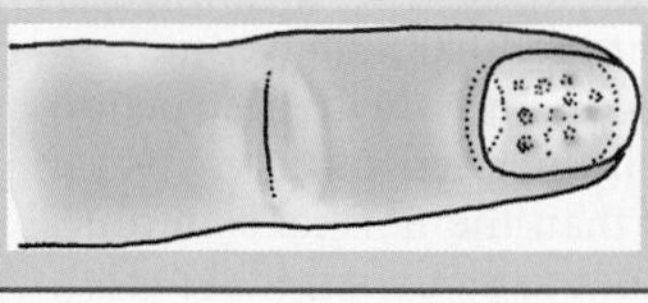	Psoriasis Alopecia areata

CHART 24-3 Best Practice for Patient Safety & Quality Care QSEN

Assessing Changes in Dark Skin

Cyanosis
- Examine lips and tongue for gray color.
- Examine nail beds, palms, and soles for blue tinge.
- Examine conjunctiva for pallor.

Inflammation
- Compare affected area with nonaffected area for increased warmth.
- Examine the skin of the affected area to determine whether it is shiny or taut or pits with pressure.
- Compare the skin color of affected area with the same area on the opposite side of the body.
- Palpate the affected area and compare it with unaffected area to determine whether texture is different (affected area may feel hard or "woody").

Jaundice
- Check for yellow tinge to oral mucous membranes, especially the hard palate.
- Examine the sclera nearest to the iris rather than the corners of the eye.

Bleeding
- Compare the affected area with the same area on the unaffected body side for swelling or skin darkening.
- If the patient has thrombocytopenia, petechiae may be present on the oral mucosa or conjunctiva.

Skin Assessment Techniques for Patients with Darker Skin

Pallor can be detected in people with dark skin by first inspecting the mucous membranes for an ash-gray color (Jarvis, 2016). If the lips and the nail beds are not heavily pigmented, they appear paler than normal for that patient. Use good lighting to assess for the absence of the underlying red tones that normally give heavily pigmented skin a healthy glow. With decreased blood flow to the skin, brown skin appears yellow-brown and very dark brown skin is ash gray.

Cyanosis can be present when gas exchange is impaired. Examine the lips, tongue, nail beds, conjunctivae, and palms and soles for subtle color changes (Jarvis, 2016). In a patient with cyanosis, the lips and tongue are gray and the palms, soles, conjunctivae, and nail beds have a bluish tinge. To support these findings, assess for other indicators of hypoxia, including tachycardia, hypotension, changes in respiratory rate, decreased breath sounds, and changes in cognition.

Inflammation in dark-skinned patients appears as excessive warmth and changes in skin consistency or texture (Jarvis, 2016). Use the back of your hand to palpate areas of suspected inflammation for increased warmth. With the fingertips, palpate for hardened areas deep in the tissue, which may give the skin a "woody" feel. Inflamed skin is tender and edematous. If edema is extensive, the skin is taut and shiny.

Skin areas where inflammation has recently resolved appear *darker* than the patient's normal skin tone. This change is due to stimulation of the melanocytes during the inflammatory process and to the increased pigment production that continues after inflammation subsides. Deep skin injury with destruction of melanocytes (e.g., deep ulcer, full-thickness burn) may heal with color changes that are *lighter* than the normal skin tone. Chronic inflammatory changes are not tender. Scarred skin feels less supple, especially over the joints. If chronic inflammatory changes are suspected, ask the patient about a history of skin problems in that area.

Jaundice in a patient with dark skin is best assessed by inspecting the oral mucosa, especially the hard palate, for yellow discoloration (Jarvis, 2016). Yellowness of the conjunctivae and adjacent sclera may be misleading because normal deposits of fat produce a yellowish hue that is visible in contrast to the dark skin around the eyes. Examine the sclera closest to the cornea for a more accurate determination of jaundice. The palms and soles of dark-skinned patients may appear yellow if they are calloused even when jaundice is not present.

Skin bleeding with purpuric lesions may not be visible with deep pigmentation. Areas of ecchymoses appear darker than normal skin; they may be tender and easily palpable, depending on whether hematoma is present. Often, the patient relates a history of trauma to the area that confirms the assessment. Petechiae are rarely visible in dark skin and may be seen only in the oral mucosa and conjunctiva.

Psychosocial Assessment

Skin changes, especially of the face, hair, and hands, often affect a person's body image. Encourage the patient to express his or her feelings about a change in appearance. Assess his or her body language for clues indicating a disturbance in self-concept. The avoidance of eye contact or the use of clothing to cover the affected areas suggests concern about appearance. Patients with chronic skin diseases often become socially isolated related to a fear of rejection by others or a belief that the skin problem is contagious.

Skin changes linked to poor hygiene are common among homeless people and among those who have reduced cognitive functioning. Assess the patient's overall appearance for excessive soiling, matted hair, body odor, or other self-care deficits. Confirm unsanitary living conditions by obtaining a social history. Patients may relate similar skin problems among family members, friends, and sexual contacts.

If skin problems related to poor hygiene are identified in older patients, also evaluate any physical limitations that might interfere with grooming. For example, visual or mobility problems can make it difficult for them to see or reach skin surfaces to clean them.

CLINICAL JUDGMENT CHALLENGE

Patient-Centered Care **QSEN**

A 55-year-old woman who has blonde hair, very light skin, and blue eyes is being seen because she noticed the recent development several light-brown, flat, irregularly shaped spots on her face just below and in front of her right ear. Although these spots do not extend into the surrounding skin, she is concerned about their appearance on her otherwise flawless complexion and is worried that they may be skin cancer. When asked about her sun exposure, she tells you that her only sun exposure is when she plays golf (4 times per week) and that she uses sunscreen on her arms, legs, and neck. She also says she wears a hat with a front brim while playing golf. When you ask about facial skin protection, she tells you that because she wears makeup, she does not use sunscreen on her face.

1. What other assessment data should you obtain?
2. What risk factors does this woman have for skin cancer?
3. Do the facial lesions have any concerning features? If so, which ones?
4. How should you counsel this woman?

Diagnostic Assessment

Laboratory Tests

When a fungal, bacterial, or viral infection of the skin is suspected, confirmation by microscopic examination is necessary. *Always wear gloves (use Standard Precautions) when examining skin that is not intact.*

Cultures for fungal infection are obtained by using a tongue blade and gently scraping scales from skin lesions into a clean container. Collect fingernail clippings and hair in a similar manner. Waiting for culture results can delay treatment of a superficial fungal infection. For this reason, the specimen is also treated with a potassium hydroxide (KOH) solution and examined microscopically. A positive fungal infection shows branched hyphae when viewed under a microscope after treatment with KOH and may eliminate the need for a culture.

For deeper fungal infections, a piece of tissue is obtained for culture. The physician obtains the specimen by punch biopsy (see the following Skin Biopsy section). Check with the laboratory for any specific instructions related to specimen handling.

Cultures for bacterial infection are obtained from intact primary lesions (bullae, vesicles, or pustules), if possible. Express material from the lesion, collect it with a cotton-tipped applicator, and place the material in a bacterial culture medium specified by the laboratory. For intact lesions, *unroofing* (lifting or puncturing of the outer surface) may be needed using a sterile small-gauge needle before the material can be easily expressed. If crusts are present, the nurse or other health care professional removes the crusts with normal saline and then swabs the underlying exudates to obtain a specimen for culture (Cross, 2014).

A biopsy of deep bacterial infections may be needed to obtain a specimen for culture. If bacterial cellulitis is suspected, the physician or advanced practice nurse can inject nonbacteriostatic saline deep into the tissue and then aspirate it back; the aspirant is sent for culture.

Cultures for viral infection are indicated if a herpes virus infection is suspected. A cotton-tipped applicator is used to obtain vesicle fluid from intact lesions. Viral culture specimen tubes must be placed on ice immediately after specimens are obtained and are transported to the laboratory as soon as possible.

The presence of a viral infection can be confirmed by *Tzanck smear* although the exact virus is not identified. A smear is obtained from the base of the lesion and examined under a microscope. The presence of multinucleated giant cells confirms a viral infection.

Other Diagnostic Tests

Other tests for diagnosis of skin problems include biopsy, special noninvasive examination techniques, and skin testing for allergy (discussed in Chapter 20).

Skin Biopsy. A small piece of skin tissue may be obtained for diagnosis or to assess the effectiveness of an intervention. Check with the health care provider to determine the number, location, and type of skin biopsies to be performed. Depending on the size, depth, and location of the skin changes, the physician may perform a punch biopsy, shave biopsy, or scalpel excision (excisional biopsy).

Punch biopsy is the most common technique. A small circular cutting instrument, or "punch," ranging in diameter from 2 to 6 mm, is used. After the site is injected with a local anesthetic, a small plug of tissue is cut and removed. The site may be closed with sutures or may be allowed to heal without suturing.

Shave biopsies remove only the portion of the skin that rises above the surrounding tissue when injected with a local anesthetic. A scalpel or razor blade is moved parallel to the skin surface to remove the tissue specimen. Shave biopsies are usually indicated for superficial or raised lesions. Suturing is not needed.

Excisional biopsy is rarely used for skin problems. When needed, larger or deeper specimens are obtained by deep excision with a scalpel followed by closure with sutures. Excisional biopsies are more uncomfortable than punch or shave biopsies while healing.

Patient Preparation. Explain to the patient what to expect and that a biopsy is a minor procedure with few complications. If a punch or shave biopsy is planned, reassure him or her that only a small amount of skin is removed and scarring is minimal. For an excisional biopsy, tell the patient that a scar similar to that of a healed surgical incision will result.

Procedure. Establish a sterile field, and assemble all needed supplies and instruments. Local anesthesia is provided by local infiltration using a small-gauge (25-gauge) needle to reduce discomfort during injection. Preparation of the biopsy site differs by health care provider preference, but usually the skin is simply wiped with alcohol.

The injection of a local anesthetic agent, which produces a burning or stinging sensation, is uncomfortable. Reassure the patient that the discomfort will subside as the anesthetic takes effect. Talking the patient through the procedure with a quiet voice along with a gentle touch may have a calming effect.

After removal, tissue specimens for pathologic study are placed in 10% formalin for fixation. Specimens for culture are placed in sterile saline solution. Bleeding of the site may be controlled by applying localized pressure, by applying a topical hemostatic agent, or by suturing.

Follow-up Care. After bleeding is controlled and any sutures are placed, the site is covered with an adhesive bandage or a dry gauze dressing. Instruct the patient to keep the dressing dry and in place for at least 8 hours. Teach him or her to clean the site daily after the dressing is removed. Tap water or saline is used to remove any dried blood or crusts. An antibiotic ointment may be prescribed to reduce the risk for infection. The site may be left open or covered for cosmetic reasons or because the site is an area often soiled. Instruct the patient to report any redness or excessive drainage. Sutures are usually removed 7 to 10 days after biopsy.

Wood's Light Examination. A handheld, long-wavelength ultraviolet (black) light or Wood's light may be used during physical examination. Exposure of some skin infections with this light produces a specific color, such as blue-green or red, that can be used to identify the infection. Hypopigmented skin is more prominent when it is viewed under black light, making evaluation of pigment changes in lighter skin easier. This examination is carried out in a darkened room and does not cause discomfort.

Diascopy. Diascopy is a painless technique to eliminate erythema caused by increased blood flow to the skin, thereby easing the inspection of skin lesions. A glass slide or lens is pressed down over the area to be examined, blanching the skin and revealing the shape of the lesions.

NCLEX EXAMINATION CHALLENGE

Safe and Effective Care Environment

What is the most important action the nurse needs to take when obtaining a specimen for a viral culture for a client who has a suspected viral skin infection?

A. Injecting the vesicle with sterile water, aspirating the fluid, adding a preservative to the specimen, and wrapping the container to protect the specimen from light.

B. Using a cotton-tipped applicator, obtain vesicle fluid from the lesion, immediately placing the specimen on ice, and transporting it to the laboratory as soon as possible.

C. Cleaning the area with an antiseptic solution, removing fluid from the center of the blister with a needle, and sending it to the laboratory.

D. Applying a gauze bandage to the area, removing it after one hour, and sending the entire gauze to the laboratory.

NURSING CONCEPTS AND CLINICAL JUDGMENT REVIEW

What might you NOTICE in a patient with adequate TISSUE INTEGRITY and body protection related to skin function?

Vital signs:
- Body temperature within normal range

Physical assessment:
- Skin intact (no rashes, abnormal lesions, open areas, or drainage)
- Skin color normal (no cyanosis, pallor, jaundice, inflammation, or areas of uneven pigmentation)
- Skin texture and elastic turgor normal (no edema, tenting, flaking, scaling, excessive oiliness, or excessive thickening)
- Oral mucous membranes moist and pink
- Nail beds pink with good capillary refill
- Fingertips and nails normal-shaped (no clubbing, nail splitting, nail separation, or increased nail thickness)
- Body hair distributed evenly over the body, no patchy areas of hair loss
- Scalp free from dandruff, no itching

Psychological assessment:
- Patient's eye contact good
- No unusual "hiding" of body areas normally visible in public
- Skin, hair, and nails clean and free of odor

GET READY FOR THE NCLEX® EXAMINATION!

KEY POINTS

Review these Key Points for each NCLEX Examination Client Needs Category

Safe and Effective Care Environment
- Assist all patients with limited mobility to change positions at least every 2 hours. **Safety** QSEN
- Wash your hands before and after touching any areas of impaired skin TISSUE INTEGRITY. **Safety** QSEN
- Use Standard Precautions when providing care to a patient who has areas of impaired skin TISSUE INTEGRITY or skin with an abnormal appearance. **Safety** QSEN
- Use lift sheets when moving patients with fragile skin. **Safety** QSEN
- Position patients who are confined to bed in a way that promotes air circulation to skinfold areas while minimizing pressure over bony prominences.

Health Promotion and Maintenance
- Encourage all patients to reduce sun exposure and exposure to ultraviolet (UV) light. **Patient-Centered Care** QSEN
- Teach patients to examine all skin areas on a monthly basis for new lesions and changes to existing lesions using the ABCDE method of checking lesions for manifestations of melanoma. **Evidence-Based Practice** QSEN
- Encourage all patients to bathe, shampoo the hair, and keep fingernails clean and trimmed.

Psychosocial Integrity
- Use effective communication when teaching patients and family members about what to expect during tests and procedures to assess skin function and skin disease. **Patient-Centered Care** QSEN
- Explain all procedures, restrictions, drugs, and follow-up care to the patient and family. **Patient-Centered Care** QSEN
- Check the cognitive function of any patient whose hygiene of the skin, hair, and nails appears inadequate.
- Reassure patients who have skin changes that are variations of normal. **Patient-Centered Care** QSEN

Physiological Integrity
- Modify techniques to assess skin changes in patients with dark skin. **Evidence-Based Practice** QSEN
- Document any known specific allergies that have skin manifestations. **Patient-Centered Care** QSEN

- Ask any patient who has started taking a newly prescribed or over-the-counter drug whether he or she has noticed any skin changes that occurred since starting the drug. **Patient-Centered Care** QSEN
- Use proper terminology to communicate skin assessment findings.
- Distinguish between normal variations and abnormal skin manifestations with regard to skin color, texture, warmth, elastic turgor, and moisture.
- Use the ABCDE method of assessing skin lesions for cancer. **Evidence-Based Practice** QSEN

25 CHAPTER

Care of Patients with Skin Problems

Janice Cuzzell and M. Linda Workman

http://evolve.elsevier.com/Iggy/

PRIORITY CONCEPTS

- TISSUE INTEGRITY
- INFECTION
- INFLAMMATION
- CELLULAR REGULATION

LEARNING OUTCOMES

Safe and Effective Care Environment

1. Use principles of infection control to prevent transmission when caring for a patient with a skin INFECTION.
2. Protect hospitalized patients from skin injury, loss of TISSUE INTEGRITY, and INFECTION.

Health Promotion and Maintenance

3. Teach all people how to protect the skin from damage and cancer development.

Psychosocial Integrity

4. Reduce the psychological impact for the patient and family regarding changes in the appearance or function of any part of the integumentary system.

Physiological Integrity

5. Use knowledge of anatomy and physiology to routinely perform a complete assessment of any skin changes, lesions, and open wounds, and document findings.
6. Work with other members of the health care team to help the patient/family experiencing pressure ulcers or other skin problems achieve desired health outcomes.
7. Coordinate nursing interventions for the patient with serious skin problems in the community.

As discussed in Chapter 24, skin TISSUE INTEGRITY helps protect the entire body. Like the wall surrounding a castle, it provides a strong barrier, especially to invasion by harmful microorganisms.

Skin problems are common, especially among older adults. Changes in skin TISSUE INTEGRITY reduce protective function, and the cause of the change is often difficult to determine. In addition to its primary functions, the skin also reflects underlying medical conditions. Thus problems may truly arise in the skin, or they may be a manifestation of systemic disease or injury.

Drugs and other interventions for any health problem can trigger a skin response. Skin problems can interfere with the management of other conditions. Age-related changes and problems caused by immobility, chronic disease, debility, and reduced immune function increase the older patient's risk for skin damage and loss of TISSUE INTEGRITY.

MINOR SKIN IRRITATIONS

PRURITUS

❖ *PATHOPHYSIOLOGY*

Pruritus (itching) is a distressing condition caused by stimulation of itch-specific nerve fibers. It may or may not occur with skin disease. Physical or chemical agents can directly trigger the nerve fibers or can activate chemical mediators (i.e., histamine), which then act on the itch receptors.

Itching is a subjective condition similar to pain, and severity of the sensation varies among patients. Regardless of the cause, patients often report that itching is worse at night when there are fewer distractions. Other conditions that make itching worse include skin dryness, increased temperature, perspiration, and emotional stress.

❖ PATIENT-CENTERED COLLABORATIVE CARE

The priority nursing interventions focus on increasing patient comfort and preventing skin injury with loss of TISSUE INTEGRITY. Patients usually try to relieve itching by scratching or rubbing the skin, a response that further stimulates the itch receptors and causes the *"itch-scratch-itch" cycle* (McCance et al., 2014). Itching with skin lesions can often be relieved by treatment of the underlying skin disorder with topical or systemic drugs. Systemic diseases, such as liver and venous disorders, can also cause itching without skin lesions. Liver disease often increases the buildup of bilirubin in the skin, which stimulates itch receptors. Pruritus can also be caused by too little or too much blood flow to an area (especially the feet and legs).

Plan care to promote comfort and prevent disruption of skin tissue integrity from vigorous scratching. Because dry skin worsens itching, emphasize interventions to prevent dry skin (Chart 25-1). Encourage patients to keep the fingernails trimmed short, with rough edges filed to reduce damage from scratching and secondary INFECTION. Wearing mittens or splints at night can help prevent scratching during sleep. If the patient cannot perform self-care, teach the family (for home care) and unlicensed assistive personnel (UAP) to trim the patient's fingernails and apply mittens or gloves. Stress the importance of not breaking the skin or digging into nail corners when trimming the nails of patients with diabetes.

A cool sleeping environment and comfort measures (e.g., cool shower, moisturizers) may help promote sleep. Using sleep-promoting herbal teas or sedating antihistamines at bedtime (when the side effect of drowsiness is welcome) may provide an uninterrupted night's sleep. Colloidal oatmeal or tar extract baths may provide temporary relief.

If antihistamines are prescribed, monitor the patient's response so that the dosage can be adjusted as needed. The effectiveness of topical steroid preparations and other topical agents is increased if the drug is applied to slightly damp skin. Using topical drugs under an occlusive dressing increases the dose being delivered. Avoid occluding treated areas unless specifically prescribed by the health care provider.

CHART 25-1 Patient and Family Education: Preparing for Self-Management

Prevention of Dry Skin

- Use a room humidifier during the winter months or whenever the furnace is in use.
- Take a complete bath or shower only every other day (wash face, axillae, perineum, and any soiled areas with soap daily).
- Use tepid water.
- Use a superfatted, nonalkaline soap instead of deodorant soap.
- Rinse the soap thoroughly from your skin.
- If you like bath oil, add the oil to the water at the end of the bath.
- Take care to avoid falls; oil makes the tub slippery.
- Pat rather than rub skin surfaces dry.
- Avoid clothing that continuously rubs the skin, such as tight belts, nylon stockings, or pantyhose.
- Maintain a daily fluid intake of 3000 mL unless contraindicated for another medical condition.
- Do not apply rubbing alcohol, astringents, or other drying agents to the skin.
- Avoid caffeine and alcohol ingestion.

URTICARIA

Urticaria (hives) is a rash of white or red edematous papules or plaques of various sizes. This problem is usually caused by exposure to allergens, which releases histamine into the skin. Blood vessel dilation and plasma protein leakage lead to formation of lesions or wheals. Some common causes of urticaria include drugs, temperature extremes, foods, INFECTION, diseases, cancer, and insect bites (Schaefer, 2011).

Management focuses on removal of the triggering substance and relief of manifestations. Because the skin reaction is caused by histamine release, antihistamines such as diphenhydramine (Benadryl) are helpful. Teach the patient to avoid overexertion, alcohol consumption, and warm environments, which further dilate blood vessels and make urticaria worse. Alcohol increases sedating effect of antihistamines, increasing the risk for falls.

TRAUMA

❖ PATHOPHYSIOLOGY

Skin trauma can vary from an aseptic surgical incision to a grossly infected, draining pressure ulcer with deep tissue destruction. Injury to the skin starts a series of actions to repair the skin and restore TISSUE INTEGRITY to this protective barrier.

Phases of Wound Healing

Wound healing occurs in three phases: inflammatory phase, proliferative phase, and maturation phase. Table 25-1 lists the key events for each stage of normal wound healing. The length of each phase depends on the type of injury and degree of loss of TISSUE INTEGRITY, the patient's overall health, and whether the wound is healing by first, second, or third intention (Fig. 25-1).

TABLE 25-1 Normal Wound Healing

Inflammatory Phase

- Begins at the time of injury or cell death and lasts 3 to 5 days.
- Immediate responses are vasoconstriction and clot formation.
- After 10 minutes, vasodilation occurs with increased capillary permeability and leakage of plasma (and plasma proteins) into the surrounding tissue.
- White blood cells (especially macrophages) migrate into the wound.
- Clinical manifestations of local edema, pain, erythema, and warmth are present.

Proliferative Phase

- Begins about the fourth day after injury and lasts 2 to 4 weeks.
- Fibrin strands form a scaffold or framework.
- Mitotic fibroblast cells migrate into the wound, attach to the framework, divide, and stimulate the secretion of collagen.
- Collagen, together with ground substance, builds tough and inflexible scar tissue.
- Capillaries in areas surrounding the wound form "buds" that grow into new blood vessels.
- Capillary buds and collagen deposits form the "granulation" tissue in the wound, and the wound contracts.
- Epithelial cells grow over the granulation tissue bed.

Maturation Phase

- Begins as early as 3 weeks after injury and may continue for a year or longer.
- Collagen is reorganized to provide greater tensile strength.
- Scar tissue gradually becomes thinner and paler in color.
- The mature scar is firm and inelastic when palpated.

The process of wound healing

▶ Healing by first intention

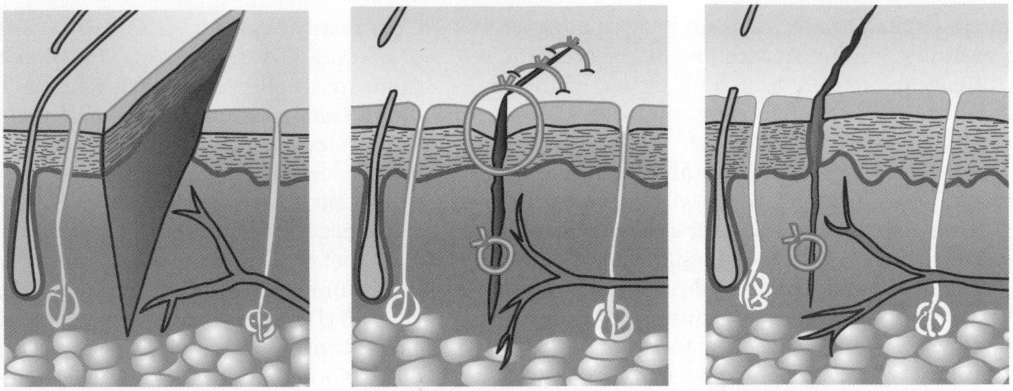

An aseptically made wound with minimal tissue destruction and minimal tissue reaction begins to heal as the edges are approximated by close sutures or staples. No open areas or dead spaces are left to serve as potential sites of infection.

▶ Healing by second intention (granulation) and contraction

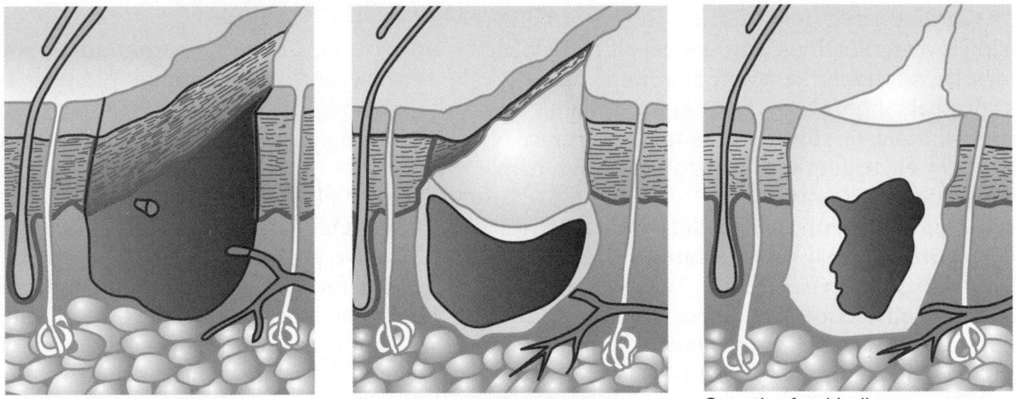

An infected or chronic wound or one with tissue damage so extensive that the edges cannot be smoothly approximated is usually left open and allowed to heal from the inside out. The nurse periodically cleans and assesses the wound for healthy tissue production. Scar tissue is extensive, and healing is prolonged.

▶ Healing by third intention (delayed closure)

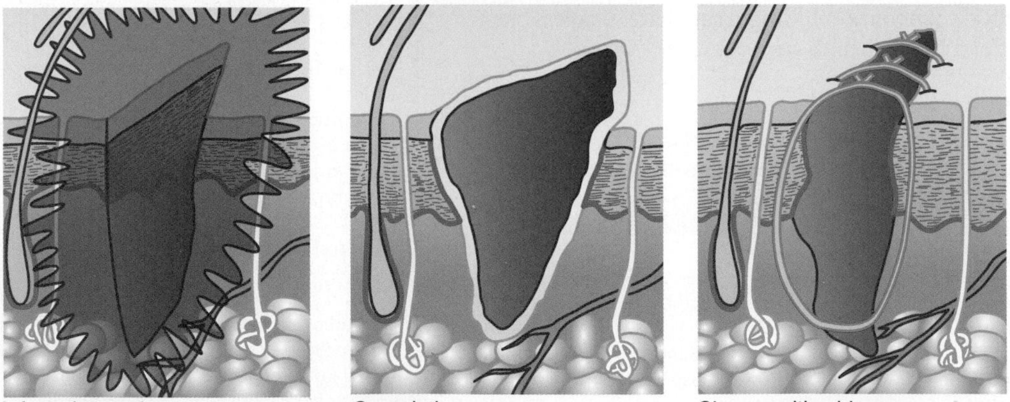

A potentially infected surgical wound may be left open for several days. If no clinical signs of infection occur, the wound is then closed surgically.

FIG. 25-1 The process of wound healing.

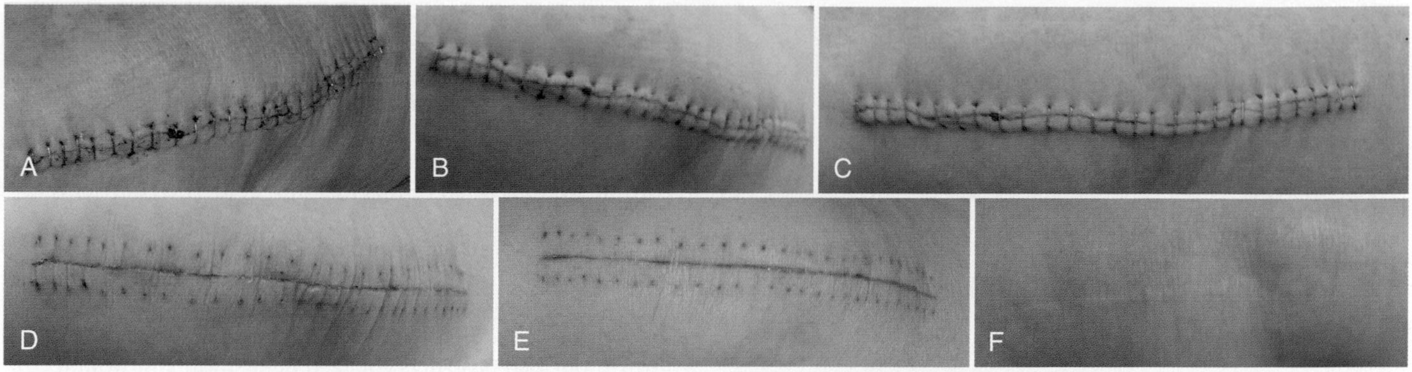

FIG. 25-2 Appearance of a normally healing surgical wound over time. **A,** Appearance at 1 day postoperative. **B,** Appearance at 1 week postoperative. **C,** Appearance at 2 weeks postoperative. **D,** Appearance at 2 months postoperative. **E,** Appearance at 6 months postoperative. **F,** Appearance at 1 year after surgery.

A wound without tissue loss, such as a clean laceration or a surgical incision, can be closed with sutures, staples, or adhesives. The wound edges are brought together with the skin layers lined up in correct anatomic position (**approximated**) and held in place until healing is complete. This type of wound represents healing by **first intention** in which the closed wound eliminates dead space and shortens the phases of tissue repair. INFLAMMATION resolves quickly, and connective tissue repair is minimal, resulting in less remodeling and a thin scar. Fig. 25-2 shows the healing of a surgical incision over time.

Deeper tissue injuries with greater loss of TISSUE INTEGRITY, such as a chronic pressure ulcer or venous stasis ulcer, result in a cavity that requires gradual filling in of the dead space with connective tissue. This represents healing by **second intention** and prolongs the repair process.

Wounds at high risk for INFECTION, such as surgical incisions into a nonsterile body cavity or contaminated traumatic wounds, may be intentionally left open for several days. After **debris** (dead tissues) and exudate have been removed (débrided) and INFLAMMATION has subsided, the wound is closed by first intention. This type of healing represents delayed primary closure (**third intention**) and results in a scar similar to that found in wounds that heal by first intention. Healing can be impaired by many factors (Table 25-2).

Mechanisms of Wound Healing

When skin injury occurs, the body restores TISSUE INTEGRITY through three processes: re-epithelialization, granulation, and wound contraction. The depth of injury and extent of tissue integrity loss determine to what degree each process contributes to wound healing.

Partial-Thickness Wounds. Partial-thickness wounds are superficial with minimal loss of TISSUE INTEGRITY from damage to the epidermis and upper dermal layers. These wounds heal by **re-epithelialization**, the production of new skin cells by undamaged epidermal cells in the basal layer of the dermis, which also lines the hair follicles and sweat glands (Fig. 25-3). Injury is followed immediately by local INFLAMMATION that causes the formation of a fibrin clot and releases growth factors that stimulate epidermal cell division (mitosis). New skin cells move into open spaces on the wound surface where the fibrin clot acts as a frame to guide cell movement. Regrowth across the open area (**resurfacing**) is only one cell layer thick at first. As healing continues, the cell layer thickens, stratifies (forms layers), and produces keratin to resemble normal skin.

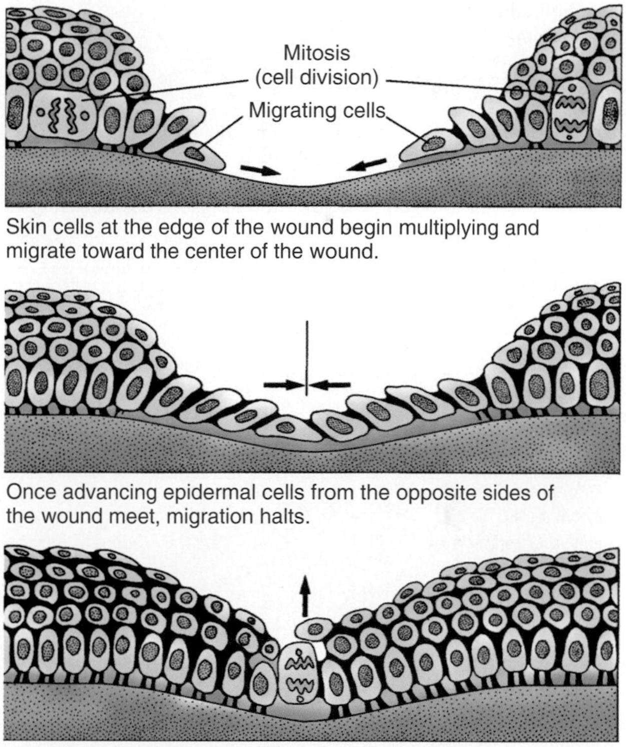

Skin cells at the edge of the wound begin multiplying and migrate toward the center of the wound.

Once advancing epidermal cells from the opposite sides of the wound meet, migration halts.

Epithelial cells continue to divide until the thickness of the new skin layer approaches normal.

FIG. 25-3 Re-epithelialization and wound contraction.

In a healthy person, healing of a partial-thickness wound takes about 5 to 7 days. This process is more rapid in skin that is hydrated, well oxygenated, and has few microorganisms.

Full-Thickness Wounds. In deep partial-thickness wounds and full-thickness wounds, loss of TISSUE INTEGRITY and damage extend into the lower layers of the dermis and subcutaneous tissue. As a result, most of the epithelial cells at the base of the wound are destroyed and the wound cannot heal by re-epithelialization alone. Removal of the damaged tissue results

TABLE 25-2 Causes of Impaired Wound Healing

CAUSE	MECHANISM
Altered Inflammatory Response	
Local	
Arteriosclerosis Diabetes Vasculitis Thrombosis Venous insufficiency Lymphedema Pharmacologic vasoconstriction Irradiated tissue Crush injuries Primary closure under tension	Reduced local tissue circulation, resulting in ischemia, impaired leukocytic response to wounding, and increased probability of wound infection
Systemic	
Leukemia Prolonged administration of high-dose anti-inflammatory drugs: • Corticosteroids • Aspirin	Systemic inhibition of leukocytic response, resulting in impaired host resistance to infection
Impaired Cellular Proliferation	
Local	
Wound infection Foreign body Necrotic tissue Repeated injury or irritation Movement of wound (e.g., across a joint) Wound desiccation or maceration	Prolonged inflammatory response, which can result in low tissue oxygen tension and further tissue destruction
Systemic	
Aging Chronic stress Nutritional deficiencies: • Calories • Protein • Vitamins • Minerals • Water Impaired oxygenation: • Pulmonary insufficiency • Heart failure • Hypovolemia Cirrhosis Uremia Prolonged hypothermia Coagulation disorders Cytotoxic drugs	Impaired cellular proliferation and collagen synthesis Decreased wound contraction

in a defect that must be filled with scar tissue (**granulation**) for healing to occur. During the second phase of healing, new blood vessels form at the base of the wound and fibroblast cells begin moving into the wound space. These cells deposit new collagen to replace the lost tissue.

Fibroblasts also begin to pull the wound edges inward along the path of least resistance (**contraction**) (see Fig. 25-3). This causes the wound to decrease in size at a uniform rate of about 0.6 to 0.75 mm/day. Complete wound closure by contraction depends on the mobility of the surrounding skin as tension is applied to it. If tension in the surrounding skin exceeds the force of wound contraction, healing will be delayed until undamaged epidermal cells at the wound edges can bridge the defect. The bridging of epithelial cells across a large area of granulation tissue results in an unstable barrier rather than near-normal skin. A venous leg ulcer is one example of a skin defect that heals poorly by contraction. Re-epithelialization of these chronic wounds often results in a thin epidermal barrier that is easily re-injured.

The natural healing processes of re-epithelialization, granulation, and contraction can slow down and even stop in the presence of INFECTION, unrelieved pressure, or mechanical obstacles. For example, dead tissue not only supports bacterial growth but also obstructs collagen deposition and wound contraction. Thus thorough wound débridement is needed for healing. In the case of chronic wounds, healing may stop spontaneously without an obvious cause. Also, infection in chronic wounds may not show the expected manifestations. Often the only manifestation is an increase in wound size or failure of the wound to decrease in size. Nonhealing chronic wounds that remain open for extended periods are of particular concern. Although rare, these wounds are at higher risk for evolving into an aggressive malignancy (Marjolin ulcer) (Yu et al., 2013).

CONSIDERATIONS FOR OLDER ADULTS

Patient-Centered Care QSEN

As skin ages, the process of wound healing is less efficient. Re-epithelialization and wound contraction slow, and replacement of connective tissue is reduced. Thus the strength of a healed wound in an older adult is reduced with poor tissue integrity and the area is at greater risk for re-injury. When inadequate nutrition, incontinence, or immobility is present, any wound in an older adult has a high risk for becoming a chronic wound. Although prevention strategies provide the best outcome, aggressive treatment of any degree of loss of skin tissue integrity, no matter how small, should be started as soon as it is discovered in an older adult (Touhy & Jett, 2014).

❖ PATIENT-CENTERED COLLABORATIVE CARE

Collaborative management of skin trauma varies with the depth and type of injury. Interventions always focus on supporting a healing environment, enhancing wound healing, preventing INFECTION, and restoring function to the area.

PRESSURE ULCERS

❖ PATHOPHYSIOLOGY

A **pressure ulcer** (PrU) is a loss of TISSUE INTEGRITY caused when the skin and underlying soft tissue are compressed between a bony prominence and an external surface for an extended period. Although they commonly occur over the sacrum, hips, and ankles, *pressure ulcers can occur on any body surface.* For example, nasal cannula tubing that is too tight can cause pressure ulcers behind the ears or in the nares (Ambutas et al., 2014).

Tissue compression from pressure restricts blood flow to the skin, resulting in reduced tissue perfusion and oxygenation and, eventually, leading to cell death. Ulcers occur most often in people with limited mobility because they cannot change their position to relieve pressure. Patients who cannot feel or communicate the pain that occurs with unrelieved pressure are more likely to develop pressure ulcers. Once formed, these chronic wounds are slow to heal, resulting in increased morbidity and health care costs. Complications include sepsis, kidney failure, infectious arthritis, and osteomyelitis.

Friction and shear are mechanical forces that impair skin TISSUE INTEGRITY and cause skin tears, which set the stage for skin breakdown (LeBlanc & Baronoski, 2014). Excessive skin moisture, such as urinary or fecal incontinence, also increases the risk for skin damage. Nutrition status is an important concern. Protein malnutrition makes normal tissue more prone to breakdown and also delays healing (Posthauer, 2012).

Mechanical Forces

Pressure occurs as a result of gravity. Dependent tissues in contact with a fixed surface experience varying degrees of pressure. Pressure is determined by the amount and distribution of weight exerted at the point of contact and the density of the contacting surface. Excessive or prolonged pressure compresses blood vessels at the point of contact, such as over bony prominences. Pressure occurs when the patient is positioned on a hard surface that does not diffuse the weight, such as when lying on a hard floor for hours after a fall or when remaining in the same position too long. Unrelieved pressure leads to ischemia, INFLAMMATION, and tissue necrosis.

Friction occurs when surfaces rub the skin and irritate or directly pull off epithelial tissue. Such forces are generated when the patient is dragged or pulled across bed linen.

Shearing forces are generated when the skin itself is stationary and the tissues below the skin (e.g., fat, muscle) shift or move (Fig. 25-4). The movement of the deeper tissue layers reduces the blood supply to the skin, leading to skin hypoxia, anoxia, ischemia, INFLAMMATION, and necrosis.

A shear injury usually occurs when a patient is in a wheelchair or in bed in a semi-sitting position and gradually slides downward. The skin over the sacrum may not slide down at the same pace as the deeper tissues, mechanically "shearing" the skin, causing blood vessels to stretch and break. Shearing leads to soft-tissue ischemia and deep tissue injury, even though no external break in skin integrity is observed.

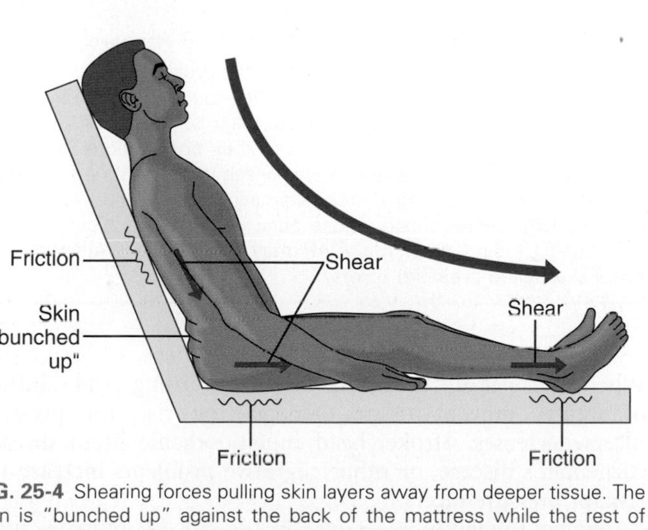

FIG. 25-4 Shearing forces pulling skin layers away from deeper tissue. The skin is "bunched up" against the back of the mattress while the rest of the bone and muscle in the area presses downward on the lower part of the mattress. Blood vessels become kinked, obstructing circulation and leading to tissue death.

CONSIDERATIONS FOR OLDER ADULTS

Patient-Centered Care QSEN

Older adults are at higher risk for skin tears and pressure ulcers because of age-related skin changes. Flattening of cells at the dermal-epidermal junction predisposes older people to skin tears from mechanical shearing forces, such as tape removal and friction from tight restraints. Skin moisture and irritation from incontinence combined with friction over bony prominences can lead to skin destruction with loss of tissue integrity and pressure ulcer formation. Patients with cognitive impairments may not readily report discomfort from inadequate pressure relief. **If pressure is unrelieved, tissue destruction progresses to full-thickness injury.** Assess patients with cognitive impairments more frequently for loss of skin tissue integrity.

Incidence and Prevalence

Pressure ulcer development is a problem found among patients in any care setting, including the home. Although new products are available for prevention and treatment, many hospitalized patients still experience pressure ulcer formation, which contributes significantly to morbidity and mortality in this patient population (Alderden et al., 2011; Lyder et al., 2012).

Health Promotion and Maintenance

Pressure ulcers can be prevented if the risk is recognized and intervention begins early (Chart 25-2) (Ackerman, 2011). Pressure ulcer prevention does not just happen even with conscientious nursing care. Deliberate and consistent interventions, as described in the Quality Improvement box, are needed to prevent hospital-acquired pressure ulcers. Key health care team members for pressure ulcer prevention and management are the certified wound care specialist and the dietitian. Involving unlicensed assistive personnel (UAP) in pressure ulcer prevention also enhances prevention program effectiveness.

A pressure ulcer prevention program consists of two steps: (1) early identification of high-risk patients, and (2) implementation of aggressive intervention for prevention with the use of pressure-relief or pressure-reduction devices. Pressure mapping with a computerized tool that measures pressure distribution during sitting or lying can identify specific body areas at risk for breakdown and can help in planning interventions for patients who are bedridden or wheelchair bound. The map is displayed in colors on the computer screen based on temperature differences. Red indicates areas of greater heat production and increased pressure loads. Blue indicates cooler areas under lower pressure. When used in combination with risk assessment tools, pressure mapping helps identify problem areas before skin changes can be seen and allows for more targeted prevention strategies.

Effective risk identification and prevention measures include patient and caregiver education. Documentation of risk assessment, implementation of prevention measures, and education of all people involved in the care of the patient at risk for pressure ulcer formation are key to the plan's success. Continuing evaluation and risk assessment are critical, especially when the patient's condition changes.

Identification of High-Risk Patients

As suggested by The Joint Commission's National Patient Safety Goals (NPSGs), all patients admitted to a health care facility or home care agency are to be assessed for pressure ulcer risk. The

CHART 25-2 Best Practice for Patient Safety & Quality Care QSEN

Preventing Pressure Ulcers

Positioning

- Pad contact surfaces with foam, silicon gel, air pads, or other pressure-relieving pads.
- Do not keep the head of the bed elevated above 30 degrees to prevent shearing.
- Use a lift sheet to move a patient in the bed. Avoid dragging or sliding him or her.
- When positioning a patient on his or her side, do not position directly on the trochanter.
- Re-position an immobile patient at least every 2 hours while in bed and at least every 1 hour while sitting in a chair.
- Do not place a rubber ring or donut under the patient's sacral area.
- When moving an immobile patient from a bed to another surface, use a designated slide board well lubricated with talc or use a mechanical lift.
- Place pillows or foam wedges between two bony surfaces.
- Keep the patient's skin directly off plastic surfaces.
- Keep the patient's heels off the bed surface using bed pillow under ankles.

Nutrition

- Ensure a fluid intake between 2000 and 3000 mL/day.
- Help the patient maintain an adequate intake of protein and calories.

Skin Care

- Perform a daily inspection of the patient's entire skin.
- Document and report any manifestations of skin infection.
- Use moisturizers daily on dry skin, and apply when skin is damp.
- Keep moisture from prolonged contact with skin:
  - Dry areas where two skin surfaces touch, such as the axillae and under the breasts.
  - Place absorbent pads under areas where perspiration collects.
  - Use moisture barriers on skin areas where wound drainage or incontinence occurs.
- ***Do not massage bony prominences.***
- Humidify the room.

Skin Cleaning

- Clean the skin as soon as possible after soiling occurs and at routine intervals.
- Use a mild, heavily fatted soap or gentle commercial cleanser for incontinence.
- Use tepid rather than hot water.
- In the perineal area, use a disposable cleaning cloth that contains a skin barrier agent.
- While cleaning, use the minimum scrubbing force necessary to remove soil.
- Gently pat rather than rub the skin dry.
- Do not use powders or talcs directly on the perineum.
- After cleansing, apply a commercial skin barrier to those areas in frequent contact with urine or feces.

QUALITY IMPROVEMENT QSEN

Use of a Team Approach to Prevent Pressure Ulcers

Armour-Burton, T., Fields, W., Outlaw, L., & Deleon, E. (2013). The healthy skin project: Changing nursing practice to prevent and treat hospital-acquired pressure ulcers. *Critical Care Nurse, 33*(3), 32-39.

The incidence of hospital-acquired pressure ulcers, defined as occurring after the first 24 hours following admission, for a 41-bed acute care unit ranged from 0% to 18.92% per quarter for 14 consecutive quarters. Although this unit had a prevention program initially in place, it relied on each patient's primary nurse for ongoing pressure ulcer risk assessment and implementation of prevention practices. This high incidence forced the staff to examine their current pressure ulcer prevention practices and design a sustainable, interdisciplinary "healthy skin project" to improve the outcomes.

Key to the "healthy skin project" was the implementation of a team approach for pressure ulcer prevention assessment and management. In addition to all nurses assigned to the unit, the team now included both a wound-liaison nurse (who has special training but was not a certified wound care nurse) and a registered dietitian. Education for all staff members was started and assessed at regular intervals. A key factor in the success of the program was the involvement of unlicensed assistive personnel (UAP) in the risk assessment and care phases of pressure ulcer prevention. Thus the responsibility of pressure ulcer prevention shifted from one person, the primary nurse, for each patient to everyone who provided care to each patient. Each patient was assessed for pressure ulcer risk every shift. Those identified at increased risk were started on evidence-based pressure-relieving and skin care algorithmic intervention. During the first 20 quarters of the project's implementation, the pressure ulcer incidence for 17 quarters was 0%. For 3 of the quarters, the incidence was 2.5%, 2.94%, and 3.33% respectively. These data suggest that consistent implementation of evidence-based strategies for pressure ulcer prevention is effective.

Commentary: Implications for Practice and Research

Although a team approach to pressure ulcer prevention is common, this project may be unique by gaining the input and participation of nonprofessional UAPs. These individuals often spend more time with patients while providing direct care, and their observations can contribute to more accurate assessment, which is the first step in pressure ulcer prevention. Research examining the degree to which engaged UAP versus those whose observations are not considered is needed to learn what role UAP may play in the prevention of hospital-acquired pressure ulcers.

use of a risk assessment tool increases the chances of identifying those patients at greater risk for skin breakdown. The Braden scale (Fig. 25-5) is a commonly used valid skin risk assessment tool. Using it helps the nurse assess and document risk categories for pressure ulcer formation (e.g., mental status, activity and mobility, nutritional status, incontinence).

Mental status changes and decreased sensation determine whether the patient is a partner in pressure ulcer prevention. When the patient understands that turning and shifting of weight prevent tissue damage, the risk for pressure ulcers decreases. Stroke, head injury, organic brain disease, Alzheimer's disease, or other cognitive problems increase the risk for pressure ulcers.

Impaired mobility is a factor in the risk for pressure ulcer formation. Patients who have unimpaired mobility and can respond to pain are at low risk for pressure ulcers. *Regardless of*

Patient's name ______	Evaluator's name ______			Date of assessment		
Sensory perception Ability to respond meaningfully to pressure-related discomfort	**1. Completely limited** Unresponsive to painful stimuli (does not moan, flinch, or grasp) because of diminished level of consciousness or sedation OR limited ability to feel pain over most of body surface	**2. Very limited** Responds only to painful stimuli; cannot communicate discomfort except by moaning or restlessness OR has a sensory impairment that limits the ability to feel pain or discomfort over half of the body	**3. Slightly limited** Responds to verbal commands but cannot always communicate discomfort or need to be turned OR has some sensory impairment that limits ability to feel pain or discomfort in one or two extremities	**4. No impairment** Responds to verbal commands; has no sensory deficit that would limit ability to feel or voice pain or discomfort		
Moisture Degree to which skin is exposed to moisture	**1. Constantly moist** Skin is kept moist almost constantly by perspiration, urine; dampness is detected every time the client is moved or turned	**2. Very Moist** Skin is often but not always moist; linen must be changed at least once a shift	**3. Occasionally moist** Skin is occasionally moist, requiring an extra linen change approximately once a day	**4. Rarely moist** Skin is usually dry; linen requires changing only at routine intervals		
Activity Degree of physical activity	**1. Bedfast** Confined to bed	**2. Chairfast** Ability to walk severely limited or nonexistent; cannot bear own weight and must be assisted into chair or wheelchair	**3. Walks occasionally** Walks occasionally during the day but for very short distances, with or without assistance; spends the majority of each shift in bed or chair	**4. Walks frequently** Walks outside the room at least twice a day and inside the room at least once every 2 hours during waking hours		
Mobility Ability to change or control body position	**1. Completely immobile** Does not make even slight changes in body or extremity position without assistance	**2. Very limited** Makes occasional slight changes in body or extremity position but unable to make frequent or significant changes independently	**3. Slightly limited** Makes frequent though slight changes in body or extremity position independently	**4. No limitations** Makes major and frequent changes in position without assistance		
Nutrition Usual food intake pattern	**1. Very poor** Never eats a complete meal; rarely eats more than a third of any food offered; eats two servings or less of protein (meat or dairy products) per day; takes fluids poorly; does not take a liquid dietary supplement OR is NPO or maintained on clear liquids or IV for more than 5 days	**2. Probably inadequate** Rarely eats a complete meal and generally eats only about half of any food offered; protein intake includes only three servings of meat or dairy products per day; occasionally will take a dietary supplement OR receives less than optimal amount of liquid diet or tube feeding	**3. Adequate** Eats over half of most meals; eats a total of four servings of protein (meat, dairy products) each day; occasionally will refuse a meal, but will usually take a supplement if offered OR is receiving tube feeding or total parenteral nutrition, which probably meets most nutritional needs	**4. Excellent** Eats most of every meal; never refuses a meal; usually eats a total of four or more servings of meat and dairy products; occasionally eats between meals; does not require supplementation		
Friction and shear	**1. Problem** Requires moderate to maximum assistance in moving; complete lifting without sliding against sheets is impossible; frequently slides down in bed or chair, requiring frequent repositioning with maximum assistance; spasticity, contractures, or agitation leads to almost constant friction	**2. Potential problem** Moves feebly or requires minimum assistance during a move; skin probably slides to some extent against sheets, chair, restraints, or other devices; maintains relatively good position in chair or bed most of the time but occasionally slides down	**3. No apparent problem** Moves in bed and in chair independently and has sufficient muscle strength to lift up completely during move; maintains good position in bed or chair at all times			
Scoring system: 15-16 = mild risk, 12-14 = moderate risk, <11 = severe risk				Total score		

FIG. 25-5 The Braden scale for predicting pressure ulcer risk. *IV,* Intravenous; *NPO,* nothing by mouth.

age, any patient who requires assistance with turning and positioning or who is unable to verbalize discomfort is at higher risk for pressure ulcers. Those confined to bed or a chair also are at higher risk than a patient who requires assistance only with ambulation.

Nutrition status is a critical risk factor for pressure ulcer development and for successful healing (Posthauer, 2012). TISSUE INTEGRITY and wound healing depend on a positive nitrogen balance and adequate serum protein levels. The patient in negative nitrogen balance not only heals more slowly but also is at risk for accelerated tissue destruction. Draining wounds contribute to protein loss and require aggressive intervention.

Nutrition assessment includes laboratory studies; evaluation of weight and weight change; ability of the patient to consume an adequate diet; and the need for vitamin, mineral, or protein supplementation. Serum prealbumin levels are often used to monitor nutrition status. *Nutrition is considered inadequate when the serum prealbumin level is less than 19.5 g/dL, albumin level is less than 3.5 g/dL, or the lymphocyte count is less than 1800/mm^3.* Because serum protein levels are affected by a number of other factors, laboratory values are valuable only when supported by additional assessment information. Other indicators of inadequate nutrition include poor daily intake of food and fluids with a weight loss greater than 5% change in 30 days or greater than 10% change in 180 days (Posthauer, 2012).

A positive nitrogen balance requires an intake of 30 to 35 calories per kilogram of body weight daily with a protein intake of 1.25 to 1.5 g/kg/day. Up to 2 g/kg/day of protein may be needed when nutritional deficits are severe or protein loss is ongoing. Vitamin and mineral supplementations are based on the patient's nutrition status. Collaborate with a dietitian for all patients at risk for a pressure ulcer to perform a thorough nutrition assessment and plan interventions for nutrition deficits (National Pressure Ulcer Advisory Panel, European Pressure Ulcer Advisory Panel, & Pan Pacific Pressure Injury Alliance, 2014).

Incontinence results in prolonged contact of the skin with substances that irritate the skin, destroy TISSUE INTEGRITY, and predispose to skin breakdown (e.g., urea, bacteria, yeast, and enzymes in urine and feces). Excessive moisture macerates skin, further increasing the risk for breakdown. Daily inspection of the skin for any areas of redness, maceration, or loss of skin TISSUE INTEGRITY is a major part of pressure ulcer prevention. Maintenance of clean, dry, intact skin also assists in ulcer prevention. Wash the skin with a pH-balanced soap to maintain the normal acid level. Use creams or lotions to lubricate and moisturize the skin. Barrier ointments protect intact skin from urine and feces when incontinence is present. Change absorbent pads or garments immediately after each incontinence episode to avoid prolonged skin contact with urine or feces.

! NURSING SAFETY PRIORITY QSEN

Action Alert

Teach all nursing care personnel and family members not to massage reddened skin areas directly or use donut-shaped pillows for pressure relief. These actions can damage capillary beds and increase tissue necrosis.

Pressure-Relieving and Pressure-Reducing Techniques

The cornerstone in the prevention and management of pressure ulcers is maintaining adequate pressure relief so that tissue pressure remains below the **capillary closing pressure**, which is the pressure needed to occlude skin capillary blood flow in a body area. The normal capillary closing pressure ranges from 12 to 32 mm Hg. An effective pressure-relieving device keeps tissue pressure *below* the capillary closing pressure for adequate tissue perfusion and oxygenation. *Most devices have a standardized guaranteed pressure-relief reading; however, these readings do not ensure that capillary blood flow for any given patient is adequate. Observe skin color, TISSUE INTEGRITY, and temperature directly to determine capillary flow adequacy.*

Devices are classified according to whether they relieve pressure or only reduce pressure. They are further classified as *dynamic* or *static*. Dynamic systems alternate inflation and deflation of the device. Static devices made of gel, water, foam, or air are in a constant state of inflation that distributes the patient pressure load over a larger area and reduces the pressure experienced by any particular area.

Pressure-relief/pressure-reduction products are available as specialty beds, mattress replacements, overlays, and assistive devices. Choosing the correct product is important in the success of the prevention plan. These factors are considered in product selection: the patient's ability to move in bed, his or her comfort level, and compatibility of the product with the care setting. Re-evaluate the product in use daily for effectiveness in reducing pressure, providing comfort, and eliminating "bottoming out." Bottoming out occurs when the product is not providing adequate pressure relief and the patient's bony prominences sink into the mattress or cushion.

Pressure-relief devices consistently reduce pressure below capillary closing pressure. These devices are recommended for patients who need:

- Prevention of skin breakdown because they cannot turn (e.g., immobility, loss of sensation)
- Prevention of extension of skin breakdown that has already occurred
- Promotion of healing for breakdown present on several turning surfaces

Pressure-reduction devices lower pressure below that of a standard hospital mattress or chair surface but do not reduce pressure consistently below the capillary closing pressure. These devices are effective for preventing pressure ulcers only when used together with a turning schedule and other skin care measures.

Frequent repositioning of bedbound patients, as described in Chart 25-2, is critical in reducing pressure over bony prominences. A good plan for positioning is the 30-degree rule. This plan ensures that the patient is positioned and propped so that whatever part of the body is elevated is tilted back to no more than a 30-degree angle to the mattress rather than resting directly on a dependent bony prominence. This rule applies to side-lying as well as head-of-bed elevation positions. The patient who requires greater head elevation because of respiratory difficulties should be tilted up above 30 degrees with pillows behind the back to keep pressure off of the sacral/coccyx area. Teach UAP the importance of proper positioning, and demonstrate how to perform it. Also teach family members to use these techniques in the home.

The patient at risk for pressure ulcers in bed is also at risk while sitting. Assess for proper chair cushioning. Collaborate with physical therapists and rehabilitation specialists for selection of these products. Periodically assist high-risk patients who are chair bound to a standing position to promote perfusion and prevent breakdown over the sacral area.

Even with an appropriate mattress or cushion, the patient needs to change or be helped to change positions periodically to prevent loss of skin TISSUE INTEGRITY. Many facilities require turning and positioning every 2 hours. *However, pressure can occur in less time, and the actual turning or repositioning schedule for each patient must be individualized.* When this action is delegated to UAP, teach them the importance of maintaining a repositioning schedule.

Use pillows and other positioning or padding devices to keep heels pressure-free at all times for high-risk patients. Assess heel positioning every 4 hours to ensure that pressure is not redistributed to other high-risk areas, such as the ankles or side of the feet. Check heels even more often when devices that hide the feet (e.g., boots, heel protectors) are used, especially if the patient has a vascular problem. Also check knees and elbows regularly, especially when the patient is in a side-lying position.

❖ PATIENT-CENTERED COLLABORATIVE CARE

◆ Assessment

History. When a patient already has a pressure ulcer, identify the cause of skin TISSUE INTEGRITY loss, as well as factors that may impair healing. Ask about the circumstances of the skin loss. Patients with chronic pressure ulcers may have a history of delayed healing or recurrence of the ulcer after healing has occurred. Assess for any of these contributing factors:

- Prolonged bedrest
- Immobility
- Incontinence
- Diabetes mellitus
- Inadequate nutrition or hydration
- Decreased sensory perception or cognitive problems
- Peripheral vascular disease

Physical Assessment/Clinical Manifestations. Inspect the entire body, including the back of the head, for areas of skin tissue integrity loss or pressure. Give special attention to bony prominences (e.g., the heels, sacrum, elbows, knees, trochanters, posterior and anterior iliac spines) and areas with excessive moisture. Make sure tubing and other medical devices are not underneath the patient and producing a pressure point. Assess the patient's general appearance for issues related to skin health, such as the proportion of weight to height. Obese patients and thin patients are at increased risk for malnutrition and pressure ulcers. Check overall cleanliness of the skin, hair, and nails. Determine whether any loss of mobility or range of joint motion has occurred. *Do not delegate this assessment to UAP.*

Wound Assessment. The appearance of pressure ulcers changes with the depth of the injury. Chart 25-3 lists the features of the six categories or stages of pressure ulceration, and Fig. 25-6 shows examples.

Assess wounds for location, size, color, extent of tissue involvement, cell types in the wound base and margins, exudate, condition of surrounding tissue, and presence of foreign bodies. Document this initial assessment to serve as a starting point for determining the intervention plan and its effectiveness. How often a wound is assessed is determined by the policies and procedures at the facility or agency. Weekly documented assessment is standard in many long-term care facilities. Daily assessment is needed when the patient is in an acute care setting. *Also assess the wound at each dressing change, comparing the existing wound features with those documented previously to determine the current state of healing or deterioration.*

For intact areas that are red (in lighter-skinned patients), press firmly with fingers at the center of the area and assess whether the area **blanches** (lightens) with pressure and

CHART 25-3 Key Features

Pressure Ulcers

Suspected Deep Tissue Injury
- The intact skin area appears purple or maroon.
- Blood-filled blisters may be present.
- Before the above-listed changes appeared, the tissue in this area may first have been painful.
- Other changes that may have preceded the discoloration include that the area may have felt more firm, boggy, mushy, warmer, or cooler than the surrounding tissue.

Stage 1
- Skin is intact.
- Area, usually over a bony prominence, is red and does not blanch with external pressure.
- For patients with darker skin that does not blanch:
  - Observable pressure-related alteration of intact skin; changes are compared with an adjacent or opposite area and include one or more of these:
    - Skin color (darker or lighted than the comparison area)
    - Skin temperature (warmth or coolness)
    - Tissue consistency (firm or boggy)
    - Sensation (pain, itching)
- The ulcer appears as a defined area of persistent redness in lightly pigmented skin, whereas in darker skin tones, the ulcer may appear with persistent red, blue, or purple hues.

Stage 2
- Skin is not intact.
- There is partial-thickness skin loss of the epidermis or dermis.
- Ulcer is superficial and may be characterized as an abrasion, a blister (open or fluid-filled), or a shallow crater.
- Bruising is *not* present.

Stage 3
- Skin loss is full thickness.
- Subcutaneous tissues may be damaged or necrotic.
- Damage extends down to but not through the underlying fascia; bone, tendon, and muscle are *not* exposed.
- The depth can vary with anatomic location; areas of thin skin (e.g., the bridge of the nose) may show only a shallow crater, whereas thicker tissue areas with larger amounts of subcutaneous fat may show a deep, crater-like appearance.
- Undermining and tunneling may or may not be present.

Stage 4
- Skin loss is full thickness with exposed or palpable muscle, tendon, or bone.
- Often includes undermining and tunneling.
- Sinus tracts may develop.
- Slough and eschar are often present on at least part of the wound.

Unstageable
- Skin loss is full thickness, and the base is completely covered with slough or eschar, obscuring the true depth of the wound.

Data from National Pressure Ulcer Advisory Panel, European Pressure Ulcer Advisory Panel, & Pan Pacific Pressure Injury Alliance. (2014). *Prevention and treatment of pressure ulcers: Quick reference guide.* Cambridge Media: Perth, Australia. Retrieved September 2014, from http://www.npuap.org/wp-content/uploads/2014/08/Quick-Reference-Guide-DIGITAL-NPUAP-EPUAP-PPPIA.pdf.

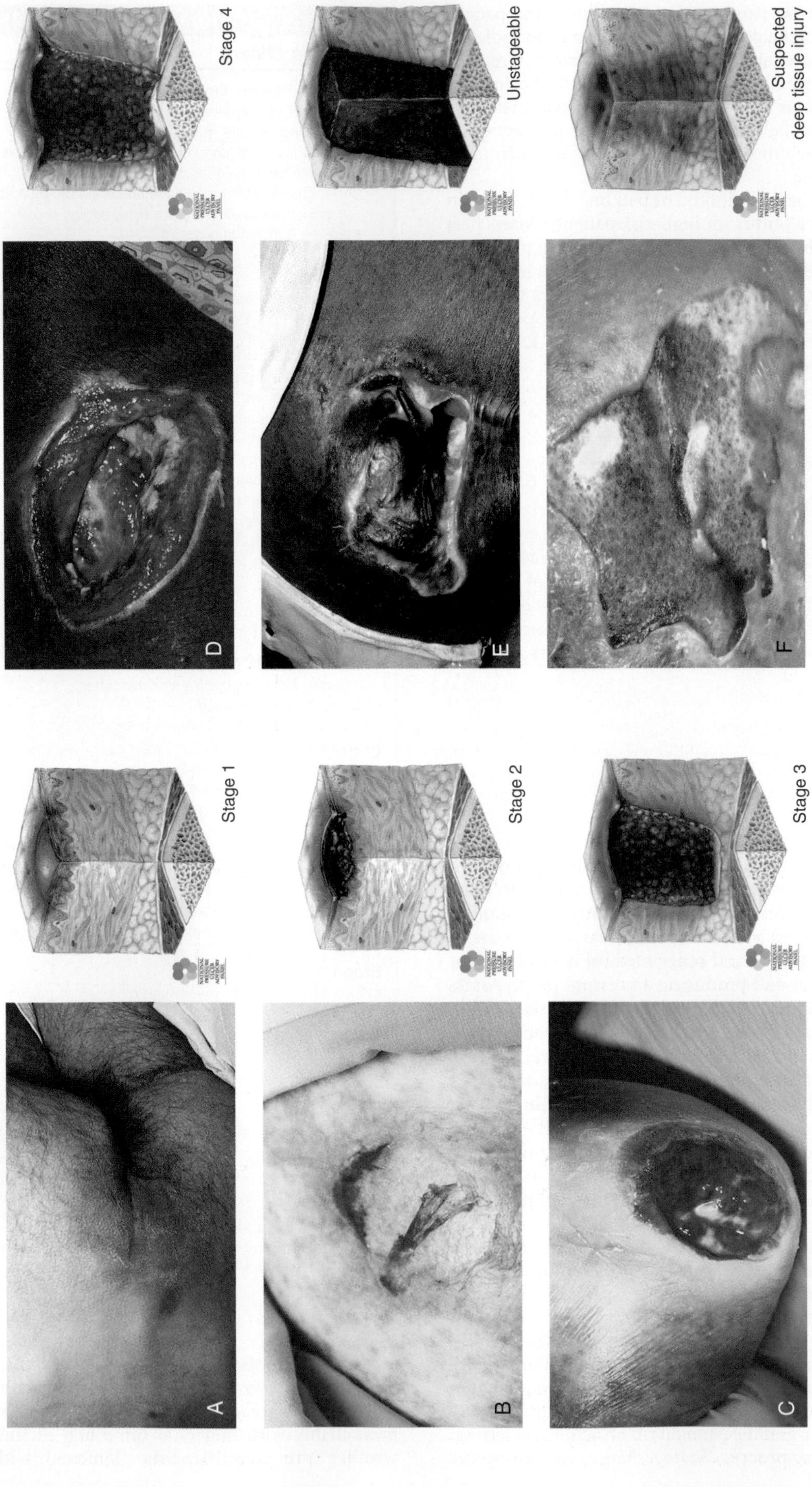

FIG. 25-6 Various stages of pressure ulcers. **A,** Stage 1 pressure ulcer. **B,** Stage 2 pressure ulcer. **C,** Stage 3 pressure ulcer. **D,** Stage 4 pressure ulcer. **E,** Unstageable ulcer. **F,** Suspected deep tissue injury.

document the response. An area that blanches with pressure and then returns to normal when pressure is removed indicates color changes related to blood flow rather than to INFLAMMATION or tissue damage. When blanching does not occur with pressure, the redness is often from skin injury. Redness and blanching may be difficult to detect in darker-skinned patients. Look for more subtle differences in the skin color over the pressure point compared with the surrounding area. In addition, compromised skin feels warmer or cooler on palpation.

Record the location and size of the wound first. Wounds are sized by length, width, and depth using millimeters or centimeters. For standardization in documentation, assess the wound as a clock face with the 12 o'clock position in the direction of the patient's head and the 6 o'clock position in the direction of the patient's feet (van Rijswijk, 2013). Using a disposable paper tape measure, always measure the length from the 12 o'clock position to the 6 o'clock position and the width between the 9 o'clock position and the 3 o'clock position. Measure depth as the distance from the deepest portion of the wound base to the skin level. Touch the bottom of the wound with a cotton-tipped applicator or swab and mark the place on the swab that is level with the skin surface to obtain wound depth. Then measure the area of the swab between the tip and the mark. When everyone uses this format, measurement is accurate and progress can be determined.

Inspect the wound margins for **cellulitis** (INFLAMMATION of the skin and subcutaneous tissue) extending beyond the area of injury. Progressive tissue destruction, seen as an increase in the size or depth of the ulcer and increased wound drainage, may indicate an increased risk for INFECTION if proper measures have been taken to relieve pressure.

Inspect the wound for the presence or absence of necrotic tissue. Because of the depth of tissue destruction, a full-thickness pressure ulcer is often covered by a layer of black, gray, or brown collagen called wound **eschar**.

In the early stages of wound healing, the eschar is dry, leathery, and firmly attached to the wound. As the inflammatory phase of wound healing begins and removal of wound debris progresses, the eschar starts to lift and separate from the tissue beneath. This nonliving eschar is a good breeding ground for any bacteria on the skin surface. As bacteria increase, they release enzymes that soften necrotic tissue, which becomes softer and more yellow. With bacterial colonization, wound exudate increases substantially; the color and odor of wound exudate indicate the major organism present. The features of wound exudate are listed in Table 25-3.

Beneath the dead tissue, granulation tissue appears. Early granulation is pale pink, progressing to a beefy red color as it grows and fills the wound. Palpate the wound to determine the granulation texture. Healthy granulation tissue is moist and has a slightly spongy texture. Wounds with a poor arterial blood supply or that have stopped healing appear dry with hard (fibrotic) granulation tissue on palpation. Venous obstruction causes a very moist ulcer surface with a deep reddish purple color from the deoxygenated blood beneath the ulcer surface.

Pressure ulcers may have more tissue destruction than is first seen on inspection. Deep, extensive tissue damage may be present under normal-appearing skin surrounding the wound, with separation of the skin layers from the underlying granulation tissue. This problem is known as **undermining**. Inspect undermined areas for gradual filling with healthy granulations and for wound-healing progress. Palpate the bony prominences for deep hardening of the surrounding soft tissue, which often occurs with deep tissue ischemia.

After ischemia has occurred, continued pressure over the area increases tissue destruction from the deep tissue layers toward the surface, resulting in the formation of tunnels. This "hidden" wound may have a small opening in the skin with purulent drainage. If such an opening is observed, use a cotton-tipped applicator to probe gently for a much larger tunnel or pocket of necrotic tissue beneath the opening. Additional tunnels may occur along the main wound. Check all wounds for tunneling and, if present, document the location and length of each tunnel.

Psychosocial Assessment. The patient with pressure ulcers may have an altered body image. Many changes in lifestyle are needed for healing. Chronic ulcers are often painful and costly to treat.

Assess the patient's and family's knowledge of the desired treatment outcomes during the healing process, as well as adherence to the prescribed treatment regimen. Also assess the patient's skills in cleaning and dressing the wound. Poor adherence to pressure ulcer care procedures may reflect an inability to cope with the pain, cost, or potential scarring associated with prolonged healing. Depending on the patient's activity level and the ulcer location, family assistance or a home care nurse may be needed to provide pressure ulcer care at home.

Teach the patient and family specific changes in ADLs to relieve pressure and promote healing. Urge increased activity whenever possible to enhance circulation to the affected tissue. Leg position changes may be needed for chronic leg ulcers, depending on whether vascular problems are present. For patients who have arterial insufficiency, keeping the legs and feet in a dependent position helps ensure adequate blood flow to the lower legs. When arterial blood flow is adequate but venous return is impaired, elevation of the legs may be needed for healing. When the patient is bedridden, frequent repositioning to relieve pressure (every 2 hours in bed, every 1 hour in a chair) can be labor intensive. In the home, repositioning, incontinence management, and dressing changes are often needed around the clock, not only increasing patient discomfort but also disrupting family routines and causing added stress.

TABLE 25-3 Types of Wound Exudate

CHARACTERISTICS	SIGNIFICANCE
Serosanguineous Exudate	
Blood-tinged amber fluid consisting of serum and red blood cells	Normal for first 48 hr after injury Sudden increase in amount precedes wound dehiscence in wounds closed by first intention
Purulent Exudate	
Creamy yellow pus	Colonization with *Staphylococcus*
Greenish blue pus causing staining of dressings and accompanied by a "fruity" odor	Colonization with *Pseudomonas*
Beige pus with a "fishy" odor	Colonization with *Proteus*
Brownish pus with a "fecal" odor	Colonization with aerobic coliform and *Bacteroides* (usually occurs after intestinal surgery)

Laboratory Assessment. An exposed wound is always *contaminated* but is not always *infected*. *Contamination* is the presence of organisms without any manifestations of infection. Normal immune defenses keep the number of bacteria to a minimum and prevent infection. *Wound INFECTION* is contamination with pathogenic organisms to the degree that organism growth and spread cannot be controlled by the body's immune defenses. Wounds that are red and indurated with moderate to heavy exudate and an odor should be cultured to identify the organism and determine antibiotic sensitivity. *The presence of purulent exudate alone does not indicate an infection because pus forms whenever necrotic tissue liquefies and separates.*

If wounds are extensive, if the patient is severely immunocompromised, or if local blood supply to the wound is impaired, bacterial growth exceeds the body's defenses against invasion into deeper tissues. The result is deep wound INFECTION and eventually bacteremia and sepsis.

Swab cultures are helpful only in identifying the types of bacteria present on the ulcer surface and may not identify bacteria in deeper tissues (Cross, 2014). Wound biopsies allow the numbers of bacteria to be analyzed, but these tests are time consuming, costly, and not always available. Clinical indicators of infection (cellulitis, progressive increase in ulcer size or depth, changes in the quantity and quality of exudate) and systemic signs of bacteremia (e.g., fever, elevated white blood cell [WBC] count) are used to diagnose an INFECTION.

Other Diagnostic Assessments. Additional laboratory studies are performed based on the suspected cause of the wound. For example, noninvasive and invasive arterial blood flow studies are indicated if arterial occlusion is suspected in delayed healing of a pressure ulcer on the heel or ankle. Blood tests to determine nutritional deficiencies (e.g., prealbumin, albumin, total protein) are helpful in managing the debilitated, malnourished patient with a pressure ulcer.

CLINICAL JUDGMENT CHALLENGE

Patient-Centered Care; Evidence-Based Practice QSEN

An 82-year-old woman, who lives alone, fell at home and lay on her right side for 10 hours on a hardwood floor before she was found. Although she broke no bones, she is very sore and does not want to move. She has an open abraded area on her right trochanter. Her other health problems include arthritis, hypertension, type 2 diabetes, osteoporosis, and gastroesophageal reflux disease.

1. Is the open area considered a pressure ulcer? Why or why not?
2. What risk factors does this patient have for pressure ulcer formation?
3. What other body areas should be inspected for possible pressure ulcer formation?
4. How will you handle her request not to move or be moved?

◆ *Analysis*

The priority NANDA-I nursing diagnoses and collaborative problems for patients with pressure ulcers include:

1. Impaired Tissue Integrity related to vascular insufficiency and trauma (NANDA-I)
2. Potential for wound deterioration related to insufficient wound management

◆ *Planning and Implementation*

The Concept Map on p. 445 addresses care issues related to patients who have or are at risk for pressure ulcers.

Managing Wounds

Planning: Expected Outcomes. The patient with a pressure ulcer is expected to progress to complete wound healing and not develop new pressure ulcers. Indicators include:

- Presence of granulation, re-epithelialization, and scar tissue formation
- Decreased wound size
- Absence of new pressure ulcers

Interventions. Wound care for pressure ulcers varies according to each patient's needs and the health care provider's preferences. Surgery may be indicated for some patients, whereas a nonsurgical approach to ulcer débridement is preferred for a patient who has adequate defenses but is too ill or debilitated for surgery.

Nonsurgical Management. General interventions for pressure ulcer care are listed in Chart 25-4. Nonsurgical intervention of pressure ulcers is often left to the discretion of the nurse, who coordinates with the health care provider and certified wound care specialist (if available) to select an appropriate method of wound dressing and management. Many agencies have guidelines for wound dressings based on wound size and depth and presence of drainage.

Dressings. A well-designed dressing helps healing by removing surface debris, protecting exposed healthy tissues, and creating a barrier until the ulcer is closed. *For a draining, necrotic ulcer, the dressing must also remove excessive exudate and loose debris without damaging healthy epithelial cells or new granulation tissue. Extensive necrosis and thick eschar require surgical or chemical removal before débridement with dressings can be*

CHART 25-4 Best Practice for Patient Safety & Quality Care QSEN

Wound Management of Pressure Ulcers

- If ulcer is covered, remove old dressings/coverings daily (unless the dressing type is to remain in place until it loosens naturally).
- Measure wound size at greatest length and width using a disposable paper tape measure or, for asymmetric ulcers, by tracing the wound onto a piece of plastic film or sheeting (plastic template) at least weekly or more often if the wound shows signs of deterioration.
- Compare all subsequent measurements against the initial measurement.
- Assess the ulcer for presence of necrotic tissue and amount of exudate.
- Assess and document the condition of the skin surrounding the pressure ulcer in terms of color, temperature, texture, moisture, and appearance.
- Remove or trim loose bits of tissue (may be done by a certified wound care specialist, physical therapist, advanced practice nurse, or other as specified by the agency and the state's nurse practice act).
- Cleanse the ulcer with saline or a prescribed solution (after diluting it as per manufacturer's directions or prescriber's instructions).
- Rinse and dry the ulcer surface.
- In collaboration with the certified wound care specialist, select and apply the dressing materials most appropriate for the volume of wound drainage.
- If possible, avoid positioning the patient on the pressure ulcer.
- Re-position at least every 1 to 2 hours to prevent ulcer extension or generation of additional pressure ulcers.
- Use prescribed pressure-relieving and pressure-reducing devices and techniques as described in Chart 27-2.

CONCEPT MAP

TISSUE INTEGRITY — INFLAMMATION — **PRESSURE ULCER** — INFECTION — CELLULAR REGULATION

HISTORY

Older adult Tom McKnight has had a loss of tissue integrity and has developed a stage 3 sacral pressure ulcer (PU) and bilateral stage 1 heel pressure ulcers. These pressure ulcers are due to significant postoperative perfusion issues from cardiac surgery and resulting immobility.

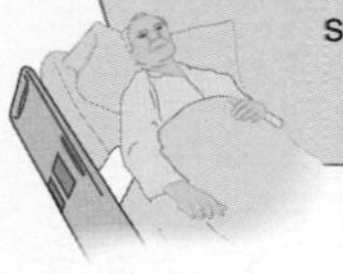

Perform and Interpret Physical Assessment

- T 100° F; P 92; R 20; BP 130/80
- Stage 3 sacral PU (moderate drainage, no necrotic tissue, red base)
- Stage 1 bilateral heels
- Midsternal chest incision–wound edges approximated, slight redness, tender to touch, no drainage
- Labs - WBC 12,000; albumin 3.0; prealbumin 12 mg/dL

Risk Factors

- Prolonged bedrest
- Immobility
- Incontinence
- Inadequate nutrition and dehydration
- Altered mental status (decreased sensory perception, cognitive problems)
- Diabetes mellitus
- Peripheral vascular disease

Data Synthesis

PATIENT PROBLEMS

Impaired TISSUE INTEGRITY related to vascular insufficiency and trauma.

Potential for wound deterioration related to insufficient wound management

Planning

EXPECTED OUTCOMES

Restoration of TISSUE INTEGRITY - demonstrate progress to complete wound healing and no new development of pressure ulcers (evidence of granulation tissue, decreased wound size, absence of new pressure ulcers).

Prevent INFECTION, INFLAMMATION, and wound deterioration - remain free of wound infection or systemic sepsis (indicators: WBC within normal range, negative blood cultures, no purulent drainage, decrease in wound size or depth, and absence of fever).

INTERVENTIONS

1 Physical Assessment/Clinical Manifestations

- Identify cause of existing PUs and factors that impair healing: prolonged bedrest, immobility, incontinence, diabetes mellitus, inadequate nutrition or hydration, decreased sensory perception, and peripheral vascular disease. *Identifies risk factors to address for minimizing or eliminating risk of developing impaired TISSUE INTEGRITY.*
- Use an evidence-based risk assessment tool (e.g., Braden) to monitor for risk of skin breakdown. Ensure tubing and other medical devices are not placed underneath the patient to produce a pressure point. *Identifies early risks to develop PU and prevents and maintains TISSUE INTEGRITY.*
- Monitor mental status and vital signs. *Assesses overall condition—confusion can be caused from infection, dehydration, and fluid & electrolyte imbalance.*
- Determine loss of mobility or a decreased range of motion (ROM). *Provides clues about mobility as a risk factor for PUs.*
- Assess wounds at each dressing change; document initial assessment as a starting point for determining the intervention plan and its effectiveness. *Indicates current state of healing or deterioration.*

2 Wound Care Assessment

- Record the location and size of wounds measuring the length, width, and depth. *Accurately measures wounds for evidence of healing and effectiveness of treatment.*
- Elevate the heels off of support surfaces. *Stops the compression of blood vessels that result in ischemia, inflammation, and tissue necrosis.*
- Inspect wounds for necrotic tissue. *Assesses the need for débridement. Dead tissue supports bacterial growth, obstructs collagen deposition, and wound contraction.*
- Coordinate with a WOCN to select the best dressing that promotes an optimal environment for healing. *Promotes evidence-based nursing care to protect new tissue and allow for wound healing.*
- Cleanse the sacral pressure ulcer with normal saline; remove existing dressing using aseptic technique. Use sterile technique for applying new dressings. *Decreases the risk of infection and promotes an environment of moist wound healing.*

3 Nursing Safety Priority: Action Alert!

Change synthetic dressings when exudate causes the adhesive seal to break and leakage to occur. *Prevents skin maceration around the wound.*

4 Assessment of Infection and Inflammation

- Monitor for signs of INFECTION (cellulitis, progressive increase in ulcer size or depth, changes in quantity and quality of exudate) and systemic signs of bacteremia (fever, elevated WBC count). *Helps prevent the slowing or stopping of wound healing.*
- Inspect wound margins for cellulitis. *Identifies signs of INFLAMMATION extending beyond area of injury which can indicate INFECTION.*
- Use Standard Precautions to care for wounds and dispose of soiled dressings and linens. *Maintains a safe environment to help prevent wound INFECTION and transmission to others.*

5 Reducing Mechanical Forces

- Obtain pressure reduction devices. *Protects against the mechanical forces of pressure, shear, friction, and moisture.*
- Perform daily inspection of the skin, especially bony prominences, skin folds, and perineal area for redness, maceration, or skin breakdown. *Prevents or minimizes mechanical forces that impair TISSUE INTEGRITY.*
- Keep skin clean and dry. *Excessive skin moisture, or urinary or fecal incontinence increases the risk for skin damage and macerates skin.*
- Wash skin with pH-balanced soap, use creams or lotions to lubricate skin, use barrier ointments with incontinence, and change absorbent pads or garments immediately. *Incontinence results in prolonged contact of the skin with irritating substances, destroys TISSUE INTEGRITY, and predisposes to skin breakdown.*

6 Nursing Safety Priority: Action Alert!

Teach all nursing care personnel and family members not to massage reddened skin areas directly or use donut-shaped pillows for pressure relief. *Prevents damage to capillary beds and decreases risk of tissue necrosis.*

7 Interpretation of Lab Values

Evaluate WBCs, prealbumin, albumin, and total protein levels. *Indicates signs of infection and protein malnutrition which makes tissue prone to breakdown and delays healing.*

Concept Map by Deanne A. Blach, MSN, RN

TABLE 25-4 Common Dressing Techniques for Wound Débridement

TECHNIQUE	MECHANISM OF ACTION
Wet-to-damp saline-moistened gauze	As with the wet-to-dry technique, necrotic debris is mechanically removed but with less trauma to healing tissue.
Continuous wet gauze	The wound surface is continually bathed with a wetting agent of choice, promoting dilution of viscous exudate and softening of dry eschar.
Topical enzyme preparations	Proteolytic action on thick, adherent eschar causes breakdown of denatured protein and more rapid separation of necrotic tissue.
Moisture-retentive dressing	Spontaneous separation of necrotic tissue is promoted by autolysis.

effective. Different dressing materials help remove debris by **mechanical débridement** (mechanical entrapment and detachment of dead tissue), by **topical chemical débridement** (topical enzyme preparations to loosen necrotic tissue), or by **natural chemical débridement** (promoting self-digestion of dead tissues by naturally occurring bacterial enzymes *[autolysis]*) (Table 25-4).

After all the dead tissue has been removed, protection of exposed healthy tissues is critical to pressure ulcer care. The ideal healing environment is a clean, *slightly* moist ulcer surface with minimal bacterial colonization. Heavy moisture from an excessively draining ulcer or a dressing that is too wet promotes the growth of organisms and causes maceration (mushiness) of healthy tissue. Likewise, if a clean ulcer surface is exposed to air or if highly absorbent dressing materials are used for prolonged periods, overdrying can dehydrate surface cells, form scabs, and convert the wound to a deeper injury. The right balance of moisture is the key to maintaining a healing environment. The type of dressing should change as wound features change with healing (Baranoski & Ayello, 2012).

Assess the ulcer for necrotic tissue and amount of exudate. Coordinate with a wound care specialist to select a dressing material that promotes an optimal environment for healing. For example, a material that does not stick to the wound surface and does not remove new epithelial cells when it is changed is used for protecting new tissue. Depending on the amount of drainage, select either a hydrophobic or a hydrophilic material:

- A **hydrophobic** (nonabsorbent, waterproof) material is useful when the wound has little drainage and needs to be protected from external contamination.
- A **hydrophilic** (absorbent) material draws excessive drainage away from the ulcer surface, preventing maceration.

A variety of synthetic materials with different absorbent properties are available. Unlike cotton gauze dressings, these may be left intact for extended periods. Biologic and synthetic skin substitutes are the newest materials being researched. Although useful, these "smart" dressings may be cost-prohibitive for many patients.

The frequency of dressing changes depends on the amount of necrotic material or exudate. Dry gauze dressings are changed when "strike through" occurs—when the outer layer of the dressing first becomes saturated with exudate. Gauze dressings used for débridement of a wet wound (allowed to become damp and then removed) are changed often enough to take off any loose debris or exudate, usually every 4 to 6 hours.

! NURSING SAFETY PRIORITY (QSEN)

Action Alert

Change synthetic dressings when exudate causes the adhesive seal to break and leakage to occur.

Before reapplying any dressing, gently clean the ulcer surface with saline or another wound cleanser as prescribed. If an antibacterial cleanser is prescribed, dilute the agent to reduce tissue toxicity and then rinse with tap water and dry the surface before applying the dressing.

Physical Therapy. Daily whirlpool treatments along with dressing changes for débridement can help remove dead tissue. The ulcerated area is immersed in or saturated with warm tap water that contains a cleansing agent. Continuous agitation of the water loosens the debris and washes away exudate and debris. During treatment, the ulcer surface is cleansed with a gauze pad. After treatment, the therapist or wound specialist often uses instruments to trim away any obvious bits of dead tissue that are still loosely attached to the ulcer surface.

Drug Therapy. Clean, healthy granulation tissue has a blood supply and is capable of providing white blood cells and antibodies to the ulcer to combat INFECTION. If extensive necrosis is present or if local tissue defenses are impaired, topical antibacterial agents are often needed to control bacterial growth (see Chart 26-5 in Chapter 26 for a list of topical antibacterial agents). Antibiotic use is avoided in the absence of infection to reduce the development of resistant bacterial strains.

Nutrition Therapy. Successful healing of pressure ulcers depends on adequate intake of calories, protein, vitamins, minerals, and water. Nutrition deficiencies are common among chronically ill patients and increase the risk for skin breakdown and delayed wound healing. Severe protein deficiency inhibits healing and impairs host INFECTION defenses.

Coordinate with the dietitian to help the patient eat a well-balanced diet, emphasizing protein, vegetables, fruits, whole grains, and vitamins. Fats also are needed to ensure formation of cell membranes. (See Chapter 60 for interventions to ensure adequate nutrition.) If the patient cannot eat sufficient amounts of food, other types of feedings may be needed to increase protein and caloric intake (see Chapter 60). Vitamin and mineral supplements are also indicated.

New Technologies. For chronic ulcers that remain open for months, new technologies have had some success. These include electrical stimulation, negative pressure wound therapy, hyperbaric oxygen therapy, topical growth factors, and skin substitutes.

Electrical stimulation is the application of a low-voltage current to a wound area to increase blood vessel growth and promote granulation. This treatment is usually performed by a certified wound care specialist. The voltage is delivered in "pulses" that may cause a "tingling" sensation. Usually this technique is performed for 1 hour a day, 5 to 7 days a week. It is not used with patients who have a pacemaker or a wound over the heart.

Negative pressure wound therapy (NPWT) can reduce or even close chronic ulcers by removing fluids or infectious materials from the wound and enhancing granulation. This technique requires that a suction tube be covered by a special sponge and sealed in place. Per manufacturer's instructions, the foam dressing is changed every 48 to 72 hours (or at least 3 times weekly). Continuous low-level negative pressure is applied through the suction tube. Duration of the treatment is determined by the wound's response. It should not be used in areas of skin cancer. Failure of NPWT is often due to the inability to maintain an adequate dressing seal (Rock, 2011).

Current evidence does not support greater effectiveness of NPWT in closing chronic wounds than more traditional methods. Serious bleeding and even deaths have occurred with NPWT, and these devices have received a warning from the Food and Drug Administration (FDA) to exclude high-risk patients from its use. Any patient who is receiving this therapy must be monitored at least every 2 hours for bleeding at or near the wound site.

! NURSING SAFETY PRIORITY QSEN

Critical Rescue

Do not use a continuous negative pressure wound therapy device with any patient who is on anticoagulant therapy; has reduced tissue health near the wound (e.g., with radiation therapy or poor nutrition); or has any exposed blood vessels, nerves, or organs in the wound area.

Hyperbaric oxygen therapy (HBOT) is the administration of oxygen under high pressure, raising the tissue oxygen concentration. This type of therapy is usually reserved for life- or limb-threatening wounds such as burns, necrotizing infections, brown recluse spider bites, osteomyelitis, and diabetic ulcers. The patient is enclosed in a large chamber and exposed to 100% oxygen at pressures greater than normal atmospheric pressure. Systemic oxygen enhances the ability of white blood cells to kill bacteria and reduce swelling. Treatment usually lasts from 60 to 90 minutes. Smaller topical oxygen delivery devices are also available. These devices are applied directly over an open wound to promote local tissue oxygenation; however, their effectiveness in promoting wound healing requires further study (Woo et al., 2012).

Topical growth factors are normal body substances that stimulate cell movement and growth. These factors are deficient in chronic wounds, and topical application is used to stimulate wound healing. For example, platelet-derived growth factor (PDGF) stimulates the movement of fibroblasts into the wound space. Use of this and other growth factors has been effective for healing of some chronic wounds, but further study is needed (Demidova-Rice et al., 2012b).

Skin substitutes are engineered products that aid in the closure of different types of wounds. These products vary widely in design and application and are used mainly for surgically débrided wounds before reconstruction with grafts or muscle flaps.

Surgical Management. Surgical management of a pressure ulcer includes removal of necrotic tissue and skin grafting or use of muscle flaps to close wounds that do not heal by re-epithelialization and contraction. Not all wounds are candidates for grafting. Those with poor blood flow are unlikely to have successful graft take and heal. The procedures are very similar to the surgical management of burn wounds. See the Surgical Management section of Managing Wound Care on pp. 483–485 of Chapter 26.

Preventing Infection and Wound Deterioration

Planning: Expected Outcomes. The patient with a pressure ulcer is expected to remain free of wound INFECTION or sepsis. Indicators include that the patient will have mild or no:

- White blood cell elevation
- Positive blood culture
- Purulent or malodorous drainage
- Increase in wound size or depth
- Fever

Interventions. Priority nursing interventions focus on preventing wound INFECTION and identifying wound infection early to prevent complications.

Monitoring the ulcer's appearance using objective criteria allows evaluation of the response to treatment and early recognition of INFECTION. If an ulcer shows no progress toward healing within 7 to 10 days or worsens, the treatment plan is re-evaluated. Chart 25-5 outlines objectives of monitoring wounds with and without tissue loss. Patients who are at highest risk for infection are those who are older, have white blood cell (WBC) disorders, are receiving steroid therapy, or have wounds with a compromised blood supply.

Preventing infection and its complications starts with monitoring the ulcer's progress. Routinely check for manifestations of wound INFECTION: increased pain, tenderness, and redness at the wound margins, edema, and purulent and malodorous drainage. Report these changes to the health care provider:

- Sudden deterioration of the ulcer, seen as an increase in the size or depth of the lesion
- Changes in the color or texture of the granulation tissue
- Changes in the quantity, color, or odor of exudate

These changes may occur with or without manifestations of bacteremia, such as fever, an elevated WBC, and positive blood cultures. Use the previously described interventions to prevent the formation of new pressure ulcers and to prevent early-stage ulcers from progressing to deeper wounds (see Chart 25-2).

Maintaining a safe environment can help prevent wound INFECTION. Because of the variety of organisms in the hospital environment, keeping an ulcer totally free of bacteria is impossible. Optimal ulcer management is based on maintaining acceptably low levels of organisms through meticulous wound care and reducing contamination with pathogenic organisms that could lead to sepsis and death. *Teach all personnel to use Standard Precautions and to properly dispose of soiled dressings and linens.*

Community-Based Care

Patients with pressure ulcers may be in acute care, subacute care, long-term care, or home care settings. If pressure ulcer therapy requires hospitalization, most patients are discharged before complete wound closure is achieved. Discharge may be to the home setting or to a long-term care facility, depending on the degree of debilitation and other patient factors.

Home Care Management. Ulcer care in the patient's home is similar to care in the hospital. Most dressing supplies and pressure-relief devices can be obtained at a pharmacy or medical supply store. If ulcer débridement is needed, a handheld shower device or forceful irrigation of the wound with a 35-mL syringe and 19-gauge angiocatheter can be substituted for whirlpool therapy.

CHART 25-5 **Best Practice for Patient Safety & Quality Care** QSEN

Monitoring the Wound

VARIABLE	FREQUENCY OF ASSESSMENT	RATIONALE
Wounds Without Tissue Loss *Examples* Surgical incisions and clean lacerations closed primarily by sutures or staples		
Observations (using first postoperative dressing change as baseline)		
Check for the presence or absence of increased: • Localized tenderness • Swelling of the incision line • Erythema of the incision line >1 cm on each side of wound • Localized heat	At least every 24 hr until sutures or staples are removed	To detect cellulitis (bacterial infections)*
Check for the presence or absence of: • Purulent drainage from any portion of the incision site • Localized fluctuance (from fluid accumulation) and tenderness beneath a *portion* of the wound when palpated	At least every 24 hr until sutures or staples are removed	To detect abscess formation related to presence of foreign body (suture material) or deeper wound infection*
Check for the presence or absence of: • Approximation (sealing) of wound edges with or without serosanguineous drainage • Necrosis of skin edges	At least every 24 hr until sutures or staples are removed	To detect potential for wound dehiscence
Wounds with Tissue Loss *Examples* Partial- or full-thickness skin loss caused by pressure necrosis, vascular disease, trauma, etc., and allowed to heal by secondary intention		
Observations ***Wound Size*** Measure wound size at greatest length and width using a disposable paper tape measure or, for asymmetric ulcers, by tracing the wound onto a piece of plastic film or sheeting (plastic template) Measure depth of full-thickness wounds using cotton-tipped applicator Compare all subsequent measurements against the initial measurement	Once per week	To detect increase in wound size and depth secondary to infectious process
Ulcer Base Check for the presence or absence of: • Necrotic tissue (loose or adherent) • Foul odor from wound when dressing is changed Note the frequency of dressing changes or dressing reinforcements owing to drainage	At least every 24 hr	To detect the need for débridement or the response to treatment (necrotic tissue) and to detect local wound infection (frequent dressing changes and foul odor)
Wound Margins Check for the presence or absence of: • Erythema and swelling extending outward >1 cm from wound margins • Increased tenderness at wound margins	At least every 24 hr or at each dressing change	To detect wound infection*
Systemic Response Check for the presence or absence of elevated body temperature or WBCs or positive blood culture	Check temperature daily; if elevated, check WBCs and blood culture	To detect bacteremia

WBCs, White blood cells.

*The wounds of patients who are severely immunosuppressed or those wounds with compromised blood supply may not exhibit a typical inflammatory response to local wound infection.

Many patients cannot change their own dressings because of wound location, distress over an altered body image, or the pain of dressing removal. Others depend on family members or support personnel because of limited physical mobility.

For some patients, drastic changes in daily activities are needed to promote healing. Patients with leg ulcers may need frequent rest periods with leg elevation to avoid or reduce edema. Immobile patients with pressure ulcers require around-the-clock repositioning as often as every 1 to 2 hours to prevent further breakdown, which takes its toll on caregivers. Explain the rationale for activity changes to the patient and family, and explore ways of coping with these changes.

Some patients may need to continue the use of special beds or mattress overlays at home. Although these items can be expensive, home use can keep the patient out of more-costly health care settings. Consider both the space and power supply when choosing a pressure-relief device for home use. Coordinate with the case manager to work with the insurance company in providing these important aids for quality patient care.

Self-Management Education. Before the patient is discharged, have the patient or caregiver demonstrate competence in removing the dressing, cleaning the wound, and applying the dressing. When choosing a dressing to be used at home, consider the patient's or caregiver's ability to apply the dressing properly. If the patient's finances are limited, address the cost of the dressing material. At times, the more expensive dressing materials that require less frequent changing may be preferred. Explain the manifestations of wound INFECTION, and remind the patient and family to report their presence to the health care provider or wound care clinic.

Encourage the patient to eat a balanced diet, including high-protein snacks. Discuss diet preferences with the patient and consult a dietitian as needed to design a food plan to promote wound healing. Vitamin and mineral supplements may be needed to prevent or treat deficiencies. If the patient is incontinent, emphasize the need to keep the skin clean and dry. If bowel and bladder training are not possible, discuss the use of absorbent underpads, briefs, and topical moisture barrier creams and ointments as methods to reduce skin exposure to urine and feces.

Health Care Resources. A home care nurse may be needed to follow wound progress after discharge. As indicated by The Joint Commission's NPSGs, the hospital nurse provides details of ulcer size and appearance and any special wound care needs in a hand-off report to the home care nurse, who can then accurately judge changes in ulcer appearance. Chart 25-6 is a guideline for a focused assessment of the patient with pressure ulcers.

To help decrease the cost of treatment, emphasize proper use of dressing materials. Clean tap water and nonsterile supplies are used for home management of chronic wounds and are less costly than sterile products. Stress the importance of properly cleaning reused items and of handwashing before touching any supplies.

The patient with activity restrictions may need daily assistance from a home care aide. Collaborate with a physical therapist or occupational therapist to help the patient and family continue rehabilitation efforts in the home.

◆ *Evaluation: Outcomes*

Evaluate the care of the patient with a pressure ulcer on the basis of the identified priority patient problems. The expected outcomes include that the patient will:

- Experience progress toward wound healing by second intention as evidenced by granulation, epithelialization, and reduction or resolution of wound size
- Re-establish skin TISSUE INTEGRITY and restore skin barrier function
- Remain INFECTION free

Specific indicators for these outcomes are listed for each priority patient problem under the Planning and Implementation section (see earlier).

CHART 25-6 Home Care Assessment

The Patient at Risk for Pressure Ulcers

Assess cardiovascular status:
- Presence or absence of peripheral edema
- Hand-vein filling in the dependent position
- Neck-vein filling in the recumbent and sitting positions
- Weight gain or loss

Assess cognition and mental status:
- Level of consciousness
- Orientation to time, place, and person
- Can the patient accurately read a seven-word sentence containing words of three syllables or fewer?

Assess condition of skin:
- Assess general skin cleanliness
- Observe all skin areas, paying particular attention to bony prominences and those areas in greatest contact with the bed and other firm surfaces
- Measure and record any areas of redness or loss of integrity
- If possible, photograph areas of concern
- Note the presence or absence of skin tenting over the sternum or the forehead
- Note the moistness of skin and mucous membranes
- If wounds are present, remove dressings (noting condition of dressings), cleanse the wound, and compare with previous notations of wound condition:
  - Presence, amount, and nature of exudate
  - Use a disposable paper tape measure to measure wound diameter and depth
  - Amount (%) and type of necrotic tissue
  - Presence of granulation/epithelium
  - Presence or absence of cellulitis
  - Presence or absence of odor

Take the patient's temperature.

Assess the patient's understanding of illness and compliance with treatment:
- Manifestations to report to health care provider
- Drug therapy plan (correct timing and dose)
- Ambulation or positioning schedule
- Dressing changes/skin care
- Nutrition modifications (24-hour diet recall)

Assess the patient's nutritional status:
- Change in muscle mass
- Lackluster nails, sparse hair
- Recent weight loss of more than 5% of usual weight
- Impaired oral intake
- Difficulty swallowing
- Generalized edema

COMMON INFECTIONS

❖ *PATHOPHYSIOLOGY*

Skin INFECTION can be bacterial, viral, or fungal. Chart 25-7 lists key features and common locations of each type.

CHART 25-7 **Key Features**

Common Skin Infections

CLINICAL MANIFESTATIONS	DISTRIBUTION
Bacterial Infections	
Folliculitis	
Isolated erythematous pustules occur singly or in groups; hairs grow from centers of many of the lesions. Occasional papules are present. There is little or no associated discomfort. There is no residual scarring.	Areas of hair-bearing skin, especially buttocks, thighs, beard area, and scalp
Furuncle	
Small, tender, erythematous nodules become pus filled and more tender over time. Lesions may be single or multiple and also recurrent. Regional lymphadenopathy is sometimes present; fever is rare. Occasional scarring results.	Areas of hair-bearing skin, especially buttocks, thighs, abdomen, posterior neck regions, and axillae
Cellulitis	
Localized area of inflammation may enlarge rapidly if not treated. Redness, warmth, edema, tenderness, and pain are present. On rare occasions, blisters are present. Cellulitis is often accompanied by lymphadenopathy and fever.	Lower legs, areas of persistent lymphedema, and areas of skin trauma (e.g., leg ulcer, puncture wound)
Viral Infections	
Herpes Simplex	
Grouped vesicles are present on an erythematous base. Vesicles evolve to pustules, which rupture, weep, and crust. Older lesions may appear as punched-out, shallow erosions with well-defined borders. Lesions are associated with itching, stinging, or pain. Secondary bacterial infection with necrosis is possible in immunocompromised patients.	Type 1 classically on the face and type 2 on the genitalia, but either may develop in any area where inoculation has occurred; recurrent infections occur repeatedly in the same skin area
Herpes Zoster (Varicella Zoster)	
Lesions are similar in appearance to herpes simplex and also progress with weeping and crusting. Grouped lesions present unilaterally along a segment of skin following the pathway of a spinal or cranial nerve (dermatomal distribution). Eruption is preceded by deep pain and itching. Postherpetic neuralgia is common in older adults. Secondary infection with necrosis is possible in immunocompromised patients.	Anterior or posterior trunk following involved dermatome; face, sometimes involving trigeminal nerve and eye
Fungal Infections	
Dermatophytosis	
Annular or serpiginous patches are present with elevated borders, scaling, and central clearing. Itching is common. Lesions may be single or multiple.	Anywhere on the body
Candidiasis	
Erythematous macular eruption occurs with isolated pustules or papules at the border (satellite lesions). Candidiasis is associated with burning and itching. Oral lesions (thrush) appear as creamy white plaques on an inflamed mucous membrane. Cracks or fissures at the corners of the mouth may be present.	Skinfold areas: perineal and perianal region, axillae, beneath breasts, and between the fingers; under wet or occlusive dressings Lesions possibly present on the oral or vaginal mucous membranes

Bacterial Infections

Bacterial skin lesions usually start at the hair follicle, where bacteria easily collect and grow in the warm, moist environment. **Folliculitis** is a superficial INFECTION involving only the upper portion of the follicle and is often caused by *Staphylococcus.* The rash is raised and red and usually shows small pustules. **Furuncles** (boils) are also caused by *Staphylococcus,* but the infection is much deeper in the follicle (Fig. 25-7). This larger, sore-looking, raised bump may or may not have a pustular "head" at its point. Cellulitis often occurs as a generalized infection with either *Staphylococcus* or *Streptococcus* and involves the deeper connective tissue.

Minor skin trauma usually occurs before the appearance of folliculitis and furuncles and may contribute to the development of cellulitis. Patients may spread the INFECTION to other parts of their bodies by scratching or rubbing the skin with fingernails. Furuncles most often occur in areas of heat and moisture, such as in the hair-bearing skinfold areas. Cellulitis

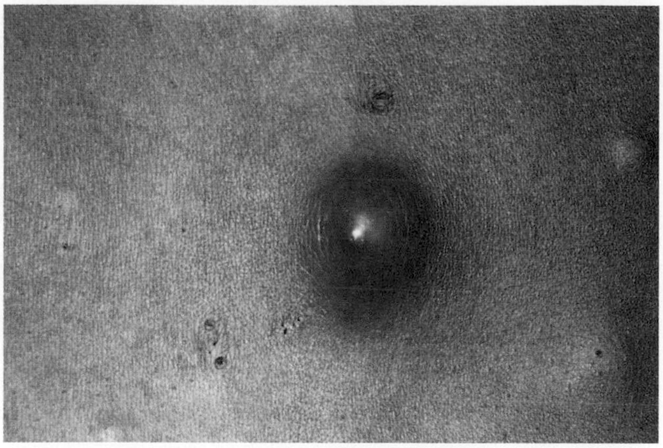

FIG. 25-7 A furuncle.

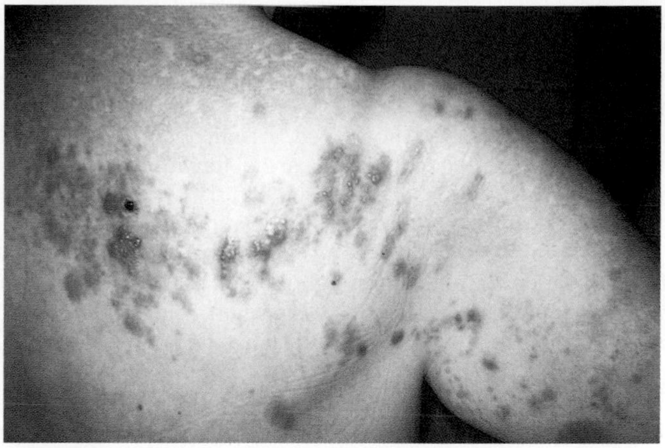

FIG. 25-8 Herpes zoster (shingles).

can occur as a result of secondary bacterial infection of an open wound, or it may be unrelated to skin trauma.

A common skin problem is INFECTION with methicillin-resistant *Staphylococcus aureus* (MRSA). This infection can range from mild folliculitis to extensive furuncles. It is easily spread to other body areas and to other people by direct contact with infected skin and by contact with clothing, linens, athletic equipment, and other objects used by a person with MRSA. The infection does not respond to cleansing with antibacterial soaps or most types of topical and many oral antibiotic therapies. If MRSA infects a wound or enters the bloodstream, deep wound infection, sepsis, organ damage, and death can occur. The incidence is highest among adults living in communal environments, such as dormitories or prisons, and among patients in hospitals or other health care settings. (See Chapter 23 for a more detailed MRSA discussion.)

Viral Infections

Herpes simplex virus (HSV) INFECTION is the most common viral infection of adult skin and has two types. Type 1 (HSV-1) infections cause the classic recurring cold sore. The severity of the disease increases with age and is worse when the patient is immunosuppressed. Genital herpes, caused by type 2 infection (HSV-2), is also recurrent (see Chapter 74).

After the first INFECTION, the virus remains in a dormant state in the nerve ganglia and the patient has no manifestations. Reactivation stimulates the virus to travel down sensory nerves to the skin, where lesions reappear. Recurrence of HSV infection in healthy people is triggered by stressors, such as dry lips, sunburn, trauma, fever, menses, and fatigue. The virus can also be spread by contact between an actively infected person and a susceptible host. *Autoinoculation,* or transfer of either viral type from one part of the body to another, is also possible.

The time span between episodes and the severity of each attack vary. Outbreaks of oral herpes simplex usually last 3 to 10 days. The patient may have tingling or burning of the lip before any lesion is evident. The patient sheds virus and is contagious for the first 3 to 5 days.

The clinical picture of HSV-1 INFECTION is isolated or grouped painful vesicles on a red base. The infection can occur anywhere on the skin and may be spread by respiratory droplets or by direct contact with an active lesion or virus-containing fluid (e.g., saliva).

Herpetic whitlow is a form of herpes simplex that occurs on the fingertips of health care personnel who come into contact with viral secretions. It can be spread easily to patients and can become severe in immunosuppressed patients.

Herpes zoster (shingles) is INFECTION caused by reactivation of the varicella-zoster virus (VZV) in patients who have previously had chickenpox. The dormant virus resides in the dorsal root ganglia of sensory nerves. Multiple lesions occur in a segmental distribution on the skin area innervated by the infected nerve (Fig. 25-8). Herpes zoster eruptions usually occur after several days of discomfort, which may vary from minor irritation and itching to severe, deep pain. The eruption usually lasts several weeks. **Postherpetic neuralgia** (severe pain persisting after the lesions have resolved) is common in older patients. Early diagnosis of shingles and prompt treatment with antiviral drugs help decrease the duration and severity of postherpetic neuralgia.

Herpes zoster occurs most often in older people or in anyone who is immunosuppressed for any reason. The disorder can be accompanied by fever and malaise. *It is contagious to people who have not previously had chickenpox and have not been vaccinated against the disease.* Keeping patients with fluid-filled blisters separated from other patients until the lesions have crusted reduces the risk for transmitting the virus to others. Complications include full-thickness skin necrosis, Bell's palsy, or eye INFECTION, and scarring if the virus is introduced into the eye.

Fungal Infections

Dermatophyte infections, especially superficial INFECTIONS, differ in lesion appearance, body location, and species of the organism. The term *tinea* is used to describe dermatophytoses; this term is then followed by the location description. For example *tinea pedis* involves the foot (athlete's foot), *tinea manus* involves the hands, *tinea cruris* involves the groin (jock itch), *tinea capitis* involves the head, and *tinea corporis* involves the rest of the body (ringworm).

Depending on the species, dermatophytes live mainly in the soil, on animals, and on humans. Superficial INFECTION can start only when the infecting organism comes in contact with impaired skin in a susceptible host. Infections are spread by direct contact with infected humans or animals. Some infections, such as tinea capitis and tinea corporis, can be transmitted by inanimate objects. For example, tinea capitis can be spread by sharing contaminated combs, hats, pillowcases, and other objects with people who have poor personal hygiene.

Candida albicans, also known as *yeast infection,* is a common fungal INFECTION of skin and mucous membranes. The organism is present almost everywhere and easily grows in a warm, moist environment. Risk factors for this infection include immunosuppression, long-term antibiotic therapy, diabetes mellitus, and obesity.

Infected skin has a moist, red, irritated appearance with itching and burning. Common areas for infection are the perineum, vagina, axillae, under the breasts, and in the mouth (where it is known as *thrush* or *oral candidiasis*).

Prevention is aimed at keeping skinfold areas clean and dry. Turning patients and positioning to enhance airflow also aid in prevention. When the INFECTION is present, meticulous cleanliness and the use of topical antifungal agents are needed.

Health Promotion and Maintenance

Preventing skin INFECTION, especially bacterial and fungal infections, involves avoiding the offending organism and practicing good hygiene to remove the organism before infection can occur. *Handwashing and not sharing personal items with others are the best ways to avoid contact with these organisms, including MRSA.* Chart 25-8 lists strategies to teach patients and family members to prevent infection spread to other body areas and to other people.

For older adults who have had chickenpox and are, therefore, at risk for shingles (herpes zoster), the vaccine *Zostavax* is available to prevent VZV reactivation and shingles. The Centers for Disease Control and Prevention (CDC) recommends the vaccine for anyone older than 50 years who has a healthy immune system. This one-time subcutaneous injection significantly reduces the incidence of shingles. Cost remains a factor in vaccination, and few insurance carriers currently include this coverage.

CHART 25-8 Patient and Family Education: Preparing for Self-Management

Preventing the Spread of MRSA

- Avoid close contact with others, including participation in contact sports, until the infection has cleared.
- Take all prescribed antibiotics exactly as prescribed for the entire time prescribed.
- Keep the infected skin area covered with clean, dry bandages.
- Change the bandage whenever drainage seeps through it.
- Place soiled bandages in a plastic bag, and seal it closed before placing it in the regular trash.
- Wash your hands with soap and warm water before and after touching the infected area or handling the bandages.
- Shower (rather than bathe) daily, using an antibacterial soap.
- Wash all uninfected skin areas before washing the infected area, or use a fresh washcloth to wash the uninfected areas.
- Use each washcloth only once before laundering, and avoid using bath sponges or puffs.
- Sleep in a separate bed from others until the infection is cleared.
- Avoid sitting on or using upholstered furniture.
- Do not share clothing, washcloths, towels, athletic equipment, shavers or razors, or any other personal items.
- Clean surfaces that may have come into contact with your infected skin, drainage, or used bandages (e.g., bathroom counters, shower/bath stalls, toilet seats) with household disinfectant or bleach water mixed daily (1 tablespoon of liquid bleach to 1 quart of water).
- Wash all soiled clothing and linens with hot water and laundry detergent. Dry clothing either in a hot dryer or outside on a clothesline in the sun.
- Urge family members and close friends to shower daily with an antibacterial soap.
- If another person assists you in changing the bandages, make certain he or she uses disposable gloves, pulls them off inside out when finished, places them with the soiled bandages in a sealed bag, and washes his or her hands thoroughly.

MRSA, Methicillin-resistant *Staphylococcus aureus.*

! NURSING SAFETY PRIORITY QSEN

Drug Alert

Zostavax is a live viral vaccine and should not be used in patients with severe immunosuppression because of the risk for viral dissemination. Always check with the prescriber before giving any live vaccines to severely immune compromised patients or those receiving biologic agents for autoimmune disease.

❖ PATIENT-CENTERED COLLABORATIVE CARE

◆ Assessment

History. Concentrate on risk factors for each type of INFECTION. If the location and appearance of lesions suggest a bacterial infection, ask about a recent history of skin trauma or recent staphylococcal or streptococcal infections. Assess living conditions, home sanitation, personal hygiene habits, and leisure or sport activities. Ask whether fever and malaise are also present.

Lesions appearing on the lips, in the mouth, or in the genital region are more likely to be a possible viral infection. Ask about:

- A history of similar lesions in the same location
- Presence of burning, tingling, or pain
- Recent stress factors that preceded the outbreak
- Recent contact with an infected person

Information that the same type of lesions has occurred before is important in helping differentiate viral from bacterial lesions. Ask whether the patient has had chickenpox in the past and about a history of shingles. Also ask whether he or she has received the shingles vaccination *Zostavax.*

Obtain information about a probable dermatophyte INFECTION based on lesion location. If tinea corporis or tinea capitis is present, assess the social and home factors that may contribute to infection, such as direct contact with an infected person, poor personal hygiene, or frequent contact with animals. If tinea cruris and tinea pedis are suspected, ask about the type and frequency of athletic activities.

Physical Assessment/Clinical Manifestations. *Because most skin infections are contagious, take precautions to prevent the spread of INFECTION when performing a physical assessment.* See Chart 25-7 for a listing of the manifestations of common skin infections.

Laboratory Assessment. When pustules are present in bacterial INFECTIONS, the infecting organism is confirmed by swab culture of the purulent material. Blood cultures may be helpful if fever and malaise are present. Various cultures and other techniques are used to identify viral and fungal infections (see Chapter 24).

◆ Interventions

Most skin INFECTIONS heal well with nonsurgical management. Surgery may be required when an infectious agent is present in deep tissue layers. *Priority nursing interventions focus on patient and family education to prevent infection spread to other body areas or to other people* (see Chart 25-8). Meticulous skin care is needed for prevention of infection spread. In some instances, drug therapy is needed.

Skin care with proper cleansing is the most effective intervention to prevent INFECTION *spread.* Teach patients with bacterial infections to bathe daily with an antibacterial soap and to not squeeze any pustules or crusts. Teach them to gently remove crusts before applying topical drugs so that the drugs can be more easily absorbed. Teach the patient to apply warm compresses to furuncles or areas of cellulitis to increase comfort. Most superficial skin infections resolve more quickly if the involved skin dries between treatments. Excessive moisture, especially if occluded by dressings, clothing, or bedding, promotes organism growth. Position bedridden patients for optimal air circulation to the area, and avoid occlusive dressings or garments.

Transmission-Based Precautions may be needed to reduce the INFECTION spread to other people. For most superficial bacterial infections, proper handwashing prevents cross-contamination. However, when hospitalized patients are colonized with antibiotic-resistant *Staphylococcus,* strict adherence to isolation procedures is necessary.

Of the dermatophyte INFECTIONS, tinea capitis, tinea corporis, and tinea pedis are most easily transmitted to others. Teach patients to avoid sharing personal items, such as hairbrushes, articles of clothing, or footwear. Repeated infections transmitted by dogs or cats indicate that the pet also needs to be treated.

Drug therapy for superficial INFECTION involves topical agents. Mild bacterial infections of the skin usually resolve with topical antibacterial treatment. Patients with extensive infections, especially if fever or lymphadenopathy is present, require systemic antibiotic therapy. The most common systemic drugs used for bacterial skin infections are the penicillins and cephalosporins. For those who are allergic to drugs from these classes, tetracyclines, macrolides, or aminoglycoside antibiotics may be used. For patients infected with MRSA or other drug-resistant organisms, drug therapy may involve IV vancomycin or oral linezolid or clindamycin.

Acyclovir (Zovirax), valacyclovir (Valtrex), or famciclovir (Famvir) is used for the treatment of viral INFECTIONS. Topical treatment decreases the numbers of active viruses on the skin surface and reduces pain in herpetic infections and localized lesions in immunocompromised patients during an initial outbreak. Topical treatment is of little benefit in recurrent infection. IV administration is limited to severe primary infections, immunosuppressed patients with manifestations of systemic infection, and recurrent outbreaks.

Topical antifungal agents are used for patients with dermatophyte or yeast INFECTIONS at least twice a day until the lesions have cleared. To prevent recurrence, therapy is usually continued for 1 to 2 weeks after clearing. In some instances, antifungal powders may also help suppress fungal growth. For widespread or resistant fungal infections, systemic antifungal agents, such as ketoconazole (Nizoral), are given.

CUTANEOUS ANTHRAX

Cutaneous anthrax is an INFECTION caused by the spores of the bacterium *Bacillus anthracis.* In the United States, the most common risk factor is contact with an infected animal. Those most at risk for cutaneous anthrax include farm workers, veterinarians, and tannery and wool workers. This organism has now become a tool for terrorism.

NCLEX EXAMINATION CHALLENGE

Health Promotion and Maintenance

Which statement made by a client with a furuncle in the groin indicates to the nurse that teaching about the care needed for this problem has been effective?

A. "I will wear tight jeans to keep the infection from spreading to other areas."
B. "I will shower with an antibacterial soap before applying the topical ointment."
C. "I will squeeze the lesion until it opens so I can remove all the pus and other material."
D. "I will shave the area around the lesion and apply cortisone cream to reduce the inflammation."

NURSING SAFETY PRIORITY QSEN

Action Alert

Consider the possibility of bioterrorism whenever lesions consistent with cutaneous anthrax appear in patients who do not have a history of exposure to infected animals.

The INFECTION can be confined to the skin, or it may be systemic. At first a raised vesicle appears on an exposed body area such as the head or arms (Fig. 25-9). The lesion may itch and often resembles an insect bite. Within a few days, the center of the vesicle becomes hemorrhagic and sinks inward, starting an area of necrosis and ulceration. The tissue around the wound swells and can become very edematous. With necrosis, an eschar forms (see Fig. 25-9). The two features that distinguish anthrax lesions from insect bites or other skin lesions are that it is painless and that eschar forms regardless of treatment. Patients may have only one lesion, or there may be multiple lesions, usually in the same body area.

Some patients develop systemic manifestations with cutaneous anthrax. The area becomes edematous and tender. Fever, chills, and enlarged lymph nodes may be present.

Diagnosis is made based on lesion features, a positive culture, or the presence of anthrax antibodies in the patient's blood. Cultures are obtained from patients who have a fever.

Oral antibiotics for 60 days are indicated for patients who have no edema or systemic manifestations and whose lesions are not located on the head or neck. The antibiotics of choice are ciprofloxacin (Cipro) or doxycycline (Doryx, Vibramycin). For patients who have a fever, have lesions on the head or neck, are pregnant, or have extensive edema, antibiotics are given IV and then followed by an oral course of 60 days.

PARASITIC DISORDERS

Parasitic skin disorders occur most often in patients with poor hygiene and in those who are homeless. Examine any patient who shows obvious signs of a self-care deficit for contagious parasitic infections.

Pediculosis

Pediculosis is a lice infestation: *pediculosis capitis* (head lice), *pediculosis corporis* (body lice), and *pediculosis pubis* (pubic, or crab, lice). Human lice are oval and 2 to 4 mm long. The female louse lays many eggs *(nits)* at the hair shaft base in hair-bearing areas.

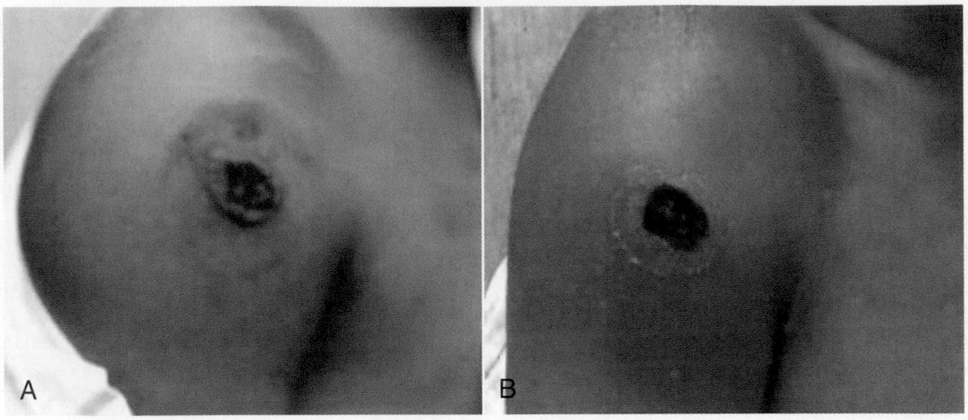

FIG. 25-9 Cutaneous anthrax. Note ulcer with vesicular ring, induration, and erythema (**A**). As eschar forms, induration lessens, surrounding desquamation occurs, but erythema persists (**B**).

The most common manifestation of pediculosis is itching (pruritus). Excoriation from scratching also may be present. Some parasites may carry disease (e.g., typhus).

Pediculosis capitis occurs more often in people with longer hair. Scalp itching from parasite bites is intense. A secondary INFECTION may also be present from scratching.

Because the louse is difficult to see, examine the scalp for visible white flecks of the nits attached to the hair shaft near the scalp. Matting and crusting of the scalp and a foul odor indicate a probable secondary INFECTION.

Pediculosis corporis is caused by lice that live and lay eggs in the seams of clothing. The parasites also cause itching. The only visible sign of infestation may be excoriations on the trunk, abdomen, or extremities.

Pediculosis pubis causes intense itching of the vulvar or perirectal region. Pubic lice are more compact and crablike in appearance than body lice and can be contracted from infested bed linens or during sexual intercourse with an infected person. Although these lice are usually found in the genital region, they can also infest the axillae, the eyelashes, and the chest.

The treatment of pediculosis is chemical killing of the parasites with topical sprays, creams, and shampoos. Agents used include permethrin (Elimite), lindane (Bio-Well, Kwell, Kwellada), or topical malathion (Ovide, Prioderm). Oral agents may also be used, such as ivermectin (Stromectol). In the case of pediculosis capitis, areas where the patient's head has rested (e.g., on pillows or chair backs) are also treated. Clothing and bed linens should be washed in hot water with detergent or dry-cleaned. The use of a fine-tooth comb helps remove nits but does not cure the INFECTION. For any louse infestation, social contacts are treated when possible.

Scabies

Scabies is a contagious skin INFECTION caused by mite infestations. It is transmitted by close contact with an infested person or infested bedding. Infestation is common among patients with poor hygiene or crowded living conditions. The scabies mite is carried by pets and is found among homeless people and institutionalized older patients. Health care personnel are at risk for contracting scabies from contact with an infected patient or his or her bed linen.

Scabies is manifested by curved or linear ridges in the skin (Fig. 25-10). The itching is very intense, and patients often report that the itching becomes unbearable at night.

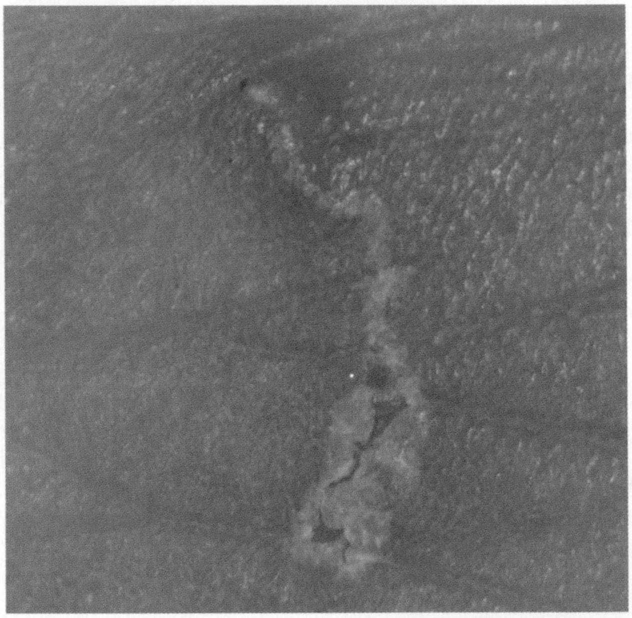

FIG. 25-10 Scabies. Note the horizontal lines indicating burrowing of the organism under the skin.

The visible horizontal white skin ridges are formed by burrowing of the mite into the outer skin layers. Examine the skin between the fingers and on the palms and inner aspects of the wrists, where these ridges are most common. A hypersensitivity reaction to the mite results in excoriated erythematous papules, pustules, and crusted lesions on the elbows, nipples, lower abdomen, buttocks, and thighs and in the axillary folds. Males can have lesions on the penis.

Infestation is confirmed by taking a scraping of a lesion and examining it under the microscope for mites and eggs. Close contacts also should be examined for possible infestation.

Treatment involves the use of scabicides, such as permethrin (Acticin), lindane (Kwell, Kildane, Scabene, Thionex), malathion (Ovide), or benzyl benzoate (Ascabiol). Laundering clothes and personal items with hot water and detergent is sufficient to eliminate the mites.

Bedbugs

A common parasite is the bedbug, *Cimex lectularius*. Infestations are increasingly common as a result of travel and resistance to pesticides. This pest does not live on humans; however, it feeds on human blood. The bite causes an itchy discomfort. The most common mode of infestation is carrying the "hitch-hiking" bug home from an infested environment such as a hotel room. This problem is not related to socioeconomic level or to a lack of cleanliness.

The adult bedbug is about the size, shape, and color of an apple seed. After feeding, it may double in size and have a red or black color. The insect bites a human host at night and sucks blood for 3 to 10 minutes. The bite area resembles a mosquito or flea bite with a raised bite mark surrounded by a wheal. The degree of itching and redness is related to how allergic the person is to the insect's saliva. All body areas are susceptible, and one insect can bite multiple times, resulting in clusters of bite marks.

Management of the patient with bedbug bites is symptomatic for discomfort from itching, usually with topical antihistamines. When the discomfort is more widespread or the allergic reaction is severe, systemic antihistamines or corticosteroids may be used. Because humans do not harbor the insect, the usual topical insecticides are not needed.

Bedbugs can live anywhere, hiding in cracks and crevices. They can live and lay their eggs in soft upholstery or in wooden crevices. Eradicating the infestation and preventing re-infestations require considerable effort and can be frustrating. Often the home environment needs the extensive eradication efforts of a licensed professional pest control company with experience in the management of bedbugs (Barnes & Murray, 2013).

COMMON INFLAMMATIONS

❖ PATHOPHYSIOLOGY

Skin INFLAMMATION can have many nonspecific manifestations, including severe itching, lesions with indistinct borders, and different distribution patterns. The cause may not be identified. Rashes from inflammation can evolve from acute to chronic conditions.

Most skin INFLAMMATIONS are related to allergic immune responses. The responses may be triggered by external skin exposure to allergens or by internal exposure to allergens and irritants. The result is tissue destruction or skin changes induced by the immune system. (A more detailed description of these immune mechanisms is presented in Chapter 17.)

The specific cause of skin INFLAMMATION is not always known. When this is the case, the catch-all diagnosis of *nonspecific eczematous dermatitis,* or *eczema,* is often used.

Contact dermatitis is an acute or chronic rash caused by direct contact with either an irritant or an allergen. Irritants cause a toxic injury to the skin. Allergens result in a cell-mediated immune reaction in the skin.

Atopic dermatitis is a chronic rash that occurs with allergies and atopic skin disease. It is made worse by dry or irritated skin, food allergies, chemicals, or stress. (Atopic reactions are described in Chapter 20.)

❖ PATIENT-CENTERED COLLABORATIVE CARE

Because all skin eruptions from INFLAMMATION appear similar, personal data are needed to identify the cause. Inflammatory skin problems differ from eczematous dermatitis in chronicity, lesion distribution, and associated manifestations. Chart 25-9 lists the manifestations of many types of inflammatory skin conditions.

CHART 25-9 Key Features

Common Inflammatory Skin Conditions

CLINICAL MANIFESTATIONS	DISTRIBUTION
Nonspecific Eczematous Dermatitis	
Evolution of lesions from vesicles to weeping papules and plaques. Lichenification occurs in chronic disease. Oozing, crusting, fissuring, excoriation, or scaling may be present. Itching is common.	Anywhere on the body; localized eczema commonly involves the hands or feet.
Contact Dermatitis	
Localized eczematous eruption with well-defined, geometric margins that are consistent with contact by an irritant or allergen. Usually seen in the acute form, but may become chronic if exposure is repeated. Allergy to plants (e.g., poison ivy or oak) classically occurs as linear streaks of vesicles or papules.	Cosmetic/perfume allergy: head and neck. Hair product allergy: scalp. Shoe/rubber allergy: dorsum of feet. Nickel allergy: earlobes. Mouthwash/toothpaste allergy: perioral region. Airborne contact allergy (e.g., paint, ragweed): generalized.
Atopic Dermatitis	
Hallmark in adults is lichenification with scaling and excoriation. Extremely itchy. Face involvement is seen as dry skin with mild to moderate erythema, perioral pallor, and skinfolds beneath the eyes (Dennie-Morgan lines). Associated with linear markings on the palms.	Face, neck, upper chest, and antecubital and popliteal fossae.
Drug Eruption	
Bright red erythematous macules and papules are found. Skin blisters in extreme cases. Lesions tend to be confluent in large areas. Moderately itchy. Fever is rare. Dehydration and hypothermia can occur with extensive involvement. Condition clears only after offending drug has been discontinued.	Generalized. Involvement begins on trunk, proceeds distally (legs are the last to be involved).

If the cause of the rash is identified, avoidance therapy is used to reverse the reaction and clear the rash. For example, if a new soap for handwashing causes contact dermatitis of the hands, teach the patient to avoid that substance. Even when the cause is unclear, certain irritants may worsen the rash and increase discomfort. Additional interventions promote comfort through suppression of INFLAMMATION.

Steroid therapy with topical, intralesional, or systemic steroids is prescribed to suppress INFLAMMATION. Because a side effect of oral corticosteroids (e.g., prednisone) is adrenal suppression, patients receiving long-term systemic therapy must taper their drug dosages rather than stop them abruptly.

Remember that corticosteroids never cure the INFLAMMATION. During active disease, these drugs reduce manifestations and relieve discomfort. Moisten dressings with warm tap water and place them over topical steroids for short periods to increase absorption. Avoid applying topical steroids under occlusive dressings unless prescribed by the health care provider.

! NURSING SAFETY PRIORITY QSEN

Drug Alert

Caution patients not to apply topical corticosteroids to potentially infected skin lesions anywhere on the body, but especially on the face. These agents suppress the local immune response and can worsen the infection.

Avoid applying oil-based ointments and pastes to the sweaty skinfold areas to prevent blocking of pores and folliculitis. Water-soluble creams are better for these areas. Lotions and gels prevent matting of the hair and are more appropriate for the scalp and other hairy areas. Thick, stiff ointments or pastes (e.g. zinc oxide pastes) are applied to localized areas because they cling to the skin where applied and resist spreading to uninvolved skin.

Antihistamines provide some relief of itching but may not keep the patient totally comfortable. The sedative effects of these drugs may be better tolerated if most of the daily dose is taken near bedtime. Teach patients to avoid driving or operating heavy machinery if these drugs are taken during the day.

Comfort measures such as cool, moist compresses and lukewarm baths with bath additives have a soothing effect, decrease INFLAMMATION, and help débride crusts and scales. Colloidal oatmeal, tar extracts, cornstarch, or oils added to baths may relieve itching.

PSORIASIS

❖ PATHOPHYSIOLOGY

Psoriasis is a chronic, autoimmune disorder affecting the skin with exacerbations and remissions. It results from overstimulation of the immune system (Langerhans' cells) in the skin that activates T-lymphocytes. These cells then target the keratinocytes, causing increased cell division (because some degree of CELLULAR REGULATION is lost) and plaque formation. Even though psoriasis cannot be cured, patients can often achieve control of manifestations with proper management.

Psoriasis lesions are scaled with underlying dermal INFLAMMATION from an abnormality in the growth of epidermal cells. Normally, basal cells take about 28 days to reach the outermost layer where they are shed. In a person with psoriasis, the rate of cell division is speeded up so that cells are shed every 4 to 5 days.

GENETIC/GENOMIC CONSIDERATIONS

Patient-Centered Care QSEN

A genetic predisposition is associated with psoriasis as indicated by the fact that when one identical (monozygotic) twin develops the disease, the second twin also develops the disease about 70% of the time. Variations in many gene sequences, labeled *PSORS1* through *PSORS13,* influence the development of this autoimmune disorder. It is likely that different variations of these gene loci also influence individual patient responses to therapy. Always ask about a family history of the disorder when assessing the patient with psoriasis (Online Mendelian Inheritance in Man [OMIM], 2014b).

Many environmental factors lead to outbreaks and influence the severity of manifestations, but these vary from person to person. Triggering factors may be local or systemic. A psoriatic lesion may appear after skin trauma (Koebner's phenomenon, in which a previously injured area is more susceptible to development of cancer or chronic skin problems) such as surgery, sunburn, or excoriation.

Patients with psoriasis often improve with more exposure to sunlight. Systemic factors that can aggravate the disease include INFECTION (severe streptococcal throat infection, *Candida* infection, upper respiratory infections), hormonal changes (e.g., puberty, menopause), stress, drugs (lithium, beta-blocking agents, indomethacin), obesity, and the presence of other diseases.

Some patients with psoriasis also develop debilitating *psoriatic arthritis.* This arthritis may lead to severe joint changes similar to those seen in rheumatoid arthritis and indicates that psoriasis is a systemic disorder (McCance et al., 2014). See Chapter 18 for more discussion of arthritis.

❖ PATIENT-CENTERED COLLABORATIVE CARE

◆ Assessment

History. Ask the patient about any family history of psoriasis, including the age at onset, a description of the disease progression, and the pattern of recurrences. Have the patient describe the current flare-up of psoriasis, including whether the onset was gradual or sudden, where the lesions first appeared, whether there have been any changes in severity over time, and whether fever and itching are present. Explore possible precipitating factors, and ask about the effectiveness of any previous interventions.

Physical Assessment/Clinical Manifestations. The appearance of psoriasis and its course vary among patients. Typically during flare-ups of the disease, lesions thicken and extend into new body areas. As psoriasis responds to treatment, lesions become thinner with less scaling.

Psoriasis vulgaris is the most common type of psoriasis, with thick, reddened papules or plaques covered by silvery white scales (Fig. 25-11). Borders between the lesions and normal skin are sharply defined. Patches are less red and moister in skinfold areas. Lesions are usually present in the same areas on both sides of the body (bilateral distribution). Common sites include the scalp, elbows, trunk, knees, sacrum, and outside surfaces of the limbs. Facial skin is rarely affected. The patient may have only a few lesions, or the entire skin surface may be affected.

Exfoliative psoriasis (erythrodermic psoriasis) is an explosively eruptive and inflammatory form with generalized erythema and scaling but no obvious lesions. Fluid loss with this severe inflammatory reaction can lead to dehydration and hypothermia or hyperthermia.

Palmoplantar pustulosis (PPP) is a type of psoriasis that forms pustules on the palms of the hands and soles of the feet along with reddened hyperkeratotic plaques. The course of the disease is cyclic, with new outbreaks of pustules occurring after older lesions have resolved. PPP is difficult to treat, and patients often have social and physical problems.

◆ Interventions

The three different approaches to therapy are based on the extent of disease, the patient's distress, and the response of the psoriasis to treatment. Patients must understand that no cure

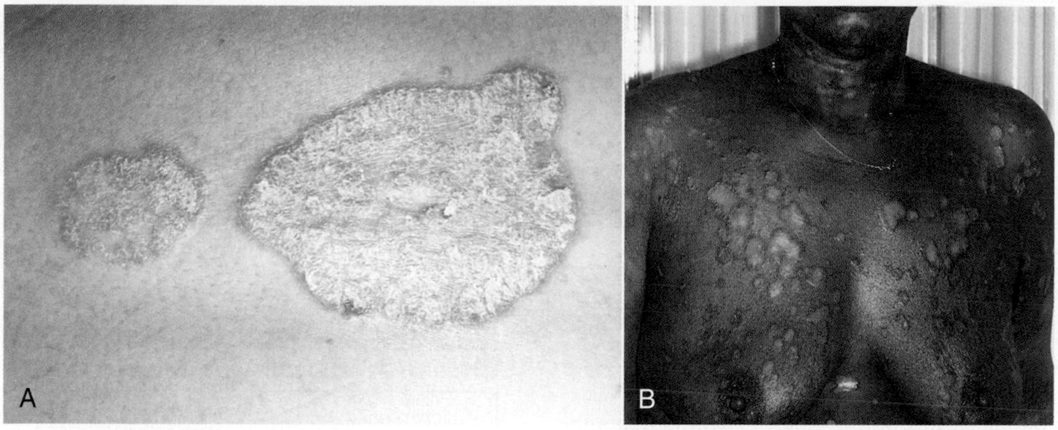

FIG. 25-11 A, Psoriasis vulgaris in a white patient. **B,** Psoriasis vulgaris in a patient with dark skin.

for psoriasis exists yet. Therapy is aimed at reducing cell proliferation and INFLAMMATION. *Priority nursing strategies include teaching the patient about the disease and its treatment and providing emotional support for the changes in body image often experienced with psoriasis.*

Topical Therapy. The topical agents used to treat psoriasis are topical steroids, topical tar and anthralin preparations, and ultraviolet (UV) light.

Corticosteroids have anti-inflammatory actions. When applied to psoriatic lesions, corticosteroids suppress cell division. The effectiveness of a topical steroid depends on its potency and ability to be absorbed into the skin. The more potent agents are used as therapy for patients with psoriasis.

Teach patients to enhance the skin penetration of these drugs by applying the steroid directly to the skin. When prescribed, using warm, moist dressings and an occlusive outer wrap of plastic (film, gloves, booties, or similar garments) may enhance absorption.

Tar preparations applied to the skin suppress cell division from impaired CELLULAR REGULATION and reduce INFLAMMATION. These drugs are available as solutions, ointments, lotions, gels, and shampoos. The ointments are messy, cause staining, and have an unpleasant odor.

Topical therapy with anthralin (Anthraforte♣, Drithocreme, Lasan), a hydrocarbon similar in action to tar, also relieves chronic psoriasis. These drugs can be used alone or in combination with coal tar baths and UV light.

Teach the patient to apply the high-potency anthralin, suspended in a stiff paste, to each lesion for short periods (not exceeding 2 hours). The drug is a strong irritant and can cause chemical burns. Remind the patient to check for local tissue reaction and to take care to prevent this drug from coming into contact with uninvolved skin.

Other topical therapies can be effective for many patients with mild to moderate psoriasis. These drugs include calcipotriene (Dovonex), a synthetic form of vitamin D that regulates skin cell division, and tazarotene (Avage, Tazorac), a derivative of vitamin A that slows cell division and reduces inflammatory responses. In some cases, calcitriol (Vectical ointment) has been helpful but is quite expensive.

Light Therapy. Ultraviolet (UV) radiation is a physical agent commonly used as a topical therapy in many skin conditions, including psoriasis. Ultraviolet B (UVB) light, which produces more energy, is responsible for the obvious biologic effects of the sun, such as burning. Although the sun is an inexpensive source of UV radiation, better availability and intensity control occur with the use of artificial light sources. These sources include lamps or cabinets containing UV tubes. *The use of commercial tanning beds is not recommended for the patient with psoriasis.*

> **! NURSING SAFETY PRIORITY (QSEN)**
>
> ***Drug Alert***
>
> Tazorac is **teratogenic** (can cause birth defects) even when used topically. Teach sexually active women of childbearing age using this drug to adhere to strict contraceptive measures.

Ultraviolet therapy is limited by exposure time and effects on the surrounding normal skin. The time of exposure is gradually increased to achieve a mild suntan effect without burning or tenderness. The patient's skin pigmentation determines the exposure times. Because of the extremely high intensity of most artificial UVB light sources, therapy is measured in seconds of exposure and patients must wear eye protection during treatment. Narrow band UVB light therapy, although intense, can shorten the time to effectiveness and reduce the number of exposures needed to maintain the response.

Light therapy with lasers can be effective in controlling mild to moderate psoriasis. Laser sources, whether administered in a continuous or pulsed exposure, allow for better focus on the lesions and reduce exposure to the surrounding normal skin.

Teach patients to inspect the skin carefully each day for signs of overexposure. If tenderness on palpation occurs and severe erythema or blister formation develops, notify the health care provider before therapy is resumed.

Psoralen and ultraviolet A (UVA) (PUVA) therapy involves the ingestion of a photosensitizing agent (psoralen) 2 hours before exposure to UVA light. Therapy sessions are limited to 2 or 3 times a week and are not given on consecutive days. Exposure is gradually increased until tanning occurs. Dosages are adjusted according to the erythema reaction of normal skin as well as the response of psoriatic lesions.

Teach the patient to check for redness with edema and tenderness. If these are present, treatment must be interrupted until they subside. Because psoralen is a strong photosensitizer, patients must wear dark glasses during treatment and for the rest of the day.

Systemic Therapy. Systemic agents are used when psoriasis does not respond to topical therapies. The most commonly used drugs are oral vitamin A derivatives—retinoids. These drugs include acitretin (Soriatane) and bexarotene (Targretin).

! NURSING SAFETY PRIORITY QSEN

Drug Alert

Both acitretin and bexarotene are teratogenic. Teach sexually active women of childbearing age using this drug to adhere to strict contraceptive measures.

A variety of biologic (immunomodulating) agents that alter the immune response and prevent overstimulation of keratinocytes from impaired CELLULAR REGULATION are now being used to manage moderate to severe plaque psoriasis. These agents may be prescribed when other drugs are not effective and when psoriatic arthritis is also present. Most of these drugs are given by intravenous infusion, intramuscular injection, or subcutaneous injection. All of these agents induce some degree of immunosuppression, and patients are at an increased risk for serious infection.

! NURSING SAFETY PRIORITY QSEN

Drug Alert

Instruct patients to discontinue the biologic agent and notify the health care provider immediately if manifestations of INFECTION occur.

Biologics currently approved for the treatment of psoriasis are listed in Chart 25-10. These drugs should NOT be used by patients who are pregnant or breast-feeding.

Other less commonly used systemic drugs for the patient whose disease is resistant to topical therapy include methotrexate (Folex, Mexate), cyclosporine (Sandimmune), and azathioprine (Imuran). The many health risks associated with these therapies must be considered along with the potential benefits, especially in older adults (Wong & Woo, 2012).

Emotional Support. Often patients' self-esteem suffers because of the presence of skin lesions. Encourage the patient and family members to express their feelings about having an incurable skin problem that can alter appearance. Support groups for people with psoriasis are available in many communities. Urge patients and families to consider participating in these groups.

The use of touch takes on an added significance for patients with psoriasis. For example, shake the patient's hand during an introduction or place a hand on the patient's shoulder when explaining a procedure. *Do not wear gloves during these social interactions. Touch, more than any other gesture, communicates acceptance of the person and the skin problem.*

? NCLEX EXAMINATION CHALLENGE

Health Promotion and Maintenance

Which precaution is most important for the nurse to teach the 32-year-old female client prescribed topical tazarotene (Tazorac) cream for psoriasis?

A. Apply a dressing over the site with each application.
B. Stop the drug use when psoriasis manifestations decrease.
C. Report symptoms of infection to the prescriber immediately.
D. Adhere to strict contraceptive measures while using the drug.

SKIN CANCER

❖ PATHOPHYSIOLOGY

Any skin cancer occurs as a result of failure of CELLULAR REGULATION over cell division. (See Chapter 21 for a discussion of the general mechanisms leading to changes in cellular regulation and cancer development.) *Overexposure to sunlight is the major cause of skin cancer, although other factors also are associated.* Because sun damage is an age-related skin finding, screening for suspicious lesions is an important part of physical assessment of the older adult. The most common skin cancers are actinic or solar keratosis, squamous cell carcinoma, basal cell carcinoma, and melanoma. Table 25-5 describes common skin cancers. A biopsy of suspicious lesions is necessary to determine whether a skin lesion is malignant.

Etiology and Genetic Risk

Actinic keratoses are premalignant lesions of the cells of the epidermis. These lesions are common in people with chronically sun-damaged skin. Progression to squamous cell carcinoma may occur if lesions are untreated.

Squamous cell carcinomas are cancers of the epidermis. They can invade locally and are potentially metastatic (Fig. 25-12). Chronic skin damage from repeated injury or irritation also

CHART 25-10 Common Examples of Drug Therapy

Plaque Psoriasis

AGENT	ROUTE	DOSE	FREQUENCY
adalimumab (Humira)	Subcutaneous	Loading dose: 80 mg Maintenance dose: 40 mg	Loading dose followed by maintenance dose every other week starting 1 week after the loading dose.
alefacept (Amevive)	Intramuscular	15 mg	Once a week for 12 weeks followed by a 12-week drug-free interval. Cycle may be repeated based on response.
etanercept (Enbrel)	Subcutaneous	50 mg	Twice weekly for 3 months followed by once-a-week injections.
infliximab (Remicade)	Intravenous	5 mg/kg	Infusions at 0, 2, and 6 weeks, then every 8 weeks.
ustekinumab (Stelara)	Subcutaneous	90 mg	Initial dose 90 mg; second dose 4 weeks later Maintenance injections of 90 mg subcutaneously every 12 weeks starting at week 16 after initial dose.

TABLE 25-5 **Common Skin Cancers**

CLINICAL MANIFESTATIONS	DISTRIBUTION	COURSE
Actinic Keratosis (Premalignant)		
Small (1-10 mm) macule or papule with dry, rough, adherent yellow or brown scale Base may be erythematous Associated with yellow, wrinkled, weather-beaten skin Thick, indurated keratoses more likely to be malignant	Cheeks, temples, forehead, ears, neck, backs of hands, and forearms	May disappear spontaneously or reappear after treatment. Slow progression to squamous cell carcinoma is possible.
Squamous Cell Carcinoma		
Firm, nodular lesion topped with a crust or with a central area of ulceration Indurated margins Fixation to underlying tissue with deep invasion	Sun-exposed areas, especially head, neck, and lower lip Sites of chronic irritation or injury (e.g., scars, irradiated skin, burns, leg ulcers)	Rapid invasion with metastasis via the lymphatics occurs in 10% of cases. Larger tumors are more prone to metastasis.
Basal Cell Carcinoma		
Pearly papule with a central crater and rolled, waxy borders Telangiectasias and pigment flecks visible on close inspection	Sun-exposed areas, especially head, neck, and central portion of face	Metastasis is rare. May cause local tissue destruction. 50% recurrence rate related to inadequate treatment.
Melanoma		
Irregularly shaped, pigmented papule or plaque Variegated colors, with red, white, and blue tones	Can occur anywhere on the body, especially where nevi (moles) or birthmarks are evident Commonly found on upper back and lower legs Soles of feet and palms in dark-skinned people	Horizontal growth phase followed by vertical growth phase. Rapid invasion and metastasis with high morbidity and mortality.

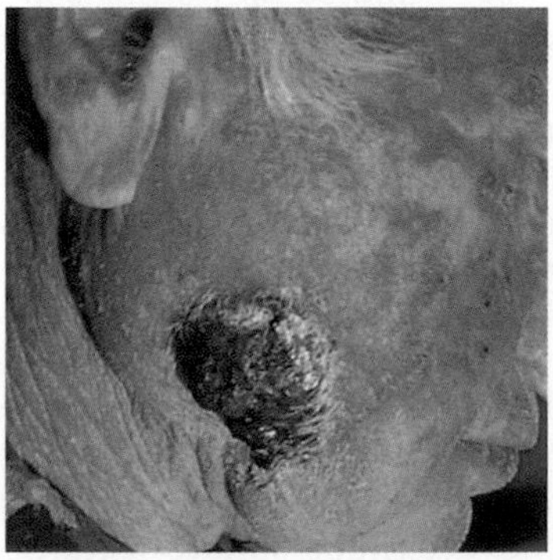
FIG. 25-12 Squamous cell carcinoma.

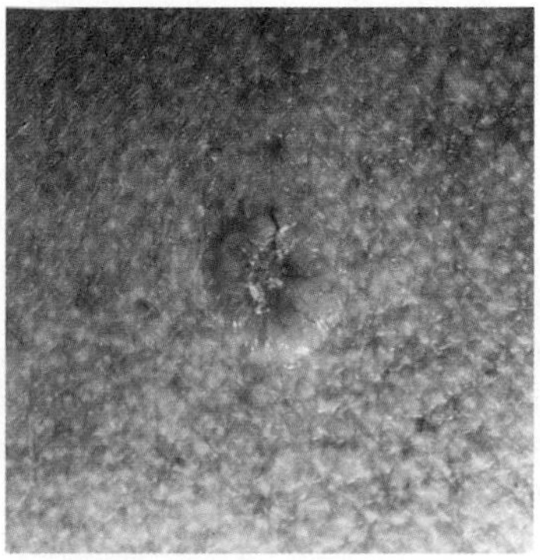
FIG. 25-13 Basal cell carcinoma.

predisposes to this malignancy. Chronic wounds that remain open for long periods are also at increased risk for malignant transformation to cancer.

Basal cell carcinomas arise from the basal cell layer of the epidermis (Fig. 25-13). Early lesions often go unnoticed, and although metastasis is rare, underlying tissue destruction can occur. Genetic predisposition and chronic irritation are risk factors; however, UV exposure is the most common cause.

Melanomas are pigmented cancers arising in the melanin-producing epidermal cells (Fig. 25-14). Most often they start as the benign growth of a **nevus** (mole) (Skin Cancer Foundation, 2014). Normal nevi have regular, well-defined borders and are uniform in color, ranging from light colors to dark brown. The lesion's surface may be rough or smooth. Nevi with irregular or spreading borders and those with multiple colors are abnormal. Other suspicious features include sudden changes in lesion size and reports of itching or bleeding.

Risk factors include genetic predisposition, excessive exposure to UV light, and the presence of one or more precursor

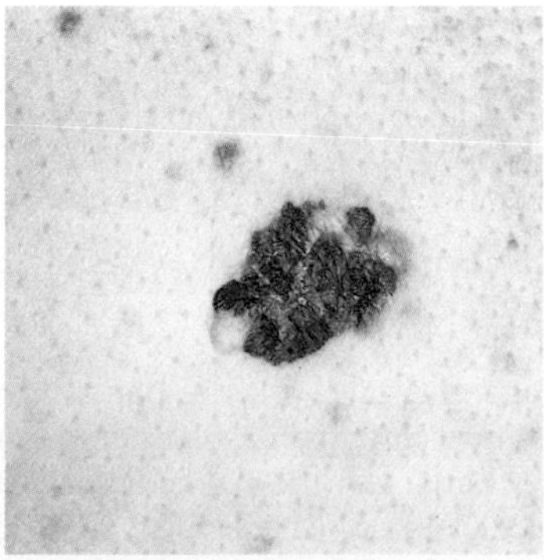
FIG. 25-14 Melanoma.

lesions that resemble unusual moles. *This skin cancer is highly metastatic, and a person's survival depends on early diagnosis and treatment.*

GENETIC/GENOMIC CONSIDERATIONS

Patient-Centered Care QSEN

Genetic mutations in the *CDKN2A* and *CDK4* have been identified for some cases of familial melanoma. These mutations in a suppressor gene result in loss of cellular regulation for cell growth. Other genetic considerations for melanoma are that some specific mutations in the genes of the actual tumor cells increase the response of these cells to targeted therapy. All melanomas should be tested for mutations of the *BRAF* and *KIT* genes (OMIM, 2014a). Always ask patients who have a diagnosed melanoma whether any other family members have ever had this disease.

Incidence and Prevalence

The incidence of skin cancer is highest among light-skinned races and people older than 60 years (American Cancer Society [ACS], 2014). Skin cancer occurs more often among those who work outdoors, live at higher altitudes or lower latitudes, or spend much time sunbathing. Occupational exposure to arsenic or other chemical carcinogens also increases risk. The incidence of melanoma has increased during the past 30 years, accounting for 4% to 5% of all cancers, although the death rate from melanoma is decreasing (ACS, 2014).

Health Promotion and Maintenance

The most effective prevention strategy for skin cancer is avoiding or reducing skin exposure to sunlight. However, even when people understand the cause of skin cancer and the seriousness of the disease, preventive behaviors are not always practiced. Common prevention practices are listed in Chart 25-11. *Teach all people to avoid tanning beds and salons.*

Secondary prevention (early detection) is critical to survival with melanoma. Teach all people to be aware of their skin markings. Keeping a total body spot and lesion map can provide baseline information about suspicious new lesions and help identify changes in existing lesions. Once a map is made, the person should systematically inspect his or her body monthly for new lesions and for changes in any existing lesions by performing thorough *skin self-examination (SSE)*. Some people find taking pictures of their skin on a regular basis makes identifying changes easier. Teach everyone to evaluate all skin lesions using the ABCDE guide for melanoma (see Chapter 24) and to consult his or her health care provider to examine any lesion having unusual features. When lesions, such as moles, are present, they should be monitored yearly by a dermatologist or other health care professional.

CHART 25-11 Patient and Family Education: Preparing for Self-Management

Prevention of Skin Cancer

- Avoid sun exposure between 11 AM and 3 PM.
- Use sunscreens with the appropriate skin protection factor for your skin type.
- Wear a hat, opaque clothing, and sunglasses when you are out in the sun.
- Keep a "body map" of your skin spots, scars, and lesions to detect when changes have occurred.
- Examine your body monthly for possibly cancerous or precancerous lesions.
- Seek medical advice if you note any of these:
  - A change in the color of a lesion, especially if it darkens or shows evidence of spreading
  - A change in the size of a lesion, especially rapid growth
  - A change in the shape of a lesion, such as a sharp border becoming irregular or a flat lesion becoming raised
  - Redness or swelling of the skin around a lesion
  - A change in sensation, especially itching or increased tenderness of a lesion
  - A change in the character of a lesion, such as oozing, crusting, bleeding, or scaling

❖ PATIENT-CENTERED COLLABORATIVE CARE

◆ Assessment

In addition to age and race, ask the patient about any family history of skin cancer and any past surgery for removal of skin growths. Recent changes in the size, color, or sensation of any mole, birthmark, wart, or scar are also significant. Ask about which geographic regions the patient has lived in and where he or she currently resides. Obtain information about occupational and recreational activities in relation to sun exposure, as well as any occupational history of exposure to chemical carcinogens (e.g., arsenic, coal tar, pitch, radioactive waste, radium). Ask whether any skin lesions are repeatedly irritated by the rubbing of clothing.

Skin that has been injured previously is at greater risk for cancer development, an effect known as *Koebner's phenomenon.* Ask the patient if he or she has ever experienced a severe skin injury that resulted in a scar. Examine all scarred skin areas for the presence of potentially cancerous lesions. A biopsy may be required to rule out cancer in a chronic open wound that fails to close with proper treatment.

Skin cancers vary in their appearance and distribution. Although most skin cancers appear in sun-exposed areas of the body, inspect the entire skin surface and any unusual lesions, particularly moles, warts, birthmarks, and scars. Also examine hair-bearing areas of the body, such as the scalp and genitalia. Palpate lesions to determine surface texture. Document the location, size, color, and features of all lesions and any reports of tenderness or itching. Use the ABCDE method of evaluating all lesions for possible melanoma (see Chapter 24).

◆ Interventions

Surgical and nonsurgical interventions are combined for the effective management of skin cancer. Treatment is determined by the size and severity of the malignancy, the location of the lesion, and the age and general health of the patient.

Surgical Management. Surgical intervention is needed to manage any type of skin cancer. It can range from local removal of small lesions to massive excision of large areas of the skin and underlying tissue for treatment of melanoma. Surgical types for skin cancer include:

- Cryosurgery—cell destruction by the local application of liquid nitrogen (−200° C) to isolated lesions, causing cell death and tissue destruction.
- Curettage and electrodesiccation—removal of cancerous cells with the use of a dermal curette to scrape away cancerous tissue, followed by the application of an electric probe to destroy remaining tumor tissue.

- Excisional biopsy—total surgical removal of small lesions for pathologic examination.
- Mohs' surgery—a specialized form of excision usually for basal and squamous cell carcinomas. Tissue is sectioned horizontally in layers, and each layer is examined histologically to determine the presence of residual tumor cells.
- Wide excision—deep skin resection often involving removal of full-thickness skin in the area of the lesion. Depending on tumor depth, subcutaneous tissues and lymph nodes may also be removed.

Nonsurgical Management. *Drug therapy* may involve topical or systemic chemotherapy, biotherapy, or targeted therapy. Topical chemotherapy with 5-fluorouracil cream is used for treatment of multiple actinic keratoses or for widespread superficial basal cell carcinoma that would require several surgical procedures to eradicate. Therapy is continued for several weeks, and the treated areas become increasingly tender and inflamed as the lesions crust, ooze, and erode. Prepare the patient for an unsightly appearance during therapy, and reassure him or her that the cosmetic result will be positive.

Systemic chemotherapeutic agents are used in the treatment of locally advanced or metastatic squamous cell skin cancer. These include a platinum based-agent (Cisplatin or Carboplatin), 5-fluorouracil, and cetuximab (Erbitux). A new drug approved for locally advanced or metastatic basal cell skin cancer is vismodegib (Erivedge).

Biotherapy with interferon, monoclonal antibodies, and targeted therapy are now accepted treatment for melanoma after surgical removal. Interferon is used for melanomas that are at stage III or higher. The patient is first started on high-dose IV interferon infusions daily for 5 days per week for 4 weeks. Maintenance doses, given subcutaneously, are then continued 3 times per week for 1 year. The patient must learn to self-inject the drug.

Monoclonal antibody therapy with ipilimumab (Yervoy), a drug that targets the *CTLA4* (cytotoxic T-lymphocyte associated antigen 4) receptor and blocks it, leads to greater T-cell lymphocyte activity. (T-cells are a type of lymphocyte that can stimulate antitumor immune responses.) The side effects of this drug include significant INFLAMMATION in many tissues, including the pituitary gland, liver, skin, GI tract, and nervous system. Some of the side effects can be life threatening (Rubin, 2012).

Targeted therapy is available for melanomas with specific mutations in the *BRAF* gene. Normally, the *BRAF* gene is involved in CELLULAR REGULATION of growth. Mutations in this gene allow melanoma to grow and metastasize. When melanoma cells are positive for a specific *BRAF* mutation *(V600E)*, the cells respond to the drug *vemurafenib* (Zelboraf). The drug inhibits an enzyme important in signaling cell division and prevents melanoma cell division. This oral drug interacts with a variety of other drugs, and allergic reactions are common.

Radiation therapy for skin cancer is limited to older patients with large, deeply invasive basal cell tumors and to those who are poor risks for surgery. Melanoma is relatively resistant to radiation therapy.

OTHER SKIN DISORDERS

Toxic Epidermal Necrolysis

Toxic epidermal necrolysis (TEN) is a rare acute drug reaction of the skin resulting in diffuse erythema and large blister formation. Mucous membranes are often involved, and systemic toxicity is evident. The most common causative drugs are chemotherapy agents, sulfonamides, pyrazolones, barbiturates, and antibiotics. Removal of the drug is usually followed by gradual healing in 2 to 3 weeks, with widespread peeling of the epidermis.

This problem can occur at any age and as a result of almost any drug therapy. However, older patients with cancer who are receiving chemotherapy, some targeted therapies, and immunotherapy are at greatest risk. Other precipitating factors include stem cell transplantation and neutropenia-induced INFECTIONS.

The drug thought to be causing a toxic reaction is discontinued, and management focuses on systemic support and prevention of secondary INFECTION. Patients are often admitted to burn units, where fluid and electrolyte balance, caloric intake, and hypothermia can be closely monitored. Topical antibacterial drugs are used to suppress bacterial growth until healing occurs.

NCLEX EXAMINATION CHALLENGE

Psychosocial Integrity

The client who has stage III metastatic melanoma and whose tumor is negative for a *BRAF* mutation asks why the treatment plan does not include the new drug *Zelboraf* (vemurafenib) that she has read about. What is the nurse's best response?

A. "Your immune system is too weak to tolerate Zelboraf."
B. "This drug is experimental and too dangerous for you to take before trying other therapies."
C. "Your melanoma does not have the gene mutation that responds to this drug, so you would not benefit from this therapy."
D. "You are young and can better tolerate the standard therapies for melanoma that have been proven effective but have strong side effects."

Stevens-Johnson Syndrome

Stevens-Johnson syndrome is often a drug-induced skin reaction caused by an immunologic mechanism, similar to toxic epidermal necrolysis. The disorder may be mild with only skin involvement, or it may be severe and systemic. The skin lesions are widely distributed, including mucous membranes, and varied in appearance (Fig. 25-15). The patient has a mix of

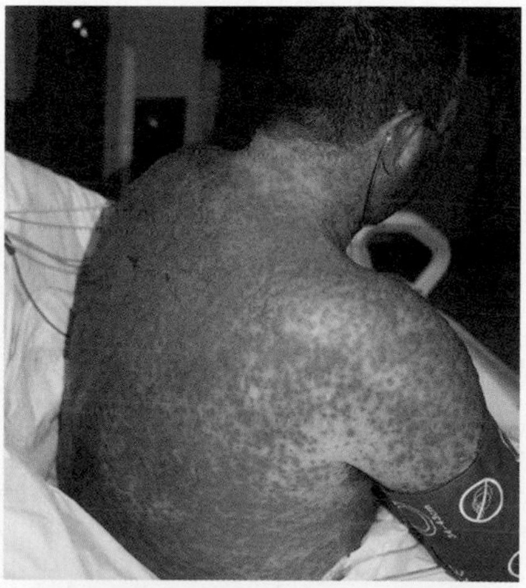

FIG. 25-15 Stevens-Johnson syndrome.

vesicles, erosions, and crusts. With severe involvement, the patient may have respiratory problems, excessive fluid loss, kidney failure, and blindness (Cooper, 2012).

Removal of the offending drug is critical. Mild forms of the disorder are usually self-limiting in 10 to 14 days unless the episode was triggered by a bacterial INFECTION. Then, antibiotics are needed. Severe problems require high doses of steroids to suppress the INFLAMMATION. Supportive care may include fluid replacement, mechanical ventilation, and even renal replacement therapy.

PLASTIC SURGERY

◆ Assessment

The two main types of plastic surgery are aesthetic and reconstructive. **Aesthetic plastic surgery** is cosmetic, with the aim of altering a person's physical appearance. This intervention is sought by those who are unsatisfied with their body image. These procedures are considered elective surgery and are not covered by insurance. **Reconstructive plastic surgery** is the correction or improvement of functional defects that have occurred

TABLE 25-6 Common Plastic Surgery Procedures

DESCRIPTION	INDICATIONS	COMPLICATIONS
Blepharoplasty		
Excision of bulging fat and redundant skin of the periorbital area with primary closure	Bags under the eyes	Hematoma Ectropion Corneal injury Visual loss (rare) Wound infection (rare)
Breast Augmentation (Augmentation Mammoplasty)		
Insertion of synthetic breast-shaped implants through a skin incision	Inadequate breast volume or contour	Hematoma or hemorrhage Wound infection (with gram-positive organisms) Phlebitis
Breast Reduction (Reduction Mammoplasty)		
Excision of excessive breast tissue and skin with primary closure	Hypertrophy of breast tissue caused by elevated hormone levels, endocrine abnormalities, or obesity Weight of large breasts can contribute to back pain	Hematoma or hemorrhage Nipple, areola, and skin flap necrosis Wound infection Fat necrosis Wound dehiscence
Dermabrasion		
Abrasive removal of the facial epidermis and portion of the dermis followed by healing by second intention	Moderate to severe acne scar Deep wrinkling Multiple actinic keratoses Hyperpigmentation (postinflammatory or after the use of estrogens)	Hypertrophic scarring Altered skin pigmentation Acne flare Wound infection (rare)
Rhinoplasty		
Removal of excessive cartilage and tissue from the nose with correction of septal defects if indicated	Disproportionate anatomy Post-traumatic nasal deformity Difficulty breathing through the nose	Hematoma or hemorrhage Ecchymosis and edema (temporary) Wound infection (with gram-positive organisms) Septal perforation Minor skin irritation
Rhytidectomy (Facelift)		
Removal of excess skin and tissue from the face at the level of the hairline followed by primary closure	Excessive wrinkling or sagging of facial skin	Hematoma or hemorrhage Facial nerve damage (temporary or permanent) Wound infection Ecchymosis and edema (temporary) Skin necrosis Hair loss
Liposuction (Suction Lipectomy)		
Removal of subcutaneous fat from localized areas of accumulation such as the hips, abdomen, neck, and arms	Disproportionate distribution of adipose tissue	Hematoma Severe pain Infection Emboli Sagging of skin (if skin is not elastic enough to contract after fat removal)

as a result of congenital problems or trauma and scarring (e.g., skin and joint contractures from burn wounds) or from other types of therapy (e.g., mastectomy for breast cancer therapy). These interventions are sought by patients who cannot perform ADLs as a result of an anatomic problem; the cost is often covered by insurance.

Regardless of whether a person is having reconstructive surgery or cosmetic surgery, body image and sense of self are always involved. These feelings may evoke emotional responses in the person, including shame, anger, resentment, and desperation. Use a sensitive, nonjudgmental approach when interacting with the person having or considering plastic surgery. It is important to avoid being directive or expressing your own opinions. Often a patient who asks the nurse "Do you think I need this surgery?" is not comfortable with his or her decision.

Address the patient's expectations of plastic surgery. Often people who seek plastic surgery have unrealistic expectations. The patient with minor deformities who is seeking perfection is sure to be disappointed. The patient who wants a procedure mainly to please a partner is also a poor candidate.

◆ *Interventions*

Many techniques to improve skin and general appearance without surgery are available. Superficial techniques for skin enhancement include chemical peels, laser resurfacing, and dermabrasion to remove or reduce small scars, fine lines, and other irregular skin surfaces. Dermal filling involves injecting substances to change the contour of a feature or an area. Generally, these fillers replace the collagen lost from the skin through aging. Injection with nerve paralyzing agents (e.g., Botulinum Toxin Type A) can improve appearance temporarily by relaxing muscles beneath the skin surface, which smoothes out some wrinkles and grooves.

Depending on the planned intervention, surgery is performed either in the ambulatory care setting with the patient under local anesthesia or in the hospital. The types and complications of common cosmetic procedures are listed in Table 25-6.

All plastic and reconstructive surgeries have a risk for complications and failure, especially bleeding, infection, and skin reattachment problems. Procedures vary depending on the location, purpose, and extent of reconstruction.

General care after surgery focuses on monitoring for typical postoperative complications (see Chapter 16). Pressure dressings may be applied at the time of surgery and left in place for several days to control hemorrhage and edema formation. Monitor dressings for bright red bleeding, and monitor changes in vital signs and level of consciousness. Positioning varies with the specific procedure performed and the surgeon's preference.

Monitor for wound INFECTION and progress toward healing. Of particular concern are any areas of skin necrosis or eschar formation near the operative site—a complication from excessive tension on the suture line as a result of edema and blood vessel obstruction. See Chart 25-5 for a listing of wound monitoring criteria. Regardless of the planned procedure, inform the patient to expect edema and discoloration of the operative site. Swelling and bruising alter the facial features and may not resolve for several weeks after surgery. The final results of surgery will not be visible until healing is complete—usually 6 months to a year or longer after surgery.

NURSING CONCEPTS AND CLINICAL JUDGMENT REVIEW

What might you NOTICE if the patient is experiencing inadequate protection as a result of loss of skin TISSUE INTEGRITY?

- Open skin areas
- Possible presence of drainage
- Sensation changes in or around the area (patient reports pain, itching, or tightness)

What should you INTERPRET and how should you RESPOND to a patient experiencing inadequate protection as a result of loss of skin TISSUE INTEGRITY?

Perform and interpret physical assessment, including:

- Assessing the wound for pain, size, depth, drainage, and presence of infection
- Assessing the skin immediately surrounding the wound for redness and swelling
- Monitoring oxygen saturation by pulse oximetry in the affected extremity (if the open area is on an extremity)
- Assessing the patient for risk factors for wound development (pressure, shear, immobility, reduced cognition, poor nutrition, advanced age, incontinence)
- Assessing the rest of the patient's skin (especially over bony prominences, between skinfolds, in the perineal area)

Respond by:

- Documenting wound features
- Cleansing the wound (obtaining cultures, if within agency policy)
- Dressing the wound if drainage is present
- Planning a turning or repositioning schedule
- Teaching UAP or family how to relieve/reduce pressure
- Collaborating with the certified wound care specialist and dietitian

On what should you REFLECT?

- Observe the patient for evidence of restored skin integrity (see Chapter 24).
- Think about what may have precipitated this loss of skin tissue integrity and what steps could be taken to either prevent a similar problem or identify it earlier.
- Think about what additional resources could improve the nursing response to this situation.

GET READY FOR THE NCLEX® EXAMINATION!

KEY POINTS

Review these Key Points for each NCLEX Examination Client Needs Category.

Safe and Effective Care Environment

- Wash your hands before and after touching any skin lesions. **Safety** QSEN
- Use Standard Precautions when providing care to a patient who has any areas of nonintact skin. **Safety** QSEN
- Ensure that the skin of incontinent patients is kept clean and dry. **Evidence-Based Practice** QSEN
- Assist all patients with limited mobility to change positions at least every 2 hours while awake. **Evidence-Based Practice** QSEN
- Use a structured approach (e.g., Braden scale or other validated tool) to evaluate the pressure ulcer risk for all patients on admission and regularly thereafter. **Evidence-Based Practice** QSEN
- Be proactive in the use of pressure-relieving devices for any patient who is identified to be at risk for pressure ulcer formation (i.e., requires prolonged bedrest, is an older adult, has some degree of immobility, is incontinent, has some degree of malnutrition, is dehydrated, has decreased sensory perception, or has an altered mental state).
- Use a lift sheet or mechanical lift to move immobilized older patients rather than pulling or dragging them across bed linens. **Safety** QSEN

Health Promotion and Maintenance

- Teach the patient with mobility problems and his or her caregivers how to reduce and relieve skin pressure in the home environment. **Patient-Centered Care** QSEN
- Encourage all patients to reduce sun exposure and exposure to ultraviolet (UV) light. **Patient-Centered Care** QSEN
- Teach patients how to examine all skin areas on a monthly basis for new lesions and changes to existing lesions. They should keep a record or "body map" of skin lesions. **Patient-Centered Care** QSEN
- Teach patients who have skin scarring from a previous skin injury to examine this area at least monthly for changes related to cancer development or chronic skin conditions. **Patient-Centered Care** QSEN
- Urge all patients to bathe, shampoo the hair, and keep fingernails clean and trimmed on a regular basis.
- Teach patients with infected skin lesions or infestations how to limit transmission to others in the home or community.
- Teach all patients the ABCDE method of evaluating a lesion for melanoma. **Patient-Centered Care** QSEN
- Assess the ability of the patient with a skin problem to see and reach the affected area and care for the problem. **Patient-Centered Care** QSEN

Psychosocial Integrity

- Assess the patient's and family's feelings about a chronic skin condition or visible scar. **Patient-Centered Care** QSEN
- Support the patient and family in coping with changes in skin integrity and in body image. **Patient-Centered Care** QSEN
- Encourage the patient with a visible wound or other skin problem to participate in the care of the wound.
- Assess and manage the patient's pain. **Patient-Centered Care** QSEN
- Allow the patient the opportunity to express feelings about a change in body image as a result of changes in the skin, hair, or nails. **Patient-Centered Care** QSEN
- Explain all procedures, restrictions, drugs, and follow-up care to the patient and family.
- Touch the patient who has skin problems to show acceptance. **Patient-Centered Care** QSEN

Physiological Integrity

- Keep skin well hydrated to promote TISSUE INTEGRITY. **Evidence-Based Practice** QSEN
- Use appropriate risk assessment tools to perform a focused skin assessment and re-assessment to determine risk for pressure ulcer development and adequacy of the skin's protective functions. **Safety** QSEN
- Keep skinfold areas clean and dry. **Evidence-Based Practice** QSEN
- Ask any patient who has started taking a newly prescribed drug if he or she has noticed whether any skin changes have occurred since starting the drug. **Patient-Centered Care** QSEN
- Avoid massaging or vigorously rubbing any area of the skin that is reddened or has been subjected to pressure. **Evidence-Based Practice** QSEN
- Encourage patients with itching to avoid scratching the skin.
- Teach patients to avoid using over-the-counter cortisone preparations on skin lesions until the cause has been identified. **Patient-Centered Care** QSEN
- Teach patients who have a skin infection how to avoid spreading the infection to other parts of their own bodies and to other people. **Safety** QSEN
- Evaluate any open skin area on a patient daily for size, depth, exudate, presence of infection, and indicators of healing. **Patient-Centered Care** QSEN
- Differentiate the manifestations for these pressure ulcer categories: stage I through stage IV, unstageable ulcers, and suspected deep tissue injury. **Evidence-Based Practice** QSEN
- Evaluate wounds for size, depth, presence of infection, and indications of healing. **Patient-Centered Care** QSEN
- Supervise skin care delegated to licensed practical nurses/licensed vocational nurses (LPNs/LVNs) or unlicensed assistive personnel (UAP). **Safety** QSEN
- Urge patients with chronic skin problems, especially those that alter appearance, to become involved in a community support group.

Care of Patients with Burns

Tammy Coffee

http://evolve.elsevier.com/Iggy/

PRIORITY CONCEPTS

- Tissue Integrity
- Infection
- Pain
- Fluid and Electrolyte Balance
- Perfusion
- Nutrition
- Mobility

LEARNING OUTCOMES

Safe and Effective Care Environment

1. Apply the principles of infection prevention to protect burn patients with open wounds.

Health Promotion and Maintenance

2. Teach everyone fire prevention strategies.

Psychosocial Integrity

3. Reduce the psychosocial impact of burn injury for the patient and family.

Physiological Integrity

4. Ensure optimal pain control for the patient with a burn injury.
5. Work with all members of the health care team to help the patient and family experiencing a burn injury achieve desired health outcomes.
6. Prioritize nursing care for the patient during the resuscitation phase of burn injury.
7. Prioritize nursing care for the patient during the acute phase of burn injury.
8. Coordinate care for the patient during the rehabilitation phase of burn injury.

Burns are complex injuries with loss of tissue integrity that cause patients to develop many physiologic, metabolic, and psychological changes. These injuries can range from a "sunburn" to major injuries involving all layers of the skin. When the skin is injured, the function of many body systems is changed. The burn patient needs comprehensive care for weeks to months to survive the injury, reduce complications, and return to his or her best functional status. For best care and patient outcomes, nurses coordinate the activities of an interdisciplinary team of health care providers.

PATHOPHYSIOLOGY OF BURN INJURY

The tissue destruction caused by a burn injury leads to local and systemic problems that affect fluid and electrolyte balance and lead to protein losses, sepsis, and changes in metabolic, endocrine, respiratory, cardiac, hematologic, and immune functioning. The extent of problems is related to age, general health, extent of injury, depth of injury, and the specific body area injured. Even after healing, the burn injury may cause late complications such as contracture formation and scarring. Thus care priorities are the prevention of infection and closure of the burn wound. A lack of or delay in wound healing is a key factor for all systemic problems and a major cause of disability and death among patients who are burned.

Skin Changes Resulting from Burn Injury

Anatomic Changes

The skin is the largest organ of the body (see Chapter 24). Each of its two major layers, the epidermis and the dermis, has several sublayers. The epidermis is the outer layer of skin. It can grow back after a burn injury because the epidermal cells surrounding sweat and oil glands and hair follicles extend into dermal tissue and regrow to heal partial-thickness wounds. Together, the sweat and oil glands and the hair follicles are the *dermal appendages,* which vary in depth in different body areas. The sweat and oil glands in the palm of the hand and the sole of the foot, for example, extend deep into the dermis. This allows for healing of deep burns in these areas. The epidermis has no blood vessels, and nutrients must diffuse from the second layer of skin, the dermis.

TABLE 26-1 **Classification of Burn Depth**

CHARACTERISTIC	SUPERFICIAL	SUPERFICIAL PARTIAL-THICKNESS	DEEP PARTIAL-THICKNESS	FULL-THICKNESS	DEEP FULL-THICKNESS
Color	Pink to red	Pink to red	Red to white	Black, brown, yellow, white, red	Black
Edema	Mild	Mild to moderate	Moderate	Severe	Absent
Pain	Yes	Yes	Yes	Yes and no	Absent
Blisters	No	Yes	Rare	No	No
Eschar	No	No	Yes, soft and dry	Yes, hard and inelastic	Yes, hard and inelastic
Healing time	3-6 days	About 2 wk	2-6 wk	Weeks to months	Weeks to months
Grafts required	No	No	Can be used if healing is prolonged	Yes	Yes
Example	Sunburn, flash burns	Scalds, flames, brief contact with hot objects	Scalds; flames; prolonged contact with hot objects, tar, grease, chemicals	Scalds; flames; prolonged contact with hot objects, tar, grease, chemicals, electricity	Flames, electricity, grease, tar, chemicals

The dermis is thicker than the epidermis and is made up of collagen, fibrous connective tissue, and elastic fibers. Within the dermis are the blood vessels, sensory nerves, hair follicles, lymph vessels, sebaceous glands, and sweat glands.

When burn injury occurs, skin can regrow as long as parts of the dermis are present. When the entire dermal layer is burned, all cells and dermal appendages are destroyed and the skin can no longer restore itself. The subcutaneous tissue lies below the dermis and is separated from the dermis by the basement membrane, a thin, noncellular protein surface. With deep burns, the subcutaneous tissues may be damaged, leaving bones, tendons, and muscles exposed.

Functional Changes

The skin has many functions when TISSUE INTEGRITY is intact (see Table 24-1 in Chapter 24). It is a protective barrier against injury and microbial invasion. Burns break this barrier, greatly increasing the risk for INFECTION.

The skin helps maintain the delicate FLUID AND ELECTROLYTE BALANCE essential for life. After a burn injury, massive FLUID loss occurs through excessive evaporation. The rate of evaporation is in proportion to the total body surface area (TBSA) burned and the depth of injury.

The skin is an excretory organ through sweating. Full-thickness burns destroy the sweat glands, reducing excretory ability.

The sensations of PAIN, pressure, temperature, and touch are triggered on the skin in normal daily activities, which allows a person to react to changes in the environment. *All burn injuries are painful.* With partial-thickness burns, nerve endings are exposed, increasing sensitivity and PAIN. With full-thickness burns, nerve endings are completely destroyed. At first, these wounds may not transmit sensation except at wound edges. Despite this destruction, patients often have dull or pressure-type of pain in these areas.

Skin exposed to sunlight activates vitamin D. Partial-thickness burns reduce the activation of vitamin D, and this function is lost completely in areas of full-thickness burns.

The internal body temperature remains within a narrow range (about 84.2° to 109.4°F [29° to 43°C]) compared with the temperatures of the external environment. Skin TISSUE INTEGRITY is important in maintaining normal body temperature. Circulating blood in the skin both provides and dissipates heat efficiently. When heat is applied to the skin, the temperature under the dermis rises rapidly. As soon as the heat source is removed, compensatory processes quickly return the area to a normal temperature. If the heat source is not removed or if it is applied at a rate that exceeds the skin's capacity to dissipate it, cells are destroyed.

Physical identity is partly determined by the skin's cosmetic quality, which contributes to each person's unique appearance. A patient who sustains a major burn often develops reduced self-image and other psychosocial problems as a result of a change in appearance.

Depth of Burn Injury

The severity of a burn is determined by how much of the body surface area is involved and the depth of the burn. The degree of TISSUE INTEGRITY loss is related to the agent causing the burn and to the temperature of the heat source, as well as to how long the skin is exposed to it.

Differences in skin thickness in various parts of the body also affect burn depth. In areas where the skin is thin (e.g., eyelids, ears, nose, genitalia, tops of the hands and feet, fingers, and toes), a short exposure to high temperatures causes a deep burn injury. The skin is thinner in older adults (Touhy & Jett, 2014), which increases their risk for greater burn severity, even at lower temperatures of shorter duration.

Burn wounds are classified as superficial-thickness wounds, partial-thickness wounds, full-thickness wounds, and deep full-thickness wounds. The partial-thickness wounds are further divided into superficial and deep subgroups. Table 26-1 lists the differences of these burns.

Burns also are described as minor, moderate, or major depending on the depth, extent, and location of injury (Table 26-2). Fig. 26-1 shows the tissue layers involved with different depths of injury.

TABLE 26-2 **Classification of Burn Injury and Burn Center Referral Criteria**

CHARACTERISTICS	COMMENTS
Minor Burns	
Partial-thickness burns less than 10% TBSA Full-thickness burns less than 2% TBSA No burns of eyes, ears, face, hands, feet, or perineum No electrical burns No inhalation injury No complicated additional injury Patient is younger than 60 years and has no chronic cardiac, pulmonary, or endocrine disorder	Patients in this category should receive emergency care at the scene and be taken to a hospital emergency department. A special expertise hospital or designated burn center is usually not necessary.
Moderate Burns	
Partial-thickness burns 15%-25% TBSA Full-thickness burns 2%-10% TBSA No burns of eyes, ears, face, hands, feet, or perineum No electrical burns No inhalation injury No complicated additional injury Patient is younger than 60 years and has no chronic cardiac, pulmonary, or endocrine disorder	Patients in this category should receive emergency care at the scene and be transferred either to a special expertise hospital or to a designated burn center.
Major Burns	
Partial-thickness burns greater than 25% TBSA Full-thickness burns greater than 10% TBSA Any burn involving the eyes, ears, face, hands, feet, perineum Electrical injury Inhalation injury Patient is older than 60 years Burn complicated with other injuries (e.g., fractures) Patient has cardiac, pulmonary, or other chronic metabolic disorders	Patients who meet *any one* of the criteria for a major burn should receive emergency care at the nearest emergency department and then be transferred to a designated burn center as soon as possible.

TBSA, Total body surface area.

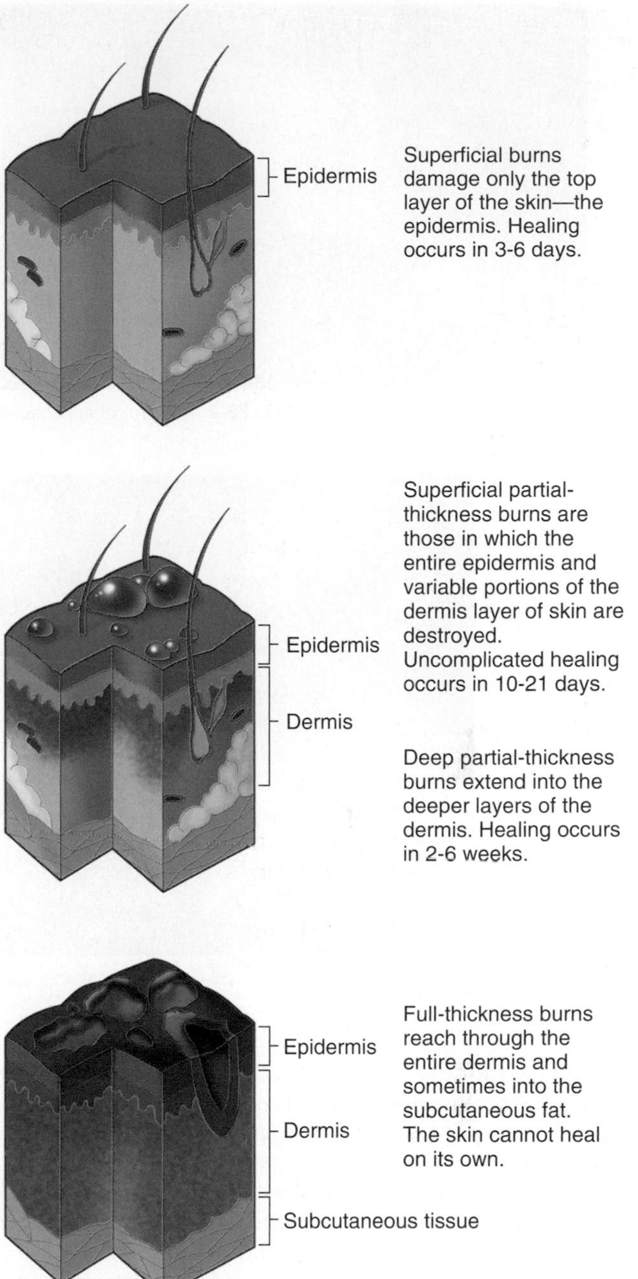

FIG. 26-1 The tissues involved in burns of various depths.

Superficial-Thickness Wounds. Superficial-thickness wounds have the least damage because the epidermis is the only part of the skin that is injured. The epithelial cells and basement membrane, needed for total regrowth, remain present.

These wounds are caused by prolonged exposure to low-intensity heat (e.g., sunburn) or short (flash) exposure to high-intensity heat. Redness with mild edema, PAIN, and increased sensitivity to heat occurs as a result. **Desquamation** (peeling of dead skin) occurs 2 to 3 days after the burn. The area heals rapidly in 3 to 6 days without a scar or other complication.

Partial-Thickness Wounds. A partial-thickness wound involves TISSUE INTEGRITY loss of the entire epidermis and varying depths of the dermis. Depending on the amount of dermal tissue damaged, partial-thickness wounds are further subdivided into superficial partial-thickness and deep partial-thickness injuries.

Superficial partial-thickness wounds are caused by injury to the upper third of the dermis, leaving a good blood supply. These wounds are pink and moist and **blanch** (lighten) when pressure is applied (Fig. 26-2). The small vessels bringing blood to this area are injured, resulting in the leakage of large amounts of plasma, which in turn lifts the heat-destroyed epidermis, causing blister formation. The blisters continue to increase in size after the burn as cell and protein breakdown occur. Small blisters are often left intact if they are not located over a joint. Large blisters usually are opened and débrided to promote healing.

Superficial partial-thickness wounds increase PAIN sensation. Nerve endings are exposed, and any stimulation (touch or temperature change) causes intense pain. With standard care, these burns heal in 10 to 21 days with no scar, but some minor pigment changes may occur.

Deep partial-thickness wounds extend deeper into the skin dermis, and fewer healthy cells remain. Blisters usually do not

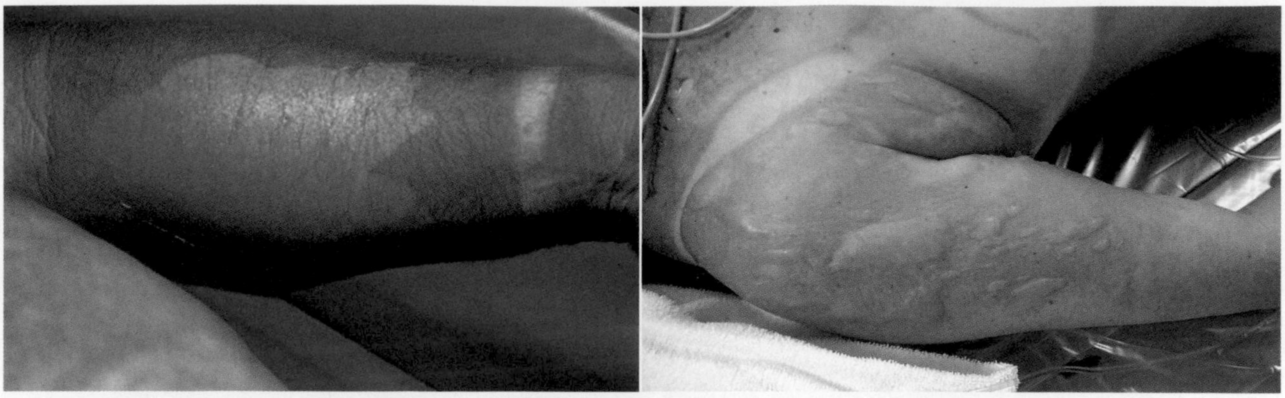

FIG. 26-2 The typical appearance of a superficial partial-thickness burn injury.

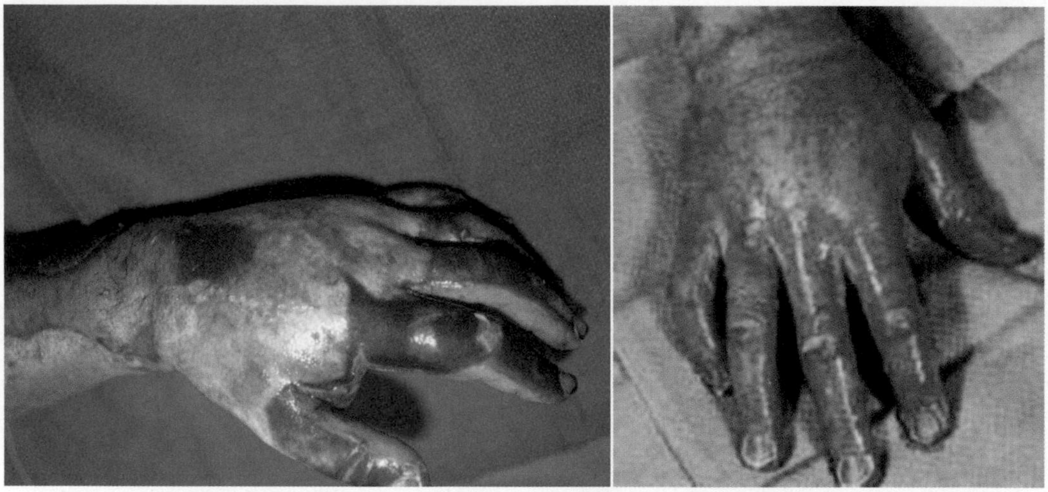

FIG. 26-3 The typical appearance of a deep partial-thickness burn injury.

form because the dead tissue layer is thick, sticks to the underlying dermis, and does not readily lift off the surface. The wound surface is red and dry with white areas in deeper parts (dry because fewer blood vessels are patent). When pressure is applied to the burn, it blanches slowly or not at all (Fig. 26-3). Edema is moderate, and PAIN is less than with superficial burns because more of the nerve endings have been destroyed.

Blood flow to these areas is reduced, and progression to deeper injury can occur from hypoxia and ischemia. Adequate hydration, nutrients, and oxygen are needed for regrowth of skin cells and prevention of conversion to deeper burns. These wounds can convert to full-thickness wounds when tissue damage increases with INFECTION, hypoxia, or ischemia. Deep partial-thickness wounds generally heal in 2 to 6 weeks, but scar formation results. Surgical intervention with skin grafting can reduce healing time.

Full-Thickness Wounds. A full-thickness wound occurs with destruction of the entire epidermis and dermis, leaving no skin cells to repopulate (Fig. 26-4). This wound does not regrow, and areas not closed by wound contraction (see Chapter 25) require grafting.

The full-thickness burn has a hard, dry, leathery *eschar* that forms from coagulated particles of destroyed skin. *The eschar is dead tissue; it must slough off or be removed from the wound before healing can occur.* These thick particles often stick to the lower tissue layers, making eschar removal difficult. Edema is severe under the eschar in a full-thickness wound. When the injury is **circumferential** (completely surrounds an extremity or the chest), blood flow and chest movement for breathing may be reduced by tight eschar. **Escharotomies** (incisions through the eschar) or **fasciotomies** (incisions through eschar and fascia) may be needed to relieve pressure and allow normal blood flow and breathing. (See p. 478 of the Surgical Management discussion in the Preventing Hypovolemic Shock and Inadequate Oxygenation section.)

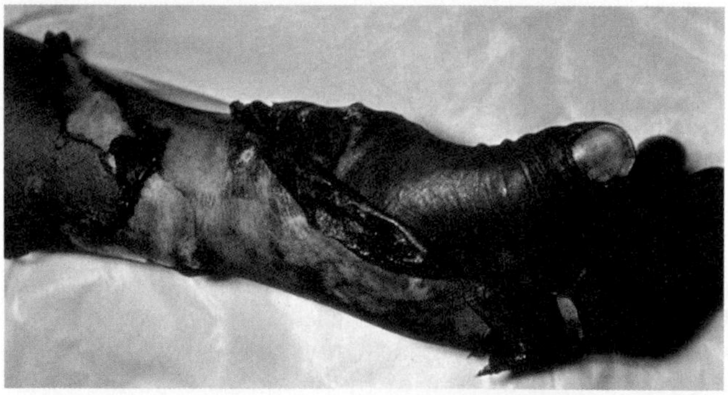

FIG. 26-4 The typical appearance of a full-thickness burn injury.

A full-thickness burn may be waxy white, deep red, yellow, brown, or black. Thrombosed and heat-coagulated blood vessels may be seen beneath the surface of the burn and leave the burned tissue without a blood supply. Sensation is reduced or absent because of nerve ending destruction. Healing time depends on establishing a good blood supply in the injured areas. This process can range from weeks to months.

Deep Full-Thickness Wounds. Deep full-thickness wounds extend beyond the skin and damage muscle, bone, and tendons. These burns occur with flame, electrical, or chemical injuries. The wound is blackened and depressed, and sensation is completely absent (Fig. 26-5). All full-thickness burns need early excision and grafting. Grafting decreases PAIN and length of stay and hastens recovery. Amputation may be needed when an extremity is involved.

Vascular Changes Resulting from Burn Injuries

Circulation to the burned skin is disrupted immediately after injury by blood vessel occlusion. Macrophages in damaged tissues release chemicals that at first cause blood vessel constriction. Blood vessel thrombosis may occur, causing necrosis, which can lead to deeper injuries in these areas.

Fluid shift occurs after initial vasoconstriction as a result of blood vessels near the burn dilating and leaking FLUIDS into the interstitial space (Fig. 26-6). This fluid shift, also known as *third spacing* or *capillary leak syndrome,* is a continuous leak of plasma from the vascular space into the interstitial space. The impaired FLUID AND ELECTROLYTE BALANCE leads to loss of plasma fluids and proteins, which decreases blood volume and blood pressure (McCance et al., 2014). Leakage of fluid and electrolytes from the vascular space continues, causing extensive edema, even in areas that were not burned. Fluid shift, with excessive weight gain, occurs in the first 12 hours after the burn and can continue for 24 to 36 hours.

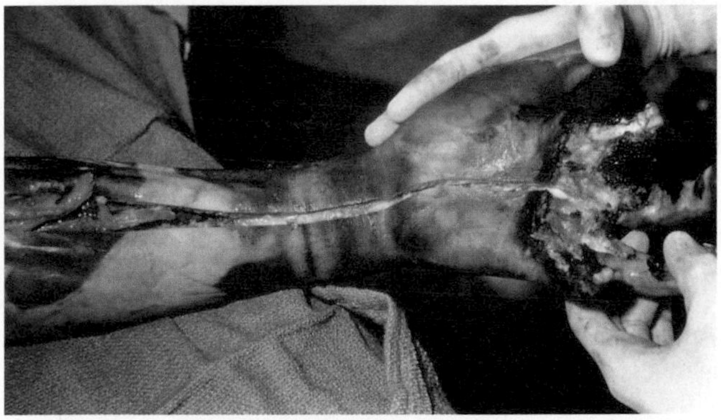

FIG. 26-5 The typical appearance of a deep full-thickness burn injury.

The amount of fluid shifted depends on the extent and severity of injury. Capillary leak occurs in both burned and unburned areas when tissue damage is extensive (i.e., more than 25% total body surface area [TBSA]). Edema develops as plasma and ELECTROLYTES escape into the interstitial space. The proteins now in the interstitial space increase the movement of *fluids* out from the vascular space.

Profound disruptions of FLUID AND ELECTROLYTE BALANCE and acid-base balance occur as a result of the fluid shift and cell damage. These imbalances often include hypovolemia, metabolic acidosis, **hyperkalemia** (high blood potassium level), and **hyponatremia** (low blood sodium level). Hyperkalemia occurs as a result of direct cell injury that releases large amounts of cellular potassium. Sodium is retained by the body as a result of the endocrine response to stress. Aldosterone secretion increases, leading to increased sodium reabsorption by the kidney. This sodium, however, quickly passes into the interstitial spaces of the burned area with the fluid shift. Thus, despite the increased amount of sodium in the body, most of the sodium is trapped in the interstitial space and a sodium deficit occurs in the blood. **Hemoconcentration** (elevated blood osmolarity, hematocrit, and hemoglobin) develops from vascular dehydration. This problem increases blood viscosity, reducing blood flow and increasing tissue hypoxia.

Fluid remobilization starts at about 24 hours after injury, when the capillary leak stops. The diuretic stage begins at about 48 to 72 hours after the burn injury as capillary membrane integrity returns and edema fluid shifts from the interstitial spaces into the intravascular space. Blood volume increases, leading to increased kidney blood flow and diuresis unless kidney damage has occurred. Body weight returns to normal over the next few days as edema subsides.

During this phase, hyponatremia develops because of increased kidney sodium excretion and the loss of sodium from wounds. **Hypokalemia** (low blood potassium level) results from potassium moving back into the cells and also being excreted in urine. Anemia often develops as a result of hemodilution, but it is generally not severe enough to require blood transfusions. Transfusions are needed only if the patient's hematocrit is less than 20% to 25% and the patient has manifestations of hypoxia. Protein continues to be lost from the wounds. Metabolic acidosis is possible because of the loss of bicarbonate in the urine and the increased rate of metabolism.

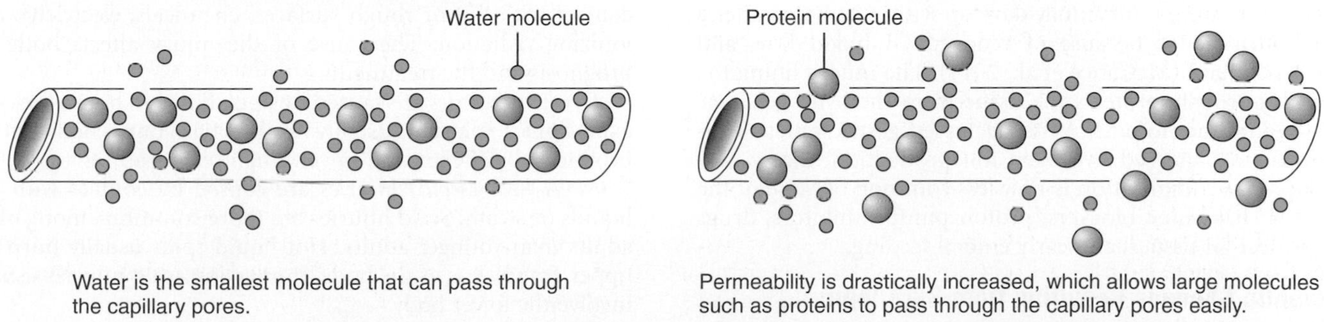

FIG. 26-6 The capillary response to burn injury (early phase). This response is also known as *capillary leak syndrome.*

Cardiac Changes Resulting from Burn Injury

Heart rate increases and cardiac output decreases because of the initial fluid shifts and hypovolemia that occur after a burn injury. Cardiac output may remain low until 18 to 36 hours after the burn injury. Cardiac output improves with fluid resuscitation and reaches normal levels before plasma volume is restored completely. Proper fluid resuscitation and support with oxygen prevent further complications.

Pulmonary Changes Resulting from Burn Injury

Direct injury to the lung from contact with flames rarely occurs. Rather, respiratory problems are caused by superheated air, steam, toxic fumes, or smoke. *Such problems are a major cause of death in patients with burns and are most likely to occur when the burn takes place indoors.* Respiratory failure with burn injuries can result from airway edema during fluid resuscitation, pulmonary capillary leak, chest burns that restrict chest movement, and carbon monoxide poisoning.

Respiratory damage from an inhalation injury can occur in the upper and major airways and the lung tissue. The upper airway is affected when inhaled smoke or irritants cause edema and obstruct the trachea. Heat can reach the upper airway, causing an inflammatory response that leads to edema of the mouth and throat with the potential of airway obstruction.

Chemicals and toxic gases produced during combustion can cause airway injury. The ciliated membranes lining the trachea normally trap foreign materials. Smoke and gases slow this activity, allowing particles to enter the bronchi. The lining of the trachea and bronchi may slough 48 to 72 hours after injury and obstruct the lower airways.

Lung tissue injuries result from toxic irritant damage to the alveoli and capillaries. Leaking capillaries cause alveolar edema, which can occur immediately or up to a week after the injury. The *fluid* that diffuses into the lung tissue spaces contains proteins that form fibrinous membranes and lead to respiratory distress. Progressive pulmonary failure develops, leading to acute pulmonary insufficiency and INFECTION.

Gastrointestinal Changes Resulting from Burn Injury

The fluid shifts and decreased cardiac output that occur after injury decrease blood flow to the GI tract. Gastric mucosal TISSUE INTEGRITY and motility are impaired. The sympathetic nervous system stress response increases secretion of epinephrine and norepinephrine, which inhibit GI motility and further reduce blood flow to the area. Peristalsis decreases, and a paralytic ileus may develop. Secretions and gases collect in the GI tract, causing abdominal distention.

Curling's ulcer (acute gastroduodenal ulcer that occurs with the stress of severe injury) may develop within 24 hours after a severe burn injury because of reduced GI blood flow and mucosal damage (McCance et al., 2014). The mucus lining the stomach normally protects the tissue from the hydrogen ions secreted into the stomach. With decreased gastric mucus production and increased hydrogen ion production, ulcers may develop. This complication is now less common because of the use of H_2 histamine blockers, proton pump inhibitors, drugs that protect GI tissues, and early enteral feeding.

Metabolic Changes Resulting from Burn Injury

A serious burn injury greatly increases metabolism by increasing secretion of catecholamines, antidiuretic hormone, aldosterone, and cortisol. With this hypermetabolism, the patient's oxygen use and calorie needs are high.

The catecholamines activate the stress response. The increased production (and loss) of heat breaks down protein and fat *(catabolism)*, rapidly uses glucose and calories, and increases urine nitrogen loss. The heat and water lost from the burn also increase metabolic rate and calorie needs. Depending on the extent of injury, the patient's calorie needs double or triple normal energy needs. These increased rates peak 4 to 12 days after the burn and can remain elevated for months until all wounds are closed.

The hypermetabolic condition also increases core body temperature. The patient loses heat through the burned areas. Core body temperature increases as a response to the adjustment in temperature regulation by the hypothalamus, resulting in a low-grade fever.

Immunologic Changes Resulting from Burn Injury

Burn injury disrupts or destroys the protective skin TISSUE INTEGRITY, increasing the risk for INFECTION. The injury activates the inflammatory response and often suppresses all types of immune functions. Antibiotic therapy and other interventions for burns further reduce immune function.

Compensatory Responses to Burn Injury

Any injury is a stressor and can disrupt homeostasis. Two compensatory (adaptive) responses have immediate benefit: the inflammatory response and the sympathetic nervous system stress response. Together these responses cause changes that result in many of the manifestations seen in the first 2 to 3 days after a burn injury.

Inflammatory compensation is helpful by triggering healing in the injured tissues and also is responsible for the serious problems that occur with the fluid shift. This compensation causes blood vessels to leak fluid into the interstitial space and white blood cells to release chemicals that trigger local tissue reactions. These responses cause the massive fluid shift, edema, and hypovolemia that are seen in the **resuscitation phase** (first 24 to 48 hours) after a burn injury. The extent of the inflammatory response depends on the burn severity. Chapter 17 explains inflammation and the inflammatory responses in detail.

Sympathetic nervous system compensation is the stress response that occurs when any physical stressors are present. Changes caused by sympathetic compensation are most evident in the cardiovascular, respiratory, and GI systems. Fig. 26-7 shows the results of sympathetic nervous system stimulation.

Etiology of Burn Injury

Burn injuries are caused by dry heat (flame), moist heat (scald), contact with hot or rough surfaces, chemicals, electricity, and ionizing radiation. The cause of the injury affects both the prognosis and the treatment.

Dry heat injuries are caused by open flame in house fires and explosions. Explosions usually result in flash burns because they produce a brief exposure to very high temperatures.

Moist heat (scald) injuries are caused by contact with hot liquids or steam. Scald injuries are more common among older adults than younger adults. Hot liquid spills usually burn the upper, front areas of the body. Immersion scald injuries usually involve the lower body.

Contact burns occur when hot metal, tar, or grease contacts the skin, often leading to a full-thickness injury. Hot metal

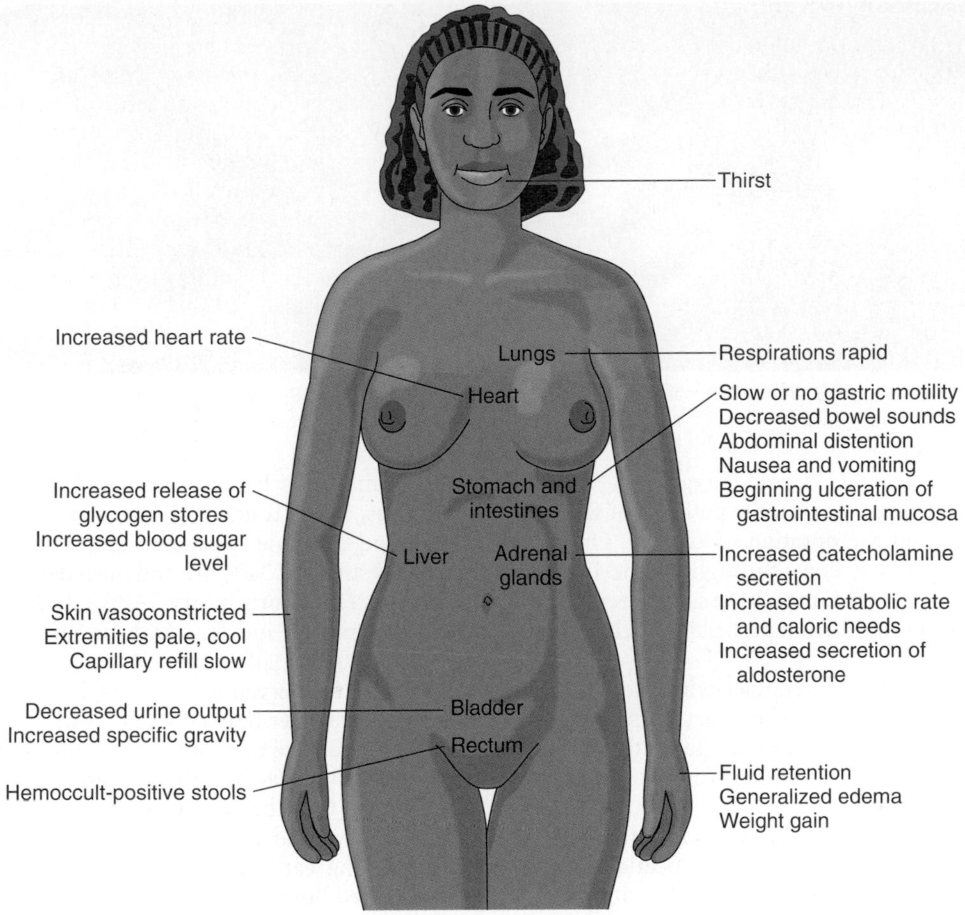

FIG. 26-7 The physiologic actions of the sympathetic nervous system compensatory responses to burn injury (early phase).

injuries occur when a body part contacts a hot surface, such as a space heater or iron. They also can occur in industrial settings from molten metals. Tar and asphalt temperatures usually are greater than 400° F, and deep injuries occur within seconds when the skin is immersed in or splashed with them. Hot grease injuries from cooking are usually deep because of the high temperature of the grease.

Chemical burns occur in home or industrial accidents or as the result of assault. Injury occurs when chemicals directly contact the skin and epithelial tissues or are ingested. The severity of the injury depends on the duration of contact, the concentration of the chemical, the amount of tissue exposed, and the action of the chemical.

Alkalis found in oven cleaners, fertilizers, drain cleaners, and heavy industrial cleaners damage the tissues by causing the skin and its proteins to liquefy. This allows for deeper spread of the chemical and more severe burns. Acids found in bathroom cleaners, rust removers, pool chemicals, and industrial drain cleaners damage TISSUE INTEGRITY by coagulating cells and skin proteins, which can limit the depth of tissue damage. Chemical disinfectants and gasoline are easily absorbed through the skin and have toxic effects on the kidneys and liver.

Electrical injuries are burns occurring when an electrical current enters the body (Fig. 26-8). These injuries have been called the "grand masquerader" of burns because the surface injuries may look small but the associated internal injuries can be huge. Tissue injury from electrical trauma results from

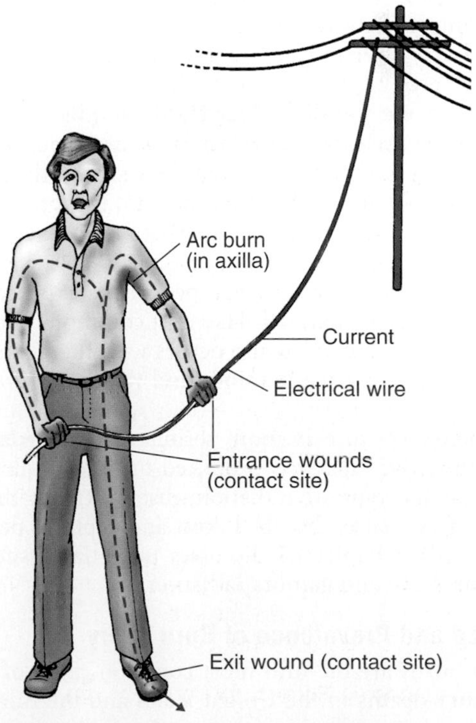

FIG. 26-8 The mechanism of electrical injury: currents passing through the body follow the path of least resistance to the ground.

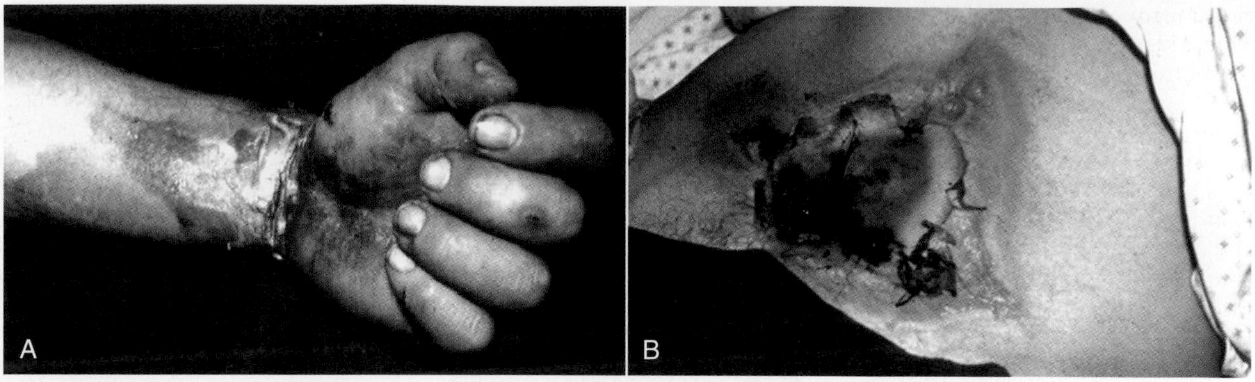

FIG. 26-9 Electrical contact sites. **A,** Possible entrance site. **B,** Possible exit site.

electrical energy being converted to heat energy. The extent of injury depends on the type of current, the pathway of flow, the local tissue resistance, and the duration of contact. Once the current penetrates the skin, it flows throughout the involved body part generating heat and damaging tissues. Deep muscle injury may be present even when superficial muscles appear normal or uninjured.

The longer the electricity is in contact with the body, the greater the damage. The duration of contact is increased by tetanic contractions of the strong flexor muscles in the forearm, which can prevent the person from releasing the electrical source.

It is difficult to know the exact path a current takes in the body. The course of flow is defined by the locations of the "contact sites," which are the entrance and exit wounds (Fig. 26-9). At first, the wounds may not be obvious. The path of the injury may involve many internal organs between the two contact sites.

Burn injuries from electricity can occur as *thermal burns, flash burns,* or *true electrical injury.* Thermal burns occur when clothes ignite from heat or flames produced by electrical sparks. External burn injuries can occur when the electrical current jumps, or "arcs," between two body surfaces. These injuries usually are severe and deep. True electrical injury occurs when direct contact is made with an electrical source. Internal damage results and can be devastating. Damage starts on the inside and goes out; deep-tissue destruction may not be apparent immediately after injury. Organs in the path of the current may become ischemic and necrotic.

Radiation injuries occur when people are exposed to large doses of radioactive material. The most common type of tissue injury from radiation exposure occurs with therapeutic radiation. This injury is usually minor and rarely causes extensive skin damage.

Radiation exposure is more serious in industrial settings where radioactive energy is produced or used. Injury severity depends on the type of radiation, distance from the source, duration of exposure, absorbed dose, and depth of penetration into the body. Chapter 22 discusses potential tissue damage from alpha, beta, and gamma radiation.

Incidence and Prevalence of Burn Injury

Fires and burns are the fifth most common cause of unintentional injury deaths in the United States and the third leading cause of fatal home injuries (American Burn Association [ABA], 2012). Although the number of fatalities and injuries caused by residential fires has declined gradually over the past several decades, many residential fire-related deaths remain preventable and continue to pose a significant public health problem.

An estimated 3400 fire and burn deaths occur each year from all sources of burn injury (ABA, 2012). Most deaths occur at the scene of the incident or during transport.

The number of deaths from burn injuries decreases with appropriate intervention. Factors that increase the risk for death include age older than 60 years, a burn greater than 40% TBSA, and the presence of an inhalation injury. When a patient has all three of these factors, the risk for death is very high. Better outcomes from burn injuries occur because of vigorous fluid resuscitation, early burn wound excision, improved critical care monitoring, early enteral NUTRITION, antibiotics, and the use of specialized burn centers.

HEALTH PROMOTION AND MAINTENANCE

Minor burns are common, and prevention involves planning and awareness. Teach all people to assess how hot the water is before bathing, showering, or immersing a body part in it. Hot water tanks should be set below 140° F (60° C). Reinforce the use of potholders when taking food from ovens. Stress the importance of never adding a flammable substance (e.g., gasoline, kerosene, alcohol, lighter fluid, charcoal starter) to an open flame. Suggest the use of sunscreen agents and protective clothing to avoid sunburn.

Teach people to reduce the risk for house fires by never smoking in bed, avoiding smoking when drinking alcohol or taking drugs that induce sleep, and keeping matches and lighters out of the reach of children or people who are cognitively impaired. When space heaters are used, stress the importance of keeping clothing, bedding, and other flammable objects away from them. Remind people to keep the screens and doors closed on the fronts of fireplaces and to have chimneys swept each year. Also remind patients using home oxygen not to smoke or have open flames in a room where oxygen is in use (Murabit & Tredget, 2012).

Leaving a burning building is critical to prevent injury or death. Teach all people to use home smoke detectors and carbon monoxide detectors and to ensure these are in good working order. The number of detectors needed depends on the size of the home. Recommendations are that each bedroom has a separate smoke detector, there should be at least one detector in the hallway of each story, and at least one detector is needed for the kitchen, each stairwell, and each home entrance. Teach everyone to develop a planned escape route with alternatives for when a main route is blocked by fire. Reinforce that no one should ever re-enter a burning building to retrieve belongings.

RESUSCITATION PHASE OF BURN INJURY

Events within the first hour after injury can make the difference between life and death for the patient with a burn injury. Immediate care focuses on maintaining an open airway, ensuring adequate breathing and circulation, limiting the extent of injury, and maintaining the function of vital organs. Chart 26-1 outlines the emergency management of a burn injury.

The **resuscitation phase** is the first phase of a burn injury. It begins at the onset of injury and continues for about 24 to 48 hours. During this phase, the injury is evaluated and the immediate problems of FLUID imbalance (loss), edema, and reduced blood flow are assessed. The priorities for management during this period are to (1) secure the airway, (2) support circulation and organ PERFUSION by fluid replacement, (3) keep the patient comfortable with analgesics, (4) prevent INFECTION through careful wound care, (5) maintain body temperature, and (6) provide emotional support.

CHART 26-1 Best Practice for Patient Safety & Quality Care (QSEN)

Emergency Management of Burns

General Management for All Types of Burns

- Assess for airway patency.
- Administer oxygen as needed.
- Cover the patient with a blanket.
- Keep the patient on NPO status.
- Elevate the extremities if no fractures are obvious.
- Obtain vital signs.
- Initiate an IV line, and begin fluid replacement.
- Administer tetanus toxoid for prophylaxis.
- Perform a head-to-toe assessment.

Specific Management

Flame Burns

- Smother the flames.
- Remove smoldering clothing and all metal objects.

Chemical Burns

- If dry chemicals are present on skin or clothing, DO NOT WET THEM.
- Brush off any dry chemicals present on the skin or clothing.
- Remove the patient's clothing.
- Ascertain the type of chemical causing the burn.
- Do not attempt to neutralize the chemical unless it has been positively identified and the appropriate neutralizing agent is available.

Electrical Burns

- At the scene, separate the patient from the electrical current.
- Smother any flames that are present.
- Initiate cardiopulmonary resuscitation.
- Obtain an electrocardiogram (ECG).

Radiation Burns

- Remove the patient from the radiation source.
- If the patient has been exposed to radiation from an unsealed source, remove his or her clothing (using tongs or lead protective gloves).
- If the patient has radioactive particles on the skin, send him or her to the nearest designated radiation decontamination center.
- Help the patient bathe or shower.

❖ PATIENT-CENTERED COLLABORATIVE CARE

◆ Assessment

History. Knowledge of circumstances surrounding the burn injury is valuable in planning the management of a burn patient. If possible, obtain information directly from the patient. If this is not possible, ask family members or witnesses to the event. Ask about the circumstances of the injury, the time and place of injury, and the source and cause of injury. Asked detailed questions about how the burn occurred and the events occurring from the time of injury until help arrived. Also obtain demographic data, health history (including pre-existing illness), drug use, any additional injuries, and PAIN information.

Demographic data include age, weight, and height. The rate of serious complications and death from burn injuries is increased among adults older than 50 years. Chart 26-2 lists the age-related differences in older adults' responses to a burn injury. The patient's preburn weight is used to calculate fluid rates, energy requirements, and drug doses. This weight is the *dry weight,* because it is the patient's weight before edema forms. Calculations based on a weight obtained after fluid replacement is started are not accurate. Height is important in determining total body surface area (TBSA), which is used to calculate NUTRITION needs.

A health history, including any pre-existing illnesses, must be known for appropriate management. Obtain specific information about the patient's history of cardiac or kidney problems, chronic alcoholism, substance abuse, and diabetes mellitus; any of these problems influence fluid resuscitation. The stress of a burn can make a mild disease process worsen. Obtain a drug history that includes allergies, current drugs, and immunization status from the patient or family. Determine the dose and time the last drug was taken. Ask whether the patient smokes or drinks alcohol daily; these factors influence treatment plans and responses.

Other injuries may occur at the time of the burn. Such injuries increase the risk for complications or death. Determine whether additional injuries such as fractures, chest injuries, and abdominal trauma are causing PAIN or discomfort.

Physical Assessment/Clinical Manifestations. Physical assessment findings in the resuscitation phase differ greatly from findings later in the course of the injury. Use a systematic approach to ensure that no problem is missed. Assessment of the respiratory system is most critical to prevent life-threatening complications.

Respiratory Assessment. Patients with major burn injuries and those with inhalation injury are at risk for respiratory problems. Respiratory manifestations common with a burn injury are listed in Table 26-3. *Thus continuous airway assessment is a nursing priority.*

Direct Airway Injury. The degree of inhalation damage depends on the fire source, temperature, environment, and types of toxic gases generated. Ask about the source of the fire, duration of exposure, and whether the fire was in an enclosed space. Inspect the mouth, nose, and pharynx. Burns of the lips, face, ears, neck, eyelids, eyebrows, and eyelashes are strong indicators that an inhalation injury may be present. Burns inside the mouth and singed nasal hairs also indicate possible inhalation injury. Black particles of carbon in the nose, mouth, and sputum; edema of the nasal septum; and a "smoky" smell to the patient's breath indicate smoke inhalation.

CHART 26-2 Nursing Focus on the Older Adult

Age-Related Changes Increasing Complications from Burn Injury

AGE-RELATED CHANGES	COMPLICATIONS AND NURSING CONSIDERATIONS
Thinner skin, sensory impairment, decreased mobility	Sensory impairment and decreased mobility increase the risk for burn injury. Thinner skin increases the depth of injury even when the exposure to the cause of injury is of shorter duration.
Slower healing time	Longer time with open areas results in a greater risk for infection, metabolic derangements, and loss of function from contracture formation and scar tissue.
More likely to have cardiac impairments	Limits the aggressiveness of fluid resuscitation. Increases the risk for shock and acute kidney injury (AKI).
Reduced inflammatory and immune responses	Increases the risk for infection and sepsis. Patient may not have a fever when infection is present.
Reduced thoracic and pulmonary compliance	Increased risk for atelectasis, hypoxia, and other pulmonary complications.
More likely to have pre-existing medical conditions such as diabetes mellitus, kidney impairment, or pulmonary impairment	Any of these disorders compromise vital organ function and can interfere with fluid resuscitation efforts or other treatments.

TABLE 26-3 Factors Determining Inhalation Injury or Airway Obstruction

- Patients who were injured in a closed space
- Patients with extensive burns or with burns of the face
- Intra-oral charcoal, especially on teeth and gums
- Patients who were unconscious at the time of injury
- Patients with singed scalp hair, nasal hairs, eyelids, or eyelashes
- Patients who are coughing up carbonaceous sputum
- Changes in voice such as hoarseness or brassy cough
- Use of accessory muscles or stridor
- Poor oxygenation or ventilation
- Edema, erythema, and ulceration of airway mucosa
- Wheezing, bronchospasm

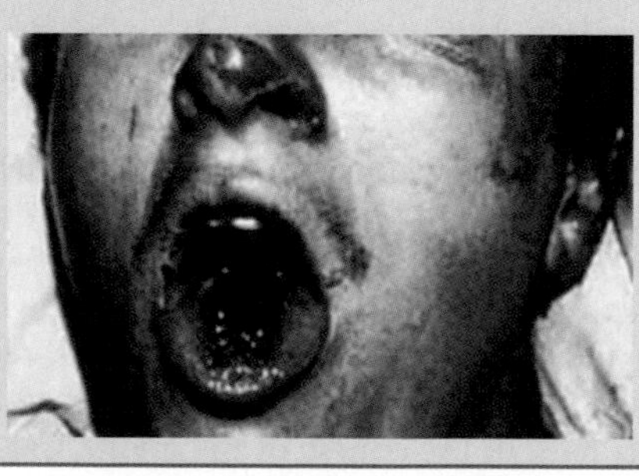

A change in respiratory pattern may indicate a pulmonary injury. The patient may:

- Become progressively hoarse
- Develop a brassy cough
- Drool or have difficulty swallowing
- Produce sounds on exhalation that include audible wheezes, crowing, and stridor

Any of these changes may mean the patient is about to lose his or her airway.

! NURSING SAFETY PRIORITY (QSEN)

Critical Rescue

For a burn patient in the resuscitation phase who is hoarse, has a brassy cough, drools or has difficulty swallowing, or produces an audible breath sound on exhalation, immediately apply oxygen and notify the Rapid Response Team.

Upper airway edema and inhalation injury are most common in the trachea and mainstem bronchi. Auscultation of these areas may reveal wheezes, which indicate partial obstruction. *Patients with severe inhalation injuries may have such rapid obstruction that, within a short time, they cannot force air through the narrowed airways. As a result, the wheezing sounds disappear. This finding indicates impending airway obstruction and demands immediate intubation.* Many patients are intubated when an inhalation injury is first suspected rather than waiting until obstruction makes intubation difficult or impossible.

Carbon Monoxide Poisoning. Carbon monoxide (CO) is one of the leading causes of death from a fire. It is a colorless, odorless, tasteless gas released in the process of combustion. Inhalation injury is a risk for carbon monoxide poisoning (Alharbi et al., 2012).

CO is rapidly transported across the lung membrane and binds tightly to hemoglobin in place of oxygen to form carboxyhemoglobin (COHb), which impairs oxygen unloading at the tissue level. Even though the oxygen-carrying capacity of the hemoglobin is reduced, the blood gas value of partial pressure of arterial oxygen (Pa_{O_2}) is normal (Laing, 2013). The vasodilating action of carbon monoxide causes the "cherry red" color (or at least the absence of cyanosis) in these patients. Manifestations vary with the concentration of COHb (Table 26-4).

Thermal (Heat) Injury. Except for steam inhalation, aspiration of scalding liquid, or explosion of flammable gases under pressure, thermal burns to the respiratory tract are usually limited to the upper airway above the glottis (nasopharynx, oropharynx, and larynx). *Heat damage of the pharynx is often severe enough to produce edema and upper airway obstruction, especially epiglottitis. The problem can occur any time during resuscitation. In the unresuscitated patient, supraglottic edema may be delayed because of the dehydration that occurs with hypovolemia. During fluid resuscitation, however, the tissues rehydrate and then swell. When it is known that the upper airways were exposed to heat, intubation may be performed as an early intervention before obstruction occurs.*

Inhaled steam can injure the lower respiratory tract down to the major bronchioles. Ulcerations, redness, and edema of the mouth and epiglottis occur first, with rapid swelling leading to upper airway obstruction. Stridor, hoarseness, and shortness of breath result.

TABLE 26-4 Physiologic Effects of Carbon Monoxide Poisoning

CARBON MONOXIDE LEVEL	PHYSIOLOGIC EFFECTS
1%-10% (normal)	Increased threshold to visual stimuli Increased blood flow to vital organs
11%-20% (mild poisoning)	Headache Decreased cerebral function Decreased visual acuity Slight breathlessness
21%-40% (moderate poisoning)	Headache Tinnitus Nausea Drowsiness Vertigo Altered mental state Confusion Stupor Irritability Decreased blood pressure, increased and irregular heart rate Depressed ST segment on ECG and dysrhythmias Pale to reddish purple skin
41%-60% (severe poisoning)	Coma Convulsions Cardiopulmonary instability
61%-80% (fatal poisoning)	Death

ECG, Electrocardiogram.

! NURSING SAFETY PRIORITY QSEN

Action Alert

When intubation has not been performed in a patient whose upper airways were exposed to heat or toxic gases, continually assess the upper airway for recognition of edema and obstruction.

Smoke Poisoning. Smoke poisoning, or chemical injury from the inhalation of combustion by-products, is a common type of inhalation injury. Toxic by-products are produced when plastics or home furnishings are burned. The products impair respiratory cell function.

Pulmonary Fluid Overload. Pulmonary edema can occur even when the lung tissues have not been damaged directly. Other damaged tissues release such large amounts of inflammatory mediators causing capillary leak that even lung capillaries leak FLUID into the pulmonary tissue spaces.

Circulatory overload from fluid resuscitation may cause congestive heart failure. This problem creates high pressure within pulmonary blood vessels that pushes fluid into the lung tissue spaces. Excess lung tissue fluid makes gas exchange difficult. *The patient is short of breath and has dyspnea in the supine position. Crackles are heard on auscultation.*

! NURSING SAFETY PRIORITY QSEN

Critical Rescue

When manifestations of pulmonary edema are present, elevate the head of the bed to at least 45 degrees, apply oxygen, and notify the burn team or the Rapid Response Team.

External Factors. Patients with burn injuries also may have breathing problems from external factors, such as tight eschar from deep circumferential chest burns. The eschar either restricts chest movement or compresses structures in the neck and throat so that airflow is impaired. Inspect the patient's chest hourly for ease of respiration, amount of chest movement, rate of breathing, and effort. If the patient is being mechanically ventilated, increased airway pressures may indicate the need for an escharotomy. Use continuous pulse oximetry to assess breathing effectiveness in maintaining blood oxygen levels.

? NCLEX EXAMINATION CHALLENGE

Physiological Integrity

For which type of burn injury is it most important for the nurse to assess the client for a respiratory injury?

A. Hot liquid scald burn
B. Liquid chemical burn
C. Electrical burn
D. Dry heat burn

Cardiovascular Assessment. Changes in the cardiovascular system begin immediately after the burn injury and include shock as a result of disrupted FLUID AND ELECTROLYTE BALANCE. *Hypovolemia shock is a common cause of death in the resuscitation phase in patients with serious injuries.* See Chapter 37 for discussion of shock.

At first, cardiac manifestations are from hypovolemia and decreased cardiac output. Monitor the degree of edema, and assess cardiac status by measuring central and peripheral pulses, blood pressure, capillary refill, and pulse oximetry. Noninvasive blood pressure readings are inaccurate in patients with large burns of the upper extremities, and invasive blood pressure monitoring may be needed. At first, the patient has tachycardia, decreased blood pressure, and decreased peripheral pulses. Peripheral capillary refill is slow or absent as blood flow decreases. With fluid resuscitation, peripheral edema increases, as does the patient's weight.

Electrocardiographic (ECG) changes can indicate damage to the heart as a result of electrical burn injuries or stress that induces a myocardial infarction. Obtain baseline ECG tracings at the time of admission, and continue the ECG monitoring throughout the resuscitation phase. Compare current ECG tracings with the initial tracings to assess whether the patient is experiencing new-onset conduction abnormalities from the burn injury or the fluid resuscitation.

Kidney/Urinary Assessment. Changes in kidney function with burn injury are related to decreased blood flow and to cellular debris. During the fluid shift, blood flow to the kidney may not be adequate for filtration. As a result, urine output is greatly decreased compared with IV fluid intake. The urine is very concentrated and has a high specific gravity.

Other substances may be present in the blood that flows through the kidney. Destroyed red blood cells release hemoglobin and potassium. When muscle damage occurs from a major burn or electrical injury, *myoglobin* is released from damaged muscle and circulates to the kidney. Most damaged cells release proteins that form uric acid. All of these large molecules in the blood may precipitate in the kidney tubular system. A "sludge" then forms that blocks kidney blood and urine flow and may cause kidney failure.

Assess kidney function by accurately measuring urine output hourly and comparing this value with fluid intake. Urine output is decreased during the first 24 hours of the resuscitation phase. Fluid resuscitation is provided at the rate needed to maintain urine output at 30 to 50 mL per hour or 0.5 mL/kg/hr. Assess response to fluid resuscitation by measuring urine specific gravity, blood urea nitrogen (BUN), serum creatinine, and serum sodium levels in addition to hourly urine output. Examine the urine for color, odor, and the presence of particles or foam.

Skin Assessment. Assess the skin to determine the size and depth of burn injury. The size of the injury is first estimated in comparison with the *total body surface area (TBSA)*. For example, a burn that involves 40% of the TBSA is a 40% burn. The size of the injury is important not only for diagnosis and prognosis but also for calculating drug doses, fluid replacement volumes, and caloric needs.

Inspect the skin TISSUE INTEGRITY to identify injured areas and changes in color and appearance. Except with electrical burns, this initial size assessment usually can be made accurately with specific assessment tools and charts.

The most rapid method for calculating the size of a burn injury in adult patients whose weights are in normal proportion to their heights is the *rule of nines* (Fig. 26-10). With this method, the body is divided into areas that are multiples of 9%. It is useful at the site of injury, but more accurate evaluations using other methods are made in the burn unit.

Because specific treatments are related to the depth of the burn injury, initial assessment of the skin includes estimations of burn depth. Criteria for depth of injury are based on appearance and associated characteristics (see Depth of Burn Injury section, p. 466).

Accurate evaluation of burn depth is performed using thermography, vital dyes, indocyanine green (ICG) video angiography, and laser Doppler imaging (LDI) that provide precise measurement of the amount of PERFUSION of the injured tissue. ICG and LDI are the most accurate of the three methods. LDI is used more frequently because it is relatively accurate, less invasive, and faster than the other methods (Park et al., 2013).

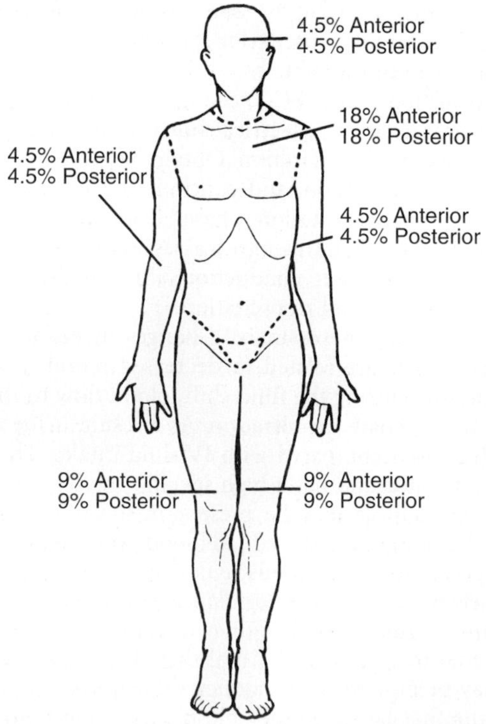

FIG. 26-10 The rule of nines for estimating burn percentage.

Gastrointestinal Assessment. Although the GI tract usually is not directly injured, changes in function occur in all burn patients. The decreased blood flow and sympathetic stimulation reduce GI motility and promote development of a paralytic ileus. Bowel sounds are usually reduced or absent in a patient with severe burns. Other indications of a paralytic ileus include nausea, vomiting, and abdominal distention. Patients with burns of 25% TBSA or who are intubated generally require a nasogastric (NG) tube inserted to prevent aspiration and remove gastric secretions. Assess the tube for placement and patency after insertion. Examine each stool and vomitus for gross blood or other material that indicates partially digested blood ("coffee ground"–appearing crumbs). Test for the presence of occult blood on any vomit or stool.

Laboratory Assessment. Certain changes in laboratory test values are found in different phases of postburn recovery and reflect tissue damage or compensatory responses. However, other changes in specific laboratory findings may suggest complications.

During the resuscitation phase and before the start of fluid resuscitation, blood analysis reflects the fluid shift and direct tissue damage. Baseline laboratory test values and early postburn expected changes are listed in Chart 26-3.

Changes in the total white blood cell (WBC) count and differential reflect immune function and inflammatory responses to the burn injury. The burn patient's total WBC count, especially the neutrophil percentage, first rises and then drops rapidly, with a "left shift" (see Chapter 17) as the immune system becomes unable to sustain its defenses. If sepsis occurs, the total WBC count may be as low as 2000 cells/mm^3.

Other laboratory tests that provide useful information about the burn patient's status include urine electrolyte assays, urine cultures, liver enzyme studies, and clotting studies. Drug and alcohol screens are obtained if drug or alcohol intoxication is suspected.

CULTURAL CONSIDERATIONS

Patient-Centered Care QSEN

For African-American patients, a sickle cell preparation is performed if sickle status is unknown. The trauma of a burn injury can trigger a sickle cell crisis in patients who have the disease and in those who carry the trait.

Imaging Assessment. Standard x-rays and scans do not provide direct assessment data about the burn wound. These assessments are not performed unless other trauma is suspected.

Other Diagnostic Assessment. Specific diagnostic studies are performed when deep organ trauma is suspected. Such studies include renal scans, computed tomography (CT), ultrasonography, bronchoscopy, and magnetic resonance imaging (MRI). When burn injuries involve the eye, an ophthalmic evaluation is performed to detect corneal damage (see Chapters 46 and 47 for specific eye and vision evaluation procedures).

CHART 26-3 Laboratory Profile

Burn Assessment During the Resuscitation Phase

TEST	NORMAL RANGE FOR ADULTS	SIGNIFICANCE OF ABNORMAL FINDINGS
Serum Studies		
Hemoglobin	12-16 g/dL (women) 14-18 g/dL (men)	Elevated as a result of fluid volume loss
Hematocrit	37%-47% (women) 42%-52% (men)	Elevated as a result of fluid volume loss
Urea nitrogen	10-20 mg/dL	Elevated as a result of fluid volume loss
Glucose	70-110 mg/dL	Elevated as a result of the stress response and altered uptake across injured tissues
Electrolytes		
Sodium	136-145 mEq/L (mmol/L)	Decreased; sodium is trapped in edema fluid and lost through plasma leakage
Potassium	3.5-5.0 mEq/L (mmol/L)	Elevated as a result of disruption of the sodium-potassium pump, tissue destruction, and red blood cell hemolysis
Chloride	98-106 mEq/L (mmol/L)	Elevated as a result of fluid volume loss and reabsorption of chloride in urine
Arterial Blood Gas Studies		
Pao_2	80-100 mm Hg	Slightly decreased
$Paco_2$	35-45 mm Hg	Slightly increased from respiratory injury
pH	7.35-7.45	Low as a result of metabolic acidosis
Carboxyhemoglobin	0%-10%	Elevated as a result of inhalation of smoke and carbon monoxide
Other		
Total protein	6.4-8.3 g/dL	Low; protein exudate is lost through the wound
Albumin	3.5-5.0 g/dL	Low; protein is lost through the wound and through vascular membranes because of increased permeability

Data from Pagana, K., & Pagana, T. (2014). *Mosby's manual of diagnostic and laboratory tests* (5th ed). St. Louis: Mosby.

◆ Analysis

The priority NANDA-I nursing diagnoses and collaborative problems for patients with burn injuries in the resuscitation phase who have sustained a burn injury greater than 25% of the TBSA include:

1. Potential for inadequate oxygenation related to upper airway edema, pulmonary edema, airway obstruction, or pneumonia
2. Risk for Shock related to increase in capillary permeability, active fluid volume loss, electrolyte imbalance, and inadequate fluid resuscitation (NANDA-I)
3. Potential for organ ischemia (brain, heart, kidney, gastrointestinal) related to hypovolemia and hypotension
4. Pain (Acute and Chronic) related to tissue injury, damaged or exposed nerve endings, débridement, dressing changes, invasive procedures, and donor sites (NANDA-I)
5. Potential for acute respiratory distress syndrome (ARDS) related to inhalation injury

◆ Planning and Implementation

Supporting Oxygenation

Planning: Expected Outcomes. With proper intervention, the patient is expected to maintain a patent airway and have adequate oxygenation. Indicators include that the patient should have either normal or nearly normal oxygen saturation, Pao_2, $Paco_2$, and arterial pH.

Interventions. Nursing and medical interventions are used to support normal pulmonary function and prevent the pulmonary problems that can result from lung injury or from fluid overload and heart failure. (Even young, healthy people can develop fluid overload and heart failure.) Specific management plans depend on the cause of the problem and the status of the respiratory tract. *Thus a priority nursing intervention is monitoring the patient's respiratory status.*

Nonsurgical Management. Interventions include airway maintenance, promotion of ventilation, monitoring gas exchange, oxygen therapy, drug therapy, positioning, and deep breathing.

Airway maintenance begins at the burn scene in an unconscious patient and may involve only a chin-lift or a head-tilt maneuver. *Remember that upper airway edema becomes pronounced 8 to 12 hours after the beginning of fluid resuscitation. Then patients often require nasal or oral intubation if crowing, stridor, or dyspnea is present.*

A bronchoscopy is performed to examine the vocal cords and airways of patients at risk for obstruction. Patients with severe smoke inhalation or poisoning may require a bronchoscopy on admission and routinely thereafter for examination of the respiratory tract, deep suctioning of the lungs, and removal of sloughing necrotic tissue. Assess the endotracheal tube hourly to ensure patency and location in intubated patients.

Other causes of airway obstruction are excessive secretions and sloughed tissue from damaged lungs. Suction as indicated based on clinical assessment. Vigorous endotracheal or nasotracheal tube suctioning is performed after chest physiotherapy and aerosol treatments. Patients report that deep endotracheal suctioning is extremely painful. Therefore suctioning the endotracheal tube often requires increased analgesia or sedation.

Promoting ventilation includes ensuring that skeletal muscle movement of the chest is adequate for ventilation. Chest movement can be restricted by eschar and by tight dressings that cover the neck, chest, and abdomen. Observe the patient for ease of respiratory movements, and loosen tight dressings as needed to assist with ventilation.

Monitor for gas exchange by using laboratory tests (e.g., arterial blood gas, carboxyhemoglobin levels) and by assessing for cyanosis, disorientation, and increased pulse rate. Additional monitoring may include chest x-ray findings, pulmonary artery catheter pressures, and central venous pressure measurement.

Cyanide poisoning may occur in patients burned in house fires. An elevated plasma lactate level is one indicator of cyanide toxicity even in patients who do not have severe burns.

Oxygen therapy with humidified oxygen by facemask, cannula, or hood is used to manage any breathing impairment in the burn patient. Arterial oxygenation less than 60 mm Hg is an indication for intubation and mechanical ventilation. Keep emergency airway equipment near the bedside. This equipment includes oxygen, masks, cannulas, manual resuscitation bags, laryngoscope, endotracheal tubes, and equipment for tracheostomy. Chapter 32 addresses specific nursing actions for patients during mechanical ventilation.

Drug therapy with antibiotics is used when pneumonia or other pulmonary INFECTIONS impair breathing. Drug selection is based on known culture and sensitivity reports or on the specific organisms common to that burn unit.

Patients with pulmonary edema and any degree of heart failure may receive beta blockers to improve left ventricular function and prevent or treat pulmonary edema. Diuretics, a mainstay of therapy for pulmonary edema from other causes, may or may not be used in the resuscitation phase, depending on the patient's blood volume and kidney function.

When a patient's activity during mechanical ventilation severely compromises respiratory mechanics, it may be necessary to use a paralytic drug, such as atracurium (Tracrium) or vecuronium (Norcuron). Paralytic drugs remove all breathing control from the patient, making mechanical ventilation easier. *These drugs do not prevent the patient from seeing and hearing or from experiencing fear, PAIN, and loss of control. Any patient receiving neuromuscular blockade drugs must also receive drugs for sedation, analgesia, and antianxiety unless clinically contraindicated.*

! NURSING SAFETY PRIORITY QSEN

Critical Rescue

As required by The Joint Commission's National Patient Safety Goals, ensure that all alarms are operative on ventilators. Check patients who are receiving neuromuscular blockage frequently, because they cannot call for help if they become extubated accidentally.

Positioning and deep breathing can improve breathing and oxygenation. Turn the patient frequently, and assist him or her out of bed to a chair as much as possible. Teach the patient to use coughing and deep-breathing exercises. Urge him or her to use incentive spirometry hourly while awake. Chest physiotherapy may be helpful to mobilize lung secretions.

Surgical Management. A tracheotomy may be needed when long-term intubation is expected. This procedure increases the risk for INFECTION in burn patients even more than in nonburned patients. Emergency tracheotomies are performed when an airway becomes occluded and oral or nasal intubation cannot be achieved.

Other surgical procedures for improving the burn patient's oxygenation include inserting chest tubes and performing an escharotomy. Chest tubes are used to re-expand the lung when a pneumothorax or hemothorax has occurred (see Chapter 32). Tight eschar on the neck, chest, or abdomen can restrict respiratory movement. Escharotomies (described on p. 479) can relieve this restriction and permit greater respiratory movement.

Preventing Hypovolemic Shock and Inadequate Oxygenation

Planning: Expected Outcomes. With appropriate intervention, the patient is expected to have blood pressure and tissue oxygenation restored to normal. Indicators include these vital signs and assessment parameters:

- Blood pressure at or near the patient's normal range
- Palpable peripheral pulses (or heard with Doppler) in all extremities
- Oxygen saturation, partial pressure of arterial oxygen (Pao_2), partial pressure of arterial carbon dioxide ($Paco_2$), and arterial pH at or near the normal ranges

Interventions. Interventions focus on increasing blood fluid volume, supporting compensation, and preventing complications. Nonsurgical management is often sufficient for achieving these aims. Surgical management may be needed for full-thickness burns.

Nonsurgical Management. FLUID volume and tissue blood flow (PERFUSION) are restored through IV fluid therapy and drug therapy. Priority nursing interventions are carrying out fluid resuscitation and monitoring for indications of effectiveness or complications.

Rapid infusion of IV fluids, known as *fluid resuscitation,* is needed to maintain sufficient blood volume for normal cardiac output, mean arterial pressure, and tissue oxygenation. Chart 26-4 lists best practices for fluid resuscitation. There are many formulas for calculating IV fluid needs, but the most commonly used one for adult patients is the Parkland Formula (4 mL/kg/%TBSA burn of crystalloid solution). Although the types and amounts of electrolytes, crystalloids, and colloids vary, the purpose of any formula is to prevent shock by maintaining blood fluid volume.

Resuscitation for a severe burn requires large FLUID loads in a short time to maintain blood flow to vital organs. All common formulas recommend that half of the calculated fluid volume for 24 hours be given in the first 8 hours after injury. The other half is given over the next 16 hours for a total of 24 hours (Culleiton & Simko, 2013b). Fluid boluses are avoided because they increase capillary pressure and worsen edema. In the second 24-hour period after a burn injury, the volume and content of the IV fluids are based on the patient's specific FLUID AND ELECTROLYTE BALANCE needs and his or her response to treatment. This resuscitation involves hourly infusion volumes that are greatly in excess of the 125 mL to 150 mL per hour common infusion rates.

FLUID replacement formulas are calculated from the time of injury and not from the time of arrival at the hospital. For example, if a burn injury occurred at 8 AM but the patient was not admitted to the hospital until 10 AM, the first 8-hour period would be completed at 4 PM (8 hours after the injury). Thus if resuscitation was delayed by 2 hours until admission to the hospital, calculated fluids would need to be given over the next 6-hour period rather than an 8-hour period. Burn resuscitation formulas are guides. The patient's response to therapy determines exact fluid requirements.

CHART 26-4 Best Practice for Patient Safety & Quality Care QSEN

Fluid Resuscitation of the Burn Patient

- Initiate and maintain at least one large-bore IV in an area of intact skin (if possible).
- Coordinate with physicians to determine the appropriate fluid type and total volume to be infused during the first 24 hours postburn.
- Administer one half of the total 24-hour prescribed volume within the first 8 hours postburn and the remaining volume over the next 16 hours.
- Assess IV access site, infusion rate, and infused volume at least hourly.
- Monitor these vital signs at least hourly:
  - Blood pressure
  - Pulse rate
  - Respiratory rate
  - Breath sounds
  - Voice quality (if not intubated)
  - Oxygen saturation
  - End-tidal carbon dioxide levels
- Assess urine output at least hourly:
  - Volume
  - Color
  - Specific gravity
  - Character
  - Presence of protein
- Assess for fluid overload:
  - Formation of dependent edema
  - Engorged neck veins
  - Rapid, thready pulse
  - Presence of lung crackles or wheezes on auscultation
- Measure additional body fluid output hourly.

The management of extensive burns requires a large-bore central venous catheter so that massive fluid loads can be given. Peripheral lines are less useful.

Monitoring patient responses is critical to determine the adequacy of resuscitation for hydration and blood PERFUSION of the brain, heart, and kidneys. Urine output is the most common and most sensitive noninvasive assessment parameter for cardiac output and tissue perfusion. *Regardless of the total amount of fluid calculated as needed for the patient, the amount of fluid given depends on how much IV fluid per hour is needed to maintain the hourly urine output at 0.5 mL/kg (about 30 mL/hr).* Adjustment of the IV fluid rate on the basis of urine output plus serum electrolyte values is known as the *titration* of fluid. In burns larger than 35% TBSA, the use of invasive cardiac and pulmonary function monitoring may be needed in addition to urine output and vital signs to guide resuscitation.

Burn patients can develop severe hypovolemic shock and need invasive cardiac monitoring. Vital parameters such as central venous pressure, pulmonary artery pressures, and cardiac output are obtained on an hourly to continuous basis.

Monitor the ECG activity of patients who have sustained large burns. Compare current ECG findings with those obtained on admission.

Drug therapy for shock prevention in burn patients is different from that for the heart failure patient. A common mistake in management is giving diuretics to increase urine output rather than changing the amount and rate of fluid infused. *Diuretics do not increase cardiac output; they actually decrease circulating volume and cardiac output by pulling fluid from the circulating blood volume to enhance diuresis.* This effect reduces blood flow to other vital organs (especially the heart, lungs, and brain) and greatly increases the risk for severe hypovolemic shock. Therefore diuretics are not generally used to improve urine output for burn patients. An exception is the patient with an electrical burn injury. In electrical burns, muscle and deep-tissue damage release the large protein *myoglobin,* which precipitates in and obstructs the renal tubules. Although the diuretic *mannitol* (Osmitrol) is often used in this situation, it should always be given after adequate urine output has been established.

NCLEX EXAMINATION CHALLENGE

Safe and Effective Care Environment

Which client response does the nurse interpret as an indication of fluid resuscitation adequacy?
A. Decreasing pulse pressure
B. Decreasing urine specific gravity
C. Decreasing core body temperature
D. Increasing respiratory rate and depth

CONSIDERATIONS FOR OLDER ADULTS

Patient-Centered Care QSEN

In older patients, especially those with cardiac disease, a complicating factor in fluid resuscitation may be heart failure or myocardial infarction. Drugs that increase cardiac output (e.g., dopamine [Intropin]) or that strengthen the force of myocardial contraction may be used along with fluid therapy. Assess the cardiac status of older adults at least every hour during fluid resuscitation.

Surgical Management. The surgical procedure for the treatment of inadequate tissue PERFUSION is *escharotomy.* An incision through the burn eschar relieves pressure caused by the constricting force of fluid buildup under circumferential burns on the extremity or chest and improves circulation. If the pressure is not relieved, arterial compression can occur with a loss of blood flow to the extremity, leading to ischemia and possible necrosis. Incisions are made along the length of the extremity and extend into the subcutaneous tissue, relieving the tourniquet effect of the eschar (Figs. 26-5 and 26-11). If tissue pressure remains elevated after escharotomy, a *fasciotomy* (a deeper incision extending through the fascia) may be needed.

Managing Pain. The PAIN with burn injuries is both chronic and acute. Many factors contribute to burn pain and may be altered to reduce pain perception. Accurate assessment of the patient's pain before and during procedures is an essential part of pain management.

Planning: Expected Outcomes. The patient's PAIN level is expected to be alleviated or reduced. Indicators include that the patient should rarely demonstrate these behaviors:

- Reporting PAIN
- Moaning and crying
- Making facial expressions of PAIN
- Losing his or her appetite

Interventions. PAIN management is tailored to the patient's tolerance for pain, coping mechanisms, and physical status. *The priority nursing actions include continually assessing the patient's pain level, using appropriate pain-reducing strategies, and preventing complications.*

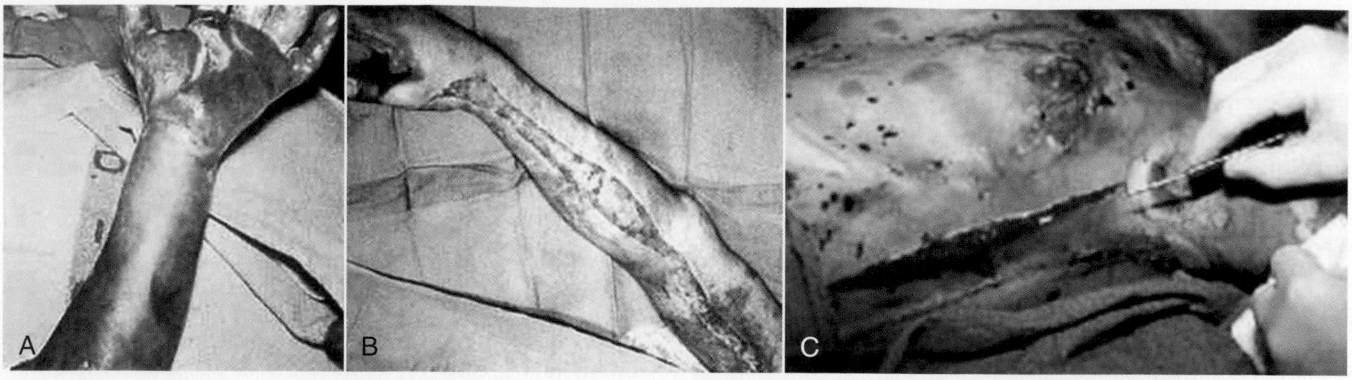

FIG. 26-11 Escharotomy to release circumferential burn eschar and improve circulation to a distal extremity. **A,** Tight circumferential eschar restricting swelling as edema forms in the tissue beneath the eschar. Edema compresses blood vessels, which inhibits blood flow to the distal extremity. **B,** An escharotomy incision allows outward swelling of edematous tissues. The restricted blood flow to the distal extremity is relieved. **C,** An anterior axillary incision is made bilaterally to relieve respiratory distress.

Nonsurgical Management. Interventions for the patient having PAIN include drug therapy, complementary therapy measures, and environmental manipulation.

Drug therapy for PAIN usually requires opioid analgesics (e.g., morphine sulfate, hydromorphone [Dilaudid], fentanyl) and non-opioid analgesics. Although these drugs may provide adequate pain relief when no procedures are being performed, they rarely offer more than moderate relief during painful procedures. They may depress respiratory function and reduce intestinal motility. Thus nonpharmacologic interventions also are needed for the burn patient.

During the resuscitation phase, the IV route is used for giving opioid drugs because of problems with absorption from the muscle and stomach (Culleiton & Simko, 2013c). When given IM or subcutaneously, these drugs remain in the tissue spaces and do not relieve PAIN. In addition, when edema is present, all the doses are rapidly absorbed at once when the fluid shift is resolving. This delayed but rapid absorption can result in lethal blood levels of opioids.

! NURSING SAFETY PRIORITY QSEN

Drug Alert

Give opioid drugs for pain only by the intravenous route during the resuscitation phase to prevent delayed rapid absorption leading to lethal blood levels.

Anesthetic agents, such as ketamine (Ketalar) and nitrous oxide, also reduce PAIN. Use strict protocols when giving these agents to prevent serious complications.

Complementary and alternative therapy measures for PAIN reduction include relaxation techniques, meditative breathing, guided imagery, music therapy, massage, and healing or therapeutic touch. Hypnosis and autohypnosis can be used by lucid, cooperative patients under the direction of trained therapists. Therapeutic touch, acupuncture, and acupressure are used to a limited extent for burn patients; the results are variable. Active music interventions for distraction have been useful in reducing patients' perceptions of pain and anxiety.

Environmental changes, such as providing a quiet environment, using nonpainful tactile stimulation, and increasing the patient's control, can increase comfort. Sleep deprivation increases patients' discomfort. Increasing sleep or rest time in a quiet environment helps reduce the adverse effects of sleep deprivation, replenishes hormone stores, helps prevent critical care unit psychosis, and restores the diurnal effects of endorphins. Coordinate with the health care team to ensure that procedures are performed during the patient's waking hours.

Tactile stimulation can reduce PAIN. Help the patient change positions every 2 hours to reduce pressure on any specific area, improve circulation to painful areas, and ease pain. Massage nonburn areas to reduce pain transmission and stimulate endorphin release. Apply heat and maintain warm room temperatures to prevent shivering.

To reduce anxiety and increase feelings of confidence and independence, encourage the patient to participate in PAIN control measures. For example, make a contract with him or her that specifies how long a painful procedure will last. This helps patients deal with the pain for that particular period. Patient-controlled analgesia (PCA) also reduces pain. Important issues and techniques for the best use of PCA include giving an initial bolus of 5 to 10 mg of morphine (or equivalent drug), increasing the PCA dose as needed to achieve pain relief, and planning for a change in dosing regimens at night (e.g., giving a bolus dose at bedtime). See Chapter 3 for a detailed discussion of combination drug therapy for pain management.

Surgical Management. Early surgical excision of the burn wound is used in many burn centers (see the Surgical Excision section on p. 484). Early excision under anesthesia reduces the PAIN from daily débridement at the bedside or during hydrotherapy.

Preventing Acute Respiratory Distress Syndrome

Planning: Expected Outcome. The patient with a burn injury is expected to:

- Not experience acute respiratory distress
- Have arterial blood gases (ABGs) within normal limits
- Maintain normal lung compliance

Interventions. Patients who develop acute respiratory distress syndrome (ARDS) from burn injuries require thorough assessments and interventions. Interventions focus on increasing lung compliance and improving partial pressure of arterial oxygen (Pa_{O_2}) levels. The priority nursing care actions are coordinating respiratory therapy strategies and monitoring the patient's response to these interventions.

CLINICAL JUDGMENT CHALLENGE

Patient-Centered Care; Safety; Evidence-Based Practice QSEN

A 50-year-old tree trimmer has been brought to hospital after coming in contact with an 8000-volt power line while trimming trees with a pole trimmer. The emergency medical technicians (EMTs) report that they recovered this man from an insulated bucket in which he was working. According to bystanders, the metal pole-saw made contact with the power line. The patient was rendered unconscious only momentarily. The EMTs report that he had pain in both arms when they transported him to the hospital. He now has pain in the neck. The patient is agitated and restless and continues to report increasing pain in both arms and hands and in the neck even though there is no area of burn on the neck. The exit wound is the right hand, including the fingers and thumb. The right arm is cyanotic and tense, and the wrist is acutely flexed and rigid in that position. There is an arc burn in the right axilla. The left arm is tense and cyanotic, and the wrist, hand, and fingers are charred.

1. What initial consideration must be given in moving the patient from the stretcher to the bed?
2. Is the patient at risk for compartment syndrome? Provide a rationale for your response. If yes, what would you expect to find on assessment that would indicate compartment syndrome?
3. A Foley catheter has been placed in this patient, and it is documented that the urine is wine pigmented. What is the etiology and potential complication if this symptom persists?
4. What interventions would you expect to be ordered to resolve myoglobinuria?

In collaboration with the physician and respiratory therapist, give positive end-expiratory pressure (PEEP) to provide a continuous positive pressure in the airways and alveoli. This procedure enhances the diffusion of oxygen across the alveolar-capillary membrane. PEEP can be combined with intermittent mandatory volume (IMV) to enhance its effectiveness.

Assess and document the patient's response so that needed ventilator changes can be made. Monitor pulse oximetry and ABG levels to assess changes in respiratory status.

NURSING SAFETY PRIORITY QSEN

Critical Rescue

Document and immediately report any signs of respiratory distress or change in respiratory patterns to the burn team and the respiratory therapist.

Neuromuscular blocking drugs (atracurium) can be used in patients receiving mechanical ventilation to reduce oxygen consumption (see the discussion of specific nursing care in the Supporting Oxygenation section, pp. 477-478).

ACUTE PHASE OF BURN INJURY

The acute phase of burn injury begins about 36 to 48 hours after injury, when the fluid shift resolves, and lasts until wound closure is complete. During this phase, the nurse coordinates interdisciplinary care that is directed toward continued assessment and maintenance of the cardiovascular and respiratory systems, as well as toward GI and NUTRITION status, burn wound care, PAIN control, and psychosocial interventions.

CLINICAL JUDGMENT CHALLENGE

Patient-Centered Care; Teamwork and Collaboration; Evidence-Based Practice QSEN

The patient who sustained an electrical injury described on the left has adequate IV access and is undergoing fluid resuscitation. While obtaining history from this patient, you find that he has not had a tetanus shot is the past 10 years. He continues to have pain in both arms and hands. On examination you note the burns are tan and dry and there are no blisters or capillary refill. The radial pulses are no longer palpable.

1. Based on the information provided about the injury and the data gathered by examination, what degree of burn injury has this patient suffered? Provide a rationale for your choice.
2. What is the preferred route for analgesic administration? Provide a rationale for your choice.
3. What additional medications do you expect to be ordered for this patient given his history?
4. The patient requires escharotomies to both his upper extremities. What steps would you take to prepare the patient for this procedure? What postprocedure care would you perform?

❖ *PATIENT-CENTERED COLLABORATIVE CARE*

◆ *Assessment*

Physical Assessment/Clinical Manifestations

Cardiopulmonary Assessment. *In the acute phase of burn injury, the priority nursing interventions are to assess the cardiovascular and respiratory systems to maintain these systems and to identify or prevent complications.* At this time, the patient may develop pneumonia that can result in respiratory failure requiring mechanical ventilation. Although cardiovascular problems related to the fluid shift should be resolved, the patient is at risk for INFECTION and sepsis, which affect cardiovascular function.

Neuroendocrine Assessment. The increased metabolic demands placed on the body after a severe burn injury can severely deplete NUTRITION stores. Weigh the patient daily without dressings or splints, and compare it with his or her preburn weight. A 2% loss of body weight indicates a mild deficit. A 10% or more weight loss requires the evaluation and modification of calorie intake. For very accurate calorie requirements, indirect calorimetry may be used. This method assesses energy expenditure by measuring oxygen consumption and carbon dioxide production. Measurements are taken while the patient is at rest—usually at least 30 minutes after the most recent dressing changes or other stressful procedures. Indirect calorimetry may be performed on admission to a burn center and then weekly until the wounds are closed.

Immune Assessment. The patient with a burn injury is at risk for INFECTION because of open wounds and reduced immune function. *Burn wound sepsis is a serious complication of burn injury, and infection is the leading cause of death during the acute phase of recovery.* Continually assess the patient for manifestations of local and systemic infections (Table 26-5), including changes in wound appearance, changes in neurologic and GI function, and subtle changes in vital signs. Monitor for manifestations of gram-positive, gram-negative, and fungal infections (Table 26-6). Enforce meticulous handwashing by all care personnel.

! NURSING SAFETY PRIORITY (QSEN)

Action Alert

Use aseptic technique in caring for wounds and during invasive monitoring to prevent INFECTION.

Musculoskeletal Assessment. Patients with a burn injury are at risk for musculoskeletal and MOBILITY problems as a result of other injuries, immobility, healing processes, and treatment. The musculoskeletal status is evaluated on admission and throughout the postburn period. Assess active and passive range of motion for all joints, including the neck. Give special attention to joints in the burn area. Ranges and limitations are documented for future reference.

◆ Analysis

During the acute phase of the burn injury, the patient may have initial problems that extend into the acute phase and may develop new problems.

The priority NANDA-I nursing diagnoses and collaborative problems for patients with burn injuries greater than 25% TBSA in the acute phase of recovery include:

1. Wound care management related to burn injury, skin grafting procedures, and immobilization
2. Risk for Infection related to open burn wounds, the presence of multiple invasive catheters, reduced immune function, and poor nutrition (NANDA-I)
3. Excessive weight loss related to increased metabolic rate, reduced calorie intake, and increased urinary nitrogen losses
4. Impaired Mobility: Physical related to open burn wounds, pain, and scars and contractures (NANDA-I)
5. Reduced self-image related to trauma, changes in physical appearance and lifestyle, and alterations in sensory and motor function

TABLE 26-5 Local and Systemic Indicators of Infection

Local Indicators	Systemic Indicators
• Conversion of a partial-thickness injury to a full-thickness injury • Ulceration of healthy skin at the burn site • Erythematous, nodular lesions in uninvolved skin and vesicular lesions in healed skin • Edema of healthy skin surrounding the burn wound • Excessive burn wound drainage • Pale, boggy, dry, or crusted granulation tissue • Sloughing of grafts • Wound breakdown after closure • Odor	• Altered level of consciousness • Changes in vital signs (tachycardia, tachypnea, temperature instability, hypotension) • Increased fluid requirements for maintenance of a normal urine output • Hemodynamic instability • Oliguria • GI dysfunction (diarrhea, vomiting, abdominal distention, paralytic ileus) • Hyperglycemia • Thrombocytopenia • Change in total white blood cell count (above normal or below normal) • Metabolic acidosis • Hypoxemia

◆ Planning and Implementation

Managing Wound Care

Planning: Expected Outcomes. With appropriate intervention, the burn patient is expected to have no wound extension and have wounds healed. Indicators include that the patient:

- Has presence of granulation, re-epithelialization, and scar tissue formation
- Has decreased wound size
- Has no new wounds

Interventions. Interventions focus on preserving skin TISSUE INTEGRITY, enhancing burn wound healing, and preventing complications.

Nonsurgical Management. Nonsurgical burn wound management involves removing exudates and necrotic tissue, cleaning the area, stimulating granulation and revascularization, and applying dressings. Restoring skin TISSUE INTEGRITY, whether by natural healing or grafting, starts with the removal of eschar and other cellular debris from the burn wound. This removal is called **débridement**, and can be performed nonsurgically through mechanical or enzymatic actions that separate eschar over time. The purpose is to prepare the wound for grafting and wound closure by a natural process. *Priority nursing interventions include assessing the wound, providing wound care, and preventing infection and other complications.*

Mechanical Débridement. Burn wounds are débrided and cleaned 1 or 2 times each day during **hydrotherapy** (the application of water for treatment). Nurses, unlicensed assistive personnel (UAP), and physical therapists perform hydrotherapy daily to débride and examine the wounds. Hydrotherapy is performed by showering the patient on a special shower table or washing only small areas of the wound at the bedside. Showering enhances wound inspection and allows water temperature

TABLE 26-6 Indications of Sepsis Caused by Different Organisms

MANIFESTATIONS	GRAM-POSITIVE	GRAM-NEGATIVE	FUNGAL
Onset	Insidious, 2-6 days	Rapid, 12-36 hr	Delayed
Cognition	Severe disorientation and lethargy	Mild disorientation	Mild disorientation
Ileus	Severe	Severe	Mild
Diarrhea	Rare	Severe	Occasional
Temperature	Fever	Hypothermia	Fever
Hypotension	Late	Early	Late
White blood cell count	Neutrophilia	Neutropenia	Neutrophilia
Platelets	Normal	Low	Low

to be kept constant. Immersion of the patient in a tub or whirlpool is no longer performed because it increases the risk for INFECTION.

Nurses and skilled technicians use forceps and scissors to remove loose, dead tissue during hydrotherapy. At most burn units, small blisters are left intact because they are a protective barrier that promotes wound healing. Larger blisters are opened. Washcloths or gauze sponges are used to débride soft, "cheesy" eschar. Wash burn areas thoroughly and gently with mild soap or detergent and water. Then rinse these areas with room-temperature water.

Enzymatic Débridement. Enzymatic débridement can occur naturally by autolysis or artificially by the application of exogenous agents. **Autolysis** is the disintegration of tissue by the action of the patient's own cellular enzymes. This process is seldom used alone in North America for larger burns because it is slow and prolongs the hospital stay, increasing the risk for INFECTION.

Topical enzyme agents, such as collagenase (Santyl), are used for rapid wound débridement. When these agents are applied to the burn wound in a once-a-day dressing change, the enzymes digest collagen in necrotic tissues.

Dressing the Burn Wound. After burn wounds are cleaned and débrided, topical antibiotics are reapplied to prevent INFECTION. Some type of dressing is then applied to the burn wound. Burn dressings include standard wound dressings, biologic dressings, synthetic dressings, and artificial skin.

Standard Wound Dressings. Standard dressings are multiple layers of gauze applied over the topical agents on the wound. The number of gauze layers depends on:

- Depth of the injury
- Amount of drainage expected
- Area injured
- Patient's MOBILITY
- Frequency of dressing changes

The gauze layers are held in place with roller-type gauze bandages applied in a distal to proximal direction or with circular net fabrics. Cover gauze dressings on the patient's extremities with elastic wraps, especially if the patient is ambulatory. Dressings are generally changed and are reapplied every 12 to 24 hours after thoroughly cleaning the areas.

Biologic Dressings. Biologic dressings are often used for temporary wound coverage and closure. These dressings are skin or membranes obtained from human tissue donors (homograft or allograft) or animals (heterograft or xenograft). When applied over open wounds, a biologic dressing adheres and promotes healing or prepares the wound for permanent skin graft coverage.

Various biologic materials are used in healing partial-thickness and granulating full-thickness wounds that are clean and free of eschar. The type of biologic dressing selected depends on the type of wound to be covered and the availability of the material.

Homografts, also called *allografts,* are human skin obtained from a cadaver and provided through a skin bank. Disadvantages to the use of homografts are the high costs and the risk for transmitting a bloodborne infection.

Heterografts, also called *xenografts,* are skin obtained from another species. Pigskin (porcine) is the most common heterograft and is compatible with human skin. Pigskin is assessed daily for adherence and need for replacement. Fig. 26-12 shows a small burn covered with a porcine dressing.

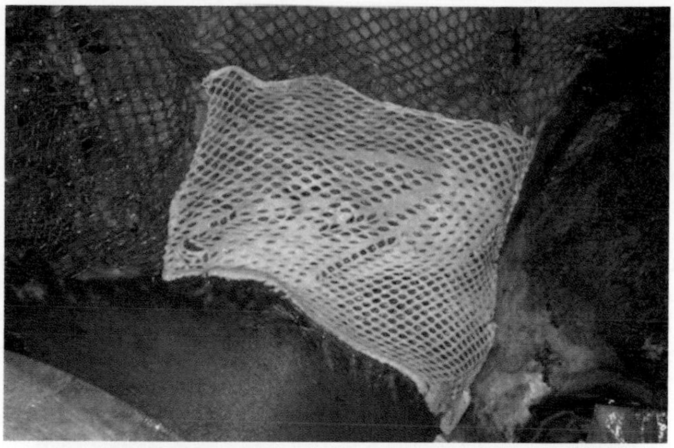

FIG. 26-12 Burn wound covered with a porcine dressing.

Cultured skin can be grown from a small specimen of epidermal cells from an unburned area of the patient's body. The cells are grown in a laboratory to produce cell sheets that can be grafted on the patient to generate a permanent skin surface. The length of time for culturing and growing the skin is long, and the cell sheets are fragile. This process is very costly.

Artificial skin is a substance with two layers—a Silastic epidermis and a porous dermis made from beef collagen and shark cartilage. After the artificial skin is applied to a clean, excised wound surface, fibroblasts move into the collagen portion and create a structure similar to normal dermis. The artificial dermis slowly dissolves and is replaced with blood vessels and connective tissue *(neodermis).* The neodermis supports a standard autograft placed over it when the Silastic layer is removed.

Biosynthetic Wound Dressings. Biosynthetic wound dressings are a combination of biosynthetic and synthetic materials. Biobrane is commonly used and effective in the treatment of clean superficial partial-thickness burns such as scalds, as a covering for meshed autografts, and as a donor site dressing. It is made up of a nylon fabric that is partially embedded into a silicone film. Collagen is incorporated into both the silicone and the nylon components. The nylon fabric comes into contact with the wound surface and adheres to it until epithelialization has occurred. The porous silicone film allows exudates to pass through.

Synthetic Dressings. Synthetic dressings are made of solid silicone and plastic membranes. They are applied directly to the surface of a prepared wound and remain in place until they fall off or are removed. Many of these dressings are transparent or translucent, and the wound can be inspected without removing the dressing. PAIN is reduced at the site because these agents also prevent contact of the wound's nerve endings with air. These dressings also are used to cover donor sites where skin was obtained for autografting.

Transparent film is the dressing commonly used for the care of donor site wounds (Fig. 26-13). This dressing type promotes faster healing with low INFECTION rates, minimal PAIN, and reduced cost.

Surgical Management. Grafting is used for wound closure when full-thickness injuries cannot close and when natural healing would result in loss of joint function, an unacceptable cosmetic appearance, or a high potential for wound recurrence. Successful skin grafting requires a clean and granulating or freshly excised wound bed. Partial-thickness (split-thickness) or full-thickness strips of skin are removed from the donor area, transferred to the ulcer, and sutured or stapled in place. Full-thickness free grafts and myocutaneous flaps are used to cover deep, massive ulcers or ulcers in which vital structures, such as bone or tendon, are exposed.

Surgical management of burn wounds involves excision and wound covering. Surgical excision is performed early in the postburn period. Autografting by taking an area of the patient's healthy skin with intact TISSUE INTEGRITY and transplanting it to an excised burn wound may be performed throughout the acute phase when wounds are ready and donor sites are available. Early grafting reduces the time patients are at risk for INFECTION and sepsis.

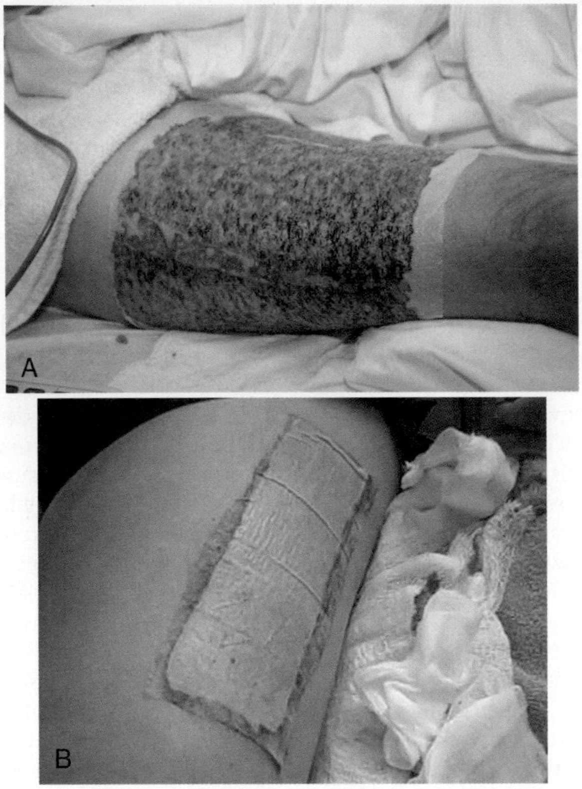

FIG. 26-13 Donor sites covered with dressings. **A,** Transparent dressing. **B,** Xeroform dressing.

Surgical Excision. Surgical excision is a common treatment for full-thickness and deep partial-thickness wounds. The patient is taken to the operating room within the first 5 days after injury and again as needed until all wounds are closed permanently.

The surgeon excises the burn wound usually by removing very thin layers of the necrotic burn surface until bleeding tissue is encountered. (Bleeding indicates that a bed of healthy dermis or subcutaneous fat has been reached.) For very deep burns, the surgeon cuts away the wound to the level of superficial fascia. Blood loss is minimal, and grafting is usually successful.

Wound Covering. Permanent skin coverage for large full-thickness injuries occurs by applying an autograft. Skin for an autograft is taken from the patient's body. The surgeon removes a piece of skin from a remote unburned area of the body and transplants it to cover the burn wound. Skin grafts are generally of split thickness, and a partial-thickness injury is formed at the site of surgical removal (the *donor site*). Grafts are placed either on a clean granulated bed or over an area from which dead tissue has just been removed.

Patients with larger burns may have only 5% to 20% of the skin surface available to use for covering the 80% to 95% burned area. Coverage for these wounds may require either repeated skin removal from the same donor site (with time allowed between harvests for healing) or meshing of the split-thickness skin grafts (Fig. 26-14). This technique allows a small graft to be stretched to cover a larger area. Healing time is slower for a meshed graft because the skin must fill in open meshed areas (interstices), as well as attach to the granulation bed.

After surgery, graft sites are immobilized with bulky cotton pressure dressings for 3 to 5 days to allow vascularization, or "take," of the newly grafted skin. Do not disturb the dressing, and encourage elevation and complete rest of the grafted area to allow blood vessels to connect the graft with the wound bed. Any activity that might cause movement of the dressing against the body and separation of the graft from the wound is prohibited.

After dressings are removed, monitor the graft for indications of failure to vascularize, nonadherence to the wound, or graft necrosis. A dusky color or sharp line of color change suggests inadequate venous or lymphatic drainage. Other techniques to monitor trends of blood flow in the graft, depending on the graft's location, include pulse oximetry, laser

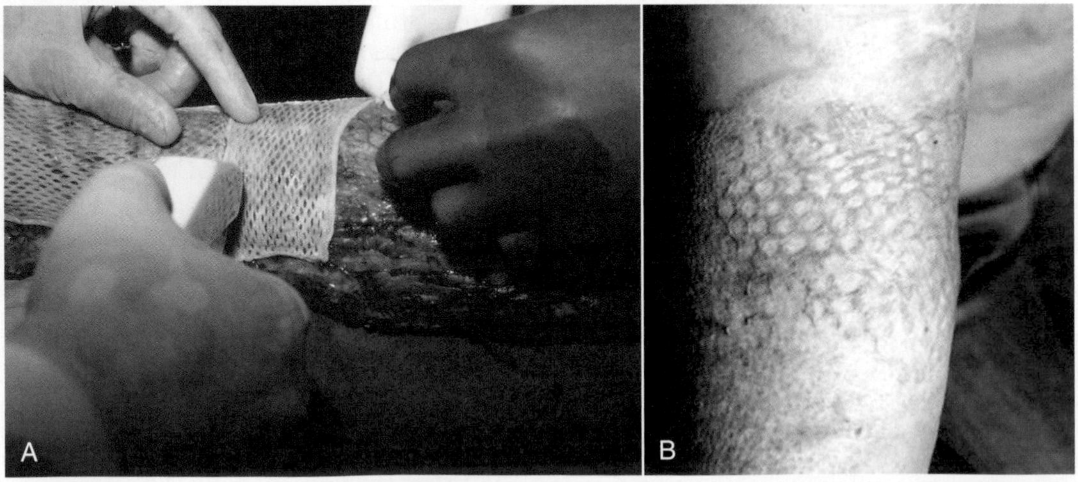

FIG. 26-14 The typical appearance of meshed autografts. **A,** Appearance of meshed autograft at application. **B,** Appearance of meshed autograft after healing.

Doppler imaging, ultrasonography, and transcutaneous oxygen determination.

Grafts and donor sites on posterior body surfaces present special problems. For the graft to become fully vascularized or for the donor sites to dry, the patient must be immobilized in a side-lying or prone position for 7 to 10 days.

An alternative to this positioning is the use of special low-pressure or air-fluidized beds, such as the Clinitron bed or KinAir bed, which not only reduce ischemia of the graft while the patient is supine but also help prevent breakdown of intact skin.

Minimizing Infection. Burn wound INFECTION occurs through **auto-contamination**, in which the patient's own normal flora overgrows and invades other body areas; and **cross-contamination**, in which organisms from other people or environments are transferred to the patient.

Planning: Expected Outcomes. The patient is expected to remain free from INFECTION and not develop sepsis. Indicators are that the patient has only mild or none of these manifestations:

- Foul-smelling discharge
- Fever
- Blood culture colonization
- Wound site colonization
- White blood cell count elevation

Interventions. Interventions focus on preventing INFECTION and removing infected tissue.

Nonsurgical Management. *Priority nursing interventions include using principles of INFECTION control to prevent transmission, providing a safe environment, and monitoring for early detection of infection.* Drug therapy, isolation therapy, and environmental management are strategies for preventing and managing infection.

Drug Therapy for Infection Prevention. Burn wound conditions promote the growth of *Clostridium tetani,* and all burn patients are at risk for this deadly INFECTION. Tetanus toxoid, 0.5 mL given IM, enhances immunity to *C. tetani* and is routinely given on admission. Administration of tetanus immune globulin (human) (HyperTet) is recommended when the patient's tetanus immunization status is not known.

Topical antimicrobial drugs are used for INFECTION prevention in burn wounds. Chart 26-5 lists commonly used agents. The expected outcome of this therapy is to reduce bacterial growth in the wound and prevent sepsis. A variety of agents can be used. Some topicals come in a form of ointments and creams (e.g., silver sulfadiazine, Sulfamylon, bacitracin) and need to be applied once or twice daily (Silverstein et al., 2011). Other products such as Acticoat, Mepilex Ag, and Aquacel Ag contain antimicrobials, which release over a period of several days and can be left on the wound for up to 7 days, thus eliminating the need for daily dressing changes.

Drug Therapy for Treatment of Infection. Systemic antibiotics are used when burn patients have symptoms of an actual INFECTION, including septicemia. Broad-spectrum antibiotics are given until the results of blood cultures and sensitivity status are available. At that time, antibiotics that are effective against the specific organism(s) causing the infection are used. Often burn patients require a higher dose of these drugs to maintain effective blood levels. Peak and trough blood levels may be used to determine treatment effectiveness and risk for toxicity.

Providing a Safe Environment. Providing a safe environment can include isolation therapy, which is used in some burn centers in the belief that it reduces cross-contamination. More often, it involves coordinating all members of the health care team in the use of asepsis and monitoring for early recognition of actual infection. Proper and consistent handwashing is the most effective technique for preventing INFECTION transmission.

Use of asepsis requires all health care personnel to wear gloves during all contact with open wounds. The use of sterile versus clean gloves for routine wound care varies by agency and is a matter of debate. Regardless of sterility, change gloves when handling wounds on different areas of the body and between handling old and new dressings.

The equipment on burn units is not shared among patients. Disposable items (e.g., pillows, dishes) are used as much as possible. Assign any equipment used in daily routine care (e.g., blood pressure cuffs, stethoscopes) to each patient for the duration of his or her stay. Daily cleaning of the equipment and general housekeeping are essential for INFECTION control. All other equipment must be cleaned after use on one patient and before use on another. Because *Pseudomonas* has been found in plants, the presence of plants and flowers is prohibited. Some burn units do not permit patients to eat raw foods (e.g., salads, fruit, pepper) to reduce exposure to organisms. Rugs and upholstered articles harbor organisms, and their use is restricted.

Visitors are restricted when the patient is immunosuppressed. Ill people, small children, and other patients should not come into direct contact with the burn patient. Some burn units recommend that all visitors wear protective clothing (gowns, gloves, masks, and shoe and hair covers) in the burn patient's room, but no data support the effectiveness of this approach.

Early detection involves careful monitoring of the burn wounds at each dressing change. Examine all wounds for these manifestations of INFECTION:

- Pervasive odor
- Color changes—focal, dark red, brown discoloration in the eschar
- Change in texture
- Purulent drainage
- Exudate
- Sloughing grafts
- Redness of wound edges extending to nonburned skin

Laboratory cultures and biopsies are recommended. Quantitative biopsies of the eschar and granulation tissue are performed routinely to monitor the growth of organisms.

Surgical Management. Infected burn wounds with colony counts at or near 10^5 colonies per gram of tissue may be life threatening, even with antibiotic therapy. Surgical excision of the wound may be needed to control these infections.

NCLEX EXAMINATION CHALLENGE

Safe and Effective Care Environment

Which action by the nurse changing the dressings on the client who has burns on the right arm, the left arm, and the upper chest is most effective at preventing auto-contamination?

A. Changing gloves after cleaning and dressing one wound area before cleaning and dressing the next wound area.
B. Using sterile gloves to remove the old dressings and changing to fresh sterile gloves before applying the new dressings.
C. Ensuring that the blood pressure cuff used on another client is thoroughly cleaned before using it on this client.
D. Warning the client's family not to bring fresh fruits and vegetables or house plants into the client's environment.

CHART 26-5 Common Examples of Drug Therapy

Burn Wounds

TOPICAL DRUG	ACTION	INTERVENTIONS
Silver sulfadiazine (Silvadene, Thermazene)	Adheres to bacterial cell membranes inhibiting DNA synthesis and bacterial replication	Watch for allergic reaction causing a drop in white blood cell count. Do not use if reaction to sulfonamide has occurred. Use on deep partial-thickness or full-thickness wounds. Monitor wounds for infection.
Collagenase (Santyl) with polysporin powder	Digests collagen in necrotic tissue	Apply once a day. Use on partial-thickness wounds with eschar. Monitor wounds for infection. May be used with barrier dressing such as Xeroform.
Mafenide acetate (Sulfamylon)	Bacteriostatic action against many gram-positive and gram-negative organisms	Premedicate for pain before application. Monitor blood gas and serum electrolyte levels. Monitor wounds for infection.
Nitrofurazone (Furacin)	Wide-spectrum antibacterial agent	Observe closely for signs of allergic reaction and evidence of superinfection.
Gentamicin sulfate (Garamycin, Gentamar)	Aminoglycoside antibacterial that inhibits bacterial protein synthesis and results in bactericidal responses	Nephrotoxic; monitor kidney function closely, especially changes in serum creatinine and blood urea nitrogen. Ototoxic; monitor hearing weekly.
Polymyxin B-bacitracin (Poly-Bac, Polysporin)	Inhibits bacterial cell wall synthesis and destroys bacterial membranes, leading to bacterial killing effects	Apply every 2-8 hours to keep area moist.
Acticoat	Releases antimicrobial silver ions when moistened with sterile water	Do not use with oil-based products or other antimicrobials. Do not use for any patient with a known sensitivity to any of the components of this drug. May dry out and adhere to wound surface; soak off to remove.
PolyMem	Dressing material containing silver granules that suppress bacterial growth	Normally leave in place for 7 days. Remove earlier if exudate is visible through outer membrane. Use on partial-thickness wounds and on donor sites. Cover with a secondary dressing. Monitor wounds for infection.
Aquacel Ag	Dressing material that releases ionic silver in a controlled manner as exudate is absorbed into dressing to support wound healing	Use on partial-thickness wounds and on donor-sites. Cover with a secondary dressing. Do not use for patients who have allergic reactions to the dressing or any of its components. Moisten with sterile water or normal saline to ease removal. Do not use with oil-based products.
Mepilex Ag	Dressing material containing silver ions that begin to inactivate wound pathogens within 30 minutes of application	Do not use along with oxidizing agents such as hydrogen peroxide. Cover with secondary dressing. May be used with partial-thickness burns, full-thickness burns, skin grafts, and donor-sites.

Minimizing Weight Loss

Planning: Expected Outcomes. The patient is expected to maintain adequate nutrient intake for meeting the body's calorie needs. Indicators include that the patient should have mild or no deviations from the normal ranges for:

- Weight/height ratio
- Food intake
- Hematocrit and hemoglobin
- Serum albumin and prealbumin
- Blood glucose

Interventions. Interventions include calculating the patient's calorie needs and providing an adequate daily source of calories and nutrients that the patient can ingest. Coordinate with a registered dietitian to meet the expected outcomes regarding the patient's NUTRITION status. Therapy begins with calculating the patient's current daily calorie needs. Several formulas and charts are used for this calculation. Nutrition requirements for a patient with a large burn area can exceed 5000 kcal/day. Not meeting this need leads to very rapid weight loss (Williams et al., 2011). In addition to a high-calorie intake, a diet high in protein is needed for wound healing. Work with the dietitian and the patient to plan additions to standard nutrition patterns.

Oral diet therapy may be delayed for several days after the injury until the GI tract is motile. Nasoduodenal tube feedings are often started soon after admission. Beginning enteral feedings early helps decrease weight loss, gut atrophy, bacterial translocation, and sepsis. This type of supplement prevents NUTRITION deficits in severely burned patients.

Encourage patients who can eat solid foods to ingest as many calories as possible. Consider the patient's preferences with diet planning and food selection. Encourage patients to request food whenever they feel they can eat, not just according to the hospital's standard meal schedule. Offer frequent high-calorie,

CHART 26-6 **Best Practice for Patient Safety & Quality Care** QSEN

Positioning to Prevent Contractures

AFFECTED BODY PART	POSITION OF FUNCTION	INTERVENTION
Head and neck	Hyperextension	No pillow. Place a towel roll under the patient's neck or shoulder. Neck splint.
Posterior neck	Flexion	Have patient turn the head from side to side.
Upper chest and chest	Shoulder retraction	Place patient in supine position. Place a folded towel under the spine, between the scapulae.
Lateral trunk	Flexion to uninvolved side	Place patient supine with arm on the affected side up over the head.
Anterior shoulder	Abduction and external rotation	Maintain the upper arm at 90 degrees of abduction from the lateral aspect of the trunk.
Posterior shoulder	Slight flexion and interior rotation	Keep the arm slightly behind the midline.
Axilla	Abduction with 10- to 15-degree forward flexion and external rotation	Support the abducted arm with suspension from IV pole or bedside table. Axilla splint.
Elbow	Extension and supination	Keep the joint in the extended position.
Wrist	30 to 45 degrees of extension	Use a splint.
Fingers		
MP joints	70 to 90 degrees of flexion	Use a splint.
PIP and DIP joints	Extension	Use a splint.
Ankle	90 degrees of dorsiflexion	Use a padded footboard or splint with heels free of pressure.
Legs	15 to 20 degrees of abduction	Place small pillow between legs.
Hip	Extension and neutral rotation	Place patient supine with lower extremity extended. Use trochanter roll. Use foam wedge along lateral aspect of thigh.

DIP, Distal interphalangeal; *MP,* metatarsophalangeal; *PIP,* proximal interphalangeal.

high-protein supplemental feedings. Keep an accurate calorie count for foods and beverages that are actually ingested by the patient.

Patients who cannot swallow but who have adequate gastric motility may meet calorie and NUTRITION needs through enteral tube feedings (see Chapter 60). Parenteral nutrition may be used when the GI tract is not functional or when the patient's nutrition needs cannot be met by oral and enteral feeding. This method is used as a last resort because it is invasive and can lead to infectious and metabolic complications.

Maintaining Mobility

Planning: Expected Outcomes. The patient with a burn injury is expected to maintain or regain an optimal MOBILITY. Indicators include that the patient has minimal limitations in these actions:

- Muscle movement
- Joint MOBILITY
- Walking
- Self-positioning

Interventions. Interventions focus on maintaining or achieving the patient's preburn range of joint motion and MOBILITY and preventing contracture formation.

Nonsurgical Management. Nonsurgical management includes the nursing interventions of positioning, range-of-motion exercises, ambulation, and pressure dressings.

Positioning is critical for patients with burn injuries because the position of comfort for the patient is often one of joint flexion, which leads to contracture development. Maintain the patient in a neutral body position with minimal flexion. Best practices for preventing contractures are listed in Chart 26-6. Splints and other devices may be used to maintain good positioning of the hands, elbows, knees, neck, and axillae.

Range-of-motion exercises to maintain MOBILITY are performed actively at least 3 times a day. If the patient cannot move a joint actively, perform passive range-of-motion exercises. Give burned hands special attention. Urge the patient to perform active range-of-motion exercises for the hand, thumb, and fingers every hour while he or she is awake.

Ambulation is started as soon as possible after the fluid shifts have resolved because it maintains MOBILITY, inhibits bone density loss, strengthens muscles, stimulates immune function, promotes ventilation, and prevents many complications. Patients with attached equipment (IV catheters, nasogastric tubes, ECG leads, extensive dressings) can ambulate with preparation and assistance. This activity is performed 2 or 3 times a day and progresses in length each time.

Compression dressings are applied after grafts heal to help prevent contractures and tight hypertrophic scars, which can inhibit MOBILITY. They also inhibit venous stasis and edema in areas with decreased lymph flow. Compression dressings may be elastic wraps or specially designed, custom-fitted, elasticized clothing that provides continuous pressure. Fig. 26-15 shows such a garment. For best effectiveness, pressure garments must be worn at least 23 hours a day, every day, until the scar tissue

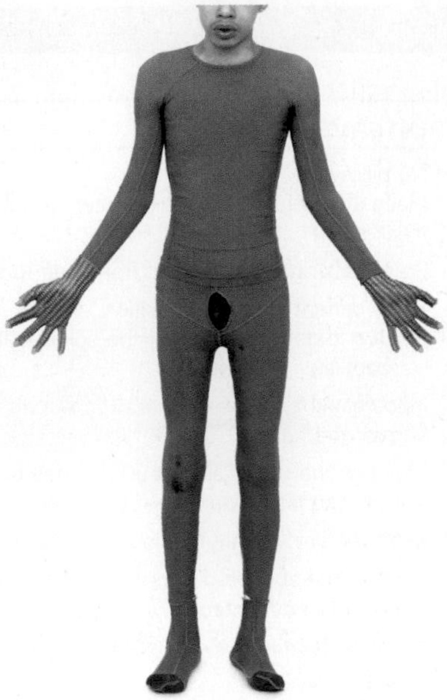

FIG. 26-15 A patient wearing full-body compression garments.

is mature (12 to 24 months). They can be uncomfortable with itchiness and increased warmth. Reinforce to the patient and family that wearing pressure garments is beneficial in saving mobility and reducing scarring.

Surgical Management. Surgical management restores MOBILITY rather than prevents immobility. Surgical release of contractures is commonly performed in the neck, axilla, elbow flexion areas, and hand. Specific surgical procedures vary for each patient.

Nursing responsibilities include interventions to prevent contractures from re-forming, as well as the care of new grafts and suture lines. Constantly reinforce the need for the patient to adhere to exercise and splinting regimens to prevent the recurrence of joint immobility.

Supporting Positive Self-Image

Planning: Expected Outcomes. After intervention, the patient with a burn injury is expected to have a positive perception of his or her own appearance, body functions, and self-worth. Indicators include that the patient should consistently demonstrate these behaviors:

- Willingness to touch the affected body part
- Adjustment to changes in body function
- Willingness to use strategies to enhance appearance and function
- Successful progression through the grieving process
- Use of support systems

Interventions. Nonsurgical and surgical interventions can assist patients who have self-image problems as a result of burn injury.

Nonsurgical Management. Understanding the stages of grief is helpful in managing care for the patient with burns. Assess which stage of grief the patient is currently experiencing, and help interpret his or her behaviors. The patient often is unaware of or is confused by his or her feelings. Reassure the patient that feelings of grief, loss, anxiety, anger, fear, and guilt are normal. The patient may be grieving the loss of body parts, appearance, role identity, social identity, and family members. Coordinate with other health care team members (e.g., psychologist/psychiatrist, social worker, clergy or religious leader) to address these issues.

Accept the physical and psychological features of the patient. Present patients and families with realistic expected outcomes for the patient's functional capacity and physical appearance. Provide information sessions and counseling for the family to identify patterns of support. Facilitate the patient's use of these systems and the development of new support systems. Make referrals to support groups. Evaluate the effectiveness and use of support resources throughout the course of recovery.

Engaging in decision making and independent activities fosters feelings of self-worth. Plan and encourage the patient's active participation in care activities. Assist family members to understand that it is more beneficial for the patient to perform these activities than to have them performed by someone else. Urge families to include the patient in family decision making to the same degree that he or she participated in this process before the injury.

Surgical Management. Reconstructive and cosmetic surgery can be performed many years after the burn injury. Restoring function and improving appearance through surgical techniques often promote the patient's positive self-image and self-worth. Many patients have unrealistic expectations of reconstructive surgery and envision an appearance identical or equal in quality to the preburn state. Teach the patient and family about expected cosmetic outcomes.

REHABILITATIVE PHASE OF BURN INJURY

Although rehabilitation efforts are started at the time of admission, the technical rehabilitative phase begins with wound closure and ends when the patient achieves his or her highest level of functioning. The emphasis is on the psychosocial adjustment of the patient, the prevention of scars and contractures, and the resumption of preburn activity, including resuming work, family, and social roles. This phase may take years or even last a lifetime as patients adjust to permanent limitations (Dahl et al., 2012).

❖ PATIENT-CENTERED COLLABORATIVE CARE

Although attention is placed first on the physical interventions for the burn injury, psychological care is equally important. Continue to provide psychosocial support to the patient and family throughout hospitalization and in the rehabilitative phase.

Obtaining information from the patient and family aids in the assessment and diagnosis of psychological problems and directs management. Explore the patient's feelings about the burn injury. It is extremely difficult for patients to concentrate on the many tasks before them when obstacles such as guilt and grief are in the forefront.

Ask whether there is a history of psychological problems. To assist with a future plan of care, assess and document the type of coping mechanisms the patient has used successfully during times of stress. Also assess the patient's family unit and the history of interaction. Consider cultural and ethnic factors when planning psychosocial interventions.

Throughout the hospitalization, the patient progresses through a variety of stages and exhibits many feelings, including denial, regression, and anger. Assess the patient's feelings at each stage so appropriate plans of care can be implemented.

TABLE 26-7 Needs to Address Before Discharge of the Patient with Burns

• Early patient assessment • Financial assessment • Evaluation of family resources • Weekly discharge planning meeting • Psychological referral • Patient and family teaching (home care) • Designation of principal learners (specific family members or significant others who will help with care) • Development of teaching plan • Training for wound care	• Rehabilitation referral • Home assessment (on-site visit) • Medical equipment • Public health nursing referral • Evaluation of community resources • Visit to referral agency • Re-entry programs for school or work environment • Long-term care placement • Environmental interventions • Auditory testing • Speech therapy • Prosthetic rehabilitation

Community-Based Care

Discharge planning for the patient with a burn injury begins at admission to the hospital or burn center. The interdisciplinary team meets regularly to evaluate the progress of each discipline and help the patient reach mutually established discharge outcomes. Table 26-7 lists common discharge needs of the patient with burns.

Psychosocial Preparation. During the recovery period and for some time after discharge, patients with severe burn injuries often have psychological problems that require intervention. Such problems include post-traumatic stress disorder, sexual dysfunction, and severe depression. Assistance is coordinated with the patient, family, and health care team. Psychosocial assistance is best provided by a professional counselor with experience in helping burn patients.

One specific area to address with the patient is the reaction of others to the sight of healing wounds and disfiguring scars. Patients with facial burns are especially subjected to stares and other negative reactions from the public. Visits from friends and short public appearances before discharge may help the patient begin adjusting to this problem. Community reintegration programs can assist the psychosocial and physical recovery of the patient with serious burns.

Home Care Management. The patient with severe burns is discharged from the acute care setting when serious complications are resolved and minimal wound areas remain open. During the first weeks at home, the patient usually needs at least daily wound care, physical therapy, NUTRITION support, symptom management, and drug therapy.

Although the patient usually views going home positively, the problems of physical care and the psychological stresses from changes in appearance, role, function, and lifestyle may overwhelm the patient and family. Successful discharge depends on extensive planning and preparation of the patient, family, and home environment through education and the involvement of appropriate support agencies and services.

Preparation for discharge includes assessment of the family and home care situation from physical and social perspectives. Consider the needs of the patient when evaluating the home for cleanliness; access to bathing facilities, electricity, and running water; stairways; number of occupants; temperature control; and safety. If the burn injuries occurred in a house fire, a new residence may need to be established.

Self-Management Education. Education about burn care and living with the consequences of burn injuries begins when the patient is admitted to the hospital or burn center. A weekly plan for patient education is outlined; a positive outcome is progression toward independence for the patient and family. Critical for this outcome is teaching patients and family members to perform such care tasks as dressing changes. Allow patients and family members to first observe dressing changes, then to assist in performing the changes, and then to change the dressings independently under your supervision.

Before discharge, all people who will be involved in the patient's home care participate in discharge planning and teaching sessions. In addition to details about dressing changes, explain:

- Indications of INFECTION
- Drug regimens
- Proper use of prosthetic and positioning devices
- Correct application and care of pressure garments
- Comfort measures to reduce pruritus
- Dates for follow-up appointments

Health Care Resources. The health care team evaluates the family's capacity and willingness to assist in caring for the patient after discharge. A visiting nurse or case manager with extensive experience in providing burn care can assist the family with care problems arising at home. This nurse can help the family determine what special equipment, supplies, or services will be needed. The frequency of home visits depends on the patient's condition and the ability of family members to function as care providers. The home care nurse may need a brief visit to the patient while in the hospital and may need to observe burn wound care.

The home care of a patient after a serious burn often involves daily physical therapy and rehabilitation sessions at special centers. Address and resolve transportation problems before the patient is discharged.

When rehabilitation is prolonged, the patient may be discharged to a rehabilitation facility. Consult with the rehabilitation team, and provide copies of the care and teaching plans used with the patient.

◆ Evaluation: Outcomes

Evaluate the care of the patient with a burn injury on the basis of the identified priority patient problems. The expected outcomes include that the patient should:

- Maintain adequate oxygenation and circulation to all vital organs
- Maintain a patent airway
- Have cardiac output restored to normal
- Have PAIN alleviated or reduced
- Experience no further loss of skin TISSUE INTEGRITY
- Have wounds healed without complications
- Remain free from INFECTION
- Not experience sepsis
- Maintain an adequate NUTRITION for meeting the body's calorie needs
- Regain and maintain an optimal ability to move purposefully
- Have a positive perception of his or her own appearance and body functions

Specific indicators for these outcomes are listed for each priority patient problem in the Planning and Implementation section (see earlier).

NURSING CONCEPTS AND CLINICAL JUDGMENT REVIEW

What might you NOTICE if the patient is experiencing INFECTION as a result of a problem of protection from a burn injury?

- Change in burn wound, including:
  Pervasive odor
  Color changes—focal, dark red, brown discoloration in the eschar
  Change in texture
  Purulent drainage
  Exudate
  Sloughing grafts
  Redness of wound edges extending to nonburned skin
- Elevated temperature
- Change in sensation in burn wound
- Change in cognition or level of consciousness

What should you INTERPRET and how should you RESPOND to a patient experiencing INFECTION as a result of a problem of protection from a burn injury?

Perform and interpret physical assessment, including:

- Taking vital signs, especially temperature
- Checking for change in cognitive status or level of consciousness
- Assessing burn wound for changes in appearance or amount/type of exudate

Interpret laboratory values:

- Elevated white blood cell count
- Positive burn wound cultures
- Positive blood cultures

Respond by:

- Documenting indicators of infection
- Notifying health care professional
- Implementing appropriate infection protocols
- Assisting the patient and family to understand the rationale for infection protocols

On what should you REFLECT?

- Observe patient for evidence of response to antimicrobial therapy and infection protocols.
- Determine whether the infection occurred by auto-contamination or cross-contamination.
- Think about what staff and patient teaching focus could help reduce the occurrence of a wound infection in the future.

GET READY FOR THE NCLEX® EXAMINATION!

KEY POINTS

Review these Key Points for each NCLEX Client Needs Category.

Safe and Effective Care Environment

- Use strict aseptic technique when caring for patients who have open burn wounds to prevent INFECTION. **Safety** QSEN
- Monitor the patient's vital signs at least every 8 hours for indications of wound INFECTION or sepsis. (For patients with greater than 25% TBSA burn, monitor vital signs more frequently.) **Safety** QSEN
- Assess burn wounds at least daily for indicators of INFECTION. **Safety** QSEN
- Give prescribed opioid analgesics by the IV route during the resuscitation phase of burn recovery. **Safety** QSEN

Health Promotion and Maintenance

- Encourage all people to have and maintain home smoke and carbon monoxide detectors.
- Warn patients who smoke about not smoking in bed or in rooms where home oxygen is in use and not smoking when taking any substance that induces sedation (drugs or alcohol). **Safety** QSEN
- Instruct patients who have reduced sensation in hands or feet to use a bath thermometer to check water temperature before bathing. **Safety** QSEN
- Teach patients to avoid exposing burned skin to the sun or to temperature extremes. **Patient-Centered Care** QSEN
- Instruct everyone to set hot water tank temperatures to the manufacturer's recommendations. **Safety** QSEN

Psychosocial Integrity

- Allow patients time to grieve over a change in body image. **Patient-Centered Care** QSEN
- Reassure patients that PAIN will be managed effectively. **Patient-Centered Care** QSEN
- Explain all procedures to the patient and family.
- Assess the patient's and family's use of coping strategies related to burn injury, treatment, possible role changes, and possible outcomes. **Patient-Centered Care** QSEN
- Support the patient and family in coping with permanent changes in appearance and function. **Patient-Centered Care** QSEN
- Encourage the burn patient with wounds and scars to participate in self-care. **Patient-Centered Care** QSEN
- Allow patients who have lost family members, homes, or jobs time to grieve for these losses.

Physiological Integrity

- Assess the burn patient's airway and adequacy of breathing before assessing any other body system. **Safety** QSEN
- Keep an endotracheal kit or tracheostomy kit at the bedside of any patient with facial burns, burns inside the mouth, singed nasal hairs, or a "smoky" smell to the breath. **Safety** QSEN
- Notify the Rapid Response Team immediately if the patient with an inhalation injury becomes more breathless or audible wheezes disappear. **Safety** QSEN
- Give analgesics, sedatives, and antianxiety drugs to patients receiving paralytic drugs during mechanical ventilation. **Patient-Centered Care** QSEN

- Give half of the fluid volume calculated for the first 24 hours after burn injury in the first 8 hours postburn. **Evidence-Based Practice** QSEN
- Use laboratory data and clinical manifestations to determine the effectiveness of fluid resuscitation during the resuscitation phase of burn injury. **Evidence-Based Practice** QSEN
- Encourage the patient to actively participate in PAIN control measures. **Patient-Centered Care** QSEN
- Position patients to prevent contractures and promote joint function. **Evidence-Based Practice** QSEN
- Assist patients to ambulate several times each day as soon as the fluid shifts have resolved.
- Coordinate with the registered dietitian to meet the nutrition needs for the patient during the acute phase of burn injury. **Teamwork and Collaboration** QSEN
- Evaluate the patient's wound healing during the acute phase of burn injury. **Patient-Centered Care** QSEN
- Use appropriate positioning and range-of-motion interventions for prevention of MOBILITY problems in the patient with burns. **Patient-Centered Care** QSEN

CONCEPT OVERVIEW

Oxygenation

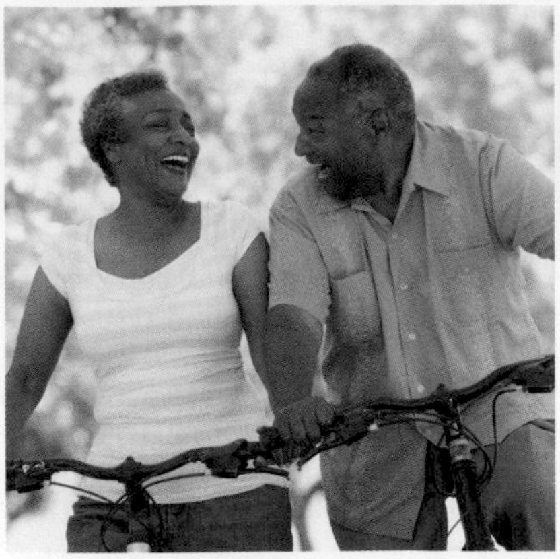

Meeting the body's need for oxygenation is dependent on the concepts of GAS EXCHANGE and PERFUSION (Giddens, 2013). All cells and tissues need oxygen to live and function. Some cells, such as brain cells and heart muscle cells, are very dependent on oxygen. Without oxygen, brain cells stop functioning and die in about 5 to 10 minutes. Other cells, such as skin cells, can live and function for many hours with low oxygen levels or even without oxygen. Skeletal muscle cells can survive for hours with low levels of oxygen but cannot function for very long without it.

The source of the oxygen for all body cells is the air we breathe into our lungs. The process of GAS EXCHANGE first occurs in the alveoli of lungs. The carbon dioxide generated in body cells as a result of metabolism diffuses from the blood into the alveoli where it is exhaled down its concentration gradient into atmospheric air. At the same time, atmospheric oxygen is inhaled into the alveoli where it then moves down its concentration gradient into capillary blood. These steps compose alveolar or pulmonary GAS EXCHANGE even though the exchange is not equal (not a one-for-one exchange between oxygen molecules and carbon dioxide molecules). Delivery of oxygen to the cells and tissues, PERFUSION, requires the pumping mechanism of the heart and the oxygen-carrying mechanism of the hemoglobin in red blood cells. Once PERFUSION delivers oxygen to the tissues, a second GAS EXCHANGE takes place with oxygen moving from capillary blood into cells at the same time that carbon dioxide leaves the cells and enters capillary blood.

In health, the need of body tissues for oxygen is balanced by the body's GAS EXCHANGE and PERFUSION systems (Fig. 1). When oxygen needs increase, such as during mild to moderate exercise, oxygen intake through the respiratory system and pulmonary GAS EXCHANGE increase to compensate (or adjust) and keep tissue oxygen PERFUSION in balance with cellular oxygen need (Fig. 2).

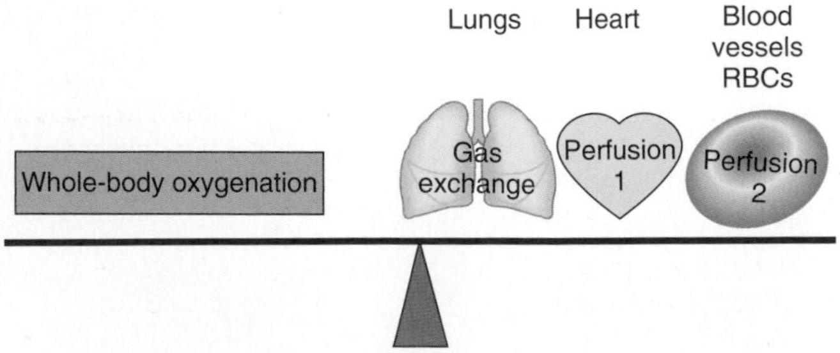

FIG. 1

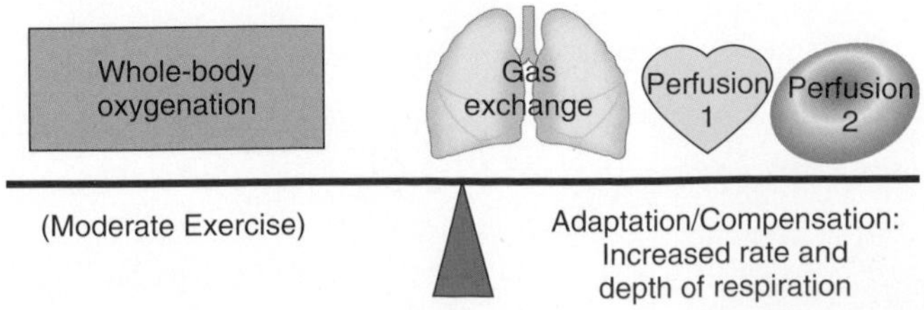

FIG. 2

When oxygen need increases as a result of heavy exercise or an illness in which metabolism is increased (and the person has a fever), all GAS EXCHANGE and PERFUSION systems must adjust by increasing their activity to match the increased oxygen need. When this compensation is perfect, the increased rate and depth of respiration, along with the increased heart rate and blood pressure, keep oxygenation in balance with oxygen need (Fig. 3).

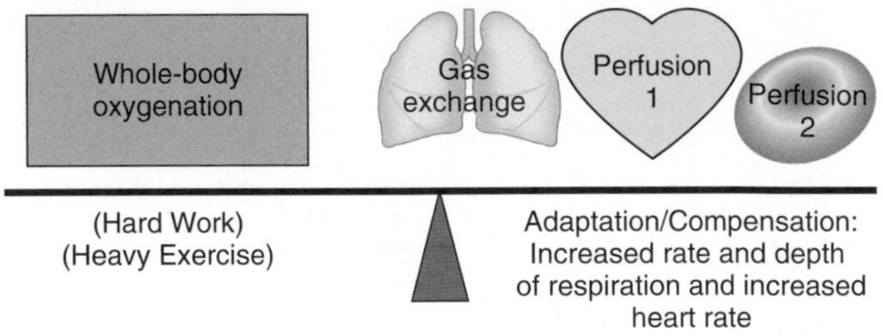

FIG. 3

Some health problems reduce the body's ability to compensate when oxygen need is greater than basic (basal) levels. For example, in a person who has asthma, the lungs may be able to take in enough oxygen to meet basic oxygen needs but cannot adjust or compensate when a greater oxygen intake is needed, such as during mild to moderate exercise (Fig. 4). In this situation, the heart and blood need to compensate *more* to increase delivery of the set amount of oxygen taken in (Fig. 5).

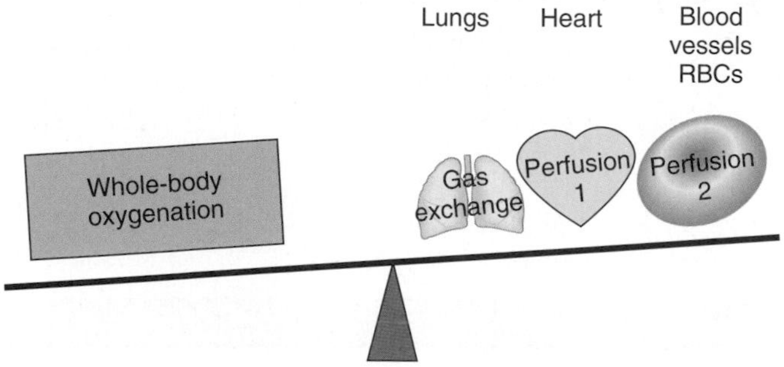

FIG. 4

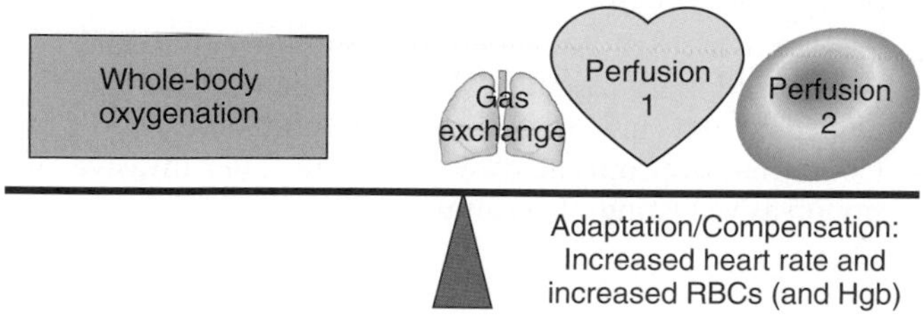

FIG. 5

In another situation, when the person has a cardiac problem and the heart rate alone cannot increase oxygen delivery during mild to moderate exercise (Fig. 6), his or her respiratory rate would have to increase more than usual to keep oxygen delivery in balance with oxygen need.

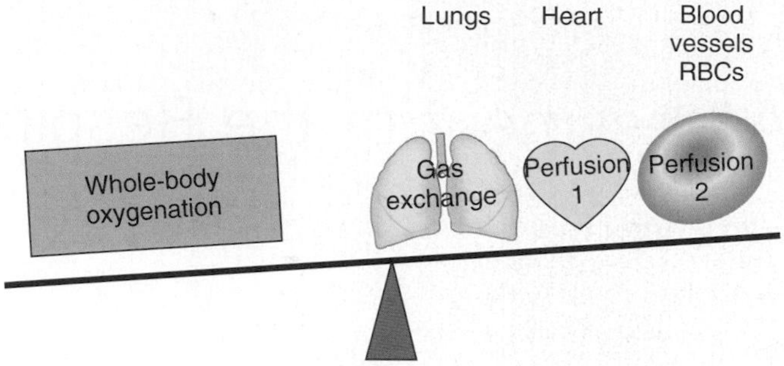

FIG. 6

What happens when any part of the oxygen intake (GAS EXCHANGE) or delivery systems (PERFUSION) has a problem that interferes with ensuring that the cells have enough oxygen? Consider a person with pneumonia who has great difficulty with pulmonary GAS EXCHANGE to the point that the body's basic oxygen need is not met. Even though the oxygen need is at a basic level, the need is unbalanced compared with pulmonary GAS EXCHANGE and oxygen PERFUSION. The person's compensation mechanisms are working (respiratory rate is increased, heart rate is increased) but are not completely effective. How could balance be restored? Interventions are needed to support the body's compensation efforts to restore balance.

The best way is to eliminate the pneumonia, which could take days even with proper drug therapy. Other ways involve (1) reducing oxygen need to the lowest possible level by having the patient rest and (2) improving pulmonary GAS EXCHANGE by increasing the percentage of oxygen in the air that he or she breathes (oxygen therapy) (Fig. 7).

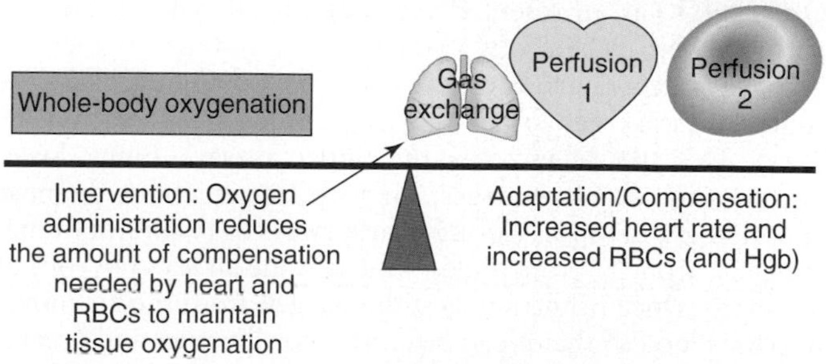

FIG. 7

27 CHAPTER

Assessment of the Respiratory System

Harry Rees

http://evolve.elsevier.com/Iggy/

PRIORITY CONCEPTS

- Gas Exchange
- Perfusion

LEARNING OUTCOMES

Health Promotion and Maintenance

1. Teach all people measures to take to protect the respiratory system, including the avoidance of tobacco use.

Psychosocial Integrity

2. Reduce the psychological impact for the patient and family regarding the assessment and testing of the respiratory system with regard to GAS EXCHANGE and PERFUSION.

Physiological Integrity

3. Perform a focused assessment of respiratory function, incorporating information about genetic risk and age-related changes affecting respiratory function.
4. Coordinate appropriate care for patients after invasive and noninvasive testing of respiratory function.

Oxygen (O_2) is an essential nutrient for all cells to live and perform their specific jobs. Oxygen intake with GAS EXCHANGE and PERFUSION depends on the respiratory system because the source of the oxygen for all body cells is the air we breathe (Fig. 27-1). This system includes the upper airways, lungs, lower airways, and alveolar air sacs. Air with oxygen enters the nose and mouth and moves through the airways or respiratory tubes (trachea, bronchi, bronchioles) and into the air sacs (alveoli) of the lungs. Once in the air sacs, the oxygen from the air moves into the blood so that it can be carried to all tissues and organs. Carbon dioxide (CO_2), the waste gas created in the tissues, moves from the blood into the lungs so it can be exhaled. All systems depend on adequate oxygen intake with GAS EXCHANGE for tissue PERFUSION. Any respiratory problem affects total body health and well-being.

HEALTH PROMOTION AND MAINTENANCE

Lung and breathing problems are common causes of death in North America (McCance et al., 2014). Some respiratory problems are chronic, and the patient has physical and lifestyle limitations. Many acute health problems, medical therapies, and surgeries adversely affect respiratory function temporarily or permanently. Exposure to inhalation irritants, especially to tobacco smoke, is the most common cause of chronic respiratory problems and physical limitations. In addition, cigarette smoking is a modifiable factor that greatly increases the risk for cardiovascular disease, stroke, and many types of cancer. Three compounds in cigarette smoke that have been implicated in the development of these serious diseases are tar, nicotine, and carbon monoxide. In the years after a patient has stopped smoking, his or her risk for respiratory-related disorders decreases significantly. Therefore assessing smoking habits, actively promoting smoking cessation, determining exposure to other inhalation irritants, and teaching people to protect the respiratory system are important nursing functions.

Assessing smoking habits begins by determining whether the patient is a current smoker or has ever smoked. The smoking history includes the number of cigarettes smoked daily, the duration of the smoking habit, and the age of the patient when smoking started even for patients who are not current smokers. Record the smoking history in **pack-years**, which is the number

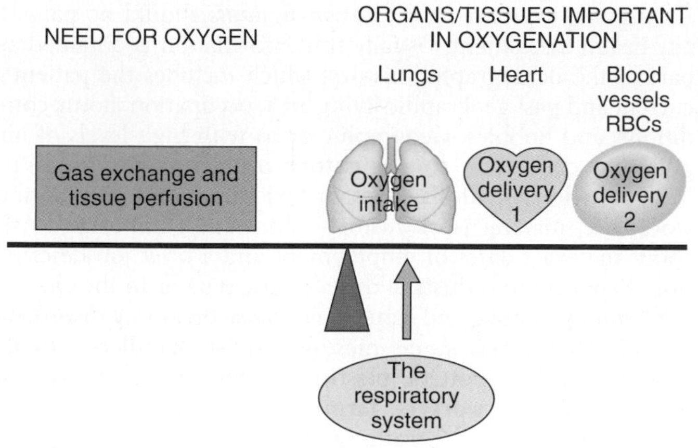

FIG. 27-1 Role of the respiratory system in the concepts of gas exchange and tissue perfusion. *RBCs,* Red blood cells.

of packs per day multiplied by the number of years the patient has smoked.

Be sure to ask those who do not currently smoke whether and to what extent they are exposed to the smoke of others. This passive smoking has two origins: direct exposure to smoke by being in the same environment with a person(s) who is actively smoking *(secondhand smoke· [SHS]);* and indirect exposure from smoke that clings to hair and clothing *(thirdhand smoke).* Both types of passive smoking contribute to health problems, especially when exposure occurs in small, confined spaces and is chronic.

Another category of cigarette smoking, particularly among younger adults, is *social smoking.* This term is used to describe people who claim to smoke cigarettes only in the presence of others, borrow rather than purchase cigarettes, prefer the company of nonsmokers, and do not smoke for stress relief (Butler et al., 2012). Often the social smoker does not consider himself or herself to be a smoker and must be asked specifically, "Do you ever smoke in social situations?" Although this type of smoking is intermittent, it can still have an adverse effect on respiratory and cardiovascular health and may lead to nicotine addiction.

Hookah or water pipe smoking is becoming more popular in North America. The highest incidence is among young people. Studies have determined that the exposure to inhaled toxins is as great or greater than with cigarette smoking. Although many cities have instituted smoking bans, water pipe smoking may be exempt, raising concerns for secondhand smoke exposure (Fiala et al., 2012).

E-cigarettes have emerged as an alternative to traditional cigarettes and are used as a method of quitting smoking. The cartridges within an e-cigarette, as well as the vapors produced, may contain nicotine or other toxins. Thus the safety for the user or the bystander has not been established. E-cigarettes are not currently an approved method of smoking cessation (Riker et al., 2012).

Promoting smoking cessation is a sensitive and sometimes uncomfortable issue for nurses and other health care professionals to approach with patients who smoke. However, this opportunity for a "teachable moment" may be the beginning support a patient needs to be successful in this healthful pursuit. Many acute care settings now have automatic smoking-cessation protocols that attach to the patient's electronic medical record

GENDER HEALTH CONSIDERATIONS

Patient-Centered Care QSEN

Gay men, lesbian women, and bisexual men and women report higher rates of smoking cigarettes, cigars, and cigarillos when compared with their heterosexual counterparts (King et al., 2012). The rate of smoking may be 2.0 to 2.5 times more likely among gay, bisexual, and transgender men than heterosexual men. Lesbian, bisexual, and transgender women may be 1.5 to 3.5 times more likely to smoke than heterosexual women, and lesbian, gay, bisexual, and transgender (LGBT) youth may pose the highest risk (American Lung Association, 2012). Concern exists that the LGBT community may not focus enough attention on prevention and smoking-cessation programs. Thus many LGBT people who smoke are highly susceptible to smoking-related health problems, such as chronic lung disease and throat and lung cancers. Therefore screening for smoking and tobacco-related health conditions is especially important when working with LGBT patients.

as soon as an active smoking history is recorded. The Centers for Medicare and Medicaid Services (CMS) no longer requires smoking cessation as part of their Core Measures. However, The Joint Commission requires documentation of screening for tobacco use and that a tobacco treatment program was offered or provided, as part of their quality measures.

Ask about the patient's desire to quit, past attempts to quit, and the methods used. Determine nicotine dependence by asking questions such as:

- How soon after you wake up in the morning do you smoke?
- Do you wake up in the middle of your sleep time to smoke?
- Do you find it difficult not to smoke in places where smoking is prohibited?
- Do you smoke when you are ill?

A variety of drug therapies are available over the counter and by prescription to help those addicted to nicotine to modify their behavior and stop smoking. Over-the-counter nicotine replacement therapies (NRTs) include nicotine-releasing transdermal patches, gums, and lozenges. Prescribed NRT products include nasal sprays and inhalers. NRT products have a success rate of smoking cessation between 50% and 70% (Grief, 2011). They have been shown to have the highest success rates when used in association with a smoking-cessation program. Chart 27-1 lists suggestions for you to use in providing support to the person interested in stopping cigarette smoking.

! NURSING SAFETY PRIORITY QSEN

Drug Alert

Teach people using drugs for nicotine replacement therapy that smoking while taking these drugs greatly increases circulating nicotine levels and the risk for stroke or heart attack.

Additional drug therapy for smoking cessation includes the oral drugs *bupropion* (Zyban) and *varenicline* (Chantix). Bupropion encourages smoking cessation by decreasing cravings and withdrawal manifestations as well as reducing the depression associated with nicotine withdrawal symptoms. Varenicline interferes with the nicotine receptors. This promotes smoking cessation by reducing the pleasure derived from nicotine and by reducing the manifestations of nicotine withdrawal.

CULTURAL CONSIDERATIONS

Patient-Centered Care QSEN

The prevalence of smoking remains higher among African Americans, blue-collar workers, and less-educated people than in the overall population of the United States. Smoking prevalence is highest among Northern Plains American Indians and Alaskan Natives. Development of culturally appropriate smoking-cessation programs as well as research examining barriers to cessation in these populations may help reduce this disparity.

CHART 27-1 Patient and Family Education: Preparing for Self-Management

Smoking Cessation

- Make a list of the reasons you want to stop smoking (e.g., your health and the health of those around you, saving money, social reasons).
- Set a date to stop smoking, and keep it. Decide whether you are going to begin to cut down on the amount you smoke or are going to stop "cold turkey." Whatever way you decide to do it, keep this important date!
- Ask for help from those around you. Find someone who wants to quit smoking and "buddy up" for support. Look for assistance in your community, such as formal smoking-cessation programs, counselors, and certified acupuncture specialists or hypnotists.
- Consult your health care provider about nicotine replacement therapy (e.g., patch, gum) or other pharmacologic therapy to assist in smoking cessation.
- Remove ashtrays and lighters from your view.
- Talk to yourself! Remind yourself of all the reasons you want to quit.
- Think of a way to reward yourself with the money you save from not smoking for a year.
- Avoid places that might tempt you to smoke. If you are used to having a cigarette after meals, get up from the table as soon as you are finished eating. Think of new things to do at times when you used to smoke (e.g., taking a walk, exercising, calling a friend).
- Find activities that keep your hands busy: needlework, painting, gardening, even holding a pencil.
- Take five deep breaths of clean, fresh air through your nose and out your mouth if you feel the urge to smoke.
- Keep plenty of healthy, low-calorie snacks, such as fruits and vegetables, on hand to nibble on. Try sugarless gum or mints as a substitute for tobacco.
- Drink at least eight glasses of water each day.
- Begin an exercise program with the approval of your health care provider. Be aware of the positive, healthy changes in your body since you stopped smoking.
- List the many reasons why you are glad that you quit. Keep the list handy as a reminder of the positive things you are doing for yourself.
- If you have a cigarette, think about what the conditions were that caused you to light it. Try and think of a strategy to avoid that (or those) conditions.
- Don't beat yourself up for backsliding; just face the next day as a new day.
- Think of each day without tobacco as a major accomplishment. It is!!

! NURSING SAFETY PRIORITY QSEN

Drug Alert

Both bupropion and varenicline carry a black box warning that use of these drugs can cause manic behavior and hallucinations. These drugs also may unmask serious mental health issues. Teach the patient prescribed either of these drugs and their families to report any change in behavior or thought processes to the prescriber immediately.

Assessing exposure to inhalation irritants should be part of any health assessment. Usually this information is obtained as part of the demographic history, which includes the patient's current and past geographic living area, occupation, home conditions, and hobbies. Geographic areas with high levels of air pollution contribute to respiratory problems. Exposures to dust, particles, chemicals, gases, or toxic fumes can occur in the workplace, making work history information important. Ask about the exact dates of employment and a brief job description. Exposure to industrial dusts of any type or to the chemicals found in smoke and fumes may cause breathing disorders. Bakers, coalminers, stone masons, cotton handlers, woodworkers, welders, potters, plastic and rubber manufacturers, printers, asbestos workers, farm workers, and steel foundry workers are at risk for breathing problems.

Ask about home conditions, such as the type of heat used (e.g., gas heater, wood-burning stove, fireplace, kerosene heater). Determine exposure to irritants (e.g., fumes, chemicals, animals, birds, air pollutants). Ask about hobbies such as painting, ceramics, model airplanes, refinishing furniture, or woodworking, which may expose the patient to harmful chemicals.

Protecting the respiratory system starts with making people aware of the sources of inhalation irritants. Teach people who live in areas with high levels of air pollution to remain indoors with windows closed on days when air quality is poor and not to engage in heavy physical activity. Teach people who have workplace or home exposure to inhalation irritants to wear masks during these exposures and to ensure the area is well ventilated.

ANATOMY AND PHYSIOLOGY REVIEW

The purpose of breathing is to ensure GAS EXCHANGE. This process has two parts: (1) oxygenation for tissue PERFUSION so that cells have enough oxygen to metabolize and generate energy; and (2) removal of carbon dioxide, the waste product of metabolism. The respiratory system also influences acid-base balance, speech, sense of smell, fluid balance, and temperature control. The lungs are also an excretory organ because they can also break down some toxins and eliminate them from the body during exhalation.

Upper Respiratory Tract

The upper airways include the nose, the sinuses, the pharynx, and the larynx (Fig. 27-2).

Nose and Sinuses

The nose is the organ of smell, with receptors from cranial nerve I *(olfactory)* located in the upper areas. The nose is rigid with a bony upper portion and a cartilaginous lower portion that can move to some extent. The septum divides the nose into two cavities that are lined with mucous membranes that have a rich blood supply. The **anterior nares** are the external openings into the nasal cavities. The posterior nares are openings from the nasal cavity into the throat.

The **turbinates** are three bones that protrude into the nasal cavities from the internal portion of the nose (see Fig. 27-2). Turbinates increase the total surface area for filtering, heating, and humidifying inspired air before it passes into the nasopharynx. Inspired air is humidified by the mucous membrane and is warmed by heat from the vascular network.

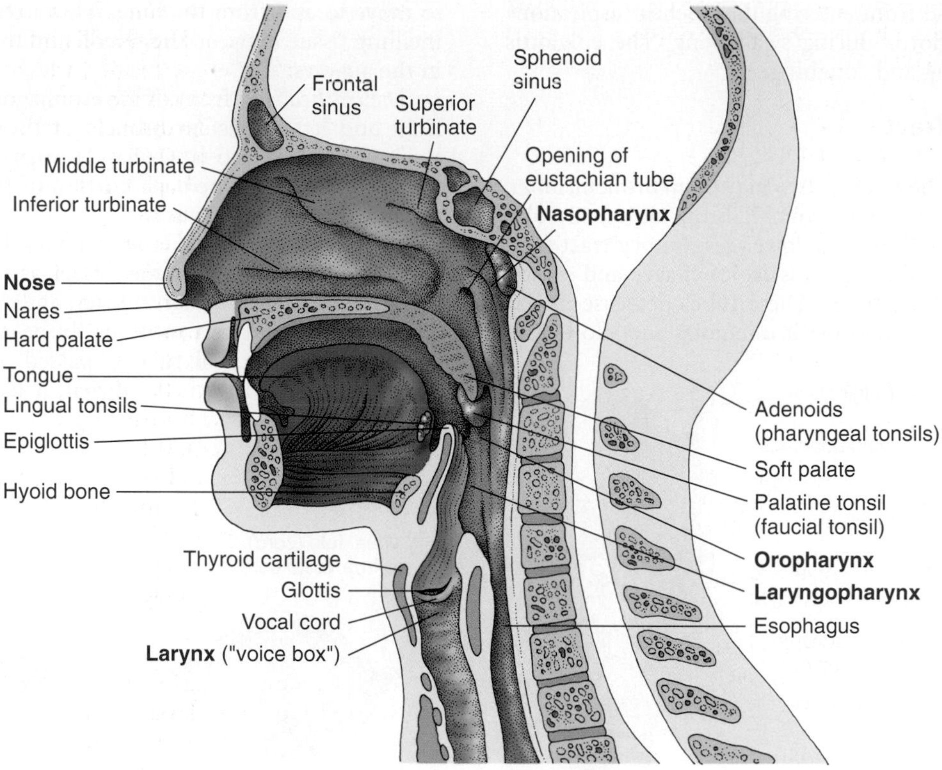

FIG. 27-2 Structures of the upper respiratory tract.

The paranasal sinuses are air-filled cavities within the bones that surround the nasal passages (Fig. 27-3). Lined with ciliated membrane, the sinuses provide resonance during speech, decrease the weight of the skull, and act as shock absorbers in the event of facial trauma.

Pharynx

The pharynx, or throat, is a passageway for both the respiratory and digestive tracts. It is located behind the oral and nasal cavities. The throat is divided into the nasopharynx, the oropharynx, and the laryngopharynx (see Fig. 27-2).

The nasopharynx is located behind the nose, above the soft palate. It contains the adenoids and the opening of the eustachian tube. The adenoids trap organisms that enter the nose or mouth. The eustachian tubes connect the nasopharynx with the middle ears and open during swallowing to equalize pressure within the middle ear.

The oropharynx is located behind the mouth, below the nasopharynx. It extends from the soft palate to the base of the tongue and is used for breathing and swallowing. The *palatine tonsils,* which are part of the immune system, are located on the sides of the oropharynx and protect against invading organisms.

The laryngopharynx is the area located behind the larynx from the base of the tongue to the esophagus. It is the dividing point between the larynx and the esophagus.

Larynx

The **larynx** is the "voice box" and is located above the trachea, just below the throat at the base of the tongue. It is composed of several cartilages (Fig. 27-4). The *thyroid cartilage* is the largest and is commonly called the "Adam's apple." The *cricoid cartilage,* which contains the vocal cords, lies below the thyroid cartilage. The *cricothyroid membrane* is located below the level of the vocal cords and joins the thyroid and cricoid cartilages. This site is used in an emergency for access to the lower airways. In this procedure, called a *cricothyroidotomy,* an opening is made between the thyroid and cricoid cartilage and results in a tracheostomy. The two *arytenoid* cartilages work with the thyroid cartilage in vocal cord movement.

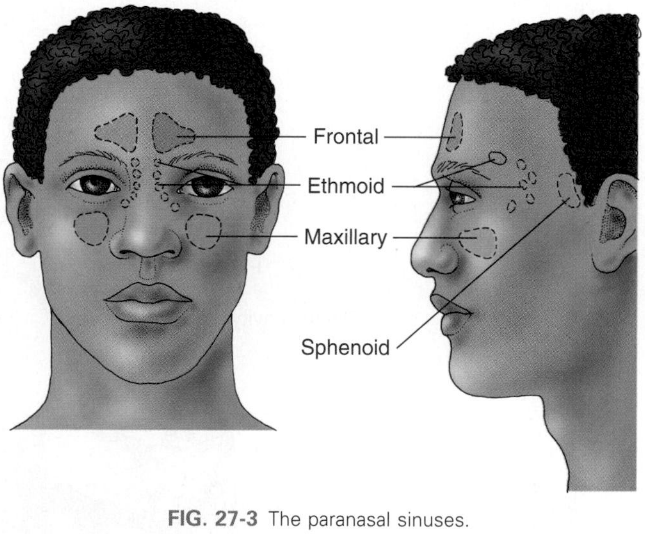

FIG. 27-3 The paranasal sinuses.

Inside the larynx are two pairs of vocal cords: the false vocal cords and the true vocal cords. The glottis is the opening between the true vocal cords (Fig. 27-5). The epiglottis is a small, elastic structure attached along one edge to the top of the larynx. It prevents food from entering the trachea (aspiration) by closing over the glottis during swallowing. The epiglottis opens during breathing and coughing.

Lower Respiratory Tract

Airways

The lower airways are the trachea; two mainstem bronchi; lobar, segmental, and subsegmental bronchi; bronchioles; alveolar ducts; and alveoli (Fig. 27-6). The lower respiratory tract *(tracheobronchial tree)* consists of muscle, cartilage, and elastic tissues forming branching tubes. These tubes decrease in size from the trachea to the respiratory bronchioles and allow gases to move to and from the lungs. GAS EXCHANGE takes place in the lung tissue between the alveoli and the lung capillaries, not in the airways.

The trachea is in front of the esophagus. It branches into the right and left mainstem bronchi at the *carina* junction. The trachea contains 6 to 10 C-shaped rings of cartilage. The open portion of the C is the back portion of the trachea and shares a wall with the esophagus.

The mainstem bronchi, or primary bronchi, begin at the carina and contain the same tissues as the trachea. The right bronchus is slightly wider, shorter, and more vertical than the left bronchus and can more easily be accidentally intubated when an endotracheal tube is passed. Also, when a foreign object is aspirated from the throat, it usually enters the right bronchus.

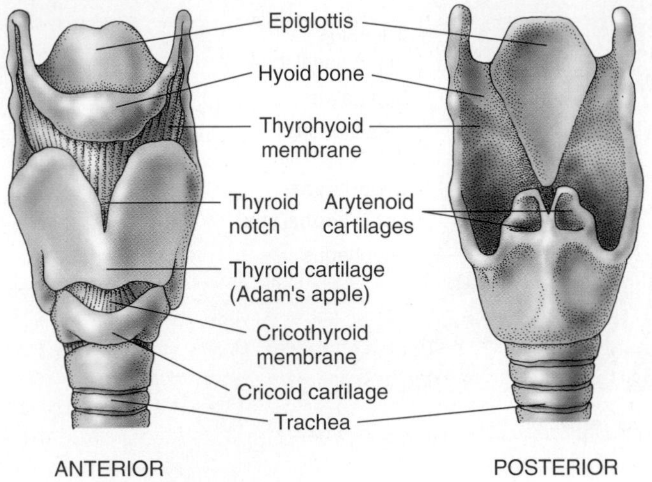

FIG. 27-4 Structures of the larynx.

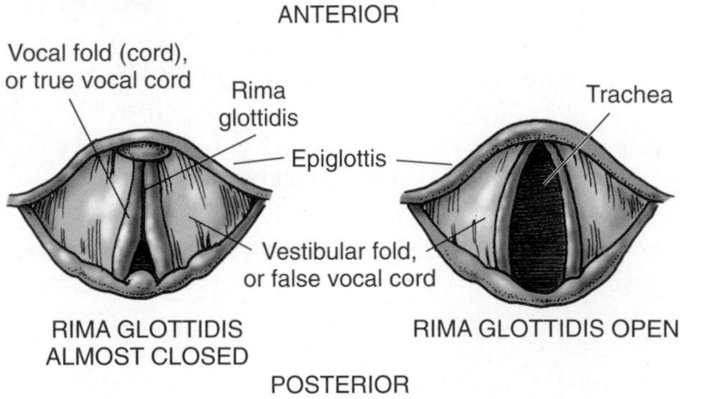

FIG. 27-5 Detail of the glottis (two vocal folds and the intervening space, the rima glottidis).

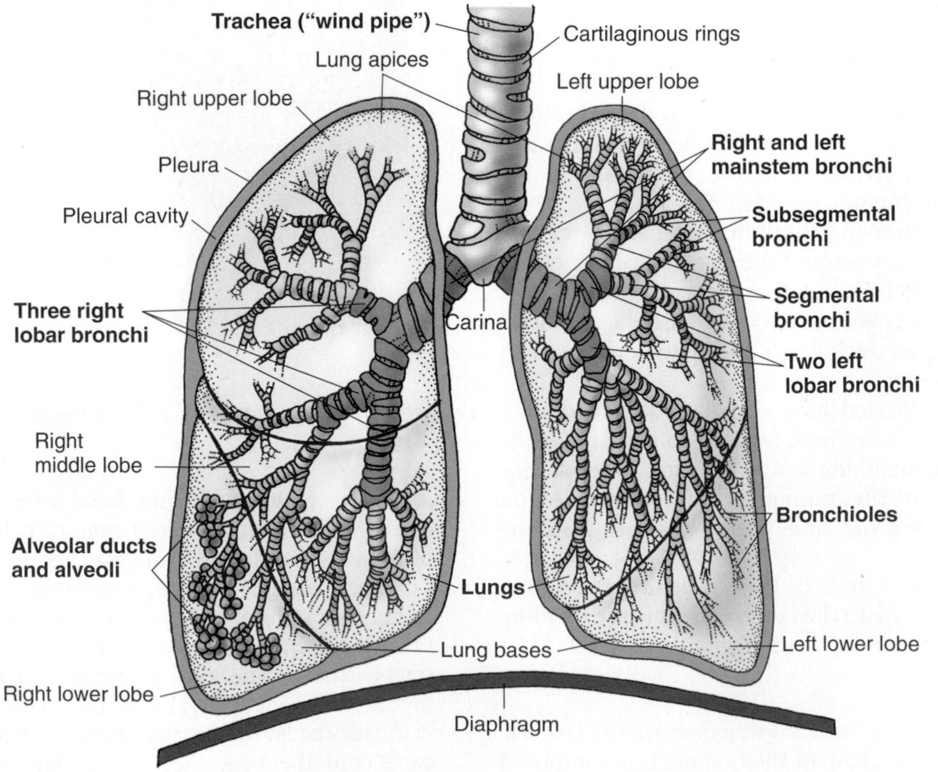

FIG. 27-6 Structures of the lower respiratory tract.

The mainstem bronchi branch into the secondary (lobar) bronchi that enter each of the five lobes of the two lungs. Each lobar bronchus branches into progressively smaller divisions. The cartilage rings of these lobar bronchi are complete and resist collapse. The bronchi are lined with a ciliated, mucus-secreting membrane that moves particles away from the lower airways.

The bronchioles branch from the secondary bronchi and divide into smaller and smaller tubes, which are the terminal and respiratory bronchioles (Fig. 27-7). These tubes have a small diameter, have no cartilage, and depend entirely on the elastic recoil of the lung to remain open.

Alveolar ducts branch from the respiratory bronchioles and resemble a bunch of grapes. Alveolar sacs arise from these ducts and contain groups of alveoli, which are the basic units of GAS EXCHANGE (see Fig. 27-7). A pair of healthy adult lungs has about 290 million alveoli, which are surrounded by lung capillaries. These numerous small alveoli normally make a large surface area for GAS EXCHANGE (about the size of a tennis court). **Acinus** is a term for the structural unit consisting of a respiratory bronchiole, an alveolar duct, and an alveolar sac.

The alveolar walls have cells called *type II pneumocytes* that secrete **surfactant,** a fatty protein that reduces surface tension in the alveoli. Without surfactant, **atelectasis** (alveolar collapse) occurs, reducing GAS EXCHANGE because the alveolar surface area is reduced.

Lungs

The lungs are elastic, cone-shaped organs located in the pleural cavity in the chest. The apex (top) of each lung extends above the clavicle; the base (bottom) of each lung lies just above the diaphragm. The lungs are composed of millions of alveoli and their related ducts, bronchioles, and bronchi. The right lung, which is larger and wider than the left, is divided into three lobes: upper, middle, and lower. The left lung is divided into only two lobes. About 60% to 65% of lung function occurs in the right lung. Any problem with the right lung interferes with GAS EXCHANGE and PERFUSION to a greater degree than a problem in the left lung.

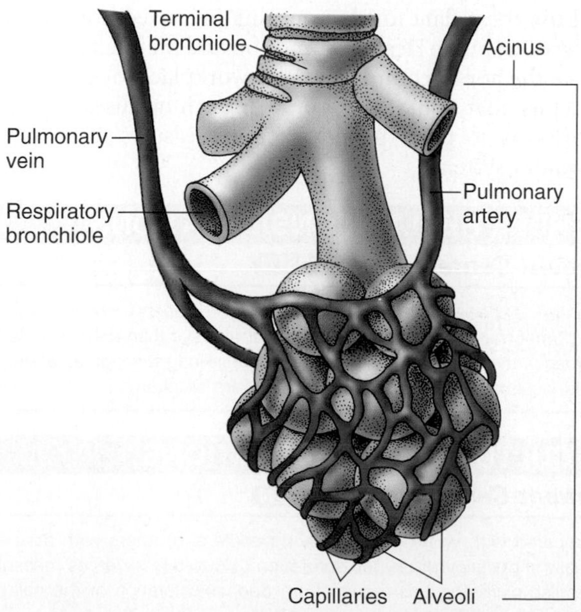

FIG. 27-7 The terminal bronchioles and the acinus.

The **pleura** is a continuous smooth membrane with two surfaces that totally enclose the lungs. The parietal pleura lines the inside of the chest cavity and the upper surface of the diaphragm. The visceral pleura covers the lung surfaces. These surfaces are lubricated by a thin fluid that allows the surfaces to glide across each other smoothly during breathing.

Blood flow in the lungs occurs through two separate systems: bronchial and pulmonary. The bronchial system carries the blood needed to oxygenate lung tissues. These arteries are part of systemic circulation and do not participate in gas exchange.

The pulmonary circulation is a highly vascular capillary network. Oxygen-poor blood travels from the right ventricle of the heart into the pulmonary artery. This artery eventually branches into arterioles to form capillary networks that are meshed around and through the alveoli—the site of GAS EXCHANGE (see Fig. 27-7). Freshly oxygenated blood travels from the capillaries to the pulmonary veins and then to the left atrium. From the left atrium, oxygenated blood flows into the left ventricle, where it is pumped throughout the systemic circulation.

Accessory Muscles of Respiration

Breathing occurs through changes in the size of and pressure within the chest cavity. Contraction and relaxation of chest muscles (and the diaphragm) cause changes in the size and pressure of the chest cavity. At times, back and abdominal muscles are used in addition to chest muscles when the work of breathing is increased.

Oxygen Delivery and the Oxygen-Hemoglobin Dissociation Curve

Oxygen delivery to the tissues requires the binding of oxygen to hemoglobin in red blood cells. Each molecule of hemoglobin can bind four oxygen molecules, which fills *(saturates)* all of its binding sites. Each red blood cell normally has hundreds of thousands of hemoglobin molecules. When blood passes through the lung alveoli, where oxygen concentration is the greatest, oxygen diffuses from the alveoli into red blood cells and binds to all those hemoglobin molecules. This oxygen-rich blood then goes to the left side of the heart and is pumped out into systemic circulation. In tissues away from the source of oxygen, hemoglobin unloads **(dissociates)** the oxygen molecules and delivers them to the tissues. Fig. 27-8 shows the oxygen-hemoglobin dissociation curve.

Tissue oxygen delivery through dissociation or unloading from hemoglobin is based on tissues' need for oxygen. The curve in Fig. 27-8 shows that the rate of this unloading changes depending on how much oxygen is already in the tissues. When blood perfuses tissues in which the oxygen levels are high, as indicated in the upper right-hand corner of the figure, hemoglobin binds oxygen very tightly and little oxygen is unloaded or dissociated from the hemoglobin into the tissues. This prevents oxygen delivery from being wasted by unloading it where it is not needed. When blood perfuses tissues in which oxygen levels are very low, as indicated in the lower left-hand corner of Fig. 27-8, hemoglobin binds oxygen less tightly and will rapidly and easily unload its remaining oxygen to provide these tissues with needed oxygen. So, how rapidly and easily hemoglobin dissociates oxygen to the tissues changes depending on oxygen need. The S-shaped curve indicates that it is harder for oxygen

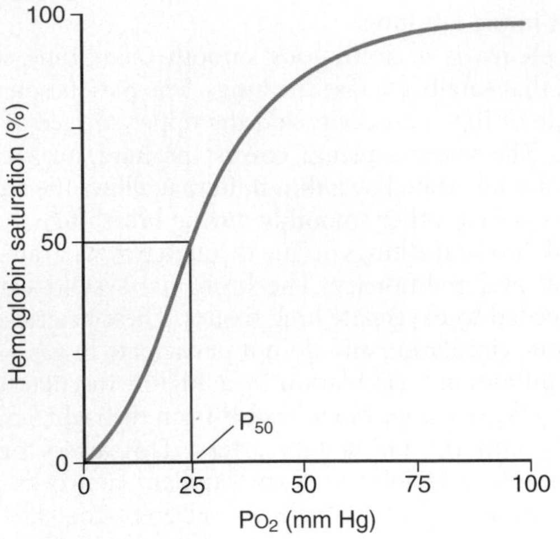

FIG. 27-8 The oxygen-hemoglobin dissociation curve. P_{50}, The partial pressure of O_2 at which hemoglobin is 50% saturated; PO_2, oxygen partial pressure.

to dissociate from hemoglobin in tissues that are well-oxygenated and much easier in tissues that are "starving" for oxygen.

The curve in Fig. 27-8 indicates that, on average, 50% of hemoglobin molecules have completely dissociated their oxygen molecules when blood perfuses tissues that have an oxygen tension (concentration) of 26 mm Hg. This is considered a "normal" point at which 50% of hemoglobin molecules are no longer saturated with oxygen.

When the need for oxygen is greater in tissues, this curve shifts to the *right,* which means the hemoglobin will dissociate oxygen faster even when the tissue oxygen tension levels are greater than 26 mm Hg. Conditions that shift the curve to the right include increased tissue temperature, increased tissue carbon dioxide concentration, and decreased tissue pH (acidosis). This means that it is easier for hemoglobin to unload oxygen to these tissues because they need it to support the higher metabolism and is a tissue protection that increases oxygen delivery to the tissues that need it the most.

When tissues have less need of oxygen because they are metabolizing more slowly than usual, the oxygen-hemoglobin dissociation curve shifts to the *left,* which means that the tissue oxygen tension level has to be even *lower* for hemoglobin to unload oxygen. Tissue conditions that cause a shift to the left include decreased tissue temperature, decreased carbon dioxide levels, decreased glucose breakdown products, and a higher tissue pH (alkalosis). This action prevents wasting oxygen delivery to tissues that are not using the oxygen they already have.

A clinical example of how these actions are helpful is one in which a person is having a myocardial infarction (heart attack). Blood flow to the area is reduced and the heart muscle is metabolizing under hypoxic conditions, which creates more carbon dioxide in the tissue and acidosis. As a result, the hemoglobin that reaches this hypoxic tissue unloads more oxygen at a faster rate to prevent ischemia and cardiac muscle cell death. What if this person believes he or she is having indigestion, which can have similar manifestations, and tries to correct the problem by taking in large amounts of bicarbonate-based antacids? The antacids increase the pH in the blood and all tissues, shifting the oxygen-hemoglobin dissociation curve to the left. As a result, the hypoxic cardiac muscle cells receive even less oxygen and more of them die.

Respiratory Changes Associated with Aging

The respiratory changes that occur with aging are described in Chart 27-2. Many additional respiratory changes in older patients result from heredity and a lifetime of exposure to environmental pollutants (e.g., cigarette smoke, bacteria, industrial fumes and irritants).

Respiratory disease is a major cause of illness and chronic disability in older patients. Although respiratory function normally declines with age, there is usually no problem keeping pace with the demands of ordinary activity. The sedentary older adult, however, often feels breathless during exercise (Touhy & Jett, 2014).

It is difficult to determine which respiratory changes in older adults are related to normal aging and which changes are caused by respiratory disease or exposure to pollutants. Age-related changes in the muscles and the cardiac and vascular system also may cause abnormal breathing, even if the lungs are normal.

NCLEX EXAMINATION CHALLENGE

Physiological Integrity

What is the effect of age-related decreased skeletal muscle strength on the effectiveness of gas exchange?

A. Reduced gas exchange as a result of decreased alveolar surface
B. Reduced gas exchange as a result of longer relaxation of bronchiolar smooth muscles
C. Reduced gas exchange as a result of decreased changes in pressures of the chest cavity
D. Reduced gas exchange as a result of failure of pulmonary circulation to fully perfuse lung tissue

ASSESSMENT METHODS

Patient History

Obtaining accurate information from the patient is important for identifying the type and severity of breathing problems. Age, gender, and race can affect the physical and diagnostic findings related to breathing (Jarvis, 2016). Many of the diagnostic studies for respiratory disorders (e.g., pulmonary function tests) use these data for determining predicted normal values. As described in the Health Promotion and Maintenance section, explore the home, community, and workplace for environmental factors that could cause or worsen lung disease. Use this opportunity to teach patients about measures to protect the respiratory system.

GENDER HEALTH CONSIDERATIONS

Patient-Centered Care QSEN

Women, especially smokers, have greater bronchial responsiveness (i.e., bronchial hyperreactivity) and larger airways than men. This factor increases the risk for a more rapid decline in lung function as a woman ages, especially in women who were or are smokers.

CULTURAL CONSIDERATIONS

Patient-Centered Care QSEN

Compared with white people, black people and others with dark skin usually show a lower oxygen saturation (3% to 5% lower) as measured by pulse oximetry; this results from deeper coloration of the nail bed and does not reflect true oxygen status.

CHART 27-2 **Nursing Focus on the Older Adult**

Changes in the Respiratory System Related to Aging

PHYSIOLOGIC CHANGE	NURSING INTERVENTIONS	RATIONALES
Alveoli		
Alveolar surface area decreases. Diffusion capacity decreases. Elastic recoil decreases. Bronchioles and alveolar ducts dilate. Ability to cough decreases. Airways close early.	Encourage vigorous pulmonary hygiene (i.e., encourage patient to turn, cough, and deep breathe) and to use incentive spirometry, especially if he or she is confined to bed or has had surgery. Encourage upright position.	Potential for mechanical or infectious respiratory complications is increased in these situations. The upright position minimizes ventilation-perfusion mismatching.
Lungs		
Residual volume increases. Vital capacity decreases. Efficiency of oxygen and carbon dioxide exchange decreases. Elasticity decreases.	Include inspection, palpation, percussion, and auscultation in lung assessments. Help patient actively maintain health and fitness. Assess patient's respirations for abnormal breathing patterns. Encourage frequent oral hygiene.	Inspection, palpation, percussion, and auscultation are needed to detect normal age-related changes. Health and fitness help keep losses in respiratory functioning to a minimum. Periodic breathing patterns (e.g., Cheyne-Stokes) can occur. Oral hygiene aids in the removal of secretions.
Pharynx and Larynx		
Muscles atrophy. Vocal cords become slack. Laryngeal muscles lose elasticity, and airways lose cartilage.	Have face-to-face conversations with patient when possible.	Patient's voice may be soft and difficult to understand.
Pulmonary Vasculature		
Vascular resistance to blood flow through pulmonary vascular system increases. Pulmonary capillary blood volume decreases. Risk for hypoxia increases.	Assess patient's level of consciousness and cognition.	Patient can become confused during acute respiratory conditions.
Exercise Tolerance		
Body's response to hypoxia and hypercarbia decreases.	Assess for subtle manifestations of hypoxia.	Early assessment helps prevent complications.
Muscle Strength		
Respiratory muscle strength, especially the diaphragm and the intercostals, decreases.	Encourage pulmonary hygiene, and help patient actively maintain health and fitness.	Regular pulmonary hygiene and overall fitness help maintain maximal functioning of the respiratory system and prevent illness.
Susceptibility to Infection		
Effectiveness of the cilia decreases. Immunoglobulin A decreases. Alveolar macrophages are altered.	Encourage pulmonary hygiene, and help patient actively maintain health and fitness.	Regular pulmonary hygiene and overall fitness help maintain maximal functioning of the respiratory system and prevent illness.
Chest Wall		
Anteroposterior diameter increases. Thorax becomes shorter. Progressive kyphoscoliosis occurs. Chest wall compliance (elasticity) decreases. Mobility of chest wall may decrease. Osteoporosis is possible, leading to chest wall abnormalities.	Discuss the normal changes of aging. Discuss the need for increased rest periods during exercise. Encourage adequate calcium intake (especially during a woman's premenopause phase).	Patients may be anxious because they must work harder to breathe. Older patients have less tolerance for exercise. Calcium intake helps prevent osteoporosis by building bone in younger patients.

Ask patients about their respiratory history (Table 27-1), including smoking history, drug use, travel, and area of residence. Document the smoking history in pack-years.

Drug use, both prescribed drugs and illicit drugs, can affect lung function. Some drugs affect the lungs when taken systemically. Ask about drugs taken for breathing problems and about drugs taken for other conditions. For example, a cough can be a side effect of some antihypertensive drugs (angiotensin-converting enzyme [ACE] inhibitors and angiotensin receptor blockers [ARBs]). Determine which over-the-counter drugs (e.g., cough syrups, antihistamines, decongestants, inhalants) the patient is using. Also assess the use of complementary and alternative therapies. Ask about past drug use. Some drugs for other conditions can cause permanent changes in lung

TABLE 27-1 Important Aspects to Assess in A Respiratory System History

- Smoking history
- Childhood illnesses:
  - Asthma
  - Pneumonia
  - Communicable diseases
  - Hay fever
  - Allergies
  - Eczema
  - Frequent colds
  - Croup
  - Cystic fibrosis
- Adult illnesses:
  - Pneumonia
  - Sinusitis
  - Tuberculosis
  - HIV and AIDS
  - Lung disease such as emphysema and sarcoidosis
  - Diabetes
  - Hypertension
  - Heart disease
- Influenza, pneumococcal (Pneumovax), and BCG vaccinations
- Surgeries of the upper or lower respiratory system
- Injuries to the upper or lower respiratory system
- Hospitalizations
- Date of last chest x-ray, pulmonary function test, tuberculin test, or other diagnostic tests and results
- Recent weight loss
- Night sweats
- Sleep disturbances
- Lung disease and condition of family members
- Geographic areas of recent travel
- Occupation and leisure activities

AIDS, Acquired immune deficiency syndrome; *BCG,* bacille Calmette-Guérin; *HIV,* human immune deficiency virus.

function. For example, patients may have pulmonary fibrosis if they received bleomycin (Blenoxane) as chemotherapy for cancer or amiodarone (Cordarone) for cardiac problems. Marijuana and illicit drugs, such as cocaine, are often inhaled and can affect lung function.

Allergies to foods, dust, molds, pollen, bee stings, trees, grass, animal dander and saliva, or drugs can affect breathing. Ask the patient to describe specific allergic responses. For example, does he or she wheeze, have trouble breathing, cough, sneeze, or have rhinitis after exposure to the allergen? Has he or she ever been treated for an allergic response? If the patient has allergies, ask about the specific cause, treatment, and the response to treatment.

! NURSING SAFETY PRIORITY QSEN

Action Alert

Document any known allergies and the specific type of allergic response in a prominent place in the patient's medical record.

Travel and geographic area of residence may reveal possible exposure to certain diseases. For example, *histoplasmosis,* a fungal disease caused by inhalation of contaminated dust, is found in the central parts of the United States and Canada. *Coccidioidomycosis* is found mostly in the western and southwestern parts of the United States, in Mexico, and in portions of Central America, as is *Hantavirus.*

Nutrition Status

Assess the patient's diet history and nutrition status to determine allergic reactions to certain foods or preservatives. Manifestations range from rhinitis, chest tightness, weakness, **dyspnea** (shortness of breath), urticaria, and severe wheezing to loss of consciousness. Ask about usual food intake and whether any breathing problems occur with eating.

Family History and Genetic Risk

Obtain a family history to assess for respiratory disorders that have a genetic component, such as cystic fibrosis, some lung cancers, and emphysema. Patients with asthma often have a family history of allergy. Ask about a history of infectious disease, such as tuberculosis, because family members may have similar environmental exposures.

Current Health Problems

Whether the breathing problem is acute or chronic, the current health problem usually includes cough, sputum production, chest pain, and shortness of breath at rest or on exertion. Explore the current illness in chronologic order. Ask about the onset of the problem, how long it lasts, the location of the problem, how often it occurs, whether the problem has become worse over time, what manifestations occur with it, which actions or interventions provide relief and which ones make it worse, and what treatments have been used.

Cough is a sign of lung disease. Ask the patient how long the cough has been present and whether it occurs at a specific time of day (e.g., on awakening in the morning) or in relation to any physical activity. Ask whether the cough produces sputum or is dry, tickling, or hacking.

Sputum production is an important manifestation associated with coughing. Check the color, consistency, odor, and amount of sputum.

Describe the consistency of sputum as thin, thick, watery, or frothy. Smokers with chronic bronchitis have mucoid sputum. Excessive pink, frothy sputum is common with pulmonary edema. Bacterial pneumonia often produces rust-colored sputum, and foul-smelling sputum often occurs with a lung abscess. **Hemoptysis** (blood in the sputum) is most often seen in patients with chronic bronchitis or lung cancer. Grossly bloody sputum may occur with tuberculosis, pulmonary infarction, lung cancer, or lung abscess.

Ask the patient to quantify sputum by describing its volume in terms such as teaspoon, tablespoon, and cup. Normally, the lungs can produce up to 90 mL of sputum per day.

Chest pain can occur with other health problems as well as with lung problems. A detailed description of chest pain helps distinguish its cause. Ask the patient whether the pain is continuous or made worse by coughing, deep breathing, or swallowing. Cardiac pain is usually intense and "crushing" and may radiate to the arm, shoulder, or neck. Pulmonary pain varies depending on the cause and most often feels like something is "rubbing" inside. The pain may appear only on deep inhalation or be present at the end of inhalation and the end of exhalation. Pulmonary pain is not made worse by touching or pressing over the area.

Dyspnea (difficulty in breathing or breathlessness) is a subjective perception and varies among patients (Baker et al., 2013). A patient's feeling of dyspnea may not be consistent with the severity of the problem. Determine the type of onset (slow or abrupt); the duration; relieving factors (position changes, drug use, activity cessation); and whether wheezing or stridor occurs with dyspnea.

Try to quantify dyspnea by asking whether this manifestation interferes with ADLs and, if so, how severely. For example, does dyspnea occur after walking one block or climbing one flight of stairs? Table 27-2 classifies dyspnea with changes in ADL performance.

TABLE 27-2 Correlation of Dyspnea Classification with Performance of ADLs

CLASSIFICATION	ADLs KEY
Class I: No significant restrictions in normal activity. Employable. Dyspnea occurs only on more-than-normal or strenuous exertion.	*4:* No breathlessness, normal.
Class II: Independent in essential ADLs but restricted in some other activities. Dyspneic on climbing stairs or on walking on an incline but not on level walking. Employable only for sedentary job or under special circumstances.	*3:* Satisfactory, mild breathlessness. Complete performance is possible without pause or assistance but not entirely normal.
Class III: Dyspnea commonly occurs during usual activities, such as showering or dressing, but the patient can manage without assistance from others. Not dyspneic at rest; can walk for more than a city block at own pace but cannot keep up with others of own age. May stop to catch breath partway up a flight of stairs. Is probably not employable in any occupation.	*2:* Fair, moderate breathlessness. Must stop during activity. Complete performance is possible without assistance, but performance may be too debilitating or time consuming.
Class IV: Dyspnea produces dependence on help in some essential ADLs such as dressing and bathing. Not usually dyspneic at rest. Dyspneic on minimal exertion; must pause on climbing one flight, walking more than 100 yards, or dressing. Often restricted to home if lives alone. Has minimal or no activities outside of home.	*1:* Poor, marked breathlessness. Incomplete performance; assistance is necessary.
Class V: Entirely restricted to home and often limited to bed or chair. Dyspneic at rest. Dependent on help for most needs.	*0:* Performance not indicated or recommended; too difficult.

ADLs, Activities of daily living.

Ask about **orthopnea,** which is a shortness of breath occurring when lying down and is relieved by sitting up. Assess for paroxysmal nocturnal dyspnea (PND), which awakens the patient from sleep with the feeling of an inability to breathe. PND also occurs while lying flat and is relieved by sitting up. It often occurs with chronic lung disease and left sided heart failure.

Physical Assessment

Assessment of the Nose and Sinuses

Inspect the patient's external nose for deformities or polyps, and inspect the nares for symmetry of size and shape. To observe the interior nose, ask the patient to tilt the head back for a penlight examination. The experienced nurse may use a nasal speculum and nasopharyngeal mirror for a more thorough inspection of the nasal cavity.

Inspect for color, swelling, drainage, and bleeding. The mucous membrane of the nose normally appears redder than the oral mucosa, but it is pale, engorged, and bluish gray in patients with allergic rhinitis. Check the nasal septum for bleeding, perforation, or deviation. Septal deviation is common and appears as an S shape, tilting toward one side or the other. A perforated septum is present if the light shines through the perforation into the opposite side; this condition is often found in cocaine users. Nasal polyps are pale, shiny, gelatinous lumps or "bags" attached to the turbinates. Block one naris at a time to check how well air moves through the unblocked side.

NCLEX EXAMINATION CHALLENGE

Physiological Integrity

For which problem does the nurse assess the client who cannot breathe through the nose because of a severe septal deviation?

A. Dry respiratory tract membranes
B. Frequent episodes of tonsillitis
C. Development of nasal polyps
D. Difficulty swallowing

Assessment of the Pharynx, Trachea, and Larynx

Assessment of the pharynx begins with inspection of the mouth. To examine the posterior pharynx, use a tongue depressor to press down one side of the tongue at a time (to avoid stimulating the gag reflex). As the patient says "ah," observe the rise and fall of the soft palate and inspect for color and symmetry, drainage, edema or ulceration, and enlarged tonsils.

Inspect the neck for symmetry, alignment, masses, swelling, bruises, and the use of accessory neck muscles in breathing. Palpate lymph nodes for size, shape, mobility with palpation, consistency, and tenderness.

Gently palpate the trachea for position, mobility, tenderness, and masses. The trachea should be in the midline. Many lung disorders cause the trachea to deviate from the midline. Tension pneumothorax, large pleural effusion, mediastinal mass, and neck tumors push the trachea *away* from the affected area. Pneumonectomy, fibrosis, and atelectasis pull it *toward* the affected area.

The larynx is usually examined by a specialist with a laryngoscope. An abnormal voice, especially hoarseness, may be heard when there are problems of the larynx.

Assessment of the Lungs and Thorax

Inspection. Inspect the front and back of the thorax with the patient sitting up. Normal landmarks of the chest front (anterior) and back (posterior) are shown in Fig. 27-9. The patient should be undressed to the waist. Observe the chest, and compare one side with the other. Work from the top (apex) and move downward toward the base, going from side to side, while inspecting for discoloration, scars, lesions, masses, and spinal curvatures. Assessing from side to side allows you to compare the findings for each lung at the same level (Jarvis, 2016).

Observe the rate, rhythm, and depth of inspirations as well as the symmetry of chest movement. Impaired movement or unequal expansion may indicate disease. Observe the type of breathing (e.g., pursed-lip or diaphragmatic breathing) and the use of accessory muscles.

Examine the shape of the patient's chest, and compare the anteroposterior (AP or front-to-back) diameter with the lateral (side-to-side) diameter. This ratio normally is about 1:1.5, depending on body build. The ratio increases to 1:1 in patients

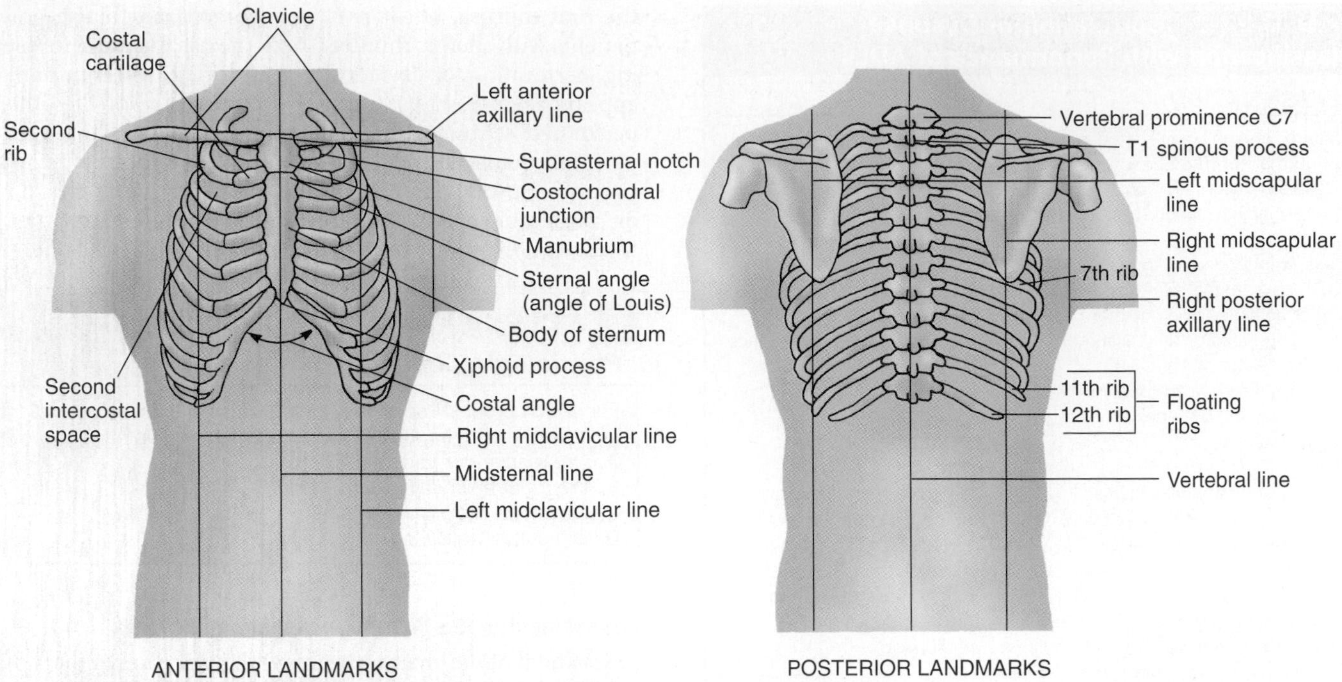

FIG. 27-9 Anterior and posterior chest landmarks.

with emphysema, which results in the typical barrel-chest appearance.

Normally the ribs slope downward. Patients with air trapping in the lungs caused by emphysema have ribs that are more horizontal. Observe or palpate the distance between the ribs *(intercostal space)*. This distance is usually one finger-breadth (2 centimeters). The distance increases in disorders that cause air trapping, such as emphysema. Observe for retraction of muscle between the ribs and at the sternal notch. Retractions are areas that get sucked inward when the patient inhales. This does not occur during normal respiratory effort. Retractions may occur when the patient is working hard to inhale around an obstruction.

Palpation. Palpate the chest after inspection to assess respiratory movement symmetry and observable abnormalities. Palpation also can help identify areas of tenderness and check vocal or tactile **fremitus** (vibration).

Assess chest expansion by placing your thumbs on the patient's spine at the level of the ninth ribs and extending the fingers sideways around the rib cage. As the patient inhales, both sides of the chest should move upward and outward together in one symmetric movement and move your thumbs apart. On exhalation, the thumbs should come back together as they return to the midline. Unequal expansion may be a result of pain, trauma, or air in the pleural cavity. Respiratory lag or slowed movement on one side indicates a pulmonary problem (Jarvis, 2016).

Palpate any abnormalities found on inspection (e.g., masses, lesions, swelling). Also palpate for tenderness, especially if the patient reports pain. Crepitus (air trapped in and under the skin, also known as *subcutaneous emphysema*) is felt as a crackling sensation beneath the fingertips. Document this finding and report it to the health care provider when it occurs around a wound site or a tracheostomy site or if a pneumothorax is suspected.

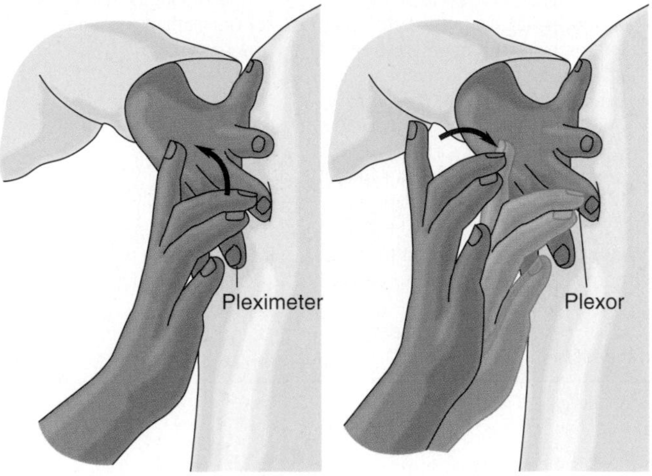

FIG. 27-10 Percussion technique.

Tactile (vocal) fremitus is a vibration of the chest wall produced when the patient speaks. This vibration can be felt on the chest wall. Fremitus is decreased if the transmission of sound waves from the larynx to the chest wall is slowed, such as when the pleural space is filled with air (pneumothorax) or fluid (pleural effusion) or when the bronchus is obstructed. Fremitus is increased with pneumonia and lung abscesses because the increased density of the chest enhances transmission of the vibrations.

Percussion. Use percussion to assess for pulmonary resonance, the boundaries of organs, and diaphragmatic excursion. Percussion involves tapping the chest wall, which sets the underlying tissues into motion and produces audible sounds (Fig. 27-10). This action produces five different sounds that help determine whether the lung tissue contains air or fluid or is solid (Table 27-3).

TABLE 27-3 **Characteristics of the Five Percussion Notes**

NOTE	PITCH	INTENSITY	QUALITY	DURATION	FINDINGS
Resonance	Low	Moderate to loud	Hollow	Long	Resonance is characteristic of normal lung tissue.
Hyperresonance	Higher than resonance	Very loud	Booming	Longer than resonance	Hyperresonance indicates the presence of trapped air, so it is commonly heard over an emphysematous or asthmatic lung and occasionally over a pneumothorax.
Flatness	High	Soft	Extreme dullness	Short	An example location is the sternum. Flatness percussed over the lung fields may indicate a massive pleural effusion.
Dullness	Medium	Medium	Thudlike	Medium	Example locations are over the liver and the kidneys. Dullness can be percussed over an atelectatic lung or a consolidated lung.
Tympany	High	Loud	Musical, drumlike	Short	Examples are the cheek filled with air and the abdomen distended with air. Over the lung, a tympanic note usually indicates a large pneumothorax.

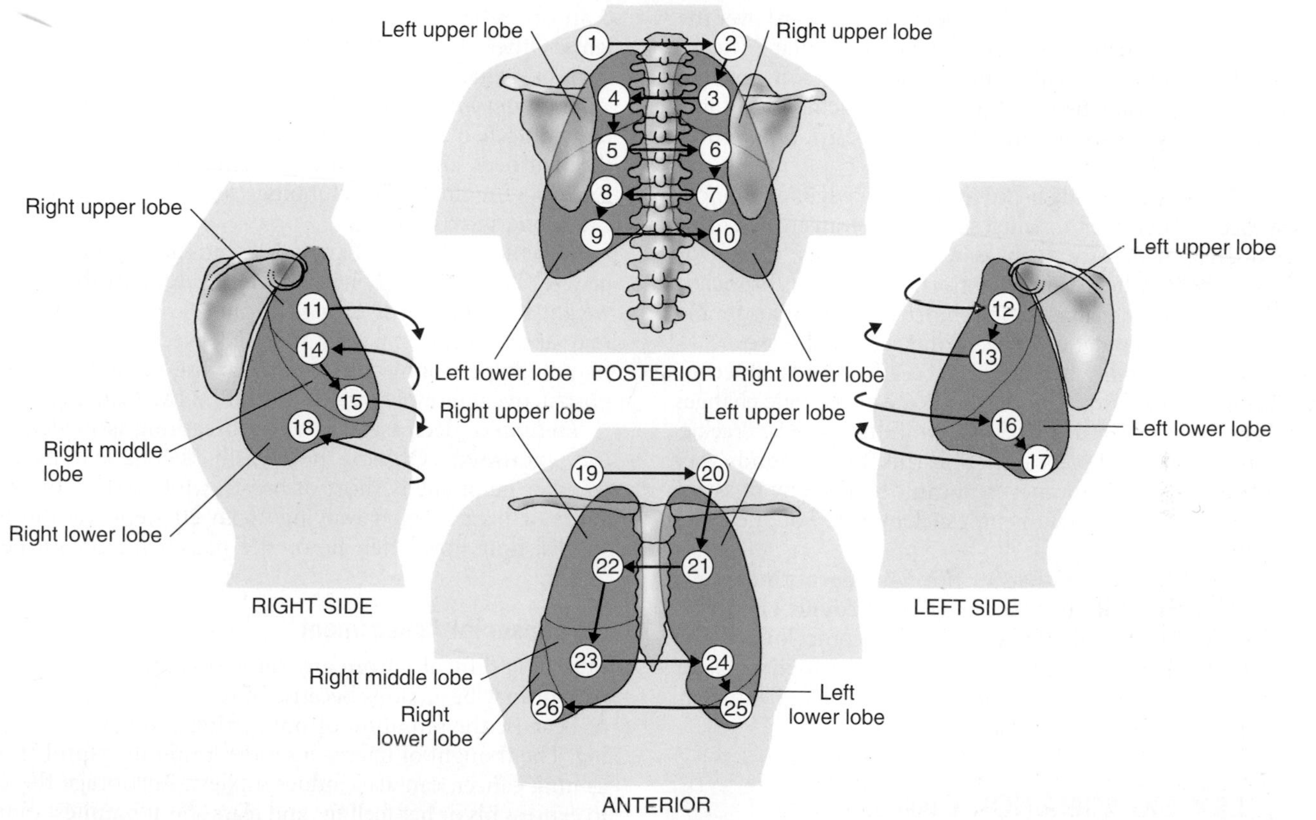

FIG. 27-11 Sequence for percussion and auscultation.

Auscultation. Auscultation includes listening with a stethoscope for normal breath sounds, abnormal *(adventitious)* sounds, and voice sounds. This technique provides information about the flow of air through the trachea and lungs and helps identify fluid, mucus, or obstruction in the respiratory system.

Begin auscultation with the patient sitting in an upright position. With the stethoscope pressed firmly against the chest wall (clothing can muffle sounds), instruct the patient to breathe slowly and deeply through an open mouth. (Breathing through the nose sets up turbulent sounds that are transmitted to the lungs.) Use a systematic approach, beginning at the lung apices and moving from side to side down through the intercostal spaces to the lung bases (Fig. 27-11). Avoid listening over bony structures. Listen to a full respiratory cycle, noting the quality and intensity of the breath sounds.

Normal breath sounds are produced as air vibrates while moving through the passages from the larynx to the alveoli. Breath sounds are identified by their location, intensity, pitch, and duration within the respiratory cycle (e.g., early or late inspiration and expiration). Normal breath sounds are known

TABLE 27-4 Characteristics of Normal Breath Sounds

	PITCH	AMPLITUDE	DURATION	QUALITY	NORMAL LOCATION
Bronchial (tubular, tracheal) 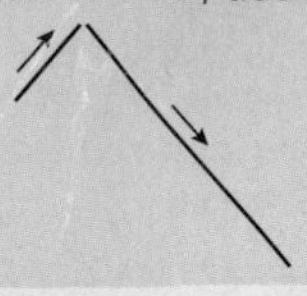	High	Loud	Inspiration < expiration	Harsh, hollow, tubular, blowing	Trachea and larynx
Bronchovesicular 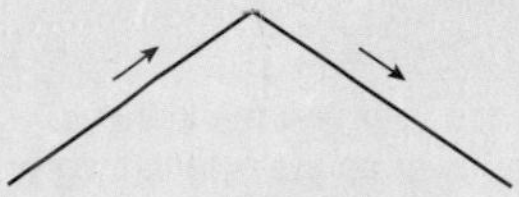	Moderate	Moderate	Inspiration = expiration	Mixed	Over major bronchi where fewer alveoli are located; posterior, between scapulae (especially on right); anterior, around upper sternum in first and second intercostal spaces
Vesicular 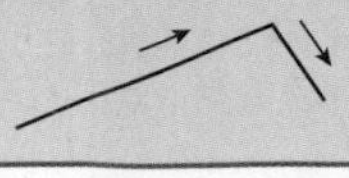	Low	Soft	Inspiration > expiration	Rustling, like the sound of the wind in the trees	Over peripheral lung fields where air flows through smaller bronchioles and alveoli

From Jarvis, C. (2016). *Physical examination and health assessment* (7th ed.). St. Louis: Saunders.

as "bronchial" or "tubular" (harsh hollow sounds heard over the trachea and mainstem bronchi), "bronchovesicular" (heard over the branching bronchi), and "vesicular" (soft rustling sounds heard in lung tissue over small bronchioles) (Table 27-4). Describe these sounds as *normal, increased, diminished,* or *absent.*

Bronchial breath sounds heard at the lung edges are abnormal and occur when the bronchial sounds are transmitted to an area of increased density, such as with atelectasis, tumor, or pneumonia. When heard in an abnormal location, bronchovesicular breath sounds may indicate normal aging or an abnormality such as consolidation and chronic airway disease.

Adventitious sounds are additional breath sounds superimposed on normal sounds, and they indicate pathologic changes in the lung. Table 27-5 describes adventitious sounds: crackle, wheeze, rhonchus, and pleural friction rub. These sounds vary in pitch, intensity, and duration and can occur in any phase of the respiratory cycle. Document exactly what you hear on auscultation.

Voice sounds (vocal resonance) through the normally air-filled lung are muffled and unclear because sound vibrations travel poorly through air. These sounds become louder and more distinct when the sound travels through a solid tissue or liquid. The presence of pneumonia, atelectasis, pleural effusion, tumor, or abscess causes increased vocal resonance.

NCLEX EXAMINATION CHALLENGE

Physiological Integrity

When auscultating the client's breath sounds, the nurse hears soft rustling sounds at the lung edges. What is the nurse's best action?

A. Listen again with the bell of the stethoscope rather than the diaphragm.
B. Ask the client to cough and spit out any collected mucus.
C. Document the finding as the only action.
D. Notify the health care provider.

Other Indicators of Respiratory Adequacy

Assess other indicators of respiratory adequacy, because GAS EXCHANGE affects all body systems. Some indicators (e.g., cyanosis) reflect immediate gas exchange and PERFUSION problems. Other changes (e.g., clubbing, weight loss) reflect long-term oxygenation problems.

Skin and mucous membrane changes (e.g., pallor, cyanosis) may indicate inadequate GAS EXCHANGE and PERFUSION. Assess the nail beds and the mucous membranes of the oral cavity. Examine the fingers for clubbing (see Fig. 30-10), which indicates long-term hypoxia.

General appearance includes muscle development and general body build. Long-term respiratory problems lead to weight loss and a loss of general muscle mass. Arms and legs may appear thin or poorly muscled. Neck and chest muscles may be hypertrophied, especially in the patient with chronic obstructive pulmonary disease (COPD) (McCance et al., 2014).

Endurance decreases whenever breathing is inadequate for GAS EXCHANGE. Observe how easily the patient moves and whether he or she is short of breath while resting or becomes short of breath when walking 10 to 20 steps. As the patient speaks, note how often he or she pauses for breath between words.

Psychosocial Assessment

Breathing difficulty from any cause often induces anxiety. The patient may be anxious because of reduced oxygen to the brain or because the sensation of not getting enough air is frightening. The thought of having a serious respiratory problem, such as lung cancer, can also induce anxiety. Encourage the patient to express his or her feelings and fears about manifestations and their possible meaning.

Assess those aspects of the patient's lifestyle that either can affect respiratory function or are affected by it. Some respiratory problems may become worse with stress. Ask about current life stresses and usual coping mechanisms.

Chronic respiratory disease may cause changes in family roles or relationships, social isolation, financial problems, and unemployment or disability. Discuss coping mechanisms to assess the patient's reaction to these stressors and identify strengths. For example, the patient may react to stress with dependence on family members, withdrawal, or failure to adhere to interventions. Assist the patient to identify available support systems.

TABLE 27-5 **Characteristics of Adventitious Breath Sounds**

ADVENTITIOUS SOUND	CHARACTER	ASSOCIATION
Fine crackles Fine rales High-pitched rales	Popping, discontinuous sounds caused by air moving into previously deflated airways; sounds like hair being rolled between fingers near the ear "Velcro" sounds late in inspiration usually associated with restrictive disorders	Asbestosis Atelectasis Interstitial fibrosis Bronchitis Pneumonia Chronic pulmonary diseases
Coarse crackles Low-pitched crackles	Lower-pitched, coarse, rattling sounds caused by fluid or secretions in large airways; likely to change with coughing or suctioning	Bronchitis Pneumonia Tumors Pulmonary edema
Wheeze	Squeaky, musical, continuous sounds associated with air rushing through narrowed airways; may be heard without a stethoscope Arise from the small airways Usually do not clear with coughing	Inflammation Bronchospasm Edema Secretions Pulmonary vessel engorgement (as in cardiac "asthma")
Rhonchus (rhonchi)	Lower-pitched, coarse, continuous snoring sounds Arise from the large airways	Thick, tenacious secretions Sputum production Obstruction by foreign body Tumors
Pleural friction rub	Loud, rough, grating, scratching sounds caused by the inflamed surfaces of the pleura rubbing together; often associated with pain on deep inspirations Heard in lateral lung fields	Pleurisy Tuberculosis Pulmonary infarction Pneumonia Lung cancer

CLINICAL JUDGMENT CHALLENGE

Patient-Centered-Care; Teamwork and Collaboration QSEN

The patient is a 68-year-old man who has had shortness of breath (SOB) for the past 2 to 3 days. His past medical history includes a 40–pack-year smoking history, COPD, and heart failure. He reports that he became concerned when he woke from sleep because he could not breathe. Your physical assessment reveals crackles in the lower lobes bilaterally. His oxygen saturation (Spo_2) is 84% without supplemental oxygen.

1. What are some areas of focus to assess as part of this patient's current history?
2. Whom should you contact and why?
3. What are some factors that may affect gas exchange for this patient?
4. What additional referrals might be appropriate for this patient?

Diagnostic Assessment

Laboratory Assessment

Several laboratory tests (Chart 27-3) are useful in assessing respiratory problems. A red blood cell (RBC) count provides data about the transport of oxygen. Hemoglobin, found in RBCs, transports oxygen to the tissues. A deficiency of hemoglobin could cause hypoxemia.

Arterial blood gas (ABG) analysis assesses GAS EXCHANGE and PERFUSION as oxygenation (partial pressure of arterial oxygen [Pao_2]), alveolar ventilation (partial pressure of arterial carbon dioxide [$Paco_2$]), and acid-base balance. Blood gas studies provide information for monitoring treatment results, adjusting oxygen therapy, and evaluating the patient's responses (Barnette & Kautz, 2013). See Chapter 12 for more details on blood gas analysis.

Sputum specimens can help identify organisms or abnormal cells. Sputum culture and sensitivity analyses identify bacterial infection and determine which specific antibiotics will be most effective. Cytologic examination can identify cancer cells. Allergic conditions may be identified by cytologic testing. Eosinophils and Curschmann's spirals (a mucus form) are often found by cytologic study in patients with allergic asthma.

Imaging Assessment

Chest x-rays with digital images are used for patients with pulmonary problems to evaluate the status of the chest and to provide a baseline for comparison with future changes. These chest x-rays are performed from **posteroanterior** (PA; back to front) and left lateral (LL) positions.

Chest x-rays are used to assess lung pathology such as with pneumonia, atelectasis, pneumothorax, and tumor. They also can detect pleural fluid and the placement of an endotracheal tube or other invasive catheters. A computer-enhanced image can be adjusted to emphasize a specific area. These images have limitations, however, and may appear normal, even when severe chronic bronchitis, asthma, or emphysema is present.

Sinus and facial x-rays are used to assess fluid levels in the sinus cavities to assist in the diagnosis of acute or chronic sinusitis.

Computed tomography (CT) assesses soft tissues with consecutive cross-sectional views of the entire chest. This type of imaging can verify the identity of a suspicious lesion or clot. Often CT scans require a contrast agent injected IV to enhance the visibility of structures such as tumors, blood vessels, and heart chambers. These scans assist in making a diagnosis. Your role in this diagnostic test is to provide information to the patient and to determine whether the patient has any sensitivity to the contrast material. Ask the patient whether he or she has a known allergy to iodine or shellfish. In addition, IV contrast

CHART 27-3 **Laboratory Profile**

Respiratory Assessment

TEST	NORMAL RANGE FOR ADULTS	SIGNIFICANCE OF ABNORMAL FINDINGS
Blood Studies		
Complete Blood Count		
Red blood cells	*Females:* 4.2-5.4 million/mm^3 *Males:* 4.7-6.1 million/mm^3	*Elevated levels* (polycythemia) often related to the excessive production of erythropoietin in response to a chronic hypoxic state, as in COPD, and from living at a high altitude. *Decreased levels* indicate possible anemia, hemorrhage, or hemolysis.
Hemoglobin, total	*Females:* 12-16 g/dL, or 7.4-9.9 mmol/L *Males:* 14-18 g/dL, or 8.7-11.2 mmol/L	Same as for red blood cells.
Hematocrit	*Females:* 37%-47%, or 0.37-0.47 SI units *Males:* 42%-52%, or 0.42-0.52 SI units	Same as for red blood cells.
White blood cell count (leukocyte count, WBC count)	*Total:* 5,000-10,000/mm^3	*Elevations* indicate possible acute infections or inflammations. *Decreased levels* may indicate an overwhelming infection, an autoimmune disorder, or immunosuppressant therapy.
Differential White Blood Cell (Leukocyte) Count		
Neutrophils	2500-8000/mm^3, or 55%-70% of total	*Elevations* indicate possible acute bacterial infection (pneumonia), COPD, or inflammatory conditions (smoking). *Decreased levels* indicate possible viral disease (influenza).
Eosinophils	50-500/mm^3, or 1%-4% of total	*Elevations* indicate possible COPD, asthma, or allergies. *Decreased levels* indicate pyogenic infections.
Basophils	25-100/mm^3, or 0.5%-1% of total	*Elevations* indicate possible inflammation; seen in chronic sinusitis, hypersensitivity reactions. *Decreased levels* may be seen in an acute infection.
Lymphocytes	1000-4000/mm^3, or 20%-40% of total	*Elevations* indicate possible viral infection, pertussis, and infectious mononucleosis. *Decreased levels* may be seen during corticosteroid therapy.
Monocytes	100-700/mm^3, or 2%-8% of total	*Elevations:* see Lymphocytes; also may indicate active tuberculosis. *Decreased levels:* see Lymphocytes.
Arterial Blood Gases		
Pao_2	80-100 mm Hg *Older adults:* values may be lower	*Elevations* indicate possible excessive oxygen administration. *Decreased levels* indicate possible COPD, asthma, chronic bronchitis, cancer of the bronchi and lungs, cystic fibrosis, respiratory distress syndrome, anemias, atelectasis, or any other cause of hypoxia.
$Paco_2$	35-45 mm Hg	*Elevations* indicate possible COPD, asthma, pneumonia, anesthesia effects, or use of opioids (respiratory acidosis). *Decreased levels* indicate hyperventilation/respiratory alkalosis.
pH	*Up to 60 yr:* 7.35-7.45 *60-90 yr:* 7.31-7.42 *>90 yr:* 7.26-7.43	*Elevations* indicate metabolic or respiratory alkalosis. *Decreased levels* indicate metabolic or respiratory acidosis.
HCO_3^-	21-28 mEq/L	*Elevations* indicate possible respiratory acidosis as compensation for a primary metabolic alkalosis. *Decreased levels* indicate possible respiratory alkalosis as compensation for a primary metabolic acidosis.
Spo_2	95%-100% *Older adults:* values may be slightly lower	*Decreased levels* indicate possible impaired ability of hemoglobin to release oxygen to tissues.

COPD, Chronic obstructive pulmonary disease; *HCO_3^-,* bicarbonate ion; *$Paco_2$,* partial pressure of arterial carbon dioxide; *Pao_2,* partial pressure of arterial oxygen; *Spo_2,* peripheral oxygen saturation.

material can be nephrotoxic. Ask about his or her kidney function and whether he or she takes drugs for type 2 diabetes. If the patient usually takes metformin, the drug is stopped at least 24 hours before contrast dye is used and is not restarted until adequate kidney function has been established (see Chapter 64).

Other Noninvasive Diagnostic Assessment

Pulse Oximetry. Pulse oximetry identifies hemoglobin saturation with oxygen. Usually hemoglobin is almost 100% saturated with oxygen in superficial tissues. The pulse oximeter uses a wave of infrared light and a sensor placed on the patient's finger, toe, nose, earlobe, or forehead (Fig. 27-12). Ideal normal pulse oximetry values are 95% to 100%. Normal values are a little lower in older patients and in patients with dark skin. To avoid confusion with the Pao_2 values from arterial blood gases, pulse oximetry readings are recorded as the Spo_2 (peripheral arterial oxygen saturation) or Sao_2.

Pulse oximetry can detect desaturation before manifestations (e.g., dusky skin, pale mucosa, pale or blue nail beds) occur. Causes for low readings include patient movement, hypothermia, decreased peripheral blood flow, ambient light (sunlight, infrared lamps), decreased hemoglobin, edema, and

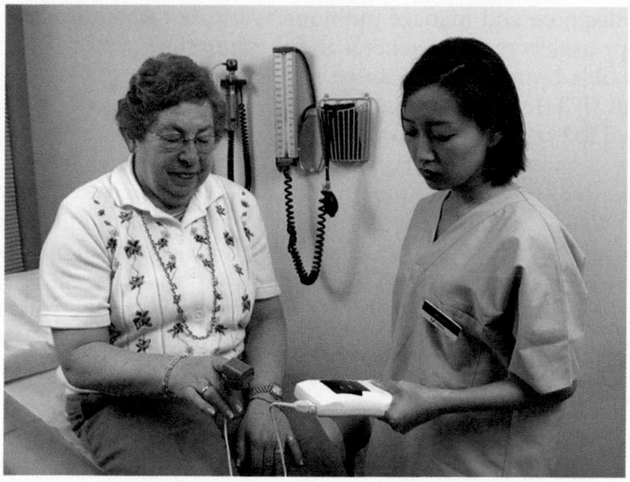

FIG. 27-12 A typical pulse oximeter.

fingernail polish. When patients have any degree of impaired peripheral blood flow, the most accurate place to test oxygen saturation is on the forehead. Covering the sensor with a fingertip cut from a glove or changing its position may help accuracy if too much ambient light is present.

Results lower than 91% (and certainly below 86%) are an emergency and require immediate assessment and treatment. When the Spo_2 is below 85%, body tissues have a difficult time becoming oxygenated. An Spo_2 lower than 70% is usually life threatening, but in some cases, values below 80% may be life threatening. Pulse oximetry is less accurate at lower values.

Capnometry and Capnography. Capnometry and capnography are methods that measure the amount of carbon dioxide present in exhaled air, which is an indirect measurement of arterial carbon dioxide levels. These noninvasive tests measure the partial-pressure of end-tidal carbon dioxide ($PETCO_2$, also known as $ETCO_2$) levels in both intubated patients and those breathing spontaneously. With capnometry, the exhaled air sample is tested with a sensor that changes the CO_2 level into a color or number for analysis. With capnography, the CO_2 level is graphed as a specific waveform along with a number. These methods provide information about CO_2 production, pulmonary perfusion, alveolar ventilation, respiratory patterns, ventilator effectiveness, and possible rebreathing of exhaled air (Carlisle, 2014).

The normal value of the partial pressure of end-tidal carbon dioxide ($PETCO_2$) ranges between 20 and 40 mm Hg. Changes in $PETCO_2$ reflect changes in breathing effectiveness and GAS EXCHANGE. These changes occur before hypoxia can be detected using pulse oximetry. The use of both pulse oximetry and $PETCO_2$ for patients at risk for respiratory problems can provide information to direct early intervention (Carlisle, 2014).

Conditions that increase $PETCO_2$ above normal levels are those that reflect inadequate GAS EXCHANGE or an increase in cellular metabolism, both of which increase production of carbon dioxide (CO_2). Conditions of inadequate gas exchange include hypoventilation, partial airway obstruction, and rebreathing exhaled air. Conditions that increase cellular metabolism include fever, acidosis, and heavy exercise.

Conditions that decrease $PETCO_2$ below normal levels are those that reflect poor pulmonary ventilation, such as pulmonary embolism, apnea, total airway obstruction, and tracheal extubation. Other causes of low $PETCO_2$ include hyperventilation not based on oxygen need in which CO_2 is "blown off" faster than it is generated in the tissues.

Pulmonary Function Tests. Pulmonary function tests (PFTs) assess lung function and breathing problems. These tests measure lung volumes and capacities, flow rates, diffusion capacity, GAS EXCHANGE, airway resistance, and distribution of ventilation. The results are interpreted by comparing the patient's data with expected findings for age, gender, race, height, weight, and smoking status.

The PFTs are useful in screening patients for lung disease even before the onset of manifestations. Repeated testing over time provides data that may be used to guide management (e.g., changes in lung function can support a decision to continue, change, or discontinue a specific therapy). Testing before surgery may identify patients at risk for lung complications after surgery. The most common reason for performing PFTs is to determine the cause of dyspnea. When performed while the patient exercises, PFTs help determine whether dyspnea is caused by lung or cardiac dysfunction or by muscle weakness.

Patient Preparation. Explain the purpose of the tests, and advise the patient not to smoke for 6 to 8 hours before testing. Depending on the reasons for testing, bronchodilator drugs may be withheld for 4 to 6 hours before the test. The patient with breathing problems often fears further breathlessness and is anxious before these "breathing" tests. Help reduce anxiety by describing what will happen during and after the testing.

Procedure. PFTs can be performed at the bedside or in the respiratory laboratory by a respiratory therapist or respiratory technician. The patient is asked to breathe through the mouth only. A nose clip may be used to prevent air from escaping. The patient performs different breathing maneuvers while measurements are obtained. Table 27-6 describes the most commonly used PFTs and their uses.

Follow-up Care. Because many breathing maneuvers are performed during PFTs, assess the patient for increased dyspnea or bronchospasm after these studies. Document any drugs given during testing.

Exercise Testing. Exercise increases metabolism and increases gas transport because energy is used. Exercise testing assesses the patient's ability to work and perform ADLs, differentiates reasons for exercise limitation, evaluates disease influence on exercise capacity, and determines whether supplemental oxygen is needed during exercise. These tests are performed on a treadmill or bicycle or by a self-paced 12-minute walking test. Exercise in the patient with normal pulmonary function is limited by circulatory factors, whereas exercise in the pulmonary patient is limited by breathing capacity, GAS EXCHANGE compromise, or both. Explain exercise testing, and assure the patient that he or she will be closely monitored by trained professionals throughout the test.

Skin Tests. Skin tests are used with other diagnostic data to identify various infectious diseases (e.g., tuberculosis), viral diseases (e.g., mononucleosis, mumps), and fungal diseases (e.g., coccidioidomycosis, histoplasmosis). Allergies and the status of the immune system also can be checked through skin testing. (See Chapters 17 and 20 for further discussion of these tests.)

Other Invasive Diagnostic Assessment

Endoscopic Examinations. Endoscopic studies to assess breathing problems include bronchoscopy, laryngoscopy, and mediastinoscopy. With *laryngoscopy,* a tube for visualization is

TABLE 27-6 Characteristics and Purposes of Pulmonary Function Tests

TEST	PURPOSE
FVC (forced vital capacity) records the maximum amount of air that can be exhaled as quickly as possible after maximum inspiration.	Indicates respiratory muscle strength and ventilatory reserve. Reduced in obstructive and restrictive diseases.
FEV_1 (forced expiratory volume in 1 sec) records the maximum amount of air that can be exhaled in the first second of expiration.	Is effort dependent and declines normally with age. It is reduced in certain obstructive and restrictive disorders.
FEV_1/FVC is the ratio of expiratory volume in 1 sec to FVC.	Indicates obstruction to airflow. This ratio is the hallmark of obstructive pulmonary disease. It is normal or increased in restrictive disease.
$FEF_{25\%-75\%}$ records the forced expiratory flow over the 25%-75% volume (middle half) of the FVC.	This measure provides a more sensitive index of obstruction in the smaller airways.
FRC (functional residual capacity) is the amount of air remaining in the lungs after normal expiration. FRC test requires use of the helium dilution, nitrogen washout, or body plethysmography technique.	Increased FRC indicates hyperinflation or air trapping, often from obstructive pulmonary disease. FRC is normal or decreased in restrictive pulmonary diseases.
TLC (total lung capacity) is the amount of air in the lungs at the end of maximum inhalation.	Increased TLC indicates air trapping from obstructive pulmonary disease. Decreased TLC indicates restrictive disease.
RV (residual volume) is the amount of air remaining in the lungs at the end of a full, forced exhalation.	RV is increased in obstructive pulmonary disease such as emphysema.
DLCO (diffusion capacity of the lung for carbon monoxide) reflects the surface area of the alveolocapillary membrane. The patient inhales a small amount of CO, holds for 10 sec, and then exhales. The amount inhaled is compared with the amount exhaled.	Is reduced whenever the alveolocapillary membrane is diminished (emphysema, pulmonary hypertension, and pulmonary fibrosis). It is increased with exercise and in conditions such as polycythemia and congestive heart disease.

inserted into the larynx to assess the function of the vocal cords, remove foreign bodies caught in the larynx, or obtain tissue samples for biopsy or culture. A *mediastinoscopy* is the insertion of a flexible tube through the chest wall just above the sternum into the area between the lungs. It is performed in the operating room with the patient under general anesthesia to examine for the presence of tumors and to obtain tissue samples for biopsy or culture. Most complications are related to the anesthetic agents and bleeding. The most common procedure is the bronchoscopy.

A **bronchoscopy** is the insertion of a tube in the airways, usually as far as the secondary bronchi, to view airway structures and obtain tissue samples for biopsy or culture. It is used to diagnose and manage pulmonary diseases. Rigid bronchoscopy usually requires general anesthesia in the operating room. Flexible bronchoscopy can be performed in the intensive care unit (ICU) with low-dose sedation. A flexible bronchoscopy is used to evaluate the airway and to assist with placing or changing an endotracheal tube, collecting specimens, and diagnosing infections. It is often used for lung cancer staging and removal of secretions that are not cleared with normal suctioning procedures. Stents can be placed during bronchoscopy to open up strictures in the trachea and bronchus.

Patient Preparation. Explain the procedure to the patient, and verify that consent for the procedure was obtained. Expected outcomes, risks, and benefits of the procedure must be discussed with the patient by the health care provider performing the procedure. Document patient allergies. Other tests before the procedure may include a complete blood count, platelet count, prothrombin time, electrolytes, and chest x-ray. The patient should be NPO for 4 to 8 hours before the procedure to reduce the risk for aspiration. Premedication with one of the benzodiazepines may be used to provide both sedation and amnesia. Opioids may also be used.

! NURSING SAFETY PRIORITY QSEN

Critical Rescue

In accordance with The Joint Commission's National Patient Safety Goals, verify the patient's identity with *two* types of identifiers (name and at least one person-specific number such as birth date, medical record number, or Social Security number) before a bronchoscopy.

Benzocaine spray as a topical anesthetic to numb the oropharynx is used cautiously, if at all. This agent may induce a condition called **methemoglobinemia**, which is the conversion of normal hemoglobin to methemoglobin (Wesley, 2014). Methemoglobin is an altered iron state that does not carry oxygen, resulting in tissue hypoxia. Other topical anesthetic sprays, such as lidocaine, appear less likely to induce this problem.

The normal blood level of methemoglobin is less than 1%. When this level increases, tissue GAS EXCHANGE is reduced. Cyanosis occurs with methemoglobin levels between 10% and 20%, and death can occur when levels reach 50% to 70%. Suspect methemoglobinemia if a patient becomes cyanotic after receiving a topical anesthetic, if he or she does not respond to supplemental oxygen, and if blood is a characteristic chocolate-brown in color. It can be reversed with oxygen and IV injection of 1% methylene blue (1 to 2 mg/kg).

! NURSING SAFETY PRIORITY QSEN

Critical Rescue

Notify the Rapid Response Team if the patient has any manifestations of methemoglobinemia (cyanosis unresponsive to oxygen therapy, chocolate-brown–colored blood) after the use of benzocaine topical anesthetic.

Procedure. The procedure can be done in a bronchoscopy suite or at the ICU bedside. The bronchoscope is inserted through either the naris or the oropharynx. Maintain IV access, and continuously monitor the patient's pulse, blood pressure, respiratory rate, and oxygen saturation. Apply supplemental oxygen.

Follow-up Care. Monitor the patient until the effects of the sedation have resolved and a gag reflex has returned. Continue to monitor vital signs, including oxygen saturation, and assess breath sounds every 15 minutes for the first 2 hours. Also assess for potential complications, including bleeding, infection, or hypoxemia.

Thoracentesis. **Thoracentesis** is the needle aspiration of pleural fluid or air from the pleural space for diagnostic or management purposes. Microscopic examination of the pleural fluid helps in making a diagnosis. Pleural fluid may be drained to relieve blood vessel or lung compression and the respiratory distress caused by cancer, empyema, pleurisy, or tuberculosis. Drugs can also be instilled into the pleural space during thoracentesis.

Patient Preparation. Patient preparation is essential before thoracentesis to ensure cooperation during the procedure and to prevent complications. Tell the patient to expect a stinging sensation from the local anesthetic agent and a feeling of pressure when the needle is pushed through the posterior chest. Stress the importance of not moving, coughing, or deep breathing during the procedure to avoid puncture of the pleura or lung.

Ask the patient about any allergy to local anesthetic agents. Verify that the patient has signed an informed consent. The entire chest or back is exposed, and the hair on the skin over the aspiration site is clipped if necessary. The site depends on the volume and location of the fluid.

Fig. 27-13 shows the best position for thoracentesis, which widens the spaces between the ribs and permits easy access to the pleural fluid. Properly position and physically support the patient during the procedure. Use pillows to make the patient comfortable and to provide physical support. When the sitting position is used for the procedure, stand in front of the patient to prevent the table from moving and the patient from falling.

Procedure. Thoracentesis is often performed at the bedside by a nurse practitioner or a physician, although CT or ultrasound may be used to guide it. The person performing the procedure and any assistants wear goggles and masks to prevent accidental eye or oral splash exposure to the pleural fluid. After the skin is prepped, a local anesthetic is injected into the selected site. Keep the patient informed of the procedure while observing for shock, pain, nausea, pallor, diaphoresis, cyanosis, tachypnea, and dyspnea.

The short 18- to 25-gauge thoracentesis needle (with an attached syringe) is advanced into the pleural space. Fluid in the pleural space is slowly aspirated with gentle suction. A vacuum collection bottle may be needed to remove larger volumes of fluid. To prevent re-expansion pulmonary edema, usually no more than 1000 mL of fluid is removed at one time. If a biopsy is performed, a second, larger needle with a cutting edge and collection chamber is used. After the needle is withdrawn, pressure is applied to the puncture site and a sterile dressing is applied. In some cases, pigtail drain catheters may be left in place to a waterseal drainage system, rather than doing a thoracentesis aspiration on a recurring basis.

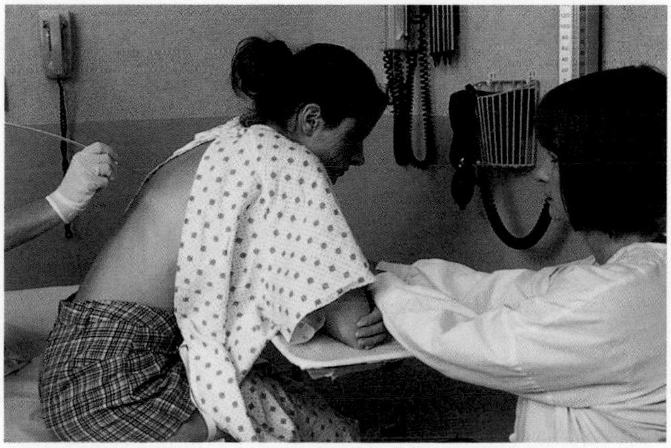

FIG. 27-13 Position for thoracentesis.

Follow-up Care. After thoracentesis, a chest x-ray is performed to rule out possible pneumothorax and **mediastinal shift** (shift of central thoracic structures toward one side). Monitor vital signs, and listen to the lungs for absent or reduced sounds on the affected side. Check the puncture site and dressing for leakage or bleeding. Assess for complications, such as reaccumulation of fluid in the pleural space, subcutaneous emphysema, infection, and tension pneumothorax. Urge the patient to breathe deeply to promote lung expansion. Document the procedure, including the patient's response; the volume and character of the fluid removed; any specimens sent to the laboratory; the location of the puncture site; and respiratory assessment findings before, during, and after the procedure.

Teach the patient about the manifestations of a **pneumothorax** (partial or complete collapse of the lung), which can occur within the first 24 hours after a thoracentesis. Manifestations include:

- Pain on the affected side that is worse at the end of inhalation and the end of exhalation
- Rapid heart rate
- Rapid, shallow respirations
- A feeling of air hunger
- Prominence of the affected side that does not move in and out with respiratory effort
- Trachea slanted more to the unaffected side instead of being in the center of the neck
- New onset of "nagging" cough
- Cyanosis

Instruct the patient to go to the nearest emergency department immediately if these manifestations occur.

Lung Biopsy. A lung biopsy is performed to obtain tissue for histologic analysis, culture, or cytologic examination. The samples are used to make a definite diagnosis of inflammation, cancer, infection, or lung disease. There are several types of lung biopsies. The site and extent of the lesion determine which one is used. Transbronchial biopsy (TBB) and transbronchial needle aspiration (TBNA) are performed during bronchoscopy. Transthoracic needle aspiration is performed through the skin (percutaneous) for areas that cannot be reached by bronchoscopy.

Patient Preparation. The patient may worry about the outcome of the biopsy and may associate the term *biopsy* with *cancer.* Explain what to expect before and after the procedure, and explore the patient's feelings. An analgesic or sedative may be prescribed before the procedure. Inform the patient undergoing percutaneous biopsy that discomfort is reduced with a local anesthetic agent but that pressure may be felt during needle insertion and tissue aspiration. Open lung biopsy is performed in the operating room with the patient under general anesthesia, and the usual preparations before surgery apply (see Chapter 14).

Procedure. Percutaneous lung biopsy is usually performed in the radiology department after an informed consent has been obtained. Fluoroscopy or CT is often used to visualize the area and guide the procedure. The patient is usually placed in the side-lying position, depending on the location of the lesion. The skin is cleansed with an antiseptic agent, and a local anesthetic is given. Under sterile conditions, a spinal-type needle is inserted through the skin into the desired area and tissue is obtained for microscopic examination. Apply a dressing after the procedure. A CT scan or chest x-ray must follow the biopsy to confirm there is no pneumothorax.

An open lung biopsy is performed in the operating room. The patient undergoes a thoracotomy in which lung tissue is exposed and appropriate tissue specimens are taken. A chest tube is placed to remove air and fluid so the lung can re-inflate, and then the chest is closed.

Follow-up Care. Monitor the patient's vital signs and breath sounds at least every 4 hours for 24 hours, and assess for signs of respiratory distress (e.g., dyspnea, pallor, diaphoresis, tachypnea). Pneumothorax is a serious complication of needle biopsy and open lung biopsy. Report reduced or absent breath sounds immediately. Monitor for hemoptysis (which may be scant and transient) or, in rare cases, for frank bleeding from vascular or lung trauma.

CLINICAL JUDGMENT CHALLENGE

Safety; Patient-Centered Care; Teamwork and Collaboration QSEN

Your patient is the 68-year-old man from the previous *Clinical Judgment Challenge* who had shortness of breath (SOB) for the past 2 to 3 days. His clinical condition deteriorated further, requiring intubation. The health care provider orders a CT scan of the chest.

1. What are your responsibilities when preparing the patient for the CT scan?
2. Why is it important to monitor your patient using capnography?
3. A large fluid collection on the left side is found during the CT scan, and a thoracentesis is planned. What are your responsibilities in preparing for and assisting with this procedure?
4. Your patient was extubated after the left thoracentesis. Within 12 hours he again develops respiratory distress, decreased breath sounds, and a trachea that appears deviated to the right. What is your assessment?

NURSING CONCEPTS AND CLINICAL JUDGMENT REVIEW

What might you NOTICE in a patient with adequate GAS EXCHANGE and tissue PERFUSION related to respiratory function?

Vital signs:
- Respiratory rate and heart rate within normal range
- Oxygen saturation of 95% or higher

Physical assessment:
- Able to speak a sentence of 12 words without stopping for breath
- Able to walk and talk without stopping for breath
- Skin color normal (no cyanosis or pallor)
- Oral mucous membrane and nail beds pink with rapid capillary refill
- Fingertips and nails normal shape, no clubbing
- Anterior to posterior diameter of chest about two-thirds the size of the lateral diameter
- Space between each rib no larger than the breadth of the patient's finger
- Usually breathes in through the nose and out through the mouth or nose
- Breathing quiet
- Air movement heard (with a stethoscope) in all lobes of both lungs
- Sputum production minimal, clear or white
- Muscle development even with no muscle loss on arms and legs
- Weight proportionate to height; does not appear underweight

Psychological assessment:
- Oriented and not confused
- Energy level good, can engage in desired work, recreational, and personal activities

Laboratory assessment:
- Red blood cell, hemoglobin, hematocrit, and white blood cell levels within normal limits for age and gender

GET READY FOR THE NCLEX® EXAMINATION!

KEY POINTS

Review these Key Points for each NCLEX Client Needs Category.

Health Promotion and Maintenance

- Assess any patient's geographic, home, occupational, and recreational exposure to inhalation irritants. **Patient-Centered Care** QSEN
- Encourage all people to use masks and adequate ventilation when exposed to inhalation irritants.
- Promote smoking cessation for people who smoke. **Patient-Centered Care** QSEN
- Support the person who chooses to stop smoking by assisting him or her to decide about drug therapy for smoking cessation and finding an appropriate smoking-cessation program. **Patient-Centered Care** QSEN

Psychosocial Integrity

- Allow the patient the opportunity to express fear or anxiety about tests of respiratory function or about a potential change in respiratory function. **Patient-Centered Care** QSEN
- Teach patients and family members about what to expect during tests and procedures to assess respiratory function and respiratory disease. **Patient-Centered Care** QSEN

Physiological Integrity

- Ask the patient about respiratory problems in any other members of the family, because some problems have a genetic component. **Patient-Centered Care** QSEN
- Ask the patient about current and past drug use (prescribed, over-the-counter, and illicit), and evaluate drug use for potential lung damage.
- Calculate the pack-year smoking history for the patient who smokes or who has ever smoked cigarettes. **Patient-Centered Care** QSEN
- Use concepts of anatomy and appropriate psychomotor skills to apply respiratory assessment techniques correctly.
- Distinguish between normal and abnormal (adventitious) breath sounds.
- Interpret arterial blood gas values to assess the patient's respiratory status.
- Assess the degree to which breathing problems interfere with the patient's ability to perform ADLs. **Patient-Centered Care** QSEN
- Document any known specific allergies that have respiratory manifestations. **Patient-Centered Care** QSEN
- Assess the airway and breathing effectiveness for any patient who has shortness of breath or any change in mental status. **Evidence-Based Practice** QSEN
- Assess the patient's respiratory status every 15 minutes for at least the first 2 hours after undergoing an endoscopic test for respiratory disorders. **Patient-Centered Care** QSEN
- Explain nursing care needs for the patient after bronchoscopy or open lung biopsy.

28 CHAPTER

Care of Patients Requiring Oxygen Therapy or Tracheostomy

Harry Rees

http://evolve.elsevier.com/Iggy/

PRIORITY CONCEPTS

- Gas Exchange
- Perfusion

LEARNING OUTCOMES

Safe and Effective Care Environment

1. Act as a patient advocate for patients receiving oxygen or who have tracheostomies.
2. Protect the patient receiving oxygen or who has a tracheostomy from injury and infection.

Health Promotion and Maintenance

3. Teach the patient and family how to avoid injury and complications related to oxygen therapy or tracheostomy in the home.

Psychosocial Integrity

4. Reduce the psychological impact of oxygen therapy or tracheostomy for the patient and family.
5. Work with other members of the health care team to ensure that patient values, preferences, and expressed needs related to a tracheostomy and oxygen therapy are respected.

Physiological Integrity

6. Apply knowledge of anatomy and physiology to perform a focused respiratory assessment and re-assessment to determine adequacy of GAS EXCHANGE, oxygenation, and tissue PERFUSION for the patient receiving oxygen therapy or who has a tracheostomy.
7. Use appropriate techniques to administer prescribed oxygen therapy.
8. Use appropriate techniques to provide tracheostomy care.

Oxygen (O_2) is an essential element that serves as a nutrient for all cells to live and perform their specific jobs. For cells to receive oxygen, GAS EXCHANGE must occur first in the lungs and then at the tissue level with PERFUSION of oxygenated blood. These processes rely on three systems—the respiratory system, the cardiovascular system, and the hematologic system—to work together to ensure sufficient oxygen for cell survival and proper function (see Fig. 27-1). Gas exchange with oxygenation and tissue perfusion needs can go unmet as a result of many problems with the lungs. When a respiratory problem interferes with adequate gas exchange, both the cardiac system and the hematologic system adjust (compensate) and work harder to restore balance and maintain oxygenation and tissue perfusion (Fig. 28-1) (McCance et al., 2014). Oxygen therapy through various delivery systems, including tracheostomy, can help improve gas exchange and tissue perfusion and reduce the burden on the cardiovascular and hematologic systems.

OXYGEN THERAPY

Oxygen (O_2) is a gas used as a drug for relief of **hypoxemia** (low levels of oxygen in the blood) and **hypoxia** (decreased tissue oxygenation). The oxygen content of atmospheric air is about 21%. Oxygen therapy is prescribed for both acute and chronic breathing problems when the oxygen needs of the patient cannot be met by atmospheric or "room air" alone. Indications for use include decreased partial pressure of arterial oxygen (Pao_2) levels or decreased arterial oxygen saturation (Sao_2). Non-respiratory conditions, such as heart failure, sepsis, fever, some poisons, and decreased hemoglobin levels or poor hemoglobin quality, can affect GAS EXCHANGE and oxygenation and are indications for oxygen therapy. These conditions increase oxygen demand, decrease the oxygen-carrying capability of the blood, or decrease cardiac output.

The purpose of oxygen therapy is to use the lowest *fraction of inspired oxygen (Fio_2)* to have an acceptable blood oxygen level without causing harmful side effects. *Although oxygen improves the Pao_2 level, it does not cure the problem or stop the disease process.* Most patients with hypoxia require an oxygen flow of 2 to 4 L/min via nasal cannula or up to 40% via Venturi mask to achieve an oxygen saturation of at least 95%. For a patient who is hypoxemic and has chronic **hypercarbia** (increased partial pressure of arterial carbon dioxide [$Paco_2$] levels), the Fio_2 delivered should be titrated to correct the

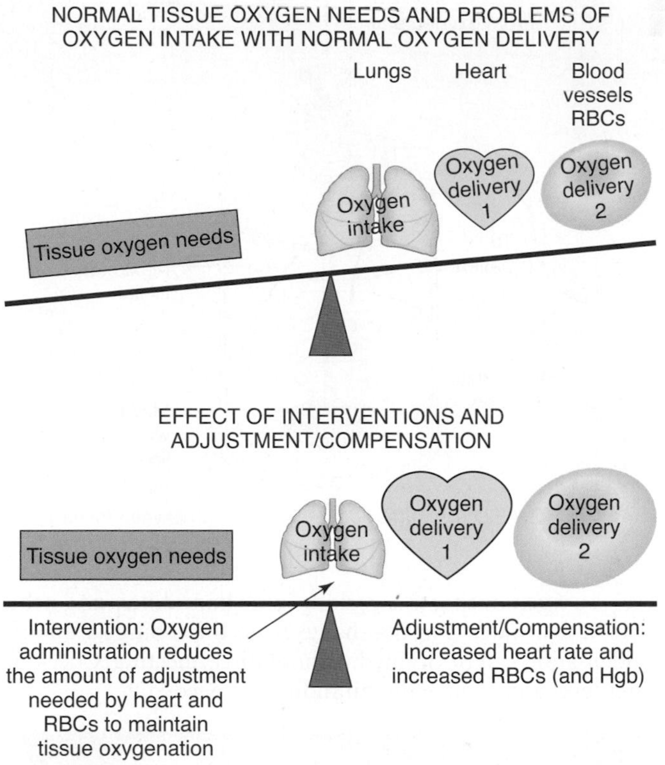

FIG. 28-1 Restoration of adequate oxygenation and tissue perfusion by oxygen delivery adjustments and oxygen therapy when respiratory problems interfere with meeting tissue oxygen needs. *Hgb,* Hemoglobin, *RBCs,* red blood cells.

CHART 28-1 Best Practice for Patient Safety & Quality Care QSEN

Oxygen Therapy

- Check the health care provider's prescription with the type of delivery system and liter flow or percentage of oxygen actually in use.
- Obtain a prescription for humidification if oxygen is being delivered at 4 L/min or more.
- Be sure the oxygen and humidification equipment are functioning properly.
- Check the skin around the patient's ears, back of the neck, and face every 4 to 8 hours for pressure points and signs of irritation.
- Ensure that mouth care is provided every 8 hours and as needed; assess nasal and oral mucous membranes for cracks or other signs of dryness.
- Pad the elastic band and change its position frequently to prevent skin breakdown.
- Pad tubing in areas that put pressure on the skin.
- Cleanse the cannula or mask by rinsing with clear, warm water every 4 to 8 hours or as needed.
- Cleanse skin under the tubing, straps, and mask every 4 to 8 hours or as needed.
- Lubricate the patient's nostrils, face, and lips with non-petroleum cream to relieve the drying effects of oxygen.
- Position the tubing so it does not pull on the patient's face, nose, or artificial airway.
- Ensure that there is no smoking and that no candles or matches are lit in the immediate area.
- Assess and document the patient's response to oxygen therapy.
- Ensure that the patient has an adequate oxygen source during any periods of transport.
- Provide the patient with ongoing teaching and reassurance to enhance his or her adherence with oxygen therapy.

hypoxemia to achieve generally acceptable oxygenation saturations in the range of 88% to 92% (Abdo & Heunks, 2012).

❖ *PATIENT-CENTERED COLLABORATIVE CARE*

◆ *Assessment*

Arterial blood gas (ABG) analysis is the best measure for determining the need for oxygen therapy and for evaluating its effects. Oxygen need is also determined by noninvasive monitoring, such as pulse oximetry and capnography (Carlisle, 2014).

◆ *Interventions*

Before starting oxygen therapy and while caring for a patient receiving oxygen therapy, you must be knowledgeable about oxygen hazards and complications. Know the rationale and the expected outcome related to oxygen therapy for each patient receiving oxygen. Chart 28-1 lists best practices for patients using oxygen therapy.

Hazards and Complications of Oxygen Therapy

Combustion. Oxygen itself does not burn, but it enhances combustion so that fire burns better in the presence of oxygen. For example, when the oxygen content of the air around a lighted cigarette is nearly 50%, the entire cigarette flames up and can catch items nearby on fire (Murabit & Tredget, 2012). Open fires, even small ones like candles or cigarettes, should not be in the same room during oxygen therapy. Take precautions during oxygen delivery, including posting a sign on the door of the patient's room. Smoking is prohibited in the patient's room, including at home, when oxygen is in use.

All electrical equipment in rooms where oxygen is in use must have grounded plugs and be plugged into grounded outlets to prevent fires from electrical arcing sparks. Frayed cords must be repaired because they can cause a spark that can ignite a flame. Flammable solutions (containing high concentrations of alcohol or oil) are not used in rooms in which oxygen is in use. (This does not include alcohol-based hand rubs.)

Oxygen-Induced Hypoventilation. For many years, oxygen was thought to induce hypoventilation in the patient with chronic lung disease who also had carbon dioxide retention (**hypercarbia**). As a result, nurses and physicians were reluctant to administer oxygen to these hypoxic patients, leading to serious problems and even deaths related to inadequate GAS EXCHANGE and PERFUSION. More recent research disproves the hypoxic drive theory and has found that patients with chronic lung disease are at risk for oxygen-induced hypercapnia but not for severely reduced respiratory effort (Makic et al., 2013). Therefore oxygen therapy is prescribed at the lowest liter flow needed to manage hypoxemia (Mac Sweeney et al., 2011). A system that delivers more precise oxygen levels (e.g., a Venturi mask) is preferred. However, some patients with chronic lung disease may not tolerate a facemask. Monitor the patient's response to therapy closely to ensure adequate gas exchange and correction of hypoxemia. Parameters to monitor include the level of consciousness, respiratory pattern and rate, and pulse oximetry. Remember, untreated or inadequately treated hypoxemia is a threat to life for any person with a breathing problem.

Oxygen Toxicity. Oxygen toxicity is related to the concentration of oxygen delivered, duration of oxygen therapy, and degree of lung disease present. In general, an oxygen level greater than 50% given continuously for more than 24 to 48 hours may damage the lungs.

The causes and manifestations of lung injury from oxygen toxicity are the same as those for acute respiratory distress syndrome (ARDS) (see Chapter 32). Initial problems include dyspnea, nonproductive cough, chest pain beneath the sternum, GI upset, and crackles on auscultation. As exposure to high levels of oxygen continues, the problems become more severe with decreased vital capacity, decreased compliance, and hypoxemia. With prolonged exposure to high oxygen levels, atelectasis, pulmonary edema, hemorrhage, and hyaline membrane formation may result. Surviving this critical condition depends on correcting the underlying disease process and decreasing the oxygen amount delivered.

The toxic effects of oxygen are difficult to manage, making prevention a priority. The lowest level of oxygen needed to maintain GAS EXCHANGE and oxygenation and prevent oxygen toxicity is prescribed. Closely monitor arterial blood gases (ABGs) during oxygen therapy, and notify the health care provider when Pa_{O_2} levels become greater than 90 mm Hg. Also monitor the prescribed oxygen level and length of therapy to identify patients at higher risk. High oxygen levels are avoided unless absolutely necessary. The use of noninvasive positive airway pressure techniques with oxygen or the use of mechanical ventilation (see Chapter 32) may reduce the amount of oxygen needed. As soon as the patient's condition allows, the prescribed amount of oxygen is decreased.

Absorptive Atelectasis. Normally, nitrogen in the air maintains patent airways and alveoli. Making up 79% of room air, nitrogen prevents alveolar collapse. When high oxygen levels are delivered, nitrogen is diluted, oxygen diffuses from the alveoli into the blood, and the alveoli collapse. Collapsed alveoli cause atelectasis (called *absorptive atelectasis*), which is detected as crackles and decreased breath sounds on auscultation.

! NURSING SAFETY PRIORITY QSEN

Action Alert

Monitor the patient receiving high levels of oxygen closely for indications of absorptive atelectasis (new onset of crackles and decreased breath sounds) every 1 to 2 hours when oxygen therapy is started and as often as needed thereafter.

Drying of the Mucous Membranes. When the prescribed oxygen flow rate is higher than 4 L/min, humidify the delivery system (Fig. 28-2). Ensure that oxygen bubbles through the water in the humidifier.

Oxygen can also be humidified via a large-volume jet nebulizer in mist form (aerosol). A heated nebulizer raises the humidity even more and is used for oxygen delivery through an artificial airway. Usually the upper airway passages warm the air during breathing, but these passages are bypassed with an artificial airway, such as an endotracheal tube.

For the patient to receive properly humidified oxygen, the humidifier or nebulizer must have a sufficient amount of sterile water and the flow rate must be adequate. Condensation often forms in the tubing. Remove this condensation as it collects by disconnecting the tubing and emptying the water. Minimize the time the tubing is disconnected because the patient does not receive oxygen during this period. Some humidifiers and nebulizers have a water trap that hangs from the tubing so that the condensation can be drained without disconnecting. Check the water level and change the humidifier as needed.

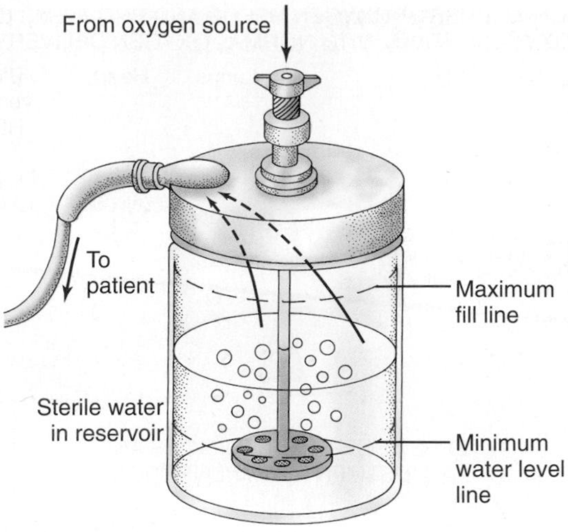

FIG. 28-2 A bubble humidifier bottle used with oxygen therapy.

! NURSING SAFETY PRIORITY QSEN

Action Alert

To prevent bacterial contamination of the oxygen delivery system, never drain the fluid from the water trap back into the humidifier or nebulizer.

Infection. The humidifier or nebulizer may be a source of bacteria, especially if it is heated. Oxygen delivery equipment such as cannulas and masks can also harbor organisms. Change equipment as per agency policy, which ranges from every 24 hours for humidification systems to every 7 days or whenever necessary for cannulas and masks.

? NCLEX EXAMINATION CHALLENGE

Physiological Integrity

Which manifestations in a client receiving oxygen therapy at 60% for more than 24 hours alert the nurse to the possibility of oxygen toxicity?

A. Oxygen saturation greater than 100%
B. Decreased rate and depth of respiration
C. Wheezing on inhalation and exhalation
D. Discomfort or pain under the sternum

Oxygen Delivery Systems. Oxygen can be delivered by many systems. Regardless of the type of delivery system used, it is important to understand its indications, advantages, and disadvantages. Use the equipment properly, and ensure appropriate equipment maintenance. Consult a respiratory therapist whenever there is a question or concern about an oxygen delivery system.

The type of delivery system used depends on:

- Oxygen concentration required by the patient
- Oxygen concentration achieved by a delivery system
- Importance of accuracy and control of the oxygen concentration

TABLE 28-1 Comparison of Low-Flow Oxygen Delivery Systems

FiO_2 DELIVERED	NURSING INTERVENTIONS	RATIONALES
Nasal Cannula		
24%-40% FiO_2 at 1-6 L/min ≈24% at 1 L/min ≈28% at 2 L/min ≈32% at 3 L/min ≈36% at 4 L/min ≈40% at 5 L/min ≈44% at 6 L/min	Ensure that prongs are in the nares properly.	A poorly fitting nasal cannula leads to hypoxemia and skin breakdown.
	Apply water-soluble jelly to nares PRN.	This substance prevents mucosal irritation related to the drying effect of oxygen; promotes comfort.
	Assess the patency of the nostrils.	Congestion or a deviated septum prevents effective delivery of oxygen through the nares.
	Assess the patient for changes in respiratory rate and depth.	The respiratory pattern affects the amount of oxygen delivered. A different delivery system may be needed.
Simple Facemask		
40%-60% FiO_2 at 5-8 L/min; flow rate must be set at least at 5 L/min to flush mask of carbon dioxide ≈40% at 5 L/min ≈45%-50% at 6 L/min ≈55%-60% at 8 L/min	Be sure mask fits securely over nose and mouth.	A poorly fitting mask reduces the FiO_2 delivered.
	Assess skin and provide skin care to the area covered by the mask.	Pressure and moisture under the mask may cause skin breakdown.
	Monitor the patient closely for risk for aspiration.	The mask limits the patient's ability to clear the mouth, especially if vomiting occurs.
	Provide emotional support to the patient who feels claustrophobic.	Emotional support decreases anxiety, which contributes to a claustrophobic feeling.
	Suggest to the health care provider to switch the patient from a mask to the nasal cannula during eating.	Use of the cannula prevents hypoxemia during eating.
Partial Rebreather Mask		
60%-75% at 6-11 L/min, a liter flow rate high enough to maintain reservoir bag two-thirds full during inspiration and expiration	Make sure that the reservoir does not twist or kink, which results in a deflated bag.	Deflation results in decreased oxygen delivered and increases the rebreathing of exhaled air.
	Adjust the flow rate to keep the reservoir bag inflated.	The flow rate is adjusted to meet the pattern of the patient.
Non-Rebreather Mask		
80%-95% FiO_2 at a liter flow high enough to maintain reservoir bag two-thirds full	Interventions as for partial rebreather mask; this patient requires close monitoring.	Rationales as for partial rebreather mask. Monitoring ensures proper functioning and prevents harm.
	Make sure that valves and rubber flaps are patent, functional, and not stuck. Remove mucus or saliva.	Valves should open during expiration and close during inhalation to prevent dramatic decrease in FiO_2. Suffocation can occur if the reservoir bag kinks or if the oxygen source disconnects.
	Closely assess the patient on increased FiO_2 via non-rebreather mask. Intubation is the only way to provide more precise FiO_2.	The patient may require intubation.

FiO_2, Fraction of inspired oxygen.

- Patient comfort
- Importance of humidity
- Patient mobility

Oxygen delivery systems are classified by the rate of oxygen delivery into either low-flow systems or high-flow systems. Low-flow systems have a low fraction of inspired oxygen (FiO_2) and therefore do not provide enough oxygen to meet the total oxygen need and air volume of the patient. So, part of the tidal volume is supplied by the patient as he or she breathes room air. The total level of oxygen inspired depends on the respiratory rate and tidal volume. High-flow systems have a flow rate that meets the entire oxygen need and tidal volume regardless of the patient's breathing pattern. These systems are used for critically ill patients and when delivery of precise levels of oxygen is needed.

If the patient needs a mask but is able to eat, request a prescription for a nasal cannula to be used at mealtimes only. Reapply the mask after the meal is completed. To increase mobility, up to 50 feet of connecting tubing can be used with connecting pieces.

Low-Flow Oxygen Delivery Systems. Low-flow systems include the nasal cannula, simple facemask, partial rebreather mask, and non-rebreather mask (Table 28-1). These systems are inexpensive, easy to use, and fairly comfortable, but the amount of oxygen delivered varies and depends on the patient's breathing pattern. The oxygen is diluted with room air (21% oxygen), which lowers the amount actually inspired.

Nasal Cannula. The nasal cannula (prongs) (Fig. 28-3), is used at flow rates of 1 to 6 L/min. Oxygen concentrations of 24% (at 1 L/min) to 44% (at 6 L/min) can be achieved. Flow rates greater than 6 L/min do not increase gas exchange because the **anatomic dead space** (places where air flows but the structures are too thick for gas exchange) is full. Also, high flow rates increase mucosal irritation.

The nasal cannula is often used for chronic lung disease and for any patient needing long-term oxygen therapy. Place the

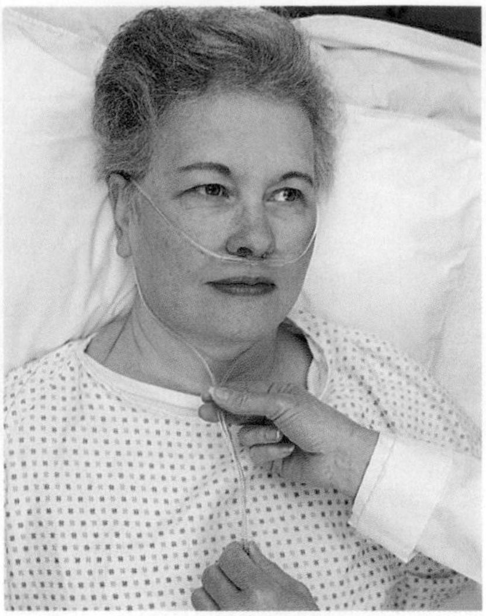

FIG. 28-3 A nasal cannula (prongs).

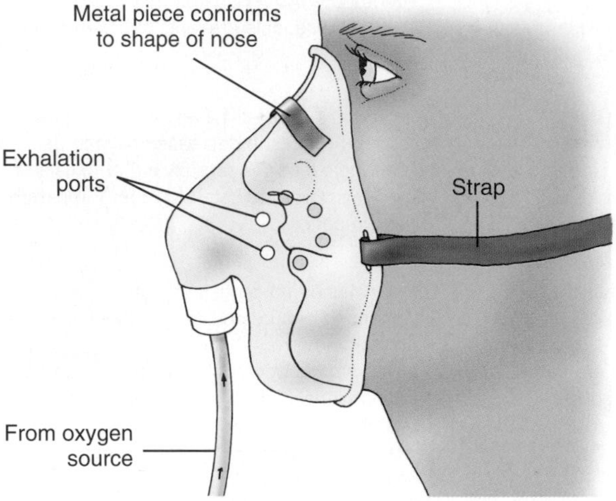

FIG. 28-4 A simple facemask used to deliver oxygen.

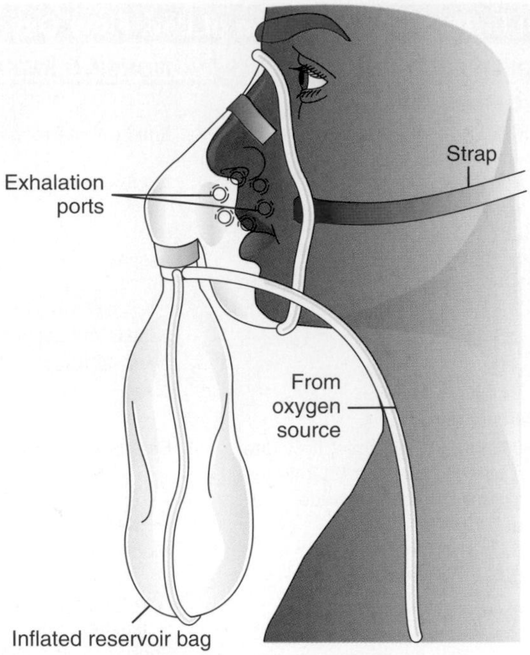

FIG. 28-5 A partial rebreather mask.

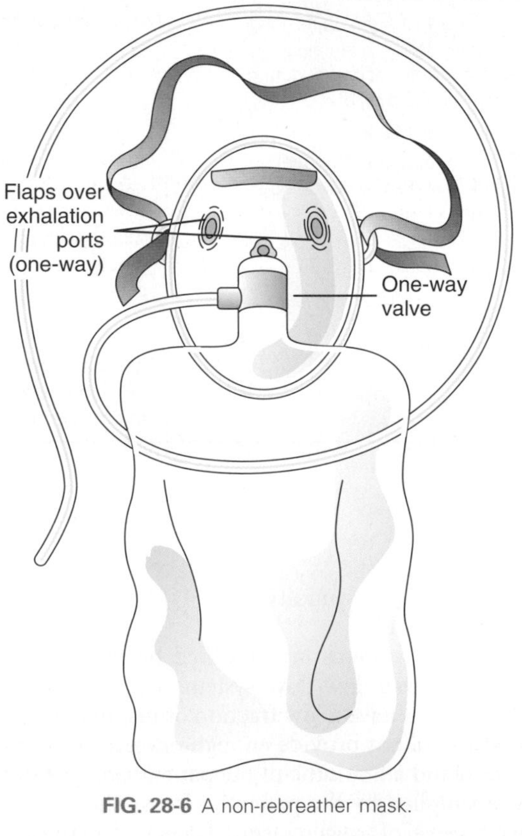

FIG. 28-6 A non-rebreather mask.

nasal prongs in the nostrils, with the openings facing the patient, following the natural anatomic curve of the nares.

Facemasks. Facemasks can deliver a wide range of oxygen flow rates and concentrations.

Simple facemasks are used to deliver oxygen concentrations of 40% to 60% for short-term oxygen therapy or in an emergency (Fig. 28-4). A minimum flow rate of 5 L/min is needed to prevent the rebreathing of exhaled air. Ensure that the mask fits well to maintain inspired oxygen levels. Care for the skin under the mask and strap to prevent skin breakdown (Ambutas et al., 2014).

Partial rebreather masks provide oxygen concentrations of 60% to 75% with flow rates of 6 to 11 L/min. It is a mask with a reservoir bag but no flaps (Fig. 28-5). With each breath, the patient rebreathes one third of the exhaled tidal volume, which is high in oxygen and increases the fraction of inspired oxygen (Fio_2). For best oxygen delivery, be sure that the bag remains slightly inflated at the end of inspiration. If needed, call the respiratory therapist for assistance.

Non-rebreather masks provide the highest oxygen level of the low-flow systems and can deliver an Fio_2 greater than 90%, depending on the patient's breathing pattern. This mask is often used with patients whose respiratory status is unstable and who may require intubation.

The non-rebreather mask has a one-way valve between the mask and the reservoir and usually has two flaps over the exhalation ports (Fig. 28-6). The valve allows the patient to draw all needed oxygen from the reservoir bag, and the flaps

TABLE 28-2 **Comparison of High-Flow Oxygen Delivery Systems**

FiO_2 DELIVERED	NURSING INTERVENTIONS	RATIONALES
Venturi Mask (Venti Mask)		
24%-50% FiO_2 with flow rates as recommended by the manufacturer, usually 4-10 L/min; provides high humidity	Perform constant surveillance to ensure an accurate flow rate for the specific FiO_2.	An accurate flow rate ensures FiO_2 delivery.
	Keep the orifice for the Venturi adaptor open and uncovered.	If the Venturi orifice is covered, the adaptor does not function and oxygen delivery varies.
	Provide a mask that fits snugly and tubing that is free of kinks.	FiO_2 is altered if kinking occurs or if the mask fits poorly.
	Assess the patient for dry mucous membranes.	Comfort measures may be indicated.
	Change to a nasal cannula during mealtime.	Oxygen is a drug that needs to be given continuously.
Aerosol Mask, Face Tent, Tracheostomy Collar		
24%-100% FiO_2 with flow rates of at least 10 L/min; provides high humidity	Assess that aerosol mist escapes from the vents of the delivery system during inspiration and expiration.	Humidification should be delivered to the patient.
	Empty condensation from the tubing.	Emptying prevents the patient from being lavaged with water, promotes an adequate flow rate, and ensures a continued prescribed FiO_2.
	Change the aerosol water container as needed.	Adequate humidification is ensured only when there is sufficient water in the canister.
T-Piece		
24%-100% FiO_2 with flow rates of at least 10 L/min; provides high humidity	Empty condensation from the tubing.	Condensation interferes with flow rate delivery of FiO_2 and may drain into the tracheostomy if not emptied.
	Keep the exhalation port open and uncovered.	If the port is occluded, the patient can suffocate.
	Position the T-piece so that it does not pull on the tracheostomy or endotracheal tube.	The weight of the T-piece pulls on the tracheostomy and causes pain or erosion of skin at the insertion site.
	Make sure the humidifier creates enough mist. A mist should be seen during inspiration and expiration.	An adequate flow rate is needed to meet the inspiration effort of the patient. If not, the patient will be "air-hungry."

FiO_2, Fraction of inspired oxygen.

prevent room air from entering through the exhalation ports (which would dilute the oxygen concentration). During exhalation, air leaves through these exhalation ports while the one-way valve prevents exhaled air from re-entering the reservoir bag. The flow rate is kept high (10 to 15 L/min) to keep the bag inflated during inhalation. Assess for this safety feature at least hourly.

! NURSING SAFETY PRIORITY QSEN

Critical Rescue

Ensure that the valve and flaps on a non-rebreather mask are intact and functional during each breath. If the oxygen source should fail or be depleted when both flaps are in place, the patient would not be able to inhale room air.

High-Flow Oxygen Delivery Systems. High-flow systems (Table 28-2) include the Venturi mask, aerosol mask, face tent, tracheostomy collar, and T-piece. These devices deliver an accurate oxygen level when properly fitted, with oxygen concentrations from 24% to 100% at 8 to 15 L/min.

Venturi masks (Venti masks) deliver the most accurate oxygen concentration without intubation. It works by pulling in a proportional amount of room air for each liter flow of oxygen. An adaptor is located between the bottom of the mask and the oxygen source (Fig. 28-7). Adaptors with holes of different sizes allow specific amounts of air to mix with the oxygen, resulting in more precise delivery of oxygen. Each adaptor requires a different flow rate. For example, to deliver 24% of oxygen, the flow rate must be 4 L/min. Another type of Venturi mask has one adaptor with a dial that is used to select the amount of oxygen desired. Humidification is not needed with the Venturi mask.

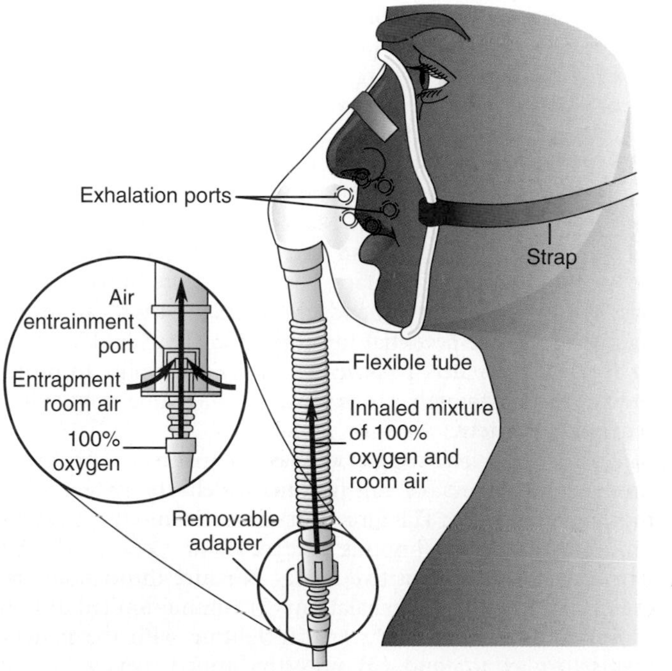

FIG. 28-7 A Venturi mask for precise oxygen delivery.

Other high-flow systems include the face tent, aerosol mask, tracheostomy collar, and T-piece. They are often used to provide

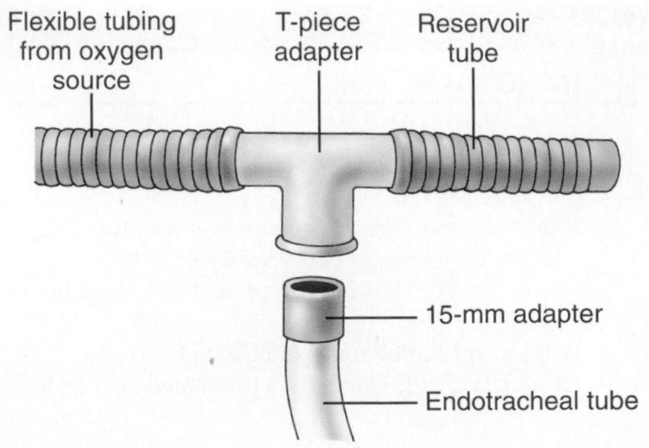

FIG. 28-8 A T-piece apparatus for attachment to an endotracheal or tracheostomy tube.

high humidity with oxygen delivery. A dial on the humidity source regulates the delivered oxygen level. A face tent fits over the chin, with the top extending halfway across the face. The oxygen level delivered varies, but the face tent, instead of a tight-fitting mask, is useful for patients who have facial trauma or burns. An aerosol mask is used when high humidity is needed. The tracheostomy collar is used to deliver high humidity and the desired oxygen to the patient with a tracheostomy. A special adaptor, called the *T-piece,* is used to deliver any desired FiO_2 to the patient with a tracheostomy, laryngectomy, or endotracheal tube (Fig. 28-8). Adjust the flow rate so that the aerosol appears on the exhalation side of the T-piece.

Noninvasive Positive-Pressure Ventilation. Noninvasive positive-pressure ventilation (NPPV) is a technique using positive pressure to keep alveoli open and improve GAS EXCHANGE without the need for airway intubation. It is now being used to manage dyspnea, hypercarbia, and acute exacerbations of chronic obstructive pulmonary disease (COPD), cardiogenic pulmonary edema, and acute asthma attacks. Although NPPV prevents the complications associated with intubation, including ventilator-associated pneumonia (VAP), risks and complications are associated with it. Masks must fit tightly in order to form a proper seal, which can lead to skin breakdown over the nose or other areas of the face. Leaks can cause uncomfortable pressure around the eyes, and gastric insufflation can lead to vomiting and the potential for aspiration. Thus NPPV should be used only on alert patients who have the ability to protect their airway, although a nasogastric (NG) tube may still be required for safety.

NPPV can deliver oxygen or may use just room air. A nasal mask, nasal pillows, or full-face mask delivery system allows mechanical delivery. The three most common modes of delivery for NPPV are (1) continuous positive airway pressure (CPAP), which delivers a set positive airway pressure throughout each cycle of inhalation and exhalation; (2) volume-limited or flow-limited, which delivers a set tidal volume with the patient's inspiratory effort; and (3) pressure-limited, which includes pressure support, pressure control, and bi-level positive airway pressure (BiPAP), which cycles different pressures at inspiration and at expiration.

For BiPAP, a cycling machine delivers a set inspiratory positive airway pressure each time the patient begins to inspire. As he or she begins to exhale, the machine delivers a lower set end-expiratory pressure. Together, these two pressures improve tidal volume, can reduce respiratory rate, and may relieve dyspnea.

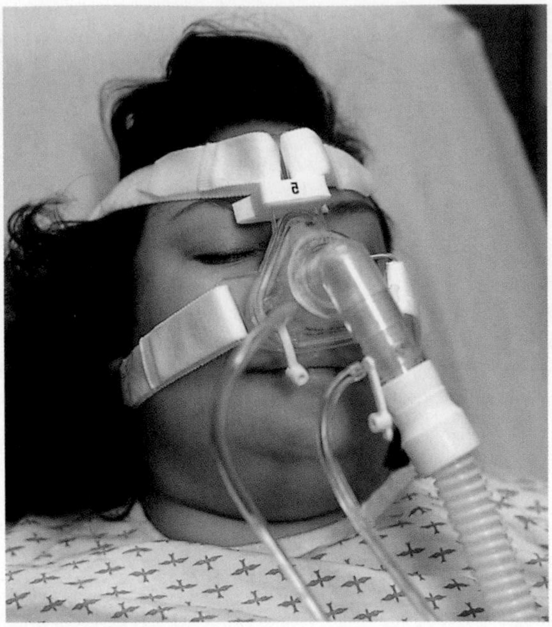

FIG. 28-9 Nasal continuous positive airway pressure (CPAP).

For CPAP, the effect is to open collapsed alveoli. Patients who may benefit from this form of oxygen or air delivery include those with atelectasis after surgery or cardiac-induced pulmonary edema or those with COPD. It is not beneficial for patients with respiratory failure following extubation. NPPV is also being used in palliative care for alleviating dyspnea, including for those patients with "do-not-intubate" orders. However, this practice is controversial. The Society of Critical Care Medicine (SCCM) recommends that goals of therapy and expected outcomes be discussed with the patient and family before initiating therapy.

NPPV is used for sleep apnea. The effect is to hold open the upper airways (Fig. 28-9). Patients using CPAP or BiPAP at home to manage sleep apnea often bring their home equipment to the hospital. They are familiar with their own machines and feel more comfortable using their own masks. The reasons for using NPPV still exist when the patient enters the hospital, and with some problems, there may be a greater need for them to continue NPPV while hospitalized.

The number of patients using NPPV therapy is increasing, and they are often cared for outside of the ICU setting. Nurses caring for the patient with NPPV must be knowledgeable about the equipment, the technique, and the potential complications. Adequate respiratory therapy support also is needed to safely manage a patient receiving NPPV.

Transtracheal Oxygen Therapy. Transtracheal oxygen (TTO) is a long-term method of delivering oxygen directly into the lungs. A small, flexible catheter is passed into the trachea through a small incision with the patient under local anesthesia. TTO avoids the irritation from nasal prongs and is less visible. A TTO team provides patient education, including the purpose of TTO and care of the catheter. Flow rates are prescribed for rest and for activity. A flow rate also is prescribed for the nasal cannula, which is used when the TTO catheter is being cleaned. Most patients using this delivery method have a 55% reduction in required oxygen flow at rest and a 30% decrease with activity.

CLINICAL JUDGMENT CHALLENGE

Patient-Centered Care; Teamwork and Collaboration; Evidence-Based Practice QSEN

Your patient is an 81-year-old male with end-stage COPD who is admitted with pneumonia and COPD exacerbation. He has a 60–pack-year smoking history and has been hospitalized many times over the past year for respiratory distress. The admitting provider orders an arterial blood gas (ABG). The patient is not using supplemental oxygen.

1. Based on your understanding of his disease process (see Chapter 30), would you expect this patient to have normal or altered ABG values, especially carbon dioxide ($Pa{CO_2}$) level?
2. The results of the ABG indicate hypoxemia ($Pa{O_2}$ of 40 mm Hg). Should you provide your patient with supplemental oxygen? Why or why not? If so, how much and which method would be best?
3. What areas will be the focus of your assessment and documentation? Provide a rationale for your choice(s).
4. Your patient has continually increasing oxygen requirements. He is now wearing a simple mask, and one of your colleagues would like to switch to a non-rebreather mask to deliver 100% oxygen. What are other good options for this patient?

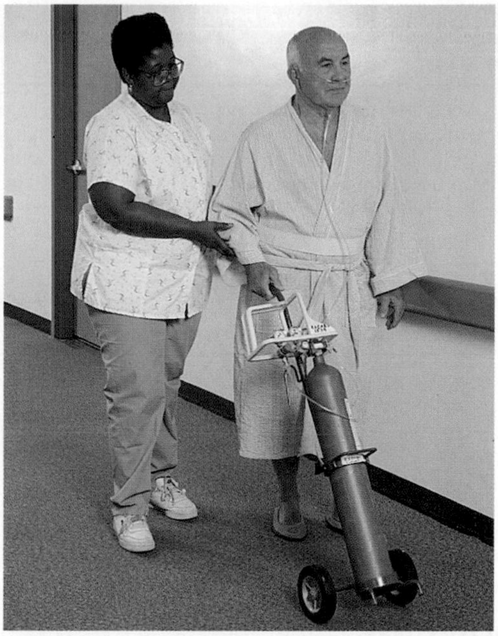

FIG. 28-10 Small E size oxygen tank (cylinder) for portability.

Community-Based Care

Home Care Management. The patient must be stable before home oxygen is considered. For Medicare to cover the cost of home oxygen therapy, the patient must have severe hypoxemia defined as a partial pressure of arterial oxygen ($Pa{O_2}$) level of less than 55 mm Hg or an arterial oxygen saturation ($Sp{O_2}$) of less than 88% on room air and at rest. The criteria vary when hypoxemia is caused by nonpulmonary problems or when oxygen is needed only at night or with exercise.

Self-Management Education. When home oxygen therapy is prescribed, begin a teaching plan about oxygen therapy. The nurse or respiratory therapist teaches the patient about the equipment needed for home oxygen therapy and the safety aspects of using and maintaining the equipment. Equipment may include the oxygen source, delivery devices, and humidity sources. Work with the discharge planner to help the patient select a durable medical equipment (DME) company to deliver oxygen equipment and select a community health nursing agency for follow-up care in the home. Re-evaluation of the need for oxygen therapy occurs on a periodic basis.

While providing discharge planning and teaching, be sensitive to the patient's emotional adjustment to oxygen therapy. Encourage the patient to share feelings and concerns. He or she may be concerned about social acceptance. Help him or her realize that adherence to oxygen therapy is important for being able to participate in ADLs and other events that bring enjoyment.

Home Care Preparation. Home oxygen therapy is provided in one of three ways: compressed gas in a tank or a cylinder, liquid oxygen in a reservoir, or an oxygen concentrator. Compressed gas in an oxygen tank (green) is the most often used oxygen source. The large H cylinder may be used as a stationary source, and the small E tank is available for transporting the patient (Fig. 28-10). Smaller cylinders are available for the patient to carry. Teach the patient and family to check the gauge daily to assess the amount of oxygen left in the tank. As a safety precaution, the tanks must always be in a stand or rack. A tank that is accidentally knocked over could suddenly decompress and move around in an uncontrolled manner.

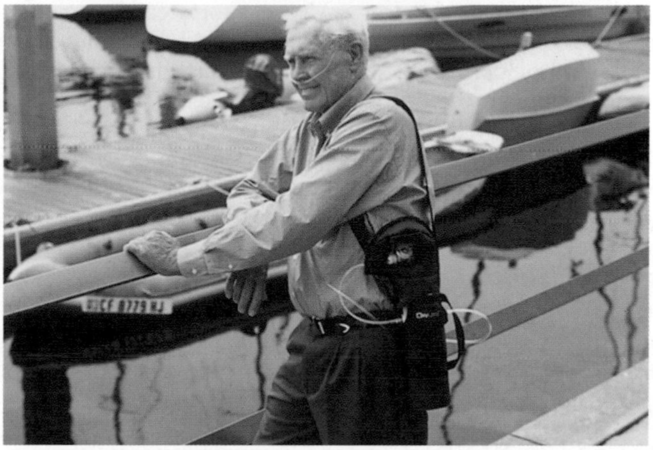

FIG. 28-11 Portable liquid oxygen.

Liquid oxygen for home use is oxygen gas that has been liquefied. A concentrated amount of oxygen is available in a lightweight and easy-to-carry container similar to a Thermos bottle (Fig. 28-11). This portable tank is filled from a large stationary liquid vessel. Liquid oxygen lasts longer than gaseous oxygen; however, it is expensive and the oxygen evaporates if it is not used continuously.

The **oxygen concentrator** or *oxygen extractor* is a machine that removes nitrogen from room air, increasing oxygen levels to more than 90%. This device is the least expensive system and does not need to be filled. It is often used in the home as a stationary system. A smaller version that can plug into DC electrical outlets can be rented for longer car or boat trips. Liquid oxygen and E tanks are used for short trips.

Regardless of the type of oxygen delivery system used, review safety issues with the patient and all family members.

NURSING SAFETY PRIORITY (QSEN)

Action Alert

Stress to the patient the importance of not smoking when he or she is using oxygen. Teach the patient and all family members that smoking materials, candles, gas burners, and fireplaces (and other open flames) are not to be used in the same room that oxygen is being used.

NCLEX EXAMINATION CHALLENGE

Health Promotion and Maintenance

For which activity does the nurse teach the client who is receiving oxygen by a transtracheal oxygen (TTO) delivery system to switch to a nasal cannula oxygen delivery system?
A. Eating a meal
B. Sleeping at night
C. Cleaning the catheter
D. Performing mouth care

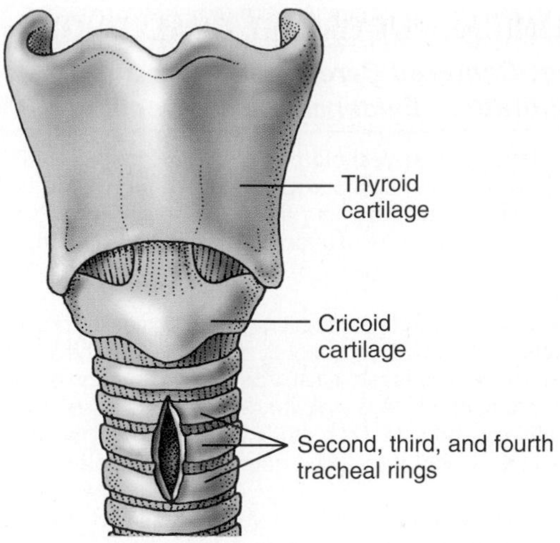

FIG. 28-12 A vertical tracheal incision for a tracheostomy.

TRACHEOSTOMY

Tracheotomy is the surgical incision into the trachea to create an airway. **Tracheostomy** is the tracheal *stoma* (opening) that results from the tracheotomy. A tracheotomy can be an emergency procedure or a scheduled surgery. Tracheostomies can be temporary or permanent. Some indications for tracheostomy include acute airway obstruction, the need for airway protection, laryngeal or facial trauma or burns, and airway involvement during head or neck surgery. Tracheostomies also are used for prolonged unconsciousness, paralysis, or the inability to be weaned from mechanical ventilation. With temporary tracheostomies, the nurse is key in evaluating patient readiness for progression toward decannulation (removal of the tracheostomy tube) (Morris et al., 2014).

❖ PATIENT-CENTERED COLLABORATIVE CARE

◆ Analysis

The priority NANDA-I nursing diagnoses and collaborative problems for patients requiring tracheostomy include:

- Impaired Gas Exchange related to weak chest muscles, obstruction, or other physical problems that interfere with ventilation and diffusion of gases (NANDA-I)
- Impaired Verbal Communication related to tracheostomy or intubation (NANDA-I)
- Imbalanced Nutrition: Less Than Body Requirements related to presence of endotracheal tube (NANDA-I)
- Potential for infection related to invasive procedures or problems with the normal protective mechanisms of the respiratory tract
- Damaged oral mucosa related to mechanical factors (endotracheal tube)

◆ Interventions

Preoperative Care. The care for the patient having a tracheotomy is similar to that for a laryngectomy (see Chapter 29). Focus on his or her knowledge deficits through teaching, and discuss tracheostomy care, communication, and speech.

Operative Procedures. Initially, the neck is extended and an endotracheal (ET) tube is placed by the anesthesia provider to maintain the airway. Incisions are made through the neck and the tracheal rings to enter the trachea (Fig. 28-12). The types of incisions and techniques vary, depending on the surgeon's preference and the reason for the surgery.

After the trachea is entered, the ET tube is removed while the tracheostomy tube is inserted. The tracheostomy tube is secured in place with sutures and tracheostomy ties or Velcro tube holders. A chest x-ray determines proper placement of the tube.

Postoperative Care. Immediately after surgery, focus care on ensuring a patent airway. Confirm the presence of bilateral breath sounds. Perform a respiratory assessment at least hourly. Assess the patient for complications from the procedure.

Complications. Major complications can arise after surgery. Table 28-3 lists manifestations, management, and prevention of complications of tracheostomy.

Tube obstruction can occur as a result of secretions or by cuff displacement. Indicators include difficulty breathing; noisy respirations; difficulty inserting a suction catheter; thick, dry secretions; and unexplained peak pressures (if a mechanical ventilator is in use). Assess the patient at least hourly for tube patency. Prevent obstruction by helping the patient cough and deep breathe, providing inner cannula care, humidifying oxygen, and suctioning. If tube obstruction occurs as a result of cuff prolapse over the end of the tracheostomy tube, the health care provider repositions or replaces the tube.

Tube dislodgement and accidental decannulation can occur when the tube is not secure. Prevent this problem by securing the tube in place to reduce movement and traction from the tubing or from accidental pulling by the patient. *Tube dislodgment in the first 72 hours after surgery is an emergency because the tracheostomy tract has not matured and replacement is difficult. The tube may end up in the subcutaneous tissue instead of in the trachea (also referred to as "false passage"). The patient will not be able to be ventilated.* Obese patients or those with short, large necks may be particularly difficult to recannulate if the tracheostomy tube is dislodged.

TABLE 28-3 **Complications of Tracheostomy**

COMPLICATIONS AND DESCRIPTION	MANIFESTATIONS	MANAGEMENT	PREVENTION
Tracheomalacia: constant pressure exerted by the cuff causes tracheal dilation and erosion of cartilage.	An increased amount of air is required in the cuff to maintain the seal. A larger tracheostomy tube is required to prevent an air leak at the stoma. Food particles are seen in tracheal secretions. The patient does not receive the set tidal volume on the ventilator.	No special management is needed unless bleeding occurs.	Use an uncuffed tube as soon as possible. Monitor cuff pressure and air volumes closely, and detect changes.
Tracheal stenosis: narrowed tracheal lumen is due to scar formation from irritation of tracheal mucosa by the cuff.	Stenosis is usually seen after the cuff is deflated or the tracheostomy tube is removed. The patient has increased coughing, inability to expectorate secretions, or difficulty in breathing or talking.	Tracheal dilation or surgical intervention is used.	Prevent pulling of and traction on the tracheostomy tube. Properly secure the tube in the midline position. Maintain proper cuff pressure. Minimize oronasal intubation time.
Tracheoesophageal fistula (TEF): excessive cuff pressure causes erosion of the posterior wall of the trachea. A hole is created between the trachea and the anterior esophagus. The patient at highest risk also has a nasogastric tube present.	Similar to tracheomalacia: Food particles are seen in tracheal secretions. Increased air in cuff is needed to achieve a seal. The patient has increased coughing and choking while eating. The patient does not receive the set tidal volume on the ventilator.	Manually administer oxygen by mask to prevent hypoxemia. Use a small, soft feeding tube instead of a nasogastric tube for tube feedings. A gastrostomy or jejunostomy may be performed by the physician. Monitor the patient with a nasogastric tube closely; assess for TEF and aspiration.	Maintain cuff pressure. Monitor the amount of air needed for inflation, and detect changes. Progress to a deflated cuff or cuffless tube as soon as possible.
Trachea–innominate artery fistula: a malpositioned tube causes its distal tip to push against the lateral wall of the tracheostomy. Continued pressure causes necrosis and erosion of the innominate artery. ***This is a medical emergency.***	The tracheostomy tube pulsates in synchrony with the heartbeat. There is heavy bleeding from the stoma. This is a life-threatening complication.	Remove the tracheostomy tube immediately. Apply direct pressure to the innominate artery at the stoma site. Prepare the patient for immediate surgical repair.	Correct the tube size, length, and midline position. Prevent pulling or tugging on the tracheostomy tube. Immediately notify the physician of the pulsating tube.

! NURSING SAFETY PRIORITY QSEN

Critical Rescue

If the tube is dislodged on an immature tracheostomy, ventilate the patient using a manual resuscitation bag and facemask while another nurse calls the Rapid Response Team.

For safety, ensure that a tracheostomy tube of the same type (including an obturator) and size (or one size smaller) is at the bedside at all times, along with a tracheostomy insertion tray. If decannulation occurs after 72 hours, extend the patient's neck and open the tissues of the stoma with a curved Kelly clamp to secure the airway. With the obturator inserted into the tracheostomy tube, quickly and gently replace the tube and remove the obturator. Check for airflow through the tube and for bilateral breath sounds. *If you cannot secure the airway, notify a more experienced nurse, respiratory therapist, or physician for assistance. Ventilate with a bag-valve mask. If the patient is in distress, call the Rapid Response Team for help.* To minimize tube dislodgment problems, many institutions have developed policies for patients with new tracheostomies and those identified at high risk (i.e., obese patients or those identified by the surgeon or anesthesiologist as high risk). One policy is to have a "difficult airway" cart available for these high-risk patients.

Pneumothorax (air in the chest cavity) can develop during the tracheotomy procedure if the chest cavity is entered. Chest x-rays after placement are used to assess for pneumothorax.

Subcutaneous emphysema occurs when there is an opening or tear in the trachea and air escapes into the fresh tissue planes of the neck. Air can progress throughout the chest and other tissues into the face. Inspect and palpate for air under the skin around the new tracheostomy.

! NURSING SAFETY PRIORITY QSEN

Critical Rescue

If the skin around a new tracheostomy is puffy and you can feel a crackling sensation when pressing on this skin, notify the physician immediately.

Bleeding in small amounts from the tracheotomy incision is expected for the first few days, but constant oozing is abnormal. Wrap gauze around the tube and pack gauze gently into the wound to apply pressure to the bleeding sites.

Infection can occur at any time. In the hospital, use sterile technique to prevent infection during suctioning and tracheostomy care. Assess the stoma site at least once every 8 hours for purulent drainage, redness, pain, or swelling. Tracheostomy dressings may be used to keep the stoma clean and dry. These dressings resemble a 4 × 4 gauze pad with an area removed to fit around the tube. If tracheostomy dressings are not available, fold standard sterile 4 × 4s to fit around the tube. *Do not cut the dressing because small bits of gauze could then be aspirated*

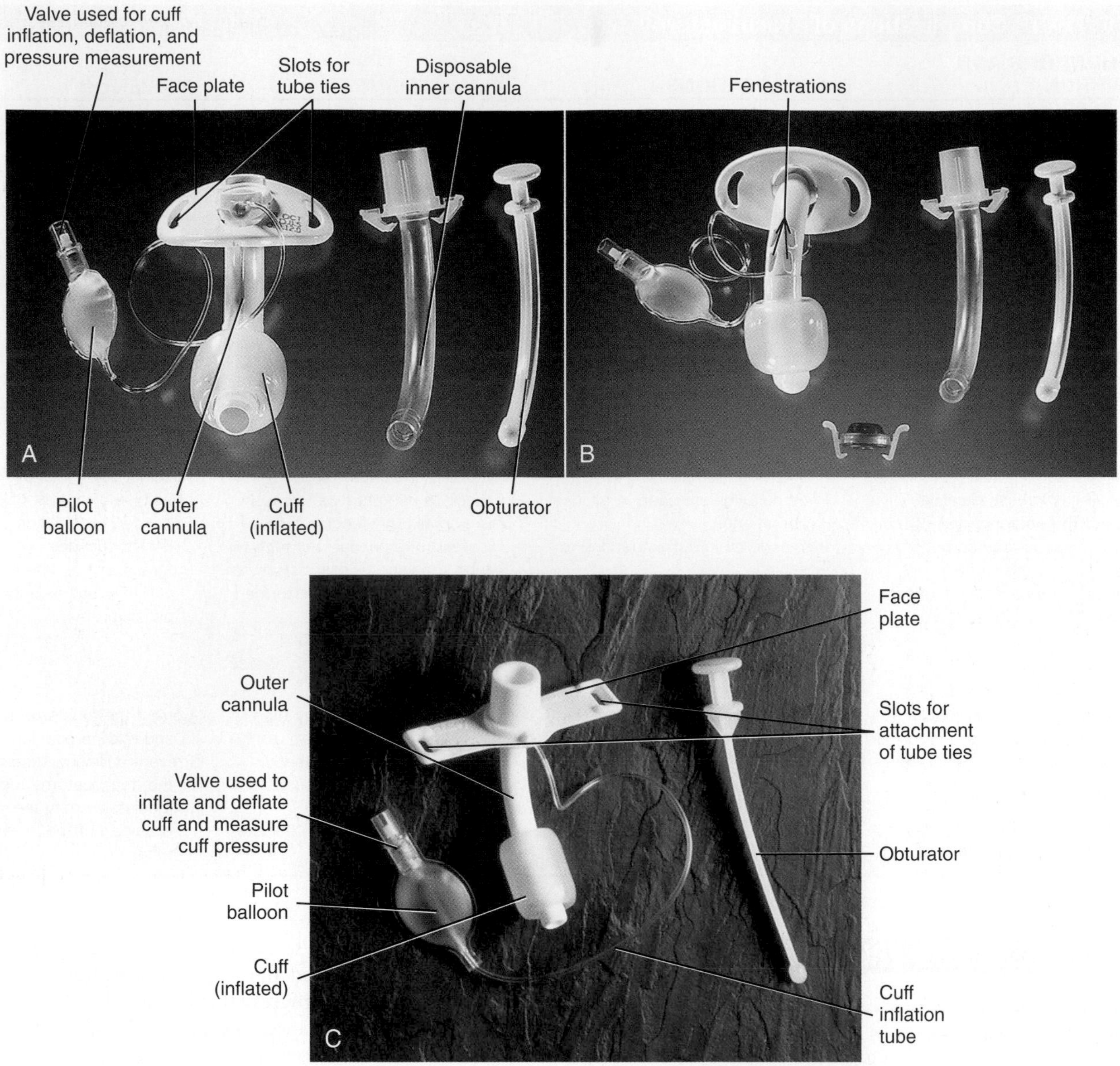

FIG. 28-13 Tracheostomy tubes. **A,** Dual-lumen cuffed tracheostomy tube with disposable inner cannula. **B,** Dual-lumen cuffed fenestrated tracheostomy tube. **C,** Single-lumen cannula cuffed tracheostomy tube.

through the tube. Change these dressings often because moist dressings provide a medium for bacterial growth. Careful wound care prevents most local infections.

Tracheostomy Tubes. Many types of tracheostomy tubes are available (Fig. 28-13). The one chosen depends on the needs of the patient. Tracheostomy tubes are available in many sizes and are made of plastic or metal. Most tubes in use today are disposable. A tracheostomy tube may have a cuff and may have an inner cannula. For patients receiving mechanical ventilation, a cuffed tube is used. A noncuffed tube is used when mechanical ventilation is not required.

For tubes with a reusable inner cannula, inspect, suction, and clean the inner cannula. During the first 24 hours after surgery, perform cannula care as often as needed, perhaps every 30 to 60 minutes. Thereafter, care is determined by the patient's needs and agency policy. In planning for self-care, teach the patient to remove the inner cannula and check for cleanliness. Also instruct him or her about suctioning and tracheostomy cleaning.

Because breathing and swallowing move the tube, a cuffed tube does not protect against aspiration. Having a cuffed tube inflated may give a false sense of security that aspiration cannot occur during feeding or mouth care. In addition, the pilot balloon does not reflect whether the correct amount of air is present in the cuff.

A fenestrated tube functions in many different ways. When the inner cannula is in place, the fenestration is closed and this tube works like a double-lumen tube. With the inner cannula removed and the plug or stopper locked in place, air can pass through the fenestration, around the tube, and up through the natural airway so that the patient can cough and speak. If the patient has trouble with these actions, he or she should be evaluated for proper tube placement, patency, size, and fenestration. *Do not cap the tube until the problem is identified and corrected.*

A fenestrated tube may or may not have a cuff. With a cuff, some air flows through the natural airway when the patient is not being mechanically ventilated.

! NURSING SAFETY PRIORITY (QSEN)

Action Alert

Always deflate the cuff before capping the tube with the decannulation cap; otherwise, the patient has no airway.

Patients with metal tracheostomy tubes scheduled for magnetic resonance imaging (MRI) need to change to a plastic tube. Metal tubes could be dislodged or heat up with exposure to the magnetic field during the scan.

Care Issues for the Patient with a Tracheostomy

Preventing Tissue Damage. Tissue damage can occur at the point where the inflated cuff presses against the tracheal mucosa. Mucosal ischemia occurs when the pressure exerted by the cuff on the mucosa exceeds the capillary perfusion pressure. To reduce the risk for tracheal damage, keep the cuff pressure between 14 and 20 mm Hg or 20 and 30 cm H_2O (ideally, 25 cm H_2O or less) (Sole et al., 2011).

Most cuffs use a high volume of air while keeping low pressure on the tracheal mucosa. Inflate the cuff to form a seal between the trachea and the cuff with the least amount of pressure. If the cuff cannot be inflated to seal well enough, a larger-diameter tube may be needed. A pressure cuff inflator can be used to inflate the cuff to a specified pressure or to check the cuff pressure (Fig. 28-14).

Check the cuff pressure at least once during each shift, especially with the minimal leak technique, and keep the pressure at 14 to 20 mm Hg or 20 to 30 cm H_2O. In rare situations, the cuff pressure is increased to maintain ventilator volumes when peak pressures are greater than 50 mm Hg (65 cm H_2O) and positive end-expiratory pressure (PEEP) is greater than 10 mm Hg (14 cm H_2O). High PEEP values can deflate the cuff over time, and more air may need to be added to maintain a proper seal. Manufacturers have guidelines for the specific volumes for each cuff size. Most cuffs are adequately inflated with less than 10 mL of air.

Although a high cuff pressure alone causes tracheal damage, other factors contribute to the risk for damage (Makic et al., 2013). The patient who is malnourished, dehydrated, hypoxic, older, or receiving corticosteroids is at risk for greater tissue damage. Tube friction and movement damage the mucosa and lead to tracheal stenosis. Reduce local airway damage by maintaining proper cuff pressures, stabilizing the tube, suctioning only when needed, and preventing malnutrition, dehydration, and hypoxia.

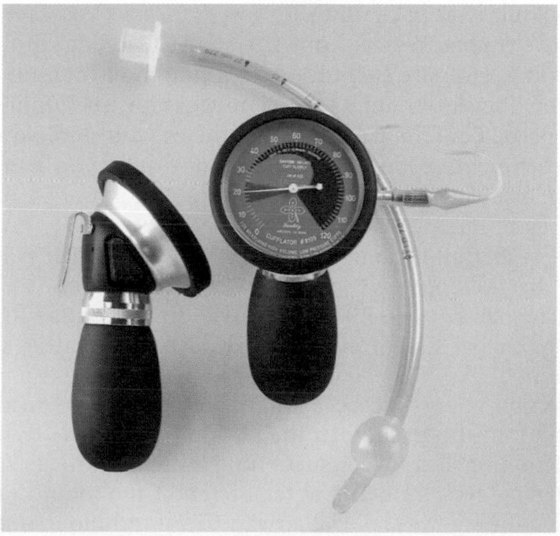

FIG. 28-14 An aneroid pressure manometer for cuff inflation and measuring cuff pressures.

Ensuring Air Warming and Humidification. The tracheostomy tube bypasses the nose and mouth, which normally humidify and warm the inspired air. If humidification and warming are not adequate, tracheal damage can occur. Thick, dried secretions can occlude the airways.

To prevent these complications, humidify the air as prescribed. Continually assess for a fine mist emerging from the tracheostomy collar or T-piece during ventilation. To increase the amount of humidity delivered, a warming device can be attached to the water source with a temperature probe in the tubing circuit. Monitor the circuit temperature hourly by feeling the tubing and by checking the probe. Ensure adequate hydration, which also helps liquefy secretions. Increasing the flow rate at the flowmeter increases the amount of delivered humidity.

! NURSING SAFETY PRIORITY (QSEN)

Action Alert

Keep the temperature of the air entering a tracheostomy between 98.6° and 100.4° F (37° and 38° C) and never exceed 104° F (40° C).

Suctioning. Suctioning maintains a patent airway and promotes GAS EXCHANGE by removing secretions when the patient cannot cough adequately. Chart 28-2 lists best practices for

CHART 28-2 Best Practice for Patient Safety & Quality Care (QSEN)

Suctioning the Artificial Airway

1. Assess the need for suctioning (routine unnecessary suctioning causes mucosal damage, bleeding, and bronchospasm).
2. Wash hands. Don protective eyewear. Maintain Standard Precautions.
3. Explain to the patient that sensations such as shortness of breath and coughing are to be expected but that any discomfort will be very brief.
4. Check the suction source. Occlude the suction source, and adjust the pressure dial to between 80 and 120 mm Hg to prevent hypoxemia and trauma to the mucosa.
5. Set up a sterile field.
6. Preoxygenate the patient with 100% oxygen for 30 seconds to 3 minutes (at least three hyperinflations) to prevent hypoxemia. Keep hyperinflations synchronized with inhalation.
7. Quickly insert the suction catheter until resistance is met. *Do not apply suction during insertion.*
8. Withdraw the catheter 0.4 to 0.8 inch (1 to 2 cm), and begin to apply suction. Apply suction and use a twirling motion of the catheter during withdrawal. *Never suction longer than 10 to 15 seconds.*
9. Hyperoxygenate for 1 to 5 minutes or until the patient's baseline heart rate and oxygen saturation are within normal limits.
10. Repeat as needed for up to three total suction passes.
11. Suction mouth as needed, and provide mouth care.
12. Remove gloves, and wash hands.
13. Describe secretions, and document patient's responses.

suctioning. Assess the patient's need for suctioning (e.g., audible or noisy secretions; crackles or wheezes heard on auscultation; restlessness; increased pulse or respiratory rates; or mucus present in the artificial airway). Other indications include patient requests for suctioning or an increase in the peak airway pressure on the ventilator.

Deep endotracheal suctioning is painful. Some unconscious or noncommunicative patients still feel pain, and this should be kept in mind during the suctioning procedure (see the Evidence-Based Practice box). At the very least, provide verbal acknowledgment of the discomfort and reassurance of when the procedure will end.

EVIDENCE-BASED PRACTICE QSEN

How Do You Know When Suctioning is Painful to a Patient?

Rahu, M., Grap, M., Cohn, J., Munro, C., Lyon, D., & Sessler, C. (2013). Facial expression as an indicator of pain in critically ill intubated adults during endotracheal suctioning. *American Journal of Critical Care, 22*(5), 412-422.

Endotracheal suctioning is often painful, and patients may require pain medication before the procedure. Patients who are not able to communicate may still feel pain during the procedure, but often this is not addressed. The investigators sought to determine whether pain in noncommunicative critically ill patients during endotracheal suctioning could be discerned by changes in facial expression.

Fifty noncommunicative patients who had endotracheal tubes were video recorded during rest phases in which no treatments or procedures were being performed and during periods of endotracheal suctioning. The video-recorded facial changes were coded using the Facial Action Coding System of the Behavioral Pain Scale. A total of 14 different facial expressions were present during suctioning that were seldom seen during rest phases. Five of the 14 accounted for 71% of the variance from expected responses as measured in stepwise multivariate analysis. These expression changes were brow raised, brow lowered, nose wrinkling, head turned right or left, and head turned up. The investigators suggest that such changes in upper facial expressions in noncommunicative critically ill patients could be used as a valid alternative to self-reports of procedural pain.

Level of Evidence: 3

The results of this quasi-experimental study in which patients served as their own controls provide significant evidence that noncommunicative critically ill patients feel pain during the suctioning procedure. The use of video-recording and the observer software analysis of facial changes strengthened the study by reducing observer bias and providing opportunity for re-examination. The Facial Action Coding System (FACS) is an established and reliable instrument useful for assessing behavioral responses to pain. The statistical analysis methods used were appropriate for the study design.

Commentary: Implications for Practice and Research

This study is important in that it was conducted under real clinical conditions using a variety of noncommunicative and intubated patients. The results indicate that the FACS could be used to standardize pain evaluation in this patient population. Additional research with larger sample sizes are needed to determine whether the instruments could be used to quantify the pain experienced by noncommunicative patients so that appropriate pain-relieving measures could be instituted. Although some limitations were present in this study, the nature of the question and the patient population do not lend themselves to randomized controlled clinical trials.

Suctioning is often performed through an artificial airway, but the nose or mouth also can be used. Suctioning of both routes is routine for the patient with retained secretions.

Suctioning through the nose has similar complications as suctioning through an artificial airway and can be painful. Slow, careful placement of the catheter following the nasopharyngeal anatomy reduces pain and trauma. Placing a nasopharyngeal airway and suctioning through it can prevent trauma to the nasal mucosa. Advance the catheter through the nasopharynx and into the laryngopharynx while the patient receives oxygen by mask or nasal cannula. Once the catheter enters the larynx, the patient may cough. On inhalation, insert the catheter into the trachea. If needed, disconnect the catheter from suction and attach it to an oxygen source so that the patient receives oxygen via the catheter.

Suctioning can cause hypoxia, mucosal trauma, infection, vagal stimulation, bronchospasm, and cardiac dysrhythmias.

Hypoxia can be caused by these factors in the patient with a tracheostomy:

- Ineffective oxygenation before, during, and after suctioning
- Use of a catheter that is too large for the artificial airway
- Prolonged suctioning time
- Excessive suction pressure
- Too frequent suctioning

Prevent hypoxia by hyperoxygenating the patient with 100% oxygen using a manual resuscitation bag attached to an oxygen source. Instruct the patient to take deep breaths 3 or 4 times with the existing oxygen delivery system before suctioning. Monitor the heart rate or use a pulse oximeter while suctioning to assess tolerance of the procedure. Assess for hypoxia (e.g., increased heart rate and blood pressure, oxygen desaturation, cyanosis, restlessness, anxiety, dysrhythmias). Oxygen saturation below 90% by pulse oximetry indicates hypoxemia. If hypoxia occurs, stop the suctioning procedure. Using the 100% oxygen delivery system, reoxygenate the patient until baseline parameters return.

Use a correct-size catheter to reduce the risk for hypoxia and still remove secretions effectively. The size should not exceed half of the size of the tracheal lumen. The standard catheter size for an adult is 12 Fr or 14 Fr.

Tissue trauma results from frequent suctioning, prolonged suctioning, excessive suction pressure, and non-rotation of the catheter. Prevent trauma to the mucosa by suctioning only when needed and lubricating the catheter with sterile water or saline before insertion. *Apply suction only during catheter withdrawal.* Use a twirling motion during withdrawal to prevent grabbing of the mucosa.

Apply suction for only 10 to 15 seconds. Estimate this time frame by holding your own breath and counting to 10 or 15 during suctioning. At the end of the 15 seconds, stop suctioning. Longer suctioning can cause alveolar collapse *(suction atelectasis)*.

Infection is possible because each catheter pass introduces bacteria into the trachea. In the hospital, use sterile technique for suctioning and for all suctioning equipment (e.g., suction catheters, gloves, saline or water). Suction the mouth or nose *after* suctioning the artificial airway. Clean technique is used at home because the number of virulent organisms in the home environment is lower than in the hospital.

NURSING SAFETY PRIORITY (QSEN)

Action Alert

Never use oral suction equipment for suctioning an artificial airway, because this can introduce oral bacteria into the lungs.

Vagal stimulation and bronchospasm are possible during suctioning. Vagal stimulation results in bradycardia, hypotension, heart block, ventricular tachycardia, or other dysrhythmias. *If vagal stimulation occurs, stop suctioning immediately and oxygenate the patient manually with 100% oxygen.* Bronchospasm may occur when the catheter passes into the airway. The patient may need a bronchodilator to relieve bronchospasm and respiratory distress. The hypoxia caused by suctioning can stimulate a variety of cardiac dysrhythmias. If the patient has cardiac monitoring in place, check the monitor during suctioning.

NCLEX EXAMINATION CHALLENGE

Safe and Effective Care Environment

During nasotracheal suctioning, the client's heart rate changes from 78 beats/min to 48 beats/min. What is the nurse's best first action?

A. Immediately stop suctioning
B. Gently pinch the client's cheek
C. Administer oxygen by mask at 2 L/min
D. Document the change as the only action

Providing Tracheostomy Care. Tracheostomy care keeps the tube free of secretions, maintains a patent airway, and provides wound care. It is performed whether or not the patient can clear secretions. Perform tracheostomy care according to agency policy, usually every 8 hours and as needed. Chart 28-3 outlines best practices for tracheostomy care.

Before tracheostomy care, assess the patient as described in Chart 28-4. The need for suctioning and tracheostomy care is determined by the secretions, the specific disorder, the ability of the patient to cough, the need for mechanical ventilation, and wound care. Using a penlight, inspect the inner lumen of a single-lumen tube to assess for secretions.

Secure tracheostomy tubes in place using either twill tape ties or commercial tube holders. Both devices require changing when soiled or at least daily to keep them clean, to prevent infection, and to assess for skin irritation under the ties. A properly secured tie or holder allows space for only one finger to be placed between the tie or holder and the neck (Morris et al., 2013). Tube movement causes irritation and coughing and may lead to decannulation. Keeping the tube secure while changing the ties or holder to prevent accidental decannulation is critical. Include the patient in tracheostomy care as a step toward self-care. Fig. 28-15 shows correct placement of a tracheostomy dressing.

NURSING SAFETY PRIORITY (QSEN)

Critical Rescue

Prevent decannulation during tracheostomy care by keeping the old ties or holder on the tube while applying new ties or holder or by keeping a hand on the tube until it is securely stable. (This is best performed with the assistance of another person.)

CHART 28-3 Best Practice for Patient Safety & Quality Care (QSEN)

Tracheostomy Care

1. Assemble the necessary equipment.
2. Wash hands. Maintain Standard Precautions.
3. Suction the tracheostomy tube if necessary.
4. Remove old dressings and excess secretions.
5. Set up a sterile field.
6. Remove and clean the inner cannula. Use half-strength hydrogen peroxide to clean the cannula and sterile saline to rinse it. If the inner cannula is disposable, remove the cannula and replace it with a new one.
7. Clean the stoma site and then the tracheostomy plate with half-strength hydrogen peroxide followed by sterile saline. Ensure that none of the solutions enters the tracheostomy.
8. Change tracheostomy ties if they are soiled. Secure new ties in place before removing soiled ones to prevent accidental decannulation. If a knot is needed, tie a square knot that is visible on the side of the neck. Only one finger should be able to be placed between the tie tape and the neck.
9. Wash hands.
10. Document the type and amount of secretions and the general condition of the stoma and surrounding skin. Document the patient's response to the procedure and any teaching or learning that occurred.

CHART 28-4 Focused Assessment

The Patient with a Tracheostomy

- Note the quality, pattern, and rate of breathing:
  - Within patient's baseline?
    Tachypnea can indicate hypoxia.
    Dyspnea can indicate secretions in the airway.
- Assess for any cyanosis, especially around the lips, which could indicate hypoxia.
- Check the patient's pulse oximetry reading.
- If oxygen is prescribed, is the patient receiving the correct amount, with the correct equipment and humidification?
- Assess the tracheostomy site:
  - Note the color, consistency, and amount of secretions in the tube or externally.
  - If the tracheostomy is sutured in place, is there any redness, swelling, or drainage from suture sites?
  - If the tracheostomy is secured with ties, what is the condition of the ties? Are they moist with secretions or perspiration? Are the secretions dried on the ties? Is the tie secure?
  - Assess the condition of the skin around the tracheostomy and neck. Be sure to check underneath the neck for secretions that may have drained to the back. Check for any skin breakdown related to pressure from the ties or related to excess secretions.
  - Assess behind the faceplate for the size of the space between the outer cannula and the patient's tissue. Are any secretions collected in this area?
- If the tube is cuffed, check cuff pressure.
- Auscultate the lungs.
- Are a second (emergency) tracheostomy tube and obturator available?

Providing Bronchial and Oral Hygiene. Bronchial hygiene promotes a patent airway and prevents infection. Turn and reposition the patient every 1 to 2 hours, support out-of-bed activities, and encourage ambulation to promote lung expansion and GAS EXCHANGE and help remove secretions. Coughing and deep breathing, combined with the chest percussion, vibration, and postural drainage, promote pulmonary hygiene (see Chapter 30).

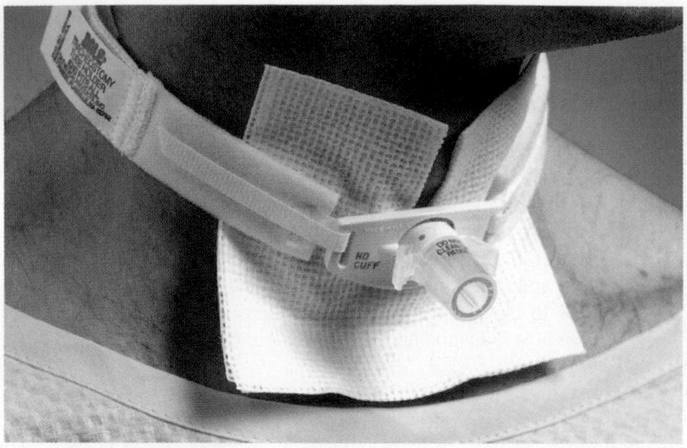

FIG. 28-15 Placement of tracheostomy gauze dressing and Velcro tracheostomy tube holder.

Good oral hygiene keeps the airway patent, prevents bacterial overgrowth, and promotes comfort. Avoid using glycerin swabs or mouthwash that contains alcohol for oral care because these products dry the mouth, change its pH, and promote bacterial growth. Instead, use a sponge tooth cleaner or soft-bristle toothbrush moistened in water for mouth care. Hydrogen peroxide solutions can help remove crusted matter but may break down healing tissue and should be used only with a physician's prescription. Help the patient rinse his or her mouth with normal saline every 4 hours while awake or as often as he or she desires.

Examine the mouth for open areas or dental problems. Ulcers and infections are treated medically. Apply lip balm or water-soluble jelly to prevent cracked lips and promote comfort. Mouth care helps promote oral health, comfort, and aesthetic appearance. Offering an opportunity for the patient or family member to perform mouth care allows participation in care and increases self-esteem.

Oral secretions can move down the trachea and collect above the inflated cuff of the endotracheal tube. When the cuff is deflated, the secretions can move into the lungs. Some endotracheal tubes have an extra lumen open to the area above the cuff, which allows suctioning of the airway above the cuff before deflating and reduces the risk for aspiration.

Ensuring Nutrition. Swallowing can be a major problem for the patient with a tracheostomy tube in place. In a normal swallow, the larynx lifts and moves forward to prevent the entering of food and saliva. The tracheostomy tube sometimes tethers the larynx in place, making it unable to move effectively. The result is difficulty in swallowing. Also, when the tracheostomy tube cuff is inflated, it can balloon backwards and interfere with food passage through the esophagus because the wall separating the back of the trachea and the front of the esophagus is thin.

Instruct the patient to keep the head of the bed elevated for at least 30 minutes after eating. Chart 28-5 outlines best practices to prevent aspiration during swallowing.

Maintaining Communication. The patient can speak when there is a cuffless tube, when a fenestrated tracheostomy tube is in place, and when the fenestrated tube is capped or covered. Until natural speech is feasible, teach him or her and the family about other communication means. A writing tablet, a board with pictures and letters, communication "flash cards" on a ring, hand signals, and a computer, as well as a call light within reach, are used to promote communication and decrease frustration from not being able to speak or be understood. Phrase questions for "yes" or "no" answers to help the patient respond easily. Move the patient closer to the nurses' station, and mark the central call light system to indicate that he or she cannot speak.

The inability to talk is a stressor for the patient. Helping communication is an important nursing action and is required by The Joint Commission's National Patient Safety Goals (NPSGs). When the patient can tolerate cuff deflation, he or she places a finger over the tracheostomy tube on exhalation, forcing air up through the larynx and mouth and allowing speech.

A device to facilitate speech for the patient with a tracheostomy is a one-way valve that fits over the tube and replaces the need for finger occlusion. The valve allows him or her to breathe in through the tracheostomy tube. On exhalation, the valve closes so that air is forced through the vocal cords, allowing speech. For this valve to assist in speech, the patient must not be connected to a ventilator, must have the cuff deflated, and must be able to breathe around the tube. Some valves have a port for supplemental oxygen without impairing the ability to speak.

Supporting Psychosocial Needs and Self-Image. Addressing psychological concerns is an important aspect of caring for patients recovering from a tracheostomy. Always keep in mind the emotional impact of an artificial airway. Acknowledge the patient's frustration with communication, and allow sufficient time for communication. When speaking to him or her, use a normal tone of voice because hearing and comprehension are not altered by the presence of a tube.

The patient may have a change in self-image because of the presence of a stoma or artificial airway, speech changes, a change in the method of eating, or difficulty with speech. Help the patient set realistic goals, starting with involvement in self-care.

Work with the family to ease the patient into a more normal social environment. Provide encouragement and positive

CHART 28-5 Best Practice for Patient Safety & Quality Care (QSEN)

Preventing Aspiration During Swallowing

- Avoid serving meals when the patient is fatigued.
- Provide smaller and more frequent meals.
- Provide adequate time; do not "hurry" the patient.
- Provide close supervision if the patient is self-feeding.
- Keep emergency suctioning equipment close at hand and turned on.
- Avoid water and other "thin" liquids.
- Thicken all liquids, including water.
- Avoid foods that generate thin liquids during the chewing process, such as fruit.
- Position the patient in the most upright position possible.
- When possible, completely (or at least partially) deflate the tube cuff during meals.
- Suction after initial cuff deflation to clear the airway and allow maximum comfort during the meal.
- Feed each bite or encourage the patient to take each bite slowly.
- Encourage the patient to "dry swallow" after each bite to clear residue from the throat.
- Avoid consecutive swallows of liquids.
- Provide controlled small volumes of liquids, using a spoon.
- Encourage the patient to "tuck" his or her chin down and move the forehead forward while swallowing.
- Allow the patient to indicate when he or she is ready for the next bite.
- If the patient coughs, stop the feeding until he or she indicates that the airway has been cleared.
- Continuously monitor tolerance to oral food intake by assessing respiratory rate, ease, pulse oximetry, and heart rate.

reinforcement while demonstrating acceptance and caring behaviors. Assess the family for the need for counseling.

After surgery, the patient may feel shy and socially isolated. He or she can wear loose-fitting shirts, decorative collars, or scarves to cover the tracheostomy tube.

Weaning. Weaning the patient from a tracheostomy tube entails a gradual decrease in the tube size and ultimate removal of the tube. Carefully monitor this process, especially after each change. The physician or advanced practice nurse performs the steps in the process.

First, the cuff is deflated as soon as the patient can manage secretions and does not need mechanical ventilation. This change allows him or her to breathe through the tube and through the upper airway. Next, the tube is changed to an uncuffed tube. If this is tolerated, the size of the tube is gradually decreased. When a small fenestrated tube is placed, the tube is capped so that all air passes through the upper airway and the fenestra, with none passing through the tube. Assess the patient to ensure adequate airflow around the tube when it is capped. The tube may be removed after he or she tolerates more than 24 hours of capping. Place a dry dressing over the stoma (which gradually heals on its own).

Another device used for the transition from tracheostomy to natural breathing is a *tracheostomy button.* The button maintains stoma patency and assists spontaneous breathing. The Kistner tracheostomy tube and Olympic tracheostomy button are examples of this type of device. To function, the button must fit properly. A disadvantage is the possibility of decannulation—the tube can dislodge from the trachea but remain in the neck tissues.

Community-Based Care

By the time of discharge, the patient should be able to provide self-care, which may include tracheostomy care, nutrition care, suctioning, and communication. Although education begins before surgery, most self-care is taught in the hospital. Teach the patient and family how to care for the tracheostomy tube. Review airway care, including cleaning and signs of infection. Teach clean suction technique, and review the plan of care.

Instruct the patient to use a shower shield over the tracheostomy tube when bathing to prevent water from entering the airway. Teach him or her to cover the airway loosely with a small cotton cloth to protect it during the day. Covering the opening filters the air entering the stoma, keeps humidity in the airway, and enhances appearance. Attractive coverings are available as cotton scarves, decorative collars, and jewelry.

Teach the patient to increase humidity in the home. Tell the patient to continue using the method of communication that began in the hospital and to wear a medical alert bracelet that identifies the inability to speak.

The health care team assesses specific discharge needs and makes referrals to home care agencies and durable medical equipment companies (for suction equipment and tracheostomy supplies). Follow-up visits occur early after discharge, and the home care nurse also is an important resource for the patient and family. This nurse initiates and coordinates the services of dietitians, nurses, speech and language pathologists, and social workers. He or she informs the patient and family of community resources that can offer support and friendship.

CLINICAL JUDGMENT CHALLENGE

Safety; Patient-Centered Care QSEN

Your patient is a 41-year-old woman with a significant closed head injury (CHI) from a motor vehicle crash (MVC). She is not anticipated to be able to be weaned from the ventilator, and the physicians have asked the patient's family for permission to create a tracheostomy. The family is concerned that the patient will not be able to speak again.

1. What is your response?
2. What are some possible concerns for patient care in the immediate postoperative period?
3. What can you do to minimize tracheal damage?
4. The patient's family is concerned that the tracheostomy will be permanent and they are worried about her image. How do you respond?

CONSIDERATIONS FOR OLDER ADULTS

Patient-Centered Care QSEN

Self-managing tracheostomy care and oxygen therapy can be difficult for the older patient who has vision problems or difficulty with upper arm movement. Teach him or her to use magnifying lenses or glasses to ensure the proper setting on the oxygen gauge. Assess his or her ability to reach and manipulate the tracheostomy. If possible, work with a family member who can provide assistance during tracheostomy care.

NURSING CONCEPTS AND CLINICAL JUDGMENT REVIEW

What might you NOTICE if the patient is experiencing inadequate GAS EXCHANGE with oxygenation and tissue PERFUSION as a result of respiratory problems?

- Respirations rapid and shallow
- Respirations noisy
- Cannot speak more than 4 or 5 words without pausing for breath
- Change in cognition, acute confusion
- Decreased oxygen saturation by pulse oximetry
- Skin cyanosis or pallor (lighter-skinned patients)
- Cyanosis or pallor of the lips and oral mucous membranes (in patients of any skin color)
- Tachycardia
- Patient appears to strain to catch breath
- Fatigue

What should you INTERPRET and how should you RESPOND to a patient experiencing inadequate GAS EXCHANGE with oxygenation and tissue PERFUSION as a result of a respiratory problem?

Perform and interpret physical assessment, including:

- Taking vital signs
- Auscultating all lung fields

- Monitoring oxygen saturation by pulse oximetry
- Checking most recent laboratory values for hematocrit, hemoglobin, and ABG levels
- Assessing cognition (Mini-Mental State Examination [MMSE])
- Assessing for the use of accessory muscles
- Assessing for the presence of thick or excessive secretions
- Assessing the patient's ability to cough and clear the airway

Respond by:

- Applying oxygen and assessing the patient's responses to this intervention
- Keeping the patient's head elevated to about 30 degrees
- Suctioning (oral, pharyngeal, endotracheal, tracheostomy), if needed
- Notifying the physician or Rapid Response Team
- Prioritizing and pacing activities to prevent fatigue

On what should you REFLECT?

- Observe the patient for evidence of restored gas exchange (see Chapter 27).
- Think about what may have made the impaired gas exchange worse and what steps could be taken to either prevent a similar episode or identify it earlier.
- Think about what additional resources could improve the nursing response to this situation.

GET READY FOR THE NCLEX® EXAMINATION!

KEY POINTS

Review these Key Points for each NCLEX Examination Client Needs Category.

Safe and Effective Care Environment

- Never allow water condensation in an oxygen delivery system to drain back into the system. **Safety** QSEN
- Use sterile technique when performing endotracheal or tracheal suctioning. **Safety** QSEN
- Inspect the oral mucous membranes each shift for anyone who has an endotracheal tube. **Safety** QSEN
- Keep a tracheostomy tube (and obturator) and tracheostomy insertion tray at the bedside for the first 72 hours after a tracheostomy has been created. **Safety** QSEN
- Never use oral suctioning equipment to suction an artificial airway. **Safety** QSEN
- Use Aspiration Precautions for any patient with an altered level of consciousness or who has an endotracheal tube (see Chart 28-5). **Safety** QSEN
- Verify safe use of appropriate oxygen delivery systems and tracheostomy equipment. **Safety** QSEN

Health Promotion and Maintenance

- Teach the patient and family about home management of oxygen therapy, including the avoidance of smoking or open flames in rooms in which oxygen is being used. **Patient-Centered Care** QSEN
- Teach the patient and family how to perform tracheostomy care (see Chart 28-3). **Patient-Centered Care** QSEN

Psychosocial Integrity

- Provide opportunity for the patient and family to express concerns about a change in breathing status or the possibility of intubation and mechanical ventilation.
- Teach family members ways to communicate with a patient who is intubated or being mechanically ventilated. **Patient-Centered Care** QSEN
- Reassure patients who are intubated that the loss of speech is temporary. **Patient-Centered Care** QSEN
- Encourage patients with permanent tracheostomies to become involved in self-care. **Patient-Centered Care** QSEN

Physiological Integrity

- Apply oxygen to anyone who is hypoxemic. **Evidence-Based Practice** QSEN
- Ensure that oxygen therapy delivered to the patient is humidified appropriately. **Evidence-Based Practice** QSEN
- Monitor arterial blood gases (ABGs) and oxygen saturation of all patients receiving oxygen therapy. **Evidence-Based Practice** QSEN
- Assess the skin under the mask and under the plastic tubing every shift for patients receiving oxygen by mask. **Patient-Centered Care** QSEN
- Assess the skin of the nares and under the elastic band every shift for patients receiving oxygen by nasal cannula. **Patient-Centered Care** QSEN
- Observe any patient receiving oxygen at greater than a 50% concentration for early manifestations of oxygen toxicity (i.e. dyspnea, nonproductive cough, chest pain, GI upset). **Patient-Centered Care** QSEN
- Use a manual resuscitation bag to ventilate the patient if the tracheostomy tube has dislodged or become decannulated. **Safety** QSEN
- Assess the new tracheostomy stoma site at least once per shift for purulent drainage, redness, pain, and swelling as indicators of infection. **Evidence-Based Practice** QSEN
- Keep the tracheal cuff pressure between 14 and 20 mm Hg to prevent tissue injury. **Safety** QSEN

CHAPTER 29

Care of Patients with Noninfectious Upper Respiratory Problems

M. Linda Workman

http://evolve.elsevier.com/Iggy/

PRIORITY CONCEPTS

- GAS EXCHANGE
- CELLULAR REGULATION

LEARNING OUTCOMES

Safe and Effective Care Environment

1. Protect patients with upper respiratory problems from hypoxia, injury, infection, and impairment in GAS EXCHANGE.

Health Promotion and Maintenance

2. Teach all people measures to take to protect the upper respiratory system from damage and cancer (loss of CELLULAR REGULATION), including the avoidance of known environmental causative agents.
3. Teach the patient and family how to manage a chronic lower respiratory disorder and avoid injury and complications in the home.

Psychosocial Integrity

4. Reduce the psychological impact for the patient and family experiencing an acute or chronic upper respiratory problem.
5. Work with other members of the health care team to ensure that values, preferences, and expressed needs of patients experiencing upper respiratory problems and reduced GAS EXCHANGE are respected.

Physiological Integrity

6. Assess and re-assess the manifestations of patients being managed for an upper respiratory problem.
7. Use laboratory data and clinical manifestations to prioritize nursing care for the patient who has an acute or chronic upper respiratory problem.
8. Prioritize nursing care needs of a patient after a nasoseptoplasty.
9. Prioritize the nursing care needs of the patient and family experiencing head and neck cancer.
10. Work with other health care professionals who help the patient and family experiencing a chronic upper respiratory problem achieve desired health outcomes.
11. Coordinate nursing interventions for the patient with a chronic upper respiratory problem in the community.

The nose, sinuses, oropharynx, larynx, and trachea are the upper airway structures. They are important for GAS EXCHANGE and perfusion by providing the entrance site for air. Problems of the upper airways, especially the larynx and trachea, can interfere with oxygen delivery. Patients with upper respiratory problems are found in the community and in all health care settings. *The nursing priority with disorders of the upper respiratory tract is to promote gas exchange by ensuring a patent airway.*

DISORDERS OF THE NOSE AND SINUSES

FRACTURE OF THE NOSE

❖ PATHOPHYSIOLOGY

Nasal fractures often result from injuries received during falls, sports activities, car crashes, or physical assaults and can interfere with GAS EXCHANGE. If the bone or cartilage is not displaced and no complications are present, treatment may not be needed. Displacement of either the bone or cartilage, however, can cause airway obstruction or cosmetic deformity and is a potential source of infection.

❖ PATIENT-CENTERED COLLABORATIVE CARE

◆ Assessment

Document any nasal problem, including deviation, malaligned nasal bridge, a change in nasal breathing, crackling of the skin *(crepitus)* on palpation, bruising, and pain. Blood or clear fluid (cerebrospinal fluid [CSF]) rarely drains from one or both nares as a result of a simple nasal fracture and, if present, indicates a serious injury (e.g., skull fracture). CSF can be differentiated from normal nasal secretions because CSF contains glucose that will test positive with a dipstick test for glucose. When CSF dries on a piece of filter paper, a yellow "halo" appears as a ring at the dried edge of the fluid. X-rays are not always useful in the diagnosis of simple nasal fractures.

◆ Interventions

The health care provider performs a simple **closed reduction** (moving the bones by palpation to realign them) of the nasal fracture using local or general anesthesia within the first 24 hours after injury. After 24 hours, the fracture is more difficult to reduce because of edema and scar formation. Then reduction may be delayed for several days until edema is gone. Simple closed fractures may not need surgical intervention. Management focuses on pain relief and cold compresses to decrease swelling.

Rhinoplasty. Reduction and surgery may be needed for severe fractures or for those that do not heal properly. **Rhinoplasty** is a surgical reconstruction of the nose. It can be performed to repair a fractured nose and also can be performed to change the shape of the nose. The patient returns from surgery with packing in both nostrils, which prevents bleeding and provides support for the reconstructed nose. As long as the packing is in place, the patient cannot breathe through the nose. A "moustache" dressing (or drip pad), often a folded 2 × 2 gauze pad, is usually placed under the nose (Fig. 29-1). A splint or cast may cover the nose for better alignment and protection. Change or teach the patient to change the drip pad as necessary.

After surgery, observe for edema and bleeding. Check vital signs every 4 hours until the patient is discharged. The patient with uncomplicated rhinoplasty is discharged the day of surgery. Instruct him or her and the family about the routine care described below.

! NURSING SAFETY PRIORITY QSEN

Action Alert

> Assessing how often the patient swallows after nasal surgery is a priority because repeated swallowing may indicate posterior nasal bleeding. Use a penlight to examine the throat for bleeding, and notify the surgeon if bleeding is present.

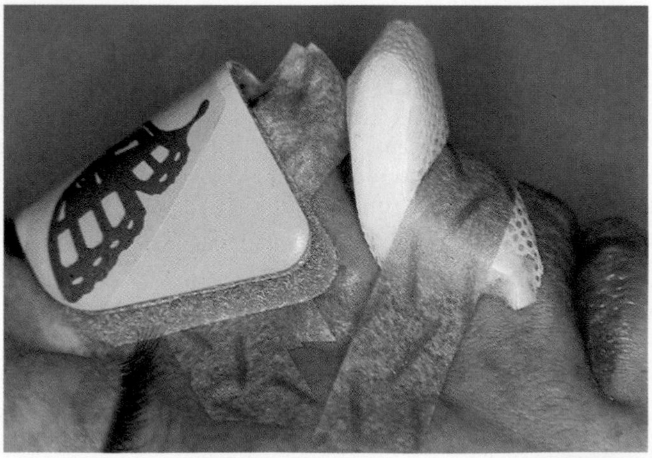

FIG. 29-1 Immediate postoperative appearance of a patient who has undergone rhinoplasty. Note the splint and gauze drip pad (moustache dressing).

Instruct the patient to stay in a semi-Fowler's position and to move slowly. Suggest that he or she rests and uses cool compresses on the nose, eyes, and face to help reduce swelling and bruising. If a general anesthetic was used, soft foods can be eaten once the patient is alert and the gag reflex has returned. Urge the patient to drink at least 2500 mL/day.

To prevent bleeding, teach the patient to limit Valsalva maneuvers (e.g., forceful coughing or straining during a bowel movement), not to sniff upward or blow the nose, and not to sneeze with the mouth closed for the first few days after the packing is removed. Instruct the patient to avoid aspirin and other NSAIDs to prevent bleeding. Antibiotics may be prescribed to prevent infection. Recommend the use of a humidifier to prevent mucosal drying. Explain that edema lasts for weeks and that the final surgical result will be evident in 6 to 12 months.

Nasoseptoplasty. Nasoseptoplasty, or **submucous resection (SMR)**, may be needed to straighten a deviated septum when chronic "stuffy" nose, snoring, sinusitis, or discomfort occurs. Slight nasal septum deviation causes no manifestations. Major deviations may obstruct the nasal passages or interfere with airflow and sinus drainage. The deviated section of cartilage and bone is removed or reshaped as an ambulatory surgical procedure. Nursing care is similar to that for a rhinoplasty.

EPISTAXIS

❖ PATHOPHYSIOLOGY

Epistaxis (nosebleed) is a common problem because of the many capillaries within the nose. Nosebleeds occur as a result of trauma, hypertension, blood dyscrasia (e.g., leukemia), inflammation, tumor, decreased humidity, nose blowing, nose picking, chronic cocaine use, and procedures such as nasogastric suctioning. Older adults tend to bleed most often from the posterior portion of the nose.

❖ PATIENT-CENTERED COLLABORATIVE CARE

The patient often reports that the bleeding started after sneezing or blowing the nose. Document the amount and color of the blood, and take vital signs. Ask the patient about the number, duration, and causes of previous bleeding episodes.

Chart 29-1 lists the best practices for emergency care of the patient with a nosebleed. An additional intervention for use at

CHART 29-1 Best Practice for Patient Safety & Quality Care QSEN

Emergency Care of a Patient with an Anterior Nosebleed

- Maintain Standard Precautions or Body Substance Precautions.
- Position the patient upright and leaning forward to prevent blood from entering the stomach and possible aspiration.
- Reassure the patient and attempt to keep him or her quiet to reduce anxiety and blood pressure.
- Apply direct lateral pressure to the nose for 10 minutes, and apply ice or cool compresses to the nose and face if possible.
- If nasal packing is necessary, loosely pack both nares with gauze or nasal tampons.
- To prevent rebleeding from dislodging clots, instruct the patient to not blow the nose for 24 hours after the bleeding stops.
- Seek medical assistance if these measures are ineffective or if the bleeding occurs frequently.

home or in the emergency department is a special nasal plug that contains an agent to promote blood clotting (sold by HemCon). The plug expands on contact with blood and compresses mucosal blood vessels.

Medical attention is needed if the nosebleed does not respond to these interventions. In such cases, the affected capillaries may be cauterized with silver nitrate or electrocautery and the nose packed. Anterior packing controls bleeding from the anterior nasal cavity.

Posterior nasal bleeding is an emergency because it cannot be easily reached and the patient may lose a lot of blood quickly (Vacca & Poirier, 2013). Posterior packing, epistaxis catheters (nasal pressure tubes), or a gel tampon is used to stop bleeding that originates in the posterior nasal region. With packing, the health care provider positions a large gauze pack in the posterior nasal cavity above the throat, threads the attached string through the nose, and tapes it to the patient's cheek to prevent pack movement. Epistaxis catheters look like very short (about 6 inches) urinary catheters (Fig. 29-2, *A*). These tubes have an exterior balloon along the tube length in addition to an anchoring balloon on the end. Placement of posterior packing or pressure tubes is uncomfortable, and the airway may be obstructed and GAS EXCHANGE impaired if the pack slips. Fig. 29-2, *B*, shows a patient with tubes in place for a posterior nasal bleed.

Observe the patient for respiratory distress and for tolerance of the packing or tubes. Humidity, oxygen, bedrest, and antibiotics may be prescribed. Opioid drugs may be prescribed for pain. Assess patients receiving opioids at least hourly for gag and cough reflexes. Use pulse oximetry to monitor for hypoxemia. The tubes or packing is usually removed after 1 to 3 days.

For posterior bleeds that do not respond to packing or tubes, additional options include cauterizing the blood vessels, ligating the vessels, or performing an embolization of the bleeding artery with interventional radiology. Potential complications of embolization include facial pain, necrosis of skin or nasal mucosa, facial nerve paralysis, and blindness (Poetker, 2013).

After the tubes or packing is removed, teach the patient and family these interventions to use at home for comfort and safety:

- Petroleum jelly can be applied sparingly to the nares for lubrication and comfort. (Excessive application could cause inhalation of the jelly into the lungs and increase the risk for pneumonia.)
- Nasal saline sprays and humidification add moisture and prevent rebleeding.
- Avoid vigorous nose blowing, the use of aspirin or other NSAIDs, and strenuous activities such as heavy lifting for at least 1 month.

NCLEX EXAMINATION CHALLENGE

Health Promotion and Maintenance

Which precaution is most important for the nurse to teach a client who is a secretary and just had nasal tubes removed after a posterior nasal bleed?

A. "Avoid NSAIDs for at least 1 week."
B. "Wait 4 weeks before returning to work."
C. "If bleeding recurs, call 911 immediately."
D. "Do not blow your nose for at least a month."

CANCER OF THE NOSE AND SINUSES

Tumors of the nasal cavities and sinuses are rare, the result of loss of CELLULAR REGULATION, and may be either benign or malignant. This type of cancer is more common among people with chronic exposure to wood dusts, dusts from textiles, leather dusts, flour, nickel and chromium dust, mustard gas, and radium. Cigarette smoking along with these exposures increases the risk (American Cancer Society [ACS], 2014).

The onset of sinus cancer is slow, and manifestations resemble sinusitis. These include persistent nasal obstruction, drainage, bloody discharge, and pain that persists after treatment of sinusitis. Lymph node enlargement often occurs on the side with tumor mass. Tumor location is identified with x-ray, CT, or MRI. A biopsy is performed to confirm the diagnosis.

Surgical removal of all or part of the tumor is the main treatment for nasopharyngeal cancers. It is usually combined with radiation therapy, especially intensity modulated radiation therapy (IMRT) (see Chapter 22). Chemotherapy may be used in conjunction with surgery and radiation for some tumors. Problems after surgery include a change in body image or speech and altered nutrition, especially when the maxilla and floor of the nose are involved in the surgery. Patients often also have changes in taste and smell.

Provide general postoperative care (see Chapter 16), including maintaining a patent airway, monitoring for hemorrhage,

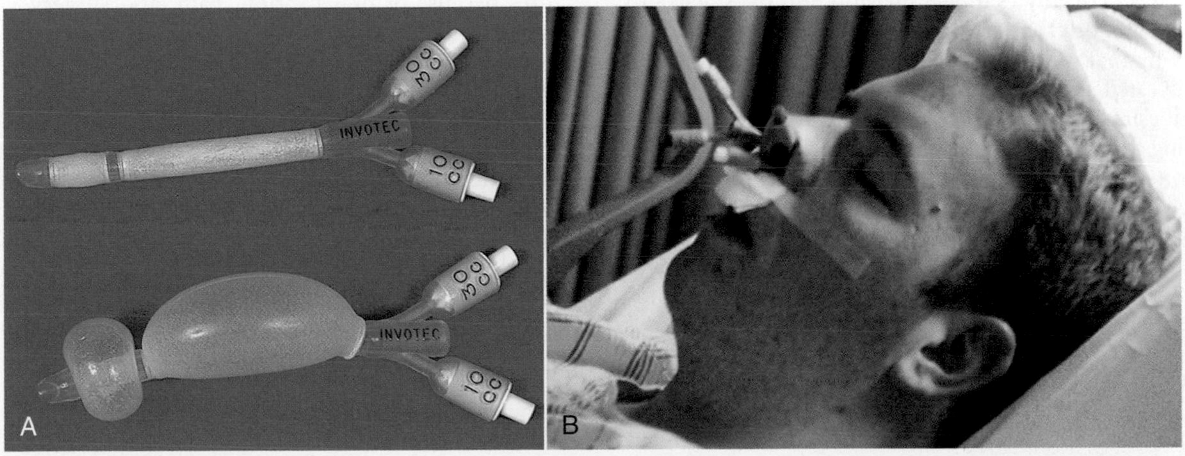

FIG. 29-2 **A,** The Ultra-Stat epistaxis catheter. **B,** Patient with epistaxis catheters in place to control a posterior nasal bleed.

providing wound care, assessing nutrition status, and performing tracheostomy care (if needed). (See Chapter 28 for tracheostomy care.) Perform careful mouth and sinus cavity care with saline irrigations using an electronic irrigation system (e.g., Waterpik, Sonicare) or a syringe. Assess the patient for pain and infection. Collaborate with the dietitian to help the patient make food selections that promote healing.

FACIAL TRAUMA

❖ PATHOPHYSIOLOGY

Facial trauma is described by the specific bones (e.g., mandibular, maxillary, orbital, nasal fractures) and the side of the face involved. Mandibular (lower jaw) fractures are the most common. *Le Fort I* is a nasoethmoid complex fracture. *Le Fort II* is a maxillary *and* nasoethmoid complex fracture. *Le Fort III* combines I and II plus an orbital-zygoma fracture, called "craniofacial disjunction" because the midface has no connection to the skull. The rich facial blood supply results in extensive bleeding and bruising.

❖ PATIENT-CENTERED COLLABORATIVE CARE

◆ Assessment

The priority action when caring for a patient with facial trauma is airway assessment for GAS EXCHANGE. Manifestations of airway obstruction are stridor, shortness of breath, dyspnea, anxiety, restlessness, hypoxia, **hypercarbia** (elevated blood levels of carbon dioxide), decreased oxygen saturation, cyanosis, and loss of consciousness. After establishing the airway, assess the site of trauma for bleeding and possible fractures. Check for soft-tissue edema, facial asymmetry, pain, or leakage of spinal fluid through the ears or nose, indicating a skull fracture. Assess vision and eye movement because orbital and maxillary fractures can entrap the eye nerves and muscles. Check behind the ears (mastoid area) for extensive bruising, known as the "battle sign," which is often associated with skull fracture and brain trauma. Because facial trauma can occur with spinal trauma and skull fractures, cranial CT, facial series, and cervical spine x-rays are obtained.

◆ Interventions

The priority action is to establish and maintain an airway for adequate GAS EXCHANGE. Anticipate the need for emergency intubation, **tracheotomy** (surgical incision into the trachea to create an airway), or **cricothyroidotomy** (creation of a temporary airway by making a small opening in the throat between the thyroid cartilage and the cricoid cartilage). Care at first focuses on establishing an airway, controlling hemorrhage, and assessing for the extent of injury. If shock is present, fluid resuscitation and identification of bleeding sites are started immediately.

Time is critical in stabilizing the patient who has head and neck trauma. Early response and treatment by special services (e.g., trauma team, maxillofacial surgeon, general surgeon, otolaryngologist, plastic surgeon, dentist) optimize the patient's recovery.

Stabilizing the fractured jaw allows the teeth to heal in proper alignment and involves **fixed occlusion** (wiring the jaws together with the mouth in a closed position). The patient remains in fixed occlusion for 6 to 10 weeks. Treatment delay, tooth infection, or poor oral care may cause jaw bone infection. This condition may then require surgical removal of dead tissue, IV antibiotic therapy, and a longer period with the jaws in a fixed position.

Extensive jaw fractures may require open reduction with internal fixation (ORIF) procedures. Compression plates and reconstruction plates with screws may be applied. Plates may be made of stainless steel, titanium, or Vitallium. If the mandibular fracture is repaired with titanium plates, the plates are permanent and do not interfere with MRI studies.

Facial fractures may be repaired with microplating surgical systems that involve bone substitutes. These shaping plates hold the bone fragments in place until new bone growth occurs. Bone cells grow into the bone substitute and re-matrix into a stable bone support. The plates may remain in place permanently or may be removed after healing.

Other fixation methods include the use of resorbable devices (plates and screws) to hold tissues in place. These devices are made from a plastic-like material that retains its integrity for about 8 weeks and then slowly biodegrades. With inner maxillary fixation (IMF), the bones are realigned and then wired in place with the bite closed. Nondisplaced aligned fractures can be repaired in a clinic or office using local dental anesthesia. General anesthesia is used to repair displaced or complex fractures or fractures that occur with other facial bone fractures.

After surgery, teach the patient about oral care with an irrigating device, such as a Waterpik or Sonicare. If the patient has inner maxillary fixation, teach self-management with wires in place, including a dental liquid diet. If the patient vomits, watch for aspiration because of the patient's inability to open the jaws to allow ejection of the emesis. Teach him or her how to cut the wires if vomiting occurs to maintain GAS EXCHANGE. If the wires are cut, instruct the patient to return to the surgeon for rewiring as soon as possible to reinstitute fixation.

! NURSING SAFETY PRIORITY (QSEN)

Action Alert

Instruct the patient to keep wire cutters with him or her at all times to prevent aspiration if vomiting occurs.

Nutrition is important and difficult for a patient with fractures because of oral fixation, pain, and surgery. Collaborate with the dietitian for patient teaching and support.

OBSTRUCTIVE SLEEP APNEA

❖ PATHOPHYSIOLOGY

Obstructive sleep apnea (OSA) is a breathing disruption during sleep that lasts at least 10 seconds and occurs a minimum of 5 times in an hour. The most common cause of sleep apnea is upper airway obstruction by the soft palate or tongue. Factors that contribute to sleep apnea include obesity, a large uvula, a short neck, smoking, enlarged tonsils or adenoids, and oropharyngeal edema.

During sleep, the muscles relax and the tongue and neck structures are displaced. As a result, the upper airway is obstructed but chest movement is unimpaired. The apnea impairs GAS EXCHANGE and increases blood carbon dioxide levels and decreases the pH. These blood gas changes stimulate neural centers. The sleeper awakens after 10 seconds or longer of apnea and corrects the obstruction, and respiration resumes. After he or she goes back to sleep, the cycle begins again, sometimes as often as every 5 minutes.

This cyclic pattern of disrupted sleep prevents the deep sleep needed for best rest. Thus the person may have excessive daytime sleepiness, an inability to concentrate, and irritability. The long-term effects of OSA include increased risk for hypertension, stroke, neurocognitive deficits, weight gain, diabetes, and pulmonary and cardiovascular disease (Woidtke, 2013).

❖ PATIENT-CENTERED COLLABORATIVE CARE

◆ Assessment

Patients are often unaware that they have sleep apnea. The disorder should be suspected for any person who has persistent daytime sleepiness or reports "waking up tired," particularly if he or she also snores heavily. Other manifestations include irritability and personality changes. Sleep apnea may be verified by family members who observe the problem when the person sleeps. A complete assessment is performed when excessive daytime sleepiness is a problem.

A beginning assessment includes having the patient complete the Epworth Sleepiness Scale (ESS) (Simmons & Pruitt, 2012). The patient is asked to score his or her likelihood of falling asleep during eight common activities or scenarios. Each is self-scored from 0 to 3. Those patients who score 18 or above are considered at risk for severe sleep apnea.

The most accurate test for sleep apnea is an overnight sleep study. In this study, the patient is directly observed while wearing a variety of monitoring equipment to evaluate depth of sleep, type of sleep, respiratory effort, oxygen saturation, and muscle movement. Monitoring devices include an electroencephalograph (EEG), an electrocardiograph (ECG), a pulse oximeter, and an electromyograph (EMG). Home-based sleep studies also are available but often not covered by insurance (Carlucci et al., 2013).

◆ Interventions

A change in sleeping position or weight loss may correct mild sleep apnea and improve GAS EXCHANGE. Position-fixing devices may prevent subluxation of the tongue and neck structures and reduce obstruction. Severe sleep apnea requires additional methods to prevent obstruction.

A common method to prevent airway collapse is the use of noninvasive positive-pressure ventilation (NPPV) to hold open the upper airways. A nasal mask or full-face mask delivery system allows mechanical delivery of either bi-level positive airway pressure (BiPAP), autotitrating positive airway pressure (APAP), or nasal continuous positive airway pressure (CPAP). With BiPAP, a machine delivers a set inspiratory positive airway pressure at the beginning of each breath. As the patient begins to exhale, the machine delivers a lower end-expiratory pressure. These two pressures hold open the upper airways. With APAP, the machine adjusts continuously, resetting the pressure throughout the breathing cycle to meet the patient's needs. Nasal CPAP delivers a set positive airway pressure continuously during each cycle of inhalation and exhalation. For any positive-pressure ventilation delivered through a facemask during sleep, a small electric compressor is required. Proper fit of the mask over the nose and mouth or just over the nose is key to successful treatment (see Fig. 28-9 in Chapter 28). Although noisy, these methods are accepted by most patients after an adjustment period.

One drug has been approved to help manage the daytime sleepiness associated with sleep apnea. Modafinil (Attenace, Provigil) is helpful for patients who have *narcolepsy* (uncontrolled daytime sleep) from sleep apnea by promoting daytime wakefulness. This drug does *not* treat the cause of sleep apnea. Sleep-inducing sedatives also are not considered first-line therapy.

Surgical intervention may involve a simple adenoidectomy, uvulectomy, or remodeling of the entire posterior oropharynx (uvulopalatopharyngoplasty [UPP]). Both conventional and laser surgeries are used for this purpose. A tracheostomy may be needed for very severe sleep apnea that is not relieved by more moderate interventions.

DISORDERS OF THE LARYNX

VOCAL CORD PARALYSIS

Vocal fold (cord) paralysis may result from injury, trauma, or diseases that affect the larynx, laryngeal nerves, or vagus nerve. Prolonged intubation with an endotracheal (ET) tube may cause temporary or permanent paralysis. Paralysis may occur in patients with neurologic disorders or with conditions that damage either the vagus nerve or the laryngeal nerves. Paralysis of both vocal cords may result from injury, brainstem stroke, or total thyroidectomy.

Vocal fold paralysis may affect both cords or only one. When only one vocal cord is involved (most common), the airway remains patent but the voice is affected. Manifestations of open bilateral vocal cord paralysis include hoarseness; a breathy, weak voice; and aspiration of food. *Bilateral closed vocal cord paralysis causes airway obstruction and is an emergency if the manifestations are severe and the patient cannot compensate. Stridor is the major manifestation.*

Securing an airway is the main intervention. Place the patient in a high-Fowler's position to aid in breathing and proper alignment of airway structures. Assess for airway obstruction.

! NURSING SAFETY PRIORITY (QSEN)

Critical Rescue

Immediately notify the Rapid Response Team if dyspnea with stridor occurs. Emergency endotracheal intubation or tracheotomy may be needed.

Various surgical procedures can improve the voice. One simple procedure for open vocal cord paralysis involves injecting polytef (Teflon) into the affected cord so it enlarges toward the unaffected cord. This technique improves closure during speaking and eating.

The patient with open cord paralysis is at risk for aspiration because the airway is open during swallowing. Teach him or her to hold the breath during swallowing to allow the larynx to rise, close, and push food back into the esophagus during swallowing. Teach the patient to tuck the chin down and tilt the forehead forward during swallowing. Indications of aspiration include immediate coughing on swallowing of liquids or solids, a "wet"-sounding voice, and "tearing up" or watery eyes on swallowing. Chest x-rays are used to diagnose aspiration pneumonia.

LARYNGEAL TRAUMA

Laryngeal trauma occurs with a crushing or direct blow injury, fracture, or prolonged endotracheal intubation. Manifestations include difficulty breathing (**dyspnea**), inability to produce sound (**aphonia**), hoarseness, and **subcutaneous emphysema** (air present in the subcutaneous tissue). Bleeding from the airway (**hemoptysis**) may occur, depending on the location of the trauma. The health care provider performs a direct visual examination of the larynx by laryngoscopy or fiberoptic laryngoscopy to determine the extent of the injury.

Management of patients with laryngeal injuries consists of assessing the effectiveness of GAS EXCHANGE and monitoring vital signs (including respiratory status and pulse oximetry) every 15 to 30 minutes. *Maintaining a patent airway is a priority.* Apply oxygen and humidification as prescribed to maintain adequate oxygen saturation. Manifestations of respiratory difficulty include tachypnea, nasal flaring, anxiety, sternal retraction, shortness of breath, restlessness, decreased oxygen saturation, decreased level of consciousness, and stridor.

! NURSING SAFETY PRIORITY (QSEN)

Critical Rescue

> If the patient has respiratory difficulty, stay with him or her and instruct other trauma team members or the Rapid Response Team to prepare for an emergency intubation or tracheotomy.

Surgical intervention is needed for lacerations of the mucous membranes, cartilage exposure, and cord paralysis. Laryngeal repair is performed as soon as possible to prevent laryngeal stenosis and to cover any exposed cartilage. An artificial airway may be needed.

OTHER UPPER AIRWAY DISORDERS

UPPER AIRWAY OBSTRUCTION

❖ PATHOPHYSIOLOGY

Upper airway obstruction is a life-threatening emergency in which airflow through nose, mouth, pharynx, or larynx is interrupted and GAS EXCHANGE is impaired. Early recognition is essential to prevent complications, including respiratory arrest. Causes of upper airway obstruction include:

- Tongue edema (surgery, trauma, angioedema as an allergic response to a drug)
- Tongue occlusion (e.g., loss of gag reflex, loss of muscle tone, unconsciousness, coma)
- Laryngeal edema
- Peritonsillar and pharyngeal abscess
- Head and neck cancer
- Thick secretions
- Stroke and cerebral edema
- Smoke inhalation edema
- Facial, tracheal, or laryngeal trauma
- Foreign-body aspiration
- Burns of the head or neck area
- Anaphylaxis

One preventable cause of airway obstruction leading to asphyxiation is inspissated (thickly crusted) oral and nasopharyngeal secretions. In this condition, poor oral hygiene leads to thickening and hardening of secretions that can completely block the airway and lead to death. Proper nursing care can eliminate this cause of airway obstruction. Patients at highest risk are those with an altered mental status and level of consciousness, are dehydrated, are unable to communicate, are unable to cough effectively, or are at risk for aspiration.

! NURSE SAFETY PRIORITY (QSEN)

Action Alert

> Assess the oral care needs of the patient with risk factors for inspissated secretions daily. Ensure that whoever provides oral care understands the importance and the correct techniques for preventing secretion buildup and airway obstruction.

❖ PATIENT-CENTERED COLLABORATIVE CARE

◆ Assessment

Airway obstruction is frightening, and prompt care is essential to prevent a partial obstruction from progressing to a complete obstruction. Partial obstruction produces general manifestations such as diaphoresis, tachycardia, and elevated blood pressure. Persistent or unexplained manifestations must be evaluated even though vague. Diagnostic procedures include chest or neck x-rays, laryngoscopic examination, and computed tomography.

Observe for hypoxia and hypercarbia, restlessness, increasing anxiety, sternal retractions, a "seesawing" chest, abdominal movements, or a feeling of impending doom from air hunger. Use pulse oximetry or end-tidal carbon dioxide ($ETCO_2$ or $PETCO_2$) for ongoing monitoring of GAS EXCHANGE. Continually assess for stridor, cyanosis, and changes in level of consciousness.

◆ Interventions

Assess for the cause of the obstruction. When the obstruction is due to the tongue falling back or excessive secretions, slightly extend the patient's head and neck and insert a nasal or an oral airway. Suction to remove obstructing secretions. If the obstruction is caused by a foreign body, perform abdominal thrusts (Fig. 29-3).

Upper airway obstruction may require emergency procedures such as cricothyroidotomy, endotracheal intubation, or tracheotomy to improve GAS EXCHANGE. Direct laryngoscopy may be performed before or with these procedures to determine the cause of obstruction or to remove foreign bodies.

Cricothyroidotomy is an emergency procedure performed by emergency medical personnel as a stab wound at the cricothyroid membrane between the thyroid cartilage and the cricoid cartilage (see Fig. 27-4 in Chapter 27). Any hollow tube—but preferably a tracheostomy tube—can be placed through the opening to hold this airway open until a tracheotomy can be performed. This procedure is used when it is the *only* way to secure an airway. Another emergency procedure to bypass an obstruction is the insertion of a 14-gauge needle directly into the cricoid space to allow airflow into and out of the lungs.

Endotracheal intubation is performed by inserting a tube into the trachea via the nose (**nasotracheal**) or mouth (**orotracheal**) by a physician, anesthesia provider, or other specially trained personnel.

Tracheotomy is a surgical procedure and takes about 5 to 10 minutes to perform. It is best performed in the operating room

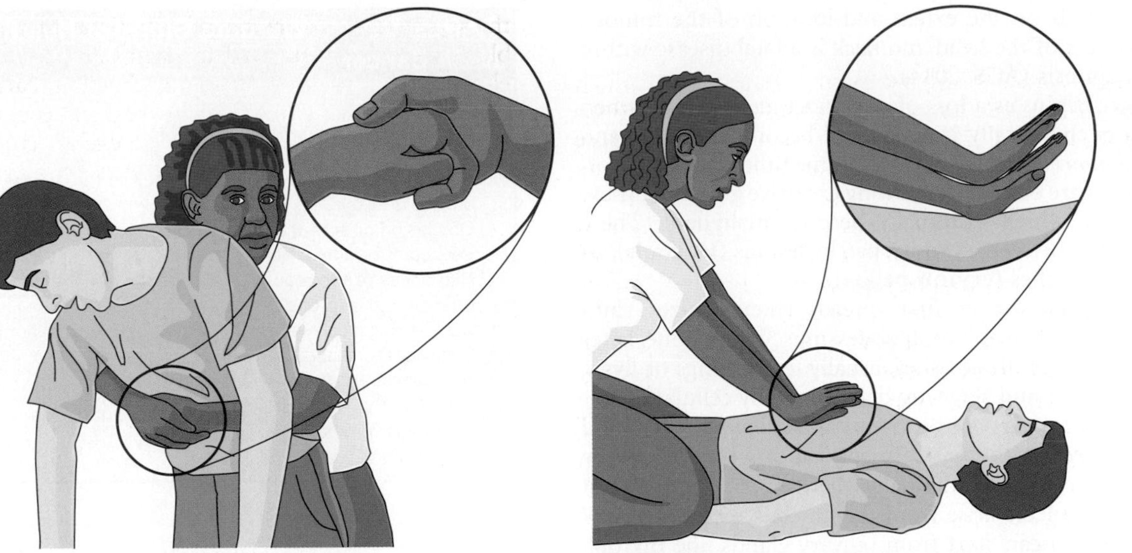

With the conscious victim standing or sitting, place your fist between the victim's lower rib cage and navel. Wrap the palm of your hand around your fist. A quick inward, upward thrust expels the air remaining in the victim's lungs, and with it the foreign body. If the first thrust is unsuccessful, repeat several thrusts in rapid succession until the foreign body is expelled or until the victim loses consciousness.

With the unconscious victim lying supine, straddle the victim's thighs. Place one hand on top of the other as shown, with the heel of the bottom hand just above the victim's navel. Quickly thrust inward and upward, toward the victim's head.

FIG. 29-3 The abdominal thrust maneuver (formerly known as the *Heimlich maneuver*) for relief of upper airway obstruction caused by a foreign body.

(OR) with the patient under local or general anesthesia but can be performed at the bedside. Local anesthesia is used if there is concern that the airway will be lost during the induction of anesthesia. A tracheotomy is reserved for the patient who cannot be easily intubated with an endotracheal tube. An emergency tracheotomy can establish an airway in less than 2 minutes. See Chapter 28 for a discussion of care of the patient with a tracheotomy.

Patients receiving mechanical ventilation for upper airway obstruction or respiratory failure may require a tracheostomy after 7 or more days of continuous intubation. In such cases, a tracheotomy is performed to prevent laryngeal injury by the endotracheal tube.

NCLEX EXAMINATION CHALLENGE

Physiological Integrity

The client is a woman with severe angioedema and tongue swelling from exposure to seafood. She has stridor, and her oxygen saturation is 70%. For which type of respiratory support does the nurse prepare?

A. Nasal BiPAP
B. Tracheotomy
C. Cricothyroidotomy
D. Endotracheal intubation

NECK TRAUMA

Neck injuries may be caused by any weapon or trauma. The patient with neck trauma may have other injuries, including cardiovascular, respiratory, intestinal, and neurologic damage. The final outcome of this type of injury depends on initial assessment and care. Consult a critical care textbook and see Chapter 43 for more detailed information.

The priority nursing care for a patient with neck trauma is assessing for and maintaining a patent airway. After airway patency is ensured, assess for bleeding or impending shock.

Perform a neurologic assessment for mental status, sensory level, and motor function. Injury to the carotid artery may result in death, stroke, or paralysis from disruption of blood flow to the brain (see Chapter 41). A carotid angiogram may be needed to rule out vascular injuries.

Esophagus injury may occur with neck trauma. Assess for chest pain and tenderness, oral bleeding, and **crepitus** (crackling sounds when palpating the skin). A barium or meglumine diatrizoate (Gastrografin) swallow may be needed to rule out an esophageal perforation injury.

Cervical spine injuries often occur at the same time as a neck injury (see Chapter 43). Obstruction can occur as a result of the initial injury or from swelling after surgery to repair the injury. Health care personnel must take great care not to make these injuries worse by causing neck movement while establishing the airway using the jaw-thrust maneuver. Prepare to assist in emergency intubation, cricothyrotomy, or tracheotomy to establish a patent airway. Interventions for patients in shock are detailed in Chapter 37.

HEAD AND NECK CANCER

❖ PATHOPHYSIOLOGY

Head and neck cancer can disrupt breathing (GAS EXCHANGE), eating, facial appearance, self-image, speech, and communication. This form of cancer can be devastating, even when cured. The care needs for patients with these problems are complex, requiring a coordinated and comprehensive team approach.

Head and neck cancers are usually squamous cell carcinomas. These slow-growing tumors are curable when treated early. The prognosis for those who have more advanced disease at diagnosis depends on the extent and location of the tumors. Untreated cancer of the head and neck is a fatal disease within 2 years of diagnosis (ACS, 2014).

The cancer begins as a loss of CELLULAR REGULATION when the mucosa is chronically irritated and becomes tougher and thicker *(squamous metaplasia)*. At the same time, genes controlling cell growth are damaged, allowing excessive growth of these abnormal cells, which eventually become malignant. These lesions may then be seen as white, patchy lesions (**leukoplakia**) or red, velvety patches (**erythroplakia**).

Head and neck cancer first spreads (**metastasizes**) into nearby structures, such as lymph nodes, muscle, and bone. Later spread is systemic to distant sites, usually to the lungs or liver.

The cancer type and stage are determined by cellular analysis. Earlier-stage cancers are described as *carcinoma in situ* and *well differentiated.* Without treatment, cancers progress to be *moderately differentiated* and, finally, *poorly differentiated.* Most head and neck cancers arise from the mucous membrane and skin, but they also can start from salivary glands, the thyroid, or other structures. Treatment is based on tumor cell type and degree of spread at diagnosis.

Etiology. The two most important risk factors for head and neck cancer are tobacco and alcohol use, especially in combination. Other risk factors include voice abuse, chronic laryngitis, exposure to chemicals or dusts, poor oral hygiene, long-term or severe gastroesophageal reflux disease, and oral infection with the human papillomavirus (ACS, 2014).

Incidence and Prevalence. The frequency of head and neck carcinoma is increasing in North America. About 60,000 new cases of oral, pharyngeal, and laryngeal cancers are diagnosed each year and account for more than 13,000 deaths per year (ACS, 2014; Canadian Cancer Society, 2014). They affect men twice as often as women and are most common in people older than 60 years.

TABLE 29-1 Warning Signs of Head and Neck Cancer

- Pain
- Lump in the mouth, throat, or neck
- Difficulty swallowing
- Color changes in the mouth or tongue to red, white, gray, dark brown, or black
- Oral lesion or sore that does not heal in 2 weeks
- Persistent or unexplained oral bleeding
- Numbness of the mouth, lips, or face
- Change in the fit of dentures
- Burning sensation when drinking citrus juices or hot liquids
- Persistent, unilateral ear pain
- Hoarseness or change in voice quality
- Persistent or recurrent sore throat
- Shortness of breath
- Anorexia and weight loss

❖ PATIENT-CENTERED COLLABORATIVE CARE

◆ Assessment

History. The patient may have difficulty speaking because of hoarseness, shortness of breath, tumor bulk, and pain. Pace the interview to avoid tiring the patient.

Ask about tobacco and alcohol use, history of acute or chronic laryngitis or pharyngitis, oral sores, and lumps in the neck. Calculate the patient's pack-years of smoking history (see Chapter 27). Ask about alcohol intake (how many drinks per day and for how many years). Also ask about exposure to pollutants.

Assess problems related to risk factors. For example, nutrition may be poor because of alcohol intake and impaired liver function. Assess dietary habits and any weight loss. Ask about any chronic lung disease, which may have an impact on GAS EXCHANGE.

Physical Assessment/Clinical Manifestations. Table 29-1 lists the warning signs of head and neck cancer. With laryngeal cancer, painless hoarseness may occur because of tumor size and an inability of the vocal cords to come together for normal speech. Vocal cord lesions form early in laryngeal cancer. Any person who has a history of hoarseness, mouth sores, or a lump in the neck for 3 to 4 weeks should be evaluated for laryngeal cancer.

Inspect the head and neck for symmetry and the presence of lumps or lesions. An advanced practice nurse or physician may perform a laryngeal examination using a laryngeal mirror or fiberoptic laryngoscope. The neck is palpated to assess for enlarged lymph nodes.

Psychosocial Assessment. Often the patient with head and neck cancer has a long-standing history of tobacco or alcohol use or both. Assess the adequacy of support systems and coping mechanisms. Document social and family support because the patient often needs extensive assistance at home after treatment. Collaborate with a social worker as needed. Assess the level of education or literacy of the patient and family to plan teaching before and after surgery.

Document any family history of cancer, as well as the patient's age, gender, occupation, and ability to perform ADLs. Ask the patient whether his or her occupation requires continual oral communication. Job retraining may be needed if treatment affects speech.

Laboratory Assessment. Diagnostic tests include a complete blood cell count, bleeding times, urinalysis, and blood chemistries. The patient with chronic alcoholism may have low protein and albumin levels from poor nutrition. Liver and kidney function tests are performed to rule out cancer spread and to evaluate the patient's ability to metabolize drugs and chemotherapy agents.

Imaging Assessment. Many types of imaging studies, including x-rays of the skull, sinuses, neck, and chest, are useful in diagnosing cancer spread, other tumors, and the extent of tumor invasion. Computed tomography (CT), with or without contrast medium, helps evaluate the tumor's exact location. Magnetic resonance imaging (MRI) can help differentiate normal from diseased tissue.

The brain, bone, and liver are evaluated with nuclear imaging, bone scans, single-photon emission computerized tomography (SPECT) scans, and positron emission tomography (PET) scans. These tests locate additional tumor sites.

Other Diagnostic Assessment. Other helpful tests include direct and indirect laryngoscopy, tumor mapping, and biopsy. *Panendoscopy* (laryngoscopy, nasopharyngoscopy, esophagoscopy, and bronchoscopy) is performed with general anesthesia to define the extent of the tumor. Tumor-mapping biopsies are performed to identify tumor location. Biopsy tissues taken at the time of the panendoscopy confirm the diagnosis, tumor type, cell features, location, and stage (see Chapter 21).

NCLEX EXAMINATION CHALLENGE
Health Promotion and Maintenance

The 62-year-old client whose brother was just diagnosed with head and neck cancer asks the nurse what he could do to reduce his risk for also developing this cancer. What is the nurse's best response?

A. "Because head and neck cancer has a strong hereditary component, participating in screening twice yearly is critical for you."
B. "Always wear sunscreen with a 50% or greater protection factor whenever you are outdoors."
C. "Avoid shouting and singing to prevent stress to your vocal cords and larynx."
D. "Stop smoking, and drink alcohol only in moderation."

◆ *Analysis*

The priority NANDA-I nursing diagnoses and collaborative problems for patients with head and neck cancer include:

1. Potential for respiratory obstruction
2. Risk for Aspiration related to edema, anatomic changes, or altered protective reflexes (NANDA-I)
3. Anxiety related to threat of death, change in role status, or change in economic status (NANDA-I)
4. Reduced self-concept related to tumor and treatment modalities

◆ *Planning and Implementation*

Preventing Respiratory Obstruction. Without treatment, head and neck cancers grow, obstruct the airway, and prevent GAS EXCHANGE leading to death. Airway obstruction also can occur as a complication of treatment modalities.

Planning: Expected Outcomes. The patient with head and neck cancer is expected to attain and maintain adequate GAS EXCHANGE and tissue oxygenation. Indicators include:

- Arterial blood gas values within the normal range
- Rate and depth of respiration within the normal range
- Pulse oximetry within the normal range

Interventions. The focus of treatment is to remove or eradicate the cancer while preserving as much normal function as possible. The physician presents the available treatment options. Surgery, radiation, chemotherapy, or biotherapy may be used alone or in combination. Considerations for treatment options include the patient's physical condition, nutrition status, and age; the effects of the tumor on body function; and the patient's personal choice. Treatment for laryngeal cancer may range from radiation therapy (for a small specific area or tumor) to total laryngopharyngectomy with bilateral neck dissections followed by radiation therapy, depending on the extent and location of the lesion. Voice-conservation procedures are used only if they do not risk incomplete removal of the tumor. Nursing care focuses on the patient's total needs, including preoperative preparation, optimal in-hospital care, discharge planning and teaching, and extensive outpatient rehabilitation.

Nonsurgical Management. Monitor GAS EXCHANGE and the respiratory system by assessing respiratory rate, breath sounds, pulse oximetry, and arterial blood gas values. Airway obstruction can occur from tumor growth, edema, or both. Teach the patient to use the Fowler's and semi-Fowler's positions for best gas exchange. Sitting upright in a reclining chair may promote more comfortable breathing. Chapters 3 and 7 provide additional information on palliation and pain control for patients who elect not to have therapy and for those whose therapy has not been effective.

Radiation therapy for treatment of small cancers in specific locations has a cure rate of at least 80%. Standard therapy uses 5000 to 7500 rad (radiation absorbed dose), usually over 6 weeks and in daily or twice-daily doses. Intensity modulated radiotherapy (IMRT) is being used increasingly to provide higher doses directly to the tumor with less damage to surrounding normal tissues. Radiation may be used alone or, more often, in combination with surgery and chemotherapy (see Chapter 22). It can be performed before or after surgery. Most patients have hoarseness, dysphagia, skin problems, and dry mouth for a few weeks after radiation therapy.

Hoarseness may become worse during therapy. Reassure the patient that voice improves within 4 to 6 weeks after completion of radiation therapy. Urge the patient to use voice rest and alternative means of communication until the effects of radiation therapy have passed.

Most patients have a sore throat and difficulty swallowing during radiation therapy to the neck. Gargling with saline or sucking ice may decrease discomfort. Mouthwashes and throat sprays containing a local anesthetic agent such as lidocaine or diphenhydramine can provide temporary relief. Analgesic drugs may be prescribed.

The skin at the site of irradiation becomes red and tender and may peel during therapy. Instruct the patient to avoid exposing this area to sun, heat, cold, and abrasive actions such as shaving. Teach the patient to wear protective clothing made of soft cotton and to wash this area gently daily with a mild soap, such as Dove (Mannix et al., 2012). Using appropriate skin care products (approved by the radiation-oncology department) can reduce the intensity of skin reactions.

If the salivary glands are in the irradiation path, the mouth becomes dry (**xerostomia**). This side effect is long-term and may be permanent. Some of the problems from reduced saliva include increased risk for dental caries, increased risk for oral infections, halitosis (bad breath), and taste changes. Fluoride gel trays and nightly fluoride treatments can reduce the incidence of tooth deterioration. The trays can be worn during radiation therapy to prevent radiation scatter from the beam deflecting off existing metal inside the mouth. Although there is no cure for xerostomia, interventions can help reduce the discomfort. Heavy fluid intake, particularly water, and humidification can help ease the discomfort. Some patients benefit from the use of artificial saliva, such as Salivart; moisturizing sprays or gels, such as Mouth Kote; or saliva stimulants, such as Salagen and cevimeline (cholinergic drugs).

Chemotherapy can be used alone or in addition to surgery or radiation for head and neck cancer. Often, chemotherapy and radiation therapy *(chemoradiation)* are used at the same time. Although the exact drugs used may vary, depending on cancer cell features, most chemotherapy regimens for head and neck cancers include cisplatin (National Comprehensive Cancer Network, 2013). The oral cavity effects of radiation are intensified with concurrent chemotherapy. These can be uncomfortable, and patients often request breaks in the treatment regimen. However, these breaks in treatment do affect the outcome of treatment and should be avoided. Intense patient education before treatment and support during treatment can improve patient adherence to the treatment plan (Mason et al., 2013). Chapter 22 discusses the general care needs of patients receiving chemotherapy.

Biotherapy in the form of epidermal growth factor receptor inhibitors (EGFRIs) may be effective for patients whose cancers overexpress the receptor. Currently, the drug approved for this purpose is cetuximab (Erbitux). Although it is a targeted therapy, this drug blocks EGFRs in normal tissues as well as those in the tumor. As a result, severe skin reactions are common and difficult for the patient (Boucher et al., 2011).

Surgical Management. Tumor size, node number, and metastasis location (TNM classification) determines the type of surgery needed for the specific head and neck cancer (see Chapter 21). Very small, early-stage tumors may be removed by laser therapy or photodynamic therapy; however, few head and neck tumors are found at this stage and most require extensive traditional surgery. Reconstruction is also determined by the tumor size and amount of tissue to be resected and reconstructed. Surgical procedures for head and neck cancers include laryngectomy (total and partial), tracheotomy, and oropharyngeal cancer resections. The major types of surgery for laryngeal cancer include cord stripping, removal of a vocal cord (**cordectomy**), partial laryngectomy, and total laryngectomy. If cancer is in the lymph nodes in the neck, the surgeon performs a nodal neck dissection along with removal of the primary tumor ("radical neck").

Preoperative Care. Teach the patient and family about the tumor. The surgeon explains the surgical procedure and obtains informed consent. Discuss and interpret the implications of such consent with the patient and family.

Explain about self-management of the airway, suctioning, pain-control methods, the critical care environment (including ventilators and critical care routines), nutrition support, feeding tubes, and plans for discharge. The patient will need to learn new methods of speech, at least during the time that mechanical ventilation is used and, depending on surgery type, perhaps forever. Help him or her prepare for this change before surgery and to practice the use of the selected form of communication (see Chart 29-2 and the discussion of Maintaining Communication in Chapter 28). Determine the communication method preferred by the patient.

A team approach for planning care and rehabilitation is critical for the best outcome. The team includes nurses, physicians, speech and language pathologists, social workers, dietitians, respiratory therapists, and occupational and physical therapists. These professionals help evaluate and prepare the patient who has head and neck cancer. Chapter 14 describes general preoperative assessment and education.

Operative Procedures. Table 29-2 lists specific information about the various surgical procedures for laryngeal cancer. Hemilaryngectomy (vertical or horizontal) and supraglottic laryngectomy are types of partial voice-conservation laryngectomies.

To protect the airway, a tracheostomy is needed. With a partial laryngectomy, the tracheostomy is usually temporary. With a total laryngectomy, the upper airway is separated from the throat and esophagus and a permanent laryngectomy stoma in the neck is created.

Neck dissection includes the removal of lymph nodes, the sternocleidomastoid muscle, the jugular vein, the 11th cranial nerve, and surrounding soft tissue. Shoulder drop is expected after extensive surgery. Physical therapy can help the patient ease the shoulder drop by using other muscle groups.

Postoperative Care. Head and neck surgery often lasts 8 hours or longer. Usually the patient spends the immediate period after surgery in the surgical intensive care unit. Monitor airway patency, vital signs, hemodynamic status, and comfort level. Monitor for hemorrhage and other general complications of anesthesia and surgery (see Chapter 16). Take vital signs hourly for the first 24 hours and then according to agency policy until the patient is stable. After the patient is transferred from the critical care unit, monitor vital signs every 4 hours or according to agency policy.

Complications after surgery include airway obstruction, hemorrhage, wound breakdown, and tumor recurrence. *The first priorities after head and neck surgery are airway maintenance and* GAS EXCHANGE. Other priorities are wound, flap, and reconstructive tissue care; pain management; nutrition; and psychological adjustment, including speech and language therapy.

CHART 29-2 **Best Practice for Patient Safety & Quality Care** QSEN

Communicating with a Patient Who Is Unable to Speak

- Assess the patient's reading skills and cognition.
- Determine in what language (languages) the patient is most fluent.
- Collaborate with a speech and language pathologist.
- If the patient requires vision-enhancing devices or hearing-enhancing devices, be sure these are available and in use.
- Provide the patient with a variety of techniques to practice before verbal skills are lost to determine with which one(s) the patient feels most comfortable. These may include:
  - Alphabet board
  - Picture board
  - Paper and pencil
  - Magic Slate
  - Hand signals/gestures
  - Computer with e-triloquist program
  - Programmable speech-generating devices (text-to-speech communication aid)
- Reinforce to the patient the technique for esophageal speech presented by the speech and language pathologist, and provide the time for practice.
- Use a normal tone of voice to talk with the patient (unless hearing is a pre-existing problem, a change in the ability to speak does not interfere with the patient's ability to hear).
- Ensure that the call-light board at the nurses' station indicates a non-speaking patient.
- Teach the patient to make noise to indicate immediate attention is needed at the bedside when he or she signals by call light. Such noises can include tapping the siderail with a spoon, making clicking noises with the tongue, using a bell, or working a noisemaker. Be sure that whatever method is selected is listed on the call-light board.
- When face-to-face with the patient:
  - Phrase questions in a "yes" or "no" format.
  - Watch the patient's face for indications of understanding or the lack of it.
  - Listen attentively to any sound the patient makes.
- If writing is selected as the method to communicate, assess whether the patient is right-handed or left-handed and ensure appropriate writing materials are within reach. Use the other arm for IV placement.
- Ensure the preferred method of communication is documented in the patient record and is communicated to all care providers.
- Encourage the family to work with the patient in the use of the selected method.
- Provide praise and encouragement.
- Do not avoid talking with the patient.
- Allow the patient to set the pace for communication.

TABLE 29-2 Surgical Procedures for Laryngeal Cancer and their Effect on Voice Quality

PROCEDURE	DESCRIPTION	RESULTING VOICE QUALITY
Laser surgery	Tumor reduced or destroyed by laser beam through laryngoscope	Normal/hoarse
Transoral cordectomy	Tumor (early lesion) resected through laryngoscope	Normal/hoarse (high cure rate)
Laryngofissure	No cord removed (early lesion)	Normal (high cure rate)
Supraglottic partial laryngectomy	Hyoid bone, false cords, and epiglottis removed Neck dissection on affected side performed if nodes involved	Normal/hoarse
Hemilaryngectomy or vertical laryngectomy	One true cord, one false cord, and one half of thyroid cartilage removed	Hoarse
Total laryngectomy	Entire larynx, hyoid bone, strap muscles, one or two tracheal rings removed Nodal neck dissection if nodes involved	No natural voice

Airway Maintenance and Gas Exchange. Immediately after surgery, the patient may need ventilatory assistance. Most patients wean easily from the ventilator after this type of surgery because the thoracic and abdominal cavities are not entered. During weaning, the patient usually uses a tracheostomy collar (over the artificial airway or open stoma) with oxygen and humidity to help move mucus secretions. Secretions may remain blood-tinged for 1 to 2 days. Use Standard Precautions, and report any increase in bleeding to the surgeon. Humidity helps remove crusts and prevents obstruction of the tube with secretions. A laryngectomy tube is used for patients who have undergone a *total laryngectomy* and need an appliance to prevent scar tissue shrinkage of the skin-tracheal border. This tube is similar to a tracheostomy tube but is shorter and wider with a larger lumen. Laryngectomy tube care is similar to tracheostomy tube care (see Chapter 28) except that the patient can change the laryngectomy tube daily or as needed. A laryngectomy button is similar to a laryngectomy tube but is softer, has a single lumen, and is very short. A button is comfortable for the patient, is easily removed for cleaning, and is available in various sizes for a custom fit. Provide alternative communication techniques because the patient cannot speak.

Coughing and deep breathing are usually effective in clearing secretions. Instruct the patient how to cough and deep breathe to clear secretions.

Oral secretions can be suctioned by the alert patient using a Yankauer or tonsillar suction or a soft red latex catheter. Teach the patient to suction *away* from the surgical side to prevent opening the wound. Using a table mirror helps the patient see the area more clearly. Provide a clean environment for the catheter.

Stoma care after a total laryngectomy is a combination of wound care and airway care. Inspect the stoma with a flashlight. Clean the suture line with sterile saline (or a prescribed solution) to prevent secretions from forming crusts and obstructing the airway. Perform suture line care every 1 to 2 hours during the first few days after surgery and then every 4 hours. The mucosa of the stoma and trachea should be bright and shiny and without crusts, similar to the appearance of the oral mucosa.

Wound, Flap, and Reconstructive Tissue Care. Tissue "flaps" may be used to close the wound and improve appearance. Flaps are skin, subcutaneous tissue, and sometimes muscle, taken from other body areas used for reconstruction after head and neck resection. After neck dissection, the surgeon places a split-thickness skin graft (STSG) over the exposed carotid artery before covering it with skin flaps or reconstructive flaps.

The first 24 hours after surgery are critical. Evaluate all grafts and flaps hourly for the first 72 hours. Monitor capillary refill, color, drainage, and Doppler activity of the major blood vessel to the area. Report changes to the surgeon immediately because surgical intervention may be needed. Position the patient so that the surgical flaps are not dependent.

Hemorrhage. Hemorrhage is a possible complication after any surgery, but it is uncommon with laryngectomy. The surgeon often places a closed surgical drain in the neck area to collect blood and drainage for about 72 hours after surgery. The drain also helps maintain the position of the reconstructed skin flaps. Any drain obstruction or equipment malfunction may cause a buildup of blood or fluid under the flaps that can impair blood flow and result in flap failure. A sudden stoppage of drainage may indicate drain obstruction by a clot. Monitor and record the amount and character of drainage. Check the patency and functioning of the drainage system. Report any drain malfunction or change in flap appearance to the surgeon. Depending on the surgeon's preference and the agency's policy, you may need to empty the drainage container or "milk" the drain.

Wound Breakdown. Wound breakdown is a complication caused by poor nutrition, a long smoking history, alcohol use, wound contamination, and radiation therapy before surgery. Manage wound breakdown with packing and local care as prescribed to keep the wound clean and to stimulate the growth of healthy granulation tissue. Wounds may be extensive, and the carotid artery may be exposed. Split-thickness skin grafts often are placed over the carotid artery for protection in the event of wound dehiscence. As the wound heals, granulation tissue covers the artery and prevents rupture. If granulation is slow and the carotid artery is at risk, another surgical flap may be made to cover the artery and close the wound.

When the carotid artery ruptures, large amounts of bright red blood spurt quickly. It is also possible for the carotid artery to have a small leak, with continuous oozing of bright red blood. Usually, a small leak leads to a complete rupture within a short time.

! NURSING SAFETY PRIORITY QSEN

Critical Rescue

If a carotid artery leak is suspected, call the Rapid Response Team and ***do not touch the area because additional pressure could cause an immediate rupture.*** If the carotid artery ruptures because of drying or infection, immediately place constant pressure over the site and secure the airway. Maintain direct manual, continuous pressure on the carotid artery, and immediately transport the patient to the operating room for carotid resection. Do not leave the patient. Carotid artery rupture has a high risk for stroke and death.

Pain Management. Pain is caused by the surgical cutting or manipulation of tissue and by nerve compression. Pain should be controlled, and the patient should still be able to participate in his or her care. Morphine (Statex ♣) often is given IV by a patient-controlled analgesia (PCA) pump for the first 1 to 2 days after surgery. As the patient progresses, liquid opioid analgesics can be given by feeding tube. Oral drugs for pain and discomfort are started only after the patient can tolerate oral intake. After discharge, the patient still requires pain management, especially if he or she is receiving radiation therapy. An adjunct to the pain regimen may be liquid NSAIDs along with opioid analgesics. Tricyclic antidepressants may also be used for the lancinating pain of nerve-root involvement.

Nutrition. Many patients with head and neck cancer have taste changes and some degree of malnutrition before cancer treatment begins (Ardilio, 2011; McLaughlin, 2013). All patients are at risk for malnutrition during treatment for head and neck cancer. A nasogastric, gastrostomy, or jejunostomy tube is placed during surgery for nutrition support while the head and neck heal. After the intestinal tract is motile, nutrients can be given via the feeding tube. The nutrition support team or dietitian assesses the patient before surgery and is available for consultation after surgery. Replacement of calories, protein, and water loss is calculated carefully for each patient (Ardilio, 2011).

The feeding tube usually remains in place for 7 to 10 days after surgery. Before removing the tube, assess the patient's ability to swallow if nutrition is to be given by mouth. Aspiration *cannot* occur after a total laryngectomy because the airway is completely separated from the esophagus. Stay with the patient during the first few swallowing attempts. Swallowing may be uncomfortable at first, and analgesics may be needed.

Speech and Language Rehabilitation. The patient's voice quality and speech are altered after surgery. Although this problem has enormous effects on the patient's ability to maintain social interactions, continue employment, and maintain a desired quality of life, it is often poorly addressed while he or she is hospitalized. Working with him or her and the family toward developing an acceptable communication method during the inpatient period is essential for a satisfactory outcome (Happ et al., 2011).

Together with the speech and language pathologist (SLP), discuss the principles of speech therapy with the patient and family early in the course of the treatment plan (see Chart 29-2). Voice and speech differences depend on the type of surgical resection (see Table 29-2). Speech production varies with patient practice, amount of tissue removed, and radiation effects, but the speech can be very understandable. Patients have reported ongoing difficulties with speech and communication to be the most distressing problem for months to years after head and neck cancer therapy (Fletcher et al., 2012; Haisfield-Wolfe et al., 2012).

The speech rehabilitation plan for patients who have a total laryngectomy at first consists of writing, using a picture board, or using a computer. The patient then uses an artificial larynx and may eventually learn esophageal speech. For success, the patient needs encouragement and support from the SLP, hospital team, and family while relearning to speak. This process can be time consuming and requires concentration each time the patient speaks. Having a **laryngectomee** (a person who has had a laryngectomy) from one of the local self-help organizations visit the patient and family is often beneficial. The International Association of Laryngectomees is very supportive, as is the American Cancer Society (ACS) Visitor Program.

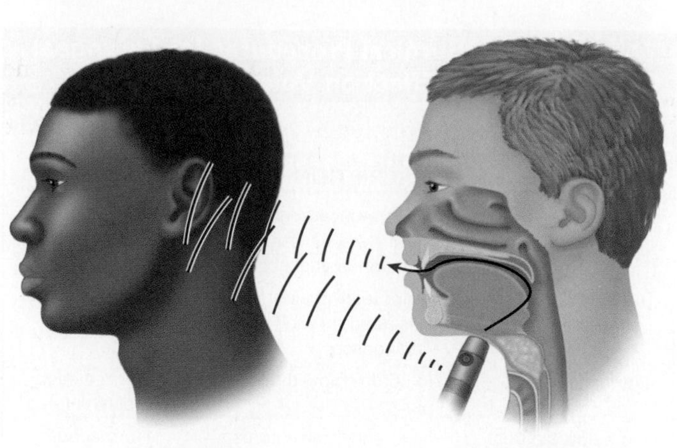

FIG. 29-4 An Electro-Larynx to generate speech after a laryngectomy.

Esophageal speech is attempted by most patients who have a total laryngectomy. Sound can be produced this way by "burping" the air swallowed or injected into the esophageal pharynx and shaping the words in the mouth. The voice produced is a monotone; it cannot be raised or lowered and carries no pitch. If patients do not have adequate hearing, esophageal speech will be difficult because they need to use their mouth to shape the words as they hear them. Hearing-impaired patients may need hearing aids.

Mechanical devices, called *electrolarynges,* may be used for communication. Most are battery-powered devices placed against the side of the neck or cheek (Fig. 29-4). The air inside the mouth and throat is vibrated, and the patient moves his or her lips and tongue as usual. The quality of speech generated with mechanical devices is robot-like.

Tracheoesophageal puncture (TEP) (formerly call a *fistula*) may be used if esophageal speech is ineffective and if the patient meets strict criteria. A small surgical puncture is created between the trachea and the esophagus using a special catheter. After the puncture heals, a silicone prosthesis (e.g., the Blom-Singer prosthesis or the Panje Voice Button) is inserted in place of the catheter. The patient covers the stoma and the opening of the prosthesis with a finger or with a special valve to divert air from the lungs, through the trachea, into the esophagus, and out of the mouth where lip and tongue movement produces speech.

Surgical Procedures for Other Head and Neck Cancers. The major types of surgeries for other head and neck cancers are called *composite resections.* These resections are a combination of surgical procedures, including partial or total glossectomies (tongue removal), partial mandibulectomies (jaw removal), and, if needed, nodal neck dissections. Tracheostomy may be planned to provide an adequate airway. (See Chapter 53 for more information about oral cancer.)

Tracheotomy. A **tracheotomy** is a surgical incision into the trachea for the purpose of establishing an airway (tracheostomy). It can be performed as an emergency procedure or as a scheduled surgical procedure. A tracheostomy can be temporary or permanent. Chapter 28 discusses the nursing care of a patient with a tracheostomy.

Preventing Aspiration

Planning: Expected Outcomes. The patient with head and neck cancer is expected to not aspirate food, gastric contents, or oral secretions into the lungs. Indicators include that the patient often or consistently demonstrates these behaviors:

- Positions self upright for eating or drinking
- Selects foods according to swallowing ability
- Chooses liquids and foods of proper consistency

Interventions. The surgical changes in the upper respiratory tract and altered swallowing mechanisms increase the patient's risk for aspiration. Aspiration can result in pneumonia, weight loss, and prolonged hospitalization. Chart 29-3 lists actions for aspiration prevention.

A nasogastric (NG) feeding tube may further increase the risk for aspiration because it keeps the lower esophageal sphincter partially open. The one exception is the patient who has undergone a total laryngectomy. In these cases, the airway is separated from the esophagus, making aspiration impossible and the patient is *not* at risk. Most patients who need enteral feeding supplementation have a percutaneous endoscopic gastrostomy (PEG) tube placed rather than an NG tube. See Chapter 60 for care of patients receiving enteral nutrition by NG or PEG tube.

A dynamic swallow study, such as a barium swallow under fluoroscopy, evaluates a patient's ability to protect the airway from aspiration and helps determine the appropriate method of swallow rehabilitation. In many cases, enteral feedings are used either because of the patient's inability to swallow or because of continued aspiration risk.

Swallowing can be a major problem for the patient who has a tracheostomy tube. Swallowing can be normal if the cranial nerves and anatomic structures are intact. In a normal swallow, the larynx rises and moves forward to protect itself from the passing stream of food and saliva. The tracheostomy tube sometimes fixes the larynx in place, resulting in difficulty swallowing.

An inflated tracheostomy tube cuff can balloon backward into the esophagus and interfere with the passage of food. The wall between the posterior trachea and the esophagus is very thin, which allows this pushing action. The patient who is cognitively intact may adapt to eating normal food when the tracheostomy tube is small and the cuff is not inflated.

The patient who has had a partial vertical or supraglottic laryngectomy *must* be observed for aspiration. It is critical to teach the patient to use alternate methods of swallowing without aspirating. The "supraglottic" method of swallowing is especially effective after a partial laryngectomy or base-of-tongue resection (Chart 29-4). To reinforce teaching and learning, place a chart in the patient's room detailing the steps. A dynamic swallow study is performed to guide rehabilitation for swallowing and to evaluate the patient's ability to protect the airway.

Minimizing Anxiety

Planning: Expected Outcomes. The patient with head and neck cancer is expected to have decreased anxiety. Indicators include that the patient often or consistently demonstrates:

- Verbalization of reduced anxiety
- Absence of distress, irritability, and facial tension
- Effective use of coping strategies

Interventions. Conferences with the physician, clinical nurse specialist, dietitian, speech and language pathologist, physical therapist, psychologist, social worker, and general nursing staff may be beneficial. Explore the reason for anxiety (e.g., fear of the unknown, lack of teaching, fear of pain, fear of death, loss of control, uncertainty). The patient and family often benefit from further information. Before the patient is scheduled for surgery (and while still at home), home care nurses or community-sponsored programs, such as the ACS, may be able to decrease fears about the disease process and surgical interventions.

Give prescribed antianxiety drugs, such as diazepam (Valium, Meval ♣), with caution because of the risk for respiratory depression and because some of these drugs are eliminated slowly. Shorter-duration drugs, such as lorazepam (Ativan), may have fewer respiratory side effects. The location of the tumor and the presence of other lung disease may cause some

CHART 29-3 Best Practice for Patient Safety & Quality Care QSEN

Prevention of Aspiration During Swallowing

- Avoid serving meals when the patient is fatigued.
- Provide smaller and more frequent meals.
- Provide adequate time; do not "hurry" the patient.
- Provide close supervision if the patient is self-feeding.
- Keep emergency suctioning equipment close at hand.
- Avoid water and other "thin" liquids.
- Thicken liquids.
- Avoid foods that generate thin liquids during the chewing process, such as fruit.
- Position the patient in the most upright position possible.
- When possible, completely (or at least partially) deflate the tube cuff during meals.
- Suction after initial cuff deflation to clear the airway and allow maximum comfort during the meal.
- Feed each bite or encourage the patient to take each bite slowly.
- Encourage the patient to "dry swallow" after each bite to clear residue from the throat.
- Avoid consecutive swallows by cup or straw.
- Provide controlled small volumes of liquids, using a spoon.
- Encourage the patient to "tuck" his or her chin down and move the forehead forward while swallowing.
- Allow the patient to indicate when he or she is ready for the next bite.
- If the patient coughs, stop the feeding until the patient indicates the airway has been cleared.
- Continuously monitor tolerance to oral food intake by assessing respiratory rate, ease, pulse oximetry, and heart rate.

CHART 29-4 Patient and Family Education: Preparing for Self-Management

The Supraglottic Method of Swallowing

1. Place yourself in an upright, preferably out-of-bed, position.
2. Clear your throat.
3. Take a deep breath.
4. Place ½ to 1 teaspoon of food into your mouth.
5. Hold your breath, or "bear down" (Valsalva maneuver).
6. Swallow twice.
7. Release your breath, and clear your throat.
8. Swallow twice again.
9. Breathe normally.

This method exaggerates the normal protective mechanisms of cessation of respiration during the swallow. The double swallow attempts to clear food that may be pooling in the pharynx, vallecula, and piriform sinuses. This method is used only after a dynamic radiographic swallow study has demonstrated that it is appropriate and safe for the patient.

degree of airway obstruction. For anxiety in these patients, drug therapy may include lorazepam (Ativan, Novo-Lorazem ♣) rather than a sedating agent.

Supporting Self-Concept

Planning: Expected Outcomes. The patient with head and neck cancer is expected to accept body image changes. Indicators include that the patient often or consistently demonstrates:

- Willingness to touch and care for the affected body part
- Willingness to use strategies to enhance appearance
- Interaction with visitors, staff, and family members

Interventions. The patient with head and neck cancer usually has a change in self-concept and self-image resulting from functional and psychological issues. Common functional issues include the presence of a stoma or artificial airway, speech changes, and a change in the method of eating. Psychological issues often include guilt, regret, and uncertainty. He or she may not be able to speak at all or may have permanent speech deficits. Help the patient set realistic goals, starting with involvement in self-care. Teach the patient alternative communication methods so he or she can communicate in the hospital and after discharge (Fletcher et al., 2012; Suzuki, 2012).

Teach the family to ease the patient into a normal social environment. Use positive reinforcement and encouragement while demonstrating acceptance and caring behaviors. The family also may benefit from counseling sessions while the patient is still in the hospital.

After surgery, the patient may feel socially isolated because of the change in voice and facial appearance. Loose-fitting, high-collar shirts or sweaters, scarves, and jewelry can be worn to cover the laryngectomy stoma, tracheostomy tube, and other changes related to surgery. Cosmetics may aid in covering disfigurement. Most surgeons try to place the incisions in the natural skinfold lines if doing so does not pose a risk for cancer recurrence.

Community-Based Care

If no complications occur, the patient is usually discharged home or to an extended-care facility within 2 weeks. At the time of discharge, he or she or a family member should be able to perform tracheostomy or stoma care and participate in nutrition, wound care, and communication methods.

The patient and family may feel more secure about discharge with a referral to support groups or a community health agency familiar with the care of patients recovering from head and neck cancer. Coordinate the efforts of the health care team in assessing the specific discharge needs and making the appropriate referrals to home care agencies. Dietitians, nurses, physical therapists, speech and language pathologists, and social workers may be needed. Coordinate the scheduling for chemotherapy or radiation therapy with the patient and family.

Home Care Management. Extensive home care preparation is needed after a laryngectomy for cancer. The convalescent period is long, and airway management is complicated. The patient or family must be able to take an active role in care.

General cleanliness of the home is assessed by the home care nurse or case manager. For the patient with severe respiratory problems, home changes to allow for one-floor living may be needed. Increased humidity is needed. A humidifier add-on to a forced-air furnace can be obtained, or a room humidifier or vaporizer may be used. Be sure to stress that meticulous cleaning of these items is needed to prevent spread of mold or other sources of infection.

A home care nurse often is involved with care after discharge and is an important resource for the patient and family. This nurse assesses the patient and home situation for problems in self-care, complications, adjustment, and adherence to the medical regimen. Chart 29-5 lists assessment areas for the patient in the home after a laryngectomy. This nurse reinforces health care teaching, self-care teaching, and smoking-cessation regimens.

Self-Management Education. Education begins before surgery, and most self-care is taught in the hospital. Teach the patient and family how to care for the stoma or tracheostomy or laryngectomy tube, depending on the type of surgery performed. Review incision and airway care, including cleaning and inspecting for signs of infection. Chart 29-6 lists self-care actions for the patient after laryngeal cancer surgery. Many of these actions also apply to any surgery for head and neck cancer.

CHART 29-5 Home Care Assessment

Patients After Laryngectomy

Assess respiratory status:
- Observe rate and depth of respiration.
- Auscultate lungs.
- Check patency of airway.
- Examine the tracheostomy drainage for amount, color, and character.
- Examine nail beds and mucous membranes for evidence of cyanosis.
- Obtain a pulse oximetry reading.

Assess condition of wound:
- Remove dressings (noting condition of dressings).
- Cleanse the wound.
- Compare with previous notations of wound condition:
  - Presence, amount, and nature of exudate
  - Presence/absence of cellulitis
  - Presence/absence of odor

Assess patient's psychosocial status:
- Ask the patient about passing the time, visitors, and trips outside the house.
- Observe whether the patient communicates responses directly or whether a family member speaks for the patient.
- Observe patient and family member interactions.
- Determine what method of communication the patient has selected, and observe the patient's skill with it.
- Observe whether the patient is wearing pajamas or is dressed in street clothes.

Take the patient's temperature at each home care visit.

Assess the patient's understanding of illness and adherence to treatment:
- Manifestations to report to the health care provider
- Medication plan (correct timing and dose)
- Ambulation or positioning schedule
- Dressing changes/skin care
- Diet modifications (24-hour diet recall)
- Skill in tracheostomy or dressing care

Assess patient's nutrition status:
- Change in muscle mass
- Lackluster nails/sparse hair
- Recent weight loss greater than 10% of usual weight
- Impaired oral intake
- Difficulty swallowing
- Generalized edema

CHART 29-6 Patient and Family Education: Preparing for Self-Management

Home Laryngectomy Care

- Avoid swimming, and use care when showering or shaving.
- Lean slightly forward and cover the stoma when coughing or sneezing.
- Wear a stoma guard or loose clothing to cover the stoma.
- Clean the stoma with mild soap and water. Lubricate the stoma with a non–oil-based ointment as needed.
- Increase humidity by using saline in the stoma as instructed, a bedside humidifier, pans of water, and houseplants.
- Obtain and wear a MedicAlert bracelet and emergency care card for life-threatening situations.

Stoma care teaching is focused on protection. Use a plastic head-and-neck cut-away model or create one from Styrofoam to use as an accurate aid for teaching about the anatomic changes resulting from surgery (Zeien, 2011). Instruct the patient to use a shower shield over the tube or stoma when bathing to prevent water from entering the airway. Teach men who use electric shavers to cover the stoma while shaving to keep hair from falling into it. Suggest that the patient wear a protective cover or stoma guard to protect the stoma during the day. For those with permanent stomas after laryngectomy or for those with permanent tracheostomies, covering the opening has two benefits: (1) to filter the air entering the stoma while keeping humidity in the airway; and (2) to enhance aesthetic appearance. Attractive coverings are available in the form of scarves, crocheted collars, and jewelry.

Instruct the patient how to increase humidity in the home. Stress the importance of keeping well hydrated to prevent secretions from thickening.

Communication involves having the patient continue the selected communication method that began in the hospital. Instruct him or her to wear a medical alert (MedicAlert) bracelet and carry a special identification card. For patients with a laryngectomy, this card is available from the local chapters of the International Association of Laryngectomees. The card instructs the reader about providing an emergency airway or resuscitating someone who has a stoma.

Smoking cessation is a difficult but important issue after head and neck cancer surgery. Stress that smoking cessation can reduce the risk for developing other cancers and can increase the rate of healing from surgery. See Chapter 27 for a detailed discussion about smoking cessation.

Psychosocial Preparation. The many changes resulting from a laryngectomy influence physical, social, and emotional functioning. Patients may perceive changes in their quality of life. Begin preparing the patient and family by scheduling a visit from a person who has adjusted to these changes.

The patient with a permanent stoma, tracheostomy tube, NG or PEG tube, and wounds has an altered body image. Stress the importance of returning to as normal a lifestyle as possible. Most patients can resume many of their usual activities within 4 to 6 weeks after surgery. A longer time is needed after a combination of radiation therapy and surgery and for those patients who also have other chronic diseases. The patient may be frustrated at times while trying to adjust to the many changes resulting from treatment of head and neck cancer.

The patient with a total laryngectomy cannot produce sounds during laughing and crying. Mucus secretions may appear unexpectedly when these emotions arise or when coughing or sneezing occurs. The mucus can be embarrassing, and the patient needs to be prepared to cover the stoma with a handkerchief or gauze. The patient who has undergone composite resections has difficulty with speech *and* swallowing. He or she may need to deal with tracheostomy and feeding tubes in public places.

Health Care Resources. Inform the patient and family of community organizations (e.g., ACS) and local laryngectomee clubs, which can offer support, information, and friendships. When the patient has problems paying for health care services, equipment, and prescriptions, a visiting nurse agency and social worker may be helpful in locating available resources.

In many areas, the local unit of the ACS or Canadian Cancer Society can help provide dressing materials and nutritional supplements to patients in need. These organizations may also provide transportation to and from follow-up visits or radiation therapy.

CLINICAL JUDGMENT CHALLENGE

Patient-Centered Care; Evidence-Based Practice; Teamwork and Collaboration QSEN

A patient who had a supraglottic partial laryngectomy with a right-sided radical neck dissection 4 weeks ago is now receiving radiation therapy. He has lost 24 pounds since his surgery, which makes him 15 pounds less than his ideal weight. He tells you that he has no appetite and that what food he does eat "has no taste." In addition, although he expresses that he is glad to be alive, he does not want friends to visit because it takes so much energy to interact with them. He also says that he can no longer play the piano because of difficulty moving his right arm and shoulder.

1. What factors are contributing to his fatigue?
2. Is the weight loss a concern? If so, what should you do about it?
3. Should you further press the issue of not wanting to visit with friends? Why or why not?
4. What other health care professionals or resources would be appropriate at this time?

◆ Evaluation: Outcomes

Evaluate the care of the patient with head and neck cancer based on the identified priority patient problems. The expected outcomes are that the patient:

- Maintains a patent airway
- Performs self-care of the artificial airway and wound
- Performs ADLs independently or with minimal assistance
- Attains or maintains adequate nutrition
- Does not aspirate gastric contents or food
- Engages in desired social interactions

Specific indicators for these outcomes are listed for priority patient problems in the Planning and Implementation section (see earlier).

NURSING CONCEPTS AND CLINICAL JUDGMENT REVIEW

What might you NOTICE if the patient is experiencing inadequate GAS EXCHANGE as a result of upper airway problems?

- Voice changes (nasal quality if the problem is above the palate, "breathy" or "whispery" if the problem is in the larynx or trachea)
- Snoring or mouth breathing
- Change in cognition or level of consciousness or acute confusion
- Decreased oxygen saturation by pulse oximetry
- Skin cyanosis or pallor (lighter-skinned patients)
- Cyanosis or pallor of the lips and oral mucous membranes (patients of any skin color)
- Tachycardia and dysrhythmia

What should you INTERPRET and how should you RESPOND to a patient experiencing inadequate GAS EXCHANGE as a result of an upper airway respiratory problem?

Perform and interpret physical assessment, including:

- Taking vital signs
- Monitoring oxygen saturation by pulse oximetry
- Assessing for the presence of thick or excessive secretions
- Assessing the patient's ability to cough and clear the airway
- Assessing nasal drainage and sputum for color and blood
- Checking most recent laboratory values for white blood cell and arterial blood gas (ABG) levels
- Assessing cognition
- Assessing hydration status

Respond by:

- Suctioning (oral, pharyngeal, endotracheal, tracheostomy), if needed
- Applying oxygen, and assessing the patient's responses to this intervention
- Keeping the patient's head elevated to about 30 degrees
- Notifying physician or Rapid Response Team
- Ensuring venous access

On what should you REFLECT?

- Observe patient for evidence of restored oxygenation (see Chapter 27).
- Think about what may have precipitated this episode and what steps could be taken to either prevent a similar episode or identify it earlier.
- Think about what additional resources could improve the nursing response to this situation.

GET READY FOR THE NCLEX® EXAMINATION!

KEY POINTS

Review these Key Points for each NCLEX Examination Client Needs Category.

Safe and Effective Care Environment

- Use sterile technique when performing endotracheal or tracheal suctioning. **Safety** QSEN
- Use Standard Precautions when caring for a patient with epistaxis. **Safety** QSEN
- Supervise care delegated to licensed practical nurses/licensed vocational nurses (LPNs/LVNs) or nursing assistants to patients who have risk factors for airway obstruction.
- Act as a patient advocate for patients who have tracheostomies or other issues that impair communication.

Health Promotion and Maintenance

- Assess the patient for risk factors for head and neck cancer.
- Encourage people who smoke to quit smoking or using tobacco in any way. **Patient-Centered Care** QSEN
- Encourage people who use alcohol to reduce their intake of alcoholic beverages.
- Use Aspiration Precautions for any patient with an altered level of consciousness or who has an endotracheal tube (see Chart 29-3). **Safety** QSEN
- Teach the patient and family how to perform tracheostomy care (see Chart 28-3 in Chapter 28). **Patient-Centered Care** QSEN
- Teach patients who have had radiation therapy to the oral cavity to have dental examinations at least every 6 months. **Patient-Centered Care** QSEN
- Teach the patient and family about home management of a laryngectomy stoma or tracheostomy. **Patient-Centered Care** QSEN

Psychosocial Integrity

- Allow the patient and family members the opportunity to express fear or anxiety regarding a cancer diagnosis or a change in breathing status.
- Teach family members ways to communicate with a patient who cannot speak after surgery for head and neck cancer. **Patient-Centered Care** QSEN
- Encourage patients with permanent tracheostomies or laryngectomies to become involved in self-care and to look at the wound and touch the affected area. **Patient-Centered Care** QSEN
- Allow the patient and family to grieve the loss of function and change in body image. **Patient-Centered Care** QSEN
- Allow time to communicate with the patient who has voice loss. **Patient-Centered Care** QSEN
- Refer patients and families to local chapters of the ACS or the Canadian Cancer Society after surgery for head and neck cancer.

Physiological Integrity

- Assess the airway patency of any patient who experiences facial or nasal trauma. **Safety** QSEN
- Perform a focused upper respiratory assessment and re-assessment to determine adequacy of GAS EXCHANGE and tissue perfusion. **Patient-Centered Care** QSEN

- Notify the Rapid Response Team when a patient experiences a posterior nasal bleed. **Safety** QSEN
- Check the airway and packing at least every hour for a patient who has posterior nasal packing placed after nasal surgery or posterior epistaxis. **Evidence-Based Practice** QSEN
- Instruct patients who have had mandibular immobilization or fixation after a mandibular fracture to keep wire cutters with them at all times. **Safety** QSEN
- Apply oxygen to any patient who develops stridor. **Safety** QSEN
- Use a manual resuscitation bag to ventilate the patient if the tracheostomy tube has dislodged or been decannulated. **Safety** QSEN
- Assess the new tracheostomy stoma site at least once per shift for purulent drainage, redness, pain, and swelling, as indicators of infection. **Safety** QSEN
- Keep the tracheal cuff pressure between 14 and 20 mm Hg to prevent tissue injury. **Evidence-Based Practice** QSEN
- Apply knowledge of anatomy to prevent aspiration in a patient with a tracheostomy. **Evidence-Based Practice** QSEN
- Use correct technique to suction via a tracheostomy or laryngectomy tube. **Evidence-Based Practice** QSEN
- Collaborate with physicians, speech and language pathologists, social workers, dietitians, respiratory therapists, and occupational and physical therapists to provide optimal care for the patient experiencing head and neck cancer. **Teamwork and Collaboration** QSEN

30 CHAPTER

Care of Patients with Noninfectious Lower Respiratory Problems

M. Linda Workman

http://evolve.elsevier.com/Iggy/

PRIORITY CONCEPTS

- Gas Exchange
- Perfusion
- Inflammation
- Cellular Regulation

LEARNING OUTCOMES

Safe and Effective Care Environment

1. Ensure safe oxygen delivery to promote gas exchange.
2. Protect patients with lower respiratory problems from injury or infection.

Health Promotion and Maintenance

3. Teach all people measures to take to protect the respiratory system from damage and cancer, including the avoidance of known environmental causative agents.
4. Teach the patient and family how to manage a chronic lower respiratory disorder and avoid injury and complications in the home.
5. Use assessment information to identify people at increased genetic risk for a respiratory disease that affects gas exchange and perfusion.

Psychosocial Integrity

6. Reduce the psychological impact for the patient and family experiencing a chronic lower respiratory problem.
7. Work with other members of the health care team to ensure that values, preferences, and expressed needs of patients experiencing lower respiratory problems are respected.

Physiological Integrity

8. Assess and re-assess the manifestations of patients being managed for a lower respiratory problem.
9. Use laboratory data and clinical manifestations to prioritize nursing care for the patient who has an acute or chronic lower respiratory problem.
10. Collaborate with other health care professionals who help patients and families experiencing a chronic lower respiratory problem achieve desired health outcomes.
11. Coordinate nursing interventions for the patient with a chronic lower respiratory problem in the community.
12. Prioritize nursing care for the patient with chest tubes.

The alveoli and the smallest airways are sites for direct gas exchange. Any problem of these tissues reduces gas exchange and interferes with perfusion. Many lower airway problems are chronic and progressive, requiring changes in lifestyle, especially for older adults. Chart 30-1 lists nursing issues for the older patient with a respiratory problem.

Chronic airflow limitation (CAL) is a group of chronic lung diseases that includes asthma, chronic bronchitis, and pulmonary emphysema. More than 10% of American adults suffer from some form of CAL, and many have moderate to severe disability from it (Centers for Disease Control and Prevention [CDC], 2012). Although CAL problems are not all reversible, good management can help maintain adequate gas exchange and improve overall health.

ASTHMA

❖ *PATHOPHYSIOLOGY*

Asthma is often a chronic condition in which reversible airflow obstruction in the airways occurs intermittently (Fig. 30-1). Airway obstruction occurs by inflammation and by airway tissue sensitivity (hyperresponsiveness) that leads to bronchoconstriction. Inflammation obstructs the airway **lumens** (i.e., the insides) (Fig. 30-2). Airway hyperresponsiveness and constriction of bronchial smooth muscle narrow the airways from the outside. Airway inflammation and sensitivity can trigger bronchiolar constriction, and many people with asthma have both problems. Severe airway obstruction impairs gas exchange and can be fatal. At least 3400 deaths

CHART 30-1 **Nursing Focus on the Older Adult**

Chronic Respiratory Disorder

- Provide rest periods between activities such as bathing, meals, and ambulation.
- Place the patient in an upright position for meals to prevent aspiration.
- Encourage nutritional fluid intake after the meal to promote increased calorie intake.
- Schedule drugs around routine activities to increase adherence to drug therapy.
- Arrange chairs in strategic locations to allow the patient with dyspnea to stop and rest while walking.
- Urge the patient to notify the health care provider promptly for any manifestation of infection.
- Encourage the patient to receive the pneumococcal vaccine and to have an annual influenza vaccination.

from acute asthma occur in the United States each year (CDC, 2014a).

Etiology and Genetic Risk

Although asthma is classified into types based on what triggers the attacks, the effect on GAS EXCHANGE is the same. INFLAMMATION of the mucous membranes lining the airways is a key event in triggering an asthma attack. It occurs in response to the presence of specific allergens; general irritants such as cold air, dry air, or fine airborne particles; microorganisms; and aspirin and other NSAIDs. Increased airway sensitivity (hyperresponsiveness) can occur with exercise, with an upper respiratory illness, and for unknown reasons.

When asthma is well controlled, the airway changes are temporary and reversible. With poor control, chronic INFLAMMATION can lead to airway damage and altered CELLULAR REGULATION with enlargement of the bronchial epithelial cells

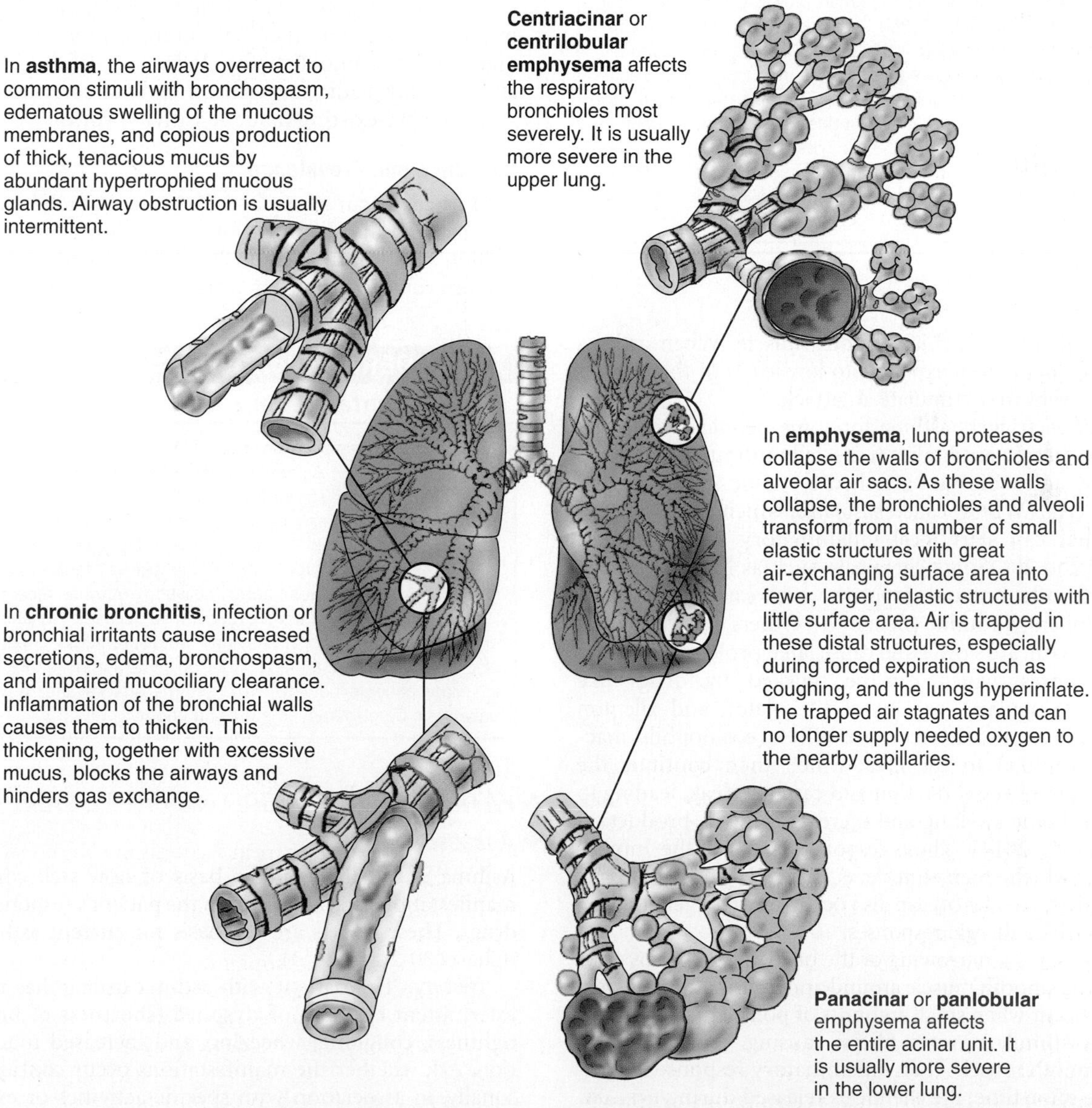

FIG. 30-1 The pathophysiology of chronic airflow limitation (CAL).

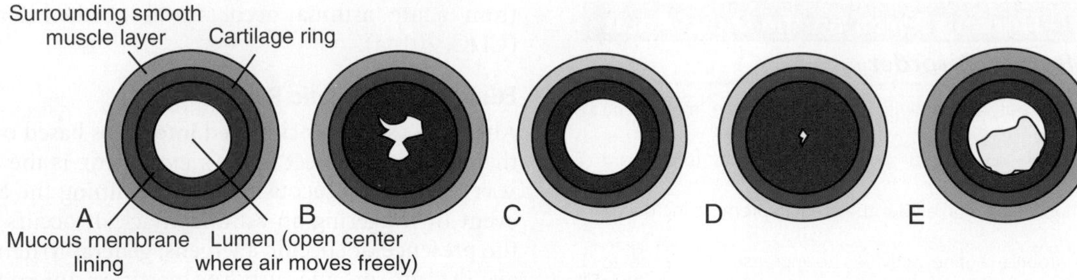

FIG. 30-2 Causes of narrowed airways. **A,** Cross section of a small airway showing the tissue layers. **B,** Mucosal swelling. **C,** Constriction of smooth muscle. **D,** Mucosal swelling and constriction of smooth muscle. **E,** Mucus plug.

GENETIC/GENOMIC CONSIDERATIONS

Patient-Centered Care QSEN

Results of genome-wide association studies (GWAS) indicate that more than 50 gene variations are associated with asthma, although asthma is a multifactorial disorder with both genetic and environmental input required for expression (Beery & Workman, 2012; Online Mendelian Inheritance in Man [OMIM], 2013b). Some variations have a greater influence for asthma expression within certain racial or ethnic groups. Also, genetic variation in the gene that controls the synthesis and activity of beta-adrenergic receptors has an impact on drug therapy for asthma. Patients who have a mutation in this gene do not respond as expected to beta agonist drugs and need an altered therapy plan. Teaching these patients about why their drug therapies are different from standard recommendations is a nursing responsibility that can assist with therapy adherence.

and changes in the bronchial smooth muscle. When asthma attacks are frequent, even exposure to low levels of the triggering agent or event may stimulate an attack.

Inflammation triggers asthma for some people when allergens bind to specific antibodies (especially immunoglobulin E [IgE]). These antibodies are attached to tissue *mast cells* and white blood cells (WBCs) called *basophils,* which are filled with chemicals that can start local inflammatory responses (see Chapters 17 and 20). Some chemicals, such as histamine, start an immediate inflammatory response, which can be blocked by drugs like diphenhydramine (Benadryl). Others, such as leukotriene and eotaxin, are slower and cause later, prolonged inflammatory responses, which can be blocked by drugs like montelukast (Singulair), zafirlukast (Accolate), and zileuton (Zyflo). Chemicals also attract more WBCs (eosinophils, macrophages, basophils) to the area, which then continue the responses of blood vessel dilation and capillary leak, leading to mucous membrane swelling and increased mucus production (McCance et al., 2014). These responses narrow the lumens even more, which then interferes with airflow and GAS EXCHANGE. INFLAMMATION can also occur through general irritation rather than allergic responses.

Bronchospasm is a narrowing of the bronchial tubes by constriction of the smooth muscle around and within the bronchial walls. It can occur when small amounts of pollutants or respiratory viruses stimulate nerve fibers, causing constriction of bronchial smooth muscle. If an inflammatory response is stimulated at the same time, the chemicals released during INFLAMMATION also trigger constriction. Severe bronchospasm alone, especially in smaller bronchioles, can profoundly limit airflow to the alveoli and greatly reduce GAS EXCHANGE.

Aspirin and other NSAIDs can trigger asthma in some people, although this response is not a true allergy. It results from increased production of leukotriene when aspirin or NSAIDs suppress other inflammatory pathways.

Gastroesophageal reflux disease (GERD) can trigger asthma in some people, who then have more asthma manifestations at night (Global Initiative for Asthma [GINA], 2014). GERD allows highly acidic stomach contents to enter the airway and make the pre-existing tissue sensitivity worse.

Incidence and Prevalence

Asthma can occur at any age. About half of adults with asthma also had the disease in childhood. Asthma affects nearly 20.8 million adults in the United States and Canada (CDC, 2012). It is more common in urban settings than in rural settings.

CONSIDERATIONS FOR OLDER ADULTS

Patient-Centered Care QSEN

Asthma occurs as a new disorder in about 3% of people older than 55 years. Another 3% of people older than 60 years have asthma as a continuing chronic disorder (CDC, 2012). Lung and airway changes as a part of aging make any breathing problem more serious in the older adult. One problem related to aging is a decrease in the sensitivity of beta-adrenergic receptors. When stimulated, these receptors relax smooth muscle and cause bronchodilation. As these receptors become less sensitive, they no longer respond as quickly or as strongly to agonists (epinephrine, dopamine) and beta-adrenergic drugs, which are often used as rescue therapy during an acute asthma attack. Thus teaching older patients how to avoid asthma attacks and to correctly use preventive drug therapy is a nursing priority.

❖ PATIENT-CENTERED COLLABORATIVE CARE

◆ Assessment

Asthma is classified on the basis of how well controlled the manifestations are, as well as on the patient's response to asthma drugs. These classes are the basis for current asthma therapy (Charts 30-2 and 30-3).

History. The patient with asthma usually has a pattern of intermittent episodes of **dyspnea** (shortness of breath), chest tightness, coughing, wheezing, and increased mucus production. Ask whether the manifestations occur continuously, seasonally, in association with specific activities or exposures, or more frequently at night. Some patients have manifestations for

CHART 30-2 Key Features

Levels of Asthma Control

CHARACTERISTIC	CONTROLLED (ALL OF THESE CHARACTERISTICS MUST BE PRESENT)	PARTLY CONTROLLED (THE PRESENCE OF ANY ONE OF THESE CHARACTERISTICS IS CONSIDERED PARTLY CONTROLLED)	UNCONTROLLED (THE PRESENCE OF THREE OR MORE CHARACTERISTICS FROM THE PARTLY CONTROLLED LIST IS CONSIDERED UNCONTROLLED ASTHMA)
Daytime manifestations	Manifestations occur twice per week or less	Manifestations occur more than twice per week	
Activity limitations	None	Any	
Nighttime manifestations	None	Any	
Reliever drug use	Reliever used twice per week or less	Reliever used more than twice per week	
PEF or FEV_1	Normal	Less than 80% of predicted or established personal best	
Treatment action	Find and maintain lowest step level that controls manifestations	Increase step until manifestations are controlled on a regular basis and then reduce step to the lowest step level that consistently controls manifestations	Increase step (step up) until control is reached and maintained

FEV_1, Forced expiratory volume in the first second; *PEF*, peak expiratory flow.

CHART 30-3 Key Features

The Step System for Medication Use in Asthma Control

STEP 1	STEP 2	STEP 3	STEP 4	STEP 5
As-needed rapid-acting $beta_2$ agonist (relief inhaler)	As-needed rapid-acting $beta_2$ agonist (relief inhaler)	As-needed rapid-acting $beta_2$ agonist (relief inhaler)	As-needed rapid-acting $beta_2$ agonist (relief inhaler)	As-needed rapid-acting $beta_2$ agonist (relief inhaler)
No daily drugs needed	Daily treatment involves the use of *one* of these two options:	Daily treatment involves the use of *one* of these four options:	Daily treatment involves the use of the Step 3 option that provided the best degree of control and was well tolerated along with one or more of these two options:	Daily treatment involves the use of the Step 4 option(s) that provided the best degree of control and was well tolerated along with either of these two options:
	Low-dose ICS*	Low-dose ICS *and* long-acting $beta_2$ agonist	Medium-dose or high-dose ICS *and* long-acting $beta_2$ agonist	Oral glucocorticosteroid (lowest dose)
	Leukotriene modifier†	Medium-dose or high-dose ICS Low-dose ICS and leukotriene modifier Low-dose ICS and sustained-release theophylline	Leukotriene modifier and sustained-release theophylline	Anti-IgE‡ treatment

Data compiled from Global Initiative for Asthma (GINA). (2014). Pocket guide for asthma management and prevention. Retrieved June 2014, from www.ginasthma.org/Guidelines/guidelines-resources.html.
*ICS = Inhaled corticosteroid.
†Leukotriene modifier = Leukotriene receptor antagonist or leukotriene synthesis inhibitor.
‡IgE = Immunoglobulin E.

4 to 8 weeks after a cold or other upper respiratory infection. The patient with atopic (allergic) asthma often has other allergic problems such as rhinitis, skin rash, or pruritus. Ask whether any family members have asthma or respiratory problems. Ask about current or previous smoking habits. If the patient smokes, use this opportunity to teach him or her about smoking cessation (see Chart 27-1 in Chapter 27). Wheezing in nonsmokers is important in the diagnosis of asthma.

Physical Assessment/Clinical Manifestations. The patient with mild to moderate asthma may have no manifestations between asthma attacks. During an acute episode, common manifestations are an audible wheeze and increased respiratory rate. At first, the wheeze is louder on exhalation. When INFLAMMATION occurs with asthma, coughing may increase.

The patient may use accessory muscles to help breathe during an attack. Observe for muscle retraction at the sternum and the suprasternal notch and between the ribs. The patient with long-standing, severe asthma may have a "barrel chest," caused by air trapping (Fig. 30-3). The anteroposterior (AP) diameter (diameter between the front and the back of the chest)

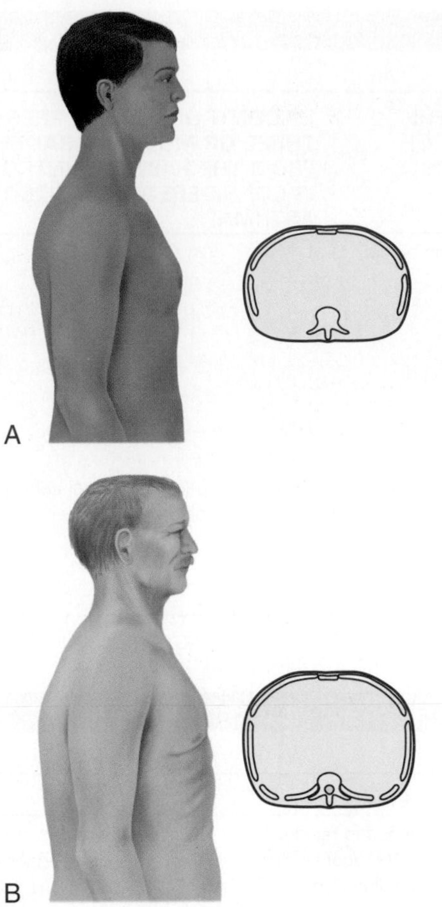

FIG. 30-3 A, Normal adult. The thorax has an oval shape with an anteroposterior-to-transverse diameter of 1 : 1.5 or 5 : 7. **B,** Barrel chest. Note equal anteroposterior-to-transverse diameter and that ribs are horizontal instead of the normal downward slope. This is associated with chronic obstructive pulmonary disease and severe asthma as a result of hyperinflation of the lungs.

increases with air trapping, giving the chest a rounded rather than an oval shape. The normal chest is about 1.5 times as wide as it is deep. In severe, chronic asthma, the AP diameter may equal or exceed the lateral diameter. Compare the AP diameter of the chest with the lateral diameter. Chronic air trapping also flattens the diaphragm and increases the space between the ribs.

Along with an audible wheeze, the breathing cycle is longer with prolonged exhalation and requires more effort. The patient may be unable to speak more than a few words between breaths. Hypoxia occurs with severe attacks. Pulse oximetry shows **hypoxemia** (poor blood oxygen levels). Examine the oral mucosa and nail beds for cyanosis. Other indicators of hypoxemia include changes in the level of cognition or consciousness and tachycardia.

Laboratory Assessment. Laboratory tests can determine asthma type and the degree of breathing impairment. Arterial blood gas (ABG) levels show the effectiveness of GAS EXCHANGE (see Chapter 12 for discussion of ABGs). The arterial oxygen level (Pao_2) may decrease during an asthma attack. Early in the attack, the arterial carbon dioxide level ($Paco_2$) may be decreased as the patient increases the breathing rate and depth. Later in an asthma episode, $Paco_2$ rises, indicating carbon dioxide retention. Allergic asthma often occurs with elevated serum eosinophil counts and immunoglobulin E (IgE) levels. The sputum may contain eosinophils and mucus plugs with shed epithelial cells (Curschmann's spirals).

Pulmonary Function Tests. The most accurate tests for measuring airflow in asthma are the pulmonary function tests (PFTs) using spirometry (O'Laughlen & Rance, 2012). Baseline PFTs are obtained for all patients diagnosed with asthma. The most important PFTs for a patient with asthma are the forced vital capacity (FVC), the forced expiratory volume in the first second (FEV_1), and the peak expiratory flow (PEF), sometimes called *peak expiratory rate flow (PERF)*. Definitions of PFTs are listed in Chapter 27. A decrease in either the FEV_1 or the PEF (PERF) of 15% to 20% below the expected value for age, gender, and size is common for the patient with asthma. Asthma is diagnosed when these values increase by 12% or more after treatment with bronchodilators. Airway responsiveness is tested by measuring the PEF and FEV_1 before and after the patient inhales the drug *methacholine,* which induces bronchospasm in susceptible people.

◆ Interventions

The purposes of asthma therapy are to control and prevent episodes, improve airflow and GAS EXCHANGE, and relieve manifestations. Asthma is best controlled when the patient is an active partner in the management plan (Pruitt, 2011). Priority nursing actions focus on patient education about implementation of the personal asthma action plan, which includes drug therapy and lifestyle management strategies to assist the patient in understanding his or her disease and its management (GINA, 2014).

Self-Management Education. Asthma often has intermittent overt manifestations. With guided self-care, patients can co-manage this disease, increasing symptom-free periods and decreasing the number and severity of attacks (Pruitt, 2011). Good management decreases hospital admissions and increases participation in patient-chosen work and leisure activities. Self-care requires extensive education for the patient to be able to self-assess respiratory status, self-manage (by adjusting the frequency and dosage of prescribed drugs), and know when to consult the health care provider.

Ideally, a personal asthma action plan is developed by the health care provider and the patient. The plan is tailored to meet the patient's personal triggers, asthma manifestations, and drug responses. It includes:

- The prescribed daily controller drug(s) schedule and prescribed reliever drug directions
- Patient-specific daily asthma control assessment questions
  - Directions for adjusting the daily controller drug schedule
  - When to contact the health care provider (in addition to regularly scheduled visits)
  - What emergency actions to take when asthma is not responding to controller and reliever drugs

Teach the patient to assess asthma severity at least daily with a peak flow meter (Fig. 30-4) and to adjust drugs according to his or her personal asthma action plan to manage INFLAMMATION and bronchospasms to prevent or relieve manifestations. Chart 30-4 describes the correct method to use the peak flow meter. The patient first establishes a baseline or "personal best" peak expiratory flow (PEF) by measuring his or her PEF twice daily for 2 to 3 weeks when asthma is well controlled and recording the results. This way, the patient will know when his or her peak flow is reduced to the point that more drugs are needed or that

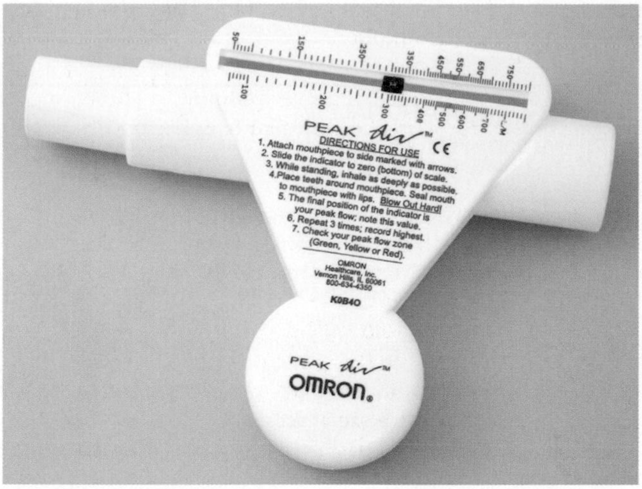

FIG. 30-4 A typical peak flowmeter. This model will show faster exhalation rates in *green,* reduced exhalation rates in *yellow,* and seriously reduced exhalation rates in *red.*

CHART 30-4 Patient and Family Education: Preparing for Self-Management

Using a Peak Flow Meter

- Set the peak flowmeter at zero.
- Use a standing position, without leaning or supporting yourself on anything, if possible.
- Take as deep a breath as you can.
- Place the mouthpiece of the meter in your mouth, taking care to wrap your lips tightly around it.
- Blow your breath out through the mouthpiece as hard and as fast as you are able. (If you cough, sneeze, or have any type of interruption while you exhale, reset the meter and perform the test again.)
- Reset and perform the test two additional times.
- The highest reading of the three is your current peak flow rate.
- Keep a record or graph of your peak flow rates and examine these for trends.

emergency assistance is needed. When the patient has established a "personal best," all other readings are compared with this value. Some meters are color-coded to help the patient interpret the results. Green zone readings are at least 80% of or above the "personal best." This is the ideal range for asthma control and indicates that no increases in drug therapy are needed. Yellow is a range between 50% and 80% of personal best. When a patient has a reading in this range, he or she needs to use the prescribed reliever drug. Within a few minutes after using the reliever drug, another PEF reading should be made to determine whether the reliever drug is working. *Frequent readings in the yellow zone or increasing use of reliever drugs indicates the need to reassess the asthma plan for the need to change controller drugs.* Red is a range below 50% of the patient's personal best, indicating serious respiratory obstruction.

! NURSING SAFETY PRIORITY (QSEN)

Action Alert

Teach the patient that if a red zone reading occurs when using the peak flowmeter to immediately use the reliever drugs and seek emergency help.

CHART 30-5 Patient and Family Education: Preparing for Self-Management

Asthma Management

- Avoid potential environmental asthma triggers, such as smoke, fireplaces, dust, mold, and weather changes of warm to cold.
- Avoid drugs that trigger your asthma (e.g., aspirin, NSAIDs, beta blockers).
- Avoid food that has been prepared with monosodium glutamate (MSG) or metabisulfite.
- If you have exercise-induced asthma, use your bronchodilator inhaler 30 minutes before exercise to prevent or reduce bronchospasm.
- Be sure you know the proper technique and correct sequence when you use metered dose inhalers.
- Get adequate rest and sleep.
- Reduce stress and anxiety; learn relaxation techniques; adopt coping mechanisms that have worked for you in the past.
- Wash all bedding with hot water to destroy dust mites.
- Monitor your peak expiratory flow rates with a flow meter at least twice daily.
- Seek immediate emergency care if you experience any of these:
  - Gray or blue fingertips or lips
  - Difficulty breathing, walking, or talking
  - Retractions of the neck, chest, or ribs
  - Nasal flaring
  - Failure of drugs to control worsening symptoms
  - Peak expiratory rate flow (PERF) declining steadily after treatment, or a flow rate 50% below your usual flow rate

Teach the patient to keep a symptom and intervention diary to learn specific triggers of asthma, early cues for impending attacks, and personal response to drugs. Stress the importance of proper use of his or her personal asthma action plan for any severity of asthma. Chart 30-5 lists areas to emphasize when teaching the patient with asthma.

Drug Therapy. Pharmacologic management of adults with asthma is based on the step category for severity and treatment (see Charts 30-2 and 30-3) (GINA, 2014). **Control therapy drugs** are drugs used to reduce airway sensitivity (responsiveness) to prevent asthma attacks from occurring. *They are used every day, regardless of symptoms.* **Reliever drugs** (also called "rescue drugs") are those used to actually stop an attack once it has started. Some patients may need drug therapy only during an asthma episode. For others, daily drugs are needed to keep asthma episodic rather than a more frequent problem. This therapy involves the use of bronchodilators and various drug types to reduce INFLAMMATION. Some drugs reduce the asthma response, and other drugs actually prevent the response. Combination drugs are two agents from different classes combined together for better response. Chart 30-6 lists the most common preferred drugs in each class for control and relief therapy of asthma. The actions, interventions, and rationales for most drugs within a single class are similar although drug dosages may differ. Be sure to consult a pharmacology text or drug handbook for more information on a specific drug.

Bronchodilators. Bronchodilators cause bronchiolar smooth muscle relaxation. They have no effect on INFLAMMATION. Thus when a patient with asthma has airflow obstruction by both bronchospasm and inflammation, at least two types of drug therapy are needed. Some bronchodilators work by stimulating the beta$_2$-adrenergic receptors on bronchial smooth muscle in the same way that the hormones *epinephrine* and *norepinephrine* do; others work by blocking the parasympathetic nervous

CHART 30-6 Common Examples of Drug Therapy

Asthma Prevention and Treatment

DRUG/USUAL DOSAGE	NURSING INTERVENTIONS	RATIONALE
Bronchodilators Cause bronchodilation through relaxing bronchiolar smooth muscle by binding to and activating pulmonary $beta_2$ receptors.		
Short-Acting Beta$_2$ Agonist (SABA) Primary use is a fast-acting reliever (rescue) drug to be used either during an asthma attack or just before engaging in activity that usually triggers an attack.		
Albuterol (Proventil, Ventolin) 1-2 inhalations every 4-6 hr (90 mcg/inhaled dose)	Teach patients to carry drug with them at all times.	The drug can stop or reduce life-threatening bronchoconstriction, which can occur anytime.
	Teach patient to monitor heart rate.	Excessive use causes systemic symptoms, especially tachycardia.
	When taking this drug with other inhaled drugs, teach patient to use this drug at least 5 minutes before the other inhaled drugs.	The bronchodilation effect of the drug allows better penetration of the other inhaled drugs.
	Teach patient the correct technique for using the MDI or DPI.	Correct technique is essential to getting the drug to the site of action.
Long-Acting Beta$_2$ Agonist (LABA) Causes bronchodilation through relaxing bronchiolar smooth muscle by binding to and activating pulmonary $beta_2$ receptors. Onset of action is slow with a long duration. Primary use is prevention of an asthma attack.		
Salmeterol (Serevent) 2 inhalations every 12 hr (25 mcg/inhalation with MDI) (50 mcg/inhalation with DPI)	Teach patient to shake inhaler (MDI) well before using.	Drug separates easily.
	Teach patient to not use this drug as a reliever drug.	Drug has slow onset of action and does not relieve symptoms.
	Teach patient the correct technique for using the MDI or DPI.	Correct technique is essential to getting the drug to the site of action.
Indacaterol (Arcapta Neohaler) 1 inhalation daily (75 mcg/inhalation with DPI) (COPD only)	Same as for salmeterol.	Same as for salmeterol.
Cholinergic Antagonist Causes bronchodilation by inhibiting the parasympathetic nervous system, allowing the sympathetic system to dominate, releasing norepinephrine that activates $beta_2$ receptors. Purpose is to both relieve and prevent asthma.		
Ipratropium (Atrovent, Apo-Ipravent) 2-4 inhalations 4-6 times daily (18 mcg/inhalation)	If patient is to use this as a reliever drug, teach him or her to carry it at all times.	The drug can stop or reduce life-threatening bronchoconstriction, which can occur anytime.
	Teach patient to shake MDI well before using.	Drug separates easily.
	Teach patient to increase daily fluid intake.	Drug causes mouth dryness.
	Teach patient to observe for and report blurred vision, eye pain, headache, nausea, palpitations, tremors, inability to sleep.	These are systemic symptoms of overdose and require intervention.
	Teach patient the correct technique for using the MDI or DPI.	Correct technique is essential to getting the drug to the site of action.
Anti-inflammatories All of these drugs help improve bronchiolar airflow by decreasing the inflammatory response of the mucous membranes in the airways. *They do not cause bronchodilation.*		
Corticosteroids Disrupt production pathways of inflammatory mediators. The main purpose is to prevent an asthma attack caused by inflammation or allergies (controller drug).		
Fluticasone (Flovent) 50 mcg by MDI twice daily; 100-250 mcg by DPI daily	Teach patient to use the drug daily, even when no symptoms are present.	Maximum effectiveness requires continued use for 48-72 hr and depends on regular use.
	Teach patient to use good mouth care and to check mouth daily for lesions or drainage.	Drug reduces local immunity and increases the risk for local infections, especially *Candida albicans* (yeast).
	Teach patient to not use this drug as a reliever drug.	Drug has slow onset of action and does not relieve symptoms.
	Teach patient the correct technique for using the MDI or DPI.	Correct technique is essential to getting the drug to the site of action.
Prednisone (Deltasone, Predone) 1-40 mg orally daily	Teach patient about expected side effects.	Knowing the side effects to expect reduces anxiety.
	Teach patient to avoid anyone who has an upper respiratory infection.	Drug reduces all protective inflammatory responses, increasing the risk for infection.
	Teach patient to avoid activities that lead to injury.	Blood vessels become more fragile, leading to bruising and petechiae.
	Teach patient to take drug with food.	Food helps reduce the drug side effect of GI ulceration.
	Teach patient not to suddenly stop taking the drug for any reason.	The drug suppresses adrenal production of corticosteroids, which are essential for life.

CHART 30-6 **Common Examples of Drug Therapy—cont'd**

Asthma Prevention and Treatment

DRUG/USUAL DOSAGE	NURSING INTERVENTIONS	RATIONALE
Cromone Stabilizes the membranes of mast cells and prevents the release of inflammatory mediators. Purpose is to prevent asthma attack triggered by inflammation or allergens.		
Nedocromil (Tilade) 4 mg by MDI every 6 hr	Teach patient to use the drug daily, even when no symptoms are present.	Drug has slow onset of action for asthma prevention and is most effective when taken consistently.
	Teach patient to not use this drug as a reliever drug.	Drug does not relieve or reverse symptoms.
	Teach patient the correct technique for using the MDI.	Correct technique is essential to getting the drug to the site of action.
Leukotriene Modifier Blocks the leukotriene receptor, preventing the inflammatory mediator from stimulating inflammation. Purpose is to prevent asthma attack triggered by inflammation or allergens.		
Montelukast (Singulair) 10 mg orally daily	Teach patient to use the drug daily, even when no symptoms are present.	Drug has slow onset of action for asthma prevention and is most effective when taken consistently.
	Teach patient not to decrease the dose of or stop taking any other asthma drugs unless instructed by the health care professional.	This drug is for long-term asthma control and does not replace other drugs, especially corticosteroids and reliever (rescue) drugs.

Data from Global Initiative for Asthma (GINA). (2014). *Pocket guide for asthma management and prevention.* Retrieved June 2014, from www.ginasthma.org/Guidelines/guidelines-resources.html; Global Initiative for Chronic Obstructive Lung Disease (GOLD). (2014). *Global strategy for the diagnosis, management, and prevention of chronic obstructive pulmonary disease.* Retrieved June 2014, from www.goldcopd.org/.

COPD, Chronic obstructive pulmonary disease; *DPI,* dry powder inhaler; *MDI,* metered dose inhaler.

system. Bronchodilators include $beta_2$ agonists and cholinergic antagonists.

$Beta_2$ agonists bind to the $beta_2$-adrenergic receptors and cause an increase in smooth muscle relaxation. Short-acting $beta_2$ agonists (SABAs) provide rapid but short-term relief. These inhaled drugs are most useful when an attack begins (as relief) or as premedication when the patient is about to begin an activity that is likely to induce an attack (GINA, 2014). Such agents include albuterol (Proventil, Ventolin), bitolterol (Tornalate), levalbuterol (Xopenex), pirbuterol (Maxair), and terbutaline (Brethaire). Teach the patient the correct technique for using an inhaled drug with a metered dose inhaler (MDI) (Chart 30-7). Fig. 30-5 shows a patient using a "spacer" with an MDI. Spacer use increases the amount of drug that is delivered to the lungs. Chart 30-8 describes the proper care and use of a dry powder inhaler (DPI).

! NURSING SAFETY PRIORITY QSEN

Action Alert

Teach the patient with asthma to always carry the relief drug inhaler with him or her and to ensure that enough drug remains in the inhaler to provide a quick dose when needed.

Dry powder inhalers indicate the amount of remaining drug. Some aerosol inhalers (MDIs) have meters that indicate the number of doses left in the canister, and others do not. It is recommended that the patient count the number of doses as they are used; however, many patients have difficulty keeping the dose count accurate.

Long-acting $beta_2$ agonists (LABAs) are also delivered by inhaler directly to the site of action—the bronchioles. Proper use of the long-acting agonists can decrease the need to use reliever drugs as often. Unlike short-acting agonists, long-acting drugs need time to build up an effect but the effects are longer lasting. Thus these drugs are useful in preventing an asthma

CHART 30-7 **Patient and Family Education: Preparing for Self-Management**

How to Use an Inhaler Correctly*

With a Spacer (Preferred Technique)

1. Before each use, remove the caps from the inhaler and the spacer.
2. Insert the mouthpiece of the inhaler into the non-mouthpiece end of the spacer.
3. Shake the whole unit vigorously 3 or 4 times.
4. Place the mouthpiece into your mouth, over your tongue, and seal your lips tightly around it.
5. Press down firmly on the canister of the inhaler to release one dose of medication into the spacer.
6. Breathe in slowly and deeply. If the spacer makes a whistling sound, you are breathing in too rapidly.
7. Remove the mouthpiece from your mouth, and, keeping your lips closed, hold your breath for at least 10 seconds and then breathe out slowly.
8. Wait at least 1 minute between puffs.
9. Replace the caps on the inhaler and the spacer.
10. At least once a day, clean the plastic case and cap of the inhaler by thoroughly rinsing in warm, running tap water; at least once a week, clean the spacer in the same manner.

Without a Spacer

1. Before each use, remove the cap and shake the inhaler according to the instructions in the package insert.
2. Tilt your head back slightly, and breathe out fully.
3. Open your mouth, and place the mouthpiece 1 to 2 inches away.
4. As you begin to breathe in deeply through your mouth, press down firmly on the canister of the inhaler to release one dose of medication.
5. Continue to breathe in slowly and deeply (usually over 5-7 sec).
6. Hold your breath for at least 10 seconds to allow the medication to reach deep into the lungs, and then breathe out slowly.
7. Wait at least 1 minute between puffs.
8. Replace the cap on the inhaler.
9. At least once a day, remove the canister and clean the plastic case and cap of the inhaler by thoroughly rinsing in warm, running tap water.

*Avoid spraying in the direction of the eyes.

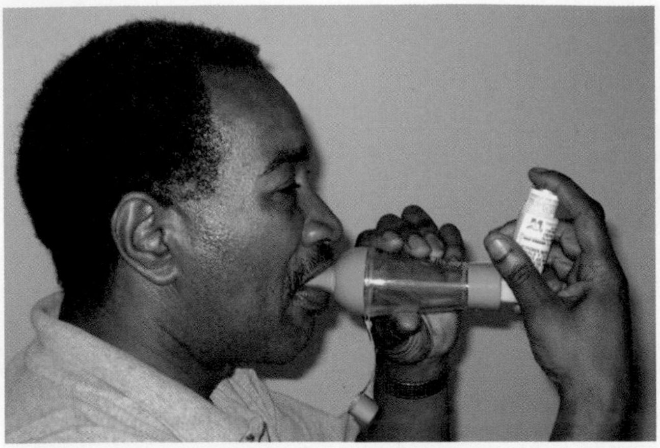

FIG. 30-5 Patient using an aerosol metered dose inhaler with a spacer.

CHART 30-8 Patient and Family Education: Preparing for Self-Management

How to Use a Dry Powder Inhaler (DPI)

For Inhalers Requiring Loading

- First load the drug by:
  - Turning the device to the next dose of drug, or
  - Inserting the capsule into the device, or
  - Inserting the disk or compartment into the device

After Loading the Drug and for Inhalers That Do Not Require Drug Loading

- Read your doctor's instructions for how fast you should breathe for your particular inhaler.
- Place your lips over the mouthpiece, and breathe in forcefully (there is no propellant in the inhaler; only your breath pulls the drug in).
- Remove the inhaler from your mouth as soon as you have breathed in.
- *Never exhale (breathe out) into your inhaler.* Your breath will moisten the powder, causing it to clump and not be delivered accurately.
- *Never wash or place the inhaler in water.*
- *Never shake your inhaler.*
- Keep your inhaler in a dry place at room temperature.
- If the inhaler is preloaded, discard the inhaler after it is empty.
- Because the drug is a dry powder and there is no propellant, you may not feel, smell, or taste it as you inhale.

attack but have no value during an acute attack. Therefore teach patients not to use LABAs alone to relieve them during an attack or when wheezing is getting worse but, instead, to use a SABA. Examples of LABAs include formoterol (Foradil) and salmeterol (Serevent). *These drugs should never be prescribed as the* ***only*** *drug therapy for asthma. Teach the patient to use these control drugs daily as prescribed, even when no manifestations are present.*

Cholinergic antagonists, also called *anticholinergic drugs,* are similar to atropine and block the parasympathetic nervous system. This action results in increased bronchodilation and decreased pulmonary secretions. The most common drug in this class is ipratropium (Atrovent), which is used as an inhalant. Most cholinergic antagonists are short acting and must be used several times a day, although long-acting agents such as tiotropium (Spiriva) are available for use once a day.

Xanthines, such as theophylline and aminophylline, are used only when other types of management are ineffective. These drugs are given systemically, and the dosage that is effective is close to the dosage that produces many dangerous side effects. Blood levels must be monitored closely to ensure the drug level is within the therapeutic range.

Anti-Inflammatory Agents. Anti-inflammatory agents decrease INFLAMMATION in the airways. Those used as inhalants have fewer systemic side effects than those taken systemically.

Corticosteroids decrease inflammation in many ways, including by reducing the production of inflammatory chemicals. Inhaled corticosteroids (ICSs) can be helpful in controlling asthma manifestations. High-potency steroid inhalers, such as fluticasone (Flovent), budesonide (Pulmicort), and mometasone (Asmanex), may be used once per day for maintenance. Systemic corticosteroids, because of severe side effects, are avoided for mild to moderate intermittent asthma and are used on a short-term basis for moderate asthma. For some patients with severe asthma, daily oral corticosteroids may be needed. *Both inhaled corticosteroids and those taken orally are controller drugs. They are not effective in reversing symptoms during an asthma attack and should not be used as reliever drugs. Teach patients to take corticosteroids on a scheduled basis, even when no manifestations are present.*

Cromones, both those that are inhaled and those that are taken orally, are useful as *controller* asthma therapy when taken on a scheduled basis. These agents reduce airway INFLAMMATION by either inhibiting the release of inflammatory chemicals (nedocromil [Tilade]) or preventing mast cell membranes from opening when an allergen binds to IgE (cromolyn sodium [Intal]). *Thus these drugs help prevent asthma attacks but are not effective in reversing symptoms during an asthma attack and should not be used alone as relief drugs.*

Leukotriene modifiers are oral drugs that work in several ways to control asthma when taken on a scheduled basis. Montelukast (Singulair) and zafirlukast (Accolate) block the leukotriene receptor. Zileuton (Zyflo) prevents leukotriene synthesis. *These drugs do not reverse symptoms during an asthma attack and should not be used alone as relief drugs.*

Exercise/Activity. Regular exercise is a recommended part of asthma therapy to maintain cardiac health, strengthen muscles, and promote GAS EXCHANGE and PERFUSION. Teach patients to examine the conditions that trigger an attack and adjust the exercise routine as needed. Some may need to use an inhaled SABA before beginning activity. For others, adjusting the environment may be needed (e.g., changing from outdoor ice-skating in cold, dry air to indoor ice-skating).

Oxygen Therapy. Supplemental oxygen by mask or nasal cannula is often used during an acute asthma attack. High flow delivery may be needed when bronchospasms are severe and limit flow of oxygen through the bronchiole tubes. Heliox, a mixture of helium and oxygen (often 50% helium and 50% oxygen), can help improve oxygen delivery to the alveoli. This gas mixture is lower in density than oxygen alone or room air and flows even when airway resistance is high.

! NURSING SAFETY PRIORITY QSEN

Action Alert

Ensure that no open flames (e.g., cigarette smoking, fireplaces, burning candles) or other combustion hazards are in rooms where oxygen is in use.

Status Asthmaticus. Status asthmaticus is a severe, life-threatening acute episode of airway obstruction that intensifies once it begins and often does not respond to usual therapy. The patient arrives in the emergency department with extremely labored breathing and wheezing. Use of accessory muscles for breathing and distention of neck veins are observed. *If the condition is not reversed, the patient may develop pneumothorax and cardiac or respiratory arrest.* IV fluids, potent systemic bronchodilators, steroids, epinephrine, and oxygen are given immediately to reverse the condition. Prepare for emergency intubation. Sudden absence of wheezing indicates complete airway obstruction and requires a tracheotomy. When breathing improves, management is similar to that for any patient with asthma.

NCLEX EXAMINATION CHALLENGE

Safe and Effective Care Environment

Which parameter indicates to the nurse that the short-acting beta-adrenergic agonist the client took 5 minutes ago for an acute asthma attack is effective?

A. SpO_2 decrease from 85% to 78%
B. Peak expiratory flow rate increase from 50% to 70%
C. The obvious use of accessory muscles during inhalation and exhalation
D. Active bubbling in the humidifier chamber of the oxygen delivery system

CHRONIC OBSTRUCTIVE PULMONARY DISEASE

PATHOPHYSIOLOGY

Chronic obstructive pulmonary diseases (COPD) include emphysema and chronic bronchitis. Although these are separate disorders with different pathologic processes, many patients with emphysema also have chronic bronchitis at the same time (Fig. 30-6).

Emphysema. The two major changes that occur with emphysema are loss of lung elasticity and hyperinflation of the lung (see Fig. 30-1). These changes result in dyspnea and the need for an increased respiratory rate.

In the healthy lung, enzymes called *proteases* are present to destroy and eliminate particulates and organisms inhaled during breathing. If these proteases are present in higher-than-normal levels, they damage the alveoli and the small airways by breaking down elastin. Over time, alveolar sacs lose their elasticity and the small airways collapse or narrow. Some alveoli are destroyed, and others become large and flabby, with less area for GAS EXCHANGE.

An increased amount of air is trapped in the lungs. Causes of air trapping are loss of elastic recoil in the alveolar walls, overstretching and enlargement of the alveoli into air-filled spaces called *bullae,* and collapse of small bronchioles. These changes greatly increase the work of breathing. The hyperinflated lung flattens the diaphragm (Fig. 30-7), weakening the effectiveness of this muscle. As a result, the patient with emphysema needs to use accessory muscles in the neck, chest wall, and abdomen to inhale and exhale. This increased effort increases the need for oxygen, making the patient have an "air hunger" sensation. Inhalation starts before exhalation is completed, resulting in an uncoordinated breathing pattern.

GAS EXCHANGE is affected by the increased work of breathing and the loss of alveolar tissue. Although some alveoli enlarge, the curves of alveolar walls decrease and less surface area is available for gas exchange. Often the patient adjusts by increasing the respiratory rate, so arterial blood gas (ABG) values may not show gas exchange problems until the patient has advanced disease. Then carbon dioxide is produced faster than it can be eliminated, resulting in carbon dioxide retention and chronic respiratory acidosis (see Chapter 12). The patient with late-stage emphysema also has a low arterial oxygen (PaO_2) level because it is difficult for oxygen to move from diseased alveoli into the blood.

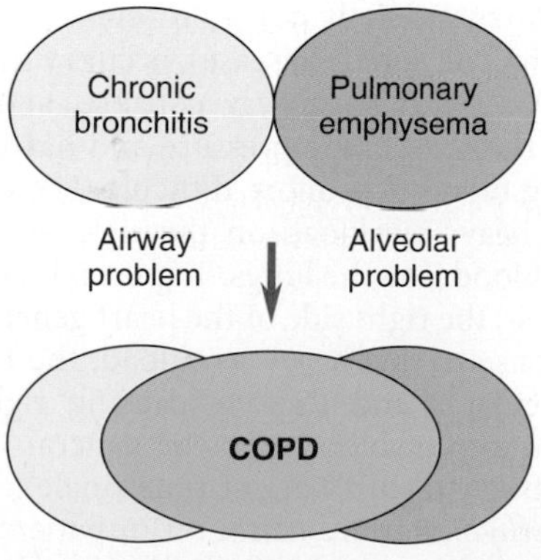

FIG. 30-6 The interaction of chronic bronchitis and emphysema in chronic obstructive pulmonary disease (COPD).

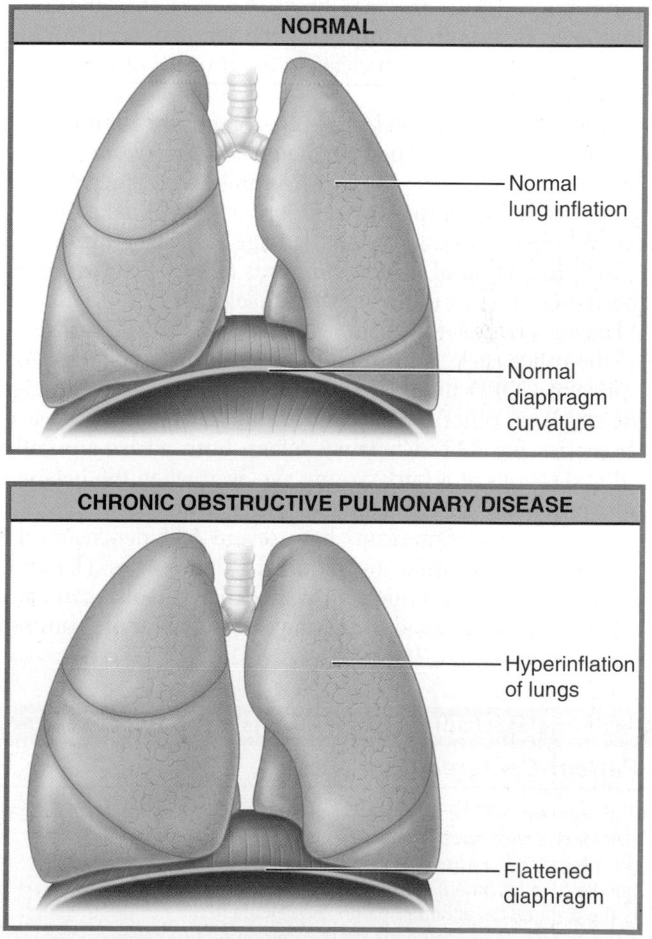

FIG. 30-7 Diaphragm shape and lung inflation in the normal patient and in the patient with chronic airflow limitation (CAL), especially chronic obstructive pulmonary disease (COPD).

Emphysema is classified as *panlobular, centrilobular,* or *paraseptal* depending on the pattern of destruction and dilation of the gas-exchanging units (acini) (see Fig. 30-1). Each type can occur alone or in combination in the same lung. Most are associated with smoking or chronic exposure to other inhaled particles such as wood smoke and biomass fuels (Global Initiative for Chronic Obstructive Lung Disease [GOLD], 2014).

Chronic Bronchitis. Bronchitis is an INFLAMMATION of the bronchi and bronchioles caused by exposure to irritants, especially cigarette smoke. The irritant triggers inflammation, vasodilation, mucosal edema, congestion, and bronchospasm. Bronchitis affects only the airways, not the alveoli.

Chronic INFLAMMATION increases the number and size of mucus glands, which produce large amounts of thick mucus. The bronchial walls thicken and impair airflow. This thickening, along with excessive mucus, blocks some of the smaller airways and narrows larger ones. Mucus provides a breeding ground for organisms and leads to chronic infection.

Chronic bronchitis impairs airflow and GAS EXCHANGE because mucus plugs and infection narrow the airways. As a result, the Pao_2 level decreases (hypoxemia) and the arterial carbon dioxide ($Paco_2$) level increases (respiratory acidosis).

Etiology and Genetic Risk. *Cigarette smoking* is the greatest risk factor for COPD. The patient with a 20–pack-year history or longer often has early-stage COPD with changes in pulmonary function tests (PFTs).

The inhaled smoke triggers the release of excessive proteases in the lungs. These enzymes break down elastin, the major component of alveoli. By impairing the action of cilia, smoking also inhibits the cilia from clearing the bronchi of mucus, cellular debris, and fluid.

Alpha$_1$-antitrypsin deficiency is a less common but important risk factor for COPD. The enzyme *alpha$_1$-antitrypsin* (AAT) is normally present in the lungs. AAT inhibits excessive protease activity so that the proteases only break down inhaled pollutants and organisms and do not damage lung structures.

The production of normal amounts of AAT depends on the inheritance of a pair of normal gene alleles for this protein. The AAT gene is recessive. Thus if one of the pair of alleles is faulty and the other allele is normal, the person makes enough AAT to prevent COPD unless there is significant exposure to cigarette smoke or other inhalation irritants. This person, however, is a carrier for AAT deficiency. When both alleles are faulty, COPD develops at a fairly young age even when the person is not exposed to cigarette smoke or other irritants.

About 100,000 Americans have severe AAT deficiency, and many more have mild to moderate deficiencies (Beery & Workman, 2012). Although an AAT deficiency also can cause problems in the skin and liver, lung diseases are more common (Kessenich & Bacher, 2014).

GENETIC/GENOMIC CONSIDERATIONS

Patient-Centered Care QSEN

The gene for AAT has many known variations, and some increase the risk for emphysema. Different variations result in different levels of AAT deficiency and is a reason why the disease is more severe for some people than for others. The most serious variation for emphysema risk is the **Z** mutation, although others also increase the risk but to a lesser degree. Table 30-1 shows the most common AAT mutations increasing the risk for emphysema. Urge patients who have any ATT deficiency to avoid smoking and other environmental pollutants.

TABLE 30-1 Characteristics Associated with the Most Common Alpha$_1$-Antitrypsin Gene Mutations

MUTATION GENOTYPE	LEVEL OF SERUM ALPHA$_1$-ANTITRYPSIN (% OF NORMAL)	DISEASE SEVERITY
M/S	80%	No detectable disease
S/S	50%-60%	Minimal to no disease expression
M/Z	50%-55%	Minimal to no disease expression
S/Z	30%-35%	Pulmonary disease, early age
Z/Z	10%-15%	Severe COPD, extrapulmonary involvement

From Workman, M.L., & Winkelman, C. (2008). Genetic influences in common respiratory disorders. *Critical Care Nursing Clinics of North America, 20*(2), 171-189.
COPD, Chronic obstructive pulmonary disease.

In addition to genetic and environmental factors, asthma also appears to be a risk factor for COPD. The incidence of COPD is reported to be 12 times greater among adults with asthma compared with adults without asthma after adjusting for smoking history (GOLD, 2014).

Incidence and Prevalence. The prevalence of chronic bronchitis and emphysema in the United States has been estimated at about 15.8 million, and more than 10% of nursing home residents have COPD (CDC, 2014b). COPD is the fourth leading cause of morbidity and mortality in the United States (GOLD, 2014).

Complications. COPD affects GAS EXCHANGE and the oxygenation of all tissues. Complications include hypoxemia, acidosis, respiratory infection, cardiac failure, dysrhythmias, and respiratory failure.

Hypoxemia and acidosis occur because the patient with COPD has reduced GAS EXCHANGE, leading to decreased oxygenation and increased carbon dioxide levels. These problems reduce cellular function.

Respiratory infection risk increases because of the increased mucus and poor oxygenation. Bacterial infections are common and make COPD manifestations worse by increasing INFLAMMATION and mucus production and inducing more bronchospasm. Airflow becomes even more limited, the work of breathing increases, and dyspnea results.

Cardiac failure, especially **cor pulmonale** (right-sided heart failure caused by pulmonary disease), occurs with bronchitis or emphysema. Air trapping, airway collapse, and stiff alveolar walls increase the lung tissue pressure and narrow lung blood vessels, making blood flow more difficult. The increased pressure creates a heavy workload on the right side of the heart, which pumps blood into the lungs. To pump blood through the narrowed vessels, the right side of the heart generates high pressures. In response to this heavy workload, the right chambers of the heart enlarge and thicken, causing right-sided heart failure with backup of blood into the general venous system. Chart 30-9 lists key features of cor pulmonale.

Cardiac dysrhythmias are common in patients with COPD. They result from hypoxemia (from decreased oxygen to the heart muscle), other cardiac disease, drug effects, or acidosis.

CHART 30-9 Key Features

Cor Pulmonale

- Hypoxia and hypoxemia
- Increasing dyspnea
- Fatigue
- Enlarged and tender liver
- Warm, cyanotic hands and feet, with bounding pulses
- Cyanotic lips
- Distended neck veins
- Right ventricular enlargement (hypertrophy)
- Visible pulsations below the sternum
- GI disturbances, such as nausea or anorexia
- Dependent edema
- Metabolic and respiratory acidosis
- Pulmonary hypertension

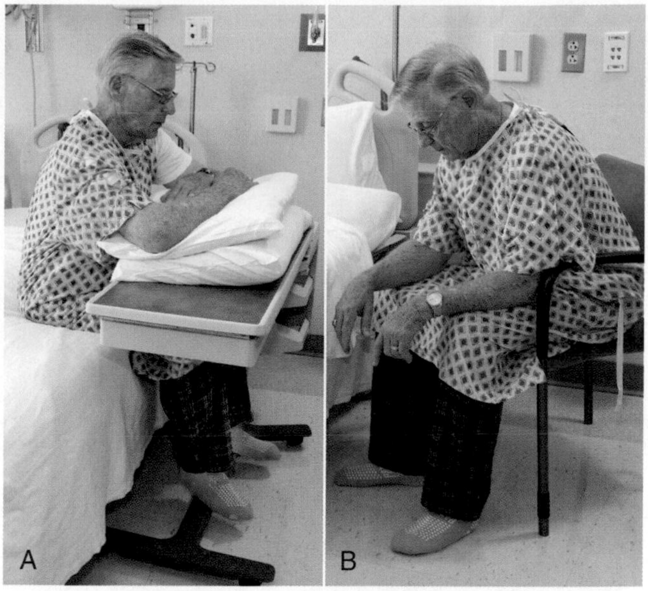

FIG. 30-8 Orthopnea positions that patients with chronic obstructive pulmonary disease (COPD) often assume to ease the work of breathing.

Health Promotion and Maintenance

The incidence and severity of COPD would be greatly reduced by smoking cessation. Urge all people who smoke to quit smoking. Chart 27-1 in Chapter 27 provides tips to teach people about smoking cessation. Also, as described in Chapter 27, teach all people specific actions to take to avoid exposure to other inhalation irritants.

❖ *PATIENT-CENTERED COLLABORATIVE CARE*

The Concept Map addresses assessment and nursing care issues related to COPD.

◆ *Assessment*

History. Ask about risk factors such as age, gender, and occupational history. COPD is seen more often in older men. Some types of emphysema occur in families, especially those with alpha$_1$-antitrypsin (AAT) deficiency.

Obtain a thorough smoking history, because tobacco use is a major risk factor. Ask about the length of time the patient has smoked and the number of packs smoked daily. Use these data to determine the pack-year smoking history.

Ask the patient to describe the breathing problems, and assess whether he or she has any difficulty breathing while talking. Does he or she speak in complete sentences, or is it necessary to take a breath between every one or two words? Ask about the presence, duration, or worsening of wheezing, coughing, and shortness of breath. Determine what activities trigger these problems. Assess any cough, and ask whether sputum is clear or colored and how much is produced each day. Ask about the time of day when sputum production is greatest. Smokers often have a productive cough when they get up in the morning; nonsmokers generally do not.

Ask the patient to compare the activity level and shortness of breath now with those of a month ago and a year ago. Ask about any difficulty with eating and sleeping. Many patients sleep in a semi-sitting position because breathlessness is worse when lying down (**orthopnea**). Ask about usual daily activities and any difficulty with bathing, dressing, or sexual activity. Document this assessment to personalize the intervention plan.

Weigh the patient, and compare this weight with previous weights. Unplanned weight loss is likely when COPD severity increases, because the work of breathing increases metabolic needs. Dyspnea and mucus production often result in poor food intake and inadequate nutrition. Ask the patient to recall a typical day's meals and fluid intake. When heart failure is present with COPD, general edema with weight gain may occur.

Physical Assessment/Clinical Manifestations. *General appearance* can provide clues about respiratory status and energy level. Observe weight in proportion to height, posture, mobility, muscle mass, and overall hygiene. The patient with increasingly severe COPD is thin, with loss of muscle mass in the extremities, although the neck muscles may be enlarged. He or she tends to be slow moving and slightly stooped. The person often sits in a forward-bending posture with the arms held forward, a position known as the *orthopneic* or *tripod position* (Fig. 30-8). When dyspnea becomes severe, activity intolerance may be so great that bathing and general grooming are neglected.

Respiratory changes occur as a result of obstruction, changes in chest size, and fatigue. Inspect the chest and assess the breathing rate and pattern. The patient with respiratory muscle fatigue breathes with rapid, shallow respirations and may have an abnormal breathing pattern in which the abdominal wall is sucked in during inspiration or may use accessory muscles in the abdomen or neck. During an acute exacerbation, the respiratory rate could be as high as 40 to 50 breaths/min and requires immediate medical attention. As respiratory muscles become fatigued, respiratory movement is jerky and appears uncoordinated.

Check the patient's chest for retractions and for asymmetric chest expansion. The patient with emphysema has limited diaphragmatic movement (excursion) because the diaphragm is flattened and below its usual resting state. Chest vibration (fremitus) is often decreased and the chest sounds hyperresonant on percussion because of trapped air.

Auscultate the chest to assess the depth of inspiration and any abnormal breath sounds. Wheezes and other abnormal sounds often occur on inspiration and expiration, although crackles are usually not present. Reduced breath sounds are common, especially with emphysema. Note the pitch and location of the sound and the point in the respiratory cycle at which the sound is heard. A silent chest may indicate serious airflow obstruction or pneumothorax.

CONCEPT MAP

GAS EXCHANGE — PERFUSION — **COPD** — INFLAMMATION — CELLULAR REGULATION

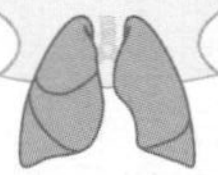

HISTORY

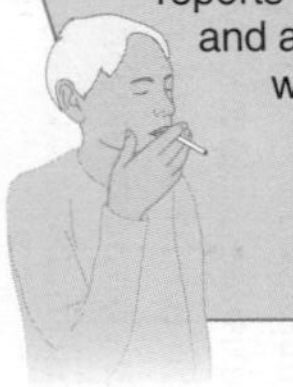

Nick Williams, age 66, is a long-time smoker admitted with an exacerbation of COPD. He reports shortness of breath and a productive cough with thick yellow sputum.

↓ Physical Assessment

ASSESSMENT DATA

ABGs-pH 7.31; PaO_2 66; $PaCO_2$ 59; HCO_3^- 26. Bilateral wheezing, dyspnea and tachypnea 28/min, O_2 sat 86%, T 100.6° F, HR 104; BP 140/88; use of accessory muscles; productive cough, thick yellow sputum; digital clubbing; barrel-shaped chest; skin cool and dry. No peripheral edema.

→ Data Synthesis

PATIENT PROBLEMS

- Hypoxemia with hypercapnia
- Weight loss related to dyspnea, excessive secretions, anorexia, and fatigue
- Anxiety related to dyspnea, a change in health status, and situational crisis
- Activity Intolerance
- Potential for pneumonia or other respiratory infections

↑ Planning

EXPECTED OUTCOMES

- Attain and maintain GAS EXCHANGE at usual baseline level: SpO_2 at least 88%, no cyanosis, maintain cognitive orientation, cough and clear secretions effectively, and maintain respiratory rate and rhythm appropriate to activity level.
- Achieve and maintain body weight within 10% of ideal: maintain appropriate weight/height ratio, maintain serum albumin or prealbumin within normal range.
- Have decreased anxiety, identify contributory factors, and perform activities to decrease or eliminate anxiety.
- Increase activity to an acceptable level: maintain baseline SpO_2 with activity, perform ADLs with no or minimal assistance, perform selected activities with minimal dyspnea or tachycardia, participate in family, work, or social activities as desired.
- Avoid serious respiratory infection: describe clinical manifestations, monitoring procedures, preventative strategies, and seek medical assistance when manifestations of respiratory infection appear.

INTERVENTIONS

1 History Assessment

- Assess ability to perform ADLs. *Good management maintains adequate GAS EXCHANGE and improves overall health.*
- Trend and monitor weight. *Monitors for unplanned weight loss when work of breathing increases metabolic needs.*
- Ask patient to recall a typical day's meals and fluid intake. *Evaluates for inadequate nutrition.*

2 Physical Assessment

- Observe weight/height proportion, posture, mobility, muscle mass, and overall hygiene. *Provides clues about GAS EXCHANGE and energy level.*
- Inspect chest size and shape; assess breath sounds, respiratory rate, pattern, depth of inspiration, presence of retractions, asymmetry of chest expansion, cyanosis and sputum production. *Determines state of respiratory distress and whether chronic symptoms are present.*
- Assess degree of dyspnea using VADS, cyanosis, delayed capillary refill, and finger clubbing. *Indicates decreased arterial oxygen levels.*
- Assess heart rate & rhythm, dependent edema or other signs and symptoms of right heart failure. *Indicates cardiac changes related to COPD-associated anatomic changes.*
- Examine nail beds and oral mucous membranes. *Indicates adequacy of GAS EXCHANGE and oxygenation of all tissues.*

3 Nursing Priority - Improving GAS EXCHANGE

- Teach patient to participate in COPD management: airway maintenance, breathing techniques, positioning, effective coughing, oxygen therapy, exercise conditioning, suctioning, hydration, use of a vibratory positive pressure device, and adhering to prescribed drug therapy. *Promotes airway maintenance to improve GAS EXCHANGE.*
- Consult with Registered Dietitian for nutritional assessment. Monitor weight and serum prealbumin levels. *Prevents loss of muscle mass and strength, lung elasticity, and alveolar-capillary surface area, which reduce GAS EXCHANGE.*
- Assist patient with strategies to manage anxiety. *Keeps patient calm during acute dyspneic episodes.*
- Assist with ADLs. Encourage patient to self-pace activities, note skin color changes, pulse rate and regularity, O_2 saturation and work of breathing, supplemental low dose O_2 for high energy activities. *Helps to manage chronic fatigue.*
- Teach patient to avoid crowds and get pneumonia and influenza vaccines. *Prevents risk for respiratory tract infections.*

4 Laboratory Assessment

- Review ABG values and monitor pulse oximetry. *Assesses changes in respiratory status and gauges treatment response to identify abnormal GAS EXCHANGE.*
- Obtain sputum samples for culture & sensitivity and white blood cell count. *Evaluates for infections and helps identify necessary treatment.*
- Review hemoglobin & hematocrit. Assess electrolytes. *Assesses for polycythemia. Evaluates for acidosis. Low electrolyte levels reduce muscle strength.*

5 Drug Therapy

Teach patient about drug management and correct techniques for inhaler use. *Helps ensure patient receives full dose of inhaled medication and ensures correct sequence is done.*

6 Psychosocial Assessment

- Assess patient's home environment, interests, hobbies, and potential factors that contribute to respiratory infections. *Helps prevent isolation due to fatigue or embarrassment from coughing and excessive sputum production.*
- Explore economic impact of disease on patient. *Evaluates patient ability to purchase and take drugs correctly.*
- Encourage the expression of concerns about lifestyle, disease progression, and use of support groups. *Urges patient to participate in a full life, and reduces anxiety and fear from feelings of breathlessness.*

Concept Map by Deanne A. Blach, MSN, RN

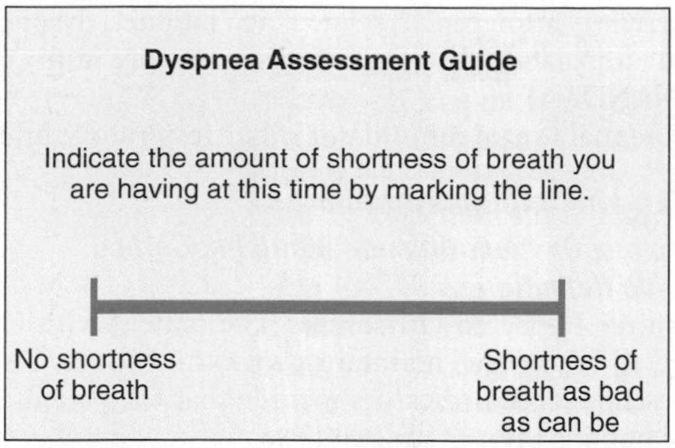

FIG. 30-9 A visual analog scale to assess dyspnea.

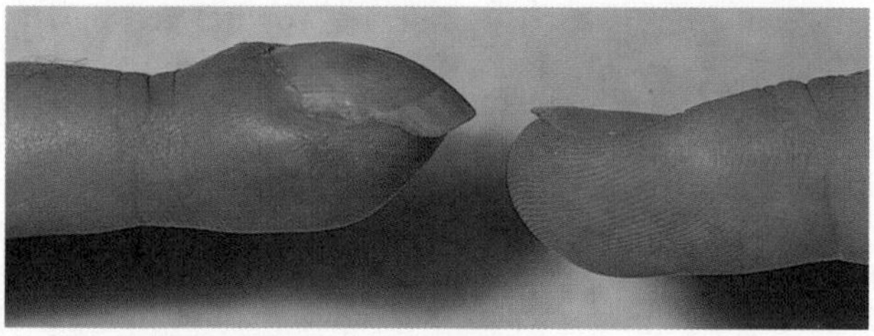

FIG. 30-10 Late digital clubbing *(on left)* compared with a normal digit *(on right).*

Assess the degree of dyspnea using a Visual Analog Dyspnea Scale (VADS), which is a straight line with verbal anchors at the beginning and end of a 100-mm line (Fig. 30-9). Ask the patient to place a mark on the line to indicate his or her perceived breathing difficulty. Document the response, and use this scale to determine the therapy effectiveness and pace the patient's activities.

Examine the patient's chest for the presence of a "barrel chest" (see Fig. 30-3). With a barrel chest, the ratio between the anteroposterior (AP) diameter of the chest and its lateral diameter is 1:1 rather than the normal ratio of 1:1.5, as a result of lung overinflation and diaphragm flattening.

The patient with chronic bronchitis often has a cyanotic, or blue-tinged, dusky appearance and has excessive sputum production. Assess for cyanosis, delayed capillary refill, and finger clubbing (Fig. 30-10), which indicate chronically decreased arterial oxygen levels.

Cardiac changes occur as a result of the anatomic changes associated with COPD. Assess the patient's heart rate and rhythm. Check for swelling of the feet and ankles (dependent edema) or other manifestations of right-sided heart failure. Examine nail beds and oral mucous membranes. In late-stage emphysema the patient may have pallor or cyanosis and is usually underweight.

Psychosocial Assessment. COPD affects all aspects of a person's life. The patient may be isolated because dyspnea causes fatigue or because of embarrassment from coughing and excessive sputum production.

Ask the patient about interests and hobbies to assess whether socialization has decreased or whether hobbies cause exposure to irritants. Ask about home conditions for exposure to smoke or crowded living conditions that promote transmission of respiratory infections.

Economic status may be affected by the disease through changes in income and health insurance coverage. Drugs, especially the metered dose inhalers (MDIs) and dry powder inhalers (DPIs), are expensive, and many patients with limited incomes may use them only during exacerbations and not as prescribed on a scheduled basis.

Anxiety and fear from feelings of breathlessness may reduce the patient's ability to participate in a full life. Work, family, social, and sexual roles can be affected. Encourage the patient and family to express their feelings about the limitations on lifestyle and disease progression. Assess their use of support groups and community services.

Laboratory Assessment. Arterial blood gas (ABG) values identify abnormal GAS EXCHANGE, oxygenation, ventilation, and acid-base status. Compare repeated ABG values to assess changes in respiratory status. Once baseline ABG values are obtained, pulse oximetry can gauge treatment response. As COPD worsens, the amount of oxygen in the blood decreases (**hypoxemia**) and the amount of carbon dioxide increases (**hypercarbia**). Chronic respiratory acidosis (increased arterial carbon dioxide [$Paco_2$]) then results; metabolic alkalosis (increased arterial bicarbonate) occurs as compensation by kidney retention of bicarbonate. This change is seen on ABGs as an elevation of HCO_3^- although pH remains lower than normal. Not all patients with COPD are CO_2 retainers, even when hypoxemia is present, because CO_2 diffuses more easily across lung membranes than does oxygen. Hypercarbia is a problem in advanced emphysema (because the alveoli are affected) rather than in bronchitis (wherein the airways are affected). For more detailed information about acidosis, see Chapter 12.

Sputum samples are obtained for culture from hospitalized patients with an acute respiratory infection. The infection is treated on the basis of manifestations and the common bacterial organisms in the local community. A WBC count helps confirm the presence of infection.

Other blood tests include hemoglobin and hematocrit to determine *polycythemia* (a compensatory increase in red blood cells [RBCs] and iron in the chronically hypoxic patient). Serum electrolyte levels are examined because acidosis can change electrolyte values. Low phosphate, potassium, calcium, and magnesium levels reduce muscle strength. In patients with a family history of COPD, serum AAT levels may be drawn.

Imaging Assessment. Chest x-rays are used to rule out other lung diseases and to check the progress of patients with respiratory infections or chronic disease. With advanced emphysema, chest x-rays show hyperinflation and a flattened diaphragm.

Other Diagnostic Assessments. COPD is classified from mild to very severe on the basis of manifestations and pulmonary function test (PFT) changes (Table 30-2; see Table 27-6 in Chapter 27). Airflow rates and lung volume measurements help distinguish airway disease (obstructive diseases) from interstitial lung disease (restrictive diseases). PFTs determine lung volumes, flow volume curves, and diffusion capacity. Each test is performed before and after the patient inhales a bronchodilator agent. Encourage the patient to express his or her feelings about testing and the potential impact of the results. Explain the preparations for the procedures (if any), whether pain or discomfort will be involved, and any needed follow-up care.

The lung volumes measured for COPD are vital capacity (VC), residual volume (RV), forced expiratory volume (FEV), and total lung capacity (TLC). Although all volumes and

TABLE 30-2 Gold Classification of COPD Severity

STAGE	MANIFESTATIONS	PULMONARY FUNCTION TEST RESULTS
0 (At risk)	±Chronic cough ±Chronic sputum production	Normal
1 (Mild)	+Chronic cough ±Sputum production	FEV_1/FVC <70% FEV_1 ≥80% of predicted
2 (Moderate)	±Dyspnea ±Chronic cough ±Sputum production	FEV_1/FVC <70% FEV_1 <80% but at least 50% of predicted
3 (Severe)	+Dyspnea +Chronic cough +Sputum production	FEV_1/FVC <70% FEV_1 <50% but at least 30% of predicted
4 (Very severe)	++Dyspnea ++Chronic cough ++Sputum production	FEV_1/FVC <70% FEV_1 <30% of predicted

Data from Global Initiative for Chronic Obstructive Lung Disease (GOLD). (2014). *Global strategy for the diagnosis, management, and prevention of chronic obstructive pulmonary disease.* Retrieved June 2014, from www.goldcopd.org/.

FEV_1, Volume of air blown out as hard and fast as possible during the first second of the most forceful exhalation after the greatest full inhalation; *FVC*, functional vital capacity.

capacities change to some degree in COPD, the RV is most affected, with increases reflecting the trapped, stale air remaining in the lungs.

A diagnosis of COPD is based mostly on the FEV_1 (the FEV in the first second of exhalation). FEV_1 can also be expressed as a percentage of the forced vital capacity (FVC). As the disease progresses, the ratio of FEV_1 to FVC becomes smaller (Smith & Tasota, 2011).

The diffusion test measures how well a test gas (carbon monoxide) diffuses across the alveolar-capillary membrane and combines with hemoglobin. In emphysema, alveolar wall destruction decreases the large surface area for diffusion of gas into the blood, leading to a decreased diffusion capacity. In bronchitis alone, the diffusion capacity is usually normal.

The patient with COPD has decreased oxygen saturation, often much lower than 90%. Changes in Spo_2 below the patient's usual saturation require medical attention.

Peak expiratory flow meters are used to monitor the effectiveness of drug therapy to relieve obstruction. Peak flow rates increase as obstruction resolves. Teach the patient to self-monitor the peak expiratory flow rates at home and adjust drugs as needed.

◆ Analysis

The priority NANDA-I nursing diagnoses and collaborative problems for patients with chronic obstructive pulmonary disease (COPD) include:

1. Hypoxemia with hypercapnia related to alveolar-capillary membrane changes, reduced airway size, ventilatory muscle fatigue, excessive mucus production, airway obstruction, diaphragm flattening, fatigue, and decreased energy
2. Weight loss related to dyspnea, excessive secretions, anorexia, and fatigue
3. Anxiety related to dyspnea, a change in health status, and situational crisis (NANDA-I)
4. Activity Intolerance related to fatigue, dyspnea, and an imbalance between oxygen supply and demand (NANDA-I)
5. Potential for pneumonia or other respiratory infections

◆ Planning and Implementation

Improving Oxygenation and Reducing Carbon Dioxide Retention

Planning: Expected Outcomes. The patient with COPD is expected to attain and maintain GAS EXCHANGE at his or her usual baseline level. Indicators include that the patient:

- Maintains Spo_2 of at least 88%
- Remains free from cyanosis
- Maintains cognitive orientation
- Coughs and clears secretions effectively
- Maintains a respiratory rate and rhythm appropriate to his or her activity level

Interventions. Most patients with COPD use nonsurgical management to improve or maintain GAS EXCHANGE. Surgical management requires that the patient meet strict criteria.

Nonsurgical Management. Nursing management for patients with COPD focuses on airway maintenance, monitoring, breathing techniques, positioning, effective coughing, oxygen therapy, exercise conditioning, suctioning, hydration, and use of a vibratory positive-pressure device. A nursing priority is to teach the patient how to be a partner in COPD management by participating in therapies to improve GAS EXCHANGE and by adhering to prescribed drug therapy.

Before any intervention, assess the breathing rate, rhythm, depth, and use of accessory muscles. The accessory muscles are less efficient than the diaphragm, and the work of breathing increases. Determine whether any factors are contributing to the increased work of breathing, such as respiratory infection. *Airway maintenance is the most important focus of interventions to improve GAS EXCHANGE.*

Monitoring. Monitoring for changes in respiratory status is key to providing prompt interventions to reduce complications. Assess the hospitalized patient with COPD at least every 2 hours, even when the purpose of hospitalization is not COPD management. Apply prescribed oxygen, assess the patient's response to therapy, and prevent complications.

If the patient's condition worsens, more aggressive therapy is needed. Noninvasive ventilation (NIV) may be useful for patients with stable, very severe COPD and daytime hypercapnia (GOLD, 2014). Intubation and mechanical ventilation may be needed for patients in respiratory failure.

Breathing Techniques. Diaphragmatic or abdominal and pursed-lip breathing may be helpful for managing dyspneic episodes. Teach the patient to use these techniques, shown in Chart 30-10, during all activities to reduce the amount of stale air in the lungs and manage dyspnea. Teach these techniques when the patient has less dyspnea.

In diaphragmatic breathing, the patient consciously increases movement of the diaphragm. Lying on the back allows the abdomen to relax. Breathing through pursed lips creates mild resistance, which prolongs exhalation and increases airway pressure. This technique delays airway compression and reduces air trapping. Pursed-lip breathing can be used during diaphragmatic or abdominal breathing.

Positioning. Placing the patient in an upright position with the head of the bed elevated can help alleviate dyspnea by increasing chest expansion and keeping the diaphragm in the

CHART 30-10 Patient and Family Education: Preparing for Self-Management

Breathing Exercises

Diaphragmatic or Abdominal Breathing

- If you can do so comfortably, lie on your back with your knees bent. If you cannot lie comfortably, perform this exercise while sitting in a chair.
- Place your hands or a book on your abdomen to create resistance.
- Begin breathing from your abdomen while keeping your chest still. You can tell if you are breathing correctly if your hands or the book rises and falls accordingly.

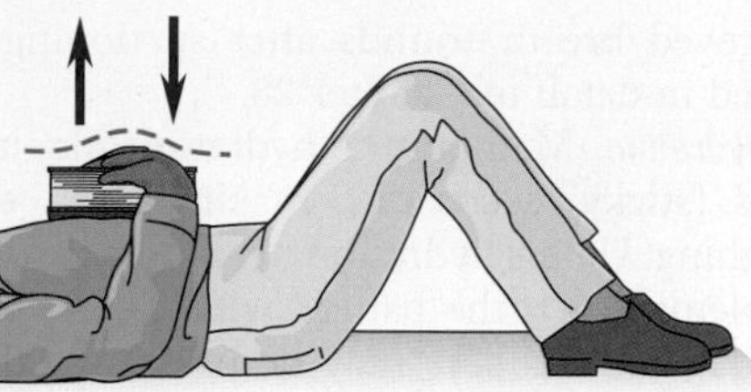

Pursed-Lip Breathing

- Close your mouth, and breathe in through your nose.
- Purse your lips as you would to whistle. Breathe out slowly through your mouth, without puffing your cheeks. Spend at least twice the amount of time it took you to breathe in.
- Use your abdominal muscles to squeeze out every bit of air you can.
- Remember to use pursed-lip breathing during any physical activity. Always inhale before beginning the activity and exhale while performing the activity. Never hold your breath.

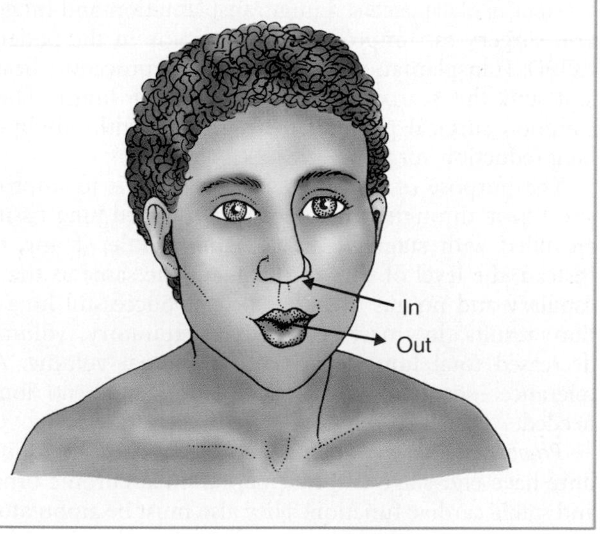

proper position to contract. This position conserves energy by supporting the patient's arms and upper body. Assist the patient who can tolerate sitting in a chair out of bed for 1-hour periods 2 or 3 times a day. This position also helps move secretions.

Effective Coughing. Coughing effectively can improve GAS EXCHANGE by helping increase airflow in the larger airways. The patient with COPD often has difficulty with removal of secretions, which results in poor gas exchange and oxygenation. Excessive mucus also increases the risk for respiratory infections.

Controlled coughing is helpful in removing excessive mucus. Teach the patient to cough on arising in the morning to eliminate mucus that collected during the night. Coughing to clear mucus before mealtimes may make meals more pleasant. Coughing before bedtime may help clear lungs for a less interrupted night's sleep.

For effective coughing, teach the patient to sit in a chair or on the side of a bed with feet placed firmly on the floor. Instruct him or her to turn the shoulders inward and to bend the head slightly downward, hugging a pillow against the stomach. The patient then takes a few breaths, attempting to exhale more fully. After the third to fifth breath (in through the nose, out through pursed lips), instruct him or her to take a deeper breath and bend forward slowly while coughing 2 or 3 times ("mini-coughs") from the same breath. On return to a sitting position, the patient takes a comfortably deep breath. The entire coughing procedure is repeated at least twice.

Oxygen Therapy. Oxygen is prescribed for relief of hypoxemia and hypoxia. The need for oxygen therapy and its effectiveness can be determined by arterial blood gas (ABG) values and oxygen saturation by pulse oximetry. The patient with COPD may need an oxygen flow of 2 to 4 L/min via nasal cannula or up to 40% via Venturi mask. Ensure that there are no open flames or other combustion hazards in rooms in which oxygen is in use. More information on oxygen therapy is found in Chapter 28.

In the past, the patient with COPD was thought to be at risk for extreme hypoventilation with oxygen therapy because of a decreased drive to breathe as blood oxygen levels rose. However, this concern has not been shown to be evidence-based and has been responsible for ineffective management of hypoxia in patients with COPD. All hypoxic patients, even those with COPD and hypercarbia, should receive oxygen therapy at rates appropriate to reduce hypoxia and bring Spo_2 levels up between 88% and 92% (Abdo & Heunks, 2012; Burt & Corbridge, 2013; Makic et al., 2013).

Drug Therapy. Drugs used to manage COPD are the same drugs as for asthma and include beta-adrenergic agents, cholinergic antagonists, xanthines, corticosteroids, and cromones (see Chart 30-6). The focus is on long-term control therapy with longer-acting drugs, such as arformoterol (Brovana), indacaterol (Arcapta Neohaler), tiotropium (Spiriva), aclidinium bromide (Tudorza Pressair), and the combination drug fluticasone furoate/vilanterol (BREO ELLIPTA). The patient with COPD is more likely to be taking systemic agents (in addition to inhaled drugs) than is the patient with asthma. An additional drug class for COPD is the mucolytics, which thin the thick secretions, making them easier to cough up and expel. Nebulizer treatments with normal saline or with a mucolytic agent such as acetylcysteine (Mucosil, Mucomyst 🍁) or dornase alfa (Pulmozyme) and normal saline help thin secretions. Guaifenesin (Organidin, Naldecon Senior EX) is a systemic mucolytic that is taken orally. A combination of guaifenesin and dextromethorphan (Mucinex DM) also raises the cough threshold.

Stepped therapy, which adds drugs as COPD progresses, is recommended for patients with chronic bronchitis or emphysema, although the patient's response to drug therapy is the best indicator of when drugs or their dosages need changing. Ideally, the patient notices changes and participates in management strategies. Teach patients and family members the correct techniques for using inhalers and to care for them properly.

Many inhalers for COPD drug therapy are dry powder inhalers. These often require having the patient "load in" each dose. The steps for this process involve opening the inhaler's capsule chamber, removing the dry powder capsule from a separate blister pack, placing the capsule in the chamber, closing the inhaler until it clicks and punctures the capsule, and then using the inhaler. Often the patient with severe COPD is older, has muscle weakness, has poor manual dexterity, and may have some problems with cognition. All of these issues can be barriers to proper use of a DPI inhaler for COPD management (Lareau & Hodder, 2012).

NCLEX EXAMINATION CHALLENGE

Health Promotion and Maintenance

A client with chronic obstructive pulmonary disease (COPD) prescribed a long-acting inhaled $beta_2$ agonist reports hating the inhaler and asks why the drug can't be taken as a pill. What is the nurse's best response?

A. "Drugs taken by inhaler work more slowly and remain in the system longer."
B. "Drugs taken by inhaler have no side effects and are less expensive."
C. "Drugs taken by mouth are more expensive because they must be sterile."
D. "Drugs taken by mouth have systemic side effects and are harder to control."

Exercise Conditioning. Exercise for conditioning and pulmonary rehabilitation can improve function and endurance in patients with COPD. Patients often respond to the dyspnea of COPD by limiting their activity, even basic ADLs. Over time, the muscles used in breathing weaken, resulting in increased dyspnea with lower activity levels.

Pulmonary rehabilitation involves education and exercise training to prevent muscle deconditioning. Each patient's exercise program is personalized to reflect his or her current limitations and planned outcomes. The simplest plan involves having the patient walk (indoors or outdoors) daily at a self-paced rate until manifestations limit further walking, followed by a rest period, and then continue walking until 20 minutes of actual walking has been accomplished. As the time during rest periods decreases, the patient can add 5 more minutes of walking time. Teach patients whose manifestations are severe to modify the exercise by using a walker with wheels or, if needed, to use oxygen while exercising. Remind patients that the exercise needs to be performed at least 2 or 3 times weekly for best improvement. Formal pulmonary rehabilitation programs can be beneficial even for patients who are severely impaired.

Additional exercise techniques to retrain ventilatory muscles include isocapneic hyperventilation and resistive breathing. Isocapneic hyperventilation, in which the patient hyperventilates into a machine that controls the levels of oxygen and carbon dioxide, increases endurance. In resistive breathing, the patient breathes against a set resistance. Resistive breathing increases respiratory muscle strength and endurance.

Suctioning. Perform suctioning only when needed—not on a routine schedule. For the patient with a weak cough, weak pulmonary muscles, and inability to expectorate effectively, perform nasotracheal suctioning. Assess the patient for dyspnea, tachycardia, and dysrhythmias during the procedure. Assess for improved breath sounds after suctioning. Suctioning is discussed in detail in Chapter 28.

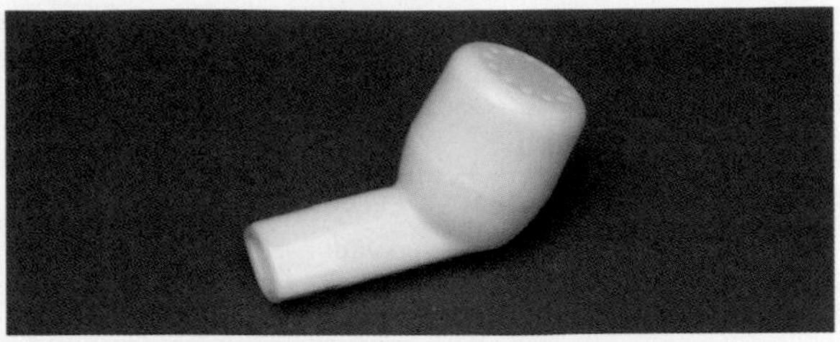

FIG. 30-11 The FLUTTER® flutter valve mucus clearance device, a type of vibratory positive-pressure device.

Hydration. Maintaining hydration may thin the thick, tenacious (sticky) secretions, making them easier to remove by coughing. Unless hydration needs to be avoided for other health problems, teach the patient with COPD to drink at least 2 to 3 L/day. Humidifiers may be useful for those living in a dry climate or those who use dry heat during the winter.

Vibratory Positive Expiratory Pressure Device. The use of a vibratory positive expiratory pressure device can help patients remove airway secretions. The device is a small, handheld plastic pipe with a short, fat stem and a perforated lid over the bowl (Fig. 30-11). A movable steel ball is inside the bowl. The patient inhales deeply and then exhales through the device, causing the ball to move and set up vibrations that are transmitted to the chest and airways. The vibrations loosen secretions and allow them to be coughed out more easily.

Surgical Management.

Lung transplantation and lung reduction surgery can improve GAS EXCHANGE in the patient with COPD. Transplantation is a relatively rare procedure because of cost and the scarce availability of donor lungs. The more common surgical procedure for patients with emphysema is lung reduction surgery.

The purpose of lung reduction surgery is to improve GAS EXCHANGE through removal of hyperinflated lung tissues that are filled with stagnant air containing little, if any, oxygen. Instead, the level of carbon dioxide is the same as that in the capillary and no gas exchange occurs. Successful lung reduction results in increased forced expiratory volume and decreased total lung capacity and residual volume. Activity tolerance increases, and oxygen therapy may no longer be needed.

Preoperative Care. Patients who are selected for this procedure have end-stage emphysema, minimal chronic bronchitis, and stable cardiac function. They also must be ambulatory; not ventilator dependent; free of pulmonary fibrosis, asthma, or cancer; and not have smoked for at least 6 months. The patient must be rehabilitated to the stage that he or she is able to walk, without stopping, for 30 minutes at 1 mile/hr and maintain a 90% or better oxygen saturation level.

In addition to standard preoperative testing, tests to determine the location of greatest lung hyperinflation and poorest lung blood flow are performed. These tests include pulmonary plethysmography, gas dilution, and perfusion scans.

Operative Procedures. Usually lung reduction is performed on both lungs, most often by the minimally invasive surgical technique of video-assisted thoracoscopic surgery (VATS) or through bronchoscopy (GOLD, 2014). Each lung is deflated separately and examined for color and texture differences. Normal lung tissue darkens to purple or gray when deflated and becomes more dense or rubbery in texture. Hyperinflated areas do not deflate and remain pink with a spongy texture. The surgeon removes as much of this tissue as possible.

Postoperative Care. After lung reduction surgery, the patient needs close monitoring for continuing respiratory problems as well as for usual postoperative complications. Bronchodilator and mucolytic therapies are maintained. Pulmonary hygiene includes incentive spirometry 10 times per hour while awake, chest physiotherapy starting on the first day after surgery, and hourly pulmonary assessment.

Preventing Weight Loss

Planning: Expected Outcomes. The patient with COPD is expected to achieve and maintain a body weight within 10% of ideal. Indicators include that the patient:

- Maintains an appropriate weight/height ratio
- Maintains serum albumin or prealbumin within the normal range

Interventions. The patient with COPD often has food intolerance, nausea, *early satiety* (feeling too "full" to eat), poor appetite, and meal-related dyspnea. The increased work of breathing raises calorie and protein needs, which can lead to protein-calorie malnutrition. Malnourished patients lose muscle mass and strength, lung elasticity, and alveolar-capillary surface area, all of which reduce GAS EXCHANGE.

Identify patients at risk for or who have this complication, and request that a registered dietitian perform a nutrition assessment. Monitor weight and other indicators of nutrition, such as serum prealbumin levels.

Dyspnea management is needed because shortness of breath interferes with eating. Teach the patient to plan the biggest meal of the day for the time when he or she is most hungry and well rested. Four to six small meals a day may be preferred to three larger ones. Remind patients to use pursed-lip and abdominal breathing and to use the prescribed bronchodilator 30 minutes before the meal to reduce bronchospasm.

Food selection can help prevent weight loss. Abdominal bloating and a feeling of fullness often prevent the patient from eating a complete meal. Collaborate with the dietitian to teach about foods that are easy to chew and not gas-forming. Advise the patient to avoid dry foods that stimulate coughing and caffeine-containing drinks that increase urine output and may lead to dehydration.

Urge the patient to eat high-calorie, high-protein foods. Dietary supplements, such as Pulmocare, provide nutrition with reduced carbon dioxide production. If early satiety is a problem, advise him or her to avoid drinking fluids before and during the meal and to eat smaller, more frequent meals.

Minimizing Anxiety

Planning: Expected Outcomes. The patient with COPD is expected to have decreased anxiety. Indicators include that the patient consistently demonstrates these behaviors:

- Identifies factors that contribute to anxiety
- Identifies activities to decrease anxiety
- States anxiety is reduced or absent

Interventions. Patients with COPD become anxious during acute dyspneic episodes, especially when excessive secretions are present. Anxiety also may cause dyspnea.

Help the patient understand that anxiety can increase dyspnea, and have a plan for dealing with anxiety. Together with the patient, develop a written plan that states exactly what he or she should do if symptoms flare. Having a plan provides confidence and control in knowing what to do, which often helps reduce anxiety. Stress the use of pursed-lip and diaphragmatic breathing techniques during periods of anxiety or panic.

Family, friends, and support groups can be helpful. Recommend professional counseling, if needed, as a positive suggestion. Stress that talking with a counselor can help identify techniques to maintain control over dyspnea and panic.

Explore other approaches to help the patient control dyspneic episodes and panic attacks, such as progressive relaxation, hypnosis therapy, and biofeedback. For some patients, antianxiety drug therapy may be needed for severe anxiety.

Improving Activity Tolerance

Planning: Expected Outcomes. The patient with COPD is expected to increase activity to a level acceptable to him or her. Indicators include that the patient:

- Maintains his or her baseline Spo_2 with activity
- Performs ADLs with no or minimal assistance
- Performs selected activities with minimal dyspnea or tachycardia
- Participates in family, work, or social activities as desired

Interventions. The patient with COPD often has chronic fatigue. During acute exacerbations, he or she may need extensive help with the ADLs of eating, bathing, and grooming. As the acute problem resolves, encourage the patient to pace activities and perform as much self-care as possible. Teach him or her to not rush through morning activities, because rushing increases dyspnea, fatigue, and hypoxemia. As activity gradually increases, assess the patient's response by noting skin color changes, pulse rate and regularity, oxygen saturation, and work of breathing. Suggest the use of oxygen during periods of high energy use, such as bathing or walking.

Energy conservation is the planning and pacing of activities for best tolerance and minimum discomfort. Ask the patient to describe a typical daily schedule. Help him or her divide each activity into its smaller parts to determine whether that task can be performed in a different way or at a different time. Teach about planning and pacing daily activities with rest periods between activities. Help the patient develop a chart outlining the day's activities and planned rest periods.

Encourage the patient to avoid working with the arms raised. Activities involving the arms decrease exercise tolerance because the accessory muscles are used to stabilize the arms and shoulders rather than to assist breathing. Many activities involving the arms can be done sitting at a table leaning on the elbows. Teach the patient to adjust work heights to reduce back strain and fatigue. Remind him or her to keep arm motions smooth and flowing to prevent jerky motions that waste energy. Work with the occupational therapist to teach about the use of adaptive tools for housework, such as long-handled dustpans, sponges, and dusters, to reduce bending and reaching.

Suggest organizing work spaces so that items used most often are within easy reach. Measures such as dividing laundry or groceries into small parcels that can be handled easily, using disposable plates to save washing time, and letting dishes dry in the rack also conserve energy. Teach the patient to not talk when engaged in other activities that require energy, such as walking. In addition, teach him or her to avoid breath-holding while performing any activity.

Preventing Respiratory Infection

Planning: Expected Outcomes. The patient with COPD is expected to avoid serious respiratory infection. Indicators include that the patient consistently demonstrates these behaviors:

- Describes clinical manifestations of respiratory infection
- Describes respiratory infection–monitoring procedures
- Uses prevention activities such as pneumonia and influenza vaccination and crowd avoidance
- Seeks medical assistance when manifestations of respiratory infection first appear

Interventions. Pneumonia is a common complication of COPD, especially among older adults. Patients who have excessive secretions or who have artificial airways are at increased risk for respiratory tract infections. Teach patients to avoid crowds, and stress the importance of receiving a pneumonia vaccination and a yearly influenza vaccine.

Community-Based Care

Home Care Management. Most patients with COPD are managed in the ambulatory care setting and cared for at home. When pneumonia or a severe exacerbation develops, the patient often returns home after hospitalization. For those with advanced disease, 24-hour care may be needed for ADLs and for monitoring. If home care is not possible, placement in a long-term care setting may be needed.

Patients with hypoxemia may use oxygen at home either as needed or continually. Continuous, long-term oxygen therapy can reverse tissue hypoxia and improve cognition and well-being. For more information on home oxygen therapy, see Chapter 28.

Collaborate with the case manager to obtain the equipment needed for care at home. Patient needs may include oxygen therapy, a hospital-type bed, a nebulizer, a tub transfer bench, and scheduled visits from a home care nurse for monitoring and evaluation.

The patient with COPD faces a lifelong disease with remissions and exacerbations. Explain to the patient and family that he or she may have periods of anxiety, depression, and ineffective coping. The person who was a smoker may also have self-directed anger.

Financial concerns often increase anxiety. The disease may worsen to the point that the patient cannot work, requiring disability benefits to help ease the financial burden. Medicare or other health insurers may help pay for home oxygen therapy and nebulizer treatments. Coordinate with the social worker or case manager to help the patient make the needed arrangements.

Self-Management Education. Patients with COPD need to know as much about the disease as possible so that they can better manage it and themselves. Patients and families should be able to discuss drug therapy, manifestations of infection, avoidance of respiratory irritants, the nutrition therapy regimen, and activity progression. Instruct them to identify and avoid stressors that can worsen the disease.

Reinforce the techniques of pursed-lip breathing, diaphragmatic breathing, positioning, relaxation therapy, energy conservation, and coughing and deep breathing. Teaching about all of the needed topics may require coordination with the home care or clinic staff.

Health Care Resources. Provide appropriate referrals as needed. Home care visits may be needed especially when home oxygen therapy is first prescribed. Chart 30-11 lists assessment areas for the patient with COPD at home. Referral to assistance programs, such as Meals on Wheels, can be helpful. Provide a list of support groups, as well as Better Breather clubs sponsored by the American Lung Association. If the patient wants to quit smoking, make the appropriate referrals.

CHART 30-11 Home Care Assessment

The Patient with Chronic Obstructive Pulmonary Disease

Assess respiratory status and adequacy of ventilation.

- Measure rate, depth, and rhythm of respirations.
- Examine mucous membranes and nail beds for evidence of hypoxia.
- Determine use of accessory muscles.
- Examine chest and abdomen for paradoxical breathing.
- Count number of words patient can speak between breaths.
- Determine need and use of supplemental oxygen. (How many liters per minute is the patient using?)
- Determine level of consciousness and presence/absence of confusion.
- Auscultate lungs for abnormal breath sounds.
- Measure oxygen saturation by pulse oximetry.
- Determine sputum production, color, and amount.
- Ask about activity level.
- Observe general hygiene.
- Measure body temperature.

Assess cardiac status.

- Measure rate, quality, and rhythm of pulse.
- Check dependent areas for edema.
- Check neck veins for distention with the patient in a sitting position.
- Measure capillary refill.

Assess nutritional status.

- Check weight maintenance, loss, or gain.
- Determine food and fluid intake.
- Determine use of nutritional supplements.
- Observe general condition of the skin.
- Assess patient's and caregiver's adherence and understanding of illness and treatment, including:
  - — Correct use of supplemental oxygen
  - — Correct use of inhalers
  - — Drug schedule and side effects
  - — Manifestations to report to the health care provider indicating the need for acute care
  - — Increasing severity of resting dyspnea
  - — Increasing severity of usual manifestations
  - — Development of new manifestations associated with poor oxygenation
  - — Respiratory infection
  - — Failure to obtain the usual degree of relief with prescribed therapies
  - — Unusual change in condition
  - — Use of pursed-lip and diaphragmatic breathing techniques
  - — Scheduling of rest periods and priority activities
  - — Participation in rehabilitation activities

◆ *Evaluation: Outcomes*

Evaluate the care of the patient with COPD based on the identified priority patient problems. The expected outcomes of care are that the patient should:

- Attain and maintain GAS EXCHANGE at a level within his or her chronic baseline values
- Achieve an effective breathing pattern that decreases the work of breathing
- Maintain a patent airway
- Achieve and maintain a body weight within 10% of his or her ideal weight

- Have decreased anxiety
- Increase activity to a level acceptable to him or her
- Avoid serious respiratory infections

Specific indicators for these outcomes are listed for each priority patient problem under the Planning and Implementation section (see earlier).

CLINICAL JUDGMENT CHALLENGE

Patient-Centered Care; Safety QSEN

The patient is a 64-year-old man with COPD who lives with his wife of 35 years. He retired 2 years ago when his disease interfered with his job as a carpenter. He also quit smoking about a year ago. Since then, his disease has remained stable; however, he now reports that he thinks his wife is preparing for widowhood by taking over all the home chores that he always performed (including driving and bill paying), limiting his interaction with friends, and making all decisions. He is angry and depressed. Routine assessment with pulmonary function testing show his FEV_1 to be 40% of his predicted value, which is an improvement over the 32% value of FEV_1 last year.

1. What severity classification is his COPD? Provide a rationale for your choice.
2. How should you respond to his statement about the wife probably preparing for widowhood?
3. Should he continue to drive and pay bills? Why or why not?
4. What psychosocial assessment of this patient and his situation should you make?
5. Should you include the wife in any part of this discussion? Why or why not?

CYSTIC FIBROSIS

PATHOPHYSIOLOGY

Cystic fibrosis (CF) is a genetic disease that affects many organs and lethally impairs lung function. Although this disorder is present from birth and usually is first seen in early childhood, almost half of all people with cystic fibrosis in the United States are adults (Cystic Fibrosis Foundation, 2014).

The underlying problem of CF is blocked chloride transport in the cell membranes (Beery & Workman, 2012). Poor chloride transport causes the formation of mucus that has little water content and is thick. The thick, sticky mucus causes problems in the lungs, pancreas, liver, salivary glands, and testes. The mucus plugs up the airways in the lungs and the glandular tissues in nonpulmonary organs, causing atrophy and organ dysfunction. Nonpulmonary problems include pancreatic insufficiency, malnutrition, intestinal obstruction, poor growth, male sterility, and cirrhosis of the liver. Additional problems of CF in young adults include osteoporosis and diabetes mellitus. Respiratory failure is the main cause of death. Improved management has increased life expectancy even among those with severe disease to about 37 years (Cystic Fibrosis Foundation, 2014).

The pulmonary problems of CF result from the constant presence of thick, sticky mucus and are the most serious complications of the disease. The mucus narrows airways, reducing airflow and interfering with GAS EXCHANGE and oxygenation. The constant presence of mucus results in chronic respiratory tract infections, chronic bronchitis, and chronic dilation of the bronchioles (bronchiectasis). Lung abscesses are common. Over time, the bronchioles distend and have increased numbers (hyperplasia) and increased size (hypertrophy) of mucus-producing cells. Complications include pneumothorax, arterial erosion and hemorrhage, and respiratory failure.

CF is most common among white people, and about 4% are carriers. It is rare among African Americans and Asians. Males and females are affected equally.

GENETIC/GENOMIC CONSIDERATIONS

Patient-Centered Care QSEN

CF is an autosomal recessive disorder in which both gene alleles must be mutated for the disease to be expressed. The CF gene (*CTFR:* cystic fibrosis transmembrane conductance regulator) produces a protein that controls chloride movement across cell membranes. The severity of CF varies greatly; however, life expectancy is always considerably reduced, with an average of 37 years. People with one mutated allele are carriers and have few or no symptoms of CF but can pass the abnormal allele on to their children. More than 1700 different mutations have been identified (OMIM, 2013c). The inheritance of different mutations is responsible for variation in disease severity. Help patients understand why their manifestations may be more or less severe than others with the disease, even within the same family.

PATIENT-CENTERED COLLABORATIVE CARE

Assessment

Usually, but not always, cystic fibrosis (CF) is diagnosed in childhood. The major diagnostic test is sweat chloride analysis (Pagana & Pagana, 2014). The sweat chloride test is positive for CF when the chloride level in the sweat ranges between 60 and 200 mEq/L (mmol/L), compared with the normal value of 5 to 35 mEq/L. Genetic testing can be performed to determine which specific mutation a person may have. Different mutations result in different degrees of disease severity.

Nonpulmonary manifestations include abdominal distention, gastroesophageal reflux, rectal prolapse, foul-smelling stools, and **steatorrhea** (excessive fat in stools). The patient is often malnourished and has many vitamin deficiencies, especially of the fat-soluble vitamins (e.g., vitamins A, D, E, K). As pancreatic function decreases, diabetes mellitus develops with loss of insulin production. The adult with severe CF is usually smaller and thinner than average.

Pulmonary manifestations caused by CF are progressive. Respiratory infections are frequent or chronic with exacerbations. Patients usually have chest congestion, limited exercise tolerance, cough, sputum production, use of accessory muscles, and decreased pulmonary function (especially forced vital capacity [FVC] and forced expiratory volume in the first second of exhalation [FEV_1]). Chest x-rays show infiltrate and an increased anteroposterior (AP) diameter.

During an acute exacerbation or when the disease progresses to end stage, the patient has increased chest congestion, reduced activity tolerance, increased crackles, increased cough, increased sputum production (often with hemoptysis), and severe dyspnea with fatigue. Arterial blood gas (ABG) studies show acidosis (low pH), greatly reduced arterial oxygen (Pao_2) levels, increased arterial carbon dioxide ($Paco_2$) levels, and increased bicarbonate levels.

With infection, the patient has fever, an elevated white blood cell count, and decreased oxygen saturation. Other

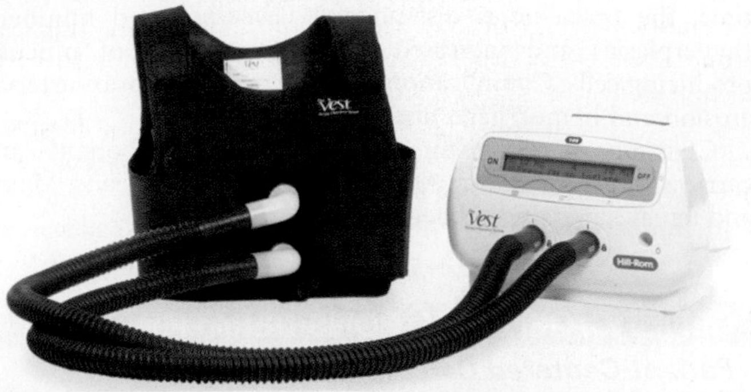

FIG. 30-12 Inflatable chest physiotherapy vest for high-frequency chest wall oscillation (HFCWO).

manifestations of infection include tachypnea, tachycardia, intercostal retractions, weight loss, and increased fatigue.

◆ *Interventions*

The patient with CF needs daily therapy to slow disease progress and enhance GAS EXCHANGE. There is no cure for CF.

Nonsurgical Management. The management of the patient with CF is complex and lifelong. Nutrition management focuses on weight maintenance, vitamin supplementation, diabetes management, and pancreatic enzyme replacement. Pulmonary management focuses on preventive maintenance and management of exacerbations. Priority nursing interventions focus on teaching about drug therapy, infection prevention, pulmonary hygiene, nutrition, and vitamin supplementation.

Preventive/maintenance therapy involves the use of positive expiratory pressure, active cycle breathing technique, and an individualized exercise program. Daily chest physiotherapy with postural drainage is beneficial for the patient with CF (Fig. 30-12). This therapy uses chest percussion, chest vibration, and dependent drainage to loosen secretions and promote drainage. Increasingly the use of a chest physiotherapy (CPT) vest is recommended (Neufeld & Keith, 2012). This system uses an inflatable vest that rapidly fills and deflates, gently compressing and releasing the chest wall up to 25 times per second, a process called high-frequency chest wall oscillation (HFCWO). The action creates mini-coughs that dislodge mucus from the bronchial walls, increase mobilization, and move it toward central airways where it can be removed by coughing or suctioning. HFCWO also thins secretions, making them easier to clear. Pulmonary function tests are monitored regularly. Daily drugs include bronchodilators, anti-inflammatories, mucolytics, and antibiotics.

Exacerbation therapy is needed when the patient with CF has increased chest congestion, reduced activity tolerance, increased or new-onset crackles, and at least a 10% decrease in FEV_1. Other exacerbation manifestations include increased sputum production with bloody or purulent sputum, increased coughing, decreased appetite, weight loss, fatigue, decreased Spo_2, and chest muscle retractions. Often infection is present, with fever, increased lung infiltrate on x-ray, and an elevated white blood cell count.

Every attempt is made to avoid mechanical ventilation for the patient with CF. Bi-level positive airway pressure (BiPAP) may be a part of daily therapy for the patient with advanced disease (Neufeld & Keith, 2012). Management focuses on airway clearance, increased GAS EXCHANGE, and antibiotic therapy. Supplemental oxygen is prescribed on the basis of Spo_2 levels. Heliox delivery of 50% oxygen and 50% helium may improve gas exchange and oxygen saturation. The respiratory therapist initiates airway clearance techniques 4 times a day. Bronchodilator and mucolytic therapies are intensified. Steroidal agents are started or increased.

Depending on the severity of the exacerbation, a 10- to 14-day course of oral antibiotics may be prescribed. For severe exacerbation, aerosolized tobramycin may be prescribed. If antibiotics are not effective or if the exacerbation is very severe, IV antibiotics are used—usually an aminoglycoside, such as tobramycin and colistin, or meropenem (Merrem).

A serious bacterial infection for patients with CF is *Burkholderia cepacia.* The organism lives in the respiratory tracts of patients with CF and is often resistant to antibiotic therapy. It is spread by casual contact from one CF patient to another. For this reason, the Cystic Fibrosis Foundation bans infected patients from participating in any foundation-sponsored events. It is also possible for *B. cepacia* to be transmitted to a CF patient during clinic and hospital visits; thus special infection control measures that limit close contact between people with CF are needed. These measures include separating infected CF patients from noninfected CF patients on hospital units and seeing them in the clinic on different days. Strict CF Foundation–approved procedures are used to clean clinic rooms and respiratory therapy equipment. Drug therapy for this infection usually includes co-trimoxazole (a combination of trimethoprim and sulfamethoxazole [Bactrim, Septra]) along with the usual drugs used for exacerbation therapy.

Teach patients about protecting themselves by avoiding direct contact of bodily fluids such as saliva and sputum. Teach them to not routinely shake hands or kiss people in social settings. Handwashing is critical because the organism also can be acquired indirectly from contaminated surfaces, such as sinks and tissues.

As life span increases for patients with CF, other problems, such as bronchiole bleeding from lung arteries, may develop. Interventional radiology may be needed to embolize the bleeding arterial branches. Patients with CF may undergo this procedure repeatedly to control hemoptysis. See Chapter 36 for information on interventional radiology vascular procedures.

Other problems that occur with CF over time include severe gastroesophageal reflux disease (GERD), osteoporosis, and sensory hearing loss. Osteoporosis increases the risk for bone fractures.

Gene therapy for CF is available for use in patients with specific gene mutations (Nakano & Tluczek, 2014). A new drug, ivacaftor (Kalydeco) has been found to be of value to patients with CF who have any one of the following specific mutations in the *CFTR* gene: G551D, G1244E, G1349D, G178R, G551S, S1251N, S1255P, S549N, or S549R. In patients with any of these mutations, the oral drug specifically targets and potentiates the CFTR channel opening so this transporter can move chloride ions across the cell membrane. This action reduces sodium and fluid absorption so that mucus is less thick and sticky. This drug has no effect in patients whose *CFTR* gene does not have any of these mutations. The most common adverse effect of the drug is an elevation of liver enzymes.

NCLEX EXAMINATION CHALLENGE
Health Promotion and Maintenance

Which precaution is most important for the nurse to teach a client who has cystic fibrosis?
A. Report a weight change of 2 pounds to your health care provider immediately.
B. Use supplemental oxygen whenever your oxygen saturation is less than 95%.
C. Eat six small meals each day instead of only three larger ones.
D. Avoid crowds and people who are ill.

Surgical Management. The surgical management of the patient with CF involves lung and/or pancreatic transplantation. The patient has reduced manifestations but is at continuing risk for lethal pulmonary infections, especially with anti-rejection drug therapy. Transplantation may extend life for some years, depending on other factors, but transplant rejection rate is high among this population, possibly caused by poor intestinal absorption of anti-rejection drugs.

Fewer lung transplants are performed compared with transplantation of other solid organs because of the scarcity of available lungs. Also, many of the people who could benefit from lung transplantation have serious problems in other organs that make this procedure even more dangerous.

Lung transplant procedures include two lobes or a single lung transplantation, as well as double-lung transplantation. The type of procedure is determined by the patient's overall condition and the life expectancy after transplantation. Usually the patient with CF has a bilateral lobe transplant from either a cadaver donor or living-related donor.

Preoperative Care. Many factors are considered before lung transplantation surgery. Recipient and donor criteria vary from one program to another, but some criteria are universal.

Recipient criteria for the patient with CF include that he or she must have severe, irreversible lung damage and still be well enough to survive the surgery. Age at transplantation is considered on an individual basis. Common exclusion criteria include a cancer diagnosis, systemic infection, human immune deficiency virus (HIV)/acquired immune deficiency syndrome (AIDS), and irreversible heart, kidney, or liver damage/disease.

Donor criteria, regardless of whether the lung tissue is obtained from a cadaver or from a living-related donor, include that the donor be infection free and cancer free, have healthy lung tissue, be a close tissue match with the recipient, and have the same blood type as the recipient. When the donor is living-related, additional criteria include an age restriction, healthy organs, and no previous chest surgery. *The two nursing priorities before surgery are teaching the patient the expected regimen of pulmonary hygiene to be used in the period immediately after surgery and assisting the patient in a pulmonary muscle strengthening/conditioning regimen.*

Operative Procedures. The patient may or may not need to be placed on cardiopulmonary bypass, depending on the exact procedure. Those having single-lung or lobe transplantation usually do not need bypass; those having double-lung transplantation usually do.

The most common incision used for lung transplantation is a transverse thoracotomy ("clamshell"). The diseased lung or lungs are removed. The new lobes, lung, or lungs are placed in the chest cavity with proper connections made to the trachea, bronchi, and blood vessels. Usually lung transplantation surgery is completed within 4 to 6 hours.

Postoperative Care. The patient is intubated for at least 48 hours, and chest tubes and arterial lines are in place. The care needed is the same as that for any thoracic surgery.

Major problem areas after lung transplantation are bleeding, infection, and transplant rejection. The patient usually remains in the ICU for several days after transplantation. Postoperative chest physiotherapy often is performed with high-frequency chest wall oscillation (HFCWO) at this time (Esguerra-Gonzalez et al., 2013).

Anti-rejection drug regimens must be started immediately after surgery, which increases the risk for infection. Combination therapy with the anti-rejection drugs, described in Chapter 17, is used for the rest of the patient's life. Corticosteroids are avoided in the first 10 to 14 days after surgery because of their negative impact on the healing process.

PULMONARY ARTERIAL HYPERTENSION

❖ PATHOPHYSIOLOGY

General pulmonary hypertension can occur as a complication of other lung disorders. Primary pulmonary arterial hypertension (PAH) (also known as *idiopathic pulmonary hypertension*) occurs in the absence of other lung disorders, and its cause is unknown; however, exposure to some drugs, such as fenfluramine/phentermine (Pondimin or "Fen-Phen") or dasatinib (Sprycel), increases the risk (World Health Organization [WHO], 2011). The disorder is rare and occurs mostly in women between the ages of 20 and 40 years (McCance et al., 2014). The familial PAH form appears to be transmitted in an autosomal dominant pattern with reduced penetrance (OMIM, 2013d).

The pathologic problem in PAH is blood vessel constriction with increasing vascular resistance in the lung. Pulmonary blood pressure rises and blood flow decreases through the lungs, leading to poor PERFUSION and GAS EXCHANGE with hypoxemia. Eventually, the right side of the heart fails *(cor pulmonale)* from the continuous workload of pumping against the high pulmonary pressures. Without treatment, death usually occurs within 2 years after diagnosis.

GENETIC/GENOMIC CONSIDERATIONS
Patient-Centered Care QSEN

About 50% of patients with pulmonary arterial hypertension have a genetic mutation in the *BMPR2* gene, which codes for a growth factor receptor (Weber et al., 2011). Excessive activation of this receptor allows increased growth of arterial smooth muscle in the lungs, making these arteries thicker. Many more people have mutations in this gene than have PAH. It is thought that these mutations increase the susceptibility to PAH when other, often unknown, environmental factors also are present. Mutations in other genes, such as the *PPH1* gene and the *SMAD9* gene, are also associated with thickening of lung arteries and increased risk for PAH (OMIM, 2013d).

Often PAH is not diagnosed until late in the disease process when the lungs and heart have already been significantly damaged. Teach people, especially women, who have a first-degree relative (parent or sibling) with PAH to have regular health checks and to consult a health care provider whenever pulmonary problems are present.

TABLE 30-3 Severity Classification for Primary Pulmonary Arterial Hypertension

CLASS	MANIFESTATIONS
I	Pulmonary hypertension diagnosed by pulmonary function tests and right-sided cardiac catheterization No limitation of physical activity Moderate physical activity does not induce dyspnea, fatigue, chest pain, or light-headedness
II	No manifestations at rest Mild to moderate physical activity induces dyspnea, fatigue, chest pain, or light-headedness
III	No or slight manifestations at rest Mild (less than ordinary) activity induces dyspnea, fatigue, chest pain, or light-headedness
IV	Dyspnea and fatigue present at rest Unable to carry out any level of physical activity without manifestations Manifestations of right-sided heart failure apparent (dependent edema, engorged neck veins, enlarged liver)

❖ PATIENT-CENTERED COLLABORATIVE CARE

◆ Assessment

The most common early manifestations are dyspnea and fatigue in an otherwise healthy adult. Some patients also have angina-like chest pain. Table 30-3 lists the classification of PAH.

Diagnosis is made from the results of right-sided heart catheterization showing elevated pulmonary pressures. Other test results suggesting PAH include abnormal ventilation-perfusion scans, pulmonary function tests (PFTs) showing reduced functional pulmonary volumes with reduced diffusion capacity, and computed tomography (CT).

◆ Interventions

Drug therapy can reduce pulmonary pressures and slow the development of cor pulmonale by dilating pulmonary vessels and preventing clot formation. Warfarin (Coumadin) is taken daily to achieve an international normalized ratio (INR) of 1.5 to 2.0. Calcium channel blockers have been used to dilate blood vessels. The two classes of drugs that have been shown to be most effective in the treatment of PAH are the endothelin-receptor antagonists and the prostacyclin agents.

Endothelin-receptor agonists, such as bosentan (Tracleer), induce blood vessel relaxation and decrease pulmonary arterial pressure. These agents, however, cause general vessel dilation and some degree of hypotension. A new endothelin receptor antagonist drug, macitentan (Opsumit), has been approved for management of adults with PAH. This oral drug is taken as a 10-mg tablet once daily, with or without food. Teach patients to take the drug with a glass of water, and teach them not to break, chew, or crush the tablet.

Because macitentan can cause birth defects, its use is contraindicated for women who are pregnant or breastfeeding. Instruct women who are sexually active and within childbearing age to use at least two reliable methods of contraception while taking this drug. In addition, the drug can harm the liver, and patients should avoid drinking alcoholic beverages while taking it.

Natural and synthetic prostacyclin agents provide the best specific dilation of pulmonary blood vessels. Continuous infusion of epoprostenol (Flolan, Veletri) or treprostinil (Remodulin) through a small IV pump reduces pulmonary pressures and increases lung blood flow (Fuentes et al., 2012). Treprostinil also can be delivered by continuous subcutaneous infusion. These continuous infusions of prostacyclin drugs can be performed by the patient at home and in other settings. These drugs also are continued when the patient is hospitalized for any reason. The unusual continuous infusion, the need to keep an IV line dedicated strictly to prostacyclin infusion, and the varied dosages of the different brands of prostacyclins contribute to a high drug error rate for administration of this drug. See the Quality Improvement box for some recommendations to reduce this error rate.

The prostacyclin agents iloprost (Ilomedin, Ventavis) and treprostinil (Tyvaso) can be delivered by inhalation (Poms & Kingman, 2011). A drug given along with prostacyclins is sildenafil (Revatio, Viagra) administered orally or IV.

While most patients with PAH need to stay on prostacyclin drugs until lung transplantation or disease progression to death, a small percentage of patients have been successfully weaned off prostacyclin drug therapy. These patients are maintained on oral bosentan, sildenafil, and warfarin therapy (Demerouti et al., 2013). The uncertain outcome of treatment and the serious nature of the disorder have been reported to increase the levels of depression and anxiety in patients diagnosed with PAH (Roberts-Collins et al., 2013).

QUALITY IMPROVEMENT (QSEN)

Continuous Prostacyclin Therapy Error Prevention

Kingman, M., & Chin, K. (2013). Safety recommendations for administering intravenous prostacyclins in the hospital. *Critical Care Nurse, 33*(5), 32-34, 36-41.

Intravenous prostacyclin drugs are most widely prescribed for management of pulmonary arterial hypertension. These drugs are categorized as *high risk* and have some unique issues, one of which is that the patient receives them by continuous infusion 24 hours daily, 7 days a week. In the hospital setting, administration of these drugs is associated with a high error rate. Two of the most common errors were flushing the dedicated prostacyclin infusion line and administering the wrong brand of prostacyclin. Because patient lives depend on continuous and correct infusion of prostacyclins, leading experts in the field were asked to generate recommendations for IV administration to reduce the error rate.

In addition to many standard recommendations for reducing drug errors, two unique ones were developed. The first involved safety strategies for ensuring the dedicated line is not flushed. The second unique recommendation involved including the patient in the administration of the prostacyclins. Most patients have been responsible for self-administration of the drug in the community setting and have been highly trained to do so correctly. Thus the recommendation is that the patient should be included in the administration (while in the hospital setting) to the "fullest extent possible," as an expert on drug administration and trouble-shooting.

Commentary: Implications for Practice and Research

This expert-generated set of recommendations for drug administration safety is a departure from the usual quality improvement (QI) project that is either unit-based or institution-based. It represents the next step in the QI process of standardizing procedures for an identified population-based problem across multiple institutions. Because it is a beginning project using a descriptive design rather than a randomized clinical trial, it was reasonable to first determine the justification for a practice change. A randomized clinical trial approach should be the next step in establishing the evidence to support a specific process or procedure to reduce drug administration errors.

! NURSING SAFETY PRIORITY QSEN

Critical Rescue

A critical nursing priority for a patient undergoing therapy with IV prostacyclin agents is to ensure that the drug therapy is never interrupted. Deaths have been reported if the drug delivery is interrupted even for a matter of minutes. Teach the patient to always have backup drug cassettes and battery packs. If these are not available or if the line is disrupted, the patient should go to the emergency department immediately.

Another critical priority is helping the patient receiving IV prostacyclin agents prevent sepsis. The central line IV setup provides an access for organisms to directly enter the bloodstream. Teach the patient to use strict aseptic technique in all aspects of using the drug delivery system. Also teach him or her to notify the pulmonologist at the first manifestation of any infection.

When the heart has undergone hypertrophy and cardiac output has fallen, the patient may be started on a regimen of digoxin (Lanoxin) and diuretics. Oxygen therapy is used when dyspnea is uncomfortable. This therapy improves function and reduces manifestations but does not cure PAH.

Surgical management of PAH involves lung transplantation. When cor pulmonale also is present, the patient may need a combined heart-lung transplantation. It is not known whether the process of pulmonary vasoconstriction can begin again in the transplanted lungs or if this is a "cure."

INTERSTITIAL PULMONARY DISEASES

The category of interstitial pulmonary diseases contains a variety of lung disorders, also called *fibrotic lung diseases,* that have some features in common. All affect the alveoli, blood vessels, and surrounding support tissue of the lungs rather than the airways. Thus these disorders are restrictive (preventing good expansion and recoil of the gas exchange unit), not obstructive. With restrictive disease, the lung tissues thicken, causing reduced GAS EXCHANGE and "stiff" lungs that do not expand well. Air trapping does not occur, and the patient does not develop a "barrel chest." Often the onset of these disorders is slow, and dyspnea is the most common manifestation.

SARCOIDOSIS

❖ PATHOPHYSIOLOGY

Sarcoidosis is a disease of INFLAMMATION of unknown cause that can affect any organ, but the lung is involved most often. It develops over time with noncancerous inflammatory growths called granulomas forming in the lungs.

Pulmonary sarcoidosis involves autoimmune responses in which the normally protective T-lymphocytes increase and cause damaging actions in the alveolar cells. No single cause for T-lymphocyte activation has been identified, although infection and genetic predisposition may play a role. Alveolar inflammation (alveolitis) occurs from the presence of immune cells in the alveoli. Chronic INFLAMMATION causes fibrosis (scar tissue formation) in the lungs. The fibrosis reduces lung compliance (elasticity) and GAS EXCHANGE. Cor pulmonale (right-sided cardiac failure) is often present because the heart can no longer pump effectively against the stiff, fibrotic lung.

The disease affects young adults. Manifestations include enlarged lymph nodes in the hilar area of the lungs, lung infiltrate on chest x-ray, skin lesions, and eye lesions. The first indication of disease may be an abnormal chest x-ray in an otherwise healthy patient. Common manifestations include cough, dyspnea, hemoptysis, and chest discomfort. In many patients, the illness resolves permanently. Others have progressive pulmonary fibrosis and severe systemic disease.

❖ PATIENT-CENTERED COLLABORATIVE CARE

Sarcoidosis is suspected in the patient who has a cough, dyspnea, and an abnormal chest x-ray but is otherwise asymptomatic. Other conditions to rule out before diagnosing sarcoidosis are lung infections and cancer. Bronchoscopy with biopsy may help diagnose this disorder (see Chapter 27).

Sarcoidosis is staged on the basis of x-ray findings. Higher stages have greater damage and more widespread disease. Pulmonary function studies often show a restrictive pattern of decreased lung volumes and impaired diffusing capacity. Irreversible lung changes occur in a small percentage of patients. Patients who have severe restrictive disease may develop pulmonary hypertension.

The focus of therapy is to reduce manifestations and prevent fibrosis. Management varies. If the patient is asymptomatic and has normal pulmonary function, no treatment is given. Decreased total lung capacity (TLC), diffusing capacity, or forced vital capacity (FVC); involvement of other organs; and hypercalcemia are indicators for treatment.

Corticosteroids are the main type of therapy. Dosages vary from 40 to 60 mg daily with tapering doses over 6 to 8 weeks, to a maintenance dose of 10 to 15 mg daily for 6 months. Further therapy may continue over 12 months. Drugs under study for management of this disease include thalidomide (Thalomid), infliximab (Remicade), and adalimumab (Humira). Follow-up and monitoring include assessment of symptom severity, pulmonary function studies, chest x-rays, a complete blood count, serum creatinine, serum calcium, and urinalysis. Teach the patient and family about side effects of steroid therapy, the need to avoid infection, and energy conservation strategies (see discussion of activity intolerance, p. 565 in the Chronic Obstructive Pulmonary Disease section).

IDIOPATHIC PULMONARY FIBROSIS

❖ PATHOPHYSIOLOGY

Idiopathic pulmonary fibrosis is a common restrictive lung disease. The patient usually is an older adult with a history of cigarette smoking, chronic exposure to inhalation irritants, or exposure to the drugs *amiodarone* (Cordarone) or *ambrisentan* (Letairis, Volibris) (WHO, 2012). Most patients have progressive disease with few remission periods. Even with proper treatment, most patients usually survive less than 5 years after diagnosis.

Pulmonary fibrosis is an example of excessive wound healing with loss of CELLULAR REGULATION. Once lung injury occurs, inflammation begins tissue repair. The INFLAMMATION continues beyond normal healing time, causing fibrosis and scarring. These changes thicken alveolar tissues, making GAS EXCHANGE difficult.

❖ PATIENT-CENTERED COLLABORATIVE CARE

The onset is slow, with early manifestations of mild dyspnea on exertion. Pulmonary function tests show decreased forced vital capacity (FVC). High resolution computed tomography (HRCT) shows a "honeycomb" pattern in affected lung tissue (Lewis & Scullion, 2012). As the fibrosis progresses, the patient becomes more dyspneic and hypoxemia becomes severe. Eventually, he or she needs high levels of oxygen and often is still hypoxemic. Respirations are rapid and shallow.

Therapy focuses on slowing the fibrotic process and managing dyspnea. Corticosteroids and other immunosuppressants are the mainstays of therapy. Immunosuppressant drugs include cytotoxic drugs such as cyclophosphamide (Cytoxan, Neosar, Procytox ♣), azathioprine (Imuran), chlorambucil (Leukeran), or methotrexate (Folex). These drugs have many side effects, including increased infection risk, nausea, and lung and liver damage, and have shown limited benefit. New studies using the combination therapy of corticosteroids, azathioprine, interferon gamma 1b, and *N*-acetylcysteine show promise of slowing disease progression. Early clinical trials using drugs that help improve CELLULAR REGULATION, such as those that belong to the class of mitogen-activated protein kinases inhibitors (MAPKIs), are being conducted. Starting any drug therapy early is critical, even though not all patients respond to therapy. Even among those who have a response to therapy, the disease eventually continues to progress and leads to death by respiratory failure. Lung transplantation is a curative therapy; however, the selection criteria, cost, and availability of organs make this option unlikely for most patients.

The patient and family need support and help with community resources after diagnosis. Nursing care focuses on assisting the patient and family in understanding the disease process and maintaining hope for control of the fibrosis (Lewis & Scullion, 2012). It is important to prevent respiratory infections. Teach the patient and family about the manifestations of infection and to avoid respiratory irritants, crowds, and people who are ill.

Home oxygen is needed by the time the patient has dyspnea because significant fibrosis has already occurred and GAS EXCHANGE is reduced. Teach about oxygen use as a continuous therapy. Fatigue is a major problem. Teach the patient and family about energy conservation measures (see discussion of activity intolerance on p. 565 in the Chronic Obstructive Pulmonary Disease section). These measures and rest help reduce the work of breathing and oxygen consumption. Encourage the patient to pace activities and accept assistance as needed.

In the later stages of the disease, the focus is to reduce the sensation of dyspnea. This is often accomplished with the use of oral, parenteral, or nebulized morphine. Provide information about hospice, which supports and coordinates resources to meet the needs of the patient and family when the prognosis for survival is less than 6 months (see Chapter 7).

OCCUPATIONAL PULMONARY DISEASE

❖ PATHOPHYSIOLOGY

Exposure to occupational or environmental fumes, dust, vapors, gases, bacterial or fungal antigens, and allergens can result in a variety of respiratory disorders. Depending on the degree, frequency, and intensity of exposure and on the specific disease, patients may have acute reversible effects or chronic lung disease. All occupational pulmonary diseases are made worse by cigarette smoking; thus smoking-cessation efforts are very important.

Many occupational diseases have an onset of manifestations long after the initial exposure to the offending agent. The patient's personal history can provide clues about the presence and cause of occupational pulmonary diseases such as occupational asthma, pneumoconiosis, diffuse interstitial fibrosis, and extrinsic allergic alveolitis. Chart 30-12 lists the key features of these disorders.

❖ PATIENT-CENTERED COLLABORATIVE CARE

Consider an occupational cause for patients with new-onset asthma or dyspnea. Ask about occupational exposure and onset of manifestations because there may or may not be a latency period between exposure and development of manifestations. Determine whether manifestations are acute or chronic. Ask about the use of inhalation protection and about cigarette smoking (see Chapter 27).

The patient who develops occupational asthma should be removed from the site of exposure, transferred to a job without exposure, and treated with asthma drugs. Nursing care is similar to the care for asthma not caused by the workplace environment. Refer the patient to a social worker, who provides information regarding compensation and pensions.

Nursing interventions for patients with occupational lung restrictive disease are the same as for those with emphysema. Hypoxemic patients require supplemental oxygen. In addition, respiratory therapies to promote sputum clearance are essential.

BRONCHIOLITIS OBLITERANS ORGANIZING PNEUMONIA

❖ PATHOPHYSIOLOGY

Bronchiolitis obliterans organizing pneumonia (BOOP) is an INFLAMMATION that reduces CELL REGULATION and allows connective tissue plugs to form in the lower airways and the tissue between the alveoli. Inflammation in the lumen triggers white blood cell clumping with uncontrolled fibroblast growth that occludes and eventually obliterates these airways and leads to restricted lung volume with decreased vital capacity. BOOP is not a true pneumonia, but the manifestations resemble respiratory infection.

The cause of BOOP is not known although many personal and environmental conditions are associated with it. Suggested triggers include infectious organisms, drugs (chemotherapy agents, certain antibiotics [sulfa-based drugs, cephalosporins, amphotericin B], antiseizure drugs, cocaine, and amiodarone), or the presence of a connective tissue disorder, such as rheumatoid arthritis or systemic lupus erythematosus. It is also associated with chest radiotherapy for breast or lung cancer.

BOOP is most common in people between ages 30 and 60 years and affects both genders. It is not associated with cigarette smoking. Depending on how fast the problem progresses and the degree to which it interferes with GAS EXCHANGE, BOOP can lead to death.

❖ PATIENT-CENTERED COLLABORATIVE CARE

An event or condition triggers excessive INFLAMMATION in the lumens of lower airways, causing dyspnea, fever, mild cough,

CHART 30-12 **Key Features**

Common Occupational Pulmonary Diseases

DISEASE AND CATEGORY	CAUSES AND MANIFESTATIONS
Occupational Asthmas	
Latency (allergic) asthma	Airway narrowing related only to workplace exposures Atopic allergic response to industrial irritants Develops after a period of exposure (from several weeks to several years) Characterized by airflow limitation Usually resolves when exposure ceases Obstructive disease
Irritant-induced asthma	Manifestations appear only in the workplace First onset usually occurs within 24 hours of exposure Common irritants are chlorine, ammonia, and phosgene Characterized by sloughing of epithelium, thickening of the basement membranes, and mucosal inflammation Early manifestations include cough, wheeze, and dyspnea High exposures can lead to pulmonary edema, ARDS, and death Most tissue changes are permanent Obstructive and restrictive disease
Pneumoconiosis	
Silicosis	Chronic fibrosis from long-term inhalation of silica dust Found among people working in mines, stone quarries, and foundries. Also found in people working in these industries: glass making, pottery, sandblasting, tile and brick making, soap and polishes, and manufacture of filters Characterized by nodule formation between alveoli leading to fibrosis Manifestations include dyspnea on exertion, fatigue, weight loss, reduced lung volume, and upper lobe fibrosis Restrictive disease
Coal Miner's Disease (Black Lung Disease)	Massive deposits of coal dust in the lungs leading to diffuse fibrosis Develops earlier among miners who smoke Early manifestations are similar to bronchitis Emphysema is a late development Restrictive disease
Diffuse Interstitial Fibrosis	
Asbestosis	Occurs among people who work in asbestos mines, building construction/remodeling, and shipyards Characterized by diffuse pleural thickening and diaphragmatic calcification Restrictive disease
Talcosis	Occurs among people who work in industries that manufacture paint, ceramics, roofing materials, cosmetics, and rubber goods Restrictive disease
Berylliosis	Occurs among people who work in industries in which metal is heated (steel mills, welding) or metal is machined, creating dust Has a genetic component for increased susceptibility to disease after beryllium exposure Restrictive disease
Extrinsic Allergic Alveolitis	
"Farmer's Lung" "Bird Fancier's Lung" "Machine Operator's Lung"	Hypersensitivity pneumonitis as an immunologic response to inhaling dust or chemical that contains bacterial or fungal antigens Characterized by formation of granulomas with central necrosis in the alveoli and surrounding blood vessels Restrictive disease

ARDS, Acute respiratory distress syndrome.

flu-like symptoms, and crackles on auscultation. In some patients, the problem resolves spontaneously. In others, it can rapidly progress to death within days. Usually manifestations are present for weeks or months and do not improve with antibiotic therapy.

Diagnosis of BOOP is difficult because manifestations are similar to many other respiratory problems. Chest x-rays and CT scans may show pulmonary tissue changes that only suggest BOOP, not confirm it. Biopsy with histologic findings is needed to confirm a BOOP diagnosis.

The most effective treatment for BOOP is corticosteroid therapy. A short course of the drug for acute disease can reduce manifestations, and the patient may never have a relapse. For those patients with more severe disease and those with any type of additional health problem, a year of corticosteroid therapy may be needed. In this population, BOOP is more of a chronic disease with some degree of permanent restrictive disease. Exacerbations can occur.

LUNG CANCER

❖ *PATHOPHYSIOLOGY*

Lung cancer is a leading cause of cancer-related deaths worldwide. In North America, more deaths from lung cancer occur each year than from prostate cancer, breast cancer, and colon cancer combined. The American Cancer Society estimates that more than 228,000 new cases of lung cancer are diagnosed each year and that more than 160,000 deaths occur each year from it (American Cancer Society [ACS], 2014). The overall 5-year survival for all patients with lung cancer is only 16%. This poor long-term survival is because most lung cancers are diagnosed at a late stage, when metastasis is present. Only 15% of patients have small tumors and localized disease at the time of diagnosis. The 5-year survival rate for this population is 52% (ACS, 2014).

Despite many advances in cancer treatment, the prognosis for lung cancer remains poor unless the tumor can be removed completely by surgery. Treatment often focuses on relieving symptoms (**palliation**) rather than cure because of metastasis.

Most primary lung cancers arise as a result of failure of CELLULAR REGULATION in the bronchial epithelium. These cancers are collectively called *bronchogenic carcinomas.* Lung cancers are classified as small cell lung cancer (SCLC) and non–small cell lung cancer (NSCLC). Chapter 21 discusses the general mechanisms and processes of cancer development.

Metastasis (spread) of lung cancer occurs by direct extension, through the blood, and by invading lymph glands and vessels. Tumors in the bronchial tubes can grow and obstruct the bronchus partially or completely. Tumors in other areas of lung tissue can grow so large that they can compress and obstruct the airway. Compression of the alveoli, nerves, blood vessels, and lymph vessels can occur and also interfere with GAS EXCHANGE. Lung cancer can spread to the lung lymph nodes, distant lymph nodes, and other tissues including bone, liver, brain, and adrenal glands.

Additional manifestations, known as *paraneoplastic syndromes,* complicate certain lung cancers. The paraneoplastic syndromes are caused by hormones secreted by tumor cells and occur most commonly with SCLC. Table 30-4 lists the endocrine paraneoplastic syndromes that may occur with lung cancer.

Staging of lung cancer is performed to assess the size and extent of the disease. These factors are related to survival. Lung cancer staging is based on the TNM system (T, primary tumor; N, number of regional lymph nodes; M, distant metastasis). See Table 21-5 in Chapter 21 for a cancer staging system. Higher numbers represent later stages and less chance for cure or long-term survival.

TABLE 30-4 Endocrine Paraneoplastic Syndromes Associated with Lung Cancer

ECTOPIC HORMONE	MANIFESTATION
Adrenocorticotropic hormone (ACTH)	Cushing's syndrome
Antidiuretic hormone	Syndrome of inappropriate antidiuretic hormone (SIADH) Weight gain General edema Dilution of serum electrolytes
Follicle-stimulating hormone (FSH)	Gynecomastia
Parathyroid hormone	Hypercalcemia
Ectopic insulin	Hypoglycemia

Incidence and Prevalence

Lung cancers occur as a result of repeated exposure to inhaled substances that cause chronic tissue irritation or INFLAMMATION interfering with CELLULAR REGULATION of cell growth. Cigarette smoking is the major risk factor and is responsible for 85% of all lung cancer deaths (ACS, 2014). The risk for lung cancer is directly related to the total exposure to cigarette smoke as determined by the number of years of smoking and number of packs of cigarettes smoked per day (pack-years). Pipe and cigar smoking also increase risk. The incidence of lung cancer decreases when smoking stops but remains higher than among people who have never smoked.

Etiology and Genetic Risk

Nonsmokers exposed to "passive," or "secondhand," smoke also have a greater risk for lung cancer than do nonsmokers who are minimally exposed to cigarette smoke. See Chapter 27 for a discussion of passive smoking risks.

Other risk factors include chronic exposure to asbestos, beryllium, chromium, coal distillates, cobalt, iron oxide, mustard gas, petroleum distillates, radiation, tar, nickel, and uranium (Held-Warmkessel & Schiech, 2014). Air pollution with hydrocarbons also increases the risk for lung cancer.

GENETIC/GENOMIC CONSIDERATIONS

Patient-Centered Care QSEN

Lung cancer development varies among people with similar smoking histories, suggesting that genetic factors can influence susceptibility. Genome-wide association studies have found specific variations in a variety of genes that increase the susceptibility to lung cancer development (OMIM, 2013a). Differences in a gene that regulates cell division, the *Tp53* gene, may be the most important genetic susceptibility link for lung cancer development. Mutations in the alleles of this gene are known to increase the susceptibility to a wide variety of cancers both with and without exposure to environmental risks, including lung cancer development among smokers and nonsmokers. Help patients understand that lung cancer susceptibility varies by genetic issues as well as by exposure to carcinogens.

Health Promotion and Maintenance

Primary prevention for lung cancer is directed at reducing tobacco smoking. Chapter 27 discusses strategies for assisting people to reduce smoking and means to protect lungs from other exposures to inhalation irritants linked to lung cancer development.

Secondary prevention by early detection involves screening of people at high risk for lung cancer development. Annual CT scans can detect cancers at stage I, when cure is probable and long-term survival (longer than 5 years) is very likely (ACS, 2014; Lehto, 2014).

❖ PATIENT-CENTERED COLLABORATIVE CARE

◆ Assessment

History. Ask the patient about risk factors, including smoking, hazards in the workplace, and warning signals (Table 30-5). Calculate the pack-year smoking history as described in Chapter 27.

Ask about the presence of lung cancer manifestations, such as hoarseness, cough, sputum production, hemoptysis, shortness of breath, or change in endurance. Assessing for and

TABLE 30-5 Warning Signals Associated with Lung Cancer

- Hoarseness
- Change in respiratory pattern
- Persistent cough or change in cough
- Blood-streaked sputum
- Rust-colored or purulent sputum
- Frank hemoptysis
- Chest pain or chest tightness
- Shoulder, arm, or chest wall pain
- Recurring episodes of pleural effusion, pneumonia, or bronchitis
- Dyspnea
- Fever associated with one or two other signs
- Wheezing
- Weight loss
- Clubbing of the fingers

documenting these manifestations provide information about the extent of nursing care and teaching the patient needs now and can be used later to determine therapy effectiveness. Many manifestations are common and may have been present for years. Ask the patient to describe any recent changes in manifestations or if position affects them.

Assess for chest pain or discomfort, which can occur at any stage of tumor development. Chest pain may be localized or on just one side and can range from mild to severe. Ask about any sensation of fullness, tightness, or pressure in the chest, which may suggest obstruction. A piercing chest pain or pleuritic pain may occur on inspiration. Pain radiating to the arm results from tumor invasion of nerve plexuses in advanced disease.

Physical Assessment/Clinical Manifestations—Pulmonary. Manifestations of lung cancer are often nonspecific and appear late in the disease. Specific manifestations depend on tumor location. Chills, fever, and cough may be related to pneumonitis or bronchitis that occurs with obstruction. Assess sputum quantity and character. Blood-tinged sputum may occur with bleeding from a tumor. Hemoptysis is a later finding in the course of the disease. If infection or necrosis is present, sputum may be purulent and copious.

Breathing may be labored or painful. Obstructive breathing may occur as prolonged exhalation alternating with periods of shallow breathing. Rapid, shallow breathing occurs with pleuritic chest pain and an elevated diaphragm. Look for and document abnormal retractions, the use of accessory muscles, flared nares, stridor, and asymmetric diaphragmatic movement on inspiration. Dyspnea and wheezing may be present with airway obstruction. Ask about the level of dyspnea at rest, with activity, and in the supine position. Determine how much the dyspnea interferes with the patient's participation in ADLs, work, recreational activities, and family responsibilities. Ask him or her to compare participation in activities during the past week with that of a month ago and a year ago.

Areas of tenderness or masses may be felt when palpating the chest wall. Increased vibrations felt on the chest wall (**fremitus**) indicate areas of the lung where airspaces are replaced with tumor or fluid. Fremitus is decreased or absent when the bronchus is obstructed. The trachea may be displaced from midline if a mass is present in the area.

Lung areas with masses sound dull or flat rather than hollow or resonant on chest percussion. Breath sounds may change with the presence of a tumor. Wheezes indicate partial obstruction of airflow in passages narrowed by tumors. Decreased or absent breath sounds indicate complete obstruction of an airway by a tumor or fluid. Increased loudness or sound intensity of the voice while listening to breath sounds indicates increased density of lung tissue from tumor compression. A pleural friction rub may be heard when INFLAMMATION also is present.

Physical Assessment/Clinical Manifestations—Nonpulmonary. Many other systems can be affected by lung cancer and have changes at the time of diagnosis. Heart sounds may be muffled by a tumor or fluid around the heart *(cardiac tamponade)*. Dysrhythmias may occur as a result of hypoxemia or direct pressure of the tumor on the heart. Cyanosis of the lips and fingertips or clubbing of the fingers may be present (see Fig. 30-10).

Bones lose density with tumor invasion and break easily. The patient may have bone pain or pathologic fractures. Handle him or her carefully. Thin bones can fracture with little pressure and without trauma. Even heavy coughing can break a rib.

Late manifestations of lung cancer usually include fatigue, weight loss, anorexia, dysphagia, and nausea and vomiting. Superior vena cava syndrome may result from tumor pressure in or around the vena cava. This syndrome is an emergency (see Chapter 22) and requires immediate intervention. The patient may have confusion or personality changes from brain metastasis. Bowel and bladder tone or function may be affected by tumor spread to the spine and spinal cord, which also can change gait.

Psychosocial Assessment. The poor prognosis for lung cancer has made it a much-feared disease. Dyspnea and pain add to the patient's fear and anxiety. The patient with a history of cigarette smoking may feel guilt and shame. Convey acceptance, and interact with the patient in a nonjudgmental way. Encourage the patient and family to express their feelings about the possible diagnosis of lung cancer.

Diagnostic Assessment. The diagnosis of lung cancer is made by examination of cancer cells. Cytologic testing of early-morning sputum specimens may identify tumor cells; however, cancer cells may not be present in the sputum. When pleural effusion is present, fluid is obtained by thoracentesis for cytology.

Most commonly, lung lesions are first identified on chest x-rays. CT examinations are then used to identify the lesions more clearly and to guide biopsy procedures.

A thoracoscopy to directly view lung tissue may be performed through a video-assisted thoracoscope entering the chest cavity via small incisions through the chest wall. Spread to mediastinal lymph nodes is assessed with a mediastinoscopy through a small chest incision.

Other diagnostic studies may be needed to determine how widely the cancer has spread. Such tests include needle biopsy of lymph nodes, direct surgical biopsy, and thoracentesis with pleural biopsy. MRI and radionuclide scans of the liver, spleen, brain, and bone help determine the location of metastatic tumors. Pulmonary function tests (PFTs) and arterial blood gas (ABG) analysis help determine the overall respiratory status. Positron emission tomography (PET) scanning is becoming the most thorough way to locate metastases. Together, these tests help determine the extent of the cancer and the best methods to treat it.

◆ Interventions for Cure

Interventions for the patient with lung cancer can have the purposes of curing the disease, increasing survival time, and enhancing quality of life through palliation. Both nonsurgical and surgical interventions are used to achieve these purposes. Some patients with lung cancer may undergo interventions for all three purposes at different stages in the disease process. Cure is most likely for patients who undergo treatment for stage I or II disease. Cure is rare for patients who undergo treatment for stage III or IV disease, although survival time is increasing.

Nonsurgical Management. *Chemotherapy* is often the treatment of choice for lung cancers, especially small cell lung cancer (SCLC). It may be used alone or as adjuvant therapy in combination with surgery for non–small cell lung cancer (NSCLC). The exact combination of drugs used depends on the response of the tumor and the overall health of the patient; however, most include platinum-based agents.

Side effects that occur with chemotherapy for lung cancer include chemotherapy-induced nausea and vomiting (CINV), **alopecia** (hair loss), open sores on mucous membranes (**mucositis**), immunosuppression with neutropenia, anemia, **thrombocytopenia** (decreased numbers of platelets), and peripheral neuropathy. Consult Chapter 22 for a thorough discussion of the nursing care needs for patients who have these side effects.

Immunosuppression with neutropenia, which greatly increases the risk for infection, is the major dose-limiting side effect of chemotherapy for lung cancer. It can be managed by the use of growth factors to stimulate bone marrow production of immune system cells. Teach the patient and family about precautions to take to reduce the patient's chances of developing an infection (see Chart 22-4 in Chapter 22). (See Chapter 22 for more information about chemotherapy and associated nursing care.)

Targeted therapy is now becoming common in the treatment of lung cancer. These agents take advantage of one or more differences in cancer cell growth or metabolism that is either not present or only slightly present in normal cells. Agents used as targeted therapies often are antibodies that work to disrupt cancer cell division in one of several ways. Some of these drugs "target" and block growth factor receptors, such as the epithelial growth factor receptor inhibitors (EGFRIs) or the vascular endothelial growth factor receptor inhibitors (VEGFRIs). When a lung cancer cell's growth depends on having the growth factors bind to their specific receptors, blocking the receptors may slow cancer cell growth. Agents most often used, along with other therapy, for targeted therapy of certain types of non–small cell lung cancer are erlotinib (Tarceva), bevacizumab (Avastin), and crizotinib (Xalkori) (Cagle & Chirieac, 2012).

Radiation therapy can be an effective treatment for locally advanced lung cancers confined to the chest. Best results are seen when radiation is used in addition to surgery or chemotherapy. Radiation may be performed before surgery to shrink the tumor and make resection easier.

Usually radiation therapy for lung cancer is performed daily for a 5- to 6-week period. Only the areas thought to have cancer are positioned in the radiation path. The immediate side effects of this treatment are skin irritation and peeling, fatigue, nausea, and taste changes. Some patients have esophagitis during therapy, making nutrition more difficult. Collaborate with a dietitian to teach patients to eat foods that are soft, bland, and high in calories. Suggest that the patient drink liquid nutrition supplements between meals to maintain weight and energy levels.

Skin care in the radiation-treated area can be difficult. Because skin in the radiation path is more sensitive to sun damage, advise patients to avoid direct skin exposure to the sun during treatment and for at least 1 year after radiation is completed. See Chapter 22 for other nursing care issues associated with radiation therapy.

Photodynamic therapy (PDT) may be used to remove small bronchial tumors when they are accessible by bronchoscopy. The patient is first injected with an agent that sensitizes cells to light. This drug enters all cells but leaves normal cells more rapidly than cancer cells. Usually, within 48 to 72 hours, most of the drug has collected in high concentrations in cancer cells. At this time, the patient goes to the operating room where, under anesthesia and intubation, a laser light is focused on the tumor. The light activates a chemical reaction within those cells retaining the sensitizing drug that induces irreversible cell damage. Some cells die and slough immediately; others continue to slough for several days.

When PDT is used in the airways, the patient usually requires a stay in the ICU for airway management. The sloughing tissue can block the airway as can airway edema from the inflammatory response of the tissues. In addition, the patient is at risk for bronchial hemorrhage, fistula formation, and hemoptysis. Patients who have undergone bronchial PDT are very sensitive to light for days to weeks after treatment.

Surgical Management. Surgery is the main treatment for stage I and stage II NSCLC. Total tumor removal may result in a cure. If complete resection is not possible, the surgeon removes the bulk of the tumor. The specific surgery depends on the stage of the cancer and the patient's overall health. Lung cancer surgery may involve removal of the tumor only, removal of a lung segment, removal of a lobe (**lobectomy**), or removal of the entire lung (**pneumonectomy**). These procedures can be performed by open thoracotomy or by thoracoscopy with minimally invasive surgery in select patients.

Preoperative Care. The focus of nursing care before surgery is to relieve anxiety and promote the patient's participation (see Chapter 14 for routine preoperative care). Encourage the patient to express fears and concerns, reinforce the surgeon's explanation of the procedure, and provide education related to what is expected after surgery. Teach about the probable location of the surgical incision or thoracoscopy openings, shoulder exercises, and the chest tube and drainage system (except after pneumonectomy).

Operative Procedures. Three types of incisions can be made depending on the location of the cancer: posterolateral, anterolateral, and median sternotomy (Fig. 30-13). The incisions are large and are held open with retractors during surgery, contributing to pain after surgery.

Surgery may consist of a lobectomy, pneumonectomy, segmental resection, or wedge resection. A segmental resection is a lung resection that includes the bronchus, pulmonary artery and vein, and tissue of the involved lung segment or segments of a lobe. A **wedge resection** is removal of the peripheral portion of small, localized areas of disease.

Removal of a lobe or entire lung can be accomplished through video-assisted thoracoscopic surgery (VATS) for select patients. The procedure involves making three small incisions in the chest for placement of the instruments. These same openings are used later for placement of drains and chest tubes. The lung section, lobe, or lung is isolated from its airway, which is surgically closed. The lobe or the lung is closed off from the rest of the lung using a double-stapling technique. The tissue is sealed in a bag to prevent leakage of tumor tissue and possible

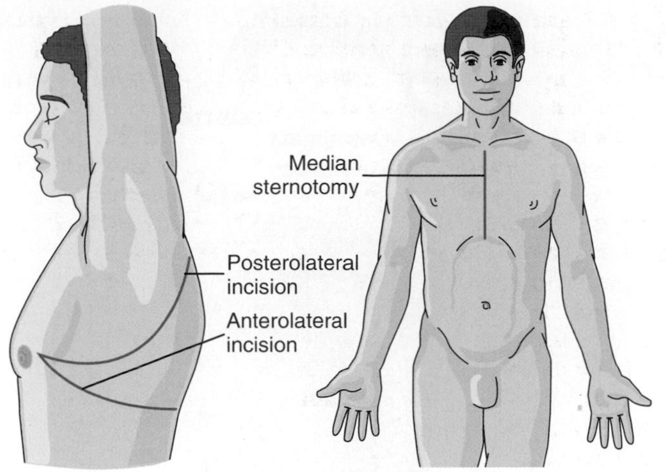

FIG. 30-13 Common incision locations for partial or total pneumonectomy.

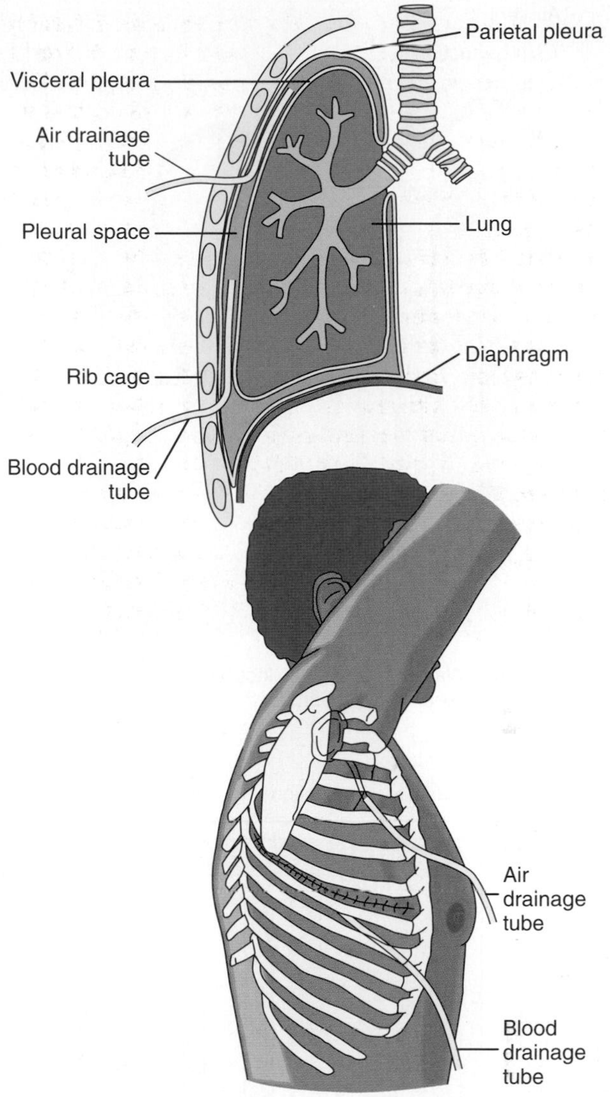

FIG. 30-14 Chest tube placement.

seeding of the cancer and is then removed whole through one of the small incisions.

Postoperative Care. Care after surgery for patients who have undergone thoracotomy (except for pneumonectomy) requires closed–chest drainage to drain air and blood that collect in the pleural space. A **chest tube**, a drain placed in the pleural space, allows lung re-expansion (Fig. 30-14). The chest tube also prevents air and fluid from returning to the chest. The drainage system consists of one or more chest tubes or drains, a collection container placed below the chest level, and a water seal to keep air from entering the chest. The drainage system may be a stationary, disposable, self-contained system (Fig. 30-15) or a smaller, portable, disposable, self-contained system that requires no connection to a vacuum source (Fig. 30-16). The nursing care priorities for the patient with a chest tube are to ensure the integrity of the system, promote comfort, ensure chest tube patency, and prevent complications.

Chest Tube Placement and Care. The tip of the tube used to drain air is placed near the front lung apex (see Fig. 30-14). The tube that drains liquid is placed on the side near the base of the lung. After lung surgery, two tubes, anterior and posterior, are used. The wounds are covered with airtight dressings.

The chest tube is connected by about 6 feet of tubing to a collection device placed below the chest. The tubing allows the patient to turn and move without pulling on the chest tube. Keeping the collection device below the chest allows gravity to drain the pleural space. When two chest tubes are inserted, they are joined by a Y-connector near the patient's body; the 6 feet of tubing is attached to the Y-connector.

Stationary chest tube drainage systems use a water seal mechanism that acts as a onc-way valve to prevent air or liquid from moving back into the chest cavity. The Pleur-evac system is a common device using a one-piece disposable plastic unit with three chambers. The three chambers are connected to one another. The tube(s) from the patient is(are) connected to the first chamber in the series of three. This chamber is the drainage collection container. The second chamber is the water seal to prevent air from moving back up the tubing system and into the chest. The third chamber, when suction is applied, is the suction regulator.

In setting up the system, chamber one (nearest to the patient) does not at first have fluid in it. The tubing from the patient penetrates shallowly into this chamber, as does the tube connecting chamber one with chamber two.

Chamber one collects the fluid draining from the patient. This fluid is measured hourly during the first 24 hours. The fluid in chamber one must never fill to the point that it comes into contact with any tubes! If the tubing from the patient enters the fluid, drainage stops and can lead to a tension pneumothorax.

Chamber two is the water seal that prevents air from reentering the patient's pleural space. As the trapped air leaves the pleural space, it will pass through chamber one (drainage

NURSING SAFETY PRIORITY (QSEN)

Action Alert

For a water seal chest tube drainage system, 2 cm of water is the minimum needed in the water seal to prevent air from flowing backward into the patient. Check the water level every shift, and add sterile water to this chamber to the level marked on the indicator (specified by the manufacturer of the drainage system).

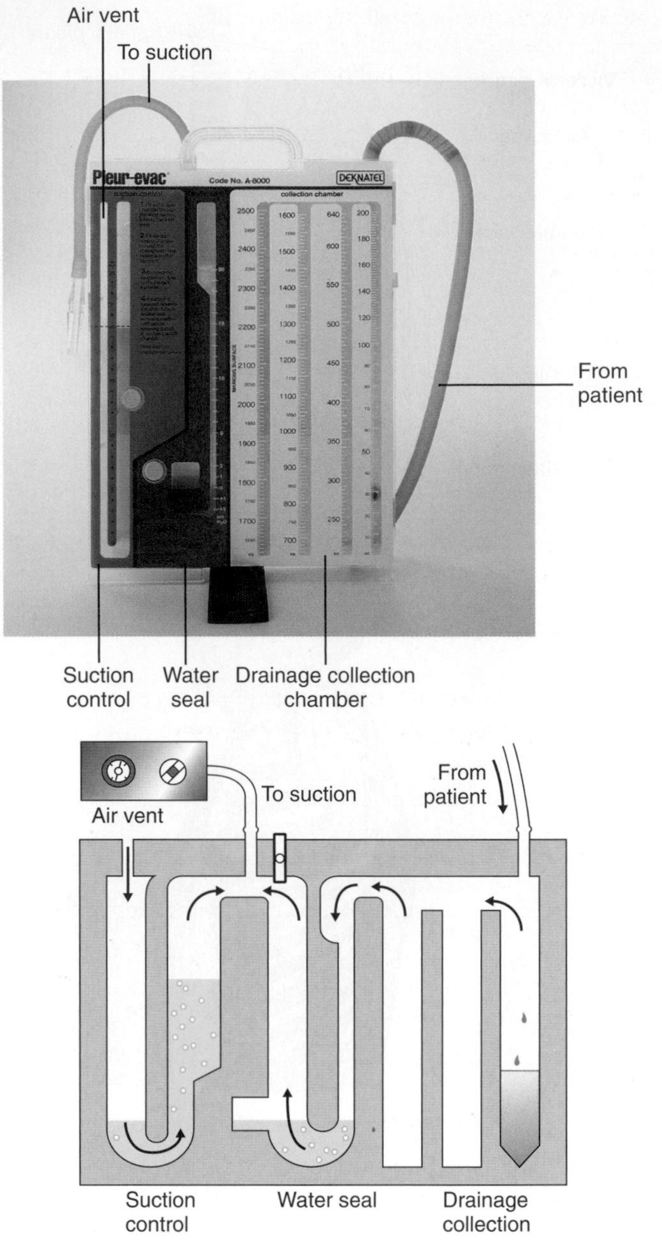

FIG. 30-15 *Left,* The Pleur-evac drainage system, a commercial three-chamber chest drainage device. *Right,* Schematic of the drainage device.

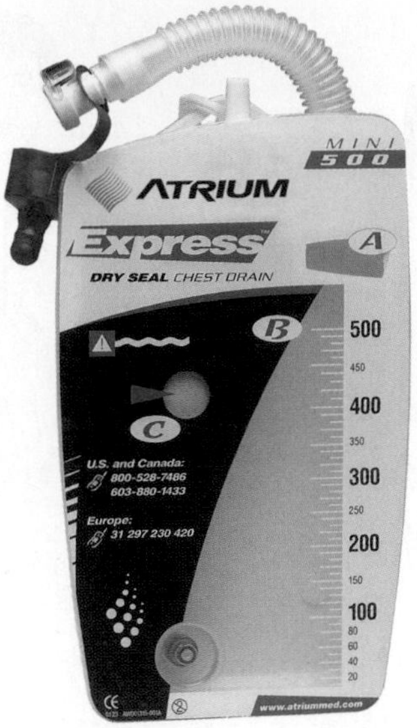

FIG. 30-16 A portable chest drainage system.

collection chamber) before entering chamber two (the water seal chamber), which should always contain at least 2 cm of water to prevent air from returning to the patient. As trapped air from the patient's pleural space passes through the water seal, which serves as a one-way valve, the water will bubble. Once all the air has been evacuated from the pleural space, bubbling of the water seal stops.

The bubbling of the water in the water seal chamber indicates air drainage from the patient. Bubbling is seen when intrathoracic pressure is greater than atmospheric pressure, such as when the patient exhales, coughs, or sneezes. When the air in the pleural space has been removed, bubbling stops. A blocked or kinked chest tube also can cause bubbling to stop. Excessive bubbling in the water seal chamber (chamber two) may indicate an air leak. The water in the narrow column of the water seal chamber normally rises 2 to 4 inches during inhalation and falls during exhalation, a process called *tidaling.* An absence of fluctuation may mean that the lung has fully re-expanded or can mean that there is an obstruction in the chest tube (Bauman & Handley, 2011).

Chamber three is the suction control of the system. There are different types of suction, most commonly wet or dry. With wet suction, the fluid level in chamber three is prescribed by the health care provider (usually –20 cm water). The chamber is connected to wall suction, which is turned up until there is gentle bubbling in the chamber. With dry suction, the health care provider prescribes the suction level to be dialed in on the device. When connected to wall suction, the regulator is set to the amount indicated by the device's manufacturer. For either type of suction, the amount of suction in the system is determined not by the wall suction unit but by the chest tube drainage device.

Chart 30-13 summarizes best safety practices when caring for a patient with a water seal chest tube drainage system. Check hourly to ensure the sterility and patency of the drainage system. Tape tubing junctions to prevent accidental disconnections, and keep an occlusive dressing at the chest tube insertion site. Keep sterile gauze at the bedside to cover the insertion site immediately if the chest tube becomes dislodged. Also keep padded clamps at the bedside for use if the drainage system is interrupted. Position the drainage tubing to prevent kinks and large loops of tubing, which can block drainage and prevent lung re-expansion.

Manipulation of the chest tube should be kept to a minimum. Do not vigorously "strip" the chest tube because this can create up to –400 cm of water negative pressure and damage lung tissue. If any tube manipulation is needed, gentle hand-over-hand "milking" of the tube, with stopping between each hand hold, is used to move blood clots and prevent obstruction. Follow surgeon prescriptions, as well as agency policies and guidelines on this action.

Assess the respiratory status and document the amount and type of drainage hourly on the collection chamber. Notify the surgeon if more than 100 mL/hr of drainage occurs. After the

CHART 30-13 **Best Practice for Patient Safety & Quality Care** QSEN

Management of Chest Tube Drainage Systems

Patient

- Ensure that the dressing on the chest around the tube is tight and intact. Depending on agency policy and the surgeon's preference, reinforce or change loose dressings.
- Assess for difficulty breathing.
- Assess breathing effectiveness by pulse oximetry.
- Listen to breath sounds for each lung.
- Check alignment of trachea.
- Check tube insertion site for condition of the skin. Palpate area for puffiness or crackling that may indicate subcutaneous emphysema.
- Observe site for signs of infection (redness, purulent drainage) or excessive bleeding.
- Check to see if tube "eyelets" are visible.
- Assess for pain and its location and intensity, and administer drugs for pain as prescribed.
- Assist patient to deep breathe, cough, perform maximal sustained inhalations, and use incentive spirometry.
- Reposition the patient who reports a "burning" pain in the chest.

Drainage System

- Do not "strip" the chest tube.
- Keep drainage system lower than the level of the patient's chest.
- Keep the chest tube as straight as possible, avoiding kinks and dependent loops.
- Ensure the chest tube is securely taped to the connector and that the connector is taped to the tubing going into the collection chamber.
- Assess bubbling in the water seal chamber; should be gentle bubbling on patient's exhalation, forceful cough, position changes.
- Assess for "tidaling."
- Check water level in the water seal chamber, and keep at the level recommended by the manufacturer.
- Check water level in the suction control chamber, and keep at the level prescribed by the surgeon (unless dry suction system is used).
- Clamp the chest tube only for brief periods to change the drainage system or when checking for air leaks.
- Check and document amount, color, and characteristics of fluid in the collection chamber, as often as needed according to the patient's condition and agency policy.
- Empty collection chamber or change the system before the drainage makes contact with the bottom of the tube.
- When a sample of drainage is needed for culture or other laboratory test, obtain it from the chest tube; after cleansing chest tube, use a 20-gauge (or smaller) needle and draw up specimen into a syringe.

Immediately Notify Physician or Rapid Response Team For:

- Tracheal deviation
- Sudden onset or increased intensity of dyspnea
- Oxygen saturation less than 90%
- Drainage greater than 70 mL/hr
- Visible eyelets on chest tube
- Chest tube falls out of the patient's chest (first, cover the area with dry, sterile gauze)
- Chest tube disconnects from the drainage system (first, put end of tube in a container of sterile water and keep below the level of the patient's chest)
- Drainage in tube stops (in the first 24 hours)

first 24 hours, assess drainage at least every 8 hours. Usually the drainage in chamber one is not emptied unless it is so full that the fluid is in danger of coming into contact with the chest drainage tube.

Check the water seal chamber for unexpected bubbling created by an air leak in the system. Bubbling is normal during forceful expiration or coughing because air in the chest is being expelled. Continuous bubbling indicates an air leak. Notify the health care provider if bubbling occurs continuously in the water seal chamber. With a prescription, gently apply a padded clamp briefly on the drainage tubing close to the occlusive dressing. If the bubbling stops, the air leak may be at the chest tube insertion site or within the chest, requiring physician intervention. Bubbling that does not stop when a padded clamp is applied indicates that the air leak is between the clamp and the drainage system. Release the clamp as soon as this assessment is made.

Mobile or portable chest tube drainage systems are "dry" chest drainage systems without a water seal to prevent air from reentering the patient's lung through the chest tube. Instead, these light-weight devices use a dynamic control "flutter" valve that prevents backflow of air. When the patient exhales, air is forced from the chest cavity into the chest tube, under pressure. This pressure forces the soft flutter valve open and air moves into the harder surrounding tube shell (which has a vent for air). Portable units allow the patient to ambulate and go home with chest tubes still in place.

NCLEX EXAMINATION CHALLENGE

Safe and Effective Care Environment

The chest tube of a client 16 hours postoperative from a lobectomy is accidentally pulled out by a portable x-ray machine. What is the nurse's best first action?

A. Clamp the tubing with padded clamps as close as possible to the insertion site.
B. Reposition the client on the nonoperative side and support the tube(s) with pillows.
C. Cover the insertion site with a sterile occlusive dressing and tape down on three sides.
D. Don sterile gloves and attempt to reinsert the chest tube at the original insertion site.

Pain Management. Most patients have intense pain after an open thoracotomy. Pain is considerably less for the patient after surgery using minimally invasive techniques. However, pain control is needed in either case for patient comfort and to assist him or her to participate in techniques to reduce the risk for complications (see Chapter 16). Give the prescribed drugs for pain, and assess the patient's responses to them. Teach patients using patient-controlled analgesia (PCA) devices to self-administer the drug before pain intensity becomes too severe. Monitor vital signs before and after giving opioid analgesics, especially for the patient who is not being mechanically ventilated. Plan care activities around the timing of analgesia to reduce pain.

Respiratory Management. Immediately after surgery the patient is mechanically ventilated. See Chapter 32 for nursing care of the patient receiving mechanical ventilation.

Once the patient is breathing on his or her own, the priorities are to maintain a patent airway, ensure adequate ventilation, and prevent complications. Assess the patient at least every 2 hours for adequacy of ventilation and GAS EXCHANGE. Check the alignment of the trachea. Assess oxygen saturation and the rate and depth of respiration. Listen to breath sounds in all lobes on the nonoperative side, particularly noting the presence of crackles. Assess the oral mucous membranes for cyanosis and the nail beds for rate of capillary refill. Perform oral suctioning as necessary.

Usually the patient receives oxygen by mask or nasal cannula for the first 2 days after surgery. Warm and humidify the oxygen. Assist the patient to a semi-Fowler's position or up in a chair as soon as possible. Encourage him or her to use the incentive spirometer every hour while awake. If coughing is permitted, help him or her cough by splinting any incision and ensuring that the chest tube does not pull with movement. Ensuring that pain is well managed increases the patient's ability to cough and deep breathe effectively.

Pneumonectomy Care. After pneumonectomy, the pleural cavity on the affected side is an empty space. The surgeon sometimes inserts a clamped chest tube for only a day. Serous fluid collection in the empty space creates adhesions that help reduce mediastinal shift toward the affected side. Closed–chest drainage is not usually used.

Complications of a pneumonectomy include empyema (purulent material in the pleural space) and development of a bronchopleural fistula (an abnormal duct that develops between the bronchial tree and the pleura). Positioning of the patient after pneumonectomy varies according to surgeon preference and the patient's comfort. Some surgeons want the patient placed on the nonoperative side immediately after a pneumonectomy to reduce stress on the bronchial stump incision. Others prefer to place the patient on the operative side to allow fluids to fill in the now empty space.

CLINICAL JUDGMENT CHALLENGE

Patient-Centered Care; Evidence-Based Practice QSEN

The patient is a 60-year-old man who has just been diagnosed with non–small cell lung cancer. He smoked cigarettes for about 25 years starting when he was 16 years old and quit when he was 41 years old. His lung cancer is at stage I in the left lower lobe. He is distraught, saying that he can't die now because he has one child in college and two in high school. He also fears chemotherapy and seems bitter that he quit smoking and got lung cancer anyway. His next statement is: "Why couldn't I get prostate cancer like most men? At least they survive. No one beats lung cancer."

1. What can you tell him about lung cancer survival?
2. What can you tell him about the benefits of having quit smoking?
3. For this cancer stage and type, what is/are the most likely therapy/therapies?
4. What resources could you recommend to help him at this time?

◆ *Interventions for Palliation*

Oxygen therapy is prescribed when the patient is hypoxemic. Even if the hypoxemia is not severe, humidified oxygen may be prescribed to relieve dyspnea and anxiety. (See Chapter 28 for issues related to home oxygen therapy.)

Drug therapy with bronchodilators and corticosteroids is prescribed for the patient with bronchospasm to decrease bronchospasm, INFLAMMATION, and edema. Mucolytics may help ease removal of thick mucus and sputum. Bacterial infections are treated with antibiotic therapy.

Radiation therapy can help relieve hemoptysis, obstruction of the bronchi and great veins (superior vena cava syndrome), difficulty swallowing from esophageal compression, and pain from bone metastasis. Radiation for palliation uses higher doses for shorter periods. Skin care issues and fatigue are the same as those occurring with radiation therapy for cure.

Thoracentesis is performed when pleural effusion is a problem for the patient with lung cancer. The excess fluid increases dyspnea, discomfort, and the risk for infection. The purpose of treatment is to remove pleural fluid and prevent its formation. **Thoracentesis** is fluid removal by suction after the placement of a large needle or catheter into the intrapleural space. Fluid removal temporarily relieves hypoxia; however, the fluid can rapidly re-form in the pleural space. When fluid development is continuous and uncomfortable, a continuously draining catheter may be placed into the intrapleural space to collect the fluid.

Dyspnea management is needed because the patient with lung cancer tires easily and is often most comfortable resting in a semi-Fowler's position. Dyspnea is reduced with oxygen, use of a continuous morphine infusion, and positioning for comfort. The severely dyspneic patient may be most comfortable sitting in a lounge chair or reclining chair.

Pain management may be needed to help the patient be as pain-free and comfortable as possible. Pain may be present in the chest or in almost any area when bone metastasis occurs. Perform a complete pain assessment with attention to onset, intensity, quality, duration, and the patient's description of the pain.

Pharmacologic management with opioid drugs as oral, parenteral, or transdermal preparations is needed. Analgesics are most effective when given around the clock. Additional PRN analgesics are used for breakthrough pain. Ongoing evaluation of pain control effectiveness is a primary nursing responsibility.

Hospice care can be beneficial for the patient in the terminal phase of lung cancer. Hospice programs provide support to the terminally ill patient and the family, meet physical and psychosocial needs, adjust the palliative care regimen as needed, make home visits, and provide volunteers for errands and respite care. (See Chapter 7 for a more complete discussion of end-of-life issues.) The American Cancer Society may provide assistance through support groups for patients and families or through the use of equipment, such as a hospital bed or bedside commode. Family members and significant others are heavily burdened at this time. They have many needs and also require much support while performing the caregiver role during this time (Grant et al., 2013).

NURSING CONCEPTS AND CLINICAL JUDGMENT REVIEW

What might you NOTICE if the patient is experiencing inadequate GAS EXCHANGE and tissue PERFUSION as a result of chronic obstructive respiratory problems?

- Respirations rapid and shallow
- Decreased oxygen saturation by pulse oximetry
- Skin cyanosis or pallor (in lighter-skinned patients)
- Cyanosis or pallor of the lips and oral mucous membranes (in patients of any skin color)
- Tachycardia
- Patient appears to work hard to inhale and exhale
- Patient is restless or anxious
- Patient's general appearance is thin relative to height
- Muscles of the neck appear thick
- Arm and leg muscles appear thin
- Fingers are clubbed
- Chest is barrel-shaped
- Ribs are spaced more than a fingerbreadth apart

What should you INTERPRET and how should you RESPOND to a patient experiencing inadequate GAS EXCHANGE and tissue PERFUSION as a result of an acute critical respiratory problem?

Perform and interpret physical assessment, including:

- Taking vital signs
- Auscultating all lung fields
- Monitoring oxygen saturation by pulse oximetry
- Assessing cognition
- Assessing for the presence and characteristics of sputum production
- Assessing the patient's ability to cough and clear the airway

Interpret laboratory values, including:

- Elevated red blood cell count, hematocrit, and hemoglobin
- Elevated white blood cell count
- Arterial blood gas values: pH lower than 7.35; HCO_3^- greater than 24 mEq/L; $Paco_2$ greater than 45 mm Hg; Pao_2 lower than 80 mm Hg

Respond by:

- Assisting the patient to an upright position, with arms resting on a table or armrests
- Performing or assisting the patient to perform chest physiotherapy/pulmonary hygiene
- Prioritizing and pacing activities to prevent fatigue
- Administering prescribed inhaled drugs
- Administering respiratory therapy treatments or collaborating with the respiratory therapist to administer these treatments
- Re-assessing respiratory status after respiratory therapy treatment
- Ensuring a fluid intake of at least 2 liters per day

On what should you REFLECT?

- Observe the patient for evidence of improved oxygenation (see Chapter 27).
- Think about what may have made the patient's dyspnea worse and what steps could be taken to prevent a similar episode.
- Think about what patient education focus could help reduce the intensity of dyspnea in the future.

GET READY FOR THE NCLEX® EXAMINATION!

KEY POINTS

Review these Key Points for each NCLEX Examination Client Needs Category.

Safe and Effective Care Environment

- Ensure there are no open flames or combustion hazards in rooms where oxygen is in use. **Safety** QSEN
- Ensure that oxygen therapy delivered to the patient is humidified. **Safety** QSEN
- Protect the patient with cystic fibrosis from hospital-acquired pulmonary infections. **Safety** QSEN
- Ensure proper function of chest tube drainage equipment. **Safety** QSEN

Health Promotion and Maintenance

- Teach patients who come into contact with inhalation irritants in their workplaces or leisure-time activities to use a mask to avoid respiratory contact with these substances. **Safety** QSEN
- Teach anyone who smokes that smoking increases the risk for development of many pulmonary problems. **Evidence-Based Practice** QSEN
- Teach patients with asthma to develop a management plan based on their identified personal best on peak expiratory rate flow testing. **Patient-Centered Care** QSEN
- Instruct patients with asthma to carry a reliever inhaler with them at all times. **Safety** QSEN
- Encourage all patients older than 50 years and anyone with a respiratory problem to receive a yearly influenza vaccination. **Patient-Centered Care** QSEN
- Teach all patients who smoke the warning signs of lung cancer. **Evidence-Based Practice** QSEN

Psychosocial Integrity

- Encourage the patient and family to express their feelings regarding the diagnosis of a chronic respiratory disease or cancer and about management/treatment regimens.
- Explain all diagnostic procedures, restrictions, and follow-up care to the patient scheduled for tests.
- Help patients use strategies to improve their appearance when alopecia occurs. **Patient-Centered Care** QSEN
- Refer patients and family members to local cancer resources and support groups. **Patient-Centered Care** QSEN

- Ensure that patient preferences are honored whenever possible. **Patient-Centered Care** QSEN

Physiological Integrity

- Assess the airway and breathing effectiveness for GAS EXCHANGE for any patient who experiences shortness of breath or any change in mental status. **Evidence-Based Practice** QSEN
- Assess the degree to which breathing problems interfere with the patient's ability to perform ADLs, work, and leisure-time activities. **Patient-Centered Care** QSEN
- Apply oxygen to anyone who is hypoxemic. **Evidence-Based Practice** QSEN
- Monitor arterial blood gases and oxygen saturation of all patients receiving oxygen therapy. **Evidence-Based Practice** QSEN
- Teach patients receiving radiation therapy how to care for the skin in the radiation path (see Chart 22-2 in Chapter 22). **Patient-Centered Care** QSEN
- Collaborate with respiratory therapists, registered dietitians, and social workers to meet the hospital and home care needs of patients with chronic lower respiratory problems. **Teamwork and Collaboration** QSEN

CHAPTER 31

Care of Patients with Infectious Respiratory Problems

Meg Blair

http://evolve.elsevier.com/Iggy/

PRIORITY CONCEPTS

- Gas Exchange
- Infection
- Inflammation

LEARNING OUTCOMES

Safe and Effective Care Environment

1. Apply principles of infection control and disease-containment activities when providing care to patients with respiratory INFECTIONS.
2. Protect patients receiving mechanical ventilation from developing ventilator-associated pneumonia.

Health Promotion and Maintenance

3. Provide information to everyone about preventing respiratory INFECTIONS.
4. Describe techniques for home care of the patient with active tuberculosis.

Psychosocial Integrity

5. Reduce the psychological impact of respiratory INFECTIONS for the patient and family.

Physiological Integrity

6. Identify adults at highest risk for contracting influenza, pneumonia, tuberculosis, and other respiratory INFECTIONS.
7. Perform focused respiratory assessment and re-assessment.
8. Recognize manifestations of infectious respiratory diseases and inadequate GAS EXCHANGE.
9. Implement appropriate interventions for the patient with a respiratory infection to ensure adequate GAS EXCHANGE and oxygenation.

DISORDERS OF THE NOSE AND SINUSES

RHINITIS

❖ PATHOPHYSIOLOGY

Rhinitis, an INFLAMMATION of the nasal mucosa, is a common problem of the nose and often involves the sinuses. It can be caused by INFECTION (viral or bacterial) or contact with allergens. An allergic rhinitis makes the mucous membranes more susceptible to bacterial invasion that may lead to INFECTION.

Allergic rhinitis *(hay fever* or *allergies)* is triggered by hypersensitivity reactions to airborne allergens. Some episodes are "seasonal," recurring at the same time of year (Krouse & Krouse, 2014). *Perennial rhinitis* occurs intermittently with no seasonal pattern or continuously whenever the person is exposed to an offending allergen such as dust, animal dander, wool, or foods (e.g., seafood). Rhinitis also occurs as a "rebound" nasal congestion from overuse of nasal decongestant drops or sprays *(rhinitis medicamentosa)* and chronic nasal inhalation of cocaine.

Acute viral rhinitis (**coryza**, or the common cold) is caused by any of over 200 viruses. It spreads from person to person by droplets from sneezing or coughing and by direct contact. Colds are most contagious in the first 2 to 3 days after symptoms appear. Colds are self-limiting unless a bacterial INFECTION occurs at the same time. Complications occur most often in immunosuppressed people and older adults.

❖ PATIENT-CENTERED COLLABORATIVE CARE

In allergic rhinitis, the presence of the allergen causes a release of histamine and other chemicals from basophils and mast cells in the nasal mucosa. These chemicals bind to blood vessel receptors, causing local blood vessel dilation and capillary leak, leading to local edema and swelling. Manifestations include headache, nasal irritation, sneezing, nasal congestion, **rhinorrhea** (watery drainage from the nose), and itchy, watery eyes.

Viral or bacterial invasion of the nasal passages causes the same local tissue responses as allergic rhinitis. Often the patient also has systemic manifestations, including a sore, dry throat; low-grade fever; and malaise.

Management of the patient with any type of rhinitis focuses on symptom relief and patient education. Teach him or her about correct use of the drug therapy prescribed.

Drug therapy commonly includes antihistamines, decongestants, and intranasal steroid spray (especially for chronic rhinitis). For severe disease, immunotherapy can be used. *Antihistamines, leukotriene inhibitors,* and *mast cell stabilizers* block or reduce the amount of chemical mediators in nasal tissues and prevent local edema and itching. *Decongestants* constrict blood vessels and decrease edema. *Antipyretics* are given if fever is present. *Antibiotics* are prescribed only when a bacterial INFECTION accompanies rhinitis. Rhinitis caused by overuse of nose drops or sprays is treated by discontinuing the drug.

CONSIDERATIONS FOR OLDER ADULTS

Patient-Centered Care QSEN

First-generation antihistamines are included as potentially inappropriate drugs for use in older adults. In this population, the drugs lead to problems with reduced clearance, higher risk for confusion, and anticholinergic effects such as dry mouth and constipation. Common drugs in this category include chlorpheniramine (Chlor-Trimeton), diphenhydramine (Benadryl), and hydroxyzine (Vistaril). Warn the older adult about these side effects.

Supportive therapy can increase the patient's comfort and help prevent spread of the INFECTION. Instruct the patient about the importance of rest (8 to 10 hours a day) and fluid intake of at least 2000 mL/day unless other health problems require fluid restriction. Humidifying the air helps relieve congestion. Humidity can be increased with a room humidifier or by breathing steamy air in the bathroom after running hot shower water. If the condition is caused by allergies, limiting exposure to the offending agent is helpful (see Chapter 20).

Teach patients to reduce the risk for spreading colds by thoroughly washing hands, especially after nose blowing, sneezing, coughing, rubbing the eyes, or touching the face. Other precautions include staying home from work, school, or places where people gather; covering the mouth and nose with a tissue when sneezing or coughing; disposing properly of used tissues immediately; and avoiding close contact with others. Stress the need to avoid close contact with people who are more susceptible to INFECTION, such as older adults, infants, and anyone who has a chronic respiratory problem. An uncomplicated cold typically subsides within 7 to 10 days.

RHINOSINUSITIS

❖ PATHOPHYSIOLOGY

Sinusitis is an INFLAMMATION of the mucous membranes of one or more of the sinuses and is usually associated with rhinitis. The preferred term for this condition is ***rhinosinusitis*** (Brook, 2013). Other conditions leading to rhinosinusitis include deviated nasal septum, nasal polyps or tumors, inhaled air pollutants or cocaine, facial trauma, and dental INFECTION. Swelling can obstruct the flow of secretions from the sinuses, which may then become infected.

Most episodes of rhinosinusitis are caused by viruses and usually develop in the maxillary and frontal sinuses, although bacterial INFECTIONS also can occur. Complications include cellulitis, abscess, and meningitis.

Diagnosis is made on the basis of the patient's history and manifestations. Other tests for rhinosinusitis include sinus x-rays, endoscopic examination, and computed tomography (CT). Bacterial sinusitis is usually indicated by purulent drainage from one or both nares, sometimes fever, and lack of response to decongestant therapy. Cultures are not usually necessary but may be useful in patients who do not respond to therapy or who develop complications.

❖ PATIENT-CENTERED COLLABORATIVE CARE

Assess for manifestations of rhinosinusitis. Common manifestations include pain over the cheek radiating to the teeth, tenderness to percussion over the sinuses, referred pain to the temple or back of the head, and general facial pain that is worse when bending forward. Additional manifestations that may accompany bacterial INFECTION include purulent nasal drainage with postnasal drip, fever, erythema, swelling, fatigue, dental pain, and ear pressure.

Treatment for bacterial rhinosinusitis includes the use of broad-spectrum antibiotics (e.g., amoxicillin [Amoxil]), analgesics for pain (e.g., acetaminophen [Tylenol, Abenol ♣, Atasol ♣, Panadol]; ibuprofen [Advil]), decongestants (e.g., phenylephrine [Neo-Synephrine]), antipyretics, steam humidification, hot and wet packs over the sinus area, and nasal saline irrigations. In some cases, nasal steroids may be prescribed. Nasal saline irrigation is an inexpensive treatment with few side effects (Thornton et al., 2011). Sleeping with the head of the bed elevated and avoiding cigarette smoke may reduce discomfort. Teach the patient to increase fluid intake unless another medical problem requires fluid restriction. If this treatment plan is not successful (no improvement seen within 48 hours), he or she may need further evaluation. Surgical intervention with endoscopic sinus surgery to relieve obstruction and promote sinus drainage may be needed if nonsurgical management fails to provide relief.

DISORDERS OF THE ORAL PHARYNX AND TONSILS

PHARYNGITIS

❖ PATHOPHYSIOLOGY

Pharyngitis, or "sore throat," is a common INFLAMMATION of the pharyngeal mucous membranes that often occurs with rhinitis and sinusitis. It accounts for up to 40 million office visits each year in the United States (Aung, 2013).

Acute pharyngitis can be caused by bacteria, viruses, other organisms, trauma, irritants, dehydration, and tobacco or alcohol use. A common bacterium causing pharyngitis is group A beta-hemolytic *Streptococcus,* but most adult cases are caused by a virus (Acerra, 2014).

❖ PATIENT-CENTERED COLLABORATIVE CARE

◆ Assessment

The patient with pharyngitis has throat soreness and dryness, throat pain, pain on swallowing *(odynophagia),* difficulty swallowing, and may have fever. Viral and bacterial pharyngitis are often difficult to distinguish on physical assessment. When inspecting a throat infected with either virus or bacteria, mild to severe redness may be seen with or without enlarged tonsils and with or without exudate. Ask about nasal discharge, which varies from thin and watery to thick and purulent. Enlargement of neck lymph nodes occurs with both viral and bacterial pharyngitis.

Bacterial INFECTIONS are often associated with enlarged red tonsils, exudate, petechiae on the soft palate, purulent discharge, and local lymph node enlargement. Chart 31-1 compares the

CHART 31-1 Key Features

Acute Viral and Bacterial Pharyngitis

FEATURE	VIRAL PHARYNGITIS	BACTERIAL PHARYNGITIS
Temperature	Low-grade or no fever	High temperature (>101° F [38.3° C] and usually 102°-104° F [38.9°-40° C])*
Ear manifestations	Retracted or dull tympanic membrane	Retracted or dull tympanic membrane
Throat manifestations	Scant or no tonsillar exudate Slight erythema of pharynx and tonsils	Severe hyperemia of pharyngeal mucosa, tonsils, tongue, and uvula Erythema of tonsils with yellow exudates Petechiae on the soft palate
Neck manifestations	Possible lymphadenopathy	Anterior cervical lymphadenopathy and tenderness
Skin manifestations	No rash	Possible scarlatiniform rash Possible petechiae on chest or abdomen or both
Dysphagia, odynophagia	Present	Present
Other symptoms	No cough Rhinitis Mild hoarseness Headache	No cough Pain on speaking and "hot potato" muffled voice Headache Arthralgia Myalgia
Laboratory data	Complete blood count usually normal White blood cell count usually ≤10,000/mm^3 Negative throat culture results	Complete blood count abnormal White blood cell count usually >12,000/mm^3* Throat culture results positive for beta-hemolytic *Streptococcus*
Onset	Gradual	Abrupt

*May not be present in adults older than 65 years.

TABLE 31-1 Complications of Group A Streptococcal Infection

• Rheumatic fever	• Sinusitis
• Acute glomerulonephritis	• Mastoiditis
• Peritonsillar abscess	• Bronchitis
• Retropharyngeal abscess	• Pneumonia
• Otitis media	• Scarlet fever

manifestations of viral and bacterial pharyngitis. Viral pharyngitis is contagious for 2 to 3 days. Symptoms usually subside within 3 to 10 days after onset, and the disease is usually self-limiting.

Bacterial pharyngitis caused by group A streptococcal INFECTION can lead to serious complications (Table 31-1), including acute glomerulonephritis and rheumatic fever. Acute glomerulonephritis may occur 7 to 10 days after the acute infection, and rheumatic fever may develop 3 to 5 weeks after the acute infection. Because rheumatic fever is rare, some experts question the need to prescribe antibiotics for all cases of pharyngitis (Acerra, 2014).

Many types of rapid antigen tests (RATs) and screens for group A beta-hemolytic streptococcal antigen are available. These tests vary in specificity and sensitivity, and the results are available in less than 15 minutes. Two common tests are the Gen-Probe and the Optical Immunoassay (OIA).

In some cases, throat cultures can be important in distinguishing viral from a group A beta-hemolytic streptococcal INFECTION. Usually 24 to 48 hours is required for results.

With either RAT or culture methods, it is essential to obtain throat specimens properly for an accurate test result. The organisms are not uniformly distributed throughout the throat and can be missed during swabbing. To obtain a specimen, rub a sterile cotton swab from a throat culture kit first over the right tonsillar area, moving across the right arch, the uvula, and then across the left arch to the left tonsillar area. Remove the swab without touching the patient's teeth, tongue, or gums. Consult with the laboratory for proper handling of the specimen. Send it to the laboratory as quickly as possible.

A complete blood count (CBC) may be performed when pharyngitis is severe or does not improve. Indications for a CBC are high fever, lethargy, or manifestations of complications.

Ask about the patient's recent contacts (within the past 10 days) with people who have been ill. Specifically ask whether he or she has been ill with manifestations of a cold or upper respiratory tract INFECTION recently. Document any history of streptococcal infections, rheumatic fever, valvular heart disease, or penicillin allergy. Ask whether the patient has had a diphtheria immunization.

◆ *Interventions*

Most sore throats in adults are viral, do not require antibiotic therapy, and respond to supportive interventions. Teach the patient to rest, increase fluid intake, humidify the air, and use analgesics for pain. Gargling several times each day with warm saline and using throat lozenges can increase comfort.

Management of bacterial pharyngitis involves antibiotics and the same supportive care as with viral pharyngitis. For streptococcal INFECTION, an oral penicillin or cephalosporin is prescribed. Drugs from the macrolide class (e.g., azithromycin or erythromycin) are used if the patient is allergic to penicillin.

! NURSING SAFETY PRIORITY (QSEN)

Action Alert

Teach patients with any bacterial INFECTION the importance of completing the entire antibiotic prescription, even when manifestations improve or subside. This action helps eradicate the organism and prevents development of resistant bacterial strains.

The patient should be re-evaluated if there is no improvement in 3 days or if manifestations are still present after completion of the antibiotic course. Any patient whose bacterial pharyngitis does not improve with antibiotics should consider human immune deficiency virus (HIV) testing.

A rare complication of pharyngitis is INFECTION of the epiglottis and supraglottic structures (**epiglottitis**). The epiglottis is a flaplike structure that closes over the trachea during swallowing to prevent aspiration. An inflamed epiglottis can swell and obstruct the airway, inhibiting GAS EXCHANGE and tissue perfusion.

! NURSING SAFETY PRIORITY QSEN

Critical Rescue

If a patient with pharyngitis develops stridor or other indications of airway obstruction, notify the Rapid Response Team. Teach patients at home to call 911 or go to the nearest emergency department if difficulty breathing, stridor, or drooling occurs.

Teach the patient with bacterial pharyngitis how to take his or her temperature every morning and evening until the INFECTION resolves. He or she is not contagious after 24 hours of effective antibiotic therapy. Family members or close contacts who also have a sore throat should be evaluated.

TONSILLITIS

❖ PATHOPHYSIOLOGY

Tonsillitis is an INFLAMMATION and INFECTION of the tonsils and lymphatic tissues located on each side of the throat. The tonsils are lymphatic tissue shaped like small almonds. They are covered by mucous membranes and have small valleys *(crypts)* across their surface. Tonsils filter organisms and protect the respiratory tract from infection (McCance et al., 2014).

Tonsillitis is a contagious airborne INFECTION that can occur in any age-group but is less common in adults. The disease usually lasts 7 to 10 days and often is caused by bacteria—most commonly *Streptococcus.* Viruses also cause tonsillitis. Chronic tonsillitis may result from an unresolved acute infection or recurrent infections.

❖ PATIENT-CENTERED COLLABORATIVE CARE

Chart 31-2 lists the manifestations of acute tonsillitis. Diagnostic tests often used to rule out other causes of the sore throat and fever include a rapid antigen test (RAT), CBC, throat culture and sensitivity (C&S) studies, and Monospot test. If respiratory manifestations are present, chest x-rays may be needed. The white blood cell (WBC) count usually is elevated in bacterial INFECTIONS and normal in viral infections.

CHART 31-2 Key Features

Acute Tonsillitis

- Sudden onset of a mild to severe sore throat
- Fever
- Muscle aches
- Chills
- Dysphagia, odynophagia (painful swallowing of food)
- Pain in the ears
- Headache
- Anorexia
- Malaise
- "Hot potato" voice (muffled voice)
- Tonsils visually swollen and red, possibly with pus
- Tonsils may be covered with a white or yellow exudate
- Purulent drainage may be expressed by pressing a tonsil
- Uvula visually edematous or inflamed
- Cervical lymph nodes usually tender and enlarged

Antibiotics, usually a non-penicillin drug, are prescribed for 7 to 10 days (Shah, 2014b). Nursing priorities include teaching the patient about supportive care and stressing the importance of completing antibiotic therapy. Teach him or her to rest, increase fluid intake, humidify the air, use analgesics for pain, gargle several times each day with warm saline, and use throat lozenges.

Surgical intervention for tonsillitis may be needed for recurrent acute or chronic INFECTIONS, a peritonsillar abscess, and enlarged tonsils or adenoids that obstruct the airway. It is usually performed after the patient has recovered from an acute tonsillitis and no infection is present (except with an acute peritonsillar abscess). The procedure also may involve adenoid removal. A variety of techniques are used to remove tonsils from adults; however, the dissection and snare technique is still the most common and is performed under general anesthesia. After surgery, nursing interventions focus on assessing for airway clearance, providing pain relief, and monitoring for excessive bleeding.

PERITONSILLAR ABSCESS

Peritonsillar abscess (PTA) is a complication of acute tonsillitis in which the INFECTION spreads from the tonsil to the surrounding tissue and forms an abscess. The most common cause of PTA is group A beta-hemolytic *Streptococcus,* although they often contain multiple organisms (Shah, 2014a).

Manifestations include a collection of pus behind the tonsil causing one-sided swelling with deviation of the uvula toward the unaffected side. The patient may drool, have severe throat pain radiating to the ear, have a muffled voice, and have difficulty swallowing. He or she may also have a tonic contraction of the muscles of chewing (trismus) and have difficulty breathing. Bad breath is present, and lymph nodes on the affected side are swollen. An ultrasound or a CT scan may be used for diagnosis (Shah, 2014a).

Ambulatory care management with antibiotic therapy and percutaneous needle aspiration and drainage of the abscess is needed. Antibiotics alone are often ineffective. Acute management may include IV opioid analgesics for severe pain and IV steroids to reduce the swelling. *Stress the importance of completing the antibiotic regimen and of coming to the emergency department quickly if manifestations of obstruction (drooling and stridor) appear.* Hospitalization is needed when the airway is endangered or when the INFECTION does not respond to antibiotic therapy. Incision and drainage of the abscess and additional antibiotic therapy may be needed. A tonsillectomy may be performed to prevent recurrence.

DISORDERS OF THE LUNGS

SEASONAL INFLUENZA

❖ PATHOPHYSIOLOGY

Seasonal influenza, or "flu," is a highly contagious acute viral respiratory INFECTION that can occur at any age. Epidemics are common and lead to complications of pneumonia or death, especially in older adults or immunocompromised patients. Between 5% and 20% of the U.S. population develop influenza each year, and up to 49,000 deaths in a single year have been attributed to it (Centers for Disease Control and Prevention

[CDC], 2014b). Hospitalization may be required. Influenza may be caused by one of several virus families, referred to as *A, B,* and *C.*

The patient with influenza often has a rapid onset of severe headache, muscle aches, fever, chills, fatigue, and weakness. Adults are contagious from 24 hours before manifestations occur and up to 5 days after they begin. Sore throat, cough, and watery nasal discharge may follow the initial manifestations for a week or longer. Infection with influenza strain B also can cause nausea, vomiting, and diarrhea (Gould, 2011). Most patients feel fatigued for 1 to 2 weeks after the acute episode has resolved.

Health Promotion and Maintenance

Vaccinations for the prevention of influenza are widely available and are recommended for adults by The Joint Commission's National Patient Safety Goals (NPSGs). The vaccine is changed every year on the basis of which specific viral strains are most likely to pose a problem during the influenza season (i.e., late fall and winter in the Northern Hemisphere). Usually the vaccines contain three or four antigens for the three or four most expected viral strains (trivalent influenza vaccine [TIV]). Influenza vaccinations can be taken as an IM injection (Fluvirin, Fluzone) or as a live attenuated influenza vaccine (LAIV) by intranasal spray (FluMist). The intranasal vaccine is live, and some people develop influenza symptoms after its use. It is recommended only for healthy people up to 49 years of age. Yearly vaccination is recommended for those older than 50 years, people with chronic illness or immune compromise, those living in institutions, people living with or caring for adults with health problems that put them at risk for severe complications of influenza, and health care personnel providing direct care to patients (CDC, 2014b).

Teach the patient who is sick to reduce the risk for spreading the flu by thoroughly washing hands, especially after nose blowing, sneezing, coughing, rubbing the eyes, or touching the face. Other precautions include staying home from work, school, or places where people gather; covering the mouth and nose with a tissue when sneezing or coughing; disposing properly of used tissues immediately; and avoiding close contact with other people. Although handwashing is a good method to prevent transmitting the virus in droplets from sneezing or coughing, many people cannot wash their hands as soon as they have coughed or sneezed. The technique recommended by the CDC for controlling flu spread is to sneeze or cough into the upper sleeve rather than into the hand (CDC, 2010a). (Respiratory droplets on the hands can contaminate surfaces and be transmitted to other people.)

❖ PATIENT-CENTERED COLLABORATIVE CARE

Viral INFECTIONS do not respond to traditional antibiotic therapy. Antiviral agents may be effective for prevention and treatment of some types of influenza. Amantadine (Symmetrel) and rimantadine (Flumadine) have been effective in the prevention and treatment of some strains of influenza A. Ribavirin (Virazole) has been used for severe influenza B. Two drugs that shorten the duration of influenza A and influenza B are zanamivir (Relenza) and oseltamivir (Tamiflu). These drugs prevent viral spread in the respiratory tract by inhibiting a viral enzyme that allows the virus to penetrate respiratory cells. To be effective, they must be taken within 24 to 48 hours after the onset of manifestations. Zanamivir should be used with caution in patients who have chronic obstructive pulmonary disease (COPD) or asthma and in older adults (Dambaugh, 2012).

Advise the patient to rest for several days and increase fluid intake unless another problem requires fluid restriction. Saline gargles may ease sore throat pain. Antihistamines may reduce the rhinorrhea. Other supportive measures are the same as those for acute rhinitis.

NCLEX EXAMINATION CHALLENGE

Safe and Effective Care Environment

The charge nurse at an assisted-living facility receives report from an emergency department (ED) nurse about one of the resident clients. The client was sent to the ED with a fever, chills, muscle aches, and headache. The ED nurse reports the client's rapid influenza report came back from the laboratory positive for influenza A. What action by the nurse at the assisted-living facility is most appropriate?

A. Prepare to administer antibiotics.
B. Have the resident eat meals in his room.
C. Provide oseltamivir (Tamiflu) to the staff.
D. Arrange a follow-up chest x-ray in 2 weeks.

PANDEMIC INFLUENZA

❖ PATHOPHYSIOLOGY

Many viral INFECTIONS among animals and birds are not usually transmitted to humans. A few notable exceptions have occurred when these animal and bird viruses mutated and became highly infectious to humans. These infections are termed **pandemic** because they have the potential to spread globally. Such pandemics include the 1918 "Spanish" influenza that resulted in 40 million to 100 million deaths worldwide. This virus, the H1N1 strain, also known as "swine flu," mutated and became highly infectious to humans. Most recently, the 2009 H1N1 influenza A resulted in a pandemic infection that spread to 215 countries. In the United States, the number of people infected with this virus during the pandemic is estimated at 61 million, resulting in more than 12,000 deaths (CDC, 2010b). A vaccine was developed in 2009 as a single antigen (monovalent) and was administered separately from the seasonal influenza vaccine. Now the trivalent seasonal vaccine contains the H1N1 antigen.

A new avian virus is the H5N1 strain, known as "avian influenza" or "bird flu," which has infected millions of birds, especially in Asia, and now has started to spread by human-to-human contact. World health officials are concerned that this strain could become a pandemic because humans have no naturally occurring immunity to this virus and it could lead to a worldwide pandemic with very high mortality rates. Another avian strain, H7N9, has appeared in China, resulting in several deaths but has not spread out of that region (CDC, 2014a).

Health Promotion and Maintenance

The prevention of a worldwide influenza pandemic of any virus is the responsibility of everyone. Health officials have been monitoring human outbreaks and testing both wild and domestic bird species throughout the world. A vaccine (Vepacel) is available but is stockpiled and not part of general influenza vaccination. The recommended early approach to disease prevention with H5N1 is early recognition of new cases and the implementation of community and personal quarantine and social-distancing behaviors to reduce exposure to the virus.

Plans for prevention and containment in North America have been developed with the cooperation of most levels of government. When a cluster of cases is discovered in an area, the stockpiled vaccine is to be made available for immunization. Because vaccination with this vaccine is a two-step process with the first IM injection followed 28 days later by a second IM injection, additional prevention measures are needed (Medication Update, 2014; Plosker, 2012).

The antiviral drugs *oseltamivir* (Tamiflu) and *zanamivir* (Relenza) should be widely distributed. These drugs are not likely to prevent the disease but may reduce the severity of the INFECTION and reduce the mortality rate. The infected patients must be cared for in strict isolation. All nonessential public activities in the area should be stopped, including public gatherings of any type, attendance at schools, religious services, shopping, and many types of employment. People should stay home and use the emergency preparedness food, water, and drugs they have stockpiled to last at least 2 weeks (see Chapter 10). Travel to and from this area should be stopped.

Urge all people to pay attention to public health announcements and early warning systems for disease outbreaks. Teach them the importance of starting prevention behaviors immediately upon notification of an outbreak. Teach all people to have a minimum of a 2-week supply of all their prescribed drugs and at least a 2-week supply of nonperishable food and water for each member of the household. They should also have a battery-powered radio (and batteries) to keep informed of updates in an active prevention situation. See Chapter 10 for more information on items to have ready in the home for disaster preparedness. *An influenza pandemic is a disaster, and containing it requires the cooperation of all people.*

❖ PATIENT-CENTERED COLLABORATIVE CARE

The care priorities for the patient with avian or any pandemic influenza are supporting the patient and preventing spread of the disease. Both are equally important. The initial manifestations of avian influenza are similar to other respiratory INFECTIONS—cough, fever, and sore throat. These progress rapidly to shortness of breath and pneumonia. In addition, diarrhea, vomiting, abdominal pain, and bleeding from the nose and gums occur. *Ask any patient with these manifestations if he or she has recently (within the past 10 days) traveled to areas of the world affected by H5N1. If such travel has occurred, coordinate with the health care team to place the patient in an airborne isolation room with negative air pressure. These precautions remain until the diagnosis of H5N1 is ruled out or the threat of contagion is over.* Diagnosis is made based on clinical manifestations and positive testing. The most rapid test currently approved for testing of H5N1 is the AVantage A/H5N1 Flu Test. It can detect a specific protein (NS1), which indicates the presence of H5N1, from nasal or throat swabs in less than 40 minutes.

When providing care to the patient with avian influenza, personal protective equipment is essential. Coordinate the protection activity by ensuring that anyone entering the patient's room for any reason wears a fit-tested respirator or a standard surgical mask. Use other Airborne Precautions and Contact Precautions as described in Chapter 23. Teach others to self-monitor for disease manifestations, especially respiratory INFECTION, for at least a week after the last contact with the patient. Use the antiviral drug *oseltamivir* (Tamiflu) or *zanamivir* (Relenza) within 48 hours of contact with the infected patient. All health care personnel working with patients suspected of having avian influenza should receive the vaccine in the recommended two-step process.

No effective treatment for this INFECTION currently exists. Antibiotics and antiviral drugs cannot kill the virus or prevent its replication. Interventions are supportive to allow the patient's own immune system to fight the infection. Oxygen is given when hypoxia or breathlessness is present. Respiratory treatments to dilate the bronchioles and move respiratory secretions are used. If hypoxemia is not improved with oxygen therapy, intubation and mechanical ventilation may be needed. Antibiotics are used to treat a bacterial pneumonia that may occur with H5N1.

In addition to the need for respiratory support, the patient with H5N1 may have severe diarrhea and need fluid therapy. The Transmission Precautions may prevent the use of a scale to determine fluid needs by weight changes. Monitor the patient's hydration status, and carefully measure intake and output. The type of fluid therapy varies with the patient's cardiovascular status and blood osmolarity. The two most important areas to monitor during rehydration are pulse rate and quality and urine output.

CLINICAL JUDGMENT CHALLENGE

Prioritization, Delegation, and Supervision

The patient is a 67-year-old man with moderate emphysema. He has just been admitted to the medical unit with a diagnosis of shortness of breath related to influenza. In the emergency department he received a chest x-ray and a nebulizer treatment with albuterol. He also had a saline lock placed, and arterial blood gases were sent to the laboratory. Vital signs before transfer were: BP, 158/92; HR, 92; RR, 32; T, 101.4° F.

The health care provider has prescribed:

- Schedule pulmonary function tests
- Obtain admission vital signs
- Tylenol 650 mg orally as needed
- Oxygen at 2 L per nasal cannula
- Nebulizer treatment with albuterol every 6 hours
- Intravenous antibiotic administration
- Use of incentive spirometer hourly
- Blood drawn for culture and sensitivity

1. Which order takes priority at this time? Provide a rationale for your choice.
2. Which action should you delegate to the unlicensed assistive personnel (UAP) who is helping you admit the patient? Provide a rationale for your choice.
3. The patient's SaO_2 is 90% on admission. What action would you take at this time? Provide a rationale for your choice.
4. The patient continues to have an elevated temperature (now 102.4° F). Which actions should you delegate to the licensed practical nurse/licensed vocational nurse (LPN/LVN) working with you and why?

PNEUMONIA

❖ PATHOPHYSIOLOGY

Pneumonia is excess fluid in the lungs resulting from an inflammatory process. The INFLAMMATION is triggered by many infectious organisms and by inhalation of irritating agents. The INFLAMMATION occurs in the interstitial spaces, the alveoli, and often the bronchioles. The process begins when organisms penetrate the airway mucosa and multiply in the alveolar spaces. White blood cells (WBCs) migrate to the area of INFECTION, causing local capillary leak, edema, and exudate. These fluids collect in and around the alveoli, and the alveolar walls thicken. Both events seriously reduce GAS EXCHANGE and lead to hypoxemia, interfering with oxygenation and possibly leading to death. Red blood cells (RBCs) and fibrin move into the alveoli, and capillary leak spreads the infection to other areas of the lung. If the organisms move into the bloodstream, septicemia results; if the infection extends into the pleural cavity, **empyema** (a collection of pus in the pleural cavity) results.

The fibrin and edema stiffen the lung, reducing compliance and decreasing the vital capacity. Alveolar collapse (atelectasis) further reduces the ability of the lung to oxygenate the blood moving through it. As a result, arterial oxygen levels fall, causing hypoxemia.

Pneumonia may occur as *lobar pneumonia* with **consolidation** (solidification, lack of air spaces) in a segment or an entire lobe of the lung or as *bronchopneumonia* with diffusely scattered patches around the bronchi. The extent of lung involvement depends on the host defenses. Bacteria multiply quickly in a person whose immune system is compromised. Tissue necrosis results when an abscess forms and perforates the bronchial wall.

Etiology

Pneumonia develops when the immune system cannot overcome the invading organisms. Organisms from the environment, invasive devices, equipment and supplies, staff, or other people can invade the body. Risk factors are listed in Table 31-2. Pneumonia can be caused by bacteria, viruses, mycoplasmas, fungi, rickettsiae, protozoa, and helminths (worms). Noninfectious causes of pneumonia include inhalation of toxic gases, chemical fumes, and smoke and aspiration of water, food, fluid (including saliva), and vomitus (Echevarria & Schwoebel, 2012). Pneumonia can be categorized as community-acquired (CAP), hospital-acquired (HAP), health care–associated (HCAP) or ventilator-associated (VAP) (Table 31-3).

Incidence and Prevalence

In the United States, 2 to 5 million cases of pneumonia occur each year and it is a major cause of death. The incidence is higher among older adults, nursing home residents, hospitalized patients, and those being mechanically ventilated. CAP is more common than HAP and occurs in late fall and winter, often as a complication of influenza.

Health Promotion and Maintenance

Patient education about vaccination is important in the prevention of pneumonia (Chart 31-3)*. The Joint Commission NPSGs require that nurses especially encourage people older than 65 years and those with a chronic health problem to receive immunization against pneumonia.* Antigens from 23 different types of pneumonia organisms are included in the pneumococcal polysaccharide vaccine (PPV23). This vaccine is usually given once; however, some experts believe that older adults and those with chronic health problems could benefit from a second vaccination if more than 5 years has passed since the first vaccination (American Lung Association [ALA], 2010a). Because pneumonia often follows influenza, especially among older adults, urge all people to receive the seasonal influenza vaccination yearly (Scott & Kardos, 2012).

Other prevention techniques include strict handwashing to avoid the spread of organisms and avoiding large gatherings of people during cold and flu season. Teach the patient who has a cold or the flu to see his or her health care provider if fever lasts more than 24 hours, if the problem lasts longer than 1 week, or if manifestations worsen.

Respiratory therapy equipment must be well maintained and decontaminated or changed as recommended. Use sterile water rather than tap water in GI tubes, and institute Aspiration Precautions as indicated, including screening patients for aspiration risk.

VAP is on the rise, but the risk can be reduced with conscientious assessment and meticulous nursing care (Echevarria &

TABLE 31-2 Risk Factors for Pneumonia

Community-Acquired Pneumonia

- Is an older adult
- Has never received the pneumococcal vaccination or received it more than 5 years ago
- Did not receive the influenza vaccine in the previous year
- Has a chronic health problem or other coexisting condition that reduces immune responses
- Has recently been exposed to respiratory viral or influenza infections
- Uses tobacco or alcohol or is exposed to high amounts of secondhand smoke

Health Care–Acquired Pneumonia

- Is an older adult
- Has a chronic lung disease
- Has presence of gram-negative colonization of the mouth, throat, and stomach
- Has an altered level of consciousness
- Has had a recent aspiration event
- Has presence of endotracheal, tracheostomy, or nasogastric tube
- Has poor nutritional status
- Has immunocompromised status (from disease or drug therapy)
- Uses drugs that increase gastric pH (histamine [H_2] blockers, antacids) or alkaline tube feedings
- Is currently receiving mechanical ventilation (ventilator-associated pneumonia [VAP])

CHART 31-3 Patient and Family Education: Preparing for Self-Management

Preventing Pneumonia

- Know whether you are at risk for pneumonia (older than 65 years, have a chronic health problem [especially a respiratory problem], or have limited mobility and are confined to a bed or chair during your waking hours).
- Have the annual influenza vaccine after discussing appropriate timing of the vaccination with your primary health care provider.
- Discuss the pneumococcal vaccine with your primary health care provider, and have the vaccination as recommended.
- Avoid crowded public areas during flu and holiday seasons.
- If you have a mobility problem, cough, turn, move about as much as possible, and perform deep-breathing exercises.
- If you are using respiratory equipment at home, clean the equipment as you have been taught.
- Avoid indoor pollutants, such as dust, secondhand (passive) smoke, and aerosols.
- If you do not smoke, do not start.
- If you smoke, seek professional help on how to stop (or at least decrease) your habit.
- Be sure to get enough rest and sleep on a daily basis.
- Eat a healthy, balanced diet.
- Drink at least 3 liters (quarts) of nonalcoholic fluids each day (unless fluid restrictions are needed because of another health problem).

TABLE 31-3 Differentiation of Types of Pneumonia

TYPE OF PNEUMONIA	DEFINITION	MANAGEMENT CONSIDERATIONS
Community acquired	Contracted outside a health care setting; acquired in the community	Most common bacterial agents: *Streptococcus pneumoniae, Haemophilus influenzae* Most common viral agents: influenza, respiratory syncytial virus (RSV) Antibiotics are often empirical based on multiple patient and environmental factors Treatment length: minimum of 5 days Prompt initiation of antibiotics required; in ED setting, first dose given before patient leaves unit for inpatient bed, or within 6 hours of presentation to the ED
Health care associated	Onset/diagnosis of pneumonia occurs <48 hours after admission in patient with specific risk factors: In hospital for >48 hours in the past 90 days Living in nursing home or assisted-living facility Received IV therapy, wound care, antibiotics, chemotherapy in the past 30 days Seen at a hospital or dialysis clinic within the past 30 days	May have multidrug-resistant organisms Hand hygiene is critical
Hospital acquired	Onset/diagnosis of pneumonia >48 hours after admission to hospital	Encourage pulmonary hygiene and progressive ambulation Provide adequate hydration Assess risk for aspiration using an evidence-based tool Monitor for early signs of sepsis Hand hygiene is critical
Ventilator associated	Onset/diagnosis of pneumonia within 48-72 hours after endotracheal intubation	Presence of ET tube increases risk for pneumonia by bypassing protective airway mechanisms and by allowing aspiration of secretions from the oropharynx and stomach; dental plaque also increases risk Initiate ventilator bundle order set, including: Elevate HOB at least 30 degrees Daily sedation "vacation" and weaning assessment DVT prophylaxis Oral care regimen Stress ulcer prophylaxis Suctioning; either as needed or continuous subglottal suction Hand hygiene is critical

Data from Echevarria, I. & Schwoebel, A. (2012). Development of an intervention model for the prevention of aspiration pneumonia in high-risk patients on a medical-surgical unit. *MEDSURG Nursing, 21*(5), 303-308; Luttenberger, K. (2010). Battling VAP from a new angle. *Nursing2010, 40*(2), 52-55; Roark, D.C. (2012). Working toward perfection on the pneumonia core measure. *Journal of Emergency Nursing, 38*, 127-129; Scott, S. & Kardos, C. (2012). Community-acquired, health care-associated, and ventilator-associated pneumonia: Three variations of a serious disease. *Critical Care Nursing Clinics of North America, 24*(3), 431-441.

DVT, Deep vein thrombosis; *ED,* emergency department; *ET,* endotracheal; *HOB,* head of bed.

Schwoebel, 2012; Roark, 2012; Scott & Kardos, 2012). The preventive care for VAP is discussed in detail in Chapter 32.

! NURSING SAFETY PRIORITY (QSEN)

Action Alert

Because pneumonia is a frequent cause of sepsis, use a sepsis screening tool to monitor patients who have pneumonia. For patients with pneumonia, always check oxygen saturation with vital signs.

❖ PATIENT-CENTERED COLLABORATIVE CARE

The Concept Map addresses assessment and nursing care issues related to patients who have pneumonia. The manifestations of pneumonia differ in older patients compared with younger patients.

◆ Assessment

History. Assess for the risk factors for INFECTION (see Table 31-2). Document age; living, work, or school environment; diet, exercise, and sleep routines; swallowing problems; presence of a nasogastrointestinal tube; tobacco and alcohol use; and past and current use of or addiction to "street" drugs. Remember that often aspiration is "silent" with no manifestations. Ask about past respiratory illnesses and whether the patient has been exposed to influenza or pneumonia or has had a recent viral infection. Ask about recent skin rashes, insect bites, and exposure to animals.

If the patient has chronic respiratory problems, ask whether respiratory equipment is used in the home. Assess whether the patient's home cleaning level is adequate to prevent INFECTION. Ask when he or she received the last influenza or pneumococcal vaccine.

Physical Assessment/Clinical Manifestations. Observe the general appearance. Many patients with pneumonia have flushed cheeks and an anxious expression. The patient may have chest pain or discomfort, myalgia, headache, chills, fever, cough, tachycardia, dyspnea, tachypnea, hemoptysis, and sputum production. Severe chest muscle weakness also may be present from sustained coughing.

Observe the patient's breathing pattern, position, and use of accessory muscles. The hypoxic patient may be uncomfortable in a lying position and will sit upright, balancing with the hands

CONCEPT MAP

COMMUNITY-ACQUIRED PNEUMONIA

INFECTION · INFLAMMATION · GAS EXCHANGE

HISTORY

60-year-old Diane Owens is admitted with CA pneumonia. She says, "My chest hurts from coughing so much." She is coughing up thick, green and rust-colored sputum. She is becoming confused and has lost her appetite.

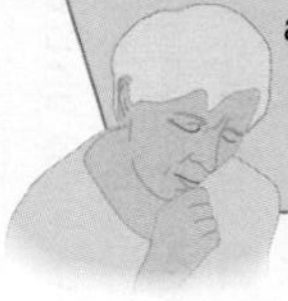

↓ Physical Assessment/ Clinical Manifestations

- Confused.
- T 99.1° F; HR 128, pulse weak; RR 24; BP 96/58 mm Hg
- Cheeks are flushed; fatigued, weak, lethargic; pain present; dyspneic; anxious
- Bilateral crackles and wheezing; fremitus over RLL; dulled percussion; unequal chest expansion on inspiration

→ Older Adult Considerations

Most common sign/symptom is acute confusion from hypoxia. Other signs/symptoms: weakness, fatigue, lethargy, poor appetite. Fever and cough may be absent. White blood cells may not be elevated until infection is severe. Greatly increased risk for sepsis and death.

↑ Planning

PATIENT PROBLEMS

- Impaired GAS EXCHANGE related to decreased diffusion at the alveolar-capillary membrane
- Potential for airway obstruction related to excessive tracheobronchial secretions, fatigue, chest discomfort, muscle weakness
- Potential for sepsis related to the presence of microorganisms in a very vascular area

↑ Data Synthesis

EXPECTED OUTCOMES

Adequate GAS EXCHANGE:
- Maintains patent airway; SaO_2 of at least 95% or in patient's normal range
- Maintains cognitive orientation
- Effective cough with absence of chest pain, crackles, or hemoptysis
- Absence of tachycardia or tachypnea, breathing discomfort with speaking, or cyanosis
- Returns to pre-pneumonia health status

INFLAMMATION:
- Absence of wheezing

INFECTION:
- Free from invading organisms in blood and sputum
- WBC and differential within normal limits
- Afebrile

INTERVENTIONS

1 Nursing Priority – Improving GAS EXCHANGE, Eliminating INFECTION
- Deliver oxygen therapy; assist with bronchial hygiene. *Promotes GAS EXCHANGE and oxygenation*
- Administer antibiotics for 5-7 days; reinforce, clarify, and provide information regarding drug therapy. *Helps to rid body of INFECTION and encourages drug compliance.*

2 Providing Safe and Effective Care

Apply principles of infection control (e.g., hand hygiene, Isolation or Airborne Precautions). *Protects client and health care providers from INFECTION transmission.*

3 Respiratory Assessment
- Perform focused respiratory assessment and re-assessment; observe breathing pattern, position, and use of accessory muscles. *Assesses for respiratory distress.*
- Assess cough and amount, color, consistency, odor produced by sputum. *Assesses for infection and inadequate GAS EXCHANGE.*
- Assess for breath sounds and document wheezes, rhonchi, crackles, and evidence of decreased breath sounds. *Crackles indicate fluid in interstitial and alveolar areas; wheezing indicates INFLAMMATION or exudate in airways; bronchial breath sounds indicate areas of density or consolidation.*

4 Vital Signs Assessment

Evaluate oxygen saturation and vital sign trends, effectiveness of antibiotics, fluids, and antipyretics.
Monitors for signs of sepsis, hypotension with orthostatic changes; rapid, weak pulse; and dysrhythmias.

5 Promoting Breathing
- Assist with coughing, deep breathing, and incentive spirometry at least every 2 hours. Encourage alert patient to drink at least 2 L of fluid daily, unless contraindicated. *Promotes removal of secretions, hydration, and ensures adequate GAS EXCHANGE and oxygenation.*
- Monitor intake & output, especially when fever and tachypnea are present. *Monitors for signs of dehydration.*

6 Diagnostic Tests
- Obtain complete blood count with differential, sputum and blood cultures. *Determines whether organisms have invaded the blood and caused sepsis.*
- Determine oxygenation status by arterial blood gas values and pulse oximetry. *Determines baseline PaO_2 and $PaCO_2$ and helps identify need for supplemental oxygen.*
- Assess electrolytes, blood urea nitrogen (BUN), and creatinine levels. *Checks for dehydration and kidney function.*
- Review chest x-rays. *Provides early diagnosis in older adults because pneumonia symptoms are often vague.*

7 Minimizing Anxiety

Assess expressions and general tenseness of facial and shoulder muscles. Listen using calm, slow approach. *Encourages calmness because pain, fatigue, and dyspnea promote anxiety.*

8 Nursing Safety Priority: Action Alert!

Teach the importance of completing the entire course of antibiotic therapy even when symptoms improve or subside. *Helps eradicate organisms and prevents drug resistance.*

Concept Map by Deanne A. Blach, MSN, RN

("tripod position"). Assess the cough and the amount, color, consistency, and odor of sputum produced.

Crackles are heard with auscultation when fluid is in interstitial and alveolar areas, and breath sounds may be diminished. Wheezing may be heard if INFLAMMATION or exudate narrows the airways. Bronchial breath sounds are heard over areas of density or consolidation. Fremitus is increased over areas of pneumonia, and percussion is dulled. Chest expansion may be diminished or unequal on inspiration.

In evaluating vital signs, compare the results with baseline values. The patient with pneumonia is often hypotensive with orthostatic changes as a result of vasodilation and dehydration, especially the older adult. A rapid, weak pulse may indicate hypoxemia, dehydration, or impending sepsis and shock. Dysrhythmias may occur as a result of cardiac tissue hypoxia. Common pneumonia manifestations and their causes are listed in Table 31-4.

Use an evidence-based pneumonia severity scale to assist in determining what treatment site is appropriate for the patient. Two such tools are the Pneumonia Severity Index (PSI) and the CURB-65. The PSI uses four risk categories (demographics, comorbid conditions, physical examination, and selected laboratory values) to determine a score reflective of the severity of the patient's pneumonia, whereas the CURB-65 relies on laboratory values (blood urea nitrogen [BUN], age, respirations, blood pressure, and presence of confusion (Scott & Kardos, 2012).

CONSIDERATIONS FOR OLDER ADULTS

Patient-Centered Care QSEN

The older adult with pneumonia has weakness, fatigue, lethargy, confusion, and poor appetite. Fever and cough may be absent, but hypoxemia is often present. The most common manifestation of pneumonia in the older adult patient is acute confusion from hypoxia. The WBC count may not be elevated until the infection is severe. Waiting to treat the disease until more typical manifestations appear greatly increases the risk for sepsis and death (Touhy & Jett, 2014).

Psychosocial Assessment. The patient with pneumonia often has pain, fatigue, and dyspnea, all of which promote anxiety. Assess anxiety by looking at his or her facial expression and general tenseness of facial and shoulder muscles. Listen to the patient carefully, and use a calm approach. Because of airway obstruction and muscle fatigue, the patient with dyspnea speaks in broken sentences. Keep the interview short if severe dyspnea or breathing discomfort is present.

Laboratory Assessment. Sputum is obtained and examined by Gram stain, culture, and sensitivity testing; however, the responsible organism often is not identified. A sputum sample is easily obtained from the patient who can cough into a specimen container. Extremely ill patients may need suctioning to obtain a sputum specimen. In these situations, a specimen is obtained by sputum trap (Fig. 31-1) during suctioning. A CBC is obtained to assess an elevated WBC count, which is a common finding except in older adults. Blood cultures may be performed to determine whether the organism has invaded the blood.

In severely ill patients, arterial blood gases (ABGs) and serum lactate levels may be assessed to determine baseline arterial oxygen and carbon dioxide levels and help identify a need for supplemental oxygen. Serum electrolyte, blood urea nitrogen (BUN), and creatinine levels also are assessed. A high BUN level may occur as a result of dehydration. Hypernatremia (high blood sodium levels) occurs with dehydration.

TABLE 31-4 Pathophysiology of Common Clinical Manifestations of Pneumonia

CLINICAL MANIFESTATION	PATHOPHYSIOLOGY
Increased respiratory rate/dyspnea	Stimulation of chemoreceptors Increased work of breathing as a result of decreased lung compliance Stimulation of J receptors Anxiety Pain
Hypoxemia	Alveolar consolidation Pulmonary capillary shunting
Cough	Fluid accumulation in the receptors of the trachea, bronchi, and bronchioles
Purulent, blood-tinged, or rust-colored sputum	A result of the inflammatory process in which fluid from the pulmonary capillaries and red blood cells moves into the alveoli
Fever	Phagocytes release pyrogens that cause the hypothalamus to increase body temperature
Pleuritic chest discomfort	Inflammation of the parietal pleura causes pain on inspiration

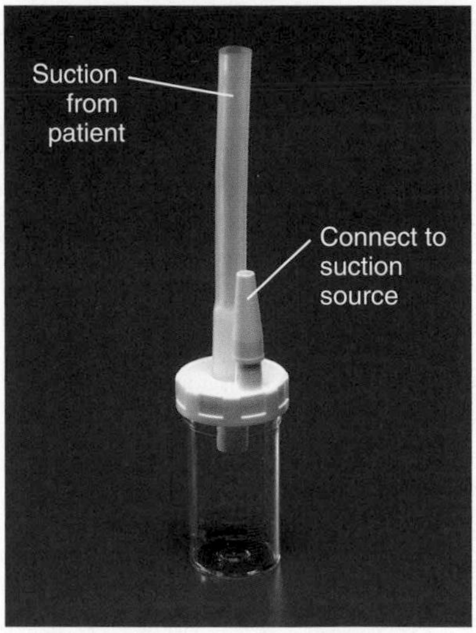

FIG. 31-1 A Lukens tube for collection of sterile sputum/mucus specimens.

Imaging Assessment. Chest x-ray is the most common diagnostic test for pneumonia but may not show changes until 2 or more days after manifestations are present. It usually appears on chest x-ray as an area of increased density. It may involve a lung segment, a lobe, one lung, or both lungs. *In the older adult, the chest x-ray is essential for early diagnosis because pneumonia manifestations are often vague* (Touhy & Jett, 2014).

Other Diagnostic Assessments. Pulse oximetry is used to assess for hypoxemia. Invasive tests such as transtracheal aspiration, bronchoscopy, or direct needle aspiration of the lung may be needed. Thoracentesis is used in patients who have an accompanying pleural effusion.

◆ *Analysis*

The priority NANDA-I nursing diagnoses and collaborative problems for patients with pneumonia include:

1. Impaired Gas Exchange related to decreased diffusion at the alveolar-capillary membrane (NANDA-I)

2. Potential for airway obstruction related to excessive tracheobronchial secretions, fatigue, chest discomfort, muscle weakness
3. Potential for sepsis related to the presence of microorganisms in a very vascular area

◆ *Planning and Implementation*

Improving Gas Exchange

Planning: Expected Outcomes. The patient with pneumonia is expected to have adequate GAS EXCHANGE and oxygenation. Indicators of adequacy are:

- Maintenance of Sao_2 of at least 95% or in the patient's normal range
- Absence of cyanosis
- Maintenance of cognitive orientation

Interventions. Interventions to improve GAS EXCHANGE and oxygenation are similar to those for the patient with chronic airflow limitation (CAL) (see Chapter 30). Nursing priorities include delivery of oxygen therapy and assisting the patient with bronchial hygiene.

Oxygen therapy is usually delivered by nasal cannula or mask unless the hypoxemia does not improve with these devices. The patient who is confused may not tolerate a facemask. Check the skin under the device and under the elastic band, especially around the ears, for areas of redness or skin breakdown. Actions for oxygen therapy are listed in Chart 28-1 in Chapter 28.

Incentive spirometry is used to improve inspiratory muscle action and to prevent or reverse atelectasis (alveolar collapse). Instruct the patient to exhale fully, then place the mouthpiece in his or her mouth, and then take a long, slow, deep breath for 3 to 5 seconds. Evaluate technique, and record the volume of air inspired. Teach the patient to perform 5 to 10 breaths per session every hour while awake.

Preventing Airway Obstruction

Planning: Expected Outcomes. The patient with pneumonia is expected to maintain a patent airway. Indicators are:

- Effective cough
- Absence of pallor or cyanosis
- Absence of crackles and wheezes on auscultation
- Pulse oximetry at or above 95%

Interventions. Interventions to avoid airway obstruction in pneumonia are similar to those for chronic obstructive pulmonary disease (COPD) or asthma. Because of fatigue, muscle weakness, chest discomfort, and excessive secretions, the patient often has difficulty clearing secretions. Help him or her cough and deep breathe at least every 2 hours. The alert patient may use an incentive spirometer to facilitate deep breathing and stimulate coughing. Encourage the alert patient to drink at least 2 liters of fluid daily to prevent dehydration unless another health problem requires fluid restriction. Monitor intake and output, oral mucus membranes, and skin turgor to assess hydration status, especially when fever and tachypnea are present.

Bronchodilators, especially $beta_2$ agonists (see Chart 30-6 in Chapter 30), are prescribed when bronchospasm is present. They are initially given by nebulizer and then by metered dose inhaler. Inhaled or IV steroids are used with acute pneumonia when airway swelling is present. Expectorants such as guaifenesin (Mucinex) may be used.

Preventing Sepsis

Planning: Expected Outcomes. The patient with pneumonia is expected to be free of the invading organism and to return to a pre-pneumonia health status. Indicators are:

- Absence of fever
- Absence of pathogens in blood and sputum cultures
- WBC count and differential within normal limits

Interventions. The key to effective treatment of pneumonia is eradication of the infecting organism. When sepsis occurs with pneumonia, the risk for death is high. Anti-infectives are given for all types of pneumonias except those caused by viruses. Which anti-infective therapy is prescribed is based on how the pneumonia was acquired (i.e., CAP, HAP, or HCAP). The exact drug or drugs and their routes of delivery are determined by the severity of the INFECTION, the organism suspected or identified, and whether the patient has other conditions or factors that increase the risk for complications. Drug therapy choices must reflect the degree of drug resistance in the specific geographic area and in that hospital setting.

The course of anti-infective therapy varies with the drug used and the organism(s) involved. Usually anti-infectives are used for 5 to 7 days for a patient with uncomplicated CAP and up to 21 days for an immunocompromised patient or one with HAP.

Drug resistance is becoming increasingly common, especially for INFECTIONS with *Streptococcus pneumoniae* (drug-resistant *Streptococcus pneumoniae* [DRSP]). It is most common in people older than 65 years and among those who became infected as a result of exposure to young children from a day-care environment.

For pneumonia resulting from aspiration of food or stomach contents, interventions focus on preventing lung damage and treating the INFECTION. Aspiration of acidic stomach contents can cause widespread INFLAMMATION, leading to acute respiratory distress syndrome (ARDS) and permanent lung damage. In these conditions, steroids and NSAIDs are used with antibiotics to reduce the inflammatory response.

NCLEX EXAMINATION CHALLENGE

Physiological Integrity

A nurse is caring for an 89-year-old client admitted with pneumonia. He has an IV of normal saline running at 100 mL/hr and antibiotics that were initiated in the emergency department 3 hours ago. He has oxygen at 2 liters/nasal cannula. What assessment finding by the nurse indicates that goals for a priority diagnosis have been met for this client?

A. The client is alert and oriented to person, place, and time.
B. Blood pressure is within normal limits and client's baseline.
C. Skin behind the ears demonstrates no redness or irritation.
D. Urine output has been >30 mL/hr per Foley catheter.

Community-Based Care

The patient needs to continue the anti-infective drugs as prescribed. An important nursing role is to reinforce, clarify, and provide information to the patient and family as needed.

Home Care Management. No special changes are needed in the home. If the home has a second story, the patient may prefer to stay on one floor for a few weeks, because stair climbing can be tiring. Toileting needs may be met by using a bedside commode if a bathroom is not located on the level the patient is using. Home care needs depend on the patient's level of fatigue, dyspnea, and family and social support.

CHART 31-4 Focused Assessment

The Patient Recovering from Pneumonia

Ask whether the patient has had any of these:	Assess the patient for:
• New-onset confusion • Chills • Fever • Persistent cough • Dyspnea • Wheezing • Hemoptysis • Increased sputum production • Chest discomfort • Increasing fatigue • Any other symptoms that have failed to resolve	• Fever • Diaphoresis • Cyanosis, especially around the mouth or conjunctiva • Dyspnea, tachypnea, or tachycardia • Adventitious or abnormal breath sounds • Weakness

The long recovery phase, especially in the older adult, can be frustrating. Fatigue, weakness, and a residual cough can last for weeks. Some patients fear they will never return to a "normal" level of functioning. Prepare them for the disease course, and offer reassurance that complete recovery will occur. After discharge, a home nursing assessment may be helpful (Chart 31-4).

Self-Management Education. Review all drugs with the patient and family, and emphasize completing anti-infective therapy. Teach the patient to notify the health care provider if chills, fever, persistent cough, dyspnea, wheezing, hemoptysis, increased sputum production, chest discomfort, or increasing fatigue recurs or fails to resolve. Instruct him or her to get plenty of rest and increase activity gradually.

An important aspect of education for the patient and family is the avoidance of upper respiratory tract INFECTIONS and viruses. Teach him or her to avoid crowds (especially in the fall and winter when viruses are prevalent), people who have a cold or flu, and exposure to irritants such as smoke. Stress the importance of following his or her health care provider's recommendations for vaccination against influenza and pneumonia. A balanced diet and adequate fluid intake are essential.

Health Care Resources. Inform patients who smoke that smoking is a risk factor for pneumonia. Provide them with information on local smoking-cessation classes and nicotine replacement options as required by The Joint Commission's NPSGs (see Chapter 27). Provide information booklets on pneumonia, and urge the patient who has not already been vaccinated against influenza or pneumonia to take this preventive measure after the pneumonia has resolved.

! NURSING SAFETY PRIORITY QSEN

Drug Alert

Warn the patient using nicotine patches or supplements of the danger of myocardial infarction if smoking is continued while using other forms of nicotine.

◆ *Evaluation: Outcomes*

Evaluate the care of the patient with pneumonia based on the identified priority patient problems. The expected outcomes are that he or she:

- Attains or maintains adequate GAS EXCHANGE
- Maintains patent airways
- Is free of the invading organism
- Returns to his or her pre-pneumonia health status

Specific indicators for these outcomes are listed for each priority patient problem under the Planning and Implementation section (see earlier).

? CLINICAL JUDGMENT CHALLENGE

Evidence-Based Practice; Patient-Centered Care QSEN

The nurse is caring for a frail, older patient in the hospital after surgery to repair a bowel obstruction. The patient has a nasogastric (NG) tube to suction, through which all her scheduled drugs are given, oxygen at 1 liter/nasal cannula at night (home order), an indwelling urinary catheter, and a saline lock. The patient is weak and fatigued, has pain not relieved by IV opioids, and is reluctant to participate in any activities.

1. What risk factors does this patient have for developing pneumonia?
2. What actions does the nurse take to decrease the patient's risk for pneumonia?
3. Two days later, the NG tube is removed and the patient is started on ice chips and other clear liquids. The patient swallows repeatedly when given sips of water. What action does the nurse perform?
4. The nurse does hourly rounds on the patient, and the patient's daughter states, "Something is just not right with mom." What action should the nurse take first? What other actions should the nurse perform?
5. The physician orders a chest x-ray, and the results show pneumonia. What actions by the nurse are most important?

SEVERE ACUTE RESPIRATORY SYNDROME (SARS)

Severe acute respiratory syndrome (SARS) is a respiratory infection first identified in China early in November 2002. The cause of SARS is a new virus from a family of virus types known as *coronaviruses.* This family of viruses causes many forms of the common cold. The new virus, known as *SARS Co-V,* is a mutated form of the coronavirus and is very virulent. It infects cells of the respiratory tract, triggering INFLAMMATION, and stays in the respiratory passageways rather than spreading into the blood.

The virus is easily spread by airborne droplets from infected people through sneezing, coughing, and talking. People at greatest risk for SARS are those in close direct contact with an infected person. The portals of entry are the mucous membranes of the eyes, nose, and mouth.

No new cases of SARS have been reported since 2004. There is no vaccination to prevent the disease, and no known effective treatment exists at this time. If such an outbreak were to occur, the same types of precautions used to prevent INFECTION spread for an avian influenza outbreak, discussed on p. 588, would be used. Patients diagnosed with or suspected of having SARS would be managed with supportive care under strict Airborne and Contact Precautions plus eye protection.

A disease similar in some respects to SARS, and also caused by a coronavirus *(MERS-CoV),* is MERS (Middle East respiratory syndrome). The first U.S. case of MERS, which originates in the Arabian peninsula, appeared in May 2014. Although SARS is considered more infectious, MERS has a higher mortality rate because patients progress to respiratory failure faster with MERS than with SARS, (Barclay, 2013; CDC, 2014d; Todd, 2014).

! NURSING SAFETY PRIORITY (QSEN)

Action Alert

When performing procedures for the patient with SARS that normally induce coughing or promote aerosolization of particles (e.g., suctioning, using a positive-pressure facemask, obtaining a sputum culture, or giving aerosolized treatments), protect yourself and other health care workers. Wear a disposable particulate mask respirator and protective eyewear during the procedures. Keep the door to the patient's room closed. Avoid touching your face with contaminated gloves. Wash your hands after you remove the gown, gloves, eyewear, and face shield and whenever you leave the patient's room. Wear gloves when disinfecting contaminated surfaces or equipment.

PULMONARY TUBERCULOSIS

❖ *PATHOPHYSIOLOGY*

Tuberculosis (TB) is a highly communicable disease caused by *Mycobacterium tuberculosis.* It is one of the most common bacterial INFECTIONS worldwide (CDC, 2014c). The organism is transmitted via **aerosolization** (i.e., an airborne route) (Fig. 31-2). When a person with active TB coughs, laughs, sneezes, whistles, or sings, droplets are airborne and may be inhaled by others. Far more people are infected with the bacillus than actually develop active TB.

The bacillus multiplies freely when it reaches a susceptible site (bronchi or alveoli). An exudative response occurs, causing pneumonitis. With the development of acquired immunity, further growth of bacilli is controlled in most initial lesions. These lesions usually resolve and leave little or no residual bacilli. Only a small percentage of people initially infected with the bacillus ever develop active TB.

Cell-mediated immunity develops 2 to 10 weeks after INFECTION and is manifested by a positive reaction to a tuberculin test. The primary infection may be so small that it does not appear on a chest x-ray. The process of infection occurs in this order:

1. The granulomatous INFLAMMATION created by the TB bacillus in the lung becomes surrounded by collagen, fibroblasts, and lymphocytes.
2. **Caseation necrosis**, which is necrotic tissue being turned into a granular mass, occurs in the center of the lesion. If this area shows on x-ray, it is the *primary* lesion.

Areas of caseation then undergo resorption, degeneration, and fibrosis. These necrotic areas may calcify *(calcification)* or liquefy *(liquefaction).* If liquefaction occurs, this material then empties into a bronchus and the evacuated area becomes a cavity *(cavitation).* Bacilli continue to grow in the necrotic cavity wall and spread via lymph channels into new areas of the lung.

A lesion also may progress by direct extension if bacilli multiply rapidly during INFLAMMATION. The lesions may extend through the pleura, resulting in pleural or pericardial effusion. **Miliary** or **hematogenous TB** is the spread of TB throughout the body when a large number of organisms enter the blood. Many tiny nodules scattered throughout the lung are seen on chest x-ray. Other body areas can become infected as a result of this spread.

Initial infection is seen more often in the middle or lower lobes of the lung. The local lymph nodes are infected and enlarged. An asymptomatic period usually follows the primary INFECTION and can last for years or decades before clinical symptoms develop. *An infected person is not infectious to others until manifestations of disease occur.*

Secondary TB is a reactivation of the disease in a previously infected person. It is more likely when defenses are lowered, such as with older adults and people with HIV disease. The upper lobes are the most common site of reactivation.

Etiology

M. tuberculosis is a slow-growing, acid-fast rod transmitted via the airborne route. People most often infected are those having repeated close contact with an infectious person who has not yet been diagnosed with TB. The risk for transmission is reduced after the infectious person has received proper drug therapy for 2 to 3 weeks, clinical improvement occurs, and acid-fast bacilli (AFB) in the sputum are reduced.

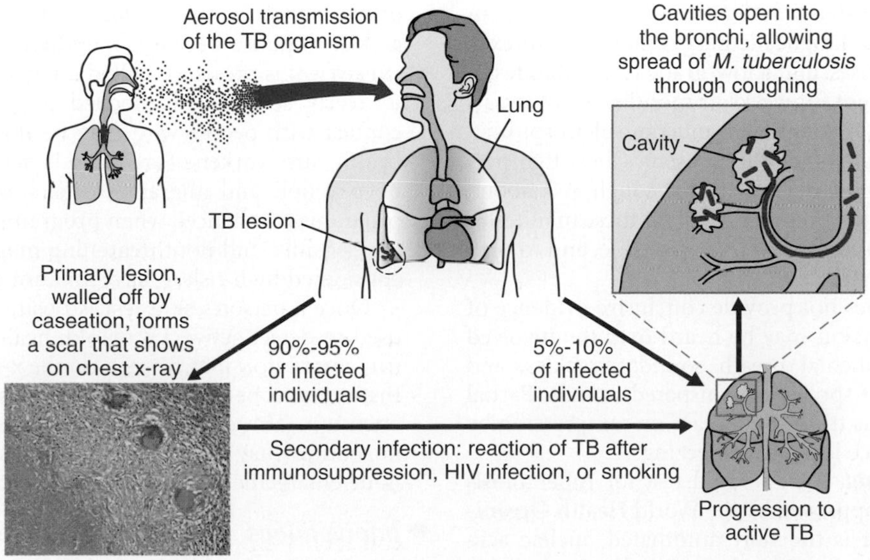

FIG. 31-2 Primary TB infection with progression to secondary infection and active disease. *HIV,* Human immune deficiency virus; *M. tuberculosis, Mycobacterium tuberculosis;* TB, tuberculosis.

Incidence and Prevalence

Worldwide, 8.7 million people were diagnosed and an additional 1.4 million people died from TB in 2012 (WHO, 2014b). The incidence of TB has been steadily decreasing in North America, although increases in incidence are seen in many other countries (ALA, 2010b). In North America, the people who are at greatest risk for development of TB are:

- Those in constant, frequent contact with an untreated person
- Those who have decreased immune function or HIV
- People who live in crowded areas such as long-term care facilities, prisons, homeless shelters, and mental health facilities
- Older homeless people
- Abusers of injection drugs or alcohol
- Lower socioeconomic groups
- Foreign immigrants (especially from Mexico, the Philippines, Vietnam, China, Japan, and Eastern Mediterranean countries [WHO, 2014b])

❖ PATIENT-CENTERED COLLABORATIVE CARE

◆ Assessment

Early detection of TB depends on subjective findings rather than on observable manifestations. TB has a slow onset, and patients are not aware of problems until the disease is advanced. *TB should be considered for any patient with a persistent cough or other manifestations compatible with TB, such as weight loss, anorexia, night sweats, hemoptysis, shortness of breath, fever, or chills.*

History. Assess the patient's past exposure to TB. Ask about his or her country of origin and travel to foreign countries where incidence of TB is high. It is important to ask about the results of any previous tests for TB. Also ask whether the patient has had bacille Calmette-Guérin (BCG) vaccine, which contains attenuated tubercle bacilli. *Anyone who has received BCG vaccine within the previous 10 years will have a positive skin test that can complicate interpretation* (Heavey, 2013). Usually the size of the skin response decreases each year after BCG vaccination. These patients should be evaluated for TB with a chest x-ray or the QuantiFERON-TB Gold test.

Physical Assessment/Clinical Manifestations. The patient with TB has progressive fatigue, lethargy, nausea, anorexia, weight loss, irregular menses, and a low-grade fever. Manifestations may have been present for weeks or months. Night sweats may occur with the fever. A cough with mucopurulent sputum, which may be streaked with blood, is present. Chest tightness and a dull, aching chest pain occur with the cough. Ask about, assess for, and document the presence of any of these manifestations to help with diagnosis, to establish a baseline, and to plan nursing interventions.

Chest examination does not provide conclusive evidence of TB. Dullness with percussion may be heard over the involved lung fields, as may bronchial breath sounds, crackles, and increased transmission of spoken or whispered sounds. Partial obstruction of a bronchus from the disease or compression by lymph nodes may produce localized wheezing.

Diagnostic Assessment. A new rapid test for tuberculosis has been developed and approved by the World Health Organization (2014b). This test is the fully automated nucleic acid amplification (NAA) test for tuberculosis. Results are available in less than 2 hours. Widespread use of this test is recommended by the CDC to replace other diagnostic methods for patients who are suspected to have TB.

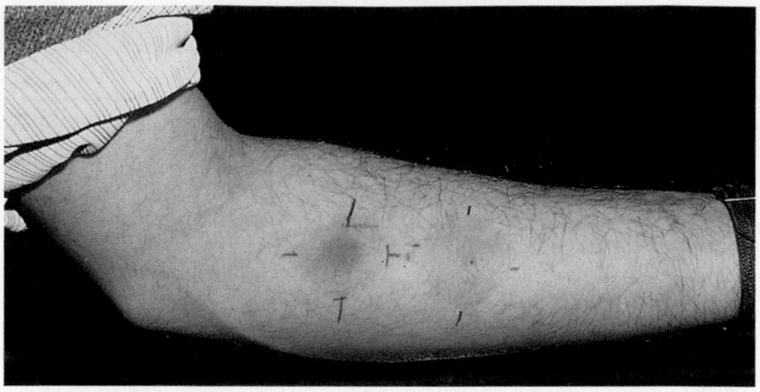

FIG. 31-3 Positive tuberculin skin test with induration.

Blood analysis by an enzyme-linked immunosorbent assay using the QuantiFERON-TB Gold (QFT-G) is a relatively rapid test for the presence of *M. tuberculosis.* Results are ready in 24 hours and are still used in acute care settings to determine whether a symptomatic patient has TB.

Sputum culture confirms the diagnosis. Enhanced TB cultures and automated mycobacterial cultures require 1 to 4 weeks to determine a positive or negative result. After drugs are started, sputum samples are obtained again to determine therapy effectiveness. Cultures are usually negative after 3 months of effective treatment.

The tuberculin test (Mantoux test) is the most commonly used reliable screening test of TB infection. A small amount (0.1 mL) of purified protein derivative (PPD) is placed intradermally in the forearm. An area of **induration** (localized swelling with hardness of soft tissue), not just redness, measuring 10 mm or greater in diameter 48 to 72 hours after injection indicates exposure to and possible INFECTION with TB (Fig. 31-3). If possible, the site is re-evaluated after 72 hours because the incidence of false-negative readings is greater at 48 hours. *A positive reaction does not mean that active disease is present but indicates exposure to TB or the presence of inactive (dormant) disease.* A reaction of 5 mm or greater is considered positive in people with HIV infection. *A reduced skin reaction or a negative skin test does not rule out TB disease or infection of the very old or anyone who is severely immunocompromised.* Failure to have a skin response because of reduced immune function when INFECTION is present is called **anergy**.

Yearly screening is needed for anyone who comes into contact with people who may be infected with TB, including health care workers. Screening is very important for foreign-born people and migrant workers. Participation in screening programs is enhanced when programs are delivered in a culturally sensitive and nonthreatening manner. Urge anyone who is considered high risk to have an annual TB screening test.

Once a person's skin test is positive for TB, a chest x-ray is used to detect active TB or old, healed lesions. Caseation and INFLAMMATION may be seen on the x-ray if the disease is active. Instruct anyone who has manifestations of TB to seek medical attention. The chest x-rays of HIV-infected patients may be normal or may show infiltrates in any lung zone and lymph node enlargement.

◆ Interventions

Combination drug therapy is the most effective method of treating TB and preventing transmission. Active TB is treated with

CHART 31-5 **Common Examples of Drug Therapy**

First-Line Treatment for Tuberculosis

DRUG/USUAL DOSAGE	PURPOSE/ACTION	NURSING INTERVENTIONS	RATIONALES
Isoniazid (INH) 200-300 mg orally daily or 600-900 mg orally twice each week	Kills actively growing mycobacteria outside the cell and inhibits the growth of dormant bacteria inside macrophages and caseating granulomas.	Teach the patient to take the drug on an empty stomach (1 hour before or 2 hours after meals) and to avoid antacids.	Food and antacids slow or prevent absorption of the drug from the GI tract.
		Teach the patient to take a daily multiple vitamin that contains the B-complex vitamins while on this drug.	Drug can deplete the body of this vitamin.
		Remind the patient to avoid drinking alcoholic beverages while on this drug.	The drug can cause liver damage. This effect is potentiated by alcohol.
		Teach the patient to report darkening of the urine, a yellow appearance to the skin or whites of the eyes, and an increased tendency to bruise or bleed.	These manifestations may indicate liver toxicity or failure.
Rifampin (RIF) 500-600 mg orally daily or twice each week	Kills slower-growing organisms, even those that reside in macrophages and caseating granulomas.	Teach the patient to expect the drug to stain the skin and urine and expect all other secretions to have a reddish orange tinge; also, soft contact lenses will become permanently stained.	This is an expected and harmless side effect of the drug and will clear some time after the patient stops taking the drug.
		Teach women using oral contraceptives to use an additional method of contraception while taking this drug and for 1 month after stopping the drug.	This drug reduces the effectiveness of oral contraceptives, increasing the risk for an unplanned pregnancy.
		Remind the patient to avoid drinking alcoholic beverages while on this drug.	The drug can cause liver damage. This effect is potentiated by alcohol.
		Teach the patient to report darkening of the urine, a yellow appearance to the skin or whites of the eyes, and an increased tendency to bruise or bleed.	These manifestations may indicate liver toxicity or failure.
		Ask the patient about all other drugs in use.	This drug interacts with many drugs.
Pyrazinamide (PZA) 1000-2000 mg orally daily or 3000-6000 mg orally twice each week	Is not inactivated by the acidic environment of macrophages and can effectively kill organisms residing within them.	Ask whether the patient has ever had gout.	This drug increases uric acid formation and will make gout worse.
		Teach the patient to drink at least 8 ounces of water when taking this tablet and to increase fluid intake.	More fluids help prevent uric acid from precipitating and causing gout or kidney problems.
		Teach the patient to wear protective clothing, a hat, and sunscreen when going outdoors in the sunlight.	The drug causes photosensitivity and greatly increases the risk for sunburn.
		Remind the patient to avoid drinking alcoholic beverages while on this drug.	The drug can cause liver damage. This effect is potentiated by alcohol.
		Teach the patient to report darkening of the urine, a yellow appearance to the skin or whites of the eyes, and an increased tendency to bruise or bleed.	These manifestations may indicate liver toxicity or failure.
Ethambutol (EMB) 750-1500 mg orally daily or 2500-5000 mg orally twice each week	Inhibits bacterial RNA synthesis, thus suppressing bacterial growth. It is slow-acting and is bacteriostatic rather than bactericidal. Thus it must be used in combination with other anti-TB drugs.	Remind the patient to avoid drinking alcoholic beverages while on this drug.	The drug induces severe nausea and vomiting when alcohol is ingested.
		Teach the patient to report any changes in vision, such as reduced color vision, blurred vision, or reduced visual fields, immediately to his or her health care provider.	The drug can cause optic neuritis, especially at high doses, and can lead to blindness. When the problem is discovered early, the eye problems are usually reversed when the drug is stopped.
		Ask whether the patient has ever had gout.	This drug increases uric acid formation and will make gout worse.
		Teach the patient to drink at least 8 ounces of water when taking this tablet and to increase fluid intake.	More fluids help prevent uric acid from precipitating and causing gout or kidney problems.

RNA, Ribonucleic acid.

a combination of drugs to which the organism is sensitive. Therapy continues until the disease is under control. The use of multiple-drug regimens destroys organisms as quickly as possible and reduces the emergence of drug-resistant organisms. First-line therapy uses isoniazid (INH) and rifampin (Rifadin) throughout the therapy; pyrazinamide is added for the first 2 months (Chart 31-5). This protocol shortens the therapy from 6 to 12 months to 6 months. Ethambutol (Myambutol) is the recommended fourth drug in first-line therapy. These drugs are now available in two-drug or three-drug combinations. One example is Rifater, which combines isoniazid, pyrazinamide, and rifampin. Variations of the first-line drugs along with other drug types are used when the patient does not tolerate the standard first-line therapy. Nursing interventions focus on patient teaching for drug therapy adherence and INFECTION control.

Strict adherence to the prescribed drug regimen is crucial for suppressing the disease. Thus your major role is teaching the patient about drug therapy and stressing the importance of taking each drug regularly, exactly as prescribed, for as long as it is prescribed. Provide accurate information in multiple formats, such as pamphlets, videos, and drug-schedule worksheets. To determine whether the patient understands how to take the drugs, ask him or her to describe the treatment regimen, side effects, and when to call the health care agency and physician.

! NURSING SAFETY PRIORITY QSEN

Drug Alert

The first-line drugs used as therapy for tuberculosis all can damage the liver. Warn the patient to not drink any alcoholic beverages for the entire duration of TB therapy. (Duration of therapy is usually 6 months but can be as long as 2 years for multidrug-resistant [MDR] TB).

The TB drugs may cause the patient to have nausea. Teach him or her to prevent nausea by taking the daily dose at bedtime. Antiemetics may also prevent this problem. Instruct him or her to eat a well-balanced diet that includes foods that are rich in iron, protein, and vitamins C and B. Collaborate with the registered dietitian for specialized needs.

The patient with TB has reduced physical stamina and also has concerns about the disease prognosis. Offer a positive outlook for the patient who adheres to the drug regimen. Tell him or her that fatigue will diminish as the treatment progresses. *With current resistant strains of TB, however, emphasize that not taking the drugs as prescribed could lead to an infection that is drug resistant.*

Some *multidrug-resistant TB* (MDR TB) strains are emerging as extensively drug-resistant (XDR TB). MDR TB is an INFECTION that resists INH and rifampin. XDR TB is resistant not only to the first-line anti-tuberculosis drugs but also to the second-line antibiotics, including the fluoroquinolones and at least one of the aminoglycosides. In 2011, there were over 690,000 cases of MDR TB worldwide with 9% being XDR TB. The most common cause of MDR TB and XDR TB is mismanagement of drug therapy, either from inappropriate selection or use of antibiotics (WHO, 2013). Patients with acquired immune deficiency syndrome (AIDS) also often have MDR TB (CDC, 2013a). Drug therapy for MDR TB and XDR TB is more limited than standard first-line therapy and requires higher doses for longer periods. A new drug combination of bedaquiline, pyrazinamide, and moxifloxacin (Sirturo) was approved in 2012 to treat multidrug-resistant TB. Another drug, delaminid (OPC-67683), is in clinical trials (Gler et al., 2012).

! NURSING SAFETY PRIORITY QSEN

Action Alert

Warn patients with extensively drug-resistant TB that absolute adherence to therapy is critical for survival and cure of the disease. These patients should receive directly observed therapy (DOT).

When teaching the patient and family with either MDR TB or XDR TB, stress that it is the organism, not the patient, that is drug resistant. So a person who acquires the INFECTION and develops TB from a person who is infected with a resistant strain of bacillus will also have drug-resistant disease. Thus teaching infection control strategies is a priority and should be constantly reinforced.

? NCLEX EXAMINATION CHALLENGE

Health Promotion and Maintenance

A client has been admitted to the hospital with suspected TB. What drugs should the nurse plan to teach the client about before discharge? **Select all that apply.**

A. Rifampin (Rifadin); contact lenses can become stained orange
B. Isoniazid (INH); report yellowing of the skin or darkened urine
C. Pyrazinamide (PZA); maintain a fluid restriction of 1200 mL/day
D. Ethambutol (Myambutol); report any changes in vision
E. Amoxicillin (Amoxil); take this drug with food or milk

Other care issues for the patient with TB include teaching about INFECTION prevention and what to expect about disease monitoring and participating in activities. TB is often treated outside the acute care setting, with the patient convalescing in the home setting. Airborne Precautions are not necessary in this setting because family members have already been exposed; however, all members of the household need to undergo TB testing. Teach the patient to cover the mouth and nose with a tissue when coughing or sneezing, to place used tissues in plastic bags, and to wear a mask when in contact with crowds until the drugs suppress infection.

Tell the patient that sputum specimens are needed usually every 2 to 4 weeks once drug therapy is initiated. When the results of three consecutive sputum cultures are negative, the patient is no longer infectious and may return to former employment. Remind him or her to avoid exposure to any inhalation irritants because these can cause further lung damage.

The hospitalized patient with active TB is placed on Airborne Precautions (see Chapter 23) in a well-ventilated room that has at least six exchanges of fresh air per minute. All health care workers must use a personal respirator when caring for the patient. When hand and clothing contamination is a risk, use Standard Precautions with appropriate contact protection (i.e., gowns and gloves). In accordance with The Joint Commission's NPSGs, perform handwashing before and after patient care. Precautions are discontinued when the patient is no longer infectious.

Community-Based Care

Home Care Management. Most patients with TB are managed outside the hospital; however, patients may be diagnosed with TB while in the hospital for another problem. Discharge may be delayed if the living situation is high risk or if nonadherence is likely. Collaborate with the case manager or social service worker in the hospital or the community health nursing agency to ensure that the patient is discharged to the appropriate environment with continued supervision.

Self-Management Education. Teach the patient to follow the drug regimen exactly as prescribed and always to have a supply on hand. Teach about side effects and ways of reducing them to promote adherence. Remind him or her that the disease is usually no longer contagious after drugs have been taken for 2 to 3 consecutive weeks and clinical improvement is seen; however, *he or she must continue with the prescribed drugs for 6 months or longer as prescribed.* **Directly observed therapy (DOT)**, in which a health care professional watches the patient swallow the drugs, may be indicated in some situations. This practice leads to more treatment successes, fewer relapses, and less drug resistance.

The patient who has weight loss and severe lethargy should gradually resume usual activities. Proper nutrition is needed to prevent INFECTION recurrence.

To help with concerns about the contagious aspect of the INFECTION, provide the patient with information about TB. A key to preventing transmission is identifying those in close contact with the infected person so that they can be tested and treated if needed. Identified contacts are assessed with a TB test and possibly a chest x-ray to determine infection status. Multidrug therapy may be indicated as a preventive strategy for heavily exposed individuals or for those who have other health problems that reduce the immune response.

Health Care Resources. Teach the patient to receive follow-up care by a health care provider for at least 1 year during and after active treatment. The American Lung Association (ALA) can provide free information to the patient about the disease and its treatment. In addition, Alcoholics Anonymous (AA) and other health care resources for patients with alcoholism are available if needed. Assist the patient who uses illicit drugs to locate a drug treatment program. In accordance with The Joint Commission's NPSGs, urge smokers to quit, and assist them in finding an appropriate smoking-cessation program (see Chapter 27).

LUNG ABSCESS

A lung abscess is a localized area of subacute INFECTION and necrosis, which is usually related to pyogenic bacteria, and occurs most often in the lung parenchyma. Patients with an abscess often have a history of pneumonia, aspiration of stomach contents, or obstruction as a result of a tumor or foreign body. Other causes of aspiration leading to lung abscesses include any condition that alters the ability to swallow, such as alcoholic blackouts, seizure disorders, neurologic deficits, and swallowing disorders. Bronchial obstruction may cause a necrotizing process in the lung that eventually becomes an abscess (Kamanger, 2013).

Multiple abscesses and cavities form in patients with tuberculosis (TB) or fungal INFECTIONS of the lung. Immunosuppressed patients, such as those receiving cancer chemotherapy or those with AIDS, are at high risk for fungal infections.

Ask the patient about any recent history of influenza, pneumonia, febrile illness, cough, and foul-smelling sputum production. Ask about the sputum color and odor and about any **pleuritic chest pain** (a stabbing pain upon taking a deep breath). Often the patient is febrile, pale, fatigued, and cachectic. Auscultation may reveal decreased breath sounds and dullness on percussion in the involved area. Bronchial breath sounds and crackles may be heard over the site of the lesion. A chest x-ray, sputum sample, and CBC are needed for diagnosis. TB testing should be considered for patients at risk for or with this problem (Zwanger, 2013).

Problems and interventions for the patient with pneumonia also apply to the patient with a lung abscess. Management involves a long course of antibiotics that target organisms acquired by aspiration (Zwanger, 2013).

PULMONARY EMPYEMA

Pulmonary empyema is a collection of pus in the pleural space most commonly caused by pulmonary INFECTION, lung abscess, or infected pleural effusion (Zwanger, 2013). Infections in other body areas also can spread to the lungs by flow of infected lymph into the pleural space. Chest surgery or trauma can introduce bacteria directly into the pleural space, leading to empyema. Blood from trauma may collect in the pleural space, promoting INFECTION.

History findings include febrile illness, pneumonia, chest pain, dyspnea, cough, and trauma. Document the character of the sputum. Chest wall motion may be reduced. If a pleural effusion is present, fremitus may be reduced or absent, percussion is flat, and breath sounds are decreased. Abnormal breath sounds, including bronchial breath sounds, egophony, and whispered pectoriloquy, also may be present. Often the patient has a fever, chills, night sweats, and weight loss.

A chest x-ray or CT scan and a sample of the pleural fluid (obtained via thoracentesis) are needed for diagnosis. Empyema fluid is thick, opaque, exudative, and foul smelling. The fluid is analyzed for color, red blood cell (RBC) count, white blood cell (WBC) count, glucose and protein levels, lactate dehydrogenase (LDH), and pH. Gram stains, acid-fast stains, culture and sensitivity, and cytology studies are also performed.

Therapy involves emptying the empyema cavity, re-expanding the lung, and controlling the INFECTION. Appropriate antibiotics are prescribed. A chest tube(s) to closed-chest drainage is used to promote lung expansion and drainage. The tube is removed when the lung is fully expanded and the infection is under control. Chest surgery may be needed for thick pus or excessive pleural thickening. Nursing interventions are similar to those for patients with a pleural effusion, pneumothorax, or infection. Chapters 30 and 32 discuss these interventions in more detail.

INHALATION ANTHRAX

❖ PATHOPHYSIOLOGY

Inhalation anthrax (respiratory anthrax) is a bacterial INFECTION caused by the gram-positive organism *Bacillus anthracis*, which lives as a spore in soil where grass-eating animals live and graze. Most cases of anthrax are on the skin (cutaneous). Inhalation anthrax accounts for only about 5% of cases, and GI anthrax accounts for about 1% of cases of the disease. When infection occurs through the lungs, the disease is nearly 100% fatal without treatment (Cunha, 2014). Inhalation anthrax is a rare natural occurrence in North America and is not spread by person-to-person contact. It is an occupational hazard of veterinarians, farmers, taxidermists, and others who come into frequent contact with animal wool, hides, bone meal, and skin (Cunha, 2014).

! NURSING SAFETY PRIORITY QSEN

Action Alert

Because inhalation anthrax is so rare, any occurrence in a person who does not have an occupational risk is considered an intentional act of bioterrorism. Report the presence of manifestations consistent with inhalation anthrax to hospital authorities immediately.

This organism first forms a **spore**—an encapsulated organism that is inactive. When many spores are inhaled deeply into the lungs, macrophages engulf them. Once inside the macrophage, the organism leaves its capsule and replicates. The active bacteria produce several toxins that are released into the infected

CHART 31-6 Key Features

Inhalation Anthrax

Prodromal Stage (Early)	Fulminant Stage (Late)
• Fever • Fatigue • Mild chest pain • Dry cough • No manifestations of upper respiratory infection • Mediastinal "widening" on chest x-ray	• Sudden onset of breathlessness • Dyspnea • Diaphoresis • Stridor on inhalation and exhalation • Hypoxia • High fever • Mediastinitis • Pleural effusion • Hypotension • Septic shock

tissues and the blood that make the INFECTION worse. Massive edema occurs along with hemorrhage and destruction of lung cells. Infected macrophages carry the organisms to the lymph nodes, and the organism spreads rapidly, causing bacteremia, sepsis, and meningitis. Lethal toxins produced by the bacteria are the most common cause of death (Cunha, 2014).

❖ *PATIENT-CENTERED COLLABORATIVE CARE*

Inhalation anthrax is a two-stage illness—prodromal and fulminant. Manifestations may not begin until as long as 8 weeks after exposure to the organism (Chart 31-6).

The prodromal stage is early and difficult to distinguish from influenza or pneumonia. Manifestations include low-grade fever, fatigue, mild chest pain, and a dry, harsh cough. *A special feature of inhalation anthrax is that it is* ***not*** *accompanied by upper respiratory manifestations of sore throat or rhinitis.* Usually the patient starts to feel better and manifestations improve in 2 to 4 days.

If the patient begins appropriate antibiotic therapy at this stage, the likelihood of survival is high. Diagnostic indicators are positive Gram stain of the serum and a mediastinal "widening" on chest x-ray as the local lymph nodes greatly enlarge. After several days, blood cultures may be positive for the organism and the genetic material of the bacteria may be detected through the amplification process of the polymerase chain reaction (PCR). Positive results for these definitive diagnostic tests may not be evident until the disease has progressed to the fulminant stage.

The fulminant stage begins after the patient feels a little better. Usually there is a sudden onset of severe illness, including respiratory distress, hematemesis (bloody vomit), dyspnea, diaphoresis, stridor, chest pain, and cyanosis. The patient has a high fever. Hemorrhagic mediastinitis and pleural effusions develop. The patient may be admitted with a decreased level of consciousness or frank shock. As the disease spreads through the blood, causing septic shock and hemorrhagic meningitis, death often occurs within 24 to 36 hours even if antibiotics are started in this stage (Cunha, 2014).

The naturally occurring organism is sensitive to common antibiotics; however, organisms grown for bioterrorism may have been altered to be resistant to these antibiotics. Therefore the antibiotics used for suspected or diagnosed inhalation anthrax include combination therapy (Chart 31-7). The same drugs are used for prophylaxis when people have been exposed to inhalation anthrax but do not yet have manifestations. A vaccine is available, but distribution is limited.

CHART 31-7 Common Examples of Drug Therapy

Prophylaxis and Treatment of Inhalation Anthrax

PROPHYLAXIS	TREATMENT
Ciprofloxacin (Cipro) 500 mg orally twice daily	Ciprofloxacin (Cipro IV) 400 mg IV every 12 hr
Or	***Or***
Doxycycline (Vibramycin) 100 mg orally twice daily	Doxycycline (Doxy 100) 100 mg IV every 12 hr
Or *(if organism is proven susceptible to penicillin)*	**Plus** *one or two of the following secondary agents (parenteral form (IV); dosage based on patient's weight and age):*
Amoxicillin (Amoxil, Trimox) 500 mg orally every 8 hr or 875 mg orally twice daily	Rifampin (RIF) Clindamycin (Cleocin) Vancomycin (Vancocin, Vancoled)
Prophylaxis must continue for 60 days (or longer if exposure was heavy).	**Treatment with IV drugs continues for at least 7 days. When the response is good and the patient improves, IV drugs are changed to oral agents and are continued for at least 60 days.**

Teach patients with any type of lower respiratory INFECTION to be especially vigilant for changes after they think they are getting well. They need to seek medical attention immediately upon having a setback that starts with breathlessness.

PERTUSSIS

Pertussis is a respiratory INFECTION caused by the bacterium *Bordetella pertussis.* It is highly contagious and spreads easily from person to person via respiratory droplets. Once considered a childhood disease, a resurgence is occurring in adults, perhaps due to waning vaccination effectiveness (Bocka, 2014; CDC, 2012). In 2010, there were 27,550 new cases in the United States (CDC, 2012).

The disease occurs in three distinct phases. During the first *(catarrhal)* phase, the patient has manifestations resembling the common cold, including a mild cough. After 1 to 2 weeks, the *paroxysmal* stage begins and the patient has severe coughing "fits" lasting several minutes, during which the coughing spasms are accompanied by turning red and/or vomiting. The patient is frequently exhausted by the coughing. The distinct "whooping" sound common in children at the end of a cough may not be present in adults. This stage can last up to 10 weeks. The recovery *(convalescent)* stage can last for months. During the course of the disease, there is a bloody, purulent, mucinous exudate in the small airways that can lead to atelectasis and pneumonia (Bocka, 2014; Schweon, 2011).

The diagnosis of pertussis can be made clinically, but sputum cultures (obtained by deep suctioning) and PCR laboratory testing are available to aid the diagnosis. Blood cultures will be negative. The CDC recommends testing for anyone who has a cough lasting longer than 3 weeks (Bocka, 2014).

COCCIDIOIDOMYCOSIS

Coccidioidomycosis is a fungal INFECTION caused by the *Coccidioides* organism that is common in the desert southwest regions of the United States, Mexico, and Central and South

America. It is also known as "valley fever," and the incidence is on the rise. The organism is present in the soil as inactive and non-reproducing microfilaments. When the soil is disturbed by excavation or dust storms, the microfilaments become airborne. As the microfilaments are inhaled, they change into the reproductively active spore form of the organism, which can lead to development of an actual pulmonary infection within 1 to 4 weeks after exposure (Buhrow, 2013).

Manifestations of the infection resemble other respiratory viral or bacterial infections with fever, cough, headache, muscle aches, chest pain, and night sweats. The presence of bone and joint pain indicates more severe infection. Often the disorder is misdiagnosed and mistreated as influenza or pneumonia. Neither antibacterial drugs nor antiviral drugs are effective in managing this infection. The disease can become widespread and cause manifestations of hemoptysis, meningitis, and involvement of the skin, adrenal glands, liver, and spleen. It also can become chronic and debilitating with low-grade fever, weight loss, fatigue, chronic cough, and chest pain.

Depending on the health of the infected person and the number of spores present in the respiratory tract, the resulting infection can be mild, moderate, severe, or widely disseminated. Most younger healthy people recover from the infection without treatment. For moderate infection, oral therapy with antifungal agents from the azole class (e.g., fluconazole [Diflucan], ketoconazole [Nizoral], voriconazole [Vfend]) is needed. For those with severe disease or women who are pregnant, IV amphotericin B may be needed. Because the infection is not spread from person to person, Isolation Precautions are not required.

In endemic areas, people working in the soil, such as farm workers or construction workers, are at highest risk for the infection. Older adults and anyone who has reduced immune competence, as well as pregnant women, also are at increased risk for developing more severe disease. Because the areas that naturally harbor this organism are often winter vacation destinations, always ask anyone with respiratory infection manifestations whether they have visited endemic regions so that the possibility of coccidioidomycosis is considered.

NURSING CONCEPTS AND CLINICAL JUDGMENT REVIEW

What might you NOTICE if the patient is experiencing inadequate GAS EXCHANGE and oxygenation as a result of a respiratory INFECTION?

- Respirations rapid and shallow
- Decreased oxygen saturation by pulse oximetry
- Tachycardia
- Skin cyanosis or pallor (in lighter-skinned patients)
- Cyanosis or pallor of the lips and oral mucous membranes (in patients of any skin color)
- Patient appears to work hard to breathe
- Patient is restless, anxious, or confused

What should you INTERPRET and how should you RESPOND to a patient experiencing inadequate GAS EXCHANGE and oxygenation as a result of a respiratory INFECTION?

Perform and interpret physical assessment, including:

- Taking vital signs
- Monitoring oxygen saturation by pulse oximetry
- Auscultating all lung fields
- Checking the accuracy of pulse oximetry readings
- Assessing cognition
- Assessing for the presence and characteristics of sputum production
- Assessing the patient's ability to cough and clear the airway

Interpret laboratory values:

- Elevated white blood cell count
- Arterial blood gas values: pH lower than 7.35, HCO_3^- at or below 24 mEq/L, $Paco_2$ at or below 45 mm Hg; Pao_2 below 90 mm Hg; serum lactate levels above 8 mg/dL

Respond by:

- Administering oxygen
- Assisting the patient to an upright position, with arms resting on a table or armrests
- Prioritizing and pacing activities to prevent fatigue
- Administering prescribed IV, oral, or inhaled drugs
- Ensuring respiratory therapy treatments are administered
- Re-assessing respiratory status after respiratory therapy treatment
- Ensuring a fluid intake of at least 2 liters per day (unless contraindicated)

On what should you REFLECT?

- Observe patient for evidence of improved gas exchange and oxygenation (see Chapter 27).
- Think about what patient teaching focus could help reduce the occurrence of a respiratory infection in the future.

GET READY FOR THE NCLEX® EXAMINATION!

KEY POINTS

Review these Key Points for each NCLEX Examination Client Needs Category.

Safe and Effective Care Environment

- Limit transmission of respiratory INFECTION spread by washing hands after blowing the nose or using a tissue. **Safety** QSEN
- Receive a yearly influenza vaccination because you are more likely to care for infected people and because you could spread influenza to people who are immunocompromised. **Safety** QSEN
- Use Airborne Precautions and Isolation Precautions for any patient who has TB manifestations until proven otherwise. **Safety** QSEN

- If possible, place the patient with a respiratory INFECTION in a private room. **Safety** QSEN
- Keep the door to the room of any patient with a respiratory INFECTION closed until the cause of the infection is identified. **Safety** QSEN

Health Promotion and Maintenance

- Teach everyone the "etiquette" of sneezing or coughing into the upper sleeve rather than the hand when a tissue is not available. **Evidence-Based Practice** QSEN
- Urge all adults older than 50 years, anyone who has a chronic respiratory problem, anyone who is immunocompromised, and anyone who lives with a person who is older or immunocompromised or has a chronic respiratory disease to receive the pneumonia vaccine and yearly influenza vaccinations. **Evidence-Based Practice** QSEN
- Urge patients to complete the anti-infective drug therapy course for any respiratory INFECTION. **Patient-Centered Care** QSEN
- Urge all people to quit smoking or using tobacco in any form. **Patient-Centered Care** QSEN
- Teach people living with patients who have TB to ensure good ventilation of the home with open windows whenever possible.
- Educate the family and the patient with tuberculosis who lives at home about the side effects of anti-tuberculosis (TB) therapy and when to notify the health care provider. **Patient-Centered Care** QSEN
- Teach all people to be prepared for an emergency or disaster by having sufficient food, water, and prescribed drugs for at least 2 weeks (see Chapter 10). **Patient-Centered Care** QSEN
- Teach all people to follow community INFECTION containment procedures if there is a possible outbreak of any pandemic influenza virus. **Patient-Centered Care** QSEN

Psychosocial Integrity

- Assess older patients with acute confusion for pneumonia (cough and fever may not be present).
- Assure the family of an older adult patient with pneumonia who is confused that the new-onset confusion is temporary. **Patient-Centered Care** QSEN
- Teach people who may be afraid of contracting inhalation anthrax that this disease is not transmitted by person-to-person contact. **Patient-Centered Care** QSEN
- Inform patients who have a positive TB test that far more people are infected with the bacillus than have active TB disease. Assess the likelihood of adherence to the drug regimen for patients with TB. **Patient-Centered Care** QSEN
- Identify patients who may require a directly observed therapy (DOT) program in which they must be directly observed by a health care professional while swallowing the drug. **Safety** QSEN

Physiological Integrity

- Assess the respiratory status of anyone suspected of having a respiratory INFECTION by taking vital signs, noting color of nail beds and mucous membranes, measuring oxygen saturation, determining ease of ventilation, determining cognition, and auscultating lung fields. **Evidence-Based Practice** QSEN
- Administer humidified oxygen therapy to patients with inadequate GAS EXCHANGE and hypoxemia. **Evidence-Based Practice** QSEN
- Assess the skin under and around a facemask or nasal cannula for evidence of skin breakdown at least every 8 hours. **Patient-Centered Care** QSEN
- Ask any patient with a respiratory INFECTION if he or she is from a foreign country or has recently visited a foreign country. Ask patients from other countries whether they have had BCG as a vaccination against TB. For patients who have had BCG, the PPD skin test is a less reliable indicator of TB. **Safety** QSEN
- Assess the patient receiving first-line drug therapy for TB for any manifestation of liver impairment (dark urine, clay-colored stools, anorexia, jaundiced sclera or hard palate). **Patient-Centered Care** QSEN
- Teach women taking rifampin or rifapentine as drug therapy for TB that these drugs reduce the effectiveness of oral contraceptives and that an additional form of birth control should be used while on this therapy. **Patient-Centered Care** QSEN

CHAPTER 32

Care of Critically Ill Patients with Respiratory Problems

Meg Blair

http://evolve.elsevier.com/Iggy/

PRIORITY CONCEPTS

- Gas Exchange
- Perfusion
- Clotting

LEARNING OUTCOMES

Safe and Effective Care Environment

1. Protect the critically ill patient with respiratory problems from injury, infection, and bleeding.
2. Ensure safe management of endotracheal tubes, tracheostomy tubes, and mechanical ventilators.

Health Promotion and Maintenance

3. Teach people at risk for pulmonary embolism techniques to reduce the risk.
4. Teach patients and family members how to avoid injury during therapy to reduce CLOTTING.

Psychosocial Integrity

5. Reduce the psychological impact for the patient and family experiencing a serious respiratory problem.

Physiological Integrity

6. Assess the respiratory status of any patient who develops sudden-onset respiratory difficulty or acute confusion.
7. Use laboratory data and clinical manifestations to evaluate the adequacy of GAS EXCHANGE with oxygenation and ventilatory interventions.
8. Prioritize nursing care for the patient experiencing a serious or critical respiratory disorder or event.
9. Work with other members of the health care team to coordinate care for the patient being mechanically ventilated.

Any respiratory problem can interfere with GAS EXCHANGE, oxygenation, and tissue PERFUSION, progressing to an emergency and death, even with prompt treatment. These problems may overwhelm the adaptive responses of the cardiac and blood oxygen delivery systems (Fig. 32-1). *Thus prompt recognition and interventions are needed to prevent serious complications and death.*

An acute injury or problem that results in severe respiratory impairment can occur at any age. Older adults, however, are more at risk for developing critical respiratory problems. The patient who is short of breath is also anxious and fearful. Be prepared to manage both the physical and emotional needs of the patient during any respiratory emergency.

PULMONARY EMBOLISM

❖ *PATHOPHYSIOLOGY*

A **pulmonary embolism (PE)** is a collection of particulate matter (solids, liquids, or air) that enters venous circulation and lodges in the pulmonary vessels. Large emboli obstruct pulmonary blood flow, leading to reduced GAS EXCHANGE, reduced oxygenation, pulmonary tissue hypoxia, decreased PERFUSION, and potential death. Any substance can cause an embolism, but a blood clot is the most common (McCance et al., 2014). PE is common and may account for as many as 100,000 deaths each year in the United States (Smithburger et al., 2013). It may be the most common preventable death in hospitalized patients but is often misdiagnosed, and patients at risk may not be provided the appropriate preventive measures (Duff et al., 2013; Hussey, 2013).

Most often, a PE occurs when inappropriate blood CLOTTING forms a venous thromboembolism (VTE) (also known as a *deep vein thrombosis* [DVT]) in a vein in the legs or the pelvis and a clot breaks off and travels through the vena cava into the right side of the heart. The clot then lodges in the pulmonary artery or within one or more of its branches. Platelets collect on the embolus, triggering the release of substances that cause blood vessel constriction. Widespread pulmonary vessel constriction and pulmonary hypertension impair GAS EXCHANGE and tissue PERFUSION. Deoxygenated blood moves into arterial circulation, causing **hypoxemia** (low arterial blood oxygen level), although some patients with PE do *not* have hypoxemia.

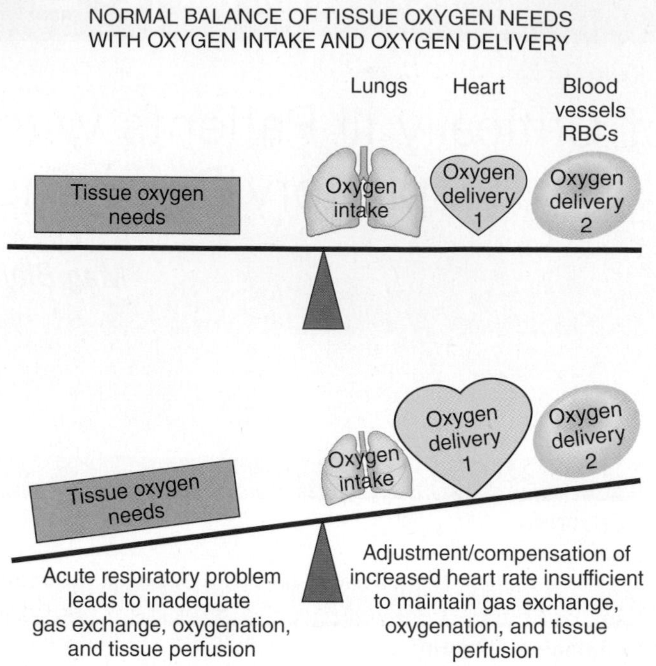

FIG. 32-1 Rapid-onset acute respiratory problems overwhelm the ability of the cardiac oxygen delivery system to adapt and restore balance. The red blood cell (RBC) oxygen delivery system cannot begin to adapt to the acute respiratory problem.

Major risk factors for VTE leading to PE are:
- Prolonged immobility
- Central venous catheters
- Surgery
- Obesity
- Advancing age
- Conditions that increase blood CLOTTING
- History of thromboembolism

Smoking, pregnancy, estrogen therapy, heart failure, stroke, cancer (particularly lung or prostate), and trauma increase the risk for VTE and PE (Hussey, 2013).

Fat, oil, air, tumor cells, amniotic fluid and fetal debris, foreign objects (e.g., broken IV catheters), injected particles, and infected clots can enter a vein and cause PE. Fat emboli from fracture of a long bone and oil emboli from diagnostic procedures do not impede lung blood flow; instead, they injure blood vessels and cause acute respiratory distress syndrome (ARDS) (Powers & Talbot, 2011). Septic clots often arise from a pelvic abscess, an infected IV catheter, and injections of illegal drugs. The effects of sepsis are more serious than the venous blockage.

Health Promotion and Maintenance

Although pulmonary embolism (PE) can occur in healthy people without warning, it occurs more often in some situations. Thus prevention of conditions that lead to PE is a major nursing concern. Preventive actions for PE are those that also prevent venous stasis and VTE. Best nursing practices for PE prevention are outlined in Chart 32-1. Also see Chapter 14 for more information about core measures during the surgical experience for VTE prevention.

Lifestyle changes can help reduce the risk for PE. Tobacco use narrows blood vessels and increases the risk for clot formation. Hormone-based contraceptives also increase blood CLOTTING. Urge patients to stop smoking cigarettes, especially women who use hormone-based contraceptives. Reducing weight and becoming more physically active can reduce risk for PE. Teach patients who are traveling for long periods to drink plenty of water, change positions often, avoid crossing their legs, and get up from the sitting position at least 5 minutes out of every hour to prevent stasis and clot formation.

For patients known to be at risk for PE, small doses of heparin or low–molecular-weight heparin (enoxaparin [Lovenox]), an indirect thrombin inhibitor, may be prescribed every 8 to 12 hours. Oral direct thrombin inhibitors may be used instead of heparin for VTE prevention in patients who have non-valvular atrial fibrillation (Golembiewski, 2011).

CHART 32-1 Best Practice for Patient Safety & Quality Care QSEN

Prevention of Pulmonary Embolism

- Start passive and active range-of-motion exercises for the extremities of immobilized and postoperative patients.
- Ambulate patients soon after surgery.
- Use antiembolism and pneumatic compression stockings and devices after surgery.
- Evaluate patient for criteria indicating the need for anticoagulant therapy.
- Avoid the use of tight garters, girdles, and constricting clothing.
- Prevent pressure under the popliteal space (e.g., do not place a pillow under the knee, use alternating pressure mattress).
- Perform a comprehensive assessment of peripheral circulation.
- Elevate the affected limb 20 degrees or more above the level of the heart to improve venous return, as appropriate.
- Change patient position every 2 hours, or ambulate as tolerated.
- Prevent injury to the vessel lumen by preventing local pressure, trauma, infection, or sepsis.
- Refrain from massaging leg muscles.
- Instruct patient not to cross legs.
- Administer prescribed prophylactic low-dose anticoagulant and antiplatelet drugs.
- Teach the patient to avoid activities that result in the Valsalva maneuver (e.g., breath-holding, bearing down for bowel movements, coughing).
- Administer prescribed drugs, such as stool softeners, that will prevent episodes of the Valsalva maneuver.
- Teach the patient and family about precautions.
- Encourage smoking cessation.

❖ PATIENT-CENTERED COLLABORATIVE CARE

◆ Assessment

Physical manifestations range from vague, non-specific discomforts to hemodynamic collapse and death. *It is important to remember that many patients with PE do not have the "classic" manifestations.* This variability in manifestations often leads to PEs being overlooked (Hussey, 2013; Smithburger et al., 2013).

Physical Assessment/Clinical Manifestations. *Respiratory manifestations* are outlined in Chart 32-2 and are mostly related to decreased GAS EXCHANGE. Assess the patient for difficulty breathing (dyspnea) and pleuritic chest pain (sharp, stabbing-type pain on inspiration). Other manifestations vary depending on the size and the type of embolism. Breath sounds may be normal or include crackles, wheezes, or a pleural friction rub. A dry or productive cough may be present; **hemoptysis** (bloody sputum) may result from pulmonary infarction.

CHART 32-2 **Key Features**

Pulmonary Embolism

Classic Manifestations	Signs
• Dyspnea, sudden onset • Sharp, stabbing chest pain • Apprehension, restlessness • Feeling of impending doom • Cough • Hemoptysis	• Tachypnea • Crackles • Pleural friction rub • Tachycardia • S_3 or S_4 heart sound • Diaphoresis • Fever, low-grade • Petechiae over chest and axillae • Decreased arterial oxygen saturation (Sao_2)

Cardiac manifestations related to decreased tissue PERFUSION include tachycardia, distended neck veins, **syncope** (fainting or loss of consciousness), cyanosis, and hypotension. Systemic hypotension results from acute pulmonary hypertension and reduced forward blood flow. Abnormal heart sounds, such as an S_3 or S_4, may occur. Electrocardiogram (ECG) changes are nonspecific and transient. T-wave and ST-segment changes may occur as can left-axis or right-axis deviations. Right ventricular dysfunction and failure are extreme manifestations. The patient may have cardiac arrest or frank shock.

! NURSING SAFETY PRIORITY QSEN

Critical Rescue

Any patient who has shortness of breath, chest pain, and or/hypotension without an obvious cause should be assessed for PE and the Rapid Response Team notified. If PE is strongly suspected, prompt categorization and management are started before diagnostic studies have been completed (McLenon, 2012; Ouellette, 2014).

Psychosocial Assessment. Manifestations of PE often occur abruptly, and the patient is anxious. Hypoxemia may stimulate a sense of impending doom and cause increased restlessness. The life-threatening nature of PE and admission to an ICU increase the patient's anxiety and fear.

Laboratory Assessment. The hyperventilation triggered by hypoxia and pain first leads to respiratory alkalosis, indicated by low partial pressure of arterial carbon dioxide ($Paco_2$) on arterial blood gas (ABG) analysis. The Pao_2-Fio_2 (fraction of inspired oxygen) ratio falls as a result of "shunting" of blood from the right side of the heart to the left without picking up oxygen from the lungs. Shunting causes the $Paco_2$ level to rise, resulting in respiratory acidosis (McCance et al., 2014). Later, metabolic acidosis results from buildup of lactic acid due to tissue hypoxia. (See Chapter 12 for a more detailed discussion of acidosis.)

Even if ABG studies and pulse oximetry show hypoxemia, these results alone are not sufficient for the diagnosis of PE (McCance et al., 2014). A patient with a small embolus may not be hypoxemic, and PE is not the only cause of hypoxemia.

Other laboratory studies performed when PE is suspected include a general metabolic panel, troponin, brain natriuretic peptide (BNP), and a D-dimer. The D-dimer, a fibrin split product, rises with fibrinolysis. When the value is normal or low, it can rule out a PE. However, even if the value is high, other diagnostic testing is needed to determine whether a PE has occurred (Pagana & Pagana, 2014; Smithburger et al., 2013).

GENETIC/GENOMIC CONSIDERATIONS

Patient-Centered Care QSEN

Factor V Leiden is an inherited thrombophilia (abnormal tendency to develop blood clots) in which the gene coding for blood clotting factor V (the *F5* gene) has a mutation that changes the nature of the factor V produced. With this genetic alteration, factor V functions normally but is not degraded as quickly as it should be. Thus clotting activity continues longer than usual, increasing the chance for developing abnormal blood clots (Lee, 2014). People can inherit either one or both abnormal gene alleles. The risk for developing clots is 8 times greater in those who inherit only one abnormal allele. The risk for developing DVT, PE, or thrombotic strokes increases greatly for people who inherit both abnormal gene alleles (one from each parent), especially if the person also smokes or uses hormone-based contraceptives. This disorder is also known as *activated protein C resistance.* Be aware that testing for factor V Leiden is recommended for people who have developed a VTE without a precipitating event and for those who have a first-degree relative with the disorder (Online Mendelian Inheritance in Man [OMIM], 2013).

Imaging Assessment. Pulmonary angiography is the "gold standard" diagnostic test but is not available in all settings. Computed tomography pulmonary angiography (CT-PA) or helical CT may also be used, which has the added advantage of diagnosing other pulmonary abnormalities causing the patient's manifestations. Ventilation-perfusion ($\dot{V}/\dot{Q}$) scans are not as widely used anymore but may be considered in certain circumstances (e.g., allergy to contrast dye). A chest x-ray may diagnose other conditions that mimic acute PE. Doppler ultrasound may be used to document the presence of VTE and to support a diagnosis of PE (Drumright et al., 2013; Kessenich & Erigo-Backman, 2012).

◆ *Analysis*

The priority NANDA-I nursing diagnoses and collaborative problems for patients with PE include:

1. Hypoxemia related to mismatch of lung perfusion and alveolar gas exchange with oxygenation
2. Hypotension related to inadequate circulation to the left ventricle
3. Potential for inadequate CLOTTING and bleeding related to anticoagulation or fibrinolytic therapy
4. Anxiety related to hypoxemia and life-threatening illness (NANDA-I)

◆ *Planning and Implementation*

Managing Hypoxemia. *When a patient has a sudden onset of dyspnea and chest pain, immediately notify the Rapid Response Team.* Reassure the patient, and elevate the head of the bed. Prepare for oxygen therapy and blood gas analysis while continuing to monitor and assess for other changes.

Planning: Expected Outcomes. The patient with PE is expected to have adequate tissue PERFUSION in all major organs. Indicators of adequate PERFUSION are that the patient has:

- ABGs within normal limits
- Pulse oximetry above 95%
- Cognitive status unimpaired compared with baseline
- Absence of pallor and cyanosis

Interventions. Nonsurgical management of PE is most common. In some cases, invasive procedures also may be needed. Best nursing care practices for the patient with PE are listed in Chart 32-3. Rapid categorization of PE severity and prompt management are required (Table 32-1).

Nonsurgical Management. Management activities for PE focus on increasing GAS EXCHANGE and oxygenation, improving lung PERFUSION, reducing risk for further clot formation, and preventing complications. Priority nursing interventions include implementing oxygen therapy, administering anticoagulation or fibrinolytic therapy to improve tissue perfusion, monitoring the patient's responses to the interventions, and providing psychosocial support.

Oxygen therapy is critical for the patient with PE. The severely hypoxemic patient may need mechanical ventilation and close monitoring with ABG studies. In less severe cases, oxygen may be applied by nasal cannula or mask. Use pulse oximetry to monitor oxygen saturation and hypoxemia.

Monitor the patient continually for any changes in status. Check vital signs, lung sounds, and cardiac and respiratory status at least every 1 to 2 hours. Document increasing dyspnea, dysrhythmias, distended neck veins, and pedal or sacral edema. Assess for crackles and other abnormal lung sounds along with cyanosis of the lips, conjunctiva, oral mucosa, and nail beds.

Drug therapy begins immediately with anticoagulants to prevent embolus enlargement and to prevent more CLOTTING. Unfractionated heparin, low–molecular-weight heparin (enoxaparin [Lovenox]), or fondaparinux (Arixtra) is usually used unless the PE is massive or occurs with hemodynamic instability. Review the patient's partial thromboplastin time (PTT)—also called *activated partial thromboplastin time* (aPTT)—before therapy is started and thereafter according to facility policy. Therapeutic PTT values usually range between 1.5 and 2.5 times the control value for this health problem. Factor anti-Xa levels may be used instead of PTT or aPTT (Riley, 2013).

Fibrinolytic drugs, such as alteplase (Activase, tPA), are used for treatment of PE when specific criteria are met such as shock, hemodynamic collapse, or instability. Fibrinolytic drugs are used to break up the existing clot. (See Chapter 38 for a discussion of fibrinolytic therapy.)

Both heparin and fibrinolytic drugs are *high alert drugs.* These drugs have a high risk to cause harm if given at too high a dose, too low a dose, or to the wrong patient.

CHART 32-3 Best Practice for Patient Safety & Quality Care QSEN

Care of the Patient with a Pulmonary Embolism

- Apply oxygen by nasal cannula or mask.
- Reassure patient that the correct measures are being taken.
- Place patient in high-Fowler's position.
- Apply telemetry monitoring equipment.
- Obtain an adequate venous access.
- Assess oxygenation continuously with pulse oximetry.
- Assess respiratory status at least every 30 minutes by:
  - Listening to lung sounds.
  - Measuring the rate, rhythm, and ease of respirations.
  - Checking skin color and capillary refill.
  - Checking position of trachea.
- Assess cardiac status by:
  - Comparing blood pressures in right and left arms.
  - Checking pulse for quality.
  - Checking cardiac monitor for dysrhythmias.
  - Checking for distention of neck veins.
- Ensure prescribed chest imaging and laboratory tests are obtained immediately (may include complete blood count with differential, platelet count, prothrombin time, partial thromboplastin time, D-dimer level, arterial blood gases).
- Examine the thorax for presence of petechiae.
- Administer prescribed anticoagulants.
- Assess for bleeding.
- Handle patient gently.
- Institute Bleeding Precautions.

! NURSING SAFETY PRIORITY QSEN

Drug Alert

Heparin comes in a variety of concentrations in vials that have differing amounts, which contributes to possible medication errors. In accordance with The Joint Commission's National Patient Safety Goals (NPSGs), check the prescribed dose carefully and ensure the correct concentration is being used to prevent overdosing or underdosing.

TABLE 32-1 Pulmonary Embolism (PE) Severity and Management Options

CATEGORY	POSSIBLE MANIFESTATIONS	MANAGEMENT OPTIONS
Massive PE Mortality may be as high as 65%	Severe hypotension (SBP <90 mm Hg for at least 15 minutes) Cardiac arrest/cardiopulmonary collapse Severe bradycardia Shock Severe dyspnea/respiratory distress	CPR Inotropic and/or vasopressor support; fluids Fibrinolytic therapy Tissue plasminogen activator (tPA) Alteplase (Activase) Unfractionated heparin initial treatment
Submassive PE	Normotension RV dysfunction on echocardiography RV dilation on echocardiography or CT Right bundle branch block ST elevation or depression T-wave inversion Elevated BNP or troponin	Treatment is controversial; some agents not approved for this group Must weigh benefits of thrombolytic therapy against risk for bleeding Thrombolytics may be preferred if patient appears to be decompensating or if there is RV dysfunction (hypokinesis) or elevation in BNP or troponin LMWH preferred agent Fondaparinux (Arixtra) Unfractionated heparin
Low-risk PE Mortality ranges from 1% to 8%	Normotension No RV dysfunction No elevation in BNP or troponin	Thrombolytics not warranted due to risk for bleeding LMWH Rivaroxaban (Xarelto)

Adapted from Jaff, M.R., McMurtry, M.S., & Archer, S.L. (2011). The use of fibrinolytics in patients with acute pulmonary embolism. *Circulation, 123,* 1788-1830.
BNP, Brain natriuretic peptide; *CPR,* cardiopulmonary resuscitation; *CT,* computed tomography; *LMWH,* low–molecular-weight heparin; *RV,* right ventricle; *SBP,* systolic blood pressure.

Heparin therapy usually continues for 5 to 10 days. Most patients are started on an oral anticoagulant, such as warfarin (Coumadin, Jantoven, Warfilone ♣), on the third day of heparin use. Therapy with both heparin and warfarin continues until the international normalized ratio (INR) reaches 2.0 to 3.0. Monitor the platelet count and INR during this time. A low–molecular-weight heparin (e.g., dalteparin [Fragmin], enoxaparin [Lovenox]) or a direct thrombin inhibitor (rivaroxaban [Xarelto]) is often used instead of warfarin. Oral anticoagulant use continues for 3 to 6 weeks, but some patients may take it indefinitely. Charts 32-4 and 32-5 list common drugs used and the laboratory tests to monitor in a patient with PE. These drugs and the associated nursing care are discussed in Chapters 36, 38, and 39.

CHART 32-4 Common Examples of Drug Therapy

Pulmonary Embolism

DRUG AND USUAL DOSAGE	PURPOSE	NURSING INTERVENTIONS	RATIONALES
Heparin sodium (Hepalean ♣) 5000-10,000 units as a bolus by IV push initially; then dose adjustment is based on PTT, often at 1300 units/hr on continuous infusion or by intermittent infusion **NOTE:** Some institutions use a weight-based algorithm.	To begin anticoagulation to minimize growth of existing clots and to prevent the development of additional clots	Monitor PTT (or factor anti-Xa) and know expected therapeutic PTT range for each patient.	Ongoing assessment helps detect side effects and prevent complications.
		Report PTT (or factor anti-Xa) results. Monitor patient for bleeding or bruising.	Reporting and monitoring enable early management of a prolonged PTT and excessive bleeding.
		Adjust infusion based on PTT (or factor anti-Xa) results and institutional protocol.	To maintain anticoagulation within consistent therapeutic levels.
		Do not use with salicylates.	An increased anticoagulation effect can occur with salicylates.
		Monitor platelets daily for thrombocytopenia.	Heparin-induced thrombocytopenia (HIT), a type of adverse reaction, can occur.
		Have the antidote *protamine sulfate* available.	Being prepared for an emergency helps prevent further complications.
		Avoid puncturing the skin, and apply pressure to venipuncture and IM injection sites.	Pressure at puncture sites helps promote clotting.
		Avoid use of firm toothbrushes, razors, and rectal manipulation.	Safety measures help prevent bleeding.
Enoxaparin (Lovenox) usually 1 mg/kg subcutaneously every 12 hr	To allow for hospital discharge before complete switch to oral anticoagulants	Monitor platelet count.	Heparin-induced thrombocytopenia (HIT), a type of adverse reaction, can occur.
		Have the antidote *protamine sulfate* available.	This drug is the only antidote for enoxaparin.
		Safety precautions are the same as for heparin.	Safety precautions are the same as for heparin.
Warfarin sodium (Coumadin, Jantoven, Warfilone sodium ♣) 10-15 mg orally once daily for 3 days initially; then dose adjustment is based on INR, usually 5-10 mg orally daily Now available as a parenteral drug for use in hospitalized patients. Dosage is the same as with the oral form of the drug.	To allow for long-term anticoagulation in at-risk patients to prevent the development of future clots	Monitor INR, and know expected therapeutic INR range for each patient.	Ongoing assessment helps detect side effects and prevent complications.
		Report INR results. Monitor the patient for bleeding or bruising.	Reporting enables early management of a prolonged INR.
		Monitor for fever and skin rash.	Adverse drug reaction can occur.
		Consult the pharmacist about potential drug interactions, and teach the patient to avoid interacting drugs.	There are many drug interactions with warfarin.
		Have the antidote *vitamin K (phytonadione)* available.	Being prepared for an emergency helps prevent further complications.
		Avoid puncturing the skin, and apply pressure to venipuncture and IM injection sites.	Pressure at puncture sites helps promote clotting.
		Avoid use of firm toothbrushes, razors, and rectal manipulation.	Safety measures help prevent bleeding.
		Teach the patient which foods are high in vitamin K (e.g., leafy dark green vegetables, herbs, spring onions, Brussels sprouts, broccoli, cabbage, asparagus).	Food sources of vitamin K will alter INR.
Alteplase (tissue plasminogen activator, recombinant; tPA; Activase) 100 mg IV infusion over 2 hr	To promote lysis of large pulmonary emboli in those patients who are hemodynamically unstable	Assess for internal and external bleeding.	Bleeding is the most common adverse effect.
		Reconstitute with sterile water without preservative immediately before use.	Recommended preparation ensures drug stability.
		Administer with caution to patients who have been receiving aspirin, dipyridamole, heparin, or other anticoagulants.	Other drugs with anticoagulation effects increase the risk for bleeding.

INR, International normalized ratio; *PTT,* partial thromboplastin time.

CHART 32-5 Laboratory Profile

Blood Tests Used to Monitor Anticoagulation Therapy

TEST	NORMAL RANGE	SIGNIFICANCE OF ABNORMAL FINDINGS
Partial thromboplastin time (PTT, aPTT [APTT])	Normal values for each local laboratory may vary. When activator reagents are used by the laboratory, the normal clotting time is shortened. Common normal ranges are 20-30 sec in some laboratories and 30-40 sec in others. Therapeutic range for PE is 1.5-2.5 times the normal value (e.g., if normal is 20-30 sec, then therapeutic range is 40-75 sec).	*Subtherapeutic times* may signify that the patient is not receiving enough heparin to prevent extension of the blood clot. An increase in the dosage or rate of infusion is usually indicated. *Therapeutic times* mean that the clotting time is increased from normal but this increase is indicated in the case of PE. *Prolonged times* in patients with PE (i.e., >75 sec) indicate that the patient is at risk for serious spontaneous bleeding. Heparin is usually held or decreased until the PTT drops back into the therapeutic range.
Prothrombin time (pro time, PT)	Common normal range is 11-12.5 sec. Therapeutic range for anticoagulant therapy in PE is 1.5-2.0 times the normal or control value in seconds. Control values can vary day to day because reagents used may vary.	*Subtherapeutic values* may signify that the patient is not receiving enough warfarin. An increase in the dosage is usually indicated. *Therapeutic values* mean that the pro time is increased from normal but this increase is indicated in the case of PE. *Prolonged values* in the treatment of PE indicate that the patient is at risk for bleeding. The warfarin dose is usually decreased or held, the patient is instructed to eat foods high in vitamin K, or an injection of vitamin K may be given.
International Normalized Ratio (INR)	The common normal range is 0.8-11. The therapeutic range for PE is 2.5-3.0, or 3.0-4.5 for recurrent PE.	*Subtherapeutic values* may signify that the patient is not receiving enough warfarin. An increase in the dosage is usually indicated. *Therapeutic values* mean that the INR is increased from normal but this increase is indicated in the case of PE. *Prolonged values* (higher than 4.5) in the treatment of PE indicate that the patient is at risk for bleeding. The warfarin dose is usually decreased or held, the patient is instructed to eat foods high in vitamin K, or an injection of vitamin K may be given.

aPTT or *APTT*, Activated partial thromboplastin time; *INR*, international normalized ratio; *PE*, pulmonary embolism.

GENETIC/GENOMIC CONSIDERATIONS

Patient-Centered Care QSEN

Many agencies perform genetic tests before starting warfarin therapy to check for variation in two specific genes. One gene, *VKORC1*, produces an enzyme that alters vitamin K so it can help activate the vitamin K–dependent clotting factors. Warfarin interferes with the activity of this enzyme. Patients who have a variation in the enzyme are resistant to the effects of warfarin, and much higher doses are needed to achieve coagulation. On the other hand, the gene *CYP2C19* produces an enzyme that metabolizes warfarin and prepares it for elimination. Patients who have a variation in this gene do not metabolize warfarin well, so higher blood levels remain and more severe side effects are possible. The dosage of warfarin needs to be much lower in patients with this gene variation. When a patient's response to warfarin therapy is either greater than expected or much less than expected, consider the possibility of a gene mutation.

Anticoagulation and fibrinolytic therapy can lead to excessive bleeding. *The antidote for heparin is protamine sulfate; the antidote for warfarin is vitamin K_1, which is available as an injectable drug, phytonadione (AquaMEPHYTON, Mephyton). Antidotes for fibrinolytic therapy include clotting factors, fresh frozen plasma, and aminocaproic acid (Amicar).* Keep antidotes to anticoagulant drugs and fibrinolytic drugs on the unit for patients undergoing these therapies.

NCLEX EXAMINATION CHALLENGE

Safe and Effective Care Environment

While assessing a client who has been receiving heparin intravenously for the past 3 days, the nurse notes the IV pump is set at twice the required setting. What orders does the nurse anticipate from the prescriber? **Select all that apply.**

A. Activated partial thromboplastin time
B. International normalized ratio
C. Prothrombin time
D. Vitamin K
E. Protamine sulfate

Surgical Management. Two surgical procedures for the management of PE are embolectomy and inferior vena cava filtration.

Embolectomy is the surgical or percutaneous removal of the embolus. It may be performed when fibrinolytic therapy cannot be used for a patient who has massive or multiple large pulmonary emboli with shock or bleeding complications. Special thrombectomy catheters that mechanically break up clots, such as the AngioJet, allow effective reduction of clots with or without the use of thrombolytic drugs (Drumright et al., 2013).

Inferior vena cava filtration with placement of a vena cava filter prevents further emboli from reaching the lungs in patients with ongoing risk for PE. Some filters can be removed when the risk for clot formation decreases, or they can be left in place permanently. Patients for whom filter placement is considered less risky than drug therapy include those with recurrent or major bleeding while receiving anticoagulants, those with septic PE, and those undergoing pulmonary embolectomy (Drumright et al., 2013). Placement of a vena cava filter is detailed in Chapter 36.

Managing Hypotension

Planning: Expected Outcomes. The patient with PE is expected to have adequate circulation and tissue PERFUSION. Indicators of adequate circulation are:

- Maintenance of pulse rate and blood pressure within the normal ranges
- Maintenance of a urine output of at least 30 mL/hr
- Absence of cyanosis

Interventions. In addition to the interventions used for hypoxemia, IV fluid therapy and drug therapy are used to increase cardiac output and maintain blood pressure.

IV fluid therapy involves giving crystalloid solutions to restore plasma volume and prevent shock (see Chapter 37). Continuously monitor the ECG and pulmonary artery and central venous/right atrial pressures of the patient receiving IV fluids because increased fluids can worsen pulmonary hypertension and lead to right-sided heart failure. Also monitor indicators of fluid adequacy including urine output, skin turgor, and moisture of mucous membranes.

Drug therapy with vasopressors is used when hypotension persists despite fluid resuscitation. Commonly used agents include norepinephrine (Levophed), epinephrine (adrenalin), or dopamine (Intropin). Agents that increase myocardial contractility (**positive inotropic agents**), including milrinone (Primacor) and dobutamine (Dobutrex), may be considered. Vasodilators, such as nitroprusside (Nipride, Nitropress), may be used to decrease pulmonary artery pressure if it is impeding cardiac contractility. Assess the patient's cardiac status hourly during therapy with any of these drugs.

Minimizing Bleeding

Planning: Expected Outcomes. The patient with PE is expected to have appropriate CLOTTING and remain free from bleeding. Indicators include that the patient:

- Does not have bruising or petechiae
- Maintains hematocrit, hemoglobin, and platelet count within the normal range

Interventions. Drug therapy that disrupts clots or prevents their formation impairs the patient's ability to start and continue the blood-CLOTTING cascade when injured, increasing the risk for bleeding. Priority nursing actions are ensuring appropriate antidotes are present on the nursing unit, protecting the patient from situations that could lead to bleeding, ensuring correct drug therapy, assessing laboratory values, and monitoring the amount of bleeding that occurs.

Assess for evidence of bleeding (e.g., oozing, bruises that cluster, petechiae, or purpura) at least every 2 hours. Examine all stools, urine, drainage, and vomitus for gross blood, and test for occult blood. Measure any blood loss as accurately as possible. Measure the patient's abdominal girth every 8 hours (increasing girth can indicate internal bleeding). Best practices to prevent bleeding are listed in Chart 32-6.

Monitor laboratory values daily. Review the complete blood count (CBC) results to determine the risk for impaired CLOTTING and whether actual blood loss has occurred. If the patient has severe blood loss, packed red blood cells may be prescribed (see Transfusion Therapy in Chapter 40). Monitor the platelet count. A decreasing count may indicate ongoing CLOTTING or heparin-induced thrombocytopenia (HIT) caused by the formation of anti-heparin antibodies.

CHART 32-6 Best Practice for Patient Safety & Quality Care QSEN

Prevention of Injury for the Patient Receiving Anticoagulant, Fibrinolytic, or Antiplatelet Therapy

- Handle the patient gently.
- Use and teach UAP to use a lift sheet when moving and positioning the patient in bed.
- Avoid IM injections and venipunctures.
- When injections or venipunctures are necessary, use the smallest-gauge needle for the task.
- Apply firm pressure to the needle stick site for 10 minutes or until the site no longer oozes blood.
- Apply ice to areas of trauma.
- Test all urine, vomitus, and stool for occult blood.
- Assess IV sites at least every 4 hours for bleeding.
- Instruct alert patients to notify nursing personnel immediately if any trauma occurs and if bleeding or bruising is noticed.
- Avoid trauma to rectal tissues:
  - Do not administer enemas.
  - If suppositories are prescribed, lubricate liberally and administer with caution.
- Instruct the patient and UAP to use an electric shaver rather than a razor.
- When providing mouth care or supervising others in providing mouth care:
  - Use a soft-bristled toothbrush or tooth sponges.
  - Do not use floss.
  - Check to make certain that dentures fit and do not rub.
- Instruct the patient not to blow the nose forcefully or insert objects into the nose.
- Ensure the patient wears shoes with firm soles whenever he or she is ambulating.
- Ensure that antidotes to anticoagulation therapy are on the unit.

UAP, Unlicensed assistive personnel.

Minimizing Anxiety

Planning: Expected Outcomes. The patient with PE is expected to have anxiety reduced to an acceptable level. Indicators include that he or she consistently demonstrates these behaviors:

- States that anxiety is reduced
- Has no distress, irritability, or facial tension
- Uses coping strategies effectively

Interventions. The patient with PE is anxious and fearful and often has pain. Interventions for reducing anxiety in those with PE include oxygen therapy (see Interventions discussion on pp. 605-606 in the Managing Hypoxemia section), communication, and drug therapy.

Communication is critical in allaying anxiety. Acknowledge the anxiety and the patient's perception of a life-threatening situation. Stay with him or her, and speak calmly and clearly, providing assurances that appropriate measures are being taken. Explain the rationale and share information when giving drugs, changing position, taking vital signs, or assessing the patient.

Drug therapy with an antianxiety drug may be prescribed if the patient's anxiety interferes with diagnostic testing, management, or adequate rest. Unless he or she is mechanically ventilated, sedating agents are avoided to reduce the risk for hypoventilation. Pharmacologic therapy is used for pain management. Care is taken to avoid suppressing the respiratory response.

CLINICAL JUDGMENT CHALLENGE

Patient-Centered Care; Safety; Evidence-Based Practice QSEN

The patient is a 70-year-old retiree who had a hip replacement 2 days ago. His hip pain kept him from participating in his usual exercise program for the past 6 months. He is a former two-pack a day smoker. At home he decreased his fluid intake because ambulating to the bathroom was so painful. He resisted getting out of bed with physical therapy yesterday. When you assess him this morning, he reports nausea, some chest pain, mild shortness of breath, and anxiety.

1. What should be your first actions? Provide a rationale for your choice(s).
2. Which of his manifestations are associated with PE, and what risk factors does he have for a PE?
3. What are the common manifestations of PE?
4. The patient is requesting something for his anxiety. Is antianxiety drug therapy appropriate at this time? Why or why not? How else might you be able to reduce his anxiety?
5. What other actions should you take?

Community-Based Care

The patient with a PE is discharged when hypoxemia and hemodynamic instability are resolved and adequate anticoagulation has been achieved. Anticoagulation therapy usually continues after discharge.

Home Care Management. Some patients are discharged to home with minimal risk for recurrence and no permanent physiologic changes. Others have heart or lung damage that requires home and lifestyle modification.

Patients with extensive lung damage may have activity intolerance from reduced GAS EXCHANGE and become fatigued easily. The living arrangements may need to be modified so that patients can spend most of the time on one floor and avoid climbing stairs. Depending on the degree of impairment, patients may require varying amounts of assistance with ADLs.

Self-Management Education. The patient with a PE may continue anticoagulation therapy for weeks, months, or years after discharge, depending on the risks for PE, and have impaired CLOTTING. Teach him or her and the family about Bleeding Precautions, activities to reduce the risk for venous thromboembolism (VTE) and recurrence of PE, complications, and the need for follow-up care (Chart 32-7).

Health Care Resources. Patients using anticoagulation therapy with warfarin are usually seen in a clinic or health care provider's office frequently for blood tests. Those who are homebound may have a visit from a home care nurse to perform these tests. Newer anticoagulation agents (dabigatran [Pradaxa] and enoxaparin [Lovenox]) do not require laboratory monitoring. Patients with severe dyspnea may need home oxygen therapy. Respiratory therapy treatments can be performed in the home. The nurse or case manager coordinates arrangements for oxygen and other respiratory therapy equipment to be available if needed at home. See Chart 32-8 for a focused assessment guide.

CHART 32-7 Patient and Family Education: Preparing for Self-Management

Preventing Injury and Bleeding

During the time you are taking anticoagulants:

- Use an electric shaver.
- Use a soft-bristled toothbrush, and do not floss.
- Do not have dental work performed without consulting your health care provider.
- Do not take aspirin or any aspirin-containing products. Read the label to be sure that the product does not contain aspirin or salicylates.
- Do not participate in contact sports or any activity likely to result in your being bumped, scratched, or scraped.
- If you are bumped, apply ice to the site for at least 1 hour.
- Avoid hard foods that would scrape the inside of your mouth.
- Eat warm, cool, or cold foods to avoid burning your mouth.
- Check your skin and mouth daily for bruises, swelling, or areas with small, reddish purple marks that may indicate bleeding.
- Notify your health care provider if you:
  - Are injured and persistent bleeding results
  - Have excessive menstrual bleeding
  - See blood in your urine or bowel movement
- Avoid anal intercourse.
- Take a stool softener to prevent straining during a bowel movement.
- Do not use enemas or rectal suppositories.
- Do not wear clothing or shoes that are tight or that rub.
- Avoid blowing your nose forcefully or placing objects in your nose. If you must blow your nose, do so gently without blocking either nasal passage.
- Avoid playing musical instruments that raise the pressure inside your head, such as brass wind instruments and woodwinds or reed instruments.
- Keep all appointments for laboratory tests.

◆ *Evaluation: Outcomes*

Evaluate the care of the patient with PE on the basis of the identified priority patient problems. The expected outcomes are that he or she:

- Attains and maintains adequate GAS EXCHANGE and oxygenation
- Does not experience hypovolemia and shock
- Remains free from bleeding episodes
- States the level of anxiety is reduced
- Uses effective coping strategies

Specific indicators for these outcomes are listed for each patient problem under the Planning and Implementation section (see earlier).

ACUTE RESPIRATORY FAILURE

❖ *PATHOPHYSIOLOGY*

A near match in the lungs between air movement or ventilation ($\dot{V}$) and blood flow or PERFUSION ($\dot{Q}$) is needed for adequate pulmonary GAS EXCHANGE. When either ventilation or perfusion is mismatched with the other in a lung or lung area, gas exchange is reduced and respiratory failure can result.

Acute respiratory failure (ARF) can be *ventilatory failure, oxygenation (GAS EXCHANGE) failure,* or a *combination of both ventilatory and oxygenation failure* and is classified by abnormal blood gas values. The critical values are:

- Partial pressure of arterial oxygen (Pao_2) less than 60 mm Hg (hypoxemic/oxygenation failure)

CHART 32-8 Home Care Assessment

The Patient After Pulmonary Embolism

Assess respiratory status:
- Observe rate and depth of ventilation.
- Auscultate lungs.
- Examine nail beds and mucous membranes for evidence of cyanosis.
- Take a pulse oximetry reading.
- Ask the patient if chest pain or shortness of breath is experienced in any position.
- Ask the patient about the presence of sputum and its color and character.

Assess cardiovascular status:
- Take vital signs, including apical pulse, pulse pressure; assess for presence or absence of orthostatic hypotension and quality and rhythm of peripheral pulses.
- Note presence or absence of peripheral edema.
- Examine hand vein filling in the dependent position.
- Examine neck vein filling in the recumbent and sitting positions.

Assess lower extremities for deep vein thrombosis:
- Examine lower legs and compare with each other for:
  - General edema
  - Calf swelling
  - Surface temperature
  - Presence of red streaks or cordlike, palpable structure
- Measure calf circumference:

Assess for evidence of bleeding:
- Examine the mouth and gums for oozing or frank bleeding.
- Examine all skin areas, especially old puncture sites and wounds, for bleeding, bruising, or petechiae.
- If the patient voids during the visit, test the urine for occult blood.

Assess cognition and mental status:
- Check level of consciousness.
- Check orientation to time, place, and person.
- Can the patient accurately read a seven-word sentence containing no words with more than three syllables?

Assess the patient's understanding of illness and adherence to treatment:
- Manifestations to report to health care provider
- Drug therapy plan (correct timing and dose)
- Bleeding Precautions
- Prevention of venous thromboembolism

- OR partial pressure of arterial carbon dioxide ($Paco_2$) more than 45 mm Hg occurring with acidemia (pH <7.35) (hypercapnic/ventilatory failure)
- AND arterial oxygen saturation (Sao_2) less than 90% in both cases

Whatever the underlying problem, the patient in acute respiratory failure is always **hypoxemic** (has low arterial blood oxygen levels) (Bekken, 2011; McLean, 2012).

Ventilatory Failure. Ventilatory failure is a problem in oxygen intake (air movement or ventilation) and blood flow (PERFUSION) that causes a ventilation-perfusion ($\dot{V}/\dot{Q}$) mismatch in which blood flow (perfusion) is normal but air movement (ventilation) is inadequate. It occurs when the chest pressure does not change enough to permit air movement into and out of the lungs. As a result, too little oxygen reaches the alveoli and carbon dioxide is retained. Perfusion is wasted in this area of no air movement from either inadequate oxygen intake or excessive carbon dioxide retention leading to poor GAS EXCHANGE and hypoxemia (McLean, 2012).

Ventilatory failure usually results from any of these problems: a physical problem of the lungs or chest wall; a defect in the respiratory control center in the brain; or poor function of the respiratory muscles, especially the diaphragm. The problem is defined by a $Paco_2$ level above 45 mm Hg plus acidemia (pH < 7.35) in patients who have otherwise healthy lungs.

TABLE 32-2 Common Causes of Ventilatory Failure

EXTRAPULMONARY CAUSES	INTRAPULMONARY CAUSES

• Neuromuscular disorders:
  • Myasthenia gravis
  • Guillain-Barré syndrome
  • Poliomyelitis
• Spinal cord injuries affecting nerves to intercostal muscles
• Central nervous system dysfunction:
  • Stroke
  • Increased intracranial pressure
  • Meningitis
• Chemical depression:
  • Opioid analgesics, sedatives, anesthetics
• Kyphoscoliosis
• Massive obesity
• Sleep apnea
• External obstruction/constriction
	• Airway disease:
	  • Chronic obstructive pulmonary disease (COPD), asthma
	• Ventilation-perfusion ($\dot{V}/\dot{Q}$) mismatch:
	  • Pulmonary embolism
	  • Pneumothorax
	  • Acute respiratory distress syndrome (ARDS)
	  • Amyloidosis
	  • Pulmonary edema
	  • Interstitial fibrosis

Many disorders can result in ventilatory failure. Causes are either **extrapulmonary** (involving nonpulmonary tissues but affecting respiratory function) or **intrapulmonary** (disorders of the respiratory tract). Table 32-2 lists causes of ventilatory failure.

Oxygenation (Gas Exchange) Failure. In oxygenation (GAS EXCHANGE) failure, chest pressure changes are normal and air moves in and out without difficulty but does not oxygenate the pulmonary blood sufficiently. It occurs in the type of $\dot{V}/\dot{Q}$ mismatch in which air movement and oxygen intake (ventilation) are normal but lung blood flow (PERFUSION) is decreased.

Many lung disorders can cause oxygenation failure. Problems include impaired diffusion of oxygen at the alveolar level, right-to-left shunting of blood in the pulmonary vessels, $\dot{V}/\dot{Q}$ mismatch, breathing air with a low oxygen level, and abnormal hemoglobin that fails to bind oxygen. In one type of $\dot{V}/\dot{Q}$ mismatch, areas of the lungs still have PERFUSION but GAS EXCHANGE does not occur, which leads to hypoxemia. An extreme example of $\dot{V}/\dot{Q}$ mismatch is when systemic venous blood (oxygen-poor) passes through the lungs without being oxygenated and is "shunted" to the left side of the heart and into the systemic arterial system. Normally, less than 5% of cardiac output contains venous blood that has bypassed oxygenation. With poor oxygenation in the lungs or a shunt that allows venous blood to bypass the lungs, even more arterial blood is not oxygenated and applying 100% oxygen does not correct the problem. A classic cause of such a $\dot{V}/\dot{Q}$ mismatch is acute respiratory distress syndrome (ARDS). Table 32-3 lists specific causes of oxygenation failure.

Combined Ventilatory and Oxygenation Failure. Combined ventilatory and oxygenation failure involves **hypoventilation** (poor respiratory movements). Impaired GAS EXCHANGE at the alveolar-capillary membrane results in poor diffusion of oxygen into arterial blood and carbon dioxide retention. The condition may or may not include poor lung perfusion. When lung PERFUSION is not adequate, $\dot{V}/\dot{Q}$ mismatch occurs and

TABLE 32-3 Common Causes of Oxygenation Failure

- Low atmospheric oxygen concentration:
  - High altitudes, closed spaces, smoke inhalation, carbon monoxide poisoning
- Pneumonia
- Congestive heart failure with pulmonary edema
- Pulmonary embolism (PE)
- Acute respiratory distress syndrome (ARDS)
- Interstitial pneumonitis-fibrosis
- Abnormal hemoglobin
- Hypovolemic shock
- Hypoventilation
- Complications of nitroprusside therapy:
  - Thiocyanate toxicity, methemoglobinemia

both ventilation and perfusion are inadequate. This type of respiratory failure leads to a more profound hypoxemia than either ventilatory failure or oxygenation failure alone.

A combination of ventilatory failure and oxygenation (GAS EXCHANGE) failure occurs in patients who have abnormal lungs, such as those who have any form of chronic bronchitis, have emphysema, have cystic fibrosis, or are having an asthma attack. The bronchioles and alveoli are diseased (causing oxygenation failure), and the work of breathing increases until the respiratory muscles cannot function effectively (causing ventilatory failure) leading to acute respiratory failure (ARF). ARF can also occur in patients who have cardiac failure along with respiratory failure and is made worse by the fact that the cardiac system cannot adapt to the hypoxia by increasing the cardiac output.

❖ PATIENT-CENTERED COLLABORATIVE CARE

◆ Assessment

The manifestations of ARF are related to the systemic effects of hypoxia, hypercapnia, and acidosis (Bekken, 2011). Assess for **dyspnea** (perceived difficulty breathing)—the hallmark of respiratory failure. Evaluate dyspnea on the basis of how breathless the patient becomes while performing common tasks. Depending on the nature of the underlying problem, the patient might not be aware of changes in the work of breathing.

Dyspnea is more intense when it develops rapidly. Slowly progressive respiratory failure may first be noticed as dyspnea on exertion (DOE) or when lying down. The patient may have **orthopnea**, finding it easier to breathe in an upright position (Bull, 2014). With chronic respiratory problems, a minor increase in dyspnea may represent severe GAS EXCHANGE problems.

Assess for a change in the patient's respiratory rate or pattern and changes in lung sounds. Pulse oximetry (Spo_2) may show decreased oxygen saturation, but end-tidal CO_2 ($ETCO_2$ or $PETCO_2$) monitoring may be more valuable for monitoring the patient with ARF (Carlisle, 2014). His or her pulse oximetry may show adequate oxygen saturation but because of increased $ETCO_2$ the patient may be close to respiratory failure. Arterial blood gas (ABG) studies are reviewed to most accurately identify the degree of hypoxia and hypercarbia.

Other manifestations of hypoxic respiratory failure include restlessness, irritability or agitation, confusion, and tachycardia. Manifestations of hypercapnic failure include decreased level of consciousness (LOC), headache, drowsiness, lethargy, and possible seizures. The effects of acidosis may lead to decreased LOC, drowsiness, confusion, hypotension, bradycardia, and weak peripheral pulses.

◆ Interventions

Oxygen therapy is appropriate for any patient with acute hypoxemia. It is used in acute respiratory failure to keep the arterial oxygen (Pao_2) level above 60 mm Hg while treating the cause of the respiratory failure. Oxygen therapy is discussed in detail in Chapter 28. If oxygen therapy does not maintain acceptable Pao_2 levels, mechanical ventilation (invasive or noninvasive) may be needed.

Drugs given systemically or by metered dose inhaler (MDI) may be prescribed to dilate the bronchioles and decrease inflammation to promote GAS EXCHANGE. Corticosteroids may be used, but their benefit has not been conclusively demonstrated. Analgesics are needed if the patient has pain. If the patient requires mechanical ventilation, he or she may need neuromuscular blockade drugs for optimal ventilator effect. Other management strategies depend on the underlying condition(s) that predisposed the patient to ARF development.

Help the patient find a position of comfort that allows easier breathing—usually a more upright position. To decrease the anxiety occurring with dyspnea, assist him or her to use relaxation, diversion, and guided imagery. Start energy-conserving measures, such as minimal self-care and no unnecessary procedures. Encourage deep breathing and other breathing exercises.

ACUTE RESPIRATORY DISTRESS SYNDROME

❖ PATHOPHYSIOLOGY

Acute respiratory distress syndrome (**ARDS**) is acute respiratory failure with these features:

- Hypoxemia that persists even when 100% oxygen is given (**refractory hypoxemia**, a cardinal feature)
- Decreased pulmonary compliance
- Dyspnea
- Noncardiac-associated bilateral pulmonary edema
- Dense pulmonary infiltrates on x-ray (ground-glass appearance)

Often ARDS occurs after an *acute lung injury (ALI)* in people who have no pulmonary disease as a result of other conditions such as sepsis, burns, pancreatitis, trauma, and transfusion. The mortality rate is about 60% depending on the underlying cause (Carroll et al., 2013). Other terms for ARDS include *adult respiratory distress syndrome* and *shock lung*.

Despite different causes of ALI in ARDS, the trigger is a systemic inflammatory response. As a result, ARDS manifestations are similar regardless of the cause. The main site of injury in the lung is the alveolar-capillary membrane, which normally is permeable only to small molecules. It can be injured during sepsis, pulmonary embolism, shock, aspiration, or inhalation injury. When injured, this membrane becomes more permeable to large molecules, which allows debris, proteins, and fluid into the alveoli. Lung tissue normally remains relatively dry, but in patients with ARDS, lung fluid increases and contains more proteins.

Other changes occur in the alveoli and respiratory bronchioles. Normally, the type II pneumocytes produce surfactant, a substance that increases lung **compliance** (elasticity) and prevents alveolar collapse. Surfactant activity is reduced in ARDS because type II pneumocytes are damaged and because the surfactant is diluted by excess lung fluids. As a result, the alveoli become unstable and tend to collapse unless they are filled with fluid. These fluid-filled and collapsed alveoli cannot participate in GAS EXCHANGE. As a result, edema forms around terminal airways, which are compressed and closed and can be destroyed. Lung volume and compliance are further reduced. As fluid continues to leak in more lung areas, fluid, protein, and blood cells collect in the alveoli and in the spaces between the alveoli. Lymph channels are compressed, and more fluid collects. Poorly inflated alveoli receive blood but cannot oxygenate it, increasing the shunt. Hypoxemia and ventilation-perfusion $\dot{V}/\dot{Q}$ mismatch result.

Transfusion-related acute lung injury (TRALI) is the sudden onset (within 6 hours of a transfusion) of hypoxemic lung disease along with infiltrates on x-ray without cardiac problems. TRALI is associated with the activation of the inflammatory response due to a recent transfusion of plasma-containing blood products such as packed red blood cells (PRBCs), platelets, and fresh frozen plasma (Benson, 2012). Other lung complications of transfusion include transfusion-associated circulatory overload (TACO) and transfusion-related immunomodulation (TRIM) (Benson, 2012).

Etiology and Genetic Risk. ALI leading to ARDS has many causes (Table 32-4). Some causes result in direct injury to lung tissue; other causes do not directly involve the lungs. As a result of sepsis, pancreatitis, trauma, and other conditions, inflammatory mediators spread to the lungs causing damage (Carroll et al., 2013; McCance et al., 2014).

ARDS also can occur from direct lung injury. Aspiration of acidic gastric contents, pneumonia, drowning, and inhaling toxic fumes are examples of conditions causing direct lung injury. With such events, surfactant production is impaired and the remaining surfactant is diluted. This situation leads to atelectasis, decreased lung compliance, and shunting (movement of blood in the lungs without GAS EXCHANGE and oxygenation) (Carroll et al., 2013; Dechert et al., 2012).

GENETIC/GENOMIC CONSIDERATIONS

Patient-Centered Care QSEN

An increased genetic risk is suspected in the development and progression of ARDS. Variations in the genes responsible for surfactant production appear to increase the predisposition to developing ARDS as does variation in the genes responsible for cytokine production during inflammatory events associated with sepsis (Dechert et al., 2012). Ask about the patient's previous responses to infection or injury. If the patient has consistently had greater-than-expected inflammatory responses, he or she may be at increased risk for ARDS after ALI and should be monitored for manifestations of the disorder.

Incidence and Prevalence. The actual incidence of ARDS is unknown because it is part of other health problems and is not systematically reported as a separate disorder. According to the ARDS Foundation, about 150,000 cases of ARDS occur yearly in North America (ARDS Foundation, 2013) although many health care professionals believe this estimate to be low.

Health Promotion and Maintenance

The nursing priority in the prevention of ARDS is early recognition of patients at high risk for the syndrome. Because patients who aspirate gastric contents are at great risk, closely assess and monitor those receiving tube feedings (because the tube keeps the gastric sphincter open) and those with problems that impair swallowing and gag reflexes. As required by The Joint Commission's NPSGs to prevent ARDS, follow meticulous infection control guidelines, including handwashing, invasive catheter and wound care, and Contact Precautions. Teach unlicensed assistive personnel (UAP) the importance of always adhering to infection control guidelines. Carefully observe patients who are being treated for any health problem associated with ARDS.

TABLE 32-4 Common Causes of Acute Lung Injury

- Shock
- Trauma
- Serious nervous system injury
- Pancreatitis
- Fat and amniotic fluid emboli
- Pulmonary infections
- Sepsis
- Inhalation of toxic gases (smoke, oxygen)
- Pulmonary aspiration (especially of stomach contents)
- Drug ingestion (e.g., heroin, opioids, aspirin)
- Hemolytic disorders
- Multiple blood transfusions
- Cardiopulmonary bypass
- Submersion in water with water aspiration (especially in fresh water)

❖ PATIENT-CENTERED COLLABORATIVE CARE

◆ Assessment

Physical Assessment/Clinical Manifestations. Assess the breathing of any patient at increased risk for ARDS. Determine whether increased work of breathing is present, as indicated by hyperpnea, noisy respiration, cyanosis, pallor, and retraction **intercostally** (between the ribs) or **substernally** (below the ribs). Document sweating, respiratory effort, and any change in mental status. *Abnormal lung sounds are **not** heard on auscultation because the edema occurs first in the interstitial spaces and not in the airways.* Assess vital signs at least hourly for hypotension, tachycardia, and dysrhythmias.

Diagnostic Assessment. The diagnosis of ARDS is established by a lowered partial pressure of arterial oxygen ($Pa{O_2}$) value (decreased GAS EXCHANGE and oxygenation), determined by arterial blood gas (ABG) measurements. Because a widening alveolar oxygen gradient (increased fraction of inspired oxygen [$Fi{O_2}$] that does not lead to increased $Pa{O_2}$ levels) develops with increased shunting of blood, the patient has a progressive need for higher levels of oxygen. He or she develops refractory hypoxemia and often needs intubation and mechanical ventilation. Sputum cultures obtained by bronchoscopy and by transtracheal aspiration are used to determine if a lung infection also is present.

The chest x-ray may show diffuse haziness or a "whited-out" (ground-glass) appearance of the lung. An ECG rules out cardiac problems and usually shows no specific changes. Hemodynamic monitoring with a pulmonary artery catheter helps diagnose ARDS. In ARDS, the pulmonary capillary wedge pressure (PCWP) is low to normal, whereas in cardiac-induced pulmonary edema, the PCWP is above 18 mm Hg. Chapter 38 explains hemodynamic monitoring in detail.

◆ Interventions

The patient with ARDS often needs intubation and mechanical ventilation with positive end-expiratory pressure (PEEP) or continuous positive airway pressure (CPAP). Best practice involves using "open lung" and lung protective ventilation strategies. Low tidal volumes (6 mL/kg of body weight) have been shown to prevent lung injury. PEEP is started at 5 cm H_2O and increased to keep oxygen saturation adequate. PEEP levels may need to be high. Pressure-controlled ventilation is preferred over volume-controlled ventilation to promote the nonfunctional alveoli to participate in GAS EXCHANGE.

Airway pressure-release ventilation (APRV) and high-frequency oscillatory ventilation are alternative modes of mechanical ventilation that improve GAS EXCHANGE with oxygenation and ventilation in patients with moderate to severe ARDS (Bortolotto & Makic, 2012). Sedation and paralysis may be needed for adequate ventilation and to reduce tissue oxygen needs. Because one of the side effects of PEEP is tension pneumothorax, assess lung sounds hourly and suction as often as needed to maintain a patent airway.

Positioning may be important in promoting GAS EXCHANGE, but the exact position is controversial. Some patients do better in the prone position, especially if it is started early in the disease course. Prone positioning may be achieved using a mechanical turning device, although the turning equipment is awkward and care in the prone position is more difficult. Automated kinetic beds are available to assist with turning. Manually turning the patient every 2 hours has been shown to improve PERFUSION; however, this intervention often is not performed as frequently as needed. Early progressive mobility also has demonstrated benefit in reducing ventilator needs, days on the ventilator, and mortality (Morris et al., 2011; Wright & Flynn, 2011).

For severe ARDS, extracorporeal membrane oxygenation (ECMO) using heart-lung bypass equipment has been a successful life support technique when the patient does not improve with more traditional management. However, the proper timing of ECMO and standardization of this therapy for best outcomes have not been established (Williams, 2013).

Drug and Fluid Therapy. Antibiotics are used to treat infections when organisms are identified. Other drugs are used to manage any underlying cause. Currently, no treatments reverse the pathologic changes in the lungs, although many interventions are under investigation. These include agents that modify the inflammatory responses and reduce oxidative stress, such as vitamins C and E, *N*-acetylcysteine, and nitric oxide, as well as surfactant replacement (Carroll et al., 2013).

Research shows that patients with ARDS who receive conservative fluid therapy have improved lung function and a shorter duration of mechanical ventilation and ICU length of stay compared with those who receive more liberal fluid therapy. Conservative fluid therapy involves infusing smaller amounts of IV fluid and the use of diuretics to maintain fluid balance, whereas liberal fluid therapy often results in an increasingly positive fluid balance and more edema (Ferri, 2013).

Nutrition Therapy. The patient with ARDS is at risk for malnutrition, which further reduces respiratory muscle function and the immune response. Consultation with a dietitian is needed, and enteral nutrition (tube feeding) or parenteral nutrition is started as soon as possible.

Case Management. Case management of the patient with ARDS focuses on the phases of ARDS rather than on day-to-day care. The course of ARDS and its management are divided into three phases:

- *Exudative phase.* This phase includes early changes of dyspnea and tachypnea resulting from the alveoli becoming fluid-filled and from pulmonary shunting and atelectasis. Early interventions focus on supporting the patient and providing oxygen.
- *Fibroproliferative phase.* Increased lung damage leads to pulmonary hypertension and fibrosis. The body attempts to repair the damage, and increasing lung involvement reduces GAS EXCHANGE and oxygenation. Multiple organ dysfunction syndrome (MODS) can occur. Interventions focus on delivering adequate oxygen, preventing complications, and supporting the lungs.
- *Resolution phase.* Usually occurring after 14 days, resolution of the injury can occur; if not, the patient either dies or has chronic disease. Fibrosis may or may not occur. Research indicates that patients surviving ARDS often have neuropsychological deficits and poor quality-of-life scores (Dechert et al., 2012; Mathay & Zemans, 2011).

CLINICAL JUDGMENT CHALLENGE

Patient-Centered Care; Teamwork and Collaboration QSEN

A 50-year-old patient is admitted to the medical-surgical floor from the emergency department with severe abdominal pain thought to be from acute pancreatitis. He has a history of drinking at least a case of beer a day. He also smokes and appears cachectic. His old chart indicates a history of COPD, but he does not take drugs for this. He does have a new productive cough. At change of shift, the nurse finds the patient dyspneic and slightly confused. Lung sounds have wheezes, and he is mildly febrile. Pulse is 120 beats/min, respirations are 32 breaths/min, and blood pressure is 118/64 mm Hg (baseline). Oximetry shows an Spo_2 of 91%.

1. What risk factors for ARDS does this patient have?
2. Explain the relationship between the lung sounds and the oximetry reading.
3. What diagnostic testing should you be prepared to obtain?

Two hours after applying oxygen at 3 liters/nasal cannula, the patient's Spo_2 is now 89%.

4. What additional measures do you anticipate for this patient?

THE PATIENT REQUIRING INTUBATION AND VENTILATION

PATHOPHYSIOLOGY

With mechanical ventilation, the patient who has severe problems of GAS EXCHANGE may be supported until the underlying problem improves or resolves. Usually mechanical ventilation is a temporary life-support technique. The need for this support may be lifelong for those with severe restrictive lung disease or chronic progressive neuromuscular disease that reduces ventilation.

Mechanical ventilation is most often used for patients with hypoxemia and progressive alveolar hypoventilation with respiratory acidosis. The hypoxemia is usually due to pulmonary shunting of blood when other methods of oxygen delivery do not provide a sufficiently high fraction of inspired oxygen (Fio_2). Mechanical ventilation may be used for patients who need ventilatory support after surgery, those who expend too much energy with breathing and barely maintain adequate GAS EXCHANGE, or those who have general anesthesia or heavy sedation.

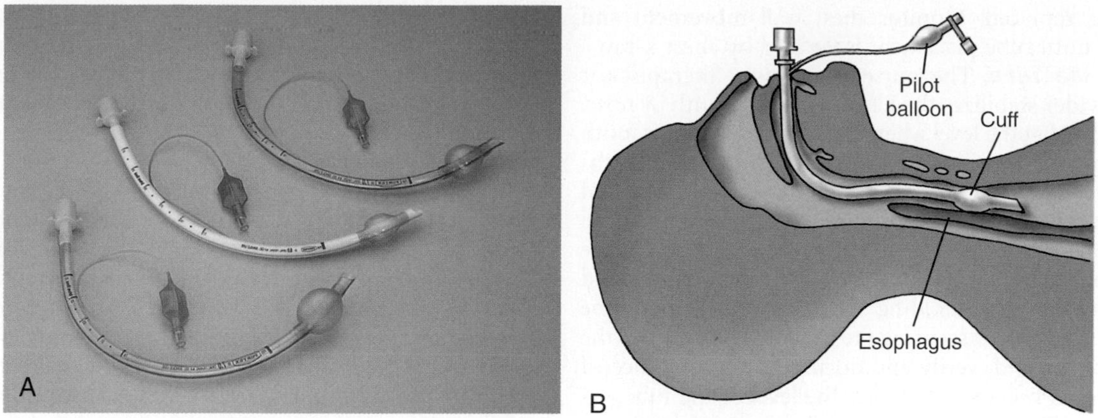

FIG. 32-2 **A,** Endotracheal tubes. **B,** Correct placement of an oral endotracheal tube.

❖ PATIENT-CENTERED COLLABORATIVE CARE

Assess the patient to be intubated in the same way as for other breathing problems. Once mechanical ventilation has been started, assess the respiratory system on an ongoing basis. Monitor and assess for problems related to the artificial airway or ventilator.

Endotracheal Intubation

The patient who needs mechanical ventilation must have an artificial airway. The most common type of airway for a short-term basis is the endotracheal (ET) tube. To reduce tracheal and vocal cord damage, a tracheostomy is considered if an artificial airway is needed for longer than 10 to 14 days (see Chapter 28). The expectations of intubation are to maintain a patent airway, provide a means to remove secretions, and provide ventilation and oxygen.

Endotracheal Tube. An ET tube is a long polyvinyl chloride tube that is passed through the mouth or nose and into the trachea (Fig. 32-2). When properly positioned, the tip of the ET tube rests about 2 cm above the **carina** (the point at which the trachea divides into the right and left mainstem bronchi). Oral intubation is a fast and easy way to establish an airway and is often performed as an emergency procedure. The nasal route is used for oral surgeries and when oral intubation is not possible but should be avoided with midface trauma or possible basilar skull fracture. This route is not used if the patient has a blood CLOTTING problem. An anesthesiologist, nurse anesthetist, or respiratory therapist usually performs the intubation.

The shaft of the tube has a radiopaque line running the length of the tube. This line shows on x-ray and is used to determine correct tube placement. Short horizontal lines (depth markings) are used to place the tube correctly at the naris or mouth (at the incisor tooth) and to identify how far the tube has been inserted.

The cuff at the distal end of the tube is inflated after placement and creates a seal between the trachea and the cuff. The seal ensures delivery of a set tidal volume when mechanical ventilation is used. The cuff is inflated using a minimal-leak technique: when the cuff is inflated to an adequate sealing volume, a minimal amount of air can pass around the cuff to the vocal cords, nose, or mouth. The patient cannot talk when the cuff is inflated.

The pilot balloon with a one-way valve permits air to be inserted into the cuff and prevents air from escaping. This balloon is a guide for determining whether air is present in the cuff, but it does not show how much or how little air is present.

The adaptor connects the ET tube to ventilator tubing or an oxygen delivery system. The endotracheal tube size is listed on the shaft of the tube. Adult tube sizes range from 7 to 9 mm. Tube size selected is based on the size of the patient.

Preparing for Intubation. Know the proper procedure for summoning intubation personnel in the facility to the bedside in an emergency situation. Explain the procedure to the patient as clearly as possible. *Basic life support measures, such as obtaining a patent airway and delivering 100% oxygen by a manual resuscitation bag with a facemask, are crucial to survival until help arrives.*

! NURSING SAFETY PRIORITY (QSEN)

Critical Rescue

For the patient requiring emergency intubation and ventilation, bring the code (or "crash") cart, airway equipment box, and suction equipment (often already on the code cart) to the bedside. Maintain a patent airway through positioning (head-tilt, chin-lift) and the insertion of an oral or nasopharyngeal airway until the patient is intubated. Delivering manual breaths with a bag-valve-mask may also be required.

During intubation, the nurse coordinates the rescue response and continuously monitors the patient for changes in vital signs, signs of hypoxia or hypoxemia, dysrhythmias, and aspiration. Ensure that each intubation attempt lasts no longer than 30 seconds, preferably less than 15 seconds. After 30 seconds, provide oxygen by means of a mask and manual resuscitation bag to prevent hypoxia and cardiac arrest. Suction as necessary (Morton & Fontaine, 2013; Urden et al., 2012).

Verifying Tube Placement. Immediately after an ET tube is inserted, placement should be verified. The most accurate ways to verify placement are by checking end-tidal carbon dioxide levels and by chest x-ray. Assess for breath sounds bilaterally, sounds over the gastric area, symmetric chest movement, and air emerging from the ET tube. If breath sounds and chest wall movement are absent on the left side, the tube may be in the right mainstem bronchus. The person intubating the patient should be able to reposition the tube without repeating the entire intubation procedure.

If the tube is in the stomach, the abdomen may be distended and must be decompressed with a nasogastric (NG) tube after the ET tube is replaced. Monitor chest wall movement and breath sounds until tube placement is verified by chest x-ray.

Stabilizing the Tube. The nurse, respiratory therapist, or anesthesia provider stabilizes the ET tube at the mouth or nose. The tube is marked at the level where it touches the incisor tooth or naris. Two people working together use a head halter technique to secure the tube. An oral airway also may be inserted or a commercial bite block placed to keep the patient from biting an oral endotracheal tube. One person stabilizes the tube at the correct position and prevents head movement while a second person applies the tube holding device. Commercial tube holders are preferred over securing the tube with tape. After the procedure is completed, verify and document the presence of bilateral and equal breath sounds and the level of the tube.

Nursing Care. *The priority nursing action when caring for an intubated patient is maintaining a patent airway.* Assess tube placement, cuff leak, breath sounds, indications of adequate GAS EXCHANGE and oxygenation, and chest wall movement regularly.

! NURSING SAFETY PRIORITY (QSEN)

Critical Rescue

If an intubated patient shows manifestations of decreased oxygenation, check for DOPE: displaced tube, obstructed tube (most often with secretions), pneumothorax, and equipment problems (Dennison et al., 2011).

Prevent the patient from pulling or tugging on the tube to avoid tube dislodgment, and check the pilot balloon to ensure that the cuff is inflated. Suctioning, coughing, and speaking can cause dislodgment. Neck flexion, neck extension, and rotation of the head also can cause the tube to move. Tongue movement also can change the tube's position. When other measures fail, obtain a prescription for soft wrist restraints and apply these for the patient who is pulling on the tube. *Restraints are used as a last resort to prevent accidental extubation.* Adequate sedation (chemical restraint) may be needed to decrease agitation or prevent extubation. Obtain permission for restraints from the patient or family. More information on airway management is found in Chapter 28.

Complications of an ET or nasotracheal tube can occur during placement, while in place, during extubation, or after extubation (either early or late). Common complications include tube obstruction, dislodgment, pneumothorax, tracheal tears, bleeding, and infection. Trauma and other problems can occur to the face; eye; nasal and paranasal areas; oral, pharyngeal, bronchial, tracheal, and pulmonary areas; esophageal and gastric areas; and cardiovascular, musculoskeletal, and neurologic systems.

? NCLEX EXAMINATION CHALLENGE

Safe and Effective Care Environment

The nurse caring for a client who is intubated and receiving mechanical ventilation notes that her oxygen saturation is 89%, her heart rate is 120 beats/min, and she is increasingly agitated and restless. On auscultation, the nurse finds that the lung sounds are diminished on one side. Which action does the nurse perform first?

A. Notify the provider, and prepare for re-intubation or repositioning the tube.
B. Document the findings, and request sedation from the provider.
C. Call respiratory therapy to obtain a set of arterial blood gases.
D. Reposition the tube, and call radiology for a stat chest x-ray.

Mechanical Ventilation

Mechanical ventilation to support and maintain GAS EXCHANGE is used in many settings, not just in critical care units. The nurse plays a pivotal role in the coordination of care and the prevention of problems. Chart 32-9 lists best practices for patient care during mechanical ventilation.

The purposes of mechanical ventilation are to improve GAS EXCHANGE and to decrease the work needed for effective breathing. It is used to support the patient until lung function is adequate or until the acute episode has passed. *A ventilator does not cure diseased lungs; it provides ventilation until the patient can resume the process of breathing on his or her own.* Remember *why* the patient is using the ventilator so that management efforts also focus on correcting the causes of the respiratory failure. If normal GAS EXCHANGE with oxygenation, ventilation, and respiratory muscle strength is achieved, mechanical ventilation can be discontinued.

Types of Ventilators. Many types of ventilators are available. The ventilator selected depends on the severity of the breathing problem and the length of time ventilator support is needed. Most ventilators are positive-pressure ventilators. During inspiration, pressure is generated that pushes air into the lungs and expands the chest. Usually an endotracheal (ET) tube or tracheostomy is needed. Positive-pressure ventilators are classified by the mechanism that ends inspiration and starts expiration. Inspiration is cycled in three major ways: pressure-cycled, time-cycled, or volume-cycled.

Pressure-cycled ventilators push air into the lungs until a preset airway pressure is reached. Tidal volumes and inspiratory time vary. These ventilators are used for short periods, such as just after surgery and for respiratory therapy. Bi-level positive airway pressure (Bi-PAP) ventilators are a newer form of pressure-cycled ventilator in which the ventilator provides a preset inspiratory pressure and an expiratory pressure similar to positive end-expiratory pressure (PEEP).

Time-cycled ventilators push air into the lungs until a preset time has elapsed. Tidal volume and pressure vary, depending on the needs of the patient and the type of ventilator.

Volume-cycled ventilators push air into the lungs until a preset volume is delivered. A constant tidal volume is delivered regardless of the pressure needed to deliver the tidal volume. A set pressure limit, however, prevents excessive pressure from being exerted on the lungs. The advantage of this type of ventilator is that a constant tidal volume is delivered regardless of changes in lung or chest wall compliance or in airway resistance.

Microprocessor ventilators are computer-managed positive-pressure ventilators. A computer is built into the ventilator to allow ongoing monitoring of ventilatory functions, alarms, and patient conditions. It often has components of volume-, time-, and pressure-cycled ventilators. This type of ventilator is more responsive to patients who have severe lung disease and those who need prolonged weaning trials. Examples include the Draeger Evita XL (Fig. 32-3) and Puritan-Bennett 840.

Modes of Ventilation. The mode of ventilation is the way in which the patient receives breaths from the ventilator. The most common modes are assist-control ventilation, synchronized intermittent mandatory ventilation, and bi-level positive airway pressure ventilation.

Assist-control (AC) ventilation is the mode used most often as a resting mode. The ventilator takes over the work of breathing for the patient. The tidal volume and ventilatory rate are

CHART 32-9 **Best Practice for Patient Safety & Quality Care** (QSEN)

Care of the Patient Receiving Mechanical Ventilation

- Assess the patient's respiratory status at least every 4 hours for the first 24 hours and then as needed:
  - Take vital signs at least every 4 hours.
  - Assess the patient's color (especially lips and nail beds).
  - Observe the patient's chest for bilateral expansion.
  - Assess the placement of the nasotracheal or endotracheal tube.
  - Obtain pulse oximetry reading.
  - Evaluate ABGs as available.
  - Maintain head of the bed more than 30 degrees when patient is supine to prevent aspiration and ventilator-associated pneumonia.
- Document pertinent observations in the patient's medical record.
- Check at least every 8 hours to be sure the ventilator setting is as prescribed.
- Check to be sure alarms are set (especially low-pressure and low-exhaled volume).
- If the patient is on PEEP, observe the peak airway pressure dial to determine the proper level of PEEP.
- Check the exhaled volume digital display to be sure the patient is receiving the prescribed tidal volume.
- Empty ventilator tubings when moisture collects. *Never empty fluid in the tubing back into the cascade.*
- Ensure humidity by keeping delivered air temperature maintained at body temperature.
- Be sure the tracheostomy cuff (or endotracheal cuff) is adequately inflated to ensure tidal volume.
- Auscultate the lungs for crackles, wheezes, equal breath sounds, and decreased or absent breath sounds.
- Check the patient's need for tracheal, oral, or nasal suctioning every 2 hours, and suction as needed.
- Assess the patient's mouth around the ET tube for pressure ulcers.
- Perform mouth care every 2 hours.
- Change tracheostomy tube holder or tape or endotracheal tube holder or tape as needed:
  - Carefully move the oral endotracheal tube to the opposite side of the mouth once daily to prevent ulcers.
  - Provide tracheostomy care every 8 hours.
- Assess ventilated patients for GI distress (diarrhea, constipation, tarry stools).
- Maintain accurate intake and output records to monitor fluid balance.
- Turn the patient at least every 2 hours, and get the patient out of bed as prescribed to promote pulmonary hygiene and prevent complications of immobility.
- Schedule treatments and nursing care at intervals for rest.
- Monitor the patient's progress on current ventilator settings, and make appropriate changes, as indicated.
- Monitor the patient for the effectiveness of mechanical ventilation in terms of his or her physiologic and psychological status.
- Monitor for adverse effects of mechanical ventilation: infection, barotrauma, reduced cardiac output.
- Position the patient to facilitate ventilation-perfusion ($\dot{V}/\dot{Q}$) matching ["good lung down"], as appropriate.
- Monitor the effects of ventilator changes on oxygenation and the patient's subjective response.
- Monitor readiness to wean.
- Explain all procedures and treatments; provide access to a call light; visit the patient frequently.
- Provide a method of communication. Request consultation with a speech-language pathologist for assistance, if necessary.
- Initiate relaxation techniques, as appropriate.
- Administer muscle-paralyzing agents, sedatives, and narcotic analgesics, as prescribed.
- Include the patient and family whenever possible (especially during suctioning and tracheostomy care).

ABGs, Arterial blood gases; *ET,* endotrachel; *PEEP,* positive end-expiratory pressure.

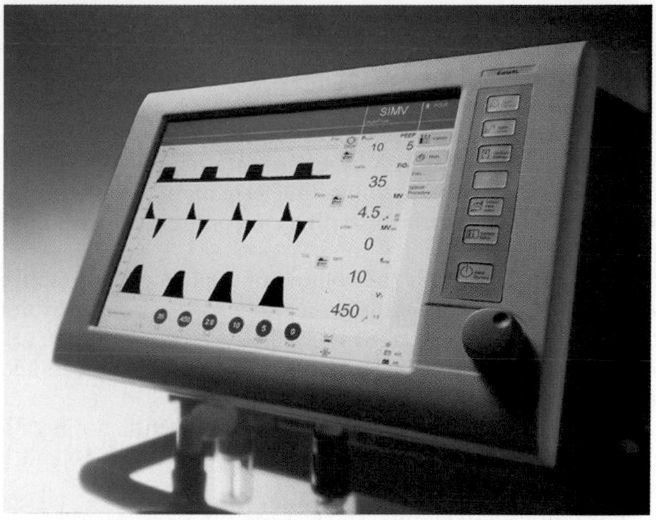

FIG. 32-3 Display signals, alarms, and control panel of a typical volume-cycled ventilator.

preset. If the patient does not trigger spontaneous breaths, a ventilatory pattern is established by the ventilator. It is programmed to respond to the patient's inspiratory effort if he or she begins a breath. In this case, the ventilator delivers the preset tidal volume while allowing the patient to control the rate of breathing.

A disadvantage of the AC mode is that the ventilator continues to deliver a preset tidal volume even when the patient's spontaneous breathing rate increases. This can cause hyperventilation and respiratory alkalosis. Investigate and correct causes of hyperventilation, such as pain, anxiety, or acid-base imbalances.

Synchronized intermittent mandatory ventilation (SIMV) is similar to AC ventilation in that tidal volume and ventilatory rate are preset. If the patient does not breathe, a ventilatory pattern is established by the ventilator. Unlike the AC mode, SIMV allows spontaneous breathing at the patient's own rate and tidal volume between the ventilator breaths. It can be used as a main ventilatory mode or as a weaning mode. When used for weaning, the number of mechanical breaths (SIMV breaths) is gradually decreased (e.g., from 12 to 2) as the patient resumes spontaneous breathing. The mandatory ventilator breaths are delivered when the patient is ready to inspire. This action coordinates breathing between the ventilator and the patient.

Bi-level positive airway pressure (BiPAP) provides noninvasive pressure support ventilation by nasal mask or facemask. It is most often used for patients with sleep apnea but also may be used for patients with respiratory muscle fatigue or impending respiratory failure to avoid more invasive ventilation methods.

Other modes of ventilation, such as pressure support and continuous flow (flow-by), are part of most microprocessor ventilators. Both types decrease the work of breathing and are used for weaning patients from mechanical ventilation. Other modes are maximum mandatory ventilation (MMV), inverse inspiration-expiration (I/E) ratio, permissive hypercarbia, airway pressure–release ventilation (APRV), proportional assist ventilation, and high-frequency oscillation. Most modes use special ventilators, tubing, or airways.

Ventilator Controls and Settings. The volume-cycled ventilator is the most widely used type in the acute care setting. Regardless of the type of volume-cycled ventilator used, the controls and types of settings are universal (see Fig. 32-3). The physician prescribes the ventilator settings, and usually the ventilator is readied or set up by the respiratory therapy department. The nurse assists in connecting the patient to the ventilator and monitors the ventilator settings in conjunction with respiratory therapy.

Tidal volume (V_T) is the volume of air the patient receives with each breath, as measured on either inspiration or expiration. The average prescribed V_T ranges between 7 and 10 mL/kg of body weight. Adding a zero to a patient's weight in kilograms gives an estimate of tidal volume.

Rate, or breaths/min, is the number of ventilator breaths delivered per minute. The rate is usually set between 10 and 14 breaths/min.

Fraction of inspired oxygen (Fio_2) is the oxygen level delivered to the patient. The prescribed Fio_2 is based on the ABG values and the patient's condition. The range is 21% to 100% oxygen.

The oxygen delivered to the patient is warmed to body temperature (98.6°F [37°C]) and humidified to 100%. This is needed because upper air passages of the respiratory tree, which normally warm and humidify air, are bypassed. Humidifying and warming prevent mucosal damage.

Peak airway (inspiratory) pressure (PIP) is the pressure used by the ventilator to deliver a set tidal volume at a given lung compliance. The PIP value appears on the display of the ventilator. It is the highest pressure reached during inspiration. Monitoring trends in PIP that reflect changes in resistance of the lungs and resistance in the ventilator. An increased PIP reading means increased airway resistance in the patient or in the ventilator tubing (bronchospasm or pinched tubing), increased secretions, pulmonary edema, or decreased pulmonary compliance (the lungs or chest wall is "stiffer" and harder to inflate). An upper pressure limit is set to prevent barotrauma. When the limit is reached, the high-pressure alarm sounds and the remaining volume is not given.

Continuous positive airway pressure (CPAP) applies positive airway pressure throughout the entire respiratory cycle for spontaneously breathing patients. Sedating drugs are given lightly or not at all when the patient is receiving CPAP so that respiratory effort is not suppressed. CPAP keeps the alveoli open during inspiration and prevents alveolar collapse during expiration. This process increases functional residual capacity (FRC) and improves GAS EXCHANGE and oxygenation.

CPAP is commonly used to help in the weaning process. During CPAP, no ventilator breaths are delivered. The ventilator just delivers oxygen and provides monitoring and an alarm system. The respiratory pattern is determined by the patient's efforts. Normal levels of CPAP are 5 to 15 cm H_2O to promote adequate GAS EXCHANGE and oxygenation. If no pressure is set, the patient receives no positive pressure. The patient is then using the ventilator as a T-piece with alarms. Modifications of CPAP include nasal CPAP and BiPAP, which are used on a temporary basis for select problems.

Positive end-expiratory pressure (PEEP) is positive pressure exerted during expiration. PEEP improves oxygenation by enhancing GAS EXCHANGE and preventing atelectasis. It is used to treat persistent hypoxemia that does not improve with an acceptable oxygen delivery level. It may be added when the arterial oxygen pressure (Pao_2) remains low with an Fio_2 of 50% to 70% or greater.

The need for PEEP indicates a severe GAS EXCHANGE problem. *It is important to lower the Fio_2 delivered whenever possible because prolonged use of a high Fio_2 can damage lungs from the toxic effects of oxygen.* PEEP prevents alveoli from collapsing because the lungs are kept partially inflated so that alveolar-capillary gas exchange is promoted throughout the ventilatory cycle. The effect should be an increase in arterial blood oxygenation so that the Fio_2 can be decreased.

PEEP is "dialed in" on the control panel. The amount of PEEP is usually 5 to 15 cm H_2O (although higher PEEP can be used) and is monitored on the peak airway pressure dial, the same dial used to read the PIP. When PEEP is added, the dial does not return to zero at the end of exhalation; rather, it returns to a baseline that is increased from zero by the amount of PEEP applied.

Flow rate is how fast each breath is delivered and is usually set at 40 L/min. *If a patient is agitated or restless, has a widely fluctuating inspiratory pressure reading, or has other signs of air hunger, the flow may be set too low. Increasing the flow should be tried before using chemical restraints.*

Other settings may be used, depending on the type of ventilator and mode of ventilation. Examples include inspiratory and expiratory cycle, waveform, expiratory resistance, and plateau.

Nursing Management. The use of mechanical ventilation involves a collaborative and complex decision-making process for the patient and family and the health care team. Address the physical and psychological concerns of the patient and family because the mechanical ventilator often causes them anxiety. Explain the purpose of the ventilator, and acknowledge the patient's and family's feelings. Encourage the patient and family to express their concerns. Act as the coach to help and support them through this experience. Patients undergoing mechanical ventilation in ICUs often experience delirium, or "ICU psychosis." These patients need frequent, repeated explanations and reassurance.

When caring for a ventilated patient, be concerned with the patient first and the ventilator second. If the ventilator alarm sounds, examine the patient for breathing, color, and oxygen saturation before assessing the ventilator. It is vital to understand why mechanical ventilation is needed. Some problems requiring ventilation, such as excessive secretions, sepsis, and trauma, require different interventions to successfully wean from the ventilator. The patient's chronic health problems, especially chronic obstructive pulmonary disease (COPD), left-sided heart failure, anemia, and malnutrition, may slow weaning from mechanical ventilation and require close monitoring and intervention.

! NURSING SAFETY PRIORITY QSEN

Action Alert

The nursing priorities in caring for the patient during mechanical ventilation are monitoring and evaluating patient responses, managing the ventilator system safely, and preventing complications.

Monitoring the Patient's Response. Monitor, evaluate, and document the patient's response to the ventilator. Assess vital signs and listen to breath sounds every 30 to 60 minutes at first.

Monitor respiratory parameters (e.g., capnography, pulse oximetry), and check ABG values (Carlisle, 2014). Monitoring provides information to guide the patient's activities, such as weaning, physical or occupational therapy, and self-care. Pace activities to ensure effective ventilation with adequate GAS EXCHANGE and oxygenation. Interpret ABG values to evaluate the effectiveness of ventilation and determine whether ventilator settings need to be changed (Lian, 2013).

Assess the breathing pattern in relation to the ventilatory cycle to determine whether the patient is tolerating or fighting the ventilator. Patient asynchrony with mechanical ventilation has many causes and reduces the effectiveness of GAS EXCHANGE (Mellott et al., 2014). Assess and record breath sounds, including bilateral equal breath sounds to ensure proper endotracheal (ET) tube placement. Determine the need for suctioning by observing secretions for type, color, and amount. Assess the area around the ET tube or tracheostomy site at least every 4 hours for color, tenderness, skin irritation, and drainage, and document the findings.

The nurse spends the most time with the patient and is most likely to be the first person to recognize changes in vital signs or ABG values, fatigue, or distress. Promptly coordinate with the physician and respiratory therapist to implement the appropriate interventions.

! NURSING SAFETY PRIORITY (QSEN)

Critical Rescue

If the patient develops respiratory distress during mechanical ventilation, immediately remove the ventilator and provide ventilation with a bag-valve-mask device. This action allows quick determination of whether the problem is with the ventilator or with the patient.

Serve as a resource for the psychological needs of the patient and family. Anxiety can reduce tolerance for mechanical ventilation. Skilled and sensitive nursing care promotes emotional well-being and synchrony with the ventilator. The patient cannot speak, and communication can be frustrating and anxiety-producing. The patient and family may panic because they believe that the voice has been lost. Reassure them that the ET tube prevents speech only temporarily.

Plan methods of communication to meet the patient's needs, such as a picture board, pen and paper, alphabet board, electronic tablet computer, or programmable speech-generating device (Grossbach et al., 2011). Finding a successful means for communication is important because the patient often feels isolated by the inability to speak. (See Chart 29-2 in Chapter 29.) Anticipate his or her needs, and provide easy access to frequently used belongings. Visits from family, friends, and pets and keeping a call light within reach are some ways of giving patients a sense of control over the environment. Urge them to participate in self-care.

Managing the Ventilator System. Ventilator settings are prescribed by the health care provider in conjunction with the respiratory therapist. Settings include tidal volume, respiratory rate, fraction of inspired oxygen (Fio_2), and mode of ventilation (assist-control [AC] ventilation, synchronized intermittent mandatory ventilation [SIMV], and adjunctive modes, such as positive end-expiratory pressure [PEEP], pressure support, or continuous flow).

Perform and document ventilator checks according to the standards of the unit or facility. Respond promptly to alarms. During a ventilator check, compare the prescribed ventilator settings with the actual settings. Check the level of water in the humidifier and the temperature of the humidifying system to ensure that they are not too high. Temperature extremes damage the airway mucosa. Remove any condensation in the ventilator tubing by draining water into drainage collection receptacles, and empty them every shift.

! NURSING SAFETY PRIORITY (QSEN)

Action Alert

To prevent bacterial contamination, do not allow moisture and water in the ventilator tubing to enter the humidifier.

Mechanical ventilators have alarm systems that warn of a problem with either the patient or the ventilator. *As required by The Joint Commission's NPSGs, alarm systems must be activated and functional at all times. If the cause of the alarm cannot be determined, ventilate the patient manually with a resuscitation bag until the problem is corrected by another health care professional.* The major alarms on a ventilator indicate either a high pressure or a low exhaled volume. Table 32-5 lists interventions for causes of ventilator alarms.

Assess and care for the ET or tracheostomy tube. Maintain a patent airway by suctioning when any of these conditions are present:

- Secretions
- Increased peak airway (inspiratory) pressure (PIP)
- Rhonchi
- Decreased breath sounds

Proper care of the ET or tracheostomy tube also ensures a patent airway. Assess tube position at least every 2 hours, especially when the airway is attached to heavy ventilator tubing that may pull on the tube. Position the ventilator tubing so that the patient can move without pulling on the ET or tracheostomy tube, possibly dislodging it. To detect changes in tube position, mark it where the tube touches the patient's teeth or nose. Give oral care per facility policy. Standardized oral care has been shown to reduce ventilator-associated pneumonia (VAP), specifically using chlorhexidine oral rinses twice daily (Kiyoshi-Teo et al., 2014; Morton & Fontaine, 2013; Urden et al., 2012).

Special attention is needed for the patient being transported while receiving mechanical ventilation. Monitor Spo_2 during transport to assess adequacy of ventilation. Assess lung sounds each time the patient is moved, transferred, or turned.

? NCLEX EXAMINATION CHALLENGE

Safe and Effective Care Environment

A student nurse is working with a client in the ICU who is intubated and being mechanically ventilated. What action by the student causes the registered nurse to intervene?

A. Repositioning the client every 2 hours
B. Providing oral care with chlorhexidine rinse
C. Checking tube placement at the client's incisor
D. Turning off ventilator alarms while working in the room

TABLE 32-5 Nursing Interventions for Various Causes of Ventilator Alarms

CAUSE	NURSING INTERVENTIONS
High-Pressure Alarm (sounds when peak inspiratory pressure reaches the set alarm limit [usually set 10-20 mm Hg above the patient's baseline PIP])	
An increased amount of secretions or a mucus plug is in the airways.	Suction as needed.
The patient coughs, gags, or bites on the oral ET tube.	Insert oral airway to prevent biting on the ET tube.
The patient is anxious or fights the ventilator.	Provide emotional support to decrease anxiety. Increase the flow rate. Explain all procedures to the patient. Provide sedation or paralyzing agent per the health care provider's prescription.
Airway size decreases related to wheezing or bronchospasm.	Auscultate breath sounds. Collaborate with respiratory therapy to provide prescribed bronchodilators.
Pneumothorax occurs.	Alert the health care provider or Rapid Response Team about a new onset of decreased breath sounds or unequal chest excursion, which may be due to pneumothorax. Auscultate breath sounds.
The artificial airway is displaced; the ET tube may have slipped into the right mainstem bronchus.	Assess the chest for unequal breath sounds and chest excursion. Obtain a chest x-ray as ordered to evaluate the position of the ET tube. After the proper position is verified, secure the tube in place.
Obstruction in tubing occurs because the patient is lying on the tubing or there is water or a kink in the tubing.	Assess the system, beginning with the artificial airway and moving toward the ventilator.
There is increased PIP associated with deliverance of a sigh.	Empty water from the ventilator tubing, and remove any kinks. Coordinate with respiratory therapist or physician to adjust the pressure alarm.
Decreased compliance of the lungs is noted; a trend of gradually increasing PIP is noted over several hours or a day.	Evaluate the reasons for the decreased compliance of the lungs. Increased PIP occurs in ARDS, pneumonia, or any worsening of pulmonary disease.
Low Exhaled Volume (or Low-Pressure) Alarm (sounds when there is a disconnection or leak in the ventilator circuit or a leak in the patient's artificial airway cuff)	
A leak in the ventilator circuit prevents breath from being delivered.	Assess all connections and all ventilator tubing for disconnection.
The patient stops spontaneous breathing in the SIMV or CPAP mode or on pressure support ventilation.	Evaluate the patient's tolerance of the mode.
A cuff leak occurs in the ET or tracheostomy tube.	Evaluate the patient for a cuff leak. A cuff leak is suspected when the patient can talk (air escapes from the mouth) or when the pilot balloon on the artificial airway is flat (see Tracheostomy Tubes section in Chapter 28).

ARDS, Acute respiratory distress syndrome; *CPAP*, continuous positive airway pressure; *ET*, endotracheal; *PIP*, peak inspiratory pressure; *SIMV*, synchronized intermittent mandatory ventilation.

Preventing Complications. Most problems are caused by the positive pressure from the ventilator. Nearly every body system is affected.

Cardiac problems from mechanical ventilation include hypotension and fluid retention. Hypotension is caused by positive pressure that increases chest pressure and inhibits blood return to the heart. The decreased blood return reduces cardiac output, causing hypotension, especially in patients who are dehydrated or need high PIP for ventilation. Teach the patient to avoid a **Valsalva maneuver** (bearing down while holding the breath).

Fluid is retained because of decreased cardiac output. The kidneys receive less blood flow, which stimulates the renin-angiotensin-aldosterone system to retain fluid. Humidified air in the ventilator system contributes to fluid retention. Monitor the patient's fluid intake and output, weight, hydration status, and manifestations of hypovolemia.

Lung problems from mechanical ventilation include:

- **Barotrauma** (damage to the lungs by positive pressure)
- **Volutrauma** (damage to the lung by excess volume delivered to one lung over the other)
- **Atelectrauma** (shear injury to alveoli from opening and closing)
- **Biotrauma** (inflammatory response–mediated damage to alveoli)
- **Ventilator-associated lung injury/Ventilator-induced lung injury (VALI/VILI)** (damage from prolonged ventilation causing loss of surfactant, increased inflammation, fluid leakage, and noncardiac pulmonary edema)
- Acid-base imbalance

Barotrauma includes pneumothorax, subcutaneous emphysema, and pneumomediastinum. Patients at highest risk for barotrauma have chronic airflow limitation (CAL), have blebs or bullae, are on PEEP, have dynamic hyperinflation, or require high pressures to ventilate the lungs (because of "stiff" lungs, as seen in acute respiratory distress syndrome [ARDS]). Ventilator-induced lung injury can be prevented by using low tidal volumes combined with moderate levels of PEEP, especially in patients with acute lung injury (ALI) or ARDS (Bortolotto & Makic, 2012). Blood gas problems can be corrected by ventilator changes and adjustment of fluid and electrolyte imbalances.

GI and nutrition problems result from the stress of mechanical ventilation. Stress ulcers occur in many patients receiving mechanical ventilation. These ulcers complicate the nutrition status and, because the mucosa are not intact, increase the risk for systemic infection. Antacids, sucralfate (Carafate, Sulcrate ♣), and histamine blockers such as ranitidine (Zantac) or proton-pump inhibitors such as esomeprazole (Nexium) may be prescribed as soon as the patient is intubated. Because many other acute or life-threatening events occur at the same time, nutrition is often neglected. Malnutrition is an extreme problem for these patients and is a cause of failing to wean from the ventilator. In malnutrition, the respiratory muscles lose mass and strength. The diaphragm, the major muscle of inspiration, is affected early. When it and other respiratory muscles are weak, ineffective breathing results, fatigue occurs, and the patient cannot be weaned.

Balanced nutrition, whether by diet, enteral feedings, or parenteral feeding, is essential during ventilation and should be started within 48 hours of intubation (Morton & Fontaine, 2013). Also, nutrition for the patient with chronic obstructive pulmonary disease (COPD) requires a reduction of dietary carbohydrates. During metabolism, carbohydrates are broken down to glucose, which then produces energy, carbon dioxide, and water. Excessive carbohydrate loads increase carbon dioxide production, which the patient with COPD may be unable to exhale. Hypercarbic respiratory failure results. Nutrition formulas with a higher fat content (e.g., Pulmocare, Nutri-Vent, Intralipid) are calorie sources to combat this problem.

Electrolyte replacement is also important because electrolytes influence muscle function. Monitor potassium, calcium, magnesium, and phosphate levels, and replace them as prescribed.

Infections are a threat for the patient using a ventilator, especially ventilator-associated pneumonia (VAP). The ET or tracheostomy tube bypasses the body's filtering process and provides a direct access for bacteria to enter the lower respiratory system. The artificial airway is colonized with bacteria within 48 hours, which promotes pneumonia development and increases morbidity. Aspiration of colonized fluid from the mouth or the stomach can be a source of infection. *Infection prevention through strict adherence to infection control, especially handwashing during suctioning and care of the tracheostomy or ET tube, is essential (Kiyoshi-Teo et al., 2014).*

To prevent VAP, implement "ventilator bundle" order sets, which typically include these actions (Morton & Fontaine, 2013; Munro & Ruggiero, 2014; Urden et al., 2012):

- Keeping the head of the bed elevated at least 30 degrees
- Performing oral care per agency policy (usually brushing teeth every 8 hours and antimicrobial rinse [chlorhexidine] every 2 hours)
- Ulcer prophylaxis
- Preventing aspiration
- Pulmonary hygiene including chest physiotherapy, postural drainage, and turning and positioning

Using the ventilator bundle has greatly reduced the overall incidence of VAP. Vigilant oral care is a key component of the VAP prevention strategy although there is considerable variation in actual practice for timing, products used, and specific application methods (Booker et al., 2013; Hiller et al., 2013; Kiyoshi-Teo et al., 2014). (See the Evidence-Based Practice box.) Additional information on pneumonia can be found in Chapter 31.

EVIDENCE-BASED PRACTICE (QSEN)

What is the Best Method and Timing of Oral Hygiene to Prevent Ventilator-Associated Pneumonia?

Hiller, B., Wilson, C., Chamberlain, D., & King, L. (2013). Preventing ventilator-associated pneumonia through oral care, product selection, and application method. *AACN Advanced Critical Care, 24*(1), 38-58.

Ventilator-associated pneumonia (VAP) is a common, costly, and preventable complication of patients receiving mechanical ventilation. During the past decade, implementation of a "ventilator bundle" care approach focusing on prevention of aspiration and prevention of oral bacterial translocation to the lower respiratory tract has been instrumental in reducing the incidence of VAP. At first, more effort was placed on preventing aspiration; however, many studies showed that improved oral care contributed significantly to VAP reduction.

The literature abounds with different methods of oral care and products used. Some methods include toothbrushing, whereas others used sponge swabs. The most commonly used product was chlorhexidine rinse, although the concentration of this solution varied. Some studies also saw a reduction in VAP using sodium chloride solutions combined with mouth swabbing or tooth brushing. Frequency of oral care ranged from twice daily to every 2 hours. Although more vigilant oral care is key to VAP prevention, a clear best practice protocol for frequency, method of care application, and specific product use has yet to be identified. In addition, the qualifications of the person performing the oral assessment and the actual oral care vary among the studies.

Level of Evidence: 1

The results are based on a systematic review and meta-analysis of previous studies related to the outcomes of implementing oral hygiene protocols to help prevent VAP among patients receiving mechanical ventilation. Results of this analysis do indicate that education for nurses and unlicensed assistive personnel (UAP) about oral care needs for the patient receiving mechanical ventilation is needed for optimal outcomes, although no particular practice methods or products emerged as superior in reducing the incidence of VAP.

Commentary: Implications for Practice and Research

For best practice, a protocol must be both effective at preventing VAP and not harmful to the patient. Thus it must demonstrate clear positive outcomes and a lack of harmful outcomes. In addition, the protocol must be viewed as valuable by the people who are supposed to be implementing it. The previous studies analyzed showed that many nurses and UAP did not understand the link between poor oral hygiene and VAP. Thus nursing education needs to stress to students and practicing nurses that good oral hygiene is not just an optional comfort measure but is actually a critical health promotion strategy. In addition, more research is needed into which solutions and solution concentrations provide adequate control of oral flora without causing harm. Chlorhexidine is a drug, and its use requires a health care provider's prescription. In some states, UAP would not be permitted to apply this topical solution in oral care. Thus studies are needed to determine the optimum frequency of chlorhexidine oral hygiene provided by nurses coupled with UAP-implemented sessions of oral hygiene using nonprescription solutions as part of the overall protocol.

Muscle deconditioning and weakness can occur because of immobility. Getting the patient out of bed and having him or her ambulate with help and perform exercises not only improves muscle strength but also boosts morale, enhances GAS EXCHANGE, and promotes oxygen delivery to all muscles. Early progressive mobility decreases ventilator days and ICU stays (Morris et al.,

2011). Early passive exercise may also be beneficial (Amidei & Sole, 2013).

Ventilator dependence is the inability to wean off the ventilator and can have both a physiologic basis and psychological basis. The longer a patient uses a ventilator, the more difficult the weaning process is because the respiratory muscles fatigue and cannot assume breathing. The health care team uses every method of weaning before a patient is declared "unweanable."

Collaborate with the physician, social worker or psychologist, and a member of the clergy to discuss with the patient and family the patient's quality of life, goals, and values. As a result of this discussion, arrange for home ventilation, nursing home placement, or withdrawal of life support (in terminal cases). Special units and facilities can maximize the rehabilitation and weaning of ventilator-dependent patients.

Weaning. **Weaning** is the process of going from ventilatory dependence to spontaneous breathing. The process is prolonged by complications. Many problems can be avoided with good nursing care. For example, turning and positioning the patient not only promote comfort and prevent skin breakdown but also improve GAS EXCHANGE and prevent pneumonia and atelectasis. Table 32-6 lists various weaning techniques.

CONSIDERATIONS FOR OLDER ADULTS

Patient-Centered Care QSEN

The older patient, especially one who has smoked or who has a chronic lung problem such as COPD, is at risk for ventilator dependence and failure to wean. Age-related changes, such as chest wall stiffness, reduced ventilatory muscle strength, and decreased lung elasticity, reduce the likelihood of weaning. The usual manifestations of ventilatory failure—hypoxemia and hypercarbia—may be less obvious in the older adult. Use other clinical measures of gas exchange and oxygenation, such as a change in mental status, to determine breathing effectiveness.

Extubation. **Extubation** is the removal of the endotracheal (ET) tube. The tube is removed when the need for intubation has been resolved. Before removal, explain the procedure. Set up the prescribed oxygen delivery system at the bedside, and bring in the equipment for emergency reintubation. Hyperoxygenate the patient, and thoroughly suction both the ET tube and the oral cavity. Then rapidly deflate the cuff of the ET tube and remove the tube at peak inspiration. Immediately instruct the patient to cough. It is normal for large amounts of oral secretions to collect. Give oxygen by facemask or nasal cannula. The fraction of inspired oxygen (FiO_2) is usually prescribed at 10% higher than the level used while the ET tube was in place.

Monitor vital signs after extubation every 5 minutes at first, and assess the ventilatory pattern for manifestations of respiratory distress. It is common for patients to be hoarse and have a sore throat for a few days after extubation. Teach the patient to sit in a semi-Fowler's position, take deep breaths every half-hour, use an incentive spirometer every 2 hours, and limit speaking. These measures help improve GAS EXCHANGE, decrease laryngeal edema, and reduce vocal cord irritation. Observe closely for respiratory fatigue and airway obstruction.

Early manifestations of obstruction are mild dyspnea, coughing, and the inability to expectorate secretions. **Stridor** is a high-pitched, crowing noise during inspiration caused by laryngospasm or edema around the glottis. It is a late manifestation of a narrowed airway and requires prompt attention. Racemic epinephrine, a topical aerosol vasoconstrictor, is given, and reintubation may be needed.

TABLE 32-6 Weaning Methods

Synchronous Intermittent Mandatory Ventilation
- The patient breathes between the machine's preset breaths/min rate.
- The machine is initially set on an SIMV rate of 12, meaning the patient receives a minimum of 12 breaths/min by the ventilator.
- The patient's respiratory rate will be a combination of ventilator breaths and spontaneous breaths.
- As the weaning process ensues, the health care provider prescribes gradual decreases in the SIMV rate, usually at a decrease of 1 to 2 breaths/min.

T-Piece Technique
- The patient is taken off the ventilator for short periods (initially 5 to 10 minutes) and allowed to breathe spontaneously.
- The ventilator is replaced with a T-piece (see Chapter 28) or CPAP, which delivers humidified oxygen.
- The prescribed FiO_2 may be higher for the patient on the T-piece than on the ventilator.
- Weaning progresses as the patient can tolerate progressively longer periods off the ventilator.
- Nighttime weaning is not usually attempted until the patient can maintain spontaneous respirations most of the day.

Pressure Support Ventilation
- PSV allows the patient's respiratory effort to be augmented by a predetermined pressure assist from the ventilator.
- As the weaning process ensues, the amount of pressure applied to inspiration is gradually decreased.
- Another method of weaning with PSV is to maintain the pressure but gradually decrease the ventilator's preset breaths/min rate.

CPAP, Continuous positive airway pressure; *FiO_2,* fraction of inspired oxygen; *PSV,* pressure support ventilation; *SIMV,* synchronized intermittent mandatory ventilation.

! NURSING SAFETY PRIORITY QSEN

Critical Rescue

When stridor or other manifestations of obstruction occur after extubation, immediately call the Rapid Response Team before the airway becomes completely obstructed.

CHEST TRAUMA

Chest injuries are responsible for about 25% of traumatic deaths in the United States each year and are a contributing factor in about 50% of deaths related to trauma (Mancini, 2012a). Many of the injured die before arriving at the hospital. A few types of chest injury require thoracotomy. Most can be treated with basic resuscitation, intubation, or chest tube placement. *The first emergency approach to all chest injuries is ABC (**a**irway, **b**reathing, **c**irculation), a rapid assessment and treatment of life-threatening conditions.* See Chapter 8 for more information on care of the trauma patient.

Pulmonary Contusion

Pulmonary contusion, a potentially lethal injury, is a common chest injury and occurs most often by rapid deceleration during car crashes. After a contusion, respiratory failure can develop immediately or over time. Hemorrhage and edema occur in and between the alveoli, reducing both lung movement and the area available for GAS EXCHANGE. The patient becomes hypoxemic and dyspneic.

Patients may be asymptomatic at first and can later develop various degrees of respiratory failure. These patients often have decreased breath sounds or crackles and wheezes over the affected area. Other manifestations include bruising over the injury, dry cough, tachycardia, tachypnea, and dullness to percussion. At first, the chest x-ray may show no abnormalities. A hazy opacity in the lobes or parenchyma may develop over several days. If there is no disruption of the parenchyma, bruise resorption often occurs without treatment (Dennison et al., 2011; Mancini, 2012a).

Management includes maintenance of ventilation and oxygenation. Provide oxygen, give IV fluids as prescribed, and place the patient in a moderate-Fowler's position. When side-lying, the "good lung down" position may be helpful. The patient in obvious respiratory distress may need mechanical ventilation with positive end-expiratory pressure (PEEP) to inflate the lungs.

A vicious cycle occurs in which more muscle effort is needed for ventilating a lung with a contusion and the patient becomes progressively hypoxemic. This situation causes him or her to tire easily, have reduced GAS EXCHANGE, and become more fatigued and hypoxemic. This condition often leads to acute respiratory distress syndrome (ARDS).

Rib Fracture

Rib fractures are a common injury to the chest wall, often resulting from direct blunt trauma to the chest. The force applied to the ribs fractures them and drives the bone ends into the chest. Thus there is a risk for deep chest injury, such as pulmonary contusion, pneumothorax, and hemothorax.

The patient has pain on movement and splints the chest defensively. Splinting reduces breathing depth and clearance of secretions. If the patient has pre-existing lung disease, the risk for atelectasis and pneumonia increases. Those with injuries to the first or second ribs, flail chest, seven or more fractured ribs, or expired volumes of less than 15 mL/kg often have a deep chest injury and a poor prognosis.

Management of uncomplicated rib fractures is simple because the fractured ribs reunite spontaneously. The chest is usually not splinted by tape or other materials. The main focus is to decrease pain so that adequate ventilation is maintained. An intercostal nerve block may be used if pain is severe. Analgesics that cause respiratory depression are avoided.

Flail Chest

Flail chest is the result of fractures of at least two neighboring ribs in two or more places causing **paradoxical chest wall movement** (inward movement of the thorax during inspiration, with outward movement during expiration) (Fig. 32-4). It usually involves one side of the chest and results from blunt chest trauma—often high-speed car crashes. Because the force required to produce a flail chest is great, it is important to assess for other possible underlying injuries (Bjerke, 2012; Poirier & Vacca, 2013).

Flail chest can also occur from bilateral separations of the ribs from their cartilage connections to each other anteriorly, without an actual rib fracture. This condition can occur as a complication of cardiopulmonary resuscitation. Other injuries to the lung tissue under the flail segment may be present. GAS EXCHANGE, coughing, and clearance of secretions are impaired. Splinting further reduces the patient's ability to exert the extra effort to breathe and may contribute later to failure to wean.

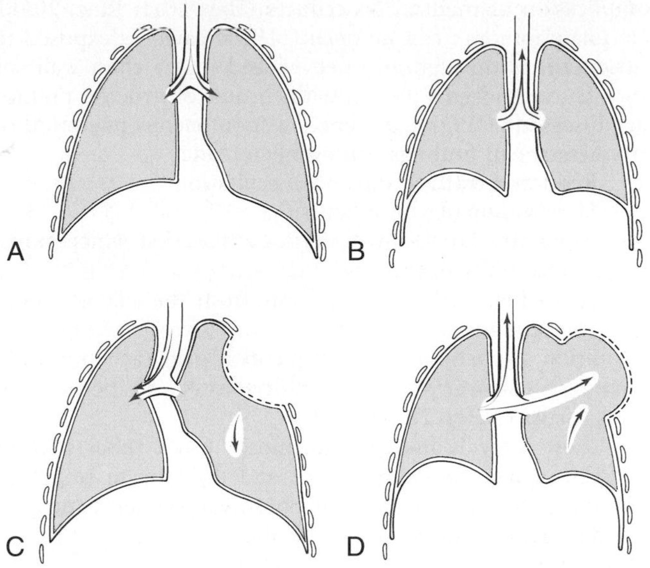

FIG. 32-4 Flail chest. Normal respiration: **A,** Inspiration; **B,** Expiration. Paradoxic motion: **C,** Inspiration—area of the lung underlying unstable chest wall sucks in on inspiration; **D,** Expiration—unstable area balloons out. Note movement of mediastinum toward opposite lung during inspiration.

Assess the patient with a flail chest for paradoxical chest movement, dyspnea, cyanosis, tachycardia, and hypotension. The patient is often anxious, short of breath, and in pain. Work of breathing is increased from the paradoxical movement of the involved segment of the chest wall (Bjerke, 2012).

Interventions include humidified oxygen, pain management, promotion of lung expansion through deep breathing and positioning, and secretion clearance by coughing and tracheal suction.

The patient with a flail chest may be managed with vigilant respiratory care. Mechanical ventilation is needed if respiratory failure or shock occurs. Monitor ABG values and vital capacity closely. With severe hypoxemia and hypercarbia, the patient is intubated and mechanically ventilated with PEEP. With lung contusion or an underlying pulmonary disease, the risk for respiratory failure increases. Usually flail chest is stabilized by positive-pressure ventilation. Surgical stabilization is used only in extreme cases of flail chest (Messing et al., 2014).

Monitor the patient's vital signs and fluid and electrolyte balance closely so that hypovolemia or shock can be managed immediately. If he or she has a lung contusion, provide oxygen as needed and give IV fluids as prescribed. Assess for and relieve pain with prescribed analgesic drugs by IV, epidural, or nerve block route. Give psychosocial support to the anxious patient by explaining all procedures, talking slowly, and allowing time for expression of feelings and concerns.

Pneumothorax

Any chest injury that allows air to enter the pleural space results in a rise in chest pressure and a reduction in vital capacity. Severity depends on the amount of lung collapse produced. Pneumothorax is often caused by blunt chest trauma and may occur with some degree of hemothorax. It can also occur as a complication of medical procedures (Day, 2011; Ruiz, 2011). The pneumothorax can be *open* (pleural cavity is exposed to outside air, as through an open wound in the chest wall) or *closed* (such as when a patient with chronic obstructive pulmonary disease [COPD] experiences a spontaneous pneumothorax). Assessment findings commonly include:

- Reduced breath sounds on auscultation
- Hyperresonance on percussion
- Prominence of the involved side of the chest, which moves poorly with respirations
- Deviation of the trachea *away* from the side of injury (tension pneumothorax)

In addition, the patient may have pleuritic pain, tachypnea, and **subcutaneous emphysema** (air under the skin in the subcutaneous tissues (Daley, 2014).

A chest x-ray is used for diagnosis. Chest tubes may be needed to allow the air to escape and the lung to re-inflate. Other care includes pain control, pulmonary hygiene, and continued assessment for respiratory failure.

Tension Pneumothorax

Tension pneumothorax, a rapidly developing and life-threatening complication of blunt chest trauma, results from an air leak in the lung or chest wall. Air forced into the chest cavity causes complete collapse of the affected lung. Air that enters the pleural space during inspiration does not exit during expiration. As a result, air collects under pressure, compressing blood vessels and limiting blood return. This process leads to decreased filling of the heart and reduced cardiac output. *If not promptly detected and treated, tension pneumothorax is quickly fatal.* Causes include blunt chest trauma, mechanical ventilation with positive end-expiratory pressure (PEEP), closed–chest drainage (chest tubes), and insertion of central venous access catheters.

Assessment findings with tension pneumothorax include:

- Asymmetry of the thorax
- Tracheal movement *away* from midline toward the *unaffected* side
- Extreme respiratory distress
- Absence of breath sounds on one side
- Distended neck veins
- Cyanosis
- Hypertympanic sound on percussion over the affected side
- Hemodynamic instability

Pneumothorax is detectable on a chest x-ray but also can be diagnosed by the patient's manifestations. ABG assays show hypoxia and respiratory alkalosis.

Initial management is an immediate **needle thoracostomy**, with a large-bore needle inserted by the health care provider into the second intercostal space in the midclavicular line of the affected side. Then a chest tube is placed into the fourth intercostal space and the other end is attached to a water seal drainage system until the lung re-inflates. Chest tubes are discussed in detail in Chapter 30.

Nursing care also involves pain control and pulmonary hygiene.

Hemothorax

Hemothorax is a common problem occurring after blunt chest trauma or penetrating injuries. A *simple* hemothorax is a blood loss of less than 1000 mL into the chest cavity; a *massive* hemothorax is a blood loss of more than 1000 mL (Mancini, 2012b).

Bleeding is caused by injury to the lung tissue, such as lung contusions or lacerations, that can occur with rib and sternal fractures. Massive internal chest bleeding in blunt chest trauma may stem from the heart, the great vessels, or the intercostal arteries.

Assessment findings vary with the size of the hemothorax. If the hemothorax is small, the patient may not have manifestations. With a large hemothorax, the patient may have respiratory distress with breath sounds reduced on auscultation. Percussion on the involved side produces a dull sound. Blood in the pleural space is visible on a chest x-ray and is confirmed by thoracentesis.

Interventions focus on removing the blood in the pleural space to normalize breathing and to prevent infection. Chest tubes are inserted to empty the pleural space; multiple chest tubes may be needed. Closely monitor the chest tube drainage. Serial chest x-rays are used to determine treatment effectiveness. Aggressive pain management and pulmonary hygiene are also part of care.

An open thoracotomy is needed when there is initial blood loss of 1000 mL from the chest or persistent bleeding at the rate of 150 to 200 mL/hr over 3 to 4 hours (Mancini, 2012b). Monitor the vital signs, blood loss, and intake and output. Assess the patient's response to the chest tubes, and infuse IV fluids and blood as prescribed. The blood lost through chest drainage can be infused back into the patient after processing if needed.

Tracheobronchial Trauma

Most tears of the tracheobronchial tree result from severe blunt trauma or rapid deceleration and often involve the mainstem bronchi. These injuries are rare, and patients often die before reaching the hospital. Injuries to the trachea usually occur at the junction of the trachea and cricoid cartilage, often by striking the neck against the dashboard or steering wheel during a car crash. Patients with tracheal lacerations develop massive air leaks, which cause air to enter the mediastinum and lead to extensive subcutaneous emphysema. Upper airway obstruction may occur, causing severe respiratory distress and stridor.

Airway management is the priority. If possible, an ET tube is placed distal to the injury. Cricothyroidotomy or tracheotomy below the level of injury may be required. A patient with a torn mainstem bronchus may develop a tension pneumothorax rapidly when intubated and ventilated with positive pressure (Dennison et al., 2011; Mancini, 2012a).

Assess for hypoxemia by ABG assays. Apply oxygen as needed. Depending on the degree of injury, the patient may need mechanical ventilation or surgical repair. Assess vital signs every 15 minutes because hypotension and shock are likely. Assess for subcutaneous emphysema and listen to the lungs every 1 to 2 hours. Decreased breath sounds or wheezing may indicate further obstruction, atelectasis, or pneumothorax. Care of the patient with a tracheostomy is discussed in Chapter 28.

NURSING CONCEPTS AND CLINICAL JUDGMENT REVIEW

What might you NOTICE if the patient is experiencing inadequate GAS EXCHANGE and tissue PERFUSION as a result of a critical respiratory problem?

- Respirations rapid and shallow
- Change in cognition, acute confusion (especially in older adults)
- Decreased oxygen saturation by pulse oximetry
- Cyanosis or pallor of the lips and oral mucous membranes
- Tachycardia
- Patient appears to strain to catch breath
- Patient is restless or anxious

What should you INTERPRET and how should you RESPOND to a patient experiencing inadequate GAS EXCHANGE and tissue PERFUSION as a result of a critical respiratory problem?

Perform and interpret physical assessment, including:

- Taking vital signs
- Auscultating all lung fields
- Monitoring oxygen saturation by pulse oximetry
- Checking the accuracy of pulse oximetry readings
- Checking most recent laboratory values for ABG levels
- Assessing chest symmetry
- Assessing accessory muscle use
- Assessing cognition
- Assessing for the presence of hemoptysis
- Assessing the patient's ability to cough and clear the airway
- Asking the patient if he or she has chest pain
- Checking for the presence of petechiae, especially over the chest

Respond by:

- Applying oxygen and assessing the patient's responses
- Keeping the patient's head elevated to about 30 degrees (unless the potential for cervical spine trauma exists)
- Suctioning (oral, pharyngeal, endotracheal, tracheostomy), if needed
- Notifying the physician or Rapid Response Team
- Staying with the patient
- Calling for the emergency cart to be brought to the patient's bedside
- Reassuring the patient that appropriate interventions are being instituted
- Preparing for intubation
- Using a manual resuscitation bag if the patient's Spo_2 falls below 60% while receiving oxygen by mask
- Starting an IV

On what should you REFLECT?

- Observe patient for evidence of restored GAS EXCHANGE and oxygenation (see Chapter 27).
- Think about what may have precipitated this episode and what steps could be taken to either prevent a similar episode or identify it earlier.
- Think about what additional resources might improve the nursing response to this situation.

GET READY FOR THE NCLEX® EXAMINATION!

KEY POINTS

Review these Key Points for each NCLEX Examination Client Needs Category.

Safe and Effective Care Environment

- Use aseptic technique when caring for a patient requiring pulmonary suctioning. **Safety** QSEN
- Identify patients in your setting who are at risk for developing a pulmonary embolism. **Safety** QSEN
- Use Bleeding Precautions for patients receiving anticlotting therapy (see Chart 32-6). **Safety** QSEN
- Keep antidotes available when patients are receiving heparin (antidote is protamine) or warfarin (antidote is phytonadione). **Safety** QSEN
- Inspect the mouth and perform oral care every 2 hours for anyone who has an endotracheal tube or is being mechanically ventilated. **Safety** QSEN
- Check and document ventilator settings hourly. **Safety** QSEN
- Ensure that alarm systems on mechanical ventilators are activated and functional at all times. **Safety** QSEN
- Ensure that bag-valve-mask device and suction equipment are at the bedside at all times. **Safety** QSEN
- Evaluate the need for chemical restraint or soft wrist restraints.

Health Promotion and Maintenance

- Teach patients ways to promote venous return and avoid venous thromboembolism (VTE), especially when traveling long distances (see Chart 32-1). **Patient-Centered Care** QSEN
- Teach patients ways to prevent injury when taking drugs that reduce CLOTTING (see Chart 32-7). **Patient-Centered Care** QSEN

Psychosocial Integrity

- Allow the patient and family members the opportunity to express feelings and concerns about a change in breathing status or the possibility of intubation and mechanical ventilation. **Patient-Centered Care** QSEN
- Use alternate ways to communicate with a patient who is intubated or being mechanically ventilated. **Patient-Centered Care** QSEN
- Reassure intubated patients that speech loss is temporary. **Patient-Centered Care** QSEN
- Remember that patients who are receiving mechanical ventilation and are being chemically paralyzed usually can hear and can feel pain. **Patient-Centered Care** QSEN
- Provide appropriate pain management. **Patient-Centered Care** QSEN

Physiological Integrity

- Use Aspiration Precautions for any patient with an altered level of consciousness, poor gag reflex, or neurologic impairment or who has an endotracheal tube. **Evidence-Based Practice** QSEN
- Check the patient with ARDS hourly for oxygen saturation, vital sign changes, or any indication of increased work of breathing such as cyanosis, pallor, and retractions. **Patient-Centered Care** QSEN
- Assess all patients with blunt chest trauma for tracheal position and bilateral breath sounds. **Patient-Centered Care** QSEN
- Notify the physician immediately for any patient who develops sudden-onset respiratory difficulty. **Safety** QSEN
- Check oxygen saturation by pulse oximetry for any patient who has trouble breathing or who develops acute confusion. **Patient-Centered Care** QSEN
- Evaluate ABG values to assess the severity of hypoxia and the patient's response to therapy. **Patient-Centered Care** QSEN
- Apply oxygen to anyone who is hypoxemic. **Evidence-Based Practice** QSEN
- Ensure that oxygen therapy delivered to the patient is humidified. **Evidence-Based Practice** QSEN
- Assess lung sounds bilaterally each hour for patients who are receiving PEEP. **Patient-Centered Care** QSEN
- Check all ventilator settings against the prescription at least once per shift. **Safety** QSEN
- Administer drugs for pain to patients who have rib fractures, and encourage deep breaths. **Patient-Centered Care** QSEN
- Evaluate nutrition status, and collaborate with the dietitian to meet the patient's nutrition needs. **Teamwork and Collaboration** QSEN
- If a patient experiences respiratory distress during mechanical ventilation, remove him or her from the ventilator and provide ventilation by bag-valve-mask device. **Safety** QSEN

CHAPTER 33

Assessment of the Cardiovascular System

Donna Ignatavicius

http://evolve.elsevier.com/Iggy/

PRIORITY CONCEPTS

- PERFUSION
- FLUID AND ELECTROLYTE BALANCE

LEARNING OUTCOMES

Safe and Effective Care Environment

1. Prioritize care for patients having invasive cardiac diagnostic tests.

Health Promotion and Maintenance

2. Identify patients at risk for cardiovascular (CV) problems.
3. Differentiate modifiable and nonmodifiable risk factors for CV disease.
4. Teach patients about evidence-based ways to decrease their risk for CV health problems.
5. Explain nursing implications related to CV changes that affect PERFUSION in older adults.

Psychosocial Integrity

6. Describe common psychological responses to CV disease.

Physiological Integrity

7. Review the anatomy and physiology of the CV system.
8. Describe the unique characteristics of heart disease in women.
9. Perform focused physical assessment for patients with CV problems.
10. Interpret laboratory test findings for patients with suspected or actual CV disease.

As the name implies, the cardiovascular (CV) system is made up of the heart and blood vessels (both arteries and veins). It is responsible for supplying oxygen to body organs and other tissues (PERFUSION). The heart muscle, called the **myocardium**, must receive sufficient oxygen to pump blood to other parts of the body. The arteries must be patent so that the pumped blood can reach the rest of the body. *Oxygen in the blood* is needed for cells to live and function properly. When diseases or other problems of the CV systems occur, oxygenation and PERFUSION decrease, often resulting in life-threatening events or a risk for these events.

The CV system works with the respiratory and hematologic systems to meet the human need for oxygenation and tissue PERFUSION (see Fig. 1 of the *Concept Overview*). Any problem in these systems requires the CV system to work harder to meet oxygenation and tissue perfusion needs.

Cardiovascular disease (CVD) continues to be the number-one cause of death in the United States. An average of one death in the United States occurs every 40 seconds from CVD (Go et al., 2013). The disease kills more people than the next four causes of death combined, including cancer, chronic lower respiratory diseases, accidents, and diabetes. *Of particular concern is that CVD is the leading cause of death for women.* In addition, the American Heart Association (AHA) estimates that more than one in three adults is living with some form of the disease. About 20% of people who experience a myocardial infarction will die within 1 year from the initial cardiac event (Go et al., 2013).

ANATOMY AND PHYSIOLOGY REVIEW

Heart

Structure

The human heart is a fist-sized, muscular organ located in the mediastinum between the lungs (Fig. 33-1). Each beat of the heart pumps about 60 mL of blood, or 5 L/min. During strenuous physical activity, it can double the amount of blood pumped

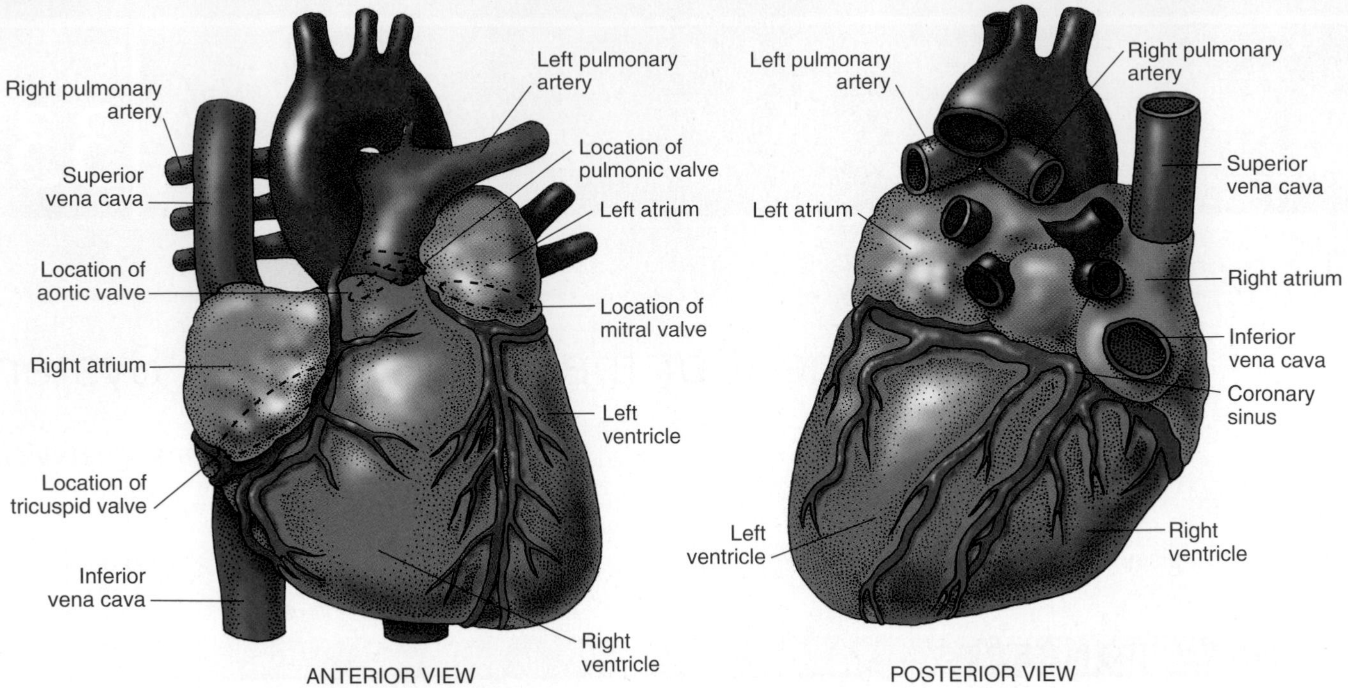

FIG. 33-1 Surface anatomy of the heart.

to meet the body's increased oxygenation needs. The heart is protected by a covering called the *pericardium*. A muscular wall (septum) separates the heart into two halves: right and left. Each half has an atrium and a ventricle (Fig. 33-2).

The *right atrium (RA)* receives *deoxygenated* venous blood, which is returned from the body through the superior and inferior venae cavae. It also receives blood from the heart muscle through the coronary sinus. Most of this venous return flows passively from the RA, through the opened tricuspid valve, and to the right ventricle during ventricular diastole, or filling. The remaining venous return is actively propelled by the RA into the right ventricle during atrial systole, or contraction.

The *right ventricle (RV)* is a muscular pump located behind the sternum. It generates enough pressure to close the tricuspid valve, open the pulmonic valve, and propel blood into the pulmonary artery and the lungs.

After blood is *reoxygenated* in the lungs, it flows freely from the four pulmonary veins into the left atrium. Blood then flows through an opened mitral valve into the left ventricle during ventricular diastole. When the left ventricle is almost full, the *left atrium (LA)* contracts, pumping the remaining blood volume into the left ventricle. With systolic contraction, the *left ventricle (LV)* generates enough pressure to close the mitral valve and open the aortic valve. Blood is propelled into the aorta and into the systemic arterial circulation. Blood flow through the heart is shown in Fig. 33-2.

Blood moves from the aorta throughout the systemic circulation to the various tissues of the body. The pressure of blood in the aorta of a young adult averages about 100 to 120 mm Hg, whereas the pressure of blood in the RA averages about 0 to 5 mm Hg. These differences in pressure produce a pressure gradient, with blood flowing from an area of higher pressure to an area of lower pressure. The heart and vascular structures are responsible for maintaining these pressures.

The four *cardiac valves* are responsible for maintaining the forward flow of blood through the chambers of the heart (see Fig. 33-2). These valves open and close when pressure and volume change within the heart's chambers. The cardiac valves are classified into two types: atrioventricular (AV) valves and semilunar valves.

The *AV valves* separate the atria from the ventricles. The *tricuspid valve* separates the RA from the RV. The *mitral (bicuspid) valve* separates the LA from the LV. During ventricular diastole, these valves act as funnels and help move the flow of blood from the atria to the ventricles. During systole, the valves close to prevent the backflow (**valvular regurgitation**) of blood into the atria.

The *semilunar valves* are the pulmonic valve and the aortic valve, which prevent blood from flowing back into the ventricles during diastole. The *pulmonic valve* separates the right ventricle from the pulmonary artery. The *aortic valve* separates the left ventricle from the aorta.

The heart muscle receives blood to meet its metabolic needs through the coronary arterial system (Fig. 33-3). The coronary arteries originate from an area on the aorta just beyond the aortic valve. All of the coronary arteries feeding the left heart originate from the left main coronary artery (LMCA). The right coronary artery (RCA) branches from the aorta to perfuse the right heart and inferior wall of the left heart.

Coronary artery blood flow to the myocardium occurs primarily during diastole, when coronary vascular resistance is minimized. *To maintain adequate blood flow through the coronary arteries,* **mean arterial pressure (MAP)** *must be at least 60 mm Hg. A MAP of between 60 and 70 mm Hg is necessary to maintain perfusion of major body organs, such as the kidneys and brain.*

The *left main artery* divides into two branches: the left anterior descending (LAD) branch and the left circumflex (LCX) branch. The LAD branch descends toward the anterior wall and the apex of the left ventricle. It supplies blood to portions of the left ventricle, ventricular septum, chordae tendineae, papillary muscle, and, to a lesser extent, the right ventricle.

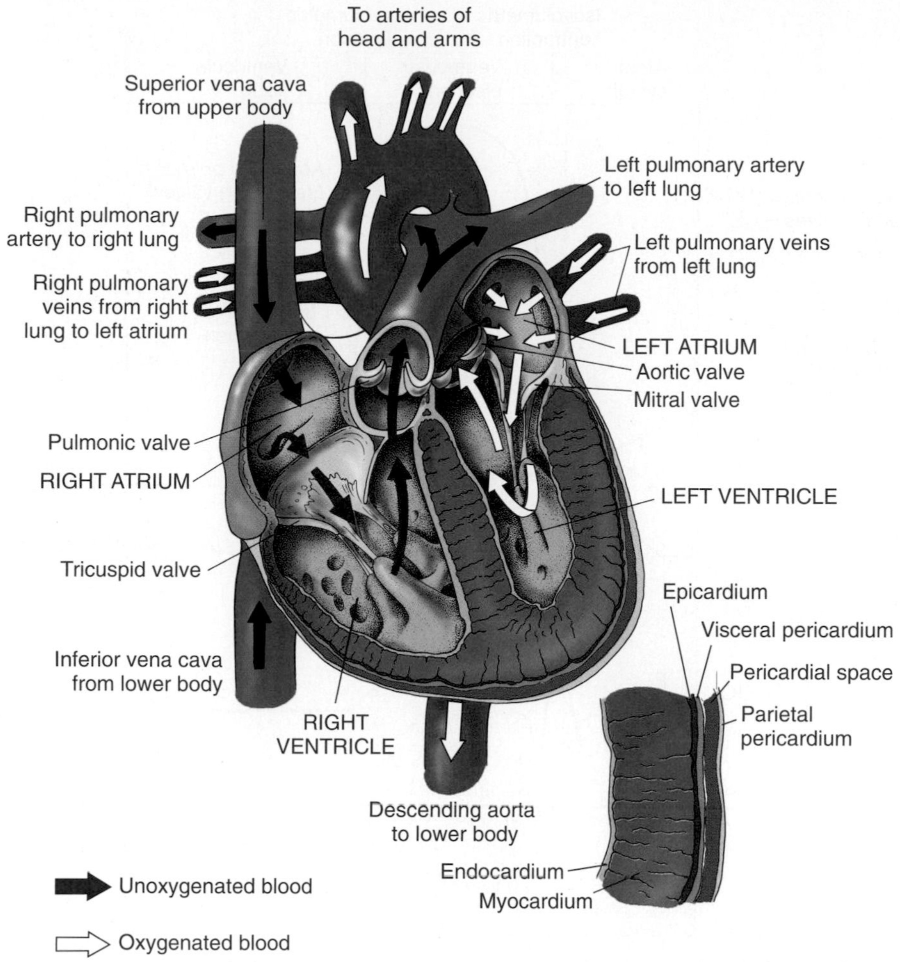

FIG. 33-2 Blood flow through the heart.

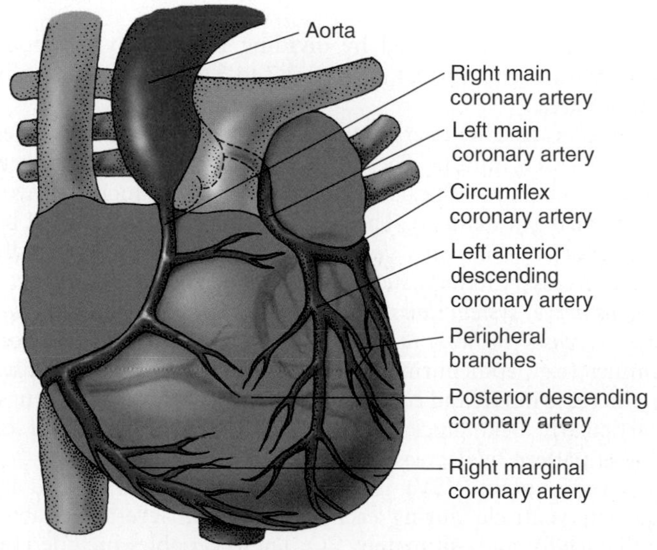

FIG. 33-3 Coronary arterial system.

The LCX branch descends toward the lateral wall of the left ventricle and apex. It supplies blood to the left atrium, the lateral and posterior surfaces of the left ventricle, and sometimes portions of the interventricular septum. In about half of people, the LCX branch supplies the sinoatrial (SA) node. In a very small number of people, it supplies the AV node. Peripheral branches arise from the LAD and LCX branches and form an abundant network of vessels throughout the entire myocardium.

The *right coronary artery (RCA)* originates from the right sinus of Valsalva, encircles the heart, and descends toward the apex of the right ventricle. The RCA supplies the RA, RV, and inferior portion of the LV. In about half of people, the RCA supplies the SA node, and in almost everyone, it supplies the AV node.

Function

The *electrophysiologic properties* of heart muscle are responsible for regulating heart rate (HR) and rhythm. Cardiac muscle cells possess the characteristics of automaticity, excitability, conductivity, contractility, and refractoriness. Chapter 34 describes these properties and cardiac conduction in detail.

Sequence of Events During the Cardiac Cycle. The phases of the cardiac cycle are generally described in relation to changes in pressure and volume in the left ventricle during filling (diastole) and ventricular contraction (systole) (Fig. 33-4). **Diastole**, normally about two thirds of the cardiac cycle, consists of relaxation and filling of the atria and ventricles. **Systole** consists of the contraction and emptying of the atria and ventricles.

Myocardial contraction results from the release of large numbers of calcium ions from the sarcoplasmic reticulum and from the blood. These ions diffuse into the myofibril sarcomere (the basic contractile unit of the myocardial cell). Calcium ions

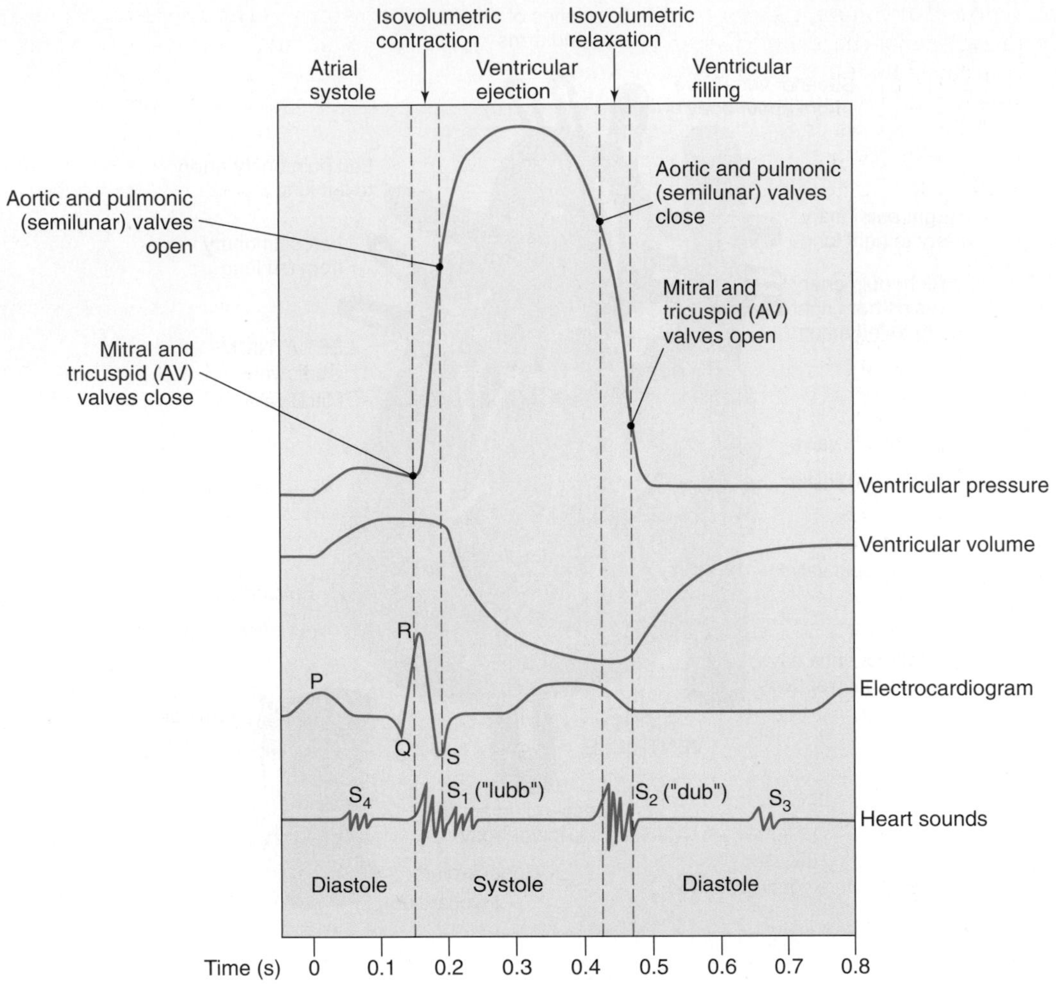

FIG. 33-4 Events of the cardiac cycle.

promote the interaction of actin and myosin protein filaments, causing these filaments to link and overlap. Cross-bridges, or linkages, are formed as the protein filaments slide over or overlap each other. These cross-bridges act as force-generating sites. The sliding of these protein filaments shortens the sarcomeres, producing myocardial contraction.

Cardiac muscle relaxes when calcium ions are pumped back into the sarcoplasmic reticulum, causing a decrease in the number of calcium ions around the myofibrils. This reduced number of ions causes the protein filaments to disengage, the sarcomere to lengthen, and the muscle to relax.

Mechanical Properties of the Heart. The electrical and mechanical properties of cardiac muscle determine the function of the cardiovascular system. The healthy heart can adapt to various pathophysiologic conditions (e.g., stress, infections, hemorrhage) to maintain PERFUSION to the various body tissues. Blood flow from the heart into the systemic arterial circulation is measured clinically as **cardiac output (CO)**, the amount of blood pumped from the left ventricle each minute. *CO depends on the relationship between heart rate (HR) and stroke volume (SV);* it is the product of these two variables:

Cardiac output = Heart rate × Stroke volume

In adults, the CO ranges from 4 to 7 L/min. Because CO requirements vary according to body size, the cardiac index is calculated to adjust for differences in body size. The **cardiac index** can be determined by dividing the CO by the body surface area. The normal range is 2.7 to 3.2 L/min/m^2 of body surface area.

Heart rate (HR) refers to the number of times the ventricles contract each minute. The normal resting HR for an adult is between 60 and 100 beats/min. Increases in rate increase myocardial oxygen demand. The HR is extrinsically controlled by the autonomic nervous system (ANS), which adjusts rapidly when necessary to regulate cardiac output. *The parasympathetic (vagus nerve) system slows the HR, whereas sympathetic stimulation increases the heart rate.* An increase in circulating catecholamines (e.g., epinephrine and norepinephrine) usually causes an increase in HR and contractility. Many cardiovascular drugs, particularly beta blockers, block this sympathetic (fight or flight) pattern by decreasing the HR.

Stroke volume (SV) is the amount of blood ejected by the left ventricle during each contraction. Several variables influence SV and, ultimately, CO. These variables include HR, preload, afterload, and contractility.

Preload refers to the degree of myocardial fiber stretch at the end of diastole and just before contraction. The stretch imposed on the muscle fibers results from the volume contained within the ventricle at the end of diastole. *Preload is determined by the amount of blood returning to the heart from both the venous system (right heart) and the pulmonary system (left heart) (left ventricular end-diastolic [LVED] volume).*

An increase in ventricular volume increases muscle-fiber length and tension, thereby enhancing contraction and improving stroke volume. This statement is derived from Starling's law of the heart: The more the heart is filled during diastole (within limits), the more forcefully it contracts. Excessive filling of the ventricles results in excessive LVED volume and pressure, however, and may result in decreased cardiac output.

Another factor affecting stroke volume, **afterload**, is the pressure or resistance that the ventricles must overcome to eject blood through the semilunar valves and into the peripheral blood vessels. The amount of resistance is directly related to arterial blood pressure and the diameter of the blood vessels.

Impedance, the peripheral component of afterload, is the pressure that the heart must overcome to open the aortic valve. The amount of impedance depends on aortic compliance and total systemic vascular resistance, a combination of blood viscosity (thickness) and arteriolar constriction. A decrease in stroke volume can result from an increase in afterload without the benefit of compensatory mechanisms, thus leading to a decrease in cardiac output.

Myocardial contractility affects stroke volume and CO and is the force of cardiac contraction independent of preload. Contractility is increased by factors such as sympathetic stimulation, calcium release, and positive inotropic drugs. It is decreased by factors such as hypoxia and acidemia.

Vascular System

The vascular system serves several purposes:

- Provides a route for blood to travel from the heart to nourish the various tissues of the body
- Carries cellular wastes to the excretory organs
- Allows lymphatic flow to drain tissue fluid back into the circulation
- Returns blood to the heart for recirculation

The vascular system is divided into the arterial system and the venous system. In the arterial system, blood moves from the larger arteries to a network of smaller blood vessels, called *arterioles*, which meet the capillary bed. In the venous system, blood travels from the capillaries to the venules and to the larger system of veins, eventually returning in the vena cava to the heart for recirculation.

Arterial System

The primary function of the arterial system is to deliver oxygen and nutrients to various tissues in the body. Nutrients are carried through arteries to arterioles, then branch into smaller terminal arterioles, and finally join with capillaries and venules to form a capillary network. Within this network, nutrients are exchanged across capillary membranes by three primary processes: osmosis, filtration, and diffusion. (See Chapter 11 for detailed discussions of these processes.)

The arterial system delivers blood to various tissues for oxygen and nourishment. At the tissue level, nutrients, chemicals, and body defense substances are distributed and exchanged for cellular waste products, depending on the needs of the particular tissue. The arteries transport the cellular wastes to the excretory organs (e.g., kidneys and lungs) to be reprocessed or removed. These vessels also contribute to temperature regulation in the tissues. Blood can be either directed toward the skin to promote heat loss or diverted away from the skin to conserve heat.

Blood pressure (BP) *is the force of blood exerted against the vessel walls.* Pressure in the larger arterial blood vessels is greater (about 80 to 100 mm Hg) and decreases as blood flow reaches the capillaries (about 25 mm Hg). By the time blood enters the right atrium, the BP is about 0 to 5 mm Hg. Volume, ventricular contraction, and vascular tone are necessary to maintain blood pressure.

BP is determined primarily by the quantity of blood flow or cardiac output (CO), as well as by the resistance in the arterioles:

$$\text{Blood pressure} = \text{Cardiac output} \times \text{Peripheral vascular resistance}$$

Any factor that increases CO or total peripheral vascular resistance increases the BP. In general, BP is maintained at a relatively constant level. Therefore an increase or decrease in total peripheral vascular resistance is associated with a decrease or an increase in CO, respectively. Three mechanisms mediate and regulate BP:

- The autonomic nervous system (ANS), which excites or inhibits sympathetic nervous system activity in response to impulses from chemoreceptors and baroreceptors
- The kidneys, which sense a change in blood flow and activate the renin-angiotensin-aldosterone mechanism
- The endocrine system, which releases various hormones (e.g., catecholamine, kinins, serotonin, histamine) to stimulate the sympathetic nervous system at the tissue level

Systolic BP is the amount of pressure/force generated by the left ventricle to distribute blood into the aorta with each contraction of the heart. It is a measure of how effectively the heart pumps and is an indicator of vascular tone. **Diastolic BP** is the amount of pressure/force against the arterial walls during the relaxation phase of the heart.

BP is regulated by balancing the sympathetic and parasympathetic nervous systems of the autonomic nervous system. Changes in autonomic activity are responses to messages sent by the sensory receptors in the various tissues of the body. These receptors, including the baroreceptors, chemoreceptors, and stretch receptors, respond differently to the biochemical and physiologic changes of the body.

Baroreceptors in the arch of the aorta and at the origin of the internal carotid arteries are stimulated when the arterial walls are stretched by an increased BP. Impulses from these baroreceptors inhibit the vasomotor center, which is located in the pons and the medulla. Inhibition of this center results in a drop in BP.

Several 1- to 2-mm collections of tissue have been identified in the carotid arteries and along the aortic arch known as **peripheral chemoreceptors**. These receptors are sensitive primarily to hypoxemia (a decrease in the partial pressure of arterial oxygen [Pa_{O_2}]). When stimulated, these chemoreceptors send impulses along the vagus nerves to activate a vasoconstrictor response and raise BP.

The central chemoreceptors in the respiratory center of the brain are also stimulated by **hypercapnia** (an increase in partial pressure of arterial carbon dioxide [Pa_{CO_2}]) and acidosis. The direct effect of carbon dioxide on the central nervous system (CNS), however, is 10 times stronger than the effect of hypoxia on the peripheral chemoreceptors.

Stretch receptors in the vena cavae and the right atrium are sensitive to pressure or volume changes. When a patient is hypovolemic, stretch receptors in the blood vessels sense a reduced volume or pressure and send fewer impulses to the CNS. This reaction stimulates the sympathetic nervous system to increase the heart rate (HR) and constrict the peripheral blood vessels.

The *kidneys* also help regulate cardiovascular activity. When renal blood flow or pressure decreases, the kidneys retain sodium and water. BP tends to rise because of fluid retention and activation of the renin-angiotensin-aldosterone mechanism (see Fig. 11-6 in Chapter 11). This mechanism results in vasoconstriction and sodium retention (and thus fluid retention). Vascular volume is also regulated by the release of antidiuretic hormone (vasopressin) from the posterior pituitary gland (see Chapter 11).

Other factors can also influence the activity of the cardiovascular system. Emotional behaviors (e.g., excitement, pain, anger) stimulate the sympathetic nervous system to increase blood pressure (BP) and heart rate (HR). Increased physical activity such as exercise also increases BP and HR during the activity. Body temperature can affect the metabolic needs of the tissues, thereby influencing the delivery of blood. In hypothermia, tissues require fewer nutrients and blood pressure falls. In hyperthermia, the metabolic requirement of the tissues is greater and BP and pulse rate rise.

Venous System

The primary function of the venous system is to complete the circulation of blood by returning blood from the capillaries to the right side of the heart. It is composed of a series of veins that are located next to the arterial system. A second superficial venous circulation runs parallel to the subcutaneous tissue of the extremity. These two venous systems are connected by communicating veins that provide a means for blood to travel from the superficial veins to the deep veins. Blood flow is directed toward the deep venous circulation.

Veins have the ability to accommodate large shifts in volume with minimal changes in venous pressure. This flexibility allows the venous system to accommodate the administration of IV fluids and blood transfusions, as well as to maintain pressure during blood loss and dehydration. Veins in the superficial and deep venous systems (except the smallest and the largest veins) have valves that direct blood flow back to the heart and prevent backflow. Skeletal muscles in the extremities provide a force that helps push the venous blood forward. The superior vena cava and inferior vena cava are valveless and large enough to allow blood flow to return easily to the heart.

Gravity exerts an increase in **hydrostatic pressure** in the capillaries when the patient is in an upright position, delaying venous return. Hydrostatic pressure is decreased in dependent areas such as the legs when the patient is lying down, and thus there is less hindrance of venous return to the heart.

Cardiovascular Changes Associated with Aging

A number of physiologic changes in the cardiovascular system occur with advancing age (Chart 33-1). Many of these changes result in a loss of cardiac reserve. Thus these changes are usually not evident when the older adult is resting. They become apparent only when the person is physically or emotionally stressed and the heart cannot meet the increased metabolic demands of the body.

ASSESSMENT METHODS

Patient History

The focus of the patient history is on obtaining information about risk factors and symptoms of cardiovascular disease. Assess *nonmodifiable* (uncontrollable) risk factors including the patient's age, gender, ethnic origin, and family history of cardiovascular disease. Ask about any chronic disease or illness that the patient may have. The incidence of conditions such as coronary artery disease (CAD) and valvular disease increases with age. The incidence of CAD also varies with the patient's gender. Men have a higher risk for CAD than women of all ages except in the oldest age-group of 80 years and older (Go et al., 2013).

GENDER HEALTH CONSIDERATIONS

Patient-Centered Care QSEN

Postmenopausal women are 2 to 3 times more likely than premenopausal women to have CAD. The incidence for the disease in women is about 10 years later than in men and 20 years later for myocardial infarction (MI) and death to occur. After an acute MI, women tend to have a higher mortality rate and suffer more complications when compared with men (Go et al., 2013).

Women with waist and abdominal obesity (greater waist-hip ratio) are more likely to experience cardiovascular disease (CVD) than are women with excess fat in their buttocks, hips, and thighs.

Heart disease is the leading cause of diabetes-related death for both men and women. Adults with diabetes have heart disease death rates 2 to 4 times higher than those without diabetes. The risk for stroke is also 2 to 4 times higher among people with diabetes. The number of premature deaths (younger than 65 years) from heart disease is greatest among American Indians and Alaska Natives and lowest among Asians (Go et al., 2013).

Modifiable (controllable) risk factors should also be assessed. *Modifiable* risk factors are personal lifestyle habits, including cigarette use, physical inactivity, obesity, and psychological variables. Ask the patient about each of these common risk factors.

Cigarette smoking is a major risk factor for CVD, specifically coronary artery disease (CAD) and peripheral vascular disease (PVD). Three compounds in cigarette smoke have been implicated in the development of CAD: tar, nicotine, and carbon monoxide. The smoking history should include the number of cigarettes smoked daily, the duration of the smoking habit, and the age of the patient when smoking started. Record the smoking history in **pack-years**, which is the number of packs per day multiplied by the number of years the patient has smoked.

Ask about the patient's desire to quit, past attempts to quit, and the methods used. Determine nicotine dependence by asking questions such as:

- How soon after you wake up in the morning do you smoke?
- Do you wake up in the middle of your sleep time to smoke?
- Do you find it difficult not to smoke in places where smoking is prohibited?
- Do you smoke when you are ill?

Three to four years after a patient has stopped smoking, his or her CVD risk appears to be similar to that of a person who has never smoked. Be sure to ask those who do not currently smoke whether they have ever smoked and when they quit. Passive smoke significantly reduces blood flow in healthy young adults' coronary arteries, and the risk for dying increases among those who are exposed to secondhand smoke (American Heart Association [AHA], 2013).

A *sedentary lifestyle* is also a major risk factor for heart disease. Regular physical activity promotes cardiovascular

CHART 33-1 **Nursing Focus on the Older Adult**

Changes in the Cardiovascular System Related to Aging

CHANGE	NURSING INTERVENTIONS	RATIONALES
Cardiac Valves		
Calcification and mucoid degeneration occur, especially in mitral and aortic valves.	Assess heart rate and rhythm and heart sounds for murmurs. Question patients about dyspnea.	Murmurs may be detected before other symptoms. Valvular abnormalities may result in rhythm changes.
Conduction System		
Pacemaker cells decrease in number. Fibrous tissue and fat in the sinoatrial node increase. Few muscle fibers remain in the atrial myocardium and bundle of His. Conduction time increases.	Assess the electrocardiogram (ECG) and heart rhythm for dysrhythmias or a heart rate less than 60 beats/min.	The sinoatrial (SA) node may lose its inherent rhythm. Atrial dysrhythmias occur in many older adults; 80% of older adults experience premature ventricular contractions (PVCs).
Left Ventricle		
The size of the left ventricle increases. The left ventricle becomes stiff and less distensible. Fibrotic changes in the left ventricle decrease the speed of early diastolic filling by about 50%.	Assess the ECG for a widening QRS complex and a longer QT interval.	Ventricular changes result in decreased stroke volume, ejection fraction, and cardiac output during exercise; the heart is less able to meet increased oxygen demands.
	Assess the heart rate at rest and with activity. Assess for activity intolerance.	Maximum heart rate with exercise is decreased. The heart is less able to meet increased oxygen demands.
Aorta and Other Large Arteries		
The aorta and other large arteries thicken and become stiffer and less distensible. Systolic blood pressure increases to compensate for the stiff arteries. Systemic vascular resistance increases as a result of less distensible arteries; therefore the left ventricle pumps against greater resistance, contributing to left ventricular hypertrophy.	Assess blood pressure. Note increases in systolic, diastolic, and pulse pressures. Assess for activity intolerance and shortness of breath. Assess the peripheral pulses.	Hypertension may occur and must be treated to avoid target organ damage.
Baroreceptors		
Baroreceptors become less sensitive.	Assess the patient's blood pressure with the patient lying and then sitting or standing. Assess for dizziness when the patient changes from a lying to a sitting or standing position. Teach the patient to change positions slowly.	Orthostatic (postural) and postprandial changes occur because of ineffective baroreceptors. Changes may include blood pressure decreases of 10 mm Hg or more, dizziness, and fainting.

fitness and produces beneficial changes in blood pressure and levels of blood lipids and clotting factors. Unfortunately, few people in the United States follow the recommended exercise guidelines: 30 minutes daily of light to moderate exercise, which is equivalent to a 30-minute brisk walk. According to the AHA (2013), fewer than two thirds of people in the United States engage in this much exercise 5 times a week and fewer engage in more vigorous physical activity to promote cardiopulmonary fitness. Encourage increased physical exercise as part of a lifestyle change to reduce the risk for CAD. Ask patients about the type of exercise they perform, how long a period they have participated in the exercise, and the frequency and intensity of the exercise.

About two thirds of American adults are **overweight** when defined as a body mass index (BMI) of 25 to 30. **Obesity**, defined as a BMI greater than 30, is particularly a problem for African-American women, Mexican Americans, and native Hawaiians, but the exact cause of this cultural difference is unknown (AHA, 2013). Obesity is also associated with hypertension, hyperlipidemia, and diabetes; all are known contributors to CVD.

The American Heart Association provides guidelines to combat obesity and improve cardiac health, including ingesting more nutrient-rich foods that have vitamins, minerals, fiber, and other nutrients but are low in calories. To get the necessary nutrients, teach patients to choose foods like vegetables, fruits, unrefined whole-grain products, and fat-free dairy products most often. Also teach patients to not eat more calories than they can burn every day (AHA, 2013).

A variety of *psychological factors* make people more vulnerable to the development of heart disease. Those who are highly competitive, overly concerned about meeting deadlines, and often hostile or angry are at higher risk for heart disease. Psychological stress, anger, depression, and hostility are all closely associated with risk for developing heart disease.

You might ask the patient "How do you respond when you have to wait for an appointment?" Chronic anger and hostility appear to be closely associated with CVD. The constant arousal of the sympathetic nervous system as a result of anger may influence blood pressure, serum fatty acids and lipids, and clotting mechanisms. Observe the patient, and assess his or her response to stressful situations.

Review the patient's medical history, noting any major illnesses such as diabetes mellitus, renal disease, anemia, high BP, stroke, bleeding disorders, connective tissue diseases, chronic pulmonary diseases, heart disease, and thrombophlebitis. These conditions can influence the patient's cardiovascular status.

Ask about previous treatment for CVD, identify previous diagnostic procedures (e.g., electrocardiography [ECG], cardiac catheterization), and request information about any medical or invasive treatment of CVD. Ask specifically about recurrent tonsillitis, streptococcal infections, and rheumatic fever, because these conditions may lead to valvular abnormalities of the heart. In addition, inquire about any known congenital heart defects. Many patients with congenital heart problems live into adulthood because of improved treatment and surgeries.

Ask patients about their drug history, beginning with any current or recent use of prescription or over-the-counter (OTC) medications or herbal/natural products. Inquire about known sensitivities to any drug and the nature of the reaction (e.g., nausea, rash). Patients should be asked whether they have recently used cocaine or any IV "street" drugs, because these substances are often associated with heart disease.

GENDER HEALTH CONSIDERATIONS

Patient-Centered Care QSEN

Ask young women whether they are taking oral contraceptives or an estrogen replacement. The incidence of myocardial infarction (MI) and stroke in women older than 35 years who take oral contraceptives is increased if they smoke, have diabetes, or have hypertension. Ask menopausal women and transgender women if they are on hormone therapy, because these drugs can also cause an increased incidence of MIs and strokes.

The *social history* includes information about the patient's living situation, including having a domestic partner, other household members, environment, and occupation. Identification of support systems is especially important in exploring the possibility that the patient might have difficulty paying for medications or treatment. People who are from a low socioeconomic (SE) group have a greater chance of having MIs than those from a higher SE status (Wright et al., 2009).

Ask about occupation, including the type of work performed and the requirements of the specific job. For instance, does the job involve physical exertion such as lifting heavy objects? Is the job emotionally stressful? What does a day's work entail? Does the patient's job require him or her to be outside in extreme weather conditions?

Nutrition History

A nutrition history includes the patient's recall of food and fluid intake during a 24-hour period, self-imposed or medically prescribed dietary restrictions or supplementations, and the amount and type of alcohol consumption. If needed, the dietitian may review the type of foods selected by the patient for the amount of sodium, sugar, cholesterol, fiber, and fat. Cultural beliefs and economic status can influence the choice of food items and therefore are seriously considered. Family members or significant others who are responsible for shopping and cooking should be included in this screening.

NCLEX EXAMINATION CHALLENGE

Health Promotion and Maintenance

The nurse is providing education to help reduce cardiovascular risks for a women's book club. Which statement made by a participant indicates a need for further teaching?

A. "We are more likely to die from cardiovascular disease than men."
B. "We need to walk or do other exercise every day for 30 minutes."
C. "We need to stay away from people who smoke."
D. "We should take hormones for menopause to decrease the risk for heart attack."

Family History and Genetic Risk

Review the family history, and obtain information about the age, health status, and cause of death of immediate family members. A positive family history for CAD in a first-degree relative (parent, sibling, or child) is a major risk factor. It is *more* important than other factors such as hypertension, obesity, diabetes, or sudden cardiac death.

GENETIC/GENOMIC CONSIDERATIONS

Patient-Centered Care QSEN

Cardiovascular disease has many contributory factors, including a genetic tendency. A significant association between familial cardiac history and cardiovascular disease is consistently demonstrated in the evidence of multiple large-scale prospective epidemiology studies (Go, et al., 2013). Although several genes have been reported to be associated with heart disease, stroke, and hypertension, the impact of each individual gene is not fully understood. Numerous genetic association studies are underway to determine more specific genetic variants that may underlie the family history (Go, et al., 2013). Additional discussions about genetic factors related to specific CV diseases are found in other chapters in this unit.

Current Health Problems

Ask the patient to describe his or her health concerns. Expand on the description of these concerns by obtaining information about their onset, duration, sequence, frequency, location, quality, intensity, associated symptoms, and precipitating, aggravating, and relieving factors. Major symptoms usually identified by patients with CVD include chest pain or discomfort, dyspnea, fatigue, palpitations, weight gain, syncope, and extremity pain.

Pain or discomfort, considered a traditional symptom of heart disease, can result from ischemic heart disease, pericarditis, and aortic dissection. Chest pain can also be due to noncardiac conditions such as pleurisy, pulmonary embolus, hiatal hernia, gastroesophageal reflux disease, neuromuscular abnormalities, and anxiety.

NURSING SAFETY PRIORITY QSEN

Action Alert

Thoroughly evaluate the nature and characteristics of the chest pain. Because pain resulting from myocardial ischemia is life threatening and can lead to serious complications, its cause should be considered ischemic (reduced or obstructed blood flow to the myocardium) until proven otherwise. When assessing for symptoms, ask the patient if he or she has "discomfort," "heaviness," "pressure," and "indigestion."

GENDER HEALTH CONSIDERATIONS

Patient-Centered Care QSEN

Some patients, especially women, do not experience pain in the chest but, instead, feel discomfort or indigestion. Women often present with a "triad" of symptoms. In addition to indigestion or feeling of abdominal fullness, chronic fatigue despite adequate rest and feelings of an "inability to catch my breath" (dyspnea) are also common in heart disease. The patient may also describe the sensation as aching, choking, strangling, tingling, squeezing, constricting, or viselike. Others with severe neuropathy may experience few or no traditional symptoms except shortness of breath, despite major ischemia.

Ask the patient to identify when the symptoms were first noticed (onset):

- Did the symptoms begin suddenly or develop gradually (manner of onset)?
- How long did the symptoms last (duration)?

If he or she has repeated painful episodes, assess how often the symptoms occur (frequency). If pain is present, ask whether it is different from any other episodes of pain. Ask the patient to describe what activities he or she was doing when it first occurred, such as sleeping, arguing, or running (precipitating factors). If possible, the patient should point to the area where the chest pain occurred (location) and describe if and how the pain radiated (spread).

In addition, ask how the pain feels and whether it is sharp, dull, or crushing (quality of pain). To understand the severity of the pain, ask the patient to grade it from 0 to 10, with 10 indicating severe pain (intensity). He or she may also report other signs and symptoms that occur at the same time (associated symptoms), such as dyspnea, diaphoresis (excessive sweating), nausea, and vomiting. Other factors that need to be addressed are those that may have made the chest pain worse (aggravating factors) or less intense (relieving factors). Chest pain can arise from a variety of sources (Table 33-1). By obtaining the appropriate information, you can help identify the source of the chest discomfort.

Dyspnea (difficult or labored breathing) can occur as a result of both cardiac and pulmonary disease. It is experienced by the patient as uncomfortable breathing or shortness of breath. When obtaining the history, ask what factors precipitate and relieve dyspnea, what level of activity produces dyspnea, and what the patient's body position was when dyspnea occurred.

Dyspnea that is associated with activity, such as climbing stairs, is referred to as **dyspnea on exertion (DOE)**. *This is usually an early symptom of heart failure and may be the only symptom experienced by women.*

The patient with advanced heart disease may experience **orthopnea** (dyspnea that appears when he or she lies flat). Several pillows may be needed to elevate the head and chest, or a recliner to prevent breathlessness may be used. *The severity of orthopnea is measured by the number of pillows or the amount of head elevation needed to provide restful sleep.* This symptom is usually relieved within a matter of minutes by sitting up or standing.

Paroxysmal nocturnal dyspnea (PND) develops after the patient has been lying down for several hours. In this position, blood from the lower extremities is redistributed to the venous system, which increases venous return to the heart. A diseased heart cannot compensate for the increased volume and is ineffective in pumping the additional fluid into the circulatory system. Pulmonary congestion results. The patient awakens abruptly, often with a feeling of suffocation and panic. He or she sits upright and dangles the legs over the side of the bed to relieve the dyspnea. This sensation may last for 20 minutes.

Fatigue may be described as a feeling of tiredness or weariness resulting from activity. The patient may report that an activity takes longer to complete or that he or she tires easily after activity. Although fatigue in itself is not diagnostic of heart disease, many people with heart failure are limited by leg fatigue during exercise. Fatigue that occurs after mild activity and exertion usually indicates inadequate cardiac output (due to low stroke volume) and anaerobic metabolism in skeletal muscle. *It can also accompany other symptoms or may be an early indication of heart disease in women.*

Ask about the time of day the patient experiences fatigue and the activities that he or she can perform. Fatigue resulting from decreased cardiac output is often worse in the evening. Ask whether the patient can perform the same activities as he or she could perform a year ago or the same activities as others of the same age. Often he or she limits activities in response to fatigue and, unless questioned, is unaware how much less active he or she has become.

A feeling of fluttering or unpleasant feeling in the chest caused by an irregular heartbeat is referred to as **palpitations**. They may result from a change in heart rate or rhythm or from an increase in the force of heart contractions. Rhythm disturbances that may cause palpitations include paroxysmal supraventricular tachycardia, premature contractions, and sinus tachycardia. Those that occur during or after strenuous physical activity, such as running and swimming, may indicate overexertion or possibly heart disease. Noncardiac factors that may precipitate palpitations include anxiety, stress, fatigue, insomnia, hyperthyroidism, and the ingestion of caffeine, nicotine, or alcohol. Ask the patient about specific factors that cause his or her palpitations.

A sudden weight increase of 2.2 pounds (1 kg) can result from excess FLUID (1 L) in the interstitial spaces. *The best indicator of fluid balance is weight.* Excess FLUID accumulation is commonly known as **edema**. It is possible for weight gains of up to 10 to 15 pounds (4.5 to 6.8 kg, or 4 to 7 L of fluid) to occur before edema is apparent. Ask whether the patient has noticed a tightness of shoes, indentations from socks, or tightness of rings.

Syncope refers to a brief loss of consciousness. The most common cause is decreased perfusion to the brain. Any condition that suddenly reduces cardiac output, resulting in decreased cerebral blood flow, can lead to a syncopal episode. Conditions such as cardiac rhythm disturbances, especially ventricular dysrhythmias, and valvular disorders, such as aortic stenosis, may trigger this symptom. **Near-syncope** refers to dizziness with an inability to remain in an upright position. Explore the circumstances that lead to dizziness or syncope.

CONSIDERATIONS FOR OLDER ADULTS

Patient-Centered Care QSEN

Syncope in the aging person may result from hypersensitivity of the carotid sinus bodies in the carotid arteries. Pressure applied to these arteries while turning the head, shrugging the shoulders, or performing a Valsalva maneuver (bearing down during defecation) may stimulate a vagal response. A decrease in blood pressure and heart rate can result, which can produce syncope. This type of syncopal episode may also result from postural (orthostatic) or postprandial (after eating) hypotension.

TABLE 33-1 Assessment of Chest Discomfort: How Various Types of Chest Pain Differ

ONSET	QUALITY AND SEVERITY	LOCATION AND RADIATION	DURATION AND RELIEVING FACTORS
Angina			
Sudden, usually in response to exertion, emotion, or extremes in temperature	Squeezing, viselike pain	Usually the left side of chest without radiation Substernal; may spread across the chest and the back and/or down the arms	Usually lasts less than 15 min; relieved with rest, nitrate administration, or oxygen therapy
Myocardial Infarction			
Sudden, without precipitating factors, often in early morning	Intense stabbing, viselike pain or pressure, severe	Substernal; may spread throughout the anterior chest and to the arms, jaw, back, or neck	Continuous or no chest discomfort; relieved with morphine, cardiac drugs, and oxygen therapy
Pericarditis			
Sudden	Sharp, stabbing, moderate to severe	Substernal; usually spreads to the left side or the back	Intermittent; relieved with sitting upright, analgesia, or administration of anti-inflammatory agents
Pleuropulmonary			
Variable	Moderate ache, worse on inspiration	Lung fields	Continuous until the underlying condition is treated or the patient has rested
Esophageal-Gastric			
Variable	Squeezing, heartburn, variable severity	Substernal; may spread to the shoulders or the abdomen	Variable; may be relieved with antacid administration, food intake, or taking a sitting position
Anxiety			
Variable, may be in response to stress or fatigue	Dull ache to sharp stabbing; may be associated with numbness in fingers	Not well located and usually does not radiate to other parts of the body as pain	Usually lasts a few minutes

Extremity pain may be caused by two conditions: ischemia from atherosclerosis and venous insufficiency of the peripheral blood vessels. Patients who report a moderate to severe cramping sensation in their legs or buttocks associated with an activity such as walking have **intermittent claudication** related to decreased arterial tissue PERFUSION. *Claudication pain is usually relieved by resting or lowering the affected extremity to decrease tissue demands or to enhance arterial blood flow.* Leg pain that results from prolonged standing or sitting is related to venous insufficiency from either incompetent valves or venous obstruction. This pain may be relieved by elevating the extremity.

Functional History

After the history of the patient's cardiovascular status is obtained, he or she may be classified according to the New York Heart Association Functional Classification (Table 33-2) or other system. The four classifications (I, II, III, and IV) depend on the degree to which ordinary physical activities (routine ADLs) are affected by heart disease. The Killip Classification provides a more objective description of the hemodynamics of heart failure and is described in Chapter 38.

Physical Assessment

A thorough physical assessment is the foundation for the nursing database and the patient's priority problems. Any changes noted during the course of illness can be compared with this initial database. Evaluate the patient's vital signs on admission to the hospital or during the initial visit to the clinic or primary care provider's office.

TABLE 33-2 New York Heart Association Functional Classification of Cardiovascular Disability

Class I
- Patients with cardiac disease but without resulting limitations of physical activity
- Ordinary physical activity does not cause undue fatigue, palpitation, dyspnea, or anginal pain

Class II
- Patients with cardiac disease resulting in slight limitation of physical activity
- They are comfortable at rest
- Ordinary physical activity results in fatigue, palpitation, dyspnea, or anginal pain

Class III
- Patients with cardiac disease resulting in marked limitation of physical activity
- They are comfortable at rest
- Less than ordinary physical activity causes fatigue, palpitation, dyspnea, or anginal pain

Class IV
- Patients with cardiac disease resulting in inability to carry on any physical activity without discomfort
- Symptoms of cardiac insufficiency or of the anginal syndrome may be present, even at rest
- If any physical activity is undertaken, discomfort is increased

Excerpted from The New York Heart Association. (1964). *Diseases of the heart and blood vessels: Nomenclature and criteria for diagnosis* (6th ed.). Boston: Little, Brown.

General Appearance

Physical assessment begins with the patient's general appearance. Assess general build and appearance, skin color, distress level, level of consciousness, shortness of breath, position, and verbal responses.

Patients can have left- or right-sided heart failure, or both. They can also be diagnosed with systolic and/or diastolic heart failure. *As a result, poor cardiac output and decreased cerebral* PERFUSION *may cause confusion, memory loss, and slowed verbal responses, especially in older adults.* Patients with chronic heart failure may also appear malnourished, thin, and cachectic. Late signs of severe right-sided heart failure are ascites, jaundice, and **anasarca** (generalized edema) as a result of prolonged congestion of the liver. Heart failure may also cause fluid retention and may be manifested by obvious generalized dependent edema. Chapter 35 differentiates right and left failure and systolic from diastolic heart failure in detail.

Skin

Skin assessment includes color and temperature. The best areas in which to assess circulation include the nail beds, mucous membranes, and conjunctival mucosa, because small blood vessels are located near the surface of the skin in those areas.

If there is normal blood flow or adequate perfusion to a given area in *light-colored skin*, it appears pink, perhaps rosy, and is warm. *Decreased* PERFUSION *is manifested as cool, pale, and moist skin. Pallor is characteristic of anemia and can be seen in areas such as the nail beds, palms, and conjunctival mucous membranes in any patient.*

A bluish or darkened discoloration of the skin and mucous membranes in *light-skinned* people is referred to as **cyanosis**. This condition results from an increased amount of deoxygenated hemoglobin. It is not an early sign of decreased perfusion but occurs later with other symptoms. *Dark-skinned patients may experience cyanosis as a graying of the same tissues.*

Central cyanosis involves decreased oxygenation of the arterial blood in the lungs and appears as a bluish tinge of the conjunctivae and the mucous membranes of the mouth and tongue. Central cyanosis may indicate impaired lung function or a right-to-left shunt found in congenital heart conditions. Because of impaired circulation, there is marked desaturation of hemoglobin in the peripheral tissues, which produces a bluish or darkened discoloration of the nail beds, earlobes, lips, and toes.

Peripheral cyanosis occurs when blood flow to the peripheral vessels is decreased by peripheral vasoconstriction. Constriction results from a low cardiac output or an increased extraction of oxygen from the peripheral tissues. Peripheral cyanosis localized in an extremity is usually a result of arterial or venous insufficiency. **Rubor** (dusky redness) that replaces pallor in a dependent foot suggests arterial insufficiency.

Skin *temperature* can be assessed for symmetry by touching different areas of the body with the dorsal (back) surface of the hand or fingers. Decreased blood flow results in decreased skin temperature. It is lowered in several clinical conditions, including heart failure, peripheral vascular disease, and shock.

Extremities

Assess the patient's hands, arms, feet, and legs for skin changes, vascular changes, clubbing, and edema. Skin mobility and turgor are affected by fluid status. Dehydration and aging reduce skin turgor, and edema decreases skin elasticity. Vascular changes in an affected extremity may include paresthesia, muscle fatigue and discomfort, numbness, pain, coolness, and loss of hair distribution from a reduced blood supply.

Clubbing of the fingers and toes is caused by *chronic* oxygen deprivation in body tissues. It is common in patients with advanced chronic pulmonary disease, congenital heart defects, and cor pulmonale (right-sided heart failure). The angle of the normal nail bed is 160 degrees. With **clubbing**, the nail straightens out to an angle of 180 degrees and the base of the nail becomes spongy. Fig. 30-12 in Chapter 30 shows late clubbing.

Peripheral edema (FLUID accumulation in the legs and feet) is a common finding in patients with cardiovascular problems. The location of edema helps determine its potential cause. Bilateral edema of the legs may be seen in those with heart failure or chronic venous insufficiency. Abdominal and leg edema can be seen in patients with heart disease and cirrhosis of the liver. Localized edema in one extremity may be the result of venous obstruction (thrombosis) or lymphatic blockage of the extremity (lymphedema). Edema may also be noted in dependent areas, such as the sacrum, when a patient is confined to bed. In other patients, edema results from third spacing when plasma proteins decrease. Dependent foot and ankle edema is also a common side effect of certain antihypertensive drugs, such as amlodipine (Norvasc).

Document the location of edema as precisely as possible (e.g., midtibial or sacral) and the number of centimeters from an anatomic landmark. The extent of edema can be assessed as mild, moderate, or severe (or 1+, 2+, 3+, or 4+). However, these values are not precise and are very unreliable. Determine whether the edema is **pitting** (the skin can be indented) (Fig. 33-5) or nonpitting.

The finger is typically used for pulse oximetry as a noninvasive method for assessing oxygenation and PERFUSION of many medical-surgical nursing patients. Correct placement of the pulse oximetry sensor is essential for accurate readings. Oxygen saturation levels of above 90% are considered normal, depending on the patient's age. Detailed information about this assessment method can be found in Chapter 27.

Blood Pressure

Arterial blood pressure is measured *indirectly* by sphygmomanometry. This technique of measurement is described in detail in nursing skills textbooks.

The 8th National High Blood Pressure Education Program Joint National Committee (JNC) on Prevention, Detection, Evaluation, and Treatment of High Blood Pressure (2013)

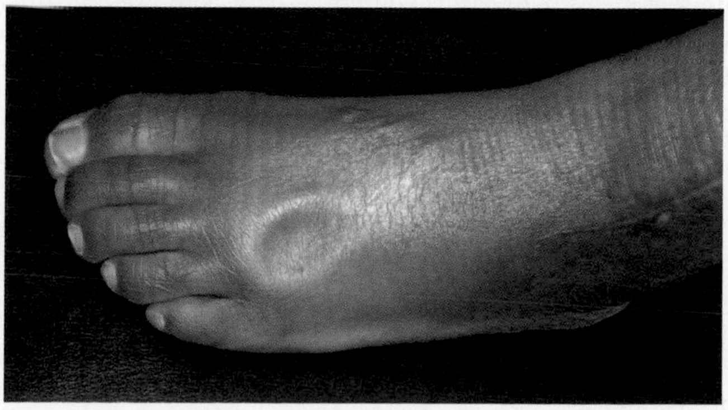

FIG. 33-5 Peripheral pitting edema.

defines **hypertension** as a systolic pressure of 140 mm Hg or higher or a diastolic pressure of 90 mm Hg or higher, or taking drugs to control blood pressure. Specific treatment goals were outlined for patients based on age and co-morbidities. Chapter 36 describes hypertension in detail.

A BP less than 90/60 mm Hg (hypotension) may not be adequate for providing enough oxygen and sufficient nutrition to body cells. In certain circumstances, such as shock, the Korotkoff sounds are less audible or are absent. In these cases, palpate the BP, use an ultrasonic device (Doppler device), or obtain a direct measurement by arterial catheter in the critical care setting. When BP is palpated, only the systolic pressure can be determined. Patients may report dizziness or light-headedness when they move from a flat, supine position to a sitting or a standing position at the edge of the bed. Normally these symptoms are transient and pass quickly; pronounced symptoms may be due to postural hypotension. **Postural (orthostatic) hypotension** *occurs when the BP is not adequately maintained while moving from a lying to a sitting or standing position. It is defined as a decrease of more than 20 mm Hg of the systolic pressure or more than 10 mm Hg of the diastolic pressure, as well as a 10% to 20% increase in heart rate.* The causes of postural hypotension include cardiovascular drugs, blood volume decrease, prolonged bedrest, age-related changes, or disorders of the ANS.

To detect orthostatic changes in BP, first measure the BP when the patient is supine. After remaining supine for at least 3 minutes, the patient changes position to sitting or standing. Normally systolic pressure drops slightly or remains unchanged as the patient rises, whereas diastolic pressure rises slightly. After the position change, wait for at least 1 minute before auscultating BP and counting the radial pulse. The cuff should remain in the proper position on the patient's arm. Observe and record any signs or symptoms of dizziness. If the patient cannot tolerate the position change, return him or her to the previous position of comfort.

Paradoxical blood pressure is an exaggerated decrease in systolic pressure by more than 10 mm Hg during the inspiratory phase of the respiratory cycle (normal is 3 to 10 mm Hg). Certain clinical conditions that potentially alter the filling pressures in the right and left ventricles may produce a paradoxical BP. Such conditions include pericardial tamponade, constrictive pericarditis, and pulmonary hypertension. During inspiration, the filling pressures normally decrease slightly. However, decreased fluid volume in the ventricles resulting from these pathologic conditions produces a marked reduction in cardiac output. The difference between the systolic and diastolic values is referred to as **pulse pressure**. This value can be used as an indirect measure of cardiac output. Narrowed pulse pressure is rarely normal and results from increased peripheral vascular resistance or decreased stroke volume in patients with heart failure, hypovolemia, or shock. It can also be seen in those with mitral stenosis or regurgitation. An increased pulse pressure may occur in patients with slow heart rates, aortic regurgitation, atherosclerosis, hypertension, and aging.

The **ankle-brachial index (ABI)** can be used to assess the vascular status of the lower extremities. A BP cuff is applied to the lower extremity just above the malleolus. The systolic pressure is measured by Doppler ultrasound at both the dorsalis pedis and posterior tibial pulses. The higher of these two pressures is then divided by the higher of the two brachial pulses to obtain the ABI.

Normal values for the ABI are 1.00 or higher because BP in the legs is usually higher than BP in the arms. ABI values less than 0.80 usually indicate moderate vascular disease, whereas values less than 0.50 indicate severe vascular compromise. Although used primarily to help identify peripheral vascular disease, the ABI may be effective as a risk factor in predicting other CV disease in women, especially coronary artery disease (Pearson, 2010).

A **toe brachial pressure index (TBPI)** may be performed instead of or in addition to the ABI to determine arterial perfusion in the feet and toes. TBPI is the toe systolic pressure divided by the brachial (arm) systolic pressure.

Venous and Arterial Pulses

Observe the *venous pulsations* in the neck to assess the adequacy of blood volume and central venous pressure (CVP). Specially educated or critical care nurses can assess jugular venous pressure (JVP) to estimate the filling volume and pressure on the right side of the heart. An increase in JVP causes **jugular venous distention (JVD)**.

Normally the JVP is 3 to 10 cm H_2O. Increases are usually caused by right ventricular failure. Other causes include tricuspid regurgitation or stenosis, pulmonary hypertension, cardiac tamponade, constrictive pericarditis, hypervolemia, and superior vena cava obstruction.

Assessment of *arterial pulses* provides information about vascular integrity and circulation. For patients with suspected or actual vascular disease, all major peripheral pulses should be assessed for presence or absence, amplitude, contour, rhythm, rate, and equality. Palpate the peripheral arteries in a head-to-toe approach with a side-to-side comparison (Fig. 33-6).

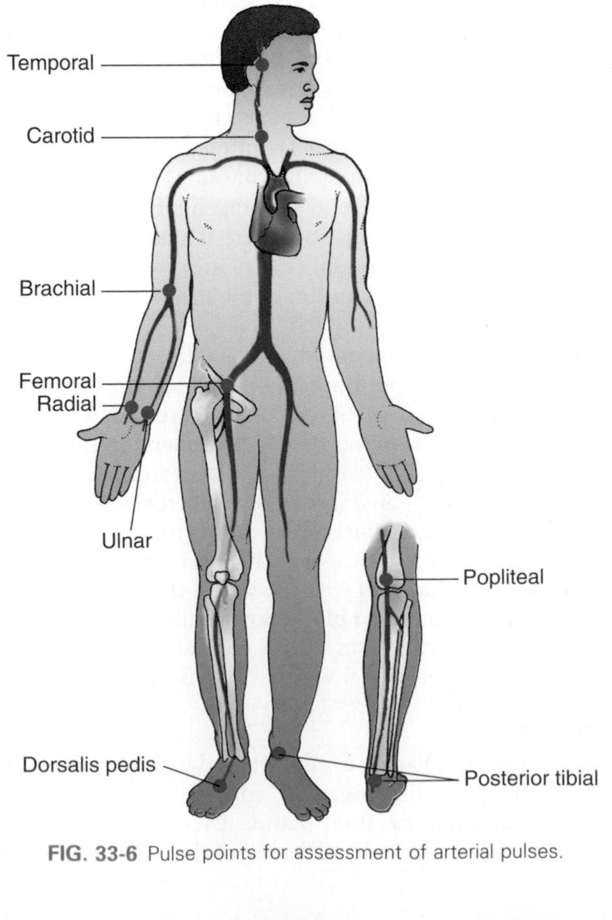

FIG. 33-6 Pulse points for assessment of arterial pulses.

A *hypokinetic* pulse is a weak pulse indicative of a narrow pulse pressure. It is seen in patients with hypovolemia, aortic stenosis, and decreased cardiac output. A *hyperkinetic* pulse is a large, "bounding" pulse caused by an increased ejection of blood. It occurs in patients with a high cardiac output (with exercise, sepsis, or thyrotoxicosis) and in those with increased sympathetic system activity (with pain, fever, or anxiety).

Auscultation of the major arteries (e.g., carotid and aorta) is necessary to assess for bruits. **Bruits** are swishing sounds that may occur from turbulent blood flow in narrowed or atherosclerotic arteries. Assess for the absence or presence of bruits by placing the bell of the stethoscope on the neck over the carotid artery while the patient holds his or her breath. Normally there are no sounds if the artery has uninterrupted blood flow. A bruit may develop when the internal diameter of the vessel is narrowed by 50% or more, but this does not indicate the severity of disease in the arteries. Once the vessel is blocked 90% or greater, the bruit often cannot be heard.

Precordium

Assessment of the precordium (the area over the heart) involves inspection, palpation, percussion, and auscultation. *In most settings, the medical-surgical nurse seldom performs precordial palpation and percussion. Critical care nurses and advanced practice nurses are qualified to perform the complete assessment.* Therefore only inspection and auscultation are described here. Begin by placing the patient in a supine position, with the head of the bed slightly elevated for comfort. Some patients may require elevation of the head of the bed to 45 degrees for ease and comfort in breathing.

Inspection. A cardiac examination is usually performed in a systematic order, beginning with inspection. Inspect the chest from the side, at a right angle, and downward over areas of the precordium where vibrations are visible. Cardiac motion is of low amplitude, and sometimes the inward movements are more easily detected by the naked eye.

Examine the entire precordium (Fig. 33-7), and note any prominent pulses. Movement over the aortic, pulmonic, and tricuspid areas is abnormal. Pulses in the mitral area (the apex of the heart) are considered normal and are referred to as the **apical impulse**, or the **point of maximal impulse (PMI)**. The PMI should be located at the left fifth intercostal space (ICS) in the midclavicular line. If it appears in more than one ICS and has shifted lateral to the midclavicular line, the patient may have left ventricular hypertrophy.

Auscultation. Auscultation evaluates heart rate and rhythm, cardiac cycle (systole and diastole), and valvular function. The technique of auscultation requires a good-quality stethoscope and extensive clinical practice. Identifying specific abnormal heart sounds is most important in critical care and telemetry.

Listen to heart sounds in a systematic order. Examination usually begins at the aortic area and progresses slowly to the apex of the heart. The diaphragm of the stethoscope is pressed tightly against the chest to listen for high-frequency sounds and is useful in listening to the first and second heart sounds and high-frequency murmurs. Repeat the progression from the base to the apex of the heart using the bell of the stethoscope, which is held lightly against the chest. The bell can screen out high-frequency sounds and is useful in listening for low-frequency gallops (diastolic filling sounds) and murmurs.

Normal Heart Sounds. The **first heart sound (S1)** is created by the closure of the mitral and tricuspid valves (atrioventricular valves) (see Fig. 33-4). When auscultated, S_1 is softer and longer; it is of a low pitch and is best heard at the lower left sternal border or the apex of the heart. It may be identified by palpating the carotid pulse while listening. S_1 marks the beginning of ventricular systole and occurs right after the QRS complex on the ECG.

S_1 can be accentuated or intensified in conditions such as exercise, hyperthyroidism, and mitral stenosis. A decrease in sound intensity occurs in patients with mitral regurgitation and heart failure. If you have difficulty hearing heart sounds, have the patient lean forward or roll to his or her left side.

The *second heart sound* (S_2) is caused mainly by the closing of the aortic and pulmonic valves (semilunar valves) (see Fig. 33-4). S_2 is characteristically shorter. It is higher pitched and is heard best at the base of the heart at the end of ventricular systole.

The splitting of heart sounds is often difficult to differentiate from diastolic filling sounds (gallops). A splitting of S_1 (closure of the mitral valve followed by closure of the tricuspid valve) occurs physiologically because left ventricular contraction

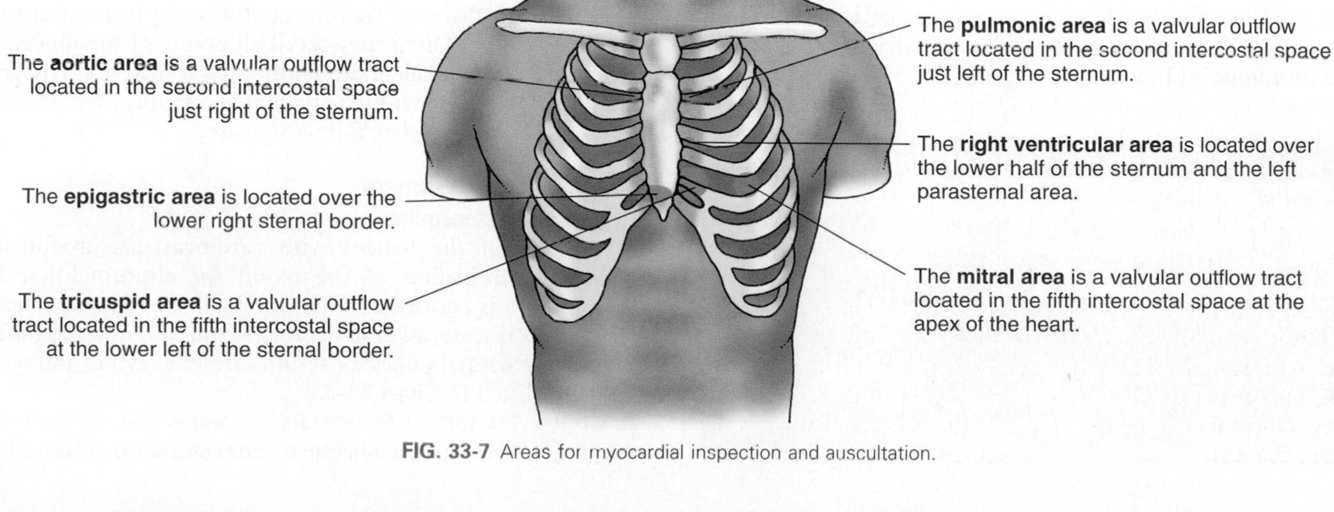

FIG. 33-7 Areas for myocardial inspection and auscultation.

occurs slightly before right ventricular contraction. Closure of the mitral valve is louder than closure of the tricuspid valve, however, so splitting is often not heard. Normal splitting of S_2 occurs because of the longer systolic phase of the right ventricle. Splitting of S_1 and S_2 can be accentuated by inspiration (due to increased venous return), and it narrows during expiration.

Abnormal Heart Sounds. Abnormal splitting of S_2 is referred to as **paradoxical splitting** and has a wider split heard on expiration. Paradoxical splitting of S_2 is heard in patients with severe myocardial depression that causes early closure of the pulmonic valve or a delay in aortic valve closure. Such conditions include myocardial infarction (MI), left bundle-branch block, aortic stenosis, aortic regurgitation, and right ventricular pacing.

Gallops and murmurs are common abnormal heart sounds that may occur with heart disease, but they can occur in some healthy people. Diastolic filling sounds (S_3 and S_4) are produced when blood enters a noncompliant chamber during rapid ventricular filling. The third heart sound (S_3) is produced during the rapid passive filling phase of ventricular diastole when blood flows from the atrium to a noncompliant ventricle. The sound arises from vibrations of the valves and supporting structures. The fourth heart sound (S_4) occurs as blood enters the ventricles during the active filling phase at the end of ventricular diastole.

S_3 is called a **ventricular gallop**, and S_4 is referred to as **atrial gallop**. These sounds can be caused by decreased compliance of either or both ventricles. Left ventricular diastolic filling sounds are best heard with the patient on his or her left side. The bell of the stethoscope is placed at the apex and at the left lower sternal border during expiration.

An S_3 heart sound is most likely to be a normal finding in those younger than 35 years. An S_3 gallop in patients older than 35 years is considered abnormal and represents a decrease in left ventricular compliance. It can be detected as an early sign of heart failure or as a ventricular septal defect.

An atrial gallop (S_4) may be heard in patients with hypertension, anemia, ventricular hypertrophy, MI, aortic or pulmonic stenosis, and pulmonary emboli. *It may be heard also with advancing age because of a stiffened ventricle.*

Murmurs reflect turbulent blood flow through normal or abnormal valves. They are classified according to their timing in the cardiac cycle: *systolic* murmurs (e.g., aortic stenosis and mitral regurgitation) occur between S_1 and S_2, whereas *diastolic* murmurs (e.g., mitral stenosis and aortic regurgitation) occur between S_2 and S_1. Murmurs can occur during presystole, midsystole, or late systole or diastole or can last throughout both phases of the cardiac cycle. They are also graded by the primary care provider according to their intensity, depending on their level of loudness (Table 33-3).

TABLE 33-3 Grading of Heart Murmurs

Grade I	Very faint
Grade II	Faint but recognizable
Grade III	Loud but moderate in intensity
Grade IV	Loud and accompanied by a palpable thrill
Grade V	Very loud, accompanied by a palpable thrill, and audible with the stethoscope partially off the patient's chest
Grade VI	Extremely loud, may be heard with the stethoscope slightly above the patient's chest, accompanied by a palpable thrill

Although you are not expected to grade murmurs as a medical-surgical nurse, describe their location based on where they are best heard. Some murmurs transmit or radiate from their loudest point to other areas, including the neck, the back, and the axilla. The configuration is described as *crescendo* (increases in intensity) or *decrescendo* (decreases in intensity). The quality of murmurs can be further characterized as harsh, blowing, whistling, rumbling, or squeaking. They are also described by pitch—usually *high* or *low*.

A **pericardial friction rub** originates from the pericardial sac and occurs with the movements of the heart during the cardiac cycle. Rubs are usually transient and are a sign of inflammation, infection, or infiltration. They may be heard in patients with pericarditis resulting from MI, cardiac tamponade, or post-thoracotomy.

Psychosocial Assessment

To most people, the heart is a symbol of their ability to exist, survive, and love. A patient with a heart-related illness, whether acute or chronic, usually perceives it as a major life crisis. The patient and family confront not only the possibility of death but also fears about pain, disability, lack of self-esteem, physical dependence, and changes in family dynamics. Assess the meaning of the illness to the patient and family by asking "What do you understand about what happened to you (or the patient)?" and "What does that mean to you?" When they perceive the stressor as overwhelming, formerly adequate support systems may no longer be effective. In these circumstances, the patient and family members attempt to cope to regain a sense or feeling of control.

Coping behaviors vary among patients and their families. Those who feel helpless to meet the demands of the situation may exhibit behaviors such as disorganization, fear, and anxiety. Ask them "Have you ever encountered such a situation before?" "How did you manage that situation?" and "To whom can you turn for help?" The answers to these questions often reassure the patient and family that they have encountered difficult situations in the past and have the ability and resources to cope with them.

A common and normal response is denial, which is a defense mechanism that enables the patient to cope with threatening circumstances. He or she may deny the current cardiovascular condition, may state that it was present but is now absent, or may be excessively cheerful. Denial becomes maladaptive when the patient is noncompliant or does not adhere to the interdisciplinary plan of care.

Family members and significant others may be more anxious than the patient. Often they recall all events of the illness, are unprotected by denial, and are afraid of recurrence. Disagreements may occur between the patient and family members over adherence to appropriate follow-up care.

Diagnostic Assessment

Laboratory Assessment

Assessment of the patient with cardiovascular dysfunction includes examination of the blood for abnormalities. The examination is performed to help establish a diagnosis, detect concurrent disease, assess risk factors, and monitor response to treatment. Normal values for serum cardiac enzymes and serum lipids are listed in Chart 33-2.

Serum Markers of Myocardial Damage. Events leading to cellular injury cause a release of enzymes from intracellular

CLINICAL JUDGMENT CHALLENGE

Safety; Teamwork and Collaboration QSEN

A middle-aged man is admitted to the cardiac unit after reports of a severe headache and flushing of the face. He is diagnosed with severe hypertension. The patient is alert and oriented; BP = 192/104 and HR = 88. You are the RN assigned to his care. There is an unlicensed nursing technician working with you.

1. What assessment data will you perform upon his arrival to the unit? Why?
2. The cardiologist prescribes IV fluids, hourly blood pressure checks, blood pressure medication, and oxygen at 2 liters per nasal cannula. What part of the patient's care will you delegate to the unlicensed nursing technician? What information will you communicate upon delegation?
3. What interventions will you implement to ensure this patient's safety?
4. The patient's wife is very concerned about her husband returning to work as owner of a roofing company. What education will you provide the patient and his wife at this time? With what health care team members will you collaborate to ensure positive patient outcomes?

storage, and circulating levels of these enzymes are dramatically elevated. Acute myocardial infarction (MI), also known as **acute coronary syndrome**, can be confirmed by abnormally high levels of certain proteins or isoenzymes. These serum studies are commonly referred to as **cardiac markers** and include troponin, creatine kinase–MB, and myoglobin.

Troponin is a myocardial muscle protein released into the bloodstream with injury to myocardial muscle. Troponins T and I are not found in healthy patients, so any rise in values indicates cardiac necrosis or acute MI. Specific markers of myocardial injury, troponins T and I, have a wide diagnostic time frame, making them useful for patients who present several hours after the onset of chest pain. Even low levels of troponin T are treated aggressively because of increased risk for death from cardiovascular disease (CVD). Obtaining cardiac markers at the bedside in the emergency department can be done as "point of care" (POC) testing for patients experiencing or at risk for acute MI, with results available within 15 to 20 minutes. These markers are evaluated in addition to clinical signs and symptoms and ECG changes when identifying at-risk patients.

Creatine kinase (CK) is an enzyme specific to cells of the brain, myocardium, and skeletal muscle. The appearance of CK in the blood indicates tissue necrosis or injury, with levels following a predictable rise and fall during a specified period. Cardiac specificity must be determined by measuring isoenzyme activity. There are three isoenzymes of CK: CK-MM is the predominant isoenzyme of skeletal muscle; CK-MB is found in myocardial muscle; and CK-BB occurs in the brain. CK-MB activity is most specific for MI and shows a predictable rise and fall during 3 days; a peak level occurs about 24 hours after the onset of chest pain.

Treatment modalities for early intervention after acute MI and acute ischemia require more rapid diagnosis of MI. An assay using monoclonal anti–CK-MB antibodies (stat CK) can detect myocardial necrosis accurately 3 hours after emergency department admission when examined with an ECG. Two subforms of CK-MB (CK-MB_1 and CK-MB_2) have also been identified. Abnormal elevations of these CK subforms may occur as

CHART 33-2 Laboratory Profile

Cardiovascular Assessment

NORMAL RANGE	SIGNIFICANCE OF ABNORMAL FINDINGS
Serum Cardiac Enzymes	
Creatine kinase (CK) *Females:* 30-135 units/L *Males:* 55-170 units/L Values higher after exercise	Elevations indicate possible brain, myocardial, and skeletal muscle necrosis or injury.
CK-MB (CK_2) 0% of total CK	Elevations occur with myocardial injury or after percutaneous transluminal angioplasty and intracoronary streptokinase infusion.
Serum Lipids	
Total lipids 400-1000 mg/dL	Elevation indicates increased risk for coronary artery disease (CAD).
Cholesterol Less than 200 mg/dL	Elevation indicates increased risk for CAD.
Triglycerides *Females:* 35-135 mg/dL *Males:* 40-160 mg/dL	Elevation indicates increased risk for CAD.
Plasma high-density lipoproteins (HDLs) *Females:* >55 mg/dL *Males:* >45 mg/dL *Older adults:* range increases with age	Elevations protect against CAD.
Plasma low-density lipoproteins (LDLs) <130 mg/dL	Elevation indicates increased risk for CAD.
HDL : LDL ratio 3 : 1	Elevated ratios may protect against CAD.
VLDL 7-32 ng/dL	Elevated level indicates risk for CAD.
C-reactive protein (CRP) <1.0 mg/dL	Elevation may indicate tissue infarction or damage.
Serum Markers	
Troponins Cardiac troponin T <0.10 ng/mL Cardiac troponin I <0.03 ng/mL	Elevations indicate myocardial injury or infarction.
Myoglobin <90 mcg/L	Elevation indicates myocardial infarction.

VLDL, Very-low-density lipoproteins.

early as 2 hours after MI. They remain elevated for up to 12 hours after MI and appear to be very sensitive and specific early diagnostic markers of MI.

Another early marker of an MI is myoglobin. **Myoglobin**, a low–molecular-weight heme protein found in cardiac and skeletal muscle, is the earliest marker detected—as early as 2 hours after an MI with rapid decline after 7 hours. Because myoglobin is not cardiac specific and is found in skeletal and cardiac muscle, its clinical usefulness is more limited than troponin.

Serum Lipids. Elevated lipid levels are considered a risk factor for coronary artery disease (CAD). **Cholesterol**, **triglycerides**, and the protein components of **high-density lipoproteins (HDLs)** and **low-density lipoproteins (LDLs)** are evaluated to assess the risk for CAD. The desired ranges for lipids are (Pagana & Pagana, 2014):

- Total cholesterol less than 200 mg/dL
- Triglycerides between 40 and 160 mg/dL for men and between 35 and 135 mg/dL for women
- HDL more than 45 mg/dL for men; more than 55 mg/dL for women ("good" cholesterol)
- LDL less than 130 mg/dL

Each of the lipoproteins contains varying proportions of cholesterol, triglyceride, protein, and phospholipid. HDL contains mainly protein and 20% cholesterol, whereas LDL is mainly cholesterol. Elevated LDL levels are positively correlated with CAD, whereas elevated HDL levels are negatively correlated and appear to be protective for heart disease. LDL pattern size is of significant importance in determining risk for CVD. LDL pattern A is associated with non–insulin resistance; normal glucose, insulin, and HDL levels; and a normal blood pressure. LDL pattern B is associated with insulin resistance; increased glucose, insulin, and triglyceride levels; and hypertension.

A fasting blood sample for the measurement of serum cholesterol levels is preferable to a nonfasting sample. If triglycerides are to be evaluated with cholesterol, the health care provider requests the specimen after a 12-hour fast

Lipoprotein-a, or Lp(a), is a modified form of LDL, the most common familial lipoprotein disorder in patients with premature coronary artery disease. Lp(a) is atherogenic (increases atherosclerotic plaques) and prothrombotic (increases clots). Therefore the desired outcome is a value less than 30 mg/dL. The patient should be fasting and avoid smoking before the test (Pagana & Pagana, 2014).

Other Laboratory Tests. **Homocysteine** is an amino acid that is produced when proteins break down. A certain amount of homocysteine is present in the blood, but elevated values may be an independent risk factor for the development of CVD. Although the relationship between homocysteine and CVD remains controversial, elevated levels of homocysteine may increase the risk for disease as much as smoking and hyperlipemia, especially in women. High-risk patients who have a personal or family history of premature heart disease should be screened. A level less than 14 mmol/dL is considered optimal, but this level increases as one ages (Pagana & Pagana, 2014).

Inflammation is a common and critical component to the development of atherothrombosis. **Highly sensitive C-reactive protein (hsCRP)** has been the most studied marker of inflammation. Any inflammatory process can produce CRP in the blood. Elevations are seen also with hypertension, infection, and smoking. A level less than 1 mg/dL is considered low risk; a level over 3 mg/dL places the patient at high risk for heart disease. The CRP is very helpful in determining treatment outcomes in patients at risk for coronary disease and in managing statin therapy after an acute myocardial infarction. The most useful time to measure CRP appears to be for risk assessment in middle-aged or older persons.

Microalbuminuria, or small amounts of protein in the urine, has been shown to be a clear marker of widespread endothelial dysfunction in cardiovascular disease (along with elevated CRP). It should be screened annually in all patients with hypertension, metabolic syndrome, or diabetes mellitus. Microalbuminuria has also been used as a marker for renal disease, particularly in patients with hypertension and diabetes.

Blood coagulation studies evaluate the ability of the blood to clot. They are important in patients with a greater tendency to form thrombi (e.g., those with atrial fibrillation, prosthetic valves, or infective endocarditis). These tests are also essential for monitoring patients receiving anticoagulant therapy (e.g., during cardiac surgery, during treatment of an established thrombus).

Prothrombin time (PT) and *international normalized ratio (INR)* are used when initiating and maintaining therapy with oral anticoagulants, such as sodium warfarin (Coumadin, Warfilone 🍁). They measure the activity of prothrombin, fibrinogen, and factors V, VII, and X. INR is the most reliable way to monitor anticoagulant status in warfarin therapy. The therapeutic ranges vary significantly based on the reason for the anticoagulation and the patient's history. The normal INR is 1.

Partial thromboplastin time (PTT) is assessed in patients who are receiving heparin (Hepalean 🍁). It measures deficiencies in all coagulation factors except VII and XIII.

Arterial blood gas (ABG) determinations are often obtained in patients with CVD. Determination of tissue oxygenation, carbon dioxide removal, and acid-base status is essential to appropriate treatment. (See Chapter 12 for a complete discussion of ABGs.)

FLUID AND ELECTROLYTE BALANCE is essential for normal cardiovascular performance. Cardiac manifestations often occur when there is an imbalance in either fluids or electrolytes in the body. For example, the cardiac effects of hypokalemia (low serum potassium level) include increased electrical instability, ventricular dysrhythmias, and an increased risk for digitalis toxicity. The effects of hyperkalemia on the myocardium include slowed ventricular conduction, peaked T waves on the ECG, and contraction followed by asystole (cardiac standstill).

Cardiac manifestations of hypocalcemia are ventricular dysrhythmias, a prolonged QT interval, and cardiac arrest. Hypercalcemia shortens the QT interval and causes AV block, digitalis hypersensitivity, and cardiac arrest. Serum sodium values reflect fluid balance and may be decreased, indicating a fluid excess in patients with heart failure (dilutional hyponatremia).

Because magnesium regulates some aspects of myocardial electrical activity, hypomagnesemia has been implicated in some forms of ventricular dysrhythmias known as *torsades de pointes*. Hypomagnesemia prolongs the QT interval, causing this specific type of ventricular tachycardia. Chapter 11 describes these electrolytes in more detail.

The *erythrocyte (red blood cell [RBC]) count* is usually decreased in rheumatic fever and infective endocarditis. It is increased in heart diseases as needed to compensate for decreased available oxygen.

Decreased *hematocrit and hemoglobin* levels (e.g., caused by hemorrhage or hemolysis from prosthetic valves) indicate anemia and can lead to angina or aggravate heart failure. Vascular volume depletion with hemoconcentration (e.g., hypovolemic shock and excessive diuresis) results in an elevated hematocrit.

The *leukocyte (white blood cell [WBC]) count* is typically elevated after an MI and in various infectious and inflammatory diseases of the heart (e.g., infective endocarditis and pericarditis). An increased WBC has been implicated as a strong independent risk factor for stroke and heart disease, particularly in postmenopausal women (Go et al., 2013).

Other Diagnostic Assessment

Posteroanterior (PA) and left lateral *x-ray* views of the chest are routinely obtained to determine the size, silhouette, and

TABLE 33-4 Indications For Cardiac Catheterization

- To confirm suspected heart disorders, including congenital abnormities, coronary artery disease, myocardial disease, valvular disease, and valvular dysfunction
- To determine the location and extent of the disease process
- To assess:
  - Stable, severe angina unresponsive to medical management
  - Unstable angina pectoris
  - Uncontrolled heart failure, ventricular dysrhythmias, or cardiogenic shock associated with acute myocardial infarction, papillary muscle dysfunction, ventricular aneurysm, or septal perforation
- To determine best therapeutic option (percutaneous transluminal coronary angioplasty, stents, coronary artery bypass graft, valvulotomy versus valve replacement)
- To evaluate effects of medical or invasive treatment on cardiovascular function, percutaneous transluminal coronary angioplasty, or coronary artery bypass graft patency

TABLE 33-5 Complications of Cardiac Catheterization

Right-Sided Heart Catheterization

- Thrombophlebitis
- Pulmonary embolism
- Vagal response

Left-Sided Heart Catheterization and Coronary Arteriography

- Myocardial infarction
- Stroke
- Arterial bleeding or thromboembolism
- Dysrhythmias

Right-Sided or Left-Sided Heart Catheterization*

- Cardiac tamponade
- Hypovolemia
- Pulmonary edema
- Hematoma or blood loss at insertion site
- Reaction to contrast medium

*In addition to those cited for each procedure.

position of the heart. In acutely ill patients, a simple anteroposterior (AP) view may be obtained at the bedside. Cardiac enlargement, pulmonary congestion, cardiac calcifications, and placement of central venous catheters, endotracheal tubes, and hemodynamic monitoring devices are assessed by x-ray.

Angiography of the arterial vessels, or **arteriography**, is an invasive diagnostic procedure that involves fluoroscopy and the use of contrast media. This procedure is performed when an arterial obstruction, narrowing, or aneurysm is suspected. The interventional radiologist performs selective arteriography to evaluate specific areas of the arterial system. For example, a coronary arteriography, which is performed during left-sided cardiac catheterization, assesses arterial circulation within the heart. It can also be performed on arteries in the extremities, mesentery, and cerebrum. Angiography is discussed under the appropriate associated diseases elsewhere in this text.

Cardiac Catheterization. The most definitive but most invasive test in the diagnosis of heart disease is cardiac catheterization. **Cardiac catheterization** may include studies of the right or left side of the heart and the coronary arteries. Some of the most common indications for cardiac catheterization are listed in Table 33-4.

Patient Preparation. Assess the patient's physical and psychosocial readiness and knowledge level about the procedure because many patients have anxiety and fear about cardiac catheterization. Review the purpose of the procedure, inform the patient about the length of the procedure, state who will be present, and describe the appearance of the catheterization laboratory. Tell the patient about the sensations he or she may experience during the procedure, such as palpitations (as the catheter is passed up to the left ventricle), a feeling of heat or a hot flash (as the medium is injected into either side of the heart), and a desire to cough (as the medium is injected into the right side of the heart). Written, electronic, or illustrated materials or DVDs may be used to assist in understanding.

The risks of cardiac catheterization are usually explained by the cardiologist. The risks vary with the procedures to be performed and the patient's physical status (Table 33-5). Although not common, several serious complications may follow coronary arteriography, such as:

- Myocardial infarction (MI)
- Stroke
- Arterial bleeding
- Thromboembolism
- Lethal dysrhythmias
- Arterial dissection
- Death

The cardiologist or interventional radiologist obtains a written informed consent from the patient or responsible party before the procedure.

The patient is admitted to the hospital on the day of the catheterization procedure. He or she may be admitted earlier if there is renal dysfunction. Fluids may be given 12 to 24 hours before the procedure for renal protection. Contrast-induced renal dysfunction can result from vasoconstriction and the direct toxic effect of the contrast agent on the renal tubules. Hydration and the administration of acetylcysteine pre- and post-study help eliminate or minimize contrast-induced renal toxicity.

Standard preoperative tests are performed, which usually include a chest x-ray, complete blood count, coagulation studies, and 12-lead ECG. The patient receives nothing by mouth after midnight or has only a liquid breakfast if the catheterization is scheduled for the afternoon. The catheterization site is antiseptically prepared with hairs clipped according to agency policy.

Before the procedure, take the patient's vital signs, auscultate the heart and the lungs, and assess the peripheral pulses. Question him or her about any history of allergy to iodine-based contrast agents. An antihistamine or steroid may be given to a patient with a positive history or to prevent a reaction. Be sure that the signed informed consent is completed, as required by The Joint Commission's National Patient Safety Goals (NPSGs). A mild sedative is usually administered before the procedure. If the patient normally takes a digitalis preparation or diuretic, it is usually withheld before the catheterization. Analysis of electrolytes, blood urea nitrogen (BUN), creatinine, coagulation profile, and complete blood count (CBC) is essential before and after the procedure, and abnormalities are discussed with the health care provider.

Procedure. The patient is taken to the cardiac catheterization laboratory (sometimes referred to as the "cath lab"), placed in the supine position on the x-ray table, and securely strapped to the table. The physician injects a local anesthetic at the insertion site. During the procedure, the patient is instructed to report any chest pain, pressure, or other symptoms to the staff.

The *right side of the heart* is catheterized first and may be the only side examined. The cardiologist inserts a catheter through the femoral vein to the inferior vena cava or through the basilic vein to the superior vena cava. The catheter is advanced through either the inferior or the superior vena cava and, guided by fluoroscopy, is advanced through the right atrium, through the right ventricle, and, at times, into the pulmonary artery. Intracardiac pressures (right atrial, right ventricular, pulmonary artery, and pulmonary artery wedge pressures) and blood samples are obtained. A contrast medium is usually injected to detect any cardiac shunts or regurgitation from the pulmonic or tricuspid valves.

In a *left-sided heart catheterization*, the cardiologist advances the catheter against the blood flow from the femoral, brachial, or radial artery up the aorta, across the aortic valve, and into the left ventricle (Fig. 33-8). Alternatively, the catheter may be passed from the right side of the heart through the atrial septum, using a special needle to puncture the septum. Intracardiac pressures and blood samples are obtained. The pressures of the left atrium, left ventricle, and aorta, as well as mitral and aortic valve status, are evaluated. The cardiologist injects contrast dye into the ventricle; digital subtraction angiography evaluates left ventricular motion. Calculations are made regarding end-systolic volume, end-diastolic volume, stroke volume, and ejection fraction.

The technique for *coronary arteriography* is the same as for left-sided heart catheterization. The catheter is advanced into the aortic arch and positioned selectively in the right or left coronary artery. Injection of a contrast medium permits viewing the coronary arteries. By assessing the flow of the medium through the coronary arteries, information about the site and severity of coronary lesions is obtained.

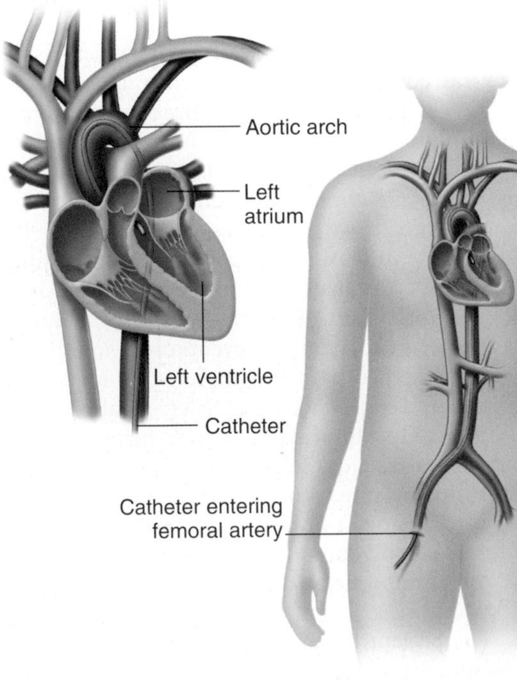

FIG. 33-8 Left-sided cardiac catheterization.

An alternative to injecting a medium into the coronary arteries is **intravascular ultrasonography (IVUS)**, which introduces a flexible catheter with a miniature transducer at the distal tip to view the coronary arteries. The transducer emits sound waves, which reflect off the plaque and the arterial wall to create an image of the blood vessel. IVUS is more reliable than angiography in indicating plaque distribution and composition, arterial dissection, and degree of stenosis of the occluded artery.

Follow-up Care. The patient recovers in a specialty area equipped with monitored beds. After cardiac catheterization, restrict the patient to bedrest and keep the insertion site extremity straight. A soft knee brace can be applied to prevent bending of the affected extremity. Some cardiologists allow the head of the bed to be elevated up to 30 degrees during the period of bedrest, whereas other cardiologists prefer that the patient remain supine. Current practice is for patients to remain in bed for 2 to 6 hours depending on the type of vascular closure device used. Various types of vascular closure devices are used to eliminate the need for manual compression after the catheterization. Examples include arteriotomy sutures and collagen plugs to seal the insertion site.

Monitor the patient's vital signs every 15 minutes for 1 hour, then every 30 minutes for 2 hours or until vital signs are stable, and then every 4 hours or according to hospital policy. Assess the insertion site for bloody drainage or hematoma formation. Complications with vascular closure devices are not common but can be very serious. Assess peripheral pulses in the affected extremity, as well as skin temperature and color, with every vital sign check. Observe for complications of cardiac catheterization (see Table 33-5).

! NURSING SAFETY PRIORITY QSEN

Critical Rescue

If the patient experiences symptoms of cardiac ischemia such as chest pain, dysrhythmias, bleeding, hematoma formation, or a dramatic change in peripheral pulses in the affected extremity, contact the Rapid Response Team or physician immediately to provide prompt intervention! Neurologic changes indicating a possible stroke, such as visual disturbances, slurred speech, swallowing difficulties, and extremity weakness, should also be reported immediately.

Because the contrast medium acts as an osmotic diuretic, monitor urine output and ensure that the patient receives sufficient oral and IV fluids for adequate excretion of the medium. Pain medication for insertion site or back discomfort may be given as prescribed.

Review home instructions and risk factor modification with the patient before discharge. Remind the patient to:

- Limit activity for several days, including avoiding lifting and exercise.
- Leave the dressing in place for at least the first day at home.
- Observe the insertion site over the next few weeks for increased swelling, redness, warmth, and pain. Bruising or a small hematoma is expected.

Electrocardiography. The electrocardiogram (ECG) is a routine part of every cardiovascular evaluation and is one of the most valuable diagnostic tests. Various forms are available: resting ECG, continuous ambulatory ECG (Holter monitoring), exercise ECG (stress test), signal-averaged ECG, and 30-day

NCLEX EXAMINATION CHALLENGE

Physiological Integrity

A client is admitted to the telemetry unit after a right-sided cardiac catheterization. What is the nurse's priority when caring for this client?

A. Assess the intensity and quality of the client's pain.
B. Position the client in a sitting position to improve breathing.
C. Check the client's arterial insertion site.
D. Apply oxygen at 2 L/min via nasal cannula.

event monitoring. The resting ECG provides information about cardiac dysrhythmias, myocardial ischemia, the site and extent of MI, cardiac hypertrophy, electrolyte imbalances, and the effectiveness of cardiac drugs. The normal ECG pattern and a detailed discussion of the interpretation of abnormal patterns are discussed in Chapter 34.

Electrophysiologic Studies. An **electrophysiologic study (EPS)** is an invasive procedure during which programmed electrical stimulation of the heart is used to cause and evaluate lethal dysrhythmias and conduction abnormalities. Patients who have survived cardiac arrest, have recurrent tachydysrhythmias, or experience unexplained syncopal episodes may be referred for EPS. Induction of the dysrhythmia during EPS helps find an accurate diagnosis and aids in effective treatment. These procedures have risks similar to those for cardiac catheterization and are performed in a special catheterization laboratory, where conditions are strictly controlled and immediate treatment is available for any adverse effects.

Exercise Electrocardiography (Stress Test). The **exercise electrocardiography** test (also known as **exercise tolerance**, or **stress test**) assesses cardiovascular response to an increased workload. The stress test helps determine the functional capacity of the heart and screens for asymptomatic coronary artery disease. Dysrhythmias that develop during exercise may be identified, and the effectiveness of antidysrhythmic drugs can be evaluated.

Patient Preparation. Because risks are associated with exercising, the patient must be adequately informed about the purpose of the test, the procedure, and the risks involved. Written consent must be obtained. Anxiety and fear are common before stress testing. Therefore assure the patient that the procedure is performed in a controlled environment in which prompt nursing and medical attention are available.

Instruct the patient to get plenty of rest the night before the procedure. He or she may have a light meal 2 hours before the test but should avoid smoking or drinking alcohol or caffeine-containing beverages on the day of the test. The cardiologist decides whether the patient should stop taking any cardiac medications. Usually cardiovascular drugs such as beta blockers or calcium channel blockers are withheld on the day of the test to allow the heart rate to increase during the stress portion of the test. Patients are advised to wear comfortable, loose clothing and rubber-soled, supportive shoes. Remind them to tell the physician if symptoms such as chest pain, dizziness, shortness of breath, and an irregular heartbeat are experienced during the test.

Before the stress test, a resting 12-lead ECG, cardiovascular history, and physical examination are performed to check for any ECG abnormalities or medical factors that might interfere with the test. Check to see that all emergency supplies such as

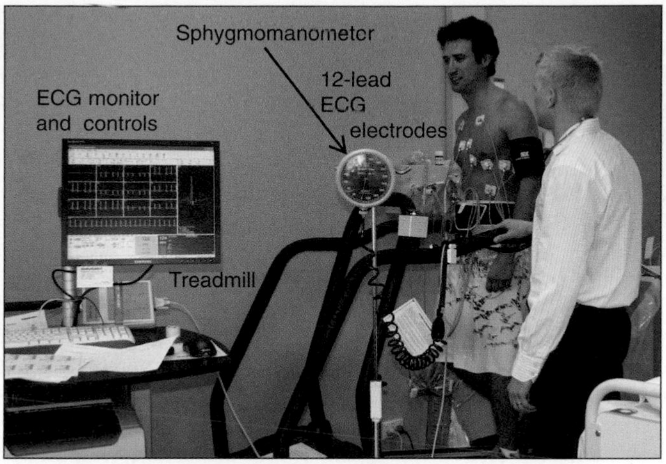

FIG. 33-9 Patient using a treadmill for a stress test.

cardiac drugs, a defibrillator, and other necessary resuscitation equipment are available in the room in which the stress test is performed. It is important to be proficient in the use of resuscitation equipment when assisting the physician because chest pain, dysrhythmias, and other ECG changes may occur.

Procedure. The technician places electrodes on the patient's chest and attaches them to a multilead monitoring system. Note baseline blood pressure (BP), heart rate (HR), and respiratory rate. The two major modes of exercise available for stress testing are pedaling a bicycle ergometer and walking on a treadmill. A bicycle ergometer has a wheel operated by pedals that can be adjusted to increase the resistance to pedaling. The treadmill is a motorized device with an adjustable conveyor belt. It can reach speeds of 1 to 10 miles/hr and can also be adjusted from a flat position to a 22-degree incline.

After the patient is shown how to use the bicycle or to walk on the treadmill, he or she begins to exercise. During the test, the BP and ECG are closely monitored as the resistance to cycling or the speed and incline of the treadmill are increased (Fig. 33-9). The patient exercises until one of these findings occurs:

- A predetermined HR is reached and maintained.
- Signs and symptoms such as chest pain, fatigue, extreme dyspnea, vertigo, hypotension, and ventricular dysrhythmias appear.
- Significant ST-segment depression or T-wave inversion occurs.
- The 20-minute protocol is completed.

Follow-up Care. After the test, the nurse or other qualified health care team member monitors the ECG and BP until the patient has completely recovered. After recovery, he or she can return home if the test was performed on an ambulatory basis. Advise him or her to avoid a hot shower for 1 to 2 hours after the test because this may cause hypotension. If he or she does not recover but continues to have pain or ventricular dysrhythmias or appears medically unstable, admission to a telemetry unit for observation is needed.

For patients who cannot exercise because of conditions such as peripheral vascular disease or arthritis, pharmacologic stress testing with agents such as dobutamine (Dobutrex) may be indicated. The nursing considerations are similar to those for the patient who has undergone an exercise ECG.

Echocardiography. As a noninvasive, risk-free test, echocardiography is easily performed at the bedside or on an ambulatory care basis. **Echocardiography** uses ultrasound waves to assess cardiac structure and mobility, particularly of the valves. It helps assess and diagnose cardiomyopathy, valvular disorders, pericardial effusion, left ventricular function, ventricular aneurysms, and cardiac tumors.

There is no special *preparation* for echocardiography. Inform the patient that the test is painless and takes 30 to 60 minutes to complete. The patient is instructed to lie quietly during the test and on his or her left side with the head elevated 15 to 20 degrees.

During an echocardiogram, a small transducer lubricated with gel to facilitate movement and conduction is placed on the patient's chest at the level of the third or fourth intercostal space near the left sternal border. The transducer transmits high-frequency sound waves and receives them as they are reflected from different structures. These echoes are usually videotaped simultaneously with the echocardiogram and can be recorded on graph paper for a permanent record.

After the images are taped, cardiac measurements that require several images can be obtained. Routine measurements include chamber size, ejection fraction, and flow gradient across the valves. There is no specific *follow-up care* for a patient who has undergone an echocardiogram.

A slightly more aggressive form of echocardiogram is a **pharmacologic stress echocardiogram** using either dobutamine or dipyridamole. This test is usually used when patients cannot tolerate exercise. Dobutamine (Dobutrex) increases the heart's contractility; dipyridamole (Persantine, Apo-Dipyridamole 🍁) is a coronary artery dilator. Patients are required to be NPO status for 3 to 6 hours before the test except for sips of water with medications. The technician ensures that IV access is present before the procedure and monitors BP and pulse continuously throughout the procedure. After the procedure, vital signs are monitored until BP returns to baseline and the pulse rate slows to less than 100 beats/min.

Transesophageal Echocardiography. Echocardiograms may also be performed transesophageally (through the esophagus). **Transesophageal echocardiography (TEE)** examines cardiac structure and function with an ultrasound transducer placed immediately behind the heart in the esophagus or stomach. The transducer provides especially detailed views of posterior cardiac structures such as the left atrium, mitral valve, and aortic arch. Preparation and follow-up are similar to that for an upper GI endoscopic examination (see Chapter 52).

Myocardial Nuclear Perfusion Imaging. The use of radionuclide techniques in cardiovascular assessment is called **myocardial nuclear perfusion imaging (MNPI)**. Cardiovascular abnormalities can be viewed, recorded, and evaluated using radioactive tracer substances. These studies are useful for detecting myocardial infarction (MI) and decreased myocardial blood flow and for evaluating left ventricular ejection. Conducting myocardial nuclear imaging tests, in conjunction with exercise or the administration of vasodilating agents, allows clearer identification of how the heart responds to stress.

Inform the patient that these tests are noninvasive. Because the amount of radioisotope is small, radiation exposure risks are minimal. If a dilating agent is to be used, advise the patient to avoid cigarettes and caffeinated food or drinks for 4 hours before administration of the vasodilator.

Common tests in nuclear cardiology include technetium (^{99m}Tc) pyrophosphate scanning, thallium imaging, and multigated cardiac blood pool imaging. Each test requires the injection of different types of radioactive isotopes into the antecubital vein. After the cells and tissues have time to take up the radioactive substances, usually 10 minutes to 2 hours, nuclear imaging can detect the difference between healthy and unhealthy tissue.

During the *technetium scan*, radioisotopes (^{99m}Tc pyrophosphate) accumulate in damaged myocardial tissue, which appears as a "hot spot" during the scan. This test helps detect the location and size of acute myocardial infarctions.

Alternatively, during the *thallium imaging scan*, necrotic or ischemic tissue does not absorb the radioisotope (thallium-201) and appears as "cold spots" on the scan. Thallium imaging is used to assess myocardial scarring and perfusion, to detect the location and extent of an acute or chronic myocardial infarction, to evaluate graft patency after coronary bypass surgery, and to evaluate antianginal therapy, thrombolytic therapy, or balloon angioplasty.

Thallium imaging may be performed during an exercise test or with the patient at rest. Thallium imaging performed during an exercise test may demonstrate perfusion deficits not apparent at rest. First, the stress test procedure is performed. After the patient reaches maximum activity level, a small dose of thallium-201 is injected IV. The patient continues to exercise for about 1 to 2 minutes, after which the scanning is performed. Nuclear cardiologists often compare the resting and stress images to differentiate between fixed and reversible defects in the myocardium.

If a patient cannot exercise on a bike or treadmill, dipyridamole (Persantine, Apo-Dipyridamole 🍁) or dobutamine hydrochloride (Dobutrex) is administered to simulate the effects of exercise. Tell the patient that these vasodilators may cause flushing, headache, dyspnea, and chest tightness for a few moments after injection.

Cardiac blood pool imaging is a noninvasive test for evaluating cardiac motion and calculating ejection fraction. It uses a computer to synchronize the patient's ECG with pictures taken by a special camera. The technician attaches the patient to an ECG and injects a small amount of ^{99m}Tc IV. The radioisotope is not taken up by tissue but remains "tagged" to red blood cells in the circulation. The camera may take pictures of the radioactive material as it makes its first pass through the heart.

During **multigated blood pool scanning**, the computer breaks the time between R waves on the ECG into fractions of a second, called "gates." The camera records blood flow through the heart during each of these gates. By analyzing the information from multiple gates, the computer can evaluate the ventricular wall motion and calculate ejection fraction (percentage of the left ventricular volume that is ejected with each contraction) and ejection velocity. Areas of decreased, absent, or paradoxical movement of the left ventricle may also be identified.

Positron emission tomography (PET) scans are used to compare cardiac perfusion and metabolic function and differentiate normal from diseased myocardium. The technician administers the first radioisotope (nitrogen-13-ammonia) and then begins a 20-minute scan to detect myocardial perfusion. Next, the technician administers a second radioisotope (fluoro-18-deoxyglucose). After a pause, a second scan is performed to detect the metabolically active myocardium, which is using glucose.

The two scans are compared. In a normal heart, performance and metabolic function will match. In an ischemic heart, there will be a mismatch—a reduction in perfusion and increased glucose uptake by the ischemic myocardium. The scanning procedure takes 2 to 3 hours, and the patient may be asked to use a treadmill or exercise bicycle in conjunction with the scan.

Depending on which test is performed, the patient may report fatigue or discomfort at the antecubital injection site. If a stress test was paired with the study, he or she will need follow-up care for the stress test.

Magnetic Resonance Imaging. Magnetic resonance imaging (MRI) is a noninvasive diagnostic option. An image of the heart or great vessels is produced through the interaction of magnetic fields, radio waves, and atomic nuclei showing hydrogen density. Simply put, the radio waves "bounce off" the body tissue being examined. Because each tissue has its own density, the computer image clearly differentiates between various types of tissues. MRI permits determination of cardiac wall thickness, chamber dilation, valve and ventricular function, and blood movement in the great vessels. Improved MRI techniques allow coronary artery blood flow to be mapped with nearly the accuracy of a cardiac catheterization.

Before an MRI, ensure that the patient has removed all metallic objects, including watches, jewelry, clothing with metal fasteners, and hair clips. Patients with pacemakers or implanted defibrillators may not be able to have an MRI because the magnetic fields can deactivate them. However, some newer MRI machines have eliminated this complication. A few patients experience claustrophobia during the 15 to 60 minutes required to complete the scan.

NURSING CONCEPTS AND CLINICAL JUDGMENT REVIEW

What might you NOTICE in a patient with adequate oxygenation and PERFUSION related to the cardiovascular system?

Physical assessment:
- Vital signs within normal limits or baseline
- No abnormal heart sounds
- Strong and equal peripheral pulses
- Even and unlabored respirations
- Regular heartbeat
- No pallor, cyanosis, or clubbing
- No syncope, fatigue, or chest pain
- No edema
- Can perform ADLs without dyspnea

Diagnostic assessment:
- No serum markers of myocardial damage
- Serum lipids within normal ranges
- Normal C-reactive protein and homocysteine
- Normal electrocardiogram (ECG)

GET READY FOR THE NCLEX® EXAMINATION!

KEY POINTS

Review these Key Points for each NCLEX Examination Client Needs Category.

Safe and Effective Care Environment
- Assess patients for allergy to iodine-based contrast media before having invasive diagnostic tests requiring an iodine-based contrast agent. **Safety** QSEN
- After invasive cardiovascular diagnostic testing, such as angiography and cardiac catheterization, monitor the insertion site for bleeding and hematoma formation. **Safety** QSEN
- Assess vital signs carefully in patients having invasive cardiovascular testing; report and document any new dysrhythmias after testing. **Informatics** QSEN

Health Promotion and Maintenance
- Identify patients at risk for cardiovascular disease, especially those with hyperlipidemia, hypertension, excess weight, physical inactivity, smoking, psychological stress, a positive family history, and diabetes. **Evidence-Based Practice** QSEN
- Teach patients how to reduce the risk for heart disease through modifiable factors such as exercise, diet modification, smoking cessation, and medications, as needed. **Patient-Centered Care** QSEN
- Inform patients that genetics and other nonmodifiable risk factors, such as family history and gender, contribute to the development of CAD.
- Assess the older adult for cardiovascular changes associated with aging as described in Chart 33-1.

Psychosocial Integrity
- Discuss with the patient any feelings or concerns he or she might have about the stress of cardiac illness, diagnostic testing, or other issues, and use therapeutic measures to decrease anxiety. **Patient-Centered Care** QSEN
- Recognize that denial is a common and normal response to help patients cope with threatening circumstances.
- Be aware that coping behaviors of those who have cardiovascular problems vary from patient to patient. **Patient-Centered Care** QSEN
- Allow the patient to express feelings about an actual or perceived loss of health or social status related to cardiovascular disease.

Physiological Integrity
- Be aware of the importance of recalling the anatomy and physiology of the cardiovascular (CV) system to best understand how to care for patients with CV health problems.
- Assess the patient's report of pain to differentiate the pain of angina and myocardial infarction (MI) from other noncardiac causes; *discomfort, indigestion, squeezing, heaviness,* and *viselike* are common terms used to describe chest pain of cardiac origin.

- Recall that syncope is a transient loss of consciousness and is common in older adults.
- Be aware that women often present with different indicators of heart disease when compared with men; examples include dyspnea, chest discomfort, indigestion, and fatigue. **Evidence-Based Practice** QSEN
- Use jugular venous pressure to assess the filling volume and pressure on the right side of the heart.
- Assess for bruits, which are swishing sounds that develop in narrowed arteries.
- Auscultate the heart for normal first and second sounds, as well as for abnormalities such as an S_3, S_4, murmur, or gallop.
- Monitor serum markers of myocardial damage and other cardiac-related laboratory tests as listed in Chart 33-2.
- Prepare patients having a cardiac catheterization for expectations of the procedure and postprocedure care.
- Assess patients having cardiac catheterizations for potential complications as listed in Table 33-5. **Safety** QSEN

CHAPTER 34

Care of Patients with Dysrhythmias

Laura Dechant

http://evolve.elsevier.com/Iggy/

PRIORITY CONCEPTS

- PERFUSION

LEARNING OUTCOMES

Safe and Effective Care Environment

1. Provide a safe environment for patients and staff when using a cardiac defibrillator.

Health Promotion and Maintenance

2. Teach patients and their families about drug therapy used for common dysrhythmias.
3. Educate patients and families about procedures and other interventions for common dysrhythmias.

Physiological Integrity

4. Identify typical physical assessment findings associated with common dysrhythmias.
5. Explain how to perform an electrocardiogram (ECG) test.
6. Analyze an ECG rhythm strip to identify normal sinus rhythm and common or life-threatening dysrhythmias.
7. Plan collaborative care for patients experiencing common dysrhythmias.
8. Explain the purpose and types of pacing used as interventions for patients with dysrhythmias to promote PERFUSION.
9. Explain the need to perform evidence-based emergency care procedures, such as cardiopulmonary resuscitation (CPR) and automated external defibrillation.
10. Teach patients with a pacemaker or implantable cardioverter/defibrillator about self-management when in the community.

Cardiac dysrhythmias are abnormal rhythms of the heart's electrical system that can affect its ability to effectively pump *oxygenated* blood throughout the body. Some dysrhythmias are life threatening, and others are not. They are the result of disturbances of cardiac electrical impulse formation, conduction, or both. When the heart does not work effectively as a pump, PERFUSION to vital organs and peripheral tissues can be impaired, resulting in organ dysfunction or failure.

Many health problems, especially coronary artery disease (CAD), electrolyte imbalances, impaired oxygenation, and drug toxicity (both legal and illicit drugs), can cause abnormal heart rhythms. Dysrhythmias can occur in people of any age but occur most often in older adults. To provide collaborative patient-centered care using best practices, a *basic* understanding of cardiac electrophysiology, the conduction system of the heart, and the principles of electrocardiography is needed as a medical-surgical nurse. Specialty nurses and advanced practice nurses have a more in-depth knowledge as they manage patients with these cardiac problems in critical care and ambulatory care settings.

REVIEW OF CARDIAC CONDUCTION SYSTEM

The cardiac conduction system consists of specialized myocardial cells (Fig. 34-1). The electrophysiologic properties of those cells regulate heart rate and rhythm and possess unique properties: automaticity, excitability, conductivity, and contractility.

Automaticity (pacing function) is the ability of cardiac cells to generate an electrical impulse spontaneously and repetitively. Normally, only primary pacemaker cells (sinoatrial [SA] node) can generate an electrical impulse. Under certain conditions, such as myocardial ischemia (decreased blood flow), electrolyte imbalance, hypoxia, drug toxicity, and infarction (cell death), any cardiac cell may produce electrical impulses independently and create dysrhythmias. Disturbances in automaticity may involve either an increase or a decrease in pacing function.

Excitability is the ability of non-pacemaker heart cells to respond to an electrical impulse that begins in pacemaker cells and to depolarize. **Depolarization** occurs when the normally negatively charged cells within the heart muscle develop a positive charge.

Conductivity is the ability to send an electrical stimulus from cell membrane to cell membrane. As a result, excitable cells depolarize in rapid succession from cell to cell until all cells have depolarized. *The wave of depolarization causes the deflections of the electrocardiogram (ECG) waveforms that are recognized as the P wave and the QRS complex.* Disturbances in conduction result when conduction is too rapid or too slow, when the pathway is totally blocked, or when the electrical impulse travels an abnormal pathway.

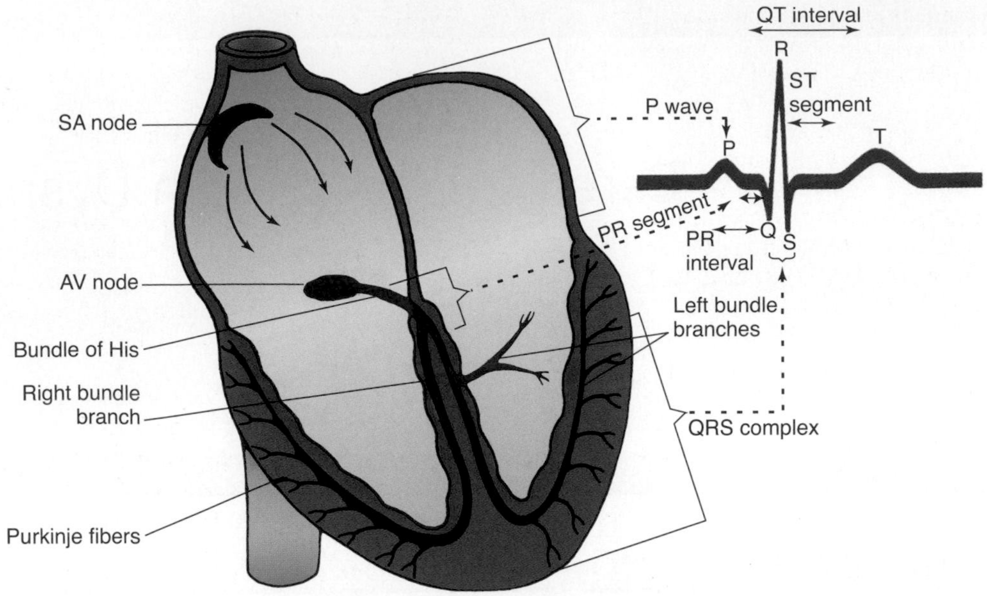

FIG. 34-1 The cardiac conduction system.

Contractility is the ability of atrial and ventricular muscle cells to shorten their fiber length in response to electrical stimulation, causing sufficient pressure to push blood forward through the heart. In other words, *contractility is the mechanical activity of the heart.*

Specialized cells of the myocardium are responsible for cardiac conduction. They consist of the sinoatrial node, atrioventricular junctional area, and bundle branch system.

Conduction begins with the **sinoatrial (SA) node** (also called the *sinus node*), located close to the surface of the right atrium near its junction with the superior vena cava. *The SA node is the heart's primary pacemaker.* It can spontaneously and rhythmically generate electrical impulses at a rate of 60 to 100 beats per minute and therefore has the greatest degree of automaticity.

The SA node is richly supplied by the sympathetic and parasympathetic nervous systems, which increase and decrease the rate of discharge of the sinus node, respectively. This process results in changes in the heart rate.

Impulses from the sinus node move directly through atrial muscle and lead to atrial depolarization, which is *reflected in a P wave on the ECG.* Atrial muscle contraction should follow. Within the atrial muscle are slow and fast conduction pathways leading to the atrioventricular (AV) node.

The **atrioventricular (AV) junctional** area consists of a transitional cell zone, the AV node itself, and the bundle of His. The AV node lies just beneath the right atrial endocardium, between the tricuspid valve and the ostium of the coronary sinus. Here T-cells (transitional cells) cause impulses to slow down or to be delayed in the AV node before proceeding to the ventricles. This delay is *reflected in the PR segment on the ECG.* This slow conduction provides a short delay, allowing the atria to contract and the ventricles to fill. The contraction is known as "atrial kick" and contributes additional blood volume for a greater cardiac output. The AV node is also controlled by both the sympathetic and the parasympathetic nervous systems. The bundle of His connects with the distal portion of the AV node and continues through the interventricular septum.

The *bundle of His* extends as a right bundle branch down the right side of the interventricular septum to the apex of the right ventricle. On the left side, it extends as a left bundle branch, which further divides.

At the ends of both the right and the left bundle branch systems are the Purkinje fibers. These fibers are an interweaving network located on the endocardial surface of both ventricles, from apex to base. The fibers then partially penetrate into the myocardium. **Purkinje cells** make up the bundle of His, bundle branches, and terminal Purkinje fibers. These cells are responsible for the rapid conduction of electrical impulses throughout the ventricles, leading to ventricular depolarization and the subsequent ventricular muscle contraction. A few nodal cells in the ventricles also occasionally demonstrate automaticity, giving rise to ventricular beats or rhythms.

ELECTROCARDIOGRAPHY

The **electrocardiogram (ECG)** provides a graphic representation, or picture, of cardiac electrical activity. The cardiac electrical currents are transmitted to the body surface. Electrodes, consisting of a conductive gel on an adhesive pad, are placed on specific sites on the body and attached to cables connected to an ECG machine or to a monitor. The cardiac electrical current is transmitted via the electrodes and through the lead wires to the machine or monitor, which displays the cardiac electrical activity.

A **lead** provides one view of the heart's electrical activity. Multiple leads, or views, can be obtained. Electrode placement is the same for male and female patients.

Lead systems are made up of a positive pole and a negative pole. An imaginary line joining these two poles is called the **lead axis**. The direction of electrical current flow in the heart is the **cardiac axis**. The relationship between the cardiac axis and the lead axis is responsible for the deflections seen on the ECG pattern:

- The baseline is the **isoelectric** line. It occurs when there is no current flow in the heart after complete depolarization and also after complete repolarization. Positive deflections occur above this line, and negative deflections occur below it. Deflections represent depolarization and repolarization of cells.

- If the direction of electrical current flow in the heart (cardiac axis) is toward the positive pole, a **positive deflection** (above the baseline) is viewed (Fig. 34-2, *A*).
- If the direction of electrical current flow in the heart (cardiac axis) is moving away from the positive pole toward the negative pole, a **negative deflection** (below the baseline) is viewed (Fig. 34-2, *B*).
- If the cardiac axis is moving neither toward nor away from the positive pole, a biphasic complex (both above and below baseline) will result (Fig. 34-2, *C*).

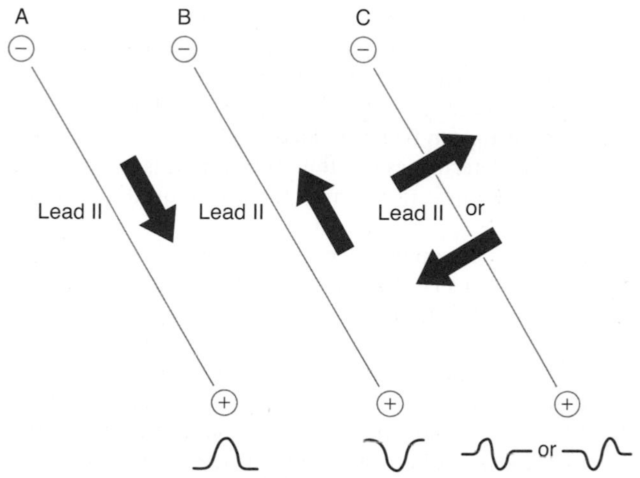

FIG. 34-2 A, The cardiac axis *(bold arrow)* is parallel to the lead axis *(the line between the negative and the positive electrodes),* going toward the positive electrode; a positive deflection is inscribed. **B,** The cardiac axis is parallel to the lead axis, going toward the negative electrode; a negative deflection is inscribed. **C,** The cardiac axis is perpendicular to the lead axis, going neither toward the positive electrode nor toward the negative electrode; a biphasic deflection is inscribed.

Lead Systems

The standard 12-lead ECG consists of 12 leads (or views) of the heart's electrical activity. Six of the leads are called *limb leads* because the electrodes are placed on the four extremities in the frontal plane. The remaining six leads are called *chest (precordial) leads* because the electrodes are placed on the chest in the horizontal plane.

Standard bipolar *limb leads* consist of three leads (I, II, and III) that each measures the electrical activity between two points and a fourth lead (right leg) that acts as a ground electrode. Of the three measuring leads, the right arm is always negative, the left leg is always positive, and the left arm can be either positive or negative.

Other lead systems include the 18-lead ECG, which adds six leads placed on the horizontal plane on the right side of the chest to view the right side of the heart. This is sometimes referred to as a "right-sided ECG." The extra leads are sometimes placed on the back. The latest evidence indicates an 80-lead ECG, which looks at the heart from 80 views instead of only 12 and gives a 360-degree view of the heart. Evaluation of this 80-lead ECG revealed an increase in diagnosing myocardial infarctions (MIs), particularly in the posterior wall and right ventricular region, which was missed in the 12-lead ECG (Franks & Lawson, 2012). This device consists of a vest which contains 58 anterior leads, 12 lateral leads, and 10 posterior leads. One limitation is that vests are available in only four sizes and therefore may not be appropriate for some patients.

Unipolar limb leads consist of a positive electrode only. The unipolar limb leads are aVR, aVL, and aVF, with *a* meaning augmented. *V* is a designation for a unipolar lead. The third letter denotes the positive electrode placement: *R* for right arm, *L* for left arm, and *F* for foot (left leg). The positive electrode is at one end of the lead axis. The other end is the center of the electrical field, at about the center of the heart (Table 34-1).

There are six unipolar (or V) *chest leads*, determined by the placement of the chest electrode. The four limb electrodes are placed on the extremities, as designated on each electrode (right arm, left arm, right leg, and left leg). The fifth (chest) electrode

TABLE 34-1 Electrode Placement for 12 Leads

LEAD	NEGATIVE ELECTRODE	POSITIVE ELECTRODE	GROUND ELECTRODE
I	Right arm or under the right clavicle	Left arm or under the left clavicle	Right leg or lowest rib, left midclavicular line
II	Right arm or under the right clavicle	Left leg or lowest rib, left midclavicular line	Right leg or under the left clavicle
III	Left arm or under the left clavicle	Left leg or lowest rib, left midclavicular line	Right leg or under the right clavicle
aVR	Average potential of left arm (or under the left clavicle) and left leg (or lowest rib, left midclavicular line)	Right arm or under the right clavicle	Right leg or lowest rib, right midclavicular line
aVL	Average potential of right arm (or under the right clavicle) and left leg (or lowest rib, left midclavicular line)	Left arm or under the left clavicle	Same as for aVR
aVF	Average potential of right arm (or under the right clavicle) and left arm (or under the left clavicle)	Left leg or lowest rib, left midclavicular line	Same as for aVR
V_1	Average potential of right arm, left arm, and left leg	Fourth intercostal space (ICS), right sternal border	Same as for aVR
V_2	Same as for V_1	Fourth ICS, left sternal border	Same as for aVR
V_3	Same as for V_1	Midway between V_2 and V_4	Same as for aVR
V_4	Same as for V_1	Fifth ICS, left midclavicular line	Same as for aVR
V_5	Same as for V_1	Horizontal to V_4, left anterior axillary line	Same as for aVR
V_6	Same as for V_1	Horizontal to V_4, left midaxillary line	Same as for aVR

on a monitor system is the positive, or exploring, electrode and is placed in one of six designated positions to obtain the desired chest lead. With a 12-lead ECG, four leads are placed on the limbs and six are placed on the chest, eliminating the need to move any electrodes about the chest.

Positioning of the electrodes is crucial in obtaining an accurate ECG. Comparisons of ECGs taken at different times will be valid only when electrode placement is accurate and identical at each test. Positioning is particularly important when working with patients with chest deformities or large breasts. Patients may be asked to move the breasts to ensure proper electrode placement.

While obtaining a 12-lead ECG, remind the patient to be as still as possible in a semi-reclined position, breathing normally. Any repetitive movement will cause artifact and could lead to inaccurate interpretation of the ECG.

Nurses are sometimes responsible for obtaining 12-lead ECGs, but more commonly, technicians are trained to perform this skill. Remind the technician to notify the nurse or physician of any suspected abnormality. A nurse may direct a technician to take a 12-lead ECG on a patient experiencing chest pain to observe for diagnostic changes, but it is ultimately the health care provider's responsibility to definitively interpret the ECG.

Continuous Electrocardiographic Monitoring

For continuous ECG monitoring, the electrodes are not placed on the limbs because movement of the extremities causes "noise," or motion artifact, on the ECG signal. Place the electrodes on the trunk, a more stable area, to minimize such artifacts and to obtain a clearer signal. If the monitoring system provides five electrode cables, place the electrodes as follows:

- Right arm electrode just below the right clavicle
- Left arm electrode just below the left clavicle
- Right leg electrode on the lowest palpable rib, on the right midclavicular line
- Left leg electrode on the lowest palpable rib, on the left midclavicular line
- Fifth electrode placed to obtain one of the six chest leads

With this placement, the monitor lead select control may be changed to provide lead I, II, III, aVR, aVL, or aVF or one chest lead. The monitor automatically alters the polarity of the electrodes to provide the lead selected.

The clarity of continuous ECG monitor recordings is affected by skin preparation and electrode quality. To ensure the best signal transmission and to decrease skin impedance, clean the skin and clip hairs if needed. Make sure the area for electrode placement is dry. The gel on each electrode must be moist and fresh. Attach the electrode to the lead cable and then to the contact site. The contact site should be free of any lotion, tincture, or other substance that increases skin impedance. Electrodes cannot be placed on irritated skin or over scar tissue. The application of electrodes may be done by unlicensed assistive personnel (UAP), but the nurse determines which lead to select and checks for correct electrode placement. Assess the quality of the ECG rhythm transmission to the monitoring system.

The ECG cables can be attached directly to a wall-mounted monitor (a hard-wired system) if the patient's activity is restricted to bedrest and sitting in a chair, as in a critical care unit. For an ambulatory patient, the ECG cable is attached to a battery-operated transmitter (a **telemetry** system) held in a pouch. The ECG is transmitted to a remote monitor via antennae located in strategic places, usually in the ceiling. Telemetry allows freedom of movement within a certain area without losing transmission of the ECG.

Most acute care facilities have monitor technicians (monitor "techs") who are educated in ECG rhythm interpretation and are responsible for:

- Watching a bank of monitors on a unit
- Printing ECG rhythm strips routinely and as needed
- Interpreting rhythms
- Reporting the patient's rhythm and significant changes to the nurse

The technical support is particularly helpful on a telemetry unit that does not have monitors at the bedside. The nurse is responsible for accurate patient assessment and management.

Some units have full-disclosure monitors, which continuously store ECG rhythms in memory up to a certain amount of time. This system allows nurses and health care providers to access and print rhythm strips for more thorough patient assessment. Routine strips, as well as any changes in rhythm, are printed and documented in the patient's record.

The health care provider is responsible for determining when monitoring can be suspended, such as during showering. He or she also determines whether monitoring is needed during off-unit testing procedures and for transportation to other facilities.

Prehospital personnel, such as paramedics and emergency medical technicians (EMTs) with advanced training, frequently monitor ECG rhythms at the scene and on the way to a health care facility. They function under medical direction and protocols but may also be communicating with a nurse in the emergency department.

The ECG strip is printed on graph paper (Fig. 34-3), with each small block measuring 1 mm in height and width. ECG recorders and monitors are standardized at a speed of 25 mm/sec. Time is measured on the horizontal axis. At this speed, each small block represents 0.04 second. Five small blocks make up one large block, defined by darker bold lines and representing 0.20 second. Five large blocks represent 1 second, and 30 large blocks represent 6 seconds. Vertical lines in the top margin of the graph paper are usually 15 large blocks apart, representing 3-second segments (Fig. 34-4).

Electrocardiographic Complexes, Segments, and Intervals

Complexes that make up a normal ECG consist of a P wave, a QRS complex, a T wave, and possibly a U wave. Segments include the PR segment, the ST segment, and the TP segment. Intervals include the PR interval, the QRS duration, and the QT interval (Fig. 34-5).

The **P wave** is a deflection representing atrial depolarization. The shape of the P wave may be a positive, negative, or biphasic (both positive and negative) deflection, depending on the lead selected. When the electrical impulse is consistently generated from the sinoatrial (SA) node, the P waves have a consistent shape in a given lead. If an impulse is then generated from a different (ectopic) focus, such as atrial tissue, the shape of the P wave changes in that lead, indicating that an ectopic focus has fired.

The **PR segment** is the isoelectric line from the end of the P wave to the beginning of the QRS complex, when the electrical impulse is traveling through the atrioventricular (AV) node, where it is delayed. It then travels through the ventricular conduction system to the Purkinje fibers.

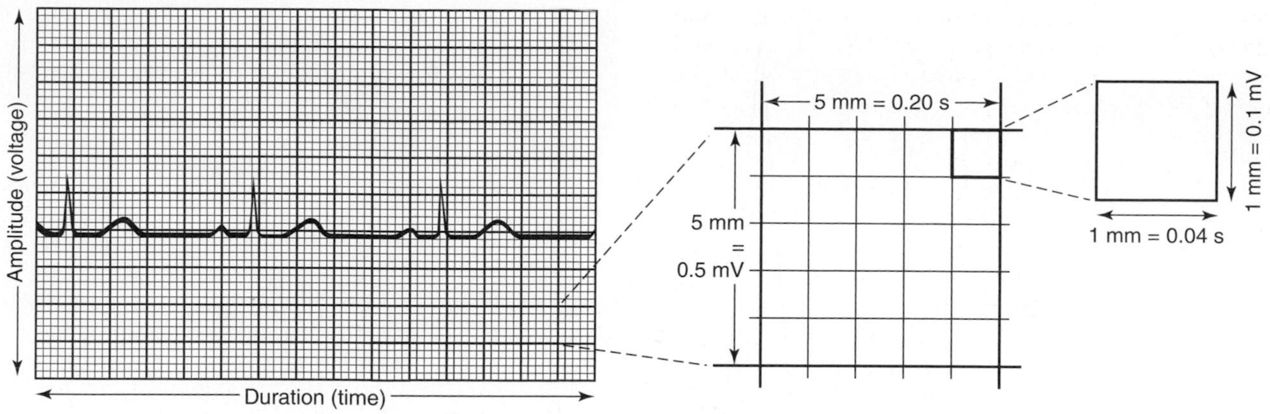

FIG. 34-3 Electrocardiographic waveforms are measured in amplitude (voltage) and duration (time).

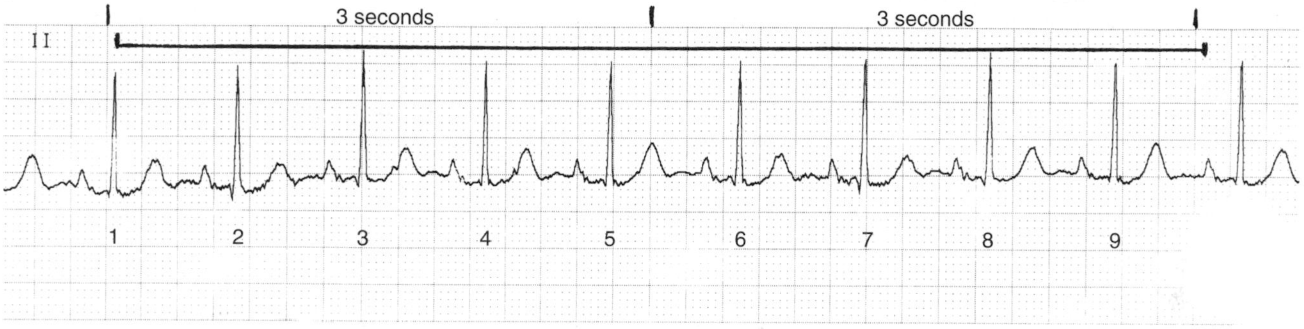

FIG. 34-4 Each segment between the dark lines *(above the monitor strip)* represents 3 seconds when the monitor is set at a speed of 25 mm per second. To estimate the ventricular rate, count the QRS complexes in a 6-second strip and then multiply that number by 10 to estimate the rate for 1 minute. In this example, there are 9 QRS complexes in 6 seconds. Therefore the heart rate can be estimated to be 90 beats per minute.

The **PR interval** is measured from the beginning of the P wave to the end of the PR segment. It represents the time required for atrial depolarization as well as the impulse delay in the AV node and the travel time to the Purkinje fibers. It normally measures from 0.12 to 0.20 second (five small blocks).

The **QRS complex** represents ventricular depolarization. The shape of the QRS complex depends on the lead selected. The Q wave is the first negative deflection and is not present in all leads. When present, it is small and represents initial ventricular septal depolarization. When the Q wave is abnormally present in a lead, it represents myocardial necrosis (cell death). The R wave is the first positive deflection. It may be small, large, or absent, depending on the lead. The S wave is a negative deflection following the R wave and is not present in all leads.

The **QRS duration** represents the time required for depolarization of both ventricles. It is measured from the beginning of the QRS complex to the J point (the junction where the QRS complex ends and the ST segment begins). It normally measures from 0.04 to 0.12 second (up to three small blocks).

The **ST segment** is normally an isoelectric line and represents early ventricular repolarization. It occurs from the J point to the beginning of the T wave. Its length varies with changes in the heart rate, the administration of medications, and electrolyte disturbances.

The **T wave** follows the ST segment and represents ventricular repolarization. It is usually positive, rounded, and slightly asymmetric. T waves may become tall and peaked, inverted (negative), or flat as a result of myocardial ischemia, potassium or calcium imbalances, medications, or autonomic nervous system effects.

The *TP segment* begins at the end of the T wave and ends at the beginning of the P wave. It is the true isoelectric interval in the ECG.

The **U wave,** when present, follows the T wave and may result from slow repolarization of ventricular Purkinje fibers. It is of the same polarity as the T wave, although generally it is smaller. It is not normally seen in all leads and is more common in lead V_3. An abnormal U wave may suggest an electrolyte abnormality (particularly hypokalemia) or other disturbance. Correct identification is important so that it is not mistaken for a P wave. If in doubt, notify the health care provider and request that a potassium level be obtained.

The **QT interval** represents the total time required for ventricular depolarization and repolarization. The QT interval is measured from the beginning of the Q wave to the end of the T wave. This interval varies with the patient's age and gender and changes with the heart rate, lengthening with slower heart rates and shortening with faster rates. It may be prolonged by certain medications, electrolyte disturbances, or subarachnoid hemorrhage. A prolonged QT interval may lead to a unique type of ventricular tachycardia called *torsades de pointes*.

Artifact is interference seen on the monitor or rhythm strip, which may look like a wandering or fuzzy baseline. It can be caused by patient movement, loose or defective electrodes,

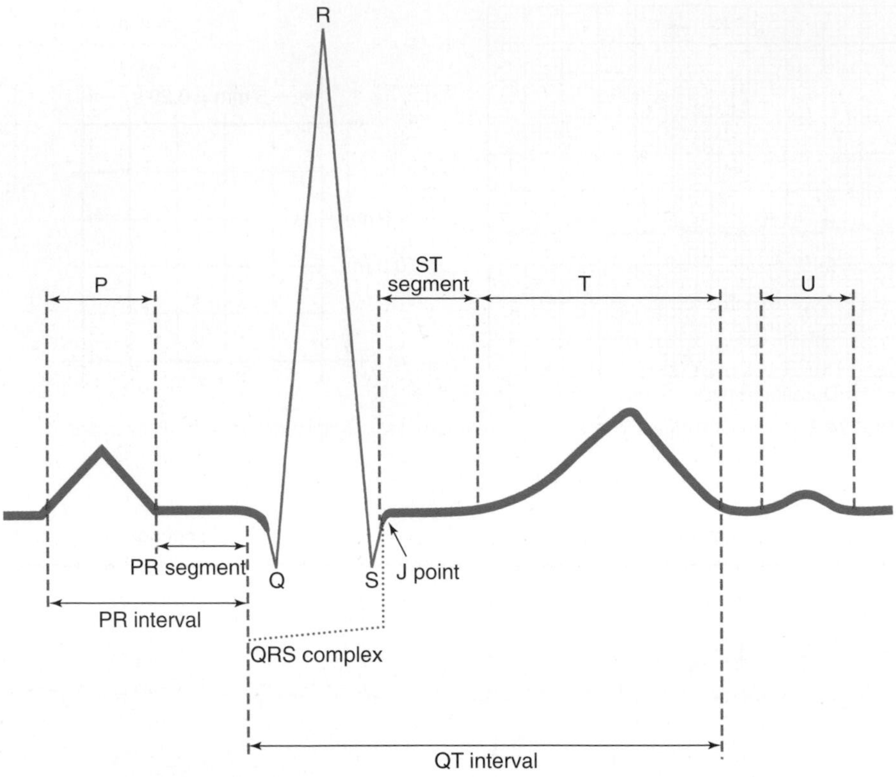

P wave:	Represents atrial depolarization.
PR segment:	Represents the time required for the impulse to travel through the AV node, where it is delayed, and through the bundle of His, bundle branches, and Purkinje fiber network, just before ventricular depolarization.
PR interval:	Represents the time required for atrial depolarization as well as impulse travel through the conduction system and Purkinje fiber network, inclusive of the P wave and PR segment. It is measured from the beginning of the P wave to the end of the PR segment.
QRS complex:	Represents ventricular depolarization and is measured from the beginning of the Q (or R) wave to the end of the S wave.
J point:	Represents the junction where the QRS complex ends and the ST segment begins.
ST segment:	Represents early ventricular repolarization.
T wave:	Represents ventricular repolarization.
U wave:	Represents late ventricular repolarization.
QT interval:	Represents the total time required for ventricular depolarization and repolarization and is measured from the beginning of the QRS complex to the end of the T wave.

FIG. 34-5 The components of a normal electrocardiogram.

improper grounding, or faulty ECG equipment, such as broken wires or cables. Some artifact can mimic lethal dysrhythmias like ventricular tachycardia (with tooth brushing) or ventricular fibrillation (with tapping on the electrode). *Assess the patient to differentiate artifact from actual lethal rhythms! Do not rely only on the ECG monitor.*

Determination of Heart Rate

The heart rate can be estimated by counting the number of QRS complexes in 6 seconds and multiplying that number by 10 to calculate the rate for a full minute. This is called the *6-second strip method* and is a quick method to determine the mean or average heart rate. This method is the least accurate; however, it is the method of choice for irregular rhythms.

For accuracy, the *big block method* is used if the QRS complexes are regular or evenly spaced. Count the number of big blocks between the same point in any two successive QRS complexes (usually R wave to R wave) and divide into 300. There are 300 big blocks in 1 minute. It is easiest to use a QRS that falls on a dark line. If little blocks are left over when counting big blocks, count each little block as 0.2, add this to the number of big blocks, and then divide that total into 300 (Fig. 34-6).

Count the number of large blocks in an interval and divide into 300 (the number of large blocks in 1 minute). For example, three large blocks equals a heart rate of 100 beats per minute ($300 \div 3 = 100$).

Another method (called the *memory method*) relies on memorizing this sequence: 300, 150, 100, 75, 60, 50, 43, 37, 33, 30. This is the big block method with the math already done. Find a QRS complex that falls on the dark line representing 0.2 second or a big block, and count backwards to the next QRS complex. Each dark line is a memorized number. This is the method most widely used in hospitals for calculating heart rates for regular rhythms.

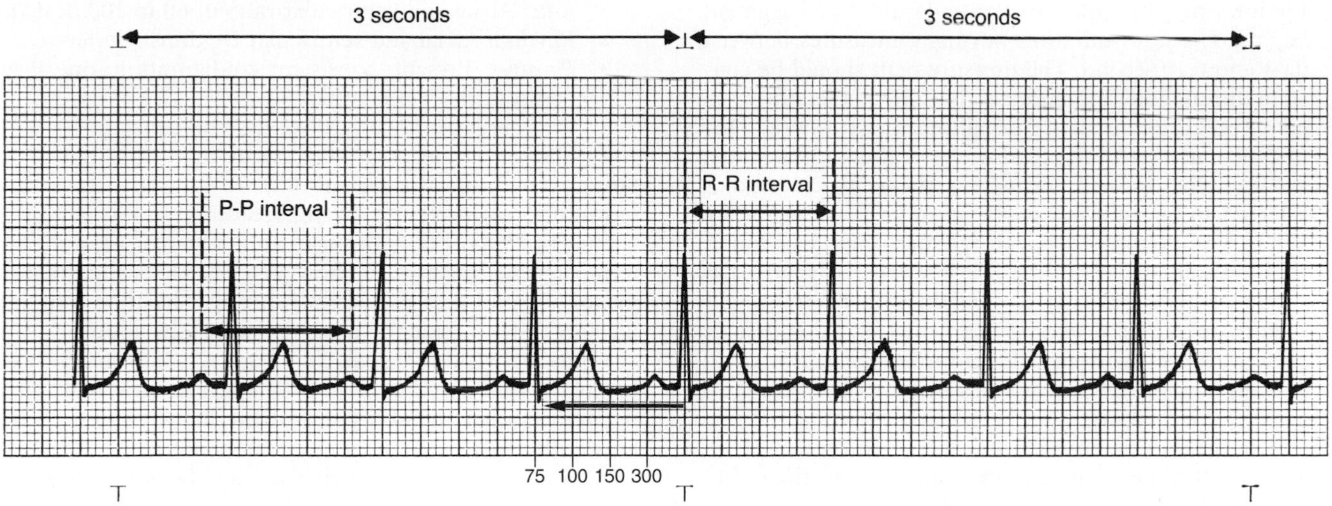

FIG. 34-6 In this example, the heart rate using the big block method is 300 ÷ 4 big blocks (between QRS complexes), or 75 beats per minute. The memory method is also demonstrated with a heart rate of 75 beats per minute.

Commercially prepared ECG rate rulers are based on these calculations and may be used for regular rhythms. Current monitoring systems will display a continuous heart rate and print the heart rate on the ECG strip. *Use caution and confirm that the rate is correct by assessing the patient's heart rate directly.* Many factors can incorrectly alter the rate displayed by the monitor.

Electrocardiographic Rhythm Analysis

Analysis of an ECG rhythm strip requires a systematic approach using an eight-step method facilitated by use of a measurement tool called an **ECG caliper** (Palmer, 2011):

1. ***Determine the heart rate.*** If the atrial and ventricular rhythms are regular, use any of the methods previously described to calculate the heart rate. If the rhythms are irregular, use the 6-second strip method for accuracy. Normal heart rates fall between 60 and 100 beats/min. A rate less than 60 beats/min is called **bradycardia**. A rate greater than 100 beats/min is called **tachycardia**.
2. ***Determine the heart rhythm.*** Assess for atrial and/or ventricular regularity. Heart rhythms can be either regular or irregular. Irregular rhythms can be regularly irregular, occasionally irregular, or irregularly irregular. Check the regularity of the atrial rhythm by assessing the PP intervals, placing one caliper point on a P wave and placing the other point on the precise spot on the next P wave. Then move the caliper from P wave to P wave along the entire strip ("walking out" the P waves) to determine the regularity of the rhythm. P waves of a different shape (ectopic waves), if present, create an irregularity and do not walk out with the other P waves. A slight irregularity in the PP intervals, varying no more than three small blocks, is considered essentially regular if the P waves are all of the same shape. This alteration is caused by changes in intrathoracic pressure during the respiratory cycle.

   Check the regularity of the ventricular rhythm by assessing the RR intervals, placing one caliper point on a portion of the QRS complex (usually the most prominent portion of the deflection) and the other point on the precise spot of the next QRS complex. Move the caliper from QRS complex to QRS complex along the entire strip (walking out the QRS complexes) to determine the regularity of the rhythm. QRS complexes of a different shape (ectopic QRS complexes), if present, create an irregularity and do not walk out with the other QRS complexes. A slight irregularity of no more than three small blocks between intervals is considered essentially regular if the QRS complexes are all of the same shape.
3. ***Analyze the P waves.*** Check that the P-wave shape is consistent throughout the strip, indicating that atrial depolarization is occurring from impulses originating from one focus, normally the SA node. Determine whether there is one P wave occurring before each QRS complex, establishing that a relationship exists between the P wave and the QRS complex. This relationship indicates that an impulse from one focus is responsible for both atrial and ventricular depolarization. The nurse may observe more than one P wave shape, more P waves than QRS complexes, absent P waves, or P waves coming after the QRS, each indicating that a dysrhythmia exists. Ask these five questions when analyzing P waves:
   - Are P waves present?
   - Are the P waves occurring regularly?
   - Is there one P wave for each QRS complex?
   - Are the P waves smooth, rounded, and upright in appearance, or are they inverted?
   - Do all the P waves look similar?
4. ***Measure the PR interval.*** Place one caliper point at the beginning of the P wave and the other point at the end of the PR segment. The PR interval normally measures between 0.12 and 0.20 second. The measurement should be constant throughout the strip. The PR interval cannot be determined if there are no P waves or if P waves occur after the QRS complex. Ask these three questions about the PR interval:
   - Are PR intervals greater than 0.20 second?
   - Are PR intervals less than 0.12 second?
   - Are PR intervals constant across the ECG strip?
5. ***Measure the QRS duration.*** Place one caliper point at the beginning of the QRS complex and the other at the

J point, where the QRS complex ends and the ST segment begins. The QRS duration normally measures between 0.04 and 0.10 second. The measurement should be constant throughout the entire strip. Check that the QRS complexes are consistent throughout the strip. When the QRS is narrow (0.10 second or less), this indicates that the impulse was not formed in the ventricles and is referred to as supraventricular or above the ventricles. When the QRS complex is wide (greater than 0.10 second), this indicates that the impulse is either of ventricular origin or of supraventricular origin with aberrant conduction, meaning deviating from the normal course or pattern. More than one QRS complex pattern or occasionally missing QRS complexes may be observed, indicating a dysrhythmia.

Ask these questions to evaluate QRS intervals:

- Are QRS intervals less than or greater than 0.12 second?
- Are the QRS complexes similar in appearance across the ECG paper?

6. ***Examine the ST segment.*** The normal ST segment begins at the isoelectric line. ST elevation or depression is significant if displacement is 1 mm (one small box) or more above or below the line and is seen in two or more leads. ST elevation may indicate problems such as myocardial infarction, pericarditis, and hyperkalemia. ST depression is associated with hypokalemia, myocardial infarction, or ventricular hypertrophy.
7. ***Assess the T wave.*** Note the shape and height of the T wave for peaking or inversion. Abnormal T waves may indicate problems such as myocardial infarction and ventricular hypertrophy.
8. ***Measure the QT interval.*** A normal QT interval should be equal to or less than one-half the distance of the R-to-R interval.

Using steps 1 through 8, you can interpret the cardiac rhythm and differentiate normal and abnormal cardiac rhythms (dysrhythmias).

OVERVIEW OF NORMAL CARDIAC RHYTHMS

Normal sinus rhythm (NSR) is the rhythm originating from the sinoatrial (SA) node (dominant pacemaker) that meets these ECG criteria (Fig. 34-7):

- *Rate:* Atrial and ventricular rates of 60 to 100 beats/min
- *Rhythm:* Atrial and ventricular rhythms regular
- *P waves:* Present, consistent configuration, one P wave before each QRS complex
- *PR interval:* 0.12 to 0.20 second and constant
- *QRS duration:* 0.04 to 0.10 second and constant

Sinus arrhythmia is a variant of NSR. It results from changes in intrathoracic pressure during breathing. In this context, the term *arrhythmia* does not mean an absence of rhythm, as the term suggests. Instead, the heart rate increases slightly during inspiration and decreases slightly during exhalation. This irregular rhythm is frequently observed in healthy adults.

Sinus arrhythmia has all the characteristics of NSR except for its irregularity. The PP and RR intervals vary, with the difference between the shortest and the longest intervals being greater than 0.12 second (three small blocks):

- *Rate:* Atrial and ventricular rates between 60 and 100 beats/min
- *Rhythm:* Atrial and ventricular rhythms irregular, with the shortest PP or RR interval varying at least 0.12 second from the longest PP or RR interval
- *P waves:* One P wave before each QRS complex; consistent configuration
- *PR interval:* Normal, constant
- *QRS duration:* Normal, constant

Sinus arrhythmias occasionally are due to nonrespiratory causes, such as digitalis or morphine. These drugs enhance vagal tone and cause decreased heart rate and irregularity unrelated to the respiratory cycle.

COMMON DYSRHYTHMIAS

Any disorder of the heartbeat is called a **dysrhythmia**. Historically, the term *arrhythmia* has been used in the literature. Although the terms are often used interchangeably, *dysrhythmia* is more accurate. Although many dysrhythmias have no clinical manifestations, many others have serious consequences if not treated.

❖ *PATHOPHYSIOLOGY*

Dysrhythmias are classified in several ways. As broad categories, they include premature complexes, bradydysrhythmias (bradycardias), and tachydysrhythmias (tachycardias). **Premature complexes** are early rhythm complexes. They occur when a

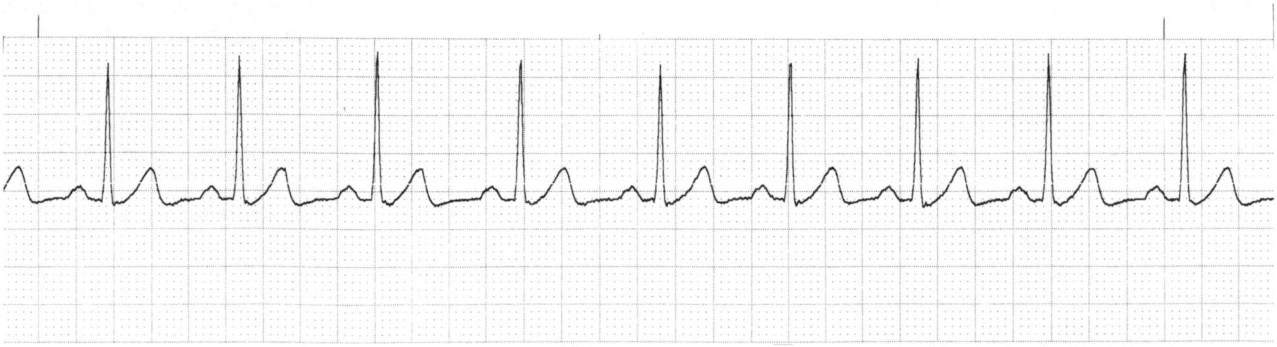

FIG. 34-7 Normal sinus rhythm. Both atrial and ventricular rhythms are essentially regular (a slight variation in rhythm is normal). Atrial and ventricular rates are both 87 beats per minute. There is one P wave before each QRS complex, and all the P waves are of a consistent morphology, or shape. The PR interval measures 0.18 second and is constant; the QRS complex measures 0.06 second and is constant.

cardiac cell or cell group, other than the sinoatrial (SA) node, becomes irritable and fires an impulse before the next sinus impulse is produced. The abnormal focus is called an *ectopic focus* and may be generated by atrial, junctional, or ventricular tissue. After the premature complex, there is a pause before the next normal complex, creating an irregularity in the rhythm. The patient with premature complexes may be unaware of them or may feel **palpitations** or a "skipping" of the heartbeat. If premature complexes, especially those that are ventricular, become more frequent, the patient may experience symptoms of decreased cardiac output.

Premature complexes may occur *repetitively in a rhythmic fashion:*

- **Bigeminy** exists when normal complexes and premature complexes occur alternately in a repetitive two-beat pattern, with a pause occurring after each premature complex so that complexes occur in pairs.
- **Trigeminy** is a repeated three-beat pattern, usually occurring as two sequential normal complexes followed by a premature complex and a pause, with the same pattern repeating itself in triplets.
- **Quadrigeminy** is a repeated four-beat pattern, usually occurring as three sequential normal complexes followed by a premature complex and a pause, with the same pattern repeating itself in a four-beat pattern.

Bradydysrhythmias occur when the heart rate is less than 60 beats per minute. These rhythms can also be significant because:

- Myocardial oxygen demand is reduced from the slow heart rate, which can be beneficial.
- Coronary perfusion time may be adequate because of a prolonged diastole, which is desirable.
- Coronary perfusion pressure may decrease if the heart rate is too slow to provide adequate cardiac output and blood pressure; this is a serious consequence.

Therefore the patient may tolerate the bradydysrhythmia well if the blood pressure is adequate. If the blood pressure is not adequate, symptomatic bradydysrhythmias may lead to myocardial ischemia or infarction, dysrhythmias, hypotension, and heart failure.

Tachydysrhythmias are heart rates greater than 100 beats per minute. They are a major concern in the adult patient with coronary artery disease (CAD). Coronary artery blood flow occurs mostly during diastole when the aortic valve is closed and is determined by diastolic time and blood pressure in the root of the aorta. Tachydysrhythmias are serious because they:

- Shorten the diastolic time and therefore the coronary perfusion time (the amount of time available for blood to flow through the coronary arteries to the myocardium).
- Initially increase cardiac output and blood pressure. However, a continued rise in heart rate decreases the ventricular filling time because of a shortened diastole, decreasing the stroke volume. Consequently, cardiac output and blood pressure will begin to decrease, reducing aortic pressure and therefore coronary PERFUSION pressure.
- Increase the work of the heart, increasing myocardial oxygen demand.

The patient with a tachydysrhythmia may have:

- Palpitations
- Chest discomfort (pressure or pain from myocardial ischemia or infarction)

CHART 34-1 Key Features

Sustained Tachydysrhythmias and Bradydysrhythmias

- Chest discomfort, pressure, or pain, which may radiate to the jaw, the back, or the arm
- Restlessness, anxiety, nervousness, confusion
- Dizziness, syncope
- Palpitations (in tachydysrhythmias)
- Change in pulse strength, rate, and rhythm
- Pulse deficit
- Shortness of breath, dyspnea
- Tachypnea
- Pulmonary crackles
- Orthopnea
- S_3 or S_4 heart sounds
- Jugular venous distention
- Weakness, fatigue
- Pale, cool, skin; diaphoresis
- Nausea, vomiting
- Decreased urine output
- Delayed capillary refill
- Hypotension

- Restlessness and anxiety
- Pale, cool skin
- Syncope ("blackout") from hypotension

Tachydysrhythmias may also lead to heart failure. Presenting symptoms of heart failure may include dyspnea, lung crackles, distended neck veins, fatigue, and weakness (see Chapter 35). Chart 34-1 summarizes key features of sustained bradydysrhythmias and tachydysrhythmias.

Etiology

Dysrhythmias occur for many reasons, including myocardial infarction (MI), electrolyte imbalances (especially potassium and magnesium), hypoxia, drug toxicity, and hypovolemia (decreased blood volume). People who use cocaine and illicit inhalants are particularly at risk for potentially fatal dysrhythmias. Stress, fear, anxiety, and caffeine can cause an increased heart rate (tachycardia or premature ventricular contractions). Nicotine and alcohol excess can lead to abnormal heart rates such as atrial fibrillation. Specific etiologies are described for each common dysrhythmia discussed in this chapter.

❖ PATIENT-CENTERED COLLABORATIVE CARE

Dysrhythmias may also be classified by their site of origin in the heart. These include common sinus, atrial, and ventricular dysrhythmias. Although there are many specific dysrhythmias that can occur, general assessment and interventions for patient care may be similar (Chart 34-2). Assess the patient's apical and radial pulses for a full minute for any irregularity, which may occur with premature beats or atrial fibrillation. If the apical pulse differs from the radial pulse rate, a **pulse deficit** exists and indicates that the heart is not pumping adequately to achieve optimal PERFUSION to the body.

Dysrhythmias are often managed with antidysrhythmic drug therapy. Specific drugs and other treatments are discussed for common dysrhythmias starting on p. 667.

Drug Classifications

When dysrhythmias are sustained and/or life threatening, drug therapy from one or more classes of antidysrhythmic agents is

CHART 34-2 **Best Practice for Patient Safety & Quality Care** QSEN

Care of the Patient with Dysrhythmias

- Assess vital signs at least every 4 hours and as needed.
- Monitor patient for cardiac dysrhythmias.
- Evaluate and document the patient's response to dysrhythmias.
- Encourage the patient to notify the nurse when chest pain occurs.
- Assess chest pain (e.g., location, intensity, duration, radiation, and precipitating and alleviating factors).
- Assess peripheral circulation (e.g., palpate for presence of peripheral pulses, edema, capillary refill, color, and temperature of extremity).
- Provide antidysrhythmic therapy according to unit policy (e.g., antidysrhythmic medication, cardioversion, or defibrillation), as appropriate.
- Monitor and document patient's response to antidysrhythmic medications or interventions.
- Monitor appropriate laboratory values (e.g., cardiac enzymes, electrolyte levels).
- Monitor the patient's activity tolerance and schedule exercise/rest periods to avoid fatigue.
- Observe for respiratory difficulty (e.g., shortness of breath, rapid breathing, labored respirations).
- Promote stress reduction.
- Offer spiritual support to the patient and/or family (e.g., contact clergy), as appropriate.

often used (Chart 34-3). The **Vaughn-Williams classification** is commonly used to categorize drugs according to their effects on the action potential of cardiac cells (classes I though IV). Other drugs also have antidysrhythmic effects but do not fit the Vaughn-Williams classification.

Class I antidysrhythmics are membrane-stabilizing agents used to decrease automaticity. The three subclassifications in this group include type IA drugs, which moderately slow conduction and prolong repolarization, prolonging the QT interval. These drugs are used to treat or to prevent supraventricular and ventricular premature beats and tachydysrhythmias, but they are not as commonly used as other drugs. An example is procainamide hydrochloride (Pronestyl). Type IB drugs shorten repolarization. These drugs are used to treat or prevent ventricular premature beats, ventricular tachycardia (VT), and ventricular fibrillation (VF). Examples include lidocaine and mexiletine hydrochloride (Mexitil). Type IC drugs markedly slow conduction and widen the QRS complex. These agents are used primarily to treat or to prevent recurrent, life-threatening ventricular premature beats, VT, and VF. Examples include flecainide acetate (Tambocor) and propafenone hydrochloride (Rythmol).

Class II antidysrhythmics control dysrhythmias associated with excessive beta-adrenergic stimulation by competing for

CHART 34-3 **Common Examples of Drug Therapy**

Common Dysrhythmias

DRUG	USUAL DOSAGE	NURSING INTERVENTIONS	RATIONALES
Class I Drugs			
Type IA			
Disopyramide phosphate (Norpace)	100-200 mg orally every 6 hr	Monitor BP.	Hypotension is a common side effect.
Used for AF, WPW syndrome, PSVT, PVCs, VT		Watch for shortness of breath and weight gain.	Disopyramide can cause heart failure in a patient with CAD.
		Monitor for widening QRS complex, prolonged QT or PR interval, or heart block.	Toxic side effects necessitate stopping disopyramide administration.
Type IB			
Lidocaine (Xylocaine) Used for PVCs, VT, VF	1-1.5 mg/kg IV bolus, then 0.5-0.75 mg/kg IV boluses every 5-10 min to a loading dose of 3 mg/kg, followed by 2-4 mg/min infusion For VF or pulseless VT: 1-1.5 mg/kg IV bolus every 3-5 min to a loading dose of 3 mg/kg, followed by 1-4 mg/min infusion	Watch for confusion, paresthesias, slurring of speech, drowsiness, or seizure activity.	CNS adverse effects predominate; they may require a decrease in dosage or discontinuation of the infusion.
Mexiletine hydrochloride (Mexitil)	200-300 mg orally every 8 hr with food	Monitor BP and heart rate.	Hypotension and bradycardia may occur.
Used for PVCs, VT, VF	125-250 mg IV bolus over 5-10 min 0.5-1.5 mg/min infusion	Assess for tremors, blurred vision, dizziness, ataxia, or confusion.	CNS adverse reactions predominate.
Tocainide hydrochloride (Tonocard)	400 mg orally every 8 hr initially	Watch for tremors.	Tremors indicate that the maximum dose is being approached.
Used for PVCs, VT, VF	Increase to 800 mg orally every 8 hr if needed Maximum of 2.4 g daily	Monitor heart rate and BP.	Bradycardia and hypotension may occur.
	Take with food	Teach patient to report shortness of breath, wheezing, chest pain, or cough, as well as dyspnea and distended neck veins or swelling of the extremities.	Pulmonary fibrosis is a serious side effect, which necessitates discontinuation of the drug; the drug may also cause CHF.

CHART 34-3 Common Examples of Drug Therapy—cont'd

Common Dysrhythmias

DRUG	USUAL DOSAGE	NURSING INTERVENTIONS	RATIONALES
Type IC			
Flecainide acetate (Tambocor) Used for AF, PSVT, life-threatening ventricular dysrhythmias	100 mg orally twice daily Maximum dose of 400 mg daily	Monitor for an increase in frequency and severity of dysrhythmias. Monitor heart rate and BP. Monitor for CHF, dizziness, visual disturbances, paresthesias, and tremors.	Flecainide can induce dysrhythmias. Bradycardia and hypotension may occur. Side effects may require a decrease in dosage or discontinuation of the drug.
Propafenone hydrochloride (Rythmol) Used for PAF, WPW syndrome, life-threatening ventricular dysrhythmias	150-300 mg orally every 8 hr	Monitor for an increase in dysrhythmias. Monitor heart rate and BP. Monitor for CNS effects, dizziness, anxiety, ataxia, insomnia, confusion, and seizures, as well as CHF and GI distress.	Propafenone can induce dysrhythmias. Bradycardia and hypotension may occur. Side effects may require a decrease in dosage or discontinuation of the drug.
Class II Drugs			
Propranolol hydrochloride (Inderal, Apo-Propranolol 🍁) Used for AF, atrial flutter, PSVT, PVCs	10-80 mg orally four times daily before meals 0.1 mg/kg slow IV bolus divided into 3 equal doses given at intervals of 2-3 min at rate of 1 mg/min	Monitor heart rate and BP. Assess for shortness of breath or wheezing. Assess for insomnia, fatigue, and dizziness.	Bradycardia and decreased BP are expected effects. Beta$_2$-blocking effects on the lungs can cause bronchospasm. Side effects may require decrease in dosage or discontinuation of the drug.
Acebutolol hydrochloride (Sectral) Used for AF, atrial flutter, PSVT, PVCs	600-1200 mg orally daily	Monitor heart rate and BP. Assess for shortness of breath or wheezing. Assess for insomnia, fatigue, and dizziness.	Bradycardia and decreased BP are expected effects. Beta$_2$-blocking effects on the lungs can cause bronchospasm. Side effects may require a decrease in dosage or discontinuation of the drug.
Esmolol hydrochloride (Brevibloc) Used for AF, atrial flutter, PSVT, PVCs	Initially, 500 mcg/kg/min over 1 min, then 50 mcg/kg/min for 4 min IV Titrate up if necessary	Monitor heart rate and BP. Assess for shortness of breath or wheezing. Assess for insomnia, fatigue, and seizures.	Bradycardia and decreased BP are expected effects. Beta$_2$-blocking effects on the lungs can cause bronchospasm. Side effects may require a decrease in dosage or discontinuation of the drug.
Sotalol hydrochloride (Betapace) Used for AF, PAF, PSVT, life-threatening ventricular dysrhythmias	Initial dose of 80 mg orally twice daily Dosage may be increased every 2-3 days, if necessary, to 240-320 mg daily in 2-3 divided doses	Assess ECG rhythm for torsades de pointes and other serious new ventricular dysrhythmias. Assess for fatigue, bradycardia, dyspnea, CHF, chest pain, hypotension, dizziness, hypoglycemia, nausea, and vomiting. Sotalol should not be administered to patients with hypokalemia or hypomagnesemia before correction of these imbalances. Sotalol is contraindicated in patients with bronchial asthma, sinus bradycardia, or second- and third-degree AV block (unless a functioning pacemaker is present), prolonged QT syndrome, cardiogenic shock, or CHF.	Sotalol may have proarrhythmic effects. Adverse reactions may warrant drug discontinuation. Hypokalemia or hypomagnesemia may prolong the QT interval and cause torsades de pointes. Sotalol has beta-blocking (class II) effects and class III effects.

Continued

CHART 34-3 **Common Examples of Drug Therapy—cont'd**

Common Dysrhythmias

DRUG	USUAL DOSAGE	NURSING INTERVENTIONS	RATIONALES
Class III Drugs			
Amiodarone hydrochloride (Cordarone) Used for AF, PAF, PSVT, life-threatening ventricular dysrhythmias	800-1600 mg orally daily in divided doses for 1-3 wk, then 600-800 mg daily for 1 mo, then 200-600 mg daily (average of 400 mg daily) Rapid loading dose: 150 mg IV over first 10 min (15 mg/min); slow loading dose: 360 mg IV over next 6 hr (1 mg/min); maintenance infusion: 540 mg IV over next 18 hr (0.5 mg/min), then 720 mg/24 hr (0.5 mg/min) For pulseless VT/Vfib: 300 mg IV/IO push; may repeat 150 mg IV/IO if necessary	Use volumetric infusion pump and polyvinyl chloride tubing with in-line filter, and infuse via central line.	Drug is irritating to peripheral vasculature; drug is more stable in glass bottle.
		Rapid-loading IV dose must not be administered faster than 10 min. Must stay with patient and monitor heart rate and BP.	Hypotension may occur. It should be treated by slowing the infusion or using other standard therapy. Cordarone should not be discontinued unless necessary.
		Continually monitor ECG rhythm during IV infusion; measure QT and QTc.	Bradycardia and AV block may occur and are treated by slowing the infusion rate and providing pacemaker therapy, if necessary. May cause a worsening of ventricular dysrhythmias.
		Assess the patient's knowledge of the treatment regimen and side effects.	Drug has major side effects, which make noncompliance a problem; patients may take the drug for 1½-3 mo before full clinical effects are apparent.
		Monitor heart rate, BP, and cardiac rhythm when initiating therapy.	Bradycardia, hypotension, and worsening dysrhythmia can occur.
		Teach patients to report any muscle weakness, tremors, or difficulty with ambulation.	Muscle-related side effects usually develop during the first week of treatment.
		Teach patients to report shortness of breath, cough, pleuritic pain, or fever.	Pulmonary side effects may indicate drug-induced pulmonary toxicity.
		Teach patients to report any visual disturbances and to wear sunglasses outdoors in the daytime if they have photophobia.	Corneal pigmentation occurs in most patients but generally does not interfere with vision; if it does, the dosage is decreased.
		Teach patients to use barrier sunscreens.	Photosensitivity reactions may occur.
		Teach patients to report any signs of thyroid problems or hepatotoxicity.	Thyroid problems or hepatotoxicity may occur, necessitating a decrease in dosage or discontinuation of the drug.
Dronedarone (Multaq) Used for AF, atrial flutter	400 mg twice daily with meals	Monitor heart rate, BP, and cardiac rhythm when initiating therapy.	Bradycardia and worsening dysrhythmia can occur.
		Monitor BUN, creatinine, and liver function panel.	May cause worsening renal function. Drug is contraindicated for patients with severe hepatic impairment.
		Teach patients to take with a meal. Do not take with grapefruit juice.	Better absorbed with food. Grapefruit juice alters drug effectiveness.
		Teach patients to notify the doctor if signs of worsening heart failure such as weight gain, dependent edema, or increasing shortness of breath.	Drug is contraindicated for patients with heart failure.
		Teach patients that if a dose is missed, take at next regularly scheduled dose. Do not double dose.	
		Advise patients to report all medications to doctor (prescription, OTC, and herbal products, especially St. John's wort).	May have serious drug interaction and cause potentially fatal dysrhythmias.

CHART 34-3 Common Examples of Drug Therapy—cont'd

Common Dysrhythmias

DRUG	USUAL DOSAGE	NURSING INTERVENTIONS	RATIONALES
Ibutilide fumarate (Corvert) Used for AF, atrial flutter	1 mg IV over 10 min for patients >60 kg; 0.01 mg/kg over 10 min for patients <60 kg May repeat dose 10 min after completion of first infusion if necessary	Stop infusion as soon as dysrhythmia is terminated, or in event of sustained or nonsustained VT, or marked prolongation of QT or QTc.	Drug may cause potentially fatal dysrhythmias.
		Observe patients with continuous ECG monitoring and measure QT or QTc for at least 4 hr after infusion or until QTc has returned to baseline.	Acute ventricular dysrhythmias must be promptly identified and treated. Patient may develop heart blocks.
		Patients with atrial fibrillation of >2-3 days' duration must be adequately anticoagulated for at least 2 wk.	Atrial fibrillation is associated with formation of thrombi in atrial chambers.
		Hypokalemia and hypomagnesemia must be corrected before Corvert infusion.	This is important to reduce potential for proarrhythmic effects.
Dofetilide (Tikosyn) Used for AF, atrial flutter	125-500 mcg orally twice daily	Teach patients to change positions slowly.	Orthostatic hypotension is a common side effect of the drug.
		Inform patients that dosages will be adjusted, depending on their creatinine clearance level.	The patient must have adequate creatinine clearance to prevent drug toxicity.
		Monitor patients on telemetry for several days; observe for and report bradycardia and hypotension.	Bradycardia and hypotension are common side effects.
Class IV Drugs			
Verapamil hydrochloride (Calan, Isoptin 🍁) Used for AF, atrial flutter, PSVT	2.5-5 mg IV over 1-2 min for narrow-complex SVT or PSVT; after 15-30 min may give 5-10 mg IV over 1-2 min, if necessary, and repeat to a maximum of 20 mg 80-120 mg orally every 6-8 hr	Monitor heart rate and BP.	Bradycardia and hypotension are common side effects.
		Teach patients to remain recumbent for at least 1 hr after IV administration.	Hypotension may occur; may be reversed with calcium chloride ($CaCl_2$), 0.5-1 g slow IV.
		Teach patients to change positions slowly when receiving oral therapy.	Dizziness and orthostatic hypotension often occur until tolerance develops.
		Teach patients to report dyspnea, orthopnea, distended neck veins, or swelling of the extremities.	Heart failure may occur, necessitating a decrease in dosage or discontinuation of the drug.
Diltiazem hydrochloride (Cardizem) Used for AF, atrial flutter, PSVT	0.25 mg/kg IV over 2 min After 15 min, give 0.35 mg/kg IV over 2 min 5-15 mg/hr IV infusion	Monitor heart rate and BP.	Bradycardia and hypotension are common side effects.
		Teach patients to remain recumbent for at least 1 hr after IV administration.	Hypotension may occur.
		Teach patients to report dyspnea, orthopnea, distended neck veins, or swelling of the extremities.	Heart failure may occur, necessitating a decrease in dosage or discontinuation of the drug.
Other Drugs			
Digoxin (Lanoxin, Novo-Digoxin 🍁) Used for CHF, AF, atrial flutter, PSVT	Rapid digitalization: 0.5-1 mg orally or IV initially; 0.125-0.5 mg orally every 6 hr or IV until a total of 1-1.5 mg is reached Maintenance: 0.125-0.25 mg orally or IV daily or every other day (may be less for older adults)	Assess apical heart rate for 1 min before each dose.	Decreased heart rate is an expected response, but bradycardia may indicate toxicity.
		Assess for sudden increase in heart rate and change of rhythm from regular to irregular, or irregular to regular.	Changes in heart rate or rhythm may indicate toxicity.
		Teach patients to report anorexia, nausea, vomiting, diarrhea, paresthesias, confusion, or visual disturbances.	Side effect can indicate toxicity.
		Monitor serum potassium levels.	Hypokalemia increases the risk for toxicity and ventricular dysrhythmias.
		Monitor serum creatinine levels.	Impaired renal function can cause toxicity; the dosage is altered if this occurs.

Contiuned

CHART 34-3 **Common Examples of Drug Therapy—cont'd**

Common Dysrhythmias

DRUG	USUAL DOSAGE	NURSING INTERVENTIONS	RATIONALES
Atropine sulfate Used for bradycardia	0.5 mg IV bolus may be repeated every 3-5 min, if necessary, to a maximum of 0.04 mg/kg (total 3 mg)	Monitor heart rate and rhythm after administration.	Increased heart rate is expected.
		Assess for chest pain after administration.	Increased heart rate may cause ischemia in patients with CAD.
		Assess for urinary retention and dry mouth after administration.	Atropine is an anticholinergic agent.
		Avoid using in patients with acute angle-closure glaucoma.	Atropine increases intraocular pressure.
Adenosine (Adenocard) Used for PSVT, WPW syndrome	6 mg rapid IV over 1-3 sec followed by 20-mL saline flush; repeat in 1-2 min at 12 mg IV over 1-3 sec with 20-mL flush	Monitor heart rate and rhythm after administration.	A short period of asystole is common after administration; bradycardia and hypotension may occur.
		Assess patients for facial flushing, shortness of breath, dyspnea, and chest pain.	These side effects commonly occur.
		Assess patients for recurrence of PSVT or ventricular ectopy.	Recurrence of PSVT is common; PVCs may occur.
Magnesium sulfate Used for torsades de pointes	1-2 g diluted in 100 mL of D_5W administered IV over 1-2 min for VF or VT 1-2 g in 50-100 mL of D_5W for 5-60 min for loading dose; 0.5-1 g/hr over 24 hr for supplementation	Assess ECG rhythm for conversion to sinus rhythm.	Hypomagnesemia may precipitate refractory VF.
		Assess patients for facial flushing, hypotension, and respiratory and CNS depression.	Magnesium sulfate causes vasodilation and respiratory and CNS depression.

AF, Atrial fibrillation; *AV,* atrioventricular; *BP,* blood pressure; *BUN,* blood urea nitrogen; *CAD,* coronary artery disease; *CHF,* congestive heart failure; *CNS,* central nervous system; *D_5W,* 5% dextrose in water; *ECG,* electrocardiogram; *EMD,* electromechanical dissociation; *IO,* intraosseous; *OTC,* over-the-counter; *PAF,* paroxysmal atrial fibrillation/flutter; *PSVT,* paroxysmal supraventricular tachycardia; *PVC,* premature ventricular complex; *SVT,* supraventricular tachycardia; *V fib,* ventricular fibrillation; *VF,* ventricular fibrillation; *VT,* ventricular tachycardia; *WPW syndrome,* Wolff-Parkinson-White syndrome.

receptor sites and thereby decreasing heart rate and conduction velocity. Beta-adrenergic blocking agents, such as propranolol (Inderal) and esmolol hydrochloride (Brevibloc), are class II drugs. They are used to treat or to prevent supraventricular and ventricular premature beats and tachydysrhythmias. Sotalol hydrochloride (Betapace, Sotacor ♣) is an antidysrhythmic agent with both non-cardioselective beta-adrenergic blocking effects (class II) and action potential duration prolongation properties (class III). It is an oral agent that may be used for the treatment of documented ventricular dysrhythmias, such as VT, that are life threatening.

Class III antidysrhythmics lengthen the absolute refractory period and prolong repolarization and the action potential duration of ischemic cells. Class III drugs include amiodarone (Cordarone) and ibutilide (Corvert) and are used to treat or prevent ventricular premature beats, VT, and VF.

Class IV antidysrhythmics slow the flow of calcium into the cell during depolarization, thereby depressing the automaticity of the sinoatrial (SA) and atrioventricular (AV) nodes, decreasing the heart rate, and prolonging the AV nodal refractory period and conduction. Calcium channel blockers, such as verapamil hydrochloride (Calan, Isoptin ♣) and diltiazem hydrochloride (Cardizem), are class IV drugs. They are used to treat supraventricular tachycardia (SVT) and atrial fibrillation (AF) to slow the ventricular response.

Other drugs, such as digoxin, atropine, adenosine, and magnesium sulfate, may be used to treat dysrhythmias. Digoxin (Lanoxin, Novo-Digoxin ♣) increases vagal tone, slowing AV nodal conduction. It is useful in treating chronic AF by controlling the rate of ventricular response. However, digoxin does not convert AF to sinus rhythm. Atropine is a parasympatholytic or vagolytic agent used to treat vagally induced symptomatic bradydysrhythmias. Adenosine is an endogenous nucleoside that slows AV nodal conduction to interrupt re-entry pathways. Magnesium sulfate is an electrolyte administered to treat refractory VT or VF because these patients may be hypomagnesemic, with increased ventricular irritability. The drug is also used for a life-threatening VT called **torsades de pointes** that can result from certain antidysrhythmics, such as amiodarone.

Sinus Dysrhythmias

The sinoatrial (SA) node in the right atrium is the pacemaker in all sinus dysrhythmias. Innervation from sympathetic and parasympathetic nerves is normally in balance to ensure a normal sinus rhythm (NSR). An imbalance increases or decreases the rate of SA node discharge either as a normal response to activity or physiologic changes or as a pathologic response to disease. Sinus tachycardia and sinus bradycardia are the two most common types of sinus dysrhythmias.

Sinus Tachycardia. Sympathetic nervous system stimulation or vagal (parasympathetic) inhibition results in an increased rate of SA node discharge, which increases the heart rate. When the rate of SA node discharge is more than 100 beats per minute, the rhythm is called **sinus tachycardia** (Fig. 34-8, *A*). From age 10 years to adulthood, the heart rate normally does not exceed 100 beats per minute except in response to activity and then usually does not exceed 160 beats per minute. Rarely does the heart rate reach 180 beats per minute.

Sinus tachycardia initially increases cardiac output and blood pressure. However, continued increases in heart rate decrease coronary PERFUSION time, diastolic filling time, and coronary perfusion pressure while increasing myocardial oxygen demand.

Increased sympathetic stimulation is a normal response to physical activity but may also be caused by anxiety, pain, stress,

A

B

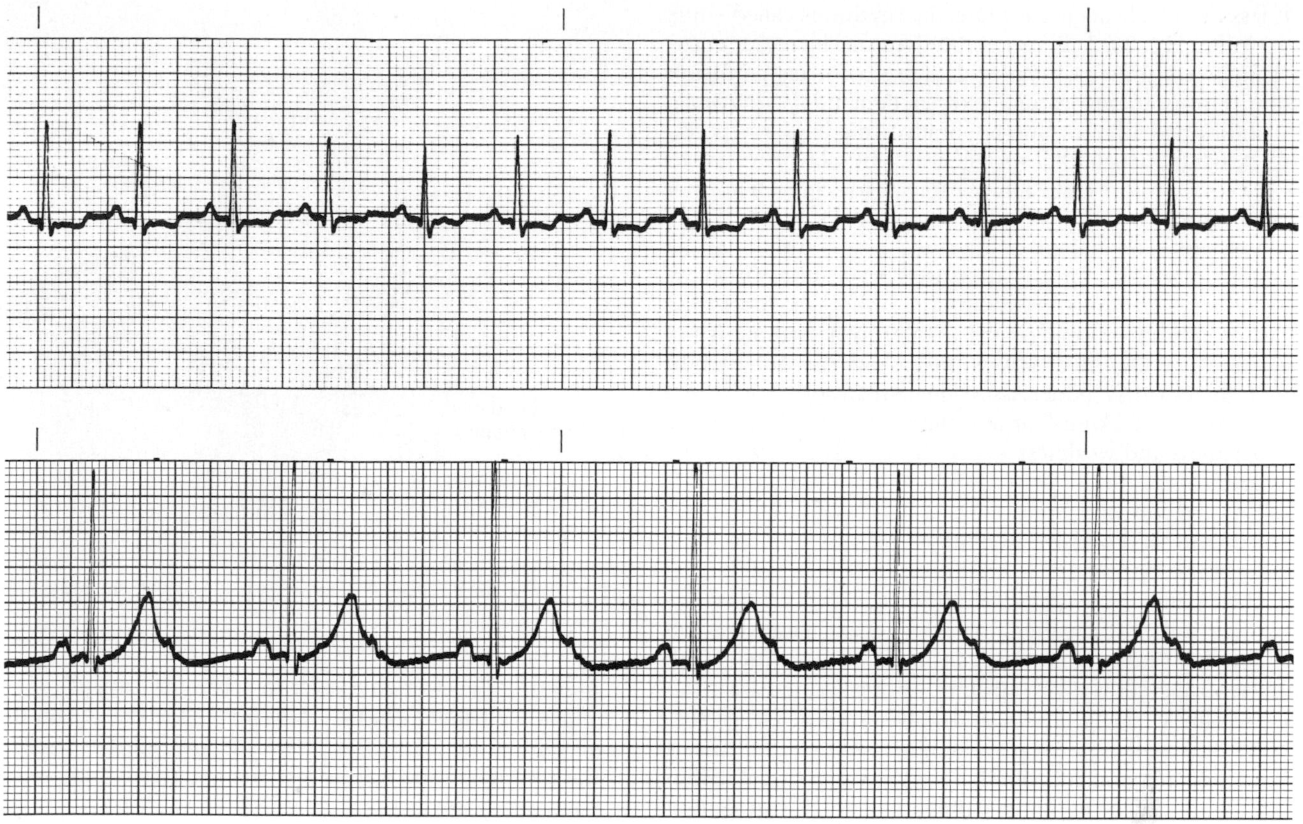

FIG. 34-8 Sinus rhythms. **A,** Sinus tachycardia (heart rate, 115 beats per minute; PR interval, 0.12 second; QRS complex, 0.08 second). **B,** Sinus bradycardia (heart rate, 52 beats per minute; PR interval, 0.18 second; QRS complex, 0.08 second).

fever, anemia, hypoxemia, and hyperthyroidism. Drugs such as epinephrine, atropine, caffeine, alcohol, nicotine, cocaine, aminophylline, and thyroid medications may also increase the heart rate. In some cases, sinus tachycardia is a compensatory response to decreased cardiac output or blood pressure, as occurs in dehydration, hypovolemic shock, myocardial infarction (MI), infection, and heart failure. Assess patients for clinical manifestations of hypovolemia and dehydration, including increased pulse rate, decreased urinary output, decreased blood pressure, and dry skin and mucous membranes.

The patient may be asymptomatic except for an increased pulse rate. However, if the rhythm is not well tolerated, he or she may have symptoms.

! NURSING SAFETY PRIORITY (QSEN)

Action Alert

For patients with sinus tachycardia, assess for fatigue, weakness, shortness of breath, orthopnea, decreased oxygen saturation, increased pulse rate, and decreased blood pressure. Also assess for restlessness and anxiety from decreased cerebral PERFUSION and for decreased urine output from impaired renal PERFUSION. The patient may also have anginal pain and palpitations. The ECG pattern may show T-wave inversion or ST-segment elevation or depression in response to myocardial ischemia.

The desired outcome is to decrease the heart rate to normal levels by treating the underlying cause. Remind the patient to remain on bedrest if the tachycardia is causing hypotension or weakness. Teach the patient to avoid substances that increase cardiac rate, including caffeine, alcohol, and nicotine. Help patients develop stress management strategies, or refer the patient to a mental health professional.

NCLEX EXAMINATION CHALLENGE

Physiological Integrity

A client who had open abdominal surgery 4 hours ago reports feeling weak and dizzy. The client's current blood pressure has decreased to 98/50, and pulse rate is 108. What is the nurse's best action at this time?

A. Document the vital signs, and continue to monitor the client.
B. Remind the client to stay in bed if feeling weak and dizzy.
C. Call the health care provider immediately.
D. Increase the client's IV rate to restore fluid volume.

Sinus Bradycardia. Excessive vagal (parasympathetic) stimulation to the heart causes a decreased rate of sinus node discharge. It may result from carotid sinus massage, vomiting, suctioning, Valsalva maneuvers (e.g., bearing down for a bowel movement or gagging), ocular pressure, or pain. Increased parasympathetic stimuli may also result from hypoxia, inferior wall MI, and the administration of drugs such as beta-adrenergic blocking agents, calcium channel blockers, and digitalis. Bradycardia may also be caused by Lyme disease and hypothyroidism.

The stimuli slow the heart rate and decrease the speed of conduction through the heart. When the sinus node discharge rate is less than 60 beats per minute, the rhythm is called **sinus bradycardia** (Fig. 34-8, *B*). Sinus bradycardia increases coronary PERFUSION time, but it may decrease coronary perfusion pressure. However, myocardial oxygen demand is *decreased*. Well-conditioned athletes who are bradycardic have a hypereffective heart in which the strong heart muscle provides an adequate stroke volume and a low heart rate to achieve a normal cardiac output.

Assessment. The patient with sinus bradycardia may be asymptomatic except for the decreased pulse rate. In many cases, the cause of sinus bradycardia is unknown. Assess the medication administration record (MAR) to determine if the patient is receiving medications that slow the conduction through the SA or AV node. Assess the patient for:

- Syncope ("blackouts" or fainting)
- Dizziness and weakness
- Confusion
- Hypotension
- Diaphoresis (excessive sweating)
- Shortness of breath
- Chest pain

Interventions. If the patient has any of these symptoms and the underlying cause cannot be determined, the treatment is to administer drug therapy with atropine 0.5 mg IV, increase intravascular volume via IV fluids, and apply oxygen. Drugs suspected of causing the bradycardia are discontinued. If the heart rate does not increase sufficiently, prepare for transcutaneous or transvenous pacing to increase the heart rate. If treatment of the underlying cause does not restore normal sinus rhythm, the patient will require permanent pacemaker implantation.

Temporary Pacing. **Temporary pacing** is a nonsurgical intervention that provides a timed electrical stimulus to the heart when either the impulse initiation or the conduction system of the heart is defective. The electrical stimulus then spreads throughout the heart to depolarize the cells, which should be followed by contraction and cardiac output. Electrical stimuli may be delivered to the right atrium or right ventricle (single-chamber pacemakers) or to both (dual-chamber pacemakers).

Temporary pacing is used for patients with symptomatic, atropine-refractory bradydysrhythmias or for patients with asystole (discussed on p. 671 in this chapter). The two basic types of *temporary* pacing are transcutaneous and transvenous pacing. ***Transcutaneous pacing*** is accomplished through the application of two large external electrodes. The electrodes are attached to an external pulse generator. The generator emits electrical pulses, which are transmitted through the electrodes and then transcutaneously to stimulate ventricular depolarization when the patient's heart rate is slower than the rate set on the pacemaker. A transvenous system consists of an external battery-operated pulse generator and pacing electrodes, or lead wires. These wires attach to the generator on one end and are threaded to the right atrium via the subclavian or femoral vein (Fig. 34-9). Electrical pulses, or stimuli, are emitted from the negative terminal of the generator, flow through a lead wire, and stimulate the cardiac cells to depolarize. The current seeks ground by returning through the other lead wire to the positive terminal of the generator, thus completing a circuit. The intensity of electrical current is set by selecting the appropriate current output, measured in milliamperes.

The two major modes of pacing are synchronous (demand) pacing and asynchronous (fixed-rate) pacing. Temporary pacing is *usually* done in the synchronous (demand) pacing mode. The pacemaker's sensitivity is set to sense the patient's own beats. When the patient's heart rate is above the rate set on the pulse generator, the pacemaker does not fire (inhibits itself). When the patient's heart rate is less than the generator setting, the pacemaker provides electrical impulses (paces).

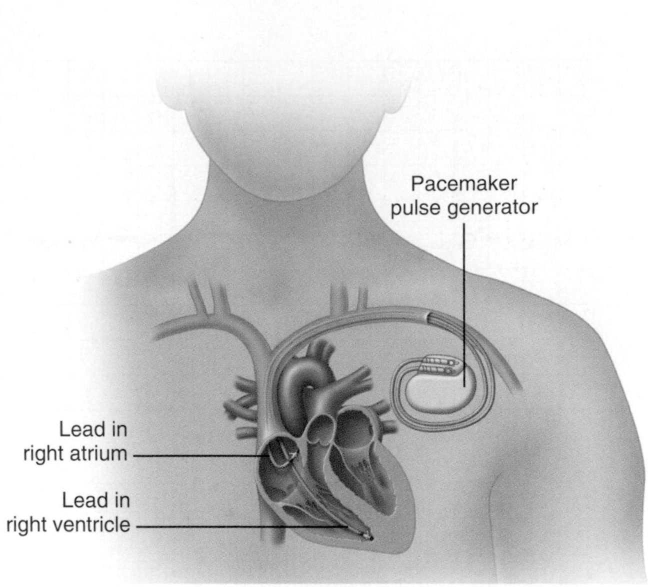

FIG. 34-9 Placement of pacemaker in chest and heart leads.

Transcutaneous pacing is used as an *emergency* measure to provide demand ventricular pacing in a profoundly bradycardic or asystolic patient until invasive pacing can be used or the patient's heart rate returns to normal. It may be used prophylactically when performing procedures or transporting patients at risk for bradydysrhythmias. However, it is used only as a temporary measure to maintain heart rate and PERFUSION until a more permanent method of pacing is used.

When a pacing stimulus is delivered to the heart, a spike (or pacemaker artifact) is seen on the monitor or ECG strip. The spike should be followed by evidence of depolarization (i.e., a P wave, indicating atrial depolarization, or a QRS complex, indicating ventricular depolarization). This pattern is referred to as *capture*, indicating that the pacemaker has successfully depolarized, or captured, the chamber.

Permanent Pacemaker. Pacemaker insertion is performed to treat conduction disorders that are not temporary, including complete heart block. These pacemakers are usually powered by a lithium battery and have an average life span of 10 years. After the battery power is depleted, the generator must be replaced by a procedure done with the patient under local anesthesia. Some pacemakers are nuclear-powered and have a life span of 20 years or longer. Other pacemakers can be recharged externally. Combination pacemaker/defibrillator devices are also available.

A biventricular pacemaker may be utilized to coordinate contractions between the right and left ventricles. In addition to pacing used in the right side of the heart, an additional lead is placed in the left lateral wall of the left ventricle through the coronary sinus. This procedure allows synchronized depolarization of the ventricles and is used in patients with moderate to severe heart failure to improve functional ability.

The electrophysiologist implants the pulse generator in a surgically made subcutaneous pocket at the shoulder in the

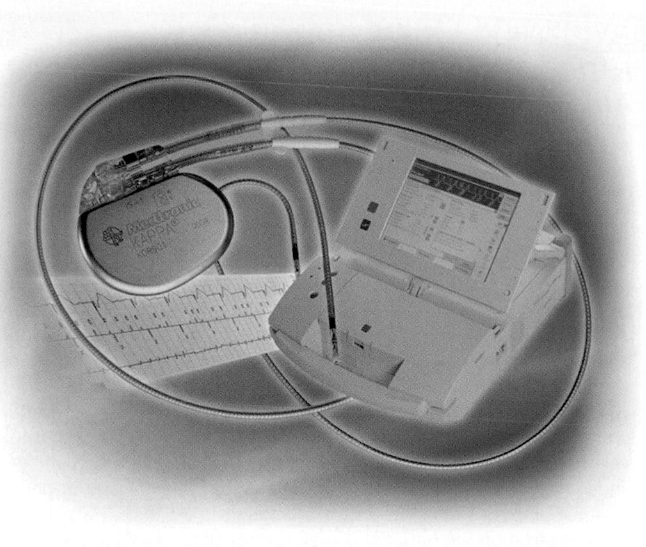

FIG. 34-10 Permanent pacemaker, programmer, and rhythm strip.

right or left subclavicular area, which may create a visible bulge. The leads are introduced transvenously via the cephalic or the subclavian vein to the endocardium on the right side of the heart. After the procedure, monitor the ECG rhythm to check that the pacemaker is working correctly. Assess the implantation site for bleeding, swelling, redness, tenderness, and infection. The dressing over the site should remain clean and dry. The patient should be afebrile and have stable vital signs. The physician prescribes initial activity restrictions, which are then gradually changed. Complications of permanent pacemakers are similar to those of temporary invasive pacing.

Pacemaker checks are done on an ambulatory care basis at regular intervals. Reprogramming may be needed if pacemaker problems develop. The pulse generator is interrogated using an electronic device to determine the pacemaker settings and battery life (Fig. 34-10). In addition, most pacemaker manufacturers offer wireless home transmitter devices. Data are then sent via landline telephone to a database, which is then accessed by the device clinic or health care provider. Stress the need to keep follow-up appointments for more detailed pacemaker checks and reprogramming, if necessary, as well as for assessment.

Atrial Dysrhythmias

In patients with atrial dysrhythmias, the focus of impulse generation shifts away from the sinus node to the atrial tissues. The shift changes the axis (direction) of atrial depolarization, resulting in a P-wave shape that differs from normal P waves. The most common atrial dysrhythmias are:

- Premature atrial complexes
- Supraventricular tachycardia
- Atrial fibrillation

Premature Atrial Complexes. A **premature atrial complex (contraction) (PAC)** occurs when atrial tissue becomes irritable. This ectopic focus fires an impulse before the next sinus impulse is due. The premature P wave may not always be clearly visible because it can be hidden in the preceding T wave. Examine the T wave closely for any change in shape, and compare with other T waves. A PAC is usually followed by a pause.

The causes of atrial irritability include:

- Stress
- Fatigue
- Anxiety
- Inflammation
- Infection
- Caffeine, nicotine, or alcohol
- Drugs such as epinephrine, sympathomimetics, amphetamines, digitalis, or anesthetic agents

PACs may also result from myocardial ischemia, hypermetabolic states, electrolyte imbalance, or atrial stretch. Atrial stretch can result from congestive heart failure, valvular disease, and pulmonary hypertension with cor pulmonale.

The patient usually has no symptoms except for possible heart palpitations. No intervention is needed except to treat causes such as heart failure. If PACs occur frequently, they may lead to more serious atrial tachydysrhythmias and therefore may need treatment. Administration of prescribed antidysrhythmic drugs may be necessary (see Chart 34-3). Teach the patient measures to manage stress and substances to avoid, such as caffeine and alcohol, that are known to increase atrial irritability.

Supraventricular Tachycardia. **Supraventricular tachycardia (SVT)** involves the rapid stimulation of atrial tissue at a rate of 100 to 280 beats per minute in adults. During SVT, P waves may not be visible, especially if there is a 1:1 conduction with rapid rates, because the P waves are embedded in the preceding T wave. *SVT may occur in healthy young people, especially women.*

SVT is usually due to a re-entry mechanism in which one impulse circulates repeatedly throughout the atrial pathway, re-stimulating the atrial tissue at a rapid rate. The term **paroxysmal supraventricular tachycardia (PSVT)** is used when the rhythm is intermittent. It is initiated suddenly by a premature complex such as a PAC and terminated suddenly with or without intervention.

Assessment. The clinical manifestations depend on the duration of the SVT and the rate of the ventricular response. In patients with a *sustained* rapid ventricular response, assess for palpitations, chest pain, weakness, fatigue, shortness of breath, nervousness, anxiety, hypotension, and syncope. Cardiovascular deterioration may occur if the rate does not sustain adequate blood pressure. In that case, SVT can result in angina, heart failure, and cardiogenic shock. With a *nonsustained* or slower ventricular response, the patient may be asymptomatic except for occasional palpitations.

Interventions. If SVT occurs in a healthy person and stops on its own, no intervention may be needed other than eliminating identified causes. If it continues, the patient should be studied in the electrophysiology study (EPS) laboratory. The preferred treatment for recurrent SVT is radiofrequency catheter ablation, described later in this chapter on p. 668. In sustained SVT with a rapid ventricular response, the desired outcomes of treatment are to decrease the ventricular response, convert the dysrhythmia to a sinus rhythm, and treat the cause.

Vagal maneuvers induce vagal stimulation of the cardiac conduction system, specifically the SA and AV nodes. Although not as common today, vagal maneuvers may be attempted to treat supraventricular tachydysrhythmias and include carotid sinus massage and Valsalva maneuvers. The results of these interventions, however, are often temporary and may cause "rebound" tachycardia or severe bradycardia. Further therapy must be initiated.

In *carotid sinus massage*, the physician massages over one carotid artery for a few seconds, observing for a change in cardiac rhythm. This intervention causes vagal stimulation, slowing SA and AV nodal conduction. Prepare the patient for the procedure. Instruct him or her to turn the head slightly away from the side to be massaged, and observe the cardiac monitor for a change in rhythm. An ECG rhythm strip is recorded before, during, and after the procedure. After the procedure, assess vital signs and the level of consciousness. Complications include bradydysrhythmias, asystole, ventricular fibrillation (VF), and cerebral damage. Because of these risks, carotid massage is not commonly performed. *A defibrillator and resuscitative equipment must be immediately available during the procedure.*

To stimulate a *vagal reflex*, the health care provider instructs the patient to bear down as if straining to have a bowel movement. Assess the patient's heart rate, heart rhythm, and blood pressure. Observe the cardiac monitor; and record an ECG rhythm strip before, during, and after the procedure to determine the effect of therapy.

Drug therapy is prescribed for some patients to convert SVT to a normal sinus rhythm (NSR). Adenosine (Adenocard) is used to terminate the acute episode and given rapidly (over several seconds) followed by a normal saline bolus.

! NURSING SAFETY PRIORITY QSEN

Drug Alert

Side effects of adenosine include significant bradycardia with pauses, nausea, and vomiting. When administering adenosine, be sure to have emergency equipment readily available!

AV nodal blocking agents, such as beta and calcium channel blockers, are also given to treat SVT. Chart 34-3 lists medications that may be used for SVT.

If symptoms of poor PERFUSION are severe and persistent, the patient may require synchronized cardioversion to immediately terminate the SVT. For long-term treatment, patients are referred to an electrophysiologist for radiofrequency catheter ablation. Synchronized cardioversion and catheter ablation are discussed in detail on p. 668 of this chapter.

Atrial Fibrillation. **Atrial fibrillation (AF)** is the most common dysrhythmia seen in clinical practice. It can impair quality of life, cause considerable morbidity and mortality, and impose a large economic burden on health care systems (Dagres & Anastasiou-Nana, 2010).

AF is associated with atrial fibrosis and loss of muscle mass. A mutation in the *lamin AC* (LMAC) gene has been linked to atrial fibrosis and dilation (Hardin & Steele, 2008). These structural changes are common in heart diseases such as hypertension, heart failure, and coronary artery disease. As AF progresses, cardiac output decreases by as much as 20 to 30 percent.

Currently, about 2.3 million people in the United States are diagnosed with AF; it is estimated that more than 12 million people will have AF by the year 2050 (Tedrow et al., 2010). The incidence of AF increases with age; AF causes serious problems in older people, leading to stroke and/or heart failure. Risk factors include hypertension (HTN), previous ischemic stroke, transient ischemic attack (TIA) or other thromboembolic event, coronary heart disease, diabetes mellitus, heart failure, and mitral valve disease.

In addition to advanced age, obesity, Caucasian race, and excessive alcohol have been identified as risk factors for AF (see the Evidence-Based Practice box). About half of obese adults may develop AF (Chilukuri et al., 2010). Caucasians are more at risk for AF than African Americans and other ethnic groups, perhaps because of the larger left atrial diameter in Caucasians (Marcus et al., 2010). AF that is temporary and reversible is associated with excessive alcohol consumption (sometimes called *"holiday heart syndrome"*).

Assessment. In patients with AF, multiple rapid impulses from many atrial foci depolarize the atria in a totally disorganized manner at a rate of 350 to 600 times per minute; ventricular response is usually 120 to 200 beats per minute. The result is a chaotic rhythm with no clear P waves, no atrial contractions, loss of atrial kick, and an irregular ventricular response (Fig. 34-11). The atria merely quiver in fibrillation (commonly called "A fib"). Often the ventricles beat with a rapid rate in response to the numerous atrial impulses. The rapid and irregular ventricular rate decreases ventricular filling and reduces cardiac output, further impairing the heart's PERFUSION ability.

EVIDENCE-BASED PRACTICE QSEN

Is There a Relationship Between Obesity and Atrial Fibrillation?

Tedrow, U.B., Conen, D., Ridker, P.M., Cook, N.R., Koplan, B.A., Manson, J.E., et al. (2010). The long- and short-term impact of elevated body mass index on the risk of new atrial fibrillation: The WHS (Women's Health Study). *Journal of the American College of Cardiology, 55*(21), 2319-2327.

There has been an increase in atrial fibrillation (AF) in recent years that is not explained by aging alone. Modifiable risk factors must be identified. Recent evidence estimates that 32.2% of adults are obese (body mass index [BMI] >30) and 6.9% of women are extremely obese (BMI >40). This study used data from the Women's Health Study (WHS) and included 34,309 women who were followed for about 12.9 years. Participants reported their weight on questionnaires at 24-, 36-, 60-, 72-, and 108-month intervals. During this time, 834 AF events were confirmed. BMI was linearly associated with AF risk, and being overweight and/or obese was associated with short-term increases in AF risk. Participants who became obese had a 41% risk for developing AF. Study limitations include the heterogeneous population with self-reported height/weight and lack of electrocardiograph (ECG) screening. The researchers concluded that weight-control strategies may reduce AF incidence.

Level of Evidence: 1

The evidence was obtained from a randomized trial of a very large longitudinal national study using multiple methods of data collection.

Commentary: Implications for Practice and Research

Obesity is a major health concern in the United States. Cases of AF are increasing. Both affect the economy of health care because of complications and hospital admissions. Nurses need to recognize AF risk factors and provide proactive education to patients at risk for obesity, cardiovascular disease, and atrial fibrillation. Further research is needed to replicate the study on different populations, to determine the economic impact on health care, and to determine if weight loss reduces the incidence of AF.

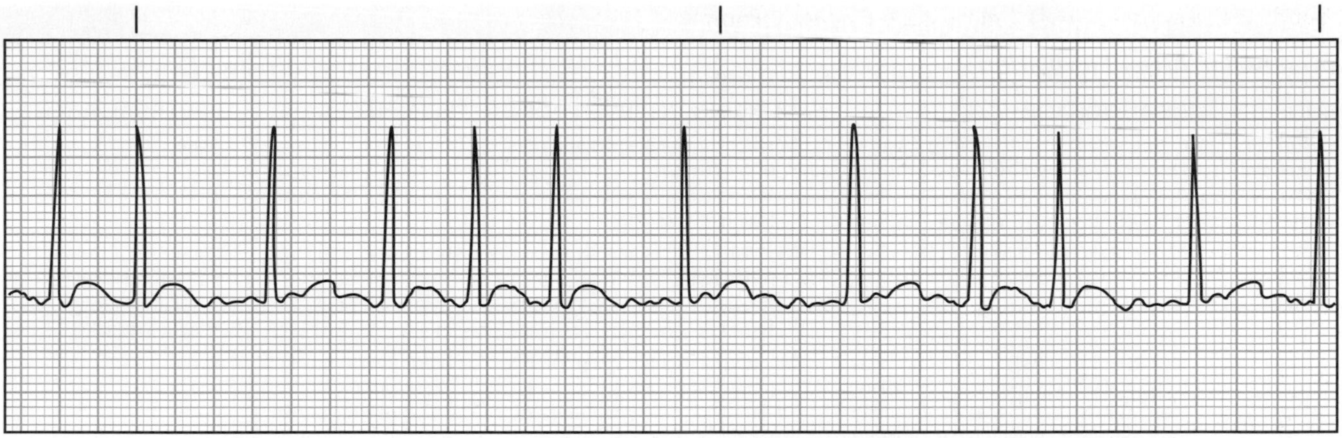

FIG. 34-11 Atrial fibrillation. Note wavy baseline with atrial electrical activity and irregular ventricular rhythm.

! NURSING SAFETY PRIORITY (QSEN)

Action Alert

The loss of coordinated atrial contractions in AF can lead to pooling of blood resulting in thrombus formation. *The patient is at high risk for pulmonary embolism!* Thrombi may form within the right atrium and then move through the right ventricle to the lungs. In addition, the patient is at risk for systemic emboli, particularly an embolic stroke, which may cause severe neurologic impairment or death. Patients with AF who have valvular disease are particularly at risk for venous thromboembolism (VTE). Monitor patients carefully for these complications discussed elsewhere in this text.

Interventions. Interventions for AF depend on the severity of the problem and the patient's response. Drug therapy is often effective for treating AF.

Drug Therapy. Traditional interventions for AF include antidysrhythmic drugs to slow the ventricular conduction or to convert the AF to normal sinus rhythm (NSR). Examples of these drugs are calcium channel blockers like diltiazem (Cardizem) or, for more difficult-to-control AF, amiodarone (Cordarone). Dronedarone (Multaq) is a new drug similar to amiodarone, yet better tolerated by patients, for maintenance of sinus rhythm after cardioversion (Cheng, 2010). However, dronedarone should not be used in patients with a history or current congestive heart failure because it can cause an exacerbation of cardiac symptoms.

Beta blockers, such as metoprolol (Toprol, Dutoprol) and esmolol (Brevibloc), may also be used to slow ventricular response. Digoxin (Lanoxin, Novo-Digoxin♣) is given for patients with heart failure and AF. These drugs are described in Chart 34-3. Carefully monitor the pulse rate of patients taking these drugs.

Health care providers use the **CHADS$_2$ scoring system** (Congestive heart failure, Hypertension, Age ≥75, Diabetes mellitus, Stroke) to determine if the patient with atrial fibrillation needs preventive anticoagulant therapy (Table 34-2). If the patient scores a 0 or 1 on the scale, aspirin is utilized as the anticoagulant of choice. Patients with a score of 2 or more are considered high risk for clot development and are placed on anticoagulants, such as heparin, enoxaparin (Lovenox), and warfarin (Coumadin). Because of the unpredictable drug response and many food-drug interactions, laboratory test monitoring (e.g., international normalized ratio [INR]) is required when a patient is taking warfarin. Teach patients the importance of avoiding high vitamin K foods and avoiding herbs, such as ginger, ginseng, goldenseal, *Ginkgo biloba*, and St. John's wort, which could interfere with the drug's action. Chapter 36 describes care of patients receiving anticoagulant therapy in detail on p. 731.

TABLE 34-2 CHADS$_2$ Scoring System for Risk of Stroke in Patients Who Have Atrial Fibrillation

RISK FACTOR	PRESENT	SCORE
History of **c**ongestive heart failure	Yes	1
	No	0
History of **h**ypertension	Yes	1
	No	0
Age ≥75 years	Yes	1
	No	0
History of **d**iabetes	Yes	1
	No	0
History of **s**troke or TIA	Yes	2
	No	0

Score of 0: Low risk—recommended 325 mg of aspirin
Score of 1: Moderate risk—recommended aspirin or warfarin
Score of 2: High risk—warfarin with INR goal of 2.0-3.0 or other anticoagulant (see Chart 34-3)

Source: Gage, B.F., Waterman, A.D., Shannon, W., Boechler, M., Rich, M.W., & Radford, M.J. (2001). Validation of clinical classification schemes for predicting stroke: Results from the National Registry of Atrial Fibrillation. *Journal of the American Medical Association, 285*(22), 2864-2870; MDCalc.com. (2013). *CHADS$_2$ score for atrial fibrillation stroke risk.* Retrieved July 2014, from www.mdcalc.com/chads2-score-for-atrial-fibrillation-stroke-risk/; QxMD.com.(2013). *HADS$_2$.* Retrieved July 2014, from www.qxmd.com/calculate-online/cardiology/chads2-stroke-risk-in-atrial-fibrillation.
INR, International normalized ratio; *TIA,* transient ischemic attack.

Because of the problems associated with warfarin, alternative anticoagulant agents such as dabigatran (Pradaxa), rivaroxaban (Xarelto), or apixaban (Eliquis) may be given on a long-term basis to prevent strokes associated with nonvalvular AF (Chart 34-4). Because these drugs achieve a steady state, there is no need for laboratory test monitoring. However, if the patient does experience severe bleeding, reversal agents are not available and prothrombin time (PT) and INR are not accurate predictors of bleeding time. These drugs should be used cautiously in patients older than 75 years because of their risk for falls (Sellers & Newby, 2011).

CHART 34-4 **Common Examples of Drug Therapy**
Nonvalvular Atrial Fibrillation

DRUG	USUAL DOSAGE	NURSING INTERVENTIONS	RATIONALES	REVERSAL AGENT
Rivaroxaban (Xarelto) (factor Xa inhibitor)	20 mg orally daily with evening meal 15 mg orally daily if CrCl <15-50 mL	Monitor for signs and symptoms of bleeding. Teach patient the importance of taking as directed.	Abrupt discontinuation may put patient at high risk for stroke.	None
Dabigatran (Pradaxa) (thrombin inhibitor)	150 mg orally twice daily	Monitor for signs and symptoms of bleeding. Teach patient the importance of taking as directed.	Abrupt discontinuation may put patient at high risk for stroke.	None Hemodialysis may remove dabigatran—limited data available.
Apixaban (Eliquis) (factor Xa inhibitor)	5 mg orally twice daily 2.5 mg orally twice daily used in patients with at least 2 of these characteristics: age ≥80 years, body weight ≤60 kg, or serum creatinine ≥1.5mg/dL	Monitor for signs and symptoms of bleeding. Teach patient the importance of taking as directed.	Abrupt discontinuation may put patient at high risk for stroke.	None

CrCl, Creatinine clearance.

! NURSING SAFETY PRIORITY QSEN
Drug Alert

Teach patients taking any type of anticoagulant drug to report bruising, bleeding nose or gums, and other signs of bleeding to their health care provider immediately. Also remind them to take aspirin with food to prevent GI distress.

NCLEX EXAMINATION CHALLENGE
Physiological Integrity

The health care provider prescribes warfarin (Coumadin) for a client with atrial fibrillation. Which foods will the nurse teach the client taking this drug to avoid? **Select all that apply.**
A. Spinach
B. Corn
C. Tomatoes
D. Brussels sprouts
E. Potatoes

Cardioversion. **Cardioversion** is a *synchronized* countershock that may be performed (1) in emergencies for unstable ventricular or supraventricular tachydysrhythmias or (2) electively for stable tachydysrhythmias that are resistant to medical therapies. If the patient has been taking digoxin, the drug is withheld for up to 48 hours before an elective cardioversion. Digoxin increases ventricular irritability and puts the patient at risk for VF after the countershock. For elective cardioversion for atrial fibrillation, the patient must take anticoagulants for 4 to 6 weeks before the procedure to prevent clots from moving from the heart to the brain or lungs. If unsure of onset of AF, a transesophageal echocardiogram (TEE) may be performed to assess for clot formation in the left atrium.

The shock depolarizes a large amount of myocardium during the cardiac depolarization. It is intended to stop the re-entry circuit and allow the sinus node to regain control of the heart. Emergency equipment must be available during the procedure. The physician, advanced practice nurse, or other qualified nurse explains the procedure to the patient and family. Assist the patient in signing a consent form unless the procedure is an emergency for a life-threatening dysrhythmia. Because he or she is usually conscious, a short-acting anesthetic agent is administered for sedation.

One electrode is placed to the left of the precordium, and the other is placed on the right next to the sternum and below the clavicle. The defibrillator should be set in the synchronized mode. This avoids discharging the shock during the T wave, which may increase ventricular irritability, causing ventricular fibrillation (VF). Charge the defibrillator to the energy level requested, usually starting at a low rate of 120 to 200 joules for biphasic machines.

! NURSING SAFETY PRIORITY QSEN
Critical Rescue

For safety before cardioversion, turn oxygen off and away from patient; fire could result. Shout "CLEAR" before shock delivery for electrical safety!

After cardioversion, assess the patient's response and heart rhythm. Therapy is repeated, if necessary, until the desired result is obtained or alternative therapies are considered. If the patient's condition deteriorates into VF after cardioversion, check to see that the synchronizer is turned off so that immediate defibrillation can be administered.

Nursing care after cardioversion includes:

- Maintaining a patent airway
- Administering oxygen
- Assessing vital signs and the level of consciousness
- Administering antidysrhythmic drug therapy, as prescribed
- Monitoring for dysrhythmias
- Assessing for chest burns from electrodes
- Providing emotional support
- Documenting the results of cardioversion

Radiofrequency Catheter Ablation. **Radiofrequency catheter ablation** is an invasive procedure that may be used to destroy an irritable focus causing a supraventricular or ventricular tachydysrhythmia. The patient must first undergo electrophysiologic studies and mapping procedures to locate the focus. Then radiofrequency waves are delivered to abolish the irritable focus. When ablation is performed in the AV nodal or His bundle area, damage may also occur to the normal conduction system, causing heart blocks and requiring implantation of a permanent pacemaker. In AF, pulmonary vein isolation and ablation creates scar tissue that blocks impulses and disconnects the pathway of the abnormal rhythm. Patients with AF with a rapid ventricular rate not responsive to drug therapy may have AV nodal ablation performed to totally disconnect the conduction from the atria to the ventricles, which requires implantation of a permanent pacemaker

Other Nonsurgical Management. *Bi-ventricular pacing* may be another alternative for patients with heart failure and conduction disorders. Bi-atrial pacing, anti-tachycardia pacing, and implantable atrial defibrillators are other methods used to suppress or resolve AF.

Patients in AF with heart failure (discussed in Chapter 35) may benefit from the *surgical* **maze procedure**, an open-chest surgical technique often performed with coronary artery bypass grafting (CABG). Before this procedure, electrophysiologic mapping studies are done to confirm the diagnosis of AF. The surgeon places a maze of sutures in strategic places in the atrial myocardium, pulmonary artery, and possibly the superior vena cava to prevent electrical circuits from developing and continuing AF. Sinus impulses can then depolarize the atria before reaching the AV node and preserve the atrial kick. Postoperative care is similar to that after other open-heart surgical procedures (see Chapter 38).

The *catheter* maze procedure is done by inserting a catheter through a leg vein into the atria and dragging a heated ablating catheter along the atria to create lines (scars) of conduction block. Patients having this minimally invasive form of the procedure have fewer complications, less pain, and a quicker recovery than those with the open, surgical maze procedure.

NCLEX EXAMINATION CHALLENGE

Physiological Integrity

A client is prescribed to take rivaroxaban (Xarelto) 20 mg orally every day. What is the nurse's priority when teaching the client about this drug?

A. "Be sure to keep laboratory appointments to check your clotting times."
B. "Take the medication every morning before breakfast."
C. "Report any signs of bleeding to your health care provider."
D. "Have vitamin K available in case you need it."

Ventricular Dysrhythmias

Ventricular dysrhythmias are potentially more life threatening than atrial dysrhythmias because the left ventricle pumps oxygenated blood throughout the body to perfuse vital organs and other tissues. The most common or life-threatening ventricular dysrhythmias include:

- Premature ventricular complexes
- Ventricular tachycardia
- Ventricular fibrillation
- Ventricular asystole

Premature Ventricular Complexes. **Premature ventricular complexes (PVCs)**, also called *premature ventricular contractions*, result from increased irritability of ventricular cells and are seen as early ventricular complexes followed by a pause. When multiple PVCs are present, the QRS complexes may be unifocal or uniform, meaning that they are of the same shape (Fig. 34-12, *A*), or multifocal or multiform, meaning that they are of different shapes (Fig. 34-12, *B*). PVCs frequently occur in repetitive rhythms, such as bigeminy (two), trigeminy (three),

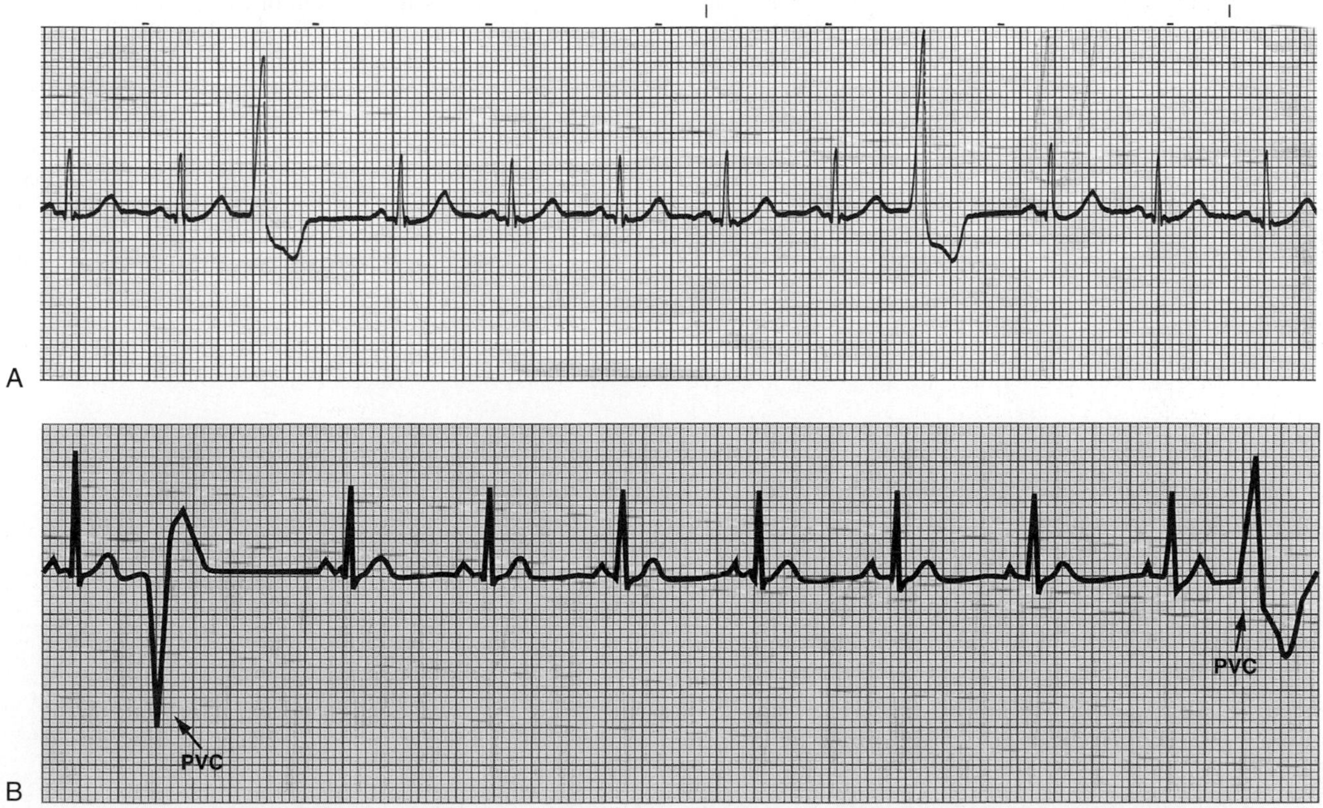

FIG. 34-12 Premature ventricular contractions. **A,** Normal sinus rhythm with unifocal premature ventricular complexes (PVCs). **B,** Normal sinus rhythm with multifocal PVCs (one negative and the other positive).

and quadrigeminy (four). Two sequential PVCs are a pair, or couplet. Three or more successive PVCs are usually called **nonsustained ventricular tachycardia (NSVT)**.

Premature ventricular contractions are common, and their frequency increases with age. They may be insignificant or may occur with problems such as myocardial infarction, chronic heart failure, chronic obstructive pulmonary disease (COPD), and anemia. PVCs may also be present in patients with hypokalemia or hypomagnesemia. Sympathomimetic agents, anesthesia drugs, stress, nicotine, caffeine, alcohol, infection, or surgery can also cause PVCs, especially in older adults. Postmenopausal women often find that caffeine causes palpitations and PVCs.

Assessment. The patient may be asymptomatic or experience palpitations or chest discomfort caused by increased stroke volume of the normal beat after the pause. Peripheral pulses may be diminished or absent with the PVCs themselves because the decreased stroke volume of the premature beats may *decrease peripheral* PERFUSION.

! NURSING SAFETY PRIORITY QSEN

Action Alert

Because other dysrhythmias can cause widened QRS complexes, assess whether the premature complexes perfuse to the extremities. Palpate the carotid, brachial, or femoral arteries while observing the monitor for widened complexes or auscultating apical heart sounds. With acute MI, PVCs may be considered as a warning, possibly triggering life-threatening ventricular tachycardia (VT) or ventricular fibrillation (VF).

Interventions. If there is no underlying heart disease, PVCs are not usually treated other than by eliminating or managing any contributing cause (e.g., caffeine, stress). Potassium or magnesium is given for replacement therapy if hypokalemia or hypomagnesemia is the cause. People with more than 5000 PVCs in a 24-hour period are usually placed on beta-adrenergic blocking agents (beta blockers) (see Chart 34-3).

Ventricular Tachycardia. **Ventricular tachycardia (VT)**, sometimes referred to as "V tach," occurs with repetitive firing of an irritable ventricular ectopic focus, usually at a rate of 140 to 180 beats/min or more (Fig. 34-13). VT may result from increased automaticity or a re-entry mechanism. It may be intermittent (nonsustained VT) or sustained, lasting longer than 15 to 30 seconds. The sinus node may continue to discharge independently, depolarizing the atria but not the ventricles, although P waves are seldom seen in sustained VT.

Ventricular tachycardia may occur in patients with ischemic heart disease, MI, cardiomyopathy, hypokalemia, hypomagnesemia, valvular heart disease, heart failure, drug toxicity (e.g., steroids), or hypotension. Patients who use cocaine or illicit inhalants are at a high risk for VT. *In patients who go into cardiac arrest, VT is commonly the initial rhythm before deterioration into ventricular fibrillation (VF) as the terminal rhythm!*

Clinical manifestations of sustained VT partially depend on the ventricular rate. Slower rates are better tolerated.

! NURSING SAFETY PRIORITY QSEN

Critical Rescue

In some patients, VT causes cardiac arrest. Assess the patient's airway, breathing, circulation, level of consciousness, and oxygenation level. For the *stable* patient with sustained VT, administer oxygen and confirm the rhythm via a 12-lead ECG. Amiodarone (Cordarone), lidocaine, or magnesium sulfate may be given.

Current Advanced Cardiac Life Support (ACLS) guidelines state that elective cardioversion is highly recommended for stable VT. The physician may prescribe an oral antidysrhythmic agent, such as mexiletine (Mexitil) or sotalol (Betapace, Sotacor♣), to prevent further occurrences. Patients who persist with episodes of stable VT may require radiofrequency catheter ablation (see p. 668 of this chapter). *Unstable* VT without a pulse is treated the same way as ventricular fibrillation as described below.

Ventricular Fibrillation. **Ventricular fibrillation (VF)**, sometimes called "V fib," is the result of electrical chaos in the ventricles and is *life threatening*! Impulses from many irritable foci fire in a totally disorganized manner so that ventricular contraction cannot occur. There are no recognizable ECG deflections (Fig. 34-14, *A*). The ventricles merely quiver, consuming a tremendous amount of oxygen. *There is no cardiac output or pulse and therefore no cerebral, myocardial, or systemic perfusion. This rhythm is rapidly fatal if not successfully ended within 3 to 5 minutes.*

VF may be the first manifestation of coronary artery disease (CAD). Patients with myocardial infarction (MI) are at great risk for VF. It may also occur in those with hypokalemia, hypomagnesemia, hemorrhage, drug therapy, rapid supraventricular

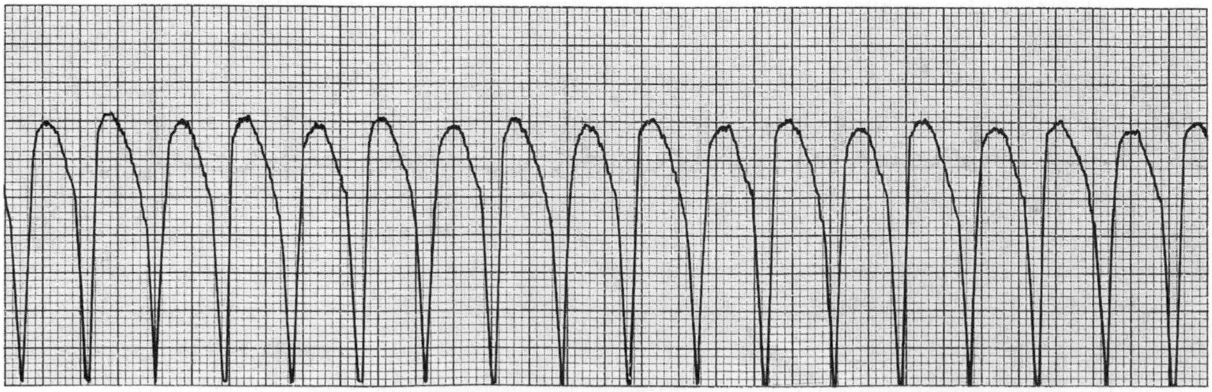

FIG. 34-13 Sustained ventricular tachycardia at a rate of 166 beats per minute.

tachycardia (SVT), or shock. Surgery or trauma may also cause VF.

Emergency Care: Ventricular Fibrillation. When VF begins, the patient becomes faint, immediately loses consciousness, and becomes pulseless and apneic (no breathing). There is no blood pressure, and heart sounds are absent. Respiratory and metabolic acidosis develop. Seizures may occur. Within minutes, the pupils become fixed and dilated and the skin becomes cold and mottled. *Death results without prompt intervention.*

The desired outcomes of collaborative care are to resolve VF promptly and convert it to an organized rhythm. *Therefore the priority is to defibrillate the patient immediately according to ACLS protocol.* If a defibrillator is not readily available, high quality CPR must be initiated and continued until the defibrillator arrives. An automated external defibrillator (AED) is frequently used because it is simple for both medical and lay personnel. Defibrillation is discussed on p. 672.

Ventricular Asystole. Ventricular asystole, sometimes called *ventricular standstill,* is the complete absence of any ventricular rhythm (Fig. 34-14, *B*). There are no electrical impulses in the ventricles and therefore *no* ventricular depolarization, no QRS complex, no contraction, no cardiac output, and no PERFUSION to the rest of the body.

Assessment. The patient in ventricular asystole has no pulse, respirations, or blood pressure. *The patient is in full cardiac arrest.* The sinoatrial (SA) node, in some cases, may continue to fire and depolarize the atria, with only P waves seen on the ECG. The sinus impulses, however, do not conduct to the ventricles, and QRS complexes remain absent. In most cases, the entire conduction system is electrically silent, with no P waves seen on the ECG.

Ventricular asystole usually results from myocardial hypoxia, which may be a consequence of advanced heart failure. It may also be caused by severe hyperkalemia and acidosis. If P waves are seen, asystole is likely because of severe ventricular conduction blocks.

Interventions. *When cardiac arrest occurs, cardiac output stops.* The underlying rhythm is usually ventricular tachycardia (VT), ventricular fibrillation (VF), or asystole. Without cardiac output, the patient is pulseless and becomes unconscious because of inadequate cerebral PERFUSION and oxygenation. Shortly after cardiac arrest, respiratory arrest occurs. Therefore cardiopulmonary resuscitation is essential to prevent brain damage and death.

Cardiopulmonary Resuscitation and Defibrillation. Cardiopulmonary resuscitation (CPR), also known as **Basic Cardiac Life Support (BCLS)**, must be initiated immediately when asystole occurs. When finding an unresponsive patient, confirm unresponsiveness and call 911 (in community or long-term care setting) or the emergency response team (in the hospital). Gather the AED or defibrillator *before initiating CPR.* Guidelines for CPR have changed from an ABC (airway-breathing-compressions) approach to the initial priorities of CAB (compressions-airway-breathing) (American Heart Association [AHA], 2010).

- Check for a carotid pulse for 5 to 10 seconds
- *If carotid pulse is absent,* start chest compressions of at least 100 compressions per minute and a compression depth of at least 2 inches. Push hard and fast!

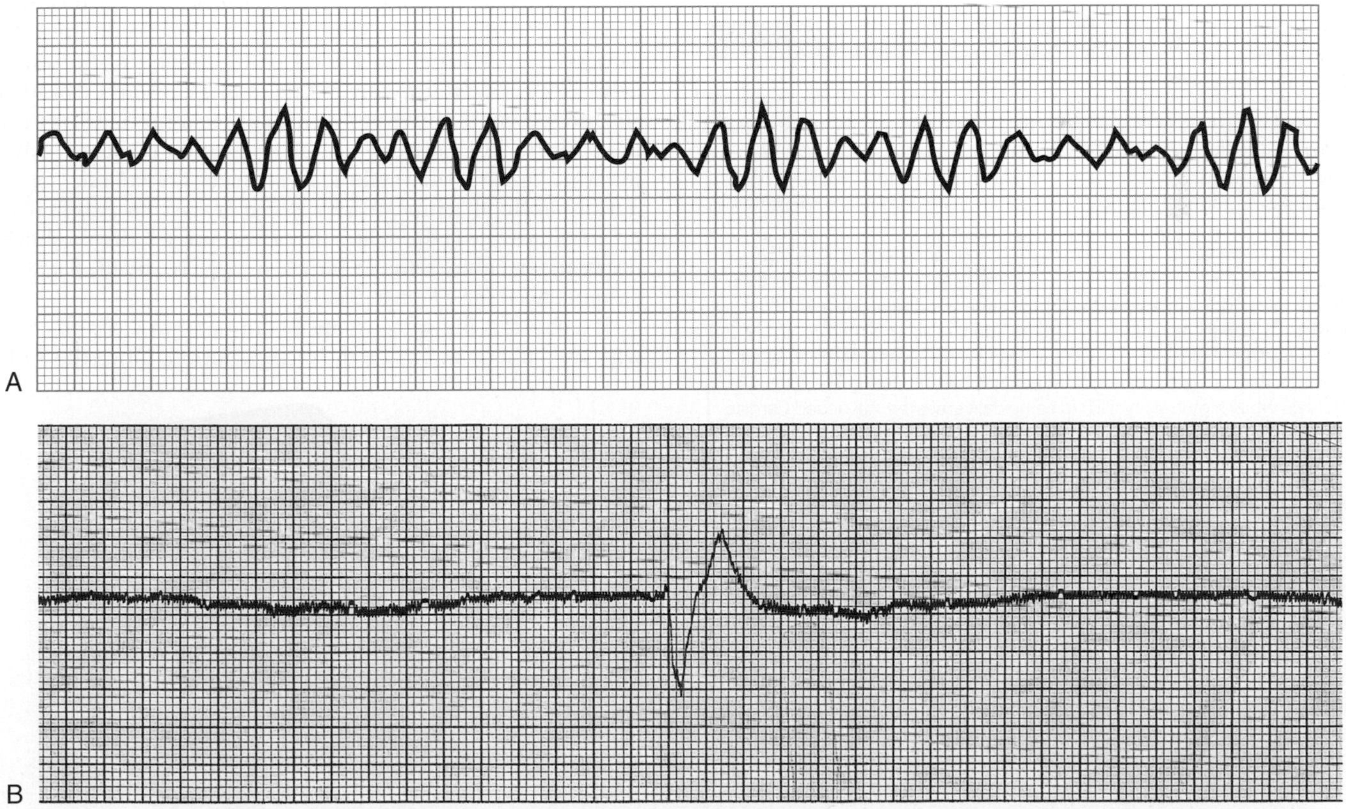

FIG. 34-14 Ventricular dysrhythmias. **A,** Coarse ventricular fibrillation. **B,** Ventricular asystole with one idioventricular complex.

- Maintain a patent airway.
- Ventilate (breathing) with a mouth-to-mask device. Give rescue breaths at a rate of 10 to 12 breaths/min. If an advanced airway is in place, one breath should be given every 6 to 8 seconds (8 to 10 breaths/min).
- Ventilation to compression ratio should be maintained at 30 compressions to 2 breaths if advanced airway is not in place

Be sure to use Standard Precautions when administering CPR. Be aware that complications of CPR include:

- Rib fractures
- Fracture of the sternum
- Costochondral separation
- Lacerations of the liver and spleen
- Pneumothorax
- Hemothorax
- Cardiac tamponade
- Lung contusions
- Fat emboli

As soon as help arrives, place a board under the patient who is not on a firm surface. To make room for the resuscitation team and the crash cart, ask that the area be cleared of movable items and unnecessary personnel. When the AED or defibrillator arrives, *do not stop chest compressions while the defibrillator is being set up*. If trained to use the AED or defibrillator, apply hands-off defibrillator pads to the patient's chest and turn on the monitor. If the patient is in VF or pulseless VT, the immediate priority is to defibrillate! **Defibrillation**, an *asynchronous* countershock, depolarizes a critical mass of myocardium simultaneously to stop the re-entry circuit, allowing the sinus node to regain control of the heart. After defibrillation, CPR is resumed. CPR must continue at all times except during defibrillation.

NURSING SAFETY PRIORITY QSEN

Critical Rescue

Early defibrillation is critical in resolving pulseless ventricular tachycardia (VT) or ventricular fibrillation (VF). It must not be delayed for any reason after the equipment and skilled personnel are present. The earlier defibrillation is performed, the greater the chance of survival! *Do not defibrillate ventricular asystole.*

Before defibrillation, loudly and clearly command all personnel to clear contact with the patient and the bed and check to see they are clear before the shock is delivered. Deliver shock and immediately resume CPR for 5 cycles or about 2 minutes. Reassess the rhythm every 2 minutes and if indicated. Charge the defibrillator to deliver an additional shock at the same energy level previously used. During the 2-minute intervals while high-quality CPR is being delivered, the Advanced Cardiac Life Support (ACLS) team administers medications and performs interventions to try and restore an organized cardiac rhythm. *Discussion of ACLS protocol is beyond the scope of this text.*

After the ACLS team initiates interventions, the role of the medical-surgical nurse is to provide information about the patient. Specific nursing responsibilities include providing a brief summary of the patient's medical condition and the events that occurred up until the time of cardiac arrest. Report the patient's initial cardiac rhythm. Remain in the room to answer questions, document the event, and assist with compressions. If family is present, provide emotional support and explanation of events in the room.

An emerging clinical practice is allowing or encouraging family presence at resuscitation attempts. This can be a positive experience for family members and significant others because it promotes closure after the death of a loved one. Although there may be staff resistance and some limits to family presence, overall it is a beneficial practice that should be considered in all resuscitation attempts.

When spontaneous circulation resumes, the patient is transported to the intensive care unit. Be ready to give hand-off report to the ICU nurse using SBAR communication or other agency system, and assist with patient transport

CLINICAL JUDGMENT CHALLENGE

Teamwork and Collaboration; Evidence-Based Practice; Safety QSEN

A 72-year-old woman is transported to the ED with a diagnosis of chest pain to rule out myocardial infarction (MI). During the initial assessment, the nurse notes the cardiac rhythm changes from sinus tachycardia to ventricular tachycardia (VT) with a pulse. Her vital signs are: blood pressure, 84/40 mm Hg; pulse, 154/min; and respirations, 30/min.

1. What is the initial treatment for this patient at this time?
2. What drugs should you anticipate administering to this patient? Why are they indicated?
3. What evidence-based precautions must be taken to promote safety for both the patient and the ACLS team?
4. If this rhythm deteriorates to ventricular fibrillation or VT without a pulse, what steps should you take? Why?

Automated External Defibrillation. The American Heart Association promotes the use of automated external defibrillators (AEDs) for use by laypersons and health care professionals responding to cardiac arrest emergencies (Fig. 34-15). These devices are found in many public places such as malls, airports, and commercial jets. The patient in cardiac arrest must be on a firm, dry surface. The rescuer places two large adhesive-patch electrodes on the patient's chest in the same positions as for defibrillator electrodes. The rescuer stops CPR and commands anyone present to move away, ensuring that no one is touching the patient. This measure eliminates motion artifact when the machine analyzes the rhythm. The rescuer presses the "analyze" button on the machine. After rhythm analysis, which may take up to 30 seconds, the machine either advises that a shock is necessary or advises that a shock is not indicated. *Shocks are recommended for VF or pulseless VT only.*

If a shock is indicated, issue a command to clear all contact with the patient and press the charge button. Once the AED is

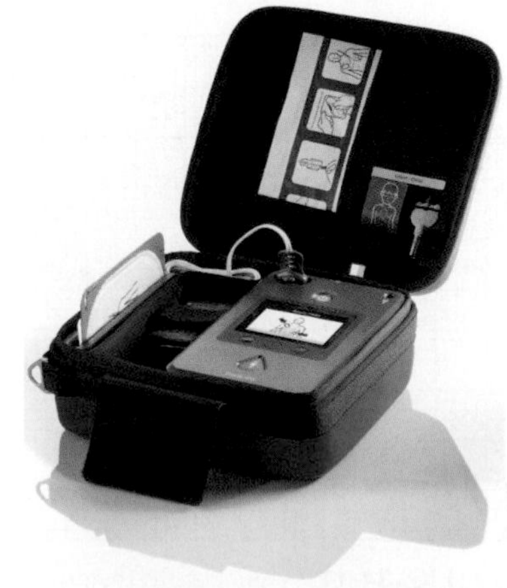

FIG. 34-15 Automated external defibrillator.

charged, press the shock button and the shock will be delivered. The shock is delivered through the patches, so it is hands-off defibrillation, which is safer for the rescuer. The rescuer then resumes CPR until the AED instructs to "stop CPR" to analyze the rhythm. If the rhythm is VF or VT and another shock is indicated, the AED will instruct the rescuer to charge and deliver another shock. Newer AEDs perform rhythm analysis and defibrillation without the need for a rescuer to press a button to analyze or to shock the victim. It is essential that Advanced Cardiac Life Support (ACLS) be provided as soon as possible. Use of AEDs allows for earlier defibrillation. Therefore there is a greater chance of successful rhythm conversion and patient survival.

Implantable Cardioverter/Defibrillator. The implantable cardioverter/defibrillator (ICD) is indicated for patients who have experienced one or more episodes of spontaneous sustained ventricular tachycardia (VT) or ventricular fibrillation (VF) not caused by an MI. Collaborate with the physician and the electrophysiology nurse to prepare the patient for this procedure. A psychological profile is done to determine whether the patient can cope with the discomfort and fear associated with internal defibrillation from the ICD. Many patients report anxiety, depression, and decreased quality of life, which improves for the majority of patients after 12 months (Hallas et al., 2010).

The leads of the device are introduced through the skin, and the generator is implanted in the left pectoral area, similar to a permanent pacemaker insertion procedure. This procedure is performed in the electrophysiology laboratory. If the patient experiences a VT or VF episode after ICD placement and the ICD therapies are not successful, the qualified nurse or health care provider promptly externally defibrillates and initiates high-quality CPR.

The generator may be activated or deactivated by the physician placing a magnet over the implantation site for a few moments. The patient requires close monitoring in the postoperative period for dysrhythmias and complications such as bleeding and cardiac tamponade. The nurse must know whether the ICD is activated or deactivated. Care of the patient is similar to that after implantation of a permanent pacemaker, discussed on p. 664 of this chapter.

Some patients use a lightweight, automated wearable cardioverter/defibrillator (WCD). This external vest-like device is worn 24 hours a day except when the patient showers or bathes. A family member must be present to call 911 and initiate CPR if the patient experiences pulseless VT or VF while in the shower. One popular brand is the Zoll Lifecore LifeVest, which is programmed to monitor for VT and VF. If the patient is conscious while experiencing VT, he or she can press a button to prevent a shock. This precaution is an advantage over implantable devices because ICDs are programmed to always deliver a shock when VT or VF occurs.

NCLEX EXAMINATION CHALLENGE

Safe and Effective Care Environment

A client in the telemetry unit is on a cardiac monitor. The monitor technician notices there are no ECG complexes and the alarm sounds. What is the first action by the nurse?

A. Begin CPR immediately.
B. Call the emergency response team.
C. Press the record button to get an ECG strip.
D. Assess the client and check lead placement.

Community-Based Care

For many patients, dysrhythmias are a disorder resulting from chronic cardiac and pulmonary diseases. Patients may be cared for in a variety of settings, including the acute care hospital, subacute unit, traditional nursing home, or their own home. They are admitted to the hospital when they experience life-threatening or potentially life-threatening dysrhythmias, often associated with an acute disorder.

Home Care Management. Patients discharged from the hospital may have considerable needs, often more related to their underlying chronic diseases than to their dysrhythmias. A case manager or care coordinator can assess the need for health care resources and coordinate access to services.

The focus of the home care nurse's interventions is assessment and health teaching. Patients and families often fear recurrence of a life-threatening dysrhythmia. Patients with an ICD may dread or fear the activation of the device. The community-based nurse provides the patient and family members with an opportunity to verbalize their concerns and fears. Provide emotional support as well as information about support groups and referrals in the community. Assess the patient for possible side effects of antidysrhythmic agents or complications from a pacemaker or ICD.

Self-Management Education. Teach the patient who has had a dysrhythmia caused by an acute problem, such as electrolyte imbalance or MI, about prevention, early recognition, and management of that disorder. Instruct the patient and family about lifestyle modifications designed to prevent, decrease, or control the occurrence of dysrhythmias, as outlined in Chart 34-5. This

CHART 34-5 Patient and Family Education: Preparing for Self-Management

How to Prevent or Decrease Dysrhythmias

For Patients at Risk for Vasovagal Attacks Causing Bradydysrhythmias

- Avoid doing things that stimulate the vagus nerve, such as raising your arms above your head, applying pressure over your carotid artery, applying pressure on your eyes, bearing down or straining during a bowel movement, and stimulating a gag reflex when brushing your teeth or putting objects in your mouth.

For Patients with Premature Beats and Ectopic Rhythms

- Take the medications that have been prescribed for you, and report any adverse effects to your physician.
- Stop smoking, avoid caffeinated beverages and energy drinks as much as possible, and drink alcohol only in moderation.
- Learn ways to manage stress and avoid getting too tired.

For Patients with Ischemic Heart Disease

- If you have an angina attack, treat it promptly with rest and nitroglycerin administration as prescribed by your physician. This decreases your chances of experiencing a dysrhythmia.
- If chest pain is not relieved after taking the amount of nitroglycerin that has been prescribed for you, seek medical attention promptly. Also, seek prompt medical attention if the pain becomes more severe or you experience other symptoms, such as sweating, nausea, weakness, and palpitations.

For Patients at Risk for Potassium Imbalance

- Know the symptoms of decreased potassium levels, such as muscle weakness and cardiac irregularity.
- Eat foods high in potassium, such as tomatoes, beans, prunes, avocados, bananas, strawberries, and lettuce.
- Take the potassium supplements that have been prescribed for you.

teaching may be provided in the acute care setting, primary care provider's office, health care clinic, or home setting.

CONSIDERATIONS FOR OLDER ADULTS

Patient-Centered Care QSEN

Older adults are at increased risk for dysrhythmias because of normal physiologic changes in their cardiac conduction system. The sinoatrial node has fewer pacemaker cells. There is a loss of fibers in the bundle branch system. Therefore older adults are at risk for sinus node dysfunction and may require pacemaker therapy. The most common dysrhythmias are premature atrial contractions, premature ventricular contractions, and atrial fibrillation. Dysrhythmias tend to be more serious in older patients because of underlying heart disease, causing cardiac decompensation. Consequently, blood flow to organs that may already be decreased because of the aging process may be further compromised, leading to multisystem organ dysfunction. Chart 34-6 highlights special considerations for older adults receiving antidysrhythmic therapy.

Patients and their families must have a thorough understanding of the prescribed *drug therapy*, including antidysrhythmic agents. Pharmacies provide written instructions with filled prescriptions. Teach patients and families the generic and trade names of their drugs, as well as the drugs' purposes, using basic terms that are easily understood. Clear instructions regarding dosage schedules and common side effects are important (see Chart 34-3). Emphasize the importance of reporting these side effects and any dizziness, nausea, vomiting, chest discomfort, or shortness of breath to the primary care provider.

Teach all patients and their family members how to take a pulse and blood pressure. Some patients may want to use technology to calculate and record their pulse rate. Several applications (apps) for handheld mobile devices (such as the iPhone) are available, but their accuracy varies. "Instant Health Rate" and "Quick Heart Rate" are examples of apps used to calculate pulse rate.

Remind patients to report any signs of a change in heart rhythm, such as a significant decrease in pulse rate, a rate more than 100 beats/min, or increased rhythm irregularity. Smart Blood Pressure (SmartBP) is a blood pressure and pulse management system that records, tracks, and analyzes data to share via an iPhone or iPad. The patient can send these readings to their health care provider as needed to maintain frequent vital sign monitoring.

Give written and verbal information to patients who have a *permanent pacemaker* about the type and settings of their pacemaker. Teach the patient to report any pulse rate lower than that set on the pacemaker. Review the proper care of the pacemaker insertion site and the importance of reporting any fever or any redness, swelling, or drainage at the pacemaker insertion site. If the surgical incision is near either shoulder, teach and demonstrate range-of-motion exercises to perform to prevent shoulder stiffness.

CHART 34-6 Nursing Focus on the Older Adult

Dysrhythmias

Special nursing considerations for the older patient with dysrhythmias are:

- Evaluate the patient with dysrhythmias immediately for the presence of a life-threatening dysrhythmia or hemodynamic deterioration.
- Assess the patient with a dysrhythmia for angina, hypotension, heart failure, and decreased cerebral and renal perfusion.
- Consider these causes of dysrhythmias when taking the patient's history: hypoxia, drug toxicity, electrolyte imbalances, heart failure, and myocardial ischemia or infarction.
- Assess the patient's level of education, hearing, learning style, and ability to understand and recall instructions to determine the best approaches for teaching.
- Assess the patient's ability to read written instructions.
- Teach the patient the generic and trade names of prescribed antidysrhythmic drugs, as well as their purposes, dosage, side effects, and special instructions for their use.
- Provide clear written instructions in basic language and easy-to-read print.
- Provide a written drug dosage schedule for the patient, considering all the drugs the patient is taking and possible drug interactions.
- Assess the patient for possible side effects or adverse reactions to drugs considering age and health status.
- Teach the patient to take his or her pulse and to report significant changes in heart rate or rhythm to the health care provider.
- Inform the patient of available resources for blood pressure and pulse checks, such as blood pressure clinics, home health agencies, and cardiac rehabilitation programs.
- Instruct the patient on the importance of keeping follow-up appointments with the health care provider and reporting symptoms promptly.
- Include the patient's family members or significant other in all teaching whenever possible.
- Teach the patient to avoid drinking caffeinated beverages, to stop smoking, to drink alcohol only in moderation, and to follow his or her prescribed diet.

! NURSING SAFETY PRIORITY QSEN

Action Alert

Teach patients who have permanent pacemakers to:

- Keep handheld cellular phones at least 6 inches away from the generator, with the handset on the ear opposite the side of the generator.
- Avoid sources of strong electromagnetic fields, such as magnets and telecommunications transmitters. These may cause interference and could change the pacemaker settings, causing a malfunction. Magnetic resonance imaging (MRI) is usually contraindicated, depending on the machine's technology.
- Carry a pacemaker identification card provided by the manufacturer and wear a medical alert bracelet at all times.

Chart 34-7 outlines the major points for patient and family teaching after the insertion of a permanent pacemaker.

Patients with an *implantable cardioverter/defibrillator (ICD)* usually continue to receive antidysrhythmic drugs after discharge from the hospital. Provide health teaching about the purposes of drug therapy, dosage schedules, special instructions, and side effects that need to be reported. If patients experience an internal defibrillator shock, remind them to sit or lie down immediately and notify the primary care provider. Some patients describe the experience of a shock as a quick thud or kick in the chest, whereas others relate severe discomfort similar to that of external defibrillation. Usually the shock is not as severe because the heart is situated between the defibrillation pads, thus requiring less electrical current to convert the dysrhythmia. Inform family members that they may feel an electrical shock if they are touching the patient during delivery of the shock but that it is not harmful. Provide information about how to access the emergency medical services (EMS) system in the community. Recommend resources for the family to learn how to perform CPR.

Remind patients with an ICD to avoid sources of strong electromagnetic fields, such as large electrical generators and radio and television transmitters. Tell the patient that these items may inhibit tachydysrhythmia detection and therapy or may cause pacing or shocks. MRI should not be used for patients with ICDs unless the patient has an MRI-conditional ICD. Handheld cellular phones must be at least 6 inches away from the generator, with the handset held to the ear opposite the side of the ICD. If the pulse generator emits a beeping sound or provides some other indicator, the patient must move away from the area as quickly as possible to prevent deactivation of the device. Teach the patient with an ICD to carry an ICD identification card and wear a medical alert bracelet. Chart 34-8 highlights the important points for health teaching.

CHART 34-7 Patient and Family Education: Preparing for Self-Management

Permanent Pacemakers

- Follow the instructions for pacemaker site skin care that have been specifically prepared for you. Report any fever or redness, swelling, or drainage from the incision site to your physician.
- Do not manipulate the pacemaker generator site.
- Keep your pacemaker identification card in your wallet, and wear a medical alert bracelet.
- Take your pulse for 1 full minute at the same time each day, and record the rate in your pacemaker diary. Take your pulse any time you feel symptoms of a possible pacemaker failure, and report your heart rate and symptoms to your physician.
- Know the rate at which your pacemaker is set and the basic functioning of your pacemaker. Know what rate changes to report to your physician.
- Do not apply pressure over your generator. Avoid tight clothing or belts.
- You may take baths or showers without concern for your pacemaker.
- Inform all health care providers that you have a pacemaker. Certain tests they may wish to perform (e.g., magnetic resonance imaging) could affect or damage your pacemaker.
- Know the indications of battery failure for your pacemaker as you were instructed, and report these findings to your health care provider if they occur.
- Do not operate electrical appliances directly over your pacemaker site because this may cause your pacemaker to malfunction.
- Do not lean over electrical or gasoline engines or motors. Be sure that electrical appliances or motors are properly grounded.
- Avoid all transmitter towers for radio, television, and radar. Radio, television, other home appliances, and antennas do not pose a hazard.
- Be aware that antitheft devices in stores may cause temporary pacemaker malfunction. If symptoms develop, move away from the device.
- Inform airport personnel of your pacemaker before passing through a metal detector, and show them your pacemaker identification card. The metal in your pacemaker will trigger the alarm in the metal detector device.
- Stay away from any arc welding equipment.
- Be aware that it is safe to operate a microwave oven unless it does not have proper shielding (old microwave ovens) or is defective.
- Report any of these symptoms to your physician if you experience them: difficulty breathing, dizziness, fainting, chest pain, weight gain, and prolonged hiccupping. If you have any of these symptoms, check your pulse rate and call your health care provider.
- If you feel symptoms when near any device, move 5 to 10 feet away from it and then check your pulse. Your pulse rate should return to normal.
- Keep all of your health care provider and pacemaker clinic appointments.
- Take all medications prescribed for you as instructed.
- Follow your prescribed diet.
- Follow instructions on restrictions on physical activity, such as no sudden, jerky movement, for 8 weeks to allow the pacemaker to settle in place.

CHART 34-8 Patient and Family Education: Preparing for Self-Management

Implantable Cardioverter/Defibrillator

- Follow the instructions for implantable cardioverter/defibrillator (ICD) site skin care that have been specifically prepared for you.
- Report to your health care provider any fever or redness, swelling, soreness, or drainage from your incision site.
- Do not wear tight clothing or belts that could cause irritation over the ICD generator.
- Do not manipulate your generator site
- Avoid activities that involve rough contact with the ICD implantation site.
- Keep your ICD identification card in your wallet, and consider wearing a medical alert bracelet.
- Know the basic functioning of your ICD device and its rate cutoff, as well as the number of consecutive shocks it can deliver.
- Avoid magnets directly over your ICD because they can inactivate the device. If beeping tones are coming from the ICD, move away from the electromagnetic field immediately (within 30 seconds) before the inactivation sequence is completed, and notify your health care provider.
- Inform all health care providers caring for you that you have an ICD implanted, because certain diagnostic tests and procedures must be avoided to prevent ICD malfunction. These include diathermy, electrocautery, and nuclear magnetic resonance tests.
- Avoid other sources of electromagnetic interference, such as devices emitting microwaves (not microwave ovens); transformers; radio, television, and radar transmitters; large electrical generators; metal detectors, including handheld security devices at airports; antitheft devices; arc welding equipment; and sources of 60-cycle (Hz) interference. Also avoid leaning directly over the alternator of a running motor of a car or boat.
- Report to your health care provider symptoms such as fainting, nausea, weakness, blackout, and rapid pulse rates.
- Take all medications prescribed for you as instructed.
- Follow instructions on restrictions on physical activity, such as not swimming, driving motor vehicles, or operating dangerous equipment.
- Follow your prescribed diet.
- Keep all health care provider and ICD clinic appointments.
- Sit or lie down immediately if you feel dizzy or faint to avoid falling if the ICD discharges.
- Post emergency telephone numbers.
- Know how to contact the local emergency medical services (EMS) systems in your community. Inform them in advance that you have an ICD so that they can be prepared if they need to respond to an emergency call for you.
- Encourage family members to learn how to perform CPR. Family members should know that if they are touching you when the device discharges, they may feel a slight shock but that this is not harmful to them.
- Follow instructions on what to do if the ICD successfully discharges, after which you feel well. This may include maintaining a diary of the date, the time, activity preceding the shock, symptoms, the number of shocks delivered, and how you feel after the shock. The physician may wish to be notified each time the device discharges.
- Avoid strenuous activities that may cause your heart rate to meet or exceed the rate cutoff of your ICD because this causes the device to discharge inappropriately.
- Notify your health care provider for information regarding access to health care if you are leaving town or are relocating.

Health Care Resources. The cardiac rehabilitation nurse typically provides written and oral information about dysrhythmias, antidysrhythmic drugs, pacemakers, and ICDs, as well as information about cardiac exercise programs, educational programs, and support groups. The office or ambulatory care nurse may also provide information about resources. Teach the patient how to contact the local chapter of the American Heart Association (www.americanheart.org) or the provincial chapter of the Heart and Stroke Foundation in Canada (www.heartandstroke.ca) for information about dysrhythmias, pacemakers, and CPR training.

Manufacturers of pacemakers and ICDs provide helpful booklets and CDs to give patients and their families a better understanding of these therapies. Teach patients how to use telephonic systems for transmission of their rhythms to the ambulatory care setting or health care provider's office. Stress the importance of keeping scheduled appointments for visits with the cardiologist and pacemaker or ICD clinic. Instruct patients to contact the local ambulance or paramedic services and emergency facilities to let them know that they have these devices implanted. Encourage the patient and family to attend pacemaker or ICD support groups.

NURSING CONCEPTS AND CLINICAL JUDGMENT REVIEW

What might you NOTICE if the patient is experiencing inadequate oxygenation and tissue PERFUSION as a result of dysrhythmias?
- Report of chest discomfort or pain
- Report of dizziness or syncope
- Shortness of breath
- Weakness and fatigue
- Decreased urine output
- Pale, cool skin
- Diaphoresis
- Anxiety or restlessness

What should you INTERPRET and how should you RESPOND to a patient experiencing inadequate oxygenation and PERFUSION as a result of dysrhythmias?

Perform and interpret physical assessment, including:
- Taking vital signs (may have hypotension and weak pulse)
- Checking for pulse deficit
- Asking if patient has palpitations
- Checking capillary refill (decreased)
- Listening to lung and heart sounds
- Assessing cognition
- Taking an ECG
- Checking oxygen saturation

Respond by:
- Applying oxygen
- Keeping the head of the bed elevated unless patient is very hypotensive
- Maintaining or starting an IV line
- Notifying the health care provider or Rapid Response Team
- Giving drug therapy as prescribed
- Initiating CPR for asystole
- Defibrillating the patient in VF
- Assisting with other procedures as needed, for example, defibrillation

On what should you REFLECT?
- Evaluate patient's response to drug therapy.
- Observe for evidence of increased oxygenation and perfusion.
- Think about what else you could have done to assist the patient with this problem.

GET READY FOR THE NCLEX® EXAMINATION!

KEY POINTS

Review these Key Points for each NCLEX Examination Client Needs Category.

Safe and Effective Care Environment
- Be very careful to protect patients and staff to prevent electrical injury when assisting with invasive pacemakers, cardioversion, and defibrillation. **Safety** QSEN
- For safety during cardioversion, turn oxygen off and away from the patient to prevent a fire. Shout "CLEAR" before shock delivery for electrical safety. **Safety** QSEN
- Teach patients who have permanent pacemakers to keep cell phones at least 6 inches away from the generator, avoid electromagnetic fields such as telecommunication transmitters, wear a medical alert bracelet at all times, and carry a pacemaker identification card. **Safety** QSEN

Health Promotion and Maintenance
- Teach patients with dysrhythmias the correct drug, dose, route, time, and side effects of prescribed drugs, and teach them to notify their primary care provider if adverse effects occur (see Chart 34-3).
- Teach patients taking anticoagulant therapy to report any signs of bruising or unusual bleeding immediately to their health care provider.
- Teach family members where to learn cardiopulmonary resuscitation (CPR) to decrease their anxiety while living with a patient with dysrhythmias or ICD/pacemaker. **Patient-Centered Care** QSEN
- Teach patients the importance of adhering to their prescribed cardiac regimen, such as checking their pulse to ascertain pacemaker function.

Physiological Integrity

- Assess patients with dysrhythmias for a decrease in cardiac output resulting in inadequate oxygenation and perfusion to vital organs (see Chart 34-2); typical assessment findings include shortness of breath, dizziness or syncope, weakness and fatigue, and irregular pulse.
- Monitor patients with dysrhythmias, including conducting a physical assessment and health history, as well as interpreting ECG rhythm strips. Report significant changes to the health care provider.
- Interpret common dysrhythmias, especially bradycardia, tachycardia, atrial fibrillation (AF) and ventricular fibrillation (VF), premature ventricular contractions (PVCs), and asystole, using the steps of ECG analysis.
- Use special considerations when caring for older adults with dysrhythmias, as described in Chart 34-6. **Patient-Centered Care** QSEN
- Recognize that noninvasive pacing is an emergency measure to provide demand ventricular pacing in patients with profound bradycardia or asystole. Teach patients to expect possible discomfort.
- Identify and intervene in life-threatening situations by providing cardiopulmonary resuscitation, electrical therapy, or drug administration. **Evidence-Based Practice** QSEN
- Be aware that automated external defibrillators (AEDs) are used by medical and lay personnel as an essential intervention for VF.
- Do not perform CPR while the patient is being defibrillated. **Safety** QSEN
- Educate patients who have permanent pacemakers or ICDs about self-management (see Charts 34-7 and 34-8).

35 CHAPTER

Care of Patients with Cardiac Problems

Laura M. Dechant

http://evolve.elsevier.com/Iggy/

PRIORITY CONCEPTS

- PERFUSION
- GAS EXCHANGE
- PAIN
- INFECTION

LEARNING OUTCOMES

Safe and Effective Care Environment

1. Evaluate the status of patients with end-stage heart disease regarding advance directives.
2. Provide the patient with heart failure (HF) and the family information on discharge to home, hospice, or other community-based setting.
3. Collaborate with the interdisciplinary team when providing care to patients with cardiac problems.

Health Promotion and Maintenance

4. Identify community resources for patients with cardiac problems and their families.
5. Provide special care needs of older adults with heart failure.
6. Teach patients about actions to maintain health and prevent worsening HF.
7. Engage patients and family members in active partnerships that promote health, safety, and self-management.

Psychosocial Integrity

8. Assess the patient and family response to living with chronic HF and possible transplantation.

Physiological Integrity

9. Explain the pathophysiology of HF.
10. Compare and contrast left-sided and right-sided HF.
11. Identify priority problems for patients with HF, including IMPAIRED GAS EXCHANGE.
12. Perform a comprehensive assessment of patients experiencing cardiac problems.
13. Explain how common drug therapies improve cardiac output, enhance peripheral PERFUSION, and prevent worsening of HF.
14. Assess patients for adverse effects of drug therapy for cardiac problems.
15. Monitor the laboratory values for patients with cardiac problems.
16. Base the plan of care on patient values, clinical expertise, and current evidence to promote safety and quality of cardiovascular care.
17. Provide emergency care for patients experiencing life-threatening complications, such as cardiac tamponade and pulmonary edema.
18. Identify the four Heart Failure Core Measures required by The Joint Commission.
19. Describe essential focused assessments used by the home care nurse for patients with heart failure.
20. Compare and contrast common valvular disorders.
21. Describe surgical management for patients with valvular disease.
22. Develop a teaching/learning plan for patients with valvular disease.
23. Differentiate between common cardiac inflammations and INFECTIONS—endocarditis, pericarditis, and rheumatic carditis.
24. Identify clinical assessment findings for patients with cardiomyopathy.
25. Plan postoperative care for patients having a heart transplant.

This chapter focuses on heart failure and its common causes in the adult population; coronary artery disease is discussed in Chapter 38. Heart failure is the most common reason for hospital stays in patients older than 65 years in the United States. When the heart is diseased, it cannot effectively pump an adequate amount of arterial blood to the rest of the body. Arterial blood carries *oxygen* and nutrients to vital organs, such as the kidneys and brain, and to peripheral tissues. When these organs and other body tissues are not adequately *perfused,* they may not function properly.

HEART FAILURE

Heart failure, sometimes referred to as ***pump failure***, is a general term for the inability of the heart to work effectively as a pump. It results from a number of acute and chronic cardiovascular problems that are discussed later in this chapter and elsewhere in the cardiovascular unit.

❖ PATHOPHYSIOLOGY

Heart failure (HF) is a common *chronic* health problem, with acute episodes often causing hospitalization. Acute coronary disease and other structural or functional problems of the heart can lead to *acute* heart failure. Both acute and chronic HF can be life threatening if they are not adequately treated or if the patient does not respond to treatment.

Types of Heart Failure

The major types of heart failure are:

- Left-sided heart failure
- Right-sided heart failure
- High-output failure

Because the two ventricles of the heart represent two separate pumping systems, it is possible for one to fail by itself for a short period. *Most heart failure begins with failure of the left ventricle and progresses to failure of both ventricles.* Typical causes of **left-sided heart (ventricular) failure** include hypertension, coronary artery disease, and valvular disease involving the mitral or aortic valve. Decreased tissue PERFUSION from poor cardiac output and pulmonary congestion from increased pressure in the pulmonary vessels indicate left ventricular failure (LVF).

Left-sided heart failure was formerly referred to as **congestive heart failure (CHF)**; however, not all cases of LVF involve fluid accumulation. In the clinical setting, though, the term *CHF* is still commonly used. Left-sided failure may be acute or chronic and mild to severe. It can be further divided into two subtypes: systolic heart failure and diastolic heart failure.

Systolic heart failure (systolic ventricular dysfunction) results when the heart cannot contract forcefully enough during systole to eject adequate amounts of blood into the circulation. Preload increases with decreased contractility, and afterload increases as a result of increased peripheral resistance (e.g., hypertension) (McCance et al., 2014). The **ejection fraction** (the percentage of blood ejected from the heart during systole) drops from a normal of 50% to 70% to below 40% with ventricular dilation. As it decreases, tissue perfusion diminishes and blood accumulates in the pulmonary vessels. Manifestations of systolic dysfunction may include symptoms of inadequate tissue PERFUSION or pulmonary and systemic congestion. Systolic heart failure is often called "forward failure" because cardiac output is decreased and fluid backs up into the pulmonary system. Because these patients are at high risk for sudden cardiac death, patients with an ejection fraction of less than 30% are considered candidates for an implantable cardioverter/defibrillator (ICD; also known as an *internal cardioverter/defibrillator*) (see Chapter 34).

In contrast, **diastolic heart failure** (heart failure with preserved left ventricular function) occurs when the left ventricle cannot relax adequately during diastole. Inadequate relaxation or "stiffening" prevents the ventricle from filling with sufficient blood to ensure an adequate cardiac output. Although ejection fraction is more than 40%, the ventricle becomes less compliant over time because more pressure is needed to move the same amount of volume as compared with a healthy heart. Diastolic failure represents about 20% to 40% of all heart failure, primarily in older adults and in women who have chronic hypertension and undetected coronary artery disease. Clinical manifestations and management of diastolic failure are similar to those of systolic dysfunction (McCance et al., 2014).

Right-sided heart (ventricular) failure may be caused by left ventricular failure, right ventricular myocardial infarction (MI), or pulmonary hypertension. In this type of heart failure (HF), the right ventricle cannot empty completely. Increased volume and pressure develop in the venous system, and peripheral edema results.

High-output heart failure can occur when cardiac output remains normal or above normal, unlike left- and right-sided heart failure, which are typically low-output states. High-output failure is caused by increased metabolic needs or hyperkinetic conditions, such as septicemia, high fever, anemia, and hyperthyroidism. This type of heart failure is not as common as other types.

Classification and Staging of Heart Failure

The American College of Cardiology (ACC) and American Heart Association (AHA) have developed evidence-based guidelines for staging and managing heart failure as a chronic, progressive disease. These guidelines do not replace the New York Heart Association (NYHA) functional classification system, which is used to describe symptoms a patient may exhibit (see Table 33-2 in Chapter 33).

The ACC/AHA staging system when compared with the NYHA system categorizes patients as:

A. Patients at high risk for developing heart failure (class I NYHA)
B. Patients with cardiac structural abnormalities or remodeling who have not developed HF symptoms (class I NYHA)
C. Patients with current or prior symptoms of heart failure (class II or III NYHA)
D. Patients with refractory end-stage heart failure (class IV NYHA)

Another method for staging HF is the Killip classification system, which is based on the heart's hemodynamic ability. Table 38-3 in Chapter 38 outlines this system.

Compensatory Mechanisms

When cardiac output is insufficient to meet the demands of the body, compensatory mechanisms work to improve cardiac output (Fig. 35-1). Although these mechanisms may initially increase cardiac output, they eventually have a damaging effect on pump function. Major compensatory mechanisms include:

- Sympathetic nervous system stimulation
- Renin-angiotensin system (RAS) activation (also called renin-angiotensin-aldosterone [RAAS] activation)
- Other chemical responses
- Myocardial hypertrophy

In heart failure (HF), *stimulation of the sympathetic nervous system* (i.e., increasing catecholamines) as a result of tissue hypoxia represents the most immediate compensatory mechanism. Stimulation of the adrenergic receptors causes an increase in heart rate (beta adrenergic) and blood pressure from vasoconstriction (alpha adrenergic).

Because cardiac output (CO) is the product of heart rate (HR) and stroke volume (SV), an increase in HR results in an immediate *increase in cardiac output.* The HR is limited, though, in its ability to compensate for decreased CO. If it becomes too rapid, diastolic filling time is limited and CO may start to

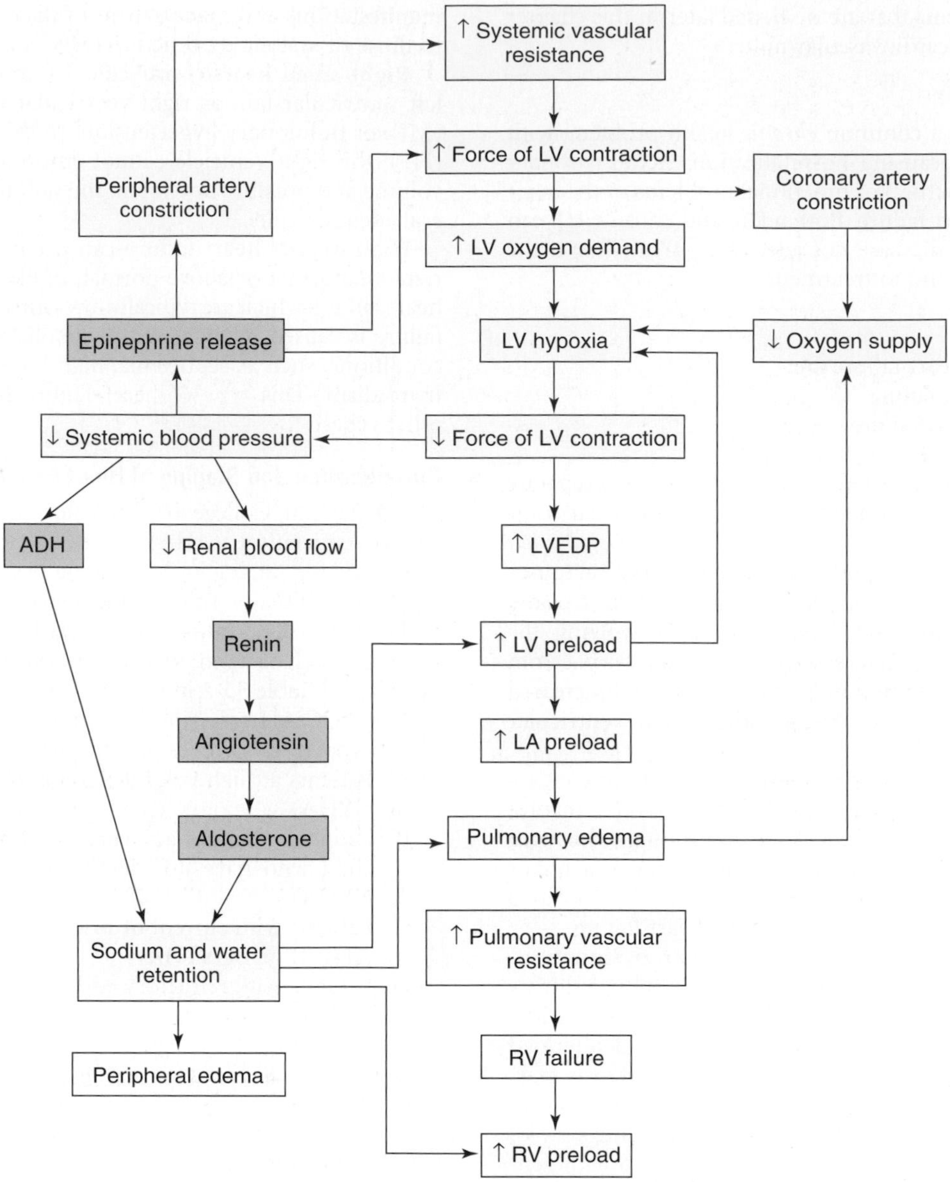

FIG. 35-1 Left-sided heart failure from elevated systemic vascular resistance. Left heart failure leads to right heart failure. Systemic vascular resistance and preload are exacerbated by renal and adrenal mechanisms. *ADH,* Antidiuretic hormone; *LA,* left atrial; *LV,* left ventricular; *LVEDP,* left ventricular end-diastolic pressure; *RV,* right ventricular.

decline. An increase in HR also significantly increases oxygen demand by the myocardium. If the heart is poorly perfused because of arteriosclerosis, HF may worsen.

Stroke volume (SV) is also *improved* by sympathetic stimulation. Sympathetic stimulation increases venous return to the heart, which further stretches the myocardial fibers causing dilation. According to Starling's law, increased myocardial stretch results in more forceful contraction. More forceful contractions increase SV and CO. After a critical point is reached within the cardiac muscle, further volume and stretch reduce the force of contraction and cardiac output.

Sympathetic stimulation also results in *arterial vasoconstriction.* Vasoconstriction has the benefit of maintaining blood pressure and improving tissue perfusion in low-output states. However, constriction of the arteries increases **afterload**, the resistance against which the heart must pump. Afterload is the major determinant of myocardial oxygen requirements. As it increases, the left ventricle requires more energy to eject its contents and SV may decline.

Reduced blood flow to the kidneys, a common occurrence in low-output states, results in *activation of the renin-angiotensin system (RAS).* Vasoconstriction becomes more pronounced in response to angiotensin II, and aldosterone secretion causes sodium and water retention. Preload and afterload increase. Angiotensin II contributes to *ventricular remodeling* resulting in progressive myocyte (myocardial cell) contractile dysfunction over time (McCance et al., 2014).

In addition to the sympathetic nervous system and RAS responses, other mechanisms are activated when a patient experiences heart failure (HF). Most of these actions contribute to worsening of the condition.

For example, in those who have had an MI, heart muscle cell injury causes an *immune response.* Pro-inflammatory cytokines, such as tumor necrosis factor (TNF) and interleukins (IL-1 and

IL-6), are released, especially with left-sided HF. These substances contribute to ventricular remodeling.

Natriuretic peptides are neurohormones that work to promote vasodilation and diuresis through sodium loss in the renal tubules. The **B-type natriuretic peptide (BNP)** is produced and released by the ventricles when the patient has fluid overload as a result of HF. It increases with age and has a greater concentration in women (Jessup et al., 2009). People who are obese have lower BNP levels compared with those who are not (Clerico et al., 2012).

Low cardiac output (CO) causes decreased cerebral perfusion. As a result, the posterior pituitary gland secretes *vasopressin* (antidiuretic hormone [ADH]). The hormone causes vasoconstriction and fluid retention, which worsen HF.

Endothelin is secreted by endothelial cells when they are stretched. As the myocardial fibers are stretched in patients with HF, this potent vasoconstrictor is released, which increases peripheral resistance and hypertension. HF worsens as a result of these actions.

Myocardial hypertrophy (enlargement of the myocardium), with or without chamber dilation, is another compensatory mechanism. The walls of the heart thicken to provide more muscle mass, which results in more forceful contractions, further increasing cardiac output. Cardiac muscle, however, may hypertrophy more rapidly than collateral circulation can provide adequate blood supply to the muscle. Often a hypertrophied heart is slightly oxygen deprived.

All the compensatory mechanisms contribute to an increase in the consumption of myocardial oxygen. When the demand for oxygen increases and the myocardial reserve has been exhausted, clinical manifestations of HF develop.

Etiology

Heart failure (HF) is caused by systemic hypertension in most cases. Some patients experiencing myocardial infarction (MI, "heart attack") also develop HF. The next most common cause is structural heart changes, such as valvular dysfunction, particularly pulmonic or aortic stenosis, which leads to pressure or volume overload on the heart. Common direct causes and risk factors for HF are listed in Table 35-1.

CONSIDERATIONS FOR OLDER ADULTS

Patient-Centered Care QSEN

Heart failure is a common problem among older adults. The use of certain drugs can contribute to the development or exacerbation of the problem in this population. For example, long-term use of NSAIDs for arthritis and other chronic pain can cause fluid and sodium retention. NSAIDs may cause peripheral vasoconstriction and increase the toxicity of diuretics and angiotensin-converting enzyme inhibitors (ACEIs). Thiazolidinediones (TZDs) (e.g., pioglitazone [Actos]) used for diabetics also cause fluid and sodium retention. Rosiglitazone (Avandia), another TZD drug, has recently been found to cause acute myocardial infarction (AMI) in patients with type 2 diabetes. These drugs should be used with caution and restrictions in the older adult population.

Right-sided HF in the absence of left-sided HF is usually the result of pulmonary problems such as chronic obstructive pulmonary disease (COPD) or pulmonary hypertension. Acute respiratory distress syndrome (ARDS) may also cause right-sided HF. These problems are discussed elsewhere in this text.

TABLE 35-1 Common Causes and Risk Factors For Heart Failure

• Hypertension	• Dysrhythmias
• Coronary artery disease	• Diabetes mellitus
• Cardiomyopathy	• Smoking/tobacco use
• Substance abuse (alcohol and illicit/prescribed drugs)	• Family history
• Valvular disease	• Obesity
• Congenital defects	• Severe lung disease
• Cardiac infections and inflammations	• Sleep apnea
	• Hyperkinetic conditions (e.g., hyperthyroidism)

TABLE 35-2 Meeting *Healthy People 2020* Objectives

Cardiac Disease

To reduce hospitalizations of older adults with heart failure as the principal diagnosis.

- For patients hospitalized for heart failure, collaborate with the case manager for discharge planning, including adequate support in the community.
- Provide a continuing plan of care for patients and their families or other caregivers when the patient is discharged from the hospital.
- If the patient is discharged to home, call to check that he or she has no impending signs and symptoms of heart failure (the case manager may make calls).
- Teach the patient and family or other caregiver about when to call the health care provider for health changes so the patient can be treated at home.
- Ensure that the interdisciplinary team provides the patient with follow-up care in the home or nursing home.

Incidence and Prevalence

Over five million people in the United States have HF, causing about 875,000 hospitalizations each year. HF is the most common reason for hospital admission for people older than 65 years. African Americans are affected more often than Euro-Americans, probably because they have more risk factors that can lead to HF (Go et al., 2013). The disease is a major cause of disability and death after MI, often due to nonadherence to the treatment plan and recommended lifestyle changes.

CONSIDERATIONS FOR OLDER ADULTS

Patient-Centered Care QSEN

Heart failure has been referred to as a U.S. epidemic, although it is a major problem worldwide. One of the U.S. *Healthy People 2020* objectives is to reduce the number of hospitalizations of older adults with HF as the principal diagnosis. Patient and family education can help meet this objective (Table 35-2). As the "baby boomer" population reaches 65 years of age, the numbers of hospital stays and deaths from HF are likely to increase dramatically.

❖ PATIENT-CENTERED COLLABORATIVE CARE

◆ Assessment

History. When obtaining a history, keep in mind the many conditions that can lead to HF. Carefully question the patient about his or her medical history, including hypertension, angina (cardiac pain), MI, rheumatic heart disease, valvular disorders, endocarditis, and pericarditis. Ask about the patient's perception of his or her activity tolerance, breathing pattern, sleeping pattern, urinary pattern, and fluid volume status, as well as his or her knowledge about HF.

Left-Sided Heart Failure. With left ventricular systolic dysfunction, cardiac output (CO) is diminished, leading to impaired tissue perfusion, anaerobic metabolism, and unusual fatigue. Assess activity tolerance by asking whether the patient can perform normal ADLs or climb flights of stairs without *fatigue* or dyspnea. Many patients with heart failure (HF) experience weakness or fatigue with activity or have a feeling of heaviness in their arms or legs. Ask about their ability to perform simultaneous arm and leg work (e.g., walking while carrying a bag of groceries). Such activity may place an unacceptable demand on the failing heart. Ask the patient to identify his or her most strenuous activity in the past week. Many people unconsciously limit their activities in response to fatigue or dyspnea and may not realize how limited they have become.

PERFUSION to the myocardium is often impaired as a result of left ventricular failure, especially with cardiac hypertrophy. The patient may report *chest discomfort* or may describe palpitations, skipped beats, or a fast heartbeat.

As the amount of blood ejected from the left ventricle diminishes, hydrostatic pressure builds in the pulmonary venous system and results in fluid-filled alveoli and pulmonary congestion, which results in a *cough.* The patient in early HF describes the cough as irritating, nocturnal (at night), and usually nonproductive. *As HF becomes very severe, he or she may begin expectorating frothy, pink-tinged sputum—a sign of life-threatening pulmonary edema.*

Dyspnea also results from increasing pulmonary venous pressure and pulmonary congestion. Carefully question about the presence of dyspnea and when and how it developed. The patient may refer to dyspnea as "trouble in catching my breath," "breathlessness," or "difficulty in breathing."

As **exertional dyspnea** develops (also called *dyspnea upon* or *on exertion [DUE/DOE]*), the patient often stops previously tolerated levels of activity because of shortness of breath. Dyspnea at rest in the recumbent (lying flat) position is known as **orthopnea.** Ask how many pillows are used to sleep or whether the patient sleeps in an upright position in a bed, recliner, or other type of chair.

Patients who describe sudden awakening with a feeling of breathlessness 2 to 5 hours after falling asleep have **paroxysmal nocturnal dyspnea (PND).** Sitting upright, dangling the feet, or walking usually relieves this condition.

Right-Sided Heart Failure. Signs of systemic congestion occur as the right ventricle fails, fluid is retained, and pressure builds in the venous system. Edema develops in the lower legs and may progress to the thighs and abdominal wall. Patients may notice that their shoes fit more tightly, or their shoes or socks may leave indentations on their swollen feet. They may have removed their rings because of swelling in their fingers and hands. Ask about weight gain. An adult may retain 4 to 7 liters of fluid (10 to 15 lb [4.5 to 6.8 kg]) before pitting edema occurs.

Reports of *nausea and anorexia* may be a direct consequence of liver engorgement (congestion) resulting from fluid retention. In *advanced* heart failure (HF), *ascites* and an increased abdominal girth may develop from severe liver congestion. Another common finding related to fluid retention is *diuresis at rest.* At rest, fluid in the peripheral tissue is mobilized and excreted and the patient describes frequent awakening at night to urinate.

CHART 35-1 Key Features

Left-Sided Heart Failure

DECREASED CARDIAC OUTPUT	PULMONARY CONGESTION
• Fatigue	• Hacking cough, worse at night
• Weakness	• Dyspnea/breathlessness
• Oliguria during the day (nocturia at night)	• Crackles or wheezes in lungs
• Angina	• Frothy, pink-tinged sputum
• Confusion, restlessness	• Tachypnea
• Dizziness	• S_3/S_4 summation gallop
• Tachycardia, palpitations	
• Pallor	
• Weak peripheral pulses	
• Cool extremities	

CHART 35-2 Key Features

Right-Sided Heart Failure

Systemic Congestion

- Jugular (neck vein) distention
- Enlarged liver and spleen
- Anorexia and nausea
- Dependent edema (legs and sacrum)
- Distended abdomen
- Swollen hands and fingers
- Polyuria at night
- Weight gain
- Increased blood pressure (from excess volume) or decreased blood pressure (from failure)

Obtain a careful nutritional history, questioning about the use of salt and the types of food consumed. Ask about daily fluid intake. Patients with HF may experience increased thirst and drink excessive fluid (4000 to 5000 mL/day) because of sodium retention.

Physical Assessment/Clinical Manifestations. Manifestations of HF depend on the type of failure, the ventricle involved, and the underlying cause. Impaired tissue perfusion, pulmonary congestion, and edema are associated with *left* ventricular failure (Chart 35-1). Conversely, systemic venous congestion and peripheral edema are associated with *right* ventricular failure (Chart 35-2).

Left-Sided Heart Failure. Left ventricular failure is associated with decreased cardiac output and elevated pulmonary venous pressure. It may appear clinically as:

- Weakness
- Fatigue
- Dizziness
- Acute confusion
- Pulmonary congestion
- Breathlessness
- Oliguria (scant urine output)

Decreased blood flow to the major body organs can cause dysfunction, especially renal failure. Nocturia may occur when the patient is at rest.

The pulse may be tachycardic, or it may alternate in strength (**pulsus alternans**). Take the apical pulse for a full minute, noting any irregularity in heart rhythm. *An irregular heart rhythm resulting from premature atrial contractions (PACs), premature ventricular contractions (PVCs), or atrial fibrillation (AF) is common in HF* (see Chapter 34). The sudden development of an irregular rhythm may further compromise CO. Carefully monitor the patient's respiratory rate, rhythm, and character, as well as oxygen saturation. The respiratory rate typically exceeds 20 breaths/min.

Assess whether the patient is oriented to person, place, and time. A short mental status examination may be used if there are concerns about orientation. Objective data are important because in daily conversation many people are skillful at covering up memory losses. Older adults are frequently disoriented or confused when the heart fails due to brain hypoxia (decreased oxygen).

Increased heart size is common with a displacement of the apical impulse to the left. A third heart sound, **S_3 gallop**, is an early diastolic filling sound indicating an increase in left ventricular pressure. This sound is often the first sign of HF. A fourth heart sound (S_4) also can occur; it is not a sign of failure but is a reflection of decreased ventricular compliance.

Auscultate for crackles and wheezes of the lungs. Late inspiratory crackles and fine profuse crackles that repeat themselves from breath to breath and do not diminish with coughing indicate HF. *Crackles are produced by intra-alveolar fluid and are often noted first in the bases of the lungs and spread upward as the condition worsens.* Wheezes indicate a narrowing of the bronchial lumen caused by engorged pulmonary vessels. Identify the precise location of crackles and wheezes and whether the wheezes are heard on inspiration, expiration, or both.

Right-Sided Heart Failure. Right ventricular failure is associated with increased systemic venous pressures and congestion. On inspection, assess the neck veins for distention and measure abdominal girth. Hepatomegaly (liver engorgement), hepatojugular reflux, and ascites may also be assessed. Abdominal fluid can reach volumes of more than 10 liters.

Assess for dependent edema. In ambulatory patients, edema commonly presents in the ankles and legs. When patients are restricted to bedrest, the sacrum is dependent and fluid accumulates there.

! NURSING SAFETY PRIORITY QSEN

Action Alert

Edema is an extremely unreliable sign of HF. Be sure that accurate daily weights are taken every morning to document fluid retention. *Weight is the most reliable indicator of fluid gain and loss!*

? NCLEX EXAMINATION CHALLENGE

Physiological Integrity

A client is diagnosed with left-sided heart failure. Which assessment findings will the nurse expect the client to have? **Select all that apply.**

A. Peripheral edema
B. Crackles in both lungs
C. Breathlessness
D. Ascites
E. Tachypnea

Psychosocial Assessment. Chronic heart failure (HF) is typically a slow, debilitating disease. Anxiety and frustration are common. Symptoms such as dyspnea increase the patient's anxiety level.

Patients with HF, especially those with advanced disease, are at high risk for depression. It is not certain whether the functional impairments contribute to the depression or depression affects functional ability. Older hospitalized patients may be depressed, particularly those who have been re-admitted for an acute episode of HF. Lifestyle changes and quality-of-life issues can also cause depression many months after the initial diagnosis of HF.

Assess patients and their families for anxiety and depression. Ask them about their usual methods of coping, as well as any history of depression. If anxiety or depression is present, notify the health care provider for further assessment. Social workers, certified clinical chaplains, or psychologists may administer specific assessment tools to determine the extent of the problem. Some patients need drug therapy and nonpharmacologic modalities, such as cognitive behavior therapy, biofeedback, or relaxation training.

Hope is a major indicator of well-being for patients with HF. Those who are hopeful tend to feel better and are more socially involved. Ask patients about their daily activities and how often they interact with the significant people in their life to help determine patient and family coping strategies.

Laboratory Assessment. Electrolyte imbalance may occur from complications of HF or as side effects of drug therapy, especially diuretic therapy. Regular evaluations of a patient's *serum electrolytes,* including sodium, potassium, magnesium, calcium, and chloride, are essential. Any impairment of renal function resulting from inadequate perfusion causes elevated blood urea nitrogen and serum creatinine and decreased creatinine clearance levels. *Hemoglobin* and *hematocrit* tests should be performed to identify HF resulting from anemia. If the patient has fluid volume excess, the hematocrit levels may be low as a result of hemodilution.

B-type natriuretic peptide (BNP) is used for diagnosing HF (in particular, diastolic HF) in patients with acute dyspnea. As discussed earlier, it is part of the body's response to decreased cardiac output from either left or right ventricular dysfunction. An increase in BNP, in conjunction with history and physical, best differentiates between the dyspnea of HF and that associated with lung dysfunction (Fard et al., 2012). However, patients with renal disease may also have elevated BNP levels (Chen et al., 2010). In the ambulatory care arena, BNP is trended over time to guide ambulatory care treatment of heart failure (DeBeradinis & Januzzi, 2012); as therapy is optimized, levels decrease. If levels increase, alternate causes such as ischemia are looked at prior to intensifying treatment.

Urinalysis may reveal proteinuria and high specific gravity. *Microalbuminuria* is an early indicator of decreased compliance of the heart and occurs before the BNP rises. It serves as an "early warning detector" that lets the health care provider know that the heart is experiencing early signs of decreased compliance, long before symptoms occur.

CONSIDERATIONS FOR OLDER ADULTS

Patient-Centered Care QSEN

Thyroxine (T_4) and thyroid-stimulating hormone (TSH) levels should be assessed in patients who are older than 65 years, have atrial fibrillation, or have evidence of thyroid disease. Heart failure (HF) may be caused or aggravated by hypothyroidism or hyperthyroidism.

Arterial blood gas (ABG) values often reveal hypoxemia (low blood oxygen level) because oxygen does not diffuse easily through fluid-filled alveoli. Respiratory alkalosis may occur because of hyperventilation; respiratory acidosis may occur because of carbon dioxide retention. Metabolic acidosis may indicate an accumulation of lactic acid.

Imaging Assessment. *Chest x-rays* can be helpful in diagnosing left ventricular failure. Typically the heart is enlarged (cardiomegaly), representing hypertrophy or dilation. Pleural effusions develop less often and generally reflect biventricular failure. *Echocardiography is considered the best tool in diagnosing heart failure.* Cardiac valvular changes, pericardial effusion, chamber enlargement, and ventricular hypertrophy can be diagnosed using this noninvasive technique. The test can also be used to determine ejection fraction.

Radionuclide studies (thallium imaging or technetium pyrophosphate scanning) can also indicate the presence and cause of HF. Multigated acquisition (MUGA) scans, also called multigated blood pool scans, provide information about left ventricular ejection fraction and velocity, which are typically low in patients with HF. These tests are discussed in Chapter 33.

Other Diagnostic Assessment. An *electrocardiogram* (ECG) is also performed. It may show ventricular hypertrophy, dysrhythmias, and any degree of myocardial ischemia, injury, or infarction. However, it is *not* helpful in determining the presence or extent of HF.

Invasive hemodynamic monitoring allows the direct assessment of cardiac function and volume status in acutely ill patients. Although medical-surgical nurses do not manage these systems on general hospital units, they should be familiar with the interpretation of some of the major hemodynamic pressures as they relate to patient assessment. These measurements can confirm the diagnosis and guide the management of HF. For example, right atrial pressure is either normal or elevated in left ventricular failure and elevated in right ventricular failure. Pulmonary artery pressure (PAP) and pulmonary artery wedge pressure (PAWP) are elevated in left-sided HF because volumes and pressures are increased in the left ventricle. Hemodynamic monitoring is described in detail in Chapter 38.

◆ Analysis

The priority NANDA-I nursing diagnoses and collaborative problems for patients with heart failure (HF) include:

1. Impaired Gas Exchange related to ventilation/perfusion imbalance (NANDA-I)
2. Decreased Cardiac Output related to altered contractility, preload, and afterload (NANDA-I)
3. Fatigue related to hypoxemia (NANDA-I)
4. Potential for pulmonary edema related to left-sided HF

◆ Planning and Implementation

The patient-centered collaborative care that patients with HF need depends on their disease stage and severity of signs and symptoms. Be sure to individualize care based on the patient's values and preferences, your clinical expertise, and best current evidence.

Improving Gas Exchange

Planning: Expected Outcomes. The expected outcome is that the patient will have an optimal spontaneous breathing pattern that increases GAS EXCHANGE and oxygenation and maintains a serum carbon dioxide level that is within normal limits.

Interventions. The purpose of collaborative care is to help promote GAS EXCHANGE and oxygenation. *Ventilation assistance* may be needed because the oxygen content of the blood is often decreased in patients who have pulmonary congestion. Monitor or have assistive personnel monitor the patient's respiratory rate, rhythm, and quality every 1 to 4 hours. Auscultate breath sounds every 4 to 8 hours.

TABLE 35-3 Commonly Used Drug Classifications for Patients with Systolic Heart Failure

Angiotensin-converting enzyme (ACE) inhibitors or angiotensin-receptor blockers (ARBs)
Diuretics:
- High-ceiling
- Potassium-sparing

Human B-type natriuretic peptides
Nitrates
Inotropics:
- Beta-adrenergic agonists
- Phosphodiesterase inhibitors
- Calcium sensitizers
- Digoxin (Lanoxin)

Beta-adrenergic blockers

! NURSING SAFETY PRIORITY QSEN

Action Alert

Provide the necessary amount of supplemental oxygen within a range prescribed by the health care provider *to maintain oxygen saturation at 90% or greater.* If the patient has dyspnea, place him or her in a high-Fowler's position with pillows under each arm to maximize chest expansion and improve oxygenation. Repositioning and performing coughing and deep-breathing exercises every 2 hours help improve oxygenation and prevent atelectasis. Collaborate with the respiratory therapist, if available, to plan the most effective methods for assisting with ventilation.

Improving Cardiac Output

Planning: Expected Outcomes. The expected outcome is that the patient will have increased cardiac output by improving stroke volume (SV) (determined by preload, afterload, and contractility) and heart rate (HR).

Interventions. Collaborative care begins with nonsurgical interventions, but the patient may need surgery if these are not successful in meeting optimal outcomes.

Nonsurgical Management. Nonsurgical management relies primarily on a variety of drugs (Table 35-3). If drug therapy is ineffective, other nonsurgical options are available. Drugs to improve stroke volume include those that reduce afterload, reduce preload, and improve cardiac muscle contractility. A major role of the nurse is to give medications as prescribed, monitor for their therapeutic and adverse effects, and teach the patient and family about drug therapy. A variety of classes of drugs that reduce afterload and preload are used to manage heart failure (see Table 35-3).

Drugs That Reduce Afterload. By relaxing the arterioles, arterial vasodilators can reduce the resistance to left ventricular ejection (afterload) and improve CO. These drugs do not cause excessive vasodilation but reverse some of the inappropriate or excessive vasoconstriction common in HF.

Angiotensin-Converting Enzyme Inhibitors (ACEIs) and Angiotensin-Receptor Blockers (ARBs). Patients with even mild heart failure (HF) resulting from left ventricular dysfunction are given a trial of ACE inhibitors or ARBs. Both ACE inhibitors (e.g., enalapril [Vasotec] and fosinopril [Monopril]) and ARBs (e.g., valsartan [Diovan], irbesartan [Avapro], and losartan [Cozaar]) improve function and quality of life for patients with HF. ACE inhibitors are the first-line drug of choice, but some health care providers prefer to start the patient on an ARB because ACE inhibitors can cause a nagging, dry cough. For patients with *acute* HF, the health care provider may prescribe an IV-push ACE inhibitor such as Vasotec IV.

The ACE inhibitors and ARBs suppress the renin-angiotensin system (RAS), which is activated in response to decreased renal blood flow. ACE inhibitors prevent conversion of angiotensin I to angiotensin II, resulting in arterial dilation and increased stroke volume. ARBs block the effect of angiotensin II receptors and thus decrease arterial resistance and arterial dilation. In addition, these drugs block aldosterone, which prevents sodium and water retention, thus decreasing fluid overload. *Both ACEIs and ARBs work more effectively for Euro-Americans than for African-American populations.* Volume-depleted patients should receive a low starting dose, or the fluid volume should be restored before beginning the prescribed drug. Monitor for hyperkalemia, a potential adverse drug effect in patients who have renal dysfunction.

! NURSING SAFETY PRIORITY QSEN

Drug Alert

ACEIs and ARBs are started slowly and cautiously. The first dose may be associated with a rapid drop in blood pressure (BP). Patients at risk for hypotension usually have an initial systolic BP less than 100 mm Hg, are older than 75 years, have a serum sodium level less than 135 mEq/L, or are volume depleted. Monitor BP every hour for several hours after the initial dose and each time the dose is increased. Immediately report to the health care provider and document a systolic blood pressure of less than 90 mm Hg (or designated protocol level). If this problem occurs, place the patient flat and elevate legs to increase cerebral perfusion and promote venous return.

Assess for orthostatic hypotension, acute confusion, poor peripheral perfusion, and reduced urine output in patients with low systolic blood pressure. Monitor serum potassium and creatinine levels to determine renal dysfunction. Additional nursing implications for selected ACE inhibitor/ARB drugs are described in Chapter 38 on p. 766 in the Drug Therapy section.

Human B-type Natriuretic Peptides. Human B-type natriuretic peptides (hBNPs) such as nesiritide (Natrecor) are often used to treat *acute* HF. Endogenous BNP is released in response to decreased CO and causes *natriuresis,* or loss of sodium in the renal tubules, as well as vasodilation. Natrecor lowers pulmonary capillary wedge pressure (PCWP) and improves renal glomerular filtration. It is given as an IV bolus over 60 seconds followed with a continuous infusion for up to 48 hours.

! NURSING SAFETY PRIORITY QSEN

Drug Alert

When giving Natrecor, monitor BP and pulse carefully because significant decreases in BP may occur. Although the patient's systolic BP may be between 90 and 100 mm Hg, he or she is usually asymptomatic. *Give Natrecor through a separate infusion line because it is incompatible with heparin and most other parenteral medications.* Expect an increase in the serum BNP after drug administration.

Interventions That Reduce Preload. Ventricular fibers contract less forcefully when they are overstretched, such as in a failing heart. Interventions aimed at reducing preload attempt to decrease volume and pressure in the left ventricle, increasing ventricular muscle stretch and contraction. Preload reduction is appropriate for HF accompanied by congestion with total body sodium and water overload.

Nutrition Therapy. In HF, nutrition therapy is aimed at reducing sodium and water retention to decrease the workload of the heart. The primary care provider may restrict sodium intake in an attempt to decrease fluid retention. Many patients need to omit table salt (no added salt) from their diet, thus reducing sodium intake to about 3 g daily.

If salt intake must be reduced further, the patient may need to eliminate all salt in cooking and high-sodium foods (e.g., ham, bacon, pickles), thus reducing sodium intake to 2 g daily. If needed, collaborate with the dietitian to help the patient select foods that meet such a restricted therapeutic diet.

Few patients are placed on severe fluid restrictions. However, patients with excessive aldosterone secretion may experience thirst and drink 3 to 5 liters of fluid each day. As a result, their fluid intake may be limited to a more normal 2 liters daily. *Supervise unlicensed assistive personnel (UAP) to ensure that they limit the prescribed intake and accurately record intake and output.*

Weigh the patient daily, or delegate this activity to UAP and supervise that it is done. Keep in mind that *1 kg of weight gain or loss equals 1 liter of retained or lost fluid.* The same scale should be used every morning before breakfast for the most accurate assessment of weight. Monitor for an expected *decrease* in weight because excess fluid is excreted from the body.

Drug Therapy. Common drugs prescribed to reduce preload are diuretics and venous vasodilators. *Morphine sulfate* is also given for patients in *acute* heart failure to reduce anxiety, decrease preload and afterload, slow respirations, and reduce the pain associated with a myocardial infarction (MI).

The health care provider adds *diuretics* to the regimen when diet and fluid restrictions have not been effective in managing the symptoms of HF. Diuretics are the first-line drug of choice in older adults with HF and fluid overload. These drugs enhance the renal excretion of sodium and water by reducing circulating blood volume, decreasing preload, and reducing systemic and pulmonary congestion.

The type and dosage of diuretic prescribed depend on the severity of HF and renal function. High-ceiling (loop) diuretics, such as furosemide (Lasix, Furoside 🍁, Novosemide 🍁), torsemide (Demadex), and bumetanide (Bumex), are most effective for treating fluid volume overload.

CONSIDERATIONS FOR OLDER ADULTS

***Patient-Centered Care* QSEN**

Loop diuretics continue to work even after excess fluid is removed. As a result, some patients, especially older adults, can become dehydrated. Observe for manifestations of dehydration in the older adult, especially acute confusion, decreased urinary output, and dizziness. Provide evidence-based interventions to reduce the risk for falls, as discussed in Chapter 2.

For those patients with *acute* HF, Lasix or Bumex can be administered by IV push (IVP). Lasix can be given in doses of 20 to 40 mg IVP and increased by 20 mg every 2 hours until the desired diuresis is obtained. The usual IVP initial dose for Bumex is 1 to 2 mg once or twice daily, but it is more often given in a continuous infusion of 10 mg over 24 hours.

The practitioner may initially use a thiazide diuretic, such as hydrochlorothiazide (HCTZ) (HydroDIURIL, Urozide 🍁) and metolazone (Zaroxolyn), for *older adults* with *mild* volume overload. Zaroxolyn is a long-acting agent and is therefore often given every second, third, or fourth day, depending on patient need and tolerance.

Unlike loop diuretics, the action of thiazides is self-limiting (i.e., diuresis decreases after edema fluid is lost). Therefore the dehydration that may occur with loop diuretics is not common with these drugs. Patients also prefer thiazides because of the gradual onset of diuresis.

As HF progresses, many patients develop diuretic resistance with refractory edema. The health care provider may choose to manage this problem by prescribing both types of diuretics. Other strategies include IV continuous infusion of furosemide or bumetanide or rotating loop diuretics.

Monitor for and prevent potassium deficiency (hypokalemia) from diuretic therapy. The primary signs of hypokalemia are nonspecific neurologic and muscular symptoms, such as generalized weakness, depressed reflexes, and irregular heart rate. A potassium supplement may be prescribed for some patients. Other practitioners prescribe a potassium-sparing diuretic, such as spironolactone (Aldactone), for patients at risk for dysrhythmias from hypokalemia. Although not as effective as other diuretics, Aldactone helps retain potassium and thus decrease the risk for ventricular dysrhythmias and is usually used in stage III/IV heart failure. Monitor for hyperkalemia and renal failure if Aldactone inhibitors are utilized, and anticipate stopping the medication if potassium or creatinine levels rise.

Patients being managed with ACE inhibitors or ARBs and diuretics at the same time may not experience hypokalemia. However, if their kidneys are not functioning well, they may develop hyperkalemia (elevated serum potassium level). Review the patient's serum creatinine level. *If the creatinine is greater than 1.8 mg/dL, notify the health care provider before administering supplemental potassium.*

The health care provider may prescribe *venous vasodilators* (e.g., nitrates) for the patient with HF who has persistent dyspnea. Significant constriction of venous and arterial blood vessels occurs to compensate for reduced CO. Constriction reduces the volume of fluid that the vascular bed can hold and increases preload. Venous vasodilators may benefit by:

- Returning venous vasculature to a more normal capacity
- Decreasing the volume of blood returning to the heart
- Improving left ventricular function

Nitrates may be administered IV, orally, or topically. IV nitrates are used most often for *acute* HF. These drugs cause primarily venous vasodilation but also a significant amount of arteriolar vasodilation. Monitor the patient's blood pressure when starting nitrate therapy or increasing the dosage. Patients may initially report headache, but assure them that they will develop a tolerance to this effect and that the headache will cease or diminish. Acetaminophen (Tylenol, Exdol 🍁) can be given to help relieve discomfort.

Unfortunately, tolerance to the vasodilating effects develops when nitrates are given around-the-clock. To prevent this tolerance, the health care provider may prescribe at least one 12-hour nitrate-free period out of every 24 hours (usually overnight). Nitrates such as isosorbide (Imdur, ISMO) are prescribed to provide nitrate-free periods and reduce the problem of tolerance. Chapter 38 discusses nitrates in more detail.

NCLEX EXAMINATION CHALLENGE

Physiological Integrity

A client has been taking furosemide (Lasix) and valsartan (Diovan) for the past year. The hospital laboratory notifies the nurse that the client's serum potassium level is 6.2 mEq/L. What is the nurse's best action at this time?

A. Assess the client's oxygen saturation level.
B. Ask the laboratory to retest the potassium level.
C. Give potassium as an IV infusion.
D. Check the client's serum creatinine.

Drugs That Enhance Contractility. Contractility of the heart can also be enhanced with drug therapy. Positive inotropic drugs are most commonly used, but vasodilators and beta-adrenergic blockers may also be administered. For *chronic* HF, low-dose beta blockers are most commonly used. Digoxin (Lanoxin) may be prescribed to improve symptoms, thereby decreasing dyspnea and improving functional activity. This older and long-used drug is not expensive. In some settings, nesiritide (Natrecor) may be administered for end-stage HF, although this drug is very expensive (see discussion of Natrecor for acute HF on p. 685).

Digoxin. Although not as commonly used today, digoxin (Lanoxin, Novodigoxin 🍁), a cardiac glycoside, has been demonstrated to provide symptomatic benefits for patients in *chronic* heart failure (HF) with sinus rhythm and atrial fibrillation. Digoxin (sometimes called "dig") therapy reduces exacerbations of HF and hospitalizations when added to a regimen of ACE inhibitors or ARBs, beta blockers, and diuretics. However, it may increase mortality due to drug toxicity, especially in older adults.

The potential benefits of digoxin include:

- Increased contractility
- Reduced heart rate (HR)
- Slowing of conduction through the atrioventricular node
- Inhibition of sympathetic activity while enhancing parasympathetic activity

Digoxin is erratically absorbed from the GI tract. Many drugs, especially antacids, interfere with its absorption. It is eliminated primarily by renal excretion. Older patients should be maintained on lower doses of the drug than younger patients.

Other Inotropic Drugs. Patients experiencing *acute* heart failure are candidates for IV drugs that increase contractility. For example, *beta-adrenergic agonists,* such as dobutamine (Dobutrex), are used for short-term treatment of *acute* episodes of HF. Dobutamine improves cardiac contractility and thus cardiac output and myocardial-systemic perfusion.

A more potent drug used for *acute* HF, milrinone (Primacor), functions as a vasodilator/inotropic medication with phosphodiesterase activity. Also known as a *phosphodiesterase inhibitor,* this drug increases cyclic adenosine monophosphate (cAMP), which enhances the entry of calcium into myocardial cells to increase contractile function. Like the beta-adrenergic agonists, Primacor is given IV.

Levosimendan (Simdax) is a calcium-sensitizing medication and a positive inotropic drug. It appears to bind to troponin C in the heart muscle and therefore increases the contraction of the heart. Simdax is used most often in patients who have had

NURSING SAFETY PRIORITY (QSEN)

Drug Alert

Increased cardiac automaticity occurs with toxic digoxin levels or in the presence of hypokalemia, resulting in ectopic beats (e.g., premature ventricular contractions [PVCs]). Changes in potassium level, especially a decrease, cause patients to be more sensitive to the drug and cause toxicity.

The clinical manifestations of **digoxin toxicity** are often vague and nonspecific and include anorexia, fatigue, blurred vision, and changes in mental status, especially in older adults. Toxicity may cause nearly any dysrhythmia, but PVCs are most commonly noted. Assess for early signs of toxicity such as bradycardia and loss of the P wave on the ECG. Carefully monitor the apical pulse rate and heart rhythm of patients receiving digoxin.

The health care provider determines the desirable heart rate (HR) to achieve. Some health care providers prefer a rate between 50 and 60 beats per minute. Report the development of either an irregular rhythm in a patient with a previously regular rhythm or a regular rhythm in a patient with a previously irregular one. Monitor serum digoxin and potassium levels (hypokalemia potentiates digoxin toxicity) to identify toxicity. Older adults are more likely than other patients to become toxic because of decreased renal excretion.

Any drug that increases the workload of the failing heart also increases its oxygen requirement. Be alert for the possibility that the patient may experience angina (chest pain) in response to digoxin.

NCLEX EXAMINATION CHALLENGE

Physiological Integrity

An older adult taking digoxin and hydrochlorothiazide (HCTZ) for chronic heart failure is admitted to the emergency department (ED) with an apical pulse of 48. A family member states that the client has reported blurred vision and loss of appetite for 2 weeks. What is the nurse's first action?

A. Call the ED physician immediately.
B. Draw a serum digoxin level.
C. Assess for signs of hypokalemia.
D. Establish the client's airway.

or are at high risk for myocardial infarction. Chapter 38 discusses inotropic drugs in more detail.

Beta-Adrenergic Blockers. Beta-adrenergic blockers (commonly referred to as "beta blockers") improve the condition of some patients in HF. Prolonged exposure to increased levels of sympathetic stimulation and catecholamines worsens cardiac function. Beta-adrenergic blockade reverses this effect, improving morbidity, mortality, and quality of life for patients in HF.

Beta blockers must be started slowly for HF. *Patients in acute HF should not be started on these drugs.* Carvedilol (Coreg), metoprolol succinate (Toprol XL), and bisoprolol (Zebeta) are approved for treatment of *chronic* HF. ***Do not confuse metoprolol tartrate with metoprolol succinate.*** Current guidelines only recommend the sustained-release formulation of metoprolol for chronic HF treatment. The first dose is extremely low. Monitor the patient either in the hospital or in the health care provider's office to assess for bradycardia or hypotension after the first dose is given.

Instruct the patient to weigh daily and to report any signs of worsening HF immediately. The health care provider gradually increases the drug dose if HF worsens. The patient is evaluated at least weekly for changes in BP, pulse, activity tolerance, and orthopnea. A modest drop in BP is acceptable if he or she remains asymptomatic and can stand without experiencing dizziness or a further drop in BP. The resting heart rate (HR) should remain between 55 and 60 and increase slightly with exercise. Activity tolerance improves, and less orthopnea is experienced. Most patients with mild and moderate HF demonstrate improved ejection fraction, decreased hospital admissions, and improvement in symptoms when beta blockers are added to their treatment regimens. The benefits of this therapy are seen over a long period rather than immediately.

For patients with *diastolic* HF, drug therapy has not been as effective. Calcium channel blockers, ACE inhibitors, and beta blockers have been used with various degrees of success.

Other Nonsurgical Options. In addition to drug therapy, other nonsurgical options, both noninvasive and invasive, may be used and include:

- Continuous positive airway pressure (CPAP)
- Cardiac resynchronization therapy (CRT)
- Investigative gene therapy

Continuous positive airway pressure (CPAP) is a respiratory treatment that improves obstructive sleep apnea in patients with HF. It also improves cardiac output (CO) and ejection fraction (EF) by decreasing afterload and preload, blood pressure (BP), and dysrhythmias. Sleep apnea is directly correlated with coronary artery disease as a result of diminished oxygen supply to the heart during apneic episodes. This respiratory problem is discussed in detail in Chapter 29.

Cardiac resynchronization therapy (CRT), also called *biventricular pacing,* uses a permanent pacemaker alone or is combined with an implantable cardioverter/defibrillator. Electrical stimulation causes more synchronous ventricular contractions to improve EF, CO, and mean arterial pressure. This modality is indicated for patients with class III or IV HF and an EF of less than 35%. CRT improves the patient's ability to perform ADLs. Chapter 34 discusses pacing in more detail.

Gene therapy may be indicated for patients in end-stage HF who are not candidates for heart transplantation. This therapy replaces damaged genes with normal or modified genes by a series of injections of growth factor into the left ventricle. Although still investigative, this therapy may result in improved exercise tolerance and regrowth of cardiac cells.

Surgical Management. Heart transplantation is still the ultimate choice for end-stage HF (see discussion on p. 702). Several surgical procedures are available to improve CO in patients who are *not* candidates for a transplant or are awaiting transplant.

Ventricular Assist Devices. Patients with debilitating end-stage heart failure are often sent home on drug therapy and referred to hospice. However, ventricular assist devices (VADs) can dramatically improve the lives of many patients. In this procedure, a mechanical pump is implanted to work with the patient's own heart (Fig. 35-2). Both left and right VADs are available, depending on the type of heart failure the patient has. Those with end stage kidney disease, severe chronic lung disease, clotting disorders, and infections that do not respond to antibiotics are not candidates for this surgery. Postoperative complications include bleeding, infective endocarditis, ventricular dysrhythmias, and stroke. Nursing care is similar to that described for cardiac surgery in Chapter 38.

Ventricular assist devices can be used short-term while awaiting heart transplantation (a "bridge-to-transplant" procedure) or long-term (destination therapy). Most patients survive with a VAD until a transplant is available. The evidence shows

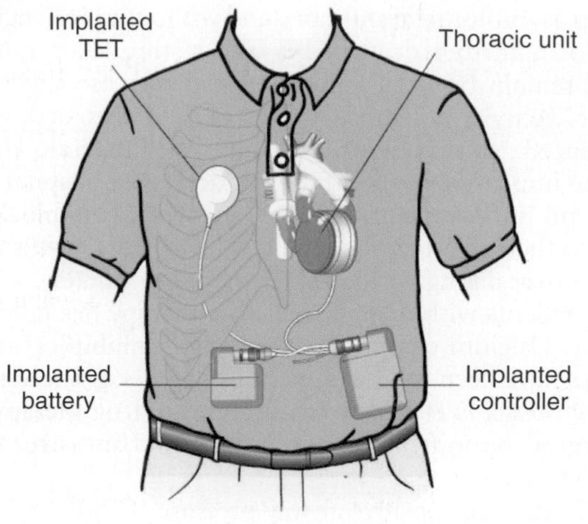

FIG. 35-2 The AbioCor Implantable Replacement Heart has four main parts that are placed inside the body. *TET,* Transtelephonic electrocardiographic transmission device.

that patients who have long-term devices live longer and have an improved quality of life (Rogers et al., 2010).

Other Surgical Therapies. Heart failure causes ventricular remodeling, or dilation, which worsens as the disease progresses. Several new therapies are used to reshape the left ventricle in patients with HF. Perioperative care is similar to that for the patient having a coronary artery bypass graft (CABG) (see Chapter 38). The most common ventricular reconstructive procedures include:

- **Partial left ventriculectomy (PLV)**
- Endoventricular circular patch cardioplasty
- Acorn cardiac support device
- Myosplint

Also known as *heart reduction surgery,* PLV (sometimes referred to as the *Batista procedure*) involves removing a triangle-shaped section of the weakened heart in the left lateral ventricle to reduce the ventricle's diameter and decrease wall tension. In *endoventricular circular patch cardioplasty,* the surgeon removes portions of the cardiac septum and left ventricular wall and grafts a circular patch (synthetic or autologous) into the opening. This procedure provides a more normal shape to the left ventricle to improve the heart's ejection fraction (EF) and cardiac output (CO).

The **Acorn cardiac support device** is a polyester mesh jacket that is placed over the ventricles to provide support and to avoid overstretching the myocardial muscle. The material for the jacket has been used for other procedures, such as vascular grafts. The jacket appears to reduce hypertrophy of the heart muscle and assists with improvement of the EF.

The **Myosplint** has recently been approved for use in the United States. Electrical stimulation of several tension pads (splints) on the outside of the ventricle changes it to a more normal shape to improve function.

Decreasing Fatigue

Planning: Expected Outcomes. The expected outcome is that the patient will have decreased fatigue and will gain energy as heart failure improves.

Interventions. The patient in severe heart failure initially requires physical and emotional rest for *energy management.* On the first day of hospitalization, he or she may sit up in a chair for meals and perform basic leg exercises while out of bed. Organize nursing care to allow periods of rest. Collaborate with the interdisciplinary team to observe and document the patient's physiologic response to activity.

As the patient's condition improves, the physical therapist (PT) starts ambulation, usually on hospital day 2. The PT or nurse checks the BP, pulse, and oxygen saturation before and after the activity. A BP change of more than 20 mm Hg or a pulse increase of more than 20 beats per minute may indicate that the activity is too stressful. Other indications of activity intolerance include dyspnea, fatigue, and chest pain. Ask a patient having any of these symptoms to rate how hard he or she has been working on a scale of 1 to 20, with 20 being the maximum perceived exertion. If the patient rates the exertion more than 12, remind him or her to slow down. If activity is tolerated, the PT steadily increases the activity level until the patient is ambulating 200 to 400 feet several times per day.

If the patient is able, the PT (or assistive nursing or PT personnel) might time him or her for 6 minutes while walking at a comfortable pace. The distance the patient can walk can be used to determine his or her functional level and activity plan.

Preventing or Managing Pulmonary Edema

Planning: Expected Outcomes. The most desirable outcome is that the patient will not develop pulmonary edema as a result of heart failure (HF). However, if the patient progresses to pulmonary edema, the expected outcome is that he or she will recover from this complication without other problems.

Interventions. Monitor for manifestations of acute pulmonary edema, a life-threatening event that can result from severe HF (with fluid overload), acute myocardial infarction (MI), mitral valve disease, and possibly dysrhythmias. In pulmonary edema, the left ventricle fails to eject sufficient blood and pressure increases in the lungs as a result. The increased pressure causes fluid to leak across the pulmonary capillaries and into the lung airways and tissues.

! NURSING SAFETY PRIORITY (QSEN)

Critical Rescue

Assess for and report early manifestations, such as crackles in the lung bases, dyspnea at rest, disorientation, and confusion, especially in older patients. Document the precise location of the crackles because the level of the fluid progresses from the bases to higher levels in the lungs when the condition worsens. The patient in acute pulmonary edema is also typically extremely anxious, tachycardic, and struggling for air. As pulmonary edema becomes more severe, he or she may have a moist cough productive of frothy, blood-tinged sputum and his or her skin may be cold, clammy, or cyanotic. Chart 35-3 lists the major clinical manifestations of this complication.

CHART 35-3 Key Features

Pulmonary Edema

- Crackles
- Dyspnea at rest
- Disorientation or acute confusion (especially in older adults as early symptom)
- Tachycardia
- Hypertension or hypotension
- Reduced urinary output
- Cough with frothy, pink-tinged sputum
- Premature ventricular contractions and other dysrhythmias
- Anxiety
- Restlessness
- Lethargy

The patient diagnosed with pulmonary edema is admitted to the acute care hospital, often in a critical care unit. Reassure the patient and family that his or her distress will decrease with proper management.

NURSING SAFETY PRIORITY (QSEN)

Critical Rescue

If the patient is not hypotensive, place him or her in a sitting (high-Fowler's) position with his or her legs down to decrease venous return to the heart. The *priority nursing action* is to administer high-flow oxygen therapy at 5 to 6 L/min by facemask or at 10 to 15 L/min by non-rebreather mask with reservoir (which may deliver up to 100% oxygen) to promote GAS EXCHANGE and PERFUSION. Apply a pulse oximeter, and titrate the oxygen flow to keep the patient's oxygen saturation above 90%. If supplemental oxygen does not resolve the patient's respiratory distress, collaborate with the respiratory therapist, physician, advanced practice nurse, or physician assistant for more aggressive therapy, such as continuous positive airway pressure (CPAP) or bi-level positive airway pressure (BiPAP) ventilation. Intubation and mechanical ventilation may be needed for some patients.

If the patient's systolic blood pressure is above 100, give sublingual nitroglycerin (NTG) to decrease afterload and preload every 5 minutes for three doses while establishing IV access for additional drug therapy. The health care provider prescribes rapid-acting diuretics, such as Lasix or Bumex. Give Lasix IV push (IVP) over 1 to 2 minutes, usually at a starting dose of 20 to 40 mg for diuretic-naive patients, and another 40 mg if needed in 30 minutes. Patients already on oral diuretic therapy should be given an amount that is the same or doubled in milligrams as initial IV diuretic therapy. Administer each increment of 40 mg of Lasix over 1 to 2 minutes to avoid ototoxicity. Bumex may be administered 1 to 2 mg IVP or as a continuous infusion to provide consistent fluid removal over 24 hours. Monitor vital signs frequently, at least every 30 to 60 minutes.

If the patient's blood pressure is adequate, IV morphine sulfate may be prescribed, 1 to 2 mg at a time, to reduce venous return (preload), decrease anxiety, and reduce the work of breathing. Monitor respiratory rate and BP closely. Other drugs, such as IV NTG and drugs to treat HF, may be administered. Monitor the patient's vital signs closely (especially BP) while these drugs are being given.

In severe cases of fluid overload and renal dysfunction or diuretic resistance, ultrafiltration may be used. The benefits of ultrafiltration include:

- Decrease in cardiac filling pressures
- Decrease in pulmonary arterial pressure
- Increase in cardiac index
- Reduction in norepinephrine, rennin, and aldosterone

Ultrafiltration can remove up to 500 mL/hr and uses a blood flow rate of 10 to 40 mL/hr. Peripheral lines are used for IV access. See Chapter 68 for discussion of this procedure and nursing implications.

Community-Based Care

Patients who are not adequately prepared for discharge or do not have adequate community support and follow-up for self-management are at high risk for repeated hospital admissions for heart failure. Collaborate with the case manager or care coordinator to assess the patient's needs for health care resources.

CLINICAL JUDGMENT CHALLENGE

Safety; Patient-Centered Care; Evidence-Based Practice; Informatics (QSEN)

A 71-year-old man is admitted to the telemetry unit with right-sided heart failure, type 2 diabetes mellitus, hypertension, and COPD. He is married but has no children. During your assessment, you observe that his color is pale, he is dyspneic, and he reports new onset of chest discomfort. Even though he has oxygen via nasal cannula at 2 L/min., you note that he seems a little confused and is oriented only to person. His oxygen saturation has decreased from 95% to 88%.

1. What lung sounds do you expect to hear and why?
2. What evidence-based actions will you plan to implement at this time based on your observations? What is the source of the evidence?
3. The patient's physician prescribes an initial dose of furosemide (Lasix) 40 mg IVP. What assessments will you perform to determine if the drug was effective?
4. What will you tell the patient's wife about his condition at this time? Should the patient's wife be present during his emergency treatment? Why or why not?
5. After two doses of Lasix, the patient's condition improves. What data will you document in the electronic medical record (EMR)?

The Heart Failure Core Measure Set must be determined for hospitals accredited by The Joint Commission. These measures include that the patient with heart failure has:

- Discharge instructions (including information on diet, activity, medications, weight monitor, and plan for worsening symptoms)
- Evaluation of left ventricular systolic function
- An ACEI or ARB for left ventricular systolic dysfunction
- Adult smoking-cessation advice/counseling (if appropriate)

An inability to obtain help in activities such as food shopping and obtaining medications is a major contributor to hospital readmission. If home support is available, the patient may be discharged home in the care of a family member or other caregiver. Home care nurses may direct the care and assess for adherence to the discharge plan; home health aides may provide assistance with ADLs for a short time. If the patient has multiple health problems or has been severely compromised by heart disease, he or she may require admission to a skilled unit for either transitional or long-term care.

Home Care Management. The focus of the home care nurse's interventions is assessment and health teaching, which are reimbursable by Medicare and other third-party payers. Chart 35-4 lists the major areas of home health assessment.

Patients with chronic HF need to make many adjustments in their lifestyles. They must adhere to the collaborative plan of care that includes dietary restrictions, activity, prescriptions, and drug therapy. They need careful, concise explanations of the self-management plan. The community-based nurse in any setting encourages the patient to verbalize fears and concerns about his or her illness and assists in exploring coping skills. Patient participation in self-management can help alleviate and control symptoms.

Self-Management Education. Health teaching is essential for promoting self-management (also called *self-care*). Many patients are re-admitted to hospitals because they do not maintain their prescribed treatment plan, including lifestyle changes. Because of the need for extensive discharge instructions, most

CHART 35-4 Home Care Assessment

The Patient with Heart Failure

Assess for signs of heart failure, including:
- Changes in vital signs (heart rate >100 beats/min at rest, new atrial fibrillation, blood pressure <90 or >150 systolic)
- Indications of poor tissue perfusion:
  - Fatigue
  - Angina
  - Activity intolerance
  - Changes in mental status
  - Pallor or cyanosis
  - Cool extremities
- Indications of congestion:
  - Presence of cough or dyspnea
  - Weight gain
  - Jugular venous distention and peripheral edema

Assess functional ability, including:
- Performance of ADLs
- Mobility and ambulation (review frequency and duration of walking, development of symptoms, and pulse rate)
- Cognitive ability

Assess nutritional status, including:
- Food and fluid intake
- Intake of sodium-rich foods
- Alcohol consumption
- Skin turgor

Assess home environment, including:
- Safety hazards, especially related to oxygen therapy
- Structural barriers affecting functional ability
- Social support (family, home health services)

Assess the patient's adherence and understanding of illness and its treatment, including:
- Signs and symptoms to report to health care provider
- Dosages, effects, and side or toxic effects of medications
- When to report for laboratory and health care provider visits
- Ability to accurately weigh self on scale
- Presence of advance directive
- Use of home oxygen, if appropriate

Assess patient and caregiver coping skills

hospitals are using teaching packets with videos, CDs, and easy-to-read information about the importance of adhering to specific self-management strategies at home. One standardized and commonly used self-management plan called *MAWDS* is outlined in Table 35-4. Medication reconciliation is also important to be sure that similar drugs are not being prescribed and that patients meet the Core Measure requirements for HF. It is important to perform a learning needs assessment and tailor education to the patient's particular need to see changes in behavior and improved outcomes (see the Evidence-Based Practice box).

Ambulatory care clinics for heart failure patients are also becoming increasingly common. Their purpose is to offer assessments, drug therapy, and health teaching. Some nurses specialize in caring for patients with health failure.

Activity Schedule. Encourage patients with heart failure to stay as active as possible and to develop a regular exercise regimen (e.g., home walking program). However, teach the patient not to overdo it. Medicare and third-party payers typically do not reimburse for cardiac rehabilitation for HF. Paying for a cardiac rehabilitation program out of pocket is expensive.

Remind patients with persistent crackles and uncontrolled edema to begin exercise after their condition stabilizes. When exercise is indicated, teach the patient to begin walking 200 to 400 feet per day. At home the patient should try to walk at least 3 times a week and should slowly increase the amount of time walked over several months. If chest pain or severe dyspnea occurs while exercising or the patient has fatigue the next day, he or she is probably advancing the activity too quickly and

TABLE 35-4 Heart Failure Self-Management Health Teaching (MAWDS)

Medications:
- Take medications as prescribed, and do not run out.
- Know the purpose and side effects of each drug.
- Avoid NSAIDs to prevent sodium and fluid retention.

Activity:
- Stay as active as possible, but don't overdo it.
- Know your limits.
- Be able to carry on a conversation while exercising.

Weight:
- Weigh each day at the same time on the same scale to monitor for fluid retention.

Diet:
- Limit daily sodium intake to 2 to 3 grams as prescribed.
- Limit daily fluid intake to 2 liters.

Symptoms:
- Note any new or worsening symptoms, and notify the health care provider immediately.

EVIDENCE-BASED PRACTICE QSEN

What is the Most Effective Education Method to Provide Heart Failure Education to Heart Failure Patients?

Boyde, M., Turner, C., Thompson, D., & Stewart, S. (2011). Educational interventions for patients with heart failure: A systematic review of randomized controlled trials. *Journal of Cardiovascular Nursing, 26*(4), E27-E35.

The purpose of this meta-analysis research was to determine the most effective educational interventions provided by nurses to improve outcomes of the heart failure population. Randomized control trials from CINAHL, MEDLINE, PsycINFO, EMBASE, and Cochrane between the years 1998 and 2008 were identified. A total of 1515 abstracts were reviewed by two independent reviewers, and a total of 19 met inclusion criteria. To be included, studies needed to have evaluation of a specific education intervention or learning activity. Interventions studied included one-on-one didactic education, video, interactive CDs, TV programs, and mailings. Although it is acknowledged that patients have different learning styles, only four studies provided learning needs assessment. The ultimate goal was not only to improve the knowledge base but also to change patient behavior and improve outcomes. Of the 19 studies, 8 evaluated self-care in which 7 showed significant improvements in self-care after intervention. Re-admission rates were evaluated in 13 studies; 4 showed decreased rates of admission, and 3 showed decreased death rates. Various outcomes were measured, and 15 studies were able to demonstrate statistically significant changes in outcomes related to the education initiative.

Level of Evidence: 1

The researchers used a systematic review of randomized controlled trials.

Commentary: Implications for Practice and Research

Gaining knowledge does not equate to a change in behavior and, therefore, improved outcomes. To impart knowledge, a learning needs assessment must be performed before tailoring an education program for the patient. It is not enough to measure the amount of knowledge transmitted; changes in behavior and outcomes need to be the endpoint of studies related to nursing education.

CHART 35-5 Patient and Family Education: Preparing for Self-Management

Beta Blocker/Digoxin Therapy

- Establish same time of day to take this medication every day.
- Continue taking this medication unless your health care provider tells you to stop.
- Do not take digoxin at the same time as antacids or cathartics (laxatives).
- Take your pulse rate before taking each dose of digoxin. Notify your health care provider of a change in pulse rate (60 to 100 beats/min is typically normal, depending on your baseline pulse rate) or rhythm, as well as increasing fatigue, muscle weakness, confusion, or loss of appetite (signs of digoxin toxicity).
- If you forget to take a dose, it may be delayed a few hours. However, if you do not remember it until the next day, you should take only your usual daily dose.
- Report for scheduled laboratory tests (e.g., potassium and digoxin levels).
- If potassium supplements are prescribed, continue the dose until told to stop by your health care provider.

should slow down. Encourage him or her to keep a diary that documents the time and duration of each exercise session, as well as HR and any symptoms that occur with exercise.

Indications of Worsening or Recurrent Heart Failure. Many patients who are re-admitted to hospitals for treatment of HF fail to seek medical attention promptly when symptoms recur.

! NURSING SAFETY PRIORITY QSEN

Action Alert

Per the HF Core Measure for discharge instructions, teach the patient and caregiver to immediately report to the health care provider the occurrence of *any* of these symptoms, which could indicate worsening or recurrent heart failure:

- Rapid weight gain (3 lb in a week or 1 to 2 lb overnight)
- Decrease in exercise tolerance lasting 2 to 3 days
- Cold symptoms (cough) lasting more than 3 to 5 days
- Excessive awakening at night to urinate
- Development of dyspnea or angina at rest or worsening angina
- Increased swelling in the feet, ankles, or hands

Drug Therapy. Provide oral, written, and video instructions about the drug regimen. Teach the caregiver and patient how to count a pulse rate, especially if the patient is on digoxin or beta blockers. Chart 35-5 lists instructions for the patient taking either of these drugs at home.

Advise the patient taking diuretics to take them in the morning to avoid waking during the night for voiding. After determining whether he or she has a weight scale and can use it, emphasize the importance of weighing each morning at the same time. Daily weights indicate whether the patient is losing or retaining fluid. Some patients are taught to use a sliding scale to adjust their daily diuretic dose depending on their daily weight, similar to the way a diabetic patient adjusts an insulin dose based on the capillary glucose level.

Teach patients taking ACEIs or ARBs to move slowly when changing positions, especially from a lying to a sitting position. Remind them to report dizziness, light-headedness, and cough to the health care provider.

Serum potassium level and renal function are monitored at least every few months for patients taking diuretics and ACE inhibitors or ARBs. Diuretics, especially loop diuretics such as Lasix and Bumex, deplete potassium and often cause hypokalemia. Conversely, ACE inhibitors, ARBs, or potassium-sparing diuretics may result in potassium retention. If serum potassium levels drop below 4.0 mEq/L, the health care provider may prescribe potassium supplements or add a potassium-sparing diuretic such as spironolactone (Aldactone) or eplerenone (Inspra). Provide information about potassium-rich foods to include in the diet for patients at risk for hypokalemia (see Chapter 11).

Nutrition Therapy. Remind patients with chronic HF to restrict their dietary sodium. In collaboration with the home care nurse or dietitian, provide written instructions on low- or restricted-sodium diets. A 3-g sodium diet is recommended for *mild to moderate* disease. Remind the patient to avoid salty foods and table salt. Patients usually find this diet acceptable and fairly easy to follow.

A 2-g sodium diet may be needed for patients with *severe* HF. They should not add salt during or after meal preparation, avoid milk and milk products, use few canned or prepared foods, and read food labels to determine sodium content. This diet is not easily tolerated for many patients, and the cost of low-sodium foods can be a financial burden.

Commercial salt substitutes typically contain potassium. Teach patients that their renal status and serum potassium level must be evaluated while using these products. Suggest that patients try lemon, spices, and herbs to enhance the flavor of low-salt foods.

Advance Directives. About 50% of deaths from HF are sudden—many without any warning or worsening of symptoms. Assess whether the patient has written advance directives. If not, provide information about them during his or her hospital stay. Because most of these deaths occur at home, it is important for the health care provider or home care nurse to discuss advance directives with the patient and family. The family should be prepared to act in agreement with the patient's wishes in the event of cardiac arrest. If resuscitation is desired, be sure that the family knows how to activate the emergency medical system (EMS) and how to provide cardiopulmonary resuscitation (CPR) until an ambulance arrives. If CPR is not desired, the patient, family, and nurse plan how the family will respond. For some patients with end-stage disease, hospice care is an option. Chapter 7 discusses hospice and end-of-life care in detail.

Health Care Resources. A home care nurse, ambulatory care clinic, or nurse-led follow-up program may be needed to assess the patient's adherence to drug and nutrition therapy and to monitor for worsening or recurrent HF. Many large hospitals use follow-up telephone calls or teleconferencing/videoconferencing devices to monitor patients at home. Teleconferencing can also assess the patient's heart and lung sounds. These follow-up processes have been very successful in decreasing repeated hospital stays for chronic HF patients.

In addition to home care support, other resources are available for patient education and family support. The American Heart Association is an excellent community resource for print and electronic pamphlets, books, newsletters, and videotapes or DVDs related to HF and heart disease. The organization also provides referrals to various local support groups for patients and their caregivers.

CHART 35-6 Key Features

Valvular Heart Disease

MITRAL STENOSIS	MITRAL REGURGITATION	MITRAL VALVE PROLAPSE	AORTIC STENOSIS	AORTIC REGURGITATION
Fatigue Dyspnea on exertion Orthopnea Paroxysmal nocturnal dyspnea Hemoptysis Hepatomegaly Neck vein distention Pitting edema Atrial fibrillation Rumbling, apical diastolic murmur	Fatigue Dyspnea on exertion Orthopnea Palpitations Atrial fibrillation Neck vein distention Pitting edema High-pitched holosystolic murmur	Atypical chest pain Dizziness, syncope Palpitations Atrial tachycardia Ventricular tachycardia Systolic click	Dyspnea on exertion Angina Syncope on exertion Fatigue Orthopnea Paroxysmal nocturnal dyspnea Harsh, systolic crescendo-decrescendo murmur	Palpitations Dyspnea Orthopnea Paroxysmal nocturnal dyspnea Fatigue Angina Sinus tachycardia Blowing, decrescendo diastolic murmur

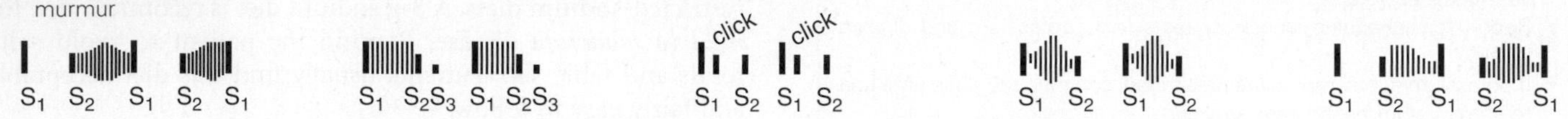

For equipment needs (e.g., home oxygen therapy, hospital bed), medical supply companies provide setup and maintenance services. Chapter 30 provides a detailed description of home oxygen therapy.

CLINICAL JUDGMENT CHALLENGE

Quality Improvement; Informatics QSEN

At a recent staff meeting, the medical-surgical nurse manager reports that the rate of repeated hospitalizations for patients with chronic heart failure has increased 50% in the past 3 months. As a staff nurse, you agree to be part of the unit quality improvement (QI) team to examine the cause(s) of the increase and make evidence-based recommendations for improving the outcomes for this patient population. Specific patient data and summaries are available for the team to review as needed.

1. Where will your team begin with this process during the first meeting of the team?
2. Formulate a PICOT clinical question using the format described in Chapter 5.
3. What Internet sites will your team use to determine best practices for decreasing repeated hospital stays and why?
4. How will your team interpret and use the evidence that you obtain? (See Chapter 5 for assistance.)
5. After your team assembles and analyzes the evidence to determine best practices, what will be done with the information?
6. How will you know if the plan of action to improve care was effective?

◆ Evaluation: Outcomes

Evaluate the care of the patient with HF on the basis of the identified patient problems. The expected outcomes include that the patient will:

- Have adequate pulmonary tissue PERFUSION
- Have increased cardiac pump effectiveness
- Take actions to manage energy
- Be free of pulmonary edema

VALVULAR HEART DISEASE

❖ PATHOPHYSIOLOGY

Acquired valvular dysfunctions include mitral stenosis, mitral regurgitation, mitral valve prolapse, aortic stenosis, and aortic regurgitation (Chart 35-6). The tricuspid valve is not affected often and may occur following endocarditis in IV drug abusers.

Mitral Stenosis

Mitral stenosis usually results from rheumatic carditis, which can cause valve thickening by fibrosis and calcification. Rheumatic fever is the most common cause of the problem. In more developed nations, congenital anomalies affect the majority of patients with mitral stenosis (Ray, 2010).

In mitral stenosis, the valve leaflets fuse and become stiff and the chordae tendineae contract and shorten. The valve opening narrows, preventing normal blood flow from the left atrium to the left ventricle. As a result of these changes, left atrial pressure rises, the left atrium dilates, pulmonary artery pressures increase, and the right ventricle hypertrophies.

Pulmonary congestion and right-sided heart failure occur first. Later, when the left ventricle receives insufficient blood volume, preload is decreased and cardiac output (CO) falls.

People with mild mitral stenosis are usually asymptomatic. As the valvular orifice narrows and pressure in the lungs increases, the patient experiences dyspnea on exertion, orthopnea, paroxysmal nocturnal dyspnea (sudden dyspnea at night), palpitations, and dry cough. Hemoptysis (coughing up blood) and pulmonary edema occur as pulmonary hypertension and congestion progress. Right-sided HF can cause hepatomegaly (enlarged liver), neck vein distention, and pitting dependent edema late in the disorder.

On palpation, the pulse may be normal, rapid, or irregularly irregular (as in atrial fibrillation). Because the development of atrial fibrillation indicates that the patient may decompensate, the physician should be notified immediately of the development of an irregularly irregular rhythm. A rumbling, apical diastolic murmur is noted on auscultation.

Mitral Regurgitation (Insufficiency)

The fibrotic and calcific changes occurring in **mitral regurgitation** (insufficiency) prevent the mitral valve from closing completely during *systole.* Incomplete closure of the valve allows the backflow of blood into the left atrium when the left ventricle contracts (Ray, 2010). During *diastole,* regurgitant output again flows from the left atrium to the left ventricle along with the normal blood flow. The increased volume must be ejected during the next systole. To compensate for the increased volume and pressure, the left atrium and ventricle dilate and hypertrophy.

The primary causes of mitral regurgitation are "degenerative" due to aging and infective endocarditis (Ray, 2010). Other causes include papillary muscle dysfunction or rupture resulting from ischemic heart disease or congenital anomalies. Rheumatic heart disease is the number-one cause in developing nations. When it results from rheumatic heart disease, it usually coexists with some degree of mitral stenosis; it affects women more often than men.

Mitral regurgitation usually progresses slowly; patients may remain symptom-free for decades. Symptoms begin to occur when the left ventricle fails in response to chronic blood volume overload. They include fatigue and chronic weakness as a result of reduced cardiac output (CO). Dyspnea on exertion and orthopnea develop later. A significant number of patients report anxiety, atypical chest pains, and palpitations. Assessment may reveal normal BP, atrial fibrillation, or changes in respirations characteristic of left ventricular failure.

When right-sided HF develops, the neck veins become distended, the liver enlarges (hepatomegaly), and pitting edema develops. A high-pitched systolic murmur at the apex, with radiation to the left axilla, is heard on auscultation. Severe regurgitation often exhibits a third heart sound (S_3).

Mitral Valve Prolapse

Mitral valve prolapse (MVP) occurs because the valvular leaflets enlarge and prolapse into the left atrium during systole. This abnormality is usually benign but may progress to pronounced mitral regurgitation in some patients.

The etiology of MVP is variable and has been associated with conditions such as Marfan syndrome and other congenital cardiac defects. MVP also has a familial tendency. Usually, however, no other cardiac abnormality is found.

Most patients with MVP are asymptomatic. However, some may report chest pain, palpitations, or exercise intolerance. Chest pain is usually atypical with patients describing a sharp pain localized to the left side of the chest. Dizziness, **syncope** ("blackouts"), and palpitations may be associated with atrial or ventricular dysrhythmias.

A normal heart rate and BP are usually found on physical examination. A midsystolic click and a late systolic murmur may be heard at the apex of the heart. The intensity of the murmur is not related to the severity of the prolapse.

Aortic Stenosis

Aortic stenosis is the most common cardiac valve dysfunction in the United States and is often considered a disease of "wear and tear." In **aortic stenosis,** the aortic valve orifice narrows and obstructs left ventricular outflow during systole. This increased resistance to ejection or afterload results in ventricular hypertrophy. As stenosis worsens, cardiac output becomes fixed and cannot increase to meet the demands of the body during exertion. Symptoms then develop. Eventually the left ventricle fails, blood backs up in the left atrium, and the pulmonary system becomes congested. Right-sided HF can occur late in the disease. *When the surface area of the valve becomes 1 cm or less, surgery is indicated on an urgent basis!*

Congenital bicuspid or unicuspid aortic valves are the primary causes for aortic stenosis in many patients. Rheumatic aortic stenosis occurs with rheumatic disease of the mitral valve and develops in young and middle-aged adults. Atherosclerosis and degenerative calcification of the aortic valve are the major causative factors in older adults. *Aortic stenosis has become the most common valvular disorder in all countries with aging populations.*

The classic symptoms of aortic stenosis result from fixed cardiac output: dyspnea, angina, and syncope occurring on exertion. When cardiac output falls in the late stages of the disease, the patient experiences marked fatigue, debilitation, and peripheral cyanosis. A narrow pulse pressure is noted when the BP is measured. A diamond-shaped, systolic crescendo-decrescendo murmur is usually noted on auscultation.

Aortic Regurgitation (Insufficiency)

In patients with **aortic regurgitation,** the aortic valve leaflets do not close properly during diastole and the *annulus* (the valve ring that attaches to the leaflets) may be dilated, loose, or deformed. This allows flow of blood from the aorta back into the left ventricle during diastole. The left ventricle, in compensation, dilates to accommodate the greater blood volume and eventually hypertrophies.

Aortic insufficiency usually results from nonrheumatic conditions such as infective endocarditis, congenital anatomic aortic valvular abnormalities, hypertension, and Marfan syndrome (a rare, generalized, systemic disease of connective tissue).

Patients with aortic regurgitation remain asymptomatic for many years because of the compensatory mechanisms of the left ventricle. As the disease progresses and left ventricular failure occurs, the major symptoms are exertional dyspnea, orthopnea, and paroxysmal nocturnal dyspnea. Palpitations may be noted with severe disease, especially when the patient lies on the left side. Nocturnal angina with diaphoresis often occurs.

On palpation, the nurse notes a "bounding" arterial pulse. The pulse pressure is usually widened, with an elevated systolic pressure and diminished diastolic pressure. The classic auscultatory finding is a high-pitched, blowing, decrescendo diastolic murmur.

❖ *PATIENT-CENTERED COLLABORATIVE CARE*

◆ *Assessment*

A patient with valvular disease may suddenly become ill or slowly develop symptoms over many years. Collect information about the patient's family health history, including valvular or other forms of heart disease to which he or she may be genetically predisposed. Question about attacks of rheumatic fever and infective endocarditis, the specific dates when these occurred, and the use of antibiotics to prevent recurrence of these diseases. Also question the patient about a history of IV drug abuse, a common cause of infective endocarditis. Discuss the patient's fatigue level and tolerated activity level, the presence of angina or dyspnea, and the occurrence of palpitations, if present.

As part of the physical assessment, obtain vital signs, inspect for signs of edema, palpate and auscultate the heart and lungs, and palpate the peripheral pulses. Assessment findings are summarized in Chart 35-6.

Echocardiography is the noninvasive diagnostic procedure of choice to visualize the structure and movement of the heart. The more invasive transesophageal echocardiography (TEE) or transthoracic echocardiography (TTE) is also performed to assess most valve problems. Exercise tolerance testing (ETT) and stress echocardiography are sometimes done to evaluate symptomatic response and assess functional capacity. With either mitral or aortic stenosis, cardiac catheterization may be indicated to assess the severity of the stenosis and its other effects on the heart.

In patients with mitral stenosis, the chest x-ray shows left atrial enlargement, prominent pulmonary arteries, and an enlarged right ventricle. In those with mitral regurgitation (insufficiency), the chest x-ray reveals an increased cardiac shadow, indicating left ventricular and left atrial enlargement.

In the later stages of aortic stenosis, the chest x-ray may show left ventricular enlargement and pulmonary congestion. Left atrial and left ventricular dilation appear on the chest x-ray of patients with aortic regurgitation (insufficiency). If HF is present, pulmonary venous congestion is also evident.

The health care provider also requests an ECG to assess abnormalities such as left ventricular hypertrophy, as seen with mitral regurgitation and aortic regurgitation, or right ventricular hypertrophy, as seen in severe mitral stenosis. Atrial fibrillation is a common finding in both mitral stenosis and mitral regurgitation and may develop in aortic stenosis because of left atrial dilation.

◆ *Interventions*

Management of valvular heart disease depends on which valve is affected and the degree of valve impairment. Some patients can be managed with yearly monitoring and drug therapy, whereas others require invasive procedures or heart surgery.

Nonsurgical Management. Nonsurgical management focuses on drug therapy and rest. During the course of valvular disease, left ventricular failure with pulmonary or systemic congestion may develop.

Drug Therapy. Diuretics, beta blockers, digoxin, and oxygen are often administered to improve the symptoms of heart failure. Nitrates are administered cautiously to patients with aortic stenosis because of the potential for syncope associated with a reduction in left ventricular volume (preload). Vasodilators such as calcium channel blockers may be used to reduce the regurgitant flow for patients with aortic or mitral stenosis.

! NURSING SAFETY PRIORITY (QSEN)

Drug Alert

Teach patients with valve disease the importance of prophylactic antibiotic therapy before any invasive dental or respiratory procedure. Prophylactic antibiotics are *not* recommended prior to gastrointestinal procedures such as upper GI endoscopy, colonoscopy, or procedures requiring genitourinary instrumentation.

A major concern in valvular heart disease is maintaining cardiac output if atrial fibrillation develops. With mitral valvular disease, left ventricular filling is especially dependent on atrial contraction. When atrial fibrillation develops, there is no longer a single coordinated atrial contraction. Cardiac output can decrease, and HF may occur. Ineffective atrial contraction may also lead to the stasis of blood and thrombi in the left atrium. Monitor the patient for the development of an irregular rhythm, and notify the primary care provider if it develops. (See Chapter 34 for a detailed explanation of atrial fibrillation.)

The primary care provider usually starts drug therapy first to control the heart rate and maintain cardiac output (<100 for heart rate is considered a controlled ventricular response). After those outcomes are met, drugs are used in an attempt to restore normal sinus rhythm (NSR). In some cases, the provider elects to convert a patient from atrial fibrillation to sinus rhythm using IV diltiazem (Cardizem, Apo-Diltiaz ♣) or amiodarone (Cordarone, Pacerone). Monitor the patient on a unit where both cardiac rhythm and BP can be closely watched. Synchronized countershock (cardioversion) may be attempted if atrial fibrillation is rapid, the patient's condition worsens, and the rhythm is unresponsive to medical treatment (see Chapter 34).

If the patient remains in atrial fibrillation, low-dose amiodarone (Cordarone) is often prescribed to slow ventricular rate. Procainamide hydrochloride (Pronestyl hydrochloride, Procanbid) may be added to the regimen. A beta-blocking agent (e.g., metoprolol) may also be considered to slow the ventricular response.

For valvular heart disease and chronic atrial fibrillation, anticoagulation with sodium warfarin (Coumadin, Warfilone ♣) is usually a part of the plan of care to prevent thrombus formation. Thrombi (clots) may form in the atria or on defective valve segments, resulting in systemic emboli. If a portion breaks off and travels to the brain, one or more strokes may occur. Assess the patient's baseline neurologic status, and monitor for changes. A transesophageal echocardiography (TEE) is often done before synchronized cardioversion to ensure that thrombi are not present that could embolize when this therapy is administered. The newer direct thrombin inhibitors *rivaroxaban* (Xarelto) and *dabigatran* (Pradaxa) are *not recommended* to anticoagulate patients with atrial fibrillation related to valvular disease.

Rest is often an important part of treatment. Activity may be limited because cardiac output (CO) cannot meet increased metabolic demands and angina or HF can result. A balance of rest and exercise is needed to prevent skeletal muscle atrophy and fatigue.

Noninvasive Heart Valve Reparative Procedures. Reparative procedures are becoming more popular because of continuing problems with thrombi, endocarditis, and left ventricular dysfunction after valve replacement. Reparative procedures do not result in a normal valve, but they usually "turn back the clock," resulting in a more functional valve and an improvement in cardiac output. Turbulent blood flow through the valve may persist, and degeneration of the repaired valve is possible.

Balloon valvuloplasty, an invasive nonsurgical procedure, is possible for stenotic mitral and aortic valves; however, careful selection of patients is needed. It may be the initial treatment of choice for people with noncalcified, mobile mitral valves. Patients selected for *aortic* valvuloplasty are usually older and are at high risk for surgical complications or have refused operative treatment. The benefits of this procedure for aortic stenosis tend to be short lived, rarely lasting longer than 6 months.

When performing *mitral* valvuloplasty, the physician passes a balloon catheter from the femoral vein, through the atrial

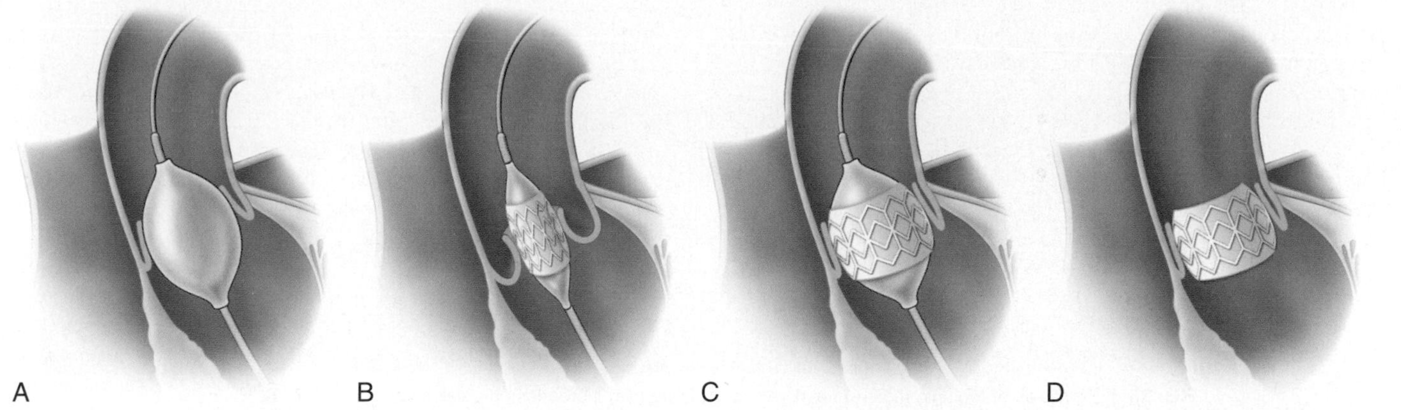

FIG. 35-3 Transcatheter aortic valve replacement (TAVR) procedure.

septum, and to the mitral valve. The balloon is inflated to enlarge the mitral orifice. For *aortic* valvuloplasty, the physician inserts the catheter through the femoral artery and advances it to the aortic valve, where it is inflated to enlarge the orifice. The procedure usually offers immediate relief of symptoms because the balloon has dilated the orifice and improved leaflet mobility. The results are comparable with those of surgical commissurotomy for appropriately selected patients.

Minimally invasive techniques have expanded. For patients who are not surgical candidates, *transcatheter aortic valve replacement (TAVR)* is an alternative option for treatment of aortic stenosis (Fig. 35-3). A bioprosthetic valve is placed percutaneously via either the transfemoral or transapical route under general anesthesia in a hybrid operating room (a combination of a catheterization laboratory and cardiovascular operating room). After initial balloon aortic valvuloplasty, the new valve, which is wrapped around a balloon on a large catheter, is inserted via the femoral artery. The patient is transvenously paced at a rate of about 200 beats per minute to mimic ventricular standstill. The balloon is then inflated and the valve deployed. In the transapical approach, a small incision is made at the apex of the heart. The catheter is then threaded through the incision and the left ventricle to gain access to the aortic valve. As in the transvenous approach, the balloon and catheter is deployed during rapid transvenous pacing. This procedure is performed by a health care team consisting of interventional cardiologists and cardiovascular surgeons. The team must be prepared to convert to an open or traditional aortic valve replacement (AVR) if necessary. Care of the patient is similar to the care of the patient undergoing CABG (see Chapter 38); however, this patient population only needs anticoagulation with aspirin and clopidogrel postprocedure.

The pulmonary valve can also be replaced percutaneously by a device from Medtronic using a similar procedure to the TAVR. The Mitraclip, approved for use in Europe and under investigation for use in the United States, is used to repair the mitral valve in patients with mitral regurgitation. Under general anesthesia, access is gained percutaneously via the femoral vein, and the catheter and Mitraclip is advanced in the left atria and then the left ventricle. The Mitraclip is then retracted and deployed to hold the leaflets of the valve together. Care is similar to the care of the patient undergoing CABG (see Chapter 38).

! NURSING SAFETY PRIORITY QSEN

Action Alert

After valvuloplasty, observe the patient closely for bleeding from the catheter insertion site and institute post-angiogram precautions. Bleeding is likely because of the large size of the catheter. Assess for signs of a regurgitant valve by closely monitoring heart sounds, CO, and heart rhythm. Because vegetations (thrombi) may have been dislodged from the valve, observe for any indication of systemic emboli (see the Infective Endocarditis section, p. 697).

Surgical Management. Surgeries for patients with valvular heart disease include invasive reparative procedures and replacement. These procedures are performed after symptoms of left ventricular failure have developed but before irreversible dysfunction occurs. Surgical therapy is the *only* definitive treatment of *aortic stenosis* and is recommended when angina, syncope, or dyspnea on exertion develops.

Invasive Heart Valve Reparative Procedures. *Direct (open) commissurotomy* is accomplished with cardiopulmonary bypass during open heart surgery. The surgeon visualizes the valve, removes thrombi from the atria, incises the fused commissures (leaflets), and débrides calcium from the leaflets, widening the orifice.

Mitral valve annuloplasty (reconstruction) is the reparative procedure of choice for most patients with acquired mitral insufficiency. To make the annulus (the valve ring that attaches to and supports the leaflets) smaller, the surgeon may suture the leaflets to an annuloplasty ring or take tucks in the patient's annulus. Leaflet repair is often performed at the same time. Elongated leaflets may be shortened, and shortened leaflets may be repaired by lengthening the chordae that bind them in place. Perforated leaflets may be patched with synthetic grafts.

Annuloplasty and leaflet repair result in an annulus of the appropriate size and in leaflets that can close completely. Thus regurgitation is eliminated or markedly reduced.

Heart Valve Replacement Procedures. The development of a wide variety of *prosthetic* (synthetic) and *biologic* (tissue) valves has improved the surgical therapy and prognosis of valvular heart disease. Each type has advantages and disadvantages. An aortic valve can be replaced only with a prosthetic valve for symptomatic adults with aortic stenosis and aortic

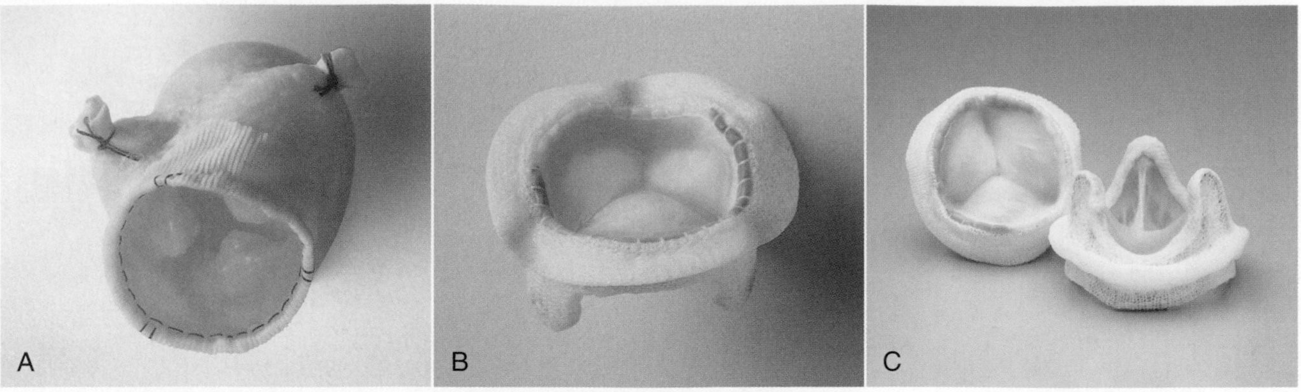

FIG. 35-4 Examples of biologic (tissue) heart valves. **A,** Freestyle, a stentless pig valve with no frame. **B,** Hancock II, a stented pig valve. **C,** Carpentier-Edwards pericardial bioprosthesis.

insufficiency. A biologic valve cannot be used because of the high pressure within the aorta.

Biologic valve replacements may be **xenograft** (from other species), such as a porcine valve (from a pig) (Fig. 35-4) or a bovine valve (from a cow). Because tissue valves are associated with little risk for clot formation, long-term anticoagulation is *not* indicated. Xenografts are not as durable as prosthetic valves and usually must be replaced every 7 to 10 years. The durability of the graft is related to the age of the recipient. Calcium in the blood, which is present in larger quantities in younger patients, breaks down the valves. The older the patient, the longer the xenograft will last. Valves donated from human cadavers and **pulmonary autographs** (relocation of the patient's own pulmonary valve to the aortic position [Ross procedure]) are also being used for valve replacement.

Patients having a valve replacement have open heart surgery similar to the procedure for a coronary artery bypass graft (CABG) (see Chapter 38). Ideally, surgery is an elective and planned procedure. Inform the patient and family about the management of postoperative pain, incision care, and strategies to prevent respiratory complications (see Chapters 14 and 16). Teach patients receiving oral anticoagulants to stop taking them before surgery, usually at least 72 hours before the procedure. Patients also need to have a preoperative dental examination. If dental caries or periodontal disease is present, these problems must be resolved before valve replacement.

Postoperative nursing interventions for patients with valve replacement are similar to those for a CABG (see Chapter 38).

! NURSING SAFETY PRIORITY (QSEN)

Critical Rescue

Patients with mitral stenosis often have pulmonary hypertension and stiff lungs. Therefore monitor respiratory status closely during weaning from the ventilator. Be especially alert for bleeding in those with aortic valve replacements because of a higher risk for postoperative hemorrhage. If heart rate or blood pressure decreases, call the Rapid Response Team or other health care provider immediately!

Patients with valve replacements are also more likely to have significant reductions in cardiac output (CO) after surgery, especially those with aortic stenosis or left ventricular failure from mitral valve disease. Carefully monitor CO, and assess for indications of heart failure. Report any manifestations of HF to the surgeon immediately, and prepare for collaborative management (see earlier discussion on heart failure in this chapter).

Community-Based Care

The patient with valvular heart disease may be discharged home on medical therapy or postoperatively after valve repair or replacement. Because fatigue is a common problem, ensure that the home environment can provide rest while moving the patient toward increased activity levels. Some older adults with aortic stenosis live in long-term care settings.

Home Care Management. A home care nurse may be needed to help the patient adhere to drug therapy and activity schedules and to detect any problems, particularly with anticoagulant therapy. Patients who have undergone surgery may require a nurse for assistance with incision care. A home care aide may assist with ADLs if the patient lives alone or is older.

Self-Management Education. The teaching plan for the patient with valvular heart disease includes:

- The disease process and the possibility of heart failure
- Drug therapy, including diuretics, vasodilators, beta blockers, calcium channel blockers, antibiotics, and anticoagulants
- The prophylactic use of antibiotics
- A plan of activity and rest to conserve energy

Because patients with defective or repaired valves are at risk for infective endocarditis, teach them to adhere to the precautions described for endocarditis. *Remind them to inform all health care providers of the valvular heart disease history. Tell providers that they require antibiotic administration before all invasive procedures and tests.* Health teaching for the patient is summarized in Chart 35-7.

Patients who have had valve replacements with prosthetic valves require lifetime prophylactic anticoagulation therapy to prevent thrombus formation. Teach patients taking anticoagulants how to manage their drug therapy successfully, including nutritional considerations (if taking warfarin) and the prevention of bleeding. For example, the patient should be taught to avoid foods high in vitamin K, especially dark green leafy vegetables, and to use an electric razor to avoid skin cuts. In addition, teach him or her to report any bleeding or excessive bruising to the health care provider.

For patients who have surgery, reinforce how to care for the sternal incision and instruct them to watch for and report any fever, drainage, or redness at the site. Most patients can usually return to normal activity after 6 weeks but should avoid heavy

CHART 35-7 Patient and Family Education: Preparing for Self-Management

Valvular Heart Disease

- Notify all your health care providers that you have a defective heart valve.
- Remind the health care provider of your valvular problem when you have any invasive dental work (e.g., extraction) or respiratory procedure.
- Request antibiotic prophylaxis before and after these procedures if the health care provider does not offer it.
- Clean all wounds and apply antibiotic ointment to prevent infection.
- Notify your health care provider immediately if you experience fever, petechiae (pinpoint red dots on your skin), or shortness of breath.

CHART 35-8 Key Features

Infective Endocarditis

- Fever associated with chills, night sweats, malaise, and fatigue
- Anorexia and weight loss
- Cardiac murmur (newly developed or change in existing)
- Development of heart failure
- Evidence of systemic embolization
- Petechiae
- Splinter hemorrhages
- Osler's nodes (on palms of hands and soles of feet)
- Janeway's lesions (flat, reddened maculae on hands and feet)
- Positive blood cultures

physical activity involving their upper extremities for 3 to 6 months to allow the incision to heal. Those who have had valvular surgery should also avoid invasive dental procedures for 6 months because of the potential for endocarditis. Those with prosthetic valves need to avoid any procedure using magnetic resonance unless the newest technology is available. Remind patients to obtain a medical alert bracelet, card, or necklace to indicate they have a valve replacement and are taking anticoagulants.

Patients with valvular heart disease may have complicated medication schedules that can potentially lead to inadequate self-management. Provide clear, concise instructions about drug therapy, and discuss the risks associated with nonadherence. Patients with a failed valve or those who do not follow the treatment plan are at high risk for heart failure. Teach them to report any changes in cardiovascular status, such as dyspnea, syncope, dizziness, edema, and palpitations.

The psychological response to valve surgery is similar to that after coronary artery bypass surgery. Patients may experience an altered self-image as a result of the required lifestyle changes or the visible medial sternotomy incision. In addition, those with prosthetic valves may need to adjust to a soft but audible clicking sound of the prosthetic valve. Encourage patients to verbalize their feelings about the prosthetic heart valve. Patients may display a variety of emotions postoperatively, especially after hospital discharge.

NCLEX EXAMINATION CHALLENGE

Physiological Integrity

A client who recently had a heart valve replacement is taking warfarin (Coumadin) as prescribed. What statement by the client indicates that the nurse will need to do additional health teaching?

A. "I will take my pulse every day, and call my doctor if it is below 60."
B. "I will eat foods that are high in vitamin K, such as kale and spinach."
C. "I will weigh myself every day in the morning using the same scale."
D. "I will take my blood pressure every day and call if it is too high or low."

Health Care Resources. The American Heart Association's *Mended Hearts, Inc.* (www.mendedhearts.org) is a community resource that provides information about valvular heart disease. A wallet-size card can be obtained to identify the patient as needing prophylactic antibiotics. An identification bracelet or necklace that states the name of the drugs the patient is taking should also be worn.

INFLAMMATIONS AND INFECTIONS

INFECTIVE ENDOCARDITIS

❖ PATHOPHYSIOLOGY

Infective endocarditis (previously called *bacterial endocarditis*) is a microbial INFECTION (e.g., viruses, bacteria, fungi) of the endocardium. The most common infective organism is *Streptococcus viridans* or *Staphylococcus aureus*.

Infective endocarditis occurs primarily in patients who abuse IV drugs, have had valve replacements, have experienced systemic INFECTION, or have structural cardiac defects. With a cardiac defect, blood may flow rapidly from a high-pressure area to a low-pressure zone, eroding a section of endocardium. Platelets and fibrin adhere to the denuded endocardium, forming a vegetative lesion. During bacteremia, bacteria become trapped in the low-pressure "sinkhole" and are deposited in the vegetation. Additional platelets and fibrin are deposited, which causes the vegetative lesion to grow. The endocardium and valve are destroyed. Valvular insufficiency may result when the lesion interferes with normal alignment of the valve. If vegetations become so large that blood flow through the valve is obstructed, the valve appears stenotic and then is very likely to *embolize* (i.e., cause emboli to be released into the systemic circulation) (McCance et al., 2010).

Possible ports of entry for infecting organisms include:

- The oral cavity (especially if dental procedures have been performed)
- Skin rashes, lesions, or abscesses
- Infections (cutaneous, genitourinary, GI, systemic)
- Surgery or invasive procedures, including IV line placement

❖ PATIENT-CENTERED COLLABORATIVE CARE

◆ Assessment

Because the mortality rate remains high, early detection of infective endocarditis is essential. Unfortunately, many patients (especially older adults) are misdiagnosed. Clinical manifestations typically occur within 2 weeks of a bacteremia (Chart 35-8).

Most patients have recurrent fevers from 99° to 103° F (37.2° to 39.4° C). As a result of physiologic changes associated with aging, however, older adults may be afebrile. The severity of symptoms may depend on the virulence of the infecting organism.

Physical Assessment/Clinical Manifestations. Assess the patient's *cardiovascular status.* Almost all patients with infective endocarditis develop murmurs. Carefully auscultate the precordium, noting and documenting any new murmurs (usually regurgitant in nature) or any changes in the intensity or quality of an old murmur. An S_3 or S_4 heart sound also may be heard.

Heart failure is the most common complication of infective endocarditis. Assess for right-sided HF (as evidenced by peripheral edema, weight gain, and anorexia) and left-sided HF (as evidenced by fatigue, shortness of breath, and crackles on auscultation of breath sounds). See discussion of HF earlier in this chapter.

Arterial embolization is a major complication in up to half of patients with infective endocarditis. Fragments of vegetation (clots) break loose and travel randomly through the circulation. When the left side of the heart is involved, vegetation fragments are carried to the spleen, kidneys, GI tract, brain, and extremities. When the right side of the heart is involved, emboli enter the pulmonary circulation.

Splenic infarction with sudden abdominal PAIN and radiation to the left shoulder can also occur. When performing an *abdominal assessment,* note rebound tenderness on palpation. The classic pain described with renal infarction is flank pain that radiates to the groin and is accompanied by hematuria (red blood cells in the urine) or pyuria (white blood cells in the urine). Mesenteric emboli cause diffuse abdominal pain, often after eating, and abdominal distention.

About a third of patients have *neurologic changes;* others have signs and symptoms of pulmonary problems. Emboli to the central nervous system cause either transient ischemic attacks (TIAs) or a stroke. Confusion, reduced concentration, and aphasia or dysphagia may occur. Pleuritic chest pain, dyspnea, and cough are symptoms of pulmonary infarction related to embolization.

Petechiae (pinpoint red spots) occur in many patients with endocarditis. Examine the mucous membranes, the palate, the conjunctivae, and the skin above the clavicles for small, red, flat lesions. Assess the distal third of the nail bed for **splinter hemorrhages**, which appear as black longitudinal lines or small red streaks.

Diagnostic Assessment. The most reliable criteria for diagnosing endocarditis include positive blood cultures, a new regurgitant murmur, and evidence of endocardial involvement by echocardiography.

A positive *blood culture* is a prime diagnostic test. Both aerobic and anaerobic specimens are obtained for culture. Some slow-growing organisms may take 3 weeks and require a specialized medium to isolate. Low hemoglobin and hematocrit levels may also be present.

Echocardiography has improved the ability to diagnose infective endocarditis accurately. Transesophageal echocardiography (TEE) allows visualization of cardiac structures that are difficult to see with transthoracic echocardiography (TTE) (see Chapter 33).

◆ *Interventions*

Care of the patient with endocarditis usually includes antimicrobials, rest balanced with activity, and supportive therapy for HF. If these interventions are successful, surgery is usually not required.

Nonsurgical Management. The major component of treatment for endocarditis is drug therapy. Other interventions help prevent the life-threatening complications of the disease.

Antimicrobials are the main treatment, with the choice of drug depending on the specific organism involved. Because vegetations surround and protect the offending microorganism, an appropriate drug must be given in a sufficiently high dose to ensure its destruction. Antimicrobials are usually given IV, with the course of treatment lasting 4 to 6 weeks. For most bacterial cases, the ideal antibiotic is one of the penicillins or cephalosporins.

Patients may be hospitalized for several days to institute IV therapy and then are discharged for continued IV therapy at home. After hospitalization, most patients who respond to therapy may continue it at home when they become afebrile, have negative blood cultures, and have no signs of HF or embolization.

Anticoagulants do not prevent embolization from vegetations. Because they may result in bleeding, these drugs are avoided unless they are required to prevent thrombus formation (clotting) on a prosthetic valve.

The patient's activities are balanced with *adequate rest.* Consistently use appropriate aseptic technique to protect the patient from contact with potentially infective organisms. Continue to assess for signs of HF (e.g., rapid pulse, fatigue, cough, dyspnea) throughout the antimicrobial regimen, and report significant changes.

Surgical Management. The cardiac surgeon may be consulted if antibiotic therapy is ineffective in sterilizing a valve, if refractory HF develops secondary to a defective valve, if large valvular vegetations are present, or if multiple embolic events occur. Current surgical interventions for infective endocarditis include:

- Removing the infected valve (either biologic or prosthetic)
- Repairing or removing congenital shunts
- Repairing injured valves and chordae tendineae
- Draining abscesses in the heart

Preoperative and postoperative care of patients having surgery involving the valves is similar to that described earlier for valve replacement (pp. 695-696).

Community-Based Care

Community-based care for patients with infective endocarditis is essential to resolve the problem, prevent relapse, and avoid complications. Patients and families need to be willing and have the knowledge, physical ability, and resources to administer IV antibiotics at home. Collaborate with the home care nurse to complete health teaching started in the hospital and to monitor patient adherence and health status as directed by The Joint Commission's National Patient Safety Goals.

In collaboration with the case manager, the home care nurse and pharmacist arrange for appropriate supplies to be available to the patient at home. Supplies include the prepared antibiotic, IV pump with tubing, alcohol wipes, IV access device, normal saline solution, and a saline flush solution drawn up in syringes. A saline lock, peripherally inserted central catheter (PICC) line, or central catheter is positioned at a venous site that is easily accessible to the patient or a family member.

Teach the patient and family how to administer the antibiotic and care for the infusion site while maintaining aseptic technique. The patient or family member should demonstrate this technique before the patient is discharged from the hospital. Emphasize the importance of maintaining a blood level of the antibiotic by administering the antibiotics as scheduled. After stabilization at home, the case manager or other nurse contacts the patient every week to determine whether he or she is adhering to the antibiotic therapy and whether any problems have been encountered.

Encourage proper oral hygiene. Advise patients to use a soft toothbrush, to brush their teeth at least twice per day, and to rinse the mouth with water after brushing. They should not use irrigation devices or floss the teeth because bacteremia may result. Teach them to clean any open skin areas well and apply an antibiotic ointment.

! NURSING SAFETY PRIORITY (QSEN)

Action Alert

Patients must remind health care providers (including their dentists) of their endocarditis. Guidelines for antibiotic prophylaxis have been revised and are recommended only if the patient with a prosthetic valve, a history of infective endocarditis, or an unrepaired cyanotic congenital heart disease undergoes invasive dental, oral, or upper respiratory procedure.

Instruct patients to note any indications of recurring endocarditis such as fever. Remind them to monitor and record their temperature daily for up to 6 weeks. Teach them to report fever, chills, malaise, weight loss, increased fatigue, sudden weight gain, or dyspnea to their primary care provider.

PERICARDITIS

PATHOPHYSIOLOGY

Acute pericarditis is an inflammation or alteration of the pericardium (the membranous sac that encloses the heart). The problem may be fibrous, serous, hemorrhagic, purulent, or neoplastic. Acute pericarditis is most commonly associated with:

- Infective organisms (bacteria, viruses, or fungi) (usually respiratory)
- Post–myocardial infarction (MI) syndrome (Dressler's syndrome)
- Post-pericardiotomy syndrome
- Acute exacerbations of systemic connective tissue disease

Chronic constrictive pericarditis occurs when chronic pericardial inflammation causes a fibrous thickening of the pericardium. It is caused by tuberculosis, radiation therapy, trauma, renal failure, or metastatic cancer. In chronic constrictive pericarditis, the pericardium becomes rigid, preventing adequate filling of the ventricles and eventually resulting in cardiac failure.

PATIENT-CENTERED COLLABORATIVE CARE

Assessment

Assessment findings for patients with *acute pericarditis* include substernal precordial PAIN that radiates to the left side of the neck, the shoulder, or the back. PAIN is classically grating and oppressive and is aggravated by breathing (mainly on inspiration), coughing, and swallowing. The PAIN is worse when the patient is in the supine position and may be relieved by sitting up and leaning forward. Ask specific questions to evaluate chest discomfort to differentiate it from the pain associated with an acute MI (see Chapter 38).

A pericardial friction rub may be heard with the diaphragm of the stethoscope positioned at the left lower sternal border. This scratchy, high-pitched sound is produced when the inflamed, roughened pericardial layers create friction as their surfaces rub together.

Patients with acute pericarditis may have an elevated white blood cell count and usually have a fever. Therefore blood culture and sensitivity may be analyzed in the laboratory. The ECG usually shows ST-T spiking in almost all leads simultaneously, and aVR with ST depression with the onset of inflammation, which returns to baseline with treatment. Atrial fibrillation is also common. Echocardiograms may be used to determine a pericardial effusion.

Patients with *chronic constrictive pericarditis* have signs of right-sided HF, elevated systemic venous pressure with jugular distention, hepatic engorgement, and dependent edema. Exertional fatigue and dyspnea are common complications. Thickening of the pericardium is seen on echocardiography or a computed tomography (CT) scan.

Interventions

The focus of collaborative management is to relieve pain and treat the cause of pericarditis before severe complications occur.

Pain Management. The health care provider usually prescribes NSAIDs for PAIN associated with pericarditis. Patients who do not obtain pain relief and who do not have bacterial pericarditis may receive corticosteroid therapy. Assist the patient to assume positions of comfort—usually sitting upright and leaning slightly forward. If the pain is not relieved within 24 to 48 hours, notify the health care provider. Colchicine 1 to 2 mg orally on Day 1 followed by 0.5 to 1 mg orally daily for 6 months has been shown to prevent pericarditis reoccurrence.

The various causes of pericarditis require specific therapies. For example, bacterial pericarditis (acute) usually requires antibiotics and pericardial drainage. The usual clinical course of acute pericarditis is short term (2 to 6 weeks), but episodes may recur. Chronic pericarditis caused by malignant disease may be treated with radiation or chemotherapy, whereas uremic pericarditis is treated by hemodialysis. The definitive treatment for chronic constrictive pericarditis is surgical excision of the pericardium (**pericardiectomy**).

Monitor all patients for **pericardial effusion**, which occurs when the space between the parietal and visceral layers of the pericardium fills with fluid. This complication puts the patient at risk for **cardiac tamponade**, or excessive fluid within the pericardial cavity.

Emergency Care: Acute Cardiac Tamponade. Acute cardiac tamponade may occur when small volumes (20 to 50 mL) of fluid accumulate rapidly in the pericardium and cause a sudden decrease in cardiac output (CO). If the fluid accumulates slowly, the pericardium may stretch to accommodate several hundred milliliters of fluid. Report any suspicion of this complication to the physician immediately. Findings of cardiac tamponade include:

- Jugular venous distention
- **Paradoxical pulse**, also known as *pulsus paradoxus* (systolic blood pressure 10 mm Hg or more higher on expiration than on inspiration) (Chart 35-9)
- Decreased heart rate, dyspnea, and fatigue
- Muffled heart sounds
- Hypotension

CHART 35-9 Best Practice for Patient Safety & Quality Care (QSEN)

Care of the Patient with Pericarditis

- Assess the nature of the patient's chest discomfort. (Pericardial pain is typically substernal. It is worse on inspiration and decreases when the patient leans forward.)
- Auscultate for a pericardial friction rub.
- Assist the patient to a position of comfort.
- Provide anti-inflammatory agents as prescribed.
- Explain that anti-inflammatory agents usually decrease the pain within 48 hours.
- Avoid the administration of aspirin and anticoagulants because these may increase the possibility of tamponade.
- Auscultate the blood pressure carefully to detect paradoxical blood pressure (pulsus paradoxus), a sign of tamponade:
  - Palpate the blood pressure, and inflate the cuff above the systolic pressure.
  - Deflate the cuff gradually, and note when sounds are first audible on expiration.
  - Identify when sounds are also audible on inspiration.
  - Subtract the inspiratory pressure from the expiratory pressure to determine the amount of pulsus paradoxus (>10 mm Hg is an indication of tamponade).
- Inspect for other indications of tamponade, including jugular venous distention with clear lungs, muffled heart sounds, and decreased cardiac output.
- Notify the physician if tamponade is suspected.

Cardiac tamponade is an emergency! The physician may initially manage the decreased cardiac output (CO) with increased fluid volume administration while awaiting an echocardiogram or x-ray to confirm the diagnosis. Unfortunately, these tests are not always helpful because the fluid volume around the heart may be too small to visualize. Hemodynamic monitoring in a specialized critical care unit usually demonstrates compression of the heart, with all pressures (right atrial, pulmonary artery, and wedge) being similar and elevated (plateau pressures).

The physician may elect to perform a **pericardiocentesis** to remove fluid and relieve the pressure on the heart. Under echocardiographic or fluoroscopic and hemodynamic monitoring, the cardiologist inserts an 8-inch (20.3-cm), 16- or 18-gauge pericardial needle into the pericardial space. When the needle is properly positioned, a catheter is inserted and all available pericardial fluid is withdrawn. A pericardial drain may be temporarily placed. Monitor the pulmonary artery, wedge, and right atrial pressures during the procedure. The pressures should return to normal as the fluid compressing the heart is removed, and the clinical manifestations of tamponade should resolve. In situations in which the cause of the tamponade is unknown, pericardial fluid specimens may be sent to the laboratory for culture and sensitivity tests and cytology.

! NURSING SAFETY PRIORITY (QSEN)

Action Alert

After the pericardiocentesis, closely monitor the patient for the recurrence of tamponade. Pericardiocentesis alone often does not resolve acute tamponade. Be prepared to provide adequate fluid volumes to increase CO and to prepare the patient for emergency sternotomy if tamponade recurs.

If the patient has a recurrence of tamponade or recurrent effusions or adhesions from chronic pericarditis, a portion or all of the pericardium may need to be removed to allow adequate ventricular filling and contraction. The surgeon may create a pericardial window, which involves removing a portion of the pericardium to permit excessive pericardial fluid to drain into the pleural space. In more severe cases, removal of the toughened encasing pericardium (pericardiectomy) may be necessary.

RHEUMATIC CARDITIS

❖ PATHOPHYSIOLOGY

Rheumatic carditis, also called *rheumatic endocarditis,* is a sensitivity response that develops after an upper respiratory tract infection with group A beta-hemolytic *Streptococci.* It occurs in almost half of patients with rheumatic fever. The precise mechanism by which the infection causes inflammatory lesions in the heart is not established; however, inflammation is evident in all layers of the heart. The inflammation results in impaired contractile function of the myocardium, thickening of the pericardium, and valvular damage.

Rheumatic carditis is characterized by the formation of Aschoff bodies (small nodules in the myocardium that are replaced by scar tissue). A diffuse cellular infiltrate also develops and may be responsible for the resulting heart failure (HF). The pericardium becomes thickened and covered with exudate, and a serosanguineous pleural effusion may develop. The most serious damage occurs to the endocardium, with inflammation of the valve leaflets developing. Hemorrhagic and fibrous lesions form along the inflamed surfaces of the valves, resulting in stenosis or regurgitation of the mitral and aortic valves (McCance et al., 2010).

❖ PATIENT-CENTERED COLLABORATIVE CARE

Rheumatic carditis is one of the major indicators of rheumatic fever. The common manifestations are:

- Tachycardia
- **Cardiomegaly** (enlarged heart)
- Development of a new murmur or a change in an existing murmur
- Pericardial friction rub
- Precordial pain
- Electrocardiogram (ECG) changes (prolonged PR interval)
- Indications of heart failure (HF)
- Evidence of an existing streptococcal infection

Primary prevention is extremely important. Teach all patients to remind their health care providers to provide appropriate antibiotic therapy if they develop the indications of streptococcal pharyngitis:

- Moderate to high fever
- Abrupt onset of a sore throat
- Reddened throat with exudate
- Enlarged and tender lymph nodes

Penicillin is the antibiotic of choice for treatment. Erythromycin (Eryc, Erythromid 🍁) is the alternative for penicillin-sensitive patients.

Once a diagnosis of rheumatic fever is made, antibiotic therapy is started immediately. Teach the patient to continue the antibiotic administration for the full 10 days to prevent re-infection. Suggest ways to manage fever, such as maintaining hydration and taking antipyretics. Encourage the patient to get adequate rest.

Explain to the patient and family that a recurrence of rheumatic carditis is most likely the result of reinfection by *Streptococcus.* Antibiotic prophylaxis is necessary for the rest of the patient's life to prevent infective endocarditis (see Infective Endocarditis, p. 697).

CARDIOMYOPATHY

❖ *PATHOPHYSIOLOGY*

Cardiomyopathy is a subacute or chronic disease of cardiac muscle, and the cause may be unknown. Cardiomyopathies are classified into four categories on the basis of abnormalities in structure and function: dilated cardiomyopathy, hypertrophic cardiomyopathy, restrictive cardiomyopathy, and arrhythmogenic right ventricular cardiomyopathy (Table 35-5). Mortality at 1 year is 20% and 70% to 80% at year 8 for patients who develop heart failure (Go et al., 2013).

Dilated cardiomyopathy (DCM) is the structural abnormality most commonly seen. DCM involves extensive damage to the myofibrils and interference with myocardial metabolism. Ventricular wall thickness is normal, but both ventricles are dilated (left ventricle is usually worse) and systolic function is impaired. Causes may include alcohol abuse, chemotherapy, infection, inflammation, and poor nutrition. Decreased CO from inadequate pumping of the heart causes the patient to experience dyspnea on exertion (DOE), decreased exercise capacity, fatigue, and palpitations.

The cardinal features of **hypertrophic cardiomyopathy (HCM)** are asymmetric ventricular hypertrophy and disarray of the myocardial fibers. Left ventricular hypertrophy leads to a stiff left ventricle, which results in diastolic filling abnormalities. Obstruction in the left ventricular outflow tract is seen in most patients with HCM. In about half of patients, HCM is transmitted as a single-gene autosomal dominant trait (McCance et al., 2010). Some patients die without any symptoms, whereas others have dyspnea on exertion (DOE), syncope, dizziness, and palpitations. Many athletes who die suddenly probably had hypertrophic cardiomyopathy.

Restrictive cardiomyopathy, the rarest of the cardiomyopathies, is characterized by stiff ventricles that restrict filling during diastole. Symptoms are similar to left or right heart failure (HF) or both. The disease can be primary or caused by endocardial or myocardial disease such as sarcoidosis

TABLE 35-5 Pathophysiology, Signs and Symptoms, and Treatment of Common Cardiomyopathies

	HYPERTROPHIC CARDIOMYOPATHY	
DILATED CARDIOMYOPATHY	**NONOBSTRUCTED**	**OBSTRUCTED**
Pathophysiology		
Fibrosis of myocardium and endocardium Dilated chambers Mural wall thrombi prevalent	Hypertrophy of all walls Hypertrophied septum Relatively small chamber size	Same as for nonobstructed except for obstruction of left ventricular outflow tract associated with the hypertrophied septum and mitral valve incompetence
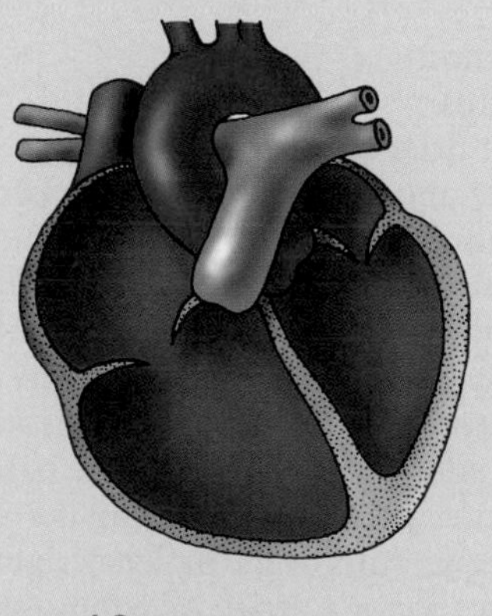		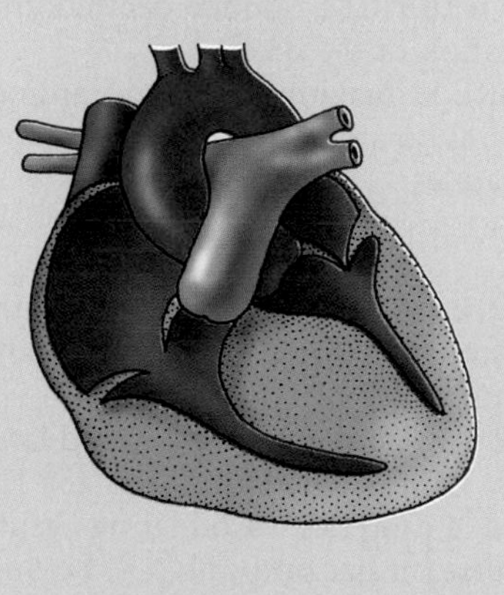
Signs and Symptoms		
Fatigue and weakness Heart failure (left side) Dysrhythmias or heart block Systemic or pulmonary emboli S_3 and S_4 gallops Moderate to severe cardiomegaly	Dyspnea Angina Fatigue, syncope, palpitations Mild cardiomegaly S_4 gallop Ventricular dysrhythmias Sudden death common Heart failure	Same as for nonobstructed except with mitral regurgitation murmur Atrial fibrillation
Treatment		
Symptomatic treatment of heart failure Vasodilators Control of dysrhythmias Surgery: heart transplant	For both: Symptomatic treatment Beta blockers Conversion of atrial fibrillation Surgery: ventriculomyotomy or muscle resection with mitral valve replacement Nitrates and other vasodilators *contraindicated* with the obstructed form	

or amyloidosis. The prognosis for this type of cardiomyopathy is poor.

Arrhythmogenic right ventricular cardiomyopathy (dysplasia) results from replacement of myocardial tissue with fibrous and fatty tissue. Although the name implies right ventricle disease, about a third of patients also have left ventricle (LV) involvement. This disease has a familial association and most often affects young adults. Some patients have symptoms, and others do not.

❖ PATIENT-CENTERED COLLABORATIVE CARE

◆ Assessment

Findings in cardiomyopathy depend on the structural and functional abnormalities. For example, left ventricular or biventricular failure is characteristic of *dilated* cardiomyopathy (DCM). Some patients with DCM are asymptomatic for months to years and have left and/or right ventricular dilation confirmed on x-ray examination or echocardiography. Others experience sudden, pronounced symptoms of left ventricular failure, such as progressive dyspnea on exertion, orthopnea, palpitations, and activity intolerance. Right-sided HF develops late in the disease and is associated with a poor prognosis. Atrial fibrillation occurs in some patients and is associated with embolism.

The clinical picture of *hypertrophic* cardiomyopathy (HCM) results from the hypertrophied septum causing a reduced stroke volume (SV) and cardiac output (CO). Most patients are asymptomatic until late adolescence or early adulthood. The primary symptoms of HCM are exertional dyspnea, angina, and syncope. The chest pain is atypical in that it usually occurs at rest, is prolonged, has no relation to exertion, and is not relieved by the administration of nitrates. A high incidence of ventricular dysrhythmias is associated with HCM. Sudden death occurs and may be the first manifestation of the disease.

Echocardiography, radionuclide imaging, and angiocardiography during cardiac catheterization are performed to diagnose and differentiate cardiomyopathies.

◆ Interventions

The treatment of choice for the patient with cardiomyopathy varies with the type of cardiomyopathy and may include both medical and surgical interventions.

Nonsurgical Management. The care of patients with dilated or restrictive cardiomyopathy is initially the same as for HF. Drug therapy includes the use of diuretics, vasodilating agents, and cardiac glycosides to increase cardiac output (CO). Because patients are at risk for sudden death, teach them to report any palpitations, dizziness, or fainting, which might indicate a dysrhythmia. Antidysrhythmic drugs or implantable cardiac defibrillators may be used to control life-threatening dysrhythmias. To block inappropriate sympathetic stimulation and tachycardia, beta blockers (e.g., metoprolol) are used. If cardiomyopathy has developed in response to a toxin (such as alcohol), further exposure to that toxin must be avoided.

Management of obstructive HCM includes administering negative inotropic agents such as beta-adrenergic blocking agents (carvedilol) and calcium antagonists (diltiazem). These drugs decrease the outflow obstruction that accompanies exercise. They also decrease heart rate (HR), resulting in less angina, dyspnea, and syncope. Vasodilators, diuretics, nitrates, and cardiac glycosides are contraindicated in patients with obstructive HCM because vasodilating and positive inotropic effects may worsen the obstruction (Sherrid & Arabadjian, 2012). Strenuous exercise is also prohibited because it can increase the risk for sudden death.

Surgical Management

Myomectomy and Ablation. The type of surgery performed depends on the type of cardiomyopathy. The most commonly used surgical treatment for obstructive HCM involves excising a portion of the hypertrophied ventricular septum to create a wider outflow tract (**ventriculomyomectomy**; also called *ventricular septal myectomy*). This procedure results in long-term improvement in activity tolerance for most patients.

Percutaneous alcohol septal ablation is another option for patients with HCM. Absolute alcohol is injected into a target septal branch of the left anterior descending coronary artery to produce a small septal infarction.

The patient with arrhythmogenic right ventricular cardiomyopathy who does not respond to drug therapy may have a radiofrequency catheter ablation or placement of an implantable defibrillator (see Chapter 34 for discussion of these procedures).

Heart Transplantation. **Heart transplantation** (surgical replacement with a donor heart) is the treatment of choice for patients with severe DCM and may be considered for patients with restrictive cardiomyopathy. The procedure may be done also for end-stage heart disease due to coronary artery disease, valvular disease, or congenital heart disease.

Preoperative Care. Criteria for candidate selection for heart transplantation include:

- Life expectancy less than 1 year
- Age generally less than 65 years
- New York Heart Association (NYHA) class III or IV
- Normal or only slightly increased pulmonary vascular resistance
- Absence of active infection
- Stable psychosocial status
- No evidence of current drug or alcohol abuse

Once the candidate is eligible and a heart is available, provide preoperative care as described in Chapter 14.

Operative Procedures. The surgeon transplants a heart from a donor with a comparable body weight and ABO compatibility into a recipient less than 6 hours after procurement. In the most common procedure (**bicaval technique**), the intact right atrium of the donor heart is preserved by anastomoses at the patient's (recipient's) superior and inferior venae cavae. In the more traditional **orthotopic** technique, cuffs of the patient's right and left atria are attached to the donor's atria. Anastomoses are made between the recipient and donor atria, aorta, and pulmonary arteries (Fig. 35-5). Because the remaining remnant of the recipient's atria contains the sinoatrial (SA) node, two unrelated P waves are visible on the ECG.

Postoperative Care. The postoperative care of the heart transplant recipient is similar to that for conventional cardiac surgery (see Chapter 38). However, the nurse must be especially observant to identify occult bleeding into the pericardial sac with the potential for tamponade (see earlier discussion of this complication on p. 699). The patient's pericardium has usually stretched considerably to accommodate the diseased, hypertrophied heart, predisposing him or her to have concealed postoperative bleeding.

The transplanted heart is denervated (disconnected from the body's autonomic nervous system) and is unresponsive to vagal

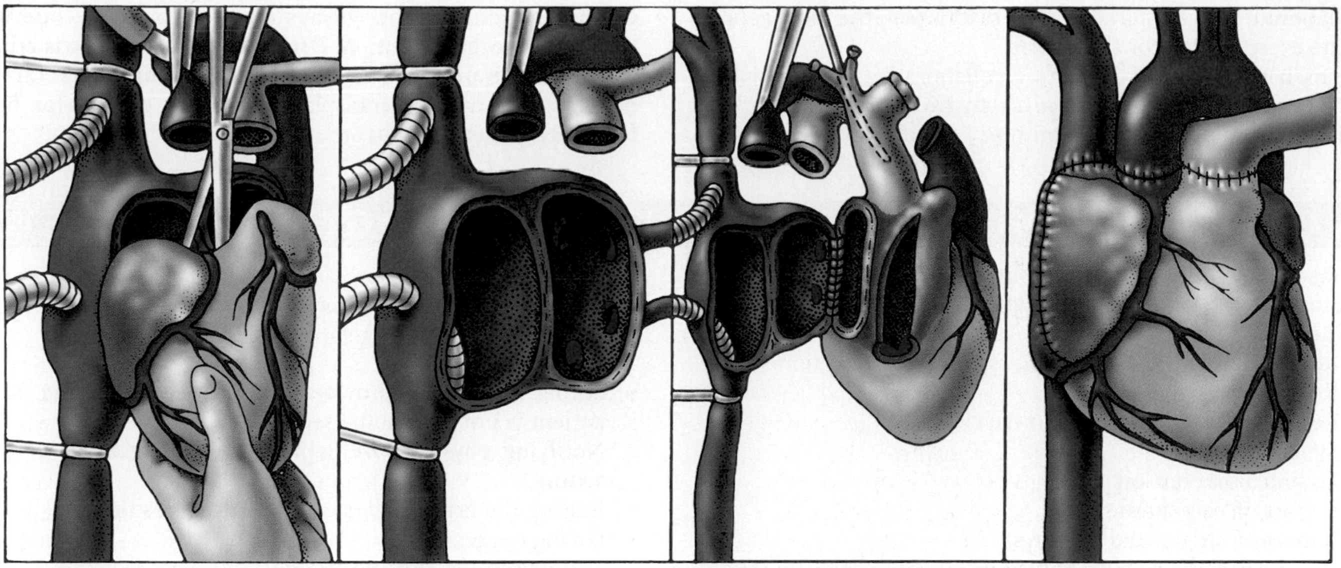
1. After the recipient is placed on cardiopulmonary bypass, the heart is removed.
2. The posterior walls of the recipient's left and right atria are left intact.
3. The left atrium of the donor heart is anastomosed to the recipient's residual posterior atrial walls, and the other atrial walls, the atrial septum, and the great vessels are joined.
POSTOPERATIVE RESULT

FIG. 35-5 One technique for heart transplantation.

stimulation. In the early postoperative phase, isoproterenol (Isuprel) may be titrated to support the HR and maintain cardiac output. Atropine, digoxin, and carotid sinus pressure are not used because they do not have their usual effects on the new heart. Denervation of the heart may cause pronounced orthostatic hypotension in the immediate postoperative phase. Caution the patient to change position slowly to help prevent this complication. Some patients also require a permanent pacemaker that is rate responsive to his or her activity level. The purpose is to increase CO and improve activity tolerance.

To suppress natural defense mechanisms (especially T- and B-cell function) and prevent transplant rejection, patients require a combination of immunosuppressants for the rest of their lives. Chapter 17 describes transplant rejection and prevention in detail.

! NURSING SAFETY PRIORITY QSEN

Critical Rescue

After surgery, perform comprehensive cardiovascular and respiratory assessments frequently according to agency or heart transplant surgical protocol. Chart 35-10 lists the signs and symptoms of rejection that are specific to heart transplant. Report any of these manifestations to the surgeon immediately! To detect rejection, the surgeon performs right endomyocardial biopsies at regularly scheduled intervals and whenever symptoms occur.

Be very careful about handwashing and aseptic technique because patients are immunosuppressed from drug therapy. *Infection is the major cause of death* and usually develops in the immediate post-transplant period or during treatment for acute rejection.

About 50% of patients survive 10 years after transplantation (Eisen, 2014). Many of the surviving patients have a form of coronary artery disease (CAD) called **coronary artery vasculopathy (CAV)**, which presents as diffuse plaque in the arteries of the donor heart. The cause is thought to involve a combination of immunologic and non-immunologic processes that result in vascular endothelial injury and an inflammatory response (Eisen, 2014). Because the heart is denervated, patients do not usually experience angina. Regularly scheduled exercise tolerance tests and angiography are required to identify CAV. Only a small percentage of patients with CAV benefit from revascularization procedures like balloon angioplasty or coronary artery bypass surgery. Stents are beginning to show some promise in managing these patients. Retransplantation may be done in select patients.

To delay the development of CAV, encourage patients to follow lifestyle changes similar to those with primary CAD (see Chapter 38). The physician may prescribe a calcium channel blocker such as diltiazem (Cardizem) to prevent coronary spasm and closure. Stress the importance of strict adherence to nutritional modifications and drug regimens. Teach the patient the importance of participating in a regular exercise program.

CHART 35-10 Best Practice for Patient Safety & Quality Care QSEN

Assessing for Clinical Manifestations of Heart Transplant Rejection

- Shortness of breath
- Fatigue
- Fluid gain (edema, increased weight)
- Abdominal bloating
- New bradycardia
- Hypotension
- Atrial fibrillation or flutter
- Decreased activity tolerance
- Decreased ejection fraction (late sign)

Collaborate with the physical therapist to plan the most appropriate exercise plan for the patient.

Discharge planning involves a collaborative, interdisciplinary approach. Patients require extensive health teaching for self-management and community resources for support. Counseling and support groups can help patients cope with their fear of organ rejection. Drug therapy adherence is crucial to prevent this problem. Continuing community-based care for patients with a heart transplant is similar to that for heart failure as discussed on p. 689.

NURSING CONCEPTS AND CLINICAL JUDGMENT REVIEW

What might you NOTICE if a patient is experiencing inadequate GAS EXCHANGE and tissue PERFUSION as a result of heart failure?

- Report of shortness of breath, especially on exertion
- Report of dizziness
- Report of weight gain within days
- Syncope
- Dyspnea on exertion
- Report of palpitations
- Report of fatigue and weakness
- Disorientation or acute confusion (especially in older adults)
- Peripheral or abdominal ascites

What should you INTERPRET and how should you RESPOND to a patient experiencing inadequate GAS EXCHANGE and tissue PERFUSION as a result of heart failure?

Perform and interpret physical assessment, including:

- Taking vital signs
- Monitoring oxygen saturation by pulse oximetry
- Performing a complete cardiovascular assessment
- Performing a complete respiratory assessment (listen for crackles or wheezes)
- Weighing patient
- Assessing cognition
- Assessing for pain or other symptoms

Respond by:

- Seeing health care provider immediately or calling 911 if patient is not in hospital setting ...OR
- Notifying physician or Rapid Response Team in hospital setting
- Raising the head of the bed to a sitting position
- Giving oxygen
- Maintaining or starting IV line
- Administering furosemide IV push (IVP) as prescribed
- Monitoring intake and output
- Giving ACE inhibitors or ARBs as prescribed IV or orally

On what should you REFLECT?

- Observe patient for increased urinary output.
- Monitor for decreased respiratory distress.
- Continue to monitor for improvement.
- Think about the possible cause(s) of the patient's heart failure.
- Think about your response to the patient.
- Develop a teaching plan for the patient to help prevent worsening or recurrent acute episodes of heart failure.

GET READY FOR THE NCLEX® EXAMINATION!

KEY POINTS

Review these Key Points for each NCLEX Examination Client Needs Category.

Safe and Effective Care Environment

- Provide information about continuing care for patients with heart failure (HF) after discharge to the community.
- Assess whether patients with end-stage HF have advance directives. If not, provide information about them.
- Collaborate with members of the health care team when developing and implementing a plan of care for patients with heart failure. **Teamwork and Collaboration** QSEN
- Teach patients about community support groups and resources such as the American Heart Association.

Health Promotion and Maintenance

- Provide teaching about self-management at home for patients with HF (see Table 35-4).
- Monitor older adults who are taking digoxin for manifestations of toxicity. Monitor potassium levels to check for hypokalemia (see Chart 35-5). **Safety** QSEN
- Teach patients taking ACE inhibitors or ARBs to change positions slowly to avoid orthostatic hypotension, especially older adults. **Safety** QSEN
- Teach the patient with valvular dysfunction, cardiac infection, or cardiomyopathy the necessity of taking preventive antibiotic therapy before any invasive procedure. **Evidence-Based Practice** QSEN

Psychosocial Integrity

- Assess the patient for depression resulting from altered self-concept and anxiety.
- Assess the patient's coping skills. **Patient-Centered Care** QSEN

Physiological Integrity

- Assess the patient for manifestations of right- and left-sided HF (see Charts 35-1 and 35-2).
- Weigh daily and record intake and output of patients with HF.
- Assess for early signs and symptoms of pulmonary edema (e.g., crackles in the lung bases, dyspnea at rest, disorientation, confusion), especially in older adults. **Safety** QSEN
- Assess for symptoms of worsening HF: rapid weight gain (3 lb in a week), a decrease in exercise tolerance lasting 2 to 3 days, cold symptoms (cough) lasting more than 3 to 5 days,

nocturia, development of dyspnea or angina at rest, or unstable angina. **Safety** QSEN

- Monitor the HF patient on beta blockers carefully for hypotension and bradycardia. **Safety** QSEN
- Monitor the pulse of patients taking digoxin before administration, and report to the health care provider a pulse that is not within the desired parameters.
- Monitor for manifestations of pulmonary edema as listed in Chart 35-3.
- Place the patient in a sitting position and provide oxygen therapy at a high flow rate (unless otherwise contraindicated) if pulmonary edema is suspected. **Evidence-Based Practice** QSEN
- Recognize that home care nurses perform and document focused physical assessments for cardiac patients as delineated in Chart 35-4. **Informatics** QSEN
- Monitor the patient with valvular dysfunction for atrial fibrillation, which may lead to hemostasis and mural thrombi. Monitor for an irregularly irregular cardiac rhythm, and administer warfarin as indicated.
- Document neurovascular status frequently because emboli from valvular disease may cause strokes. **Informatics** QSEN
- Differentiate major types of cardiomyopathy as described in Table 35-5.
- Observe for symptoms of heart transplant rejection as listed in Chart 35-10.
- Provide care for patients with pericarditis as outlined in Chart 35-9.

36 CHAPTER

Care of Patients with Vascular Problems

Donna D. Ignatavicius

http://evolve.elsevier.com/Iggy/

PRIORITY CONCEPTS

- Perfusion
- Clotting
- Pain
- Inflammation

LEARNING OUTCOMES

Safe and Effective Care Environment

1. Collaborate with interdisciplinary health care team members when providing care for patients with PERFUSION and CLOTTING problems.
2. Prioritize care for patients with hypertension.

Health Promotion and Maintenance

3. Identify risk factors for vascular problems.
4. Teach patients about lifestyle modifications to prevent vascular problems.

Physiological Integrity

5. Explain the INFLAMMATION process that is associated with the development of arteriosclerosis and atherosclerosis.
6. Interpret essential laboratory data related to risk for atherosclerosis.
7. Discuss the role of nutrition therapy in the management of patients with arteriosclerosis.
8. Describe the differences between essential and secondary hypertension.
9. Develop an evidence-based plan of care for a patient with essential hypertension.
10. Document a teaching plan for patients receiving drug therapy for hypertension.
11. Compare common assessment findings present in patients with peripheral arterial and peripheral venous disease.
12. Identify when venous thromboembolism (VTE) and complications of VTE occur.
13. Plan evidence-based nursing interventions to help prevent VTE.
14. Explain the nurse's role in monitoring patients who are receiving anticoagulants.
15. Compare assessment findings associated with Raynaud's phenomenon and Buerger's disease.

The *peripheral* vascular system is essential for transporting blood to and from distal tissues in the extremities. When peripheral blood vessels are diseased or damaged, especially in the legs, arterial blood flow is impaired, preventing distal areas like the feet from having adequate PERFUSION. The result can be ischemia and necrosis (cell death). Venous disease causes blood to back up into the distal areas and can lead to edema and thromboses (clots) that can become emboli, a life-threatening complication.

ARTERIOSCLEROSIS AND ATHEROSCLEROSIS

❖ PATHOPHYSIOLOGY

Arteriosclerosis is a thickening, or hardening, of the arterial wall that is often associated with aging. **Atherosclerosis,** a type of arteriosclerosis, involves the formation of plaque within the arterial wall and is the leading risk factor for cardiovascular disease. Usually the disease affects the larger arteries, such as coronary artery beds; aorta; carotid and vertebral arteries; renal, iliac, and femoral arteries; or any combination of these.

The exact pathophysiology of atherosclerosis is not known, but the condition is thought to occur from blood vessel damage that causes INFLAMMATION (see the discussion of inflammation in Chapter 17) (Fig. 36-1). After the vessel becomes inflamed, a fatty streak appears on the intimal surface (inner lining) of the artery. Through the process of cellular proliferation, collagen migrates over the fatty streak, forming a fibrous plaque. The fibrous plaque is often elevated and protrudes into the vessel lumen, partially or completely obstructing blood flow through the artery. Plaques are either stable or unstable. Unstable plaques are prone to rupture and are often clinically silent until they rupture (McCance et al., 2014).

In the final stage, the fibrous plaques become calcified, hemorrhagic, ulcerated, or thrombosed and affect all layers of the vessel. The rate of progression of the process may be influenced by genetic factors; certain chronic diseases (e.g., diabetes

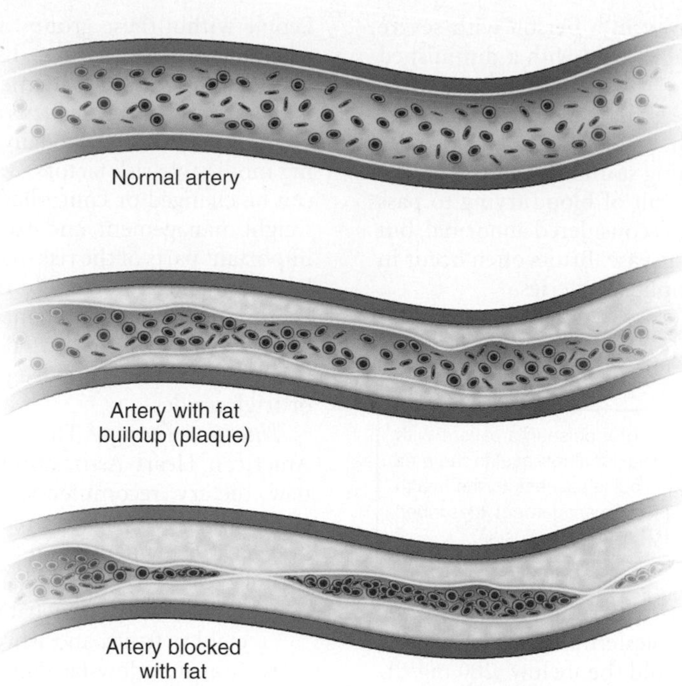

FIG. 36-1 Pathophysiology of atherosclerosis.

mellitus); and lifestyle habits, including smoking, eating habits, and level of exercise.

When *stable* plaque ruptures, thrombosis (blood clot) and constriction obstruct the vessel lumen, causing inadequate perfusion and oxygenation to distal tissues. *Unstable* plaque rupture causes more severe damage. After the rupture occurs, the exposed underlying tissue causes platelet adhesion and rapid thrombus formation. The thrombus may suddenly block a blood vessel, resulting in ischemia and infarction (e.g., myocardial infarction) (McCance et al., 2014).

Endothelial (intimal) injury of the major arteries of the body can be caused by many factors. Elevated levels of **lipids** (fats) like low-density lipoprotein cholesterol (LDL-C) and decreased levels of high-density lipoprotein cholesterol (HDL-C) can cause chemical injuries to the vessel wall. (Chapter 33 discusses lipids in detail.) Chemical injury can also be caused by elevated levels of toxins in the bloodstream, which may occur with renal failure or by carbon monoxide circulating in the bloodstream from cigarette smoking. The vessel wall can be weakened by the natural process of aging or by diseases such as hypertension.

Genetic predisposition and diabetes have a major effect on the development of atherosclerosis. Some patients have familial **hyperlipidemia**, an elevation of serum lipid levels. In these people, the liver makes excessive cholesterol and other fats. However, some people with hereditary atherosclerosis have a normal blood cholesterol level. The reason for the development and progression of plaque in these patients is not understood (McCance et al., 2014).

Adult patients of any age with severe diabetes mellitus frequently have premature and severe atherosclerosis from microvascular damage. The premature atherosclerosis occurs because diabetes promotes an increase in LDL-C and triglycerides (lipids) in plasma. In addition, arterial damage may result from the effect of hyperglycemia.

Other factors are indirectly related to atherosclerosis development. A list of risk factors is found in Table 36-1.

TABLE 36-1 Risk Factors for Atherosclerosis

• Low HDL-C	• Sedentary lifestyle
• High LDL-C	• Smoking
• Increased triglycorides	• Stress
• Genetic predisposition	• African-American or Hispanic ethnicity
• Diabetes mellitus	• Older adult
• Obesity	

HDL-C, High-density lipoprotein cholesterol; *LDL-C,* low-density lipoprotein cholesterol.

It is not known exactly how many people have atherosclerosis, but small plaques are almost always present in the arteries of young adults. The incidence can be better quantified by assessing the number of cardiovascular diseases (CVDs) that result from atherosclerosis. An estimated 81 million U.S. adults have one or more types of CVD (Go et al., 2013). About half of those with CVD are older than 60 years, and many more are middle-aged. The number of people affected by atherosclerosis is likely to increase as the population ages.

❖ PATIENT-CENTERED COLLABORATIVE CARE

◆ Assessment

Physical Assessment/Clinical Manifestations. The assessment of a patient with atherosclerosis includes a complete cardiovascular assessment because associated heart disease is often present. Because of the high incidence of hypertension in patients with atherosclerosis, assess the blood pressure in both arms.

Palpate pulses at all of the major sites on the body, and note any differences. *Palpate each carotid artery separately to prevent blocking blood flow to the brain!* Also feel for temperature differences in the lower extremities, and check capillary filling. Prolonged capillary filling (>3 seconds in young to middle-aged adults; >5 seconds in older adults) generally indicates poor circulation, *although this indicator is not the most reliable indicator of* PERFUSION. An extremity in a person with severe atherosclerotic disease may be cool or cold with a diminished or absent pulse.

Many patients with vascular disease have a bruit in the larger arteries, which can be heard with a stethoscope or Doppler probe. A **bruit** is a turbulent, swishing sound, which can be soft or loud in pitch. It is heard as a result of blood trying to pass through a narrowed artery. A bruit is considered abnormal, but it does not indicate the severity of disease. Bruits often occur in the carotid, aortic, femoral, and popliteal arteries.

! NURSING SAFETY PRIORITY QSEN

Critical Rescue

A decrease in intensity or a complete loss of a pulse in a patient with atherosclerosis may indicate an arterial occlusion (blockage) in the area supplied by the artery. Immediately report pulselessness to the health care provider and document for emergency management (described later in this chapter under Acute Peripheral Arterial Occlusion).

Laboratory Assessment. Patients with atherosclerosis often have elevated lipids, including cholesterol and triglycerides. Total serum *cholesterol* levels should be below 200 mg/dL. Elevated cholesterol levels are confirmed by HDL and LDL measurements. Increased low-density lipoprotein cholesterol (LDL-C) ("bad" cholesterol) levels indicate that a person is at an increased risk for atherosclerosis. Low high-density lipoprotein cholesterol (HDL-C) ("good" cholesterol) levels also indicate an increased risk. In general, a desirable LDL-C level is one below 130 mg/dL for healthy people and below 70 mg/dL for those diagnosed with CVD or who are diabetic. A desirable HDL-C level is 45 mg/dL or above for men and 55 mg/dL for women (Pagana & Pagana, 2014). These values differ based on age and comorbidities.

Triglyceride level may also be elevated with atherosclerosis and is an emerging lipid risk factor by the classic Adult Treatment Panel Report No. 3 (ATP III) released by the National Heart, Lung, and Blood Institute (National Cholesterol Education Program, 2002). A level of 160 mg/dL or above indicates **hypertriglyceridemia** in men. Women should have a level below 135 mg/dL (Pagana & Pagana, 2014). Elevated triglycerides are considered a marker for other lipoproteins. They also suggest metabolic syndrome, which increases the risk for coronary heart disease (see Table 38-1 and discussion in Chapter 38).

◆ *Interventions*

Atherosclerosis progresses for years before clinical manifestations occur. Adults who are at risk for the disease can often be identified through cholesterol screening and history. Because of the high incidence in the United States, low-risk people 20 years of age and older are advised to have their total serum cholesterol level evaluated at least once every 5 years. More frequent measurements are suggested for people with multiple risk factors and those older than 40 years.

People with multiple risk factors are grouped into high-risk patient categories termed "coronary heart disease equivalents." These groups include:

- Patients with diabetes but without signs of vascular disease
- Patients with a Framingham Heart Study 10-year absolute risk score of over 20% for coronary heart disease events
- Patients identified with multiple metabolic risk factors

People within these groups are at the same risk level as those who already have vascular disease.

Interventions for patients with atherosclerosis or those at high risk for the disease focus on lifestyle changes. Teach patients about the need to make daily changes by avoiding or minimizing modifiable risk factors. *Modifiable risk factors* are those that can be changed or controlled by the patient, such as smoking, weight management, and exercise. Nutrition is one of the most important parts of the risk-reduction plan. Chapter 38 describes how to manage modifiable risk factors in detail in the Health Promotion and Maintenance section, p. 759. If lipoprotein levels do not improve after lifestyle changes, the health care provider may prescribe drug therapy to lower cholesterol and/or triglycerides.

Nutrition Therapy. The American College of Cardiology and American Heart Association (ACC/AHA) recently published new dietary recommendations for lowering LDL-C levels (Eckel et al., 2014). These recommendations were based on the best current evidence from randomized controlled trials and include:

- Consume a dietary pattern that emphasizes intake of vegetables, fruits, and whole grains.
- Consume low-fat dairy products, poultry, fish, legumes, nontropical (e.g., canola) vegetable oils, and nuts.
- Limit intake of sweets, sugar-sweetened beverages, and red meats.
- Aim for a dietary pattern that includes 5% to 6% of calories from saturated fat.
- Reduce percent of calories from *trans* fat.

These guidelines are similar to the Dietary Approaches to Stop Hypertension (DASH), which also recommend daily sodium, potassium, and fiber amounts (National Heart, Lung, and Blood Institute, 2012). In collaboration with the dietitian as needed, teach the patient about the types of fat content in food. Meats and eggs contain mostly saturated fats and are high in cholesterol. Instruct patients about increasing dietary fiber to 30 g each day, which is consistent with DASH guidelines.

Physical Activity. The ACC/AHA also recommends that adults engage in aerobic physical activity 3 or 4 times a week to reduce LDL-C levels. Each session should last for 40 minutes on average and involve moderate-to-vigorous physical activity (Eckel et al., 2014).

Drug Therapy. For patients with elevated total and LDL-C levels that do not respond adequately to dietary intervention, the health care provider prescribes a cholesterol-lowering agent. Drug choice and dosing depend on the serum cholesterol level, the degree to which the level needs to be decreased, and the patient's age (Stone et al., 2014). Because most of these drugs can produce major side effects, they are generally given only when nonpharmacologic management has been unsuccessful.

A class of drugs known as *3-hydroxy-3-methylglutaryl coenzyme A (HMG-CoA) reductase inhibitors (statins)* successfully reduces total cholesterol in most patients when used for an extended period. Examples include lovastatin (Mevacor), simvastatin (Zocor), and pitavastatin (Livalo), which lower both LDL-C and triglyceride levels (Table 36-2).

The American College of Cardiology/American Heart Association recently published new recommendations for treatment of high cholesterol to reduce atherosclerotic cardiovascular disease (ASCVD) in adults (Stone et al., 2014). These evidence-based recommendations are highlighted in Table 36-3.

TABLE 36-2 Commonly Used Drugs for Lowering LDL-C Levels

HMG-CoA Reductase Inhibitors (Statins)	Combination Drugs
• Lovastatin (Mevacor) • Atorvastatin (Lipitor) • Simvastatin (Zocor) • Fluvastatin (Lescol) • Rosuvastatin (Crestor) • Pravastatin (Pravachol) • Pitavastatin (Livalo)	• Ezetimibe and simvastatin (Vytorin) • Amlodipine and atorvastatin (Caduet) • Niacin and lovastatin (Advicor)

HMG-CoA, 3-hydroxy-3-methylglutaryl coenzyme A.

! NURSING SAFETY PRIORITY QSEN

Drug Alert

Statins reduce cholesterol synthesis in the liver and increase clearance of LDL-C from the blood. Therefore they are contraindicated in patients with active liver disease or during pregnancy because they can cause muscle myopathies and marked decreases in liver function. Statins also have the potential for interactions with other drugs, such as warfarin, cyclosporine, and selected antibiotics. Statins are discontinued if the patient has muscle cramping or elevated liver enzyme levels. Some patients also report abdominal bloating, flatulence, diarrhea, and/or constipation as side effects of these drugs. Remind patients to have laboratory testing follow-up as prescribed by their health care provider (Lilley et al., 2014).

Teach patients taking statin drugs, especially those taking atorvastatin, lovastatin, and simvastatin, to *avoid grapefruit and grapefruit juice in their diet.* Grapefruit contains a group of chemicals called *furanocoumarins* that bind to and inactivate the enzyme *CYP3A4.* This enzyme is important for metabolism of many drugs, including statins. If it is inactivated, too much of the statin drug can remain in the patient's bloodstream, causing possible kidney failure, heart failure, GI bleeding, or even death (Bailey et al., 2013).

A different type of lipid-lowering agent, ezetimibe (Zetia), may be used in place of or in combination with statin-type drugs. This drug inhibits the absorption of cholesterol through the small intestine. Vytorin is a combination drug containing ezetimibe and simvastatin. This drug works two ways—by reducing the absorption of cholesterol and by decreasing the amount of cholesterol synthesis in the liver. Other statin combinations have been developed to improve lipid levels, such as Advicor—a combination of niacin and lovastatin. Aspirin and pravastatin are combined as Pravigard. Amlodipine (Norvasc) and atorvastatin are combined as Caduet to decrease blood pressure while decreasing triglycerides (TGs), increasing HDL, and lowering LDL. Combining drugs may improve adherence for the patient who is often taking multiple drugs.

Complementary and Alternative Therapies. Nicotinic acid or niacin (Niaspan), a B vitamin, may lower LDL C and very-low-density lipoprotein (VLDL) cholesterol levels and increase HDL-C levels in some patients, although the evidence supporting its use is lacking. It is used as a single agent or in combination with an acid-binding resin drug or a statin. Low doses are recommended because many patients experience flushing and a very warm feeling all over. Higher doses can result in an elevation of hepatic enzymes.

Lovaza (omega-3 ethyl esters) is approved by the Food and Drug Administration (FDA) as an adjunct to diet to reduce TGs that are greater than 500 mg/dL. This drug also decreases plaque growth and INFLAMMATION and reduces clot formation.

TABLE 36-3 Selected 2013 ACC/AHA Recommendations for the Treatment of Serum Cholesterol to Reduce Atherosclerotic Cardiovascular Disease Risk in Adults

Primary Prevention

- All people with LDL-C equal to or greater than 190 mg/dL should be evaluated for secondary causes of hyperlipidemia and treated with statin therapy.
- Adults with diabetes mellitus who are 40 to 75 years of age should be treated with high-intensity statin therapy.
- Adults 40 to 75 years of age with LDL-C of 70 to 189 mg/dL without clinical signs of ASCVD or diabetes should be treated with moderate- to high-intensity statin therapy.

Secondary Prevention

- High-intensity statin therapy should be initiated or continued as first-line treatment in adults 75 years of age or younger who have clinical manifestations of ASCVD, unless contraindicated.
- In people older than 75 years, the potential for ASCVD risk-reduction benefits, adverse drug effects, and drug-drug interactions should be evaluated.

Data from Stone, N.J., Robinson, J., Lichtenstein, A.H., Merz, N.B., Blum, C.B., Eckel, R.H., et al. (2014). 2013 ACC/AHA guidelines on the treatment of blood cholesterol to reduce atherosclerotic cardiovascular risk in adults: A report of the American College of Cardiology/American Heart Association Task Force on Practice Guidelines. *Circulation, 129*(25 Suppl 2), S1-S45.

ASCVD, Atherosclerotic cardiovascular disease; *LDL-C,* low-density lipoprotein cholesterol.

? NCLEX EXAMINATION CHALLENGE

Health Promotion and Maintenance

A client diagnosed with atherosclerosis has been prescribed lovastatin (Mevacor). Which statement by the client indicates a need for further teaching?

A. "I won't need to change my diet because now I'm taking a pill."
B. "I'll follow up with my nurse practitioner on a regular basis."
C. "I need to quit smoking as soon as I possibly can."
D. "I shouldn't drink grapefruit juice while on this drug."

HYPERTENSION

Hypertension, or high blood pressure (BP), is the most common health problem seen in primary care settings and can cause stroke, myocardial infarction (heart attack), kidney failure, and death if not treated early and effectively. The Eighth Joint National Committee (JNC 8) on Prevention, Detection, Evaluation, and Treatment of High Blood Pressure recently published its *2014 Evidence-Based Guidelines for the Management of High Blood Pressure in Adults* based on the results of randomized controlled trials, the gold standard for establishing recommendations for best clinical practice (James et al., 2014). These new guidelines replace the JNC 7 recommendations and hypertension classifications.

According to JNC 8, in the general population ages 60 years and older, the desired BP is below 150/90. For people younger than 60 years, the desired BP is below 140/90. Patients whose blood pressures are above these desired goals should be treated with drug therapy (James et al., 2014). Adult patients with specific risk factors for developing hypertension should be treated at any age, as described later under Drug Therapy.

❖ PATHOPHYSIOLOGY

To best understand the pathophysiology of hypertension, a review of normal blood pressure and how it is normally maintained is essential.

Mechanisms That Influence Blood Pressure. The systemic arterial blood pressure is a product of cardiac output (CO) and total peripheral vascular resistance (PVR). Cardiac output is determined by the stroke volume (SV) multiplied by heart rate (HR) ($CO = SV \times HR$). Control of peripheral vascular resistance (i.e., vessel constriction or dilation) is maintained by the autonomic nervous system and circulating hormones, such as norepinephrine and epinephrine. Consequently, any factor that increases peripheral vascular resistance, heart rate, or stroke volume increases the systemic arterial pressure. Conversely, any factor that decreases peripheral vascular resistance, heart rate, or stroke volume decreases the systemic arterial pressure and can cause decreased PERFUSION to body tissues.

Stabilizing mechanisms exist in the body to exert an overall regulation of systemic arterial pressure and to prevent circulatory collapse. Four control systems play a major role in maintaining blood pressure:

- The arterial baroreceptor system
- Regulation of body fluid volume
- The renin-angiotensin-aldosterone system
- Vascular autoregulation

Arterial baroreceptors are found primarily in the carotid sinus, aorta, and wall of the left ventricle. They monitor the level of arterial pressure and counteract a rise in arterial pressure through vagally mediated cardiac slowing and vasodilation with decreased sympathetic tone. Therefore reflex control of circulation elevates the systemic arterial pressure when it falls and lowers it when it rises. Why baroreceptor control fails in hypertension is not clear (McCance et al., 2014).

Changes *in fluid volume* also affect the systemic arterial pressure. For example, if there is an excess of sodium and/or water in a person's body, the blood pressure rises through complex physiologic mechanisms that change the venous return to the heart, producing a rise in cardiac output. If the kidneys are functioning adequately, a rise in systemic arterial pressure produces diuresis (excessive voiding) and a fall in pressure. Pathologic conditions change the pressure threshold at which the kidneys excrete sodium and water, thereby altering the systemic arterial pressure.

The *renin-angiotensin-aldosterone* system also regulates blood pressure (see discussion in Chapter 11). The kidney produces renin, an enzyme that acts on angiotensinogen (a plasma protein substrate) to split off angiotensin I, which is converted by an enzyme in the lung to form angiotensin II. Angiotensin II has strong vasoconstrictor action on blood vessels and is the controlling mechanism for aldosterone release. Aldosterone then works on the collecting tubules in the kidneys to reabsorb sodium. Sodium retention inhibits fluid loss, thus increasing blood volume and subsequent blood pressure.

Inappropriate secretion of renin may cause increased peripheral vascular resistance in patients with hypertension. When the blood pressure is high, renin levels should decrease because the increased renal arteriolar pressure usually inhibits renin secretion. However, for most people with essential hypertension, renin levels remain normal.

The process of *vascular autoregulation,* which keeps perfusion of tissues in the body relatively constant, appears to be important in causing hypertension. However, the exact mechanism of how this system works is poorly understood.

Classifications of Hypertension. Hypertension can be essential (primary) or secondary. **Essential hypertension** is the most common type and is not caused by an existing health problem. However, a number of risk factors can increase a person's likelihood of becoming hypertensive. Continuous BP elevation in patients with essential hypertension results in damage to vital organs by causing medial hyperplasia (thickening) of the arterioles. As the blood vessels thicken and PERFUSION decreases, body organs are damaged. These changes can result in myocardial infarctions, strokes, peripheral vascular disease (PVD), or kidney failure.

Specific disease states and drugs can increase a person's susceptibility to hypertension. A person with this type of elevation in blood pressure has **secondary hypertension.**

Malignant hypertension is a severe type of elevated blood pressure that rapidly progresses. A person with this health problem usually has symptoms such as morning headaches, blurred vision, and dyspnea and/or symptoms of uremia (accumulation in the blood of substances ordinarily eliminated in the urine). Patients are often in their 30s, 40s, or 50s with their systolic blood pressure greater than 200 mm Hg. The diastolic blood pressure is greater than 150 mm Hg or greater than 130 mm Hg when there are pre-existing complications. Unless intervention occurs promptly, a patient with malignant hypertension may experience kidney failure, left ventricular heart failure, or stroke.

Etiology and Genetic Risk. *Essential* hypertension can develop when a patient has any one or more of the risk factors listed in Table 36-4.

Kidney disease is one of the most common causes of *secondary* hypertension. Hypertension can develop when there is any sudden damage to the kidneys. Renovascular hypertension is associated with narrowing of one or more of the main arteries carrying blood directly to the kidneys, known as *renal artery stenosis (RAS).* Many patients have been able to reduce the use of their antihypertensive drugs when the narrowed arteries are dilated through angioplasty with stent placement.

Dysfunction of the adrenal medulla or the adrenal cortex can also cause secondary hypertension. *Adrenal-mediated hypertension* is due to primary excesses of aldosterone, cortisol, and catecholamines. In *primary aldosteronism,* excessive aldosterone causes hypertension and hypokalemia (low potassium levels). It usually arises from benign adenomas of the adrenal cortex.

TABLE 36-4 Etiology of Hypertension

Essential (Primary)	Secondary
• Family history of hypertension	• Kidney disease
• African-American ethnicity	• Primary aldosteronism
• Hyperlipidemia	• Pheochromocytoma
• Smoking	• Cushing's disease
• Older than 60 years or postmenopausal	• Coarctation of the aorta
• Excessive sodium and caffeine intake	• Brain tumors
• Overweight/obesity	• Encephalitis
• Physical inactivity	• Pregnancy
• Excessive alcohol intake	• Drugs:
• Low potassium, calcium, or magnesium intake	• Estrogen (e.g., oral contraceptives)
• Excessive and continuous stress	• Glucocorticoids
	• Mineralocorticoids
	• Sympathomimetics

Pheochromocytomas are tumors that originate most commonly in the adrenal medulla and result in excessive secretion of catecholamines, resulting in life-threatening high blood pressure. In *Cushing's syndrome,* excessive glucocorticoids are excreted from the adrenal cortex. The most common cause of Cushing's syndrome is either adrenocortical hyperplasia or adrenocortical adenoma (tumor).

Drugs that can cause secondary hypertension include estrogen, glucocorticoids, mineralocorticoids, sympathomimetics, cyclosporine, and erythropoietin. The use of estrogen-containing oral contraceptives is likely the most common cause of secondary hypertension in women. Drugs that cause hypertension are discontinued to reverse this problem.

Incidence and Prevalence. Hypertension is a worldwide epidemic. In the United States, one in every three adults has high blood pressure or is being treated for hypertension (Go et al., 2013). The disease can shorten life expectancy.

GENDER HEALTH CONSIDERATIONS

Patient-Centered Care QSEN

A higher percentage of men than women have hypertension until age 45 years. From 45 to 54 years, women have a slightly higher percentage of hypertension than men. After age 54 years, women have a much higher percentage of the disease (Go et al., 2013). The causes for these differences are not known.

CULTURAL CONSIDERATIONS

Patient-Centered Care QSEN

The prevalence of hypertension in African Americans in the United States is among the highest in the world and is constantly increasing. When compared with Euro-Americans, they develop high BP earlier in life, making them much more likely to die from strokes, heart disease, and kidney disease (Go et al., 2013). The exact reasons for these differences are not known, but genetics and environmental factors may play a role. Efforts to raise awareness of hypertension through education within African-American communities, including the importance of receiving treatment and controlling blood pressure, have been somewhat successful. Geographic differences still exist (Go et al., 2013).

Health Promotion and Maintenance

Control of hypertension has resulted in major decreases in cardiovascular morbidity and mortality. The U.S. *Healthy People 2020* campaign includes a number of objectives related to hypertension to decrease cardiovascular mortality (Table 36-5).

The *2013 ACA/AHA Guidelines on Lifestyle Management to Reduce Cardiovascular Risk* outlines evidence-based dietary and exercise practices to help lower blood pressure (Eckel et al., 2014). These guidelines are similar to the Dietary Approaches to Stop Hypertension (DASH) and include:

- Consume a dietary pattern that emphasizes intake of vegetables, fruits, and whole grains.
- Consume low-fat dairy products, poultry, fish, legumes, nontropical vegetable oils, and nuts.
- Limit intake of sweets, sugar-sweetened beverages, and red meats.
- Lower sodium intake to no more than 2400 mg per day; a limit of 1500 mg of sodium per day is preferred.
- Engage in aerobic physical activity 3 or 4 times a week. Each session should last for 40 minutes on average and involve moderate-to-vigorous physical activity.

TABLE 36-5 Meeting *Healthy People 2020* Objectives

Heart Disease and Stroke

Selected objectives retained from *Healthy People 2010:*
- Increase the proportion of adults with high blood pressure who are taking action to help control their blood pressure.
- Increase the proportion of adults who have had their blood pressure measured within the preceding 2 years and can state whether their blood pressure was normal or high.

Selected objectives retained but modified from *Healthy People 2010:*
- Reduce the proportion of persons in the population with hypertension.
- Increase the proportion of adults with prehypertension who meet the recommended guidelines for:
  a. Body mass index (BMI)
  b. Saturated fat consumption
  c. Sodium intake
  d. Physical activity
  e. Moderate alcohol consumption
- Increase the proportion of adults with hypertension who meet the [above] recommended guidelines.

New objectives for *Healthy People 2020:*
- Increase the proportion of adults with hypertension who are taking the recommended medications to decrease their blood pressure.

Data from www.healthypeople.gov/2020.

In addition to following specific dietary and physical activity guidelines, teach patients ways to decrease other modifiable risk factors for hypertension, such as smoking and excessive alcohol intake. Risk factor prevention and lifestyle changes are discussed in more detail in Chapter 38.

❖ PATIENT-CENTERED COLLABORATIVE CARE

◆ Assessment

History. During history taking, review the patient's risk factors for hypertension. Collect data on the patient's age; ethnic origin or race; family history of hypertension; average dietary intake of calories, sodium- and potassium-containing foods, and alcohol; and exercise habits. Also assess any past or present history of kidney or cardiovascular disease and current use of drug therapy or illicit drugs.

Physical Assessment/Clinical Manifestations. When a diagnosis of hypertension is made, most people have no symptoms. However, some patients experience headaches, facial flushing (redness), dizziness, or fainting as a result of the elevated blood pressure. Obtain blood pressure readings in both arms. Two or more readings may be taken at each visit (Fig. 36-2). Some patients have high blood pressure due to anxiety associated with visiting a health care provider. Be sure to take an accurate blood pressure by using an appropriate-size cuff. Anderson et al. (2010) found that forearm blood pressure measurements are as accurate as upper arm blood pressures, especially in patients who are obese.

To detect postural (orthostatic) changes, take readings with the patient in the supine (lying) or sitting position and at least 2 minutes later when standing. **Orthostatic hypotension** is a decrease in blood pressure (20 mm Hg systolic and/or 10 mm Hg diastolic) when the patient changes position from lying to sitting.

Funduscopic examination of the eyes to observe vascular changes in the retina is done by a skilled health care practitioner.

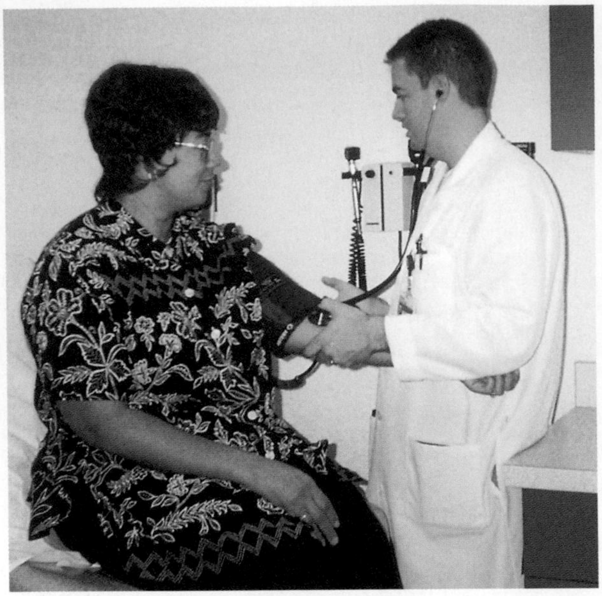

FIG. 36-2 Blood pressure screening during history and physical examination.

The appearance of the retina can be a reliable index of the severity and prognosis of hypertension.

Physical assessment is helpful in diagnosing several conditions that produce secondary hypertension. The presence of abdominal bruits is typical of patients with renal artery stenosis. Tachycardia, sweating, and pallor may suggest a pheochromocytoma (adrenal medulla tumor). Coarctation of the aorta is evidenced by elevation of blood pressure in the arms, with normal or low blood pressure in the lower extremities. Femoral pulses are also delayed or absent.

Psychosocial Assessment. Assess for psychosocial stressors that can worsen hypertension and affect the patient's ability to adhere to treatment. Evaluate job-related, economic, and other life stressors, as well as the patient's response to these stressors. Some patients may have difficulty coping with the lifestyle changes needed to control hypertension. Be sure to assess past coping strategies.

Diagnostic Assessment. Although no laboratory tests are diagnostic of essential hypertension, several laboratory tests can assess possible causes of secondary hypertension. Kidney disease can be diagnosed by the presence of protein and red blood cells in the urine, elevated levels of blood urea nitrogen (BUN), and elevated serum creatinine levels. The creatinine clearance test directly indicates the glomerular filtration ability of the kidneys. The normal value is 107 to 139 mL/min for men and 87 to 107 mL/min for women (Pagana & Pagana, 2014). Decreased levels indicate acute or chronic kidney disease.

Urinary test results are positive for the presence of catecholamines in patients with a pheochromocytoma (tumor of the adrenal medulla). An elevation in levels of serum corticoids and 17-ketosteroids in the urine is diagnostic of Cushing's disease.

No specific x-ray studies can diagnose hypertension. Routine chest radiography may help recognize cardiomegaly (heart enlargement).

An electrocardiogram (ECG) determines the degree of cardiac involvement. Left atrial and ventricular hypertrophy is the first ECG sign of heart disease resulting from hypertension. Left ventricular remodeling can be detected on the 12-lead ECG (see Chapter 38 for discussion of remodeling).

◆ Analysis

The priority collaborative problems for patients with hypertension include:

1. Need for health teaching related to the plan of care for hypertension management
2. Risk for nonadherence related to side effects of drug therapy and necessary changes in lifestyle

◆ Planning and Implementation

Health Teaching

Planning: Expected Outcomes. The patient with hypertension is expected to verbalize his or her individualized plan of care for hypertension (see the Concept Map on Hypertension).

Interventions. Lifestyle changes are considered the foundation of hypertension control. If these changes are unsuccessful, the primary care provider considers the use of antihypertensive drugs. There is no surgical treatment for essential hypertension. However, surgery may be indicated for certain causes of secondary hypertension, such as kidney disease, coarctation of the aorta, and pheochromocytoma.

Lifestyle Changes. In collaboration with the health care team, teach the patient to (Baldwin, 2011):

- Restrict sodium intake in the diet per the ACA/AHA guidelines
- Reduce weight, if overweight or obese
- Use alcohol sparingly (no more than 1 drink a day for women and 2 drinks a day for men [1 drink = 12 oz. beer, 5 oz. wine, or 1.5 oz. liquor such as vodka or gin.])
- Exercise 3 or 4 days a week for 40 minutes each day per the ACA/AHA guidelines
- Use relaxation techniques to decrease stress
- Avoid tobacco and caffeine

Strategies to help patients make these changes are discussed in Chapter 38.

Complementary and Alternative Therapies. Garlic and coenzyme Q_{10} have been used for a number of health problems, but evidence to support their use to prevent hypertension is controversial. Evidence by consensus and case reports does support garlic's cholesterol-lowering ability and its ability to decrease blood pressure in patients with hypertension (National Center for Complementary and Alternative Medicine, 2013). Teach patients to check with their health care provider before starting garlic or any herbal therapy because of possible side effects and interactions with other herbs, foods, or drugs. Garlic can damage the liver and cause bleeding in some patients, especially if they have invasive procedures such as surgery.

Some patients have also had success with biofeedback, meditation, and acupuncture as part of their overall management plan. These methods may be most useful as adjuncts for patients who experience continuous and severe stress.

Drug Therapy. Drug therapy is individualized for each patient, with consideration given to culture, age, other existing illness, severity of blood pressure elevation, and cost of drugs and follow-up. Once-a-day drug therapy is best, especially for the older adult, because the more doses required each day, the higher the risk that a patient will not follow the treatment regimen. However, many patients with hypertension need two or more drugs to adequately control blood pressure.

In the largest hypertensive trial done to date, Antihypertensive and Lipid Lowering Treatment to Prevent Heart Attack Trial (ALLHAT), the use of diuretics has been practically

CONCEPT MAP

PAIN — CLOTTING — **HYPERTENSION** — PERFUSION

HISTORY

Mike Jones is an older adult admitted for control of his blood pressure. He has a history of hypertension and type 2 diabetes. He takes captopril (Captoten) 50 mg BID, metformin (Glucaphage) 850 mg daily, gemfibrozil (Lopid) 600 mg BID, and hydrochlorothiazide (HCTZ) 20 mg daily.

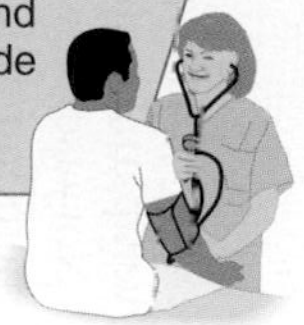

Physical Assessment/ Clinical Manifestations

- BP 170/86 mm Hg; HR 80; Chol - 240; LDL-C 150; HDL-C 40; triglycerides - 400; HgA,C 7%; BS 170
- Face is flushed, patient is dizzy
- Recently divorced, consumes lots of canned goods, lives alone on fixed income

Risk Factors HTN

- Family history of CV and PVD; African-American male
- Type 2 diabetes, alcoholism
- Postoperative pain
- 45 lbs overweight
- Divorced, shares custody of 2 teenagers with ex-wife

Data Synthesis

Patient Problems

- Need for health teaching related to the plan of care for hypertension management
- Risk for nonadherence related to side effects of drug therapy and necessary changes in lifestyle

Planning

EXPECTED OUTCOMES

- Verbalize plan to change lifestyle to reduce modifiable factors of hypertension
- Patient with diabetes will target BP of <130/90 mm Hg; patient without diabetes will target BP of <120/80 mm Hg
- Lab goals:
  - Cholesterol: <200 mg/dL
  - LDL-C: <70 mg/dL with CVD or DM
  - HDL-C: >40 mg/dL
  - Triglycerides <150 mg/dL
  - HgA_{1C}: 6%
  - BS <130 mg/dL

INTERVENTIONS

1 **Data Collection**

Assess risk factors: age, ethnicity, family history, diet history, alcohol consumption, drug use, history of renal or CV disease. *Reviews modifiable and nonmodifiable risk factors that decrease PERFUSION and provides a foundation for teaching lifestyle changes.*

2 **Physical Assessment**

- Assess BP in both arms with accurately sized BP cuff. *Determines orthostatic changes; increased incidence of hypertension in patients with atherosclerosis.*
- Palpate all pulses and note differences; palpate each carotid artery separately. *Prevents blocking PERFUSION to the brain.*
- Check temperature differences in lower extremities; check capillary filling. *Assesses for heart disease that is often present in patients with DM.*

3 **Lifestyle Modifications**

- Teach the patient to restrict sodium, identify potassium-rich foods, control weight, consume alcohol sparingly, increase exercise, use relaxation techniques, and avoid tobacco and caffeine. *Educates about decreasing modifiable risk factors to control hypertension and stresses the importance of lifestyle choices.*
- Identify ways to encourage drug adherence. *Encourages the patient without physical symptoms, economic restraints, or forgetfulness, the importance of taking medications as prescribed to prevent decreased PERFUSION*

4 **Psychosocial Assessment**

Evaluate economic and other life stressors as well as patient's response to stressors. Assess past coping strategies. *Determines the patient's coping ability and gauges probability of treatment compliance; stressors can worsen hypertension and affect the patient's ability to follow treatment*

5 **Interpretation of Lab Values**

Review and intervene with abnormal lab values: total cholesterol, HDL-C, LDL-C triglycerides, blood sugar. *Monitors lipid levels; patients with DM can have increased lipid levels leading to early severe atherosclerosis, arterial damage, and CAD.*

6 **Drug Therapy**

- Administer antihypertensive and antihyperlipoproteinemic drugs as prescribed. *Controls hypertension and lipid levels; medications are instituted if lifestyle changes prove unsuccessful.*
- Monitor for signs of orthostatic hypotension. *Promotes safety in the older patient who is at greatest risk for postural hypotension because of perfusion changes associated with aging.*

7 **Nursing Safety Priority: Drug Alert!**

Monitor K^+ levels and assess for irregular pulse and muscle weakness, which may indicate decreased K^+. Patients taking potassium-depleting diuretics should eat foods high in K^+; supplements may be needed. *Helps prevent electrolyte imbalance which can cause cardiac dysrhythmias.*

8 **Complementary and Alternative Therapies**

Help the patient explore complementary and alternative therapies. *Gives the patient alternatives to replace or supplement conventional therapies. Garlic and Q_{10} may prevent/treat hypertension and have short-term lipid-lowering abilities; biofeedback, meditation, and acupuncture may help with continuous and severe stress.*

Concept Map by Deanne A. Blach, MSN, RN

unmatched in preventing the cardiovascular complications of hypertension. The *2014 Evidence-Based Guidelines for the Management of High Blood Pressure in Adults* presented by JNC 8 recommends the use of one or more of these four classes of drugs: thiazide-type diuretics, calcium channel blockers (CCBs), angiotensin-converting enzyme inhibitors (ACEIs), and angiotensin II receptor blockers (ARBs). Patients who do not respond to these first-line drugs may be placed on an aldosterone receptor antagonist (blocker), beta-adrenergic blocker, or renin inhibitor. Examples of commonly used drug classes for hypertension are listed in Chart 36-1. JNC 8 recommendations for pharmacologic management are summarized in Table 36-6.

Diuretics. Diuretics are the first type of drugs for managing hypertension. Three basic types of diuretics are used to decrease blood volume and lower blood pressure in order of how commonly they are typically prescribed:

- Thiazide (low-ceiling) diuretics, such as hydrochlorothiazide (HydroDIURIL, Microzide, Oretic, Urozide ♣), inhibit sodium, chloride, and water reabsorption in the distal tubules while promoting potassium, bicarbonate, and magnesium excretion. However, they decrease calcium excretion, which helps prevent kidney stones and bone loss. Because of the low cost and high effectiveness of thiazide-type diuretics, they are usually the drugs of choice for patients with uncomplicated hypertension. These drugs can be prescribed as a single agent or in combination with other classes of drugs.

! NURSING SAFETY PRIORITY QSEN

Drug Alert

Teach men that they may experience decreased libido (desire for sex) and decreased sexual performance when taking thiazides. Thiazides should be used with caution in patients with diabetes mellitus because they can interfere with serum glucose control. Caution is also indicated for patients with gout or a history of significant hyponatremia (decreased serum sodium level) because these problems can worsen when thiazides are taken.

- Loop (high-ceiling) diuretics, such as furosemide (Lasix, Furoside ♣) and torsemide (Demadex), inhibit sodium, chloride, and water reabsorption in the ascending loop of Henle and promote potassium excretion.

CONSIDERATIONS FOR OLDER ADULTS

***Patient-Centered Care* QSEN**

Loop diuretics are not used commonly for older adults because they can cause dehydration and orthostatic hypotension. These complications increase the patient's risk for falls. Teach families to monitor for and report patient dizziness, falls, or confusion to the health care provider as soon as possible and discontinue the medication.

- Potassium-sparing diuretics, such as spironolactone (Aldactone, Novospiroton ♣), triamterene (Dyrenium), and amiloride (Midamor), act on the distal renal tubule to inhibit reabsorption of sodium ions in exchange for potassium, thereby *retaining* potassium in the body. When used, they are typically in combination with another diuretic or antihypertensive drug to *conserve* potassium.

TABLE 36-6 Selected 2014 Evidence-Based Recommendations for the Management of High Blood Pressure in Adults (JNC 8)

- In the general population ages 60 years and older, start drug therapy to lower blood pressure at systolic blood pressure (SBP) equal to or greater than 150 mm Hg or diastolic blood pressure (DBP) equal to or greater than 90 mm Hg. The goal is to decrease blood pressure (BP) to below 150/90.
- In the general population younger than 60 years, start drug therapy to lower blood pressure at SBP equal to or greater than 140 mm Hg or DBP equal to or greater than 90 mm Hg. The goal is to decrease blood pressure to below 140/90.
- In people ages 18 years and older with chronic kidney disease (CKD), start drug therapy to lower BP to less than 140/90.
- In the general *nonblack* population, including those with diabetes mellitus, initial drug therapy should include a thiazide-type diuretic, calcium channel blocker (CCB), angiotensin-converting enzyme inhibitor (ACEI), or angiotensin receptor blocker (ARB).
- In the general *black* population, including those with diabetes mellitus, initial drug therapy should include a thiazide-type diuretic or CCB.
- If the goal BP is not reached within a month of treatment, increase drug dosage or add a second drug from one of the recommended classes.

Data from James, P.A., Oparil, S., Carter, B.L., Cushman, W.C., Dennison-Himmelfarb, C., Handler, J., et al. (2014). 2014 evidence-based guidelines for the management of high blood pressure in adults: Report from the panel members appointed to the Eighth National Committee (JNC 8). *Journal of the American Medical Association, 311*(5), 507-520. Retrieved December 2013, from http://jama.jamanetwork.com/article.aspx?articleid=1791497.

Frequent voiding caused by any type of diuretic may interfere with daily activities. Teach patients to take their diuretic in the morning rather than at night to prevent nocturia (voiding during the night).

! NURSING SAFETY PRIORITY QSEN

Drug Alert

The most frequent side effect associated with *thiazide and loop diuretics* is hypokalemia (low potassium level). Monitor serum potassium levels, and assess for irregular pulse, dysrhythmias, and muscle weakness, which may indicate hypokalemia. Teach patients taking potassium-depleting diuretics to eat foods high in potassium, such as bananas, potatoes, and orange juice. Most people also need a potassium supplement to maintain adequate serum potassium levels.

Assess for hyperkalemia (high potassium level) for patients taking potassium-sparing diuretics, such as spironolactone. Like hypokalemia, an increased potassium level can also cause weakness, irregular pulse, and cardiac dysrhythmias. In some cases, patients may have painful muscle spasms (cramping) in their legs. These electrolyte imbalances are described in detail in Chapter 11.

Other Antihypertensive Drugs. Calcium channel blockers, such as verapamil hydrochloride (Calan, Nu-Verap ♣) and amlodipine (Norvasc), lower blood pressure by interfering with the transmembrane flux of calcium ions. This results in vasodilation, which *decreases* blood pressure. These drugs also block SA and AV node conduction, resulting in a decreased heart rate. Calcium channel blockers are most effective in older adults and African Americans (Go et al., 2013).

Some calcium channel blockers (CCBs), especially felodipine (Plendil, Renedil ♣) and nifedipine (Adalat, Apo-Nifed ♣), react with grapefruit and grapefruit juice. Grapefruit contains

CHART 36-1 Common Examples of Drug Therapy

Hypertension Management

DRUG/USUAL DOSAGE	PURPOSE/ACTION	NURSING INTERVENTIONS	RATIONALES
Diuretics			
Hydrochlorothiazide (HCTZ) (Microzide, Oretic, Urozide 🍁) 25-100 mg orally daily	Low-ceiling diuretic that inhibits Na^+, Cl^-, and water reabsorption in the distal tubules of the kidney.	Teach patient to eat foods high in K^+ and have follow-up laboratory tests to monitor electrolyte levels.	Drug causes K^+ and Mg^{2+} excretion.
		Teach older adults to rise slowly from chair or bed.	Drug causes diuresis, which can cause orthostatic hypotension.
		Use with caution for patients with diabetes.	Drug can affect glucose control.
		Use with caution for patients with gout.	Drug can cause uric acid retention.
Furosemide (Lasix, Furoside 🍁) 40-600 mg orally daily	High-ceiling diuretic that inhibits Na^+, Cl^-, and water reabsorption in the kidney's loop of Henle.	Report to the health care provider weakness or dizziness or new-onset confusion.	Drug can cause hypovolemia, dehydration, and hypokalemia.
		Same as for HCTZ, except safer to give to patients with diabetes and gout.	Same as for HCTZ.
Spironolactone (Aldactone, Novo-Spiroton 🍁) 50-400 mg orally daily	Acts on distal tubules of kidneys to inhibit reabsorption of Na^+ in exchange for K^+.	Teach patients to *decrease* intake of foods high in potassium and have follow-up laboratory tests for electrolyte levels.	Drug causes K^+ retention in the body.
		Teach patients to report weakness and irregular pulse to health care provider.	These symptoms may indicate hyperkalemia.
Calcium Channel Blockers			
Verapamil (Calan, Nu-Verap 🍁) Up to 480 mg orally in 3 divided doses; *Extended-release* form (ER) also available as 240-480 mg orally daily	Interferes with flux of calcium ions to cause vasodilation, which lowers blood pressure (BP).	Monitor pulse and blood pressure before taking each day; do not take without contacting health care provider if pulse is less than 60 or systolic BP is below 100 mm Hg.	Drug slows SA and AV conduction in the heart, thus decreases heart rate; vasodilation causes decreased blood pressure.
		Teach patients and their families that patients should avoid grapefruit juice and grapefruits when taking calcium channel blockers.	Grapefruit and its juice can enhance the action of the drug causing organ dysfunction or death.
Amlodipine (Norvasc) 5-10 mg orally daily	Same as above for verapamil.	Same as above for verapamil, but safe to drink grapefruit juice.	Same as above for verapamil, but safe to drink grapefruit juice.
Angiotensin-Converting Enzyme (ACE) Inhibitors			
Lisinopril (Prinivil, Zestril) 10-80 mg orally daily	Blocks action of ACE in converting angiotensin I to angiotensin II (vasoconstrictor).	Report nagging cough to health care provider.	Cough is a common and annoying side effect, and drug should be discontinued if it occurs.
		Monitor blood pressure carefully, especially orthostatic checks; remind patients to move slowly from sitting to standing to prevent dizziness and possible falls. Do not give drug without checking with health care provider if systolic blood pressure is below 100.	Drug prevents vasoconstriction by angiotensin II, resulting in vasodilation and decreased blood pressure.
Enalapril (Vasotec) 10-40 mg orally daily or in divided doses; also available in IV form	Same as above for lisinopril.	Monitor blood pressure as described above for lisinopril.	Same as above for lisinopril.
Angiotensin II Receptor Blockers (ARBs)			
Valsartan (Diovan) 80-320 mg orally daily	Blocks binding of angiotensin II to receptor sites in vascular smooth muscle and adrenal glands.	Teach patients to avoid foods high in potassium.	ARBs can cause hyperkalemia, especially when combined with other antihypertensive drugs.
		Monitor blood pressures to ensure that hypotension does not occur. Do not take drug without checking with a health care provider if systolic BP is below 100.	Vasodilation causes decreased blood pressure.
Losartan (Cozaar) 25-100 mg orally daily or in divided doses twice a day	Same as above for valsartan.	Same as above for valsartan.	Same as above for valsartan.

Continued

CHART 36-1 **Common Examples of Drug Therapy—cont'd**

Hypertension Management

DRUG/USUAL DOSAGE	PURPOSE/ACTION	NURSING INTERVENTIONS	RATIONALES
Aldosterone Receptor Antagonists			
Eplerenone (Inspra) 25-50 mg orally daily	Blocks aldosterone binding at receptor sites in kidney, heart, blood vessels, and brain to inhibit sodium reabsorption by the kidneys.	Teach patients to follow up with laboratory tests as scheduled; decrease intake of high-potassium foods.	Drug can cause increases in K^+ and triglycerides and a decreased Na^+.
		Avoid taking the drug with grapefruit, grapefruit juice, and St. John's wort.	Grapefruit, grapefruit juice, and St. John's wort increase the risk for adverse drug events (including death) when taking eplerenone due to enhancing the drug's action.
		Avoid taking the drug with itraconazole (Sporanox) and ketoconazole (Nizoral).	These drugs interact with eplerenone.
		Check with the pharmacist about interactions with other drugs or herbs that the patient is taking.	Drug interacts with many other drugs and herbs and is either not prescribed or drug dosage is adjusted.
Beta-Adrenergic Blockers			
Metoprolol (Toprol, Toprol XL, Lopressor, Betaloc 🍁) 100-400 mg orally daily or in divided doses (one dose daily for XL form)	Cardioselective drugs block $beta_1$ receptors in the heart and peripheral blood vessels.	Monitor carefully for orthostatic hypotension; teach patients to rise slowly from the sitting position to prevent dizziness; do not take drug without contacting the health care provider if systolic BP is below 100.	Orthostatic hypotension is a common adverse effect of the drug and can contribute to falls and confusion, especially in older adults.
		Monitor pulse rate every day; do not take drug without contacting the health care provider if pulse is below 60.	The $beta_1$-blocking action of the drug decreases the rate, contractility, and output of the heart.
		Teach the patient that the drug can cause fatigue, depression, and sexual dysfunction; report any of these problems to the health care provider.	The drug has many side and adverse effects because of its potent action.
		Use the drug with caution in patients who are diabetic.	Because of the sympathetic blocking action of the drug, glucose production may be affected.
Atenolol (Tenormin, Apo-Atenol 🍁) 50-100 mg orally daily	Same as above for metoprolol.	Same as above for metoprolol.	Same as above for metoprolol.
Renin Inhibitors			
Aliskiren (Tekturna) 150-300 mg orally daily	Inhibits renin production, which prevents conversion of angiotensinogen to angiotensin I; decreased vasoconstriction, peripheral resistance, and cardiac output result.	Teach patients that side effects (cough and diarrhea) are not common; in a few cases, respiratory distress has occurred.	Drug is relatively safe with few side effects.

AV, Atrioventricular; **SA**, sinoatrial.

a group of chemicals called *furanocoumarins* that bind to and inactivate the enzyme *CYP3A4*. This enzyme is important for metabolism of many drugs, including some CCBs. If it is inactivated, too much of the CCB drug can remain in the patient's bloodstream causing possible kidney failure, heart failure, GI bleeding, or even death (Bailey et al., 2013).

A newer CCB, clevidipine butyrate (Cleviprex), is available only in IV form and must be administered using an infusion pump. This drug is indicated when oral therapy is not possible and is most often used for hypertensive urgency or severe hypertension. The most common side effects are headache and nausea. Monitor the patient's blood pressure frequently to check for hypotension. A dosage increase of 1 to 2 mg/hr generally produces an additional 2- to 4-mm Hg decrease in systolic blood pressure (Lilley et al., 2014).

Angiotensin-converting enzyme inhibitors (ACE inhibitors or ACEIs), known as the "pril" drugs, are also used as single or combination agents in the treatment of hypertension. These drugs block the action of the angiotensin-converting enzyme as it attempts to convert angiotensin I to angiotensin II, one of the most powerful vasoconstrictors in the body. This action also decreases sodium and water retention and lowers peripheral vascular resistance, both of which lower blood pressure. ACE inhibitors include captopril (Capoten), lisinopril (Prinivil,

Zestril), and enalapril (Vasotec). *The most common side effect of this group of drugs is a nagging, dry cough.* Teach patients to report this problem to their health care provider as soon as possible. If a cough develops, the drug is discontinued.

! NURSING SAFETY PRIORITY (QSEN)

Drug Alert

Instruct the patient receiving an ACE inhibitor for the first time to get out of bed slowly to avoid the severe hypotensive effect that can occur with initial use. Orthostatic hypotension may occur with subsequent doses, but it is usually less severe. If dizziness continues or there is a significant decrease in the systolic blood pressure (more than a change of 20 mm Hg), notify the health care provider or teach the patient to notify his or her provider. *The older patient is at the greatest risk for postural hypotension because of the cardiovascular changes associated with aging.*

Angiotensin II receptor antagonists, also called *angiotensin II receptor blockers (ARBs)* or the *-sartan drugs,* make up a group of drugs that selectively block the binding of angiotensin II to receptor sites in the vascular smooth muscle and adrenal tissues by competing directly with angiotensin II but not inhibiting ACE. Examples of drugs in this group are candesartan (Atacand), valsartan (Diovan), losartan (Cozaar), and azilsartan (Edarbi). ARBs can be used alone or in combination with other antihypertensive drugs. These drugs are excellent options for patients who report a nagging cough associated with ACE inhibitors. In addition, these drugs do not require initial adjustment of the dose for older adults or for any patient with renal impairment. Like the ACEs, the ARBs are not as effective in African Americans unless these drugs are taken with diuretics or another category such as a beta blocker or calcium channel blocker (Go et al., 2013).

Aldosterone receptor antagonists block the hypertensive effect of the mineralocorticoid hormone *aldosterone.* Aldosterone increases sodium reabsorption by the kidney and is a significant contributor to hypertension, cardiac and vascular remodeling, and heart failure. Eplerenone (Inspra) lowers blood pressure by blocking aldosterone binding at the mineralocorticoid receptor sites in the kidney, heart, blood vessels, and brain. Generally well tolerated, eplerenone has dose-related adverse effects of hypertriglyceridemia, hyponatremia, and hyperkalemia. Teach patients taking eplerenone to avoid grapefruit or grapefruit juice in their diet to prevent severe complications, including death. Using ACE inhibitors or ARBs at the same time increases the risk for hyperkalemia. Therefore monitor potassium levels carefully, initially every 2 weeks for the first few months and then monthly thereafter.

! NURSING SAFETY PRIORITY (QSEN)

Drug Alert

When taking eplerenone, itraconazole (Sporanox) and ketoconazole (Nizoral) should not be taken. Drug interactions are common. Patients taking erythromycin, fluconazole (Diflucan), saquinavir (Fortovase), and verapamil (Calan) can take eplerenone but with a reduction in dosage by half to 25 mg daily. Teach patients that grapefruit juice and the popular herb *St. John's wort* can also increase the chance of adverse effects. Similar to all antihypertensives, remind patients not to get up quickly, drive, or climb stairs until they adjust to the effects of the drug.

Beta-adrenergic blockers, identified by the ending -olol, are categorized as cardioselective (working only on the cardiovascular system) and non-cardioselective. Cardioselective beta blockers, affecting only beta$_1$ receptors, may be prescribed to lower blood pressure by blocking beta receptors in the heart and peripheral vessels. By blocking these receptors, the drugs decrease heart rate and myocardial contractility. Teach patients about common side effects of beta blockers, including fatigue, weakness, depression, and sexual dysfunction. The potential for side effects depends on the "selective" blocking effects of the drug. Atenolol (Tenormin, Apo-Atenol ♣), bisoprolol (Zebeta), and metoprolol (Lopressor, Toprol, Toprol-XL, Betaloc ♣) are cardioselective beta blockers given for hypertension.

Patients with diabetes who take beta blockers may not have the usual manifestations of hypoglycemia because the sympathetic nervous system is blocked. The body's responses to hypoglycemia such as gluconeogenesis may also be inhibited by certain beta blockers.

Beta blockers are often the drug of choice for hypertensive patients with ischemic heart disease (IHD) because the heart is the most common target of end-organ damage with hypertension. If this drug is not tolerated, a long-acting calcium channel blocker can be used. In patients with unstable angina or myocardial infarction (MI), beta blockers or calcium channel blockers should be used initially in combination with ACE inhibitors or ARBs, with addition of other drugs if needed to control the blood pressure (see Chapter 38).

Renin inhibitors are effective for mild to moderate hypertension. Aliskiren (Tekturna) is an example and can be used alone or with a thiazide diuretic. Renin is an enzyme produced in the kidneys that causes vasoconstriction, increases peripheral resistance, and increases cardiac output. The result is an increase in blood pressure. Renin inhibitors prevent renin from producing this action. Side effects are minimal and not common, although respiratory distress may occur.

? NCLEX EXAMINATION CHALLENGE

Physiological Integrity

A client is prescribed enalapril (Vasotec) for control of hypertension. What health teaching will the nurse provide before the client begins therapy?

A. "You may develop a higher pulse rate."
B. "You may notice some swelling in your feet."
C. "You may develop a nagging cough."
D. "Your diet should include foods high in sodium."

Promoting Adherence to the Plan of Care

Planning: Expected Outcomes. The patient with hypertension is expected to adhere to the plan of care, including making necessary lifestyle changes.

Interventions. Patients who require medications to control essential hypertension usually need to take them for the rest of their lives. Some patients stop taking them because they have no symptoms and have troublesome side effects.

In the hospital setting, collaborate with the pharmacist, as needed, to discuss the outcomes of therapy with the patient, including potential side effects. Assist the patient in tailoring the therapeutic regimen to his or her lifestyle and daily schedule.

Patients who do not adhere to antihypertensive treatment are at a high risk for target organ damage and **hypertensive**

CHART 36-2 Best Practice for Patient Safety & Quality Care QSEN

Emergency Care of Patients with Hypertensive Urgency or Crisis

Assess

- Severe headache
- Extremely high blood pressure (BP)
- Dizziness
- Blurred vision
- Shortness of breath
- Epistaxis (nosebleed)
- Severe anxiety

Intervene

- Place patient in a semi-Fowler's position.
- Administer oxygen.
- Start IV of 0.9% normal saline (NS) solution slowly to prevent fluid overload (which would increase blood pressure).
- Administer IV beta blocker or nicardipine (Cardene IV) or other infusion drug as prescribed; when stable, switch to oral antihypertensive drug.
- Monitor BP every 5 to 15 minutes until the diastolic pressure is below 90 and not less than 75; then monitor BP every 30 minutes to ensure that BP is not lowered too quickly.
- Observe for neurologic or cardiovascular complications, such as seizures; numbness, weakness, or tingling of extremities; dysrhythmias; or chest pain (possible indicators of target organ damage).

crisis, a severe elevation in blood pressure (greater than 180/120), which can cause organ damage in the kidneys or heart (target organs) (Chart 36-2). Patients in hypertensive crisis are admitted to critical care units, where they receive IV antihypertensive therapy such as nitroprusside (Nipride), nicardipine (Cardene IV), fenoldopam (Corlopam), or labetalol (Normodyne). These drugs act quickly as vasodilators to decrease blood pressure (BP) by no more that 25% within 2 to 6 hours. Provide oxygen to the patient, and monitor oxygen saturation levels. When the patient's blood pressure stabilizes, oral antihypertensive drugs are given (Day, 2011).

Community-Based Care

Home Care Management. Hypertension is a chronic illness. Allow patients to verbalize feelings about the disease and its treatment. Emphasize that their involvement in the collaborative plan of care can lead to control of the disease and can prevent complications.

Some patients do not adhere to their drug therapy regimen at home because they have no symptoms or they simply forget to take their drugs. Others may think they are not sick enough to need medication. Some patients may assume that once their blood pressure returns to normal levels, they no longer need treatment. They may also stop taking their drugs because of side effects or cost. Develop a plan with the patient and family, and identify ways to encourage adherence to the plan of care.

Self-Management Education. Health teaching is essential to help patients become successful in managing their blood pressure. Provide oral and written information about the indications, dosage, times for administration, side effects, and drug interactions for antihypertensives. Stress that medication must be taken as prescribed; when all of it has been consumed, the prescription must be renewed on a continual basis. Suddenly stopping drugs such as beta blockers can result in angina (chest pain), myocardial infarction (MI), or rebound hypertension. Urge patients to report unpleasant side effects such as excessive fatigue, cough, or sexual dysfunction. In many instances, an alternative drug can be prescribed to minimize certain side effects.

Teach the patient to obtain an ambulatory blood pressure monitoring (ABPM) device for use at home so that the pressure can be checked. Evaluate the patient's and family's ability to use this device. If weight reduction is a desired outcome, suggest having a scale in the home for weight monitoring. For patients who do not want to self-monitor, are not able to self-monitor, or have "white-coat" syndrome when they go to their health care provider (causing elevated BP), continuous ABPM may be used. The monitor is worn for 24 hours or longer while patients perform their normal daily activities. Blood pressure is automatically taken every 15 to 30 minutes and recorded for review later. The advantage of this technique is that the health care provider can view the changes in BP readings throughout the 24-hour period to get a picture of a true BP value. Research strongly supports 24-hour ambulatory blood pressure monitoring as a first-line procedure to determine the need for antihypertensive therapy (Verdecchia et al., 2009).

Instruct the patient about sodium restriction, weight maintenance or reduction, alcohol restriction, stress management, and exercise. If necessary, also explain about the need to stop using tobacco, especially smoking.

Health Care Resources. A home care nurse may be needed for follow-up to monitor the blood pressure. Evaluate the patient's or family's ability to obtain accurate BP measurements, and assess adherence with treatment. The American Heart Association (www.aha.org), the Red Cross, or a local pharmacy may be used for free blood pressure checks if patients cannot buy equipment to monitor their blood pressure. Health fairs are also available in most locations.

◆ *Evaluation: Outcomes*

Evaluate the care of the patient with hypertension on the basis of the identified patient problems. The expected outcomes are that the patient will:

- Verbalize understanding of the plan of care, including drug therapy and any necessary lifestyle changes
- Report adverse drug effects, such as coughing, dizziness, or sexual dysfunction, to the health care provider immediately
- Consistently adhere to the plan of care, including regular follow-up health care provider visits

PERIPHERAL ARTERIAL DISEASE

Peripheral vascular disease (PVD) includes disorders that change the natural flow of blood through the arteries and veins of the peripheral circulation, causing decreased PERFUSION to body tissues. It affects the legs much more frequently than the arms. Generally, a diagnosis of PVD implies arterial disease (peripheral arterial disease [PAD]) rather than venous involvement. Some patients have both arterial and venous disease. The cost of the disease is very high and is expected to increase as baby boomers age and obesity in the United States continues to be a major health problem.

❖ *PATHOPHYSIOLOGY*

PAD is a result of systemic atherosclerosis. It is a chronic condition in which partial or total arterial occlusion (blockage)

CLINICAL JUDGMENT CHALLENGE

Patient-Centered Care; Teamwork and Collaboration; Evidence-Based Practice QSEN

A nursing home administrator reports having severe headache and facial flushing for the past 3 weeks. He does not smoke but is overweight. Both of his parents have hypertension and cardiac disease. One of his nurses takes his blood pressure, which is 210/116. He states that he will see his primary care provider as soon as possible. At the physician's office, his heart rate is 88 beats/min, blood pressure is 190/110, and respiratory rate is 24 breaths/min.

1. What additional information will you need from his past and current family and personal history?
2. What physical assessment data will you collect as the office nurse?
3. What type of drug therapy may be prescribed for this patient? What are your nursing responsibilities when giving these drugs?
4. What health teaching will you provide for the patient? What evidence do you have to support your answer?
5. What members of the health care team may be involved in this patient's care?
6. What community resources are available to assist this patient to self-manage his hypertension?

decreases PERFUSION to the extremities. The tissues below the narrowed or obstructed arteries cannot live without an adequate *oxygen* and nutrient supply. PAD in the legs is sometimes referred to as *lower extremity arterial disease (LEAD).*

Obstructions are classified as inflow or outflow, according to the arteries involved and their relationship to the inguinal ligament (Fig. 36-3). *Inflow* obstructions involve the distal end of the aorta and the common, internal, and external iliac arteries. They are located above the inguinal ligament. *Outflow* obstructions involve the femoral, popliteal, and tibial arteries and are below the superficial femoral artery (SFA). Gradual inflow occlusions may not cause significant tissue damage. Gradual outflow occlusions typically do.

Atherosclerosis is the most common cause of chronic arterial obstruction; therefore the risk factors for atherosclerosis apply to PAD as well. Common risk factors include hypertension, hyperlipidemia, diabetes mellitus, cigarette smoking, obesity, high cholesterol and lipid levels, and familial predisposition. Advancing age also increases the risk for disease related to atherosclerosis. Patients with PAD have an increased risk for developing chronic angina, MI, or stroke and are much more likely to die within 10 years compared with those who do not have the disease (Go et al., 2013).

About 10 to 12 million people in the United States have PAD, most of them older than 65 years. African Americans are affected more often than any other group, most likely because they have many risk factors such as diabetes and hypertension (Go et al., 2013).

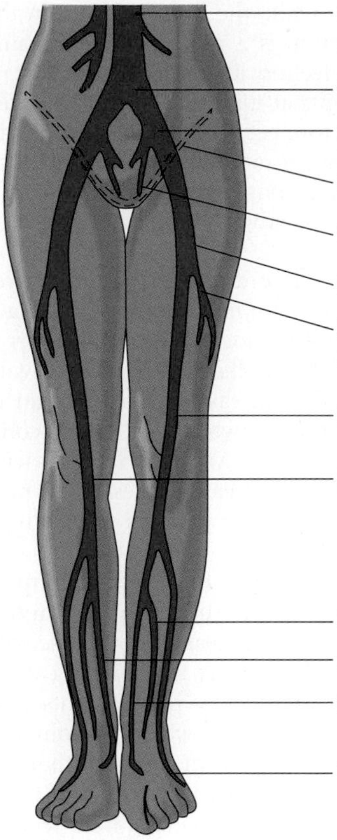

FIG. 36-3 Common locations of inflow and outflow lesions.

CHART 36-3 Key Features

Chronic Peripheral Arterial Disease

Stage I: Asymptomatic
- No claudication is present.
- Bruit or aneurysm may be present.
- Pedal pulses are decreased or absent.

Stage II: Claudication
- Muscle pain, cramping, or burning occurs with exercise and is relieved with rest.
- Symptoms are reproducible with exercise.

Stage III: Rest Pain
- Pain while resting commonly awakens the patient at night.
- Pain is described as numbness, burning, toothache-type pain.
- Pain usually occurs in the distal portion of the extremity (toes, arch, forefoot, or heel), rarely in the calf or the ankle.
- Pain is relieved by placing the extremity in a dependent position.

Stage IV: Necrosis/Gangrene
- Ulcers and blackened tissue occur on the toes, the forefoot, and the heel.
- Distinctive gangrenous odor is present.

❖ PATIENT-CENTERED COLLABORATIVE CARE

◆ Assessment

The clinical course of chronic PAD can be divided into four stages (Chart 36-3). Patients do not experience symptoms in the early stages of disease. Most patients are not diagnosed until they develop leg pain.

Physical Assessment/Clinical Manifestations. Most patients initially seek medical attention for a classic leg pain known as **intermittent claudication** (a term derived from a word meaning "to limp"). Usually they can walk only a certain distance before a cramping, burning muscle discomfort or PAIN forces them to stop. The pain stops after rest. When patients resume walking, they can walk the same distance before it returns. Thus the pain is considered reproducible. As the disease progresses, they can walk only shorter and shorter distances before pain recurs. Ultimately, it may occur even while at rest.

Rest pain, which may begin while the disease is still in the stage of intermittent claudication, is a numbness or burning sensation, often described as feeling like a toothache that is severe enough to awaken patients at night. It is usually located in the toes, the foot arches, the forefeet, the heels, and, rarely, in the calves or ankles. Patients can sometimes get PAIN relief by keeping the limb in a dependent position (below the heart). Those with rest pain often have advanced disease that may result in limb loss.

Patients with **inflow disease** have discomfort in the lower back, buttocks, or thighs. Patients with *mild* inflow disease have discomfort after walking about two blocks. This discomfort is not severe but causes them to stop walking. It is relieved with rest. Patients with *moderate* inflow disease experience pain in these areas after walking about one or two blocks. The discomfort is described as being more like PAIN, but it eases with rest most of the time. *Severe* inflow disease causes severe pain after walking less than one block. These patients usually have rest pain.

Patients with **outflow disease** describe burning or cramping in the calves, ankles, feet, and toes. Instep or foot discomfort indicates an obstruction below the popliteal artery. Those with *mild* outflow disease experience discomfort after walking about five blocks. This discomfort is relieved by rest. Patients with *moderate* outflow disease have pain after walking about two blocks. Intermittent rest pain may be present. Those with *severe* outflow disease usually cannot walk more than one-half block and usually experience rest PAIN. They may hang their feet off the bed at night for comfort and report more frequent rest pain than do those with inflow disease.

Specific findings for PAD depend on the severity of the disease. Observe for loss of hair on the lower calf, ankle, and foot; dry, scaly, dusky, pale, or mottled skin; and thickened toenails. With severe arterial disease, the extremity is cold and gray-blue (cyanotic) or darkened. Pallor may occur when the extremity is elevated. Dependent **rubor** (redness) may occur when the extremity is lowered (Fig. 36-4). Muscle atrophy can result from prolonged chronic arterial disease.

CULTURAL CONSIDERATIONS

Patient-Centered Care QSEN

Only severe cyanosis is evident in the skin of dark-skinned patients. To detect cyanosis, assess the skin and nail beds for a dull, lifeless color. The soles of the feet and the toenails are less pigmented and allow detection of cyanosis or duskiness in the lower extremities.

Palpate all pulses in both legs. The most sensitive and specific indicator of arterial function is the quality of the posterior tibial pulse, because the pedal pulse is not palpable in a small percentage of people. The strength of each pulse should be compared bilaterally.

Note early signs of ulcer formation or complete ulcer formation, a complication of PAD. Arterial and venous stasis ulcers differ from diabetic ulcers (Chart 36-4). Initially, **arterial ulcers** are painful and develop on the toes (often the great toe), between the toes, or on the upper aspect of the foot. With prolonged occlusion, the toes can become gangrenous. Typically, the ulcer is small and round with a "punched out" appearance and well-defined borders. Skin lesions are discussed in further detail in Chapter 25.

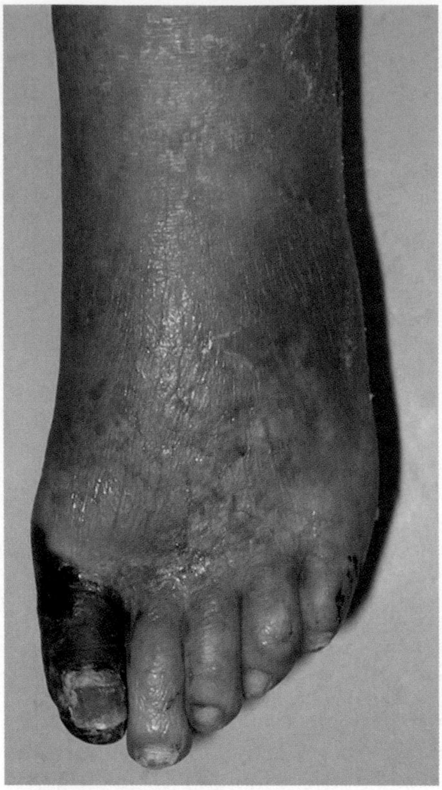

FIG. 36-4 Dependent rubor in the left leg of a patient with peripheral arterial disease.

Imaging Assessment. *Magnetic resonance angiography (MRA)* is commonly used to assess blood flow in the peripheral arteries. A contrast medium such as gadolinium is used to help visualize blood flow through peripheral arteries. This test is often the only one used to diagnose PAD, although a computed tomography angiography (CTA) may also be performed.

Other Diagnostic Assessment. Using a Doppler probe, *segmental systolic blood pressure measurements* of the lower extremities at the thigh, calf, and ankle are an inexpensive, noninvasive method of assessing PAD. Normally, blood pressure readings in the thigh and calf are higher than those in the upper extremities. With the presence of arterial disease, these pressures are lower than the brachial pressure.

With *inflow* disease, pressures taken at the thigh level indicate the severity of disease. Mild inflow disease may cause a difference of only 10 to 30 mm Hg in pressure on the affected side compared with the brachial pressure. Severe inflow disease can cause a pressure difference of more than 40 to 50 mm Hg. The ankle pressure is normally equal to or more than the brachial pressure.

To evaluate *outflow* disease, compare ankle pressure with the brachial pressure, which provides a ratio known as the **ankle-brachial index (ABI)**. The value can be derived by dividing the ankle blood pressure by the brachial blood pressure. *An ABI of less than 0.90 in either leg is diagnostic of PAD. Patients with diabetes are known to have a falsely elevated ABI.*

Doppler-derived maximal systolic acceleration is a newer technique that has demonstrated successful evaluations of peripheral arterial disease in patients with diabetes (Van Tongeren et al., 2010).

Exercise tolerance testing (by chemical stress test or treadmill) may give valuable information about claudication (muscle

CHART 36-4 Key Features

Lower Extremity Ulcers

FEATURE	ARTERIAL ULCERS	VENOUS ULCERS	DIABETIC ULCERS
History	Patient reports claudication after walking about 1-2 blocks Rest pain usually present Pain at ulcer site Two or three risk factors present	Chronic nonhealing ulcer No claudication or rest pain Moderate ulcer discomfort Patient reports of ankle or leg swelling	Diabetes Peripheral neuropathy No reports of claudication
Ulcer location and appearance	End of the toes Between the toes Deep Ulcer bed pale, with even edges Little granulation tissue 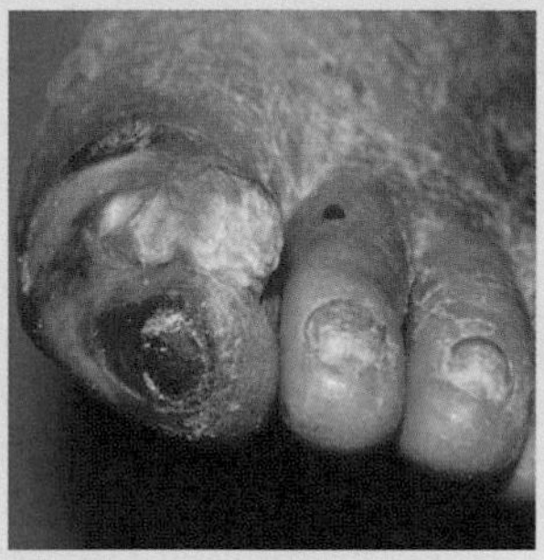	Ankle area Brown pigmentation Ulcer bed pink Usually superficial, with uneven edges Granulation tissue present 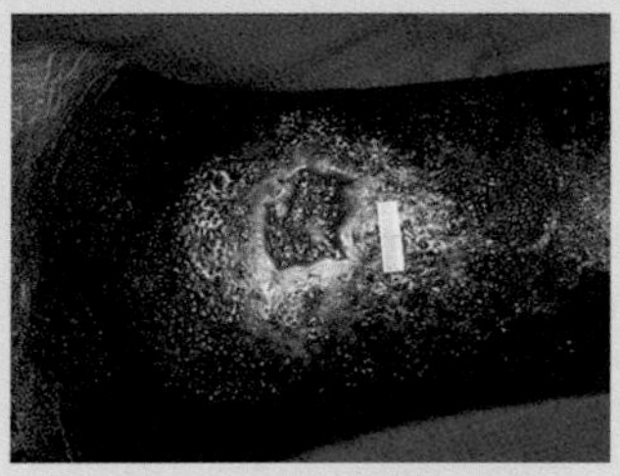	Plantar area of foot Metatarsal heads Pressure points on feet Deep Pale, with even edges Little granulation tissue 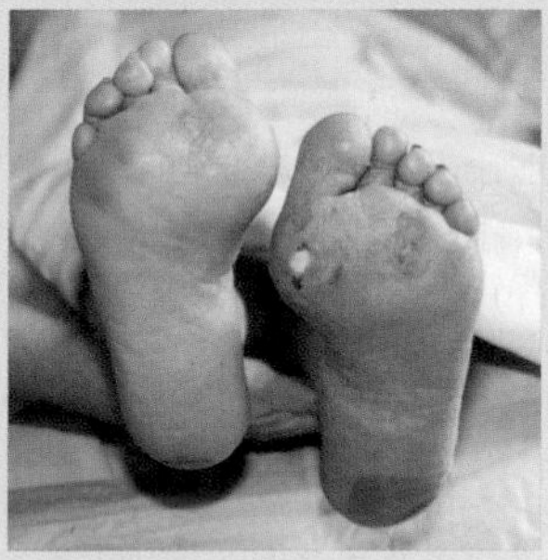
Other assessment findings	Cool or cold foot Decreased or absent pulses Atrophy of skin Hair loss Pallor with elevation Dependent rubor Possible gangrene When acute, neurologic deficits noted	Ankle discoloration and edema Full veins when leg slightly dependent No neurologic deficit Pulses present May have scarring from previous ulcers	Pulses usually present Cool or warm foot Painless
Treatment	Treat underlying cause (surgical, revascularization) Prevent trauma and infection Patient education, stressing foot care	Long-term wound care (Unna boot, damp-to-dry dressings) Elevate extremity Patient education Prevent infection	Rule out major arterial disease Control diabetes Patient education regarding foot care Prevent infection

Photograph of arterial ulcer from Bonow, R.O., Mann, D.L., Zipes, D.P., & Libby, P. (2011). *Braunwald's heart disease: A textbook of cardiovascular medicine* (9th ed.). Philadelphia: Saunders. Photograph of venous ulcer from Bryant, R., & Nix, D. (2012). *Acute and chronic wounds: Current management concepts* (4th ed.). Philadelphia: Saunders. Photograph of diabetic ulcer from Bryant, R., & Nix, D. (2007). *Acute and chronic wounds: Current management concepts* (3rd ed.). Philadelphia: Saunders.

pain) without rest PAIN. The technician obtains resting pulse volume recordings and asks the patient to walk on a treadmill until the symptoms are reproduced. At the time of symptom onset or after about 5 minutes, the technician obtains another pulse volume recording. Normally, there may be an increased waveform with minimal, if any, drop in the ankle pressure. In patients with arterial disease, the waveforms are decreased (dampened) and there is a decrease in the ankle pressure of 40 to 60 mm Hg for 20 to 30 seconds in the affected limb. If the return to normal pressure is delayed (longer than 10 minutes), the results suggest abnormal arterial flow in the affected limb.

Plethysmography can also be performed to evaluate arterial flow in the lower extremities. The measurement provides graphs or tracings of arterial flow in the limb. If an occlusion is present, the waveforms are decreased to flattened, depending on the degree of occlusion.

◆ *Interventions*

Collaborative management of PAD may include nonsurgical interventions and/or surgery. The patient must first be assessed to determine if the altered tissue PERFUSION is due to arterial disease, venous disease, or both.

Nonsurgical Management. Exercise, positioning, promoting vasodilation, drug therapy, and invasive nonsurgical procedures are used to increase *arterial* flow to the affected leg(s).

Using Exercise and Positioning. *Exercise* may improve arterial blood flow to the affected leg through buildup of the collateral circulation. **Collateral circulation** provides blood to the affected area through smaller vessels that develop and compensate for the occluded vessels. Exercise is individualized for each patient, but people with severe rest pain, venous ulcers, or gangrene should not participate. Others with PAD can benefit from exercise that is started gradually and slowly increased. Instruct the patient to walk until the point of claudication, stop and rest, and then walk a little farther. Eventually, he or she can walk longer distances as collateral circulation develops. Collaborate with the health care provider and physical therapist in determining an appropriate exercise program. Exercise rehabilitation has been used to relieve symptoms but requires a motivated patient. Supervised sessions are generally not reimbursed by health care insurance.

Positioning to promote circulation has been somewhat controversial. Some patients have swelling in their extremities. Teach them to avoid raising their legs above the heart level because extreme elevation slows arterial blood flow to the feet. In severe cases, patients with PAD and swelling may sleep with the affected leg hanging from the bed or sit upright in a chair for comfort.

! NURSING SAFETY PRIORITY (QSEN)

Action Alert

Instruct all patients with the disease to avoid crossing their legs and avoid wearing restrictive clothing (e.g., garters to hold up nylon stockings, particularly common among older women), which interfere with blood flow. Teach them the importance of inspecting their feet daily for color or other changes.

Promoting Vasodilation. Vasodilation can be achieved by providing warmth to the affected extremity and preventing long periods of exposure to cold. Encourage the patient to maintain a warm environment at home and to wear socks or insulated shoes at all times. *Caution him or her to never apply direct heat to the limb such as with the use of heating pads or extremely hot water. Sensitivity is decreased in the affected limb. Burns may result.*

Encourage patients to prevent exposure of the affected limb to the cold because cold temperatures cause vasoconstriction (decreasing of the diameter of the blood vessels) and therefore decrease arterial PERFUSION. Patients should also drink adequate fluids to prevent increased blood viscosity.

Emotional stress, caffeine, and nicotine also can cause vasoconstriction. *Emphasize that complete abstinence from smoking or chewing tobacco is essential to prevent vasoconstriction.* The vasoconstrictive effects of each cigarette may last up to 1 hour after the cigarette is smoked.

? NCLEX EXAMINATION CHALLENGE

Physiological Integrity

The nurse is caring for a client with lower extremity peripheral arterial disease. Which statement made by the client regarding self-management requires further health teaching?

A. "I need to quit smoking as soon as I can."
B. "I will elevate my legs above the level of my heart."
C. "I will use a heating pad to promote circulation."
D. "I will avoid crossing my legs at all times."

Drug Therapy. For patients with chronic PAD, prescribed drugs include hemorheologic and antiplatelet agents. Pentoxifylline (Trental) is a hemorheologic agent that increases the flexibility of red blood cells. It decreases blood viscosity by inhibiting platelet aggregation and decreasing fibrinogen and thus increases blood flow in the extremities. Many patients report limited improvement in their daily lives after taking pentoxifylline. However, those with extremely limited endurance for walking have reported improvement to the point that they can perform some activities (e.g., walk to the mailbox or dining room) that were previously impossible.

Antiplatelet agents, such as aspirin (acetylsalicylic acid, Ancasal 🍁) and clopidogrel (Plavix), are commonly used. Aspirin 325 or 81 mg daily may be recommended for patients with chronic PAD. However, clopidogrel is better than aspirin for reducing the risk for myocardial infarction (MI), ischemic stroke, and vascular death. Patients with PAD and no contraindications to antiplatelet therapy should receive either aspirin or clopidogrel. Some patients receive both drugs (dual antiplatelet therapy).

Remind patients not to eat grapefruit or drink grapefruit juice while on clopidogrel. Grapefruit contains a group of chemicals called *furanocoumarins* that bind to and inactivate the enzyme *CYP3A4*. This enzyme is important for metabolism of many drugs, including clopidogrel. If it is inactivated, too much of the drug can remain in the patient's bloodstream causing possible kidney failure, heart failure, GI bleeding, or even death (Bailey et al., 2013).

Patients who experience disabling intermittent claudication may also benefit from phosphodiesterase inhibitors such as cilostazol (Pletal). This drug can also increase HDL-C levels. Teach patients taking the drug that it may cause headaches and GI disturbances, especially flatulence (gas) and diarrhea.

Controlling hypertension can improve tissue PERFUSION by maintaining pressures that are adequate to perfuse the periphery but not constrict the vessels. Teach about the effect of blood pressure on the circulation, and instruct in methods of control. For example, patients taking beta blockers may have drug-related claudication or a worsening of symptoms. The health care provider closely monitors those who are receiving beta blockers. If the patient has high serum lipids, lipid-lowering drugs such as statins are used (see earlier discussion of statins under Drug Therapy for Atherosclerosis, p. 712).

Invasive Nonsurgical Procedures. A nonsurgical but invasive approach for improving arterial flow is the use of **percutaneous vascular intervention,** also called **percutaneous transluminal coronary angioplasty (PTCA).** This procedure requires an arterial puncture in the patient's groin. One or more arteries are dilated with a balloon catheter advanced through a cannula, which is inserted into or above an occluded or stenosed artery. When the procedure is successful, it opens the vessel and improves arterial blood flow. Patients who are candidates for percutaneous procedures such as PTA must have occlusions or stenoses that are accessible to the catheter. Reocclusion may occur, and the procedure may be repeated. Some patients are occlusion-free for up to 3 to 5 years, whereas others may experience reocclusion within a year.

During percutaneous vascular intervention, intravascular stents (wire meshlike devices) are usually inserted to ensure adequate blood flow in a stenosed vessel. Candidates for stents are patients with stenosis of the common or external iliac arteries. Stents are also available to effectively treat superficial femoral artery disease. Patients have these procedures in same-day surgery or ambulatory care centers.

Another arterial technique to improve blood flow to ischemic legs in people with PAD is mechanical rotational abrasive **atherectomy.** The Rotablator device is designed to scrape plaque from inside the artery while minimizing damage to the vessel surface.

! NURSING SAFETY PRIORITY (QSEN)

Critical Rescue

The priority for nursing care following a PTA or atherectomy is to observe for bleeding at the arterial puncture site, which is sealed with a special collagen plug. Monitor for manifestations of impending hypovolemic shock, including a decrease in blood pressure, increased pulse rate, and decreased urinary output. Perform frequent checks of the distal pulses in both legs to ensure adequate PERFUSION and oxygenation.

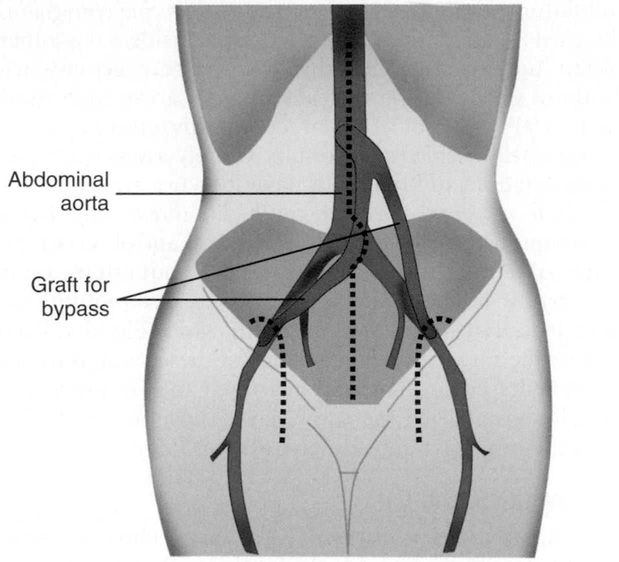

FIG. 36-5 In aortoiliac and aortofemoral bypass surgery, a midline incision into the abdominal cavity is required, with an additional incision in each groin.

Most patients receive anticoagulant or antiplatelet therapy, such as heparin or clopidogrel (Plavix), before and/or during the procedure. An antiplatelet drug may also be prescribed for 1 to 3 months or longer after the procedure to prevent arterial clotting.

Surgical Management. Patients with severe rest pain or claudication that interferes with the ability to work or threatens loss of a limb become surgical candidates. **Arterial revascularization** is the surgical procedure most commonly used to increase arterial blood flow in an affected limb.

Surgical procedures are classified as *inflow* or *outflow.* Inflow procedures involve bypassing arterial occlusions above the superficial femoral arteries (SFAs). Outflow procedures involve surgical bypassing of arterial occlusions at or below the SFAs. For those who have both inflow and outflow problems, the inflow procedure (for larger arteries) is done before the outflow repair.

Inflow procedures include aortoiliac, aortofemoral, and axillofemoral bypasses. Outflow procedures include femoropopliteal and femorotibial bypasses. Inflow procedures are more successful, with less chance of reocclusion or postoperative ischemia. Outflow procedures are less successful in relieving ischemic pain and are associated with a higher incidence of reocclusion.

Graft materials for bypasses are selected on an individual basis. For outflow procedures, the preferred graft material is the patient's own **(autogenous)** saphenous vein. However, some patients experience coronary artery disease and may need this vein for coronary artery bypass. When the saphenous vein is not usable, the cephalic or basilic arm veins may be used. Grafts made of synthetic materials have also been used when autogenous veins were not available.

Preoperative Care. Preparing the patient for surgery is similar to procedures described for general or epidural anesthesia (see Chapter 14). Documentation of vital signs and peripheral pulses provides a baseline of information for comparison during the postoperative phase. Depending on the surgical procedure, the patient may have one or more IV lines, urinary catheter, central venous catheter, and/or arterial line. To prevent postoperative infection, antibiotic therapy is typically given before the procedure.

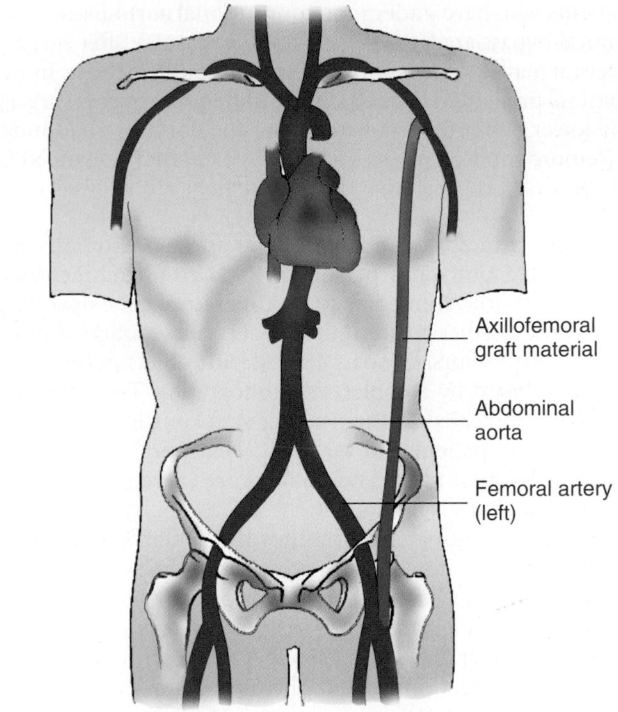

FIG. 36-6 An axillofemoral bypass graft

Operative Procedures. The anesthesia provider places the patient under general, epidural, or spinal anesthesia. Epidural or spinal induction is preferred for older adults to decrease the risk for cardiopulmonary complications in this age-group. If arterial bypass is to be accomplished by autogenous grafts, the surgeon removes the veins through an incision. The blocked artery is then exposed through an incision, and the replacement vein or synthetic graft material is sutured above and below the occlusion to increase blood flow around the occlusion.

For conventional open *aortoiliac* and *aortofemoral* bypass (AFB) surgery, the surgeon makes a midline incision into the abdominal cavity to expose the abdominal aorta, with additional incisions in each groin (Fig. 36-5). Graft material is tunneled from the aorta to the groin incisions, where it is sutured in place.

In an open *axillofemoral* bypass (Fig. 36-6), the surgeon makes an incision beneath the clavicle and tunnels graft material subcutaneously with a catheter from the chest to the iliac crest, into a groin incision, where it is sutured in place. Neither the thoracic nor the abdominal cavity is entered. For that reason, the axillofemoral bypass is used for high-risk patients who cannot tolerate a procedure requiring abdominal surgery.

Minimally invasive surgical techniques are beginning to be performed by vascular surgeons in large urban medical centers using robotic-assisted laparoscopic procedures. These newer surgical techniques require extensive training and do not shorten surgical time.

Postoperative Care. Thorough and ongoing nursing assessment for postoperative arterial revascularization patients is crucial to detect complications. Deep breathing every 1 to 2 hours and using an incentive spirometer are essential to prevent respiratory complications.

Patients who have undergone conventional aortoiliac or aortofemoral bypass are NPO status for at least 1 day after surgery to prevent nausea and vomiting, which could increase intra-abdominal pressure. Those who have undergone bypass surgery of the lower extremities not involving the aorta or abdominal wall (femoropopliteal or femorotibial bypass) may remain NPO until the first postoperative day, when they are allowed clear liquids.

Warmth, redness, and edema of the affected extremity are often expected outcomes of surgery as a result of increased arterial PERFUSION. Immediately postoperatively, the operating suite or postanesthesia care unit (PACU) nurse marks the site where the distal (dorsalis pedis or posterior tibial) pulse is best palpated or heard by Doppler ultrasonography. This information is communicated to the nursing staff on the critical care unit where the patient will be sent. "Hand-off" reporting is essential to promote safety and quality care (as required by The Joint Commission's National Patient Safety Goals).

To promote graft patency, monitor the patient's blood pressure and notify the surgeon if the pressure increases or decreases beyond the patient's baseline. Hypotension may indicate hypovolemia, which can increase the risk for CLOTTING. Range of motion of the operative leg is usually limited, with no bending of the hip and knee. Consult with the surgeon on a case-by-case basis regarding limitations of movement, including turning. Patients having open procedures may be restricted to bedrest for 24 hours or longer after surgery to prevent disruption of the suture lines. Patients having minimally invasive surgical (MIS) procedures may be ambulatory and eat within the day of surgery. Pain and surgical complications tend to occur less often in patients who have MIS procedures.

! NURSING SAFETY PRIORITY (QSEN)

Critical Rescue

Graft occlusion (blockage) is a postoperative emergency that can occur within the first 24 hours after arterial revascularization. Monitor the patient for and report severe continuous and aching pain, which may be the first indicator of postoperative graft occlusion and ischemia. Many people experience a throbbing PAIN caused by the increased blood flow to the extremity. Because this sensation is different from ischemic pain, be sure to assess the type of pain that is experienced. Pain from occlusion may be masked by patient-controlled analgesia (PCA). Some patients have ischemic pain that is not relieved by PCA.

Monitor the patency of the graft by checking the extremity every 15 minutes for the first hour and then hourly for changes in color, temperature, and pulse intensity. Compare the operative leg with the unaffected one. *If the operative leg feels cold; becomes pale, ashen, or cyanotic; or has a decreased or absent pulse, contact the surgeon immediately!*

Emergency **thrombectomy** (removal of the clot), which the surgeon may perform at the bedside, is the most common treatment for acute graft occlusion. Thrombectomy is associated with excellent results in prosthetic grafts. Results of thrombectomy in autogenous vein grafts are not as successful and often necessitate graft revision and even replacement.

Local intra-arterial thrombolytic (clot-dissolving) therapy with an agent such as tissue plasminogen activator (t-PA) or an infusion of a platelet inhibitor such as abciximab (ReoPro) may be used for acute graft occlusions. This therapy is provided in select settings in which health care providers are experts in its use. Other antiplatelet drugs such as the glycoprotein IIb/IIIa inhibitors *tirofiban (Aggrastat)* and *eptifibatide (Integrilin)* may be used as alternatives. The physician considers these therapies when the surgical alternative (e.g., thrombectomy with or without graft revision or replacement) carries high morbidity or mortality rates or when surgery for this type of occlusion has traditionally yielded poor results. Closely assess the patient for manifestations of bleeding if thrombolytics are used.

Graft or wound infections can be life threatening. Use sterile technique when providing incisional care, and observe for symptoms of infection. Assess the area for induration, erythema, tenderness, warmth, edema, or drainage. Also monitor for fever and leukocytosis (increased serum white blood cell count). Notify the surgeon promptly if any of these symptoms occur.

Patients having conventional open bypass procedures are usually hospitalized for 5 to 7 days. Those having MIS procedures usually have shorter stays of 2 or 3 days.

Community-Based Care

Peripheral arterial disease (PAD) is a chronic, long-term problem with frequent complications. Patients may benefit from a case manager who can follow them across the continuum of care. The desired outcome is that the patient can be maintained in the home.

Management at home often requires an interdisciplinary team approach, including several home care visits. Chart 36-5 outlines the assessment highlights for home care patients with peripheral vascular disease (PVD).

Instruct patients on methods to promote vasodilation. Teach them to avoid raising their legs above the level of the heart unless venous stasis is also present. Provide written and oral instructions on foot care and methods to prevent injury and ulcer development (Chart 36-6).

Patients who have had surgery require additional instruction on incision care (see Chapter 16). Encourage all patients to avoid smoking and to limit dietary fat intake to 5% to 6% of the total daily calories (Eckel et al., 2014). Remind them to drink adequate fluids to prevent dehydration.

Patients with chronic arterial obstruction may fear recurrent occlusion or further narrowing of the artery. They often fear that they might lose a limb or become debilitated in other ways.

CHART 36-5 Home Care Assessment

The Patient with Peripheral Vascular Disease

Assess tissue perfusion to affected extremity(ies), including:
- Distal circulation, sensation, and motion
- Presence of pain, pallor, paresthesias, pulselessness, paralysis, poikilothermy (coolness)
- Ankle-brachial index

Assess adherence to therapeutic regimen, including:
- Following foot care instructions
- Quitting smoking
- Maintaining dietary restrictions
- Participating in exercise regimen
- Avoiding exposure to cold and constrictive clothing

Assess ability to manage wound care and prevent further injury, including:
- Use of compression stockings or compression pumps as directed
- Use of various dressing materials
- Signs and symptoms to report to nurse

Assess coping ability of patient and family members.

Assess home environment, including:
- Safety hazards, especially related to falls

CHART 36-6 Patient and Family Education: Preparing for Self-Management

Foot Care for the Patient with Peripheral Vascular Disease

- Keep your feet clean by washing them with a mild soap in room-temperature water.
- Keep your feet dry, especially the ankles and between the toes.
- Avoid injury to your feet and ankles. Wear comfortable, well-fitting shoes. Never go without shoes.
- Keep your toenails clean and filed. Have someone cut them if you cannot see them clearly. Cut your toenails straight across.
- To prevent dry, cracked skin, apply a lubricating lotion to your feet.
- Prevent exposure to extreme heat or cold. Never use a heating pad on your feet.
- Avoid constricting garments.
- If a problem develops, see a podiatrist or physician.
- Avoid extended pressure on your feet or ankles, such as occurs when you lean against something.

Indeed, chronic PAD may worsen, especially in those with diabetes mellitus. Reassure them that participation in prescribed exercise, nutrition therapy, and drug therapy, along with cessation of smoking, can limit further formation of atherosclerotic plaques.

Patients with arterial compromise may need assistance with ADLs if activity is limited by PAIN. They may need to limit or avoid stair climbing, depending on the severity of disease. Patients who have undergone surgery or need to limit activity usually need temporary help with daily activities by the family or other caregiver.

Patients who must limit activity because of PAD may benefit from the assistance of a home care aide. Those who have undergone surgery may require a home care nurse to assist with incision care. In collaboration with the case manager, arrange for home care resources before discharge.

ACUTE PERIPHERAL ARTERIAL OCCLUSION

❖ PATHOPHYSIOLOGY

Although chronic peripheral arterial disease (PAD) progresses slowly, the onset of **acute arterial occlusions** is sudden and dramatic. An **embolus** (piece of clot that travels and lodges in a new area) is the most common cause of peripheral occlusions, although a local thrombus may be the cause. Occlusion may affect the upper extremities, but it is more common in the lower extremities. Emboli originating from the heart are the most common cause of acute arterial occlusions. Most patients with an embolic occlusion have had an acute myocardial infarction (MI) and/or atrial fibrillation within the previous weeks.

❖ PATIENT-CENTERED COLLABORATIVE CARE

Patients with an acute arterial occlusion describe severe pain below the level of the occlusion that occurs even at rest. The affected extremity is cool or cold, pulseless, and mottled. Small areas on the toes may be blackened or gangrenous due to lack of PERFUSION. *Those with acute arterial insufficiency often present with the "six P's" of ischemia:*

- Pain
- Pallor
- Pulselessness
- Paresthesia
- Paralysis
- Poikilothermy (coolness)

The health care provider must initiate treatment promptly to avoid permanent damage or loss of an extremity. Anticoagulant therapy with unfractionated heparin (UFH, Hepalean ♣) is usually the first intervention to prevent further clot formation. A bolus of up to 10,000 units may be prescribed. The patient may undergo angiography.

A surgical *thrombectomy* or *embolectomy* with local anesthesia may be performed to remove the occlusion. The physician makes a small incision, which is followed by an **arteriotomy** (a surgical opening into an artery). A catheter is inserted into the artery to retrieve the embolus. It may be necessary to close the artery with a synthetic or autologous (patient's own blood vessel) patch graft.

! NURSING SAFETY PRIORITY QSEN

Critical Rescue

After an arterial thrombectomy, observe the affected extremity for improvement in color, temperature, and pulse every hour for the first 24 hours or according to the postoperative surgical protocol. Monitor patients for manifestations of new thrombi or emboli, especially pulmonary emboli (PE). Chest pain, dyspnea, and acute confusion (older adults) typically occur in patients with PE. Notify the health care provider or Rapid Response Team immediately if these symptoms occur.

PAIN should significantly diminish after the surgical procedure, although mild incisional pain remains. Watch closely for complications caused by reperfusing the artery after thrombectomy or embolectomy, which include spasms and swelling of the skeletal muscles. Swelling of the skeletal muscles can result in compartment syndrome.

Compartment syndrome occurs when tissue pressure within a confined body space becomes elevated and restricts blood flow. The resulting ischemia can lead to tissue damage and eventually tissue death. Assess the motor and sensory function of the affected extremity. Monitor for increasing pain, swelling, and tenseness. Report any of these symptoms to the health care provider immediately. **Fasciotomy** (surgical opening into the tissues) may be necessary to prevent further injury and save the limb.

The use of *systemic thrombolytic therapy* for acute arterial occlusions has been disappointing because bleeding complications often outweigh the benefits obtained. Catheter-directed intra-arterial thrombolytic therapy with *fibrinolytics,* such as alteplase (Activase) or t-PA, has emerged as an alternative to surgical treatment in selected settings. A catheter is placed percutaneously (through the skin) into the artery with or without ultrasound guidance by the vascular surgeon or interventional radiologist. The tip of the catheter is embedded in the clot to directly deliver the thrombolytic infusion for 24 to 36 hours until the clot dissolves.

During infusion, monitor the patient for complications such as bleeding and hemorrhagic stroke. Maintain a normal blood pressure for the patient by monitoring fluids to prevent a potential stroke. As the clot dissolves, the patient typically experiences severe pain that requires patient-controlled analgesia (PCA).

! NURSING SAFETY PRIORITY (QSEN)

Drug Alert

When *fibrinolytics* are given, assess for signs of bleeding, bruising, or hematoma. For patients receiving any *platelet inhibitor,* monitor platelet counts for the first 3, 6, and 12 hours after the start of the infusion or per agency protocol. If the platelet count decreases to below 100,000/mm^3, the infusion needs to be readjusted or discontinued. If any of these complications occur, notify the physician or Rapid Response Team immediately.

ANEURYSMS OF CENTRAL ARTERIES

❖ PATHOPHYSIOLOGY

An **aneurysm** is a permanent localized dilation of an artery, which enlarges the artery to at least 2 times its normal diameter. It may be described as *fusiform* (a diffuse dilation affecting the entire circumference of the artery) or *saccular* (an outpouching affecting only a distinct portion of the artery). Aneurysms may also be described as *true* or *false.* In true aneurysms, the arterial wall is weakened by congenital or acquired problems. False aneurysms occur as a result of vessel injury or trauma to all three layers of the arterial wall. *Dissecting aneurysms* differ from aneurysms in that they are formed when blood accumulates in the wall of an artery.

Aneurysms tend to occur at specific anatomic sites (Fig. 36-7), most commonly in the abdominal aorta. They often occur at a point where the artery is not supported by skeletal muscles or on the lines of curves or flexion in the arterial tree. This chapter discussed aneurysms of the central arteries. Brain aneurysms are discussed in Chapter 45.

An aneurysm forms when the middle layer (media) of the artery is weakened, producing a stretching effect in the inner layer (intima) and outer layers of the artery. As the artery widens, tension in the wall increases and further widening occurs, thus enlarging the aneurysm and increasing the risk for arterial rupture. Elevated blood pressure can also increase the rate of aneurysmal enlargement and risk for early rupture. When *dissecting* aneurysms occur, the aneurysm enlarges, blood is lost, and blood flow to organs is diminished.

Abdominal aortic aneurysms (AAAs) account for most aneurysms, are commonly asymptomatic, and frequently rupture. Most of these are located between the renal arteries and the aortic bifurcation (dividing area).

Thoracic aortic aneurysms (TAAs) are not quite as common and are frequently misdiagnosed. They are typically discovered when advanced imaging is used to assess other conditions. TAAs commonly develop between the origin of the left subclavian artery and the diaphragm. They are located in the descending, ascending, and transverse sections of the aorta. They can also occur in the aortic arch and are very difficult to manage surgically.

Aneurysms can cause symptoms by exerting pressure on surrounding structures or by rupturing. *Rupture is the most frequent complication and is life threatening because abrupt and massive hemorrhagic shock results.* Thrombi within the wall of an aneurysm can also be the source of emboli in distal arteries below the aneurysm.

Atherosclerosis is the most common cause of aneurysms, with hypertension, hyperlipidemia, and cigarette smoking being contributing factors. Age, gender, and family history also play a role (McCance et al., 2014). Syphilis (a sexually transmitted disease), Marfan syndrome (a connective tissue disease), and Ehlers-Danlos syndrome (a rare genetic disorder) are other causes of AAAs. Chronic INFLAMMATION (aortitis) and blunt trauma, usually from motor vehicle crashes, can cause aneurysms in the descending thoracic aorta (Hiratzka et al., 2010).

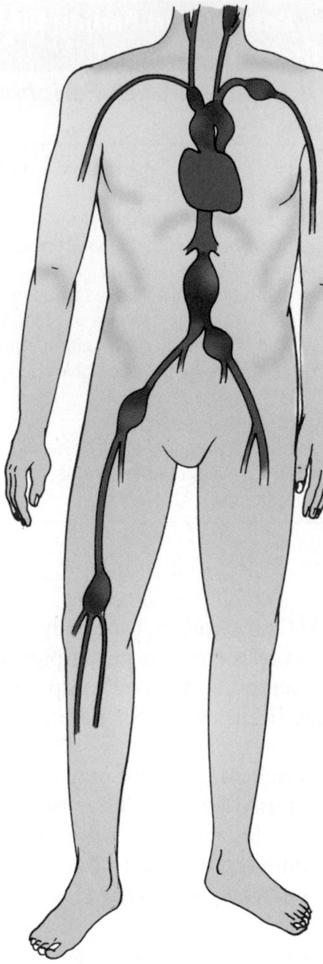

FIG. 36-7 Common anatomic sites of arterial aneurysms.

❖ PATIENT-CENTERED COLLABORATIVE CARE

◆ Assessment

Most patients with abdominal or thoracic aneurysms are asymptomatic when their aneurysms are first discovered by routine examination or during an imaging study performed for another reason. However, a few patients do have symptoms that bring them to their health care provider or the emergency department.

Physical Assessment/Clinical Manifestations. Assess patients with a known or suspected *abdominal aortic aneurysm (AAA)* for abdominal, flank, or back pain. Pain is usually described as steady with a gnawing quality, unaffected by movement, and lasting for hours or days.

A pulsation in the upper abdomen slightly to the left of the midline between the xyphoid process and the umbilicus may be present. A detectable aneurysm is at least 5 cm in diameter. *Auscultate for a bruit over the mass, but avoid palpating the mass because it may be tender and there is risk for rupture!* If expansion and impending rupture of an AAA are suspected, assess for severe PAIN of sudden onset in the back or lower abdomen, which may radiate to the groin, buttocks, or legs.

Patients with a rupturing AAA are critically ill and are at risk for hypovolemic shock due to hemorrhage. Clinical manifestations include hypotension, diaphoresis, decreased level of consciousness, oliguria (scant urine output), loss of pulses distal to the rupture, and dysrhythmias. Retroperitoneal hemorrhage is manifested by hematomas in the flanks (lower back). Rupture into the abdominal cavity causes abdominal distention.

When *a thoracic aortic aneurysm* is suspected, assess for back PAIN and manifestations of compression of the aneurysm on adjacent structures. Signs include shortness of breath, hoarseness, and difficulty swallowing. TAAs are not often detected by physical assessment, but occasionally a mass may be visible above the suprasternal notch. Assess the patient with suspected rupture of a thoracic aneurysm for sudden and excruciating back or chest pain. Hypovolemic shock also occurs with TAA.

Imaging Assessment. *Computed tomography (CT) scanning* with contrast is the standard tool for assessing the size and location of an abdominal or thoracic aneurysm. *Ultrasonography* is also used.

◆ *Interventions*

The size of the aneurysm and the presence of symptoms determine patient management. The nurse's role is to perform frequent patient assessments, including blood pressure, pulse, and peripheral circulation checks.

Nonsurgical Management. The desired outcome of nonsurgical management is to monitor the growth of the aneurysm and maintain the blood pressure at a normal level to decrease the risk for rupture. Patients with hypertension are treated with antihypertensive drugs to decrease the rate of enlargement and the risk for early rupture.

For those with small or asymptomatic aneurysms, frequent ultrasound or CT scans are necessary to monitor the growth of the aneurysm. Emphasize the importance of following through with scheduled tests to monitor the growth. Also explain the clinical manifestations of aneurysms that need to be promptly reported.

Surgical Management. Surgical management of an aneurysm may be an elective or an emergency procedure. *For patients with a rupturing abdominal aortic or a thoracic aneurysm, emergency surgery is performed.* Patients with smaller aneurysms that are producing symptoms are advised to have elective surgery. Those with smaller aneurysms that are not causing symptoms are treated nonsurgically until symptoms occur or the aneurysm enlarges.

The most common surgical procedure for AAA has traditionally been a resection or repair (**aneurysmectomy**). However, the mortality rate for elective resection is high and markedly increases for emergency surgery. Endovascular stent grafts have improved mortality rates and shortened the hospital stay for select patients who need AAA repair.

The repair of AAAs with **endovascular stent grafts** is the procedure of choice for almost all patients on an elective or emergent basis. Stents (wirelike devices) are inserted percutaneously (through the skin), avoiding abdominal incisions and therefore decreasing the risk for a prolonged postoperative recovery. Postoperative care is similar to care required after an arteriogram (angiogram).

Different designs of endovascular stent grafts are used, depending on the anatomic involvement of the aneurysm. The stent graft is flexible with either Dacron or polytetrafluoroethylene (PTFE) material. It is inserted through a skin incision into the femoral artery by way of a catheter-based system. The catheter is advanced to a level above the aneurysm away from the renal arteries. The graft is released from the catheter, and the stent graft is placed with a series of hooks. This procedure is done in collaboration with the vascular surgeon, interventional radiologist, operating suite team, and, at some centers, vascular medicine physician.

Complications for stent repair include:

- Conversion to open surgical repair
- Bleeding
- Aneurysm rupture
- Peripheral embolization
- Misplacement of the stent graft

The endovascular repair of AAAs has decreased the length of hospital stay for patients requiring repair of abdominal aneurysms. However, the patient needs to be closely monitored, in the hospital and at home, for the development of complications after the procedure. Expert nursing care is required to allow for early identification of problems, and complications require timely surgical intervention. In addition, coordination and collaboration with the health care team are required for discharge planning and follow-up care for patients at home.

Community-Based Care

Most patients are discharged to home after aneurysm repair. However, in the absence of family or other support systems, the postoperative patient may be discharged to a transitional care or long-term care facility for rehabilitation.

If discharged to home, the patient must follow instructions regarding activity level and incisional care. Because stair climbing may be restricted initially, he or she may need a bedside commode if the bathroom is inaccessible. Teach the patient who has undergone surgical repair about activity restrictions, wound care, and pain management. Patients may not perform activities that involve lifting heavy objects (usually more than 15 to 20 pounds [6.8 to 9.1 kg]) for 6 to 12 weeks postoperatively. Advise them to use caution for activities that involve pulling, pushing, or straining. Those who usually engage in vigorous activities should discuss them with their health care provider. Most patients are restricted from driving a car for several weeks after discharge.

For patients who have not undergone surgical aneurysm repair, the teaching plan emphasizes the importance of compliance with the schedule of frequent ultrasound scanning to monitor the size of the aneurysm.

! NURSING SAFETY PRIORITY QSEN

Action Alert

Teach patients receiving treatment for hypertension about the importance of continuing to take prescribed drugs. Instruct them about the signs and symptoms that must promptly be reported to the health care provider, which include:

- Abdominal fullness or pain or back pain
- Chest or back pain
- Shortness of breath
- Difficulty swallowing or hoarseness

In collaboration with the case manager or social worker, assess the availability of transportation to and from appointments for patients needing ultrasound monitoring. Those who have undergone surgery may require the services of a home care nurse for initial assistance with dressing changes. A home care aide may be needed to assist with ADLs, depending on the patient's support system.

ANEURYSMS OF THE PERIPHERAL ARTERIES

Although femoral and popliteal aneurysms are not common, they may be associated with an aneurysm in another location of the arterial tree (see Fig. 36-7). To detect a popliteal aneurysm, assess for a pulsating mass in the popliteal space. To detect a femoral aneurysm, observe a pulsatile mass over the femoral artery. *To prevent its rupture, do not palpate the mass!* Evaluate both extremities because more than one femoral or popliteal aneurysm may be present.

The patient may have symptoms of limb ischemia (decreased PERFUSION), including diminished or absent pulses, cool to cold skin, and pain. PAIN also may be present if an adjacent nerve is compressed. The recommended treatment for either type of aneurysm, regardless of the size, is surgery because of the risk for thromboembolic complications.

To treat a femoral aneurysm, the surgeon removes the aneurysm and restores circulation using a synthetic or an autogenous saphenous vein graft-stent repair. Most surgeons prefer to bypass rather than resect a popliteal aneurysm.

After surgery, monitor for lower limb ischemia. Palpate pulses below the graft to assess graft patency. Often, Doppler ultrasonography is necessary to assess blood flow when pulses are not palpable. *Report sudden development of pain or discoloration of the extremity immediately to the physician because it may indicate graft occlusion.*

AORTIC DISSECTION

❖ PATHOPHYSIOLOGY

Aortic dissection was previously referred to as a *dissecting aneurysm.* However, because this condition is more accurately described as a *dissecting hematoma,* the term *aortic dissection* is more commonly used. Aortic dissection is not common but is a life-threatening problem.

Aortic dissection is thought to be caused by a sudden tear in the aortic intima, opening the way for blood to enter the aortic wall. Degeneration of the aortic media may be the primary cause for this condition, with hypertension being an important contributing factor. It is often associated with connective tissue disorders such as Marfan syndrome. It occurs also in middle-aged and older people, peaking in adults in their 50s and 60s. Men are more commonly affected than women (Hiratzka et al., 2010).

The circulation of any major artery arising from the aorta can be impaired in patients with aortic dissection; therefore this condition is highly lethal and represents an emergency situation. Although the ascending aorta and descending thoracic aorta are the most common sites, dissections can also occur in the abdominal aorta and other arteries.

❖ PATIENT-CENTERED COLLABORATIVE CARE

◆ Assessment

The most common symptom is PAIN. It is described as "sharp," "tearing," "ripping," and "stabbing" and tends to move from its point of origin. Depending on the site of dissection, the patient may feel pain in the anterior chest, back, neck, throat, jaw, or teeth at a level of 10 on a 0-to-10 PAIN intensity scale.

Diaphoresis (excessive sweating), nausea, vomiting, faintness, and apprehension are also common. Blood pressure is usually elevated unless complications such as cardiac tamponade or rupture have occurred. In these cases, the patient becomes rapidly hypotensive. A decrease or absence of peripheral pulses is common, as is aortic regurgitation, which is characterized by a musical murmur best heard along the right sternal border. Neurologic deficits such as an altered level of consciousness, paraparesis, and strokes also can occur.

Chest x-ray, computed tomography (CT), magnetic resonance imaging (MRI), and aortic angiography may be used to confirm the diagnosis. However, MRI scanning is very time-consuming and may not be the test of choice. Transthoracic echocardiography (TTE) or transesophageal echocardiography (TEE) may be performed at the bedside for patients who cannot be moved (Braverman, 2010).

◆ Interventions

The expected outcomes for emergency care for a patient with an aortic dissection are elimination of PAIN and reduction of systolic blood pressure to 100 to 120 mm Hg. Make sure that the patient has two large-bore IV catheters to infuse 0.9% sodium chloride and give medication. Insert an indwelling urinary catheter. The physician prescribes IV morphine sulfate to relieve PAIN and an IV beta blocker, such as esmolol (Brevibloc), to lower heart rate and blood pressure (Carlson, 2012). If this regimen is not effective, nicardipine hydrochloride (Cardene) or other antihypertensive may be used.

Subsequent treatment depends on the location of the dissection. Patients receive continued medical treatment for uncomplicated distal dissections and surgical treatment for proximal dissections. For those receiving long-term medical treatment, the systolic blood pressure must be maintained at or below 130 to 140 mm Hg. Beta blockers (e.g., propranolol) and calcium channel antagonists (e.g., amlodipine) are prescribed to assist with blood pressure maintenance once the patient is stabilized.

Patients having surgical intervention for a proximal dissection typically require cardiopulmonary bypass (CPB) (see Chapter 38). The surgeon removes the intimal tear and sutures edges of the dissected aorta. Usually a synthetic graft is used.

OTHER ARTERIAL HEALTH PROBLEMS

Fewer health problems affect peripheral and central arteries. Examples of some of these problems are summarized in Table 36-7.

PERIPHERAL VENOUS DISEASE

To function properly, veins must be patent (open) with competent valves. Vein function also requires the assistance of the surrounding muscle beds to help pump blood toward the heart. If one or more veins are not operating properly, they become distended and clinical manifestations occur.

Three health problems alter the blood flow in veins:

- Thrombus formation *(venous thrombosis)* can lead to pulmonary embolism (PE), a life-threatening complication. **Venous thromboembolism** (VTE) is the current term that includes both deep vein thrombosis and PE.

TABLE 36-7 Assessment and Interventions for Other Arterial Health Problems

DISEASE/HEALTH PROBLEM	ASSESSMENT	COLLABORATIVE MANAGEMENT	NURSING CARE
Buerger's Disease	Claudication in feet and lower extremities worse at night; causes ischemia and fibrosis of vessels in extremities with increased sensitivity to cold. Ulcerations and gangrene occur on digits. Cause unknown but is associated with smoking.	Vasodilating drugs, such as nifedipine (Procardia); management of ulceration and gangrene; chronic pain management modalities.	Teach patient about smoking cessation, avoid cold by wearing gloves and warm clothes, manage stress, avoid caffeine; teach patient taking nifedipine to avoid grapefruit and grapefruit juice to prevent severe adverse effects, including possible death; teach patients on vasodilators about side effects such as facial flushing, hypotension, headaches.
Raynaud's Phenomenon/ Disease	Painful vasospasms of arteries and arterioles in extremities, especially digits; causes red-white-blue skin color changes on exposure to cold or stress; cause unknown, occurs more in women, and may be autoimmune because it is associated with many rheumatic diseases like systemic lupus erythematosus.	Same as above	Same as above
Subclavian Steal	Occurs in upper extremities as result of subclavian artery occlusion or stenosis causing ischemia in the arm and pain; paresthesias and dizziness are also common; BP difference in arms and presence of subclavian bruit on the affected side.	Surgical interventions for cyanosis or unrelenting pain, such as endarterectomy, bypass, or dilation of subclavian artery.	Monitor patient closely for new signs and symptoms; postoperative, check pulses and observe for ischemic changes, including severe pain or color changes (e.g., cyanosis).
Thoracic Outlet Syndrome	Compression of subclavian artery by rib or muscle that is more common in women and those who have to keep arms moving or above their heads (e.g., golfers, swimmers); also present with trauma; causes neck, arm, and shoulder pain with numbness and possible cyanosis.	Physical therapy for exercise program, avoiding aggravating positions; surgery as last resort for severe pain.	Health teaching about avoiding activities and positions that aggravate pain; monitor for new signs and symptoms; neurovascular assessments; postoperative care if needed.

- Defective valves lead to *venous insufficiency* and *varicose veins,* which are not life threatening but are problematic.
- Skeletal muscles do not contract to help pump blood in the veins. This problem can occur when weight bearing is limited or muscle tone decreases.

VENOUS THROMBOEMBOLISM

❖ PATHOPHYSIOLOGY

Venous thromboembolism (VTE) is one of health care's greatest challenges and includes both thrombus and embolus complications. A **thrombus** (also called a *thrombosis*) is a blood clot believed to result from an endothelial injury, venous stasis, or hypercoagulability. The thrombosis may be specifically attributable to one element, or it may involve all three elements. It is often associated with an inflammatory process. When a thrombus develops, INFLAMMATION occurs around the clot, thickening the vein wall and consequently possibly leading to embolization (the formation of an **embolus**). Pulmonary embolism (PE) is the most common type of embolus and is discussed in detail in Chapter 32.

Thrombophlebitis refers to a thrombus that is associated with INFLAMMATION. **Phlebothrombosis** is a thrombus without inflammation. Thrombophlebitis can occur in superficial veins. However, it most frequently occurs in the deep veins of the lower extremities.

Deep vein thrombophlebitis, commonly referred to as **deep vein thrombosis (DVT),** is the most common type of thrombophlebitis. Deep vein thrombophlebitis (thrombosis) is more serious than superficial thrombophlebitis because it presents a greater risk for PE. In PE, a dislodged blood clot travels to the pulmonary artery—a medical emergency! DVT develops most often in the legs but can occur also in the upper arms as a result of increased use of central venous devices.

Thrombus formation has been associated with stasis of blood flow, endothelial injury, and/or hypercoagulability, known as **Virchow's triad.** The precise cause of these events remains unknown; however, a few predisposing factors have been identified.

The highest incidence of clot formation occurs in patients who have undergone hip surgery, total knee replacement, or open prostate surgery. Other conditions that seem to promote thrombus formation are ulcerative colitis, heart failure, cancer, oral contraceptives, and immobility. Complications of immobility occur during prolonged bedrest such as when a patient is confined to bed for an extensive illness. People who sit for long periods (e.g., on an airplane or at a computer) are also at risk. **Phlebitis** (vein INFLAMMATION) associated with invasive procedures such as IV therapy can also predispose patients to thrombosis.

A systematic literature review by Anthony (2013) found a valid and reliable model for placing patients in high- and low-risk groups for DVT. This model is highly predictive of DVT development. During the nursing assessment, one point is given for each of nine characteristics, which include:

- Active cancer, paralysis, or casting of an extremity
- Bedridden for more than 3 days
- Major surgery with general anesthesia during the previous 3 months
- Localized tenderness along the deep venous system
- Swelling of the entire leg
- Calf swelling of greater than 3 cm larger when compared with the other leg
- Pitting edema in one leg
- Dilated superficial veins in one leg
- Previously documented DVT

A score of 2 or more indicates that a DVT is likely to occur.

Millions of people in the United States are affected by deep vein thrombosis each year, and many die from pulmonary embolism. The largest number of deaths occur in older adults.

Health Promotion and Maintenance

In the *community,* if a person has a history of any type of VTE, these precautions should be taken:

- Avoid oral contraceptives.
- Drink adequate fluids to avoid dehydration.
- Exercise legs during long periods of bedrest or sitting.

The Joint Commission's VTE Core Measure Set requires that hospitals report data on 6 areas related to VTE prophylaxis and management (Table 36-8). If VTE is not prevented or adequately managed, the hospital may not be paid by the third party payer (e.g., Medicare) for the patient's care. In the *inpatient setting,* all patients must be assessed for risk for VTE on admission. For those at moderate to high risk, initiate these interventions to prevent VTE:

- Patient education
- Leg exercises
- Early ambulation
- Adequate hydration
- Graduated compression stockings
- Intermittent pneumatic compression, such as sequential compression devices (SCDs)
- Venous plexus foot pump
- Anticoagulant therapy

TABLE 36-8 Venous Thromboembolism (VTE) Core Measure Set

CORE MEASURE	ASSESSMENT OF MEASURE
VTE-1	**VTE Prophylaxis:** Number of patients who received VTE prophylaxis or have documented why no VTE prophylaxis was given the day of or the day after hospital admission or surgery
VTE-2	**ICU VTE:** Number of patients who received VTE prophylaxis on ICU admission or have documented why no VTE prophylaxis was given the day of admission, transfer, or surgery
VTE-3	**VTE Patients with Anticoagulant Overlap Therapy:** Number of patients diagnosed with confirmed VTE who received overlap of parenteral anticoagulant and warfarin
VTE-4	**VTE Patients Receiving Unfractionated Heparin:** Number of patients receiving heparin with dosages/platelet count monitoring by protocol or nomogram
VTE-5	**VTE Warfarin Therapy Discharge Instructions:** Number of patients who received written instructions that address these four criteria: • Compliance issues • Dietary advice • Follow-up monitoring • Information about potential for adverse drug reactions/interactions
VTE-6	**Hospital-Acquired Potentially Preventable VTE:** Number of patients who developed VTE while hospitalized

Data from www.jointcommission.org/venous_thromboembolism/.
ICU, Intensive care unit.

❖ PATIENT-CENTERED COLLABORATIVE CARE

◆ Assessment

People with DVT may have symptoms or may be asymptomatic. *The classic signs and symptoms of DVT are calf or groin tenderness and pain and sudden onset of unilateral swelling of the leg.* PAIN in the calf on dorsiflexion of the foot (positive Homans' sign) appears in only a small percentage of patients with DVT, and false-positive findings are common (Anthony, 2013). *Therefore checking a Homans' sign is not advised because it is an unreliable tool!* Examine the area described as painful, comparing this site with the other limb. *Gently* palpate the site, observing for **induration** (hardening) along the blood vessel and for warmth and edema. Redness may also be present (Fig. 36-8).

Although diagnostic tests are available, physical examination findings are often adequate for diagnosis. If a definitive diagnosis is lacking from physical assessment findings alone, diagnostic tests may be performed.

The preferred diagnostic test for DVT is *venous duplex ultrasonography,* a noninvasive ultrasound that assesses the flow of blood through the veins of the arms and legs. *Doppler flow studies* may also be useful in the diagnosis, but they are more sensitive in detecting proximal rather than distal DVT. Normal venous circulation creates audible signals, whereas thrombosed veins produce little or no sound. The accuracy of the scanning depends on the technical skill of the health care professional performing the test. If the test is negative but a DVT is still

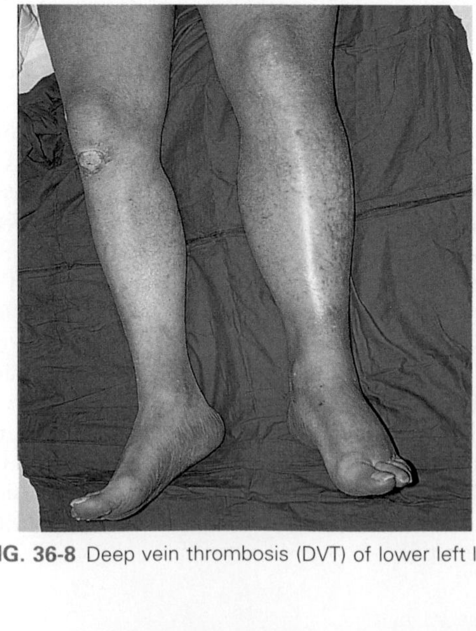

FIG. 36-8 Deep vein thrombosis (DVT) of lower left leg.

suspected, a venogram may be needed to make an accurate diagnosis.

Impedance plethysmography assesses venous outflow and can detect most DVTs that are located above the popliteal vein. It is not helpful in locating clots in the calf and is less sensitive than Doppler studies.

Magnetic resonance direct thrombus imaging (MRI), another noninvasive test, is useful in finding a DVT in the proximal deep veins and is better than traditional venography in finding DVT in the inferior vena cava or pelvic veins.

A D-dimer test is a global marker of coagulation activation and measures fibrin degradation products produced from fibrinolysis (clot breakdown). The test is used for the diagnosis of DVT when the patient has few clinical signs and stratifies patients into a high-risk category for reoccurrence. Useful as an adjunct to noninvasive testing, a negative D-dimer test can exclude a DVT without an ultrasound.

Physical and diagnostic assessment of patients with pulmonary embolism is described in Chapter 32.

◆ Interventions

The focus of managing thrombophlebitis is to prevent complications such as pulmonary emboli, prevent further thrombus formation, and prevent an increase in size of the thrombus. Patients with deep vein thrombosis (DVT) may be hospitalized for treatment, although this practice is changing as a result of the use of newer drugs.

Nonsurgical Management. DVT is usually treated medically using a combination of rest and drug therapy. Prevention of DVT and other types of venous thromboembolism (VTE) is crucial for patients at risk. Preventive measures are listed on p. 730 in the Health Promotion and Maintenance section.

Rest. Supportive therapy for DVT has typically included bedrest and elevation of the extremity. However, a review and synthesis of the literature showed that outcomes are not different if the patient is allowed to ambulate (Gay et al., 2009). Ambulation did not cause pulmonary embolus, and the DVT did not worsen any more with ambulation than with bedrest. Allowing patients to ambulate may decrease their fear and anxiety about dislodging the clot and life-threatening complications.

Teach the patient to elevate his or her legs when in bed and chair. To help prevent chronic venous insufficiency, instruct patients with active and resolving DVT to wear knee- or thigh-high sequential or graduated compression stockings for an extended period. Be sure to select the correct stocking size for the patient according to the sizing chart provided.

Some health care providers prescribe intermittent or continuous warm, moist soaks to the affected area. *To prevent the thrombus from dislodging and becoming an embolus, do not massage the affected extremity.* Monitor all patients for signs and symptoms of pulmonary embolism (PE), which include shortness of breath, chest pain, and acute confusion (in older adults). Emboli may also travel to the brain or heart, but these complications are not as common as PE. Chapter 32 describes PE manifestations in detail.

Drug Therapy. *Anticoagulants are the drugs of choice for actual DVT and for patients at risk for DVT.* However, these drugs are known to cause medical complications and even death. Therefore The Joint Commission's National Patient Safety Goals (NPSGs) include the need for agencies to reduce the likelihood of patient harm associated with the use of anticoagulant therapy.

The conventional treatment has been IV unfractionated heparin followed by oral anticoagulation with warfarin (Coumadin). However, unfractionated heparin can be problematic because each patient's response to the drug is unpredictable and hospital admission is usually required for laboratory monitoring and dose adjustments. The use of low–molecular-weight heparin (LMWH) has changed the management of both DVT and PE.

Unfractionated Heparin Therapy. Some patients with a confirmed diagnosis of an existing blood clot are started on a regimen of IV unfractionated heparin (UFH, Hepalean ♣) therapy. UFH is an anticoagulant agent that at low doses interacts with antithrombin III to produce selective inhibition of clotting factors IIa (thrombin) and Xa. At higher doses, it inhibits practically all CLOTTING factors. The ultimate result is inhibition of fibrin formation. The health care provider prescribes UFH to prevent the formation of further clots, which often develop in the presence of an existing clot, and to prevent enlargement of the existing clot. Over a long period, the existing clot is slowly absorbed by the body.

Before UFH administration, a baseline prothrombin time (PT), activated partial thromboplastin time (APTT or aPTT), international normalized ratio (INR), complete blood count (CBC) with platelet count, urinalysis, stool for occult blood, and creatinine level are required. Notify the physician if the platelet count is below 100,000 to 120,000/mm^3, depending on agency protocol.

UFH is initially given in a bolus IV dose of about 80 to 100 units/kg of body weight in a prefilled syringe or 5000 units followed by continuous infusion via an infusion pump. The infusion is regulated by a reliable electronic pump that protects against accidental free flow of solution. The physician or clinical pharmacist prescribes concentrations of UFH (in 5% dextrose in water) and the number of units or milliliters per hour needed to maintain a therapeutic aPTT (usually 18-20 units/kg/hr or at least 30,000 units over 24 hours). aPTT is measured at least daily, and results are reported to the health care provider as soon as results are available to allow adjustment of heparin dosage. Therapeutic levels of aPTTs are usually 1½ to 2 times normal control levels.

! NURSING SAFETY PRIORITY QSEN

Critical Rescue

Notify the physician if the aPTT value is greater than 70 seconds, or follow hospital protocol for reporting critical laboratory values. Assess patients for signs and symptoms of bleeding, which include hematuria, frank or occult blood in the stool, ecchymosis (bruising), petechiae, an altered level of consciousness, or pain. If bleeding occurs, stop the anticoagulant immediately and call the health care provider or Rapid Response Team!

UFH can also decrease platelet counts. Mild reductions are common and are resolved with continued heparin therapy. Severe platelet reductions, although rare, result from the development of antiplatelet bodies within 6 to 14 days after the beginning of treatment. Platelets aggregate into "white clots" that can cause thrombosis, usually in the form of an acute arterial occlusion. The provider discontinues heparin administration if severe **heparin-induced thrombocytopenia (HIT)** (platelet count <150,000), or "white clot syndrome," occurs. Low–molecular-weight heparin is used more commonly today because of the complications involved with unfractionated heparin.

CHART 36-7 Best Practice for Patient Safety & Quality Care QSEN

The Patient Receiving Anticoagulant Therapy

- Carefully check the dosage of anticoagulant to be administered, even if the pharmacy prepared the drug.
- Monitor the patient for signs and symptoms of bleeding, including hematuria, frank or occult blood in the stool, ecchymosis, petechiae, altered mental status (indicating possible cranial bleeding), or pain (especially abdominal pain, which could indicate abdominal bleeding).
- Monitor vital signs frequently for decreased blood pressure and increased pulse (indicating possible internal bleeding).
- Have antidotes available as needed (e.g., protamine sulfate for heparin; vitamin K for warfarin [Coumadin, Warfilone]).
- Monitor activated partial thromboplastin time (aPTT) for patients receiving unfractionated heparin. Monitor prothrombin time (PT)/international normalized ratio (INR) for patients receiving warfarin or low–molecular-weight heparin (LMWH).
- Apply prolonged pressure over venipuncture sites and injection sites.
- When administering *subcutaneous* heparin, apply pressure over the site and do not massage.
- Teach the patient going home while taking an anticoagulant to:
  - Use only an electric razor
  - Take precautions to avoid injury; for example, do not use tools such as hammers or saws, where accidents commonly occur
  - Report signs and symptoms of bleeding, such as blood in the urine or stool, nosebleeds, ecchymosis, or altered mental status
  - Take the prescribed dosage of drug at the precise time that it was prescribed to be taken
  - Not stop taking the drug abruptly; the physician usually tapers the anticoagulant gradually

Bivalirudin (Angiomax), lepirudin (Refludan), and argatroban injection are *highly selective direct thrombin inhibitors* that may be used as alternatives to heparin or for patients who have had HIT. Like heparin, these drugs increase the risk for bleeding. Monitor hemoglobin, hematocrit, aPTT, platelet count, urinalysis, fecal occult blood test, and blood pressure for indications of this complication. An oral anticoagulant like warfarin (Coumadin) may also be substituted for heparin if necessary.

Ensure that protamine sulfate, the antidote for heparin, is available if needed for excessive bleeding. Chart 36-7 highlights information important to nursing care and patient education associated with anticoagulant therapy.

To *prevent* DVT, unfractionated heparin may be given in low doses subcutaneously for high-risk patients, especially after orthopedic surgery. Commonly used alternatives to unfractionated heparin include:

- Low–molecular-weight heparin (e.g., enoxaparin [Lovenox]) (drug class of choice after orthopedic surgery)
- Selective factor Xa inhibitors (e.g., fondaparinux [Arixtra]; rivaroxaban [Xarelto] used most often for orthopedic surgery)
- Warfarin (Coumadin, Warfilone ♣)

Low–Molecular-Weight Heparin. Subcutaneous low–molecular-weight heparins (LMWHs) such as enoxaparin (Lovenox), dalteparin (Fragmin), and ardeparin (Normiflo) have a consistent action and are preferred for prevention and treatment of DVT. Danaparoid (Orgaran) is also classified as an LMWH but is actually a heparinoid. LMWHs bind less to plasma proteins, blood cells, and vessel walls, resulting in a longer half-life and more predictable response. These drugs inhibit thrombin formation because of reduced factor IIa activity and enhanced inhibition of factor Xa and thrombin.

Some patients taking LMWH may be safely managed at home with visits from a home care nurse. Candidates for home therapy must have stable DVT or PE, low risk for bleeding, adequate renal function, and normal vital signs. They must be willing to learn self-injection or have a family member, friend, or home care nurse administer the subcutaneous injections.

Some health care providers place the patient on a regimen of IV unfractionated heparin (UFH) for several days and then follow up with an LMWH. In this case, the UFH is discontinued at least 30 minutes before the first LMWH injection. The usual dose of enoxaparin is 1 mg/kg of body weight, not to exceed 90 mg, and is repeated every 12 hours. If the patient's creatinine level is greater than 2 mg/dL (indicating renal insufficiency), the health care provider lowers the dose. Dalteparin can be given once daily at 200 units/kg of body weight and does not require dose adjustment for renal insufficiency. The usual dose of ardeparin is 50 units/kg of body weight and is given every 12 hours.

Assess all stools for occult blood. The aPTTs are not checked on an ongoing basis because the doses of LMWH are not adjusted.

Warfarin Therapy. If the patient is receiving continuous UFH, warfarin (Coumadin), an oral anticoagulant, may be *added* at least 5 days later. Patients receiving LMWH are placed on the oral drug after the first dose. This anticoagulant drug overlap is necessary because heparin and warfarin work differently. Warfarin works in the liver to inhibit synthesis of the four vitamin K–dependent clotting factors and takes 3 to 4 days before it can exert therapeutic anticoagulation. The heparin continues to provide therapeutic anticoagulation until this effect is achieved. IV heparin is then discontinued.

According to the National Patient Safety Goals, therapeutic levels of warfarin must be monitored by measuring the international normalized ratio (INR) at frequent intervals. Because prothrombin times are often inconsistent and misleading, the INR was developed. Most laboratories report both results. Most patients receiving warfarin should have an INR between 1.5 and 2.0 to prevent future DVT and to minimize the risk for stroke or hemorrhage (Pagana & Pagana, 2014). For patients with additional cardiovascular problems or pulmonary embolus, the desired INR is higher, up to 3.5 or 4.0. The health care provider specifies the desired INR level to obtain. Be aware of the critical value for INR according to agency policy (ranges between 4.5 and 6.0). Notify the health care provider immediately if your patient's INR is at a critical value.

After obtaining the patient's baseline INR, warfarin therapy should be started with low doses, at least 5 mg, and gradually titrated up according to the INR. Patients usually receive this drug for 3 to 6 months or longer after an episode of DVT if no precipitating factors were discovered, with recurrence, or if there are continuing risk factors.

! NURSING SAFETY PRIORITY QSEN

Drug Alert

For patients taking warfarin, assess for any bleeding, such as hematuria or blood in the stool. *Ensure that vitamin K, the antidote for warfarin, is available in case of excessive bleeding* (see Chart 36-7). Report any bleeding to the health care provider, and document in the patient's health record. Teach patients to avoid foods with high concentrations of Vitamin K, especially dark green leafy vegetables. These foods interfere with the action of warfarin.

NCLEX EXAMINATION CHALLENGE

Physiological Integrity

The nurse is providing care to a client who has started warfarin after being diagnosed with a deep vein thrombosis. What health teaching will the nurse provide to the client related to self-management of warfarin therapy?

A. "You must have your partial thromboplastin time checked every 2 weeks."
B. "Massage the injection site after the warfarin is injected."
C. "Eat plenty of dark green leafy vegetables while taking warfarin."
D. "Report any signs of bleeding to your primary care provider."

Thrombolytic Therapy. Thrombolytic therapy using fibrinolytics is not commonly prescribed unless it is the treatment of last resort.

Surgical Management. A deep vein thrombus is rarely removed surgically unless there is a massive occlusion that does not respond to medical treatment and the thrombus is of recent (1 to 2 days) onset. **Thrombectomy** is a common surgical procedure for removing the clot. Preoperative and postoperative care of patients undergoing thrombectomy is similar to the care for those undergoing arterial surgery (see pp. 723-725 in the Peripheral Arterial Disease section).

For patients with recurrent deep vein thrombosis (DVT) or pulmonary emboli that do not respond to medical treatment and for patients who cannot tolerate anticoagulation, **inferior vena cava filtration** may be indicated. The surgeon usually inserts a filter device, or "umbrella," into the femoral vein. The device is meant to trap emboli in the inferior vena cava before they progress to the lungs. Holes in the device allow blood to pass through, thus not significantly interfering with the return of blood to the heart. There are several new filter brands available and designed to allow for removal if and when DVT risks diminish.

Preoperative care is similar to that provided for patients receiving local anesthesia (see Chapter 14). If they have recently been taking anticoagulants, collaborate with the physician about interrupting this therapy in the preoperative period to avoid hemorrhage.

Postoperatively, inspect the groin insertion site for bleeding and signs or symptoms of infection. Other postoperative nursing care is similar to that for any patient undergoing local anesthesia (see Chapter 16).

Community-Based Care

Patients recovering from thrombophlebitis or DVT are ambulatory when they are discharged from the hospital. The primary focus of planning for discharge is to educate the patient and family about anticoagulation therapy.

Teach patients recovering from DVT to stop smoking and avoid the use of oral contraceptives to decrease the risk for recurrence. Alternative forms of birth control may be used. Most patients are discharged on a regimen of warfarin (Coumadin, Warfilone ♣) or low–molecular-weight heparin (LMWH). The VTE Core Measures and the Joint Commission's National Patient Safety Goals require that the patients be given written discharge instructions about anticoagulant therapy that address:

CHART 36-8 Patient and Family Education: Preparing for Self-Management

Foods and Drugs That Interfere with Warfarin (Coumadin)

Eat small amounts of foods rich in vitamin K each day, including any of these:	If possible, avoid:
• Broccoli	• Allopurinol
• Cauliflower	• NSAIDs
• Spinach	• Acetaminophen
• Kale	• Vitamin E
• Other green leafy vegetables	• Histamine blockers
• Brussels sprouts	• Cholesterol-reducing drugs
• Cabbage	• Antibiotics
• Liver	• Oral contraceptives
	• Antidepressants
	• Thyroid drugs
	• Antifungal agents
	• Other anticoagulants
	• Corticosteroids
	• Herbs, such as St. John's wort, garlic, ginseng, *Ginkgo biloba*

- Drug compliance issues (need to take drug as prescribed)
- Dietary advice (e.g., foods to avoid)
- Follow-up monitoring (e.g., Coumadin clinic, INR testing)
- Information about potential for adverse drug reactions/interactions (e.g., bleeding, bruising)

Instruct patients and their families to avoid potentially traumatic situations, such as participation in contact sports. Provide written and oral information about the signs and symptoms of bleeding (see Chart 36-7). Reinforce the need to report any of these manifestations to the health care provider immediately.

The anticoagulant effect of warfarin may be reversed by omitting one or two doses of the drug or by the administration of vitamin K. In case of injury, teach patients to apply pressure to bleeding wounds and to seek medical assistance immediately. Encourage them to carry an identification card or wear a medical alert bracelet that states that they are taking warfarin or any other anticoagulant.

Instruct patients to tell their dentist and other health care providers before receiving treatment or prescriptions that they are taking warfarin. Prothrombin times are affected by many prescription and over-the-counter drugs such as NSAIDs. Teach patients to avoid high-fat and vitamin K–rich foods, such as cabbage, cauliflower, broccoli, asparagus, turnips, spinach, kale, fish, and liver (Chart 36-8). Remind them to drink adequate fluids to stay well hydrated, avoid alcohol (which can cause dehydration), and avoid sitting for prolonged periods.

If possible, in collaboration with the case manager (CM) or other discharge planner, arrange for the patient to obtain a device to self-monitor INR at home. Some insurance companies do not pay for the INR monitoring device. Clinical studies show that self-monitoring of the INR and self-adjusting of anticoagulation therapy result in better anticoagulation control, improve patient satisfaction, and improve quality of life (Michaels & Regan, 2013). The device used to self-monitor is similar to a glucometer for glucose testing and requires a fingerstick blood sample applied to a test strip or plastic cuvette, which is then inserted into the machine. Self-monitoring can be used either for the testing alone or for self-management, in which the patient uses the test results to adjust drug dosages based on a dosing protocol. If the patient cannot use a monitoring device, teach a family member or other caregiver how to perform the procedure. If the patient lives alone, collaborate with the CM to arrange for follow-up laboratory appointments to have blood drawn at frequent intervals—usually every week until the patient's values are stabilized. Communication with the primary care provider is essential while patients are receiving warfarin.

Patients receiving subcutaneous LMWH injections at home need instruction on self-injection. Teach the appropriate caregiver and family members or friends, if necessary, to administer the injections.

Patients who have experienced DVT may fear recurrence of a thrombus. They may also be concerned about treatment with warfarin and the risk for bleeding. Assure them that the prescribed treatment will help resolve this problem and that ongoing assessment of prothrombin times and INR values decreases the risks for bleeding.

VENOUS INSUFFICIENCY

❖ PATHOPHYSIOLOGY

Venous insufficiency occurs as a result of prolonged venous hypertension that stretches the veins and damages the valves. Valvular damage can lead to a backup of blood and further venous hypertension, resulting in edema and decreased tissue perfusion. With time, this stasis (stoppage) results in venous stasis ulcers, swelling, and cellulitis.

The veins cannot function properly when thrombosis occurs or when valves are not working correctly. Venous hypertension can occur in people who stand or sit in one position for long periods (e.g., teachers, office personnel). Obesity can also cause chronically distended veins, which lead to damaged valves. Thrombus formation can contribute to valve destruction. Chronic venous insufficiency also often occurs in patients who have had thrombophlebitis. In severe cases, venous ulcers develop.

Venous leg ulcers are a major cause of death, PAIN, and health care costs. Most venous ulcer care is delivered in the community setting by home care nurses or through self-management.

❖ PATIENT-CENTERED COLLABORATIVE CARE

◆ Assessment

Venous insufficiency may result in edema of both legs. There may be **stasis dermatitis** or reddish brown discoloration along the ankles, extending up to the calf. In people with long-term venous insufficiency, **stasis ulcers** often form. They can result from the edema or from minor injury to the limb. Ulcers typically occur over the malleolus, more often medially (inner ankle) than laterally (outer ankle). The ulcer usually has irregular borders. In general, these ulcers are chronic and difficult to heal (see Chart 36-4). Many people live with ulcers for years, and recurrence is common. Some may lose one or both legs if ulcers are not controlled.

◆ Interventions

The focus of treating venous insufficiency is to decrease edema and promote venous return from the affected leg. Patients are not usually hospitalized for venous insufficiency alone unless it is complicated by an ulcer or another disorder is occurring at the same time.

Nonsurgical Management. Treatment of chronic venous insufficiency is nonsurgical unless it is complicated by a venous stasis ulcer that requires surgical débridement. The desired outcomes of managing venous stasis ulcers are to heal the ulcer, prevent infection, and prevent stasis with recurrence of ulcer formation. Collaborate with the wound care nurse or wound, ostomy, and continence nurse (WOCN) to make recommendations for ulcer care. A dietitian can suggest dietary supplements, such as zinc and vitamins A and C, as well as high-protein foods, to promote wound healing.

Patients with chronic venous insufficiency wear graduated compression stockings, which fit from the middle of the foot to just below the knee or to the thigh. Stockings should be worn during the day and evening. Explain the purpose and importance of wearing the compression stockings. Be sure to use the sizing chart that comes with the stockings to select the best fit. Teach patients to not roll them down and to report if they become too tight or uncomfortable.

Teach the patient to elevate his or her legs for at least 20 minutes 4 or 5 times per day. When the patient is in bed, remind him or her to elevate the legs above the level of the heart (Chart 36-9).

Coordinate with the physician about the use of intermittent sequential pneumatic compression or foot plexus pumps for patients with past or present venous stasis ulcers. If an open venous ulcer is present, the device may be applied over a dressing such as an Unna boot. Instruct the patient to apply the pump as directed during the period of healing. Because of the high incidence of venous ulcer recurrence, encourage patients with chronic venous insufficiency whose ulcers have healed to continue compression therapy for life.

CHART 36-9 Patient and Family Education: Preparing for Self-Management

Venous Insufficiency

Graduated Compression Stockings (GCSs)

- Wear stockings as prescribed, usually during the day and evening.
- Put the stockings on upon awakening and before getting out of bed.
- When applying the stockings, do not "bunch up" and apply like socks. Instead, place your hand inside the stocking and pull out the heel. Then place the foot of the stocking over your foot and slide the rest of the stocking up. Be sure that rough seams on the stocking are on the outside, not next to your skin.
- Do not push stockings down for comfort, because they may function like a tourniquet and further impair venous return.
- Put on a clean pair of stockings each day. Wash them by hand (not in a washing machine) in a gentle detergent and warm water.
- If the stockings seem to be "stretched out," replace them with a new pair.

Dos and Don'ts

- Elevate your legs for at least 20 minutes 4 or 5 times a day. When in bed, elevate your legs above the level of your heart.
- Avoid prolonged sitting or standing.
- Do not cross your legs. Crossing at the ankles is acceptable for short periods.
- Do not wear tight, restrictive pants. Avoid girdles and garters.

Venous stasis ulcers are slightly more manageable than ulcers resulting from arterial disease. They are chronic in nature, with some patients having the same ulcer for years. Ulcers often heal, only to recur in the same area several years later.

Two types of occlusive dressings are used for venous stasis ulcers: oxygen-permeable dressings and oxygen-impermeable dressings. Because the role of atmospheric oxygen in wound healing is controversial, opinions vary with regard to which type of dressing is preferred. An oxygen-permeable polyethylene film and an oxygen-impermeable hydrocolloid dressing (e.g., DuoDERM) are common. Hydrocolloid dressings are left in place for a minimum of 3 to 5 days for best effect. Use medical aseptic technique when changing dressings. If the wound is infected, use Contact Precautions in addition to Standard Precautions.

Artificial skin products can be used for difficult-to-heal venous leg ulcers. These first-generation products are very expensive but are laying the foundation in the field, with costs anticipated to come down in the future. Except for cultured epithelial autografts, artificial skins are only temporary. Artificial skin serves as a biologic cover to secrete growth factors to promote more growth factor secretion from the patient's own skin to speed the wound healing process.

If the patient is ambulatory, an **Unna boot** may be used. An Unna boot dressing is constructed of gauze that has been moistened with zinc oxide. Apply the boot to the affected limb, from the toes to the knee, after the ulcer has been cleaned with normal saline solution. It is then covered with an elastic wrap and hardens like a cast. This promotes venous return and prevents stasis. The Unna boot also forms a sterile environment for the ulcer. The physician or advanced practice nurse changes the boot about once a week. Instruct the patient to report increased pain, which indicates that the boot may be too tight.

The health care provider may prescribe topical agents, such as Accuzyme, to chemically débride the ulcer, eliminating necrotic tissue and promoting healing. Remind patients that they may temporarily feel a burning sensation when the agent is applied. If an infection or cellulitis develops, systemic antibiotics are necessary.

Surgical Management. Surgery for chronic venous insufficiency is not usually performed because it is not successful. Attempts at transplanting vein valves have had limited success. Surgical débridement of venous ulcers is similar to that performed for arterial ulcers.

NCLEX EXAMINATION CHALLENGE

Health Promotion and Maintenance

The nurse is caring for a client with chronic venous stasis ulcers. Which statement by the client indicates a need for further health teaching?

A. "I'll wear compression stockings at night."
B. "I'll keep my affected leg above my heart."
C. "I'll eat protein and vitamin C foods to help heal the ulcer"
D. "I'll change my dressing every 3 to 5 days as needed."

Community-Based Care

The desired outcome for the patient with chronic venous insufficiency is to be managed in the home. For patients with frequent acute complications and repeated hospital admissions, case management can help meet appropriate clinical and cost outcomes.

Help patients plan for opportunities and facilities that allow for elevation of the lower extremities in and outside the home. In addition, collaborate with the wound specialist to plan care of the ulcers at home.

If the physician prescribes graduated compression stockings, teach patients to apply these stockings before they get out of bed in the morning and to remove them just before going to bed at night (see Chart 36-9). Also advise them that they will probably need to wear these stockings for the rest of their lives.

To improve circulation and aid in weight reduction, collaborate with the physical therapist to prescribe an exercise program on an individual basis. Encourage all patients to maintain an optimal weight and consult with the dietitian to plan a weight-reduction diet.

Patients with venous stasis disease, especially those with venous stasis ulcers, may require long-term emotional support to assist them in meeting long-term needs. They may also need assistance in coping with necessary lifestyle adjustments, such as possible changes in occupation.

Patients with venous stasis ulcers may need the assistance of a home care nurse to perform dressing changes. Those with Unna boots need weekly transportation to their health care provider for dressing changes. Collaborate with the case manager to arrange for a sequential compression device in the home if the health care provider prescribes one.

VARICOSE VEINS

❖ *PATHOPHYSIOLOGY*

Varicose veins are distended, protruding veins that appear darkened and tortuous. They can occur in anyone, but they are common in adults older than 30 years whose occupations require prolonged standing or heavy physical activity. Varicose veins are frequently seen also in patients with systemic problems (e.g., heart disease), obesity, high estrogen states, and a family history of varicose veins.

Both *superficial* and *deep* veins can become distended. As the vein wall weakens and dilates, venous pressure increases and the valves become incompetent (defective), causing venous reflux (Armstrong, 2013). The incompetent valves enhance the vessel dilation, and the veins become tortuous and distended. The severity of the disease depends on the extent of the distention and reflux. **Telangiectasias** (spider veins) are dilated *intradermal* veins less than 1 to 3 mm in diameter that are visible on the skin surface. Most patients are not bothered by them but may consider them unattractive. Most telangiectasias do not develop into the more severe varicose vein disease.

More advanced disease causes venous distention (bulging), edema, a feeling of fullness in the legs, and pruritus (itching). As a result, signs and symptoms of venous insufficiency may occur, including venous stasis ulcers, brown pigmentation from extravasated red blood cells (also called *skin staining*), and pain.

Varicose veins and reflux are diagnosed by simple ultrasonography or duplex ultrasonography. Informal assessments of venous reflux can be made with the patient lying down to determine the direction of flow within a vein. For the duplex ultrasound procedure, the patient is upright and BP cuffs are placed at the thigh, calf, and ankle. The cuffs are serially inflated and deflated while the scanner tests for reflux. A reflux time greater than 0.5 second in the saphenous vein is considered abnormal (Armstrong, 2013).

❖ *PATIENT-CENTERED COLLABORATIVE CARE*

The overall purpose of management for patients with varicose veins is to improve and maintain optimal venous return to the heart and prevent disease progression. Conservative measures are the treatment of choice, including the three *Es*: elastic compression hose, exercise, and elevation. Graduated compression stockings (GCSs) rely on graduated external pressure to improve venous return by applying pressure to the muscles. They are available in many grades or strengths, ranging from 8 to 50 mm Hg pressure. Exercise increases venous return by helping the muscles pump blood back to the heart. Teach patients to avoid high-impact exercises such as horseback riding and running. Daily walks and ankle flexion exercises while sitting are common exercises that are helpful in promoting circulation. Elevating the extremities as much as possible allows gravity to work with the valves in promoting venous return and prevent reflux.

Patients who continue to have pain or unsightly veins despite using the three Es may opt for more invasive approaches. Surgical ligation and/or removal of veins ("stripping") were the procedures of choice for many years. Sclerotherapy to occlude the affected vessel is also an option.

However, newer, less-invasive treatments are more common today. They are less painful and have a shorter recovery time. A common procedure is an endovenous ablation, which occludes the varicose vein, most commonly the saphenous vein. Using ultrasound guidance, the clinician advances a catheter into the vein and injects an anesthetic agent around it. Then the vessel is ablated (occluded) while the catheter is slowly removed. The two modalities for ablation are (1) endovenous laser treatment (EVLT) using laser heat and (2) radiofrequency ablation (RFA) using a radiofrequency heating element.

After the procedure, teach the patient the importance of using a GCS or other form of compression (such as elastic compression bandages) for 24 hours a day, except for showers, for at least the first week. Follow-up ultrasonography ensures that the treated vein is closed. The patient is monitored carefully for the first 6 to 8 weeks to determine how healing has progressed. Some patients require continued use of the three Es for many years, depending on the severity of their disease.

Assess the affected limb for vascular status, including any changes in color or temperature of the leg. Monitor for PAIN, edema, and paresthesias that could indicate complications such as DVT or nerve damage. Nerve damage is usually temporary and minimal; it usually resolves within a few months (Armstrong, 2013).

VASCULAR TRAUMA

Many types of trauma can result in vascular injury. Vascular injuries include punctures, lacerations, and transections. Acute blunt or penetrating trauma may result in a false aneurysm or hematoma. Arteriovenous fistulas may be seen after penetrating injuries. The more common causes of penetrating injuries to the blood vessels are gunshot and knife wounds.

Blunt trauma can result from high-speed automobile crashes as a result of the shearing force of rapid deceleration. Vascular trauma can also occur during arterial puncture for arteriographic or hemodynamic studies in which a dissection, hematoma, or occlusive lesion occurs.

The history and physical examination aid in establishing the diagnosis of vascular injury. Ask the patient or family about the mechanism of injury, the site of injury, the amount of blood loss, and symptoms present after the injury. Assess for circulatory, sensory, and motor impairment. Be aware that, despite significant trauma, impairment may not be apparent, especially if deep vessels have been injured. Arteriography can provide essential information about the vascular injury.

Management of vascular injuries is often initiated in a hospital emergency department. Careful patient triage is crucial. The most important principles in the management of vascular trauma are establishing a patent airway, controlling bleeding, and restoring blood flow. Emergency or urgent surgical intervention is needed for ischemia to maximize successful revascularization.

The method of repair varies with the type of vascular injury. Techniques include vein bypass grafting, lateral suture repair, thrombectomy (excision of blood clot), resection with end-to-end anastomosis, and vein patch grafting. Vascular repair can sometimes be done via angiographic access (covered stent sealing an injury or embolizing a branch artery where appropriate).

NURSING CONCEPTS AND CLINICAL JUDGMENT REVIEW

What might you NOTICE if the patient is experiencing inadequate GAS EXCHANGE and tissue PERFUSION as a result of vascular problems?

- Redness and swelling in lower leg (venous)
- Pallor, cyanosis (darkened), mottling, or rubor in lower leg (arterial)
- Report of pain/cramping in lower legs or hands (at rest or during activity)
- Ulcers on ankles, feet, or digits
- Pulsating mass in abdomen (abdominal aortic aneurysm)
- Decreased level of consciousness (LOC), diaphoresis, decreased urine output (rupturing aortic aneurysm)

What should you INTERPRET and how should you RESPOND to a patient experiencing inadequate GAS EXCHANGE and tissue PERFUSION as a result of peripheral vascular disease?

Perform and interpret physical assessment, including:

- Taking vital signs
- Assessing peripheral pulses
- Assessing capillary refill
- Checking for sensation and temperature
- Completing a pain assessment
- Assessing ulcer

Respond by:
- Notifying physician immediately or calling Rapid Response Team if aortic rupture suspected
- Monitoring vital signs
- Giving oxygen if aneurysm rupture suspected
- Starting an IV line if aneurysm rupture suspected
- Documenting abnormal peripheral vascular assessment findings
- Elevating legs if swollen unless arterial blood flow is poor

On what should you REFLECT?
- Think about how you responded.
- Continue to monitor patient for changes in peripheral blood flow, including pulse assessments.
- Observe patient for decreased report of pain.

GET READY FOR THE NCLEX® EXAMINATION!

KEY POINTS

Review these Key Points for each NCLEX Examination Client Needs Category.

Safe and Effective Care Environment

- Plan care for the patient with atherosclerosis and hypertension, in collaboration with the health care team, including the dietitian, pharmacist, and primary health care provider as needed. **Teamwork and Collaboration** QSEN
- To reduce the risk for injury, caution patients about orthostatic hypotension when taking antihypertensive drugs. **Safety** QSEN
- Monitor blood pressure carefully in patients who have hypertension; be aware that they may develop a hypertensive crisis, a life-threatening medical emergency (see Chart 36-2).

Health Promotion and Maintenance

- In collaboration with the dietitian, assist the patient to incorporate healthy eating behaviors to lower cholesterol and saturated fats and increase fresh fruits, vegetables, and fiber in the diet. For overweight patients, assist in a weight-reduction plan. **Teamwork and Collaboration** QSEN
- Teach patients to engage in 40 minutes of moderate-to-vigorous physical activity 3 or 4 times a week to lower blood pressure and LDL-C levels.
- Assess the patient for modifiable and nonmodifiable risk factors for vascular disease, and teach health promotion behaviors to the patient and family. Pay particular attention to the patient with a family history of cardiovascular disease (see Table 36-1). **Patient-Centered Care** QSEN

Physiological Integrity

- Remember that risk factors such as smoking increase the pathophysiologic process of atherosclerosis (see Table 36-1).
- Remember that atherosclerosis occurs when fatty plaques occlude arteries and prevent adequate PERFUSION to vital body tissues.
- Monitor total cholesterol, HDL-C, and LDL-C levels to assess patient risk for atherosclerosis.
- Teach patients taking any of the statins in Table 36-2 to report any adverse effects including muscle cramping to their health care provider. Monitor the patient's liver enzymes carefully.
- Teach patients to decrease saturated and *trans* fats in their diet; instruct them to consume a diet rich in fruits, vegetables, and whole grains; and instruct them to include legumes, poultry, fish, and low-fat dairy products. Remind them to limit sweets, red meats, and sugar-sweetened beverages. **Evidence-Based Practice** QSEN
- Hypertension is categorized as either essential or secondary; the risk factors and causes for each type are described in Table 36-4. Essential hypertension is called *primary hypertension* and is not caused by another health problem or drug. *Secondary hypertension* is caused by other health problems or drug therapy.
- Closely observe the patient receiving anticoagulants or fibrinolytics for signs of bleeding, and monitor appropriate laboratory values for desired outcome values (see Chart 36-7). **Safety** QSEN
- Monitor for decreased serum potassium levels when patients are taking thiazide or loop diuretics; hypokalemia could cause life-threatening cardiac dysrhythmias (see Chart 36-1). **Safety** QSEN
- Teach patients to move slowly when changing position if taking any of the antihypertensive drugs listed in Chart 36-1. **Safety** QSEN
- Recognize that clinical manifestations of peripheral vascular disease (PVD) depend on whether it affects the arteries or veins. In addition to pallor, rubor, or cyanosis, key features of chronic peripheral arterial disease are listed in Chart 36-3.
- Vasodilating drugs or surgery is used for arterial vascular diseases.
- Deep vein thrombosis (DVT) is the most common type of peripheral vascular problem. When symptoms are present, they include swelling, redness, localized pain, and warmth.
- Be aware that DVT can lead to pulmonary embolism, a life-threatening emergency!
- Teach patients to prevent VTE by leg exercises, early ambulation, adequate hydration, graduated compression stockings (GCSs), sequential compression devices (SCDs), and anticoagulant therapy.
- Monitor aPTT values for patients receiving unfractionated heparin; monitor INR for patients receiving warfarin (Coumadin). **Safety** QSEN
- Assess for venous and arterial ulcers as described in Chart 36-4.
- Teach foot care for patients with PVD as outlined in Chart 36-6.
- Teach patients about precautions for anticoagulant therapy as described in Chart 36-7. Teach about food and drugs that interfere with warfarin (Coumadin) as listed in Chart 36-8. **Evidence-Based Practice** QSEN

- Monitor for indications of aneurysm rupture: diaphoresis, nausea, vomiting, pallor, hypotension, tachycardia, severe pain, and decreased level of consciousness. **Safety** QSEN
- Varicose veins can cause severe pain and reflux requiring the three *Es*: elastic compression hose, exercise, and elevation. Endovascular ablation can occlude the affected vessel with minimal pain and the risk for few complications. Post-procedure compression with graduated stockings or other elastic bandages is essential for this procedure to be successful.
- Raynaud's and Buerger's disease affect the digits of the fingers and toes as outlined in Table 36-7.

Care of Patients with Shock

M. Linda Workman

http://evolve.elsevier.com/Iggy/

PRIORITY CONCEPTS

- Perfusion
- Clotting
- Inflammation
- Infection

LEARNING OUTCOMES

Safe and Effective Care Environment

1. Evaluate patient risk for hypovolemic shock or sepsis and septic shock.
2. Apply principles of infection control to prevent INFECTION and sepsis in susceptible patients, especially older adults.

Health Promotion and Maintenance

3. Teach all people how to prevent and recognize hypovolemic shock or sepsis.

Psychosocial Integrity

4. Reduce the psychological impact for the patient and family regarding the assessment and management of hypovolemic or septic shock.

Physiological Integrity

5. Use laboratory data and clinical manifestations of PERFUSION to determine the effectiveness of therapy for hypovolemic shock and sepsis.
6. Prioritize the nursing care for the patient experiencing any stage of hypovolemic shock.
7. Prioritize the nursing care for the patient with sepsis or septic shock, especially when impaired CLOTTING is present.

OVERVIEW

All organs, tissues, and cells need a continuous supply of oxygen to function properly. The lungs first bring oxygen into the body through ventilation and gas exchange, and the cardiovascular system (heart, blood, and blood vessels) delivers oxygen by PERFUSION to all tissues and removes cellular wastes (Fig. 37-1). **Shock** is widespread abnormal cellular metabolism that occurs when gas exchange with oxygenation and tissue perfusion needs are not met sufficiently to maintain cell function (McCance et al., 2014). It is a condition rather than a disease and is the "whole-body" response that occurs when too little oxygen is delivered to the tissues. All body organs are affected by shock and either work harder to adapt and compensate for reduced gas exchange or perfusion (see Fig. 37-1) or fail to function because of hypoxia. Shock is a "syndrome" because the problems resulting from it occur in a predictable sequence.

Any problem that impairs oxygen PERFUSION to tissues and organs can start the syndrome of shock and lead to a life-threatening emergency. Shock is often a result of cardiovascular problems. Patients in acute care settings are at higher risk, but shock can occur in any setting. For example, older patients in long-term care settings are at risk for sepsis and shock related to urinary tract infections. When the body's adaptive adjustments (compensation) or health care interventions are not effective and shock progresses, severe hypoxia can lead to cell loss, multiple organ dysfunction syndrome (MODS), and death.

Shock is classified by the type of impairment causing it into the categories of hypovolemic shock, cardiogenic shock, distributive shock (which includes septic shock, neurogenic shock, and anaphylactic shock), and obstructive shock. Table 37-1 describes this classification and common causes of shock.

Most manifestations of shock are similar regardless of what starts the process or which tissues are affected first. These manifestations result from physiologic adjustments *(compensatory mechanisms)* that the body makes in the attempt to ensure continued PERFUSION of vital organs. These adjustment actions are triggered by the sympathetic nervous system's stress response activating the endocrine and cardiovascular systems. Manifestations unique to any one type of shock result from specific tissue dysfunction. The common features of shock are listed in Chart 37-1.

Review of Oxygenation and Tissue Perfusion

Oxygenation with gas exchange and PERFUSION depend on how much oxygen from arterial blood perfuses the tissue. Perfusion

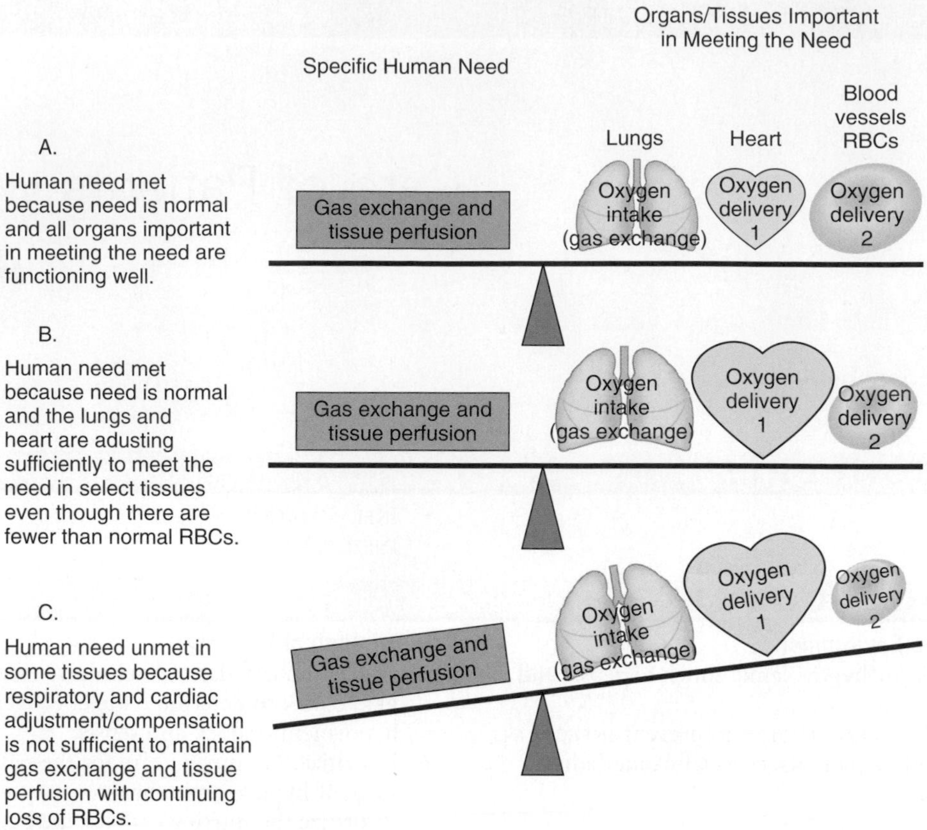

FIG. 37-1 Gas exchange and tissue perfusion affected by hypovolemic shock and adjustment/compensation. *RBCs,* Red blood cells.

is related to mean arterial pressure (MAP). The factors that influence MAP include:

- Total blood volume
- Cardiac output
- Size and integrity of the vascular bed, especially capillaries

Total blood volume and cardiac output are directly related to MAP, so increases in either total blood volume or cardiac output *raise* MAP. Decreases in either total blood volume or cardiac output *lower* MAP.

The size of the vascular bed is inversely (negatively) related to MAP. This means that increases in the size of the vascular bed *lower* MAP and decreases *raise* MAP (Fig. 37-2). The small arteries and veins connected to capillaries can increase in diameter by relaxing the smooth muscle in vessel walls (**dilation**) or decrease in diameter by contracting the muscle (**vasoconstriction**). When blood vessels dilate and total blood volume remains the same, blood pressure decreases and blood flow is slower. When blood vessels constrict and total blood volume remains the same, blood pressure increases and blood flow is faster.

Blood vessels are innervated by the sympathetic nervous system. Some nerves continuously stimulate vascular smooth muscle so that the blood vessels are normally partially constricted, a condition called **sympathetic tone**. Increases in sympathetic stimulation constrict smooth muscle even more, raising MAP. Decreases in sympathetic tone relax smooth muscle, dilating blood vessels and lowering MAP.

PERFUSION (blood flow) to organs varies and adjusts to changes in tissue oxygen needs. The body can selectively increase blood flow to some areas while reducing flow to others. The skin and skeletal muscles can tolerate low levels of oxygen for hours without dying or being damaged. Other organs (e.g., heart, brain, liver, pancreas) do not tolerate **hypoxia** (low levels of tissue oxygenation), and a few minutes without oxygen results in serious damage and cell death.

Types of Shock

Types of shock vary because shock is a manifestation of a pathologic condition rather than a disease state (see Table 37-1). *More than one type of shock can be present at the same time.* For example, trauma caused by a car crash may trigger hemorrhage (leading to hypovolemic shock) and a myocardial infarction (leading to cardiogenic shock).

Hypovolemic shock occurs when too little circulating blood volume decreases MAP, resulting in inadequate total body PERFUSION and oxygenation. Common problems leading to hypovolemic shock are poor CLOTTING with hemorrhage and dehydration. A complete discussion of the pathophysiology and management of hypovolemic shock begins on p. 741.

Cardiogenic shock occurs when the heart muscle is unhealthy and pumping is impaired. Myocardial infarction is the most common cause of direct pump failure. Other causes are listed in Table 37-1. Any type of pump failure decreases cardiac output and MAP. Chapter 38 discusses the pathophysiology and care for the person with shock from myocardial infarction.

Distributive shock occurs when blood volume is not lost from the body but is distributed to the interstitial tissues where it cannot perfuse organs. It can be caused by blood vessel dilation, pooling of blood in venous and capillary beds, and increased capillary leak. All these factors decrease mean arterial

TABLE 37-1 Causes and Types of Shock by Functional Impairment

Hypovolemic Shock

Overall Cause

Total body fluid decreased (in all fluid compartments).

Specific Cause or Risk Factors

- Hemorrhage
  - Trauma
  - GI ulcer
  - Surgery
  - Inadequate clotting
    - Hemophilia
    - Liver disease
    - Cancer therapy
    - Anticoagulation therapy
- Dehydration
  - Vomiting
  - Diarrhea
  - Heavy diaphoresis
  - Diuretic therapy
  - Nasogastric suction
  - Diabetes insipidus

Cardiogenic Shock

Overall Cause

Direct pump failure (fluid volume not affected).

Specific Cause or Risk Factors

- Myocardial infarction
- Cardiac arrest
- Ventricular dysrhythmias
- Cardiac amyloidosis
- Cardiomyopathies
- Myocardial degeneration

Distributive Shock

Overall Cause

Fluid shifted from central vascular space (total body fluid volume normal or increased).

Specific Cause or Risk Factors

- Neural-induced
  - Pain
  - Anesthesia
  - Stress
  - Spinal cord injury
  - Head trauma
- Chemical-induced
  - Anaphylaxis
  - Sepsis
  - Capillary leak
    - Burns
    - Extensive trauma
    - Liver impairment
    - Hypoproteinemia

Obstructive Shock

Overall Cause

Cardiac function decreased by noncardiac factor (indirect pump failure). Total body fluid is not affected although central volume is decreased.

Specific Cause or Risk Factors

- Cardiac tamponade
- Arterial stenosis
- Pulmonary embolus
- Pulmonary hypertension
- Constrictive pericarditis
- Thoracic tumors
- Tension pneumothorax

CHART 37-1 Key Features

Shock

Cardiovascular Manifestations

- Decreased cardiac output
- Increased pulse rate
- Thready pulse
- Decreased blood pressure
- Narrowed pulse pressure
- Postural hypotension
- Low central venous pressure
- Flat neck and hand veins in dependent positions
- Slow capillary refill in nail beds
- Diminished peripheral pulses

Respiratory Manifestations

- Increased respiratory rate
- Shallow depth of respirations
- Increased $Paco_2$
- Decreased Pao_2
- Cyanosis, especially around lips and nail beds

Gastrointestinal Manifestations

- Decreased motility
- Diminished or absent bowel sounds
- Nausea and vomiting
- Constipation

Neuromuscular Manifestations

Early

- Anxiety
- Restlessness
- Increased thirst

Late

- Decreased central nervous system activity (lethargy to coma)
- Generalized muscle weakness
- Diminished or absent deep tendon reflexes
- Sluggish pupillary response to light

Kidney Manifestations

- Decreased urine output
- Increased specific gravity
- Sugar and acetone present in urine

Integumentary Manifestations

- Cool to cold
- Pale to mottled to cyanotic
- Moist, clammy
- Mouth dry; pastelike coating present

$Paco_2$, Partial pressure of arterial carbon dioxide; *Pao_2*, partial pressure of arterial oxygen.

pressure (MAP) and may be started either by nerve changes *(neural-induced)* or by the presence of some chemicals *(chemical-induced)*.

Neural-induced distributive shock is a loss of MAP that occurs when sympathetic nerve impulses are decreased and blood vessel smooth muscles relax, causing vasodilation and poor perfusion. Shock results when vasodilation is widespread. Problems leading to loss of sympathetic tone are listed in Table 37-1.

Chemical-induced distributive shock has three common origins: anaphylaxis, sepsis, and capillary leak syndrome. It occurs when certain body chemicals or foreign substances in the blood and vessels start widespread changes in blood vessel walls. The chemicals are usually **exogenous** (originate outside the body), but this type of shock also can be induced by substances normally found in the body, such as excessive amounts of histamine.

Anaphylaxis is an extreme type I allergic reaction. It begins within seconds to minutes after exposure to a specific allergen in a susceptible person. The result is widespread loss of blood vessel tone, with decreased blood pressure and decreased cardiac output. Table 20-2 (in Chapter 20) lists common allergens that can cause anaphylaxis. Chapter 20 describes the pathophysiology, prevention, and care of the patient with anaphylactic shock.

Sepsis is a widespread infection that triggers whole-body INFLAMMATION. It leads to distributive shock when infectious microorganisms are present in the blood and is most commonly called **septic shock**. A complete discussion of the pathophysiology, prevention, and care for the patient with sepsis and septic shock begins on p. 748.

Capillary leak syndrome is the response of capillaries to the presence of body chemicals that enlarge capillary pores and allow fluid to shift from the capillaries into the interstitial tissues. Once in the interstitial tissue, these fluids are stagnant and cannot deliver oxygen or remove tissue waste products. Problems causing fluid shifts include severe burns, liver disorders, ascites, peritonitis, large wounds, kidney disease, hypoproteinemia, and trauma.

Obstructive shock is caused by problems that impair the ability of the normal heart to pump effectively. The heart itself remains normal, but conditions outside the heart prevent either adequate filling of the heart or adequate contraction of the healthy heart muscle. The most common cause of obstructive shock is cardiac tamponade (Table 37-1). Care of the person with cardiac tamponade is presented in Chapter 35 (pericarditis) and Chapter 38.

Although the causes and initial manifestations associated with the different types of shock vary, eventually the effects of hypotension and **anaerobic cellular metabolism** (metabolism without oxygen) result in the common key features of shock listed in Chart 37-1.

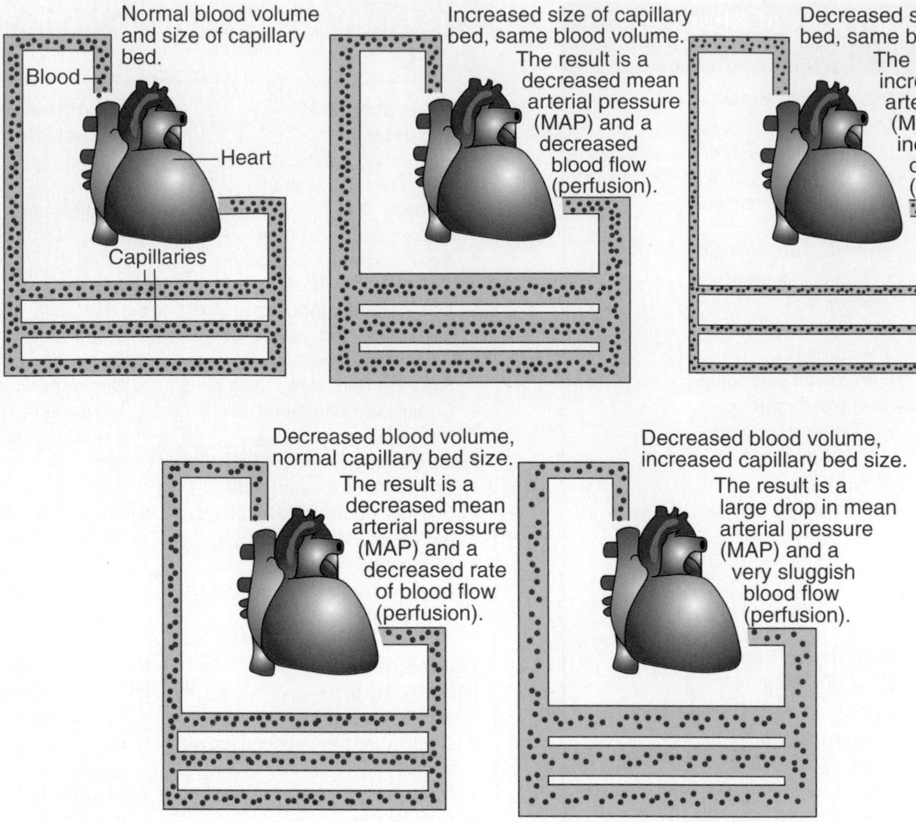

FIG. 37-2 Interaction of blood volume and the size of the capillary bed affecting mean arterial pressure (MAP).

HYPOVOLEMIC SHOCK

❖ *PATHOPHYSIOLOGY*

The basic problem of hypovolemic shock is a loss of blood volume from the vascular space, resulting in a decreased mean arterial pressure (MAP) (see Fig. 37-2) and a loss of oxygen-carrying capacity from the loss of circulating red blood cells (RBCs). The reduced MAP slows blood flow, decreasing tissue PERFUSION. The loss of RBCs decreases the ability of the blood to oxygenate the tissue it does reach. These oxygenation and perfusion problems lead to *anaerobic* (without oxygen) cellular metabolism.

The main trigger leading to hypovolemic shock is a sustained decrease in MAP from decreased circulating blood volume. A decrease in MAP of 5 to 10 mm Hg below the patient's normal baseline value is detected by pressure-sensitive nerve receptors *(baroreceptors)* in the aortic arch and carotid sinus. This information is transmitted to brain centers, which stimulate adjustments *(compensatory mechanisms)* to help ensure continued blood flow and oxygen delivery to vital organs while limiting blood flow to less vital areas. The movement of blood into selected areas while bypassing others ("shunting") results in some shock manifestations.

If the events that caused the initial decrease in MAP are halted now, compensatory mechanisms provide adequate oxygenation and PERFUSION without intervention. If events continue and MAP decreases further, some tissues function under anaerobic conditions. This condition increases lactic acid levels and other harmful metabolites (e.g., protein-destroying enzymes, oxygen free radicals) (McCance et al., 2014). These substances cause acid-base imbalances with tissue-damaging effects and depressed heart muscle activity. These effects are temporary and reversible if the cause of shock is corrected within 1 to 2 hours after onset. When shock conditions continue for longer periods without help, the resulting acid-base imbalance and increased metabolites cause so much cell damage in vital organs that they are unable to perform their critical functions. When this problem, known as multiple organ dysfunction syndrome (MODS), occurs to the extent that vital organs die, recovery from shock is no longer possible (see the section on the Refractory Stage of Shock on p. 742). Table 37-2 summarizes the progression of shock.

Stages of Shock

The syndrome of shock progresses in four stages when the conditions that cause shock remain uncorrected and poor cellular oxygenation continues. These stages are:

1. Initial stage
2. Nonprogressive stage
3. Progressive stage
4. Refractory stage

Initial Stage of Shock. The initial (early) stage of shock is present when the patient's baseline MAP is decreased by less than 10 mm Hg. Compensatory mechanisms are so effective at returning systolic pressure to normal during this stage that oxygen PERFUSION to vital organs is maintained. The cellular change in this stage is increased anaerobic metabolism in some tissues with production of lactic acid, although overall metabolism is still aerobic. The compensation responses of vascular constriction and increased heart rate are effective, and both cardiac output and MAP are maintained within the normal range. Because vital organ function is not disrupted, the

TABLE 37-2 Adaptive Responses and Events During Hypovolemic Shock

Initial Stage
- Decrease in mean arterial pressure (MAP) of 5-10 mm Hg from baseline value
- Increased sympathetic stimulation
  - Mild vasoconstriction
  - Increased heart rate

Progressive Stage
- Decrease in MAP of >20 mm Hg from baseline value
- Anoxia of nonvital organs
- Hypoxia of vital organs
- Overall metabolism is anaerobic
  - Moderate acidosis
  - Moderate hyperkalemia
  - Tissue ischemia

Nonprogressive Stage
- Decrease in MAP of 10-15 mm Hg from baseline value
- Continued sympathetic stimulation
  - Moderate vasoconstriction
  - Increased heart rate
  - Decreased pulse pressure
- Chemical compensation
  - Renin, aldosterone, and antidiuretic hormone secretion
    Increased vasoconstriction
    Decreased urine output
    Stimulation of the thirst reflex
- Some anaerobic metabolism in nonvital organs
  - Mild acidosis
  - Mild hyperkalemia

Refractory Stage
- Severe tissue hypoxia with ischemia and necrosis
- Release of myocardial depressant factor from the pancreas
- Buildup of toxic metabolites
- Multiple organ dysfunction syndrome (MODS)
- Death

manifestations of shock are difficult to detect at this stage. *A heart and respiratory rate increased from the patient's baseline level or a slight* ***increase*** *in diastolic blood pressure may be the only manifestation of this stage of shock.*

Nonprogressive Stage. The nonprogressive (compensatory) stage of shock occurs when MAP decreases by 10 to 15 mm Hg from baseline. Kidney and hormonal compensatory mechanisms are activated because cardiovascular responses alone are not enough to maintain MAP and supply oxygen to vital organs.

The ongoing decrease in MAP triggers the release of renin, antidiuretic hormone (ADH), aldosterone, epinephrine, and norepinephrine to start kidney compensation. Urine output decreases, sodium reabsorption increases, and widespread blood vessel constriction occurs. ADH increases water reabsorption in the kidney, further reducing urine output, and increases blood vessel constriction in the skin and other less vital tissue areas. Together these actions compensate for shock by maintaining the fluid volume within the central blood vessels.

Tissue hypoxia occurs in nonvital organs (e.g., skin, GI tract) and in the kidney, but it is not great enough to cause permanent damage. Acid-base and electrolyte changes occur in response to the buildup of metabolites. Changes include **acidosis** (low blood pH) and **hyperkalemia** (increased blood potassium level).

Manifestations of this stage include changes resulting from decreased tissue PERFUSION. Subjective changes include thirst and anxiety. Objective changes include restlessness, tachycardia, increased respiratory rate, decreased urine output, falling systolic blood pressure, rising diastolic blood pressure, narrowing pulse pressure, cool extremities, and a 2% to 5% decrease in oxygen saturation. *Comparing these changes with the values and manifestations obtained earlier is critical to identifying this stage of shock.*

If the patient is stable and compensatory mechanisms are supported by medical and nursing interventions, he or she can remain in this stage for hours without having permanent damage. *Stopping the conditions that started shock and providing supportive interventions can prevent the shock from progressing.* The effects of this stage are reversible when nurses recognize the problem and coordinate the health care team to start appropriate interventions.

Progressive Stage of Shock. The progressive stage of shock occurs when there is a sustained decrease in MAP of more than 20 mm Hg from baseline. Compensatory mechanisms are functioning but can no longer deliver sufficient oxygen, even to vital organs. Vital organs develop hypoxia, and less vital organs become **anoxic** (no oxygen) and **ischemic** (cell dysfunction or death from lack of oxygen). As a result of poor PERFUSION and a buildup of metabolites, some tissues die.

Manifestations of the progressive stage of shock include a *worsening* of changes resulting from decreased tissue PERFUSION. The patient may express a sense of "something bad" (impending doom) about to happen. He or she may seem confused, and thirst increases. Objective changes are a rapid, weak pulse; low blood pressure; pallor to cyanosis of oral mucosa and nail beds; cool and moist skin; anuria; and a 5% to 20% decrease in oxygen saturation. Laboratory data at this stage may show a low blood pH, along with rising lactic acid and potassium levels.

! NURSING SAFETY PRIORITY (QSEN)

Critical Rescue

The progressive stage of shock is a life-threatening emergency. Vital organs can tolerate this situation for only a short time before developing multiple organ dysfunction syndrome (MODS) and being damaged permanently. Immediate interventions are needed to reverse the effects of this stage of shock. The patient's life usually can be saved if the conditions causing shock are corrected within 1 hour or less of the onset of the progressive stage. Continuously monitor and compare with earlier findings to assess therapy effectiveness and determine when therapy changes are needed.

Refractory Stage of Shock and Multiple Organ Dysfunction Syndrome. The refractory stage of shock occurs when too much cell death and tissue damage result from too little oxygen reaching the tissues. Vital organs have extensive damage and cannot respond effectively to interventions, and shock continues. So much damage has occurred with release of metabolites and enzymes that damage to vital organs continues despite interventions.

The sequence of cell damage caused by massive release of toxic metabolites and enzymes is termed **multiple organ dysfunction syndrome (MODS)**. Once the damage has started, the sequence becomes a vicious cycle as more dead and dying cells open and release metabolites. These trigger small clots (microthrombi) to form, which block tissue PERFUSION and damage more cells, continuing the devastating cycle. Liver, heart, brain, and kidney function are lost first. The most profound change is damage to the heart muscle.

Manifestations are a rapid loss of consciousness; nonpalpable pulse; cold, dusky extremities; slow, shallow respirations; and unmeasurable oxygen saturation. *Therapy is not effective in saving the patient's life, even if the cause of shock is corrected and MAP temporarily returns to normal.*

Etiology

Hypovolemic shock occurs when too little circulating blood volume causes a MAP decrease that prevents total body PERFUSION and oxygenation. Problems leading to hypovolemic shock are listed in Table 37-1.

Hypovolemic shock from external hemorrhage is common after trauma and surgery. Hypovolemic shock from internal hemorrhage occurs with blunt trauma, GI ulcers, and poor control of surgical bleeding. Hemorrhage leading to hypovolemia also can be caused by any problem that reduces the levels of CLOTTING factors (see Table 37-1). Hypovolemia as a result of dehydration can be caused by any problem that decreases fluid intake or increases fluid loss (see Table 37-1).

Incidence and Prevalence

The exact incidence of hypovolemic shock is not known because it is a response rather than a disease. It is a common complication among hospitalized patients in emergency departments and after surgery or invasive procedures.

Health Promotion and Maintenance

Hypovolemic shock from most causes can be prevented. Teach all people to prevent dehydration by having an adequate fluid intake during exercise and when in hot, dry environments. Urge people to prevent trauma and hemorrhage by using proper safety equipment and seat belts and being aware of hazards in the home or workplace.

Recognizing hypovolemic shock is a major nursing responsibility. Keep in mind that just being a patient in the acute care setting is a risk factor. Also identify patients at risk for dehydration, and assess for early manifestations. This is especially important for those who have reduced cognition or reduced mobility or who are on NPO status.

Assess all patients with invasive procedures or trauma for obvious or occult impaired CLOTTING with bleeding. Compare pulse quality and rate with baseline. Compare urine output with fluid intake. Check vital signs of patients who have persistent thirst. Assess for shock in any patient who develops a change in mental status, an increase in pain, or an increase in anxiety.

Teach patients who have invasive procedures in an ambulatory setting the manifestations of shock. Stress the importance of seeking immediate help for obvious heavy bleeding, persistent thirst, decreased urine output, light-headedness, or a sense of impending doom (a feeling that something bad is happening or going to happen).

❖ PATIENT-CENTERED COLLABORATIVE CARE

The Concept Map on p. 744 addresses assessment and nursing care issues related to hypovolemic shock.

◆ Assessment

History. Ask about risk factors related to hypovolemic shock. If the patient is alert, question him or her directly. If the patient is not alert, collect information from family members. *Age* is important because shock from trauma is more common in young adults and other types of shock are more common in older adults. Ask about recent illness, trauma, procedures, or chronic health problems that may lead to shock (e.g., GI ulcers, general surgery, hemophilia, liver disorders, prolonged vomiting or diarrhea). Ask about the use of drugs such as aspirin, other NSAIDs, and diuretics that may cause changes leading to hypovolemic shock.

Ask about fluid intake and output during the previous 24 hours. *Information about urine output is especially important because urine output is reduced during the first stages of shock, even when fluid intake is normal.*

Assess the patient for factors that can lead to shock. Areas to examine for poor CLOTTING and hemorrhage include the gums, wounds, and sites of dressings, drains, and vascular accesses. Also check *under* the patient for blood. Observe for any swelling or skin discoloration that may indicate an internal hemorrhage.

Physical Assessment/Clinical Manifestations. Most manifestations of hypovolemic shock are caused by the changes resulting from compensatory efforts. **Compensatory mechanisms** are physiologic responses that try to keep an adequate PERFUSION to vital organs. Shock may be first evident as changes in cardiovascular function. As shock progresses, changes in the renal, respiratory, integumentary, musculoskeletal, and central nervous systems become evident. Ensure that vital sign measurements are accurate, and monitor them for trends indicating shock.

! NURSING SAFETY PRIORITY (QSEN)

Action Alert

Assign a registered nurse rather than a licensed practical nurse/licensed vocational nurse (LPN/LVN) or unlicensed assistive personnel (UAP) to assess the vital signs of a patient who is at risk for or suspected of having hypovolemic shock.

Cardiovascular changes that occur with hypovolemic shock start with decreased mean arterial pressure (MAP) leading to compensatory responses. Assess the central and peripheral pulses for rate and quality. In the initial stage of shock, the pulse rate increases to keep cardiac output and MAP at normal levels, even though the actual **stroke volume** (amount of blood pumped out from the heart) per beat is decreased. *Increased heart rate is the first manifestation of shock.* Because stroke volume is decreased, the peripheral pulses are difficult to palpate and are blocked with light pressure. As shock progresses, peripheral pulses may be absent.

When assessing the blood pressure (BP), consider the patient's normal baseline blood pressure. Although a blood pressure of 90/50 mm Hg may indicate severe shock in one person, it may be the normal blood pressure for another healthy adult.

! NURSING SAFETY PRIORITY (QSEN)

Action Alert

Because changes in systolic blood pressure are not always present in the initial stage of shock, use changes in pulse rate and quality as the main indicators of shock presence or progression.

CONCEPT MAP

INFECTION · CLOTTING · HYPOVOLEMIC SHOCK · INFLAMMATION · PERFUSION

HISTORY

A 59 year-old involved in a motor vehicle crash comes to the ED in a confused and restless state with HR 120 (weak and thready), RR 24, BP 102/76 mm Hg. No open wounds, abdomen distended, hypoactive bowel sounds.

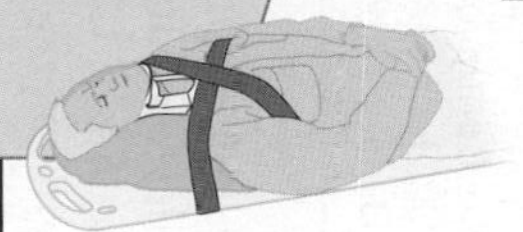

Physical Assessment/ Clinical Manifestations

Subjective signs: Thirst, anxiety

Objective signs: Restlessness, rapid, weak pulse, ↑ RR, ↓ U/O, ↓ systolic BP, ↑ diastolic BP (narrowing pulse pressure), cool extremities, ↓ O_2 sat, pallor, cyanosis, ↓ pH, ↑ lactic acid, ↑ K^+

Causes

- Hemorrhage after blunt trauma
- Hemorrhage that reduces levels of clotting factors.

Data Synthesis

Patient Problems

- Hypoxia related to hypovolemia
- Inadequate PERFUSION related to active fluid volume loss and hypotension
- Anxiety related to potential for death and decreased cerebral PERFUSION
- Acute confusion related to decreased cerebral PERFUSION

Planning

EXPECTED OUTCOMES

Maintain normal aerobic cellular metabolism as evidenced by:

- Clear thought processes
- MAP <10 mm Hg from baseline
- BP, HR, RR, ABGs, O_2 saturation return to baseline
- U/O significantly >30 mL/hr
- No development of complications by supportive and drug therapies

INTERVENTIONS

1 Nursing Priority – Ensuring a Patent Airway

- Administer oxygen; monitor and respond to: ↑ RR, shallow depth; ↓ $PaCO_2$; ↓ PaC_2; cyancsis, especially around lips and nail beds. *Monitors for progression of shock and inadequate* PERFUSION.
- Assess oxygen saturation through pulse oximetry. *Indicates life-threatening emergency when O_2 saturation is below 70%.*

2 Nursing Safety Priority: Critical Rescue!

Do not leave the patient. RN (not LPN or UAP) must assess vital signs. *An unstable patient requires the assessment skills of an RN.*

3 Assessment of Vital Signs in Shock

Monitor vital signs at least every 15 minutes until shock is controlled and patient's condition improves. Assess pulse (rate, regularity, quality), blood pressure, pulse pressure, central venous pressure, respiratory rate, skin and mucosal color, oxygen saturation, cognition, and urine output. *Determines the patient's condition and the effectiveness of therapy.*

4 Nursing Safety Priority: Action Alert!

Use changes in pulse rate and quality as the main indicators of shock presence or progression. *Changes in systolic blood pressure are not always present in the initial stage of shock.*

5 Minimizing Bleeding

- Apply direct pressure for overt bleeding. Check *under* the patient for blood. Observe for swelling or skin discoloration. *Discoloration may indicate internal hemorrhage.*
- Prepare the patient for surgical intervention. *Corrects internal bleeding for the patient's survival.*

6 Fluid Replacement Therapy

Increase the rate of IV fluid delivery: crystalloids, colloids, and/or blood products. *Restores fluid volume and improves perfusion to vital organs which is the primary intervention for hypovolemic shock.*

7 Nursing Safety Priority: Action Alert!

Use only normal saline for infusion with blood or blood products. *Calcium in Ringer's lactate induces clotting of the infusing blood.*

8 Drug Therapy

Administer drugs for shock, vasoconstrictors, inotropic agents, and/or drugs that enhance cardiac perfusion when volume loss is severe and the patient does not respond sufficiently to fluid replacement and blood products. *Increases likelihood to recover from shock by increasing venous return, improving cardiac contractility, or improving cardiac* PERFUSION *by dilating the coronary vessels.*

9 Nursing Safety Priority: Drug Alert!

Monitor the patient closely. *Drugs that dilate coronary blood vessels, such as nitroprusside, can cause systemic vasodilation and increase shock if the patient is volume depleted. Drugs that increase heart muscle contraction increase heart oxygen consumption and can cause angina or infarction.*

Concept Map by Deanne A. Blach, MSN, RN

With vasoconstriction, diastolic pressure increases but systolic pressure remains the same. As a result, the difference between the systolic and diastolic pressures *(pulse pressure)* is smaller or "narrower." Monitor blood pressure for changes from baseline levels and for changes from the previous measurement. For accuracy, use the same equipment on the same extremity. Validate an abnormal electronic BP reading with a manual BP reading.

Systolic pressure decreases as shock progresses and cardiac output decreases. A reduced systolic pressure narrows the pulse pressure even further. When shock continues and interventions are not adequate, compensation fails and both systolic and diastolic pressures decrease and blood pressure is difficult to hear. Palpation or a Doppler device may be needed to detect the systolic blood pressure.

Oxygen saturation is assessed through pulse oximetry. Pulse oximetry values between 90% and 95% occur with the nonprogressive stage of shock, and values between 75% and 80% occur with the progressive stage of shock. *Any value below 70% is considered a life-threatening emergency and may signal the refractory stage of shock.*

Respiratory changes with shock are an adaptive response to help maintain oxygenation when tissue PERFUSION is decreased. Assess the rate and depth of respiration. Respiratory rate increases during shock to ensure that oxygen intake is increased so that it can be delivered to critical tissues. When shock progresses to the stage at which lactic acidosis is present, the respiratory depth also increases.

Kidney and urinary changes occur with shock to compensate for decreased MAP by saving body water through decreased filtration and increased water reabsorption. Assess urine for volume, color, specific gravity, and the presence of blood or protein. *Decreased urine output is a sensitive indicator of early shock. Measure urine output at least every hour. In severe shock, urine output may be absent.* Of the four vital organs (heart, brain, liver, and kidney), only the kidney can tolerate hypoxia and anoxia for up to 1 hour without permanent damage. When hypoxia or anoxia persists beyond this time, patients are at risk for acute kidney injury (AKI) and kidney failure.

Skin changes occur because of reduced blood flow in the skin. An early compensatory mechanism is skin blood vessel constriction, which reduces skin PERFUSION. This allows more blood to perfuse the vital organs, which cannot tolerate low oxygen levels.

Assess the skin for temperature, color, and moisture. With shock, it feels cool or cold to the touch and is moist. Color changes appear first in oral mucous membranes and in the skin around the mouth. In dark-skinned patients, pallor or cyanosis is best assessed in the oral mucous membranes. Other color changes are noted first in the skin of the extremities and then in the central trunk area. The skin feels clammy or moist to the touch, not because sweating increases but because the normal fluid lost through the skin does not evaporate well on cool skin. As shock progresses, skin becomes mottled. Lighter-skinned patients have an overall grayish blue color and darker-skinned patients appear darker, without an underlying reddish glow.

Evaluate capillary refill time by pressing on the patient's fingernail until it blanches and then observing how fast the nail bed resumes color when pressure is released. Normally these capillaries resume color as soon as pressure is released. With shock, capillary refill is slow or may be absent. Capillary refill is not a reliable indicator for peripheral blood flow in older patients or those with anemia, diabetes, or peripheral vascular disease.

Central nervous system (CNS) changes with shock first manifest as thirst. Thirst is caused by stimulation of the thirst centers in the brain in response to decreased blood volume.

Assess the patient's level of consciousness (LOC) and orientation. CNS changes with shock are caused by cerebral hypoxia. In the initial and nonprogressive stages, patients may be restless or agitated and may be anxious or have a feeling of impending doom that has no obvious cause. As hypoxia progresses, confusion and lethargy occur. Lethargy progresses to somnolence and loss of consciousness as cerebral hypoxia worsens with shock progression.

Skeletal muscle changes during shock include weakness and pain in response to tissue hypoxia and anaerobic metabolism, which are later manifestations. Weakness is generalized and has no specific pattern. Deep tendon reflexes are decreased or absent.

Assess muscle strength by having the patient squeeze your hand and by trying to keep his or her arms flexed while you attempt to straighten them. Assess deep tendon reflexes by lightly tapping the patellar tendons and Achilles tendons with a reflex hammer and observing the degree of responsive movement.

Psychosocial Assessment. *Changes in mental status and behavior occur early in shock.* Observe the patient closely, and document behavior. Assess mental status by evaluating LOC and noting whether the patient is asleep or awake. If the patient is asleep, attempt to awaken him or her and document how easily he or she is aroused. If the patient is awake, determine whether he or she is oriented to person, place, and time. Avoid asking questions that can be answered with a "yes" or a "no" response. Consider these points during assessment:

- Is it necessary to repeat questions to obtain a response?
- Does the response answer the question asked?
- Does the patient have difficulty making word choices?
- Is the patient irritated or upset by the questions?
- Can the patient concentrate on a question long enough to answer, or is the attention span limited?

Talk with the family to determine whether the patient's behavior and cognition are typical or represent a change.

NCLEX EXAMINATION CHALLENGE

Physiological Integrity

Which manifestations of shock are a result of compensatory mechanisms to maintain circulating blood volume?

A. Edema and weight gain
B. Confusion and lethargy
C. Decreased urine output and thirst
D. Increased pulse and respiratory rates

Laboratory Assessment. Although no single test confirms or rules out shock, changes in laboratory data may support the diagnosis. Chart 37-2 lists laboratory changes occurring with hypovolemic shock. As shock progresses, arterial blood gas values become abnormal. The pH decreases, the partial pressure of arterial oxygen (Pao_2) decreases, and the partial pressure of arterial carbon dioxide ($Paco_2$) increases. Other laboratory changes occur with specific causes of hypovolemic shock.

Hematocrit and hemoglobin levels decrease if shock is caused by poor CLOTTING and hemorrhage. When shock is

CHART 37-2 Laboratory Profile

Hypovolemic Shock

TEST	NORMAL RANGE FOR ADULTS	SIGNIFICANCE OF ABNORMAL FINDINGS
pH (arterial)	7.35-7.45	Decreased: insufficient tissue oxygenation causing anaerobic metabolism and acidosis
Pao_2	80-100 mm Hg	Decreased: anaerobic metabolism
$Paco_2$	35-45 mm Hg	Increased: anaerobic metabolism
Lactic acid (arterial)	3-7 mg/dL 0.3-0.8 mmol/L	Increased: anaerobic metabolism with buildup of metabolites
Hematocrit	*Females:* 37%-47% *Males:* 42%-52%	Increased: fluid shift, dehydration Decreased: hemorrhage
Hemoglobin	*Females:* 12-16 g/dL *Males:* 14-18 g/dL	Increased: fluid shift, dehydration Decreased: hemorrhage
Potassium	3.5-5.0 mEq/L or mmol/L	Increased: dehydration, acidosis

Pagana, K., & Pagana, T. (2014). *Mosby's manual of diagnostic and laboratory tests* (5th ed.). St. Louis: Mosby.

$Paco_2$, Partial pressure of arterial carbon dioxide; *Pao_2*, partial pressure of arterial oxygen.

caused by dehydration or a fluid shift, hematocrit and hemoglobin levels are elevated.

◆ *Analysis*

The priority NANDA-I nursing diagnoses and collaborative problems for patients with hypovolemic shock include:

- Hypoxia related to hypovolemia
- Inadequate perfusion related to active fluid volume loss and hypotension
- Anxiety related to potential for death and decreased cerebral perfusion (NANDA-I)
- Acute Confusion related to decreased cerebral perfusion (NANDA-I)

CLINICAL JUDGMENT CHALLENGE

Patient-Centered Care; Evidence-Based Practice; Safety QSEN

Your patient is a 40-year-old woman who is returned to your ambulatory care unit after having a cholecystectomy (gall bladder removal) performed as minimally invasive surgery by laparoscopy. After moving her from the stretcher to her bed, you take her vital signs. Her pulse is 118 and thready, blood pressure is 88/72, respiratory rate is 28, and pulse oxymetry is 88%. When you call her name, she opens her eyes but does not answer any questions.

1. What should you do first?
2. What manifestations of shock are present based on the information you currently have?
3. How would you classify this stage of shock? Provide a rationale for your evaluation.
4. What other assessment data should you obtain?
5. Given the type of surgery she has undergone, where would you expect bleeding to occur and what manifestations would indicate possible bleeding?
6. She still has an IV in her left hand infusing dextrose 5% in 0.45% saline. The post-surgical orders indicate that it should be removed when she is stable. Should you remove it now? Why or why not?

CHART 37-3 Best Practice for Patient Safety & Quality Care QSEN

The Patient in Hypovolemic Shock

- Ensure a patent airway.
- Insert an IV catheter, or maintain an established catheter.
- Administer oxygen.
- Elevate the patient's feet, keeping his or her head flat or elevated to no more than a 30-degree angle.
- Examine the patient for overt bleeding.
- If overt bleeding is present, apply direct pressure to the site.
- Administer drugs as prescribed.
- Increase the rate of IV fluid delivery.
- Do not leave the patient.

◆ *Interventions*

Medical and nursing interventions for patients in hypovolemic shock focus on reversing the shock, restoring fluid volume to the normal range, and preventing complications. Monitoring is critical to determine whether the patient is responding to therapy or whether shock is progressing and a change in intervention is needed. Surgery may be needed to correct the cause of shock. Chart 37-3 lists best practices for patients in hypovolemic shock.

Nonsurgical Management. The purposes of shock management are to maintain tissue oxygenation, increase vascular volume, and support compensatory mechanisms. Oxygen therapy, fluid replacement therapy, and drug therapy are useful.

Oxygen therapy is used at any stage of shock and is delivered by mask, hood, nasal cannula, endotracheal tube, or tracheostomy tube. It is given in liters per minute (L/min) by cannula or percentage concentration with a mask.

IV therapy for fluid resuscitation is a primary intervention for hypovolemic shock. Crystalloids and colloids are often used for volume replacement. Crystalloid solutions contain nonprotein substances (e.g., minerals, salts, sugars). Colloid solutions contain large molecules of proteins or starches (see Chapter 11).

Crystalloid fluids help maintain an adequate fluid and electrolyte balance. Two common solutions are normal saline and Ringer's lactate. Normal saline (0.9% sodium chloride in water) is a replacement solution used to increase plasma volume and can be infused with any blood product. Ringer's lactate contains sodium, chloride, calcium, potassium, and lactate. This isotonic solution expands volume, and the lactate buffers acidosis.

! NURSING SAFETY PRIORITY QSEN

Action Alert

Use only normal saline for infusion with blood or blood products because the calcium in Ringer's lactate induces clotting of the infusing blood.

Protein-containing colloid fluids help restore osmotic pressure and fluid volume. Blood and blood products are used when shock is caused by blood loss. These fluids include whole blood, packed red blood cells, and plasma.

Whole blood and packed red blood cells (PRBCs) increase hematocrit and hemoglobin levels along with fluid volume. PRBCs are given for moderate blood loss because they restore

CHART 37-4 **Common Examples of Drug Therapy**

Hypovolemic Shock

DRUGS	NURSING INTERVENTIONS	RATIONALES
Vasoconstrictors	**Improve mean arterial pressure by increasing peripheral resistance, increasing venous return, and increasing myocardial contractility.**	
Dopamine (Intropin, Revimine 🍁) Norepinephrine (Levophed) Phenylephrine HCl	Assess patient for chest pain.	Drugs increase myocardial oxygen consumption.
	Monitor urine output hourly.	Higher doses decrease kidney perfusion and urine output.
	Assess blood pressure every 15 min.	Hypertension is a manifestation of overdose.
	Assess the patient for headache.	Headache is an early manifestation of drug excess.
	Assess every 30 min for extravasation; check extremities for color and perfusion.	If the drug gets into the tissues, it can cause severe vasoconstriction, tissue ischemia, and tissue necrosis.
	Assess for chest pain.	Drug can cause rapid onset of vasoconstriction in the myocardium and impair cardiac oxygenation.
Inotropic Agents	**Directly stimulate beta adrenergic receptors on the heart muscle, improving contractility**	
Dobutamine (Dobutrex) Milrinone (Primacor)	Assess for chest pain.	Drugs increase myocardial oxygen consumption and can cause angina or infarction.
	Assess blood pressure every 15 min.	Hypertension is a manifestation of overdose.
Agents Enhancing Myocardial Perfusion	**Improve myocardial perfusion by dilating coronary arteries rapidly for a short time.**	
Sodium nitroprusside (Nitropress, Nipride 🍁)	Protect drug container from light.	Light degrades drug quickly.
	Assess blood pressure at least every 15 min.	Drug can cause systemic vasodilation and hypotension, especially in older adults.

the red blood cell deficit and improve oxygen-carrying capacity without adding excessive fluid volume. Massive transfusion therapy, defined as 10 units of PRBCs given within the first 6 hours of severe hemorrhage, can improve outcomes and prevent death from acute traumatic coagulopathy (Day et al., 2013). See Chapter 40 for nursing care during transfusion therapy.

Plasma, an acellular blood product containing clotting factors, is given to restore osmotic pressure when hematocrit and hemoglobin levels are normal. Plasma protein fractions (e.g., Plasmanate) and synthetic plasma expanders (e.g., hetastarch [hydroxyethyl starch, Hespan]) increase volume and are used for hypovolemic shock before a cause is identified.

Drug therapy is used in addition to fluid therapy when the volume lost is severe and the patient does not respond sufficiently to fluid replacement and blood products. Drugs for shock increase venous return, improve cardiac contractility, or improve cardiac PERFUSION by dilating the coronary vessels. Chart 37-4 lists common drugs used to treat shock.

! NURSING SAFETY PRIORITY QSEN

Drug Alert

Monitor the patient closely because drugs that dilate coronary blood vessels, such as nitroprusside, can cause systemic vasodilation and increase shock if the patient is volume depleted. Drugs that increase heart muscle contraction increase heart oxygen consumption and can cause angina or infarction.

Monitoring vital signs and level of consciousness is a major nursing action to determine the patient's condition and the effectiveness of therapy. Monitor these vital signs:

- Pulse (rate, regularity, and quality)
- Blood pressure
- Pulse pressure
- Central venous pressure (CVP)
- Respiratory rate
- Skin and mucosal color
- Oxygen saturation
- Cognition
- Urine output

Assess these parameters at least every 15 minutes until the shock is controlled and the patient's condition improves. Hemodynamic monitoring in critical care settings includes intra-arterial monitoring, mixed venous oxygen saturation (Svo_2), pulmonary artery monitoring, and pulmonary capillary wedge pressures.

Insertion of a CVP catheter allows pressure to be monitored in the patient's right atrium or superior vena cava while providing venous access. A decrease in CVP from baseline levels reflects hypovolemic shock with reduced venous return to the right atrium.

Intra-arterial catheters allow continuous blood pressure monitoring and are an access for arterial blood sampling. They are inserted into an artery (radial, brachial, femoral, or dorsalis pedis). The catheter is attached to pressure tubing and a transducer, which converts arterial pressure into an electrical signal seen as a waveform on an oscilloscope and as a numeric value.

Surgical Management. Surgical intervention in addition to nonsurgical management may be needed to correct the cause of shock. Such procedures include vascular repair, surgical hemostasis of major wounds, closure of bleeding ulcers, and chemical scarring (chemosclerosis) of varicosities.

Community-Based Care

Hypovolemic shock is a complication of another condition and is resolved before patients are discharged from the acute care setting. Because surgery and many other invasive procedures now occur on an ambulatory care basis, more patients at home are at increased risk for hypovolemic shock. Teach patients and family members the early manifestations of shock (increased thirst, decreased urine output, light-headedness, sense of apprehension) and to seek immediate medical attention if they appear.

NCLEX EXAMINATION CHALLENGE

Safe and Effective Care Environment

Which change in laboratory value or clinical manifestations in a client with hypovolemic shock indicates to the nurse that current therapy may need to be changed?

A. Urine output increases from 5 mL/hour to 6 mL/hour
B. Pulse pressure decreases from 28 mm Hg to 22 mm Hg
C. Serum potassium level increases from 3.6 mEq/L to 3.9 mEq/L
D. Core body temperature increases from 98.2°F (36.8°C) to 98.8°F (37.1°C)

SEPSIS AND SEPTIC SHOCK

❖ PATHOPHYSIOLOGY

Sepsis leading to septic shock is a complex type of distributive shock that usually begins as a bacterial or fungal infection and progresses to a critical emergency over a period of days. The progression of sepsis to septic shock is outlined in Fig. 37-3. *As progression occurs, the pathologic problems occur faster and to a greater degree. Thus control of sepsis and prevention of severe sepsis and septic shock are easier to achieve early in the process. Failure to recognize and intervene in early sepsis is a major factor for progression to septic shock and death.*

Infection

When INFECTION is confined to a local area, it should not lead to sepsis and shock. In the person whose immune system and inflammatory responses are effective, the presence of organism invasion first starts a helpful, local response of INFLAMMATION to confine and eliminate the organism and to prevent the infection from becoming worse or widespread.

The white blood cells (WBCs) in the area of invasion secrete cytokines to trigger local inflammation and bring more WBCs to kill the invading organisms. The results of this response constrict the small veins and dilate the arterioles in the area, which increases PERFUSION to locally infected tissues.

Capillary leak occurs, allowing plasma to leak into the tissues. This response causes swelling. The duration of INFLAMMATION depends on the size and severity of the INFECTION, but usually it subsides within a few days, when the infection has been managed by these responses. A benefit of inflammation is that it is limited only to the area of infection and stops as soon as it is no longer needed. The patient does not have fever, tachycardia, decreased oxygen saturation, or reduced urine output.

Sepsis and Systemic Inflammatory Response Syndrome

Sepsis is the presence of infection systemic manifestations (Dellinger et al., 2013). Infectious organisms have entered the bloodstream. As their numbers increase, widespread INFLAMMATION, known as *systemic inflammatory response syndrome (SIRS)*, is triggered as a result of INFECTION escaping local control. With the organisms and their toxins in the bloodstream and entering other body areas, inflammation is an enemy, leading to extensive hormonal, tissue, and vascular changes and oxidative stress that further impair oxygenation and tissue PERFUSION. The WBCs produce many pro-inflammation cytokines, especially interleukin-1 (IL-1), interleukin-6 (IL-6), and tumor necrosis factor-alpha (TNF-A or TNF-α) (Abbas et al., 2012). (See Chapter 17 for a discussion of cytokines.) As a result, there is widespread vasodilation and blood pooling (Schell-Chaple & Lee, 2014). The patient has mild hypotension, a low urine output, and an increased respiratory rate. These responses result in a hypodynamic state with decreased cardiac output. Body temperature varies depending on the duration of the sepsis and on WBC function. Some patients have a low-grade fever and others have a high fever. Still others may have a below-normal body temperature. Fever and hypotension result from SIRS. The reduced urine output and increased respiratory rate are compensatory responses to impaired oxygenation and perfusion. Often the patient has the elevated WBC count expected with a systemic infection.

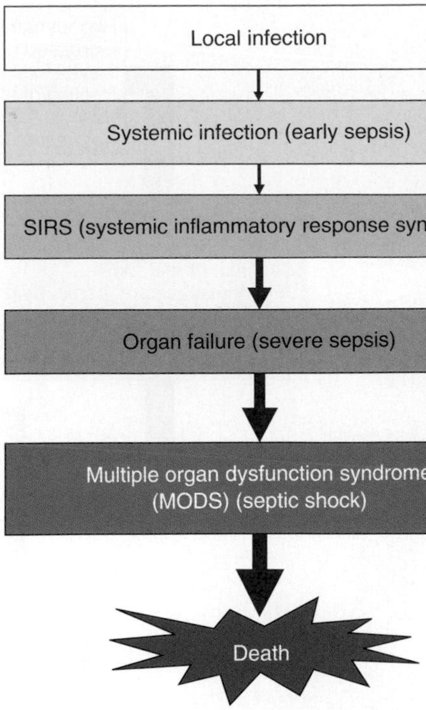

FIG. 37-3 Common progression of events leading to septic shock and multiple organ dysfunction syndrome (MODS).

Inappropriate CLOTTING with microthrombi forming in some organ capillaries causes hypoxia and reduces organ function. This problem is hard to detect, but if sepsis is stopped at this point, the organ damage is completely reversible. The microthrombi increase hypoxic conditions, which then generate more toxic metabolites. These damage more cells and increase the production of pro-inflammatory cytokines, leading to an amplification of SIRS and a vicious repeating cycle of poor oxygenation and PERFUSION (Fig. 37-4). Although these manifestations are subtle, they indicate sepsis and SIRS and will progress unless intervention begins now.

Unfortunately, this early hypodynamic state has a relatively short duration and manifestations are so subtle that the condition is often missed or misdiagnosed. When early sepsis and SIRS are identified and treated aggressively at this stage, the cycle of progression is stopped and the outcome is good. When sepsis and SIRS are not identified and treated at this stage, it progresses to severe sepsis, which is much harder to control. Nurses, as well as all other health care professionals, have a responsibility to identify cues that indicate sepsis before it becomes severe (Kleinpell et al., 2013). Identifying criteria have been established (Table 37-3) and must be used to ensure interventions are instituted at this stage.

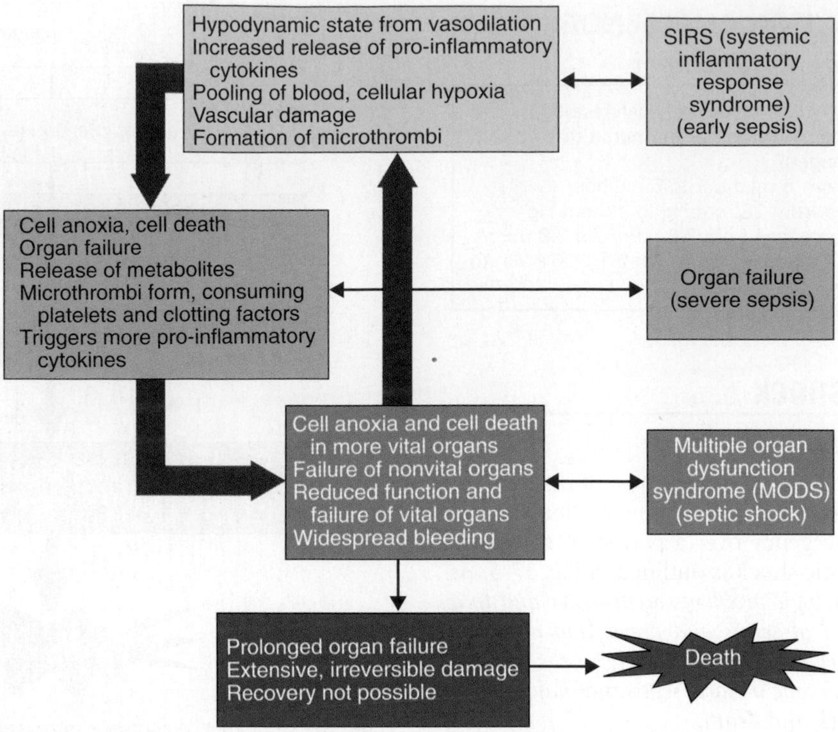

FIG. 37-4 Vicious cycle of systemic inflammatory response syndrome (SIRS) and multiple organ dysfunction syndrome (MODS) in septic shock.

TABLE 37-3 Sepsis with Systemic Inflammatory Response Syndrome (SIRS) Criteria

Suspected or identified infection with some of the following:

- Temperature of more than 101°F (38.3°C) or less than 96.8°F (36°C)
- Heart rate of more than 90 beats per minute
- Respiratory rate of more than 20 breaths per minute
- Abnormal WBC count (>12,000/mm^3 or <4000/mm^3)
- Normal WBC count with >10% bands
- Plasma C-reactive protein >2 standard deviations above normal
- Plasma prolactin >2 standard deviations above normal
- Arterial hypotension (SBP <90 mm Hg; MAP <70 mm Hg)
- Arterial hypoxemia (PaO_2/FiO_2 <300)
- Urine output <0.5 mL/kg/hr for 2 hours despite adequate fluid resuscitation
- Creatinine increase >0.5 mg/dL
- INR >1.5 or aPTT >60
- Absent bowel sounds
- Platelet count <100,000/mm^3
- Total bilirubin >4 mg/dL
- Elevated lactic acid (lactate) levels
- Decreased capillary refill or presence of mottling
- Hyperglycemia (plasma glucose >140 mg/dL or 7.7 mmol/L) in absence of diabetes
- Unexplained change in mental status
- Significant edema or positive fluid balance

Adapted from Dellinger, R.P., Levy, M., Rhodes, A., Annane, D., Gerlach, H., Opal, S.M., et al. (2013). Surviving sepsis campaign: International guidelines for management of severe sepsis and septic shock: 2012. *Critical Care Medicine, 41*(2), 580-637.

aPTT, Activated partial thromboplastin time; *FiO_2,* fraction of inspired oxygen; *INR,* international normalized ratio; *MAP,* mean arterial pressure; *PaO_2,* partial pressure of arterial oxygen; SBP, systolic blood pressure; *WBC,* white blood cell.

! NURSING SAFETY PRIORITY QSEN

Critical Rescue

Notify the health care provider or the Rapid Response Team for any patient who has vital signs or other conditions that meet the sepsis with SIRS criteria.

Severe Sepsis

Severe sepsis is sepsis plus sepsis-induced organ dysfunction or tissue hypoperfusion (Dellinger et al., 2013). It represents the progression of sepsis with an amplified SIRS (see Fig. 37-4). All tissues are involved and are hypoxic to some degree. Some organs are experiencing cell death and dysfunction at this time. Microthrombi formation is widespread with clots forming where they are not needed. This process uses up or consumes much of the available platelets and clotting factors, a condition known as *disseminated intravascular coagulation (DIC).* The amplified SIRS and cytokine release increase capillary leakiness, injure cells, and increase cell metabolism. Damage to endothelial cells reduces anticlotting actions and triggers the formation of even more small clots, increasing DIC. Anaerobic metabolism continues, and cell uptake of oxygen is poor. The continued stress response triggers the continued release of glucose from the liver and causes hyperglycemia. The more severe the response, the higher the blood glucose level (Kleinpell et al., 2013; Schell-Chaple & Lee, 2014).

Despite the severity of this stage and the fact that it may be present for 24 hours or more, it is often missed. One of the reasons it may be missed is that the cardiac function is hyperdynamic in this phase. The pooling of blood and the widespread capillary leak stimulate the heart, and cardiac output is *increased* with a more rapid heart rate and an elevated systolic blood pressure. In addition, the patient's extremities may feel warm and there is little or no cyanosis. Even though the patient may "look" better, the pathologic changes occurring at the tissue level are serious and have caused significant damage. The WBC count at this time may no longer be elevated. The reason for this is that a prolonged sepsis stage may have exceeded the bone marrow's ability to keep producing and releasing new mature neutrophils and other WBCs. The WBC count may be extremely low, especially the segmented neutrophils (segs).

Clinical manifestations of this stage include a lower oxygen saturation, rapid respiratory rate, decreased to absent urine output, and a change in the patient's cognition and affect. Appropriate and aggressive interventions at this stage can still prevent septic shock, although mortality after a patient reaches this stage is much higher than for sepsis and SIRS. *At this point, the down-hill course leading to septic shock is extremely rapid.*

Septic Shock

Septic shock is sepsis-induced hypotension persisting despite adequate fluid resuscitation. It is the stage of sepsis and SIRS when multiple organ dysfunction syndrome (MODS) with organ failure is evident and poor CLOTTING with uncontrolled bleeding occurs (see Fig. 37-4). *Even with appropriate intervention, the death rate among patients in this stage of sepsis is very high* (Dellinger et al., 2013). Severe hypovolemic shock and hypodynamic cardiac function are present as a result of an inability of the blood to clot because the platelets and clotting factors were consumed earlier. Vasodilation and capillary leak continue from vascular endothelial cell disruption, and cardiac contractility is poor from cellular ischemia. The clinical manifestations resemble the late stage of hypovolemic shock.

Etiology

The major cause of sepsis is a bacterial infection that escapes local control, although in immunocompromised patients, fungal infections also cause sepsis. Common organisms causing sepsis include gram-negative bacteria (*Pseudomonas aeruginosa, Escherichia coli,* and *Klebsiella pneumoniae*) and gram-positive bacteria (*Staphylococcus* and *Streptococcus*). Patients especially at risk for sepsis are those who are immunocompromised in any way and those who have central lines. Central lines in place even for short periods create a direct access point for microorganisms and can lead to central line–associated bloodstream infections (CLABSIs) (Dumont & Nesselrodt, 2012; Earhart, 2013). Table 37-4 lists some of the health problems that increase the risk for sepsis and septic shock.

TABLE 37-4 Conditions Predisposing to Sepsis and Septic Shock

• Malnutrition	• Infection with resistant microorganisms
• Immunosuppression	• Receiving cancer chemotherapy
• Large, open wounds	• Alcoholism
• Mucous membrane fissures in prolonged contact with bloody or drainage-soaked packing	• Diabetes mellitus
• GI ischemia	• Chronic kidney disease
• Exposure to invasive procedures	• Transplantation recipient
• Cancer	• Hepatitis
• Older than 80 years	• HIV/AIDS

AIDS, Acquired immune deficiency syndrome; *HIV,* human immune deficiency virus.

Incidence and Prevalence

Sepsis and septic shock are common events in the United States and throughout the world (Dellinger et al., 2013). Although sepsis management has improved, the incidence is increasing as a result of more drug-resistant organisms and the fact that patients are discharged from the hospital "quicker and sicker" (Lopez-Bushnell et al., 2014). Sepsis takes time to develop, and the patient may be discharged before manifestations are obvious.

Health Promotion and Maintenance

Prevention is the best management strategy for sepsis and septic shock. Evaluate all patients for their risk for sepsis, especially older adults because the death rate from sepsis in people older than 65 years is nearly twice that of younger adults. Table 37-4 lists some of the health problems that increase the risk for septic shock. Use aseptic technique during invasive procedures and when working with nonintact skin and mucous membranes in immunocompromised patients. Remove indwelling urinary catheters and IV access lines as soon as they are no longer needed. Ensure that patients receiving mechanical ventilation are weaned from the ventilator as soon as possible (Kleinpell et al., 2013).

Because sepsis can be a complication of many conditions found in acute care settings, always consider its possibility.

QUALITY IMPROVEMENT QSEN

Improving Nurse Recognition of Sepsis Indicators in the Emergency Department

Kilburn, F., Baily, P., & Price, D. (2013). Sepsis: Recognizing the next event. *Nursing2013, 43*(10), 14-16.

After prevention, the greatest positive factor for surviving sepsis is early recognition of the condition, which leads to implementation of the evidence-based interventions through early goal-directed therapy (EGDT). Recognition of the condition while patients are being seen in the emergency department (ED) can be challenging; however, delay of diagnosis significantly increases the risk for death (Dellenger et al., 2013). One rural Midwestern emergency department found that of the 42 patients admitted through the ED who were diagnosed after admission with sepsis or systemic inflammatory response syndrome (SIRS), 21 had two or more defining criteria while in the ED. Of these 21, only 3 were actually recognized and diagnosed in the ED. The Quality Management department determined that the greatest obstacle to early recognition of SIRS or sepsis was the seven-page assessment document that, although comprehensive, was time-consuming and minimally used by the ED nurses.

The stakeholders in the process developed a shorter, clearer, and more user-friendly SIRS and sepsis protocol consisting of a recognition and treatment order set based on the 2012 sepsis guidelines. In the first 3 months after developing this tool and incorporating it into the triage nurse admission data set, there was a 37% increase in the recognition of patients meeting SIRS and sepsis criteria in the ED.

Commentary: Implications for Practice and Research

Evidence-based practice has demonstrated that early recognition of patients with SIRS or sepsis is the first step in improving survival from this devastating condition. The implementation of a more user-friendly protocol in one ED has improved the step of recognition at one facility. Research measuring the final survival and cost outcomes based on speed of implementing EGDT is needed to determine how well early recognition is turned into early intervention through communication and teamwork.

Early detection of sepsis before progression to septic shock is a major nursing responsibility. The nurse is the health care professional most in contact with the patient and is in a unique position to detect subtle changes in appearance and behavior that can indicate sepsis. Use the assessment techniques described below for changes in vital signs, laboratory findings, appearance, and behavior to identify early any characteristics of sepsis and sepsis progression at least every shift for potentially infected, seriously ill patients (Kleinpell & Schorr, 2014). Using an evidence-based protocol to identify patients in the emergency department who may be in early sepsis on admission can improve the timing of implementing an appropriate sepsis bundle intervention (see the Quality Improvement box).

Early detection can be made by patients and families, as well as by health care personnel. This is especially important for patients discharged to home after invasive procedures or surgery. Teach patients the manifestations of local infection (local redness, pain, swelling, purulent drainage, loss of function) and of early sepsis (fever, urine output less than intake, lightheadedness). Teach them how to use a thermometer and to take the temperature twice a day and whenever they are not feeling well. Urge those with manifestations of early sepsis to immediately contact their health care provider. Teach them that if antibiotics are prescribed, to take these drugs as prescribed and to complete the entire course.

❖ PATIENT-CENTERED COLLABORATIVE CARE

◆ Assessment

Sepsis and septic shock differ from other types of shock in many ways. The entire syndrome may occur over many hours to days, and the manifestations are less obvious. The chance for recovery is good when the patient is recognized as having sepsis with SIRS and appropriate interventions are started within 6 hours. Septic shock, on the other hand, has a rapid downhill course and chances for recovery are relatively poor. Nurses identifying patients in the earlier stages of sepsis can make the greatest difference in survival.

History. Age is important because sepsis develops more easily among older, debilitated patients who are immunosuppressed (Touhy & Jett, 2014). Chart 37-5 lists factors that increase the older adult's risk for shock. Ask about the patient's medical history including recent illness, trauma, invasive procedures, or chronic conditions that may lead to sepsis. Check which drugs the patient has used in the past week. Some drugs may directly cause changes leading to shock. Also, a drug regimen may indicate a disorder or problem that can contribute to sepsis. These drugs include aspirin, corticosteroids, antibiotics, and cancer therapy drugs.

Physical Assessment/Clinical Manifestations. Manifestations of sepsis and septic shock occur over many hours, and some change during the progression. See Table 37-3 for a listing of specific manifestations and laboratory changes that often occur with sepsis and septic shock.

Cardiovascular changes differ in the different stages of sepsis and septic shock. Cardiac output and blood pressure are low in early sepsis and very low in septic shock. In severe sepsis, cardiac output is higher as are heart rate and blood pressure, although this is an indication of a worsening condition rather than an improvement. Increased cardiac output is reflected by tachycardia, increased stroke volume, a normal systolic blood pressure, and a normal central venous pressure (CVP). Increased cardiac output and vasodilation make the skin color appear normal with pink mucous membranes, and the skin is warm to the touch. This situation is temporary, and eventually the cardiac output is greatly reduced.

With progression, disseminated intravascular coagulation (DIC) occurs as a result of excessive CLOTTING with formation of thousands of small clots in the tiny capillaries of the liver, kidney, brain, spleen, and heart. DIC reduces PERFUSION and oxygenation and decreases oxygen saturation, causing hypoxia and ischemia.

The huge number of small clots uses clotting factors and fibrinogen faster than they can be produced, which eventually leads to poor CLOTTING. This increases the risk for hemorrhage, which occurs in the septic shock stage. Coupled with the continued capillary leak, the bleeding causes hypovolemia and a dramatic decrease in cardiac output, blood pressure, and pulse pressure. The manifestations of this phase are the same as those of the later stages of hypovolemic shock.

Respiratory changes are first caused by compensatory mechanisms that try to maintain oxygenation with a rate increase. As tissue hypoxia becomes more profound and acidosis is present, the depth of respiration also increases. The lungs are susceptible to damage, and the complication of acute respiratory distress syndrome (ARDS) may occur in septic shock. ARDS in septic shock is caused by the continued systemic inflammatory response syndrome (SIRS) increasing the formation of oxygen free radicals, which damage lung cells. *ARDS in a patient with septic shock has a high mortality rate.*

Skin changes differ at different stages of sepsis. In the hyperdynamic stage, the skin is warm and no cyanosis is evident. With progression to septic shock and compromised circulation, the skin is cool and clammy with pallor, mottling, or cyanosis. In DIC, petechiae and ecchymoses can occur anywhere. Blood may ooze from the gums, other mucous membranes, and venipuncture sites, as well as around IV catheters.

A kidney/urinary change of low urine output compared with fluid intake indicates shock. When a patient who has no known kidney or bladder problem suddenly starts having a low urine output, be suspicious of severe sepsis or septic shock. Reduced output is caused by capillary leak, low circulating volume, and hormonal changes. Kidney function decreases, and serum creatinine levels increase.

CHART 37-5 Nursing Focus on the Older Adult

Risk Factors for Shock

Hypovolemic Shock
- Diuretic therapy
- Diminished thirst reflex
- Immobility
- Use of aspirin-containing products
- Use of complementary therapies such as *Ginkgo biloba*
- Anticoagulant therapy

Cardiogenic Shock
- Diabetes mellitus
- Presence of cardiomyopathies

Distributive Shock
- Diminished immune response
- Reduced skin integrity
- Presence of cancer
- Peripheral neuropathy
- Strokes
- Being in a hospital or extended-care facility
- Malnutrition
- Anemia

Obstructive Shock
- Pulmonary hypertension
- Presence of cancer

Psychosocial Assessment. The indicator that patients may be in the beginning of severe sepsis is often a change in affect or behavior. Compare the patient's current behavior, verbal responses, and general affect with those assessed earlier in the day or the day before. They may seem just slightly different in their reactions to greetings, comments, or jokes. They may be less patient than usual or act restless or fidgety. Patients may make statements such as "I feel as if something is wrong, but I don't know what." If behavior is changed from prior assessments, consider the possibility of severe sepsis and shock.

Laboratory Assessment. No single laboratory test confirms the presence of sepsis and septic shock, although the hallmark of sepsis is an increasing serum lactate level, a normal or low total white blood cell (WBC) count, and a decreasing segmented neutrophil level with a rising band neutrophil level (left shift, see Chapter 17). The presence of bacteria in the blood supports the diagnosis of sepsis although this finding may not be present. Obtain specimens of urine, blood, sputum, and any drainage for culture to identify the causative organisms. Blood cultures should be taken before antibiotic therapy is started provided that this action does not delay antibiotic therapy by more than 45 minutes (Dellinger et al., 2013). Other abnormal laboratory findings that occur with septic shock include changes in the white blood cell (WBC) count; the differential leukocyte count may show a left shift. Hematocrit and hemoglobin levels usually do not change until late in septic shock. At that point, the hematocrit and hemoglobin levels, fibrinogen levels, and platelet count are low from disseminated intravascular coagulation (DIC). The serum lactate level is above normal, and the serum bicarbonate levels are lower than normal. Unfortunately, these parameters may take time to change and cannot be relied on as sensitive indicators of the patient's worsening condition.

Another indicator of sepsis and septic shock is a low blood level of activated protein C. Protein C is an enzyme that prevents inappropriate clot formation. It is activated when it binds to healthy vascular endothelial cells. In severe sepsis, the injured endothelial cells cannot activate protein C and thousands of small clots form in the capillaries of vascular organs. Decreasing levels of activated protein C indicate the beginning of severe sepsis even before other manifestations are evident.

Other biologic indicators of severe sepsis and septic shock are changes in plasma D-dimer levels and cytokine (interleukin-6 [IL-6] and interleukin-10 [IL-10]) levels. Plasma D-dimer levels rise during sepsis as the fibrin in clots is broken down. IL-6 is a pro-inflammatory cytokine, and IL-10 is an anti-inflammatory cytokine. In sepsis, IL-6 levels rise and IL-10 levels either remain normal or decrease. These indicators have a lag time, and changes may not be present soon enough to identify sepsis with SIRS before severe sepsis or septic shock develops.

Because the results of blood cultures may not be available until the patient's condition has progressed to severe sepsis or septic shock, other biomarkers for sepsis and SIRS are needed to help identify the condition when it can be managed and cured. Two such markers are increasing lactic acid levels and increasing prolactin levels.

The actual diagnosis of sepsis is difficult to make, yet the best outcome depends on an early diagnosis and the implementation of appropriate aggressive interventions within 6 hours. In general, sepsis is considered to exist when an infection is present along with some of the additional established criteria listed in Table 37-3.

TABLE 37-5 Bundles for Resuscitation and Management of Severe Sepsis

Surviving Sepsis Care Bundle

Within the first 3 hours of suspecting severe sepsis:

1. Measure serum lactate levels.
2. Obtain blood cultures *before* administering antibiotics.
3. Administer broad-spectrum antibiotics.
4. If either hypotension or a serum lactate level greater than 4 mmol/L (36 mg/dL) is present, administer 30 mL/kg crystalloids intravenously.

Within 6 hours of initial manifestations of suspected septic shock:

5. Administer prescribed vasopressors for hypotension that does not respond to initial fluid resuscitation measures to maintain MAP ≥65 mm Hg.
6. If arterial hypotension persists despite fluid volume resuscitation (indicating septic shock) or lactic acid remains ≥4 mmol/L (36 mg/dL), institute these assessments:
   - Measure central venous pressure.
   - Measure central venous oxygen saturation.
7. Re-measure lactic acid (lactate) level if initial value was elevated.

Data from Dellinger, R.P., Levy, M., Rhodes, A., Annane, D., Gerlach, H., Opal, S.M., et al. (2013). Surviving sepsis campaign: International guidelines for management of severe sepsis and septic shock: 2012. *Critical Care Medicine, 41*(2), 580-637; Kleinpell, R., Aitken, L., & Schorr, C. (2013). Implications of the new international sepsis guidelines for nursing care. *American Journal of Critical Care, 22*(3), 212-222.
MAP, Mean arterial pressure.

NCLEX EXAMINATION CHALLENGE
Safe and Effective Care Environment

Which clinical manifestation in a client alerts the nurse to the probability of septic shock instead of hypovolemic shock?
A. Hypotension
B. Pale, clammy skin
C. Decreased urine output
D. Oozing of blood at the IV site

◆ *Planning and Implementation*

The priority problem for patients with septic shock is potential for multiple organ dysfunction syndrome (MODS).

Planning: Expected Outcomes. With appropriate interventions, the patient with sepsis or septic shock is expected to have normal aerobic cellular metabolism. Indicators include:

- Arterial blood gases (pH, $Pa{O_2}$, and $Pa{CO_2}$) within the normal range
- Maintenance of a urine output of at least 20 mL/hr
- Maintenance of mean arterial blood pressure within 10 mm Hg of baseline
- Absence of multiple organ dysfunction syndrome (MODS)

Interventions. Interventions for sepsis and septic shock focus on identifying the problem as early as possible, correcting the conditions causing it, and preventing complications. The use of a sepsis resuscitation bundle for treatment of sepsis within 6 hours is the standard of practice. A *bundle* is a group of two or more specific interventions that have been shown to be effective when applied together or in sequence. The sepsis management bundle is presented in Table 37-5. Target outcomes of implementing the bundle are obtaining and maintaining a central venous pressure of 8 mm Hg or higher, central venous oxygen saturation of at least 70%, and return of lactic acid levels to normal (Kleinpell et al., 2013).

Oxygen therapy is useful whenever poor tissue PERFUSION and poor oxygenation are present. Oxygen is delivered in the same ways as for hypovolemic shock. However, the patient with septic shock is more likely to be mechanically ventilated. Care of the patient being mechanically ventilated is discussed in detail in Chapter 32.

Drug therapy to enhance cardiac output and restore vascular volume is essentially the same as that used in hypovolemic shock (see Chart 37-4). In addition, drug therapy is needed to combat sepsis, adrenal insufficiency, hyperglycemia, and clotting problems.

Although septic shock can be caused by any organism, the most common agents are gram-negative bacteria. In accordance with the recommendations of The Joint Commission's National Patient Safety Goals (NPSGs), IV antibiotics with known activity against gram-negative bacteria are given before organisms are identified, preferably within 1 hour of a sepsis diagnosis. Multiple drugs with wide activity are prescribed, based on the site of infection and the most common geographic infections, until the actual causative organism is known.

The stress of severe sepsis can cause adrenal insufficiency. Adrenal support may involve providing the patient with low-dose corticosteroids during the treatment period. Drugs used for this purpose are IV hydrocortisone and oral fludrocortisone (Florinef).

Patients with sepsis or septic shock usually have elevated blood glucose levels (>180 mg/dL), which is associated with a poor outcome. Insulin therapy is used to maintain blood glucose levels between 110 mg/dL and 150 mg/dL. Keeping the blood glucose level below 110 mg/dL is associated with increased mortality.

During severe sepsis, patients have microvascular abnormalities and form many small clots. Heparin therapy with fractionated heparin is used to limit inappropriate CLOTTING and to prevent the excessive consumption of clotting factors.

Blood replacement therapy is used when poor CLOTTING with hemorrhage occurs and may include clotting factors, platelets, fresh frozen plasma (FFP), or packed red blood cells. Chapter 40 discusses in detail the care of the patient during blood replacement. The use of platelet transfusion is recommended ahead of other blood products for patients with septic shock to improve CLOTTING (Dellinger et al., 2013).

Community-Based Care

Identified sepsis should be resolved before patients are discharged from the acute care setting. Because more patients are receiving treatment on an ambulatory care basis and are being discharged earlier from acute care settings, more patients at home are at increased risk for sepsis.

Home Care Management. Evaluate the home environment for safety regarding infection hazards. Note the general cleanliness, especially in the kitchen and bathrooms. Chart 37-6 lists focused patient and environmental assessment data to obtain during a home visit.

Self-Management Education. Protecting frail patients from infection and sepsis at home is an important nursing function. Teach about the importance of self-care strategies, such as good hygiene, handwashing, balanced diet, rest and exercise, skin care, and mouth care. If patients or family members do not know how to take a temperature or read a thermometer, teach them and obtain a return demonstration. Teach patients and families to notify the health care provider immediately if fever or other signs of infection appear. General recommendations for Infection Precautions for patients at risk for sepsis are listed in Chart 22-4 in Chapter 22.

CHART 37-6 Home Care Assessment

The Patient at Risk for Sepsis

- Assess the patient for any clinical manifestations of infection, including:
  - Temperature, pulse, respiration, and blood pressure
  - Color of skin and mucous membranes
  - The mouth and perianal area for fissures or lesions
  - Any nonintact skin area for the presence of exudates, redness, increased warmth, swelling
  - Any pain, tenderness, or other discomfort anywhere
  - Cough or any other symptoms of a cold or the flu
  - Urine; or ask patient whether urine is dark or cloudy, has an odor, or causes pain or burning during urination
- Assess patient's and caregiver's adherence to and understanding of infection prevention techniques.
- Assess home environment, including:
  - General cleanliness
  - Kitchen and bathroom facilities, including refrigeration
  - Availability and type of soap for handwashing
  - Presence of pets, especially cats, rodents, or reptiles

◆ Evaluation: Outcomes

Evaluate the care of the patient with sepsis or septic shock. The expected outcome is that the patient will maintain normal aerobic cellular metabolism. Specific indicators for these outcomes are listed for the priority patient problem under the *Planning and Implementation* section (see earlier).

CLINICAL JUDGMENT CHALLENGE

Patient-Centered Care; Evidence-Based Practice; Safety QSEN

The patient is a 70-year-old man undergoing chemotherapy for lymphoma who was brought to the hospital by his wife because he was confused. His vital signs are: T = 95.7°F (35.4°C); P = 112; R = 28; BP = 96/50; SpO_2 = 84%. His health history includes type 2 diabetes, a myocardial infarction 10 years ago (he now has an "on-demand" pacemaker), and hypertension. In addition to chemotherapy, his current oral medications include metformin (Glucophage) 850 mg twice daily, losartan (Cozaar) 50 mg daily, and aspirin 81 mg daily. When you ask whether there have been any changes lately, the wife tells you that he had a "touch" of fungal pneumonia 6 weeks ago and still has a cough with sputum. He has been very uncomfortable for the past week with a "boil" near his rectum. When you assess his perianal region, you find a large raised red bump with an open area draining purulent fluid.

1. What risk factors does this man have for sepsis? Explain why each factor increases his risk.
2. What stage of the sepsis spectrum is he at this time and why?
3. Should you apply oxygen to him before he is seen by the health care provider? Why or why not?

The health care provider evaluates the patient and orders: IV with dextrose 5% in normal saline; IV amikacin (Amikin); cultures of the urine, blood, sputum, his central line, and any open skin areas; complete blood count with differential; and blood values for glucose and lactic acid.

4. Which intervention do you perform first and why?
5. What do you do next and why?

NURSING CONCEPTS AND CLINICAL JUDGMENT REVIEW

What might you NOTICE if the patient is experiencing inadequate oxygenation and tissue PERFUSION as a result of hypovolemic shock?

- Pulse rapid and thready
- Pulse pressure narrowed
- Respirations rapid and shallow
- Oxygen saturation by pulse oximetry decreased
- Skin cyanosis or pallor (for lighter-skinned patients)
- Skin cool and clammy
- Cyanosis or pallor of the lips and oral mucous membranes (for patients of any skin color)
- Patient is restless or anxious
- Patient has a urine output that is less than expected compared with fluid intake
- Patient states he or she is thirsty

What should you INTERPRET and how should you RESPOND to a patient experiencing inadequate oxygenation and tissue PERFUSION as a result of hypovolemic shock?

Perform and interpret physical assessment, including:

- Taking vital signs
- Auscultating all lung fields
- Monitoring oxygen saturation by pulse oximetry
- Assessing cognition
- Checking incisions, body orifices, and under the patient for signs of active bleeding
- Assessing the skin for bruises and petechiae
- Examining all body areas for swelling or discoloration that could indicate internal bleeding

Interpret laboratory values:

- Arterial blood gas values: pH lower than 7.35
- Elevated serum lactate levels
- Hemorrhage
  Decreased hematocrit and hemoglobin
  Decreased total red blood cells and platelets
- Dehydration
  Elevated red blood cell count, hematocrit, and hemoglobin
  Elevated white blood cell count

Respond by:

- Applying oxygen
- Assisting the patient to shock position (head and chest flat or elevated to no more than 30 degrees; legs elevated)
- Notifying the Rapid Response Team
- Ensuring placement of venous access
- Increasing IV fluid infusion rate

On what should you REFLECT?

- Observe patient for evidence of improved circulation and oxygenation (see Chapter 33).
- Think about what may have caused the hypovolemia.
- Think about how you may have identified the problem sooner.

GET READY FOR THE NCLEX® EXAMINATION!

KEY POINTS

Review these Key Points for each NCLEX Examination Client Needs Category.

Safe and Effective Care Environment

- Ensure vital sign measurements are accurate, and monitor them for changes indicating the presence of shock. **Safety** QSEN
- Identify patients at high risk for infection due to age, disease, or the environment. **Safety** QSEN
- Use the recommended criteria to assess for the presence of sepsis (see Table 37-3). **Evidence-Based Practice** QSEN
- Use strict aseptic techniques when performing invasive procedures, administering IV medications, changing dressings, and handling nonintact skin. **Safety** QSEN
- Use good handwashing techniques before providing any care to a patient who is either immunocompromised or immune deficient. **Safety** QSEN
- Assign a registered nurse rather than a licensed practical nurse/licensed vocational nurse (LPN/LVN) or unlicensed assistive personnel (UAP) to assess the vital signs of a patient who is at risk for or suspected of having hypovolemic shock. **Safety** QSEN
- Use only normal saline for infusion with blood or blood products.

Health Promotion and Maintenance

- Teach all people how to avoid dehydration. **Patient-Centered Care** QSEN
- Teach all people to use safety devices to avoid trauma. **Patient-Centered Care** QSEN
- Instruct all patients going home after surgery or invasive procedures to seek immediate attention for persistent manifestations of early shock. **Patient-Centered Care** QSEN
- Teach all patients who have a local infection to seek medical attention when manifestations of systemic infection appear. **Patient-Centered Care** QSEN

Psychosocial Integrity

- Assess all patients at risk for shock for a change in affect, reduced cognition, altered level of consciousness, and increased anxiety. **Patient-Centered Care** QSEN
- Stay with the patient in shock. **Patient-Centered Care** QSEN
- Reassure patients who are in shock that the appropriate interventions are being instituted. **Patient-Centered Care** QSEN

Physiological Integrity

- Be aware of the role of the systemic inflammatory response syndrome (SIRS) in the manifestations and progression of sepsis and septic shock. **Safety** QSEN

- Assess the immunocompromised patient every shift for infection. **Safety** QSEN
- Assess the skin integrity of the patient with reduced immune function at least every shift. **Patient-Centered Care** QSEN
- Immediately assess vital signs of patients who have a change in level of consciousness, increased thirst, or anxiety. **Evidence-Based Practice** QSEN
- Assess for changes in pulse rate and quality or a decrease in urine output rather than blood pressure as an indicator of shock. **Evidence-Based Practice** QSEN
- Give oxygen to any patient in shock. **Evidence-Based Practice** QSEN
- Assess hourly urine output to evaluate the adequacy of treatment for hypovolemic shock. **Evidence-Based Practice** QSEN
- Before administering prescribed antibiotics, obtain blood cultures and cultures of urine, wound drainage, and sputum for any patient suspected to have sepsis. **Evidence-Based Practice** QSEN
- Administer prescribed antibiotics within 1 hour of a diagnosis of sepsis. **Evidence-Based Practice** QSEN

CHAPTER 38

Care of Patients with Acute Coronary Syndromes

Laura M. Dechant

http://evolve.elsevier.com/Iggy/

PRIORITY CONCEPTS

- Perfusion
- Pain

LEARNING OUTCOMES

Safe and Effective Care Environment

1. Explain the role of the interdisciplinary team in cardiac rehabilitation.

Health Promotion and Maintenance

2. Differentiate between modifiable and nonmodifiable risk factors for coronary artery disease (CAD).

Psychosocial Integrity

3. Assess patient and family responses to acute coronary events, especially myocardial infarction (MI).

Physiological Integrity

4. Compare and contrast the clinical manifestations of stable angina, unstable angina, and MI.
5. Interpret physical and diagnostic assessment findings in patients who have CAD.
6. Prioritize nursing care for patients who have chest PAIN.
7. Teach patients and families about drug therapy for CAD.
8. Explain the nursing care for patients who have thrombolysis for an MI.
9. Develop a plan of care for the patient who has a percutaneous coronary intervention (PCI) to promote PERFUSION.
10. Plan postoperative care for the patient who has coronary artery bypass graft (CABG) surgery based on patient preferences, clinical expertise, and current evidence.
11. Identify the postoperative needs of adults having CABG surgery.

Coronary artery disease (CAD), also called *coronary heart disease (CHD)* or simply *heart disease,* is the single largest killer of American men and women in all ethnic groups. When the arteries that supply the **myocardium** (heart muscle) are diseased, the heart cannot pump blood effectively to adequately perfuse vital organs and peripheral tissues. The organs and tissues need oxygen in arterial blood for survival. When PERFUSION is impaired, the patient can have life-threatening clinical manifestations and possibly death.

The incidence of CAD has declined over the past decade (Go et al., 2013). This decline is due to many factors, including increasingly effective treatment and an increased awareness and emphasis on reducing major cardiovascular risk factors (e.g., hypertension, smoking, high cholesterol). Some coronary events occur in patients without common risk factors.

❖ *PATHOPHYSIOLOGY*

Coronary artery disease (CAD) is a broad term that includes chronic stable angina and acute coronary syndromes. It affects the arteries that provide blood, oxygen, and nutrients to the myocardium. When blood flow through the coronary arteries is partially or completely blocked, ischemia and infarction of the myocardium may result. Ischemia occurs when *insufficient oxygen* is supplied to meet the requirements of the myocardium. **Infarction** (necrosis, or cell death) occurs when severe ischemia is prolonged and decreased PERFUSION causes irreversible damage to tissue.

Chronic Stable Angina Pectoris

Angina pectoris is chest PAIN caused by a temporary imbalance between the coronary arteries' ability to supply oxygen and the cardiac muscle's demand for *oxygen*. **Ischemia** (lack of oxygen) that occurs with angina is limited in duration and does not cause permanent damage of myocardial tissue.

Angina may be of two main types: stable angina and unstable angina. **Chronic stable angina (CSA)** is chest discomfort that occurs with moderate to prolonged exertion in a pattern that is familiar to the patient. The frequency, duration, and intensity of symptoms remain the same over several months. CSA results in only slight limitation of activity and is usually associated with a *fixed* atherosclerotic plaque. It is usually relieved by nitroglycerin or rest and often is managed with drug therapy. Rarely does

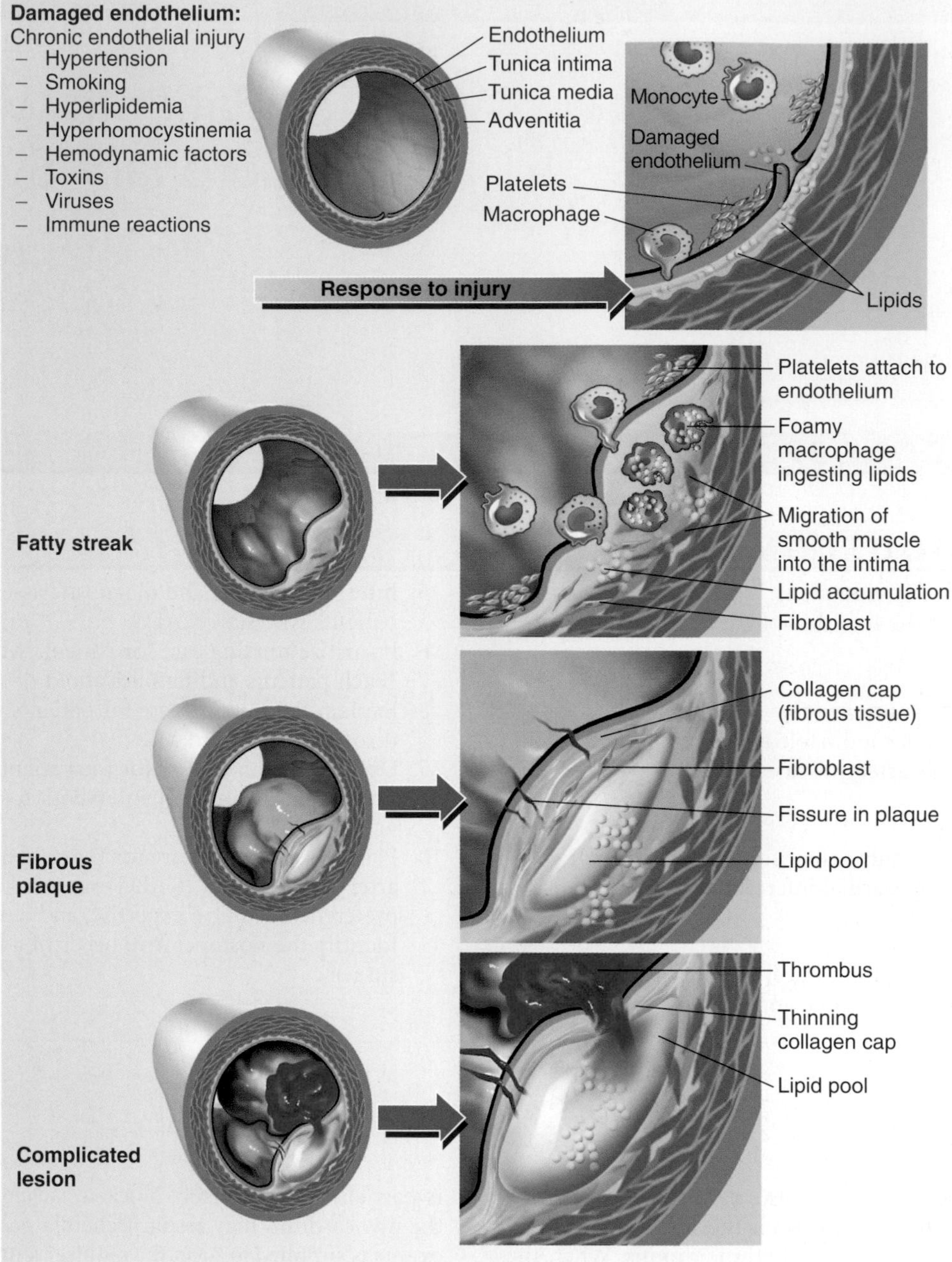

FIG. 38-1 A cross section of an atherosclerotic coronary artery.

CSA require aggressive treatment. *Unstable* angina is discussed in the following Acute Coronary Syndrome section.

Acute Coronary Syndrome

The term **acute coronary syndrome (ACS)** is used to describe patients who have either *unstable* angina or an acute myocardial infarction. In ACS, it is believed that the atherosclerotic plaque in the coronary artery *ruptures,* resulting in platelet aggregation ("clumping"), thrombus (clot) formation, and vasoconstriction (Fig. 38-1). The amount of disruption of the atherosclerotic plaque determines the degree of coronary artery obstruction (blockage) and the specific disease process. The artery has to have at least 40% plaque accumulation before it starts to block blood flow (McCance et al., 2014).

Historically, an acute myocardial infarction (MI) was diagnosed by the presence of ST-segment elevation on the 12-lead electrocardiogram (ECG) (see discussion of the normal ECG in Chapter 34). However, all patients do not present with this finding. Instead, they are classified into one of three categories according to the presence or absence of ST-segment elevation on the ECG and positive serum troponin markers:

- ST-elevation MI (STEMI) (traditional manifestation)
- Non–ST-elevation MI (NSTEMI) (common in women)
- Unstable angina pectoris

Unstable Angina Pectoris. *Unstable angina* (the most commonly used term) is chest pain or discomfort that occurs at rest or with exertion and causes severe activity limitation. An increase in the number of attacks and in the intensity of the pressure indicates unstable angina. The pressure may last longer than 15 minutes or may be poorly relieved by rest or nitroglycerin. Unstable angina describes a variety of disorders, including *new-onset angina, variant (Prinzmetal's) angina,* and *pre-infarction angina. Patients with unstable angina present with ST changes on a 12-lead ECG but do not have changes in troponin or creatine kinase (CK) levels.*

New-onset angina describes the patient who has his or her first angina symptoms, usually after exertion or other increased demands on the heart. **Variant (Prinzmetal's) angina** is chest pain or discomfort resulting from coronary artery spasm and typically occurs after rest. **Pre-infarction angina** refers to chest pain that occurs in the days or weeks before an MI.

Myocardial Infarction. The most serious acute coronary syndrome is myocardial infarction (MI), often referred to as *acute MI* or *AMI.* Undiagnosed or untreated angina can lead to this very serious health problem. **Myocardial infarction (MI)** occurs when myocardial tissue is abruptly and severely deprived of oxygen. When blood flow is quickly reduced by 80% to 90%, ischemia develops. Ischemia can lead to injury and necrosis of myocardial tissue if blood flow is not restored. Patients presenting with **non–ST-segment elevation myocardial infarction (NSTEMI)** typically have ST and T-wave changes on a 12-lead ECG. This indicates myocardial ischemia. Cardiac enzymes may be initially normal but elevate over the next 3 to 12 hours. Causes of NSTEMI include coronary vasospasm, spontaneous dissection, and sluggish blood flow due to narrowing of the coronary artery.

Patients presenting with **ST-elevation myocardial infarction (STEMI)** typically have ST elevation in two contiguous leads on a 12-lead ECG. This indicates myocardial infarction/necrosis. STEMI is attributable to rupture of the fibrous atherosclerotic plaque leading to platelet aggregation and thrombus formation at the site of rupture (McCance et al., 2014). *The thrombus causes an abrupt 100% occlusion to the coronary artery, is a medical emergency, and requires immediate revascularization of the blocked coronary artery.*

Often MIs begin with infarction of the subendocardial layer of cardiac muscle. This layer has the longest myofibrils in the heart, the *greatest* oxygen *demand*, and the *poorest* oxygen *supply.* Around the initial area of infarction (zone of necrosis) in the subendocardium are two other zones: (1) the zone of injury—tissue that is injured but not necrotic; and (2) the zone of ischemia—tissue that is oxygen deprived. This pattern is illustrated in Fig. 38-2.

GENDER HEALTH CONSIDERATIONS

Patient-Centered Care QSEN

Many women with symptomatic ischemic heart disease or abnormal stress testing do not have normal coronary angiography. Studies implicate microvascular disease or endothelial dysfunction or both as the causes for risk for CAD in women. Endothelial dysfunction is the inability of the arteries and arterioles to dilate due to lack of nitric oxide production by the endothelium. Nitric oxide is a relaxant of vascular smooth muscle.

Women typically have smaller coronary arteries and frequently have plaque that breaks off and travels into the small vessels to form an embolus (clot). Positive remodeling, or outward remodeling (lesions that protrude outward), is more common in women (McCance et al., 2014). This outpouching may be missed on coronary angiography.

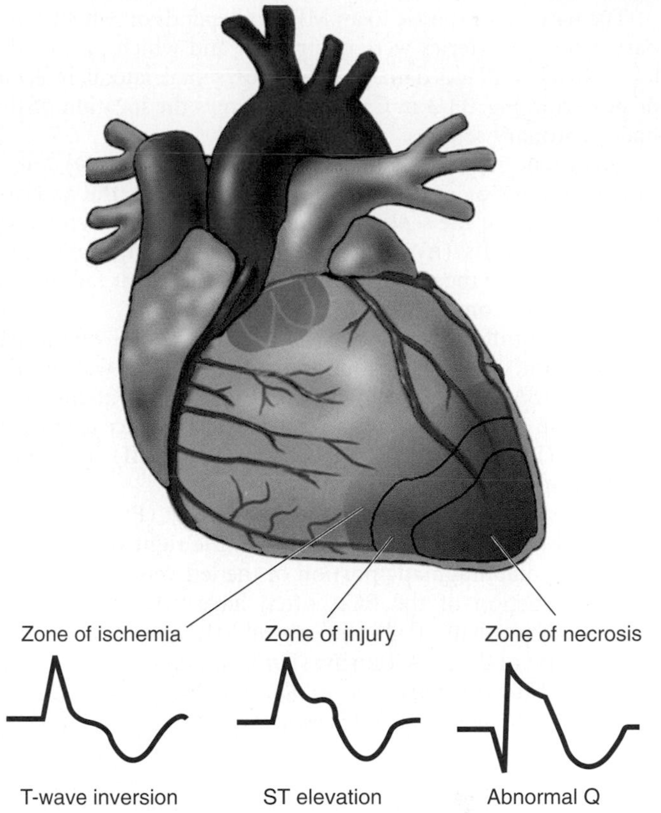

FIG. 38-2 Electrocardiographic changes and patterns associated with myocardial infarction.

Infarction is a dynamic process that does not occur instantly. Rather, it evolves over a period of several hours. Hypoxemia from ischemia may lead to local vasodilation of blood vessels and acidosis. Potassium, calcium, and magnesium imbalances, as well as acidosis at the cellular level, may cause changes in normal conduction and contractile functions. Catecholamines (epinephrine and norepinephrine) released in response to hypoxia and pain may increase the heart's rate, contractility, and afterload. These factors increase *oxygen* requirements in tissue that is already oxygen deprived. This may lead to life-threatening ventricular dysrhythmias. The area of infarction may extend into the zones of injury and ischemia. The actual extent of the zone of infarction depends on three factors: collateral circulation, anaerobic metabolism, and workload demands on the myocardium.

Obvious physical changes do not occur in the heart until 6 hours after the infarction, when the infarcted region appears blue and swollen. *These changes explain the need for intervention within the first 4 to 6 hours of symptom onset!* After 48 hours, the infarcted area turns gray with yellow streaks as neutrophils invade the tissue and begin to remove the necrotic cells. By 8 to 10 days after infarction, granulation tissue forms at the edges of the necrotic tissue. Over a 2- to 3-month period, the necrotic area eventually develops into a shrunken, thin, firm scar. Scar tissue permanently changes the size and shape of the entire left ventricle, called **ventricular remodeling.** Remodeling may decrease left ventricular function, cause heart failure, and increase morbidity and mortality. The scarred tissue does not contract, nor does it conduct electrically. Thus this area is often the cause of chronic ventricular dysrhythmias surrounding the infarcted zone (McCance et al., 2014).

The patient's response to an MI also depends on which coronary artery or arteries were obstructed and which part of the left ventricle wall was damaged: anterior, septal, lateral, inferior, or posterior. Fig. 33-3 in Chapter 33 shows the location of the major coronary arteries.

Obstruction of the left anterior descending (LAD) artery causes *anterior* or *septal* MIs because it perfuses the anterior wall and most of the septum of the left ventricle. Patients with anterior wall MIs (AWMIs) have the highest mortality rate because they are most likely to have left ventricular failure and dysrhythmias from damage to the left ventricle.

The circumflex artery supplies the lateral wall of the left ventricle and possibly portions of the posterior wall or the sinoatrial (SA) and atrioventricular (AV) nodes. Patients with obstruction of the circumflex artery may experience a *posterior* wall MI (PWMI) or a *lateral* wall MI (LWMI) and sinus dysrhythmias.

In most people, the right coronary artery (RCA) supplies most of the SA and AV nodes, as well as the right ventricle and inferior or diaphragmatic portion of the left ventricle. Patients with obstruction of the RCA often have **inferior wall MIs (IWMI)**. About half of all inferior wall MIs are associated with an occlusion of the RCA, causing significant damage to the right ventricle. *Thus it is important to obtain a "right-sided" ECG to assess for right ventricular involvement.*

Etiology and Genetic Risk

Atherosclerosis is the primary factor in the development of CAD. Numerous risk factors, both nonmodifiable and modifiable, contribute to atherosclerosis and subsequently to CAD (see Chapter 36).

Nonmodifiable risk factors are personal characteristics that cannot be altered or controlled. These risk factors, which interact with each other, include age, gender, family history, and ethnic background. People with a family history of CAD are at high risk for developing the disease.

CULTURAL CONSIDERATIONS

Patient-Centered Care QSEN

Several groups have a higher genetic risk for CAD than others. For example, African-American and Hispanic women have higher CAD risk factors than white women of the same socioeconomic status. Of American Indians and Alaskan Natives 18 years of age and older, about 46.7% have one or more CAD risk factors (hypertension [HTN], smoking, high cholesterol, excess weight, or diabetes mellitus). The leading cause of death for both men and women in the Euro-American population is cardiovascular disease, even though they may not have genetic predispositions to developing cardiovascular risk factors (Go et al., 2013).

GENDER HEALTH CONSIDERATIONS

Patient-Centered Care QSEN

Age is the most important risk factor for developing CAD in women. The older a woman is, the more likely she will have the disease. When compared with men, women are usually 10 years older when they have CAD. In addition, women who have MIs have a greater risk for dying during hospitalization. When they are older than 40 years, women are more likely than men to die within 1 year after their MI. If women do survive, they are less likely to participate in cardiac rehabilitation programs (Go et al., 2013).

Modifiable risk factors are lifestyle choices that can be controlled by the patient (with possible medical intervention), such as:

- Elevated serum lipid levels
- Smoking/tobacco use
- Limited physical activity
- Hypertension
- Diabetes mellitus
- Obesity
- Excessive alcohol
- Excessive stress/decreased coping skills

These risk factors are described in more detail in Chapters 33 and 36.

Incidence and Prevalence

The average age of a person having a first MI is 64.7 years for men and 72.2 years for women (Go et al., 2013). Every 34 seconds, a person in the United States has a major coronary event, and every minute, an American will die from CAD (Go et al., 2013). Many people die from coronary heart disease without being hospitalized. Most of these are sudden deaths caused by cardiac arrest.

GENDER HEALTH CONSIDERATIONS

Patient-Centered Care QSEN

Premenopausal women have a lower incidence of MI than men. However, for postmenopausal women in their 70s or older, the incidence of MI equals that of men. Family history is also a risk factor for women; those whose parents had CAD are more susceptible to the disease. Women with abdominal obesity (androidal shape) and metabolic syndrome (described on p. 760) are also at increased risk for CAD. Because lesbian and bisexual women have a higher incidence of overweight and obesity than women who are not lesbian or bisexual, they should be considered an especially high-risk group for CAD. The reasons for these trends are not known (Pettinato, 2012).

Many patients who survive MIs are not able to return to work. CAD is the leading cause of premature, permanent disability in the United States and the world.

Health Promotion and Maintenance

Ninety-five percent of sudden cardiac arrest victims die before reaching the hospital, largely because of ventricular fibrillation ("v fib"). To help combat this problem, automatic external defibrillators (AEDs) are found in many public places, such as in shopping centers and on airplanes. Employees are taught how to use these devices if a sudden cardiac arrest occurs. Some patients with diagnosed CAD have AEDs in their homes or at work. The procedure for using this device is described on p. 671 in Chapter 34.

Health promotion efforts are directed toward controlling or altering modifiable risk factors for CAD. For patients at risk for coronary artery disease (CAD), especially MI, assess specific risk factors and implement an individualized health teaching plan. Teach people who have one or more of these risk factors the importance of modifying or eliminating them to decrease their chances of CAD (Chart 38-1). Chapter 36 describes health teaching and evidence-based interventions for preventing and

CHART 38-1 Patient and Family Education: Preparing for Self-Management

Prevention of Coronary Artery Disease

Smoking/Tobacco Use
- If you smoke or use tobacco, quit.
- If you don't smoke or use tobacco, don't start.

Diet
- Consume sufficient calories for your body to include:
  - 5% to 6% from saturated fats
  - Avoiding *trans* fatty acids
- Limit your cholesterol intake to less than 200 mg/day.
- Limit your sodium intake as specified by your health care provider, or under 1500 mg/day, if possible.

Cholesterol
- Have your lipid levels checked regularly.
- If your cholesterol and LDL-C levels are elevated, follow your health care provider's advice, including taking statin medications as indicated.

Physical Activity
- If you are middle-aged or older or have a history of medical problems, check with your health care provider before starting an exercise program.
- Exercise periods should be at least 40 minutes long with 10-minute warm-up and 5-minute cool-down periods.
- If you cannot exercise moderately 3 to 4 times each week, walk daily for 30 minutes at a comfortable pace.
- If you cannot walk 30 minutes daily, walk any distance you can (e.g., park farther away from a site than necessary; use the stairs, not the elevator, to go one floor up or two floors down).

Diabetes Mellitus
- Manage your diabetes with your health care provider.

Hypertension
- Have your blood pressure checked regularly.
- If your blood pressure is elevated, follow your health care provider's advice.
- Continue to monitor your blood pressure at regular intervals.

Obesity
- Avoid severely restrictive or fad diets.
- Restrict intake of saturated fats, sweets, sweetened beverages, and cholesterol-rich foods.
- Increase your physical activity.

LDL-C, Low-density lipoprotein–cholesterol.

managing atherosclerosis and hypertension. Smoking cessation is discussed in Chapter 27.

Using Complementary and Alternative Therapies

Teach patients that adding omega 3 fatty acids from fish and plant sources has been effective for some patients in reducing lipid levels, stabilizing atherosclerotic plaques, and reducing sudden death from an MI. The preferred source of omega-3 acids is from fish 3 times a week or a daily fish oil nutritional supplement (1-2 g/day) containing eicosapentaenoic acid (EPA) and docosahexaenoic acid (DHA) (American Heart Association [AHA], 2013). Plant sources (flaxseed, flaxseed oil, walnuts, and canola oil) contain α-linolenic acid, and the conversion of α-linolenic acid to EPA and DHA is not as efficient in patients who consume a typical Western diet. Lovaza (omega-3 fatty acids) is a medication used to reduce very high triglycerides (>500 mg/dL) levels. However, it has not been proven to prevent MIs or stroke.

Garlic supplements may also have a small effect on reducing lipid levels, but they have not been shown to prevent MI. Patients often take a number of other supplements, such as vitamin E, coenzyme Q10, Pantesin, and vitamin B complex to decrease the risk for heart disease. However, studies do not show that these substances are helpful in reducing coronary artery disease.

TABLE 38-1 Indicators of Risk Factors for Metabolic Syndrome

RISK FACTOR	INDICATOR
Hypertension	**Either** blood pressure of 130/85 mm Hg or higher **or** taking antihypertensive drug(s)
Decreased HDL-C (usually with high LDL-C) level	**Either** HDL-C <45 mg/dL for men or <55 mg/dL for women **or** taking an anticholesterol drug
Increased level of triglycerides	**Either** 160 mg/dL or higher for men or 135 mg/dL or higher for women **or** taking an anticholesterol drug
Increased fasting blood glucose (due to diabetes, glucose intolerance, or insulin resistance)	**Either** 100 mg/dL or higher **or** taking antidiabetic drug(s)
Large waist size (excessive abdominal fat causing central obesity)	40 inches (102 cm) or greater for men or 35 inches (89 cm) or greater for women

HDL-C, High-density lipoprotein–cholesterol; *LDL-C,* low-density lipoprotein–cholesterol.

Managing Metabolic Syndrome

Metabolic syndrome, also called *syndrome X,* has been recognized as a risk factor for cardiovascular (CV) disease and is being aggressively researched. Patients who have three of the factors in Table 38-1 are diagnosed with **metabolic syndrome**. This health problem increases the risk for developing diabetes and CAD. About a third of adults older than 20 years in the United States have metabolic syndrome (Go et al., 2013). This increase is likely due to physical inactivity and the current obesity epidemic. Management is aimed at reducing risks, managing hypertension, and preventing complications.

NCLEX EXAMINATION CHALLENGE

Health Promotion and Maintenance

An older client has a history of coronary artery disease. Which modifiable risk factors will the nurse assess to guide the client's teaching plan? **Select all that apply.**

A. Older age
B. Tobacco use
C. Female
D. High-fat diet
E. Family history
F. Obesity

❖ PATIENT-CENTERED COLLABORATIVE CARE

◆ Assessment

History. If symptoms of CAD are present at the time of the interview, delay collecting data until interventions for symptom relief, vital sign instability, and dysrhythmias are started and discomfort resolves. If the patient had PAIN, ask about how he or she has managed the discomfort and other symptoms and which drugs he or she may be taking. When the patient is pain-free, obtain information about family history and modifiable risk factors, including eating habits, lifestyle, and physical activity levels. Ask about a history of smoking and how much alcohol is consumed each day. Collaborate with the dietitian to assess current body mass index (BMI) and weight as needed.

Physical Assessment/Clinical Manifestations. *Rapid assessment of the patient with chest pain or other presenting symptoms is crucial.* It is important to differentiate among the types of chest PAIN and to identify the source. Question the patient to determine the characteristics of the discomfort. Patients may deny pain, however, and report that they feel "pressure." Appropriate questions to ask concerning the discomfort include onset, location, radiation, intensity, duration, and precipitating and relieving factors.

CULTURAL CONSIDERATIONS

Patient-Centered Care QSEN

African Americans and women tend to delay seeking treatment for MI and therefore have higher mortality rates than Euro-Americans. One contributing factor to this delay is a greater incidence of dyspnea as an acute symptom among these groups rather than the classic PAIN more typical of other groups (Go et al., 2013).

If PAIN is present, ask the patient if the pain is in the chest, epigastric area, jaw, back, shoulder, or arm. Ask him or her to rate the pain on a scale of 0 to 10, with 10 being the highest level of discomfort. Some patients describe the discomfort as tightness, a burning sensation, pressure, or indigestion. A complete pain assessment is described in Chapter 3.

GENDER HEALTH CONSIDERATIONS

Patient-Centered Care QSEN

Many women of any age experience atypical angina. **Atypical angina** manifests as indigestion, pain between the shoulders, an aching jaw, or a choking sensation that occurs with exertion. These symptoms typically manifest during stressful circumstances or during activities of daily living. Women may curtail activity as a result of angina, and health care providers need to ask about changes in routine. Symptoms in women typically include fatigue, sleep disturbance, and dyspnea (Go et al., 2013).

Chart 38-2 compares and contrasts angina and infarction PAIN. Because angina pain is ischemic pain, it usually improves when the imbalance between oxygen supply and demand is resolved. For example, rest reduces tissue demands and nitroglycerin improves oxygen supply. Discomfort from a myocardial infarction (MI) does not usually resolve with these measures. Ask about any associated symptoms, including *nausea, vomiting, diaphoresis, dizziness, weakness, palpitations, and shortness of breath.*

Assess *blood pressure* and *heart rate.* Interpret the patient's cardiac rhythm and presence of *dysrhythmias.* Sinus tachycardia with premature ventricular contractions (PVCs) frequently occurs in the first few hours after an MI.

Next assess *distal peripheral pulses* and *skin temperature.* The skin should be warm with all pulses palpable. In the patient with unstable angina or MI, poor cardiac output may be manifested by cool, diaphoretic ("sweaty") skin and diminished or absent pulses. *Auscultate for an S_3 gallop, which often indicates heart failure—a serious and common complication of MI.* In adults, the S_3 heart sound is heard with the bell of the stethoscope over the apex of the heart (Jarvis, 2016).

CHART 38-2 Key Features

Angina and Myocardial Infarction

ANGINA	MYOCARDIAL INFARCTION
• Substernal chest discomfort: ▪ Radiating to the left arm ▪ Precipitated by exertion or stress (or rest in variant angina) ▪ Relieved by nitroglycerin or rest ▪ Lasting less than 15 min • Few, if any, associated symptoms	• Pain or discomfort: ▪ Substernal chest pain/pressure radiating to the left arm ▪ Pain or discomfort in jaw, back, shoulder, or abdomen ▪ Occurring without cause, usually in the morning ▪ Relieved only by opioids ▪ Lasting 30 min or more • Frequent associated symptoms: ▪ Nausea/vomiting ▪ Diaphoresis ▪ Dyspnea ▪ Feelings of fear and anxiety ▪ Dysrhythmias ▪ Fatigue ▪ Palpitations ▪ Epigastric distress ▪ Anxiety ▪ Dizziness ▪ Disorientation/acute confusion ▪ Feeling "short of breath"

CONSIDERATIONS FOR OLDER ADULTS

Patient-Centered Care QSEN

The presence of associated symptoms without chest discomfort is significant. In up to 40% of all patients with MI, primarily older women and patients with diabetes, chest pain or discomfort may be mild or absent. Instead, they have associated symptoms. Some older patients may think they are having indigestion and therefore not recognize that they are having an MI. Others report shortness of breath as the only symptom. The major manifestation of MI in people older than 80 years may be disorientation or acute confusion because of poor cardiac output and due to inadequate coronary perfusion.

In some older adults with MI, absence of chest pain may be due to cognitive impairment or inability to verbalize pain sensation. However, in most cases it is probably the result of increased collateral circulation. Silent myocardial ischemia increases the incidence of new coronary events and should be treated aggressively.

Assess the *respiratory rate* and breath sounds for signs of heart failure. An increased respiratory rate is common because of anxiety and pain, but *crackles or wheezes* may indicate *left-sided* heart failure. Assess for the presence of jugular venous distention and peripheral edema.

The patient with MI may experience a *temperature elevation* for several days after infarction. Temperatures as high as 102° F (38.9° C) may occur in response to myocardial necrosis, indicating the inflammatory response.

Psychosocial Assessment. *Denial* is a common early reaction to chest discomfort associated with angina or MI. On average, the patient with an acute MI waits more than 2 hours before seeking medical attention. Often he or she rationalizes that symptoms are due to indigestion or overexertion. In some situations, denial is a normal part of adapting to a stressful event. However, denial that interferes with identifying a symptom such as chest discomfort can be harmful. Explain the importance of reporting any discomfort to the health care provider.

Fear, depression, anxiety, and anger are other common reactions of many patients and their families. Assist in identifying these feelings. Encourage them to explain their understanding of the event, and clarify any misconceptions.

Laboratory Assessment. Although there is no single ideal test to diagnose MI, the most common laboratory tests include troponins T and I and creatine kinase-MB (CK-MB). These cardiac markers are specific for MI and cardiac necrosis. Troponins T and I rise quickly. CK-MB is the most specific marker for MI but does not peak until about 24 hours after the onset of pain. These tests are described in more detail in Chapter 33. If serial enzymes are negative, the patient has a nuclear medicine test such as those described in the next section.

Imaging Assessment. Unless there is associated cardiac dysfunction (e.g., valve disease) or heart failure, a chest x-ray is not diagnostic for angina or MI. A chest x-ray may be performed to assist with ruling out aortic dissection, which may mimic a MI. If the x-ray demonstrates a widened mediastinum, further testing for aortic dissection with either transesophageal echography (TEE) or computed tomography (CT) scan is needed.

Thallium scans use radioisotope imaging to assess for ischemia or necrotic muscle tissue related to angina or myocardial infarction (MI). Areas of decreased or absent perfusion, referred to as *cold spots,* identify ischemia or infarction. Thallium may be used with the exercise tolerance test. Dipyridamole (Persantine) thallium scanning (DTS) may also be used.

Contrast-enhanced cardiovascular magnetic resonance (CMR) imaging may also be done as a noninvasive approach to detect CAD. *Echocardiography* may be used to visualize the structures of the heart.

Use of the 64-slice **computed tomography coronary angiography (CTCA)** has been found to be helpful in diagnosing coronary artery disease in symptomatic patients identified as having a "low- or intermediate-pretest probability" risk for CAD. This new generation of high-speed computed tomography (CT) scanners is becoming a highly reliable, noninvasive way to evaluate CAD (Weustink et al., 2010).

Other Diagnostic Assessment. *Twelve-lead electrocardiograms (ECGs)* allow the health care provider to examine the heart from varying perspectives. By identifying the lead(s) in which ECG changes are occurring, the health care provider can identify both the occurrence and the location of ischemia (angina) or necrosis (infarction). In addition to the traditional 12-lead ECG, the health care provider may request a "right-sided" or 18-lead ECG to determine whether ischemia or infarction has occurred in the right ventricle. *The ECG should be obtained within 10 minutes of patient presentation with chest discomfort!*

An ischemic myocardium does not repolarize normally. Thus 12-lead ECGs obtained during an angina episode reveal ST depression, T-wave inversion, or both. **Variant angina**, caused by coronary vasospasm (vessel spasm), usually causes elevation of the ST segment during angina attacks. These ST and T-wave changes usually subside when the ischemia is resolved and pain is relieved. However, the T wave may remain flat or inverted for a period of time. If the patient is not experiencing angina at the moment of the test, the ECG is usually normal unless he or she has evidence of an old MI.

When infarction occurs, one of two ECG changes is usually observed: ST-elevation MI (STEMI), or non–ST-elevation MI (NSTEMI). An abnormal Q wave (wider than 0.04 seconds or more than one-third the height of the QRS complex) may develop, depending on the amount of myocardium that has necrosed. Women having an MI often present with an NSTEMI.

The Q wave may develop because necrotic cells do not conduct electrical stimuli. Hours to days after the MI, the ST-segment and T-wave changes return to normal. However, when the Q wave exists, it may become permanent. The Q waves may disappear after a number of years, but their absence does not necessarily mean that the patient has not had an MI.

After the acute stages of an unstable angina episode, the health care provider often requests an *exercise tolerance test (stress test)* on a treadmill to assess for ECG changes consistent with ischemia, evaluate medical therapy, and identify those who might benefit from invasive therapy. Pharmacologic stress-testing agents such as dobutamine (Dobutrex) may be used instead of the treadmill. Treadmill exercise testing is only moderately accurate for women when compared with men. The results are also not as reliable in tall, obese men when compared with short, thinner men. In women with suspected CAD, stress echocardiography or single photon emission computed tomography (SPECT) should be performed.

Cardiac catheterization may be performed to determine the extent and exact location of coronary artery obstructions. It allows the cardiologist and cardiac surgeon to identify patients who might benefit from percutaneous coronary intervention (PCI) or from coronary artery bypass grafting (CABG). Each of these diagnostic tests is described in detail in Chapter 33.

◆ Analysis

The patient with coronary artery disease (CAD) may have either stable angina or acute coronary syndrome (ACS). If ACS is suspected or cannot be completely ruled out, the patient is admitted to a telemetry unit for continuous monitoring or to a critical care unit if hemodynamically unstable.

The priority NANDA-I nursing diagnoses and collaborative problems for most patients with CAD include:

1. Acute Pain related to imbalance between myocardial oxygen supply and demand (NANDA-I)
2. Inadequate tissue perfusion (cardiopulmonary) related to interruption of arterial blood flow
3. Activity Intolerance related to fatigue caused by imbalance between oxygen supply and demand (NANDA-I)
4. Ineffective Coping related to effects of acute illness and major changes in lifestyle (NANDA-I)
5. Potential for dysrhythmias

6. Potential for heart failure
7. Potential for recurrent symptoms and extension of injury

◆ Planning and Implementation

Astute assessment skills, timely analysis of troponin, and analysis of the 12-lead ECG (or 18-lead ECG for a suspected right ventricular infarction) are essential to ensure appropriate patient care management. This is particularly important since the average time a patient waits before seeking treatment is over 2 hours. This delay lessens the 4- to 6-hour window of opportunity for the most advantageous treatment with percutaneous intervention.

Managing Acute Pain. Patients with *diabetes mellitus* and coronary artery disease (CAD) may not experience chest PAIN or pressure because of diabetic neuropathy. In this patient population, the onset of ACS may be signaled by new onset of atrial fibrillation. With new-onset atrial fibrillation, a cardiac workup should be done to rule out ACS.

Planning: Expected Outcomes. The expected outcome is that the patient will verbalize a report of decreased PAIN and discomfort as a result of prompt collaborative interventions.

Interventions. The purpose of patient-centered collaborative care is to eliminate discomfort by providing PAIN relief measures, decreasing myocardial oxygen demand, and increasing myocardial oxygen supply.

Emergency Care: Myocardial Infarction. Evaluate any report of pain, obtain vital signs, ensure an IV access, and notify the health care provider of the patient's condition. Chart 38-3 summarizes the emergency interventions for the patient with symptoms of CAD.

Pain relief helps increase the oxygen supply and decrease myocardial oxygen demand. The American Heart Association (AHA) recommends several pain management strategies, including morphine sulfate and oxygen. *Give morphine as the priority in managing pain in patients having an ACS!*

Drug Therapy. At home or in the hospital, the patient may take nitroglycerin to relieve episodic anginal pain. Aspirin 325 mg, an antiplatelet drug, may also be taken daily to prevent clots that further block coronary arteries.

Nitroglycerin (NTG), a nitrate often referred to as "nitro," increases collateral blood flow, redistributes blood flow toward the subendocardium, and dilates the coronary arteries. In addition, it decreases myocardial oxygen demand by peripheral vasodilation, which decreases both preload and afterload.

! NURSING SAFETY PRIORITY (QSEN)

Drug Alert

Before administering NTG, ensure that the patient has not taken any phosphodiesterase inhibitors for erectile dysfunction such as sildenafil (Viagra, Revatio) or tadalafil (Cialis) within the past 24 to 48 hours. Concomitant use of NTG with these inhibitors can cause profound hypotension. Remind patients not to take these medications within 24 to 48 hours of one another.

Teach the patient to hold the NTG tablet under the tongue and drink 5 mL (1 teaspoon) of water, if necessary, to allow the tablet to dissolve. NTG spray is also available and is more quickly absorbed. Pain relief should begin within 1 to 2 minutes and should be clearly evident in 3 to 5 minutes. After 5 minutes, recheck the patient's pain intensity and vital signs. If the blood pressure (BP) is less than 100 mm Hg systolic or 25 mm Hg lower than the previous reading, lower the head of the bed and notify the health care provider.

If the patient is experiencing some but not complete relief and vital signs remain stable, another NTG tablet or spray may be used. In 5-minute increments, a total of three doses may be administered in an attempt to relieve angina PAIN. If the patient uses NTG spray instead of the tablet, teach him or her to sit upright and spray the dose under the tongue. NTG topical patches should be placed below the nipple line to decrease discomfort.

Angina usually responds to NTG. The patient typically states that the PAIN is relieved or markedly diminished. When simple measures, such as taking three sublingual nitroglycerin tablets one after the other, do not relieve chest discomfort, the patient may be experiencing an MI.

! NURSING SAFETY PRIORITY (QSEN)

Critical Rescue

If the patient is experiencing an MI, prepare him or her for transfer to a specialized unit where close monitoring and appropriate management can be provided. If the patient is at home or in the community, call 911 for transfer to the closest emergency department.

In a specialized unit, the health care provider may prescribe IV NTG for management of the chest PAIN. Begin the drug infusion slowly, checking the BP and pain level every 3 to 5 minutes. The nitroglycerin dose is increased until the pain is relieved, the BP falls excessively, or the maximum prescribed dose is reached (Chart 38-4).

When PAIN or other symptoms have subsided and the patient is stabilized, the health care provider may change the drug to an oral or topical nitrate. During administration of long-term

CHART 38-3 Best Practice for Patient Safety & Quality Care (QSEN)

Emergency Care of the Patient with Chest Discomfort

- Assess airway, breathing, and circulation (ABCs). Defibrillate as needed.
- ***Provide continuous ECG monitoring.***
- Obtain the patient's description of pain or discomfort.
- Obtain the patient's vital signs (blood pressure, pulse, respiration).
- Assess/provide vascular access.
- Consult chest pain protocol or notify the physician or Rapid Response Team for specific intervention.
- Obtain a 12-lead ECG within 10 minutes of report of chest pain.
- Provide pain-relief medication and aspirin (non–enteric coated) as prescribed.
- Administer oxygen therapy to maintain oxygen saturation ≥95%.
- Remain calm. Stay with the patient if possible.
- Assess the patient's vital signs and intensity of pain 5 minutes after administration of medication.
- Remedicate with prescribed drugs (if vital signs remain stable), and check the patient every 5 minutes.
- Notify the physician if vital signs deteriorate.

ECG, Electrocardiogram.

CHART 38-4 Common Examples of Drug Therapy

Coronary Artery Disease (Nitrates, Beta Blockers, and Antiplatelet Agents)

DRUG	USUAL DOSAGE	NURSING INTERVENTIONS	RATIONALES
Nitrates			
Nitroglycerin (Nitrostat, NitroQuick)	0.3-0.4 mg sublingually every 5 min; up to 3 tablets over 15 min	Instruct patients to lie down with the head of the bed at a level of comfort when taking the sublingual form.	Hypotension can be dramatic, immediate, and intensified by the upright position.
Nitrolingual translingual spray	0.4 mg/metered spray	Monitor BP. Pay attention to orthostatic changes.	A decrease in BP occurs with vasodilation.
		Instruct patients to allow the sublingual tablet to dissolve and to avoid swallowing the tablet.	The sublingual dose is absorbed through the sublingual mucous membranes.
		Check the expiration date on sublingual tablets and sprays. Tablets should be replaced every 3-5 mo.	The efficacy of the tablets decreases with time.
		Determine whether pain is relieved.	Additional medication may be required to relieve pain.
		Monitor for headache.	Vasodilation is generalized.
		Do not administer to patients taking drugs used to treat sexual dysfunction (e.g., sildenafil, tadalafil, vardenafil).	Very serious (possibly fatal) interactions may occur.
Isosorbide dinitrate (Isordil, Iso-Bid)	2.5 mg sublingually every 4-6 hr; 5-40 mg orally four times daily 40-80 mg sustained-release tablet every 8-12 hr	Instruct patients taking sublingual forms to lie down before administration.	The hypotensive effect can be dramatic and immediate with sublingual administration.
		Monitor BP, and assess for dizziness.	A decrease in BP occurs with vasodilation.
Isosorbide mononitrate (Imdur)	60-mg extended-release tablet daily	Schedule sustained-release form with an 8- to 12-hr dose-free interval.	Tolerance may develop.
Nitroglycerin patch (Minitran, Nitro-Dur, Nitrek)	Transdermally started at 5 mg/24 hr (10-cm^2 system)	Remove the patch from the patient before defibrillation.	The patient may develop a burn.
		Rotate application sites.	Rotation prevents skin irritation.
		Apply the patch to a clean, dry, hairless area.	The drug is better absorbed when the skin is clean, dry, and hairless.
		Remove patch after 12-14 hr each day.	Removal prevents drug tolerance.
Beta Blockers			
Carvedilol (Coreg, Coreg CR)	12.5-25 mg orally twice daily for Coreg; 40-80 mg orally once daily for Coreg CR	Assess heart rate before administration.	Beta-blocking effects cause a decrease in heart rate.
		Monitor BP.	The hypotensive effect is due to a decrease in cardiac output, suppressed renin activity, and beta-blocking effects.
		Observe for signs of heart failure.	Heart failure may occur as a result of a decrease in cardiac output.
		Assess for shortness of breath and wheezing.	Beta$_2$-blocking effects in the lungs can cause bronchoconstriction.
Metoprolol (Lopressor, Toprol XL, Betaloc 🍁), a cardioselective beta-adrenergic blocker	*Angina:* 25-100 mg orally daily *MI:* 100 mg orally twice daily; 5 mg IV over 2 min may be repeated twice for a total of 15 mg	Assess heart rate before administration; do not administer if heart rate <50-60 beats/min.	Beta blockers may cause further decreases in heart rate.
		Monitor BP, and hold for systolic <90-100 mm Hg.	Decreased BP pressure is an anticipated effect.
		Assess patients for cough, shortness of breath, edema, and weight gain.	These are indications of heart failure.
Antiplatelet Agents			
Aspirin (Empirin, Apo-ASA 🍁, Ecotrin)	81-325 mg orally daily	Suggest that patients take the daily dose with food.	Gastric irritation may occur.
		Question patients about ringing in the ears.	Tinnitus may occur with aspirin toxicity.
		Emphasize to patients that aspirin is an important cardiac medication and should be continued unless they are told to stop.	Studies document significantly better survival rates for patients with coronary artery disease receiving aspirin.

Continued

CHART 38-4 **Common Examples of Drug Therapy—cont'd**

Coronary Artery Disease (Nitrates, Beta Blockers, and Antiplatelet Agents)

DRUG	USUAL DOSAGE	NURSING INTERVENTIONS	RATIONALES
P2Y12 Platelet Inhibitors			
Clopidogrel (Plavix) ***Do not confuse Plavix with Paxil***	*Acute coronary syndrome or after stent implantation:* 300-600 mg orally loading dose, then 75-150 mg daily	Teach patients to take drug with food. Inform patients to report any unusual bleeding or bruising.	Drug can cause diarrhea and other GI disturbances. Drug prevents platelet aggregation, thus slowing down clot formation.
Prasugrel (Effient)	*Acute coronary syndrome or after stent implantation:* 60 mg orally loading dose, then 10 mg daily	Inform patients to report any unusual bleeding or bruising.	Contraindicated in patients with history of prior stroke or >75 yrs of age, due to increased risk for bleeding. If patient weighs <60 kg, consider lowering dose to 5 mg daily.
Ticagrelor (Brilinta)	*Acute coronary syndrome or after stent implantation:* 180 mg load with 325 mg aspirin, then 90 mg daily with 81 mg of aspirin	Inform patients to report any unusual bleeding or bruising. Teach patients to avoid over-the-counter pain relievers that contain aspirin. Teach patients to take no more than 100 mg of aspirin in a 24 hour period.	May cause dyspnea or bradycardia that is self-limiting. May not work as effectively with high-dose aspirin; use 81 mg of aspirin.

BP, Blood pressure; *MI,* myocardial infarction.

oral and topical nitrates, an 8- to 12-hour nitrate-free period should be maintained to prevent tolerance. The patient may initially report a headache. Give acetaminophen (Tylenol, Exdol ♣) before the nitrate to ease some of this discomfort.

The health care provider usually prescribes *morphine sulfate (MS)* to relieve discomfort that is unresponsive to nitroglycerin. Morphine relieves MI PAIN, decreases myocardial oxygen demand, relaxes smooth muscle, and reduces circulating catecholamines. It is usually administered in 2- to 10-mg doses IV every 5 to 15 minutes until the maximum prescribed dose is reached or the patient experiences relief or signs of toxicity. Monitor for adverse effects of morphine, which include respiratory depression, hypotension, bradycardia, and severe vomiting. Treatment for morphine toxicity is naloxone (Narcan) 0.2 to 0.8 mg IV, vasopressor drugs, IV fluids, and oxygen therapy. Monitor the patient's vital signs and cardiac rhythm every few minutes.

These strategies are often enough to relieve the PAIN. If they are not adequate, additional interventions identified in the Improving Cardiopulmonary Tissue Perfusion section below may be attempted.

Other Interventions. Several other interventions may be used with drug therapy to relieve chest PAIN. Supplemental oxygen increases the amount of oxygen available to myocardial tissue. Therefore oxygen is usually prescribed and administered at a flow of 2 to 4 L/min by nasal cannula titrated to maintain an arterial oxygen saturation (Sao_2) of 95% or higher. If the BP is stable, assist the patient in assuming any position of comfort. Placing the patient in semi-Fowler's position often enhances comfort and tissue oxygenation. A quiet, calm environment and explanations of interventions often reduce anxiety and help relieve chest pain. If needed, remind the patient to take several deep breaths to increase oxygenation.

Improving Cardiopulmonary Tissue Perfusion

Planning: Expected Outcomes. The primary outcome is that the patient will have increased myocardial PERFUSION as evidenced by an adequate cardiac output, normal sinus rhythm, and vital signs within normal limits.

CLINICAL JUDGMENT CHALLENGE

Patient-Centered Care; Evidence-Based Practice; Informatics QSEN

An 82-year-old man living alone at home had a sudden onset of chest pain. He called 911 and was taken to the emergency department (ED).

1. As his ED nurse, what is your first action in response to his report of chest pain? What evidence supports this decision?
2. The physician prescribes IV nitroglycerin for pain. What assessment will you perform prior to administering this drug and why? For what adverse effects will you monitor during and after morphine administration?
3. What other drugs might the physician prescribe at this time and why?
4. The physician prescribed oxygen at 3 L/min via nasal cannula. What is the purpose of this intervention for managing chest pain?
5. What will you document in the electronic health record about this patient's care?

Interventions. Because myocardial infarction (MI) is a dynamic process, restoring PERFUSION to the injured area (usually within 4 to 6 hours for NSTEMI and 60 to 90 minutes for STEMI) often limits the amount of extension and improves left ventricular function. Complete, sustained reperfusion of coronary arteries after an ACS has decreased mortality rates.

Drug Therapy. *Aspirin (ASA)* therapy is recommended by the American College of Cardiology (ACC) and the American Heart Association (AHA) (Cayla et al., 2012). It inhibits both platelet aggregation and vasoconstriction, thereby decreasing the likelihood of thrombosis. *If the patient has new-onset angina at home, teach him or her to chew aspirin 325 mg (4 "baby aspirins" that are 81 mg each) immediately and call 911!* The antiplatelet effect of ASA begins within 1 hour of use and continues for several days. In the hospital setting, The Joint Commission

Acute Myocardial Infarction Core Measure Set requires that aspirin be given upon arrival to the emergency department or when an MI occurs in the hospital. Administer 162 to 325 mg non–enteric-coated aspirin every day to all patients with suspected CAD unless absolutely contraindicated. Instruct the patient to chew and swallow the drug and continue taking the drug as prescribed unless adverse effects occur.

! NURSING SAFETY PRIORITY QSEN

Drug Alert

For patients taking aspirin every day, observe for bleeding tendencies, such as nosebleeds or blood in the stool. Aspirin should be discontinued if bleeding occurs.

Glycoprotein (GP) IIb/IIIa inhibitors target the platelet component of the thrombus. Abciximab (ReoPro), eptifibatide (Integrilin), or tirofiban (Aggrastat) may be administered IV to prevent fibrinogen from attaching to activated platelets at the site of a thrombus. These medications are used in unstable angina and NSTEMI. They are also given before and during percutaneous coronary intervention (PCI) to maintain patency of an artery with a large clot and are given with fibrinolytic agents after STEMI. If the GP IIb/IIIa inhibitors are used with a fibrinolytic agent, the dose of the thrombolytic is reduced by 25% to 50% to decrease the risk for bleeding.

! NURSING SAFETY PRIORITY QSEN

Drug Alert

When giving GP IIb/IIIa inhibitors, assess the patient closely for bleeding or hypersensitivity reactions. If either occurs, notify the health care provider or Rapid Response Team immediately. Monitor the platelet level 4 hours after starting the drug and daily after that. Notify the cardiologist if the patient experiences a significant decrease in platelet count per agency protocol.

Once-a-day *beta-adrenergic blocking agents* (e.g., metoprolol XL [Toprol XL], carvedilol CR [Coreg CR]), sometimes just called *beta blockers (BBs),* decrease the size of the infarct, the occurrence of ventricular dysrhythmias, and mortality rates in patients with MI. The physician usually prescribes a cardioselective beta-blocking agent within the first 1 to 2 hours after an MI if the patient is hemodynamically stable. Beta blockers slow the heart rate and decrease the force of cardiac contraction (see Chart 38-4). Thus these agents prolong the period of diastole and increase myocardial PERFUSION while reducing the force of myocardial contraction. With beta blockade, the heart can perform more work without ischemia. During beta-blocking therapy, monitor for:

- Bradycardia
- Hypotension
- Decreased level of consciousness (LOC)
- Chest discomfort

Assess the lungs for crackles (indicative of heart failure) and wheezes (indicative of bronchospasm). Hypoglycemia, depression, nightmares, and forgetfulness are also problems with beta blockade, especially in older patients. Many of these side effects decrease with time. Unless contraindicated, all patients experiencing NSTEMI and STEMI should be discharged on beta blocker therapy.

! NURSING SAFETY PRIORITY QSEN

Drug Alert

Do not give beta blockers if the pulse is below 55 or the systolic BP is below 100 without first checking with the health care provider.

Health care providers frequently prescribe *angiotensin-converting enzyme inhibitors (ACEIs)* or *angiotensin receptor blockers (ARBs)* within 48 hours of ACS if ejection fraction is equal to or less than 40% to prevent ventricular remodeling and the development of heart failure. Both ACEIs and ARBs increase survival after an MI. Monitor the patient for decreased urine output, hypotension, and cough. Check for changes in serum potassium, creatinine, and blood urea nitrogen. (Chapter 36 provides a more detailed discussion of ACEIs and ARBs.)

For patients with angina, the health care provider may prescribe calcium channel blockers (CCBs) to promote vasodilation and myocardial PERFUSION. These drugs are indicated for patients with variant angina or for those who are hypertensive and continue to have angina despite therapy with beta blockers (unstable angina). They are *not* indicated after AMI. Monitor the patient for hypotension and peripheral edema, and review the frequency of angina episodes.

Calcium channel blockers are also used for chronic stable angina (CSA). When they are not successful in managing CSA, *ranolazine (Ranexa)* may be added to the drug regimen. This drug has anti-angina and anti-ischemic properties and is often effective in relieving the pain associated with CSA.

Reperfusion Therapy. As time passes, myocardial tissue can become increasingly ischemic and necrotic. Therefore, based on the location and skill set within the health care institution, one of two reperfusion strategies are employed to open a blocked artery in a patient experiencing AMI: thrombolytic therapy or percutaneous coronary intervention (PCI).

Thrombolytic Therapy. *Thrombolytic therapy* using **fibrinolytics** dissolves thrombi in the coronary arteries and restores myocardial blood flow. Examples of these agents, which target the fibrin component of the coronary thrombosis, include:

- Tissue plasminogen activator (t-PA, alteplase [Activase]) (IV or intracoronary)
- Reteplase (Retavase) (IV or intracoronary)
- Tenecteplase (TNK) (IV push [IVP])

Intracoronary fibrinolytics may be delivered during cardiac catheterization. Thrombolytic agents are most effective when administered within the first 6 hours of a coronary event. They are used in men and women, young and old.

Thrombolytic therapy is given in a unit where the patient can be continuously monitored. It is indicated for chest pain of longer than 30 minutes' duration that is unrelieved by nitroglycerin, with *indications of STEMI by the ECG.* It is *not* indicated for the NSTEMI patient population. The goal is to start the infusion of fibrinolytics within 30 minutes of ED admission. Contraindications include recent abdominal surgery or stroke, because bleeding may occur when fresh clots are lysed (broken down or dissolved). Table 38-2 lists the current contraindications to thrombolytic therapy.

TABLE 38-2 Contraindications to Thrombolytic Therapy

Absolute
- Any prior intracranial hemorrhage
- Known structural cerebral vascular lesion (e.g., arteriovenous malformations)
- Known malignant intracranial neoplasm (primary or metastatic)
- Ischemic stroke within 3 months EXCEPT acute ischemic stroke within 3 hours
- Suspected aortic dissection
- Active bleeding or bleeding diathesis (excluding menses)
- Significant closed-head or facial trauma within 3 months

Relative
- History of chronic, severe, poorly controlled hypertension
- Severe uncontrolled hypertension on presentation (SBP >180 mm Hg or DBP >110 mm Hg)*
- History of prior ischemic stroke within 3 months, dementia, or known intracranial pathology not covered in contraindications
- Traumatic or prolonged (≥10 minutes) CPR or major surgery (within 3 weeks)
- Recent (within 2-4 weeks) internal bleeding
- Noncompressible vascular punctures
- For streptokinase/anistreplase: prior exposure (>5 days ago) or prior allergic reaction to these agents
- Pregnancy
- Active peptic ulcer
- Current use of anticoagulants; the higher the INR, the higher risk for bleeding

CPR, Cardiopulmonary resuscitation; *DBP,* diastolic blood pressure; *INR,* international normalized ratio; *MI,* myocardial infarction; *SBP,* systolic blood pressure.
*Could be an absolute contraindication in low-risk patients with MI.

! NURSING SAFETY PRIORITY (QSEN)

Drug Alert

During and after thrombolytic administration, immediately report any indications of bleeding to the health care provider or Rapid Response Team. Observe for signs of bleeding by:
- Documenting the patient's neurologic status (in case of intracranial bleeding)
- Observing all IV sites for bleeding and patency
- Monitoring clotting studies
- Observing for signs of internal bleeding (Monitor hemoglobin, hematocrit, and blood pressure.)
- Testing stools, urine, and emesis for occult blood

Patients who weigh less than 143 pounds (65 kg) may need to have their dose of thrombolytic adjusted to lessen the likelihood of bleeding.

Percutaneous Coronary Intervention. For some patients having an ACS, primary percutaneous coronary intervention (PCI) may be used to reopen the clotted coronary artery and restore PERFUSION. Percutaneous intervention has been associated with excellent return of blood flow through the coronary artery when it can be performed by an interventional cardiologist within 2 to 3 hours of the onset of symptoms. Many community hospitals can now perform emergent PCI. When primary PCI is not available, patients should receive immediate thrombolytic agents if they are appropriate candidates and then be transferred to a facility that can perform PCI. This procedure is described in detail on p. 772 of this chapter. After PCI with stent placement, the patient requires dual antiplatelet therapy, explained later in the chapter.

Patients who receive fibrinolytics require PCI for more definitive treatment such as stent placement. Therefore, if criteria for PCI are met, it is more advantageous to go directly to the catheterization laboratory where definitive treatment, not just clot resolution, can be performed.

Monitor the patient for indications that the clot has been lysed (dissolved) and the artery reperfused. These indications include:
- Abrupt cessation of pain or discomfort
- Sudden onset of ventricular dysrhythmias
- Resolution of ST-segment depression/elevation or T-wave inversion
- A peak at 12 hours of markers of myocardial damage

After clot lysis with thrombolytics, large amounts of thrombin are released into the system, increasing the risk for vessel reocclusion. To maintain the patency of the coronary artery after thrombolytic therapy, the health care provider usually prescribes aspirin and IV heparin, a *high-alert drug*. Maintain the heparin infusion via pump for 3 to 5 days as prescribed, and monitor the activated partial thromboplastin time (aPTT). The target aPTT range is usually 1½ to 2½ times the control sample. The heparin antifactor Xa assay (heparin assay) test may be used instead of the aPTT in some clinical facilities. Low–molecular-weight heparin (LMWH) (enoxaparin [Lovenox]) may be substituted for IV heparin. Therapeutic dosing of LMWH in this patient population should be based on weight (1 mg/kg). Chapter 36 describes care of the patient receiving heparin or LMWH in detail.

? NCLEX EXAMINATION CHALLENGE

Physiological Integrity

A client weighing 174 pounds had thrombolytic therapy followed by a one-time dose of IV Lovenox 30 mg. The physician prescribes Lovenox 1 mg/kg subcutaneously after the IV administration. The nurse will give ____ mg of Lovenox to the client.

Increasing Activity Tolerance

Planning: Expected Outcomes. The patient is expected to increase activity without chest PAIN and the need for supplemental oxygen as a result of a collaborative cardiac rehabilitation program.

Interventions. Activity intolerance is reduced by a planned program of cardiac rehabilitation implemented primarily by the nurse and physical therapist and continued after discharge.

Cardiac rehabilitation is the process of actively assisting the patient with cardiac disease in achieving and maintaining a vital and productive life while remaining within the limits of the heart's ability to respond to increases in activity and stress. It can be divided into three phases. *Phase 1* begins with the acute illness and ends with discharge from the hospital. *Phase 2* begins after discharge and continues through convalescence at home. *Phase 3* refers to long-term conditioning.

In the acute phase (phase 1), promote rest and ensure limited mobility. Assistance may be needed for some ADLs, such as ambulation to the bathroom. Patients progress at their own rate to increasing levels of activity depending on their clinical status, age, and physical capabilities.

The next step in phase 1 is independent ambulation of the patient in the room and to the bathroom. Encourage progressive ambulation in the hallway, usually 50, 100, and then 200 feet 3 times a day. In addition, the patient may begin showering for 5 or 10 minutes with warm water. A chair should be available to facilitate rest and maintain balance.

! NURSING SAFETY PRIORITY QSEN

Action Alert

During cardiac rehabilitation, assess the patient's heart rate, blood pressure (BP), respiratory rate, and level of fatigue with each higher level of activity. Decreases greater than 20 mm Hg in the systolic BP, changes of 20 beats per minute in the pulse rate, and/or reports of dyspnea or chest pain indicate intolerance of activity. If these manifestations develop, notify the health care provider and do not advance the patient to the next level. Older adults with CAD often have needs and concerns different from those of younger adults, as described in Chart 38-5.

All patients with ACS should be referred to a phase 2 cardiac rehabilitation program upon discharge from the hospital. Collaborate with the case manager to plan for the patient's continuing care.

Promoting Effective Coping

Planning: Expected Outcomes. The patient is expected to learn to cope with the cardiac event and identify effective coping strategies with the help of support systems.

Interventions. Assess the patient's level of anxiety while allowing expressions of any apprehension, and attempt to define its origin. Simple, repeated explanations of therapies, expectations, and surroundings, as well as patient progress, may help relieve anxiety.

Identify the patient's current *coping* mechanisms. The most common are denial, anger, and depression. Denial allows the patient to decrease a threat and use problem-focused coping mechanisms. The patient may avoid discussing what has happened and yet comply with treatment regimens. This type of denial decreases anxiety and should not be discouraged. *However, denial that results in a patient who refuses to follow treatment regimens can be harmful.* Because this behavior is usually due to extreme anxiety or fear, threats only worsen the behavior. Remain calm, and avoid confronting the patient. Clearly indicate when a behavior is not acceptable and is potentially harmful as a result of noncompliance.

Anger may represent an attempt to regain control of life. Encourage the patient to verbalize the source of frustration, and provide opportunities for decision making and control. Collaborate with the certified spiritual chaplain or social worker in the hospital to help the patient cope with the situation based on his or her preferences, values, and beliefs. Help the patient identify support systems, such as family, friends, church, or social group.

Depression may be a response to grief and loss of function. Listen as the patient verbalizes feelings of loss, being careful not to offer false or general reassurances. Acknowledge depression, but encourage the patient to perform ADLs and other activities within restrictions.

Identifying and Managing Dysrhythmias

Planning: Expected Outcomes. The most desired outcome for the patient is that he or she will be free of dysrhythmias. If dysrhythmias occur, they will be identified and managed early to prevent complications or death.

Interventions. *Dysrhythmias are the leading cause of prehospital death in most patients with ACS.* Even in the early period of hospitalization, most patients with ACS experience some abnormal cardiac rhythm. When a dysrhythmia develops:

- Identify the dysrhythmia.
- Assess hemodynamic status.
- Evaluate for discomfort.

Dysrhythmias are treated when they cause hemodynamic compromise, increase myocardial oxygen requirements, or predispose the patient to lethal ventricular dysrhythmias.

Typical dysrhythmias for the patient with an *inferior* ACS are bradycardias and second-degree AV blocks resulting from ischemia of the AV node. These rhythms tend to be intermittent. Monitor the cardiac rhythm and rate and the hemodynamic status. If the patient becomes hemodynamically unstable, a temporary pacemaker may be necessary.

The patient with an *anterior* ACS is likely to exhibit premature ventricular contractions (PVCs) caused by ventricular irritability. Third-degree or bundle branch block is a serious complication in this patient because it indicates that a large portion of the left ventricle is involved. The health care provider may insert a pacemaker. Observe the patient closely to detect the development of heart failure. Appropriate interventions for dysrhythmias are described in Chapter 34.

Monitoring for and Managing Heart Failure

Planning: Expected Outcomes. The most desired outcome for the patient is that he or she will be free of heart failure. However, if it occurs, the outcome is that the heart failure will be identified and treated early to prevent further complications.

Interventions. Decreased cardiac output related to heart failure is a relatively common complication after an MI resulting from left ventricular dysfunction, rupture of the intraventricular septum, papillary muscle rupture with valvular

CHART 38-5 Nursing Focus on the Older Adult

Coronary Artery Disease

- Recognize that chest pain may not be evident in the older patient. Examples of associated symptoms are unexplained dyspnea, confusion, or GI symptoms.
- Although older adults have a greater reduction in mortality rate from myocardial infarction (MI) with the use of thrombolytics, they also have the most severe side effects. Monitor older patients receiving thrombolytics extremely carefully.
- Dysrhythmia may be a normal age-related change rather than a complication of MI. Determine whether the dysrhythmia is causing significant symptoms. Then notify the physician.
- If beta blockers are used, assess the patient carefully for the development of side effects. Exacerbation of the depression some older adults have is a significant problem with beta blockade.
- Plan slow, steady increases in activity. Older adults with minimal previous exercise show particular benefit from a gradual increase in activity.
- Older adults should plan longer warm-up and cool-down periods when participating in an exercise program. Their pulse rates may not return to baseline until 30 minutes or longer after exercise.

dysfunction, or right ventricular infarction. The most severe form of acute heart failure, *cardiogenic shock,* discussed later in this chapter, causes most in-hospital deaths after an ACS. The type of management used to increase cardiac output depends on the location of the ACS and the type of heart failure that resulted from the infarction.

Managing Left Ventricular Failure. When a patient with ACS experiences damage to the left ventricle, rupture of the intraventricular septum, or tear of a papillary muscle, the amount of blood that the heart can eject is reduced. When volume and pressure are markedly increased in the pulmonary vasculature, pulmonary complications can develop.

Assess for manifestations of left ventricular failure and pulmonary edema by listening for crackles and identifying their location in the lung fields. Wheezing, tachypnea, and frothy sputum may also occur with pulmonary edema. Auscultate the heart, paying particular attention to the presence of an S_3 heart sound.

! NURSING SAFETY PRIORITY QSEN

Critical Rescue

Monitor for, report, and document these signs of inadequate organ PERFUSION that may result from decreased cardiac output:

- A change in orientation or mental status
- Urine output less than 0.5-1 mL/kg/hr
- Cool, clammy extremities with decreased or absent pulses
- Unusual fatigue
- Recurrent chest pain

In specialized units, hemodynamic monitoring requiring the insertion of a pulmonary artery catheter may be started to assess the patient's preload, afterload, and cardiac output.

Hemodynamic Monitoring. Hemodynamic monitoring is an invasive system used in critical care areas to provide quantitative information about vascular capacity, blood volume, pump effectiveness, and tissue PERFUSION. It directly measures pressures in the heart and great vessels. These procedures are usually performed for more seriously ill patients and can provide more accurate measurements of blood pressure, heart function, and volume status. Although medical-surgical nurses do not manage these systems on general hospital units, they should be familiar with the interpretation of some of the major hemodynamic pressures as they relate to patient assessment.

Hemodynamic monitoring does involve significant risks, although complications are uncommon. Therefore informed consent is required. After obtaining consent, the critical care nurse prepares a pressure-monitoring system. The components of this system are a catheter with an infusion system, a transducer, and a monitor. The catheter receives the pressure waves (mechanical energy) from the heart or the great vessels. The transducer converts the mechanical energy into electrical energy, which is displayed as waveforms or numbers on the monitor. Patency of the catheter is maintained with a slow continuous flush of normal saline, usually infused at 3 to 4 mL/hr under pressure to prevent the backup of blood and occlusion of the catheter.

To prepare the transducer, balance and calibrate it according to hospital policy and the manufacturer's specifications. Finally, identify the phlebostatic axis (Chart 38-6) and level the transducer to it. The physician inserts a balloon-tipped catheter percutaneously through a large vein, usually the internal jugular or subclavian, and directs it to the right atrium (RA). When the catheter tip reaches the RA, the physician inflates the balloon. The catheter advances with the flow of blood through the tricuspid valve, into the right ventricle, past the pulmonic valve, and into a branch of the pulmonary artery. The balloon is deflated after the catheter tip reaches the pulmonary artery. Waveforms are viewed on the monitor as the pulmonary artery catheter is advanced (Fig. 38-3). A chest x-ray is used to check the location of the catheter.

CHART 38-6 Best Practice for Patient Safety & Quality Care QSEN

Identification of the Phlebostatic Axis

1. Position the patient supine.
2. Palpate the fourth intercostal space at the sternum.
3. Follow the fourth intercostal space to the side of the patient's chest.
4. Determine the midway point between anterior and posterior.
5. Find the intersection between the midway point and the line from the fourth intercostal space, and mark it with an X in indelible ink. This is the phlebostatic axis.

A pulmonary artery catheter is a multi-lumen catheter with the capacity to measure right atrial and indirect left atrial pressures or pulmonary artery wedge pressure (PAWP), also known as the **pulmonary artery occlusive pressure (PAOP).** A cardiac output measurement may also be obtained, as well as cardiac index and systemic and pulmonary vascular resistance.

Right atrial pressure is measured by a pressure sensor on the catheter inside the RA. Normal RA pressure ranges from 1 to 8 mm Hg. *Increased RA pressures may occur with right ventricular failure, whereas low RA pressures usually indicate hypovolemia.*

Normal pulmonary artery pressure (PAP) ranges from 15 to 26 mm Hg systolic/5 to 15 mm Hg diastolic (mean, 15) and is constantly visible on the monitor. When the balloon at the catheter tip is inflated, the catheter advances and wedges in a branch of the pulmonary artery. The tip of the catheter can sense pressures transmitted from the left atrium, which reflect left ventricular end-diastolic pressure (LVEDP). The pressure measured during balloon inflation is called the **pulmonary artery wedge pressure (PAWP).** PAWP closely reflects left atrial pressure and LVEDP in patients with normal left ventricular function, normal heart rates, and no mitral valve disease. The PAWP is a mean pressure and normally ranges between 4 and 12 mm Hg.

Elevated PAWP measurements may indicate left ventricular failure, hypervolemia, mitral regurgitation, or intracardiac shunt. A decreased PAWP is seen with hypovolemia or afterload reduction. Individual values may be less important than the trend in values.

The critical care nurse obtains and records RA pressure, PAP, and PAWP at appropriate intervals (usually every 1 to 4 hours). Single values of these measurements are less significant than the trend of values combined with the patient's clinical manifestations. They help health care providers identify heart failure and guide the administration of fluids and vasoactive drugs. During pressure recording, it is important that the transducer be at the level of the phlebostatic axis. The patient is usually supine with

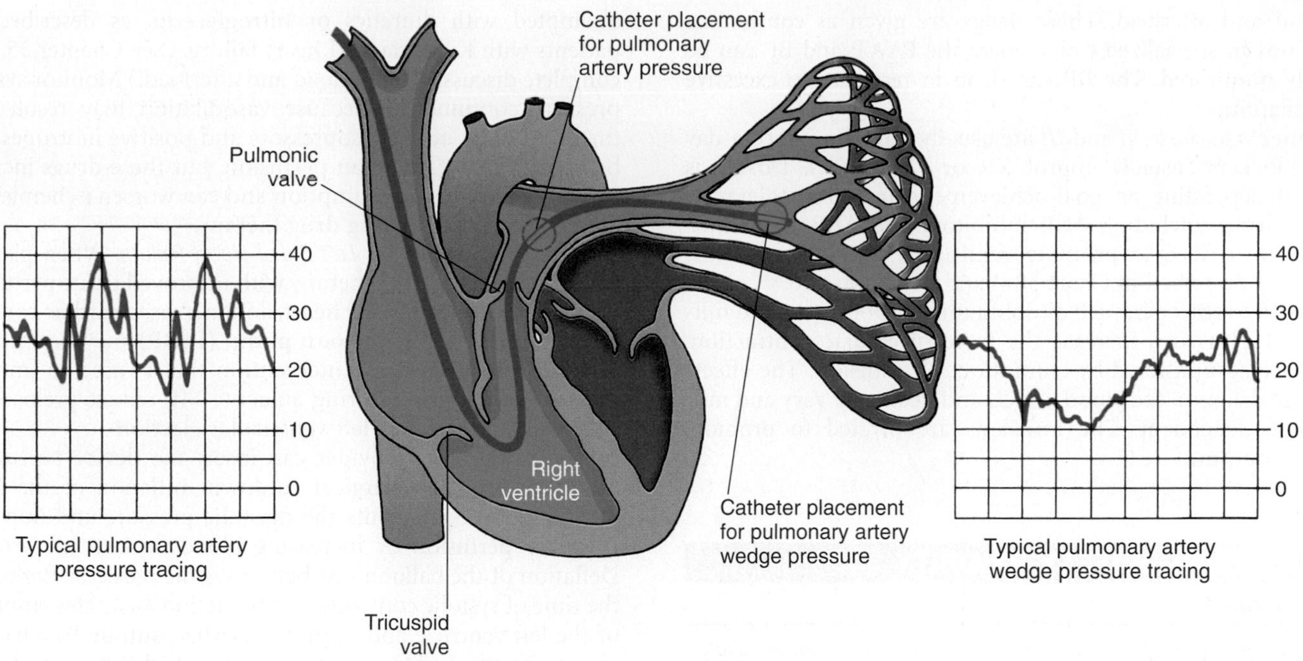

FIG. 38-3 Cardiac pressure waveforms can be seen on the monitor.

the head elevated up to 45 degrees during hemodynamic readings, although the position may not affect results. If the balloon remains in the wedge position after PAWP measurement, try to change the catheter's position by asking the patient to cough or by changing his or her position. *If these methods are not successful, notify the physician immediately.*

Change the occlusive sterile dressing over the catheter according to hospital policy. Inspect the insertion site for redness, induration, swelling, drainage, and intactness of the sutures. Detailed discussion of the management and care of patients with pulmonary artery catheters can be found in textbooks on critical care nursing.

Be sure to assess for a number of complications associated with pulmonary artery catheters. For example, pulmonary infarction or pulmonary rupture may occur if the catheter remains in the wedge position. Air embolism is possible if the balloon has ruptured and repeated attempts are made to inflate it. Ventricular dysrhythmias may occur during insertion or if the catheter tip slips back into the right ventricle and irritates the myocardium. Thrombus and embolus formation may occur at the catheter site. Infection may result, and bleeding may be pronounced if the infusion system becomes disconnected.

Direct measurement of *arterial BP* is done by invasive arterial catheter in critically ill patients. The physician or specially trained health care professional inserts an intra-arterial catheter into the radial or femoral artery. After the catheter is inserted, it is attached to pressure tubing. A normal saline flush solution is infused constantly under pressure to maintain the integrity of the system. A transducer attached to the tubing allows continuous direct monitoring of the arterial BP. Direct measurements of BP are usually 10 to 15 mm Hg greater than indirect (cuff) measurements. The arterial catheter may also be used to obtain blood samples for arterial blood gas values and other blood tests.

Because the arterial vasculature is a high-pressure system, frequent assessment of the arterial site and infusion system is essential. *Note any bleeding around the intra-arterial catheter or any loose connections, and correct the situation immediately.* Collateral circulation must be assessed by Doppler before and while the arterial catheter is in place. Carefully monitor color, pulse, and temperature distal to the insertion site for any early signs of circulatory compromise. Complications of systemic intra-arterial monitoring include pain, infection, arteriospasm, or obstruction at the site with the potential for distal infarction, air embolism, and hemorrhage.

TABLE 38-3 Killip Classification of Heart Failure

CLASS	DESCRIPTION
I	Absent crackles and S_3
II	Crackles in the lower half of the lung fields and possible S_3
III	Crackles more than halfway up the lung fields and frequent pulmonary edema
IV	Cardiogenic shock

Classification of Post–Myocardial Infarction Heart Failure. Several classification systems may be used to categorize heart failure after an MI. For example, the classic Killip system identifies four classes based on prognosis (Table 38-3). This system complements the ACC/AHA heart failure classification of function assessment discussed in Chapter 35.

Patients with *class I* heart failure often respond well to reduction in preload with IV nitrates and diuretics. Monitor the urine output hourly, check vital signs hourly, continue to assess for signs of heart failure, and review the serum potassium level.

Patients with *class II* and *class III* heart failure may require diuresis and more aggressive medical intervention, such as afterload reduction and/or enhancement of contractility. IV nitroprusside or nitroglycerin may be used to decrease both preload and afterload. These drugs are given as continuous infusions in specialized units where the PAWP and BP can be closely monitored. The BP can drop in response to excessive vasodilation.

Patients in *classes II* and *III* are usually started on once-a-day beta blockers (usually Toprol XR or Coreg CR). Dosing is titrated depending on goal achievement and drug tolerance. Other drugs, including ACE inhibitors and ARBs, are commonly prescribed to promote ventricular remodeling. These drugs are described in Chart 38-4 and in Chapter 36.

Positive inotropes, such as dobutamine (Dobutrex) and milrinone (Primacor), increase the force of cardiac contraction. They are administered by continuous IV infusion. The effects of these drugs on the blood vessels and heart rate vary and may be dose dependent. The infusions are titrated to promote cardiac output.

! NURSING SAFETY PRIORITY QSEN

Drug Alert

Use caution when giving positive inotropes because of the potential risk for increasing myocardial oxygen consumption and further decreasing cardiac output. Monitor the patient frequently, paying particular attention to the development of chest pain.

Class IV heart failure is cardiogenic shock. In **cardiogenic shock**, necrosis of more than 40% of the left ventricle occurs. Most patients have a stuttering pattern of chest pain, resulting in piecemeal extension of the ACS.

! NURSING SAFETY PRIORITY QSEN

Critical Rescue

Monitor for, report, and document manifestations of cardiogenic shock immediately. These signs and symptoms include:

- Tachycardia
- Hypotension
- Systolic BP less than 90 mm Hg or 30 mm Hg less than the patient's baseline
- Urine output less than 0.5-1 mL/kg/hr
- Cold, clammy skin with poor peripheral pulses
- Agitation, restlessness, or confusion
- Pulmonary congestion
- Tachypnea
- Continuing chest discomfort

Early detection is essential because undiagnosed cardiogenic shock has a high mortality rate!

Drug Therapy. Medical interventions aim to relieve pain and decrease myocardial oxygen requirements through preload and afterload reduction (see Chart 38-4 and Chart 38-7). The health care provider prescribes IV morphine, which is used to decrease pulmonary congestion and relieve pain. Oxygen is administered. Intubation and mechanical ventilation may be necessary.

Use the information gained from hemodynamic monitoring to titrate drug therapy. Preload reduction may be cautiously attempted with diuretics or nitroglycerin, as described for patients with Killip class III heart failure. (See Chapter 35 for a complete discussion of preload and afterload.) Monitor systolic pressure continuously because vasodilation may result in a further decline in BP. Vasopressors and positive inotropes may be used to maintain organ perfusion, but these drugs increase myocardial oxygen consumption and can worsen ischemia. Use extreme caution in giving drug therapy.

Other Interventions for Left-Sided Heart Failure. When patients do not respond to drug therapy with improved tissue perfusion, decreased workload of the heart, and increased cardiac contractility, an **intra-aortic balloon pump (IABP)** may be inserted. The IABP is an invasive intervention that is used to improve myocardial perfusion during an acute MI, reduce preload and afterload, and facilitate left ventricular ejection.

The health care provider can insert the device percutaneously or through a surgical cutdown. Inflation of the IABP during diastole augments the diastolic pressure and improves coronary perfusion by increasing blood flow to the arteries. Deflation of the balloon just before systole reduces afterload at the time of systolic contraction. This action facilitates emptying of the left ventricle and improves cardiac output. The balloon catheter is attached to a pump console, which is triggered by an ECG tracing and arterial waveform.

In patients undergoing high-risk percutaneous coronary intervention (PCI) or those at risk for cardiogenic shock, a *percutaneous ventricular assist device* may be used. These devices are temporary to decrease the myocardial workload and oxygen consumption of the heart and increase cardiac output and peripheral perfusion.

Immediate reperfusion is an invasive intervention that shows some promise for managing cardiogenic shock. The patient is taken to the cardiac catheterization laboratory, and an emergency left-sided heart catheterization is performed. If he or she has a treatable occlusion or occlusions, the interventional cardiologist performs a percutaneous coronary intervention in the catheterization laboratory or the patient is transferred to the operating suite for a coronary artery bypass graft (CABG).

Managing Right Ventricular Failure. Conditions other than left ventricular failure may result in decreased cardiac output after an ACS. In about a third of patients with inferior MIs, right ventricular infarction and failure develop. In this instance, the right ventricle fails independently of the left. Decreased cardiac output with a paradoxical pulse, clear lungs, and jugular venous distention occurs when the patient is in semi-Fowler's position.

A right ventricular MI may be documented by echocardiography and by an ECG using right-sided precordial leads. The desired outcome of management is to improve right ventricular stroke volume by increasing right ventricular fiber stretch or preload. To enhance right ventricular preload, give sufficient fluids (as much as 200 mL/hr) to increase right atrial pressure to 20 mm Hg. In the critical care unit, *monitor the pulmonary artery wedge pressure (PAWP)—attempting to maintain it below 15 to 20 mm Hg—and auscultate the lungs to assess for left-sided heart failure. If symptoms of this complication occur, notify the health care provider immediately.*

Monitoring for and Managing Recurrent Symptoms and Extension of Injury

Planning: Expected Outcomes. The most desired outcome is that the patient will not have recurrent symptoms or an

CHART 38-7 Common Examples of Drug Therapy

Commonly Used Intravenous Vasodilators and Inotropes

DRUG	USUAL DOSAGE	NURSING INTERVENTIONS	RATIONALES
Nitrates			
Nitroprusside sodium (Nipride, Nitropress)	IV only by infusion device Begin with 0.4-0.5 mcg/kg/min May increase gradually to 10 mcg/kg/min	Monitor BP every 2-5 min when initiating therapy. If BP drops excessively, elevate the legs, decrease the dose, and increase fluids per unit policy. Monitor PAWP, SVR, BP, heart rate, urine output frequently. Titrate medication to obtain the desired effect.	This agent is a potent, rapidly reversible vasodilator acting on both peripheral venous and arterial musculature. BP may drop in 2 min.
		Protect from light.	This agent is light sensitive.
		Maintain dose at less than 3 mcg/kg/min if possible.	Doses higher than 3 mcg/kg/min are associated with thiocyanate or cyanide toxicity.
		In patients requiring doses higher than 3 mcg/kg/min for longer than 24-36 hr, monitor for metabolic acidosis, confusion, or hyperreflexia. Examine blood thiocyanate level.	These are indications of the toxic effects of cyanide.
Nitroglycerin (Tridil)	IV only by infusion device Begin with 5 mcg/kg/min and gradually increase in increments of 5 every 3-5 min If no response after 20 mcg/kg/min, increase by 10-20 mcg until desired response	Monitor BP every 1-3 min when initiating therapy. If BP drops excessively, elevate the legs and decrease the dose according to unit policies. Monitor RAP, PAWP, SVR, BP, heart rate, and urine output frequently. Titrate medication to obtain the desired effect.	This agent dilates coronary arteries. It is a more potent systemic vasodilator than an arterial vasodilator. BP may drop in 1 min.
		Intermittent administration of IV nitroglycerin should be considered.	Tolerance may develop rapidly to nitroglycerin administered by continuous IV.
		Monitor patients for headache.	Headache is a frequent side effect of initial nitroglycerin therapy.
Milrinone (Primacor)	IV bolus 50 mcg/kg given over 10 min; start infusion of 0.375-0.75 mcg/kg/min; reduce dose in renal impairment	Assess BP and pulse every 5 min. If systolic BP drops 30 mm Hg, stop infusion and call health care provider.	Hypotension is a common adverse effect.
		Monitor I&O and weight.	The drug causes diuresis.
Fenoldopam (Corlopam)	0.01-1.6 mcg/kg/min IV	Assess BP and pulse every 5 min, then every 1 hr × 2, then every 4 hr, or according to agency policy. Monitor I&O, and assess for signs of dehydration. Observe IV site for extravasation.	Same as for milrinone.
Sympathomimetics			
Dopamine (Intropin)	IV only by infusion device Starting dose 2-5 mcg/kg/min Titrate up to 50 mcg/kg/min	Determine the reason for use and the expected result. Observe the patient's heart rate, ECG, BP, PAWP, SVR, cardiac output, and urine output every 5 min to every 1 hr. Titrate the dose carefully to maintain the dose range and obtain the desired effect. Infuse through a central catheter. Monitor patients for ectopy and angina.	This agent is a dose-dependent activator of alpha, beta, and dopaminergic receptors. 2-5 mcg/kg/min stimulates dopaminergic receptors, which promotes renal and mesenteric blood flow. 5 mcg/kg/min stimulates beta receptors. This increases heart rate and contractility more than 10-15 mcg/kg/min; alpha effects predominate. This causes peripheral constriction. Extravasation can cause tissue necrosis and sloughing. These are adverse effects.
Dobutamine (Dobutrex)	IV only by infusion device, 2-10 mcg/kg/min. May increase to 40 mcg/kg/min.	Observe patients continuously during administration. Titrate the drug on the basis of adequate tissue perfusion: mentation, skin temperature, peripheral pulses, PAWP, cardiac output, SVR, and urine output.	This agent is a very strong $beta_1$-receptor activator and a moderately strong $beta_2$-receptor activator.
		Monitor for atrial and ventricular ectopy.	Dysrhythmias are an adverse effect.

BP, Blood pressure; *ECG,* electrocardiogram; *I&O,* input and output; *PAWP,* pulmonary artery wedge pressure; *RAP,* right atrial pressure; *SVR,* systemic vascular resistance.

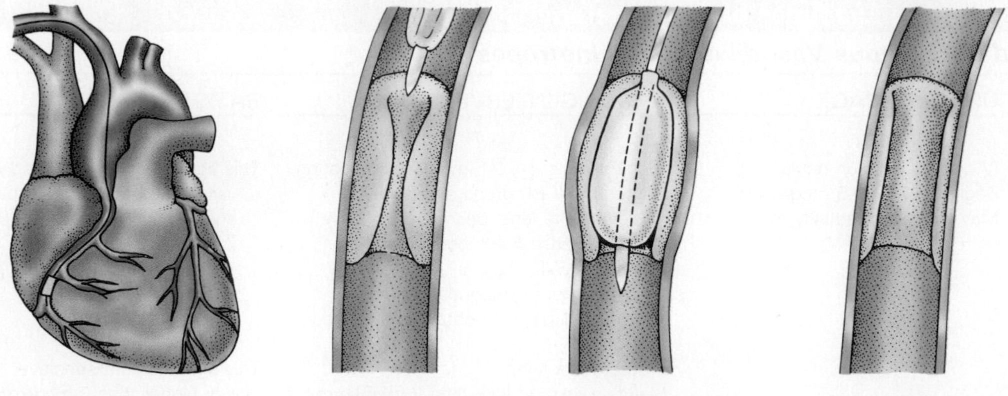

FIG. 38-4 Percutaneous coronary intervention.

extension of myocardial injury. If these problems occur, they will be identified and treated early to prevent further complications or death.

Interventions. *Recurrent discomfort despite medical therapy is one of the major indications for surgical management of CAD.* Patients who continue to have chest discomfort despite medical therapy or who have ischemia during a stress test may require invasive correction by PCI or CABG to resolve angina or prevent MI. Before invasive treatment, a left-sided cardiac catheterization with coronary angiogram is performed to document that the lesions are correctable and that left ventricular pump function is adequate.

Percutaneous Coronary Intervention. **Percutaneous coronary intervention (PCI)** is an invasive but nonsurgical technique that is performed within 90 minutes of an acute MI (AMI) diagnosis. Hospitals are required to report how many patients with AMI receive a PCI within that time frame per the AMI Core Measure Set. It is performed to reduce the frequency and severity of discomfort for patients with angina and to bridge patients to coronary artery bypass graft (CABG) surgery. It combines clot retrieval, coronary angioplasty, and stent placement. Under fluoroscopic guidance, the cardiologist performs initial coronary angiography. In the STEMI patient, if a clot is seen, a clot retrieval device is inserted over the guidewire and the clot is removed. Once the clot is removed in the STEMI patient or area of narrowing is identified in the NSTEMI patient, a balloon-tipped catheter is introduced through a guidewire to the coronary artery occlusion. The physician activates a compressor that inflates the balloon (angioplasty) to force the plaque against the vessel wall, thus dilating the wall, and reduces or eliminates the occluding clot. Balloon inflation may be repeated until angiography indicates a decrease in the stenosis (narrowing) to less than 50% of the vessel's diameter (Fig. 38-4). The balloon catheter is then withdrawn, and a balloon catheter with stent is introduced. Once the stent and balloon are in position, the stent is deployed by the balloon inflation. The balloon is deflated and the stent stays in place acting as scaffolding to hold the diseased artery open. **Stents** are expandable metal mesh devices that are used to maintain the patent lumen created by angioplasty or atherectomy. Bare metal or drug-eluting stents (DES) (drug-coated) may be used. By providing a supportive scaffold, these devices prevent closure of the vessel from arterial dissection or vasospasm. Fig. 38-5 shows a stent positioned in a coronary artery.

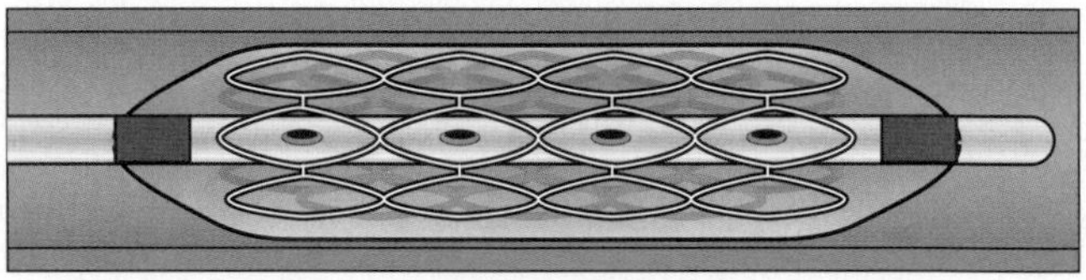

FIG. 38-5 A coronary stent open after balloon inflation.

Patients who are most likely to benefit from PCI have single- or double-vessel disease with discrete, proximal, noncalcified lesions or clots. This procedure often does not work for complex clots. When identifying which lesions are treatable with PCI, the cardiologist considers the clot's complexity and location, as well as the amount of myocardium at risk. Although treating lesions located in the left main artery places a large amount of myocardial tissue at risk if the vessel closes quickly, these lesions are now being treated more with PCI. In the past, coronary artery bypass grafting (CABG) was the intervention used for these patients. PCI may also be used for the patient with an evolving acute MI, either alone or with thrombolytic therapy or glycoprotein (GP) IIb/IIIa inhibitor, to reperfuse the damaged myocardium.

Without stent placement, the artery often reoccludes due to the artery's normal elasticity and memory. Patients who undergo PCI are required to take dual antiplatelet therapy (DAT) consisting of aspirin and a P2Y12 inhibitor (see Chart 38-4). Before the procedure, the patient receives an initial dose of a P2Y12 platelet inhibitor (clopidogrel [Plavix]) or ticagrelor [Brilinta]) and aspirin. If prasugrel (Effient) is the preferred P2Y12 platelet inhibitor, it is given immediately after PCI. If there are any concerns that the patient may require CABG, the P2Y12 inhibitor may be held until after the procedure. The inhibition of the platelets is permanent and increases the risk for postoperative bleeding. Patients should wait 5 (clopidogrel and ticagrelor) to 7 (prasugrel) days before undergoing CABG. If the patient has received thrombolytic therapy, clopidogrel (Plavix) is the preferred drug.

During the procedure, the patient may receive boluses of IV heparin or a continuous infusion of bivalirudin (Angiomax). Heparin is used to maintain an elevated activated clotting time and prevent clotting on wires and catheters during the procedure. Heparin is discontinued before removal of the catheters. Bivalirudin (Angiomax) is a direct thrombin inhibitor and is frequently used as an alternative to IIb/IIIa inhibitors and heparin. Bivalirudin has a short half-life (25 minutes) and is less dependent on renal function. IV or intracoronary nitroglycerin or diltiazem (Cardizem) is given to prevent coronary vasospasm. PCI initially reopens the vessel in most appropriately selected patients. Within the first 24 hours, however, a small percentage of patients have re-stenosis. At 6 months, a larger number have one or more blockages.

! NURSING SAFETY PRIORITY QSEN

Critical Rescue

After PCI, monitor for potential problems including acute closure of the vessel (causes chest pain), bleeding from the insertion site, and reaction to the contrast medium used in angiography. Also monitor for and document hypotension, hypokalemia, and dysrhythmias. Document and report any of these findings to the physician or Rapid Response Team immediately!

The health care provider also prescribes a long-term nitrate and beta blocker, and an ACE inhibitor or ARB is added for patients who have had primary angioplasty after an MI. Some patients may experience hypokalemia after the procedure and require careful monitoring and potassium supplements. The nursing interventions for patients receiving these drugs are described in Chart 38-4. Provide careful explanations of drug therapy and any recommended lifestyle changes.

Other Procedures. Other techniques being used to ensure continued patency of the vessel are laser angioplasty (the laser breaks up the clot) and atherectomy. **Atherectomy** devices can either excise and retrieve plaque or emulsify it. One of the advantages of this procedure is that it creates a less bulky vessel with better elastic recoil. Another procedure that may be performed is rheolytic thrombectomy (e.g., AngioJet, Vortex), which uses low-pressure, high-speed saline jets to break up the clot. The EndiCOR X-SIZER lances and aspirates a clot simultaneously.

Injecting vascular endothelial growth factor (VEGF) during angioplasty has increased PERFUSION to the wall of the heart. Also, VEGF helps initiate new blood vessel growth and development, which results in increased blood supply to cardiac muscle.

Traditional Coronary Artery Bypass Graft Surgery. Over 500,000 traditional open **coronary artery bypass graft (CABG)** surgeries are performed in the United States each year (Go et al., 2013). It is the most common type of cardiac surgery and the most common procedure for older adults. Almost half of all CABGs are done for patients older than 65 years. The occluded coronary arteries are bypassed with the patient's own venous or arterial blood vessels or synthetic grafts. The internal mammary artery (IMA) is the current graft of choice because it has an excellent patency rate many years after the procedure.

CABG is indicated when patients do not respond to medical management of CAD or when disease progression is evident. Because of the development of drug-eluting stents (DESs), patients who previously had no option other than CABG have been able to have their vessels revascularized without surgery. The decision for surgery is based on the patient's symptoms and the results of cardiac catheterization. Candidates for surgery are patients who have:

- Angina with greater than 50% occlusion of the left main coronary artery that cannot be stented
- Unstable angina with severe two-vessel disease, moderate three-vessel disease, or small-vessel disease in which stents could not be introduced
- Ischemia with heart failure
- Acute MI with cardiogenic shock
- Signs of ischemia or impending MI after angiography or percutaneous transluminal coronary angioplasty (PTCA)
- Valvular disease
- Coronary vessels unsuitable for PCI

The vessels to be bypassed should have proximal clots blocking more than 70% of the vessel's diameter but with good distal runoff. Bypass of less occluded vessels may result in poor perfusion through the graft and early obstruction. CABG is most effective when adequate ventricular function remains and the ejection fraction is close to or greater than 50%. Patients with lower ejection fractions are subject to develop more complications.

For most patients, the risk is low and the benefits of bypass surgery are clear. Surgical treatment of CAD does not appear to affect the life span. Left ventricular function is the most important long-term indicator of survival. CABG improves the quality of life for most patients. Most are pain-free at 1 year after surgery and remain so at 5 years after the procedure. The percentage of patients experiencing some PAIN increases sharply after 5 years.

Preoperative Care. CABG surgery may be planned as an elective procedure or performed as an emergency. It may be done as a *traditional* operative technique or performed as a *minimally invasive surgical (MIS)* technique, discussed later on p. 777. Patients undergoing elective surgery are admitted on the morning of surgery. Preoperative preparations and teaching are completed during prehospitalization interviews. Teach patients that their drugs will be changed after surgery. Ensure that the necessary drugs have been administered before surgery.

Familiarize the patient and family with the cardiac surgical–critical care unit (sometimes referred to as the "open heart" unit), and prepare them for postoperative care. If the procedure is elective, demonstrate and have the patient return a demonstration of how to splint the chest incision, cough, deep breathe, and perform arm and leg exercises. Stress that:

- The patient should report any PAIN to the nursing staff.
- Most of the pain will be in the site where the vessel was harvested. (With the use of endovascular vessel harvesting [EVH] and one or two small incisions, the pain and edema are less than for previously performed procedures.)
- Analgesics will be given for pain.
- Coughing and deep breathing are essential to prevent pulmonary complications.
- Early ambulation is important to decrease the risk for venous thrombosis and possible embolism.

For the traditional surgical procedure, explain that the patient will have a sternal incision; possibly a large leg incision; one, two, or three chest tubes; an indwelling urinary catheter; pacemaker wires; and hemodynamic monitoring. An endotracheal tube will be connected to a ventilator for several hours postoperatively. Tell the patient and family that the patient will not be able to talk while the endotracheal tube is in place. When describing the postoperative course, emphasize that close monitoring and the use of sophisticated equipment are standard treatment.

Preoperative anxiety is common. An appropriate nursing assessment should identify the level of anxiety and the coping methods patients have used successfully in the past. Some patients may find it helpful to define their fears. Common sources of fear include fear of the unknown, fear of bodily harm, and fear of death.

In elective procedures, patients may benefit from detailed information about the surgery, depending on individual preferences and cultural practices. Others may feel overwhelmed by so much material. Some patients need to discuss their feelings in detail or describe the experiences of people they know who have undergone CABG. Assess patients' anxiety level and help them cope.

Operative Procedures. Coronary artery bypass surgery is performed with the patient under general anesthesia for both cardiopulmonary bypass and off-pump surgery. For the *traditional operative procedure,* the cardiac surgical team begins the procedure with a median sternotomy incision and visualization of the heart and great vessels. Another surgical team may begin harvesting the vein if it is to be used for the graft. Synthetic grafts may be used instead.

Cardiopulmonary bypass (CPB) is used to provide oxygenation, circulation, and hypothermia during induced cardiac arrest. Blood is diverted from the heart to the bypass machine, where it is heparinized, oxygenated, and returned to the circulation through a cannula placed in the ascending aortic arch or femoral artery (Fig. 38-6). During bypass, the patient's core temperature remains between 95° F (35° C) (cold cardioplegia) and normal temperature (warm cardioplegia). Although cooling decreases the rate of metabolism and demand for oxygen, keeping the heart "warm" decreases postoperative complications that were more common when cold cardioplegia was used. The heart is perfused with a potassium solution, which decreases myocardial oxygen consumption and causes the heart to stop during diastole. This process ensures a motionless operative field and prevents myocardial ischemia.

Once the heart is arrested, the grafting procedure can begin. The surgeon uses the internal mammary artery (IMA), a saphenous vein, and/or a radial artery to bypass blockages in the coronary arteries (Fig. 38-7). The distal end of the vessel graft is dissected and attached below the clot in the coronary artery. If the surgeon uses a venous graft or the radial artery, it is anastomosed (sutured) proximally to the aorta and distally to the coronary artery just beyond the occlusion, thus improving myocardial perfusion. After flow rates through the grafts are measured, the heart is rewarmed slowly. The cardioplegic solution is flushed from the heart. The heart regains its rate and rhythm, or it may be defibrillated to return it to a normal rhythm. When the procedure is completed, the patient may be rewarmed (if cold cardioplegia was used) and weaned from the bypass machine while the grafts are observed for patency and leakage. The surgeon may place atrial and ventricular pacemaker wires and mediastinal and pleural chest tubes. Finally, the surgeon closes the sternum with wire sutures.

Postoperative Care. After traditional surgery, the patient is transported to a post–open heart surgery unit and undergoes mechanical ventilation for 3 to 6 hours. He or she requires highly skilled nursing care from a nurse qualified to provide post–cardiac surgery care, including routine postoperative care described in Chapter 16. *Be sure to use sterile technique when changing sternal or donor-site dressings.*

Connect the mediastinal tubes to water seal drainage systems, and ground the epicardial pacer wires by connecting them to the pacemaker generator. Monitor pulmonary artery and arterial pressures, as well as the heart rate and rhythm, which are displayed on a monitor.

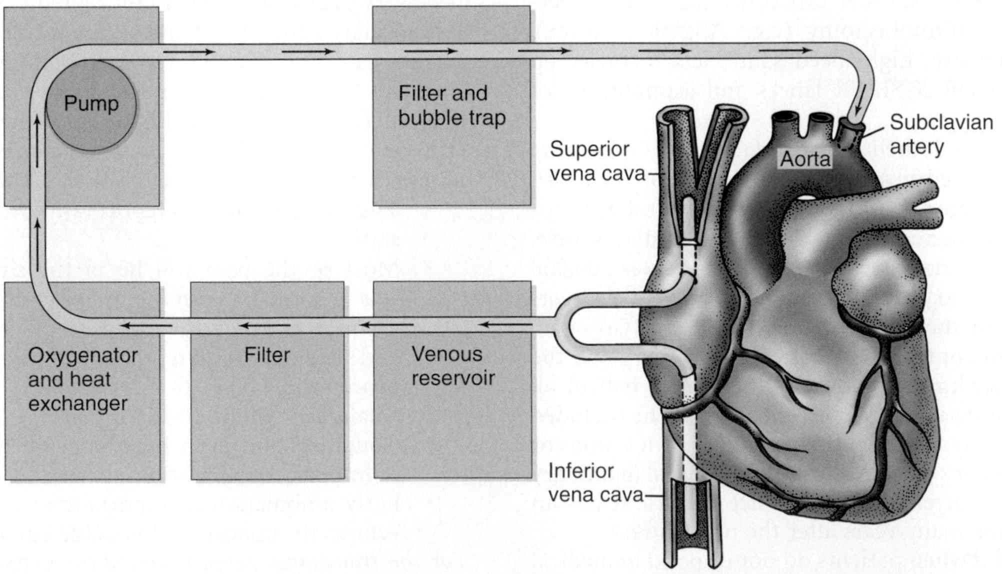

FIG. 38-6 Heart-lung bypass circuitry used during cardiopulmonary bypass.

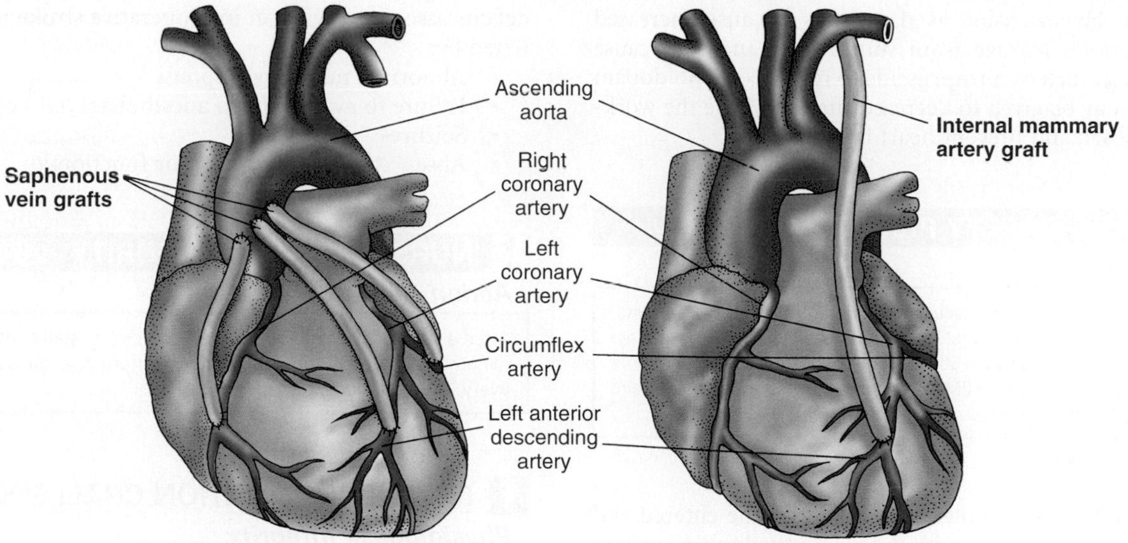

FIG. 38-7 Two methods of coronary artery bypass grafting. The procedure used depends on the nature of the coronary artery disease, the condition of the vessels available for grafting, and the patient's health status.

Closely assess the patient for dysrhythmias, such as bradydysrhythmias, atrial fibrillation, or heart block. Manage symptomatic dysrhythmias according to unit protocol or the health care provider's prescription. Hypoxemia and hypokalemia are frequent causes of ventricular dysrhythmias. If the patient has symptomatic bradydysrhythmias or heart block, turn on the pacemaker and adjust the pacemaker settings as prescribed. Monitor for, report, and document other complications of CABG, including:

- Fluid and electrolyte imbalance
- Hypotension
- Hypothermia
- Hypertension
- Bleeding
- Cardiac tamponade
- Decreased level of consciousness
- Anginal pain

Managing Fluid and Electrolyte Imbalance. Assessing fluid and electrolyte balance is a high priority in the early postoperative period. Edema is common. However, decisions concerning fluid administration are made on the basis of BP, pulmonary artery wedge pressure (PAWP), right atrial pressure, cardiac output, cardiac index, systemic vascular resistance, blood loss, and urine output. An experienced specialized nurse interprets the assessment findings and adjusts fluid administration on the basis of standing unit policies or specific prescription from the physician.

Serum electrolytes (especially calcium, magnesium, and potassium) may be decreased postoperatively and are monitored carefully. Because the serum potassium level can fluctuate dramatically, electrolyte levels are checked frequently, since imbalances can cause dysrhythmias. Potassium and magnesium depletions are common and may result from hemodilution or diuretic therapy. Calcium replacement is based on the *ionized* serum calcium. The desired potassium level is 4.0 mEq/L, and the magnesium level should be 2.2 mEq/L.

If the serum potassium level is decreased, the health care provider may prescribe IV potassium replacement. The dose of potassium given exceeds the usual recommended level of no more than 20 mEq of potassium per hour. For potassium replacement, as much as 40 to 80 mEq may be mixed in 100 mL of IV solution and given at a rate up to 40 mEq per hour. The drug must be given through a central catheter and controlled by an infusion pump. The patient is placed on a cardiac monitor for intense, focused nursing observation.

Managing Other Complications. Hypotension (systolic BP <90 mm Hg) is a major problem because it may result in the collapse of the coronary graft. Decreased preload (decreased PAWP) can result from hypovolemia or vasodilation. If the patient is hypovolemic, it might be appropriate to increase fluid administration or administer blood. The health care provider may manage the patient with volume replacement followed by vasopressor therapy to increase the BP. However, if hypotension is the result of left ventricular failure (increased PAWP), IV inotropes might be needed.

Hypothermia is a common problem after surgery. Although warm cardioplegia is now the usual operative procedure used, it is not uncommon for the body temperature to drift downward after the patient leaves the surgical suite. Monitor the body temperature, and institute rewarming procedures if the temperature drops below 96.8° F (36° C). Rewarming may be accomplished with warm blankets, lights, or thermal blankets. The danger of rewarming patients too quickly is that they may begin shivering, resulting in metabolic acidosis, increased myocardial oxygen consumption, and hypoxia. To prevent shivering, rewarming should proceed at a rate no faster than 1.8° F (1° C) per hour. Discontinue the procedure when the body temperature approaches 98.6° F (37° C) and the patient's extremities feel warm.

Hypothermia is a significant risk for the patient after CABG surgery because it promotes vasoconstriction and *hypertension.* Other factors contributing to hypertension in the CABG patient include CPB, drug therapy, and increased sympathetic nervous system activity.

After surgery, many patients experience *hypertension* (hypertension is defined as a systolic BP greater than 140 to

150 mm Hg). Hypertension is dangerous because increased pressure promotes leakage from suture lines and may cause bleeding. Drugs such as nitroprusside (Nipride) or fenoldopam (Corlopam) may be given to decrease afterload, ease the workload of the heart, and prevent heart failure.

! NURSING SAFETY PRIORITY QSEN

Action Alert

Bleeding after CABG surgery occurs to a limited extent in all patients. Measure mediastinal and pleural chest tube drainage at least hourly. Report drainage amounts over 150 mL per hour to the surgeon. Patients with internal mammary artery (IMA) grafts may have more chest drainage than those with saphenous vein grafts (from the leg).

To access the IMA, the pleural space has to be entered and requires a pleural chest tube with the mediastinal tubes, making pulmonary assessment crucial. An autotransfusion of chest drainage to assist with volume management when 500 mL has accumulated or 4 hours has elapsed may be done, depending on the clinical pathway or the health care provider's protocol. Maintain the patency of the mediastinal and pleural chest tubes. One effective way of promoting chest tube drainage is to prevent a dependent loop from forming in the tubing.

If the patient is bleeding and the mediastinal tubes are not kept patent, fluid (blood) may accumulate around the heart. The myocardium is then compressed, and **cardiac tamponade** results. The fluid compresses the atria and ventricles, preventing them from filling adequately and thus reducing cardiac output.

! NURSING SAFETY PRIORITY QSEN

Critical Rescue

Assess for, document, and report manifestations of cardiac tamponade immediately, including:

- Sudden cessation of previously heavy mediastinal drainage
- Jugular venous distention but clear lung sounds
- Pulsus paradoxus (BP more than 10 mm Hg higher on expiration than on inspiration)
- An equalizing of PAWP and right atrial pressure
- Cardiovascular collapse

Prepare the patient for echocardiogram or chest x-ray to confirm the diagnosis. Pericardiocentesis (withdrawal of fluid from the pericardium via a large needle) may not be appropriate for tamponade after coronary artery bypass graft (CABG) because the blood in the pericardium may have clotted. Volume expansion and emergency sternotomy with drainage are the treatments of choice.

The patient may also demonstrate *changes in level of consciousness,* which may be permanent or transient (temporary, short-term). Transient changes related to anesthesia, cardiopulmonary bypass (CPB), air emboli, or hypothermia occur in many patients. Assess for neurologic deficits, which may include slowness to arouse, memory loss, and new-onset confusion.

Patients with transient neurologic deficits usually return to baseline neurologic status within 4 to 8 hours. *Permanent* deficits associated with an intraoperative stroke may be manifested by:

- Abnormal pupillary response
- Failure to awaken from anesthesia
- Seizures
- Absence of sensory or motor function

! NURSING SAFETY PRIORITY QSEN

Action Alert

After a CABG, check the patient's neurologic status every 30 to 60 minutes until he or she has awakened from anesthesia. Then check every 2 to 4 hours or per agency policy.

? NCLEX EXAMINATION CHALLENGE

Physiological Integrity

The nurse assesses a client who had a coronary artery bypass graft yesterday. Which assessment finding will the nurse report to the surgeon immediately?

A. Incisional pain
B. Blood pressure of 136/76
C. Decreased level of consciousness
D. Apical pulse of 88

Managing Pain. Differentiate between *sternotomy pain,* which is expected after CABG, and *anginal pain,* which might indicate graft failure. Typical sternotomy PAIN is localized, does not radiate, and often becomes worse when the patient coughs or breathes deeply. He or she may describe the pain as sharp, aching, or burning. Pain may stimulate the sympathetic nervous system, which increases the heart rate and vascular resistance while decreasing cardiac output. Administer enough of the prescribed analgesic in adequate doses to control pain. During the process of weaning the patient from mechanical ventilation, however, it may be necessary to use short-acting analgesics and to limit pain medication because of the respiratory depressant effects of analgesia.

Transfer from the Special Care Unit. Mechanical ventilation is usually provided for 3 to 6 hours after surgery until the patient is breathing adequately and is hemodynamically stable. During the first day, the patient usually has pacemaker wires, hemodynamic monitoring lines, and mediastinal tubes removed. He or she is then transferred to an intermediate care unit. *All CABG patients, especially those with IMA grafts, are at high risk for atelectasis, the number-one complication.* Encourage them to splint, cough, turn, and deep breathe to expectorate secretions. Early ambulation after surgery is essential. Two hours after extubation (removal of the endotracheal tube), patients should be dangled as tolerated and turned side to side. Within 4 to 8 hours after extubation, help patients out of bed into a chair. By the first day after surgery, they should be out of bed in a chair and ambulating 25 to 100 feet 3 times a day as tolerated. Continue to monitor for decreased cardiac output, pain, dysrhythmias, decreased oxygen saturation, and infection during these activities.

Many patients have supraventricular dysrhythmias (especially atrial fibrillation) during the postoperative period, usually on the second or third postoperative day. Examine the monitor

! NURSING SAFETY PRIORITY (QSEN)

Action Alert

Monitor the neurovascular status of the donor arm of patients whose radial artery was used as a graft in CABG. Assess the hand color, temperature, pulse (both ulnar and radial), and capillary refill every hour initially. In addition, check the fingertips, hand, and arm for sensation and mobility at least every 4 hours. IV nitroglycerin is often given for the first 24 hours postoperatively to promote vasodilation in the donor arm and therefore maintain circulation.

pattern for atrial fibrillation. When auscultating the heart, listen for an irregular rhythm.

Sternal wound infections develop between 5 days and several weeks after surgery in a small number of patients and are responsible for increased costs and longer hospital stays. Be alert for **mediastinitis** (infection of the mediastinum) by observing for:

- Fever continuing beyond the first 4 days after CABG
- Instability (bogginess) of the sternum
- Redness, induration, swelling, or drainage from suture sites
- An increased white blood cell count

The health care provider may perform a needle biopsy to confirm a sternal infection. Surgical débridement, antibiotic wound irrigation, and IV antibiotics are usually indicated. If sternal osteomyelitis has developed, 4 to 6 weeks of IV antibiotics are required. Prophylactic use of mupirocin (Bactroban) intranasally may be prescribed to decrease the incidence of sternal wound infection.

Postpericardiotomy syndrome is a source of chest discomfort for some post–cardiac surgery patients. The syndrome is characterized by pericardial and pleural pain, pericarditis, a friction rub, an elevated temperature and white blood cell count, and dysrhythmias. Postpericardiotomy syndrome may occur days to weeks after surgery and seems to be associated with blood remaining in the pericardial sac. Observe for the development of pericardial or pleural pain. For most patients, the syndrome is mild and self-limiting. However, they may require treatment similar to that for pericarditis. Be prepared to detect acute cardiac (pericardial) tamponade.

Minimally Invasive Direct Coronary Artery Bypass. The **minimally invasive direct coronary artery bypass (MIDCAB)** (also known as *"keyhole" surgery*) may be indicated for patients with a lesion of the left anterior descending (LAD) artery. In one of the most common MIDCAB procedures, a 2-inch left thoracotomy incision is made and the fourth rib is removed. Then the left internal mammary artery (IMA) is dissected and attached to the still-beating heart below the level of the lesion. Cardiopulmonary bypass (CPB) is not required.

After surgery, assess for chest pain and ECG changes (Q waves and ST-segment and T-wave changes in leads V_2 to V_6) because occlusion of the IMA graft occurs acutely in only a small percentage of patients. *If there is any question of acute graft closure, immediately notify the health care provider.* Patients tend to have more incisional PAIN after MIDCAB than after traditional CABG surgery, but it can usually be managed with oxycodone or codeine. Because they have a thoracotomy incision and a chest tube or smaller-lumen vacuum chest device, patients are encouraged to cough, deep breathe, and use an incentive spirometer for a week postoperatively. Most patients spend less than 6 hours in a critical care unit and are discharged in 2 or 3 days.

Endovascular (Endoscopic) Vessel Harvesting. Regardless of whether the traditional CABG or the MIDCAB is performed, the donor vessel may be obtained using an endoscope rather than a large surgical incision. The radial artery or a vein in the leg may be taken using this method. Instead of a large, painful incision, the patient has one or two very small incisions in the leg or arm. This procedure has decreased hospital length of stay, postoperative complications, and pain.

Transmyocardial Laser Revascularization. **Transmyocardial laser revascularization** is a procedure for patients with unstable angina and inoperable CAD with areas of reversible myocardial ischemia. After a single-lung intubation, a left anterior thoracotomy is performed and the heart is visualized. A laser is used to create 20 to 24 long, narrow channels through the left ventricular muscle to the left ventricle. These channels will eventually allow oxygenated blood to flow during diastole from the left ventricle to nourish the muscle. After surgery, the patient is transported to a critical care unit, where hemodynamic monitoring is used to assess for anginal episodes and bleeding disturbances.

Off-Pump Coronary Artery Bypass. Off-pump coronary artery bypass (OPCAB) is a procedure in which open heart surgery is performed without the use of a heart-lung bypass machine. Advantages include shorter hospital stays and decreased mortality rate, risk for infection, and cost. The disadvantage of OPCAB is that it requires cardiac surgeons to have increased skill to master the technique.

Robotic Heart Surgery. Robotic heart surgery is a new step toward less invasive open heart surgery. Surgeons operate endoscopically through very small incisions in the chest wall. Use of robotics provides surgeons with capabilities that simplify the surgical process, eliminate tremors that can exist with human hands, increase the ability to reach otherwise inaccessible sites, and improve depth perception and visual acuity.

Other advantages of robotic procedures include shorter hospital stays (average stay is 2 to 3 days), less PAIN because of smaller incisions, no need for heart-lung bypass machine, less anxiety for the patient, and greater patient acceptance. The use of robotics also allows surgeons to perform telesurgery, performing heart procedures over long distances.

Disadvantages include computer failure, limited numbers of surgeons skilled in these techniques, and the length of surgery time (the time is about 50 minutes longer than the conventional surgery).

Community-Based Care

Home Care Management. Case management is most appropriate for patients who meet high-cost, high-volume, and high-risk criteria. Patients with coronary artery disease (CAD) clearly meet all these criteria. Clinical pathways and case management programs for those with CAD are used in most U.S. hospitals. By focusing on cardiovascular risk reduction and improving the continuity of care, health care professionals have reduced the length and cost of hospital stays. Posthospital case management should reduce hospital readmission rates and improve patient health.

Patients who have experienced a myocardial infarction (MI), angina, or coronary artery bypass graft (CABG) surgery are usually discharged to home or to a transitional care setting with drug therapy and specific activity prescriptions. Depending on the procedure, hospital stays may be 3 to 5 days for patients with MI or those undergoing CABG and only 1 to 3 days for those undergoing percutaneous coronary intervention (PCI) or newer surgeries. Therefore patients are still recovering when they are discharged from the hospital and need continuing care.

Patients should not be discharged to home alone. Assess whether the patient has family or friends to provide assistance. In some cases, a home care nurse may be needed (Chart 38-8). Older adults are often living alone when coronary events occur and may have a greater need for home assistance after CABG surgery (Chart 38-9). A patient who was a resident in a long-term care facility may be returned there after hospitalization for unstable angina, MI, or CABG surgery.

Cardiac rehabilitation is available in most communities for patients after an MI or CABG surgery, but only a small percentage participate in structured rehabilitation programs. Dolansky et al. (2010) found that although post–acute care (PAC) is available for older adults, only 50% of patients who had a myocardial infarction (MI) received PAC. Only 44% of patients who had cardiac surgery participated in post–acute care. Cossette et al. (2012) found that a stepwise nursing intervention post-discharge significantly increased enrollment in cardiac rehabilitation programs over standard of care (see the Evidence-Based Practice box).

CHART 38-8 Home Care Assessment

The Patient Who Has Had a Myocardial Infarction

Assess cardiovascular function, including:
- Current vital signs (compare with previous to identify changes)
- Recurrence of discomfort (characteristics, frequency, onset)
- Indications of heart failure (weight gain, crackles, cough, dyspnea)
- Adequacy of tissue perfusion (mentation, skin temperature, peripheral pulses, urine output)
- Indications of serious dysrhythmia (very irregular pulse, palpitations with fainting or near fainting)

Assess coping skills, including:
- Is patient displaying denial, anger, or fear?
- Is caregiver providing adequate support?
- Are patient and caregiver disagreeing about treatment?

Assess functional ability, including:
- Activity tolerance (examine the patient's activity diary: review distance, duration, frequency, and symptoms occurring during exercise)
- Activities of daily living (is any assistance needed?)
- Household chores (who performs them?)
- Does patient plan to return to work? When?

Assess nutritional status, including:
- Food intake (review patient's intake of fats and cholesterol)

Assess patient's understanding of illness and treatment, including:
- How to treat chest discomfort
- Signs and symptoms to report to health care provider
- Dosage, effects, and side effects of medications
- How to advance and when to limit activity
- Modification of risk factors for coronary artery disease

CHART 38-9 Nursing Focus on the Older Adult

Coronary Artery Bypass Graft Surgery

- Be aware that perioperative mortality rates are higher for the older patient than for the patient younger than 60 years.
- Monitor neurologic and mental status carefully because older adults are more likely to have transient neurologic deficits after coronary artery bypass graft (CABG) surgery than younger adults are.
- Observe for side effects of cardiac drugs because older patients are more likely to develop toxic effects from positive inotropes (dobutamine) and potent antihypertensives (nitroglycerin or nitroprusside).
- Monitor the patient closely for dysrhythmias because older adults are more likely to have dysrhythmias such as atrial fibrillation or supraventricular tachycardia after CABG surgery.
- Be aware that recuperation after CABG surgery is slower for older patients and that their average hospital stay is longer.
- Teach the patient and family that during the first 2 to 5 weeks after discharge, fatigue, chest discomfort, and lack of appetite may be particularly bothersome for older adults.
- Teach the patient to let someone know where he or she is walking outside.

EVIDENCE-BASED PRACTICE QSEN

Can Nursing Interventions Tailored to the Acute MI Population Increase Enrollment in Cardiac Rehabilitation?

Cossette, S., Frasure-Smith, N., Dupuis, J., Juneau, M., & Guertin, M. (2012). Randomized controlled trial of tailored nursing interventions to improve cardiac rehabilitation enrollment. *Nursing Research, 61*(2), 111-120.

Cardiac rehabilitation, which is widely available, can reduce recurrence of coronary events by 25%. Due to the decreased length of stay, the nurse has limited time to provide important post-discharge education. In a randomized control trial, adults who experienced acute myocardial infarction (AMI) were contacted at three separate encounters: face to face prior to discharge, telephone call at 3 days post-discharge, and telephone call or face to face meeting at 10 days. The first call focused on the current condition of the patient, symptomology, activity, and patient's concerns. At the second call, the patient's current condition was reviewed and education and discussion about risk factor modification occurred. In addition to cardiac rehabilitation review, risk factor and lifestyle modification were the focus of the third call. The control group received the standard of care that included standard discharge instructions with encouragement to follow up with health care provider.

All participants completed baseline questionnaires: Revised Illness Perception Questionnaire, Family Care Climate Questionnaire—Patient Version, and State-Trait Anxiety Inventory. In addition, all participants received follow-up phone calls from a research assistant at 6 weeks post-discharge. A total of 242 participants were enrolled, and results revealed 45% of patients in the intervention group versus 24% of the control group enrolled in cardiac rehabilitation program (defined as attendance at one session prior to end of 6 weeks post-discharge). The time to mean first visit (day 20 post-discharge) did not differ between the groups. The intervention did not impact modification of risk factors. Limitations included lack of data on continued attendance, cost-effectiveness of the intervention, and long-term outcomes.

Level of Evidence: 1

The study was a large randomized controlled trial.

Commentary: Implications for Practice and Research

In view of the low percentages of older adults who attend cardiac rehabilitation, nurses can provide the necessary intervention to encourage attendance. Collaborate with the case manager or discharge planner to ensure that follow-up on lifestyle modification occurs after discharge because the patient is focused on immediate discharge needs at the time of discharge. More studies need to be completed to determine the nursing interventions that may be valuable post-discharge in the AMI patient population that not only improve outcomes but also are cost-effective.

MI, Myocardial infarction.

The most frequently cited reasons for nonparticipation are lack of insurance coverage, a physician's decision that it is unnecessary, and the patient's decision that it is not necessary. Those who participate in these programs report greater improvement in exercise tolerance and improved ability to control stress. However, no difference in their return to work has been seen.

Self-Management Education. The need for health teaching depends in part on the treatment plan or type of procedure that the patient received. Because hospital stays are short and patients are quite ill during hospitalization, most in-hospital education programs concentrate on the skills essential for self-care after discharge.

As part of home visits or a cardiac rehabilitation program, identify the additional educational needs of the patient and family and their readiness to learn. Develop a teaching plan, which usually includes education about the normal anatomy and physiology of the heart, the pathophysiology of angina and MI, risk factor modification, activity and exercise protocols, cardiac drugs, and when to seek medical assistance. Teach patients that myocardial healing after an MI begins early and is usually complete in 6 to 8 weeks. Remind those who have undergone traditional CABG that the sternotomy should heal in about 6 to 8 weeks, but upper body exercise needs to be limited for several months.

Patients who have undergone CABG require instruction on incision care for the sternum and the graft site. Teach them to inspect the incisions daily for any redness, swelling, or drainage. The leg of a saphenous vein donor site is often edematous. Instruct patients to avoid crossing legs, to wear elastic stockings until the edema subsides, and to elevate the surgical limb when sitting in a chair. Teach patients who have had a radial artery graft to open and close the hand vigorously 10 times every 2 hours.

Risk Factor Modification. Modification of risk factors is a necessary part of a patient's management and involves changing his or her health maintenance patterns. Such modifications may include tobacco cessation, altered dietary patterns, regular exercise, BP control, and blood glucose control.

For patients who use tobacco, explain its negative effects, especially cigarette smoking. Many patients choose to quit smoking soon after an MI. Chapter 30 also provides information on this lifestyle change.

The mainstays of cholesterol control are nutritional therapy and anti-hyperlipidemic agents, as described in Chapter 36. Teach patients to avoid adding salt when beginning a meal. A reduction of 80 mg/day of sodium can reduce the systolic blood pressure (SBP) by 5 mm Hg and 3 mm Hg for the diastolic blood pressure (DBP). Maintain adequate dietary potassium, calcium, and magnesium intake. Increasing potassium may reduce the SBP by 8 mm Hg. Booklets and cookbooks that can assist the patient in learning to cook with reduced fats, oils, and salt are available from the American Heart Association (AHA).

Collaborate with the physical therapist to establish an activity and exercise schedule as part of rehabilitation, depending on the cardiac procedure that was performed. Instruct the patient to remain near home during the first week after discharge and to continue a walking program. Patients may engage in light housework or any activity done while sitting and that does not precipitate angina. During the second week, they are encouraged to increase social activities and possibly to return to work part-time. By the third week, they may begin to lift objects as heavy as 15 pounds (e.g., 2 gallons of milk) but should avoid lifting or pulling heavier objects for the first 6 to 8 weeks. Chart 38-10 lists suggested instructions for activity level.

CHART 38-10 Patient and Family Education: Preparing for Self-Management

Activity for the Patient with Coronary Artery Disease

- Begin by walking the same distance at home as in the hospital (usually 400 feet) 3 times each day.
- Carry nitroglycerin with you.
- Check your pulse before, during, and after the exercise.
- Stop the activity for a pulse increase of more than 20 beats/min, shortness of breath, angina, or dizziness.
- Exercise outdoors when the weather is good.
- Gradually increase the walking until the distance is ¼ mile twice daily (usually the end of the second week).
- After an exercise tolerance test and with your physician's approval, walk at least 3 times each week, increasing the distance by ½ mile every other week, until the total distance is 2 miles.
- Avoid straining (lifting, push-ups, pull-ups, and straining at bowel movements).

Patients may begin a simple walking program by walking 400 feet twice a day at the rate of 1 mile/hr the first week after discharge and increasing the distance and rate as tolerated, usually weekly, until they can walk 2 miles at 3 to 4 miles/hr. Teach them to take their pulse reading before, halfway through, and after exercise. Teach the patient to stop exercising if the target pulse rate is exceeded or if dyspnea or angina develops.

After a limited exercise tolerance test, the physical therapist or nurse encourages the patient to join a formal exercise program, ideally one that assists him or her in monitoring cardiovascular progress. The program should include 5- to 7-minute warm-up and cool-down periods, as well as 30 minutes of aerobic exercise. The patient should engage in aerobic exercise a minimum of 3 (and preferably 5) times a week.

Complementary and Alternative Therapies. Additional therapies can aid in reducing the patient's anxiety about progressive activity both in the immediate postoperative period and during the rehabilitation phase. Many patients who have had cardiac surgery or other invasive procedures use complementary and alternative therapies. However, they often do not share with their health care providers that they use these therapies. Techniques such as progressive muscle relaxation, guided imagery, music therapy, pet therapy, and therapeutic touch may decrease anxiety, reduce depression, and increase compliance with activity and exercise regimens after heart surgery.

Sexual Activity. Sexual activity is often a subject of great concern to patients and their partners. Inform the patient and his or her partner that engaging in their usual sexual activity is unlikely to damage the heart. Patients can resume sexual intercourse on the advice of the health care provider, usually after an exercise tolerance assessment. In general, those who can walk one block or climb two flights of stairs without symptoms can usually safely resume sexual activity.

Suggest that initially these patients have intercourse after a period of rest. They might try having intercourse in the morning when they are well rested or wait 1½ hours after exercise or a heavy meal. The position selected should be comfortable for both the patient and his or her partner so that no undue stress is placed on the heart or suture line.

Drug Therapy. Assess patients with diabetes mellitus for their ability to control hyperglycemia. Review the prescribed dosage of insulin or oral antidiabetic drugs with the patient and family. The patient and/or family should demonstrate accurate testing of blood for glucose levels and the technique for insulin administration, if used.

Teach the patient about the type of prescribed cardiac drugs, the benefit of each drug, potential side effects, and the correct dosage and time of day to take each drug. Drug regimens vary considerably. Many patients with angina are discharged while taking aspirin, a beta blocker, a calcium channel blocker, an anti-hyperlipidemic agent, and a nitrate. Those who have experienced an MI may require aspirin, a beta blocker, an anti-hyperlipidemic agent (statin drug), and an ACEI and/or an ARB. The Joint Commission Acute MI Core Measure Set requires hospitals to report whether patients with an MI are discharged on these drugs. Determine whether the patient can comply with the instructions.

! NURSING SAFETY PRIORITY QSEN

Drug Alert

Use of sublingual or spray nitroglycerin (NTG) deserves special attention. *Teach the patient to carry NTG at all times.* Keep the tablets in a glass, light-resistant container. The drug should be replaced every 3 to 5 months before it loses its potency or stops producing a tingling sensation when placed under the tongue. Chart 38-11 gives instructions for management of chest discomfort at home.

Seeking Medical Assistance. Teach patients to notify their health care provider if they have:

- Heart rate remaining less than 50 after arising
- Wheezing or difficulty breathing
- Weight gain of 3 pounds in 1 week or 1 to 2 pounds overnight
- Persistent increase in NTG use
- Dizziness, faintness, or shortness of breath with activity

Remind them to always call 911 for transportation to the hospital if they have:

- Chest discomfort that does not improve after 5 minutes or 1 sublingual NTG tablet or spray
- Extremely severe chest or epigastric discomfort with weakness, nausea, or fainting
- Other associated symptoms that are particular to them, such as fatigue and nausea

CHART 38-11 Patient and Family Education: Preparing for Self-Management

Management of Chest Pain at Home

- Keep fresh nitroglycerin available for immediate use.
- At the first indication of chest discomfort, cease activity and sit or lie down.
- Place one nitroglycerin tablet or spray under your tongue, allowing the tablet to dissolve.
- Wait 5 minutes for relief.
- If no relief results, call 911 for transportation to a health care facility.
- While waiting for emergency medical services (EMS), repeat the nitroglycerin and wait 5 more minutes.
- If there is no relief, repeat and wait 5 more minutes.
- Carry a medical identification card or wear a bracelet or necklace that identifies a history of heart problems.

Health Care Resources. The American Heart Association (AHA) is an excellent source for booklets, films, CDs, DVDs, cookbooks, and professional service referrals for the patient with coronary artery disease (CAD). Many local chapters have their own cardiac rehabilitation programs.

Within the community, cardiac rehabilitation programs may be affiliated with local hospitals, community centers, or other facilities, such as clinics. Many shopping malls open before shopping hours to allow a measured walking program indoors. This opportunity is particularly popular with older patients because it provides a good support group and allows for an appropriate place to exercise in inclement weather.

Mended Hearts is a nationwide program with local chapters that provides education and support to coronary artery bypass graft (CABG) patients and their families. Smoking-cessation programs and clinics and weight-reduction programs are located within the community. Many hospitals also sponsor health fairs, BP screening, and risk factor modification programs.

? CLINICAL JUDGMENT CHALLENGE

Teamwork and Collaboration; Safety QSEN

A 55-year-old woman had a MIDCAB surgical procedure and is scheduled to begin cardiac rehabilitation on an ambulatory care basis. Her daughter plans to take her to the physical therapist for this program 3 days a week. The patient wants to return to her job as a nursing educator in a local community college as soon as possible.

1. What are the expected outcomes for this patient as a result of cardiac rehabilitation?
2. What is the role of the physical therapist in cardiac rehabilitation?
3. With what other members of the health care team will the nurse collaborate to ensure the patient's continuity of care?
4. What community resources might this patient use after the completion of her cardiac rehabilitation program?
5. For what surgical complications is she still at risk?

◆ *Evaluation: Outcomes*

Evaluate the care of the patient with CAD based on the identified priority patient problems. The expected outcomes are that the patient will:

- State that discomfort or other symptoms are alleviated
- Have adequate blood flow through the coronary vasculature to ensure heart function
- Walk 200 feet 4 times a day without discomfort, shortness of breath, or other symptoms of CAD
- Identify support systems and other sources to assist in effective coping with the cardiac event
- Be free of complications, such as dysrhythmias and heart failure

NURSING CONCEPTS AND CLINICAL JUDGMENT REVIEW

What might you NOTICE if the patient is experiencing inadequate GAS EXCHANGE and tissue PERFUSION as a result of coronary artery disease?

- Report of pain (chest, shoulder, arm, jaw, back, or abdomen)
- Report of persistent indigestion
- Dyspnea
- Diaphoresis
- Report of nausea
- Vomiting
- Anxious behavior
- Report of palpitations
- Report of fatigue
- Disorientation or acute confusion (especially in older adults)

What should you INTERPRET and how should you RESPOND to a patient experiencing inadequate GAS EXCHANGE and tissue PERFUSION as a result of coronary artery disease?

Perform and interpret physical assessment, including:

- Taking vital signs
- Monitoring oxygen saturation by pulse oximetry
- Taking 12-lead ECG
- Assessing level of consciousness and cognition
- Conducting complete pain assessment
- Drawing blood for laboratory assessment (e.g., troponins)
- Auscultating breath sounds for crackles or wheezes (left-sided heart failure)
- Auscultating heart for abnormal heart sounds
- Assessing for peripheral edema (right-sided heart failure)

Respond by:

- Calling 911 if patient is not in hospital setting OR notifying physician or Rapid Response Team in hospital setting
- Ensuring that patient rests
- Giving oxygen
- Giving nitroglycerin tablet
- Maintaining or starting IV line
- Administering morphine sulfate if MI suspected or diagnosed

On what should you REFLECT?

- Observe patient for decreased report of pain and associated symptoms.
- Continue to monitor oxygen.
- Continue to monitor for dysrhythmias and vital signs.
- Think about what could have precipitated this coronary event.
- Think about how you responded.
- Develop teaching plan for the patient to help prevent further episodes.

GET READY FOR THE NCLEX® EXAMINATION!

KEY POINTS

Review these Key Points for each NCLEX Examination Client Needs Category.

Safe and Effective Care Environment

- Collaborate with members of the interdisciplinary health care team members (e.g., physical therapist, case manager, home care providers) when caring for patients preparing for or participating in cardiac rehabilitation. **Teamwork and Collaboration** QSEN

Health Promotion and Maintenance

- Assess the patient for risk factors for coronary artery disease (CAD). Examples of modifiable risk factors that can be managed or controlled include obesity, smoking, high serum lipids, and hypertension; examples of nonmodifiable risk factors that cannot be altered include older age, being African American, and having a family history of CAD.
- Teach patients about the importance of decreasing their risk for CAD (see Chart 38-1). **Safety** QSEN

Psychosocial Integrity

- Allow patients to verbalize and express feelings of fear, anxiety, anger, denial, and grief regarding their CAD.
- Address the needs of the family and significant others, and provide teaching and information regarding the disease process. Clarify any misconceptions.

Physiological Integrity

- Teach patients that angina is the PAIN associated with decreased blood flow to the heart muscle. An MI indicates necrosis of heart muscle tissue (see Chart 38-2).
- Identify and interpret diagnostic values for cardiac markers, such as troponins and myoglobin, and other indicators of CAD.
- Monitor patients receiving thrombolytics and anticoagulants, such as heparin, for bleeding and bruising. **Safety** QSEN
- For patients undergoing invasive cardiac procedures, assess for signs and symptoms of active bleeding.
- Interpret and assess the patient with CAD for dysrhythmias.
- Evaluate the patient for PAIN characteristics (e.g., type, location, duration, cause, intensity, and measures taken to relieve symptoms).
- Teach patients and their families about drug therapy, including how to use nitroglycerin if they have chest or other cardiac-related PAIN (see Chart 38-4).
- After percutaneous cardiac intervention, monitor the patient for potential complications such as chest PAIN, bleeding from the insertion site, hypotension, hypokalemia, and

dysrhythmias. Document and report any of these findings immediately. **Safety** QSEN

- Identify and assess for complications for post–cardiac surgery patients, especially fluid and electrolyte imbalance, bleeding, hypothermia, hypertension, and angina PAIN.
- Provide emergency care for the patient with chest PAIN as described in Chart 38-3.
- For patients having coronary artery bypass graft (CABG) surgery, be sure to manage PAIN adequately, assess fluid and electrolyte balance, and monitor for potential complications. Examples of complications include fluid and electrolyte imbalances (especially hypokalemia), hypothermia, hypertension, bleeding, and neurologic deficits. **Evidence-Based Practice** QSEN

CHAPTER 39

Assessment of the Hematologic System

M. Linda Workman

http://evolve.elsevier.com/Iggy/

PRIORITY CONCEPTS

- CLOTTING
- PERFUSION

LEARNING OUTCOMES

Safe and Effective Care Environment

1. Protect the patient with a potential hematologic problem from injury.

Health Promotion and Maintenance

2. Teach all people how to protect the hematologic system.

Psychosocial Integrity

3. Reduce the psychological impact for the patient and family regarding the assessment and testing of the hematologic system.

Physiological Integrity

4. Explain the relationship between hematologic problems and the concepts of CLOTTING and PERFUSION.
5. Perform a focused assessment of the hematologic system, incorporating information about genetic risk and age-related changes affecting hematologic function, especially CLOTTING and PERFUSION.
6. Use knowledge of anatomy, physiology, laboratory analysis, and human development to determine whether hematologic assessment findings are normal or abnormal.
7. Explain the effects of anticoagulants, fibrinolytics, and inhibitors of platelet activity on CLOTTING and PERFUSION.
8. Prioritize nursing care for the patient after bone marrow aspiration or biopsy.

The hematologic system includes the blood, blood cells, lymph, and organs involved with blood formation or blood storage. This system is important for oxygenation (gas exchange) and tissue PERFUSION because the blood is the oxygen delivery system (Fig. 39-1). All systems depend on the blood for oxygen perfusion, and any problem of the hematologic system affects total body health. This chapter, together with Chapter 17, reviews the normal physiology of the hematologic system and assessment of hematologic status.

ANATOMY AND PHYSIOLOGY REVIEW

Bone Marrow

Bone marrow is responsible for blood formation. It produces red blood cells (RBCs, erythrocytes), white blood cells (WBCs, leukocytes), and platelets. Bone marrow also is involved in the immune responses (see Chapter 17).

Each day the bone marrow normally releases about 2.5 billion RBCs, 2.5 billion platelets, and 1 billion WBCs per kilogram of body weight. In adults, cell-producing marrow is present only in flat bones (sternum, skull, pelvic and shoulder girdles) and the ends of long bones. With aging, fatty tissue replaces active bone marrow and only a small portion of the remaining marrow continues to produce blood in older adults (Touhy & Jett, 2014).

The bone marrow first produces **blood stem cells**, which are immature, unspecialized (undifferentiated) cells that are capable of becoming any type of blood cell, depending on the body's needs (Fig. 39-2) (McCance et al., 2014).

The next stage in blood cell production is the *committed stem cell* (or *precursor* cell). A committed stem cell enters one growth pathway and can at that point specialize (differentiate) into only one cell type. Committed stem cells actively divide but require the presence of a specific growth factor for specialization. For example, erythropoietin is a growth factor specific for the RBC. Other growth factors control WBC and platelet growth (see Chapters 17, 22, and 40 for discussion of growth factors and cytokines).

Blood Components

Blood is composed of plasma and cells. Plasma is an extracellular fluid. It is similar to the interstitial fluid found between tissue cells, but plasma contains much more protein. The three major types of plasma proteins are albumin, globulins, and fibrinogen.

Albumin maintains the osmotic pressure of the blood, preventing the plasma from leaking into the tissues (see Chapter 11). *Globulins* have many functions, such as transporting other substances and, as antibodies, protecting the body against

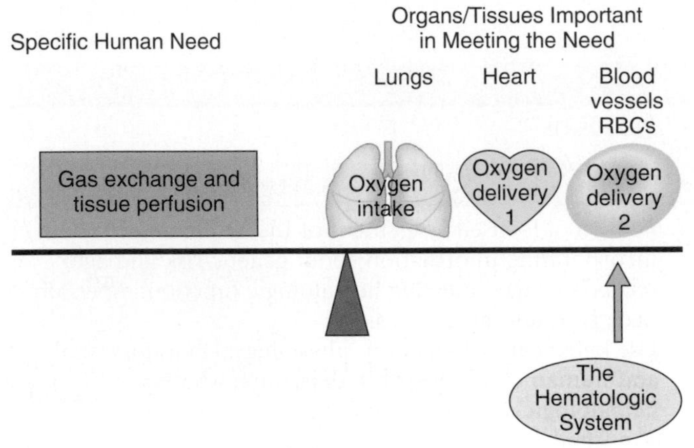

FIG. 39-1 Role of the hematologic system in gas exchange and tissue perfusion. *RBCs,* Red blood cells.

infection. *Fibrinogen* is activated to form fibrin, which is critical in the blood CLOTTING process.

The blood cells include RBCs, WBCs, and platelets. These cells differ in structure, site of maturation, and function.

Red blood cells (**erythrocytes**) are the largest proportion of blood cells. Mature RBCs have no nucleus and have a biconcave disk shape. Together with a flexible membrane, this feature allows RBCs to change their shape without breaking as they pass through narrow, winding capillaries. The number of RBCs a person has varies with gender, age, and general health, but the normal range is from 4,200,000 to 6,100,000/mm^3.

As shown in Figs. 39-2 and 39-3, RBCs start out as stem cells, enter the myeloid pathway, and progress in stages to mature erythrocytes. Healthy, mature, circulating RBCs have a life span of about 120 days. As RBCs age, their membranes become more fragile. These old cells are trapped and destroyed in the tissues, spleen, and liver. Some parts of destroyed RBCs (e.g., iron, hemoglobin) are recycled and used to make new RBCs.

The RBCs produce hemoglobin (Hgb). Each normal mature RBC contains hundreds of thousands of hemoglobin molecules. Each hemoglobin molecule needs iron to be able to transport up to four molecules of oxygen. *Therefore iron is an essential part of hemoglobin.* Hemoglobin also carries carbon dioxide. RBCs also help maintain acid-base balance.

The most important feature of hemoglobin is its ability to combine loosely with oxygen. Only a small drop in tissue oxygen levels increases the transfer of oxygen from hemoglobin to tissues, known as **oxygen dissociation**. See Chapter 27 for a discussion of oxygen dissociation.

The total number of RBCs a person has is carefully controlled to ensure that enough are present for good PERFUSION with oxygen and for CLOTTING without having too many cells that could "thicken" the blood and slow its flow. RBC production or **erythropoiesis** (selective growth of stem cells into mature erythrocytes) must be properly balanced with RBC destruction or loss. When balanced, this process helps tissue perfusion by ensuring adequate delivery of oxygen. The trigger

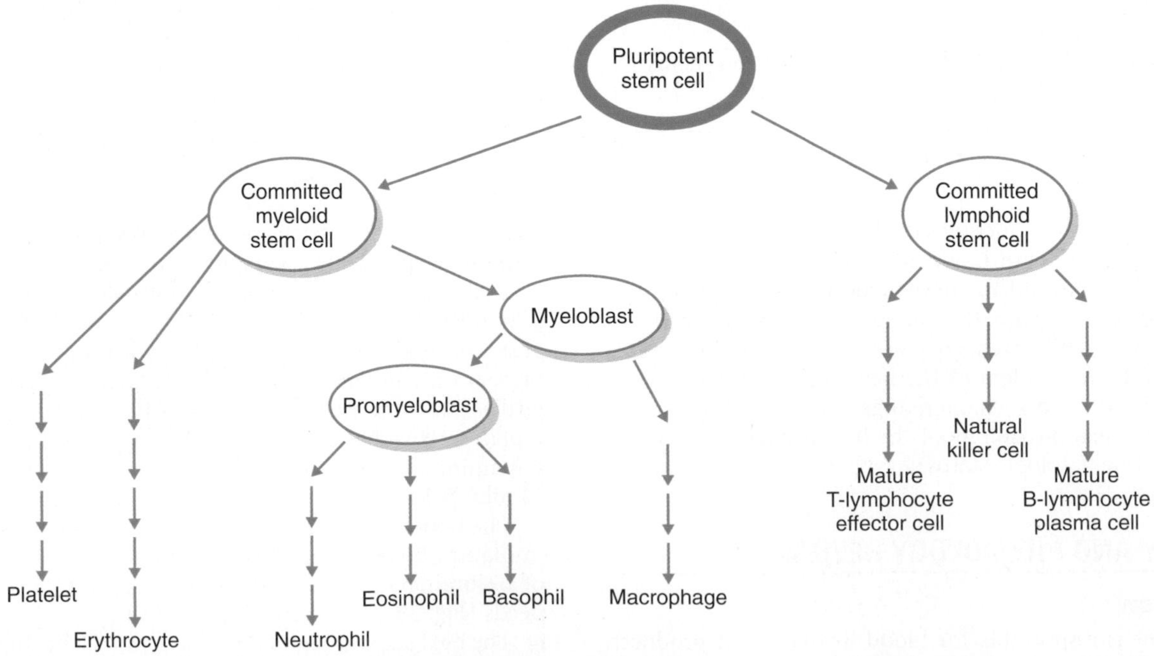

FIG. 39-2 Bone marrow cell growth and blood cell differentiation pathways.

for RBC production is an increase in the tissue need for oxygen. The kidney produces the RBC growth factor *erythropoietin* at the same rate as RBC destruction or loss occurs to maintain a constant normal level of circulating RBCs. When tissue oxygen is less than normal (**hypoxia**), the kidney releases more erythropoietin, which then increases RBC production in the bone marrow. When tissue oxygen is normal or high, erythropoietin levels fall, slowing RBC production. Synthetic erythrocyte stimulating agents (ESAs) such as Procrit, Epogen, and EPO have the same effect on bone marrow as the naturally occurring erythropoietin.

Many substances are needed to form hemoglobin and RBCs, including iron, vitamin B_{12}, folic acid, copper, pyridoxine, cobalt, and nickel. A lack of any of these substances can lead to anemia, which results in unmet tissue oxygen needs because of a reduction in the number or function of RBCs.

White blood cells (WBCs, leukocytes) also are formed in the bone marrow. The many types of WBCs all have specialized functions that provide protection through inflammation and immunity (Table 39-1). WBC function is presented in Chapter 17.

Platelets are the third type of blood cells. They are the smallest blood cells, formed in the bone marrow from megakaryocyte precursor cells. When activated, platelets stick to injured blood vessel walls and form platelet plugs that can stop the flow of blood at the injured site. They also produce substances important to blood CLOTTING and aggregate (clump together) to perform most of their functions. Platelets help keep small blood vessels intact by initiating repair after damage.

Production of platelets is controlled by the growth factor *thrombopoietin*. After platelets leave the bone marrow, they are stored in the spleen and then released slowly to meet the body's needs. Normally, 80% of platelets circulate and 20% are stored in the spleen.

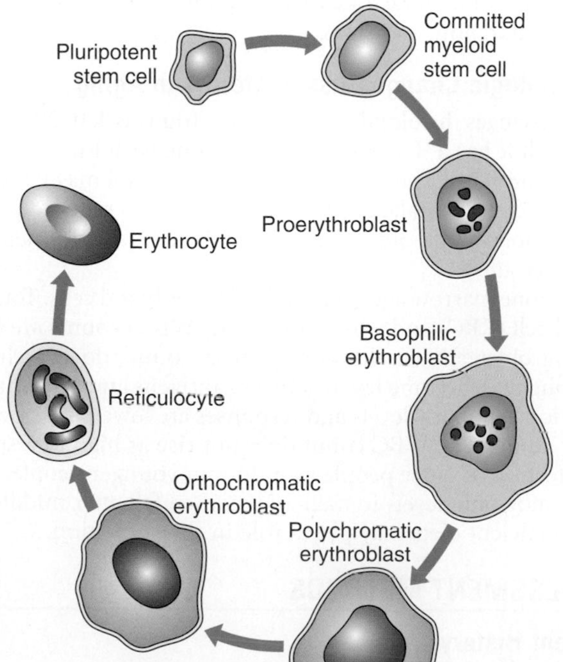

FIG. 39-3 Erythrocyte (red blood cell) growth pathway.

Accessory Organs of Blood Formation

The spleen and liver are important accessory organs for blood production. They help regulate the growth of blood cells and form factors that ensure proper blood CLOTTING.

The spleen contains three types of tissue: white pulp, red pulp, and marginal pulp. These tissues all help balance blood cell production with blood cell destruction and assist with immunity. White pulp is filled with white blood cells (WBCs) and is a major site of antibody production. As whole blood filters through the white pulp, bacteria and old RBCs are removed. Red pulp is the storage site for RBCs and platelets. Marginal pulp contains the ends of many blood vessels.

The spleen destroys old or imperfect RBCs, breaks down the hemoglobin released from these destroyed cells, stores platelets, and filters antigens. Anyone who has had a splenectomy has reduced immune functions and has an increased risk for infection and sepsis.

The liver produces prothrombin and other blood CLOTTING factors. Also, proper liver function is important in forming vitamin K in the intestinal tract. (Vitamin K is needed to produce clotting factors VII, IX, and X and prothrombin.) Large amounts of whole blood and blood cells can be stored in the liver. The liver also stores extra iron within the protein *ferritin*.

Hemostasis and Blood Clotting

Hemostasis is the multi-stepped process of controlled blood CLOTTING. It results in localized blood clotting in damaged blood vessels to prevent excessive blood loss while blood continues to PERFUSE all other areas. This complex function balances blood clotting actions with anti-clotting actions. When

TABLE 39-1 Functions of Specific Leukocytes

LEUKOCYTE	FUNCTION
Inflammation	
Neutrophil	Nonspecific ingestion and phagocytosis of microorganisms and foreign protein
Macrophage	Nonspecific recognition of foreign proteins and microorganisms; ingestion and phagocytosis
Monocyte	Destruction of bacteria and cellular debris; matures into macrophage
Eosinophil	Weak phagocytic action; releases vasoactive amines during allergic reactions
Basophil	Releases histamine and heparin in areas of tissue damage
Antibody-Mediated Immunity	
B-lymphocyte	Becomes sensitized to foreign cells and proteins
Plasma cell	Secretes immunoglobulins in response to the presence of a specific antigen
Memory cell	Remains sensitized to a specific antigen and can secrete increased amounts of immunoglobulins specific to the antigen on re-exposure
Cell-Mediated Immunity	
T-lymphocyte helper/inducer T-cell	Enhances immune activity through the secretion of various factors, cytokines, and lymphokines
Cytotoxic-cytolytic T-cell	Selectively attacks and destroys non-self cells, including virally infected cells, grafts, and transplanted organs
Natural killer cell	Nonselectively attacks non-self cells, especially body cells that have undergone mutation and become malignant; also attacks grafts and transplanted organs

injury occurs, hemostasis starts the formation of a platelet plug and continues with a series of steps that eventually cause the formation of a fibrin clot. Three sequential processes result in blood clotting: platelet aggregation with platelet plug formation; the blood clotting cascade; and the formation of a complete fibrin clot.

Platelet aggregation begins forming a platelet plug by having platelets clump together, a process essential for blood CLOTTING. Platelets normally circulate as individual small cells that do not clump together until activated. Activation causes platelet membranes to become sticky, allowing them to clump together. When platelets clump, they form large, semi-solid plugs in blood vessels, disrupting local blood flow. *These platelet plugs are not clots and last only a few hours. Thus they cannot provide complete hemostasis but only start the hemostatic process.*

Substances that activate platelets and cause clumping include adenosine diphosphate (ADP), calcium, thromboxane A_2, and collagen. Platelets secrete some of these substances, and other activating substances are external to the platelet. Platelet plugs start the cascade action that ends with local blood CLOTTING and are important at most steps within the cascade. When too few platelets are present, blood clotting is impaired, increasing the risk for excessive bleeding.

Blood clotting is a cascade triggered by the formation of a platelet plug, which then rapidly amplifies the cascade (Pezzotti & Freuler, 2012). The final result is much larger than the triggering event. Thus the cascade works like a landslide—a few small pebbles rolling down a steep hill can dislodge large rocks, trees, and soil, causing an enormous movement of earth. Just like landslides, cascade reactions are hard to stop once set into motion.

Intrinsic factors are conditions, such as circulating debris or venous stasis, within the blood itself that can activate platelets and trigger the blood CLOTTING cascade (Fig. 39-4). Continuing the cascade to blood clotting requires sufficient amounts of all the clotting factors and cofactors (Table 39-2).

Extrinsic factors outside of the blood can also activate platelets. The most common extrinsic event is trauma that damages blood vessels and exposes collagen. Collagen then activates platelets to form a platelet plug within seconds. The blood clotting cascade is started sooner by this pathway because some intrinsic pathway steps are bypassed. Other blood vessel changes that can activate platelets include inflammation, bacterial toxins, or foreign proteins.

Whether the platelet plugs are formed because of abnormal blood (intrinsic factors) or by exposure to inflamed or damaged blood vessels (extrinsic factors), the end result of the cascade is the same: *formation of a fibrin clot and local blood CLOTTING (coagulation).* The cascade, from the formation of a platelet plug to the formation of a fibrin clot, depends on the presence of specific clotting factors, calcium, and more platelets at every step.

Clotting factors (see Table 39-2) are inactive enzymes that become activated in a sequence. The last part of the sequence is the activation of fibrinogen into fibrin. At each step, the activated enzyme from the previous step activates the next enzyme. The last two steps in the cascade are the activation of thrombin from prothrombin and the conversion (by thrombin) of fibrinogen into fibrin. Only fibrin molecules can begin the formation of a true clot.

Fibrin clot formation is the last phase of blood clotting. Fibrinogen is an inactive protein made in the liver. The activated enzyme *thrombin* removes the end portions of fibrinogen, converting it to active fibrin that can link together to form fibrin threads. Fibrin threads make a meshlike base to form a blood clot.

After the fibrin mesh is formed, clotting factor XIII tightens up the mesh, making it more dense and stable. More platelets stick to the threads of the mesh and attract other blood cells and proteins to form an actual blood clot. As this clot tightens (retracts), the serum is squeezed out and clot formation is complete.

Anti-Clotting Forces

Because blood CLOTTING occurs through a rapid cascade process, in theory it keeps forming fibrin clots whenever the cascade is set into motion until all blood throughout the entire body has coagulated and PERFUSION stops. Therefore, whenever the blood clotting cascade is started, anti-clotting forces are also started to limit clot formation only to damaged areas so that normal perfusion is maintained everywhere else. When blood clotting and anti-clotting actions are balanced, clotting occurs only where it is needed and normal perfusion is maintained. The anti-clotting forces both ensure that activated clotting factors are present only in limited amounts and also cause fibrinolysis to prevent over-enlargement of the fibrin clot. **Fibrinolysis** is the process that dissolves fibrin clot edges with special enzymes (Fig. 39-5). The process starts by activating plasminogen to plasmin. Plasmin, an active enzyme, then digests fibrin, fibrinogen, and prothrombin, controlling the size of the fibrin clot.

When the blood clotting cascade is activated, certain anti-clotting substances are also activated, such as protein C, protein S, and antithrombin III. Protein C and protein S increase the breakdown of clotting factors V and VIII. Antithrombin III inactivates thrombin and clotting factors IX and X. These actions prevent clots from becoming too large or forming in an area where CLOTTING is not needed. Deficiency of any anti-clotting factor increases the risk for pulmonary embolism, myocardial infarction, and strokes.

Hematologic Changes Associated with Aging

Aging changes the blood components (Touhy & Jett, 2014). The older adult has a decreased blood volume with lower levels of plasma proteins. The lower plasma protein level may be related to a low dietary intake of proteins, as well as to reduced protein production by the older liver. Chart 39-1 lists assessment tips for older adults.

As bone marrow ages, it produces fewer blood cells. Total red blood cell (RBC) and white blood cell (WBC) counts are lower among older adults, although platelet counts do not change. Lymphocytes become less reactive to antigens and lose immune function. Antibody levels and responses are lower and slower in older adults. The WBC count does not rise as high in response to infection in older people as it does in younger people.

Hemoglobin levels in men and women fall after middle age. Iron-deficient diets may play a role in this reduction.

ASSESSMENT METHODS

Patient History

Age and gender are important to consider when assessing the patient's hematologic status. Bone marrow function and immune activity decrease with age.

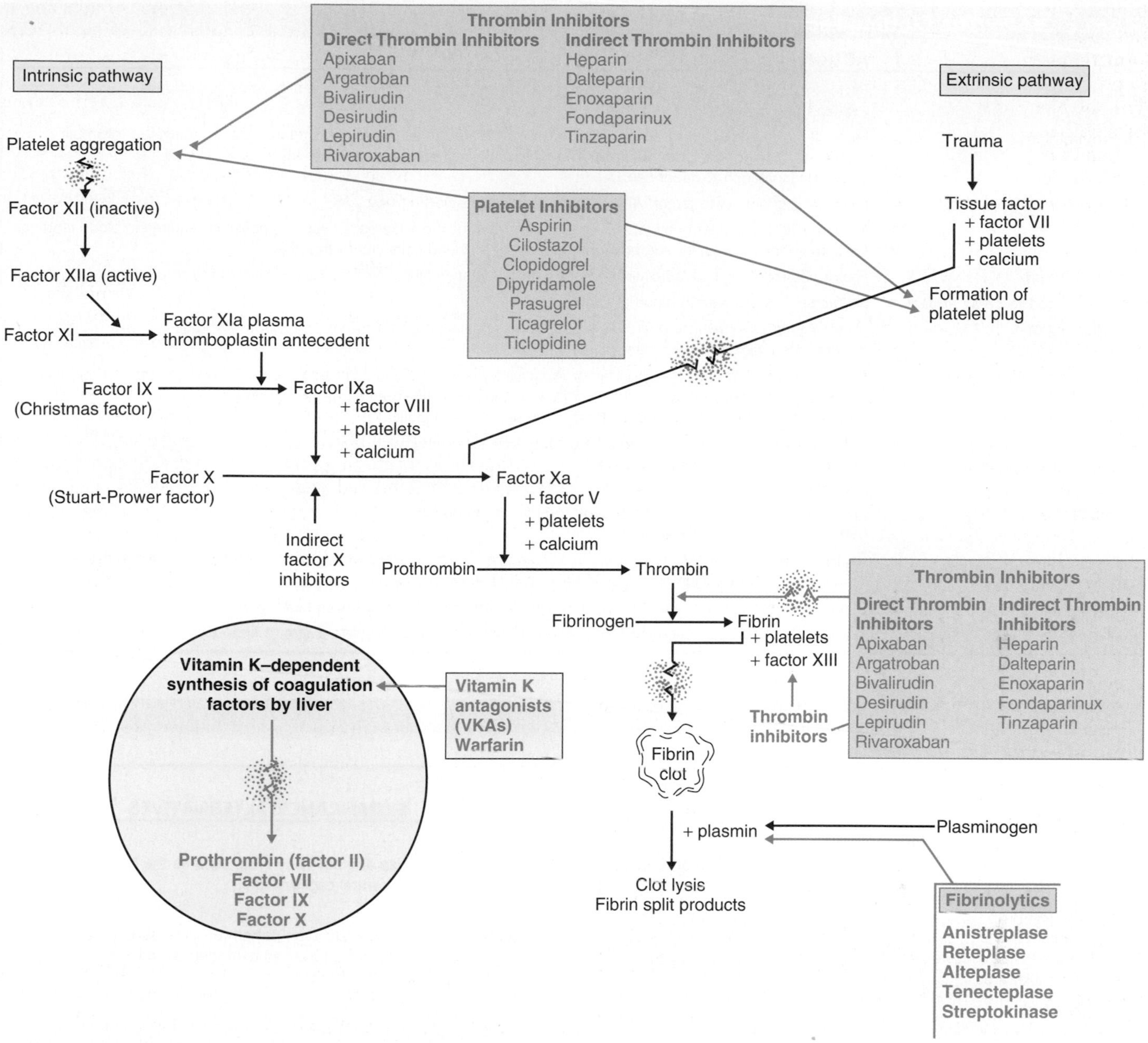

FIG. 39-4 Summary of the blood clotting cascade.

GENDER HEALTH CONSIDERATIONS

Patient-Centered Care QSEN

At all ages, women have lower blood cell counts than do men. This difference is greater during menstrual years because menstrual blood loss may occur faster than blood cell production. This difference also may be related to blood dilution caused by fluid retention from female hormones. Always assess for RBC adequacy in a woman hospitalized for any reason.

Liver function, the presence of known immunologic or hematologic disorders, current drug use, dietary patterns, and socioeconomic status are important to assess. Because the liver makes CLOTTING factors, ask about manifestations that may indicate liver problems, such as jaundice, anemia, and gallstones. Previous radiation therapy for cancer may impair hematologic function if marrow-forming bones were in the radiation path.

Ask about the patient's occupation and hobbies and whether the home is located near an industrial setting. This information may identify exposure to agents that affect bone marrow and hematologic function.

Check all drugs that the patient is using or has used in the past 3 weeks. Ask about the use of drugs listed in Table 39-3 that are known to change hematologic function. Check a drug handbook to determine whether other drugs the patient takes can affect hematologic function.

Ask the patient about use of blood "thinners" and NSAIDs, which change blood CLOTTING activity. Such drugs include anticoagulants, fibrinolytics, and platelet inhibitors. Many patients refer to these drugs as "blood thinners" although they do not

TABLE 39-2 The Clotting Factors

FACTOR	ACTION
I: Fibrinogen	Factor I is converted to fibrin by the enzyme *thrombin*. Individual fibrin molecules form fibrin threads, which are the mesh for clot formation and wound healing.
II: Prothrombin	Factor II is the inactive thrombin. Prothrombin is activated to thrombin by clotting factor X. Activated thrombin converts fibrinogen (clotting factor I) into fibrin and activates factors V and VIII. Synthesis is vitamin K–dependent.
III: Tissue thromboplastin	Factor III interacts with factor VII to initiate the extrinsic clotting cascade.
IV: Calcium	Calcium (Ca^{2+}), a divalent cation, is a cofactor for most of the enzyme-activated processes required in blood clotting. Calcium enhances platelet aggregation and makes red blood cells clump together.
V: Proaccelerin	Factor V is a cofactor for activated factor X, which is essential for converting prothrombin to thrombin.
VI: Discovered to be an artifact	No factor VI is involved in blood clotting.
VII: Proconvertin	Factor VII activates factors IX and X, which are essential in converting prothrombin to thrombin. Synthesis is vitamin K–dependent.
VIII: Antihemophilic factor	Factor VIII together with activated factor IX activates factor X. Factor VIII also combines with another protein (von Willebrand's factor) to help platelets adhere to capillary walls in areas of tissue injury. A lack of factor VIII is the basis for classic hemophilia (hemophilia A).
IX: Plasma thromboplastin component (Christmas factor)	Factor IX, when activated, activates factor X to convert prothrombin to thrombin. A lack of factor IX causes hemophilia B. Synthesis is vitamin K–dependent.
X: Stuart-Prower factor	Factor X, when activated, converts prothrombin into thrombin. Synthesis is vitamin K–dependent.
XI: Plasma thromboplastin antecedent	Factor XI, when activated, assists in the activation of factor IX. However, a similar factor must exist in tissues. People who are deficient in factor XI have mild bleeding problems.
XII: Hageman factor	Factor XII is critically important in the intrinsic pathway for the activation of factor XI.
XIII: Fibrin-stabilizing factor	Factor XIII assists in forming cross-links among the fibrin threads to form a strong fibrin clot.

CHART 39-1 Nursing Focus on the Older Adult

Hematologic Assessment

FINDINGS IN HEMATOLOGIC DISORDERS	NORMAL CHANGES IN THE OLDER ADULT	SIGNIFICANCE/ALTERNATIVES
Nail Beds (for Capillary Refill)		
Pallor or cyanosis may indicate a hematologic disorder.	Thickened or discolored nails make viewing color of nail beds impossible.	Use another body area, such as the lip, to assess central capillary refill.
Hair Distribution		
Thin or absent hair on the trunk or extremities may indicate poor circulation to a particular area.	Progressive loss of body hair is a normal facet of aging.	A relatively even pattern of hair loss that has occurred over an extended period is not significant.
Skin Moisture		
Skin dryness may indicate any of a number of hematologic disorders.	Skin dryness is a normal result of aging.	Skin moisture is not usually a reliable indicator of an underlying pathologic condition in the older adult.
Skin Color		
Skin color changes, especially pallor and jaundice, are associated with some hematologic disorders.	Pigment loss and skin yellowing are common changes associated with aging.	Pallor in an older adult may not be a reliable indicator of anemia. Laboratory testing is required. Yellow-tinged skin in an older adult may not be a reliable indicator of increased serum bilirubin levels. Laboratory testing is required.

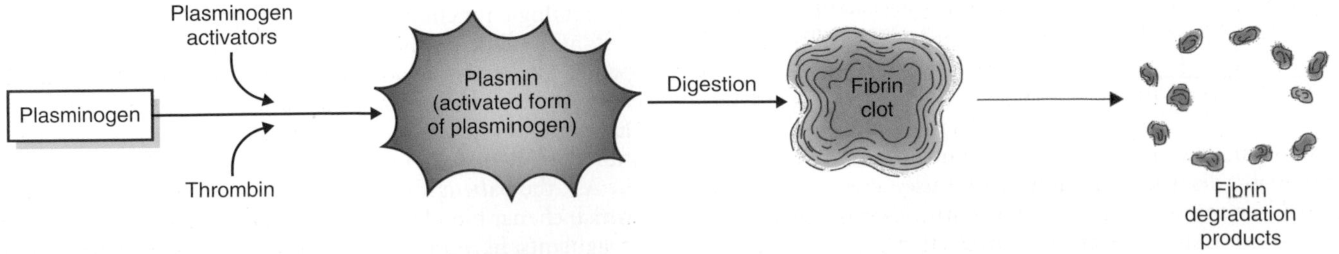

FIG. 39-5 The process of fibrinolysis.

TABLE 39-3 Drugs Impairing the Hematologic System

Drugs Causing Bone Marrow Suppression	Drugs Causing Hemolysis	Drugs Disrupting Platelet Action
• Altretamine • Amphotericin B • Azathioprine • Chemotherapeutic agents • Chloramphenicol • Chromic phosphate • Colchicine • Didanosine • Eflornithine • Foscarnet sodium • Ganciclovir • Interferon alfa • Pentamidine • Sodium iodide • Zalcitabine • Zidovudine	• Acetohydroxamic acid • Amoxicillin • Chlorpropamide • Doxapram • Glyburide • Mefenamic acid • Menadiol diphosphate • Methyldopa • Nitrofurantoin • Penicillin G benzathine • Penicillin V • Primaquine • Procainamide hydrochloride • Quinidine polygalacturonate • Quinine • Sulfonamides • Tolbutamide • Vitamin K	• Aspirin • Carbenicillin • Carindacillin • Dipyridamole • Ibuprofen • Meloxicam • Naproxen • Oxaprozin • Pentoxifylline • Sulfinpyrazone • Ticarcillin • Ticlopidine • Valproic acid

change blood thickness (viscosity) (Karch, 2012). Fig. 39-4 shows where in the blood clotting cascade these agents work.

Anticoagulant drugs work by interfering with one or more steps involved in the blood CLOTTING cascade. Thus these agents *prevent* new clots from forming and limit or prevent extension of formed clots. *Anticoagulants do not break down existing clots.* These drugs are classified as direct thrombin inhibitors, indirect thrombin inhibitors, and vitamin K antagonists.

Direct thrombin inhibitors (DTIs) can be given by the parenteral route and orally. The parenteral drugs include lepirudin (Refludan), desirudin (Iprivask), bivalirudin (Angiomax), argatroban (ARGATROBAN, Acova ♣), rivaroxaban (Xarelto), and apixaban (Eliquis). The drugs prevent the conversion of prothrombin (factor X) to its active form, thrombin (factor Xa). Less thrombin disrupts the CLOTTING cascade by reducing the amount of fibrinogen that is converted to active fibrin (Karch, 2012; Straznitskas & Giarratano, 2014).

Indirect thrombin inhibitors include the heparins and heparinoids. These drugs include enoxaparin (Lovenox), dalteparin (Fragmin), tinzaparin (Innohep), and fondaparinux (Arixtra). All are given parenterally. The lower molecular weight drugs are preferred for home use. The drugs cause anticoagulation by binding to and increasing the activity of antithrombin III (AT III). By activating antithrombin III, coagulation factor Xa (thrombin) is indirectly inhibited (Karch, 2012).

Vitamin K antagonists (VKAs) decrease the synthesis of vitamin K in the intestinal tract, which then reduces the production of vitamin K–dependent CLOTTING factors II, VII, IX, and X, along with the anticoagulant proteins C and S (Karch, 2012). When the clotting factors are reduced, anticoagulation results. The most commonly used VKA is warfarin (Coumadin, Jantoven), an oral agent.

Fibrinolytic drugs (also known as *thrombolytic drugs* or "clot busters") selectively break down fibrin threads present in formed blood clots. The mechanism to start fibrin degradation is activation of the inactive tissue protein *plasminogen* to its active form, *plasmin*. Plasmin directly attacks and degrades the fibrin molecule. Common fibrinolytic drugs include alteplase (Activase), reteplase (Retavase), tenecteplase (TNKase), and urokinase (Abbokinase, Kinlytic). All are administered by the IV route. Urokinase is approved for use only in patients who have a massive pulmonary embolism.

The use of fibrinolytic drugs results in the best clot breakdown with less disruption of blood CLOTTING. These drugs are the first-line therapy for problems caused by small, localized formed clots such as myocardial infarction (MI), limited arterial thrombosis, and thrombotic strokes. For some problems, such as MI, these drugs are usually given only within the first 6 hours after the onset of symptoms. This time limitation is not related to drug activity because fibrinolytic agents can break down clots older than 6 hours. Rather, the tissue that has been anoxic for more than 6 hours as a result of an acute event is not likely to benefit from this therapy, making the risks to the patient greater than the advantages.

Platelet inhibitors or antiplatelet drugs prevent either platelet activation or aggregation (clumping). The most widely used drug for this effect is aspirin, which inhibits the production of substances that activate platelets, such as thromboxane. Other drugs change the platelet membrane, reducing its "stickiness," or prevent activators from binding to platelet receptors by inhibiting a variety of enzymes important to platelet activation (Karch, 2012). These drugs include cilostazol (Pletal), clopidogrel (Plavix), dipyridamole (Persantine), prasugrel (Effient), ticagrelor (Brilinta), and ticlopidine (Ticlid). Another group of drugs that inhibits platelets by binding to certain membrane proteins include abciximab (ReoPro), eptifibatide (Integrilin), and tirofiban (Aggrastat), which are all administered parenterally. In addition, many complementary therapy agents, such as St. John's wort and *Ginkgo biloba*, inhibit platelet activity.

Nutrition Status

Diet can alter cell quality and affect CLOTTING. Ask patients to recall what they have eaten during the past week. Use this information to assess possible iron, protein, mineral, or vitamin deficiencies. Diets high in fat and carbohydrates and low in protein, iron, and vitamins can cause many types of anemia and decrease the functions of all blood cells. Diets high in vitamin K, found in leafy green vegetables, may increase the rate of blood clotting. Assess the amount of salads and other raw vegetables that the patient eats and whether supplemental vitamins and calcium are used.

Ask about alcohol consumption because chronic alcoholism causes nutrition deficiencies and impairs the liver, both of which reduce blood CLOTTING.

Ask about personal resources, such as finances and social support. A person with a low income may have a diet deficient in iron and protein because foods containing these substances are more expensive.

Family History and Genetic Risk

Assess family history because many disorders affecting blood and blood CLOTTING are inherited. Ask whether anyone in the family has had hemophilia, frequent nosebleeds, postpartum hemorrhages, excessive bleeding after tooth extractions, or heavy bruising after mild trauma. Ask whether any family member has sickle cell disease or sickle cell trait. Although sickle cell disease is seen most often among African Americans, anyone can have the trait.

NCLEX EXAMINATION CHALLENGE

Health Promotion and Maintenance

Why is it important for the nurse to teach the client starting on the anticoagulant *warfarin* (Coumadin) to limit his or her intake of leafy green vegetables?

A. These foods contain vitamin K, which can increase the effects of warfarin.
B. These foods contain vitamin K, which can reduce the effects of warfarin.
C. These foods enhance aspirin activity and increase the risk for bleeding in the person who also takes warfarin.
D. These foods reduce aspirin activity and increase the risk for pulmonary embolism in the person who also takes warfarin.

Current Health Problems

Ask about lymph nodes swelling, excessive bruising or bleeding, and whether the bleeding was spontaneous or induced by trauma. Ask about the amount and duration of bleeding after routine dental work. Ask women to estimate the number of pads or tampons used during the most recent menstrual cycle and whether this amount represents a change from the usual pattern of flow. Ask whether clots are present in menstrual blood. If menstrual clots occur, ask her to estimate clot size using coins or fruit for comparison.

Assess and record whether the patient has shortness of breath on exertion, palpitations, frequent infections, fevers, recent weight loss, headaches, or paresthesias. Any or all of these symptoms may occur with hematologic disease.

The most common manifestation of anemia is fatigue as a result of decreased oxygen delivery to cells. Cells use oxygen to produce the high-energy chemical *adenosine triphosphate (ATP)* needed to perform most cellular work. When oxygen delivery to cells is reduced, cellular work decreases and fatigue increases. Ask patients about feeling tired, needing more rest, or losing endurance during normal activities. Ask them to compare their activities during the past month with those of the same month a year ago. Determine whether other manifestations of anemia, such as vertigo, tinnitus, and a sore tongue, are present.

Physical Assessment

Assess the whole body because blood problems may reduce oxygen delivery and tissue PERFUSION to all systems (Jarvis, 2016). Some assessment findings associated with hematologic problems are less reliable when seen in the older adult (see Chart 39-1). Equipment needed for hematologic assessment includes gloves, a stethoscope, a blood pressure cuff, and a penlight. Remember to gently handle the patient suspected of having a hematologic problem to avoid causing bruising, petechiae, or excessive bleeding.

Skin Assessment

Inspect the skin and mucous membranes for pallor or jaundice. Assess nail beds for pallor or cyanosis. Pallor of the gums, conjunctivae, and palmar creases (when the palm is stretched) indicates decreased hemoglobin levels and poor tissue oxygenation. Assess the gums for active bleeding in response to light pressure or brushing the teeth with a soft-bristled brush, and assess any lesions or draining areas. Inspect for petechiae and large bruises *(ecchymoses)*. **Petechiae** are pinpoint hemorrhagic lesions in the skin. Bruises may cluster together. For hospitalized patients, determine whether there is bleeding around nasogastric tubes, endotracheal tubes, central lines, peripheral IV sites, or Foley catheters. Check the skin turgor, and ask about itching because dry skin from poor perfusion itches. Assess body hair patterns. Areas with poor circulation, especially the lower legs and toes, may have sparse or absent hair, although this may be a normal finding in an older adult.

CULTURAL CONSIDERATIONS

Patient-Centered Care QSEN

Pallor and cyanosis are more easily detected in people with darker skin by examining the oral mucous membranes and the conjunctiva of the eye. Jaundice can be seen more easily on the roof of the mouth. Petechiae may be visible only on the palms of the hands or the soles of the feet. Bruises can be seen as darker areas of skin and palpated as slight swellings or irregular skin surfaces. Ask the patient about pain when skin surfaces are touched lightly or palpated. (Chapter 24 provides tips for assessing darker skin.)

Head and Neck Assessment

Check for pallor or ulceration of the oral mucosa. The tongue is smooth in pernicious anemia and iron deficiency anemia or smooth and beefy red in other nutrition deficiencies. These manifestations may occur with fissures at the corners of the mouth. Assess for scleral jaundice.

Inspect and palpate all lymph node areas. Document any lymph node enlargement, including whether palpation of the enlarged node causes pain and whether the enlarged node moves or remains fixed with palpation.

Respiratory Assessment

When blood problems reduce oxygen delivery, the lungs work harder to make adjustments that can maintain tissue PERFUSION. Assess the rate and depth of respiration while the patient is at rest and during and after mild physical activity (e.g., walking 20 steps in 10 seconds). Note whether the patient can complete a 10-word sentence without stopping for a breath. Assess whether the patient is fatigued easily, has shortness of breath at rest or on exertion, or needs extra pillows to breathe well at night. Anemia can cause these manifestations as a result of respiratory changes made as adjustments to the reduced tissue oxygen levels.

Cardiovascular Assessment

When blood problems reduce oxygen delivery, the heart works harder to make adjustments to maintain tissue PERFUSION. Pulses may become weak and thready. Observe for distended neck veins, edema, or indications of phlebitis. Use a stethoscope to listen for abnormal heart sounds and irregular rhythms. Assess blood pressure (BP). Systolic BP tends to be lower than normal in patients with anemia and higher than normal when the patient has excessive red blood cells.

Kidney and Urinary Assessment

The kidneys have many blood vessels, and bleeding problems may cause gross or occult *hematuria* (blood in the urine). Inspect urine for color. Hematuria may appear as grossly bloody red or dark brownish gold urine. Test the urine for proteins with a urine test dipstick because blood contains protein and blood in the urine increases its protein content. Keep in mind that the person with chronic kidney disease (CKD) produces less natural erythropoietin and often is anemic.

Musculoskeletal Assessment

Rib or sternal tenderness may occur with leukemia (blood cancer) when the bone marrow overproduces cells, increasing the pressure in the bones. Examine the skin over superficial bones, including the ribs and sternum, by applying firm pressure with the fingertips. Assess the range of joint motion, and document any swelling or joint pain.

Abdominal Assessment

The normal adult spleen is usually *not* palpable, but an enlarged spleen occurs with many hematologic problems. An enlarged spleen may be detected by palpation, but this is usually performed by the health care provider because an enlarged spleen is tender and ruptures easily.

> **! NURSING SAFETY PRIORITY** (QSEN)
>
> ***Action Alert***
>
> Do not palpate the splenic area of the abdomen for any patient with a suspected hematologic problem. An enlarged spleen ruptures easily and can lead to hemorrhage and death.

Palpating the edge of the liver in the right upper quadrant of the abdomen can detect enlargement, which often occurs with hematologic problems. The normal liver may be palpable as much as 4 to 5 cm below the right costal margin but is usually not palpable in the epigastrium.

A common cause of anemia among older adults is a chronically bleeding GI ulcer or intestinal polyp. If the ulcer is located in the stomach or the small intestine, obvious blood may not be visible in the stool or such a small amount is passed each day that the patient is not aware of it. Obtain a stool specimen for occult blood testing.

Central Nervous System Assessment

Assessing cranial nerves and testing neurologic function are important in hematologic assessment because some problems cause specific changes. Vitamin B_{12} deficiency impairs nerve function, and severe chronic deficiency may cause permanent neurologic degeneration. Many neurologic problems can develop in patients who have leukemia, because leukemia can cause bleeding, infection, or tumor spread within the brain. When the patient with a suspected bleeding disorder has any head trauma, expand the assessment to include frequent neurologic checks and checks of cognitive function (see Chapter 41).

Psychosocial Assessment

Regardless of the type of hematologic problem, each person brings his or her own coping style to the illness. Develop a rapport with the patient and learn what coping mechanisms he or she has used successfully in the past.

Ask the patient and family members about social support networks and financial resources. A problem in these areas can interfere with the patient's adherence to therapy.

Diagnostic Assessment

Laboratory Tests

Laboratory test results often provide the most definitive information about hematologic problems. Chart 39-2 lists laboratory data used to assess hematologic function. When a venipuncture is necessary, apply pressure to the site for at least 5 minutes on a patient suspected of having a hematologic problem to prevent bleeding and hematoma formation.

Tests of Cell Number and Function. *A peripheral blood smear* is made by taking a drop of blood and spreading it over a slide. It can be read by an automated calculator or by a technologist with a microscope. This rapid test provides information on the sizes, shapes, and proportions of different blood cell types within the peripheral blood.

A complete blood count (CBC) includes a number of studies: red blood cell (RBC) count, white blood cell (WBC) count, hematocrit, and hemoglobin level. The RBC count measures circulating RBCs in 1 mm^3 of blood. The WBC count measures all leukocytes present in 1 mm^3 of blood. To determine the percentages of different types of leukocytes circulating in the blood, a WBC count with differential leukocyte count is performed (see Chapter 17). The hematocrit (Hct) is the percentage of red blood cells in the total blood volume. The hemoglobin (Hgb) level is the total amount of hemoglobin in blood.

The CBC can measure other features of the RBCs. The mean corpuscular volume (MCV) measures the average volume or size of individual RBCs and is useful for classifying anemias. When the MCV is elevated, the cell is larger than normal *(macrocytic),* as seen in megaloblastic anemias. When the MCV is decreased, the cell is smaller than normal *(microcytic),* as seen in iron deficiency anemia. The mean corpuscular hemoglobin (MCH) is the average amount of hemoglobin by weight in a single RBC. The mean corpuscular hemoglobin concentration (MCHC) measures the average amount of hemoglobin by percentage in a single RBC. When the MCHC is decreased, the cell has a hemoglobin deficiency and is *hypochromic* (a lighter color), as in iron deficiency anemia. These three tests can help determine possible causes of low RBC counts that are not related to blood loss (Rauen, 2012).

Reticulocyte count is helpful in determining bone marrow function. A reticulocyte is an immature RBC that still has its nucleus. An elevated reticulocyte count indicates that RBCs are being produced and released by the bone marrow before they mature. Normally only about 2% of circulating RBCs are reticulocytes. An elevated reticulocyte count is desirable in an anemic patient or after hemorrhage because this indicates that the bone marrow is responding to a decrease in the total RBC level. An elevated reticulocyte count without a precipitating cause usually indicates health problems, such as polycythemia vera (a malignant condition in which the bone marrow overproduces RBCs).

A platelet count, also known as a *thrombocyte count,* reflects the number of platelets in circulation. The normal range is 150,000 to 400,000/mm^3. When this value is low *(thrombocytopenia),* the person is at greater risk for bleeding because platelets are critical for blood clotting. Patients who have values between 40,000/mm^3 and 80,000/mm^3 may have prolonged bleeding from trauma, dental work, and surgery. Patients who have platelet values below 20,000/mm^3 may have spontaneous bleeding that is very difficult to stop.

Hemoglobin electrophoresis detects abnormal forms of hemoglobin, such as hemoglobin S in sickle cell disease. Hemoglobin A is the major type of hemoglobin in an adult.

Leukocyte alkaline phosphatase (LAP) is an enzyme produced by normal mature neutrophils. Elevated LAP levels occur during episodes of infection or stress. An elevated neutrophil

CHART 39-2 Laboratory Profile

Hematologic Assessment

TEST	REFERENCE RANGE	INTERNATIONAL REFERENCE UNITS	SIGNIFICANCE OF ABNORMAL FINDINGS
Red blood cell (RBC) count	*Females:* 4.2-5.4 million/μL *Males:* 4.7-6.1 million/μL	$4.2\text{-}5.4 \times 10^{12}$ cells/L $4.7\text{-}6.1 \times 10^{12}$ cells/L	*Decreased levels* indicate possible anemia or hemorrhage. *Increased levels* indicate possible chronic hypoxia or polycythemia vera.
Hemoglobin (Hgb)	*Females:* 12-16 g/dL *Males:* 14-18 g/dL	7.4-9.9 mmol/L 8.7-11.2 mmol/L	Same as for RBC.
Hematocrit (Hct)	*Females:* 37%-47% *Males:* 42%-52%	0.37-0.47 fraction 0.42-0.52 fraction	Same as for RBC.
Mean corpuscular volume (MCV)	80-95 fL	Same as reference range	*Increased levels* indicate macrocytic cells, possible anemia. *Decreased levels* indicate microcytic cells, possible iron deficiency anemia.
Mean corpuscular hemoglobin (MCH)	27-31 pg	Same as reference range	Same as for MCV.
Mean corpuscular hemoglobin concentration (MCHC)	32-36 g/dL	32%-36%	*Increased levels* may indicate spherocytosis or anemia. *Decreased levels* may indicate iron deficiency anemia or a hemoglobinopathy.
White blood cell (WBC) count	5000-10,000/mm³	$5.0\text{-}10.0 \times 10^9$ cells/L	*Increased levels* are associated with infection, inflammation, autoimmune disorders, and leukemia. *Decreased levels* may indicate prolonged infection or bone marrow suppression.
Reticulocyte count	0.5%-2.0% of RBCs	0.005-0.20 fraction	*Increased levels* may indicate chronic blood loss. *Decreased levels* indicate possible inadequate RBC production.
Total iron-binding capacity (TIBC)	250-460 mcg/dL	45-82 μmol/L	*Increased levels* indicate iron deficiency. *Decreased levels* may indicate anemia, hemorrhage, hemolysis.
Iron (Fe)	*Females:* 60-160 mcg/dL *Males:* 80-180 mcg/dL	11-29 μmol/L 14-32 μmol/L	*Increased levels* indicate iron excess, liver disorders, hemochromatosis, megaloblastic anemia. *Decreased levels* indicate possible iron deficiency anemia, hemorrhage.
Serum ferritin	*Females:* 10-150 ng/mL *Males:* 12-300 ng/mL	10-150 mcg/L 12-300 mcg/L	Same as for iron.
Platelet count	150,000-400,000/mm³	$150\text{-}400 \times 10^9$/L	*Increased levels* may indicate polycythemia vera or malignancy. *Decreased levels* may indicate bone marrow suppression, autoimmune disease, hypersplenism.
Hemoglobin electrophoresis	Hgb A_1: 95%-98% Hgb A_2: 2%-3% Hgb F: 0.8%-2% Hgb S: 0% Hgb C: 0% Hgb E: 0%	Same as reference range	*Variations* indicate hemoglobinopathies.
Direct Coombs' and indirect Coombs' test	Negative	Negative	*Positive findings* indicate antibodies to RBCs.
Prothrombin time (PT)	11-12.5 sec 85%-100%	Patient PT/normal PT INR 0.8-1.1	*Increased time* indicates possible deficiency of clotting factors V and VII. *Decreased time* may indicate vitamin K excess.

Data from Pagana, K., & Pagana, T. (2014). *Mosby's manual of diagnostic and laboratory tests* (5th ed.). St. Louis: Mosby.
fL, Femtoliter; *INR,* international normalized ratio; *pg,* picograms.

count without an elevation in LAP level occurs with some types of leukemia.

Coombs' tests, both direct and indirect, are used for blood typing. The direct test detects antibodies against RBCs that may be attached to a person's RBCs. Although healthy people can make these antibodies, in certain diseases (e.g., systemic lupus erythematosus, mononucleosis) these antibodies are directed against the patient's own RBCs. Excessive amounts of these antibodies can cause hemolytic anemia (Pagana & Pagana, 2014).

The indirect Coombs' test detects the presence of circulating antiglobulins. The test is used to determine whether the patient has serum antibodies to the type of RBCs that he or she is about to receive by blood transfusion (Pagana & Pagana, 2014).

Serum ferritin, transferrin, and the total iron-binding capacity (TIBC) tests measure iron levels. Abnormal levels of iron and TIBC occur with problems such as iron deficiency anemia.

The serum ferritin test measures the amount of free iron present in the plasma, which represents 1% of the total body iron stores. Therefore the serum ferritin level provides a means to assess total iron stores. People with serum ferritin levels within 10 g of the normal range for their gender have adequate iron stores; people with levels 10 g or more lower than the normal range have inadequate iron stores and have difficulty recovering from any blood loss.

Transferrin is a protein that transports dietary iron from the intestines to cell storage sites. Measuring the amount of iron that can be bound to serum transferrin indirectly determines whether an adequate amount of transferrin is present. This test is the total iron-binding capacity (TIBC) test. Normally, only about 30% of the transferrin is bound to iron in the blood. TIBC increases when a person is deficient in serum iron and stored iron levels. Such a value indicates that an adequate amount of transferrin is present but less than 30% of it is bound to serum iron.

Tests Measuring Bleeding and Coagulation. Tests that measure bleeding and coagulation provide information that reflects the effectiveness of different aspects of blood CLOTTING. These tests are used to diagnose specific hematologic health problems, determine drug therapy effectiveness, and identify risk for excessive bleeding or clotting.

Prothrombin time (PT) measures how long blood takes to clot, reflecting the level of clotting factors II, V, VII, and X and how well they are functioning. When enough of these clotting factors are present and functioning, the PT shows blood CLOTTING between 11 and 12.5 seconds or within 85% to 100% of the time needed for a control sample of blood to clot. PT is prolonged when one or more of these clotting factors are deficient.

The PT test is now used less often to assess how fast blood clots, because control blood is taken from different people and may not be the same even in one laboratory from one day to the next. To reduce PT errors as a result of control blood variation or in some of the chemicals used in the test, the international normalized ratio is used to assess clotting time.

International normalized ratio (INR) measures the same process as the PT by establishing a normal mean or standard for PT. The INR is calculated by dividing the patient's PT by the established standard PT. A normal INR ranges between 0.7 and 1.8. When using the INR to monitor warfarin therapy, the desired outcome is usually to maintain the patient's INR between 2.0 and 3.0 regardless of the actual PT in seconds. The desired INR range for any patient, however, is individualized for specific patient factors and medical conditions.

The partial thromboplastin time (PTT) assesses the intrinsic CLOTTING cascade and the action of factors II, V, VIII, IX, XI, and XII. PTT is prolonged whenever any of these factors is deficient, such as in hemophilia or disseminated intravascular coagulation (DIC). Because factors II, IX, and X are vitamin K–dependent and are produced in the liver, liver disease can prolong the PTT. Desired therapeutic ranges for anticoagulation are usually between 1.5 and 2.0 times normal values but can be greater depending on the reason the person is receiving anticoagulation therapy.

The anti-factor Xa test measures the amount of anti-activated factor X (anti-Xa) in blood, which is affected by heparin. It is used mainly to monitor heparin levels in patients treated with either standard unfractionated heparin or low–molecular-weight heparin. For people not receiving heparin in any form, the reference range is less than 0.1 IU/mL. The usual therapeutic range for patients receiving standard heparin is 0.5 to 1.0 IU/mL, and the usual therapeutic range for patients receiving low–molecular-weight heparin is 0.3 to 0.7 IU/mL. Test results are affected by age, gender, health history, and the specific laboratory technique used for the test.

Platelet aggregation, or the ability to clump, is tested by mixing the patient's plasma with an agonist substance that should cause clumping. The degree of clumping is noted. Aggregation can be impaired in von Willebrand's disease and during the use of drugs such as aspirin, anti-inflammatory agents, psychotropic agents, and platelet inhibitors.

NCLEX EXAMINATION CHALLENGE

Physiological Integrity

Which blood test result for a client being assessed for a hematologic problem indicates to the nurse that chronic anemia is likely?

A. International normalized ratio (INR) is 0.9
B. Platelet count of 180,000/mm^3
C. Reticulocyte value of 14%
D. Hematocrit of 27%

Imaging Assessment

Assessment of the patient with a suspected hematologic problem can include radioisotopic imaging. Isotopes are used to evaluate the bone marrow for sites of active blood cell formation and sites of iron storage. Radioactive colloids are used to determine organ size and liver and spleen function.

The patient is given a radioactive isotope by IV about 3 hours before the procedure. Once in the nuclear medicine department, he or she must lie still for about an hour during the scan. No special patient preparation or follow-up care is needed for these tests.

Standard x-rays may be used to diagnose some hematologic problems. For example, multiple myeloma causes classic bone destruction, with a "Swiss cheese" appearance on x-ray.

Bone Marrow Aspiration and Biopsy

Bone marrow aspiration or biopsy, which are similar invasive procedures, helps evaluate the patient's hematologic status when other tests show abnormal findings that indicate a possible problem in blood cell production or maturation. Results provide information about bone marrow function, including the production of all blood cells and platelets. In a bone marrow aspiration, cells and fluids are suctioned from the bone marrow. In a bone marrow biopsy, solid tissue and cells are obtained by coring out an area of bone marrow with a large-bore needle.

A health care provider's order and a signed informed consent are obtained before either procedure is performed. Bone marrow aspiration may be performed by a physician, an advanced practice nurse, or a physician assistant, depending on the agency's policy and regional law. The procedure may be performed at the patient's bedside, in an examination room, or in a laboratory.

After learning what specific tests will be performed on the marrow, check with the hematology laboratory to determine how to handle the specimen. Some tests require that heparin or other solutions be added to the specimen.

Patient Preparation. Most patients are anxious before a bone marrow aspiration, even those who have had one in the past. You can help reduce anxiety and allay fears by providing accurate information and emotional support. Some patients like to have their hand held during the procedure.

Explain the procedure, and reassure the patient that you will stay during the entire procedure. Occasionally a friend or family member is permitted to be present to provide emotional support. Tell the patient that the local anesthetic injection will feel like a stinging or burning sensation. Tell him or her to expect a heavy sensation of pressure and pushing while the needle is being inserted. Sometimes a crunching sound can be heard or scraping sensation felt as the needle punctures the bone. Explain that a brief sensation of painful pulling will be experienced as the marrow is being aspirated by mild suction in the syringe. If a biopsy is performed, the patient may feel more discomfort as the needle is rotated into the bone.

Assist the patient onto an examining table, and expose the site (usually the iliac crest). If this site is not available or if more marrow is needed, the sternum may be used. If the iliac crest is the site, place the patient in the prone or side-lying position. Depending on the tests to be performed on the specimen, a laboratory technician may also be present to ensure proper handling of the specimen.

Procedure. The procedure usually lasts from 5 to 15 minutes. The type and the amount of anesthesia or sedation depend on the physician's preference, the patient's preference and previous experience with bone marrow aspiration and biopsy, and the setting.

A local anesthetic agent is injected into the skin around the site. The patient may also receive a mild tranquilizer or a rapid-acting sedative, such as midazolam (Versed), lorazepam (Ativan, Apo-Lorazepam ♣, Novo-Lorazem ♣), or etomidate (Amidate). Some patients do well with guided imagery or autohypnosis.

! NURSING SAFETY PRIORITY QSEN

Action Alert

Aspiration or biopsy procedures are invasive, and sterile technique must be observed.

The skin over the site is cleaned with a disinfectant. For an aspiration, the needle is inserted with a twisting motion and the marrow is aspirated by pulling back on the plunger of the syringe. When sufficient marrow has been aspirated to ensure accurate analysis, the needle is rapidly withdrawn while the tissues are supported at the site. For a biopsy, a small skin incision is made and the biopsy needle is inserted through the skin opening. Pressure and several twisting motions are needed to ensure coring and loosening of an adequate amount of marrow tissue. Apply external pressure to the site until hemostasis is ensured. A pressure dressing or sandbags may be applied to reduce bleeding at the site.

Follow-Up Care. The nursing priority after a bone marrow aspiration or biopsy is prevention of excessive bleeding. Cover the site with a dressing after bleeding is controlled, and closely observe it for 24 hours for manifestations of bleeding and infection. A mild analgesic (aspirin-free) may be given for discomfort, and ice packs can be placed over the site to limit bruising. Instruct the patient to inspect the site every 2 hours for the first 24 hours and to note the presence of active bleeding or bruising. Advise him or her to avoid contact sports or any activity that might result in trauma to the site for 48 hours.

Information obtained from bone marrow aspiration or biopsy reflects the degree and quality of bone marrow activity present. The counts made on a marrow specimen can indicate whether different cell types are present in the expected quantities and proportions. In addition, bone marrow aspiration or biopsy can confirm the spread of cancer cells from other tumor sites.

? CLINICAL JUDGMENT CHALLENGE

Safety; Patient-Centered Care QSEN

A 52-year-old man is scheduled for a bone marrow aspiration because his white blood cell count has been persistently abnormal and his father died from chronic lymphocytic leukemia (CLL). He is very anxious this morning, and you remember him from one of his earlier visits in which you drew his blood. At that visit, he started vomiting when you placed the needle in his vein. He tells you that he is very worried about the results and the pain of the procedure. He also tells you that his daughter has a dance recital tonight and he very much wants to attend this event.

1. Is this patient a candidate for autohypnosis? Why or why not?
2. Is there any reason(s) for him to think he may also have CLL? If so, what might this be?
3. What will you tell him about attending the dance recital?

NURSING CONCEPTS AND CLINICAL JUDGMENT REVIEW

What might you NOTICE in a patient with adequate tissue PERFUSION related to normal hematologic function?

Vital signs:
- Heart rate and respiratory rate within normal range
- Blood pressure within normal range

Physical assessment:
- Able to speak a sentence of 12 words without stopping for breath
- Able to walk and talk without stopping for breath
- Skin color normal (no cyanosis, pallor, or jaundice)
- Oral mucous membrane and nail beds pink with rapid capillary refill
- Gums pink, no petechiae or bleeding
- Appropriate distribution of body hair, especially on legs and feet
- Warm hands and feet, no dependent edema
- Skin clear with no large bruises or petechiae
- Lower eyelid conjunctivae red
- Urine output just about equal to fluid intake
- Urine clear and yellow

Psychological assessment:
- Oriented and not confused
- Energy level good; able to engage in desired work, recreational, and personal activities

Laboratory assessment:
- Red blood cell, hemoglobin, hematocrit, white blood cell, and platelet levels within normal limits for age and gender
- Reticulocyte count less than 2%

GET READY FOR THE NCLEX® EXAMINATION!

KEY POINTS

Review these Key Points for each NCLEX Examination Client Needs Category.

Safe and Effective Care Environment

- Verify that a patient having a bone marrow aspiration or biopsy has signed an informed consent statement. **Safety** QSEN
- Handle patients with suspected hematologic problems gently to avoid bleeding or bruising. **Safety** QSEN
- Do not palpate the splenic area of any patient suspected of having a hematologic problem. **Safety** QSEN
- Maintain pressure over a venipuncture site for at least 5 minutes to prevent excessive bleeding. **Safety** QSEN

Health Promotion and Maintenance

- Teach people to avoid unnecessary contact with environmental chemicals or toxins. If contact cannot be avoided, teach people to use safety precautions.
- Instruct patients about the importance of eating a diet with adequate amounts of foods that are good sources of iron, folic acid, and vitamin B_{12}. **Patient-Centered Care** QSEN

Psychosocial Integrity

- Teach patients and family members about what to expect during procedures to assess hematologic function, including restrictions, drugs, and follow-up care. **Patient-Centered Care** QSEN
- Ask patients about their activity level and whether they are satisfied with the energy they have for activities. **Patient-Centered Care** QSEN
- Support the patient during a bone marrow aspiration or biopsy. **Patient-Centered Care** QSEN

Physiological Integrity

- Interpret blood cell counts and CLOTTING tests to assess hematologic status. **Evidence-Based Practice** QSEN
- Be aware of these facts for hematologic function:
  - Tissue oxygenation and perfusion rely on normal hematologic function for oxygen delivery.
  - The most common manifestation of a hematologic problem is fatigue.
  - A platelet plug and a fibrin clot are not the same.
  - Both CLOTTING forces and anti-CLOTTING forces are needed to maintain adequate PERFUSION.
  - Women have reduced red blood cell, hematocrit, and hemoglobin levels at all ages compared with men.
- Use the lip rather than nail beds to assess capillary refill on older adults. **Evidence-Based Practice** QSEN
- Rely on laboratory tests rather than skin color changes in older adults to assess anemia or jaundice. **Evidence-Based Practice** QSEN
- Assess the patient's endurance in performing ADLs. **Patient-Centered Care** QSEN
- Apply an ice pack to the needle site after a bone marrow aspiration or biopsy. **Patient-Centered Care** QSEN
- Check the needle insertion site at least every 2 hours after a bone marrow aspiration or biopsy. If the patient is going home, teach the patient and family how to assess the site for bleeding and when to seek help. **Patient-Centered Care** QSEN
- Instruct patients to avoid activities that may traumatize the site after a bone marrow aspiration or biopsy.

40 CHAPTER

Care of Patients with Hematologic Problems

Katherine I. Byar

http://evolve.elsevier.com/Iggy/

PRIORITY CONCEPTS

- Gas Exchange
- Perfusion
- Clotting
- Immunity
- Infection

LEARNING OUTCOMES

Safe and Effective Care Environment

1. Use principles of infection control to prevent INFECTION when caring for a patient with a hematologic problem who also has reduced IMMUNITY.
2. Protect patients who have a hematologic problem with impaired CLOTTING from injury.

Health Promotion and Maintenance

3. Teach all people to take measures to protect the hematologic system from damage and cancer, including the avoidance of known environmental causative agents.
4. Teach the patient with hematologic problems and the family how to avoid injury and complications in the home.
5. Use assessment information to identify people at increased genetic risk for a hematologic problem.

Psychosocial Integrity

6. Reduce the psychological impact for the patient and family regarding changes in the function of the hematologic system.
7. Work with other members of the health care team to ensure that the values, preferences, and expressed needs of patients with a hematologic problem are respected.

Physiological Integrity

8. Assess and reassess the manifestations of patients being managed for a hematologic problem.
9. Use appropriate strategies to relieve pain and promote comfort for patients experiencing a hematologic problem.
10. Use laboratory data and clinical manifestations to prioritize nursing care for the patient who has an acute or chronic hematologic problem.
11. Collaborate with other health care professionals who help patients and families experiencing an acute or chronic hematologic problem achieve desired health outcomes.
12. Coordinate nursing interventions for the patient with a hematologic disorder in the community.
13. Prioritize nursing responsibilities during transfusion therapy.

Any condition that impairs the production or function of blood cells or that causes the abnormal destruction of any type of blood cell can result in a hematologic problem. Problems of the hematologic system can affect many tissues and organs by interfering with GAS EXCHANGE and tissue PERFUSION. The type and severity of the disorder determine the impact it has on patient health. This chapter discusses mild hematologic disorders and those that are potentially life threatening, such as sickle cell disease and hematologic malignancies.

RED BLOOD CELL DISORDERS

Red blood cells (RBCs), also known as **erythrocytes**, are the major cell in the blood. As discussed in Chapter 39, tissue GAS EXCHANGE for oxygenation depends on keeping the circulating number of RBCs within the normal range for the person's age and gender and on maintaining normal RBC function. RBC disorders include problems in production, function, and destruction. Problems may result in poor function of RBCs, decreased numbers of RBCs (anemia), or an excess of RBCs (polycythemia).

Anemia is a reduction in either the number of RBCs, the amount of hemoglobin, or the **hematocrit** (percentage of packed RBCs per deciliter of blood). It is a clinical indicator, not a specific disease, because it occurs with many health problems. Anemia can result from dietary problems, genetic disorders, bone marrow disease, or excessive bleeding. GI bleeding is the most common reason for anemia in adults.

There are many types and causes of anemia (Table 40-1). Some are caused by a deficiency in one of the components needed to make fully functional RBCs. Other anemias are caused by decreased RBC production or increased RBC

TABLE 40-1 Common Causes of Anemia

TYPE OF ANEMIA	COMMON CAUSES
Sickle cell disease	Autosomal recessive inheritance of two defective gene alleles for hemoglobin synthesis
Glucose-6-phosphate dehydrogenase (G6PD) deficiency anemia	X-linked recessive deficiency of the enzyme *G6PD*
Autoimmune hemolytic anemia	Abnormal immune function in which a person's immune reactive cells fail to recognize his or her own red blood cells as self cells
Iron deficiency anemia	Inadequate iron intake caused by: • Iron-deficient diet • Chronic alcoholism • Malabsorption syndromes • Partial gastrectomy Rapid metabolic (anabolic) activity caused by: • Pregnancy • Adolescence • Infection
Vitamin B_{12} deficiency anemia	Dietary deficiency Failure to absorb vitamin B_{12} from intestinal tract as a result of: • Partial gastrectomy • Pernicious anemia • Malabsorption syndromes
Folic acid deficiency anemia	Dietary deficiency Malabsorption syndromes Drugs: • Oral contraceptives • Anticonvulsants • Methotrexate
Aplastic anemia	Exposure to myelotoxic agents: • Radiation • Benzene • Chloramphenicol • Alkylating agents • Antimetabolites • Sulfonamides • Insecticides Viral infection (unproven): • Epstein-Barr virus • Hepatitis B • Cytomegalovirus

destruction. Despite the many causes, manifestations (Chart 40-1) and the nursing care needed are similar for all types of anemia.

ANEMIAS RESULTING FROM INCREASED DESTRUCTION OF RED BLOOD CELLS

SICKLE CELL DISEASE

❖ PATHOPHYSIOLOGY

Sickle cell disease (SCD), which used to be called *sickle cell anemia,* is a genetic disorder that results in chronic anemia, pain, disability, organ damage, increased risk for INFECTION, and early death. There is great variation among patients in how severe the disease is and when complications start.

This disorder results in the formation of abnormal hemoglobin chains. In healthy adults, the normal hemoglobin

CHART 40-1 Key Features

Anemia

Integumentary Manifestations

- Pallor, especially of the ears, the nail beds, the palmar creases, the conjunctivae, and around the mouth
- Cool to the touch
- Intolerance of cold temperatures
- Nails become brittle and become concave over time

Cardiovascular Manifestations

- Tachycardia at basal activity levels, increasing with activity and during and immediately after meals
- Murmurs and gallops heard on auscultation when anemia is severe
- Orthostatic hypotension

Respiratory Manifestations

- Dyspnea on exertion
- Decreased oxygen saturation levels

Neurologic Manifestations

- Increased somnolence and fatigue
- Headache

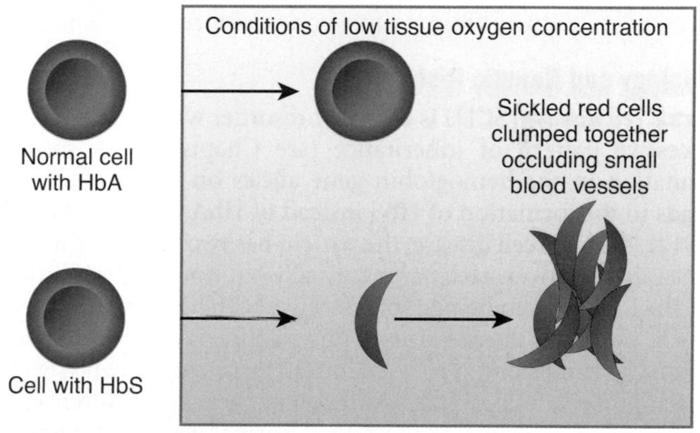

FIG. 40-1 Red blood cell actions under conditions of low tissue oxygenation. (*HbA,* Hemoglobin A; *HbS,* hemoglobin S.)

(**hemoglobin A [HbA]**) molecule has two alpha chains and two beta chains of amino acids. Normal adult red blood cells usually contain 98% to 99% HbA, with a small percentage of a fetal form of hemoglobin (HbF).

In SCD, at least 40% (and often much more) of the total hemoglobin is composed of an abnormal beta chain (**hemoglobin S [(HbS])**). HbS is sensitive to low oxygen content of the RBCs. When RBCs having large amounts of HbS are exposed to decreased oxygen conditions, the abnormal beta chains contract and pile together within the cell, distorting the cell into a sickle shape. Sickled cells become rigid and clump together, causing the RBCs to become "sticky" and fragile. The clumped masses of sickled RBCs block blood flow (Fig. 40-1), known as a *vaso-occlusive event (VOE).* VOE leads to further tissue **hypoxia** (reduced oxygen supply) and more sickle-shaped cells, which then leads to more blood vessel obstruction and ischemia in the affected tissues. Repeated episodes of ischemia cause progressive organ damage from anoxia and infarction. Conditions that cause sickling include hypoxia, dehydration, INFECTION, venous stasis, pregnancy, alcohol consumption, high altitudes, low or high environmental or body temperatures, acidosis, strenuous exercise, emotional stress, and anesthesia.

Usually sickled cells go back to normal shape when the precipitating condition is removed, the blood oxygen level is normalized, and proper tissue PERFUSION resumes. Although the cells then appear normal, some of the hemoglobin remains twisted, decreasing cell flexibility. The cell membranes are damaged over time, and cells are permanently sickled. The membranes of cells with HbS are more fragile and more easily broken. The average life span of an RBC containing 40% or more of HbS is about 10 to 20 days, much less than the 120-day life span of normal RBCs. This reduced RBC life span causes **hemolytic** (blood cell–destroying) anemia in patients with sickle cell disease.

The patient with SCD has periodic episodes of extensive cellular sickling, called **crises**. The crises have a sudden onset and can occur as often as weekly or as seldom as once a year. Many patients are in good health much of the time, with crises occurring only in response to conditions that cause local or systemic **hypoxemia** (deficient oxygen in the blood).

Repeated VOEs in large blood vessels cause long-term damage to tissues and organs. Most damage results from tissue hypoxia, anoxia, ischemia, and cell death. Organs begin to have small infarcted areas and scar tissue formation, and eventually organ failure results. Tissues most often affected are the spleen, liver, heart, kidney, brain, joints, bones, and retina.

Etiology and Genetic Risk

Sickle cell disease (SCD) is a genetic disorder with an autosomal recessive pattern of inheritance (see Chapter 4). A specific mutation in the hemoglobin gene alleles on chromosome 11 leads to the formation of HbS instead of HbA (Parsh & Kumar, 2012). In sickle cell disease, the patient has two HbS gene alleles, one inherited from each parent, usually resulting in 80% to100% of the hemoglobin being HbS. Because both hemoglobin alleles are S, sickle cell disease is sometimes abbreviated "SS." Patients with SCD often have severe manifestations even when triggering conditions are mild. If a patient with SCD has children, each child will inherit one of the two abnormal gene alleles and at least have sickle cell trait.

Sickle cell trait occurs when one normal gene allele and one abnormal gene allele for hemoglobin are inherited and only half of the hemoglobin chains are abnormal. Sickle cell trait is abbreviated "AS." The patient is a carrier of the HbS gene allele (Fig. 40-2) and can pass the trait on to his or her children. However, the patient has only mild manifestations of the disease when precipitating conditions are present because less than 40% of the hemoglobin is abnormal.

Incidence and Prevalence

Sickle cell trait and different forms of SCD occur in people of all races and ethnicities but is most common among African Americans in the United States. About 72,000 people have SCD, occurring in 1 in 500 African Americans. About 1 in 12 to 1 in 15 (8%) African Americans are carriers of one sickle cell gene allele and have AS (United States National Library of Medicine, 2014).

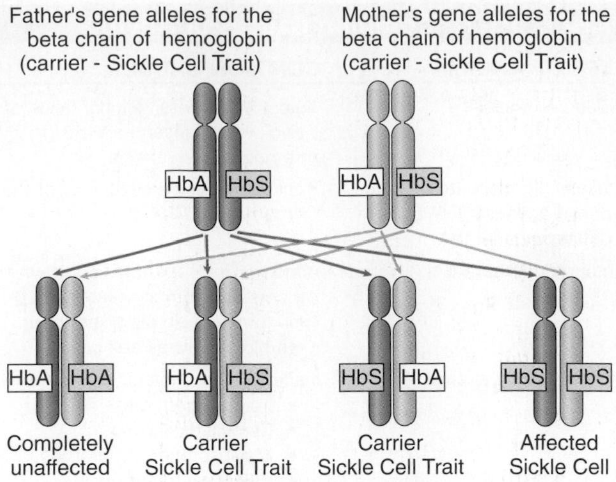

FIG. 40-2 Possible transmission of sickle cell disease and sickle cell trait when both parents are carriers. (*HbA*, Hemoglobin A; *HbS*, hemoglobin S.)

❖ PATIENT-CENTERED COLLABORATIVE CARE

◆ Assessment

History. An adult with sickle cell disease (SCD) usually has a long-standing diagnosis of the disorder. Those with sickle cell trait usually have no manifestations or abnormal laboratory findings other than the presence of hemoglobin S. This person may be unaware that he or she has a hematologic problem until an acute illness is present or when anesthesia is administered.

Ask about previous crises, what led to the crises, severity, and usual management. Explore recent contact with ill people and activities to determine what caused the current crisis. Ask about manifestations of INFECTION.

Review all activities and events during the past 24 hours, including food and fluid intake, exposure to temperature extremes, drugs taken, exercise, trauma, stress, recent airplane travel, and ingestion of alcohol or other recreational drugs. Ask about changes in sleep and rest patterns, ability to climb stairs, and any activity that induces shortness of breath. Determine the patient's perceived energy level using a scale ranging from 0 to 10 (0 = not tired with plenty of energy; 10 = total exhaustion) to assess the degree of fatigue.

Physical Assessment/Clinical Manifestations. *Pain is the most common manifestation of SCD crisis.* Others vary with the site of tissue damage.

Cardiovascular changes, including the risk for high-output heart failure, occur because of the anemia. Assess the patient for shortness of breath and general fatigue or weakness. Other problems may include murmurs, the presence of an S_3 heart sound, and increased jugular-venous pulsation or distention. Assess the cardiovascular status by comparing peripheral pulses, temperature, and capillary refill in all extremities. Extremities distal to blood vessel occlusion are cool to the touch with slow capillary refill and may have reduced or absent pulses. Heart rate may be rapid and blood pressure may be low to average with anemia.

Priapism is a prolonged penile erection that can occur in men who have SCD. The cause is excessive vascular engorgement in erectile tissue. The condition is very painful and can last for hours. During the priapism episode, the patient usually cannot urinate.

Skin changes include pallor or cyanosis because of poor GAS EXCHANGE from decreased PERFUSION and anemia. Examine the lips, tongue, nail beds, conjunctivae, palms, and soles of the feet at least every 8 hours for subtle color changes. With cyanosis, the lips and tongue are gray and the palms, soles, conjunctivae, and nail beds have a bluish tinge.

Another skin manifestation of SCD is jaundice. Jaundice results from RBC destruction and release of bilirubin. To assess for jaundice in patients with darker skin, inspect the roof of the mouth for a yellow appearance. Examine the sclera closest to the cornea to assess jaundice more accurately. Jaundice often causes intense itching.

Many adults with SCD have ulcers on the lower legs that are caused by poor PERFUSION, especially on the outer sides and inner aspect of the ankle or the shin (Ladizinski et al., 2012). These lesions often become necrotic or infected, requiring débridement and antibiotic therapy. Inspect the legs and feet for ulcers or darkened areas that may indicate necrotic tissue.

Abdominal changes include damage to the spleen and liver, which often occurs early from many episodes of hypoxia and ischemia. In crisis, abdominal pain is diffuse and steady, involving the back and legs. The liver or spleen may feel firm and enlarged with a nodular or "lumpy" texture in later stages of the disease.

Kidney and urinary changes are common as a result of poor PERFUSION and decreased tissue GAS EXCHANGE. Chronic kidney disease occurs as a result of anoxic damage to the kidney nephrons. Early damage makes the kidneys less effective at filtration and reabsorption. The urine contains protein, and the patient may not concentrate urine. Eventually, the kidneys fail, resulting in little or no urine output.

Musculoskeletal changes occur because arms and legs are often sites of blood vessel occlusion. Joints may be damaged from hypoxic episodes and have necrotic degeneration. Inspect the arms and legs, and record any areas of swelling, temperature, or color difference. Ask patients to move all joints. Record the range of motion and any pain with movement.

Central nervous system (CNS) changes may occur in SCD. During crises, patients may have a low-grade fever. If the CNS has infarcts or repeated episodes of hypoxia, patients may have seizures or manifestations of a stroke. Assess for the presence of "pronator drift," bilateral hand grasp strength, gait, and coordination. See Chapter 41 for details of neurologic assessment.

Psychosocial Assessment. Often behavioral changes are early manifestations of cerebral hypoxia from poor PERFUSION. Observe the patient, and document behavior. Ask family members whether the current behavior and mental status are usual for the patient.

SCD is a painful, life-limiting disorder that can be passed on to one's children. Assess the patient's psychosocial needs in terms of new factors that might contribute to a crisis, established support systems, use of coping patterns, and disease progression.

Laboratory Assessment. The diagnosis of SCD is based on the percentage of hemoglobin S (HbS) on electrophoresis. A person who has AS usually has less than 40% HbS, and the patient with SCD may have 80% to 100% HbS. This percentage does not change during crises. Another indicator of SCD is the number of RBCs with permanent sickling. This value is less than 1% among people with no hemoglobin disease, is 5% to 50% among people with AS, and may be 90% among patients with SCD.

Other laboratory tests can indicate complications of the disease, especially during crises. The hematocrit of patients with SCD is low (between 20% and 30%) because of RBC shortened life span and RBC destruction. This value decreases even more during crises or during stress (aplastic crisis). The reticulocyte count is high, indicating anemia of long duration. The total bilirubin level may be high because damaged RBCs release iron and bilirubin.

The total white blood cell (WBC) count is usually high in patients with SCD. This elevation is related to chronic inflammation caused by tissue hypoxia and ischemia.

Imaging Assessment. Bone changes occur as a result of chronically stimulated marrow and low bone oxygen levels. The skull may show changes on x-ray as a result of bone surface cell destruction and new growth, giving the skull a "crew cut" appearance on x-ray. X-rays of joints may show necrosis and destruction. Ultrasonography, CT, positron emission tomography (PET), and MRI may show soft-tissue and organ changes from poor PERFUSION and chronic inflammation.

Other Diagnostic Assessment. Electrocardiographic (ECG) changes document cardiac infarcts and tissue damage. Specific ECG changes are related to the area of the heart damaged. Echocardiograms may show cardiomyopathy and decreased cardiac output (low ejection fraction).

NCLEX EXAMINATION CHALLENGE

Safe and Effective Care Environment

Which new assessment finding in a client with sickle cell disease who currently is in crisis does the nurse report immediately to the health care provider?

A. Pain in the right hip with limited range of motion
B. Slow capillary refill in the toes of the right foot
C. Yellow appearance of the roof of the mouth
D. Facial drooping on the right side

◆ *Analysis*

The priority NANDA-I nursing diagnoses and collaborative problems for patients with sickle cell disease include:

1. Acute Pain and Chronic Pain related to poor tissue oxygenation and joint destruction (NANDA-I)
2. Potential for infection, sepsis, multiple organ dysfunction, and death

◆ *Interventions*

Managing Pain. The pain with sickle cell crisis is the result of tissue injury caused by poor PERFUSION and tissue GAS EXCHANGE from obstructed blood flow. Mild pain episodes can be managed at home. However, pain is often severe enough to require hospitalization and opioid analgesics. Acute pain episodes have a sudden onset, usually involving the chest, back, abdomen, and extremities. Complications of SCD can cause severe, chronic pain, requiring large doses of opioid analgesics.

Ask whether the pain is typical of past pain episodes. If not, other pain causes or disease complications must be explored. Ask the patient to rate pain on a scale ranging from 0 to 10, and evaluate the effectiveness of interventions based on the ratings.

Concerns about substance abuse can lead to inadequate pain treatment in these patients. Opioid addiction is rare, occurring in only 2% to 5% of patients with SCD. Pain management is based on past pain history, previous drug use, disease complications, and current pain assessment. Health care providers need to be aware of their own attitudes when caring for this population. If substance abuse occurs, management of addiction is incorporated into the overall treatment plan. Addicted patients in acute pain crisis still need opioids (Jenerette & Leak, 2012).

CHART 40-2 Best Practice for Patient Safety & Quality Care (QSEN)

Care of the Patient in Sickle Cell Crisis

- Administer oxygen.
- Administer prescribed pain medication.
- Hydrate the patient with normal saline IV and with beverages of choice (without caffeine) orally.
- Remove any constrictive clothing.
- Encourage the patient to keep extremities extended to promote venous return.
- Do not raise the knee position of the bed.
- Elevate the head of the bed no more than 30 degrees.
- Keep room temperature at or above 72° F (22.2° C).
- Avoid taking blood pressure with external cuff.
- Check circulation in extremities every hour:
  - Pulse oximetry of fingers and toes
  - Capillary refill
  - Peripheral pulses
  - Toe temperature

Drug therapy for patients in acute sickle cell crisis often starts with at least 48 hours of IV analgesics. (Chart 40-2 lists best practices for nursing care of the patient in sickle cell crisis.) Morphine and hydromorphone (Dilaudid) are given IV on a routine schedule or by infusion pump using patient-controlled analgesia (PCA) (Myers & Eckes, 2012). Once relief is obtained, the IV dose can be tapered and the drug given orally. Avoid "as needed" (PRN) schedules because they do not provide adequate relief. Moderate pain may be managed with oral doses of opioids or NSAIDs. (See Chapter 3 for more information on pain management.)

Hydroxyurea (Droxia) may reduce the number of sickling and pain episodes by stimulating fetal hemoglobin (HbF) production. Increasing the level of HbF reduces sickling of red blood cells in patients with sickle cell disease. However, this drug is associated with an increased incidence of leukemia. Long-term complications should be discussed with the patient before this therapy is started. Hydroxyurea also suppresses bone marrow function including IMMUNITY, and regular follow-up to monitor complete blood counts (CBCs) for drug toxicity is important.

! NURSING SAFETY PRIORITY (QSEN)

Action Alert

Hydroxyurea is **teratogenic** (can cause birth defects). Teach sexually active women of childbearing age using this drug to adhere to strict contraceptive measures while taking hydroxyurea and for 1 month after the drug is discontinued.

Hydration by the oral or IV route helps reduce the duration of pain episodes. Urge the patient to drink water or juices. Because the patient is often dehydrated and his or her blood is hypertonic, hypotonic fluids are usually infused at 250 mL/hr for 4 hours. Once the patient's blood osmolarity is down to the normal range of 270 to 300 mOsm, the IV rate is reduced to 125 mL/hr if more hydration is needed.

Complementary therapies and other measures, such as keeping the room warm, using distraction and relaxation techniques, positioning with support for painful areas, aroma therapy, therapeutic touch, and warm soaks or compresses, all help reduce pain perception.

? CLINICAL JUDGMENT CHALLENGE

Ethical/Legal

A 27-year-old African-American man in sickle cell crisis is a patient on your unit. During report, one of the nurses from the previous shift mentions that she withheld the IV opioid pain medication during the night because she had taken care of this patient a year ago and feels that he is a "drug seeker."

1. What is your first action?
2. How should you approach your colleague?
3. Can a patient with sickle cell disease become addicted to opioids?
4. What can you do to prevent an incident like this one from happening again?

Preventing Sepsis, Multiple Organ Dysfunction, and Death. The patient with SCD is at greater risk for bacterial INFECTION because of decreased spleen function resulting from anoxic damage. Interventions focus on preventing infection, controlling infection, and starting treatment early for specific infections. The patient with a fever should have diagnostic testing for sepsis including CBC with differential, blood cultures, reticulocyte count, urine culture, and a chest x-ray. Usually these patients are started on prophylactic antibiotics.

Prevention and early detection strategies are used to protect the patient in sickle cell crisis from INFECTION. Frequent, thorough handwashing is of the utmost importance. Any person with an upper respiratory tract infection who enters the patient's room must wear a mask. Use strict aseptic technique for all invasive procedures.

Continually assess the patient for INFECTION, and monitor the daily CBC with differential WBC count. Inspect the mouth every 8 hours for lesions indicating fungal or viral infection. Listen to the lungs every 8 hours for crackles, wheezes, or reduced breath sounds. Inspect voided urine for odor and cloudiness, and ask about urgency, burning, or pain on urination. Take vital signs at least every 4 hours to assess for fever, or supervise this action when performed by others.

Drug therapy by prophylaxis with twice-daily oral penicillin reduces the number of pneumonia and other streptococcal infections. Urge the patient to receive yearly influenza vaccinations and to receive the pneumonia vaccine. Drug therapy for an actual INFECTION depends on the sensitivity of the specific organism, as well as on the extent of the infection.

Continued blood vessel occlusion by clumping of sickled cells increases the risk for multiple organ dysfunction. Acute chest syndrome, in which a vaso-occlusive event (VOE) causes infiltration and damage to the pulmonary system, is a major cause of death in adults with SCD. Thus preventing heart and lung damage is a priority. Management focuses on prevention of VOEs and promotion of PERFUSION.

Assess the patient admitted in sickle cell crisis for adequate PERFUSION to all body areas. Remove restrictive clothing, and instruct the patient to avoid flexing the knees and hips.

Hydration is needed because dehydration increases cell sickling and must be avoided. Assist him or her in maintaining adequate hydration. The patient in acute crisis needs an oral or IV fluid intake of at least 200 mL/hr.

Oxygen is given during crises because lack of oxygen is the main cause of sickling. Ensure that oxygen therapy is nebulized to prevent dehydration. Monitor oxygen saturation.

CHART 40-3 Patient and Family Education: Preparing for Self-Management

Prevention of Sickle Cell Crisis

- Drink at least 3 to 4 liters of liquids every day.
- Avoid alcoholic beverages.
- Avoid smoking cigarettes or using tobacco in any form.
- Contact your health care provider at the first sign of illness or infection.
- Be sure to get a "flu shot" every year.
- Ask your health care provider about taking the pneumonia vaccine.
- Avoid temperature extremes of hot or cold.
- Be sure to wear socks and gloves when going outside on cold days.
- Avoid planes with unpressurized passenger cabins.
- Avoid travel to high altitudes (e.g., cities like Denver and Santa Fe).
- Ensure that any health care professional who takes care of you knows you have sickle cell disease, especially the anesthesia provider and radiologist.
- Consider genetic counseling.
- Avoid strenuous physical activities.
- Engage in mild, low-impact exercise at least 3 times a week when you are not in crisis.

If saturation is low, evaluation of arterial blood gases (ABGs) and a chest x-ray may be needed.

Transfusion with RBCs can be helpful to increase HbA levels and dilute HbS levels, although they must be prescribed cautiously to prevent iron overload from repeated transfusions. Monitor the patient for transfusion complications (discussed on pp. 822-823 in the Acute Transfusion Reactions section).

In some treatment centers, hematopoietic stem cell transplantation (HSCT) is performed to correct abnormal hemoglobin permanently. Because HSCT is expensive and may result in life-threatening complications, its risks and benefits need to be considered for each patient.

Community-Based Care

Sickle cell disease (SCD) becomes worse over time, and a true remission is rare, although the number of crisis episodes may be reduced. Care focuses on teaching the patient and family how to prevent crises and complications (Chart 40-3). The patient with SCD may receive care in acute care, subacute care, extended or assistive care, and home care settings.

Teach the patient to avoid specific activities that lead to hypoxia and hypoxemia. Stress the recognition of the early manifestations of crisis so that interventions can be started early to prevent pain, complications, and permanent tissue damage. Teach the patient and family about the correct use of opioid analgesics at home. Counsel patients about the hereditary aspects of SCD, and provide information about birth control methods and pregnancy options. Many patients and family members can be helped by local support groups. Provide information about the closest local chapter of the Sickle Cell Foundation. Often local children's hospitals have sickle cell support groups that include adults with the disease.

GENDER HEALTH CONSIDERATIONS

Patient-Centered Care **QSEN**

Pregnancy in women with SCD may be life threatening. Barrier methods of contraception (cervical cap, diaphragm, or condoms with or without spermicides) are often recommended for women with SCD. The use of hormone-based contraceptives is controversial, because these drugs may increase clot formation, especially among smokers, predisposing them to crises. Urge women using hormone-based contraceptives to not smoke.

GLUCOSE-6-PHOSPHATE DEHYDROGENASE DEFICIENCY ANEMIA

❖ PATHOPHYSIOLOGY

More than 200 forms of **hemolytic** (blood cell–destroying) anemia are present from birth as a result of defects or deficiencies of one or more enzymes in red blood cells (RBCs). Most of these enzymes are needed to complete some critical step in RBC energy production. The most common type of inherited hemolytic anemia is the deficiency of the enzyme *glucose-6-phosphate dehydrogenase* (G6PD). This disease is inherited as an X-linked recessive disorder with more severe expression in males and mild partial expression in carrier females. It affects about 10% of all African Americans and also may occur in Sephardic Jews, Greeks, Iranians, Chinese, Filipinos, and Indonesians (McCance et al., 2014).

G6PD stimulates reactions in glucose metabolism important for energy in RBCs because they contain no other way to produce adenosine triphosphate (ATP). Cells with reduced amounts of G6PD break more easily during exposure to some drugs (e.g., sulfonamides, aspirin, quinine derivatives, chloramphenicol, dapsone, high doses of vitamin C, and thiazide diuretics) and exposure to benzene and other toxins.

New RBCs have some G6PD, but the enzyme diminishes as the cells age. The patient usually does not have manifestations until exposed to triggering agents or until a severe INFECTION develops. After exposure to a precipitating cause, acute RBC breakage begins and lasts 7 to 12 days. During this acute phase, anemia and jaundice develop. The hemolytic reaction is limited because only older RBCs, containing less G6PD, are destroyed.

❖ PATIENT-CENTERED COLLABORATIVE CARE

Prevention is the most important therapeutic measure. Men who belong to the high-risk groups should be tested for this problem before being given drugs that can cause the hemolytic reaction.

Hydration is important during an episode of hemolysis to prevent debris and hemoglobin from collecting in the kidney tubules, which can lead to acute kidney injury (AKI). Osmotic diuretics, such as mannitol (Osmitrol), may help prevent this complication. Transfusions are needed when anemia is present and kidney function is normal (see Transfusion Therapy section, p. 819).

IMMUNOHEMOLYTIC ANEMIA

The most common types of hemolytic anemias in North America are the immunohemolytic anemias, also referred to as *autoimmune hemolytic anemias* (McCance et al., 2014). The pathophysiology is abnormal IMMUNITY that results in the excessive destruction of red blood cell membranes *(lysis)* followed by accelerated erythropoiesis. Acquired hemolytic syndromes result from increased RBC destruction occurring from trauma, viral infection, malaria, exposure to certain chemicals or drugs, and autoimmune reactions.

In immunohemolytic anemia, immune system products (e.g., antibodies) attack a person's own RBCs for unknown reasons. Regardless of the cause, RBCs are viewed as non-self by the immune system and then are attacked and destroyed.

The two types of immunohemolytic anemia are warm antibody anemia and cold antibody anemia. **Warm antibody anemia** occurs with immunoglobulin G (IgG) antibody excess. These antibodies are most active at 98.6° F (37° C) and may be triggered by drugs, chemicals, or other autoimmune problems. **Cold antibody anemia** has complement protein fixation on immunoglobulin M (IgM) and occurs most at 86° F (30° C). This problem often occurs with a Raynaud's-like response in which the arteries in the hands and feet constrict profoundly in response to cold temperatures or stress.

Management depends on disease severity. Steroid therapy to suppress IMMUNITY is temporarily effective in most patients. Splenectomy and more intense immunosuppressive therapy with chemotherapy drugs may be used if steroid therapy fails. Plasma exchange therapy with antibody removal is effective for patients who do not respond to chemotherapy drugs.

ANEMIAS RESULTING FROM DECREASED PRODUCTION OF RED BLOOD CELLS

Anemias caused by decreased RBC production occur in response to many problems. Some are caused by failure of the bone marrow to produce healthy RBCs. Anemias also are caused by failure of the body to make or absorb a substance needed for RBC production. Many substances needed for RBC production are ingested as part of a healthy diet. For some patients with anemia resulting from a dietary deficiency, diet therapy is sufficient to manage anemia.

CONSIDERATIONS FOR OLDER ADULTS

Patient-Centered Care QSEN

Older patients often have restricted diets and may be unable to eat meat because of tooth loss or economic reasons and thus are at risk for iron deficiency anemia. Ask about a family history of anemia. B_{12} deficiency anemia often occurs in patients 50 to 80 years of age and may result from an inherited genetic mutation. Because manifestations are vague, the disorder can easily be overlooked (Orton, 2012).

Iron deficiency anemia is the most common anemia worldwide, especially among women, older adults, and people with poor diets. It can result from blood loss, poor GI absorption of iron, and an inadequate diet (McCance et al., 2014). The problem is a decreased iron supply for the developing RBC.

Adults usually have between 2 and 6 g of iron, depending on the size of the person and the amount of hemoglobin in the cells. With chronic iron deficiency, RBCs are small (**microcytic**) and the patient has mild symptoms of anemia, including weakness and pallor. Other manifestations include fatigue, reduced exercise tolerance, and fissures at the corners of the mouth. Serum ferritin values are less than 10 ng/mL (normal range is 12 to 300 ng/mL).

Any adult with iron deficiency should be evaluated for abnormal bleeding, especially from the GI tract. Management of iron deficiency anemia involves increasing the oral intake of iron from food sources (e.g., red meat, organ meat, egg yolks, kidney beans, leafy green vegetables, and raisins). If iron losses are mild, oral iron supplements, such as ferrous sulfate, are started until the hemoglobin level returns to normal. Instruct patients to take the iron supplement between meals for better absorption and to reduce GI distress. When iron deficiency anemia is severe, iron solutions (iron dextran [Dexferrum, INFeD, Pri-Dextra]; ferumoxytol [Feraheme]) can be given parenterally.

Vitamin B_{12} deficiency anemia results in failure to activate the enzyme that moves folic acid into precursor RBC cells so that cell division and growth into functional RBCs can occur. These precursor cells then undergo improper DNA synthesis and increase in size. Only a few are released from the bone marrow. This type of anemia is called *megaloblastic* or **macrocytic anemia** because of the large size of these abnormal cells.

Causes of vitamin B_{12} deficiency include vegan diets or diets lacking dairy products, small bowel resection, chronic diarrhea, diverticula, tapeworm, or overgrowth of intestinal bacteria. Anemia resulting from failure to absorb vitamin B_{12} (**pernicious anemia**) is caused by a deficiency of **intrinsic factor** (a substance normally secreted by the gastric mucosa), which is needed for intestinal absorption of vitamin B_{12}.

Vitamin B_{12} deficiency anemia may be mild or severe, usually develops slowly, and manifestations include pallor and jaundice, **glossitis** (a smooth, beefy-red tongue) (Fig. 40-3), fatigue, and weight loss. Patients with pernicious anemia may also have **paresthesias** (abnormal sensations) in the feet and hands and poor balance (Simmons, 2012).

When anemia is caused by a dietary deficiency, the focus of management is to increase the intake of foods rich in vitamin B_{12} (animal proteins, fish, eggs, nuts, dairy products, dried beans, citrus fruit, and leafy green vegetables). Vitamin supplements may be prescribed when anemia is severe. Patients who have pernicious anemia are given vitamin B_{12} injections weekly at first and then monthly for the rest of their lives. Oral B_{12} preparations and nasal spray or sublingual forms of cobalamin may be used to maintain vitamin levels after the patient's deficiency has first been corrected by the traditional injection method (Orton, 2012).

Folic acid deficiency can also cause anemia with manifestations similar to those of vitamin B_{12} deficiency. However, nervous system functions remain normal because folic acid deficiency does not affect nerve function. The disease develops slowly.

Common causes of folic acid deficiency are poor nutrition, malabsorption, and drugs. Poor nutrition, especially a diet lacking green leafy vegetables, liver, yeast, citrus fruits, dried beans, and nuts, is the most common cause. Malabsorption syndromes, such as Crohn's disease, are the second most

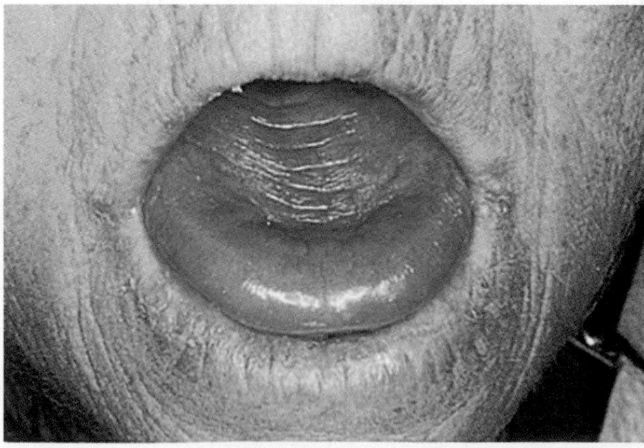

FIG. 40-3 Glossitis, a smooth tongue as a result of vitamin B_{12} deficiency anemia.

common cause. Anticonvulsants and oral contraceptives can contribute to folic acid deficiency and anemia.

Prevention begins by identifying high-risk patients, such as older, debilitated patients with alcoholism; patients at risk for malnutrition; and those with increased folic acid requirements. A diet rich in foods containing folic acid and vitamin B_{12} prevents a deficiency. This type of anemia is managed with scheduled folic acid replacement therapy.

Aplastic anemia is a deficiency of circulating red blood cells (RBCs) because of failure of the bone marrow to produce these cells. It is caused by an injury to the immature precursor cell for red blood cells. Although aplastic anemia sometimes occurs alone, it usually occurs with **leukopenia** (a reduction in white blood cells [WBCs]) and **thrombocytopenia** (a reduction in platelets), a condition known as **pancytopenia**. Disease onset may be slow or rapid.

The most common type of the disease is caused by long-term exposure to toxic agents, drugs (see Table 39-3 in Chapter 39), ionizing radiation, or infection, but often the cause is unknown. The disease also may follow viral infection. The most common hereditary form of the disease is Fanconi's anemia.

The patient has manifestations of severe anemia. A complete blood count (CBC) shows severe macrocytic anemia, leukopenia, and thrombocytopenia. A bone marrow biopsy may show replacement of cell-forming marrow with fat. Infection is common.

Blood transfusions are used only when the anemia causes disability or when bleeding is life threatening because of low platelet counts. Unnecessary transfusion increases the chances for developing immune reactions to platelets and shortens the life span of the transfused cell. This therapy is discontinued as soon as the bone marrow begins to produce RBCs.

Hematopoietic stem cell transplantation with donor cells is the most successful method of treatment for aplastic anemia that does not respond to other therapies. Cost, availability, and complications limit this treatment. For those patients who are unable to undergo such treatment or lack a suitable donor, immunosuppressive therapy remains the treatment of choice.

Immunosuppressive therapy helps patients who have the types of aplastic anemia with a disease course similar to that of autoimmune problems. Drugs such as prednisone, antithymocyte globulin (ATG), and cyclosporine A (Sandimmune) have resulted in partial or complete remissions. For moderate aplastic anemia, daclizumab (Zenapax) has improved both blood counts and transfusion requirements. Splenectomy may be needed for patients with an enlarged spleen that is either destroying normal RBCs or suppressing their development. (See discussion of surgical management for autoimmune thrombocytopenic purpura on p. 818.)

DISORDERS OF EXCESS RED BLOOD CELLS OR IRON

POLYCYTHEMIA VERA

❖ PATHOPHYSIOLOGY

In polycythemia, the number of red blood cells (RBCs) in the blood is *greater* than normal. The blood of a patient with polycythemia is **hyperviscous** (thicker than normal blood). The problem may be temporary (because of other conditions) or chronic.

Polycythemia vera (PV) is a disease with a sustained increase in blood hemoglobin levels to 18 g/dL, an RBC count of 6 million/mm^3, or a hematocrit of 55% or greater. PV is a cancer of the RBCs with three major hallmarks: massive production of RBCs, excessive leukocyte production, and excessive production of platelets. More than 90% of patients with PV show a mutation of the *JAK2* kinase gene in the affected cells (McCance et al., 2014). Extreme **hypercellularity** (cell excess) of the peripheral blood occurs in people with PV.

The patient's facial skin and mucous membranes have a dark, purple or cyanotic, flushed (**plethoric**) appearance with distended veins. Intense itching caused by dilated blood vessels, and poor PERFUSION is common. The thick blood moves more slowly and places increased demands on the heart, resulting in hypertension. In some areas, blood flow may be so slow that stasis occurs. Vascular stasis causes **thrombosis** (CLOTTING) within the smaller vessels, occluding them, which leads to tissue hypoxia, anoxia and, later, to infarction and necrosis. Tissues most at risk for this problem are the heart, spleen, and kidneys, although damage can occur in any organ or tissue.

Because the actual number of cells in the blood is greatly increased and the cells are not completely normal, cell life spans are shorter. The shorter life spans and increased cell production cause a rapid turnover of circulating blood cells. This rapid turnover increases the amount of cell debris (released when cells die) in the blood, adding to the general "sludging" of the blood. This debris includes uric acid and potassium, which cause the manifestations of gout and hyperkalemia (elevated serum potassium level).

Even though the number of RBCs is greatly increased, their oxygen-carrying capacity is impaired, and patients have poor GAS EXCHANGE with severe hypoxia. Bleeding problems are common because of platelet impairment.

❖ PATIENT-CENTERED COLLABORATIVE CARE

Polycythemia vera is a malignant disease that progresses in severity over time. If left untreated, few people with PV live longer than 2 years after diagnosis. With management by repeated phlebotomy with apheresis (2 to 5 times per week), the patient may live 10 to 15 years or longer. (**Apheresis** is the withdrawal of whole blood and removal of some of the patient's blood component, in this case RBCs. The plasma is then reinfused back into the patient.) Increasing hydration and promoting venous return help prevent clot formation. Therapy for PV also includes the use of anticoagulants. Chart 40-4 lists health tips for patients with PV.

CHART 40-4 Patient and Family Education: Preparing for Self-Management

Polycythemia Vera

- Drink at least 3 liters of liquids each day.
- Avoid tight or constrictive clothing, especially garters and girdles.
- Wear gloves when outdoors in temperatures lower than 50° F (10° C).
- Keep all health care–related appointments.
- Contact your health care provider at the first sign of infection.
- Take anticoagulants as prescribed.
- Wear support hose or stockings while you are awake and up.
- Elevate your feet whenever you are seated.
- Exercise slowly and only on the advice of your physician.
- Stop activity at the first sign of chest pain.
- Use an electric shaver.
- Use a soft-bristled toothbrush to brush your teeth.
- Do not floss between your teeth.

Aggressive IV chemotherapy is no longer recommended because of its increased risk for inducing leukemia. Aspirin therapy may be used to decrease clot formation but increases the risk for GI bleeding. Hydroxyurea, an oral chemotherapy drug, may be prescribed for severe manifestations of the disease. Interferon-alfa therapy has also shown some benefit in controlling RBC production.

NCLEX EXAMINATION CHALLENGE

Health Promotion and Maintenance

Which intervention is most important for the nurse to teach the client with polycythemia vera to prevent injury as a result of the increased bleeding tendency?

A. Use a soft-bristled toothbrush.
B. Drink at least 3 liters of liquids per day.
C. Wear gloves and socks outdoors in cool weather.
D. Exercise slowly and only on the advice of the physician.

HEREDITARY HEMOCHROMATOSIS

Hereditary hemochromatosis is an autosomal recessive disorder in which a mutation in both alleles of the *HFE* gene cause increased intestinal absorption of dietary iron (Beery & Workman, 2012). The excess iron is deposited in a variety of tissues and organs, including the liver, spleen, heart, joints, skin, and pancreas. The iron deposits can damage the organs, leading to organ failure. Usually the disease is more common in men and manifestations appear in men during their 40s. Women have manifestations later because the loss of menstrual blood before menopause helps remove excess iron. The most common clinical manifestations are abdominal pain, liver enlargement, hyperglycemia, and a gradual darkening of the skin. Later problems include diabetes, liver cirrhosis, endocrine gland failure, heart disease, and death.

The disorder is usually diagnosed on the basis of clinical manifestations and altered iron levels. Genetic testing is available to determine carrier status. When the disorder is identified early before organ damage, management is simple and can prevent severe organ damage and early death. Phlebotomy and removal of 500 mL of blood at a time, occurring as often as twice weekly at first, is performed to reduce the overall iron load of the blood. The desired outcome is to reduce blood ferritin levels to less than 9 to 50 micrograms per liter. Once this level has been achieved, phlebotomy frequency can be reduced to once every 2 to 4 months for maintenance.

MYELODYSPLASTIC SYNDROMES

❖ PATHOPHYSIOLOGY

Myelodysplastic syndromes (MDS) are a group of disorders caused by the formation of abnormal cells in the bone marrow. These abnormal cells are usually destroyed shortly after they are released into the blood. As a result, patients with MDS have a decrease in all blood cell types. Anemia is the most common problem with MDS, although **neutropenia** (low white blood cell count [WBC]) and **thrombocytopenia** (low platelets) are also often present.

MDS most often occurs in people ages 60 years or older. MDS has cancer-like features and is considered to be a *precancerous* state. Like cancer, it arises from a single population of abnormal cells. About 30% of all patients with MDS do eventually develop acute leukemia (McCance et al., 2014). There are a number of subtypes of MDS with different prognoses and responses to therapy. Patients are categorized into risk groups (i.e., low, intermediate [1 and 2], high) based on the severity of **pancytopenia** (low counts of all blood cell types), cytogenetic abnormalities, and numbers of blast cells (immature WBC cells) found in the bone marrow (Kurtin, 2012).

The exact cause of MDS is not clear. Risk factors include normal physiologic changes associated with aging, chemical exposures (pesticides, benzene), tobacco smoke, and exposure to radiation or chemotherapy drugs. Diagnosis is made by examination of the chromosomes and the genes within the chromosomes (cytogenetic testing) of the bone marrow cells. Peripheral blood smears are used to assess the level of cell maturation and the proportion of abnormal cells.

❖ PATIENT-CENTERED COLLABORATIVE CARE

The only potentially curative treatment for MDS is an allogeneic hematopoietic stem cell transplantation, which is often not an option because of the advanced age of many patients (Kurtin, 2012). Several alternate management strategies have demonstrated some promise. For low-risk and intermediate-1–risk MDS, the antitumor immunomodulatory agent *lenalidomide* (Revlimid) is approved for patients whose dysplastic cells have the chromosome abnormality of a deleted *5q*. Two other agents approved for intermediate-2–risk and high-risk MDS are azacitidine (Vidaza) and decitabine (Dacogen) (Kurtin, 2012). These drugs often require at least 3 to 6 months to achieve a clinical response; therefore supportive care is necessary.

Supportive care includes blood transfusions for anemia and platelet transfusions when platelet levels are very low. Erythropoiesis-stimulating agents (ESAs), such as epoetin alfa (Epogen, Procrit) or darbepoetin alfa (Aranesp), may be given in addition to transfusions.

WHITE BLOOD CELL DISORDERS

As discussed in Chapter 17, white blood cells (WBCs), or **leukocytes**, provide protection from INFECTION and cancer development. This protection depends on maintaining normal numbers and ratios of the different mature circulating WBCs. When any one type of WBC is present in either abnormal amounts (too high or too low), IMMUNITY, GAS EXCHANGE, and CLOTTING are altered to some degree, placing patients at risk for many complications. This section covers the changes and nursing care for patients with disorders involving overgrowth of specific types of WBCs. (See Chapter 19 for the problems and care needs for patients with immune deficiency.)

LEUKEMIA

❖ PATHOPHYSIOLOGY

Leukemia is cancer with uncontrolled production of immature WBCs ("blast" cells) in the bone marrow. As a result, the bone marrow becomes overcrowded with immature, nonfunctional cells and production of normal blood cells is greatly decreased. Leukemia may be **acute**, with a sudden onset, or **chronic**, with a slow onset and manifestations that persist for years.

Leukemias are classified by cell type. Leukemic cells coming from the lymphoid pathways (see Fig. 17-3 in Chapter 17) are typed as **lymphocytic** or **lymphoblastic**. Leukemic cells coming from the myeloid pathways are typed as **myelocytic** or **myelogenous**. Several subtypes exist for each of these diseases, which are classified according to the degree of maturity of the abnormal cell and the specific cell type involved. These are identified as M0 through M8. M3 is a subtype (referred to as *acute promyelocytic leukemia* [APL]) that has a specific treatment different from other AMLs. It is identified by a translocation of chromosomes 15 and 17. *Biphenotypic leukemia* is acute leukemia that shows both lymphocytic and myelocytic features.

With leukemia, cancer most often occurs in the stem cells or early precursor leukocyte cells, causing excessive growth of a specific type of immature leukocyte. In some chronic leukemias, the cancerous cells may be more mature. These cells are abnormal, and their excessive production in the bone marrow stops normal bone marrow production, leading to anemia, thrombocytopenia, and leukopenia. Often the number of immature, abnormal WBCs ("blasts") in the blood is greatly elevated, and these cells cannot provide infection protection. Leukemic cells can also be found in the spleen, liver, lymph nodes, and central nervous system. Without treatment, the patient will die of INFECTION or hemorrhage. For patients with acute leukemia, these changes occur rapidly and, without intervention, progress to death. Chronic leukemia may be present for years before changes appear.

Etiology and Genetic Risk

The exact cause of leukemia is unknown, although many genetic and environmental factors are involved in its development. The basic problem involves damage to genes controlling cell growth. This damage then changes cells from a normal to a **malignant** (cancer) state. Analysis of the bone marrow of a patient with acute leukemia shows abnormal chromosomes about 50% of the time (McCance et al., 2014). Possible risk factors for the development of leukemia include ionizing radiation, viral infection, exposure to chemicals and drugs, disorders such as myelodysplastic syndrome or Fanconi's anemia, genetic factors, immunologic factors, environmental factors, and the interaction of these factors.

Ionizing radiation exposures such as radiation therapy for cancer treatment or heavy accidental exposures increase the risk for leukemia development, particularly acute myelogenous leukemia (AML). Chemicals and drugs have been linked to leukemia development because of their ability to damage DNA. Previous treatment for cancer with some chemotherapy drugs (e.g., melphalan, doxorubicin, etoposide, and cyclophosphamide) poses risks for leukemia development about 5 to 8 years after treatment. Table 39-3 in Chapter 39 lists chemicals and drugs that damage the hematologic system.

Genetic and IMMUNITY factors influence leukemia development. There is an increased incidence of the disease among patients with genetic conditions such as Down syndrome, Bloom syndrome, Klinefelter syndrome, and Fanconi's anemia. Immune deficiencies may promote the development of leukemia. Chronic lymphocytic leukemia appears to have a familial or genetic predisposition.

Incidence and Prevalence

Leukemia accounts for 2% of all new cases of cancer and 4% of all deaths from cancer (American Cancer Society [ACS], 2014). The incidence depends on many factors, including the type of WBC affected, age, gender, race, and geographic locale.

TABLE 40-2 Classification of Leukemia Types

LEUKEMIA TYPE	FEATURES
Acute myelogenous leukemia (AML)	Most common in adults Has 8 subtypes
Acute promyelocytic leukemia (APL)	Subtype of AML Most curable of adult leukemias
Acute lymphocytic leukemia (ALL)	Forms about 10% of adult-onset leukemias Often is Philadelphia chromosome–positive
Chronic myelogenous leukemia (CML)	Forms about 20% of adult-onset leukemias Occurs most often after age 50 years Usually is Philadelphia chromosome–positive Has three phases: • *Chronic*—slow growing with mild manifestations that respond to therapy • *Accelerated*—more rapid growing with more severe manifestations, increased blast cells, and failure to respond to therapy • *Blast*—very aggressive leukemia with high percentage of blast and promyelocytes that spread to other organs
Chronic lymphocytic leukemia (CLL)	Most common chronic leukemia in adults; occurs most often after age 50 years Is associated with a genetic predisposition Survival time can extend to 10 years or more in patients diagnosed with early-stage disease

In the United States, about 49,000 new cases of leukemia occur each year (ACS, 2014). Leukemia is classified into four different types based on the cell type affected and how fast the disease progresses (Table 40-2).

❖ PATIENT-CENTERED COLLABORATIVE CARE

◆ Assessment

History. Ask the patient about exposure to risk factors and related genetic factors. Age is important because the risk for adult-onset leukemia increases with age. Occupation and hobbies may reveal exposure to agents that increase the risk for leukemia. Previous illnesses and the medical history may reveal exposure to ionizing radiation or drugs that increase risk.

Changes in IMMUNITY increase the risk for INFECTION in the patient with leukemia. Even when the blood count shows a normal or high level of WBCs, these cells are immature and cannot protect the patient from infection. Ask about the frequency and severity of infections, such as colds, influenza, pneumonia, bronchitis, or unexplained fevers, during the past 6 months.

Platelet function is reduced with leukemia, interfering with CLOTTING. Ask about any excessive bleeding episodes, such as:

- A tendency to bruise easily or longer after minor trauma
- Nosebleeds
- Increased menstrual flow
- Bleeding from the gums
- Rectal bleeding
- Hematuria (blood in the urine)

If the patient has experienced such an episode, ask whether this type and extent of bleeding is his or her usual response to injury or represents a change.

CHART 40-5 **Key Features**

Acute Leukemia

Integumentary Manifestations
- Ecchymoses
- Petechiae
- Open infected lesions
- Pallor of the conjunctivae, nail beds, palmar creases, and around the mouth

Gastrointestinal Manifestations
- Bleeding gums
- Anorexia
- Weight loss
- Enlarged liver and spleen

Renal Manifestations
- Hematuria

Musculoskeletal Manifestations
- Bone pain
- Joint swelling and pain

Cardiovascular Manifestations
- Tachycardia at basal activity levels
- Orthostatic hypotension
- Palpitations

Respiratory Manifestations
- Dyspnea on exertion

Neurologic Manifestations
- Fatigue
- Headache
- Fever

The patient with leukemia often has weakness and fatigue from anemia and from the increased metabolism of the leukemic cells. Ask whether any of these problems have occurred:

- Headaches
- Behavior changes
- Increased somnolence; decreased alertness; fatigue
- Decreased attention span
- Muscle weakness
- Loss of appetite
- Weight loss

A 24-hour activity history may reveal activity intolerance, changes in behavior, and unexplained fatigue. Determine how long the patient has had any of these debilitating problems.

Physical Assessment/Clinical Manifestations. Leukemia affects all blood cells, and blood influences the health and function of all organs and systems. Thus many body areas and systems may be affected (Chart 40-5). The following manifestations occur with acute leukemia and chronic leukemia in the blast phase.

Cardiovascular changes often are related to adjustments needed when PERFUSION and GAS EXCHANGE are reduced from anemia. The heart rate is increased, and blood pressure is decreased. **Murmurs** (abnormal blood flow sounds in the heart) and **bruits** (abnormal blood flow sounds over arteries) may be heard. Capillary refill is slow. When the WBC count is greatly elevated and blood is highly viscous, blood pressure is elevated with a bounding pulse.

Respiratory changes are related to reduced GAS EXCHANGE from anemia and to INFECTION. Respiratory rate increases as anemia becomes more severe. If a respiratory infection is present, the patient may have coughing and dyspnea. Abnormal breath sounds are heard on auscultation.

Skin changes include pallor and coolness to the touch as a result of reduced PERFUSION from anemia. Pallor is most evident on the face, around the mouth, and in the nail beds. The conjunctiva of the eye also is pale, as are the creases on the palm of the hand. Petechiae may be present on any area of skin surface, especially the legs and feet. The petechiae may be unrelated to any obvious trauma. Inspect for skin infections or injured areas that have failed to heal. Inspect the mouth for gum bleeding and any sore or lesion that may indicate infection.

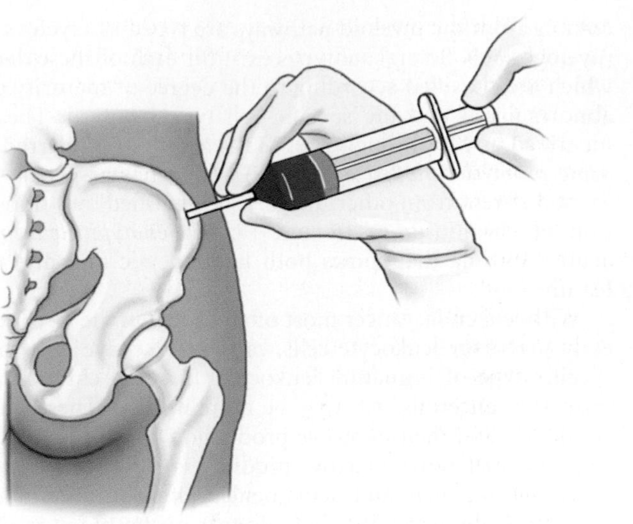

FIG. 40-4 Bone marrow aspiration from the posterior iliac crest. (*GVHD,* Graft-versus-host disease.)

Intestinal changes may be related to an increased bleeding tendency and to fatigue. Weight loss, nausea, and anorexia are common. Examine the rectal area for fissures, and test stool for occult blood. Many patients with leukemia have reduced bowel sounds and are constipated because reduced blood flow to intestinal tissue leads to decreased peristalsis. Enlargement of the liver and spleen and abdominal tenderness also may be present from leukemic cells trapped in these organs.

Central nervous system (CNS) changes include cranial nerve problems, headache, and papilledema from leukemic invasion of the CNS. Seizures and coma also may occur.

Miscellaneous changes can include bone and joint tenderness as the marrow is damaged and the bone reabsorbs. Leukemic cells invade lymph nodes, causing enlargement.

Psychosocial Assessment. The patient with newly diagnosed leukemia is very anxious and fearful of the disease outcome. Spend time with the patient and family to assess what the diagnosis means to them and what they expect in the future (Albrecht, 2014).

A diagnosis of leukemia has serious consequences for a person's lifestyle. Hospitalization for initial treatment often lasts weeks and may result in boredom, loneliness, isolation, and financial stress. Assess coping patterns, including activities that the patient finds enjoyable and methods that help him or her relax. After initial therapy, the patient may resume work, depending on the occupation. Often the patient must make adjustments for changes in functional status. He or she usually is hospitalized repeatedly for complications.

Laboratory Assessment. The patient with acute leukemia usually has decreased hemoglobin and hematocrit levels, a low platelet count, and an abnormal white blood cell (WBC) count. The WBC count may be low, normal, or elevated. The patient with a high WBC count consisting of mostly blast cells at diagnosis has a poorer prognosis.

The definitive test for leukemia is an examination of cells obtained from bone marrow aspiration and biopsy (Fig. 40-4). The bone marrow is full of leukemic **blast phase cells** (immature cells that are dividing). The proteins (**antigens**) on the surfaces of the leukemic cells are "markers" that help diagnose the type of leukemia and may indicate prognosis. These include the T11 protein, terminal deoxynucleotidyl transferase (TDT), the common acute lymphoblastic leukemia antigen (CALLA), and the CD33 antigen.

Blood CLOTTING times and factors are usually abnormal with acute leukemia. Reduced levels of fibrinogen and other clotting factors are common. Whole-blood clotting time (Lee-White clotting test) is prolonged, as is the activated partial thromboplastin time (aPTT).

Chromosome analysis (cytogenetic studies) of the leukemic cells may identify marker chromosomes to help diagnose the type of leukemia, predict the prognosis, and determine therapy effectiveness. An example is the Philadelphia chromosome, which is important in the diagnosis and treatment of some chronic myelogenous leukemia (CML) and adult acute lymphocytic leukemia (ALL). The Philadelphia chromosome is an abnormal chromosome caused by a translocation of the *ABL* gene from chromosome 9 onto the *BCR* gene of chromosome 22. The new protein produced by this mutation inhibits cell apoptosis and DNA repair, leading to further genetic abnormality (Simoneau, 2013).

Imaging Assessment. Specific manifestations determine the need for specific tests. In a patient with dyspnea, a chest x-ray is needed to determine whether leukemic infiltrates are present in the lung. Skeletal x-rays may help determine whether loss of bone minerals and bone density is present.

NCLEX EXAMINATION CHALLENGE

Physiological Integrity

The blood of a client who has chronic myelogenous leukemia shows a high percentage of blast cells and promyelocytes. What is the nurse's correct interpretation of this test result?

A. The client's risk for infection is decreasing.
B. The disease has become more aggressive.
C. The drug therapy for the disease is effective.
D. The type of leukemia is now lymphocytic rather than myelogenous.

◆ *Analysis*

The priority NANDA-I nursing diagnoses and collaborative problems for patients with acute myelogenous leukemia (AML), the most common type of acute leukemia seen in adults, include:

1. Risk for Infection related to decreased immune response and chemotherapy (NANDA-I)
2. Risk for Injury related to thrombocytopenia and chemotherapy (NANDA-I)
3. Fatigue related to decreased tissue oxygenation and increased energy demands (NANDA-I)

◆ *Planning and Implementation*

Preventing Infection

Planning: Expected Outcomes. The patient with leukemia is expected to remain free from infection. Indicators include:

- Absence of fever and foul-smelling or purulent drainage
- Absence of cough, chest pain, and dyspnea
- Absence of urinary frequency, urgency, or pain and burning
- Intact skin and mucous membranes

Interventions. *INFECTION is a major cause of death in the patient with leukemia* because the white blood cells are immature and cannot function or the cells are depleted from chemotherapy, and sepsis is a common complication. Infection occurs through both **auto-contamination** (normal flora overgrows and penetrates the internal environment) and **cross-contamination** (organisms from another person or the environment are transmitted to the patient). The most common sources of infection are the skin, respiratory tract, and intestinal tract.

Gram-negative bacteria are the most common cause of infection, although infections from other causes do occur. Interventions aim to halt infection and control infections early. Chart 40-6 lists areas to assess for the patient at risk for infection.

CHART 40-6 Focused Assessment

Patients at Risk for Infection

General Condition
- Age
- History of allergies
- History of chemotherapy, radiation therapy, or other immunosuppressive therapies, such as steroid use
- Chronic diseases
- History of febrile neutropenia and associated symptoms
- Nutrition status
- Functional status—problems with immobility
- Tobacco use—cigarettes, pipe, cigars, oral
- Recreational drug use
- Alcohol use
- Prescribed and over-the-counter drug use
- Baseline and ongoing vital signs—blood pressure, heart rate, respiratory rate, and temperature

Skin and Mucous Membranes
- Thorough inspection of all skin surfaces with attention to axillae, anorectal area, and under breasts; inspection of skin for color, vascularity, bleeding, lesions, edema, moist areas, excoriation, irritation, erythema; general condition of hair and nails, pressure areas, swelling, pain, tenderness, biopsy or surgical sites, wounds, enlarged lymph nodes, catheters, or other devices
- Inspection of oral cavity, including lips, tongue, mucous membranes, gingiva, teeth, and throat—color, moisture, bleeding, ulcerations, lesions, exudate, mucositis, stomatitis, plaque, swelling, pain, tenderness, taste changes, amount and character of saliva, ability to swallow, changes in voice, dental caries, patient's oral hygiene routine
- History of current skin or mucous membrane problems

Head, Eyes, Ears, Nose
- Pain, tenderness, exudate, crusting, enlarged lymph nodes

Cardiopulmonary
- Respiratory rate and pattern, breath sounds (presence/absence, adventitious sounds), quantity and characteristics of sputum, shortness of breath, use of accessory muscles, dysphagia, diminished gag reflex, tachycardia, blood pressure

Gastrointestinal
- Pain, diarrhea, bowel sounds, character and frequency of bowel movements, constipation, rectal bleeding, hemorrhoids, change in bowel habits, sexual practices, erythema, ulceration

Genitourinary
- Dysuria, frequency, urgency, hematuria, pruritus, pain, vaginal or penile discharge, vaginal bleeding, burning, lesions, ulcerations, characteristics of urine

Central Nervous System
- Cognition, level of consciousness, personality, behavior

Musculoskeletal
- Tenderness, pain, loss of function

Drug Therapy for Acute Leukemia. Drug therapy for patients with AML is divided into three distinctive phases: induction, consolidation, and maintenance.

Induction therapy is intense and consists of combination chemotherapy started at the time of diagnosis. The purpose of this therapy is to achieve a rapid, complete remission of all manifestations of disease. A combination of chemotherapeutic agents is usually prescribed. However, agencies and physicians differ in drugs used and the treatment schedule. One example of aggressive induction therapy is continuous IV cytosine arabinoside for 7 days together with an anthracycline for the first 3 days, sometimes referred to as a "7 plus 3" regimen. This therapy results in severe bone marrow suppression with neutropenia, making the patient even more at risk for infection. For acute promyelocytic leukemia, the agent *tretinoin* (Vesanoid) is added to the chemotherapy regimen.

Prolonged hospitalizations are common while the patient is neutropenic. Recovery of bone marrow function requires at least 2 to 3 weeks, during which the patient must be protected from life-threatening INFECTIONS. Other side effects of drugs used for induction therapy include nausea, vomiting, diarrhea, **alopecia** (hair loss), **stomatitis** (mouth sores), kidney toxicity, liver toxicity, and cardiac toxicity. (See Chapter 22 for information on effects of anticancer agents.) Older patients have a greater infection-related death rate during this phase than do younger patients. Patients with APL are at greater risk for sepsis with disseminated intravascular coagulation (DIC) during induction therapy than are patients with other subtypes of AML.

Consolidation therapy consists of another course of either the same drugs used for induction at a different dosage or a different combination of chemotherapy drugs. This treatment occurs early in remission, and its intent is to cure. Consolidation therapy may be either a single course of chemotherapy or repeated courses. Hematopoietic stem cell transplantation also may be considered, depending on the disease subtype and the patient's response to induction therapy.

Maintenance therapy may be prescribed for months to years after successful induction and consolidation therapies for acute lymphocytic leukemia (ALL) and acute promyelocytic leukemia (APL). The purpose is to maintain the remission achieved through induction and consolidation. Not all types of leukemia respond to maintenance therapy.

Drug Therapy for Chronic Leukemia. Imatinib mesylate (Gleevec) is a common first-line drug therapy for CML that is Philadelphia chromosome–positive. This oral drug is well tolerated and has been effective at inducing remission for early stages of CML. Other drugs approved for first-line therapy or for patients whose disease is resistant or intolerant to imatinib are dasatinib (Sprycel) or nilotinib (Tasigna) (Byar & Workman, 2012). Other drugs used to treat CML include interferon-alfa, which reduces the growth of leukemic cells, but its use is limited because of side effects, such as flu-like manifestations and fevers. Patient responses to therapy are evaluated on the basis of hematologic, cytogenetic, and molecular criteria.

Chronic lymphocytic leukemia (CLL) is the most prevalent form of leukemia in adults, affecting women more often than men. Cytogenetic testing is important in the prognosis. Partial deletion of chromosome 13 is associated with a benign disease course, whereas a deletion of chromosome 11 or of chromosome 17 (*p53* mutation) is associated with a poor prognosis. Treatment of CLL with standard chemotherapy can cause remissions but does not cure the disease. The decision to initiate therapy is based on disease stage, manifestations, and disease activity. Rituximab (Rituxan) is often combined with standard chemotherapy drugs or used as a single agent. Another drug approved for CLL is bendamustine (Treanda), which may be used alone or along with rituximab. Other monoclonal antibodies approved for CLL are ofatumumab (Arzerra) and alemtuzumab (Campath). Current investigational therapies for CLL include ibrutinib, oblimersen (Genasense), flavopiridol (Alvocidib), and lenalidomide (Revlimid).

Hematopoietic stem cell transplantation in patients with CLL is an option that offers curative potential or prolonged disease-free survival. However, it comes with considerable risk for mortality and is not an appropriate alternative for all patients.

Drug Therapy for Infection. Drug therapy is the main defense against INFECTIONS that develop in patients undergoing therapy for AML. Drugs used depend on the sensitivity of the organism causing the infection, as well as infection severity. Drugs for infection include antibacterial, antiviral, and antifungal agents.

Infection Protection. A major focus in caring for the patient with leukemia is protection from INFECTION. All personnel must use extreme care during all nursing procedures. Frequent, thorough handwashing is of the utmost importance. Anyone with an upper respiratory tract infection who enters the patient's room must wear a mask. Observe strict asepsis when changing dressings or accessing a central venous catheter. Maintain strict aseptic technique in the care of these catheters at all times.

If possible, ensure that the patient is in a private room to reduce cross-contamination. Other precautions are used, such as not allowing standing water in vases, denture cups, or humidifiers in the patient's room, because they are breeding grounds for organisms.

Some facilities place the immunosuppressed patient in a room with a high-efficiency particulate air (HEPA) filtration or laminar airflow system. These systems decrease the number of airborne pathogens. It is not known whether these systems benefit patients.

Continually assess the patient for the presence of INFECTION. This task is difficult because manifestations are not obvious in the patient with leukopenia. The patient with leukopenia may have a severe infection without pus and with only a low-grade fever.

Monitor the patient's daily CBC with differential WBC count and absolute neutrophil count (ANC). Inspect the mouth during every shift for lesions and mucosa breakdown. Assess the lungs every 8 hours for crackles, wheezes, and reduced breath sounds. Assess urine for odor and cloudiness. Ask about any urgency, burning, or pain on urination. Take vital signs at least every 4 hours to assess for fever.

! NURSING SAFETY PRIORITY (QSEN)

Critical Rescue

A temperature elevation of even 1° F (or 0.5° C) above baseline is significant for a patient with leukopenia and indicates INFECTION until it has been proven otherwise. Report this finding to the health care provider at once.

Many hospital units that specialize in the care of patients with neutropenia have specific protocols for antibiotic therapy if infection is suspected. Usually the health care provider is notified immediately and specific specimens are obtained for culture. Obtain blood for bacterial and fungal cultures from peripheral IV sites and from the central venous catheter (Myers & Reyes, 2011). Obtain urine specimens, sputum specimens, and specimens from open lesions for culture. Chest x-rays are taken. After the specimens are obtained, the patient begins IV antibiotics.

Skin care is important for preventing INFECTION in the patient with leukemia because the skin may be the only intact defense. Teach him or her about hygiene, and urge daily bathing. If the patient is immobile, turn him or her every hour and apply skin lubricants.

Perform pulmonary hygiene every 2 to 4 hours. Listen to the lungs for crackles, wheezes, and reduced breath sounds. Urge the patient to cough and deep breathe or to perform sustained maximal inhalations every hour while awake.

Hematopoietic Stem Cell Transplantation. Hematopoietic stem cell transplantation (HSCT), sometimes called *bone marrow transplantation (BMT),* is standard treatment for the patient with leukemia who has a closely matched donor and who is in temporary remission after induction therapy. It is used also for lymphoma, multiple myeloma, aplastic anemia, sickle cell disease, and many solid tumors.

The bone marrow is the actual site of production of leukemic cells. It can be difficult to ensure that all leukemic cells have been eradicated during induction therapy. Therefore before an HSCT, additional chemotherapy with or without total body irradiation is given to purge (condition or clean) the marrow of leukemic cells. *These treatments are lethal to the bone marrow, and without replacement of stem cells by transplantation, the patient would die of INFECTION or hemorrhage.*

After conditioning, new healthy stem cells are given to the patient. The new cells go to the marrow and then begin the process of hematopoiesis, which results in normal, properly functioning blood cells and, ideally, a permanent cure.

Many hospitals have transplant units. With long-term survival increasing after HSCT, nurses can expect to be caring for these people—if not during the actual transplantation or recovery period, then after the recovery period—in a variety of health care settings.

HSCT started with the use of **allogeneic bone marrow transplantation** (transplantation of bone marrow from a sibling or matched unrelated donor) and has advanced to the use of human leukocyte antigen (HLA)–matched stem cells from the umbilical cords of unrelated donors. Transplants are classified by the source of stem cells (Table 40-3). Stem cells for transplantation may be obtained by bone marrow harvest, peripheral stem cell apheresis, or umbilical cord blood stem cell banking. Transplantation has five phases: stem cell obtainment, conditioning regimen, transplantation, engraftment, and post-transplantation recovery.

Obtaining the Stem Cells. Stem cells are taken either from the patient directly (*autologous stem cells*), an HLA-identical twin (*syngeneic stem cells*), or from an HLA-matched person (*allogeneic stem cells*). For allogeneic transplant, the best results occur when the donor is an HLA-identical sibling; however, transplant also can be successful between those with closely but not perfectly matched HLA types. The chance of matching with any given sibling is 25%. Donor registries keep records of potential donors who can provide stem cells for patients who do not have a family member HLA match. The chance of matching with an unrelated donor is 1 in 5000.

TABLE 40-3 Classification of Transplants

TYPE OF TRANSPLANT	SOURCES OF STEM CELLS
Autologous	
Self-donation	Bone marrow harvest Peripheral stem cell pheresis Umbilical cord blood
Syngeneic	
Patient's HLA identical twin	Bone marrow harvest Peripheral stem cell pheresis
Allogeneic	
HLA-matched relative	Bone marrow harvest
Unrelated HLA-matched donor	Peripheral stem cell pheresis
Mismatched or partially HLA-matched family member or unrelated donor (donor registries)	Umbilical cord blood

HLA, Human leukocyte antigen.

CULTURAL CONSIDERATIONS

Patient-Centered Care QSEN

About 70% of people on the bone marrow donor lists are white. The chance of finding an HLA-matched unrelated donor is estimated at 30% to 40% for white people, but for African Americans the chance is less than 20% because there are fewer African Americans among registered donors. Although blood types are common in all racial groups, tissue types can be very different among racial and ethnic groups. Nationally, efforts are made to publicize the need for donors from all cultural backgrounds. Help in this effort by providing accurate information and dispelling myths.

Bone marrow harvesting occurs after a suitable donor is identified by tissue typing. The procedure occurs in the operating room, where marrow is removed through multiple aspirations from the iliac crests, although this technique is used less often today. About 500 to 1000 mL of marrow is aspirated, and the donor's marrow regrows within a few weeks. The marrow is then filtered and, if autologous, is treated to rid the marrow of any remaining cancer cells. Allogeneic marrow is transfused into the recipient immediately. Autologous marrow is frozen for later use.

Monitor the donor for fluid loss, assess for complications of anesthesia, and manage pain. During surgery, donors may lose a large amount of fluid in addition to the volume of marrow taken. Donors are hydrated with saline infusions before and immediately after surgery. Occasionally the donor may need an RBC transfusion. Assess the harvest sites to ensure that the dressings are dry and intact and that the donor is not bleeding excessively.

Marrow donation is usually a same-day surgical procedure. Teach the donor to inspect the harvest sites for bleeding and to take analgesics for pain. Pain at the harvest sites (hips) is common and is managed with oral non–aspirin-containing analgesics. Some donors may require opioid analgesics for pain control.

Peripheral blood stem cell (PBSC) harvesting requires three phases: mobilization, collection by apheresis, and reinfusion. **PBSCs** are stem cells that have been released from the bone marrow and circulate within the blood. Although there are fewer stem cells in peripheral blood than in bone marrow, their numbers can be artificially increased. During the mobilization

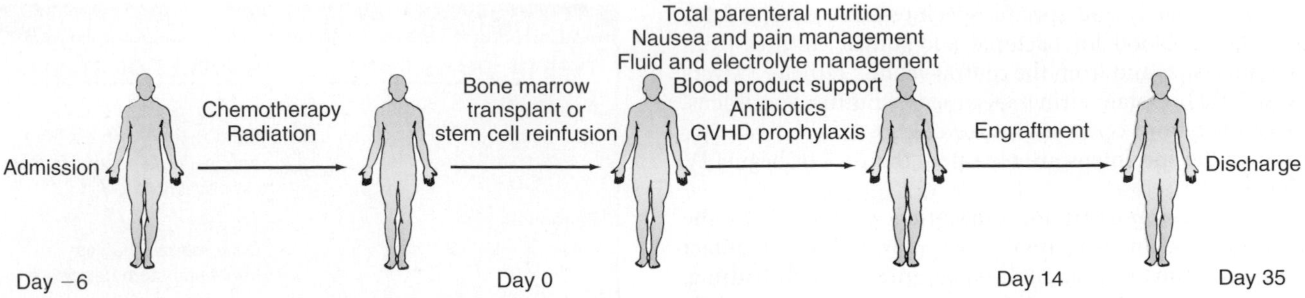

FIG. 40-5 Timing and steps of allogeneic bone marrow transplantation.

phase, chemotherapy or hematopoietic growth factors are given to the patient for an autologous collection, depending on the cancer type, and hematopoietic growth factors alone are given to the donor for an allogeneic or syngeneic collection. These agents increase the numbers of stem cells and WBCs in the peripheral blood. A new agent approved for some other types of hematologic malignancies to mobilize stem cells before harvesting in combination with hematopoietic growth factors is plerixafor (Mozobil). This drug has been shown to decrease the number of apheresis collections needed (Slater, 2012).

After mobilization, the stem cells are then collected by **apheresis** (withdrawing whole blood, filtering out the cells, and returning the plasma to the patient). One to five apheresis procedures, each lasting 2 to 4 hours, are needed to obtain enough stem cells for transplantation. The cells are frozen and stored for reinfusion after the patient's conditioning regimen is completed.

Monitor the patient or donor closely during apheresis. Complications include catheter clotting and hypocalcemia (caused by anticoagulants). Low calcium levels may cause numbness or tingling in the fingers and toes, abdominal or muscle cramping, or chest pain. Oral calcium supplements may be used to manage these symptoms. Monitor vital signs at least every hour during apheresis. The patient may become hypotensive from fluid loss during the procedure.

Cord blood harvesting involves obtaining stem cells from umbilical cord blood of newborns. This blood has a high concentration of stem cells. These cells are obtained through a simple blood draw from the placenta after birth and before the placenta detaches. The blood is then sent to the Cord Blood Registry for processing and storage. The stem cells may be used later for an unrelated recipient or stored in case the infant develops a serious illness later in life and needs them.

Conditioning Regimen. Fig. 40-5 outlines the timing and steps involved in transplantation. The day the patient receives the stem cells is day T-0. Before transplantation, the conditioning days are counted in reverse order from T-0, just like a rocket countdown. After transplantation, days are counted in order from the day of transplantation.

The patient first undergoes a conditioning regimen, which varies with the diagnosis and type of transplant to be received. The conditioning regimen serves two purposes: (1) to "wipe out" the patient's own bone marrow, thus preparing him or her for optimal graft take; and (2) to give higher-than-normal doses of chemotherapy and/or radiotherapy to rid the person of cancer cells *(myeloablation)*. Usually a period of 5 to 10 days is required. The regimen usually includes high-dose chemotherapy and, less commonly, total-body irradiation (TBI). Each conditioning regimen is individually tailored, with the patient's specific disease, overall health, and previous treatment considered.

Because of the problems and risk for death associated with this conditioning regimen, a non-myeloablative approach may be used instead. Non-myeloablative regimens use lower doses of chemotherapy and/or lower dose of TBI that allow for recovery of a recipient's own immune system. The use of non-myeloablative conditioning regimens decreases the chemotherapy side effects but relies on the development of graft-versus-host disease (GVHD) for the control of the cancer. There are many variations of non-myeloablative conditioning regimens. In contrast, myeloablative conditioning regimens use high doses of chemotherapy with or without radiation therapy to completely destroy a recipient's bone marrow, allowing for replacement by a new immune system.

During conditioning, bone marrow and normal tissues respond immediately to the chemotherapy and radiation. *The patient has all of the expected side effects associated with both therapies (see Chapter 22). When chemotherapy is given in high doses, these side effects are more intense than those seen with standard doses.*

Late effects from the conditioning regimen may occur as late as 3 to 10 years after transplantation. These problems include veno-occlusive disease (VOD), skin toxicities, cataracts, lung fibrosis, second cancers, cardiomyopathy, endocrine complications, and neurologic complications.

Transplantation. Day T-0 is the day of transplantation. The transplantation itself is very simple. Frozen marrow, PBSCs, or umbilical cord blood cells are thawed and then infused through the patient's central catheter like an ordinary blood transfusion.

! NURSING SAFETY PRIORITY QSEN

Action Alert

Do not use blood administration tubing to infuse stems cells because the cells could get caught in the filter, resulting in the patient receiving fewer stem cells.

Side effects of all types of stem cell transfusions are similar. The patient may have fever and hypertension in response to the preservative used in stem cell storage. To prevent these reactions, acetaminophen (Tylenol), hydrocortisone, and diphenhydramine (Benadryl) are given before the infusion. Antihypertensives or diuretics may be needed to treat fluid volume changes.

Engraftment. The transfused PBSCs and marrow cells circulate briefly in the peripheral blood. The stems cells find their way to the marrow-forming sites of the patient's bones and establish residency there.

Engraftment, the successful "take" of the transplanted cells in the patient's bone marrow, is key to the whole transplantation process. For the stem cells to "rescue" the patient after his or her own bone marrow have been wiped out, the stem cells must survive and grow in the patient's bone marrow sites. The average time to engraftment for PBSC cells is 14 days. For bone marrow, the average time is 21 days. To aid engraftment, growth factors, such as granulocyte colony-stimulating factor or granulocyte-macrophage colony-stimulating factor, may be given. When engraftment occurs, the patient's WBC, RBC, and platelet counts begin to rise. Engraftment syndrome (ES) with fever and weight gain may occur at this time (Thoele, 2014).

Monitoring of engraftment involves checking the patient's blood for *"chimerism,"* which is the presence of blood cells that show a different genetic profile or marker from those of the patient. Mixed chimerism is the presence of both the patient's cells and those from the donor. Progressive chimerism with increasing percentages of donor cells indicates engraftment. Regressive chimerism with increasing percentages of the patient's cells indicates graft failure. When engraftment is successful, only the donor's cells are present.

Prevention of Complications. The period after transplantation is difficult. INFECTION and poor CLOTTING with bleeding are severe problems because the patient remains without any IMMUNITY until the transfused cells grow and engraft. Care for this patient is the same as for the patient during induction therapy for AML. Helping the patient maintain hope through this long recovery period is difficult. Complications are often severe and life threatening. Help the patient have a positive attitude and be involved in his or her own recovery.

In addition to the problems related to the period of **pancytopenia** (too few circulating blood cells), other complications of HSCT include failure to engraft, development of graft-versus-host disease (GVHD), and veno-occlusive disease (VOD).

Failure to engraft occurs when the donated stem cells fail to grow in the bone marrow and function properly. This issue is discussed in advance with the patient and the donor. Failure to engraft occurs more often with transplants using allogeneic stem cells than with those using autologous stem cells. The causes include too few cells transplanted, attack or rejection of donor cells by the recipient's remaining immune system cells, infection of transplanted cells, and unknown biologic factors. *If the transplanted cells fail to engraft, the patient will die unless another transplant with stem cells is successful.*

Graft-versus-host disease (GVHD) occurs mostly in allogeneic transplants but also can occur in autologous transplants (Baker & McKiernan, 2011). The immunocompetent cells of the donated marrow recognize the patient's (recipient) cells, tissues, and organs as foreign and start an immunologic attack against them. The graft is actually trying to attack the host tissues and cells.

Although all host tissues can be attacked and harmed, the tissues usually damaged are the skin, eyes, intestinal tract, liver, female genitalia, lungs, immune system, and musculoskeletal system (Johnson, 2013). Fig. 40-6 shows the typical skin appearance of GVHD. About 25% to 50% of all allogeneic HSCT recipients have some degree of GVHD, and more than 15% of the patients who develop GVHD die of its complications. The presence of some GVHD indicates successful engraftment.

Management of GVHD involves limiting the activity of donor T-cells by using drugs to suppress IMMUNITY such as cyclosporine, tacrolimus, methotrexate, corticosteroids, mycophenolate mofetil (Cellcept, MMF), and antithymocyte globulin (ATG) (Baker & McKiernan, 2011). Care is taken to avoid suppressing the new immune system to the extent that either INFECTION risk increases or the new cells stop engrafting.

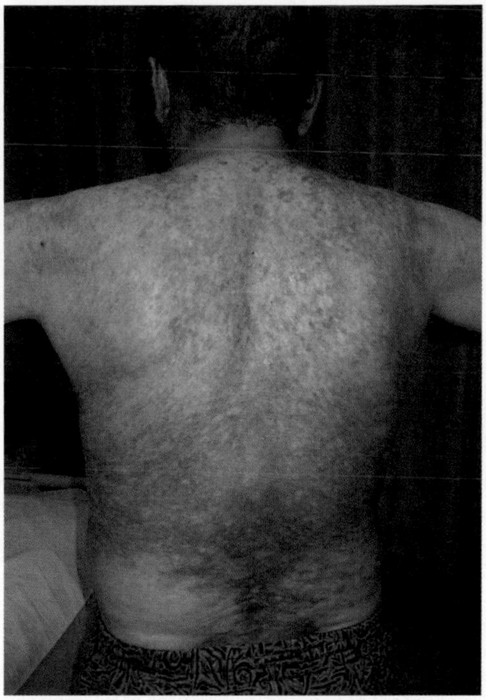

FIG. 40-6 Typical skin manifestations of graft-versus-host disease (GVHD).

Veno-occlusive disease (VOD) is the blockage of liver blood vessels by CLOTTING and inflammation (phlebitis) and occurs in about one fifth of patients with HSCT. Problems usually begin within the first 30 days after transplantation. Patients who received high-dose chemotherapy, especially with alkylating agents, are at risk for life-threatening liver complications. Manifestations include jaundice, pain in the right upper quadrant, ascites, weight gain, and liver enlargement.

Because there is no way of opening the liver vessels, treatment is supportive. Early detection improves the chance for survival. Fluid management is also crucial. Assess the patient

CLINICAL JUDGMENT CHALLENGE

Safety; Teamwork and Collaboration QSEN

The patient is a 44-year-old chemical plant foreman who developed acute myelogenous leukemia 6 months ago. His initial therapy was successful, and he is scheduled to have a stem cell transplant with his identical twin brother as the donor. His brother lives in the same city and is a professor at a local university. The patient is very grateful that his brother will donate bone marrow and states that he is certain that he has no risk for infection during the procedure because his brother is his identical twin.

1. What type of class of stem cell transplant would this procedure be considered?
2. Is the patient correct in assuming that he has no risk for infection because the donor is his twin brother? Provide a rationale for your response.
3. Which, if any, complications of stem cell transplantation are reduced or eliminated by having an identical sibling donate the stem cells?
4. Which, if any, complications (and why) are still possible even with a donor who is an identical sibling?

CHART 40-7 Best Practice for Patient Safety & Quality Care QSEN

The Patient with Thrombocytopenia

- Handle the patient gently.
- Use a lift sheet when moving and positioning in bed.
- Avoid IM injections and venipunctures.
- When injections or venipunctures are necessary, use the smallest-gauge needle for the task.
- Apply firm pressure to the needle stick site for 10 minutes or until the site no longer oozes blood.
- Apply ice to areas of trauma.
- Test all urine and stool for the presence of occult blood.
- Observe IV sites every 2 hours for bleeding.
- Avoid trauma to rectal tissues:
  - Do not give enemas.
  - Administer well-lubricated suppositories with caution.
  - Advise patient not to have anal intercourse.
- Measure abdominal girth daily.
- Advise the patient to use an electric shaver.
- Teach the patient to avoid mouth trauma:
  - Use soft-bristled toothbrush or tooth sponges.
  - Do not floss between teeth.
  - Avoid dental work, especially extractions.
  - Avoid hard foods.
  - Make sure that dentures fit and do not rub.
- Encourage the patient not to blow the nose or insert objects into the nose.
- Advise the patient to avoid contact sports.
- Teach the patient to wear shoes with firm soles when ambulating.

daily for weight gain, fluid retention, increases in abdominal girth, and hepatomegaly.

Minimizing Injury. Bone marrow production of platelets is severely limited with acute myelogenous leukemia (AML), leading to thrombocytopenia. The patient is at great risk for poor CLOTTING with excessive bleeding in response to minimal trauma. Thrombocytopenia can also be caused by induction therapy for AML or high-dose chemotherapy for transplantation.

Planning: Expected Outcomes. The patient with leukemia is expected to remain free from bleeding. Indicators include:

- Maintenance of hematocrit and hemoglobin within normal limits
- Absence of visible bleeding, petechiae, or ecchymosis
- Absence of evidence of occult bleeding (e.g., abdominal swelling, tarry stools)

Interventions. The platelet count is decreased as a side effect of chemotherapy. During the period of greatest bone marrow suppression (the **nadir**), the platelet count may be less than 10,000/mm^3. The patient is at extreme risk for bleeding once the platelet count falls below 50,000/mm^3, and spontaneous bleeding may occur when the count is lower than 20,000/mm^3.

Bleeding Precautions are used to protect the patient at increased risk for injury from bleeding (Chart 40-7). Assess at least every 4 hours for evidence of bleeding: oozing, enlarging bruises, petechiae, or purpura. Inspect all stools, urine, drainage, and vomit for blood, and test for occult blood. Measure any blood loss as accurately as possible, and measure the abdominal girth daily. Increases in abdominal girth can indicate internal hemorrhage. Institute the Bleeding Precautions listed in Chart 40-7. Platelet levels return to normal more slowly than do either WBCs or RBCs, and the patient remains at bleeding risk for weeks after discharge.

Monitor laboratory values daily, especially CBC results, to assess bleeding risk, as well as actual blood loss. The patient with a platelet count below 10,000/mm^3 may need a platelet transfusion. For the patient with severe blood loss, packed RBCs may be prescribed (see discussion on p. 822 in the Red Blood Cell Transfusions section).

Conserving Energy. Production of red blood cells is limited in leukemia, causing anemia and fatigue. Also, leukemic cells have high rates of metabolism, increasing fatigue in the anemic patient. Anemia may also occur as a side effect of chemotherapy.

Planning: Expected Outcomes. The patient with leukemia is expected to have no increase in fatigue. Indicators include that the patient consistently demonstrates these behaviors:

- Participates in self-care
- Recognizes manifestations of fatigue
- Changes activity level to match energy level

Interventions. Interventions to reduce fatigue focus on conserving energy and improving RBC counts.

Nutrition therapy is needed to assist the patient to eat enough calories to meet at least basal energy requirements. However, increasing food intake can be difficult with fatigue. Collaborate with a dietitian to provide small, frequent meals high in protein and carbohydrates.

Blood transfusions are sometimes indicated for the patient with fatigue. Transfusions with packed RBCs increase the blood's oxygen-carrying capacity and replace missing RBCs. (See Chart 40-12 on p. 820 for nursing care during transfusions.)

Drug therapy with colony-stimulating growth factors may reduce the severity and duration of anemia and neutropenia after intensive chemotherapy. For anemia, erythropoiesis-stimulating agents (ESAs) that boost production of RBCs may be used. These agents now carry a warning for causing hypertension and increasing the risk for myocardial infarction. ESAs must be given with care and should be avoided in patients with myeloid malignancies. They are not used unless the hemoglobin level is lower than 10 mg/dL and are stopped when this level is reached. Assess for side effects such as hypertension, headaches, fever, **myalgia** (muscle aches), and rashes. (See Chapter 22 for information on hematopoietic growth factors.)

Activity management helps conserve the patient's energy (Chart 40-8). Examine the patient's schedule of prescribed and routine activities. Assess those activities that do not have a direct positive effect on the patient's condition in terms of their usefulness. If the benefit of an activity is less than its worsening of fatigue, coordinate with other members of the health care team about eliminating or postponing it. Activities that may be postponed include physical therapy and invasive diagnostic tests not needed for assessment or treatment of current problems.

? NCLEX EXAMINATION CHALLENGE

Safe and Effective Care Environment

The client is 3 weeks post-transplant from an allogeneic stem cell transplantation for acute lymphocytic leukemia. There is now some peeling of the client's skin on the palms of the hands and the soles of the feet. Which additional assessment data support the nurse's suspicion of possible graft-versus-host disease (GVHD)?

A. The client's temperature is slightly below normal.
B. Today's platelet count is 5,000/mm^3 and the WBCs are low.
C. The client has had 6 to 10 watery stools daily for 3 days.
D. The client's urine output is less than 800 mL in 24 hours.

CHART 40-8 Best Practice for Patient Safety & Quality Care (QSEN)

Conserving Energy

- Reassure the patient that fatigue is temporary and energy levels will improve over a period of weeks to months. Stress that a return to previous energy levels may take as long as a year.
- Teach the patient that shortness of breath and palpitations are symptoms of over-activity.
- Instruct the patient to stop activity when shortness of breath or palpitations are present.
- Space care activities at least an hour apart, and avoid the time right before or right after meals.
- Schedule care activities at times when the patient has more energy (e.g., immediately after naps).
- Perform complete bed bath only every other day. In between complete baths, ensure cleansing of face, hands, axillae, and perineum.
- In collaboration with other members of the health care team, cancel or reschedule non-essential tests and activities.
- Provide four to six small, easy-to-eat meals instead of three larger ones.
- Urge the patient to drink small amounts of protein shakes or other nutritional supplements.
- During periods of extreme fatigue, encourage the patient to allow others to perform personal care.
- Help the patient identify one or two lead visitors (those designated as allowed to visit at any time and who do not disturb the patient).
- Selectively limit non–lead visitors when the patient is resting or sleeping.
- Remind families that, although independence is important, independence in ADLs during extreme fatigue can be detrimental to the patient's health.
- Monitor oxygen saturation and respiratory rate during any activity to determine patient responses and activity tolerance.

Community-Based Care

The patient with leukemia is discharged after induction chemotherapy and recovery of blood cell production. Follow-up care continues on an ambulatory care basis. Although many transplant centers discharge patients after engraftment, some centers also give high-dose chemotherapy and stem cell infusion on an ambulatory care basis. This plan involves daily clinic visits and frequent follow-up by nurses in the home care setting.

Home Care Management. Planning for home care for the patient with leukemia begins as soon as remission is achieved. Assess the available support systems. Many patients need a visiting nurse to assist with dressing changes for central venous catheters, infusions, and to answer questions. Home transfusion therapy for blood components may be needed.

Coordination of the home care team is critical for the patient receiving stem cell transplantation in the home setting. Potential candidates are evaluated in advance. Criteria include a knowledgeable caregiver, a clean home environment, location near the hospital, telephone access, and emotional stability of the patient and caregiver.

Home care nurses give chemotherapy and monitor for complications. Nurses visit the patient once or twice per day and spend between 4 and 8 hours per day in the home. The patient receives the stem cell transplant infusion in the ambulatory care clinic. Nursing care is similar to that provided in the hospital. If complications such as sepsis or veno-occlusive disease (VOD) occur, the patient is admitted to the inpatient facility.

Self-Management Education. Instruct the patient and family about the importance of continuing therapy and medical follow-up. Many patients go home with a central venous catheter in place and need instructions about its care. Chart 40-9 lists guidelines for central venous catheter care at home. These guidelines may be altered depending on the home setting, assistance available, and agency policy.

CHART 40-9 Patient and Family Education: Preparing for Self-Management

Home Care of the Central Venous Catheter

- To maintain patency, flush the catheter briskly with saline once a day and after completing infusions.
- Change the Luer-Lok cap on each catheter lumen weekly.
- Change the dressing as often as prescribed:
  - Use clean technique with thorough handwashing.
  - Clean the exit site with alcohol and povidone-iodine (Betadine) or with chlorhexidine.
  - Apply antibacterial ointment to the site, if prescribed.
  - Cover the site with dry sterile gauze dressing, taped securely, or with transparent adherent dressing.
- To prevent tension, always tape the catheter to yourself.
- Look for and report any signs of infection (redness, swelling, or drainage at the exit site).
- In case of a break or puncture in the catheter lumen, immediately clamp the catheter between yourself and the opening. *Notify your physician immediately.*

Protecting the patient from infection at home is just as important as it was during hospitalization. (See Chart 40-6 for focused assessment for the patient at risk for INFECTION.) Teach about proper hygiene and the need to avoid crowds or others with infections. Neither the patient nor any household member should receive live virus immunization (poliomyelitis, measles, or rubella) for 2 years after transplantation. Instruct the patient to continue mouth care regimens at home. Stress to the patient that he or she should immediately notify the physician if a fever or any other indications of infection develop. Chart 40-10 lists guidelines for infection prevention.

Many patients return home still at risk for bleeding because platelet recovery is slower than recovery of other cells. Reinforce safety and bleeding precautions, and emphasize that these precautions must be followed until the platelet count remains above 50,000/mm^3. Teach the patient and family to assess for petechiae, avoid trauma and sharp objects, apply pressure to wounds for 10 minutes, and report blood in the stool or urine or headache that does not respond to acetaminophen. Chart 40-11 lists guidelines for patients at risk for bleeding.

Psychosocial Preparation. A diagnosis of leukemia threatens self-esteem and the family role. The patient faces the possibility of death, and treatment causes major changes in self-image. Changes occur in body image, level of independence, and lifestyle. Some feel threatened by the environment, seeing everything as infectious. Patients who are cared for in protective isolation may feel lonely and isolated. Help the patient and family define priorities, understand the illness and its treatment, and find hope. Make referrals to support groups sponsored by organizations such as the American Cancer Society or the Leukemia and Lymphoma Society of America.

One problem that lasts for a long period after transplantation is severe fatigue. Although the acute period after transplantation requires energy conservation with reduced activity, in the later recovery period, exercise provides benefits and fatigue reduction (see the Evidence-Based Practice box) (Albrecht,

CHART 40-10 Patient and Family Education: Preparing for Self-Management

Prevention of Infection

- Avoid crowds and other gatherings of people who might be ill.
- Do not share personal toilet articles, such as toothbrushes, toothpaste, washcloths, or deodorant sticks, with others.
- If possible, bathe daily.
- Wash the armpits, groin, genitals, and anal area at least twice a day with an antimicrobial soap.
- Clean your toothbrush daily by either running it through the dishwasher or rinsing it in liquid laundry bleach and then rinsing it with running water.
- Wash your hands thoroughly with an antimicrobial soap before you eat or drink, after touching a pet, after shaking hands with anyone, as soon as you come home from any outing, and after using the toilet.
- Eat a low-bacteria diet, and avoid salads, raw fruits and vegetables, and undercooked meat.
- Wash dishes between uses with hot, sudsy water, or use a dishwasher.
- Do not drink water that has been standing for longer than 15 minutes.
- Do not reuse cups and glasses without washing.
- Avoid changing pet litter boxes. If unavoidable, use gloves or wash hands immediately.
- Avoid keeping turtles and reptiles as pets.
- Do not feed pets raw or undercooked meat.
- Take your temperature at least twice a day.
- Report any of these manifestations of infection to your physician immediately:
  - Temperature greater than 100° F (38° C)
  - Persistent cough (with or without sputum)
  - Pus or foul-smelling drainage from any open skin area or normal body opening
  - Presence of a boil or abscess
  - Urine that is cloudy or foul smelling, or burning on urination
- Take all drugs as prescribed.
- Do not dig in the garden or work with houseplants.
- Avoid travel to areas of the world with poor sanitation or inadequate health care facilities.

CHART 40-11 Patient and Family Education: Preparing for Self-Management

The Patient at Risk for Bleeding

- Use an electric shaver.
- Use a soft-bristled toothbrush, and do not floss.
- Do not have dental work done without consulting your doctor.
- Do not take aspirin or any aspirin-containing products. Read the label to be sure the products do not contain aspirin or salicylates.
- Wear shoes or slippers with a sole to avoid foot injury.
- Do not participate in contact sports or any activity likely to result in your being bumped, scratched, or scraped.
- If you are bumped, apply ice to the site for at least 1 hour.
- Notify your physician if you:
  - Experience an injury and persistent bleeding results
  - Have excessive menstrual bleeding
  - See blood in your urine or bowel movement
  - Have a headache that does not respond to acetaminophen
- Avoid anal intercourse.
- Take a stool softener to prevent straining during a bowel movement.
- Do not use enemas or rectal suppositories.
- Avoid bending over at the waist.
- Do not wear clothing or shoes that are tight or that rub.
- Avoid blowing your nose or placing objects in your nose. If you must blow your nose, do so gently without blocking either nasal passage.

EVIDENCE-BASED PRACTICE QSEN

Exercise for Less Fatigue

Chiffelle, R., & Kenny, K. (2013). Exercise for fatigue management in hematopoietic stem cell transplantation recipients. *Clinical Journal of Oncology Nursing, 17*(3), 241-242.

Fatigue associated with cancer therapy has been recognized as one of the most distressing and debilitating side effects. The fatigue experienced by patients after hematopoietic stem cell transplantation (HSCT) has been found to be more severe and persist much longer than that associated with more standard therapy. Exercise, even during the treatment period, has been shown to reduce the perception of fatigue and its negative effects on performance of desired activities in patients undergoing standard chemotherapy or radiation. It is not known whether exercise would be beneficial in reducing the long-term fatigue frequently experienced after HSCT or even could have harmful effects.

Level of Evidence: 1

The results are based on a systematic review and meta-analysis of 25 previous studies related to assessing the evidence for recommending an exercise intervention for relief of cancer-related fatigue (CRF) in patients receiving traditional cancer treatments and those whose treatment additionally involved HSCT. The studies analyzed included 6 other systematic reviews, 16 randomized controlled clinical trials, 6 nonrandomized controlled trials, and 1 qualitative study. Results of this analysis do indicate that exercise for patients after HSCT is at least not harmful and has some benefit in reducing the distress of fatigue. Although not all patients universally had fatigue reduction, none experienced an increase in fatigue with exercise.

Commentary: Implications for Practice and Research

For best practice, interventions must be both effective and not harmful. Therefore this meta-analysis contributes substantial evidence that some exercise in patients after HSCT is not harmful and does provide some reduction of the distress associated with CRF. Because many patients and their families believe that the patient is much more fragile after HSCT, some are hesitant to increase activity in any way. Nurses can be instrumental in helping patients and families get past the mental barrier of fear regarding activity and can recommend low-impact exercise. However, the type of exercise (e.g., walking, cycling, low-impact aerobics) and the best timing for implementing an exercise intervention to have maximum benefit have yet to be determined.

2014; Chiffelle & Kenny, 2013). Help the patient and family understand the benefits of low-impact exercise.

Health Care Resources. The patient with limited social support may need help at home until strength and energy return. A home care aide may suffice for some patients, whereas for others a visiting nurse may be needed. The patient may also need equipment for ADLs and ambulation. Assess financial resources. Cancer treatment is expensive, and you will need to coordinate with the social services department to ensure that insurance is adequate. If the patient is uninsured, explore other sources, such as drug company–sponsored compassionate aid programs. The Leukemia and Lymphoma Society of America also offers limited financial help.

Prolonged outpatient contact and follow-up are necessary, and patients need transportation to the outpatient facility. Many local units of the American Cancer Society offer free transportation to patients with cancer, including leukemia.

◆ *Evaluation: Outcomes*

Evaluate the care of the patient with leukemia based on the identified priority patient problems. The expected outcomes include that the patient will:

- Remain free of infection and sepsis
- Not experience episodes of bleeding
- Be able to balance activity and rest
- Use energy conservation techniques

Specific indicators for these outcomes are listed for each priority patient problem in the Planning and Implementation section (see earlier).

MALIGNANT LYMPHOMAS

Lymphomas are cancers of the lymphoid tissues with abnormal overgrowth of lymphocytes. Lymphomas are cancers of committed lymphocytes rather than stem cell precursors (as in leukemia). This growth occurs as solid tumors in lymphoid tissues scattered throughout the body, especially the lymph nodes and spleen, rather than in the bone marrow. The two major adult forms of lymphoma are Hodgkin's lymphoma (HL) and non-Hodgkin's lymphoma (NHL).

HODGKIN'S LYMPHOMA

❖ *PATHOPHYSIOLOGY*

Hodgkin's lymphoma (HL) is a cancer that can affect any age-group. However, it appears to peak in two different age-groups: (1) teens and young adults, and (2) adults in their 50s and 60s (McCance et al., 2014). HL affects younger men and women equally, but the disease is more prevalent in men in the older group.

The exact cause of HL is uncertain. Possible causes of HL include viral infections (i.e. Epstein-Barr virus [EBV], human T-cell leukemia/lymphoma virus [HTLV], and human immune deficiency virus [HIV]) and exposure to chemicals. Most cases of the disease, however, occur in people without known risk factors.

This cancer usually starts in a single lymph node or a single chain of nodes. These nodes contain a specific cancer cell type, the **Reed-Sternberg cell**, a marker for HL. HL often spreads predictably from one group of lymph nodes to the next, unlike non-Hodgkin's lymphoma.

❖ *PATIENT-CENTERED COLLABORATIVE CARE*

◆ *Assessment*

The most common assessment finding is a large but painless lymph node or nodes. The patient may also have constitutional manifestations ("B symptoms") that include: fevers (>101.5° F [>38.6° C]); heavy night sweats; and unplanned weight loss (>10% of normal body weight). The presence of these manifestations often means a poorer prognosis. Many patients have no manifestations at time of diagnosis, and specific manifestations often depend on the site and extent of disease.

Diagnosis and subtype are established when biopsy reveals Reed-Sternberg cells (McCance et al., 2014). HL is then classified into one of several different subtypes.

After diagnosis, staging is performed to determine the extent of disease. This process is detailed and must be accurate because the treatment regimen is determined by the extent of disease. Staging usually includes a history and physical examination, CBC, electrolyte panel, kidney and liver function tests, erythrocyte sedimentation rate (ESR), bone marrow aspiration and biopsy, and computed tomography (CT) of the neck, chest, abdomen, and pelvis. Positron emission tomography (PET) may be used to assess for disease not detected by CT. PET scans are helpful after treatment to assess disease response to therapy. After staging procedures are complete, the stage of the disease is determined by the Ann Arbor Staging Criteria (Table 40-4).

TABLE 40-4 Ann Arbor Staging Criteria for Hodgkin's Lymphoma

STAGE	MANIFESTATION CRITERIA
Ia	Disease is present only in a single lymph node region or in only one non–lymph node site.
Ib	Disease location is the same as Ia. In addition, the patient has some or all of these manifestations: persistent fever, night sweats, weight loss of more than 10% of normal body weight.
IIa	Disease is present in two or more separate lymph node regions on the same side of the diaphragm or in two non–lymph node sites on the same side of the diaphragm.
IIb	Disease location is the same as IIa. In addition, the patient has some or all of these manifestations: persistent fever, night sweats, weight loss of more than 10% of normal body weight.
IIIa	Disease extends to lymph node regions on both sides of the diaphragm.
IIIb	Disease location is the same as IIIa. In addition, the patient has some or all of these manifestations: persistent fever, night sweats, weight loss of more than 10% of normal body weight.
IIIc	Same as IIIb along with disease present in the spleen.
IV	Disease is present in many body areas, including in one or more non-nodal tissues and organs.

◆ *Interventions*

HL is one of the most treatable types of cancer. For stages I and II disease, the treatment is external radiation of involved lymph node regions. With more extensive disease, radiation and combination chemotherapy are used to achieve remission. (See Chapter 22 on general care of patients receiving radiation and chemotherapy.)

Nursing management of the patient undergoing treatment for HL focuses on the acute side effects of therapy, especially:

- Drug-induced pancytopenia with increased risk for INFECTION, anemia, and bleeding
- Severe nausea and vomiting
- Skin problems at the site of radiation
- Constipation or diarrhea
- Permanent sterility for male patients receiving radiation to the lower abdomen or pelvic region in combination with specific chemotherapy drugs (The patient is informed and given the option to store sperm in a sperm bank *before* treatment.)
- Secondary cancer development and the need for long-term follow-up

NON-HODGKIN'S LYMPHOMA

❖ PATHOPHYSIOLOGY

Non-Hodgkin's lymphoma (NHL) includes all lymphoid cancers that do not have the Reed-Sternberg cell. There are over 60 subtypes of NHL divided into either indolent or aggressive lymphomas. NHL generally spreads through the lymphatic system in a less orderly fashion than HL. About 70,000 new cases are diagnosed each year in North America (ACS, 2014). The disease is more common in men and older adults.

The exact cause of NHL is unknown although the incidence is higher among patients with solid organ transplantation, immunosuppressive drug therapy, and HIV disease. Chronic infection from *Helicobacter pylori* is associated with a type of lymphoma called *mucosa-associated lymphoid tissue (MALT) lymphoma,* and Epstein-Barr viral infection has been associated with Burkitt's lymphoma. There is an increased incidence of NHL among people exposed to pesticides, insecticides, and dust.

Patients usually have swollen lymph nodes (lymphadenopathy) or tumor spread to other organs (e.g., GI tract, skin, bone marrow, sinuses, thyroid, central nervous system) at the time of diagnosis. Enlarged lymph nodes may be the only manifestation of lymphoma. Painless swelling of the cervical, axillary, inguinal, and femoral nodes is most often seen. The diagnosis of NHL is made only after the biopsy of an involved lymph node is reviewed by a hematopathologist.

Lymphoma is not a single disease but, rather, a group of diseases. The specific subtype of lymphoma must be classified because management varies with the subtype. Classification is based on cytology, immunophenotyping by flow cytometry, and genetic (chromosomal changes and molecular rearrangements) and clinical features. NHLs are broadly classified as B-cell or T-cell lymphomas, depending on the lymphocyte type that gave rise to the cancer. B-cell lymphomas are most common.

Classification of NHL is more complicated than that for Hodgkin's lymphoma and is based on the World Health Organization (WHO) classification system. In addition, lactate dehydrogenase (LDH) levels and beta-2 microglobulin levels are also evaluated to measure tumor growth rates and calculate prognosis. (High LDH levels and high beta-2 microglobulin levels are associated with a poorer prognosis.) Cerebrospinal fluid is evaluated when lymphoma is present in the CNS, around the spinal column, brain, or testes, and when HIV-related lymphoma is diagnosed.

Patients with **indolent** (slow-growing) lymphomas usually have painless lymph node swelling at diagnosis. Those with more aggressive B-cell lymphomas may have large masses at diagnosis and manifestations. Constitutional manifestations ("B symptoms"), as seen in Hodgkin's lymphoma, occur in about one third of patients with aggressive lymphomas and rarely in indolent lymphomas. Bone marrow involvement in indolent lymphomas is common.

❖ PATIENT-CENTERED COLLABORATIVE CARE

Treatment options for patients with NHL vary based on the subtype of the tumor, international prognostic index (IPI) score, stage of the disease, performance status, and overall tumor burden. Special consideration for patients with additional health problems is important, especially among older adult patients. Many new therapies have evolved over the past decade for various subtypes of NHL. These therapies include combinations of chemotherapy drugs alone or in combination with monoclonal antibodies (e.g., rituximab and alemtuzumab), localized radiation therapy, radiolabeled antibodies (^{131}I tositumomab and ^{90}Y ibritumomab tiuxetan), hematopoietic stem cell transplantation, and investigational agents (Byar & Workman, 2012).

Nursing care needs are similar to those for patients with HL, with additional organ-specific problems if the disease is widespread. With the use of biotherapy for NHL, close monitoring for infusion-related reactions is needed during and after the delivery of monoclonal antibodies (see Chapter 22 for general care of patients undergoing treatment with biotherapy). Patient and family education are important in the management and prevention of complications.

CLINICAL JUDGMENT CHALLENGE

Prioritization, Delegation, and Supervision QSEN

The patient is a 52-year-old woman who has undergone an autologous stem cell transplantation for non-Hodgkin's lymphoma. She is recovering, and her white blood cell count is improving but is still very low. She remains on neutropenic precautions. The LPN reports that the patient's heart rate, respiratory rate, temperature, and blood pressure are elevated.

1. Which vital sign finding would you report to the health care provider immediately and why?
2. You must assign an unlicensed assistive personnel (UAP) to help care for this patient. Of the four UAP available, one is newly pregnant and has worked on this unit for 3 years, one has had cold symptoms for 3 days, one has not yet cared for a patient on neutropenic precautions, and one has a fear of people with cancer. Which UAP should you avoid assigning to this patient? Provide a rationale for your choice.
3. A nursing student tearfully reports to you, "I took some flowers into the patient's room to cheer him up and he told me that he didn't think he was supposed to have flowers. I took them out of the room right away and then I realized I had made a mistake." How should you respond to this student?
4. The student asks you whether a book still wrapped in shrink wrap just now brought in by a friend of the patient can be taken to the patient's room. How will you help the student know what to do in this situation?

MULTIPLE MYELOMA

❖ PATHOPHYSIOLOGY

Multiple myeloma is a white blood cell (WBC) cancer that involves a mature B-lymphocyte called a *plasma cell,* which secretes antibodies. These cells are overgrown in the bone marrow. When these cells become cancerous, they produce excessive antibodies (gamma globulins). Thus the disorder is called a "gammopathy." When myeloma cells are overproduced, fewer red blood cells (RBCs), WBCs, and platelets are produced, leading to anemia and increased risk for INFECTION and bleeding.

In addition to the excess antibodies, multiple myeloma cells also produce excess cytokines (see Chapter 17) that increase cancer cell growth and destroy bone. The excess antibodies are in the blood, increasing the serum protein levels and clogging blood vessels in the kidney and other organs. Without treatment, the disease causes progressive bone destruction, bleeding problems, kidney failure, immunosuppression, and death.

Multiple myeloma accounts for about 11,000 deaths per year in the United States (ACS, 2014). The disease is most common in people older than 65 years. The incidence is higher in American blacks than in whites, with a much higher incidence in men.

The cause of multiple myeloma is unknown. Possible risk factors include radiation exposure, chemical exposure, and INFECTION with human herpes virus-8 (HHV-8). This cancer can be distinguished by changes in immunoglobulin structure that begin within a single clone of cells even before transformation to cancer occurs. When the specifically altered immunoglobulin is present in a high enough quantity, the type can be recognized as a unique "spike" pattern on a serum electrophoresis test of plasma proteins. Because one clone of cells develops into cancer cells, the abnormal immunoglobulin produced by these cells is a *monoclonal* paraprotein.

❖ PATIENT-CENTERED COLLABORATIVE CARE

◆ Assessment

Some patients have no symptoms at time of the diagnosis. An elevation of serum total protein or a detection of a monoclonal protein (also known as *paraprotein*) in the blood or urine may be the only finding. Other common manifestations include fatigue, anemia, bone pain, pathologic fractures, recurrent bacterial INFECTIONS, and kidney dysfunction.

A positive finding of a serum monoclonal protein is not sufficient to make a diagnosis of multiple myeloma. About 1% of the population produce a monoclonal protein in the blood but do not have multiple myeloma. This condition is labeled ***m**onoclonal **g**ammopathy of **u**ndetermined **s**ignificance* or *MGUS*, which is a premalignant condition. Follow-up of patients with MGUS is important because a small percentage eventually will develop multiple myeloma. Multiple myeloma is distinguished from MGUS by having more than 10% of the bone marrow infiltrated with plasma cells, the presence of a monoclonal protein in the serum or urine, and the presence of osteolytic bone lesions.

The staging system for multiple myeloma divides patients into stages and prognostic groups on the basis of the serum beta-2 microglobulin and albumin levels. Other factors that help determine prognosis include age, performance status, serum creatinine, serum albumin, serum calcium, lactate dehydrogenase (LDH) level, C-reactive protein, hemoglobin level, platelet count, quantitative immunoglobulins, beta-2 microglobulin, serum free light chains, serum protein electrophoresis (SPEP) with immunofixation, 24-hour urine for SPEP, and cytogenetic abnormalities found in the bone marrow biopsy (Kurtin & Faiman, 2013).

The patient usually first notices fatigue, easy bruising, and bone pain. Bone fractures, hypertension, INFECTION, hypercalcemia, and fluid imbalance may occur as the disease progresses. Diagnosis is made by x-ray findings of bone thinning with areas of bone loss that resemble Swiss cheese, high immunoglobulin and plasma protein levels, and the presence of Bence-Jones protein (protein composed of incomplete antibodies) in the urine. A bone marrow biopsy is performed to diagnose the disease and to determine chromosome changes. An abnormality of chromosome 11 predicts a longer survival, and absence of chromosome 13 is a poor prognostic factor.

◆ Interventions

Treatment options vary. For minimal disease, watchful waiting may be an option instead of chemotherapy. Standard treatment for multiple myeloma is the use of proteasome inhibitors, such as bortezomib (Velcade) or carfilzomib (Kyprolis), and immunomodulating drugs, such as thalidomide (Thalomid) or lenalidomide (Revlimid). All these agents, which are types of targeted cancer therapy (see Chapter 22), may be used alone or in combination with steroids, such as dexamethasone (Decadron). Drug selection is based on whether the patient is eligible for an autologous stem cell transplant. If eligible, drug therapy is used to reduce tumor burden before transplantation. For patients who are not eligible for an autologous stem cell transplantation, standard chemotherapy drugs such as melphalan, prednisone, vincristine, cyclophosphamide, doxorubicin, and carmustine are usually effective in controlling but not curing the disease.

Side effects and severe toxicities can occur with these agents. Myelosuppression is an expected side effect of many myeloma therapies. A nursing priority is to teach the patient about the manifestations. The risk for thromboembolic events is increased with the use of thalidomide and lenalidomide. Peripheral neuropathy can be challenging, causing pain and poor quality of life. GI side effects, such as nausea, vomiting, diarrhea, and constipation, are severe and can be life threatening if not managed properly.

Despite therapy, multiple myeloma remains largely incurable (Kurtin & Faiman, 2013). Best outcomes are seen with autologous hematopoietic stem cell transplantation, although few patients are able to pursue this option (Mangan et al., 2013). Because most patients with multiple myeloma have bone pain, analgesics and alternative approaches for pain management, such as relaxation techniques, aromatherapy, or hypnosis, are used for pain relief. The bone disease of multiple myeloma is treated with bisphosphonates (pamidronate [Aredia], zoledronic acid [Zometa], denosumab [Xgeva]), which inhibit bone resorption and can help reduce the skeletal complications.

COAGULATION DISORDERS

Coagulation disorders are bleeding disorders with increased bleeding resulting from defects in one or more components regulating blood CLOTTING. Bleeding disorders may be spontaneous or traumatic, localized or generalized, lifelong or acquired. They can arise from a defect in the clotting processes at the vascular, platelet, or clotting factor level.

PLATELET DISORDERS

As discussed in Chapter 39, CLOTTING always starts with platelets sticking together (aggregation) and forming a platelet plug. Any condition that either reduces the number of platelets or interferes with their ability to adhere (stick to one another, blood vessel walls, collagen, or fibrin threads) can result in increased bleeding. Platelet disorders are inherited, acquired, or temporarily induced by drugs that limit platelet production or inhibit aggregation.

Platelet numbers below that needed for blood CLOTTING is called **thrombocytopenia**. It may occur as a result of other conditions or treatments that suppress general bone marrow activity. The problem also can occur from limited platelet formation or an increased rate of platelet destruction in the spleen. The two thrombocytopenic conditions affecting adults are *autoimmune thrombocytopenic purpura* and *thrombotic thrombocytopenic purpura*.

AUTOIMMUNE THROMBOCYTOPENIC PURPURA

❖ PATHOPHYSIOLOGY

Autoimmune thrombocytopenic purpura is also called *idiopathic thrombocytopenic purpura (ITP)*. The number of circulating platelets is greatly reduced in ITP, even though platelet production is normal.

Patients with this disorder make an antibody against the surface of their own platelets (an antiplatelet antibody). This antibody coats the platelet surfaces, making destruction by macrophages easier (see Chapter 17). The spleen has many macrophages, and the blood vessels of the spleen are long and twisted. These conditions increase destruction of antibody-coated platelets in the spleen. When platelet destruction exceeds platelet production, the number of circulating platelets decreases and CLOTTING is impaired.

The trigger for the production of autoantibodies is unknown, but viral INFECTION is suspected. ITP is most common among women between the ages of 20 and 50 years and among people who have other autoimmune disorders (McCance et al., 2014; Radovich, 2011).

❖ PATIENT-CENTERED COLLABORATIVE CARE

◆ Assessment

Manifestations of ITP are at first seen in the skin and mucous membranes: large **ecchymoses** (bruises) or a petechial rash on the arms, legs, upper chest, and neck; mucosal bleeding occurs easily. If the patient has had significant blood loss, anemia may also be present.

A rare complication is intracranial bleeding–induced stroke. Assess for neurologic function and mental status (see Chapter 41).

ITP is diagnosed by a low platelet count and increased megakaryocytes in the bone marrow. Antiplatelet antibodies may be detected in the blood. If the patient has any episodes of bleeding, hematocrit and hemoglobin levels may be low.

◆ Interventions

As a result of the decreased platelet count, the patient is at great risk for poor CLOTTING and increased bleeding. Interventions include therapy for the underlying condition and protection from bleeding episodes. Management is often limited to those patients with platelet counts lower than 50,000/mm^3, those who are bleeding, and those who are at high risk for bleeding.

Drug therapy to control ITP includes drugs that suppress immune function. Drugs such as corticosteroids, azathioprine (Imuran), eltrombopag, rituximab (Rituxan), and romiplostim are used to inhibit production of antiplatelet autoantibodies. IV immunoglobulin and IV anti-Rho can help prevent the destruction of antibody-coated platelets, although anti-Rho carries a Black Box Warning for increased risk for intravascular hemolysis and death. Aggressive therapy involves low doses of chemotherapy drugs.

Platelet transfusions are used when platelet counts are less than 10,000/mm^3 or the patient has an acute life-threatening bleeding episode. Transfusions are not performed routinely because the donated platelets are just as rapidly destroyed by the spleen as the patient's own platelets. (See discussion on p. 822 in the Platelet Transfusions section.)

Maintaining a safe environment helps protect the patient from bleeding. Closely monitor the amount of bleeding that is occurring. (For nursing care actions, see the discussion of Minimizing Injury on p. 812 in the Leukemia section.)

Surgical management with a splenectomy may be needed for the patient who does not respond to drug therapy. (The spleen is the site of excessive platelet destruction.)

Depending on the size of the spleen and the risk for bleeding, splenectomy may be performed as an open abdominal surgery or as minimally invasive surgery by laparoscopy. Nursing care after surgery is the same as for any other abdominal surgery (see Chapter 16). After splenectomy, the patient is at increased risk for INFECTION because the spleen performs many protective immune functions, especially antibody generation. For this reason, vaccinations against pneumococcal, meningococcal, and *Haemophilus influenzae* are recommended either 2 weeks before a planned splenectomy or 2 weeks after the surgery. Teaching patients about their increased risk for infection, avoiding crowds and people who are ill, and consulting with the health care provider is a nursing priority.

THROMBOTIC THROMBOCYTOPENIC PURPURA

In thrombotic thrombocytopenic purpura (TTP), platelets clump together abnormally in the capillaries and too few platelets remain in circulation. The patient has inappropriate CLOTTING, yet the blood fails to clot when trauma occurs. The cause of TTP appears to be an autoimmune reaction in small blood vessel cells (endothelial cells) that starts platelet aggregation and clotting there. Tissues become ischemic, leading to kidney failure, myocardial infarction, and stroke. Untreated, this disorder is often fatal within 3 months.

Management of the patient with TTP focuses on preventing platelet clumping and stopping the autoimmune process. Plasma removal and the infusion of fresh frozen plasma reduce the clumping caused by elements of the patient's blood. Drugs that inhibit platelet clumping, such as aspirin, alprostadil (Prostin), and plicamycin, also may be helpful. Immunosuppressive therapy reduces the intensity of this disorder.

CLOTTING FACTOR DISORDERS

Coagulation or bleeding disorders can result from a CLOTTING factor defect. Defects include the inability to produce a specific clotting factor, production of low quantities of a clotting factor, or production of a less active form of a clotting factor.

Most clotting factor disorders are genetic problems of one clotting factor. A damaged liver also leads to a clotting disorder by reducing the amount of clotting factors produced. Common disorders that result from defects at the clotting factor level include hemophilias A and B and von Willebrand's disease. Disseminated intravascular coagulation (DIC) often occurs with septic shock (see Chapter 37).

HEMOPHILIA

❖ PATHOPHYSIOLOGY

Hemophilia is a hereditary bleeding disorder with two forms resulting from different CLOTTING factor deficiencies. Hemophilia A (classic hemophilia) is a deficiency of factor VIII and accounts for 80% of cases of hemophilia. Hemophilia B (Christmas disease) is a deficiency of factor IX and accounts for 20% of cases. The incidence of both disorders is 1 in 10,000 (Hitch, 2013; McCance et al., 2014).

GENETIC/GENOMIC CONSIDERATIONS

Patient-Centered Care QSEN

Hemophilia is an X-linked recessive trait. Women who are **carriers** (can pass on the gene without expressing bleeding problems) have a 50% chance of passing the hemophilia gene to their daughters (who then are carriers) and to their sons (who then have hemophilia). Hemophilia A affects mostly males, none of whose sons will have the gene for hemophilia and all of whose daughters will be carriers. About 30% of patients with hemophilia have no family history and their disease may be the result of a new gene mutation (Beery & Workman, 2012). Ensure that the family is referred to the appropriate level of genetic counseling.

The clinical pictures of hemophilias A and B are identical. The patient has abnormal bleeding in response to any trauma because of a deficiency of the specific CLOTTING factor. Hemophiliacs form platelet plugs at the bleeding site, but the clotting factor deficiency impairs the formation of stable fibrin clots. This allows excessive bleeding, which may be mild, moderate, or severe, depending on the degree of factor deficiency.

❖ *PATIENT-CENTERED COLLABORATIVE CARE*

Assessment of the patient with hemophilia shows:

- Excessive bleeding from minor cuts, bruises, or abrasions (from abnormal platelet function)
- Joint and muscle hemorrhages that lead to disabling long-term problems and may require joint replacement
- A tendency to bruise easily
- Prolonged and potentially fatal hemorrhage after surgery

The laboratory test results for a patient with hemophilia show a prolonged activated partial thromboplastin time (aPTT), a normal bleeding time, and a normal prothrombin time (PT). The most common problem that occurs with hemophilia is degenerating joint function as a result of chronic bleeding into the joints, especially the hip and knee.

The bleeding problems of hemophilia A are managed by either regularly scheduled infusions of synthetic factor VIII or the infusion of this substance only when injury or bleeding occurs. The cost of factor VIII replacement is prohibitive for many people with hemophilia. The source of factor VIII varies (Table 40-5), and the traditional sources, derived from pooled human serum, are no longer recommended because of the risk for transfusion-related INFECTIONS (National Hemophilia Foundation, 2014).

TABLE 40-5 Antihemophilic Drugs

DRUG TYPES	SOURCES
High purity antihemophilic factor • Alphanate • Humate-P • Koate-DIV	Pooled human serum
Monoclonal antibody purified antihemophilic factor • Hemofil-M • Monarc-M • Monoclate-P	Pooled human serum
Recombinant antihemophilic factor • Helixate FS • Kogenate FS • Recombinate	Recombinant DNA technology
B-domain deleted (BDD) recombinant antihemophilic factor • ReFacto	Recombinant DNA technology
Recombinant antihemophilic factor plasma/albumin-free method (rAHF-PFM) • Advate	Recombinant DNA technology
Recombinant antihemophilic factor plasma/albumin-free method • Xyntha	Recombinant DNA technology
Porcine factor VIII • Hyate: C	Animal serum

HEPARIN-INDUCED THROMBOCYTOPENIA

Heparin-induced thrombocytopenia (HIT) is a serious IMMUNITY-mediated CLOTTING disorder with an unexplained drop in platelet count after heparin treatment. The occurrence is increasing because of the increased use of heparin. Unlike other clotting disorders, HIT is an immune-mediated drug reaction that is caused by heparin-dependent platelet-activating immunoglobulin G (IgG) antibodies in which heparin binds with platelet factor 4 (PF4). This drug binding leads to the development of a highly reactive immune complex that activates the platelets. Once activated, platelets release procoagulants and PF4, which neutralizes heparin and increases thrombin generation from prothrombin.

HIT can occur in patients receiving any type of heparin, although it is more common after exposure to unfractionated heparin. The incidence is higher among patients with risk factors of (1) duration of heparin use longer than 1 week, (2) exposure to unfractionated heparin, (3) postsurgical thromboprophylaxis, and (4) being female.

Manifestations of HIT include venous thromboembolism (VTE) such as deep vein thrombosis and pulmonary embolism. The diagnosis is based on the patient's exposure to heparin, which can be up to 100 days before the event. Thrombocytopenia after heparin exposure is the hallmark sign of HIT. Clinical, as well as laboratory, findings need to be interpreted to properly diagnose this disorder.

Once HIT is diagnosed, anticoagulation therapy is started. Drug management for HIT management is with a direct thrombin inhibitor such as argatroban (Argatroban), lepirudin (Refludan), and bivalirudin (Angiomax).

TRANSFUSION THERAPY

Any blood component may be removed from a donor and transfused into a recipient. Blood components may be transfused individually or collectively, with varying degrees of benefit to the recipient. Table 40-6 lists indications for transfusion therapy.

Pretransfusion Responsibilities

Nursing actions during transfusions focus on prevention or early recognition of adverse transfusion reactions. Preparation of the patient for transfusion is critical, and blood product administration procedures must be carefully followed. Before infusing any blood product, review the agency's policies and procedures. Chart 40-12 lists best practices for transfusion therapy.

A health care provider's prescription is needed to administer blood components. The prescription specifies the type of component, the volume, and any special conditions. Verify the

TABLE 40-6 Indications for Treatment with Blood Components

COMPONENT	VOLUME	INFUSION TIME	INDICATIONS
Packed red blood cells (PRBCs)	200-250 mL	2-4 hr	Anemia; hemoglobin <6 g/dL, 6-10 g/dL, depending on symptoms
Washed red blood cells (WBC-poor PRBCs)	200 mL	2-4 hr	History of allergic transfusion reactions Hematopoietic stem cell transplant patients
Platelets			
Pooled	About 300 mL	15-30 min	Thrombocytopenia, platelet count <20,000 Patients who are actively bleeding with a platelet count <50,000
Single donor	200 mL	30 min	History of febrile or allergic reactions
Fresh frozen plasma	200 mL	15-30 min	Deficiency in plasma coagulation factors Prothrombin or partial thromboplastin time 1.5 times normal
White blood cells (WBCs)	400 mL	1 hr	Sepsis, neutropenic infection not responding to antibiotic therapy

CHART 40-12 Best Practice for Patient Safety & Quality Care QSEN

Transfusion Therapy

NURSING ACTIONS	RATIONALES
Before Infusion	
1. Assess laboratory values.	Many institutions have specific guidelines for blood product transfusions (e.g., platelet count <20,000 or hemoglobin <6 g/dL).
2. Verify the medical prescription.	Legally, a physician's prescription is required for transfusions. The prescription should state the type of product, dose, and transfusion time.
3. Assess the patient's vital signs, urine output, skin color, and history of transfusion reactions.	Determine whether the patient can tolerate infusion. Baseline information may be needed to help identify transfusion reactions.
4. Obtain venous access. Use a central catheter or at least a 19-gauge needle if possible.	The larger-bore needle allows cells to flow more easily without occluding the lumen of the catheter.
5. Obtain blood products from a blood bank. Transfuse as soon as possible after first performing **all the required safety checks.** QSEN	Once a blood product has been released from the blood bank, the product should be transfused as soon as possible (e.g., red blood cell transfusions should be completed within 4 hours of removal from refrigeration).
6. With another registered nurse, verify the patient by name and number, check blood compatibility, and note expiration time.	Human error is the most common cause of ABO incompatibility reactions.
During Infusion	
7. Administer the blood product using the appropriate filtered tubing.	Filters are needed to remove aggregates and possible contaminants.
8. Dilute blood products with only normal saline solution.	Hemolysis occurs if some other IV solution is used.
9. Remain with the patient during the first 15 to 30 minutes of the infusion.	Hemolytic reactions occur most often within the first 50 mL of the infusion.
10. Infuse the blood product at the prescribed rate.	Fluid overload is a potential complication of rapid infusion.
11. Monitor vital signs.	Vital sign changes often indicate transfusion reactions.
After Infusion	
12. When the transfusion is completed, discontinue infusion and dispose of the bag and tubing properly.	Bloodborne pathogens may be spread inadvertently through improper disposal.
13. Document.	The patient record should indicate the type of product infused, product number, volume infused, time of infusion, and any adverse reactions.

prescription for accuracy and completeness. In many hospitals, a separate consent form must be obtained from the patient before a transfusion is performed.

A blood specimen is obtained for type and crossmatch (testing of the donor's blood and the recipient's blood for compatibility). The procedures for obtaining this specimen are specified by hospital policy. Usually a new type-and-crossmatch specimen is required at least every 72 hours.

Both Y-tubing and straight tubing sets are used for blood component infusion (Fig. 40-7). A blood filter (about 170 μm) to remove sediment from the stored blood products is included with blood administration sets and must be used to transfuse most, but not all, blood products.

Use normal saline as the solution to administer with blood products, although this practice is not evidence-based (Kessler, 2013). Ringer's lactate and dextrose in water are not used for infusion with blood products because they may cause clotting or hemolysis of blood cells, although there is not sufficient evidence of hemolysis when using hypotonic fluids (Elgin et al., 2011; Kessler, 2013; Kessler et al., 2012; Tolich et al., 2013).

! NURSING SAFETY PRIORITY QSEN

Action Alert

Never add to or infuse other drugs with blood products because they may clot the blood during transfusion.

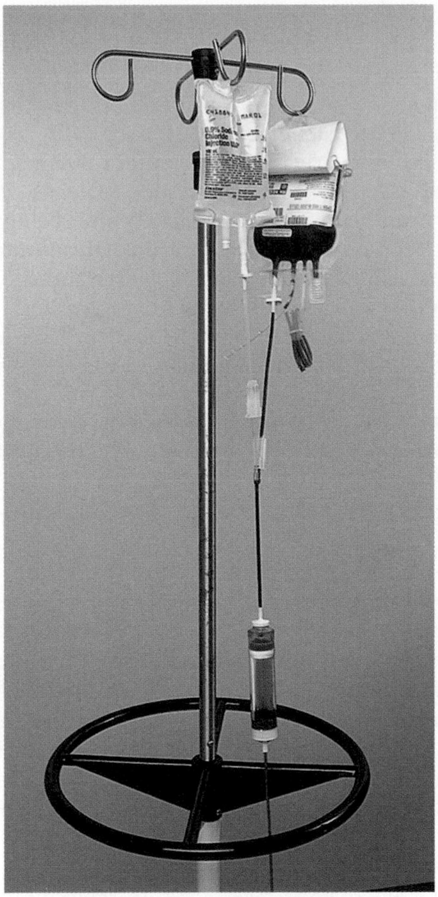

FIG. 40-7 Blood administration setup.

Before the transfusion, in compliance with recommendations by The Joint Commission's National Patient Safety Goals (NPSGs), the priority action is to determine that the blood component delivered is correct and that identification of the patient is correct. Check the physician's prescription together with another registered nurse to determine the patient's identity and whether the hospital identification band name and number are identical to those on the blood component tag. According to The Joint Commission's National Patient Safety Goals, *the patient's room number is not an acceptable form of identification.* Some facilities use a bar code–point of care (BC-POC) system, similar to drug dispensing systems, in an attempt to improve patient safety and reduce identification errors.

! NURSING SAFETY PRIORITY (QSEN)

Action Alert

The nurse who will be actually administering the blood products must be one of the two professionals comparing the patient's identification with the information on the blood component bag.

Examine the blood bag label, the attached tag, and the requisition slip to ensure that the ABO and Rh types are compatible with those of the patient. Check the expiration date, and inspect the product for discoloration, gas bubbles, or cloudiness, which are all indicators of bacterial growth or hemolysis.

CHART 40-13 Best Practice for Patient Safety & Quality Care (QSEN)

The Older Adult Receiving a Transfusion

- Assess the patient's circulatory, kidney, and fluid status before initiating the transfusion.
- Use no larger than a 19-gauge needle.
- Try to use blood that is less than 1 week old. (Older blood cell membranes are more fragile, break easily, and release potassium into the circulation.)
- Take vital signs (especially pulse, blood pressure, and respiratory rate) every 15 minutes throughout the transfusion. Changes in these parameters can indicate fluid overload and may also be the only indicators of adverse transfusion reactions.
  - Overload
    - Rapid bounding pulse
    - Hypertension
    - Swollen superficial veins
  - Transfusion Reaction
    - Rapid thready pulse
    - Hypotension
    - Increased pallor, cyanosis
- Administer blood slowly, taking 2 to 4 hours for each unit of whole blood, packed red blood cells, or plasma.
- Avoid concurrent fluid administration into any other IV site.
- If possible, allow 2 full hours after the administration of 1 unit of blood before administering the next unit.

Transfusion Responsibilities

Before starting the transfusion, explain the procedure to the patient. Assess vital signs and temperature immediately before starting the infusion. Begin the infusion slowly. *Remain with the patient for the first 15 to 30 minutes.* Any severe reaction usually occurs with infusion of the first 50 mL of blood. Ask the patient to report unusual sensations such as chills, shortness of breath, hives, or itching. Assess vital signs 15 minutes after starting the infusion for indications of a reaction. If there are none, the rate can be increased to transfuse 1 unit in 2 hours (depending on the patient's cardiac status and the facility's policy for rate of administration). Take vital signs every hour during the transfusion or as specified by the agency's policy. Some facilities are now continuously monitoring patients during transfusions using a wireless remote monitoring device (Card et al., 2012).

Blood components without large amounts of RBCs can be infused more quickly. The identification checks are the same as for RBC transfusions. It may be necessary to infuse blood products at a slower rate for older patients. Best practices related to the nursing care needs of older patients during transfusion therapy are listed in Chart 40-13.

Electrolyte imbalances are possible as a result of transfusions, especially with packed red blood cells or with whole blood. During transfusions, some cells are damaged, releasing potassium and raising the patient's serum potassium level above normal (hyperkalemia). This problem is more likely when the blood being transfused has been frozen or is several weeks old.

Types of Transfusions

At one time, transfusion with whole blood was the most common form of transfusion therapy. Today, whole-blood transfusions are extremely rare (AABB [formerly called the American Association of Blood Banks], 2013). When a whole-blood donation is made, it is centrifuged on arrival at the

TABLE 40-7 Compatibility Chart for Red Blood Cell Transfusions

	RECIPIENT			
DONOR	A	B	AB	O
A	X		X	
B		X	X	
AB			X	
O	X	X	X	X

blood-banking facility and separated in to various components. The individual components are then transfused according to patients' specific needs.

Red Blood Cell Transfusions

RBCs are given to replace cells lost from trauma or surgery. Patients with problems that destroy RBCs or impair RBC maturation also may receive RBC transfusions. Packed RBCs, supplied in 250-mL bags, are a concentrated source of RBCs and are the most common component given to RBC-deficient patients.

Blood transfusions are actually transplantations of tissue from one person to another. Therefore the donor and recipient blood must be carefully checked for compatibility to prevent lethal reactions (Table 40-7). Compatibility is determined by two different antigen systems (cell surface proteins): the ABO system antigens and the Rh antigen, present on the membranes of RBCs.

RBC antigens are inherited. For the ABO system, a person inherits one of these:

- A antigen (type A blood)
- B antigen (type B blood)
- Both A and B antigens (type AB blood)
- Neither A nor B antigens (type O blood)

People develop circulating antibodies against the blood type antigens they did not inherit. For example, a person with type A blood forms antibodies against type B blood. A person with type O blood has not inherited either A or B antigens and will form antibodies against RBCs with either A or B antigens. If RBCs that have an antigen are infused into a recipient who does not share that antigen, the infused blood is recognized by the recipient's antibodies as non-self and the recipient then has a reaction to the transfused products.

The Rh antigen system is slightly different. An Rh-negative person is born without the Rh-antigen on his or her RBCs and does not form antibodies unless specifically sensitized to it. Sensitization can occur with RBC transfusions from an Rh-positive person or from exposure during pregnancy and birth. Once an Rh-negative person has been sensitized and antibodies develop, any exposure to Rh-positive blood can cause a transfusion reaction. Antibody development can be prevented by giving anti-Rh-immunoglobulin (RHoGAM) as soon as exposure to the Rh antigen is suspected. *People who have Rh-positive blood can receive an RBC transfusion from an Rh-negative donor, but Rh-negative people should not receive Rh-positive blood.*

Platelet Transfusions

Platelets are given to patients with platelet counts below 10,000/mm^3 and to patients with thrombocytopenia who are actively bleeding or are scheduled for an invasive procedure. Platelet transfusions are pooled from as many as 10 donors and do not have to be of the same blood type as the patient has. For patients who are having a hematopoietic stem cell transplantation (HSCT) or who need multiple platelet transfusions, platelets from a single donor may be prescribed, which reduces the chances of allergic reactions.

Platelet infusion bags usually contain 300 mL for pooled platelets and 200 mL for single-donor platelets. Platelets are fragile and must be infused immediately after being brought to the patient's room, usually over a 15- to 30-minute period. A special transfusion set with a smaller filter and shorter tubing is used. Additional platelet filters help remove white blood cells (WBCs) from the platelets for patients who have a history of febrile reactions or who need multiple platelet transfusions.

! NURSING SAFETY PRIORITY QSEN

Action Alert

When infusing platelets, do not use the standard blood administration set because the filter traps the platelets and the longer tubing increases platelet adherence to the lumen.

Take the vital signs before the infusion, 15 minutes after the infusion starts, and at its completion. A patient who has had a transfusion reaction in the past may be given diphenhydramine (Benadryl) and acetaminophen (Tylenol) before the transfusion to reduce the fever and severe chills (rigors) that often occur during platelet transfusions.

Plasma Transfusions

Plasma infusions may be given fresh to replace blood volume and CLOTTING factors. More often, plasma is frozen immediately after donation, forming **fresh frozen plasma (FFP)**. Infuse FFP immediately after thawing while the clotting factors are still active.

ABO compatibility is required for transfusion of plasma products because the plasma contains the donor's ABO antibodies that could react with the recipient's RBC antigens. The infusion bag contains about 200 mL. Infuse FFP as rapidly as the patient can tolerate, generally over a 30- to 60-minute period, through a regular Y set or straight filtered tubing.

Granulocyte (White Blood Cell) Transfusions

Rarely, neutropenic patients with INFECTIONS receive white blood cell (WBC) replacement transfusions. WBC surfaces have many antigens that can cause severe reactions when infused into a patient whose immune system recognizes these antigens as non-self.

WBCs are suspended in 400 mL of plasma and should be infused slowly, usually over a 45- to 60-minute period depending on the concentration of cells being infused. Agency policies often require stricter monitoring of patients receiving WBCs because reactions are more common. A physician may need to be present in the hospital unit, and vital signs may need to be taken every 15 minutes throughout the transfusion. Amphotericin B infusion should be separated from WBC transfusions by 4 to 6 hours.

Acute Transfusion Reactions

Patients can develop any of these transfusion reactions: febrile, hemolytic, allergic, or bacterial reactions; circulatory overload; or transfusion-associated graft-versus-host disease (GVHD). To prevent complications, remain alert during transfusions to detect early reactions and initiate appropriate management.

Febrile transfusion reactions occur most often in the patient with anti-WBC antibodies, which can develop after multiple transfusions, white blood cell transfusions, and platelet transfusions. The patient develops chills, tachycardia, fever, hypotension, and tachypnea. Giving leukocyte-reduced blood or single-donor HLA-matched platelets reduces the risk for this type of reaction. WBC filters may be used to trap WBCs and prevent their infusion into the patient.

Hemolytic transfusion reactions are caused by blood type or Rh incompatibility. When blood containing antigens different from the patient's own antigens is infused, antigen-antibody complexes are formed in his or her blood. These complexes destroy the transfused cells and start inflammatory responses in the blood vessel walls and organs. The reaction may be mild, with fever and chills, or life threatening, with disseminated intravascular coagulation (DIC) and circulatory collapse (McCance et al., 2014). Other manifestations include:

- Apprehension
- Headache
- Chest pain
- Low back pain
- Tachycardia
- Tachypnea
- Hypotension
- Hemoglobinuria
- A sense of impending doom

The onset of a hemolytic reaction may be immediate or may not occur until subsequent units have been transfused (Kessler et al., 2012).

Allergic transfusion reactions (anaphylactic transfusion reactions) are most often seen in patients with other allergies. They may have urticaria, itching, bronchospasm, or anaphylaxis. Onset usually occurs during or up to 24 hours after the transfusion. Patients with an allergy history can be given leukocyte-reduced or washed RBCs in which the WBCs, plasma, and immunoglobulin A have been removed, reducing the possibility of an allergic reaction.

Bacterial transfusion reactions occur from infusion of contaminated blood products, especially those contaminated with a gram-negative organism. Manifestations include tachycardia, hypotension, fever, chills, and shock. The onset of a bacterial transfusion reaction is rapid. (See Chapter 37 for care of the patient with septic shock.)

Circulatory overload can occur when a blood product is infused too quickly, especially in an older adult. This is most common with whole-blood transfusions or when the patient receives multiple packed RBC transfusions. Manifestations include:

- Hypertension
- Bounding pulse
- Distended jugular veins
- Dyspnea
- Restlessness
- Confusion

You can both manage and prevent this complication by monitoring intake and output, infusing blood products more slowly, and giving diuretics. (See Chapter 11 for management of patients with fluid overload.)

Transfusion-associated graft-versus-host disease (TA-GVHD) is a rare but life-threatening problem that occurs more often in an immunosuppressed patient. Its cause in immunosuppressed patients is similar to that of GVHD that occurs with allogeneic stem cell transplantation, discussed on p. 811, in which donor T-cell lymphocytes attack host tissues.

Manifestations usually occur within 1 to 2 weeks and include thrombocytopenia, anorexia, nausea, vomiting, chronic hepatitis, weight loss, and recurrent INFECTION.

TA-GVHD has an 80% to 90% mortality rate but can be prevented by using irradiated blood products. Irradiation destroys T-cells and their cytokine products.

Transfusion-related acute lung injury (TRALI) is a life-threatening event that occurs most often when donor blood contains antibodies against the recipient's neutrophil antigens, HLA, or both (Kessler et al., 2012). Common manifestations are a rapid onset of dyspnea and hypoxia within 6 hours of the transfusion.

Acute pain transfusion reaction or APTR is a recently identified but rare event that can occur during or shortly after transfusion of any blood product. Its actual pathophysiology has not yet been elucidated. The manifestations are severe chest pain, back pain, joint pain, hypertension, and redness of the head and neck (Hardwick et al., 2013). Most patients also have anxiety. The reaction does not appear to be life threatening, and most patients respond well with drugs for pain and rigors. Although the manifestations are general, diagnosis can be supported with a positive direct antibody test (DAT), indicating that some degree of hemolysis has occurred but is not widespread. APTR management focuses on patient support and drugs to control or reduce manifestations.

Interventions for transfusion reactions occurring during transfusion (hemolytic reactions, allergic reactions, and bacterial reactions) begin with stopping the transfusion and removing the blood tubing. (For hemolytic and suspected bacterial reactions, return the component bag, labels, and all tubing to the blood bank or laboratory.) Notify the Rapid Response Team. If the patient has no other IV access, keep the access and flush with normal saline. *Do not flush the contents of the blood transfusion tubing, which would allow more of the reaction-causing blood to enter the patient.* Usually oxygen is applied and diphenhydramine (Benadryl) is administered by IV push. If manifestations of shock are present, fluid resuscitation and hemodynamic monitoring are needed. Blood pressure support with vasopressors may be needed (see Chapter 37). Other drug therapy is supportive, such as antipyretics for fever, antibiotics for suspected bacterial contamination, and meperidine for rigors.

Autologous Blood Transfusions

Autologous blood transfusions involve collection and infusion of the patient's own blood. This type of transfusion eliminates compatibility problems and reduces the risk for transmitting bloodborne diseases. The four types of autologous blood transfusions are preoperative autologous blood donation, acute normovolemic hemodilution, intraoperative autologous transfusion, and postoperative blood salvage.

Autologous blood donation before surgery is the most common type of autologous blood transfusion. It involves collecting whole blood from the patient (who must meet certain criteria), dividing it into components, and storing it for later use. As long as hematocrit and hemoglobin levels are within a safe range, the patient can donate blood on a weekly basis until the prescribed amount of blood is obtained. Fresh packed RBCs may be stored for 40 days. For patients with rare blood types, blood may be frozen for up to 10 years.

Acute normovolemic hemodilution involves withdrawal of a patient's RBCs and volume replacement just before a surgical procedure. The goal is to decrease RBC loss during surgery. The blood is stored at room temperature for up to 6 hours and reinfused after surgery. This type of autologous transfusion is not used with anemic patients or those with poor kidney function.

Intraoperative autologous transfusion and blood salvage after surgery are the recovery and reinfusion of a patient's own blood from an operative field or from a bleeding wound. Special devices collect, filter, and drain the blood into a transfusion bag. This blood is used for trauma or surgical patients with severe blood loss. The salvaged blood must be reinfused within 6 hours.

Transfuse autologous blood products using the guidelines previously described. Although the patient receiving autologous blood is not at risk for some types of transfusion reactions, circulatory overload or bacterial transfusion reactions can still occur and are managed in the same way they are managed in transfusions derived from donors.

NCLEX EXAMINATION CHALLENGE

Safe and Effective Care Environment

The nurse who just came on duty observes that the client, whose blood type is AB negative, is receiving a transfusion with type O negative packed red blood cells. What is the nurse's best first action?

A. Call the blood bank.
B. Take and record the client's vital signs.
C. Stop the transfusion and keep the IV open.
D. Document the observation as the only action.

NURSING CONCEPTS AND CLINICAL JUDGMENT REVIEW

What might you NOTICE if the patient is experiencing inadequate GAS EXCHANGE and PERFUSION as a result of hematologic problems?

- Skin cyanosis or pallor (in patients with light skin)
- Cyanosis or pallor of the lips and oral mucous membranes
- Tachycardia
- Tachypnea and dyspnea
- Slow capillary refill
- Cool to cold extremities
- Change in cognition, acute confusion
- Decreased oxygen saturation
- Decreased urine output
- Presence of bruises or petechiae
- Bleeding of gums, at IV sites, at injection sites

What should you INTERPRET and how should you RESPOND to this patient experiencing inadequate GAS EXCHANGE and PERFUSION as a result of a hematologic problem?

Perform and interpret physical assessment, including:

- Taking vital signs
- Monitoring oxygen saturation by pulse oximetry
- Checking for blood in stool, urine, emesis
- Checking for bleeding in the mouth, around IV sites, drains, urinary catheters
- Checking most recent laboratory values for hematocrit and hemoglobin levels and platelet and RBC counts
- Assessing cognition

Respond by:

- Applying oxygen
- Keeping the patient's head elevated to about 30 degrees
- Handling the patient gently
- Keeping the patient warm (blankets)
- Applying firm pressure to areas actively bleeding
- Notifying physician or Rapid Response Team
- Instituting Bleeding Precautions
- Maintaining or initiating IV therapy
- Preparing to administer blood or blood products
- Prioritizing and pacing activities to prevent fatigue

On what should you REFLECT?

- Observe patient for evidence of restored tissue perfusion (see Chapter 39)
- Think about what may have precipitated this episode and what steps could be taken to identify it earlier.

GET READY FOR THE NCLEX® EXAMINATION!

KEY POINTS

Review these Key Points for each NCLEX Examination Client Needs Category.

Safe and Effective Care Environment

- Use aseptic technique during all central line dressing changes or any invasive procedure. **Safety** QSEN
- Use good handwashing techniques before providing any care to a patient who is either immunocompromised or immune deficient. **Safety** QSEN
- Modify the environment to protect patients who have thrombocytopenia. **Safety** QSEN
- Use Bleeding Precautions for any patient with thrombocytopenia or pancytopenia (see Chart 40-7). **Safety** QSEN
- Ensure informed consent is obtained before any invasive procedure or transfusion. **Safety** QSEN
- Verify with another registered nurse prescriptions for transfusion of blood products. **Safety** QSEN
- Use at least two forms of identification for the patient who is to receive a blood product transfusion (e.g., name, birthdate, identification number). **Safety** QSEN

Health Promotion and Maintenance

- Teach patients with sickle cell disease to avoid conditions that are known to trigger crises. **Patient-Centered Care** QSEN

- Teach people to avoid unnecessary contact with environmental chemicals or toxins. If contact cannot be avoided, teach people to use safety precautions.
- Identify patients at high risk for INFECTION because of disease or therapy. **Patient-Centered Care** QSEN
- Teach the patient and family about the manifestations of INFECTION and when to seek medical advice. **Patient-Centered Care** QSEN
- Instruct patients who have anemia as a result of dietary deficiency which foods are good sources of iron, folic acid, and vitamin B_{12}. **Patient-Centered Care** QSEN
- Teach precautions to take to avoid injury (see Chart 40-11) to patients at risk for poor CLOTTING and increased bleeding. **Patient-Centered Care** QSEN

Psychosocial Integrity

- Allow the patient the opportunity to express his or her feelings regarding the diagnosis of leukemia or lymphoma or the treatment regimen. **Patient-Centered Care** QSEN
- Explain all procedures, restrictions, drugs, and follow-up care to the patient and family. **Patient-Centered Care** QSEN
- Offer alternative therapies for relaxation, pain reduction, and distraction, such as massage, music therapy, and guided imagery. **Patient-Centered Care** QSEN
- Reassure patients having pain that using opioid analgesics for needed pain relief is not drug abuse. **Patient-Centered Care** QSEN

Physiological Integrity

- Pace nonurgent health care activities to reduce the risk for fatigue among patients with anemia or pancytopenia. **Patient-Centered Care** QSEN
- Assess patients in the induction phase of chemotherapy, those after HSCT, and anyone with neutropenia every 8 hours for manifestations of INFECTION. **Evidence-Based Practice** QSEN
- Assess the skin integrity of the perianal region of a patient with leukemia or profound neutropenia after every bowel movement. **Patient-Centered Care** QSEN
- Administer analgesics on a schedule rather than PRN. **Evidence-Based Practice** QSEN
- Use normal saline as the solution infusing with blood products.
- Transfuse blood products more slowly to older patients or those who have a cardiac problem. **Patient-Centered Care** QSEN
- Remain with the patient during the first 15 minutes of infusion of any blood product. **Safety** QSEN
- Do not administer any drugs with infusing blood products. **Evidence-Based Practice** QSEN
- Make referrals to support groups sponsored by organizations such as the Sickle Cell Foundation Support Group, American Cancer Society, Leukemia and Lymphoma Society of America, and the National Hemophilia Foundation. **Teamwork and Collaboration** QSEN

CONCEPT OVERVIEW

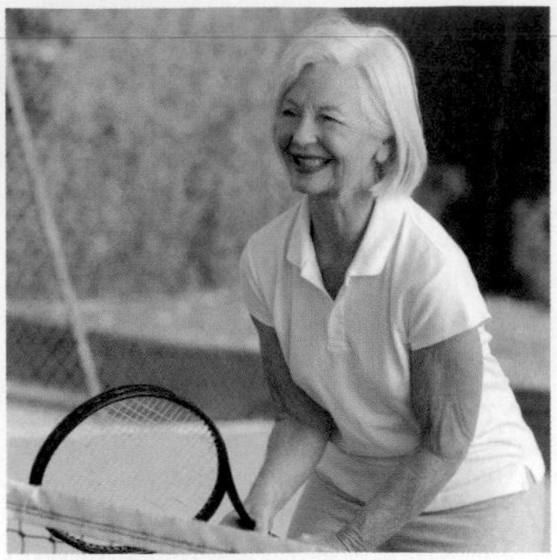

Mobility, Sensory Perception, and Cognition

The term *mobility* means movement. When referring to physical MOBILITY, it means the ability of the body to purposely move (Giddens, 2013). MOBILITY is needed for ADL performance and many body functions, including digestion, elimination, circulation, and muscle integrity. In some cases, it helps keep a person *safe* by being able to move to prevent injury.

MOBILITY is accomplished primarily through the integration of the neurologic and musculoskeletal body systems. Risk factors for decreased MOBILITY are typically acute and chronic health problems that cause pain or injury (Giddens, 2013).

SENSORY PERCEPTION refers to receiving sensory input from the cells of the skin (feeling), eyes (seeing), and ears (hearing) and accurately interpreting this input in the neurons of the central nervous system (CNS). Therefore SENSORY PERCEPTION is also needed to keep the body *safe*. For example, if a person cannot feel water temperature, a burn may result. If vision is impaired, a fall may occur.

COGNITION refers to mental processes and intellectual function and is controlled by certain neurons in the gray matter of the brain. These cells are very sensitive to serum glucose and oxygen levels. If either of these substances falls below the amounts needed, the cells cannot function properly, resulting in diminished cognitive ability and a decreased level of consciousness.

One or all of these three concepts may be impaired as a result of disease, injury, surgery, or drugs. Problems of the neurologic, sensory, and musculoskeletal systems most commonly affect the need for MOBILITY, SENSORY PERCEPTION, and COGNITION. The interrelationship of these concepts can be compared to a computer and its parts.

As seen in Fig. 1, the computer's central processing unit (CPU), or processor, is the brain of the machine (the *cognitive* center). Much like the spinal cord, it works with the motherboard to send and receive messages (input and output). The connected pins and wires function like the spinal nerves. Peripherals such as the mouse and keyboard are similar in function to the peripheral nervous system (PNS) (SENSORY PERCEPTION) and musculoskeletal system (MOBILITY). When all of these parts are working properly, the computer functions without any problems.

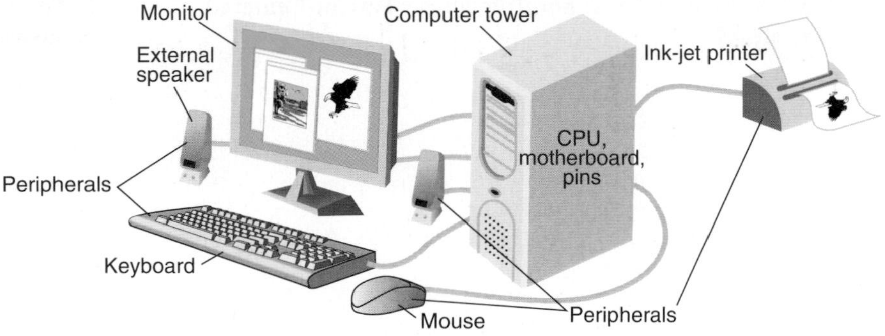

FIG. 1

However, when the CPU (brain) does not work properly (decreased COGNITION), the motherboard (spinal cord) and/or peripherals (PNS and muscles) may not function as they should (decreased MOBILITY and SENSORY PERCEPTION). If the motherboard (spinal cord) is broken, no information is sent to or from any of the other parts of the computer. In both cases, there is no display on the monitor (Fig. 2).

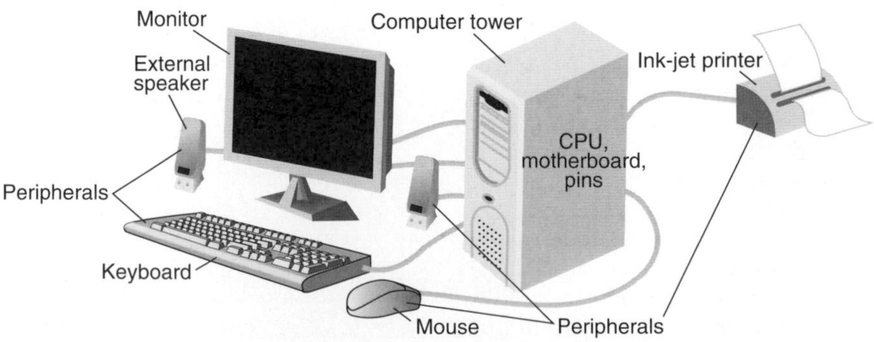

FIG. 2

CHAPTER 41

Assessment of the Nervous System

Rachel L. Gallagher

http://evolve.elsevier.com/Iggy/

PRIORITY CONCEPTS

- COGNITION
- MOBILITY
- SENSORY PERCEPTION

LEARNING OUTCOMES

Safe and Effective Care Environment

1. Collaborate with health care team members to establish priorities in neurologic assessment.

Health Promotion and Maintenance

2. Identify factors such as risky behaviors or lifestyle choices that place patients at risk for neurologic health problems.
3. Detect neurologic health problems early with health screening and physical assessment strategies.

Psychosocial Integrity

4. Explain psychological responses to neurologic health problems.

Physiological Integrity

5. Document findings from the neurologic history and physical examination to identify new and chronic changes in COGNITION, MOBILITY, and SENSORY PERCEPTION.
6. Perform a comprehensive and a rapid focused neurologic examination to manage conditions and promote patient safety related to impaired neurologic function.
7. Use interventions to provide assistance in the performance of activities of daily living when neurologic conditions interfere with self-care.
8. Reduce complications from diagnostic testing by determining risk factors for adverse reaction to contrast media.
9. Review neurologic anatomy and physiology to identify changes that result in health alterations.
10. Describe common physiologic changes associated with aging that affect the nervous system.

The major divisions of the nervous system are the central nervous system (CNS) and peripheral nervous system (PNS). The PNS is further divided into the somatic and autonomic systems. These systems work together to control COGNITION, MOBILITY, and SENSORY PERCEPTION. The nervous system interacts with the endocrine system to balance fluid and electrolytes. In addition, through the autonomic nervous system (ANS), it innervates many other body systems including the reproductive and digestive organs to promote their function. For example, the sacral spinal nerves (part of the ANS) stimulate the detrusor muscle to contract when the urinary bladder is full, contributing to elimination.

Health problems involving trauma and diseases of the nervous system can impair fluid and electrolyte balance, thermoregulation, elimination, and many other functions. One of the earliest and most sensitive functions that signal new-onset brain disorders is COGNITION, a term used to refer to all the processes in human thought. The primary role of the nurse is to help restore these human needs or assist the patient adapt to their deficits and avoid complications from dysfunction.

ANATOMY AND PHYSIOLOGY REVIEW

The CNS is composed of the brain and the spinal cord. The brain is contained within the cranium; the brain's role is to direct the regulation and function of the nervous system and other systems of the body. The spinal cord is lodged in the vertebral canal. From the brain, the spinal cord descends down the middle of the back and is surrounded and protected by the bony vertebral column. The spinal cord is surrounded by a clear fluid called *cerebrospinal fluid (CSF)* that protects the delicate nerve tissues against damage from banging against the inside of the vertebrae.

The PNS is composed of 12 pairs of cranial nerves, 31 pairs of spinal nerves, and the autonomic nervous system. The autonomic nervous system is further subdivided into sympathetic and parasympathetic fibers.

The nervous system contains two types of cells: neurons, which transmit or conduct nerve impulses; and neuroglia cells, which have an interdependent role with the neuron.

Nervous System Cells: Structure and Function

Two types of cells make up the nervous system: neurons and neuroglia cells. The basic unit of the nervous system, the **neuron**, transmits impulses, or "messages." Some neurons are **motor** (causing purposeful physical movement or MOBILITY), and some are **sensory** (resulting in the ability to perceive stimulation through one's sensory organs or SENSORY PERCEPTION). Some process information and some retain information. When a neuron receives an impulse from another neuron, the effect may be excitation or inhibition. Each neuron has a *cell body,* or *soma;* short, branching processes called *dendrites;* and a single *axon* (Fig. 41-1).

Afferent neurons, also known as *sensory neurons,* are specialized to send impulses toward the CNS, away from the PNS. *Efferent* neurons are motor nerve cells that carry signals from the CNS to the cells in the PNS. Each dendrite synapses with another cell body, axon, or dendrite and sends impulses along the efferent and afferent neuron pathways.

Many axons are covered by a **myelin sheath**—a white, lipid covering. Myelinated axons appear whitish and therefore are also called **white matter.** Nonmyelinated axons have a grayish cast and are called **gray matter.** Myelinated axons have gaps in the myelin called *nodes of Ranvier.* The nodes of Ranvier play a major role in impulse conduction (see Fig. 41-1). When the myelin is impaired, the impulses cannot travel from the brain to the rest of the body, such as in patients with multiple sclerosis.

The enlarged distal end of each axon is called the *synaptic* or *terminal knob.* Within the synaptic knobs are the mechanisms for manufacturing, storing, and releasing a transmitter substance. Each neuron produces a specific **neurotransmitter** chemical (e.g., acetylcholine or serotonin) that can either enhance or inhibit the impulse but cannot do both. Other substances, although not specifically identified as neurotransmitters, are considered probable transmitters or neuromodulators.

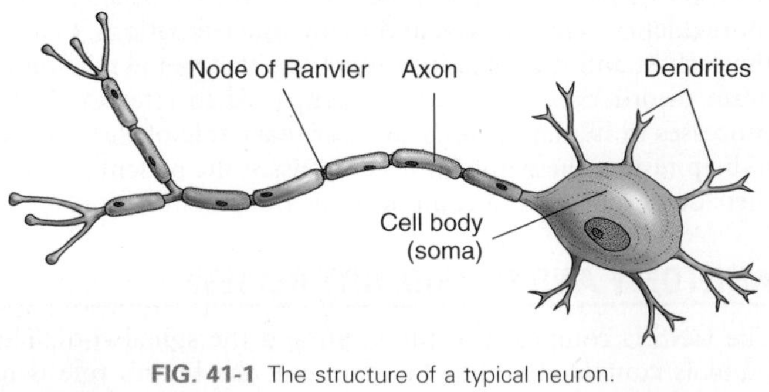

FIG. 41-1 The structure of a typical neuron.

Impulses are transmitted to their eventual destination through synapses, or spaces between neurons. There are two distinct types of synapses: *neuron to neuron* and *neuron to muscle* (or gland). Between the terminal knob and the next cell is a small space called the *synaptic cleft.* The knob, the cleft, and the portion of the cell to which the impulse is being transmitted make up the **synapse.**

Neuroglia cells, which vary in size and shape, provide protection, structure, and nutrition for the neurons. They are classified into four types: astroglial cells, ependymal cells, oligodendrocytes, and microglial cells. These cells are also part of the blood-brain barrier and help regulate cerebrospinal fluid (CSF).

Central Nervous System: Structure and Function

The central nervous system (CNS) is composed of the *brain,* which directs the regulation and function of the nervous system and all other systems of the body, and the *spinal cord,* which starts reflex activity and transmits impulses to and from the brain.

Brain

The **meninges** form the protective covering of the brain and the spinal cord. The outside layer is the *dura mater.* The **subdural space** is located between the dura mater and the middle layer, the *arachnoid.* The *pia mater* is the most inner layer. Situated between the arachnoid and pia mater is the **subarachnoid space,** where CSF circulates. A potential space, referred to as the *epidural space,* is located between the skull and the outer layer of the dura mater. This area also extends down the spinal cord and is used for the delivery of epidural analgesia and anesthesia.

The dura mater also lies between the cerebral hemispheres and the cerebellum and is called the *tentorium.* It helps decrease or prevents the transmission of force from one hemisphere to another and protects the lower brainstem when head trauma occurs. Clinical references may be made to a lesion (e.g., a tumor) as being **supratentorial** (above the tentorium) or **infratentorial** (below the tentorium).

Major Parts of the Brain. The brain consists of three main areas—the brainstem, the cerebellum, and the forebrain. The *brainstem* connects the rest of the brain with the CNS. It is concerned primarily with life support and basic functions such as movement.

The *cerebellum* is concerned with coordination of movement and works together with the brainstem to focus on the functionality of the muscles. This structure is found below the occipital lobe and adjacent to the brainstem.

The *forebrain* lies above the brainstem and cerebellum and is the most advanced in evolution. This area of the brain is further divided into three areas—the diencephalon, the cerebrum, and the cerebral cortex.

The *diencephalon,* which lies below the cerebrum, includes the thalamus, hypothalamus, and epithalamus (Fig. 41-2). The **thalamus** is the major "relay station," or "central switchboard," for the CNS. The **hypothalamus** plays a major role in autonomic nervous system control (controlling temperature and other functions) and COGNITION. The epithalamus contains the roof of the third ventricle and the pineal gland. The

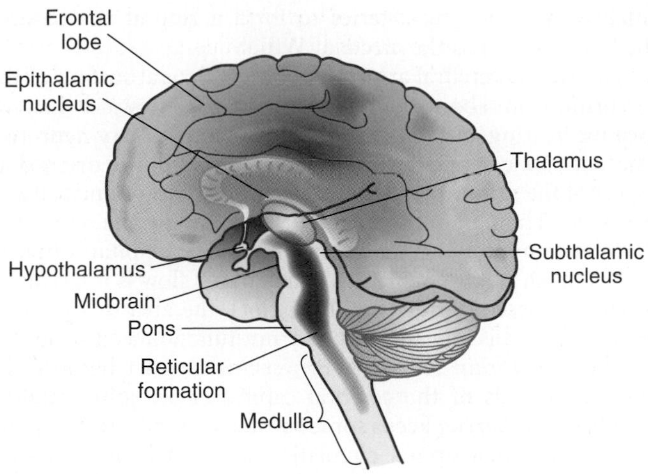

FIG. 41-2 The structures of the brainstem and diencephalon.

epithalamus connects the pathways to regulate emotion. Pathways through the epithalamus also contribute to smooth voluntary motor function.

The *cerebrum* is the largest part of the brain and controls intelligence, creativity, and memory. The "gray matter" of the cerebrum is the central cortex—the center that receives information from the thalamus and all the lower areas of the brain. The cerebrum consists of two halves, referred to as the *right hemisphere* and the *left hemisphere,* which are joined by the corpus callosum. The *left* hemisphere is the dominant hemisphere in most people (even in many left-handed people). Within the deeper structures of the cerebrum are the right and left lateral ventricles. At the base of the cerebrum near the ventricles is a group of neurons called the *basal ganglia,* which help regulate motor function.

The *cerebral cortex* is part of the cerebrum and is involved with almost all of the higher functions of the brain. This part of the brain processes and communicates all information coming from the peripheral nervous system (PNS). It also translates the impulses into understandable feelings and thoughts. The cerebral cortex is so complex that it is further divided into four lobes—the frontal lobe, parietal lobe, temporal lobe, and occipital lobe.

The frontal lobe is found at the front of the head near the temples and forehead. It processes voluntary muscle movements and higher functioning actions such as thought and speech. It also helps control mood, planning for the future, setting goals, and making judgments. The parietal lobe is found behind the frontal lobe. It processes spatial awareness and receives and processes information about temperature, taste, touch, and movement coming from the rest of the body. Reading and arithmetic are also processed in this lobe. The temporal lobes are located in the area of the brain parallel to the ears. They process hearing, memory, and language functions. The occipital lobe is located in the posterior of the brain and assists in the processing of visual information.

Located in the frontal lobe, the **motor cortex** controls voluntary movement. Corticospinal tracts, also called *pyramidal tracts,* begin in the motor cortex and travel through the brain before crossing in the medulla. This crossing explains how right motor cortex damage affects the movement in the left side of the body and vice versa, such as in many patients who have cerebral strokes. The cerebrum is divided into lobes by sulci (fissures). These lobes work together and are connected by nerve fibers. The name and main functions of cerebral lobes are listed in Table 41-1.

TABLE 41-1 Cerebral Lobe Main Functions

Frontal Lobe
- The primary motor area (also known as the *motor "strip"* or *cortex*)
- Broca's speech center on the dominant side
- Voluntary eye movement
- Access to current sensory data
- Access to past information or experience
- Affective response to a situation
- Regulates behavior based on judgment and foresight
- Judgment
- Ability to develop long-term goals
- Reasoning, concentration, abstraction

Parietal Lobe
- Understand sensory input such as texture, size, shape, and spatial relationships
- Three-dimensional (spatial) perception
- Important for singing, playing musical instruments, and processing nonverbal visual experiences
- Perception of body parts and body position awareness
- Taste impulses for interpretation

Temporal Lobe
- Auditory center for sound interpretation
- Complicated memory patterns
- Wernicke's area for speech

Occipital Lobe
- Primary visual center

Limbic Lobe
- Emotional and visceral patterns connected with survival
- Learning and memory

Two important speech areas of the cerebrum are Broca's area and Wernicke's area. **Broca's area** (speech area), also located in the frontal lobe, is responsible for the formation of words, or speech. **Wernicke's area** (language area) is located in the temporal lobe and allows processing of words into coherent thought and understanding of written or spoken words.

The *hypophysis (pituitary gland)* has two lobes, each releasing specific hormones into the circulation under the regulation of the hypothalamus. The pituitary is often referred to as the "master gland" because of its control of numerous hormonal functions. However, the hypothalamus actually controls its functions.

The *cerebellum* receives immediate and continuous information about the condition of the muscles, joints, and tendons. Cerebellar function enables a person to:

- Keep an extremity from overshooting an intended target
- Move from one skilled movement to another in an orderly sequence
- Predict distance or gauge the speed with which one is approaching an object
- Control voluntary movement
- Maintain equilibrium

Unlike the motor cortex, cerebellar control of the body is **ipsilateral** (situated on the same side). The right side of the cerebellum controls the right side of the body, and the left cerebellum controls the left side of the body.

The brainstem includes the midbrain, pons, and medulla. The functions of these structures are presented in Table 41-2. Throughout the brainstem are special cells that constitute the **reticular activating system (RAS)**, which controls awareness and alertness. For example, this tissue awakens a person from sleep when presented with a stimulus such as loud noise or pain or when it is time to awaken. The reticular formation area has many connections with the cerebrum, the rest of the brainstem, and the cerebellum.

Circulation in the Brain. Circulation in the brain originates from the carotid and vertebral arteries (Fig. 41-3). The internal carotid arteries branch into the anterior cerebral artery (ACA) and middle cerebral artery (MCA), the largest ones. The two posterior vertebral arteries become the basilar artery, which then divides into two posterior cerebral arteries. The anterior, middle, and posterior cerebral arteries are joined together by small communicating arteries to form a ring at the base of the brain known as the **circle of Willis.**

The *middle* cerebral artery supplies the lateral surface of the cerebrum from about the mid-temporal lobe upward (i.e., the area for hearing and upper body motor and sensory neurons). The *anterior* cerebral artery supplies the midline, or medial, aspect of the same area (i.e., the lower body motor and sensory neurons). The *posterior* cerebral arteries supply the area from the mid-temporal region down and back (occipital lobe), as well as much of the brainstem. When blood flow is interrupted in any of these arteries (e.g., by a clot), the area of the brain being supplied is affected and may not function as it should.

The *blood-brain barrier (BBB)* seems to exist because the endothelial cells of the cerebral capillaries are joined tightly together. This barrier keeps some substances in the bloodstream out of the cerebrospinal circulation and out of brain tissue. Substances that can pass through the BBB include oxygen, glucose, carbon dioxide, alcohol, anesthetics, and water. Large molecules such as albumin, any substance bound to albumin, and many antibiotics are prevented from crossing the barrier.

Cerebrospinal fluid (CSF) also circulates, surrounds, and cushions the brain and spinal cord. While moving through the subarachnoid space, the fluid is continuously produced by the choroid plexus, reabsorbed by the arachnoid villi, and then channeled into the superior sagittal sinus. Expanded areas of subarachnoid space, where there are large amounts of CSF, are called *cisterns.* The largest one is the lumbar cistern, the site of lumbar puncture, from the level of the second lumbar vertebra to the second sacral vertebra (L2-S2).

TABLE 41-2 Brainstem Functions

Medulla
- Cardiac-slowing center
- Respiratory center
- Cranial nerves IX (glossopharyngeal), X (vagus), XI (accessory), and XII (hypoglossal) emerge from the medulla, as do portions of cranial nerves VII (facial) and VIII (vestibulocochlear)

Pons
- Cardiac acceleration and vasoconstriction centers
- Pneumotaxic center helps control respiratory pattern and rate
- Four cranial nerves originate from the pons: V (trigeminal), VI (abducens), VII (facial), and VIII (vestibulocochlear)

Midbrain
- Contains the cerebral aqueduct or aqueduct of Sylvius
- Location of periaqueductal gray, which may abolish pain when stimulated
- Cranial nerve nuclei III (oculomotor) and IV (trochlear) located here

Spinal Cord

The spinal cord controls body movement (MOBILITY); regulates organ function; processes sensory information from the extremities, trunk, and many internal organs; and transmits information to and from the brain. It contains H-shaped **gray matter** (neuron cell bodies) that is surrounded by **white matter**

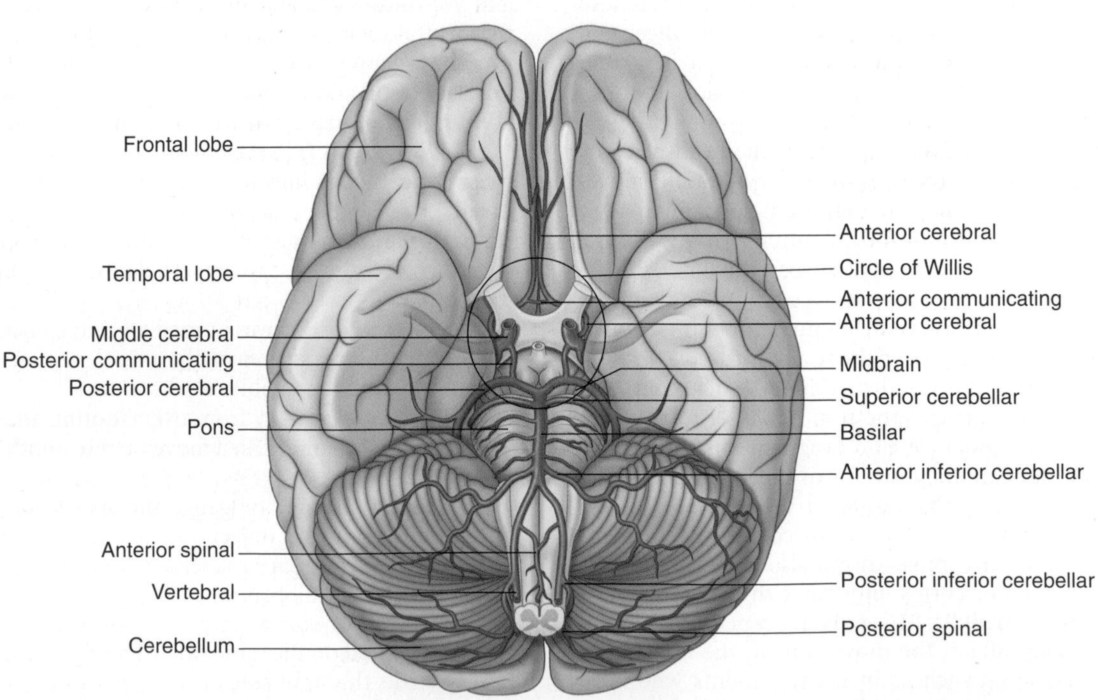

FIG. 41-3 Cerebral circulation and the circle of Willis at the base of the brain.

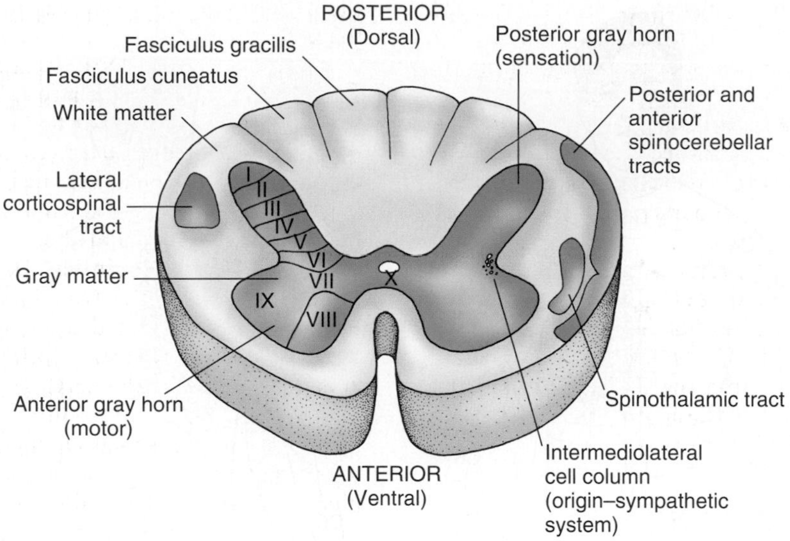

FIG. 41-4 A cross section of the spinal cord showing the common tracts.

(myelinated axons). The white matter is divided into posterior, lateral, and anterior columns. Groups of cells in the white matter (ascending and descending tracts) have been fairly well identified (Fig. 41-4).

Ascending Tracts. **Ascending tracts** originate in the spinal cord and end in the brain. Three groups of ascending tracts are important for understanding the patient with neurologic problems: spinothalamic tracts, spinocerebellar tracts, and fasciculi gracilis and cuneatus (posterior white columns).

As the name indicates, *spinothalamic* tracts begin in the spinal cord with most ending in the thalamus. These tracts carry SENSORY PERCEPTION of pain, temperature, light touch, and pressure. The axon fibers from the cells cross to the opposite side and then continue up to the thalamus. Some branches end in the medulla and pons.

Spinocerebellar tracts begin in the spinal cord and end in the cerebellum. The *posterior* spinocerebellar tract transmits impulses of **proprioception** (awareness of position and movements of body parts) or movement, mostly from the lower extremities. The impulses enter the posterior gray horn and synapse with tracts contained in the spinal cord. Spinocerebellar axons then connect on the *same,* or ipsilateral, side. These axons begin at the second lumbar level and ascend to the medulla and then, with additional synapses to neurons, to the cerebellum.

The *anterior* spinocerebellar tract begins lower in the lumbar spine than does the posterior tract. These fibers cross immediately and ascend as an opposite-side tract, transmitting proprioceptive impulses from the lower extremities. The fibers cross again in the midbrain on their way to the cerebellum. Because these fibers have crossed the midline twice, the sensations end on the side on which they started.

The *posterior white columns* transmit this information to the thalamus:

- The sensory perception of the position, location, and proprioception or orientation and movement of the body and its parts including muscles, joints, and tendons
- Vibratory sense
- Light touch from the skin
- Localization

Most of the fibers ascend on the *same* side as their origin to the medulla, where they cross and then synapse in the thalamus, with termination in the parietal lobe. This tract allows a person to feel an exact point of pressure on the skin. Recognition of pressure includes the shape of an object (with eyes closed), movement across the skin (a number being written), and awareness of two points of touch close together (two-point discrimination).

Descending Tracts. **Descending tracts** *begin* in the brain and *end* in the spinal cord. The major descending tract of importance for understanding neurologic problems is the lateral *corticospinal,* or *pyramidal,* tract. The corticospinal tract originates in the motor cortex of the frontal lobe and portions of the parietal lobe. The lateral tract fibers cross to the opposite side at the level of the medulla. After crossing, the fibers descend and synapse with interneurons of the gray matter in the spinal cord. These few fibers connect directly with lower motor neurons (LMNs). The cervical spine has a high concentration of fibers synapsing with interneurons, which possibly reflects the complexity of hand and finger movements.

The motor neurons of the other descending tracts and the basal ganglia used to be referred to as an *extrapyramidal system.* It was thought that pyramidal neurons caused voluntary muscle activity and that extrapyramidal neurons caused automatic or involuntary muscle action. However, all of the descending tracts and the basal ganglia are necessary for MOBILITY. The term *extrapyramidal* is still often used clinically, meaning *abnormal spontaneous movement.*

Peripheral Nervous System: Structure and Function

The peripheral nervous system (PNS) is composed of the spinal nerves, cranial nerves, and autonomic nervous system.

There are 31 pairs of spinal nerves (8 cervical, 12 thoracic, 5 lumbar, 5 sacral, and 1 coccygeal) exiting from the spinal cord. Each of the nerves has a posterior and an anterior branch. The posterior branch carries sensory information (SENSORY PERCEPTION) to the cord *(afferent pathway).* The anterior branch transmits motor impulses (MOBILITY) to the muscles of the body *(efferent pathway).*

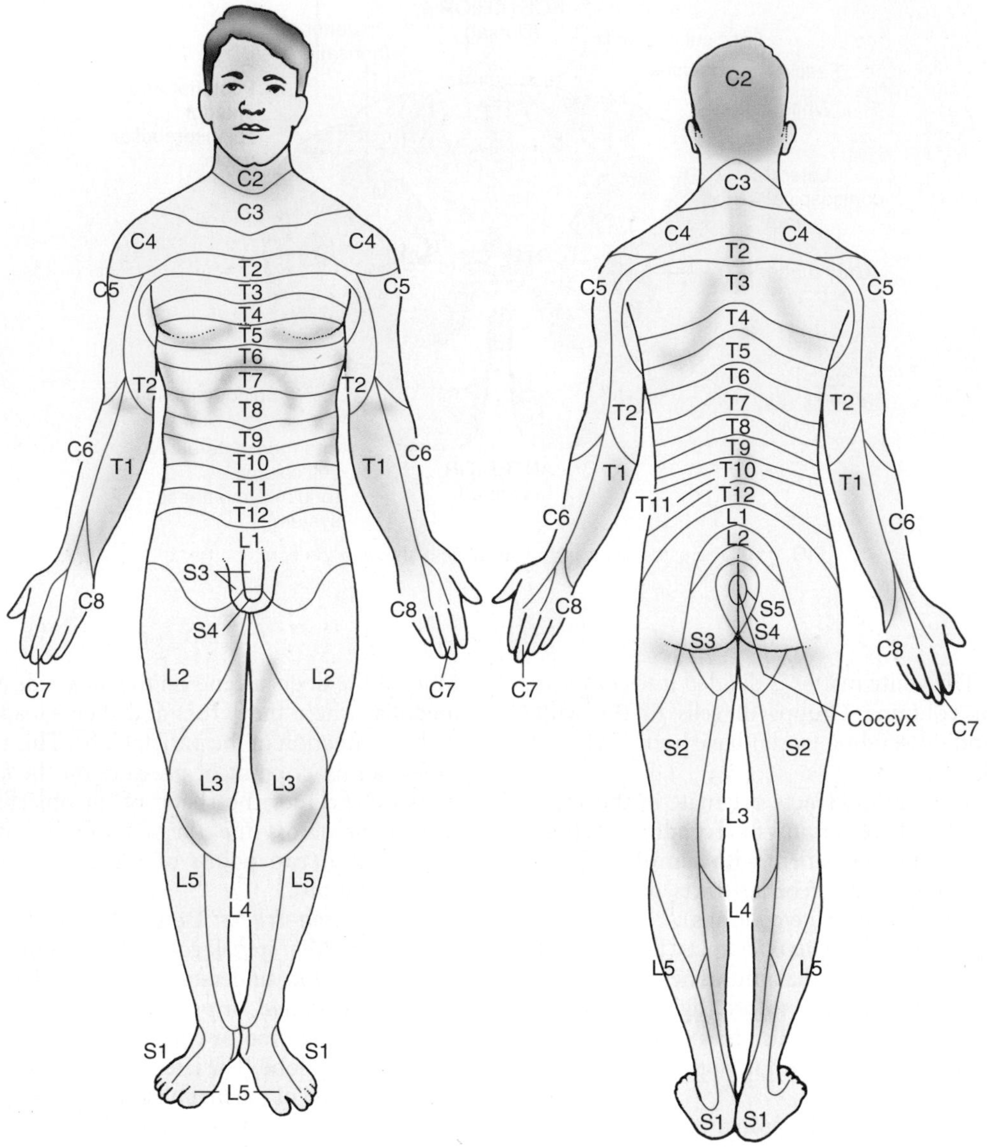

FIG. 41-5 Dermatomes (cutaneous innervation of spinal nerves). *C*, Cervical; *L*, lumbar; *S*, sacral; *T*, thoracic.

Each spinal nerve is responsible for the muscle innervation and sensory reception of a given area of the body. The cervical and thoracic spinal nerves are relatively close to their areas of responsibility, whereas the lumbar and sacral spinal nerves are some distance from theirs. Because the spinal cord ends between L1 and L2, the axons of the lumbar and sacral cord extend downward before exiting at the appropriate intervertebral foramen. The area controlled by each spinal nerve is roughly reflected in the dermatomes. **Dermatomes** represent sensory input from spinal nerves to specific areas of the skin (Fig. 41-5). For example, the patient with an injury to cervical spinal nerves C6 and C7 has sensory changes in the thumb, index finger, middle finger, middle of the palm, and back of the hand.

Sensory receptors throughout the body monitor and transmit impulses of pain, temperature, touch, vibration, pressure, visceral sensation, and proprioception. Sensory receptors also monitor and transmit the sensory perceptions of the special senses—vision, taste, smell, and hearing.

The cell bodies of the anterior spinal nerves are located in the anterior gray matter (anterior horn) of each level in the spinal cord. The anterior motor neurons are also referred to as *lower motor neurons.* As each nerve axon leaves the spinal cord, it joins other spinal nerves to form **plexuses** (clusters of nerves). Plexuses continue as trunks, divisions, and cords and finally branch into individual peripheral nerves.

The **reflex arc** is a closed circuit of spinal and peripheral nerves and therefore requires no control by the brain (Fig. 41-6).

Reflexes consist of sensory input from:

- Skeletal muscles, tendons, skin, organs, and special senses
- Small cells in the spinal cord lying between the posterior and anterior gray matter (interneurons)
- Anterior motor neurons, along with the muscles they innervate

There are 12 *cranial nerves.* Their number, name, origin, type, and function are summarized in Table 41-3. Cranial nerve function is an important part of the nursing assessment of the patient with a neurologic problem. For example, cranial nerves II, III, IV, and VI are important for assessment of the patient with a stroke or traumatic brain injury.

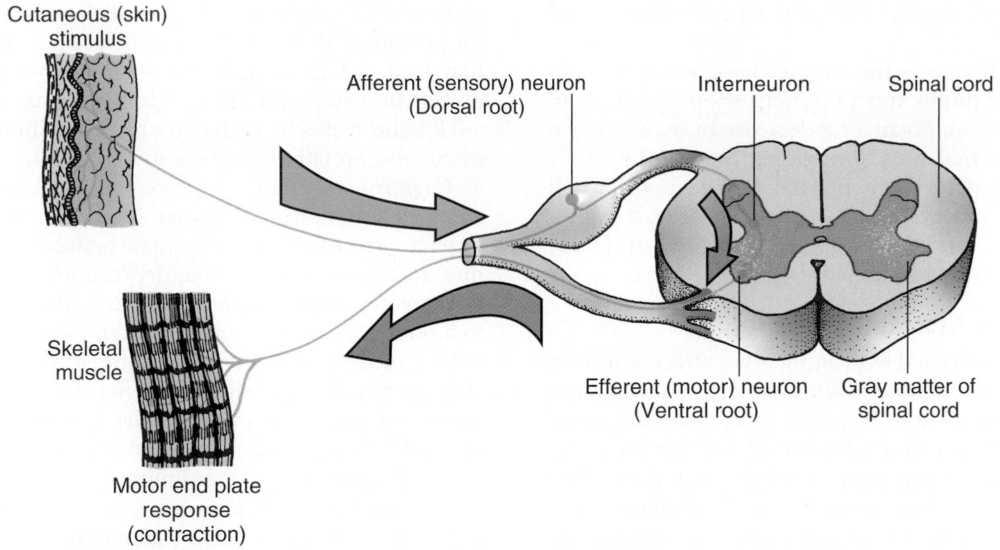

FIG. 41-6 An example of reflex activity. Stimulation of skin results in involuntary muscle contraction (reflex arc).

TABLE 41-3 Origins, Types, and Functions of the Cranial Nerves

CRANIAL NERVE	ORIGIN	TYPE	FUNCTION
I: Olfactory	Olfactory bulb	Sensory	Smell
II: Optic	Midbrain	Sensory	Central and peripheral vision
III: Oculomotor	Midbrain	Motor to eye muscles	Eye movement via medial and lateral rectus and inferior oblique and superior rectus muscles; lid elevation via the levator muscle
		Parasympathetic-motor	Pupil constriction; ciliary muscles
IV: Trochlear	Lower midbrain	Motor	Eye movement via superior oblique muscles
V: Trigeminal	Pons	Sensory	Sensory perception from skin of face and scalp and mucous membranes of mouth and nose
		Motor	Muscles of mastication (chewing)
VI: Abducens	Inferior pons	Motor	Eye movement via lateral rectus muscles
VII: Facial	Inferior pons	Sensory	Pain and temperature from ear area; deep sensations from the face; taste from anterior two thirds of the tongue
		Motor	Muscles of the face and scalp
		Parasympathetic-motor	Lacrimal, submandibular, and sublingual salivary glands
VIII: Vestibulocochlear	Pons-medulla junction	Sensory	Hearing Equilibrium
IX: Glossopharyngeal	Medulla	Sensory	Pain and temperature from ear; taste and sensations from posterior one third of tongue and pharynx
		Motor	Skeletal muscles of the throat
		Parasympathetic-motor	Parotid glands
X: Vagus	Medulla	Sensory	Pain and temperature from ear; sensations from pharynx, larynx, thoracic and abdominal viscera
		Motor	Muscles of the soft palate, larynx, and pharynx
		Parasympathetic-motor	Thoracic and abdominal viscera; cells of secretory glands; cardiac and smooth muscle innervation to the level of the splenic flexure
XI: Accessory	Medulla (anterior gray horn of the cervical spine)	Motor	Skeletal muscles of the pharynx and larynx and sternocleidomastoid and trapezius muscles
XII: Hypoglossal	Medulla	Motor	Skeletal muscles of the tongue

Autonomic Nervous System: Structure and Function

The **autonomic nervous system (ANS)** is composed of two parts: the sympathetic nervous system (SNS) and the parasympathetic nervous system. ANS functions are not usually under conscious control but may be altered in some people by using biofeedback and other methods.

The SNS cells originate in the gray matter of the spinal cord from T1 through L2 or L3. This part of the ANS is considered *thoracolumbar* because of its anatomic location. The SNS stimulates the functions of the body needed for "fight or flight" (e.g., heart and respiratory rate). It also inhibits certain functions not needed in urgent and stressful situations.

The parasympathetic cells originate in the gray matter of the sacral area of the spinal cord (from S2 through S4) plus portions of cranial nerves III, VII, IX, and X *(craniosacral)*. The parasympathetic nervous system can slow body functions when needed and contribute to digestion and reproduction ("feed and breed").

Parasympathetic fibers to the organs have some sensory ability in addition to motor function. Sensory perceptions of irritation, stretching of an organ, or a decrease in tissue oxygen are transmitted to the thalamus through pathways not yet fully understood. Because pain from internal organs is often felt below the body wall innervated by the spinal nerve, it is presumed that there are connections between the viscera and body structure that relay pain sensation.

Neurologic Changes Associated with Aging

Neurologic changes associated with aging often affect MOBILITY and SENSORY PERCEPTION. *Motor changes* in late adulthood can cause slower movement and response time and decreased sensory perception (Chart 41-1). Any problems that affect the nerves, bones, muscles, or joints also affect motor and therefore ADL ability. Determining functional status—a combination of COGNITION, MOBILITY, and SENSORY PERCEPTION—is a recommended core measure for patients with complex chronic conditions (www.cms.gov).

Sensory changes in older adults can also affect their daily activities. Pupils decrease in size, which restricts the amount of light entering the eye, and adapt more slowly. Older adults need increased lighting to see. Chapter 48 describes collaborative care for persons with hearing loss. Touch sensation decreases, which may lead to falls because the older person may not feel small objects or a step underfoot. Vibration sense may be lost in the ankles and feet. These changes can contribute to falls. (See the discussion on fall prevention in Chapter 2.)

Cognitive functions of perceiving, registering, storing, and using information often change as a normal part of aging. Therefore it is important to differentiate between these expected findings and those of dementia, depression, and delirium. Failure to correctly diagnosis pathologic cognitive problems may lead to a poor patient outcome. For example, unsafe driving can be both a cause and a result of cognitive changes. The cognitive changes may be reversible, allowing the person to continue to drive once the condition is resolved, or irreversible, indicating the health care provider may need to assist with advice or efforts to stop the person from continuing to drive (Iverson et al., 2010).

Intellect does not decline as a result of aging. However, a person with certain health problems may have a decrease in cognitive level. *Cognitive decline is frequently caused by drug interactions or toxicity or by an inadequate oxygen supply to the brain.* Some older adults may need more time than a younger person to process questions, learn and process new information, solve problems, or complete analogies.

CHART 41-1 Nursing Focus on the Older Adult

Changes in the Nervous System Related to Aging

PHYSIOLOGIC CHANGES	NURSING IMPLICATIONS	RATIONALES
Slower processing time	Provide sufficient time for the affected older adult to respond to questions and/or direction.	Allowing adequate time for processing helps differentiate normal findings from neurologic deterioration.
Recent memory loss	Reinforce teaching by repetition, using written teaching, and employing memory aids like electronic alarms or applications for electronic devices that provide recurrent alerts.	Greatest loss of brain weight is in the white matter of the frontal lobe. Intellect is not impaired, but the learning process is slowed. Repetition helps the patient learn new information and recall it when needed.
Decreased sensory perception of touch	Remind the patient to look where his or her feet are placed when walking. Instruct the patient to wear shoes that provide good support when walking. If the patient is unable, change his or her position frequently (every hour) while he or she is in bed or the chair.	Decreased sensory perception may cause the patient to fall.
Change in perception of pain	Ask the patient to describe the nature and specific characteristics of pain. Monitor additional assessment variables to detect possible health problems.	Accurate and complete nursing assessment ensures that the interventions will be appropriate for the older adult (see Chapter 2).
Change in sleep patterns	Ascertain sleep patterns and preferences. Ask if sleep pattern interferes with ADLs. Adjust the patient's daily schedule to his or her sleep pattern and preference as much as possible (e.g., evening versus morning bath).	Older adults require as much as younger adults. It is more common for older adults to fall asleep early and arise early.
Altered balance and/or decreased coordination	Instruct the patient to move slowly when changing positions. If needed, advise the patient to hold on to handrails when ambulating. Assess the need for an ambulatory aid, such as a cane.	The patient may fall if moving too quickly. Assistive and adaptive aids provide support and prevent falls.
Increased risk for infection	Monitor carefully for infection.	Older adults often have structural deterioration of microglia, the cells responsible for cell-mediated immune response in the central nervous system (CNS).
Changes in sleep patterns	Assess sleep habits. Provide usual bedtime routines. Decrease noise and light at night.	Age-related changes include more time in bed spent awake before falling asleep, reduced sleep time, daytime napping, and changes in circadian rhythm leading to "early to bed and early to rise."

Subtle memory changes can occur for many older people. Long-term memory seems better than recall (recent) or immediate (registration) memory. Older adults may need more time to retrieve information. These changes may be partly due to the loss of cerebral neurons, which is associated with the aging process.

Biorhythms vary among people. Circadian responses are reduced in older adults, and the sleep-wake cycle may become less responsive to stimuli that signal patterns of sleep. Older adults may experience changes in sleep architecture and sleeping patterns (Touhy & Jett, 2014). For example, older adults are more likely to go bed earlier and experience an earlier awakening compared with younger adults. They are also more likely to experience more periods of wakefulness lasting 30 or more minutes during the night. On average, an older person needs as much sleep as a younger person but is more likely to nap in the afternoon.

Sleep deprivation at any age can lead to significant changes in COGNITION. Sleep deprivation, common in many inpatient settings, is related to both the earlier onset and greater severity of delirium. Lack of sleep can worsen symptoms of mild dementia. Sleep deprivation can also interfere with normal immune function and wound healing. Interrupted sleep and sleep deprivation can also impair physical function and self-management. Sleep and rest are both necessary for health. Nurses can review sleep habits and promote a good sleep environment, including periods of rest and do-not-disturb during patient care (see the Quality Improvement box).

QUALITY IMPROVEMENT QSEN

Unit-based Quality Improvement Project Promotes Patient Sleep

Faraklas, I., Holt, B., Tran, S., Lin, H., Saffle, J., & Cochran, A. (2013). Impact of a nursing-driven sleep hygiene protocol on sleep quality. *Journal of Burn Care and Research, 34*(2), 249-254.

Sleep is important to cognition. In this report, a nurse-driven protocol and the use of a sound meter to monitor noise was used to evaluate patient perceptions of sleep in acutely ill and burned adults. Noise reduction, reduced lighting, and prioritizing and clustering care activities to minimize sleep interruptions between midnight and 5 AM were phased in over several months in a single unit. When the protocol was fully implemented, patient self-reports indicated an improvement in falling asleep and going back to sleep compared with self-reports before the protocol was implemented. Because it is a nurse-driven protocol, it can be implemented and adapted in quick cycles to meet quality improvement goals. For example, other studies confirm that the use of a sound meter can contribute to noise reduction. The cost of sound meters is small (less than $25), and they can be placed in high impact areas, including alarm stations or where staff commonly converse. The sound meter detects decibels providing immediate feedback to staff about high noise levels that can disrupt patient sleep.

Commentary: Implications for Practice and Research

Steps to improve patient sleep can be implemented without increasing the workload of nurses or increasing the cost of care. Both light reduction and clustering care activities require thoughtful planning and collaboration with health care team members so that the period of planned uninterrupted rest for a patient is recognized. The immediate feedback from a device to monitor decibels is helpful to noise reduction. Although this is a single unit report, the protocol can be used in a variety of inpatient settings. Phasing in interventions of light reduction, noise monitoring, and clustering activities contributes to successful changes in practice.

Mental status may be impaired as a result of infection, hypoxia, and hypoglycemia or hyperglycemia. These conditions are usually easily assessed and managed. During an acute change in mental status, assess the adult for peripheral oxygenation (Spo_2), serum glucose (fingerstick), and potential infection (e.g., fever, urine with sediment or odor, sputum production, red or draining wound). *Often a decrease in mental status is a key early sign of an infectious process in the older patient, and a urinary tract infection is a common site.*

ASSESSMENT METHODS

Patient History

Obtain information from the patient about health problems and function as outlined in Chart 41-2. During your introduction, note the patient's appearance and assess his or her speech, affect, and movement. If he or she seems to have cognitive deficits or has trouble speaking or hearing, ask a family member or significant other to stay during the interview to help obtain an accurate history. Be sure that glasses, contact lenses, and hearing aids are available if the patient wears any of these aids.

Ask the patient about his or her medical history to determine its association with the current health problem. Inquire about the ability to perform ADLs. Knowing the level of daily activity helps establish a baseline for later comparison as the patient improves or worsens. Ask whether the patient is right-handed or left-handed. This information is important for several reasons:

- The patient may be somewhat stronger on the dominant side, which is expected.
- The effects of cerebral injury or disease are more pronounced if the dominant hemisphere is involved.

Ask about family medical history such as stroke or myocardial infarction (MI) (heart attack). Some diseases occur more often in certain groups of people and may be caused by a genetic influence or other reason. For example, it has been long established that Huntington disease is inherited. A number of other neurologic diseases have a genetic basis, such as neuromuscular disorders, migraine headaches, and epilepsy. These genetic risks are described with specific neurologic diseases found later in this unit.

Physical Assessment

Compare each assessment with the patient's baseline, as well as between right and left sides and between upper and lower extremities. *Two types of neurologic assessments may be performed—a complete assessment and a focused assessment.* Some focused assessments are specifically designed to be rapid to ease repetition when recurrent neurologic assessments are needed to monitor the patient's condition over time. The type chosen depends on the information needed, the time available with the patient, and your clinical skill level. Advanced practice registered nurses (APRNs) and other health care providers usually perform the complete assessment, with selected parts done by the nurse. It is important that you understand each component of the assessment and what the results might indicate.

Complete Neurologic Assessment

A complete neurologic assessment includes a history (see Chart 41-2) and evaluation of mental status (consciousness and cognition), cranial nerves (see Table 41-3), MOBILITY and motor

CHART 41-2 Best Practice for Patient Safety & Quality Care QSEN

Establishing a Nursing Database: History

Demographic Data
- Age
- Gender

Past Medical History
- Patient's medical history
- Family's medical history
- Previous injuries or congenital problems
- Sleep disorders (e.g., insomnia, sleep apnea)
- Chronic diseases:
  - Hypertension and cardiovascular disease
  - Diabetes mellitus and thyroid disorders
  - Lung disease and conditions that cause hypoxemia
- Previous neurologic problems:
  - Headaches
  - Seizures
  - Head or spine trauma
  - Eye problems
  - Brain injury from stroke or trauma

Current History
- Current symptoms:
  - Blurred vision
  - Headache
  - Speech or swallowing difficulty
  - Numbness, tingling
  - Weakness, clumsiness
  - Bowel or bladder difficulties
  - Nausea or vomiting
  - Personality changes
  - Seizures
  - Disorientation or other change in mental status
- Allergies:
  - Food
  - Medications
  - Environment
- Pain tolerance:
  - Medications taken for pain
  - Behaviors to reduce pain
- Medications:
  - Prescribed
  - Illicit
  - Over-the-counter
- ADLs

Social History
- Usual recreational activities
- Level of physical activity each day
- Hobbies
- Alcohol consumption and use of recreational drugs
- Smoking, use of any tobacco products
- Sleep habits:
  - Changes in pattern, duration, or intensity
- Work history:
  - Exposure to toxic agents
- Ethnic and cultural background
- Handedness (right or left)
- Educational background

system function (e.g., range, strength, posture, abnormal movements), deep tendon reflexes, sensation (e.g., pain, touch, temperature, vibration, and position), and cerebellar function (gait, balance, and coordination). Although not all components of a complete assessment are completed by the nurse, noting abnormalities at baseline or with disease progression is important. During any neurologic assessment, look for asymmetry, such as subtle unequal movement in the facial muscles.

The complete neurologic assessment is used by the health care provider to consider whether a single lesion or more than one site in the nervous system may be contributing to abnormal physical assessment findings. A complete neurologic assessment will also help establish if a lesion or injury is in the CNS, PNS, or both. If the lesion or injury is in the CNS, a complete neurologic assessment can further help the health care provider determine if abnormalities are in the cortex, below the cortex, or multifocal. These findings, along with patient history, help determine the urgency of treatment. For example, a sudden unilateral loss in motor function and sensation is an emergency requiring a stroke center and staff with expertise to diagnose and intervene during a "**brain attack**." A gradual unilateral loss or a variable loss (with waxing and waning symptoms) may be less urgent and not require stroke center expertise. Generally, the nurse completes a focused or rapid assessment to detect concerning changes.

Assessment of Mental Status. Mental status assessment is generally divided into assessment of *consciousness* and *cognition*. Consciousness is the ability to be aware of the environment, an object, and oneself; consciousness is often documented as level of consciousness (LOC). Consciousness usually refers to the degree of alertness or the amount of stimulation needed to engage a patient's attention and can range from *alert* to *coma*. When alert, the patient is awake and easily engaged. A patient in coma appears to be asleep and does not rouse or react despite vigorous or noxious simulation.

! NURSING SAFETY PRIORITY QSEN

Action Alert

Be aware that a change in level of consciousness and orientation is an early and reliable indication that central neurologic function has declined! The patient who is described as ***alert*** is awake and responsive. A patient may be alert but not oriented to person, place, or time. Patients who are less than alert are labeled *lethargic, stuporous,* or *comatose*. A ***lethargic*** patient is drowsy but is easily awakened. One who is arousable only with vigorous or painful stimulation is ***stuporous***. The ***comatose*** patient is unconscious and cannot be aroused.

After determining alertness, the next step is to evaluate orientation. Once the patient's attention is engaged, ask him or her questions to determine orientation. Varying the sequence of questioning on repeated assessments prevents the patient from memorizing the answers. Responses that indicate orientation include ability to answer questions about person, place, and time such as:
- The patient's ability to relate the onset of symptoms
- The name of his or her physician/nurse practitioner/nurse
- The year and month
- His or her address
- The name of the referring physician or health care agency

Time of day, drug therapy, and the need for sleep, glucose, or oxygen may affect these responses, so be sure to link any changes in orientation with respiratory status, changes in drug regimens or use of intermittent drugs, time of day/sleep deprivation, or current serum glucose values. Education, occupation, interest, culture, anxiety, and depression affect performance during assessment of mental status. What is considered "normal" may not be so for a particular patient, so adaptation of questions suggested for mental status assessment may be necessary. Be alert to both *sudden* and *subtle* changes, particularly when changes are noted by family members or others who know the patient.

NCLEX EXAMINATION CHALLENGE

Physiological Integrity

During a client's neurologic assessment, the nurse finds that he is arousable after light touch combined with a loud voice. How does the nurse document this client's level of consciousness?
A. Stuporous
B. Lethargic
C. Comatose
D. Drowsy

COGNITION is intellectual function. It is processes of thought that embody perception, attention, visuospatial recognition, language, learning, memory and executive functions of comprehension, insight, problem solving, reasoning, decision making, creativity, and metacognition (Giddens, 2013). Cognition typically is evaluated in a rapid or focused manner using tests of memory and attention that require verbal or written ability (Chart 41-3). *Loss of memory, especially recent memory, tends to be an early sign of neurologic problems.* Three types of memory can be tested: long-term (remote) memory, recall (recent) memory, and immediate memory.

Remote, or long-term, **memory** can be tested by asking patients about their birth date, schools attended, the city of birth, or anything from the past that can be verified. Nurses often ask the name of the patient's contact person listed on the admission form.

Recall (recent) **memory** can be tested during the history and checked on the medical record:
- The accuracy of the medical history
- Dates of clinic or physician appointments
- The time of admission
- Health care providers seen within the past few days
- Mode of transportation to the hospital or clinic

Immediate (new) **memory** is tested by giving the patient three unrelated words, such as "apple," "street," and "chair," and asking him or her to repeat the words to make sure they were heard. After about 5 minutes, while continuing with the examination, ask the patient to repeat the words. An alternative to this method is to give a three-step command and observe whether it is carried out correctly. For example, "Pick up the paper, fold it in half, and draw a square on it."

To assess *attention,* ask the patient to repeat a series of three numbers, such as 4, 7, and 3. The series is increased by one number with each successful repetition until seven or eight digits are achieved. If the patient has difficulty at any level (cannot repeat the series), repeat the numbers. If the patient cannot repeat, stop the procedure. Next, ask the patient to repeat the numbers backward, starting again with three digits and increasing by one each time. Normally, a person should be able to repeat five to eight digits forward and four to six backward. The serial-seven test to determine attention may also be used. The patient is asked to count backward from 100 by 7 (the examiner stops when the patient reaches 65 successfully). An alternative approach is to ask the person to subtract by three or to add forward by five. Clinical judgment and assessment skills are used when deciding which of these tests to use.

CHART 41-3 Best Practice for Patient Safety & Quality Care QSEN

Assessment of Cognition

Perform assessment at the following care interactions:
- On admission to and discharge from an institutional care setting
- Upon transfer from one care setting to another
- Every 8 to 12 hours throughout hospitalization
- Following major changes in pharmacotherapy
- With behavior that is unusual for the person and/or inappropriate to the situation

Assess and document (noting "sometimes," "frequently," or "always" as observed):
- Does the patient respond to voice; require being shaken awake to communicate; doze off during a conversation or when no activities occur; or not respond to voice or touch?
- Is speech clear and understandable; disoriented to person, place, or time; inappropriate; or incomprehensible/garbled?
- Can the patient name the place, reason for admission or visit, month, and age?
- Can the patient follow one-step commands: open/close eyes; make fist/let go?
- Can the patient switch to a different topic or activity versus loses the thread of the conversation or is easily distracted (inattention)?
- Can the patient recognize a familiar object and its purpose or a familiar person and name relationship?
- Can the patient respond relevantly and quickly?
- Does the patient have unrealistic thoughts or act distrustful of others (e.g., does not dare to take his/her medicine; says that people are "listening," etc.)?
- Is the patient cooperative, euphoric, hostile, anxious, withdrawn, or guarded?
- Is the patient's appearance, behavior, or facial expression appropriate for the situation?

Other assessments of COGNITION include examining language and executive function. Many *language* skills can be assessed during the initial interview. Language skills include understanding the spoken or written word and being able to speak or write. The patient demonstrates understanding by following directions on admission (e.g., getting undressed). If he or she hesitates, it may be the patient does not understand the vocabulary or word. When speech hesitation or performance hesitation occurs, point to objects and ask the patient to name them, such as the door or bed. Speech is assessed as being normal, slow, garbled, difficult to find words, or other impairments. If the change in speech is new and represents a deterioration from a previous ability to communicate, this change must be urgently reported to the health care provider because it may indicate a stroke, new onset of confusion, or other serious neurologic condition (Rattray et al., 2011).

The health care provider or speech-language pathologist (SLP) completes additional language tests such as reading comprehension. This is done by writing a simple command and giving it to the patient (e.g., "close your eyes"). Written language can be tested by asking the patient to write a sentence. The clinician must remember that some patients cannot read or write or may speak a language different from that of the clinician. In this case, modify the examination accordingly such as having the patient copy something that has been drawn (e.g., a cross, circle, diamond, or square).

Executive function allows for flexibility, adaptability, and goal directedness; it determines the contents of consciousness, supervises voluntary action, and is future oriented. Several approaches are used to assess executive function. Although most tests of executive function are not done by the nurse, it is important to identify and document altered executive function because this type of impairment can place the patient at risk for harm. To identify whether such a risk exists and to ensure that the need for further specialized evaluation is recognized, begin to assess the patient's judgment during the interview. Did he or she make rational decisions in dealing with his or her symptoms? Ask questions such as "What would you do if stopped for speeding?" and "What would you do if there was a fire in the wastepaper basket?" Asking the meaning of proverbs (e.g., "A stitch in time saves nine" or "A rolling stone gathers no moss") provides information about insight and abstraction. These questions might also elicit important information about a new onset of a confusional state. People from countries other than the United States or young adults may be unfamiliar with abstract proverbs. Finally, ask the patient to follow a two-step motor process such as "Show me two fingers with your right hand" (you can illustrate with your right hand) and then ask him or her to do the same thing with the other hand (removing the visual cue of your hand before asking for step two). Consult a professional interpreter to assist with language and culturally appropriate phrasing before making an evaluation of executive function to ensure that both sudden and subtle changes are identified accurately.

There are several rapid tests of COGNITION useful in clinical settings. One example is the Brief Interview for Mental Status (BIMS), commonly used in long-term care settings (Saliba et al., 2012). The BIMS consists of three categories. The first category is "repetition of three words." The nurse tells the patient that he or she will hear three words and then be asked to repeat them. Allow five seconds to pass between stating the words and asking for repetition. Then the three words are verbally repeated and placed into a category (e.g., blue, a color) by the assessor but not yet retested. Next, "temporal orientation" is evaluated by asking the patient to identify the year, month, and day of week. The third category of assessment is "recall." The patient is asked to name the same three words used earlier and the assessor determines if the words are recalled independently, after coaching by naming the category, or not recalled at all. Patients can achieve scores of 0 to 15 by adding across the three categories. Scores below 8 indicate severe cognitive impairment (Saliba et al., 2012). Cognitive impairment can be permanent or temporary.

An example of permanent cognitive impairment is **dementia**, an irreversible and degenerative condition described in Chapter 42. Two screening tools useful for identifying dementia that can be completed quickly are the clock drawing test and the Mini-Cog, and each require less than 3 minutes to complete. An example of a longer test is the Mini-Mental State Examination (3MS; average time to administer, 17 minutes) (Holsinger et al., 2012).

Another consideration in assessing cognition is delirium. **Delirium**, an acute confusional state, is characterized by a new and sudden cognitive impairment (Touhy & Jett, 2014). Symptoms tend to fluctuate over the course of a day and include disturbances in consciousness, attention, memory deficits, and perceptual disturbances. Delirium can also be manifested by delusional (paranoid) thoughts and behavior. Delirium is a medical emergency and specifically places geriatric patients at risk for harm and prolonged cognitive impairment. Once a patient is identified as having delirium, reassessment should be done every shift.

Early identification and targeted interventions for delirium can decrease the occurrence and severity of delirium. Delirium is associated with significant consequences such as distress (including post-traumatic distress syndrome), prolonged hospital stay, increased morbidity and mortality, and institutionalization (Touhy & Jett, 2014). Two tests to detect new onset of delirium are the Confusion Assessment Method (CAM) and the NEECHAM Confusional Scale (Adamis et al., 2010). The CAM-ICU is used for nonverbal patients (Barr et al., 2013).

Assessment of Cranial Nerves. Cranial nerves are typically tested to establish a baseline from which to compare progress or deterioration. However, they are not routinely tested unless the patient has a suspected problem affecting one or more of the cranial nerves (see Table 41-3). Adding the specific cranial nerves to be tested to the documentation record of a patient with a problem affecting the cranial nerves helps ensure continued comparison and assessment.

Testing pupils is a common cranial nerve test performed by nurses. Pupil constriction is a function of cranial nerve III, the oculomotor nerve. Pupils should be equal in size, round and regular in shape, and react to light and accommodation (**PERRLA**). Estimate the size of both pupils using a millimeter ruler or a pupillometer. Patients who have had eye surgery for cataracts or glaucoma often have irregularly shaped pupils. Those using eye drops for either cataracts or glaucoma may have unequal pupils if only one eye is being treated, and the pupillary response may be altered.

To test for pupil constriction, ask the patient to close his or her eyes and dim the room lights. Bring a penlight in from the side of the patient's head, and shine the light in the eye being tested as soon as the patient opens his or her eyes. The pupil being tested should constrict (**direct response**). The other pupil should also constrict slightly (**consensual response**). To test accommodation, relight the room and ask the patient to focus on a distant object and then immediately look at an object 4 to 5 inches from the nose. The eyes should converge, and the pupils should constrict. Pinpoint, dilated, and nonreactive pupils are late signs of neurologic deterioration (Jarvis, 2016).

Assessment of Motor Function. Throughout the physical assessment, observe the patient for involuntary tremors or movements. Describe these movements as accurately as possible, such as "pill-rolling with the thumbs and fingers at rest" or "intention tremors of both hands" (tremors that occur when the patient tries to do something). These abnormalities can indicate certain diseases, such as multiple sclerosis, or the effects of selected psychotropic drugs. In addition, assess the patient for motor movements that indicate irritability, hyperactivity, or slowed movements. Measure the patient's hand *strength* by asking him or her to grasp and squeeze two fingers of each of your hands. Then compare the grasps for equality of strength. As another means of evaluating strength, try to withdraw the fingers from the patient's grasp and compare the ease or difficulty. He or she should release the grasps on command—another assessment of consciousness and the ability to follow commands.

Collaborate with the physical therapist to test the patient's strength. To test strength against resistance, ask the patient to resist the examiner's bending or straightening of the arm, hand, leg, or foot being tested (Fig. 41-7). A five-point rating scale is commonly used (see Chapter 49, Table 49-2). Always evaluate and compare strength on each side. Compare previous results with current findings, and report all decreases to the health care providers.

Cerebral motor or *brainstem* integrity may also be assessed. Ask the patient to close his or her eyes and hold the arms perpendicular to the body with the palms up for 15 to 30 seconds. If there is a cerebral or brainstem reason for muscle weakness, the arm on the weak side will start to fall, or "drift," with the palm pronating (turning inward). This is called a **pronator drift**. The same can be done for the lower extremities, with the patient lying on his or her stomach with the legs bent upward at the knees. However, it is easier for most patients to sit on the side of the bed and extend the legs outward.

Decortication is abnormal motor movement seen in the patient with lesions that interrupt the corticospinal pathways (Fig. 41-8, *A*). The patient's arms, wrists, and fingers are flexed with internal rotation and plantar flexion of the legs. **Decerebration** is abnormal movement with rigidity characterized by extension of the arms and legs, pronation of the arms, plantar flexion, and opisthotonos (body spasm in which the body is bowed forward) (Fig. 41-8, *B*). Decerebration is usually associated with dysfunction in the brainstem area.

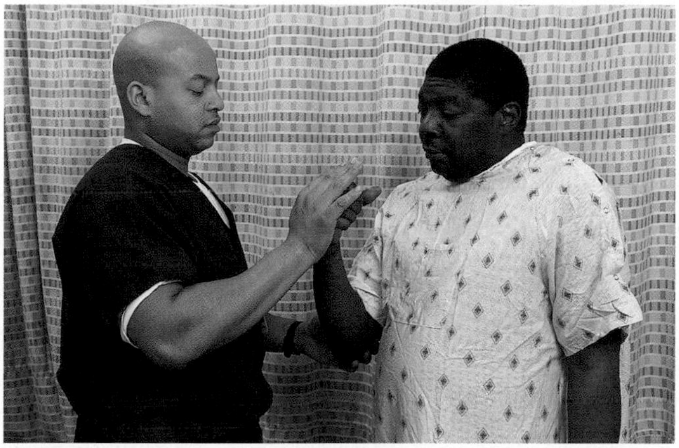

FIG. 41-7 Testing for strength against resistance.

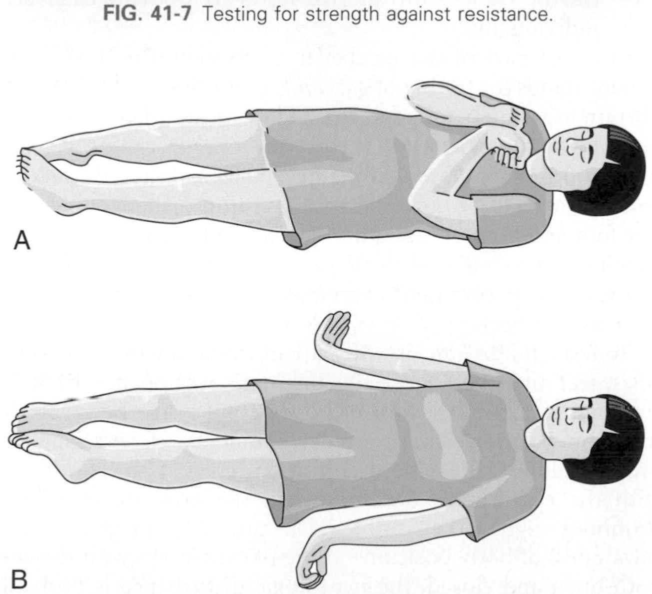

FIG. 41-8 Posturing. **A,** Decorticate posturing. **B,** Decerebrate posturing.

Assessment of Reflex Activity. The health care provider, including the APRN, may assess deep tendon reflexes (DTRs) and superficial (cutaneous) reflexes. The **deep tendon reflexes** of the biceps, triceps, brachioradialis, and quadriceps muscles and of the Achilles tendon can be tested as part of the complete neurologic assessment (Jarvis, 2016). Striking the tendon with the reflex hammer should cause contraction of the muscle. The appropriate muscle contraction indicates an intact reflex arc. The tendon is tapped quickly but not with too much force. If the patient is tensing the muscle, the reflexes will not respond. Having the patient interlock his or her hands and pull outward will help decrease muscle tensing so the reflex can be tested.

The **cutaneous (superficial) reflexes** usually tested are the plantar reflexes and sometimes the abdominal reflexes. The plantar reflex is tested with a pointed (but not sharp) object, such as the handle end of the reflex hammer or the rounded end of bandage scissors. The normal response is plantar flexion of all toes. **Babinski's sign**, a dorsiflexion of the great toe and fanning of the other toes, is abnormal in anyone older than 2 years and represents the presence of central nervous system (CNS) disease. The term "positive Babinski's sign" (abnormal response) and "negative Babinski's sign" (normal response) are clinically used terms but are not correct. Health care providers may also use the terms "upgoing" or "downgoing" to refer to the toes of the stimulated foot. "Upgoing" toes are an abnormal response that indicates the presence of pathology in the CNS. Babinski's sign can occur with drug and alcohol intoxication, after a seizure, or in patients with multiple sclerosis or liver disease.

To test the abdominal reflex, stroke the patient's abdomen in all four quadrants diagonally toward the umbilicus. The umbilicus should deviate toward the stimulus, but obesity may mask the reflex. The abdominal reflex can be absent in both upper and lower motor neuron disease.

Hyperactive reflexes indicate possible upper motor neuron disease, tetanus, or hypocalcemia. *Hypoactive* reflexes may result from lower motor neuron disease (damage to the spinal cord), disease of the neuromuscular junction, muscle disease, or health problems such as diabetes mellitus, hypothyroidism, or hypokalemia.

Asymmetry of reflexes is an important finding because it probably indicates a disease process. The results of reflex testing are recorded by the use of a stick figure and a scale of 0 to 4 (Fig. 41-9). A score of 2 is considered normal, although scores of 1 (hypoactive) or 3 (stronger than normal) may be normal for a particular patient. **Clonus** (also called *myoclonus*) is the sudden, brief, jerking contraction of a muscle or muscle group often seen in seizures.

Assessment of Sensory Function. The assessment of sensory function is done for patients with problems affecting the spinal cord or spinal nerves, such as trauma, intervertebral disk disease, Guillain-Barré syndrome (GBS), tumor, infection, stenosis, or transverse myelitis. The sensory assessment includes pain, superficial and deep sensation, light touch, and proprioception. *Pain and light touch are the most commonly assessed.*

The acuity level of the patient determines how often the sensory assessment is done. For example, patients with acute spinal cord trauma or ascending GBS are assessed every hour until stable and then every 4 hours. As the condition improves, sensory assessment may be needed only once each shift. Findings are documented according to agency protocol. A special spinal cord assessment flow sheet may be used to document

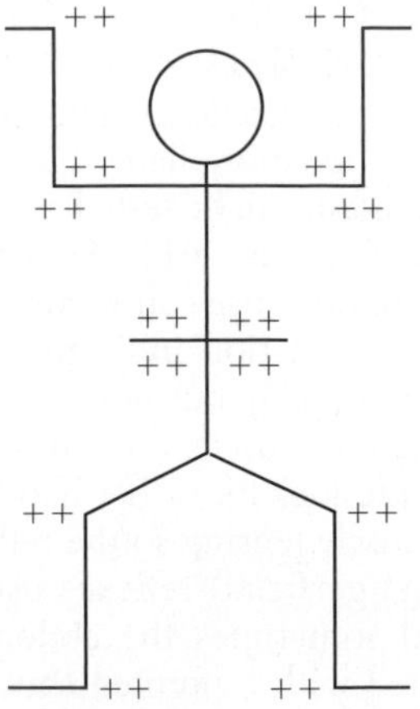

0	Absent, no response
1 (+)	Weaker than normal, hypoactive
2 (++)	Normal
3 (+++)	Stronger or more brisk than normal
4 (++++)	Hyperactive
	(Note: 1 and 3 may be normal for some individuals)

FIG. 41-9 A stick figure and scale for recording reflex activity.

sensory and/or motor findings for the patient with a spinal cord injury.

Pain and temperature sensation are transmitted by the same nerve endings. Therefore if one sensation is tested and found to be intact, it can safely be assumed that the other is intact. Testing temperature sensation can usually be accomplished using a cold reflex hammer and the warm touch of the hand for patients with known or suspected spinal problems.

Assess for *pain perception* with any sharp or dull object, such as the tips of a cotton-tipped applicator. While the patient's eyes are open, demonstrate what will be done. Then ask him or her to keep eyes closed and to indicate whether the touch is sharp or dull. The sharp and dull ends should be changed at random so he or she does not anticipate the next type of stimulus for SENSORY PERCEPTION. Not all areas need to be tested unless a spinal cord injury has occurred. If testing begins on the hands and feet, there is no need to test the other parts of the extremities because the tracts transmitting pain and temperature sensations are intact. Compare reactions on each side. A sensation reported as dull when the stimulus was actually sharp requires further testing. A patient with sensory loss as a result of diabetes mellitus or peripheral vascular disease may or may not be aware of the loss until tested. Some patients with chronic illness may report that they have had sensory losses for a long time. Prior to testing for pain, the nurse must check to determine whether the patient is on anticoagulant therapy. If the patient is on anticoagulant therapy, then any testing with a sharp object must be avoided—this can cause bleeding.

Light *touch discrimination* is likely to be normal if pain and temperature sensory tracts are intact. Touch discrimination and two-point discrimination may be assessed as part of a complete neurologic examination by the physician or APRN.

For testing **touch discrimination**, the patient closes his or her eyes. The practitioner touches the patient with a finger and asks that he or she point to the area touched. This procedure is repeated on each extremity at random rather than at sequential points. Next, the practitioner touches the patient on each side of the body on corresponding sites at the same time. The patient should be able to point to both sites.

The clinician then touches the patient in two places on the same extremity with two objects, such as cotton-tipped applicators. A person can normally identify two points fairly close together depending on the location of the stimuli. When an area is heavily innervated, the *two-point discrimination will feel closer.*

Abnormal sensory findings may have a CNS or a peripheral nervous system (PNS) cause. The neuropathies of diabetes, malnutrition, and vascular problems have a PNS cause. Damage to a specific spinal nerve may not result in significant sensory loss because the spinal nerves overlap. Injury to several nearby spinal nerves is manifested as decreased or absent SENSORY PERCEPTION in the dermatomes of those nerves.

CNS problems can occur within the spinal cord, the brainstem, the cerebellum, and the cerebral cortex. Sensory deficits from spinal cord damage vary with the location of the damage. Involvement of only the posterior column leads to lost proprioception (position sense) below the level of the damage on the same side or on both sides (if both the right and left posterior columns are involved). A lesion involving only the right spinothalamic tract results in a loss of pain and temperature sensations below the lesion on the *left* side. Problems in the brainstem, thalamus, and cortex generally result in loss of sensation on the **contralateral** (opposite) side of the body. Cerebellar lesions result in sensory deficits on the *same* side of the body.

Assessment of Cerebellar Function. Most of the assessment of cerebellar function can be performed with the patient sitting on the side of the bed or examining table. Fine *coordination* of muscle activity is tested. If cerebellar problems are suspected or diagnosed, ask the patient to perform these tasks with his or her eyes closed:

- Run the heel of one foot down the shin of the other leg and repeat with the other leg (the patient should be able to do this smoothly and keep the heel on the shin).
- Place the hands palm-up and then palm-down on each thigh, repeating as fast as possible (this can normally be done rapidly).
- With arms out at the side, touch the finger to the nose 2 or 3 times, with eyes open and then with eyes closed (this can be done with alternating arms or with each arm individually).

For the last part of the cerebellar assessment, the *ambulatory* patient stands for testing of *gait and equilibrium.* Gait and equilibrium are usually tested at the end or beginning of the entire neurologic assessment. Ask the patient to walk across the room, turn, and return. Observe for uneven steps, difficulty walking, and so forth. To evaluate balance, ask him or her to stand on one foot and then on the other. Tiptoe walking and heel-to-toe walking can also demonstrate gait problems. For patients with sciatic nerve involvement, pain may worsen when they walk on their toes or heels.

To test equilibrium, ask the patient to stand with arms at the sides, feet and knees close together, and eyes open. Check for swaying, and then ask him or her to close his or her eyes and maintain position. The examiner should be close enough to prevent falling if the patient cannot stay erect. If he or she sways with the eyes closed but not when the eyes are open (the **Romberg sign**), the problem is probably **proprioceptive** (awareness of body position). If the patient sways with the eyes both open and closed, the neurologic disturbance is probably *cerebellar* in origin.

QUALITY IMPROVEMENT QSEN

System-Wide Project Standardizes Assessments and Communication for Neuroscience Patients

Iacono L.A., Wells C., & Mann-Finnerty, K. (2014). Standardizing neurological assessments. *The Journal of Neuroscience Nursing, 46*(2), 125-132.

The nursing and physician leadership team at a large urban hospital identified an opportunity to improve neurologic assessment by adopting standard assessment tools. Problems during transitions in care, particularly when reporting neurologic deterioration to health care team members, alerted staff to the need to address issues in quality and safety. Assessment tools were identified and evaluated. Modifications were made to three tools to capture team-generated key components to a neurologic assessment and to improve the process for describing neurologic deterioration. The Basic Neurological Check (addressing alertness, orientation, facial palsy, and four-limb strength), the National Institutes of Health Stroke Scale (NIHSS) Neurological Check (specific for patients with stroke or suspected stroke), and the Coma Neurological Check (based on the Glasgow Coma Scale) were then incorporated into electronic documentation. An algorithm to help health care providers and nurses determine which neurologic tool to use was made available and folded into training. Mandatory training about the use of the tools was implemented. Ongoing education during orientation for new nurses as well as in-depth training of nurse educators and assistant managers to provide reinforcement and feedback also took place. Three short videos, one for each of the selected neurologic tools, were developed for staff viewing. Following implementation, nurses and physicians report that observations were more consistent and changes were more measurable. Use of the standardized neurologic assessment tools in the neuroscience patient population has helped in early identification of neurologic symptoms. Nurses verbalized more confidence in their ability to identify clinical important symptoms so that early intervention can occur. The authors emphasized the role of nurse educators in training and reinforcement of learning and outcome measures.

Commentary: Implications for Practice and Research

This quality improvement project began in a stroke unit and then was expanded to all units where patients with neurologic conditions received care. This is an example of a team working together to solve a system-wide problem. Both practice and communication issues were identified as contributing to delayed recognition of clinical deterioration in neuroscience patients and in confusion or error during hand-offs. The use of nurse educators as champions was an effective strategy of adoption and ongoing achievement of goals for care.

If the patient cannot perform any of these activities smoothly, the problem is manifested on the same side as the cerebellar lesion. If both lobes of the cerebellum are involved, the incoordination affects both sides of the body (bilateral).

Rapid Neurologic Assessment

A rapid neurologic assessment, or "neuro check," is completed when the patient is admitted to a health care facility on an emergent basis. It is also part of ongoing patient assessment and performed in the event of a sudden change in neurologic status. The typical record contains data related to alertness, orientation, movement of arms and legs, and pupil size and reaction to light. *Be sure to document all aspects of the rapid neurologic assessment.* One example of a rapid neurologic assessment is the National Institutes of Health Stroke Scale, described in Chapter 45 (Table 45-2). (See the Quality Improvement box.)

GLASGOW COMA SCALE*

Eye Opening	
Spontaneous	**4**
To sound	**3**
To pain	**2**
Never	**1**
Motor Response	
Obeys commands	**6**
Localizes pain	**5**
Normal flexion (withdrawal)	**4**
Abnormal flexion	**3**
Extension	**2**
None	**1**
Verbal Response	
Oriented	**5**
Confused conversation	**4**
Inappropriate words	**3**
Incomprehensible sounds	**2**
None	**1**

* The highest possible score is 15

FIG. 41-10 The Glasgow Coma Scale.

A second example of standard rapid neurologic assessment is the Glasgow Coma Scale (GCS) (Fig. 41-10). The GCS is used in many acute care settings to establish baseline data in each of these areas: eye opening, motor response, and verbal response. The patient is assigned a numeric score for each of these areas. The lower the score, the lower the patient's neurologic function. For patients who are intubated and cannot talk, record their score with a "t" after the number for verbal response.

The GCS is easy to teach and has demonstrated a consistent score among trained assessors. The reliability of the GCS is based on recording the patient's "best" response. If the patient does not follow commands or is unresponsive to voice, then the nurse proceeds to increasingly noxious (painful) stimuli to elicit an eye and motor response. Typically, the patient's response to central pain (brain response) is assessed first. On the basis of this response, peripheral pain may then be assessed. Failure to apply painful stimuli appropriately may lead to an incorrect conclusion about the patient's neurologic status. If the patient responds fully to voice or light touch, there is no need to progress to more vigorous or painful stimuli.

Start with the least noxious irritation or pressure and proceed to more painful stimulation if the patient does not respond. Begin each phase of the assessment by speaking in a normal voice. If no response is obtained, use a loud voice. If the patient does not respond, gently shake him or her. The shaking should be similar to that used in attempting to wake up a child. If that is unsuccessful, apply painful stimuli using one of these methods:

- Supraorbital (above eyes) pressure by placing a thumb under the orbital rim in the middle of the eyebrow and

pushing upward. Do not use this technique if the patient has orbital or facial fractures.
- Trapezius muscle squeeze by pinching or squeezing the trapezius muscle located at the angle of the shoulder and neck muscle.
- Mandibular (jaw) pressure to the jaw by using your index and middle fingers to pinch the lower jaw.
- Sternal (breastbone) rub by making a fist and rubbing/twisting your knuckles against the sternum.

The tissue in these areas is tender, and bruising is not unusual. Therefore do not use this technique for older adults or for patients who may experience severe bruising (e.g., recipients of anticoagulant therapy). Peripheral pain is assessed with pressure at the base of the nail on one finger and one toe and both on the right and left.

The patient may respond to painful stimuli in several ways. Although the initial response to pain may be abnormal flexion or extension, continued application of pain for no more than 20 to 30 seconds may demonstrate that he or she can localize or withdraw. If the patient does not respond after 20 to 30 seconds, stop applying the painful stimulus.

! NURSING SAFETY PRIORITY QSEN

Critical Rescue

A decrease of 2 or more points in the Glasgow Coma Scale total is clinically significant and should be communicated to the health care provider immediately. Other findings requiring urgent communication with the health care provider include a new finding of abnormal flexion or extension, particularly of the upper extremities (decerebrate or decorticate posturing); pinpoint, dilated, and nonreactive pupils; and sudden or subtle changes in mental status. Remember, changes in cognition are the earliest signs of changes in neurologic status. Early recognition of neurologic changes and communicating changes to the health care provider provide the best opportunity to prevent complications and preserve function.

Psychosocial Assessment

Depression can result in cognitive and behavioral changes that are similar to delirium or dementia. Depression is a common mental health disorder that is often missed in a variety of health care settings, especially in settings that care for older adults (Touhy & Jett, 2014). Consider using a depression screening tool like the Center for Epidemiological Studies Depression-Revised (CESD-R) or the Geriatric Depression Scale (short form) to identify patients with depressive symptoms, and consider referring them to the appropriate provider (both primary care and mental health care) if the screening is positive.

Patients vary in their responses to a suspected or actual health problem, often depending on whether it is acute or chronic. Response is also influenced by MOBILITY, SENSORY PERCEPTION, and/or COGNITION; these abilities can be temporarily or permanently altered as a result of neurologic disease or injury. For example, patients who have a mild stroke and no lasting neurologic deficits are less likely to be severely depressed than patients who experience a loss of independent movement or impaired communication as a result of a stroke.

Age may also be a factor in how a patient accepts the illness. For instance, a young adult who has a motorcycle crash causing a traumatic brain injury (TBI) may react differently from an older adult who has a spinal injury. In some cases, the patient's emotional responses result from the health problem itself, especially for TBI patients.

Men may feel differently about their illness than women. Male patients who have had strokes are depressed more often than women who have had strokes. Discussions of these response differences can be found in the following chapters on specific neurologic health problems.

Regardless of what the health problem is, do not assume that everyone reacts the same way to his or her illness or injury. Consider the cultural background of the patient because this will influence his or her reaction to pain or injury. Patients experience the grieving process and may fluctuate between denial, anger, and depression. Encourage patients to express their feelings. Refer them to the appropriate support services if needed. Assess support systems, including family members and friends, if available. Document your assessment and interventions.

Diagnostic Assessment

Laboratory Assessment

Fluid, electrolyte, and glucose abnormalities can cause neurologic impairment. The basic metabolic panel and serum calcium, phosphorus, and magnesium are evaluated. Both anemia and malnutrition can contribute to neurologic disorders so a complete blood count and serum levels of albumin and minerals/vitamins (particularly B vitamins) are collected. Collection of arterial blood to evaluate pH, oxygen, and carbon dioxide levels may be done because these three results, when either too high or too low, will alter neurologic status. Serum evaluation may be required to determine the presence of a **toxidrome** from prescribed or illicit drugs. For patients with a neurologic problem resulting from an infection, cultures are necessary to identify the pathogen. Although the cause of infection must be determined for any patient, this is especially true for those with existing CNS disease. The blood-brain barrier is often not intact in neurologic disease, and the patient is more likely to get an infection of the nervous system, such as meningitis or encephalitis.

Imaging Assessment

Plain X-Rays. Plain *x-rays* of the skull and spine are used to determine bony fractures, curvatures, bone erosion, bone dislocation, and possible calcification of soft tissue, which can damage the nervous system. Several views are taken—anteroposterior, lateral, oblique, and, when necessary, special views of the facial bones. *In head trauma and multiple injuries, one of the first priorities is to rule out cervical spine fracture.*

Explain that the x-ray procedure for the skull and spine is similar to that for a chest x-ray. The patient must remain still during the procedure. Remind him or her that the exposure to radiation is minimal. If the patient is in traction and a portable x-ray unit is not available, the nurse may need to accompany him or her to assist with positioning. Any patient who cannot walk from a wheelchair to the x-ray table should be transferred to the radiology department on a stretcher. Hospitals may have specific procedures for transferring patients in wheelchairs or on stretchers to the radiology department. Check with your hospital on this procedure. For example, with a patient who is confused or disoriented, the hospital radiology department staff may require two or more hospital personnel to assist with the transfer. The patient is positioned for each of the desired views and is asked to not move just before each x-ray. Follow-up care is not required.

In general, for any image that involves being placed in a scanner, the nurse needs to be aware of special circumstances that can either prevent the procedure from taking place or can interfere with the procedure. If the patient is alert and claustrophobic, two options are available: one is a mild sedative such as diazepam (Valium) to calm the patient; the other option is an open scanner. The nurse must determine whether the patient has any metal prosthetics, such as heart valves or shrapnel in the part of the body to be scanned. If the patient does have any type of metal object in the body part to be examined, the nurse must notify radiology immediately because the procedure may need to be cancelled. If the patient does have a metal prosthetic or device, the nurse should ask the patient or significant other if the patient carries a medical alert card from the manufacturer. Medical device manufacturers issue cards to physicians for their patients to carry with the device number and instructions if radiologic diagnostic testing is needed.

Cerebral Angiography. Cerebral angiography (arteriography) is done to visualize the cerebral circulation to detect blockages in the arteries or veins in the brain, head, or neck. It remains the gold standard for the diagnosis of intracranial vascular disease and is required for any transcatheter therapy or for surgical intervention. Angiography may be used to identify aneurysms, traumatic injuries, strictures/occlusions, tumors, blood vessel displacement from edema, and arteriovenous (AV) malformations. Chart 41-4 lists the precautions that must be taken for patients having any test using an iodine-based contrast agent. Risk factors for adverse events must be determined before scheduling the test. Patients sensitive to iodine may be sensitive to iodinated contrast agents; as well, patients with a history of hypersensitivity in general (e.g., multiple food allergies or asthma) are more likely to have an adverse reaction compared with the general population. Seafood allergies are no longer considered an indicator of iodinated contrast allergy. Table 41-4 describes patient preparation and follow-up nursing care for cerebral angiography and other imaging tests.

The patient is placed on an examining table and made as comfortable as possible. At this time, dentures and hearing aids must be removed. He or she is then connected to cardiac monitoring throughout the procedure. Deep or moderate sedation is usually not used, although the patient may be given medication for relaxation.

The interventional radiologist or other specially trained physician numbs the area at the groin and inserts a catheter into the femoral artery. Under fluoroscopic guidance, the catheter is advanced into a carotid or vertebral artery. Then the physician injects iodinated contrast material into each vessel while recording images from different angles over the head and neck. After all the vessels have been imaged, the radiologist reviews all the images and consults with the referring physician to decide whether the patient could benefit from a therapeutic radiologic procedure or surgery to treat the problem. An arterial closure device is typically used to seal the artery and prevent bleeding.

The x-ray images are stored on a computer. With older equipment, a two-dimensional picture of the vessels is produced. Most radiographic systems now come with software to create three-dimensional images of the blood vessels in the head and/or neck. These systems can also display a "subtracted image" made from two images—one just before the contrast was injected and one with the contrast in the artery. The risks of the procedure are contrast reaction (including hives and flushing), thrombosis (clotting), and bleeding from the entry site. Patients with known contrast sensitivity are pre-treated with steroids.

CHART 41-4 Best Practice for Patient Safety & Quality Care QSEN

Precautions for the Use of Iodine-Based or Gadolinium Contrast for Diagnostic Testing

Special precautions are taken for patients who will receive an iodinated or high osmolar contrast agent as part of their diagnostic test. These measures include:

- Following agency guidelines regarding informed consent.
- Screening patients at risk for developing contrast-induced kidney damage:
  - Ask the patient about all allergies (food, drug, environmental antigens), asthma, and prior reaction to contrast agents.
  - Review for the presence of these conditions:
    - Pre-existing renal disease such as a diagnosis of chronic kidney disease
    - Diabetic nephropathy
    - Heart failure
    - Dehydration
    - Older age
    - Drugs that interfere with renal perfusion such as metformin or NSAIDs
    - Administration of contrast media in the previous 72 hours
- Evaluating current kidney function. Patients with a serum creatinine greater than or equal to 1.5 mg/dL OR a calculated glomerular filtration rate (GFR) of less than 60 mL/min are at highest risk for kidney damage from contrast.
- Communicating with the health care provider before diagnostic testing when risk factors and allergic reaction to iodinated contrast are present.
  - Consider including a discussion of the patient's serum creatinine as a component of the "time-out" process prior to a diagnostic procedure.
  - Document the date, time, and name of the health care provider with whom communication of risk occurred and what actions were prescribed, if any.
  - Some diagnostic tests can be completed with a lower volume of contrast or an alternate agent.
  - Medications that are associated with kidney damage may be held for 24-48 hours before AND after the test.
- Providing adequate hydration before and after contrast administration:
  - Collaborate with the health care provider to determine whether hydration before the diagnostic test, typically with intravenous normal saline, is used. Bicarbonate with normal saline or an intravenous dose of *N*-acetylcysteine may be used in a high-risk patient.
  - Determine the optimal post-diagnostic intake and output. Provide sufficient hydration to flush out the contrast with oral or IV fluids over the 4-5 hours following the test.
- Re-evaluating serum creatinine and glomerular filtration rate (GFR) 24-48 hours after the diagnostic test. Communicate an increase of serum creatinine 0.5 mg/dL above baseline and a decrease in GFR >25% to the health care provider. Document communication and follow-up interventions, if any. Generally, the peak creatinine rise is at 48-72 hours after the administration of contrast.

Computed Tomography. Computed tomography (CT) scanning is an accurate, quick, easy, noninvasive, painless, and least-expensive method of diagnosing neurologic problems (see Table 41-4). Using x-rays (i.e., ionizing radiation), pictures are taken at many horizontal levels, or slices, of the brain or spinal cord (Schmidt, 2012). A computer then generates three-dimensional detailed anatomic pictures of tissues, typically the brain, spinal cord, or peripheral neuromuscular system in

TABLE 41-4 **Preparation and Follow-Up for Selected Diagnostic Procedures**

TEST	PATIENT CARE PREPARATION	PATIENT CARE FOLLOW-UP
Sonography or Ultrasonography	No preparation is needed. This diagnostic imaging approach is noninvasive and not painful. A light and moderate touch with a probe occurs along the neck/carotid vessels.	The gel used to enhance probe images can be immediately wiped off or removed with water.
Cerebral angiography	Determine whether the patient is allergic to iodinated contrast agents, and follow the guideline in Chart 41-4. To minimize risk for aspiration, assess for the presence of nausea or recent vomiting and medicate as needed. Ensure that the patient is NPO 4 to 6 hours before the test. Reinforce these important points: • Your head is immobilized during the procedure. • Do not move during the procedure. • Contrast dye is injected through a catheter placed in the femoral artery. You will feel a warm or hot sensation when the dye is injected—this is normal. • You will be able to talk to the physician—let him or her know if you are in pain or have any concerns. Assess and document neurologic signs, vital signs, and neurovascular checks.	Follow agency policy regarding care of the injection site, which may include: • Check dressing for bleeding and swelling around site. • Apply ice pack to site. • Keep the extremity straight and immobilized. • Maintain pressure dressing for 2 hours. Check the extremity for adequate circulation to include skin color and temperature, pulses distal to the injection site, and capillary refill. If bleeding is present, maintain manual pressure on the site and notify the physician immediately. Assess vital signs with neurologic examination. Increase oral or IV fluid intake unless contraindicated. Document assessments and interventions.
Computed tomography (CT) with and without contrast CT angiography (CTA) CT myelogram	Follow the guidelines listed in Chart 41-4 if a contrast agent is to be given. Determine whether the patient is claustrophobic and whether a closed CT scan is used. Inform the radiology staff or physician to determine if pre-procedure sedation is necessary. Instruct the patient to remove hairpins, hairpieces, or wigs. Inform the patient that the scanner may make noise or knocking sounds. Reassure the patient that he or she will be able to communicate with the technician throughout the procedure. If contrast is used, the patient may feel a warm or cool sensation after the dye is injected. Occasionally the patient may report a slight metallic taste. A lumbar puncture is performed before an intrathecal contrast-enhanced CT.	Monitor the patient for a delayed allergic response if contrast medium was used.
Positron emission tomography (PET)	Follow preparation as listed for CT. Instruct the patient to withhold caffeine, alcohol, and tobacco for 24 hours before the test. Ensure that the patient has been NPO status for 4 to 12 hours before the procedure (if the patient is diabetic, no insulin is given before the test). Do not give any glucose solutions and any other drugs that alter glucose metabolism. Insert two IV lines.	The radioisotope is eliminated in the urine; no special precautions required. Encourage the patient to increase fluid intake unless contraindicated.
Single-photon emission computed tomography (SPECT)	Patient preparation is similar to that for PET/CT. Determine whether the patient has recently had other nuclear medicine screenings, which may leave traces of the radiopharmaceutical agent. Follow the guidelines listed in Chart 41-4 regarding use of a contrast agent.	The patient can return to his or her previous activity level.
Magnetic resonance imaging (MRI) Magnetic resonance angiography (MRA) Magnetic resonance spectroscopy (MRS)	Follow the information for CT scan. No metal objects may enter the MRI room. Ask the patient about any metal implants including any type of pacemaker device, implantable pumps, or stimulating devices. Instruct the patient to remove all metal objects (jewelry, earrings, body piercings, hairpins, watches, rings, pens). Check with the radiologist regarding tattoos. Do not enter the MRI room unless you have checked with the radiology technician and are sure that neither you nor the patient has any metal device. Ensure all equipment and supplies are free of metal. Gadolinium contrast is to be avoided in patients with low renal function (i.e., glomerular filtration rate <30 mL/min/1.73 m^2.)	No special post-procedure or follow-up care is required. Avoid risk for nephrogenic systemic fibrosis following gadolinium for contrast by restricting its use to patients with normal renal function or using an alternate medium during MRI with contrast diagnostic imaging.

TABLE 41-4 Preparation and Follow-Up for Selected Diagnostic Procedures—cont'd

TEST	PATIENT CARE PREPARATION	PATIENT CARE FOLLOW-UP
Lumbar puncture	Explain the procedure, noting that some discomfort may be felt when the local anesthetic is injected or that pain may occur in the leg(s) when the spinal needle is inserted. Place the patient in the fetal position, and remind him or her to remain still. If needed, keep the patient from moving.	Obtain vital signs and complete neurologic checks. Follow agency policy regarding bedrest and remaining flat. Encourage the patient to increase fluid intake unless contraindicated. Monitor for complications, especially increased intracranial pressure (severe headache, nausea, vomiting, photophobia, and change in level of consciousness). Observe the needle insertion site for leakage. Notify the physician if it occurs. Provide drug for headache. Notify the physician if drug does not relieve pain.
Electroencephalogram (EEG)	Ensure that hair is clean and without conditioners, hair creams, lotions, sprays, or styling gels. Avoid the use of sedatives or stimulants in the 12-24 hours preceding the EEG. Instruct the patient not to fast before the test because hypoglycemia can affect the recording. Ensure a quiet room with signage to inform visitors of EEG recording in progress. Instruct the patient or family members about the reasons for periodic or continuous monitoring. The reasons for EEG monitoring include: • Determining the general activity of the cerebral hemispheres. • Determining the origin of seizure activity (epilepsy). • Determining cerebral function in epilepsy and other pathologic conditions such as tumors, abscesses, cerebrovascular disease, hematomas, injury, metabolic diseases, degenerative brain disease, and drug intoxication. • Differentiating between organic and hysterical or feigned blindness or deafness. • Monitoring cerebral activity during surgical anesthesia or sedation in the intensive care unit. • Diagnosing sleep disorders. If the EEG is related to a sleep disorder diagnosis, the patient may be asked to sleep less the night before the EEG. • Assisting in the determination of brain death.	The gel and glue used for placing electrodes can be washed out immediately after the test ends. Acetone or witch hazel will dissolve the paste. Advise the patient who has had a sleep-deprived EEG not to drive home.

neurologic testing. A contrast medium may be used to enhance the image. CT scans distinguish bone, soft tissue (e.g., the brain, vascular system, and ventricular system), and fluids such as cerebrospinal fluid (CSF) or blood. Tumors, infarctions, hemorrhage, hydrocephalus, and bone malformations can also be identified.

The patient is placed on a movable table in a head-holding device. He or she must remain completely still during the test, which may be difficult. The table is positioned in the machine—a large, donut-shaped structure. Depending on the scan, the patient may be completely enclosed or in a more open situation. A noncontrast series of pictures are taken first. Then, if needed, the patient is withdrawn from the scanner and given an injection of the iodinated contrast medium. The scan is then repeated. Each set of head scans takes less than 5 minutes in newer scanners. Spinal studies take about 10 minutes per body section (cervical, thoracic, lumbar) and are less likely to require contrast injection.

Most patients with new neurologic symptoms have both a pre-contrast and post-contrast study of the head. Contrast-enhanced CT is especially useful in locating and identifying tumor types and abscesses. For situations in which bleeding is the only concern (e.g., in trauma patients), contrast scans are not usually required.

After a standard CT scan, imaging software digitally removes images of soft tissue so that only images of bone remain. Through the use of this technology, bone deformities, trauma, and birth defects are more easily identified.

CT angiography involves administering contrast dye IV before the CT scan. It is used to identify blockages or narrowing of blood vessels, aneurysms, and other blood vessel abnormalities.

An intrathecal contrast-enhanced CT scan is performed to diagnose disorders of the spine and spinal nerve roots. A lumbar puncture is performed so that a small amount of spinal fluid can be removed and mixed with contrast dye and injected. The patient is positioned to allow for the contrast medium to move around the spinal cord and nerve roots as needed. The patient may have a headache after the procedure. Follow facility policy regarding patient positioning after the procedure.

Magnetic Resonance Imaging. Magnetic resonance imaging (MRI or MR) has advantages over CT in the diagnostic imaging of the brain, spinal cord, and nerve roots. It does not use ionizing radiation but, instead, relies on magnetic fields. Multiple sets of images are taken that are used to determine normal and abnormal anatomy. Images may be enhanced with the use of gadolinium, a non–iodine-based contrast medium. MRIs of the spine have largely replaced CT scans and myelography for evaluation. Bony structures cannot be viewed with MR; CT scans are the best way to see bones. Some facilities have a *functional MRI (fMRI)* machine that can assess blood flow to the brain rather than merely show its anatomic structure.

In addition to the traditional MRI, a *magnetic resonance angiography (MRA), magnetic resonance spectroscopy (MRS)*, or *diffusion imaging (DI)* may be requested. MRA is used to evaluate blood flow and blood vessel abnormalities such as an arterial blockage, intracranial aneurysms, and AV malformations. MRS is used to detect abnormalities in the brain's biochemical processes, such as that which occurs in epilepsy, Alzheimer's disease, and brain attack (stroke). DI uses MRI techniques to evaluate ischemia in the brain to determine the location and severity of a stroke.

Newer, open-sided units ("open MRI") now produce adequate images for those patients who do not want standard MRI scanners. MRI has been contraindicated for patients with cardiac pacemakers, other implanted pumps or devices, and ion-containing metal aneurysm clips. However, extensive trials are testing ways to safely scan some patients with pacemakers. Other implanted devices, such as vascular stents, intravascular catheter (IVC) filters, and metal antiembolic devices, may be scanned immediately or after a certain period of time, depending on manufacturers' recommendations. MRI may also be contraindicated in patients who are confused or agitated, have unstable vital signs, are on continuous life support, or have older tattoos (which contain lead). New physiologic monitoring systems made specifically for the scanner allow some patients who are unstable to be scanned. A comprehensive online list of medical devices tested for MRI safety and compatibility can be found at *www.mrisafety.com*. Medical personnel must remove any medical devices they are carrying or wearing and ensure that only approved devices are allowed in the MRI room (see Table 41-4).

Positron Emission Tomography. Positron emission tomography (PET) is a diagnostic tool that is not available in all medical centers (see Table 41-4). Its benefit over a CT scan or MRI is that it provides information about the *function* of the brain, specifically glucose and oxygen metabolism and cerebral blood flow. Current CT scanners provide information about the *structure* of the central nervous system (CNS). The newest PET machines are combination CT-PET scanners that fuse images together to produce better information about the type and location of brain dysfunction.

The physician or nuclear medicine technologist injects the patient with IV deoxyglucose, which is tagged to an isotope. The isotope emits activity in the form of positrons, which are scanned and converted into a color image by computer. The more active a given part of the brain, the greater the glucose uptake. This test is used to evaluate drug metabolism and detect areas of metabolic alteration that occur in dementia, epilepsy, psychiatric and degenerative disorders, neoplasms, and Alzheimer's disease. The level of radiation is equivalent to that of five or six x-rays but much less than exposure during CT.

Teach the patient that he or she will be NPO the night before morning testing and 4 hours before afternoon testing. Patients with diabetes have their test in the morning before taking their antidiabetic drugs. During this 2- to 3-hour procedure, the patient may be blindfolded and have earplugs inserted for all or part of the test. He or she is asked to perform certain mental functions to activate different areas of the brain. Older adults and patients with mental health/behavioral health problems may be too anxious to have a PET scan.

Single-Photon Emission Computed Tomography. The limitation of PET may be overcome through the use of **single-photon emission computed tomography (SPECT)**. This test uses a radiopharmaceutical agent that enables radioisotopes to cross the blood-brain barrier. The agent is administered by IV injection. Gamma-emitting radionuclides have longer half-lives, therefore eliminating the need for a cyclotron near the scanner. Although SPECT is less expensive than PET, the resolution of the images is limited. SPECT is particularly useful in studying cerebral blood flow, amnesia, neoplasms, head trauma, or persistent vegetative state. The test is contraindicated in women who are breast-feeding.

The patient is injected with the material about 1 hour before the actual scan by the radiologist, certified nuclear medicine technologist, or specially trained RN. The patient is positioned on an x-ray table in a quiet dark room for the actual scans. Several gamma cameras scan his or her head. When completed, the images are downloaded to a computer.

Magnetoencephalography. **Magnetoencephalography (MEG)** is a noninvasive imaging technique used to measure the magnetic fields produced by electrical activity in the brain via extremely sensitive devices such as superconducting quantum interference devices (SQUIDs). MEG is somewhat similar to electroencephalography (EEG). The advantage is greater accuracy because of the minimal distortion of the signal. This allows for more usable and reliable localization of brain function. The brain can be observed "in action" rather than just viewing a still MRI image. These machines are not widely available because of their extremely high cost.

NCLEX EXAMINATION CHALLENGE

Physiological Integrity

A client with possible Parkinson disease is scheduled to have magnetic resonance imaging (MRI). The daughter asks the nurse how this test is different from a computed tomography (CT) scan. What is the nurse's best response?

A. "The MRI scan provides better contrast between normal tissue and pathologic tissue."
B. "They are not different; both use ionizing radiation."
C. "The MRI will not require contrast material and has no special precautions."
D. "The CT scan does not provide a view of deep brain structures like the region where Parkinson originates.

Other Diagnostic Assessment

Electromyography. **Electromyography (EMG)** is used to identify nerve and muscle disorders as well as spinal cord disease. (See Chapter 44 for a description of patient preparation, procedure, and follow-up care.) Electromyography and electroneurography or nerve conduction velocity studies (NCVSs) are usually used together and are referred to as *electromyoneurography*.

Electroencephalography. **Electroencephalography (EEG)** records the electrical activity of the cerebral hemispheres. Each graphic recording represents electrical impulses within the brain. The frequency, amplitude, and characteristics of the brain waves are recorded. For example, a cerebral tumor or infarct may have abnormally slow waveforms. EEGs are used both as a diagnostic test and to provide sustained monitoring, and the indications for testing and monitoring are listed in Table 41-4.

Abnormal results on an EEG test may be due to:

- An abnormal structure in the brain, such as a brain tumor
- Attention problems
- Tissue death due to a blockage in blood flow (cerebral infarction)
- Drug or alcohol intoxication
- Inflammation of the brain (encephalitis)
- Ischemia to brain tissue from low blood flow to the brain during a migraine or a surgical procedure like a carotid endarterectomy
- Seizure disorder
- Sleep disorder or sleep deprivation

Fasting is avoided before EEG testing because hypoglycemia can alter the test results. The patient is placed on a reclining chair or bed. According to an internationally accepted procedure, 16 or more electrodes are applied to the scalp with a jelly-like substance and connected to the machine. The physician or EEG technician places glue over the electrodes to prevent slippage. The patient must lie still with his or her eyes closed during the initial recording. The rest of the test engages the patient in certain activities: hyperventilation, photic stimulation, and sleep. A portable EEG may be performed at the bedside if necessary, but the preference is for the EEG to be done in a very quiet room.

Hyperventilation produces cerebral vasoconstriction and alkalosis, which increases the likelihood of seizure activity. The patient is asked to breathe deeply 20 times per minute for 3 minutes. In *photic stimulation,* a flashing bright light is placed in front of the patient. Frequencies of 1 to 20 flashes per second are used with the patient's eyes open and then closed. If the patient's seizures are photosensitive in origin, seizure activity may be seen on the EEG. A *sleep* EEG may be performed to aid in the detection of abnormal brain waves that are seen only when the patient is sleeping, such as with frontal lobe epilepsy (Pagana & Pagana, 2014).

During an EEG test, which takes 45 to 120 minutes, the recording can be stopped about every 5 minutes to allow the patient to move. If the patient moves during the recording, movement creates a change in the brain waves and the technician will note movements on the graph. Examples of unintentional movement that can affect the recordings are tongue movement, eye blinking, and muscle tensing. The technician may induce or request certain movements or sensory stimulation and record these events on the EEG record to link changes in brain waves with motor activity or sensory stimulation; these intentional movements are also documented on the EEG recording.

Evoked Potentials. **Evoked potentials** (also called *evoked response*) measure the electrical signals to the brain generated by sound, touch, or light. These tests are used to assess sensory nerve problems and confirm neurologic conditions including multiple sclerosis, brain tumor, acoustic neuroma (small tumors of the inner ear), and spinal cord injury. Evoked potentials are also used to test sight and hearing (especially in infants and young children), monitor brain activity in comatose patients, and confirm brain death (Wijdicks et al., 2010). During evoked potentials, a second set of electrodes is attached to the part of the body that will experience sensation. A stimulus is applied, and the amount of time it takes for the impulse generated by the stimulus to reach the brain is recorded. Under normal circumstances, the process of signal transmission is instantaneous.

Auditory evoked potentials (also called *brainstem auditory evoked response*) are used to assess high-frequency hearing loss, diagnose any damage to the acoustic nerve and auditory pathways in the brainstem, and detect acoustic neuromas. The patient sits in a soundproof room and wears headphones. Clicking sounds are delivered one at a time to one ear while a masking sound is sent to the other ear.

Visual evoked potentials detect loss of vision from optic nerve damage (in particular, damage caused by multiple sclerosis). The patient sits close to a screen and is asked to focus on the center of a shifting checkerboard pattern. Only one eye is tested at a time. The other eye is either kept closed or covered with a patch.

Somatosensory evoked potentials measure response from stimuli to the peripheral nerves and can detect nerve or spinal cord damage or nerve degeneration from multiple sclerosis and other degenerating diseases. Tiny electrical shocks are delivered by electrode to a nerve in an arm or leg.

Cerebral Blood Flow Evaluation. **Cerebral blood flow (CBF)** can be measured in many areas of the brain with the use of radioactive substances. It is particularly useful in evaluating cerebral vasospasm. Explain the test, and ask the physician if central nervous system (CNS) depressants and stimulants should be withheld for 24 hours before the test.

Lumbar Puncture. **Lumbar puncture (spinal tap)** is the insertion of a spinal needle into the subarachnoid space between the third and fourth (sometimes the fourth and fifth) lumbar vertebrae (see Table 41-4).

A lumbar puncture (LP) is used to:

- Obtain cerebrospinal fluid (CSF) pressure readings with a manometer
- Obtain CSF for analysis
- Check for spinal blockage caused by a spinal cord lesion
- Inject contrast medium or air for diagnostic study
- Inject spinal anesthetics
- Inject selected drugs

Because of the danger of sudden release of CSF pressure, a lumbar puncture is not done for patients with symptoms indicating severely increased ICP. The procedure is also not performed in patients with skin infections at or near the puncture site because of the danger of introducing infective organisms into the CSF.

Before an LP is performed, position the patient in a fetal side-lying position to separate the vertebrae and move the spinal nerve roots away from the area to be accessed. The health care provider then cleans the skin site thoroughly. The injection site is determined, and a local anesthetic is injected. In a few minutes, a spinal needle is inserted between the third and fourth lumbar vertebrae. Instruct the patient to inform the provider if there is shooting pain or a tingling sensation. After determining proper placement in the subarachnoid space by removing the stylet and seeing CSF, the patient is asked to relax as much as possible so the pressure reading will be accurate. Opening and

! NURSING SAFETY PRIORITY QSEN

Action Alert

Be sure that the patient does not move during a lumbar puncture. If the patient is restless or cannot cooperate, two people may need to assist instead of one. The patient may need a sedative to reduce movement. Consider patient needs for additional assistance or sedation before beginning the procedure.

closing pressure readings are taken and recorded. Three to five test tubes of CSF are usually collected and numbered sequentially. After specimen collection, the needle is withdrawn, slight pressure is applied, and an adhesive bandage strip is placed over the insertion site.

Examination of CSF has been a useful diagnostic tool for some time. Recent technical advances are increasing the number of analyses that can be done on CSF. The normal characteristics of CSF and some of the more common abnormalities are given in Table 41-5. Gram-stain smears can test for particular types of meningitis, such as tubercular meningitis. CSF can be cultured, and sensitivity studies determine the best choice of antibiotic if an infection is diagnosed. A specific test for neurosyphilis is the fluorescent treponemal antibody absorption (FTA-ABS) test. Cytologic studies of CSF can identify tumor cells.

Complications of lumbar puncture, although not common, include brainstem herniation (discussed in Chapter 45), infection, CSF leakage, and hematoma formation.

Transcranial Doppler Ultrasonography. Intracranial hemodynamics can be evaluated through the use of the transcranial Doppler (TCD). It uses sound waves to measure blood flow through the arteries. The test is particularly valuable in evaluating cerebral vasospasm or narrowing of arteries. TCD is safe, can be used repeatedly for the same patient, and is an inexpensive alternative to angiography.

Muscle and Nerve Biopsies. *Muscle* or *nerve biopsies* are used to diagnose neuromuscular disorders. They may also reveal if a person is a carrier of a defective gene that could be passed on to children. Under local anesthesia, an incision is made into the skin or a hollow needle is inserted through the skin to remove a small sample of muscle or nerve. A CT scan or MRI is performed before a *brain biopsy.* This procedure involves injection of a local anesthetic into the scalp, drilling a small hole through the skull, and inserting a hollow needle into the site of the lesion. Muscle, nerve, and brain biopsy samples are analyzed under a microscope to identify abnormalities.

TABLE 41-5 Significance of Cerebrospinal Fluid Findings

FINDINGS	SIGNIFICANCE
Pressure	
More than 20 cm H_2O	Indicates increased spinal pressure, most often from bleeding, tumors, or infection within the central nervous system (CNS)
Color/Appearance	
Clear, colorless	Normal
Pink-red to orange	Red blood cells present
Yellow	Bilirubin present owing to hemolysis of red blood cells; possible causes include subarachnoid hemorrhage, jaundice, increased cerebrospinal fluid (CSF) protein, hypercarotenemia, or hemoglobinemia
Brown	Methemoglobin present, indicating previous meningeal hemorrhage
Unclear or hazy	Cell count is elevated
Cells	
0-5 small lymphocytes/mm^3	Normal
More than 5 lymphocytes/mm^3	Reaction to infection, tumor, chemical substance, or blood
Proteins	
Total	
15-45 mg/dL *(up to 70 mg/dL in older adults)*	Normal
45-100 mg/dL	Paraventricular tumor
50-200 mg/dL	Viral infection
More than 500 mg/dL	Bacterial infection, Guillain-Barré syndrome
Less than 15 mg/dL	Meningismus, pseudotumor cerebri, hyperthyroidism, normal finding after lumbar puncture
Immune Gamma Globulin (IgG, the most important protein)	
3%-12% of total protein	Normal
More than 12% of total protein	Multiple sclerosis, neurosyphilis, or viral infection
Albumin/Globulin Ratio	
8:1	Normal
Glucose	
50-75 mg/dL or 60%-70% of blood glucose level	Normal
Less than 50 mg/dL (usually accompanied by the presence of pathologic organisms)	May occur with bacterial, fungal, or viral meningitis; CNS leukemia; or cancer
Other Characteristics	
Lactic Acid	
10-25 mg/dL	Normal
More than 25 mg/dL	Systemic acidosis or increased CSF glucose metabolism
Glutamine	
6-15 mg/dL	Normal
More than 15 mg/dL	Hepatic coma or cirrhosis of liver
Lactate Dehydrogenase	
10% of serum level or 2.0-7.2 units/mL	Normal
More than 10% of serum level	Bacterial meningitis, inflammatory diseases of CNS

NURSING CONCEPTS AND CLINICAL JUDGMENT REVIEW

What might you NOTICE in a patient with adequate COGNITION, MOBILITY, and SENSORY PERCEPTION?

Physical assessment:
- Alert and oriented, intact short-term and long-term memory, appropriate judgment, and adequate attention span
- Communicates clearly
- Moves all four extremities without assistance and normal strength
- Performs ADLs independently
- Walks, with or without assistive devices, using normal gait
- No deficits in or unusual sensory perception
- Pupils equal in size, round and regular in shape, and reactive to light and accommodation (PERRLA)

Diagnostic assessment:
- Normal ECG
- Normal CSF
- Normal EEG
- Normal CT scan of brain
- Normal MRI scan of spinal cord

GET READY FOR THE NCLEX® EXAMINATION!

KEY POINTS

Review these Key Points for each NCLEX Examination Client Needs Category.

Safe and Effective Care Environment

- Perform a neurologic examination that may be either comprehensive or focused as determined by patient needs. **Patient-Centered Care** QSEN
- Identify key changes in the examination that need to be communicated urgently to the health care provider or other team members. **Teamwork and Collaboration** QSEN
- Collaborate with the health care provider, physical therapist, and speech-language pathologist to establish priorities in neurologic assessment. **Teamwork and Collaboration** QSEN

Health Promotion and Maintenance

- Evaluate the presence of risk factors that place patients at risk for neurologic health problems such as behaviors that result in serious harm (e.g., driving recklessly) and lifestyle choices. **Evidence-Based Practice** QSEN
- Detect neurologic changes early with health screening and physical assessment strategies that reflect the prioritized assessment. Recall that a deterioration in level of consciousness (e.g., from alert to lethargic) is the most sensitive and reliable indicator of an adverse neurologic change. Include a daily evaluation for acute confusion or delirium in hospital settings. **Evidence-Based Practice** QSEN
- Consider loss of short-term memory as a potential early sign of neurologic problems. Use findings from diagnostic imaging tests to help evaluate potential neurologic impairment (Tables 41-4 and 41-5).

Psychosocial Integrity

- Assess the reaction of the person to neurologic disease. The psychological responses to neurologic health problems can vary by age, gender, and cultural background. **Patient-Centered Care** QSEN
- Encourage patients to express their feelings, and refer them to appropriate support services as needed.

Physiological Integrity

- Take a patient history, including information listed in Chart 41-2. **Patient-Centered Care** QSEN
- Evaluate the patient's cognitive abilities on admission and regularly thereafter, using a systematic approach (Chart 41-3). **Evidence-Based Practice** QSEN
- Use the Glasgow Coma Scale for patients with new traumatic brain injury.
- Use the BIMS, CAM, CAM-ICU, or other validated tool to detect delirium, an acute confusional state.
- Assess motor and sensory function to reduce harm from acute deterioration or chronic deficits. This type of assessment is also needed for discharge planning.
- Include assessment of gait, balance, and coordination to determine risk for falls. **Safety** QSEN
- Check cranial nerve III by examining pupils for size, shape, and reaction to light. Pupils should be equal in size, round and regular in shape, and become smaller in bright light. Changes in eye signs can indicate new neurologic deterioration in nonverbal patients. **Evidence-Based Practice** QSEN
- Accommodation occurs when the eyes converge and pupils constrict as an object is moved from several feet away to within 4 to 5 inches of the nose.
- Promote independence in consultation with physical and occupational therapists and the use of assistive devices like a walker or brace. **Teamwork and Collaboration** QSEN
- Assist with the performance of daily living activities when the neurologic condition interferes with self-care. **Patient-Centered Care** QSEN
- Reduce complications for patients having neurologic diagnostic testing by providing adequate teaching and preparation as outlined in Table 41-4. **Evidence-Based Practice** QSEN
- Use serum creatinine or estimated glomerular filtration rate to identify patients with reduced kidney function. Older adults and patients with chronic kidney disease, diabetes, or heart failure are at high risk for kidney damage from iodinated and gadolinium contrast media. Provide adequate fluid intake before and after diagnostic testing to flush contrast after a diagnostic test (see Chart 41-4).
- Teach patients having an EEG to follow the precautions listed in Table 41-4.
- Check for bleeding after patients have an angiography. If bleeding is observed, call the radiologist immediately.

- Before MRI, check for implanted devices such as pacemakers, vascular stents, pumps, and aneurysm clips.
- Link abnormal neurologic function with anatomy and physiology to anticipate impaired function, prognosis, and safe, effective interventions. **Evidence-Based Practice** QSEN
- Cerebrospinal fluid (CSF) is clear and colorless with few cells. Significant changes include the presence of cells, color, and turbidity (Table 41-5).
- Use findings from diagnostic imaging tests and anatomic location of injury to locate potential neurologic impairment for a focused examination (Tables 41-1, 41-2, and 41-3).
- Decerebrate or decorticate posturing and pinpoint or dilated nonreactive pupils are late signs of neurologic deterioration.
- Recognize that older adults do not normally experience deterioration in COGNITION and memory but do experience physical and physiological changes that affect MOBILITY and SENSORY PERCEPTION (Chart 41-1). **Patient-Centered Care** QSEN
- Provide a safe environment when memory loss is part of the older adult's health status by using memory aids and assistive technology to meet teaching or self-care goals. **Safety** QSEN
- Provide safe opportunities for MOBILITY, including physical activity like walking, when caring for older adults. Mobility and physical activity promote COGNITION.

CHAPTER 42

Care of Patients with Problems of the Central Nervous System: The Brain

Rachel L. Gallagher

http://evolve.elsevier.com/Iggy/

PRIORITY CONCEPTS

- Cognition
- Pain
- Mobility
- Infection

LEARNING OUTCOMES

Safe and Effective Care Environment

1. Plan with the interdisciplinary team for transitions in care including discharge to home or other setting for patients with chronic problems of the brain.
2. Implement interventions to protect patients with chronic brain conditions from injury and infection, including pain management.
3. Provide written instructions about drug therapy for chronic health problems to patients and caregivers when transitioning to a new care setting.

Health Promotion and Maintenance

4. Teach patients with chronic headaches about preventive and management approaches to therapy.
5. Develop a teaching plan about drug therapy for patients with epilepsy.
6. Teach patients about vaccination to prevent meningitis.

Psychosocial Integrity

7. Include family members, patient preferences, and values in planning care, including strategies to reduce the psychosocial impact of chronic brain conditions on patients and family members.
8. Identify community resources to support caregivers or patients with chronic neurodegenerative diseases to promote cognition and mobility.

Physiological Integrity

9. Compare and contrast assessment and management for migraine and cluster headaches.
10. Differentiate the common types of seizures, including presenting clinical manifestations.
11. Prioritize evidence-based care for patients with a seizure disorder, including appropriate seizure precaution interventions.
12. Identify nursing priorities for patients with bacterial meningitis and encephalitis.
13. Identify the genetic and environmental influences on development of Parkinson disease (PD), dementia (Alzheimer's disease [AD]), and Huntington disease (HD).
14. Document a collaborative plan of care for patients with chronic brain conditions like PD, dementia, and HD based on patient values and preferences.
15. Prevent or reduce common risk factors that contribute to functional decline and decreased quality of life in adults and older adults with chronic brain disorders.

This chapter discusses five chronic and two acute neurologic conditions. All of these neurologic disorders interfere with self-management and independence; many of them contribute to chronic pain and reduced mobility. Care of patients with chronic neurologic disorders requires coordination by nurses and significant collaboration with other members of the interdisciplinary health care team. The patient and family are the center of the collaborative team in making decisions about the plan of care (Quality and Safety Education for Nurses [QSEN], 2014).

HEADACHES

Almost everyone has had a headache at some time in his or her life. Some headaches are related to sinus congestion, allergies, or stress and are temporary. Others can be very serious and potentially life threatening. For example, an abnormal neurologic assessment together with symptoms of a cluster headache may indicate a serious neurologic problem. Patients with these symptoms are referred immediately to their health care provider or the emergency department.

Although there are many types and causes of headaches, the focus of this section is on two common types that cause people to seek medical attention: migraine headaches and cluster headaches. Patients are usually managed in the ambulatory care setting by the primary health care provider. However, it is not unusual for the person in severe pain to seek treatment in the emergency department. Refer to Chart 42-1 for questions to determine the pattern of headaches when assessing a patient.

CHART 42-1 Determining a Pattern of Headaches

Ask the patient:

- When do the headaches occur?
- How do they start?
- How often?
- How long do they last?
- Do you have the same type of headache all the time?
- Where do you feel the headache pain?
- Does the headache pain spread to other areas of the head?
- How does the headache pain feel: throbbing, stabbing, pounding, squeezing, or something else?
- Do you ever have accompanying symptoms with your headache, such as nausea, vomiting, diarrhea, dizziness, changes in vision, weakness?
- Do certain foods, alcohol, or other things trigger the headaches?
- Have there been any recent changes in your headaches?
- How do you treat the headaches? Does this treatment work?
- How often and what drug or herbal remedy do you take?
- Has a headache ever been severe enough to go to the emergency room for treatment?
- Have you ever been hospitalized for headache treatment?
- Have you ever seen a specialist (neurologist) for your headache?
- What do think might be causing your headaches?
- Is there a family history of headaches?
- Do you have to stop what you are doing or miss work when you get a headache?

! NURSING SAFETY PRIORITY QSEN

Action Alert

Encourage patients to keep a headache diary to help identify the type of headache they are experiencing and the response to medication or other intervention. Teach them to notify their health care provider if the quality, intensity, or nature of the headache increases or changes. Encourage them to report whether the headache is associated with new or unusual visual changes and whether the prescribed drug is no longer effective.

MIGRAINE HEADACHE

❖ PATHOPHYSIOLOGY

A **migraine headache** is a common clinical syndrome characterized by recurrent episodic attacks of head PAIN that serve no protective purpose. Migraine headache pain is usually described as throbbing and unilateral. Migraine can be accompanied by associated symptoms such as nausea or sensitivity to light, sound, or head movement. Migraine disorders are further characterized by multiple subtypes (McCance et al., 2014). Migraine pain and associated symptoms can last 4 to 72 hours. Migraines tend to be familial, and women are affected more commonly than men. Women diagnosed with migraines are more likely to have major depressive disorder (Modgill et al., 2012). Migraine sufferers are also at risk for stroke and epilepsy (McCance et al., 2014).

The cause of migraine headaches is not clear but includes a combination of neuronal hyperexcitability and vascular, genetic, hormonal, and environmental factors. In general, experts suggest that migraines are a neurogenic process with secondary cerebral vasodilation followed by a sterile brain tissue inflammation. Patients may inherit a condition of neuronal hyperexcitability from ion channel variations, particularly calcium and sodium-potassium pump channels, as well as from genetic variations in serotonin and dopamine receptors. Following stimulation of these hyper-excitable neuronal pathways, vascular changes occur. Pain-sensing cells in the blood vessels of the brain initiate the attack. Activation of the trigeminal nerve pathways contributes to the cascade of events that activate **nociceptors**. Substances that increase sensitivity to pain such as glutamate are synthesized through the trigeminal pathway (McCance et al., 2014). As cerebral arteries dilate, **prostaglandins** are released (chemicals that cause inflammation and swelling). Vasodilation, in turn, allows prostaglandins and other intravascular molecules to leak (**extravasate**), contributing to widespread tissue swelling and the sensation of throbbing pain.

Many patients find that certain factors, or *triggers*, such as caffeine, red wine, and monosodium glutamate (MSG), tend to cause migraine headache attacks. Each patient is different regarding which environmental factors trigger headaches. For some patients, stress or a change in weather can lead to an attack. These stimuli are thought to initiate the cascade of events that cause migraines by activating hyper-excitable neurons. Neurons involved in the initiation and propagation of migraines may have an early sensitization to neurotransmitters such that patients become increasingly susceptible to triggers and to the cascade of events that culminate in migraine PAIN. Thus care includes not only managing pain but also disrupting the migraine cascade to decrease sensitization and recurrent attacks.

❖ PATIENT-CENTERED COLLABORATIVE CARE

◆ Assessment

Migraines fall into three categories: migraines with aura, migraines without aura, and atypical migraines. An **aura** is a sensation such as visual changes that signals the onset of a headache or seizure. In a migraine, the aura occurs immediately before the migraine episode. *Most headaches are migraines without aura.* The key features of migraines are listed in Chart 42-2. **Atypical migraines** are less common and include menstrual and cluster migraines. The stages of migraine may include:

- Prodromal (or prodrome) phase, in which the patient has specific symptoms such as food cravings or mood changes
- Aura phase (if present), which generally involves visual changes, flashing lights, or **diplopia** (double vision)
- Headache phase, which may last a few hours to a few days
- Termination phase, in which the intensity of the headache decreases
- Postprodrome phase, in which the patient is often fatigued, may be irritable, and has muscle pain

The diagnosis of migraine headache is based on the patient's history and on physical, neurologic, and psychological assessment. The typical migraine is described as a unilateral, frontotemporal, *throbbing* PAIN in the head that is often worse behind one eye or ear. It is often accompanied by a sensitive scalp, anorexia, **photophobia** (sensitivity to light), **phonophobia** (sensitivity to noise), and nausea with or without vomiting. Patients tend to have the same clinical manifestations each time they have a migraine headache. Some may have to refrain from regular activities for several days if they cannot control or relieve the PAIN in its early stage.

Some physicians recommend screening patients with migraines using the Minnesota Multiphasic Personality Inventory–2 to identify personality traits and possible mental health/behavioral health problems like depression that may contribute to the headache experience (Rausa et al., 2013).

CHART 42-2 Key Features

Migraine Headaches

Phases of Migraine with Aura (Classic Migraine)

First, or Prodrome, Phase

- Aura develops over a period of several minutes and lasts no longer than 1 hour.
- Well-defined transient focal neurologic dysfunction exists.
- Pain may be preceded by:
  - Visual disturbances
    - Flashing lights
    - Lines or spots
    - Shimmering or zigzag lights
- A variety of neurologic changes, including:
  - Numbness, tingling of the lips or tongue
  - Acute confusional state
  - Aphasia
  - Vertigo
  - Unilateral weakness
  - Drowsiness

Second Phase

- Headache is accompanied by nausea and vomiting.
- Pain usually begins in the temple. It increases in intensity and becomes throbbing within 1 hour.

Third Phase

- Pain changes from throbbing to dull.
- Headache, nausea, and vomiting usually last from 4 to 72 hours. (Older patients may have aura without pain, known as a *visual migraine*.)

Migraine Without Aura (Common Migraine)

- Migraine begins without an aura before the onset of the headache.
- Pain is aggravated by performing routine physical activities.
- Pain is unilateral and pulsating.
- One of these symptoms is present:
  - Nausea and/or vomiting
  - **Photophobia** (light sensitivity)
  - **Phonophobia** (sound sensitivity)
- Headache lasts for 4 to 72 hours.
- Migraine often occurs in the early morning, during periods of stress, or in those with premenstrual tension or fluid retention.

Atypical Migraine

- Status migrainous:
  - Headache lasts longer than 72 hours.
- Migrainous infarction:
  - Neurologic symptoms are not completely reversible within 7 days.
  - Ischemic infarct is noted on neuroimaging.
- Unclassified:
  - Headache does not fulfill all of the criteria to be classified a migraine.

Neuroimaging such as magnetic resonance imaging (MRI) may be indicated if the patient has other neurologic findings, a history of seizures, findings not consistent with a migraine, or a change in the severity of the symptoms or frequency of the attacks.

Neuroimaging is also recommended in patients older than 50 years with a new onset of headaches, especially women. Women with a history of migraines with visual symptoms may have an increased risk for stroke, particularly if a migraine with visual symptoms occurred in the past year. Teach women older than 50 years who have migraines about the risk factors for cardiovascular disease. Encourage them to notify their health care provider if they experience symptoms such as facial drooping, arm weakness, or difficulties with speech.

TABLE 42-1 Commonly Used Drugs for Migraine Headache

Nonspecific Analgesics

- Acetaminophen
- Isometheptene
- Butalbital

Nonsteroidal Anti-Inflammatory Drugs (NSAIDs)

- Ibuprofen
- Naproxen

Ergotamine Preparations

- Ergotamine with caffeine (oral or suppository) (Cafergot, Migergot)
- Ergotamine sublingual (SL) (Ergomar SL)
- Medihaler ergotamine (oral inhalation aerosol)
- Dihydroergotamine (DHE) nasal spray (Migranal)

Beta Blockers

- Propranolol
- Timolol

Calcium Channel Blockers

- Verapamil (Calan)

Triptan Preparations

- Almotriptan (Axert)
- Eletriptan (Relpax)
- Rizatriptan (Maxalt)
- Zolmitriptan (Zomig)
- Sumatriptan (Imitrex)
- Frovatriptan (Frova)

Isometheptene Combination

- Midrin

Antiepileptic Drugs (AEDs)

- Divalproex (Depakote)
- Topiramate (Topamax)

◆ Interventions

The priority for care of the patient having migraines is pain management. This outcome may be achieved by abortive and preventive therapy. Drug therapy, trigger management, and complementary and alternative therapies are the major approaches to care. Provide detailed patient and family education regarding the collaborative plan of care. Effective physician/patient communication is increasingly important in managing the symptoms of migraines. Tools to help patients communicate with their health care provider and partner with their provider to manage PAIN are best practices in migraine diagnosis and treatment (Marcus, 2014).

Abortive Therapy. Abortive therapy is aimed at alleviating PAIN during the aura phase (if present) or soon after the headache has started. *Drug therapy* is prescribed to manage migraine headaches. Some of the drugs being used have major side effects, contraindications, and nursing implications. The health care provider must consider any other medical conditions that the patient has when prescribing drug therapy. In general, the patient is started on a low dose that is increased until the desired clinical effect is obtained. Table 42-1 lists commonly used drugs for migraine headaches. Many new drugs are being investigated for this painful and often debilitating health problem.

Mild migraines may be relieved by acetaminophen (APAP) (Tylenol, Abenol ♣). NSAIDs such as ibuprofen (Motrin) and naproxen (Naprosyn) may also be prescribed. In the United States, the Food and Drug Administration (FDA) has approved several over-the-counter (OTC) anti-inflammatory drugs for migraines, including Advil Migraine Capsules, Motrin Migraine Pain Caplets, and Excedrin Migraine Tablets or Caplets (contain APAP, aspirin, and caffeine). Caffeine narrows blood vessels by blocking adenosine, which dilates vessels and increases inflammation. Antiemetics may be prescribed to relieve nausea and vomiting. Metoclopramide (Reglan, Clopra) may be administered with NSAIDs to promote gastric emptying and decrease vomiting.

For more *severe* migraines, drugs such as triptan preparations, ergotamine derivatives, and isometheptene combinations are needed. A potential side effect of these drugs is **rebound headache**, also known as **medication overuse headache**, in which another headache occurs after the drug relieves the initial migraine.

Triptan preparations relieve the headache and associated symptoms by activating the 5-HT (serotonin) receptors on the cranial arteries, the basilar artery, and the blood vessels of the dura mater to produce a vasoconstrictive effect. Examples are listed in Table 42-1. For many patients, these drugs are highly effective for PAIN, nausea, vomiting, and light and sound sensitivity with few side effects. Most are contraindicated in patients with actual or suspected ischemic heart disease, cerebrovascular ischemia, hypertension, and peripheral vascular disease and in those with Prinzmetal's angina because of the potential for coronary vasospasm. Patients respond differently to drugs, and several types or combinations may be tried before the headache is relieved.

! NURSING SAFETY PRIORITY QSEN

Drug Alert

Teach patients taking triptan drugs to take them as soon as migraine symptoms develop. Instruct patients to report angina (chest pain) or chest discomfort to their health care providers immediately to prevent cardiac damage from myocardial ischemia. Remind them to use contraception (birth control) while taking the drugs because the drugs may not be safe for women who are pregnant. Teach them to expect common side effects that include flushing, tingling, and a hot sensation. These annoying sensations tend to subside after the patient's body gets used to the drug. Triptan drugs should not be taken with selective serotonin reuptake inhibitor (SSRI) antidepressants or St. John's wort, an herb used commonly for depression (Lilley et al., 2014).

Ergotamine preparations such as Cafergot are taken at the start of the headache. The patient may take up to six tablets in 24 hours or use a rectal suppository. Dihydroergotamine (DHE) may be given IV, IM, or as a nasal spray (Migranal) with an antiemetic if PAIN control and relief of nausea are not achieved with other drugs. DHE should not be given within 24 hours of a triptan drug.

Midrin is a combination drug containing APAP, isometheptene, and dichloralphenazone. It is the most common *isometheptene combination* given for treating migraines and is an excellent option when ergotamine preparations are not tolerated or do not work.

Other drugs that have been prescribed to relieve migraine PAIN include opioids and barbiturates. *These drugs should be avoided if at all possible because they are addictive. Some opioids actually cause a migraine.*

Preventive Therapy. Prevention drugs and other strategies are used when a migraine occurs more than twice per week, interferes with ADLs, or is not relieved with acute treatment. Unless otherwise contraindicated, the health care provider may initially prescribe an NSAID, a beta-adrenergic blocker, a calcium channel blocker, or an antiepileptic drug (AED). Propranolol (Inderal, Apo-Propranolol ♣, Novopranol ♣) and timolol (Blocadren, Apo-Timol ♣) are the only *beta blockers* approved for migraine prevention. Verapamil (Calan, Apo-Verap ♣), a *calcium channel blocking agent*, may also be used for some patients. The calcium channel and beta blockers are thought to reduce the activity of hyper-excitable neurons and act on the neurogenic causes of migraine. Both calcium channel blockers and beta blockers interfere with vasodilation, a contributing cause of migraine PAIN. Both beta-adrenergic blockers and calcium channel blocking drugs can lower blood pressure and decrease pulse rate.

! NURSING SAFETY PRIORITY QSEN

Drug Alert

Teach patients who take beta-adrenergic blockers or calcium channel blockers how to take their pulse. Encourage them to report bradycardia or adverse reactions such as fatigue and shortness of breath to their health care provider as soon as possible.

Topiramate (Topamax) is one of the most common *antiepileptic drugs (AEDs)* used for migraines, but it should be used in low doses of 25 to 100 mg daily. The mechanism of action is not clear, but this drug may inhibit the sodium channels, channels that may be hyper-excitable in patients with migraine. Reports of suicides have been associated with this drug when it is used in larger doses of 400 mg daily, most often with patients who have bipolar disorder.

For chronic migraine, onabotulinumtoxinA (Botox) is the only therapy approved for adults. Doses of 75 to 260 units are administered in seven specific areas of the head and neck by the health care provider. Monthly treatments for up to five treatment cycles are considered safe and effective (Diener et al., 2014; Carod-Artel, 2014).

In addition to drug therapy, *trigger avoidance and management* are important interventions for preventing migraine episodes. For example, some patients find that avoiding tyramine-containing products, such as pickled products, caffeine, beer, wine, preservatives, and artificial sweeteners, reduces their headaches. Others have identified specific factors that trigger an attack for them. Help patients identify triggers that could cause migraine episodes, and teach them to avoid them once identified (Chart 42-3). For example, at the beginning of a migraine attack, the patient may be able to reduce PAIN by lying down and darkening the room. He or she may want both eyes covered and a cool cloth on the forehead. If the patient falls asleep, he or she should remain undisturbed until awakening.

Complementary and Alternative Therapies. Many patients use complementary and alternative therapies as adjuncts to drug therapy. Yoga, meditation, massage, exercise, and biofeedback are helpful in preventing or treating migraines for some patients. Vitamin B_{12} (riboflavin), coenzyme *Q10*, and magnesium supplement to maintain normal serum values have a role in migraine prevention (Mauskop, 2012).

Acupuncture and acupressure may be effective in relieving PAIN for some patients. Some plastic surgeons have resected the

CHART 42-3 Patient and Family Education: Preparing for Self-Management

Factors That May Trigger a Migraine Attack

Teach patients to avoid factors that may trigger a migraine attack.

Foods Commonly Associated with Migraines
- Alcoholic drinks: beer, wine, and hard liquor
- Aged cheese or other foods with tyramine
- Caffeine found in beverages such as coffee, tea, cola OR caffeine withdrawal
- Chocolate
- Foods with yeast such as pastry and fresh breads
- Monosodium glutamate (MSG)
- Nitrates (meats), pickled or fermented foods
- Nuts
- Artificial sweeteners
- Smoked fish

Drugs Associated with Migraines
- Cimetidine (Tagamet)
- Estrogens
- Nitroglycerin
- Nifedipine (Procardia, Nifed 🍁)

Other Factors That Can Trigger a Migraine Attack
- Anger, conflict
- Fatigue
- Hormonal fluctuations, such as menstruation, pregnancy, and menopause
- Light glare
- Missed meals, hypoglycemia
- Psychological stress
- Sleep problems
- Smells, such as tobacco smoke
- Travel to different altitudes

trigeminal nerve to relieve chronic migraine pain. A number of herbs are also used for headaches, both for prevention and pain management. Teach patients that all herbs and nutritional remedies should be approved by their health care provider before use because they could interact with prescribed medication. At this time, there is insufficient evidence to support any herb or natural remedy, but some patients have had positive results.

NCLEX EXAMINATION CHALLENGE

Health Promotion and Maintenance

The nurse is preparing a teaching plan for a client with migraine headaches. Which of these foods or food additives may trigger a migraine headache?

A. Salt
B. Sugar
C. Tyramine
D. Glutamine

CLUSTER HEADACHE

❖ PATHOPHYSIOLOGY

Cluster headaches are manifested by brief (30 minutes to 2 hours), intense unilateral PAIN that generally occurs in the spring and fall without warning. It is classified as the *most common chronic short-duration headache* with pain lasting less than 4 hours. Also referred to as *trigeminal autonomic cephalalgia,* it is far less common than migraines. Cluster headaches typically develop in men between 20 and 50 years of age. The cause and mechanism of cluster headaches are not known but have been attributed to vasoreactivity and neurogenic inflammation (McCance et al., 2014). Neuroimaging studies suggest that cluster headaches are related to an overactive and enlarged hypothalamus.

❖ PATIENT-CENTERED COLLABORATIVE CARE

◆ Assessment

Question the patient about prescribed drugs for both the prevention and relief of the headache, as well as OTC drugs and herbal preparations he or she may be taking. Interventions used by the patient may include relaxation techniques, meditation, acupuncture, massage therapies, and avoidance of the known headache trigger. Ask the patient to recall a typical week's activities and any recent changes in lifestyle. Explore the relationship of cluster headache onset with emotional and behavioral precipitating factors such as bursts of anger, prolonged anticipation, excessive physical activity, and excitement. Ask him or her to identify bedtimes and waking times to help assess changes in activity or lack of continuity in the sleep-wake cycle.

The PAIN of these unilateral (one-sided) oculotemporal or oculofrontal headaches is often described as excruciating, boring, and *nonthrobbing*. The intense pain is felt deep in and around the eye. The headaches occur at about the same time of day for about 4 to 12 weeks (hence the term *cluster*), followed by a period of remission for 9 months to a year. This episodic form is the most common, although there is a chronic, intractable form in which there may not be a remission for more than a year.

The PAIN may radiate to the forehead, temple, or cheek. It may also radiate, but to a lesser extent, to the ear and neck. The temporal artery may be prominent and tender. The patient often paces, walks, or sits and rocks during an attack. A cluster is the only headache type in which this behavior occurs. During periods of remission, alcohol does not cause a headache (as it does during the headache period). The onset of the pain is associated with relaxation, napping, or rapid eye movement (REM) sleep.

The headache usually occurs with:
- **Ipsilateral** (same side) tearing of the eye
- **Rhinorrhea** ("runny nose") or congestion
- **Ptosis** (drooping eyelid)
- Eyelid edema
- Facial sweating
- **Miosis** (constriction of pupils)

The ptosis may become permanent. Assess for possible bradycardia, flushing or pallor of the face, increased intraocular pressure, and increased skin temperature. Nausea and vomiting may also occur. The patient may become restless and agitated from the intense pain of the headache.

◆ Interventions

Explain the need for and importance of a consistent sleep-wake cycle. The health care provider typically prescribes some of the same types of drugs used for migraines, such as triptans, ergotamine preparations, calcium channel blockers, and antiepileptic drugs (see discussion of drug therapy in the Migraine Headache section). Additional drugs include lithium and corticosteroids. OTC civamide (a capsaicin isomer), available as a nasal spray, oral melatonin, and oral glucosamine are also used by some patients. Provide health teaching about drug therapy (Lilley et al., 2014).

During the periods of attack, teach the patient to wear sunglasses and to sit facing away from the window to help decrease exposure to light and glare. For a cluster migraine, the health care provider may prescribe oxygen via high-flow mask at 12 L/min. High-flow oxygen to manage a cluster migraine is typically administered with the patient in a sitting position. Administer the oxygen for 15 to 20 minutes; most patients report relief within 15 minutes. High-flow oxygen is thought to inhibit activity of the carotid bodies and reduce the vasoreactivity of cerebral blood vessels to neurogenic stimuli. Patients may use oxygen at home. Teach them about the precautions that must be taken when oxygen is used (see Chapter 28).

Surgical intervention may be recommended for patients with *chronic* drug-resistant cluster headaches. Invasive ambulatory care procedures, such as *percutaneous stereotactic rhizotomy (PSR),* are performed with varying success rates. Information about this procedure is found in Chapter 44 in the Trigeminal Neuralgia section. Long-term high-frequency electrical stimulation of the posterior hypothalamus, also known as *deep brain stimulation,* may reduce or eliminate PAIN (see procedure discussion on p. 871 in the Parkinson Disease section). It has not been approved by the FDA but is being investigated. Both of these procedures have major complications that can cause permanent brain or nerve damage. Therefore they are done as a last resort.

SEIZURES AND EPILEPSY

❖ PATHOPHYSIOLOGY

A **seizure** is an abnormal, sudden, excessive, uncontrolled electrical discharge of neurons within the brain that may result in a change in level of consciousness (LOC), motor or sensory ability, and/or behavior. A single seizure may occur for no known reason. Some seizures are caused by a pathologic condition of the brain, such as a tumor. In this case, once the underlying problem is treated, the patient is often asymptomatic.

Epilepsy is defined by the National Institute of Neurological Disorders and Stroke as two or more seizures experienced by a person. It is a chronic disorder in which repeated unprovoked seizure activity occurs. It may be caused by an abnormality in electrical neuronal activity; an imbalance of neurotransmitters, especially gamma aminobutyric acid (GABA); or a combination of both (McCance et al., 2014).

Types of Seizures

The International Classification of Epileptic Seizures recognizes three broad categories of seizure disorders: generalized seizures, partial seizures, and unclassified seizures.

Five types of **generalized seizures** may occur in adults and involve *both* cerebral hemispheres. The *tonic-clonic seizure* lasting 2 to 5 minutes begins with a **tonic phase** that causes stiffening or rigidity of the muscles, particularly of the arms and legs, and immediate loss of consciousness. **Clonic** or **rhythmic** jerking of all extremities follows. The patient may bite his or her tongue and may become incontinent of urine or feces. Fatigue, acute confusion, and lethargy may last up to an hour after the seizure.

Occasionally, only tonic or clonic movement may occur. A *tonic seizure* is an abrupt increase in muscle tone, loss of consciousness, and autonomic changes lasting from 30 seconds to several minutes. The *clonic seizure* lasts several minutes and causes muscle contraction and relaxation.

The *myoclonic seizure* causes a brief jerking or stiffening of the extremities that may occur singly or in groups. Lasting for just a few seconds, the contractions may be symmetric (both sides) or asymmetric (one side).

In an *atonic (akinetic) seizure,* the patient has a sudden loss of muscle tone, lasting for seconds, followed by **postictal** (after the seizure) confusion. In most cases, these seizures cause the patient to fall, which may result in injury. This type of seizure tends to be most resistant to drug therapy.

Partial seizures, also called *focal* or *local* seizures, begin in a part of *one* cerebral hemisphere. They are further subdivided into two main classes: complex partial seizures and simple partial seizures. In addition, some partial seizures can become generalized tonic-clonic, tonic, or clonic seizures. Partial seizures are most often seen in adults and generally are less responsive to medical treatment when compared with other types.

Complex partial seizures may cause loss of consciousness (**syncope**), or "black out," for 1 to 3 minutes. Characteristic automatisms may occur as in absence seizures. The patient is unaware of the environment and may wander at the start of the seizure. In the period after the seizure, he or she may have **amnesia** (loss of memory). Because the area of the brain most often involved in this type of epilepsy is the temporal lobe, complex partial seizures are often called *psychomotor* seizures or *temporal lobe* seizures.

CONSIDERATIONS FOR OLDER ADULTS

Patient-Centered Care QSEN

Complex partial seizures are most common among older adults. These seizures are difficult to diagnose because symptoms appear similar to dementia, psychosis, or other neurobehavioral disorders, especially in the **postictal stage** (after the seizure). New-onset seizures in older adults are typically associated with conditions such as hypertension, cardiac disease, diabetes mellitus, stroke, dementia, and recent brain injury (Lin et al., 2012).

The patient with a *simple partial seizure* remains conscious throughout the episode. He or she often reports an **aura** (unusual sensation) before the seizure takes place. This may consist of a "déjà vu" (already seen) phenomenon, perception of an offensive smell, or sudden onset of PAIN. During the seizure, the patient may have one-sided movement of an extremity, experience unusual sensations, or have autonomic symptoms. Autonomic changes include a change in heart rate, skin flushing, and epigastric discomfort.

Unclassified, or **idiopathic, seizures** account for about half of all seizure activity. They occur for no known reason and do not fit into the generalized or partial classifications.

Etiology and Genetic Risk

Primary or *idiopathic epilepsy* is not associated with any identifiable brain lesion or other specific cause; however, genetic factors most likely play a role in its development. *Secondary seizures* result from an underlying brain lesion, most commonly a tumor or trauma. They may also be caused by:

- Metabolic disorders
- Acute alcohol withdrawal

- Electrolyte disturbances (e.g., hyperkalemia, water intoxication, hypoglycemia)
- High fever
- Stroke
- Head injury
- Substance abuse
- Heart disease

Seizures resulting from these problems are not considered epilepsy. Various risk factors can trigger a seizure, such as increased physical activity, emotional stress, excessive fatigue, alcohol or caffeine consumption, or certain foods or chemicals.

GENDER HEALTH CONSIDERATIONS

Patient-Centered Care QSEN

Management of women with epilepsy is challenging. Hormonal changes from menstrual cycling and the interaction of oral contraceptives with antiepileptic drugs (AEDs) require the health care provider and patient to be aware of a variety of guidelines and to more frequently monitor drug effectiveness. There are potential teratogenic risks associated with AEDs. Despite the considerable risk for teratogenicity with AEDs use in pregnancy, more than 90% of pregnancies are uneventful (Babtain, 2012). AEDs can also contribute to osteoporosis in menopausal women. As a result, coordination between the neurologist, the woman's health care provider, and the patient is required for safe, effective care. Nurses can facilitate patient education, communication, and collaboration to promote safe, effective care.

❖ *PATIENT-CENTERED COLLABORATIVE CARE*

◆ *Assessment*

Question the patient or family about how many seizures the patient has had, how long they last, and any pattern of occurrence. Ask the patient or family to describe the seizures that the patient has had. Clinical manifestations vary depending on the type of seizure experienced, as described earlier. Ask about the presence of an aura before seizures begin (**preictal phase**). Question whether the patient is taking any prescribed drugs or herbs or has had head trauma or high fever. Assess any alcohol and/or illicit drug history. Ask about any other medical condition such as a previous stroke or hypertension.

If the seizure is a new symptom, ask the patient or family if any loss of consciousness or brain injury has occurred, both in the recent and distant past. Oftentimes, patients may have had a head or brain injury sufficient to cause a loss of consciousness but may not remember this at the time of the seizure, especially if it was during their childhood.

Diagnosis is based on the history and physical examination. A variety of diagnostic tests are performed to rule out other causes of seizure activity and to confirm the diagnosis of epilepsy. Typical diagnostic tests include an electroencephalogram (EEG), computed tomography (CT) scan, MRI, or positron emission tomography (PET) scan. These tests are described in Chapter 41. Laboratory studies are performed to identify metabolic or other disorders that may cause or contribute to seizure activity.

◆ *Interventions*

Removing or treating the underlying condition or cause of the seizure manages *secondary* epilepsy and seizures that are not considered epileptic. *In most cases, primary epilepsy is successfully managed through drug therapy.*

Nonsurgical Management. Most seizures can be completely or almost completely controlled through the administration of **antiepileptic drugs (AEDs)**, sometimes referred to as *anticonvulsants,* for specific types of seizures.

Drug Therapy. Drug therapy is the major component of management (Chart 42-4). The health care provider introduces one antiepileptic drug (AED) at a time to achieve seizure control. If the chosen drug is not effective, the dosage may be increased or another drug introduced. At times, seizure control is achieved only through a combination of drugs. The dosages are adjusted to achieve therapeutic blood levels without causing major side effects.

Teach patients to take their drugs on time to maintain therapeutic blood levels and maximum effectiveness. Emphasize the importance of taking their AEDs as prescribed. Instruct patients that they can build up sensitivity to the drugs as they age. If sensitivity occurs, tell them they will need to have blood levels of this drug checked frequently to adjust the dose. In some cases, the antiseizure effects of drugs can decline and lead to an increase in seizures. Because of this potential for "drug decline and sensitivity," patients need to keep their scheduled laboratory appointments to check serum drug levels.

Be aware of drug-drug and drug-food interactions. For instance, warfarin (Coumadin, Warfilone 🍁) should not be given with phenytoin (Dilantin). Document side and adverse effects of the prescribed drugs, and report to the health care provider. Patients should be taught that some citrus fruits, such as grapefruit juice, can interfere with the metabolism of these drugs. This interference can raise the blood level of the drug and cause the patient to develop drug toxicity.

Self-Management Education. Provide self-management education for the patient and family (Chart 42-5). Ask them what they understand about the disorder, and correct any misinformation. As new information is presented, be sure that the patient and family can understand it. Refer patients and families to the Epilepsy Foundation of America for more information and community support groups. Encourage patients and their significant others to utilize information from the Epilepsy Foundation website (www.epilepsy.com).

Emphasize that AEDs must not be stopped even if the seizures have stopped. Discontinuing these drugs can lead to the recurrence of seizures or the life-threatening complication of status epilepticus (discussed below). Some patients may stop therapy because they do not have the money to purchase the drugs. Refer limited-income patients to the social services department for assistance or to a case manager to locate other resources.

A balanced diet, proper rest, and stress-reduction techniques usually minimize the risk for breakthrough seizures. Encourage the patient to keep a seizure diary to determine whether there are factors that tend to be associated with seizure activity. Patients should follow state law concerning allowances for driving a motor vehicle.

All states prohibit discrimination against people who have epilepsy. Patients who work in occupations in which a seizure might cause serious harm to themselves or others (e.g., construction workers, operators of dangerous equipment, pilots) may need other employment. They may need to decrease or modify strenuous or potentially dangerous physical activity to avoid harm, although this varies with each person. Various local, state, and federal agencies can help with finances, living arrangements, and vocational rehabilitation.

CHART 42-4 Common Examples of Drug Therapy

Epilepsy

DRUG	INDICATION FOR USE	NURSING INTERVENTIONS
Carbamazepine (Tegretol, Tegretol-XR, Carbatrol)	Partial, generalized tonic-clonic seizures	Monitor for headache, dizziness, diplopia or blurred vision, N/V, and leukopenia. Monitor CBC. Do not crush or chew sustained-release capsules.
Clonazepam (Klonopin)	Absence, myoclonic, and akinetic seizures	Monitor results of liver function tests.
Clorazepate dipotassium	Adjunctive management of partial seizures	Give with food. Monitor blood pressure.
Diazepam (Valium, Apo-Diazepam 🍁), lorazepam (Ativan), Diastat (diazepam rectal gel delivery system)	Status epilepticus	Monitor **a**irway, **b**reathing, **c**irculation (ABCs).
Divalproex (Depakote), valproic acid (Depakene)	All types of seizures	Monitor for hair loss, tremor, increased liver enzymes, bruising, and N/V. Monitor CBC, PT, PTT, and AST.
Ethosuximide (Zarontin)	Absence seizures	Watch for N/V, skin rash, lethargy, and anorexia. Monitor CBC and liver function tests. (Drug used infrequently.)
Felbamate (Felbatol)	Adjunctive therapy for intractable complex partial seizures	Note that aplastic anemia and liver failure are major sequelae of treatment. Patient must sign consent for use, acknowledging risk for aplastic anemia and liver failure. Monitor CBC. Monitor liver function tests. Watch for anorexia and weight loss.
Gabapentin (Neurontin)	Partial seizures	Watch for increased appetite and weight gain. Monitor for ataxia, irritability, dizziness, and fatigue.
Lamotrigine (Lamictal)	Partial seizures	Watch for diplopia, headaches, dizziness, drowsiness, ataxia, N/V, and life-threatening rash when given with valproic acid.
Levetiracetam (Keppra)	Adjunct management of partial seizures	Monitor renal function carefully. Notify health care provider for gait or coordination problems.
Oxcarbazepine (Trileptal)	Partial seizures	Monitor for hyponatremia.
Phenobarbital (Barbita, Luminal)	Generalized tonic-clonic seizures, partial seizures	Note that this is less desirable than other antiepileptic drugs (AEDs) because of sedation. Be aware that overdose can be fatal. Monitor for drowsiness, sleep disturbances, impaired cognition, and depression.
Phenytoin (Dilantin), fosphenytoin (Cerebyx)	All types, except absence, myoclonic, and atonic seizures; for status epilepticus	Monitor for gastric distress, gingival hyperplasia, anemia, ataxia, and nystagmus. Check CBC and calcium levels; monitor for therapeutic drug levels (10-20 mcg/mL) and toxic levels (>30 mcg/mL). For IV phenytoin, flush catheter with saline before and after administration. For fosphenytoin, use phenytoin equivalent for dosing.
Primidone (Mysoline, Sertan 🍁)	Partial seizures, generalized tonic-clonic seizures	Monitor for vertigo and lethargy. Watch for drug interactions with phenobarbital and isoniazid.
Tiagabine (Gabitril)	Partial seizures	Monitor for dizziness, weakness, nervousness, psychomotor slowing, nystagmus, and paresthesias. Administer with food.
Topiramate (Topamax)	Adjunctive therapy for intractable partial seizures	Monitor for ataxia, confusion, dizziness, and fatigue. Be aware of increased risk for renal calculi.
Valproate (Depakote), valproate sodium injection (Depacon)	Simple and complex absence seizures Adjunct therapy for partial complex and generalized tonic-clonic seizures	Monitor for hair loss, tremor, increased liver enzymes, bruising, and N/V. Monitor CBC, PT, PTT, AST.
Zonisamide (Zonegran)	Adjunctive therapy for partial seizures	Monitor CBC, platelets, and renal function. Assess mental status, especially memory.

AST, Aspartate aminotransferase; *CBC,* complete blood count; *N/V,* nausea and vomiting; *PT,* prothrombin time; *PTT,* partial thromboplastin time.

Seizure Precautions. Precautions are taken to prevent the patient from injury if a seizure occurs. Specific seizure precautions vary depending on health care agency policy.

Siderails are rarely the source of significant injury, and the effectiveness of the use of padded siderails to maintain safety is debatable. Padded siderails may embarrass the patient and the family. Follow agency policy about the use of siderails because they may be classified as a restraint device. Other methods to

! NURSING SAFETY PRIORITY (QSEN)

Action Alert

Seizure precautions include ensuring that oxygen and suctioning equipment with an airway are readily available. If the patient does not have an IV access, insert a saline lock, especially if he or she is at significant risk for generalized tonic-clonic seizures. The saline lock provides ready access if IV drug therapy must be given to stop the seizure.

CHART 42-5 Patient and Family Education: Preparing for Self-Management

Health Teaching for the Patient with Epilepsy

- Drug therapy information:
  - Name, dosage, time of administration
  - Actions to take if side effects occur
  - Importance of taking drug as prescribed and not missing a dose
  - What to do if a dose is missed or cannot be taken
  - Importance of having blood drawn for therapeutic or toxic levels as requested by the health care provider
- Do not take any medication, including over-the-counter drugs, without asking your health care provider.
- Wear a medical alert bracelet or necklace, or carry an identification card indicating epilepsy.
- Follow up with your neurologist, physician, or other health care provider as directed.
- Be sure a family member or significant other knows how to help you in the event of a seizure and knows when your health care provider or emergency medical services should be called.
- Investigate and follow state laws concerning driving and operating machinery.
- Avoid alcohol and excessive fatigue.
- Contact the Epilepsy Foundation (www.epilepsy.com) or other organized epilepsy group for additional information. Epilepsy Canada (www.epilepsy.ca) also provides resources and support.

CHART 42-6 Best Practice for Patient Safety & Quality Care QSEN

Care of the Patient During a Tonic-Clonic or Complete Partial Seizure

- Protect the patient from injury.
- Do not force anything into the patient's mouth.
- Turn the patient to the side to keep the airway clear.
- Loosen any restrictive clothing the patient is wearing.
- Maintain the patient's airway and suction oral secretions as needed.
- Do not restrain or try to stop the patient's movement; guide movements if necessary.
- Record the time the seizure began and ended.
- At the completion of the seizure:
  - Take the patient's vital signs.
  - Perform neurologic checks.
  - Keep the patient on his or her side.
  - Allow the patient to rest.
  - Document the seizure (see Chart 42-7).

protect the patient, such as placing a mattress on the floor, may be used instead of siderails.

Padded tongue blades do not belong at the bedside and should NEVER be inserted into the patient's mouth because the jaw may clench down as soon as the seizure begins! Forcing a tongue blade or airway into the mouth is more likely to chip the teeth and increase the risk for aspirating tooth fragments than prevent the patient from biting the tongue. Furthermore, improper placement of a padded tongue blade can obstruct the airway.

Seizure Management. The actions taken during a seizure should be appropriate for the type of seizure (Chart 42-6). For example, for a simple partial seizure, observe the patient and document the time that the seizure lasted. Redirect the patient's attention away from an activity that could cause injury. Turn the patient on the side during a generalized tonic-clonic or complex partial seizure because he or she may lose consciousness. If possible, turn the patient's head to the side to prevent aspiration and allow secretions to drain. Remove any objects that might injure the patient.

It is not unusual for the patient to become cyanotic during a generalized tonic-clonic seizure. The cyanosis is generally self-limiting, and no treatment is needed. Some health care providers prefer to give the high-risk patient (e.g., older adult, critically ill, or debilitated patient) oxygen by nasal cannula or facemask during the postictal phase. He or she is not restrained because this may cause injury and may worsen the situation, causing more seizure activity. For any type of seizure, carefully observe the seizure and document assessment findings (Chart 42-7).

CHART 42-7 Focused Assessment

Seizures: Nursing Observations and Documentation

- How often the seizures occur:
  - Date, time, and duration of the seizure
- Description of each seizure:
  - Tonic, clonic
  - Staring spells, blinking
  - Automatism
- Whether more than one type of seizure occurs
- Sequence of seizure progression:
  - Where the seizure began
  - Body part first involved
- Observations during the seizure:
  - Changes in pupil size and any eye deviation
  - Level of consciousness
  - Presence of apnea, cyanosis, and salivation
  - Incontinence of bowel or bladder during the seizure
  - Eye fluttering
  - Movement and progression of motor activity
  - Lip smacking or other automatism
  - Tongue or lip biting
- How long the seizures last
- When the last seizure took place
- Whether the seizures are preceded by an aura:
  - Dizziness, numbness, or visual disturbances
  - Gustatory (taste) or auditory disturbances
- What the patient does after the seizure:
  - Feels drowsy or weak
  - May resume normal behavior
  - May be unaware that the seizure took place
- How long it takes for the patient to return to pre-seizure status

Emergency Care: Acute Seizure and Status Epilepticus Management. Seizures occurring in greater intensity, number, or length than the patient's usual seizures are considered *acute.* They may also appear in clusters that are different from the patient's typical seizure pattern. Treatment with lorazepam (Ativan, Apo-Lorazepam 🍁) or diazepam (Valium, Meval 🍁, Vivol 🍁, Diastat [rectal diazepam gel]) may be given to stop the clusters to prevent the development of status epilepticus. IV phenytoin (Dilantin) or fosphenytoin (Cerebyx) may be added.

Status epilepticus is a medical emergency and is a prolonged seizure lasting longer than 5 minutes or repeated seizures over the course of 30 minutes. It is a potential complication of all types of seizures. *Seizures lasting longer than 10 minutes can cause death!* Common causes of status epilepticus include:

- Sudden withdrawal from antiepileptic drugs
- Infection
- Acute alcohol or drug withdrawal

NURSING SAFETY PRIORITY (QSEN)

Critical Rescue

Convulsive status epilepticus must be treated promptly and aggressively! Establish an airway and notify the health care provider or Rapid Response Team immediately if this problem occurs! Establishing an airway is the priority for this patient's care. Intubation by an anesthesia provider or respiratory therapist may be necessary. Administer oxygen as indicated by the patient's condition. If not already in place, establish IV access with a large-bore catheter, and start 0.9% sodium chloride. The patient is usually placed in the intensive care unit for continuous monitoring and management.

- Head trauma
- Cerebral edema
- Metabolic disturbances

Blood is drawn to determine arterial blood gas levels and to identify metabolic, toxic, and other causes of the uncontrolled seizure. Brain damage and death may occur in the patient with tonic-clonic status epilepticus. Left untreated, metabolic changes result, leading to hypoxia, hypotension, hypoglycemia, cardiac dysrhythmias, or lactic (metabolic) acidosis. Further harm to the patient occurs when muscle breaks down and myoglobin accumulates in the kidneys, which can lead to renal failure and electrolyte imbalance. *This is especially likely in the older adult.*

The drugs of choice for treating status epilepticus are IV-push lorazepam (Ativan, Apo-Lorazepam ♣) or diazepam (Valium). Diazepam rectal gel (Diastat) may be used instead. Lorazepam is usually given as 4 mg over a 2-minute period. This procedure may be repeated, if necessary, until a total of 8 mg is reached.

To prevent additional tonic-clonic seizures or cardiac arrest, a loading dose of IV phenytoin (Dilantin) is given and oral doses administered as a follow-up after the emergency is resolved. Initially, give phenytoin at no more than 50 mg/min using an infusion pump. An alternative to phenytoin is fosphenytoin (Cerebyx), a water-soluble phenytoin prodrug. It is compatible with most IV solutions. It also causes fewer cardiovascular complications than phenytoin and can be given in an IV dextrose solution. After administration, fosphenytoin converts to phenytoin in the body. Therefore the FDA requires the dosage to be written as a phenytoin equivalent (PE): 150 mg of fosphenytoin equals 100 mg of phenytoin. Give fosphenytoin at a rate of 100 to 150 mg/min IV piggyback (Lilley et al., 2014).

Serum drug levels are checked every 6 to 12 hours after the loading dose and then 2 weeks after oral phenytoin has started. Teach the patient about the side and adverse effects of any AED that is prescribed (see Chart 42-4).

NCLEX EXAMINATION CHALLENGE

Safe and Effective Care Environment

A client with a history of seizures is placed on seizure precautions. What emergency equipment will the nurse provide at the bedside? **Select all that apply.**

A. Oropharyngeal airway
B. Oxygen
C. Nasogastric tube
D. Suction setup
E. Padded tongue blade

Surgical Management. Patients who cannot be managed effectively with drug therapy may be candidates for surgery, including vagal nerve stimulation (VNS) and conventional surgical procedures. VNS has been very successful for many patients with epilepsy.

Vagal Nerve Stimulation. Vagal nerve stimulation (VNS) may be performed for control of continuous simple or complex partial seizures. Patients with generalized seizures are not candidates for surgery because VNS may result in severe neurologic deficits. The stimulating device (much like a cardiac pacemaker) is surgically implanted in the left chest wall. An electrode lead is attached to the left vagus nerve, tunneled under the skin, and connected to a generator. The procedure usually takes 2 hours with the patient under general anesthesia. The stimulator is activated by the physician either in the operating room or, more commonly, 2 weeks after surgery. Programming is adjusted gradually over a period of time. The pattern of stimulation is individualized to the patient's tolerance. The generator runs continuously, stimulating the vagus nerve according to the programmed schedule.

The patient can activate the VNS with a handheld magnet when experiencing an aura, thus aborting the seizure. Patients experience a change in voice quality, which signifies that the vagus nerve has been stimulated. They usually report a relief in intensity and duration of seizures and an improved quality of life.

Observe for complications after the procedure such as hoarseness (most common), cough, dyspnea, neck pain, or dysphagia (difficulty swallowing). Teach the patient to avoid MRIs, microwaves, shortwave radios, and ultrasound diathermy (a physical therapy heat treatment).

Conventional Surgical Procedures. A small percentage of patients with epilepsy cannot be fully controlled with drug therapy or VNS. When all other options are exhausted, conventional surgery may be needed to improve the patient's quality of life. The largest group of conventional surgical candidates includes those with complex partial seizures in the frontal or temporal lobe.

Before surgery, the patient is admitted to a special inpatient observation unit. While there, he or she has continuous electroencephalogram (EEG) recording, close observation, and in many hospitals, video monitoring at all times except during personal care activities. The patient is taken off all AEDs. After the seizure area is identified, electrodes may be surgically implanted into the brain tissue to identify the extent of the focal area. This step is followed by additional continuous EEG and video monitoring, as well as close observation by the nursing staff. The area is surgically removed if vital areas of brain function will not be affected.

Preoperative care is similar to that described for patients undergoing a craniotomy (see Chapter 45). Preoperative diagnostic tests include MRI and single-photon emission computed tomography (SPECT)/positron emission tomography (PET) scans as described in Chapter 41. An intracarotid amobarbital test (Wada test) and neuropsychological testing are also done. The Wada test assesses hemispheric lateralization of language and memory after injection of amobarbital, a short-acting anesthetic. This procedure establishes the safety of surgery to preserve language memory. Neuropsychological testing evaluates memory, visuospatial function, language function, and intelligence quotient (IQ) to identify deficiencies in the brain that might correspond to areas believed to be the epileptic region. It is also used to compare preoperative and postoperative COGNITION.

Another surgical approach, the *partial corpus callosotomy,* may be used to treat tonic-clonic or atonic seizures in patients who are not candidates for other surgical procedures. The surgeon sections the anterior two thirds of the corpus callosum, preventing neuronal discharges from passing between the two hemispheres of the brain. This surgery usually reduces the number and severity of the seizures, making them more likely to respond to more conventional drug therapy. This procedure is not as commonly done as other surgeries but is very successful for some patients.

INFECTIONS

MENINGITIS

❖ PATHOPHYSIOLOGY

Meningitis is an inflammation of the meninges, specifically the pia mater and arachnoid. Bacterial and viral organisms are most often responsible for meningitis, although fungal and protozoal meningitis also occur. Cancer and some drugs, notably NSAIDs, antibiotics, and intravenous immunoglobulins, can also cause sterile meningitis. Regardless of cause of meningitis, the symptoms are similar.

The organisms responsible for meningitis enter the central nervous system (CNS) via the bloodstream or are directly introduced into the CNS. Direct routes of entry occur as a result of penetrating trauma, surgical procedures on the brain or spine, or a ruptured brain **abscess**. A basilar skull fracture may lead to meningitis as a result of the direct communication of cerebrospinal fluid (CSF) with the ear or nasal passages, manifested by **otorrhea** (ear discharge) or **rhinorrhea** (nasal discharge, or "runny nose") that is actually CSF. The infecting organisms follow the tract created by skull damage to enter the CNS and circulate in the CSF. The patient with an INFECTION in the head (i.e., eye, ear, nose, mouth) or neck has an increased risk for meningitis because of the proximity of anatomic structures. Infections linked to meningitis include otitis media, acute or chronic sinusitis, and tooth abscess; there are also reports of rare infection from a tongue piercing leading to meningitis. The immunocompromised patient (e.g., one without a spleen) receiving treatment for cancer, taking immunosuppressant drugs to manage autoimmune disease or solid organ transplant, and older adults) is also at increased risk for meningitis. The infecting organism may spread to both cranial and spinal nerves, causing irreversible neurologic damage. Increased intracranial pressure (ICP) may occur as a result of blockage of the flow of CSF, change in cerebral blood flow, or thrombus (blood clot) formation.

Viral meningitis, the most common type, is sometimes referred to as *aseptic meningitis* because no organisms are typically isolated from culture of the CSF. Common viral organisms causing meningitis are enterovirus, herpes simplex virus–2 (HSV-2), varicella zoster virus (VZV) (also causes chickenpox and shingles), mumps virus, and the human immune deficiency virus (HIV). The severity of symptoms can vary by the infecting viral agent. For example, the herpes simplex virus alters cellular metabolism, which quickly results in necrosis of the cells. HSV-2 meningitis may be accompanied by genital infections. Other viruses cause an alteration in the production of enzymes or neurotransmitters. While these alterations result in cell dysfunction, neurologic defects are more likely to be temporary and a full recovery occurs as the inflammation resolves. Treatment may include the administration of antiviral agents.

Cryptococcus neoformans meningitis is the most common *fungal* INFECTION that affects the central nervous system (CNS) of patients with acquired immune deficiency syndrome (AIDS). Fulminant invasive fungal sinusitis is also a recognized cause of fungal meningitis. The clinical manifestations vary because the compromised immune system affects the inflammatory response. For example, some patients have fever and others do not. Treatment is symptomatic and includes IV antifungal agents.

The most frequently involved organisms responsible for bacterial meningococcal meningitis are *Streptococcus pneumoniae (pneumococcal disease)* and *Neisseria meningitidis. N. meningitidis* meningitis is also known as *meningococcal meningitis. Meningococcal meningitis is a medical emergency with a fairly high mortality rate, often within 24 hours.* Unlike other types, this disorder is highly contagious. Outbreaks of meningococcal meningitis are most likely to occur in areas of high population density, such as college dormitories, military barracks, and crowded living areas.

! NURSING SAFETY PRIORITY (QSEN)

Action Alert

People ages 16 through 21 years have the highest rates of INFECTION from life-threatening *N. meningitidis* meningococcal infection. The Centers for Disease Control and Prevention (CDC) recommends an initial meningococcal vaccine between ages 11 and 12 years with a booster at age 16 years (www.cdc.gov). Adults are advised to get an initial or booster vaccine if living in a shared residence (residence hall, military barracks, group home), traveling or residing in countries in which the disease is common, or are immunocompromised due to a damaged or surgically removed spleen or a serum complement deficiency. If the patient's baseline vaccination status is unclear and the immediate risk for exposure to *N. meningitidis* infection is high, the CDC recommends vaccination. It is safe to receive a booster as early as 8 weeks after the initial vaccine.

❖ PATIENT-CENTERED COLLABORATIVE CARE

◆ Assessment

Perform a complete neurologic and neurovascular assessment to detect clinical manifestations associated with a diagnosis of meningitis or suspected meningitis as outlined in Chart 42-8. Signs and symptoms of meningitis result from meningeal irritation. Clinical manifestations of meningitis include fever, **nuchal rigidity** (neck stiffness), **photophobia** (light sensitivity), **phonophobia** (noise sensitivity), headache, **myalgia** (muscle aches), nausea, and vomiting. Confusion and altered consciousness may be present. A maculopapular rash is seen when the causative organism is an enterovirus. A petechial rash is associated with *N. meningitidis* meningitis. Although the classic nuchal rigidity (stiff neck) and positive Kernig's and Brudzinski's signs have been traditionally used to diagnose meningitis, these findings occur in only a small percentage of patients with a definitive diagnosis. Older adults, patients who are immunocompromised, and those who are receiving antibiotics may not have fever. Assess the patient for complications, including increased ICP. Left untreated, increased ICP can lead to herniation of the brain and death (see Chapter 45).

CHART 42-8 Key Features

Meningitis

- Decreased (or change in) level of consciousness
- Disoriented to person, place, and year
- Pupil reaction and eye movements:
  - Photophobia
  - Nystagmus
  - Abnormal eye movements
- Motor response:
  - Normal early in disease process
  - Hemiparesis, hemiplegia, and decreased muscle tone possible later
  - Cranial nerve dysfunction, especially CN III, IV, VI, VII, VIII
- Memory changes:
  - Attention span (usually short)
  - Personality and behavior changes
  - Bewilderment
- Severe, unrelenting headaches
- Generalized muscle aches and pain
- Nausea and vomiting
- Fever and chills
- Tachycardia
- Red macular rash (meningococcal meningitis)

Seizure activity may occur when meningeal inflammation spreads to the cerebral cortex. Inflammation can also result in abnormal stimulation of the hypothalamic area where excessive amounts of antidiuretic hormone (ADH) (vasopressin) are produced. Excess vasopressin results in water retention and dilution of serum sodium caused by increased sodium loss by the kidneys. This syndrome of inappropriate antidiuretic hormone (SIADH, Chapter 62) may lead to further increases in ICP.

Systemic inflammation (systemic inflammatory response syndrome or **SIRS**), a reaction to either endotoxin produced by infecting bacteria or activation of the immune cells by infecting organisms, can cause a rapidly falling blood pressure and tachycardia. Coagulopathy can occur as a result of systemic inflammation. Assess the patient's vascular status by:

- Observing the color and temperature of the extremities
- Determining the presence of peripheral pulses
- Identifying any indicators of abnormal bleeding

Thrombi may block circulation in the small vessels of the hands and feet, leading to gangrene. Coagulopathy from SIRS may lead to disseminated intravascular coagulation (DIC).

The most significant laboratory test used in the diagnosis of meningitis is the analysis of the *cerebrospinal fluid (CSF)*. Patients older than 60 years, those who are immunocompromised, or those who have signs of increased ICP usually have a CT scan before the lumbar puncture. If there will be a delay in obtaining the CSF, blood is drawn for culture and sensitivity. A broad-spectrum antibiotic should be given before the lumbar puncture. The CSF is analyzed for cell count, differential count, and protein. Glucose concentrations are determined, and culture, sensitivity, and Gram stain studies are performed. Table 42-2 compares the CSF findings in bacterial and viral meningitis.

Counterimmunoelectrophoresis (CIE) may be performed to determine the presence of viruses or protozoa in the CSF. CIE is also indicated if the patient has received antibiotics before the CSF was obtained. To identify a bacterial source of INFECTION, specimens for Gram stains and culture are obtained from the urine, throat, and nose when indicated.

TABLE 42-2 Cerebrospinal Fluid Findings in Bacterial and Viral Meningitis

FINDING	BACTERIAL MENINGITIS	VIRAL MENINGITIS
Appearance	Cloudy, turbid	Clear
White blood cells	Increased	Increased
Protein	Increased	Slightly increased
Glucose	Decreased	Most often normal, but may be decreased
CSF pressure	Elevated	Normal or elevated

CSF, Cerebrospinal fluid.

A complete blood count (CBC) is performed. The white blood cell (WBC) count is usually elevated well above the normal value. Serum electrolyte values are also assessed so as to assess and maintain fluid and electrolyte balance.

X-rays of the chest, air sinuses, and mastoids are obtained to determine the presence of INFECTION. A CT or MRI scan may be performed to identify increased ICP, hydrocephalus, or the presence of a brain abscess.

◆ Interventions

Prevent meningitis by teaching people to obtain vaccination. Vaccines are available to protect against Haemophilus influenzae *type B (Hib), pneumococcal, mumps, varicella, and meningococcal organisms. Although many of these vaccines were developed to prevent respiratory illness, they have also reduced CNS infections. Mandatory vaccination programs for school enrollment and proof of vaccination as a prerequisite for group home or dormitory experiences have significantly reduced the incidence of meningitis.*

Maintain thorough handwashing. Teach visitors to wash hands before and after entering a patient's room. Preventing the transmission of infection through hand cleaning is a National Patient Safety Goal (The Joint Commission, 2014).

The most important nursing interventions for patients with meningitis are accurately monitoring and documenting their neurologic status. Best practices for nursing care are listed in Chart 42-9.

! NURSING SAFETY PRIORITY QSEN

Action Alert

For the patient with meningitis, assess his or her neurologic status and vital signs at least every 4 hours or more often if clinically indicated. *The priority for care is to monitor for early neurologic changes that may indicate increased ICP, such as decreased level of consciousness (LOC).* The patient is also at risk for seizure activity. Care should be provided as discussed in Interventions on pp. 859-863 in the Seizures and Epilepsy section.

Cranial nerve testing is included as part of the routine neurologic assessment because of possible cranial nerve involvement. Particular attention is given to cranial nerves III, IV, VI, VII, and VIII, nerves involved in pupillary shape and accommodation to light (see Chapter 41). *A sixth cranial nerve defect (inability to move the eyes laterally) may indicate the development of* **hydrocephalus** *(excessive accumulation of CSF within the brain's ventricles).* Other indicators of hydrocephalus include signs of increased ICP and urinary incontinence. Urinary incontinence results from decreasing LOC.

CHART 42-9 Best Practice for Patient Safety & Quality Care (QSEN)

Care of the Patient with Meningitis

- Prioritize care to maintain airway, breathing, circulation.
- Take vital signs and perform neurologic checks every 2 to 4 hours, as required.
- Perform cranial nerve assessment, with particular attention to cranial nerves III, IV, VI, VII, and VIII, and monitor for changes.
- Manage pain with drug and nondrug methods.
- Perform vascular assessment, and monitor for changes.
- Give drugs and IV fluids as prescribed, and document the patient's response.
- Record intake and output carefully to maintain fluid balance and prevent fluid overload.
- Monitor body weight to identify fluid retention early.
- Monitor laboratory values closely; report abnormal findings to the physician or nurse practitioner promptly.
- Position carefully to prevent pressure ulcers.
- Perform range-of-motion exercises every 4 hours as needed.
- Decrease environmental stimuli:
  - Provide a quiet environment.
  - Minimize exposure to bright lights from windows and overhead lights.
  - Maintain bedrest with head of bed elevated 30 degrees.
- Maintain Transmission-Based Precautions per hospital policy (for bacterial meningitis).
- Monitor for and prevent complications:
  - Increased intracranial pressure
  - Vascular dysfunction
  - Fluid and electrolyte imbalance
  - Seizures
  - Shock

To avoid life-threatening complications, the health care provider prescribes a broad-spectrum antibiotic until the results of the culture and Gram stain are available. After this information is available, the appropriate anti-infective drug to treat the specific type of meningitis is given. Treatment of bacterial meningitis generally requires a 2-week course of IV antibiotics. Drug therapy should begin within 1 to 2 hours after it is prescribed. Monitor and document the patient's response.

Drugs may be used to treat increased ICP or seizures, including mannitol, a hyperosmolar agent for ICP, and antiepileptic drugs (AEDs). Controversy exists as to whether steroids are helpful in the treatment of all adults with meningitis. They are, however, recommended for patients with *S. pneumoniae* meningitis.

People who have been in close contact with a patient with *N. meningitidis* should have prophylaxis (preventive) treatment with rifampin (Rifadin, Rofact ♣), ciprofloxacin (Cipro), or ceftriaxone (Rocephin). Preventive treatment with rifampin may be prescribed for those in close contact with a patient with *H. influenzae* meningitis (Lilley et al., 2014).

Perform a complete vascular assessment every 4 hours or more often, if indicated, to detect early vascular compromise. Thrombotic or embolic complications are most often seen in circulation to the hand. Assess the patient's temperature, color, pulses, and capillary refill in the fingernails. If vascular compromise is not noticed and left untreated, gangrene can develop quickly, possibly leading to loss of the involved arm. The health care team monitors the patient for other complications, including septic shock, coagulation disorders, acute respiratory distress syndrome, and septic arthritis. These health problems are discussed elsewhere in this textbook.

Standard Precautions are appropriate for all patients with meningitis unless the patient has a bacterial type that is transmitted by droplets, such as *N. meningitides* and *H. influenzae.*

! NURSING SAFETY PRIORITY (QSEN)

Action Alert

Place the patient with bacterial meningitis that is transmitted by droplets on Droplet Precautions *in addition to* Standard Precautions. When possible, place the patient in a private room. Stay at least 3 feet from the patient unless wearing a mask. Patients who are transported outside of the room should wear a mask (see Chapter 23). Teach visitors about the need for these precautions and how to follow them.

ENCEPHALITIS

❖ PATHOPHYSIOLOGY

Encephalitis is an inflammation of the brain tissue and often the surrounding meninges. It affects the cerebrum, the brainstem, and the cerebellum. A viral agent most often causes the disease, although bacteria, fungi, or parasites may also be involved (e.g., malaria). The virus travels to the central nervous system (CNS) via the bloodstream, along peripheral or cranial nerves, or in the meninges (e.g., varicella zoster). Therefore viral encephalitis can be life threatening or lead to persistent neurologic problems such as learning disabilities, epilepsy, memory deficits, or fine motor deficits.

After the virus invades the brain tissue, it begins to reproduce, causing an inflammatory response. Unlike in meningitis, this response does not cause exudate (pus) formation. Inflammation extends over the cerebral cortex, the white matter, and the meninges, causing degeneration of the neurons of the cortex. Demyelination of axons occurs in the involved area because the white matter is destroyed. This destruction leads to hemorrhage, edema, necrosis (cell death), and the development of small lacunae (hollow cavities) within the cerebral hemispheres. Widespread edema can cause compression of blood vessels leading to a further increase in intracranial pressure (ICP). Death may occur from herniation and increased ICP.

Arboviruses can be transmitted to humans through the bite of an infected mosquito or tick. The most common types of encephalitis caused by arboviruses are Eastern or Western equine encephalitis, St. Louis encephalitis, California encephalitis, and West Nile virus.

West Nile virus has gained attention in the United States because it has spread rapidly throughout the country and is a potentially serious illness. This INFECTION is typically mild, and usually the patient is asymptomatic. However, a small percentage of patients develop severe disease. The incubation period is 2 to 15 days after being bitten by an infected mosquito. Other possible sources of transmission include blood products, breast milk, or an organ transplant. Diagnostic tests to determine the presence of West Nile virus include enzyme-linked immunosorbent assay and West Nile virus–specific immunoglobulin M (IgM) antibody in the blood or CSF.

In mild cases of *West Nile virus,* the patient has no symptoms or has mild flu-like symptoms (e.g., fever, body aches, nausea, vomiting). Some people develop serious symptoms that may include high fever, severe headache, decreased level of consciousness, tremors, vision loss, seizures, and muscle weakness or paralysis. These manifestations may last for several weeks, and neurologic deficits may be permanent. A few patients die from the disease, especially those older than 50 years with a weakened immune system (Overstreet, 2011).

Echovirus, coxsackievirus, poliovirus, herpes zoster, and viruses that cause mumps and chickenpox are the common *enteroviruses* associated with encephalitis. *Herpes simplex virus type 1* (HSV1) encephalitis is the most common nonepidemic type of encephalitis in North America. Patients with this disease often have a history of cold sores. The mortality rates for HSV1 encephalitis are very high compared with those for other types of encephalitis.

Amebic meningoencephalitis is caused by the amebae *Naegleria* and *Acanthamoeba.* Both are found in warm freshwater areas and can enter the nasal mucosa of people swimming in ponds or lakes. The amebae may also be found in soil and decaying vegetation. Although this INFECTION has not often been seen in the past, the incidence in North America is increasing, perhaps because ponds and lakes are becoming more polluted.

❖ PATIENT-CENTERED COLLABORATIVE CARE

◆ Assessment

The typical patient with encephalitis has a high fever and reports nausea, vomiting, and a stiff neck. Assess for other clinical manifestations, including possible:

- Changes in mental status (e.g., agitation)
- Motor dysfunction (e.g., dysphagia [difficulty swallowing])
- Focal (specific) neurologic deficits
- Photophobia (light sensitivity) and phonophobia (noise sensitivity)
- Fatigue
- Symptoms of increased ICP (e.g., decreased LOC)
- Joint pain
- Headache
- Vertigo

Assess LOC using the Glasgow Coma Scale (see Chapter 41) or other agency-approved assessment tool. The patient may be lethargic, stuporous, or comatose. Mental status changes are more extensive in the patient with encephalitis than with meningitis. Changes include acute confusion, irritability, and personality and behavior changes (especially noted in the presence of herpes simplex). Signs of meningeal irritation include the presence of nuchal (neck) rigidity and motor changes that vary from a mild weakness to hemiplegia. The patient may have muscle tremors, spasticity, an ataxic gait (postencephalitic Parkinsonism), myoclonic jerks, and increased deep tendon reflexes. Seizure activity is common.

Observe for cranial nerve involvement, such as ocular palsies (paralysis), facial weakness, and nystagmus (involuntary lateral eye movements). The herpes zoster lesion affects cranial and spinal nerve root ganglia, which is clinically manifested by a rash, severe PAIN, itching, burning, or tingling in the areas innervated by these nerves.

Lumbar puncture (LP) is done to analyze the CSF for the specific offending organism. A polymerase chain reaction (PCR) test may be used to detect viral DNA or ribonucleic acid (RNA) in the CSF. Specificity and sensitivity in diagnosing encephalitis are excellent, especially with herpes simplex virus (HSV). The test is rapid and noninvasive, replacing the brain biopsy for diagnosis.

An electroencephalogram is done to evaluate brain wave activity to detect seizures. Brain imaging in the form of a CT scan with and without contrast is performed to evaluate elevated intracranial pressure (ICP) or obstructive hydrocephalus.

CHART 42-10 Patient and Family Education: Preparing for Self-Management

Protecting the Patient and Family from West Nile Virus

- Limit your time outside between dusk and dawn when mosquitoes are out.
- Wear protective clothing, including long sleeves and pants.
- Use an insect repellent containing DEET when outdoors.
- Remove areas of standing water from flower pots, trash cans, and rain gutters.
- Check window and door screens for holes that need repair.
- Keep hot tubs and pools clean and properly chlorinated.

! NURSING SAFETY PRIORITY (QSEN)

Critical Rescue

In severe cases of encephalitis, the patient may have increased ICP resulting from cerebral edema, hemorrhage, and necrosis of brain tissue. If the patient is nonverbal or comatose at baseline, then monitoring vital signs and pupils becomes essential for detecting worsening neurologic status and increased ICP. Changes in vital signs that require an immediate notification of the health care provider are a widened pulse pressure, new bradycardia, and irregular respiratory effort. Pupils that become increasingly dilated and less responsive to light are also communicated urgently. Left untreated, increased ICP leads to herniation of the brain tissue and possibly death (see Chapter 45).

◆ Interventions

Teach people who live in mosquito-infested areas to protect themselves and their families from West Nile virus infections. Chart 42-10 lists measures for preventing this infection. There is no curative treatment for West Nile viral encephalitis.

Acyclovir (Zovirax) is the antiviral drug of choice for the treatment of herpes encephalitis and is associated with a significantly lower mortality rate than vidarabine (Vira-A). Drug therapy is most effective if begun early, before the patient becomes stuporous or comatose. This neurologic decline usually occurs within 4 to 6 days after the initial neurologic symptoms. No specific drug therapy is available for INFECTION by arboviruses or enteroviruses.

Nursing interventions for encephalitis are similar to those for meningitis with the exception of drug therapy. Supportive nursing care and prompt recognition and treatment of increased ICP are essential components of management. *Maintain a patent airway to prevent the development of atelectasis or pneumonia, which can lead to further brain hypoxia (lack of oxygen).*

Provide supportive nursing care for the patient who is immobile, stuporous, or comatose. Delegate and supervise unlicensed assistive personnel (UAP) to turn, cough, and deep breathe the patient at least every 2 hours. Perform deep tracheal suctioning even in the presence of increased ICP if respiratory status is compromised. Assess vital signs and neurologic signs every 2 hours or more frequently if clinically indicated. Elevate the head of the bed 30 to 45 degrees unless contraindicated (e.g., after lumbar puncture or in the patient with severe hypotension). Keep the patient's room darkened and quiet to promote comfort and decrease agitation. Remind UAP to provide safety measures such as keeping the bed in the lowest position.

Provide patient and family support. Families need health teaching to understand how to care for their loved ones. They are often fearful that the patient may not return to his or her baseline. Collaborate with a certified chaplain, social worker, or case manager to provide additional emotional support and counseling.

Patients with encephalitis and permanent neurologic deficits are usually discharged to a rehabilitation setting or a long-term care facility. Those with minimal neurologic problems are discharged to the home setting.

PARKINSON DISEASE

❖ PATHOPHYSIOLOGY

Parkinson disease (PD), also referred to as *Parkinson's disease* and *paralysis agitans,* is a progressive neurodegenerative disease that is the one of the most common neurologic disorders of older adults. It is a debilitating disease affecting motor ability and is characterized by four cardinal symptoms: tremor, muscle rigidity, **bradykinesia** or **akinesia** (slow movement/no movement), and postural instability. Most people have *primary,* or idiopathic, disease. A few patients have *secondary* parkinsonian symptoms from conditions such as brain tumors and certain anti-psychotic drugs.

Motor activity occurs as a result of integrating the actions of the cerebral cortex, basal ganglia, and cerebellum. The basal ganglia are a group of neurons located deep within the cerebrum at the base of the brain near the lateral ventricles. When the basal ganglia are stimulated, muscle tone in the body is inhibited and voluntary movements are refined. The secretion of two major neurotransmitters accomplishes this process: dopamine and acetylcholine (ACh).

Dopamine is produced in the substantia nigra, as well as in the adrenal glands, and is transmitted to the basal ganglia along a connecting neural pathway for secretion when needed. *ACh* is produced and secreted by the basal ganglia, as well as in the nerve endings in the periphery of the body. ACh-producing neurons transmit *excitatory* messages throughout the basal ganglia. Dopamine *inhibits* the function of these neurons, allowing control over voluntary movement. This system of checks and balances allows for refined, coordinated movement, such as picking up a pencil and writing.

Widespread degeneration of the *substantia nigra* then leads to a decrease in the amount of dopamine in the brain. When dopamine levels are decreased, a person loses the ability to refine voluntary movement. The large numbers of excitatory ACh-secreting neurons remain active, creating an imbalance between excitatory and inhibitory neuronal activity. The resulting excessive excitation of neurons prevents a person from controlling or initiating voluntary movement (McCance et al., 2014).

Not only does PD interfere with movement as a result of dopamine loss in the brain, it also reduces the sympathetic nervous system influence on the heart and blood vessels. This loss results in the orthostatic hypotension frequently seen in the patient with PD.

TABLE 42-3 Stages of Parkinson Disease

Stage 1: Initial Stage • Unilateral limb involvement • Minimal weakness • Hand and arm trembling	**Stage 3: Moderate Disease** • Postural instability • Increased gait disturbances
Stage 2: Mild Stage • Bilateral limb involvement • Masklike face • Slow, shuffling gait	**Stage 4: Severe Disability** • Akinesia • Rigidity **Stage 5: Complete ADL Dependence**

PD is separated into stages according to the symptoms and degree of disability. Stage 1 is mild disease with unilateral limb involvement, whereas the patient with stage 5 disease is completely dependent in all ADLs. Other classifications refer simply to mild, moderate, and severe disease (Table 42-3).

Although the exact cause of PD is not known, it is probably due to environmental and genetic factors. Exposure to pesticides, herbicides, and industrial chemicals and metals and drinking well water, being older than 40 years, and having reduced estrogen levels are known risk factors for the development of PD.

GENETIC/GENOMIC CONSIDERATIONS

Patient-Centered Care QSEN

Primary Parkinson disease (PD) often has a familial tendency. The disease is associated with a variety of mitochondrial DNA (mtDNA) variations that often involve deletions in the genetic sequences that are used in CNS mitochondria, the energy powerhouses of cells. These variations ultimately cause destruction of neurons that produce dopamine in the substantia nigra. Mitochondrial dysfunction is a common observation in PD and other neurodegenerative diseases, indicating there is a disorder of energy regulation that contributes to cell death (Coskun et al., 2012).

As the population ages, the number of people affected by PD is expected to dramatically increase. About 50% more men than women currently have the disease.

❖ PATIENT-CENTERED COLLABORATIVE CARE

◆ Assessment

Collect data related to the time and progression of symptoms noticed by the patient or the family. The older adult, who may assume that these behaviors are normal changes associated with aging, may ignore early signs and symptoms such as *resting* tremors, bradykinesia (slowed movement), and problems with muscular rigidity. Tremors are usually noticed in the upper extremities first and may increase with stress. Slow voluntary movements and reduced automatic movements may be manifested by a change in the patient's handwriting. Some patients report "freezing" because they feel that they are stuck to the floor. Chart 42-11 summarizes the clinical manifestations of Parkinson disease. Assess the patient for *rigidity,* or resistance to passive movement of the extremities, which is classified as:

- *Cogwheel,* manifested by a rhythmic interruption of the muscle movement
- *Plastic,* defined as mildly restrictive movement
- *Lead pipe,* or total resistance to movement

CHART 42-11 **Key Features**

Parkinson Disease

- Posture:
  - Stooped posture
  - Flexed trunk
  - Fingers abducted and flexed at the metacarpophalangeal joint
  - Wrist slightly dorsiflexed
- Gait:
  - Slow and shuffling
  - Short, hesitant steps
  - Propulsive gait
  - Difficulty stopping quickly
- Motor:
  - **Bradykinesia** (slow movement)
  - Muscular rigidity
  - Akinesia
  - Tremors
  - "Pill-rolling" movement
  - Masklike face
  - Difficulty chewing and swallowing
  - Uncontrolled drooling, especially at night
  - Fatigue
  - Difficulty getting into and out of bed
  - Reduced arm swinging on one side of the body when walking
  - Micrographia (change in handwriting or handwriting gets smaller)
- Speech:
  - Soft, low-pitched voice
  - **Dysarthria** (slurred speech)
  - **Echolalia** (automatic repetition of what another person says) and repetition of sentences
  - **Hypophonia** (soft voice), change in voice volume or articulation
- Autonomic dysfunction:
  - Orthostatic hypotension
  - Excessive perspiration
  - Oily skin
  - Seborrhea
  - Flushing
  - Changes in skin texture
  - Blepharospasm (eyelid spasm)
- Psychosocial assessment:
  - Emotionally labile
  - Depressed
  - Paranoid
  - Easily upset
  - Rapid mood swings
  - Impaired cognition (i.e., dementia or delirium)
  - Delayed reaction time
  - Sleep disturbances

Rigidity is present early in the disease process and progresses over time. Observe the patient's ability to relax a muscle or move a selected muscle group.

Changes in facial expression or a *masklike face* with wide-open, fixed, staring eyes is caused by rigidity of the facial muscles (Fig. 42-1). This rigidity can lead to difficulties in chewing and swallowing, particularly if the pharyngeal muscles are involved. As a result, the patient may have inadequate nutrition. Uncontrolled drooling may occur. Some patients develop dementia later as the disease progresses. In addition to changes in voluntary movement, many patients experience autonomic nervous system symptoms, such as excessive perspiration and orthostatic hypotension. Orthostatic hypotension is likely related to loss of sympathetic innervation in the heart and blood vessel response.

Patients can also develop emotional changes such as depression, irritability, pessimism, fear, and insecurity. These symptoms may develop because patients fear that they will not be able to cope with new situations.

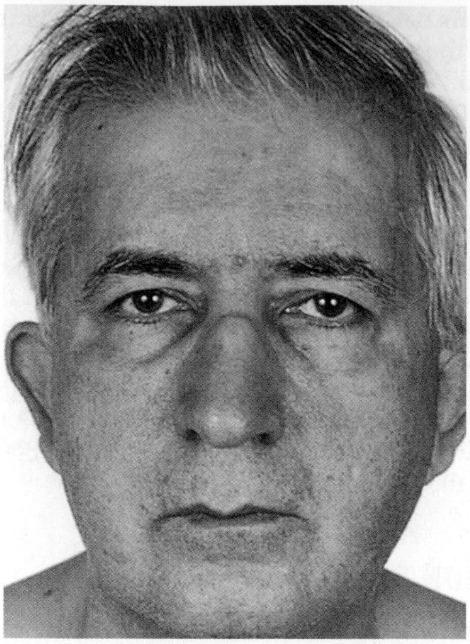

FIG. 42-1 The masklike facial expression typical of patients with Parkinson disease.

Changes in speech pattern are common in PD patients. They may speak very softly, slur or repeat their words, use a monotone voice or a halting speech, hesitate before speaking, or exhibit a rapid speech pattern.

Bowel and bladder problems are commonly seen in PD due to malfunction of the autonomic nervous system, which regulates smooth muscle activity. Patients can exhibit symptoms of either urinary incontinence or difficulty urinating. Constipation can occur due to the slow motility of the GI tract or because of poor dietary habits and poor fluid intake.

The diagnosis of PD is made based on clinical findings after other neurologic diseases are eliminated as possibilities. There are no specific diagnostic tests. Analysis of cerebrospinal fluid (CSF) may show a decrease in dopamine levels, although the results of other studies are usually normal. Other diagnostic tests may be done such as an MRI, single-photon emission computed tomography (SPECT), or a positron emission tomography (PET) to rule out other CNS health problems.

◆ *Interventions*

In addition to the health care provider, physical and/or occupational therapist, speech-language pathologist, dietitian, and case manager, collaborate with the patient and family to develop a patient-centered plan of care. In some cases, palliative surgery may be performed to assist the patient to remain mobile for as long as possible. Chart 42-12 summarizes best practices for nursing management of the patient with PD.

Nonsurgical Management. Care for the patient with Parkinson disease includes drug therapy, exercise programs or physical therapy, strategies and collaboration to promote self-management, and psychosocial support. Ultimately, the goals of care are to preserve MOBILITY, COGNITION, and quality of life.

Drug Therapy. Drugs are prescribed to treat the symptoms of PD with the purpose of increasing the patient's functional abilities. An equally important desired outcome is to prescribe

CHART 42-12 Best Practice for Patient Safety & Quality Care (QSEN)

Care of the Patient with Parkinson Disease

- Allow the patient extra time to respond to questions.
- Administer medications promptly on schedule to maintain continuous therapeutic drug levels.
- Provide medication for pain, tingling in limbs, as needed.
- Monitor for side effects of medications, especially orthostatic hypotension, hallucinations, and acute confusional state (delirium).
- Collaborate with physical and occupational therapists to keep the patient as mobile and as independent as possible in ADLs.
- Allow the patient time to perform ADLs and mobility skills.
- Implement interventions to prevent complications of immobility, such as constipation, pressure ulcers, and contractures.
- Schedule appointments and activities late in the morning to prevent rushing the patient, or schedule them at the time of the patient's optimal level of functioning.
- Teach the patient to speak slowly and clearly. Use alternative communication methods, such as a communication board. Refer to speech-language pathologist.
- Monitor the patient's ability to eat and swallow. Monitor actual food and fluid intake. Collaborate with the dietitian.
- Provide high-protein, high-calorie foods or supplements to maintain weight.
- Recognize that Parkinson disease affects the patient's body image. Focus on the patient's strengths.
- Assess for depression and anxiety.
- Assess for insomnia or sleeplessness.

drugs with minimal long-term side effects. Many questions and controversies remain about which drugs to use, when to start therapy, and how to prevent complications. Drug administration is closely monitored, and the health care provider adjusts the dosage or changes therapy as the patient's condition requires. Teach the patient and family how to monitor for and report adverse effects of drug therapy.

Dopamine agonists mimic dopamine by stimulating dopamine receptors in the brain. They are typically the most effective during the first 3 to 5 years of use. The benefit of these agents is fewer incidents of **dyskinesias** (problems with movement) and "wearing off" phenomenon (loss of response to the drug) when compared with other drugs. This problem is characterized by periods of good MOBILITY ("on") alternating with periods of poor MOBILITY ("off"). Patients report that their most distressing symptom is "off time."

Examples of dopamine agonists are apomorphine (Apokyn [a morphine derivative]), pramipexole (Mirapex), and ropinirole (Requip). Another drug in this class, rotigotine, is available as a continuous transdermal patch (Neupro) to maintain a consistent level of dopamine.

! NURSING SAFETY PRIORITY (QSEN)

Drug Alert

Dopamine agonists are associated with adverse effects such as orthostatic (postural) hypotension, hallucinations, sleepiness, and drowsiness. Remind patients to avoid operating heavy machinery or driving if they have any of these symptoms. Teach them to change from a lying or sitting position to standing by moving slowly. The health care provider should not prescribe drugs in this class to older adults because of their severe adverse drug effects.

Almost all patients are on Sinemet, a combination *levodopa-carbidopa* drug, at some point in their disease. It may be the initial drug of choice if the patient's presenting symptoms are severe or interfere with work or school. Both an immediate-release (IR) and controlled-release (CR) form of Sinemet in varying doses are available. The levodopa agents are less expensive than the dopamine agonists and are better at improving motor function. Long-term use leads to dyskinesia (inability to perform voluntary movement). Teach the patient and family to give the drug before meals to increase absorption and transport across the blood-brain barrier.

Catechol O–methyltransferases (COMTs) are enzymes that inactivate dopamine. Therefore COMT *inhibitors* block this enzyme activity, thus prolonging the action of levodopa. One example is entacapone (Comtan), which is often used in combination with levodopa. Stalevo is a combination of levodopa, carbidopa, and entacapone. The benefit of these combinations is that the disease is treated in several ways with one drug. However, they are not beneficial for those patients who need more specific dosages of individual drugs.

Monamine oxidase type B (MAO-B) inhibitors (MAOIs) are more popular for use in patients with early or mild symptoms of PD. Entacapone (Comtan) and selegiline (Deprenyl, Eldepryl) are often given with levodopa for early or mild disease. A newer MAOI-B for PD is rasagiline mesylate (Azilect), which can be given as a single drug or with levodopa. This drug has been reported to decrease "freezing" episodes (Cranwell-Bruce, 2010).

The MAOI-B drugs work by slowing the main type (B) of monamine oxidase in the brain, increasing dopamine concentrations and helping reduce the clinical manifestations of PD. They may also protect neurons in the brain (Cranwell-Bruce, 2010).

! NURSING SAFETY PRIORITY (QSEN)

Drug Alert

Teach patients taking MAOIs about the need to avoid foods, beverages, and drugs that contain tyramine, including cheese and aged, smoked, or cured foods and sausage. Remind them to also avoid red wine and beer to prevent severe headache and life-threatening hypertension (Lilley et al., 2014). Patients should continue these restrictions for 14 days after the drug is discontinued.

When other drugs are no longer effective, bromocriptine mesylate (Parlodel), a *dopamine receptor agonist,* may be prescribed to promote the release of dopamine. It may be used alone or in combination with carbidopa/levodopa (Sinemet). Some providers may prescribe Parlodel early in the course of treatment. It is especially useful in the patient who has experienced side effects such as dyskinesias or orthostatic hypotension while receiving Sinemet.

Amantadine (Symmetrel) is an *antiviral drug* that has anti-Parkinson benefits. It may be given early in disease to reduce symptoms. It is also prescribed with Sinemet to reduce dyskinesias. Rivastigmine (Exelon) is a *cholinesterase inhibitor* that is used only when patients with PD have dementia. This drug works to improve the transmission of acetylcholine in the brain by delaying its destruction by the enzyme *acetylcholinesterase.*

For severe motor symptoms such as tremors and rigidity, one of the older *anticholinergic* drugs may be prescribed, but they are rarely used as primary drugs of choice for Parkinson disease

(PD) (Cranwell-Bruce, 2010). Examples are benztropine (Cogentin), trihexyphenidyl HCl (Artane), and procyclidine (Kemadrin). *These drugs should be avoided in older adults because they can cause acute confusion, urinary retention, constipation, dry mouth, and blurred vision. Newer and safer drugs are now available for this age-group.*

For the patient on any long-term drug therapy regimen, drug tolerance or *drug toxicity* often develops. Drug toxicity may be evidenced by changes in COGNITION such as delirium (acute confusion) or hallucinations and decreased effectiveness of the drug. Delirium may be difficult to assess in the patient who is already suffering from chronic dementia as a result of PD or another disease. If possible, compare the patient's current cognitive and behavioral status with his or her baseline before drug therapy began.

When drug tolerance is reached, the drug's effects do not last as long as previously. The treatment of PD drug toxicity or tolerance includes:

- A reduction in drug dosage
- A change of drug or in the frequency of administration
- A drug holiday (particularly with levodopa therapy)

During a **drug holiday**, which typically lasts up to 10 days, the patient receives no drug therapy for PD. Carefully monitor the patient for symptoms of PD during this time, and document assessment findings.

Many patients are on additional drugs to help relieve symptoms associated with the disease. For example, muscle spasms may be relieved by baclofen (Kemstro), drooling can be minimized by sublingual atropine sulfate (Atropair), and insomnia may require a sleeping aid like zolpidem tartrate (Ambien). If patients also become moderately to severely depressed, an antidepressant such as short-acting venlafaxine (Effexor) may be prescribed. This complicated drug regimen may be confusing to patients. A review by Vervloet and colleagues (2012) supports electronic reminders as effective in helping to educate patients and maintain drug adherence.

Other Interventions. *A freezing gait and postural instability are major problems for patients with PD.* Nontraditional exercise programs, such as yoga and tai chi, may help elevate mood, as well as improve MOBILITY, in the early stage of the disease. Early in the disease process, collaborate with physical and occupational therapists to plan and implement a program to keep the patient flexible, prevent falling, and retain mobility by incorporating active and passive range-of-motion (ROM) exercises, muscle stretching, and out-of-bed activity. Remind the patient to avoid concentrating on his or her feet when walking to prevent falls.

In collaboration with the rehabilitation team, encourage the patient to participate as much as possible in self-management, including ADLs. The team makes the environment conducive to independence in activity and as stress-free and safe as possible. Occupational and physical therapists provide training in ADLs and the use of adaptive devices, as needed, to facilitate independence. The occupational therapist (OT) evaluates the patient for the need for adaptive devices (e.g., special utensils for eating).

Patients with PD tend to not sleep well at night because of drug therapy and the disease itself. Some patients nap for short periods during the day and may not be aware that they have done so. This sleep misperception may put the patient at risk for injury. For example, he or she may fall asleep while driving an automobile. Therefore teach the patient and family to monitor the patient's sleeping pattern and discuss whether he or she can operate machinery or perform other potentially high-risk tasks safely.

Collaborate with the dietitian, if needed, to evaluate the patient's food intake and ability to eat. The patient's intake of calcium, vitamin K, and other nutrients is evaluated, especially in the patient who has difficulty swallowing or is susceptible to injury from falling. The dietitian considers the patient's bowel habits and adjusts the diet if constipation occurs. If the patient has trouble swallowing, collaborate with the speech-language pathologist (SLP) for an extensive swallowing evaluation. Based on these findings and the patient interview, an individualized nutritional plan is developed. Usually a soft diet and thick, cold fluids, such as milk shakes, are more easily tolerated.

Small, frequent meals or a commercial powder, such as Thick-It, added to liquids may assist the patient who has difficulty swallowing. Elevate the patient's head to allow easier swallowing and prevent aspiration. Remind UAP and teach the family to be careful when serving or feeding the patient. The SLP can be very helpful in recommending specific feeding strategies. Be sure that UAP record food intake daily or as needed. The patient loses weight because of altered food intake and the increased number of calories burned secondary to muscle rigidity. Teach the family to weigh the patient once a week so that adjustments to the diet can be made as indicated. As the disease progresses and swallowing becomes more of a problem, supplemental feedings become the main source of nutrition to maintain weight, with meals and other foods taken as the patient can tolerate.

Collaborate with the SLP if the patient has speech difficulties. Together with the interdisciplinary health care team, patient, and family, develop a communication plan. The SLP teaches exercises to strengthen muscles used for breathing, speech, and swallowing. Remind the patient to speak slowly and clearly and to pause and take deep breaths at times during each sentence. Teach the family the importance of avoiding unnecessary environmental noise to increase the listener's ability to hear and understand the patient. Ask the patient to repeat words that the listener does not understand. Have the listener watch the patient's lips and nonverbal expressions for cues as to the meaning of conversation. Remind the patient to organize his or her thoughts before speaking and use facial expression and gestures, if possible, to assist with communication. In addition, he or she should exaggerate words to increase the listener's ability to understand. If the patient cannot communicate verbally, he or she can use alternative methods of communication, such as a communication board, mechanical voice synthesizer, computer, or handheld mobile device. The SLP assesses the ability to use these devices before a decision is made about which method to use. Some older patients may not want to use electronic methods to communicate.

Psychosocial Support. Although not all patients with PD have dementia, impaired COGNITION and memory deficits are common. Some patients also experience changes in gait and tremors that are uncontrollable. In the late stages of the disease, they cannot move without assistance, have difficulty talking, have minimal facial expression, and may drool. Patients often state that they are embarrassed and tend to avoid social events or groups of people. They should not be forced into situations in which they feel ashamed of their appearance. Encourage patients to undertake activities that do not require small-muscle dexterity, such as light, modified aerobic exercises.

Collaborate with the social worker or case manager to help the family with financial and health insurance issues, as well as respite care or permanent placement if needed. Refer the patient and family to social and state agencies, as well as support groups as needed (e.g., the National Parkinson Foundation [www.pdf.org]).

Teach the family to emphasize the patient's abilities or strengths and provide positive reinforcement when he or she meets expected outcomes. The patient, the family or significant other, and the rehabilitation team mutually set realistic expected outcomes that can be achieved.

The long-term management of PD presents a special challenge in the home care setting. A case manager may be required to coordinate interdisciplinary care and provide support for the patient and family. Impaired MOBILITY affects the patient's daily lifestyle, including sexuality. The case manager or home care nurse uses a holistic approach to ensure that psychosocial, as well as physical, needs are addressed.

As the disease progresses and drug effectiveness decreases, refer the family to a palliative care organization or hospice. Referral sources can be obtained from the Center to Advance Palliative Care (www.capc.org), which advocates applying the principles of palliative care to chronic disease. Chapter 7 discusses palliative and hospice care in detail.

CLINICAL JUDGMENT CHALLENGE

Informatics QSEN

A 68-year-old man reports shaking of his arms, hands, and head that he cannot control. He has also noticed that he walks more slowly now and thought it was part of the aging process. He is afraid that he won't be able to continue his job as an auto body worker, and he says he can't live on his monthly Social Security income. His mother had Parkinson disease for many years and died of complications before she was 70. He decided he should see his family practice physician to discuss the changes he is experiencing. He is accompanied by his wife of 45 years; they have two children who live out of town.

1. As the patient's intake nurse, what questions might you include in his history?
2. What physical assessment will you perform and why?
3. The physician places the patient on Sinemet. You realize that you need to look up information about this drug to provide accurate health teaching. What reliable resources might you use?
4. What health teaching will you need to provide for this patient and his wife regarding his drug and other aspects of his illness?

Surgical Management. Several options are available if surgery for the patient with PD is needed. Surgery is a last resort when drugs are not effective in symptom management. The most common surgeries are stereotactic pallidotomy and thalamotomy, although newer surgical procedures are being tried. Deep brain stimulation may also be done.

Stereotactic Pallidotomy/Thalamotomy. **Stereotactic pallidotomy** (opening into the pallidum within the corpus striatum) can be a very effective treatment for controlling the symptoms associated with PD. First, the target area within the pallidum is identified by a CT or MRI scan. Next, the stereotactic head frame is placed on the patient. IV sedation is given, and a burr hole is made into the cranium. An electrode or cylindric rod is inserted into the target area. The target area receives a mild electrical stimulation, and the patient's reaction is assessed for reduction of tremor and rigidity. If this result does not occur or if unexpected visual, motor, or sensory symptoms appear, the probe is repositioned. When the probe is in the ideal location, a permanent lesion (scarring) is made to destroy the tissue. The patient is monitored in the postanesthesia care unit (PACU) for about 1 hour and is then returned to the inpatient unit for continuing postoperative care.

As an alternative to stereotactic pallidotomy, the surgeon may perform a **thalamotomy** (opening into the thalamus of the brain for the stimulation) for treatment of tremor through thermocoagulation (high-frequency currents to destroy tissue) of brain cells. This procedure is effective for a limited number of patients. Because bilateral procedures have increased surgical complication rates, only unilateral (one-sided) surgery is done to benefit the side of the body that is most affected by the disease.

Deep Brain Stimulation. Deep brain stimulation (DBS) is approved as a treatment for Parkinson disease. In DBS, electrodes are implanted into the brain and connected to a small electrical device called a *pulse generator* that delivers electrical current. The generator is placed under the skin similar to a cardiac pacemaker device. The generator is externally programmed to deliver an electrical current to decrease involuntary movements known as **dyskinesias**, resulting in a reduced need for levodopa and related drugs. DBS also helps to alleviate fluctuations of symptoms and to reduce tremors, slowness of movements, and gait problems (National Institute of Neurological Disorders and Stroke [NINDS], 2014).

Fetal Tissue Transplantation. Fetal tissue transplantation is an experimental and highly controversial ethical and political treatment. Fetal substantia nigra tissue, either human or pig, is transplanted into the caudate nucleus of the brain. Preliminary reports suggest that patients show clinical improvement in motor symptoms without dyskinesias after receiving the transplanted tissue. Long-term results are yet to be seen or studied.

DEMENTIA

❖ *PATHOPHYSIOLOGY*

Dementia is a loss of brain function that is chronic and progressive. Dementia affects the ability to learn new information. It also impairs language, judgment, and behavior. Alzheimer's disease (AD) is the most common type of dementia, accounting for most of the chronic confusional states that occur in people older than 65 years. Vascular dementia is the second most common dementia and is associated with stroke. When dementia occurs in people in their 40s and 50s, it is referred to as *early dementia, Alzheimer type,* or *presenile dementia.* Although symptoms of dementia can vary greatly, at least two of these cognitive functions must be significantly impaired for a diagnosis of dementia:

- Memory
- Communication and language
- Attention span or ability to focus and pay attention
- Reasoning and judgment
- Visual perception

People with dementia often have problems with short-term memory such as keeping track of keys or personal items, paying bills, preparing meals, remembering appointments, or traveling out of the neighborhood. Many dementias are progressive and result in a chronic confusional state. Severe physical deterioration occurs over time, and death is usually associated with complications of immobility.

The brain of the older adult usually weighs less and occupies less space in the cranial vault than does the brain of a younger person. Other changes in the brain that occur with aging include widening of the cerebral sulci, narrowing of the gyri, and enlargement of the ventricles. In the presence of AD and vascular dementia, these normal changes are greatly accelerated. Brain weight is reduced further. Marked atrophy of the cerebral cortex and loss of cortical neurons occur. The cerebral sulci and fissures, as well as the ventricles, are enlarged more than those of persons of the same age without AD. These areas of the brain are particularly affected:

- Precentral gyrus of the frontal lobe
- Superior temporal gyrus
- Hippocampus
- Substantia nigra

Microscopic changes of the brain found in people with AD include neurofibrillary tangles, amyloid-rich senile or neuritic plaques, and granulovascular degeneration. **Neurofibrillary tangles** are a classic finding at autopsy in the brains of patients with AD. They consist of tangled masses of fibrous tissue throughout the neurons (McCance et al., 2014).

Neuritic plaques are composed of degenerating nerve terminals and are found particularly in the hippocampus, an important part of the limbic system. Deposited within the plaques are increased amounts of an abnormal protein called *beta amyloid.* These peptides have a tendency to accumulate and form the neurotoxic plaques found in the brain (McCance et al., 2014).

Although *vascular degeneration* occurs in the normally aging brain, its presence is significantly increased in patients with dementia. Vascular degeneration accounts for at least partial loss of the ability of nerve cells to function properly. Cell deterioration and death may lead to hemorrhage. This pathologic change contributes to the mortality associated with this disorder.

In addition to the structural changes in the brain associated with AD and other dementias, abnormalities in the neurotransmitters (acetylcholine [ACh], norepinephrine, dopamine, and serotonin) may occur. High levels of beta amyloid are associated with significantly reduced ACh, which leads to a decrease in the amount of acetyltransferase in the hippocampus. This loss is major because the decrease in acetyltransferase interferes with cholinergic innervation to the cerebral cortex. This results in impaired COGNITION, recent memory, and the ability to acquire new memories. The specific role of reduced neurotransmitters in the development of AD is not well understood.

Etiology and Genetic Risk

The exact cause of AD is unknown. It is well established that *age, gender (women more than men), and family history are the most important risk factors.* Several other theories and risk factors have been studied, including chemical imbalances, environmental agents, immunologic changes, and ethnicity/race. Compared with Euro-Americans, African Americans have a greater risk for developing the disease and Hispanics tend to develop the disease earlier than other groups. The cause of these differences is not yet known.

Environmental agents, especially certain viruses such as herpes zoster and herpes simplex, and toxic metals such as zinc and copper have also been suggested as causes. Patients who have experienced a head injury or repeated head trauma (e.g., boxers) may be more at risk for AD and at an earlier age than others.

> **GENETIC/GENOMIC CONSIDERATIONS**
>
> ***Patient-Centered Care*** QSEN
>
> There is little doubt that many patients with AD had a genetic predisposition to the development of the disease. The inheritance pattern is highly complex with both isolated and interactive genes identified from multiple sites such as the beta-amyloid precursor *(APP),* the presenilin1 *(PSEN1),* and presenilin2 *(PRESN2)* genes—all involved in the formation of the distinctive plaque and neurofibrillary tangles in AD. Other genes implicated in AD are apolipoprotein E *(APOE)* and clusterin *(CLU)* genes that code for products in lipid metabolism and inflammation. A third family of genes associated with AD progression is responsible for endocytosis and vesicle trafficking—intracellular processes that help deliver neurotransmitters. These genes are phosphatidylinositol-binding clathrin assembly protein *(PICALM)* and Bridging Integrator 1 *(BIN1)* (Bettens et al., 2013). The genetic studies in AD are an example of how genetics, genomics, and proteomics are not only finding genes associated with the condition but also illustrating the mechanisms of pathology in complex conditions.

Incidence and Prevalence

There is a significant increase in both the incidence and prevalence of AD after 65 years of age, although it may affect anyone older than 40 years. The number of people in the United States with AD is estimated at 4.5 million and expected to triple in the next three decades (Mayeux & Stern, 2012). AD has a significant impact on health care costs, including direct and indirect medical and social service costs.

Health Promotion and Maintenance

There are no proven ways to prevent AD or other dementias. Current research activities are focusing on eating a balanced diet, eating dark-colored fruits and vegetables, using soy products, and consuming sufficient amounts of folate and vitamins B_{12}, C, and E. These substances have been reported to decrease the risk for developing AD, but study results are inconclusive and inconsistent. Walking, swimming, and other exercise not only increase tone and muscle strength but also may decrease mental decline in AD, as well as other dementias. Avoiding lifestyle factors that contribute to stroke risk, including untreated hypertension, is also advocated.

❖ PATIENT-CENTERED COLLABORATIVE CARE

◆ Assessment

History. The patient with dementia and Alzheimer's disease (AD) often presents with cognitive impairment, although many other disorders, drugs, and environmental factors can cause changes in COGNITION. A thorough history and physical examination are necessary to differentiate AD from other, possibly reversible causes of cognitive impairment (Table 42-4). Obtain information from family members or significant others because the patient may be unaware of the problems, denying their existence or covering them up. Family members often do not recognize or may deny early changes in their loved one as well.

The most important information to be obtained is the onset, duration, progression, and course of the symptoms. Question the patient and the family about changes in memory or increasing forgetfulness and about the ability to perform ADLs. Ask

TABLE 42-4 Causes of Cognitive Impairment in the Older Adult

Neurologic Causes
- Vascular insufficiency
- Infections
- Trauma
- Tumors
- Normal-pressure hydrocephalus

Cardiovascular Causes
- Myocardial infarction
- Dysrhythmias
- Heart failure
- Cardiogenic shock
- Endocarditis
- Stroke

Pulmonary Causes
- Infection
- Pneumonia
- Hypoventilation

Metabolic Causes
- Electrolyte imbalance
- Acidosis/alkalosis
- Hypoglycemia/hyperglycemia
- Kidney failure
- Fluid volume deficit
- Urinary tract infection
- Hepatic failure

Drug Intoxication
- Misuse of prescribed medications
- Side effects of medications
- Incorrect use of over-the-counter medications
- Ingestion of heavy metals

Nutritional Deficiencies
- B vitamins
- Vitamin C
- Hypoproteinemia

Environmental Causes
- Hypothermia/hyperthermia
- Unfamiliar environment
- Sensory deprivation/overload

Psychological Causes
- Depression
- Anxiety
- Pain
- Fatigue
- Grief
- Paranoia

CHART 42-13 Key Features

Alzheimer's Disease

Early (Mild), or Stage I (first symptoms up to 4 years)
- Independent in ADLs
- No social or employment problems initially
- Denies presence of symptoms
- Forgets names; misplaces household items
- Short-term memory loss; difficulty recalling new information
- Subtle changes in personality and behavior
- Loss of initiative; less engaged in social relationships
- Mild impaired cognition, problems with judgment
- Decreased performance, especially when stressed
- Unable to travel alone to new destinations
- Decreased sense of smell

Middle (Moderate), or Stage II (2 to 3 years)
- Impairment of all cognitive functions
- Problems with handling or unable to handle money and finances
- Disorientation to time, place, and event
- Possible depression, agitated
- Increasingly dependent in ADLs
- Visuospatial deficits: difficulty driving, gets lost
- Speech and language deficits: less talkative, decrease in use of vocabulary, increasingly non-fluent, and eventually aphasic
- Incontinent
- Wandering; trouble sleeping

Late (Severe), or Stage III
- Completely incapacitated; bedridden
- Totally dependent in ADLs
- Motor and verbal skills lost
- General and focal neurologic deficits
- Agnosia (loss of facial recognition)

about current employment status, work history, and ability to fulfill household responsibilities, including cleaning, grocery shopping, and preparing meals. Inquire about changes in driving ability, ability to handle routine financial transactions, and language and communication skills. In addition, document any changes in personality and behavior. Assessing functional status for complex chronic conditions such as dementia is a recommended core measure by the Centers for Medicare and Medicaid Services (www.cms.gov).

There is increasing evidence that an altered sense of smell is associated with the development of AD. Therefore ask about changes in the ability to smell or changes in the sense of smell. The history taking concludes with a review of the patient's medical history. Of particular importance is a history of head trauma, viral illness, or exposure to metal or toxic waste, as well as any family history of AD or Down syndrome.

Physical Assessment/Clinical Manifestations

Stages of Alzheimer's Disease. The clinical manifestations associated with AD can be grouped into three broad stages based on the progress of the disease (Chart 42-13). The patient does not necessarily progress from one stage to the next in an orderly fashion. A stage may be bypassed, or he or she may exhibit symptoms of one or several stages. Each patient exhibits different disease stages and clinical manifestations. Consequently, most authorities now use broader terms such as *early (mild), middle (moderate),* and *late (severe)* stages.

The primary focus of the neurologic assessment of patients with AD is to identify abnormalities in COGNITION, including language, personality, and behavior. Physical manifestations of neurologic impairment (seizures, tremors, or ataxia) tend to occur late in the disease process.

Changes in Cognition. **Cognition** refers to the ability of the brain to process, store, retrieve, and use information. Therefore assess the patient for deficits in these abilities:
- Attention and concentration
- Judgment and perception
- Learning and memory
- Communication and language
- Speed of information processing

One of the first symptoms of AD is short-term memory impairment. New memory and defects in information retrieval result from dysfunction in the hippocampal, frontal, or parietal region. Alterations in communication abilities, such as **apraxia** (inability to use words or objects correctly), **aphasia** (inability to speak or understand), **anomia** (inability to find words), and **agnosia** (loss of sensory comprehension), are due to dysfunction of the temporal and parietal lobes. Frontal lobe impairment causes problems with judgment, an inability to make decisions, decreased attention span, and a decreased ability to concentrate. As the disease progresses to a later stage, the patient loses all cognitive abilities, is totally unable to communicate, and becomes less aware of the environment.

To more clearly identify the nature and extent of the patient's cognitive impairment, the neurologist or psychologist administers several neuropsychological tests. The tests selected depend on clinician preference and the ability of the patient to participate in testing. All of the tests focus on cognitive ability and may be repeated over time to measure changes. Folstein's Mini-Mental State Examination (MMSE) is an example of a tool used to determine the onset and severity of cognitive impairment.

Orientation to Time
"What is the date?"

Registration
"Listen carefully, I am going to say three words. You say them back after I stop. Ready? Here they are... HOUSE (pause), CAR (pause), LAKE (pause). Now repeat those words back to me." [Repeat up to 5 times, but score only the first trial.]

Naming
"What is this?" [Point to a pencil or pen.]

Reading
"Please read this and do what it says." [Show examinee the words on the stimulus form.]

CLOSE YOUR EYES

A

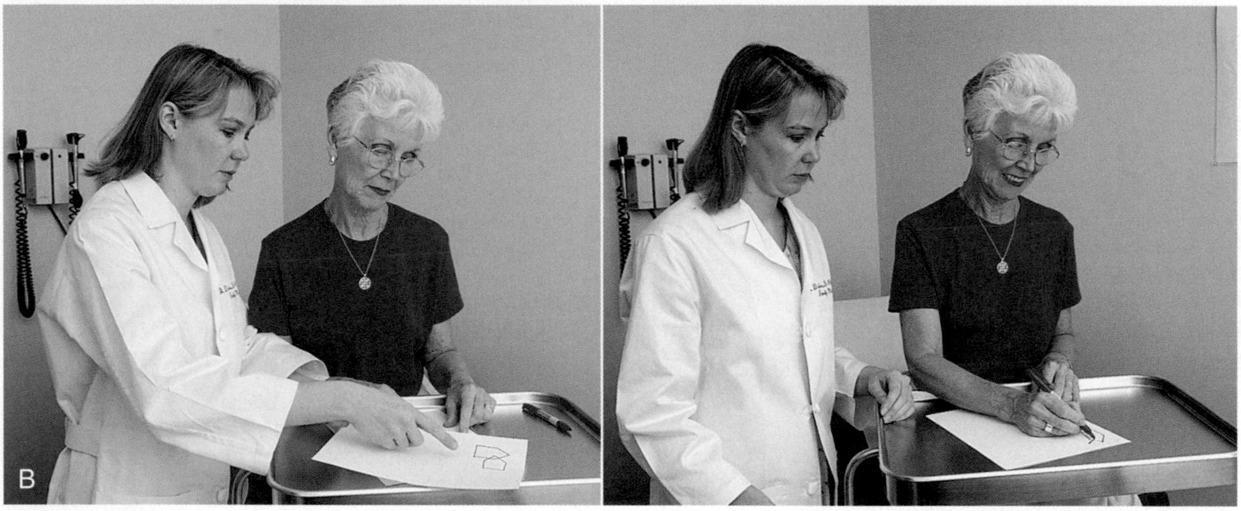

FIG. 42-2 A, Examples of questions that are asked on the Mini-Mental State Examination (MMSE). **B,** Copying is one of the tasks on the MMSE.

The MMSE is also known as the "mini-mental exam." The MMSE assesses five major areas—orientation, registration, attention and calculation, recall, and speech-language (including reading). Fig. 42-2 lists examples of the questions asked on this test. The patient performs certain cognitive tasks that are scored and added together for a total score of 0 to 30. The lower the score is, the greater the severity of the dementia. It is not unusual for a patient with advanced AD to score below 5.

Although the MMSE is used frequently by specialists and researchers outside of the acute care setting, it is a copyrighted tool and the patient must be able to read. For the patient who cannot read or for a quicker screening test, the "set test" can be used. The patient is asked to name 10 items in each of four sets or categories: fruits, animals, colors, and towns (FACT). Other categories can be used, if needed. The patient receives 1 point for each item for a possible maximum score of 40. Patients who score above 25 do not have dementia. Although this assessment is easy to administer, it should not be used for patients with hearing impairments or speech and language problems. Another brief tool to screen for dementia that has validity and reliability in acute care settings is the Short Blessed Test (www.mybraintest.org). In long-term care settings, the federally required Brief Interview for Mental Status (BIMS) is required as part of the Minimum Data Set 3.0 for Nursing Homes (Saliba et al., 2012).

Changes in Behavior and Personality. One of the most difficult aspects of AD and dementia that families and caregivers cope with is the behavioral changes that can occur in advanced disease. Assess the patient for:

- Aggressiveness, especially verbal and physical abusive tendencies
- Rapid mood swings
- Increased confusion at night or when light is not adequate (**sundowning**) or in excessively fatigued patients

The patient may wander and become lost or may go into other rooms to rummage through another's belongings. Hoarding or hiding objects is also common. For example, patients may hoard washcloths in the long-term care setting.

For some patients with dementia, emotional and behavioral problems occur with the primary disease. They may experience paranoia (suspicious behaviors), delusions, hallucinations, and depression. Document these behaviors, and ensure the patient's safety. (Refer to a mental health/behavior health nursing textbook for a complete discussion of these disorders.)

Although drug therapy is not effective in treating dementia, certain drugs may help control the emotional and psychiatric manifestations (e.g., depression, anxiety, paranoia, aggression) associated with the primary disease.

Changes in Self-Management Skills. Observe for changes in the patient's self-management skills, such as:

- Decreased interest in personal appearance
- Selection of clothing that is inappropriate for the weather or event
- Loss of bowel and bladder control
- Decreased appetite or ability to eat

Over time, the patient becomes less mobile and muscle contractures develop. He or she eventually becomes totally immobile and requires total physical care. The patient is then unable to meet the human needs of MOBILITY and COGNITION.

Psychosocial Assessment. In people with dementia, the cognitive changes and biochemical and structural dysfunctions affect personality and behavior. In the early stage, patients often recognize that they are experiencing memory or cognitive changes and may attempt to hide the problems. They begin the grieving process because of anticipated loss, experiencing denial, anger, bargaining, and depression at varying times. Older patients typically think the changes are part of "old age."

When the patient and family receive the diagnosis, one or more family members may desire genetic testing. Support the patient's/family's decisions regarding testing, and assist them in finding credible resources for testing and professional genetics counseling.

As the disease progresses, patients begin to display major changes in emotional and behavioral affect. Of particular importance is the need for an assessment of the patients' reactions to changes in routine or environment. For example, a hospital admission is very traumatic for most patients with dementia. It is not unusual for them to exhibit a catastrophic response or overreact to any change by becoming excessively aggressive or abusive. This is referred to as *traumatic relocation syndrome.*

As patients become unaware of their behavior, the focus of the psychosocial assessment shifts to the family or significant others. The health care team assesses their ability to cope with the chronicity and progression of the disease and identifies possible support systems.

Laboratory and Imaging Assessment. No laboratory test can confirm the diagnosis of AD. Definitive diagnosis is made on the basis of brain tissue examination at autopsy, which confirms the presence of neurofibrillary tangles and neuritic plaques.

Genetic testing, specifically for *apolipoprotein E4 (Apo E4),* may be helpful as an ancillary test (not a predictive test) for the differential diagnosis of AD. *Amyloid beta protein precursor (soluble)* (sBPP) may be measured for patients to diagnose AD and other types of dementia. A decrease in the patient's sBPP in the cerebrospinal fluid (CSF) supports the diagnosis because the amyloid tends to deposit in the brain and is not circulating in the CSF (Pagana & Pagana, 2014).

A variety of other laboratory tests may be performed to rule out other treatable causes of dementia or delirium, including:

- Complete blood count (CBC)
- Serum electrolyte levels, blood urea nitrogen, and glucose
- Vitamin B_{12} levels
- Folate levels
- Blood ammonia levels
- Blood gas analysis
- Cerebrospinal fluid (CSF) analysis
- Urinalysis
- Thyroid and liver function tests
- Serologic test for syphilis
- Toxicity screening tests; heavy metal screen
- Alcohol screening tests

A CT, PET, or SPECT scan may be performed to rule out other causes of disease. The CT scan typically shows cerebral atrophy and ventricular enlargement, wide sulci, and shrunken gyri in the later stages of the disease. An MRI scan can also rule out other causes of neurologic disease. The PET and SPECT scans show a significant decrease in metabolic activity in the brains of people with AD.

◆ Analysis

The priority NANDA-I nursing diagnoses and collaborative problems for patients with Alzheimer's disease (AD) include:

1. Chronic Confusion related to neuronal degeneration in the brain (NANDA-I)
2. Risk for Injury related to wandering or elder abuse (NANDA-I)
3. Caregiver Role Strain related to the patient's prolonged progression of disability and the patient's increasing care needs (NANDA-I)

◆ Planning and Implementation

The priority for interdisciplinary care is safety! Chronic confusion and physical deficits place the patient with AD at a high risk for injury.

Managing Chronic Confusion

Planning: Expected Outcomes. In the very early stages of the disease, the patient with dementia is expected to maintain the ability to perform complex mental processes. As the disease progresses, patients cannot meet this outcome. Instead, the desired outcome is to maintain cognitive function for as long as possible to keep patients safe and increase their quality of life.

Interventions. Although drug therapy may be used for patients with dementia or AD, nonpharmacologic interventions are the main focus of patient-centered collaborative management. Teach family members and significant others about the importance of being consistent in following the plan of care.

Nonpharmacologic Management. The health care provider should answer the patient's questions truthfully concerning the diagnosis of dementia or AD. In this way, the patient can more fully participate in the interdisciplinary plan of care. Interventions are the same whether he or she is cared for at home, in an adult day-care center, in an assisted-living center, in a long-term care facility, or in a hospital admitted with another medical condition. The patient with memory problems always benefits best from a structured and consistent environment (Seitz et al., 2012).

Many factors, including physical illness and environmental factors, can exacerbate (worsen) the clinical manifestations of AD (Table 42-5). The patient with dementia frequently has other medical problems such as cardiovascular disease, arthritis,

TABLE 42-5 Factors That Can Worsen Alzheimer's Disease and Dementia

• Stroke	• Impaired hepatic function
• Subdural hematoma	• Infection
• Space-occupying lesion (tumor)	• Impaired vision and hearing
• Decrease in blood supply to the brain	• Sudden changes in surroundings
• Myocardial infarction	• Pain and discomfort
• Dysrhythmias	• Drugs
• Hypoglycemia	• Physical or chemical restraint
• Impaired renal function	

renal insufficiency, and pulmonary disease. Changes in vision and hearing also may be present. Managing these conditions helps the patient's functional abilities.

Approaches to managing the patient who has Alzheimer's disease include:

- Cognitive stimulation and memory training
- Structuring the environment
- Orientation and validation therapy
- Promoting self-management
- Promoting bowel and bladder continence
- Promoting communication

The purpose of *cognitive stimulation and memory training* is to reinforce or promote desirable cognitive function and facilitate memory. An individualized cognitive therapy program may provide some benefit to the patient. Training in communication can help nurses and health care team members interact with better effect and compassion (Eggenberger et al., 2013; Johnson et al., 2013).

As the disease progresses, the patient may experience **prosopagnosia**, an inability to recognize oneself and other familiar faces. Encourage the family to provide pictures of family members and close friends that are labeled with the person's name on the picture. In addition, advise the family to reminisce with the patient about pleasant experiences from the past (Subramaniam & Woods, 2012). Use *reminiscence therapy* while assisting the patient with ADLs or performing a treatment or assessment. Refer to a personal item in the room to help the patient begin to talk about its meaning in the present and in the past.

It is not unusual for the patient to talk to his or her image in the mirror. This behavior should be allowed as long as it is not harmful. If the patient becomes frightened by the mirror image, remove or cover the mirror. In some long-term care or assisted-living settings, a picture of the patient is placed on the room door to help with facial recognition and to help the patient locate his or her room. This picture also helps the staff locate the patient in case of elopement (running away).

Teach the family to keep environmental distractions and noise to a minimum. The patient's home, hospital room, or nursing home room should not have pictures on the wall or other decorations that could be misinterpreted as people or animals that could harm the patient. An abstract painting or wallpaper might look like a fire or an explosion and scare the patient. The room should have adequate, nonglare lighting and no potentially frightening shadows.

In addition to disturbed sleep, other negative effects of high noise levels include decreased nutritional intake, changes in blood pressure and pulse rates, and feelings of increased stress and anxiety. The patient with AD is especially susceptible to these changes and needs to have as much undisturbed sleep at night as possible. Fatigue increases confusion and behavioral manifestations such as agitation and aggressiveness.

! NURSING SAFETY PRIORITY QSEN

Action Alert

When a patient with Alzheimer's disease is in a new setting or environment, collaborate with the staff and admitting department to select a room that is in the quietest area of the unit and away from obvious exits, if possible. A private room may be needed if the patient has a history of agitation or wandering. The television should remain off unless the patient turns it on or requests that it be turned on.

Objects such as furniture, a hairbrush, and eyeglasses should be kept in the same place. Establish a daily routine, and follow it as much as possible. Arrange for a communication board for scheduled activities and other information to promote orientation such as the day of the week, the month, and the year. Pictures of people familiar to the patient can also be placed on this board.

Explain changes in routine to the patient before they occur, repeating the explanation immediately before the changes take place. Clocks and single-date calendars also help the patient maintain day-to-day orientation to the environment in the early stages of the disease process. *For the patient with early disease, reality orientation is usually appropriate.* Teach family members and health care staff to frequently reorient the patient to the environment. Remind the patient what day and time it is, where he or she is, and who you are.

For the patient in the later stages of AD or dementia, reality orientation does not work and often increases agitation. *The health care team uses validation therapy for the patient with moderate or severe AD. In* **validation therapy**, *the staff member recognizes and acknowledges the patient's feelings and concerns.* For example, if the patient is looking for his or her mother, ask him or her to talk about what Mother looks like and what she might be wearing. This response does not argue with the patient but also does not reinforce the patient's belief that Mother is still living.

As the disease progresses, altered thought processes affect the *ability to perform ADLs.* Encourage the patient to perform as much self-care as possible and to maintain independence in daily living skills as long as possible. For example, in the home setting, complete clothing outfits that can be easily removed and put on (e.g., shirt, slacks, underwear, and socks) and placed on a single hanger are preferred for patient selection. When possible, the patient should participate in meal preparation, grocery shopping, and other household routines. Many patients cannot make purposeful movements as the disease progresses.

? NCLEX EXAMINATION CHALLENGE

Psychosocial Integrity

A client with moderate dementia asks the nurse to find her brother who is deceased. What is the nurse's best response?

A. "Your brother died over 20 years ago."
B. "We can call him in a little while if you want."
C. "What did your brother look like?"
D. "I'll ask your daughter to find him for you when she comes in."

Collaborate with the occupational and physical therapists to provide a complete evaluation and assistance in helping the patient become more independent. Adaptive devices, such as grab bars in the bathtub or shower area, an elevated commode, and adapted eating utensils, may enable him or her to maintain independence in grooming, toileting, and feeding. The physical therapist prescribes an exercise program to improve physical health and functionality.

The patient may remain continent of bowel and bladder for long periods if taken to the bathroom or given a bedpan or urinal every 2 hours. Toileting may be needed more often during the day and less frequently at night. Unlicensed assistive personnel (UAP) or home caregiver encourages the patient to drink adequate fluids to promote optimal voiding. A patient

EVIDENCE-BASED PRACTICE QSEN

Does the Use of Sitters Improve the Care of Older Adults with Dementia in Acute Care Settings?

Moyle, W., Borbasi, S., Wallis, M., Olorenshaw, R., & Gracia, N. (2011). Acute care management of older people with dementia: A qualitative perspective. *Journal of Clinical Nursing, 20*(3-4), 420-428.

This Australian study explored management for older people with dementia in an acute hospital setting using a descriptive qualitative approach. A total of 13 nurses participated in semi-structured audio-taped interviews. All nurses worked in acute medical or surgical wards in a large South East Queensland, Australia, hospital. The authors identified an inconsistent approach to care in that the most common intervention—providing a sitter—emphasized safety at the expense of well-being and dignity. Using untrained staff (i.e., a sitter or "patient observers") to monitor a patient with dementia is a risk management strategy that reduces the use of restraints but does not incorporate other evidence-based approaches to care such as reminiscent therapy, mobility activities, or family member presence. The use of sitters does not individualize care, a hallmark of nursing care.

Level of Evidence: 3

The research was a small qualitative study.

Commentary: Implications for Practice and Research

Although this study occurred in Australia, sitters are commonly used in the United States. It may be that sitters need to be trained in communication and assisting in activities of daily living to provide safe and compassionate care that recognizes the dignity of hospitalized patients with dementia. The study needs to be repeated in the United States using a larger sample size.

may refuse to drink enough fluids because of a fear of incontinence. Assure the patient that he or she will be toileted on a regular schedule to prevent incontinent episodes.

When patients with dementia are in the hospital or other unfamiliar place, avoid the use of restraints, including siderails. Serious injury can occur when a patient with dementia attempts to get out of bed with either limb restraints or siderail use. Use frequent surveillance, toileting every 2 hours, and other strategies to prevent falls. Restraint reduction has been associated with a reduced length of stay and fewer injuries (Kwok et al., 2012). In some cases, sitters may be used to help prevent patient injury (see the Evidence-Based Practice box). Chapter 2 discusses fall prevention in detail.

Maintain a clear path between the bed and bathroom at all times. For patients who are too weak to walk to the bathroom, a bedside commode may be used. Some patients may void in unusual places, such as the sink or a wastebasket. As a reminder of where they should toilet, place a picture of the commode on the bathroom door.

Use **redirection** by attracting the patient's attention to promote communication. Keep the environment as free from distractions as possible. Speak directly to the patient in a distinct manner. Sentences should be clear and short. Remind the patient to perform one task at a time, and allow sufficient time for completion. It may be necessary to break each task down into many small steps (Chart 42-14).

As the disease progresses, the patient is unable to perform tasks when asked. Show the patient what needs to be done, or provide cues to remind him or her how to perform the task. When possible, explain and demonstrate the task that the patient is asked to perform.

CHART 42-14 Best Practice for Patient Safety & Quality Care QSEN

Promoting Communication with the Patient with Advanced Dementia or Alzheimer's Disease

- Ask simple, direct questions that require only a "yes" or "no" answer if the patient can communicate.
- Provide instructions with pictures in a place that the patient will see if he or she can read them.
- Use simple, short sentences and one-step instructions.
- Use gestures to help the patient understand what is being said.
- Validate the patient's feelings.
- Limit choices; too many choices cause frustration and increased confusion.
- Never assume that the patient is totally confused and cannot understand what is being communicated.
- Try to anticipate the patient's needs and interpret nonverbal communication.

Patients with dementia disorders typically have specific speech and language problems, such as:

- **Aphasia** (difficulty speaking and understanding language)
- **Anomia** (difficulty findings words to name an object)
- **Apraxia** (difficulty recognizing words)

Recognize that emotional and physical behaviors may be a form of communication. Interpret the meaning of these behaviors to address them. For example, restlessness may indicate urinary retention, PAIN, INFECTION, or hypoxia (lack of oxygen to the brain).

Drug Therapy. **Cholinesterase inhibitors** are drugs approved for treating AD symptoms. They work to improve cholinergic neurotransmission in the brain by delaying the destruction of acetylcholine (ACh) by the enzyme *acetylcholinesterase.* This action slows the onset of cognitive decline in some patients. None of these drugs alters the course of the disease. Examples include donepezil (Aricept), galantamine (Reminyl), and rivastigmine (Exelon).

Memantine (Namenda) is the first of a new class of drugs that is a low to moderate affinity ***N*-methyl-D-aspartate (NMDA) receptor antagonist.** Overexcitation of NMDA receptors by the neurotransmitter *glutamate* may play a role in AD. This drug therefore blocks excess amounts of glutamate that can damage nerve cells. It is indicated for advanced AD and has been shown to slow the pace of deterioration. Namenda may help maintain patient function for a few months longer. Some patients also have improved memory and thinking skills. This drug can be given with donepezil (Aricept), a cholinesterase inhibitor.

Some patients with AD develop depression and may be treated with **antidepressants**. Selective serotonin reuptake inhibitors (SSRIs), such as paroxetine (Paxil) and sertraline (Zoloft), are usually prescribed. Tricyclic antidepressants, such as amitriptyline (Elavil, Levate 🍁), should not be used because of their anticholinergic effect, especially for older adults. Anticholinergic drugs frequently cause serious side effects, including increased confusion, urinary retention, and constipation.

Psychotropic drugs, also called *antipsychotic* or *neuroleptic drugs,* should be reserved for patients with emotional and behavioral health problems that sometimes accompany dementia, such as hallucinations and delusions. In clinical practice, however, these drugs are sometimes incorrectly used for agitation, combativeness, or restlessness. Psychotropic drugs are considered chemical restraints because they decrease MOBILITY and patients' self-management ability. Therefore most geriatricians recommend that these drugs be used as a last resort and with caution in low doses for a specific emotional or behavioral health problem. The specific drug prescribed depends on side effects, the condition of the patient, and expected outcomes. Follow agency policy and The Joint Commission standards concerning the use of chemical restraints.

Preventing Injury

Planning: Expected Outcomes. The patient with dementia is expected to remain free from physical harm and not injure anyone else.

Interventions. Many patients with dementia tend to wander and may easily become lost. In later stages of the disease, some patients may become severely agitated and physically or verbally abusive to others. Teach the family the importance of a patient identification badge or bracelet. The badge should include how to contact the primary caregiver. In an inpatient setting, check the patient frequently and place him or her in a room that can be monitored easily. The room should be away from exits and stairs. Some health care agencies place large stop signs or red tape on the floor in front of exits. Others have installed alarm systems to indicate when a patient is opening the door or getting out of a bed or chair.

Teach the family to enroll the patient in the Safe Return Program—a national, government-funded program of the Alzheimer's Association (www.alz.org) that assists in the identification and safe, timely return of people with dementia. The program includes registration of the patient and a 24-hour hotline to be called to assist in finding a lost patient. If a patient wanders and becomes lost, the family (or health care institution) should immediately notify the police department. An up-to-date picture of the patient makes it easier for local authorities, the public, and neighbors to identify the missing patient. Devices using radio wave beacons and a global positioning system (GPS) have been developed to help families and law enforcement officials find a lost patient more easily. These devices include shoes with a GPS unit implanted, jewelry that is hard to remove, and bracelets. Caution families that these devices are not foolproof. Just like cell phones, there are some areas where the signal from the patient may not be picked up easily if at all.

Restlessness may be decreased if the patient is taken for frequent walks. If the patient begins to wander, redirect him or her. For example, if the patient insists on going shopping for clothes, the patient is redirected to his or her closet to select clothing that will not be recognized as his or her own. This type of activity can be repeated a number of times because the patient has lost short-term memory. Best practices for preventing and managing wandering are listed in Chart 42-15.

In any setting, keep the patient busy with structured activities. In a health care agency, an activity therapist or volunteer may work with patients as a group or individually to determine the type of activity that is appropriate for the stage of the disease. Puzzles, board games, and art activities are often appropriate. Music and art therapy are nonpharmacologic approaches to managing patients with dementia (Seitz et al., 2012).

Patients with dementia may be injured because they cannot recognize objects or situations as harmful. Remove or secure all potentially dangerous objects (e.g., knives, drugs, cleaning solutions). Patients are often unaware that their driving ability is impaired and usually want to continue this activity even if their driver's license has been suspended or they are unsafe. Automobile keys must be secured, but the patient should be told why they were taken. (See Chapter 2 for more discussion on older adult driving.)

Late in the disease process, the patient may experience seizure activity. If he or she is cared for at home, teach caregivers what action to take when a seizure occurs. (See discussion of Interventions on pp. 859-863 in the Seizures and Epilepsy section.)

Talking calmly and softly and attempting to redirect the patient to a more positive behavior or activity are effective strategies when he or she is agitated. Use calm, positive statements, and reassure the patient that he or she is safe. Statements such as "I'm sorry that you are upset," "I know it's hard," and "I will have someone stay with you until you feel better" may help.

Actions to *avoid* when the patient is agitated include raising the voice, confrontation, arguing, reasoning, taking offense, or explaining. Teach the caregiver to not show alarm or make sudden movements out of the person's view. If the patient remains agitated, ensure his or her safety and leave the room after explaining that you will return later. Frequent visual checks must be done during this time. If the patient is connected to any type of tubing or other device, he or she may try to disconnect it or pull it out. These devices should be used cautiously in the patient with dementia. If IV access, for example, is needed,

CHART 42-15 Best Practice for Patient Safety & Quality Care (QSEN)

Approaches to Prevent and Manage Wandering in Hospitalized Patients

- Identify the patients most at risk for wandering through observation and history provided by family.
- Provide appropriate supervision, including frequent checks (especially at shift-change times).
- Place the patient in an area that provides maximum observation, but not in the nurses' station.
- Use family members, friends, volunteers, and sitters as needed to monitor the patient.
- Keep the patient away from stairs or elevators.
- Do not change rooms to prevent increasing confusion.
- Avoid physical or chemical restraints.
- Assess and treat pain.
- Use re-orientation methods and validation therapy, as appropriate.
- Provide frequent toileting and incontinence care as needed.
- If possible, prevent overstimulation, such as excessive noise; use soft music and nonglare lighting if possible.

! NURSING SAFETY PRIORITY (QSEN)

Action Alert

In inpatient health care agencies, use physical restraints such as waist belts and geri-chairs with lapboards only as a last resort because they often increase patient restlessness and cause agitation. Federal regulations in long-term care facilities in the United States mandate that all residents have the right to be free of both physical and chemical restraints. All health care agencies accredited by The Joint Commission are required to use alternatives to restraints before resorting to any physical or chemical restraint.

TABLE 42-6 Minimizing Behavioral Problems for Patients with Alzheimer's Disease at Home

Carefully evaluate the patient's environment.
- Ensure environment is safe:
  - Remove small area rugs.
  - Consider replacing tile floors with non-slippery floors.
  - Arrange furniture and room decorations to maximize the patient's safety when walking.
  - Minimize clutter in all rooms in and outside of the house.
  - Install nightlights in patient's room, bathroom, and hallway.
  - Install and maintain smoke alarms, fire alarms, and natural gas detectors.
- Install safety devices in the bathroom such as handles for changing position (sit-to-stand).
- Install alarm system or bells on outside doors; place safety locks on doors and gates.
- Ensure that door locks cannot be easily opened by the patient.

Assist the patient to remain oriented.
- Place single-date calendars in patient's room and in kitchen.
- Use large-face clocks with a neutral background.

Communicate with the patient based on his or her ability to understand.
- Explain activity immediately before the patient needs to carry it out.
- Break complex tasks down to simple steps.

Encourage the patient to be as independent as possible in ADLs.
- Place complete outfits for the day on hangers; have the patient select one to wear.
- Develop and maintain a predictable routine (e.g., meals, bedtime, morning routine).

When a problem behavior occurs, divert patient to another activity.

Minimize excessive stimulation.
- Take the patient on outings when crowds are small.
- If crowds cannot be avoided, minimize the amount of time the patient is present in a crowd. For example, at family gatherings, provide a quiet room for the patient to rest throughout the visit.

Arrange for a day-care program to maintain interaction and provide respite for home caregiver.

Register the patient with the Alzheimer's Association Safe Return Program (www.alz.org).

the catheter or cannula is placed in an area that the patient cannot easily see or it should be covered.

Another way to manage this problem is to provide a diversion. For example, if the patient is doing an activity or holding an item such as a stuffed animal or other special item, he or she might be less likely to pay attention to medical devices. Additional strategies to minimize behavioral problems, especially at home, are listed in Table 42-6.

Drugs may be used only if other modalities fail to control the patient's agitation and the behavior may lead to the patient or other being harmed. For example, atypical psychotics like risperidone (Risperdal), quetiapine (Seroquel), and olanzapine (Zyprexa) can help with aggressive and unsafe behaviors, although not all patients respond to these drugs. Lorazepam (Ativan) should be used with particular caution because of significant sedation and reports of increased confusion.

Patients who are cared for at home are at high risk for neglect or abuse. The Joint Commission requires all patients to be assessed for neglect and abuse on admission to a health care facility. Patients with mild dementia may not report these concerns for fear of retaliation. Those with severe dementia may not have the ability to report the abuse. Asking questions such as "Who cooks for you?" "Do you get help when you need it?" or "Do you wait long for help to the bathroom?" may be less stressful for the patient to answer.

NCLEX EXAMINATION CHALLENGE

Safe and Effective Care Environment

The nurse is caring for a client with dementia. Which nursing intervention is most appropriate when caring for this client?

A. Provide a large clock and calendar at the nurses' station.
B. Use removable restraints like a roll-waist belt to prevent wandering.
C. Use incontinence pads or absorbent underwear to prevent complications from incontinence.
D. Place the patient in a room close to the nurses' station for frequent observation.

Managing Caregiver Role Strain

Planning: Expected Outcomes. The family or other caregivers of the patient with dementia are expected to plan time to care for themselves to promote a reasonable quality of life and satisfaction (Van Mierlo et al., 2012).

Interventions. The patient with moderate or severe dementia requires continual 24-hour supervision and caregiving. Severe cognitive changes leave the patient unable to manage finances, property, or personal care. The family needs to seek legal counsel regarding the patient's competency and the need to obtain guardianship or a durable medical power of attorney when necessary. Refer the family to the local Alzheimer's or dementia support group for literature and information concerning the disease and related problems (Corbett et al., 2012).

Family members and other caregivers must be aware of their own health and stress levels. Signs of stress include anger, social withdrawal, anxiety, depression, lack of concentration, sleepiness, irritability, and health problems. When signs of stress occur, the caregiver should be referred to his or her health care provider or should seek one on his or her own. It is not unusual for the caregiver to refuse to accept help from others, even for a few brief hours. Initially, the caregiver may be more comfortable accepting help for just a few minutes a day so he or she could shower, enjoy a cup of tea, or take a brief walk. Some caregivers find that eventually they need to place their loved one into a respite setting or unit so that they can re-energize.

Refer all families to their local chapter of the Alzheimer's Association (www.alz.org) in the United States or to the Alzheimer Society of Canada (www.alzheimer.ca). These organizations provide information and support services to patients and their families, including seminars, audiovisual aids, and publications.

Community-Based Care

Home Care Management. AD is a chronic, progressive condition that eventually leaves the patient completely disoriented and totally dependent on others for all aspects of care. In the early stages, patients may be cared for at home with little need for outside intervention. Whenever possible, the patient and family should be assigned a case manager who can assess their needs for health care resources and find the best placement throughout the continuum of care.

The patient usually begins to withdraw from friends and social events as memory impairment and personality and behavior changes occur. The family may begin to decrease their own social activities as the demands of the patient's care take

CHART 42-16 Best Practice for Patient Safety & Quality Care QSEN

Reducing Caregiver Stress

- Maintain realistic expectations for the person with Alzheimer's disease (AD).
- Take each day one at a time.
- Try to find the positive aspects of each incident or situation.
- Use humor with the person who has AD.
- Use the resources of the Alzheimer's Association, including attending local support group meetings.
- Explore alternative care settings early in the disease process for possible use later.
- Establish advance directives with the AD patient early in the disease process.
- Set aside time each day for rest or recreation away from the patient, if possible.
- Seek respite care periodically for longer periods of time.
- Take care of yourself by watching your diet, exercising, and getting plenty of rest.
- Be realistic about what you or they can do, and accept help from family, friends, and community resources.
- Use relaxation techniques.

more of their time. Emphasize to the family the importance of maintaining their own social contacts and leisure activities. Many family members experience caregiver stress, which affects their physical, mental, and emotional health. Chart 42-16 lists strategies for reducing caregiver stress. Chapter 2 discusses caregiver role strain and interventions in more detail.

It is now possible in most areas of the United States and Canada for families to arrange respite care. The patient may be placed in a respite facility or nursing home for the weekend or for several weeks to give the family a rest from the constant care demands. The family may also be able to obtain respite care in the home through a home care agency or assisted-living facility. Remind the family that respite care is for a short period—it is not permanent placement. Some health care agencies have opened adult day-care centers or specialty units for patients with AD. In the day-care center, patients spend all or part of the day at the facility and participate in activities as their condition permits. Although these centers are usually open only on weekdays, this arrangement allows the caregiver to work or participate in other activities. If patients require 24-hour care, they may be placed in a specialty unit of a long-term care or assisted-living facility.

Teach the family how to be prepared in case the patient becomes restless, agitated, abusive, or combative. In addition, the family can learn how to use reality orientation or validation therapy, depending on the stage of the disease.

Self-Management Education. Usually patients with AD and dementia are cared for in the home until late in the disease process unless they can afford private-pay care. Because health insurance coverage in the United States and family finances may not be sufficient to cover the services of a private duty nurse or home care aide, family members typically provide the care. The patient plan of care developed by the nurse or case manager, in conjunction with the family, must be reasonable and realistic for the family to implement.

Review how to assist with bathing, dressing, toileting, and other self-management activities. The occupational therapist teaches the family and the patient how to use adaptive equipment, such as a brace, a sling, a cane, or modified eating utensils. The patient may have difficulty chewing, swallowing, or tasting foods and may not be able to eat without assistance.

The family and the dietitian should develop a diet plan to increase the patient's nutritional intake. In the late stage of AD, the patient's intake often decreases and he or she loses weight.

Provide information to the family on what to do in the event of a seizure and how to protect the patient from injury. Instruct them to notify the health care provider if the seizure is prolonged or if the patient's seizure pattern changes.

Review with the family or other caregiver the name, time, and route of administration; the dosage; and the side effects of all drugs. Remind the family to check with the health care provider before using any over-the-counter drugs or herbs because they may interact with prescribed drug therapy.

Emphasis is placed on the need for the patient to have an established exercise program to maintain MOBILITY for as long as possible, as well as to prevent complications of immobility. In collaboration with the family, the physical therapist (PT) develops an individualized exercise program. The PT may continue to work with the patient at home until goals are achieved, depending on the payer source.

Remind the family or other caregiver to take special precautions to maintain the patient safely at home. The environment must be uncluttered, consistent, and structured. All hazardous items (e.g., cooking range and oven, power tools) are removed, secured, or "locked out." All electrical sockets not in use should be covered with safety plugs. Teach families to install handrails and grab bars in the bathroom. Handrails should be along all stairways, and a guardrail should be placed around porches or open stairwells. Because the patient may have a tendency to wander, especially at night, the family may want to install alarms to all outside doors, the basement, and the patient's bedroom. All outside and basement doors should have deadbolt locks to prevent the patient from going outside unsupervised. Remind the family to adjust the temperature of the water to prevent accidental burns. Nightlights should be used in the patient's bedroom, hallway, and bathroom to prevent fear and to help with orientation.

Health Care Resources. When the patient can no longer be cared for at home, referral to an assisted-living or long-term care facility may be needed. Early in the course of the disease, advise the family that placement might be needed in the late stages of the disease or sooner. This allows the family to begin to search for an appropriate facility before a crisis develops and immediate placement is needed. A number of facilities specialize in the care of patients with AD and other dementias. These units generally have a high staff-to-patient ratio and are architecturally designed to meet the special needs of this type of patient. The national office of the Alzheimer's Association publishes an outline of criteria for a dementia unit. In the advanced stage of the disease, the patient may need referral to hospice services for total care. (See the discussion of end-of-life and hospice care in Chapter 7.)

◆ *Evaluation: Outcomes*

Evaluate the care of the patient with dementia based on the identified priority patient problems. The expected outcomes include that the patient and/or family will:

- Remain free from injury and have a safe home environment
- Sleep through the night and be awake at appropriate times

- Meet basic human needs (e.g., nutrition, MOBILITY)
- Have a positive perception of his or her health status and life circumstances

Specific indicators for these outcomes are listed in the Planning and Implementation section (see earlier).

CLINICAL JUDGMENT CHALLENGE

Patient-Centered Care QSEN

A middle-aged man brings his 90-year old mother to the neurologist for re-evaluation of her Alzheimer's disease (AD). The patient was diagnosed with AD 2 years ago and continues to live alone most of the time in her home. One of her sons stays with her at night, but she cannot bathe herself or prepare meals. She forgets to eat and take her medications for hypertension. Her weight is 98 pounds and she is 5′4″ tall.

1. As the nurse in the neurologist office, what questions might you ask the son about his mother's health?
2. What health assessment will you perform?
3. To promote the patient's safety, what options might you recommend for her caregiving?
4. What interventions are needed to improve the patient's nutritional status?
5. What health teaching is needed for the son at this time?

HUNTINGTON DISEASE

PATHOPHYSIOLOGY

Huntington disease (HD) is a hereditary disorder transmitted as an autosomal dominant trait at the time of conception. HD is called an *autosomal dominant disorder* because only one copy of the defective gene, inherited from one parent, is necessary to produce the disease. This movement disorder causes both neurologic and behavioral symptoms that usually begin between the ages of 30 and 50 years and worsen during the next one to two decades. Patients typically die from pneumonia, heart failure, or other complication of immobility (Huntington's Disease Society of America [HDSA], 2014).

GENETIC/GENOMIC CONSIDERATIONS

Patient-Centered Care QSEN

Huntington disease is a single gene disorder caused by a mutation in the HD gene *(IT15)* located on chromosome 4. The mutation is a multiple repeat of the specific base triplet *cytosine, adenine, guanine (CAG),* increasing the length of the gene. An autosomal dominant trait with high penetrance means that a person who inherits just one mutated allele has nearly a 100% chance of developing the disease (McCance et al., 2014). This gene mutation has different expressions, depending on whether it is inherited from the mother or the father. People who inherit the mutation from their father have an earlier onset and a shorter life expectancy than do those who inherit from their mother. In addition, there is some variation in the disease, depending on the size (length) of the mutation. The longer the mutation, the more severe the disease is at an earlier age.

It is estimated that 30,000 people in the United States have HD, and another 20,000 to 50,000 are thought to carry the gene (HDSA, 2014). Men and women are equally affected at a highly productive time in life. The clinical onset of HD is gradual. The two main symptoms of the disease are progressive mental status changes, leading to dementia, and **choreiform movements** (rapid, jerky movements) in the limbs, trunk, and facial muscles. Dementia is related to the destruction of neurons within the cerebral cortex. It may also be associated with excessive amounts of dopamine found within the cerebral cortex and limbic systems of those affected. Two structures within the basal ganglia are involved in the development of HD: the caudate nucleus and the putamen. Both structures have close connections to the cerebral cortex and are closely associated with neurotransmitters. Neurotransmitters are secreted at the synapse, or junction, of one neuron with another, and it is through their specific excitation or inhibition of neurons that fine, controlled, integrated motor activity occurs.

In HD, there is a decrease in the amount of *gamma-aminobutyric acid (GABA),* an inhibitory neurotransmitter in the basal ganglia. GABA depletion causes increased activity of the thalamus and other parts of the brain. There may also be an increase in *glutamate,* a major excitatory neurotransmitter. The result of these chemical changes in the brain is brisk, jerky, purposeless movements, particularly of the hands, face, tongue, and legs, which the patient cannot stop (McCance et al., 2014).

There are three stages of HD, each lasting roughly 5 years, corresponding to the average 15-year course of the disease. Stage 1 is the onset of neurologic or psychological symptoms. Stage 2 is characterized by an increasing dependence on others for care. Stage 3 results in loss of independent function.

The diagnosis of HD is made on the basis of a family history of the disease and clinical assessment. The triad of dominant inheritance, choreoathetosis (neuromuscular symptoms), and dementia is the hallmark of the disease. The symptoms exhibited by the patient vary in range and severity, age of onset, and rate of progression. Observe for clinical manifestations, which include chorea (jerky movements), poor balance, hesitant or explosive speech, dysphagia (difficulty swallowing), impaired respiration, and bowel and bladder incontinence. Mental status changes include decreased attention span, poor judgment, memory loss, personality changes, and dementia (later in the disease process). Perform a complete neurologic assessment.

PATIENT-CENTERED COLLABORATIVE CARE

There is no known cure or treatment for HD. The only way to prevent transmission of the gene is for those affected to avoid having biologic children. Genetic counseling is important for children of patients with the disease. People at risk for the disease can be tested to determine whether the gene mutation is present. Before the testing procedure is undertaken, counseling is necessary to ensure that the patient has voluntarily decided in favor of testing and is not being pressured by family or friends. In addition, counseling helps determine whether the benefits of knowing the results outweigh the risks of a positive result (e.g., depression or suicide).

The first drug to be approved to decrease chorea associated with HD is tetrabenazine (Xenazine). It is given orally and is thought to work by depleting the monoamines (e.g., dopamine, serotonin) from nerve terminals. In some patients, it may increase the risk for suicide ideations and depression. Be sure to teach them and their families to report early signs of depression, including sleeplessness, decreasing appetite, and mood changes.

In other patients, psychotropic agents may be used to manage movement abnormalities that interfere with ADLs or are functionally disabling. They are also used to help control agitation, hallucinations, or psychotic delusions. Drug therapy may be used to treat other symptoms such as depression, anxiety, or obsessive-compulsive behaviors. Many of the drugs used to treat HD may cause side effects that may be difficult to differentiate from signs of HD.

A number of clinical trials are being conducted to find other drugs or supplements that may decrease HD symptoms. Examples include the CoQ10 enzyme, growth factors, glutamate blockers, and antidepressants, such as sertraline (Zoloft).

The care of the patient with HD is managed by the collaborative efforts of the family and health care team and includes:

- Speech-language pathologist (SLP) who helps with communication, swallowing, and drooling
- Dietitian who plans meals based on the SLP's recommendations and the patient's likes and dislikes
- Physical and occupational therapists who determine exercise conditioning and assistive devices
- Nurses or home health care aides who provide supportive care
- Case manager and social worker who coordinate care and help with referrals to community resources (e.g., Huntington's Disease Society of America [www.hdsa.org]) and health care agencies for placement as needed

NURSING CONCEPTS AND CLINICAL JUDGMENT REVIEW

What might you NOTICE if the patient is experiencing PAIN, impaired MOBILITY, *or* altered COGNITION as a result of an acute or chronic brain disorder?

- Headache
- Acute or chronic confusion
- Sleepiness or lethargy
- Inability to perform ADLs
- Inability to ambulate or alteration in gait
- Reduced nutritional intake resulting in weight loss
- Inability to communicate effectively
- Report of photophobia or phonophobia
- One or more seizures
- Extremity tremors, rigidity, or jerky movements

What should you INTERPRET and how should you RESPOND to a patient experiencing PAIN, impaired MOBILITY, and altered COGNITION as a result of an acute CNS INFECTION or chronic brain disorder?

Perform and interpret physical assessment, including:

- Assessing neurologic status, especially level of consciousness (LOC)
- Taking vital signs (high fever may indicate infection)
- Performing a comprehensive pain assessment
- Assessing ability to communicate
- Assessing nutritional status

Respond by:

- Notifying health care provider or Rapid Response Team if seizure or sudden change in LOC or onset of an acute confusional state
- Ensuring an adequate airway
- Protecting patient from injury
- Managing pain
- Giving oxygen (during a seizure and for status epilepticus)
- Reorienting patient
- Assisting with ADLs if needed
- Collaborating with health care team members (e.g., PT, OT, SLP, dietitian)

On what should you REFLECT?

- Think about how you responded.
- Continue to monitor for improving mental status and changes in LOC.
- Assess triggers or other causes for acute event.
- Develop teaching plan for patient and family for self-management.
- Think about what resources the patient and family may need.

GET READY FOR THE NCLEX® EXAMINATION!

KEY POINTS

Review these Key Points for each NCLEX Examination Client Needs Category.

Safe and Effective Care Environment

- Provide a written summary of events during hospitalization and an oral report to the receiving caregiver during all transitions in care (e.g., from hospital to rehabilitation or home).
- Implement best practices for fall prevention and prevent injury from impaired cognition and immobility with frequent observation and interventions described in Table 42-6 and Charts 42-9, -12, -14, and -15. **Safety** QSEN
- Ensure that drugs have been reviewed with the patient and caregivers with each administration and that discharge drugs have been reconciled with a list of problems or indications. Provide written information about all home-going drugs. **Informatics** QSEN
- Collaborate with the health care team in discharge planning and health teaching for patients who have chronic seizures or neurodegenerative diseases such as PD, dementia, and HD. **Teamwork and Collaboration** QSEN
- Ensure a safe environment for a patient with seizure precautions by ensuring that suction and oxygen are available and that frequent observation occurs to detect seizure activity early. **Safety** QSEN
- Implement interventions for seizures as listed in Chart 42-6. Patients with status epilepticus have a life-threatening complication. Lorazepam and diazepam are the major drugs used for this emergency. **Evidence-Based Practice** QSEN
- For the patient with a chronic brain disorder, provide an environment that maximizes their MOBILITY, including consultation with physical and occupational therapy. **Teamwork and Collaboration** QSEN

Health Promotion and Maintenance

- Teach patients with migraine headaches about triggers that could cause an attack, such as tyramine in wine, pickled products, and aged cheeses; nitrates and nitrites in processed and grilled meats; and other dietary or environmental triggers. **Patient-Centered Care** QSEN
- Teach patients with cluster headaches about precipitating factors, such as anger episodes, excitement, and excessive physical activity.
- In addition to prescribed drug therapy, encourage patients with headaches to use complementary and alternative therapies to help relieve PAIN, such as ice, darkened room, and relaxation techniques. **Patient-Centered Care** QSEN
- Teach the patient with epilepsy to maintain seizure-free health or reduced seizure activity through using prescribed antiepileptic drugs (AEDs) and follow-up medical care. Additional instructions for the patient and family are listed in Chart 42-5.
- Document vaccination status and provide vaccination to prevent some types of infectious meningitis, particularly meningococcal vaccination to people who are in areas of high population density, such as university residences, military barracks, and crowded living areas. Vaccination is a core measure of health care effectiveness. **Evidence-Based Practice** QSEN

Psychosocial Integrity

- Remind caregivers of patients with chronic neurologic diseases, such as dementia, to find ways to cope with their own stress to remain physically and psychologically healthy, as suggested in Chart 42-16. **Patient-Centered Care** QSEN
- Teach caregivers of patients with dementia to use validation therapy rather than reality orientation. Acknowledge the patient's feelings and concerns.
- Involve families who care for patients with neurodegenerative diseases like Parkinson disease, dementia, or Huntington disease to develop a culturally appropriate continuing plan of care that reflects patient values and preferences.
- Adapt communication techniques for the patient with dementia as outlined in Chart 42-14. **Patient-Centered Care** QSEN
- Assist patients and family members to identify community resources that can assist with education and caregiver support, including consultation with social services or a case manager.

Physiological Integrity

- Assess patients with classic migraine headaches as listed in Chart 42-2.
- Compare migraine to cluster headache, recalling that the PAIN of cluster headaches is usually accompanied by ipsilateral (same side) eye tearing, rhinorrhea, congestion, ptosis, facial sweating, eyelid edema, and/or miosis. Migraine pain is characterized by throbbing pain that is unilateral and can be accompanied by nausea, light sensitivity, and worsening symptoms with movement.
- Recognize that generalized seizures, such as the tonic-clonic seizure, involve both cerebral hemispheres. Partial seizures, also called *focal* or *local seizures,* usually involve only one hemisphere.
- During a seizure, document the patient's body movements and other assessments as described in Chart 42-7. **Informatics** QSEN
- Monitor for side and adverse effects of antiepileptic drugs (AEDs) as listed in Chart 42-4. **Safety** QSEN
- For patients who have had one or more seizures, place on "seizure precautions," which includes having oxygen delivery and suctioning equipment available and starting or maintaining IV access. **Safety** QSEN
- Assess for clinical manifestations of meningitis as listed in Chart 42-8. For patients with meningitis and encephalitis, carefully monitor neurologic status, including vital signs and neurologic and vascular checks. Observe for signs and symptoms of increased intracranial pressure (ICP), and communicate changes in level of consciousness immediately to the health care provider. **Safety** QSEN
- Assess for key features of Parkinson disease as described in Chart 42-11. Monitor for drug toxicity when patients are taking medications for Parkinson disease, especially levodopa combinations such as Sinemet. Delirium and decreased drug effectiveness are the most common indicators of toxicity. **Safety** QSEN
- Communicate worsening neurologic assessment findings immediately following electrode placement for deep brain stimulation and injection of stem cells when used to control symptoms of Parkinson disease.
- Document cognitive and functional abilities of the patient with dementia, recognizing that it is a progressive condition (e.g., Alzheimer stages are listed in Chart 42-13).
- For patients with dementia, recall that a few drugs improve function and COGNITION (cholinesterase inhibitors, such as donepezil [Aricept]) or slow the disease process (Memantine) but they do not cure the disease.
- Remember that Huntington disease is a chronic, hereditary illness that is transmitted as an autosomal dominant trait at the time of conception. Refer patients with the disease for genetic counseling. **Patient-Centered Care** QSEN
- Foster a collaborative communication, establish outcomes for care with health care team members, and review them regularly. Document communication to reduce complications and promote quality of life in patients. **Informatics** QSEN

43 CHAPTER

Care of Patients with Problems of the Central Nervous System: The Spinal Cord

Rachel L. Gallagher

http://evolve.elsevier.com/Iggy/

PRIORITY CONCEPTS

- MOBILITY
- SENSORY PERCEPTION
- PAIN
- INFLAMMATION
- TISSUE INTEGRITY
- PALLIATION
- SEXUALITY

LEARNING OUTCOMES

Safe and Effective Care Environment

1. Use best practices to teach strategies that reduce back and neck injury and PAIN.
2. Prioritize the nursing care of the patient with an acute spinal cord injury (SCI).
3. Collaborate with other health care team members to manage care for patients with spinal cord problems.
4. Establish patient values and preferences, including integration of advance directives, PALLIATION, and managing distressing symptoms for patients with progressively debilitating spinal cord conditions.

Health Promotion and Maintenance

5. Identify with the patient behaviors that promote optimal weight.
6. Communicate with health care team members to establish outcomes for care and strategies to promote independence in ADLs.
7. Identify community resources for patients with spinal cord health problems and their families.

Psychosocial Integrity

8. Describe the impact of spinal cord conditions on the patient's SEXUALITY.
9. Use therapeutic communication to assess the need for emotional, mental, and social support of patients with spinal cord health problems and their families.

Physiological Integrity

10. Perform a comprehensive assessment of the patient with a spinal cord injury.
11. Establish priorities in care for the patient with spinal cord–related problems of MOBILITY, SENSORY PERCEPTION, elimination, and skin TISSUE INTEGRITY.
12. Apply knowledge of pathophysiology when caring for a patient having autonomic dysreflexia.
13. Explain the pathophysiology of multiple sclerosis (MS) and amyotrophic lateral sclerosis (ALS).
14. Explain the role of drug therapy in managing patients with spinal cord problems.
15. Develop an evidence-based postoperative plan of care for patients having spinal cord surgery, including monitoring for complications.

The spinal cord relays messages to and from the brain. Besides injuries, the spinal cord can develop tumors, infections such as meningitis and poliomyelitis, inflammatory and autoimmune diseases, and degenerative diseases such as amyotrophic lateral sclerosis (ALS) and spinal muscular atrophy. The spinal cord itself may be damaged, or the spinal nerves leading from the cord to the extremities may be affected, often by chronic INFLAMMATION. In some cases, both the spinal cord and the nerves are involved. Symptoms vary but often include problems with MOBILITY, SENSORY PERCEPTION, and PAIN. As a result, the patients' ability to perform ADLs, their skin TISSUE INTEGRITY, elimination patterns, and SEXUALITY are often affected. Health care team members with expertise in symptom management can provide significant contributions to this population's quality of life by providing PALLIATION of symptoms that are chronic and often progressive. Health care team members also can promote a safe environment, preventing complications from impaired mobility and sensory perception (Forrest et al., 2012). (See the Quality Improvement box.)

QUALITY IMPROVEMENT (QSEN)

Reducing Falls and Harm from Falls

Forrest, G., Huss, S., Patel, V., Jeffries, J., Myers, D., Barber, C., et al. (2012). Falls on an inpatient rehabilitation unit: Risk assessment and prevention. *Rehabilitation Nursing, 37*(2), 56-61.

This quality improvement project had a twofold purpose. The first was to determine if a common measure of function used in a rehabilitation setting identified patients at increased risk for a fall. The second purpose was to determine if a comprehensive plan for fall reduction that used the functional assessment results to guide interventions was effective at reducing falls.

The strength of this project is the interdisciplinary team that designed the process of both assessment and care. This report also details the application of a quality improvement process to refine interventions as data became available about the usefulness of a functional assessment in identifying high-risk patients. Functional impairment was found to be associated with more falls. It is important to note that functional impairment was most often associated with Guillain-Barré, spinal cord injury, myopathy, and peripheral neuropathy. Neurologic diagnoses were then used to revise the screening tool that identified patients at increased risk for falls and develop novel interventions. Over time, falls were reduced by 50%—a significant improvement in patient safety.

Commentary: Implications for Practice and Research

This report illustrates several steps of a Plan-Do-Study-Act cycle in developing and sustaining a quality improvement project. First, the authors used information in the literature about fall reduction and then adapted that information to develop a protocol that met their patient population needs and hospital resources. Adding functional assessment provided essential information about high-risk patients in this setting. The report also illustrates the need for ongoing feedback to sustain adherence to quality improvement (protocol) interventions that were successful in reducing falls.

BACK PAIN

Back pain affects as many of 80% of adults at some time in their life. It can be recurrent, and subsequent episodes tend to increase in severity. The prevalence of both acute and chronic back pain varies with age, lifestyle factors including obesity and osteoporosis, and certain types of physical activity such as heavy physical work and lifting. Low back pain is the leading cause of work disability (Costa-Black et al., 2010).

The lumbosacral (lower back) and cervical (neck) vertebrae are most commonly affected because these are the areas where the vertebral column is the most flexible. *Acute* back PAIN is usually self-limiting. If the pain continues for 3 months or if repeated episodes of pain occur, the patient has *chronic* back pain.

LOW BACK PAIN (LUMBOSACRAL BACK PAIN)

❖ *PATHOPHYSIOLOGY*

Low back pain (LBP) occurs along the lumbosacral area of the vertebral column. Acute pain is caused by muscle strain or spasm, ligament sprain, disk (also spelled "disc") degeneration (osteoarthritis), or herniation of the center of the disk, the nucleus pulposus, past the lateral vertebral border. A **herniated nucleus pulposus (HNP)** in the lumbosacral area can press on the adjacent spinal nerve (usually the sciatic nerve), causing severe burning or stabbing pain down into the leg or foot (Fig. 43-1). Herniated disks occur most often between the fourth and fifth lumbar vertebrae (L4-5) but may occur at other levels. The specific area of symptoms depends on the level of herniation.

In addition to PAIN, there may be both muscle spasm and numbness and tingling (paresthesia) in the affected leg because spinal nerves have both motor and sensory fibers. The HNP may press on the spinal cord itself, causing leg weakness. Bowel and bladder incontinence or retention may occur with motor nerve involvement and because sacral spinal nerves have parasympathetic nerve fibers that help control bowel and bladder function.

Back pain may also be caused by **spondylolysis**, a defect in one of the vertebrae usually in the lumbar spine. **Spondylolisthesis** occurs when one vertebra slips forward on the one below it, often as a result of spondylolysis. This problem causes pressure on the nerve roots, leading to pain in the lower back and into the buttocks. Pain or numbness may also occur in the leg and foot. **Spinal stenosis**, a narrowing of the spinal canal, nerve root canals, or intervertebral foramina is typically seen in people older than 50 years. This narrowing may be caused by infection, trauma, herniated disk, arthritis, and disk degeneration. Most adults older than 50 years have some degree of degenerative disk disease, although they may not be symptomatic.

Low back pain is most prevalent during the third to sixth decades of life but can occur at any time. Acute back PAIN usually results from injury or trauma such as during a fall, vehicular crash, or lifting a heavy object. The mechanisms of injury include repetitive flexion and/or extension and

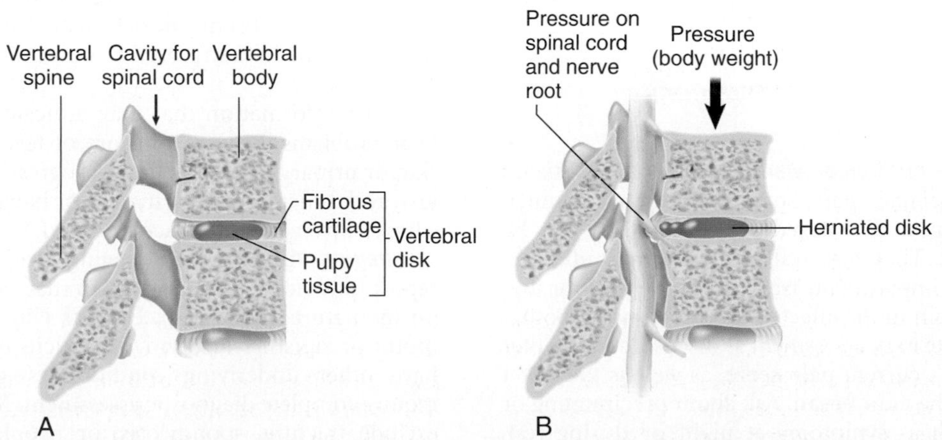

FIG. 43-1 Sagittal section of vertebrae showing (**A**) a normal disk and (**B**) a herniated disk.

CHART 43-1 Nursing Focus on the Older Adult

Factors Contributing to Low Back Pain

- Changes in support structures
  - Spinal stenosis
  - Hypertrophy of the intraspinal ligaments
  - Osteoarthritis
  - Osteoporosis
- Changes in vertebral support and malalignment
  - Scoliosis
  - Lordosis
- Vascular changes
  - Diminished blood supply to the spinal cord or cauda equina caused by arteriosclerosis
  - Blood dyscrasias
- Intervertebral disk degeneration

hyperflexion or hyperextension with or without rotation. Obesity places increased stress on the vertebral column and back muscles, contributing to risk for injury. Smoking has been linked to disk degeneration, possibly caused by constriction of blood vessels that supply the spine. Congenital spinal conditions like scoliosis can also lead to LBP. Older adults are at high risk for both acute and chronic LBP. Vertebral fracture from osteoporosis contributes to LBP. Petite, Euro-American women are at high risk for both bone loss and subsequent vertebral fractures. Chart 43-1 provides a list of specific factors that can cause low back pain in the older adult. Vertebral compression fractures are discussed in detail in Chapter 51.

Health Promotion and Maintenance

Many of the problems related to acute back PAIN can be prevented by recognizing the factors that contribute to tissue injury and taking appropriate preventive measures. For example, good posture and exercise can significantly decrease the incidence of low back pain. The U.S. Occupational Safety and Health Administration (OSHA) mandated that all industries develop and implement a plan to decrease musculoskeletal injuries among their workers. One way to meet this requirement is to develop an ergonomic plan for the workplace. **Ergonomics** is an applied science in which the workplace is designed to increase worker comfort (thus reducing injury) while increasing efficiency and productivity. An example is a celling lift designed to help nurses assist patients to get out of bed. A variety of equipment can be used to decrease injury related to moving patients. Professional guidelines and legislative rules promote safe patient handling for health care workers (www.nursingworld.org/rnnoharm). Chart 43-2 summarizes various ways to help prevent LBP related to lifting objects and handling patients (ANA, 2013; Nelson et al., 2008).

CHART 43-2 Patient and Family Education: Preparing for Self-Management

Prevention of Low Back Pain and Injury

- Use safe manual handling practices, with specific attention to bending, lifting, and sitting.
- Assess the need for assistance with your household chores or other activities.
- Participate in a regular exercise program, especially one that promotes back strengthening, such as swimming and walking.
- Do not wear high-heeled shoes.
- Use good posture when sitting, standing, and walking.
- Avoid prolonged sitting or standing. Use a footstool and ergonomic chairs and tables to lessen back strain. Be sure that equipment in the workplace is ergonomically designed to prevent injury.
- Keep weight within 10% of ideal body weight.
- Ensure adequate calcium intake. Consider vitamin D supplementation if serum levels are low.
- Stop smoking. If you are not able to stop, cut down on the number of cigarettes or decrease the use of other forms of tobacco.

❖ *PATIENT-CENTERED COLLABORATIVE CARE*

◆ *Assessment*

Physical Assessment/Clinical Manifestations. *The patient's primary concern is continuous pain.* Some patients have so much pain that they walk in a stiff, flexed posture or they may be unable to bend at all. They may walk with a limp, indicating possible sciatic nerve impairment. Walking on the heels or toes often causes severe pain in the affected leg, the back, or both.

Conduct a complete PAIN assessment as discussed in Chapter 3. Record the patient's current pain score, as well as the worst and best score since the PAIN began. Ask about precipitating or relieving factors such as symptoms at night or during rest. Determine if a recent injury to the back has occurred. It is not unusual for the patient to say "I just turned around and felt my back go out."

Inspect the patient's back for vertebral alignment and tenderness. Examine the surrounding anatomy and lower extremities for secondary injury (Patton & Thibodeau, 2014). Patients report stabbing, continuous PAIN in the muscle closest to the affected disk. They often describe a sharp, burning posterior thigh or calf pain that may radiate to the ankle or toes along the path of one or more spinal nerves. Pain usually does not extend the entire length of the limb. Patients may also report the same type of pain in the middle of one buttock. The pain is often aggravated by sneezing, coughing, or straining. Driving a vehicle is particularly painful.

Ask whether **paresthesia** (tingling sensation) or numbness is present in the involved leg. Both extremities may be checked for SENSORY PERCEPTION by using a cotton ball and a paper clip for comparison of light and deep touch. The patient may feel sensory perception in both legs but may experience a stronger sensation on the unaffected side. Ask about urinary and fecal continence and difficulty in urination or constipation.

If the sciatic nerve is compressed, severe pain occurs when the patient's leg is held straight and lifted upward. Foot, ankle, and leg weakness may accompany lower back pain. To complete the neurologic assessment, evaluate the patient's muscle tone and strength. Muscles in the extremity or lower back can atrophy as a result of severe chronic back pain. The patient has difficulty with movement, and certain movements create more pain than others.

Other information that may indicate more serious neurologic problems includes a history of fever and chills, recurrent skin or urinary tract infections, progressive motor and sensory loss, and difficulty with urination or having a bowel movement (due to involvement of sacral nerves).

Imaging Assessment. Imaging studies for patients who report mild nonspecific back PAIN may not be done depending on the nature of the pain. Patients with severe or progressive motor or SENSORY PERCEPTION deficits or who are thought to have other underlying conditions (e.g., cancer, infection) require complete diagnostic assessment. X-rays of the spine can exclude fracture, spondylosis, or neoplasm as the causative agent. Flexion-extension views can be very useful to show instability of the spine. The imaging studies of choice are magnetic resonance imaging (MRI) or computerized tomography (CT) scanning. The MRI is usually the first test of choice because it is noninvasive. A CT myelogram is done when a better delineation of the bony anatomy and the specific nerve root involvement is needed.

Electro-diagnostic testing, such as electromyography (EMG) and nerve-conduction studies, may help distinguish motor neuron diseases from peripheral neuropathies and **radiculopathies** (spinal nerve root involvement). These tests are especially useful in chronic diseases of the spinal cord or associated nerves. Chapter 41 describes these tests in more detail.

◆ *Interventions*

Management of patients with back PAIN varies with the severity and chronicity of the problem. Most patients with acute LBP experience a spontaneous resolution of pain and other symptoms over the short term (i.e., less than 3-6 months). Other patients need a brief treatment regimen of at-home exercise or physical therapy and drugs to manage pain. In general, return to work, if safe, is beneficial for recovery and well-being. When motor function is abruptly lost, surgery may be needed. Some patients have continuous or intermittent chronic pain that must be managed for an extended period. Referral to an interdisciplinary team that specializes in pain or back pain can provide expert long-term management.

Nonsurgical Management. Nonsurgical conservative management of LBP includes positioning, drug therapy, physical therapy, weight control, and smoking cessation.

Acute Low Back Pain. The **Williams position** is typically more comfortable and therapeutic for the patient with LBP from a bulging or herniated disk. In this *position*, the patient lies in the semi-Fowler's position with a pillow under the knees to keep them flexed or sits in a recliner chair. This position relaxes the muscles of the lower back and relieves pressure on the spinal nerve root. Most patients also find that they need to change position frequently. Prolonged standing, sitting, or lying down increases back PAIN. If the patient must stand for a long time for work or other reason, shoe insoles or special floor pads may help decrease pain.

The health care provider prescribes acetaminophen or NSAIDs; muscle relaxants may also be used for acute LBP. Opioid analgesics are no more effective than non-opioid analgesics and should be avoided if at all possible. If they must be used, the course of therapy should be short to prevent adverse drug events. Short-term oral steroids in tapering doses may be prescribed for some patients to rapidly reduce INFLAMMATION.

Some patients may need an epidural injection for pain relief. A corticosteroid and an anesthetic are injected to reduce INFLAMMATION in the affected area. During a facet joint injection, fluoroscopy is used to insert a needle into the epidural space surrounding the facet and a corticosteroid is injected to coat the nerve roots and outside lining of the joints.

Chronic Low Back Pain. Patients having chronic low back PAIN (LBP) are treated with NSAIDs, opioids, and/or antidepressants (as adjunctive therapy). In a recent systematic review of drug treatment, the authors reported NSAIDs and opioids provided somewhat higher relief in pain in the short term as compared with placebo. However, these drugs are associated with significant adverse drug effects. Further, there were no differences in outcomes between antidepressants and placebo in patients with nonspecific chronic LBP (Kuijpers et al., 2011).

CHART 43-3 Patient and Family Education: Preparing for Self-Management

Typical Exercises for Chronic or Postoperative Low Back Pain

Extension Exercises

- **Stomach lying:** Lie face down with a pillow under your chest; lift legs straight up (alternate legs) (may not be tolerated).
- **Upper trunk extension:** Lie face down with your arms at your sides, and lift your head and neck.
- **Prone push-ups:** Lie face down on a mat and, keeping your body stiff, push up to extend your arms.

Flexion Exercises

- **Pelvic tilt:** Lying on your back with your knees bent, tighten your abdominal muscles to push your lower back against the mat.
- **Semi-sit-ups:** Lying on your back with your knees bent, raise your upper body at a 45-degree angle and hold this position for 5 to 10 seconds.
- **Knee to chest:** Lying on your back with your knees bent, tighten your abdominal muscles to push your lower back against the mat. Now bring one or both knees to your chest and hold this position for 5 to 10 seconds.

! NURSING SAFETY PRIORITY (QSEN)

Drug Alert

Teach older adults and their families to monitor for the adverse drug effects of opioids, including constipation, drowsiness, and acute confusion. Opioids can put older adults at increased risk for falls and injury. Instruct them to notify their health care provider to report these changes, and suggest a lower dose or change to a non-opioid pain drug.

Some patients with back PAIN may have temporary relief from *heat or cold* application. Heat increases blood flow to the affected area and promotes the healing of injured nerves. Moist heat from heat packs or hot towels applied for 20 to 30 minutes at least 4 times per day is often recommended. Hot showers or baths may also be beneficial, although data are insufficient to support the use of *superficial* heat/cold applications for low back pain (van Middelkoop et al., 2011).

The physical therapist (PT) may provide *deep* heat therapy, such as ultrasound treatments and diathermy. Some patients may receive **phonophoresis**, which is the application of a topical drug (e.g., Xylocaine, hydrocortisone) followed by continuous ultrasound for 10 minutes. **Iontophoresis** is a similar procedure in which a small electrical current and dexamethasone are typically used. Both procedures push the medication into the subcutaneous tissue and provide longer-lasting pain relief.

The PT also works with the patient to develop an individualized exercise program. The type of exercises prescribed depends on the location and nature of the injury and the type of PAIN. The patient does not begin exercises until acute pain is reduced by other means. Several specific exercises for strengthening muscles to manage LBP are listed in Chart 43-3. A systematic review of 37 studies showed that there is low-quality evidence for the effectiveness of exercise for low back pain (van Middelkoop et al., 2010). Water therapy combined with exercise is helpful for some patients with chronic pain. The water also provides muscle resistance during exercise to prevent atrophy.

Weight reduction may help reduce chronic lower back PAIN by decreasing the strain on the vertebrae caused by excess weight. If the patient's weight exceeds the ideal by more than 10%, caloric restriction is recommended. Health care providers must be sensitive when reinforcing the need for patients to lose weight to prevent or to lessen chronic back pain. Behavioral approaches to weight loss and positive reinforcement are important for the nutrition plan.

Complementary and Alternative Therapies. The patient may find that nontraditional and complementary therapies provide short-term pain relief. Patients with low back muscle injuries or mild nerve involvement may find relief of pain from chiropractic therapies, although there is insufficient evidence to support consistent use of this intervention (Parkinson et al., 2013). The purpose of chiropractic or spinal manipulative therapy (SMT) is to promote alignment and prevent or treat pressure on nerve roots (Bergman & Peterson, 2011).

Imagery, acupuncture, music therapy, massage, and herbal medicines are examples of other possible pain-relief therapies for acute and chronic back pain. A systematic review of research on the effectiveness of complementary and alternative medicine (CAM) for chronic back pain supported the use of acupressure and herbal therapies for short-term pain relief (Rubinstein et al., 2010).

As many as 20% of patients with back pain may use or be prescribed weighted traction, an intervention that applies a weighted pulley system and a girdle or other device to create a pulling force along the vertebrae. However, a recent review of the evidence for this therapy suggests that weighted traction provides little or no effect on pain intensity, function, or return to work (Wegner et al., 2013).

Surgical Management

Surgery is usually performed if conservative measures fail to relieve back PAIN or if neurologic deficits continue to progress. An orthopedic surgeon and/or neurosurgeon perform these surgeries. Two major types of surgery are used depending on the severity and exact location of pain: minimally invasive surgery (MIS) and conventional open surgical procedures. MIS is not done if the disk is pressing into the spinal cord (central cord involvement).

Preoperative Care. Preoperative care for the patient preparing for lumbar surgery is similar to that for any patient undergoing surgery (see Chapter 14). Teach the patient about postoperative expectations, including:

- Techniques to get into and out of bed
- Turning and moving in bed
- Reporting immediately new SENSORY PERCEPTION, such as numbness and tingling, or new motor impairment that may occur in the affected leg or in both legs
- Home care activities and restrictions

Many patients are discharged to home within 23 to 48 hours after surgery. Therefore, before surgery, teach family members or other caregiver how to assist the patient and what restrictions the patient must follow at home.

A bone graft is done if the patient has a *spinal fusion*. The surgeon explains from where the bone for grafting will be obtained. The patient's own bone is used whenever possible, but additional bone from a bone bank may be needed. The surgeon provides verbal and written information about the type and the source of bone for surgery. Be sure that the patient signs an informed consent form before surgery. While the bone graft heals, the patient may wear a back orthotic device for 4 to 6 weeks after surgery, but this is not common practice today. Provide information about the importance of wearing the brace as instructed during the healing process, how to take it off and put it on while maintaining spinal alignment, and how to clean it.

Operative Procedures. *Minimally invasive surgeries (MISs)* have the advantage of being associated with minimal muscle injury, decreased blood loss, and decreased postoperative pain. The primary advantage of these surgical procedures is a shortened hospital stay and the possibility of an ambulatory care (same-day) procedure. Spinal cord and nerve complications are also less likely. Several specific procedures are commonly performed.

A local anesthetic is given for the *microscopic (or surgical) endoscopic diskectomy (MED)* or *percutaneous endoscopic diskectomy (PED)*. The surgeon uses x-ray fluoroscopy to insert an endoscope (arthroscope) next to the affected disk. A special cutting tool or laser probe is threaded through the cannula for removal or destruction of the *disk pieces* that are compressing the nerve root. A newer procedure combines the PED with *laser thermodiskectomy* to also shrink the herniated disk before removal. Inpatient hospitalization is not necessary for this procedure.

A *microdiskectomy* involves microscopic surgery directly through a 1-inch incision. This procedure allows easier identification of anatomic structures, improved precision in removing small fragments, and decreased tissue trauma and pain.

Laser-assisted laparoscopic lumbar diskectomy combines a laser with modified standard disk instruments inserted through the laparoscope using an umbilical ("belly button") incision. The procedure may be used to treat herniated disks that are bulging but do not involve the vertebral canal. The primary risks of this surgery are infection and nerve root injury. The patient is typically discharged in 23 hours but may go home sooner.

The most common *conventional open procedures* are diskectomy, laminectomy, and spinal fusion. These procedures involve a surgical incision to expose anatomic landmarks for extensive muscle and soft-tissue dissection. In patients with fragile vertebrae following major spine surgery, vertebroplasty (insertion of acrylic bone cement) is sometimes performed at the levels above and below surgery. This procedure strengthens adjacent vertebral bodies that will be more stressed. Major complications from spine surgery include nerve injuries, **diskitis** (disk INFLAMMATION), and dural tears (tears in the dura covering the spinal cord).

As the name implies, a *diskectomy* is removal of a herniated disk. A *laminectomy* involves removal of part of the laminae and facet joints to obtain access to the disk space. When repeated laminectomies are performed or the spine is unstable, the surgeon may perform a **spinal fusion (arthrodesis)** to stabilize the affected area. Chips of bone are removed, typically from the iliac crest, or obtained from donor bone and are grafted between the vertebrae for support and to strengthen the back. Metal implants (usually titanium pins, screws, plates, or rods) may be required to ensure the fusion of the spine. Before closing, the surgeon may give an **intrathecal** (spinal) or epidural dose of long-acting morphine (Duramorph) to decrease postoperative pain.

Interbody cage fusion is a newer spinal implant. A cagelike device is implanted into the space where the disk was removed.

Bone graft tissue is packed around the device. As with instrumentation and fusion, the bone graft grows into and around the cage and creates a stable spine at that level.

An adjunct for patients for whom fusion may be difficult is the placement of an implantable **direct current stimulation (DCS)** device to promote bone fusion. External bone stimulators may also be effective for healing bone fusions.

Postoperative Care. Postoperative care depends on the type of surgery that was performed. In the postanesthesia care unit (PACU), vital signs and level of consciousness are monitored frequently, the same as for any surgery. Best practices for PACU nursing care are discussed in Chapter 16.

Minimally Invasive Surgery. Patients go home the same day or the day after surgery with a Band-Aid or Steri-Strips over their small incision. Those having a microdiskectomy may also have a clear or gauze dressing over the bandage. Most patients notice less PAIN immediately after surgery, but mild oral analgesics are needed while nerve tissue heals over the next few weeks. In collaboration with the health care provider and physical therapist, teach the patient to follow the prescribed exercise program, which begins immediately after discharge. Patients should start walking routinely every day. Complications of MIS are rare.

Conventional Open Surgery. Early postoperative nursing care focuses on preventing and assessing complications that might occur in the first 24 to 48 hours (Chart 43-4). As for any patient undergoing surgery, take vital signs at least every 4 hours during the first 24 hours to assess for fever and for hypotension, which could indicate bleeding or severe pain. Perform a neurologic assessment every 4 hours. Of particular importance are movement, strength, and SENSORY PERCEPTION in the lower extremities.

Carefully check the patient's ability to void. PAIN and a flat position in bed make voiding difficult, especially for men. An inability to void may indicate damage to the sacral spinal nerves, which control the detrusor muscle in the bladder. Opioid analgesics have also been associated with difficulty voiding. The patient with a diskectomy or laminectomy typically gets out of bed with assistance on the evening of surgery, which may help with voiding.

PAIN control may be achieved with patient-controlled analgesia (PCA) with morphine. The route is changed to oral administration after the patient is able to take fluids or the next morning.

! NURSING SAFETY PRIORITY QSEN

Critical Rescue

For the patient after back surgery, inspect the surgical dressing for blood or any other type of drainage. Clear drainage may mean cerebrospinal fluid (CSF) leakage. The loss of a large amount of CSF may cause the patient to report having a sudden headache. Report signs of any drainage on the dressing to the surgeon immediately. Bulging at the incision site may be due to a CSF leak or a hematoma, both of which should also be reported to the surgeon.

Empty the surgical drain, usually a Jackson-Pratt or Hemovac, and record the amount of drainage every 8 hours. The surgeon usually removes the drain in 24 to 36 hours.

Correct turning of the patient in bed is especially important. Teach the patient to log roll every 2 hours from side to back and vice versa. In **log rolling**, the patient turns as a unit while his or her back is kept as straight as possible. A turning sheet may be used for obese patients. Either turning method may require additional assistance, depending on how much the patient can assist and on his or her weight. Instruct the patient to keep his or her back straight when getting out of bed. He or she should sit in a straight-back chair with the feet resting comfortably on the floor. As with all surgical patients, prevent atelectasis and iatrogenic pneumonia with deep breathing. Follow best practices to avoid venous thromboembolism (VTE) postoperatively with early MOBILITY and intermittent sequential compression or pneumatic devices per The Joint Commission's Core Measures.

When a spinal fusion is performed in addition to a laminectomy, more care is taken with MOBILITY and positioning. The nurse or unlicensed assistive personnel (UAP) assist with log rolling the patient every 2 hours. For the conventional fusion, inspect both the iliac and spinal incision dressings for drainage

CHART 43-4 Best Practice for Patient Safety & Quality Care QSEN

Assessing and Managing the Patient with Major Complications of Lumbar Spinal Surgery

COMPLICATION	ASSESSMENT/INTERVENTIONS
Cerebrospinal fluid (CSF) leakage	Observe for clear fluid on or around the dressing. If leakage occurs, place patient flat. Report CSF leakage immediately to the surgeon. (The patient is usually kept on flat bedrest for several days while the dural tear heals.)
Fluid volume deficit	Monitor intake and output; monitor drain output, which should not be more than 250 mL in 8 hours during the first 24 hours. Monitor vital signs carefully for hypotension and tachycardia.
Acute urinary retention	Assist the patient to the bathroom or a bedside commode as soon as possible postoperatively. Assist male patients to stand at the bedside as soon as possible postoperatively.
Paralytic ileus	Monitor for flatus or stool. Assess for abdominal distention, nausea, and vomiting.
Fat embolism syndrome (FES) (more common in people with spinal fusion)	Observe for and report chest pain, dyspnea, anxiety, and mental status changes (particularly common in older adults). Note petechiae around the neck, upper chest, buccal membrane, and conjunctiva. Monitor arterial blood gas values for decreased PaO_2.
Persistent or progressive lumbar radiculopathy (nerve root pain)	Report pain not responsive to opioids. Document the location and nature of pain. Administer analgesics as prescribed.
Infection (e.g., wound, diskitis, hematoma)	Monitor the patient's temperature carefully (a slight elevation is normal). Increased temperature elevation or a spike after the second postoperative day is possibly indicative of infection. Report increased pain or swelling at the wound site or in the legs. Give antibiotics as prescribed if infection is confirmed. Use clean technique for dressing changes.

and make sure they are intact. Remind the patient to avoid prolonged sitting or standing.

Community-Based Care

The patient with back PAIN who does not undergo surgery is typically managed at home. If back surgery is performed, the patient is usually discharged to home with support from family or significant others. For older adults without a community support system, a short-term stay in a nursing home or transitional care unit may be needed. Collaborate with the case manager or discharge planner, patient, and family to determine the most appropriate placement.

Home Care Management. After *conventional open back surgery,* the patient may have activity restrictions such as limited daily stair climbing. Driving, lifting objects heavier than 5 pounds, pushing, and pulling (e.g., dog walking) are also restricted during home recovery for many weeks. However, daily walking is encouraged. The duration of home-based recovery depends on the nature of the job and the extent and type of surgery. Most patients return to work after 6 weeks; some patients may not return for 3 to 6 months if their jobs are physically strenuous.

Patients having any of the *MIS procedures* may resume normal activities within a few days up to 3 weeks after surgery, depending on the specific procedure that was done and the condition of the patient. He or she may take a shower on the third or fourth day after surgery. Teach the patient to remove the outer clear or gauze dressing, if any is in place, but leave the Steri-Strips in place for removal by the surgeon or until they fall off. Instruct the patient to contact the surgeon immediately if clear drainage seeps from the incision. Clear drainage usually indicates a meningeal tear and cerebrospinal fluid is leaking.

Self-Management Education. The patient with an acute episode of back PAIN typically returns to his or her usual activities but may fear a recurrence. Remind the patient that he or she may never have another episode if caution is used. However, continuous or repeated pain can be frustrating and tiring. Encourage the patient and family members to plan short-term goals and take steps toward recovering each day.

After surgery, in collaboration with the physical therapist, instruct the patient to:

- Continue with a weight-reduction diet, if needed.
- Stop smoking, if applicable.
- Perform strengthening exercises as instructed.

The physical therapist reviews and demonstrates the principles of body mechanics and muscle-strengthening exercises. The patient is then asked to demonstrate these principles (Chart 43-5). Formal physical therapy usually begins about 2 weeks after surgery. Teach the patient the importance of keeping all appointments and following the prescribed exercise plan.

The health care provider may want the patient to continue taking anti-inflammatory drugs or, if muscle spasm is present, muscle relaxants. Remind the patient and family about the possible side effects of drugs and what to do if they occur.

In a few patients, back surgery is not successful. This situation, referred to as **failed back surgery syndrome (FBSS)**, is a complex combination of organic, psychological, and socioeconomic factors. Repeated surgical procedures often discourage these patients, who must continue PAIN management after multiple operations. Nerve blocks, implantable spinal cord stimulators (neurostimulators), and other chronic pain management modalities may be needed on a long-term basis.

CHART 43-5 Best Practice for Patient Safety & Quality Care QSEN

Prevention of Musculoskeltal Injuries

Use Best Practices to Prevent Back Injury when Moving Objects

- Avoid lifting objects of more than 10 pounds without assistance or aid until the surgeon approves.
- Push objects rather than pull them.
- Do not twist your back during movement.
- Use handles or grips to prevent unintended shifting of the object during movement.
- Avoid prolonged sitting or standing. Use a footstool to lessen back strain.
- Sit in chairs with good support.
- Avoid shoulder stooping; maintain proper posture.
- Do not walk or stand in high-heeled shoes for prolonged periods (for women).

Use Best Practices to Prevent Back Injury when Moving a Person

- Establish an interdisciplinary team responsible for reviewing and implementing OSHA guidelines for the prevention of musculoskeletal disorders. Originally developed for nursing homes, these guidelines provide guidance for education and practice and programs for health care workers and other stakeholders involved in patient handling, transfers, and movement.
- Build and support a culture of safety in health care settings that protects staff as well as patients from injury.
- Improve communication channels among nurses, physical therapists, and family caregivers to facilitate safe patient handling and movement tasks.
- Develop policies and procedures for the therapeutic use of patient handling equipment:
  - Select equipment that first provides safety of patients, staff, and family caregivers.
  - Train all staff and family caregivers in the proper and safe operation of all ergonomic-appropriate equipment.
  - Encourage patient participation in the use of assistive equipment like sit and stand lifts that are used as an ambulation aid.
- Develop competency-based assessments that demonstrate proficiency for use of all patient handling approaches and equipment.
- Encourage quality improvement projects and research that support safe and effective patient handling and movement while maximizing patient-assisted or patient-independent movement. For example, investigate the cost-effectiveness of ergonomic interventions.

Spinal cord stimulation is an *invasive* technique that provides PAIN control by applying an electrical field over the spinal cord. A trial with a percutaneous epidural stimulator is conducted to determine whether or not permanent placement is appropriate. If the trial is successful, electrodes are surgically placed in the epidural space and connected to an external or implanted programmable generator. The patient is taught to program and adjust the device to maximize comfort. Spinal cord stimulation can be extremely effective in select patients but is reserved for intractable neuropathic pain syndromes that have been unresponsive to other treatments.

Ziconotide (Prialt) is a drug used for severe chronic back pain. It is given by intrathecal (spinal) infusion with a surgically implanted pump. It is the first available drug in a new class called *N-type calcium channel blockers (NCCBs).* NCCBs seem to selectively block calcium channels on those nerves that usually transmit pain signals to the brain. Ziconotide is also used for patients with cancer, acquired immune deficiency syndrome (AIDS), and unremitting pain from other nervous system disorders.

! NURSING SAFETY PRIORITY QSEN

Critical Rescue

For patients who have a spinal cord stimulator implanted in the epidural space, assess neurologic status below the level of insertion frequently. Monitor for early changes in SENSORY PERCEPTION, movement, and muscle strength. Ensure that the patient can void without difficulty. *If any changes occur, document and report them immediately to the surgeon!*

! NURSING SAFETY PRIORITY QSEN

Drug Alert

Ziconotide can be given with opioid analgesics but should *not* be given to patients with severe mental health/behavioral health problems because it can cause psychosis. *If symptoms such as hallucinations and delusions occur, teach patients to stop the drug immediately and notify their health care provider.*

NCLEX EXAMINATION CHALLENGE

Physiological Integrity

When providing discharge teaching to a client after a lumbar laminectomy, the nurse teaches the client to engage in which activities?

A. Evening showers with hot water
B. Vigorous stair climbing
C. Return to work within 1-2 weeks
D. Daily walking

Health Care Resources. Assist the patient in identifying support systems (e.g., family, church groups, clubs) after back surgery or FBSS. For example, a spouse may help the patient with exercises or perform the exercises with the patient. Members of a church group may help run errands and do household chores. The patient with back pain may continue physical therapy on an ambulatory basis after discharge. For unresolved PAIN, the patient may be referred to pain specialists or clinics, which are usually found in large metropolitan hospitals. A case manager may be assigned to the patient to help with resource management and utilization.

CERVICAL NECK PAIN

PATHOPHYSIOLOGY

Cervical neck PAIN most often results from a bulging or herniation of the nucleus pulposus (HNP) in an intervertebral disk, illustrated in Fig. 43-1. The disk tends to herniate laterally where the annulus fibrosus is weakest and the posterior longitudinal ligament is thinned. The result is spinal nerve root compression with resulting motor and sensory manifestations, typically in the neck, upper back (over the shoulder), and down the affected arm. The disk between the fifth and sixth cervical vertebrae (C5-6) is affected most often.

If the disk does not herniate, nerve compression may be caused by osteophyte (bony spur) formation from osteoarthritis. The osteophyte presses on the intervertebral foramen, which results in a narrowing of the disk and pressure on the nerve root. As with sciatic nerve compression, the patient with cervical nerve compression may have either continuous or intermittent chronic pain. When the disk herniates centrally, pressure on the spinal cord occurs.

Cervical PAIN—acute or chronic—may also occur from muscle strain, ligament sprain resulting from aging, poor posture, lifting, tumor, rheumatoid arthritis, osteoarthritis, or infection. The typical history of the patient includes a report of pain when moving the neck, which radiates to the shoulder and down the arm. The pain may interrupt sleep and may be accompanied by a headache or numbness and tingling in the affected arm. To determine the exact cause of the pain, a number of diagnostic tests may be used, including:

- Plain x-rays (show general arthritis changes and bony alignment)
- Computerized tomography (CT) scan (shows spinal bones, nerves, disks, and ligaments)
- Magnetic resonance imaging (MRI) (provides images of the spinal tissue, bones, spinal cord, nerves, ligaments, musculature, and disks)
- Bone scan (shows bone changes by injecting radioactive tracers, which attach to areas of increased bone production or show increased vascularity associated with tumor or infection)
- Myelogram/post-myelogram CT (evaluates nerve root lesions and any other mass lesion or infection of the meninges or spinal cord)
- Electromyography/nerve conduction studies (help differentiate cervical radiculopathy, ulnar or radial neuropathy, carpal tunnel syndrome, or other peripheral nerve problems)

PATIENT-CENTERED COLLABORATIVE CARE

Conservative treatment for acute neck PAIN is the same as described for low back pain except the exercises focus on the shoulders and neck. The physical therapist teaches the patient the correct techniques for performing "shoulder shrug," "shoulder squeeze," and "seated rowing." Some health care providers prescribe a soft collar to stabilize the neck, especially at night. Using the collar longer than 10 days can lead to decreased muscle strength and range of motion. For that reason, some health care providers do not recommend collars for cervical disk problems. Therapeutic manipulation (chiropractic interventions) alone or in combination with other interventions does not appear to cause harm, does not consistently reduce pain or disability, but does benefit some patients (Mior et al., 2013).

If conservative treatment is ineffective, surgery may be required, most often using a *conventional open surgical approach*. A neurosurgeon usually performs this surgery because of the complexity of the nerves and other structures in that area of the spine. Depending on the cause and the location of the herniation, either an anterior or posterior approach is used. An anterior cervical diskectomy and fusion (ACDF) is commonly performed. The patient is fitted with a large neck brace before surgery. Routine preoperative and postoperative care is the same as described in Chapters 14 and 16.

! NURSING SAFETY PRIORITY QSEN

Critical Rescue

The priority for care in the immediate postoperative period after an ACDF is maintaining an airway and ensuring that the patient has no problem with breathing. Swelling from the surgery can narrow the trachea, causing a partial obstruction. Surgery can also interfere with cranial innervation for swallowing, resulting in a compromised airway or aspiration.

CHART 43-6 **Best Practice for Patient Safety & Quality Care** QSEN

Care of the Patient After an Anterior Cervical Diskectomy and Fusion

Postoperative Interventions

- Assess **a**irway, **b**reathing, and **c**irculation (first priority!).
- Check for bleeding and drainage at the incision site.
- Monitor vital signs and neurologic status frequently.
- Check for swallowing ability.
- Monitor intake and output.
- Assess the patient's ability to void (may be a problem secondary to opiates or anesthesia).
- Manage pain adequately.
- Assist the patient with ambulation within a few hours of surgery, if he or she is able.

Discharge Teaching

- Be sure that someone stays with the patient for the first few days after surgery.
- Review drug therapy.
- Teach care of the incision.
- Review activity restrictions:
  - No lifting
  - No driving until physician permission
  - No strenuous activities
- Walk every day.
- Call the surgeon if symptoms of pain, numbness, and tingling worsen or if swallowing becomes difficult.
- Wear brace or collar per surgeon's prescription

CHART 43-7 **Key Features**

Postoperative Complications of Anterior Cervical Diskectomy and Fusion

- Hoarseness due to laryngeal injury; may be temporary or permanent
- Temporary dysphagia; may last few days to several months; usually not severe
- Esophageal, tracheal, or vertebral artery injury
- Wound infection
- Injury to the spinal cord or nerve roots
- Dura mater tears with associated cerebrospinal fluid leaks
- Pseudoarthrosis caused by nonunion of fusion
- Graft and screw loosening if a fusion was performed

Chart 43-6 summarizes best practices for postoperative care and discharge planning. Complications of ACDF can occur from the brace or the surgery itself. The initial brace is worn for 4 to 6 weeks, depending on the patient. When it is removed, a soft collar is worn for several more weeks, or longer if needed. Potential complications of the anterior surgical approach can be found in Chart 43-7.

Some patients may be candidates for minimally invasive surgery (MIS), such as percutaneous cervical diskectomy through an endoscope, with or without laser thermodiskectomy to shrink the herniated portion of the disk. The care for these patients is very similar to that for the patient with low back pain who has MIS (see discussion of surgical management of patients with low back pain on pp. 888-889). Patients may also benefit from the placement of an artificial disk, a surgical option that preserves movement of the vertebrae. Artificial disks are newly approved by the U.S. Food and Drug Administration (FDA); there is evidence of their safety but the long-term effects on patient health are not yet established.

SPINAL CORD INJURY

Caring for a patient with an SCI requires both a patient-centered and family-centered collaborative approach and involves every health care team member to help meet the patient's expected outcomes. Optimally, patients with a new SCI are quickly transported to a model SCI System Center. Because of the complexity of a spinal cord injury, discharge planning needs to begin the day of admission. The rehabilitation team must be consulted on the day of admission.

❖ *PATHOPHYSIOLOGY*

Loss of motor function (MOBILITY), SENSORY PERCEPTION, reflex activity, and bowel and bladder control often result from an SCI. In addition, the patient may experience significant behavior and emotional problems as a result of changes in functional ability, body image, role performance, and self-concept. Addressing family member concerns and changes in family dynamics is also important to effective care

The SCIs are classified as complete or incomplete. A **complete spinal cord injury** is one in which the spinal cord has been damaged in a way that eliminates all innervation below the level of the injury. Injuries that allow some function or movement below the level of the injury are described as an **incomplete spinal cord injury**. Incomplete injuries are more common than complete SCIs.

Mechanisms of Injury

When enough force is applied to the spinal cord, the resulting damage causes many neurologic deficits. Sources of force include direct injury to the vertebral column (fracture, dislocation, and subluxation [partial dislocation]) or penetrating injury from violence (gunshot or knife wounds). Although in some cases the cord itself may remain intact, at other times the cord undergoes a destructive process caused by a contusion (bruise), compression, laceration, or transaction (severing of the cord, either complete or incomplete) (Nayduch, 2010).

The causes of SCI can be divided into primary and secondary mechanisms of injury. Five *primary* mechanisms may result in an SCI:

- Hyperflexion
- Hyperextension
- Axial loading, or vertical compression
- Excessive rotation
- Penetrating trauma

A **hyperflexion** injury occurs when the head is suddenly and forcefully accelerated (moved) forward, causing extreme flexion of the neck (Fig. 43-2). This type of injury often occurs in head-on vehicle collisions and diving accidents. Flexion injury to the lower thoracic and lumbar spine may occur when the trunk is suddenly flexed on itself, such as occurs in a fall on the buttocks. The posterior ligaments can be stretched or torn, or the vertebrae may fracture or dislocate. Either process may damage the spinal cord, causing hemorrhage, edema, and necrosis.

Hyperextension injuries occur most often in vehicle collisions in which the vehicle is struck from behind or during falls when the patient's chin is struck (Fig. 43-3). The head is suddenly accelerated and then decelerated. This stretches or tears

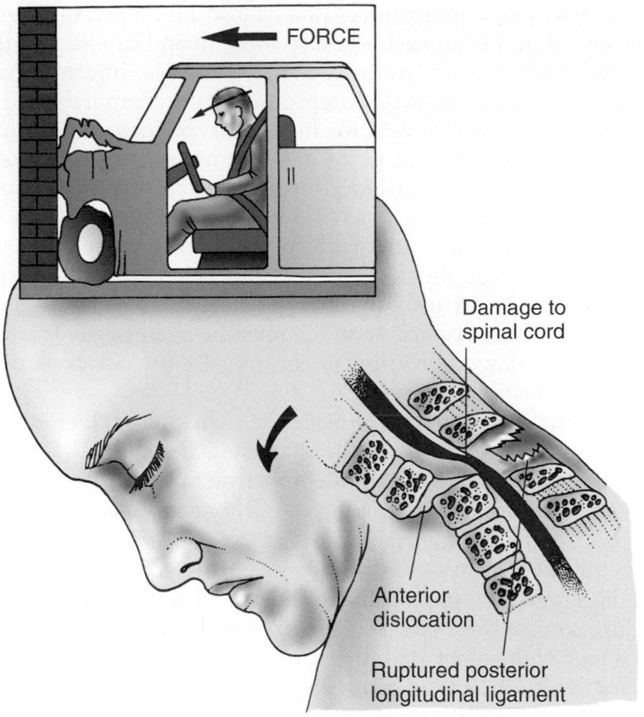

FIG. 43-2 Hyperflexion injury of the cervical spine.

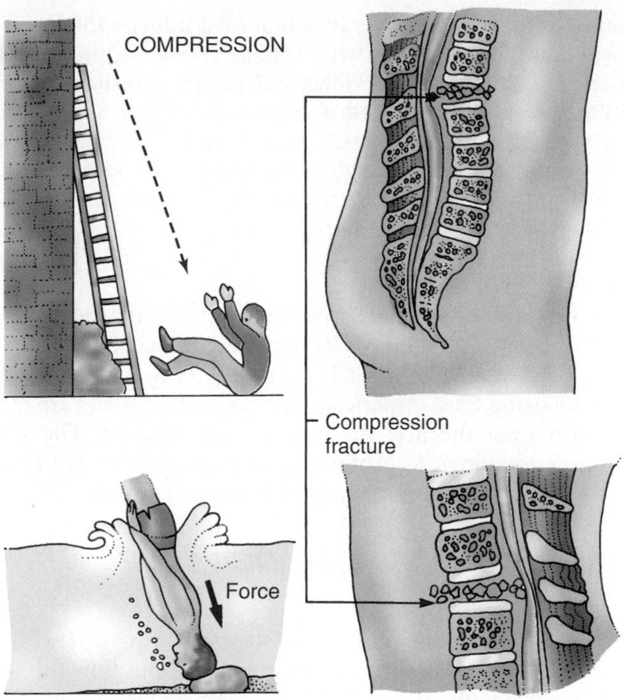

FIG. 43-4 Axial loading (vertical compression) injury of the cervical spine and the lumbar spine.

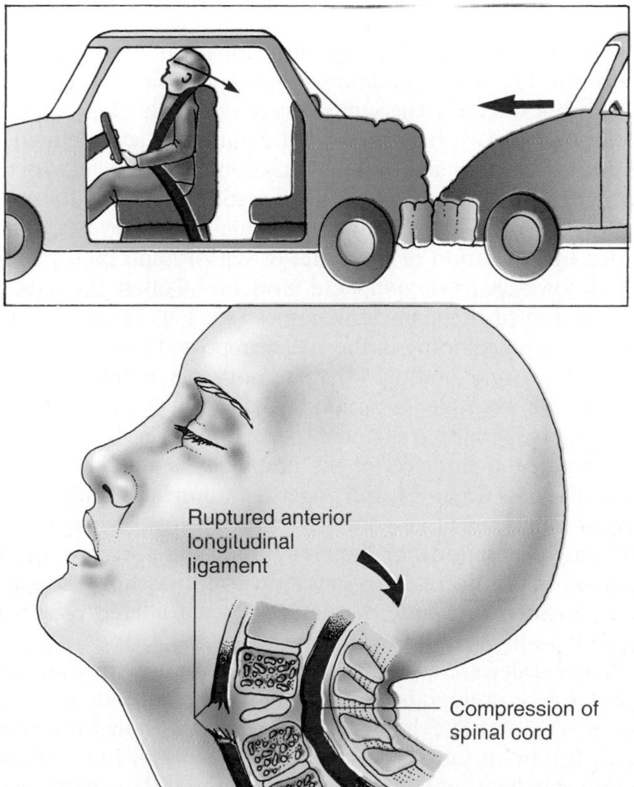

FIG. 43-3 Hyperextension injury of the cervical spine.

the anterior longitudinal ligament, fractures or subluxates the vertebrae, and perhaps ruptures an intervertebral disk. As with flexion injuries, the spinal cord may easily be damaged.

Diving accidents, falls on the buttocks, or a jump in which a person lands on the feet can cause many of the injuries attributable to **axial loading** (vertical compression) (Fig. 43-4). A blow to the top of the head can cause the vertebrae to shatter. Pieces of bone enter the spinal canal and damage the cord. **Rotation** injuries are caused by turning the head beyond the normal range.

Penetrating trauma to the spinal cord is classified by the speed of the object (e.g., knife, bullet) causing the injury. Low-speed or low-impact injuries cause damage directly at the site or local damage to the spinal cord or spinal nerves. In contrast, high-speed injuries that occur from gunshot wounds cause both direct and indirect damage.

Secondary injury worsens the primary injury. Secondary injuries include:

- Hemorrhage
- Ischemia (lack of oxygen, typically from reduced/absent blood flow)
- Hypovolemia (decreased circulating blood volume)
- Impaired tissue perfusion form neurogenic shock (a *medical emergency*)
- Local edema

Hemorrhage into the spinal cord may be manifested by contusion or petechial leaking into the central gray matter and later into the white matter. Systemic hemorrhage can result in shock and decrease perfusion to the spinal cord. Edema occurs with both primary and secondary injuries, contributing to capillary compression and cord ischemia. In neurogenic shock, loss of blood vessel tone (dilation) after *severe* cord injury may result in hypoperfusion (McCance et al., 2014).

Etiology

Trauma is the leading cause of spinal cord injuries (SCIs), with more than 35% resulting from vehicle crashes. Other leading causes are falls, acts of violence (usually gunshot wounds [GSWs]), and sport-related accidents (National Spinal Cord Injury Statistical Center, 2013). SCIs from falls are particularly likely among older adults. Spinal cord damage in adults can also result from nontraumatic vertebral fracture and diseases such as benign or malignant tumors.

Incidence and Prevalence

According to the National Spinal Cord Injury Statistical Center (2013), about 12,000 new SCIs occur every year in the United States. Almost 80% of all SCIs occur in young males, with the majority being Euro-American. Cervical cord injuries are more common than thoracic or lumbar cord injuries. The most common neurologic level of injury is C5. In paraplegia, T12 and L1 are the most common levels (Juknis et al., 2012).

❖ PATIENT-CENTERED COLLABORATIVE CARE

◆ Assessment

History. When obtaining a history from a patient with an acute SCI, gather as much data as possible about how the accident occurred and the probable mechanism of injury. Questions include the location and position of the patient immediately after the injury, the symptoms that occurred immediately with the injury, and the changes that have occurred subsequently. If possible, ask Emergency Medical Transport (EMT) rescue personnel about the type of immobilization devices used and whether any problems occurred during stabilization and transport to the hospital. Review the patient's medical record regarding the treatment given at the scene of injury or in the emergency department (ED) (e.g., drugs, IV fluids). Communicate with the ED nurse as he or she "hands off" the patient. Use the situation, background, assessment, recommendation (SBAR) communication technique to collect valuable information for continuing patient care per The Joint Commission's National Patient Safety Goals. (See Chapter 1 for how to use SBAR.)

Obtain the patient's medical history, including a history of osteoporosis or arthritis of the spine, congenital deformities, cancer, and previous injury or surgery of the neck or back. These health problems may cause or contribute to an SCI. A detailed history of any respiratory problems is particularly important if the patient has experienced a cervical SCI.

Physical Assessment/Clinical Manifestations

Initial Assessment. Assessing the ABCs (airway, breathing, and circulation) is the priority for any trauma patient. Therefore the first priority for the patient with an SCI is to assess the patient's airway, breathing pattern, and circulation status. The airway may be compromised because of foreign body obstruction from the tongue or teeth due to facial trauma, injury to the larynx, or mandibular (jaw) fracture. After an airway is established, assess the patient's breathing pattern. The patient with a cervical SCI is at high risk for respiratory compromise because the cervical spinal nerves (C3-5) innervate the phrenic nerve, controlling the diaphragm. A significant head injury, pneumothorax (air in the chest cavity), hemothorax (blood in the chest cavity), and/or fractured ribs may also cause respiratory distress or failure. Endotracheal intubation with mechanical ventilation may be necessary to prevent respiratory arrest.

To assess for circulation, evaluate pulse, blood pressure, and peripheral perfusion such as pulse strength and capillary refill. In the patient with traumatic SCI, multiple injuries may contribute to circulatory compromise from hemorrhage or hemorrhagic shock. Assess for indications of intra-abdominal *hemorrhage* or hemorrhage or bleeding around fracture sites. Indicators of significant blood loss compromising circulation include hypotension and tachycardia with a weak and thready pulse. In patients with known or potential cervical spinal cord injury, neurologic shock with profound vasodilation and bradycardia can occur resulting in hypotension. All symptoms of circulatory compromise or shock must be aggressively treated to preserve tissue perfusion to the spinal cord. Shock is discussed in detail in Chapter 37.

Use the Glasgow Coma Scale (see Chapter 41) or other agency-approved assessment tool to assess the patient's *level of consciousness (LOC).* Cognitive impairment as a result of an associated traumatic brain injury (TBI) or substance abuse can occur in patients with traumatic SCIs. Perform a detailed assessment of the patient's motor function and SENSORY PERCEPTION to determine the level of injury and establish baseline data for future comparison. The level of injury is the lowest neurologic segment with intact or normal motor and sensory function. **Tetraplegia** (also called *quadriplegia*) (paralysis) and **quadriparesis** (weakness) involve all four extremities, as seen with cervical cord and upper thoracic injury. **Paraplegia** (paralysis) and **paraparesis** (weakness) involve only the lower extremities, as seen in lower thoracic and lumbosacral injuries or lesions.

Spinal shock, also called **spinal shock syndrome**, occurs immediately as the cord's response to the injury. The patient has complete but temporary loss of motor, sensory, reflex, and autonomic function that often lasts less than 48 hours but may continue for several weeks (McCance et al., 2014). Muscle spasticity, reflex activity, and bladder function begin in patients with cervical or high thoracic injuries when spinal shock is resolved. Spinal shock is NOT the same as neurogenic shock.

Sensory and Motor Assessment. Neurologic level defined by the American Spinal Injury Association (ASIA) refers to the highest neurologic level of normal function and is not the same as the anatomic level of injury. The neurologic level is determined by evaluation of the zones of sensory and motor function, known as *dermatomes* and *myotomes.* Follow the sensory distribution of the skin dermatomes (see Fig. 41-5), with the examination beginning in the area of reported loss of SENSORY PERCEPTION and ending where sensory perception becomes normal. For example, sensation of the top of the foot and calf of the leg is spinal skin segment (dermatome) levels L3, L4, and L5. The area at the level of the umbilicus is T10, the clavicle (collarbone) is C3 or C4, and finger sensation is C7 and C8. The patient may report a complete sensory loss, **hypoesthesia** (decreased sensation), or **hyperesthesia** (increased sensation). In acute SCI, a decrease in sensation from baseline, especially in a proximal (upward) dermatome, is considered reason to urgently notify the neurosurgeon.

Many scales are available to measure motor function after SCI. ASIA recommends a six-point grading scale, with 0 being no movement and 5 being normal strength against full resistance. It is important to test all muscle groups for function. For example, patients with spinal injuries at the fifth or sixth cervical vertebra often can flex but not extend their arms. Extensive training is needed to fully assess a patient with SCI (Furlan et al., 2011b). New loss of motor function in a patient with recent SCI is an emergency and requires immediate communication with the neurosurgeon.

The advanced practice nurse or health care provider may also test deep tendon reflexes (DTRs), including the biceps (C5), triceps (C7), patella (L3), and ankle (S1). It is not unusual for these reflexes, as well as all movement or sensation, to be absent immediately after the injury because of spinal shock. After shock has resolved, the reflexes may return if the lesion is incomplete.

Cardiovascular and Respiratory Assessment. *Cardiovascular* dysfunction results from disruption of sympathetic fibers of the autonomic nervous system (ANS), especially if the injury is above the sixth thoracic vertebra. Bradycardia, hypotension, and hypothermia occur because of loss of sympathetic input. These changes may lead to cardiac dysrhythmias. *A systolic blood pressure below 90 mm Hg requires treatment because lack of perfusion to the spinal cord could worsen the patient's condition.* In addition, the lack of sympathetic or hypothalamic control causes the patient to lose thermoregulatory functions. As a result, the body tends to assume the temperature of the environment and attempts to compensate by increasing extracellular fluid.

A patient with a cervical SCI is at risk for *breathing* problems resulting from an interruption of spinal innervation to the respiratory muscles. In collaboration with the respiratory therapist (RT), if available, perform a complete respiratory assessment, including pulse oximetry for arterial oxygen saturation every 8 to 12 hours. An oxygen saturation 92% or less and adventitious breath sounds may indicate a complication like atelectasis or pneumonia. Hypercarbia measured by end-tidal carbon dioxide in an intubated patient may indicate circulatory or worsening respiratory failure. The RT should also evaluate vital capacity and minute volume and repeat the tests daily and during periods of worsening oxygenation during the acute phase. Early tracheostomy is recommend if the patient is likely to need prolonged (i.e., more than 7 days) mechanical ventilation.

Gastrointestinal and Genitourinary Assessment. Assess the patient's *abdomen* for manifestations of internal bleeding, distention, or paralytic ileus. Hemorrhage may result from the trauma, or it may occur later from a stress ulcer or the administration of steroids. Monitor for abdominal pain and changes in bowel sounds. Paralytic ileus may develop within 72 hours of hospital admission. During the period of spinal shock, peristalsis decreases, leading to a loss of bowel sounds and to gastric distention. This disruption of the autonomic nervous system may lead to a hypotonic bowel.

Consult with the registered dietitian for assessment to initiate early nutrition to meet caloric and protein needs. Assess serum glucose levels to avoid complications from hypoglycemia and sustained hyperglycemia. Assess the patient for swallowing difficulties such as weak gag reflex, drooling, or cough with oral intake. Collaborate with the speech-language specialist to evaluate swallowing for patients with cervical and high thoracic injury before starting oral intake and plan for appropriate diet and treatment when **dysphagia** is present. Monitor intake and output.

Autonomic dysfunction initially causes an areflexic (neurogenic) bladder (no reflex ability for bladder contraction), which later leads to urinary retention. Assess for bladder distention and urine stasis. The patient with an indwelling urinary catheter has increased risk for urinary tract infection. Start a bowel regimen congruent with best practices for paralyzed patients. Maintain bladder and bowel programs for patients with established SCI. One source for best practices is the Paralyzed Veterans of America (www.pva.org).

Assessment of Patients for Long-Term Complications. Assess for skin TISSUE INTEGRITY with each turn or repositioning. Monitor for signs of VTE with vital signs. Monitor intake and output to maintain a normal volume of intravascular fluid (**euvolemia**). Assess glycemic and nutritional status including intake of protein, vitamins (A, C, E), zinc, and iron. Nursing management for neurogenic bowel care is usually started in rehabilitation. In patients with established SCI, assess baseline ability and encourage their participation in self-care and management (Furlan et al., 2011a). Encourage family participation in care, and support their effort to keep the patient engaged in family life.

Bones become *osteopenic* and *osteoporotic* without weight-bearing exercise, placing the long-term SCI patient at risk for fractures. Another complication of prolonged immobility is **heterotopic ossification (HO)** (bony overgrowth, often into muscle). Assess for swelling, redness, warmth, and decreased range of motion (ROM) of the involved extremity. The hip is the most common place where HO occurs (Zychowicz, 2013). Changes in the bony structure are not visible until several weeks after initial symptoms appear.

Laboratory and Imaging Assessment. The health care provider requests laboratory studies for the patient with an SCI to establish baseline data or to prepare for surgery. Arterial blood gas analysis is done to monitor the respiratory status of a patient at risk for respiratory insufficiency. The findings should be within normal limits unless the patient has a history of heavy smoking or pre-injury pulmonary disease. Respiratory failure is indicated by decreased oxygen levels, increased carbon dioxide levels, and respiratory acidosis. A complete blood count can help determine hemorrhage; blood in the urine may be another significant indication of hemorrhage. Check laboratory values for a low hemoglobin count, leukocytosis (increased white blood cells [WBCs]), lymphocytopenia (decreased lymphocytes), and thrombocytopenia (decreased platelets), which can occur in patients with cervical spine injuries. These abnormalities may be related to lack of autonomic innervation to the hematopoietic (blood-cell producing) system. Observe patients for clinical signs and symptoms of these changes, such as an increased bleeding tendency.

Computed tomography (CT) is obtained as soon as possible, especially for the patient who has sustained multiple trauma. Magnetic resonance imaging (MRI) is performed to determine the degree and extent of damage to the spinal cord and to detect the presence of blood and bone within the spinal column. The health care provider may also request a series of x-rays of the spine to identify vertebral fractures, subluxation, or dislocation.

◆ Analysis

The priority NANDA-I nursing diagnoses and collaborative problems for patients with an acute spinal cord injury (SCI) include:

1. Risk for respiratory distress/failure related to aspiration or diaphragmatic denervation (e.g., impaired phrenic nerve impulses in patients with cervical injury)
2. Potential for cardiovascular instability related to loss or interruption of sympathetic innervation or hemorrhage

3. Potential for secondary spinal cord injury related to hypoperfusion, edema, or delayed spinal column stabilization
4. Impaired Physical Mobility related to spinal compression and edema (NANDA-I)
5. Spastic or flaccid bladder and bowel related to direct neurologic damage or disruption in nerve impulses
6. Risk for Compromised Resilience from injury requiring need for life change (NANDA-I)

◆ Planning and Implementation

The desired outcomes of patient-centered collaborative care following acute SCI are to stabilize the vertebral column, manage damage to the spinal cord, and prevent secondary injuries. Systemic hypothermia is an experimental approach to provide neuroprotection in the first 24 to 48 hours after SCI wherein the patient is cooled to 32° to 34° C (89° to 93.2° F) (Ahmad et al., 2013). Therapeutic hypothermia is described in Chapter 34 in conjunction with treatment for cardiac arrest. Although stem cell therapies have significant potential to treat SCI, they are not yet established as an intervention to restore damaged neurons or neuron function.

Many patients with previous spinal cord injuries (SCIs) are admitted to the acute care or long-term care setting for complications of immobility, such as pressure ulcers or fractures resulting from osteoporosis. Pressure ulcers contribute to local infection, including osteomyelitis and septicemia. Priorities in care may need to be re-evaluated as complications occur and resolve.

Nursing management strategies that promote high level of patient participation in care are associated with patient outcomes of higher life satisfaction, MOBILITY, and return to occupation (Bailey et al., 2012). Preventing complications of immobility and infection following SCI is an effort that requires patient, family, and health care team communication, collaboration, and individualized intervention.

Managing the Airway and Improving Breathing

Planning: Expected Outcomes. The patient with an SCI is expected to have a patent airway and adequate ventilation.

Interventions. *Airway management is the priority for a patient with cervical spinal cord injury!* Patients with injuries at or above T6 are especially at risk for respiratory complications and pulmonary embolus during the first 5 days after injury. These complications are due to impaired functioning of the intercostal muscles and decreased MOBILITY. Depending on the level of injury, intubation or tracheotomy with mechanical ventilation may be needed.

! NURSING SAFETY PRIORITY (QSEN)

Action Alert

Assess breath sounds every 2 to 4 hours during the first few days after SCI, and document and report any adventitious or diminished sounds. Monitor vital signs with pulse oximetry. Watch for changes in respiratory pattern or airway obstruction, and intervene when there are decreases in pulse oximetry values.

Respiratory secretions are managed with manually assisted coughing, pulmonary hygiene, and suctioning. Implement strategies to prevent ventilator-associated pneumonia (VAP) when the patient needs continuous mechanical ventilation as discussed in Chapter 32.

Teach the patient who is tetraplegic to coordinate his or her cough effort with an assistant. The nurse, or other assistant, places his or her hands on the upper abdomen over the diaphragm and below the ribs. Hands are placed one over the other, with fingers interlocked and away from the skin. If the patient is obese, an alternate hand placement is one hand on either side of the rib cage. Have the patient take a breath and cough during exhalation. The assistant locks his or her elbows and pushes inward and upwards as the patient coughs. This technique is sometimes called "assisted coughing," "quad cough," or "**cough assist**." Repeat the coordinated effort, with rest periods as needed, until the airway is clear.

Encourage the patient to use an incentive spirometer. The nurse and respiratory therapist perform a respiratory assessment at least every 8 hours to determine the effectiveness of these strategies. In some cases it may be necessary to perform oral or nasal suctioning if the patient cannot clear the airway of secretions effectively.

Monitoring for Neurogenic Shock and Hemorrhagic/Hypovolemic Shock

Planning: Expected Outcomes. The patient is expected to not develop neurogenic shock. If signs and symptoms of this potentially life-threatening complication occur, the patient is expected to receive prompt intervention.

Interventions. Maintain adequate hydration through IV therapy and oral fluids as appropriate, depending on the patient's overall condition. Carefully observe for manifestations of **neurogenic shock**, which may occur within 24 hours after injury most commonly in patients with injuries above T6. This potentially life-threatening problem results from disruption in the communication pathways between upper motor neurons and lower motor neurons.

! NURSING SAFETY PRIORITY (QSEN)

Critical Rescue

Monitor the patient with acute spinal cord injury at least hourly for:

- Pulse oximetry (SpO_2) <90% or symptoms of aspiration (e.g., stridor, garbled speech, or inability to clear airway)
- Symptomatic bradycardia, including reduced level of consciousness and deceased urine output
- Hypotension with systolic blood pressure (SBP) <90 or mean arterial pressure (MAP) <65 mm Hg

Notify the physician immediately if these symptoms occur, because this problem is an emergency! Respiratory compromise from aspiration may be treated with intubation or bronchial endoscopy. Neurogenic shock is treated symptomatically by providing fluids to the circulating blood volume, adding vasopressor intravenous therapy, and providing supportive care to stabilize the patient.

Preventing Secondary Spinal Cord Injury

Planning: Expected Outcomes. The patient with an *acute* SCI is expected to demonstrate adequate spinal cord stabilization as evidenced by no further deterioration in neurologic status.

Interventions. If the patient has a fractured vertebra, the primary concern of the health care team is to reduce and immobilize the fracture to prevent further damage to the spinal cord from bone fragments. Nonsurgical techniques include external fixation or orthotic devices, but surgery is usually needed to stabilize the spine and prevent further spinal cord damage.

CHART 43-8 **Best Practice for Patient Safety & Quality Care** QSEN

Assessing Motor Function in the Patient with a Spinal Cord Injury

- To assess C4-5, apply downward pressure while the patient shrugs his or her shoulders upward.
- To assess C5-6, apply resistance while the patient pulls up his or her arms.
- To assess C7, apply resistance while the patient straightens his or her flexed arms.
- To assess C8, make sure the patient is able to grasp an object and form a fist.
- To assess L2-4, apply resistance while the patient lifts his or her legs from the bed.
- To assess L5, apply resistance while the patient dorsiflexes his or her feet.
- To assess S1, apply resistance while the patient plantarflexes his or her feet.

Assess the patient's neurologic status, particularly focusing on sensory and motor function, vital signs, pulse oximetry, and PAIN, at least every 1 to 4 hours depending on the patient's overall condition. See Chart 43-8 for elements of a focused motor assessment related to spinal cord injury. *Document your assessments carefully and in detail, particularly changes in motor or sensory function. Failure to do so may prevent other staff members from quickly recognizing deterioration in neurologic status.*

Regardless of the level of SCI, keep the patient in proper body alignment to prevent further cord injury or irritability. Devices such as traction, orthoses, or collars may be used to keep the spine immobilized during healing and rehabilitation.

Spinal Immobilization and Stabilization. During the immediate care of the patient with a suspected or confirmed cervical spine injury, a hard cervical collar, such as the Miami J or Philadelphia, is placed immediately and maintained until a specific order indicates it can be removed. A daily inspection of skin beneath the collar is recommended while a health care provider assists with maintaining neck alignment when the collar is removed. Padding at pressure points beneath and at the edges of the collar, particularly at the occiput, may be necessary to sustain TISSUE INTEGRITY. Until the spinal column is stabilized, a jaw-thrust maneuver is preferable to a head-tilt maneuver to open the airway should the patient need an airway intervention. Maintain spinal alignment at all times with log rolling to change position from supine to side-lying. Log rolling may also be prescribed in the initial period following surgical stabilization. Provide ongoing spinal alignment by using a slider board to transfer the patient between surfaces such as placement on a computerized tomography (CT) scanner table.

The patient may be placed in fixed skeletal traction to realign the vertebrae, facilitate bone healing, and prevent further injury, often after surgical stabilization. The most commonly used device for immobilization of the *cervical spine* is the halo fixation device, which is worn for 8 to 12 weeks. The device is affixed by the physician into the outer aspect of the skull. For patients not having surgery, the addition of traction helps reduce the fracture.

The **halo fixator** is a static traction device (Fig. 43-5). Four pins (or screws) are inserted into the skull. The metal halo ring may be attached to a plastic vest or cast when the spine is stable, allowing increased patient MOBILITY.

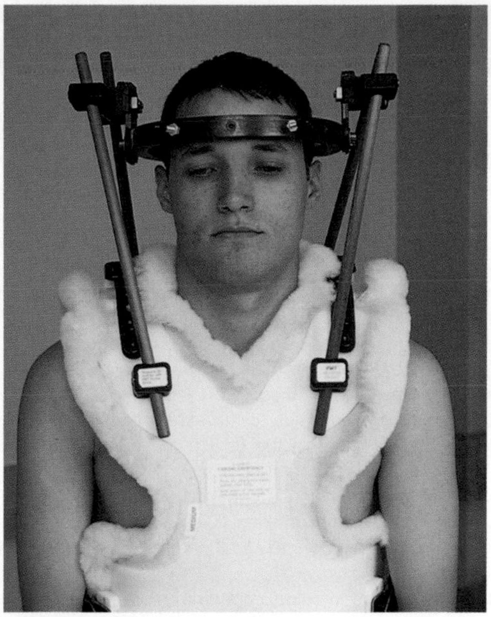

FIG. 43-5 Halo fixation device with jacket.

! NURSING SAFETY PRIORITY QSEN

Action Alert

Never move or turn the patient by holding or pulling on the halo device. Do not adjust the screws holding it in place. Check the patient's skin frequently to ensure that the jacket is not causing pressure. Pressure is avoided if one finger can be inserted easily between the jacket and the patient's skin. Monitor the patient's neurologic status for changes in movement or decreased strength. A special wrench is needed to loosen the vest in emergencies such as cardiopulmonary arrest. Tape the wrench to the vest for easy and consistent accessibility. Do not use sharp objects (e.g., coat hangers, knitting needles) to relieve itching under the vest; skin damage and infection will slow recovery.

Common complications of the halo device are pin loosening, local infection, and scarring. More serious complications include osteomyelitis (cranial bone infection), subdural abscess, and instability. Hospital policy is followed for pin site care, which may specify the use of solutions such as saline. Vaseline dressings may also be used. *Monitor vital signs for indications of possible infection (e.g., fever, purulent drainage from the pin sites), and report any changes to the physician immediately. Discharge teaching related to halo fixator management is described in* Chart 43-9.

Nonsurgical treatment of *thoracic and lumbosacral injuries* is often challenging. Most health care providers choose to refer the patient for surgery and then immobilize the spine with lightweight, custom-fit thoracic lumbar sacral orthoses (TLSOs) to prevent prolonged periods of immobility.

? NCLEX EXAMINATION CHALLENGE

Safe and Effective Care Environment

A client was admitted this morning with an incomplete cervical spinal cord injury and is placed in a halo fixator. Halo fixation is used to reduce motion of the cervical spine. Which assessment finding will the nurse report immediately to the health care provider?

A. A new-onset heart rate of 48 beats/min
B. Mean arterial pressure of 90 mm Hg
C. Pain level of 2 on a 0-to-10 pain scale
D. Oxygen saturation of 95% on room air

CHART 43-9 Patient and Family Education: Preparing for Self-Management

*Use of a Halo Device**

- Be aware that the weight of the halo device alters balance. Be careful when leaning forward or backward.
- Wear loose clothing, preferably with hook and loop (Velcro) fasteners or large openings for head and arms.
- Bathe in the bathtub, or take a sponge bath. (Some physicians allow showers.)
- Wash under the lambs wool liner of the vest to prevent rashes or sores; use powders or lotions sparingly under the vest.
- Have someone change the liner if it becomes odorous.
- Support the head with a small pillow when sleeping to prevent unnecessary pressure and discomfort.
- Try to resume usual activities to the extent possible; keep as active as possible. (The weight of the device may cause fatigue or weakness.) However, avoid contact sports and swimming.
- Do not drive because vision is impaired with the device.
- Keep straws available for drinking fluids.
- Cut meats and other food into small pieces to facilitate chewing and swallowing.
- Before going outside in cold temperatures, wrap the pins with cloth to prevent the metal from getting cold.
- Have someone clean the pin sites as recommended by physician or hospital protocol.
- Observe the pin sites daily for redness, drainage, or loosening; report changes to the physician.
- Increase fluids and fiber in the diet to prevent constipation.
- Use a position of comfort during sexual activity.

*Home care instructions may vary depending on hospital or physician preference.

Drug Therapy. *Dextran*, a plasma expander, may be used to increase capillary blood flow within the spinal cord and to prevent or treat hypotension. *Atropine sulfate* is used to treat bradycardia if the pulse rate falls below 50 to 60 beats per minute. Hypotension, if severe, is treated with continuous intravenous sympathomimetic agents such as *dopamine* or other vasoactive agent.

Centrally-acting skeletal muscular relaxants, such as *tizanidine* (Zanaflex, Sirdalud), may help control severe muscle spasticity. However, these drugs cause severe drowsiness and sedation in most patients and may not be effective in reducing spasticity. As an alternative to these drugs, *intrathecal baclofen (ITB) (Lioresal)* therapy may be prescribed. This drug is administered through a programmable, implantable infusion pump and intrathecal catheter directly into the cerebrospinal fluid. The pump is surgically placed in a subcutaneous pouch in the lower abdomen. Monitor for common adverse effects, which include sedation, fatigue, dizziness, and changes in mental status. *Seizures and hallucinations may occur if ITB is suddenly withdrawn.*

Other drugs to prevent or treat complications of immobility may be needed *later* during the rehabilitative phase. For example, celecoxib (Celebrex) may be prescribed to prevent or treat **heterotopic ossification** (bony overgrowth). Calcium and bisphosphonates may prevent the osteoporosis that results from lack of weight-bearing or resistance activity. Osteoporosis can cause fractures in later years. Early and continued exercise may help decrease the incidence of these complications.

Surgical Management. Surgery within 24 hours of injury to stabilize the vertebral spinal column, particularly if there is evidence of spinal cord compression, results in decreased secondary complications (Stahel et al., 2012). Emergent surgery also removes bone fragments, hematomas, or penetrating objects such as a bullet. Typical procedures include wiring and spinal fusion for cervical injuries and the insertion of steel or metal rods (e.g., Harrington rods) to stabilize thoracic and lumbar spinal injuries. During a cervical fusion, the surgeon reduces the fracture by placing the bone ends in proper alignment. Metal wiring is then used to secure bone chips (bone graft) taken from the patient's hip. The patient wears a halo vest to immobilize the spine during the healing process. For thoracic and lumbar fusions, metal or steel rods (e.g., Harrington rods) are used to keep the bone ends in alignment after fracture reduction. After surgery, the patient usually wears a molded plastic support (cervical or thoracic-lumbar or both) to keep the injured and operative areas immobilized during recovery. Postoperative care occurs as described in Chapter 16.

! NURSING SAFETY PRIORITY QSEN

Action Alert

After surgical spinal fusion, assess the patient's neurologic status and vital signs at least every hour for the first 4 to 6 hours and then, if the patient is stable, every 4 hours. Assess for complications of surgery, including worsening of motor or sensory function at or above the site of surgery.

Managing Impaired Mobility

Planning: Expected Outcomes. The patient with an SCI is expected to be free from complications of immobility and perform ADLs as independently as possible with or without assistive/adaptive devices.

Interventions. The patient with an SCI is especially at risk for pressure ulcers (impaired skin TISSUE INTEGRITY), venous thromboembolism (VTE), contractures, orthostatic hypotension, and fractures related to osteoporosis. Patients with high SCIs are also at risk for orthostatic hypotension. Frequent and therapeutic positioning not only helps prevent complications but also provides alignment to prevent further spinal cord injury or irritability. Assess the condition of the patient's skin, especially over pressure points, with each turn or repositioning. Reduce pressure on any reddened area, and monitor it with the next turn. Reposition patients frequently (every 1-2 hours). When sitting in a chair, the patient is repositioned or taught to reposition himself or herself more often than every hour. Paraplegic patients usually perform frequent "wheelchair push-ups" to relieve skin pressure. Use a pressure-reducing mattress and wheel chair or chair pad to help prevent skin breakdown. Prevent pressure ulcers using best practices as described in Chapter 25. Prevent VTE including using interventions of intermittent pneumatic compression stockings and low–molecular-weight heparin (LMWH). Document pressure ulcer and VTE prophylaxis in accordance with Core Measures developed by the Centers for Medicare and Medicaid Services and The Joint Commission (www.jointcommision.org).

Contractures may be prevented or minimized with splints. Consult with the PT and occupational therapist (OT) for optimal scheduling for placing/removing splints (typically individually molded to the patient's extremity), trigger points to relieve spasticity, and positioning to maintain joint function. Administer antispasmodic drugs, and monitor the patient's response.

Patients with cervical cord injuries are especially at high risk for orthostatic (postural) hypotension, but anyone who is immobilized may have this problem. If the patient changes from a lying position to a sitting or standing position too quickly, he or she may experience hypotension, which could result in dizziness and falls. Because of interrupted sympathetic innervation caused by the spinal cord injury, the blood vessels do not constrict quickly enough to push blood up into the brain. The resulting vasodilation causes dizziness or light-headedness and possible falls with syncope ("blackout"). Consult with the registered dietitian to optimize diet for general health and to reduce osteoporosis from reduced daily weight-bearing activities. Provide out-of-bed activity in collaboration with the PT and OT. Resistance exercise, if it can be performed, promotes bone health.

Promote self-management with regular communication with the patient, family, and interdisciplinary health care team members. Help identify and set realistic expected outcomes on the basis of the patient's MOBILITY and functional level. Even patients with a cervical SCI often learn how to perform most ADLs independently in specialized rehabilitation programs, and the majority of patients with SCI return home.

Managing Risk for Autonomic Dysreflexia

Planning: Expected Outcomes. The patient with an SCI is expected to be free from episodes of autonomic dysreflexia (AD). If this complication of a high SCI occurs, the patient is expected to receive prompt interventions

Interventions. **Autonomic dysreflexia (AD),** sometimes referred to as *autonomic hyperreflexia,* is a potentially life-threatening condition in which noxious visceral or cutaneous stimuli cause a sudden, massive, uninhibited reflex sympathetic discharge in people with high-level SCI. AD primarily affects men more than women. The signs and symptoms of AD are listed in Chart 43-10 (Gunduz & Binak, 2012). The sudden rise in blood pressure can result in end-organ damage, including stroke.

People with a cervical or high-thoracic SCI face lifelong abnormalities in systemic arterial pressure control (Krassioukov, 2012). Be aware that the sudden rise in blood pressure in AD is usually associated with bradycardia. Normal systolic blood pressure (SBP) for SCI above T6 is 90 to 110 mm Hg; a SBP 20 to 40 mm Hg above the reference range for patients with established SCI may be a sign of AD. Patients with AD may display no symptoms other than an elevated blood pressure.

CHART 43-10 Key Features

Autonomic Dysreflexia

- Sudden, significant rise in systolic and diastolic blood pressure, accompanied by bradycardia
- Profuse sweating above the level of lesion—especially in the face, neck, and shoulders; rarely occurs below the level of the lesion because of sympathetic cholinergic activity
- Goose bumps above or possibly below the level of the lesion
- Flushing of the skin above the level of the lesion—especially in the face, neck, and shoulders
- Blurred vision
- Spots in the patient's visual field
- Nasal congestion
- Onset of severe, throbbing headache
- Flushing about the level of the lesion with pale skin below the level of the lesion
- Feeling of apprehension

The causes of AD are typically gastrointestinal (GI), gynecologic-urologic (GU), and vascular stimulation as well as skin and bone injury. Conditions associated with AD onset are bladder distention, urinary tract infection, epididymitis or scrotal compression, bowel distention or impaction from constipation, or irritation of hemorrhoids. PAIN, circumferential constriction of the thorax, abdomen, or an extremity (e.g., tight clothing), contact with hard or sharp objects, and temperature fluctuations can also cause AD.

Certain procedures and pathologic conditions are also associated with AD. Anticipate the need for frequent assessment to detect AD early and intervene before blood pressure becomes dangerously elevated. For example, INFLAMMATION or injury in the GI system from gallstones, ulcers, gastritis, appendicitis, or other pathology is associated with the onset of AD. Stimulation of the GU system from menses, vaginitis, sexual penetration, ejaculation, and pregnancy (especially labor) can lead to AD. Venous thromboembolism can also cause AD. Acute and deep skin or mucosal injury from insect bites, blistering, pressure ulcers, and invasive instrumentation (e.g., cystoscopy, urodynamic testing, central line placement, and surgical procedures) can initiate AD. Heterotopic bone (i.e., bone tissue formed outside of the skeleton due to derangements in bone metabolism in patients confined to bed) and fractures can lead to AD. There have been case reports of ingrown toenails leading to AD.

Awareness of the causes of AD assists the nurse in prioritizing assessment and using best practices to avoid conditions that contribute to the onset and severity of AD. For example, proper bladder and bowel care to prevent fecal impaction and bladder distention are essential. *AD is a neurologic emergency and must be promptly treated to prevent a hypertensive stroke!* Chart 43-11 lists emergency care for autonomic dysreflexia.

Managing Urinary and Bowel Elimination

Planning: Expected Outcomes. The patient with an SCI is expected to achieve control of elimination of urine and stool without complications, if possible.

CHART 43-11 Best Practice for Patient Safety & Quality Care QSEN

Emergency Care of the Patient Experiencing Autonomic Dysreflexia: Immediate Interventions

- Place patient in sitting position (first priority!), or return to previous safe position.
- Page/notify care provider.
- Assess for and treat the cause:
- Check for urinary retention or catheter blockage:
- Check the urinary catheter tubing (if present) for kinks or obstruction.
- If a urinary catheter is not present, check for bladder distention and catheterize immediately if indicated:
- Consider using anesthetic ointment on tip of catheter before catheter insertion to reduce urethral irritation.
- Determine if a urinary tract infection or bladder calculi (stones) are contributing to genitourinary irritation.
- Check the patient for fecal impaction or other colorectal irritation, using anesthetic ointment at rectum. Disimpact if needed.
- Examine skin for new or worsening pressure ulcer symptoms.
- Monitor blood pressures every 10 to 15 minutes.
- Give nifedipine or nitrate as prescribed:
- Patients with recurrent autonomic dysreflexia may receive an alpha blocker prophylactically.

Interventions. Patients with SCIs have reflex or neurogenic loss of bowel and bladder control. Many can become continent if they rigorously adhere to an established program. The type of program depends on the usual elimination pattern and whether the injury involved cervical or lower motor neurons (LMNs). A urologic evaluation may be needed to identify bladder type.

Patients with injuries to the lumbosacral area usually have a flaccid bladder and bowel. Patients with a **flaccid bladder** may achieve emptying of the bladder by performing a Valsalva maneuver or tightening the abdominal muscles. These techniques are not successful for all LMN injuries. To determine the effectiveness of these maneuvers, use a bedside **bladder ultrasound** or bladder scan device to measure bladder residual. This use of this device is discussed in Chapter 65.

Some patients rely on intermittent catheterization 2 or 3 times daily to empty the bladder. Obese patients and those with thoracic and cervical SCIs may need an indwelling urinary catheter for a period of time. External urinary catheters connected to a leg bag may be used for men.

The patient with *any* SCI is at risk for long-term kidney complications, such as hydronephrosis, acute and chronic kidney disease, and kidney stones. Urinary tract infections (UTIs) are common because organisms are introduced into the urinary tract by urinary catheters. Patients with an SCI may not be aware of the infection because they cannot feel dysuria, urgency, or back pain. They must rely on other signs and symptoms, such as foul-smelling urine or fever.

Teach the patient that the essential elements of a bowel program include stool softeners, fluid intake sufficient to result in clear, light yellow urine (unless medically contraindicated), high-fiber diet, and a consistent time for elimination. *Rectal digital stimulation is done only if requested by the health care provider because it could cause a vagal response, manifested by severe bradycardia and syncope.*

Adjusting to Major Life Change, Promoting Resilience

Planning: Expected Outcomes. The patient with an SCI is expected to adapt to a significant life change.

Interventions. Information obtained from the psychosocial assessment is used by the interdisciplinary team to identify strategies to help the patient adjust to the disability. Help the patient set realistic goals and verbalize feelings about the injury and his or her future. Invite the patient to ask questions, and answer them openly and honestly. Questions about prognosis and potential for complete recovery are referred to the health care provider because the timing and extent of recovery are different for each patient.

Collaborate with the case manager or discharge planner for a review of the patient's insurance and financial status. Many insurance policies cover rehabilitation services but for a limited time each year. The discharge coordinator or financial counselor may be able to assist the patient or family to locate other sources for adapting the home or funding an adapted car, such as private foundations and community organizations.

Community-Based Care

Case managers are ideal care coordinators to act as SCI patient advocates. In some settings, case managers begin working with patients in the emergency department to establish a positive image of SCI rehabilitation. Rehabilitation begins in the acute or critical care unit when patients are hemodynamically stable. They are usually transferred from the acute care setting to a rehabilitation setting, where they learn more about self-care, MOBILITY skills, and bladder and bowel retraining. One promising therapy in rehabilitation is functional electrical stimulation (FES). FES uses small electrical pulses to paralyzed muscles to restore or improve their function. FES is commonly used for exercise but also to assist with breathing, grasping, transferring, standing, and walking.

Psychosocial adaptation is one of the critical factors in determining the success of rehabilitation. The case manager or acute care nurse can help the patient and family members prepare for discharge or transfer to a rehabilitation hospital. Assist in verbalizing feelings and fears about body image, self-concept, role performance, self-esteem, and SEXUALITY. The patient should be told about the expected reactions of those outside the security of the hospital environment. Role-playing or anticipating responses to potential problems is helpful. For example, the patient can practice answering questions from children about why he or she is in a wheelchair or cannot move certain parts of the body.

Particularly among young men, who are the most common patients with SCI, SEXUALITY is a major issue. Many patients are concerned about their ability to have sexual intercourse and have children. Most hospitals do not have psychological social workers or counselors to discuss sexuality issues. Rehabilitation programs often include a sexuality/intimacy counselor as part of the interdisciplinary team approach to patient care.

Home Care Management. If the patient is discharged home or returns home for a weekend visit from the rehabilitation setting, the environment must be assessed to ensure that it is free from hazards and can accommodate the patient's special needs (e.g., a wheelchair). The occupational or physical therapist, in collaboration with rehabilitation and the home care nurse, usually assesses the patient's temporary or permanent home environment. Ease of accessibility is particularly important at the entrance of the home as well as the bathroom, kitchen, and bedroom. The height of the patient's bed may need to be adjusted to allow a smooth transfer into and out of the bed.

All adaptive devices that the patient will use at home should be requested and delivered to the rehabilitation facility. This enables the nurse and other therapists to ensure that the items fit correctly and that the patient and family know how to use them correctly.

Self-Management Education. The teaching plan for the patient with an SCI includes:

- Mobility skills
- Pressure ulcer prevention
- ADL skills
- Bowel and bladder program
- Education about sexuality and referral for counseling to promote sexual health
- Prevention of autonomic dysreflexia with appropriate bladder, bowel, and skin care practices and recognition of early signs or symptoms of autonomic dysreflexia

This information should be reinforced with written handouts, CDs, DVDs, or other patient education material that the patient and family members can use after discharge to the home. Chart 43-12 provides information about aging for middle-aged and older adults with a spinal cord injury.

A full-time caregiver or personal assistant is sometimes required if the patient with tetraplegia returns home. The caregiver may be a family member or a nursing assistant employed to help provide care and companionship. A patient who is

CHART 43-12 **Nursing Focus on the Older Adult**

What Patients Need to Know About Aging with Spinal Cord Injury

NURSING INTERVENTION	RATIONALES
Follow guidelines for adult vaccination, particularly influenza and pneumococcus vaccination recommendations.	Respiratory complications are the most common cause of death after spinal cord injury (SCI). The vaccine to prevent herpes zoster (shingles) can help prevent skin breakdown.
For women, have Papanicolaou (Pap) smears and mammograms as recommended by the American Cancer Society or your health care provider.	Limitations in movement may make breast self-examination difficult.
Take measures to prevent osteoporosis, such as increasing calcium intake, avoiding caffeine, and not smoking. Exercise against resistance can maintain muscle strength and slow bone loss.	Women older than 50 years often lose bone density, which can result in fractures. Men can also have osteoporotic fractures as a result of immobility.
Practice meticulous skin care, including frequent repositioning, using pressure-reduction surfaces in bed and chairs/wheelchairs, and applying skin protective products like Mepilex.	As a person ages, skin becomes dry and less elastic, predisposing the patient to pressure ulcers.
Take measures to prevent constipation, such as drinking adequate fluids, eating a high-fiber diet, adding a stool softener or bowel stimulant daily, and establishing a regular time for bowel elimination.	Constipation is a problem for most patients with SCI, and bowel motility can slow, contributing to constipation later in life.
Modify activities if joint pain occurs; use a powered rather than a manual wheelchair. Ask the health care provider about treatment options.	Arthritis occurs in more than half of people older than 65 years. Patients with SCI are more likely to develop arthritis as a result of added stress on the upper extremities when using a wheelchair.

paraplegic is often able to function without assistance after an appropriate rehabilitation program.

ADL training for the patient with an SCI includes a structured exercise program to promote strength and endurance. The occupational therapist instructs the patient in the correct use of all adaptive equipment. In collaboration with the therapists, instruct family members or the caregiver in transfer skills, feeding, bathing, dressing, positioning, and skin care as discussed briefly in this chapter and in more detail in Chapter 6.

! NURSING SAFETY PRIORITY QSEN

Drug Alert

Teach the SCI patient and his or her family or other caregiver about the name, purpose, dosage, timing of administration, and side effects of all *drugs*. Make sure they understand the possible interaction of prescribed drugs with over-the-counter drugs or alcohol and illegal drugs.

SEXUALITY is associated with sexual and reproductive function. Sexual function after spinal cord injury depends on the level and extent of injury. Incomplete lesions allow some control over SENSORY PERCEPTION and motor ability. Complete lesions disconnect the messages from the brain to the rest of the body, and vice versa. However, men with injuries above T6 are often able to have erections by stimulating reflex activity. For example, stroking the penis will cause an erection. Ejaculation is less predictable and may be mixed with urine. However, urine is sterile, so the patient's partner will not get an infection. To prevent AD, prophylactic administration of a vasodilator may be needed prior to intercourse (Courtois et al., 2012).

Women with an SCI have a different challenge because they have indwelling urinary catheters more commonly than men with an SCI. However, some women do become pregnant and have full-term children. For others, ovulation stops in response to the injury. In this case, alternate methods for pregnancy, such as *in vitro* fertilization, may be an option. Some women also report vaginal dryness. Recommend a water-soluble lubricant for both partners to promote comfort.

For patients who choose not to have intercourse, intimate pleasure can be achieved in other ways, including kissing, hugging, fondling, masturbation, and oral sex. Variations in positioning may be needed to accommodate weak or paralyzed parts of the body. An understanding partner can help the patient adjust to his or her physical changes.

CLINICAL JUDGMENT CHALLENGE

Safety; Evidence-Based Practice; Teamwork and Collaboration QSEN

A 52-year-old man who has had a T-10 spinal cord injury for 10 years is admitted for septicemia. He has a 3 × 2–centimeter discoloration on his left buttock that is classed as an unstageable pressure ulcer. He has an indwelling urinary catheter. The patient has been living alone and states that he has no family or friends. He has had a variety of health problems and wishes he would die. An antidepressant was prescribed for the patient 3 years ago, but he does not take it because it makes him tired.

1. What priority problems does this patient have at this time? Which problems need immediate action and why? What other data do you need to help formulate your answer?
2. With what members of the interdisciplinary and nursing team should you collaborate to provide quality care for this patient?
3. What may be causing the patient's septicemia? What are the evidence-based interventions for the care of patients with septicemia? Use a reliable electronic database to help you answer this question.
4. Use the SBAR method to communicate your concerns about this patient to another nurse who will be continuing his care.

Health Care Resources. Refer the patient and family to local, state or province, and national organizations for more information and support for patients with SCI. These organizations include the National Spinal Cord Injury Association (www.spinalcord.org) in the United States and Spinal Cord Injury Canada (www.sci-can.ca). Many excellent consumer-oriented books, journals, and DVDs are also available. Support groups may help the patient and family adjust to a changed lifestyle and provide solutions to commonly encountered problems.

The primary purpose of rehabilitation is to enable patients to function independently in their communities. However,

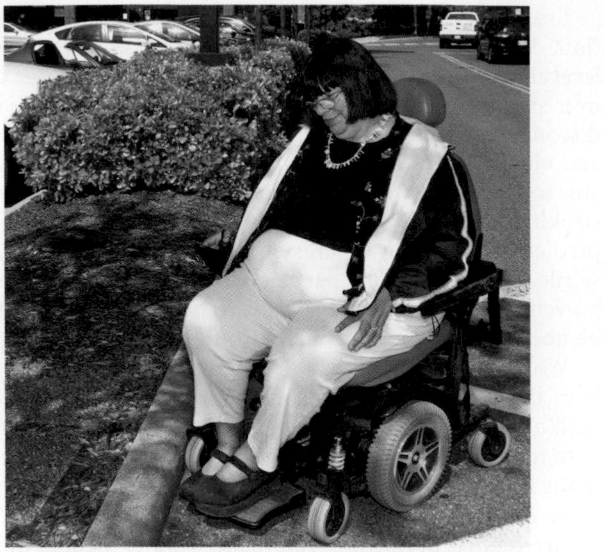

FIG. 43-6 Community physical barrier example: A curb prevents the patient in a wheelchair from getting onto the sidewalk.

many physical barriers still exist in some communities that prevent the patient in a wheelchair from finding a parking place, using sidewalks, and attending activities or utilizing resources (Fig. 43-6). The use of Photovoice (sometimes referred to as *Photo Voice*) projects can be very helpful in making positive changes in the community for people who are disabled.

Photovoice is a combination of photographs, videos, and storytelling that allows disabled people in the community to "voice our individual and collective experiences" in an organized way. This process can allow groups of patients with SCIs to work together to record and discuss their community's strengths and concerns. The collective desired outcome for Photovoice is to influence policymakers to make changes that remove or change their community's barriers. Newman (2010) described a Photovoice project to create a database of community environmental barriers and facilitators in a large city in the southeastern United States. Over 500 facilitators and over 500 barriers were identified. The authors produced a YouTube video and concluded that this type of community-based participatory project was extremely valuable to help wheelchair-bound SCI patients.

◆ Evaluation: Outcomes

Evaluate the care of the patient with an SCI based on the identified priority patient problems. The expected outcomes are that the patient:

- Exhibits no deterioration in neurologic status
- Maintains a patent airway, a physiologic breathing pattern, and adequate ventilation
- Is free from complications of immobility
- Performs basic ADLs as independently as possible with or without the use of assistive/adaptive devices
- Achieves control of regular elimination of stool and urine
- Adapts to a significant life change

SPINAL CORD TUMORS

❖ PATHOPHYSIOLOGY

Primary spinal cord tumors make up only a small percentage of all central nervous system neoplasms. Most spinal cord tumors are secondary or metastatic. Common primary cancers that metastasize (spread) to the spinal cord are lungs, breasts, prostate, colon, and uterus. Spinal cord tumors, whether primary or secondary, occur most often in the thoracic area, but they can occur in the lumbar and cervical areas. Signs and symptoms depend on the location of the tumor and its speed of growth. In addition, tumors in the spinal area can involve the vertebrae, and this location for bone cancer is usually as a result of metastasis from other areas of the body.

The pathologic effects of a spinal cord tumor are more often related to compression of the cord rather than the tumor itself. As the tumor expands, it compresses the cord or the spinal nerve roots. A large tumor may affect the blood supply to the cord causing ischemia or obstruct the normal flow of cerebrospinal fluid (CSF). Venous occlusion by the tumor may lead to spinal cord congestion and infarction (tissue death).

The appearance of neurologic signs and symptoms is related to the rate of tumor growth. With a slow-growing tumor, the cord may become significantly misshapen and displaced but the patient has surprisingly few symptoms. However, a rapidly growing tumor quickly leads to spinal cord compression, edema, and the development of neurologic symptoms, such as numbness and paralysis.

Primary spinal cord tumors can be extradural or intramedullary. Their cause is unknown. **Intramedullary tumors** are within the cord in the central gray matter or glial cells of the spinal cord. Intramedullary tumors are usually cancerous and grow rapidly and invasively. **Extramedullary tumors**, representing 90% of primary spinal cord tumors, are found within the spinal dura but outside the cord. They are further defined anatomically as extradural and intradural tumors. *Extradural or epidural* tumors occur between the vertebrae and the spinal dura. They develop in the surrounding bone and cause destruction of the vertebral bodies. *Intradural* tumors are located within the dura and originate from the pia-arachnoid, spinal roots, or ligaments. Most extramedullary tumors (e.g., schwannomas, neurofibromas, and meningiomas) do not exhibit the signs of uncontrolled growth and organ invasion of cancerous tumors.

❖ PATIENT-CENTERED COLLABORATIVE CARE

◆ Assessment

The clinical manifestations of a spinal cord tumor depend on its location (Chart 43-13) and rate of growth. The most common problem is non-mechanical back PAIN. Pain results from spinal cord compression, infiltration of the spinal tracts, or irritation of the spinal roots. Assess the quality, severity, and intensity of the pain. In addition, ask the patient to describe factors that worsen and relieve the pain. **Radicular** (nerve root) pain is stabbing or dull, with intermittent episodes of sharp, piercing pain. The pain may increase during coughing, straining, or sneezing. Lying flat may increase the pain as a consequence of stretching the involved spinal nerve roots.

Involvement of the corticospinal tract may lead to MOBILITY problems. Assess for weakness, clumsiness, spasticity, and hyperactive reflexes, and compare responses on both sides of the body. Other presenting signs include ataxia (staggered gait), hypotonia (decreased muscle tone), and a positive Babinski's reflex. Spastic paralysis occurs most often, although a flaccid paralysis may be present in a tumor that affects the spinal roots, an intramedullary tumor in the lumbosacral area, or an extramedullary tumor.

CHART 43-13 Key Features

Spinal Cord Tumors

General Manifestations
- Pain
- Sensory loss or impairment
- Motor loss or impairment
- Sphincter disturbance (bladder before bowel)

Cervical Manifestations

High Cervical
- Respiratory distress
- Diaphragm paralysis
- Occipital headache
- Quadriparesis
- Stiff neck
- Nystagmus
- Cranial nerve dysfunction

Low Cervical
- Pain in the arms and the shoulders
- Weakness
- Paresthesia
- Motor loss
- Horner's syndrome
- Increased reflexes

Thoracic Manifestations
- Sensory loss
- Spastic paralysis
- Positive Babinski's sign
- Bladder and bowel dysfunction
- Pain in the chest and the back
- Muscle atrophy
- Muscle weakness in the legs
- Foot drop

Lumbosacral Manifestations
- Low back pain
- Paresis
- Spastic paralysis
- Sensory loss
- Bladder and bowel dysfunction
- Sexual dysfunction
- Decreased-to-absent ankle and knee reflexes

Determine SENSORY PERCEPTION on each side of the body, and compare the responses. Early symptoms include a slowly progressive numbness or tingling, PAIN, and temperature loss. The sensory deficit is further marked by a decreased touch perception, an inability to sense vibration, and a loss of position sense. The patient often reports a tight, bandlike feeling around the trunk.

Loss of bladder control often occurs before a loss of bowel control. Assess for urinary hesitancy, dribbling, incontinence, urgency, or acute retention. Bowel dysfunction is manifested by constipation. Keep in mind that the patient is often embarrassed to admit to bladder or bowel dysfunction.

A lesion in the sacral area may cause a decrease in genital sensation and thus affect the patient's sexual function and enjoyment. Men may be unable to have an erection or to ejaculate.

Diagnostic Assessment. Radiographic examinations or scans of the spine are obtained to detect a narrowing of the spinal canal, destruction of the vertebrae, or the presence of calcification. An MRI scan with and without contrast medium provides more detail of the pathologic condition of the spinal cord than either a CT scan or myelography. Electromyography (EMG) may help make a differential diagnosis to rule out multiple sclerosis (MS) or amyotrophic lateral sclerosis (ALS) or when spinal cord symptoms indicate an incomplete block. It indicates the level, extent, and boundaries of a tumor. This test is being performed less today because of newer imaging techniques.

A biopsy may be done to diagnose the specific type of tumor using a CT/MRI–guided needle. If the tumor is malignant, a biopsy assists in determining the cancer's type, which will subsequently determine treatment options. A biopsy is not needed for tumors that result from metastases if cancer has been diagnosed in another site of the body.

◆ *Interventions*

Nursing care of the patient with a spinal cord tumor focuses on careful monitoring of vital signs and neurologic status at least every 4 hours or more often if clinically indicated.

! NURSING SAFETY PRIORITY (QSEN)

Critical Rescue

For the patient with a spinal cord tumor, report any change in motor and sensory status immediately to the physician or Rapid Response Team. Swelling or tumor invasion can damage the spinal nerves that help control the diaphragm, and respiratory failure can result.

The primary management of a spinal cord tumor is *surgery.* The desired outcome of surgical intervention is to remove as much of the tumor as possible. Often this is not possible and other treatment is needed (e.g., radiation therapy). *Emergency surgery is performed if the patient has a rapid loss of motor and sensory function or a loss of bladder and bowel control. Surgical decompression may be performed to maintain bladder, bowel, or motor function and to preserve quality of life—even with a poor prognosis.*

The neurosurgeon performs a laminectomy and surgical total or partial resection of the tumor to remove the source of spinal cord compression. Depending on the extent of the tumor, a spinal fusion may be necessary. Experts in palliative care can provide interventions to relieve pain. Rarely, a cordotomy or a palliative sectioning of sensory roots is done to control intractable pain.

After surgery, assess the patient's vital signs and neurologic status every 1 to 2 hours until they are stable and then every 4 hours. Help turn the patient as a unit (log roll) and reposition every 2 hours. Inspect the incision site for drainage, especially for cerebrospinal fluid (CSF), and signs of infection. Carefully monitor the patient with a cervical cord tumor for respiratory compromise. Postoperative nursing care for a patient undergoing a laminectomy is discussed on pp. 888-889 in the Back Pain section of this chapter.

Radiation therapy may be necessary, depending on the tumor type. It is usually used with low-grade malignant tumors that are not completely removed, with metastatic tumors, or with recurrent tumors when there is no other treatment option. The spinal cord cannot tolerate high doses of radiation. Overexposure to radiation may lead to spinal damage, which can develop as long as 6 to 12 months after therapy. Radiation overdose is manifested by progressive spinal cord degeneration and neurologic deficits. With time, the patient experiences spastic paralysis, loss of SENSORY PERCEPTION, and bowel and bladder dysfunction. Death may occur. Care of the patient undergoing radiation therapy is described in detail in Chapter 22.

The use of chemotherapy in the treatment of spinal cord tumors is very limited. The drugs that are given tend to be alkylating agents, which are effective for some CNS tumors because they cross the barrier formed in the CNS by unique capillary characteristics and glial cells similar to the blood-brain barrier in the skull. Chemotherapy may also be used as an adjunctive therapy for tumors that have metastasized to the spinal cord from other primary sites, such as the breast. Meningeal involvement may benefit from intrathecal (spinal) chemotherapy. Chapter 22 describes the general nursing care associated with giving chemotherapy.

Community-Based Care

Collaborate with the patient and his or her family members or significant others to identify and suggest ways to eliminate potential hazards in the home. If needed, make a referral to a home care nurse, social worker, or case manager to assess the need for structural alterations to the home. Alterations may be needed to accommodate ambulatory aids (e.g., a walker) and to help the patient perform ADLs.

Depending on the prognosis, some patients are discharged from the acute care hospital to a rehabilitation setting, where they can learn to function as independently as possible. Chapter 6 describes rehabilitation in detail.

The teaching plan for the patient with a spinal cord tumor depends on his or her level of dysfunction. With decompression of the tumor, the severity of the patient's symptoms often lessens. Deficits that may remain include MOBILITY and SENSORY PERCEPTION. Learning mobility skills can enable the patient to negotiate movement on sidewalks, carpeting, and other flooring surfaces. The patient must also be able to negotiate sidewalk curbs independently. The physical or occupational therapist instructs the patient in the correct use of all adaptive equipment. Review the individualized bowel and bladder program with the patient, family member, or other caregiver. Chapter 6 describes these programs and the rehabilitation process in detail.

The interventions related to SEXUALITY are usually focused on education in the acute care setting. The nurse answers questions and corrects any misinformation. Unless the nurse has had specific training or experience in sexual counseling of people with spinal cord tumors or injuries, more detailed questions should be directed to a sexual counselor.

The prognosis for the patient with malignant tumors or metastatic tumors is poor. Determine what the physician and family members have told the patient about diagnosis and prognosis. Encourage the patient to verbalize feelings and fears about prognosis, body image, self-concept, role performance, and self-esteem.

Refer patients and family members to local, state or province, and national organizations for people with spinal cord injuries. These groups often have information and support groups for patients with spinal cord tumors. Refer patients with a malignancy to the American Cancer Society (www.cancer.org). Referral to support groups may also assist families with helping the patient adapt to lifestyle changes. The Canadian Cancer Society (www.cancer.ca) offers similar services.

MULTIPLE SCLEROSIS

Multiple sclerosis (MS) is a life-long inflammatory disease of unknown etiology that affects the brain and spinal cord. It is one of the leading causes of neurologic disability in young adults. This chronic disease is characterized by periods of remission and **exacerbation** (flare), which is commonly referred to as a *relapsing-remitting course.* Patients progress at different rates and over different lengths of time. However, as the severity and duration of the disease progress, the periods of exacerbation become more frequent. Patients with MS have a normal life expectancy as long as the effects of the disease are treated.

A major concern reported by most patients is how long it takes to establish a diagnosis of MS. Many patients go to several health care providers, are given varying diagnoses and treatment, and/or are told that their symptoms are related to stress and anxiety. Often times, young adults will present with weakness, fatigue, or changes in vision and are diagnosed with exhaustion and advised to get more sleep. The patient and family are often relieved to have a definite diagnosis but may express anger and frustration that it took a long time to start appropriate treatment. Therefore establish open and honest communication with the patient, and allow him or her to share frustrations, anger, and anxiety.

❖ PATHOPHYSIOLOGY

Multiple sclerosis is characterized by an inflammatory process causing **demyelination** and axonal injury. Diffuse random or patchy areas of *plaque* in the white matter of the CNS is the definitive finding. Initially, remyelination takes place to some degree, and clinical symptoms decrease. Over time, however, new lesions develop and neuronal injury and atrophy occurs. Myelin is responsible for the electrochemical transmission of impulses between the brain and spinal cord and the rest of the body, and demyelination can result in slowed or stopped impulse transmission. The white fiber tracts that connect the neurons in the brain and spinal cord are generally involved in MS. The areas particularly affected include optic nerves, pyramidal tracts, posterior columns, brainstem nuclei, and the ventricular region of the brain. Eventually, with repeated exacerbations of the disease, damage to the axons becomes permanent.

The four major types of MS include (McCance et al., 2014):

- Relapsing-remitting
- Primary progressive
- Secondary progressive
- Progressive-relapsing

The classic picture of the **relapsing-remitting** type of **MS (RRMS)** occurs in most cases of multiple sclerosis. The course of the disease may be mild or moderate, depending on the degree of disability. Symptoms develop and resolve in a few weeks to months, and the patient returns to baseline. During the relapsing phase, the patient reports loss of function and the continuing development of new symptoms.

Primary progressive MS (PPMS) involves a steady and gradual neurologic deterioration without remission of symptoms. The patient has progressive disability with no acute attacks. Patients with this type of MS tend to be between 40 and 60 years of age at onset of the disease.

Secondary progressive MS (SPMS) begins with a relapsing-remitting course that later becomes steadily progressive. About half of all people with RRMS developed SPMS within 10 years. The current addition of disease-modifying drugs as part of disease management may decrease the development of SPMS.

Progressive-relapsing MS (PRMS) is characterized by frequent relapses with partial recovery but not a return to baseline. This type of MS is seen in only a small percentage of patients. Progressive, cumulative symptoms and deterioration occur over several years.

Etiology

The exact cause of MS remains unknown and is very complex. Research continues on viral, immunologic, genetic, and environmental etiologic factors. Viruses are well recognized as causes of demyelination and INFLAMMATION. Therefore it may be possible that a virus or other infectious agent is the triggering factor in MS. Although a number of viruses have been studied, no single virus has been identified as causing MS in genetically predisposed people. The environment may also contribute to the development of MS. The disease is seen more often in the colder climates of the northeastern, Great Lakes, and Pacific northwestern states, as well as in Canada. MS is common in areas inhabited by people of northern European ancestry (National Multiple Sclerosis Society, 2013a).

GENETIC/GENOMIC CONSIDERATIONS

Patient-Centered Care QSEN

Large genome studies of families have helped identify familial patterns of multiple sclerosis (MS). For example, having a first-degree relative such as a parent or sibling with MS increases a person's risk for developing the disease. Recent research also confirms the association of MS with the interleukin (IL)-7 and IL-2 receptor genes. Other interleukin genes, B-lymphocytes, and B-cells play a role in more progressive forms of the disease (McCance et al., 2014). These data help guide development of targeted drug therapies that may cure or better manage MS.

Incidence and Prevalence

MS usually occurs in people between the ages of 20 and 40 years, but cases may occur in those younger than 15 years and older than 50 years. About 400,000 people in the United States have MS, and women are affected about twice as often as men. The disease affects over 2 million people worldwide. Although MS tends to occur more frequently among whites, it affects people of all races (Frankel & James, 2011).

❖ PATIENT-CENTERED COLLABORATIVE CARE

◆ Assessment

History. Multiple sclerosis (MS) often looks like other neurologic diseases, which can make the diagnosis difficult and prolonged. As a result, patients often see many health care providers and undergo a variety of diagnostic tests and treatments. Obtaining a thorough history is essential for accurate diagnosis. Ask about a history of vision, MOBILITY, and SENSORY PERCEPTION changes, all of which are early indicators of MS. Symptoms are often vague and nonspecific in the early stages of the disease and may disappear for months or years before returning. Ask about the progression of symptoms. Pay particular attention to whether the symptoms are intermittent or are becoming progressively worse. Document the date (month and year) when the patient first noticed the clinical manifestations.

Next, ask about factors that aggravate the symptoms, such as fatigue, stress, overexertion, temperature extremes, or a hot shower or bath. Ask the patient and the family about any personality or behavioral changes that have occurred (e.g., euphoria [very elated mood], poor judgment, attention loss). In addition, determine whether there is a family history of MS or autoimmune disease.

Physical Assessment/Clinical Manifestations. Multiple sclerosis produces a wide variety of manifestations (Chart 43-14). Any myelinated fibers of the brain and spinal cord may be affected. To determine a patient's specific manifestations, perform a comprehensive neurologic assessment as described in Chapter 41.

First, assess the patient's ability to move. The patient often reports increased fatigue and stiffness of the extremities, particularly the legs. Fatigue is one of the most disabling manifestations, affecting almost all patients with MS. Unlike fatigue in

CHART 43-14 Key Features

Multiple Sclerosis

- Muscle weakness and spasticity
- Fatigue
- Intention tremors
- Dysmetria (inability to direct or limit movement)
- Numbness or tingling sensations (paresthesia)
- Hypalgesia (decreased sensitivity to pain)
- Ataxia (decreased motor coordination)
- Dysarthria (slurred speech)
- Dysphagia (difficulty swallowing)
- Diplopia (double vision)
- Nystagmus (involuntary eye movements)
- Scotomas (changes in peripheral vision)
- Decreased visual and hearing acuity
- Tinnitus (ringing in the ears), vertigo (dizziness)
- Bowel and bladder dysfunction
- Alterations in sexual function, such as impotence
- Cognitive changes, such as memory loss, impaired judgment, and decreased ability to solve problems or perform calculations
- Depression

other patients, MS fatigue is associated with continuous sensitivity to temperature.

Flexor spasms at night may awaken the patient from sleep. Further examination reveals increased or hyperactive deep tendon reflexes, positive Babinski's reflex, and absent abdominal reflexes. Gait may be unsteady because of leg weakness and spasticity due to cerebral motor strip damage.

Significant *cerebellar* findings include **intention tremor** (tremor when performing an activity), **dysmetria** (inability to direct or limit movement), and dysdiadochokinesia (inability to stop one motor impulse and substitute another). Motor movements are often clumsy. The patient may lose balance easily and may exhibit signs of poor coordination.

During examination of the *cranial nerves* and brainstem function, ask the patient if he or she has or has had episodes of tinnitus (ringing in the ears), vertigo (dizziness), and hearing loss. Assess for facial weakness and dysphagia. Speech problems include dysarthria, such as slurred words resulting from weak muscles of the tongue, lips, cheek, or mouth. Scanning is also a type of dysarthria common in MS. Scanning is an abnormal speech pattern with long pauses between words or syllables.

Typical clinical findings from assessment of the patient's visual acuity, visual fields, and pupils include:

- Blurred vision
- **Diplopia** (double vision)
- Decreased visual acuity
- **Scotomas** (changes in peripheral vision)
- **Nystagmus** (involuntary rapid eye movements)

Sensory findings include hypalgesia (diminished sensitivity to pain), paresthesia, facial pain, and decreased temperature perception. The patient may report numbness, tingling, burning, or crawling sensations. Some patients with RRMS, especially women, report pain (Newland, et al., 2010) (see the Evidence-Based Practice box). Perform a complete pain assessment for all patients with MS as described in Chapter 3.

If demyelination of the *spinal cord* has occurred, the patient may experience bowel and bladder dysfunctions. The patient may have an areflexic bladder or may experience frequency, urgency, or nocturia. Ask the patient if he or she has constipation or incontinence. Inquire about problems with SEXUALITY,

EVIDENCE-BASED PRACTICE QSEN

Are There Differences in Pain Between Women with Multiple Sclerosis and Healthy Women?

Newland, P.K., Riley, M.A., Fearing, A.D., Neath, A.A., & Gibson, D. (2010). Pain in women with relapsing-remitting multiple sclerosis and healthy women: Relationship to demographic variables. *MEDSURG Nursing, 19*(3), 177-182.

The purpose of this descriptive study was to determine if there is a relationship among aspects of pain and demographic variables in women with relapsing-remitting multiple sclerosis (RRMS) and healthy women. The researcher used data from a previous study consisting of 40 women with RRMS and 40 healthy women in the Midwest. Subjects were volunteers from one hospital. They were primarily Caucasian, married, and highly educated.

Findings revealed that pain prevalence was higher in women with RRMS when compared with healthy women. As years of education increased, prevalence and intensity of pain decreased. Pain also increased significantly in women who did not work. Conversely, for healthy women there was not a significant relationship with years of experience and pain prevalence or intensity.

Level of Evidence: 4

The study was a descriptive study that used a small convenience sample but with comparative groups.

Commentary: Implications for Practice and Research

When caring for patients with MS, especially women, medical-surgical nurses need to assess for the presence and intensity of their pain. When providing health teaching, patients may have special learning needs due to possible cognitive impairment. In addition, if possible, women should be encouraged to work or stay active to prevent increased pain.

This research used only Caucasian women in the study. Therefore the findings cannot be generalized to men or to any other racial or ethnic group. The research needs to be duplicated using male patients with MS and/or using a larger sample size of both men and women to compare with healthy men and women of mixed racial/ethnic origin.

including impotence, difficulty sustaining an erection, and decreased vaginal secretions.

Psychosocial Assessment. Assess the patient for mental status changes. Cognitive changes are usually seen late in the course of the disease and include decreased short-term memory, concentration, and ability to perform calculations; inattentiveness; and impaired judgment.

After the initial diagnosis of MS, the patient is often anxious. Apathy and emotional lability are common problems that occur later. Depression may occur at the time of diagnosis and can also occur later with disease progression. The patient may be euphoric or giddy, either as a result of the disease itself or because of the drugs used to treat the disease. Assess the patient's previously used coping and stress-management skills in preparing him or her for a chronic, usually debilitating disease. Secondary depression is the most frequent mental health disorder diagnosed in people with MS.

Assess the impact of bowel and bladder problems. Managing fecal incontinence or constipation can be time-consuming and embarrassing. The authors of a single site study found that elimination problems affected quality of life as much as MOBILITY difficulties (Norton & Chelvanayagam, 2010).

SEXUALITY can be affected in people with multiple sclerosis, and sexual dysfunction can have a major impact on quality of life. Assess the patient's fatigue level and pattern, since fatigue contributes to sexual dysfunction. Be sensitive when asking about the patient's sexual practices and orientation. Women report impaired genital sensation, diminished orgasm, and loss of sexual interest. Men most often report difficulty in achieving and maintaining an erection and delayed ejaculation. If able, answer the patient's questions, or refer the patient to a counselor or urologist with experience in the field of sexuality, intimacy, and disability.

MS affects the entire family due to the unpredictability and uncertainty of the course of the disease. Chronic fatigue and PAIN may also prevent the patient from participating in family and community activities. CNS stimulants such as amantadine (Symmetrel), aerobic exercise as tolerated, and energy-conservation strategies may help manage fatigue. Assess coping strategies of family members or other caregivers, and help them identify support systems that can assist them as they live with the patient with MS.

Laboratory Assessment. No single specific laboratory test is definitively diagnostic for MS. However, the collective results of a variety of tests are usually conclusive. Abnormal cerebrospinal fluid (CSF) findings include an elevated protein level and a slight increase in the white blood cell count. CSF electrophoresis reveals an increase in the myelin basic protein and the presence of increased immunoglobulins, especially immunoglobulin G (IgG). IgG bands are seen in most patients with MS.

Other Diagnostic Assessment. MRI of the brain and spinal cord demonstrates the presence of plaques and is considered diagnostic for MS. MRI with contrast shows active plaques and reveals older lesions not associated with current symptoms.

A complete history and physical examination is necessary to exclude other disease diagnoses. In general, assessment of cranial nerve function, coordination, strength, reflexes, and sensation are needed to diagnose MS, and a variety of neurologic tests are used to evaluate the many areas in which dysfunction from MS plaques can occur. Results of visual, auditory, and brainstem evoked potential studies are often abnormal. Electromyography (EMG) findings may be grossly abnormal in people with advanced disease.

◆ *Interventions*

The purpose of management is to modify the disease's effects on the immune system, prevent exacerbations, manage symptoms, and improve function. As with other spinal cord diseases, care of the patient with MS requires the collaborative efforts of the interdisciplinary team.

The patient with MS is often weak and easily fatigued. The Concept Map on p. 907 illustrates the priority problems and interventions for the patient with MS. Teach the patient the importance of planning activities and allowing sufficient time to complete activities. For example, the patient should check that all items needed for work are gathered before leaving the house. Items used on a daily basis should be easily accessible.

Drug Therapy. Current therapies are based on emerging evidence that MS is an autoimmune disorder. A variety of drugs are used to treat and control the disease, decrease specific symptoms, and attempt to slow its progression.

One or more of these drugs is recommended for treatment of relapsing types of MS:

- Interferon-beta-1a (Avonex or Rebif)—immunomodulators that *modify* the course of the disease and have antiviral effects

CONCEPT MAP

MULTIPLE SCLEROSIS

MOBILITY · SENSORY PERCEPTION · PAIN

HISTORY

40-year-old Carolyn Brown is admitted with progressive relapsing MS (PRMS) after a fall. She was diagnosed last year after several years of vague and nonspecific symptoms. Married with two school-age children, she is having difficulty managing ADLs. Her marriage is struggling due to these health issues. She is experiencing generalized weakness, muscle spasms, and urinary incontinence.

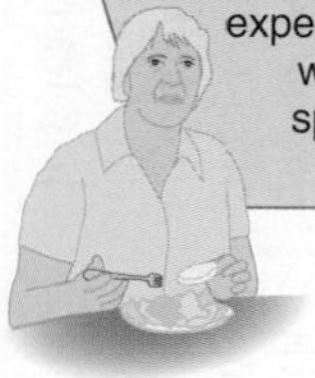

Physical Assessment

Subjective Data: "I am so tired, I can hardly get around....and my legs are so stiff, I fall. I just gradually get worse. I sometimes choke when I'm eating." The patient reports weakness, muscle spasms, trouble with balance, and has periods of double vision and vertigo.

Objective Data: Slightly slurred speech. Intention tremor with eating or writing.

Medical Diagnosis

Ms. Brown has been diagnosed with PRMS – frequent relapses with partial recovery. Progressive, cumulative symptoms occur over many years from inflammatory damage to myelin in the brain and spinal cord.

Data Synthesis

PATIENT PROBLEMS

MOBILITY – Difficulty managing ADLs related to generalized weakness, muscle spasms, fatigue, loss of balance, and falls

SENSORY PERCEPTION – Urinary incontinence, dysarthria, dysphagia, pain

Knowledge Deficit related to drug therapy and safety [MOBILITY, SENSORY PERCEPTION]

SEXUALITY and Psychosocial Issues – Life management of chronic illness

Planning

EXPECTED OUTCOMES

- Participate in regular exercise to maintain mobility
- Maximize independence in ADLs
- Manage urinary and bowel elimination
- Adhere to drug regimen to avoid complications
- Remain free of complications from ineffective airway clearance
- Use effective coping strategies for patient and family to reduce stress and enhance relationships

INTERVENTIONS

1 History and Physical Assessment

Assess history of onset and severity of signs/symptoms. Ask about their progression and about factors that aggravate or reduce symptoms. Complete a neurological assessment. *A focused history and physical assessment guides effective nursing care.*

2 Nursing Safety Priority: Action Alert!

Assist the cognitively impaired patient with orientation by placing a calendar in the room. Encourage written lists or recorded messages. Suggest keeping frequently used items in familiar places, and using mobile device "apps" for re-orientation or reminders. *Cognitive impairment impacts patient safety. Orientation helps the patient to function as safely as possible in the environment.*

3 SENSORY PERCEPTION Management

- Instruct the patient to wear an eye patch, alternating between eyes every few hours. *Relieves diplopia.*
- Teach scanning techniques. *Compensates for peripheral vision loss.*
- Encourage patient to see an ophthalmologist. *Manages changes in visual acuity that may be aided by corrective lenses.*

4 Maintaining Mobility

Collaborate with a physical/occupational therapist to maintain mobility and promote independence with ADLs. Teach patient to conserve energy and balance activities with periods of rest. Avoid common aggravating factors such as fatigue, stress, overexertion, or temperature extremes. *Maintain mobility by managing MS fatigue, the most disabling symptom. Fatigue level and pattern can contribute to immobility, dysfunction, and depression.*

5 Elimination Management

Assess for urinary hesitancy, dribbling, incontinence, urgency, and constipation. Use a bladder scanner to assess for urinary retention. Implement necessary interventions such as catheterization, bladder pacemaker, or drug therapy. Use best practices to prevent hospital acquired UTIs. *Promotes urinary continence and bowel evacuation. Dysfunction can have a major impact on quality of life.*

6 Drug and Complementary Therapies

- Review and provide written instructions of drug therapies for PAIN, inflammation, and incontinence. *Ensures patient understands drug mechanisms of action for safe administration.*
- Discuss complementary therapies such as massage, yoga, meditation, acupuncture, reflexology, and aromatherapy. *May help the patient to maintain MOBILITY and independence.*

7 Managing Dysarthria and Dysphagia

Collaborate with a speech-language pathologist for evaluation and treatment of slurred speech and swallowing difficulty. *Avoids complications resulting in ineffective airway clearance of secretions and aspiration.*

8 Maintaining Psychosocial Integrity

Assist patient in verbalizing concerns about body image, self-concept, role performance, self-esteem, and sexuality. *Helps patient cope with anxiety and depression over the progression of the disease. Depression is the most frequent mental health disorder diagnosed with MS.*

Concept Map by Deanne A. Blach, MSN, RN

- Interferon-beta-1b (Betaseron, Extavia)—another immunomodulator with antiviral properties
- Glatiramer acetate (Copaxone)—a synthetic protein that is similar to myelin-based protein
- Mitoxantrone (Novantrone)—an antineoplastic agent and anti-inflammatory used to resolve relapses but with risks for leukemia and cardiotoxicity
- Natalizumab (Tysabri)—the first monoclonal antibody approved for MS that binds to WBCs to prevent further damage to the myelin
- Fingolimod (Gilenya), teriflunomide (Aubagio), or dimethyl fumarate (Tecfidera)—newer oral immunomodulating drugs
- Mitoxantrone (Novantrone) for patients with worsening disease or increased frequency of relapses
- Corticosteroid (methylprednisolone [Solu-Medrol], dexamethasone, or prednisone) for acute exacerbation or onset
- Other immunosuppressants (e.g., cyclophosphamide, methotrexate, azathioprine, cladribine, and cyclosporine) can reduce symptoms of MS and suppress the number of circulating immune cells to slow the autoimmune process and neuronal damage

The interferons and glatiramer acetate are subcutaneous injections that patients can self-administer.

! NURSING SAFETY PRIORITY QSEN

Drug Alert

Teach patients how to give and rotate the site of interferon-beta and glatiramer acetate injections because local injection site (skin) reactions are common. The first dose of these drugs is given under medical supervision to monitor for allergic response, including anaphylactic shock. Teach patients receiving these drugs to avoid crowds and people with infections. Remind them to report any sign or symptom associated with infection immediately to their health care provider.

Natalizumab, a humanized monoclonal antibody, is a controversial drug because it can cause many adverse events. It is given as an IV infusion in an infusion clinic under careful supervision. The patient is monitored carefully for allergic or anaphylactic reaction when each dose is given because the drug tends to build up in the body. *Patients receiving this drug are at a high risk for* progressive multifocal leukoencephalopathy (PML). This opportunistic viral infection leads to death or severe disability. Monitor for neurologic changes, especially changes in mental state, such as disorientation or acute confusion. PML is confirmed by an MRI and examining the cerebrospinal fluid for the causative pathogen. Natalizumab also causes damage to hepatic cells. Carefully monitor liver enzymes and teach patients to have frequent laboratory tests to assess for changes.

Mitoxantrone (Novantrone), a chemotherapy drug, has been shown to be effective in reducing neurologic disability. It also decreases the frequency of clinical relapses in patients with secondary progressive, progressive-relapsing, or worsening relapsing-remitting MS.

Fingolimod (Gilenya) was the first oral immunomodulator approved for the management of MS. The capsules may be taken with or without food. Teach patients to monitor their pulse every day because the drug can cause bradycardia, especially within the first 6 hours after taking it (Duddy et al., 2011). Two newer oral immunomodulating drugs have been approved for MS—teriflunomide (Aubagio) and dimethyl fumarate (Tecfidera). Like fingolimod, these drugs inhibit immune cells and have antioxidant properties that protect brain and spinal cord cells. Teach the patient that the two most common side effects of all the oral drugs are facial flushing and GI disturbances (Lilley et al., 2014). Remind the patient to keep follow-up appointments for laboratory monitoring of the white blood cell (WBC) count because the oral drugs can cause a decrease in WBCs, which can predispose the patient to infection.

Another oral drug, dalfampridine (also known as fampridine) (Ampyra), was approved several years ago to improve walking ability in patients with MS. However, half of patients taking the drug have experienced seizures. The FDA has issued a warning to limit patients who are eligible to take the drug. For example, patients older than 50 years, those with renal impairment, and those with a history of seizures should not take dalfampridine. For these reasons, the drug is not widely prescribed.

Immunosuppressive therapy with a combination of cyclophosphamide (Cytoxan) and methylprednisolone (Solu-Medrol) may be used for some patients to stabilize the disease process and decrease INFLAMMATION. IV adrenocorticotropic hormone (ACTH) may be given instead of methylprednisolone and tapered gradually over 2 to 4 weeks.

Promoting Mobility and Managing Symptoms. The symptoms of MS include spasticity, tremor, worsening of symptoms triggered by increased body temperature (i.e., Uhthoff phenomenon), pain, cognitive impairment, dysphagia, dysarthria, bladder and bowel dysfunction, oculomotor symptoms (e.g. diplopia, nystagmus), sexual dysfunction, and fatigue. Referral to rehabilitative services can help manage functional deficits from MS symptoms. A multidisciplinary approach is important to provide pharmacotherapy, physiotherapy, and psychotherapy as well as attain patient-centered goals for care.

For spasticity, the health care provider may prescribe baclofen (Lioresal), tizanidine (Zanaflex), diazepam (Valium, Apo-Diazepam), or dantrolene sodium (Dantrium) to lessen muscle spasticity. Dalfampridine (Ampyra), a potassium channel blocker, is a new oral drug that can be prescribed to improve walking ability and speed. Dalfampridine is not given to patients with a history of seizures or renal disease.

Severe muscle spasticity may be treated with intrathecal baclofen (ITB) administered through a surgically implanted pump. Paresthesia may be treated with carbamazepine (Tegretol) or tricyclic antidepressants. Propranolol hydrochloride (Inderal) and clonazepam (Klonopin) have been used to treat cerebellar ataxia. If fatigue cannot be controlled through the use of nonpharmacologic measures, amantadine hydrochloride (Symmetrel) may be prescribed.

In collaboration with physical and occupational therapists, plan an exercise program that includes range-of-motion (ROM) exercises and stretching and strengthening exercises to manage spasticity and tremor. Beta-blockers (e.g., propranolol [Inderal]) and neurosurgery (e.g., thalamotomy or deep brain stimulation) can provide some relief from tremors.

Emphasize the importance of avoiding rigorous activities that increase body temperature. Increased body temperature may lead to increased fatigue, diminished motor ability, and decreased visual acuity resulting from changes in the conduction abilities of the injured axons.

PAIN and paresthesia are often problems for the MS patient. Antispasmodics, antiepileptic drugs (AEDs), analgesics, NSAIDs, tranquilizers, or antidepressants may be used, depending on the cause of the pain and the patient's response. Teach patients about side and adverse effects for drugs that they may need to help increase their quality of life.

Cognitive impairment may occur early in the disease process. Many patients have some degree of neuropsychological dysfunction during the course of their disease. Areas affected include attention, memory, problem solving, auditory reasoning, handling distractions, visual perception, and use of speech.

! NURSING SAFETY PRIORITY QSEN

Action Alert

For the patient with MS who has cognitive impairment, assist with orientation by placing a single-date calendar in his or her room. Give or encourage the patient to use written lists or recorded messages. To maintain an organized environment, encourage him or her to keep frequently used items in familiar places. Applications for handheld devices like mobile phones and electronic tablets can also be used for re-orientation, reminders, and behavioral cues.

If the patient experiences dysarthria (slurred speech), refer him or her to the speech-language pathologist (SLP) for evaluation and treatment. It is not unusual for the patient with dysarthria also to have dysphagia (difficulty swallowing). The SLP performs a swallowing evaluation, but further diagnostic testing may be indicated.

The patient may experience a variety of bladder problems. Bladder dysfunction (detrusor hyperreflexia) may be treated with anticholinergic agents. Other measures include an intermittent self-catheterization program, indwelling urinary catheter, or insertion of a bladder pacemaker. When the patient activates the control on the pacemaker, the bladder is stimulated and voiding is initiated. Patients with MS are at increased risk for urinary tract infections. Prophylactic antibiotics may be prescribed by the health care provider. Remind the patient to drink plenty of fluids unless contraindicated by other medical conditions.

Bowel symptoms can include constipation that can be treated with increased physical activity, adequate fluid intake of 1.5 to 2 liters daily, and increased dietary fiber to 25 to 35 g daily. Osmotic agents such as magnesium oxide may be used. Prokinetic agents such as lubiprostone may be used to increase motility. Enemas or suppositories may also be used.

An eye patch that is alternated from eye to eye every few hours usually relieves **diplopia** (double vision). For peripheral visual deficits, teach scanning techniques by having the patient move his or her head from side to side. Changes in visual acuity may be assisted by corrective lenses.

Sexual dysfunction may benefit from counseling. Prostaglandin-5 inhibitors (sildenafil, vardenafil, tadalafil) can be used to help men with erectile dysfunction. Penile prostheses are also used for men. The EROS Clitoral Therapy Device is a FDA-approved therapy for women with impaired sexual response.

Patients with MS who experience fatigue may limit their professional and social interactions. Depression can be manifested by fatigue, so screen for both of these symptoms. There are no licensed therapies for MS-related fatigue. Physiotherapy and occupational therapy can help reduce effort and fatigue. Depression can be managed with cognitive therapy and antidepressant drugs.

Complementary and Alternative Therapies. Patients with MS have reported a number of complementary and alternative medicine (CAM) therapies that have been successful in decreasing their symptoms. Consultation with a health care provider certified in palliative care may also provide strategies for effective symptom management. Some of the CAM therapies used by patients with MS are:

- Reflexology
- Massage
- Yoga
- Relaxation and meditation
- Acupuncture
- Aromatherapy

Marijuana has been used by some patients to relieve the PAIN of muscle spasms and is now legal for medical use in over 20 U.S. states and in Canada.

Community-Based Care

Home Care Management. To help the patient maintain maximum strength, function, and independence, continuity of care by an interdisciplinary team in both the rehabilitation and home setting is necessary. Admission to a rehabilitation center is brief but provides a program to improve functional ability. In collaboration with the case manager and occupational therapist, assess the patient's home before discharge for any hazards. Any items that might interfere with MOBILITY (e.g., scatter rugs) are removed. In addition, care must be taken to prevent injury resulting from vision problems. Teach the patient and family to keep the home environment as structured and as free from clutter as possible. As the disease progresses, the home may need to be adapted for wheelchair accessibility. Adaptation in the kitchen, bedroom, and bathroom may also be needed to promote self-management. Any necessary assistive/adaptive device should be readily available before discharge from the hospital.

Self-Management Education and Health Care Resources. The health care provider explains to the patient and family the development of MS and the factors that may exacerbate the symptoms. Emphasize the importance of avoiding overexertion, stress, extremes of temperatures (fever, hot baths, use of sauna baths and hot tubs, overheating, and excessive chilling), humidity, and people with infections. Explain all medications to be taken on discharge, including the time and route of administration, dosage, purpose, and side effects. Teach the patient how to differentiate expected side effects from adverse or allergic reactions, and provide the name of a resource person to call if questions or problems occur. Provide written instructions as a resource for the patient and caregivers at home.

The physical therapist develops an exercise program appropriate for the patient's tolerance level at home. The patient is instructed in techniques for self-care, daily living skills, and the use of required adaptive equipment, such as walkers and electric carts. Include information related to bowel and bladder management, skin care, nutrition, and positioning techniques. Chapter 6 describes in detail these aspects of chronic illness and rehabilitation.

Teach patients about conservation strategies that balance periods of rest and activity, including regular social interactions. Remind them to use assistive devices and modify the environment to avoid fatigue. Explore strategies to manage stress and avoid undue stress. Often patients are anxious and worry about how long the remission will last or when the disease will progress.

Because personality changes are not unusual, teach the family or significant others strategies to enable them to cope with these changes. For example, the family may develop a nonverbal signal to alert the patient to potentially inappropriate behavior. This action avoids embarrassment for the patient.

Resources required by the patient depend on the course of the disease and the complications that occur. Patients often are able to live completely independently, but they may need some assistance. In severe disease, placement in an assisted-living or long-term care facility may be the best alternative. The population of young and middle-aged residents in these settings is increasing as people with chronic, disabling diseases live longer. Refer the patient and family members or significant others to the local chapter of the National Multiple Sclerosis Society (www.nationalmssociety.org). Other community resources include meal delivery services (e.g., Meals on Wheels), transportation services for the disabled, and homemaker services.

AMYOTROPHIC LATERAL SCLEROSIS

❖ PATHOPHYSIOLOGY

Amyotrophic lateral sclerosis (ALS), also known as **Lou Gehrig's disease**, is an upper and lower motor neuron disease of adult onset. It is characterized by progressive weakness, muscle wasting, and spasticity that eventually lead to paralysis. Beginning in one area of the body, motor weakness and deterioration spread until the entire body is involved, including the ability to talk, swallow, and breathe. As a result of loss of lower motor neurons (LMNs) found in the spinal cord and brainstem, the muscles to which they connect weaken, atrophy, and die.

Loss or death of upper neurons (found in the brain) breaks their connections with LMNs, and spasticity occurs in the muscles. Death typically occurs within 3 years of diagnosis due to respiratory failure (McCance et al., 2014). There is no known cause, no cure, no specific treatment, no standard pattern of progression, and no method of prevention. Unlike with many other neural degenerative diseases, the sensory and autonomic nervous systems are not involved. Cognitive and behavioral dysfunction may occur, although the exact cause and extent of this has not been established.

Amyotrophic lateral sclerosis commonly affects people between the ages of 40 and 60 years, but it may also begin in younger and older age-groups. The incidence increases with each decade of life. ALS affects about 5 of every 100,000 people worldwide and is more common in men than in women. The cause of the disease is unknown but is likely due to multiple genetic and cell biologic hits and interactions of genetic, viral, and environmental factors (Ludolph et al., 2012).

❖ PATIENT-CENTERED COLLABORATIVE CARE

◆ Assessment

The clinical manifestations of ALS include fatigue, muscle atrophy, and weakness. Early symptoms are listed in Chart 43-15.

CHART 43-15 Key Features

Early Clinical Manifestations of Amyotrophic Lateral Sclerosis

- Tongue atrophy
- Weakness of the hands and arms
- Beginning muscle atrophy of the arms
- **Fasciculations** (twitching) of the face or tongue
- Difficulty controlling crying or laughing (emotional incontinence)
- Nasal quality of speech
- **Dysarthria** (slurred speech)
- **Dysphagia** (difficulty swallowing)
- Fatigue while talking
- Stiff or clumsy gait
- Abnormal reflexes

In addition to motor changes, cognitive changes may affect the thinking and planning processes. As the disease progresses, muscle atrophy, particularly of the trapezius and sternocleidomastoid muscles, develops. Eventually the respiratory muscles become involved, leading to respiratory compromise, pneumonia, and death.

Diagnosis is based on clinical and diagnostic test findings and by ruling out other causes of the motor changes. There is no specific test to diagnose ALS, but creatine kinase (CK) is increased. The electromyogram (EMG) demonstrates fibrillations and fasciculations of the muscles. The use of ultrasound to visualize fasciculation particularly in deep muscles can lead to earlier diagnosis (de Carvalho & Swash, 2011). A muscle biopsy specimen typically demonstrates small, angulated, atrophic fibers. Other diagnostic studies reveal motor strength deficits in serial muscle testing; abnormal pulmonary function test results, such as a decreased vital capacity (<2 L); and dysphagia (difficulty swallowing).

◆ Interventions

There is no known cure for ALS, but an interdisciplinary approach is needed for maintaining optimum functioning and end-of-life care. Interdisciplinary care can prolong survival and enhance quality of life in this population (Miller et al., 2009).

Riluzole (Rilutek) is the only drug approved by the Food and Drug Administration for use with ALS patients (Miller et al., 2012). It is not a cure, but it does extend survival time. Remind patients to take the drug when the stomach is empty. Teach the patient how to detect signs and symptoms of liver toxicity, such as vomiting and jaundice, that the drug may cause. Instruct them to have frequent liver enzyme tests, such as alanine aminotransferase (ALT) and aspartate aminotransferase (AST), as directed by the health care provider.

The health care provider also prescribes drug therapy for PAIN, fatigue, spasticity, excessive secretions, sleep disturbances, and other complications as they occur (Andersen et al., 2012). The interdisciplinary health care team collaborates with the patient and family to develop an individualized plan of care and PALLIATION of symptoms. The physical therapist and occupational therapist evaluate the patient's home and recommend modifications as the disease progresses. An exercise program is developed, and special equipment is obtained as needed to help with ADLs and MOBILITY. Other interventions are directed toward preventing complications of immobility and promoting comfort.

The speech-language pathologist (SLP) evaluates the patient for speech and swallowing problems and makes recommendations as needed. The SLP teaches patients various adaptive strategies, such as techniques to help them speak louder and more clearly. He or she works with the patient and family to develop a communication system to be used when the patient can no longer verbally communicate.

A nutrition consult may be needed to help with planning meals that the patient can swallow when dysphagia occurs. The family is taught how to ensure that the patient obtains sufficient nutrients, fiber, and fluids. When the patient can no longer swallow, a feeding tube may be placed, depending on the patient's decision or advance directives. The dietitian can recommend the appropriate enteral feedings.

For symptomatic treatment of dyspnea and/or intractable PAIN, opioids alone or in combination with benzodiazepines if anxiety is present may be prescribed. Titrating the dose against the clinical symptoms is less likely to cause life-threatening respiratory depression. For PALLIATION of terminal restlessness and confusion because of hypercapnia, neuroleptics may be used (e.g., chlorpromazine [Thorazine, Chlorpromanyl ♣] 12.5 mg orally, IV, or rectally every 4 to 12 hours).

As the patient's condition worsens, he or she will require respiratory support. Intermittent positive-pressure ventilation (IPPV) or bi-level positive airway pressure (BiPAP) may be used to aid breathing during sleep or full time. Some patients may be a candidate for diaphragmatic pacing (Scherer & Bedlack, 2012). **Diaphragmatic pacing**, also known as *phrenic nerve pacing*, is a pacemaker-like application of electrical impulses to the diaphragm, resulting in inhalation. Another option is invasive mechanical ventilation. None of these options prolong life. For this reason, many patients elect not to be placed on a mechanical ventilator, according to their wishes or advance directives. Teach the patient about the need for advance directives, such as a living will. Chapter 7 discusses end-of-life issues and hospice services in detail.

! NURSING SAFETY PRIORITY QSEN

Action Alert

Refer the patient with amyotrophic lateral sclerosis to palliative care for symptom management. The palliative team collaborates with the health care provider to ensure that the patient has effective interventions to manage pain, fatigue, and dyspnea. Focusing care on symptom management is not restricted to patients who are at the end of life and can significantly improve quality of life in complexly ill patients and their family caregivers.

Other community resources include clinics and other support services run by the ALS Association (www.alsa.org) or the Muscular Dystrophy Association (www.mda.org).

NURSING CONCEPTS AND CLINICAL JUDGMENT REVIEW

What might you NOTICE if the patient is experiencing impaired MOBILITY and SENSORY PERCEPTION as a result of spinal cord health problems?

- Weakness or paralysis of one or more extremities
- Report of decreased sensation in one or more extremities
- Muscle spasticity or flaccidity
- Forward bent position when ambulating
- Limp or altered gait
- Bladder incontinence or retention
- Bowel incontinence or retention
- Report of pain at or above the site of injury along the spinal column and/or in one or more extremities
- Difficulty breathing

What should you INTERPRET and how should you RESPOND to a patient experiencing inadequate MOBILITY and SENSORY perception as a result of spinal cord health problems?

Perform and interpret physical assessment, including:

- Assessing airway patency and breathing pattern
- Assessing use of accessory muscles, pattern of respiratory effort, and rate and depth of breathing
- Assessing level of consciousness
- Taking vital signs
- Performing a complete physical assessment
- Performing a complete neurologic assessment

Respond by:

- Establishing an airway as needed
- Stabilizing the spine by positioning until surgery or other treatment is provided
- Preparing for imaging assessment tests
- Inserting an indwelling urinary catheter
- Collaborating with the health care team, especially the physical therapist and the occupational therapist, if needed

On what should you REFLECT?

- Monitor the patient for changes in condition, including deterioration of neurologic status.
- Consider how to best collaborate with the health care team when caring for patients with spinal cord injury or illness.
- Think about family reaction to the injury or illness and what additional resources could have been used or should be used in the future.

GET READY FOR THE NCLEX® EXAMINATION!

KEY POINTS

Review these Key Points for each NCLEX Examination Client Needs Category.

Safe and Effective Care Environment

- Use safe object and patient handling practices to prevent back injury as described in Chart 43-5. **Safety** QSEN
- Assess airway and breathing *first* for patients with an acute SCI. **Evidence-Based Practice** QSEN
- Integrate team meetings into care of patients with long-term or degenerating spinal cord conditions.
- Identify patient and family values and preferences as the foundation for regular communication and collaboration with health care team members, including the physician, physiatrist, advanced practice provider, physical therapist, occupational therapist, sexual counselor, registered dietitian, respiratory therapist, and case manager. **Teamwork and Collaboration** QSEN
- Ask the patient about advance directives and palliative care/ symptom management to promote patient-centered care. **Patient-Centered Care** QSEN

Health Promotion and Maintenance

- Use community resources and behavioral strategies to assist overweight and obese patients in losing weight to reduce back PAIN and strain.
- Collaborate with physical and occupation therapy to promote self-management, including the provision of adaptive/ assistive devices for independence in ADLs. **Teamwork and Collaboration** QSEN
- Include community resources in discharge planning and teaching for patients with SCI, MS, ALS, and cancer that involves the spine or vertebrae. There are specialty organizations for each of these spinal conditions.

Psychosocial Integrity

- Refer patients to appropriate resources, such as a sexual counselor or urologist, for sexual dysfunction resulting from illness or disease. Counsel them as needed about SEXUALITY. **Teamwork and Collaboration** QSEN
- Recognize that spinal cord injury and progressive neurologic diseases, such as MS, require the patient and family to make major adjustments to roles and goals. **Patient-Centered Care** QSEN
- Include the family in planning for rehabilitation and discharge when spinal disorders occur or worsen.
- Determine patient and family coping strategies to help patients adjust to spinal trauma or disease. **Patient-Centered Care** QSEN

Physiological Integrity

- Assess PAIN level in patients with back injury, including the nature of the pain and location.
- Provide complete neurologic assessment of patients with spinal cord health problems, with ongoing focused motor assessment as described in Chart 43-8.
- Implement effective drug and non-drug interventions for back PAIN, including analgesics, NSAIDs, and adjunctives such as heat and exercise.
- Implement interventions to prevent complications associated with immobility, including turning; VTE prophylaxis; early ambulation or transfers out of bed; and airway and breathing management such as bedside suctioning equipment, incentive spirometry, and Aspiration Precautions. **Safety** QSEN
- Monitor patients with cervical spinal injuries for manifestations of autonomic dysreflexia (see Chart 43-10). Provide a bowel and bladder regimen to prevent retention of stool and urine because these common problems can initiate autonomic dysreflexia. **Evidence-Based Practice** QSEN
- Provide emergency care for patients who experience autonomic dysreflexia as listed in Chart 43-11. **Safety** QSEN
- Explain that the pathophysiology of MS is a demyelination syndrome of the brain and spinal neurons.
- Explain the pathophysiology of ALS is unknown. Neurons that conduct nerve impulses from the spinal or brain to muscles degenerate. Without motor neuron input, the muscles atrophy and the patient becomes weak and then paralyzed.
- Monitor respiratory status carefully in patients with ALS. Patients experience respiratory failure as the disease progresses. **Safety** QSEN
- Assess patients with multiple sclerosis for clinical manifestations as listed in Chart 43-14. Fatigue is the most common symptom.
- For patients who have surgery to manage vertebral or spinal cord conditions, observe the incision site for bleeding and cerebrospinal fluid leakage (clear fluid).
- Log roll during repositioning, especially during acute spinal cord injury or following surgical fusion of vertebrae.
- Provide postoperative care and discharge teaching for patients having cervical neck surgery as listed in Chart 43-6.

CHAPTER 44

Care of Patients with Problems of the Peripheral Nervous System

Rachel L. Gallagher

http://evolve.elsevier.com/Iggy/

PRIORITY CONCEPTS

- Mobility
- Sensory Perception
- Pain
- Inflammation
- Gas Exchange

LEARNING OUTCOMES

Safe and Effective Care Environment

1. Collaborate with interdisciplinary health care team members when providing care for patients with Guillain-Barré syndrome (GBS) and myasthenia gravis (MG) to avoid pain or complications from reduced sensory perception.

Health Promotion and Maintenance

2. Provide information to patients and families on common side effects and administration of drugs for peripheral nervous system (PNS) disorders to ensure safety.
3. Identify community resources for PNS disorders for patients and families.

Psychosocial Integrity

4. Plan interventions for patients with GBS and MG for promoting communication based on patient preferences.

Physiological Integrity

5. Describe how to perform focused neurologic assessments for patients with PNS disorders.
6. Compare and contrast the pathophysiology of GBS and MG, including the roles of inflammation and autoimmunity.
7. Prioritize evidence-based nursing interventions for the patient with GBS or MG to maintain mobility, reduce pain, and promote gas exchange.
8. Differentiate between a myasthenic crisis and a cholinergic crisis. Assess patients having a thymectomy for postoperative complications.
9. Plan and implement evidence-based postoperative care for the patient undergoing peripheral nerve repair.
10. Compare trigeminal neuralgia and facial paralysis assessment findings.

There are over 100 peripheral nerve disorders. Although only a few require treatment in an acute care setting, many peripheral nerve disorders are present in patients admitted with an unrelated diagnosis. For example, neuropathies caused by systemic diseases like diabetes, chronic kidney disease, or cancers are common and interfere with mobility, alter sensory perception, and cause pain. Generally, peripheral nervous system disorders have symptoms that start gradually and then get worse. Often symptoms include:

- Pain, burning, or tingling
- Muscle weakness
- Either increased or reduced sensitivity to touch

The peripheral nervous system (PNS) is composed of the spinal nerves, cranial nerves, and part of the autonomic nervous system. Its function is to provide communication from the brain and spinal cord to other parts of the body. *Neuropathy* or *peripheral neuropathy (PN)* is a global word that refers to any disease, disorder, or damage to the PNS. These health problems may be acute, such as Guillain-Barré syndrome (GBS), or chronic, such as myasthenia gravis (MG). Secondary PN may result from disorders such as peripheral vascular disease and diabetes mellitus. These health problems are discussed elsewhere in this text.

GUILLAIN-BARRÉ SYNDROME

❖ PATHOPHYSIOLOGY

Guillain-Barré syndrome (GBS) is an acute inflammatory polyradiculoneuropathy that affects the axons and/or myelin of the peripheral nervous system, causing motor weakness and abnormalities in sensory perception. It is an uncommon disorder, affecting males slightly more than females and peaking after age 55 years (Sejvar et al., 2011).

GBS may be referred to by a variety of other names, such as *acute idiopathic polyneuritis, acute inflammatory demyelinating polyneuropathy (AIDP), acute motor axonal neuropathy (AMAN),* and *acute motor and sensory axonal neuropathy* (Arcila-Londono & Lewis, 2012). In some forms of GBS, primarily the axons are affected. In other forms, **demyelination** (destruction of the myelin sheath) of the peripheral nerves occurs. Symptoms are the same: progressive motor weakness and abnormal SENSORY PERCEPTION. In demyelinating GBS, symptoms typically begin in the legs and spread to the arms and upper body. This is referred to as an *ascending paralysis.* Paralysis can increase in intensity until the muscles cannot be used at all and the patient is almost totally immobile. As a result, some patients require mechanical ventilation because of a weak or paralyzed diaphragm and accessory muscles for respiration. Healing occurs in reverse; the neurons affected last are the first to recover.

GBS is the result of immune-mediated pathology. Antibodies attack the myelin sheath that surrounds the axons of the peripheral nerves. On microscopic examination, groups of lymphocytes are seen at the points of myelin breakdown. In some instances, secondary damage to the cell body, the neurilemma, or the axon occurs. Neurilemma and axonal injury can delay recovery or result in permanent neurologic defects. Segmental demyelination (the destruction of myelin between the nodes of Ranvier) is the major pathologic finding in most variants of GBS. This destruction slows the transmission of impulses from node to node. Damaged motor neurons result in weakness. Damaged sensory nerves send fewer messages to the brain, affecting the patient's SENSORY PERCEPTION.

Three stages make up the *acute* course of GBS:

- The *acute or initial period* (1 to 4 weeks), which begins with the onset of the first symptoms and ends when no further deterioration occurs
- The *plateau period* (several days to 2 weeks)
- The *recovery phase* (gradually over 4 to 6 months, maybe up to 2 years), which is thought to coincide with remyelination and axonal regeneration (Some patients do not completely recover and have permanent neurologic deficits, referred to as *chronic GBS.*)

GBS is associated with bacterial infection, especially infection with *Campylobacter jejuni.* Influenza, Epstein-Barr, and cytomegalovirus viral infections have also been associated with GBS. There are other anecdotal and case reports from patients with surgery, trauma, and pregnancy who also developed GBS, but numbers are not sufficient to establish a causal relationship. There are also reports of some vaccines increasing the risk for GBS slightly, but epidemiologic evidence is weak (Centers for Disease Control and Prevention [CDC], 2014). It is believed that the precipitating infection or event sensitizes the T-cells to the patient's myelin, resulting in production of a demyelinating autoantibody.

❖ PATIENT-CENTERED COLLABORATIVE CARE

◆ Assessment

Obtain a complete health history. Ask the patient to describe GBS symptoms in chronologic order, if possible. Inquire about the presence of PAIN, numbness, and **paresthesias** (unpleasant sensations such as burning, stinging, and prickly feeling).

Although features vary, most people report a sudden onset of muscle weakness (Chart 44-1). The common symptoms of GBS are loss of reflexes in the arms and legs; low blood pressure or poor blood pressure control; muscle weakness or paralysis; numbness; uncoordinated movement, clumsiness, and falls; blurred or double vision; difficulty moving facial muscles; and palpitations (Simmons, 2010). Typically, the disease does not affect level of consciousness, cognition, or pupillary constriction or dilation. The clinical variations of GBS reflect the areas of earliest or most severe involvement (Arcila-Londono & Lewis, 2012).

CHART 44-1 Key Features

Guillain-Barré Syndrome

Motor Manifestations
- Ascending symmetric muscle weakness → flaccid paralysis without muscle atrophy
- Decreased or absent deep tendon reflexes (DTRs)
- Respiratory compromise (dyspnea, diminished breath sounds, decreased tidal volume, reduced peripheral oxygenation [Spo_2] and vital capacity) and respiratory failure
- Loss of bowel and bladder control (less common)
- Ataxia

Sensory Manifestations
- Paresthesias
- Pain (cramping)

Cranial Nerve Manifestations
- Facial weakness
- Dysphagia
- Diplopia
- Difficulty speaking

Autonomic Manifestations
- Labile blood pressure
- Cardiac dysrhythmias
- Tachycardia

With any of the variants, *cranial nerve* involvement most often affects the facial nerve (cranial nerve [CN] VII). Assess the patient's ability to smile, frown, whistle, or drink from a straw. Assess the patient for dysphagia (difficulty swallowing), which involves CNs V, VII, X, XI, and XII. The patient's inability to cough, gag, or swallow results from the involvement of CNs IX and X. Monitor the patient closely for varying blood pressure (hypertensive and hypotensive episodes or orthostatic hypotension), bradycardia, heart block, and, possibly, asystole. These symptoms are part of *autonomic dysfunction,* which is linked to vagus nerve (CN X) deficit. Assess CN XI (accessory) by asking the patient to shrug the shoulders. Hypoglossal nerve (CN XII) deficit is manifested by an inability to stick the tongue out straight.

In addition to determining the usual roles and responsibilities, occupation, motivation, and available support systems, assess the patient's ability to cope with this devastating illness and the accompanying fear and anxiety. In general, GBS is self-limiting and the paralysis is temporary. It is not unusual for the patient to have depression throughout the recovery period or feel significant powerlessness.

Although no single clinical or laboratory finding confirms the diagnosis of GBS, the health care provider may perform a lumbar puncture (LP) to evaluate *cerebrospinal fluid (CSF).* An increase in CSF protein level can occur from inflammatory plasma proteins, myelin breakdown, and damage to nerve roots. However, high protein levels may not occur until after 1 to 2 weeks of illness, reaching a peak in 4 to 6 weeks. The CSF lymphocyte count is normal.

Peripheral blood tests may show a moderate *leukocytosis* early in the illness. The number of leukocytes rapidly returns to normal if there are no complications or concurrent illness.

Electrophysiologic studies (EPSs) demonstrate demyelinating neuropathy. The degree of abnormality found on testing does not always correlate with clinical severity. Within 3 weeks of symptoms, nerve conduction velocities are depressed. In some cases, denervated potentials (fibrillations) develop later in the illness. Electromyographic (EMG) findings, which reflect peripheral nerve function, are normal early in the illness.

Electrophysiologic changes appear only after denervation of muscle has been present for 4 weeks or longer. Nerve conduction velocity (NCV) testing is performed with the EMG. Nerve damage or disease may still exist despite normal NCV results. A magnetic resonance imaging (MRI) or computed tomography (CT) scan may be requested to rule out other causes of motor weakness. These tests are described in Chapter 41.

Respiratory function manifested by poor GAS EXCHANGE is often compromised in patients with GBS. Therefore vital capacity or tidal volume may be decreased and respiratory rate increased. Arterial blood gas (ABG) values may be abnormal with a decreased partial pressure of arterial oxygen (Pao_2), increased partial pressure of arterial carbon dioxide ($Paco_2$), or decreased pH.

◆ Interventions

Managing Drug Therapy and Plasmapheresis. The health care provider follows the most recent best practice guidelines from the American Academy of Neurology (Patwa et al., 2012) for the treatment of GBS. The patient may receive either plasma exchange (also known as *plasmapheresis* or *apheresis*) or IV immunoglobulin (IVIG). There is no benefit to combining these treatments (Rajabally, 2012). Corticosteroids are not used unless medically necessary to treat other associated diseases.

Plasmapheresis removes the circulating antibodies thought to be responsible for the disease. In this procedure, plasma is selectively separated from whole blood. The blood cells are returned to the patient without the plasma. Plasma usually replaces itself, or the patient is transfused with a colloidal substitute such as albumin. Fresh frozen plasma is generally not used because of the associated risk for infection and allergic pulmonary edema. Plasmapheresis should be done within several days after the onset of the illness, although some patients benefit up to 30 days after the onset of symptoms. The patient usually receives three or four treatments, 1 to 2 days apart. Some patients may require a second round of treatment if they deteriorate after the first plasmapheresis.

Nursing interventions for the patient undergoing plasmapheresis include providing information and reassurance, weighing the patient before and after the procedure, and caring for the shunt or venous access site and preventing complications described in Chart 44-2 (Kaplan, 2012).

! NURSING SAFETY PRIORITY QSEN

Action Alert

If a shunt is used for plasmapheresis, be sure to:
- Check shunt patency by assessing the presences of bruit or thrill every 2 to 4 hours
- Keep double bulldog clamps at the bedside
- Observe the access site for bleeding or ecchymosis (bruising)

IVIG has been shown to be as effective as plasmapheresis and is immediately available in most settings. Side effects of immunoglobulin therapy range from minor discomforts (e.g., chills, mild fever, myalgia, and headache) to major complications (e.g., anaphylaxis, aseptic meningitis, retinal necrosis, acute renal failure). Infuse IVIG slowly when it is started. Observe for and document side and adverse effects, and report their occurrence to the health care provider. The rate of administration can be increased based on the patient's tolerance and on agency protocol.

CHART 44-2 Best Practice for Patient Safety & Quality Care QSEN

Preventing and Managing Complications of Plasmapheresis

COMPLICATION	NURSING INTERVENTIONS
Treatment-Related Complications	
Citrate-induced hypocalcemia	Monitor electrolytes before and after therapy. Communicate abnormal results appropriately to the health care provider. Anticipate calcium replacement therapy (Chapter 11).
Urticarial (skin) reactions from proteins in replacement fluids	Obtain order and administer diphenhydramine (Benadryl) or corticosteroid as premedications when urticaria occurred with previous exchange.
Depletion coagulopathy	Monitor complete blood count and coagulation panel before and after treatment. Communicate abnormal values to the health care provider in an urgent time frame.
Risk for infection from immunoglobulin depletion	Assess and document vital signs, including temperature 3 times daily. Report symptoms of infection, fever, or abnormal vital signs to the health care provider promptly.
Fluid shift or depletion	Monitor fluid status and vital signs during treatment and at least twice in the first hour following treatment.
Sensitivity reaction (including potential anaphylaxis with incorrect crossmatch or administration) when fresh frozen plasma is used in replacement fluid	Follow institution policy for safe, effective administration of blood products like fresh frozen plasma.
Site-Related Complications	
Trauma to skin and blood vessels from large-bore needles for access or catheter-related trauma	Teach the patient rationale for and how to monitor access site as described below.
Bleeding, phlebitis, or infection at access site	Anchor tubing securely during treatment. Minimize patient agitation, if present, during treatment. Assess access site immediately following cessation of treatment and at regular intervals (every 4 hours or more often). Assessment includes appearance of site or dressing, palpation of thrill, and auscultation of bruit.
Clotting at access site	Report loss of thrill or bruit, uncontrolled or large volume bleeding, and presence of redness (particularly along venous pathway), drainage, and swelling to provider immediately.

Managing Respiratory and Cardiac Status. Frequent and focused monitoring of both the respiratory and cardiovascular systems can prevent complications from GBS as well as identify patients in need of critical rescue interventions.

Inability to maintain an airway is a high risk and potentially fatal consequence of rapidly ascending GBS. The priority nursing intervention of *airway management* is to promote airway patency and adequate GAS EXCHANGE. Consider implementing Aspiration Precautions that include elevating the head of the bed to 45 degrees or higher and testing for dysphagia prior to restarting oral drugs or nutrition. Have suctioning equipment available and follow institution procedure for oral or oral-tracheal suctioning if the airway becomes compromised with secretions or food. Monitor the color, consistency, and amount of secretions obtained. Chest physiotherapy, often performed by the respiratory therapist (RT), and frequent position changes are combined with breathing exercises (coughing and deep breathing) and the use of an incentive spirometer to prevent pneumonia and atelectasis. Oxygen may be administered by nasal cannula at a flow rate prescribed by the health care provider.

! NURSING SAFETY PRIORITY QSEN

Action Alert

In the initial phase of Guillain-Barré syndrome, monitor the patient closely with each interaction for signs of respiratory distress, such as dyspnea, air hunger, adventitious breath sounds, decreased oxygen saturation, and cyanosis. In addition, assess respiratory rate, rhythm, and depth every 1 to 2 hours. In collaboration with the respiratory therapist (RT), check vital capacity every 2 to 4 hours and auscultate the lungs at 4-hour intervals. Monitor the patient's ability to cough and swallow for any change. Assess cognitive status, especially in older adults; a decline in mental status often indicates hypoxia.

Monitor ABG values or end-tidal carbon dioxide for signs of respiratory failure; pulse oximetry reveals decreasing oxygen saturation. A decrease in vital capacity to less than 15 to 20 mL/kg (or less than two thirds of the patient's normal) and the inability to clear secretions may be indications for elective intubation.

Both the sympathetic and parasympathetic systems may be affected. A patient with acute GBS may require cardiac monitoring because of the risk for dysrhythmias. Monitor trends in vital signs closely. Report significant changes in heart rate and blood pressure to the health care provider in an urgent time frame. Hypertension is treated with a beta blocker or nitroprusside (Nitropress). Hypotension is treated with IV fluids and placing the patient in a supine position unless he or she is in extreme respiratory distress. Atropine may be prescribed to treat bradycardia.

Improving Mobility and Preventing Complications of Immobility. Collaborate with the patient, family, physical and occupational therapists (PT/OT), speech-language pathologist (SLP), and dietitian to develop interventions that prevent complications of immobility and to address deficits in self-care. Assess the patient's motor (muscle) strength every 2 to 4 hours as part of the neurologic assessment. The interventions prescribed for MOBILITY and self-management and to prevent complications depend on the degree of motor deficit. The PT and OT provide assistive devices and instructions for their use.

To ensure safety, assist the patient with walking, transfers from bed to chair, position changes, and maintenance of proper body alignment until he or she is able to perform these activities independently. Encourage maximum independence. Perform active or passive range-of-motion (ROM) exercises at least daily, or delegate this activity to unlicensed assistive personnel (UAP) with supervision. Teach family members these techniques. See Chapter 6 for detailed discussion of ways to promote self-management and prevent complications of immobility. Monitor the patient's responses, including fatigue level. Provide adequate rest periods between activities.

Decreased gastric motility, dysphagia, and depression can cause malnutrition. Collaborate with the dietitian to develop caloric and protein intake goals. The patient may require assistance with feeding. If he or she cannot safely swallow food or liquids, enteral nutrition is prescribed. Weigh the patient 3 times a week, and monitor serum prealbumin each week to evaluate nutritional status.

Immobility and malnutrition place patients at risk for pressure ulcers. Assess skin integrity at least daily and with any assisted MOBILITY intervention. While bedbound, ensure the patient is turned a minimum of every 2 hours. Consider the use of pressure-relieving supports after a turn or special mattress or overlay. Document the skin assessment daily. Consult with the skin or wound care expert when changes occur that contribute to pressure ulcer formation (see Chapter 25).

Because venous thromboembolism (VTE) and pulmonary emboli are common complications of immobility, the health care provider may prescribe prophylactic anticoagulant therapy, such as subcutaneous low–molecular-weight heparin. Sequential pneumatic compression devices for legs may be used to promote venous return. Ensure documentation of starting and maintaining VTE prophylaxis; this is a Joint Commission Core Measure of high-quality health care delivery in acute and critical care units.

Managing Pain. Assess the severity and nature of the patient's PAIN, which is often worse at night. The patient may have paresthesia or hyperesthesia (extreme sensitivity to touch), deep muscle aches, and muscle stiffness. The typical pain experienced is severe and requires opioids at least initially for management. Other drugs that are given include gabapentin (Neurontin) or tricyclic antidepressants (Cranwell-Bruce, 2011).

! NURSING SAFETY PRIORITY QSEN

Drug Alert

Older adults should not receive tricyclic drugs because they cause serious anticholinergic effects such as urinary retention, blurred vision, and confusion. These adverse drug events can contribute to cognitive impairment, falls, and injury (see Chapter 2).

Other pain control measures include frequent repositioning, massage, ice, heat, relaxation techniques, guided imagery, hypnosis, and distractions (e.g., music, visitors). Chapter 3 discusses these modalities and other pain-relief measures in detail.

? NCLEX EXAMINATION CHALLENGE

Physiological Integrity

A client is admitted to the critical care unit with possible Guillain-Barré syndrome. Which symptom of neurologic impairment will require priority nursing interventions? **Select all that apply.**

A. New adventitious breath sounds
B. A respiratory rate of 12
C. Rapid, shallow breathing pattern
D. A peripheral oxygen saturation (SpO_2) of 90%
E. New-onset nausea following a position change

Promoting Communication. The patient may have difficulty communicating because the muscles required for the production of speech are weak or he or she may be mechanically ventilated. In either case, collaborate with the speech-language pathologist to develop a communication system. A simple technique involves eye blinking or moving a finger to indicate "yes" and "no." A communication board or flash cards can be used with the letters of the alphabet or a list of common requests, such as the need to be repositioned or the need for pain medication. Computer or handheld mobile devices may also be used, depending on functional ability.

Providing Psychosocial Support. Teach the patient and family about the illness, and explain all diagnostic tests and treatments. Assess the patient and family for verbal and nonverbal behaviors that indicate powerlessness, anxiety, fear, and isolation (Simmons, 2010). Encourage the patient to verbalize feelings about the illness and its effects, if possible, while fostering hope. Assess previous decision-making patterns, roles, and responsibilities. To help identify personal factors that influence coping ability, ask the patient and/or family to describe their usual lifestyles and the situations in which they coped effectively. Sleep disturbances related to PAIN and altered autonomic function may affect the patient's sleep-wake cycle. Allow for regularly scheduled rest periods (Simmons, 2010).

Refer patients who need further psychosocial support to the social worker, certified hospital chaplain or appropriate spiritual resource, and local support groups. If necessary, obtain a psychological consultation for further evaluation and intervention.

Community-Based Care

The severity and course of GBS are variable, which makes the prognosis difficult to predict. The most likely residual deficits at discharge are related to MOBILITY, self-management, altered SENSORY PERCEPTION, and disturbed self-concept. For patients who have total quadriparesis (weakness in all four extremities) or respiratory paralysis, the course of the rehabilitation phase is even more variable and may require weeks to years. The expected outcome of the recovery phase is to move from dependence to independence (Khan & Amatya, 2012).

Planning for discharge begins on admission. Include a family member in the education process throughout the patient's hospitalization and in the discharge process. Provide them with both oral and written instructions to improve adherence to the plan of care and promote continuity during care transitions. The patient may transition to home or skilled care. In collaboration with the discharge planner or case manager (CM), the nurse communicates patient status and summarizes the hospital stay to provide safe transitions in care to a rehabilitation or long-term care setting. If the patient is discharged to home, consider referral to a home health care agency or support group. If assistive devices are needed at home, the CM in collaboration with the interdisciplinary health care team makes certain that the necessary equipment has been delivered after evaluating the home setting. Home care management for patients with GBS is similar to that for those who have had a stroke or spinal cord injury, depending on the nature of the neurologic deficit.

Self-help and support groups for patients with chronic illness are common. Refer the patient and family to these groups, if indicated. For example, the Guillain-Barré Syndrome Foundation International (www.gbs-cidp.org) provides resources and information for patients and their families. The psychosocial adjustment needed may be minimal or dramatic, depending on the patient's residual deficit, age, gender, usual roles and responsibilities, usual coping strategies, available support systems, and occupation. Help the patient identify other support systems, such as church members, friends, or spiritual resources.

? CLINICAL JUDGMENT CHALLENGE

Patient-Centered Care; Safety QSEN

A female patient is admitted to the critical care unit with Guillain-Barré syndrome. She has ascending paralysis to the level of the waist.

1. What is the priority for this patient's care?
2. What health teaching will you provide for this patient about her disease?
3. What options for treatment will she have during this acute phase?
4. What other care will you include in your health teaching?

MYASTHENIA GRAVIS

❖ PATHOPHYSIOLOGY

Myasthenia gravis (MG) is an acquired autoimmune disease characterized by muscle weakness. There are two types of MG: ocular and generalized. About two thirds of patients initially present with reports about vision that arise from disturbances of the ocular muscles. MG may take many forms—from mild disturbances of the cranial and peripheral motor neurons to a rapidly developing, generalized weakness that may lead to death from respiratory failure. MG can present at any age, and the incidence is slightly higher among men. It is a progressive disease.

MG is caused by distorted acetylcholine receptors (AChRs) in the muscle motor end plate membranes. Antibodies are attached to the AChRs. As a result, nerve impulses are reduced at the neuromuscular junction; nerve impulses do not result in muscle contraction. MG and hyperplasia (abnormal growth) of the thymus gland are related because **thymoma** (encapsulated thymus gland tumor) occurs in a few cases.

There are five main classes and several subclasses of MG (Liang & Han, 2013):

- Class I: Any ocular muscle weakness; may have weakness of eye closure; all other muscle strength is normal
- Class II: Mild weakness affecting other than ocular muscles; may also have ocular muscle weakness of any severity:
  - Class IIa: Predominantly affecting limb, axial muscles, or both; may also have lesser involvement of oropharyngeal muscles
  - Class IIb: Predominantly affecting oropharyngeal, respiratory muscles, or both; may also have lesser or equal involvement of limb, axial muscles, or both
- Class III: Moderate weakness affecting other than ocular muscles; may also have ocular weakness of any severity:
  - Class IIIb: Predominantly affecting oropharyngeal, respiratory muscles, or both; may also have lesser or equal involvement of limb, axial muscles, or both;
- Class IV: Severe weakness affecting other than ocular muscles; may also have ocular muscle weakness of any severity:
  - Class IVa: Predominantly affecting limb, axial muscles, or both; may also have lesser involvement of oropharyngeal muscles

- Class IVb: Predominantly affecting oropharyngeal, respiratory muscles, or both; may also have lesser or equal involvement of limb, axial muscles, or both; use of a feeding tube to avoid aspiration and maintain nutrition
- Class V: Defined by the need for intubation, with or without mechanical ventilation, except when used during routine postoperative management

❖ PATIENT-CENTERED COLLABORATIVE CARE

◆ Assessment

Physical Assessment/Clinical Manifestations. In addition to the biographic data and history, ask the patient about specific muscle weakness (Abbott, 2010). Although the onset of MG is usually insidious (slow), some instances of fairly rapid development have been caused by infection, pregnancy, or anesthesia. A temporary increase in weakness may be noted after vaccination, menstruation, and exposure to extremes in environmental temperature. The course of the disease may have periods of exacerbation or flares when symptoms worsen. Ask the patient when symptoms worsen, specifically noting the affected muscle groups and any limitation or inability in performing ADLs. Anticipate worsening symptoms with repetitive muscle use. Determine the reason for admission to plan care. Patients with MG are typically hospitalized for diagnostic evaluation, myasthenic or cholinergic crisis resulting in respiratory failure, or periods of exacerbation when GAS EXCHANGE is threatened.

Additional areas of inquiry include any history of **ptosis** (drooping eyelids), **diplopia** (double vision), or **dysphagia** (difficulty chewing or swallowing) and the type of diet best tolerated. Assess the patient about a history of respiratory difficulty, choking, or voice weakness. Other areas of assessment include asking about any difficulty holding up the head, brushing teeth, combing hair, or shaving. Assess for the presence of paresthesias or aching in weakened muscles. Finally, ask about a history of thymus gland tumor. The most common symptoms of MG are related to involvement of the levator palpebrae or extraocular muscles (Chart 44-3). These symptoms may last only a few days at the onset and then resolve, only to return weeks or months later. Pupillary responses to light and accommodation are usually normal.

For most patients, the muscles of facial expression, chewing, and speech are affected (**bulbar** involvement). Note the patient's smile, which may be transformed into a snarl. The jaw may hang so that the patient must prop it up with the hand. Chewing and swallowing difficulties, choking, and regurgitation of fluids through the nose may lead to considerable weight loss. Ask about the patient's nutritional intake and any recent weight loss. He or she may have more difficulty eating after talking. After extended conversations, the voice may become weaker or exhibit a nasal twang. In some patients, the tongue has fissures (ulcers).

Less often involved are the muscles of the shoulders, the flexors of the neck, and the hip flexors. Because limb weakness is more often *proximal* (closer to the body), the patient may have difficulty climbing stairs, lifting heavy objects, or raising the arms overhead. Neck weakness may be mild or severe enough to cause difficulty in holding the head erect. Among the trunk muscles, the erector spinae are most commonly affected, causing difficulty maintaining a sitting or walking posture.

In the most advanced cases of MG, all muscles are weakened, including those associated with respiratory function and the control of bladder and bowel. In these severe cases, ask about bowel and bladder function. Assess respiratory rate, depth, pattern, and Spo_2 frequently to ensure adequate GAS EXCHANGE.

Muscle atrophy, although rarely severe, occurs in a small percentage of patients with MG. The tendon reflexes should be assessed, but they are not often affected. Assess for pain, although this is seldom a major concern. Some patients report that their weakened muscles ache. If present, paresthesias (painful tingling sensations) affecting the muscles of the face, hands, and thighs are not associated with any loss of sensation. Lost or decreased sensations of smell and taste have been reported. Consciousness is not altered.

In **Eaton-Lambert syndrome**, a form of myasthenia often seen with small cell carcinoma of the lung, the muscles of the trunk and the pelvic and shoulder girdles are most commonly affected. Although weakness increases after exertion, muscle strength may temporarily increase during the first few contractions, followed by rapid decline. Diagnosis is confirmed by electromyography (EMG). Management differs somewhat from that of other types of MG. Treatment includes removing the tumor, managing the cancer, and administering drug therapy to release acetylcholine (ACh). Additional therapies may include plasmapheresis and immunosuppressive therapy (discussed later).

Diagnostic Assessment. Because the incidence of MG is rare, diagnosis may be delayed or missed (Abbott, 2010). An experienced clinician can diagnose the disease from the history and physical examination findings. MG may be immediately confirmed by the patient's response to cholinergic drugs. A standard series of laboratory studies is usually performed for patients with known or suspected MG. *Thyroid function* should be tested because **thyrotoxicosis** (excessive thyroid hormone) is present in a small number of myasthenic patients. *Serum protein electrophoresis* evaluates the patient for immunologic disorders. Immunologic-based diseases, such as rheumatoid arthritis, systemic lupus erythematous, and polymyositis, may be associated with the disease (Pagana & Pagana, 2014).

Several types of antibodies are found in the majority of patients with MG and include forms directed against the acetylcholine receptor (AChR) and the enzyme *muscle-specific receptor tyrosine kinase* (MuSK). However, whereas a positive antibody test confirms the diagnosis, a negative finding does not rule out the disease.

Some patients with MG have a thymoma, and therefore patients are assessed for this condition. The thymus, an H-shaped gland located in the upper mediastinum beneath the

CHART 44-3 Key Features

Myasthenia Gravis

Motor Manifestations
- Progressive (proximal) muscle weakness that worsens with repetitive use and usually improves with rest
- Poor posture
- Ocular palsies
- Ptosis; incomplete eyelid closure
- Diplopia
- Respiratory compromise
- Loss of bowel and bladder control
- Fatigue

Sensory Manifestations
- Muscle achiness
- Paresthesias
- Decreased sense of smell and taste

sternum, is where B- and T-cells interact, refining self-recognition of these white blood cells. It is hypothesized that thymic abnormalities cause the breakdown in tolerance that causes the immune-mediated attack on AChR in myasthenia gravis. A thymoma can be seen on a chest *x-ray* or a *CT scan.*

The most common electrodiagnostic test performed to detect MG is *repetitive nerve stimulation (RNS)* of proximal nerves. Each nerve studied is electrically stimulated 6 to 10 times at 2 or 3 Hertz. The compound muscle action potential (CMAP) is recorded with surface electrodes over muscle. In MG, there is a progressive decline in CMAP amplitude (force, or strength) with the first 4 or 5 stimuli. This test diagnoses most cases of generalized MG but far fewer cases of ocular MG.

During *electromyography* (EMG) to diagnose MG, a recording electrode is placed into skeletal muscle and the electrical activity of skeletal muscle can be monitored in a way similar to electrocardiography (ECG) (Pagana & Pagana, 2014). A progressive decrease in the amplitude of the electrical waveform is a classic sign of MG. This study can be combined with nerve conduction studies and may be called an *electromyoneurography.* It can be performed at the bedside by a technician.

Single-fiber EMG (SFEMG) is a newer and most sensitive form of electromyography in detecting defects of neuromuscular transmission. This test compares the stability of the firing of one muscle fiber with that of another fiber innervated by the same motor neuron. The time interval between the two firings normally shows a minor degree of variability, called *jitter.* Defective transmission increases jitter or actually blocks successive discharges. This test can diagnose almost all cases of generalized and ocular MG.

Pharmacologic tests with the cholinesterase inhibitors *edrophonium chloride (Tensilon)* and *neostigmine bromide (Prostigmin)* may be performed. This older test is often referred to as a *Tensilon challenge test.* Tensilon is used most often for testing because of its rapid onset and brief duration of action. This drug inhibits the breakdown of ACh at the postsynaptic membrane, which increases the availability of ACh for excitation of postsynaptic receptors. To perform the test, the health care provider first estimates the strength of cranial muscles. Initially, 2 mg (0.2 mL) is injected IV; if this is tolerated, an additional 8 mg (0.8 mL) is injected after 30 seconds. Within 30 to 60 seconds of the first dose, most myasthenic patients show a marked improvement in muscle tone that lasts 4 to 5 minutes. False-positive test results may be caused by increased muscle effort by the patient. False-negative findings may be seen if the tested muscle is extremely weak or refractory to the drug.

Tensilon testing may be used also to help determine whether increasing weakness in the previously diagnosed myasthenic patient is due to a **cholinergic crisis** (too much cholinesterase inhibitor drugs) or a **myasthenic crisis** (too little cholinesterase inhibitor drugs). In a cholinergic crisis, muscle tone does not improve after giving Tensilon. Instead, weakness may actually increase, and **fasciculations** (muscle twitching) may be seen around the eyes and face.

! NURSING SAFETY PRIORITY QSEN

Drug Alert

The Tensilon test can cause cardiac dysrhythmias and cardiac arrest, but these reactions rarely occur. Be sure that atropine sulfate, the antidote for Tensilon, is available in case these complications occur.

◆ *Interventions*

MG is one of the most treatable neurologic disorders. The classic presentation of MG is muscle weakness that increases when the patient is fatigued and limits his or her MOBILITY and ability to participate in activities. Management for this disease falls into two categories:

- Treatment that affects the symptoms of MG without influencing the actual course of the disease (anticholinesterases or cholinergic drugs)
- Therapeutic efforts for inducing remission, such as the administration of immunosuppressive drugs or corticosteroids, plasmapheresis, and thymectomy (removal of the thymus gland)

Nonsurgical Management. *Although not all patients with MG have respiratory compromise, ongoing assessment and maintenance of respiratory gas exchange are nursing care priorities.*

Providing Respiratory Support. Both myasthenic crisis and cholinergic crisis increase muscle weakness and the patient's risk for respiratory compromise. The diaphragm and intercostal muscles may be affected, which inhibits the patient's ability to maintain adequate GAS EXCHANGE, breathe deeply, and cough effectively. In addition, dysphagia may result in the aspiration of foods, fluids, or saliva, which worsens the respiratory problems. Because of their respiratory muscle involvement, many of these patients have an increased risk for lung infections.

The patient who cannot cough effectively may require oropharyngeal or nasopharyngeal suctioning. If needed, teach the assisted-cough technique, similar to that used by patients who are quadriplegic. Collaborate with the respiratory therapist (RT) to provide chest physiotherapy consisting of postural drainage, percussion, and vibration to mobilize secretions and improve GAS EXCHANGE.

! NURSING SAFETY PRIORITY QSEN

Critical Rescue

Keep a bag-valve-mask setup (e.g., Ambu), equipment for oxygen administration, and suction equipment at the bedside of the patient with myasthenia gravis in case of respiratory distress.

Because breathing difficulty or the inability to breathe easily is frightening, be aware of the patient's mental and emotional status during periods of respiratory compromise. Monitor his or her response to drug therapy for muscle weakness. Monitor for pulmonary congestion that can lead to respiratory complications like pneumonia and atelectasis.

Noninvasive mechanical ventilation (NIMV) can be used to support patients with acute respiratory failure from MG crisis while awaiting improvement from IV immunoglobulin (IVIG) therapy or plasma exchange. Chapter 32 explains further about NIMV.

Promoting Mobility. Assess the patient's muscle strength before and after periods of activity. Provide assistance as necessary to prevent the patient from becoming fatigued. Schedule him or her for tests, treatments, and other activities early in the day or during the energy peaks after giving the prescribed drugs. Assist the patient in planning the periods of rest.

During periods of maximum weakness, provide assistance with positioning and activity. Assess for skin breakdown with each repositioning intervention. Pressure-reducing devices or mattresses are used to help prevent pressure ulcers. Collaborate with the physical and occupational therapists to develop a program for the patient to assist with MOBILITY, self-care, and energy conservation techniques. Chapter 6 discusses rehabilitation as one strategy to improve functional ability after a period of immobility, and Chapter 25 describes strategies to prevent and manage pressure ulcers.

Administering Drug Therapy. Two groups of drugs are typically prescribed for the treatment of myasthenia gravis (MG): anticholinesterases and immunosuppressants. Be sure to *give these drugs on time to maintain blood levels and thus improve muscle strength.* Monitor and document the patient's response to drug therapy. Provide information for the patient and the family about the indications for, effectiveness of, and side effects of the drugs used in the treatment of MG.

Cholinesterase Inhibitor Drugs. *Cholinesterase (ChE) inhibitor drugs are the first-line management of MG.* These drugs are also referred to as *anticholinesterase drugs* or *antimyasthenics.* They enhance neuromuscular impulse transmission by preventing the decrease of ACh by the enzyme *ChE.* This increases the response of the muscles to nerve impulses and improves muscle strength. The ChE inhibitor drug of choice is pyridostigmine (Mestinon, Regonol). Expect a day-to-day variation in dosage depending on the patient's changing symptoms.

Administer ChE inhibitors with a small amount of food to help alleviate GI side effects.

! NURSING SAFETY PRIORITY (QSEN)

Drug Alert

Instruct the patient to eat meals 45 minutes to 1 hour after taking ChE inhibitors to avoid aspiration. This is especially important if the patient has bulbar involvement. Drugs containing magnesium, morphine or its derivatives, curare, quinine, quinidine, procainamide, or hypnotics or sedatives should be avoided because they may increase the patient's weakness. Antibiotics such as neomycin and certain tetracyclines impair transmitter release and also increase myasthenic symptoms (Lilley et al., 2014).

A potential adverse effect of ChE inhibitors is cholinergic crisis. Sudden increases in weakness accompanied by hypersalivation, sweating, and increased bronchial secretions help identify this as a cholinergic crisis rather than a myasthenic crisis. A cholinergic crisis is more likely to be associated with nausea, vomiting, and diarrhea. Teach the patient and family to monitor for these two types of crises:

1. Myasthenic crisis—an exacerbation (flare-up or worsening) of the myasthenic symptoms caused by not enough anticholinesterase drugs
2. Cholinergic crisis—an acute exacerbation of muscle weakness caused by too many anticholinesterase drugs

Because myasthenic and cholinergic crises have many common characteristics, the type of crisis the patient is experiencing must be identified for effective treatment to be provided (Table 44-1). Monitor carefully for early detection of these emergencies if the patient is in a health care setting.

Emergency Care: Myasthenic Crisis. Myasthenic crisis is often caused by some type of infection. For other patients, increasing muscle weakness leads to an overdose of anticholinesterase drugs. As a result, the patient may experience a *mixed* crisis. The Tensilon test (described on p. 919), although not always conclusive, is an important procedure for differentiation. *Tensilon produces a temporary improvement in myasthenic crisis but worsening or no improvement of symptoms in cholinergic crisis.*

TABLE 44-1 Characteristics of Myasthenic and Cholinergic Crises

MYASTHENIC CRISIS	CHOLINERGIC CRISIS	FEATURES COMMON TO BOTH
Increased pulse and respiration Rise in blood pressure Bowel and bladder incontinence Decreased urine output Absence of cough and swallow reflex Improvement of symptoms with Tensilon test*	Flaccid paralysis Hypersecretion: salivation, tearing, and sweating Nausea Vomiting Diarrhea Abdominal cramps Miosis, blurred vision Pallor Worsening of symptoms with Tensilon test	Apprehension Restlessness Dyspnea Dysphagia (difficult swallowing) Generalized weakness Respiratory failure

*Tensilon test: Edrophonium (Tensilon) is given intravenously; muscle movement improves immediately in patients with myasthenia or myasthenia crisis.

The priority for nursing management of the patient in myasthenic crisis is maintaining adequate respiratory function to promote GAS EXCHANGE. The acutely ill patient may need intensive nursing care for monitoring. He or she may require mechanical ventilation or other technologic support. Cholinesterase-inhibiting drugs are withheld because they increase respiratory secretions and are usually ineffective for the first few days after the crisis begins. Drug therapy is restarted gradually and at lower dosages.

Emergency Care: Cholinergic Crisis. In *cholinergic* crisis, do not give anticholinesterase drugs while the patient is maintained with mechanical ventilation. Atropine 1 mg IV may be given and repeated, if necessary. When atropine is prescribed, observe the patient carefully. Secretions can be thickened by the drug, which causes more difficulty with airway clearance and possibly the development of mucus plugs. Unless complications such as pneumonia or aspiration develop, the patient in crisis improves rapidly after the appropriate drugs have been given. Continue to provide assistance as necessary because he or she tires easily after minimal exertion.

Immunosuppressants. Immunosuppression may be accomplished with the use of corticosteroids, methotrexate, a chemotherapeutic agent, or rituximab, a biologic agent effective against B-cells (Diaz-Manera et al., 2012). B-cells are lymphocytes active in antibody formation (see Chapter 17). For ocular MG, corticosteroid treatment that does not cause significant systemic complications may significantly reduce the prevalence of generalized myasthenia gravis after 2 years on the drug. IV immunoglobulins (IVIGs) may also be used for acute disease management or as a long-term option for disease refractory to other treatment.

Other Interventions. **Plasmapheresis** is a method by which antibodies are removed from the plasma to decrease symptoms. This is used as short-term management of an exacerbation. Six exchanges occur over a 2-week period with follow-up exchanges weekly or monthly as needed, usually as an ambulatory care patient. Nursing management of the patient undergoing plasmapheresis is presented in the earlier discussion of Guillain-Barré syndrome, p. 915, and Chart 44-2.

Generalized weakness and fatigue affect the patient's ability to participate in ADLs. Impaired fine motor control and shoulder weakness, which results in difficulty raising the arms, can compound the problem. Self-care deficits may be complete or partial depending on the severity of the illness or the patient's response to drugs.

Assess the patient's ability to perform ADLs. Although he or she is encouraged to perform activities as independently as possible, assistance is provided as needed to avoid frustration and fatigue. *For maximizing independence and making attempts at self-management successful, plan activities to follow the administration of medication.* Monitor and document the patient's response to or tolerance of activity, providing periods of rest after an activity. *Rest is critical because repetitive movement can precipitate a crisis.* Occupational and physical therapists evaluate patients for assistive-adaptive devices. In collaboration with the nurse, they also teach the patient and family energy conservation techniques and ideas for making work and self-management easier after discharge from the hospital.

Weakness of the speech and facial muscles often results in dysarthric (slurred) and nasal speech. In collaboration with the speech-language pathologist (SLP), determine the patient's ability to communicate. Instruct the patient to speak slowly while attempting to lip-read. Repeat what the patient says to check that it is correct. Questions that can be answered with "yes" or "no" or by gestures may be used along with other communication systems such as eye blinking, notebook and pencil, computer, handheld mobile devices, and picture, letter, or word boards.

The patient with myasthenia gravis (MG) may have difficulty maintaining an adequate intake of food and fluid because the muscles needed for chewing and swallowing become weakened and tire easily. In collaboration with the dietitian, occupational therapist, and speech-language pathologist, evaluate the patient's nutritional status and his or her ability to receive adequate oral nutrition. High-calorie snacks are often well tolerated. Monitor the effectiveness of the nutrition program by recording the patient's calorie counts, intake and output, serum prealbumin levels, and daily weights (Chart 44-4). If he or she cannot swallow, a feeding tube may be used.

The patient's inability to completely close the eyes may lead to corneal abrasions and further decrease vision and comfort. During the day, apply artificial tears to keep the corneas moist and free from abrasion. A lubricant gel and shield may be applied to the eyes at bedtime to provide more extensive coverage. To help relieve diplopia, cover the eyes with a patch for 2 to 3 hours at a time, one eye at a time. At times, patients tape their eyes shut at night.

Surgical Management. For patients with MG, **thymectomy** (removal of the thymus gland) is usually performed early in the disease. The procedure is not always immediately effective. Those who have surgery within 2 years of the onset of myasthenic symptoms show the most improvement, but many patients do not experience a change in status despite thymectomy.

Provide routine preoperative care as discussed in Chapter 14. Because there is no way to predict whether remission or improvement will occur, it is important to avoid making promises but be optimistic. Immediately before surgery, pyridostigmine (Mestinon) may be given with a small amount of water to keep the patient stable during and after surgery. If steroids have been used, they are also given before surgery and are tapered during the postoperative period. Antibiotics are administered immediately before or during the surgery. Plasmapheresis may be used before and after surgery to decrease circulating antibodies.

CHART 44-4 Best Practice for Patient Safety & Quality Care QSEN

Improving Nutrition in Patients with Myasthenia Gravis

- Assess the patient's gag reflex and ability to chew and swallow.
- Provide frequent oral hygiene as needed.
- Collaborate with the dietitian, speech-language pathologist, and occupational therapist to plan and implement meals that the patient can eat and enjoy.
- Cut food into small bites or request a soft or edentulous diet, and encourage the patient to eat slowly.
- Observe the patient for choking, nasal regurgitation, and aspiration.
- Provide high-calorie snacks or supplements (e.g., puddings).
- Keep the head of the bed elevated during meals and for 30 to 60 minutes after the patient eats.
- Consider thickening liquids to avoid choking or aspiration.
- Monitor caloric and food intake.
- Weigh the patient daily.
- Monitor serum prealbumin levels.
- Administer anticholinesterase drugs as prescribed, usually 45 to 60 minutes before meals.

One of two surgical approaches may be used: the transcervical incision (minimal access technique) or the sternal split. The *transcervical approach* is becoming more popular because it allows more rapid recovery with less discomfort after surgery, especially if done using the video-assisted thoracoscopic surgery (VATS) technique. However, this procedure is used only for patients who do not have a thymoma. Only a small dressing and an IV line are needed after surgery.

The older *sternal split* procedure is preferred when patients have a thymoma. It allows the surgeon to directly see the mediastinum and areas around the thymus. When thymoma is present, all surrounding involved structures (i.e., the pericardium, the innominate vein, a portion of the superior vena cava, and a portion of the lung) are removed. A single chest tube is placed in the anterior mediastinum. The patient is usually admitted to the critical care unit after surgery. Thymoma should be considered as a potentially malignant tumor requiring prolonged follow-up. The presence of myasthenic weakness can still complicate its management.

Although patients with adequate respiratory effort and GAS EXCHANGE may be extubated immediately after surgery, most require a gradual weaning from the ventilator. Prolonged ventilatory assistance is rare. *After the patient is extubated, pay special attention to respiratory status and maintaining a patent airway.* Encourage the patient to turn, breathe deeply 3 to 6 times every 15 to 30 minutes in the hours after extubation, and use incentive spirometry.

For the sternal surgical technique, provide chest tube care (see Chapter 32). Both surgical approaches require sterile technique for wound care. Observe the patient for signs of infection, such as increasing or purulent drainage; redness, warmth, or swelling around the wound; and elevated temperature. Patient and family teaching about follow-up care is needed before discharge from the hospital.

NURSING SAFETY PRIORITY QSEN

Critical Rescue

For the patient having a thymectomy, monitor respiratory effort and promote effective GAS EXCHANGE. Observe for signs of pneumothorax or hemothorax, including:
- Chest pain
- Sudden shortness of breath
- Diminished or delayed chest wall expansion
- Diminished or absent breath sounds
- Restlessness or a change in vital signs (decreasing blood pressure or a weak, rapid pulse)

If respiratory distress or symptoms of ineffective gas exchange occur, provide oxygen to the patient and raise the head of the bed to at least 45 degrees. Then report any of these signs and symptoms to the surgeon or Rapid Response Team immediately!

Community-Based Care

The patient with myasthenia gravis (MG) may be cared for in a variety of settings, including the home, long-term acute care facility, rehabilitation setting, or skilled nursing facility. The patient discharged from the hospital may require the assistance of a family member, home care nurse, physical therapist (PT), occupational therapist (OT), and/or home care aide.

Home Care Management. Patients with MG are often managed at home. Unless the patient requires new assistive devices, little preparation of the home setting is required. In collaboration with physical and occupational therapists, the case manager (CM) and nurse make certain that the necessary equipment has been delivered and properly installed. Teach the patient and family members how to use the equipment safely. If the patient becomes wheelchair dependent, the discharge planner, CM, or OT checks on any necessary modifications to the home (e.g., the installation of ramps or widening of doorways) that have been completed. Home health care can provide assistance in transitioning from acute to home care.

Self-Management Education. The patient and family need to know about the disease and the drugs used for treatment. Discuss the episodic nature of the disease, including factors that increase the risk for exacerbation, such as infection, stress, surgery, hard physical exercise, sedatives, and enemas or strong cathartics (Table 44-2). Teach the patient the importance of collaborating with the health care team to monitor muscle strength, ability to perform ADLs, and the need to evaluate and adjust drug therapy.

Stress the importance of lifestyle adaptations such as avoiding heat (e.g., sauna, hot tubs, sunbathing), crowds, overeating, erratic changes in sleep habits, or emotional extremes. Teach the signs of exacerbation, such as increased weakness, increased diplopia, ptosis, and problems with chewing or swallowing. Remind the patient to plan activities to allow for rest periods and to conserve energy.

Provide the drug regimen in a written format that includes the names, purposes, dosages, scheduled dosage times, and side effects of the drugs. Explain that the drugs are normally taken before activities such as eating, participating in sports, or working. Stress the importance of maintaining therapeutic blood levels by taking the medications on time and as prescribed and not missing or postponing doses (Chart 44-5). In addition, inform the patient of the side effects of anticholinesterase drugs and drugs that can worsen symptoms, such as corticosteroids, narcotics, antidysrhythmics, and antimalarials.

TABLE 44-2 Factors Precipitating or Worsening Myasthenia Gravis

- Various drugs, including:
  - Strong cathartics
  - Antidysrhythmics
  - Beta-blocking agents
  - Aminoglycosides and other antibiotics
  - Antirheumatic drugs
  - Antispasmodics, including quinine
  - Antihistamines
  - Opioids
  - Phenytoin (Dilantin)
  - Antidepressants (tricyclics)
- Rheumatoid arthritis
- Alcohol
- Hormonal changes
- Stress
- Infection
- Seasonal temperature changes
- Heat
- Surgery
- Enemas

CHART 44-5 Patient and Family Education: Preparing for Self-Management

Helpful Hints for Teaching Patients with Myasthenia Gravis About Drug Therapy

- Keep prescribed drugs and a glass of water at your bedside if you are weak in the morning.
- Wear a watch with an alarm function (or beeper) to remind you to take your drugs.
- Post your drug schedule so others know it.
- Plan strenuous activities, when possible, when the drug peaks.
- Keep a secure supply of drugs in your car or at work.
- Check with your health care provider before using any over-the-counter drugs.

Check with the pharmacist before starting or stopping drugs. In preparing the patient for discharge, explain the signs and symptoms of myasthenic and cholinergic crises and the need to contact the health care provider whenever either type of crisis is suspected.

NURSING SAFETY PRIORITY QSEN

Action Alert

Because respiratory compromise often occurs in myasthenic patients, encourage family members to learn resuscitation procedures. A manual resuscitation bag, suctioning equipment, and oxygen should be available in the home for patients susceptible to crises. Teach family members in the proper use of equipment.

The episodic and progressive nature of MG, the potential or actual loss of independence, and body image changes (e.g., the inability to smile) affect the patient's adjustment. During discharge planning, the CM considers factors such as age, gender, usual roles and responsibilities, available support systems, occupation, and financial status. Because the patient's and family's need for psychosocial adjustment may range from minimal to dramatic, the CM remains sensitive to their needs and provides information and support. Encourage family members or significant others to discuss their feelings with one another.

Health Care Resources. In collaboration with the health care provider, patient, and family, the staff nurse or CM may initiate referrals to home care agencies and to local self-help groups for people who have chronic illnesses and their families. The

Myasthenia Gravis Foundation (www.myasthenia.org) provides education and research programs and assistance with financial aid and community resources. Support groups are also available. Teach the patient the importance of obtaining and wearing a medical alert (MedicAlert) bracelet or necklace and to carry a medical alert identification card at all times.

PERIPHERAL NERVE TRAUMA

❖ PATHOPHYSIOLOGY

The peripheral nerves are subject to injuries associated with mechanical injury, vehicular crashes, sports, the injection of particular drugs, military conflicts or wars, and acts of violence (e.g., knife or gunshot wounds). Most commonly affected are the median, ulnar, and radial nerves of the arms and the peroneal, femoral, and sciatic nerves of the legs (Fig. 44-1). Specific mechanisms of injury to a peripheral nerve include:

- Partial or complete severance
- Contusion, stretching, constriction, or compression
- Ischemia
- Electrical, thermal, or radiation exposure

Six degrees of peripheral nerve injury can occur (Novak, 2012):

- First-degree nerve injury (neuropraxia) involves a temporary conduction block with demyelination of the nerve at the site of injury. EMG study results are normal above and below the level of injury, and no denervation muscle changes are present. Once the nerve has remyelinated at that area, complete recovery occurs. Recovery may take up to 12 weeks.
- Second-degree nerve injury (axonotmesis) results from a more severe trauma or compression. This causes degeneration distal to the level of injury and proximal axonal degeneration to at least the next node of Ranvier. In more severe traumatic injuries, the proximal degeneration may extend beyond the next node of Ranvier. EMG studies demonstrate denervation changes in the affected muscles. In cases of reinnervation, motor unit potentials (MUPs) are present. Axonal regeneration occurs at the rate of 1 mm/day or 1 inch/month and can be monitored by the physiatrist or physical therapist.
- Third-degree injury is more severe than a second-degree injury and causes degeneration. EMG studies demonstrate denervation changes with fibrillations in the affected muscles. In cases of reinnervation, MUPs are present. Regeneration occurs at 1 mm/day. However, with the increased severity of the injury, regenerating axons may not reinnervate their original motor and sensory targets. The pattern of recovery is mixed and incomplete. Reinnervation occurs only if sensory fibers grow into a different area within the nerve's sensory distribution. If

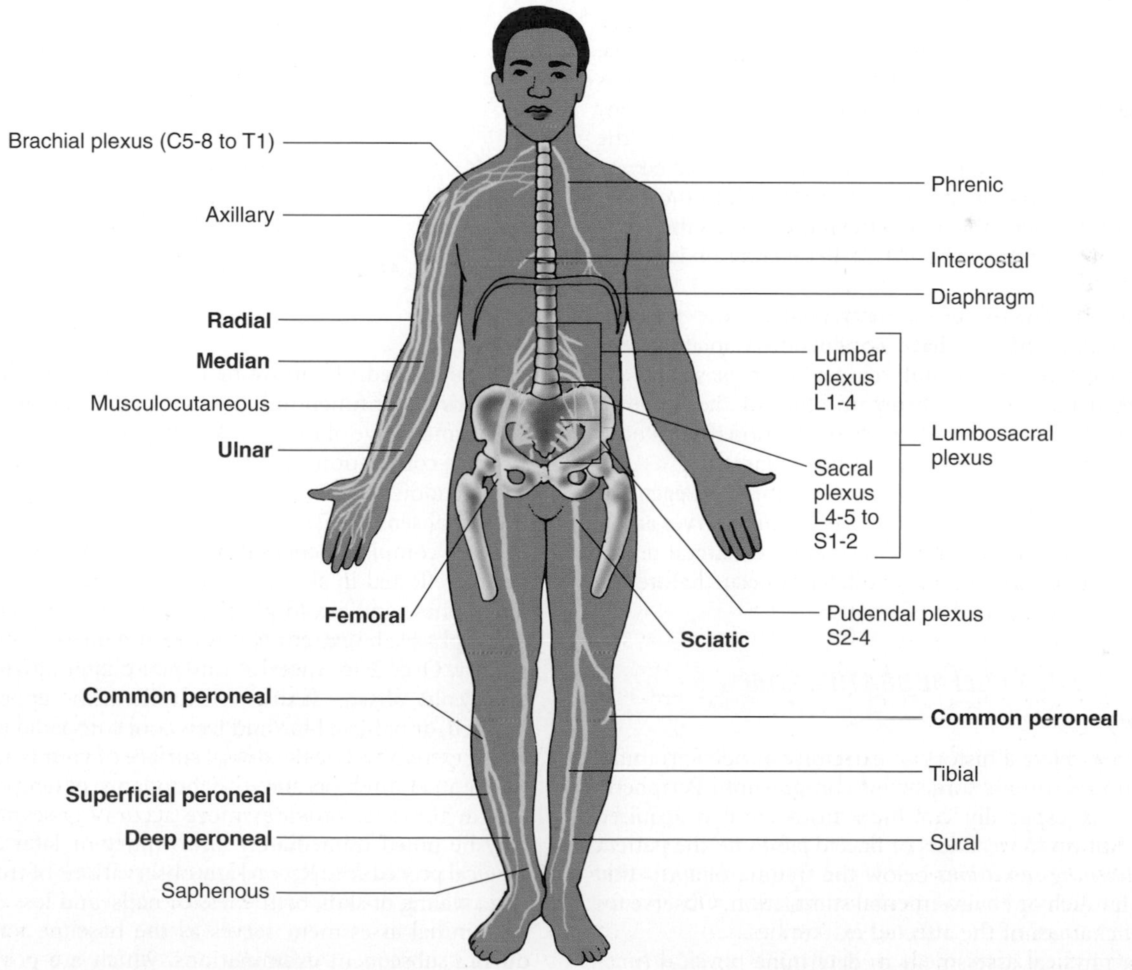

FIG. 44-1 Distribution of selected peripheral nerves in the body. The nerves most commonly affected by trauma are highlighted in bold type.

the muscle target is a long distance from the site of injury, nerve regeneration may occur. The muscle may not be completely reinnervated because of the long period of denervation.

- Fourth-degree injury results in a large scar at the site of nerve injury and prevents any axons from advancing distal to the level of nerve injury. EMG studies reveal denervation changes in the affected muscles. No improvement in motor function is noted, and the patient requires surgery to restore neural continuity, thus permitting axonal regeneration and motor and sensory reinnervation.
- Fifth-degree injury is a complete transection (cutting across) of the nerve. Similar to a fourth-degree injury, it requires surgery to restore neural continuity. EMG findings are the same as those for a fourth-degree injury.
- Sixth-degree injury describes a mixed nerve injury that combines the other degrees of injury. This commonly occurs when some fascicles of the nerve are working normally while other fascicles may be recovering. Other fascicles may require surgical intervention to permit axonal regeneration.

Injuries to the peripheral nerves may result in loss of motor function (reduced MOBILITY), sensory function (impaired SENSORY PERCEPTION), or both. After a nerve is cut or damaged, the nerve distal to the injury degenerates and retracts within 24 hours. Motor and sensory dysfunction below the injury coincides with the loss of electrical excitability. Recovery occurs as Schwann cells of the neurilemma regenerate from both the proximal and distal stumps. Dividing mitotically, these cells form neurilemmal cords, which act as guidelines for the regenerating axon. Tiny unmyelinated sprouts are generated at the proximal axon and grow daily. Some can cross a transected gap through guidance by the neurilemma and reattach to the distal stump. The better aligned the union, the more normal the physical functional ability return (Fig. 44-2). Reinnervation is always a slow process.

Successfully realigned nerves remyelinate, grow to their former size, and eventually have conduction velocities near their former capacity. Successful reinnervation is slowed by infection and increasing age. Disorganization of the nerve or mismatched realignments may result in functional weakness, unintentional muscle movements, and poor sensation.

Some SENSORY PERCEPTION may return before the regeneration process can occur. This return occurs because nerves above the injured neurons are stimulated to produce collateral innervation to the affected areas. These collaterals occur before the injured axon has regenerated sufficiently.

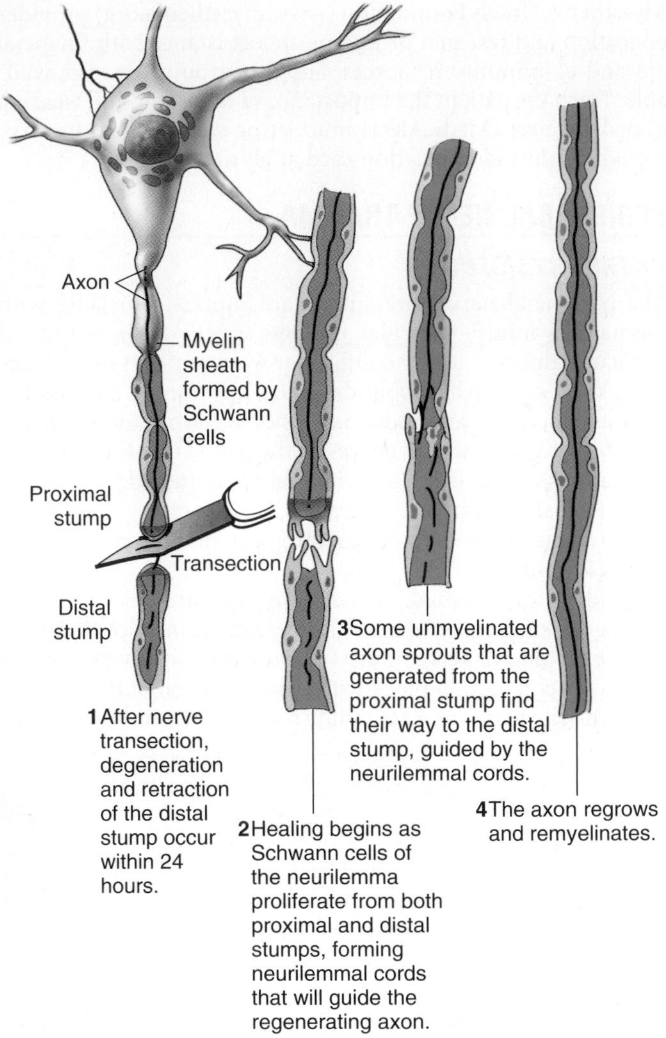

FIG. 44-2 Regeneration of peripheral nerve after injury.

❖ PATIENT-CENTERED COLLABORATIVE CARE

◆ Assessment

The patient may relate a history of extremity or pelvic trauma, penetrating injury, recent surgery, or compression. Peripheral nerve trauma is especially common from combat-acquired injuries. In addition to weakness or flaccid *paralysis,* the patient may report *burning sensations* below the trauma or PAIN that increases with touch or environmental stimulation. Observe for skin and nail changes of the affected extremities.

Perform a physical assessment to determine physical function. In acute trauma, the injury should first be evaluated by the health care provider to determine whether movement is contraindicated. If movement is not contraindicated, the patient's motor function is assessed by putting the limb through the normal range of motion. Any abnormal movements, tremor, atrophy, contractions, paresis or paralysis, and weak or absent deep tendon reflexes are documented. Ask the patient about abnormal sensations.

After complete denervation, the extent of vasomotor function is reflected in skin temperature, skin color, and edema. A warm phase and a cold phase have been identified. During the **warm phase**, the extremity is warm and the skin appears flushed or rosy. Over 2 to 3 weeks, this phase is gradually superseded by a **cold phase**, during which the skin appears cyanotic, mottled, or reddish blue and feels cool compared with the unaffected extremity. Use the dorsal surface of your hand to compare skin temperatures because the abundance of temperature receptors in this area provides more accurate assessments. Edema may be noted immediately after injury or later as a result of surgical procedures. Record any observations of trophic changes (e.g., scaling of skin, brittleness of nails, and loss of body hair). This initial assessment serves as the baseline for comparison during subsequent examinations, which are performed every 2 to 4 hours or less frequently as the patient's condition indicates.

◆ Interventions

Interventions for the patient with peripheral nerve trauma depend on the location as well as the type and degree of injury. If the nerve trauma results from a primary lesion, such as a tumor, the underlying problem is addressed first (Walsh, 2012).

The health care provider may prescribe immobilization of the involved area by splint, cast, or traction to provide the rest needed to limit and resolve any INFLAMMATION. The purpose of surgical management is to restore the function of the damaged nerve. There are usually no special preoperative interventions for the patient undergoing peripheral nerve repair. Chapter 14 describes the general care of the patient before surgery.

If the nerve is lacerated or transected, surgery may be indicated. Restorative procedures include resecting and suturing to realign the severed nerve ends, nerve grafts, and nerve and tendon transplants.

The timing of procedures to repair nerves has been controversial. In the past, a repair delay of 3 to 8 weeks after injury allowed associated injuries to heal, after which the surgeon could better assess the extent of nerve damage. Although microsurgery and the use of lasers now allow primary nerve repair at the time of injury, the surgeon's judgment in selecting the optimal time and surgical procedure remains crucial.

After an injury, the two severed nerve segments contract and may form scar tissue. Before surgical anastomosis, the surgeon dissects these stumps to remove any damaged nerve tissue. This further decreases the lengths of the ends to be joined. To compensate for this shortening and to avoid excessive tension on the sutured nerve, the involved extremity is positioned in exaggerated flexion. The surgeon aligns the segments under magnification, bringing the nerve fiber ends together, and then sutures the nerve tissue.

After suturing, the extremity is placed in a cast to maintain the flexed position and to avoid tension on the suture line. Ten to 14 days after nerve repair, the entire dressing is removed, the joint flexion is eased, and a new splint may be applied for an additional 2 weeks. At that time, a removable splint may be applied and physical therapy begun. Protection of the nerve sutures is continued for a minimum of 6 weeks.

If a large segment of nerve has been damaged and direct anastomosis would be impossible without stretching the nerve, the surgeon may insert a *nerve graft.* Motor and sensory axons may regenerate through the graft, joining the nerve segments through the two sites of anastomosis. The results of grafting are not usually as favorable as with direct anastomosis. Immobilization by splints or casts to facilitate healing of the surgical sites is essential.

Splints are usually held in place with elastic wrapping or hook-and-loop (Velcro) closures, which can become too tight if edema develops.

! NURSING SAFETY PRIORITY (QSEN)

Critical Rescue

Perform frequent neurovascular assessments after surgical nerve repair, including checking the skin around the splints and casts (hourly, initially) for tightness, warmth, and color. If the patient reports discomfort, tingling, or coolness or if the color is blanched, the cast or splint may be too tight (constricted). *Inform the health care provider immediately about constriction and any indication of drainage under a splint or cast!*

Skin care is essential. Atrophy of the epidermis and underlying tissue causes the skin to become more fragile and more susceptible to injury and breakdown. Decreased skin nutrition and vascularity associated with denervation cause delayed healing, which further worsens the problem. Thoroughly examine the skin for signs of irritation or injury, and assist or instruct the patient to wash and dry the involved areas carefully. If the skin is dry, lanolin or cocoa butter may be used as a lubricant. *Because sensation may be absent or inhibited, teach the patient to protect the involved areas from temperature extremes and other sources of potential trauma.*

Physical or occupational therapy is the major approach for rehabilitation after surgical repair. Reinforce and help the patient perform the exercises learned in these therapy sessions. Because the regeneration of nerves and subsequent return of sensory and motor function may be extremely slow and produce PAIN, the patient may become discouraged and depressed. If the disability is permanent, he or she needs encouragement and assistance to cope with the changes in body image, self-esteem, and lifestyle.

RESTLESS LEGS SYNDROME

❖ PATHOPHYSIOLOGY

Restless legs syndrome (RLS) is characterized by leg paresthesias (burning, prickly sensation) associated with an irresistible urge to move. Over 10% of the population in the United States have the problem, and women are affected twice as often as men (National Institute of Neurological Disorders and Stroke, 2013a). RLS occurs most often in middle-aged and older adults. Stress can exacerbate this condition. RLS is related to a dysfunction in the brain circuits that use the neurotransmitter *dopamine.* Many of those affected with *primary RLS* have a positive family history, indicating a possible genetic basis. The incidence is higher in patients who have diabetes mellitus type 2; chronic kidney disease; iron deficiency; Parkinson disease; peripheral neuropathy; use of certain medications such as caffeine, calcium channel blockers, lithium, or neuroleptics; and withdrawal from sedatives. Although not a cause of hospitalization, restless leg syndrome may be a comorbidity that complicates recovery from other conditions.

❖ PATIENT-CENTERED COLLABORATIVE CARE

◆ Assessment

The patient reports intense burning or "crawling-type" sensations in the legs and therefore feels the need to move them repeatedly. These symptoms are worse in the evening and at night and when the patient is still for a period of time. Patients feel they need to move to relieve the symptoms. Many move their legs periodically while sleeping. For that reason, they often refer to themselves as "night walkers."

◆ Interventions

The management of RLS is symptomatic and involves treating the underlying cause or contributing factor, if known. Both nonpharmacologic measures and drug therapy are used. Teach patients to avoid as many risk factors as possible or make lifestyle modifications. Examples are avoiding caffeine and alcohol, quitting smoking, losing weight, and exercising.

Strategies to relieve the symptoms of RLS include walking, stretching, moderate exercise, or a warm bath. Refer them to

The Restless Legs Foundation (www.rls.org) as an excellent resource for information and patient and family support.

Many of the drugs prescribed for RLS are also used for either Parkinson disease (PD) or epilepsy. *Dopamine agonists* such as pramipexole (Mirapex) and ropinirole (Requip) are oral drugs used extensively. Gabapentin enacarbil (Horizant) is an *antiepileptic drug (AED)* that is also approved by the U.S. Food and Drug Administration (FDA) for RLS. These agents are usually taken at bedtime because they may cause daytime sleepiness. Teach patients to be cautious of driving or operating heavy equipment when taking these drugs (Silber, 2013). Correcting iron and magnesium deficiencies can reduce RLS symptoms, and ongoing supplementation of these minerals may be needed.

Some patients have had success with *Sinemet,* a combination of levodopa and carbidopa. This drug is often given with other medications to be more effective in reducing the symptoms of the disease. Other classes of drugs for managing RLS include *benzodiazepines, such as diazepam (Valium), and opioids* as a last resort. Two other AEDs, carbamazepine (Tegretol) and gabapentin (Neurontin), have been particularly effective and are taken in divided doses throughout the day. For insomnia from RLS, *melatonin* may be effective for many people, especially older adults. However, the focus of treatment should be on RLS, not insomnia. Teach patients to inform their health care providers when adding these supplements.

DISEASES OF THE CRANIAL NERVES

Patients with cranial nerve disease may be seen in any practice setting. The cranial nerves may be affected in association with other disorders of the nervous system or as a result of trauma. The most common disorders, those affecting cranial nerves V (trigeminal) and VII (facial), are discussed here.

TRIGEMINAL NEURALGIA

❖ *PATHOPHYSIOLOGY*

Trigeminal neuralgia (TN) is also known as *tic douloureux.* The trigeminal nerve has three branches: the first branch controls sensation in a person's eye, upper eyelid, and forehead; the second branch controls sensation in the lower eyelid, cheek, nostril, upper lip, and upper gum; and the third branch controls sensations in the jaw, lower lip, lower gum, and some of the muscles used for chewing.

According to the National Institute of Neurological Disorders and Stroke (2013b), trigeminal neuralgia has these characteristics:

- Affects the trigeminal (fifth cranial) nerve
- Occurs more often in people older than 50 years and in women more often than men
- Causes a specific type of facial pain, which occurs in sudden, intense facial spasms
- Is usually provoked by minimal stimulation of a trigger zone (like dental procedures)
- Is unilateral (one-sided) and confined to the area innervated by the trigeminal nerve, most often the second and third branches (Fig. 44-3)
- Is familial due to an inherited pattern of blood vessel formation

The cause of trigeminal neuralgia is thought to be related to impaired inhibitory mechanisms in the brainstem caused by excessive firing of irritated fibers in the trigeminal nerve.

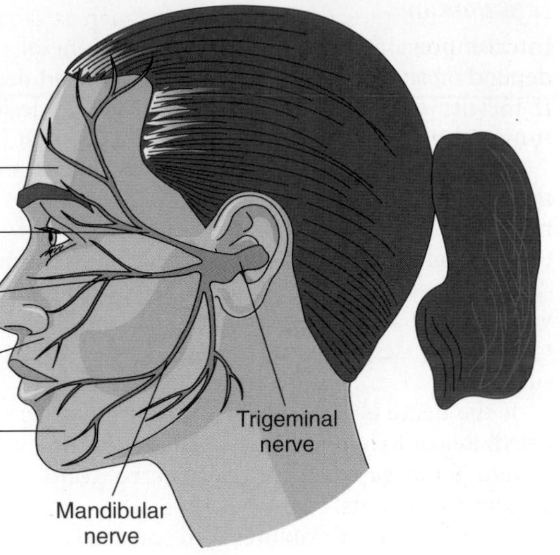

FIG. 44-3 Distribution of the trigeminal nerve and its three divisions: ophthalmic, maxillary, and mandibular.

Trauma and infection of the teeth, jaw, or ear may be contributing factors. Patients younger than 30 years with pain in more than one branch of the trigeminal nerve may be further evaluated to rule out the possibility of a tumor or multiple sclerosis.

❖ *PATIENT-CENTERED COLLABORATIVE CARE*

◆ *Assessment*

TN is a chronic PAIN syndrome. It can be categorized into two types of pain: classic and atypical. When describing trigeminal pain, patients use terms such as "excruciating," "sharp," "shooting," "piercing," "burning," and "jabbing." Atypical pain descriptions may include migraine-like headache. Between bursts of pain, which last from seconds to minutes, there is usually no pain. Often no sensory or motor deficits are found on examination. Pain can be initiated by light touch, a change in facial expression (e.g., smiling), or chewing. The fear of precipitating agonizing attacks often causes patients to avoid talking, smiling, eating, or attending to hygienic needs such as shaving, washing the face, and brushing the teeth. The pain can cause uncontrollable facial twitching. The course of TN involves bouts of classic pain for several weeks or months followed by spontaneous remissions. The length of these remissions may vary from days to years, but attack-free periods tend to become shorter as the patient grows older.

The patient suspected of TN usually has a CT scan and MRI to determine whether there is a reversible cause of trigeminal compression or INFLAMMATION. The diagnosis is made based on patient history and the results of these imaging tests.

◆ *Interventions*

The priority for care of the patient with TN is pain management. Specific interventions are determined by the amount of pain he or she is experiencing. Drug therapy is the first choice, but surgery can provide satisfactory pain relief in patients who do not respond to drug management or who experience profound adverse drug reactions (Ibrahim, 2012).

Drug Therapy and Radiosurgery. The first choice for drug therapy is carbamazepine (CBZ, Tegretol), an antiepileptic drug

(AED) (Ibrahim, 2012). Other drugs, such as gabapentin (Neurontin), pregabalin (Lyrica), and baclofen (Lioresal, Kemstro), a muscle relaxant, may be used. Some patients also achieve pain relief with complementary therapies, such as acupuncture (Lui et al., 2010).

Microvascular decompression, radiosurgery techniques such as a peripheral chemical nerve block with ropivacaine, or stereotactic radiation treatments with the Gamma Knife are surgical approaches to disrupt trigeminal neuralgia. These minimally invasive procedures prevent the complications of major surgery. Surgical interventions are often combined with drug therapy for pain management of this challenging condition.

In some cases, a **percutaneous stereotactic rhizotomy (PSR)** is performed as an ambulatory care procedure under general anesthesia. The surgeon passes a hollow needle through the inside of the patient's cheek into the trigeminal nerve fibers. A heating current (radiofrequency thermocoagulation) goes through the needle to destroy some of the fibers. As an option to heat, a balloon microcompression of the trigeminal nerve root may be performed. A glycerol injection may also be used as an option, but it is not done as commonly as thermocoagulation.

The entire nerve is not destroyed. The advantages of this procedure include long-term pain relief, absence of facial paralysis, and preservation of the sensation of touch. Puncturing the internal carotid artery is a possible complication. The affected side is permanently insensitive to pain.

After the PSR procedure, apply an ice pack to the PSR operative site on the cheek and jaw for 3 to 4 hours. Perform a focused cranial nerve assessment to assess whether other nerves have been damaged (e.g., facial nerve). Discourage the patient from chewing on the affected side until paresthesias resolve. A soft diet is usually prescribed.

! NURSING SAFETY PRIORITY (QSEN)

Action Alert

Teach the patient who has had percutaneous stereotactic rhizotomy to avoid rubbing the eye on the affected side because the protective mechanism of pain will no longer warn of injury. Instruct him or her to inspect the eye daily for redness or irritation and report to the health care provider any change or blurred vision. Stress the importance of regular dental examinations because the absence of pain may not warn the patient of potential problems.

Surgical Management. In addition to the general preoperative care provided to all patients, the surgeon thoroughly explains the surgical benefits and any expected neurologic deficits. Ensure that the patient understands the procedure to be performed and any risks or complications.

In some patients, a small artery compresses the trigeminal nerve as it enters the pons. Surgical relocation of this artery (**microvascular decompression**) may relieve the pain of TN without compromising facial sensation. This procedure is more invasive, requiring a craniotomy. Though not common, complications include aseptic meningitis, cerebrospinal fluid leak, ataxia, **ipsilateral** (same side) hearing loss, and facial nerve damage. Older adults and patients with other medical problems may not be candidates for this procedure.

In addition to general post-craniotomy care for patients as described in Chapter 45, monitor the patient who has microvascular decompression for signs of complications including headache, cranial nerve dysfunction, and bleeding. Assess his or her corneal reflex, extraocular muscles, and facial nerve, and report abnormal findings to the surgeon. Document all changes promptly.

Psychosocial considerations for the patient with trigeminal neuralgia include disappointment with ineffective drug protocols or surgical procedures, as well as the fear that the pain may recur with any activity. The patient may fail to move the face in an attempt to prevent pain. This behavior may be misinterpreted by others as withdrawal or depression. Refer patients and their families to the TNA—Facial Pain Association (www.fpa-support.org) for more information and support. TNA of Canada (www.catna.ca) is the national organization in Canada that advocates and informs patients and their families about trigeminal neuralgia.

FACIAL PARALYSIS

❖ *PATHOPHYSIOLOGY*

Facial paralysis, or **Bell's palsy**, is an acute paralysis of cranial nerve VII but may also affect cranial nerves V (trigeminal) and VIII (vestibulocochlear [auditory]). The condition is also known as *cranial polyneuritis.* Although the incidence may be slightly higher among people with diabetes, Bell's palsy occurs in all ages; however, it is more commonly seen in young adults.

Acute maximum paralysis occurs over 2 to 5 days in almost all patients with this condition. PAIN behind the ear or on the face may occur a few hours or even days before paralysis. The disorder involves a drawing sensation and paralysis of all facial muscles on the affected side. The patient cannot close his or her eye, wrinkle the forehead, smile, whistle, or grimace. Tearing may stop or become excessive. The face appears masklike and sags. Taste is usually impaired to some degree, but this symptom seldom persists beyond the second week of paralysis. Tinnitus (ringing in the ears) may also occur. Most patients go into remission within 3 months.

The cause of Bell's palsy is believed to be the result of INFLAMMATION triggered by a formerly dormant herpes simplex virus type 1 (HSV-1). Infection, immunosuppression, or exposure to cold may trigger the HSV-1 re-activation. Patients are rarely hospitalized, but the nurse may encounter them in clinics, office settings, or emergency departments.

❖ *PATIENT-CENTERED COLLABORATIVE CARE*

Medical management usually includes corticosteroids, 30 to 60 mg daily, during the first week after the onset of symptoms. Antiviral drugs such as acyclovir (Zovirax), famciclovir (Famvir), or valacyclovir (Valtrex) may be prescribed for 7 to 10 days after symptoms begin. Mild analgesics may help relieve the PAIN. Nursing care is directed toward managing the major neurologic deficits and providing psychosocial support. Because the eye does not close, the cornea must be protected from drying and subsequent ulceration or abrasion. Teach the patient to manually close the eyelid at intervals and to instill artificial tears during the day. An ointment to supply moisture can be used at night. The eye may be patched or taped closed at bedtime.

The patient may be unable to chew, sip fluids through a straw, or control drooling on the affected side, creating difficulties at mealtimes. Encourage the patient to eat and drink using the unaffected side of the mouth. High-calorie snacks may supplement meals, and patients may require a soft diet. Explain how to use massage; the application of warm, moist heat; and facial exercises to manage pain and paralysis. In some cases, physical therapy is prescribed. As muscle tone improves, teach the patient to grimace, wrinkle the brow, force the eyes closed, whistle, and blow air out of the cheeks 3 or 4 times daily for 5 minutes.

Nerve block to manage pain may be performed, but it is not common. Surgery is reserved for patients with complete, severe Bell's palsy to decompress the facial nerve. In some cases, cosmetic surgery is done.

Although most patients recover fully within a few weeks or months, some may experience permanent neurologic deficits. For chronic PAIN, gabapentin (Neurontin) may be prescribed. Patients with Bell's palsy may require psychosocial support because body image and self-esteem are affected. Provide both information and psychosocial support. Refer patients and their families to the Bell's Palsy Research Foundation for information (www.angelfire/az/BellsPalsy.com). The Bell's Palsy Association in the United Kingdom is also a good source of web-based information (www.bellspalsy.org.uk).

NCLEX EXAMINATION CHALLENGE

Safe and Effective Care Environment

The nurse is caring for a client with Bell's palsy. Which potential problem requires assessment by the nurse to ensure client safety?
A. Risk for falls from balance impairment
B. Risk for communication difficulties from impaired hearing
C. Risk for eye ulceration or abrasion from inability to close eyelid
D. Risk for adverse drug effects from pain management therapy

NURSING CONCEPTS AND CLINICAL JUDGMENT REVIEW

What might you NOTICE if a patient is experiencing impaired MOBILITY, altered SENSORY PERCEPTION, or PAIN as a result of acute or chronic peripheral nervous system disorders?

- Report of muscle weakness in face, arms, or legs
- Inability to swallow or clear the upper airway
- Changes in respiratory rate and pattern indicating respiratory compromise or failure
- Loss of sensation in face or extremities
- Report of burning, tingling sensations in face or extremities
- Report of pain in extremities or face
- Ptosis and either dry eye or excessive tearing

What should you INTERPRET and how should you RESPOND to a patient experiencing impaired MOBILITY, and/or SENSORY PERCEPTION, and/or PAIN as a result of peripheral nervous system disorders?

Perform and interpret physical assessment, including:

- Completing a neurologic assessment
- Assessing a patient's airway and breathing ability
- Performing a comprehensive pain assessment (see Chapter 3)

Respond by:

- Notifying health care provider or contacting Rapid Response Team if patient has problems with breathing or experiences a sudden change in neurologic status
- Establishing an airway and promoting ease in breathing (e.g., put patient in sitting position, provide oxygen, set up suction)
- Having emergency equipment like ventilator and tracheostomy set available for patient who has respiratory compromise
- Assisting with ADLs as needed
- Providing analgesics and other pain-relief measures

On what should you REFLECT as you assess and manage care for a patient with problems of the peripheral nervous system?

- Continue to observe patient for changes in functional ability and gas exchange.
- Consider multiple approaches to managing pain.
- Think about ways to promote independence in mobility and self-care.
- Think about health care team members with whom you will need to collaborate to improve mobility.
- Consider how to provide a safe environment for patients with decreased sensory perception.
- Develop a teaching plan for the patient and family for continuing care.

GET READY FOR THE NCLEX® EXAMINATION!

KEY POINTS

Review these Key Points for each NCLEX Examination Client Needs Category.

Safe and Effective Care Environment

- Collaborate with members of the interdisciplinary team, including the health care provider, physical and occupational therapists, speech-language pathologist, and dietitian, to establish goals for care and individualized interventions for patients with Guillain-Barré syndrome (GBS) and myasthenia gravis (MG). **Teamwork and Collaboration** QSEN

Health Promotion and Maintenance

- Reinforce the need for patients with MG to take their drugs on time. **Safety** QSEN
- Assess patient response to drugs to control PAIN related to peripheral nerve conditions; opioids, AEDs, and antidepressants have the potential to cause significant adverse effects.
- Refer patients with peripheral nervous system (PNS) disorders to community support groups and health care organizations, such as The Restless Legs Syndrome Foundation and the Myasthenia Gravis Foundation.

Psychosocial Integrity

- Provide alternatives to promote communication for patients with GBS and MG, including speaking slowly, lip-reading, and using communication boards or electronic technology. **Patient-Centered Care** QSEN

Physiological Integrity

- Assess for changes related to GAS EXCHANGE and functional ability for patients with PNS disorders.
- Recall that patients with GBS have ascending paralysis, sensory changes, cranial nerve involvement, and autonomic manifestations as a result of demyelination of neurons (see Chart 44-1).
- Note that patients with MG have an autoimmune disease in which muscle weakness, including ocular symptoms, is the result of attacks on the acetylcholine receptors at neuromuscular junctions (see Chart 44-3).
- Teach patients about factors that can worsen (exacerbate) MG as listed in Table 44-2. **Evidence-Based Practice** QSEN
- Remember that the priority for care for patients with GBS and MG is respiratory monitoring and airway management. **Safety** QSEN
- Prevent complications of immobility for patients with GBS and MG, such as pressure ulcers and venous thromboembolic events.
- Teach patients on cholinesterase inhibitor drugs and their families about clinical manifestations of cholinergic and myasthenic crises as listed in Table 44-1. **Safety** QSEN
- For patients having a thymectomy, maintain adequate GAS EXCHANGE and observe for complications such as pneumothorax or hemothorax (e.g., chest pain, shortness of breath). **Evidence-Based Practice** QSEN
- Perform frequent neurovascular assessments for patients having a peripheral nerve repair.
- Teach patients with restless legs syndrome to minimize risk factors for the disorder, including exercising, losing weight, and quitting smoking. **Evidence-Based Practice** QSEN
- Recall that trigeminal neuralgia (TN) affects primarily the fifth cranial nerve (although others may be involved) and does not typically involve paralysis or changes in sensation other than excruciating pain along the cranial nerve tract. Facial paralysis (Bell's palsy) affects cranial nerve VII and involves unilateral facial muscle paralysis.
- Prioritize pain management for the care of the patient with TN. **Patient-Centered Care** QSEN

45 CHAPTER

Care of Critically Ill Patients with Neurologic Problems

Chris Winkelman and Rachel L. Gallagher

http://evolve.elsevier.com/Iggy/

PRIORITY CONCEPTS

- Mobility
- Sensory Perception
- Cognition
- Perfusion

LEARNING OUTCOMES

Safe and Effective Care Environment

1. Prioritize airway, breathing, and circulation during the initial care of a patient with acute and critical neurologic illness to avoid complications from inadequate gas exchange or low perfusion
2. Explain the importance of collaborating with health care team members when planning and providing care for critically ill patients with neurologic problems.
3. Discuss strategies to provide safe, effective transitions in care following acute management of patients with a stroke, traumatic brain injury (TBI), or brain tumor.

Health Promotion and Maintenance

4. Develop a teaching plan about risk factors for having a stroke.
5. Describe strategies to prevent secondary brain injury.

Psychosocial Integrity

6. Discuss how to support the patient and family coping with life changes that result from stroke, TBI, or brain tumor.

Physiological Integrity

7. Perform a neurologic assessment of patients who are experiencing acute neurologic events of stroke, TBI, or cranial surgery, with a focus on changes in cognition, mobility, and sensory perception.
8. Prioritize evidence-based care for a patient with acute neurologic changes indicating a stroke or TBI.
9. Assess the patient after fibrinolytic therapy for ischemic stroke for potential adverse effects.
10. Describe elements of care for common patient responses to acute stroke, TBI, or brain tumor.
11. Explain the role of chemotherapy, radiation, and surgery in the management of patients with a brain tumor.

Many acute neurologic problems are associated with high mortality and severe morbidity and create significant and enduring impact upon patients, their families, and the wider society. Early recognition and comprehensive care of adult patients with acute neurologic compromise by the nurse can reduce mortality and disability. Acute neurologic problems from stroke, brain trauma, and malignancy cause varying degrees of impaired mobility, sensory perception, cognition, and perfusion.

TRANSIENT ISCHEMIC ATTACK

Ischemic strokes often follow warning signs such as a **transient ischemic attack (TIA)**. Temporary neurologic dysfunction resulting from a *brief* interruption in cerebral blood flow is easy to ignore or miss, particularly if symptoms resolve by the time the patient reaches the emergency department (ED). Typically, symptoms of a TIA resolve within 30 to 60 minutes (Chart 45-1). TIAs may damage the brain tissue with repeated insults, as seen on MRI or CT scan. Single TIAs indicate a high stroke risk; recurrent and multiple TIAs increase the risk for permanent brain damage.

Upon admission to the ED, a complete neurologic assessment is performed and laboratory tests, electrocardiogram (ECG), and CT scan are performed. If no neurologic deficit is identified, the patient may be admitted for further diagnostic testing to evaluate the risk for stroke, including an MRI of carotid and cerebral blood vessels and brain tissue. Treatment focuses on preventing another TIA or stroke and may include:

- Reducing high blood pressure, the most common risk factor for stroke, by adding or adjusting drugs to lower blood pressure
- Taking aspirin or another antiplatelet drug (e.g., clopidogrel [Plavix]) to prevent strokes (Aw & Sharma, 2012)
- Controlling diabetes and keeping blood sugar levels in a target range, typically 100-180 mg/dL
- Promoting lifestyle changes such as quitting smoking, eating heart-healthy foods, and being more active

As part of the discharge processes to meet The Joint Commission's National Patient Safety Goals and Core Measures for Venous Thromboembolism (VTE), ensure that the patient taking antiplatelet drugs is aware of precautions and actions to

CHART 45-1 Key Features

Transient Ischemic Attack

Symptoms resolve typically within 30 to 60 minutes.

Visual Deficits
- Blurred vision
- Diplopia (double vision)
- Blindness in one eye
- Tunnel vision

Motor Deficits
- Weakness (facial droop, arm or leg drift, hand grasp)
- Ataxia (gait disturbance)

Sensory Perception Deficits
- Numbness (face, hand, arm, or leg)
- Vertigo

Speech Deficits
- Aphasia
- Dysarthria (slurred speech)

take if bleeding occurs. Anticoagulant therapy is discussed in detail in Chapter 36 under the VTE section. Reinforce the need to follow up with the health care provider and to complete any diagnostic tests requested on an ambulatory care basis.

STROKE (BRAIN ATTACK)

PATHOPHYSIOLOGY

A **stroke** is caused by an interruption of PERFUSION to any part of the brain. The National Stroke Association uses the term **brain attack** to convey the urgency for acute stroke care similar to that provided for acute myocardial infarction. *A stroke is a medical emergency, and it should be treated immediately to reduce permanent disability.* About 14% of patients in hospitals in the United States have a stroke while in the hospital (Mink & Miller, 2011a).

Stroke is the third leading cause of death in the United States and is considered a major cause of disability worldwide. According to the Centers for Disease Control and Prevention (CDC), about 137,000 Americans die each year from stroke (CDC, 2013b) On average, one American dies from stroke every 4 minutes (CDC, 2013b).

Pathophysiologic Changes in the Brain

The brain cannot store oxygen or glucose and therefore must receive a constant flow of blood to provide these substances for normal function. In addition, blood flow is important for the removal of metabolic waste (e.g., carbon dioxide, lactic acid). If blood supply to any part of the brain is interrupted for more than a few minutes, cerebral tissue dies (**infarction**). The result is disability, depending on the location and amount of brain tissue affected. Brain metabolism and blood flow after a stroke are affected around the infarction as well as in the **contralateral** (opposite side) hemisphere. Effects of a stroke on the contralateral (nonaffected) side may be due to brain edema or global changes in PERFUSION in the brain. As a result of brain edema, patients may develop increased intracranial pressure and secondary brain damage.

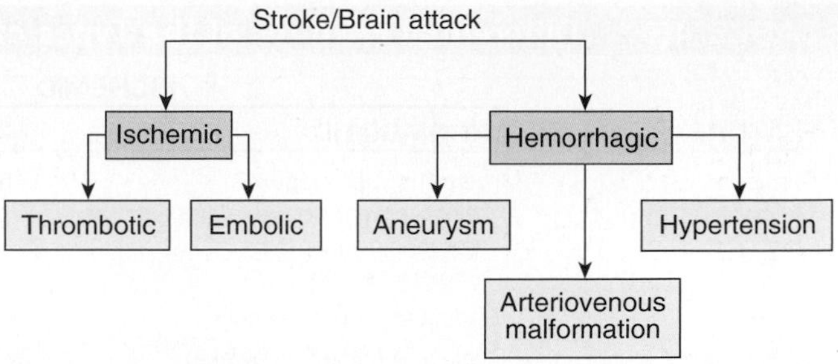

FIG. 45-1 Types of stroke/brain attack.

Types of Strokes

Strokes are generally classified as ischemic (occlusive) or hemorrhagic (Fig. 45-1). Acute ischemic strokes are either thrombotic or embolic in origin (Table 45-1). Most strokes are ischemic.

Ischemic Stroke. An acute **ischemic stroke** is caused by the occlusion (blockage) of a cerebral artery by either a thrombus or an embolus. A stroke that is caused by a **thrombus** (clot) is referred to as a **thrombotic stroke**, whereas a stroke caused by an **embolus** (dislodged clot) is referred to as an **embolic stroke**.

Thrombotic strokes account for more than half of all strokes and are commonly associated with the development of atherosclerosis in either intracranial or extracranial arteries (usually the carotid arteries). Atherosclerosis is the process by which fatty plaques develop on the inner wall of the affected arterial vessel. Chapter 36 describes this health problem, including its pathophysiology, in detail.

Rupture of one or more plaques promotes clot formation. When the clot is of sufficient size, it interrupts blood flow to the brain tissue supplied by the vessel, causing an ischemic (occlusive) stroke. The **bifurcation** (point of division) of the common carotid artery and the vertebral arteries at their junction with the basilar artery are the most common sites involved in atherosclerotic plaque formation. Because of the gradual nature of clot formation when atherosclerotic plaque is present, thrombotic strokes tend to have a *slow* onset, evolving over minutes to hours.

An *embolic stroke* is caused by a thrombus or a group of thrombi that break off from one area of the body and travel to the cerebral arteries via the carotid artery or vertebrobasilar system. The usual source of emboli is the heart. Emboli can occur in patients with atrial fibrillation, heart valve disease, mural thrombi after a myocardial infarction (MI), or a prosthetic heart valve. Another source of emboli may be plaque or clot that breaks off from the carotid sinus or internal carotid artery. Emboli tend to become lodged in the smaller cerebral blood vessels at their point of bifurcation or where the lumen narrows.

The middle cerebral artery (MCA) is most commonly involved in an embolic stroke. As the emboli occlude the vessel, ischemia develops and the patient experiences the clinical manifestations of the stroke. However, the occlusion may be temporary if the embolus breaks into smaller fragments, enters smaller blood vessels, and is absorbed. For these reasons, embolic strokes are characterized by the *sudden* development and rapid occurrence of neurologic deficits. The symptoms may resolve over several hours or a few days. Conversion of an occlusive stroke to a hemorrhagic stroke may occur because the arterial vessel wall is also vulnerable to ischemic damage from blood

TABLE 45-1 **Differential Features of the Types of Stroke**

	ISCHEMIC		
FEATURE	**THROMBOTIC**	**EMBOLIC**	**HEMORRHAGIC**
Evolution	Intermittent or stepwise improvement between episodes of worsening symptoms Completed stroke	Abrupt development of completed stroke Steady progression	Usually abrupt onset
Onset	Gradual (minutes to hours)	Sudden	Sudden, may be gradual if caused by hypertension
Level of consciousness	Preserved (patient is awake)	Preserved (patient is awake)	Deepening stupor or coma
Contributing associated factors	Hypertension Atherosclerosis	Cardiac disease	Hypertension Vessel disorders
Prodromal symptoms	Transient ischemic attack		
Neurologic deficits	Deficits during the first few weeks Slight headache Speech deficits Visual problems Confusion	Maximum deficit at onset Paralysis Expressive aphasia	Focal deficits Severe, frequent
Cerebrospinal fluid	Normal; possible presence of protein	Normal	Bloody
Seizures	No	No	Usually
Duration	Improvements over weeks to months Permanent deficits possible	Rapid improvements	Variable Permanent neurologic deficits possible

supply interruption. Sudden hemodynamic stress may result in vessel rupture, causing bleeding directly within the brain tissue.

Hemorrhagic Stroke. The second major classification of stroke is hemorrhagic stroke. In this type of stroke, vessel integrity is interrupted and bleeding occurs into the brain tissue or into the subarachnoid space.

Intracerebral hemorrhage (ICH) describes bleeding into the brain tissue generally resulting from severe or sustained hypertension. Elevated blood pressure (BP) leads to changes within the arterial wall that leave it likely to rupture. Damage to the brain occurs from bleeding, causing edema, distortion, and displacement, which are direct irritants to brain tissue. Cocaine use is one example of a trigger for sudden, dramatic blood pressure elevation leading to hemorrhagic stroke.

Subarachnoid hemorrhage (SAH) is much more common and results from bleeding into the subarachnoid space—the space between the pia mater and arachnoid layers of the meninges covering the brain. This type of bleeding is usually caused by a ruptured aneurysm or arteriovenous malformation (Mink & Miller, 2011b). It can also be caused by trauma.

An **aneurysm** is an abnormal ballooning or blister along a normal artery, which usually develops in a weak spot on the artery wall, typically along the posterior circulation such as the basilar artery, vertebral artery, or the superior cerebral artery. Larger aneurysms are more likely to rupture than smaller ones.

An **arteriovenous malformation (AVM)** is an uncommon abnormality that occurs during embryonic development. It is a tangled collection of malformed, thin-walled, dilated vessels without a capillary network (Fig. 45-2). Normally the capillary network lowers the pressure between the arterial and venous systems. In the absence of the capillary network, the thin-walled veins are subjected to arterial pressure. The abnormal vessels may eventually rupture, causing bleeding into the intracerebral tissue or spaces.

Vasospasm, a sudden and periodic constriction of a cerebral artery, often follows SAH or bleeding from an aneurysm or AVM rupture. Blood flow to distal areas of the brain supplied by the damaged cerebral vessel is markedly diminished. Reduced

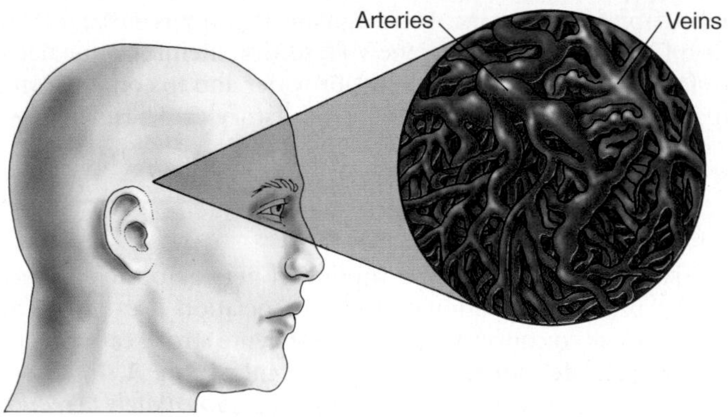

FIG. 45-2 Appearance of an arteriovenous malformation. Note the dilated, entangled blood vessels.

PERFUSION from vasospasm contributes to secondary cerebral ischemia and infarction and further neurologic dysfunction.

Etiology and Genetic Risk

As with many health problems, the causes of stroke are likely a combination of genetic and environmental risk factors. Major risk factors increase the likelihood of strokes and can be divided into those that can be modified and those that cannot (nonmodifiable factors) (see Health Promotion and Maintenance section on p. 933). Many of these factors have a familial or genetic predisposition and are discussed elsewhere in this text. For example, the first-order relative (mother, father, sister, brother) stroke risk increases with a strong family history of hypertension, atherosclerotic disease, and a diagnosis of aneurysm. Relatives of a patient with an aneurysm, regardless of vessel location, may be at higher risk for intracranial aneurysms and should consider diagnostic testing and follow-up.

Incidence and Prevalence

It is estimated that there are more than 4.7 million stroke survivors in the United States. About 795,000 Americans have strokes each year, but deaths have declined over the past 15 years. The number of strokes occurring in the younger adult population is increasing (Lee et al., 2012). Strokes are associated with illicit drug use because many street drugs cause hypercoagulability, spasm of cerebral vessels, or hypertensive crisis.

Health Promotion and Maintenance

Risk factors that contribute to stroke are divided into three groups: risk factors that cannot be changed, risk factors that can be changed with medical treatment, and risk factors that can be changed by lifestyle modification.

People with predisposing health conditions should be aware that lifestyle habits contribute to stroke. Many of these factors contribute to other health problems. Teach them the importance of seeking professional health care and adhering to the recommended treatment plan. Recommend a diet high in fruits and vegetables and low in saturated fats. Light to moderate alcohol consumption may reduce the risk for stroke, but a higher consumption may increase it. Chart 45-2 describes common risk factors that can be changed (modifiable).

CULTURAL CONSIDERATIONS

Patient-Centered Care QSEN

American Indian/Alaskan Native groups have the highest prevalence of stroke. Black men and women have more strokes than white men and women. Hispanic or Latino men have more strokes than non-Hispanic men. About half of the excess stroke risk in blacks between ages 45 and 65 years is attributable to traditional risk factors such as elevated systolic blood pressure and socioeconomic factors. These data suggest a critical need to study the role that nontraditional risk factors play in stroke development and severity in this group (Howard et al., 2011; Lakoski et al., 2011).

NCLEX EXAMINATION CHALLENGE

Health Promotion and Maintenance

Which statements by a client or family member about preventing stroke indicate a need for further teaching by the nurse? **Select all that apply.**

A. "I will adjust my aspirin drug dose depending on whether I have pain."
B. "I have cut down on smoking to only a half-pack daily."
C. "I need to walk at least 30 minutes most days of the week."
D. "I need to consider salt content in the foods I eat at restaurants."
E. "I don't need to worry about fat calories in what I eat—my heart is fine!"

CHART 45-2 Patient and Family Education: Preparing for Self-Management

Common Modifiable Risk Factors for Developing a Stroke

- Smoking
- Substance use (particularly cocaine)
- Obesity
- Sedentary lifestyle
- Oral contraceptive use
- Heavy alcohol use
- Use of phenylpropanolamine (PPA), found in antihistamine drugs

PATIENT-CENTERED COLLABORATIVE CARE

Assessment

History. Although an accurate history is important in the diagnosis of a stroke, *the first priority is to ensure the patient is transported to a stroke center.* A stroke center is designated by The Joint Commission for its ability to rapidly recognize and effectively treat strokes. At the center, the patients are evaluated for their eligibility to receive fibrinolytic therapy. Obtaining a history should not delay the patient's arrival to either the stroke center or interventional radiology within the stroke center. A focused history to determine if the patient has had a recent bleeding event or is taking an anticoagulant is an important part of the rapid stroke assessment protocol.

A more extensive history, after either fibrinolytic therapy or determination that the patient is unable to receive this therapy, assists in identifying the cause of the stroke and the area of brain involved. If possible, obtain a history of the patient's activity when the stroke began. Hemorrhagic strokes tend to occur during activity. Next ask the patient or a family member how the symptoms progressed. Be sure to document the history of the stroke's onset. Symptoms of a hemorrhagic stroke tend to occur abruptly, whereas thrombotic strokes generally have a more gradual progression. Determine the severity of the symptoms, such as whether they worsened after the initial onset or began to improve.

During the interview, observe the patient's level of consciousness (LOC) and assess for indications of cognitive or memory impairments and difficulties with speech or hearing. When LOC is suddenly decreased or altered, immediately determine if hypoglycemia or hypoxia is present because these conditions may mimic emergent neurologic disorders. Hypoglycemia and hypoxia are easily treated and reversed, unlike brain injury from poor PERFUSION or trauma.

Question the patient or family member about the presence of SENSORY PERCEPTION deficits or motor changes, visual problems, problems with balance or gait, and changes in reading or writing abilities.

In addition, ask about the patient's medical history with specific attention directed toward a history of head trauma, diabetes, hypertension, heart disease, anemia, and obesity. Obtain a list of current medications, including prescribed drugs, over-the-counter (OTC) drugs, herbal and nutritional supplements, and recreational (illicit) drugs. To complete the history, obtain data about the patient's social history, including education, employment, travel, leisure activities, and personal habits (e.g., smoking, diet, exercise pattern, drug and alcohol use).

The patient with a SAH, particularly when the hemorrhage is from a leaking aneurysm, often reports the onset of a sudden, severe headache described as "the worst headache of my life." Additional symptoms of SAH or cerebral aneurysmal and AVM bleeding are nausea and vomiting, photophobia, cranial neuropathy, stiff neck, and change in mental status. There may also be a family history of aneurysms.

Physical Assessment/Clinical Manifestations. First-responder personnel (e.g., paramedics, emergency medical technicians) perform an initial neurologic examination using well-established stroke assessment tools.

Nurses also perform a complete neurologic assessment on admission to the ED. The National Institutes of Health Stroke Scale (NIHSS) is a commonly used valid and reliable assessment tool that nurses complete as soon as possible after the patient

! NURSING SAFETY PRIORITY QSEN

Critical Rescue

In the ED, assess the stroke patient within 10 minutes of arrival. This same standard applies to patients already hospitalized for other medical conditions who have a stroke. The priority is assessment of ABCs—**a**irway, **b**reathing, and **c**irculation. Many hospitals have designated stroke teams and centers that are expert in acute stroke assessment and management.

arrives in the ED (Table 45-2). The NIHSS includes 11 areas of assessment (Mink & Miller, 2011a).

As the patients are transitioned from the ED to other settings, the most important area to assess is the patient's level of consciousness (LOC). Use the Glasgow Coma Scale (see Fig. 41-10) to frequently monitor for changes in LOC throughout the patient's acute care. Specific patient manifestations of stroke should also be monitored. Stroke symptoms depend on the extent and location of the ischemia and the arteries involved as described in Chart 45-3.

Stroke symptoms can appear at any time of the day or night (Beal, 2010). The five most common symptoms are (CDC, 2013b):

- Sudden confusion or trouble speaking or understanding others
- Sudden numbness or weakness of the face, arm, or leg
- Sudden trouble seeing in one or both eyes
- Sudden dizziness, trouble walking, or loss of balance or coordination
- Sudden severe headache with no known cause

Cognitive Changes. The patient may have a variety of cognitive problems in addition to changes in LOC. LOC varies depending on the extent of increased intracranial pressure (ICP) caused by the stroke and on the location of the stroke. Assess for:

- Denial of the illness
- Spatial and proprioceptive (awareness of body position in space) dysfunction
- Impairment of memory, judgment, or problem-solving and decision-making abilities
- Decreased ability to concentrate and attend to tasks

Dysfunction in one or more of these areas may be severe depending on the hemisphere involved (Chart 45-4).

The *right* cerebral hemisphere is more involved with visual and spatial awareness and **proprioception** (sense of body position). A person who has a stroke involving the right cerebral hemisphere is often unaware of any deficits and may be disoriented to time and place. Personality changes include impulsivity (poor impulse control) and poor judgment. The *left* cerebral hemisphere, the dominant hemisphere in all but about 15% to 20% of the population, is the center for language, mathematic skills, and analytic thinking. Therefore a left hemisphere stroke results in **aphasia** (inability to use or comprehend language), **alexia** or **dyslexia** (reading problems), **agraphia** (difficulty with writing), and **acalculia** (difficulty with mathematic calculation). A complete assessment of these problems is performed by a speech-language pathologist (SLP).

Motor Changes. The motor examination provides information about which part of the brain is involved. A *right* **hemiplegia** (paralysis on one side of the body) or **hemiparesis** (weakness on one side of the body) indicates a stroke involving the *left* cerebral hemisphere because the motor nerve fibers cross in the medulla before entering the spinal cord and periphery. On the other hand, a *left* hemiplegia or hemiparesis indicates a stroke in the *right* cerebral hemisphere. If the brainstem or cerebellum is affected, the patient may experience hemiparesis or quadriparesis and **ataxia** (gait disturbance).

In collaboration with the physical therapist (PT) and occupational therapist (OT), assess the patient's muscle tone. The patient with **hypotonia**, or **flaccid paralysis**, cannot overcome the forces of gravity, and the extremities tend to fall to the side. The extremities feel heavy, and muscle tone is inadequate for balance, equilibrium, or protective mechanisms. **Hypertonia** (**spastic paralysis**) tends to cause fixed positions or contractures of the involved extremities. Range of motion (ROM) of

CHART 45-3 Key Features

Stroke Syndromes

Middle Cerebral Artery Strokes

- Contralateral hemiparesis: arm > leg
- Contralateral sensory perception deficit
- Homonymous hemianopsia
- Unilateral neglect or inattention
- Aphasia, anomia, alexia, agraphia, and acalculia
- Impaired vertical sensation
- Spatial deficit
- Perceptual deficit
- Visual field deficit
- Altered level of consciousness: drowsy to comatose

Posterior Cerebral Artery Strokes

- Perseveration (word or action repetition)
- Aphasia, amnesia, alexia, agraphia, visual agnosia, and ataxia
- Loss of deep sensation
- Decreased touch sensation
- Stupor, coma

Internal Carotid Artery Strokes

- Contralateral hemiparesis
- Sensory perception deficit
- Hemianopsia, blurred vision, blindness
- Aphasia (dominant side)
- Headache
- Bruit

Anterior Cerebral Artery Strokes

- Contralateral hemiparesis: leg > arm
- Bladder incontinence
- Personality and behavior changes
- Aphasia and amnesia
- Positive grasp and sucking reflex
- Perseveration
- Sensory perception deficit (lower extremity)
- Memory impairment
- Apraxic gait

Vertebrobasilar Artery Strokes

- Headache and vertigo
- Coma
- Memory loss and confusion
- Flaccid paralysis
- Areflexia, ataxia, and vertigo
- Cranial nerve dysfunction
- Disconjugate gaze
- Visual deficits (uniorbital) and homonymous hemianopsia
- Sensory loss: numbness

TABLE 45-2 NIH Stroke Scale

CATEGORY AND MEASUREMENT	SCORE*
1a. Level of Consciousness (LOC) 0 = Alert; keenly responsive. 1 = Not alert; but arousable by minor stimulation to obey, answer, or respond. 2 = Not alert; requires repeated stimulation to attend or is obtunded and requires strong or painful stimulation to make movements (not stereotyped). 3 = Responds only with reflex motor or autonomic effects or totally unresponsive, flaccid, and areflexic.	_____
1b. LOC Questions 0 = Answers two questions correctly. 1 = Answers one question correctly. 2 = Answers neither question correctly.	_____
1c. LOC Commands 0 = Performs two tasks correctly. 1 = Performs one task correctly. 2 = Performs neither task correctly.	_____
2. Best Gaze 0 = Normal. 1 = Partial gaze palsy; gaze is abnormal in one or both eyes, but forced deviation or total gaze paresis is not present. 2 = Forced deviation, or total gaze paresis not overcome by the oculocephalic maneuver.	_____
3. Visual 0 = No visual loss. 1 = Partial hemianopia. 2 = Complete hemianopia. 3 = Bilateral hemianopia (blind including cortical blindness).	_____
4. Facial Palsy 0 = Normal symmetrical movements. 1 = Minor paralysis (flattened nasolabial fold, asymmetry on smiling). 2 = Partial paralysis (total or near-total paralysis of lower face). 3 = Complete paralysis of one or both sides (absence of facial movement in the upper and lower face).	_____
5. Motor (Arm) 0 = No drift; limb holds 90 (or 45) degrees for full 10 seconds. 1 = Drift; limb holds 90 (or 45) degrees, but drifts down before full 10 seconds; does not hit bed or other support. 2 = Some effort against gravity; limb cannot get to or maintain (if cued) 90 (or 45) degrees, drifts down to bed, but has some effort against gravity. 3 = No effort against gravity; limb falls. 4 = No movement. Untestable = Amputation or joint fusion.	Right arm: _____ Left arm: _____
6. Motor (Leg) 0 = No drift; leg holds 30-degree position for full 5 seconds. 1 = Drift; leg falls by the end of the 5-second period but does not hit bed. 2 = Some effort against gravity; leg falls to bed by 5 seconds, but has some effort against gravity. 3 = No effort against gravity; leg falls to bed immediately. 4 = No movement. Untestable = Amputation or joint fusion.	Right leg: _____ Left leg: _____
7. Limb Ataxia 0 = Absent. 1 = Present in one limb. 2 = Present in two limbs. Untestable = Amputation or joint fusion.	_____
8. Sensory 0 = Normal; no sensory loss. 1 = Mild-to-moderate sensory loss; patient feels pinprick is less sharp or is dull on the affected side; or there is a loss of superficial pain with pinprick, but patient is aware of being touched. 2 = Severe-to-total sensory loss; patient is not aware of being touched in the face, arm, and leg.	_____
9. Best Language 0 = No aphasia; normal. 1 = Mild-to-moderate aphasia; some obvious loss of fluency or facility of comprehension, without significant limitation on ideas expressed or form of expression. 2 = Severe aphasia; all communication is through fragmentary expression; great need for inference, questioning, and guessing by the listener. 3 = Mute, global aphasia; no usable speech or auditory comprehension.	_____

Continued

TABLE 45-2 NIH Stroke Scale—cont'd

CATEGORY AND MEASUREMENT	SCORE*
10. Dysarthria 0 = Normal. 1 = Mild-to-moderate dysarthria; patient slurs at least some words and, at worst, can be understood with some difficulty. 2 = Severe dysarthria; patient's speech is so slurred as to be unintelligible in the absence of or out of proportion to any dysphasia, or is mute/anarthric. Untestable = Intubated or other physical barrier.	_____
11. Extinction and Inattention (Neglect) 0 = No abnormality. 1 = Visual, tactile, auditory, spatial, or personal inattention or extinction to bilateral simultaneous stimulation in one of the sensory modalities. 2 = Profound hemi-inattention or extinction to more than one modality; does not recognize own hand or orients to only one side of space.	_____

Modified from National Institutes of Health Stroke Scale, 2013. www.ninds.nih.gov/doctors/NIH_stroke_scale.pdf.
*The patient can have a score of 0 to 40, with 0 having no neurologic deficits and 40 being the most deficits.

CHART 45-4 Key Features

Left and Right Hemisphere Strokes

FEATURE	LEFT HEMISPHERE*	RIGHT HEMISPHERE
Language	Aphasia Agraphia Alexia	Impaired sense of humor
Memory	Possible deficit	Disorientation to time, place, and person Inability to recognize faces
Vision	Inability to discriminate words and letters Reading problems Deficits in the right visual field	Visual spatial deficits Neglect of the left visual field Loss of depth perception
Behavior	Slowness Cautiousness Anxiety when attempting a new task Depression or a catastrophic response to illness Sense of guilt Feeling of worthlessness Worries over future Quick anger and frustration Intellectual impairment	Impulsiveness Lack of awareness of neurologic deficits Confabulation Euphoria Constant smiling Denial of illness Poor judgment Overestimation of abilities (risk for injury)
Hearing	No deficit	Loss of ability to hear tonal variations

*Location for speech in all but 5% to 20% of people.

the joints is restricted, and shoulder subluxation may easily occur from either spasticity or flaccidity. Also assess head and trunk control, balance, coordination, and gait. The patient who has had a stroke may also be unable to use an object correctly (**agnosia**) or carry out a purposeful motor activity or speech (**apraxia**).

Loss of neurologic control by the cerebral cortex causes a spastic (upper motor neuron) uninhibited bladder. Bowel function may also be affected. Assess the patient for incontinence (most common) or retention of urine and stool. Some patients have both problems.

Sensory Changes. The sensory examination evaluates the patient's response to touch and painful stimuli. In addition to diminished motor function, decreased sensation typically occurs on the affected side of the body.

Evaluate for indications of **unilateral body neglect syndrome**, which is particularly common with strokes in the *right* cerebral hemisphere. In this syndrome, the patient is unaware of the existence of his or her left or paralyzed side. The typical picture is that of the patient sitting in a wheelchair and leaning to the left with the arm caught in the wheelchair wheel. When questioned, the patient often states that everything is fine and believes that he or she is sitting up straight in the chair. The patient may wash or dress only one side of the body or eat from only one side of a plate.

Another important part of the nursing assessment focuses on visual ability. Infarction or ischemia involving the carotid artery may cause pupil constriction or dilation, **ptosis** (eyelid drooping), visual field deficits, or pallor and petechiae of the conjunctiva. **Amaurosis fugax**, a brief episode of blindness in one eye, results from retinal ischemia caused by ophthalmic or carotid artery insufficiency. **Hemianopsia**, or blindness in half of the visual field, results from damage to the optic tract or occipital lobe. Usually this deficit occurs as **homonymous hemianopsia**, in which there is blindness in the same side of both eyes (Fig. 45-3). The patient with this condition must turn his or her head to scan the complete range of vision. Otherwise, he or she does not see half of the visual field. For example, the patient eats only half of a meal because that is the only portion seen. Patients with brainstem or cerebellar damage may have abnormal eye movements, such as **nystagmus** (involuntary movements of the eyes).

Cranial Nerve Function. Assess the patient's ability to chew, which reflects the function of cranial nerve (CN) V. Assessment of the patient's ability to swallow reflects the function of CNs IX and X. In addition, note any facial paralysis or paresis (CN VII), absent gag reflex (CN IX), or impaired tongue movement (CN XII). The patient who has difficulty chewing or swallowing foods and liquids (**dysphagia**) is at risk for aspiration pneumonia and may become constipated or dehydrated from inadequate fluid intake.

Cardiovascular Assessment. Patients with embolic strokes may have a heart murmur, dysrhythmias (most often atrial fibrillation), or hypertension. It is not unusual for the patient to be admitted to the hospital with a blood pressure greater than 180 to 200/110 to 120 mm Hg. Although a somewhat higher blood pressure of 150/100 mm Hg is needed to maintain

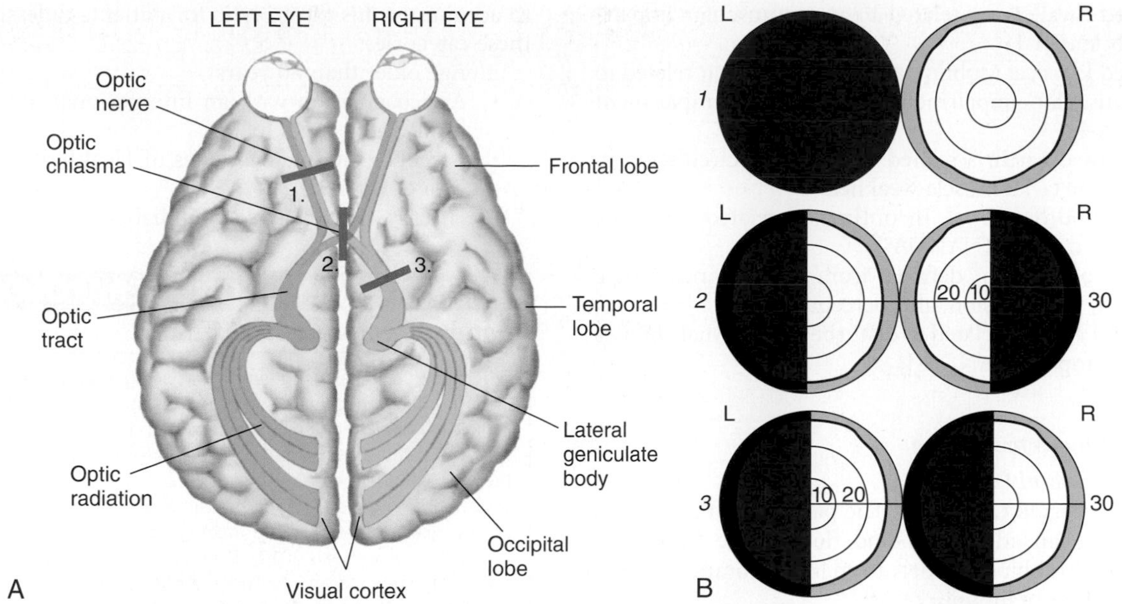

FIG. 45-3 A, Site of lesions causing visual loss. *1,* Total blindness left eye; *2,* Bitemporal hemianopia; *3,* Left homonymous hemianopia. **B,** Visual fields corresponding to lesions shown in **A.** *1,* Total blindness left eye; *2,* Bitemporal hemianopia; *3,* Left homonymous hemianopia.

cerebral PERFUSION after an acute ischemic stroke, pressures above these values may lead to another stroke.

Psychosocial Assessment. The typical patient with a stroke is older than 60 years, is hypertensive, and has varying degrees of motor weakness and level of consciousness. Language and cognitive deficits, as well as behavior and memory problems, may also occur.

Assess the patient's reaction to the illness, especially in relation to changes in body image, self-concept, and ability to perform ADLs. In collaboration with the patient's family and friends, identify any problems with coping or personality changes.

Ask about the patient's financial status and occupation, because they may be affected by the residual neurologic deficits of the stroke. Patients who do not have disability or health insurance may worry about how their family will cope financially with the disruption in their lives. Early involvement of social services, certified hospital chaplain, or psychological counseling may enhance coping skills.

Assess for **emotional lability,** especially if the frontal lobe of the brain has been affected. In such cases, the patient laughs and then cries unexpectedly for no apparent reason. Explain these uncontrollable emotions to the family or significant others so they do not feel responsible for these reactions.

Laboratory Assessment. Clinical history and presentation are usually enough to identify a stroke once it has occurred. No definitive laboratory tests confirm its diagnosis. Elevated hematocrit and hemoglobin levels are often associated with a severe or major stroke as the body attempts to compensate for lack of oxygen to the brain. An elevated white blood cell (WBC) count may indicate the presence of an infection, possibly subacute bacterial endocarditis, or a response to physiologic stress or inflammation. Cardiac enzymes may be elevated in patients who have a cardiac cause for their stroke.

The health care provider typically requests a prothrombin time (PT) or international normalized ratio (INR) and a partial thromboplastin time (PTT) to establish baseline information in case anticoagulation therapy is started. These diagnostic tests may also provide supportive evidence that a hemorrhagic stroke has occurred.

Imaging Assessment. Brain imaging is the most important tool for confirming the diagnosis of a stroke. *CT* without contrast is the standard for initial diagnosis (Mink & Miller, 2011b). Cerebral aneurysms or AVM may also be identified. For a patient with an ischemic or occlusive stroke, the head CT is usually initially negative, indicating a thrombotic or embolic stroke rather than intracerebral hemorrhage. After the first 24 hours, CT shows progressive changes of ischemia, infarction, and associated cerebral edema. This test establishes baseline information for future comparison in case the patient's condition deteriorates. In addition, the scan enables the physician to identify pathologic changes that may mimic a stroke, such as a brain tumor or cerebral hematoma, both of which may be unrelated to cerebrovascular disease.

MRI demonstrates ischemic brain injury earlier than CT. *Magnetic resonance angiography (MRA)* and multimodal techniques such as perfusion-weighted imaging enhance the sensitivity of the MRI to detect early changes in the brain, including confirming blood flow. *Ultrasonography* (carotid duplex scanning) and *echocardiography* help determine additional cardiovascular risks.

Other Diagnostic Assessment. To assist in the determination of a cardiac cause of a stroke, the health care provider may request a 12-lead electrocardiogram (ECG) and an evaluation of cardiac enzymes. As with other cardiovascular diseases, it is not unusual to find these changes on the ECG: inverted T wave, ST depression, and prolongation of the QT interval in the cardiac cycle.

◆ Analysis

The priority NANDA-I nursing diagnoses and collaborative problems for patients with a stroke include:

1. Inadequate perfusion to the brain related to interruption of arterial blood flow and a possible increase in ICP

2. Impaired Swallowing related to neuromuscular impairment (NANDA-I)
3. Impaired Physical Mobility and self-care deficit related to neuromuscular impairment or cognitive impairment (NANDA-I)
4. Aphasia or dysarthria related to decreased circulation in the brain or facial muscle weakness
5. Urinary and/or Bowel Incontinence related to reflex bladder and bowel (NANDA-I)
6. Sensory perception deficits from altered neurologic reception, transmission, and perception
7. Unilateral Neglect related to disturbed perceptual abilities or hemianopsia (NANDA-I)

◆ Planning and Implementation

Improving Cerebral Perfusion

Planning: Expected Outcomes. The patient with a stroke is expected to have an adequate blood flow to the brain and through the cerebral blood vessels to maintain brain function and prevent further brain injury.

Interventions. Interventions for patients experiencing strokes are determined primarily by the type and extent of the stroke. For patients having ischemic strokes, the standard of practice is to start two IV lines with non-dextrose isotonic saline (Hughes, 2011). Consider placing the patient in a supine position with a low head-of-bed elevation to maximize cerebral PERFUSION. The immediate primary role of the nurse is to manage the patient receiving treatment and continuously assess for increasing intracranial pressure.

Nonsurgical Management. Nursing interventions are initially aimed at monitoring for neurologic changes or complications associated with stroke and its treatment. The two major treatment modalities for patients with acute ischemic stroke are systemic fibrinolytic therapy and endovascular interventions. Regardless of the immediate management approach used, once the patient is stable, provide ongoing supportive care. Provide interventions to prevent and/or monitor for early signs of complications, such as hyperglycemia, urinary tract infection, and pneumonia. Implement interventions to prevent patient falls. These health problems are discussed in appropriate chapters in this textbook.

Fibrinolytic Therapy. For select patients with ischemic strokes, early intervention with systemic fibrinolytic therapy ("clot-busting drug") is the standard of practice to improve blood flow to or through the brain. The success of fibrinolytic therapy for a stroke depends on the interval between the time symptoms begin and available treatment. It also depends on where the treatment is given. Hospitals with stroke centers or specialized stroke teams who care for numerous stroke patients have lower mortality rates than those hospitals that care for fewer of these patients (Hughes, 2011).

Intravenous (systemic) fibrinolytic therapy (also called *thrombolytic therapy*) for an acute ischemic stroke dissolves the cerebral artery occlusion to re-establish blood flow and prevent cerebral infarction. Alteplase (Activase) is the only drug approved at this point for the treatment of acute ischemic stroke. It is a fibrinolytic that activates plasminogen to degrade the thrombus. The most important factor in whether or not to give alteplase is the time between symptom onset and time seen in the stroke center. In 2009, the American Stroke Association recommended an expanded time interval from 3 to 4.5 hours to administer this fibrinolytic for patients unless they fall into these categories:

- Age older than 80 years
- Anticoagulation with an international normalized ratio less than or equal to 1.7
- Baseline National Institutes of Health Stroke Scale score greater than 25
- History of both stroke and diabetes

GENDER HEALTH CONSIDERATONS

Patient-Centered Care QSEN

Previous studies have suggested that being a female is a risk factor for delay in recognizing early symptoms of stroke and may contribute to ineligibility for fibrinolytic therapy. Current data show that women arrive at the ED at the same speed as men after acute ischemic stroke, so the delay in treatment does not appear to be related to transport time once the emergency medical transport system is called. Woman may be less likely to demonstrate focal symptoms, leading to diagnostic or treatment delay (Beal, 2010). Women have greater functional impairments at 3 months and 12 months after stroke and stroke treatment despite similar pre-stroke functional ability and admission score of stroke severity (Knauft et al., 2010).

Fibrinolytic therapy is explained to the patient and/or family member, and informed consent is obtained. The dosage of the drug is based on the patient's actual weight. Each hospital has strict protocols for mixing and administering the fibrinolytic drug and for monitoring the patient before and after fibrinolytic drug administration.

! NURSING SAFETY PRIORITY QSEN

Drug Alert

In addition to frequent monitoring of vital signs, carefully observe for signs of intracerebral hemorrhage and other signs of bleeding during administration of fibrinolytic drug therapy. Other best practice interventions are listed in Chart 45-5.

NCLEX EXAMINATION CHALLENGE

Physiological Integrity

A client begins to have severe epistaxis after completing a dose of alteplase. In order of priority, what are the nurse's actions?
A. Obtain vital signs.
B. Assess the airway, and set up suction at bedside.
C. Draw blood for anticoagulation studies.
D. Call the health care provider.

Endovascular Interventions. Endovascular procedures include intra-arterial thrombolysis using drug therapy, mechanical **embolectomy** (clot removal), and carotid stent placement. *Intra-arterial thrombolysis* has the advantage of delivering the fibrinolytic agent directly into the thrombus within 6 hours of the stroke's onset. It is particularly beneficial for some patients who have an occlusion of the middle cerebral artery or those who arrive in the ED after the window for rtPA. If the patient arrives in less than 8 hours, the interventional neuroradiologist may perform mechanical embolectomy using special instrumentation systems that can remove the clot by suction or other

CHART 45-5 Best Practice for Patient Safety & Quality Care QSEN

Nursing Interventions During and After IV Administration of Alteplase

- Perform a double check of the dose. Use a programmable pump to deliver the initial dose of 0.9 mg/kg (maximum dose 90 mg) over 60 minutes with 10% of the dose given as a bolus over 1 minute. Do not manually push this drug.
- Admit the patient to a critical care or specialized stroke unit.
- Perform neurologic assessments, including vital signs, every 10 to 15 minutes during infusion and every 30 minutes after that for at least 6 hours; monitor hourly for 24 hours after treatment. Be consistent regarding the device used to obtain blood pressures because blood pressures can vary when switching from a manual to a noninvasive automatic to an intra-arterial device.
- If systolic blood pressure is 180 mm Hg or greater or diastolic is 105 mm Hg or greater, give antihypertensive drugs as prescribed.
- To prevent bleeding, do not place invasive tubes, such as nasogastric (NG) tubes or indwelling urinary catheters, until the patient is stable.
- Discontinue the infusion if the patient reports severe headache or has severe hypertension, bleeding, nausea, and/or vomiting; notify the health care provider immediately.
- Obtain a follow-up CT scan after treatment before starting antiplatelet or anticoagulant drugs.

method (Mink & Miller, 2011a). Patients having either fibrinolytic therapy or endovascular interventions are admitted to the critical care setting for intensive collaborative monitoring.

Carotid artery angioplasty with stenting is common to *prevent* or, in some cases, help manage an acute ischemic stroke. This interventional radiology procedure is usually done under moderate sedation. It may be performed by a cardiovascular surgeon or interventional radiologist. A technique using a distal/embolic protection device has made this procedure very safe. The device is placed beyond the stenosis through a catheter inserted into the femoral artery (groin). The device catches any clot debris that breaks off during the procedure. Placement of a carotid stent is performed to open a blockage in the carotid artery typically at the division of the common carotid artery into the internal and external carotid arteries. Throughout the procedure, the patient's neurologic and cardiovascular statuses are assessed.

! NURSING SAFETY PRIORITY QSEN

Action Alert

Before discharge after carotid stent placement, teach the patient to report these symptoms to the health care provider as soon as possible:

- Severe headache
- Change in level of consciousness or COGNITION (e.g., drowsiness, new-onset confusion)
- Muscle weakness or motor dysfunction
- Severe neck pain
- Neck swelling
- Hoarseness or difficulty swallowing (due to nerve damage)

When the stroke is hemorrhagic and the cause is related to an AVM or cerebral aneurysm, the patient is evaluated for the optimal procedure to stop bleeding. The goal of treatment is to embolize abnormal vessels or the aneurysm itself. Some procedures can be used to prevent bleeding in an AVM or aneurysm that is discovered *prior* to symptom onset or SAH. Procedures occur in the interventional radiology suite or operating room. The different approaches used by the interventional neuroradiologist or neurosurgeon to embolize the vessel defect and nursing implications during postprocedure recovery are summarized in Table 45-3. How a brain aneurysm or AVM is treated depends on the size of the aneurysm, whether it has ruptured (bled), where in the brain it is located, and the age and overall health of the patient. Fig. 45-4 illustrates a common approach to manage an intact (non-ruptured) AVM.

Following endovascular procedures, a rare postprocedure complication, hyperperfusion syndrome, has a high morbidity and mortality rate. This syndrome is thought to be the result of an impaired autoregulation of cerebral blood flow that results from long-standing decreased cerebral PERFUSION pressure resulting from carotid artery disease. The signs and symptoms include severe temporal headache, hypertension, seizures, and focal neurologic deficits. This syndrome may be associated with intracranial hemorrhage and may occur within 1 hour postprocedure up to 24 hours or even 1 week later (Oran & Oran, 2010).

Monitoring for Increased Intracranial Pressure. The patient is most at risk for increased ICP resulting from edema during the first 72 hours after onset of the stroke. Some patients may have worsening of their neurologic status starting within 24 to 48 hours after their endovascular procedure from increased ICP (Chart 45-6). Reassess patients with stroke and with endovascular treatment of stroke symptoms every 1 to 4 hours depending on severity of the condition. Use the approved assessment strategy and documentation tools.

! NURSING SAFETY PRIORITY QSEN

Critical Rescue

Be alert for symptoms of increased ICP in the stroke patient, and report any deterioration in the patient's neurologic status to the health care provider immediately! *The first sign of increased ICP is a declining level of consciousness (LOC).*

The best head-of-bed (HOB) positioning has not yet been determined; more studies are needed to determine best practice. A reduced head elevation of less than 25 degrees can improve perfusion pressure to damaged brain in ischemic conditions like most strokes. However, a HOB elevation greater than 30 degrees can improve oxygenation and reduce aspiration risk. Provide oxygen therapy to prevent hypoxia for patients with oxygen saturation less than 93%. Maintain the head in a midline, neutral position to help promote venous drainage from the brain. In collaboration with other team members, avoid sudden and acute hip or neck flexion during positioning. Extreme hip flexion may increase intrathoracic pressure, leading to decreased cerebral venous outflow and elevated ICP. Extreme neck flexion also interferes with venous drainage from the brain and intracranial dynamics.

Additional nursing considerations include avoiding the clustering of nursing procedures (e.g., giving a bath followed immediately by changing the bed linen). When multiple activities are clustered in a narrow time period, the effect on ICP can be dramatic elevation. Hyperoxygenating the patient before suctioning may also be appropriate to avoid even transient hypoxemia and resultant ICP elevation from dilation of cerebral arteries. Coughing and suctioning increase ICP. Careful attention to airway management can reduce unnecessary increases in ICP.

TABLE 45-3 Surgical and Interventional Radiologic Procedures to Manage Intracranial Aneurysms and Arteriovenous Malformations

PROCEDURE	DESCRIPTION	NURSING IMPLICATIONS
Surgical ligation or resection	A neurosurgeon performs a full or micro-craniectomy. Once the defective vessels are located, they are separated from brain tissue and removed. A graft may be placed to preserve blood flow of the parent vessel. Surgical elimination of arteriovenous malformation (AVM) or aneurysm depends on the size of the defect, the risk for major brain damage during resection, the absence of bleeding, and the condition of the patient preoperatively.	Ligation and clip placement can be done simultaneously. Preoperative and postoperative care are similar to that for patients undergoing a craniotomy as described in this chapter. Perioperative care described in Chapters 14-16 is also essential.
Clip	Clips are small devices, similar to a paperclip, that are clamped over the aneurysm base to isolate it from the parent vessel circulation. The neurosurgeon performs a full craniotomy or micro-craniotomy to visualize the aneurysm in the operating room. A contrast agent is injected into the vessel to determine the degree of aneurysm occlusion and parent vessel patency. Micro-Doppler ultrasonography can also be used to evaluate the placement of the clips intraoperatively.	Older clips have metal components, preventing use of magnetic resonance imaging postprocedure. It is possible for clips to move, and movement is greatest immediately postplacement. Movement may occur as late as 2-5 years after placement. Patients require care as outlined under the perioperative chapters with close neurologic assessment to detect early rebleeding or migration of the clip. Changes in cognition or new focal neurologic deficits must be communicated urgently to the neurosurgeon.
Coil —With stent assist —With balloon assist	Detachable coils are placed under fluoroscopy to occlude the aneurysm without interrupting main vessel flow. Coils are platinum, and some are coated with polymers to promote fibrosis. Stents are used to enhance vessel stability and are an adjunct prior to vessel rupture. Balloon-assisted coil placement is thought to enhance endovascular remodeling and decrease postprocedure rebleeding when the aneurysm is intact before the procedure.	Up to 20% of patients experience bleeding or rebleeding after coil placement, with the greatest risk for bleeding occurring in the year following the procedure. As a result, patients are advised to avoid drugs that interfere with clotting during recovery. Patients return for re-evaluation typically at 3, 6, and 12 months to determine the extent of embolization. Full embolization is the goal for this type of procedure; it is possible to undergo a second placement of coils to achieve best results. Teach the patient to maintain an ongoing relationship with the neurosurgeon to evaluate the effectiveness of the procedure over time. Perform frequent neurologic assessments in the first 24 hours postprocedure to detect intracranial bleeding early.
Flow diversion	These stent-like devices look like a braided cylindric mesh and are delivered under fluoroscopy to the neck of an aneurysm, shifting blood flow away from the vessel defect and resulting in a thrombosed (clotted) aneurysm over 5-6 months. An example is the pipeline embolization device (PED).	These are the newest devices for treatment of intracranial aneurysms. Full embolization takes 5-12 months, so ongoing monitoring by the neurosurgery staff in community health settings (office or clinic) is common postprocedure. Encourage the patient to avoid strenuous activity or situations that create hypertension while the prolonged embolization occurs.
Liquid polymer embolization	This procedure is reserved for AVMs. It is used either preoperatively to reduce the size of the AVM or as a permanent treatment for a small AVM. Treatment can occur once or over several stages to achieve maximum AVM reduction.	This procedure is often used prior to surgical ligation or stereotactic surgery to reduce the size of the AVM and decrease the number of branches of the tangled, defective vessel. Help the patient understand that this procedure may not provide definitive treatment if it is either staged or planned to precede surgery. Perform frequent neurologic assessment in the 24 hours postprocedure to detect early signs of bleeding.
Stereotactic surgery	Under the simultaneous supervision of the neurosurgeon, radiologist, and physicist, microwave or radio beams are directed to the defective vessel(s) to obliterate the defect.	Stereotactic surgery requires that the patient undergo extensive diagnostic study and be placed in a brace that will hold the head fixed while the beam is directed toward the abnormal vessel. Swelling around the beam site may alter neurologic status. Perform neurologic assessment with each opportunity to take vital signs, and inform the neurosurgeon of any deterioration in consciousness or new focal weakness or sensory changes.

A quiet environment is particularly important for the patient experiencing a headache, which is common with a cerebral hemorrhage or increased ICP. The patient may have **photophobia** (sensitivity to light). Therefore keep the room lights very low.

Close physiologic monitoring of blood pressure, heart rhythm, oxygen saturation, blood glucose, and body temperature may prevent secondary brain injury and promote good outcomes after stroke. High quality evidence is not available on how to manage blood pressure in patients with hemorrhagic strokes, but for many patients, severe hypertension is the cause of their stroke (Mink & Miller, 2011b). Assessing vital signs (VS) regularly and communicating concerning changes from baseline promote quality and safety for both individualized and system-wide outcomes.

Monitor vital signs closely, at least every 1 to 2 hours. Notify the health care provider if the blood pressure or core temperature does not meet a prescribed range of values. Although the optimal blood pressure range after stroke is controversial, the health care provider may allow the patient with *acute ischemic stroke* to be slightly hypertensive with a systolic blood pressure (SBP) between 140 and 150 mm Hg to promote cerebral tissue

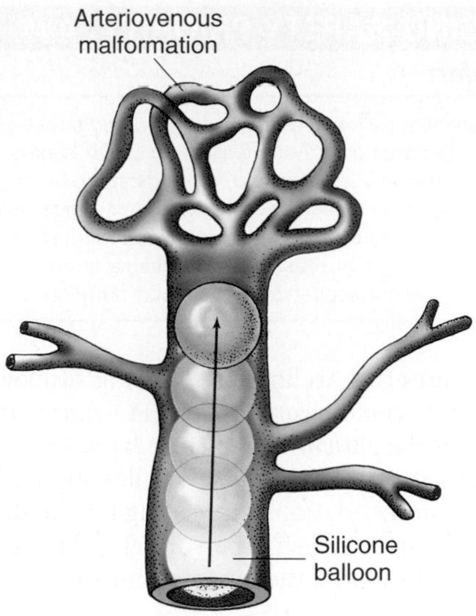

FIG. 45-4 Embolization procedure to treat an arteriovenous malformation. The liquid embolic agent causes vessel thrombosis.

CHART 45-6 Key Features
Increased Intracranial Pressure (ICP)

- Decreased level of consciousness (LOC) (lethargy to coma)
- Behavior changes: restlessness, irritability, and confusion
- Headache
- Nausea and vomiting (may be projectile)
- Change in speech pattern
  - Aphasia
  - Slurred speech
- Change in sensorimotor status
  - Pupillary changes: dilated and nonreactive pupils ("blown pupils") or constricted and nonreactive pupils
  - Cranial nerve dysfunction
  - Ataxia
- Seizures (usually within first 24 hours after stroke)
- Cushing's triad
  - Severe hypertension
  - Widened pulse pressure
  - Bradycardia
- Abnormal posturing:
  - Decerebrate (extensor)
  - Decorticate (flexion)

PERFUSION. A SBP greater than 180 mm Hg or a diastolic BP greater than 110 mm Hg is generally considered dangerous, contributing to a risk for hemorrhagic stroke or rebleeding of an aneurysm (if present). Carefully monitor the patient's temperature because fever may extend the area of injury in the brain.

! NURSING SAFETY PRIORITY (QSEN)
Critical Rescue

If the stroke patient's SBP is more than 180 mm Hg, notify the health care provider immediately and anticipate prescription of an IV antihypertensive medication. Monitor the patient's BP and mean arterial pressure (MAP) every 5 minutes until the SBP is between 140 and 150 mm Hg to maintain brain PERFUSION. Avoid a sudden SBP drop to less than 120 mm Hg with drug administration.

Monitoring for Other Complications. Monitor the patient with an aneurysm or arteriovenous malformation (AVM) as well as patients following repair of these vessel malformations for signs and symptoms of hydrocephalus and vasospasm. **Hydrocephalus** (increased cerebrospinal fluid [CSF] within the ventricular and subarachnoid spaces) may occur as a result of blood in the CSF. This prevents CSF from being reabsorbed properly by the arachnoid villi. Cerebral edema, which interferes with the flow of CSF out from the ventricular system, may also develop. Eventually the ventricles become enlarged. If hydrocephalus is left untreated, increased intracranial pressure (ICP) results. Observe for clinical manifestations of hydrocephalus, which are similar to those of ICP elevation, including a change in the LOC. Clinical findings may also include headache, pupil changes, seizures, poor coordination, gait disturbances (if ambulatory), and behavior changes.

If blood is in the subarachnoid space, the patient is at risk for cerebral vasospasm. Clinical manifestations of vasospasm may include decreased LOC, motor and reflex changes, and increased neurologic deficits (e.g., cranial nerve dysfunction, motor weakness, and aphasia). The symptoms may fluctuate with the occurrence and degree of vasospasm present. Hemorrhage-related cerebral vasospasm can result in permanent vascular changes and irreversible neurologic impairment.

Rebleeding or rupture is a common complication for the patient with an aneurysm or AVM. Recurrent hemorrhage may occur within 24 hours of the initial bleed or rupture and up to 7 to 10 days later. About 20% of patients experience a second episode of bleeding after a repair of vessel malformations. Assess for severe headache, nausea and vomiting, a decreased LOC, and additional neurologic deficits. Potential consequences of a second cerebral hemorrhagic event may be catastrophic.

Patients admitted to a critical care unit are observed for dysrhythmias with cardiac monitoring. The nurse performs a cardiac assessment, with particular attention to identify the presence of cardiac murmurs or atrial fibrillation (AF). Cardiac valve disorders, manifested by a murmur or AF, place the patient at increased risk for emboli.

Both hyperglycemia and hypoglycemia are associated with new, secondary brain damage. Too high or too low blood sugar values increase the area of primary brain damage and contribute to greater disability from stroke. Monitor the patient's finger stick blood sugars (FSBS) frequently. Perform an FSBS when there is any unexplained decrease in level of consciousness for the patient admitted with a central nervous system injury or insult. Ensure daily communication with the health care team members to share desired glycemic outcomes and interventions to achieve them.

Ongoing Drug Therapy. Ongoing drug therapy depends on the type of stroke and the resulting neurologic dysfunction. In general, the purposes of drug therapy are to prevent further thrombotic episodes (anticoagulation) and to protect the neurons from hypoxia.

The use of aspirin or other antiplatelet drug is considered for treatment following acute ischemic strokes or for preventing future strokes when risk factors of prodromal symptoms (TIA) occur (Bousser, 2012). Sodium heparin and other anticoagulants, such as warfarin (Coumadin, Warfilone 🍁), are used in the presence of atrial fibrillation. *Anticoagulants are high-alert drugs that can cause bleeding, including intracerebral hemorrhage.*

An *initial* dose of 325 mg of aspirin (Ecotrin, Ancasal 🍁) is recommended within 24 to 48 hours after stroke onset. Aspirin should not be given within 24 hours of rtPA administration. Low-dose aspirin is an antiplatelet drug and reduces blood clotting by reducing platelet adhesiveness (clumping). Aspirin can cause bruising, hemorrhage, and liver disease over a long-term period. Teach the patient to report any unusual bruising or bleeding to the health care provider.

A calcium channel blocking drug that crosses the blood-brain barrier such as nimodipine (Nimotop) may be given to treat or prevent cerebral vasospasm after a subarachnoid hemorrhage. Vasospasm, which usually occurs between 4 and 14 days after the stroke, slows blood flow to the area and worsens ischemia. Nimodipine works by relaxing the smooth muscles of the vessel wall and reducing the incidence and severity of the spasm. Neurologic functioning may improve, and further deterioration from ischemia is then prevented. In addition, this drug dilates collateral vessels to ischemic areas of the brain.

Stool softeners, analgesics for pain, and antianxiety drugs may also be prescribed as needed for symptom management. Stool softeners also prevent the Valsalva maneuver during defecation to prevent increased ICP.

Surgical Management. Few patients are candidates for immediate surgery once a stroke occurs. A neurosurgeon may perform a decompressive craniectomy (explained on p. 956) to manage refractory intracranial hypertension in a patient with a massive stroke.

Following recovery from a stroke or to prevent a TIA from progressing to a stroke, the patient may have surgery to improve cerebral circulation. In an **extracranial-intracranial bypass**, the surgeon performs a craniotomy (surgical opening into the brain through the skull) and bypasses the blocked artery by making a graft or a bypass from the first artery to the second artery. This procedure establishes blood flow around the blocked artery and re-establishes blood flow to the involved areas. The two most common techniques are the superficial temporal artery–to–middle cerebral artery (STA-MCA) graft and the occipital–to–posterior inferior cerebellar artery (PICA) bypass.

Whenever possible, an AVM is also totally removed via a craniotomy. The surgeon cuts and separates the group of vessels and removes the defect. Radiosurgery (Gamma Knife) can also be used by the neurosurgeon. Radiation delivered during surgery results in fibrous thickening of the endothelial lining of the vessels to prevent further vessel enlargement and ultimately eliminate the lesion from the cerebral circulation. Improved microsurgical techniques have significantly reduced morbidity and mortality rates, and these procedures are becoming the treatment of choice in many medical centers.

Managing Impaired Swallowing

Planning: Expected Outcomes. The patient with a stroke is expected to avoid aspiration and have adequate nutrition to promote health and prevent complications, including major weight loss.

Interventions. Aspiration is a frequent complication for patients with dysphagia (difficulty swallowing) (Hughes, 2011). Many of these aspirations are "silent" and are not recognized until pulmonary complications occur.

Observe the patient for facial drooping, drooling, impaired voluntary cough, hoarseness, incomplete mouth closure, or cranial nerve palsies. Next check the gag and cough reflexes. If the patient does not pass this swallowing screen, collaborate with the speech-language pathologist (SLP) to conduct a bedside swallowing evaluation. He or she may recommend a modified barium swallow (video fluoroscopy) to identify specific structures that are impaired during swallowing. *Ensure that the patient remains completely NPO status until the SLP determines that the patient can tolerate liquids or foods without aspirating.* Based on the complete swallowing evaluation, the SLP makes recommendations for feeding for the staff to follow. Remind all unlicensed assistive personnel (UAP) and the family about the need to follow these precautions exactly as they are written.

> **! NURSING SAFETY PRIORITY** QSEN
>
> ***Action Alert***
>
> The best practice for all *suspected* and *diagnosed* stroke patients is to maintain a NPO status until their swallowing ability is assessed. Before the patient is given any liquids, food, or medication, he or she must be screened for the ability to swallow. Follow agency guidelines for screening or use an evidence-based bedside swallowing screening tool to determine if dysphagia is present. If dysphagia is present, develop a plan of care to prevent aspiration and support nutrition.

Some patients can swallow without difficulty but are at risk for aspiration because they are easily distracted and impulsive. These patients require a distraction-free environment with minimal disruption from television, visitors, or environmental noise. Observe for indications of fatigue, because it can significantly interfere with the patient's desire and ability to eat.

Studies indicate that as many as 50% of patients are malnourished at 2 to 3 weeks after a severe stroke. To avoid this complication, collaborate with the dietitian to provide an accurate, comprehensive nutritional assessment on admission and throughout the hospital stay (Perry et al., 2013). Implement nutritional interventions, such as an early gastrostomy or oral nutrition, by at least the third or fourth hospital day to prevent weight loss, an altered immune status, increased length of stay, and increased mortality (Hughes, 2011).

For patients who can tolerate oral foods and liquids, follow the SLP's recommendations for thickened liquids, head positioning, and patient teaching to prevent aspiration. Teach UAP and family members how to follow these instructions, and have them readily available for reference.

> **NCLEX EXAMINATION CHALLENGE**
>
> ***Physiological Integrity***
>
> A client with a confirmed acute ischemic stroke is comatose but breathing spontaneously. The client has an advance directive requesting limited resuscitation and is not a candidate for fibrinolytic therapy. What is the nurse's priority action on admission?
>
> A. Ask for palliative care consultation to assist with end-of-life decision making.
> B. Consult with the speech-language pathologist about alternative strategies for communication.
> C. Evaluate swallowing ability with an institution-specific, evidence-based protocol.
> D. Assess vital signs and determine if the advance directives need to be communicated to the health care provider.

Improving Mobility and Promoting Self-Care

Planning: Expected Outcomes. The patient with a stroke is expected to ambulate and provide self-care independently, with or without one or more assistive-adaptive devices.

Interventions. Patients who have had a stroke often have flaccid or spastic paralysis. It is not unusual for the patient to eventually have a flaccid arm and spastic leg on the affected side because the affected leg often regains function more quickly than the arm. Patients begin rehabilitation as soon as possible to regain function and prevent complications of immobility, such as pneumonia, atelectasis, and pressure ulcers.

! NURSING SAFETY PRIORITY (QSEN)

Action Alert

Be sure to support the affected flaccid arm of the stroke patient, and teach UAP to avoid pulling on it. Position the arm on a pillow while the patient is sitting to prevent it from hanging freely, which could cause shoulder subluxation. The physical or occupational therapist provides a sling-like device to support the arm during ambulation.

Another major complication of impaired MOBILITY is the development of venous thromboembolism (VTE), especially deep vein thrombosis (DVT) that can lead to a pulmonary embolism (PE). This risk is highest in older patients and those with a severe stroke. Per The Joint Commission's Core Measures for VTE, provide care to prevent this complication by applying intermittent sequential pneumatic devices, changing the patient's position frequently, and ambulating the patient if possible. Report any indications of DVT to the health care provider, and document assessments in the patient's record. Chapter 36 discusses VTE prevention in detail.

The rehabilitation therapists evaluate the patient's ability to perform MOBILITY skills, basic ADLs, and household tasks that will be performed at home. After a thorough evaluation, collaborate with them to develop a plan of care to promote patient independence, with or without assistive or adaptive devices. Therapy begins in the hospital setting and continues after discharge in most cases. Chapter 6 describes interventions for rehabilitation, including improving MOBILITY and promoting self-care.

Promoting Effective Communication

Planning: Expected Outcomes. The patient with a stroke is expected to receive, interpret, and express spoken, written, and nonverbal messages, if possible. However, some patients may need to develop strategies for alternative methods of communication, such as pictures or nonverbal language.

Interventions. Language or speech problems are usually the result of a stroke involving the dominant hemisphere. The left cerebral hemisphere is the speech center in most patients. Speech and language problems may be the result of aphasia or dysarthria. Whereas aphasia is caused by cerebral hemisphere damage, **dysarthria** (slurred speech) is due to a loss of motor function to the tongue or to the muscles of speech, causing facial weakness and slurred speech. Involvement of the speech-language pathologist (SLP) as early as possible in the hospitalization greatly increases the patient's chances for optimal recovery. Remind patients to practice their exercises for dysarthria to strengthen their facial and oral muscles.

Aphasia can be classified in a number of ways. Most commonly, it is classified as expressive, receptive, or mixed (Table 45-4). **Expressive (Broca's, or motor) aphasia** is the result of damage in Broca's area of the frontal lobe. It is a motor speech problem in which the patient generally understands what is said but cannot communicate verbally. He or she also has difficulty writing but may be able to write. Rote speech and automatic speech such as responses to a greeting are often intact. The

TABLE 45-4 Types of Aphasia

Expressive (or nonfluent)
- Referred to as *Broca's*, or *motor, aphasia*
- Difficulty speaking
- Difficulty writing

Receptive
- Referred to as *Wernicke's*, or *sensory, aphasia*
- Difficulty understanding spoken words
- Difficulty understanding written words
- Speech often meaningless
- Made-up words

Mixed
- Combination of difficulty understanding words and speech
- Difficulty with reading and writing

Global
- Profound speech and language problems
- Often no speech or sounds that cannot be understood

patient is aware of the deficit and may become frustrated and angry. Reassure patients, and remind them to talk slowly.

Receptive (Wernicke's, or sensory) aphasia is due to injury involving Wernicke's area in the temporoparietal area. The patient cannot understand the spoken and often the written word. Although he or she may be able to talk, the language is often meaningless. Neologisms (made-up words) are common parts of speech.

Usually the patient has some degree of dysfunction in the areas of both expression and reception. This is known as *mixed aphasia.* Reading and writing ability are equally affected. Few patients have just expressive *or* receptive aphasia. In most cases, though, one type is dominant.

To help communicate with the patient with aphasia, use these guiding principles:

- Present one idea or thought in a sentence (e.g., "I am going to help you get into the chair.").
- Use simple one-step commands rather than ask patients to do multiple tasks.
- Speak slowly but not loudly; use cues or gestures as needed.
- Avoid "yes" and "no" questions for patients with expressive aphasia, because they often give automatic responses that may be incorrect.
- Use alternative forms of communication if needed, such as a computer, communication board, or flash cards (often with pictures).

For more specific communication strategies for your patient, collaborate with the SLP.

Promoting Continence

Planning: Expected Outcomes. The patient with a stroke is expected to control elimination of urine and stool.

Interventions. The patient may be incontinent of urine and stool because of an altered level of consciousness, impaired innervation to the bladder and rectum, and/or the inability to communicate the need to urinate or defecate. Before beginning a patient education program to correct these problems, the cause must first be established. Typically, the patient who has had a stroke can regain both bowel and bladder control in time. To begin a bladder training program, place the patient on the bedpan or the commode or offer the urinal every 2 hours. Encourage a total fluid intake to maintain dilute urine and a balanced intake and output. A bedside bladder ultrasound is used to check for residual urine after voiding in the early phase of the bladder training program to ensure that the patient is emptying the bladder. Retained urine can lead to a urinary tract infection.

Before establishing a bowel training program, determine the patient's normal time for bowel elimination and any routine that helps promote a stool. This routine is followed, if possible, and the patient is placed on the commode or toilet at the same time as the previous schedule at home. Encourage the patient to drink apple or prune juice and to consume high-fiber foods to help promote bowel elimination. A stool softener (Colace) may be prescribed. Suppositories may also assist in re-establishing a bowel routine. Chapter 6 provides a discussion of bowel and bladder training programs.

If the patient has an indwelling urinary catheter, it should be removed as soon as hourly urine output is no longer essential to therapeutic decisions. The patient with a fever or an older adult who becomes increasingly confused should always be evaluated for a urinary tract infection.

Managing Changes in Sensory Perception

Planning: Expected Outcomes. The major concern of patients with SENSORY PERCEPTION deficits is adapting to neurologic deficits. Therefore the patient with a stroke is expected to adapt to sensory perception changes in vision, proprioception (position sense), and sensation and to be free from injury.

Interventions. Patients with right hemisphere brain damage typically have difficulty with visual-perceptual or spatial-perceptual tasks. They have problems with depth and distance perception and with discrimination of right from left or up from down. Because of these problems, they have difficulty performing routine ADLs. Caregivers help the patient adapt to these disabilities by using frequent verbal and tactile cues and by breaking down tasks into discrete steps. Always approach the patient from the unaffected side, which should face the door of the room.

Place objects within the patient's field of vision. A mirror may help visualize more of the environment. If the patient has **diplopia** (double vision), a patch may be placed over the affected eye. Remind the nursing staff to ensure a safe environment by removing clutter from the room.

The patient with a left hemisphere lesion generally has memory deficits and may show significant changes in the ability to carry out simple tasks. To assist with memory problems, re-orient the patient to the month, year, day of the week, and circumstances surrounding hospital admission. Establish a routine or schedule that is as structured, repetitious, and consistent as possible. Provide information in a simple, concise manner. A step-by-step approach is often most effective because the patient can master one step before moving to the next. When possible, ask the family to bring in pictures and other familiar objects.

The patient may be unable to plan and execute tasks in an organized manner. **Apraxia**, or the inability to perform previously learned motor skills or commands, may be present. Typically, the patient with apraxia exhibits a slow, cautious, and hesitant behavior style. The physical therapist (PT) assists the patient in compensating for loss of position sense.

Managing Unilateral Body Neglect

Planning: Expected Outcomes. The patient with stroke is expected to adjust and use techniques to compensate for unilateral (one-sided) body neglect.

Interventions. Unilateral neglect, or neglect syndrome, occurs most commonly in patients who have had a right cerebral stroke. However, it can occur in any patient who experiences hemianopsia, in which the vision of one or both eyes is affected. This problem places the patient at additional risk for injury, especially falls, because of an inability to recognize his or her physical impairment or because of a lack of proprioception (position sense).

Teach the patient to touch and use both sides of the body. For example, encourage the patient to wash both the affected and unaffected sides of the body. When dressing, remind the patient to dress the affected side first. If hemianopsia is present, teach the patient to turn his or her head from side to side to expand the visual field. This scanning technique is also useful when the patient is eating or ambulating.

Community-Based Care

The patient with a stroke may be discharged to home, a rehabilitation center, or a skilled nursing facility (SNF), depending on the extent of the disability and the availability of family or caregiver support. Some patients have no significant neurologic dysfunction and are able to return home and live independently or with minimal support. Other patients are able to return home but require ongoing assistance with ADLs and supervision to prevent accidents or injury. The case or care manager coordinates speech/language, physical, and/or occupational therapy services to continue in the home or on an ambulatory care basis. Patients admitted to a rehabilitation unit/facility or SNF require continued or more complex nursing care as well as extensive physical, occupational, recreational, speech-language, or cognitive therapy, which is coordinated by a case manager. The expected outcome for rehabilitation is to maximize the patient's abilities in all aspects of life. Some patients who have strokes have severe brain damage with profound neurologic impairments and require palliative care.

Home Care Management. Collaborate with the case manager to plan the patient's discharge. Coordinate with rehabilitation therapists to identify needs for assistive or adaptive and safety equipment. The extent of this assessment depends on the patient's disabilities. Teach the patient and family to ensure that the home is free from scatter rugs or other obstacles in the walking pathways. The bathtub and toilet should be equipped with grab bars. Anti-skid patches or strips should be placed in the bathtub to prevent slipping. The PT or OT works with the patient and the family or significant others to obtain all needed assistive devices and home modifications *before* the patient is discharged from the hospital, rehabilitation setting, or SNF. Appointments for ambulatory care speech, physical, and occupational therapy are arranged before discharge for continuing care.

Self-Management Education. As part of the discharge process, teach the family about depression that may occur within the 3 months after a stroke. The strongest predictors of post-stroke depression (PSD) are a history of depression, severe stroke, and post-stroke physical or cognitive impairment. Patients may not exhibit typical signs of depression because of their cognitive, physical, and emotional impairments. PSD is associated with increased morbidity and mortality, especially in older men.

The three areas that should be included in patient and family education are disease prevention, disease-specific information, and self-management (American Heart Association, 2014).

EVIDENCE-BASED PRACTICE (QSEN)

What Are the Best Practices for Teaching Patients and Their Families About Strokes?

Cameron, V. (2013). Best practices for stroke patient and family education in the acute care setting: A literature review. *MEDSURG Nursing, 22*(3), 51-55.

Many patients have strokes and are admitted to the acute care setting. Nurses need to know the most effective methods for educating these patients and their families before they are discharged from the hospital. The researcher conducted an integrative interdisciplinary review of the literature published between 2003 and 2012 to determine the best practices for patient and family education. Three areas of health teaching are needed: stroke prevention, stroke-specific education, and self-management skills. Best practices for these areas include:

- Be flexible and adapt to the health and learning needs of the patient (e.g., aphasia is/is not present).
- Use multiple types of education materials (written, audiovisual, interactive strategies).
- Focus on key points, and be repetitive; as many as five or six repetitions are associated with retention.
- Group meetings may be beneficial to patient understanding, motivation, and quality of life.
- Use reading materials with a low literacy level, large font type, and short (15 minute) learning sessions.
- Identify sources of emotional support, encourage social support, and locate community education groups for caregivers to enhance their well-being.

Level of Evidence: 1

This study provided a systematic review of literature to determine best practices for teaching patients with strokes and their families about the disease and self-management.

Commentary: Implications for Practice and Research

This review did not use statistical analysis to generate recommendations for patient and family education, an approach common to integrative reviews. The strategies are practical and accessible to nurses and health care team members in both hospital and community care settings. Nurses need to consider the specific limitations, health needs, and health literacy of patients with strokes to modify their approach to health teaching as needed.

The teaching plan includes lifestyle changes, drug therapy, ambulation/transfer skills, communication skills, safety precautions, nutritional management, activity levels, and self-management skills. Health teaching should focus on tasks that must be performed by the patient and the family after hospital discharge. Provide both written and verbal instruction in all these areas (see the Evidence-Based Practice box). Return demonstrations assist in evaluating the family members' competency in tasks required for the patient's care (Fig. 45-5).

Teach patients to take their prescribed drugs to prevent another stroke and control hypertension. Instruct the patient and the family the name of each drug, the dosage, the timing of administration, how to take it, and possible side effects. In collaboration with the PT and OT, teach the patient how to climb stairs safely, if he or she is able; transfer from the bed to a chair; get into and out of a car; and use any aids for MOBILITY. The patient and family members are also taught how to use any equipment needed to increase independence in self-management skills. Provide important information regarding what to do in an emergency and who to call for nonemergency questions.

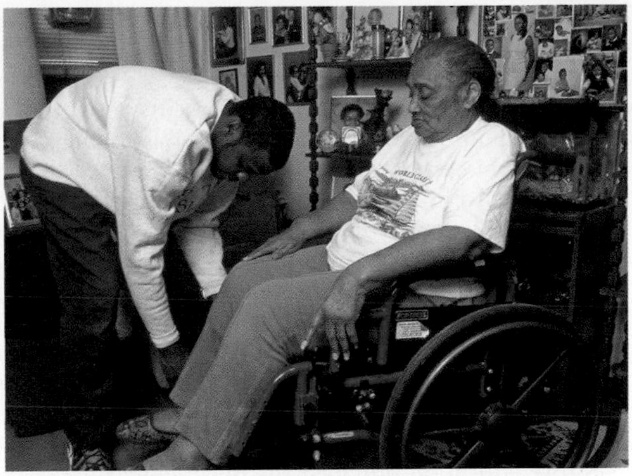

FIG. 45-5 Son adjusting his mother's wheelchair.

Families may feel overwhelmed by the continuing demands placed on them. Depending on the location of the lesion, the patient may be anxious, slow, cautious, and hesitant and lack initiative (left hemisphere lesions). As a result of right hemisphere lesions, he or she may be impulsive and seemingly unaware of any deficit. Family members and other caregivers need to spend time away from the patient on a routine basis to continue to provide full-time care without sacrificing their own physical and emotional health. Refer the family to social services or other community resources for further support, counseling, and possible respite care.

Health Care Resources. Available resources include a variety of publications from the American Heart Association (www.americanheart.org), including *Stroke: A Guide for Families* and *Stroke: Why Do They Behave That Way?* The National Stroke Association (www.stroke.org) also provides publications and videotapes for caregivers and patients. *Recovering After a Stroke: A Patient and Family Guide* is available from the Agency for Healthcare Research and Quality (www.ahrq.gov). Refer the patient and family members or significant others to local stroke support groups.

For patients who require symptom management or end-of-life care, refer the family to palliative care or hospice services. Chapter 7 gives a detailed description of end-of-life care and advance directives.

◆ *Evaluation: Outcomes*

Evaluate the care of the patient with stroke based on the identified priority patient problems. The expected outcomes are that the patient:

- Maintains blood pressure and blood sugar within a safe, prescribed range
- Performs self-care and MOBILITY activities independently, with or without assistive devices
- Learns to adapt to SENSORY PERCEPTION changes
- Adjusts and uses techniques to compensate for one-sided neglect
- Communicates effectively or develops strategies for effective communication
- Has adequate nutrition and avoids aspiration
- Controls elimination of urine and stool

There are eight core measures associated with the care of stroke patients (The Joint Commission, 2014). These core measures form the basis of not only individual patient goals but also system-wide goals of care. As a result, continuous quality improvement efforts are based on these core measures. Certification as a Stroke Center is tied to consistent performance in achieving satisfactory core measures. The core measures may have additional implications in terms of reimbursement in the future. The eight core measures for Ischemic Stroke Care are:

1. Venous thromboembolism (VTE) prophylaxis
2. Discharge with antithrombotic therapy
3. Anticoagulation therapy for atrial fibrillation/flutter
4. Thrombolytic therapy (in the presence of a thrombotic stroke of <4 hours from symptom onset)
5. Antithrombotic therapy is evaluated by end of hospital day (e.g., diagnostic testing for therapeutic range of values following thrombolytic or anticoagulant therapy)
6. Discharged on statin medication
7. Stroke education provided and documented
8. Assessed for rehabilitation

Comprehensive stroke centers are required to collect data for the eight stroke core measures and submit monthly data points every quarter through the Certification Measure Information Process (CMIP). Nurses not only provide direct care to patients with ischemic stroke but also contribute to the peer review process to evaluate and monitor the care provided to patients with ischemic stroke.

TRAUMATIC BRAIN INJURY

PATHOPHYSIOLOGY

Traumatic brain injury (TBI) is damage to the brain from an external mechanical force and not caused by neurodegenerative or congenital conditions. TBI can lead to temporary and permanent impairment of cognitive, physical, and psychosocial functions.

Various terms are used to describe the brain injuries that occur when a mechanical force is applied either directly or indirectly to the brain. A force produced by a blow to the head is a *direct* injury, whereas a force applied to another body part with a rebound effect to the brain is an *indirect* injury. The brain responds to these forces by movement within the rigid cranial vault. It may also rebound or rotate on the brainstem, causing diffuse axonal injury (shearing injuries). The brain may be contused (bruised) or lacerated/torn as it moves over the inner surfaces of the cranium, which are irregularly shaped and sharp.

Movement or distortion within the cranial cavity is possible because of multiple factors. The first factor is how the brain is supported by cerebrospinal fluid (CSF) within the cranial cavity. When external force is applied to the head, the brain can be injured by the internal surfaces of the skull and meninges. The second factor is the consistency of brain tissue, which is very fragile and prone to injury. Brain injury occurs from both initial forces on the head and brain and as a result of secondary derangements of physiologic stability.

The type of force and the mechanism of injury contribute to traumatic brain injury. An *acceleration* injury is caused by an external force contacting the head, suddenly placing the head in motion. A *deceleration* injury occurs when the moving head is suddenly stopped or hits a stationary object (Fig. 45-6). These forces may be sufficient to cause the cerebrum to rotate about the brainstem, resulting in shearing, straining, and distortion of the brain tissue, particularly of the axons in the brainstem and cerebellum. Small areas of hemorrhage (contusion, intracranial hemorrhage) may develop around the blood vessels that sustain the impact of these forces (stress), with destruction of adjacent brain tissue. Particularly affected are the basal nuclei and the hypothalamus.

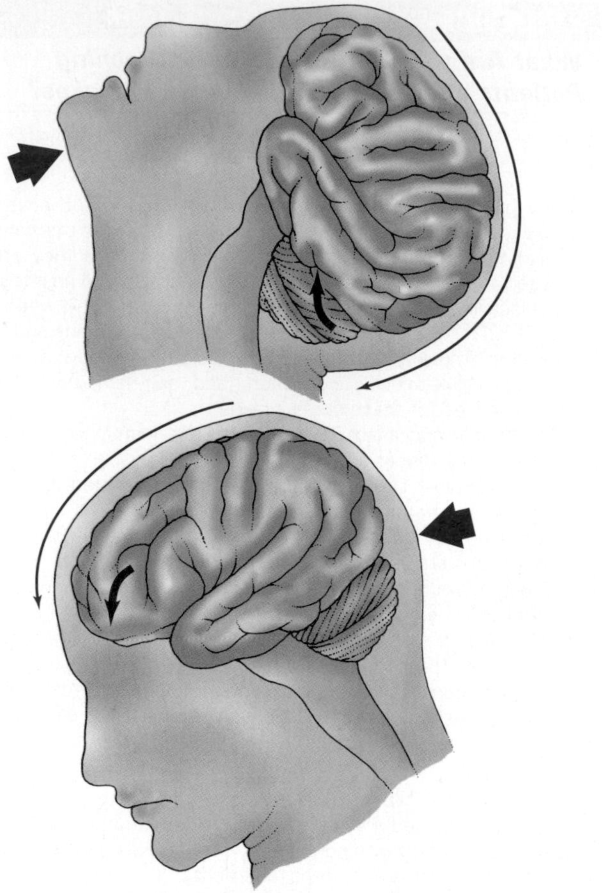

FIG. 45-6 Head movement during acceleration-deceleration injury, which is typically seen in motor vehicle crashes.

Primary Brain Injury

Primary brain damage occurs at the time of injury and results from the physical stress (force) within the tissue caused by blunt force. A primary brain injury may be categorized as focal or diffuse. A *focal* brain injury is confined to a specific area of the brain and causes localized damage that can often be detected with a CT scan or MRI. *Diffuse* injuries are characterized by damage throughout many areas of the brain. They initially may be at a microscopic level and not initially detectable by CT scan. MRI has greater ability to detect microscopic damage, but these areas may not be imaged until necrosis occurs.

Primary brain injuries are also classed as either open or closed. An **open traumatic brain injury** occurs when the skull is fractured or when it is pierced by a penetrating object. The integrity of the brain and the dura is violated, and there is exposure to environmental contaminants. Damage may occur to the underlying vessels, dural sinus, brain, and cranial nerves. In a **closed traumatic brain injury**, the integrity of the skull is not violated.

Open Versus Closed Traumatic Brain Injury. The types of skull fractures associated with *open traumatic brain injury* are linear, depressed, open, and comminuted. A *linear fracture* is a simple, clean break in which the impacted area of bone bends inward and the area around it bends outward. Linear fractures

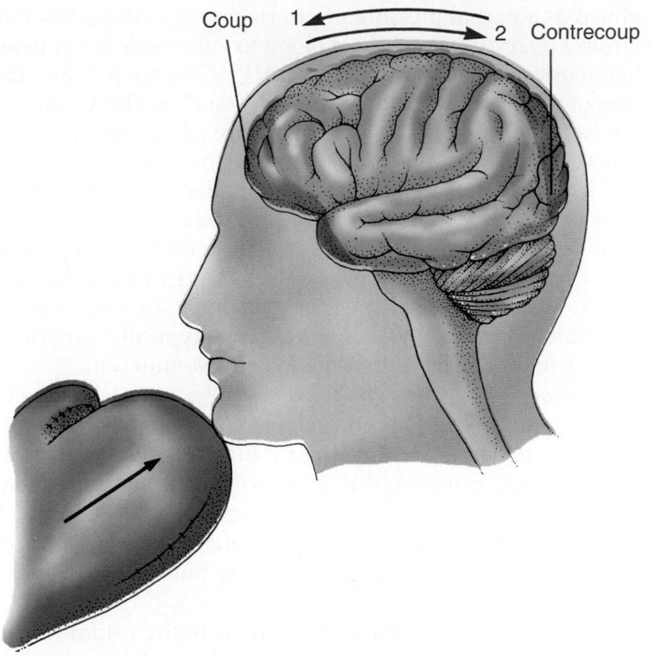

FIG. 45-7 Coup (site of impact) injury to frontal area of brain, and contre-coup injury to frontal and temporal areas of the brain.

are the most common type of skull fracture. In a *depressed fracture,* the bone is pressed inward into the brain tissue to at least the thickness of the skull. In an *open fracture,* the scalp and dura are lacerated, creating a direct opening to the brain tissue. A *comminuted fracture* involves fragmented bone with depression into the brain tissue.

A unique skull fracture is a *basilar fracture.* It occurs at the base of the skull, usually extending into the anterior, middle, or posterior fossa, and can result in cerebrospinal fluid (CSF) leakage from the nose or ears. A CSF leak increases the risk for a central nervous system (CNS) infection. A basilar skull fracture is associated with an increased risk for hemorrhage caused by damage to the internal carotid artery. Basilar skull fractures can also damage cranial nerves (CNs) I, II, VII, and VIII.

Most penetrating injuries to the brain are caused by gunshot wounds (GSWs) and knife injuries. The degree of injury to brain tissue depends on the velocity (speed), mass, shape, and direction of impact. High-velocity injuries produce the greatest damage to brain tissue. As with any open wound, the patient with a penetrating injury is at high risk for infection from the object that pierced the skull and from other environmental contaminants.

Closed traumatic brain injuries are caused by blunt force. The blunt force can be direct or a result of a blast shock wave. These forces can lead to contusions and lacerations of the brain. A **contusion** is a bruising of the brain tissue and is most commonly found at the site of impact (**coup injury**) or in a line opposite the site of impact (**contrecoup injury**) (Fig. 45-7). Contusions and lacerations are most commonly located at the base of the frontal and temporal lobes. A **laceration** causes actual tearing of the cortical surface vessels, which may lead to secondary hemorrhage and significant cerebral edema and inflammation. This condition is more serious than a contusion.

When damage to the brain is severe but without local injury such as a contusion or laceration, a closed traumatic brain injury may be diagnosed as diffuse axonal injury or widespread injury to the white matter of the brain. **Diffuse axonal injury (DAI)** is usually related to high-speed acceleration/deceleration, typically seen in motor vehicle crashes. This type of brain injury causes shearing of large nerve fibers and stretching of blood vessels in many areas of the brain. In addition to bleeding, a DAI can trigger a biochemical cascade of toxic substances in the brain during the days following the initial injury. DAI occurs throughout the brain, and the frontal and temporal lobes are particularly susceptible. Damage may also be found in the corpus callosum, midbrain, cerebellum, and upper brainstem. DAI can also occur in focal but important nerve centers (white matter tracts) causing visual field loss or weakness on one side of the body. Depending on severity, small areas of hemorrhage and changes in the lateral ventricles may be seen with a CT or MRI, but there is no specific or sensitive test to definitively diagnose DAI. The most prominent manifestation of DAI is impaired cognitive function, resulting in disorganization, impaired memory, and varying degrees of inattentiveness. Severe DAI may present with immediate coma, and most survivors require long-term care.

Mild, Moderate, and Severe Traumatic Brain Injury. TBI is further defined as mild, moderate, or severe. Generally, the determination of severity of TBI is the result of the Glasgow Coma Scale (GCS) score immediately following resuscitation, the presence (or absence) of brain damage imaged by CT or MRI following the trauma, an estimation of the force of the trauma, and symptoms in the injured person.

Mild Traumatic Brain Injury. The terms *mild traumatic brain injury (MTBI)* and *concussion* are used synonymously (Thompson & Mauk, 2011). MTBI is characterized by a blow to the head, transient confusion or feeling dazed or disoriented, and one or more of these conditions: (1) loss of consciousness for up to 30 minutes, (2) loss of memory for events immediately before or after the accident, and (3) focal neurologic deficit(s) that may or not be transient. Loss of consciousness does not have to occur for a person to be diagnosed with MTBI. With MTBI, there is no evidence of brain damage on a CT or MRI imaging scan. Subsequent to a new MTBI, symptoms can include a wide array of physical and cognitive problems that range from headache and dizziness to changes in behavior listed on Chart 45-7. These symptoms usually resolve within 72 hours. In some cases the symptoms persist and may last days, weeks, or months. For other patients, severe physical and cognitive problems remain despite relatively mild initial symptoms and normal diagnostic test findings. Persistent symptoms following MTBI are also referred to as **post-concussion syndrome.**

The incidence of *MTBI* is difficult to estimate because most cases are not reported. Further, the symptoms and diagnostic terminology (international classification diagnostic [ICD] codes) used for mild traumatic brain injury are not well established in the practice community. For example, some providers use the word *concussion* for a temporary and reversible change in COGNITION OR SENSORY PERCEPTION from a blow to the head. A concussion is a MTBI. Regardless of terminology, MTBI accounts for at least 75% of all traumatic brain injuries in the United States. Estimating incidence and prevalence is also complicated because patients may not seek medical care. Some patients may not perceive any health problem from the injury. Others do not have any health insurance to assist with costs of diagnosis and care or may feel guilty or embarrassed over the circumstances of the injury.

CHART 45-7 Key Features

Mild Traumatic Brain Injury

Physical Findings
- Appears dazed or stunned
- Loss of consciousness <30 minutes (unresponsive after injury)
- Headache
- Nausea
- Vomiting
- Balance or gait problems
- Dizziness
- Visual problems
- Fatigue
- Sensitivity to light
- Sensitivity to noise

Cognitive Findings
- Feeling mentally foggy
- Feeling slowed down
- Difficulty concentrating
- Difficulty remembering
- Amnesia about the events around the time of injury

Sleep Disturbances
- Drowsiness
- Sleeping less than usual
- Sleeping more than usual
- Trouble falling asleep

Emotional Changes
- Irritability
- Sadness
- Nervousness
- More "emotional"

Moderate Traumatic Brain Injury. A moderate TBI is characterized by a period of loss of consciousness (LOC) for 30 minutes to 6 hours and a GCS score of 9 to 12. Often but not always, focal or diffuse brain injury can be seen with a diagnostic CT or MRI scan. Post-traumatic amnesia (memory loss) may last up to 24 hours. Moderate TBI may occur with either closed or open brain injury. A short acute or critical care stay may be needed for close monitoring and to prevent secondary injury from brain edema, intracranial bleeding, or inadequate cerebral PERFUSION. Additional secondary injury results from complex inflammatory processes, also known as the *biomolecular cascade* that occurs in the CNS immediately, hours, or days after primary injury (Thompson & Mauk, 2011).

Severe Traumatic Brain Injury. A severe TBI is defined by a GCS score of 3 to 8 and loss of consciousness for longer than 6 hours. Focal and diffuse damage to the brain, cerebrovascular vessels, and/or ventricles are common. Both open and closed head injuries can cause severe TBI, and injury can be focal or diffuse. When the damage is present in a localized area of the brain, it is usually extensive. CT and MRI scans can capture images of tissue damage quite early in the course of this illness. Patients with severe TBI require management in critical care, including monitoring of hemodynamics, neurologic status, and possibly, intracranial pressure (ICP). Patients with severe TBI are also at high risk for secondary brain injury from cerebral edema, hemorrhage, reduced PERFUSION, and the biomolecular cascade.

Secondary Injury

Secondary injury to brain injury includes any processes that occur *after* the initial injury and worsen or negatively influence patient outcomes. Secondary injuries result from physiologic, vascular, and biochemical events that are an extension of the primary injury. The most common secondary injuries result from hypotension and hypoxia, intracranial hypertension, and cerebral edema. Damage to the brain tissue occurs primarily because the delivery of oxygen and glucose to the brain is interrupted.

Hypotension and Hypoxia. Both hypotension, defined as a mean arterial pressure less than 70 mm Hg, and hypoxemia, defined as a partial pressure of arterial oxygen (Pao_2) less than 80 mm Hg, restrict the flow of blood to vulnerable brain tissue. Hypotension may be related to shock (Chapter 37) or other states of reduced blood flow to the brain such as clot formation. Hypoxia can be due to respiratory failure, asphyxiation, or loss of airway and impaired ventilation (Chapter 32). These problems may occur as a direct result of moderate to severe brain injury or secondary to systemic injuries and comorbidities. Low blood flow and hypoxemia contribute to cerebral edema, creating a cycle of deteriorating PERFUSION and hypoxic damage. Patients with hypoxic damage related to moderate or severe brain injury face a poor prognosis and typically experience memory impairment and reduced cognitive function.

Increased Intracranial Pressure. The cranial contents include brain tissue, blood, and cerebrospinal fluid (CSF). These components are encased in the relatively rigid skull. Within this space, there is little room for any of the components to expand or increase in volume. A normal level of ICP is 10 to 15 mm Hg. Periodic increases in pressure occur with straining during defecation, coughing, or sneezing but do not harm the uninjured brain.

As a result of brain injury, the increase in the volume of one component must be compensated for by a decrease in the volume of one of the other components. As a first response to an increase in the volume of any of these components, the CSF is shunted or displaced from the cranial compartment to the spinal subarachnoid space or the rate of CSF absorption is increased. An additional response, if needed, is a decrease in cerebral blood volume by movement of cerebral venous blood into the sinuses. As long as the brain can compensate for the increase in volume and remain compliant, increases in ICP are minimal.

Increased ICP is the leading cause of death from head trauma in patients who reach the hospital alive. It occurs when compliance no longer takes place and the brain cannot accommodate further volume changes. As ICP increases, cerebral perfusion decreases, leading to brain tissue ischemia and edema. If edema remains untreated, the brain may herniate downward toward the brainstem or laterally from a unilateral lesion within one cerebral hemisphere, causing irreversible brain damage and possibly death (**brain herniation syndromes**).

Three types of edema may contribute to increased ICP: vasogenic edema, cytotoxic edema, and interstitial edema. *Vasogenic edema* is caused by an abnormal permeability of the walls of the cerebral vessels, which allows protein-rich plasma infiltrate to leak into the extracellular space of the brain. The fluid collects primarily in the white matter. *Cytotoxic edema* may occur as a result of a hypoxic insult, which causes a disturbance in cellular metabolism and active ion transport. The brain is quickly depleted of available oxygen, glucose, and glycogen and converts to anaerobic metabolism. Derangements in cell membrane function result in cell edema, cell dysfunction, and cell death. Cytotoxic edema may lead to vasogenic edema and a further increase in ICP. *Interstitial edema* occurs with fluid accumulation between the cells of the brain. Interstitial edema is *associated with* elevated blood pressure or increased CSF pressure. Interstitial edema develops rapidly in the perivascular and periventricular white space and can be controlled through measures to reduce blood pressure or decrease CSF pressures.

Besides providing oxygen to decrease ischemic injury, sustaining mean arterial pressure or systolic blood pressure within a therapeutic range, and draining cerebral spinal fluid, the staff nurse manages increased intracranial pressure with attention to balancing fluid intake and output and promoting normal serum electrolyte values. When intracranial pressure monitoring is used, a desired outcome of therapy includes maintaining **cerebral perfusion pressure (CPP)**. The CPP is the pressure gradient over which the brain is perfused. CPP is determined by subtracting the mean ICP from the mean arterial pressure. *Maintenance of a CPP above 70 mm Hg is generally accepted as an expected outcome of therapy.* ICP monitoring also includes evaluating the shape and quality of the ICP waveform to determine whether compliance is compromised as manifested by an abnormal ICP waveform. Some specialized units also monitor jugular venous oxygenation saturation to evaluate the amount of hemoglobin saturated by oxygen as it drains from the cranium. A value that falls outside the range of 55% to 70% indicates inadequate delivery of oxygen to brain tissue.

Hemorrhage. Hemorrhage, which causes a brain hematoma (collection of blood) or clot, may occur as part of the primary injury and begin at the moment of impact. It may also arise later from vessel damage. Classically, bleeding is caused by vascular damage from the shearing force of the trauma or direct physical damage from skull fractures or penetrating injury. *All hematomas are potentially life threatening because they act as space-occupying lesions and are surrounded by edema.* Three major types of hemorrhage after TBI are epidural, subdural, and intracerebral hemorrhage. Subarachnoid hemorrhage may also occur.

An **epidural hematoma** results from arterial bleeding into the space between the dura and the inner skull (Fig. 45-8). It is often caused by a fracture of the temporal bone, which houses the middle meningeal artery. Patients with epidural hematomas have "lucid intervals" that last for minutes during which time the patient is awake and talking. This follows a momentary unconsciousness that occurs within minutes of the injury.

A **subdural hematoma (SDH)** results from venous bleeding into the space beneath the dura and above the arachnoid (see Fig. 45-8). It occurs most often from a tearing of the bridging veins within the cerebral hemispheres or from a laceration of brain tissue. *Bleeding from this injury occurs more slowly than from an epidural hematoma.* SDHs are subdivided into acute, subacute, and chronic. An acute SDH presents within 48 hours after impact; the subacute SDH, between 48 hours and 2 weeks; and the chronic SDH, from 2 weeks to several months after injury. SDHs have the highest mortality rate because they often are unrecognized until the patient presents with severe neurologic compromise.

Traumatic **intracerebral hemorrhage** (ICH) is the accumulation of blood within the brain tissue caused by the tearing of small arteries and veins in the subcortical white matter (see Fig. 45-8). It often acts as a space-occupying lesion (like a tumor) and may be potentially devastating, depending on its location. ICH may also produce significant brain edema and ICP elevations. A traumatic brainstem hemorrhage occurs as a result of a blow to the back of the head, fractures, or torsion injuries to the brainstem. Brainstem injuries have a very poor prognosis.

Hydrocephalus. Hydrocephalus is an abnormal increase in CSF volume. It may be caused by impaired reabsorption of CSF at the arachnoid villi (from subarachnoid hemorrhage or meningitis), called a **communicating hydrocephalus**. It may also be caused by interference or blockage with CSF outflow from the ventricular system (from cerebral edema, tumor, or debris). The ventricles may dilate from the relative increase in CSF

! NURSING SAFETY PRIORITY (QSEN)

Critical Rescue

After the initial interval, symptoms of neurologic impairment from hemorrhage can progress very quickly with potentially life-threatening ICP elevation and irreversible structural damage to brain tissue. Monitor the patient suspected of epidural bleeding frequently (every 5-10 minutes) for changes in neurologic status. The patient can become quickly and increasingly symptomatic. *A loss of consciousness from an epidural or subdural hematoma is a neurosurgical emergency!* Notify the health care provider or Rapid Response Team immediately if these changes occur. Carefully document your assessments.

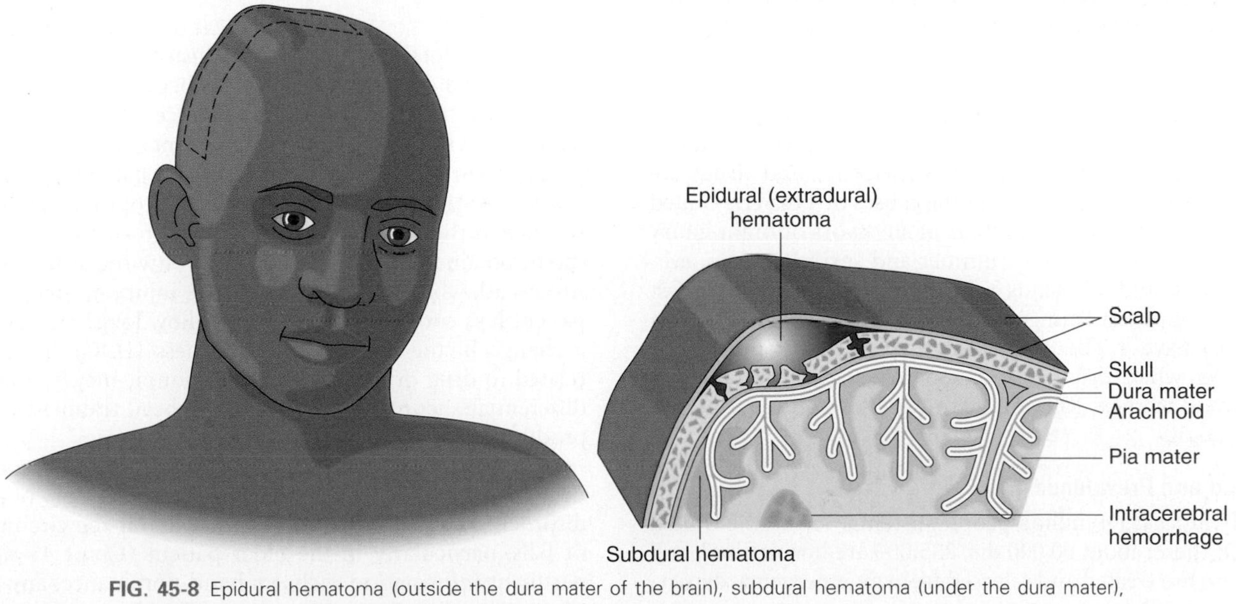

FIG. 45-8 Epidural hematoma (outside the dura mater of the brain), subdural hematoma (under the dura mater), and intracerebral hemorrhage (within the brain tissue).

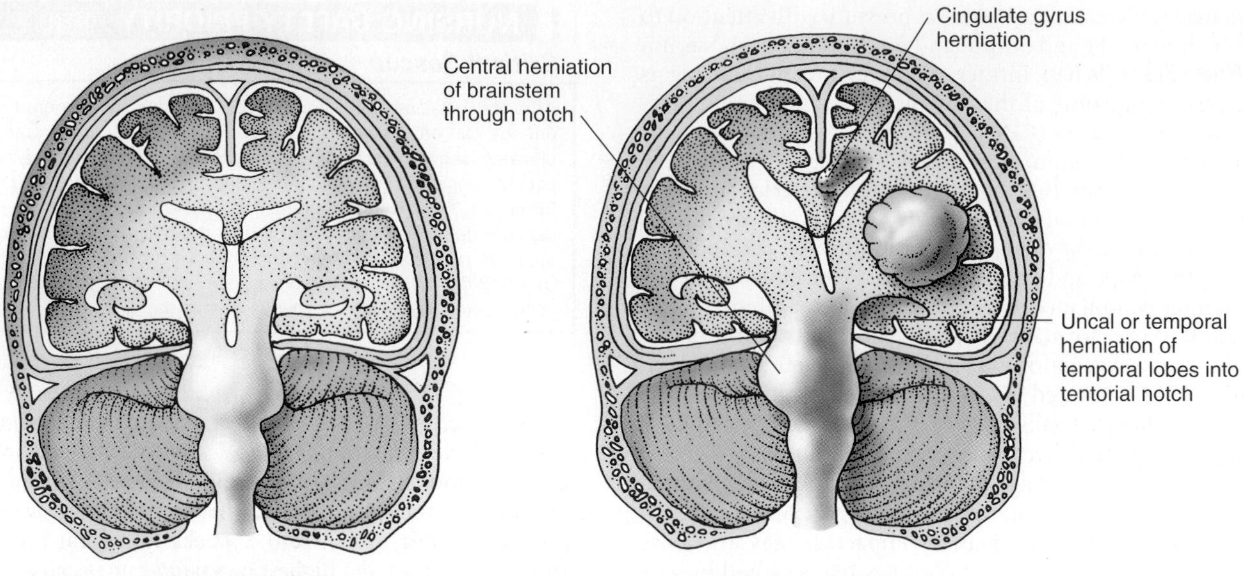

FIG. 45-9 Herniation syndromes.

volume. Ultimately, if not treated, this increase may lead to increased ICP.

Brain Herniation. In the presence of increased ICP, the brain tissue may shift and herniate downward. Of the several types of herniation syndromes (Fig. 45-9), uncal herniation is one of the most clinically significant because it is life threatening. It is caused by a shift of one or both areas of the temporal lobe, known as the **uncus**. This shift creates pressure on the third cranial nerve. Late findings include dilated and nonreactive pupils, ptosis (drooping eyelids), and a rapidly deteriorating level of consciousness. Central herniation is caused by a downward shift of the brainstem and the diencephalon from a supratentorial lesion. It is clinically manifested by Cheyne-Stokes respirations, pinpoint and nonreactive pupils, and potential hemodynamic instability. All herniation syndromes are potentially life threatening, and the physician must be notified immediately when they are suspected.

Etiology

The most common causes of TBI in the United States are falls and motor vehicle crashes, followed by colliding with a stationary or moving object (CDC, 2013a). Alcohol and drugs are significant contributing factors to the causes of TBI. The United States is seeing increasing numbers of survivors of brain injury from wartime blast injuries. Summer and spring months, evenings, nights, and weekends are associated with the greatest number of injuries. Young males are more likely than young females to have a TBI. Men tend to play more sports, take more risks when driving, and consume larger amounts of alcohol than women. Falls are the most common cause of TBI in older adults.

Incidence and Prevalence

Annually, at least 1.4 million people sustain a TBI in the United States. Of these, about 50,000 die, 235,000 are hospitalized, and 1.1 million are treated and released from an emergency department (CDC, 2013a).

Health Promotion and Maintenance

Nurses can educate the public on ways to decrease the incidence of TBI by using safe driving practices such as not driving while impaired and wearing seat belts. Teach people at risk about how alcohol and illicit drug use affect driving ability. Promote the use of helmets for skateboarding and bicycle and motorcycle riding. Help prevent falls by providing a safe environment, especially for older adults. People need to be aware of environmental factors that may increase the likelihood of falls such as inadequate lighting and loose rugs. When possible, install safety equipment in bathtubs and showers. Evaluate balance and coordination as part of a falls prevention strategy inside the hospital and at home.

❖ PATIENT-CENTERED COLLABORATIVE CARE

◆ Assessment

History. Obtaining an accurate history from a patient who has sustained a TBI may be difficult because of either the seriousness of the injury or the presence of **amnesia** (loss of memory). It is not unusual for the patient to experience amnesia for events before or after the injury. The patient with a serious brain injury may be unconscious or in a confused and combative state. If the patient cannot provide information, the history can be obtained from first responders or witnesses to the injury. Always ask when, where, and how the injury occurred. Did the patient lose consciousness; if so, for how long? Has there been a change in the level of consciousness (LOC)? If trauma is related to drug or alcohol consumption, it may be difficult to differentiate neurologic changes from head trauma from those produced by intoxication.

Determine whether the patient had fluctuating consciousness or seizure activity and whether there is a history of a seizure disorder. Obtain precise information about the circumstances of falls, particularly in the older patient (Chart 45-8). Other pertinent information includes hand dominance, any diseases of or injuries to the eyes, and any allergies to drugs or food.

CHART 45-8 Nursing Focus on the Older Adult

Traumatic Brain Injury

- Brain injury is the fifth leading cause of death in older adults.
- The 65- to 75-year age-group has second highest incidence of brain injury of all age-groups.
- Falls and motor vehicle crashes are the most common causes of brain injury.
- Factors that contribute to high mortality are:
  - Falls causing subdural hematomas (closed head injuries), especially chronic subdural hematomas
  - Poorly tolerated systemic stress, which is increased by admission to a high-stimuli environment
  - Medical complications, such as hypotension, hypertension, and cardiac problems
  - Decreased protective mechanisms, which make patients susceptible to infections (especially pneumonia)
  - Decreased immunologic competence, which is further diminished by brain injury

Inquire about a history of alcohol or drug use and abuse because these substances may interfere with the neurologic baseline assessment. Consider whether the patient is a victim of violence if he or she lives in residential care. The Joint Commission and the Centers for Medicare and Medicaid Services require that all patients be screened for abuse and neglect when they are admitted to any type of health care facility.

Physical Assessment/Clinical Manifestations. No two brain injuries are alike. The patient with a TBI may have a variety of manifestations depending on the severity of injury and the resulting increase in intracranial pressure (ICP) (see Chart 45-6). Assess for signs of increased ICP, hypotension, hypoxemia (decreased blood level of oxygen), or **hypercarbia** ($Paco_2$ >40-45 mm Hg or increased partial pressure of carbon dioxide in arterial blood). Hypercarbia can cause cerebral vasodilation and contribute to elevated ICP. Determination of hypercarbia in an intubated patient can be done with an end-tidal carbon dioxide ($EtCO_2$) monitor. The early detection of changes in the patient's neurologic status enables the health care team to prevent or treat potentially life-threatening complications. Subtle changes in blood pressure, consciousness, and pupillary reaction to light can be very informative about neurologic deterioration.

Airway and Breathing Pattern Assessment. *The first priority is the assessment of the patient's ABCs—airway, breathing, and circulation.* Because TBI is occasionally associated with cervical spinal cord injuries, all patients with head trauma are treated as though they have cord injury until radiography proves otherwise. *Older adults are especially prone to cervical injuries at the first or second vertebral level, a life-threatening problem.* Assess for indicators of spinal cord injury, such as loss of motor function (MOBILITY) and SENSORY PERCEPTION, tenderness along the spine, and abnormal head tilt.

Injuries to the brainstem may cause a change in the patient's breathing pattern, such as Cheyne-Stokes respirations, central neurogenic hyperventilation, and/or apnea. In the unconscious patient, an artificial airway provides protection from aspiration as well as a route for oxygenation. Mechanical ventilation may be needed to support inadequate respiratory effort.

Spine Precautions. Patients with blunt trauma to the head or neck are typically transported from the scene of the injury to the hospital with a rigid cervical collar and a long spine board. The goal is to prevent new and secondary spine injury if there is unstable vertebrae or ligament damage. Spine precautions require placing the patient supine and aligning the spinal column in a neutral position so there is no rotation, flexion, or extension. The long spine board is removed as soon as possible upon arrival to the emergency department (ED) or intensive care unit (ICU); some EDs require this to be done within 20 minutes of arrival. The rigid cervical collar is maintained until definitive diagnostic studies to rule out cervical spine injury are completed (see Chapter 43). Skin breakdown and pressure ulcer formation are concerns when either the spine board or rigid collar are used.

! NURSING SAFETY PRIORITY QSEN

Critical Rescue

The upper cervical spinal nerves innervate the diaphragm to control breathing. Monitor TBI patients for respiratory problems and diaphragmatic breathing, as well as diminished or absent reflexes in the airway (cough and gag). Hypoxia and hypercapnia are best detected through arterial oxygen levels (partial pressure of arterial oxygen [PaO_2]), oxygen saturation (Spo_2), and end-tidal volume carbon dioxide measurement ($EtCO_2$). Observe chest wall movement and listen to breath sounds. Report any sign of respiratory problems immediately to the physician!

Once the spine board is removed, spinal precautions are maintained until the provider indicates it is safe to bend or rotate the cervical, thoracic, and lumbar spine. Spinal precautions include: (1) bedrest; (2) no neck flexion with a pillow or roll; (3) no thoracic or lumbar flexion with head of bed elevation/bed controls (reverse Trendelenburg is acceptable); (4) manual control of the cervical spine anytime the rigid collar is removed; and (5) using a "log roll" procedure to reposition the patient. Log roll allows for maintaining the neutral anatomic alignment of the entire vertebral column while turning or moving the patient. A patient with known or suspected spine injury requires preplanning and the assistance of three or more qualified people to move the patient. One person is assigned to maintain manual control of the cervical spine, and one person is positioned on each side of the torso to turn the patient while preventing segmental rotation, flexion, extension, and/or lateral bending of the chest or abdomen during transfer of the patient. A fourth person may be assigned to check skin integrity and/or change linens and position padding. Neurologic function must be assessed after each position change.

A rigid cervical collar is used to maintain cervical spine ("c-spine") precautions as well as cervical spine immobilization with a confirmed cervical injury. If the collar is ill-fitting or soiled, it may be changed according to hospital guidelines while a second qualified person maintains c-spine immobilization.

Spine clearance is a clinical decision made by the health care provider, often in collaboration with the radiologist. Spine clearance includes determining the absence of acute bony, ligamentous, and neurologic abnormalities of the cervical spine based on history, physical examination, and/or negative radiologic studies.

Vital Signs Assessment. The mechanisms of autoregulation are often impaired as the result of a TBI. The more serious the injury, the more severe is the impact on *autoregulation* or the ability of cerebral vasculature to modify systemic pressure such that blood flow to the brain is sufficient. Monitor the patient's blood pressure and pulse. The patient may have hypotension or hypertension. **Cushing's triad**, a classic but late sign of increased ICP, is manifested by severe hypertension, a widened pulse pressure (increasing difference between systolic and diastolic values), and bradycardia. This triad of cardiovascular changes usually indicates imminent death.

Hypotension and tachycardia suggest hypovolemic shock. A decrease in blood volume may lead to decreased CPP and secondary brain ischemia and injury. Hypovolemic shock is usually due to bleeding outside the cranial vault such as traumatic injuries to the abdomen or chest. Cardiac dysrhythmias may result from chest trauma, bruising of the heart, or interference with the autonomic nervous system from primary or secondary injuries to the brain or spinal cord. Chapter 43 describes acute spinal cord injury manifestations and management.

Neurologic Assessment. Many hospitals use the Glasgow Coma Scale to document neurologic status (see Fig. 42-10). A change of 2 points is considered clinically important; urgent notification of the provider is advised if the change is a 2-point deterioration of GCS values.

The most important variable to assess with any brain injury is LOC! A decrease or change in LOC is typically the first sign of deterioration in neurologic status. A decrease in arousal or increased sleepiness should result in an increased aggressiveness and/or frequency in assessment. *Early* indicators of a change in LOC include behavior changes (e.g., restlessness, irritability) and disorientation, which are often subtle in nature.

Use a bright light to assess pupillary size and reaction to light. Facial trauma may swell eyelids, making this assessment difficult. Consider whether drugs that affect pupillary dilation and constriction, such as anticholinergics or adrenergics, have been used recently. Cycloplegics (eye drops to dilate the pupil) are used by ophthalmologists to evaluate eye and orbit injuries; these drugs also alter pupillary response to light.

! NURSING SAFETY PRIORITY QSEN

Critical Rescue

Check pupils of TBI patients for size and reaction to light, particularly if the patient is unable to follow directions to assess changes in level of consciousness. Report and document any changes in pupil size, shape, and reactivity to the health care provider immediately because they could indicate an increase in ICP.

Pupillary changes or eye signs differ depending on which areas of the brain are damaged. *Pinpoint and nonresponsive pupils are indicative of brainstem dysfunction at the level of the pons.* Of particular importance is the **ovoid pupil**, which is regarded as the midstage between a normal-size pupil and a dilated pupil. In some agencies, a portable automated pupillometer is used to measure pupil size and reaction rather than manual examination.

Asymmetric (uneven) pupils, loss of light reaction, or unilateral or bilateral dilated pupils are treated as herniation of the brain from increased ICP until proven differently. *Pupils that are fixed (nonreactive) and dilated are a poor prognostic sign. Patients with this problem are sometimes referred to as having "blown" pupils.*

Check gross vision if the patient's condition permits. Have the patient read any printed material (e.g., your name tag) or count the number of fingers that you hold within the patient's visual field. Loss of vision is usually caused by either direct injury to the eye or injury to the occipital lobe. Visual loss may be temporary or permanent.

If the patient can participate, the health care provider or neurosurgical nurse tests *cranial nerves* (CNs) III, IV, and VI by asking the patient to following the sketch of an "H" in the visual field. Extraocular movements may be diminished because of injury or increased ICP. Damage to the optic chiasm or optic tract may cause visual-field deficits or **diplopia** (double vision). In the unconscious patient, additional oculocephalic and oculovestibular tests are performed to test the integrity of the brainstem and of CNs III, VI, and VII.

Monitor for additional late signs of increased ICP. These manifestations include severe headache, nausea, vomiting (often projectile), and seizures. The provider may evaluate for papilledema (seen by ophthalmoscopic examination). **Papilledema,** *also known as a* **choked disc,** *is edema and hyperemia (increased blood flow) of the optic disc. It is always a sign of increased ICP.* Headache and seizures are a response to the injury and may or may not be associated with increased ICP. Always remember that the patient with a brain injury is at risk for potentially devastating ICP elevations during the first hours after the event and that this risk decreases over the course of 1 to 3 days.

Assess for bilateral *motor* responses. The patient's motor loss or dysfunction usually appears contralateral (opposite side) to the site of the lesion, similar to a stroke. For example, a left-sided hemiparesis reflects an injury to the right cerebral hemisphere. Deterioration in motor function or the development of abnormal posturing (**decerebrate** or **decorticate posturing**) or flaccidity is another indicator of progressive brain injury (see Fig. 41-11 in Chapter 41). These changes are due to dysfunction within the pyramidal (motor) tracts of the spinal cord. Assess for brainstem or cerebellar injury, which may cause **ataxia** (loss of balance), decreased or increased muscle tone, and weakness. Remember that absence of motor function may also be an indicator of a spinal cord injury.

Carefully observe the patient's ears and nose for any signs of cerebrospinal fluid (CSF) leaks that result from a basilar skull fracture. Suspicious ear or nose fluid can be analyzed by the laboratory for glucose and electrolyte content. CSF placed on a white absorbent paper or linen can be distinguished from other fluids by the "halo" sign, a clear or yellowish ring surrounding a spot of blood. Although other body fluids can be used, a halo sign is most reliable when blood is in the center of the absorbent material since tears and saliva can also cause a clear ring in some conditions.

Palpate the patient's head gently to detect the presence of fractures or hematomas. Look for areas of ecchymosis (bruising), tender areas of the scalp, and lacerations. *Battle sign* or mastoid ecchymosis is bruising behind the ears and lower jaw indicating a fracture of the middle cranial fossa of the skull. *Raccoon's eyes* are purplish discoloration around eyes that can follow fracture of the skull's base. When CT scans are used with head and brain injury, these fractures are often visualized before bruising appears.

Psychosocial Assessment. Patients with mild brain injury may still have symptoms of disability 1 year or longer after injury, but long-term effects are not common. Patients with moderate to severe TBI may have varying degrees of psychosocial changes that persist for a lifetime. Personality changes manifested by temper outbursts, depression, risk-taking

NCLEX EXAMINATION CHALLENGE

Safe and Effective Care Environment

An alert and oriented person is admitted to the emergency department with a GCS of 10, indicating a moderate brain injury. Which assessment finding will the nurse report immediately to the health care provider?

A. Photophobia accompanied by headache
B. New onset of dizziness when lying quietly in bed
C. A brisk pupillary reaction to light
D. New difficulty in responsiveness or sudden drowsiness

behavior, and denial of disability can occur. The patient may become talkative and develop a very outgoing personality. Memory, especially recent or short-term memory, is often affected. The patient may report difficulties in concentrating or the ability to learn new information and may have problems with insight and planning. Aggressive behavior, agitation, and sleep disorders may interfere with the ability to return to work or school. The ability to communicate and understand the spoken and written language may be altered. Changes in MOBILITY and SENSORY PERCEPTION may necessitate rehabilitation or use of assistive devices. All these changes in health status may lead to difficulties within the family structure and with social and work-related interactions. Behavioral interventions are used by cognitive and brain injury rehabilitation specialists to help both the patient and family members develop adaptive strategies.

Assess family dynamics, particularly if the patient is discharged to the family's care directly from the acute care hospital. The family or significant others must also cope with changes in the patient's physical appearance and cognitive abilities. Family members may feel guilty or angry about not being able to prevent the injury or blame the patient for the personal choices that contributed to the event. The family or significant others may feel overwhelmed by the complexity of care required and the long recovery period. Help both the family and the patient identify coping strategies to deal with the role changes caused by the injury.

Laboratory Assessment. There are no established serum tests to diagnose a primary brain injury. Detection of the protein *S-100B* in serum is showing some promise as an indicator of brain injury (Defazio et al., 2013; Müller et al., 2011). Several laboratory tests are used to guide interventions and to prevent secondary brain insult. The health care provider requests arterial blood gases, complete blood count (CBC), serum glucose, osmolarity, and electrolyte levels. These tests are performed to monitor hemodynamic status, identify electrolyte imbalance, determine oxygen-carrying capacity, and detect infection. Electrolyte imbalances, hypoxia, hypovolemia, and reduced blood pressure from infection or shock can contribute to secondary injury, as well as increase the risk for seizures. A toxicology screen and an electrocardiogram (ECG) are often requested.

Imaging Assessment. The health care provider immediately requests CT of the brain to identify the extent and scope of injury. This diagnostic test can identify the presence of an injury that requires surgical intervention, such as an epidural or subdural hematoma. *Radiography* and *CT scanning* of the cervical spine and the skull are done to rule out fractures and dislocations. An *MRI* may be done to detect subtle changes in brain tissue and show more specific detail of the brain injury. MRI is particularly useful in the diagnosis of diffuse axonal injury, but it is not recommended for patients with ICP monitoring devices.

Other Diagnostic Assessment. As the patient's condition stabilizes, the physician may request other diagnostic tests to identify the extent of injury to the brain. For example, the integrity of the cerebral vessels is measured through the use of ultrasonography. *Evoked potentials* (electroencephalogram recordings with sensory stimuli) provide information on cerebral function and may be useful in predicting the patient's outcome.

◆ Interventions

The patient with a *severe* TBI is admitted to the critical care unit or a trauma center. Patients with *moderate* TBI are admitted to either the general nursing unit or the critical care unit, where they are closely observed for at least 24 hours. Those with *mild* TBI may be sent home from the emergency department with instructions for home-based observation and primary care provider follow-up.

Nonsurgical Management. *As with any critically injured patient, priority is given to maintaining a patent airway, breathing, and circulation.* Specific nursing interventions for the patient with a TBI are directed toward preventing or detecting secondary brain injury or the conditions that contribute to secondary brain injury such as increased ICP, promoting fluid and electrolyte balance, and monitoring the effects of treatments and drug therapy. Providing health teaching and emotional support for the patient and family are vital parts of the plan of care.

Preventing and Detecting Secondary Brain Injury. Take and record the patient's *vital signs* every 1 to 2 hours or more often based on patient acuity. The health care provider may prescribe IV fluids or drug therapy to prevent severe hypertension or hypotension. Dysrhythmias and nonspecific ST-segment or T-wave changes may occur, possibly in response to stimulation of the autonomic nervous system or an increase in the level of circulating catecholamines such as epinephrine. Document and report cardiac dysrhythmias, hypotension, and hypertension to the health care provider. Obtain the target range for blood pressure and heart rate from the health care provider.

The patient with a brain injury may develop a fever as a result of systemic trauma, blood in the cranium, or a generalized inflammatory response to brain injury. Fever as a consequence of infection may develop later in the course of the disease. A third cause of fever is a central fever caused by hypothalamic damage. It is manifested by an absence of sweating and no diurnal (night and day) variation. This type of fever is high and lasts several days to weeks. In addition, it responds better to cooling (e.g., cool air hypothermia, sponge bath) than to the administration of antipyretic drugs such as acetaminophen (Tylenol, Ace-Tabs ♣). *Fever from any cause is associated with higher morbidity and mortality rates.*

Therapeutic hypothermia may be started regardless of the presence of fever. The purpose of **therapeutic hypothermia** is to rapidly cool the patient to a core temperature of 89.6° and 93.2° F (32° to 34° C) for 24 to 48 hours after the primary injury. Rewarming to a normal core temperature requires specialized knowledge and skill because rapid fluid and electrolyte shifts can cause cardiac dysrhythmias and changes to systemic and cerebral pressures. The rationale for therapeutic hypothermia is to reduce brain metabolism and prevent the cascade of molecular and biochemical events that contribute to secondary brain injury in moderate to severe TBI.

Arterial blood gas (ABG), oxygen saturation (Spo_2), and end-tidal carbon dioxide ($EtCO_2$) values are all used to evaluate respiratory status and guide mechanical ventilation therapy. *Hyperventilation* for the intubated patient during the first 24 hours after brain injury is usually avoided because it may produce ischemia by causing cerebral vasoconstriction. The result is a decrease in cerebral blood volume. In acute elevations of ICP or neurologic deterioration, however, brief periods of hyperventilation may be used. After the first 24 hours, when a patient is mechanically ventilated and intracranial hypertension persists, the health care provider may adjust mechanical ventilation settings to reduce arterial carbon dioxide. Other interventions are used first, including diversion of CSF and manipulation of fluid intake and output. When mechanical ventilation adjustments are used, the goal is to maintain the partial pressure of arterial carbon dioxide ($Paco_2$) at 35 to 38 mm Hg. *Carbon dioxide is a very potent vasodilator that can contribute to increases in ICP.*

Prevent intermittent and sustained hypoxemia. Monitor peripheral oxygen saturation continuously in moderate to severe TBI. Hypoxemia damages brain tissue and contributes to cerebral vasodilation and increased ICP. Arterial oxygen levels (Pao_2) are maintained between 80 and 100 mm Hg to prevent secondary injury. If the patient is intubated, provide 100% oxygen before each pass of the endotracheal suction catheter. Avoid overly aggressive hyperventilation with endotracheal suctioning because of the potential for hypocarbia. Cerebral ischemia caused by even transiently decreased oxygen and either high or low carbon dioxide levels contributes to secondary brain injury. Lidocaine given IV or endotracheally may be used to suppress the cough reflex; coughing increases ICP.

Patients with moderate or severe brain injury are at risk for losing airway patency. Absence of a cough and/or gag reflex, pooled oral and nasal secretions in the pharynx, and inability to position oneself to facilitate pulmonary secretion removal all contribute to the need to manage the airway in the non-intubated brain-injured adult. Pulmonary secretions may be thick because of the diuretics or fluid intake restriction that may be used to prevent cerebral edema. Collaborate with the respiratory therapist to provide humidified air and chest physiotherapy as needed based on patient assessment. If the patient has an ICP monitor present, pay close attention to the ICP response and moderate or stop suctioning, chest vibration, or repositioning when ICP increases.

! NURSING SAFETY PRIORITY QSEN

Action Alert

Position the TBI patient to avoid extreme flexion or extension of the neck and to maintain the head in the midline, neutral position. Log roll the patient during turning to avoid extreme hip flexion, and keep the head of the bed elevated at least 30 degrees or as recommended by the health care provider.

Generally, HOB elevation in patients with TBI is elevated at 30 to 45 degrees to prevent aspiration. However, if increasing head elevation significantly lowers systemic blood pressure, the patient does not benefit from drainage of venous blood or CSF out of the skull from this position. If hypotension accompanies an elevated backrest position, the patient may be harmed. Adjust head elevation to sustain CPP >70 mm Hg when possible. Avoid sudden vertical changes of the head of the bed in the older patient because the dura is tightly adhered to the skull and may pull away from the brain, leading to a subdural hematoma.

Patients with *severe* TBI often die. As the physiologic deterioration begins, keep in mind that the patient may be a potential organ donor. *Before* brain death is declared, contact the local organ procurement organization. Determine if the patient consented to be an organ donor. This information is typically on a driver's license or other state-issued card or advance directive. The patient's wishes should be followed unless he or she has a medical condition that prevents organ donation. The organ donor agency representative or physician discusses the possibility of organ donation with the family. Some families may not agree with the patient's decision, which can cause an ethical dilemma. Many health care agencies have an ethics specialist of committee members who can help with these situations.

Determining Brain Death. In 2010, the American Academy of Neurology guidelines for determining brain death were updated. Four prerequisites must be met to establish a brain death diagnosis (Wijdicks et al., 2010):

- Coma of known cause as established by history, clinical examination, laboratory testing, and neuroimaging
- Normal or near-normal core body temperature (higher than 96.8° F (36° C)
- Normal systolic blood pressure (higher than or equal to 100 mm Hg)
- At least one neurologic examination (some states and health care systems require two)

No consensus has been reached on who is qualified to perform head-to-toe brain death neurologic examinations, but neurologists and critical care intensivists typically do them. Neuroimaging tests are not required to confirm brain death but are desirable. Examples of tests that may be done include cerebral angiography, bedside electroencephalography (EEG), and cerebral computed tomographic angiography (CTA).

Drug Therapy. Mannitol (Osmitrol), an osmotic diuretic, is used to treat cerebral edema by pulling water out of the extracellular space of the edematous brain tissue. It is most effective when given in boluses rather than as a continuous infusion. Furosemide (Lasix), a loop diuretic, is often used as adjunctive therapy to reduce the incidence of rebound from mannitol. It also enhances the therapeutic action of mannitol, reduces edema and blood volume, decreases sodium uptake by the brain, and decreases the production of CSF at the choroid plexus. *Glucocorticoids* (dexamethasone [Decadron, Dexasone] and methylprednisolone sodium succinate [Solu-Medrol, Medrol]) have no benefit in the management of increased ICP caused by brain injury or infarction.

Administer *mannitol* through a filter in the IV tubing or, if given by IV push, draw it up through a filtered needle to eliminate microscopic crystals. For the patient receiving either osmotic or loop diuretics, monitor for intake and output, severe dehydration, and indications of acute renal failure, weakness, edema, and changes in urine output. Serum electrolyte and osmolarity levels are measured every 6 hours. Mannitol is used to obtain a serum osmolarity of 310 to 320 mOsm/L, depending on physician preference and the desired outcome of therapy. Insert an indwelling urinary catheter to maintain strict measurement of output. Check the patient's serum and urine osmolarity daily.

Sedative agents like dexmedetomidine (Precedex, Dexdor) or propofol (Diprivan) can be used as continuous IV infusions to manage agitation and ventilatory asynchrony. They have a short duration of action and can be stopped for a daily neurologic examination. However, when a patient requires sedation for management of ICP hypertension, stopping these drugs is not advised until periods of ICP elevation are infrequent and not sustained.

Opioids such as morphine sulfate or fentanyl may be used with ventilated patients to decrease agitation and control restlessness if the agitation is caused by pain. Fentanyl has fewer effects on blood pressure and heart rate than morphine and may therefore be a safer agent to manage pain. These agents may be reversed with naloxone (Narcan), but opioid reversal should be avoided if at all possible to reduce risk for withdrawal and rebound pain and agitation.

Antiepileptic drugs, such as phenytoin (Dilantin), to prevent seizures are not recommended routinely. However, they may be given as an option to prevent early-onset seizure activity that may occur with some types of specific brain injury. Acetaminophen (Tylenol, Ace-Tabs 🍁) and aspirin (acetylsalicylic acid [ASA], Ancasal 🍁) are given to patients who are febrile (temperature greater than 101° F [38.3° C]) to reduce fever.

Inducing Barbiturate Coma. Barbiturate coma (coma induced by barbiturates) has been used for intracranial hypertension (increased ICP) that cannot be controlled by other means. Either pentobarbital sodium (Nembutal, Novopentobarb 🍁) or thiopentone is the drug of choice. These drugs decrease the metabolic demands of the brain and cerebral blood flow, stabilize cell membranes, decrease the formation of vasogenic edema, and produce a more uniform blood supply. The health care provider adjusts the dosage to maintain complete unresponsiveness. As a consequence, it is difficult to recognize subtle or obvious neurologic changes. The patient requires mechanical ventilation, sophisticated hemodynamic monitoring, and ICP monitoring. Complications of barbiturate coma include decreased GI motility, cardiac dysrhythmias from hypokalemia, hypotension, and fluctuations in body temperature.

Maintaining Fluid and Electrolyte Management. The patient with TBI is at risk for diabetes insipidus (DI) and the syndrome of inappropriate antidiuretic hormone (SIADH) because the pituitary gland may be injured or compressed from cerebral edema (see Chapter 62). In the patient with multiple trauma, fluid overload can occur and cerebral edema can worsen from the rapid administration of IV fluids or plasma expanders. Fluid management is titrated to optimize volume resuscitation but minimize brain swelling and ICP elevation. ICP is also influenced by the response to diuretic therapy and laboratory values. Monitor serum and urine osmolarity and electrolytes at least daily when IV fluids and diuretics are used for management of the TBI patient.

Managing Nutritional Status. The patient with a brain injury may have changes in these areas:

- Coma or impaired ability to feed oneself
- Dysphagia, including swallowing difficulties or pocketing food and being unaware of the presence of food within the oral cavity
- Sense of smell
- Sense of taste

As a result, he or she is at risk for acute or chronic nutritional deficits that may interfere with the healing process. Weigh the patient daily to assess fluid and nutritional intake. Collaborate with the dietitian to determine whether caloric needs are being met.

A small-lumen nasogastric or nasoduodenal tube or a percutaneous endoscopic gastrostomy (PEG) tube can be used to provide enteral nutrition. Parenteral nutrition can be used if the patient is unable to meet caloric or protein intake goals because of GI dysfunction, which is common during acute care and immediately following trauma. Communicate with the health care provider before a nasogastric tube is placed. Do not insert anything into nasal passages in the presence of a cribriform plate fracture since this type of fracture can allow passage of the tube into the brain.

For the patient who can take food and fluids by mouth, ensure that mealtime is a pleasant experience. Position the patient to maximize swallowing ability. The speech-language pathologist (SLP) identifies strategies to prevent food from accumulating in the cheek of the affected side. In general, patients who have swallowing problems can tolerate or swallow soft or semisoft foods and liquids (mechanical soft or dental diet, junior baby foods, custards, scrambled eggs) better than thin liquids (water, juice, milk). Powdered thickener (e.g., Thick-It) may be added to increase liquid consistency to aid in swallowing effort. Commercial dietary supplements (e.g., Ensure) may be needed to meet the patient's caloric and protein requirements. Collaborate with the dietitian and SLP to create a nutritional plan appropriate for the patient with dysphagia.

Managing Sensory Perception, Cognitive, and Behavioral Changes. If a large lesion of the parietal lobe is present, the patient may experience a loss of sensation for pain, temperature, touch, and proprioception (position sense), which prevents an appropriate response to environmental stimuli. A hazard-free environment is necessary to prevent injury (e.g., from burns if the patient's coffee is too hot). In collaboration with the rehabilitation therapist, integrate a sensory stimulation program into the comatose or stuporous patient's routine care activities. Sensory stimulation is done to facilitate a meaningful response to the environment. Present visual, auditory, or tactile stimuli one at a time, and explain the purpose and the type of stimulus presented. For example, show a picture of the patient's mother and say, "This is a picture of your mother." The picture is shown several times, and the same words are used to describe the picture. If auditory tapes or DVDs are used, they should be no longer than 10 to 15 minutes. If the stimulus is presented for a longer period, it simply becomes "white" noise, or meaningless background noise.

Patients with a mild brain injury may be disoriented and have a short-term memory loss. Always introduce yourself before any interaction. Keep explanations of procedures and activities short and simple, and give them immediately before and throughout patient care. To the extent possible, maintain a sleep-wake cycle with scheduled rest periods. Orient the patient to time (day, month, and year) and place, and explain the reason for the hospitalization. Reassure the patient that he or she is safe. Ask the family to bring in familiar objects, such as pictures. Provide orientation cues within the environment, such as a large clock with numbers or a single-date calendar.

An overwhelming majority of brain injury survivors have altered COGNITION. Cognitive impairments interfere with the brain-injured patient's ability to function effectively in school,

TABLE 45-5 Advantages and Disadvantages of Intracranial Pressure Monitoring Devices

MONITORING DEVICE	ADVANTAGES	DISADVANTAGES
Intraventricular catheter (IVC)	Allows accurate measurement of intracranial pressure (ICP) Allows drainage or sampling of cerebrospinal fluid (CSF) Allows instillation of contrast media Provides reliable evaluation of cerebral compliance	Provides additional site for potential infection Most invasive method for monitoring ICP Must be balanced and recalibrated frequently Catheter can become occluded by blood or tissue Insertion can be difficult with small or collapsed ventricles CSF leakage can occur around insertion site
Subarachnoid bolt or screw	Lower infection rates than with IVC Quickly and easily placed Can be used with small or collapsed ventricles Does not penetrate brain parenchyma	Tendency for dampened waveform Less accurate at high ICP May become occluded by blood or tissue Must be balanced and recalibrated frequently (i.e., every 4 hours and whenever patient is repositioned) Baseline drift Does not provide for CSF sampling
Subdural/epidural catheter or sensor	Least invasive Decreased risk for infection Easily and quickly placed	Increasing baseline drift over time; therefore accuracy and reliability are questionable Does not provide for CSF sampling or drainage
Fiberoptic transducer-tipped catheter	Can be placed in subdural or subarachnoid space, in ventricle, or into brain tissue Easily transported Requires calibrating only once (during insertion) Baseline drift to 1 mm Hg/day Decreased risk for infection Less waveform artifact No need to adjust transducer to patient's position Easy to insert	Does not provide for CSF sampling or drainage Cannot be recalibrated after placement Probe needs periodic replacement Fragile fiberoptic cable easily damaged and broken

at work, and in his or her personal life. *Cognitive rehabilitation* is a way of helping brain-injured patients regain function in areas that are essential for a return to independence and a reasonable quality of life. However, these services are not widely available or accessible.

The patient may be at risk for seizure activity. Keep the bed in low position, and have oxygen and suction available at the bedside. For patients who exhibit poor judgment or who dislodge therapeutic lines, consider the use of hand mittens. Be sure to follow the agency's policy for caring for patients in restraints, if needed. Provide opportunities for toileting. Encourage self-care to promote function at discharge.

Surgical Management. The physician may elect to insert an intracranial pressure (ICP) monitoring device to evaluate the patient's ICP more closely (Table 45-5). All devices are inserted through a *burr hole* (also known as a *keyhole craniotomy*). Strict sterile technique is observed during placement of ICP monitoring devices, and the site is maintained subsequently with attention to sterile technique. Each device is connected to an electronic transducer and a bedside monitor that displays pressure waves and provides a digital value of the pressure. *Be sure to provide ongoing head-to-toe assessments even though the patient's ICP is being invasively monitored!*

In extreme cases in which the patient's ICP cannot be controlled, the physician may elect to perform a **decompressive craniectomy** (removal of a section of the skull) or craniotomy (skull opening followed by immediate skull closure) to remove ischemic brain tissue or the tips of the temporal lobes. The removal of a portion of the skull and/or nonvital brain tissue allows additional space for edema without increasing ICP. Following a craniectomy, information about side-lying restrictions may be placed in the plan of care and repeated in a sign at the head of bed; patients do not lie on the side from with the skull fragment was removed. The patient must wear protective gear (bike or football helmet) when out of bed because an injury to the head where the skull fragment is missing will cause significant brain injury. The skull fragment can be frozen and re-implanted as late as 3 years after removal; re-implantation is planned as the patient becomes ambulatory.

A craniotomy without brain tissue removal may be performed to remove an epidural or subdural clot (hematoma). Care of the patient with a craniotomy is discussed on p. 960 under Postoperative Care in the Brain Tumors section.

Community-Based Care

The patient with a *mild* brain injury recovers at home after discharge from the emergency department (ED) or hospital (Chart 45-9). The patient with a *severe* brain injury requires long-term case management and ongoing rehabilitation after hospitalization. A number of specialized brain injury rehabilitation facilities are available in the United States and Canada. Communicate the patient's plan of care, including drug therapy (use best practices for drug reconciliation and transitions in care), to the receiving nurse or provider during each transition in care.

Home Care Management. The major desired outcome for rehabilitation after brain injury is to maximize the patient's ability to return to his or her highest level of functioning. Activities such as occupational therapy (OT), physical therapy (PT), and speech-language therapy may continue in the home after discharge from the hospital or rehabilitation facility. Adaptation of the home environment to accommodate the patient safely may be needed. For example, smoke and fire alarms must function properly because the patient with a brain injury often loses the sense of smell. Home evaluations and referrals to outside agencies are completed before discharge.

Self-Management Education. Collaborate with the case manager (CM) to provide the patient and family with both

CHART 45-9 Patient and Family Education: Preparing for Self-Management

Mild Brain Injury

- Initial neurologic assessment occurs hourly until the patient returns to baseline. The frequency of ongoing assessment for mild traumatic brain injury (MTBI) is not established.
- For a headache, give acetaminophen (Tylenol) every 4 hours as needed.
- Avoid giving the person sedatives, sleeping pills, or alcoholic beverages for at least 24 hours unless the physician instructs otherwise.
- Do not allow the person to engage in strenuous activity for at least 48 hours.
- While assessment of balance is a component of advanced nursing or medical practice, the caregiver should be aware that balance disturbances cause safety concerns and he or she should provide for monitored or assisted movement.
- If any of these symptoms occur, take the person back to the emergency department immediately:
  - Severe headache
  - Persistent or severe nausea or vomiting
  - Blurred vision
  - Drainage from the ear or nose
  - Weakness
  - Slurred speech
  - Progressive sleepiness
  - Worsening headache
  - Unequal pupil size
- Keep follow-up appointments with the health care provider.

written and verbal instructions for discharge. The teaching plan includes a review of seizure safety at home and strategies to adapt to sensory dysfunction. Discuss issues related to personality or behavior problems that may arise and how to cope with them. Explain the purpose, dosage, schedule, and route of administration of drug therapy. Teach the family to encourage the patient to participate in activities as tolerated. Demonstrations and return demonstrations of care activities help family members become more skillful. Stress the importance of regular follow-up visits with therapists and other health care providers.

Patients with personality and behavior problems respond best to a structured and consistent environment. Instruct the family to develop a home routine that provides structure, repetition, and consistency. Remind the family about the importance of reinforcing positive behaviors rather than negative behaviors.

! NURSING SAFETY PRIORITY (QSEN)

Action Alert

Teach the patient who has sustained a *mild* brain injury, sometimes called a *concussion*, that symptoms that disturb sleep, enjoyment of daily activities, work performance, mood, memory, and ability to learn new material and cause changes in personality require follow-up care. Provide the patient and family with education materials that will alert them to symptoms and management options. A good source of written instructions is *Heads Up: What to Expect After a Concussion—Patient Discharge Instruction Sheet and Getting Better (after concussion)* from the Centers for Disease Control and Prevention (CDC, 2013a).

Most patients with *moderate to severe* TBI are discharged with varied physical and cognitive disabilities. Changes in personality and behavior are very common. The family must learn to cope with the patient's increased fatigue, irritability, temper outbursts, depression, and memory problems. These patients often require constant supervision at home, and families may feel socially isolated. Teach the family about the importance of regular respite care, either in a structured day-care respite program for the patient or through relief provided by a friend or neighbor. Family members, particularly the primary caregiver, may become depressed and have feelings of loneliness. In addition, they may feel angry with the patient because of the physical, financial, and emotional responsibilities that his or her care has placed on them. To help the family cope with these problems, suggest that they join and actively participate in a local brain injury support group.

Health Care Resources. Collaborate with the CM to refer families and patients to local chapters of the Brain Injury Association of America (BIAA) (www.biausa.org) and the National Brain Injury Foundation (www.nbif.org) for information and support. The BIAA has a number of helpful publications on preventing and living with TBI. Other resources include religious, spiritual, and cultural leaders.

BRAIN TUMORS

Brain tumors can arise anywhere within the brain structures and are named according to the cell or tissue where they are located; however, cerebral tumors are the most common. *Primary* tumors originate within the CNS and rarely metastasize (spread) outside this area. *Secondary* brain tumors result from metastasis from other areas of the body, such as the lung, breast, kidney, and GI tract.

❖ *PATHOPHYSIOLOGY*

Complications of Cerebral Tumors

Regardless of location, the tumor expands and invades, infiltrates, compresses, and displaces normal brain tissue. This leads to one or more of these complications:

- Cerebral edema/brain tissue inflammation
- Increased intracranial pressure (ICP)
- Neurologic deficits
- Hydrocephalus
- Pituitary dysfunction

Cerebral edema (vasogenic edema) results from changes in capillary endothelial tissue permeability that allows plasma to seep into the extracellular spaces. This leads to *increased ICP* and, depending on the location of the tumor, brain herniation syndromes. A variety of *neurologic deficits* result from edema, infiltration, distortion, and compression of surrounding brain tissue. The cerebral blood vessels may become compressed because of edema and increased ICP. This compression leads to ischemia (decreased blood flow) of the area supplied by the vessel. In addition, the tumor may enter the walls of the vessel, causing it to rupture and hemorrhage into the tumor bed or other brain tissue. Some patients who have brain tumors have seizure activity from interference with the brain's normal electrical activity.

Increased ICP may also result from *hydrocephalus* (increased cerebrospinal fluid [CSF]) related to obstruction of the flow of CSF or displacement of the lateral ventricles by the expanding lesion. Typically, a tumor obstructs the aqueduct of Sylvius or one of the ventricles or pushes into the subarachnoid space.

TABLE 45-6 Classification of Brain Tumors

Benign	Malignant
• Acoustic neuroma (schwannoma)	• Astrocytoma (a *glioblastoma multiforme* is a Grade 4 astrocytoma)
• Choroid plexus papilloma	• Oligodendroglioma
• Meningioma	• Ependymoma
• Pituitary adenoma	• Medulloblastoma
• Astrocytoma	• Chondrosarcoma
• Grade 1 (may undergo changes and become malignant)	• Glioma
• Chondroma	• Lymphoma
• Craniopharyngioma	
• Hemangioblastoma	

Pituitary dysfunction may occur as the tumor compresses the pituitary gland and causes the syndrome of inappropriate antidiuretic hormone (SIADH) or diabetes insipidus (DI). These disorders result in severe fluid and electrolyte imbalances and can be life threatening. (See Chapters 42 and 62 for a complete description.)

Classification of Tumors

Brain tumors are usually classified as benign, malignant (cancerous), or metastatic (Table 45-6). They may or may not be treated, depending on their location. Benign (noncancerous) tumors are generally associated with a favorable outcome. Malignant or metastatic tumors require more aggressive intervention including surgery, radiation, and/or chemotherapy.

A second classification system is based on location. **Supratentorial** tumors are located within the cerebral hemispheres. Located beneath the tentorium (fold of dura mater) is the **infratentorial** area—the area of the brainstem structures and cerebellum.

A third classification system depends on the cellular or anatomic origins of the tumor. The nervous system is composed of two types of cells: (1) neurons, which are responsible for nerve impulse conduction; and (2) neuroglial cells, which provide support, nourishment, and protection for neurons. Four specific types of neuroglial cells are astrocytes, oligodendroglia, ependymal cells, and microglia. When classifying gliomas according to this system, tumors are named by their cell type. For example, an astrocytoma is a tumor of astrocytes. Gliomas are *malignant* tumors.

Meningiomas, the most common *benign* tumors, arise from the coverings of the brain (the meninges). This tumor is capsular, globular, and well outlined and causes compression and displacement of nearby brain tissue. Although complete removal of the tumor is possible, it tends to recur.

Pituitary tumors that occur in the anterior lobe account for up to one fourth of brain tumors and may cause endocrine dysfunction. The most common type of pituitary tumor is the adenoma. These tumors are *benign* and often occur in young and middle-aged adults. The presenting symptoms include visual disturbances and hypopituitary signs, such as loss of body hair, diabetes insipidus (DI), infertility, visual field defects, and headaches.

Acoustic neuromas arise from the sheath of Schwann cells in the peripheral portion of cranial nerve VIII. They are also referred to as *cerebellar pontine angle (CPA) tumors* to describe their anatomic location. Acoustic neuromas compress brain tissue and tend to surround nearby cranial nerves (VII, V, IX, X), making surgical removal difficult without causing permanent cranial nerve dysfunction. Women are twice as likely as men to have acoustic neuromas. Common symptoms include hearing loss, **tinnitus** (ringing in the ears), and dizziness or vertigo.

Metastatic, or secondary, tumors account for many brain tumors. Cancer cells from the lung, breast, colon, pancreas, and kidney can travel to the brain via the blood and the lymphatic system. Multiple metastatic lesions are fairly common.

Brain tumors are also grouped by grade, which refers to the microscopic tissue evaluated by the histologist:

- Grade I: The tissue is benign; the cells look nearly like normal brain cells, and they grow slowly.
- Grade II: The tissue is malignant; the cells look less like normal cells than do the cells in a Grade I.
- Grade III: The malignant tissue has cells that look very different from normal cells; the abnormal cells are actively growing (anaplastic).
- Grade IV: The malignant tissue has cells that look most abnormal and tend to grow quickly.

Etiology and Genetic Risk

The exact cause of brain tumors is unknown. Several areas under investigation include genetic mutations and a variety of environmental factors. The use of cellular phones has been investigated as a cause of brain tumors, but findings are not confirmed. Brain tumors account for a small percentage of all cancer deaths. Primary brain tumors are relatively uncommon; many more patients have metastatic lesions (Cahill & Armstrong, 2011). Malignant brain tumors are seen primarily in patients 40 to 70 years of age, and the survival rate is low compared with that of other cancers.

❖ PATIENT-CENTERED COLLABORATIVE CARE

◆ Assessment

When possible, obtain a history from both the patient and the family, including current signs and symptoms. A complete neurologic assessment is needed to establish baseline data and to determine the nature and extent of neurologic deficits.

The clinical manifestations of brain tumors vary with the site of the tumor (Chart 45-10). In general, assess for these symptoms of a brain tumor:

- Headaches that are usually more severe on awakening in the morning
- Nausea and vomiting
- Visual symptoms
- Seizures or convulsions
- Facial numbness or tingling
- Loss of balance or dizziness
- Weakness or paralysis in one part or one side of the body
- Difficulty thinking, speaking, or articulating
- Changes in mentation or personality
- **Papilledema** (swelling of the optic disc) indicating increased ICP

Neurologic deficits result from the destruction, distortion, or compression of brain tissue. *Supratentorial (cerebral)* tumors usually result in paralysis, seizures, memory loss, cognitive impairment, language impairment, or vision problems. *Infratentorial* tumors produce ataxia, autonomic nervous system dysfunction, vomiting, drooling, hearing loss, and vision impairment. As the tumor grows, ICP increases and the symptoms become progressively more severe.

CHART 45-10 **Key Features**

Common Brain Tumors

Cerebral Tumors
- Headache (most common feature)
- Vomiting unrelated to food intake
- Changes in visual acuity and visual fields; diplopia (visual changes caused by papilledema)
- Hemiparesis or hemiplegia
- Hypokinesia (decreased motor ability)
- Hyperesthesia, paresthesia, decreased tactile discrimination
- Seizures
- Aphasia
- Changes in personality or behavior

Brainstem Tumors
- Hearing loss (acoustic neuroma)
- Facial pain and weakness
- Dysphagia, decreased gag reflex
- Nystagmus
- Hoarseness
- Ataxia and dysarthria (cerebellar tumors)

Diagnosis is based on the history, neurologic assessment, clinical examination, and results of neurodiagnostic testing. Noninvasive diagnostic studies such as *CT, MRI,* and *skull films* are conducted first. These tests identify the size, location, and extent of the tumor. The MRI may be used for initial diagnostic evaluation and is a more sensitive diagnostic study, whereas the CT is often used for follow-up during the course of illness.

Cerebral angiography is usually not indicated to diagnose a brain tumor but may be used to provide additional information about blood supply to the tumor. *Electroencephalography (EEG), lumbar puncture (LP), brain scan,* and *positron emission tomography (PET)* may be indicated to provide further information about the size, location, and characteristics of the tumor. *To prevent brain herniation, LP should not be performed if the patient is exhibiting signs of ICP elevation.* Laboratory tests may also be requested to evaluate endocrine function, renal status, and electrolyte balance.

◆ *Interventions*

Interventions depend on the type, size, and location of the tumor. For example, a small benign tumor may be periodically monitored through CT and MRI scanning to assess its growth. Malignant tumors may be managed by chemotherapy, radiation, and/or surgery.

Nonsurgical Management. The desired outcomes of treatment of brain tumors are to decrease tumor size, improve quality of life, and improve survival time. The type of treatment selected depends on the tumor size and location, patient symptoms and general condition, and whether the tumor has recurred. In addition to traditional interventions, a number of experimental treatment modalities are being investigated. These include blood-brain barrier disruption, recombinant DNA, monoclonal antibodies, new chemotherapeutic drugs, and immunotherapy. Traditional *radiation therapy* may be used alone, after surgery, or in combination with chemotherapy and surgery. Chapter 22 discusses radiation treatment for patients with cancer.

Drug Therapy. The health care provider may prescribe a variety of drugs to treat the tumor, manage the patient's symptoms, and prevent complications. *Chemotherapy* may be given

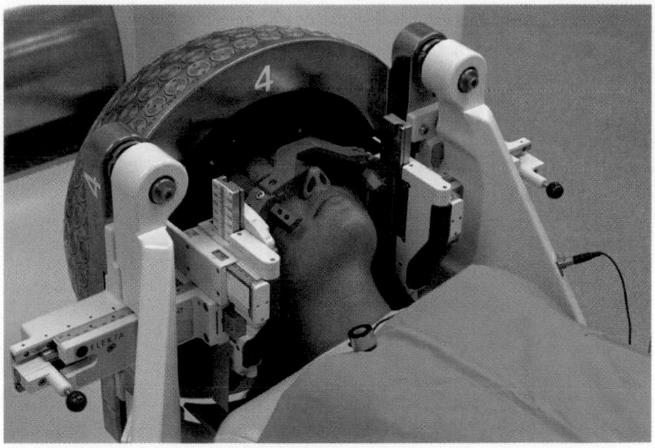

FIG. 45-10 A gamma knife treatment. The treatment beams are widely dispersed over the surface of the head to prevent damage to healthy brain tissue. The beams are intense only at the point of target.

alone, in combination with radiation and surgery, and with tumor progression. Although these drugs may control tumor growth or decrease tumor burden, the benefit does not last. Chemotherapy usually involves more than one agent that may be given orally, IV, intra-arterially, and/or intrathecally through an Ommaya reservoir placed in a cranial ventricle. In electrochemotherapy, electric voltage carries agents into the tumor. When given systemically, the drug must be lipid-soluble to cross the blood-brain barrier.

Commonly used oral drugs are lomustine (CCNU), temozolomide (Temodar), procarbazine (Matulane), and methotrexate (MTX). Vincristine (Oncovin) may be given IV in combination with other drugs. Monitor for side effects of these drugs, which are similar to those of any chemotherapeutic drug. Chapter 22 describes general nursing implications for care of a patient receiving chemotherapy.

Direct drug delivery to the tumor is an emerging practice. Disk-shaped drug (Gliadel) wafers may be placed directly into the cavity created during surgical tumor removal (interstitial chemotherapy). The major drug in the wafer is carmustine (BCNU). This therapy is usually given for newly diagnosed high-grade malignant gliomas, but recurrent tumors may also be treated with this method. Other drugs used are molecularly targeted. Examples include erlotinib (Tarceva), gefitinib (Iressa), and bevacizumab (Avastin) (Lilley et al., 2014).

Analgesics, such as codeine and acetaminophen (Tylenol, Ace-Tabs 🍁), are given for headache. Dexamethasone (Decadron) is usually given to control cerebral edema. Phenytoin (Dilantin) or other antiepileptic drugs may be given to prevent or treat seizure activity. Proton pump inhibitors are given to decrease gastric acid secretion and prevent the development of stress ulcers.

Stereotactic Radiosurgery. Stereotactic radiosurgery (SRS) is an alternative to traditional surgery. Several techniques are used, including the modified linear accelerator (LINAC) using accelerated x-rays, a particle accelerator using beams of protons (cyclotron), and isotope seeds implanted in the tumor (brachytherapy).

The gamma knife is an SRS procedure that uses a single high dose of ionized radiation to focus multiple beams of gamma radiation produced by the radioisotope *cobalt-60* to destroy intracranial lesions selectively without damaging surrounding healthy tissue (Fig. 45-10). Combining neurodiagnostic imaging tools—including MRI, CT, magnetic resonance angiography (MRA), and angiography—with the gamma knife allows for precise localization of deep-seated or anatomically difficult lesions. Treatment usually takes less than an hour, and patients require only overnight hospitalization. Advantages of this technique include its:

- Noninvasive nature
- Lower risk when compared with traditional craniotomy
- Surgical precision
- Decreased cost
- Decreased morbidity
- Deceased length of hospital stay
- Rapid recovery time

A disadvantage is that the device requires an uncomfortable rigid head frame. In another system, called the *CyberKnife,* no frame is needed. A third stereotactic system is the Novalis system. This radiosurgery system utilizes a small computer-controlled micro Multi Leaf Collimator (mMLC) that can produce many complicated shapes with a wide range of tumor area. Both procedures are used primarily for brain tumors or arteriovenous malformations (AVMs) that are in a difficult location and therefore not removable by craniotomy. These procedures may also be used with patients who decline conventional surgery, for patients whose age and physical condition do not allow general anesthesia, as an adjunct to radiation therapy, and for recurrent or residual AVM or tumors after embolization or craniotomy.

Surgical Management. A **craniotomy** (incision into the cranium) may be performed to remove the tumor, to improve symptoms related to the lesion, or to decrease the tumor size (debulk). The challenge for the neurosurgeon is to remove the tumor as completely as possible without damaging normal tissue. Complete removal is possible with some benign tumors, which results in a "surgical cure." Postoperatively, the patient may be admitted to the critical care unit or neurosurgical unit for frequent observation.

Preoperative Care. The patient having a craniotomy is typically very anxious about having his or her head opened and the brain exposed. Concerns are centered on the possibility of increased neurologic deficits after the surgery and the patient's self-image when part or all of the head is shaved. Provide reassurance that the surgeon will spare vital parts of the brain while removing or decreasing the size of the tumor. Teach the patient and family about what to expect immediately after surgery and throughout the recovery period. Some patients require short-term or long-term rehabilitation.

Check that the patient has not had alcohol, tobacco, anticoagulants, or NSAIDs for at least 5 days before surgery. Some neurosurgeons require a week or longer. Be sure that the patient has been NPO status for at least 8 hours. Other preoperative care is similar to that for any patient having surgery, as described in Chapter 14.

Operative Procedures. Surgery is performed under local or general anesthesia or sedation. Small tumors that are easily located may be removed by *minimally invasive surgery (MIS).* For example, the trans-nasal approach using endoscopy can be performed for pituitary tumors. The patient has a short hospital stay and few complications after surgery. Stereotactic surgery using a rigid head frame can be done for tumors that are easily reached. This procedure requires only burr holes and local anesthesia because the brain has no sensory neurons for pain. Laser surgery can also be done.

For a *craniotomy,* the surgeon makes an incision along or behind the hairline after placing the patient's head in a skull fixation device. Several burr holes are drilled into the skull, and a saw is used to remove a piece of bone (bone flap) to expose the tumor area. The flap is stored carefully until the end of the procedure. The tumor is located using imaging technology and removed or debulked. After the tumor removal, the bone flap is replaced and held by small screws or bolts. A drain or monitoring device may be inserted. The surgeon creates a soft dressing "cap" over the top of the head to keep the surgical area clean.

Postoperative Care. The focus of postoperative care is to monitor the patient to detect changes in status and to prevent or minimize complications, especially increased intracranial pressure (ICP).

! NURSING SAFETY PRIORITY QSEN

Action Alert

Assess neurologic and vital signs every 15 to 30 minutes for the first 4 to 6 hours after a craniotomy and then every hour. If the patient is stable for 24 hours, the frequency of these checks may be decreased to every 2 to 4 hours, depending on the agency's policy or the patient's condition. *Report immediately and document new neurologic deficits, particularly a decreased level of consciousness (LOC), motor weakness or paralysis, aphasia (speech and/or language problems), decreased sensation, and reduced pupil reaction to light!* Personality changes such as agitation, aggression, or passivity can also indicate worsening neurologic status.

Managing the Patient. Periorbital (around the eye) edema and ecchymosis of one or both eyes are not unusual and are treated with cold compresses to decrease swelling. Irrigate the affected eye with warm saline solution or artificial tears to improve patient comfort. The patient in the critical care unit has routine cardiac monitoring because dysrhythmias may occur as a result of brain–autonomic nervous system–cardiac interactions or fluid and electrolyte imbalance.

Regardless of setting, ensure recording of the patient's intake and output for the first 24 hours. Anticipate fluid restriction to 1500 mL daily if there is pituitary involvement in either the tumor or surgical site. Reposition the patient, but do not turn him or her onto the operative site. Delegate or provide repositioning and deep breathing every 2 hours. To prevent the development of VTE, maintain intermittent sequential pneumatic devices until the patient ambulates.

For patients who have undergone *supratentorial* surgery, elevate the head of the bed 30 degrees or as tolerated to promote venous drainage from the head. *Position the patient to avoid extreme hip or neck flexion and maintain the head in a midline, neutral position to prevent increased ICP.* Turn the patient side to side or supine to prevent pressure ulcers and prevent pneumonia.

Keep the patient with an *infratentorial* (brainstem) craniotomy flat and positioned side-lying, alternating sides every 2 hours, for 24 to 48 hours. This position prevents pressure on the neck-area incision site. It also prevents pressure on the internal tumor excision site from higher cerebral structures. Make sure that the patient remains NPO status for 24 hours, because edema around the medulla and lower cranial nerves may cause vomiting and aspiration.

Check the head dressing every 1 to 2 hours for signs of drainage. Mark the area of drainage once during each shift for baseline comparison, although this practice varies by health care agency. A small or moderate amount of drainage is expected. Some patients may have a Hemovac, Jackson-Pratt, or other surgical drain in place for 24 hours after surgery. Measure the drainage every 8 hours, and record the amount and color. A typical amount of drainage is 30 to 50 mL every 8 hours. Follow the manufacturer's and neurosurgeon's instructions to maintain suction within the drain.

NURSING SAFETY PRIORITY QSEN

Critical Rescue

After craniotomy, monitor the patient's dressing for excessive amounts of drainage. Report a saturated head dressing or drainage greater than 50 mL/8 hrs immediately to the surgeon! Observe for manifestations of hypovolemic shock, and position the patient flat to maintain blood pressure if needed.

The usual laboratory studies monitored postoperatively include complete blood count (CBC), serum electrolyte levels and osmolarity, and coagulation studies. The patient's hematocrit and hemoglobin concentration may be abnormally low from blood loss during surgery or elevated if the blood was replaced. Hyponatremia (low serum sodium) may occur as a result of fluid volume overload, syndrome of inappropriate antidiuretic hormone (SIADH), or steroid administration.

Hypokalemia (low serum potassium) may cause cardiac irritability. Weakness, a change in LOC, and confusion are symptoms of hyponatremia and hypokalemia. Hypernatremia may be caused by meningitis, dehydration, or diabetes insipidus (DI). It is manifested by muscle weakness, restlessness, extreme thirst, and dry mouth. Additional signs of dehydration such as decreased urinary output, thick lung secretions, and hypotension may be present. *Untreated hypernatremia can lead to seizure activity. DI should be considered if the patient voids large amounts of very dilute urine with an increasing serum osmolarity and electrolyte concentration.*

Often the patient is mechanically ventilated for the first 24 to 48 hours after surgery to help manage the airway and maintain optimal oxygen levels. If the patient is awake or attempting to breathe at a rate other than that set on the ventilator, drugs such as dexmedetomidine (Precedex) or propofol (Diprivan) and fentanyl are given to treat pain and anxiety, as well as to promote rest and comfort. Suction the patient as needed. *Remember to hyperoxygenate the patient carefully before, during, and after suctioning!*

Drugs routinely given postoperatively include antiepileptic drugs, histamine blockers or proton pump inhibitors for stress ulcer prophylaxis, and glucocorticoids, such as dexamethasone (Decadron) to reduce intracranial edema. Give acetaminophen for fever or mild pain. Some surgeons may prescribe antibiotics to prevent infection.

NCLEX EXAMINATION CHALLENGE

Physiological Integrity

A client returns from the postanesthesia care unit (PACU) after a craniotomy for removal of a left parietal lobe tumor. How will the nurse position the client after surgery?

A. Flex the client's knees to decrease intra-abdominal pressure and cerebral hypertension.
B. Keep the client on the left side to prevent surgical site bleeding or cerebrospinal fluid leakage.
C. Elevate the client's head to at least 30 degrees to promote cerebral venous drainage.
D. Hyperextend the client's neck to maintain the airway and prevent aspiration regardless of supine or side-lying positioning.

TABLE 45-7 Postoperative Complications of Craniotomy

- Increased intracranial pressure (ICP)
- Hematomas
  - Subdural hematoma
  - Epidural hematoma
- Subarachnoid hemorrhage
- Hypovolemic shock
- Hydrocephalus
- Respiratory complications
  - Atelectasis
  - Hypoxia
  - Pneumonia
  - Neurogenic pulmonary edema
- Wound infection
- Meningitis
- Fluid and electrolyte imbalances
  - Dehydration
  - Hyponatremia
  - Hypernatremia
- Seizures
- Cerebrospinal fluid (CSF) leak
- Cerebral edema

Preventing and Managing Postoperative Complications. Postoperative complications are listed in Table 45-7. The major complications of supratentorial surgery are increased ICP from cerebral edema or hydrocephalus and hemorrhage.

Symptoms of *increased ICP* include severe headache, deteriorating LOC, restlessness, irritability, and dilated or pinpoint pupils that are slow to react or nonreactive to light. Treatment of increased ICP is the same as that described on p. 948 under Interventions in the Traumatic Brain Injury section.

Hydrocephalus (increased CSF in the brain) is caused by obstruction of the normal CSF pathway from edema, an expanding lesion such as a hematoma, or blood in the subarachnoid space. Rapidly progressive hydrocephalus produces the classic symptoms of increased ICP. Slowly progressive hydrocephalus is manifested by headache, decreased LOC, irritability, blurred vision, and urinary incontinence. An intraventricular catheter (ventriculostomy) may be placed to drain CSF during surgery or emergently postoperatively for rapidly deteriorating neurologic function. If long-term treatment is required for chronic hydrocephalus, a surgical shunt is inserted to drain CSF to another area of the body. A major complication of the shunting procedure is a subdural hematoma from the tearing of bridging veins. An external lumbar drain may also be used temporarily. Additional information about shunts may be found in neuroscience nursing textbooks.

Subdural and epidural *hematomas and intracranial hemorrhage* are manifested by severe headache, a rapid decrease in LOC, progressive neurologic deficits, and herniation syndromes (brain tissue shifting, often downward). Bleeding into the posterior fossa may lead to sudden cardiovascular and respiratory arrest. Treatment of a hematoma requires surgical removal. An intracranial hemorrhage is treated with aggressive medical management (e.g., osmotic diuretics, ICP monitoring, CPP management).

Respiratory complications include atelectasis, pneumonia, and neurogenic pulmonary edema. Prevent atelectasis and pneumonia by turning the patient frequently and encouraging him or her to take frequent deep breaths to expand the lungs each hour. Humidified air and incentive spirometry are also useful techniques. Other treatment modalities include endotracheal or oral tracheal suctioning and chest physiotherapy.

However, these measures may cause an increase in ICP. Although not common, *neurogenic pulmonary edema* is a life-threatening complication of traumatic brain injury (TBI), brain tumors, and brain surgery. Its symptoms are the same as those of acute pulmonary edema, but there are no associated cardiac problems. In spite of aggressive treatment, most patients with neurogenic pulmonary edema do not survive.

Wound infections occur more often in older and debilitated patients and in patients with a history of diabetes, long-term steroid use, obesity, and previous infections. The patient may contribute to the problem by rubbing or scratching the wound. If infection is present, the wound appears reddened and puffy. It may begin to separate, is sensitive to touch, and feels warm. The patient may or may not be febrile. Treatment is based on the degree and extent of the infection. A localized infection may be treated by cleaning it with an antiseptic and applying a topical antibiotic. For more severe infections, systemic antibiotic administration is needed. If the underlying bone is involved, it may need to be removed.

Meningitis is an inflammation of the meninges and may occur as a result of surgery or wound infection, a cerebrospinal fluid (CSF) leak, or contamination during surgery. (See the Meningitis section in Chapter 42 for a more complete explanation of this condition.)

Complications related to *fluid and electrolyte imbalance* include DI, SIADH, and cerebral salt wasting (CSW). DI is seen most often after supratentorial surgery, especially procedures involving the pituitary gland or hypothalamus. Failure of the posterior pituitary gland to release antidiuretic hormone (ADH) leads to failure of the renal tubules to reabsorb water. The patient's urine output increases dramatically (it may be up to 10 L/day), and the urine specific gravity drops to below 1.005. Urine osmolarity decreases, whereas serum osmolarity increases. The patient may become dehydrated and hypovolemic shock may develop rapidly if this condition is left untreated. Fluid therapy to replace urinary losses and prevent dehydration may be accomplished by having the patient increase oral intake or use IV fluids. Hormonal replacement may also be necessary, especially if fluid loss is greater than 6 L/24 hr. Aqueous vasopressin is short-acting, lasting only 6 to 8 hours. Desmopressin acetate (DDAVP) may be administered for long-term replacement therapy.

Syndrome of inappropriate antidiuretic hormone (SIADH) occurs when the posterior pituitary gland releases too much ADH, causing water retention. The urine output decreases dramatically, with a urine output of less than 20 mL/hr. Sodium concentration in the urine is normal or elevated, whereas the serum sodium level falls. Other indications of SIADH are loss of thirst, weight gain, irritability, muscle weakness, and decreased LOC. SIADH is treated by fluid restriction, which is usually sufficient to correct the hyponatremia. Conivaptan (Vaprisol) and tolvaptan are vasopressin receptor antagonists used to increase water diuresis without serum electrolyte loss and may be useful in hypervolemic hyponatremic conditions. Slow, controlled IV infusion of hypertonic sodium may be needed for severe hyponatremia (<118 mEq/L).

Cerebral salt wasting (CSW) is thought to result from the influence of atrial natriuretic factor (ANF). ANF cells are located in the hypothalamus and the right atrium and regulate fluid volume. CSW is believed to be the primary cause of hyponatremia in the neurosurgical population. It is characterized by hyponatremia, decreased serum osmolarity, and decreased blood volume. Serum vasopressin and ANF levels can differentiate CSW and SIADH. CSW is treated with the replacement of sodium and isotonic fluid volume.

Patients with complications related to fluid and electrolyte imbalance undergo strict measurement of their intake and output. Be sure that an accurate weight measurement is taken every day at the same time with the same scale. Carefully assess for indications of fluid overload or dehydration during treatment. Serum electrolyte levels and osmolarity are measured daily (or more often if clinically indicated).

Community-Based Care

The patient with a brain tumor is managed at home if possible. Maintaining a reasonable quality of life is an important outcome for recovery and rehabilitation. Unless the patient has a significant degree of disability, no special preparation for home care is needed. Patients with hemiparesis need assistance to ensure that their home is accessible according to their method of MOBILITY (e.g., cane, walker, and wheelchair). The environment should be made safe to prevent falls. For example, teach caregivers to remove scatter rugs and to place grab bars in the bathroom.

Information about the selection of rehabilitation or chronic care facility, if needed, can be obtained from the case manager (CM) or discharge planner. The selected facility should have experience in providing care for neurologically impaired patients. A psychologist should be available to provide input in the evaluation of the cognitive disabilities that the patient may have.

It is very important that the patient and family fully understand the importance of any recommended follow-up health care appointments. The discharge summary should state the name of the person who has been given the follow-up information.

Health teaching includes drug therapy and who to call if adverse drug events occur. Remind the patient to avoid taking any over-the-counter drugs unless approved by the health care provider.

Teach the patient to maintain a program of regular physical exercise within the limits of any disabilities. Referral to the dietitian may be needed to ensure adequate caloric intake for the patient receiving radiation or chemotherapy.

Seizures are a potential complication that can occur at any time for as long as 1 year or more after surgery. Provide the patient and the family with information about seizure precautions and what to do if a seizure occurs.

Refer the patient and the family or significant others to the American Brain Tumor Association (www.abta.org) or the National Brain Tumor Foundation (www.braintumor.org). The American Cancer Society (www.cancer.org) is also an appropriate community resource for patients with malignant tumors. Home care agencies are available to provide both the physical and rehabilitative care that the patient may need at home. Hospice services and palliative care may be needed if he or she is terminally ill. (See Chapter 7 for additional information about end-of-life care.) Brain tumor support groups may also be a valuable asset to the patient and family.

BRAIN ABSCESS

A **brain abscess** is a purulent infection of the brain in which pus forms in the extradural, subdural, or intracerebral area of the brain. The causative organisms are usually bacteria that invade the brain directly or indirectly. Cerebral abscesses may be a complication of meningitis.

❖ PATHOPHYSIOLOGY

In general, organisms from the ear, sinus, or mastoid area enter the brain by traveling along the wall of the cerebral veins, and therefore they may spread to any area of the brain. The typical source is a lung infection, although it is common not to find the source of infection. Bacteria may travel from a nearby infected area such as an ear infection or a sinus infection or enter the body with a bullet, knife wound, or neurosurgery. At times, the organisms (especially those from the ear) destroy the bone, form a tract, and enter the brain directly. A portion of an abscess from a distant organ, such as the heart or tonsils, may break off and enter the systemic circulation. These septic emboli contain organisms that may become lodged in a cerebral vessel and produce a localized infection. Penetrating trauma, open head injuries, and neurosurgical procedures provide a potential means for the direct entry of an organism into the brain.

The organisms cause a local infection, and acute inflammation surrounds the involved area. Within a few days, necrosis of the tissue takes place, pus forms, and the tissue liquefies. This process is followed by the development of cerebral edema from localized vascular congestion and tissue swelling in response to inflammation. During the next few weeks, the area becomes encapsulated. The abscess usually occurs deep within the cerebral hemisphere and involves the white matter of the brain. In a few cases, it spreads through the brain tissue to the subarachnoid space and ventricular system. The organism varies with the source of the abscess. Streptococci are the most common organisms and are often found with other anaerobes such as *Bacteroides.* Enterobacteriaceae such as *Escherichia coli* and proteus organisms may also be combined with streptococcus. Yeast and fungi also cause cerebral abscess formation, particularly in patients who are immunosuppressed. *Toxoplasma gondii* is one of the most commonly seen central nervous system (CNS) opportunistic infections in the acquired immune deficiency syndrome (AIDS) population.

Most brain abscesses occur in the frontal and temporal lobes. A few affected patients have more than one abscess. Mortality rates vary up to more than one half of patients with abscesses. Those that occur in immunosuppressed patients are associated with a higher mortality rate.

❖ PATIENT-CENTERED COLLABORATIVE CARE

◆ Assessment

Physical Assessment/Clinical Manifestations. The clinical manifestations of a brain abscess begin slowly and are similar to some of the manifestations of meningitis. The patient may have headache, fever, and neurologic deficits or nonspecific signs and symptoms (Chart 45-11). Perform ongoing neurologic assessments. The patient may be mildly lethargic or somewhat confused. The pupillary response to light is normal in the early stages. As increased intracranial pressure (ICP) progresses, the pupils may become sluggish, unequal, dilated, and nonresponsive to light. The patient's level of consciousness (LOC) declines to a state in which he or she loses the ability to interact with the environment. Airway and respiratory function may also be altered.

CHART 45-11 Key Features

Brain Abscess

- Headache
- Fever
- Pain
- Motor deficits, such as hemiplegia
- Ataxia
- Sensory impairment (varies)
- Aphasia
- Seizure activity
- Visual field changes (e.g., decreased peripheral vision, nystagmus)
- *If severe,* signs of increased intracranial pressure (ICP), such as decreased level of consciousness (LOC), severe headache, bradycardia, widened pulse pressure

Examination of the patient's visual fields often reveals a **temporal field blindness** (decrease in peripheral vision laterally). If the abscess affects the cerebral hemispheres, nystagmus (involuntary eye movements) may be evident. Motor examination reveals a generalized weakness. More significant motor problems, such as hemiplegia, may be apparent in the presence of a frontal lobe abscess. An ataxic gait is seen with a cerebellar abscess. Sensory impairment varies, although the patient often exhibits no SENSORY PERCEPTION deficits. The patient may have varying degrees of aphasia (impaired communication ability) if he or she has a frontal or temporal lobe abscess. Seizure activity may occur because of irritation of the cortical tissue. Late in the disease process, more severe symptoms of increased ICP occur and include severe headache, decreased LOC (possibly coma), a widened pulse pressure, bradycardia, and irregular respirations. The patient with AIDS often presents with systemic infection, CNS involvement, and lymphoma.

Some patients may have atypical presentations, including older adults (age-related compromise in immune function), those receiving steroid therapy or immune-modulating drugs, and patients with later stages of human immune deficiency virus (HIV) infection (immune system compromise). In the earlier stages, the inflammatory response is responsible for much of the clinical presentation, particularly if cerebral abscess formation results from meningitis. The risk is that the patient may progress to severe abscess formation before the onset of "classic" manifestations.

Diagnostic Assessment. The white blood cell (WBC) count and erythrocyte sedimentation rate (ESR) are usually elevated, indicating the presence of infection. If the abscess is encapsulated, the WBC count may be normal. Obtain specimens for aerobic and, when possible, anaerobic cultures of the blood, ear, nose, and throat to determine the primary source of infection.

The health care provider requests a CT scan to determine the presence of cerebritis, hydrocephalus, or a midline shift. MRI is also useful in detecting the presence of an abscess early in the course of the disease. An EEG can localize the lesion in most cases and shows high-voltage, slow-wave activity; electrocerebral silence may be noted in the area of the abscess. Radiography of the sinuses and the mastoid is often indicated. A lumbar puncture may be performed if meningitis is also suspected and the patient does not have ICP elevation. A needle biopsy is performed to identify the cause of the infection.

◆ Interventions

Drug therapy is recommended if the patient has several abscesses, a small abscess (less than 2 cm), an abscess deep in the brain, an abscess and meningitis, a shunt for hydrocephalus (in some cases the shunt may need to be removed temporarily or replaced) or *Toxoplasma gondii* infection in a person with HIV. Drug therapy is prescribed by the physician to treat the abscess. Antibiotic dosing may be maximized to ensure adequate CNS penetration. Antibiotics are particularly useful in the early stages (cerebritis) of abscess formation. A combination of antibiotics is used, particularly if the infection resulted from septic emboli. Antiepileptic drugs such as phenytoin (Dilantin) may be used to prevent seizures. The drug regimen is strictly followed to maintain therapeutic blood levels. Give analgesics to treat headache.

The physician may surgically drain an encapsulated abscess via a burr hole to reduce the mass effect of the lesion. In certain cases, a craniotomy may be performed to remove the abscess. The decision to perform surgery is based on the patient's general condition, the stage of abscess development, and the site of the abscess. Provide routine preoperative and postoperative care for the patient undergoing a craniotomy, as discussed in this chapter under Surgical Management in the Brain Tumors section.

The patient with a brain abscess is discharged to home if few or no neurologic deficits are present. Patients with severe dysfunction are usually transferred to long-term care or a rehabilitation facility. Some patients have permanent neurologic deficits.

ACQUIRED HYPOXIC-ANOXIC BRAIN INJURY

Acquired hypoxic-anoxic brain injury is brain damage caused by a reduced or absent supply of oxygen. Common causes include cardiac arrest, asphyxiation from a suicide attempt (i.e., hanging), near-drowning, drug use and overdose, accidental electrocution, and severe asthma. Neurons in the brain experience ischemia, injury, and cell death within 4 minutes of a reduced oxygen supply to the brain. The reduction of oxygen can be a primary event such as asphyxiation or a secondary event such as loss of airway during a drug overdose or decreased cerebral PERFUSION from increased intracranial pressure (Smania et al., 2013). Generally hypoxic-anoxic brain injury is global with decreases in COGNITION, MOBILITY, and sensation that occur with the event and persist in an unpredictable manner following resuscitation. An MRI provides the most sensitive diagnostic test for determining hypoxic-anoxic brain injury (Muttikkal & Wintermark, 2013).

Initial interventions are generally supportive with a focus on airway, breathing, and circulation to restore the oxygen. Therapeutic hypothermia, described earlier in this chapter on p. 953, is useful when anoxia is related to a witnessed cardiac arrest. Frequent neurologic assessment is undertaken to detect and prevent secondary injury as discussed with severe traumatic brain injury in this chapter. It is not uncommon for patients to experience increased intracranial pressure from cerebral edema in the days following the initial anoxic event. Increased intracranial pressure and cerebral edema are managed similarly to severe traumatic brain injury. Because it is difficult to predict whether brain function will be restored and the course of recovery, patients and family often require emotional support to deal with uncertainty. Early physical and specialized neurocognitive rehabilitation can promote functional outcomes following this type of brain injury.

NURSING CONCEPTS AND CLINICAL JUDGMENT REVIEW

What might you NOTICE if the patient is experiencing changes in cerebral PERFUSION, MOBILITY, SENSORY PERCEPTION, and COGNITION as a result of severe acute neurologic health problems affecting the brain?

- Decreased level of consciousness (LOC)
- Inability to communicate (aphasia)
- Impaired swallowing (dysphagia)
- Weakness or paralysis of one side of the body (hemiparesis or hemiplegia)
- Alteration in gait
- Inability to perform ADLs
- Report of nausea and vomiting
- Report of impaired visual acuity or fields
- Ptosis (eyelid drooping)
- Unilateral body neglect
- Report of decreased peripheral sensation
- Inability to make appropriate judgments; confusion
- Impaired memory
- Report of severe headache

What should you INTERPRET and how should you RESPOND to a patient experiencing impaired PERFUSION, MOBILITY, SENSORY PERCEPTION, and COGNITION as a result of severe neurologic health problems affecting the brain?

Perform and interpret physical assessment, including:

- Assess airway, breathing, and circulation status.
- Assess neurologic status, especially LOC and mental state.
- Take vital signs, and establish blood pressure goals.
- Assess neurologic status with particular attention to level of consciousness and cognition.
- Assess functional status.
- Assess for swallowing and nutrition status.

Respond by:

- Notifying health care provider or Rapid Response Team of changes in the Glasgow Coma Scale value of 2 or more points, a reduction in level of consciousness or pupil reactivity to light, hypertension, hypotension, widened pulse pressure, dysrhythmias, fever, and hypoxemia (low Spo_2) urgently
- Ensuring an adequate airway
- Giving oxygen if Spo_2 <92%
- Establishing IV access
- Communicating and collaborating with health care team members efficiently to meet patient's needs
- Assisting with ADLs and mobility as needed
- Providing a safe environment to prevent harm from altered sensory perception

On what should you REFLECT?
- Evaluate the effectiveness and timeliness of health care team responses, including your own.
- Determine strategies to efficiently monitor neurologic status.
- Monitor for indications of secondary brain insult as the patient is treated.
- Plan health teaching for the patient and family.
- Initiate actions to provide emotional and spiritual support for the patient and family.
- Consider whether the patient preferences and values been incorporated into care.

GET READY FOR THE NCLEX® EXAMINATION!

KEY POINTS

Review these Key Points for each NCLEX Examination Client Needs Category.

Safe and Effective Care Environment
- When caring for a patient with a stroke or traumatic brain injury (TBI), assess airway, breathing, and circulation status first and implement interventions to maintain them.
- Collaborate with the interdisciplinary team members including physicians, physical therapists, respiratory therapists, occupational therapists, social workers, and dietitians to ensured shared priorities in care. **Teamwork and Collaboration** QSEN
- Develop electronic care pathways and document patient progress using interdisciplinary patient-centered plans for care based on patient values for the patient recovering from neurologic critical illness. **Informatics** QSEN

Health Promotion and Maintenance
- Identify risk factors for new or recurrent stroke and teach patients and families about modifiable risk factors for stroke as listed in Chart 45-2. **Evidence-Based Practice** QSEN
- Prevent secondary brain injury by protecting the airway, promoting an appropriate range of blood pressure and mean arterial pressure, maintaining fluid and electrolyte balance, promptly treating fever, avoiding sustained hypoglycemia and hyperglycemia, addressing hypoxia and hypercarbia, positioning the patient appropriately, and managing intracranial hypertension with prescribed interventions.
- Teach patients and families about community organizations, such as the National Stroke Association and the Brain Injury Association of America.

Psychosocial Integrity
- Assess the emotional reactions of families to a TBI, stroke, or brain cancer diagnosis, and help them cope by providing information and including them in planning for care. **Patient-Centered Care** QSEN

Physiological Integrity
- Perform a comprehensive, rapid, or focal neurologic assessment at regular intervals to identify changes in status. **Evidence-Based Practice** QSEN
- Recall that decreased level of consciousness is the most sensitive indicator of adverse outcome or complication from stroke, TBI, brain tumor, or craniotomy.
- Recall the differences between a transient ischemic attack and a brain attack (stroke) as described in Table 45-1 and Chart 45-1.
- Monitor patients with critical neurologic health problems for manifestations of increasing intracranial pressure (ICP) as described in Chart 45-6.
- Assess the patient's ability to swallow before providing oral intake if a stroke is suspected or diagnosed. **Safety** QSEN
- Assess patients with strokes for SENSORY PERCEPTION changes such as unilateral neglect and impaired vision; help patients adapt to these changes, such as turning their head from side to side to see the entire meal tray. **Patient-Centered Care** QSEN
- Provide alternate means of communication when expressive and/or receptive aphasia is present in patients who have had a stroke or brain injury in consultation with the speech-language expert. **Teamwork and Collaboration** QSEN
- Monitor the patient on fibrinolytic therapy or anticoagulants for bleeding and abnormal coagulation studies. Best practices for fibrinolytic therapy administration are listed in Chart 45-5. **Safety** QSEN
- Teach patients with mild traumatic brain injury and their families to monitor for neurologic changes as listed in Charts 45-7 and 45-9.
- Assess for manifestations of brain tumors as listed in Chart 45-10.
- Recognize that the desired outcome for the patient with a brain tumor is to remove it if possible. Other methods may be used to decrease its size, including chemotherapy and radiation.
- Administer antibiotic therapy to provide the most effective management of patients with brain abscess.

46 CHAPTER

Assessment of the Eye and Vision

M. Linda Workman

http://evolve.elsevier.com/Iggy/

PRIORITY CONCEPTS

- Sensory Perception

LEARNING OUTCOMES

Safe and Effective Care Environment

1. Prevent injury or infection of the eye to preserve visual SENSORY PERCEPTION.

Health Promotion and Maintenance

2. Teach all people about eye health and the use of eye protection equipment and strategies.

Psychosocial Integrity

3. Reduce the psychological impact for the patient and family regarding the assessment and testing of the eyes and vision.

Physiological Integrity

4. Use knowledge of anatomy, physiology, pathophysiology, and psychomotor skills when assessing the eye and vision.
5. Perform a focused assessment of visual SENSORY PERCEPTION, incorporating information about genetic risk and age-related changes affecting the eye and vision.

The eye and the brain work together to allow visual SENSORY PERCEPTION. Many people consider vision to be the most important sensory perception. It is used to assess surroundings, allow independence, warn of danger, appreciate beauty, work, play, and interact with others.

Vision begins with the eye, where light is changed into nerve impulses. These impulses are sent to the brain, where images are fully perceived (McCance et al., 2014). Many systemic conditions, as well as eye problems, change vision temporarily or permanently. Changes in the eye and vision can provide information about the patient's general health status and problems that might occur in self-care.

ANATOMY AND PHYSIOLOGY REVIEW

Structure

The eyeball, a round, ball-shaped organ, is located in the front part of the eye orbit. The **orbit** is the bony socket of the skull that surrounds and protects the eye along with the attached muscles, nerves, vessels, and tear-producing glands.

Layers of the Eyeball

The eye has three layers (Fig. 46-1). The external layer is the **sclera** (the "white" of the eye) and the transparent cornea on the front of the eye.

The middle layer, or **uvea,** is heavily pigmented and consists of the choroid, the ciliary body, and the iris. The choroid, a dark brown membrane between the sclera and the retina, lines most of the sclera. It has many blood vessels that supply nutrients to the retina.

The ciliary body connects the choroid with the iris and secretes aqueous humor. The **iris** is the colored portion of the external eye; its center opening is the **pupil**. The muscles of the iris contract and relax to control pupil size and the amount of light entering the eye.

The innermost layer is the **retina**, a thin, delicate structure made up of sensory photoreceptors that begin the transmission of impulses to the optic nerve (McCance et al., 2014). The retina contains blood vessels and two types of photoreceptors called *rods* and *cones.* The rods work at low light levels and provide peripheral vision. The cones are active at bright light levels and provide color and central vision.

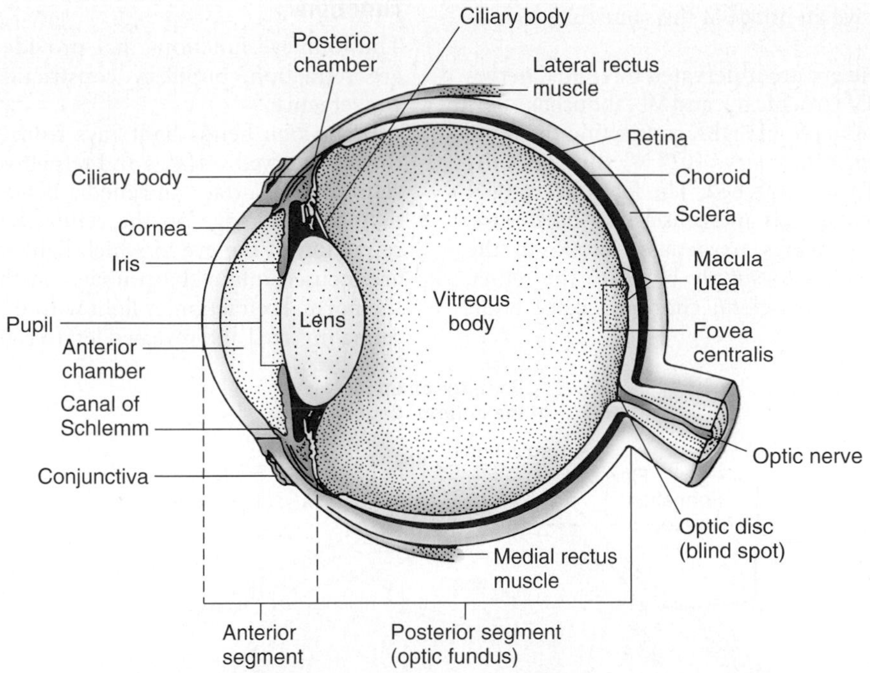

FIG. 46-1 Anatomic features of the eye.

The **optic fundus** is the area at the inside back of the eye that can be seen with an ophthalmoscope. This area contains the **optic disc**—a pink or white depressed area where the nerve fibers that synapse with the photoreceptors join together to form the optic nerve and exit the eyeball. The optic disc contains only nerve fibers and no photoreceptor cells. To one side of the optic disc is a small, yellowish pink area called the *macula lutea.* The center of the macula is the *fovea centralis,* where vision is most acute.

Refractive Structures and Media

Light waves pass through the cornea, aqueous humor, lens, and vitreous humor on the way to the retina. Each structure bends *(refracts)* the light waves to focus images on the retina. Together, these structures are the eye's *refracting media.*

The **cornea** is the clear layer that forms the external bump on the front of the eye (see Fig. 46-1). The **aqueous humor** is a clear, watery fluid that fills the anterior and posterior chambers of the eye. This fluid is continually produced by the ciliary processes and passes from the posterior chamber, through the pupil, and into the anterior chamber. This fluid drains through the canal of Schlemm into the blood to maintain a balanced intraocular pressure (IOP), the pressure within the eye (Fig. 46-2).

The **lens** is a circular, convex structure that lies behind the iris and in front of the vitreous body. It is transparent and bends the light rays entering through the pupil to focus properly on the retina. The curve of the lens changes to focus on near or distant objects. A *cataract* is a lens that has lost its transparency.

The **vitreous body** is a clear, thick gel that fills the large vitreous chamber (the space between the lens and the retina). This gel transmits light and maintains eye shape.

The eye is a hollow organ and must be kept in the shape of a ball for vision to occur. To maintain this shape, the vitreous humor gel in the posterior segment and the aqueous humor in the anterior segment must be present in set amounts that apply pressure inside the eye to keep it inflated. This pressure is the **intraocular pressure** or **IOP**. IOP has to be just right. If the pressure is too low, the eyeball is soft and collapses, preventing light from getting to the photoreceptors on the retina in the back of the eye. If the pressure becomes too high, the extra pressure compresses capillaries in the eye as well as nerve fibers. Pressure on retinal blood vessels prevents blood from flowing through them; therefore the photoreceptors and nerve fibers become hypoxic. Compression of the fine nerve fibers prevents intracellular fluid flow, which also reduces nourishment to the distal portions of these thin nerve fibers. The increased pressure and resulting hypoxia of photoreceptors and their synapsing nerve fibers is a condition called *glaucoma.* Continued hypoxia in the retina results in photoreceptor necrosis and death and permanent nerve fiber damage. When extensive photoreceptor and nerve fiber loss occur, vision is lost and the person is permanently blind.

External Structures

The eyelids are thin, movable skinfolds that protect the eyes and keep the cornea moist. The upper lid is larger than the lower one. The **canthus** is the place where the two eyelids meet at the corner of the eye.

The **conjunctivae** are the mucous membranes of the eye. The palpebral conjunctiva is a thick membrane with many blood vessels that lines the under surface of each eyelid. The thin, transparent bulbar conjunctiva covers the entire front of the eye.

Tears are produced by a small **lacrimal gland**, which is located in the upper outer part of each orbit (Fig. 46-3). Tears flow across the front of the eye, toward the nose, and into the inner canthus. They drain through the **punctum** (an opening at the nasal side of the lid edges) into the lacrimal duct and sac and then into the nose through the nasolacrimal duct.

Muscles, Nerves, and Blood Vessels

Six voluntary muscles rotate the eye and coordinate eye movements (Fig. 46-4 and Table 46-1). Coordinated eye movements ensure that both eyes receive an image at the same time so only a single image is seen.

The muscles around the eye are innervated by cranial nerves (CNs) III (oculomotor), IV (trochlear), and VI (abducens). The **optic nerve** (CN II) is the nerve of sight, connecting the optic disc to the brain. The trigeminal nerve (CN V) stimulates the blink reflex when the cornea is touched. The facial nerve (CN VII) innervates the lacrimal glands and muscles for lid closure.

The ophthalmic artery brings oxygenated blood to the eye and the orbit. It branches to supply blood to the retina. The ciliary arteries supply the sclera, choroid, ciliary body, and iris.

Function

The four eye functions that provide clear images and vision are refraction, pupillary constriction, accommodation, and convergence.

Refraction bends light rays from the outside into the eye through curved surfaces and refractive media and finally to the retina. Each surface and media bend (refract) light differently to focus an image on the retina. **Emmetropia** is the perfect refraction of the eye in which light rays from a distant source are focused into a sharp image on the retina. Fig. 46-5 shows the normal refraction of light within the eye. Images fall on the retina inverted and reversed left to right. For example, an object

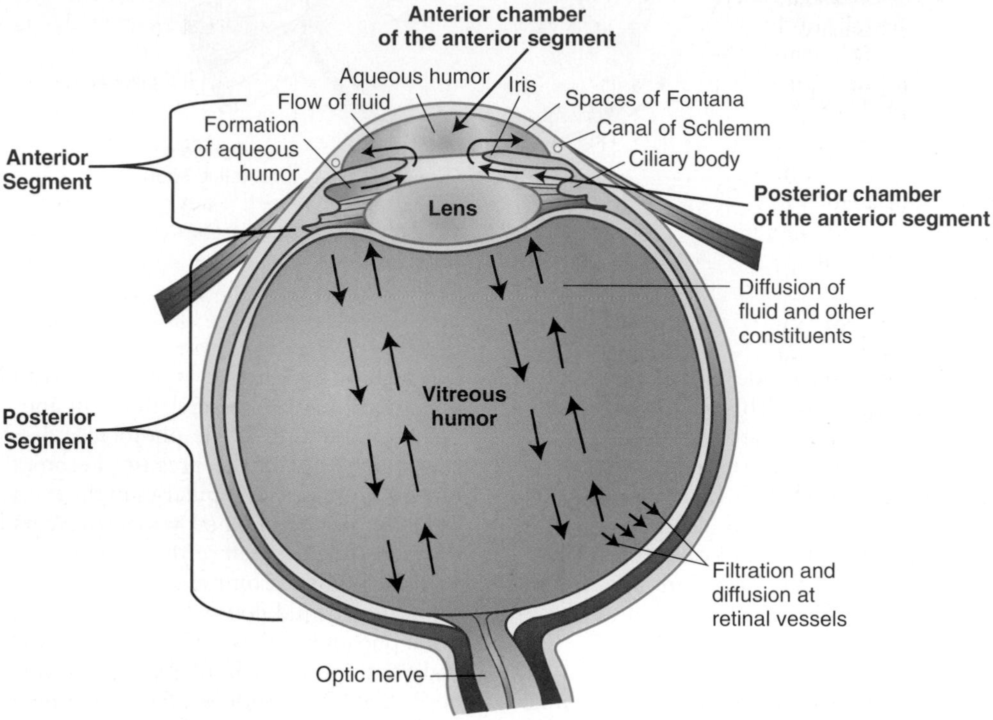

FIG. 46-2 Flow of aqueous humor.

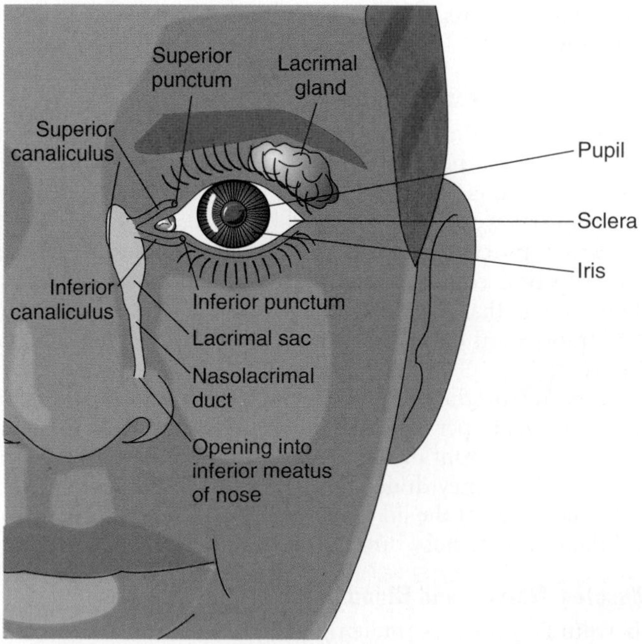

FIG. 46-3 Front view of the eye and adjacent structures.

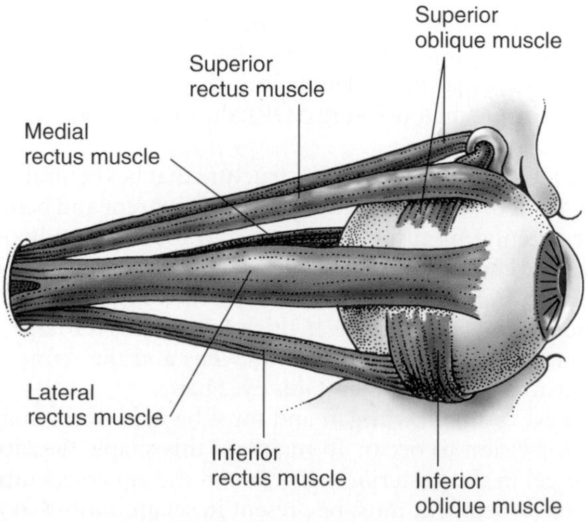

FIG. 46-4 The extraocular muscles.

in the lower nasal visual field strikes the upper outer area of the retina.

Errors of refraction are common. **Hyperopia** (farsightedness) occurs when the eye does not refract light enough. As a result, images actually converge behind the retina (see Fig. 46-5). With hyperopia, distant vision is normal but near vision is poor. It is corrected with a convex lens in eyeglasses or contact lenses.

Myopia (nearsightedness) occurs when the eye overbends the light and images converge in front of the retina (see Fig. 46-5). Near vision is normal, but distance vision is poor. Myopia is corrected with a biconcave lens in eyeglasses or contact lenses.

Astigmatism is a refractive error caused by unevenly curved surfaces on or in the eye, especially of the cornea. These uneven surfaces distort vision.

Pupillary constriction and dilation control the amount of light that enters the eye. If the level of light to one or both eyes is increased, both pupils constrict (become smaller). The amount of constriction depends on how much light is available and how well the retina can adapt to light changes. Pupillary constriction is called **miosis**, and pupillary dilation is called **mydriasis** (Fig. 46-6). Drugs can alter pupillary constriction.

TABLE 46-1 Functions of Ocular Muscles

Superior Rectus Muscle
- Together with the lateral rectus, this muscle moves the eye diagonally upward toward the side of the head.
- Together with the medial rectus, this muscle moves the eye diagonally upward toward the middle of the head.

Lateral Rectus Muscle
- Together with the medial rectus, this muscle holds the eye straight.
- Contracting alone, this muscle turns the eye toward the side of the head.

Medial Rectus Muscle
- Contracting alone, this muscle turns the eye toward the nose.

Inferior Rectus Muscle
- Together with the lateral rectus, this muscle moves the eye diagonally downward toward the side of the head.
- Together with the medial rectus, this muscle moves the eye diagonally downward toward the middle of the head.

Superior Oblique Muscle
- Contracting alone, this muscle pulls the eye downward.

Inferior Oblique Muscle
- Contracting alone, this muscle pulls the eye upward.

Accommodation allows the healthy eye to focus images sharply on the retina whether the image is close to the eye or distant. The process of maintaining a clear visual image when the gaze is shifted from a distant to a near object is known as **accommodation**. The healthy eye can adjust its focus by changing the curve of the lens.

Convergence is the ability to turn both eyes inward toward the nose at the same time. This action helps ensure that only a single image of close objects is seen.

Eye Changes Associated with Aging

Changes inside the eye cause visual acuity to decrease with age (Touhy & Jett, 2014). Age-related changes of the nervous system and in the eye support structures also reduce visual function (Chart 46-1).

Structural changes occur with aging, including decreased eye muscle tone that reduces the ability to keep the gaze focused on a single object. The lower eyelid may relax and fall away from the eye *(ectropion)*, leading to dry eye manifestations.

Arcus senilis, an opaque, bluish white ring within the outer edge of the cornea, is caused by fat deposits (see Fig. 24-4 in Chapter 24). This change does not affect vision.

The clarity and shape of the cornea change with age. The cornea flattens, and the curve of its surface becomes irregular. This change causes or worsens astigmatism and blurs vision.

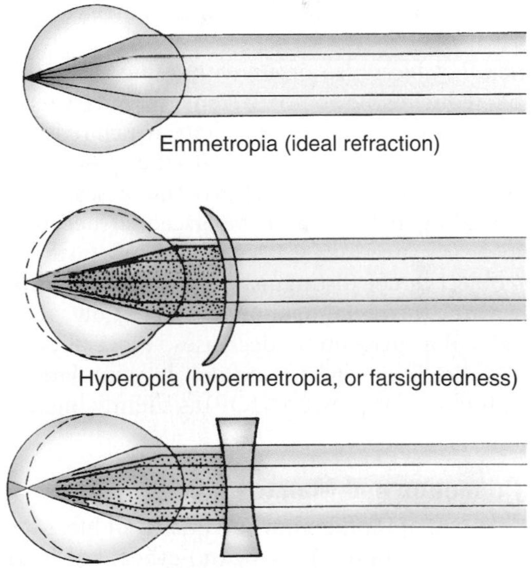

FIG. 46-5 Refraction and correction in emmetropia, hyperopia, and myopia.

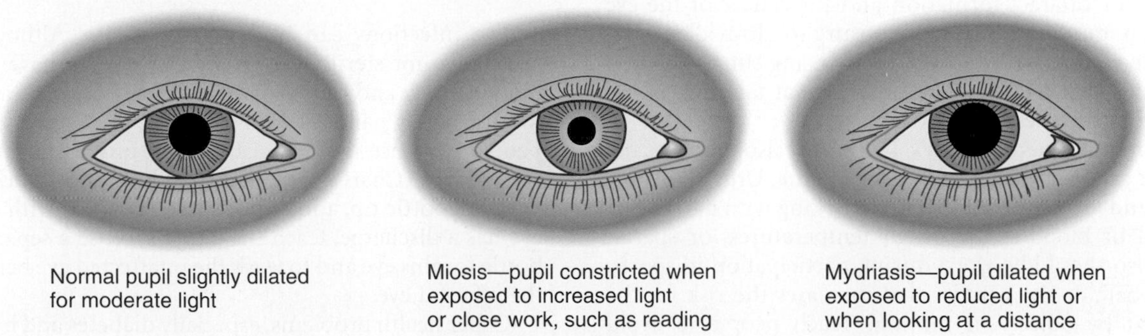

FIG. 46-6 Miosis and mydriasis.

CHART 46-1 Nursing Focus on the Older Adult

Changes in the Eye and Vision Related to Aging

STRUCTURE/ FUNCTION	CHANGE	IMPLICATION
Appearance	Eyes appear "sunken."	Do not use eye appearance as an indicator for hydration status.
	Arcus senilis forms.	Reassure patient that this change does not affect vision.
	Sclera yellows or appears blue.	Do not use sclera to assess for jaundice.
Cornea	Cornea flattens, which blurs vision.	Encourage older adults to have regular eye examinations and wear prescribed corrective lenses for best vision.
Ocular muscles	Muscle strength is reduced, making it more difficult to maintain an upward gaze or maintain a single image.	Reassure patient that this is a normal happening and to re-focus gaze frequently to maintain a single image.
Lens	Elasticity is lost, increasing the near point of vision (making the near point of best vision farther away).	Encourage patient to wear corrective lenses for reading.
	Lens hardens, compacts, and forms a cataract.	Stress the importance of yearly vision checks and monitoring.
Iris and Pupil	Decrease in ability to dilate results in small pupil size and poor adaptation to darkness.	Teach about the need for good lighting to avoid tripping and bumping into objects.
Color vision	Discrimination among greens, blues, and violets decreases.	The patient may not be able to use color-indicator monitors of health status.
Tears	Tear production is reduced, resulting in dry eyes, discomfort, and increased risk for corneal damage or eye infections.	Teach about the use of saline eyedrops to reduce dryness. Teach patient to increase humidity in the home.

Fatty deposits cause the sclera to develop a yellowish tinge. A bluish color may be seen as the sclera thins. With age, the iris has less ability to dilate, which leads to difficulty in adapting to dark environments. Older adults may need additional light for reading and other "close up" work and to avoid tripping over objects.

Functional changes also occur with aging. The lens yellows with aging, reducing the ability to transmit and focus light. The lens hardens, shrinks, and loses elasticity, which reduces accommodation. The **near point of vision** (the closest distance at which the eye can see an object clearly) increases. Near objects, especially reading material, must be placed farther from the eye to be seen clearly (**presbyopia**). The **far point** (farthest point at which an object can be distinguished) decreases. Together these changes narrow the visual field of an older adult.

General color perception decreases, especially for green, blue, and violet. More light is needed to stimulate the visual receptors. Intraocular pressure (IOP) is slightly higher in older adults.

Health Promotion and Maintenance

Vision is important for function and quality of life. Many vision and eye problems can be avoided, and others can be corrected or managed if discovered early. Teach all people about eye protection methods, adequate nutrition, and the importance of regular eye examinations.

The risks for cataract formation and for cancer of the eye (ocular melanoma) increase with exposure to ultraviolet (UV) light. Teach people to protect the eyes by using sunglasses that filter UV light whenever they are outdoors, at tanning salons, and when work involves UV exposure.

Vision can be affected by injury. Eye injury also increases the risk for both cataract formation and glaucoma. Urge all people to wear eye and head protection when working with particulate matter, fluid or blood spatter, high temperatures, or sparks. Protection also should be worn during participation in sports, such as baseball, or any activity that increases the risk for the eye being hit by objects in motion. Teach people to avoid rubbing the eyes to avoid trauma to outer eye surfaces.

CHART 46-2 Patient and Family Education: Preparing for Self-Management

Using Eyedrops

- Check the eyedrop name, strength, expiration date, color, and clarity.
- If both eyes are to receive the same drug and one eye is infected, use two separate bottles and label each bottle with "right" or "left" for the correct eye.
- Wash your hands.
- Remove the cap from the bottle.
- Tilt your head backward, open your eyes, and look up at the ceiling.
- Using your nondominant hand, gently pull the lower lid down against your cheek, forming a small pocket.
- Hold the eyedrop bottle (with the cap off) like a pencil, with the tip pointing down, with your dominant hand.
- Rest the wrist holding the bottle against your mouth or upper lip.
- Without touching any part of the eye or lid with the tip of the bottle, gently squeeze the bottle and release the prescribed number of drops into the pocket of your lower lid.
- Release the lower lid and gently close your eye without squeezing the lids.
- Gently press and hold the corner of the eye nearest the nose to close off the punctum and prevent the drug from being absorbed systemically.
- Gently blot away any excess drug or tears with a tissue.
- Keep the eye closed for about 1 minute.
- Place the cap back on the bottle, and store it as prescribed.
- Wash your hands again.

Eye infections can lead to vision loss. Although the eye surface is not sterile, the sclera and cornea have no separate blood supply and thus are at risk for infection. Teach everyone to wash their hands before touching the eye or eyelid. Teach people who use eyedrops about the proper technique to use these drugs (Chart 46-2), which includes not touching the eye with the bottle tip, and to not share eyedrops with others. If an eye has a discharge, teach the patient to use a separate eyedrop bottle for this eye and to wash the unaffected eye before washing the affected eye.

Other health problems, especially diabetes and hypertension, can seriously affect visual SENSORY PERCEPTION. Teach patients with these health problems about the importance of controlling blood glucose levels and managing blood pressure to reduce the risk for vision loss. Yearly evaluation by an ophthalmologist is needed to slow or prevent eye complications.

Teach all people who have a refractive error to have an eye examination yearly. Young adults without vision problems may need an eye examination only every 3 to 5 years. Adults older than 40 years should have an eye examination yearly that includes assessment of intraocular pressure and visual fields, because the risk for both glaucoma and cataract formation increases with age.

! NURSING SAFETY PRIORITY QSEN

Action Alert

Teach people to see a health care provider *immediately* when an eye injury occurs or an eye infection is suspected.

? NCLEX EXAMINATION CHALLENGE

Health Promotion and Maintenance

For which client does the nurse recommend annual evaluation by an ophthalmologist?

A. 35-year-old man with asthma
B. 21-year-old man with psoriasis
C. 24-year-old woman with diabetes
D. 38-year-old woman who has lost 50 pounds

ASSESSMENT METHODS

Patient History

Collect information to determine whether problems with the eye or vision have an impact on ADLs or other daily functions. *Age* is an important factor to consider when assessing visual SENSORY PERCEPTION and eye structure. The incidence of glaucoma and cataract formation increases with aging. Presbyopia commonly begins in the 40s.

Gender may be important. Retinal detachments occur more often in men, and dry eye syndromes occur more often in women.

Occupation and leisure activities can affect visual SENSORY PERCEPTION. Ask about how the eye is used at work. In occupations such as computer programming, constant exposure to monitors may lead to eyestrain. Machine operators are at risk for eye injury because of the high speeds at which particles can be thrown at the eye. Chronic exposure to infrared or ultraviolet light may cause photophobia and cataract formation. Teach the patient about the use of eye protection during work.

Ask whether the patient wears eye protection when participating in sports. A blow to the head near the eye, such as with a baseball, can damage external structures, the eye, the connections with the brain, or the area of the brain where vision is perceived.

Systemic health problems can affect vision. Check whether the patient has any condition listed in Table 46-2. Ask about past accidents, injuries, surgeries, or blows to the head that may have led to the present problem. Specifically ask about previous laser surgeries.

Drugs can affect vision and the eye (see Table 46-2). Ask about the use of any prescription or over-the-counter drugs, especially decongestants and antihistamines, which tend to dry the eye and may increase intraocular pressure. Document the name, strength, dose, and scheduling for all drugs the patient uses. Ocular effects from drugs include itching, foreign body sensation, redness, tearing, **photophobia** (sensitivity to light), and the development of cataracts or glaucoma.

TABLE 46-2 Systemic Conditions and Common Drugs Affecting the Eye and Vision

SYSTEMIC CONDITIONS AND DISORDERS	DRUGS
Diabetes mellitus	Antihistamines
Hypertension	Decongestants
Lupus erythematosus	Antibiotics
Sarcoidosis	Opioids
Thyroid problems	Anticholinergics
Acquired immune deficiency syndrome	Cholinergic agonists
Cardiac disease	Adrenergic agonists
Multiple sclerosis	Adrenergic antagonists (beta blockers)
Pregnancy	Oral contraceptives
	Chemotherapy agents
	Corticosteroids

Nutrition History

Some eye problems are caused by or made worse with vitamin deficiencies. Ask the patient about food choices. For example, vitamin A deficiency can cause eye dryness, keratomalacia, and blindness. Some nutrients and antioxidants, such as lutein and beta carotene, help maintain retinal function. A diet rich in fruit and red, orange, and dark green vegetables is important to eye health. Teach all people to eat about 10 servings of these foods daily.

Family History and Genetic Risk

Ask about a family history of eye problems because some conditions have a familial tendency and some genetic problems lead to visual impairment. When a patient tells you that other relatives, especially first-degree relatives (parents, siblings, and children), have eye problems, document the gender of the affected person, the relationship to the patient, the exact nature of the problem, and the age that the problem was first noted.

Current Health Problems

Ask the patient about the onset of visual changes. Did the change occur rapidly or slowly? Determine whether the manifestations are present to the same degree in both eyes. Ask these questions if eye injury or trauma is involved:

- How long ago did the injury occur?
- What was the patient doing when it happened?
- If a foreign body was involved, what was its source?
- Was any first aid administered at the scene? If so, what actions were taken?

! NURSING SAFETY PRIORITY QSEN

Critical Rescue

Notify the ophthalmologist immediately for any patient who has a sudden or persistent loss of visual SENSORY PERCEPTION within the past 48 hours, eye trauma, a foreign body in the eye, or sudden ocular pain.

Physical Assessment

Inspection

Look for head tilting, squinting, or other actions that indicate the patient is trying to attain clear vision. For example, patients with double vision may cock the head to the side to focus the two images into one or they may close one eye to see clearly.

Assess for symmetry in the appearance of the eyes. Check the eyes to determine whether they are equal distance from the nose, are the same size, and have the same degree of prominence. Assess the eyes for their placement in the orbits and for symmetry of movement. **Exophthalmos** (*proptosis*) is protrusion of the eye. **Enophthalmos** is the sunken appearance of the eye.

Examine the eyebrows and eyelashes for hair distribution, and determine the direction of the eyelashes. Eyelashes normally point outward and away from the eyelid. Assess the eyelids for **ptosis** (drooping), redness, lesions, or swelling. The lids normally close completely, with the lid edges touching. When the eyes are open, the upper lid covers a small portion of the iris. The edge of the lower lid lies at the iris. No sclera should be visible between the eyelid and the iris.

Scleral and corneal assessment require a penlight. Examine the sclera for color; it is usually white. A yellow color may indicate jaundice or systemic problems. In dark-skinned people, the normal sclera may appear yellow and small, pigmented dots may be visible (Jarvis, 2016).

The cornea is best seen by directing a light at it from the side. The cornea should be transparent, smooth, shiny, and bright. Any cloudy areas or specks may indicate injury.

Assess the blink reflex by bringing a fist quickly toward the patient's face. Patients with vision will blink.

Pupillary assessment involves examining each pupil separately and comparing the results. The pupils are usually round and of equal size. About 5% of people normally have a noticeable difference in the size of their pupils, which is known as **anisocoria** (Jarvis, 2016). Pupil size varies in people exposed to the same amount of light. Pupils are smaller in older adults. People with myopia have larger pupils. People with hyperopia have smaller pupils. The normal pupil diameter is between 3 and 5 mm. Smaller pupils reduce vision in low light conditions.

Observe pupils for response to light. Increasing light causes constriction, whereas decreasing light causes dilation. Constriction of both pupils is the normal response to direct light and to accommodation. Assess pupillary reaction to light by asking the patient to look straight ahead while you quickly bring the beam of a penlight in from the side and direct it at the right pupil. Constriction of the right pupil is a direct response to shining the penlight into that eye. Constriction of the left pupil when light is shined at the right pupil is known as a **consensual response**. Assess the responses for each eye. (You may see the abbreviation "PERRLA" in a patient's medical record, which stands for pupils equal, round, reactive to light, and accommodative.)

Evaluate each pupil for speed of reaction. The pupil should immediately constrict when a light is directed at it—a *brisk* response. If the pupil takes more than 1 second to constrict, the response is *sluggish*. Pupils that fail to react are *nonreactive* or *fixed*. Compare the reactivity speed of right and left pupils, and document any difference.

Assess for accommodation by holding your finger about 18 cm from the patient's nose and move it toward the nose. The patient's eyes normally converge during this movement, and the pupils constrict equally.

Vision Testing

Visual SENSORY PERCEPTION is measured by first testing each eye separately and then testing both eyes together. Patients who wear corrective lenses are tested both without and with their lenses.

Visual acuity tests measure both distance and near vision. The Snellen eye chart measures distance vision. This chart has letters, numbers, pictures, or a single letter presented in various positions. The chart with one letter in different positions is used for patients who cannot read, who do not speak the language used at the facility, or who cannot speak but do have adequate cognition. Have the patient stand or sit 20 feet from the chart, cover one eye, and use the other eye to read the line that appears most clear. If the patient can do this accurately, ask him or her to read the next lower line. Repeat this sequence to the last line on which the patient can correctly identify most characters. Repeat the procedure with the other eye. Record findings as a comparison between what the patient can read at 20 feet and the distance that a person with normal vision can read the same line. For example, *20/50* means that the patient sees at 20 feet from the chart what a healthy eye sees at 50 feet.

For patients who cannot see the 20/400 character, assess visual acuity by holding fingers in front of their eyes and asking them to count the number of fingers. Acuity is recorded as "count fingers vision at 5 feet," or the farthest distance at which fingers are counted correctly.

Patients who cannot count fingers are tested for hand motion (HM) acuity. Stand about 2 to 3 feet in front of the patient. Ask him or her to cover the eye not being tested. Direct a light onto your hand from behind the patient. Demonstrate the three possible directions in which the hand can move during the test (stationary, left-right, or up-down). Move your hand slowly (1 second per motion), and ask the patient, "What is my hand doing now?" Repeat this procedure 5 times. Visual acuity is recorded as HM at the farthest distance at which most of the hand motions are identified correctly.

If the patient cannot detect hand motion, assess light perception (LP). Ask the patient first to cover the left eye. In a darkened room, direct the beam of a penlight at the patient's right eye from a distance of 2 to 3 feet for 1 to 2 seconds. Instruct the patient to say "on" when the beam of light is perceived and "off" when it is no longer detected. If the patient identifies the presence or absence of light 3 times correctly, acuity is documented as LP.

Near vision is tested for patients who have difficulty reading without using glasses or other means of vision correction. Use a small, handheld miniature eye chart called a *Rosenbaum Pocket Vision Screener* or a *Jaeger card.* Ask the patient to hold the card 14 inches away from his or her eyes and read the characters. Test each eye separately and then together. Document the lowest line on which the patient can identify more than half the characters.

Visual field testing determines the degree of peripheral vision. It can be performed with a computerized machine or with a "confrontation test" for a rapid check of peripheral vision. Perimetry is a computerized test. During this test, the patient is asked to look straight ahead into a viewer and then indicate, by pressing a control button, when a moving light enters the peripheral vision. This process maps the person's peripheral vision and any deficits.

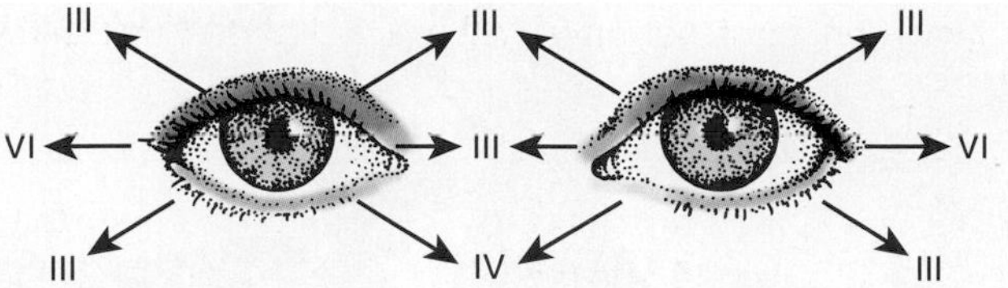

FIG. 46-7 Checking extraocular movements in the six cardinal positions indicates the functioning of cranial nerves III, IV, and VI.

During the confrontation test, sit facing the patient and ask him or her to look directly into your eyes while you look into the patient's eyes. Cover your right eye and have the patient cover his or her left eye so that you both have the same visual field. Then move a finger or an object from a nonvisible area into the patient's line of vision. The patient with normal peripheral vision notices the object at about the same time you do. Repeat this examination by covering your left eye and the patient covering his or her right eye. Document any areas in which you can see but the patient cannot.

Extraocular muscle function is assessed using the corneal light reflex and the six cardinal positions of gaze. These tests assess smoothness of eye movements and the function of cranial nerves III, IV, and VI.

The corneal light reflex determines alignment of the eyes. After asking the patient to stare straight ahead, shine a penlight at both corneas from a distance of 12 to 15 inches. The bright dot of light reflected from the shiny surface of the cornea should be in a symmetric position (e.g., at the 1 o'clock position in the right eye and at the 11 o'clock position in the left eye). An asymmetric reflex indicates a deviating eye and possible muscle weakness.

Use the six cardinal positions of gaze to assess muscle function (Fig. 46-7). The eye will not turn to a particular position if the muscle is weak or if the controlling nerve is affected. Ask the patient to hold his or her head still and to move only the eyes to follow a small object. Move the object to the patient's right (lateral), upward and right (temporal), down and right, left (lateral), upward and left (temporal), and down and left (see Fig. 46-7). While the patient moves the eyes to these positions, note whether both eyes move in a parallel manner and any deviation of movement. Nystagmus, an involuntary and rapid twitching of the eyeball, is a normal finding for the far lateral gaze. It may also be caused by abnormal nerve function or problems with the inner ear.

Color vision is usually tested using the *Ishihara chart,* which shows numbers composed of dots of one color within a circle of dots of a different color (Fig. 46-8). Test each eye separately by asking the patient what numbers he or she sees on the chart. Reading the numbers correctly indicates normal color vision.

Psychosocial Assessment

A patient with changes in visual SENSORY PERCEPTION may be anxious about possible vision loss. Patients with severe visual defects may be unable to perform ADLs. Dependency from reduced vision can affect self-esteem. Ask the patient how he or she feels about the vision changes, and assess coping techniques. Assess the family to determine available support. Provide information about local resources and services for reduced vision.

Diagnostic Assessment

Laboratory Assessment

Cultures of corneal or conjunctival swabs and scrapings help diagnose infections. Obtain a sample of the exudate for culture before antibiotics or topical anesthetics are instilled. Take swabs from the conjunctivae and any ulcerated or inflamed areas.

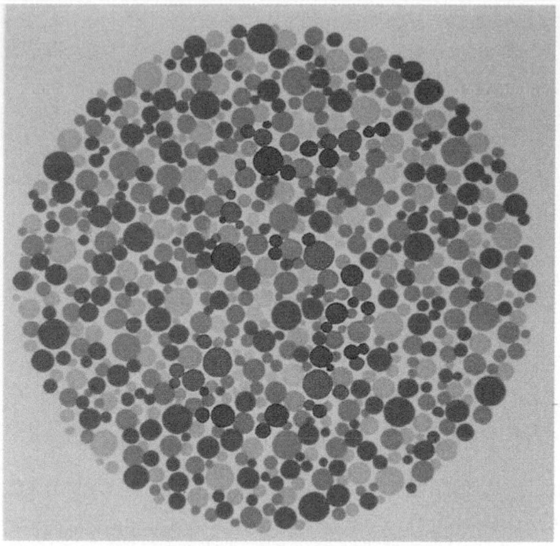

FIG. 46-8 An Ishihara chart for testing color vision.

Imaging Assessment

CT is useful for assessing the eyes, the bony structures around the eyes, and the extraocular muscles. It can also detect tumors in the orbital space. Contrast dye is used unless trauma is suspected. Tell the patient that this test is not painful but does require being in a confined space and keeping the head still.

MRI is often used to examine the orbits and the optic nerves and to evaluate ocular tumors. MRI cannot be used to evaluate injuries involving metal in the eyes. *Metal in the eye is an absolute contraindication for MRI.*

Radioisotope scanning is used to locate tumors and lesions. This test requires that the patient sign an informed consent. The patient receives a tracer dose of the radioactive isotope, either orally or by injection, and must then lie still. The scanner measures the radioactivity emitted by the radioactive atoms concentrated in the area being studied. Sedation may be used for patients who are anxious. No special follow-up care is required.

Ultrasonography is used to examine the orbit and eye with high-frequency sound waves. This noninvasive test helps diagnose trauma, intraorbital tumors, proptosis, and choroidal or retinal detachments. It is also used to determine the length of the eye and any gross outline changes in the eye and the orbit in patients with cloudy corneas or lenses that reduce direct examination of the fundus.

Inform the patient that this test is painless because the test is performed either with the eyes closed or, when the eyes must remain open, anesthetic eyedrops are instilled first. He or she sits upright with the chin in the chin rest. The probe is touched against the patient's anesthetized cornea, and sound waves are bounced through the eye. The sound waves create a reflective pattern on a computer screen that can be examined for abnormalities. No special follow-up care is needed. Remind the patient not to rub or touch the eye until the anesthetic agent has worn off.

Other Diagnostic Assessment

Many tests are used to examine specific eye structures when patients have specific risks, manifestations, or exposures. These

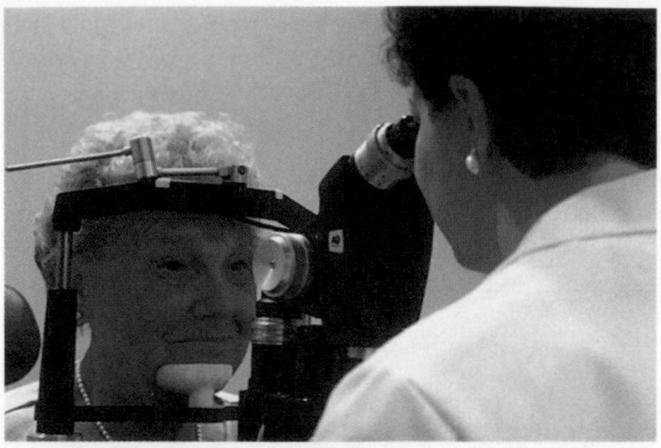

FIG. 46-9 Slit-lamp ocular examination.

tests are performed only by physicians, optometrists, or advanced practice nurses.

Slit-lamp examination magnifies the anterior eye structures (Fig. 46-9). The patient leans on a chin rest to stabilize the head. A narrow beam (slit) of light is aimed so that only a segment of the eye is brightly lighted. The examiner can then locate the position of any abnormality in the cornea, lens, or anterior vitreous humor.

Corneal staining consists of placing fluorescein or other topical dye into the conjunctival sac. The dye outlines irregularities of the corneal surface that are not easily visible. This test is used for corneal trauma, problems caused by a contact lens, or the presence of foreign bodies, abrasions, ulcers, or other corneal disorders.

This procedure is noninvasive and is performed under aseptic conditions. The dye is applied topically to the eye, and the eye is then viewed through a blue filter. Nonintact areas of the cornea stain a bright green color.

Tonometry measures intraocular pressure (IOP) using a tonometer. This instrument applies pressure to the outside of the eye until it equals the pressure inside the eye. Normal IOP readings have always been considered to range from 10 to 21 mm Hg; however, this number is not absolute and must be considered along with corneal thickness. The thickness of the cornea affects how much pressure must be applied before indentation occurs. For example, a person with a thicker cornea will have a higher tonometer reading that may falsely indicate increased IOP. A person with a thinner-than-normal cornea may have a low tonometer reading even when higher IOP is present.

About 5% of patients with healthy eyes have a slightly higher pressure. Tonometer readings are indicated for all patients older than 40 years. Adults with a family history of glaucoma should have their IOP measured once or twice a year. The most common method to measure IOP by an ophthalmologist is the Goldman's applanation tonometer used with a slit lamp (Fig. 46-10). This method involves direct eye contact. Another instrument, the Tono-Pen (Fig. 46-11), is designed for use by patients in the home to measure IOP daily.

Intraocular pressure varies throughout the day and may peak at any time of the day. Therefore always document the time of IOP measurement, and teach patients who are measuring IOP at home to perform the measurement at the same time or times each day.

Ophthalmoscopy allows viewing of the eye's external and interior structures with an instrument called an *ophthalmoscope.* This examination can be performed by any nurse but usually is performed by a physician, advanced practice nurse, or physician assistant. It is easiest to examine the fundus when the room is dark, because the pupil dilates. Stand on the same side as the eye being examined. Tell the patient to look straight ahead at an object on the wall behind you. Hold the ophthalmoscope firmly against your face, and align it so that your eye sees through the sight hole (Fig. 46-12).

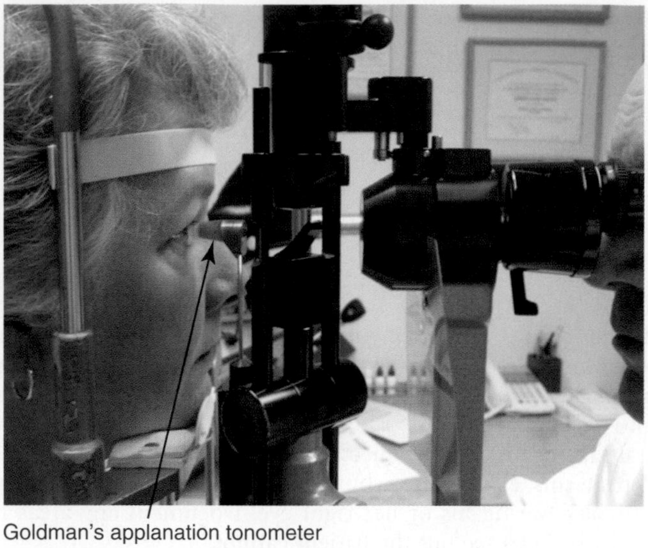

FIG. 46-10 Use of Goldman's applanation tonometer and a slit lamp to measure intraocular pressure (IOP).

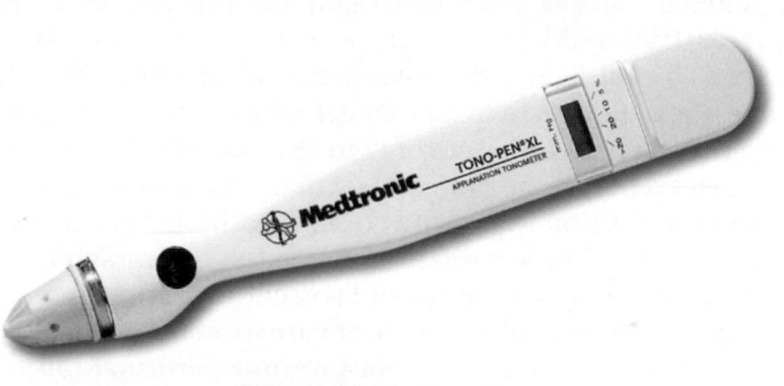

FIG. 46-11 The Tono-Pen.

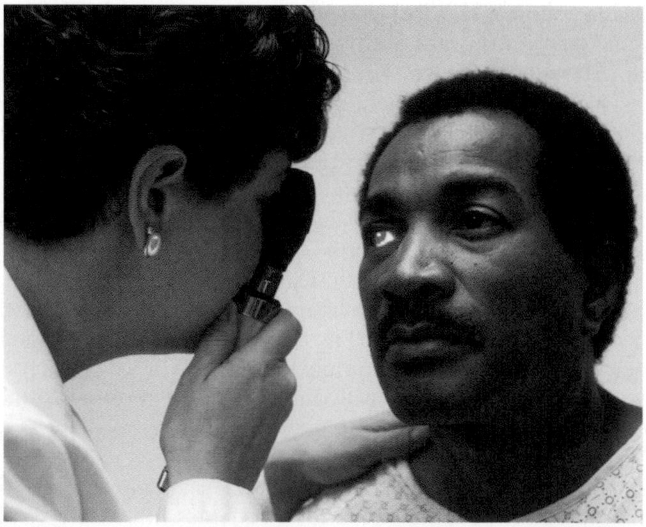

FIG. 46-12 Proper technique for direct ophthalmoscopic visualization of the retina.

TABLE 46-3 Structures Assessed By Direct Ophthalmoscopy

Red Reflex
- Presence or absence

Optic Disc
- Color
- Margins (sharp or blurred)
- Cup size
- Presence of rings or crescents

Optic Blood Vessels
- Size
- Color
- Kinks or tangles
- Light reflection
- Narrowing
- Nicking at arteriovenous crossings

Fundus
- Color
- Tears or holes
- Lesions
- Bleeding

Macula
- Presence of blood vessels
- Color
- Lesions
- Bleeding

When using the ophthalmoscope, move toward the patient's eye from about 12 to 15 inches away and to the side of his or her line of vision. As you direct the ophthalmoscope at the pupil, a red glare (**red reflex**) should be seen in the pupil as a reflection of the light on the retina. An absent red reflex may indicate a lens opacity or cloudiness of the vitreous. Move toward the patient's pupil while following the red reflex. The retina should then be visible through the ophthalmoscope. Examine the optic disc, optic vessels, fundus, and macula. Table 46-3 lists the features that can be observed in each structure.

The use of an ophthalmoscope may make a confused patient or one who does not understand the language more anxious. When working with a patient who does not speak the language used at the facility, use an interpreter, when possible, to ensure the patient's understanding and cooperation with the examination.

! NURSING SAFETY PRIORITY QSEN

Action Alert

Avoid using an ophthalmoscope with a confused patient.

Fluorescein angiography, which is performed by a physician or advanced practice nurse, provides a detailed image of eye circulation. Digital pictures are taken in rapid succession after the dye is given IV. This test helps assess problems of retinal circulation (e.g., diabetic retinopathy, retinal hemorrhage, and macular degeneration) or diagnose intraocular tumors.

Explain the procedure to the patient, and instill mydriatic eyedrops (cause pupil dilation) 1 hour before the test. Chart 46-3 lists the best practice for correct eyedrop instillation. Check that the informed consent has been signed by the patient. Warn that the dye may cause the skin to appear yellow for several hours after the test. The stain is eliminated through the urine, which turns green.

Encourage patients to drink fluids to help eliminate the dye. Remind them that any staining of the skin will disappear in a few hours. Instruct the patient to wear dark glasses and avoid direct sunlight until pupil dilation returns to normal, because the bright light will cause eye pain.

CHART 46-3 Best Practice for Patient Safety & Quality Care QSEN

Instillation of Eyedrops

- Check the name, strength, expiration date, color, and clarity of the eyedrops to be instilled.
- Check to see whether only one eye is to have the drug or if both eyes are to receive the drug.
- If both eyes are to receive the same drug and one eye is infected, use two separate bottles and carefully label each bottle with "right" or "left" for the correct eye.
- Wash your hands.
- Put on gloves if secretions are present in or around the eye.
- Explain the procedure to the patient.
- Have the patient sit in a chair, and you stand behind the patient.
- Ask the patient to tilt the head backward, with the back of the head resting against your body and looking up at the ceiling.
- Gently pull the lower lid down against the patient's cheek, forming a small pocket.
- Hold the eyedrop bottle (with the cap off) like a pencil, with the tip pointing down.
- Rest the wrist holding the bottle against the patient's check.
- Without touching any part of the eye or lid with the tip of the bottle, gently squeeze the bottle and release the prescribed number of drops into the pocket you have made with the patient's lower lid.
- Gently release the lower lid.
- Tell the patient to close the eye gently (without squeezing the lids tightly).
- Gently press and hold the corner of the eye nearest the nose to close off the punctum and prevent the drug from being absorbed systemically.
- Without pressing on the lid, gently blot away any excess drug or tears with a tissue.
- Remove your gloves, and place the cap back on the bottle.
- Ask the patient to keep the eye closed for about 1 minute.
- Wash your hands again.

Electroretinography graphs the retina's response to light stimulation. This test is helpful in detecting and evaluating blood vessel changes from disease or drugs. The graph is obtained by placing an electrode on an anesthetized cornea. Lights at varying speeds and intensities are flashed, and the neural response is graphed. The measurement from the cornea is identical to the response that would be obtained if electrodes were placed directly on the retina.

Gonioscopy is a test performed when a high IOP is found and determines whether open-angle or closed-angle glaucoma is present. It uses a special lens that eliminates the corneal curve, is painless, and allows visualization of the angle where the iris meets the cornea.

Laser imaging of the retina and optic nerve creates a three-dimensional view of the back of the eye. It is often used for those people with ocular hypertension or who are at risk for glaucoma from other problems. This computerized examination assesses the thickness and contours of the optic nerve and retina for changes that indicate damage as a result of high IOP. It can be used serially for a person at risk for glaucoma to detect early changes and indicate when intervention is needed.

CLINICAL JUDGMENT CHALLENGE

Patient-Centered Care; Safety QSEN

The patient is a 56-year-old woman whose primary care provider has referred her to an ophthalmologist because she is having manifestations of glaucoma. She has never been evaluated by an ophthalmologist, even though she has used reading glasses for about 10 years. She seems very anxious and tells you that she cannot stand to have her eyes touched directly. She also tells you that her mother developed an eye infection and lost the vision in that eye after she had her intraocular pressure tested by an instrument with small feet that scratched her eye.

1. Will this patient's eyes be "touched" during a typical assessment of intraocular pressure?
2. What will you tell her about this procedure?
3. What assurance can you give her that she will not develop an infection from this evaluation?
4. Should you relay this patient's concerns to the ophthalmologist? Why or why not?

NURSING CONCEPTS AND CLINICAL JUDGMENT REVIEW

What might you NOTICE in a patient with adequate visual SENSORY PERCEPTION?

Physical assessment:

- Eyes are symmetric on the face on a line just about even with the tops of the ears.
- Eyes are clear with no drainage or open areas.
- Patient does not squint or tilt the head.
- Patient does not close one eye to read or see at a distance.
- Patient startles when a sudden move is made at the face.
- Patient blinks 5 to 10 times per minute.
- Pupils are the same size in each eye.
- Both pupils constrict when a light is shined at only one eye.
- Patient comments on the presence of art or unusual visual objects in the immediate environment.
- Patient walks without hesitation into a room without bumping into objects in his or her path.

Psychological assessment:

- Patient is oriented and not confused.
- Patient makes eye contact when speaking.

GET READY FOR THE NCLEX® EXAMINATION!

KEY POINTS

Review these Key Points for each NCLEX Examination Client Needs Category.

Safe and Effective Care Environment

- Wash your hands before moving a patient's eyelids or instilling drugs into the eye. **Safety** QSEN
- If a patient has discharge from one eye, examine the eye without the discharge first. **Safety** QSEN
- Wear gloves when examining an eye with drainage. **Safety** QSEN
- Avoid using an ophthalmoscope on a confused patient. **Safety** QSEN

Health Promotion and Maintenance

- Teach patients not to rub their eyes. **Patient-Centered Care** QSEN
- Identify patients at risk for eye injury as a result of work environment or leisure activities. **Patient-Centered Care** QSEN
- Urge all patients to wear eye protection when they are performing yard work, working in a woodshop or metal shop, using chemicals, or are in any environment in which drops or particulate matter is airborne. **Safety** QSEN
- Teach everyone to wear sunglasses outdoors in bright sunlight. **Patient-Centered Care** QSEN

Psychosocial Integrity

- Provide opportunities for the patient and family to express their concerns about a possible change in visual SENSORY PERCEPTION. **Patient-Centered Care** QSEN
- Explain all diagnostic procedures, restrictions, and follow-up care to the patient scheduled for tests. **Patient-Centered Care** QSEN

Physiological Integrity

- Ask the patient about vision problems in any other members of the family, because some vision problems have a genetic component. **Patient-Centered Care** QSEN
- Test the vision of both eyes immediately of any person who experiences an eye injury or any sudden change in vision. **Patient-Centered Care** QSEN

CHAPTER 47

Care of Patients with Eye and Vision Problems

M. Linda Workman

http://evolve.elsevier.com/Iggy/

PRIORITY CONCEPTS

- SENSORY PERCEPTION
- INFECTION

LEARNING OUTCOMES

Safe and Effective Care Environment

1. Protect the patient with eye and vision problems from injury or INFECTION.
2. Ensure that all members of the health care team are aware of a patient's visual limitations and need for assistance.

Health Promotion and Maintenance

3. Teach people when annual eye examinations with measurement of intraocular pressure are important to receive.
4. Teach patients and family members how to correctly instill ophthalmic drops and ointment into the eye.
5. Teach patients with glaucoma the relationship between increased intraocular pressure (IOP) and their eye problems.
6. Teach the patient with reduced visual SENSORY PERCEPTION and family how to alter the home environment for patient safety.

Psychosocial Integrity

7. Reduce the psychological impact for the patient and family experiencing a potential change in visual SENSORY PERCEPTION.
8. Work with other members of the health care team to ensure that the values, preferences, and expressed needs of patients with reduced visual SENSORY PERCEPTION are respected.

Physiological Integrity

9. Prioritize care and educational needs for the patient after cataract surgery with lens replacement.
10. Prioritize care and educational needs for patients with primary open-angle glaucoma.
11. Collaborate with other health care professionals to help patients and families experiencing reduced visual sensory perception achieve their desired health outcomes.
12. Coordinate interventions for the patient with reduced visual SENSORY PERCEPTION in the community.

Many factors and problems can affect visual SENSORY PERCEPTION. Problems may have a gradual onset, such as the most common form of glaucoma or cataracts, whereas others may have a sudden onset. Any temporary or permanent change in visual sensory perception requires the patient to make some changes in function or lifestyle.

EYELID DISORDERS

The eyelid is composed of skin and small muscles to protect the eye surface and spread tears. Vision is affected by problems that change the structure, function, or position of the eyelid.

Entropion and Ectropion

An **entropion** is the turning inward of the eyelid causing the lashes to rub against the eye. It can be caused by eyelid muscle spasms or by scarring and deformity of the eyelid after trauma and is seen more often among older adults because of age-related loss of tissue support.

The patient reports "feeling something in my eye." Pain and tears may also be present. The conjunctiva is red, and corneal abrasion may result from constant irritation.

Surgery corrects eyelid position by either tightening the orbicular muscles and moving the eyelid to a normal position or by preventing inward rotation of the eyelid. After surgery, the eye is covered with a patch and the patient is discharged.

Demonstrate instillation of eyedrops, and evaluate the patient's ability to instill the drops. Teach the patient how to clean the suture line with a cotton swab and the prescribed solution. A small amount of antibiotic ointment may be applied (Fig. 47-1). Chart 47-1 describes how to apply ophthalmic ointment. Chart 47-2 lists common drugs for eye inflammation and INFECTION.

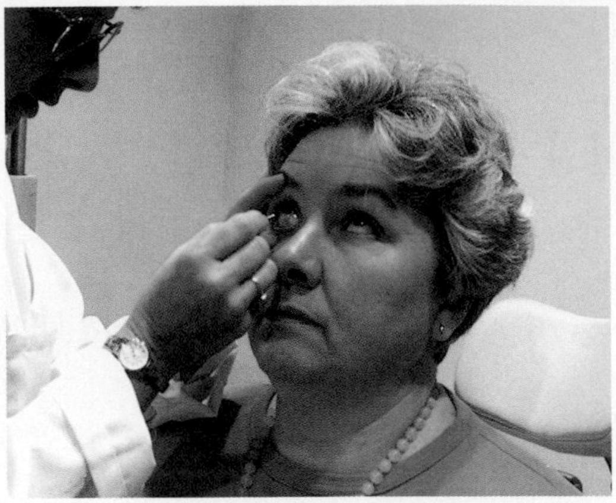

FIG. 47-1 Application of ophthalmic ointment.

! NURSING SAFETY PRIORITY (QSEN)

Drug Alert

Check the route of administration for ophthalmic drugs. Most are administered by the eye instillation route, not the oral route. Administering these drugs orally can cause systemic side effects in addition to not having a therapeutic effect on the eye.

An **ectropion** is the turning outward and sagging of the eyelid caused by muscle relaxation or weakness, which often occurs with aging. This lid position reduces the washing action of tears, leading to corneal drying and ulceration.

Patients often have constant tears and a sagging lower eyelid. Surgery can restore lid alignment. After surgery, the eye is covered with a patch and the patient is discharged. Nursing care is the same as for an entropion.

Hordeolum

A **hordeolum**, or *stye*, is INFECTION of the eyelid sweat glands (external hordeolum) or of the eyelid sebaceous gland (internal hordeolum). A red, swollen, painful area occurs on the skin surface side of the eyelid. The most common causative organisms are *Staphylococcus aureus, Staphylococcus epidermidis,* and *Streptococcus.* Visual SENSORY PERCEPTION is not affected.

Management includes applying warm compresses 4 times a day and an antibacterial ointment. When the lesion opens, the purulent material drains and the pain subsides.

Nursing interventions include instructing the patient how to apply compresses to the eye (Chart 47-3) and how to instill antibiotic ointment (see Chart 47-1). Remind the patient to remove the ointment from the eyes before driving or operating machinery.

Chalazion

A **chalazion** is an inflammation of a sebaceous gland in the eyelid. It begins with redness and tenderness, followed by a gradual *painless* swelling. Later, redness and tenderness are not present. Most chalazia protrude on the inside of the eyelid. The patient has eye fatigue, light sensitivity, and excessive tears.

Management includes applying warm compresses 4 times a day, followed by instillation of ophthalmic antibiotic ointment. If the chalazion is large enough to affect vision or is cosmetically displeasing, it may be removed surgically. Instruct the patient to immediately report increasing redness, purulent drainage, or reduced vision to the ophthalmologist.

CHART 47-1 Best Practice for Patient Safety & Quality Care (QSEN)

Instillation of Ophthalmic Ointment

- Check the name, strength, and expiration date of the ointment to be instilled. Be sure it is an ophthalmic (eye) preparation and not a general topical ointment.
- Check whether only one eye or both eyes are to receive the drug.
- If both eyes are to receive the same drug and one eye is infected, use two separate tubes and carefully label each tube with "right" or "left" for the correct eye.
- Wash your hands and put on gloves.
- Explain the procedure to the patient.
- Ask the patient to tilt the head backward and look up at the ceiling.
- Gently pull the lower lid down against the patient's cheek, forming a small pocket.
- Hold the tube (with the cap off) like a pencil, with the tip down.
- Rest the wrist holding the tube against the patient's cheek.
- Without touching any part of the eye or lid with the tip of the tube, gently squeeze the tube and release a small thin strip of ointment into the pocket of the lower lid. Start at the nose side of the pocket, and move toward the outer edge of the pocket.
- Gently release the lower lid.
- Tell the patient to close the eye without squeezing the lid.
- While the eye is closed, gently wipe away excess ointment.
- Remind the patient that vision in that eye will be blurred and to not drive or operate heavy machinery until the ointment is removed.
- Remove your gloves, and place the cap back on the tube.
- Ask the patient to keep the eye closed for about 1 minute.
- Wash your hands again.
- To remove ointment, wear gloves if drainage is present.
- Then ask the patient to close the eye; wipe the closed lids with a clean tissue from the corner of the eye nearest the nose outward. If you are wiping the same eye twice, use a different area of the tissue or use a new one.

KERATOCONJUNCTIVITIS SICCA

The lacrimal system moistens the eye surface with tears and removes tears from the eye. Problems arise from reduced tear production, INFECTION, or inflammation in the lacrimal system.

Keratoconjunctivitis sicca, or dry eye syndrome, results from changes in tear production, tear composition, or tear distribution. Drugs (e.g., antihistamines, beta-adrenergic blocking agents, anticholinergic drugs) also can reduce tear production. Diseases associated with dry eye syndrome include rheumatoid arthritis, leukemia, sarcoidosis, and Sjögren's syndrome. Radiation or chemical burns to the eye also decrease tear production. Injury to cranial nerve VII inhibits tears. Eye dryness may follow vision-enhancing surgery.

The patient has a foreign body sensation in the eye, burning and itching eyes, and *photophobia* (sensitivity to light). The corneal light reflex is dulled. Tears contain mucus strands.

Management depends on symptom severity. Cyclosporine (Restasis) eyedrops may be prescribed to increase tear production. Artificial tears (HypoTears, Refresh) also can be used to reduce daytime dryness. A lubricating ointment (Lacri-Lube SOP, Refresh P.M.) is used at night. If the dry eye syndrome is caused by an abnormal eyelid position, surgery may be needed.

CONJUNCTIVAL DISORDERS

The conjunctiva is a thin mucous membrane that covers and protects the eye. Because of its location, the conjunctiva is subject to trauma and INFECTION.

CHART 47-2 Common Examples of Drug Therapy

Eye Inflammation and Infection

DRUG	NURSING INTERVENTIONS*†	RATIONALES
Topical Anesthetics		
Proparacaine HCl, or proxymetacaine (AK-Taine, Alcaine, Ocu-Caine, Ophthetic) Tetracaine HCl, cocaine HCl (Pontocaine)	Remind the patient not to rub or touch the eye while it is anesthetized. Patch the eye if the patient leaves the facility before the anesthetic wears off. Instruct the patient not to use discolored solution. Teach the patient to store the bottle tightly closed.	Touching may injure the eye. The use of a patch prevents injury, such as corneal abrasion. Discoloration is a sign of altered drug composition. Air may cause drug contamination and oxidation.
Topical Steroids		
Prednisolone acetate (Ocu-Pred, Ophtho-Tate 🍁) Prednisolone phosphate (Inflamase) Dexamethasone (Dexair, Dexotic, Maxidex) Betamethasone (Betnesol) Fluorometholone (Fluor-Op, Liquifilm)	Tell the patient to shake the bottle vigorously before use. Teach the patient to check for corneal ulceration (pain, reduced vision, secretions). Warn the patient not to share eyedrops with others.	Drug is a suspension; shaking is required to distribute the drug evenly in the solution. Steroid use predisposes the patient to local infection. Disease transmission is possible when sharing eyedrops.
Anti-Infective Agents		
Gentamicin (Genoptic, Gentak Alcomicin 🍁) Tobramycin (Tobrex) Ciprofloxacin (Ciloxan) Erythromycin (Ilotycin) Chlortetracycline (Aureomycin) Sulfisoxazole (Gantrisin) Ofloxacin (Ocuflox) Levofloxacin (Quixin) Bacitracin; Polymyxin B (Polysporin, Polytracin ophthalmic, AK-Poly-Bac)	Teach the patient the importance of using the drug exactly as prescribed, even if he or she needs to use it hourly. Teach the patient how to clean exudate from the eyes before using drops. Reinforce the importance of completing the prescribed drug regimen.	Bacterial and fungal eye infections worsen rapidly and can lead to blindness if not treated adequately. Cleansing decreases the risk for contaminating the drug and increases contact of the conjunctiva with the drug. Adherence is critical to maintain a therapeutic level of drug.
Antibiotic-Steroid Combinations		
Tobramycin with dexamethasone (TobraDex) Neomycin sulfate with polymyxin B sulfate and dexamethasone (Maxitrol)	This is the same as for the general anti-infective agents alone and for the steroids alone.	This is the same as for the general anti-infective agents alone and for the steroids alone.
Topical Antiviral Agents		
Trifluridine (Viroptic) Vidarabine (Vira-A)	Teach the patient to refrigerate the drug and protect it from light. Teach the patient to assess for itching lids and burning eyes.	Drug stability is affected by warm temperatures and light. Sensitivity to these drugs is common.
Antifungal Agents		
Amphotericin B Natamycin (Natacyn)	Teach the patient to assess for itching lids and burning eyes.	Sensitivity to these drugs is common.
Nonsteroidal Anti-Inflammatory Agents		
Flurbiprofen (Ocufen) Diclofenac (Voltaren) Bromfenac (Xibrom) Ketorolac (Acular)	Teach the patient to check for bleeding in the eye. Teach the patient not to wear soft contact lenses during therapy with these drugs.	These drugs disrupt platelet aggregation. These drugs interact with contact lens materials and increase the risk for infection.

*When instilling eyedrops, teach patients to use nasal punctal occlusion to reduce the risk for systemic absorption and side effects.
†When more than one topical ophthalmic drug is prescribed, teach patients to separate the instillation of each drug by 5-10 minutes (or package recommendations).

Conjunctivitis

Conjunctivitis is an inflammation with or without INFECTION of the conjunctiva. Inflammation occurs from exposure to allergens or irritants. Infectious conjunctivitis occurs with bacterial or viral infection and is easily transmitted from person to person.

Allergic conjunctivitis manifestations are edema, a sensation of burning, a "bloodshot" eye appearance, excessive tears, and itching (Watkinson, 2013). Management includes vasoconstrictor and corticosteroid eyedrops (see Chart 47-2). Instruct patients to avoid using makeup near the eye until all manifestations are gone.

Bacterial conjunctivitis, or "pink eye," is most often caused by *S. aureus.* Manifestations are blood vessel dilation, edema, tears, and discharge. The discharge is watery at first and then becomes thicker, with shreds of mucus.

Cultures of the drainage may be obtained to identify the organism. Ophthalmic antibiotics are prescribed to eliminate the infection. Nursing interventions focus on preventing INFECTION spread to the other eye or to other people. Remind the patient to wash his or her hands after touching the eye and before using eyedrops. Warn him or her not to touch the unaffected eye without first washing the hands and to avoid sharing washcloths and towels with others. Instruct patients to discard

CHART 47-3 Patient and Family Education: Preparing for Self-Management

Application of an Ocular Compress

- Wash your hands.
- Fold a clean washcloth into fourths.
- Soak the washcloth with running tap water that is warm to your inner wrist. (If cool compresses are needed, follow the same steps using cold running tap water.)
- Place the cloth over your closed eye.
- Keep the cloth in place with light pressure until the cloth cools (or warms, if cool compresses are prescribed).
- Refold the washcloth so that a different "fourth" will be held against the eye.
- Resoak the cloth with running tap water.
- Repeat applications 3 times for as many times each day as prescribed by your health care provider.

eye makeup and applicators used at the time the infection developed. Contact lenses worn during the infection need to be discarded to avoid reinfection.

Trachoma

Trachoma is a chronic conjunctivitis caused by *Chlamydia trachomatis.* It scars the conjunctiva and is a common cause of preventable blindness worldwide. The incidence is highest in warm, moist climates where sanitation is poor.

At first the disease resembles bacterial conjunctivitis with manifestations of tears, photophobia, and eyelid edema. Follicles form on the upper eyelid conjunctiva. As the disease progresses, the eyelid scars and turns inward, causing the eyelashes to damage the cornea.

Antibiotic therapy is used when the organism is identified. The most effective antibiotic is oral azithromycin (Zithromax). The infection also can be eliminated early in the disease with a 4-week course of tetracycline eye ointment. Nursing interventions focus on INFECTION control. Patient teaching is the same as for conjunctivitis.

! NURSING SAFETY PRIORITY QSEN

Action Alert

Teach patients who are prescribed oral antibiotics or antibiotic ointments to complete the entire course of antibiotics. Stopping antibiotic therapy too soon promotes INFECTION recurrence and development of antibiotic-resistant bacteria.

CORNEAL DISORDERS

For a sharp retinal image, the cornea must be transparent and intact. Corneal problems may be caused by irritation or INFECTION (keratitis) with ulceration of the corneal surface, degeneration of the cornea (keratoconus), or deposits in the cornea. All corneal problems reduce visual SENSORY PERCEPTION, and some can lead to blindness.

CORNEAL ABRASION, ULCERATION, AND INFECTION

❖ *PATHOPHYSIOLOGY*

A **corneal abrasion** is a scrape or scratch injury of the cornea. This painful condition can be caused by a small foreign body, trauma, or contact lens use (Corneal Abrasion, 2013). Other problems contributing to corneal injury are malnutrition, dry eye syndromes, and some cancer therapies. The abrasion allows organisms to enter, leading to corneal INFECTION. Bacterial, protozoal, and fungal infections can lead to **corneal ulceration**, which is a deeper injury. *This problem is an emergency because the cornea has no separate blood supply and infections that can permanently impair vision develop rapidly.* Use of homemade contact lens solutions and the use of large-volume solution containers that can easily become contaminated have led to a sharp rise in the incidence of corneal ulcers infected with *Pseudomonas aeruginosa* and fungi.

❖ *PATIENT-CENTERED COLLABORATIVE CARE*

The patient with a corneal disorder has pain, reduced vision, photophobia, and eye secretions. Cloudy or purulent fluid may be present on the eyelids or lashes. Wear gloves when examining the eye.

The cornea looks hazy or cloudy with a patchy area of ulceration. When fluorescein stain is used, the patchy areas appear green. Microbial culture and corneal scrapings are used to determine the causative organism. Anti-infective therapy is started before the organism is identified because of the high risk for vision loss. For culture, obtain swabs from the ulcer and its edges. For corneal scrapings, the cornea is anesthetized with a topical agent and a physician or advanced practice nurse removes samples from the ulcer center and edge.

Antibiotics, antifungals, and antivirals are prescribed to eliminate the organisms. A broad-spectrum antibiotic is prescribed first and may be changed when culture results are known. Steroids may be used with antibiotics to reduce the eye inflammation. Drugs can be given topically as eyedrops, injected subconjunctivally, or injected IV. Chart 46-3 in Chapter 46 lists best practices for instilling eyedrops. The nursing priorities are to begin the drug therapy, to ensure patient understanding of the drug therapy regimen, and to prevent INFECTION spread.

Often the anti-infective therapy involves instilling eyedrops *every hour* for the first 24 hours. Teach the patient or family member how to instill the eyedrops correctly. (See Chart 46-2 in Chapter 46.)

If the eye INFECTION occurs only in one eye, teach the patient not to use the drug in the unaffected eye. Instruct him or her to wash hands after touching the affected eye and before touching or doing anything to the healthy eye. If both eyes are infected, separate bottles of drugs are needed for each eye. Teach the patient to clearly label the bottles "right eye" and "left eye" and not to switch the drugs from eye to eye. Also teach him or her to completely care for one eye, then wash the hands, and using the drugs designated for the other eye, care for that eye. Remind the patient not to wear contact lenses during the entire time that these drugs are being used because the eye is more vulnerable to infection or injury and because the drugs can cloud or damage the contact lenses.

! NURSING SAFETY PRIORITY QSEN

Action Alert

Stress the importance of applying the drug as often as prescribed, even at night. Stopping the infection at this stage can save the vision in the infected eye. Instruct the patient to make and keep all follow-up appointments; usually the patient is seen again in 24 hours or less.

Drug therapy may continue for 3 or more weeks to ensure eradication of the INFECTION. Warn patients to avoid using makeup around the eye until the infection has cleared (Corneal Abrasion, 2013). Instruct patients to discard all open containers of contact lens solutions and bottles of eyedrops because these may be contaminated. Patients should not wear contact lenses for weeks to months until the infection is gone and the ulcer is healed.

KERATOCONUS AND CORNEAL OPACITIES

❖ PATHOPHYSIOLOGY

The cornea can permanently lose it shape, become scarred or cloudy, or become thinner, reducing useful visual SENSORY PERCEPTION. **Keratoconus**, the degeneration of the corneal tissue resulting in abnormal corneal shape, can occur with trauma or may be an inherited disorder (Fig. 47-2). Inadequately treated corneal INFECTION and severe trauma can scar the cornea and lead to severe visual impairment that can be improved only by surgical interventions.

❖ PATIENT-CENTERED COLLABORATIVE CARE

For a misshaped cornea that is still clear, surgical management involves a corneal ring implant that adjusts the shape of the cornea. With this procedure, the shape of the cornea is changed by placing a flexible ring in the outer edges of the cornea (outside of the optical zone).

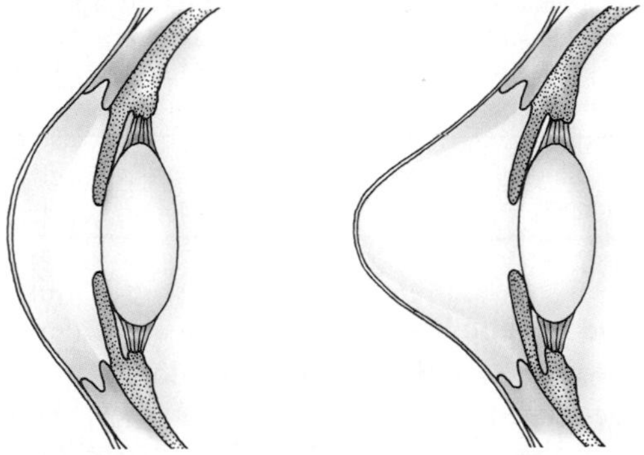

FIG. 47-2 Profile of a normal cornea and one with keratoconus.

The procedure is performed under local anesthesia. Improvement to best vision is immediate. Removal, replacement, or adjustment of ring tightness can enhance refraction, especially when the patient's vision changes further as a result of aging. Because the ring is placed outside of the optical zone, the risk for corneal clouding or scarring is low.

Surgery to improve clarity for a permanent corneal disorder that obscures vision is a **keratoplasty** (corneal transplant), in which the diseased corneal tissue is removed and replaced with tissue from a human donor cornea. This process improves vision by removing corneal deformities and replacing them with healthy corneal tissue.

Preoperative care may be short, with little time for teaching because transplantation is performed when the donor cornea becomes available. Examine the eyes for manifestations of INFECTION, and report any redness, drainage, or edema to the ophthalmologist. Instill prescribed antibiotic eyedrops and obtain IV access before surgery.

Operative procedures are *keratoplasties* and are usually performed with local anesthesia in an ambulatory surgical setting. The transplant may involve the entire depth of corneal tissue (penetrating keratoplasty) or only certain layers of the corneal tissue (lamellar keratoplasty). The nerves around the eye are anesthetized so that the patient cannot move the eye or see out of the eye. The center 7 to 8 mm of the diseased cornea is removed with an instrument that works like a cookie cutter (Fig. 47-3). The same instrument is used to cut the tissue graft from the donor cornea so that the graft will be a perfect fit. The donor cornea is sutured into place on the eye. The procedure takes about an hour, and the patient is discharged to home within 1 to 2 hours.

Postoperative care involves extensive patient teaching. Local antibiotics are injected or instilled. Usually the eye is covered with a pressure patch and a protective shield until the patient returns to the surgeon.

Instruct the patient to lie on the nonoperative side to reduce intraocular pressure (IOP). If a patch is to be used for more

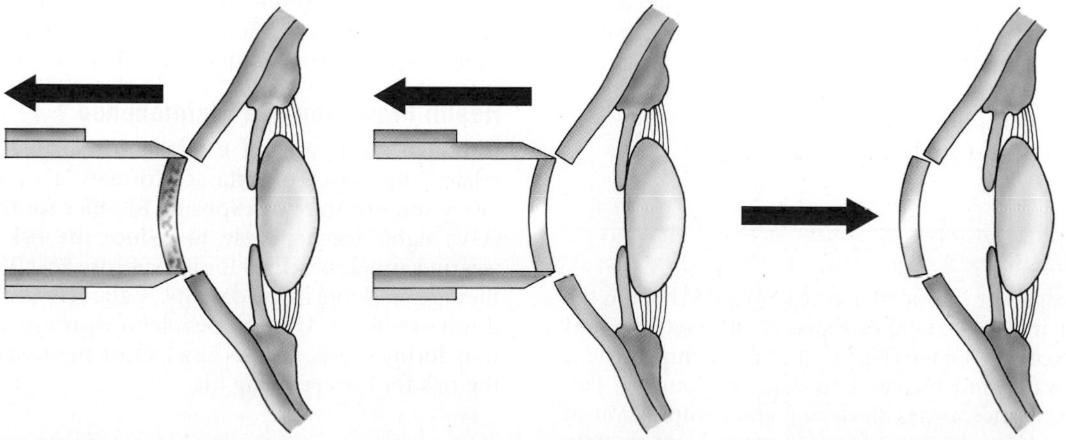

FIG. 47-3 The steps involved in corneal transplantation (penetrating keratoplasty).

TABLE 47-1 Activities That Increase Intraocular Pressure

• Bending from the waist • Lifting objects weighing more than 10 lbs • Sneezing, coughing • Blowing the nose • Straining to have a bowel movement	• Vomiting • Having sexual intercourse • Keeping the head in a dependent position • Wearing tight shirt collars

than a day, teach the patient or family member how to apply it. Instruct the patient to wear the shield at night for the first month after surgery and whenever he or she is around small children or pets. Instruct him or her *not* to use an ice pack on the eye. Complications after surgery include bleeding, wound leakage, INFECTION, and graft rejection. Teach the patient how to instill eyedrops. Teach him or her to examine the eye (or have a family member do the examination) daily for the presence of infection or graft rejection. Stress that the presence of purulent discharge, a continuous leak of clear fluid from around the graft site (not tears), or excessive bleeding needs to be reported immediately to the surgeon. Other complications include decreased vision, increased reddening of the eye, pain, increased sensitivity to light, and the presence of light flashes or "floaters" in the field of vision. Teach the patient to report any of these manifestations to the surgeon if they develop after the first 48 hours and persist for more than 6 hours.

The eye should be protected from any activity that can increase the pressure on, around, or inside the eye. Teach the patient to avoid jogging, running, dancing, and any other activity that promotes rapid or jerky head motions for several weeks after surgery. Other activities that may raise intraocular pressure (IOP) and should be avoided are listed in Table 47-1.

Graft rejection can occur and starts as inflammation in the cornea near the graft edge that moves toward the center. Vision is reduced, and the cornea becomes cloudy. Topical corticosteroids and other immunosuppressants are used to stop the rejection process. If rejection continues, the graft becomes opaque and blood vessels branch into the opaque tissue.

Eye donation is a common procedure and needed for corneal transplantation. If a deceased patient is a known eye donor, follow these recommended steps:

- Raise the head of the bed 30 degrees.
- Instill prescribed antibiotic eyedrops.
- Close the eyes, and apply a *small* ice pack.

CATARACT

❖ PATHOPHYSIOLOGY

The lens is a transparent, elastic structure suspended behind the iris that focuses images onto the retina. A **cataract** is a lens opacity that distorts the image (Fig. 47-4). With aging, the lens gradually loses water and increases in density (Touhy & Jett, 2014). Lens density increases with drying and compression of older lens fibers and production of new fibers and lens crystals. With time, as lens density increases and transparency is lost, visual SENSORY PERCEPTION is greatly reduced. Both eyes may have cataracts, but the rate of progression in each eye is different.

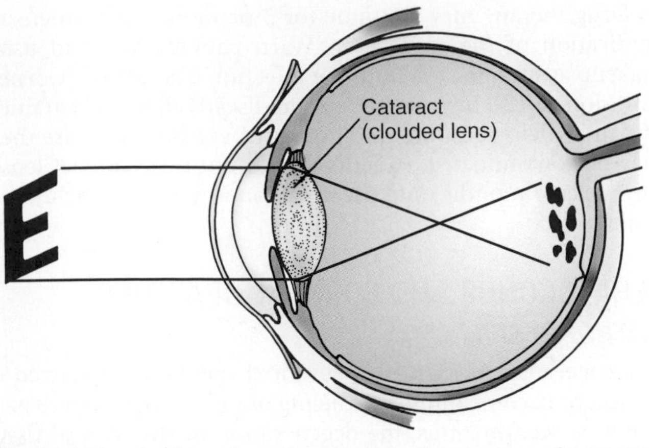

FIG. 47-4 The visual impairment produced by the presence of a cataract.

TABLE 47-2 Common Causes of Cataracts

Age-Related Cataracts • Lens water loss and fiber compaction **Traumatic Cataracts** • Blunt injury to eye or head • Penetrating eye injury • Intraocular foreign bodies • Radiation exposure, therapy **Toxic Cataracts** • Corticosteroids • Phenothiazine derivatives • Miotic agents	**Associated Cataracts** • Diabetes mellitus • Hypoparathyroidism • Down syndrome • Chronic sunlight exposure **Complicated Cataracts** • Retinitis pigmentosa • Glaucoma • Retinal detachment

Etiology and Genetic Risk

Cataracts may be present at birth or develop at any time. They may be age-related or caused by trauma or exposure to toxic agents. They also occur with other diseases and eye disorders (Table 47-2).

Incidence and Prevalence

About 25 to 27 million people in North America have cataracts (National Eye Institute, 2012). The age-related cataract is the most common type. Some degree of cataract formation is expected in all people older than 70 years.

Health Promotion and Maintenance

Although most cases of cataracts in North America are age-related, the onset of cataract formation occurs earlier with heavy sun exposure or exposure to other sources of ultraviolet (UV) light. Teach people to reduce the risk for cataract by wearing sunglasses that limit exposure to UV light whenever they are outdoors in the daytime. Cataracts also may result from direct eye injury. Urge all people to wear eye and head protection during sports, such as baseball, or any activity that increases the risk for the eye being hit.

❖ PATIENT-CENTERED COLLABORATIVE CARE

◆ Assessment

History. Age is important because cataracts are most prevalent in the older adult. Ask about these predisposing factors:

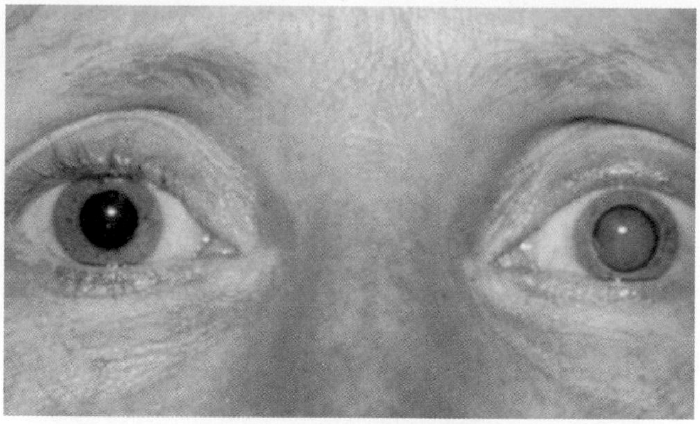

FIG. 47-5 The appearance of an eye with a mature cataract.

- Recent or past trauma to the eye
- Exposure to radioactive materials, x-rays, or UV light
- Systemic disease (e.g., diabetes mellitus, hypoparathyroidism)
- Prolonged use of corticosteroids, chlorpromazine, beta blockers, or miotic drugs
- Intraocular disease (e.g., recurrent uveitis)
- Family history of cataracts

Ask the patient to describe his or her vision. For example, you might say "Tell me what you can see well and what you have difficulty seeing."

Physical Assessment/Clinical Manifestations. Early manifestations of cataracts are slightly blurred vision and decreased color perception. At first the patient may think his or her glasses or contact lenses are smudged. As lens cloudiness continues, blurred and double vision occur and the patient may have difficulty with ADLs. Without surgical intervention, visual impairment progresses to blindness. *No pain or eye redness is associated with age-related cataract formation.*

Visual SENSORY PERCEPTION is tested using an eye chart and brightness acuity testing (see Chapter 46). Examine the lens with an ophthalmoscope, and describe any observed densities by size, shape, and location. As the cataract matures, the opacity makes it difficult to see the retina and the red reflex may be absent. When this occurs, the pupil is bluish white (Fig. 47-5).

Psychosocial Assessment. Loss of vision is gradual, and the patient may not be aware of it until reading or driving is affected. The patient often has anxiety about loss of independence. Encourage the patient and family to express concerns about reduced vision.

◆ Planning and Implementation

The priority problem for the patient with cataracts is reduced visual SENSORY PERCEPTION, which is a safety risk. Patients often live with reduced vision for years before the cataract is removed. Interventions for safety and independence before surgery are on pp. 993-994 in Patient-Centered Collaborative Care in the Reduced Visual Sensory Perception section.

Improving Vision

Planning: Expected Outcomes. The patient with cataracts is expected to recognize when ADLs cannot be performed safely and independently and then is expected to have cataract surgery. This procedure is covered by Medicare for patients who are 65 years or older.

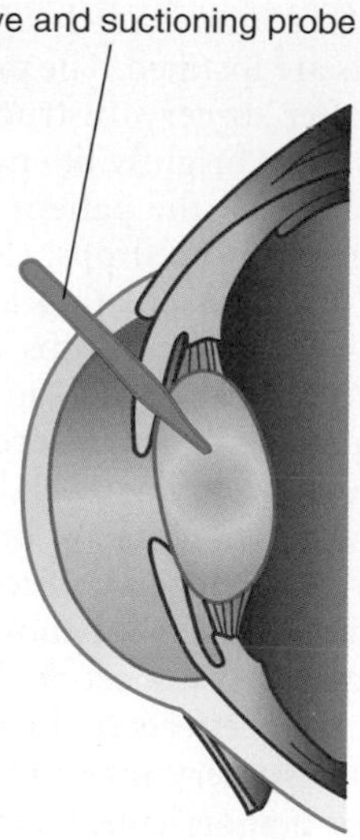

FIG. 47-6 Cataract removal by phacoemulsification.

Interventions. Surgery is the only "cure" for cataracts and should be performed as soon as possible after vision is reduced to the extent that ADLs are affected.

Preoperative Care. The ophthalmologist provides the patient with accurate information so that he or she can make informed decisions about treatment and obtains informed consent. Reinforce this information, and teach about the nature of cataracts, their progression, and their treatment.

Assess how the reduced vision affects ADLs, especially dressing, eating, and ambulating. Stress that care after surgery requires the instillation of different types of eyedrops several times a day for 2 to 4 weeks. Careful assessment of eye appearance is also needed. If the patient is unable to perform these tasks, help him or her make arrangements for this care.

Ask whether the patient takes any drugs that affect blood clotting, such as aspirin, warfarin (Coumadin), clopidogrel (Plavix), and dabigatran (Pradaxa). Communicate this information to the surgeon because, for some patients, these drugs may need to be discontinued before cataract surgery.

A series of ophthalmic drugs are instilled just before surgery to dilate the pupils and cause vasoconstriction. Other eyedrops are instilled to induce paralysis to prevent lens movement. When the patient is in the surgical area, a local anesthetic is injected into the muscle cone behind the eye for anesthesia and eye paralysis.

Operative Procedures. The lens is extracted by *phacoemulsification* (Fig. 47-6), in which a probe is inserted through the capsule and high-frequency sound waves break the lens into small pieces, which are then removed by suction. The replacement intraocular lens (IOL) is placed inside the capsule to be positioned so that light rays are focused in the retina. The IOL is a small, clear, plastic lens. Different types are available, and one is selected by the surgeon and patient to allow correction of a specific refractive error. Some patients have distant vision restored to 20/20 and may need glasses only for reading or close work. Some replacement lenses have multiple focal planes and may correct vision to the extent that glasses or contact lenses may not be needed.

Postoperative Care. Immediately after surgery, antibiotic and steroid ointments are instilled. The patient usually is discharged within an hour after surgery. Instruct him or her to wear dark glasses outdoors or in brightly lit environments until the pupil responds to light. Teach the patient and family members how to instill the prescribed eyedrops. (See Chart 46-2 in Chapter 46.) Work with them in creating a written schedule for the timing and the order of eyedrops administration. Stress the importance of keeping all follow-up appointments.

Remind the patient that mild eye itching is normal, as is a "bloodshot appearance." The eyelid may be slightly swollen. However, significant swelling or bruising is abnormal. Cool compresses may be beneficial. Discomfort at the site is controlled with acetaminophen (Abenol ♣, Tylenol) or acetaminophen with oxycodone (Endocet ♣, Percocet, Tylox). Aspirin is avoided because of its effects on blood clotting.

Pain early after surgery may indicate increased intraocular pressure (IOP) or hemorrhage. Instruct patients to contact the surgeon if pain occurs with nausea or vomiting.

To prevent increases in IOP, teach the patient and family about activity restrictions. Activities that can cause a sudden rise in IOP are listed in Table 47-1.

INFECTION is a potential and serious complication. Teach the patient and family to observe for increasing eye redness, a decrease in vision, or an increase in tears and photophobia. Creamy white, dry, crusty drainage on the eyelids and lashes is normal. However, yellow or green drainage indicates infection and must be reported.

Patients experience a dramatic improvement in vision within a day of surgery. Remind them that final best vision will not occur until 4 to 6 weeks after surgery.

! NURSING SAFETY PRIORITY (QSEN)

Action Alert

Instruct the patient who has had cataract surgery to immediately report any reduction of vision after surgery in the eye that had the cataract removed.

Community-Based Care

The patient is usually discharged within an hour after cataract surgery. Nursing interventions focus on helping the patient and family plan the eyedrop schedule and daily home eye examination.

Home Care Management. If the patient has difficulty instilling eyedrops, a supportive neighbor, friend, or family member can be taught the procedure. Adaptive equipment that positions the bottle of eyedrops directly over the eye can also be purchased (Fig. 47-7).

Self-Management Education. The best outcome of cataract removal requires close adherence to the eyedrop regimen after surgery. Providing the patient or family with accurate information and demonstration of needed skills are nursing priorities. Before discharge, review these indications of complications after cataract surgery with the patient and family:

- Sharp, sudden pain in the eye
- Bleeding or increased discharge
- Green or yellow, thick drainage
- Lid swelling
- Reappearance of a bloodshot sclera after the initial appearance has cleared

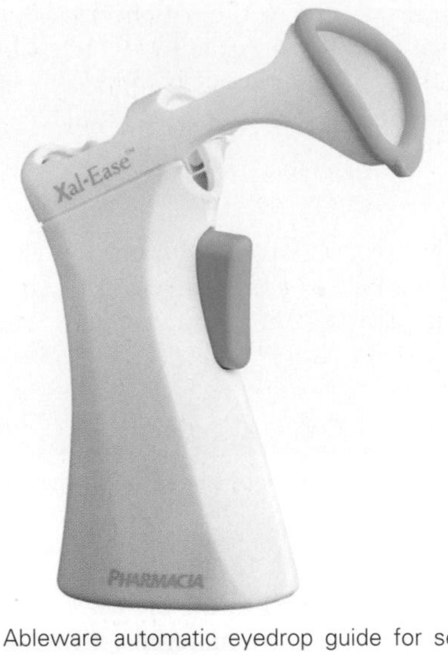

FIG. 47-7 The Ableware automatic eyedrop guide for self-administering eyedrops.

CHART 47-4 Focused Assessment

The Patient After Cataract Surgery

Assess the eye and vision:
- Visual acuity in both eyes using a handheld eye chart
- Visual fields of both eyes
- Compare operative eye with nonoperative eye for presence or absence of:
  - Redness
  - Tearing
  - Drainage

Ask the patient about:
- Pain in or around the operative eye
- Any change in vision (decreased or improved) in the operative eye
- Whether any of these has been noticed in the operative eye:
  - Dark spots
  - Increase in the number of floaters
  - Bright flashes of light

Assess the home environment for:
- Safety hazards (especially tripping and falling hazards)
- Level of room lighting

Assess patient adherence with and understanding of treatment and limitations, such as:
- Manifestations to report
- Drug regimen
- Activity restrictions
- Ability to perform ADLs

- Decreased vision
- Flashes of light or floating shapes

Remind the patient to avoid activities that might increase IOP (see Table 47-1). Some patients are prescribed to wear a light eye patch at night to prevent accidental rubbing. Instruct the patient to avoid getting water in the eye for 3 to 7 days after surgery.

Teach the patient about activity restrictions. Cooking and light housekeeping are permitted, but vacuuming should be avoided for several weeks because of the forward flexion involved and the rapid, jerky movements required. Advise him or her to refrain from driving until vision is not blurry. Chart 47-4 lists items to cover in the focused assessment of a patient at home after cataract surgery.

Health Care Resources. If the patient lives alone and has no support, arrange for a home care nurse to assess him or her and the home situation. If the patient is unable to instill eyedrops independently, a friend, neighbor, or family member can be taught this technique.

◆ Evaluation: Outcomes

Evaluate the care of the patient with cataracts on the basis of improving visual SENSORY PERCEPTION. The expected outcomes include that the patient after cataract surgery will:

- Have improved visual sensory perception
- Recognize manifestations of complications

Specific indicators for these outcomes are listed under the Planning and Implementation section (see earlier).

NCLEX EXAMINATION CHALLENGE

Health Promotion and Maintenance

The client who had cataract surgery with a lens implant 1 week ago remarks to the home care nurse that after his daughter left to go to her home in another state yesterday, he combined all of his prescribed eyedrops together in one container so he had fewer drops to administer. What is the nurse's best response?

A. "This is not a good idea because not all of the drugs are on the same schedule."
B. "That is a good idea; just remember to not touch the dropper to your eye when giving yourself the drops."
C. "Call your surgeon immediately and get new prescriptions because together these drugs can lower your blood pressure."
D. "Call your surgeon immediately and get new prescriptions to use one at a time because these drugs cannot be mixed together."

GLAUCOMA

❖ PATHOPHYSIOLOGY

Glaucoma is a group of eye disorders resulting in increased IOP (intraocular pressure). As described in Chapter 46, the eye is a hollow organ. For proper eye function, the gel in the posterior segment (vitreous humor) and the fluid in the anterior segment (aqueous humor) must be present in set amounts that apply pressure inside the eye to keep it ball-shaped.

In adults the volume of the vitreous humor does not change. The aqueous humor, however, is continuously made from blood plasma by the ciliary bodies located behind the iris and just in front of the lens (see Fig. 46-2 in Chapter 46). The fluid flows through the pupil into the bulging area in front of the iris. At the outer edges of the iris beneath the cornea, blood vessels collect fluid and return it to the blood. Usually about 1 mL of aqueous humor is always present, but it is continuously made and reabsorbed at a rate of about 5 mL daily. *A normal IOP requires a balance between production and outflow of aqueous humor (McCance et al., 2014). If the IOP becomes too high, the extra pressure compresses retinal blood vessels and photoreceptors and their synapsing nerve fibers. This compression results in poorly oxygenated photoreceptors and nerve fibers. These sensitive nerve tissues become ischemic and die. When too many have died, vision is lost permanently.* Tissue damage starts in the periphery and moves inward toward the fovea centralis. Untreated, glaucoma can lead to complete loss of visual SENSORY PERCEPTION. Glaucoma is usually painless, and the patient may be unaware of gradual vision reduction.

TABLE 47-3 Common Causes of Glaucoma

Primary Glaucoma	Secondary Glaucoma
• Aging • Heredity • Central retinal vein occlusion	• Uveitis • Iritis • Neovascular disorders • Trauma • Ocular tumors • Degenerative disease • Eye surgery
Associated Glaucoma • Diabetes mellitus • Hypertension • Severe myopia • Retinal detachment	

There are several causes and types of glaucoma (Table 47-3), classified as primary, secondary, or associated. The most common type is primary glaucoma.

Primary open-angle glaucoma (POAG), the most common form of primary glaucoma, usually affects both eyes and has no manifestations in the early stages. Outflow of aqueous humor through the chamber angle is reduced. Because the fluid cannot leave the eye at the same rate it is produced, IOP gradually increases. **Primary angle-closure glaucoma** (PACG or *acute glaucoma*) has a sudden onset and is an emergency. The problem is a forward displacement of the iris, which presses against the cornea and closes the chamber angle, suddenly preventing outflow of aqueous humor.

Glaucoma is a common cause of blindness in North America. It is usually age-related, occurring in about 3.5 million people in North America (National Eye Institute, 2012).

❖ PATIENT-CENTERED COLLABORATIVE CARE

Primary open-angle glaucoma (POAG) develops slowly, with gradual loss of visual fields that may go unnoticed because central vision at first is unaffected. At times, vision is foggy and the patient has mild eye aching or headaches. Late manifestations occur after irreversible damage to optic nerve function and include seeing halos around lights, losing peripheral vision, and having decreased visual SENSORY PERCEPTION that does not improve with eyeglasses. The Concept Map on p. 986 addresses collaborative care issues for patients with glaucoma.

◆ Assessment

Physical Assessment/Clinical Manifestations. Ophthalmoscopic examination shows cupping and atrophy of the optic disc. It becomes wider and deeper and turns white or gray. In POAG the visual fields first show a small loss of peripheral vision that gradually progresses to a larger loss.

Manifestations of acute angle-closure glaucoma include a sudden, severe pain around the eyes that radiates over the face. Headache or brow pain, nausea, and vomiting may occur. Other manifestations include seeing colored halos around lights and sudden blurred vision with decreased light perception. The sclera may appear reddened and the cornea foggy. Ophthalmoscopic examination reveals a shallow anterior chamber, cloudy aqueous humor, and a moderately dilated, nonreactive pupil.

Diagnostic Assessment. An elevated intraocular pressure (IOP) is measured by tonometry. In open-angle glaucoma, the tonometry reading is between 22 and 32 mm Hg (normal is 10 to 21 mm Hg). In angle-closure glaucoma, the tonometry reading may be 30 mm Hg or higher. Visual field testing by

CONCEPT MAP

SENSORY PERCEPTION

PRIMARY OPEN-ANGLE GLAUCOMA (POAG)

INFECTION

HISTORY

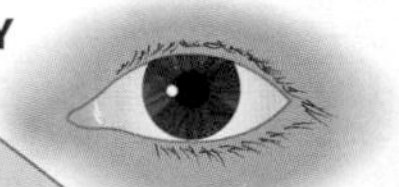

80 year-old Donald Vincent has just been diagnosed with POAG. He states he has been having a gradual loss of vision, including foggy vision, with occasional eye aches. He has recently had the prescription changed on his eyeglasses but still has vision issues.

Objective Data

Subjective Data

OBJECTIVE DATA

- PERRL with reduced accommodation
- Tonometry reading – 28 mm Hg (N = 10-21 mm Hg)
- Cupping and atrophy of the optic disk noted
- Peripheral vision decreased
- Patient instills 1 drop of travoprost ophthalmic solution (Travatan) 0.004% to the left eye daily

SUBJECTIVE DATA

"Everything is a little bit deteriorated. I have a little double vision sometimes. I can't read very much, that's why I like to watch the news on TV. I can't see far away, I just see a figure walking, not the facial features. I have to use a magnifying glass to read the label on the eyedrop bottle."

Data Synthesis

Data Synthesis

PATIENT PROBLEMS

- Altered SENSORY PERCEPTION due to loss of vision
- Knowledge Deficit: Medications
- Compromised safety
- Loss of independence

Planning

EXPECTED OUTCOMES

SENSORY PERCEPTION: Prevent blindness from glaucoma by early detection, lifelong treatment, and close monitoring with follow-up care.

SAFETY: Remain as independent as possible while ensuring safety.

INFECTION: Avoid infection by instilling eye drops correctly.

INTERVENTIONS

1 **Physical Assessment/Clinical Manifestations**

Perform an eye exam; glaucoma will show cupping and atrophy of the optic disc. *Measures visual fields to determine the extent of peripheral vision loss (SENSORY PERCEPTION).*

2 **Medication Administration**

- Demonstrate how to apply eyedrops and evaluate the patient's ability to self-administer. If needed, suggest adaptive equipment that positions the bottle directly over the eye. *Provides psychomotor demonstration for verifying the skill is done correctly. Adaptive equipment used for SENSORY PERCEPTION loss.*
- Teach the patient that most eye medications initially cause tearing and mild burning with blurred vision; the sclera may become red and itchy. *Helps the patient understand these are expected effects and not to be alarmed.*
- Emphasize instilling eyedrops on time, not skipping doses, and when more than one drug is required, wait 5-10 minutes between drops. *Reinforces verbal and written instructions; prevents one drug from "washing out" or diluting the other.*

3 **Nursing Safety Priority: Drug Alert!**

Teach the correct technique to instill eyedrops (punctal occlusion). *Prevents drugs for glaucoma from being systemically absorbed, causing serious side effects.*

4 **Providing Safe and Effective Care**

Teach principles of infection control (e.g., hand hygiene), and teach the patient not to touch the tip of the eyedrop container to any part of the eye. *Protects the patient from transmission of INFECTION.*

5 **Blindness Prevention Strategy**

Encourage the patient to keep follow-up appointments to monitor intraocular pressure (IOP). *Monitors IOP; if it becomes too high, the extra pressure can cause sensitive nerve tissues to become ischemic and die, leading to permanent blindness.*

6 **Travoprost (Travatan) Side Effects**

Teach the patient to report emergent signs of allergy – hives, difficulty breathing, angioedema. Stop using drops and call the provider for serious side effects: redness, swelling, itching, eye pain, discharge, increased light sensitivity, visual changes, or chest pain. *Educates the patient and prevents medication complications.*

7 **Psychosocial Integrity**

Encourage the patient and family to express concerns about reduced vision. *Helps the patient and family to cope with fear of blindness and anxiety about loss of independence.*

8 **Health Promotion and Maintenance**

Teach the patient and family how to alter the home for patient safety. *Minimizes patient risk of injury from lack of vision.*

Concept Map by Deanne A. Blach, MSN, RN

perimetry is performed, as is visualization by gonioscopy to determine whether the angle is open or closed. Usually the optic nerve is imaged to determine to what degree nerve damage is present. All of these diagnostic assessment techniques are described in Chapter 46.

◆ *Interventions*

Nonsurgical Management. Loss of visual SENSORY PERCEPTION from glaucoma can be prevented by early detection, lifelong treatment, and close monitoring. Use of ophthalmic drugs that reduce ocular pressure delays or prevents damage. Chart 47-5 lists ways to assist the patient with reduced vision to remain as independent as possible.

Drug therapy for glaucoma works to reduce IOP in several ways. Eyedrop drugs can reduce the production, increase the absorption of aqueous humor, or constrict the pupil so that the ciliary muscle is contracted, allowing better circulation of the aqueous humor to the site of absorption. *These drugs do not improve lost vision but prevent more damage by decreasing IOP.* The prostaglandins agonists drugs reduce IOP by dilating blood vessels in the trabecular mesh, which then collects and drains aqueous humor at a faster rate. The adrenergic agonists and beta-adrenergic blockers reduce IOP by limiting the production of aqueous humor and by dilating the pupil, which improves the flow of the fluid to its absorption site. Cholinergic agonists reduce IOP by limiting the production of aqueous humor and by making more room between the iris and the lens, which improves fluid outflow. Carbonic anhydrase inhibitors directly and strongly inhibit production of aqueous humor. They do not affect the flow or the absorption of the fluid. Most eyedrops cause tearing, mild burning, blurred vision, and a reddened sclera for a few minutes after instilling the drug. Specific nursing interventions are listed in Chart 47-6.

The priority nursing intervention for the patient on drug therapy for glaucoma is teaching. The benefit of drug therapy occurs only when the drugs are used on the prescribed schedule, usually every 12 hours. Teach patients the importance of instilling the drops on time and not skipping doses. When more than one drug is prescribed, teach him or her to wait 5 to 10 minutes between drug instillations to prevent one drug from "washing out" or diluting another drug. Stress the need for good handwashing, keeping the eyedrop container tip clean, and avoiding touching the tip to any part of the eye. Also teach the technique of punctal occlusion (placing pressure on the corner of the eye near the nose) immediately after eyedrop instillation to prevent systemic absorption of the drug (Fig. 47-8).

CHART 47-5 Nursing Focus on the Older Adult

Promote Independent Living in Patients with Impaired Vision

Drugs

- Having a neighbor, relative, friend, or visiting nurse visit once a week to measure the proper drugs for each day may be helpful.
  - If the patient is to take drugs more than once each day, it is helpful to use a container of a different shape (with a lid) each time. For example, if the patient is to take drugs at 9 AM, 1 PM, and 9 PM, the 9 AM drugs would be placed in a round container, the 1 PM drugs in a square container, and the 9 PM drugs in a triangular container.
  - It is helpful to place each day's drug containers in a separate box with raised letters on the side of the box spelling out the day.
- "Talking clocks" are available for the patient with low vision.
- Some drug boxes have alarms that can be set for different times.

Communication

- Telephones with large, raised block numbers may be helpful. The best models are those with black numbers on a white phone or white numbers on a black phone.
- Telephones that have a programmable automatic dialing feature ("speed dial") are very helpful. Programmed numbers should include those for the fire department, police, relatives, friends, neighbors, and 911.

Safety

- It is best to leave furniture the way the patient wants it and not move it.
- Throw rugs are best eliminated.
- Appliance cords should be short and kept out of walkways.
- Lounge-style chairs with built-in footrests are preferable to footstools.
- Nonbreakable dishes, cups, and glasses are preferable to breakable ones.
- Cleansers and other toxic agents should be labeled with large, raised letters.
- Hook-and-loop (Velcro) strips at hand level may help mark the locations of switches and electrical outlets.

Food Preparation

- Meals on Wheels is a service that many older adults find helpful. This service brings meals at mealtime, cooked and ready to eat. The cost of this service varies, depending on the patient's ability to pay.
- Many grocery stores offer a "shop by telephone" service. The patient can either complete a computer booklet indicating types, amounts, and brands of items desired, or the store will complete this booklet over the telephone by asking the patient specific information. The store then delivers groceries to the patient's door (many stores also offer a "put away" service) and charges the patient's bank card.
- A microwave oven is a safer means of cooking than a standard stove, although many older patients are afraid of microwave ovens. If the patient has and will use a microwave oven, others can prepare meals ahead of time, label them, and freeze them for later use. Also, many microwavable complete frozen dinners that comply with a variety of dietary restrictions are available.
- Friends or relatives may be able to help with food preparation. Often relatives do not know what to give an older person for birthdays or other gift-giving occasions. One suggestion is a homemade prepackaged frozen dinner that the patient enjoys.

Personal Care

- Handgrips should be installed in bathrooms.
- The tub floor should have a nonskid surface.
- Male patients should use an electric shaver rather than a razor.
- Choosing a hairstyle that is becoming but easy to care for (avoiding parts) helps in independent living.
- Home hair care services may be available.

Diversional Activity

- Some patients can read large-print books, newspapers, and magazines (available through local libraries and vision services).
- Books, magazines, and some newspapers are available on audiotapes or discs.
- Patients experienced in knitting or crocheting may be able to create items fashioned from straight pieces, such as afghans.
- Card games, dominoes, and some board games that are available in large, high-contrast print may be helpful for patients with low vision.

CHART 47-6 Common Examples of Drug Therapy (Eyedrops)

Glaucoma

CATEGORY/DRUG	NURSING IMPLICATIONS	RATIONALES
Prostaglandins Agonists		
Bimatoprost (Lumigan) Latanoprost (Xalatan) Tafluprost (Zioptan) Travoprost (Travatan) Unoprostone (Rescula)	Teach the patient to check the cornea for abrasions or trauma.	Drugs should not be used when the cornea is not intact.
	Remind the patient that, over time, the eye color darkens and eyelashes elongate in the eye receiving the drug.	Knowing the side effects in advance reassures the patient that their presence is expected and normal.
	If only one eye is to be treated, teach the patient *not* to place drops in the other eye to try to make the eye colors similar.	Using the drug in an eye with normal IOP can cause a *lower*-than-normal IOP, which reduces vision.
	Warn the patient that using more drops than prescribed reduces drug effectiveness.	Drug action is based on blocking receptors, which can increase in number when the drug is overused.
Adrenergic Agonists		
Apraclonidine (Iopidine) Brimonidine tartrate (Alphagan) Dipivefrin hydrochloride (Propine)	Ask whether the patient is taking any antidepressants from the MAO inhibitor class, such as phenelzine (Nardil) or tranylcypromine (Parnate).	These enzyme inhibitors increase blood pressure as do the adrenergic agonists. When taken together, the patient may experience hypertensive crisis.
	Teach the patient to wear dark glasses outdoors and also indoors when lighting is bright.	The pupil dilates (mydriasis) and remains dilated, even when there is plenty of light, causing discomfort.
	Teach the patient not to use the eyedrops with contact lenses in place and to wait 15 minutes after using the drug to put in the lenses.	These drugs are absorbed by the contact lens, which can become discolored or cloudy.
Beta-Adrenergic Blockers		
Betaxolol hydrochloride (Betoptic) Carteolol (Cartrol, Ocupress) Levobunolol (Betagan) Timolol (Betimol, Istalol, Timoptic) Timoptic GFS (gel-forming solution) (Timoptic-XE, Timolol-GFS)	Ask whether the patient has moderate to severe asthma or COPD.	If these drugs are absorbed systemically, they constrict pulmonary smooth muscle and narrow airways.
	Warn diabetic patients to check their blood glucose levels more often when taking these drugs.	These drugs induce hypoglycemia and also mask the hypoglycemic symptoms.
	Teach patients who also take oral beta blockers to check their pulse at least twice per day and to notify the health care provider if the pulse is consistently below 58 beats per minute.	These drugs potentiate the effects of systemic beta blockers and can cause an unsafe drop in heart rate and blood pressure.
Cholinergic Agonists		
Carbachol (Carboptic, Isopto Carbachol, Miostat) Echothiophate (Phospholine Iodide) Pilocarpine (Adsorbocarpine, Akarpine, Isopto Carpine, Ocu-Carpine, Ocusert, Piloptic, Pilostat)	Teach the patient not to use more eyedrops than are prescribed and to report increased salivation or drooling to the health care provider.	These drugs are readily absorbed by conjunctival mucous membranes and can cause systemic side effects of headache, flushing, increased saliva, and sweating.
	Teach the patient to use good light when reading and to take care in darker rooms.	The pupil of the eye will not open more to let in more light, and it may be harder to see objects in dim light. This problem can increase the risk for falls.
Carbonic Anhydrase Inhibitors		
Brinzolamide (Azopt) Dorzolamide (Trusopt)	Ask whether the patient has an allergy to sulfonamide antibacterial drugs.	Drugs are similar to the sulfonamides, and if a patient is allergic to the sulfonamides, an allergy is likely with these drugs, even as eyedrops.
	Teach the patient to shake the drug before applying.	Drug separates on standing.
	Teach the patient not to use the eyedrops with contact lenses in place and to wait 15 minutes after using the drug to put in the lenses.	These drugs are absorbed by the contact lens, which can become discolored or cloudy.
Combination Drugs		
Brimonidine tartrate and timolol maleate (Combigan) Latanoprost and timolol (Xalcom)	Same as for each drug alone.	Same as for each drug alone.

COPD, Chronic obstructive pulmonary disease; *IOP*, intraocular pressure; *MAO*, monamine oxidase.

! NURSING SAFETY PRIORITY QSEN

Drug Alert

Most eyedrops used for glaucoma therapy can be absorbed systemically and cause systemic problems. It is critical to teach punctal occlusion to patients using eyedrops for glaucoma therapy.

Systemic osmotic drugs may be given for angle-closure glaucoma to rapidly reduce IOP. These agents include oral glycerin and IV mannitol (Osmitrol).

Surgical Management. Surgery is used when drugs for open-angle glaucoma are not effective at controlling IOP. Two common procedures are laser trabeculoplasty and trabeculectomy. A *laser trabeculoplasty* burns the trabecular meshwork, scarring it and causing the meshwork fibers to tighten. Tight fibers increase the size of the spaces between the fibers, improving outflow of aqueous humor and reducing IOP. *Trabeculectomy* is a surgical procedure that creates a new channel for fluid outflow. Both are ambulatory surgery procedures.

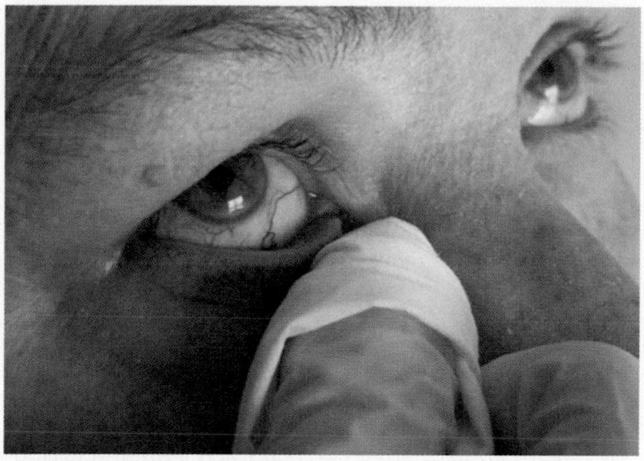

FIG. 47-8 Applying punctal occlusion to prevent systemic absorption of eyedrops.

If glaucoma fails to respond to common approaches, an implanted shunt procedure may be used. A small tube or filament is connected to a flat plate that is positioned on the outside of the eye in the eye orbit. (The plate is not visible on the front part of the eye.) The open part of the fine tube is placed into the front chamber of the eye. The fluid then drains through or around the tube into the area around the flat plate where it collects and is reabsorbed into the bloodstream. Potential complications of glaucoma surgery include choroidal hemorrhage and choroidal detachment.

NCLEX EXAMINATION CHALLENGE

Safe and Effective Care Environment

Which assessment is most important for the nurse to perform before instilling travoprost (Travatan) into the client's eye?

A. Measuring the client's blood pressure
B. Measuring the client's intraocular pressure
C. Checking the cornea for abrasions or open areas
D. Assessing heart rate and rhythm for 1 full minute

RETINAL DISORDERS

MACULAR DEGENERATION

❖ *PATHOPHYSIOLOGY*

Macular degeneration is the deterioration of the macula (the area of central vision) and can be age-related or exudative. Age-related macular degeneration (AMD) has two types. The most common type is *dry* AMD, caused by gradual blockage of retinal capillaries, allowing retinal cells in the macula to become ischemic and necrotic. Central vision declines, and patients describe mild blurring and distortion at first. Eventually the person loses all central vision. About 2.5 million older adults in the United States and Canada have dry AMD (National Eye Institute, 2012). This loss of visual SENSORY PERCEPTION affects independence, well-being, and quality of life. It is often the reason an older adult leaves his or her independent living environment and moves into an assisted-living facility (Touhy & Jett, 2014).

Dry AMD is more common and progresses at a faster rate among smokers than among nonsmokers. Other risk factors include hypertension, female gender, short stature, family history, and a long-term diet poor in carotene and vitamin E.

Another cause of AMD is the growth of new blood vessels in the macula, which have thin walls and leak blood and fluid (*wet* AMD). Exudative macular degeneration is also a type of wet macular degeneration but can occur at any age. The condition can occur in only one eye or in both eyes. The person with dry AMD can also develop exudative macular degeneration. Patients with exudative degeneration have a sudden decrease in vision after a detachment of pigment epithelium in the macula. Newly formed blood vessels invade this injured area and cause fluid and blood to collect under the macula (like a blister), with scar formation and visual distortion.

❖ *PATIENT-CENTERED COLLABORATIVE CARE*

Dry AMD has no cure. Management is focused on slowing the progression of the vision loss and helping the patient maximize remaining vision (Kerr, 2013). The risk for dry AMD can be reduced by increasing long-term dietary intake of antioxidants, vitamin B_{12}, and the carotenoids *lutein* and *zeaxanthin*. The same dietary therapy slows the progression of dry AMD.

Central vision loss reduces the ability to read, write, recognize safety hazards, and drive. Suggest alternatives (e.g., large-print books, public transportation) and referrals to community resources that provide adaptive equipment. See pp. 992-994 of Patient-Centered Collaborative Care in the Reduced Visual Sensory Perception section for discussion of patient care needs.

Management of patients with exudative or wet AMD is geared toward slowing the process and identifying further changes in visual perception. Fluid and blood may resorb in some patients. Laser therapy to seal the leaking blood vessels can limit the extent of the damage. Ocular injections with the vascular endothelial growth factor inhibitors (VEGFIs), such as bevacizumab (Avastin) or ranibizumab (Lucentis), can improve vision for the patient with wet AMD.

NCLEX EXAMINATION CHALLENGE

Health Promotion and Maintenance

Which precaution is most important for the nurse to teach a 62-year-old client newly diagnosed with early-stage dry age-related macular degeneration?

A. Quit smoking
B. Quit drinking alcoholic beverages
C. Eat more dark green, red, and yellow vegetables
D. Wear dark glasses whenever he or she is outside or in bright interior lighting environments

RETINAL HOLES, TEARS, AND DETACHMENTS

❖ *PATHOPHYSIOLOGY*

A **retinal hole** is a break in the retina. These holes can be caused by trauma or can occur with aging. A **retinal tear** is a more jagged and irregularly shaped break in the retina. It can result from traction on the retina. A **retinal detachment** is the separation of the retina from the epithelium. Detachments are classified by the type and cause of their development.

❖ *PATIENT-CENTERED COLLABORATIVE CARE*

The onset of a retinal detachment is usually sudden and painless. Patients may suddenly see bright flashes of light (photopsia) or floating dark spots in the affected eye. During the initial phase of the detachment or if the detachment is partial, the patient may describe the sensation of a curtain being pulled over part of the visual field. The visual field loss corresponds to the area of detachment.

On ophthalmoscopic examination, detachments are seen as gray bulges or folds in the retina. Sometimes a hole or tear may be seen at the edge of the detachment.

If a retinal hole or tear is discovered before it causes a detachment, the defect may be closed or sealed. Closure prevents fluid from collecting under the retina and reduces the risk for a detachment. Treatment involves creating a scar that will bind the retina and choroid together around the break. Common methods to create the scar are with laser photocoagulation or with a freezing probe (cryopexy).

Spontaneous reattachment of a totally detached retina is rare. Surgical repair is needed to place the retina in contact with the underlying structures. A common repair procedure is scleral buckling.

Preoperative Care

The patient is usually anxious and fearful about a possible permanent loss of vision. *Nursing priorities include providing information and reassurance to allay fears.*

Instruct the patient to restrict activity and head movement before surgery to prevent further tearing or detachment. An eye patch is placed over the affected eye to reduce eye movement. Topical drugs are given before surgery to inhibit pupil constriction and accommodation.

Operative Procedures

The surgery is performed with the patient under general anesthesia. In scleral buckling, the ophthalmologist repairs wrinkles or folds in the retina and indents the eye surface to relieve the tugging pressure on the retina. The indentation or "buckling" is performed by placing a small piece of silicone against the outside of the sclera and holding it in place with an encircling band. This device keeps the retina in contact with the choroid for reattachment. Any fluid under the retina is drained.

A gas or silicone oil placed inside the eye can be used to promote retinal reattachment. These agents float up and against the retina to hold it in place until healing occurs.

Postoperative Care

After surgery an eye patch and shield usually are applied. Monitor the patient's vital signs, and check the eye patch and shield for any drainage.

Activity after surgery varies. If gas or oil has been placed in the eye, teach the patient to keep his or her head in the position prescribed by the surgeon to promote reattachment. Teach the patient to report any sudden increase in pain or pain occurring with nausea to the surgeon immediately. Remind the patient to avoid activities that increase intraocular pressure (IOP) (see Table 47-1).

Instruct the patient to avoid reading, writing, and close work, such as sewing, in the first week after surgery because these activities cause rapid eye movements and detachment. Teach him or her the manifestations of INFECTION and detachment (sudden reduced visual acuity, eye pain, pupil that **does not constrict** in response to light) and to notify the surgeon immediately if these manifestations occur.

CLINICAL JUDGMENT CHALLENGE

Safety; Patient-Centered Care QSEN

The patient is a 68-year-old retired college professor who was recently widowed. He lives alone with a cat. His main leisurely activities are reading, using the computer, and listening to classical music. While hiking with a friend, he pulled himself along a rope bridge, assuming a variety of positions. At the far end of the bridge, he stood up and noticed that the vision in his right eye was greatly reduced to the extent that he could see only the bottom half of the visual field. His friend insisted that the patient go immediately to the emergency department. Once there, a large partial retinal detachment is diagnosed. It is treated within the hour with laser therapy and the injection of a gas to the affected eye. He is permitted to go home and instructed to sit upright with his head bent slightly downward for the next 24 hours and then to return to the ophthalmology office. He tells you that he really likes wine and sometimes drinks as much as two bottles in an evening.

1. Should he drive himself home? Why or why not?
2. Is drinking permitted at this time? Why or why not?
3. What will you tell him about a sleeping position?
4. What suggestions and precautions do you have for him about caring for the cat?
5. Which of the leisure-time activities can he perform this evening and which ones should he avoid? Provide a rationale for your choices.

RETINITIS PIGMENTOSA

Several types of retinal disorders can cause progressive degeneration of the retina and lead to loss of visual SENSORY PERCEPTION. Retinitis pigmentosa (RP) is a condition in which retinal nerve cells degenerate and the pigmented cells of the retina grow and move into the sensory areas of the retina, causing further degeneration.

GENETIC/GENOMIC CONSIDERATIONS

Patient-Centered Care QSEN

Different forms of retinitis pigmentosa can be inherited as an autosomal dominant (AD) trait, an autosomal recessive (AR) trait, or an X-linked recessive trait (Online Mendelian Inheritance in Man [OMIM], 2014). Mutations in more than 20 genes have been identified as being responsible for retinitis pigmentosa, and gene testing for more than 800 mutations of the AR and AD forms of the problem is commercially available.

The earliest manifestation of RP is night blindness, often occurring in childhood. Over time, decreased acuity progresses to total blindness. Examination of the retina shows heavy pigmentation in a lacy pattern. Cataracts may accompany this disorder.

No current therapy is effective in preventing the degenerative process. Management strategies focus on protecting active retinal cells and slowing the progression of disease. Teach patients with RP to avoid drugs that are known to adversely affect retinal cells, such as isotretinoin (Accutane) and drugs for erectile dysfunction (e.g., sildenafil [Viagra]). Also remind them to wear eyeglasses that provide ultraviolet protection. The ingestion of 15,000 international units of vitamin A daily is recommended to slow the progression of the disorder, as is the daily ingestion of docosahexaenoic acid (DHA), an omega-3 fatty acid and antioxidant. Additional supplements that may slow the progression of RP include beta carotene, lutein, and zeaxanthin. When macular edema is present, oral acetazolamide (Diamox) can reduce the edema. Cataract surgery and lens replacement is recommended when cataracts further reduce vision. Other treatments under investigation include retinal transplantation, stem cell therapy, and gene therapy (Foundation Fighting Blindness, 2012).

REFRACTIVE ERRORS

❖ PATHOPHYSIOLOGY

The ability of the eye to focus images on the retina depends on the length of the eye from front to back and the refractive power of the lens system. **Refraction** is the bending of light rays. Problems in either eye length or refraction can result in refractive errors.

Myopia is nearsightedness, in which the eye over-refracts the light and the bent images fall in front of, not on, the retina. **Hyperopia**, also called *hypermetropia,* is farsightedness, in which refraction is too weak, causing images to be focused behind the retina. **Presbyopia** is the age-related problem in which the lens loses its elasticity and is less able to change shape to focus the eye for close work. As a result, images fall behind the retina. This problem usually begins in people in their 30s and 40s. **Astigmatism** occurs when the curve of the cornea is uneven. Because light rays are not refracted equally in all directions, the image does not focus on the retina.

❖ PATIENT-CENTERED COLLABORATIVE CARE

Refractive errors are diagnosed through a process known as **refraction**. The patient is asked to view an eye chart while lenses of different strengths are systematically placed in front of the eye. With each lens strength, he or she is asked whether the lenses sharpen or worsen vision. The strength of the lens needed to focus the image on the retina is expressed in measurements called *diopters.*

Nonsurgical Management

Refractive errors are corrected with eyeglass lenses or contact lenses that focus light rays on the retina (see Fig. 46-5 in Chapter 46). Hyperopic vision is corrected with a convex lens that moves the image forward. Myopic vision is corrected with a biconcave lens to move the image back to the retina.

Surgical Management

Surgery can correct some refractive errors and enhance vision. The most common vision-enhancing surgery is laser in-situ keratomileusis (LASIK). This procedure can correct nearsightedness, farsightedness, and astigmatism. The superficial layers of the cornea are lifted temporarily as a flap, and powerful laser pulses reshape the deeper corneal layers. After reshaping is complete, the corneal flap is placed back into its original position.

Usually both eyes are treated at the same time, which is convenient for the patient, although this practice has some risks. Many patients have improved vision within an hour after surgery, and complete healing to best vision takes up to 4 weeks. The outer corneal layer is not damaged, and pain is minimal.

Complications of LASIK include INFECTION, corneal clouding, chronic dry eyes, and refractive errors. Some patients have developed blurred vision, halos around lights, and other refractive errors months to years after this surgery as a result of excessive laser-thinning of the cornea. The cornea then becomes unstable and does not refract appropriately.

Another procedure, corneal ring placement, can enhance vision for nearsightedness, although this procedure is usually performed for keratoconus. For more information about the procedure, see surgical intervention for keratoconus on pp. 981-982.

TRAUMA

Trauma to the eye or orbital area can result from almost any activity. Care varies depending on the area of the eye affected and whether the globe of the eye has been penetrated.

Foreign Bodies

Eyelashes, dust, dirt, and airborne particles can come in contact with the conjunctiva or cornea and irritate or abrade the surface. If nothing is seen on the cornea or conjunctiva, the eyelid is everted to examine the conjunctivae. The patient usually has a feeling of something being in the eye and may have blurred vision. Pain occurs if the corneal surface is injured. Tearing and photophobia may be present.

Visual SENSORY PERCEPTION is assessed before treatment. The eye is examined with fluorescein, followed by irrigation with normal saline (0.9%) to gently remove the particles. Best practices for ocular irrigation are listed in Chart 47-7.

CHART 47-7 Best Practice for Patient Safety & Quality Care QSEN

Ocular Irrigation

1. Assemble equipment:
   - Normal saline IV (1000-mL bag)
   - Macrodrip IV tubing
   - IV pole
   - Eyelid speculum
   - Topical anesthetic (proparacaine hydrochloride)
   - Gloves
   - Collection receptacle (emesis basin works well)
   - Towels
   - pH paper
2. Quickly obtain a history from the patient while flushing the tubing with normal saline:
   - Nature and time of the injury
   - Type of irritant or chemical (if known)
   - Type of first aid administered at the scene
   - Any allergies to the "caine" family of medications
3. Evaluate the patient's visual acuity *before* treatment:
   - Ask the patient to read your name tag with the affected eye while covering the good eye.
   - Ask the patient to "count fingers" with the affected eye while covering the good eye.
4. Put on gloves.
5. Place a strip of pH paper in the cul-de-sac of the patient's affected eye to test the pH of the agent splashed into the eye and to know when it has been washed out.
6. Instill proparacaine hydrochloride eyedrops as prescribed.
7. Place the patient in a supine position with the head turned slightly toward the affected eye.
8. Have the patient hold the affected eye open, or position an eyelid speculum.
9. Direct the flow of normal saline across the affected eye from the nasal corner of the eye toward the outer corner of the eye.
10. Assess the patient's comfort during the procedure.
11. If both eyes are affected, irrigate them simultaneously using separate personnel and equipment.

If an eye patch is applied after the foreign body is removed, tell the patient how long the patch must be left in place. Follow-up with the ophthalmologist is needed.

Lacerations

Lacerations are caused by sharp objects and projectiles. The injury occurs most commonly to the eyelids and cornea, although any part of the eye can be lacerated.

The patient should receive medical attention as soon as possible. Initially the eye is closed and a small ice pack is applied to decrease bleeding. Minor lacerations of the eyelid can be sutured in an emergency department, an urgent care center, or an ophthalmologist's office. A microscope is needed in the operating room if the patient has a laceration that involves the eyelid margin, affects the lacrimal system, involves a large area, or has jagged edges.

Corneal lacerations are an emergency because eye contents may prolapse through the laceration. Manifestations include severe eye pain, photophobia, tearing, decreased vision, and inability to open the eyelid. If the laceration is the result of a penetrating injury, an object may be seen protruding from the eye.

! NURSING SAFETY PRIORITY QSEN

Action Alert

An object protruding from the eye is removed only by an ophthalmologist because it may be holding the eye structures in place. Improper removal can cause structures to prolapse out of the eye.

Antibiotics are given to reduce the risk for INFECTION. Depending on the depth of the laceration, scarring may develop. If the scar alters vision, a corneal transplant may be needed later. If the eye contents have prolapsed through the laceration or if the injury is severe, **enucleation** (surgical eye removal) may be indicated.

Penetrating Injuries

A penetrating eye injury often leads to permanent loss of visual SENSORY PERCEPTION. Glass, high-speed metal or wood particles, BB pellets, and bullets are common causes of penetrating injuries. The particles can enter the eye and lodge in or behind the eyeball.

The patient has eye pain and reports "I suddenly felt something hit my eye." A wound may be visible. Depending on where the object enters and rests within the eye, vision may be affected.

X-rays and CT scans of the orbit are usually performed. *MRI is contraindicated because the procedure may move any metal-containing projectile and cause more injury.*

Surgery is usually needed to remove the foreign object, and sometimes vitreal removal is needed. IV antibiotics are started before surgery, and a tetanus booster is given if necessary.

OCULAR MELANOMA

❖ PATHOPHYSIOLOGY

Melanoma is the most common malignant eye tumor in adults (American Cancer Society, 2014). This tumor occurs most often in the uveal tract among people in their 30s and 40s and is associated with exposure to ultraviolet (UV) light. Because of its rich blood supply, a melanoma can spread by extension through the sclera or invasion into nearby tissue and the brain.

❖ PATIENT-CENTERED COLLABORATIVE CARE

Manifestations of melanoma may not be readily apparent; the tumor may be discovered during a routine examination. Blurred vision may occur if the macular area is invaded. Vision is reduced if the tumor grows inward toward the center of the eye and alters the visual pathway. Increased intraocular pressure (IOP) can result if the tumor obstructs flow of aqueous humor. Iris color changes when the tumor infiltrates the iris. Sudden loss of a visual field may result from tumor invasion that causes retinal detachment.

Diagnostic tests for a melanoma depend on the size and tumor growth rate. Ultrasonography or MRI is performed to determine the tumor's location and size. Treatment depends on the tumor's size and growth rate, as well as the condition of the other eye. Small iris lesions are monitored until growth is observed. Tumors of the choroid are treated by surgical enucleation or by radiation therapy with a radioactive plaque.

Enucleation (surgical removal of the entire eyeball) is the most common surgery for ocular melanoma and is performed under general anesthesia. After the eye is removed, a ball implant is inserted as a base for the socket prosthesis, which is fitted about 1 month after surgery.

Radiation therapy is an "eye-sparing" procedure that can reduce the size and thickness of melanomas and sometimes eliminates the tumor completely. The radioactive plaque—a round, flat disk about the size of a dime and containing a radioactive material—is sutured to the sclera overlying the tumor site. The length of time the plaque remains sutured to the sclera depends on the size of the tumor and the dose of radiation to be delivered (usually 3 to 6 days).

Complications of radiation therapy include vascular changes, retinopathy, glaucoma, necrosis of the sclera, and cataract formation. Vitreous hemorrhage may develop as the tumor becomes smaller and pulls or breaks blood vessels.

While the plaque is in place, an eye patch may or may not be used. Cycloplegic eyedrops and an antibiotic-steroid combination are given. Teach the patient how to instill eyedrops.

REDUCED VISUAL SENSORY PERCEPTION

❖ PATHOPHYSIOLOGY

Different forms of reduced visual SENSORY PERCEPTION may affect color, light, image, eye movement, and acuity. Reduced vision may be temporary, such as when cataracts obscure vision but surgery has not yet been performed. Patients are legally blind if their best visual acuity with corrective lenses is 20/200 or less in the better eye or if the visual field is 20 degrees or less.

Blindness can occur in one or both eyes. When one eye is affected, the field of vision is narrowed and depth perception is impaired.

❖ PATIENT-CENTERED COLLABORATIVE CARE

Priorities for nursing involve safety and teaching the patient with reduced visual SENSORY PERCEPTION some techniques to make better use of existing vision. Moving the head slightly up and down can enhance a three-dimensional effect. When shaking hands or pouring water, the patient can line up the object and move toward it. He or she should choose a position that favors the eye with better vision. For example, people with vision in the right eye should position people and items on their right.

Nursing interventions for the patient with reduced sight focus on communication, safety, ambulation, self-care, and

CHART 47-8 Best Practice for Patient Safety & Quality Care QSEN

Care of the Patient with Reduced Vision

- Always knock or announce your entrance into the patient's room or area and introduce yourself.
- Ensure that all members of the health care team also use this courtesy of announcement and introduction.
- Ensure that the patient's reduced vision is noted in the medical record, is communicated to all staff, is marked on the call board, and is identified on the door of the patient's room.
- Determine to what degree the patient can see anything.
- Orient the patient to the environment, counting steps with him or her to the bathroom.
- Assist the patient in placing objects on the bedside table or in the bed and around the bed and room, and do not move them without the patient's permission.
- Remove all objects and clutter between the patient's bed and the bathroom.
- Ask the patient what type of assistance he or she prefers for grooming, toileting, eating, and ambulating, and communicate these preferences with the staff.
- Describe food placement on a plate in terms of a clock face.
- Open milk cartons; open salt, pepper, and condiment packages; and remove lids from cups and bowls.
- Unless the patient also has a hearing problem, use a normal tone of voice when speaking.
- When walking with the patient, offer him or her your arm and walk a step ahead.

support. Chart 47-8 lists ways to help patients with reduced vision to function as independently as possible.

Communication is important in helping the patient remain independent and connected to the world. Many adaptive devices are available to help the person with reduced vision maintain independence. Many cities have auditory traffic signals so that people with reduced vision can know when it is safe to cross a street. Curbs in these areas may have high-contrast color paint to let the person know when to step up or down. Libraries have large-print books and books on disc. "Talking" clocks, watches, and timers are available. Playing cards, games, restaurant menus, calendars, and instruction booklets are available in large print sizes using bold black print, sans-serif fonts, and white or yellow backgrounds (Russo & Bowden, 2013). Computer keyboards with high contrast and larger letters on the keys are available, as are large screens. Direct the patient with reduced vision to the local resources to obtain adaptive items and to learn how to use them (Warren, 2013).

Safety is a major issue for the person with reduced vision. For most patients, home is the place where they feel most safe because they are familiar with room and item location. For example, they may have counted the number of footsteps needed to move from one area to another. Stress to family members not to change item locations without input from the patient. Teach family members with vision to make these home adaptations to increase the patient's independence and safety:

- Using tape and a heavy black marker, mark the 350-degree temperature setting on the oven and mark the 70-degree temperature setting on the heating or cooling thermostat.
- Paint or mark light switches in a deep color that contrasts with the surrounding wall.
- Label canned goods with large, bold, black letters on white tape.
- Teach the patient to feel for the crease in paper milk cartons that indicates the place to open the spout.
- Differentiate different drugs by altering the shape of a bottle. Rubber bands can be wound around a bottle to change its texture. Raised symbols can be glued to caps to make identification easier.

The patient with reduced visual SENSORY PERCEPTION is most at risk for safety problems in an unfamiliar or changing environment. When he or she must be hospitalized, promote safety and independence by orienting him or her to the new environment.

Many people with reduced vision had sight at some time and have background knowledge regarding size and shape that can be used when providing information. When talking with a person who has limited vision, use a normal tone of voice unless he or she also has a hearing problem.

First orient the patient to the immediate environment, including the size of the room. Use one object in the room, such as a chair or hospital bed, as the focal point for the description. Guide the person to the focal point, and orient him or her to the environment from that point. For example, you might say "To the left of the bed is a chair." Then describe all other objects in relation to the focal point. Go with the patient to the bathroom so that he or she can learn this location. Highlight the location of the toilet, sink, and toilet paper. Use specific descriptors, and avoid gestures or vague language (Warren, 2013). For example, say "the wall to the right of the door" instead of "over there."

! NURSING SAFETY PRIORITY QSEN

Action Alert

Never leave the patient with reduced vision in the center of an unfamiliar room.

Patients with reduced vision prefer to establish the location of important objects, such as the call light, water pitcher, and clock. Once their location has been fixed, do not move these items without the patient's consent. Do not move the location of chairs, stools, and wastebaskets without consulting the patient.

At mealtime, set up food on the tray using clock placement. For example, "There is sliced ham at the 6 o'clock position; peas are located at the 3 o'clock position; to the right of the plate is coffee; salt and pepper are next to the coffee."

Ambulation with a patient who has reduced vision is best when he or she holds your arm at the elbow. Keep the arm close to your body so that the patient can detect your direction of movement. Alert him or her when obstacles are in the path ahead.

Patients may use a cane to detect obstacles, such as furniture, walls, or curbs. The cane is held several inches off the floor and sweeps the ground where the foot will be placed next. The laser cane sends out signals to help detect obstacles.

Self-care and the ability to control the environment are important. Knock on the door before entering the hospital room or any other environment of a patient with reduced vision. State your name and the reason for visiting when entering the room. Coordinate with other members of the health care team to ensure this etiquette is used consistently. Mark the door to the room to indicate it is occupied by a person with reduced visual SENSORY PERCEPTION.

Support is needed, especially when the reduced vision occurs suddenly and may be permanent. The reactions are similar to the reaction to loss of a body part. Allow the newly blind person a period of grieving for the "dead" (nonseeing) eye. He or she may feel hopeless and angry. The ability to cope may begin within days, but some patients mourn for months or years.

Patients benefit from the honest support that you can provide. They need to hear that it is normal to mourn, to cry, and to feel the loss. Help them move toward acceptance by encouraging the mastery of one task at a time and by providing positive reinforcement for each success.

NCLEX EXAMINATION CHALLENGE

Safe and Effective Care Environment

Which action by a nurse is most likely to increase accurate communication with a client who has low vision?

A. Speaking slowly and loudly
B. Enhancing the talk using hand gestures
C. Being very specific with descriptions and directions
D. Marking the door of the client's room to indicate his or her vision status

NURSING CONCEPTS AND CLINICAL JUDGMENT REVIEW

What might you NOTICE if the patient is experiencing reduced visual SENSORY PERCEPTION?

Assessment:

- Patient squints or tilts the head when viewing objects or print at a distance.
- Patient closes one eye to read or see at a distance.
- Patient moves reading materials either very close to his or her face or as far away from the face as he or she can reach.
- Patient may not startle when a sudden move is made at the face.
- Pupils are unequal and may not react to light.
- Eyes do not focus on a distant object and track it as it is moved closer to the face.
- Red reflex may be absent or present in only one eye.
- Patient does not make eye contact and turns head toward sounds rather than sights.
- Patient walks with hesitation into a room or bumps into objects in his or her path.
- Patient may seem confused about time and place.

What should you INTERPRET and how should you RESPOND to a patient experiencing reduced visual SENSORY PERCEPTION?

Interpret by:

- Assessing visual acuity with an eye chart, counting fingers, hand motion, or light perception
- Asking the patient to describe the objects in the room and their colors
- Asking the patient what he or she can see well and what is more difficult to see

Respond by:

- Orienting the patient to the immediate surroundings
- Offering your arm for the patient to hold when he or she is moving to a different location
- Not leaving the patient alone in the center of a strange room
- Asking him or her what assistance is needed for independent activity
- Assessing the immediate environment for safety hazards and removing the hazard

On what should you REFLECT?

- Consider what environmental changes could make the unit safer or more manageable for a person with reduced vision.

GET READY FOR THE NCLEX® EXAMINATION!

KEY POINTS

Review these Key Points for each NCLEX Examination Client Needs Category.

Safe and Effective Care Environment

- Use aseptic technique when performing an eye examination or instilling drugs into the eye. **Safety** QSEN
- Apply the principles of INFECTION control when caring for a patient with an eye infection. **Safety** QSEN
- Avoid performing an ophthalmoscopic examination on a confused patient. **Safety** QSEN
- Orient the patient with reduced vision to his or her immediate surroundings, including how to call for help and where the bathroom is located. **Safety** QSEN
- Identify the room of a patient with reduced vision. **Safety** QSEN
- Never administer a topical ophthalmic liquid or ointment by the oral route. **Safety** QSEN

Health Promotion and Maintenance

- Identify people at risk for visual SENSORY PERCEPTION problems as a result of work environment or leisure activities, and teach them specific ways to protect the eyes. **Patient-Centered Care** QSEN
- Encourage all patients to wear eye protection when they are performing yard work, are working in a woodshop or metal shop, are using chemicals, or are in any environment in which drops or particulate matter is airborne.
- Encourage all adult patients older than 40 years and those with chronic disorders that affect the eye and vision to have an eye examination with measurement of intraocular pressure every year. **Patient-Centered Care** QSEN
- Encourage everyone to use polarizing sunglasses whenever outdoors in the daytime. **Patient-Centered Care** QSEN
- Teach all patients to wash their hands before and after touching the eyes. **Patient-Centered Care** QSEN

- Teach family members who have good vision to make the adaptations for the patient's home listed on p. 993 to increase the patient's independence and safety. **Patient-Centered Care** QSEN

Psychosocial Integrity

- Teach patients and family members about what to expect during procedures to correct visual SENSORY PERCEPTION and eye problems.
- Provide opportunities for the patient and family to express concerns about a change in visual SENSORY PERCEPTION.
- Refer the patient with reduced visual SENSORY PERCEPTION to local services, resources, and support groups for the blind and those with low vision. **Patient-Centered Care** QSEN
- Teach the patient with reduced visual SENSORY PERCEPTION techniques for performing ADLs and self-care independently. **Patient-Centered Care** QSEN
- Use a normal tone of voice to talk with a patient who has a vision problem and normal hearing.
- Knock on the door before entering the room of a patient with reduced visual SENSORY PERCEPTION and introduce yourself. **Patient-Centered Care** QSEN

Physiological Integrity

- Ask the patient about vision problems in any other members of the family, because many vision problems have a genetic component. **Evidence-Based Practice** QSEN
- Teach patients the proper techniques for self-instillation of eyedrops and eye ointment. **Safety** QSEN
- Stress the importance of completing an antibiotic regimen for an eye INFECTION. **Evidence-Based Practice** QSEN
- When instilling more than one type of eyedrop into the same eye, wait 5 to 10 minutes (or as directed by the manufacturer) between instillations. **Evidence-Based Practice** QSEN
- Teach patients who are at risk for increased intraocular pressure (IOP) what activities to avoid (see Table 47-1). **Patient-Centered Care** QSEN
- Teach patients with an INFECTION of the eye or eyelid not to rub the eye (to avoid infecting the other eye). **Evidence-Based Practice** QSEN
- Instruct the patient who has cataract surgery to report immediately any reduction in vision after initial improvement in vision in the eye that had cataract surgery. **Patient-Centered Care** QSEN
- Stress the importance of using antiglaucoma eyedrop agents exactly as prescribed to prevent IOP from increasing and to prevent complications of glaucoma drug therapy. **Patient-Centered Care** QSEN
- Never attempt to remove any object protruding from the eye. **Safety** QSEN
- Use and teach punctal occlusion technique when administering antiglaucoma eyedrops. **Safety** QSEN
- Work with the physician, occupational therapist, social worker, and other health care professionals to increase the patient's independence and safety within the home and the community. **Teamwork and Collaboration** QSEN

48 CHAPTER

Assessment and Care of Patients with Ear and Hearing Problems

M. Linda Workman

http://evolve.elsevier.com/Iggy/

PRIORITY CONCEPTS

- Sensory Perception

LEARNING OUTCOMES

Safe and Effective Care Environment

1. Protect the patient with ear and hearing problems from injury and infection.

Health Promotion and Maintenance

2. Teach all people how to protect the ear and hearing.
3. Teach patients who need them how to use hearing assistive devices.

Psychosocial Integrity

4. Reduce the psychological impact for the patient and family experiencing a potential change in auditory sensory perception.
5. Work with other members of the health care team to ensure that the values, preferences, and expressed needs of the patient with reduced auditory sensory perception are respected.

Physiological Integrity

6. Perform a focused assessment of the ear and auditory sensory perception, incorporating information about anatomy and physiology, genetic risk, environmental risk, and age-related changes affecting the ear and hearing.
7. Use laboratory data and clinical manifestations to evaluate and prioritize the nursing care needs for the patient with a problem of the ear or hearing.
8. Prioritize the nursing care and educational needs of the patient with Ménière's disease.
9. Prioritize nursing care and educational needs for the patient after ear surgery.
10. Collaborate with other health care professionals to help patients and families experiencing reduced auditory sensory perception achieve desired health outcomes.

Together, the ear and the brain allow auditory sensory perception. Hearing is one of the five senses important for cognition and communicating with others. It is used to assess surroundings, allow independence, warn of danger, appreciate music, work, play, and interact with other people.

Ear and hearing problems are common among adults of all ages. Assessment of the ear and hearing is an important skill for nurses in any care environment. Many ear and hearing problems develop over long periods and may be affected by drugs or systemic health problems. Auditory sensory perception problems reduce the ability to fully communicate with the world and can lead to confusion, mistrust, and social isolation.

ANATOMY AND PHYSIOLOGY REVIEW

Structure

The ear has three divisions: the external ear, the middle ear, and the inner ear. Each part is important to hearing.

External Ear

The external ear develops in the embryo at the same time as the kidneys and urinary tract. Thus any person with a defect of the external ear should be examined for possible problems of the kidney and urinary systems.

The *pinna* is the part of the external ear that is composed of cartilage covered by skin and attached to the head at about a 10-degree angle at the level of the eyes. The external ear extends from the pinna through the external ear canal to the *tympanic membrane* (eardrum) (Fig. 48-1). The external ear includes the *mastoid process,* which is the bony ridge located over the temporal bone behind the pinna. The ear canal is slightly S-shaped and lined with cerumen-producing glands, oil glands, and hair follicles. Cerumen (ear "wax") helps protect and lubricate the ear canal. The distance from the opening of the ear canal to the eardrum in an adult is 1 to 1½ inches (2.5 to 3.75 cm).

Middle Ear

The eardrum separates the external ear and the middle ear. The middle ear consists of a compartment called the *epitympanum.*

Located in the epitympanum are the top opening of the eustachian tube and three small bones known as the *bony ossicles,* which are the *malleus* (hammer), the *incus* (anvil), and the *stapes* (stirrup) (Fig. 48-2). The bony ossicles are joined loosely, thereby moving with vibrations created when sound waves hit the eardrum.

The eardrum is a thick sheet of tissue; is transparent, opaque, or pearly gray; and moves when air is injected into the external canal. The landmarks on the eardrum include the *annulus,* the *pars flaccida,* and the *pars tensa.* These correspond to the parts of the malleus that can be seen through the transparent eardrum. The eardrum is attached to the first bony ossicle, the malleus, at the umbo (Fig. 48-3). The umbo is seen through the eardrum membrane as a white dot and is one end of the long process of the malleus. The pars flaccida is that portion of the eardrum above the short process of the malleus. The pars tensa is that portion surrounding the long process of the malleus.

The middle ear is separated from the inner ear by the round window and the oval window. The eustachian tube begins at the floor of the middle ear and extends to the throat. The tube opening in the throat is surrounded by adenoid lymphatic tissue (Fig. 48-4). The eustachian tube allows the pressure on both sides of the eardrum to equalize. Secretions from the middle ear drain through the tube into the throat.

Inner Ear

The inner ear is on the other side of the oval window and contains the semicircular canals, the cochlea, the vestibule, and the

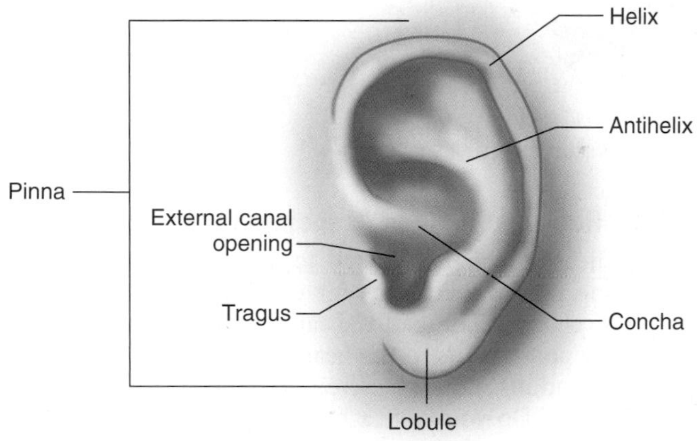

FIG. 48-1 Anatomic features of the external ear.

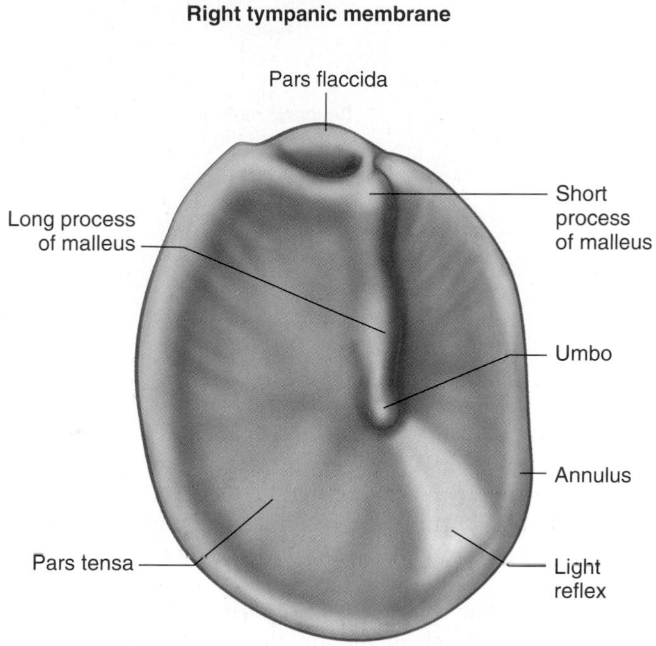

FIG. 48-3 Landmarks on the tympanic membrane.

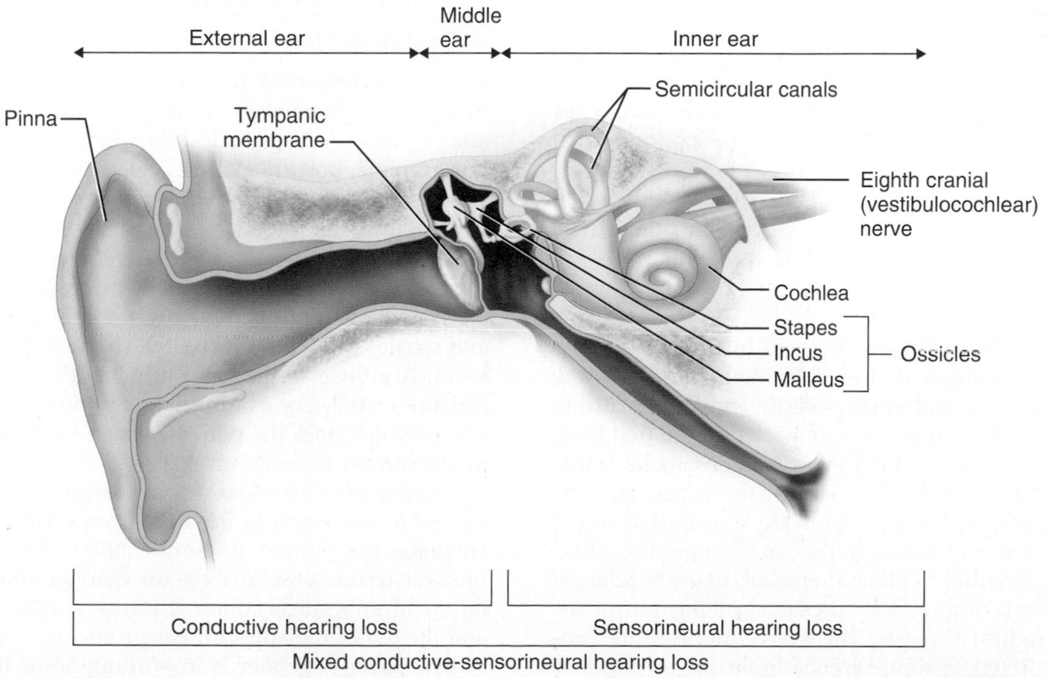

FIG. 48-2 Anatomic features of the middle and inner ear and areas involved in the three types of hearing loss.

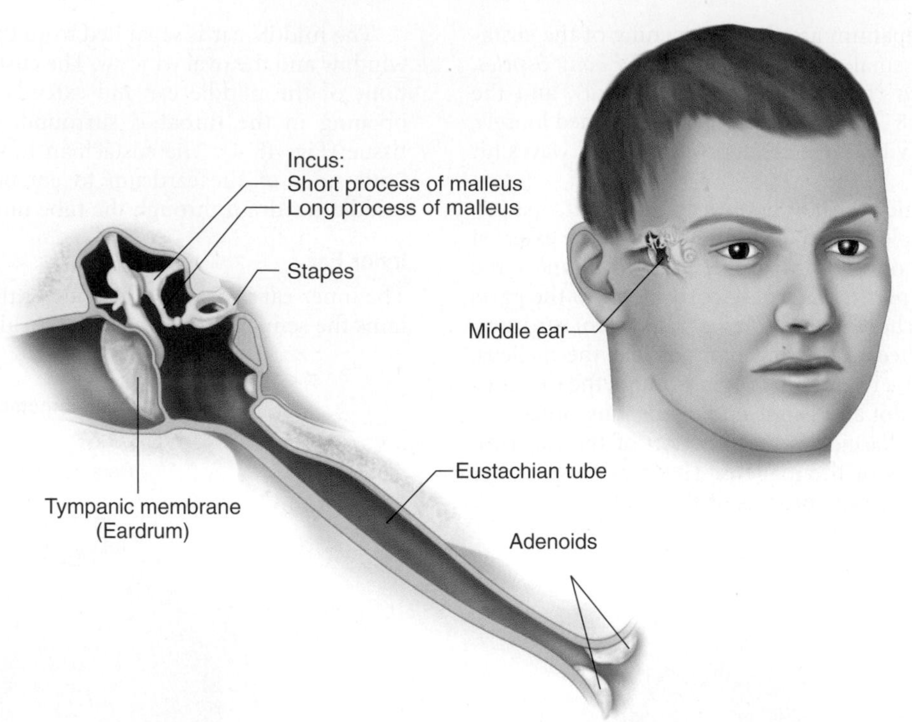

FIG. 48-4 Anatomic features and attached structures of the middle ear.

distal end of the eighth cranial nerve (see Fig. 48-2). The *semicircular canals* are tubes made of cartilage and contain fluid and hair cells. These canals are connected to the sensory nerve fibers of the vestibular portion of the eighth cranial nerve. The fluid and hair cells within the canals help maintain the sense of balance.

The *cochlea,* the spiral organ of hearing, is divided into the scala tympani, the scala media, and the scala vestibuli. The scala media is filled with *endolymph,* and the scala tympani and scala vestibuli are filled with *perilymph.* These fluids protect the cochlea and the semicircular canals by allowing these structures to "float" in the fluids and be cushioned against abrupt head movements.

The *organ of Corti* is the receptor of hearing located on the membrane of the cochlea. The cochlear hair cells detect vibration from sound and stimulate the eighth cranial nerve.

The *vestibule* is a small, oval-shaped, bony chamber between the semicircular canals and the cochlea. It contains the utricle and the saccule, organs that are important for balance.

Function

Auditory SENSORY PERCEPTION is the main function of the ear and occurs when sound is delivered through the air to the external ear canal. The sound waves strike the movable eardrum, creating vibrations. The eardrum is connected to the first bony ossicle, which allows the sound wave vibrations to be transferred from the eardrum to the malleus, the incus, and the stapes. From the stapes, the vibrations are transmitted to the cochlea. Receptors at the cochlea transduce (change) the vibrations into action potentials. The action potentials are conducted to the brain as nerve impulses by the cochlear portion of the eighth cranial (auditory) nerve. The nerve impulses are processed and interpreted as sound by the brain in the auditory cortex of the temporal lobe.

Ear and Hearing Changes Associated with Aging

Ear and hearing changes related to aging are listed in Chart 48-1, along with implications for care of older patients who have these changes. Some of the ear changes are harmless, and others may pose threats to the hearing ability of older adults.

All older adults should be screened for hearing acuity, starting by asking "Do you have a hearing problem now?" Family members may have noticed behaviors that suggest changes in a patient's hearing.

ASSESSMENT METHODS

Patient History

Hearing assessment begins while observing the patient listening to and answering questions (Jarvis, 2016). The patient's posture and responses can provide information about hearing acuity. For example, posture changes, such as tilting the head to one side or leaning forward when listening to another person speak, may indicate the presence of a hearing problem. Other indicators of hearing difficulty include frequently asking the speaker to repeat statements or frequently saying "What?" or "Huh?" Notice whether the patient responds to whispered questions and startles when an unexpected sound occurs in the environment. Also assess whether the patient's responses match the question asked. For example, when you ask the patient "How old are you?" does the patient respond with an age or does he or she say "No, I don't have a cold."

During the interview, sit in adequate light and face the patient to allow him or her to see you speak. Use short, simple language the patient is comfortable with rather than long medical terms. Obtain data on demographics, personal and family history, socioeconomic status, current health problems, and the use of remedies for ear problems.

The patient's gender is important. Some hearing disorders, such as otosclerosis, are more common in women. Other

CHART 48-1 **Nursing Focus on the Older Adult**

Age-Related Changes in the Ear and Hearing

EAR OR HEARING CHANGE	NURSING ADAPTATIONS AND ACTIONS
Pinna becomes elongated because of loss of subcutaneous tissues and decreased elasticity.	Reassure the patient that this is normal. When positioning a patient on the side, do not "fold" the ear under the head.
Hair in the canal becomes coarser and longer, especially in men.	Reassure the patient that this is normal. More frequent ear irrigation may be needed to prevent cerumen clumping.
Cerumen is drier and impacts more easily, reducing hearing function.	Teach the patient to irrigate the ear canal weekly or whenever he or she notices a change in hearing.
Tympanic membrane loses elasticity and may appear dull and retracted.	Do not use this finding as the only indication of otitis media.
Hearing acuity decreases (in some people).	Assess hearing with the voice test or the watch test. If a deficit is present, refer the patient to a specialist to determine hearing loss and appropriate intervention. Do not assume all older adults have a hearing loss!!
The ability to hear high-frequency sounds is lost first. Older adults may have particular problems hearing the *f, s, sh,* and *pa* sounds.	Provide a quiet environment when speaking (close the door to the hallway), and face the patient. If the patient wears glasses, be sure he or she is using them to enhance speech understanding. Speak slowly and in a deeper voice, and emphasize beginning word sounds. Some patients with a hearing loss that is not corrected may benefit from wearing a stethoscope while listening to you speak.

disorders, such as Ménière's disease, are more common in men. Age is also an important factor in hearing loss.

Personal history includes past or current manifestations of ear pain, ear discharge, **vertigo** (spinning sensation), **tinnitus** (ringing), decreased hearing, and difficulty understanding people when they talk. Ask the patient about:

- Ear trauma or surgery
- Past ear infections
- Excessive cerumen
- Ear itch
- Any invasive instruments routinely used to clean the ear (e.g., Q-tip, match, bobby pin, key)
- Type and pattern of ear hygiene
- Exposure to loud noise or music
- Air travel (especially in unpressurized aircraft)
- Swimming habits and the use of ear protection when swimming
- History of health problems that can decrease the blood supply to the ear such as heart disease, hypertension, or diabetes
- History of vitiligo (a pigment disorder that may include a loss of melanin-containing cells in the inner ear, resulting in hearing loss)
- History of smoking
- History of vitamin B_{12} and folate deficiency

If the patient uses foreign objects to clean the ear canal, explain the danger in using these objects. They can scrape the skin of the canal, push cerumen up against the eardrum, and even puncture the eardrum. If the patient says that cerumen buildup is a problem, teach him or her to use an ear irrigation syringe and proper solutions to remove it. Chart 48-2 describes techniques to teach patients how to remove cerumen safely.

! NURSING SAFETY PRIORITY (QSEN)

Action Alert

Teach patients the safe way to clean their ears, stressing that nothing smaller than his or her own fingertip should be inserted into the canal.

CHART 48-2 **Patient and Family Education: Preparing for Self-Management**

Self–Ear Irrigation for Cerumen Removal

- *Do not attempt to remove earwax or irrigate the ears if you have ear tubes or if you have blood, pus, or other drainage from the ear.*
- Use an ear syringe designed for the purpose of wax removal (available at most drugstores).
- The safest type of ear syringe to use is one that has a right-angle or "elbow" in the tip.
- Irrigating your ears in the shower is an easy method.
- Always use tap water that feels just barely warm to you. Water that is warmer or colder can make you feel dizzy and nauseated.
- If your earwax is thick and sticky, you may need to place a few warm commercial eardrops that soften earwax (or baby oil or mineral oil) into the ear an hour or so before you irrigate the ear.
- Fill the syringe with the lukewarm tap water.
- If you are using a syringe with an elbow tip, place only the last part of the tip into your ear and aim it toward the roof of your ear canal.
- If you are using a straight-tipped syringe, insert the tip only about ½ to ¾ inch into your ear canal, aiming toward the roof of the canal.
- Hold your head at a 30-degree angle to the side you are irrigating.
- Use one hand to hold the syringe and the other to push the plunger or squeeze the bulb.
- Apply gentle but firm continuous pressure, allowing the water to flow against the top of the canal.
- *Do not use blasts or bursts of sudden pressure.*
- The ear canal should fill, and water will begin to flow out, bringing earwax and debris with it.
- If a dental water-pressure irrigator is used, put it on the lowest possible setting.
- This process should not be painful! If pain occurs, decrease the pressure. If pain persists, stop the irrigation.
- Continue the irrigation until at least a cup of solution has washed into and out from your ear canal. (You may have to refill the syringe.)
- Tilting your head at a 90-degree angle to the side should allow most, if not all, of the water to drain out of your ear.
- Repeat the procedure on the other ear.
- If you feel that water is still in the canal, hold a hair dryer on a low setting near the ear.
- Irrigate your ears weekly to monthly, depending on how fast your earwax collects.

If the patient uses a hearing aid, assess whether hearing is improved with its use. Obtain the date of the last hearing test, the type of test given, and the results. Ask about problems that may impair auditory SENSORY PERCEPTION such as allergies, upper respiratory infections, hypothyroidism, atherosclerosis, head trauma, and recent head, facial, or dental surgery. A thorough drug history is important because many drugs are **ototoxic** (damaging to the ear), especially many antibiotics, some diuretics, NSAIDs, and many chemotherapy agents. Use a drug handbook to determine whether any of the patient's prescribed drugs are known to affect auditory SENSORY PERCEPTION.

Ask about the patient's occupation and hobbies that involve exposure to loud noise or music. Assess whether protective ear devices are used. Also ask whether any devices are consistently inserted into the ear, such as ear plugs or earpiece headsets, and for how long each day they are used. Use this opportunity to teach the patient about protecting the ears from loud noises by wearing protective ear devices, such as over-the-ear headsets or foam ear inserts, when persistent loud noises are in the environment. Also suggest the use of earplugs when engaging in water sports to prevent ear infections.

Family History and Genetic Risk

Family history, as well as personal history, is important in determining genetic risk for hearing loss. Although most hearing loss as a result of a genetic mutation is seen in childhood, some genetic problems can lead to progressive hearing loss in adults. For example, most people with Down syndrome develop hearing loss as adults. People with osteogenesis imperfecta have bilateral and progressive hearing loss by their 30s.

GENETIC/GENOMIC CONSIDERATIONS

Patient-Centered Care QSEN

Mutations in several different genes are associated with hearing loss. One type of hearing loss among adults has a genetic basis with a mutation in gene *GJB2* (Online Mendelian Inheritance in Man [OMIM], 2014). This mutation causes poor production of the protein *connexin-26,* which has a role in the function of cochlear hair cells. Other genetic variations in some of the genes for drug-metabolizing enzymes (cytochrome p450) family) slow the metabolism and excretion of drugs, including ototoxic drugs. This allows ototoxic drugs to remain in the body longer, thus increasing the risk for hearing loss.

Ask the patient:

- Who in your family has hearing problems?
- Are the hearing problems present in men and women equally, or are they present more in one gender?
- At what age was hearing loss diagnosed in your relative(s)?
- Are both ears affected?

Current Health Problems

Assess current ear-related problems by asking about any ear "trouble," ear pain, or discharge, including earwax. Ask about a change in hearing, such as **hyperacusis** (the intolerance for sound levels that do not bother other people), or **tinnitus** (ringing in the ears). If a change in hearing is reported, ask whether one or both ears are involved and if the change was sudden or gradual. Also ask about problems with dizziness, sensations of being "off-balance," or vertigo.

Physical Assessment

Begin the examination by having the patient sit or lie down. Remove any hearing aids before the examination. After the examination, inspect the hearing aid for cracks, debris, and a proper fit. A complete ear examination is usually performed by a physician, advanced practice nurse, or physician assistant. The brief assessment of the ear and hearing usually performed by a medical-surgical nurse is described next.

External Ear and Mastoid Assessment

Inspect the entire external ear for shape, location of attachment to the head, and condition of all visible ear structures. The normal pinna has no skin tags or deformity. It should be attached to the side of the head at a posterior angle of 10 degrees or less. The normal external canal is dry, clean, free from lesions, and not reddened.

Abnormalities of the pinna include swelling, nodules, and lesions (Jarvis, 2016). In chronic gout, collections of uric acid crystals result in hard, irregular, painless nodules called *tophi* on the pinna. Other nodules on the pinna might also be from basal cell carcinoma or rheumatoid arthritis. Small, crusted, ulcerated, or indurated lesions on the pinna that fail to heal could be squamous cell carcinoma.

Inspect the mastoid process for redness and swelling. To assess for tenderness, gently tap with one finger over the mastoid process, compress the tragus with one finger, and gently move the pinna forward and backward. Any tenderness suggests an inflammation in either the external ear or the mastoid.

Assess for and record these problems:

- Furuncles
- Large amounts of cerumen
- Scaliness
- Redness
- Swelling of the ear
- Drainage and its character

Otoscopic Assessment

The purpose of a brief otoscopic examination is to assess the patency of the external canal, identify lesions or excessive cerumen in the canal, and assess whether the tympanic membrane (eardrum) is intact or inflamed (Jarvis, 2016). An instrument called an **otoscope** is used to examine the ear. Many types are available. It consists of a light, a handle, a magnifying lens, and a pressure bulb for injecting air into the external canal to test mobility of the eardrum (Fig. 48-5). Specula of various diameters attach to the head of the otoscope. Select the largest speculum that most comfortably fits the patient's external canal.

NURSING SAFETY PRIORITY QSEN

Action Alert

Do not use an otoscope to examine the ears of any patient who is unable to hold his or her head still during the examination or who is confused.

If the patient has pain during the external ear examination, cautiously attempt an otoscopic examination. The speculum will cause extreme pain if it comes in contact with inflamed tissue in the external canal.

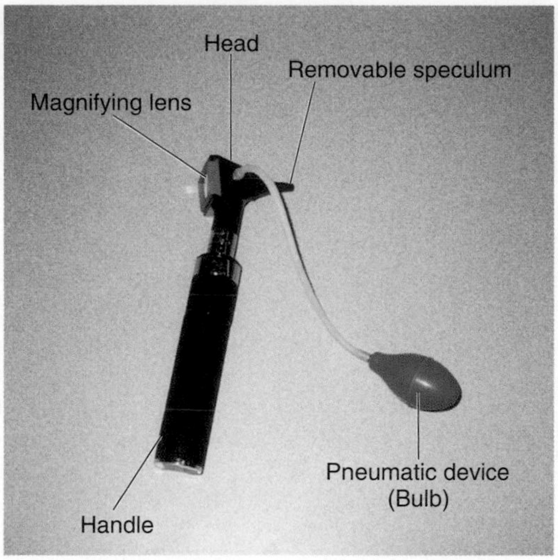

FIG. 48-5 Functional components of an otoscope.

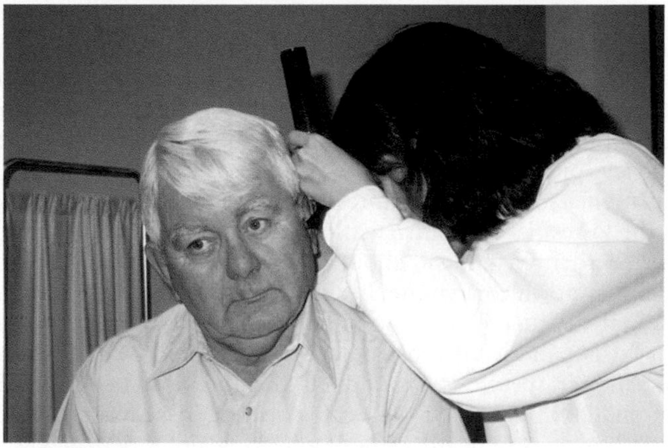

FIG. 48-6 Proper technique for an otoscopic examination.

Tilt the patient's head slightly away, and hold the otoscope upside down, like a large pen (Fig. 48-6). This position permits your hand to lie against the patient's head for support. If the patient moves, both your hand and the otoscope also move, preventing damage to the canal or eardrum. Hold the otoscope in your dominant hand, and gently pull the pinna up and back with your other hand to straighten the canal. View the ear canal while you slowly insert the speculum. Use caution to avoid causing pain by touching the speculum on the walls of the canal.

NURSING SAFETY PRIORITY QSEN

Action Alert

Observe the ear canal through the otoscope as you insert the speculum into the external canal to avoid the risk for perforating the eardrum.

After the otoscope is comfortably in the external canal, assess for lesions and the amount, consistency, and color of cerumen and hair. The normal external canal is skin-colored, intact, and without lesions. It contains various amounts of soft cerumen and small, fine hairs.

Assess the eardrum for intactness and color. *The normal eardrum is always intact.* The eardrum is shiny, transparent or opaque, pearly gray, and without lesions. Redness is seen in otitis media. Reflection of the otoscope's light from the normal eardrum is the **light reflex**, and it appears as a clearly outlined triangle of light. On the right eardrum, the light reflex appears in the right lower quadrant. On the left eardrum, the light reflex appears in the left lower quadrant. The light reflex is termed **diffuse** when the light reflex is spotty or multiple because of a changed eardrum shape.

CULTURAL CONSIDERATIONS

Patient-Centered Care QSEN

Cerumen is generally moist and tan or brown in white people and black people. It is dry and light brown to gray in Asians and American Indians. The color of the lining of the external ear canal varies with the patient's skin tone. Variations should not be mistaken for indications of problems. Patients with more moist earwax form cerumen impactions more easily than patients with drier, flaky earwax and require more frequent ear irrigations.

General Hearing Assessment

Several rapid and simple tests for acuity of auditory SENSORY PERCEPTION can be performed at the patient's bedside. Although these tests do not determine the true extent or type of hearing loss, they can indicate a patient's functional hearing ability.

The *voice test* for hearing is conducted by asking the patient to block one external ear canal while standing 1 to 2 feet (30 to 60 cm) away. Quietly whisper a statement, and then ask the patient to repeat it. Test each ear separately. If the patient does not respond correctly, use a louder whisper. If you suspect the patient is lip-reading, use your hand to block the view of your mouth or stand behind him or her while whispering. More complex hearing tests, performed by audiologists, physicians, advanced practice nurses, specialty nurses, and physician assistants, can determine the type and extent of hearing loss.

Sound is transmitted by air conduction and bone conduction. Air conduction of sound is normally more sensitive than bone conduction. If auditory SENSORY PERCEPTION is decreased, the hearing loss is categorized as:

- **Conductive hearing loss**, resulting from obstruction of sound wave transmission such as a foreign body in the external canal, a retracted or bulging tympanic membrane, or fused bony ossicles.
- **Sensorineural hearing loss**, resulting from a defect in the cochlea, the eighth cranial nerve, or the brain. Exposure to loud noise or music causes this type of hearing loss by damaging the cochlear hair.
- **Mixed conductive-sensorineural hearing loss**, resulting from both conductive and sensorineural hearing loss.

Audioscopy testing involves the use of a handheld device to generate tones of varying intensities to test hearing. Auditory SENSORY PERCEPTION can be measured at a 40-decibel (dB) intensity at frequencies of 500, 1000, 2000, and 4000 cycles per second (cps), or hertz (Hz).

Tuning fork tests for hearing are the Weber and Rinne tests. These tests are useful, although limited, in distinguishing between conductive and sensorineural hearing losses. The frequency range of the tuning fork used for these tests corresponds to that of normal speech.

The Weber tuning fork test is performed by placing a vibrating tuning fork on the middle of the patient's head and asking him or her to indicate in which ear the sound is louder. The normal test result is sound heard equally in both ears. The term *lateralization* is used if the sound is louder in one ear. For example, lateralization to the right means that the sound is heard louder in the right ear.

The Rinne tuning fork test compares hearing by air conduction with hearing by bone conduction. Sound is normally heard 2 to 3 times longer by air conduction than by bone conduction. Perform this test by placing the vibrating tuning fork stem on the mastoid process (bone conduction) and asking the patient to indicate when the sound is no longer heard. When the patient no longer hears the sound, bring the fork quickly in front of the pinna (air conduction) without touching the patient. He or she should then indicate when this sound is no longer heard. The patient normally continues to hear the sound 2 to 3 times longer in front of the pinna after not hearing it with the tuning fork touching the mastoid process.

Psychosocial Assessment

The patient may become frustrated and depressed by an inability to hear well. Reduced or lost hearing may lead to social isolation. Be sensitive to the patient, and conduct the interview at a pace appropriate for that person.

Ask about social and work relationships to determine whether the patient is isolated because of hearing problems. Encourage the patient to express feelings related to hearing loss and discuss any changes in ADLs that have been made as a result of a change in hearing. Ask family members whether hearing problems have changed the patient's interactions.

NCLEX EXAMINATION CHALLENGE

Safe and Effective Care Environment

With which client does the nurse avoid performing an otoscopic examination?

A. 34-year-old woman who is pregnant
B. 90-year-old woman who is visually impaired
C. 75-year-old man with dizziness and vertigo
D. 70-year-old man with advanced Alzheimer's disease

Diagnostic Assessment

Laboratory Assessment

Laboratory tests are helpful only when an external or internal ear infection is suspected. For an external ear infection, the typical causative organisms are known and this infection is managed without obtaining cultures. If the usual antibiotic therapy is not successful at clearing the infection, microbial culture and antibiotic sensitivity tests may be performed.

Imaging Assessment

CT, with or without contrast enhancement, shows the structures of the ear in great detail. CT is especially helpful in diagnosing acoustic tumors.

MRI most accurately reflects soft-tissue changes. Patients with older internal metal vascular clips cannot have MRI. Newer clips are made from titanium and are not a contraindication for MRI.

Specific Auditory Assessment

Audiometry. Audiometry is the most reliable method of measuring the acuity of auditory SENSORY PERCEPTION. It is performed by audiologists, audiology technicians, or nurses with special training. **Frequency** is the highness or lowness of tones (expressed in hertz). The greater the number of vibrations per second, the higher the frequency (pitch) of the sound. The fewer the number of vibrations per second, the lower the frequency (pitch).

TABLE 48-1 Decibel Intensity and Safe Exposure Time for Common Sounds

SOUND	DECIBEL INTENSITY (dB)	SAFE EXPOSURE TIME*
Threshold of hearing	0	
Whispering	20	
Average residence or office	40	
Conversational speech	60	
Car traffic	70	>8 hr
Motorcycle	90	8 hr
Chain saw	100	2 hr
Rock concert, front row	120	3 min
Jet engine	140	Immediate danger
Rocket launching pad	180	Immediate danger

*For every 5-dB increase in intensity, the safe exposure time is cut in half.

Intensity of sound is expressed in decibels (dB). **Threshold** is the lowest level of intensity at which pure tones and speech are heard by a patient about 50% of the time. The lowest intensity at which a young, healthy ear can detect sound about 50% of the time is 0 dB. Sound at 110 dB is so intense (loud) that it is painful for most people with normal hearing. Conversational speech is around 60 dB, and a soft whisper is around 20 dB (Table 48-1). With a hearing loss of 45 to 50 dB, speech cannot be heard without a hearing aid. A person with a hearing loss of 90 dB may not be able to hear speech even with a hearing aid.

Pure tones are generated by an audiometer to determine hearing acuity. The two types of audiometry are pure-tone audiometry and speech audiometry.

Pure-Tone Audiometry. Pure-tone audiometry generates tones that are presented to the patient at frequencies for hearing speech, music, and other common sounds. The results of pure-tone audiometry are graphed on an audiogram. For some patients, the hearing of one ear is "masked" while the hearing of the other ear is tested.

Pure-tone air-conduction testing determines whether a patient hears normally or has a hearing loss. It tests air-conduction hearing sensitivity (through earphones) at frequencies ranging from 125 to 8000 Hz. The intensities for pure tones generally range from 10 to 110 dB.

The patient sits in a sound-isolated room so that background noise does not interfere with the test. Earphones are placed over his or her ears, and tones of varying frequencies and intensities are delivered through the earphones, testing one ear at a time. The patient presses a button or raises a hand to indicate when he or she hears a tone.

Pure-tone bone-conduction testing determines whether the hearing loss detected by air-conduction testing is due to conductive or sensorineural factors or to a combination of the two. It is used only when air-conduction testing results are abnormal. Testing is similar to air-conduction testing except that a bone-conduction vibrator, placed firmly behind the ear on the mastoid process, is used instead of earphones.

Interpretation of audiometric evaluation determines whether hearing is within normal limits or shows a hearing impairment and, if present, whether the hearing loss is conductive, sensorineural, or mixed. The type of loss is determined by an experienced clinician who examines the shape of the audiogram after completion of pure-tone air-conduction and bone-conduction audiometry.

Speech Audiometry. In speech audiometry, the patient's ability to hear spoken words is measured. The speech reception threshold and speech discrimination are assessed.

Speech reception threshold is the minimum loudness at which a patient can repeat simple words. This test determines how intense (or loud) a simple speech stimulus must be before the patient can hear it well enough to repeat it correctly at least 50% of the time. In one common test, lists of two-syllable words called **spondee** are used (i.e., words in which there is equal stress on each syllable, such as *airplane, railroad,* and *cowboy*).

Speech discrimination testing determines the patient's ability to discriminate among similar sounds or among words that contain similar sounds. This test assesses the patient's *understanding* of speech. An auditory SENSORY PERCEPTION loss decreases sensitivity to sound and impairs understanding of what is being said.

A standard format contains lists of 25 to 50 *monosyllabic* (one-syllable) words, such as *carve, day, toe,* and *ran,* and phonemically balanced words, and with equal word difficulty between lists. The lists are presented to the patient through earphones at a selected loudness level, generally about 30 to 40 dB above the speech reception threshold, or at the patient's most comfortable listening level. The score indicates the percentage of words repeated correctly.

Tympanometry. Tympanometry assesses mobility of the eardrum and structures of the middle ear by changing air pressure in the external ear canal. The progression or resolution of serous otitis and otitis media can be accurately monitored with this procedure.

This test is helpful in distinguishing middle ear problems, such as otosclerosis, ossicular disarticulation, otitis media, and perforation of the eardrum. It is also useful for assessing patency of the eustachian tube and for checking recovery of middle ear function after surgery.

Auditory Brainstem-Evoked Response. Auditory brainstem-evoked response (ABR) assesses hearing in patients who are unable to indicate their recognition of sound stimuli during standard hearing tests. It helps diagnose conductive and sensorineural hearing losses. Electrodes are placed on the scalp during the test. After the test, the patient's hair should be cleansed to remove the electrode gel.

Assessment of Balance

Electronystagmography (ENG) is a test to assess for central and peripheral disease of the vestibular system in the ear by detecting and recording **nystagmus** (involuntary eye movements). This response is accurate because the eyes and ears depend on each other for balance. Electrodes are taped to the skin near the eyes, and one or more procedures (caloric testing, changing gaze position, or changing head position) are performed to stimulate nystagmus. Failure of nystagmus to occur with cerebral stimulation suggests an abnormality in the vestibulocochlear apparatus, the cerebral cortex, the auditory nerve, or the brainstem.

To prepare the patient for ENG:

- Explain the procedure and its purpose. The examiners will be asking the patient to name names or do simple mathematics problems during the test to ensure he or she stays alert.
- Tell the patient to fast for several hours before the test and to avoid caffeine-containing beverages for 24 to 48 hours before the test.
- Tell patients with pacemakers that they should not have the test because pacemaker signals interfere with the sensitivity of ENG.
- Carefully introduce oral fluids after the test to prevent nausea and vomiting.

Caloric testing evaluates the vestibular (inner ear) portion of the auditory nerve. Water or air that is warmer or cooler than body temperature is infused into the ear. A normal response is the onset of vertigo and nystagmus within 20 to 30 seconds. Prepare the patient for caloric testing by:

- Explaining the procedure and its purpose
- Telling the patient to fast for several hours before the test
- Explaining that he or she will be on bedrest after the procedure with careful introduction of oral fluids to prevent nausea and vomiting

DISORDERS OF THE EAR AND HEARING

Although ear and hearing disorders are often easily managed, early recognition and intervention are necessary to prevent additional damage and to promote a maximum level of wellness. Without proper intervention, auditory SENSORY PERCEPTION can be affected.

CONDITIONS AFFECTING THE EXTERNAL EAR

The external ear is subject to outside factors that can cause problems. Disorders include congenital malformation, trauma, and infectious or noninfectious lesions of the pinna, auricle, or auditory canal. Abnormalities of the external ear range from crumpling or falling forward of the pinna to complete absence of the ear canal. Trauma can damage or destroy the auricle and external canal. Surgical reconstruction can re-form the pinna with skin grafts and plastic prostheses. Trauma to the auricle resulting in a hematoma requires the removal of blood via needle aspiration to prevent calcification and hardening, which is often referred to as a *cauliflower* or *boxer's ear.*

Benign cysts or polyps of the auricle or external canal are surgically removed if they block the canal and affect hearing. Cancer cells, usually basal cell carcinoma, can occur on the pinna. Usually treatment consists of simple excision. When the lesion becomes larger, its location near the skull and facial nerve makes treatment more difficult.

EXTERNAL OTITIS

❖ PATHOPHYSIOLOGY

External otitis is a painful condition caused when irritating or infective agents come into contact with the skin of the external ear. The result is either an allergic response or inflammation with or without infection. Affected skin becomes red, swollen, and tender to touch or movement. Swelling of the ear canal can lead to temporary hearing loss from obstruction. Allergic external otitis is often caused by contact with cosmetics, hair sprays, earphones, earrings, or hearing aids. The most common infectious organisms are *Pseudomonas aeruginosa, Streptococcus, Staphylococcus,* and *Aspergillus.*

External otitis occurs more often in hot, humid environments, especially in the summer, and is known as **swimmer's ear** because it occurs most often in people involved in water sports. Patients who have traumatized their external ear canal with sharp or small objects (e.g., hairpins, cotton-tipped applicators) or with headphones also are more susceptible to external otitis.

Necrotizing or *malignant otitis* is the most virulent form of external otitis. Organisms spread beyond the external ear canal into the ear and skull. Death from complications such as meningitis, brain abscess, and destruction of cranial nerve VII is possible.

❖ PATIENT-CENTERED COLLABORATIVE CARE

Manifestations of external otitis range from mild itching to pain with movement of the pinna or tragus, particularly when upward pressure is applied to the external canal. Patients report feeling as if the ear is plugged and hearing is reduced. The temporary hearing loss can be severe when inflammation obstructs the canal and prevents sounds from reaching the eardrum.

Treatment focuses on reducing inflammation, edema, and pain. Nursing priorities include comfort measures, such as applying heat to the ear for 20 minutes 3 times a day. This can be accomplished by using towels warmed with water and then wrapped in a plastic bag or by using a heating pad placed on a low setting. Teach the patient that minimizing head movements reduces pain.

Topical antibiotic and steroid therapies are most effective in decreasing inflammation and pain. Review best practices for instilling eardrops with the patient, as shown in Chart 48-3. Observe the patient self-administer the eardrops to make sure that proper technique is used. Oral or IV antibiotics are used in severe cases, especially when infection spreads to surrounding tissue or area lymph nodes are enlarged.

Analgesics, including opioids, may be needed for pain relief during the initial days of treatment. NSAIDs, such as acetylsalicylic acid (aspirin, Entrophen 🍁) and ibuprofen (Advil), or acetaminophen (Tylenol, Abenol 🍁) may relieve less severe pain.

After the inflammation has subsided, a solution of 50% rubbing alcohol, 25% white vinegar, and 25% distilled water may be dropped into the ear to keep it clean and dry and to prevent recurrence. Teach the patient to use preventive measures for minimizing ear canal moisture, trauma, or exposure to materials that lead to local irritation or contact dermatitis.

CHART 48-3 Best Practice for Patient Safety & Quality Care QSEN

Instillation of Eardrops

- Gather the solutions to be administered.
- Check the labels to ensure correct dosage and time.
- Wear gloves to remove and discard any ear packing.
- Wash your hands.
- Perform a gentle otoscopic examination to determine whether the eardrum is intact.
- Irrigate the ear if the eardrum is intact (see Chart 48-4).
- Place the bottle of eardrops (with the top on tightly) in a bowl of warm water for 5 minutes.
- Tilt the patient's head in the opposite direction of the affected ear, and place the drops in the ear.
- With his or her head tilted, ask the patient to gently move the head back and forth 5 times.
- Insert a cotton ball into the opening of the ear canal to act as packing.
- Wash your hands again.

PERICHONDRITIS

Perichondritis is an infection of the **perichondrium**, a tough, fibrous tissue layer that surrounds the cartilage and shapes the pinna. This tissue supplies blood to the ear cartilage. Infection can be caused by opening an area of pus or localized infection, insect bites, trauma, and cartilage ear piercing. When infection occurs between the perichondrium and the cartilage, blood flow to the cartilage can be reduced, leading to necrosis and pinna deformity. This can occur as a complication of high helical ear piercing and may require removal of necrotic tissue.

The purposes of management are to eliminate the infection and ensure that the perichondrium stays in direct contact with the cartilage. In addition to systemic antibiotic therapy, a wide incision is made and suction drainage is used to remove pus and other fluid.

CERUMEN OR FOREIGN BODIES

❖ PATHOPHYSIOLOGY

Cerumen (earwax) is the most common cause of an impacted canal. A canal can also become impacted as a result of foreign bodies that can enter or be placed in the external ear canal, such as vegetables, beads, pencil erasers, and insects. Although uncomfortable, cerumen or foreign bodies are rarely emergencies and can be carefully removed by a health care professional. Cerumen impaction in the older adult is common, and removal of the cerumen from older adults often improves hearing.

❖ PATIENT-CENTERED COLLABORATIVE CARE

Patients with a cerumen impaction or a foreign body in the ear may have a sensation of fullness in the ear, with or without hearing loss, and may have ear pain, itching, dizziness, or bleeding from the ear. The object may be visible with direct inspection.

When the occluding material is cerumen, management options include watchful waiting, manual removal, and the use of ceruminolytic agents followed by either manual irrigation or the use of a low-pressure electronic oral irrigation device. The canal can be irrigated with a mixture of water and hydrogen peroxide at body temperature (Fig. 48-7), following best practices for proper irrigation (Chart 48-4). Removal of a cerumen obstruction by irrigation is a slow process and may take more than one sitting. When it is the cause of hearing loss, cerumen removal may improve hearing. Between 50 and 70 mL of solution is the maximum amount that the patient usually can tolerate at one sitting.

If the cerumen is thick and dry or cannot be removed easily, use a ceruminolytic product such as Cerumenex to soften the wax before trying to remove it. Another way to soften cerumen is to add 3 drops of glycerin or mineral oil to the ear at bedtime and 3 drops of hydrogen peroxide twice a day for several days. Then the cerumen is more easily removed by irrigation. In some cases, a small curette or cerumen spoon may be used by a health

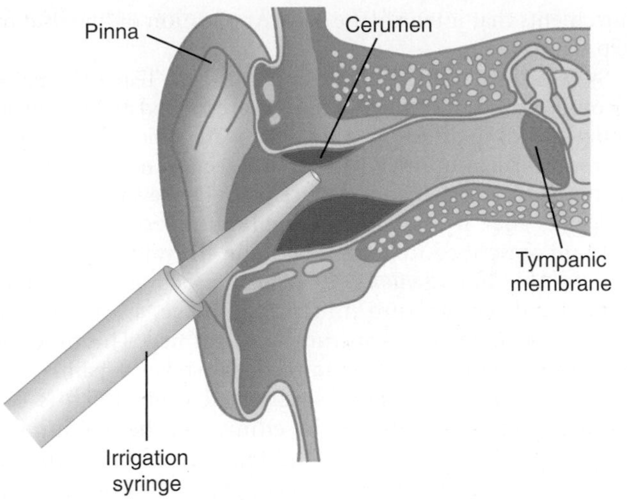

FIG. 48-7 Irrigation of the external canal. Cerumen and debris can be removed from the ear by irrigation with warm water. The stream of water is aimed above or below the impaction to allow back-pressure to push it out rather than further down the canal.

CHART 48-4 Best Practice for Patient Safety & Quality Care QSEN

Ear Irrigation

- Wash your hands.
- Use an otoscope to locate the impaction; ascertain that the eardrum is intact and that the patient does not have otitis media.
- Gather the equipment: basin, irrigation syringe, otoscope, towel.
- Warm tap water (or other prescribed solution) to body temperature.
- Fill a syringe with the warmed irrigating solution.
- Place a towel around the patient's neck.
- Place a basin under the ear to be irrigated.
- Place the tip of the syringe at an angle so that the fluid pushes to one side of and not directly on the impaction (to loosen it without moving it deeper into the canal).
- Apply gentle but firm continuous pressure, allowing the water to flow against the top of the canal.
- Do not use blasts or bursts of sudden pressure.
- If pain occurs, reduce the pressure. If pain persists, stop the irrigation.
- Watch the fluid return for cerumen plug removal.
- Continue to irrigate the ear with about 70 mL of fluid.
- If the cerumen does not drain out, wait 10 minutes and repeat the irrigation procedure.
- Monitor the patient for signs of nausea.
- If the patient becomes nauseated, stop the procedure.
- If the cerumen cannot be removed by irrigation, place mineral oil into the ear 3 times a day for 2 days to soften dry, impacted cerumen, after which irrigation may be repeated.
- After completion of the irrigation, have the patient turn his or her head to the side just irrigated to drain any remaining irrigation fluid.
- Wash your hands.

! NURSING SAFETY PRIORITY QSEN

Action Alert

Do not irrigate an ear with an eardrum perforation or otitis media because this may spread the infection to the inner ear. Also, do not irrigate the ear when the foreign object is vegetable matter, because this material expands when wet, making the impaction worse. For vegetable matter, the object needs to be physically removed by an experienced health care professional.

CHART 48-5 Nursing Focus on the Older Adult

Cerumen Impaction

- Assess the hearing of all older patients using simple voice tests.
- Perform a gentle otoscopic inspection of the external canal and eardrum of any older patient who has a problem with hearing acuity, especially the patient who wears a hearing aid.
- Use ear irrigation to remove any impacted cerumen.
- Make certain that the irrigating fluid is about 98.6° F (37° C) to reduce the chance for stimulating the vestibular sense.
- Use no more than 5 to 10 mL of irrigating fluid at a time.
- If nausea, vomiting, or dizziness develops, stop the irrigation immediately.
- Teach the patient how to irrigate his or her own ears.
- Obtain a return demonstration of ear irrigation from the patient, observing for specific areas in which the patient may need assistance.
- Encourage the patient to wash the external ears daily using a soapy, wet washcloth over the index finger (best done in the shower or while washing the hair).

care professional to scoop out the wax. Improper use of the curette can damage the canal or the eardrum.

Discourage the use of cotton swabs and ear candles (hollow tubes coated in wax inserted into the ear and then lighted at the far end) to clean the ears or remove cerumen. Chart 48-2 describes steps to teach patients regarding ear hygiene and self–ear irrigation. Refer to Chart 48-5 for nursing care considerations of older adult patients with cerumen impaction.

Insects are killed before removal unless they can be coaxed out by a flashlight. A topical anesthetic can be placed in the ear canal for pain relief. Mineral oil or diluted alcohol instilled into the ear can suffocate the insect, which is then removed with ear forceps.

If the patient has local irritation, an antibiotic or steroid ointment may be applied to prevent infection and reduce local irritation. Hearing acuity is tested if hearing loss is not resolved by removal of the object.

Surgical removal of the foreign object may be performed through the ear canal by a health care provider using a wire bent at a 90-degree angle. The wire is looped around the object, and the object is pulled out. Because this procedure is painful, general anesthesia is needed.

CONDITIONS AFFECTING THE MIDDLE EAR

OTITIS MEDIA

❖ *PATHOPHYSIOLOGY*

The common forms of otitis media are acute otitis media, chronic otitis media, and serous otitis media. Each type affects the middle ear but has different causes and pathologic changes. If otitis progresses or is untreated, permanent conductive hearing loss may occur.

Acute otitis media and chronic otitis media are similar. An infecting agent in the middle ear causes inflammation of the mucosa, leading to swelling and irritation of the ossicles within the middle ear, followed by purulent inflammatory exudate. Acute disease has a sudden onset and lasts 3 weeks or less. Chronic otitis media often follows repeated acute episodes, has a longer duration, and causes greater middle ear injury. It may be a result of the continuing presence of a biofilm in the middle ear. A *biofilm* is a community of bacteria working together to overcome host defense mechanisms to continue to survive and proliferate (see Chapter 23 for more information about biofilms). Therapy for complications associated with chronic otitis media usually involves surgical intervention.

The eustachian tube and mastoid, connected to the middle ear by a sheet of cells, are also affected by the infection. If the eardrum membrane perforates, the infection can thicken and scar the eardrum and middle ear if left untreated. Necrosis of the ossicles destroys middle ear structures and causes hearing loss.

❖ PATIENT-CENTERED COLLABORATIVE CARE

◆ Assessment

The patient with acute or chronic otitis media has ear pain. Acute otitis media causes more intense pain from increased pressure in the middle ear. Conductive hearing is reduced and distorted as sound wave transmission is obstructed. The patient may notice tinnitus in the form of a low hum or a low-pitched sound. Headaches and systemic manifestations such as malaise, fever, nausea, and vomiting can occur. As the pressure on the middle ear pushes against the inner ear, the patient may have dizziness.

Otoscopic examination findings vary, depending on the stage of the condition. The eardrum is initially retracted, which allows landmarks of the ear to be seen clearly. At this early stage, the patient has only vague ear discomfort. As the condition progresses, the eardrum's blood vessels dilate and appear red (Fig. 48-8). Later, the eardrum becomes red, thickened, and bulging, with loss of landmarks. Decreased eardrum mobility is evident on inspection with a pneumatic otoscope. Pus may be seen behind the membrane.

With progression, the eardrum spontaneously perforates and pus or blood drains from the ear (Fig. 48-9). Then the patient notices a marked decrease in pain as the pressure on middle ear structures is relieved. Eardrum perforations often heal if the underlying problem is controlled. Simple central perforation does not interfere with hearing unless the ossicles are damaged or the perforation is large. Repeated perforations with extensive scarring cause hearing loss.

◆ Interventions

Nonsurgical Management. Management can be as simple as putting the patient in a quiet environment. Bedrest limits head movements that intensify the pain. Application of low heat may help reduce pain.

Systemic antibiotic therapy is prescribed. Teach the patient to complete the antibiotic therapy as prescribed and to not stop taking the drug when manifestations are relieved. Analgesics such as aspirin, ibuprofen (Advil), and acetaminophen (Tylenol, Abenol 🍁) relieve pain and reduce fever. For severe pain, opioid analgesics may be prescribed. Antihistamines and decongestants are prescribed to decrease fluid in the middle ear.

Surgical Management. If pain persists after antibiotic therapy and the eardrum continues to bulge, a **myringotomy** (surgical opening of the eardrum) is performed. This procedure drains middle ear fluids and immediately relieves pain.

The procedure is a small surgical incision, which is often performed in an office or clinic setting, and the incision heals rapidly. Another approach is the removal of fluid from the middle ear with a needle. For relief of pressure caused by serous otitis media and for those patients who have repeated episodes of otitis media, a small **grommet** (polyethylene tube) may be surgically placed through the eardrum to allow continuous drainage of middle ear fluids (Fig. 48-10).

Priority care after surgery includes teaching the patient to keep the external ear and canal clean and dry while the incision is healing. Instruct him or her to not wash the hair or shower for several days. Other instructions after surgery are listed in Chart 48-6.

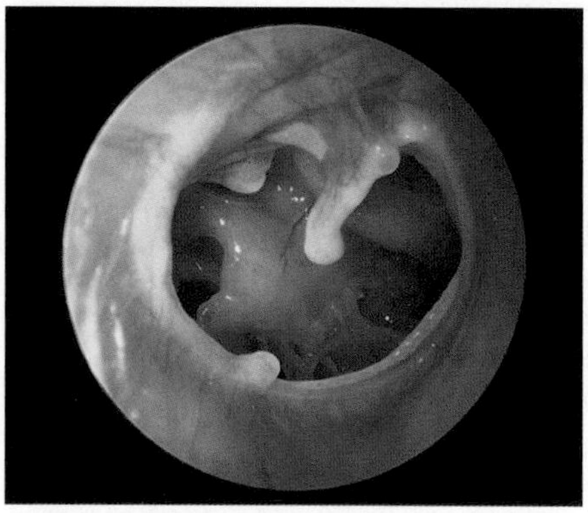

FIG. 48-9 Otoscopic view of a perforated tympanic membrane.

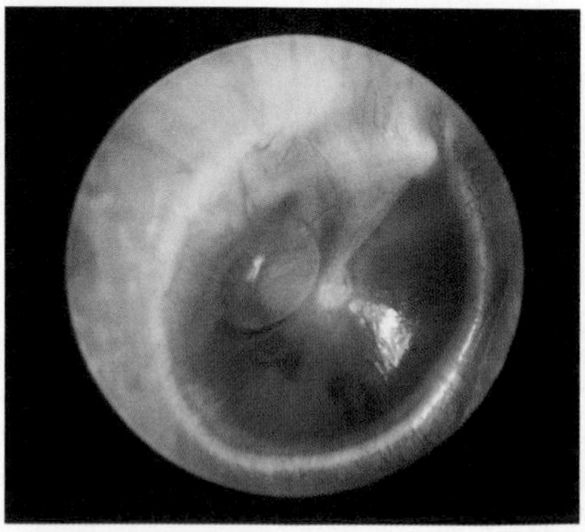

FIG. 48-8 Otoscopic view of otitis media.

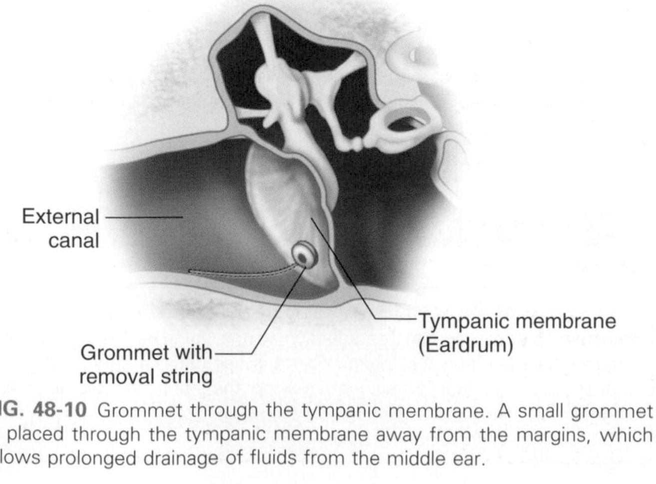

FIG. 48-10 Grommet through the tympanic membrane. A small grommet is placed through the tympanic membrane away from the margins, which allows prolonged drainage of fluids from the middle ear.

CHART 48-6 Patient and Family Education: Preparing for Self-Management

Recovery from Ear Surgery

- Avoid straining when you have a bowel movement.
- Do not drink through a straw for 2 to 3 weeks.
- Avoid air travel for 2 to 3 weeks.
- Avoid excessive coughing for 2 to 3 weeks.
- Stay away from people with respiratory infections.
- When blowing your nose, blow gently, without blocking either nostril, with your mouth open.
- Avoid getting your head wet, washing your hair, and showering for 1 week.
- Keep your ear dry for 6 weeks by placing a ball of cotton coated with petroleum jelly (e.g., Vaseline) in your ear. Change the cotton ball daily.
- Avoid rapidly moving the head, bouncing, and bending over for 3 weeks.
- Change your ear dressing every 24 hours or as directed.
- Report excessive drainage immediately to your physician.

MASTOIDITIS

❖ *PATHOPHYSIOLOGY*

The lining of the middle ear is continuous with the lining of the mastoid air cells, which are embedded in the temporal bone. **Mastoiditis** is an infection of the mastoid air cells caused by progressive otitis media. Antibiotic therapy is used to treat the middle ear infection before it progresses to mastoiditis. If mastoiditis is not managed appropriately, it can lead to brain abscess, meningitis, and death.

❖ *PATIENT-CENTERED COLLABORATIVE CARE*

The manifestations of mastoiditis include swelling behind the ear and pain when moving the ear or the head. Pain is *not* relieved by myringotomy. Cellulitis develops on the skin or external scalp over the mastoid process, pushing the ear sideways and down. The eardrum is red, dull, thick, and immobile. Perforation may or may not be present. Lymph nodes behind the ear are tender and enlarged. Patients may have low-grade fever, malaise, and ear drainage. Hearing loss occurs, and CT scans show fluid in the air cells of the mastoid process.

Interventions focus on halting the infection before it spreads to other structures. IV antibiotics are used but do not easily penetrate the infected bony structure of the mastoid. Cultures of the ear drainage determine which antibiotics should be most effective. Surgical removal of the infected tissue is needed if the infection does not respond to antibiotic therapy within a few days. A simple or modified radical mastoidectomy with tympanoplasty is the most common treatment. All infected tissue must be removed so that the infection does not spread to other structures. A tympanoplasty is then performed to reconstruct the ossicles and the eardrum to restore hearing (see pp. 1012-1013 for care after tympanoplasty.)

TRAUMA

Trauma and damage may occur to the eardrum and ossicles by infection, by direct damage, or through rapid changes in the middle ear pressure. Objects placed in the external canal exert pressure on the eardrum and cause perforation. If the objects continue through the canal, the ossicles may be damaged. Blunt injury to the skull and ears can also damage or fracture middle ear structures. Slapping the external ear increases the pressure in the ear canal and can tear the eardrum. Excessive nose blowing and rapid changes of pressure *(barotrauma)* can increase pressure within the middle ear leading to damaged ossicles and a perforated eardrum.

Most eardrum perforations heal within a week or two without treatment. Repeated perforations heal more slowly, with scarring. Depending on the amount of damage to the ossicles, auditory SENSORY PERCEPTION may or may not return. Hearing aids can improve hearing in this type of hearing loss. Surgical reconstruction of the ossicles and eardrum through a tympanoplasty or a myringoplasty may also improve hearing. (See later discussion of nursing care on p. 1013 in the Tympanoplasty section.)

Nursing care priorities focus on teaching about trauma prevention. Caution patients to avoid inserting objects into the external canal and to follow the steps in Chart 48-2 for ear hygiene. Stress the importance of using ear protectors when blunt trauma is likely.

NEOPLASMS

Middle ear tumors are rare, and the most common type is the *glomus jugulare,* a benign vascular lesion. Malignant ear tumors also can occur. The growth of any lesion within the middle ear area disrupts conductive auditory SENSORY PERCEPTION, erodes the ossicles, and may affect the inner ear and cranial nerves.

Patients have progressive hearing loss and tinnitus. Infection and pain are rare. Otoscopic examination shows a bulging eardrum or a mass extending to the external ear canal. The blood vessels of the *glomus jugulare* tumor give the mass a reddish color and a visible pulsation.

Diagnosis is made by physical examination, tomography, and angiography. Tumors are removed by surgery, which often destroys hearing in the affected ear. Depending on the extent of the tumor, surgery can performed through the ear canal or may involve opening the cranium to remove the tumor.

Benign tumors are removed because, with continued growth, other structures can be affected, further damaging the facial or trigeminal nerve. When possible, reconstruction of the middle ear structures is performed later to restore conductive hearing.

CONDITIONS AFFECTING THE INNER EAR

TINNITUS

Tinnitus (continuous ringing or noise perception in the ear) is a common ear problem that can occur in one or both ears. Diagnostic testing cannot confirm tinnitus; however, testing is performed to assess hearing and rule out other disorders.

Manifestation range from mild ringing, which can go unnoticed during the day, to a loud roaring in the ear, which can interfere with thinking and attention span. Some patients feel as if the constant ringing could drive them mad. Factors that contribute to tinnitus include age, sclerosis of the ossicles, Ménière's disease, certain drugs (aspirin, NSAIDs, high-ceiling diuretics, quinine, aminoglycoside antibiotics), exposure to loud noise, and other inner ear problems (Ruppert & Fay, 2012).

The problem and its management vary with the underlying cause. When no cause can be found or the disorder is untreatable, therapy focuses on ways to mask the tinnitus with background sound, noisemakers, and music during sleeping hours. Ear mold hearing aids can amplify sounds to drown out the tinnitus during the day. A drug that is helpful to some patients is pramipexole (Mirapex), an antiparkinson drug. The American Tinnitus Association assists patients in coping with tinnitus. Refer patients with tinnitus to local and online support groups to help them cope with this problem.

NCLEX EXAMINATION CHALLENGE

Physiological Integrity

The client who has tinnitus is taking these drugs daily: 1 multiple vitamin, losartan (Cozaar) 50 mg, aspirin 650 mg, and diphenhydramine (Benadryl) 25 mg. Which drug alerts the nurse to a possible cause of tinnitus?

A. Aspirin
B. Losartan
C. Multiple vitamin
D. Diphenhydramine

VERTIGO AND DIZZINESS

Vertigo and dizziness are common manifestations of many ear disorders. **Dizziness** is a disturbed sense of a person's relationship to space. Vertigo is often used interchangeably with dizziness, but the definition and cause are somewhat different. True **vertigo** is a sense of whirling or turning in space.

Because the visual system, the vestibular system, and the proprioceptive system (muscles and nerve endings) combine to give input to the brain about balance, problems in any of these areas lead to a disturbed sense of balance. Problems that cause vertigo include Ménière's disease, labyrinthitis, acoustic neuromas, motion sickness, and drug or alcohol ingestion.

Manifestations of vertigo include nausea, vomiting, falling, nystagmus, hearing loss, and tinnitus. Until the cause of the vertigo can be identified, each manifestation is treated. Teach patients these strategies to reduce manifestations:

- Restrict head motion and change position slowly
- Take drugs that reduce the vertigo effects, such as over-the counter dimenhydrinate (Dramamine, Gravol 🍁) or prescription drugs such as diazepam (Valium, Apo-Diazepam 🍁), meclizine (Antivert, Bonamine 🍁), and scopolamine (Transderm Scop, Transderm-V 🍁)

LABYRINTHITIS

Labyrinthitis is an infection of the labyrinth, which may occur as a complication of acute or chronic otitis media that spreads to the inner ear. Labyrinthitis also may result from the growth of a **cholesteatoma** (benign overgrowth of squamous cell epithelium) from the middle ear into the semicircular canal. It may follow middle ear or inner ear surgery and may follow a viral upper respiratory infection or mononucleosis.

Manifestations include auditory SENSORY PERCEPTION loss, tinnitus, nystagmus to the affected side, and vertigo with nausea and vomiting. Labyrinthitis is usually a self-limiting condition. If it does not resolve with supportive therapy, management includes systemic antibiotics. Teach the patient to complete the antibiotic therapy as prescribed and to not stop taking the drug when manifestations are no longer present because inadequate treatment may lead to meningitis. Advise patients to stay in bed in a darkened room until manifestations are reduced. Antiemetics and antivertiginous drugs, such as dimenhydrinate (Dramamine, Gravol 🍁) and meclizine (Antivert, Bonamine 🍁), relieve nausea and dizziness.

MÉNIÈRE'S DISEASE

❖ *PATHOPHYSIOLOGY*

Ménière's disease has three features: tinnitus, one-sided sensorineural auditory SENSORY PERCEPTION loss, and vertigo, occurring in attacks that can last for several days (Haynes, 2014). (Some patients have continuous manifestations of varying intensity rather than intermittent attacks.) Patients are almost totally incapacitated during an attack, and recovery takes hours to days. The pathology of Ménière's disease is an excess of endolymphatic fluid that distorts the entire inner-canal system. This distortion decreases hearing by dilating the cochlear duct, causes vertigo because of damage to the vestibular system, and stimulates tinnitus. At first, hearing loss is reversible, but repeated damage to the cochlea from increased fluid pressure leads to permanent hearing loss.

❖ *PATIENT-CENTERED COLLABORATIVE CARE*

◆ *Assessment*

Ménière's disease usually first occurs in people between the ages of 20 and 50 years. It is more common in men and affects about 615,000 people in the United States (Alm, 2012). Severe, debilitating attacks alternate with symptom-free periods. Patients often have certain manifestations before an attack of vertigo, such as headaches, increasing tinnitus, and fullness in the affected ear.

Patients describe the tinnitus as a continuous, low-pitched roar or a humming sound, which worsens just before and during an attack. Hearing loss occurs first with the low-frequency tones but progresses to include all levels and, with repeated attacks, can become permanent. The vertigo with periods of whirling may even cause patients to fall. It is so intense that even while lying down, the patient often holds the bed or ground to keep from falling. Severe vertigo usually lasts 3 to 4 hours, but he or she may feel dizzy long after the attack. Nausea and vomiting are common. Other manifestations include rapid eye movements (**nystagmus**) and severe headaches.

◆ *Interventions*

Nonsurgical Management. Teach patients to move the head slowly to prevent worsening of the vertigo. Nutrition and lifestyle changes can reduce the amount of endolymphatic fluid. Encourage patients to stop smoking because of the blood vessel constricting effects.

Nutrition therapy with a hydrops diet may stabilize body fluid levels to prevent excess endolymph accumulation. The basic structure of this diet involves:

- Distributing food and fluid intake evenly throughout the day and from day to day
- Avoiding foods or fluids with a high salt content
- Drinking adequate amounts of fluids daily
- Avoiding caffeine-containing fluids and foods
- Limiting alcohol intake to one serving per day
- Avoiding monosodium glutamate (MSG)

Coordinate with a dietitian for more information about diet therapy for reduction of Ménière's manifestations.

Drug therapy may reduce the vertigo and vomiting and restore normal balance. Mild diuretics are prescribed to decrease endolymph volume, which reduces vertigo, hearing loss, tinnitus, and aural fullness. Nicotinic acid has been found to be useful because of its vasodilatory effect. Antihistamines, such as diphenhydramine hydrochloride (Benadryl, Allerdryl ♣) and dimenhydrinate (Dramamine, Gravol ♣), and antivertiginous drugs, such as meclizine (Antivert, Bonamine ♣), help reduce the severity of or stop an acute attack. Antiemetics, such as chlorpromazine hydrochloride (Thorazine, Novo-Chlorpromazine♣), droperidol (Inapsine), promethazine (Phenergan), and ondansetron (Zofran), help reduce the nausea and vomiting. Diazepam (Valium, Apo-Diazepam ♣) calms the patient; reduces vertigo, nausea, and vomiting; and allows the patient to rest quietly during an attack. Intratympanic therapy with gentamycin and steroids can prevent manifestations; however, this therapy results in some hearing loss.

Pressure pulse treatments, such as the Meniett device, which use a tympanostomy tube to apply low-pressure micropulses to the inner ear several times daily, have helped reduce episodes in some patients with Ménière's disease (National Institute on Deafness and other Communication Disorders [NIDCD], 2010). This action displaces inner ear fluid and prevents or relieves manifestations.

An experimental technique to control dizziness is in clinical trials. This technique involves the use of an implant placed behind the affected ear that blocks abnormal activity of the eighth cranial nerve (Alm, 2012).

Surgical Management. When medical therapy is ineffective and the patient's general function is decreased significantly, surgery may be performed. The choice of the surgical procedure depends on the degree of usable hearing, the severity of the spells, and the condition of the opposite ear. The most radical procedure involves resection of the vestibular nerve or total removal of the labyrinth (**labyrinthectomy**), performed through the ear canal. This procedure results in total auditory SENSORY PERCEPTION loss on the operative side.

Another procedure performed early in the course of the disease is endolymphatic decompression with drainage and a shunt. The effectiveness of this procedure varies. The endolymphatic sac is drained, and a tube is inserted for continued fluid drainage. Some patients report relief of vertigo with retention of their hearing. Vertigo is present immediately after surgery from movement of the vestibule of the inner ear during surgery. Reassure the patient that the vertigo is a temporary result of the surgical procedure, not the disease.

NCLEX EXAMINATION CHALLENGE

Health Promotion and Maintenance

Which lifestyle modification does the nurse suggest to the client with Ménière's disease to reduce the frequency or intensity of acute episodes?

A. Quitting cigarette smoking
B. Avoiding aspirin-containing drugs
C. Reducing the amount of saturated fats in the diet
D. Avoiding crowds and people who have upper respiratory infections

ACOUSTIC NEUROMA

An **acoustic neuroma** is a benign tumor of cranial nerve VIII that often damages other structures as it grows. Depending on the size and exact location of the tumor, damage to hearing, facial movements, and sensation can occur (McCance et al., 2014). An acoustic neuroma can cause many neurologic manifestations as the tumor enlarges in the brain.

Manifestations begin with tinnitus and progress to gradual sensorineural hearing loss. Later, patients have constant mild to moderate vertigo. As the tumor enlarges, nearby cranial nerves are damaged.

The tumor is diagnosed with CT scanning and MRI. Cerebrospinal fluid assays show increased pressure and protein.

Surgical removal can be performed in a variety of ways. Usually a craniotomy is performed, and usually the remaining hearing is lost. Care is taken to preserve the function of the facial nerve (cranial nerve VII). Care after craniotomy is discussed in Chapter 45. Acoustic neuromas rarely recur after surgical removal.

HEARING LOSS

❖ PATHOPHYSIOLOGY

Loss of auditory SENSORY PERCEPTION is common and may be conductive, sensorineural, or a combination of the two (see Fig. 48-2). Conductive hearing loss occurs when sound waves are blocked from contact with inner ear nerve fibers because of external ear or middle ear disorders. If the inner ear sensory nerve that leads to the brain is damaged, the hearing loss is *sensorineural.* Combined hearing loss is *mixed conductive-sensorineural.*

The differences in conductive and sensorineural hearing loss are listed in Table 48-2. Disorders that cause conductive hearing loss are often corrected with minimal or no permanent damage. Sensorineural hearing loss is often permanent.

Etiology and Genetic Risk

Conductive hearing loss can be caused by any inflammation or obstruction of the external or middle ear. Changes in the

TABLE 48-2 Comparison of Features for Conductive and Sensorineural Hearing Loss

CONDUCTIVE HEARING LOSS	SENSORINEURAL HEARING LOSS
Causes	
Cerumen	Prolonged exposure to noise
Foreign body	Presbycusis
Perforation of the tympanic membrane	Ototoxic substance
	Ménière's disease
Edema	Acoustic neuroma
Infection of the external ear or middle ear	Diabetes mellitus
	Labyrinthitis
Tumor	Infection
Otosclerosis	Myxedema
Assessment Findings	
Evidence of obstruction with otoscope	Normal appearance of external canal and tympanic membrane
Abnormality in tympanic membrane	Tinnitus common
	Occasional dizziness
Speaking softly	Speaking loudly
Hearing best in a noisy environment	Hearing poorly in loud environment
Rinne test: air conduction greater than bone conduction	Rinne test: air conduction less than bone conduction
Weber test: lateralization to affected ear	Weber test: lateralization to unaffected ear

eardrum such as bulging, retraction, and perforations may damage middle ear structures and lead to conductive hearing loss. Tumors, scar tissue, and overgrowth of soft bony tissue (**otosclerosis**) on the ossicles from previous middle ear surgery also lead to conductive hearing loss.

Sensorineural hearing loss occurs when the inner ear or auditory nerve (cranial nerve VIII) is damaged. Prolonged exposure to loud noise damages the hair cells of the cochlea (NIDCD, 2012). Many drugs are toxic to the inner ear structures, and their effects on hearing can be transient or permanent, dose related, and affect one or both ears. When ototoxic drugs are given to patients with reduced kidney function, increased ototoxicity can occur because drug elimination is slower, especially among older patients.

Presbycusis is a sensorineural auditory SENSORY PERCEPTION loss that occurs with aging (McCance et al., 2014). It is caused by degeneration of cochlear nerve cells, loss of elasticity of the basilar membrane, or a decreased blood supply to the inner ear. Deficiencies of vitamin B_{12} and folic acid increase the risk for presbycusis. Other causes include atherosclerosis, hypertension, infections, fever, Ménière's disease, diabetes, and ear surgery (Touhy & Jett, 2014). Trauma to the ear, head, or brain also contributes to sensorineural hearing loss.

Incidence and Prevalence

Because hearing loss may be gradual and affect only some aspects of hearing, many adults are unaware that their hearing is impaired. The incidence of adult hearing loss in the United States is estimated to be 36 to 46 million, or 17% of the population, and dramatically increases among people in their 70s and 80s (NIDCD, 2014; Oyler, 2012).

Health Promotion and Maintenance

With special care to the ears, hearing can be preserved at maximum levels. Address barriers to the use of hearing protection, exposure to loud music, and other modifiable risk factors that affect hearing. Encourage everyone to have simple hearing testing performed as part of their annual health assessment.

Teach everyone the danger in using objects such as bobby-pins, Q-tips, or toothpicks to clean the ear canal. These can scrape the skin of the canal, push cerumen up against the eardrum, and puncture the eardrum. If cerumen buildup is a problem, teach the person the proper technique to remove it (see Chart 48-2).

Teach all people to use protective ear devices, such as over-the-ear headsets or foam ear inserts, when exposed to persistent loud noises. Suggest using earplugs when engaging in water sports to prevent ear infections, as well as using an over-the-counter product such as Swim-Ear to assist with drying the ears after swimming.

❖ PATIENT-CENTERED COLLABORATIVE CARE

◆ Assessment

History. Ask patients how long they have noticed a change in hearing and whether the changes were sudden or gradual. Age is important, because some ear and hearing changes occur with aging. Ask about exposures to loud or continuous noises, as well as current or previous use of ototoxic drugs. Also ask about a history of ear infections and whether eardrum perforation occurred. Ask patients about any direct trauma to the ears. Because some types of hearing loss have a genetic basis, ask whether any family members are hearing impaired. When pain occurs with acute-onset hearing loss, ask about recent upper respiratory infection and allergies affecting the nose and sinuses.

CHART 48-7 Focused Assessment

The Patient with Suspected Hearing Loss

Assess whether the patient has any of these ear problems:
- Pain
- Feeling of fullness or congestion
- Dizziness or vertigo
- Tinnitus
- Difficulty understanding conversations, especially in a noisy room
- Difficulty hearing sounds
- The need to strain to hear
- The need to turn the head to favor one ear or the need to lean forward to hear

Assess visible ear structures, particularly the external canal and tympanic membrane:
- Position and size of the pinna
- Patency of the external canal; presence of cerumen or foreign bodies, edema, or inflammation
- Condition of the tympanic membrane: intact, edema, fluid, inflammation

Assess functional ability, including:
- Frequency of asking people to repeat statements
- Withdrawal from social interactions or large groups
- Shouting in conversation
- Failing to respond when not looking in the direction of the sound
- Answering questions incorrectly

The patient with hearing loss from peripheral neuropathy may have other systemic diseases, including human immune deficiency virus (HIV) disease or diabetes. Patients undergoing cancer chemotherapy or interferon therapy are at risk for neuropathic hearing loss.

Physical Assessment/Clinical Manifestations. Chart 48-7 lists focused assessment techniques for patients with suspected loss of auditory SENSORY PERCEPTION. The loss may be sudden or gradual and often affects both ears. The ability to hear high-frequency consonants—especially *s, sh, f, th,* and *ch* sounds—is lost first. Patients may state that they have no problem with hearing but cannot understand specific words and that other people are mumbling. Vertigo and continuous tinnitus may be present.

Tuning fork tests help diagnose hearing loss. With the Weber test, the patient can usually hear sounds well in the ear with a conductive hearing loss because of bone conduction. With the Rinne test, the patient reports that sound transmitted by bone conduction is louder and more sustained than that transmitted by air conduction.

Otoscopic examination is used to assess the ear canal, eardrum, and middle ear structures that can be seen through the eardrum. Findings vary, depending on the cause of the hearing loss. Perform the examination as described earlier on pp. 1000-1001, and document the findings.

Psychosocial Assessment. For people with a loss of auditory SENSORY PERCEPTION, communication can be a struggle and they may isolate themselves because of the difficulty in talking and listening. Social isolation can lead to depression (Spyridakou, 2012). Be sensitive to emotional changes that may be related to reduced hearing and a decline in conversational skills. Encourage the patient and family to express their feelings and concerns about an actual or potential hearing loss.

Laboratory Assessment. No laboratory test diagnoses hearing loss. However, some laboratory findings can indicate problems that affect hearing. White blood cell counts are assessed in the patient with otitis media.

Imaging Assessment. Imaging assessment can determine some problems affecting hearing ability. Skull x-rays determine bony involvement in otitis media and the location of otosclerotic lesions. CT and MRI are used to determine soft-tissue involvement and the presence and location of tumors.

Other Diagnostic Assessment. Audiometry can help determine whether hearing loss is only conductive or whether it has a sensorineural component. This is important in determining possible causes of the hearing loss and in planning interventions.

◆ Analysis

The priority NANDA-I nursing diagnoses and collaborative problems for the patient with any degree of hearing impairment include:

1. Difficulty hearing related to obstruction, infection, damage to the middle ear, or damage to the auditory nerve
2. Impaired Verbal Communication related to difficulty hearing (NANDA-I)

◆ Planning and Implementation

Increasing Hearing

Planning: Expected Outcomes. The patient with impaired auditory SENSORY PERCEPTION is expected to either have an increase in functional hearing or maintain existing hearing levels. Indicators include:

- No or minimal loss of high-pitch tones
- No or minimal loss of ability to distinguish conversation from background noise
- Turning toward sound
- Identifying discrete sounds

Interventions. Interventions are expected to identify the problem, halt the pathologic processes, and increase usable hearing. Nursing care priorities focus on teaching the patient about the use of an appropriate assistive device, providing support to the patient and family to maintain or increase communication, and assisting patients to find support services.

Nonsurgical Management. Interventions include early detection of impaired auditory SENSORY PERCEPTION, use of appropriate therapy, and use of assistive devices to augment the patient's usable hearing.

Early detection helps correct the problem causing the hearing loss. Assess for indications of hearing loss, as listed in Chart 48-7.

Drug therapy is focused on correcting the underlying problem or reducing the side effects of problems occurring with hearing loss. Antibiotic therapy is used to manage external otitis and other ear infections. Teach the patient the importance of taking the drug or drugs exactly as prescribed and completing the entire course. Caution him or her to not stop the drug just because manifestations have improved. By treating the infection, antibiotics reduce local edema and improve hearing. When pain is also present, analgesics are used. Many ear disorders induce vertigo and dizziness with nausea and vomiting. Antiemetic, antihistamine, antivertiginous, and benzodiazepine drugs can help reduce these problems.

Assistive devices are useful for patients with permanent hearing loss. Portable amplifiers can be used while watching television to avoid increasing the volume and disturbing others. Telephone amplifiers increase telephone volume, allowing the caller to speak in a normal voice. Flashing lights activated by the ringing telephone or a doorbell alert patients visually. Some patients may have a service dog to alert them to sounds (ringing telephones or doorbells, cries of other people, and potential dangers). Provide information about agencies that can assist the hearing-impaired person.

Small, portable audio amplifiers can assist in communicating with patients with hearing loss who do not use a hearing aid. Using amplifiers or allowing patients to use a stethoscope for listening helps you communicate with anyone who requires additional volume to hear speech.

A hearing aid is a small electronic amplifier that assists patients with conductive hearing loss but is less effective for sensorineural hearing loss. Most common hearing aids are small. Some are attached to a person's glasses and are visible to other people. Another type fits into the ear and is less noticeable. Newer devices fit completely in the canal with only a fine, clear filament visible. The cost of smaller hearing aids varies with size and quality. Some people benefit from classes that explain the best use and care of these devices.

Remind patients that hearing with a hearing aid is different from natural hearing. Teach the patient to start using the hearing aid slowly, at first wearing it only at home and only during part of the day. Listening to television and the radio and reading aloud can help the patient get used to new sounds. A difficult aspect of a hearing aid is the amplification of background noise. The patient must learn to concentrate and filter out background noises. In a study of hearing aid users, the most desired feature for a hearing aid is its functionality in noisy settings (see the Evidence-Based Practice box).

Teach the patient how to care for the hearing aid (Chart 48-8). Hearing aids are delicate devices that should be handled only by people who know how to care for them properly.

Cochlear implantation may help patients with sensorineural hearing loss. Although a superficial surgical procedure is needed

CHART 48-8 Patient and Family Education: Preparing for Self-Management

Hearing Aid Care

- Keep the hearing aid dry.
- Clean the ear mold with mild soap and water while avoiding excessive wetting.
- Using a toothpick, clean debris from the hole in the middle of the part that goes into your ear.
- Turn off the hearing aid when not in use.
- Check and replace the battery frequently.
- Keep extra batteries on hand.
- Keep the hearing aid in a safe place.
- Avoid dropping the hearing aid or exposing it to temperature extremes.
- Adjust the volume to the lowest setting that allows you to hear, to prevent feedback squeaking.
- Avoid using hair spray, cosmetics, oils, or other hair and face products that might come into contact with the receiver.
- If the hearing aid does not work:
  - Change the battery.
  - Check the connection between the ear mold and the receiver.
  - Check the on/off switch.
  - Clean the sound hole.
  - Adjust the volume.
  - Take the hearing aid to an authorized service center for repair.

EVIDENCE-BASED PRACTICE QSEN

What Do People with Reduced Hearing Want Most from a Hearing Aid?

Bridges, J., Lataille, A., Buttorff, C., White, S., & Niparko, J. (2012). Consumer preference for hearing aid attributes: A comparison of rating and conjoint analysis methods. *Trends in Amplification, 16*(1), 40-48.

The number of older adults with hearing loss is increasing, although only about one in five hearing-impaired people uses a hearing aid. Several drawbacks from hearing aid use include cost, appearance, and the quality of amplification, particularly the utility of the device in noisy environments. The purpose of this study was to determine what hearing aid factors or attributes are preferred by users. There were 75 subjects with documented hearing loss followed in the ambulatory care setting of a large medical center. With the exception of income, the cohort strongly represented the typical hearing aid user (male, older). This group had a higher-than-typical education level and income level. The study built upon previous studies that identified the seven hearing aid attributes (i.e., performance in quiet settings, comfort, feedback, frequency of battery replacement, purchase price, water and sweat resistance, and performance in noisy settings) that were important in the choice and use of different models of hearing aids.

Subjects were asked to rate these attributes on a Likert-like scale and were asked to perform eight pair-comparison conjoint tasks. In addition to descriptive statistics, data were analyzed using ordinary least squares (OLS) and logit models.

Although all positive attributes (e.g., good performance, lower cost, longer battery life) were considered desirable, the attribute considered by a large margin to be most desirable and most likely to help the person continue usual activities was improved performance in noisy environments. Both methods of measurement and analysis had similar results. This result was confirmed by the subjects indicating that they would be willing to pay $2000 to $4000 more for a hearing aid that had good performance in noisy environments.

Level of Evidence: 3

This quasi-experimental study did not include randomization or a true control group. However, the identified variables were evidence-based from previous studies and the methods of statistical analysis were appropriate for the research questions posed.

Commentary: Implications for Practice and Research

A limitation to the generalizability of this study is the higher-than-average levels of income and education among the subject population. The results of this study indicated that the attribute of improving hearing in a noisy environment is very important in hearing aid selection, even when the cost of hearing aids with this attribute is considerably greater than for hearing aids that performed less well in this area. These results indicate that people with hearing loss would prefer to maintain all their social and work activities, including those in environments in which noise affects communication. Nurses and other health care professionals may have been underestimating the degree and effect of social isolation experienced by people who have reduced or lost auditory sensory perception. Until technologic advances in hearing aid performance in noisy environments are more affordable, research into the types of social activities that can be satisfying to the person with reduced hearing is needed.

to implant the device, the procedure does not enter the inner ear and thus is not considered a surgical correction for hearing impairment. A small computer converts sound waves into electronic impulses. Electrodes are placed near the internal ear, with the computer attached to the external ear. The electronic impulses then directly stimulate nerve fibers. Some patients have a 50% return of their hearing with this method (Holmes et al., 2012).

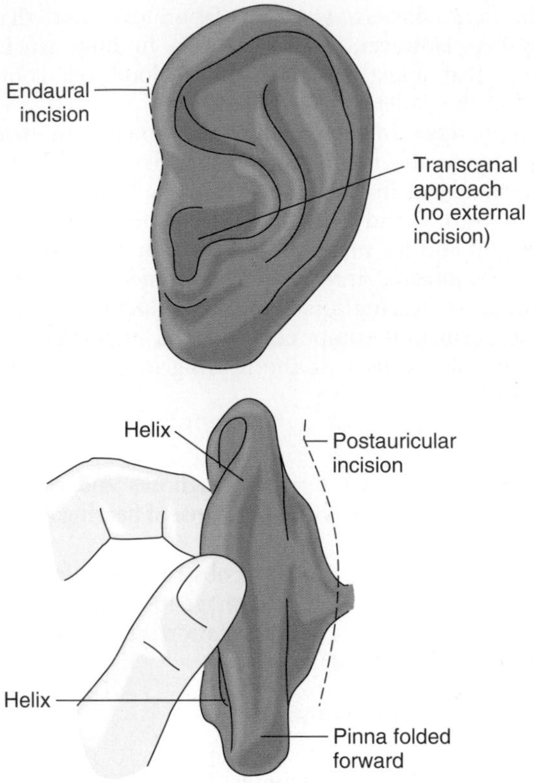

FIG. 48-11 Surgical approaches for repair of the ear and hearing structures.

Surgical Management. Many surgical interventions are available for patients with specific disorders leading to hearing loss.

Tympanoplasty. Tympanoplasty reconstructs the middle ear to improve conductive hearing loss. The procedures vary from simple reconstruction of the eardrum (**myringoplasty**) to replacement of the ossicles within the middle ear (**ossiculoplasty**).

Preoperative Care. The patient requires specific instructions before surgery. Systemic antibiotics reduce the risk for infection. Teach the patient to follow other measures to decrease the risks for infection, such as avoiding people with upper respiratory infections, getting adequate rest, eating a balanced diet, and drinking adequate amounts of fluid.

Assure the patient that hearing loss immediately after surgery is normal because of canal packing and that hearing will improve when it is removed. Stress that forceful coughing increases middle ear pressure and must be avoided.

Operative Procedures. Surgery is performed only when the middle ear is free of infection. If an infection is present, the graft is more likely to become infected and not heal. Surgery of the eardrum and ossicles requires the use of a microscope and is a delicate procedure. Local anesthesia can be used, although general anesthesia is often used to prevent the patient from moving.

The surgeon can repair the eardrum with many materials, including muscle fascia, a skin graft, and venous tissue. If the ossicles are damaged, more extensive surgery is needed for repair or replacement. The ossicles can be reached in several ways—through the ear canal, with an endaural incision, or by an incision behind the ear (Fig. 48-11).

CHART 48-9 Patient and Family Education: Preparing for Self-Management

Prevention of Ear Infection or Trauma

- Do not use small objects, such as cotton-tipped applicators, matches, toothpicks, keys, or hairpins, to clean your external ear canal.
- Wash your external ear and canal daily in the shower or while washing your hair.
- Blow your nose gently.
- Do not block one nostril while blowing your nose.
- Sneeze with your mouth open.
- Wear sound protection around loud or continuous noises.
- Avoid or wear head and ear protection during activities with high risk for head or ear trauma, such as wrestling, boxing, motorcycle riding, and skateboarding.
- Keep the volume on head receivers at the lowest setting that allows you to hear.
- Frequently clean objects that come into contact with your ear (e.g., headphones, telephone receivers).
- Avoid environmental conditions with rapid changes in air pressure.

The surgeon removes diseased tissue and cleans the middle ear cavity. The patient's cartilage or bone, cadaver ossicles, stainless steel wire, or special polymers (Teflon) are used to repair or replace the ossicles.

Postoperative Care. An antiseptic-soaked gauze, such as iodoform gauze (NU GAUZE), is packed in the ear canal. If a skin incision is used, a dressing is placed over it. Keep the dressing clean and dry, using sterile technique for changes. Keep the patient flat, with the head turned to the side and the operative ear facing up for at least 12 hours after surgery. Give prescribed antibiotics to prevent infection.

Patients often report hearing improvement after removal of the canal packing. Until that time, communicate as with a hearing-impaired patient, directing conversation to the unaffected ear. Instruct the patient in care and activity restrictions (see Chart 48-6).

Stapedectomy. A partial or complete stapedectomy with a prosthesis can correct some hearing loss, especially in patients with hearing loss related to otosclerosis. Although hearing usually improves after primary stapes surgery, some patients redevelop conductive hearing loss after surgery and revision surgery is needed.

Preoperative Care. To prevent infection, the patient must be free from external otitis at surgery. Teach the patient to follow measures that prevent middle ear or external ear infections (Chart 48-9).

Review with the patient the expected outcomes and possible complications of the surgery. Hearing is initially worse after a stapedectomy. The success rate of this procedure is high. However, there is always a risk for failure that might lead to total deafness on the affected side. Other possible complications include vertigo, infection, and facial nerve damage.

Operative Procedures. A stapedectomy is usually performed through the external ear canal with the patient under local anesthesia. After removal of the affected ossicles, a piston-shaped prosthesis is connected between the incus and the footplate (Fig. 48-12). Because the prosthesis vibrates with sound as the stapes did, most patients have restoration of functional hearing.

Postoperative Care. Remind the patient that improvement in hearing may not occur until 6 weeks after surgery. Drugs for pain help reduce discomfort, and antibiotics are used to prevent infection. Teach the patient about the precautions in Chart 48-6.

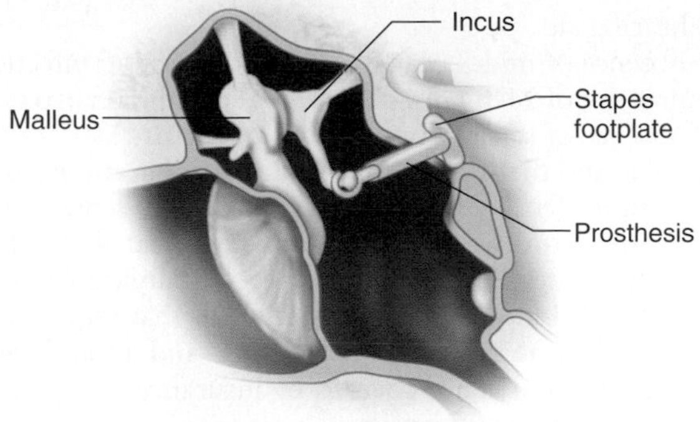

FIG. 48-12 Prosthesis used with stapedectomy. The stapes is removed, leaving the footplate. A metal or plastic prosthesis is connected to the incus and inserted through the hole to act as an artificial stapes.

The surgical procedure is performed in an area where cranial nerves VII, VIII, and X can be damaged by trauma or by swelling after surgery. *Assess for facial nerve damage or muscle weakness. Indications include an asymmetric appearance or drooping of features on the affected side of the face. Ask the patient about changes in facial perception of touch and in taste.* Vertigo, nausea, and vomiting usually occur after surgery because of the nearness to inner ear structures.

Antivertiginous drugs, such as meclizine (Antivert, Bonamine ♣), and antiemetic drugs, such as droperidol (Inapsine), are given. Take care to prevent falls.

! NURSING SAFETY PRIORITY QSEN

Action Alert

Prevent injury by assisting the patient with ambulation during the first 1 to 2 days after stapedectomy. Keep top bed siderails up, and remind the patient to move the head slowly to avoid vertigo.

Totally Implanted Devices. Totally implanted devices, such as the Esteem, can improve bilateral moderate to severe sensorineural hearing loss without any visible part (Barbara et al., 2011). These devices have three totally implanted components: a sound processor, a sensor, and a computer. Vibrations of the eardrum and ossicles are picked up by the sensor and converted to electric signals that are processed by the sound processor. The processor is programmed to the patient's specific hearing pathology. The processor filters out some background noise and amplifies the desired sound signal. The signal is transferred to the computer, which then converts the processed signal into vibrations that are transmitted to the inner ear for auditory SENSORY PERCEPTION.

Patient criteria for totally implantable devices include:

- Bilateral stable sensorineural hearing loss
- Speech discrimination score of 40% or higher
- Healthy tympanic membrane, eustachian tube, and ossicles of the middle ear
- Large enough ear cavity to fit the device components

- At least 30 days experience with an appropriate hearing aid
- Absence of middle ear, inner ear, or mastoid infection
- Absence of Ménière's disease or recurring vertigo
- Absence of sensitivity to device materials

The devices and the surgery may lead to complications, including temporary facial paralysis, changes in taste sensation, and ongoing or new-onset tinnitus. Unlike cochlear implants, the middle ear is entered and it is considered a surgical procedure. Care before and after surgery is similar to that required with stapedectomy. The cost of the implant and procedure can exceed $30,000 and is not covered by insurance.

Maximizing Communication

Planning: Expected Outcomes. The patient with reduced auditory SENSORY PERCEPTION is expected to become proficient in hearing compensation behaviors to maintain or improve communication. Indicators include that the patient consistently demonstrates these behaviors:

- Uses hearing assistive devices
- Uses sign language, lip-reading, closed captioning, or video description (for television viewing)
- Accurately interprets messages
- Uses nonverbal language
- Exchanges messages accurately with others

Interventions. Nursing priorities focus on facilitating communication and reducing anxiety.

Use best practices that are listed in Chart 48-10 for communicating with a hearing-impaired patient. Ask the patient what type of communication tools he or she is most comfortable using, and then use that format (Shuler et al., 2013). Do not shout at the patient, because the sound may be projected at a higher frequency, making him or her less able to understand. Communicate by writing (if he or she is able to see, read, and write) or pictures of familiar phrases and objects. Many television programs are now closed captioned or video described (subtitled). When available, use the assistive devices described on p. 1011 to increase communication.

Lip-reading and *sign language* can increase communication. In lip-reading, patients are taught special cues to look for when lip-reading and how to understand body language. However, the best lip-reader still misses more than half of what is being said. Because hearing is assisted by even minimal lip-reading, urge patients to wear their eyeglasses when talking with someone to see lip movement.

CHART 48-10 Best Practice for Patient Safety & Quality Care (QSEN)

Communicating with a Hearing-Impaired Patient

- Position yourself directly in front of the patient.
- Make sure that the room is well lighted.
- Get the patient's attention before you begin to speak.
- Move closer to the better-hearing ear.
- Speak clearly and slowly.
- Do not shout (shouting often makes understanding more difficult).
- Keep hands and other objects away from your mouth when talking to the patient.
- Have conversations in a quiet room with minimal distractions.
- Have the patient repeat your statements, not just indicate assent.
- Rephrase sentences and repeat information to aid understanding.
- Use appropriate hand motions.
- Write messages on paper if the patient is able to read.

Sign languages, such as American Sign Language (ASL), combine speech with hand movements that signify letters, words, and phrases. These languages take time and effort to learn, and many people are unable to use them effectively (Richardson, 2014).

Managing anxiety can increase the effectiveness of communication efforts. One source of anxiety is the possibility of permanent hearing loss. Provide accurate information about the likelihood of hearing returning. When the hearing impairment is likely to be permanent, reassure patients that communication and social interaction can be maintained.

To reduce anxiety and prevent social isolation, assist patients to use resources and communication to make social contact satisfying. Identify the patient's most satisfying activities and social interactions, and determine the effort necessary to continue them. The patient can alter activities to improve satisfaction. Instead of large gatherings, the patient might choose smaller groups. A meal at home with friends can substitute for dining in a noisy restaurant.

Community-Based Care

Lengthy hospitalization is rare for ear and hearing disorders. If surgery is needed and the procedure is completed without complications, it may be performed in an ambulatory surgery center.

Home Care Management. Patients who have persistent vertigo are in danger of falling. Assess the home for potential hazards and to determine whether family or significant others are available to assist with meal preparation and other ADLs. A nurse case manager can coordinate with the home care nurse to assist patients and their families in determining how to maintain adequate self-care abilities, maintain a safe environment, decide about assistance needs, and provide needed care.

Self-Management Education. Provide written instructions to the patient and family about how to take drugs and when to return for follow-up care. Teach patients how to instill eardrops (see Chart 48-3) and irrigate the ears (see Chart 48-2), and obtain a return demonstration.

To prevent infection after surgery, instruct patients to follow the suggestions in Chart 48-9. Teach patients who use a hearing aid how to use it effectively.

Health Care Resources. If patients do not have family or friends to help before or after surgery, a referral to a home care agency is needed. Help with meal preparation, cleaning, and personal hygiene can be arranged by the case manager.

Follow-up hearing tests are scheduled when the lesions are well healed, in about 6 to 8 weeks. Audiograms done before and after treatment are compared, and evaluation for further intervention to improve hearing begins. A complication of surgery is continued disability or complete loss of hearing in the affected ear. Surgery is performed first on the ear with the greatest hearing loss. If the surgery does not improve hearing, patients must decide to either attempt surgical correction of the other ear or continue to use an amplification device. When the underlying disorder causing the hearing impairment is progressive, this decision is difficult. Support patients by listening to their concerns and giving additional information when needed.

Costs to the person with a hearing impairment can be extensive. Information and support can come from public and private agencies that specialize in counseling patients with disorders affecting auditory SENSORY PERCEPTION.

◆ *Evaluation: Outcomes*

Evaluate the care of the patient with hearing loss or hearing impairment based on the identified priority patient problems. The expected outcomes include that the patient will:

- Have at least partial improvement of hearing
- Have minimal anxiety
- Use appropriate hearing compensation behaviors
- Communicate effectively in most situations

Specific indicators for these outcomes are listed for each priority problem under the Planning and Implementation section (see earlier).

CLINICAL JUDGMENT CHALLENGE

Ethical/Legal

The patient is a 78-year-old man whose hearing loss has progressed to the extent that hearing aids are no longer helpful. His only other health problems are early-stage prostate cancer (for which he is undergoing "watchful waiting") and type 2 diabetes mellitus (which is well controlled by diet and exercise). He lives alone in a condominium complex with many amenities. His son has voiced concern that his father should not live alone but should go into assisted living. The patient insists that this is not necessary because he can still drive, cook, and take care of himself. He also states that he has many friends in the condo complex and wants to remain active within the social groups there.

1. What should be your question when you meet with the father and the son?
2. Are there any major concerns for the father's immediate safety or health because of the hearing loss?
3. Are there any ethical or legal considerations in play here? If so, which one(s)?
4. What accommodations or environmental alterations can you recommend that would make it easier for the father to continue to live alone?
5. What other health care professionals should you consult with or bring in to this situation?

NURSING CONCEPTS AND CLINICAL JUDGMENT REVIEW

What might you NOTICE if the patient has auditory SENSORY PERCEPTION problems?

- Person tilts head to one side or leans forward to listen when another person speaks.
- Person watches the lips of a speaker closely.
- Person does not startle when a loud or unexpected sound occurs in the environment.
- Person frequently asks the speaker to repeat statements or questions.
- Person does not verbally interact with those around him or her.
- When a sentence is whispered to the person, he or she does not accurately repeat it back to the speaker.
- Person responds inappropriately to questions.

How should you RESPOND to a patient who has auditory SENSORY PERCEPTION problems?

- Reduce the background sound when speaking to the person (close the door to the hall, use a private area, turn off televisions and radios).
- Speak slowly, distinctly, and with a deeper tone.
- Face the patient while speaking.
- Ensure that all members of the health care team are aware of the patient's impairment and use an appropriate method to communicate with him or her.
- Determine whether the patient can communicate by sign language.
- Identify safety issues specific for the patient with a hearing impairment.
- Use a certified medical interpreter when taking a history from, explaining procedures to, or teaching the patient who has a hearing impairment.

GET READY FOR THE NCLEX® EXAMINATION!

KEY POINTS

Review these Key Points for each NCLEX Examination Client Needs Category.

Safe and Effective Care Environment

- Use Contact Precautions with any patient who has drainage from the ear canal. **Safety** QSEN
- Use a separate speculum cover for each ear when conducting an otoscopic examination. **Safety** QSEN
- Slowly and gently introduce the otoscopic speculum into the external ear canal during assessment. **Safety** QSEN
- Do not perform an otoscopic examination on a confused patient. **Safety** QSEN
- Use the suggestions presented in the Patient History section (p. 998) to enhance communication with a patient who has an impairment of auditory SENSORY PERCEPTION. **Safety** QSEN
- Protect the patient with vertigo or dizziness from injury by assisting with ambulation. **Safety** QSEN
- Follow the guidelines in Chart 48-4 when irrigating the ear canal. **Safety** QSEN

Health Promotion and Maintenance

- Teach patients the proper way to clean the pinna and external ear canal and how to remove cerumen from the external canal. **Evidence-Based Practice** QSEN

- Identify patients at risk for hearing impairment as a result of work environment or leisure activities. **Patient-Centered Care** QSEN
- Encourage all patients, even if they already have a hearing impairment, to use ear protection in loud environments. **Patient-Centered Care** QSEN
- Inform all patients who smoke that smoking increases the risk for development of hearing problems. **Evidence-Based Practice** QSEN
- Teach patients how to properly care for their hearing aids. **Patient-Centered Care** QSEN
- Instruct patients to avoid closing off one naris when blowing the nose. **Patient-Centered Care** QSEN
- Remind patients who engage in water sports and who are at risk for external otitis to wear earplugs when in the water. **Patient-Centered Care** QSEN
- Teach patients the proper techniques for self-instillation of eardrops and ear irrigation. **Patient-Centered Care** QSEN

Psychosocial Integrity

- Allow the patient the opportunity to express fear or anxiety about a change in hearing status. **Patient-Centered Care** QSEN
- Explain all diagnostic and therapeutic procedures, restrictions, and follow-up care to the patient and family. **Patient-Centered Care** QSEN
- Refer patients newly diagnosed with hearing impairment or any chronic ear problem to appropriate local resources and support groups.
- Teach family members ways to communicate with a hearing-impaired patient with and without a hearing aid. **Patient-Centered Care** QSEN
- Assess the degree to which hearing problems interfere with the patient's ability to interact with others. **Patient-Centered Care** QSEN
- Remind patients having ear surgery that hearing in the affected ear may be reduced immediately after surgery because of packing, swelling, or surgical manipulation. **Patient-Centered Care** QSEN

Physiological Integrity

- Ask the patient about hearing problems in any other members of the family, because many hearing problems have a genetic component. **Patient-Centered Care** QSEN
- Check the hearing of any patient receiving an ototoxic drug for more than 5 days. **Evidence-Based Practice** QSEN
- Ask the patient about current and past drug use (prescribed, over-the-counter), and check with a pharmacist to evaluate for ototoxicity. **Patient-Centered Care** QSEN
- Avoid ear canal irrigation if the eardrum is perforated or if the canal contains vegetative matter. **Safety** QSEN
- Stress the importance of completing an antibiotic regimen for an ear infection. **Evidence-Based Practice** QSEN
- Remind patients to move the head slowly after ear surgery to prevent dizziness or vertigo. **Patient-Centered Care** QSEN
- Use upper siderails for any patient experiencing dizziness or vertigo. **Safety** QSEN
- Work with the case manager, home care nurse, speech-language pathologist, and occupational therapist to ensure safety and optimal function for the patient with a hearing or balance problem in the community setting. **Teamwork and Collaboration** QSEN

CHAPTER 49

Assessment of the Musculoskeletal System

Donna D. Ignatavicius

http://evolve.elsevier.com/Iggy/

PRIORITY CONCEPTS

- MOBILITY
- PAIN
- SENSORY PERCEPTION

LEARNING OUTCOMES

Safe and Effective Care Environment

1. Collaborate with the physical and occupational therapists to perform a complete musculoskeletal assessment, including functional status, as needed.

Health Promotion and Maintenance

2. Explain how physiologic aging changes of the musculoskeletal system affect care of older adults.

Psychosocial Integrity

3. Assess the patient's and family's reaction to change in body image caused by a major musculoskeletal health problem.

Physiological Integrity

4. Recall the basic anatomy and physiology of the musculoskeletal system.
5. Assess patients for MOBILITY, gait, motor skills, PAIN, SENSORY PERCEPTION, and the use of assistive devices.
6. Interpret assessment findings in a patient with a musculoskeletal health problem.
7. Explain the use of laboratory testing for a patient with a musculoskeletal health problem.
8. Develop a teaching plan to educate the patient and family about diagnostic procedures.

The musculoskeletal system is the second largest body system. It includes the bones, joints, and skeletal muscles, as well as the supporting structures needed to move them. MOBILITY (movement) is a basic human need that is essential for performing ADLs. When a patient cannot move to perform ADLs or other daily routines, self-esteem and a sense of self-worth can be diminished.

Disease, surgery, and trauma can affect one or more parts of the musculoskeletal system, often leading to decreased mobility. When MOBILITY is impaired for a long time, other body systems can be affected. For example, prolonged immobility can lead to skin breakdown, constipation, and thrombus formation. If nerves are damaged by trauma or disease, patients may also have problems with SENSORY PERCEPTION, also known as *sensation*.

ANATOMY AND PHYSIOLOGY REVIEW

Skeletal System

The skeletal system consists of 206 bones and multiple joints. The growth and development of these structures occur during childhood and adolescence and are not discussed in this text. Common physical skeletal differences among selected racial/ethnic groups are listed in Table 49-1.

Bones

Types and Structure. Bone can be classified in two ways—by shape and by structure. **Long bones**, such as the femur, are cylindric with rounded ends and often bear weight. **Short bones**, such as the phalanges, are small and bear little or no weight. **Flat bones**, such as the scapula, protect vital organs and

TABLE 49-1 Musculoskeletal Differences in Selected Racial/Ethnic Groups

GROUP	MUSCULOSKELETAL DIFFERENCES
African Americans	Greater bone density than Europeans, Asians, and Hispanics. Accounts for decreased incidence of osteoporosis.
Amish	Greater incidence of dwarfism than in other populations.
Chinese Americans	Bones are shorter and smaller with less bone density. Increased incidence of osteoporosis.
Egyptian Americans	Shorter in stature than Euro-Americans and African Americans.
Filipino/Vietnamese	Short in stature; adult height about 5 feet.
Irish Americans	Taller and broader than other Euro-Americans. Less bone density than African Americans.
Navajo American Indians	Taller and thinner than other American Indians.

often contain blood-forming cells. Bones that have unique shapes are known as **irregular bones**. The carpal bones in the wrist and the small bones in the inner ear are examples of **irregular bones**. The sesamoid bone is the least common type and develops within a tendon; the patella is a typical example.

The second way bone is classified is by *structure* or composition. As shown in Fig. 49-1, the outer layer of bone, or cortex, is composed of dense, compact bone tissue. The inner layer, in the medulla, contains spongy, cancellous tissue. Almost every bone has both tissue types but in varying quantities. The long bone typically has a shaft, or diaphysis, and two knoblike ends, or epiphyses.

The structural unit of the cortical compact bone is the haversian system, which is detailed in Fig. 49-1. The haversian system is a complex canal network containing microscopic blood vessels that supply nutrients and oxygen to bone, as well as lacunae, which are small cavities that house **osteocytes** (bone cells). The canals run vertically within the hard cortical bone tissue.

The softer **cancellous** tissue contains large spaces, or trabeculae, which are filled with red and yellow marrow. **Hematopoiesis** (production of blood cells) occurs in the red marrow. The yellow marrow contains fat cells, which can be dislodged and enter the bloodstream to cause fat embolism syndrome (FES), a life-threatening complication. Volkmann's canals connect bone marrow vessels with the haversian system and periosteum, the outermost covering of the bone. In the deepest layer of the periosteum are osteogenic cells, which later differentiate into **osteoblasts** (bone-forming cells) and **osteoclasts** (bone-destroying cells).

Bone also contains a matrix consisting chiefly of collagen, mucopolysaccharides, and lipids. Deposits of inorganic calcium salts (carbonate and phosphate) in the matrix provide the hardness of bone.

Bone is a very vascular tissue. Its estimated total blood flow is between 200 and 400 mL/min. Each bone has a main nutrient artery, which enters near the middle of the shaft and branches into ascending and descending vessels. These vessels supply the cortex, the marrow, and the haversian system. Very few nerve

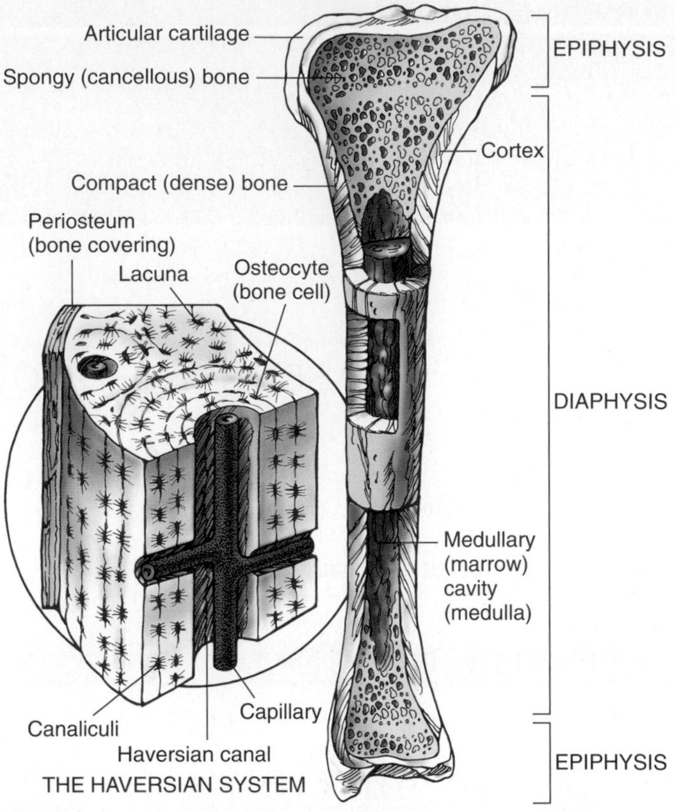

FIG. 49-1 The structure of a typical long bone. The cortex, or outer layer, is composed of dense, compact tissue. The microscopic structure of this compact cortical tissue is the haversian system.

fibers are connected to bone. Sympathetic nerve fibers control dilation of blood vessels. Sensory nerve fibers transmit pain signals experienced by patients who have primary lesions of the bone, like bone tumors.

Function. The skeletal system:

- Provides a framework for the body and allows the body to be weight bearing, or upright
- Supports the surrounding tissues (e.g., muscle and tendons)
- Assists in movement through muscle attachment and joint formation
- Protects vital organs, such as the heart and lungs
- Manufactures blood cells in red bone marrow
- Provides storage for mineral salts (e.g., calcium and phosphorus)

After puberty, bone reaches its maturity and maximum growth. Bone is a dynamic tissue. It undergoes a continuous process of formation and **resorption**, or destruction, at equal rates until the age of 35 years. In later years, bone resorption increases, decreasing bone mass and predisposing patients to injury, especially older women.

Numerous minerals and hormones affect bone growth and metabolism, including:

- Calcium
- Phosphorus
- Calcitonin
- Vitamin D
- Parathyroid hormone (PTH)
- Growth hormone
- Glucocorticoids

- Estrogens and androgens
- Thyroxine
- Insulin

Bone accounts for about 99% of the *calcium* in the body and 90% of the *phosphorus.* In healthy adults, the serum concentrations of calcium and phosphorus maintain an inverse relationship. As calcium levels rise, phosphorus levels decrease. When serum levels are altered, calcitonin and PTH work to maintain equilibrium. If the calcium in the blood is decreased, the bone, which stores calcium, releases calcium into the bloodstream in response to PTH stimulation.

Calcitonin is produced by the thyroid gland and *decreases* the serum calcium concentration if it is increased above its normal level. Calcitonin inhibits bone resorption and increases renal excretion of calcium and phosphorus as needed to maintain balance in the body.

Vitamin D and its metabolites are produced in the body and transported in the blood to promote the absorption of calcium and phosphorus from the small intestine. They also seem to enhance PTH activity to release calcium from the bone. A decrease in the body's vitamin D level can result in osteomalacia (softening of bone) in the adult. Vitamin D metabolism and osteomalacia are described in Chapter 50.

When serum calcium levels are lowered, *parathyroid hormone* (PTH, or parathormone) secretion increases and stimulates bone to promote osteoclastic activity and *release* calcium to the blood. PTH reduces the renal excretion of calcium and facilitates its absorption from the intestine. If serum calcium levels increase, PTH secretion diminishes to preserve the bone calcium supply. This process is an example of the feedback loop system of the endocrine system.

Growth hormone secreted by the anterior lobe of the pituitary gland is responsible for increasing bone length and determining the amount of bone matrix formed before puberty. During childhood, an increased secretion results in gigantism and a decreased secretion results in dwarfism. In the adult, an increase causes acromegaly, which is characterized by bone and soft-tissue deformities (see Chapter 62).

Adrenal glucocorticoids regulate protein metabolism, either increasing or decreasing catabolism to reduce or intensify the organic matrix of bone. They also aid in regulating intestinal calcium and phosphorus absorption.

Estrogens stimulate osteoblastic (bone-building) activity and inhibit PTH. When estrogen levels decline at menopause, women are susceptible to low serum calcium levels with increased bone loss (osteoporosis). *Androgens,* such as testosterone in men, promote anabolism (body tissue building) and increase bone mass.

Thyroxine is one of the principal hormones secreted by the thyroid gland. Its primary function is to increase the rate of protein synthesis in all types of tissue, including bone. *Insulin* works together with growth hormone to build and maintain healthy bone tissue.

Joints

A **joint** is a space in which two or more bones come together. This is also referred to as *articulation* of the joint. The major function of a joint is to provide movement and flexibility in the body.

There are three types of joints in the body:

- Synarthrodial, or completely immovable, joints (e.g., in the cranium)

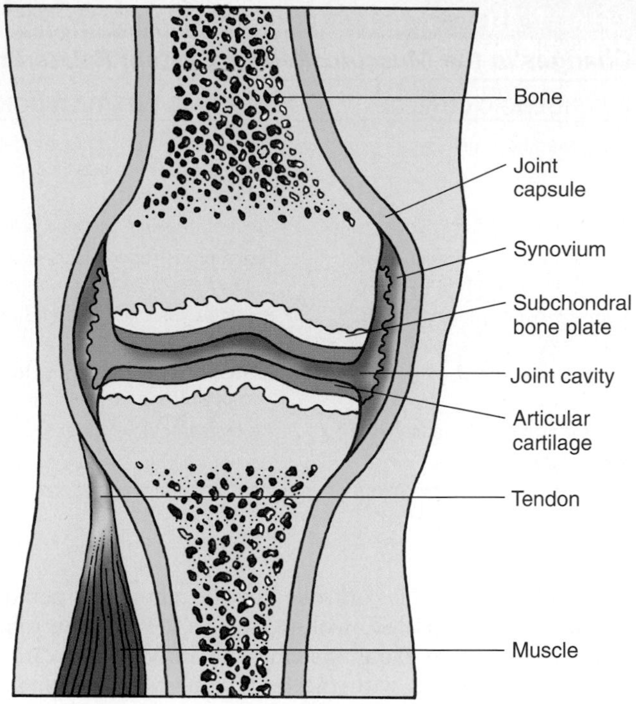

FIG. 49-2 The structure of a synovial joint. Synovium lines the joint capsule but does not extend into the articular cartilage.

- Amphiarthrodial, or slightly movable, joints (e.g., in the pelvis)
- Diarthrodial (synovial), or freely movable, joints (e.g., the elbow and knee)

Although any of these joints can be affected by disease or injury, the synovial joints are most commonly involved as discussed in Chapter 18.

The diarthrodial, or synovial, joint is the most common type of joint in the body. **Synovial joints** are the only type lined with synovium, a membrane that secretes synovial fluid for lubrication and shock absorption. As shown in Fig. 49-2, the synovium lines the internal portion of the joint capsule but does not normally extend onto the surface of the cartilage at the spongy bone ends. Articular cartilage consists of a collagen fiber matrix impregnated with a complex ground substance. Patients with inflammatory types of arthritis often have synovitis (synovial inflammation) and breakdown of the cartilage. Bursae, small sacs lined with synovial membrane, are located at joints and bony prominences to prevent friction between bone and structures adjacent to bone. These structures can also become inflamed, causing bursitis.

Synovial joints are described by their anatomic structures. *Ball-and-socket* joints (shoulder, hip) permit movement in any direction. *Hinge* joints (elbow) allow motion in one plane—flexion and extension. The knee is often classified as a hinge joint, but it rotates slightly, as well as flexes and extends. It is best described as a *condylar* type of synovial joint. The gliding movement of the wrist is characteristic of the *biaxial* joint. *Pivot* joints permit rotation only, as in the radioulnar area.

Muscular System

There are three types of muscle in the body: smooth muscle, cardiac muscle, and skeletal muscle. Smooth, or non-striated, involuntary muscle is responsible for contractions of organs

CHART 49-1 **Nursing Focus on the Older Adult**

Changes in the Musculoskeletal System Related to Aging

PHYSIOLOGIC CHANGE	NURSING INTERVENTIONS	RATIONALES
Decreased bone density	Teach safety tips to prevent falls. Reinforce need to exercise, especially weight-bearing exercise.	Porous bones are more likely to fracture. Exercise slows bone loss.
Increased bone prominence	Prevent pressure on bone prominences.	There is less soft tissue to prevent skin breakdown.
Kyphotic posture: widened gait, shift in the center of gravity	Teach proper body mechanics; instruct the patient to sit in supportive chairs with arms.	Correction of posture problems prevents further deformity; the patient should have support for bony structures.
Cartilage degeneration	Provide moist heat, such as a shower or warm, moist compresses.	Moist heat increases blood flow to the area.
Decreased range of motion (ROM)	Assess the patient's ability to perform ADLs and mobility.	The patient may need assistance with self-care skills.
Muscle atrophy, decreased strength	Teach isometric exercises.	Exercises increase muscle strength.
Slowed movement	Do not rush the person; be patient.	The patient may become frustrated if hurried.

and blood vessels and is controlled by the autonomic nervous system. Cardiac or striated involuntary muscle is also controlled by the autonomic nervous system. The smooth and cardiac muscles are discussed with the body systems to which they belong in the assessment chapters.

In contrast to smooth and cardiac muscle, skeletal muscle is striated voluntary muscle controlled by the central and peripheral nervous systems. The junction of a peripheral motor nerve and the muscle cells that it supplies is sometimes referred to as a **motor end plate**. Muscle fibers are held in place by connective tissue in bundles, or fasciculi. The entire muscle is surrounded by dense fibrous tissue, or fascia, which contains the muscle's blood, lymph, and nerve supply.

The main function of skeletal muscle is *movement* of the body and its parts. When bones, joints, and supporting structures are adversely affected by injury or disease, the adjacent muscle tissue is often involved, limiting mobility. During the aging process, muscle fibers decrease in size and number, even in well-conditioned adults. Atrophy results when muscles are not regularly exercised, and they deteriorate from disuse.

Supporting structures for the muscular system are very susceptible to injury. They include **tendons** (bands of tough, fibrous tissue that attach muscles to bones) and **ligaments**, which attach bones to other bones at joints.

MUSCULOSKELETAL CHANGES ASSOCIATED WITH AGING

Osteopenia, or decreased bone density (bone loss), occurs as one ages. Many older adults, especially white, thin women, have severe osteopenia, a disease called *osteoporosis*. This condition causes postural and gait changes and predisposes the person to fractures. Chapter 50 discusses this health problem in detail.

Synovial joint cartilage can become less elastic and compressible as a person ages. As a result of these cartilage changes and continued use of joints, the joint cartilage becomes damaged, leading to osteoarthritis (OA). Genetic defects in cartilage may also contribute to joint disease. The most common joints affected are the weight-bearing joints of the hip, knee, and cervical and lumbar spine, but joints in the shoulder and upper extremity, feet, and hands also can be affected. Refer to Chapter 18 for a complete discussion of OA.

As one ages, muscle tissue atrophies. Increased activity and exercise can slow the progression of atrophy and restore muscle strength (Touhy & Jett, 2014). Musculoskeletal changes cause decreased coordination, loss of muscle strength, gait changes, and a risk for falls with injury. (See Chapter 2 for discussion on fall prevention.) Chart 49-1 lists the major anatomic and physiologic changes and implications for nursing care.

ASSESSMENT METHODS

Patient History

In the assessment of a patient with an actual or potential musculoskeletal problem, a detailed and accurate history is helpful in identifying priority problems and nursing interventions. The history reveals information about the patient that can direct the physical assessment.

Accidents, illnesses, lifestyle, and drugs may contribute to a patient's current problem. Young men are at the greatest risk for trauma related to motor vehicle crashes. Older adults are at the greatest risk for falls that result in fractures and soft-tissue injury. When taking a personal health history, question the patient about any traumatic injuries and sports activities, no matter when they occurred. An injury to the lumbar spine 30 years ago may have caused a patient's current low back pain. A motor vehicle crash or sports injury can cause osteoarthritis years after the event.

Previous or current illness or disease may affect musculoskeletal status. For example, a patient with diabetes who is treated for a foot ulcer is at high risk for acute or chronic osteomyelitis (bone infection). In addition, diabetes slows the healing process. Ask the patient about any previous hospitalizations and illnesses or complications. Inquire about his or her ability to perform ADLs independently or if assistive/adaptive devices are used.

Current lifestyle also contributes to musculoskeletal health. Weight-bearing activities such as walking can reduce risk factors for osteoporosis and maintain muscle strength (McCance et al., 2014). High-impact sports, such as excessive jogging or running, can cause musculoskeletal injury to soft tissues and bone. Tobacco use slows the healing of musculoskeletal injuries. Excessive alcohol intake can decrease vitamins and nutrients the person needs for bone and muscle tissue growth.

When assessing a patient with a possible musculoskeletal alteration, inquire about occupation or work life. A person's occupation can cause or contribute to an injury. For instance, fractures are not uncommon in patients whose jobs require manual labor, such as housekeepers, mechanics, and industrial workers. Certain occupations, such as computer-related jobs, may predispose a person to carpal tunnel syndrome (entrapment of the median nerve in the wrist) or neck pain. Construction workers and health care workers may experience back injury from prolonged standing and excessive lifting. Amateur and professional athletes often experience acute musculoskeletal injuries (e.g., joint dislocations and fractures) and chronic disorders (e.g., joint cartilage trauma), which can lead to osteoarthritis.

Ask about allergies, particularly allergy to dairy products, and previous and current use of drugs—prescribed, over-the-counter, and illicit. Allergy to dairy products could cause decreased calcium intake. Some drugs, such as steroids, can negatively affect calcium metabolism and promote bone loss. Other drugs may be taken to relieve musculoskeletal pain. Inquire about herbs, vitamin and mineral supplements, or biologic compounds that may be used for arthritis and other musculoskeletal problems, such as glucosamine and chondroitin. Complementary and alternative therapies are commonly used by patients with various types of arthritis and **arthralgias** (joint aching). Chapter 18 discusses these therapies in detail.

Nutrition History

A brief review of the patient's nutrition history helps determine any risks for inadequate nutrient intake. For example, most people, especially women, do not get enough calcium in their diet. Determine if the patient has had a significant weight gain or loss.

Ask the patient to recall a typical day of food intake to help identify deficiencies and excesses in the diet. Lactose intolerance is a common problem that can cause inadequate calcium intake. People who cannot afford to buy food are especially at risk for undernutrition. Some older adults and others are not financially able to buy the proper foods for adequate nutrition.

Inadequate protein or insufficient vitamin C or D in the diet slows bone and tissue healing. Obesity places excess stress and strain on bones and joints, with resulting trauma to joint cartilage. In addition, obesity inhibits MOBILITY in patients with musculoskeletal problems, which predisposes them to complications such as respiratory and circulatory problems. People with eating disorders such as anorexia nervosa and bulimia nervosa are also at risk for osteoporosis related to decreased intake of calcium and vitamin D.

Family History and Genetic Risk

Obtaining a family history assists in identifying disorders that have a familial or genetic tendency. Osteoporosis (age-related bone loss) and gout, for instance, often occur in several generations of a family. Osteogenic sarcoma, a type of bone cancer, may be genetically influenced by *Tp53* gene mutation (Nussbaum et al., 2007). Positive family history of these types of disorders can increase risks to the patient. Chapters 18 and 50 provide a more complete description of musculoskeletal problems that have strong genetic links.

Current Health Problems

The most common reports of persons with a musculoskeletal problem are PAIN and weakness, either of which can impair MOBILITY. Collect data pertinent to the patient's presenting health problem:

- Date and time of onset
- Factors that cause or exacerbate (worsen) the problem
- Course of the problem (e.g., intermittent or continuous)
- Clinical manifestations (as expressed by the patient) and the pattern of their occurrence
- Measures that improve clinical manifestations (e.g., heat, ice)

Assessment of PAIN can present many challenges. Pain can be related to bone, muscle, or joint problems. It may be described as acute or chronic, depending on the onset and duration. Pain with movement could indicate a fracture and/or muscle or joint injury. Assess the intensity of pain by using a pain scale and asking the patient to rate the level he or she is experiencing. Quality of pain may be described as dull, burning, aching, or stabbing. Determine the location of pain and areas to which it radiates. With any assessment, it is always best if the patient describes the pain in his or her own words and points to its location, if possible. Chapter 3 describes acute and chronic pain in detail.

Weakness may be related to individual muscles or muscle groups. Determine if weakness occurs in proximal or distal muscles or muscle groups. Proximal weakness (near trunk of body) may indicate **myopathy** (a problem in muscle tissue), whereas distal weakness (in extremities) may indicate **neuropathy** (a problem in nerve tissue). Muscle weakness in the lower extremities may increase the risk for falls and injury. Weakness in the upper extremities may interfere with ADLs.

Assessment of the Skeletal System

Although bones, joints, and muscles are usually assessed simultaneously in a head-to-toe approach, each subsystem is described separately for emphasis and understanding. For physical assessment of the musculoskeletal system, use inspection, palpation, and range of motion (ROM). A general assessment is described in this chapter. More specific assessment techniques are discussed in the musculoskeletal problem chapters in this unit.

General Inspection

Observe the patient's posture, gait, and general mobility for gross deformities and impairment. Note unusual findings, and coordinate with the physical or occupational therapist for an in-depth physical assessment.

Posture and Gait. **Posture** includes the person's body build and alignment when standing and walking. Assess the curvature of the spine and the length, shape, and symmetry of extremities. Fig. 49-3 illustrates several common spinal deformities. Inspect muscle mass for size and symmetry.

Most patients with musculoskeletal problems eventually have a problem with *gait*. The nurse or therapist evaluates the patient's balance, steadiness, and ease and length of stride. Any limp or other asymmetric leg movement or deformity is noted. An abnormality in the stance phase of gait is called an **antalgic** gait. When part of one leg is painful, the patient shortens the stance phase on the affected side. An abnormality in the swing phase is called a **lurch**. This abnormal gait occurs when the muscles in the buttocks and/or legs are too weak to allow the person to change weight from one foot to the other. In this case, the shoulders are moved either side-to-side or front-to-back for help in shifting the weight from one leg to the other. Some patients, such as those with chronic hip pain and muscle atrophy from arthritic disorders, have a combination of an antalgic gait and lurch.

Mobility and Functional Assessment. In collaboration with the physical or occupational therapist, assess the patient's need for ambulatory devices, such as canes and walkers, during transfer from bed to chair and while walking and climbing stairs. Observe his or her ability to perform ADLs, such as dressing and bathing. PAIN and deformity may limit physical MOBILITY and function. Coordinate with the physical and occupational therapists to assess the patient's functional status. A complete discussion of functional assessment is found in Chapter 6.

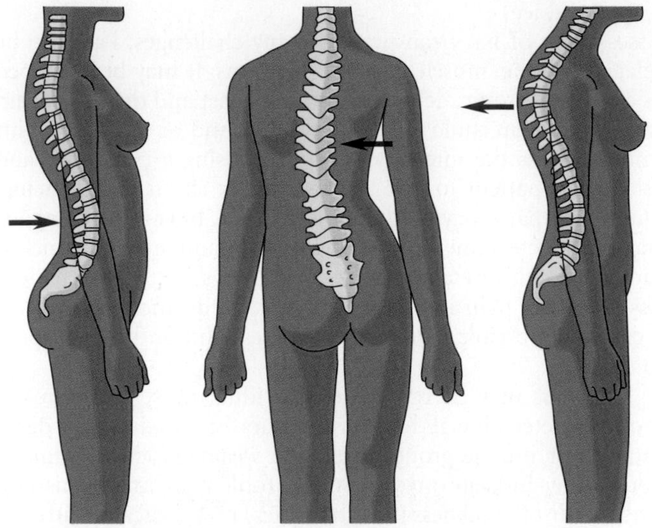

FIG. 49-3 Common spinal deformities.

Assess major bones, joints, and muscles by inspection, palpation, and determination of ROM. Pay special attention to areas that are affected or may be affected, according to the patient's history or current problem.

A **goniometer** is a tool that may be used by rehabilitation therapists or nurses to provide an exact measurement of flexion and extension or joint ROM. Active range of motion (AROM) can be evaluated by asking the patient to move each joint through the ROM himself or herself. If the patient cannot actively move a joint through range of motion, ask him or her to relax the muscles in the extremity. Hold the part with one hand above and one hand below the joint to be evaluated and allow passive range of motion (PROM) to evaluate joint MOBILITY. Movements shown in Fig. 49-4 may be used to evaluate active and passive ROM. Circumduction is a movement that can also be evaluated in the shoulder by having the patient move the arm in circles from the shoulder joint. As long as the patient can function to meet personal needs, a limitation in ROM may not be significant. For each anatomic location, observe the skin for color, elasticity, and lesions that may relate to musculoskeletal dysfunction. For instance, redness or warmth may indicate an inflammatory process and/or pressure injury to skin.

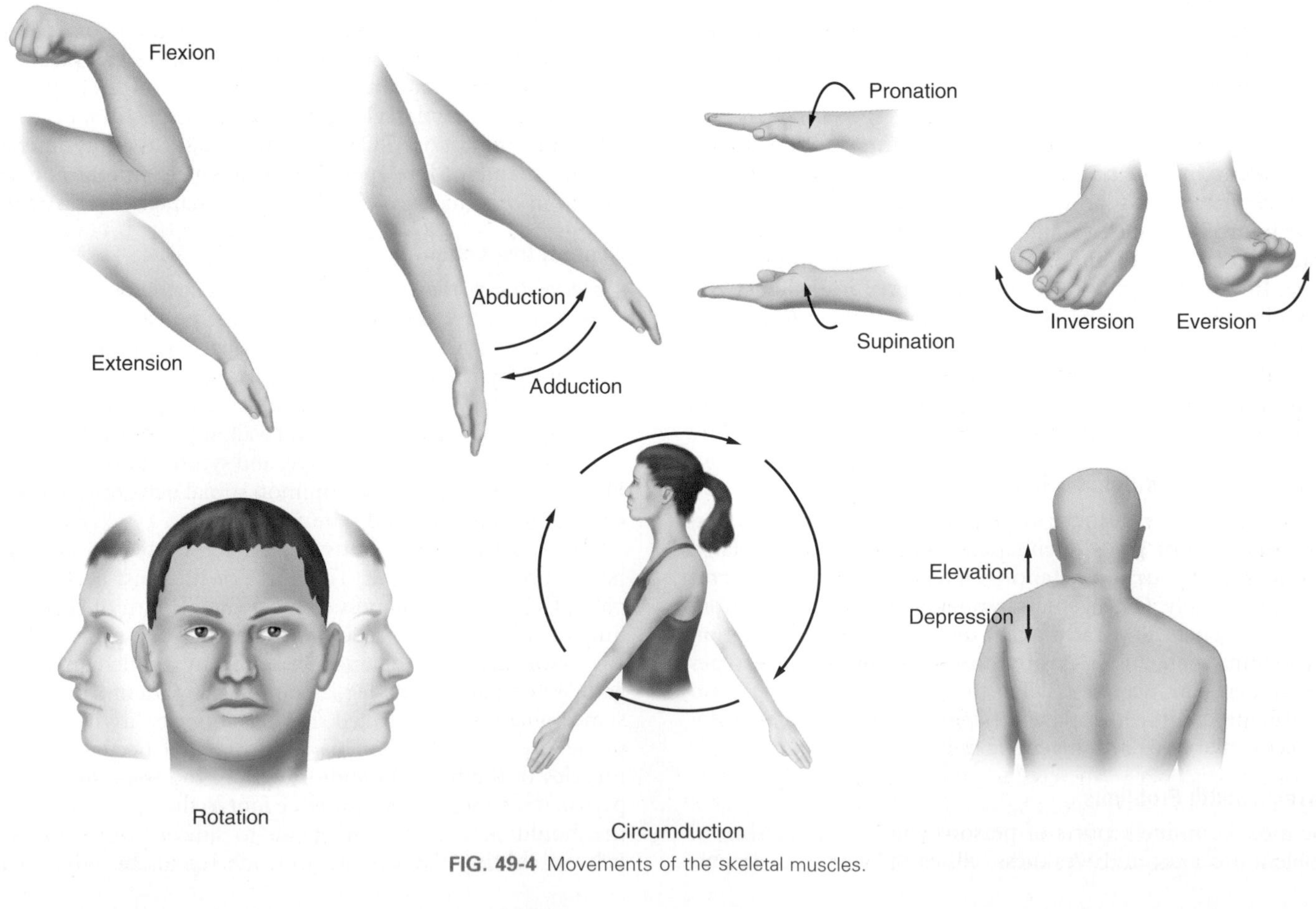

FIG. 49-4 Movements of the skeletal muscles.

NCLEX EXAMINATION CHALLENGE

Health Promotion and Maintenance

A nurse is performing a musculoskeletal assessment on an older adult living independently in a senior housing apartment. What normal physiologic changes of aging does the nurse expect? **Select all that apply.**

A. Muscle contractures
B. Slowed movement
C. Lordosis
D. Antalgic gait
E. Decreased coordination

Specific Assessments

If the patient has PAIN or weakness in the *face* or *neck*, inspect and palpate this area for tenderness and masses. Ask the patient to open his or her mouth while palpating the temporomandibular joints (TMJs). Common abnormal findings are tenderness or PAIN, **crepitus** (a grating sound), and a spongy swelling caused by excess synovium and fluid.

Inspect and palpate each vertebra of the spine in the neck. Proceed cautiously and gently if PAIN is present. Clinical findings may include malalignment; tenderness; or inability to flex, extend, and rotate the neck as expected. Muscle and nerve pain often accompany neck pain if spinal nerves are involved.

The thoracic spine, lumbar spine, and sacral spine are evaluated in the same manner as the neck. Spinal alignment problems are common (see Fig. 49-3). Place both hands over the posterior iliac crests with the thumbs over the lumbosacral area. Apply pressure with the thumbs along the lumbosacral spine to elicit tenderness. Many patients do not have discomfort until the area is palpated. **Lordosis** is a common finding in adults who have abdominal obesity. During screening for **scoliosis**, ask the patient to flex forward from the hips and inspect for a lateral curve in the spine.

If the extremities are affected by a musculoskeletal problem, assess arms or legs at the same time for side-to-side comparisons. For example, inspect and palpate both shoulders for size, swelling, deformity, poor alignment, tenderness or PAIN, and MOBILITY. A shoulder injury may prevent the patient from combing his or her hair with the affected arm, but severe arthritis may inhibit movement in both arms. Assess the elbows and wrists in a similar way.

Because the hand has multiple joints in a single digit, assessment of hand function is perhaps the most critical part of the examination. If the hands are affected, inspect and palpate the metacarpophalangeal (MCP), proximal interphalangeal (PIP), and distal interphalangeal (DIP) joints. The same digits are compared on the right and left hands (Fig. 49-5). Determine the range of motion (ROM) for each joint by observing active movement. If movement is not possible, evaluate passive motion. For a quick and easy assessment of ROM, ask the patient to make a fist and then appose each finger to the thumb. If he or she can perform these maneuvers, ROM of the hand is not seriously restricted.

Evaluation of the hip joint relies primarily on determination of its degree of mobility, because the joint is deep and difficult to inspect or palpate. *The patient with hip pain usually experiences it in the groin or has pain that radiates to the knee.* The knee is readily accessible for physical assessment, particularly when the patient is sitting and the knee is flexed. Fluid accumulation,

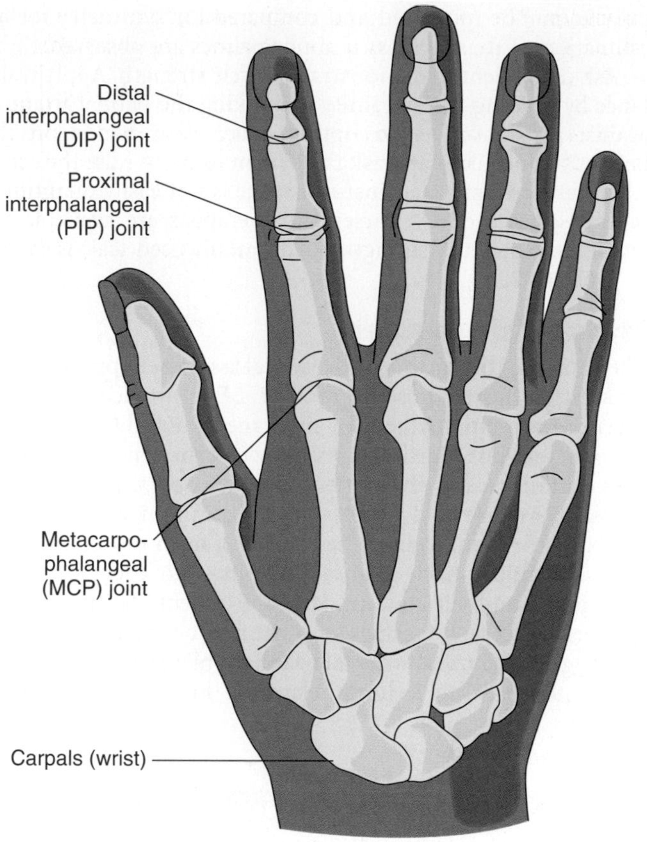

FIG. 49-5 The small joints of the hand.

or **effusion**, is easily detected in the knee joint. Limitations in movement with accompanying PAIN are common findings. The knees may be poorly aligned, as in **genu valgum** ("knock-knee") or **genu varum** ("bowlegged") deformities.

The ankles and feet are often neglected in the physical examination. However, they contain multiple bones and joints that can be affected by disease and injury. Observe and palpate each joint and test for ROM if feet are affected by musculoskeletal problems.

Neurovascular Assessment

While completing a physical assessment of the musculoskeletal system, perform an assessment of peripheral vascular and nerve integrity. Beginning with the injured side, always compare one extremity with the other.

NURSING SAFETY PRIORITY QSEN

Action Alert

Perform a complete **neurovascular assessment** (also called a "circ check"), which includes *palpation of pulses in the extremities below the level of injury and assessment of sensation, movement, color, temperature, and pain in the injured part.* If pulses are not palpable, use a Doppler to find pulses in the extremities. See Chart 51-3 in Chapter 51 for more details about neurovascular assessment.

Assessment of the Muscular System

During the skeletal assessment, notice the size, shape, tone, and strength of major skeletal muscles. The circumference of each muscle may be measured and compared for symmetry for an estimation of muscle mass if abnormalities are observed.

Ask the patient to demonstrate muscle strength. Apply resistance by holding the extremity and asking thc patient to move against resistance. As an option, place your hands on the patient's upper arms and ask the patient to try to raise the arms. Although movement against resistance is not easily quantified, several scales used by nurses and therapists are available for grading the patient's strength. A commonly used scale is shown in Table 49-2.

Psychosocial Assessment

The data from the history and physical assessment provide clues for anticipating psychosocial problems. For instance, prolonged absence from employment or permanent disability may cause job or career loss. Further stress may be experienced if chronic pain continues and the patient cannot cope with numerous stressors. Anxiety and depression are common when patients have chronic pain. Deformities resulting from musculoskeletal disease or injury, such as an amputation, can affect a person's body image and self-concept. Help the patient identify support systems and coping mechanisms that may be useful if he or she has long-term musculoskeletal health problems. Encourage him or her to verbalize feelings related to loss and body image changes. Refer the patient for psychological or spiritual counseling if needed and if it is culturally appropriate.

Diagnostic Assessment

Laboratory Assessment

Chart 49-2 lists the common laboratory tests used in assessing patients with musculoskeletal disorders. There is no special

TABLE 49-2 Common Scale for Grading Muscle Strength

RATING	DESCRIPTION
5	Normal: ROM unimpaired against gravity with full resistance
4	Good: can complete ROM against gravity with some resistance
3	Fair: can complete ROM against gravity
2	Poor: can complete ROM with gravity eliminated
1	Trace: no joint motion and slight evidence of muscle contractility
0	Zero: no evidence of muscle contractility

ROM, Range of motion.

CHART 49-2 Laboratory Profile

Musculoskeletal Assessment

TEST	NORMAL RANGE FOR ADULTS	SIGNIFICANCE OF ABNORMAL FINDINGS
Serum calcium	9.0-10.5 mg/dL (2.25-2.75 mmol/L) *Older adults:* decreased	*Hypercalcemia* (increased calcium) • Metastatic cancers of the bone • Paget's disease • Bone fractures in healing stage *Hypocalcemia* (decreased calcium) • Osteoporosis • Osteomalacia
Serum phosphorus (phosphate)	3.0-4.5 mg/dL (0.97-1.45 mmol/L) *Older adults:* decreased	*Hyperphosphatemia* (increased phosphorus) • Bone fractures in healing stage • Bone tumors • Acromegaly *Hypophosphatemia* (decreased phosphorus) • Osteomalacia
Alkaline phosphatase (ALP)	30-120 units/L *Older adults:* slightly increased	*Elevations* may indicate: • Metastatic cancers of the bone • Paget's disease • Osteomalacia
Serum muscle enzymes Creatine kinase (CK-MM)	Total CK: *Men:* 55-170 units/L *Women:* 30-135 units/L	*Elevations* may indicate: • Muscle trauma • Progressive muscular dystrophy • Effects of electromyography
Lactic dehydrogenase (LDH)	Total LDH: 100-190 units/L LDH_1: 17%-27% LDH_2: 27%-37% LDH_3: 18%-25% LDH_4: 3%-8% LDH_5: 0% to 5%	*Elevations* may indicate: • Skeletal muscle necrosis • Extensive cancer • Progressive muscular dystrophy
Aspartate aminotransferase (AST)	0-35 units/L *Older adults:* slightly increased	*Elevations* may indicate: • Skeletal muscle trauma • Progressive muscular dystrophy
Aldolase (ALD)	3.0-8.2 units/dL	*Elevations* may indicate: • Polymyositis and dermatomyositis • Muscular dystrophy

patient preparation or follow-up care for any of these tests. Teach the patient about the purpose of the test and the procedure that can be expected. Additional tests performed for patients with connective tissue diseases, such as rheumatoid arthritis, are described in Chapter 18.

Disorders of bone and the parathyroid gland are often reflected in an alteration of the serum calcium or phosphorus level. Therefore these electrolytes, especially calcium, are monitored. A decrease in serum calcium could indicate bone density loss.

Alkaline phosphatase (ALP) is an enzyme normally present in blood. The concentration of ALP increases with bone or liver damage. In metabolic bone disease and bone cancer, the enzyme concentration rises in proportion to the osteoblastic activity, which indicates bone formation. The level of ALP is normally slightly increased in older adults (Pagana & Pagana, 2014).

The major *muscle enzymes* affected in skeletal muscle disease or injuries are:

- Creatine kinase (CK-MM)
- Aspartate aminotransferase (AST)
- Aldolase (ALD)
- Lactic dehydrogenase (LDH)

As a result of damage, the muscle tissue releases additional amounts of these enzymes, which increases serum levels.

The serum CK level begins to rise 2 to 4 hours after muscle injury and is elevated early in muscle disease, such as muscular dystrophy. The CK molecule has two subunits: M (muscle) and B (brain). Three isoenzymes have been identified. Skeletal muscle CK (CK-MM, or CK_3) is the only isoenzyme that rises in concentration with damage to skeletal muscle, such as trauma, surgery, and neuromuscular disease. This test is 90% accurate because it is affected by exercise and certain drugs, such as anticoagulants, furosemide, and statins (Kress et al., 2008).

AST is moderately elevated (3 to 5 times normal) in certain muscle diseases, such as muscular dystrophy. The levels of the isoenzymes *aldolase A (ALD-A)* and LDH_5 also increase in patients with these disorders.

Imaging Assessment

The skeleton is very visible on *standard x-rays.* Anteroposterior and lateral projections are the initial screening views used most often. Other approaches, such as oblique or stress views, depend on the part of the skeleton to be evaluated and the reason for the x-ray.

Radiography. Bone density, alignment, swelling, and intactness can be seen on x-ray. The conditions of joints can be determined, including the size of the joint space, the smoothness of articular cartilage, and synovial swelling. Soft-tissue involvement may be evident but not clearly differentiated.

Inform the patient that the x-ray table is hard and cold, and instruct him or her to remain still during the filming process. Coordinate with the radiology department or clinic to keep older adults and those at risk for hypothermia as warm as possible (e.g., by using blankets).

Myelography involves the injection of contrast medium into the subarachnoid space of the spine, usually by spinal puncture. The vertebral column, intervertebral disks, spinal nerve roots, and blood vessels can be visualized. Although this test is still performed, CT and MRI have often replaced such invasive and potentially painful and risky diagnostic techniques. The post-test care is similar to that for lumbar puncture, except that the patient is usually placed with the head of the bed elevated 30 to 50 degrees to prevent the contrast medium from getting into the brain (see Chapter 41).

An **arthrogram** is an x-ray study of a joint after contrast medium (air or solution) has been injected to enhance its visualization. Double-contrast arthrography, which uses both air and solution, may be performed when a traumatic injury is suspected. The physician can often determine bone chips, torn ligaments, or other loose bodies within the joint. This test is not used commonly because of newer advances in diagnostic imaging. Most joints are now studied by MRI and magnetic resonance (MR) arthrography.

CT has gained wide acceptance for detecting musculoskeletal problems, particularly those of the vertebral column and joints. The scanned images can be used to create additional images from other angles or to create three-dimensional images and view complex structures from any position. The nurse or radiology technologist should ask the patient about iodine-based contrast allergies.

Nuclear Scans. The **bone scan** is a radionuclide test in which radioactive material is injected for viewing the entire skeleton. It may be used primarily to detect tumors, arthritis, osteomyelitis, osteoporosis, vertebral compression fractures, and unexplained bone pain. Bone scans are used less commonly today as more sophisticated MRI equipment becomes more available. However, it may be very useful for detecting hairline fractures in patients with unexplained bone pain and diffuse metastatic bone disease.

The **gallium** and **thallium scans** are similar to the bone scan but are more specific and sensitive in detecting bone problems. Gallium citrate (^{67}Ga) is the radioisotope most commonly used. This substance also migrates to brain, liver, and breast tissue and therefore is used in examination of these structures when disease is suspected.

For patients with osteosarcoma, thallium (^{201}Tl) is better than gallium or technetium for diagnosing the extent of the disease. Thallium has traditionally been used for the diagnosis of myocardial infarctions but can be used for additional evaluation of cancers of the bone.

Because bone takes up gallium slowly, the nuclear medicine physician or technician administers the isotope 4 to 6 hours before scanning. Other tests that require contrast media or other isotopes cannot be given during this time.

Instruct the patient that the radioactive material poses no threat because it readily deteriorates in the body. Because gallium is excreted through the intestinal tract, it tends to collect in feces after the scanning procedure.

Depending on the tissue to be examined, the patient is taken to the nuclear medicine department 4 to 6 hours after injection. The procedure takes 30 to 60 minutes, during which time the patient must lie still for accurate test results to be achieved. The scan may be repeated at 24, 48, and/or 72 hours. Mild sedation may be necessary to facilitate relaxation and cooperation during the procedure for confused older adults or those in severe pain.

No special care is required after the test. The radioisotope is excreted in stool and urine, but no precautions are taken in handling the excreta. Remind the patient to push fluids to facilitate urinary excretion.

Magnetic Resonance Imaging. MRI, with or without the use of contrast media, is commonly used to diagnose musculoskeletal disorders. It is more accurate than CT and myelography for many spinal and knee problems. MRI is most appropriate for

CHART 49-3 Best Practice for Patient Safety & Quality Care QSEN

Preparing the Patient for Magnetic Resonance Imaging

- Is the patient pregnant?
- Does the patient have ferromagnetic fragments or implants, such as an older-style aneurysm clip?
- Does the patient have a pacemaker, stent, or electronic implant?
- Does the patient have chronic kidney disease? (Gadolinium contrast agents may cause severe systemic complications if the kidneys do not function.)
- Can the patient lie still in the supine position for 45 to 60 minutes? (May require sedation.)
- Does the patient need life-support equipment available?
- Can the patient communicate clearly and understand verbal communication?
- Did the patient get any tattoo *more than* 35 years ago? (If so, metal particles *may* be in the ink.)
- Is the patient claustrophobic? (Ask this question for closed MRI scanners; open MRIs do not cause claustrophobia.)

joints, soft tissue, and bony tumors that involve soft tissue. CT is still the test of choice for injuries or pathology that involves only bone.

The image is produced through the interaction of magnetic fields, radio waves, and atomic nuclei showing hydrogen density. Simply put, the radio waves "bounce" off the body tissues being examined. Because each tissue has its own density, the computer image clearly distinguishes normal and abnormal tissues. For some tissues, the cross-sectional image is better than that produced by radiography or CT. The lack of hydrogen ions in cortical bone makes it easily distinguishable from soft tissues. The test is particularly useful in identifying problems with muscles, tendons, and ligaments.

Ensure that the patient removes all metal objects and checks for clothing zippers and metal fasteners. Although joint implants made of titanium or stainless steel are usually safe, depending on the age of the MRI equipment, pacemakers, stents, and surgical clips usually are not. Chart 49-3 lists questions that the nurse or technician should consider in preparing the patient for MRI. Open MRIs prevent the claustrophobia that occurs with the older, encased machines.

MR arthrography combines arthrography and magnetic resonance imaging. It is particularly useful for diagnosing problems of the shoulder. The patient's shoulder is injected with gadolinium contrast medium under fluoroscopy. Then the patient is taken for an MRI where the shoulder is examined. This test is particularly useful for diagnosing the type and degree of rotator cuff tears (Smith & Smith, 2010).

Ultrasonography. Sound waves produce an image of the tissue in ultrasonography. An ultrasound procedure may be used to view:

- Soft-tissue disorders, such as masses and fluid accumulation
- Traumatic joint injuries
- Osteomyelitis
- Surgical hardware placement

A jelly-like substance applied to the skin over the site to be examined promotes the movement of a metal probe. No special preparation or post-test care is necessary. A quantitative ultrasound (QUS) may be done for determining fractures or bone density. Bone density testing is discussed in Chapter 50.

Other Diagnostic Assessment

Biopsies. In a **bone biopsy**, the physician extracts a specimen of the bone tissue for microscopic examination. This invasive test may confirm the presence of infection or neoplasm, but it is not commonly done today. One of two techniques may be used to retrieve the specimen: needle (closed) biopsy or incisional (open) biopsy.

! NURSING SAFETY PRIORITY QSEN

Action Alert

After a bone biopsy, watch for bleeding from the puncture site and for tenderness, redness, or warmth that could indicate infection. Mild analgesics may be used.

Muscle biopsy is done for the diagnosis of atrophy (as in muscular dystrophy) and inflammation (as in polymyositis). The procedure and care for patients undergoing muscle biopsy are the same as those for patients undergoing bone biopsy.

Electromyography. Although not commonly used today, electromyography (EMG) may be performed to evaluate diffuse or localized muscle weakness. EMG is usually accompanied by nerve conduction studies for determining the electrical potential generated in an individual muscle. This test helps in the diagnosis of neuromuscular, lower motor neuron, and peripheral nerve disorders.

Inform the patient that EMG may cause temporary discomfort, especially when the patient is subjected to episodes of electrical current. For selected patients, mild sedation is prescribed. The physician may also prescribe a temporary discontinuation of skeletal muscle relaxants several days before the procedure to prevent drugs from affecting the test results.

Arthroscopy. **Arthroscopy** may be used as a diagnostic test or a surgical procedure. An arthroscope is a fiberoptic tube inserted into a joint for direct visualization of the ligaments, menisci, and articular surfaces of the joint. The knee and shoulder are most commonly evaluated. In addition, synovial biopsy and surgery to repair traumatic injury can be done through the arthroscope as an ambulatory care or same-day surgical procedure.

Patient Preparation. Arthroscopy is performed on an ambulatory care basis or as same-day surgery. The patient must have mobility in the joint being examined. Those who cannot move the joint or who have an infected joint are not candidates for the procedure.

If the procedure is done for surgical repair, the patient may have a physical therapy consultation before arthroscopy to learn the exercises that are necessary after the test. ROM exercises are also taught but may not be allowed immediately after arthroscopic surgery. The nurse in the surgeon's office or at the surgical center can teach these exercises or reinforce the information provided by the physical therapist. The nurse also reinforces the explanation of the procedure and post-test care and ensures that the patient has signed an informed consent.

Procedure. The patient is usually given local, light general, or epidural anesthesia, depending on the purpose of the procedure. As shown in Fig. 49-6, the arthroscope is inserted through a small incision less than ¼-inch (0.6 cm) long. Multiple incisions may be required to allow inspection at a variety of angles. After the procedure, a dressing may be applied, depending on the amount of manipulation during the test or surgery.

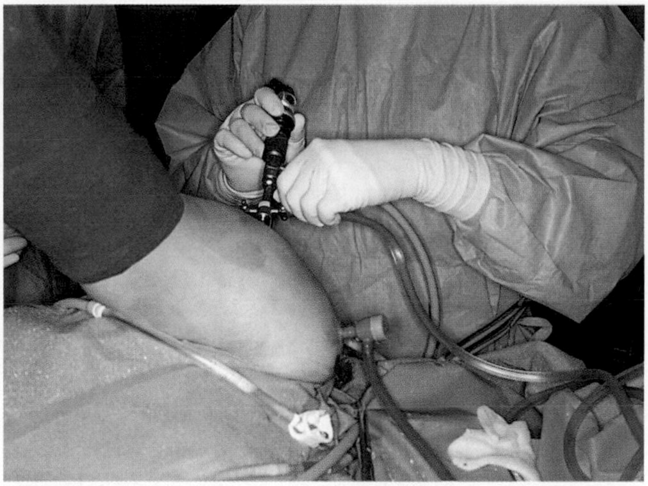

FIG. 49-6 An arthroscope is used in the diagnosis of pathologic changes in the joints. This patient is undergoing arthroscopy of the shoulder.

Postprocedure Care. The immediate care after an arthroscopy is the same for patients having the procedure for diagnostic purposes as for those having it for surgical intervention.

NURSING SAFETY PRIORITY QSEN

Action Alert

The priority for postprocedure care after arthroscopy is to assess the neurovascular status of the patient's affected limb every hour or according to agency or surgeon protocol. Monitor and document distal pulses, warmth, color, capillary refill, PAIN, movement, and sensation of the affected extremity.

Encourage the patient to perform exercises as taught before the procedure, if appropriate. For the mild discomfort experienced after the diagnostic arthroscopy, the surgeon prescribes a mild analgesic, such as acetaminophen (Tylenol, Ace-Tabs ♣). If postoperative, the patient may have short-term activity restrictions, depending on the musculoskeletal problem. Ice is often used for 24 hours, and the extremity should be elevated for 12 to 24 hours. When arthroscopic surgery is performed, the health care provider usually prescribes an opioid-analgesic combination, such as oxycodone and acetaminophen (Percocet, Tylox).

Although complications are not common, monitor and teach the patient to observe for:

- Swelling
- Increased joint pain attributable to mechanical injury
- Thrombophlebitis
- Infection

Severe joint or limb PAIN after discharge may indicate a possible complication. Teach the patient to contact the physician immediately. The surgeon usually sees the patient about 1 week after the procedure to check for complications.

NCLEX EXAMINATION CHALLENGE

Safe and Effective Care Environment

A client returns to the postanesthesia care unit (PACU) after an arthroscopy for a shoulder rotator cuff tear. What is the nurse's priority when caring for this client?

A. Perform passive range-of-motion exercises.
B. Keep the affected arm immobilized.
C. Ensure that the patient uses the patient-controlled analgesia (PCA) pump.
D. Check the neurovascular status of the affected arm.

NURSING CONCEPTS AND CLINICAL JUDGMENT REVIEW

What might you NOTICE in a patient with adequate MOBILITY and SENSORY PERCEPTION related to the musculoskeletal system?

Physical assessment:

- No gross deformities or impairments in posture or gait
- Adequate size, strength, and symmetry of muscle for age
- Can perform ADLs independently
- Can perform other routine daily activities independently
- Can ambulate with or without assistive devices
- No pain or tenderness on palpation or passive range-of-motion (ROM) of joints
- Active ROM of joints within normal limits for age
- No crepitus when moving joints
- No swelling of joints or extremities
- Equal size and alignment of extremities
- Equal sensation in extremities

Diagnostic assessment:

- Muscle enzymes (e.g., CK-MM, ALD) within normal limits for age
- Bone density adequate for age and gender
- Joint changes within normal limits for age

GET READY FOR THE NCLEX® EXAMINATION!

KEY POINTS

Review these Key Points for each NCLEX Examination Client Needs Category.

Safe and Effective Care Environment

- Collaborate with the physical and/or occupational therapist to perform a complete musculoskeletal assessment, including gait, muscle strength, and ADL ability, as indicated. **Teamwork and Collaboration** QSEN

Health Promotion and Maintenance

- Be aware that older adults have physiologic changes that affect their musculoskeletal system, such as decreased bone density and joint cartilage degeneration (see Chart 49-1). **Patient-Centered Care** QSEN

Psychosocial Integrity

- Assess the patient's support systems and coping mechanisms when musculoskeletal trauma or disease affects his or her body image. **Patient-Centered Care** QSEN
- Ask about the patient's occupation, because heavy manual labor may cause back injury and other musculoskeletal trauma.

Physiological Integrity

- Assess the patient's pain intensity, quality, duration, and location.
- Assess the patient's mobility, including gait, posture, and muscle strength.
- Interpret the patient's laboratory values that are related to musculoskeletal disease (see Chart 49-2).
- Teach the patient that mild discomfort can be expected during electromyography, a test to assess the electrical potential of muscles and their innervation.
- Instruct the patient to report swelling, infection, and increased pain after an arthroscopy.
- Ask the patient questions to ensure safety before an MRI (see Chart 49-3). **Safety** QSEN
- Ask the patient about allergy to contrast media before diagnostic testing such as CT scans.
- Evaluate the neurovascular status of the patient's affected extremity after an arthroscopic procedure as the *priority for care*. **Safety** QSEN

CHAPTER 50

Care of Patients with Musculoskeletal Problems

Donna D. Ignatavicius

http://evolve.elsevier.com/Iggy/

PRIORITY CONCEPTS

- Pain
- Mobility
- Inflammation
- Infection

LEARNING OUTCOMES

Safe and Effective Care Environment

1. Coordinate with health care team members when planning and providing high quality care for patients with musculoskeletal problems.
2. Teach the patient and family about home safety when the patient has a metabolic bone problem such as osteoporosis.

Health Promotion and Maintenance

3. Identify community resources for patients with musculoskeletal problems that impair mobility.
4. Develop a patient-centered teaching plan for all age-groups about ways to decrease the risk for osteoporosis.
5. Assess the genetic risk for patients who have parents with muscular dystrophy.

Psychosocial Integrity

6. Assess the patient's and family's responses to a bone cancer diagnosis and treatment options.

Physiological Integrity

7. Educate the patient and family about common drugs used for bone diseases, such as calcium supplements and bisphosphonates, to promote patient safety.
8. Compare and contrast osteoporosis and osteomalacia.
9. Identify key features of Paget's disease of the bone.
10. Prioritize care for patients with osteomyelitis.
11. Identify collaborative management options for treating patients with primary and metastatic bone cancer.
12. Describe common disorders of the foot, including hallux valgus and plantar fasciitis, that can affect mobility.
13. Explain the role of the nurse when caring for an adult patient with muscular dystrophy.

Musculoskeletal disorders include metabolic bone diseases (e.g., osteoporosis and Paget's disease), bone tumors, and a variety of deformities and syndromes. Older adults are at the greatest risk for most of these problems, although *primary* bone cancer is most often found in adolescents and young adults. As technology advances and patients survive longer with primary cancers, metastatic lesions have become more prevalent among older adults. Almost all musculoskeletal health problems can cause the patient to have difficulty meeting the human need of mobility. This chapter focuses on selected disorders not covered in Chapter 18 on arthritis and other connective tissue diseases.

METABOLIC BONE DISEASES

OSTEOPOROSIS

❖ PATHOPHYSIOLOGY

Osteoporosis is a chronic metabolic disease in which bone loss causes decreased density and possible fracture. It is often referred to as a "silent disease" or "silent thief" because the first sign of osteoporosis in most people follows some kind of a fracture (Kamienski et al., 2011). The spine, hip, and wrist are most often at risk, although any bone can fracture (National Osteoporosis Foundation [NOF], 2010).

Osteoporosis is a major health problem in the world. The estimated cost for osteoporosis-related health care alone in the United States is more than $18 billion each year with continual cost increases each year. By 2040, that number is expected to double or triple as baby boomers become older adults (NOF, 2010).

Bone is a dynamic tissue that is constantly undergoing changes in a process referred to as **bone remodeling**. Osteoporosis and **osteopenia** (low bone mass) occur when osteoclastic (bone resorption) activity is greater than osteoblastic (bone building) activity. The result is a decreased **bone mineral density (BMD)**. BMD determines bone strength and peaks between 25 and 30 years of age. Before and during the peak years, osteoclastic activity and osteoblastic activity work at the same rate. After the peak years, bone resorption activity exceeds bone-building activity and bone density decreases. BMD decreases most rapidly in postmenopausal women as serum estrogen levels diminish. Although estrogen does not build bone, it helps prevent bone loss. Trabecular, or cancellous (spongy), bone is lost first, followed by loss of cortical (compact) bone. This results in thin, fragile bone tissue that is at risk for fracture.

Standards for the diagnosis of osteoporosis are based on BMD testing that provides a T-score for the patient. A T-score represents the number of standard deviations above or below the average BMD for young, healthy adults. *Osteopenia is present when the T-score is at −1 and above −2.5. Osteoporosis is diagnosed in a person who has a T-score at or lower than −2.5.* Medicare reimburses for BMD testing every 2 years in people ages 65 years and older who (NOF, 2010):

- Are estrogen deficient
- Have vertebral abnormalities
- Receive long-term steroid therapy
- Have primary hyperparathyroidism
- Are being monitored while on osteoporosis drug therapy

Osteoporosis can be classified as generalized or regional. *Generalized* osteoporosis involves many structures in the skeleton and is further divided into two categories—primary and secondary. *Primary* osteoporosis is more common and occurs in postmenopausal women and in men in their seventh or eighth decade of life. Even though men do not experience the rapid bone loss that postmenopausal women have, they do have decreasing levels of testosterone (which builds bone) and altered ability to absorb calcium. This results in a slower loss of bone mass in men, especially those older than 75 years. *Secondary* osteoporosis may result from other medical conditions, such as hyperparathyroidism; long-term drug therapy, such as with corticosteroids; or prolonged immobility, such as that seen with spinal cord injury (Table 50-1). Treatment of the secondary type is directed toward the cause of the osteoporosis when possible.

Regional osteoporosis, an example of secondary disease, occurs when a limb is immobilized related to a fracture, injury, or paralysis. Immobility for longer than 8 to 12 weeks can result in this type of osteoporosis. Bone loss also occurs when people spend prolonged time in a gravity-free or weightless environment (e.g., astronauts).

Etiology and Genetic Risk

Primary osteoporosis is caused by a combination of genetic, lifestyle, and environmental factors. Chart 50-1 lists the major factors that contribute to the development of this disease.

TABLE 50-1 Causes of Secondary Osteoporosis

Diseases/Conditions	Drugs (Chronic Use)
• Diabetes mellitus • Hyperthyroidism • Hyperparathyroidism • Cushing's syndrome • Growth hormone deficiency • Metabolic acidosis • Female hypogonadism • Paget's disease • Osteogenesis imperfecta • Rheumatoid arthritis • Prolonged immobilization • Bone cancer • Cirrhosis • HIV/AIDS • Chronic airway limitation	• Corticosteroids • Anti-epileptic drugs (AEDs) (e.g., phenytoin) • Barbiturates (e.g., phenobarbital) • Ethanol (alcohol) • Drugs that induce hypogonadism (decreased levels of sex hormones) • High levels of thyroid hormone • Cytotoxic agents • Immunosuppressants • Loop diuretics • Aluminum-based antacids

AIDS, Acquired immune deficiency syndrome; HIV, human immune deficiency virus.

CHART 50-1 Best Practice for Patient Safety & Quality Care QSEN

Assessing Risk Factors for Primary Osteoporosis

Assess for:
- Older age in both genders and all races
- Parental history of osteoporosis, especially mother
- History of low-trauma fracture after age 50 years
- Low body weight, thin build
- Chronic low calcium and/or vitamin D intake
- Estrogen or androgen deficiency
- Current smoking (active or passive)
- High alcohol intake (3 or more drinks a day)
- Lack of physical exercise or prolonged immobility

GENETIC/GENOMIC CONSIDERATIONS

Patient-Centered Care **QSEN**

The genetic and immune factors that cause osteoporosis are very complex. Strong evidence demonstrates that genetics is a significant factor, with a heritability of 50% to 90% (Chang et al., 2010). Many genetic changes have been identified as possible causative factors, but there is no agreement about which ones are most important or constant in all patients. For example, changes in the vitamin D_3 receptor *(VDR)* gene and calcitonin receptor *(CTR)* gene have been found in some patients with the disease. Receptors are essential for the uptake and use of these substances by the cells.

The bone morphogenetic protein-2 *(BMP-2)* gene has a key role in bone formation and maintenance. Some osteoporotic patients who had fractures have changes in their *BMP-2* gene. Alterations in growth hormone-1 (GH-1) have been discovered in petite Asian-American women, those who are predisposed to developing osteoporosis.

Hormones, tumor necrosis factor (TNF), interleukins, and other substances in the body help control osteoclasts in a very complex pathway. The identification of the importance of the cytokine receptor activator of nuclear factor kappa-B ligand *(RANKL)*, its receptor *RANK*, and its decoy receptor osteoprotegerin *(OPG)* has helped researchers understand more about the activity of osteoclasts in metabolic bone disease. Disruptions in the *RANKL, RANK,* and *OPG* system can lead to increased osteoclast activity in which bone is rapidly broken down (McCance et al., 2014).

EVIDENCE-BASED PRACTICE QSEN

What Do Men Know About Their Risk of Osteoporosis?

Doheny, M.O., Sedlak, C.A., Estok, P.J., & Zeller, R.A. (2011). Bone density, health beliefs, and osteoporosis preventing behaviors in men. *Orthopaedic Nursing, 30*(4), 266-272.

The researchers conducted an experimental, two-group longitudinal study to examine the effect of dual-energy x-ray absorptiometry (DXA) results on osteoporosis preventing behaviors (OPB), health beliefs, and knowledge of osteoporosis of men ages 50 years or older. The sample was obtained through a community call for volunteers, and the participants were randomly assigned to either the control or experimental group. At the beginning of the study, all 196 subjects received information on osteoporosis diagnosis and management and completed a series of questionnaires. All subjects also had a free DXA test in which 50 men were found to be osteopenic or osteoporotic. Knowledge about osteoporosis was not a predictor of calcium intake or exercise. Although the osteoporotic men increased their calcium and increased their exercise, the amount of each intervention was below the national recommendations. Health beliefs predicted both calcium intake and exercise.

Level of Evidence: 2

This study used an experimental design over a period of time to determine changes in behavior.

Commentary: Implications for Practice and Research

Very little research has been done on the diagnosis and management of osteoporosis in men. This study used an experimental design to examine multiple factors. Nurses and other health care professionals need to educate men older than 50 years about the risk for and prevention of osteoporosis. The cost of DXA screening is far less than the financial, social, and health care costs of osteoporosis.

The subjects in the convenience sample were fairly well educated, almost all were white, and most were married. Further studies are needed using more diverse samples to allow generalization of the findings of this research.

GENDER HEALTH CONSIDERATIONS

Patient-Centered Care QSEN

Primary osteoporosis most often occurs in women after menopause as a result of decreased estrogen levels. Women lose about 2% of their bone mass every year in the first 5 years after natural or surgical (ovary removal) menopause. Obese women can store estrogen in their tissues for use as necessary to maintain a normal level of serum calcium.

Men also develop osteoporosis after the age of 50 years because their testosterone levels decrease. Testosterone is the major sex hormone that builds bone tissue. Men are often underdiagnosed, even when they become older adults (Swislocki et al., 2010; Voda, 2009b). In a large experimental study, Doheny et al. (2011) found that men lacked knowledge about osteoporosis and their risk for the disease (see the Evidence-Based Practice box).

The relationship of osteoporosis to nutrition is well established. For example, excessive caffeine in the diet can cause calcium loss in the urine. A diet lacking enough calcium and vitamin D stimulates the parathyroid gland to produce parathyroid hormone (PTH). PTH triggers the release of calcium from the bony matrix. Activated vitamin D is needed for calcium uptake in the body. Malabsorption of nutrients in the GI tract also contributes to low serum calcium levels. Institutionalized or homebound patients who are not exposed to sunlight may be at a higher risk because they do not receive adequate vitamin D for the metabolism of calcium.

Calcium loss occurs at a more rapid rate when phosphorus intake is high. (Chapter 11 describes the usual relationship between calcium and phosphorus in the body.) People who drink large amounts of carbonated beverages each day (over 40 ounces) are at high risk for calcium loss and subsequent osteoporosis, regardless of age or gender.

Protein deficiency may also reduce bone density. Because 50% of serum calcium is protein bound, protein is needed to use calcium. However, excessive protein intake may increase calcium loss in the urine. For instance, people who are on high-protein, low-carbohydrate diets, like the Atkins diet, may consume too much protein to replace other food not allowed. Dietary protein intake in healthy adults is recommended at 0.8 grams per kilogram of body weight. Protein is needed for bone healing when a fracture occurs.

Excessive alcohol and tobacco use are other risk factors for osteoporosis. Although the exact mechanisms are not known, these substances promote acidosis, which in turn increases bone loss. Alcohol also has a direct toxic effect on bone tissue, resulting in decreased bone formation and increased bone resorption. For those people who have excessive alcohol intake, alcohol calories decrease hunger and the need to take in adequate amounts of nutrients.

Incidence and Prevalence

Osteoporosis is a potential health problem for more than 44 million Americans. About 10 million people in the United States have the disease, and about 34 million people 50 years of age and older have osteopenia and are at risk for development of osteoporosis. Women remain the largest group affected by osteoporosis, although some men, especially those older than 75 years, also have the disease.

CULTURAL CONSIDERATIONS

Patient-Centered Care QSEN

Body build, weight, and race/ethnicity seem to influence who gets the disease. Osteoporosis occurs most often in older, lean-built Euro-American and Asian women, particularly those who do not exercise regularly. However, African Americans are at risk for decreased vitamin D, which is needed for adequate calcium absorption in the small intestines. Dietary preferences or intolerances or the inability to afford high-nutrient food may influence anyone's rate of bone loss. For example, many blacks have lactose intolerance and cannot drink regular milk or eat other dairy-based foods (NOF, 2010). Lactose-free milk (e.g., Lactaid) or soy milk provides calcium. Milk and cheese are good sources of protein, a nutrient needed to bind calcium for use by the body.

Osteoporosis results in more than 1.5 million fragility fractures each year (NOF, 2010). A woman who experiences a hip fracture has a 4 times greater risk for a second fracture. Fractures as a result of osteoporosis and falling can decrease a patient's MOBILITY and quality of life. The mortality rate for older patients with hip fractures is very high, especially within the first 6 months, and the debilitating effects can be devastating.

Health Promotion and Maintenance

Peak bone mass is achieved by about 30 years of age in most women. *Building strong bone as a young person may be the best defense against osteoporosis in later adulthood.* Young women need to be aware of appropriate health and lifestyle practices that can prevent this potentially disabling disease. Teaching should begin with young women because they begin to lose bone after 30 years of age. Nurses can play a vital role in patient education for women of any age to prevent and manage osteoporosis.

The focus of osteoporosis prevention is to decrease modifiable risk factors. For example, teach patients who do not include enough dietary calcium which foods to eat, such as dairy products and dark green leafy vegetables. Teach them to read food labels for sources of calcium content. Explain the importance of sun exposure (but not so much as to get sunburned) and adequate vitamin D in the diet. The National Osteoporosis Foundation recommends taking a vitamin D_3 supplement for all adults. Patients being treated for osteopenia or osteomalacia (vitamin D deficiency) may be prescribed high therapeutic doses up to 20,000 international units a week (NOF, 2010).

Teach the need to limit the amount of carbonated beverages consumed each day. Remind patients who have sedentary lifestyles about the importance of exercise and what types of exercise builds bone tissue. Weight-bearing exercises, such as regularly scheduled walking, are preferred. Teach high-risk people to avoid activities that cause jarring, such as horseback riding and jogging, to prevent potential vertebral compression fractures.

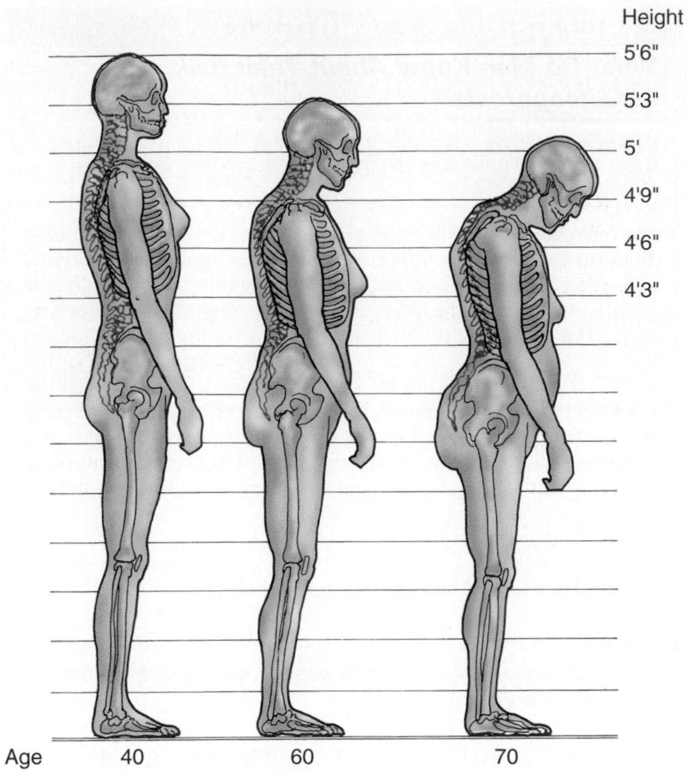

FIG. 50-1 A normal spine at age 40 years and osteoporotic changes at ages 60 and 70 years. These changes can cause a loss of as much as 6 inches in height and can result in the so-called *dowager's hump (far right)* in the upper thoracic vertebrae.

❖ PATIENT-CENTERED COLLABORATIVE CARE

◆ Assessment

A complete health history with assessment of risk factors is important in the prevention, early detection, and treatment of osteoporosis. Patients who have risk factors for osteoporosis are at increased risk for fractures when falls occur. Include a fall risk assessment in the health history, especially for older adults. Assess for fall risk factors as described in Chapter 2. The Joint Commission's National Patient Safety Goals (NPSGs) specify the need to reduce risk for harm to patients resulting from falls. People with osteoporosis are at an increased risk for fracture if a fall occurs.

Physical Assessment/Clinical Manifestations. When performing a musculoskeletal assessment, inspect and palpate the vertebral column. The classic "dowager's hump," or kyphosis of the dorsal spine, is often present (Fig. 50-1). The patient may state that he or she has gotten shorter, perhaps as much as 2 to 3 inches (5 to 7.5 cm) within the previous 20 years. Take or delegate height and weight measurements, and compare with previous measurements if they are available.

The patient may have back pain, which often occurs after lifting, bending, or stooping. The pain may be sharp and acute in onset. Pain is worse with activity and is relieved by rest. Palpation of the vertebrae, particularly the lower thoracic and lumbar vertebrae, can increase the patient's discomfort. Therefore palpation should be gentle.

Back pain accompanied by tenderness and voluntary restriction of spinal movement suggests one or more compression vertebral fractures—the most common type of osteoporotic fracture. Movement restriction and spinal deformity may result in constipation, abdominal distention, reflux esophagitis, and respiratory compromise in severe cases. The most likely area for spinal fracture is between T8 and L3.

Fractures are also common in the distal end of the radius (wrist) and the upper third of the femur (hip). Ask the patient to locate all areas that are painful, and observe for signs and symptoms of fractures, such as swelling and malalignment. Fractures are discussed in Chapter 51.

Psychosocial Assessment. Women associate osteoporosis with menopause, getting older, and becoming less independent. The disease can result in suffering, deformity, and disability that can affect the patient's well-being and life satisfaction. The quality of life may be further impacted by pain, insomnia, depression, and **fallophobia** (fear of falling) (Touhy & Jett, 2014).

Assess the patient's concept of body image, especially if he or she is severely kyphotic. For example, the patient may have difficulty finding clothes that fit properly. Social interactions may be avoided because of a change in appearance or the physical limitations of being unable to sit in chairs in restaurants, movie theaters, and other places. Changes in sexuality may occur as a result of poor self-esteem or the discomfort caused by positioning during intercourse.

Because osteoporosis poses a risk for fractures, teach the patient to be extremely cautious about activities. As a result, the threat of fracture can create anxiety and fear and result in further limitation of social or physical activities. Assess for these feelings to assist in treatment decisions and health teaching. For example, the patient may not exercise as prescribed for fear that a fracture will occur.

Laboratory Assessment. No definitive laboratory tests confirm a diagnosis of primary osteoporosis, although a number of *biochemical markers* can provide information about bone resorption and formation activity. Although not commonly tested, these biochemical markers are sensitive to bone changes and can be used to monitor effectiveness of treatment for osteoporosis. *Bone-specific alkaline phosphatase (BSAP)* is found in the cell membrane of the osteoblast and indicates bone formation status. *Osteocalcin* is a protein substance in bone and increases during bone resorption activity. Pyridinium (PYD) cross-links are released into circulation during bone resorption. *N-telopeptide (NTX)* and *C-telopeptide (CTX)* are proteins released when bone is broken down. Some laboratories require a 24-hour urine collection for testing, whereas others use a double-voided specimen. Some markers, like NTX and CTX, can also be measured in the blood using immunoassay techniques. Increased levels of any of these markers indicate a risk for osteoporosis. Increased levels are found in patients with osteoporosis, Paget's disease, and bone tumors (Pagana & Pagana, 2014).

Serum calcium and vitamin D_3 levels should be routinely monitored (at least once a year) for all women and men older than 50 years who are at a high risk for the disease. These results determine the need for drug supplements.

A battery of tests can be performed to rule out secondary osteoporosis or other metabolic bone diseases, such as osteomalacia and Paget's disease. These include measurements of serum calcium, vitamin D, and phosphorus. Urinary calcium levels may also be assessed.

Imaging Assessment. Conventional x-rays of the spine and long bones show decreased bone density but only after a 25% to 40% bone loss has occurred. Fractures can also be seen on x-ray.

The most commonly used screening and diagnostic tool for measuring bone mineral density (BMD) is **dual x-ray absorptiometry** (**DXA**, or **DEXA**). The spine and hip are most often assessed when central DXA (cDXA) scan is performed. Many physicians recommend that women in their 40s have a baseline screening DXA scan so that later bone changes can be detected and compared. DXA is a painless scan that emits less radiation than a chest x-ray. *It is the best tool currently available for a definite diagnosis of osteoporosis.* A height is taken prior to performing the test. The patient stays dressed but is asked to remove any metallic objects such as belt buckles, coins, keys, or jewelry that might interfere with the test. The results are displayed on a computer graph, and a T-score is calculated. No special follow-up care for the test is required. However, the patient needs to discuss the results with the primary care provider for any decisions about possible preventive or management interventions.

A peripheral DXA (pDXA) scan assesses BMD of the heel, forearm, or finger. It is often used for large-scale screening purposes. The pDXA is commonly used for screening at community health fairs, skilled nursing facilities, and women's health centers.

Peripheral quantitative ultrasound (pQUS) is an effective and low-cost peripheral screening tool that can detect osteoporosis and predict risk for hip fracture. The heel, tibia, and patella are most commonly tested. The procedure requires no special preparation, is quick, and has no radiation exposure or specific follow-up care (Pagana & Pagana, 2014). The National Osteoporosis Foundation recommends that men older than 70 years have the pQUS as a screening tool for the disease (NOF, 2010).

◆ Analysis

The most common problem for patients with osteoporosis or osteopenia is *potential for fractures related to weak, porous bone tissue.*

◆ Planning and Implementation

Planning: Expected Outcomes. The expected outcome is that the patient avoids fractures by preventing falls, managing risk factors, and adhering to preventive or treatment measures for bone loss.

Interventions. Because the patient is predisposed to fractures, nutritional therapy, exercise, lifestyle changes, and drug therapy are used to slow bone resorption and form new bone tissue. Self-management education (SME) can help prevent osteoporosis or slow the progress.

Nutrition Therapy. The nutritional considerations for the treatment of a patient with a diagnosis of osteoporosis are the same as those for preventing the disease. Teach patients about the adequate amounts of protein, magnesium, vitamin K, and trace minerals that are needed for bone formation. Calcium and vitamin D intake should be increased. Teach patients to avoid excessive alcohol and caffeine consumption. For the patient who has sustained a fracture, adequate intake of protein, vitamin C, and iron is important to promote bone healing. People who are lactose intolerant can choose a variety of soy and rice products that are fortified with calcium and vitamin D. In addition, calcium and vitamin D are added to many fruit juices, bread, and cereal products.

A variety of nutrients are needed to maintain bone health. *The promotion of a single nutrient will not prevent or treat osteoporosis.* Help the patient develop a nutritional plan that is most beneficial in maintaining bone health; the plan should emphasize fruits and vegetables, low-fat dairy and protein sources, increased fiber, and moderation in alcohol and caffeine (NOF, 2010).

Lifestyle Changes. Exercise is important in the prevention and management of osteoporosis. It also plays a vital role in PAIN management, cardiovascular function, and an improved sense of well-being.

In collaboration with the health care provider, the physical therapist may prescribe exercises for strengthening the abdominal and back muscles for those at risk for vertebral fractures. These exercises improve posture and support for the spine. Abdominal muscle tightening, deep breathing, and pectoral stretching are stressed to increase lung capacity. Exercises for the extremity muscles include muscle-tightening, resistive, and range-of-motion (ROM) exercises. Encourage active ROM exercises, which improve joint MOBILITY and increase muscle tone, as well as prescribed exercise activities. Swimming provides overall muscle exercise.

In addition to exercises for muscle strengthening, a general weight-bearing exercise program should be implemented. Teach patients that walking for 30 minutes 3 to 5 times a week is the single most effective exercise for osteoporosis prevention.

In addition to nutrition and exercise, other lifestyle changes may be needed. Teach the patient to avoid tobacco in any form, especially cigarette smoking. Remind women not to consume more than one alcoholic drink per day (5 ounces each); instruct men not to have more than two alcoholic drinks per day.

Hospitals and long-term care facilities have risk management programs to assess for the risk for falls. For those patients at high risk, communicate this information to other members of the health care team, using colored armbands or other easy-to-recognize methods (National Patient Safety Goals). Chapter 2 discusses fall prevention in health care agencies and at home in more detail.

NCLEX EXAMINATION CHALLENGE

Health Promotion and Maintenance

Which statement by the client regarding lifestyle changes to prevent osteoporosis indicates a need for further teaching by the nurse?

A. "I should get rid of the scatter rugs and clutter in my house."
B. "I will cut down to only three martinis at night."
C. "I plan to increase calcium and vitamin D_3 foods in my diet."
D. "I am going to walk every day for at least 30 minutes."

Drug Therapy. Drug therapy is used when the BMD T-score for the hip is below −2.0 with no other risk factors or when the T-score is below −1.5 with one or more risk factors or previous fracture (NOF, 2010). The health care provider may prescribe calcium and vitamin D_3 supplements, bisphosphonates, or estrogen agonist/antagonists (formerly called *selective estrogen receptor modulators*) or a combination of several drugs to treat or prevent osteoporosis (Chart 50-2). Estrogen and combination hormone therapy are not used solely for osteoporosis prevention or management because they can increase other health risks such as breast cancer and myocardial infarction.

Calcium and Activated Vitamin D (D_3). Intake of *calcium* alone is not a treatment for osteoporosis, but calcium is an important part of a *prevention* program to promote bone health. Most people cannot or do not have enough calcium in their diet, and therefore calcium supplements are needed. Calcium carbonate, found in over-the-counter (OTC) drugs such as Os-Cal, is one of the most cost-effective supplement formulas. Calcium citrate, available OTC as Citracal, is often recommended for those who have gastric upset when taking a calcium supplement. Teach patients to take calcium supplements with food and 6 to 8 ounces of water, although Citracal can be taken anytime. It is best to divide the daily dose, with at least one third of the daily dose being taken in the evening. Teach women to start taking supplements in young adulthood to assist in maintaining peak bone mass. Instruct patients of any age to take calcium supplements that also contain a small amount of activated vitamin D (D_3), such as Os-Cal Ultra.

Because vitamin D is needed for calcium absorption by the body, vitamin D_3 supplementation is often indicated. Both calcium and vitamin D_3 are OTC supplements. Remind patients to take these drugs under the supervision of a health care provider. **Hypercalcemia** (excess serum calcium) can cause serious damage to the urinary system and other body systems. Teach patients to drink plenty of fluids to prevent urinary calculi (stones). Remind them to have regular laboratory assessments of their calcium and vitamin D_3 serum levels. Chapter 11 describes the clinical manifestations of hypercalcemia.

Bisphosphonates. Bisphosphonates (BPs) slow bone resorption by binding with crystal elements in bone, especially spongy, trabecular bone tissue. They are the most common drugs used for osteoporosis, but some are also approved for Paget's disease and hypercalcemia related to cancer. Three Food and Drug Administration (FDA)–approved BPs—alendronate (Fosamax), ibandronate (Boniva), and risedronate (Actonel, Atelvia)—are commonly used for the *prevention and treatment* of osteoporosis (Lilley et al., 2014). These drugs are available as oral preparations, with ibandronate (Boniva) also available as an IV preparation.

After taking any of these drugs for 3 years, the patient has a DXA scan. If bone density has improved or is maintained, the primary care provider may discontinue the bisphosphonate until the next scan in another 3 years. At that time, the provider will determine if the drug needs to be restarted. For some patients, long-term bisphosphonate use may cause osteonecrosis (discussed below) or a long-bone fracture.

NURSING SAFETY PRIORITY QSEN

Drug Alert

Do not confuse Fosamax with Flomax, a selective alpha-adrenergic blocker used for benign prostatic hyperplasia (BPH).

Oral BPs are commonly associated with a serious problem called **esophagitis** (inflammation of the esophagus). Esophageal ulcers have also been reported with the use of BPs, especially when the tablet is not completely swallowed.

NURSING SAFETY PRIORITY QSEN

Drug Alert

To promote safety, teach patients to take bisphosphonates (BPs) early in the morning with 8 ounces of water and wait 30 to 60 minutes in an upright position before eating. If chest discomfort occurs, a symptom of esophageal irritation, instruct patients to discontinue the drug and contact their health care provider. Patients with poor renal function, hypocalcemia, or gastroesophageal reflux disease (GERD) should not take BPs.

The most recent additions to the bisphosphonates are IV zoledronic acid (Reclast) and IV pamidronate (Aredia). For management of osteoporosis, Reclast is needed only once a year and Aredia is given every 3 to 6 months. Both drugs have been linked to a complication called jaw **osteonecrosis** (also known as *avascular necrosis,* or *bone death*) in which infection and necrosis of the mandible or maxilla occur (Lilley et al., 2014). The incidence of this serious problem is low but can be a complication of this infusion therapy.

NURSING SAFETY PRIORITY QSEN

Drug Alert

Teach patients to have an oral assessment and preventive dentistry before beginning any bisphosphonate therapy. To promote safety, instruct them to inform any dentist who is planning invasive treatment, such as a tooth extraction or implant, that they are taking a BP drug (Cohen, 2010).

Estrogen Agonist/Antagonists. Formerly called the *selective estrogen receptor modulators (SERMs)*, estrogen agonist/antagonists are a class of drugs designed to mimic estrogen in some parts of the body while blocking its effect elsewhere. Raloxifene (Evista) is currently the only approved drug in this class and is used for *prevention and treatment* of osteoporosis in postmenopausal women. Raloxifene increases bone mineral density (BMD), reduces bone resorption, and reduces the incidence of osteoporotic vertebral fractures. The drug should not be given to women who have a history of thromboembolism.

Monoclonal Antibodies. A newer type of drug is denosumab (Prolia, Xgeva), a monoclonal antibody that has been approved

CHART 50-2 Common Examples of Drug Therapy

Osteoporosis

DRUG AND USUAL DOSAGE	PURPOSE OF DRUG	NURSING INTERVENTIONS	RATIONALES
Supplements			
Calcium (with vitamin D if needed) (e.g., Os-Cal, Citracal) 1-1.5 g in divided doses orally daily	Increases calcium intake (and vitamin D if needed)	Give a third of daily dose at bedtime. Push fluids.	Calcium is most readily utilized by the body when the patient is fasting and immobile. Increased fluid intake aids in preventing the formation of calcium-based urinary stones.
		Assess for a history of urinary stones.	Calcium supplements are not given to patients who are susceptible to urinary stone formation.
		Monitor serum calcium level.	Hypercalcemia, or calcium excess, is a side effect of calcium supplementation.
		Monitor urinary calcium level (no more than 4 mg/kg in 24 hr).	The kidneys attempt to excrete excess calcium.
		Observe for signs of hypercalcemia.	Hypercalcemia can result in urinary stones, cardiac dysrhythmias, and an increase or decrease in skeletal muscle tone.
Bisphosphonates			
Alendronate (Fosamax) or (Fosamax plus D) **For Prevention:** 5 mg orally daily or 35 mg orally weekly (available as tablet or liquid) **For Treatment:** 10 mg orally daily or 70 mg orally weekly with 2800-5600 international units of vitamin D	Prevents bone loss and increases bone density	Take on an empty stomach, first thing in the morning with a full glass of water. Take 30 minutes before food, drink, or other drugs. Remain upright, sitting or standing, for 30 minutes after administration. Take liquid (75 mL) and follow with 2 ounces of water.	Difficulty swallowing, esophagitis, esophageal ulcers, and gastric ulcers can result from alendronate therapy. Any of these should be reported to a health care provider as soon as possible.
Risedronate (Actonel) or (Actonel with Calcium) 5 mg orally daily, 35 mg orally every week, or 150 mg monthly	Same as for alendronate	Follow interventions for alendronate.	Same as for alendronate.
		Observe for CNS side/adverse effects, such as drowsiness, anxiety, agitation.	Drug can also cause CNS effects that may not be tolerated.
Ibandronate (Boniva) 150 mg orally once every month or 3.375 mg IV every 3 months	Same as for alendronate	Take on the same day each month. Take on an empty stomach, first thing in the morning with a full glass of water. Take 60 minutes before food, drink, or other drugs. Remain upright for 1 hour after administration.	Same as for alendronate.
Zoledronic acid (Reclast, Zometa) **For Prevention:** 5 mg IV once every 2 years **For Treatment:** 5 mg IV once a year	Same as for other bisphosphonates	Infuse over 15-30 minutes.	The drug should not be infused too quickly to prevent rare complications such as atrial fibrillation.
		Make sure the patient has a dental examination before starting the drug.	The drug can cause jaw or maxillary osteonecrosis, particularly if oral hygiene is poor.
		Do not give to patients who are sensitive to aspirin.	The patient may experience bronchoconstriction.
		Check serum creatinine before and after administering the drug.	The drug can cause renal insufficiency or kidney failure.
Estrogen Agonist/Antagonists*			
Raloxifene (Evista) 60 mg orally daily	Prevents bone loss and increases bone density	Teach patient signs and symptoms of VTE.	Raloxifene can cause increased risk for VTE, especially in the first 4 months of therapy.
		Monitor liver function tests (LFTs) in collaboration with health care provider.	Raloxifene can cause increased LFT values or worsen hepatic disease (should not be given to patient who has liver disease).

CNS, Central nervous system; *VTE,* venous thromboembolism.
*Formerly Selective Estrogen Receptor Modulators (SERMs).

for treatment of osteoporosis when other drugs are not effective (Lilley et al., 2014). The drug binds to a protein that is essential for the formation, function, and survival of osteoclasts and is given subcutaneously twice a year. By preventing the protein from activating its receptor, the drug decreases bone loss and increases bone mass and strength. The most common side effects of denosumab are back pain, high cholesterol, urinary tract infection, and muscle pain. The drug can also cause a decrease in serum calcium levels. Therefore patients who already have a low calcium level should not take the drug. Like other drugs used for osteoporosis, denosumab can cause fractures, especially of the femur, and jaw osteonecrosis.

CLINICAL JUDGMENT CHALLENGE

Patient-Centered Care; Evidence-Based Practice QSEN

A 71-year-old Caucasian (Euro-American) woman has been diagnosed with osteoporosis for over 15 years. She has been on calcium and vitamin D_3 supplements since her diagnosis and has been taking risedronate (Actonel) on and off for the past 12 years. According to her most recent DXA scan, the patient continues to lose bone density despite being on drug therapy. Last year she sustained a fracture of her humerus after she tripped over her small dog. When reviewing her history, you note that her mother and older sister had osteoporosis for many years. Her sister recently died less than a year after fracturing her hip. The patient expresses her fear of having another fracture and wants to be considered for Prolia therapy.

1. What risk factors does this patient have for osteoporosis? What other information do you need to do a complete assessment?
2. Is this patient a good candidate for beginning denosumab? Why or why not? Will you need more information? If so, what do you need to know?
3. If the patient begins the new drug, what health teaching will she need?
4. How will you respond to her fear of having more fractures?

Community-Based Care

Patients with osteoporosis are usually managed at home unless they have major fragility fractures. Osteoporosis disease-management programs managed by nurse practitioners have helped diagnose and treat the disease. Greene and Dell (2010) reported that over a 6-year period, a large osteoporosis disease-management program resulted in a 263% increase in the number of DXA scans done each year, a 153% increase in the number of patients treated with drug therapy, and a 38.1% decrease in the expected hip fracture rate.

Refer patients to the National Osteoporosis Foundation (www.nof.org) in the United States for information regarding the disease and its treatment. The Osteoporosis Society of Canada (www.osteoporosis.ca) has similar services. Large health care systems often have osteoporosis specialty clinics and support groups for patients with osteoporosis.

OSTEOMALACIA

❖ PATHOPHYSIOLOGY

Osteomalacia is loss of bone related to a vitamin D deficiency. It causes softening of the bone resulting from inadequate deposits of calcium and phosphorus in the bone matrix. Normal remodeling of the bone is disrupted, and calcification does not occur. Osteomalacia is the adult equivalent of **rickets**, or vitamin D deficiency, in children.

Vitamin D deficiency is the most important factor in development of osteomalacia. In its natural form, vitamin D is activated by the ultraviolet radiation of the sun and obtained from certain foods as a nutritional supplement. In combination with calcium and phosphorus, the vitamin is necessary for bone formation.

Osteomalacia may be confused with osteoporosis because of similar characteristics shared by the two disease processes. Table 50-2 compares and contrasts osteoporosis and osteomalacia.

In addition to primary disease related to lack of sunlight exposure or dietary intake, vitamin D deficiency caused by various health problems may result in osteomalacia (Table 50-3). Malabsorption of vitamin D from the small bowel is a common complication of partial or total gastrectomy and bypass or resection surgery of the small intestine. Disease of the small bowel, such as Crohn's disease, may cause decreased vitamin and mineral absorption.

TABLE 50-2 Differential Features of Osteoporosis and Osteomalacia

CHARACTERISTIC	OSTEOPOROSIS	OSTEOMALACIA
Definition	Decreased bone mass	Demineralized bone
Pathophysiology	Lack of calcium	Lack of vitamin D
Radiographic findings	Osteopenia, fractures	Pseudofractures, Looser's zones, fractures
Calcium level	Low or normal	Low or normal
Phosphate level	Normal	Low or normal
Parathyroid hormone	Normal	High or normal
Alkaline phosphatase	Normal	High

TABLE 50-3 Causes of Osteomalacia

Vitamin D Disturbance
- Inadequate production
- Lack of sunlight exposure
- Dietary deficiency
- Abnormal metabolism
- Drug therapy
  - Phenytoin (Dilantin)
  - Fluoride
  - Barbiturates
- Liver disease
- Renal disease
- Inadequate absorption
  - Postgastrectomy
  - Malabsorption syndrome
- Inflammatory bowel disease

Kidney Disease
- Chronic kidney disease
- Acute tubular disorders
  - Acidosis
  - Hypophosphatemia

Familial Metabolic Error
- Hypophosphatemia

Liver and pancreatic disorders disrupt vitamin D metabolism and decrease its production. Chronic kidney disease (CKD) interferes with the synthesis of calcitriol, the most active vitamin metabolite. Osteomalacia can also be caused by bone tumors (oncogenic or tumor-induced osteomalacia).

Conditions that contribute to phosphate depletion (hypophosphatemia) lead to osteomalacia because they stimulate movement from bone and prevent calcium uptake in the bone. Osteomalacia is also an adverse effect of long-term therapy with certain drugs such as antiepileptic drugs (AEDs) and barbiturates. The exact mechanism for the drug effects is not known. Genetic deviations in vitamin D or phosphate metabolism may contribute to bone changes seen in osteomalacia.

Osteomalacia is not common in the United States and Western Europe. However, it is more common in less affluent nations and in countries where famine is common. Newcomers from these countries may seek health care in the United States. Older adults are most at risk. This group may have inadequate exposure to sunlight or intake of vitamin D–fortified foods. People who adhere to very restrictive vegan diets without adequate supplement of vitamin D can also be at risk. Assess for the risk for osteomalacia in anyone who has poor nutritional intake related to homelessness, who severely abuses drugs or alcohol, or who is very poor.

Health Promotion and Maintenance

To prevent or help treat osteomalacia, teach patients to increase vitamin D through dietary intake, sun exposure, and drug supplements. Instruct the at-risk patient about foods high in vitamin D, such as milk and food that has had it added. Remind patients that cheese and yogurt rarely contain vitamin D although they are rich in calcium. Instruct them to read food labels for nutrient content. Remind patients, especially those who are homebound, about the importance of daily sun exposure (at least 5 minutes each day) for the most important source of vitamin D.

Some people are lactose intolerant or do not use dairy products because of their vegan diets. However, many products are available for people who avoid dairy products. Soy and rice milk, tofu, and soy products are substitutes, but they are expensive. Teach patients to choose those products that are fortified with vitamin D. Other foods rich in the vitamin are eggs, swordfish, chicken, and liver, as well as enriched cereals and bread products. The at-risk patient should also take vitamin D supplements as prescribed by his or her health care provider.

❖ PATIENT-CENTERED COLLABORATIVE CARE

◆ Assessment

Collect important data for the patient with osteomalacia or suspected osteomalacia, including age, ability to be exposed to sunlight, and skin pigmentation. The older adult who has been homebound or chronically institutionalized is at the greatest risk. People who have dark skin and who may consume minimal protein are more at risk than light-skinned people with the same dietary habits. Dark-skinned people may avoid the sun and need protein for calcium binding. Take a thorough nutritional history to determine the intake of foods containing vitamin D and calcium. Coordinate the assessment with the dietitian.

Assessment includes any history of chronic disease processes of the GI tract including inflammatory bowel disease, gastric or intestinal bypass surgery, or any problem that interferes with absorption from the GI tract. A history of renal or liver dysfunction may lead to ineffective metabolism of vitamin D. Drugs such as phenytoin (Dilantin) or fluoride preparations may also interfere with metabolism of vitamin D.

Osteomalacia and osteoporosis may occur at the same time (see Table 50-2). In the early stages of osteomalacia, the manifestations are nonspecific. Muscle weakness and bone pain may be misdiagnosed as arthritis or another connective tissue disorder. In some cases, proximal muscle weakness in the shoulder and pelvic girdle area is the only presenting symptom.

Muscle weakness in the lower extremities may cause a waddling and unsteady gait, which contributes to falls and subsequent fractures. Hypophosphatemia leads to an inadequate production of muscle cell adenosine triphosphate, thus resulting in a decrease in muscle cell energy. If hypocalcemia is present, muscle cramping may occur with weakness.

In collaboration with the physical therapist, assess muscle strength and observe the patient's gait. Document concerns about muscle cramps and bone pain. Skeletal discomfort is often vague and generalized. The spine, ribs, pelvis, and lower extremities are most often affected. The patient usually describes the pain as aggravated by activity and worse at night.

Palpate the affected bones for tenderness. Bone tenderness may occur when pressure is applied to the tibia or rib cage. Skeletal malalignment, like long-bone bowing or spinal deformity, may be similar to that seen in osteoporosis. In extreme cases, the pelvis narrows, so vaginal childbirth is difficult. If osteomalacia is untreated, vertebral, rib, and long-bone fractures may occur. The patient may be misdiagnosed as having bone cancer or osteoporosis.

X-rays of bone in patients with osteomalacia reveal a decrease in the cancellous bone and lack of osteoid sharpness. The classic diagnostic finding specific to the disease, however, is the presence of radiolucent bands (Looser's lines or zones). Looser's zones represent stress fractures that have not mineralized. They often appear symmetrically in the medial area of the femoral neck, ribs, and pelvis and may progress to complete fractures with minimal trauma. Bone biopsy of these areas may be needed for complete diagnosis. DXA scan may assist in diagnosis of osteomalacia.

◆ Interventions

The major treatment for osteomalacia is vitamin D in an active form, such as ergocalciferol. Vitamin D is needed to adequately absorb and utilize calcium in the body.

Nurses play a vital role in educating other health care professionals about the need to screen patients for low vitamin D levels. For all at-risk patients, teach them about which high calcium and vitamin D foods to eat and the importance of adequate daily sunlight. Additional health teaching is discussed above in the Health Promotion and Maintenance section.

PAGET'S DISEASE OF THE BONE

❖ PATHOPHYSIOLOGY

Paget's disease, or **osteitis deformans**, is a chronic metabolic disorder in which bone is excessively broken down (osteoclastic activity) and re-formed (osteoblastic activity). The result is bone that is structurally disorganized, causing bones to be weak with increased risk for bowing of long bones and fractures. Two types of Paget's disease can occur—familial and sporadic.

Three pathophysiologic phases of the disorder have been described: active, mixed, and inactive. In the first phase (the active phase), a rapid increase in osteoclasts (cells that break down bone) causes massive bone destruction and deformity. The osteoclasts of pagetic bone are large and multinuclear, unlike the osteoclasts of normal bone tissue.

In the mixed phase, the osteoblasts (bone-forming cells) react to compensate in forming new bone. The result is bone that is vascular, structurally weak, and deformed. Paget's disease occurs in one bone or in multiple sites. The most common areas of involvement are the vertebrae, femur, skull, clavicle, humerus, and pelvis.

GENETIC/GENOMIC CONSIDERATIONS

Patient-Centered Care QSEN

Because Paget's disease is often present in identical twins, an autosomal dominant pattern has been suggested. The disease has been noted in up to 30% of people with a positive family history for Paget's disease. Several complex genetic factors have been identified in families with the disease (Najat et al., 2009), including mutations in the:

- *RANKL/RANK/OPG* system, which is needed for osteoclast development and activity (see p. 1030 in the Osteoporosis section)
- Valosin-containing gene of complement binding protein (valosin-containing protein [*VCP*]), an important inflammatory factor
- Sequestosome 1 (*SQSTM1*) or *p62*, an expressed adaptor protein that can bind to ubiquitin and the atypical protein kinase C

Teach patients the importance of genetics in familial Paget's disease, and refer them to the appropriate genetics counseling resource. Ask the patient if genetic testing is desired.

When the osteoblastic activity exceeds the osteoclastic activity, the inactive phase occurs. The newly formed bone becomes sclerotic and very hard (McCance et al., 2014).

Paget's disease is second only to osteoporosis as one of the most common bone diseases in the United States, affecting about one million people. The disease is seen more frequently in people ages 50 years and older and in those of European heritage. The reason for this pattern is not known. The risk for developing Paget's disease increases as a person ages, particularly in those 80 years old and older. Men are affected twice as often as women (National Institute of Arthritis and Musculoskeletal and Skin Diseases, 2013).

❖ PATIENT-CENTERED COLLABORATIVE CARE

◆ Assessment

Physical Assessment/Clinical Manifestations. Most patients are asymptomatic, and the disease may be confined to one bone. It may be accidentally discovered during a routine laboratory or x-ray examination. In more severe disease, the manifestations are diverse and potentially fatal (Chart 50-3).

Ask the patient about a history of fracture and current bone pain. Bone PAIN, usually described as mild to moderate, may cause the patient to seek medical attention. The most common sites for pain are the hip and pelvis, but even the bones in the ear may be affected, causing hearing loss. The pain is usually described as aching, poorly defined, deep, and worsened by pressure. It is most noticeable at night or when the patient is resting. Patients may report redness and warmth at affected sites. These manifestations may be related to increased vascularity and blood flow.

The PAIN associated with the disorder may result from metabolic bone activity, secondary arthritis, impending fracture, or nerve impingement. Arthritis often occurs at the joints (cartilage) of the affected bones, resulting from bowing in the long bones of the leg. Some patients have joint replacements as a result of very painful weight-bearing joints. Nerve impingement is particularly common in the lumbosacral area of the vertebral column, presenting as back PAIN that radiates along one or both legs.

Observe posture, stance, and gait to identify gross bony deformities. Because of the enlargement of the vertebrae, loss of normal spinal curvature, and lower extremity malalignment, the patient may have decreased height. Assess for kyphosis or scoliosis of the spinal column. Note any long-bone bowing in the legs with subsequent varus (bow-leg) deformity. Long bones of the arms may also develop bowing. Flexion contracture in the hip joint is often present. Any of these deformities may be asymmetric. This weakened bone is at risk for fracture from even a minor injury. All of these problems interfere with the patient's need for independent mobility.

When performing a musculoskeletal assessment in a patient with Paget's disease, pay particular attention to the size and shape of the skull, which is typically soft, thick, and enlarged. Pressure from an enlarged temporal bone may lead to deafness and vertigo (dizziness). Basilar (in the occipital area) complications can compress any of the cranial nerves and result in neurologic problems. Assess the patient for changes in vision, swallowing, hearing, and speech. Platybasia, or basilar invagination, causes brainstem (vital sign center) damage that threatens life. In some cases, the bony enlargement of the skull blocks cerebrospinal fluid (CSF), resulting in hydrocephalus.

Fragility (pathologic) fractures may be the presenting clinical manifestation of the disorder. The femur and the tibia are most often affected, and fracture of these bones can result from minimal trauma. The fracture line is usually perpendicular to the long axis of the bone, and healing is unpredictable because of abnormal metabolic activity within the bone.

Although rare, bones affected by Paget's disease may develop malignant changes. The most dreaded complication of Paget's disease is cancer, most commonly osteogenic sarcoma. It affects the femur, humerus, and old fracture sites and has a grave prognosis because of early metastasis to the lung or extensive local invasion. When severe bone PAIN is present in a patient with Paget's disease, bone cancer is suspected.

Assess the skin for its color and temperature. In people with Paget's disease, the skin is typically flushed and warm because of increased blood flow. In addition, assess the patient's energy level because apathy, lethargy, and fatigue are common.

Other less common manifestations of Paget's disease include hyperparathyroidism and gout. Secondary hyperparathyroidism leads to an increase in serum and urinary calcium levels. In severe cases, serum calcium excess results from prolonged immobilization. Calcium deposits occur in joint spaces or as stones in the urinary tract. **Hyperuricemia** (serum uric acid excess) and gout occur because the increased metabolic activity of bone creates an increase in nucleic acid catabolism. Therefore kidney stones are more common in people with Paget's disease.

In a few cases, increased blood flow causes the heart to work harder to increase cardiac output, resulting in heart failure if not treated. Cardiac complications tend to occur only when more than a third of the skeleton is involved.

Diagnostic Assessment. Increases in *serum alkaline phosphatase (ALP)* and urinary hydroxyproline levels are the primary laboratory findings indicating possible Paget's disease. Overactive osteoblasts cause an altered ALP level. ALP can be further evaluated by alkaline phosphatase isoenzymes. The isoenzyme testing can further break ALP into three fractions—liver, bone, and intestinal. Elevated bone isoenzymes can help in a more definitive diagnosis of Paget's disease. Serum isoenzyme levels of bone ALP are used to monitor effectiveness of treatment (Pagana & Pagana, 2014).

The 24-hour *urinary hydroxyproline* level reflects bone collagen turnover and indicates the degree of disease severity. The higher the hydroxyproline, the more severe is the disease.

The *calcium* levels in blood and urine may be low, normal, or elevated. The immobilized patient is more likely to have an

CHART 50-3 Key Features

Paget's Disease of the Bone

Musculoskeletal Manifestations

- Bone and joint pain (may be in a single bone) that is aching, poorly described, and aggravated by walking
- Low back and sciatic nerve pain
- Bowing of long bones
- Loss of normal spinal curvature
- Enlarged, thick skull
- Pathologic fractures
- Osteogenic sarcoma (bone cancer)

Skin Manifestations

- Flushed, warm skin

Other Manifestations

- Apathy, lethargy, fatigue
- Hyperparathyroidism
- Gout
- Urinary or renal stones
- Heart failure from fluid overload

increase in calcium levels as a result of calcium moving from bone into the blood.

Paget's disease often causes an elevated *uric acid* because nucleic acid from overactive bone metabolism increases. This finding may be misinterpreted as primary gout.

X-rays are also used to diagnose Paget's disease. They reveal characteristic changes including the presence of osteolytic lesions and enlarged bones with radiolucent, or punched-out, appearance. Decrease in joint space may be seen with arthritic changes in joints. Malalignment deformities, fractures, and secondary arthritic changes may be present.

Radionuclide bone scan may be most sensitive in detecting Paget's disease. A radiolabeled bisphosphonate is injected IV and shows pagetic bone in areas of high bone turnover activity. This test can determine the extent of Paget's disease in the skeleton. CT and MRI are useful in the detection of cancerous tumors, changes in the skull, and spinal cord or nerve compression (Pagana & Pagana, 2014).

◆ Interventions

Nonsurgical or surgical management may be necessary to reduce pain and promote MOBILITY. Nonsurgical interventions are used first.

Drug Therapy. The primary intervention for Paget's disease is drug therapy. The purpose of *drug therapy* in Paget's disease is to relieve pain and to decrease bone resorption.

Management of mild to moderate pain may include the use of aspirin or NSAIDs such as ibuprofen (Motrin, Apo-Ibuprofen 🍁). When the calcium level is more than twice the normal value and the disease is widespread, the health care provider usually prescribes more potent drugs, such as selected bisphosphonates. Treatment with these agents for Paget's disease requires dosages and duration of therapy different from those for osteoporosis. Chart 50-2 includes information about some of these commonly used drugs.

Oral bisphosphonates are a first-line treatment choice for Paget's disease when alkaline phosphatase levels are at least twice the normal serum level. Alendronate (Fosamax), risedronate (Actonel), etidronate (Didronel), or tiludronate (Skelid) is given in tablet form. When oral agents are not effective, pamidronate (Aredia) or zoledronic acid (Reclast, Zometa) is administered IV (Lilley et al., 2014). Aredia is given once every 3 months, and Reclast is given once a year as a single IV dose. These drugs are usually highly effective. To reduce the risk for hypocalcemia, patients should receive 1500 mg of calcium daily in divided doses and 800 international units of vitamin D_3 daily for at least 2 weeks after zoledronic acid infusion unless they are prone to kidney stones. Chart 50-2 provides additional information about caring for patients receiving bisphosphonates.

Denosumab (Prolia) is a monoclonal antibody that is also approved for Paget's disease. The drug binds to a protein that is essential for the formation, function, and survival of osteoclasts and is given subcutaneously twice a year. By preventing the protein from activating its receptor, the drug decreases bone loss and increases bone mass and strength. This drug is discussed in the Osteoporosis section of this chapter.

Calcitonin is a hormone that seems to reduce bone resorption and, subsequently, relieve pain. The drug often causes a dramatic decrease in the alkaline phosphatase level in a few weeks. Calcitonin is approved for subcutaneous administration in treating Paget's disease because the nasal spray is not effective. The drug binds to osteoclast receptors, therefore slowing bone breakdown (Lilley et al., 2014). The drug may be used for those patients who do not tolerate bisphosphonates. Side effects of calcitonin include nausea, flushing, and skin rash. Skin testing may be done before administration of the first dose.

Other Interventions. In addition to administering drugs, implement physical measures to reduce pain and increase MOBILITY. These measures may include application of heat and gentle massage. An exercise program may be started with the help of a physical therapist. Exercise may be difficult because of pain and danger of fracture. Non-impact exercise should be used, but the patient may benefit from strengthening and weight-bearing exercises. In collaboration with the physical therapist, teach the patient about ROM and gentle stretching. Additional interventions for pain relief, such as relaxation techniques, are discussed in Chapter 3.

Measures to promote bone health are also important and include a diet rich in calcium and vitamin D. Nutrition therapy for bone health is described on p. 1033 in the discussion of Interventions in the Osteoporosis section.

Provide the patient with information to contact the U.S. local chapter of The Paget Foundation (www.paget.org) and the Arthritis Foundation (www.arthritis.org). The Arthritis Society in Canada (www.arthritis.ca) is also an excellent service. These resources provide information and support for the patient and family or significant others.

NCLEX EXAMINATION CHALLENGE

Physiological Integrity

A client is starting on risedronate (Actonel) for treatment of Paget's disease. What precaution does the nurse include in the client's health teaching about this drug?

A. "This drug can cause serious infections."
B. "Monitor the drug injection site for redness or itching."
C. "Drink a full glass of water after taking the drug."
D. "Do not take calcium and vitamin D while on the drug."

OSTEOMYELITIS

INFECTION in bony tissue can be a severe and difficult-to-treat problem. Bone infection can result in chronic recurrence of infection, loss of function and mobility, amputation, and even death.

❖ PATHOPHYSIOLOGY

Bacteria, viruses, or fungi can cause INFECTION in bone, known as **osteomyelitis**. Invasion by one or more pathogenic microorganisms stimulates the inflammatory response in bone tissue. The INFLAMMATION produces an increased vascular leak and edema, often involving the surrounding soft tissues. Once inflammation is established, the vessels in the area become thrombosed and release exudate (pus) into bony tissue. Ischemia of bone tissue follows and results in necrotic bone. This area of necrotic bone separates from surrounding bone tissue, and **sequestrum** is formed. The presence of sequestrum prevents bone healing and causes superimposed infection, often in the form of bone abscess. As shown in Fig. 50-2, the cycle repeats itself as the new infection leads to further inflammation, vessel thromboses, and necrosis.

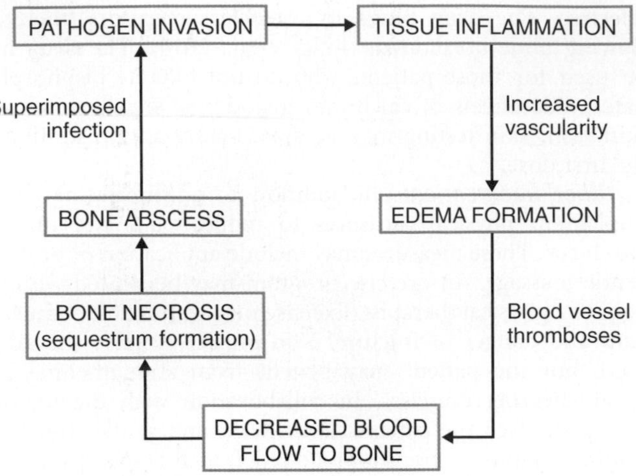

FIG. 50-2 Infection cycle of osteomyelitis.

Osteomyelitis is categorized as *exogenous*, in which infectious organisms enter from outside the body as in an open fracture, or **endogenous** (**hematogenous**), in which organisms are carried by the bloodstream from other areas of infection in the body. A third category is *contiguous*, in which bone infection results from skin infection of adjacent tissues. Osteomyelitis can be further divided into two major types: acute osteomyelitis and chronic osteomyelitis.

Each type of bone infection has its own causative factors. Pathogenic microbes favor bone that has a rich blood supply and a marrow cavity. **Acute hematogenous infection** results from bacteremia, underlying disease, or nonpenetrating trauma. Urinary tract infections, particularly in older men, tend to spread to the lower vertebrae. Long-term IV catheters (e.g., Hickman catheters) can be primary sources of INFECTION. Patients undergoing long-term hemodialysis and IV drug users are also at risk for osteomyelitis. *Salmonella* infections of the GI tract may spread to bone. Patients with sickle cell disease and other hemoglobinopathies often have multiple episodes of salmonellosis, which can cause bone infection (McCance et al., 2014).

Poor dental hygiene and periodontal (gum) INFECTION can be causative factors in **contiguous** osteomyelitis in facial bones. Minimal nonpenetrating trauma can cause hemorrhages or small-vessel occlusions, leading to bone necrosis. Regardless of the source of infection, many infections are caused by *Staphylococcus aureus.* Treatment of infection may be complicated further by the presence of methicillin-resistant *Staphylococcus aureus* (MRSA) or other multiple drug-resistant organisms (MDRO), which is very common in hospitalized and other institutionalized patients. One of the major desired outcomes in health care settings today is to reduce the number of MRSA infections from any source.

CONSIDERATIONS FOR OLDER ADULTS

Patient-Centered Care QSEN

Malignant external otitis media involving the base of the skull is sometimes seen in older adults with diabetes. The most common cause of contiguous spread in older adults, however, is found in those who have slow-healing foot ulcers. Multiple organisms tend to be responsible for the resulting osteomyelitis (McCance et al., 2014).

CHART 50-4 Key Features

Acute and Chronic Osteomyelitis

Acute Osteomyelitis	Chronic Osteomyelitis
• Fever; temperature usually above 101° F (38.3° C) • Swelling around the affected area • Erythema of the affected area • Tenderness of the affected area • Bone pain that is constant, localized, and pulsating; intensifies with movement	• Foot ulcer(s) (most commonly) • Sinus tract formation • Localized pain • Drainage from the affected area

Penetrating trauma leads to acute osteomyelitis by direct inoculation. A soft-tissue infection may be present as well. Animal bites, puncture wounds, skin ulcerations, and bone surgery can result in bone INFECTION. The most common offending organism is *Pseudomonas aeruginosa*, but other gram-negative bacteria may be found.

If bone infection is misdiagnosed or inadequately treated, **chronic osteomyelitis** may develop, especially in older adults who have foot ulcers. Inadequate care management results when the treatment period is too short or when the treatment is delayed or inappropriate. About half of cases of chronic osteomyelitis are caused by gram-negative bacteria. Although bacteria are the most common causes of osteomyelitis, viruses and fungal organisms also may cause INFECTION.

❖ PATIENT-CENTERED COLLABORATIVE CARE

◆ Assessment

Bone PAIN, with or without other manifestations, is a common concern of patients with bone INFECTION. The pain is described as a constant, localized, pulsating sensation that worsens with movement.

The patient with *acute* osteomyelitis has fever, usually with temperature greater than 101° F (38.3° C). *Older adults may not have an extreme temperature elevation because of lower core body temperature and compromised immune system that occur with normal aging.* The area around the infected bone swells and is tender when palpated. Erythema (redness) and heat may also be present. When vascular compromise is severe, patients may not feel discomfort because of nerve damage from lack of blood supply.

When vascular insufficiency is suspected, assess circulation in the distal extremities. Ulcerations may be present on the feet or hands, indicating inadequate healing ability as a result of poor circulation.

Fever, swelling, and erythema are less common in those with *chronic* osteomyelitis. Ulceration resulting in sinus tract formation, localized pain, and drainage is more characteristic of chronic infection (Chart 50-4).

The patient with osteomyelitis may have an elevated white blood cell (leukocyte) count, which may be double the normal value. The erythrocyte sedimentation rate (ESR) may be normal early in the course of the disease but rises as the condition progresses. It may remain elevated for as long as 3 months after drug therapy is discontinued.

If bacteremia is present, a potentially life-threatening complication that could lead to septic shock, a blood culture identifies the offending organisms to determine which antibiotics should be used in treatment. Both aerobic and anaerobic blood cultures are collected before drug therapy begins.

Although bone changes cannot be detected early with standard x-rays, changes in blood flow can be seen early in the course of the disease by radionuclide scanning or MRI.

◆ Interventions

The specific treatment protocol depends on the type and number of microbes present in the infected tissue. If other measures fail to resolve the infectious process, surgical management may be needed.

Nonsurgical Management. The health care provider starts antimicrobial (e.g., antibiotic) therapy as soon as possible. In the presence of copious wound drainage, Contact Precautions are used to prevent the spread of the offending organism to other patients and health care personnel. Teach patients, visitors, and staff members how to use these precautions. (See Chapter 23 for a discussion of Contact Precautions.)

More than one agent may be needed to combat multiple types of organisms. The hospital or home care nurse gives the drugs at specifically prescribed times so that therapeutic serum levels are achieved. Observe for the actions, side effects, and toxicity of these drugs. *Teach family members or other caregivers in the home setting how to administer antimicrobials if they are continued after hospital discharge or are used only at home.*

The optimal drug regimen for patients with chronic osteomyelitis is not well established. Prolonged therapy for more than 3 months may be needed to eliminate the infection. Because of the cost of lengthy hospital stays, patients are typically cared for in the home or long-term care (LTC) setting with long-term vascular access catheters, such as the peripherally inserted central catheter (PICC), for drug administration. After discontinuation of IV drugs, oral therapy may be needed for weeks or months. Patients and families must understand the complications of inadequate treatment or failure to follow up with health care providers. Teach them that drug therapy must be continued over a long period to be effective.

! NURSING SAFETY PRIORITY QSEN

Drug Alert

Even when symptoms of osteomyelitis appear to be improved, teach the patient and family that the full course of IV and oral antimicrobials must be completed to ensure that the infection is resolved.

In addition to systemic drug therapy, the wound may be irrigated, either continuously or intermittently, with one or more antibiotic solutions. A medical technique in which beads made of bone cement are impregnated with an antibiotic and packed into the wound can provide direct contact of the antibiotic with the offending organism.

Drugs are also needed to control PAIN. Patients experience acute and chronic pain and must receive a regimen of drug therapy for control. Chapter 3 describes pharmacologic and nonpharmacologic interventions for both acute and chronic pain.

A treatment to increase tissue perfusion for patients with chronic, unremitting osteomyelitis is the use of a hyperbaric chamber or portable device to administer hyperbaric oxygen (HBO) therapy. These devices are usually available in large tertiary care centers and may not be accessible to all patients who might benefit from them. With HBO therapy, the affected area is exposed to a high concentration of oxygen that diffuses into the tissues to promote healing. In conjunction with high-dose drug therapy and surgical débridement, HBO has proven very useful in treating a number of anaerobic infections. Other wound-management therapies are described in Chapter 25.

Surgical Management. Antimicrobial therapy alone may not meet the desired outcome of treatment. Surgical techniques may be used to minimize the disfigurement that can be a devastating result of severe osteomyelitis. Surgery is reserved for patients with chronic osteomyelitis.

Because bone cannot heal in the presence of necrotic tissue, a *sequestrectomy* may be performed to débride the necrotic bone and allow revascularization of tissue. The excision of dead and infected bone often results in a sizable cavity, or bone defect. Bone *grafts* to repair bone defects are also widely used.

When infected bone is extensively resected, reconstruction with *microvascular bone transfers* may be done. This procedure is reserved for larger skeletal defects. The most common donor sites are the patient's fibula and iliac crest. The bone graft may have an attached muscle or skin flap, if necessary. The steps of the procedure are similar to those of bone grafting in that débridement of dead or necrotic bone is done before bone transfer.

Nursing care of the patient after surgery is similar to that for any postoperative patient (see Chapter 16). However, the important difference is that neurovascular (NV) assessments must be done frequently because the patient experiences increased swelling after the surgical procedure. Elevate the affected extremity to increase venous return and thus control swelling. Assess and document the patient's NV status, including:

- Pain
- Movement
- Sensation
- Warmth
- Temperature
- Distal pulses
- Capillary refill (not as reliable as the above indicators)

! NURSING SAFETY PRIORITY QSEN

Critical Rescue

After surgery to treat osteomyelitis, frequently check for signs of neurovascular compromise, including the six *P*s: **p**ain that cannot be controlled, **p**ressure, paresis or **p**aralysis (weakness or inability to move), **p**aresthesia (abnormal, tingling sensation), **p**allor, and **p**ulselessness. If any of these findings occur, report them immediately to the surgeon.

If the bony defect is small, a *muscle flap* may be the only surgery required. Local muscle flaps are used in the treatment of chronic osteomyelitis when soft tissue does not fill the dead space, or cavity, that results from bone débridement. The flap provides wound coverage and enhances blood flow to promote healing. A split-thickness skin graft is often applied several days after the muscle flap.

When the previously described surgical procedures are not appropriate or successful and as a last resort, the affected limb may need to be amputated. The physical and psychological care for a patient who has undergone an amputation is discussed in Chapter 51.

BENIGN BONE TUMORS

❖ PATHOPHYSIOLOGY

Benign (noncancerous) bone tumors are often asymptomatic and may be discovered on routine x-ray examination or as the cause of pathologic fractures. The cause of benign bone tumors is not known. Tumors may arise from several types of tissue. The major classifications include *chondrogenic* tumors (from cartilage), *osteogenic* tumors (from bone), and *fibrogenic* tumors (from fibrous tissue and found most often in children). Although many specific benign tumors have been identified, only the common ones are described here.

The most common benign bone tumor is the *osteochondroma*. Although its onset is usually in childhood, the tumor grows until skeletal maturity and may not be diagnosed until adulthood. The tumor may be a single growth or multiple growths and can occur in any bone. The femur and the tibia are most often involved.

The *chondroma*, or endochondroma, is a lesion of mature hyaline cartilage affecting primarily the hands and the feet. The ribs, sternum, spine, and long bones may also be involved. Chondromas are slow growing and often cause pathologic fractures after minor injury. They are found in people of all ages, occur in both men and women, and can affect any bone.

The origin of the *giant cell tumor* remains uncertain. This lesion is aggressive and can be extensive and may involve surrounding soft tissue. Although classified as benign, giant cell tumors can metastasize (spread) to the lung. The peak incidence occurs in patients in their 30s.

❖ PATIENT-CENTERED COLLABORATIVE CARE

Assess for PAIN, the most common manifestation of benign bone tumors. Pain can range from mild to moderate. It can be caused by direct tumor invasion into soft tissue, compressing peripheral nerves, or by a resulting pathologic fracture.

In addition, observe and palpate the suspected involved area. When the tumor affects the lower extremities or the small bones of the hands and feet, local swelling may be detected as the tumor enlarges. In some cases, muscle atrophy or muscle spasm may be present. Carefully palpate the bone and muscle to detect these changes and elicit tenderness.

Routine x-rays and tomography are used to find bone tumors. Tumors are characterized by sharp margins, intact cortices, and smooth, uniform periosteal bone.

CT is less useful except in complex anatomic areas, such as the spinal column and sacrum. The test is helpful in evaluating the extent of soft-tissue involvement. MRI may be especially helpful in viewing problems of the spinal column.

The health care provider uses drug therapy and surgery in combination when possible. Non-drug pain-relief measures are also used. Depending on the patient's preference and tolerance, measures such as heat or cold may help relieve pain.

In addition to prescribing analgesics to reduce pain, the health care provider usually prescribes one or more NSAIDs to inhibit prostaglandin synthesis that increases pain and INFLAMMATION. Give these drugs after meals or with food to reduce GI side effects. Teach patients to report any signs of bleeding to the primary health care provider immediately.

The most common surgical procedure used for benign bone tumors is removal. If the tumor is small, surgery may not be needed. When the tumor is very extensive, as in a giant cell tumor, it is removed with care to restore or maintain the function of the adjacent joint, most often the knee. In some cases, the knee is replaced with a prosthetic device and, less often, is fused (**arthrodesis**). Bone grafting may be needed. The collaborative care for patients undergoing total knee replacement is discussed in Chapter 18.

BONE CANCER

Cancerous bone tumors may be primary or secondary (those that originate in other tissues and metastasize to bone). *Primary tumors* occur most often in people between 10 and 30 years of age and make up a small percentage of bone cancers. As for other forms of cancer, the exact cause of bone cancer is unknown but genetic and environmental factors are likely causes. *Metastatic lesions* most often occur in the older age-group and account for most bone cancers (McCance et al., 2014).

Previous radiation therapy in the anatomic area is a big risk factor. For example, bone cancer of the ribs in the path of radiation for breast cancer is fairly common.

❖ PATHOPHYSIOLOGY

Osteosarcoma, or osteogenic sarcoma, is the most common type of *primary* malignant bone tumor. More than 50% of cases occur in the distal femur, followed in decreasing order of occurrence by the proximal tibia and humerus.

The tumor is relatively large, causing acute pain and swelling. The involved area is usually warm because the blood flow to the site increases. The center of the tumor is sclerotic from increased osteoblastic activity. The periphery is soft, extending through the bone cortex in the classic sunburst appearance associated with the neoplasm. An inward spread into the medullary canal is also common. Osteosarcoma typically **metastasizes** (spreads), which results in death.

Although *Ewing's sarcoma* is not as common as other tumors, it is the most malignant. Like other primary tumors, it causes PAIN and swelling. In addition, systemic manifestations, particularly low-grade fever, leukocytosis, and anemia, characterize the lesions. The pelvis and the lower extremity are most often affected. Pelvic involvement is a poor prognostic sign. It often extends into soft tissue. Death results from metastasis to the lungs and other bones. Although the tumor can be seen in patients of any age, it usually occurs in children and young adults in their 20s. Men are affected more often than women (McCance et al., 2014). The reason for this pattern is not known.

In contrast to the patient with osteosarcoma, the patient with *chondrosarcoma* experiences dull PAIN and swelling for a long period. The tumor typically affects the pelvis and proximal femur near the diaphysis. Arising from cartilaginous tissue, it destroys bone and often calcifies. The patient with this type of tumor has a better prognosis than one with osteogenic sarcoma. Chondrosarcoma occurs in middle-aged and older people, with a slight predominance in men.

Arising from fibrous tissue, *fibrosarcomas* can be divided into subtypes, of which malignant fibrous histiocytoma (MFH) is the most malignant. Usually the clinical presentation of MFH is gradual, without specific symptoms. Local tenderness, with or without a palpable mass, occurs in the long bones of the lower extremity. As with other bone cancers, the lesion can metastasize to the lungs (McCance et al., 2014).

Primary tumors of the prostate, breast, kidney, thyroid, and lung are called *bone-seeking* cancers because they spread to the bone more often than other primary tumors. The vertebrae, pelvis, femur, and ribs are the bone sites commonly affected. Simply stated, primary tumor cells, or seeds, are carried to bone through the bloodstream. *Fragility fractures caused by metastatic bone are a major concern in patient care management.*

❖ PATIENT-CENTERED COLLABORATIVE CARE

◆ Assessment

The data collected for the patient suspected of having a malignant bone tumor are similar to the data needed for the patient with a benign growth. In addition, ask whether the patient has had previous radiation therapy for cancer and determine the status of the patient's general health.

The clinical manifestations seen in the patient with primary bone cancer or metastatic disease vary, depending on the specific type of lesion. Usually the patient has a group of nonspecific concerns, including pain, local swelling, and a tender, palpable mass. Marked disability and impaired MOBILITY may occur in those with advanced metastatic bone disease.

In a patient with Ewing's sarcoma, a low-grade fever may occur because of the systemic features of the neoplasm. For this reason, it is often confused with osteomyelitis. Fatigue and pallor resulting from anemia are also common.

In performing a musculoskeletal assessment, inspect the involved area and palpate the mass for size and tenderness. In collaboration with the physical and occupational therapists, assess the patient's ability to perform MOBILITY tasks and ADLs.

Patients with malignant bone tumors may be young adults whose productive lives are just beginning. They need strong support systems to help cope with the diagnosis and its treatment. Family, significant others, and health care professionals are major components of the needed support. Determine what systems or resources are available.

Patients often experience a loss of control over their lives when a diagnosis of cancer is made. As a result, they become anxious and fearful about the outcome of their illness. Coping with the diagnosis becomes a challenge. As patients progress through the grieving process, there may be initial denial. Identify the anxiety level, and assess the stage or stages of the grieving process. Explore any maladaptive behavior, indicating ineffective coping mechanisms. Chapter 22 further describes the psychosocial assessment for patients with cancer.

The patient with a malignant bone tumor typically shows elevated serum alkaline phosphatase (ALP) levels, indicating the body's attempt to form new bone by increasing osteoblastic activity. The patient with Ewing's sarcoma or metastatic bone cancer often has anemia. In addition, leukocytosis is common with Ewing's sarcoma. The progression of Ewing's sarcoma may be evaluated by elevated serum lactic dehydrogenase (LDH) levels.

In some patients with bone metastasis from the breast, kidney, or lung, the serum calcium level is elevated. Massive bone destruction stimulates release of the mineral into the bloodstream. In patients with Ewing's sarcoma and bone metastasis, the erythrocyte sedimentation rate (ESR) may be elevated because of secondary tissue inflammation (Pagana & Pagana, 2014).

As with benign bone tumors, routine x-rays and CT reveal malignant lesions. Metastatic lesions may increase or decrease bone density, depending on the amount of osteoblastic and osteoclastic activity. CT is helpful in determining the extent of soft-tissue damage. The patient may have an MRI for difficult-to-visualize areas such as the vertebrae.

In some cases a needle bone biopsy may be performed, usually under fluoroscopy to guide the surgeon. Needle biopsy is an ambulatory care procedure with rare complications. After biopsy, the cancer is staged for size and degree of spread. One popular method is the TNM system, based on tumor size and number (T), the presence of cancer cells in lymph nodes (N), and metastasis (spread) to distant sites (M) (see Chapter 21 for further discussion).

Another method is to correlate the tumor grade (high or low), tumor site (intracompartmental or extracompartmental), and presence of metastatic disease (positive or negative). Staging guides the health care team in their decision regarding patient-centered collaborative care.

◆ Interventions

Because the pain is often due to direct primary tumor invasion, treatment is aimed at reducing the size of or removing the tumor. The expected outcome of treating metastatic bone tumors is palliative rather than curative. Palliative therapies may prevent further bone destruction and improve patient function. A combination of nonsurgical and surgical management is used. Collaborate with members of the interdisciplinary health care team to plan high quality care to achieve positive patient outcomes.

Nonsurgical Management. In addition to analgesics for local PAIN relief, chemotherapeutic agents and radiation therapy are often administered to shrink the tumor. In patients with spinal involvement, bracing and immobilization with cervical traction may reduce back pain. Interventional radiology techniques are used to decrease vertebral pain and treat compression fractures (see Chapter 51).

Drug Therapy. The physician may prescribe *chemotherapy* to be given alone or in combination with radiation or surgery. Certain proliferating tumors, such as Ewing's sarcoma, are sensitive to cytotoxic drugs. Others, such as chondrosarcomas, are often totally drug resistant. Chemotherapy seems to work best for small, metastatic tumors and may be administered before or after surgery. In most cases the physician prescribes a combination of agents. At present, there is no one universally accepted protocol of chemotherapeutic agents. The drugs selected are determined in part by the primary source of the cancer in metastatic disease. For example, when metastasis occurs from breast cancer, estrogen and progesterone blockers may be used. Chapter 22 describes the general nursing care of patients who receive chemotherapy. *Remember that all chemotherapeutic agents are categorized as high-alert medications* (Institute for Safe Medication Practices, 2013).

Other drugs are given for specific metastatic cancers, depending on the location of the primary site. For example, biologic agents, such as cytokines, are given to stimulate the immune system to recognize and destroy cancer cells, especially in patients with renal cancer. Zoledronic acid (Zometa) and pamidronate (Aredia) are two IV bisphosphonates that are approved for bone metastasis from the breast, lung, and prostate (Lilley et al., 2014). These drugs help protect bones and prevent fractures. Inform patients that osteonecrosis of the jaw may also occur, especially in those who have invasive dental procedures. Monitor associated laboratory tests, such as serum creatinine and electrolytes, because these drugs can be toxic to the kidneys. Bisphosphonates are described earlier in the Osteoporosis section.

Denosumab (Prolia) is a monoclonal antibody that is also approved for metastatic bone disease (Lilley et al., 2014). The drug binds to a protein that is essential for the formation, function, and survival of osteoclasts and is given subcutaneously twice a year. By preventing the protein from activating its receptor, the drug decreases bone loss and increases bone mass and strength. This drug is discussed earlier in the Osteoporosis section.

Radiation Therapy. Radiation, either brachytherapy or external radiation, is used for selected types of malignant tumors. For patients with Ewing's sarcoma and early osteosarcoma, radiation may be the treatment of choice in reducing tumor size and thus pain.

For patients with metastatic disease, radiation is given primarily for palliation. The therapy is directed toward the painful sites to provide a more comfortable life. One or more treatments are given, depending on the extent of disease. With precise planning, radiation therapy can be used with minimal complications. The general nursing care for patients receiving radiation therapy is described in Chapter 22.

Interventional Radiology. Interventional radiologists can perform several noninvasive procedures to help relieve PAIN in the patient with metastasis to the spinal column. Two types of *thermal ablation techniques, radiofrequency ablation (RFA)* and *cryoablation*, can be done under moderate sedation or general anesthesia. RFA kills the targeted tissue with heat using a small needle inserted into the tumor. Most patients have pain relief or control after this ambulatory care procedure. Cryoablation is similar to RFA, but the radiologist uses an extremely cold gas through a probe into the tumor. Although this procedure has been available for years, newer surgical equipment allows a small incision and the patient can return to usual daily activities in a day or two.

The radiologist may also perform a *vertebroplasty* if the patient with spinal metastasis has pathologic compression fractures. After making a small incision, bone cement is injected through a needle into the fractured area. The cement hardens within 15 minutes. Like thermal ablation, this procedure is done in an ambulatory care setting and the patient is placed under moderate sedation.

Surgical Management. Primary bone tumors are usually reduced or removed with surgery, and surgery may be combined with radiation or chemotherapy.

Preoperative Care. In addition to the nature, progression, and extent of the tumor, the patient's age and general health state are considered. Chemotherapy may be administered preoperatively.

As for any patient preparing for cancer surgery, the patient with bone cancer needs psychological support from the nurse and other members of the health care team. Assess the level of the patient's and family's understanding about the surgery and related treatments. As an advocate, encourage the patient and family to discuss concerns and questions and provide information regarding hospital routines and procedures. Spiritual support is important to some patients. They may prefer to contact a member of the clergy or a spiritual leader or talk with a clergy member affiliated with the hospital. Offer assistance in arranging for spiritual assistance if requested.

Anticipate postoperative needs as much as possible before the patient undergoes surgery. Remind the patient what to expect postoperatively and how to help ensure adequate recovery.

Operative Procedures. Wide or radical resection procedures are used for patients with bone sarcomas to salvage the affected limb. Wide excision is removal of the lesion surrounded by an intact cuff of normal tissue and leads to cure of low-grade tumors only. A radical resection includes removal of the lesion, the entire muscle, bone, and other tissues directly involved. It is the procedure used for high-grade tumors.

Large bone defects that result from tumor removal may require either:

- Total joint replacements with prosthetic implants, either whole or partial
- Custom metallic implants
- Allografts from the iliac crest, rib, or fibula

As an alternative to total replacement, an allograft may be implanted with internal fixation for those patients who do not have metastases. This is a common procedure for sarcomas of the proximal femur. Allograft procedures for the knee are also performed, particularly in young adults. Preoperative chemotherapy is given to enhance the likelihood of success. **Allografts** with adjacent tendons and ligaments are harvested from cadavers and can be frozen or freeze-dried for a prolonged period. The graft is fixed with a series of bolts, screws, or plates.

Postoperative Care. The surgical incision for a limb salvage procedure is often extensive. A pressure dressing with wound suction is typically maintained for several days. The patient who has undergone a limb salvage procedure has some degree of impaired physical mobility and a self-care deficit. The nature and extent of the alterations depend on the location and extent of the surgery.

! NURSING SAFETY PRIORITY QSEN

Action Alert

For patients who have allografts, observe for signs of hemorrhage, infection, and fracture. Report these complications to the surgeon immediately.

After upper extremity surgery, the patient can engage in active-assistive exercises by using the opposite hand to help achieve motions such as forward flexion and abduction of the shoulder. Continuous passive motion (CPM) using a CPM machine may be initiated as early as the first postoperative day for either upper extremity or lower extremity procedures.

After lower extremity surgery, the emphasis is on strengthening the quadriceps muscles by using passive and active motion when possible. Maintaining muscle tone is an important prerequisite to weight bearing, which progresses from toe touch or partial weight bearing to full weight bearing by 3 months postoperatively. Coordinate the patient's plan of care for ambulation and muscle strengthening with the physical therapist.

The patient who has had a bone graft may have a cast or other supportive device for several months. Weight bearing is prohibited until there is evidence that the graft is incorporated into the adjacent bone tissue.

During the recovery phase, the patient may also need assistance with ADLs, particularly if the surgery involves the upper extremity. Assist if needed, but at the same time encourage the patient to do as much as possible unaided. Some patients need assistive/adaptive devices for a short period while they are healing. Coordinate the patient's plan of care for promoting independence in ADLs with the occupational therapist.

Surrounding tissues, including nerves and blood vessels, may be removed during surgery. Vascular grafting is common, but the lost nerve(s) is (are) usually not replaced. Assess the neurovascular status of the affected extremity and hand or foot every 1 to 2 hours immediately after surgery. Splinting or casting of the limb may also cause neurovascular (NV) compromise and needs to be checked for proper placement.

In addition to needing emotional support to cope with physical disabilities, the patient may need help coping with the surgery and its effects. Help identify available support systems as soon as possible.

As a result of most of the surgical procedures, the patient experiences an altered body image. Suggest ways to minimize cosmetic changes. For example, a lowered shoulder can be covered by a custom-made pad worn under clothing. The patient can cover lower extremity defects with pants.

Advocate for the patient and the family to promote the physician-patient relationship. For instance, the patient may not completely understand the medical or surgical treatment plan but may hesitate to question the physician. The nurse's intervention can increase communication, which is essential in successful management of the patient with cancer.

CLINICAL JUDGMENT CHALLENGE

Patient-Centered Care; Teamwork and Collaboration; Safety QSEN

A 77-year-old widower reports pain in his back and abdomen. He had a radical prostatectomy for prostate cancer 5 years ago and was thought to be cancer-free until this time. A chest x-ray revealed bone metastasis in his vertebral spine. The patient is admitted to the cancer center for intensive treatment.

1. What other patient history information do you need to provide quality care for this patient and why?
2. What treatment options does this patient have to manage his bone cancer? What is the purpose of treating the cancer at this time?
3. For what major complications might this patient be most at risk, and how will you plan to help prevent them? *(Hint: see Chapter 22.)*
4. With what health care team members will you collaborate and why?
5. What are the major considerations for discharge planning?

Community-Based Care

After medical treatment for a primary malignant tumor, the patient is usually managed at home with follow-up care. The patient with metastatic disease may remain in the home or, when home support is not available, may be admitted to a long-term care facility for extended or hospice care. Coordinate the patient's discharge plan and continuity of care with the case manager and other health care team members, depending on the patient's needs.

Home Care Management. In collaboration with the occupational therapist, evaluate the patient's home environment for structural barriers that may hinder MOBILITY. The patient may be discharged with a cast, walker, crutches, or a wheelchair. Assess the patient's support system for availability of assistance if needed.

Accessibility to eating and toileting facilities is essential to promote ADL independence. Because the patient with metastatic disease is susceptible to pathologic fractures, potential hazards that may contribute to falls or injury should be removed.

Self-Management Education. For the patient receiving intermittent chemotherapy or radiation on an ambulatory care basis, emphasize the importance of keeping appointments. Review the expected side and toxic effects of the drugs with the patient and family. Teach how to treat less serious side effects and when to contact the health care provider. If the drugs are administered at home via long-term IV catheter, explain and demonstrate the care involved with daily dressing changes and potential catheter complications. Chapter 13 describes the health teaching required for a patient receiving infusion therapy at home.

If the patient has undergone surgery, he or she has a wound and limited MOBILITY. Teach the patient, family, and/or significant others how to care for the wound. Help the patient learn how to perform ADLs and mobility activities independently for self-management. Coordinate with the physical and occupational therapists to assist in ADL teaching, and provide or recommend assistive and adaptive devices, if necessary. The physical therapist also teaches the proper use of ambulatory aids, such as crutches, and exercises.

PAIN management can be a major challenge, particularly for the patient with metastatic bone disease. Discuss the various options for pain relief, including relaxation and music therapy. Emphasize the importance of those techniques that worked during hospitalization. See Chapter 3 for cancer pain assessment and management.

The patient with bone cancer may fear that the malignancy will return. Acknowledge this fear, but reinforce confidence in the health care team and medical treatment chosen. Mutually establish realistic outcomes regarding returning to work and participating in recreational activities. Encourage the patient to resume a functional lifestyle, but caution that it should be gradual. Certain activities, such as participating in sports, may be prohibited.

Help the patient with advanced metastatic bone disease prepare for death. The nurse and other support personnel assist the patient through the stages of death and dying. Identify resources that can help the patient write a will, visit with distant family members, or do whatever he or she thinks is needed for a peaceful death. Chapter 7 describes end-of-life care in detail.

Health Care Resources. In addition to family and significant others, cancer support groups are helpful to the patient with bone cancer. Some organizations, such as *I Can Cope*, provide information and emotional support. Others, such as *CanSurmount*, are geared more toward patient and family education. The American Cancer Society (www.cancer.org) and the Canadian Cancer Society (www.cancer.ca) can also provide education and resources for patients and families.

The hospital staff nurse, discharge planner, or case manager also ensures that follow-up care, including nursing care and physical or occupational therapy, is available in the home. The patient with terminal cancer may choose to become part of a hospice program as described in Chapter 7.

DISORDERS OF THE HAND

Dupuytren's Contracture

Dupuytren's contracture, or deformity, is a slowly progressive thickening of the palmar fascia, resulting in flexion contracture of the fourth (ring) and fifth (little) fingers of the hand. The third or middle finger is occasionally affected. Although

Dupuytren's contracture is a common problem, the cause is unknown. It usually occurs in older Euro-American men, tends to occur in families, and can be bilateral.

When function becomes impaired, surgical release is required. A partial or selective fasciectomy (cutting of fascia) is performed. After removal of the surgical dressing, a splint may be used. Nursing care is similar to that for the patient with carpal tunnel repair (see Chapter 51).

Ganglion

A **ganglion** is a round, benign cyst, often found on a wrist or foot joint or tendon. The synovium surrounding the tendon degenerates, allowing the tendon sheath tissue to become weak and distended. Ganglia are painless on palpation, but they can cause joint discomfort after prolonged joint use or minor trauma or strain. The lesion can rapidly disappear and then recur. Ganglia are most likely to develop in people between 15 and 50 years of age. With local or regional anesthesia in a physician's office or clinic, the fluid within the cyst can be aspirated through a small needle. A cortisone injection may follow. If the cyst is very large, it is removed using a small incision. Patients should avoid strenuous activity for 48 hours after surgery and report any signs of INFLAMMATION to their health care provider.

DISORDERS OF THE FOOT

Foot Deformities

The **hallux valgus** deformity is a common foot problem in which the great toe drifts laterally at the first metatarsophalangeal (MTP) joint (Fig. 50-3). The first metatarsal head becomes enlarged, resulting in a **bunion.** As the deviation worsens, the bony enlargement causes pain, particularly when shoes are worn. Women are affected more often than men. Hallux valgus often occurs as a result of poorly fitted shoes—in particular, those with narrow toes and high heels. Other causes include osteoarthritis, rheumatoid arthritis, and family history.

For some patients who are of advanced age or are not surgical candidates, custom-made shoes can be made to fit the deformed feet and provide comfort and support. A plaster mold is made to conform to each foot from which shoes can be made. Teach the patient to consult with a podiatrist or foot clinic to be evaluated for custom shoes.

The surgical procedure, a simple **bunionectomy,** involves removal of the bony overgrowth and bursa and realignment. When other toe deformities accompany the condition or if the bony overgrowth is large, several **osteotomies,** or bone resections, may be performed. Fusions may also be performed. Screws or wires are often inserted to stabilize the bones in the great toe and first metatarsal during the healing process. If both feet are affected, one foot is usually treated at a time. Surgery usually is performed as a same-day procedure.

Most patients are allowed partial weight bearing while wearing an orthopedic boot or shoe. Walking is difficult because the feet bear body weight. The healing time after surgery may be more than 6 to 12 weeks because the feet receive less blood flow than other parts of the body because of their distance from the heart.

Often patients have hammertoes and hallux valgus deformities at the same time. As shown in Fig. 50-4, a **hammertoe** is the dorsiflexion of any MTP joint with plantar flexion of the proximal interphalangeal (PIP) joint next to it. The second toe is most often affected. As the deformity worsens, uncomfortable corns may develop on the dorsal side of the toe and calluses may appear on the plantar surface. Patients are uncomfortable when wearing shoes and walking.

Hammertoe may be treated by surgical correction of the deformity with osteotomies (bone resections) and the insertion of wires or screws for fixation. The postoperative course is similar to that for the patient with hallux valgus repair. The patient uses crutches until full weight bearing is allowed several weeks after surgery.

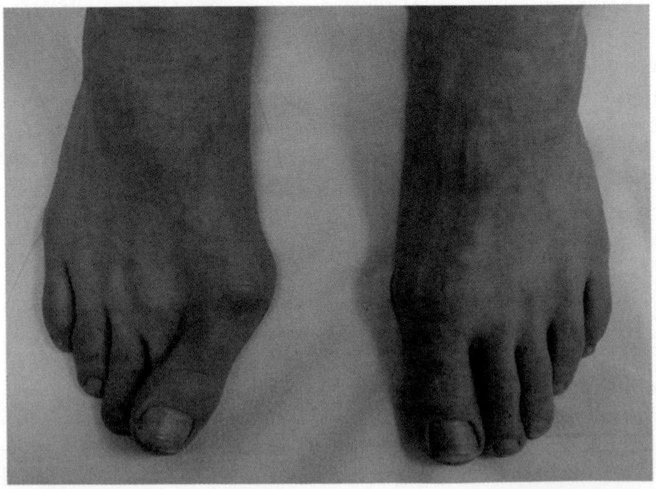

FIG. 50-3 Appearance of hallux valgus with a bunion.

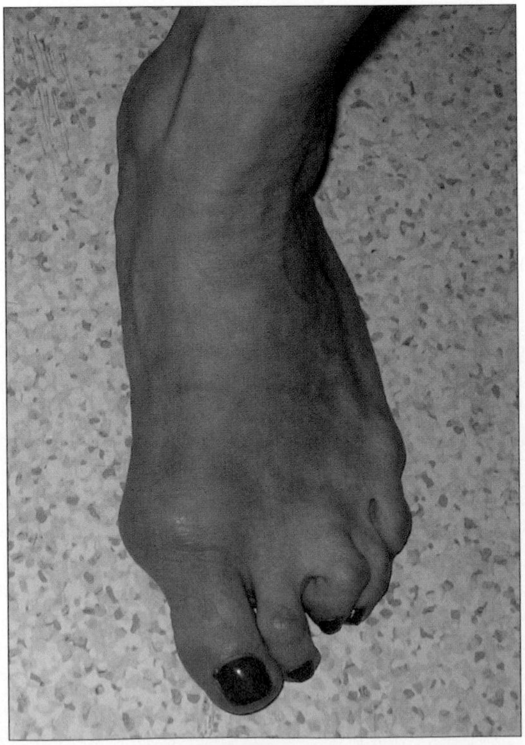

FIG. 50-4 Hammertoe of the second metatarsophalangeal joint.

Morton's Neuroma

In the patient with **Morton's neuroma**, or plantar digital neuritis, a small tumor grows in a digital nerve of the foot. The patient usually describes the PAIN as an acute, burning sensation in the web space. The pain involves the entire surface of the third and fourth toes. Management involves surgical removal of the neuroma and application of a pressure dressing. Ambulation is usually permitted immediately after surgery.

Plantar Fasciitis

Plantar fasciitis is an INFLAMMATION of the plantar fascia, which is located in the area of the arch of the foot. It is often seen in middle-aged and older adults, as well as in athletes, especially runners. Obesity is also a contributing factor. Patients report severe PAIN in the arch of the foot, especially when getting out of bed. The pain is worsened with weight bearing. Although most patients have unilateral plantar fasciitis, the problem can affect both feet (McCance et al., 2014).

Most patients respond to conservative management, which includes rest, ice, stretching exercises, strapping of the foot to maintain the arch, shoes with good support, and orthotics. NSAIDs or steroids may be needed to control PAIN and INFLAMMATION. If conservative measures are unsuccessful, endoscopic surgery to remove the inflamed tissue may be required. Teach the patient about the importance of adhering to the treatment plan and coordinating care with the physical therapist for instruction in exercise.

Other Problems of the Foot

Table 50-4 lists other common foot problems and how they are managed. Although patients are usually not hospitalized for these conditions, the nurse may recognize a foot disorder and alert the physician. Even small deformities or other foot deformities can be very annoying and painful for the patient and may hinder ambulation, as well as interfere with ADLs.

TABLE 50-4 Treatment of Common Foot Problems

DESCRIPTION/CAUSE	TREATMENT
Corn	
Induration and thickening of the skin caused by friction and pressure; painful conical mass	Surgical removal by podiatrist
Callus	
Flat, poorly defined mass on the sole over a bony prominence caused by pressure	Padding and lanolin creams; overall good skin hygiene
Ingrown Nail	
Nail sliver penetration of the skin, causing inflammation	Removal of sliver by podiatrist; warm soaks; antibiotic ointment
Hypertrophic Ungual Labium	
Chronic hypertrophy of nail lip caused by improper nail trimming; results from untreated ingrown nail	Surgical removal of necrotic nail and skin; treatment of secondary infection

SCOLIOSIS

❖ PATHOPHYSIOLOGY

Scoliosis occurs when the vertebrae rotate and begin to compress. The spinal column begins to move into a lateral curve, most commonly in the right lateral thoracic area (see Fig. 49-3 in Chapter 49). As the degree of curvature increases, damage to the vertebral bodies results. The degree of the curvature increases during periods of growth, such as in adolescence. Curvature of greater than 50 degrees results in an unstable spine, and curvature of greater than 60 degrees in the thoracic spine results in compromise of cardiopulmonary function.

The exact cause of scoliosis is not well understood, yet it affects about 6 million people in the United States. The process may result from some problem in the balance mechanism located in the central nervous system. Females are affected more often than males, and onset is often in adolescence (Voda, 2009a). School health nurses screen children for scoliosis during the middle school years. Information about caring for children with scoliosis is found in most pediatric nursing textbooks. Scoliosis that occurs in childhood or early adolescence may persist into adulthood. Adults often develop scoliosis as a result of spinal degeneration.

Three types of scoliosis can be described: congenital, neuromuscular, and idiopathic; the most common curve pattern in adults is idiopathic scoliosis and the cause is unknown (Voda, 2009a). Congenital scoliosis occurs during embryonic development. Neuromuscular scoliosis can result from a neuromuscular condition in childhood or adulthood, such as cerebral palsy or spinal cord tumors. Untreated scoliosis can lead to back pain, deformity, and cardiopulmonary complications.

❖ PATIENT-CENTERED COLLABORATIVE CARE

◆ Assessment

A complete history of the patient with spinal deformity should include onset of problem, in adolescence or adulthood, and what treatments may have been used in the past. Patients who had surgery for scoliosis during adolescence are returning with progressive, debilitating back pain from degenerative disk disease below the level of vertebral fusion. A loss of lumbar curvature, or **lordosis**, described as "flat back" syndrome, may also be present (Voda, 2009a). Complete a thorough pain assessment for patients reporting back pain.

Observe the patient from the front and back, while standing and during forward flexion from the hips. Physical examination usually reveals asymmetry of hip and shoulder height, prominence of the thoracic ribs and scapula on one side, and visible curve in the spinal column. Observation from the side may reveal kyphosis of the thoracic spine. Assess for leg length differences as well.

Methods of managing adult scoliosis differ from those used for children. The adult spinal column is less flexible and therefore less likely to respond to exercises, weight reduction, bracing, and casting for correction of the deformity. In the adult, the disorder is progressive and can result in an additional one degree of deviation each year.

◆ Interventions

Adults with less than 50 degrees of curvature of the spine may be treated conservatively with moist heat, pain medication, and exercise. Those with greater than 50 degrees of curvature may require surgical intervention to prevent shortness of breath and fatigue, osteoarthritis, and severe back pain (Voda, 2009a).

The traditional open *surgical* reconstructive procedure consists of surgical fusion and insertion of instrumentation, including plates, screws, or rods to stabilize the spine. The surgeon performs spinal fusion by packing cancellous bone chips, usually from the iliac crest, between the affected vertebrae for support and stabilization. Both an anterior and a posterior approach may be needed. If so, the surgeon may perform both procedures during the same operative day or may stage them 7 to 10 days apart. The metal instrumentation supports the spine and immobilizes the fused area during healing.

! NURSING SAFETY PRIORITY QSEN

Action Alert

The priority for nursing care after open spinal reconstructive surgery for scoliosis is to assess the patient's respiratory status and encourage deep breathing. Teach the patient how to use the incentive spirometer to prevent atelectasis.

Either an anterior or posterior surgical thoracic or abdominal approach may be used. For anterior thoracic surgery, a chest tube is in place for about 72 hours; for anterior abdominal surgery, the patient has a nasogastric tube for 24 hours. Chapter 16 discusses general postoperative care for patients who have general anesthesia. Other nursing care is similar to that for the patient undergoing a laminectomy or spinal fusion, including teaching the patient how to log roll, keeping the body in alignment. The traditional surgery for treating scoliosis has a high percentage of complications and results in major scarring.

Several newer minimally invasive surgical (MIS) procedures are being performed at major neurosurgery centers to treat degenerative and idiopathic adult scoliosis. These surgeries are done in stages, usually several days apart, using special endoscopic instrumentation that does not require large incisions. The advantages of these procedures include shorter hospital stays, far fewer complications, less pain, and very small incisions (Voda, 2009a).

Teach patients and their families about home care, including how to care for the wound; body mechanics to prevent bending, twisting, and lifting; and how to adapt to achieve ADLs independently. Some patients may require home care nursing, physical therapy, or a home health aide for a short time after discharge if a traditional surgical approach was used (Voda, 2009a). Collaborate with the case manager to make the appropriate arrangements for continuity of care to meet the patient's needs.

For some patients, a return to work in about 3 to 6 weeks is realistic. Other surgical procedures may prevent the patient from performing these activities until 3 to 6 months postoperatively. Refer patients and their families to the National Scoliosis Foundation (www.scoliosis.org) for information and support services.

PROGRESSIVE MUSCULAR DYSTROPHIES

Many types of **muscular dystrophy (MD)** have been categorized as slowly progressive or rapidly progressive. The slowly progressive types are most commonly seen in adults. Most pediatric nursing books describe the care for patients with MD in detail. Four forms of MD are often seen in adults. Each type has its own distinct characteristics and causes, but all are progressive (Table 50-5).

The exact pathophysiologic mechanisms are unknown, but several causes are possible. These include:

- Poor blood flow to muscle resulting in reduced tissue oxygenation
- Disturbance in nerve-muscle interaction
- Loss of cell membrane integrity as a result of increased enzyme activity

Regardless of the type of MD, the primary problem is progressive muscle weakness. The major cause of death is respiratory failure caused by profound respiratory muscle weakness. Cardiac failure also occurs because dystrophin activity is needed for cardiac muscle contraction and maintenance (McCance et al., 2014).

Diagnosis of MD is often difficult because the clinical manifestations are similar to those of other muscular disorders. Muscle biopsy often confirms the diagnosis. Muscle weakness

TABLE 50-5 Differential Features of Common Muscular Dystrophies Seen in Adults

ONSET	GENETIC LINK	CLINICAL MANIFESTATIONS	PROGRESSION
Becker (Benign X-Linked) Dystrophy			
5-25 yr	Sex-linked recessive; expression in males	Wasting of pelvic and shoulder muscles; normal cardiac and mental function	Gradual progression; inability to walk 25 yr after onset; usually normal life span
Limb-Girdle Dystrophy			
Usually 20s or 30s	Usually autosomal dominant; expression in either gender	Upper extremity and neck muscles and lower extremity and hip muscle weakness	Extremely variable; severe disability within 10-20 yr after onset; life span shortened by 10-20 yr
Facioscapulohumeral (Landouzy-Dejerine) Dystrophy			
Usually in 20s	Autosomal dominant; expression in either gender	Facial and shoulder girdle muscle involvement	Usually benign; normal life span
Myotonic (Steinert) Dystrophy			
Birth to 40s	Autosomal dominant; expression in either gender	Muscle atrophy with multiple organ involvement (e.g., heart, lungs, smooth muscle, and endocrine system)	Usually gradual if onset in adulthood

GENETIC/GENOMIC CONSIDERATIONS

Patient-Centered Care QSEN

The major pathologic change that occurs in most types of MD is the production or faulty action of a muscle protein called **dystrophin**. The purpose of this protein is to maintain muscle integrity by sending signals to coordinate smooth, synchronous muscle fiber contraction. The coding of this protein is by a large gene that has many parts located on the X chromosome. Different mutations of the gene where dystrophin is located determine the degree of muscle weakness. Because this protein connects with other substances for final muscle action, genetic mutations of these other substances can make dystrophin fail to work properly.

The most common forms of MD are Duchenne MD (DMD) and Becker MD (BMD). Both are X-linked recessive disorders. Women who are *carriers* (able to pass on the gene without having the disorder) have a 50% chance of passing the MD gene to their daughters, who are then carriers, and to their sons, who then have the disease. These types of MD, then, affect only males. In DMD, most patients die very young and therefore do not have children. In BMD, the patient lives longer and may have children. None of these men's sons will have the disease, but their daughters will be carriers (Nussbaum et al., 2007). Refer carriers for genetic testing and counseling.

and trophic changes are characteristic of all types of MD. Serum muscle enzyme values, such as aldolase and creatine kinase, may be elevated, and electromyographic (EMG) findings are often abnormal (Pagana & Pagana, 2014).

Collaborative care of the patient with MD is supportive and involves the entire health care team. Physical and occupational therapy help the patient maintain as much function, MOBILITY, and independence as possible. A neurologist is often the specialist who diagnoses and treats patients with MD. Refer the patient and family to the local chapter of the Muscular Dystrophy Association (www.mda.org) for support services and information.

Major organ or body system involvement is medically managed, but the life span is often shortened from these manifestations of the disease. With the exception of steroids, no drug has been found to slow the progression of the disorder, although immunosuppressive agents, anabolic steroids, and growth factors have been tried.

Nursing interventions focus on making the patient as comfortable as possible, providing supportive care, and reinforcing techniques and exercises taught in the physical therapy program. The nurse's role in caring for a patient with cardiac or other organ involvement is the same as for any patient with dysfunction of these systems.

NURSING CONCEPTS AND CLINICAL JUDGMENT REVIEW

What might you NOTICE if the patient has impaired MOBILITY as a result of chronic musculoskeletal disorders?

- Spinal deformity (e.g., kyphosis, lateral deviation)
- Bone malalignment (e.g., leg bowing)
- Muscle weakness
- Bone swelling or deformity
- Fracture
- Joint inflammation
- Flushed skin (Paget's disease)
- Fever (bone infection)
- Report of pain
- Report of weight loss

What should you INTERPRET and how should you RESPOND to a patient with impaired MOBILITY as a result of chronic musculoskeletal disorders?

Perform and interpret focused physical assessment findings, including:

- Ability to ambulate (with or without assistive device)
- ADLs ability
- Body weight
- Pain intensity and quality
- Neurovascular assessment findings
- Ability to cope with decreased mobility

Respond by:

- Providing pain control interventions, including drugs and nonpharmacologic measures
- Collaborating with members of the health care team, including physical therapist (PT), occupational therapist (OT), dietitian, as needed
- Teaching about drugs that may be needed for long-term use, including side and toxic effects
- Explaining about the need for adequate calcium and vitamin D for healthy bones and bone healing
- Assisting with ADLs and ambulation as needed, but encouraging independence when possible
- Implementing measures to prevent patient falls in the inpatient and home setting
- Encouraging the patient to discuss feelings related to disorders causing impaired mobility
- Referring patients to appropriate community resources, such as the National Osteoporosis Foundation and Paget Disease Foundation

On what should you REFLECT?

- Monitor the patient's response to pain control interventions.
- Prevent and monitor the patient for falls.
- Evaluate the patient's knowledge of nutrition and drug therapy.
- Evaluate the patient's coping ability related to disease diagnosis and treatment.
- Think about what else you might do to promote mobility.
- Decide whether you need to provide alternative interventions or additional health teaching.

GET READY FOR THE NCLEX® EXAMINATION!

KEY POINTS

Review these Key Points for each NCLEX Examination Client Needs Category.

Safe and Effective Care Environment

- Coordinate with health care team members when assessing patients with osteoporosis for risk for falls. **Safety** QSEN
- In coordination with the physical and occupational therapists, educate the patient and family on home safety when the patient has a metabolic bone disease, such as osteoporosis. **Teamwork and Collaboration** QSEN
- Refer to The Joint Commission for information about National Patient Safety Goals related to fall injury prevention.

Health Promotion and Maintenance

- Teach patients at risk for osteoporosis to minimize risk factors, such as stopping smoking, decreasing alcohol intake, exercising regularly, and increasing dietary calcium.
- Remind patients at risk for osteoporosis to have regular screening tests, such as the DXA scan.
- Instruct older adults to have at least 5 minutes of sun per day and to eat vitamin D–fortified foods to prevent osteomalacia.
- Assess the genetic risk for patients who have parents with muscular dystrophy, and refer them for genetic testing and counseling if the patient desires. **Patient-Centered Care** QSEN
- Refer patients with musculoskeletal problems to appropriate community resources, such as the Paget Disease Foundation and the National Osteoporosis Foundation.

Psychosocial Integrity

- Assess the patient's and family's responses to a diagnosis of bone cancer and treatment options. Be aware that they will progress through the grieving process.

Physiological Integrity

- Remind patients taking bisphosphonates (BPs) to take them early in the morning, at least 30 to 60 minutes before breakfast, with a full glass of water and to remain sitting upright during that time to prevent esophagitis, a common complication of BP therapy.
- Most patients are unaware that they have osteoporosis until they experience a fracture, the most common complication of the disease.
- Osteomalacia, the result of a deficiency in vitamin D, can be caused by the factors listed in Table 50-3.
- Priority care for patients with osteomyelitis is to treat the INFECTION and maintain Contact Precautions for open wounds. For patients having surgical intervention, assess the affected extremity for neurovascular status to ensure adequate tissue perfusion.
- For patients who have surgery for bone cancer, report postoperative manifestations of infection, dislocation, or neurovascular compromise to the surgeon promptly.
- Assess for key features of Paget's disease as summarized in Chart 50-3.
- Remember that bone tumors can be benign or malignant.
- Remember that severe chronic PAIN is a priority for patients with metastatic bone disease.
- Be aware that even minor hand and foot problems can be very painful. Common foot problems are described in Table 50-4.
- In collaboration with the health care team (physical therapist, occupational therapist, neurologist), provide supportive care for patients with muscular dystrophy and bone cancer.
- Recognize that most major types of muscular dystrophy are genetic and manifest usually in childhood. Care is supportive.
- Foot disorders can be treated with custom-made shoes or surgery to repair deformities. Recall that foot disorders are painful, and a plan for pain management is essential.

CHAPTER 51

Care of Patients with Musculoskeletal Trauma

Donna D. Ignatavicius

http://evolve.elsevier.com/Iggy/

PRIORITY CONCEPTS

- MOBILITY
- SENSORY PERCEPTION
- PAIN
- PERFUSION
- INFECTION

LEARNING OUTCOMES

Safe and Effective Care Environment

1. Explain the importance of collaborating with the health care team when providing care for patients with fractures and amputations.

Health Promotion and Maintenance

2. Identify community resources about amputations for patients and their families.
3. Teach the public about ways to prevent fractures and other musculoskeletal injuries.
4. Plan discharge teaching for patients with fractures and amputations.

Psychosocial Integrity

5. Describe how to assess the patient's and family's reaction to changes in body image and SENSORY PERCEPTION resulting from amputation.

Physiological Integrity

6. Compare and contrast open versus closed fractures and their potential complications.
7. Assess patients with musculoskeletal trauma to prioritize interventions for their care.
8. Delineate nursing care needed to maintain casts for patients with fractures.
9. Plan nursing care needed to maintain traction and external fixation for patients with fractures.
10. Implement measures to prevent complications of fractures, including INFECTION and decreased PERFUSION.
11. Develop an evidence-based postoperative plan of care, including health teaching, for a patient after fracture repair.
12. Describe emergency care for people who have a traumatic amputation.
13. Plan postoperative care, including health teaching, after an elective amputation.
14. Describe the patient-centered care needed to manage complex regional PAIN syndrome.
15. Plan care for patients with common types of soft tissue injuries, such as carpal tunnel syndrome.

Musculoskeletal trauma accounts for about two thirds of all injuries and is one of the primary causes of disability in the United States. It ranges from simple muscle strain to multiple bone fractures with severe soft-tissue damage.

Fractures and other musculoskeletal trauma impair a patient's MOBILITY in varying degrees, depending on the severity and extent of the injury. These injuries also affect SENSORY PERCEPTION and PAIN because of pressure on nerve endings from edema. In some cases, peripheral nerves are directly damaged as a result of musculoskeletal injury.

FRACTURES

❖ PATHOPHYSIOLOGY

A **fracture** is a break or disruption in the continuity of a bone that often affects MOBILITY and SENSORY PERCEPTION. It can occur anywhere in the body and at any age. All fractures have the same basic pathophysiologic mechanism and require similar patient-centered collaborative care, regardless of fracture type or location.

Classification of Fractures

A fracture is classified by the extent of the break:

- *Complete fracture.* The break is across the entire width of the bone in such a way that the bone is divided into two distinct sections.
- *Incomplete fracture.* The fracture does not divide the bone into two portions because the break is through only part of the bone.

A fracture is described by the extent of associated soft-tissue damage as **open** (or **compound**) or **closed** (or **simple**). The skin surface over the broken bone is disrupted in a *compound*

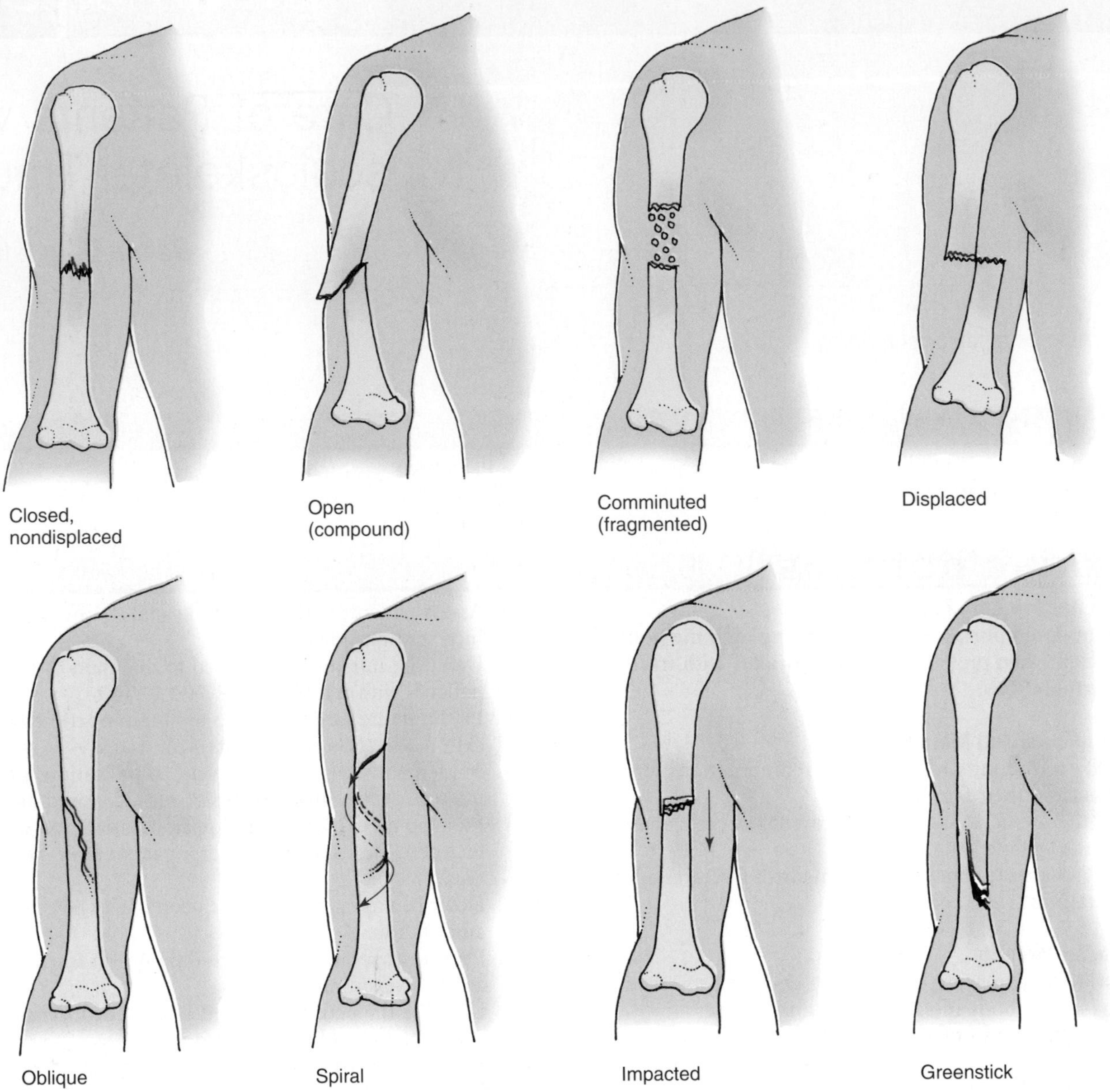

FIG. 51-1 Common types of fractures.

fracture, which causes an external wound. These fractures are often graded to define the extent of tissue damage. A *simple* fracture does not extend through the skin and therefore has no visible wound.

Fig. 51-1 shows common types of fractures. In addition to being identified by type, fractures are described by their cause. A **pathologic (spontaneous) fracture** occurs after minimal trauma to a bone that has been weakened by disease. For example, a patient with bone cancer or osteoporosis can easily have a pathologic fracture. A **fatigue (stress) fracture** results from excessive strain and stress on the bone. This problem is commonly seen in recreational and professional athletes. **Compression fractures** are produced by a loading force applied to the long axis of cancellous bone. They commonly occur in the vertebrae of older patients with osteoporosis and are extremely painful.

Stages of Bone Healing

When a bone is fractured, the body immediately begins the healing process to repair the injury and restore the body's equilibrium. Fractures heal in five stages that are a continuous process and not single stages.

- In stage one, within 24 to 72 hours after the injury, a hematoma forms at the site of the fracture because bone is extremely vascular.
- Stage two occurs in 3 days to 2 weeks when granulation tissue begins to invade the hematoma. This then prompts the formation of fibrocartilage, providing the foundation for bone healing.
- Stage three of bone healing occurs as a result of vascular and cellular proliferation. The fracture site is surrounded by new vascular tissue known as a *callus* (within 3 to 6

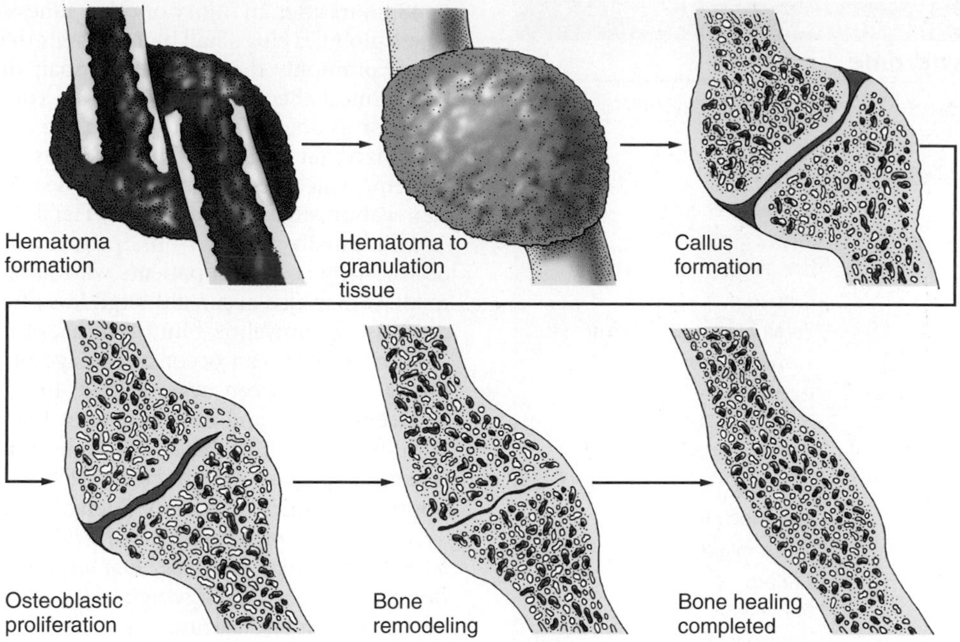

FIG. 51-2 The stages of bone healing.

weeks). **Callus** formation is the beginning of a nonbony union.

- As healing continues in stage four, the callus is gradually resorbed and transformed into bone. This stage usually takes 3 to 8 weeks.
- During the fifth and final stage of healing, consolidation and remodeling of bone continue to meet mechanical demands. This process may start as early as 4 to 6 weeks after fracture and can continue for up to 1 year, depending on the severity of the injury and the age and health of the patient. Fig. 51-2 summarizes the stages of bone healing.

In young, healthy adult bone, healing takes about 4 to 6 weeks. In the older person who has reduced bone mass, healing time is lengthened. Complete healing often takes 3 months or longer in people who are older than 70 years. Other factors also affect healing. Examples include the severity of the trauma, the type of bone injured, how the fracture is managed, infections at the fracture site, and ischemic or avascular necrosis (AVN), also called **osteonecrosis**.

CONSIDERATIONS FOR OLDER ADULTS

Patient-Centered Care QSEN

Bone healing is often affected by the aging process. Bone formation and strength rely on adequate nutrition. Calcium, phosphorus, vitamin D, and protein are necessary for the production of new bone (see Chapter 50). For women, the loss of estrogen after menopause decreases the body's ability to form new bone tissue. Chronic diseases can also affect the rate at which bone heals. For instance, peripheral vascular diseases, such as arteriosclerosis, reduce arterial circulation to bone. Thus the bone receives less oxygen and fewer nutrients, both of which are needed for repair.

Complications of Fractures

Regardless of the type or location of the fracture, several limb- and life-threatening acute and chronic complications can result from the injury. Clinical manifestations of beginning complications must be treated early to prevent serious consequences. In some cases, careful monitoring and assessment can prevent these complications:

- Acute compartment syndrome
- Crush syndrome
- Hypovolemic shock
- Fat embolism syndrome
- Venous thromboembolism
- Infection
- Chronic complications, such as ischemic necrosis and delayed union

Acute Compartment Syndrome. Compartments are areas in the body in which muscles, blood vessels, and nerves are contained within fascia. Most compartments are located in the extremities. **Fascia** is an inelastic tissue that surrounds groups of muscles, blood vessels, and nerves in the body. **Acute compartment syndrome (ACS)** is a serious condition in which increased pressure within one or more compartments reduces circulation to the area. The most common sites for this problem in patients with musculoskeletal trauma are the compartments in the lower leg (tibial fractures) and forearm (Hershey, 2013).

The pathophysiologic changes of increased compartment pressure are sometimes referred to as the *ischemia-edema cycle.* Capillaries within the muscle dilate, which raises capillary (arterial) pressure and venous pressure (Hershey, 2013). Capillaries become more permeable because of the release of histamine by the ischemic muscle tissue, and venous drainage decreases (Friedrich & Shin, 2012). As a result, plasma proteins leak into the interstitial fluid space and edema occurs. Edema increases pressure on nerve endings and causes pain. PERFUSION to the area is reduced, and further ischemia results. SENSORY PERCEPTION deficits or paresthesia generally appears before changes in vascular or motor signs. The color of the tissue pales, and pulses begin to weaken but rarely disappear. The affected area is usually palpably tense, and PAIN occurs with passive motion of the extremity. If the condition is not treated, cyanosis, tingling,

CHART 51-1 Key Features

Compartment Syndrome

PHYSIOLOGIC CHANGE	CLINICAL FINDINGS
Increased compartment pressure	No change
Increased capillary permeability	Edema
Release of histamine	Increased edema
Increased blood flow to area	Pulses present Pink tissue
Pressure on nerve endings	Pain
Increased tissue pressure	Referred pain to compartment
Decreased tissue perfusion	Increased edema
Decreased oxygen to tissues	Pallor
Increased production of lactic acid	Unequal pulses Flexed posture
Anaerobic metabolism	Cyanosis
Vasodilation	Increased edema
Increased blood flow	Tense muscle swelling
Increased tissue pressure	Tingling Numbness
Increased edema	Paresthesia
Muscle ischemia	Severe pain unrelieved by drugs
Tissue necrosis	Paresis/paralysis

numbness, paresis, necrosis, and severe pain can occur. Chart 51-1 summarizes the sequence of pathophysiologic events in compartment syndrome and the associated clinical assessment findings.

The pressure to the compartment can be from an external or internal source, but fracture is present in 75% of all cases of ACS (Hershey, 2013). Tight, bulky dressings and casts are examples of *external* pressure. Blood or fluid accumulation in the compartment is a common source of *internal* pressure. The injury or trauma causing the problem is above the compartment involved, which decreases blood flow to the more distal area of injury. ACS is not limited to patients with musculoskeletal problems. It can also occur in those with severe burns, extensive insect bites or snakebites, or massive infiltration of IV fluids. In these situations, edema increases internal pressure in one or more compartments.

Problems resulting from compartment syndrome include infection, persistent motor weakness in the affected extremity, contracture, and myoglobinuric renal failure. In extreme cases, amputation becomes necessary (Hershey, 2013).

Infection from necrosis may become severe enough that amputation of the limb is needed. *Motor weakness* from injured nerves is not reversible, and the patient may require an orthotic device for assistance in mobility. Volkmann's *contractures* of the forearm, which can begin within 12 hours of the pressure increase, result from shortening of the ischemic muscle and from nerve involvement.

Hypovolemic Shock. Bone is very vascular. Therefore bleeding is a risk with bone injury. In addition, trauma can cut nearby arteries and cause hemorrhage, resulting in rapidly developing hypovolemic shock. (The pathophysiology of hypovolemic shock is described in Chapter 37.)

Fat Embolism Syndrome. Fat embolism syndrome (FES) is another serious complication in which fat globules are released from the yellow bone marrow into the bloodstream within 12 to 48 hours after an injury or other illness (mechanical theory). These globules clog small blood vessels that supply vital organs, most commonly the lungs, and impair organ PERFUSION. The biochemical theory for FES may be considered as a separate cause or as an additive process to the mechanical theory. The embolized fat degrades into free fatty acids and C-reactive protein, which results in capillary leakage, lipid and platelet aggregation, and clot formation (Hershey, 2013).

FES usually results from fractures or fracture repair but occasionally is seen in patients who have a total joint replacement. It may also occur, although less often, in those with pancreatitis, osteomyelitis, blunt trauma, or sickle cell disease.

The problem can occur at any age or in either gender, but young men between ages 20 and 40 years and older adults between ages 70 and 80 years are at the greatest risk. Patients with fractured hips have the highest risk, but FES is also common in those with fractures of the pelvis within 24 to 72 hours after injury or surgery (Hershey, 2013).

The earliest manifestations of FES are a low arterial oxygen level (hypoxemia), dyspnea, and tachypnea (increased respirations). Headache, lethargy, agitation, confusion, decreased level of consciousness, seizures, and vision changes may follow (Hershey, 2013). Nonpalpable, red-brown **petechiae**—a macular, measles-like rash—may appear over the neck, upper arms, and/or chest. This rash is a classic manifestation but is usually the last sign to develop (Hershey, 2013).

Abnormal laboratory findings include:

- Decreased Pa_{O_2} level (often below 60 mm Hg)
- Increased erythrocyte sedimentation rate (ESR)
- Decreased serum calcium levels
- Decreased red blood cell and platelet counts
- Increased serum level of lipids

These changes in blood values are poorly understood, but they aid in diagnosis of the condition.

The chest x-ray often shows bilateral infiltrates but may be normal. The chest CT often reveals a patchy distribution of opacities. An MRI of the brain can show evidence of neurologic deficits from hypoxemia. FES can result in respiratory failure or death, often from pulmonary edema. When the lungs are affected, the complication may be misdiagnosed as a pulmonary embolism from a blood clot (Chart 51-2).

Venous Thromboembolism. Venous thromboembolism (VTE) includes deep vein thrombosis (DVT) and its major complication, pulmonary embolism (PE). It is the most common complication of lower extremity surgery or trauma and the most often fatal complication of musculoskeletal surgery. Factors that make patients with fractures most likely to develop VTE include:

- Cancer or chemotherapy
- Surgical procedure longer than 30 minutes
- History of smoking
- Obesity
- Heart disease
- Prolonged immobility
- Oral contraceptives or hormones
- History of VTE complications
- Older adults (especially with hip fractures)

The pathophysiology and management of VTE are described in Chapter 36.

Infection. Whenever there is trauma to tissues, the body's defense system is disrupted. Wound infections are the most common type of INFECTION resulting from orthopedic trauma.

CHART 51-2 Key Features

Pulmonary Emboli: Fat Embolism Versus Blood Clot Embolism

FAT EMBOLISM	BLOOD CLOT EMBOLISM
Definition	
Obstruction of the pulmonary vascular bed by fat globules	Obstruction of the pulmonary artery by a blood clot or clots
Origin	
95% from fractures of the long bones; occurs usually within 48 hr of injury	85% from deep vein thrombosis in the legs or pelvis; can occur anytime
Assessment Findings	
Altered mental status (earliest sign) Increased respirations, pulse, temperature Chest pain Dyspnea Crackles Decreased SaO_2 Petechiae (50%-60%) Retinal hemorrhage (not common) Mild thrombocytopenia	Same as for fat embolism, except no petechiae
Treatment	
Bedrest Gentle handling Oxygen Hydration (IV fluids) Possibly steroid therapy Fracture immobilization	Preventive measures (e.g., leg exercises, antiembolism stockings, SCDs) Bedrest Oxygen Possibly mechanical ventilation Anticoagulants Thrombolytics Possible surgery: pulmonary embolectomy, vena cava umbrella

SaO_2, Arterial oxygen saturation; *SCD*, sequential compression device.

They range from superficial skin infections to deep wound abscesses. Infection can also be caused by implanted hardware used to repair a fracture surgically, such as pins, plates, or rods. Clostridial infections can result in gas gangrene or tetanus and can prevent the bone from healing properly.

Bone INFECTION, or **osteomyelitis**, is most common with open fractures in which skin integrity is lost and after surgical repair of a fracture (see Chapter 50 for discussion of osteomyelitis). For patients experiencing this type of trauma, the risk for hospital-acquired infections is increased. These infections are common, and many are from multidrug-resistant organisms, such as methicillin-resistant *Staphylococcus aureus* (MRSA). Reducing MRSA infections is a primary desired outcome for all health care agencies.

Chronic Complications. Avascular necrosis and delayed bone healing are later complications of musculoskeletal trauma. Blood supply to the bone is disrupted causing decreased PERFUSION and death of bone tissue. This problem is most often a complication of hip fractures or any fracture in which there is displacement of bone. Surgical repair of fractures also can cause necrosis because the hardware can interfere with circulation. Patients on long-term corticosteroid therapy, such as prednisone, are also at high risk for ischemic necrosis.

Delayed union is a fracture that has not healed within 6 months of injury. Some fractures never achieve union; that is, they never completely heal *(nonunion)*. Others heal incorrectly *(malunion)*. These problems are most common in patients with tibial fractures, fractures that involve many treatment techniques (e.g., cast, traction), and pathologic fractures. Union may also be delayed or not achieved in the older patient. If bone does not heal, he or she typically has chronic pain and immobility from deformity.

Etiology and Genetic Risk

The primary cause of a fracture is trauma from a motor vehicle crash or fall, especially in older adults. The trauma may be a direct blow to the bone or an indirect force from muscle contractions or pulling forces on the bone. Sports, vigorous exercise, and malnutrition are contributing factors. Bone diseases, such as osteoporosis, increase the risk for a fracture in older adults (see Chapter 50). Genetic factors that increase risk for fracture are discussed with these specific health problems throughout this text.

Incidence and Prevalence

The incidence of fractures depends on the location of the injury. Rib fractures are the most common type in the adult population. Femoral shaft fractures occur most often in young and middle-aged adults. The incidence of proximal femur (hip) fractures is highest in older adults. Humeral fractures are common in adults; the older the person, usually the more proximal is the fracture. Wrist (Colles') fractures are typically seen in middle and late adulthood and usually result from a fall. Middle-aged and older adults, especially women, have a higher incidence of osteoporosis, which increases the risk for fragility fractures.

Health Promotion and Maintenance

Airbags and seat belts have decreased the number of severe injuries and deaths, but they have increased the number of leg and ankle fractures, especially in older adults. Health teaching should also focus on other risks for musculoskeletal injury, including:

- Osteoporosis screening and self-management education
- Fall prevention
- Home safety assessment and modification, if needed
- Dangers of drinking and driving
- Drug safety (prescribed, over-the-counter, and illicit)
- Older adults and driving
- Helmet use when riding bicycles, motorcycles, all-terrain vehicles (ATVs), and skateboards

These educational interventions are discussed throughout this book and in other texts. Fall prevention is discussed in detail in Chapter 2 as part of care for older adults.

❖ *PATIENT-CENTERED COLLABORATIVE CARE*

◆ *Assessment*

History. If the patient is in severe PAIN, delay the interview until he or she is more comfortable. Then ask about the cause of the fracture, which helps in developing an individualized plan of care. Certain types of force (e.g., incisional, crush, acceleration or deceleration), shearing, and friction lead to most musculoskeletal injuries. As a result, several body systems are often affected.

Incisional injuries, as from a knife wound, and *crush* injuries cause hemorrhage and decrease blood flow to major organs. *Acceleration or deceleration* injuries cause direct trauma to the spleen, brain, and kidneys when these organs are moved from their fixed locations in the body. *Shearing and friction* damage the skin and cause a high level of wound contamination.

Asking about the events leading to the injury helps identify which forces have been experienced and therefore which body systems or parts of the body to assess. For example, a forward fall often results in Colles' fracture of the wrist because the person tries to catch himself or herself with an outstretched hand. Knowing the mechanism of injury also helps determine whether other types of injury, such as head and spinal cord injury, might be present.

A drug history, including substance use, is important regardless of the patient's age. For example, a young adult may have had an excessive amount of alcohol, which contributed to a motor vehicle crash or to a fall at the work site. Many older adults also consume alcohol and an assortment of prescribed and over-the-counter drugs, which can cause dizziness and loss of balance.

A medical history may identify possible causes of the fracture and gives clues as to how long it will take for the bone to heal. Certain diseases such as bone cancer and Paget's disease cause fragility fractures that often do not achieve total healing or union.

Ask about the patient's occupation and recreational activities. Some occupations are more hazardous than others. For instance, construction work is potentially more physically dangerous than office work. Certain hobbies and recreational activities are also extremely hazardous, such as skiing. Contact sports, such as football and ice hockey, often result in musculoskeletal injuries, including fractures. Other activities do not have such an obvious potential for injury but can cause fractures nonetheless. For instance, daily jogging or running can lead to fatigue fractures.

Physical Assessment/Clinical Manifestations. The patient with a fracture often has trauma to other body systems. Therefore assess all major body systems *first* for life-threatening complications, including head, chest, and abdominal trauma. Some fractures can cause internal organ damage resulting in hemorrhage. When a pelvic fracture is suspected, assess vital signs, skin color, and level of consciousness for indications of possible hypovolemic shock. Check the urine for blood, which indicates possible damage to the urinary system, often the bladder. If the patient cannot void, suspect that the bladder or urethra has been damaged. Complete assessment of these areas is described elsewhere in this text.

The most common manifestation of fractures is moderate to often severe PAIN. Patients with severe or multiple fractures of the arms, legs, or pelvis have severe pain. Vertebral compression factures are also extremely painful. Patients *with a fractured hip may have groin pain or pain referred to the back of the knee or lower back.* Pain is usually due to muscle spasm and edema, which result from the fracture.

For fractures of the shoulder and upper arm, the physical assessment is best done with the patient in a sitting or standing position, if possible, so that shoulder drooping or other abnormal positioning can be seen. Support the affected arm and flex the elbow to promote comfort during the assessment. For more distal areas of the arm, perform the assessment with the patient in a supine position so that the extremity can be elevated to reduce swelling.

! NURSING SAFETY PRIORITY QSEN

Action Alert

Patients with one or more fractured ribs have severe pain when they take deep breaths. Monitor respiratory status, which may be severely compromised from PAIN or pneumothorax (air in the pleural cavity). Assess the patient's pain level and manage pain *before* continuing the physical assessment.

Place the patient in a supine position for assessment of the legs and pelvis. A patient with an impacted hip fracture may be able to walk for a short time after injury, although this is not recommended.

When inspecting the site of a possible fracture, look for a change in bone alignment. The bone may appear deformed, a limb may be internally or externally rotated, and/or one or more bones may also be dislocated (out of their joint capsules). Observe for extremity shortening or a change in bone shape.

If the skin is intact (closed fracture), the area over the fracture may be **ecchymotic** (bruised) from bleeding into the underlying soft tissues. **Subcutaneous emphysema**, the appearance of bubbles under the skin because of air trapping, may be present but is usually seen later.

! NURSING SAFETY PRIORITY QSEN

Action Alert

Swelling at the fracture site is rapid and can result in marked neurovascular compromise due to decreased arterial PERFUSION. *Gently perform a thorough neurovascular assessment, and compare extremities.* Assess skin color and temperature, sensation, mobility, pain, and pulses distal to the fracture site. If the fracture involves an extremity and the patient is not in severe pain, check the nails for capillary refill by applying pressure to the nail and observing for the speed of blood return. If nails are brittle or thick, assess the skin next to the nail. Checking for capillary refill is not as reliable as other indicators of perfusion. Chart 51-3 describes the procedure for a neurovascular assessment, which evaluates **c**irculation, **m**ovement, and **s**ensation (SENSORY PERCEPTION) (CMS function).

? CLINICAL JUDGMENT CHALLENGE

***Patient-Centered Care; Evidence-Based Practice* QSEN**

A 63-year-old woman fell while standing on a step ladder to reach an item on the top shelf of her closet. After calling 911, she sat in a recliner chair while protecting her swollen right arm. When the paramedics arrived, the woman was drowsy but could be awakened. She had no other apparent injury or problem. Upon arrival at the emergency department (ED), you greet the patient and help her transfer into a room. The patient continues to become very drowsy at times but stated that she did not "hit her head" when she fell.

1. What are your priority evidence-based assessments for the patient when coming into the ED?
2. What history questions will you ask the patient once her pain is controlled?
3. The patient has a fractured right distal radius and reports that she is still in pain even though the emergency medical technician (EMT) gave her IV fentanyl. How will you respond to this patient, and what action will you take?
4. The patient's husband comes to the ED and asks you if his wife's history of bone loss may have caused the fracture. How will you answer him?

CHART 51-3 **Best Practice for Patient Safety & Quality Care** QSEN

Assessment of Neurovascular Status in Patients with Musculoskeletal Injury

ASSESSMENT METHOD	NORMAL FINDINGS
Skin Color	
Inspect the area distal to the injury.	No change in pigmentation compared with other parts of the body.
Skin Temperature	
Palpate the area distal to the injury (the dorsum of the hands is most sensitive to temperature).	The skin is warm.
Movement	
Ask the patient to move the affected area or the area distal to the injury (active motion).	The patient can move without discomfort.
Move the area distal to the injury (passive motion).	No difference in comfort compared with active movement.
Sensation	
Ask the patient if numbness or tingling is present (paresthesia).	No numbness or tingling.
Palpate with a paper clip (especially the web space between the first and second toes or the web space between the thumb and forefinger).	No difference in sensation in the affected and unaffected extremities. (Loss of sensation in these areas indicates peroneal nerve or median nerve damage.)
Pulses	
Palpate the pulses distal to the injury.	Pulses are strong and easily palpated; no difference in the affected and unaffected extremities.
Capillary Refill (Least Reliable)	
Press the nail beds distal to the injury until blanching occurs (or the skin near the nail if nails are thick and brittle).	Blood returns (return to usual color) within 3 sec (5 sec for older patients).
Pain	
Ask the patient about the location, nature, and frequency of the pain.	Pain is usually localized and is often described as stabbing or throbbing. (Pain out of proportion to the injury and unrelieved by analgesics might indicate compartment syndrome.)

Psychosocial Assessment. The psychosocial status of a patient with a fracture depends on the extent of the injury, possible complications, coping ability, and the availability of support systems. Hospitalization is not required for a single, uncomplicated fracture, and the patient returns to usual daily activities within a few days. Examples include a single fracture of a bone in the finger, wrist, foot, or toe.

In contrast, a patient suffering severe or multiple traumas may be hospitalized for weeks and may undergo many surgical procedures, treatments, and prolonged rehabilitation. These disruptions in lifestyle can create a high level of stress.

The stresses that result from a long-term condition affect relationships between the patient and family members or friends. Assess the patient's feelings, and ask how he or she coped with previously experienced stressful events. Body image and sexuality may be altered by deformity, treatment modalities for fracture repair, or long-term immobilization. Assess the availability of needed support systems, such as family, church, or community groups, who can help patients during the acute and rehabilitation phases when multiple or severe fractures occur. Active patients of any age or those who are older and live alone may become depressed during the healing process. Acute and chronic PAIN can decrease energy levels and may also cause sadness, depression, and/or anxiety.

Laboratory Assessment. No special laboratory tests are available for assessment of fractures. Hemoglobin and hematocrit levels may often be low because of bleeding caused by the injury. If extensive soft-tissue damage is present, the erythrocyte sedimentation rate (ESR) may be elevated, which indicates the expected inflammatory response. If this value and the white blood cell (WBC) count increase during fracture healing, the patient may have a bone INFECTION. During the healing stages, serum calcium and phosphorus levels are often increased as the bone releases these elements into the blood.

Imaging Assessment. The health care provider requests standard *x-rays* to confirm a diagnosis of fracture. These reveal the bone disruption, malalignment, or deformity. If the x-ray does not show a fracture but the patient is symptomatic, the x-ray is usually repeated with additional views.

The *CT* scan is useful in detecting fractures of complex structures, such as the hip and pelvis. It also identifies compression fractures of the spine. *MRI* is useful in determining the amount of soft-tissue damage that may have occurred with the fracture.

◆ *Analysis*

The priority NANDA-I nursing diagnoses and collaborative problems for patients with fractures include:

1. Acute Pain related to one or more fractures, soft-tissue damage, muscle spasm, and edema (NANDA-I)
2. Potential for neurovascular compromise related to tissue edema and/or bleeding
3. Risk for Infection related to a wound caused by an open fracture (NANDA-I)
4. Impaired Physical Mobility related to need for bone healing and/or pain (NANDA-I)

◆ *Planning and Implementation*

Managing Acute Pain

Planning: Expected Outcomes. The patient with a fracture is expected to state that he or she has adequate PAIN control after fracture reduction and immobilization.

CHART 51-4 **Best Practice for Patient Safety & Quality Care** (QSEN)

Emergency Care of the Patient with an Extremity Fracture

1. Assess the patient's airway, breathing, and circulation, and perform a quick head-to-toe assessment.
2. Remove the patient's clothing (cut if necessary) to inspect the affected area while supporting the area above and below the injury. Do not remove shoes because this can cause increased trauma.
3. Remove jewelry on the affected extremity in case of swelling.
4. Apply direct pressure on the area if there is bleeding and pressure over the proximal artery nearest the fracture.
5. Keep the patient warm and in a supine position.
6. Check the neurovascular status of the area distal to the fracture, including temperature, color, sensation, movement, and capillary refill. Compare affected and unaffected limbs.
7. Immobilize the extremity by splinting; include joints above and below the fracture site. Recheck circulation after splinting.
8. Cover any open areas with a dressing (preferably sterile).

Interventions. A fracture can happen anywhere and may be accompanied by multiple injuries to vital organs. Patient-centered collaborative care depends on the severity and extent of the injury and the number of fractures the patient has.

Emergency Care: Fracture. For any patient who experiences trauma in the community, first call 911 and assess for airway, breathing, and circulation (ABCs, or primary survey). Then provide lifesaving care if needed before being concerned about the fracture (Chart 51-4). If cardiopulmonary resuscitation (CPR) is needed, ensure circulation first, followed by airway and breathing (see Chapter 34).

If the person is clothed, cut away clothing from the fracture site, and remove any jewelry from the affected extremity. Control any bleeding by direct pressure on the area and digital pressure over the artery above the fracture. To prevent shock, place the patient in a supine position and keep him or her warm.

After a head-to-toe assessment (secondary survey) and patient stabilization by the prehospital team, pain is managed with IV opioids such as fentanyl, hydromorphone (Dilaudid), or morphine sulfate. Cardiac monitoring for patients who are older than 50 years is established before drug administration. To prevent further tissue damage, reduce pain, and increase circulation, the prehospital or emergency team immobilizes the fracture by splinting. An air splint or any object or device that extends to the joints above and below the fracture to immobilize it can be used as a **splint**. Sterile gauze is placed loosely over open areas to prevent further contamination of the wound.

In the emergency department (ED), physician's office, or urgent care center, fracture management begins with reduction and immobilization of the fracture while attending to continued pain assessment and management.

Bone reduction, or realignment of the bone ends for proper healing, is accomplished by a closed method or an open (surgical) procedure. In some cases, dislocated bones are also reduced, such as when the distal tibia and fibula are dislocated with a fractured ankle. Immobilization is achieved by the use of bandages, casts, traction, internal fixation, or external fixation.

The health care provider selects the treatment method based on the type, location, and extent of the fracture. These interventions prevent further injury and reduce pain.

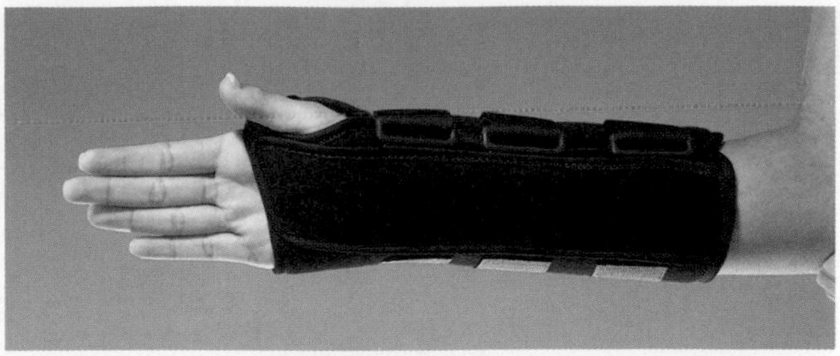

FIG. 51-3 A universal wrist and forearm splint used for immobilization.

Nonsurgical Management. Nonsurgical management includes closed reduction and immobilization with a bandage, splint, cast, or traction. For some small, closed incomplete bone fractures in the hand or foot, reduction is not required. Immobilization with an orthotic device or special orthopedic shoe or boot may be the only management during the healing process.

For each modality, the primary nursing concern is assessment and prevention of neurovascular dysfunction or compromise. Assess the patient's neurovascular status every hour for the first 24 hours and every 1 to 4 hours thereafter, depending on the injury (see Chart 51-3). The patient usually reports discomfort that is unrelieved by analgesics if the bandage, splint, or cast is too tight. Elevate the fractured extremity higher than the heart, and apply ice for the first 24 to 48 hours as needed to reduce edema.

Closed Reduction and Immobilization. Closed reduction is the most common nonsurgical method for managing a simple fracture. While applying a manual pull, or traction, on the bone, the health care provider moves the bone ends so that they realign. Moderate sedation and/or analgesia is used during this procedure to decrease PAIN. The nurse monitors the patient's oxygen saturation (and possibly end-tidal carbon dioxide [$EtCO_2$] level) to ensure adequate rate and depth of respirations during the procedure. An x-ray confirms that the bone ends are approximated (aligned) before the bone is immobilized, and a splint is usually applied to keep the bone in alignment.

Splints and Orthopedic Boots/Shoes. For certain areas of the body, such as the scapula (shoulder) and clavicle (collarbone), a commercial immobilizer may be used to keep the bone in place during healing. Because upper extremity bones do not bear weight, splints may be sufficient to keep bone fragments in place for a closed fracture. Fig. 51-3 shows a wrist splint for fracture immobilization. Thermoplastic, a durable, flexible material for splinting, allows custom fitting to the patient's body part. Splints for lower extremities are also custom-fitted using flexible materials and held in place with elastic bandages (e.g., ACE wrap). When possible, splints are preferred over casts to prevent the complications that can occur with casting. Splints also allow room for extremity swelling without causing decreased arterial PERFUSION.

For foot or toe fractures, orthopedic shoes may be used to support the injured area during healing. For ankles or the lower part of the leg, padded orthopedic boots supported by multiple Velcro straps to hold the boot in place may be used. These devices are especially useful when the patient is allowed to bear weight on the affected leg.

Casts. For more complex fractures or fractures of the lower extremity, the physician or orthopedic technician may apply a cast to hold bone fragments in place after reduction. A **cast** is a rigid device that immobilizes the affected body part while

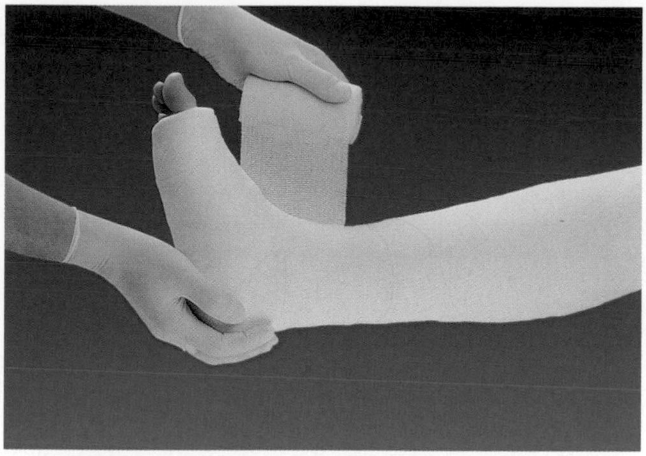

FIG. 51-4 Application of a fiberglass synthetic cast.

allowing other body parts to move. It also allows early mobility and reduces pain. Although its most common use is for fractures, a cast may be applied for correction of deformities (e.g., clubfoot) or for prevention of deformities (e.g., those seen in some patients with rheumatoid arthritis).

Fiberglass is the most common material used for casting and is typically the preferred method for immobilization with a cast (Fig. 51-4) (Satryb et al., 2011). Fiberglass can dry and become rigid within minutes and decreases the risk for skin breakdown. Waterproof casting is designed to get wet in the shower or pool and is used most commonly for athletes, especially during the summer (Satryb et al., 2011). Plaster is the traditional material used for casts but is not as commonly used today for management of most fractures. It requires application of a well-fitted stockinette under the material. If the stockinette is too tight, it may impair circulation. If it is too loose, wrinkles can lead to the development of pressure ulcers. Padding is applied over the stockinette, followed by wet plaster rolls wrapped around the extremity or other body part. The cast feels hot because an immediate chemical reaction occurs, but it soon becomes damp and cool. This type of cast takes at least 24 hours to dry, depending on the size and location of the cast. A wet cast feels cold, smells musty, and is grayish. The cast is dry when it feels hard and firm, is odorless, and has a shiny white appearance.

If the skin under the cast is open, the health care provider, orthopedic technician, or specially trained nurse cuts a window in the cast so that the wound can be observed and cared for. The piece of cast removed to make the window must be retained and replaced after wound care to prevent localized edema in the area. This is most important when a window is cut from a cast on an extremity. Tape or elastic bandage wrap may be used to keep the "window" in place. A window is also an access for taking pulses, removing wound drains, or preventing abdominal distention when the patient is in a body or spica cast.

If the cast is too tight, it may be cut with a cast cutter to relieve pressure or allow tissue swelling. The health care provider may choose to **bivalve** the cast (i.e., cut it lengthwise into two equal pieces) if bone healing is almost complete. Either half of the cast can be removed for inspection or for provision of care. The two halves are then held in place by an elastic bandage wrap (Satryb et al., 2011).

When a patient is in bed with an *arm cast,* teach him or her to elevate the arm above the heart to reduce swelling. The hand should be higher than the heart. Ice may be prescribed for the first 24 to 48 hours. When the patient is out of bed, the arm is supported with a sling placed around the neck to alleviate fatigue caused by the weight of the cast. The sling should distribute the weight over a large area of the shoulders and trunk, not just the neck. Some health care providers prefer that the patient not use a sling after the first few days in an arm cast, particularly a short-arm cast. This encourages normal movement of the mobile joints and enhances bone healing. For many wrist fractures, a splint is used to immobilize the area instead of a cast to accommodate for edema formation.

A *leg cast* allows MOBILITY and requires the patient to use ambulatory aids such as crutches. A cast shoe, sandal, or boot that attaches to the foot or a rubber walking pad attached to the sole of the cast assists in ambulation (if weight bearing is allowed) and helps prevent damage to the cast. Teach the patient to elevate the affected leg on several pillows to reduce swelling and to apply ice for the first 24 hours or as prescribed. Table 51-1 describes specific casts that are used for various parts of the body.

Before the cast is applied, explain its purpose and the procedure for its application. With a plaster cast, warn the patient about the heat that will be felt immediately after the wet cast is applied. Do not cover the new cast. Allow for air-drying.

! NURSING SAFETY PRIORITY QSEN

Action Alert

When moving a patient with a wet plaster cast, handle it with the palms of the hands to prevent indentations and resulting areas of pressure on the skin. Turn the patient every 1 to 2 hours to allow air to circulate and dry all parts of the cast. Be sure to remind unlicensed assistive personnel (UAP) and the family that the cast is wet and requires special handling. If the health care provider requests that the cast be elevated to reduce swelling, use a cloth-covered pillow instead of one encased in plastic, which could cause the cast to retain heat and prevent drying. Elevation of the casted extremity reduces edema but may impair arterial circulation to the affected limb. Therefore performing a neurovascular assessment of the limb distal to (below) the cast is very important.

! NURSING SAFETY PRIORITY QSEN

Action Alert

Check to ensure that any type of cast is not too tight, and frequently monitor neurovascular status—usually every hour for the first 24 hours after application if the patient is hospitalized. You should be able to insert a finger between the cast and the skin. Teach the patient to apply ice for the first 24 to 36 hours to reduce swelling and inflammation.

Once the plaster cast is dry, inspect it at least once every 8 hours for drainage, cracking, crumbling, alignment, and fit. Plaster casts act like sponges and absorb drainage, whereas synthetic casts act like a wick pulling drainage away from the drainage site. Padding can also absorb wound drainage. Document the presence of any drainage on the cast. However, the evidence is not clear on whether drainage should be circled on the cast because it may increase anxiety and is not a reliable indicator of drainage amount. *Immediately report to the health care provider any sudden increases in the amount of drainage or change in the integrity of the cast.* After swelling decreases, it is not uncommon for the cast to become too loose and need replacement. If the patient is not admitted to the hospital, provide instructions regarding cast care.

TABLE 51-1 Types of Casts Used for Musculoskeletal Trauma

TYPE AND CHARACTERISTICS OF CAST	USE
Upper Extremity Casts	
Short-arm cast (SAC) (extends from below the elbow to and including part of the hand)	Stable fractures of the wrist (metacarpals, carpals, or distal radius)
Long-arm cast (LAC) (includes the upper arm to and including part of the hand)	Unstable fractures of the wrist, distal humerus, radius, or ulna
Hanging-arm cast (same as LAC but heavier, with added loop at the mid-forearm)	Fractures of the humerus that cannot be aligned by LAC (light traction is possible while the patient is in bed or by an attached strap that extends around the neck)
Thumb spica (gauntlet) cast (similar to SAC with the thumb casted in abduction)	Fractures of the thumb
Shoulder spica cast (the shoulder is casted in abduction with the elbow flexed)	Unstable fractures of the shoulder girdle or humerus; dislocations of the shoulder
Lower Extremity Casts	
Short-leg cast (SLC) (from below the knee to the base of the toes)	Fractures of the ankle, metatarsals, or foot
Long-leg cast (LLC) (from the mid-upper thigh to the base of the toes)	Unstable fractures of the tibia, fibula, or ankle
Walking cast (a walking device on the bottom of SLC or LLC)	Same as for SLC or LLC
Leg cylinder (similar to SLC, but the ankle and foot are not casted)	Stable fractures of the tibia, fibula, or knee
Long-leg cylinder (similar to LLC, but the ankle and foot are not casted)	Stable fractures of the distal femur, proximal tibia, or knee
Cast Braces (or Brace Casts) (not as common)	
Patellar weight-bearing cast (similar to SLC or leg cylinder)	Mid-shaft or distal shaft fractures of the femur
External polycentric knee hinge cast (a hinge connects the lower and upper leg and allows 90 degrees of knee flexion)	Same as for the patellar weight-bearing cast

During hospitalization, assess for other complications resulting from casting that can be serious and life threatening, such as INFECTION, circulation impairment, and peripheral nerve damage. If the patient returns home after cast application, teach him or her how to monitor for these complications and when to notify the health care provider.

INFECTION most often results from the breakdown of skin under the cast (pressure necrosis). If pressure necrosis occurs, the patient typically reports a very painful "hot spot" under the cast and the cast may feel warmer in the affected area. Teach the patient or family to smell the area for mustiness or an unpleasant odor that would indicate infected material. If the infection progresses, a fever may develop.

Circulation impairment causing decreased PERFUSION and *peripheral nerve damage* can result from tightness of the cast. Teach the patient to assess for circulation at least daily, including the ability to move the area distal to the extremity, numbness, and increased PAIN.

The patient with a cast may be immobilized for a prolonged period, depending on the extent of the fracture and the type of cast. Assess for complications of immobility, such as skin breakdown, pneumonia, atelectasis, thromboembolism, and constipation. Before the cast is removed, inform the patient that the cast cutter will not injure the skin but that heat may be felt during the procedure.

Because of prolonged immobilization, a joint may become contracted, usually in a fixed state of flexion. Osteoarthritis and osteoporosis may develop from lack of weight bearing. Muscle can also atrophy from lack of exercise during prolonged immobilization of the affected body part, usually an extremity.

Traction. **Traction** is the application of a pulling force to a part of the body to provide reduction, alignment, and rest. It is also used as a last resort to decrease muscle spasm (thus relieving pain) and prevent or correct deformity and tissue damage. A patient in traction is often hospitalized, but in some cases, home care is possible even for skeletal traction.

Traction may be classified as running traction or balanced suspension. In *running* traction, the pulling force is in one direction and the patient's body acts as countertraction. Moving the body or bed position can alter the countertraction force. *Balanced suspension* provides the countertraction so that the pulling force of the traction is not altered when the bed or patient is moved. This allows for increased movement and facilitates care (Table 51-2).

Although not used as often today, the two most common types of traction are skin and skeletal traction. *Skin traction* involves the use of a Velcro boot (Buck's traction) (Fig. 51-5), belt, or halter, which is usually secured around the affected leg. The primary purpose of skin traction is to decrease painful muscle spasms that accompany hip fractures. A weight is used as a pulling force, which is limited to 5 to 10 pounds (2.3 to 4.5 kg) to prevent injury to the skin.

In *skeletal traction,* screws are surgically inserted directly into bone (e.g., Halo traction). These allow the use of longer traction time and heavier weights—usually 15 to 30 pounds (6.8 to 13.6 kg). Skeletal traction aids in bone realignment. Pin site care is an important part of nursing management to prevent infection.

The nurse may set up or assist in the setup of traction if specially educated. In larger or specialty hospitals or units,

! NURSING SAFETY PRIORITY QSEN

Action Alert

When patients are in traction, weights usually are not removed without a prescription. They should not be lifted manually or allowed to rest on the floor. Weights should be freely hanging at all times. Teach this important point to UAP on the unit, to other personnel such as those in the radiology department, and to visitors. Inspect the skin at least every 8 hours for signs of irritation or inflammation. When possible, remove the belt or boot that is used for skin traction every 8 hours to inspect under the device.

TABLE 51-2 Types of Traction Used for Musculoskeletal Trauma

TYPE AND CHARACTERISTICS OF TRACTION	USE
Upper Extremity Traction	
Sidearm skin or skeletal traction (the forearm is flexed and extended 90 degrees from the upper part of the body)	Fractures of the humerus with or without involvement of the shoulder and clavicle
Overhead or 90-90 traction, skin or skeletal (the elbow is flexed and the arm is at a right angle to the body over the upper chest)	Same as above (depends on the physician's preference)
Plaster traction (pins inserted through the bone are fixed in the cast)	Fractures of the wrist
Lower Extremity Traction	
Buck's extension traction (skin) (the affected leg is in extension)	Fractures of the hip or femur preoperatively Prevention of hip flexion contractures Hip dislocation
Russell's traction (similar to Buck's traction, but a sling under the knee suspends the leg)	Fractures of the hip or distal end of the femur
Balanced skin or skeletal traction (the limb is usually elevated in a Thomas splint with Pearson's attachment, or a Böhler-Braun splint is used)	Fractures of the femur or pelvis (acetabulum)
Spinal Column and Pelvic Traction	
Cervical halter (a strap under the chin)	Cervical muscle spasms, strain/sprain, or arthritis
Cervical skeletal (e.g., halo brace)	Cervical fractures of the spine; muscle spasms
Pelvic belt (a strap around the hips at the iliac crests is attached to weights at the foot of the bed)	Pain, strain, sprain, or muscle spasms in the lower back
Pelvic sling (a wide strap around the hips is attached to an overhead bar to keep the pelvis off the bed)	Pelvic fractures; other pelvic injuries

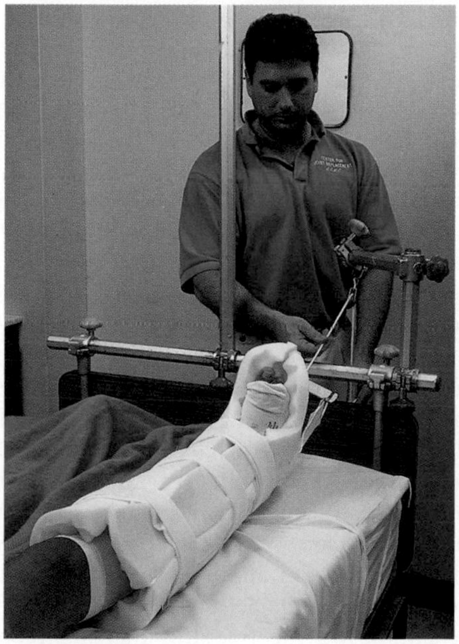

FIG. 51-5 Skin traction with a hook-and-loop fastener (Velcro) boot, commonly used for hip fractures.

orthopedic technicians or physician assistants often set up traction. Once traction is applied, maintain the correct balance between traction pull and countertraction force.

Check traction equipment frequently to ensure its proper functioning. Inspect all ropes, knots, and pulleys at least every 8 to 12 hours for loosening, fraying, and positioning. Check the weight for consistency with the health care provider's prescription. Sometimes one of the weights is accidentally removed by a staff member or visitor who bumps into it. Replace the weights if they are not correct, and notify the health care provider or orthopedic technician.

If the patient reports severe pain from muscle spasm, the weights may be too heavy or the patient may need realignment. Report the pain to the health care provider if body realignment fails to reduce the discomfort. Assess neurovascular status of the affected body part to detect circulatory compromise and tissue damage. The circulation is usually monitored every hour for the first 24 hours after traction is applied and every 4 hours thereafter.

NCLEX EXAMINATION CHALLENGE

Physiological Integrity

A client has a new synthetic leg cast for a tibial fracture. What health care teaching does the nurse include for the client's self-management at home? **Select all that apply.**

A. "Keep your leg elevated, preferably above your heart, as much as possible."
B. "Apply ice on the cast for the first 24 hours to increase blood flow for healing."
C. "Report severe numbness or inability to move your toes to your health care provider."
D. "Take your pain medication as needed according to the prescription directions."
E. "Don't cover the cast with anything because it will stay wet for 24 hours."

Drug Therapy. After fracture treatment, the patient often has pain for a prolonged time during the healing process. The health care provider commonly prescribes opioid and non-opioid analgesics, anti-inflammatory drugs, and muscle relaxants.

For patients with chronic, severe PAIN, opioid and non-opioid drugs are alternated or given together to manage pain both centrally in the brain and peripherally at the site of injury. For severe or multiple fractures, patient-controlled analgesia (PCA) with morphine, fentanyl, or hydromorphone (Dilaudid) is used. *Meperidine (Demerol) should never be used for older adults because it has toxic metabolites that can cause seizures and other complications. Most hospitals no longer use this drug for patients of any age.* Oxycodone and oxycodone with acetaminophen (Percocet) are common oral opioid drugs that are very effective for most patients with fracture pain. NSAIDs are given to decrease associated tissue inflammation.

For patients who have less severe injury, the analgesic may be given on an as-needed basis. Collaborate with the patient regarding the best times for the strong analgesics to be given (e.g., before a complex dressing change, after physical therapy sessions, and at bedtime). Assess the effectiveness of the analgesic and its side effects. Constipation is a common side effect of opioid therapy, especially for older adults. Assess for frequency of bowel movements, and administer stool softeners as needed. Encourage fluids and activity as tolerated. Chapter 3 discusses the various methods of PAIN management, including epidural analgesia and patient-controlled analgesia.

Some patients experience a long-term, intense burning PAIN and edema that are associated with *complex regional pain syndrome (CRPS)*. This syndrome often results from fractures and other musculoskeletal trauma and is discussed on p. 1075 later in this chapter.

Surgical Management. For some types of fractures, closed reduction is not sufficient. Surgical intervention may be needed to realign the bone for the healing process.

Preoperative Care. Teach the patient and family what to expect during and after the surgery. The preoperative care for a patient undergoing orthopedic surgery is similar to that for anyone having surgery with general or epidural anesthesia. (See Chapter 14 for a thorough discussion of preoperative nursing care.)

Operative Procedures. Open reduction with internal fixation (ORIF) is one of the most common methods of reducing and immobilizing a fracture. External fixation with closed reduction is used when patients have soft-tissue injury (open fracture). Although nurses do not decide which surgical technique is used, understanding the procedures enhances patient teaching and care.

Because ORIF permits early MOBILITY, it is often the preferred surgical method. **Open reduction** allows the surgeon to directly view the fracture site. **Internal fixation** uses metal pins, screws, rods, plates, or prostheses to immobilize the fracture during healing. The surgeon makes one or more incisions to gain access to the broken bone(s) and implants one or more devices into bone tissue after each fracture is reduced. A cast, boot, or splint is placed to maintain immobilization during the healing process, depending on the body part affected.

After the bone achieves union, the metal hardware may be removed, depending on the location and type of fracture. Hardware is removed most frequently in ankle fractures, depending on the severity of the injury. If the metal implants are not bothersome, they remain in place. Specific types of internal fixation devices are discussed later in the Selected Fractures of Specific Sites section.

An alternative modality for the management of fractures is the external fixation apparatus, as shown in Fig. 51-6. **External fixation** is a system in which pins or wires are inserted through the skin and affected bone and then connected to a rigid external frame. The system may be used for upper or lower extremity fractures or for fractures of the pelvis, especially for open fractures when wound management is needed. After a fixator is removed, the patient may be placed in a cast or splint until healing is complete.

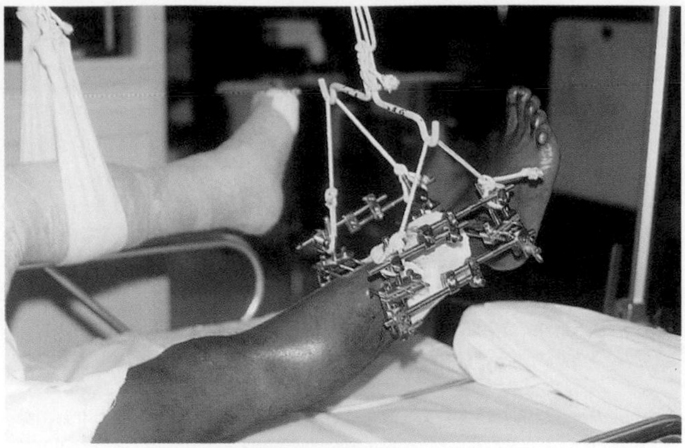

FIG. 51-6 The Hex-Fix external fixation system for tibia-fibula fractures.

External fixation has several advantages over other surgical techniques:

- There is minimal blood loss compared with internal fixation.
- The device allows early ambulation and exercise of the affected body part while relieving pain.
- The device maintains alignment in closed fractures that will not maintain position in a cast and stabilizes comminuted fractures that require bone grafting.

In open fractures, in which skin and tissue trauma accompany the fracture, the device permits easy access to the wound while the bone heals. This method is usually preferred over the use of a window in a cast for wound care.

A disadvantage of external fixation is an increased risk for pin site INFECTION. Pin site infections can lead to osteomyelitis, which is serious and difficult to treat (see Chapter 50).

Postoperative Care. The postoperative care for a patient undergoing ORIF or external fixation is similar to that provided for any patient undergoing surgery (see Chapter 16). Because bone is a vascular, dynamic body tissue, the patient is at risk for complications specific to fractures and musculoskeletal surgery. IV ketorolac (Toradol) is often given in the postanesthesia care unit (PACU) or soon after discharge to the post-surgical area to reduce inflammation and pain. Aggressive pain management starts as soon as possible after surgery to prevent the development of chronic pain and promote early mobility.

Additional information about postoperative care is found beginning on p. 1066 in the Selected Fractures of Specific Sites section. Depending on the fractures that are repaired, some ORIF procedures are performed as same-day surgeries. Patients stay in the hospital up to 23 hours after surgery.

For patients with an **external fixator**, pay particular attention to the pin sites for signs of inflammation or infection. In the first 48 to 72 hours, *clear* fluid drainage or weeping is expected. Although no standardized method or evidence-based protocol for pin site care has been established, recommendations have been made based on the evidence available regarding pin site care. Because the pins go through the skin and into bone, the risk for infection is high. Monitor the pin sites at least every 8 to 12 hours for drainage, color, odor, and severe redness, which indicate inflammation and possible infection. Follow agency policy for how to clean the pin site areas.

The patient with an external fixator may have a disturbed body image. The frame may be large and bulky, and the affected area may have massive tissue damage with dressings.

Be sensitive to this possibility in planning care. Teach about alterations to clothing that may be required while the fixator is in place.

The Ilizarov technique of circular external fixation is sometimes used to treat new fractures (closed, comminuted fractures and open fractures with bone loss), as well as malunion or nonunion of fractures. It may also be used to treat congenital bone deformities, especially in "little people" (e.g., dwarfs).

The circular external fixation device is used to gently pull apart the cortex of the bone and stimulate new bone growth. Unlike the traditional fixator, the Ilizarov external fixator promotes rotation, angulation, lengthening, or widening of bone to correct bony defects and allows for healing of any soft-tissue defect. The nursing care associated with this device is similar to the care of the patient with other external fixation systems with one major exception. If the device is being used for filling bone gaps, teach the patient how to manually turn the four-sided nuts (also called *clickers*) up to 4 times a day. Daily distraction rates vary, but 1 mm daily is common. Screening and teaching are particularly important because the patient adjusts and cares for the apparatus over a long period of up to 6 months to 1 year. PAIN control is a priority outcome for patients using this device.

Procedures for Nonunion. Some management techniques are not successful because the bone does not heal. Several additional options are available to the physician to promote bone union, such as electrical bone stimulation, bone grafting, and ultrasound fracture treatment.

For selected patients, *electrical bone stimulation* may be successful. This procedure is based on research showing that bone has electrical properties that are used in healing. The exact mechanism of action is unknown. A noninvasive, external **electrical bone stimulation** system delivers a small continuous electrical charge directed toward the non-healed bone. There are no known risks with this system, although patients with pacemakers cannot use this device on an arm. Implanted direct-current stimulators are placed directly in the fracture site and have no external apparatus. Both systems require several months of treatment.

Another method of treating nonunion is *bone grafting.* A bone graft may also replace diseased bone or increase bone tissue for joint replacement. In most cases, chips of bone are taken from the iliac crest or other site and are packed or wired between the bone ends to facilitate union. Allografts from cadavers may also be used. These grafts are frozen or freeze-dried and stored under sterile conditions in a bone bank.

Bone banking from living donors is becoming increasingly popular. If qualified, patients undergoing total hip replacement may donate their femoral heads to the bank for later use as bone grafts for others. Careful screening ensures that the bone is healthy and that the donor has no communicable disease. The bone cannot be donated without written consent.

One of the newest modalities for fracture healing is **low-intensity pulsed ultrasound** (Exogen therapy). Used for slow-healing fractures or for new fractures as an alternative to surgery, ultrasound treatment has had excellent results. The patient applies the treatment for about 20 minutes each day. It has no contraindications or adverse effects.

Physical Therapy. Many patients with musculoskeletal trauma, including fractures, are referred by their health care provider for rehabilitation therapy with a physical therapist (PT). The timing for this referral depends on the nature, severity, and treatment modality of the fracture(s).

For example, some patients who have an ORIF for one or more ankle fractures may begin therapy when the incisional staples or Steri-Strips are removed and an orthopedic boot is fitted. Based on the initial evaluation, the PT performs gentle manipulative exercises to increase range of motion. The therapist may also begin to help the patient with laterality, a concept to help the brain identify the injured foot from the uninjured foot. Computer programs and mirror-box therapy can help reprogram the brain as part of cognitive retraining. In mirror-box therapy for an injured foot, the patient covers his or her affected foot while looking at and moving the uninjured foot in front of the mirror. The brain perceives the foot in the mirror as the injured foot.

Stimulation by touch also helps the brain acknowledge the injured foot. The PT teaches the patient to have someone frequently touch the injured area and use various materials and objects against the skin to desensitize it. These interventions decrease the risk for complex regional pain syndrome, discussed later in this chapter.

When weight bearing begins about 6 weeks after surgery, the PT teaches the patient how to begin with toe-touch or partial weight bearing using crutches or a walker. Muscle strengthening exercises of the affected leg help with ambulation because atrophy begins shortly after injury.

The PT also assists with PAIN control and edema reduction by using ice/heat packs, electrical muscle stimulation ("e-stim"), and special treatments such as dexamethasone iontophoresis. **Iontophoresis** is a method for absorbing dexamethasone, a synthetic steroid, through the skin near the painful area to decrease inflammation and edema. A small device delivers a minute amount of electricity via electrodes that are placed on the skin. The patient may describe the sensation as a pinch or slight sting. The electrical current increases the ability of the skin to absorb the drug from a topical patch into the affected soft tissue.

The success of rehabilitation is affected by the patient's motivation and willingness to perform prescribed exercises and activities between PT visits. Rehabilitation for ankle surgery, for example, may take several months, depending on the severity of the injury and the age and general health of the patient.

Preventing and Monitoring for Neurovascular Compromise

Planning: Expected Outcomes. The patient with a fracture is expected to have no compromise in neurovascular status as evidenced by adequate circulation, movement, and SENSORY PERCEPTION (CMS). If severe compromise occurs, the patient is expected to have early and prompt emergency treatment to prevent severe tissue damage.

Interventions. Perform neurovascular (NV) assessments (also known as "circ checks" or CMS assessments) frequently before and after fracture treatment. Patients who have extremity casts, splints with elastic bandage wraps, and open reduction with internal fixation (ORIF) or external fixation are especially at risk for NV compromise. If blood flow to the distal extremity is impaired, the patient reports increased PAIN and decreased SENSORY PERCEPTION and movement. If these symptoms are allowed to progress, patients are at risk for acute compartment syndrome (ACS).

Early recognition of the signs and symptoms of ACS can prevent loss of function or loss of a limb. Identify patients who may be at risk, and monitor them closely. ACS can begin in 6 to 8 hours after an injury or take up to 2 days to appear. If it is suspected, notify the health care provider immediately, and if possible, implement interventions to relieve the pressure. For example, for the patient with tight, bulky dressings, loosen the bandage or tape. If the patient has a cast, follow agency protocol about who may cut the cast.

> **! NURSING SAFETY PRIORITY (QSEN)**
>
> ***Critical Rescue***
>
> Monitor for early signs of ACS. Assess for the "six Ps" including **p**ain, **p**ressure, **p**aralysis, **p**aresthesia, **p**allor, and **p**ulselessness (rare). PAIN is increased even with passive motion and may seem out of proportion to the degree of injury. Analgesics that had controlled pain become less effective. Numbness and tingling or paresthesias are often one of the first signs of the problem. The affected extremity then becomes pale and cool as a result of decreased arterial perfusion to the affected area. Capillary refill is an important assessment of PERFUSION but may not be reliable in an older adult because of arterial insufficiency. Losses of movement and function and decreased pulses or pulselessness are late signs of ACS! Fortunately, ACS is not common, but it creates an emergency situation when it does occur.

In a few cases, compartment pressure may be monitored on a one-time basis with a handheld device with a digital display, or pressure can be monitored continuously. Monitoring is recommended for comatose or unresponsive high-risk patients with multiple trauma and fractures.

If ACS is verified, the surgeon may perform a **fasciotomy**, or opening in the fascia, by making an incision through the skin and subcutaneous tissues into the fascia of the affected compartment. This procedure relieves the pressure and restores circulation to the affected area. No consensus exists on what pressure requires fasciotomy (normal is 0 to 8 mm Hg). Compartment pressures must be considered in relation to the patient's hemodynamic status. After fasciotomy, the open wound is packed and dressed daily or more often until secondary closure occurs, usually in 4 to 5 days, depending on the patient's healing ability. Some surgeons use negative pressure wound therapy (e.g., Wound Vac) over a fasciotomy to decrease edema until the wound is closed. For other patients, a skin graft may be used to promote healing.

Preventing Infection

Planning: Expected Outcomes. The patient with a fracture is expected to be free of wound or bone INFECTION as evidenced by no fever, no increase in white blood cell count, and negative wound culture (if wound is present).

Interventions. When caring for a patient with an open fracture, use clean or aseptic technique for dressing changes and wound irrigations. Check agency policy for specific protocols. *Immediately notify the health care provider if you observe inflammation and purulent drainage.* Other infections, such as pneumonia and urinary tract infection, may occur several days after the fracture. Monitor the patient's vital signs every 4 to 8 hours because increases in temperature and pulse often indicate systemic infection.

> **CONSIDERATIONS FOR OLDER ADULTS**
>
> ***Patient-Centered Care (QSEN)***
>
> Older adults may not have a temperature elevation even in the presence of severe infection. An acute onset of confusion (delirium) often suggests an infection in the older adult patient.

For most patients with an open fracture, the health care provider prescribes one or more broad-spectrum antibiotics prophylactically and performs surgical débridement of any wounds as soon as possible after the injury. First-generation cephalosporins, clindamycin (Cleocin), and gentamycin are commonly used. In addition to systemic antibiotics, local antibiotic therapy through wound irrigation is commonly prescribed, especially during débridement.

A very effective treatment is negative pressure wound therapy (e.g., vacuum-assisted closure [VAC] system) as a method of increasing the rate of wound healing for open fractures. This device allows quicker wound closure, which decreases the risk for INFECTION.

When the bone is surgically repaired, hardware and/or bone grafts have typically been implanted. However, they are limited in their use. The U.S. Food and Drug Administration (FDA) approved the use of recombinant human bone morphogenetic protein-2 (rhBMP-2) for tibial and spinal fractures. This implanted genetically engineered substance increases wound healing, decreases hardware failure, and decreases the risk for infection.

Improving Physical Mobility

Planning: Expected Outcomes. The patient with a fracture is expected to increase physical MOBILITY and be free of complications associated with impaired mobility. The patient is also expected to move purposefully in his or her own environment independently with or without an ambulatory device unless restricted by traction or other modality.

Interventions. The interventions necessary for this diagnosis can be grouped into two types: those that help increase MOBILITY and those that prevent complications of impaired mobility.

Promoting Mobility. The use of crutches or a walker increases MOBILITY and assists in ambulation. The patient may progress to using a walker or cane after crutches.

Crutches are the most commonly used ambulatory aid for many types of lower extremity musculoskeletal trauma (e.g., fractures, sprains, amputations). In most agencies, the physical therapist or emergency department/ambulatory care nurse fits the patient for crutches and teaches him or her how to ambulate with them. Reinforce those instructions, and evaluate whether the patient is using the crutches correctly.

Walking with crutches requires strong arm muscles, balance, and coordination. For this reason, crutches are not often used for older adults. Walkers and canes are preferred for the older adult. Crutches can cause upper extremity bursitis or axillary nerve damage if they are not fitted or used correctly. For that reason, the top of each crutch is padded. To prevent pressure on the axillary nerve, there should be two to three fingerbreadths between the axilla and the top of the crutch when the crutch tip is at least 6 inches (15 cm) diagonally in front of the foot. The crutch is adjusted so that the elbow is flexed no more than 30 degrees when the palm is on the handle (Fig. 51-7). The distal tips of each crutch are rubber to prevent slipping.

There are several types of gaits for walking with crutches. The most common one for musculoskeletal injury is the three-point gait, which allows little weight bearing on the affected leg. The procedure for these gaits is discussed in fundamentals of nursing books.

A *walker* is most often used by the older patient who needs additional support for balance. The physical therapist assesses the strength of the upper extremities and the unaffected leg. Strength is improved with prescribed exercises as needed.

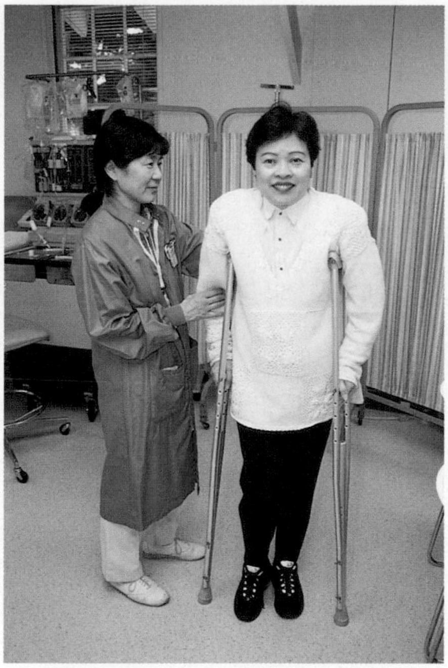

FIG. 51-7 Assisting the patient with crutch walking. Note how the therapist guards the patient and how the patient's elbows are at no more than 30 degrees of flexion.

A *cane* is sometimes used if the patient needs only minimal support for an affected leg. The straight cane offers the least support. A hemi-cane or quad-cane provides a broader base for the cane and therefore more support. The cane is placed on the *unaffected* side and should create no more than 30 degrees of flexion of the elbow. The top of the cane should be parallel to the greater trochanter of the femur or stylus of the wrist. Chapter 6 and fundamentals textbooks describe these ambulatory devices in more detail.

Preventing Complications of Immobility. The nurse plays a vital role in preventing and assessing for complications in immobilized patients with fractures. Additional information about nursing care for preventing problems associated with immobility is found in Chapter 6.

Community-Based Care

The patient with an *uncomplicated* fracture is usually discharged to home from the emergency department or urgent care center. Older adults with hip or other fractures or patients with multiple traumas are hospitalized and then transferred to home, a rehabilitation setting, or a long-term care facility for rehabilitation. Collaborate with the case manager or the discharge planner in the hospital to ensure continuity of care. Be sure to communicate the plan of care clearly to the health care agency receiving the patient.

Home Care Management. If the patient is discharged to home, the nurse, therapist, or case manager (CM) may assess the home environment for structural barriers to mobility, such as stairs. Be sure that the patient has easy access to the bathroom. Ask about scatter rugs, waxed floors, and walkway areas that could increase the risk for falls. If the patient needs to use a wheelchair or ambulatory aid, make sure that he or she can use it safely and that there is room in the house to ambulate with these devices. The physical therapist may teach the patient how to use stairs, but older adults or those using crutches may

CHART 51-5 Patient and Family Education: Preparing for Self-Management

Care of the Extremity After Cast Removal

- Remove scaly, dead skin carefully by soaking; do not scrub.
- Move the extremity carefully. Expect discomfort, weakness, and decreased range of motion.
- Support the extremity with pillows or your orthotic device until strength and movement return.
- Exercise slowly as instructed by your physical therapist.
- Wear support stockings or elastic bandages to prevent swelling (for lower extremity).

experience difficulty performing this task. Depending on the age and condition of the patient, a home health care nurse may make one or two visits to check that the home is safe and that the patient and family are able to follow the interdisciplinary plan of care.

Self-Management Education. The patient with a fracture may be discharged from the hospital, emergency department, office, or clinic with a bandage, splint, cast, or external fixator. Provide verbal and written instructions on the care of these devices. Chart 51-5 describes care of the affected extremity after removal of the cast.

The patient may also need to continue wound care at home. Instruct the patient and family about how to assess and dress the wound to promote healing and prevent INFECTION. Teach them how to recognize complications and when and where to seek professional health care if complications occur. Additional educational needs depend on the type of fracture and fracture repair.

Encourage patients and their families to ensure adequate foods high in protein and calcium that are needed for bone and tissue healing. For patients with lower extremity fractures, less weight bearing on long bones can cause anemia. The red bone marrow needs weight bearing to simulate red blood cell production. Encourage foods high in iron content. Teach the patient to take a daily iron-added multivitamin (take with food to prevent possible nausea).

Health Care Resources. Arrange for follow-up care at home. A social worker may need to help the patient apply for funds to pay medical bills. If there is severe bone and tissue damage, be realistic and help the patient and family understand the long-term nature of the recovery period. Multiple treatment techniques and surgical procedures required for complications can be mentally and emotionally draining for the patient and family. A vocational counselor may be needed to help the patient find a different type of job, depending on the extent of the fracture.

An older or incapacitated patient may need assistance with ADLs, which can be provided by home care aides if family or other caregiver is not available. In collaboration with the case manager, anticipate the patient's needs and arrange for these services.

◆ *Evaluation: Outcomes*

Evaluate the care of the patient with one or more fractures based on the identified priority patient problems. The expected outcomes include that the patient:

- States that he or she has adequate PAIN control
- Has adequate blood flow to maintain tissue PERFUSION and function

- Is free of INFECTION
- Is free of physiologic consequences of impaired MOBILITY
- Ambulates or moves independently with or without an assistive device (if not restricted by traction or other device)

NCLEX EXAMINATION CHALLENGE

Physiological Integrity

A client returns to the same-day surgical unit after having an ankle open reduction internal fixation (ORIF). What is the nurse's priority action when caring for this client?

A. Monitor the client's vital signs frequently.
B. Assess the client's abdomen for bowel sounds.
C. Keep the client's affected leg on a pillow.
D. Encourage the client to drink fluids.

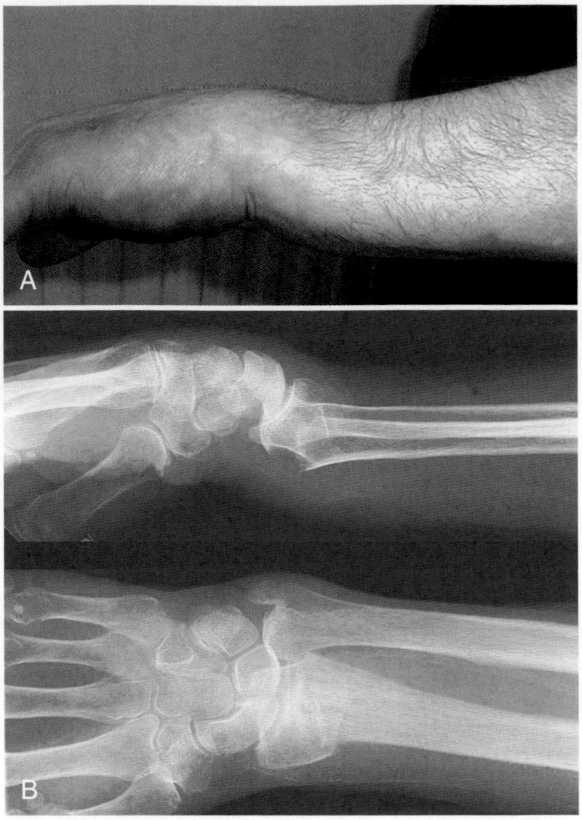

FIG. 51-8 Colles' wrist fracture showing "dinner fork" deformity.

SELECTED FRACTURES OF SPECIFIC SITES

Upper Extremity Fractures

In addition to the general care discussed in the previous section, management of upper extremity fractures includes specific interventions related to the location and nature of the injury.

Fractures of the *proximal humerus,* particularly impacted or displaced fractures, are common in the older adult. An impacted injury is usually treated with a sling or other device for immobilization. A displaced fracture often requires ORIF with pins or a prosthesis. Humeral shaft fractures are generally corrected by closed reduction and a hanging-arm cast or splint. If necessary, the fracture is repaired surgically (with an intramedullary rod or metal plate and screws) or with external fixation.

The most common upper extremity (UE) fracture is the *distal radius fracture (DRF),* which occurs in both younger and older adults. Younger adults experience this injury from high-energy (high-impact) trauma as a result of motor vehicle crashes and sports. Older adults, particularly women with osteopenia, typically have low-impact DRFs as a result of falls (Voda, 2011).

Various names are used to classify DRFs, including Colles' and Smith fractures. A Colles' fracture can occur when a person attempts to break a fall by landing on the heel of the hand when the wrist is extended. The resulting deformity is often called a "dinner fork" injury (Fig. 51-8). Seen less commonly, a Smith fracture occurs from a fall on a flexed wrist (Voda, 2011).

Initial nursing interventions for a patient with a DRF include:

- Removing jewelry on the affected hand and wrist before edema worsens (Walsh, 2013)
- Performing a neurovascular assessment of the affected UE
- Immobilizing the affected wrist and hand
- Elevating the affected UE
- Applying ice to the affected area
- Managing pain

After initial stabilization, the most common treatment for a DRF is closed reduction. The health care provider realigns the bone ends while the patient is moderately sedated. A splint is applied and held in place with an elastic bandage. The splint may be replaced several days later with a cast after edema decreases.

For more complicated DRFs, an ORIF with pins and plates may be performed. The patient may have surgery in an ambulatory care or same-day surgical setting using general anesthesia, a peripheral nerve block, or a combination of both. The nerve block is often given as a single injection of levobupivacaine (Chirocaine) or bupivacaine (Marcaine), which provides pain relief for 12 to 20 hours (Guarin, 2013). Teach patients having a peripheral nerve block (e.g., supraclavicular block) that temporarily they will not be able to move their affected arm. Also observe, report, and document signs and symptoms of pneumothorax, including tachypnea, decreased breath sounds, or respiratory distress (Guarin, 2013).

For all patients who experience a DRF, assess for nerve compression, especially the radial and median nerves. Be sure to perform frequent neurovascular assessment with special attention to the presence of decreased SENSORY PERCEPTION (e.g., numbness) or decreased movement.

Fractures of the *metacarpals* and *phalanges (fingers)* are usually not displaced, which makes their treatment less difficult than that of other fractures. Metacarpal fractures are immobilized for 3 to 4 weeks. Phalangeal fractures are immobilized in finger splints for 10 to 14 days.

Lower Extremity Fractures

Fractures of the Hip

Hip fracture is the most common injury in older adults and one of the most frequently seen injuries in any health care setting or community. It has a high mortality rate as a result of multiple complications related to surgery, depression, and prolonged immobility. Over half of older adults experiencing a hip fracture are unable to live independently, and many die within the first year (Sweitzer et al., 2013).

Hip fractures include those involving the upper third of the femur and are classified as **intracapsular** (within the joint

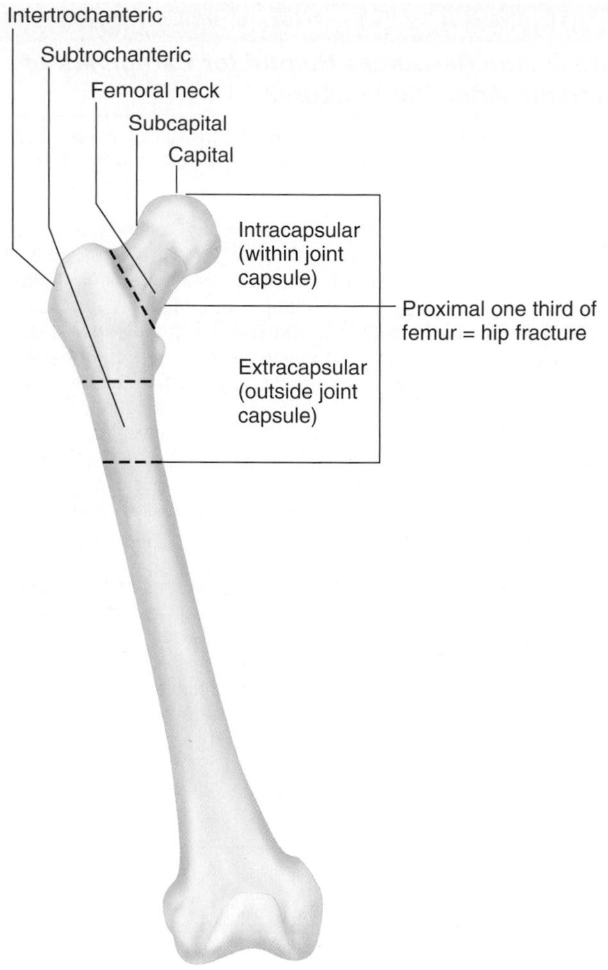

FIG. 51-9 Types of hip fractures.

capsule) or **extracapsular** (outside the joint capsule). These types are further divided according to fracture location (Fig. 51-9). In the area of the femoral neck, disruption of the blood supply to the head of the femur is a concern, which can result in ischemic or avascular necrosis (AVN) of the femoral head. AVN causes death and necrosis of bone tissue and results in pain and decreased mobility. This problem is most likely in patients with displaced fractures.

Osteoporosis is the biggest risk factor for hip fractures (see Chapter 50). This disease weakens the upper femur (hip), which causes it to break and then causes the person to fall. The number of people with hip fracture is expected to continue to increase as the population ages, and the associated health care costs will be tremendous.

The treatment of choice is surgical repair by ORIF, when possible, to reduce PAIN and allow the older patient to be out of bed and ambulatory. Skin (Buck's) traction may be applied before surgery to help decrease pain associated with muscle spasm. Depending on the exact location of the fracture, an ORIF may include an intramedullary rod, pins, prostheses (for femoral head or femoral neck fractures), or a compression screw. Figs. 51-10 and 51-11 illustrate examples of these devices. Epidural or general anesthesia is used. Occasionally a patient will be so debilitated that surgery cannot be done. In these cases, nonsurgical options include pain management and bedrest to allow natural fracture healing.

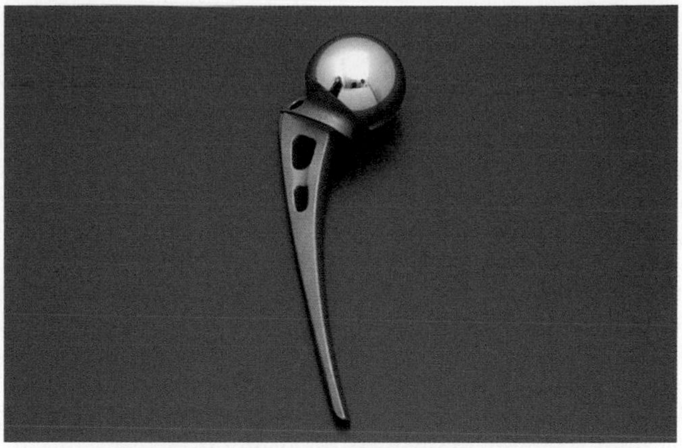

FIG. 51-10 A hip prosthesis used for fractures.

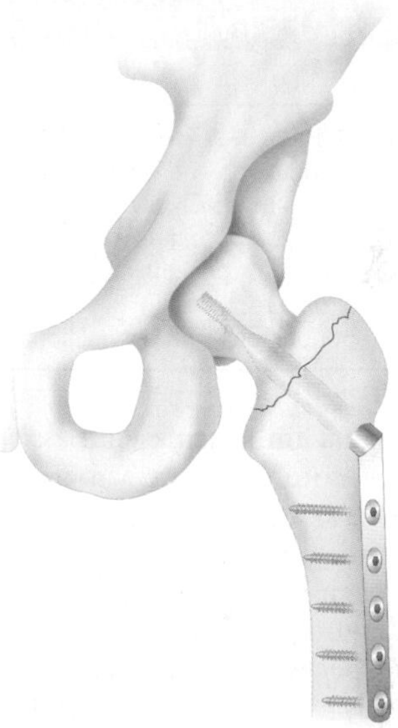

FIG. 51-11 A compression hip screw used for open reduction with internal fixation (ORIF) of the hip.

CONSIDERATIONS FOR OLDER ADULTS

Patient-Centered Care QSEN

Teach older adults about the risk factors for hip fracture including physiologic aging changes, disease processes, drug therapy, and environmental hazards. Physiologic changes include sensory changes such as diminished visual acuity and hearing; changes in gait, balance, and muscle strength; and joint stiffness. Disease processes like osteoporosis, foot disorders, and changes in cardiac function increase the risk for hip fracture. Drugs, such as diuretics, antihypertensives, antidepressants, sedatives, opioids, and alcohol, are factors that increase the risks for falling in older adults. Use of three or more drugs at the same time drastically increases the risk for falls. Throw rugs, loose carpeting, inadequate lighting, uneven walking surfaces or steps, and pets are environmental hazards that also cause falls.

The older adult with hip fracture usually reports groin pain or pain behind the knee on the affected side. In some cases, the patient has pain in the lower back or has no pain at all. However, the patient is not able to stand. X-ray or other imaging assessment confirms the diagnosis.

Patients usually receive IV morphine after admission to the emergency department and PCA morphine or epidural analgesia after surgery. In some cases, a femoral nerve block may also be performed during surgery to help relieve pain for up to 24 hours after surgery (Guarin, 2013). Meperidine (Demerol) should not be used due to its toxic metabolites that can cause seizures and other adverse drug events, especially in the older adult population. Chapter 3 discusses the nursing care associated with pain management in detail.

After a hip repair, older adults frequently experience acute confusion, or delirium. They may pull at tubes or the surgical dressing or attempt to climb out of bed, possibly falling and causing self-injury. Other patients stay awake all night and sleep during the day. Keep in mind that some patients have a quiet delirium. Monitor the patient frequently to prevent falls. Ask the family or other visitors to let staff know if the patient is attempting to get out of bed. Chapter 2 describes fall prevention strategies and delirium management in detail.

! NURSING SAFETY PRIORITY (QSEN)

Action Alert

Patients who have an ORIF are at risk for hip dislocation or subluxation. Be sure to prevent hip adduction and rotation to keep the operative leg in proper alignment. Regular pillows or abduction devices can be used for patients who are confused or restless. If straps are used to hold the device in place, check the skin for signs of pressure. Perform neurovascular assessments to ensure that the device is not interfering with arterial circulation or peripheral nerve conduction.

The patient begins ambulating with assistance the day after surgery to prevent complications associated with immobility (e.g., pressure ulcers, atelectasis, venous thromboembolism). Early MOBILITY and ambulation also decrease the chance of INFECTION and increase surgical site healing.

Special considerations for the patient having a hip repair also include careful inspection of skin including areas of pressure, especially the heels. Use of skin traction to reduce muscle spasms may increase the period of bedrest before surgery. Decreased MOBILITY after surgery can increase the risk for pressure injury in this area within 24 hours.

! NURSING SAFETY PRIORITY (QSEN)

Action Alert

Be sure that the patient's heels are up off the bed at all times. Inspect the heels and other high-risk bony prominence areas every 8 to 12 hours. Delegate turning and repositioning every 1 to 2 hours to unlicensed assistive personnel (UAP), and supervise this nursing activity.

Other postoperative interventions to prevent complications, such as venous thromboembolism, are similar to those for total hip replacement (see Chapter 16).

Many patients recover fully from hip fracture repair and regain their functional ability. They are typically discharged to their home, rehabilitation unit or center, or a skilled nursing facility for physical and occupational therapy. However, some patients are not able to return to their pre-fracture ADLs and MOBILITY level. Family caregivers often have unexpected responsibilities caring for patients during their recovery. Hip fracture resource centers can be very useful in providing caregiver support (see the Evidence-Based Practice box).

EVIDENCE-BASED PRACTICE (QSEN)

Are Online Resources Helpful for Caregivers of Patients After Hip Fracture?

Nahm, E-S., Resnick, B., Plummer, L., & Park, B.K. (2013). Use of discussion boards in an online hip fracture resource center for caregivers. *Orthopaedic Nursing, 32*(2), 89-96.

Family caregivers (CGs) are important for the successful recovery of patients who have hip fracture repair. In a previous study the authors found that CGs lacked knowledge in understanding how to provide care during the rehabilitation and recovery phase. The purpose of this qualitative study was to explore the experiences of CGs while they were using an online hip resource center over an 8-week period. The majority of the 27 caregivers in the study were female and white. Most had some college education, and their average age was 55.5 years. Each CG posted comments related to specific topics posted on the online discussion boards. Examples of topics included the roles of therapists, awareness of bone health, and caregiver stress. Three coders recorded and analyzed the data using well-established coding rules to ensure validity and reliability.

The analysis revealed common themes, such as need for adjustment to the fracture event, and three categories: types of care provided by the CGs, strategies used by CGs to prevent fractures, and coping mechanisms used to handle stress. The researchers concluded that discussion boards (DBs) can serve as a useful medium for CGs to share their experiences. They also noted that DBs can assist health care providers identify ways to support CGs.

Level of Evidence: 4

This study was a well-designed qualitative study to gain specific information about the needs of caregivers of patients with hip fractures.

Commentary: Implications for Practice and Research

Although this study was limited to a small sample size, the researchers were very careful to ensure validity and reliability of the coding process for data analysis. Additional studies with larger sample sizes that are more diverse are needed to provide generalization of results. Nurses caring for patients having surgical hip repair need to help families locate resources to provide information and support during the patients' rehabilitation and recovery period.

Other Fractures of the Lower Extremity

Other fractures of the lower extremity may or may not require hospitalization. However, if the patient has severe or multiple fractures, especially with soft-tissue damage, hospital admission is usually required. Patients who have surgery to repair their injury may also be hospitalized. Coordinate care with the physical therapist regarding mobility, transfers, positioning, and ambulation. Collaborate with the case manager regarding placement after discharge. Most patients go home unless there is no support system or additional rehabilitation is needed. Health teaching and ensuring continuity of care are essential.

Fractures of the *lower two thirds of the femur* usually result from trauma, often from a motor vehicle crash. A femur fracture is seldom immobilized by casting because the powerful muscles of the thigh become spastic, which causes displacement of bone ends. Extensive hemorrhage can occur with femur fracture.

Surgical treatment is ORIF with nails, rods, or a compression screw. In a few cases in which extensive bone fragmentation or severe tissue trauma is found, external fixation may be employed. Healing time for a femur fracture may be 6 months or longer.

Skeletal traction, followed by a full-leg brace or cast, may be used in nonsurgical treatment.

Trauma to the lower leg most often causes fractures of both the *tibia* and the *fibula,* particularly the lower third, and is often referred to as a "tib-fib" fracture. The major treatment techniques are closed reduction with casting, internal fixation, and external fixation. If closed reduction is used, the patient may wear a cast for 6 to 10 weeks. Because of poor PERFUSION to parts of the tibia and fibula, delayed union is not unusual with this type of fracture. Internal fixation with nails or a plate and screws, followed by a long-leg cast for 4 to 6 weeks, is another option. When the fractures cause extensive skin and soft-tissue damage, the initial treatment may be external fixation, often for 6 to 10 weeks, usually followed by application of a cast until the fracture is completely healed. The patient uses ambulatory aids, usually crutches.

Ankle fractures are described by their anatomic place of injury. For example, a bimalleolar (Pott's) fracture involves the medial malleolus of the tibia and the lateral malleolus of the fibula. The small talus that makes up the rest of the ankle joint may also be broken. An ORIF is usually performed using two incisions—one on the medial (inside) aspect of the ankle and one on the lateral (outer) side. Several screws or nails are placed into the tibia, and a compression plate with multiple screws keeps the fibula in alignment. Weight bearing is restricted until the bone heals.

Treatment of fractures of the foot or phalanges (toes) is similar to that of other fractures. Phalangeal fractures may be more painful but are not as serious as most other types of fractures. Crutches are used for ambulation if weight bearing is restricted, but many patients can ambulate while wearing an orthopedic shoe or boot while the bone heals.

Fractures of the Chest and Pelvis

Chest trauma may cause fractures of the ribs or sternum. The major concern with rib and sternal fractures is the potential for puncture of the lungs, heart, or arteries by bone fragments or ends. *Assess airway, breathing, and circulation status* ***first*** *for any patient having chest trauma!* Fractures of the lower ribs may damage underlying organs, such as the liver, spleen, or kidneys. These fractures tend to heal on their own without surgical intervention. Patients are often uncomfortable during the healing process and require analgesia. They also have a high risk for pneumonia because of shallow breathing caused by pain on inspiration. Encourage them to breathe normally if possible.

Because the pelvis is very vascular and is close to major organs and blood vessels, associated internal damage is the major focus in fracture management. After head injuries, pelvic fractures are the second most common cause of death from trauma. In young adults, pelvic fractures typically result from motor vehicle crashes or falls from buildings. Falls are the most common cause in older adults. The major concern related to pelvic injury is venous oozing or arterial bleeding. Loss of blood volume leads to hypovolemic shock.

Assess for internal abdominal trauma by checking for blood in the urine and stool and by monitoring the abdomen for the development of rigidity or swelling. The trauma team may use peritoneal lavage, CT scanning, or ultrasound for assessment of hemorrhage. Ultrasound is noninvasive, rapid, reliable, and cost-effective and can be done at the bedside.

There are many classification systems for pelvic fractures. A system that is particularly useful divides fractures of the pelvis into two broad categories: non–weight-bearing fractures and weight-bearing fractures.

When a *non–weight-bearing* part of the pelvis is fractured, such as one of the pubic rami or the iliac crest, treatment can be as minimal as bedrest on a firm mattress or bed board. This type of fracture can be quite painful, and the patient may need stool softeners to facilitate bowel movements because of hesitancy to move. Well-stabilized fractures usually heal in 2 months.

A *weight-bearing* fracture, such as multiple fractures of the pelvic ring creating instability or a fractured acetabulum, necessitates external fixation or ORIF or both. Progression to weight bearing depends on the stability of the fracture after fixation. Some patients can fully bear weight within days of surgery, whereas others managed with traction may not be able to bear weight for as long as 12 weeks. For complex pelvic fractures with extensive soft-tissue damage, external fixation may be required.

Compression Fractures of the Spine

Most vertebral fractures are associated with osteoporosis, metastatic bone cancer, and multiple myeloma. Compression fractures result when trabecular or cancellous bone within the vertebra becomes weakened and causes the vertebral body to collapse. The patient has severe PAIN, deformity (kyphosis), and occasional neurologic compromise. As discussed in the Osteoporosis section of Chapter 50, the patient's quality of life is reduced by the impact of this problem.

Nonsurgical management includes bedrest, analgesics, nerve blocks, and physical therapy to maintain muscle strength. Vertebral compression fractures (VCFs) that remain painful and impair mobility may be surgically treated with **vertebroplasty** or kyphoplasty. These procedures are minimally invasive techniques in which bone cement is injected through the skin (percutaneously) directly into the fracture site to provide stability and immediate pain relief. **Kyphoplasty** includes the additional step of inserting a small balloon into the fracture site and inflating it to contain the cement and to restore height to the vertebra. This procedure is preferred because it reduces the complication of leaking of bone cement outside the vertebral body and it may restore height to decrease kyphosis.

Minimally invasive surgeries can be done in an operating or interventional radiology suite by a surgeon or interventional radiologist. They can be done with moderate sedation or general anesthesia. IV ketorolac (Toradol) may be given before the procedure to reduce inflammation. Large-bore needles are placed into the fracture site using fluoroscopy or CT guidance. Then the deflated balloon is inserted through the needles and inflated in the fracture site, and the cement is injected.

Patients may have the procedures in an ambulatory care setting and return home after 2 to 4 hours or be admitted to the hospital for an overnight stay. Chart 51-6 describes the preoperative and postoperative care for percutaneous interventions for vertebral compression fractures.

Before discharge, teach the patient to report any signs or symptoms of infection from puncture sites. Remind him or her to not soak in a bath for 1 week, use analgesics as needed, resume activity, and contact the health care provider for questions or concerns.

AMPUTATIONS

An **amputation** is the removal of a part of the body. Advances in microvascular surgical procedures, better use of antibiotic

CHART 51-6 Best Practice for Patient Safety & Quality Care QSEN

Nursing Care for Patients Having Vertebroplasty or Kyphoplasty

Provide *preoperative care* including:

- Check the patient's coagulation laboratory test results; platelet count should be more than 100,000/mm^3.
- Make sure that all anticoagulant drugs were discontinued as requested by the physician.
- Assess and document the patient's neurologic status, especially extremity movement and sensation.
- Assess the patient's pain level.
- Assess the patient's ability to lie prone for at least 1 hour.
- Establish an IV line, and take vital signs.

Provide *postoperative care* including:

- Place the patient in a flat supine position for 1 to 2 hours or as requested by the physician.
- Monitor and record vital signs and frequent neurologic assessments; report any change immediately to the physician.
- Apply an ice pack to the puncture site if needed to relieve pain.
- Assess the patient's pain level, and compare it with the preoperative level; give mild analgesic as needed.
- Monitor for complications such as bleeding at the puncture site or shortness of breath; report these findings immediately if they occur.
- Assist the patient with ambulation.

Before discharge, teach the patient and family the following:

- The patient should avoid driving or operating machinery for the first 24 hours because of drugs used during the procedure.
- Monitor the puncture site for signs of infection, such as redness, pain, swelling, or drainage.
- Keep the dressing dry, and remove it the next day.
- The patient should begin usual activities, including walking the next day, and should slowly increase activity level over the next few days.

therapy, and improved surgical techniques for traumatic injury and bone cancer have reduced the number of elective amputations. The psychosocial aspects of the procedure are as devastating as the physical impairments that result. The loss is complete and permanent and causes a change in body image and self-esteem. Collaborate with members of the health care team, including prosthetists, rehabilitation therapists, psychologists, case managers, and physiatrists (rehabilitation physicians), when providing care to the patient who has an amputation.

❖ PATHOPHYSIOLOGY

Types of Amputation

Amputations may be elective or traumatic. Most are *elective* and are related to complications of peripheral vascular disease and arteriosclerosis. These complications result in ischemia in distal areas of the lower extremity. Diabetes mellitus is often an underlying cause. Amputation is considered only after other interventions have not restored circulation to the lower extremity, sometimes referred to as *limb salvage procedures* (e.g., percutaneous transluminal angioplasty [PTA]). These procedures are discussed elsewhere in this text.

Traumatic amputations most often result from accidents or war and are the primary cause of *upper extremity* amputation. A person may clean lawn mower blades or a snow blower without disconnecting the machine. A motor vehicle crash or industrial machine accident may also cause an amputation. The number of traumatic amputations also increases during war as a result of hidden land mines and bombs (e.g., in Iraq and Afghanistan). Multiple limbs or parts of limbs may be amputated as a result of these devices. Thousands of veterans of war in the United States are amputees and have had to adjust to major changes in their lifestyles.

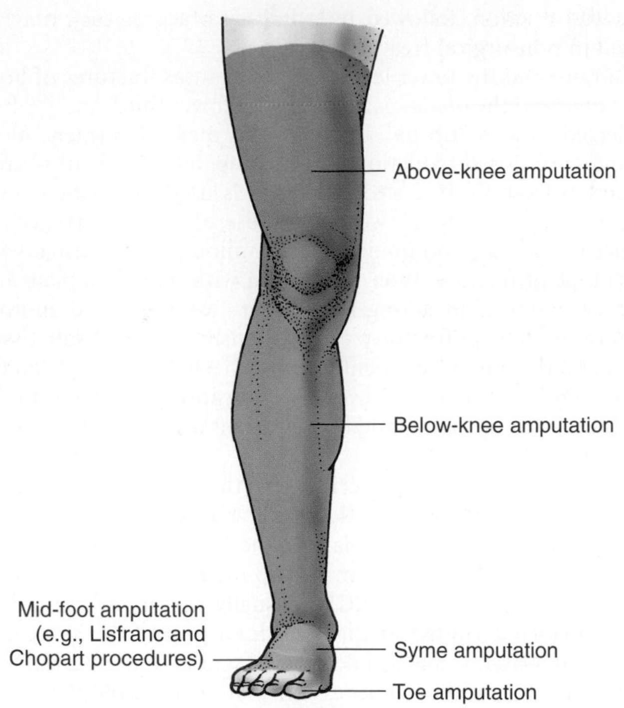

FIG. 51-12 Common levels of lower extremity amputation.

Levels of Amputation

Elective lower extremity (LE) amputations are performed much more frequently than upper extremity amputations. Several types of LE amputations may be performed (Fig. 51-12).

The loss of any or all of the small toes presents a minor disability. Loss of the great toe is significant because it affects balance, gait, and "push off" ability during walking. Midfoot amputations and the Syme amputation are common procedures for peripheral vascular disease. In the Syme amputation, most of the foot is removed but the ankle remains. The advantage of this surgery over traditional amputations below the knee is that weight bearing can occur without the use of a prosthesis and with reduced pain.

An intense effort is made to preserve knee joints with below-the-knee amputation (BKA). When the cause for the amputation extends beyond the knee, above-knee or higher amputations are performed. Hip disarticulation, or removal of the hip joint, and hemipelvectomy (removal of half of the pelvis with the leg) are more common in younger patients than in older ones who cannot easily handle the cumbersome prostheses required for ambulation. The higher the level of amputation, the more energy is required for mobility. These higher-level procedures are typically done for cancer of the bone, osteomyelitis, or trauma as a last resort.

An amputation of any part of the upper extremity is generally more incapacitating than one of the leg. The arms and hands are necessary for ADLs such as feeding, bathing, dressing, and driving a car. In the upper extremity, as much length as possible is saved to maintain function. Early replacement with a prosthetic device is vital for the patient with this type of amputation.

CULTURAL CONSIDERATIONS

Patient-Centered Care QSEN

The incidence of lower extremity amputations is greater in black and Hispanic populations because the incidence of major diseases leading to amputation, such as diabetes and arteriosclerosis, is greater in these populations (Lowe & Tariman, 2008). Limited access to health care or lack of health insurance for these minority groups may also play a major role in limb loss. Language barriers may also be an obstacle to seeking health care providers.

Complications of Amputation

The most common complications of elective or traumatic amputations are:

- Hemorrhage
- INFECTION
- Phantom limb PAIN
- Neuroma
- Flexion contractures

When a person loses part or all of an extremity either by surgery or by trauma, major blood vessels are severed, which causes *bleeding*. If the bleeding is uncontrolled, the patient is at risk for hypovolemic shock and possibly death.

As with any surgical procedure or trauma, INFECTION can occur in the wound or the bone (osteomyelitis). The older adult who is malnourished and confused is at the greatest risk because excreta may soil the wound or he or she may remove the dressing and pick at the incision. Preventing infection is a major emphasis in hospitals and other health care settings.

PAIN is a frequent complication of amputation. Sensation is felt in the amputated part immediately after surgery and usually diminishes over time. When this sensation persists and is unpleasant or painful, it is referred to as **phantom limb pain (PLP)**. PLP is more common in patients who had chronic limb pain before surgery and less common in those who have traumatic amputations. The patient reports pain in the removed body part shortly after surgery, usually after an above-the-knee amputation (AKA). The pain is often described as intense burning, crushing, or cramping. Some patients report that the removed part is in a distorted, uncomfortable position. They experience numbness and tingling, referred to as *phantom limb sensation*, as well as pain. Others state that the most distal area of the removed part feels as if it is retracted into the residual limb end. For most patients, the PAIN is triggered by touching the residual limb or by temperature or barometric pressure changes, concurrent illness, fatigue, anxiety, or stress. Routine activities such as urination can trigger the pain. If pain is long-standing, especially if it existed before the amputation, any stimulus can cause it, including touching any part of the body.

Neuroma—a sensitive tumor consisting of damaged nerve cells—forms most often in amputations of the upper extremity but can occur anywhere. The patient may or may not have pain. It is diagnosed by sonography and can be treated either surgically or nonsurgically. Surgery to remove the neuroma may be performed, but it often regrows and is more painful than before the surgery. Nonsurgical modalities include peripheral nerve blocks, steroid injections, and cognitive therapies such as hypnosis.

Flexion contractures of the hip or knee are seen in patients with amputations of the lower extremity. This complication must be avoided so that the patient can ambulate with a prosthetic device. Proper positioning and active range-of-motion exercises help prevent this complication.

Health Promotion and Maintenance

The typical patient undergoing elective amputation is a middle-aged or older man with diabetes and a lengthy history of smoking. He most likely has not cared for his feet properly, which has resulted in a nonhealing, infected foot ulcer and possibly gangrene. Therefore adherence to the disease management plan may help prevent the need for later amputation. Lifestyle habits like maintaining a healthy weight, regular exercise, and avoiding smoking can help prevent chronic diseases like diabetes and poor blood circulation.

The second largest group who have amputations comprise young men who have motorcycle or other vehicular crashes or who are injured by industrial equipment or by combat or accidents in war. These men may either experience a traumatic amputation or undergo a surgical amputation because of a severe crushing injury and massive soft-tissue damage. Teach young male adults the importance of taking safety precautions to prevent injury at work and to avoid speeding or driving while drinking alcohol. An increasing number of young women also tend to speed and drive while drinking, which endangers themselves and others around them.

❖ *PATIENT-CENTERED COLLABORATIVE CARE*

◆ *Assessment*

Physical Assessment/Clinical Manifestations. Monitor neurovascular status in the affected extremity that will be amputated. When the patient has peripheral vascular disease, check circulation in both legs. Assess skin color, temperature, sensation, and pulses in both affected and unaffected extremities. Capillary refill can be difficult to determine in the older adult related to thickened and opaque nails. In this situation, the skin near the nail bed can be used (see Chart 51-3). Capillary refill may not be as reliable as other indicators. Observe and document any discoloration of the skin, edema, ulcerations, presence of necrosis, and hair distribution on the lower extremities.

Psychosocial Assessment. People react differently to the loss of a body part. Be aware that an amputation of only a portion of one finger, especially the thumb, can be traumatic to the patient. The thumb is needed for hand activities. Therefore the loss must not be underestimated. Patients undergoing amputation face a complete, permanent loss. Evaluate their psychological preparation for a planned amputation, and expect them to go through the grieving process. Adjusting to a traumatic, unexpected amputation is often more difficult than accepting a planned one. The young patient may be bitter, hostile, and depressed. In addition to loss of a body part, the patient may lose a job, the ability to participate in favorite recreational activities, or a social relationship if other people cannot accept the body change.

The patient has an altered self-concept. The physical alteration that results from an amputation affects body image and self-esteem. For example, a patient may think that an intimate relationship with a partner is no longer possible. An older adult may feel a loss of independence. Assess the patient's feelings about himself or herself to identify areas in which he or she needs emotional support. Consult with the certified hospital chaplain, other spiritual leader, or hospital social worker if the patient is hospitalized. Counseling resources are also available in the community.

Attempt to determine the patient's willingness and motivation to withstand prolonged rehabilitation after the amputation. Asking questions about how he or she has dealt with previous life crises can provide clues. Adjustment to the amputation and rehabilitation is less difficult if the patient is willing to make needed changes.

In addition to assessing the patient's psychosocial status, assess the family's reaction to the surgery or trauma. Their response usually correlates directly with the patient's progress during recovery and rehabilitation. Expect the family to grieve for the loss, and allow them time to adjust to the change.

Assess the patient's and family's coping abilities, and help them identify personal strengths and weaknesses. Assess the patient's religious, spiritual, and cultural beliefs. Certain groups require that the amputated body part be stored for later burial with the rest of the body or be buried immediately. Other cultural customs and rituals may apply, depending on the group with which the patient associates.

Diagnostic Assessment. The surgeon determines which tests are performed to assess for viability of the limb based on blood flow. A large number of noninvasive techniques are available for this evaluation. For complete accuracy, the health care provider does not rely on any single test.

One procedure is measurement of segmental limb blood pressures, which can also be used by the nurse at the bedside. In this test, an **ankle-brachial index (ABI)** is calculated by dividing ankle systolic pressure by brachial systolic pressure. A normal ABI is 0.9 or higher.

Blood flow in an extremity can also be assessed by other noninvasive tests, including Doppler ultrasonography or laser Doppler flowmetry and transcutaneous oxygen pressure ($TcPO_2$). The ultrasonography and laser Doppler measure the speed of blood flow in the limb. The $TcPO_2$ measures oxygen pressure to indicate blood flow in the limb and has proved reliable for predicting healing.

◆ Interventions

A traumatic amputation requires rapid emergency care to possibly save the severed body part for reattachment and to prevent hemorrhage.

Emergency Care: Traumatic Amputation. For a person who has a traumatic amputation in the community, first call 911. Assess the patient for airway or breathing problems. Examine the amputation site, and apply direct pressure with layers of dry gauze or other cloth, using clean gloves if available. Many nurses carry gloves and first aid kits for this type of emergency. Elevate the extremity above the patient's heart to decrease the bleeding. Do not remove the dressing to prevent dislodging the clot.

The fingers are the most likely part to be amputated and replanted. The current recommendation for prehospital care is to wrap the completely severed finger in dry sterile gauze (if available) or a clean cloth. Put the finger in a watertight, sealed plastic bag. *Place the bag in ice water, never directly on ice, at 1 part ice and 3 parts water.* Avoid contact between the finger and the water to prevent tissue damage. Do not remove any semidetached parts of the digit. Be sure that the part goes with the patient to the hospital.

Collaborative Care for the Patient with an Amputation. Patient care depends on the type and location of the amputation. For example, an above-the-knee amputation (AKA) has the potential for more postoperative complications than does a partial foot amputation. Regardless of where the amputation occurs, collaborate with the rehabilitation therapists to improve ambulation and/or enable the patient to be independent in ADLs. For many amputations, prostheses can be used to substitute for the missing body part.

Patients undergoing lower extremity amputation today are not usually confined to a wheelchair. Advancements in the design of prosthetics have enabled them to become independent. Therefore complications from extended bedrest are not common, even for older adults.

Assessing Tissue Perfusion and Managing Pain. *The nurse's primary focus is to monitor for signs indicating that there is sufficient tissue* PERFUSION *and no hemorrhage.* The skin flap at the end of the residual (remaining) limb should be pink in a light-skinned person and not discolored (lighter or darker than other skin pigmentation) in a dark-skinned patient. The area should be warm but not hot. Assess the closest proximal pulse for presence and strength, and compare it with that in the other extremity. If the patient has bilateral vascular disease, however, comparison of limbs may not be an accurate way of measuring blood flow. Use a Doppler device to determine if the affected side is being perfused.

All patients experience PAIN as a result of either a traumatic or surgical (elective) amputation. Some patients also report pain in the missing body part (PLP). Be sure to determine which type the patient has, because they are managed very differently.

! NURSING SAFETY PRIORITY (QSEN)

Action Alert

If the patient reports PLP, recognize that the PAIN is real and should be managed promptly and completely! It is not therapeutic to remind the patient that the limb cannot be hurting because it is missing. To prevent increased pain, handle the residual limb carefully when assessing the site or changing the dressing.

Opioid analgesics are not as effective for PLP as they are for residual limb pain. IV infusions of calcitonin (Miacalcin, Calcimar) during the week after amputation can reduce phantom limb pain. The health care provider prescribes other drugs on the basis of the type of PLP the patient experiences. For instance, beta-blocking agents such as propranolol (Inderal, Apo-Propranolol ♣, Detensol ♣) are used for constant, dull, burning pain. Antiepileptic drugs such as pregabalin (Lyrica) and gabapentin (Neurontin) may be used for knifelike or sharp burning pain. Antispasmodics such as baclofen (Lioresal) may be prescribed for muscle spasms or cramping. Some patients improve with antidepressant drugs.

Other pain management modalities are described in Chapter 3. Incorporate them into the plan of care if agreeable with the patient by collaborating with specialists who are trained to perform them. For example, physical therapists often use massage, heat, transcutaneous electrical nerve stimulation (TENS), and ultrasound therapy for pain control. Consult with the certified hospital chaplain or social worker to provide emotional support. A psychologist may be needed to provide psychotherapy.

NCLEX EXAMINATION CHALLENGE

Psychosocial Integrity

A client who had an elective above-the-knee amputation (AKA) reports pain in the foot that was amputated. What is the nurse's best response to the client's pain?

A. "The pain will go away in a few days or so."
B. "That's phantom limb pain and every amputee has that."
C. "On a scale of 0 to 10, how would you rate your pain?"
D. "The pain is not real, so we don't treat it."

Preventing Infection. The surgeon typically prescribes a broad-spectrum prophylactic antibiotic immediately before elective surgery to prevent INFECTION. These may be continued for patients with *traumatic* amputations or for those who have open wounds on the residual limb. The initial pressure dressing and drains are usually removed by the surgeon 36 to 48 hours after surgery. Inspect the incision or wound for signs of infection. Record the appearance, amount, and odor of drainage, if present. The surgeon may want the incision open to air until staples or sutures are removed or may want the residual limb to have a continuous soft or rigid dressing made of fiberglass. A soft dressing is secured by an elastic bandage wrapped firmly around the residual limb.

Promoting Mobility and Preparing for Prosthesis. Collaborate with the physical therapist to begin exercises as soon as possible after surgery. If the amputation is planned, the therapist may work with the patient before surgery to start muscle-strengthening exercises and evaluate the need for ambulatory aids, such as crutches. If the patient can practice with these devices before surgery, learning how to ambulate after surgery is much easier.

For patients with AKAs or BKAs, teach range-of-motion (ROM) exercises for prevention of flexion contractures, particularly of the hip and knee. A trapeze and an overhead frame aid in strengthening the arms and allow the patient to move independently in bed. Teach the patient how to perform range-of-motion exercises. Be sure to turn the patient every 2 hours, or teach the patient to turn independently. Move the patient slowly to prevent muscle spasms (Pullen, 2010).

A firm mattress is essential for preventing contractures with a leg amputation. Assist the patient into a prone position every 3 to 4 hours for 20- to 30-minute periods if tolerated and not contraindicated. This position may be uncomfortable initially but helps prevent hip flexion contractures. Instruct the patient to pull the residual limb close to the other leg and contract the gluteal muscles of the buttocks for muscle strengthening. After staples are removed, the physical therapist may begin resistive exercises, which should also be done at home.

For above- and below-the-knee amputations, teach the patient how to push the residual limb down toward the bed while supporting it on a soft pillow at first. Then instruct him or her to continue this activity using a firmer pillow and then progress to a harder surface. This activity helps prepare the residual limb for prosthesis and reduces the incidence of phantom limb pain and sensation (Pullen, 2010).

Elevation of a lower-leg residual limb on a pillow while the patient is in a supine position is controversial. Some practitioners advocate avoiding this practice at all times because it promotes hip or knee flexion contracture. Others allow elevation for the first 24 to 48 hours to reduce swelling and subsequent discomfort. Inspect the residual limb daily to ensure that it lies completely flat on the bed.

Before an elective amputation, the patient often sees a certified prosthetist-orthotist (CPO) so that planning can begin for the postoperative period. Arrangements for replacing an arm part are especially important so that the patient can achieve self-management. Some patients are fitted with a temporary prosthesis at the time of surgery. Others, particularly older patients with vascular disease, are fitted after the residual limb has healed.

The patient being fitted for a leg prosthesis should bring a sturdy pair of shoes to the fitting. The prosthesis will be adjusted to that heel height.

Several devices help shape and shrink the residual limb in preparation for the prosthesis. Rigid, removable dressings are preferred because they decrease edema, protect and shape the limb, and allow easy access to the wound for inspection. The Jobst air splint, a plastic inflatable device, is sometimes used for this purpose. One of its disadvantages is air leakage and loss of compression. Wrapping with elastic bandages can also be effective in reducing edema, shrinking the limb, and holding the wound dressing in place.

For wrapping to be effective, reapply the bandages every 4 to 6 hours or more often if they become loose. *Figure-eight wrapping prevents restriction of blood flow. Decrease the tightness of the bandages while wrapping in a distal-to-proximal direction.* After wrapping, anchor the bandages to the highest joint, such as above the knee for BKAs (Fig. 51-13).

The design of and materials for prostheses have improved dramatically over the years. Computer-assisted design and manufacturing (CAD-CAM) is used for a custom fit. One of the most important developments in lower extremity prosthetics is the ankle-foot prosthesis, such as the Flex-Foot for more active amputees.

Promoting Body Image and Lifestyle Adaptation. The patient often experiences feelings of inadequacy as a result of losing a body part, especially the older adult who was in poor health before surgery and men who are often the main providers for their families. If possible, arrange for him or her to meet with a rehabilitated amputee who is about the same age as the patient.

Use of the word *stump* for referring to the remaining portion of the limb (residual limb) continues to be controversial. Patients have reported feeling as if they were part of a tree when the term was used. However, some rehabilitation specialists who routinely work with amputees believe the term is appropriate because it forces the patient to realize what has happened and promotes adjustment to the amputation. *Assess the patient to determine what term he or she prefers.*

Assess the patient's verbal and nonverbal references to the affected area. Some patients behave euphorically (extremely happy) and seem to have accepted the loss. *Do not jump to the conclusion that acceptance has occurred.* Ask the patient to describe his or her feelings about changes in body image and self-esteem. He or she may verbalize acceptance but refuse to look at the area during a dressing change. This inconsistent behavior is not unusual and should be documented and shared with other health care team members.

A patient who seems to adjust to the amputation during hospitalization may realize that it is difficult to cope with the

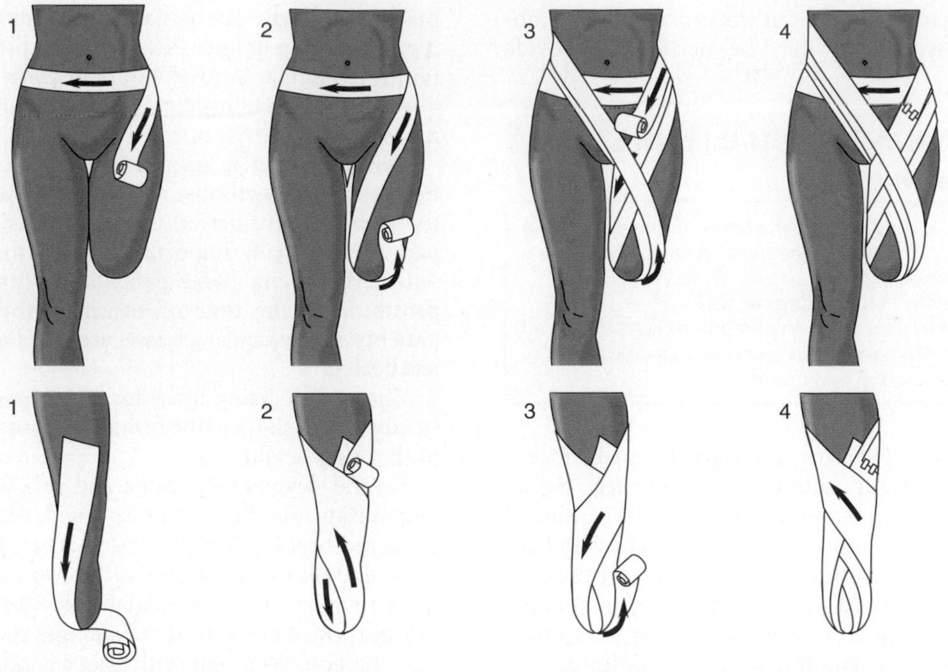

FIG. 51-13 A common method of wrapping an amputation stump. *Top,* Wrapping for above-knee amputation. *Bottom,* Wrapping for below-knee amputation.

loss after discharge from the hospital. Teach the patient and family about available resources and support from organizations such as the Amputee Coalition of America (ACA) (www.amputee-coalition.org) and the National Amputation Foundation (NAF) (www.nationalamputation.org). The NAF was originally started for veterans but has since expanded to offer services to civilians.

With advancements in prostheses and surgical techniques, most patients can return to their jobs and other activities. Professional athletes who use prostheses are often quite successful in sports. Patients with amputations ski, hike, golf, bowl, and participate in other physically demanding activities. Many amputees participate actively in organized and recreational sports.

If a job or career change is necessary, collaborate with a social worker or vocational rehabilitation specialist to evaluate the patient's skills. A supportive family or significant other is important for the adjustment to this change. The patient may also think that an intimate relationship is no longer possible because of physical changes. Discuss sexuality issues with the patient and his or her partner as needed. Professional assistance from a sex therapist, intimacy coach, or psychologist may be needed.

Help the patient and family set realistic desired outcomes and take one day at a time. Help them recognize personal strengths. If the desired outcomes are not realistic, frustration and disappointment may decrease motivation during rehabilitation. Basic principles of rehabilitation are discussed in Chapter 6.

Community-Based Care

The patient is discharged directly to home or to a skilled facility or rehabilitation facility, depending on the extent of the amputation. When rehabilitation is not feasible as in the debilitated or demented older adult, he or she may be discharged to a long-term care facility. Coordinate this transfer with the case manager or discharge planner to ensure continuity of care.

At home, the patient with a leg amputation needs to have enough room to use a wheelchair if the prosthesis is not yet available. He or she must be able to use toileting facilities and have access to areas necessary for self-management, such as the kitchen. Structural home modifications may be required before the patient goes home.

After the sutures or staples are removed, the patient begins residual limb care. A home care nurse may be needed to teach the patient and/or family how to care for the limb and the prosthesis if it is available (Chart 51-7). The limb should be rewrapped 3 times a day with an elastic bandage applied in a

CLINICAL JUDGMENT CHALLENGE

Patient-Centered Care; Teamwork and Collaboration; Informatics QSEN

A 45-year-old man attempted to remove excess grass from his electric lawn mower blades while the mower continued to run. As a result, he severed part of his right hand. The amputated hand parts are mangled and cannot be salvaged. His wife called 911, and he was admitted to the emergency department (ED). He rates his pain as a 9 on a 0-to-10 pain intensity scale on admission.

1. As his nurse, what is your priority action when assessing this patient?
2. What other assessments will you perform and document in the electronic medical record (EMR)?
3. A hand surgeon evaluates the patient and finds that he will require surgery to débride and close the wound. What preoperative teaching will the patient require?
4. His wife is very concerned that he will lose his job if he cannot return to work soon. What is your best response at this time?
5. With what members of the health care team will you consult and collaborate?

CHART 51-7 **Home Care Assessment**

The Patient with a Lower Extremity Amputation in the Home

- Assess the residual limb for:
  - Adequate circulation
  - Infection
  - Healing
  - Flexion contracture
  - Dressing/elastic wrap
- Assess the patient's ability to perform ADLs in the home.
- Evaluate the patient's ability to use ambulatory aids and to care for the prosthetic device (if available).
- Assess the patient's nutritional status.
- Assess the patient's ability to cope with body image change.

figure-eight manner (see Fig. 51-13). For many patients, a shrinker stocking or sock is easier to apply. After the limb is healed, it is cleaned each day with the rest of the body during bathing with soap and water. Teach the patient and/or family to inspect it every day for signs of inflammation or skin breakdown.

! NURSING SAFETY PRIORITY QSEN

Action Alert

Collaborate with the prosthetist to teach the patient about prosthesis care after amputation to ensure its reliability and proper function. These devices are custom made, taking into account the patient's level of amputation, lifestyle, and occupation. Proper teaching regarding correct cleansing of the socket and inserts, wearing the correct liners, assessing shoe wear, and a schedule of follow-up care is essential before discharge. This information may need to be reviewed by the home care nurse.

COMPLEX REGIONAL PAIN SYNDROME

❖ PATHOPHYSIOLOGY

Complex regional pain syndrome (**CRPS**), formerly called **reflex sympathetic dystrophy** (**RSD**), is a poorly understood dysfunction of the central and peripheral nervous systems that leads to severe, chronic PAIN. Genetic factors may play a role in the development of this devastating complication. CRPS most often results from fractures or other traumatic musculoskeletal injury and commonly occurs in the feet and hands. In some cases, specific nerve injuries are present, but in others, no injury can be identified. A triad of clinical manifestations is present, including abnormalities of the autonomic nervous system (changes in color, temperature, and sensitivity of skin over the affected area, excessive sweating, edema), motor symptoms (paresis, muscle spasms, loss of function), and SENSORY PERCEPTION symptoms (intense burning pain that becomes intractable [unrelenting]).

Over time, spotty and diffuse osteoporosis can be seen on x-ray examination. Timing of diagnosis is important because the syndrome is more difficult to treat when diagnosed in the later stages.

❖ PATIENT-CENTERED COLLABORATIVE CARE

The first priority of management is pain relief. Little research has been done to demonstrate the best practices for caring for a patient with CRPS (Hsu, 2009). Therefore a combination of interventions is used. Nurses play an important role in patient management, which includes drug therapy and a variety of nonpharmacologic modalities. Many classes of drugs may be used to manage the intense pain. These include topical analgesics, antiepileptic drugs, antidepressants, corticosteroids, bisphosphonates, and analgesics. Chapter 3 discusses pain management in detail.

In collaboration with the physical and occupational therapists, assist in maintaining adequate ROM and function. The skin of a patient with CRPS tends to alternate between warm, swollen, and red to cool, clammy, and bluish. Skin care needs to be gentle with minimal stimulation.

Peripheral or spinal cord neurostimulation using an external or internal implanted device delivers electrical pulses to block pain from getting to the brain where pain is perceived. The external or acupuncture method requires weekly sessions or a short-term continuous trial before the device is surgically implanted. Complications of implantable neurostimulators include spinal cord damage from hematoma or edema formation or other neurologic dysfunction.

A chemical sympathetic nerve block may be used. This procedure can be done by an IV infusion of phentolamine (Regitine), a drug that blocks sympathetic receptors, or by injecting an anesthetic agent next to the spine to block sympathetic nerves.

Minimally invasive surgical **sympathectomy**, or cutting of the sympathetic nerve branches via endoscopy through a small axillary incision, may be required. Topical skin adhesive is used to close the very small incision. The patient is discharged to home a few hours later with a follow-up examination the next day with the health care provider. Usual activities can resume a few days later.

Assist the patient in coping with CRPS because it often has a profound psychological effect. A referral for psychological counseling or psychotherapy may be indicated. The Reflex Sympathetic Dystrophy Syndrome Association (RSDSA) (www.rsds.org) and National Pain Association (www.nationalpainassociation.org) are available to help patients and their families organize or locate support groups and other resources.

? NCLEX EXAMINATION CHALLENGE

Physiological Integrity

The nurse is concerned that a client who had an ankle open reduction and internal fixation is at risk for complex regional pain syndrome. What assessment findings at the affected area are common when a client has this complication? **Select all that apply.**

A. Burning pain
B. Increase in sweating
C. Muscle weakness
D. Absent pedal pulse
E. Edema

KNEE INJURIES

In addition to the bone and muscle problems already discussed, trauma can cause cartilage, ligament, and tendon injury. Many musculoskeletal injuries are the result of playing sports (professional and recreational) or doing other strenuous physical activities. The popularity of all-terrain vehicles (ATVs) and skateboarding has increased injuries in younger patients. Sports

CHART 51-8 Best Practice for Patient Safety & Quality Care QSEN

Emergency Care of Patients with Sports-Related Injuries

- Do not move the victim until spinal cord injury is ascertained (see Chapter 43 for assessment of spinal cord injury).
- Rest the injured part; immobilize the joint above and below the injury by applying a splint if needed.
- Apply ice intermittently for the first 24 to 48 hours (heat may be used thereafter).
- Elevate the affected limb to decrease swelling.
- Use compression for the first 24 to 48 hours (e.g., elastic wrap).
- Always assume the area is fractured until x-ray studies are done.
- Assess neurovascular status in the area distal to the injury.

injuries have become so common that large metropolitan hospitals have sports medicine clinics and physicians who specialize in this field.

The principles of injury to one part of the body are similar to those of other sports injuries and accidents. For example, a tendon rupture in a knee is cared for in the same manner as a tendon rupture in the wrist. Chart 51-8 lists general emergency measures for sports-related injuries. All patients require frequent neurovascular monitoring.

Because the knee is most often injured, it is discussed as a typical example of other areas of the body. Trauma to the knee results in **internal derangement**, a broad term for disturbances of an injured knee joint. When surgery is required to resolve the problem, most surgeons prefer to perform the procedure through an arthroscope when possible. A description of arthroscopy is presented in Chapter 49.

Patellofemoral pain syndrome (PFPS) is the most common diagnosis in patients who have knee PAIN. It occurs most often in people who are runners or who overuse their knee joints. For that reason, it is sometimes referred to as "runner's knee." Patients with this problem describe pain as being behind or around their patella (knee cap) in one or both knees. Swelling is not common although stiffness may be present, especially when the knee is flexed. Management usually involves rest, physical therapy, bracing or splinting, and mild analgesics. For patients who have pain lasting for more than 12 months, arthroscopic surgery is performed.

The patient with a **torn meniscus** (medial or lateral) typically has pain, swelling, and tenderness in the knee. A clicking or snapping sound can often be heard when the knee is moved. For a locked knee resulting from the tear, the treatment may be manipulation followed by splinting or casting for 3 to 6 weeks. If the problem recurs, a partial or total **meniscectomy** is performed through an arthroscope as a same-day surgical procedure. As described in Chapter 49, an arthroscope is a metal tubular instrument used for examination or surgery of joints. One or more small incisions (less than ¼-inch [0.6-cm] long) are made in the knee for insertion of the arthroscope. The surgeon threads a cutting device through the arthroscope for removal of the torn cartilage while the knee is irrigated. The surgeon may use a laser during the procedure, depending on the type and severity of the injury. A bulky pressure dressing is applied after the procedure, and the affected leg is wrapped in elastic bandages.

As for any postoperative patient, check the surgical dressing for bleeding and monitor vital signs after the patient is admitted

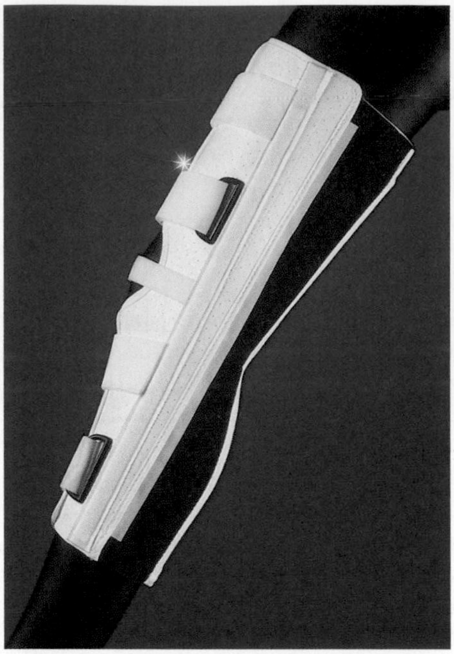

FIG. 51-14 A knee immobilizer.

to the same-day surgical unit. Perform neurovascular checks as outlined in Chart 51-3, usually every hour for the first few hours and then every 4 hours. Teach the patient and family what signs and symptoms to watch for after surgery and when to notify the health care provider.

The patient begins exercises immediately after surgery to strengthen the leg, prevent venous thromboembolism, and reduce swelling. Quadriceps setting, in which the patient straightens the leg while pushing the knee against the bed, is done in sets of 10 or more. Straight-leg raises are also performed. ROM exercises are usually not started for several days.

To prevent bending the affected knee, the health care provider often requests a knee immobilizer, such as the one shown in Fig. 51-14. Elevate the leg on one or two pillows according to the physician's preference, and apply ice to reduce postoperative swelling. Full weight bearing is restricted for several weeks, depending on the amount of cartilage removed. The patient is usually discharged from the hospital with crutches in less than 23 hours.

The cruciate and collateral ligaments in the knee are predisposed to injury, often from sports or vehicular crashes. The most common ligament injury is an *anterior cruciate ligament (ACL) tear*. Athletes often get these injuries during skiing, skating, or gymnastics. Women have ACL tears more often than men, possibly related to hormonal influences, biomechanical factors, and anatomic differences. Proper athletic shoes and learning how to land when jumping can help prevent this injury.

When the ACL is torn, the patient feels a snap and the knee gives way because of ACL laxity. Within hours, the knee is swollen, stiff, and painful. Examination by the health care provider shows positive ligament laxity. The diagnosis of an ACL tear is best confirmed by MRI (Pagana & Pagana, 2014).

Treatment may be nonsurgical or surgical, depending on the severity of the injury and the activity of the patient. Exercises, bracing, and limits on activities while the ligament heals may be sufficient. If medical management is not effective or the tear is severe, surgery may be needed.

The surgeon repairs the tear by reattaching the torn portions of the ligament through arthroscopy. The leg is placed in a brace or immobilizer. If the ligament cannot be repaired, reconstructive surgery may be performed with autologous grafts. A ligament from another part of the body is used to replace the torn knee ligament. Another option is artificial knee implants such as the GORE-TEX ligament.

Complete healing of knee ligaments after surgery can take 6 to 9 months or longer. These patients may use a continuous passive motion (CPM) machine at home. Teach the patient how to use and care for the machine. CPM use is discussed in Chapter 16 with the postoperative care of the patient who has had a total knee replacement.

CARPAL TUNNEL SYNDROME

❖ PATHOPHYSIOLOGY

Carpal tunnel syndrome (CTS) is a common condition in which the median nerve in the wrist becomes compressed, causing PAIN and numbness. The carpal tunnel is a rigid canal that lies between the carpal bones and a fibrous tissue sheet. A group of tendons surround the synovium and share space with the median nerve in the carpal tunnel. When the synovium becomes swollen or thickened, this nerve is compressed.

The median nerve supplies motor, sensory, and autonomic function for the first three fingers of the hand and the palmar aspect of the fourth (ring) finger. Because the median nerve is close to other structures, wrist flexion causes nerve impingement and extension causes increased pressure in the lower portion of the carpal tunnel.

CTS usually presents as a chronic problem. Acute cases are rare. Excessive hand exercise, edema or hemorrhage into the carpal tunnel, or thrombosis of the median artery can lead to acute CTS. *Patients with hand burns or a Colles' fracture of the wrist are particularly at risk for this problem.* In most cases, the cause may not result in nerve deficit for years.

CTS is also a common complication of certain metabolic and connective tissue diseases. For example, **synovitis** (inflammation of the synovium) occurs in patients with rheumatoid arthritis (RA). The hypertrophied synovium compresses the median nerve. In other chronic disorders such as diabetes mellitus, inadequate blood supply can cause median nerve neuropathy or dysfunction, resulting in CTS.

CTS is the most common type of **repetitive stress injury (RSI)**. RSIs are the fastest growing type of occupational injury. People whose jobs require repetitive hand activities such as pinching or grasping during wrist flexion (e.g., factory workers, computer operators, jackhammer operators) are predisposed to CTS. It can also result from overuse in sports activities such as golf, tennis, or racquetball.

In a few cases, CTS may be a familial or congenital problem that manifests in adulthood. Space-occupying growths such as ganglia, tophi, and lipomas can also result in nerve compression.

Women, especially those older than 50 years, are much more likely than men to experience CTS, probably due to the higher prevalence of diseases such as RA in women. The problem usually affects the dominant hand but can occur in both hands simultaneously. CTS is beginning to be found in children and adolescents as a result of the increased use of computers and handheld devices.

CHART 51-9 Best Practice for Patient Safety & Quality Care (QSEN)

Health Promotion Activities to Prevent Carpal Tunnel Syndrome

- Become familiar with federal and state laws regarding workplace requirements to prevent repetitive stress injuries such as carpal tunnel syndrome (CTS).
- When using equipment or computer workstations that can contribute to developing CTS, assess that they are ergonomically appropriate, including:
  - Specially designed wrist rest devices
  - Geometrically designed computer keyboards
  - Chair height that allows good posture
- Take regular short breaks away from activities that cause repetitive stress, such as working at computers.
- Stretch fingers and wrists frequently during work hours.
- Stay as relaxed as possible when using equipment that causes repetitive stress.

Health Promotion and Maintenance

Most businesses recognize the hazards of repetitive motion as a primary cause of occupational injury and disability. Both men and women in the labor force are experiencing increasing numbers of RSIs. Occupational health nurses have played an important role in ergonomic assessments and in the development of ergonomically designed furniture and various aids to decrease CTS and other musculoskeletal injuries.

U.S federal and state legislation has been passed to ensure that all businesses, including health care organizations (HCOs), provide *ergonomically appropriate workstations* for their employees (Occupational Safety and Health Administration [OSHA]). The Joint Commission also requires that hospitals and other HCOs provide a safe work environment for all staff. In Canada, each province requires the work setting to have joint health and safety committees in which employees are actively involved in setting safety standards (Canadian Centre for Occupational Health and Safety). Chart 51-9 lists best practices for preventing CTS in the health care setting.

❖ PATIENT-CENTERED COLLABORATIVE CARE

◆ Assessment

A medical diagnosis is often made based on the patient's history and report of hand pain and numbness and without further assessment. Ask about the nature, intensity, and location of the PAIN. Patients often state that the pain is worse at night as a result of flexion or direct pressure during sleep. The pain may radiate to the arm, shoulder and neck, or chest.

In addition to reports of numbness, patients with carpal tunnel syndrome (CTS) may also have **paresthesia** (painful tingling). *Sensory* changes usually occur weeks or months before *motor* manifestations.

The health care provider performs several tests for abnormal sensory findings. Phalen's wrist test, sometimes called **Phalen's maneuver**, produces paresthesia in the median nerve distribution (palmar side of the thumb, index and middle fingers, and half of the ring finger) within 60 seconds due to increased internal carpal pressure. The patient is asked to relax the wrist into flexion or to place the back of the hands together and flex both wrists at the same time. The Phalen's test is positive in most patients with CTS (Jarvis, 2016) (Fig. 51-15).

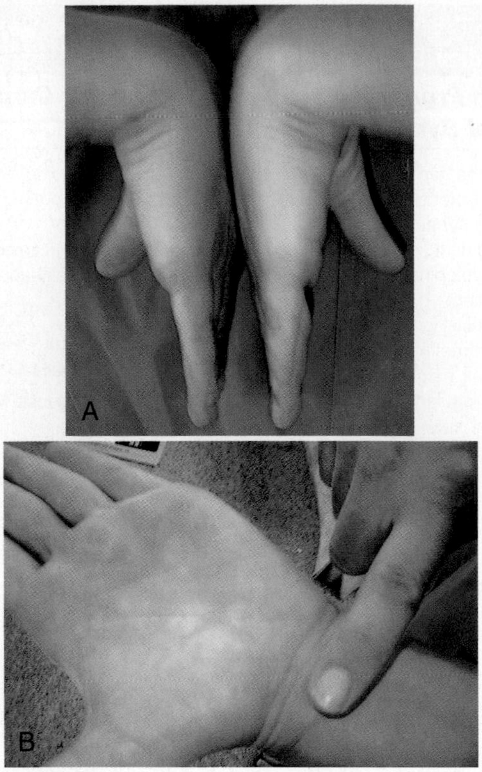

FIG. 51-15 Testing the patient for positive Phalen's sign (A) and Tinel's sign (B).

The same sensation can be created by tapping lightly over the area of the median nerve in the wrist (**Tinel's sign**). If the test is unsuccessful, a blood pressure cuff can be placed on the upper arm and inflated to the patient's systolic pressure (tourniquet). This often causes pain and tingling (Jarvis, 2016).

Motor changes in CTS begin with a weak pinch, clumsiness, and difficulty with fine movements. These changes progress to muscle weakness and wasting, which can impair self-management. If desired, test for pinching ability and ask the patient to perform a fine-movement task, such as threading a needle. Strenuous hand activity worsens the pain and numbness (McCance et al., 2014).

In addition to inspecting for muscle atrophy and task performance, observe the wrist for swelling. Gently palpate the area and note any unusual findings. Autonomic changes may be evidenced by skin discoloration, nail changes (e.g., brittleness), and increased or decreased hand sweating.

◆ Interventions

The health care provider uses conservative measures before surgical intervention. However, CTS can recur with either type of treatment. Management depends on the patient, but established best practices have not been determined (Uchiyama et al., 2010).

Nonsurgical Management. Aggressive drug therapy and immobilization of the wrist are the major components of nonsurgical management. Teach the patient the importance of these modalities in the hope of preventing surgical intervention.

NSAIDs are the most commonly prescribed drugs for the relief of PAIN and inflammation, if present. In addition to or instead of systemic medications, the physician may inject corticosteroids directly into the carpal tunnel. If the patient responds to the injection, several additional weekly or monthly injections are given. Teach him or her to take NSAIDs with or after meals to reduce gastric irritation.

A splint or hand brace may be used to immobilize the wrist during the day, during the night, or both. Many patients experience temporary relief with these devices. The occupational therapist places the wrist in the neutral position or in slight extension.

Laser or ultrasound therapy may also be helpful. Some patients report fewer symptoms after beginning yoga or other exercise routine.

Surgical Management. Surgery is necessary in about half of patients with CTS. Surgery can relieve the pressure on the median nerve by providing nerve decompression. Major surgical complications are rare after CTS surgery. In some cases, however, CTS recurs months to years after surgery.

The nurse in the physician's office or same-day surgical center reinforces the teaching provided by the surgeon regarding the nature of the surgery. Postoperative care is reviewed so the patient knows what to expect. Chapter 14 describes general preoperative care in detail.

Whatever the cause of nerve compression, the surgeon removes it either by cutting or by laser. The most common surgery is the endoscopic carpal tunnel release (ECTR). In this procedure, the surgeon makes a very small incision (less than ½ inch [1.2 cm]) through which the endoscope is inserted. The surgeon then uses special instruments to free the trapped median nerve. Although ECTR is less invasive and costs less than the open procedure, the patient may have a longer period of postoperative pain and numbness compared with recovery from open carpal tunnel release (OCTR). A recent systematic review showed that surgical treatment seems to be more effective than conservative measures over the long term. However, there was no evidence that one type of procedure, open or endoscopic, was more effective than the other (Huisstede et al., 2010).

After surgery, monitor vital signs and check the dressing carefully for drainage and tightness. If ECTR has been performed, the dressing is very small. The surgeon may require that the patient's affected hand and arm be elevated above heart level for several days to reduce postoperative swelling. Check the neurovascular status of the fingers every hour during the immediate postoperative period, and encourage the patient to move them frequently. Offer pain medication, and assure him or her that a prescription for analgesics will be provided before discharge.

Hand movements, including lifting heavy objects, may be restricted for 4 to 6 weeks after surgery. The patient can expect weakness and discomfort for weeks or perhaps months. Teach him or her to report any changes in neurovascular status, including increased PAIN, to the surgeon's office immediately (Huisstede et al., 2010).

Remind the patient and family that the surgical procedure might not be a cure. For instance, synovitis may recur with rheumatoid arthritis and may recompress the median nerve. Multiple surgeries and other treatments are common with CTS.

The patient may need assistance with self-management activities during recovery. Ensure that assistance in the home is available before discharge; this is usually provided by the family or significant others.

TENDINOPATHY AND JOINT DISLOCATION

Other injuries can affect any synovial joint. The nursing management of each of these is similar to the collaborative care previously discussed for knee injuries. One of the most common injuries seen in general and sports medicine is Achilles tendon–related injuries (tendinopathy). *Rupture of the Achilles tendon* is common in adults who participate in strenuous sports or in women who wear high heels regularly. It can also occur after taking fluoroquinolone antibiotics, such as levofloxacin (Levaquin) and ciprofloxacin (Cipro) (Barry, 2010).

In the older adult, quadriceps tendon rupture may occur from a fall down several steps. Most cases of Achilles tendinopathy can be treated with RICE (see Chart 51-8):

- **R**est
- **I**ce
- **C**ompression
- **E**levation

Some evidence supports the use of NSAIDs, and changes in activity and shoes may be helpful (Chang et al., 2010). Ultrasound treatments may also be effective.

For severe damage and as a last resort, the tendon is surgically repaired and the leg is immobilized in a cast or brace for at least 6 to 8 weeks. If the tendon is beyond repair, a **tendon transplant** (also known as *tendon reconstruction*) may be performed. A tendon is removed from one part of the body and transplanted to the affected area, or a cadaver donor is used.

Dislocation of a joint occurs when the ends of two or more bones are moved away from each other. If the dislocation is not complete, the joint is partially dislocated, or **subluxed**. It can occur in any diarthrodial (synovial) joint but is most common in the shoulder, hip, knee, and fingers. This injury is usually the result of trauma but can be congenital or pathologic and can result from joint disease, such as arthritis.

The typical manifestations of dislocation are:

- Pain
- Decreased mobility
- Alteration in contour of the joint
- Deviation in length of the extremity
- Rotation of the extremity

The health care provider performs a closed reduction of the joint and moves the joint surfaces back into their normal anatomic position. The patient requires light anesthetic or moderate sedation. The joint is immobilized by a cast, splint, brace, or immobilizer until healing occurs.

Recurrent dislocations are common in the knee and shoulder. For this problem, the joint may be fixed with wires or other device to prevent further displacement. A cast, splint, or traction is applied for 3 to 6 weeks.

STRAINS AND SPRAINS

A **strain** is excessive stretching of a muscle or tendon when it is weak or unstable. Strains are sometimes referred to as *muscle pulls*. Falls, lifting a heavy item, and exercise often cause this injury.

Strains are classified according to their severity:

- A first-degree (mild) strain causes mild inflammation but little bleeding. Swelling, ecchymosis (bruising), and tenderness are usually present.
- A second-degree (moderate) strain involves tearing of the muscle or tendon fibers without complete disruption. Muscle function may be impaired.
- A third-degree (severe) strain involves a ruptured muscle or tendon with separation of muscle from muscle, tendon from muscle, or tendon from bone. Severe pain and disability result from severe strains.

Management usually involves cold and heat applications, exercise, and activity limitations. The health care provider may prescribe anti-inflammatory drugs to decrease inflammation and pain. Muscle relaxants may also be used. In third-degree strains, surgical repair of the ruptured muscle or tendon may be needed.

A **sprain** is excessive stretching of a ligament. Twisting motions from a fall or sports activity typically cause the injury. Sprains are also classified according to severity. Pain and swelling result from ligament injuries. The treatment for *mild (first-degree)* sprains includes RICE (rest, ice, compression, elevation) (see Chart 51-8).

Second-degree sprains require immobilization, such as elastic bandage and an air stirrup ankle brace or splint, and partial weight bearing while the tear heals. For severe ligament damage (*third-degree* sprain), immobilization for 4 to 6 weeks is necessary. Arthroscopic surgery may be done, particularly for chronic joint instability.

ROTATOR CUFF INJURIES

The musculotendinous, or rotator, cuff of the shoulder functions to stabilize the head of the humerus in the glenoid cavity during shoulder abduction. Young adults usually sustain a tear of the cuff by substantial trauma, such as may occur during a fall, while throwing a ball, or with heavy lifting. Older adults tend to have small tears related to aging, repetitive motions, or falls, and the tears are usually painless.

The patient with a torn rotator cuff has shoulder PAIN and cannot easily abduct the arm at the shoulder. When the arm is abducted, he or she usually drops the arm because abduction cannot be maintained (drop arm test). Pain is more intense at night and with overhead activities. Partial-thickness tears are more painful that full-thickness tears, but full-thickness tears result in more weakness and loss of function. Muscle atrophy is commonly seen, and MOBILITY is reduced. Diagnosis is confirmed with x-rays, MRI, ultrasonography, and/or CT scans.

The health care provider usually treats the patient with partial-thickness tears conservatively with NSAIDs, intermittent steroid injections, physical therapy, and activity limitations while the tear heals. Physical therapy treatments may include ultrasound, electrical stimulation, ice, and heat (Smith & Smith, 2010).

For patients who do not respond to conservative treatment in 3 to 6 months or for those who have a complete (full-thickness) tear, the surgeon repairs the cuff using mini-open or arthroscopic procedures. An interscalene nerve block may be used to extend analgesia for an open repair (Guarin, 2013). If a peripheral nerve block is used, remind the patient that the arm will feel numb and cannot be moved for up to 20 or more hours after surgery. Observe, report, and document complications of respiratory distress and neurovascular compromise.

After surgery the affected arm is usually immobilized for several weeks. Pendulum exercises are started on the third or fourth postoperative day and progress to active exercises in about 2 weeks. Patients then begin rehabilitation in the ambulatory care occupational therapy department. Teach them that they may not have full function for several months.

NURSING CONCEPTS AND CLINICAL JUDGMENT REVIEW

What might you NOTICE if the patient has impaired MOBILITY and SENSORY PERCEPTION as a result of acute musculoskeletal trauma?

- Extremity swelling, bleeding, bruising, shortening, malalignment, and/or rotation
- Report of severe pain
- Break in skin integrity
- Report of decreased or unusual sensation in extremity
- Inability or decreased ability to move extremity
- Difficulty breathing (rib trauma)
- Severe kyphosis (compression fractures)

What should you INTERPRET and how should you RESPOND to a patient with impaired MOBILITY and SENSORY PERCEPTION as a result of acute musculoskeletal trauma?

Perform and interpret focused physical assessment findings, including:

- ABC (airway, breathing, circulation) ability (first action!)
- Pain intensity and quality
- Vital signs
- Neurovascular assessment ("circ check")

Respond by:

- First, establishing ABCs if problem exists
- If skin is not intact, covering wound with dry, sterile dressing, if available, using clean cloth as an option; applying pressure to proximal pulse if patient is bleeding; for traumatic amputation, applying direct pressure to the residual body part
- Implementing measures to prevent hypovolemic shock if patient is bleeding, including having patient lie flat, keeping him or her warm, and elevating the bleeding part
- Splinting the extremity (in community setting) to prevent movement and further damage
- If in hospital setting, assisting health care provider in splinting
- Providing pain control interventions by drug therapy as soon as possible
- Providing emotional assurance for the patient by being present and comforting

On what should you REFLECT?

- Monitor the patient's response to pain control interventions.
- Think about what else you could do to prevent complications.
- Determine what health teaching will be needed, depending on the treatment that is provided (e.g., surgery, cast).

GET READY FOR THE NCLEX® EXAMINATION!

KEY POINTS

Review these Key Points for each NCLEX Examination Client Needs Category.

Safe and Effective Care Environment

- Collaborate with physical and occupational therapists for care of patients with extremity fractures to improve MOBILITY and muscle strength. **Teamwork and Collaboration** QSEN
- Collaborate with the prosthetist, physical and occupational therapists, psychologist, and sex therapist or intimacy coach for care of patients with amputations to improve MOBILITY, muscle strength, ADLs, and self-image. **Teamwork and Collaboration** QSEN

Health Promotion and Maintenance

- Teach people to avoid musculoskeletal injury by treating or preventing osteoporosis (see Chapter 50), being cautious when walking to prevent a fall, wearing supportive shoes, avoiding dangerous sports or activities, and decreasing time spent doing repetitive stress activities, such as using a computer keyboard.
- Several community organizations, such as the Amputee Coalition of America, are available to help patients and their families cope with the loss of a body part.
- Teach patients and their family members and significant others how to care for casts or traction at home.
- Reinforce teaching for ambulating with crutches, walkers, or canes.
- Provide special care for older adults with hip fractures, including preventing heel pressure ulcers and promoting early ambulation to prevent complications of immobility.
- Teach exercises to patients with leg amputation to prevent hip flexion contractures.

Psychosocial Integrity

- Be aware that patients with severe musculoskeletal trauma may have a prolonged hospitalization and recovery period.
- For patients with severe trauma or amputation, assess coping skills and encourage verbalization. **Patient-Centered Care** QSEN
- Recognize that the patient having an amputation may need to adjust to an altered lifestyle; however, new custom prosthetics improve mobility.
- Help the patient with an amputation or other musculoskeletal trauma and family to set realistic expected outcomes and take one day at a time.

Physiological Integrity

- Be aware that open fractures cause a higher risk for infection than do closed fractures; use strict aseptic technique when providing wound management.
- Assess the risk for and implement interventions to prevent complications of immobility in patients having musculoskeletal injury or surgery (e.g., pressure ulcers, venous thromboembolism [VTE]).
- Assess patients with fractures for complications, such as VTE, INFECTION, and acute compartment syndrome.
- Recognize that fat embolism syndrome is different from pulmonary (blood clot) embolism as outlined in Chart 51-2.
- Provide emergency care of the patient with a fracture as described in Chart 51-4.

- Identify the patient at risk for acute compartment syndrome; loosen bandages, or request that the patient's cast be cut if neurovascular compromise is noted. **Evidence-Based Practice** QSEN
- As a priority, document neurovascular status frequently in patients with musculoskeletal injury, traction, or cast as described in Chart 51-3 and manage PAIN adequately. **Informatics** QSEN
- Provide evidence-based appropriate cast care, depending on the type of cast (plaster or synthetic); check for pressure necrosis under the cast by feeling for heat, assessing the patient's pain level, and smelling the cast for an unpleasant odor. **Evidence-Based Practice** QSEN
- Provide pin care for patients with skeletal traction or external fixation; assess for manifestations of INFECTION at the pin sites.
- Provide postoperative care for the patient having a fracture repair, including promoting MOBILITY and monitoring for complications of immobility.
- Provide care for patients having a vertebroplasty or kyphoplasty as described in Chart 51-6.
- Provide emergency care for a patient having a traumatic amputation in the community: Call 911, assess the patient for ABCs, apply direct pressure on the amputation site, and elevate the extremity above the patient's heart to decrease bleeding. For finger parts, wrap the amputated part with a clean cloth and place in a sealed bag, which is lowered into ice water. **Evidence-Based Practice** QSEN
- Observe for postoperative hemorrhage and INFECTION in the patient having an amputation.
- Postoperatively, assess for and promptly manage phantom limb PAIN in the patient who has an amputation; collaborate with specialists to incorporate complementary and alternative therapies and drug therapy into the patient's plan of care.
- Provide emergency care for patients with a sports-related injury as outlined in Chart 51-8.
- Recall that carpal tunnel syndrome (CTS) is the most common type of repetitive stress injury (RSI) caused by certain occupations such as computer operators and factory workers.
- Many acute musculoskeletal injuries are initially treated by RICE: rest, ice, compression, and elevation.
- The priority for managing complex regional pain syndrome (CRPS) is prompt and effective PAIN relief. Consult with PT, OT, and the pharmacist/pain specialist to determine the most effective pain management plan based on the patient's and family's preferences, values, and beliefs. **Patient-Centered Care** QSEN

CONCEPT OVERVIEW

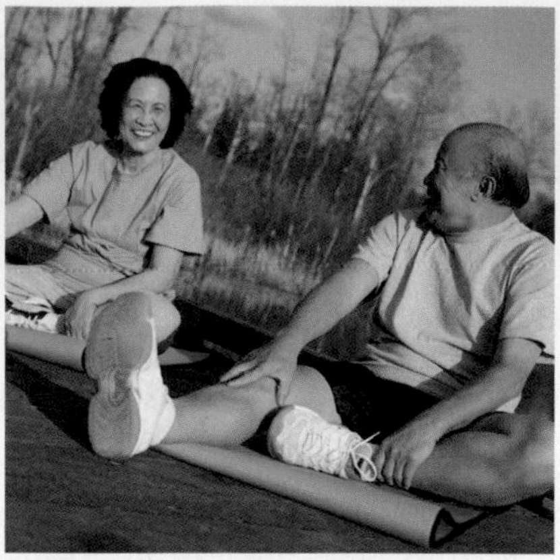

Metabolism

The word *metabolism* means to change or transform. Humans transform the energy stored within food into the types of energy needed to make the body work. Thus maintaining homeostasis of metabolism involves balancing the concepts of NUTRITION and ELIMINATION—in this instance, bowel elimination (Giddens, 2013).

As shown in Fig. 1, NUTRITION is complex and involves ingesting all of the macronutrients and micronutrients needed for optimal cellular metabolism (Giddens, 2013). As humans, we ingest many types of foods that contain proteins, carbohydrates, fats, vitamins, and minerals. Once inside the GI tract, the processes of digestion break down food into its basic elements, which then are absorbed into the blood and delivered to cells. Through metabolism, cells convert these basic elements into chemical energy, mostly adenosine triphosphate (ATP). Different cells then use metabolism to further transform ATP into heat energy, mechanical energy, chemical energy, and electrical energy. The transformation of chemical energy into other types of energy within the human body is *irreversible.* It is lost from the body in the form of heat and work. Thus bringing food into the body on a daily basis is important in meeting the human needs of nutrition and metabolism.

Heat energy helps maintain the core body temperature at or near 98.6° F—the ideal temperature for important physiologic reactions. When environmental temperatures are low, more NUTRITION intake is needed to maintain body temperature. When environmental temperatures are high, less food is needed to maintain body temperature. Therefore, in general, more calories need to be consumed per day in the winter than in the summer.

Mechanical energy is used for cell and tissue movement, cell shape changes, and whole body movement. *Electrical energy* generates the action potentials that allow nerves to transmit impulses and muscles to contract. *Chemical energy* is used to drive every chemical reaction in the body. As long as it remains alive, the body continuously needs to change food into these different energies.

Bowel ELIMINATION is the excretion of waste products so that the body rids itself of those food components that cannot be absorbed into the blood and converted into energy, such as fiber and cellulose (Giddens, 2013). If these components remained in the GI tract, they would soon fill it to the point that no nutrients could be ingested.

Consider Fig. 1 as representing the entire NUTRITION, metabolism, and bowel ELIMINATION of a person throughout his or her lifetime. The energy ingested in the form of food exactly matches the energy transformed by metabolism and is used for all the different types of internal and external "work" of the body. When this ideal situation exists, the person always has the right amount of nutrients and neither stores excess nutrients nor breaks down body tissues to use for energy.

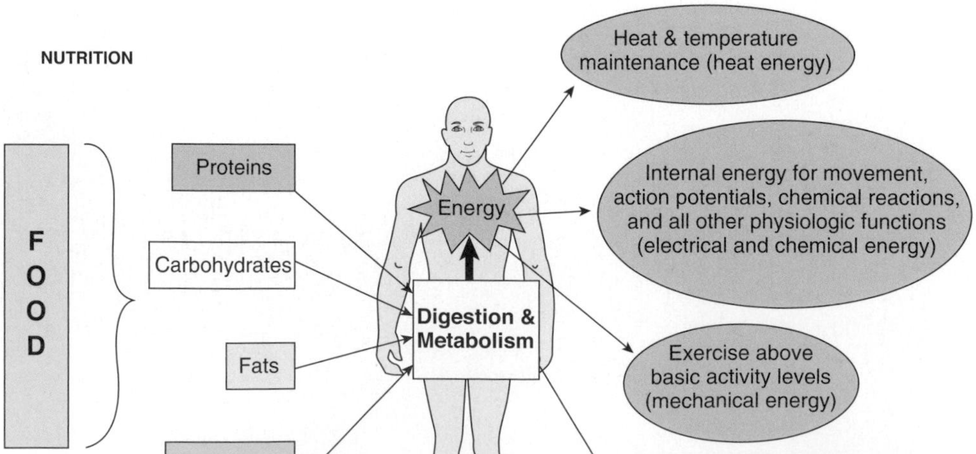

FIG. 1

In Fig. 2, the person is not ingesting enough nutrients to meet metabolic energy needs. As a result, the different types of work are less efficient and the person metabolizes his or her own body tissues to provide needed energy. If this situation continues, it will lead to death.

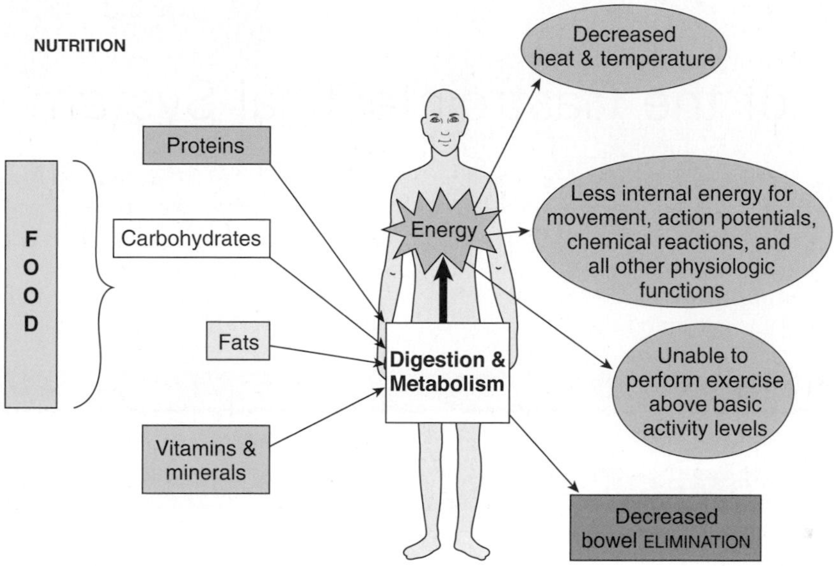

FIG. 2

In Fig. 3, the person's NUTRITION intake is greater than is needed to meet energy needs. As a result, these extra energy compounds are converted first into glycogen and eventually into fat. Although fat represents stored energy, excessive fat can harm the body. Thus excessive NUTRITION is not necessarily adequate or healthy and does not represent a balanced metabolic state. In addition, when NUTRITION is excessive, metabolism and work energies are not increased. Only heat and bowel ELIMINATION increase.

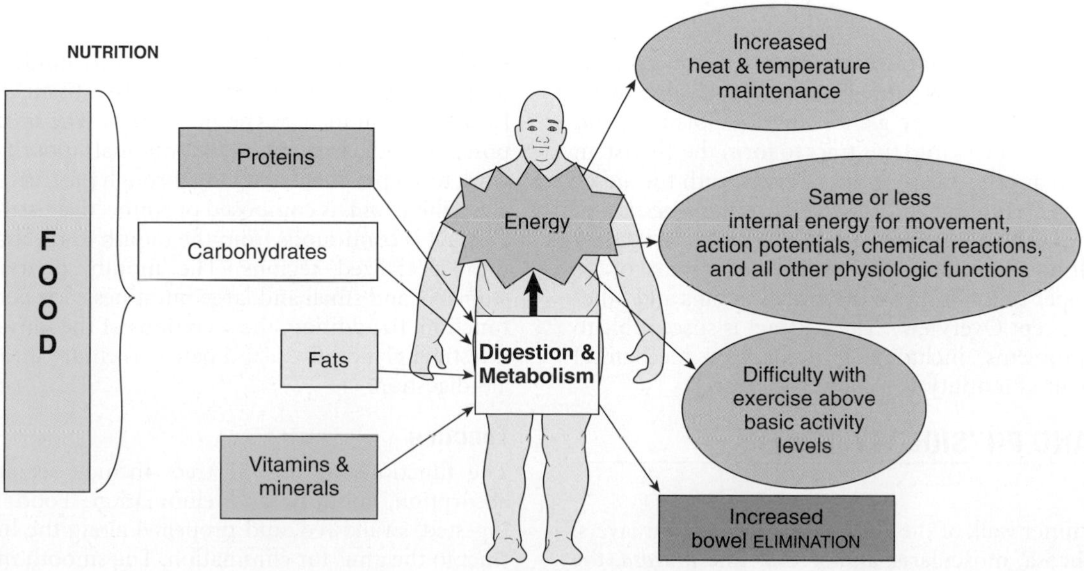

FIG. 3

52 CHAPTER

Assessment of the Gastrointestinal System

Donna D. Ignatavicius

http://evolve.elsevier.com/Iggy/

PRIORITY CONCEPTS

- NUTRITION
- ELIMINATION

LEARNING OUTCOMES

Safe and Effective Care Environment

1. Assess patients for complications of esophagogastroduodenoscopy (EGD).

Health Promotion and Maintenance

2. Identify factors that place patients at risk for GI problems.
3. Teach pre-test and post-test care for diagnostic GI testing to patients and families to promote safety and comfort.

Psychosocial Integrity

4. Identify common psychological responses to GI health problems and diagnostic testing.

Physiological Integrity

5. Briefly review the anatomy and physiology of the GI system.
6. Describe NUTRITION and ELIMINATION changes associated with aging.
7. Perform focused physical assessment for patients with suspected or actual GI health problems.
8. Explain and interpret common laboratory tests for a patient with a GI health problem.
9. Describe care for patients having selected GI diagnostic tests.

The GI system includes the GI tract (alimentary canal), consisting of the mouth, esophagus, stomach, small and large intestines, and rectum. The salivary glands, liver, gallbladder, and pancreas secrete substances into this tract to form the GI system (Fig. 52-1). The main functions of the GI tract, with the aid of organs such as the pancreas and the liver, are the *digestion* of food to meet the body's *nutritional* needs and the ELIMINATION of waste resulting from digestion. Adequate NUTRITION is required for proper functioning of the body's organs and other cells (see the Concept Overview). The GI tract is susceptible to many health problems, including structural or mechanical alterations, impaired motility, infection, and cancer.

ANATOMY AND PHYSIOLOGY REVIEW

Structure

The **lumen**, or inner wall, of the GI tract consists of four layers: mucosa, submucosa, muscularis, and serosa. The *mucosa,* the innermost layer, includes a thin layer of smooth muscle and specialized exocrine gland cells. It is surrounded by the *submucosa,* which is made up of connective tissue. The *submucosa* layer is surrounded by the muscularis. The *muscularis* is composed of both circular and longitudinal smooth muscles, which work to keep contents moving through the tract. The outermost layer, the *serosa,* is composed of connective tissue. Although the GI tract is continuous from the mouth to the anus, it is divided into specialized regions. The mouth, pharynx, esophagus, stomach, and small and large intestines each perform a specific function. In addition, the secretions of the salivary, gastric, and intestinal glands; liver; and pancreas empty into the GI tract to aid digestion.

Function

The functions of the GI tract include secretion, digestion, absorption, motility, and elimination. Food and fluids are ingested, swallowed, and propelled along the lumen of the GI tract to the anus for elimination. The smooth muscles contract to move food from the mouth to the anus. Before food can be

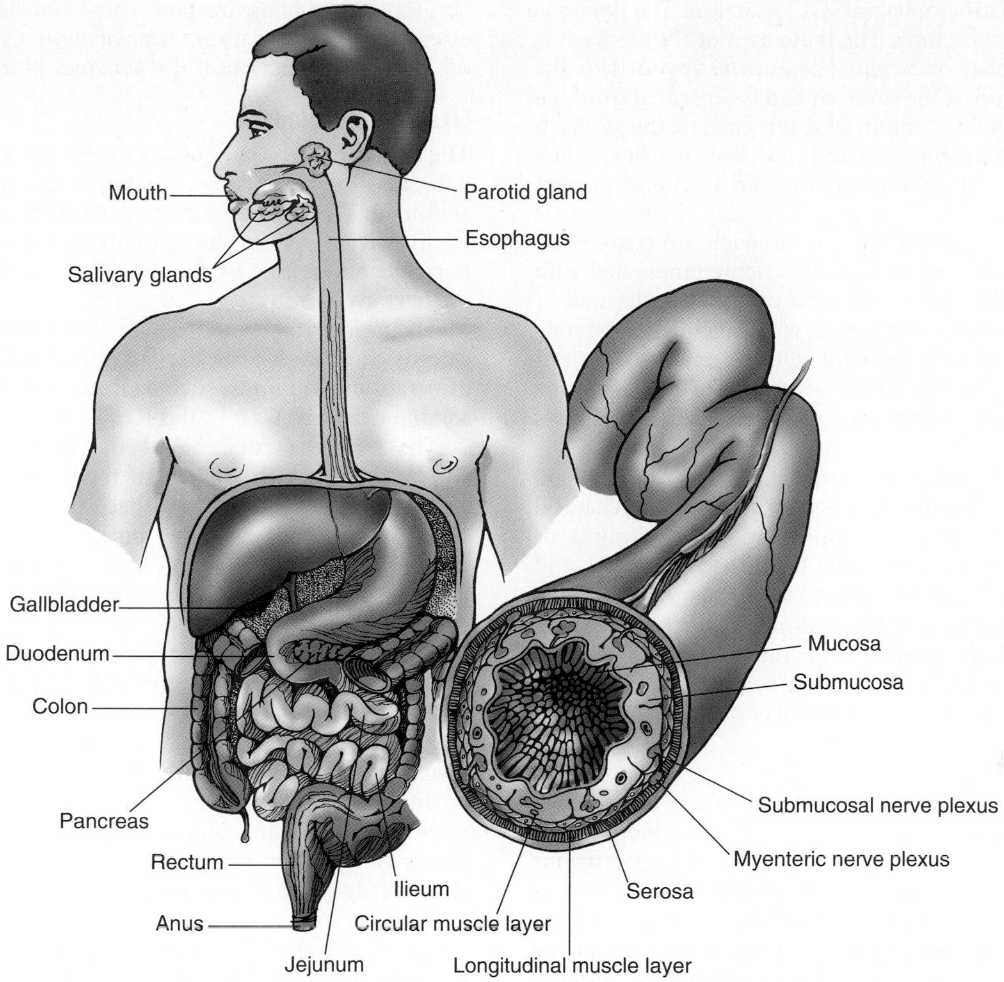

FIG. 52-1 The gastrointestinal system (GI tract) can be thought of as a tube (with necessary structures) extending from the mouth to the anus for a 25-foot length. The structure of this tube *(shown enlarged)* is basically the same throughout its length.

absorbed, it must be broken down to a liquid, called **chyme**. **Digestion** is the mechanical and chemical process in which complex foodstuffs are broken down into simpler forms that can be used by the body. During digestion, the stomach secretes hydrochloric acid, the liver secretes bile, and digestive enzymes are released from accessory organs, aiding in food breakdown. After the digestive process is complete, absorption takes place. **Absorption** is carried out as the nutrients produced by digestion move from the lumen of the GI tract into the body's circulatory system for uptake by individual cells (Jarvis, 2016).

Oral Cavity

The oral cavity (mouth) includes the buccal mucosa, lips, tongue, hard palate, soft palate, teeth, and salivary glands. The buccal mucosa is the mucous membrane lining the inside of the mouth. The tongue is involved in speech, taste, and **mastication** (chewing). Small projections called *papillae* cover the tongue and provide a roughened surface, permitting the movement of food in the mouth during chewing. The hard palate and the soft palate together form the roof of the mouth.

Adults have 32 permanent teeth: 16 each in upper and lower arches. The different types of teeth function to prepare food for digestion by cutting, tearing, crushing, or grinding the food. Swallowing begins after food is taken into the mouth and chewed. Saliva is secreted in response to the presence of food in the mouth and begins to soften the food. Saliva contains mucin and an enzyme called *salivary amylase* (also known as *ptyalin*), which begins the breakdown of carbohydrates.

Esophagus

The esophagus is a muscular canal that extends from the pharynx (throat) to the stomach and passes through the center of the diaphragm. Its primary function is to move food and fluids from the pharynx to the stomach. At the upper end of the esophagus is a sphincter referred to as the **upper esophageal sphincter (UES)**. When at rest, the UES is closed to prevent air into the esophagus during respiration. The portion of the esophagus just above the gastroesophageal (GE) junction is referred to as the **lower esophageal sphincter (LES)**. When at rest, the LES is normally closed to prevent reflux of gastric contents into the esophagus. If the LES does not work properly, gastroesophageal reflux disease (GERD) can develop (see Chapter 54).

Stomach

The stomach is located in the midline and left upper quadrant (LUQ) of the abdomen and has four anatomic regions (McCance et al., 2014). The *cardia* is the narrow portion of the stomach that is below the gastroesophageal (GE) junction. The *fundus* is the area nearest to the cardia. The main area of the stomach is referred to as the *body* or *corpus.* The *antrum* (pylorus) is the distal (lower) portion of the stomach and is separated from the duodenum by the pyloric sphincter. Both ends of the stomach are guarded by sphincters (cardiac [LES] and pyloric), which aid in the transport of food through the GI tract and prevent backflow.

Smooth muscle cells that line the stomach are responsible for gastric motility. The stomach is also richly innervated with intrinsic and extrinsic nerves. **Parietal cells** lining the wall of the stomach secrete hydrochloric acid, whereas chief cells secrete pepsinogen (a precursor to pepsin, a digestive enzyme). Parietal cells also produce **intrinsic factor**, a substance that aids in the absorption of vitamin B_{12}. Absence of the intrinsic factor causes pernicious anemia.

After ingestion of food, the stomach functions as a food reservoir where the digestive process begins, using mechanical movements and chemical secretions. The stomach mixes or churns the food, breaking apart the large food molecules and mixing them with gastric secretions to form chyme, which then empties into the duodenum. The *intestinal phase* begins as the chyme passes from the stomach into the duodenum, causing distention. It is assisted by secretin, a hormone that inhibits further acid production and decreases gastric motility.

Pancreas

The pancreas is a fish-shaped gland that lies behind the stomach and extends horizontally from the duodenal C-loop to the spleen (Jarvis, 2016). The pancreas is divided into portions known as the *head,* the *body,* and the *tail* (Fig. 52-2).

Two major cellular bodies (exocrine and endocrine) within the pancreas have separate functions. The *exocrine* part consists of cells that secrete enzymes needed for digestion of carbohydrates, fats, and proteins (trypsin, chymotrypsin, amylase, and lipase). The *endocrine* part of the pancreas is made up of the islets of Langerhans, with alpha cells producing glucagon and beta cells producing insulin. These hormones produced are essential in the regulation of *metabolism.* Chapter 64 describes the endocrine function of the pancreas in detail.

Liver and Gallbladder

The *liver* is the largest organ in the body (other than skin) and is located mainly in the right upper quadrant (RUQ) of the abdomen. The right and left hepatic ducts transport bile from the liver. It receives its blood supply from the hepatic artery and portal vein, resulting in about 1500 mL of blood flow through the liver every minute.

The *liver* performs more than 400 functions in three major categories: storage, protection, and metabolism. It *stores* many minerals and vitamins, such as iron, magnesium, and the fat-soluble vitamins A, D, E, and K.

The *protective* function of the liver involves phagocytic **Kupffer cells**, which are part of the body's reticuloendothelial system. They engulf harmful bacteria and anemic red blood cells. The liver also detoxifies potentially harmful compounds (e.g., drugs, chemicals, alcohol). Therefore the risk for drug toxicity increases with aging because of decreased liver function.

The liver functions in the *metabolism* of proteins considered vital for human survival. It breaks down amino acids to remove ammonia, which is then converted to urea and is excreted via the kidneys (McCance et al., 2014). In addition, it synthesizes several plasma proteins, including albumin, prothrombin, and fibrinogen. The liver's role in carbohydrate metabolism involves storing and releasing glycogen as the body's energy requirements change. The organ also synthesizes, breaks down, and temporarily stores fatty acids and triglycerides.

The liver forms and continually secretes bile, which is essential for the breakdown of fat. The secretion of bile increases in response to gastrin, secretin, and cholecystokinin. Bile is secreted into small ducts that empty into the common bile duct and into the duodenum at the sphincter of Oddi. However, if the sphincter is closed, the bile goes to the gallbladder for storage.

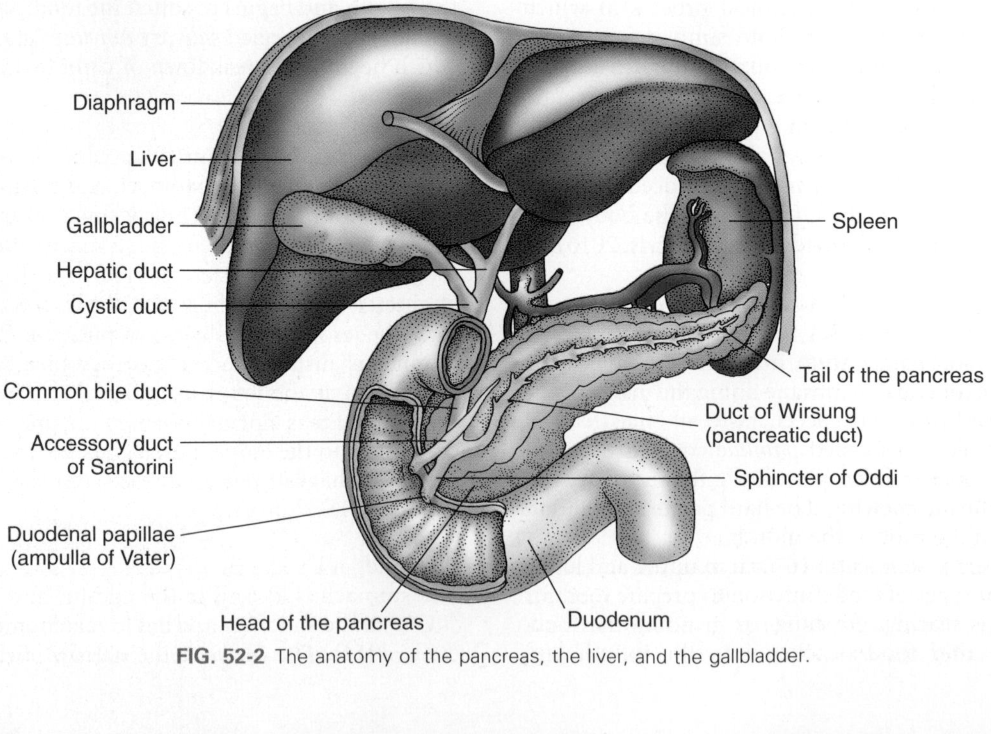

FIG. 52-2 The anatomy of the pancreas, the liver, and the gallbladder.

The *gallbladder* is a pear-shaped, bulbous sac that is located underneath the liver. It is drained by the cystic duct, which joins with the hepatic duct from the liver to form the common bile duct (CBD). The gallbladder collects, concentrates, and stores the bile that has come from the liver. It releases the bile into the duodenum via the CBD when fat is present.

Small Intestine

The small intestine is the longest and most convoluted portion of the digestive tract, measuring 16 to 19 feet (5 to 6 m) in length in an adult. It is composed of three different regions: duodenum, jejunum, and ileum. The *duodenum* is the first 12 inches (30 cm) of the small intestine and is attached to the distal end of the pylorus. The common bile duct and pancreatic duct join to form the ampulla of Vater, emptying into the duodenum at the duodenal papilla. This papillary opening is surrounded by muscle known as the **sphincter of Oddi**. The 8-foot (2.5-m) portion of the small intestine that follows the sphincter of Oddi is the *jejunum*. The last 8 to 12 feet (2.5 to 4 m) of the small intestine is called the *ileum*. The ileocecal valve separates the entrance of the ileum from the cecum of the large intestine (McCance et al., 2014).

The inner surface of the small intestine has a velvety appearance because of numerous mucous membrane fingerlike projections. These projections are called *intestinal villi*. In addition to the intestinal villi, the small intestine has circular folds of mucosa and submucosa, which increase the surface area for digestion and absorption.

The small intestine has three main *functions:* movement (mixing and peristalsis), digestion, and absorption. Because the intestinal villi increase the surface area of the small intestine, it is the major organ of absorption of the digestive system. The small intestine mixes and transports the chyme to mix with many digestive enzymes. It takes an average of 3 to 10 hours for the contents to be passed by peristalsis through the small intestine. Intestinal enzymes aid in the digestion of proteins, carbohydrates, and lipids.

Large Intestine

The large intestine extends about 5 to 6 feet in length from the ileocecal valve to the anus and is lined with columnar epithelium that has absorptive and mucous cells. It begins with the *cecum*, a dilated, pouchlike structure that is inferior to the ileocecal opening. At the base of the cecum is the vermiform appendix, which has no known digestive function. The large intestine then extends upward from the cecum as the colon. The colon consists of four divisions: ascending colon, transverse colon, descending colon, and sigmoid colon (McCance et al., 2014). The sigmoid colon empties into the rectum.

Following the sigmoid colon, the large intestine bends downward to form the rectum. The last 1 to 1½ inches (3 to 4 cm) of the large intestine is called the *anal canal*, which opens to the exterior of the body through the anus. Sphincter muscles surround the anal canal.

The large intestine's *functions* are movement, absorption, and ELIMINATION. Movement in the large intestine consists mainly of segmental contractions, like those in the small intestine, to allow enough time for the absorption of water and electrolytes. In addition, peristaltic contractions are triggered by colonic distention to move the contents toward the rectum, where the material is stored until the urge to defecate occurs. Absorption of water and some electrolytes occurs in the large intestine to reduce the fluid volume of the chyme. This process creates a more solid material, the feces, for elimination.

GASTROINTESTINAL CHANGES ASSOCIATED WITH AGING

Physiologic changes occur in the GI system as people age, especially ages 65 years and older. Changes in digestion and ELIMINATION that can affect NUTRITION are common (McCance et al., 2014). For example, decreased gastric hydrochloric acid (HCl) can lead to decreased absorption of essential minerals like iron. Chart 52-1 lists common GI changes and nursing implications when caring for older adults.

ASSESSMENT METHODS

Patient History

The purpose of the health history is to determine the events related to the current health problem (Chart 52-2). Focus questions about changes in appetite, weight, and stool. Determine the patient's pain experience.

Collect data about the patient's age, gender, and culture. This information can be helpful in assessing who is likely to have particular GI system disorders. For instance, older adults are more at risk for stomach cancer than are younger adults. Younger adults are more at risk for inflammatory bowel disease (IBD). The exact reasons for these differences continue to be studied.

Question the patient about previous GI disorders or abdominal surgeries. Ask about prescription medications being taken, including how much, when the drugs are taken, and why they have been prescribed. Inquire if the patient takes over-the-counter (OTC) drugs, herbs, and/or supplements. In particular, ask whether aspirin, NSAIDs (e.g., ibuprofen), laxatives, herbal preparations, or enemas are routinely taken. Large amounts of aspirin or NSAIDs can predispose the patient to peptic ulcer disease and GI bleeding. Long-term use of laxatives or enemas can cause dependence and result in constipation and electrolyte imbalance. Some herbal preparations, especially ayurvedic herbs, can affect appetite, absorption, and ELIMINATION. Determine if the patient smokes or has ever smoked cigarettes, cigars, or pipes. Smoking is a major risk factor for most GI cancers. Chewing tobacco is a major cause of oral cancer.

Finally, investigate the patient's travel history. Ask whether he or she has traveled outside of the country recently. This information may provide clues about the cause of symptoms like diarrhea.

Nutrition History

A NUTRITION history is important when assessing GI system function. Many conditions manifest themselves as a result of alterations in intake and absorption of nutrients. The purpose of a nutritional assessment is to gather information about how well the patient's needs are being met. Inquire about any special diet and whether there are any known food allergies. Ask the patient to describe the usual foods that are eaten daily and the times that meals are taken.

Health problems can also affect NUTRITION, so explore any changes that have occurred in eating habits as a result of illness. **Anorexia** (loss of appetite for food) can occur with GI disease. Assess changes in taste and any difficulty or pain with swallowing (dysphagia) that could be associated with esophageal

CHART 52-1 **Nursing Focus on the Older Adult**

Changes in the Gastrointestinal System Related to Aging

PHYSIOLOGIC CHANGE	DISORDERS RELATED TO CHANGE	NURSING INTERVENTIONS	RATIONALES
Stomach			
Atrophy of the gastric mucosa is characterized by a decrease in the ratio of gastrin-secreting cells to somatostatin-secreting cells. This change leads to decreased hydrochloric acid levels (hypochlorhydria).	Decreased hydrochloric acid levels lead to decreased absorption of iron and vitamin B_{12} and to proliferation of bacteria. Atrophic gastritis occurs as a consequence of bacterial overgrowth.	Encourage bland foods high in vitamins and iron. Assess for epigastric pain.	Bland foods help prevent gastritis. Assessment helps detect gastritis.
Large Intestine			
Peristalsis decreases, and nerve impulses are dulled.	Decreased sensation to defecate can result in postponement of bowel movements, which leads to constipation and impaction.	Encourage a high-fiber diet and 1500 mL of fluid intake daily (if not contraindicated). Encourage as much activity as tolerated.	These interventions increase the sensation of needing to defecate.
Pancreas			
Distention and dilation of pancreatic ducts change. Calcification of pancreatic vessels occurs with a decrease in lipase production.	Decreased lipase level results in decreased fat absorption and digestion. Steatorrhea, or excess fat in the feces, occurs because of decreased fat digestion.	Encourage small, frequent feedings. Assess for diarrhea.	Small, frequent feedings help prevent steatorrhea. Diarrhea may be steatorrhea. Excessive diarrhea can lead to dehydration.
Liver			
A decrease in the number and size of hepatic cells leads to decreased liver weight and mass. This change and an increase in fibrous tissue lead to decreased protein synthesis and changes in liver enzymes. Enzyme activity and cholesterol synthesis are diminished.	Decreased enzyme activity depresses drug metabolism, which leads to accumulation of drugs—possibly to toxic levels.	Assess for adverse effects of all drugs.	Assessment can help detect drug toxicity.

CHART 52-2 **Best Practice for Patient Safety and Quality Care** QSEN

Questions for Gastrointestinal Health History

- What is your typical daily food intake? Do you take any supplements? If so, what are they?
- How is your appetite? Any recent change?
- Have you lost or gained weight recently? If so, was the weight loss or gain intentional?
- Are you on a special diet?
- Do you have any difficulty chewing or swallowing?
- Do you wear dentures? How well do they fit?
- Do you ever experience indigestion or "heartburn"? How often? What seems to cause it? What helps it?
- Have you had any GI disorders or surgeries? If so, what are they?
- Is there a family history of GI health problems?
- What medications are you taking? Be sure to include prescription and over-the-counter (OTC) drugs.
- Do you smoke or have you ever smoked? Do you chew or have you ever chewed tobacco?
- Do you drink alcoholic beverages? If so, how many each week?
- Do you have pain, diarrhea, gas, or any other problems? Do any specific foods cause the problem?
- Have you traveled out of the country recently? If so, where?
- What is your usual bowel elimination pattern? Frequency? Character? Discomfort? Laxatives?
- Do you have any pain or bleeding associated with bowel movements?
- Have you experienced any changes in your usual bowel pattern or stool?
- Have you ever had an endoscopy or a colonoscopy?

CULTURAL CONSIDERATIONS

Patient-Centered Care QSEN

Cultural and religious patterns are important in obtaining a complete nutritional history. Ask if certain foods pose a problem for the patient. For example, the spices or hot pepper used in cooking in many cultures can aggravate or precipitate GI tract symptoms such as indigestion. Note religious patterns such as fasting or abstinence.

Many black people are lactose intolerant. A much smaller percentage of white people also have this problem. Lactose intolerance causes bloating, cramping, and diarrhea as a result of lack of the enzyme *lactase* (McCance et al., 2014). Lactase is needed to convert lactose in milk and other dairy products to glucose and galactose.

disorders. Also ask if abdominal pain or discomfort occurs with eating and whether the patient has experienced any nausea, vomiting, or **dyspepsia** (indigestion or heartburn). Unknown food allergies often cause these symptoms. Inquire about any unintentional weight loss, because some cancers of the GI tract may present in this manner. Assess for alcohol and caffeine consumption, because both substances are associated with many GI disorders, such as gastritis and peptic ulcer disease.

The patient's socioeconomic status may have a profound impact on his or her NUTRITION. For example, people who have limited budgets, such as some older adults or the unemployed, may not be able to purchase foods required for a balanced diet.

In addition, they may substitute less expensive and perhaps less effective OTC medications or herbs for prescription drugs. Necessary medical care may be delayed, and patients may not seek health care until conditions are well advanced.

Family History and Genetic Risk

Ask about a family history of GI disorders. Some GI health problems have a genetic predisposition. For example, familial adenomatous polyposis (FAP) is an inherited autosomal dominant disorder that predisposes the patient to colon cancer (McCance et al., 2014). Specific genetic risks are discussed with the GI problems in later chapters.

Current Health Problems

Because GI clinical manifestations are often vague and difficult for the patient to describe, it is important to obtain a chronologic account of the current problem, symptoms, and any treatments taken. Furthermore, ask about the location, quality, quantity, timing (onset, duration), and factors that may aggravate or alleviate each symptom (see Chart 52-2).

For example, a change in bowel habits is a common assessment finding. Obtain this information from the patient:

- Pattern of bowel movements
- Color and consistency of the feces
- Occurrence of diarrhea or constipation
- Effective action taken to relieve diarrhea or constipation
- Presence of frank blood or tarry stools
- Presence of abdominal distention or gas

An unintentional weight gain or loss is another symptom that needs further investigation. Assess the patient's:

- Normal weight
- Weight gain or loss
- Period of time for weight change
- Changes in appetite or oral intake

Pain is a common concern of patients with GI tract disorders. The mnemonic PQRST may be helpful in organizing the current problem assessment (Jarvis, 2016):

P: Precipitating or palliative. What brings it on? What makes it better? Worse? When did you first notice it?

Q: Quality or quantity. How does it look, feel, or sound? How intense/severe is it?

R: Region or radiation. Where is it? Does it spread anywhere?

S: Severity scale. How bad is it (on a scale of 0 to 10)? Is it getting better, worse, or staying the same?

T: Timing. Onset—Exactly when did it first occur? Duration—How long did it last? Frequency—How often does it occur?

Abdominal pain is often vague and difficult to evaluate. Ask the patient to describe the type of pain, such as burning, gnawing, or stabbing. The location of the pain can be determined by asking him or her to point to the involved site. Ask about the relationship of food intake to the onset or worsening of pain. For example, a high-fat meal may cause gallbladder pain.

Changes in the skin may result from several GI tract disorders, such as liver and biliary system obstruction. Ask about whether these clinical manifestations have occurred, or assess whether they are present:

- Skin discolorations or rashes
- Itching
- Jaundice (yellowing of skin caused by bilirubin pigments)
- Increased bruising
- Increased tendency to bleed

Physical Assessment

Physical assessment involves a comprehensive examination of the patient's nutritional status, mouth, and abdomen. Nutritional assessment is discussed in detail in Chapter 60. Oral assessment is described in Chapter 53.

In preparation for examination of the *abdomen,* ask the patient to empty his or her bladder and then to lie in a supine position with knees bent, keeping the arms at the sides to prevent tensing of the abdominal muscles.

The abdominal examination usually begins at the patient's right side and proceeds in a systematic fashion (Fig. 52-3):

- Right upper quadrant (RUQ)
- Left upper quadrant (LUQ)
- Left lower quadrant (LLQ)
- Right lower quadrant (RLQ)

Table 52-1 lists the organs that lie in each of these areas.

If areas of pain or discomfort are noted from the history, this area is examined last in the examination sequence. This sequence should prevent the patient from tensing abdominal muscles because of the pain, which would make the examination difficult. Examine any area of tenderness cautiously, and instruct the patient to state whether it is too painful. Observe his or her face for signs of distress or pain.

The abdomen is assessed by using the four techniques of examination, but in a sequence different from that used for other body systems: inspection, auscultation, percussion, and then palpation. This sequence is preferred so that palpation and percussion do not increase intestinal activity and bowel sounds. As a nurse generalist, perform inspection, auscultation, and light palpation. Percussion and deep palpation may be done by

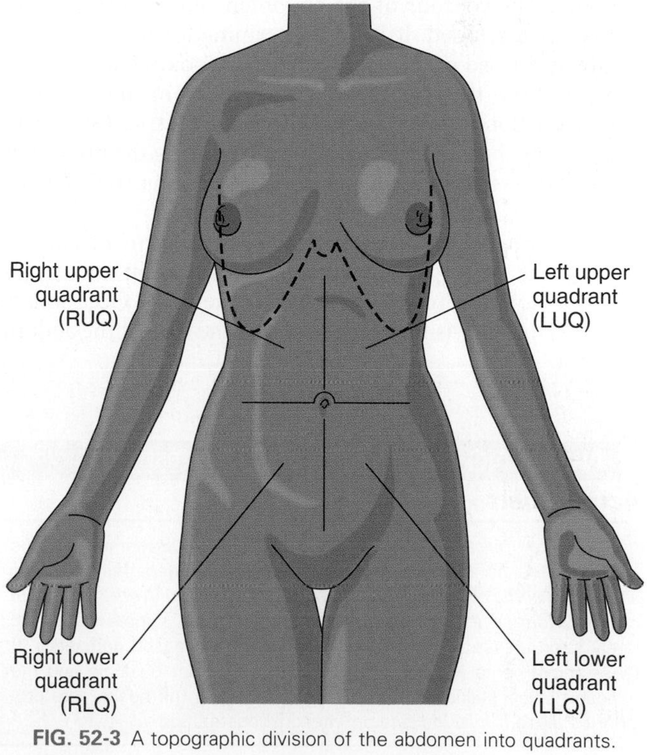

FIG. 52-3 A topographic division of the abdomen into quadrants.

TABLE 52-1 Location of Body Structures in Each Abdominal Quadrant and Midline

Right Upper Quadrant (RUQ)	Left Upper Quadrant (LUQ)
• Most of the liver • Gallbladder • Duodenum • Head of the pancreas • Hepatic flexure of the colon • Part of the ascending and transverse colon	• Left lobe of the liver • Stomach • Spleen • Body and tail of the pancreas • Splenic flexure of the colon • Part of the transverse and descending colon

Midline
- Abdominal aorta
- Uterus (if enlarged)
- Bladder (if distended)

Right Lower Quadrant (RLQ)	Left Lower Quadrant (LLQ)
• Cecum • Appendix • Right ureter • Right ovary and fallopian tube • Right spermatic cord	• Part of the descending colon • Sigmoid colon • Left ureter • Left ovary and fallopian tube • Left spermatic cord

primary health care providers, including advanced practice nurses (APNs), or specialty nurses. If appendicitis or an abdominal aneurysm is suspected, palpation is not done.

Inspection

Inspect the skin, and note any of these findings:
- Overall asymmetry of the abdomen
- Presence of discolorations or scarring
- Abdominal distention
- Bulging flanks
- Taut, glistening skin

Observe the shape of the abdomen by observing its contour and symmetry. The contour of the abdomen can be rounded, flat, concave, or distended. It is best determined when standing at the side of the bed or treatment table and looking down on the abdomen. View the abdomen at eye level from the side. Note whether the contour is symmetric or asymmetric. Asymmetry of the abdomen can indicate problems affecting the underlying body structures (see Table 52-1). Note the shape and position of the umbilicus for any deviations.

Finally, observe the patient's abdominal movements, including the normal rising and falling with inspiration and expiration, and note any distress during movement. Occasionally, pulsations may be visible, particularly in the area of the abdominal aorta.

! NURSING SAFETY PRIORITY (QSEN)

Action Alert

If a bulging, pulsating mass is present during assessment of the abdomen, do not touch the area because the patient may have an abdominal aortic aneurysm, a life-threatening problem. Notify the health care provider of this finding immediately! Peristaltic movements are rarely seen unless the patient is thin and has increased peristalsis. If these movements are observed, note the quadrant of origin and the direction of peristaltic flow. Report this finding to the health care provider because it may indicate an intestinal obstruction.

Auscultation

Auscultation of the abdomen is performed with the diaphragm of the stethoscope, because bowel sounds are usually high pitched. Place the stethoscope lightly on the abdominal wall while listening for bowel sounds in all four quadrants, beginning in the RLQ at the ileocecal valve area.

Bowel sounds are created as air and fluid move through the GI tract. They are normally heard as relatively high-pitched, irregular gurgles every 5 to 15 seconds, with a normal frequency range of 5 to 30 per minute (Jarvis, 2016). Bowel sounds are characterized as normal, hypoactive, or hyperactive. They are diminished or absent after abdominal surgery or in the patient with peritonitis or paralytic ileus.

For many years, nurses have been taught to count the number of bowel sounds in each quadrant as part of routine and postoperative abdominal assessment to assess for peristalsis. However, the best, most reliable method for assessing the return of peristalsis after abdominal surgery is to ask the patient if he or she has passed flatus within the past 8 hours or a stool within the past 12 to 24 hours.

Increased bowel sounds, especially loud, gurgling sounds, result from increased motility of the bowel (**borborygmus**). These sounds are usually heard in the patient with diarrhea or gastroenteritis or above a complete intestinal obstruction.

When auscultating the abdomen, also listen for vascular sounds or **bruits** ("swooshing" sounds) over the abdominal aorta, the renal arteries, and the iliac arteries. A bruit heard over the aorta usually indicates the presence of an aneurysm. *If this sound is heard, do not percuss or palpate the abdomen. Notify the health care provider of your findings!*

Percussion

Percussion may be used by APNs and other health care providers to determine the size of solid organs; to detect the presence of masses, fluid, and air; and to estimate the size of the liver and spleen. The percussion notes normally heard in the abdomen are termed *tympanic* (the high-pitched, loud, musical sound of an air-filled intestine) or *dull* (the medium-pitched, softer, thudlike sound over a solid organ, such as the liver).

The liver and spleen can be percussed. An enlarged liver is called **hepatomegaly**. Dullness heard in the left anterior axillary line indicates enlargement of the spleen (**splenomegaly**). Mild to moderate splenomegaly can be detected before the spleen becomes palpable.

Palpation

The purpose of palpation is to determine the size and location of abdominal organs and to assess for the presence of masses or tenderness. Palpation of the abdomen consists of two types: light palpation and deep palpation. Only physicians and APNs, such as clinical nurse specialists and nurse practitioners, should perform deep palpation. Deep palpation is used to further determine the size and shape of abdominal organs and masses.

The technique of *light palpation* is used to detect large masses and areas of tenderness. Place the first four fingers of the palpating hand close together and then place them lightly on the abdomen and proceed smoothly and systematically from quadrant to quadrant. Depress the abdomen to a depth of ½ to 1 inch (1.25 to 2.5 cm). Proceed with a rotational movement of the palpating hand. Note any areas of tenderness or guarding because these areas will be examined last and cautiously during deep palpation. While performing light palpation, notice signs

NCLEX EXAMINATION CHALLENGE

Physiological Integrity

The nurse auscultates a client's abdomen and hears a loud bruit near the umbilicus. What is the nurse's best action based on this assessment finding?

A. Document the assessment finding in the medical record.
B. Palpate the abdomen lightly in all four quadrants.
C. Report the finding to the health care provider.
D. Place the client in a semi-Fowler's position.

of rigidity, which, unlike voluntary guarding, is a sign of peritoneal inflammation.

Psychosocial Assessment

Psychosocial assessment focuses on how the GI health problem affects the patient's life and lifestyle. Remember that patients are often reluctant to discuss elimination problems, which may be very personal and embarrassing. The interview focus is on whether usual activities have been interrupted or disturbed, including employment. Question the patient about recent stressful events. Emotional stress has been associated with the development or exacerbation (flare-up) of irritable bowel syndrome (IBS) and other GI disorders. If the patient is diagnosed with cancer, he or she is expected to experience the phases of the grieving process. Patients may be depressed, angry, or in denial. More specific psychosocial assessments are included in later GI chapters as part of each disease discussion.

Diagnostic Assessment

Laboratory Assessment

To make an accurate assessment of the many possible causes of GI system abnormalities, laboratory testing of blood, urine, and stool specimens may be performed.

Serum Tests. A *complete blood count (CBC)* aids in the diagnosis of anemia and infection. It also detects changes in the blood's formed elements. In adults, GI bleeding is the most frequent cause of anemia. It is associated with GI cancer, peptic ulcer disease, diverticulitis, and inflammatory bowel disease.

Because the liver is the main site of all proteins involved in coagulation, *prothrombin time (PT)* is useful in evaluating the levels of these clotting factors. PT measures the rate at which prothrombin is converted to thrombin, a process that depends on vitamin K–associated clotting factors. Severe acute or chronic liver damage leads to a prolonged PT secondary to impaired synthesis of clotting proteins (Pagana & Pagana, 2014).

Many *electrolytes* are altered in GI tract dysfunction. For example, calcium is absorbed in the GI tract and may be measured to detect malabsorption. Excessive vomiting or diarrhea causes sodium or potassium depletion, thus requiring replacement.

Assays of serum enzymes are important in the evaluation of liver damage. *Aspartate aminotransferase (AST)* and *alanine aminotransferase (ALT)* are two enzymes found in the liver and other organs. These enzymes are elevated in most liver disorders, but they are highest in conditions that cause necrosis, such as severe viral hepatitis and cirrhosis.

Elevations in serum *amylase* and *lipase* may indicate acute pancreatitis. In this disease, serum amylase levels begin to elevate within 24 hours of onset and remain elevated for up to 5 days. Serum amylase and lipase are not elevated when *extensive* pancreatic necrosis is present because there are few pancreatic cells manufacturing the enzymes (Pagana & Pagana, 2014).

Bilirubin is the primary pigment in bile, which is normally conjugated and excreted by the liver and biliary system. It is measured as total serum bilirubin, conjugated (direct) bilirubin, and unconjugated (indirect) bilirubin. These measurements are important in the evaluation of jaundice and in the evaluation of liver and biliary tract functioning. Elevations in direct and indirect bilirubin levels can indicate impaired secretion.

The serum level of *ammonia* may also be measured to evaluate hepatic function. Ammonia is normally used to rebuild amino acids or is converted to urea for excretion. Elevated levels are seen in conditions that cause severe hepatocellular injury, such as cirrhosis of the liver or fulminant hepatitis (Pagana & Pagana, 2014).

Two primary *oncofetal antigens—CA19-9* and *CEA*—are evaluated to diagnose cancer, monitor the success of cancer therapy, and assess for the recurrence of cancer in the GI tract. These antigens may also be increased in benign GI conditions. Chart 52-3 lists blood tests commonly used by the health care provider in the diagnosis of GI disorders.

Additional serum tests are described in other chapters of this GI health unit.

Urine Tests. The presence of amylase can be detected in the urine. In acute pancreatitis, renal clearance of amylase is increased. Amylase levels in the urine remain high even after serum levels return to normal. This becomes an important finding in patients who are symptomatic for 3 days or longer (Pagana & Pagana, 2014).

Urine *urobilinogen* is a form of bilirubin that is converted by the intestinal flora and excreted in the urine. Its measurement is useful in the evaluation of hepatic and biliary obstruction, because the presence of bilirubin in the urine often occurs before jaundice is seen.

Stool Tests. The American Cancer Society screening guidelines (2014) recommend yearly guaiac fecal occult blood test (gFOBT) or yearly fecal immunochemical test (FIT) at unspecified intervals to detect colorectal cancer early when it can be treated. These tests use a take-home, multi-sample method rather than having the test done during a digital rectal examination.

The traditionally used **FOBT** (e.g., Hemoccult II) requires an active component of guaiac and is therefore more likely than the FIT (e.g., HemeSelect) to yield false-positive results. In addition, patients having the guaiac-based test must avoid certain foods before the test, such as raw fruits and vegetables and red meat. Vitamin C–rich foods, juices, and tablets must also be avoided. Anticoagulants, such as warfarin (Coumadin), and NSAIDs should be discontinued for 7 days before testing begins. Patient compliance is likely to be higher with the FIT method because drugs and food do not interfere with the test results.

Stool samples may also be collected to test for *ova and parasites* to aid in the diagnosis of parasitic infection. They may also be tested for *fecal fats* when **steatorrhea** (fatty stools) or malabsorption is suspected. Fat is normally absorbed in the small intestine in the presence of biliary and pancreatic secretions. In malabsorption, fat is abnormally excreted in the stool.

Other common stool tests—stool cytotoxic assay and stool culture—detect the presence of infectious agents, especially

CHART 52-3 Laboratory Profile

Gastrointestinal Assessment

TEST (SERUM)	NORMAL RANGE FOR ADULTS	SIGNIFICANCE OF ABNORMAL FINDINGS
Calcium (total)	9.0-10.5 mg/dL (values decrease in older adults)	*Decreased* values indicate possible: Malabsorption Kidney failure Acute pancreatitis
Potassium	3.5-5.0 mEq/L or 3.5-5.0 mmol/L	*Decreased* values indicate possible: Vomiting Gastric suctioning Diarrhea Drainage from intestinal fistulas
Albumin	3.5-5.0 g/dL	*Decreased* values indicate possible: Hepatic disease
Alanine aminotransferase (ALT)	4-36 units/L (may be slightly higher in older adults)	*Increased* values indicate possible: Liver disease Hepatitis Cirrhosis
Aspartate aminotransferase (AST)	0-35 units/L (may be slightly higher in older adults)	*Increased* values indicate possible: Liver disease Hepatitis Cirrhosis
Alkaline phosphatase	30-120 units/L (may be slightly higher in older adults)	*Increased* values indicate possible: Cirrhosis Biliary obstruction Liver tumor
Bilirubin (total)	0.3-1.0 mg/dL	*Increased* values indicate possible: Hemolysis Biliary obstruction Hepatic damage
Conjugated (direct) bilirubin	0.1-0.3 mg/dL	*Increased* values indicate possible: Biliary obstruction
Unconjugated (indirect) bilirubin	0.2-0.8 mg/dL	*Increased* values indicate possible: Hemolysis Hepatic damage
Ammonia	10-80 mg/dL	*Increased* values indicate possible: Hepatic disease such as cirrhosis
Xylose absorption	20-57 mg/dL (60-minute plasma) 30-58 mg/dL (20-minute plasma)	*Decreased* values in blood and urine indicate possible: Malabsorption in the small intestine
Serum amylase	30-220 units/L	*Increased* values indicate possible: Acute pancreatitis
Serum lipase	0-160 units/L	*Increased* values indicate possible: Acute pancreatitis
Cholesterol	<200 mg/dL	*Increased* values indicate possible: Pancreatitis Biliary obstruction *Decreased* values indicate possible: Liver cell damage
Carbohydrate antigen 19-9 (CA19-9)	<37 units/mL	*Increased* values indicate possible: Cancer of the pancreas, stomach, colon Acute pancreatitis Inflammatory bowel disease
Carcinoembryonic antigen (CEA)	<5 ng/mL	*Increased* values indicate possible: Colorectal, stomach, pancreatic cancer Ulcerative colitis Crohn's disease Hepatitis Cirrhosis

Clostridium difficile. Patients who are suspected of having *C. difficile* are usually symptomatic. Prolonged antibiotic therapy, especially in older adults, depresses the natural intestinal flora, causing an overgrowth of the pathogen. The bacterium releases a toxin that causes colonic epithelium necrosis resulting in severe diarrhea that is easily transmitted from person to person via the fecal-oral route.

A stool culture takes a longer time to get results and is not the test of choice. Instead, the cytotoxic assay is considered the most reliable because it has a high sensitivity (Keske & Letizia,

2010). However, the results may not be available for up to 3 days. The most common test to detect *C. difficile* is the enzyme-linked immunosorbent assay (ELISA) toxin A+B. It is easy to use, and the results are usually available in 2 to 6 hours (Keske & Letizia, 2010).

Imaging Assessment

Radiographic examinations and similar diagnostic procedures are useful in detecting structural and functional disorders of the GI system. Teach the patient how to prepare for the examination, provide an explanation of the procedure, and teach the required postprocedure care.

A *plain film of the abdomen* may be the first x-ray study that the health care provider requests when diagnosing a GI problem. This film can reveal abnormalities such as masses, tumors, and strictures or obstructions to normal movement. Patterns of bowel gas appear light on the abdominal film and can be useful in detecting an obstruction (ileus). No preparation is required except to wear a hospital gown and remove any jewelry or belts, which may interfere with the film.

When abdominal pain is severe or when bowel perforation is suspected, an *acute abdomen series* may be requested. This procedure consists of a chest x-ray, supine abdomen film, and an upright abdomen film. The chest x-ray may reveal a hiatal hernia, and an upright abdomen film may show air in the peritoneum from a bowel perforation. Today CT and MRI scans or ultrasound scans are used more often than abdominal x-rays.

An **upper GI radiographic series** is an x-ray visualization from the mouth to the duodenojejunal junction. It may be done to detect disorders of structure or function of the esophagus (barium swallow), stomach, or duodenum. An extension of the upper GI series, the *small bowel follow-through* (SBFT), continues tracing the barium through the small intestine—up to and including the ileocecal junction—to detect disorders of the jejunum or ileum. These tests are seldom performed today because endoscopy procedures allow for direct visualization of the internal GI tract.

A double-contrast barium enema examination, also known as a lower GI series, is an x-ray of the large intestine. The 2014 American Cancer Society screening guidelines include this test every 5 years as an option to determine the presence of colorectal cancer and polyps for people older than 50 years. The other options include:

- Flexible sigmoidoscopy every 5 years, or
- CT colonography (virtual colonoscopy) every 5 years, or
- Colonoscopy every 10 years

Patient preparation is similar to that for colonoscopy. After the study is completed, the patient expels the barium. The radiology nurse or technician teaches the patient to drink plenty of fluids to assist in eliminating the barium and prevent an intestinal obstruction. A laxative is given to help remove the barium from the intestinal tract. Stools are chalky white for about 24 to 72 hours, until all barium is passed. If the patient has positive results, he or she is scheduled for a colonoscopy.

Percutaneous transhepatic cholangiography (PTC) is an x-ray of the biliary duct system using an iodinated dye instilled via a percutaneous needle inserted through the liver into the intrahepatic ducts. This procedure may be performed when a patient has jaundice or persistent upper abdominal pain, even after cholecystectomy, but is rarely done as a diagnostic procedure today. Better information about dilated biliary ducts can be obtained using ultrasound scans and endoscopic retrograde cholangiopancreatography (ERCP) (discussed on p. 1094).

CT, also referred to as a *CT scan,* provides a noninvasive cross-sectional x-ray view that can detect tissue densities and abnormalities in the abdomen, including the liver, pancreas, spleen, and biliary tract. It may be performed with or without contrast medium. If contrast medium is to be used, ask about allergies to seafood and iodine. The patient is NPO for at least 4 hours before the test if a contrast medium is to be used. IV access will be required for injection of the contrast medium. Advise the patient that he or she may feel warm and flushed upon injection. The patient who is mildly claustrophobic may require a mild sedative to tolerate the study. The radiologic technician instructs the patient to lie still and to hold his or her breath when asked, as the technician takes a series of images. The test takes about 30 minutes.

Like other parts of the body, the abdomen and its organs may also be evaluated by *MRI, such as magnetic resonance cholangiopancreatography (MRCP).* For many patients with abdominal symptoms, this may be the first diagnostic test requested by the health care provider.

NCLEX EXAMINATION CHALLENGE

Health Promotion and Maintenance

A client is provided with materials to obtain three fecal occult blood tests (Hemoccult). What health teaching does the nurse provide? **Select all that apply**.

A. "Avoid red meat and raw vegetables for a week before getting the samples."
B. "Drink a gallon of GoLYTELY before you collect the first sample."
C. "Do not take food or fluids for 24 hours before the test."
D. "Do not take ibuprofen for a week before obtaining the samples."
E. "Avoid vitamin C tablets, foods, and juices a week before getting the samples."

Other Diagnostic Assessment

Endoscopy is direct visualization of the GI tract using a flexible fiberoptic endoscope. It is commonly requested to evaluate bleeding, ulceration, inflammation, tumors, and cancer of the esophagus, stomach, biliary system, or bowel. Obtaining specimens for biopsy and cell studies (e.g., *Helicobacter pylori*) is also possible through the endoscope. There are several types of endoscopic examinations. The patient must sign an informed consent form before having these invasive studies.

One of the challenges with endoscopic procedures is proper cleaning of equipment between patients to prevent the transmission of bacterial biofilms and *C. difficile* (see Chapter 23). Teach patients that these infections are possible but are not common (Muscarella, 2010).

Esophagogastroduodenoscopy. **Esophagogastroduodenoscopy (EGD)** is a visual examination of the esophagus, stomach, and duodenum. This procedure has largely replaced upper GI series testing. If GI bleeding is found during an EGD, the physician can inject a sclerotherapy or other type agent into the affected area to stop the bleeding. If the patient has an esophageal stricture, it can be dilated during an EGD. In addition, gastric lesions and celiac disease can be diagnosed using this procedure.

Teach the patient preparing for an upper GI endoscopic examination to remain NPO for 6 to 8 hours before

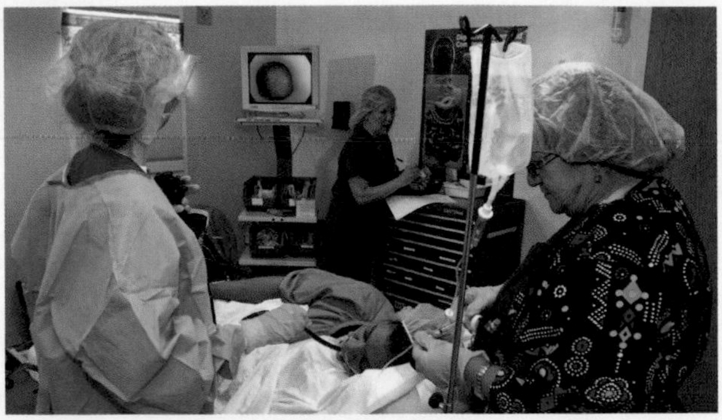

FIG. 52-4 Esophagogastroduodenoscopy allows visualization of the esophagus, the stomach, and the duodenum. If the esophagus is the focus of the examination, the procedure is called *esophagoscopy.* If the stomach is the focus, the procedure is called *gastroscopy.*

the procedure. Usual drug therapy for hypertension or other diseases may be taken the morning of the test. However, diabetic patients should consult their health care provider for special instructions. Patients are also usually asked to avoid anticoagulants, aspirin, or other NSAIDs for several days before the test unless it is absolutely necessary. Tell the patient that a flexible tube will be passed down the esophagus while he or she is under moderate sedation. Midazolam hydrochloride (Versed), fentanyl (Fentanyl, Sublimaze), and/or propofol (Diprivan) are commonly used drugs for sedation. *These drugs can depress the rate and depth of the patient's respirations.* Atropine may be administered to dry secretions. In addition, a local anesthetic is sprayed to inactivate the gag reflex and facilitate passage of the tube. Explain that this anesthetic will depress the gag reflex and that swallowing will be difficult. If the patient has dentures, they are removed.

After the drugs are given, the patient is placed in a position with the head of the bed elevated. A bite block is inserted to prevent biting down on the endoscope and to protect the teeth. The physician passes the tube through the mouth and into the esophagus (Fig. 52-4). The procedure takes about 20 to 30 minutes.

During the test, the endoscopy nurse monitors the patient's respirations for rate and depth and the oxygen saturation level via pulse oximetry. Some agencies require the use of capnography to monitor the amount of carbon dioxide that the patient exhales (Welliver, 2012). Shallow respirations decrease the amount of carbon dioxide that the patient exhales. *If the patient's respiratory rate is below 10 breaths per minute or the exhaled carbon dioxide level falls below 20%, the nurse typically uses a stimulus such as a sternal rub to encourage deeper and faster respirations.*

After the test, the endoscopy nurse or technician checks vital signs frequently (usually every 30 minutes) until the sedation begins to wear off. The siderails of the bed are raised during this time. The patient remains NPO until the gag reflex returns (usually in 30 to 60 minutes). Intravenous fluids that were started before the procedure are discontinued when the patient is able to tolerate oral fluids without nausea or vomiting.

! NURSING SAFETY PRIORITY QSEN

Action Alert

The priority for care to promote patient safety after esophagogastroduodenoscopy is to prevent aspiration. Do not offer fluids or food by mouth until you are sure that the gag reflex is intact! Monitor for signs of perforation, such as pain, bleeding, or fever.

Because the EGD is most often performed as an ambulatory care (outpatient) procedure requiring moderate sedation, be sure that the patient has someone to drive him or her home. Remind the patient to not drive for at least 12 to 18 hours after the procedure because of sedation. Teach him or her that a hoarse voice or sore throat may persist for several days after the test. Throat lozenges can be used to relieve throat discomfort. A few patients may also experience bruising around their eyes (periorbital ecchymosis), which usually resolves in about a week (Tas, 2013).

Endoscopic Retrograde Cholangiopancreatography. **Endoscopic retrograde cholangiopancreatography (ERCP)** includes visual and radiographic examination of the liver, gallbladder, bile ducts, and pancreas to identify the cause and location of obstruction. It is commonly used today for therapeutic purposes rather than for diagnosis. After a cannula is inserted into the common bile duct, a radiopaque dye is instilled and then several x-ray images are obtained. The physician may perform a **papillotomy** (a small incision in the sphincter around the ampulla of Vater) to remove gallstones. If a biliary duct stricture is found, plastic or metal stents may be inserted to keep the ducts open. Biopsies of tissue are also frequently taken during this test.

The patient prepares for this test in the same manner as for an EGD, including being NPO for 6 to 8 hours before the test. The patient requires IV access for moderate sedation drugs. Ask about prior exposure to x-ray contrast media and any sensitivities or allergies. If the patient has dentures, they are removed.

Ask the patient if he or she has an implantable medical device, such as a cardiac pacemaker. Electrocautery cannot be used with this type of device (Bruesehoff, 2010). Perform medication reconciliation to determine if the patient is taking anticoagulants, NSAIDs, antiplatelet drugs, or antihyperglycemic agents. The physician decides which of these drugs are safe to take and whether any will need to be stopped before the test.

The endoscopic procedure and nursing care for a patient having an ERCP are similar to those for the EGD procedure, except that the endoscope is advanced farther into the duodenum and into the biliary tract. Once the cannula is in the common duct, contrast medium is injected and x-rays are taken to view the biliary tract. A tilt table assists in distributing the contrast medium to all areas to be assessed. The patient is placed in a left lateral position for viewing the common bile duct. Once the cannula is placed, he or she is put in a prone position. After examination of the biliary tree, the cannula is directed into the pancreatic duct for examination. The ERCP lasts from 30 minutes to 2 hours, depending on the treatment that may be done.

After the test, assess vital signs frequently, usually every 15 minutes, until the patient is stable. To prevent aspiration, check to ensure that the gag reflex has returned before offering fluids or food. Discontinue intravenous fluids that were started before the procedure when the patient is able to tolerate oral fluids without nausea or vomiting.

Colicky abdominal pain can result from air instilled during the procedure. Instruct the patient to report abdominal pain, fever, nausea, or vomiting that fails to resolve after returning

! NURSING SAFETY PRIORITY (QSEN)

Action Alert

Teach the patient and family to monitor for severe postprocedure complications at home, including cholangitis (gallbladder inflammation), bleeding, perforation, sepsis, and pancreatitis. The patient has severe pain if any of these complications occur. Fever is present in sepsis. These problems do not occur immediately after the procedure; they may take several hours to 2 days to develop.

home. Be sure that the patient has someone to drive him or her home if the test was done on an ambulatory care basis. Remind the patient to not drive for at least 12 to 18 hours after the procedure because of sedation.

Small Bowel Capsule Endoscopy. Small bowel endoscopy, or **enteroscopy**, provides a view of the small intestine. Capsule video endoscopy (M2A) is a small bowel enteroscopy that visualizes the entire small bowel, including the distal ileum. It is used to evaluate and locate the source of GI bleeding. Before the development of the M2A Capsule Endoscope, viewing the small intestine was inadequate. The capsule battery lasts around 8 hours, so it is not used to view the colon.

Prepare the patient by explaining the procedure, the purpose, and what to expect during the testing. The patient must fast (water only) for 8 to 10 hours before the test and be NPO for the first 2 hours of the testing.

At the time of the procedure, the patient's abdomen is marked for the location of the sensors, and the eight-lead sensors (Sensor Array) are applied. The patient wears an abdominal belt that houses a data recorder to capture the transmitted images. After the capsule is swallowed with a glass of water, the patient may return to normal activity for the remainder of the study. He or she can resume a normal diet 4 hours after swallowing the capsule. At the end of the procedure, the patient returns to the facility with the capsule equipment for downloading to a central computer. The procedure lasts about 8 hours.

Because the M2A Capsule Endoscope is a single-use device that moves through the GI tract by peristalsis and is excreted naturally, explain to the patient that the capsule will be seen in the stool. No other follow-up is necessary.

Colonoscopy. **Colonoscopy** is an endoscopic examination of the entire large bowel. The American Cancer Society recommends that, beginning at age 50 years, all healthy men and women should have a colonoscopy every 10 years or choose another equally effective recommended screening option (ACS, 2014). The colonoscopy, however, is considered the gold standard test for detecting colon cancer. Those at high risk for cancer (e.g., family history) or those who had polyps removed should have the test more often. The physician may also obtain tissue biopsy specimens or remove polyps through the colonoscope. A colonoscopy can also evaluate the cause of chronic diarrhea or locate the source of GI bleeding. A sclerotherapy drug may be injected at the site to manage bleeding.

An alternative to this invasive procedure is the *CT colonography (virtual colonoscopy),* which is not invasive and uses a CT scanner to view the colon. Patient preparation for this alternative is the same as that for the traditional colonoscopy and should be performed every 5 years.

Patient Preparation. Patients who have their first colonoscopy are often very anxious. Provide information about the procedure, and reassure them that pain will be controlled with medication as needed (Mikocka-Walus et al., 2012).

To help cleanse the bowel, teach the patient to stay on a clear liquid diet the day before the scheduled colonoscopy. Instruct him or her to avoid red, orange, or purple (grape) beverages and to drink an abundant amount of Gatorade or other sports drink to replace electrolytes that are lost during bowel preparation. The patient should be NPO (except water) 4 to 6 hours before the procedure.

Remind patients to avoid aspirin, anticoagulants, and antiplatelet drugs for several days before the procedure. Diabetic patients should check with their health care provider about drug therapy requirements on the day of the test because they are NPO.

The patient may be required to drink an oral liquid preparation for cleaning the bowel (e.g., sodium phosphate [Phospho-Soda]) the evening before the examination and may repeat that procedure the morning of the study. Some physicians prescribe a gallon of GoLYTELY to cleanse the bowel the day before. *This regimen should not be used for older adults to prevent excessive fluid and electrolyte loss.* All solutions should be chilled to improve their taste. Remind the patient to drink them quickly to prevent nausea. Watery diarrhea usually begins in about an hour after starting the bowel preparation process. In some cases, the patient may also require laxatives, suppositories (e.g., bisacodyl [Dulcolax]), or one or more small-volume cleansing enemas (e.g., Fleet's).

Up to 25% of patients do not have an adequate bowel preparation, which prevents complete visualization of the entire colon. An integrative review of studies on bowel preparation procedures showed that split-dose preparations (the day before and the morning of the test) were better than bowel preparations done only on the day before the test (Van Dongen, 2012).

Procedure. IV access is necessary for the administration of moderate sedation. The physician prescribes drugs to aid in relaxation, usually IV midazolam hydrochloride (Versed), propofol (Diprivan), and/or an opiate, such as Fentanyl. Complementary and alternative therapies, such as Reiki, have been found to decrease the amount of pain medication needed during the procedure (Bourque et al., 2012).

Initially, the patient is placed on the left side with the knees drawn up while the endoscope is placed into the rectum and moved to the cecum. Air may be instilled for better visualization. The entire procedure lasts about 30 to 60 minutes. Atropine sulfate is kept available in case of bradycardia resulting from vasovagal response.

During the test, the endoscopy nurse monitors the patient's respirations for rate and depth and the oxygen saturation level via pulse oximetry. Shallow respirations decrease the amount of carbon dioxide that the patient exhales. *If the patient's respiratory rate is below 10 breaths per minute or the exhaled carbon dioxide level falls below 20%, the nurse typically uses a stimulus such as a sternal rub to encourage deeper and faster respirations.*

Follow-Up Care. Check vital signs every 15 minutes until the patient is stable. Keep the siderails up until the patient is fully alert, and maintain NPO status. Ask the patient to lie on his or her left side to promote comfort and encourage passing flatus (see the Evidence-Based Practice box). Observe for signs of perforation (causes severe pain) and hemorrhage, such as a rapid drop in blood pressure. Reassure the patient that a feeling of fullness, cramping, and passage of flatus are expected for several hours after the test. Fluids are permitted after the patient passes flatus to indicate that peristalsis has returned. Discontinue intravenous fluids that were started before the procedure when the patient is able to tolerate oral fluids without nausea or vomiting.

EVIDENCE-BASED PRACTICE QSEN

What Position Is Best for Patients after Undergoing a Colonoscopy?

Devitt, J., Shellman, L., Gardner, K., & Wernett, L. (2011). Using positioning after a colonoscopy for patient comfort management. *Gastroenterology Nursing, 34*(2), 93-100.

This study compared the effect of patient positioning on comfort and passage of flatus after a colonoscopy. After having a colonoscopy, 512 patients were randomly assigned to one of three body positions: left lateral, right lateral, and supine (168-174 patients per position). The patients' position, pain, bloating, and passage of flatus were assessed and rated every 15 minutes.

The results of the study found significant differences in pain and passage of flatus among the three groups of patients. The researchers concluded that patients who were positioned in the left lateral position had less discomfort and quicker passage of flatus when compared with the other two groups.

Level of Evidence: 2

This study used a large sample of patients who were randomly assigned to one of three study groups.

Commentary: Implications for Practice and Research

Nurses caring for patients who have a colonoscopy should teach patients about the need to be in a left lateral position after the procedure. Although the study used a convenience sample, patients were randomly assigned to one of three groups to compare the effect of body position on comfort and flatus passage. The study used a large sample size from which a conclusion can be generalized for best practice in nursing and health care.

If a polypectomy or tissue biopsy was performed, there may be a *small* amount of blood in the first stool after the colonoscopy. Complications of colonoscopy are not common. However, splenic injury may occur during the procedure and is difficult to diagnose (Bittler, 2011). *Report excessive bleeding or severe pain to the health care provider immediately* (Chart 52-4).

As with other endoscopic procedures, the patient will need someone to provide transportation home if the procedure was done in an ambulatory care setting. Remind the patient to avoid driving for 12 to 18 hours after the procedure because of the effects of sedation.

Virtual Colonoscopy. A noninvasive imaging procedure to obtain multi-dimensional views of the entire colon is the *CT colonography,* most popularly known as the **virtual colonoscopy.** The bowel preparation and dietary restrictions are similar to those for traditional colonoscopy. However, if a polyp is detected during a virtual colonoscopy or bleeding is found, the patient must have a follow-up invasive colonoscopy for treatment. Therefore the advantage of the traditional colonoscopy is that both diagnostic testing and minor surgical procedures can be done at the same time.

Sigmoidoscopy. Proctosigmoidoscopy, often referred to as a *sigmoidoscopy,* is an endoscopic examination of the rectum and sigmoid colon using a flexible scope. The purpose of this test is to screen for colon cancer, investigate the source of GI bleeding, or diagnose or monitor inflammatory bowel disease. If sigmoidoscopy is used as an alternative to colonoscopy for colorectal cancer screening, it is recommended that screening begin at 50 years of age and should be done every 5 years thereafter (American Cancer Society, 2014). Patients at high risk for cancer may require more frequent screening.

The patient should have a clear liquid diet for at least 24 hours before the test. A cleansing enema or sodium biphosphate (Fleet's) enema is usually required the morning of the procedure. A laxative may also be prescribed the evening before the test.

The patient is placed on the left side in the knee-chest position. No moderate sedation is required. The endoscope is lubricated and inserted into the anus to the required depth for viewing. Tissue biopsy may be performed during this procedure, but the patient cannot feel it. The examination usually lasts about 30 minutes.

Inform the patient that mild gas pain and flatulence may be experienced from air instilled into the rectum during the examination. If a biopsy was obtained, a small amount of bleeding may be observed. Instruct the patient that excessive bleeding should be reported immediately to the health care provider.

CHART 52-4 Best Practice for Patient Safety & Quality Care QSEN

Care of the Patient after a Colonoscopy

- Do not allow the patient to take anything by mouth until sedation wears off and he or she is alert and passes flatus.
- Take vital signs every 15 to 30 minutes until the patient is alert.
- Keep patient in left lateral position to promote passing of flatus.
- Keep the top siderails up until the patient is alert.
- Assess for rectal bleeding or severe pain.
- Remind the patient that fullness and mild abdominal cramping are expected for several hours.
- Assess for manifestations of bowel perforation, including *severe* abdominal pain and guarding. Fever may occur later.
- Assess for manifestations of hypovolemic shock, including dizziness, light-headedness, decreased blood pressure, tachycardia, pallor, and altered mental status (may be the first sign in older adults).
- If the procedure is performed in an ambulatory care setting, arrange for another person to drive the patient home.

CLINICAL JUDGMENT CHALLENGE

Safety; Evidence-Based Practice QSEN

A 50-year-old man has his first screening colonoscopy today. You are assigned as his preprocedure and postprocedure nurse. When you take the patient's vital signs before the procedure, his blood pressure is 148/86 mm Hg. The patient states that he has a history of hypertension that is being well controlled with medication and diet. He tells you that he took his amlodipine (Norvasc) this morning with a small amount of water.

1. Why do you suspect his blood pressure is increased? What other assessment data will you collect?
2. What actions might you consider to decrease his blood pressure?
3. After the procedure, the patient asks for something to drink. How will you respond to him and why? What evidence supports this decision?
4. What evidence-based position should the patient be in after the procedure and why?
5. The patient tells you that he had a polyp removed. What health teaching about colorectal cancer screening will you provide?

Gastric Analysis. Although not commonly performed, gastric analysis measures the hydrochloric acid and pepsin content for evaluation of aggressive gastric and duodenal disorders (e.g., Zollinger-Ellison syndrome). There are two tests in gastric analysis: basal gastric secretion and gastric acid stimulation. Basal gastric secretion measures the secretion of hydrochloric acid between meals. If only small amounts of secretion are collected, a follow-up gastric stimulation test is given.

The patient is NPO for at least 12 hours before the test. Teach patients to avoid alcohol, tobacco, and drugs that may affect gastric secretion for 24 hours before the study. A nasogastric (NG) tube is inserted, and gastric residual contents are aspirated and discarded.

The NG tube is attached to suctioning equipment for collecting the contents at 15-minute intervals for 1 hour. Samples are collected and labeled with basal acid output (BAO), time, and volume of each specimen.

For the gastric acid stimulation test, the NG tube is left in place and a drug that stimulates gastric acid secretion (e.g., pentagastrin or betazole dihydrochloride [Histalog]) is given. Fifteen minutes after injection of the drug, specimens are again collected at 15-minute intervals for 1 hour. Samples are collected and labeled with maximal acid output (MAO), time, and volume of each specimen. Depressed levels of gastric secretion suggest the presence of gastric cancer. Increased levels of gastric secretion may indicate one or more duodenal ulcers (see Chapter 55).

After the test is completed, the NG tube is removed and the patient can resume normal eating patterns. No other follow-up is necessary.

Ultrasonography. Ultrasonography (US) is a technique in which high-frequency, inaudible vibratory sound waves are passed through the body via a transducer. The echoes created by the sound waves are then recorded and converted into images for analysis. US is commonly used to view soft tissues, such as the liver, the spleen, the pancreas, and the biliary system. The advantages of this test are that it is painless and noninvasive and requires no radiation.

The patient may be fasting, depending on the abdominal organs to be examined. Inform the patient that it will be necessary to lie still during the study.

The patient is usually placed in a supine position. The technician applies insulating gel to the end of the transducer and on the area of the abdomen under study. This gel allows airtight contact of the transducer with the skin. The technician moves the transducer back and forth over the skin until the desired images are obtained. The study takes about 15 to 30 minutes. No follow-up care is necessary.

Endoscopic Ultrasonography. Endoscopic ultrasonography (EUS) provides images of the GI wall and high-resolution images of the digestive organs. The ultrasonography is performed through the endoscope. This procedure is useful in diagnosing the presence of lymph node tumors, mucosal tumors, and tumors of the pancreas, stomach, and rectum. The patient preparation and follow-up care are similar to the preparation and follow-up care for both endoscopy and ultrasonography.

Liver-Spleen Scan. A liver-spleen scan uses IV injection of a radioactive material that is taken up primarily by the liver and secondarily by the spleen. The scan evaluates the liver and the spleen for tumors or abscesses, organ size and location, and blood flow.

Teach the patient about the need to lie still during the scanning. Assure the patient that the injection has only small amounts of radioactivity and is not dangerous. Ask female patients of childbearing age if they may be pregnant or are currently breast-feeding. The radionuclide can be found in breast milk, and radiation from x-rays or scans should be avoided in pregnancy.

The technician or the physician gives the radioactive injection through an IV line, and a wait of about 15 minutes is necessary for uptake. The patient is placed in many different positions while the scanning takes place. Tell the patient that the radionuclide is eliminated from the body through the urine in 24 hours. Careful handwashing after toileting decreases the exposure to any radiation present in the urine.

NURSING CONCEPTS AND CLINICAL JUDGMENT REVIEW

What might you NOTICE in a patient with adequate nutrition and ELIMINATION related to the GI system?

Physical assessment:
- No nausea or vomiting
- Sufficient appetite
- No intentional weight loss
- No dyspepsia (indigestion)
- No jaundice
- Abdomen soft and not tender
- Normoactive bowel sounds present is all quadrants
- No change in bowel habits
- No abdominal pain
- Normal brown, formed stool
- No frequent diarrhea or constipation

Diagnostic assessment:
- No occult blood in stool
- Normal liver enzymes, such as ALT
- Normal bilirubin levels
- Serum and urine amylase within normal limits
- Serum ammonia level within normal limit
- Serum albumin within normal limit
- Electrolytes within normal limits

GET READY FOR THE NCLEX® EXAMINATION!

KEY POINTS

Review these Key Points for each NCLEX Examination Client Needs Category.

Safe and Effective Care Environment

- Remember that the priority for care is to check for the return of the gag reflex after an upper endoscopic procedure before offering fluids or food; aspiration may occur if the gag reflex is not intact. **Safety** QSEN

Health Promotion and Maintenance

- If an endoscopic procedure on an ambulatory care basis is scheduled, remind the patient to have someone available to drive him or her home because of the effects of moderate sedation. **Safety** QSEN
- Teach patients having invasive colon diagnostic procedures to follow instructions carefully for the bowel preparation before testing; the bowel must be clear to allow visualization of the colon.
- Instruct the patient to drink plenty of fluids and take a laxative as prescribed to eliminate barium if used during diagnostic testing. **Evidence-Based Practice** QSEN

Psychosocial Integrity

- Remember that problems of digestion, nutrition, and elimination can markedly affect lifestyle.
- Recall that patient responses to GI health problems such as cancer or peptic ulcer can include anger, denial, and depression.

Physiological Integrity

- The GI tract is continuous from the mouth to the anus. It is responsible for food digestion and bowel elimination; the secretions of the liver, pancreas, and gallbladder empty into the GI tract to aid in digestion.
- Perform a focused abdominal assessment using inspection, auscultation, and light palpation.
- Do not palpate or auscultate any abdominal pulsating mass because it could be a life-threatening aortic aneurysm. **Safety** QSEN
- Be aware that aging causes changes in the GI system as summarized in Chart 52-1. **Patient-Centered Care** QSEN
- Assess and report any major complications of GI testing to the health care provider.
- Review and interpret laboratory results, and report abnormal findings to the health care provider (see Chart 52-3).
- Monitor vital signs carefully for the patient having any endoscopic procedure and moderate sedation.
- Assess patients who have endoscopies for bleeding, fever, and severe pain. **Safety** QSEN
- For patients who have had a colonoscopy, check for passage of flatus before allowing fluids or food (see Chart 52-4).

CHAPTER 53

Care of Patients with Oral Cavity Problems

Cherie R. Rebar, Nicole Heimgartner, Laura Willis

http://evolve.elsevier.com/Iggy/

PRIORITY CONCEPTS

- INFECTION
- NUTRITION
- GAS EXCHANGE
- PAIN

LEARNING OUTCOMES

Safe and Effective Care Environment

1. Use principles of INFECTION control when caring for a patient with oral cavity problems to promote safety.
2. Collaborate with health care professionals to help patients and families experiencing oral cavity problems achieve their desired health outcomes.
3. Identify appropriate community resources for patients with oral cavity problems.

Health Promotion and Maintenance

4. Teach all people how to prevent oral cancer and maintain good oral health.
5. Develop a teaching plan for patients with stomatitis to promote digestion and NUTRITION and to minimize PAIN.
6. Teach patients with oral cancer about community-based resources.

Psychosocial Integrity

7. Reduce the psychological impact for the patient and family regarding changes in the appearance or function of any part of the oral cavity.
8. Refer patients with oral cancer to appropriate support groups.

Physiological Integrity

9. Perform a complete assessment of any oral cavity changes, lesions, and wounds.
10. Prioritize postoperative care for patients undergoing surgery for oral cancer to maintain GAS EXCHANGE and prevent aspiration.
11. Describe collaborative interventions to promote NUTRITION for postoperative patients having extensive oral surgery.
12. Identify methods to help patients communicate effectively after oral surgery.
13. Plan care for patients who have disorders of the salivary glands.
14. Identify evidence-based practice for teaching or providing oral care for patients.
15. Coordinate continuity of care between the hospital and community-based agencies for patients having oral surgery.

Digestion of food begins in the oral cavity. Within the mouth, teeth tear, grind, and crush food into small particles to promote swallowing. The enzymes in saliva begin the breakdown of carbohydrates. If a person cannot take food or fluid into the mouth, cannot chew food, or cannot swallow, the basic human need for NUTRITION may not be met by use of the GI tract. Adequate intake of fluids and nutrients into the body is vital to promote function of every body organ and system.

The pharynx (throat) is located just behind the mouth and has a role in both digestion and GAS EXCHANGE (oxygenation). The pharynx is the portal between the mouth and the GI tract, where nutrients are broken down. The pharynx also is a portal for GAS EXCHANGE, as inhaled air passes through the nose, into the pharynx, and down into the trachea. A blockage of the posterior oral cavity, such as a tumor, can interfere with GAS EXCHANGE and digestion.

Oral cavity disorders, then, can severely affect NUTRITION and GAS EXCHANGE, as well as speech, body image, and self-esteem. These disorders commonly affect people who (World Health Organization, 2014):

- Have developmental delays or mental health disorders
- Are homeless or have less (decreased) access to care
- Reside in institutions
- Use tobacco and/or alcohol
- Consume an unhealthy diet
- Have an oral cancer

This chapter discusses the most common oral health problems. As a nurse, you will play an important role in maintaining and restoring oral health through nursing interventions, including patient and family education. Chart 53-1 lists ways to help maintain a healthy oral cavity.

CHART 53-1 Patient and Family Education: Preparing for Self-Management

Maintaining a Healthy Oral Cavity

- Perform self-examination of your mouth every week; report any unusual finding or any noted change.
- Be sure to eat a well-balanced diet.
- Brush and floss your teeth every day. Set and maintain a consistent routine. Keeping floss where you can see it (e.g., on the countertop by the sink) will encourage you to stick to your routine.
- Manage your stress as much as possible; learn how to maintain your emotional health by using healthy coping mechanisms.
- Avoid contact with agents that may cause inflammation of the mouth, such as mouthwashes that contain alcohol.
- If possible, avoid drugs that may cause inflammation of the mouth or reduce the flow of saliva.
- Be aware of any changes in the occlusion of your teeth, mouth pain, or swelling; seek medical attention promptly if these occur.
- See your dentist regularly; have problems attended to promptly.
- If you wear dentures, make sure they are in good repair and fit properly.

STOMATITIS

❖ PATHOPHYSIOLOGY

Stomatitis is a broad term that refers to inflammation within the oral cavity and may present in many different ways. Painful single or multiple ulcerations (called *aphthous ulcers* or "canker sores") that appear as inflammation and erosion of the protective lining of the mouth are one of the most common forms of stomatitis. The sores cause PAIN, and open areas place the person at risk for bleeding and INFECTION. Mild erythema (redness) may respond to topical treatments. Extensive stomatitis may require treatment with opioid analgesics and/or antifungal medications, depending on the source of inflammation. Stomatitis is classified according to the cause of the inflammation. *Primary stomatitis,* the most common type, includes **aphthous** (noninfectious) **stomatitis,** herpes simplex stomatitis, and traumatic ulcers. *Secondary stomatitis* generally results from INFECTION by opportunistic viruses, fungi, or bacteria in patients who are immunocompromised. It can also result from drugs, such as chemotherapy. (See Chapter 22 for discussion of chemotherapy-induced stomatitis.)

A common type of secondary stomatitis is caused by *Candida albicans. Candida* is sometimes present in small amounts in the mouth, especially in older adults. Long-term antibiotic therapy destroys other normal flora and allows the *Candida* to overgrow. The result can be **candidiasis,** also called *moniliasis,* a fungal INFECTION that is very painful. Candidiasis is also common in those undergoing immunosuppressive therapy, such as chemotherapy, radiation, and steroids.

CONSIDERATIONS FOR OLDER ADULTS

Patient-Centered Care QSEN

Older adults are especially at high risk for candidiasis because aging causes a decrease in immune function. The risk increases for patients who are diabetic, malnourished, or under emotional stress. Many older adults take multiple medications that can contribute to oral dryness and decreased salivation, as well. Those who wear dentures may use soft denture liners that provide comfort but can also be colonized by *C. albicans,* contributing to denture stomatitis. In addition, older adults who have poor oral hygiene are at high risk for mouth infections and aspiration pneumonia. All health care professionals in any health care setting should be educated in and aware of best practices for oral care for older adults. Improved oral care could greatly improve patient outcomes, especially for older intubated adults in critical care settings.

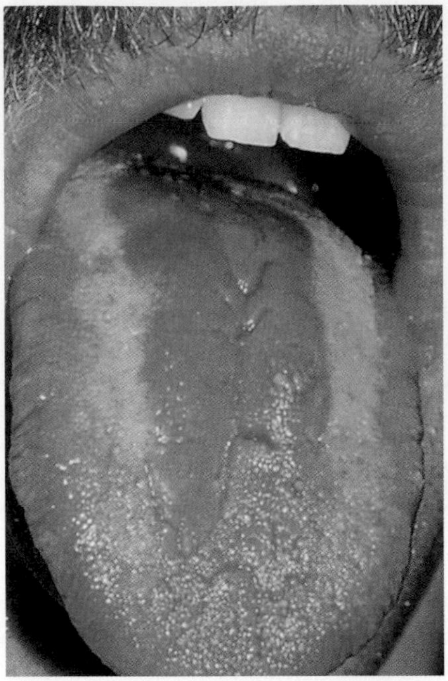

FIG. 53-1 Oral candidiasis.

Stomatitis can result from INFECTION, allergy, vitamin deficiency (complex B vitamins, folate, zinc, iron), systemic disease, and irritants such as tobacco and alcohol. Infectious agents, such as bacteria and viruses, may have a role in the development of recurrent stomatitis. Certain foods such as coffee, potatoes, cheese, nuts, citrus fruits, and gluten may trigger allergic responses that cause aphthous ulcers. In some cases, strict diets have resulted in the improvement of ulcers.

❖ PATIENT-CENTERED COLLABORATIVE CARE

◆ Assessment

When performing an oral assessment, ask about a history of recent infections, NUTRITION changes, oral hygiene habits, oral trauma, and stress. Also collect a drug history, including over-the-counter (OTC) drugs and NUTRITION and herbal supplements. Document the course of the current outbreak, and determine if stomatitis has occurred frequently. Ask the patient if the lesions interfere with swallowing, eating, or communicating.

The symptoms of stomatitis range in severity from a dry, painful mouth to open ulcerations, placing the patient at risk for INFECTION. These ulcerations can alter NUTRITION status because of difficulty with eating or swallowing. When they are severe, stomatitis and edema have the potential to obstruct the airway.

In oral candidiasis, white plaque-like lesions appear on the tongue, palate, pharynx (throat), and buccal mucosa (inside the cheeks) (Fig. 53-1). When these patches are wiped away, the underlying surface is red and sore. Patients may report pain, but others describe the lesions as dry or hot.

While examining the mouth, wear gloves, use a penlight to ensure adequate lighting, and use a tongue blade to aid examining the oral cavity. Assess the mouth for lesions, coating, and cracking. Document characteristics of the lesions including their location, size, shape, odor, color, and drainage.

If lesions are seen along the pharynx and the patient reports **dysphagia** (pain on swallowing), the lesions might extend down the esophagus. To establish a definitive diagnosis, the primary care provider may prescribe additional swallowing studies.

The physical assessment also includes palpating the cervical and submandibular lymph nodes for swelling. Advanced practice nurses and other primary care providers usually perform this part of the examination.

! NURSING SAFETY PRIORITY QSEN

Action Alert

When assessing the patient with stomatitis, be alert for signs and symptoms of dysphagia, such as coughing or choking when swallowing, a sensation of food "sticking" in the pharynx, or difficulty initiating the swallowing process. If dysphagia is suspected, document all findings and report these to the health care provider because dysphagia can cause numerous problems, including airway obstruction, aspiration pneumonia, and malnutrition.

◆ *Interventions*

Interventions for stomatitis are targeted toward health promotion and reduced risk for INFECTION through careful *oral hygiene* (see the Evidence-Based Practice box) and food selection. When providing mouth care for the patient, you may delegate oral care to unlicensed assistive personnel (UAP). Because you are accountable for the delegated task, remind UAP to use a soft-bristled toothbrush or disposable foam swabs to stimulate gums and clean the oral cavity and to use toothpaste that is free of sodium lauryl sulfate (SLS), if possible, because this ingredient has been associated with stomatitis. Teach the patient to rinse the mouth every 2 to 3 hours with a sodium bicarbonate solution or warm saline solution (may be mixed with hydrogen peroxide). He or she should avoid most commercial mouthwashes because they have high alcohol content, causing a burning sensation in irritated or ulcerated areas. Health food stores sell more natural mouthwashes that are not alcohol-based. Teach the patient to check the labels for alcohol content. Frequent, gentle mouth care promotes débridement of ulcerated lesions and can prevent superinfections. Chart 53-2 lists measures for special oral care.

Drug therapy used for stomatitis includes antimicrobials, immune modulators, and symptomatic topical agents. Complementary and alternative therapies may also be tried.

Antimicrobials, including antibiotics, antivirals, and antifungals, may be necessary for control of INFECTION. Tetracycline syrup may initially be prescribed, especially for recurrent aphthous ulcers (RAUs). The patient rinses for 2 minutes and swallows the syrup, thus obtaining both topical and systemic therapy. Minocycline swish/swallow and chlorhexidine mouthwashes may also be used.

A regimen of IV acyclovir (Zovirax) is prescribed for immunocompromised patients who contract herpes simplex stomatitis. Patients with healthy immune systems may be given acyclovir in oral or topical form.

CHART 53-2 Best Practice for Patient Safety & Quality Care QSEN

Care of the Patient with Problems of the Oral Cavity

- Remove dentures if the patient has severe stomatitis or oral pain.
- Encourage the patient to perform oral hygiene or provide it after each meal and as often as needed.
- Increase mouth care to every 2 hours or more frequently if stomatitis is not controlled.
- Use a soft toothbrush or gauze for oral care.
- Encourage frequent rinsing of the mouth with warm saline, sodium bicarbonate (baking soda) solution, or a combination of these solutions.
- Teach the patient to avoid commercial mouthwashes, particularly those with high alcohol content, and lemon-glycerin swabs.
- Assist the patient in selecting soft, bland, and nonacidic foods.
- Apply topical analgesics or anesthetics as prescribed by the health care provider, and monitor their effectiveness.

EVIDENCE-BASED PRACTICE QSEN

Does Providing Standard or Comprehensive Oral Care Result in the Best Outcomes for ICU Patients?

Prendergast, V., Jakobsson, U., Renvert, S., & Hallberg, I. (2012). Effects of a standard versus comprehensive oral care protocol among intubated neuroscience ICU patients: Results of a randomized controlled trial. *Journal of Neuroscience Nursing, 44*(3), 134-146.

Evidence shows that proper oral care is essential to prevent infections such as aspiration pneumonia and ventilator-associated pneumonia (VAP). In this study, a 2-year randomized clinical trial (RCT) involving 56 patients was conducted to compare the effect of standard oral care (manual toothbrushing) with that of comprehensive oral care (tongue scraping, electric toothbrushing, and moisturizing) on oral health of intubated neuroscience ICU patients.

Oral health was evaluated based on a standardized tool (Eilers' Oral Assessment Guide) at certain points during patients' hospitalizations. The results of this RCT demonstrated that comprehensive oral care protocols were more effective in maintaining oral health throughout intubation and after extubation when compared with standard oral care protocols.

Level of Evidence: 2

The study was a randomized controlled trial (RCT), which was also part of a larger RCT, comparing the effects of standard versus comprehensive oral care on ventilator-associated pneumonia among patients in a neuroscience ICU.

Commentary: Implications for Practice and Research

The findings of this research clearly indicate that delivery of comprehensive oral care was more effective than delivery of standard oral care in maintaining oral health of neuroscience patients who were intubated in the ICU setting. The review of literature also indicated that existing information about the specific ways in which to deliver oral care to this patient population is lacking. Be aware of best practices to deliver the most effective, evidence-based care to yield optimal patient outcomes. Further studies using larger and more diverse subjects need to be conducted.

For fungal infections like yeast, nystatin (Mycostatin) oral suspension swish/swallow is most commonly prescribed. Ice pop troches (lozenges) of the antifungal preparation allow the drug to slowly dissolve, and the cold provides an analgesic effect. Topical triamcinolone in benzocaine (Kenalog in

Orabase) and oral dexamethasone elixir used as a swish/expectorate preparation are commonly used for stomatitis, especially RAU.

Immune-modulating agents that may be prescribed as second-line therapy include:

- Topical amlexanox (Aphthasol)
- Topical granulocyte-macrophage colony-stimulating factor (GM-CSF)
- Thalidomide

The exact mechanism for how these drugs work is not clear. However, they may inhibit release of mediators that contribute to the inflammation seen in patients with RAU.

Over-the-counter (OTC) benzocaine anesthetics (e.g., Orabase, Anbesol) and camphor phenol (Campho-Phenique) can also control PAIN. Viscous lidocaine may also be prescribed to use as a gargle or mouthwash. "Magic mouthwash," a mixture of lidocaine, Benadryl, Maalox, Carafate, glucocorticoids, and other ingredients, is also commonly prescribed for those with oral pain due to cancer treatments.

! NURSING SAFETY PRIORITY (QSEN)

Drug Alert

Teach patients to use viscous lidocaine with extreme caution because its anesthetizing effect may cause burns from hot liquids in the mouth and/or increase the risk for choking.

Dietary changes may also help decrease PAIN. Cool or cold liquids can be very soothing, whereas hard, spicy, salty, and acidic foods or fluids can further irritate the ulcers. Include foods high in protein and vitamin C to promote healing, including scrambled eggs, bananas, custards, puddings, and ice cream, unless the patient has lactose intolerance.

? NCLEX EXAMINATION CHALLENGE

Physiological Integrity

Viscous lidocaine is prescribed for a client. What client teaching does the nurse provide?

A. "Be certain your food's temperature is not too hot."
B. "This medication will kill bacteria found within your mouth."
C. "You may use this drug as many times during the day as you wish."
D. "Viscous lidocaine is the most effective medication to treat fungal infections."

ORAL TUMORS

Oral cavity tumors can be benign, precancerous, or cancerous. Whether benign or malignant, tumors of the mouth affect many daily functions, including swallowing, chewing, and speaking. PAIN accompanying the tumor can also limit daily activities and self-care. Oral tumors affect body image, especially if treatment involves removal of the tongue or part of the mandible (jaw) or requires a tracheostomy.

PREMALIGNANT LESIONS

Leukoplakia presents as slowly developing changes in the oral mucous membranes causing thickened, white, firmly attached patches that cannot easily be scraped off. These patches appear slightly raised and sharply rounded. Most of these lesions are benign. However, a small percentage of them become cancerous. Although leukoplakia can be found anywhere on the oral mucosa, lesions on the lips or tongue are more likely to progress to cancer.

Leukoplakia results from mechanical factors that cause long-term oral mucous membrane irritation, such as poorly fitting dentures, chronic cheek nibbling, or broken or poorly repaired teeth. In addition, oral hairy leukoplakia (OHL) can be found in patients with human immune deficiency virus (HIV) INFECTION. The Joint Commission (TJC) Core Measures TOB-1 requires asking about tobacco use, because tobacco products (smoked, dipped, or chewed) have also been implicated in the development of leukoplakia, sometimes referred to as "smoker's patch." Oral leukoplakia can be confused with oral candidal INFECTION. However, unlike candidal infection, leukoplakia cannot be removed by scraping.

Leukoplakia is the most common oral lesion among adults. OHL is associated with Epstein-Barr virus (EBV) and can be an early manifestation of HIV INFECTION. When associated with HIV infection, the appearance of OHL is highly correlated with progression from HIV infection to acquired immune deficiency syndrome (AIDS). Leukoplakia not associated with HIV infection is more often seen in people older than 40 years. The incidence of leukoplakia is two times higher in men than in women; however, this ratio is changing because increasing numbers of women are smoking.

Erythroplakia appear as red, velvety mucosal lesions on the surface of the oral mucosa. There are more malignant changes in erythroplakia than in leukoplakia; therefore erythroplakia is often considered "precancerous" in presentation. As such, these lesions should be regarded with suspicion and analyzed by biopsy. Erythroplakia is most commonly found on the floor of the mouth, tongue, palate, and mandibular mucosa. It can be difficult to distinguish from inflammatory or immune reactions.

ORAL CANCER

Dentists and physicians systematically screen patients for oral cancer. Oral assessment has become a part of the routine dental examination. People should visit a dentist at least twice a year for professional dental hygiene and oral cancer screening, which includes inspecting and palpating the mouth for lesions.

Prevention strategies for oral cancer include minimizing sun and tanning bed exposure, tobacco cessation, and decreasing alcohol intake. Most dentists use digital technology instead of x-rays when performing the annual or biannual dental examination, because excessive, prolonged radiation from x-rays has been associated with head and neck cancer (Oral Cancer Foundation [OCF], 2014). Teach patients to follow the guidelines in Chart 53-1 to maintain oral health.

❖ PATHOPHYSIOLOGY

More than 90% of oral cancers are *squamous cell carcinomas* that begin on the surface of the epithelium. Over a period of many years, premalignant (or dysplastic) changes begin. Cells begin to vary in size and shape. Alterations in the thickness of the lining of the epithelium develop, resulting in atrophy. These tumors usually grow slowly, and the lesions may be large before the onset of symptoms unless ulceration is present. *Mucosal erythroplasia is the earliest sign of oral carcinoma. Oral lesions that appear as red, raised, eroded areas are suspicious for cancer.*

A lesion that does not heal within 2 weeks or a lump or thickening in the cheek is a symptom that warrants further assessment (OCF, 2013).

Squamous cell cancer can be found on the lips, tongue, buccal mucosa, and oropharynx. The major risk factors in its development are increasing age, tobacco use, and alcohol use. Most oral cancers occur in people older than 40 years. Tobacco use in any form (e.g., smoking or chewing tobacco) can increase the risk for cancer. A person who frequently consumes alcohol and uses tobacco in any form is at the highest risk.

GENETIC/GENOMIC CONSIDERATIONS

Patient-Centered Care QSEN

Genetic changes in patients with oral cancer have been found, especially the mutation of the *TP53* gene (McCance et al., 2014). The *TP53* gene is nicknamed the "guardian of the genome" because tumor protein *p53* is essential for cell division regulation and prevention of tumor formation (National Institutes of Health, 2014). Because mutations in this gene are linked to various cancers, always ask about a personal and family history of ***any*** type of cancer when assessing the patient with oral cavity problems.

An increased rate of squamous cell cancer is found in people with occupations such as textile workers, plumbers, and coal and metal workers, mainly due to prolonged exposure to polycyclic aromatic hydrocarbons (PAHs). People with **periodontal** (gum) **disease** in which mandibular (jaw) bone loss has occurred are especially at risk for cancer of the mouth. Additional factors, such as sun exposure, poor NUTRITION habits, poor oral hygiene, and INFECTION with the human papilloma virus (HPV16) may also contribute to oral cancer (OCF, 2013).

Research indicates a correlation between specific strains of the human papilloma virus (HPV) and oral cancer. Oral cancer associated with HPV appears in the tonsillar area or along the base of the tongue in younger people. Because HPV-positive oral cancers account for a large number of oral cancer diagnoses, routine oral assessment is essential. Oral cavity inspection combined with neck palpation is recommended yearly to aid in early detection (OCF, 2013).

Basal cell carcinoma of the mouth occurs primarily on the lips. The lesion is asymptomatic and resembles a raised scab. With time, it evolves into a characteristic ulcer with a raised, pearly border. Basal cell carcinomas do not metastasize (spread) but can aggressively involve the skin of the face. The major risk factor for this type of cancer is excessive sunlight exposure.

Basal cell carcinoma occurs as a result of the failure of basal cells to mature into keratinocytes. It is the second most common type of oral cancer, but it is much less common than squamous cell carcinoma.

Kaposi's sarcoma is a malignant lesion in blood vessels, appearing as a raised, purple nodule or plaque, which is usually painless. In the mouth, the hard palate is the most common site of Kaposi's sarcoma, but it can be found also on the gums, tongue, or tonsils. It is most often associated with AIDS. (See Chapter 19 for a complete discussion of Kaposi's sarcoma.)

As a group, oral cancers account for about 3% of all cancers in men and 2% of all cancers in women in the United States. Over 42,000 new cases are diagnosed each year, with almost 8000 deaths (OCF, 2013). Most cancers occur in middle-aged and older people, although in recent years, younger adults have been affected, probably as a result of sun exposure and HPV.

CHART 53-3 Key Features

Oral Cancer

- Bleeding from the mouth
- Poor appetite
- Difficulty chewing
- Difficulty swallowing
- Poor nutrition status and weight loss
- Thick or absent saliva
- Painless oral lesion that is red, raised, or eroded
- Thickening or lump in cheek

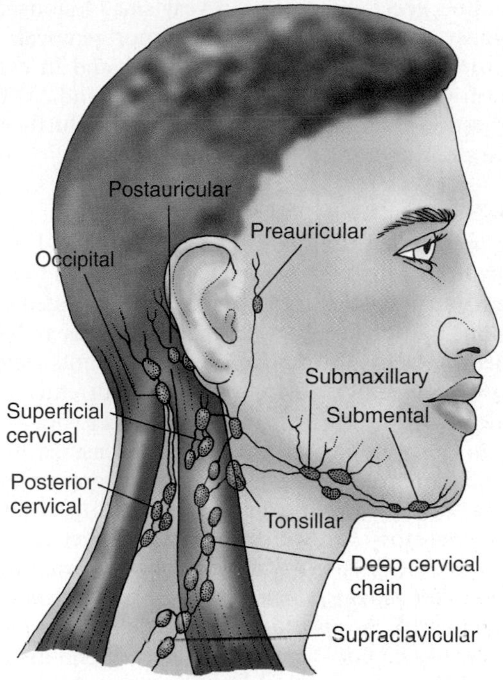

FIG. 53-2 The lymph nodes of the cervical region.

❖ PATIENT-CENTERED COLLABORATIVE CARE

◆ Assessment

Begin by assessing the patient's routine oral hygiene regimen and use of dentures or oral appliances, which might add to discomfort or mechanically irritate the mucosa. Ask about oral bleeding, which might indicate an ulcerative lesion or periodontal (gum) disease. Determine the patient's past and current appetite and NUTRITION state, including difficulty with chewing or swallowing. A continuing trend of weight loss may be related to metastasis, heavy alcohol intake, difficulty in eating or chewing, or an underlying health problem (Chart 53-3).

An examination of the oral cavity requires adequate lighting. Thoroughly inspect the oral cavity for any lesions, evidence of PAIN, or restriction of movement. Gently using a tongue blade and penlight, examine all areas of the mouth. Carefully note any change in speech caused by tongue movement. Notice any change in voice or swallowing, and assess for thick or absent saliva. After inspection, the advanced practice nurse, specialty nurse, or other health care provider uses bimanual palpation of any visible nodules to determine size and fixation. The cervical lymph nodes are also palpated (Fig. 53-2).

The functioning and appearance of the mouth are strongly linked with body image and quality of life. Therefore it is important to assess the impact of oral lesions on the patient's self-concept. In addition, assess for any educational or cultural needs that might affect health teaching or treatment. Evaluate the patient's support system and past coping mechanisms.

OralCDx is a diagnostic procedure usually performed by a dentist during a routine dental examination. The procedure involves brushing of a lesion and is helpful in determining whether the lesion is precancerous (OralCDx, 2013). However, biopsy is the definitive method for diagnosis of oral cancer. The physician obtains a needle biopsy specimen of the abnormal tissue to assess for malignant or premalignant changes. Incisional biopsies may also be performed. An intraoral biopsy can be done under local anesthesia. In very small lesions, an excisional biopsy can permit complete tumor removal. MRI is useful in detecting perineural involvement and in evaluating thickness in cancers of the tongue. Both CT and MRI can be used to determine spread to the liver or lungs if further staging of the disease is warranted.

◆ Interventions

Both the presence of tumors of the oral cavity and the effects of their treatment threaten the integrity of the oral mucosa and the patient's airway. Oral cavity lesions can be treated by surgical excision, by nonsurgical treatments such as radiation or chemotherapy, or by a combination of treatments (referred to as *multimodal therapy*). Chemotherapy is currently not used independently in the treatment of oral cancers but is used in addition to other modes of treatment to sensitize malignant cells to radiation, to shrink a malignancy before surgery, or to decrease the potential for malignancy (OCF, 2013). Multimodal therapy is the most costly treatment option yet is more frequently used (OCF, 2013). *If the patient has extensive tumor involvement and copious, tenacious (thick and "stringy") secretions, maintaining an open airway is your priority for care to promote* GAS EXCHANGE. Other nursing interventions focus on restoring and maintaining oral health.

Nonsurgical Management. Implement interventions to *manage the patient's airway* by increasing air exchange, removing secretions, and preventing aspiration as needed. Assess for dyspnea resulting from the tumor obstruction or from excessive secretions. Assess the quality, rate, and depth of respirations. Auscultate the lungs for adventitious sounds, such as wheezes caused by aspiration. Listen for stridor caused by partial airway obstruction. Promote deep breathing to help produce an effective cough to mobilize the patient's secretions.

To promote GAS EXCHANGE, place the patient in a semi-Fowler's or high-Fowler's position. If the patient is able to swallow and gag reflexes are intact, it is beneficial to encourage fluids to liquefy secretions for easier removal. Chest physiotherapy also increases air exchange as well as promotes effective coughing. If available, collaborate with the respiratory therapist about performing this procedure. If needed, use oral suction equipment with a dental tip or a tonsil tip (Yankauer catheter) to remove secretions that obstruct the airway. Teach the patient and family to use the catheters as needed.

If edema occurs with oral cavity lesions, the patient may receive steroids to reduce inflammation. Antibiotics may be prescribed if INFECTION is present because it can increase inflammation and edema. A cool mist supplied by a face tent may assist with oxygen transport and control of edema.

It is important to work with the patient to *establish an oral hygiene routine.* Perform oral hygiene every 2 hours for ulcerated lesions, INFECTION, or in the immediate postoperative period. Modifications might be needed because of oral

! NURSING SAFETY PRIORITY (QSEN)

Action Alert

Aspiration Precautions prevent or reduce the risk factors for aspiration. Assess the patient's level of consciousness (LOC), gag reflex, and ability to swallow. To prevent aspiration, place the patient sitting upright at 90 degrees (high-Fowler's position). As a precaution, keep suction equipment nearby. For patients at high risk, assess the gag reflex before giving any fluids. Remind UAP to feed patients at risk for aspiration in small amounts. Teach visitors to speak with you before offering any type of food or drink to the patient. Provide thickened liquids as an aid to prevent aspiration. Referral to the speech/language pathologist can be beneficial for patients who are experiencing aspiration with swallowing. A swallow study may be needed to fully assess the risk for aspiration.

discomfort, bleeding, or edema. Oral care with a soft-bristled toothbrush is preferred. If the platelet count falls below 40,000/mm^3, switch the patient to an ultrasoft "chemobrush." The use of "Toothettes" or a disposable foam brush is discouraged because these products may not adequately control bacteremia-promoting plaque and may further dry the oral mucosa. Lubricant can be applied to moisten the lips and oral mucosa as needed.

Teach patients and their families that the patient should avoid using commercial mouthwashes and lemon-glycerin swabs. Commercial mouthwashes contain alcohol, and lemon-glycerin swabs are acidic. These substances can cause a burning sensation and contribute to dry oral mucous membranes. Encourage frequent rinsing of the mouth with sodium bicarbonate solution or warm saline (see also Chart 53-2). Follow hospital or health care provider protocol if available.

Radiation therapy for oral cancers can be given by external beam or interstitial implantation to reduce the size of the tumor before surgery. *External-beam* radiation passes through the skin or mucous membrane to the tumor site. Typically, treatments are given as five daily treatments per week, with a 2-day break each week, over a 6- to 9-week period. Each treatment lasts only about 10 to 15 minutes, with more time being dedicated to undertaking special precautions to minimize the dose of radiation to the brain or spinal cord (OCF, 2013).

Another option is the implantation of radioactive substances (*interstitial radiation therapy* or *brachytherapy*) either to boost the dosage or to deliver a radiation dose close to the tumor bed. This form of implant therapy can be curative in early-stage lesions in the floor of the mouth or anterior tongue. It may also add a boost of radiation to a tumor that received external-beam radiation.

With the exception of radioactive seeds, which have a low level of emission, patients receiving interstitial radiation are usually hospitalized for the duration of treatment. *Place patients on radiation transmission precautions while the materials are active or in place.* Patients need to be placed in a private room with lead-lined walls or moveable panels. When permitted, visitors may stay only 30 minutes or less each day and must sit or stand away from the patient in designated areas. Pregnant women and children younger than 18 years should not be permitted to visit. A tracheostomy may be required with interstitial implants because of edema and increased oral secretions. (See Chapter 22 for general nursing care of patients undergoing radiation therapy.)

Teach the patient undergoing *chemotherapy* and family members about the side effects of these agents, which vary with each drug. Give antiemetics as prescribed, and provide other comfort measures as needed. (See Chapter 22 for general care of patients receiving chemotherapy.)

NURSING SAFETY PRIORITY QSEN

Drug Alert

Patients who are undergoing radiation and/or chemotherapy treatment may experience a decreased ability to tolerate prescribed and over-the-counter medications due to being immunocompromised. Teach patients about expected side effects, and remind them to not take any medication (including over-the-counter medications, herbs, or vitamin supplements) without first discussing them with their health care provider.

One of the most recent advances in the use of drugs for oral cancer is targeted therapy. Hormone-like substances known as *growth factors (GFs)* occur in the body's cells. Oral tumor cells, along with other types of cancers, grow quickly because they have more GF receptors than does normal healthy tissue. One of these GFs is called *epidermal growth factor (EGF)*, which has been associated with oral cancers. Newer drugs that can target and block EGF receptors (EGF-R) are being tested, and more than a dozen have been approved, including cetuximab (Erbitux), erlotinib (Tarceva), and panitumumab (Vectibix). (Chapter 22 describes targeted molecular therapy.)

NCLEX EXAMINATION CHALLENGE

Physiological Integrity

A male client is admitted with a diagnosis of oral cancer. Which statement by the nursing assistant indicates a need for further teaching by the nurse about this client's oral care?

A. "I need to do oral care at least every 2 hours."
B. "I'll use a soft-bristled toothbrush to prevent bleeding."
C. "I'll remind him to use mouthwash after brushing."
D. "I'll tell him to rinse his mouth frequently with sodium bicarbonate."

Surgical Management. The physician can often remove small, noninvasive lesions of the oral cavity in an ambulatory surgical center with local anesthesia. The surgical defect is usually small enough to be closed by sutures. These smaller lesions may also be responsive to carbon dioxide laser therapy or **cryotherapy** (extreme cold application), as well as photodynamic therapy. These procedures can be performed as an ambulatory care procedure in a surgical center but may require general anesthesia.

Small oral cancers are equally responsive to radiation or photodynamic therapy and to surgery. More invasive lesions (stages III and IV) require more extensive surgical excision and result in a greater loss of function and disfigurement. Not all lesions can be excised by the peroral approach (through the mouth). The goal of surgical resection is removal of the tumor with a surgical margin that is free of cancer cells.

Preoperative Care. Before excision of a lesion in the oral cavity, assess and document the patient's level of understanding of the disease process, the rationale for the surgery, and the planned intervention. Problems associated with cancer therapy can be reduced or optimally managed by collaborating with the patient and family regarding preparation and instruction. Reinforce information as needed. Include family members or other caregivers in the health teaching unless culturally inappropriate.

For small, local excisions, postoperative restrictions include a liquid diet for a day and then advancing as tolerated. There are no activity limitations, and postoperative analgesics are prescribed.

Instructions for the patient undergoing large surgical resections may include but are not limited to these expectations after surgery:

- Placement of a temporary tracheostomy, oxygen therapy, and suctioning
- Temporary loss of speech because of the tracheostomy
- Frequent monitoring of postoperative vital signs
- NPO status until intraoral suture lines are healed
- Need to have IV lines in place for drug delivery and hydration
- Postoperative drug therapy and activity (out of bed on the day or surgery or first postoperative day)
- Possibility of surgical drains

Because communication is interrupted, assess the patient's ability to read, write, and draw pictures to communicate. In coordination with the patient, select the method of communication to use after surgery with staff and family members (e.g., Magic Slate, handheld mobile device, computer, picture board, or pad and pencil). Preprinted flashcards may be used to communicate the patient's needs, such as "I am tired," "I am in pain," or "I am hungry." Urge the patient to practice the chosen method before surgery to reduce frustration after surgery.

Operative Procedures. Three factors influence the extent of surgery performed for oral cancers: the size and location of the tumor, tumor invasion into the bone, and whether there has been metastasis (cancer spread) to neck lymph nodes. Small, noninvasive tumors can be removed perorally (through the mouth). Otherwise, an external approach may be used. The most extensive oral operations are composite resections, which combine partial or total **glossectomy** (tongue removal) and partial **mandibulectomy** (jaw removal). In the **commando** (co-mandible) **procedure** (COMbined neck dissection, MANDibulectomy, and Oropharyngeal resection), the surgeon removes a segment of the mandible with the oral lesion and performs a radical neck dissection (see Chapter 29).

Metastasis to cervical lymph nodes usually indicates a poor prognosis for patients with cancer of the oral cavity. In those with cervical node metastasis, a neck dissection may also be performed. A radical neck dissection usually involves the removal of all cervical lymph nodes on the affected side, along with cranial nerve XI (the accessory nerve), the internal jugular vein, and the sternocleidomastoid (front neck) muscle. Modified and selective neck dissections may be performed in patients with minimal lymph node involvement.

Postoperative Care. The patient may have a temporary or permanent tracheostomy, requiring intensive nursing care to promote airway clearance. In addition, care must be taken to protect the surgical incision site from mechanical damage and INFECTION (see Chapter 29). Nursing interventions to relieve PAIN or discomfort and promote NUTRITION are also important. Older adults are a special risk for surgery and need to be monitored very carefully (Chart 53-4).

Ensure that the predetermined method of communication is available for the patient, family members, and staff. When the patient has an adequate airway and can effectively clear secretions by coughing, the tracheostomy tube may be removed.

CHART 53-4 Focused Assessment

The Postoperative Older Adult with Oral Cancer

- Assess the mouth and surrounding tissues for candidiasis, mucositis, and pain; assess for loss of appetite and taste.
- Monitor the patient's weight.
- Monitor nutrition and fluid intake.
- Assess for difficulty in eating or speech.
- Assess pain status and measures used to control pain.
- Monitor the patient's response to medications.
- Identify psychosocial problems, such as depression, anxiety, and fear.
- Assess the patient's overall physiologic condition and how this may affect pharmacologic therapy.

! NURSING SAFETY PRIORITY QSEN

Action Alert

After extensive excision or resection for oral cancer, the most important nursing intervention is maintaining the patient's airway to promote GAS EXCHANGE! Upon awakening from anesthesia, the patient may not recall, or realize, that a tracheostomy tube is in place and may initially panic because of the inability to speak. Remind the patient why he or she cannot speak, and provide reassurance that the vocal cords are intact (unless a total laryngectomy has been performed, in which case the loss of voice is permanent).

When the tube is removed, an airtight dressing is placed over the site and the tracheostomy incision heals without the need for sutures.

Patients who have undergone extensive resection may have slurred speech or difficulty in speaking as a result of nerve damage or tongue removal. Collaborate with the speech-language pathologist if speech is altered.

Protect the incision site to avoid infection. Provide gentle mouth care for cleaning away thick secretions and stimulating the flow of saliva. The delivery of oral care depends on the nature and extent of the surgical procedure. Give oral care at least every 4 hours in the early postoperative phase. The presence of unusual odors from the mouth can indicate INFECTION; therefore continual assessment of the oral cavity is very important. In the early postoperative phase, take care to avoid disruption of the suture line during oral hygiene.

Elevate the head of the bed to assist in decreasing edema by gravity. If skin grafting was done, inspect the donor site (generally on the anterior thigh) every 8 hours for bleeding or signs of INFECTION. (See Chapter 29 for specific nursing care of the patient with a radical neck dissection.)

To provide optimal *pain relief* in the postoperative period, rely on subjective and objective data to assess the need for analgesics and their effectiveness. The desired outcome of drug therapy during this period is relief of PAIN while allowing the patient to function at an optimal level. Those who have undergone surgery for oral cancer describe their PAIN as throbbing or pounding. IV morphine is usually the initial pain medication given with acetaminophen or ibuprofen to decrease inflammation. Tylox or Percocet (oxycodone plus acetaminophen) may be used for systemic relief of moderate pain after the IV morphine is discontinued.

Patients who have undergone extensive resections of the oral cavity remain on NPO status for several days. This time allows healing in the oral cavity before food comes in contact with the incision. Nasogastric feeding or total parenteral NUTRITION may be needed until oral nutrition can begin (see Chapter 60).

! NURSING SAFETY PRIORITY QSEN

Action Alert

When oral fluid intake is started, assess for and document signs of difficulty swallowing, aspiration, or leakage of saliva or fluids from the suture line. Monitor daily weights and hydration. NUTRITION supplementation may be used to improve the patient's quality of life. Patients who have weight loss or who are having difficulty maintaining hydration may be candidates for the placement of a gastrostomy tube. Coordinate NUTRITION care with the dietitian.

Encourage the patient to perform swallowing exercises. Collaborate with the speech-language pathologist to assist with swallowing techniques. Thickened fluids may be needed to prevent aspiration. A swallowing impairment may be temporary or permanent.

Community-Based Care

Continuing care for the patient with an oral tumor depends on the severity of the tumor, its collaborative care, and available support systems. Most patients are maintained at home during follow-up care. Ongoing NUTRITION management remains a vital part of the treatment plan. In addition, the patient and family may benefit from a community-based support group for cancer patients.

Home Care Management. If radiation therapy is part of the patient's treatment plan, home care considerations include health teaching and management strategies. Complications due to radiation to the head or neck can be acute or delayed. Acute effects include treatment-related mucositis, stomatitis, and alterations in taste. Long-term effects such as **xerostomia** (excessive mouth dryness) and dental decay require ongoing oral care, the use of saliva substitutes, and follow-up dental visits. Although ongoing dental care is important, the possible adverse effects that radiation has on bone make elective oral surgical procedures, such as tooth extraction, impossible in the area of the radiation. Fatigue is a common side effect of radiation and chemotherapy.

The patient whose tracheostomy tube has been removed is often placed on a soft diet by mouth before discharge. Occasionally, however, patients are discharged from the hospital while still requiring tracheostomy suction, oral suction, and nasogastric feedings. Suction equipment, NUTRITION supplies, and nursing care can be provided by home care companies. (See Chapter 60 for home care preparation for the patient receiving home parenteral nutrition and Chapter 28 for home care preparation for the patient with a tracheostomy.)

Self-Management Education. Before hospital discharge, teach the patient and family about drug therapy, NUTRITION therapies, any treatments (e.g., tracheostomy care, suture line care, dressing changes), and early symptoms of INFECTION (Chart 53-5). Alterations in taste and dysphagia make maintaining adequate nutrition a challenge for the oral cancer patient. Alterations in taste occur when the taste buds are included in the radiation treatment field. Taste sensation may begin to return several weeks after the completion of treatment. Some types of chemotherapy can also affect the patient's taste. Sometimes the loss of taste is permanent.

CHART 53-5 Patient and Family Education: Preparing for Self-Management

Care of the Patient with Oral Cancer at Home

- Follow the treatment plan for cancer therapies.
- Remember that taste sensation may be decreased; add non-spicy seasonings to food to better enjoy it.
- Use a thickening agent for liquids if dysphagia is present.
- Eat soft foods if stomatitis occurs.
- Inspect the mouth every day for changes, such as redness or lesions.
- Continue meticulous oral hygiene at home using a chemobrush and frequent rinsing; clean brush after every use.
- Use saliva substitute as prescribed.
- Avoid sun or tanning bed exposure if radiation is part of therapy.
- Clean with a gentle, nondeodorant soap, such as Ivory.

Changes in taste include dislike of meat, such as beef or pork, and metallic tastes in the mouth. Teach patients to add seasonings to foods, to use gravies or sauces to make foods more palatable, and to use high-protein foods such as cheeses, milk, eggs, puddings, and legumes in place of meat. Instruct patients with dysphagia in swallowing exercises. Recommend thickened liquids because thin liquids, such as water, are difficult to control during swallowing. Collaborate with the dietitian to teach the family how to assess the NUTRITION intake of the patient who is just beginning to eat. Liquid dietary supplements are usually recommended at this time. If bleeding or stomatitis is present, recommend soft foods to prevent further injury to the mucous membranes.

Teach the patient or family members to inspect the oral cavity daily for areas of redness, which can indicate the onset of stomatitis. Meticulous oral hygiene should be continued at home, especially with adjuvant chemotherapy or radiation. Reinforce the oral hygiene routine, emphasizing the need for frequent mouth rinsing to reduce the number of microorganisms and to maintain adequate hydration. The patient should use a chemobrush (an extra-soft type of toothbrush), rinse the chemobrush with hydrogen peroxide and water or with a diluted bleach solution after each use, and change chemobrushes weekly. The brush may also be cleaned in a dishwasher.

Saliva production is greatly reduced as a consequence of radiation. The resulting xerostomia (dry mouth) causes the inability to eat dry foods and may be permanent. Teach the patient regarding the use of saliva substitutes.

Skin reactions are also a common side effect of radiation. Instruct the patient to avoid sun exposure, to avoid perfumed lotions and powders, and to cleanse the face and neck area with a gentle nondeodorant soap. Teach male patients to use an electric razor for shaving and to avoid alcohol-based aftershave lotions to prevent further skin irritation.

Health Care Resources. Patients who have undergone composite resection often require community services because they have both physical and psychosocial needs. Depression related to a change in body image is common. Excision of a portion of the jaw can leave a facial defect that may be difficult to hide. Assess for depression and other behavioral responses. A social worker or other health care professional may be needed for patient and family counseling. Those who have undergone a total glossectomy may be able to speak with special training and the use of an intraoral prosthesis created by a maxillofacial prosthodontist. The prosthesis is similar to dentures.

Collaborate with the case manager to provide assistance in obtaining special equipment or NUTRITION resources needed by the patient at home. The case manager assesses the patient's financial needs and makes referrals to government, community, and religious organizations as needed. Refer the patient to the American Cancer Society (ACS) (www.cancer.org), the Oral Cancer Foundation (www.oralcancerfoundation.org), and/or the Canadian Cancer Society (www.cancer.ca/en/region-selector-page/) for local support groups and resources, including additional information. The ACS often provides dressing supplies and transportation to and from follow-up visits or medical treatments.

NCLEX EXAMINATION CHALLENGE

Safe and Effective Care Environment

A client has completed chemotherapy and radiation therapy for an oral tumor and is being discharged to home. Which client statements require further teaching by the nurse? **Select all that apply.**

A. "Radiation therapy will not affect my sense of taste."
B. "I am likely to be fatigued after radiation."
C. "It is important for me to keep my oral cavity very clean."
D. "I will avoid tanning beds and sun exposure."
E. "I am eager to use my perfume soon after radiation therapy."
F. "My chemobrush should be replaced monthly."

CLINICAL JUDGMENT CHALLENGE

Teamwork and Collaboration; Patient-Centered Care QSEN

A 50-year-old businessman has just undergone oral surgery to remove a large oral tumor. Documentation of assessment of the oral cavity shows that the patient has poor oral hygiene. You are preparing to teach the patient methods of self-care management.

1. As the patient's nurse, what is your priority for his care immediately after surgery?
2. As you develop his plan of care, for what complications is this patient most at risk?
3. What would you teach the patient that would be most helpful to improve his oral hygiene?
4. Considering that he is a businessman, what psychosocial or sociocultural concerns would you anticipate he may experience?
5. What follow-up care is most important for this patient?

DISORDERS OF THE SALIVARY GLANDS

ACUTE SIALADENITIS

❖ PATHOPHYSIOLOGY

Acute sialadenitis, the inflammation of a salivary gland, can be caused by infectious agents, irradiation, or immunologic disorders. Salivary gland inflammation can have a bacterial or viral cause, such as INFECTION with cytomegalovirus (CMV). The most common bacterial organisms are *Staphylococcus aureus, Staphylococcus pyogenes, Streptococcus pneumoniae,* and *Escherichia coli.* This disorder most commonly affects the parotid or submandibular gland in adults.

A decrease in the production of saliva (as in dehydrated or debilitated patients or in those who are on NPO status postoperatively for an extended time) can lead to acute sialadenitis. The bacteria or viruses enter the gland through the ductal opening in the mouth. Systemic drugs, such as phenothiazines and the tetracyclines, can also trigger an episode of acute sialadenitis. Untreated infections of the salivary glands can evolve into abscesses, which can rupture and spread INFECTION into the tissues of the neck and the mediastinum.

Patients who receive radiation for the treatment of cancers of the head and neck or thyroid may develop decreased salivary flow, predisposing them to acute or persistent sialadenitis. The effect of radiation on the salivary glands is rapid and dose related. Immunologic disorders such as HIV INFECTION can cause enlargement of the parotid gland that results from secondary infection. Sjögren's syndrome, an autoimmune disorder, is characterized by chronic salivary gland enlargement and inflammation that cause a very dry mouth (see Chapter 20).

❖ PATIENT-CENTERED COLLABORATIVE CARE

During the initial interview, assess for any predisposing factors for sialadenitis, such as ionizing radiation to the head or neck area. Collect a thorough drug history, and ask about systemic illnesses, such as HIV infection.

Dehydration can be assessed by examining the oral membrane for dryness and the skin for turgor. Other assessment findings include PAIN and swelling of the face over the affected gland. Assess facial function because the branches of cranial nerve VII (the facial nerve) lie close to the salivary glands. Fever and general malaise also occur, and purulent drainage can often be massaged from the affected duct in the oral cavity.

Collaborative care includes the administration of IV fluids and measures such as these to treat the underlying cause and increase the flow of saliva:

- Hydration
- Application of warm compresses
- Massage of the gland
- Use of a saliva substitute
- Use of **sialagogues** (substances that stimulate the flow of saliva)

Sialagogues include lemon slices and citrus-flavored and other fruit-flavored candy. Massage is accomplished by milking the edematous gland with the fingertips toward the ductal opening. Elevation of the head of the bed promotes gravity drainage of the edematous gland.

Acute sialadenitis is best prevented by adherence to routine oral hygiene. This practice prevents INFECTION from ascending to the salivary glands from the mouth.

POST-IRRADIATION SIALADENITIS

The salivary glands are sensitive to ionizing radiation, such as from radiation therapy or radioactive iodine treatment of thyroid cancers. Exposure of the glands to radiation produces a type of sialadenitis known as **xerostomia** (very dry mouth caused by a severe reduction in the flow of saliva) within 24 hours. Radiation to the salivary glands can also produce PAIN and edema, which generally abate after several days.

Xerostomia may be temporary or permanent, depending on the dose of radiation and the percentage of total salivary gland tissue irradiated. Little can be done to relieve the patient's dry mouth during the course of radiation therapy. Frequent sips of water and frequent mouth care, especially before meals, are the most effective interventions. After the course of radiation therapy has been completed, saliva substitutes may provide moisture for 2 to 4 hours at a time. Over-the-counter solutions are available, or methylcellulose (Cologel), glycerin, and saline may be mixed to form a solution.

SALIVARY GLAND TUMORS

Of all oral tumors, those of the salivary glands are relatively rare. Initially, malignant tumors present as slow-growing, painless masses. Involvement of the facial nerve results in facial weakness or paralysis (partial or total) on the affected side.

Collect information about any prior radiation exposure, because radiation to the head and neck areas is associated with the occurrence of salivary gland tumors. Salivary gland tumors present as localized, firm masses. Submandibular and minor salivary gland tumors may be tender or painful. Tumor invasion of the hypoglossal nerve causes impaired movement of the tongue, and a loss of sensation can follow. *Pay particular attention to assessment of the facial nerve because of its proximity to the salivary glands.* Assess the patient's ability to:

- Wrinkle the brow
- Raise the eyebrows
- Squeeze and hold the eyes shut while you gently pull upwards on the eyebrows and cheeks beneath the orbit to check for symmetry
- Wrinkle the nose
- Pucker the lips
- Puff out the cheeks
- Grimace or smile

Be aware of any asymmetry when the patient performs these motions. The treatment of choice for both benign and malignant tumors of the salivary glands is surgical excision. However, radiation therapy is often used for salivary gland cancers that are large, have recurred, show evidence of residual disease after excision, or are highly malignant.

Patients who have undergone **parotidectomy** (surgical removal of the parotid glands) or submandibular gland surgery are at risk for weakness or loss of function of the facial nerve because the nerve courses directly through the gland. Facial nerve repair with grafting can be done at the time of surgery. A combination of surgery followed by radiation is common for advanced disease. Care for patients after parotidectomy is similar to that required for those having oral cancer surgery, described on pp. 1105-1106.

NURSING CONCEPTS AND CLINICAL JUDGMENT REVIEW

What might you NOTICE if the patient has inadequate digestion and GAS EXCHANGE as a result of oral cavity problems?

- Dysphagia (difficulty swallowing)
- Dyspnea
- Stridor or wheezes
- Changes in speech or voice
- Copious, thickened oral secretions
- Excessive coughing during meals

What should you INTERPRET and how should you RESPOND to a patient experiencing inadequate digestion and GAS EXCHANGE as a result of oral cavity problems?

Perform and interpret focused physical assessment findings, including:

- Breath sounds
- Oxygen saturation by pulse oximetry

- Ability to cough and clear the airway
- Ability to manage excessive oral secretions
- Ability to chew food and swallow

Respond by:
- Placing the patient with the head elevated to at least 30 degrees
- Applying oxygen as needed
- Suctioning the oral cavity as needed
- Encouraging deep breathing and coughing every 2 hours
- Increasing fluids to liquefy secretions, depending on swallowing ability
- Notifying the respiratory therapist or Rapid Response Team if interventions are not successful in restoring gas exchange (oxygenation).

On what should you REFLECT?
- Observe patient for evidence of increased gas exchange (oxygenation), including increased ease of breathing.
- Observe patient for evidence of increased ability to swallow.
- Observe patient for evidence of increased ability to manage oral secretions.
- Consider follow-up interventions to manage patient, including coordinating care with dietitian and speech-language pathologist.
- Think about what else you might do to promote digestion and nutrition.

GET READY FOR THE NCLEX® EXAMINATION!

KEY POINTS

Review these key points for each NCLEX Examination Client Needs Category.

Safe and Effective Care Environment
- Be aware that airway management is the priority for care for patients having surgery for oral cancer. **Safety** QSEN
- Place patients having oral cancer surgery in a high-Fowler's position to facilitate breathing and prevent aspiration. **Safety** QSEN
- Be sure to assess for swallowing ability to prevent aspiration by checking the gag reflex before offering liquids or food to the patient who has had oral cancer surgery. **Safety** QSEN
- Plan continuity of care to meet patients' needs when they are transferred from the hospital to community-based agencies. **Teamwork and Collaboration** QSEN

Health Promotion and Maintenance
- Teach patients to seek medical or dental attention for oral lesions that do not heal; these lesions could be oral carcinomas.
- Remind patients to visit their dentist regularly for dental hygiene and oral examination.
- Follow the best practice recommendations for maintaining oral health as listed in Chart 53-1.
- Instruct patients to avoid harsh commercial mouthwashes if they have oral lesions.
- In keeping with The Joint Commission (TJC) Core Measures TOB-2, teach patients to avoid tobacco, alcohol, and sun exposure to decrease their chance of having oral cancer.
- Instruct patients with acute sialadenitis to use sialagogues to stimulate saliva, such as citrus foods or candies.

Psychosocial Integrity
- Identify the patient's and family's response to an oral cancer diagnosis.
- Assist the patient and family in identifying and using coping mechanisms to deal with possible changes in body image and altered self-esteem. **Patient-Centered Care** QSEN
- Recognize that patients with stomatitis are often unable to eat or swallow without discomfort.
- Refer patients with oral cancer to support groups, such as those available through the American Cancer Society.

Physiological Integrity
- Remember that stomatitis usually manifests as painful single or multiple ulcerations within the mouth.
- Recognize that stomatitis can be caused by a variety of organisms; *Candida* INFECTIONS are very common in patients who receive antibiotic therapy and in those who are immunocompromised.
- Provide gentle oral care for patients with oral lesions, including using chemobrushes and warm saline or sodium bicarbonate solution. **Safety** QSEN
- Be aware that patients with stomatitis receive antimicrobials, anti-inflammatory agents, immune modulators, and topical agents for relief of symptoms, including PAIN. **Evidence-Based Practice** QSEN
- Differentiate leukoplakia and erythroplakia: leukoplakia presents as thin, white patches; and erythroplakia presents as red, velvety lesions.
- Be aware that patients with oral cancer may have chemotherapy, radiation, surgery, or a combination of these treatment methods.
- Be aware that sialadenitis can occur as a result of radiation therapy.
- For patients with salivary gland tumors, assess for facial nerve involvement.
- Remember that a parotidectomy involves the removal of the salivary glands; postoperative care is similar to that for patients who have oral cancer surgery.

54 CHAPTER

Care of Patients with Esophageal Problems

Cherie R. Rebar, Nicole Heimgartner, Laura Willis

http://evolve.elsevier.com/Iggy/

PRIORITY CONCEPTS

- INFECTION
- NUTRITION
- PAIN

LEARNING OUTCOMES

Safe and Effective Care Environment

1. Collaborate with health care team members when providing care to patients with esophageal health problems that impair swallowing or limit NUTRITION.

Health Promotion and Maintenance

2. Teach patients about lifestyle changes that decrease gastroesophageal reflux disease (GERD) and the PAIN associated with hiatal hernias.
3. Describe special considerations for the older adult with GERD.
4. Teach patients with esophageal health problems about community-based resources.

Psychosocial Integrity

5. Reduce the psychological impact for the patient and family who have received a diagnosis and treatment of esophageal cancer.

Physiological Integrity

6. Perform focused assessments for patients with esophageal health problems.
7. Evaluate the impact of esophageal cancer on the patient's NUTRITION status, including the risk for aspiration.
8. Apply knowledge of pathophysiology to anticipate complications of GERD and esophageal surgical procedures.
9. Teach patients how to reduce the physiological impact of esophageal health problems.
10. Develop an evidence-based teaching plan for the patient and family about postoperative care after esophageal surgery.
11. Plan community-based care for patients diagnosed with esophageal cancer.

Partially digested food is moved by the esophagus from the mouth to the stomach. If food cannot reach the stomach, the patient cannot meet the basic human need for NUTRITION. Nutrients in food are necessary for normal body cell function. Common problems of the esophagus that can interfere with digestion and NUTRITION are caused by inflammation, structural defects or obstruction, and cancer. Patient-centered collaborative care requires dietary and lifestyle changes, as well as medical and surgical therapies.

GASTROESOPHAGEAL REFLUX DISEASE

❖ PATHOPHYSIOLOGY

Gastroesophageal reflux disease (GERD) is the most common upper GI disorder in the United States. It occurs most often in middle-aged and older adults but can affect people of any age. **Gastroesophageal reflux (GER)** occurs as a result of backward flow of stomach contents into the esophagus. GERD is the chronic and more serious condition that arises from persistent GER.

Reflux produces symptoms by exposing the esophageal mucosa to the irritating effects of gastric or duodenal contents, resulting in inflammation. A person with acute symptoms of inflammation is often described as having mild or severe **reflux esophagitis** (McCance et al., 2014).

The reflux of gastric contents into the esophagus is normally prevented by the presence of two high-pressure areas that remain contracted at rest. A 1.2-inch (3-cm) segment at the proximal end of the esophagus is called the *upper esophageal sphincter (UES),* whereas another small portion at the gastroesophageal junction (near the cardiac sphincter) is called the **lower esophageal sphincter (LES)**. The function of the LES is supported by its anatomic placement in the abdomen, where the surrounding pressure is significantly higher than in the low-pressure thorax. Sphincter function is also supported by the acute angle (angle of His) that is formed as the esophagus enters the stomach.

The most common cause of GERD is excessive relaxation of the LES, which allows the reflux of gastric contents into the esophagus and exposure of the esophageal mucosa to acidic gastric contents. Patients who are overweight or obese are at highest risk for development of GERD because increased weight increases intra-abdominal pressure, which contributes to reflux of stomach contents into the esophagus. Nighttime reflux tends to cause prolonged exposure of the esophagus to acid because lying supine decreases peristalsis and the benefit of gravity. **Hiatal hernias** also increase the risk for development of GERD due to the creation of increased intra-abdominal pressure. *Helicobacter pylori* may contribute to reflux (McCance et al., 2014) by causing gastritis and thus poor gastric emptying. This increases frequency of GER events and acid exposure to the esophagus.

A person having reflux may be asymptomatic. However, the esophagus has limited resistance to the damaging effects of the acidic GI contents. The pH of acid secreted by the stomach ranges from 1.5 to 2.0, whereas the pH of the distal esophagus is normally neutral (6.0 to 7.0).

Refluxed material is returned to the stomach by a combination of gravity, saliva, and peristalsis. The inflamed esophagus cannot eliminate the refluxed material as quickly as a healthy one, and therefore the length of exposure increases with each reflux episode. Hyperemia (increased blood flow) and **erosion** (ulceration) occur in the esophagus in response to the chronic inflammation. Gastric acid and pepsin injure tissue. Minor capillary bleeding often occurs with erosion, but hemorrhage is rare.

During the process of healing, the body may substitute **Barrett's epithelium** (columnar epithelium) for the normal squamous cell epithelium of the lower esophagus. Although this new tissue is more resistant to acid and therefore supports esophageal healing, it is considered premalignant and is associated with an increased risk for cancer in patients with prolonged GERD. The fibrosis and scarring that accompany the healing process can produce **esophageal stricture** (narrowing of the esophageal opening). The stricture leads to progressive difficulty swallowing. Uncontrolled esophageal reflux also increases risk for other complications such as asthma, laryngitis, dental decay, cardiac disease, and serious concerns for hemorrhage and aspiration pneumonia.

Gastric distention caused by eating very large meals or delayed gastric emptying predisposes the patient to reflux. Certain foods and drugs, as well as smoking and alcohol, influence the tone function of the LES (Table 54-1).

Patients who have a nasogastric tube also have decreased esophageal sphincter function. The tube keeps the cardiac sphincter open and allows acidic contents from the stomach to enter the esophagus. Other factors that increase intra-abdominal and intragastric pressure (e.g., pregnancy, wearing tight belts or girdles, bending over, ascites) overcome the gastroesophageal pressure gradient maintained by the LES and allow reflux to occur. Many patients with obstructive sleep apnea report frequent episodes of GERD. People with hiatal hernias often have reflux because the upper portion of the stomach protrudes through the diaphragm into the thorax, which allows acid to reach the esophagus (see later discussion of hiatal hernia).

TABLE 54-1 Factors Contributing to Decreased Lower Esophageal Sphincter Pressure

- Caffeinated beverages, such as coffee, tea, and cola
- Chocolate
- Citrus fruits
- Tomatoes and tomato products
- Smoking and use of other tobacco products
- Calcium channel blockers
- Nitrates
- Peppermint, spearmint
- Alcohol
- Anticholinergic drugs
- High levels of estrogen and progesterone
- Nasogastric tube placement

❖ PATIENT-CENTERED COLLABORATIVE CARE

◆ Assessment

Ask the patient about a history of heartburn or atypical chest PAIN associated with the reflux of GI contents. Ask whether he or she has been newly diagnosed with asthma or has experienced morning hoarseness or pneumonia, because these symptoms may indicate severe reflux reaching the pharynx or mouth or pulmonary aspiration.

Physical Assessment/Clinical Manifestations. **Dyspepsia**, also known as "indigestion," and regurgitation are the main symptoms of GERD, although symptoms may vary in severity (Chart 54-1). Symptoms associated with "indigestion" may include abdominal discomfort, feeling uncomfortably full, nausea, and burping. Because indigestion might not be viewed as a serious concern, patients may delay seeking treatment. The symptoms typically worsen when the patient bends over, strains, or lies down. If the indigestion is severe, the PAIN may radiate to the neck or jaw or may be referred to the back, mimicking cardiac pain. Patients may come to the emergency department (ED) fearing that they are having a myocardial infarction ("heart attack").

With severe GERD, PAIN generally occurs after each meal and lasts for 20 minutes to 2 hours. Discomfort may worsen when the patient lies down. Drinking fluids, taking antacids, or maintaining an upright posture usually provides prompt relief.

Regurgitation (backward flow into the throat) of food particles or fluids is common. Risk for aspiration is increased if regurgitation occurs when the patient is lying down. Even if the patient is in an upright position, he or she may experience warm fluid traveling up the throat without nausea. If the fluid reaches the level of the pharynx, he or she notes a sour or bitter taste in the mouth. A reflex salivary hypersecretion known as **water brash** occurs in response to reflux. Water brash is different from regurgitation. The patient reports a sensation of fluid in the throat, but unlike with regurgitation, there is no bitter or sour taste.

CHART 54-1 Key Features

Gastroesophageal Reflux Disease

- Dyspepsia (indigestion)
- Regurgitation (may lead to aspiration or bronchitis)
- Coughing, hoarseness, or wheezing at night
- Water brash (hypersalivation)
- Dysphagia
- Odynophagia (painful swallowing)
- Epigastric pain
- Generalized abdominal pain
- Belching
- Flatulence
- Nausea
- Pyrosis (heartburn)
- Globus (feeling of something in back of throat)
- Pharyngitis
- Dental caries (severe cases)

Ask the patient if he or she experiences **eructation** (belching), **flatulence** (gas), and bloating after eating; these are other common manifestations. Nausea and vomiting rarely occur; unplanned weight loss is not common.

Assess for crackles in the lung, which can be an indication of associated aspiration. Patients who have had long-term regurgitation may experience coughing, hoarseness, or wheezing at night, which may be associated with bronchitis.

Chronic GERD can cause **dysphagia** (difficulty swallowing). Dysphagia usually indicates a narrowing of the esophagus because of stricture or inflammation. Assess the patient for degree of dysphagia, whether ingesting solids and/or liquids induces dysphagia, and whether dysphagia occurs intermittently or with each swallowing effort.

Odynophagia (painful swallowing) can also occur with chronic GERD, but it is rare in people with uncomplicated reflux disease. Severe and long-lasting chest PAIN may be present if esophageal spasms cause the muscle to contract with excess force. The resulting PAIN can be agonizing and may last for hours.

Other manifestations include atypical chest PAIN, symptoms of asthma, and chronic cough that occurs mostly at night or when the patient is lying down. Cough and symptoms of asthma occur when refluxed acid is spilled over into the tracheobronchial tree. *Atypical chest pain* is thought to be caused by stimulation of PAIN receptors in the esophageal wall and by esophageal spasm. This type of chest PAIN can mimic angina and needs to be carefully distinguished from cardiac PAIN.

CONSIDERATIONS FOR OLDER ADULTS

Patient-Centered Care QSEN

Older adults are at risk for developing severe complications associated with GERD due to age-related physiologic changes, medication side effects, and an increased prevalence of hiatal hernias (Solomon & Reynolds, 2012). Instead of heartburn associated with GERD, this population experiences more severe complications of the disease such as atypical chest pain; ear, nose, and throat infections; and pulmonary problems, such as aspiration pneumonia, sleep apnea, and asthma. Barrett's esophagus and esophageal erosions are also more common in older adults (Chait, 2010).

Diagnostic Assessment. A definitive diagnostic test for GERD does not exist; however, health care providers may use one or more options to attempt to establish a diagnosis when GERD is suspected (The Ohio State University Wexner Medical Center [OSUWMC], 2014).

Patients may drink a solution and then have x-rays performed as part of a *barium swallow,* which shows hiatal hernias, strictures, and other structural or anatomic esophageal problems. Although this test, when conducted by itself, does not confirm GERD, it can be helpful when used in combination with other diagnostic procedures.

Upper endoscopy (also called **esophagogastroduodenoscopy [EGD]**) involves insertion of an endoscope (a flexible plastic tube equipped with a light and lens) down the throat, which allows the health care provider to see the esophagus and look for abnormalities. A biopsy can be taken while the patient undergoes endoscopy (see Chapter 52) (OSUWMC, 2013). This test requires the use of moderate sedation during the procedure, and patients must have someone accompany them home after recovery.

A **pH monitoring examination** is the most accurate method of diagnosing GERD. This involves either (1) placing a small catheter through the nose into the distal esophagus or (2) temporarily attaching a small capsule to the wall of the esophagus during an upper endoscopy (the 48-hour Bravo esophageal ph test). The patient is asked to keep a diary of activities and symptoms over 24 to 48 hours (depending on diagnostic method), and the pH is continuously monitored and recorded. Ambulatory pH monitoring is especially useful in diagnosing patients with atypical symptoms. A wireless monitoring device may be used to promote patient comfort (OSUWMC, 2014).

Although not as common, *esophageal manometry,* or motility testing, may be performed when the diagnosis is uncertain. Water-filled catheters are inserted in the patient's nose or mouth and slowly withdrawn while measurements of LES pressure and peristalsis are recorded. When used alone, manometry is not sensitive or specific enough to establish a diagnosis of GERD (National Institutes of Health, 2013). A Gastric Emptying Study can also be done while a patient is in the radiology/nuclear medicine department. He or she is given a meal mixed with radiolucent dye, and imaging is performed to determine how well the stomach empties over the next few hours. If food stays too long in the stomach, it can reflux back into the esophagus, causing symptoms (OSUWMC, 2014). Imaging of the lungs can also be conducted 24 hours later to visualize whether the patient has aspirated stomach contents.

◆ *Interventions*

Nonsurgical Management. The purpose of treatment for GERD is to relieve symptoms, treat esophagitis, and prevent complications such as strictures or Barrett's esophagus. For most patients, GERD can be controlled by NUTRITION therapy, lifestyle changes, and drug therapy. *The most important role of the nurse is patient and family education. Teach the patient that GERD is a chronic disorder that requires ongoing management. The disease should be treated more aggressively in older adults (Chait, 2010).*

Nonpharmacologic Interventions. *NUTRITION therapy* is used to relieve symptoms in patients with relatively mild GERD. Ask about the patient's basic meal patterns and food preferences. Coordinate with the dietitian, patient, and family about how to adapt to changes in eating that may decrease reflux symptoms.

Teach the patient to limit or eliminate foods that decrease LES pressure and that irritate inflamed tissue, causing heartburn, such as peppermint, chocolate, alcohol, fatty foods (especially fried), caffeine, and carbonated beverages. The patient should also restrict spicy and acidic foods (e.g., orange juice, tomatoes) until esophageal healing can occur. Patients who are smartphone users may find different types of applications ("apps") that can help them follow a healthier diet, such as MyFitnessPal (www.myfitnesspal.com). In keeping with The Joint Commission Core Measures, teach patients that smoking and alcohol use should also be avoided, because these can also decrease LES pressure. Explore the possibility and methods for smoking cessation, and make appropriate referrals. Ask the patient about his or her use of alcoholic beverages, and if appropriate, assist the patient in finding alcohol-cessation programs.

Large meals increase the volume of and pressure in the stomach and delay gastric emptying. Remind the patient to eat four to six small meals each day rather than three large ones. Encourage patients to avoid eating at least 3 hours before going

CHART 54-2 Patient and Family Education: Preparing for Self-Management

Health Promotion and Lifestyle Changes to Control Reflux

- Eat four to six small meals a day.
- Limit or eliminate fatty foods, coffee, tea, cola, and chocolate.
- Reduce or eliminate from your diet any food or spice that increases gastric acid and causes pain.
- Limit or eliminate alcohol and tobacco, and reduce exposure to secondhand smoke.
- Do not snack in the evening, and do not eat for 2 to 3 hours before you go to bed.
- Eat slowly and chew your food thoroughly to reduce belching.
- Remain upright for 1 to 2 hours after meals, if possible.
- Elevate the head of your bed 6 to 12 inches using wooden blocks, or elevate your head using a foam wedge. Never sleep flat in bed.
- If you are overweight, lose weight.
- Do not wear constrictive clothing.
- Avoid heavy lifting, straining, and working in a bent-over position.
- Chew "chewable" antacids thoroughly, and follow with a glass of water.

to bed because reflux episodes are most damaging at night. Advise the patient to eat slowly and chew thoroughly to facilitate digestion and prevent eructation (belching).

The control of GERD involves *lifestyle changes* to promote health and control reflux (Chart 54-2). Teach the patient to elevate the head by 6 to 12 inches for sleep to prevent nighttime reflux. This can be done by placing blocks under the head of the bed or by using a large, wedge-style pillow instead of a standard pillow. Teach the patient to sleep in the right side-lying position to promote oxygenation and frequent swallowing to clear the esophagus. Assist the patient in examining approaches to weight reduction. Decreasing intra-abdominal pressure often reduces reflux symptoms. Teach the patient to avoid wearing constrictive clothing, lifting heavy objects or straining, and working in a bent-over or stooped position. Emphasize that these general adaptations are an essential and effective part of disease management and can produce prompt results in uncomplicated cases.

Obese patients often have obstructive sleep apnea, as well as GERD. Those who receive continuous positive airway pressure (CPAP) treatment report improved sleeping and decreased episodes of reflux at night. See Chapter 29 for a discussion of CPAP.

Some drugs lower LES pressure and *cause* reflux, such as oral contraceptives, anticholinergic agents, sedatives, NSAIDs (e.g., ibuprofen), nitrates, and calcium channel blockers. The possibility of eliminating those drugs causing reflux should be explored with the health care provider.

Drug Therapy. Drug therapy for GERD management includes three major types—antacids, histamine blockers, and proton pump inhibitors. These drugs, which are also used for peptic ulcer disease, have one or more of these functions (see Chapter 55, Chart 55-3):

- Inhibit gastric acid secretion
- Accelerate gastric emptying
- Protect the gastric mucosa

In uncomplicated cases of GERD, *antacids* may be effective for *occasional* episodes of heartburn. Antacids act by elevating the pH level of the gastric contents, thereby deactivating pepsin. They are not helpful in controlling frequent symptoms because their length of action is too short and their nighttime effectiveness is minimal. These drugs also *increase* LES pressure and therefore are not given for long-term use.

Antacids containing aluminum hydroxide or magnesium hydroxide may be used. Maalox and Mylanta consist of a combination of these two agents. Patients often tolerate them better because they produce fewer side effects, such as constipation and diarrhea. Liquid forms of these medications are preferred, since they coat the esophagus to provide pain relief and to buffer acid. Teach the patient to take the antacid 1 hour before and 2 to 3 hours after each meal.

Gaviscon, a combination of alginic acid and sodium bicarbonate, is often a very effective drug for GERD. It forms thick foam that floats on top of the gastric contents and theoretically decreases the incidence of reflux. If reflux occurs, the foam enters the esophagus first and buffers the acid in the refluxed material. Remind the patient to take this drug when food is in the stomach.

Histamine receptor antagonists, commonly called *histamine blockers,* such as famotidine (Pepcid) and ranitidine (Zantac), decrease acid, are long acting, have fewer side effects, and allow less-frequent dosing. Although these drugs do not affect the occurrence of reflux directly, they do reduce gastric acid secretion, improve symptoms, and promote healing of inflamed esophageal tissue. With these drugs available over the counter (OTC) and widely advertised for heartburn, many patients self-medicate before seeking professional assistance from their primary care provider. Encourage patients to speak with their primary care provider to determine whether long-term use of these medications is appropriate.

Proton pump inhibitors (PPIs), such as omeprazole (Prilosec), rabeprazole (AcipHex), pantoprazole (Protonix), and esomeprazole (Nexium), are the *main* treatment for more severe GERD. Some PPIs are available as OTC drugs. These agents provide effective, long-acting inhibition of gastric acid secretion by affecting the proton pump of the gastric parietal cells. PPIs reduce gastric acid secretion and can be given in a single daily dose. If once-a-day dosing fails to control symptoms, twice-daily dosing may be used (National Guideline Clearinghouse [NGC], 2013). A newer PPI, omeprazole/sodium bicarbonate (Zegerid), is the first immediate-release PPI and is designed for short-term use. Another newer PPI, dexlansoprazole (Kapidex), is a dual-release (delayed-release) drug that is available in several dosages but tends to be associated with more side and adverse effects than some of the other PPIs.

Some PPIs, such as Nexium and Protonix, may be administered in IV form for short-term use to treat or to prevent stress ulcers that can result from surgery. PPIs promote rapid tissue healing, but recurrence is common when the drug is stopped. Long-term use may mask reflux symptoms, and stopping the drug determines if reflux has been resolved. Long-term use may also cause community-acquired pneumonia and GI infections such as those caused by *Clostridium difficile.*

CONSIDERATIONS FOR OLDER ADULTS

Patient-Centered Care QSEN

Research has also found that long-term use of proton pump inhibitors may increase the risk for hip fracture, especially in older adults. PPIs can interfere with calcium absorption and protein digestion and therefore reduce available calcium to bone tissue. Decreased calcium makes bones more brittle and likely to fracture, especially as people age (Chait, 2010).

NCLEX EXAMINATION CHALLENGE

Physiological Integrity

A client with gastroesophageal reflux disease (GERD) is prescribed to start pantoprazole (Protonix) 40 mg every day. Which statement by the client requires further teaching by the nurse?

A. "When I feel better, I can stop taking this drug."
B. "I'll take this drug at 8 AM every morning."
C. "This drug can cause headache and dizziness."
D. "I should not crush the drug because it has a delayed release."

Endoscopic Therapies. The Stretta procedure, a nonsurgical method, can replace surgery for GERD when other measures are not effective. Patients who are very obese or have severe symptoms may not be candidates for this procedure. In the Stretta procedure, the physician applies radiofrequency (RF) energy through the endoscope using needles placed near the gastroesophageal junction. The RG energy decreases vagus nerve activity, thus reducing discomfort for the patient. Postoperative instructions for patients who have undergone the Stretta procedure can be found in Chart 54-3.

Surgical Management. A very small percentage of patients with GERD require anti-reflux surgery. It is usually indicated for otherwise healthy patients who have failed to respond to medical treatment or have developed complications related to GERD. Various surgical procedures may be used through conventional open techniques or laparoscope.

Laparoscopic Nissen fundoplication (LNF) is a minimally invasive surgery (MIS) and is the standard surgical approach for treatment of severe GERD (Buckley & Roberts, 2014). Information about this procedure can be found in the next section (Hiatal Hernia) in the Surgical Management discussion. Patients who have surgery are encouraged to continue following the basic anti-reflux regimen of antacids and NUTRITION therapy because the rate of recurrence is high (University of Michigan Health System, 2012).

HIATAL HERNIA

Hiatal hernias, also called *diaphragmatic hernias*, involve the protrusion of the stomach through the esophageal hiatus of the diaphragm into the chest. The esophageal hiatus is the opening in the diaphragm through which the esophagus passes from the thorax to the abdomen. Most patients with hiatal hernias are asymptomatic, but some may have daily symptoms similar to those with GERD (McCance et al., 2014).

❖ *PATHOPHYSIOLOGY*

The two major types of hiatal hernias are sliding hernias (which are most common) and paraesophageal (rolling) hernias. The esophagogastric junction and a portion of the fundus of the stomach slide upward through the esophageal hiatus into the chest, usually as a result of weakening of the diaphragm (Fig. 54-1). The hernia generally moves freely and slides into

CHART 54-3 Patient and Family Education: Preparing for Self-Management

Postoperative Instructions for Patients Having Stretta Procedure

- Remain on clear liquids for 24 hours after the procedure.
- After the first day, consume a soft diet, such as custard, pureed vegetables, mashed potatoes, and applesauce.
- Avoid nonsteroidal anti-inflammatory drugs (NSAIDs) and aspirin for 10 days.
- Continue drug therapy as prescribed, usually proton pump inhibitors.
- Use liquid medications whenever possible.
- Do not allow nasogastric tubes for at least 1 month because the esophagus could be perforated.
- Contact the health care provider immediately if these problems occur:
  - Chest or abdominal pain
  - Bleeding
  - Dysphagia
  - Shortness of breath
  - Nausea or vomiting

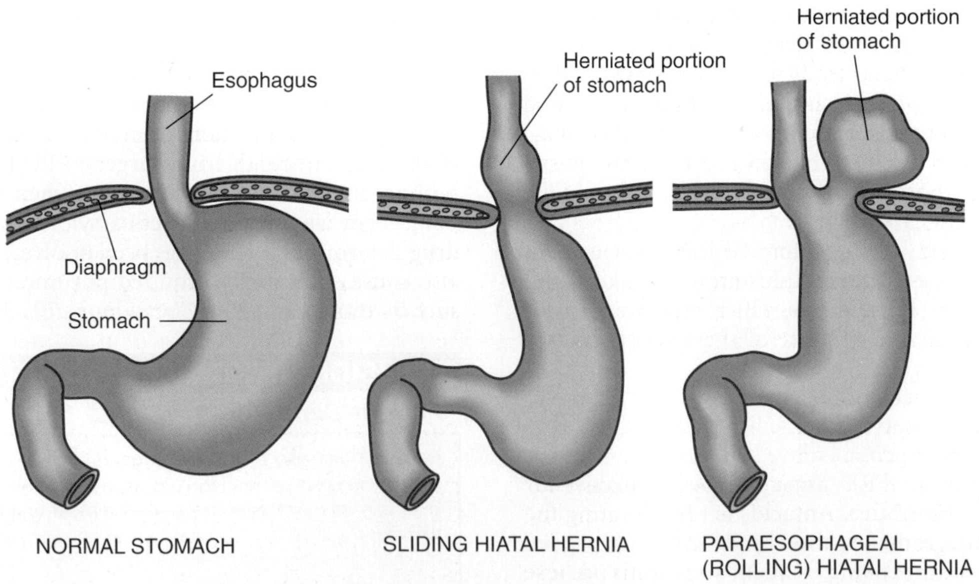

FIG. 54-1 A comparison of the normal stomach and sliding and paraesophageal (rolling) hiatal hernias.

and out of the chest during changes in position or intra-abdominal pressure. Although **volvulus** (twisting of a GI structure) and obstruction do occur rarely, the major concern for a sliding hernia is the development of esophageal reflux and associated complications (see Gastroesophageal Reflux Disease section earlier in this chapter). The development of reflux is related to chronic exposure of the lower esophageal sphincter (LES) to the low pressure of the thorax, which significantly reduces the effectiveness of the LES. Symptoms associated with decreased LES pressure are worsened by positions that favor reflux, such as bending or lying supine. Coughing, obesity, and ascites also increase reflux symptoms.

With *rolling hernias,* also known as *paraesophageal hernias,* the gastroesophageal junction remains in its normal intra-abdominal location but the fundus (and possibly portions of the stomach's greater curvature) rolls through the esophageal hiatus and into the chest beside the esophagus (see Fig. 54-1). The herniated portion of the stomach may be small or quite large. In rare cases, the stomach completely inverts into the chest. Reflux is not usually present because the LES remains anchored below the diaphragm. However, the risks for volvulus (twisting of a GI structure), obstruction (blockage), and strangulation (stricture) are high. The development of iron deficiency anemia is common because slow bleeding from venous obstruction causes the gastric mucosa to become engorged and ooze. Significant bleeding or hemorrhage is rare.

Rolling hernias are thought to develop from an anatomic defect occurring when the stomach is not properly anchored below the diaphragm rather than from muscle weakness. They can also be caused by previous esophageal surgeries, including sliding hernia repair.

❖ PATIENT-CENTERED COLLABORATIVE CARE

◆ Assessment

Ask the patient if he or she has heartburn, regurgitation (backward flow of food into the throat), PAIN, dysphagia (difficulty swallowing), and eructation (belching). Assess general physical appearance and NUTRITION status. Note the location, onset, duration, and quality of PAIN, as well as factors that relieve it or make it worse. The primary symptoms of sliding hiatal hernias are associated with reflux. Auscultate the lungs because pulmonary symptoms similar to asthma may be triggered by episodes of aspiration, particularly at night. A detailed history is crucial in attempting to differentiate angina from noncardiac chest PAIN caused by reflux. Symptoms resulting from hiatal hernia typically worsen after a meal or when the patient is in a supine position (Chart 54-4).

In those with rolling hernias, assess for symptoms related to stretching or displacement of thoracic contents by the hernia. Patients may report a feeling of fullness after eating or have breathlessness or a feeling of suffocation if the hernia interferes with breathing. Some may experience chest PAIN associated with reflux that mimics angina.

The *barium swallow study with fluoroscopy* is the most specific diagnostic test for identifying hiatal hernia. Rolling hernias are usually clearly visible, and sliding hernias can often be observed when the patient moves through a series of positions that increase intra-abdominal pressure. To visualize sliding hernias, an esophagogastroduodenoscopy (EGD) may be performed to view both the esophagus and gastric lining (see Chapter 52).

CHART 54-4 Key Features

Hiatal Hernias

Sliding Hiatal Hernias	Paraesophageal Hernias
• Heartburn	• Feeling of fullness after eating
• Regurgitation	• Breathlessness after eating
• Chest pain	• Feeling of suffocation
• Dysphagia	• Chest pain that mimics angina
• Belching	• Worsening of manifestations in a recumbent position

◆ Interventions

Patients with hiatal hernias may be managed either medically or surgically. Collaborative care is based on the severity of symptoms and the risk for serious complications. Sliding hiatal hernias are most commonly treated medically. Large rolling hernias can become strangulated or obstructed; therefore early surgical repair is preferred.

Nonsurgical Management. The collaborative interventions for patients with hiatal hernia are similar to those for GERD and include drug therapy, NUTRITION therapy, and lifestyle changes. The health care provider typically recommends antacids and a proton-pump inhibitor such as lansoprazole (Prevacid), omeprazole (Prilosec), or esomeprazole (Nexium) in an attempt to control reflux and its symptoms (Harvard Health Publications, 2011). NUTRITION therapy is also important and follows the guidelines discussed earlier for GERD.

! NURSING SAFETY PRIORITY QSEN

Action Alert

The most important role of the nurse in caring for a patient with a hiatal hernia is health teaching. Encourage the patient to avoid eating in the late evening and to avoid foods associated with reflux. Teach the patient and family that the patient should follow a restricted diet and should exercise regularly. Reducing body weight is beneficial because obesity increases intra-abdominal pressure and worsens both the hernia and the symptoms of reflux. Teach about positioning, including:

- Sleep at night with the head of the bed elevated 6 inches
- Remain upright for several hours after eating
- Avoid straining or excessive vigorous exercise
- Refrain from wearing clothing that is tight or constrictive around the abdomen

Surgical Management. Surgery may be required when the risk for complications is high or when damage from chronic reflux becomes severe.

Preoperative Care. If the surgery is not urgent, the surgeon instructs patients who are overweight to lose weight before surgery. They are also advised to quit or significantly reduce smoking. As part of preoperative teaching, reinforce the surgeon's instructions and prepare the patient for what to expect after surgery.

Operative Procedures. Several types of hiatal hernia repair procedures are used, each of which involves reinforcement of the lower esophageal sphincter (LES) by fundoplication. The surgeon wraps a portion of the stomach fundus around the distal esophagus to anchor it and reinforce the LES (Fig. 54-2).

Laparoscopic Nissen fundoplication (LNF) is a minimally invasive surgery commonly used for hiatal hernia repair (Buckley & Roberts, 2014). Complications after LNF occur less

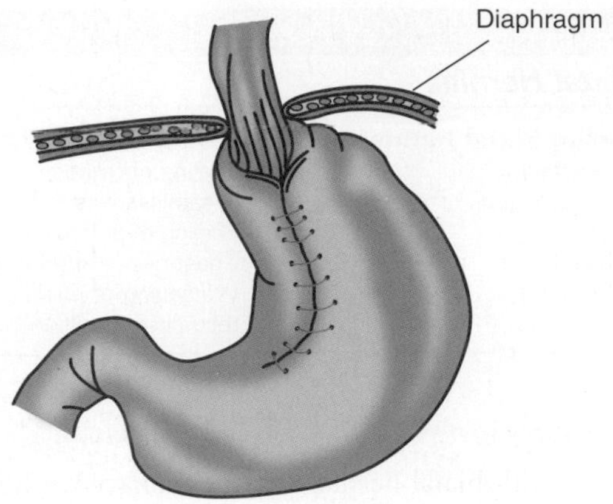

FIG. 54-2 Open surgical approach for Nissen fundoplication for gastroesophageal reflux disease or hiatal hernia repair.

frequently compared with those seen in patients having the more traditional open surgical approach. A small percentage of patients are not candidates for LNF and therefore require a conventional open fundoplication.

For the trans-thoracic surgical approach, teach the patient about chest tubes. Inform the patient that a nasogastric tube will be inserted during surgery and will remain in place for several days. Oral intake is started gradually with clear liquids after peristalsis is re-established or to stimulate peristalsis. Instruct the patient how to deep breathe and use the incentive spirometer. These measures are essential to prevent postoperative respiratory complications. The high incision makes deep breathing extremely painful. Teach the patient about postoperative pain, and assure him or her that adequate postoperative analgesic will be given promptly. PAIN levels must be continuously monitored.

In paraesophageal repair (a laparoscopic surgery), several ½-inch incisions are made in the abdomen, through which the hernia is closed and is typically reinforced using mesh. Less commonly, a conventional open procedure is used in which the surgeon uses a high trans-thoracic approach that requires a large chest incision for access to the surgical area.

Postoperative Care. Patients having the *LNF procedure* or paraesophageal repair via laparoscope are at risk for bleeding and infection, although these problems are not common. *The nursing care priority is to observe for these complications and provide health teaching as described in* Chart 54-5.

Postoperative care after *conventional open repair* closely follows that required after any esophageal surgery. Complications after open surgery are more common and potentially serious. Carefully assess for complications of open fundoplication surgery, described next, and report any complications to the health care provider (Chart 54-6).

! NURSING SAFETY PRIORITY (QSEN)

Action Alert

The primary focus of care after conventional surgery for a hiatal hernia repair is the prevention of respiratory complications. Elevate the head of the patient's bed at least 30 degrees to lower the diaphragm and promote lung expansion. Assist the patient out of bed and begin ambulation as soon as possible. Be sure to support the incision during coughing to reduce PAIN and to prevent excessive strain on the suture line, especially with obese patients.

CHART 54-5 Patient and Family Education: Preparing for Self-Management

Postoperative Instructions for Patients Having Laparoscopic Nissen Fundoplication (LNF) or Paraesophageal Repair via Laparoscope

- Stay on a soft diet for about a week, including mashed potatoes, puddings, custard, and milkshakes; avoid carbonated beverages, tough foods, and raw vegetables that are difficult to swallow.
- Remain on anti-reflux medications as prescribed for at least a month.
- Do not drive for a week after surgery; do not drive if taking opioid pain medication.
- Walk every day, but do not do any heavy lifting.
- Remove small dressings 2 days after surgery, and shower; do not remove Steri-Strips until 10 days after surgery.
- Wash incisions with soap and water, rinse well, and pat dry; report any redness or drainage from the incisions to your surgeon.
- Report fever above 101° F (38.3° C), nausea, vomiting, or uncontrollable bloating or pain. For patients older than 65 years, report elevations above 100° F (37.8° C).
- Schedule an appointment for follow-up with your surgeon in 3 to 4 weeks.

CHART 54-6 Best Practice for Patient Safety & Quality Care (QSEN)

Assessment of Postoperative Complications Related to Fundoplication Procedures

COMPLICATION	ASSESSMENT FINDINGS
Temporary dysphagia	The patient has difficulty swallowing when oral feeding begins.
Gas bloat syndrome	The patient has difficulty belching to relieve distention.
Atelectasis, pneumonia	The patient experiences dyspnea, chest pain, or fever.
Obstructed nasogastric tube	The patient experiences nausea, vomiting, or abdominal distention. The nasogastric tube does not drain.

Incentive spirometry and deep breathing are routinely used after surgery to maintain patency of the airways and lung expansion. Adequate PAIN control with analgesics is essential for postoperative deep breathing and coughing. Patients with a smoking history or chronic airway limitation (e.g., chronic obstructive pulmonary disease, asthma) require more aggressive management by the respiratory therapist to prevent atelectasis and pneumonia. Patients with large hiatal hernias are at the highest risk for developing respiratory complications.

The patient having the conventional surgery usually has a large-bore (diameter) nasogastric (NG) tube to prevent the fundoplication wrap from becoming too tight around the esophagus. Initially the NG drainage should be dark brown with old blood. The drainage should become normal yellowish green within the first 8 hours after surgery. Check the NG tube every 4 to 8 hours for proper placement in the stomach. The tube should be properly anchored so it is not displaced, because re-insertion could perforate the fundoplication. Follow the surgeon's directions for care of the patient with an NG tube.

Monitor patency of the NG tube to keep the stomach decompressed. This prevents retching or vomiting, which can strain or rupture the stomach sutures. The NG tube is irritating.

Therefore provide frequent oral hygiene to increase comfort. Assess the patient's hydration status regularly, including accurate measures of intake and output. Adequate fluid replacement helps thin respiratory secretions.

After open fundoplication, the patient may begin clear fluids when peristalsis is re-established or in an effort to stimulate peristalsis. Some surgeons create a temporary gastrostomy for feeding to allow for undisturbed healing of the repair. The patient gradually progresses to a near-normal diet during the first 4 to 6 weeks. Some foods, especially caffeinated or carbonated beverages and alcohol, are either restricted or eliminated. The food storage area of the stomach is reduced by the surgery, and meals need to be both smaller and more frequent.

Carefully supervise the first oral feedings because temporary dysphagia is common. Continuous dysphagia usually indicates that the fundoplication is too tight, and dilation may be required.

Another common complication of this surgery is *gas bloat syndrome,* in which patients are unable to voluntarily eructate (belch). The syndrome is usually temporary but may persist, even in those who have the laparoscopic approach. Teach the patient to avoid drinking carbonated beverages and to avoid eating gas-producing foods (especially high-fat foods), chewing gum, and drinking with a straw.

Other patients have *aerophagia* (air swallowing) from attempting to reverse or clear acid reflux. Teach them to relax consciously before and after meals, to eat and drink slowly, and to chew all food thoroughly. Air in the stomach that cannot be removed by belching can be extremely uncomfortable. Frequent position changes and ambulation are often effective interventions for eliminating air from the GI tract. If gas PAIN is still present, patients are taught to take simethicone, which dissolves in the mouth.

Community-Based Care

Patients undergoing one of the open surgical repairs require activity restrictions during the 3- to 6-week postoperative recovery period. For laparoscopic surgery, activity is typically restricted for a shorter time and the patient can return to his or her usual lifestyle more quickly, usually in a few days to a week.

For long-term management, teach the patient and family about appropriate NUTRITION modifications. The use of stool softeners or bulk laxatives is recommended for the first postoperative weeks until healing is complete. Instruct the patient to avoid straining and to prevent constipation. Teach him or her to inspect the healing incision daily and to notify the health care provider if swelling, redness, tenderness, discharge, or fever occurs. According to The Joint Commission National Patient Safety Goals for 2014, advise the patient to avoid contact with people with a respiratory INFECTION and to contact the health care provider if symptoms of a cold or influenza develop. Continuous coughing can cause the incision or the fundoplication to dehisce ("break open"). Per The Joint Commission Core Measures to decrease tobacco use, advise the patient to avoid smoking. Provide information about smoking-cessation methods, if appropriate.

If needed, collaborate with the dietitian to educate the patient and family about dietary changes. Encourage the patient to eat smaller and more frequent meals. Few ongoing diet restrictions are needed, but overeating or eating the wrong types of foods can produce discomfort if the patient cannot belch. Instruct the patient to report reflux symptoms to the health care provider.

Although severe surgical complications are rare, conditions such as gas bloat syndrome and dysphagia may continue. Prepare the patient for these problems and for the potential that reflux may not be completely controlled or may occur again. Although surgery controls the condition, a cure is rare and lifestyle modifications need to be ongoing.

ESOPHAGEAL TUMORS

❖ PATHOPHYSIOLOGY

Although esophageal tumors can be benign, most are malignant (cancerous) and the majority arise from the epithelium. Squamous cell carcinomas of the esophagus are located in the upper two thirds of the esophagus. Adenocarcinomas are more commonly found in the distal third and at the gastroesophageal junction and are now the most common type of esophageal cancer (McCance et al., 2014). Esophageal tumors grow rapidly because there is no serosal layer to limit their extension. Because the esophageal mucosa is richly supplied with lymph tissue, there is early spread of tumors to lymph nodes. Esophageal tumors can protrude into the esophageal lumen and can cause thickening or invade deeply into surrounding tissue. In rare cases, the lesion may be confined to the epithelial layer (in situ). In most cases, the tumor is large and well established on diagnosis. More than half of esophageal cancers **metastasize** (spread throughout the body).

Primary risk factors associated with the development of esophageal cancer are smoking and obesity. The compounds in tobacco smoke may be responsible for the genetic mutations seen in many squamous cell carcinomas of the esophagus. "Obesity poses a sixteen-fold increased risk of esophageal adenocarcinoma" (American Cancer Society [ACS], 2012, p. 29). Increased abdominal pressure associated with obesity is linked to reflux as well as Barrett's esophagus (a pre-malignant condition). Both conditions can contribute to changes in cellular structure in the esophagus increasing the potential for adenocarcinoma of the esophagus (ACS, 2012). In addition to these primary risk factors, malnutrition, untreated gastroesophageal reflux disease (GERD), and excessive alcohol intake are also associated with esophageal cancer. **Barrett's esophagus** results

GENETIC/GENOMIC CONSIDERATIONS

Patient-Centered Care QSEN

Certain genetic factors may have a role in the development of esophageal cancers. It is thought that these cancers result from mutations in tumor suppressor genes. Tumor suppressor genes are normal genes that control cell growth and division. When this type of gene is mutated and does not work properly, cells are unable to stop growing and dividing and tumors can result. (See Chapter 21 for a more complete discussion.)

Overexpression and mutations of the *Tp53, Tp16,* and *Tp17* tumor suppressor genes have been found in people with esophageal cancer (Nussbaum et al., 2007). In addition, the presence of the mutated *Tp53* gene may be an indication of advanced disease, especially in patients with adenocarcinomas.

Overexpression of *cyclin D1,* a protein that promotes cell growth and division, has also been found in patients with esophageal squamous cell cancers. Cyclins are products of oncogenes, which are normal genes involved in cell division and are controlled by suppressor genes. Prolonged exposure to carcinogens, such as tobacco, can cause oncogenes to escape the control of suppressor genes, leading to overexpression of cyclins and uncontrolled cell growth (cancer).

NCLEX EXAMINATION CHALLENGE

Health Promotion and Maintenance

Over the past 3 months, a client with a history of gastroesophageal reflux disease and obesity has implemented lifestyle changes. What lifestyle changes does the nurse recognize as important for the client to decrease chances of development of cancer of the esophagus? **Select all that apply.**

A. Lost 10 pounds
B. Sleeps with two pillows
C. Has quit eating processed foods
D. Drinks a glass of wine every night
E. Uses a nicotine patch instead of smoking

from exposure to acid and pepsin, which leads to the replacement of normal distal squamous mucosa with columnar epithelium as a response to tissue injury. This tissue undergoes dysplasia (cell appearance changes) and, ultimately, becomes cancerous. In parts of the world where esophageal cancer is more common, the incidence of squamous cell carcinoma appears to be linked to high levels of nitrosamines (which are found in pickled and fermented foods) and foods high in nitrate. Diets that are chronically deficient in fresh fruits and vegetables have also been implicated in the development of squamous cell carcinoma.

❖ *PATIENT-CENTERED COLLABORATIVE CARE*

◆ *Assessment*

History. Assess for risk factors related to the development or symptoms of esophageal cancer, such as gender, history of alcohol consumption, tobacco use, dietary habits, and other esophageal problems (e.g., dysphagia, reflux). In the United States, adenocarcinoma of the esophagus is more common than squamous cell carcinoma (National Cancer Institute at the National Institutes of Health, 2013). Men, regardless of race or ethnicity, have higher incidence and mortality rates associated with esophageal cancer (National Cancer Institute, 2013). Ask the patient about consumption of smoked and/or pickled foods, changes in appetite, changes in taste, or weight loss.

Physical Assessment/Clinical Manifestations. Cancer of the esophagus is a silent tumor in its early stages, with few observable signs. By the time the tumor causes symptoms, it usually has spread extensively.

Dysphagia *(difficulty swallowing) is the most common symptom of esophageal cancer, but it may not be present until the esophageal opening has gotten much smaller.* Dysphagia is persistent and progressive when **stricture** (narrowing) occurs. It is initially associated with swallowing solids, particularly meat, and then progresses rapidly over a period of weeks or months to difficulty in swallowing soft foods and liquids. Late in the disease, even saliva can cause choking. Patients usually report a sensation of food sticking in the throat or in the substernal area. Careful assessment of dysphagia is important because dysphagia associated with other esophageal disorders is not usually continuous. Weight loss often accompanies dysphagia and can exceed 20 pounds over several months.

Odynophagia (painful swallowing) is reported by many patients as a steady, dull, substernal PAIN that may radiate. It occurs most often when the patient drinks cold liquids. The presence of severe or persistent PAIN often indicates tumor invasion of the mediastinal structures. Assess for regurgitation,

CHART 54-7 Key Features

Esophageal Tumors

- Persistent and progressive dysphagia (most common feature)
- Feeling of food sticking in the throat
- Odynophagia (painful swallowing)
- Severe, persistent chest or abdominal pain or discomfort
- Regurgitation
- Chronic cough with increasing secretions
- Hoarseness
- Anorexia
- Nausea and vomiting
- Weight loss (often more than 20 pounds)
- Changes in bowel habits (diarrhea, constipation, bleeding)

vomiting, **halitosis** (foul breath), and chronic hiccups, which often accompany advanced disease. In most patients, pulmonary problems develop. Assess for chronic cough, increased secretions, and a history of recent infections. Tumors in the upper esophagus may involve the larynx and thus cause hoarseness. Chart 54-7 summarizes the common clinical manifestations of esophageal tumors.

Psychosocial Assessment. The diagnosis of esophageal cancer causes high patient anxiety. The disease is accompanied by distressing symptoms and is often terminal. The fear of choking can place unusual stress, especially at mealtimes. The loss of pleasure and social aspects of eating may affect relationships with family and friends. Assess the patient's response to the diagnosis and prognosis. Ask about his or her usual coping strengths and resources. Assess the impact of the disease on the patient's usual daily activity routine. Determine the availability of support systems and the potential financial impact of the disease and its treatment. Refer the patient and family members to psychological counseling, pastoral care, and/or the social worker or case manager as needed. Chapter 7 describes end-of-life care for patients in the terminal stage of the disease.

Diagnostic Assessment. A *barium swallow* study with fluoroscopy may be the first diagnostic test requested to evaluate dysphagia. In a barium swallow, the margins of a tumor may be seen. The definitive diagnosis of esophageal cancer is made by *esophageal ultrasound (EUS)* with fine needle aspiration to examine the tumor tissue. An *esophagogastroduodenoscopy (EGD)* may also be performed to inspect the esophagus and obtain tissue specimens for cell studies and disease staging. A complete cancer staging workup is performed to determine the extent of the disease and plan appropriate therapy.

Positron emission tomography (PET) may identify metastatic disease with more accuracy than a CT scan. PET can also help evaluate response to chemotherapy to treat the cancer.

◆ *Analysis*

The most specific common problem for patients with esophageal cancer is *decreased* NUTRITION *intake related to impaired swallowing and possible metastasis.* Many patients with cancer also have pain and are fearful because of the diagnosis of cancer. Chapter 22 describes problems that are typically seen with any patient with cancer.

◆ *Planning and Implementation*

Promoting Nutrition

Planning: Expected Outcomes. The major concern for a patient with esophageal cancer is weight loss secondary to dysphagia. Therefore he or she is expected to maintain adequate nutrient intake and weight either orally or via an alternative method.

Interventions. Interventions to maintain or improve NUTRITION status focus on treatments that remove or shrink the obstructive tumor. Methods to reduce the effects of treatment that can impact NUTRITION are also a priority. Surgery is the most definitive intervention for esophageal cancer.

Nonsurgical treatment options for cancer of the esophagus that can assist in both disease and NUTRITION management include:

- Nutrition therapy
- Swallowing therapy
- Chemotherapy
- Radiation therapy
- Chemoradiation
- Targeted therapies
- Photodynamic therapy
- Esophageal dilation
- Endoscopic therapies

Nonsurgical Management. The treatment of esophageal cancer often involves a combination of therapies. Patients with cancer of the esophagus experience many physical problems, and symptom management becomes essential.

Nutrition and Swallowing Therapy. The purpose of NUTRITION therapy is to administer food and fluids to support the patient who is malnourished or at high risk for becoming malnourished. Conduct a screening assessment to provide information about the patient's NUTRITION status. The dietitian determines the caloric needs of the patient to meet daily requirements. Be sure the patient is weighed daily before breakfast on the same scale each day. To keep the esophagus patent, careful positioning is essential for a patient who is experiencing frequent reflux or who has tubes. Teach the patient to remain upright for several hours after meals and to avoid lying completely flat. Remind unlicensed assistive personnel (UAP) and other health care team members to keep the head of the bed elevated to a 30-degree angle or more to prevent reflux.

Semisoft foods and thickened liquids are preferred because they are easier to swallow. Record the amount of food and fluid intake every day to monitor progress in meeting desired NUTRITION outcomes. Liquid NUTRITION supplements (e.g., Boost, Ensure) are used between feedings to increase caloric intake. Ongoing efforts are made to preserve the ability to swallow, but enteral feedings (tube feedings) may be needed temporarily when dysphagia is severe. In patients with complete esophageal obstruction or life-threatening fistulas, the surgeon may create a gastrostomy or jejunostomy for feeding. Encourage the patient and family to meet with the dietitian for diet teaching and planning. Chapter 60 describes care for patients receiving enteral feeding.

Collaborate with the speech-language pathologist (SLP) to assist the patient with oral exercises to improve swallowing *(swallowing therapy)* and with the occupational therapist (OT) for feeding therapy. Ask the patient to suck on a lollipop to enhance tongue strength. Teach the patient to reach for food particles on the lips or chin using the tongue. In preparation for swallowing, remind the patient to position the head in forward flexion (chin tuck). Then tell him or her to place food at the back of the mouth. Monitor him or her for sealing of the lips and for tongue movements while eating. Check for pocketing of food in the cheeks after swallowing.

! NURSING SAFETY PRIORITY (QSEN)

Critical Rescue

When the patient with an esophageal tumor is eating or drinking, monitor for signs and symptoms of aspiration, such as choking or coughing. Food aspiration can cause airway obstruction, pneumonia, or both, especially in older adults. In coordination with the SLP, teach family members and caregivers how to feed the patient, if needed. Teach them how to monitor for aspiration and implement appropriate measures if choking occurs.

Chemotherapy and Radiation. The use of *chemotherapy* in the treatment of esophageal cancer has been only moderately effective. It can be given as a primary treatment if the patient is not a candidate for surgery or given for palliation (control of symptoms). In most cases, however, chemotherapy is given in combination with radiation therapy to provide the patient the best chance of cure. The rationale for this approach is to shrink the primary tumor and eliminate any other tumor that may be in the local lymph nodes, improving the odds for a complete surgical resection. The most commonly used paired chemotherapeutic agents for esophageal cancer are carboplatin and paclitaxel (Taxol) or cisplatin and 5-fluorouracil (5-FU). These drugs are often combined with radiation because they make the tumor cells more sensitive to radiation effects (American Cancer Society [ACS], 2014a). Because chemotherapeutic drugs affect healthy cells as well as cancer cells, they have many side effects that cause discomfort to the patient. Chapter 22 describes chemotherapy in detail and discusses the role of the nurse in caring for patients receiving these drugs.

Radiation therapy to manage esophageal cancer is only moderately effective and can be used alone or in combination with other treatments. Radiation alone can provide palliation of symptoms by shrinking the tumor. It is contraindicated for patients with tracheoesophageal fistula, mediastinitis, mediastinal hemorrhage, or infiltration of the cancer to the trachea or bronchus. Normal esophageal tissue is very sensitive to the effects of radiation. Although high doses of radiation demonstrate the best results for tumor shrinkage, esophageal stricture or stenosis can result in many patients, which then requires esophageal dilation. Chapter 22 describes radiation methods and the general nursing care for the patient having radiation therapy.

Chemoradiation is a treatment for esophageal cancer that involves the use of chemotherapy at the same time as radiation therapy. One cycle of chemotherapy is given during the first week of radiation and another is delivered during the fifth week of radiation. Additional drug cycles are given after radiation therapy is complete.

Other Therapies. Targeted therapies may be used in combination with radiation and chemotherapy. Unlike chemotherapy, these therapies interfere with cancer cell growth in a variety of ways with less impact on healthy cells. Many of these drugs focus on proteins that are involved in signaling cells when to grow and divide. A key to success with targeted therapy is that the cancer cells must overexpress the targeted protein. Thus each patient's cancer cells are first examined for the overexpression to determine if targeted therapy is appropriate and which drug to use. Trastuzumab (Herceptin) is a commonly used drug that is used for patients whose esophageal cancer tests positive for an excess of the *HER2* protein on the cell surface. It is given by IV injection once every 3 weeks, in addition to chemotherapy (ACS, 2014b). Chapter 22 describes targeted therapies in detail, including nursing implications for patient safety and quality care.

Photodynamic therapy (PDT) is used as a palliative treatment for patients with advanced esophageal cancer who are not candidates for surgery. It may be used also as a cure for patients who have very small, localized tumors. The patient is injected with porfimer sodium (Photofrin), a light-sensitive drug that collects in cancer cells. Two days after the injection, a fiberoptic probe with a light at the tip is threaded into the esophagus through an endoscope. The light activates the Photofrin, destroying only cancer cells. PDT is far less invasive than surgery and is performed on an ambulatory care basis under moderate sedation. Endoscopy nurses observe the patient's rate and depth of respirations and monitor the patient's oxygen saturation and end-tidal (exhaled) carbon dioxide to ensure adequate oxygenation.

The side effects of Photofrin are rare but include nausea, fever, and constipation. Before the procedure, the patient is given written guidelines concerning photosensitivity measures. Remind the patient to avoid exposure to sunlight for 1 to 3 months. Sunglasses and protective clothing that covers all exposed body areas are essential. The patient may experience chest PAIN secondary to tissue damage and will require PAIN relief with opioid analgesics for a short time. Teach the patient to follow a clear liquid diet for 3 to 5 days after the procedure and advance to full liquids as tolerated. Warn the patient that tissue particles may release from the tumor site and be present in the sputum. Chapter 22 describes in detail the health teaching needed to promote patient safety associated with PDT.

Esophageal dilation may be performed as necessary throughout the course of the disease to achieve temporary but immediate relief of dysphagia. It is usually performed on an ambulatory care basis. Dilators are used to tear soft tissue, thereby widening the esophageal lumen (opening). In most cases, malignant tumors can be dilated safely, but perforation remains a significant risk. Large metal stents may be used to keep the esophagus open for longer periods. A stent covered with graft material can be used to seal a perforation. Bacteremia can also occur. To reduce the risk for endocarditis, antibiotics are given. The treatment is repeated as often as needed to preserve the patient's ability to swallow. Prolonged stent embedment into benign esophageal tissue can cause ulceration, bleeding, fistula, dysphagia, and formation of new stricture if the stent is not removed (Patel & Siddiqui, 2013).

When patients are not candidates for surgery or the tumor is too large to remove surgically, laser therapy or electrocoagulation using endoscopy may be performed as a palliative measure. Both of these methods destroy some cancer cells and reduce tumor size to improve swallowing. The procedures are done in ambulatory care settings or same-day surgery centers using moderate sedation.

Surgical Management. The purposes of surgical resection vary from palliation to cure. **Esophagectomy** is the removal of all or part of the esophagus. An **esophagogastrostomy** involves the removal of part of the esophagus and proximal stomach. The remaining stomach may be "pulled up" to take the place of the esophagus, or a section of the jejunum or colon may be placed as a conduit. Conventional open surgical techniques are lengthy and are associated with many complications or death. Fistula formation between the trachea and esophagus, abscess, and respiratory complications are common.

For patients with early-stage cancer, a laparoscopic-assisted **minimally invasive esophagectomy (MIE)** may be performed. However, most patients require the conventional open surgery because of tumor size and metastasis by the time they are diagnosed with the disease.

Preoperative Care. Preoperative preparation for patients undergoing esophagectomy or esophagogastrostomy can be quite extensive, especially before conventional techniques. Advise the patient to stop smoking 2 to 4 weeks before surgery to enhance pulmonary function. Patient preparation may include 5 days to 2 to 3 weeks of NUTRITION support to decrease the risk for postoperative complications. Ideally this supplementation is given orally, but many patients require tube feeding or parenteral NUTRITION. Teach the patient and family to monitor the patient's weight and intake and output. A preoperative evaluation may be required to treat dental disease. Teach the patient to use meticulous oral care 4 times daily to decrease the risk for postoperative INFECTION.

Preoperative nursing care focuses on teaching and on psychological support regarding the surgical procedure and preoperative and postoperative instructions. Teach the patient about:

- The number and sites of all incisions and drains
- The placement of a jejunostomy tube for initial enteral feedings
- The need for chest tubes if the pleural space is entered
- The purpose of the nasogastric tube
- The need for IV infusion

Teach the patient about routines for turning, coughing, deep breathing, and chest physiotherapy. Emphasize the crucial nature of postoperative respiratory care. If colon interposition (resecting a piece of colon and creating an esophagus) is planned, the patient also has a complete bowel preparation before surgery.

The patient facing a serious illness and extensive surgery can be expected to have feelings of grief and anxiety. Encourage the patient to talk about personal feelings and fears, and involve the family or significant others in all preoperative teaching and discussions. A social worker, certified hospital chaplain, or case manager can be extremely helpful in providing continuity of care and support to the entire family.

Operative Procedures. In the MIE procedure, the surgeon makes four or five small incisions in the chest and abdomen using a video-assisted thoracoscope and laparoscope. The lower esophagus and gastric fundus are removed. The remaining portion of the esophagus is then anastomosed (reconnected) to the stomach.

For most patients, the surgeon performs an open subtotal or total esophagectomy because tumors are often large and involve distant lymph nodes. For a subtotal (partial) removal, the diseased portion of the esophagus is removed and the cervical portion is anastomosed (connected) to the stomach (Fig. 54-3). A **pyloromyotomy** is done by cutting and suturing the pylorus. Finally, a jejunostomy tube may be placed for postoperative enteral feeding.

For patients with early-stage tumors of the lower third of the esophagus, a transhiatal esophagectomy is the preferred surgical approach. The surgery is performed through an upper midline cervical incision. With this approach, the pleural space is not entered, reducing respiratory complications. For patients with tumors in the upper esophagus, a radical neck dissection and laryngectomy may also be needed if the disease has spread to the larynx. Chapter 29 discusses the care of patients having these procedures.

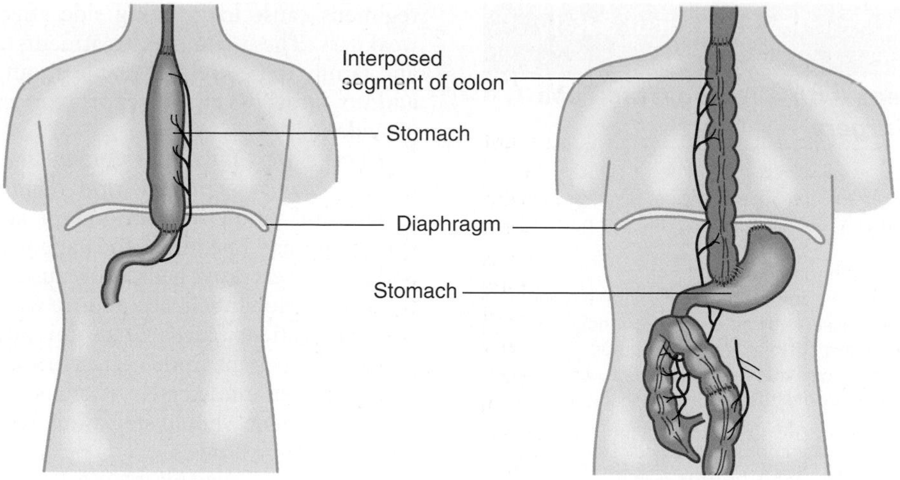

FIG. 54-3 Open surgical approaches to the treatment of esophageal cancer.

The surgeon may perform a **colon interposition** when the tumor involves the stomach or the stomach is otherwise unsuitable for anastomosis. A section of right or left colon is removed and brought up into the thorax to substitute for the esophagus (see Fig. 54-3).

Postoperative Care. The patient requires intensive postoperative care and is at risk for multiple serious complications. The patient having an MIE has the same risk for postoperative complications as one having the open procedure. The advantages of MIE, though, include:

- Less blood loss during surgery; fewer blood transfusions
- Decreased healing and recovery time
- Decreased trauma to the body
- No large incisions
- Less postoperative PAIN
- Shorter hospital stay (5 to 7 days rather than 7 to 10 days)

! NURSING SAFETY PRIORITY QSEN

Action Alert

Respiratory care is the highest postoperative priority for patients having an esophagectomy. For those who had traditional surgery, intubation with mechanical ventilation is needed for at least the first 16 to 24 hours. Pulmonary complications include atelectasis and pneumonia. The risk for postoperative pulmonary complications is increased in the patient who has received preoperative radiation. Once the patient is extubated, begin deep breathing, turning, and coughing every 1 to 2 hours. Assess the patient for decreased breath sounds and shortness of breath every 1 to 2 hours. Provide incisional support and adequate analgesia for effective coughing.

Remind nursing and other staff to keep the patient in a semi-Fowler's or high-Fowler's position to support ventilation and prevent reflux. The health care provider prescribes prophylactic antibiotics and supplemental oxygen. *Ensure the patency of the chest tube drainage system, and monitor for changes in the volume or color of the drainage.*

Cardiovascular complications, particularly hypotension during surgery, can occur as a result of pressure placed on the posterior heart and usually respond well to IV fluid administration.

! NURSING SAFETY PRIORITY QSEN

Action Alert

Monitor for manifestations of fluid volume overload, particularly in older patients and in those who have undergone lymph node dissection. Assess for edema, crackles in the lungs, and increased jugular venous pressure. In the immediate postoperative phase, the patient is often admitted to the intensive care unit. Critical care nurses assess hemodynamic parameters such as cardiac output, cardiac index, and systemic vascular resistance every 2 hours to monitor for myocardial ischemia. Observe for atrial fibrillation that results from irritation of the vagus nerve during surgery, and manage according to agency protocol.

The patient with poor NUTRITION or prior radiation or chemotherapy is at risk for INFECTION. For those who undergo more radical surgical procedures, there is a serious risk for leakage at the anastomosis (surgical connection) sites. This situation is especially true with colon interpositions because several sites are stressed by the effects of tension, poor blood supply, and delayed healing. *Mediastinitis* (inflammation of the mediastinum) resulting from an anastomotic leak can lead to fatal sepsis.

Wound management is another major postoperative concern for conventional surgery because the patient typically has multiple incisions and drains. *Provide direct support to the incision during turning and coughing to prevent dehiscence.* Wound INFECTION can occur 4 to 5 days after surgery. Leakage from the site of anastomosis is a dreaded complication that can appear 2 to 10 days after surgery. If an anastomotic leak occurs, all oral intake is discontinued and is not resumed until the site of the leak has healed.

! NURSING SAFETY PRIORITY QSEN

Critical Rescue

After esophageal surgery, carefully assess for fever, fluid accumulation, signs of inflammation, and symptoms of early shock (e.g., tachycardia, tachypnea). Report any of these findings to the surgeon **or** Rapid Response Team immediately!

CHART 54-8 Best Practice for Patient Safety & Quality Care QSEN

Managing the Patient with a Nasogastric Tube after Esophageal Surgery

- Check for tube placement every 4 to 8 hours.
- Ensure that the tube is patent (open) and draining; drainage should turn from bloody to yellowish green by the end of the first postoperative day.
- Secure the tube well to prevent dislodgment.
- Do not irrigate or reposition the tube without a physician's request.
- Provide meticulous oral and nasal hygiene every 2 to 4 hours.
- Keep the head of the bed elevated to at least 30 degrees.
- When the patient is permitted to have a small amount of water, place him or her in an upright position and observe for dysphagia (difficulty swallowing).
- Observe for leakage from the anastomosis site, as indicated by fever, fluid accumulation, and manifestations of early shock (tachycardia, tachypnea, altered mental status).

A nasogastric (NG) tube is placed intraoperatively to decompress the stomach to prevent tension on the suture line. Monitor the NG tube for patency, and carefully secure the tube to prevent dislodgment, which can disrupt the sutures at the anastomosis. *Do not irrigate or reposition the NG tube in patients who have undergone esophageal surgery unless requested by the surgeon!* The initial nasogastric drainage is bloody but should change to a greenish yellow color by the end of the first postoperative day. The continued presence of blood may indicate internal bleeding at the suture line. Commonly, an antacid will be prescribed to support the patient's healing. Provide oral hygiene for the patient every 2 to 4 hours while the tube is in place, or delegate and supervise this activity (Chart 54-8).

NUTRITION management of the patient who has undergone esophageal surgery is an early postoperative concern. After conventional surgery, on the second postoperative day, initial feedings usually begin through the jejunostomy tube (J tube). Do not aspirate for residual, because this increases the risk for mucosal tearing. Feedings are slowly increased over the next several days. Feeding by this method can be discontinued once the patient is taking adequate oral NUTRITION.

Before beginning oral feedings, a cine-esophagram study is performed to detect any anastomotic leaks, strictures, or signs of aspiration. If no leaks are seen, a liquid diet is started. If liquids are well tolerated, the patient's diet is advanced to include semi-solid foods and then solid foods.

Place the patient in an upright position, and supervise all initial swallowing efforts. The food storage area of the stomach has been radically decreased, and gravity is the only defense against reflux. *Teach the patient and/or family the importance of the patient eating six to eight small meals per day. Fluids should be taken between, rather than with, meals to prevent diarrhea.* Diarrhea can occur 20 minutes to 2 hours after eating and can be managed with loperamide (Imodium) before meals. The diarrhea is thought to be the result of *vagotomy syndrome,* which develops as a result of interrupted vagal fibers to the abdominal organs during surgery.

Community-Based Care

Patients with esophageal cancer have many challenges to face once they are discharged home. The combination treatment regimens cause long-lasting side effects, such as fatigue and weakness. These complex treatments also require the patient and family to be knowledgeable about symptom management and to know when to report concerns to the health care provider.

Home Care Management. *Once the patient is discharged to home, ongoing respiratory care remains a priority.* Give the patient and family instructions for ambulation and incentive spirometer use. Encourage the patient to be as active as possible and to avoid excessive bedrest because this can lead to complications of immobility. In accordance with The Joint Commission National Patient Safety Goals for 2014, teach the family to protect the patient from INFECTION and to contact the health care provider immediately if signs of respiratory INFECTION develop. Patients should stay away from people with infections and avoid large crowds.

Self-Management Education. Remind the patient and family to wash their hands frequently, and teach them to inspect the incisions daily for redness, tenderness, swelling, odor, and discharge because proper wound healing is still a concern at the time of discharge. Instruct them to report a temperature greater than 101° F (38.3° C), or 100° F (37.8° C) for older adults, which may be a sign of INFECTION. Prepare written instructions about the signs of anastomosis leakage. *Teach the patient or family to immediately report to the health care provider the presence of fever and a swollen, painful neck incision.*

NUTRITION support is important. Encourage the patient to continue increasing oral feedings as tolerated. Remind him or her to eat small, frequent meals containing high-calorie, high-protein foods that are soft and easily swallowed. Teach the value of using supplemental milkshakes between meals, and instruct the patient to eat slowly. Patients who have undergone esophageal resection can lose up to 10% of their body weight. Teach the patient to monitor his or her weight at home and to report a weight loss of 5 pounds or more in 1 month. If sufficient oral intake is not possible, the patient and family may need instruction about tube feedings or parenteral NUTRITION at home.

Emphasize the importance of remaining upright after meals. Dysphagia or odynophagia may recur because of stricture, reflux, or cancer recurrence. These symptoms should be promptly reported to the health care provider. Despite radical surgery, the patient with cancer of the esophagus often still has a terminal illness and a relatively short life expectancy. Emphasis is placed on maximizing quality of life. Realistic planning is important as the patient's condition eventually worsens, and the patient and family are assisted to plan for the future together. Assist family members in exploring formal and informal sources of support. Help the family or significant others arrange for hospice care when it is needed. Chapter 7 describes end-of-life care, including hospice.

Health Care Resources. Referrals to community or home care organizations assist the family in providing care in the home. The patient may need transportation to the radiation treatment center 5 times per week for up to 6 weeks. Oncology nursing care may be needed to monitor and evaluate the patient who is receiving chemotherapy at home through venous access devices or portable infusion pumps. Inform the patient and family about the services available through the American Cancer Society (www.cancer.org), including support groups and transportation. Familiarize the family with area hospice services for future planning. Coordinate resource referrals with the case manager or home care agency.

◆ *Evaluation: Expected Outcomes*

Evaluate the care of the patient with esophageal cancer based on the identified priority patient problems. The major expected outcome is that the patient will be able to consume adequate NUTRITION and maintain a stable weight.

CLINICAL JUDGMENT CHALLENGE

Teamwork and Collaboration; Safety; Evidence-Based Practice QSEN

A 55-year-old patient has undergone a partial esophagectomy. He has a history of alcoholism and states that he quit drinking when he found out about his diagnosis. Just prior to discharge, you are preparing to teach him and his family about self-management.

1. For what postoperative complications will you monitor, and why could they occur after this surgery?
2. Of all potential postoperative complications, which signs and symptoms should the patient and family be instructed to *immediately* report?
3. Why is the patient's history of alcoholism significant? What referrals would you provide to support his choice to discontinue using alcohol?
4. The patient's life partner tells you that the patient is the family's primary provider of income. His life partner is concerned that the patient may not recover well enough to return to work. How might you respond to his concern?
5. To what community agencies would you refer the patient and his family?

ESOPHAGEAL DIVERTICULA

Diverticula are sacs resulting from the herniation of esophageal mucosa and submucosa into surrounding tissue. They may develop anywhere along the length of the esophagus. No environmental risk factors are known to be involved in their development. The incomplete or late opening of swallowing muscles can cause high pressure in the hypopharynx and lead to *Zenker's diverticula,* the most common form. This type occurs most often in older adults. Patients report dysphagia (difficulty swallowing), regurgitation (reflux), nocturnal cough, and halitosis (bad breath). They can also be at risk for perforation because the mucosa is without the protection of the normal esophageal muscle layer.

Esophageal diverticula are diagnosed most often by *esophagogastroduodenoscopy (EGD).* This procedure must be performed with strict care because of the risk for perforation. NUTRITION therapy and positioning are the major interventions for controlling symptoms related to diverticula. Collaborate with the dietitian to assist the patient in exploring variations in the size and frequency of meals and in food texture and consistency. Semisoft foods and smaller meals are often best tolerated and may reduce or relieve the symptoms of pressure and reflux. Nocturnal reflux associated with diverticula is managed by teaching the patient to sleep with the head of the bed elevated and to avoid the supine position for at least 2 hours after eating. Advise the patient to avoid vigorous exercise after meals. Teach him or her to avoid restrictive clothing and frequent stooping or bending.

Surgical management is aimed at removing the diverticula. Postoperatively, the patient is NPO status for several days to promote healing. During that period, the patient receives IV fluids for hydration and tube feedings; after that, he or she is given oral fluid and food. Provide PAIN relief measures, and monitor for complications such as bleeding or perforation. *A nasogastric (NG) tube is placed during surgery for decompression and is not irrigated or repositioned unless specifically requested by the surgeon.*

Community-based care includes teaching the patient and family about:

- Nutrition therapy
- Positioning guidelines to prevent reflux
- Warning signs of complications, such as bleeding or infection

TABLE 54-2 Common Causes of Esophageal Perforation

• Straining	• Instrument or tubes
• Seizures	• Chemical injury
• Trauma	• Complications of esophageal surgery
• Foreign objects	• Ulcers

ESOPHAGEAL TRAUMA

Trauma to the esophagus can result from blunt injuries, chemical burns, surgery or endoscopy (rare), or the stress of continuous severe vomiting (Table 54-2). Trauma may affect the esophagus directly, impairing swallowing and NUTRITION, or it may create problems in related structures such as the lungs or mediastinum. The incidence of most forms of esophageal trauma is low in adults. When excessive force is exerted on the esophageal mucosa, it may perforate or rupture, allowing the caustic acid secretions to enter the mediastinal cavity. These tears are associated with a high mortality rate related to shock, respiratory impairment, or sepsis.

Chemical injury is usually a result of the accidental or intentional ingestion of caustic substances. The damage to the mouth and esophagus is rapid and severe. Acid burns tend to affect the superficial mucosal lining, whereas alkaline substances cause deeper penetrating injuries. Strong alkalis can cause full perforation of the esophagus within 1 minute. Additional problems may include aspiration pneumonia and hemorrhage. Esophageal strictures may develop as scar tissue forms.

Patients with esophageal trauma are initially evaluated and treated in the emergency department. Assessment focuses on the nature of the injury and the circumstances surrounding it. *Assess for airway patency, breathing, chest pain, dysphagia, vomiting, and bleeding as the priorities for patient care.* If the risk for extending the damage is not excessive, an endoscopic study may be requested to evaluate tears or perforation. A CT scan of the chest can be done to assess for the presence of mediastinal air.

After the injury, keep the patient NPO to prevent further leakage of esophageal secretions. Esophageal and gastric suction can be used for drainage and to rest the esophagus. Esophageal rest is maintained for more than a week after injury to allow for initial healing of the mucosa. Total parenteral NUTRITION (TPN) is prescribed to provide calories and protein for wound healing while the patient is not eating.

To prevent sepsis, the health care provider prescribes broad-spectrum antibiotics. High-dose corticosteroids may be administered to suppress inflammation and prevent strictures (esophageal narrowing). In addition, opioid and non-opioid analgesics are prescribed for PAIN management. When caustic burns involve the mouth, topical agents such as lidocaine (Xylocaine Viscous) may be used for analgesia and local anti-inflammatory action.

If nonsurgical management is not effective in healing traumatized esophageal tissue, the patient may need surgery to remove the damaged tissue. Those with severe injuries may require resection of part of the esophagus with a gastric pull-through and repositioning or replacement by a bowel segment; also, gastrostomy tube (G-tube) placement may be needed to meet NUTRITION needs while healing.

NURSING CONCEPTS AND CLINICAL JUDGMENT REVIEW

What might you NOTICE if the patient has inadequate digestion and NUTRITION as a result of chronic esophageal problems?

- Dysphagia (difficulty swallowing)
- Odynophagia (painful swallowing)
- Dyspepsia (indigestion)
- Regurgitation (reflux)
- Eructation (belching)
- Chronic cough
- Choking
- Halitosis (foul breath)
- Weight loss
- Vomiting
- Chest pain

What should you INTERPRET and how should you RESPOND to a patient experiencing inadequate digestion and NUTRITION as a result of chronic esophageal problems?

Perform and interpret focused physical findings, including:

- Assessing ability to chew and swallow food
- Assessing chest pain (dyspepsia) for quality, location, and intensity
- Assessing body weight change
- Auscultating lungs
- Assessing readiness to learn

Respond by:

- Providing semi-solid or thickened liquids if solid foods cannot be swallowed comfortably
- Collaborating with the dietitian and occupational therapist (OT) for swallowing evaluation and training
- Monitoring for aspiration of secretions or food
- Teaching lifestyle changes, such as foods to avoid, smoking and alcohol cessation, weight reduction (if obese), and importance of drug therapy to control symptoms
- Monitoring weight
- Monitoring for increased dysphagia

On what should you REFLECT?

- Evaluate for rapid weight changes (decrease if obese, and increase if severe weight loss has occurred).
- Monitor for manifestations of aspiration.
- Observe patient for improvement in GI symptoms.
- Evaluate effectiveness of health teaching.
- Consider ways to promote digestion and nutrition.

GET READY FOR THE NCLEX® EXAMINATION!

KEY POINTS

Review these Key Points for each NCLEX Examination Client Needs Category.

Safe and Effective Care Environment

- Consult with the dietitian, patient, and family regarding NUTRITION restrictions for patients with GERD. **Teamwork and Collaboration** QSEN
- Collaborate with the health care team for the patient with impaired swallowing and/or limited NUTRITION. **Teamwork and Collaboration** QSEN
- Teach the patient and family to recognize the symptoms of dysphagia. **Safety** QSEN
- Remain with the dysphagic patient during meals to prevent or assist with choking episodes. **Safety** QSEN

Health Promotion and Maintenance

- Teach the patient oral exercises aimed at improving swallowing.
- Stress the importance of recognizing and controlling reflux through NUTRITION therapy and medications to avoid further esophageal damage that could lead to Barrett's esophagus.
- Teach the patient to elevate the head of the bed by 6 inches for sleep to prevent nighttime reflux.
- Instruct the patient to sleep in the right side-lying position to minimize the effects of nighttime episodes of reflux.
- Teach the patient with esophageal cancer to monitor his or her body weight and to notify the health care provider of weight loss.
- Teach the patient to avoid alcoholic beverages, smoking, and other substances as listed in Chart 54-2 because they lead to increased gastroesophageal reflux.
- Teach the patient to prevent gas bloat syndrome by avoiding drinking carbonated beverages, eating gas-producing foods, chewing gum, and drinking with a straw.
- Review postprocedure instructions for patients having the Stretta procedure for GERD as outlined in Chart 54-3.

Psychosocial Integrity

- Allow the patient the opportunity to express fear or anxiety regarding the diagnosis of esophageal cancer and related treatment regimen of surgery, chemotherapy, and radiation. **Patient-Centered Care** QSEN
- Explain all procedures, restrictions, drug therapy, and follow-up care to the patient and family.
- Refer the patient or family members to psychological counseling, hospice, pastoral care, and the case manager as needed. **Teamwork and Collaboration** QSEN

Physiological Integrity

- For patients with GERD, teach the importance of strict adherence to anti-reflux agents in preventing esophageal damage (see Chapter 55, Chart 55-3).
- Be aware that laparoscopic Nissen fundoplication (LNF) and laparoscopic paraesophageal repairs are common surgical procedures for patients with GERD and hiatal hernia.
- Assess for complications and provide postoperative care for patients having the LNF procedure, as described in Chart 54-6. **Safety** QSEN
- Be sure to frequently monitor the NUTRITION status of the patient with esophageal cancer.
- Teach the patient having open conventional esophageal surgery about incisions, drains, and jejunostomy tube placement before he or she undergoes surgery for esophageal cancer.
- For the patient with a nasogastric (NG) tube, check the NG tube every 4 to 8 hours for proper placement and anchorage; follow guidelines as outlined in Chart 54-8.
- Assess the patient after esophageal surgery for pulmonary and cardiac complications of surgery, and report changes to the health care provider. **Safety** QSEN
- Assess patients for key features of esophageal tumors as listed in Chart 54-7.

55 CHAPTER

Care of Patients with Stomach Disorders

Lara Carver

http://evolve.elsevier.com/Iggy/

PRIORITY CONCEPTS

- Nutrition
- Pain
- Inflammation
- Infection

LEARNING OUTCOMES

Safe and Effective Care Environment

1. Describe the importance of collaborating with members of the health care team when caring for patients with gastric (stomach) disorders.

Health Promotion and Maintenance

2. Identify community resources for patients with gastric disorders.
3. Develop a teaching plan for patients about complementary and alternative therapies that have been used to help manage gastritis and peptic ulcer disease (PUD).
4. Plan interventions to promote GI health and prevent gastritis.

Psychosocial Integrity

5. Identify the need for end-of-life care for patients with advanced gastric cancer.

Physiological Integrity

6. Compare assessment findings of acute and chronic gastritis.
7. Compare and contrast assessment findings associated with gastric and duodenal ulcers.
8. Identify the most common medical complications that can result from PUD.
9. Describe the purpose and adverse effects of drug therapy for gastritis and PUD.
10. To promote patient safety and quality care, monitor patients with PUD and gastric cancer for signs of upper GI bleeding.
11. Prioritize evidence-based interventions for patients with upper GI bleeding.
12. To prevent complications, develop a collaborative preoperative and postoperative plan of care for the patient undergoing gastric surgery.

Although only a few diseases affect the stomach, they can be very serious and in some cases life threatening. The most common disorders include gastritis, peptic ulcer disease, and gastric cancer. Each of these health problems can result in impaired or altered *digestion* and NUTRITION. In addition, INFLAMMATION and INFECTION associated with these problems can cause PAIN. The stomach is part of the upper GI system that is responsible for a large part of the digestive process. Patient-centered collaborative care for stomach disorders often includes therapies to meet the patient's need for adequate nutrition.

GASTRITIS

Gastritis is the INFLAMMATION of gastric mucosa (stomach lining). It can be scattered or localized and can be classified according to cause, cellular changes, or distribution of the lesions. Gastritis can be erosive (causing ulcers) or nonerosive. Although the mucosal changes that result from *acute* gastritis typically heal after several months, this is not true for *chronic* gastritis.

❖ PATHOPHYSIOLOGY

Prostaglandins provide a protective mucosal barrier that prevents the stomach from digesting itself by a process called acid **autodigestion**. If there is a break in the protective barrier, mucosal injury occurs. The resulting injury is worsened by histamine release and vagus nerve stimulation. Hydrochloric acid can then diffuse back into the mucosa and injure small vessels. This back-diffusion causes edema, hemorrhage, and erosion of the stomach's lining. The pathologic changes of gastritis include vascular congestion, edema, acute inflammatory cell infiltration, and degenerative changes in the superficial epithelium of the stomach lining.

Types of Gastritis

INFLAMMATION of the gastric mucosa or submucosa after exposure to local irritants or other causes can result in **acute gastritis**. The early pathologic manifestation of gastritis is a thickened, reddened mucous membrane with prominent **rugae**, or folds. Various degrees of mucosal necrosis and inflammatory reaction occur in acute disease. The diagnosis cannot be based solely on clinical symptoms. Complete regeneration and healing usually occur within a few days. If the stomach muscle is not involved, complete recovery usually occurs with no residual evidence of gastric inflammatory reaction. If the muscle is affected, hemorrhage may occur during an episode of acute gastritis.

Chronic gastritis appears as a patchy, diffuse (spread out) INFLAMMATION of the mucosal lining of the stomach. As the disease progresses, the walls and lining of the stomach thin and atrophy. With progressive gastric atrophy from chronic mucosal injury, the function of the parietal (acid-secreting) cells decreases and the source of intrinsic factor is lost. Intrinsic factor is critical for absorption of vitamin B_{12}. When body stores of vitamin B_{12} are eventually depleted, **pernicious anemia** results. The amount and concentration of acid in stomach secretions gradually decrease until the secretions consist of only mucus and water.

Chronic gastritis is associated with an increased risk for gastric cancer. The persistent INFLAMMATION extends deep into the mucosa, causing destruction of the gastric glands and cellular changes. Chronic gastritis may be categorized as type A, type B, or atrophic (McCance et al., 2014).

Type A (nonerosive) chronic gastritis refers to an INFLAMMATION of the glands as well as the fundus and body of the stomach. Type B chronic gastritis usually affects the glands of the antrum but may involve the entire stomach. In atrophic chronic gastritis, diffuse inflammation and destruction of deeply located glands accompany the condition. Chronic atrophic gastritis affects all layers of the stomach, thus decreasing the number of cells. The muscle thickens, and inflammation is present. Chronic atrophic gastritis is characterized by total loss of fundal glands, minimal inflammation, thinning of the gastric mucosa, and intestinal metaplasia (abnormal tissue development). These cellular changes can lead to peptic ulcer disease (PUD) and gastric cancer (McCance et al., 2014).

Etiology and Genetic Risk

The onset of INFECTION with *Helicobacter pylori* can result in acute gastritis. *H. pylori* is a gram-negative bacterium that penetrates the mucosal gel layer of the gastric epithelium. Although less common, other forms of bacterial gastritis from organisms such as staphylococci, streptococci, *Escherichia coli,* or salmonella can cause life-threatening problems such as sepsis and extensive tissue necrosis (death).

Long-term NSAID use creates a high risk for acute gastritis. NSAIDs inhibit prostaglandin production in the mucosal barrier. Other risk factors include alcohol, coffee, caffeine, and corticosteroids. Acute gastritis is also caused by local irritation from radiation therapy and accidental or intentional ingestion of corrosive substances, including acids or alkalis (e.g., lye and drain cleaners).

Type A chronic gastritis has been associated with the presence of antibodies to parietal cells and intrinsic factor. Therefore an autoimmune cause for this type of gastritis is likely. Parietal cell antibodies have been found in most patients with pernicious anemia and in more than one half of those with type A gastritis. A genetic link to this disease, with an autosomal dominant pattern of inheritance, has been found in the relatives of patients with pernicious anemia (McCance et al., 2014).

The most common form of chronic gastritis is **type B gastritis**, caused by *H. pylori* infection. A direct correlation exists between the number of organisms and the degree of cellular abnormality present. The host response to the *H. pylori* infection is activation of lymphocytes and neutrophils. Release of inflammatory cytokines, such as interleukin (IL)-1, IL-8, and tumor necrosis factor (TNF)–alpha, damages the gastric mucosa (McCance et al., 2014).

Chronic local irritation and toxic effects caused by alcohol ingestion, radiation therapy, and smoking have been linked to chronic gastritis. Surgical procedures that involve the pyloric sphincter, such as a pyloroplasty, can lead to gastritis by causing reflux of alkaline secretions into the stomach. Other systemic disorders such as Crohn's disease, graft-versus-host disease, and uremia can also precipitate the development of chronic gastritis.

Atrophic gastritis is a type of chronic gastritis that is seen most often in older adults. It can occur after exposure to toxic substances in the workplace (e.g., benzene, lead, nickel) or *H. pylori* infection, or it can be related to autoimmune factors. Atrophic gastritis can lead to two types of cancer: gastric cancer and gastric mucosa-associated lymphoid tissue (MALT) lymphoma. See p. 1138 for a more detailed explanation of gastric cancer.

Health Promotion and Maintenance

Gastritis is a very common health problem in the United States. A balanced diet, regular exercise, and stress-reduction techniques can help prevent it (Chart 55-1). A balanced diet includes following the recommendations of the U.S. Department of Agriculture (USDA) and limiting intake of foods and spices that can cause gastric distress, such as caffeine, chocolate, mustard, pepper, and other strong or hot spices. Alcohol and tobacco should also be avoided. Regular exercise maintains peristalsis, which helps prevent gastric contents from irritating the gastric mucosa. Stress-reduction techniques can include aerobic exercise, meditation, reading, and/or yoga, depending on individual preferences.

Excessive use of aspirin and other NSAIDs should also be avoided. If a family member has *H. pylori* INFECTION or has had it in the past, patient testing should be considered. This test can identify the bacteria before they cause gastritis.

❖ *PATIENT-CENTERED COLLABORATIVE CARE*

◆ *Assessment*

Symptoms of *acute* gastritis range from mild to severe. The patient may report epigastric discomfort or PAIN, anorexia,

CHART 55-1 Patient and Family Education: Preparing for Self-Management

Gastritis Prevention

- Eat a well-balanced diet.
- Avoid drinking excessive amounts of alcoholic beverages.
- Use caution in taking large doses of aspirin, other NSAIDs (e.g., ibuprofen), and corticosteroids.
- Avoid excessive intake of coffee (even decaffeinated).
- Be sure that foods and water are safe, to avoid contamination.
- Manage stress levels using complementary and alternative therapies such as relaxation and meditation techniques.
- Stop smoking.
- Protect yourself against exposure to toxic substances in the workplace such as lead and nickel.
- Seek medical treatment if you are experiencing symptoms of esophageal reflux (see Chapter 54).

CHART 55-2 **Key Features**

Gastritis

Acute Gastritis	Chronic Gastritis
• Rapid onset of epigastric pain or discomfort	• Vague report of epigastric pain that is relieved by food
• Nausea and vomiting	• Anorexia
• Hematemesis (vomiting blood)	• Nausea or vomiting
• Gastric hemorrhage	• Intolerance of fatty and spicy foods
• Dyspepsia (heartburn)	• Pernicious anemia
• Anorexia	

cramping, nausea, and vomiting (Chart 55-2). Assess for abdominal tenderness and bloating, **hematemesis** (vomiting blood), or **melena** (dark, sticky feces, as evidence of blood in the stool). Symptoms last only a few hours or days and vary with the cause. Aspirin/NSAID–related gastritis may result in **dyspepsia** (heartburn). Gastritis or food poisoning caused by endotoxins, such as staphylococcal endotoxin, has an abrupt onset. Severe nausea and vomiting often occur within 5 hours of ingestion of the contaminated food. *In some cases gastric hemorrhage is the presenting symptom, which is a life-threatening emergency.*

Chronic gastritis causes few symptoms unless ulceration occurs. Patients may report nausea, vomiting, or upper abdominal discomfort. Periodic epigastric pain may occur after a meal. Some patients have anorexia (see Chart 55-2).

Esophagogastroduodenoscopy (EGD) via an endoscope with biopsy is the gold standard for diagnosing gastritis. (See Chapter 52 for discussion of nursing care associated with this diagnostic procedure.) The physician performs a biopsy to establish a definitive diagnosis of the type of gastritis. If lesions are patchy and diffuse, biopsy of several suspicious areas may be necessary to avoid misdiagnosis. A *cytologic examination* of the biopsy specimen is performed to confirm or rule out gastric cancer. Tissue samples can also be taken to detect *H. pylori* INFECTION using *rapid urease testing*. The results of these tests are more reliable if the patient has discontinued taking antacids for at least a week (Pagana & Pagana, 2014).

Interventions

Patients with gastritis are not often seen in the acute care setting unless they have an exacerbation ("flare-up") of acute or chronic gastritis that results in fluid and electrolyte imbalance, bleeding, or increased PAIN. Collaborative care is directed toward supportive care for relieving the symptoms and removing or reducing the cause of discomfort.

Acute gastritis is treated symptomatically and supportively because the healing process is spontaneous, usually occurring within a few days. When the cause is removed, PAIN and discomfort usually subside. If bleeding is severe, a blood transfusion may be necessary. Fluid replacement is prescribed for patients with severe fluid loss. Surgery, such as partial gastrectomy, pyloroplasty, and/or vagotomy, may be needed for patients with major bleeding or ulceration. Treatment of *chronic* gastritis varies with the cause. The approach to management includes the elimination of causative agents, treatment of any underlying disease (e.g., uremia, Crohn's disease), avoidance of toxic substances (e.g., alcohol, tobacco), and health teaching.

Eliminating the causative factors, such as *H. pylori* INFECTION if present, is the primary treatment approach. Drugs and nutritional therapy are also used. In the *acute* phase the health care provider prescribes drugs that block and buffer gastric acid secretions to relieve pain.

H_2-receptor antagonists, such as famotidine (Pepcid) and nizatidine (Axid), are typically used to block gastric secretions. Sucralfate (Carafate, Sulcrate ♣), a *mucosal barrier fortifier*, may also be prescribed. *Antacids* used as buffering agents include aluminum hydroxide combined with magnesium hydroxide (Maalox) and aluminum hydroxide combined with simethicone and magnesium hydroxide (Mylanta). Antisecretory agents (**proton pump inhibitors [PPIs]**) such as omeprazole (Prilosec) or pantoprazole (Protonix) may be prescribed to suppress gastric acid secretion (see Chart 55-3).

! NURSING SAFETY PRIORITY QSEN

Drug Alert

Teach the patient to monitor for symptom relief and side effects of drugs to treat gastritis and to notify the health care provider of any adverse effects or worsening of gastric distress. The dose, frequency, or type of drug may need to be changed if symptoms of gastric irritation appear or persist. *Remind patients not to take additional over-the-counter (OTC) drugs such as Pepcid AC or Axid AR if they are taking similar prescribed drugs.*

Patients with *chronic* gastritis may require vitamin B_{12} for prevention or treatment of pernicious anemia. If *H. pylori* is found, the health care provider treats the infection. Current practice for INFECTION treatment is described on p. 1134 in the discussion of Drug Therapy in the Peptic Ulcer Disease section.

The nurse, primary care provider, or pharmacist teaches patients to avoid drugs and other irritants that are associated with gastritis episodes, if possible. These drugs include corticosteroids, erythromycin (E-Mycin, Erythromid ♣), ASA (aspirin), and NSAIDs such as naproxen (Naprosyn) and ibuprofen (Motrin, Advil, Amersol ♣, Novo-Profen ♣). NSAIDs are also available as OTC drugs and should not be used. Teach patients to read all OTC drug labels because many preparations contain aspirin or other NSAID.

Instruct the patient to limit intake of any foods and spices that cause distress, such as those that contain caffeine or high acid content (e.g., tomato products, citrus juices) or those that are heavily seasoned with strong or hot spices. Bell peppers and onions are also commonly irritating foods. Most patients seem to progress better with a bland, non-spicy diet and smaller, more frequent meals. Alcohol and tobacco should also be avoided.

Teach the patient about various techniques that reduce stress and discomfort, such as progressive relaxation, cutaneous stimulation, guided imagery, and distraction. Table 55-1 lists commonly used complementary and alternative therapies for gastritis and peptic ulcer disease.

PEPTIC ULCER DISEASE

A **peptic ulcer** is a mucosal lesion of the stomach or duodenum. **Peptic ulcer disease (PUD)** results when mucosal defenses become impaired and no longer protect the epithelium from the effects of acid and pepsin.

TABLE 55-1 Commonly Used Complementary and Alternative Therapies for Gastritis and Peptic Ulcer Disease (PUD)

Herbs and Vitamins	Homeopathy
• Cranberry	• Carbo vegetabilis
• DGL (deglycyrrhizinated licorice)	• Ipecacuanha
• Ginger	• Nux vomica
• Probiotics	• Pulsatilla
• Slippery elm	
• Vitamin C	

❖ *PATHOPHYSIOLOGY*

Types of Ulcers

Three types of ulcers may occur: gastric ulcers, duodenal ulcers, and stress ulcers (less common). Most gastric and duodenal ulcers are caused by *H. pylori* INFECTION. Although it is not certain about how *H. pylori* is transmitted, it is believed to be spread through contaminated food or water. Studies have also suggested that contact with stool, vomit, and sometimes saliva of an infected person can spread the infection (National Digestive Diseases Information Clearinghouse, 2012).

As a response to the bacteria, cytokines, neutrophils, and other substances are activated and cause epithelial cell necrosis. These bacteria produce substances that damage the mucosa. Urease produced by *H. pylori* breaks down urea into ammonia, which neutralizes the acidity of the stomach. Urease can be detected through laboratory testing to confirm the *H. pylori* infection. Also, the helical shape of *H. pylori* allows the bacterium to burrow into the mucus layer of the stomach and become undetectable by the body's immune cells. Although this bacterium does not cause illness in most people, it is a major risk factor for peptic and duodenal ulcers and gastric cancer (McCance et al., 2014).

Gastric ulcers usually develop in the antrum of the stomach near acid-secreting mucosa. When a break in the mucosal barrier occurs (such as that caused by *H. pylori* INFECTION), hydrochloric acid injures the epithelium. Gastric ulcers may then result from back-diffusion of acid or dysfunction of the pyloric sphincter (Fig. 55-1). Without normal functioning of the pyloric sphincter, bile refluxes (backs up) into the stomach. This reflux of bile acids may break the integrity of the mucosal barrier, which leads to mucosal INFLAMMATION. Toxic agents and bile then destroy the membrane of the gastric mucosa.

Gastric emptying is often delayed in patients with gastric ulceration. This causes regurgitation of duodenal contents, which worsens the gastric mucosal injury. Decreased blood flow to the gastric mucosa may also alter the defense barrier and thereby allow ulceration to occur. Gastric ulcers are deep and penetrating, and they usually occur on the lesser curvature of the stomach, near the pylorus (Fig. 55-2).

Most *duodenal ulcers* occur in the upper portion of the duodenum. They are deep, sharply demarcated lesions that penetrate through the mucosa and submucosa into the muscularis propria (muscle layer). The floor of the ulcer consists of a necrotic area residing on granulation tissue and surrounded by areas of fibrosis (McCance et al., 2014).

The main feature of a duodenal ulcer is high gastric acid secretion, although a wide range of secretory levels are found. In patients with duodenal ulcers, pH levels are low (excess acid) in the duodenum for long periods. Protein-rich meals, calcium,

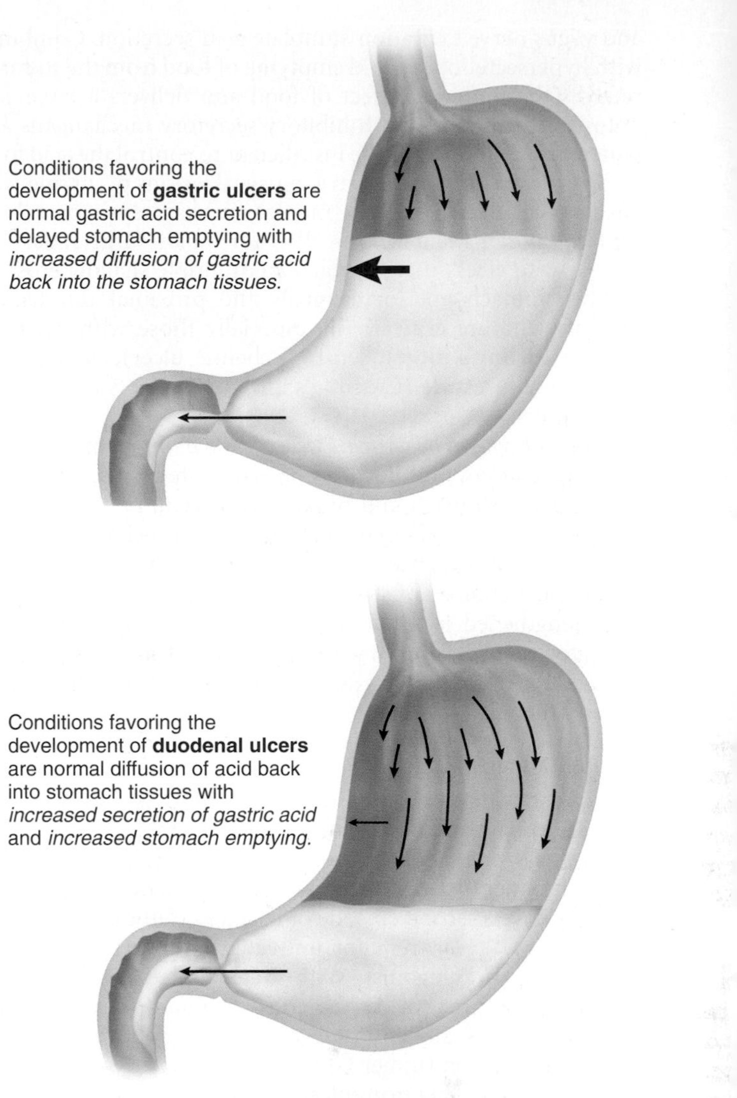

FIG. 55-1 The pathophysiology of peptic ulcer.

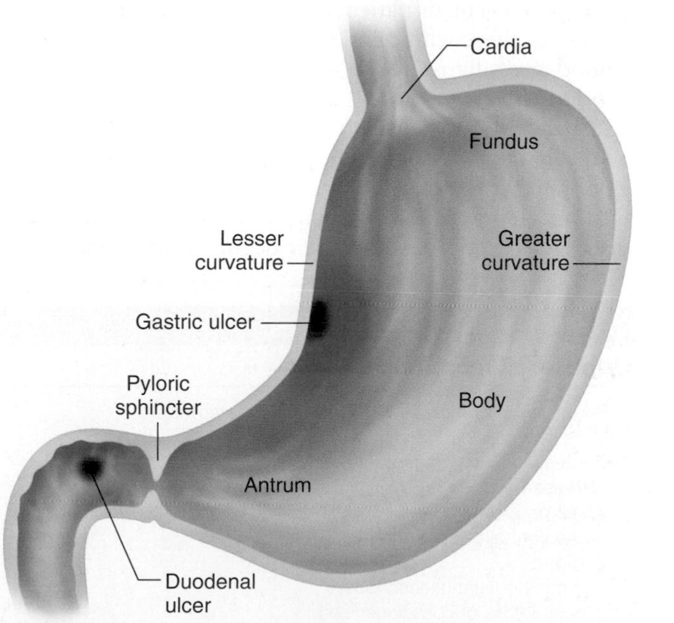

FIG. 55-2 The most common sites for peptic ulcers.

and vagus nerve excitation stimulate acid secretion. Combined with hypersecretion, a rapid emptying of food from the stomach reduces the buffering effect of food and delivers a large acid bolus to the duodenum. Inhibitory secretory mechanisms and pancreatic secretion may be insufficient to control the acid load.

Stress ulcers are acute gastric mucosal lesions occurring after an acute medical crisis or trauma, such as sepsis or a head injury. In the patient who is NPO for major surgery, gastritis may lead to **stress ulcers**, which are multiple shallow erosions of the stomach and occasionally the proximal duodenum. Patients who are critically ill, especially those with extensive burns (**Curling's ulcer**), sepsis (ischemic ulcer), or increased intracranial pressure (**Cushing's ulcer**), are also susceptible to these ulcers.

Bleeding caused by gastric erosion is the main manifestation of acute stress ulcers. Multifocal lesions associated with stress ulcers occur in the stomach and proximal duodenum. These lesions begin as areas of ischemia and evolve into erosions and ulcerations that may progress to massive hemorrhage. Little is known of the exact etiology of stress ulcers. Stress ulcers are associated with lengthened hospital stay and increased mortality rates. Therefore most patients who have major trauma or surgery receive IV drug therapy (e.g., PPI) to prevent stress ulcer development.

Complications of Ulcers

The most common complications of PUD are hemorrhage, perforation, pyloric obstruction, and intractable disease. *Hemorrhage is the most serious complication.* It tends to occur more often in patients with *gastric* ulcers and in older adults. Many patients have a second episode of bleeding if underlying INFECTION with *H. pylori* remains untreated or if therapy does not include an H_2 antagonist. With massive bleeding the patient vomits bright red or coffee-ground blood (**hematemesis**). Hematemesis usually indicates bleeding at or above the duodenojejunal junction (upper GI bleeding) (Chart 55-3).

Minimal bleeding from ulcers is manifested by occult blood in a dark, "tarry" stool (**melena**). The digestion of blood within the duodenum and small intestine may result in this black stool. Melena may occur in patients with gastric ulcers but is more common in those with duodenal ulcers. Gastric acid digestion of blood typically results in a granular dark vomitus *(coffee-ground appearance)*.

Gastric and duodenal ulcers can perforate and bleed (Fig. 55-3). *Perforation* occurs when the ulcer becomes so deep that the entire thickness of the stomach or duodenum is worn away. The stomach or duodenal contents can then leak into the peritoneal cavity. Sudden, sharp PAIN begins in the midepigastric region and spreads over the entire abdomen. The amount of pain correlates with the amount and type of GI contents spilled. The classic pain causes the patient to be apprehensive. The abdomen is tender, rigid, and boardlike (**peritonitis**). The patient often assumes a "fetal" position to decrease the tension on the abdominal muscles. He or she can become severely ill within hours. Bacterial septicemia and hypovolemic shock follow. Peristalsis diminishes, and paralytic ileus develops. *Peptic ulcer perforation is a surgical emergency and can be life threatening!*

CHART 55-3 Key Features

Upper GI Bleeding

- Bright red or coffee-ground vomitus (hematemesis)
- Melena (tarry or dark, sticky) stools
- Decreased blood pressure
- Increased heart rate
- Weak peripheral pulses
- Acute confusion (in older adults)
- Vertigo
- Dizziness or light-headedness
- Syncope (loss of consciousness)
- Decreased hemoglobin and hematocrit

NCLEX EXAMINATION CHALLENGE

Safe and Effective Care Environment

The nurse has been assigned to provide care for four clients at the beginning of the day shift. In what order does the nurse assess these clients?

A. A client planned for an esophagogastroduodenoscopy (EGD) at 1 PM (1300)
B. A client requesting pain medication 2 days after a partial gastrectomy
C. A client with peptic ulcer disease experiencing a sudden onset of acute stomach pain
D. A client who is NPO for tests to rule out gastric cancer

Pyloric (gastric outlet) obstruction (blockage) occurs in a small percentage of patients and is manifested by vomiting caused by stasis and gastric dilation. Obstruction occurs at the pylorus (the gastric outlet) and is caused by scarring, edema, INFLAMMATION, or a combination of these factors.

Symptoms of obstruction include abdominal bloating, nausea, and vomiting. When vomiting persists, the patient may have hypochloremic (metabolic) alkalosis from loss of large quantities of acid gastric juice (hydrogen and chloride ions) in the vomitus. Hypokalemia may also result from the vomiting or metabolic alkalosis.

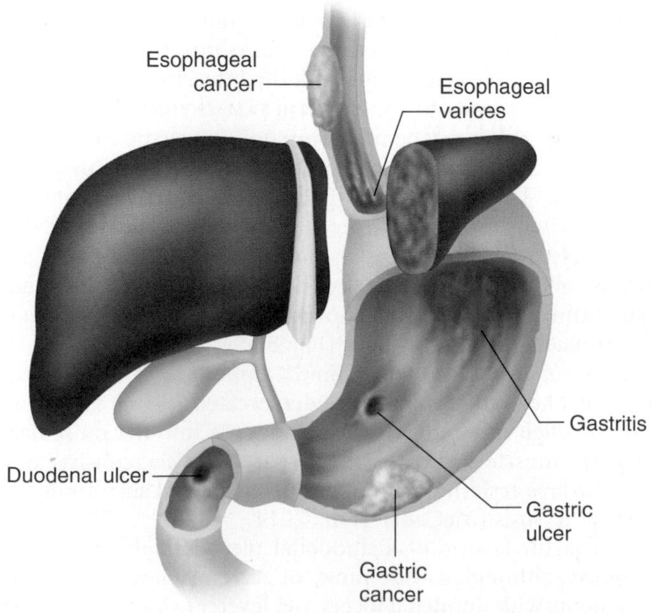

FIG. 55-3 Common causes of upper GI bleeding.

Many patients with ulcers have a single episode with no recurrence. However, *intractability* may develop from complications of ulcers, excessive stressors in the patient's life, or an inability to adhere to long-term therapy. He or she no longer responds to conservative management, or recurrences of symptoms interfere with ADLs. In general, the patient continues to have recurrent pain and discomfort despite treatment. Those who fail to respond to traditional treatments or who have a relapse after discontinuation of therapy are referred to a gastroenterologist.

Etiology and Genetic Risk

Peptic ulcer disease is caused most often by bacterial INFECTION with *H. pylori* and NSAIDs. NSAIDs (e.g., ibuprofen) break down the mucosal barrier and disrupt the mucosal protection mediated systemically by cyclooxygenase (COX) inhibition. COX-2 inhibitors (celecoxib [Celebrex]) are less likely to cause mucosal damage but place patients at high risk for cardiovascular events, such as myocardial infarction. In addition, NSAIDs cause decreased endogenous prostaglandins, resulting in local gastric mucosal injury (Lilley et al., 2014). GI complications from NSAID use can occur at any time, even after long-term uncomplicated use. NSAID-related ulcers are difficult to treat, even with long-term therapy, because these ulcers have a high rate of recurrence.

Certain substances may contribute to gastroduodenal ulceration by altering gastric secretion, which produces localized damage to mucosa and interferes with the healing process. For example, corticosteroids (e.g., prednisone), theophylline (Theo-Dur), and caffeine stimulate hydrochloric acid production. Patients receiving radiation therapy may also develop GI ulcers. Other risk factors for PUD are the same as for gastritis (see Chart 55-1).

Incidence and Prevalence

PUD affects millions of people across the world. However, health care provider visits, hospitalizations, and the mortality rate for PUD have decreased in the past few decades. The use of proton pump inhibitors and *H. pylori* treatment may explain these declines.

❖ PATIENT-CENTERED COLLABORATIVE CARE

◆ Assessment

History. Collect data related to the causes and risk factors for peptic ulcer disease (PUD). Question the patient about factors that can influence the development of PUD, including alcohol intake and tobacco use. Note if certain foods such as tomatoes or caffeinated beverages precipitate or worsen symptoms. Information regarding actual or perceived daily stressors should also be obtained.

A history of current or past medical conditions focuses on GI problems, particularly any history of diagnosis or treatment for *H. pylori* INFECTION. Review all prescription and OTC drugs the patient is taking. Specifically inquire whether the patient is taking corticosteroids, chemotherapy, or NSAIDs. Also ask whether he or she has ever undergone radiation treatments. Assess whether the patient has had any GI surgeries, especially a partial gastrectomy, which can cause chronic gastritis.

A history of GI upset, PAIN and its relationship to eating and sleep patterns, and actions taken to relieve pain are also important. Inquire about any changes in the character of the pain, because this may signal the development of complications. For example, if pain that was once intermittent and relieved by food and antacids becomes constant and radiates to the back or upper quadrant, the patient may have ulcer perforation. However, many people with active duodenal or gastric ulcers report having no ulcer symptoms.

Physical Assessment/Clinical Manifestations. Physical assessment findings may reveal epigastric tenderness, usually located at the midline between the umbilicus and the xiphoid process. *If perforation into the peritoneal cavity is present, the patient typically has a rigid, boardlike abdomen accompanied by rebound tenderness and pain.* Initially, auscultation of the abdomen may reveal hyperactive bowel sounds, but these may diminish with progression of the disorder.

Dyspepsia *(indigestion) is the most commonly reported symptom associated with PUD.* It is typically described as sharp, burning, or gnawing PAIN. Some patients may perceive discomfort as a sensation of abdominal pressure or of fullness or hunger. Older adults often have more nausea and vomiting rather than abdominal discomfort (DeRanieri, 2013). Specific differences between gastric and duodenal ulcers are listed in Table 55-2.

Gastric ulcer PAIN often occurs in the upper epigastrium with localization to the left of the midline and is aggravated by food. *Duodenal* ulcer pain is usually located to the right of or below the epigastrium. The pain associated with a duodenal ulcer occurs 90 minutes to 3 hours *after* eating and often awakens the patient at night (McCance et al., 2014). Pain may also be exacerbated (made worse) by certain foods (e.g., tomatoes, hot spices, fried foods, onions, alcohol, caffeine drinks) and certain drugs (e.g., NSAIDs, corticosteroids). Perform a comprehensive pain assessment.

Nausea and vomiting may be symptoms accompanying ulcer disease, most commonly with pyloric sphincter dysfunction. It may result from gastric stasis associated with pyloric obstruction. Appetite is generally maintained in patients with a peptic ulcer unless pyloric obstruction is present.

To assess for fluid volume deficit that occurs from bleeding, take orthostatic blood pressures and monitor for signs and symptoms of dehydration. Also assess for dizziness, especially when the patient is upright, because this is a symptom of fluid volume deficit. Older adults often experience dizziness when they get out of bed and are at risk for falls.

NCLEX EXAMINATION CHALLENGE

Physiological Integrity

When taking a history of a client diagnosed with a gastric ulcer, which assessment findings does the nurse expect? **Select all that apply**.

A. Vomiting
B. Weight loss
C. Epigastric pain at night
D. Relief of epigastric pain after eating
E. Melena

Psychosocial Assessment. Assess the impact of ulcer disease on the patient's lifestyle, occupation, family, and social and leisure activities. Evaluate the impact that lifestyle changes will have on the patient and family. This assessment may reveal information about the patient's ability to adhere to the prescribed treatment regimen and to obtain the needed social support to alter his or her lifestyle.

TABLE 55-2 **Differential Features of Gastric and Duodenal Ulcers**

FEATURE	GASTRIC ULCER	DUODENAL ULCER
Age	Usually 50 yr or older	Usually 50 yr or older
Gender	Male/female ratio of 1.1 : 1	Male/female ratio of 1 : 1
Blood group	No differentiation	Most often type O
General nourishment	May be malnourished	Usually well nourished
Stomach acid production	Normal secretion or hyposecretion	Hypersecretion
Occurrence	Mucosa exposed to acid-pepsin secretion	Mucosa exposed to acid-pepsin secretion
Clinical course	Healing and recurrence	Healing and recurrence
Pain	Occurs 30-60 min after a meal; at night: rarely Worsened by ingestion of food	Occurs 1½-3 hr after a meal; at night: often awakens patient between 1 and 2 AM Relieved by ingestion of food
Response to treatment	Healing with appropriate therapy	Healing with appropriate therapy
Hemorrhage	Hematemesis more common than melena	Melena more common than hematemesis
Malignant change	Perhaps in less than 10%	Rare
Recurrence	Tends to heal, and recurs often in the same location	60% recur within 1 yr; 90% recur within 2 yr
Surrounding mucosa	Atrophic gastritis	No gastritis

Laboratory Assessment. There are three simple, noninvasive tests to detect *H. pylori* in the patient's blood, breath, or stool. Although the breath and stool tests are considered more accurate, *serologic testing* for *H. pylori* antibodies is the most common method to confirm *H. pylori* INFECTION. The *urea breath test* involves swallowing a capsule, liquid, or pudding that contains urea with a special carbon atom. After a few minutes the patient exhales, and if the special carbon atom is found, the bacterium is present. The *stool antigen test* is performed on a stool sample provided by the patient and is tested for *H. pylori* antigens. Patients who have venous bleeding from a peptic ulcer may have *decreased hemoglobin and hematocrit* values. The *stool* may also be positive for occult (not seen) blood if bleeding is present (Pagana & Pagana, 2014).

Imaging Assessment. If perforation is suspected, the health care provider may request a *chest and abdomen x-ray series,* but other diagnostic tests are more helpful in diagnosis.

Other Diagnostic Assessment. *The major diagnostic test for PUD is esophagogastroduodenoscopy (EGD), which is the most accurate means of establishing a diagnosis.* Direct visualization of the ulcer crater by EGD allows the health care provider to take specimens for *H. pylori* testing and for biopsy and cytologic studies for ruling out gastric cancer. The rapid urease test can confirm a quick diagnosis because urease is produced by the bacteria in the gastric mucosa. EGD may be repeated at 4- to 6-week intervals while the health care provider evaluates the progress of healing in response to therapy. Chapter 52 describes this test in more detail.

GI bleeding may be tested using a *nuclear medicine scan.* No special preparation is required for this scan. The patient is injected with a contrast medium (usually Tc99m), and the GI system is scanned for the presence of bleeding after a waiting period. A second scan may be done 1 to 2 days after the bleeding is treated to determine if the interventions were effective.

◆ *Analysis*

The priority NANDA-I nursing diagnoses and collaborative problems for patients with peptic ulcer disease (PUD) include:

1. Acute Pain or Chronic Pain related to gastric and/or duodenal ulceration (NANDA-I)
2. Upper GI bleeding related to perforation

◆ *Planning and Implementation*

Managing Acute Pain or Chronic Pain

Planning: Expected Outcomes. The patient with PUD is expected to report PAIN control as evidenced by no more than a 3 on a 0-to-10 pain intensity scale.

Interventions. PUD causes significant discomfort that impacts many aspects of daily living. Interventions to manage PAIN focus on drug therapy and dietary changes.

Drug Therapy. The primary purposes of drug therapy in the treatment of PUD are to (1) provide PAIN relief, (2) eliminate *H. pylori* INFECTION, (3) heal ulcerations, and (4) prevent recurrence. Several different regimens can be used. In selecting a therapeutic drug regimen, the health care provider considers the efficacy of the treatment, the anticipated side effects, the ability of the patient to adhere to the regimen, and the cost of the treatment.

Although numerous drugs have been evaluated for the treatment of *H. pylori* INFECTION, no single agent has been used successfully against the organism. A common drug regimen for *H. pylori* infection is PPI–triple therapy, which includes a proton pump inhibitor (PPI) such as lansoprazole (Prevacid) plus two antibiotics such as metronidazole (Flagyl, Novonidazol 🍁) and tetracycline (Ala-Tet, Panmycin, Nu-Tetra 🍁) or clarithromycin (Biaxin, Biaxin XL) and amoxicillin (Amoxil, Amoxi 🍁) for 10 to 14 days. Some health care providers may prefer to use quadruple therapy, which contains combination of a proton pump inhibitor (PPI), any two commonly used antibiotics as described above, with the addition of bismuth (Pepto-Bismol). Bismuth therapy is often used in patients who are allergic to penicillin-based medications.

CONSIDERATIONS FOR OLDER ADULTS

Patient-Centered Care QSEN

Many older adults have *H. pylori* infection that is undiagnosed because of vague symptoms associated with physiologic changes of aging and comorbidities that mask dyspepsia. Because the average age of gastric cancer diagnosis is 70 years, it is important to teach older adults about the symptoms of PUD and to consider *H. pylori* screening. Early detection and aggressive treatment can prevent PUD and gastric cancer.

Hyposecretory drugs reduce gastric acid secretions and are therefore used for both peptic ulcer disease (PUD) and gastritis management. The primary prescribed drugs include proton pump inhibitors and H_2-receptor antagonists (Chart 55-4).

Proton pump inhibitors (PPIs) is the drug class of choice for treating patients with acid-related disorders. Examples include omeprazole (Prilosec), lansoprazole (Prevacid), rabeprazole (Aciphex), pantoprazole (Protonix), and esomeprazole (Nexium). These drugs suppress the H,K–ATPase enzyme

CHART 55-4 Common Examples of Drug Therapy

Peptic Ulcer Disease

DRUG AND USUAL DOSAGE	PURPOSE OF DRUG	NURSING INTERVENTIONS	RATIONALES
Antacids			
Magnesium hydroxide with aluminum hydroxide (Maalox, Mylanta) 50-80 mEq orally 1 hr and 3 hr after meals and at bedtime	Increases pH of gastric contents by deactivating pepsin	Give 2 hr after meals and at bedtime.	Hydrogen ion load is high after ingestion of foods.
		Use liquid rather than tablets.	Suspensions are more effective than chewable tablets.
		Do not give other drugs within 1-2 hr of antacids.	Antacids interfere with absorption of other drugs.
		Assess patients for a history of renal disease.	Hypermagnesemia may result. These antacids have a high sodium content. These antacids contain magnesium, which cannot be excreted by poorly functioning kidneys, thus causing toxicity.
		Assess the patient for a history of heart failure.	Inadequate renal perfusion from heart failure decreases the ability of the kidneys to excrete magnesium, thus causing toxicity.
		Observe the patient for the side effect of diarrhea.	Magnesium often causes diarrhea.
Aluminum hydroxide (Amphojel) 50-80 mEq orally 1 hr and 3 hr after meals and at bedtime		Give 1 hr after meals and at bedtime.	Hydrogen ion load is high after ingestion of food.
		Use liquid rather than tablets if palatable.	Suspensions are more effective than chewable tablets.
		Do not give other drugs within 1-2 hr of antacids.	Antacids interfere with absorption of other drugs.
		Observe patients for the side effect of constipation. If constipation occurs, consider alternating with magnesium antacid.	Aluminum causes constipation, and magnesium has a laxative effect.
		Use for patients with renal failure.	Aluminum binds with phosphates in the GI tract. This antacid does not contain magnesium.
H_2 Antagonists (Blockers)			
Ranitidine (Zantac) 150 mg orally twice daily or 300 mg orally at bedtime; 50 mg IV every 6 hr or 8 mg/hr IV (continuous) Famotidine (Pepcid) 40 mg orally once daily or in two divided doses; 20 mg IV every 12 hr Nizatidine (Axid) 150 mg orally twice daily or 300 mg at bedtime	Decreases gastric acid secretions by blocking histamine receptors in parietal cells	Give single dose at bedtime for treatment of GI ulcers, heartburn, and PUD. **NOTE:** IV famotidine or IV ranitidine may also be given to prevent surgical stress ulcers.	Bedtime administration suppresses nocturnal acid production.
Mucosal Barrier Fortifiers			
Sucralfate (Carafate, Sulcrate 🍁) 1 g orally four times daily or 2 g twice daily	Binds with bile acids and pepsin to protect stomach mucosa	Give 1 hr before and 2 hr after meals and at bedtime.	Food may interfere with drug's adherence to mucosa.
		Do not give within 30 min of giving antacids or other drugs.	Antacids may interfere with effect.
Bismuth Subsalicylate (Pepto-Bismol) 525 mg (30 mL) orally four times daily	Stimulates mucosal protection and prostaglandin production Inhibits *H. pylori* from binding to mucosal lining	Patients cannot take aspirin while on this drug. **NOTE:** May cause the stools to be discolored black.	Aspirin is a salicylic acid and will lead to overdose of aspirin.

Continued

CHART 55-4 Common Examples of Drug Therapy—cont'd

Peptic Ulcer Disease

DRUG AND USUAL DOSAGE	PURPOSE OF DRUG	NURSING INTERVENTIONS	RATIONALES
Proton Pump Inhibitors			
Omeprazole (Prilosec, Losec 🍁) 20-40 mg orally daily	Suppresses H,K–ATPase enzyme system of gastric acid secretion Indications for short-term and long-term use for PUD, symptomatic heartburn, and *H. pylori* treatment	Have patients take capsule whole; do not crush. Give 30 minutes before the main meal of the day.	Delayed-release capsules allow absorption after granules leave the stomach. The proton pump is activated by the presence of food. Therefore the drug needs a chance to work before the patient eats.
Lansoprazole (Prevacid) 15-30 mg orally daily		Give 30 min before the main meal of the day.	The proton pump is activated by the presence of food. Therefore the drug needs a chance to work before the patient eats.
Rabeprazole (Aciphex) 20 mg orally once daily		Take after the morning meal. Do not crush capsule.	Drug promotes healing and symptom relief of duodenal ulcers. Drug is a sustained-release capsule.
Pantoprazole (Protonix) 40 mg orally or IV daily for 7-10 days		Do not crush. IV form must be given on a pump with a filter and in a separate line. Do not give Protonix IV with other IV drugs. **NOTE:** This medication may have several adverse drug interactions. Be aware of the patient's other medications.	Drug is enteric-coated. Given IV, drug precipitates easily. The IV form is not compatible with most other drugs. This medication will alter how other drugs are metabolized, either increasing or decreasing their effectiveness.
Esomeprazole (Nexium) 20 or 40 mg orally daily (or IV daily for 7-10 days)		Assess for hepatic impairment. Do not give Nexium IV with other IV drugs. **NOTE:** This medication may have several adverse drug interactions. Be aware of the patient's other medications.	Patients with severe hepatic problems need a low dose. The IV form is not compatible with most other drugs. This medication will alter how other drugs are metabolized, either increasing or decreasing the effectiveness.
Prostaglandin Analogs			
Misoprostol (Cytotec) 200 mcg orally four times daily	Synthetic prostaglandin that stimulates mucosal protection and decreases gastric acid secretions Helps resist mucosal injury in patients taking NSAIDs and/or high-dose corticosteroids	Avoid magnesium-containing antacids. **NOTE:** Do not use in pregnant women.	Both misoprostol and magnesium-containing antacids can cause diarrhea. Can cause abortion, premature birth, or birth defects.
Antimicrobials			
Clarithromycin (Biaxin) 500 mg orally three times daily	Treats *H. pylori* infection	Be aware that the drug should be given with caution to patients with renal impairment; monitor renal function lab values.	The drug can increase the patient's BUN level and should be monitored.
Amoxicillin (Amoxil) 1 g orally twice daily	Treats *H. pylori* infection	Teach patients to take the drug with food or immediately after a meal.	The drug can cause GI disturbances, including nausea, vomiting, and diarrhea.
Tetracycline 500 mg orally four times daily	Treats *H. pylori* infection	Teach patients to take the drug at least 1 hour before meals or 2 hours after meals. Teach patients to avoid direct sunlight and wear sunscreen when outdoors.	Dairy products and other foods may interfere with drug absorption. The drug can cause the skin to burn due to photosensitivity.
Metronidazole (Flagyl) 250 mg orally three times daily and at bedtime	Treats *H. pylori* infection	Teach patients to take the drug with food. Teach patients to avoid alcohol during drug therapy and for at least 3 days after therapy is completed.	The drug can cause GI disturbances, especially nausea. The patient can experience a drug-alcohol reaction, including severe nausea, vomiting, and headache.

system of gastric acid production, and several of them are available as over-the-counter (OTC) drugs (Lilley et al., 2014).

Omeprazole, lansoprazole, and esomeprazole are each available as delayed-release capsules designed to release their contents after they pass through the stomach. Omeprazole and lansoprazole may be dissolved in a sodium bicarbonate solution and given through any feeding tube. Bicarbonate protects the dissolved omeprazole and lansoprazole granules in gastric acid. Therefore the drugs are still absorbed correctly. These capsules can also be opened. The enteric-coated capsules can be put in apple juice or orange juice and given through a large-bore feeding tube. Rabeprazole (Aciphex) and pantoprazole (Protonix) are enteric-coated tablets that quickly dissolve after the tablet has moved through the stomach and should not be crushed before giving them. Several of the PPIs are also available in an IV form, which may be helpful for patients who are NPO.

Some patients use these PPIs for years and perhaps a lifetime. However, these drugs should not be used for a prolonged period because, over time, they may contribute to osteoporotic-related fractures, especially spinal fractures in older women (Kwok et al., 2010). Omeprazole (Prilosec and Prilosec OTC) reduces the effect of clopidogrel (Plavix), an antiplatelet drug. Teach patients to tell their health care provider if they are taking clopidogrel. PPIs should not be discontinued abruptly to prevent rebound activation of the proton pump. Therefore, a step-down approach over several days is recommended (Zarowitz, 2011).

H_2-receptor antagonists are drugs that block histamine-stimulated gastric secretions. These drugs may also be used for indigestion and gastritis. Lower-dose forms are available in over-the-counter (OTC) products. H_2-receptor antagonists block the action of the H_2 receptors of the parietal cells, thus inhibiting gastric acid secretion. Two of the most common drugs are famotidine (Pepcid) and nizatidine (Axid) and are available as Pepcid OTC and Axid AR in OTC form. These drugs are typically administered in a single dose at bedtime and are used for 4 to 6 weeks in combination with other therapy.

Antacids buffer gastric acid and prevent the formation of pepsin. They may help small duodenal ulcers heal but are usually not used alone as drug therapy. Liquid suspensions are the most therapeutic form, but tablets may be more convenient and enhance adherence. The most widely used preparations are mixtures of aluminum hydroxide and magnesium hydroxide. This combination overcomes the unpleasant GI side effects of either of these preparations when used alone. Mylanta and Maalox are examples of this type of combination antacid formulation. The aluminum and magnesium hydroxide combination products neutralize well at small doses. These products must be administered cautiously to patients with renal impairment because elimination is reduced and excessive amounts are retained in the body.

! NURSING SAFETY PRIORITY (QSEN)

Drug Alert

Teach the patient that to achieve a therapeutic effect, sufficient antacid must be ingested to neutralize the hourly production of acid. For optimal effect, take antacids about 2 hours after meals to reduce the hydrogen ion load in the duodenum. Antacids may be effective from 30 minutes to 3 hours after ingestion. If taken on an empty stomach, they are quickly evacuated. Thus the neutralizing effect is reduced (Lilley et al., 2014).

Calcium carbonate (Tums) is a potent antacid, but it triggers gastrin release, causing a rebound acid secretion. Therefore its use in acid inhibition is not recommended.

Antacids can interact with certain drugs such as phenytoin (Dilantin), tetracycline (Ala-Tet, Nu-Tetra ♣), and ketoconazole (Nizoral) and interfere with their effectiveness. Ask what other drugs the patient is using before a specific antacid is prescribed. Other drugs are given 1 to 2 hours before or after the antacid. Inform the patient that flavored antacids, especially wintergreen, should be avoided. The flavoring increases the emptying time of the stomach. Thus the desired effect of the antacid is negated.

Teach the patient with past or present heart failure to avoid antacids with high sodium content, such as aluminum hydroxide, magnesium hydroxide, sodium bicarbonate, and simethicone combination products (Gelusil and Mylanta). Magaldrate (Riopan) has the lowest sodium concentration.

Sucralfate (Carafate) is a *mucosal barrier fortifier* (protector) that forms complexes with proteins at the base of a peptic ulcer. This protective coat prevents further digestive action of both acid and pepsin. Sucralfate does not inhibit acid secretion. Rather, it binds bile acids and pepsins, reducing injury from these substances. The drug may be used in conjunction with H_2-receptor antagonists and antacids but should not be administered within 1 hour of the antacid. Sucralfate is given on an empty stomach 1 hour before each meal and at bedtime. The main side effect of this drug is constipation.

Bismuth subsalicylate (Pepto-Bismol) inhibits *H. pylori* from binding to the mucosal lining and stimulates mucosal protection and prostaglandin production. Teach patients they cannot take aspirin while on this drug because aspirin is a salicylic acid and could cause an overdose of salicylates. Patients should also be taught that this medication may cause the stools to be discolored black. This discoloration is temporary and harmless.

Nutrition Therapy. The role of diet in the management of ulcer disease is controversial. There is no evidence that dietary restriction reduces gastric acid secretion or promotes tissue healing, although a bland diet may assist in relieving symptoms. Food itself acts as an antacid by neutralizing gastric acid for 30 to 60 minutes. An increased rate of gastric acid secretion, called *rebound,* may follow.

! NURSING SAFETY PRIORITY (QSEN)

Action Alert

Teach the patient with peptic ulcer disease to avoid substances that increase gastric acid secretion. This includes caffeine-containing beverages (coffee, tea, cola). Both caffeinated and decaffeinated coffees should be avoided, because coffee contains peptides that stimulate gastrin release (McCance et al., 2014).

Teach the patient to exclude any foods that cause discomfort. A bland, nonirritating diet is recommended during the acute symptomatic phase. Bedtime snacks are avoided because they may stimulate gastric acid secretion. Eating six smaller meals daily may help, but this regimen is no longer a regular part of therapy. No evidence supports the theory that eating six meals daily promotes healing of the ulcer. This practice may actually stimulate gastric acid secretion. Patients should avoid alcohol and tobacco because of their stimulatory effects on gastric acid secretion.

Complementary and Alternative Therapies. Teach patients about complementary and alternative therapies that can reduce stress, including hypnosis and imagery. For example, the use of yoga and meditation techniques has demonstrated a beneficial effect on anxiety disorders. Many have suggested that GI disorders result from the dysfunction of both the GI tract itself and the brain. This means that emotional stress is thought to worsen GI disorders such as peptic ulcer disease. Yoga may alter the activities of the central and autonomic nervous systems.

Many herbs, such as powders of slippery elm and marshmallow root, quercetin, and licorice, are used commonly by patients with gastritis and PUD. These herbs may help heal inflamed tissue and increase blood flow to the gastric mucosa. Other substances include zinc, vitamin C, essential fatty acids, acidophilus, vitamin A, and glutamine. Table 55-1 provides a list of therapies that have been used by many patients with gastric disorders. Many of them have been scientifically supported in animal studies but have not been thoroughly studied in humans.

! NURSING SAFETY PRIORITY QSEN

Action Alert

Teach the patient who has peptic ulcer disease to seek immediate medical attention if experiencing any of these symptoms:

- Sharp, sudden, persistent, and severe epigastric or abdominal PAIN
- Bloody or black stools
- Bloody vomit or vomit that looks like coffee grounds

Managing Upper GI Bleeding

Planning: Expected Outcomes. The patient with upper GI bleeding (often called *upper GI hemorrhage* or *UGH*) is expected to have bleeding promptly and effectively controlled and vital signs within normal limits.

Interventions. Blood loss from PUD results in high morbidity and mortality. Fluid volume loss secondary to vomiting can lead to dehydration and electrolyte imbalances. Interventions aimed at managing complications associated with PUD include prevention and/or management of bleeding, perforation, and gastric outlet obstruction. In some cases surgical treatment of complications becomes necessary.

Nonsurgical Management. Because prevention or early detection of complications is needed to obtain a positive clinical outcome, monitor the patient carefully and immediately report changes to the health care provider. The type of intervention selected will depend on the type and severity of the complication.

Emergency: Upper GI Bleeding. The patient who is actively bleeding has a life-threatening emergency. He or she needs supportive therapy to prevent hypovolemic shock and possible death.

! NURSING SAFETY PRIORITY QSEN

Critical Rescue

*The first priority for care of the patient with upper GI bleeding is to maintain **a**irway, **b**reathing, and **c**irculation (ABCs).* Provide oxygen and other ventilatory support as needed. Start two large-bore IV lines for replacing fluids and blood. Monitor vital signs, hematocrit, and oxygen saturation.

The purpose of managing hypovolemia is to expand intravascular fluid in a patient who is volume depleted. Carefully monitor the patient's fluid status, including intake and output. *Fluid replacement in older adults should be closely monitored to prevent fluid overload.* Serum electrolytes are also assessed because depletions from vomiting or nasogastric suctioning must be replaced. Volume replacement with isotonic solutions (e.g., 0.9% normal saline solution, lactated Ringer's solution) should be started immediately. The health care provider may prescribe blood products such as packed red blood cells to expand volume and correct a low hemoglobin and hematocrit. For patients with active bleeding, fresh frozen plasma may be given if the prothrombin time is 1.5 times higher than the mid-range control value.

Continue to monitor the patient's hematocrit, hemoglobin, and coagulation studies for changes from the baseline measurements. With mild bleeding (less than 500 mL), slight feelings of weakness and mild perspiration may be present. When blood loss exceeds 1 L/24 hr, manifestations of shock may occur, such as hypotension, chills, palpitations, diaphoresis, and a weak, thready pulse.

A combination of several different treatments, including nasogastric tube (NGT) placement and lavage, endoscopic therapy, interventional radiologic procedures, and acid suppression, can be used to control acute bleeding and prevent rebleeding. If the patient is actively bleeding at home, he or she is usually admitted to the emergency department for GI lavage. If the patient is already a patient in the hospital, lavage can be done at the bedside. After the bleeding has stopped, H_2-receptor antagonists, proton pump inhibitors, and antacids are the primary drugs used.

Nasogastric Tube Placement and Lavage. Upper GI bleeding often requires the primary care provider or nurse to insert a large-bore nasogastric tube (NGT) to:

- Determine the presence or absence of blood in the stomach
- Assess the rate of bleeding
- Prevent gastric dilation
- Administer lavage

Although not performed as commonly today, **gastric lavage** requires the insertion of a large-bore NGT with instillation of a room-temperature solution in volumes of 200 to 300 mL. There is no evidence that sterile saline or sterile water is better than tap water for this procedure. Follow agency protocol for the solution that is required. The solution and blood are repeatedly withdrawn manually until returns are clear or light pink and without clots. Instruct the patient to lie on the left side during this procedure. The NGT may remain in place for a few days or be removed after lavage.

Endoscopic Therapy. Endoscopic therapy via an esophagogastroduodenoscopy (EGD) can assist in achieving homeostasis during an acute hemorrhage by isolating the bleeding artery to embolize (clot) it. A physician can insert instruments through the endoscope during the procedure to stop bleeding in three different ways: (1) inject chemicals into the bleeding site; (2) treat the bleeding area with heat, electric current, or laser; or (3) close the affected blood vessels with a band or clip. During the EGD, a specialized endoscopy nurse and technician assist the physician with the procedure.

Pre-EGD nursing care involves inserting one or two large-bore IV catheters if they are not in place. A large catheter allows the patient to receive IV moderate sedation (e.g., midazolam

[Versed] and an opioid) and possibly a blood transfusion. Keep the patient NPO for 4 to 6 hours before the procedure. This prevents the risk for aspiration and allows the endoscopist to view and treat the ulcer. A patient must sign a consent form before the EGD *after* the physician informs him or her about the procedure.

NURSING SAFETY PRIORITY QSEN

Action Alert

After esophagogastroduodenoscopy (EGD), monitor vital signs, heart rhythm, and oxygen saturation frequently until they return to baseline. In addition, frequently assess the patient's ability to swallow saliva. The patient's gag reflex may initially be absent after an EGD because of anesthetizing (numbing) the throat with a spray before the procedure. *After the procedure, do not allow the patient to have food or liquids until the gag reflex is intact!*

Endoscopic therapy is beneficial for most patients with active bleeding. However, ulcers that continue to bleed or continue to rebleed despite endoscopic therapy may require an interventional radiologic procedure or surgical repair.

Interventional Radiologic Procedures. For patients with persistent, massive upper GI bleeding or those who are not surgical candidates, catheter-directed embolization may be performed. This endovascular procedure is usually done if endoscopic procedures are not successful or available. A femoral approach is most often used, but brachial access may be used. An arteriogram is performed to identify the arterial anatomy and find the exact location of the bleeding. The physician injects medication or other material into the blood vessels to stop the bleeding. Post-arteriogram nursing care should be provided after the procedure as described in Chapter 36.

Acid Suppression. Aggressive acid suppression is used to prevent rebleeding. When acute bleeding is stopped and clot formation has taken place within the ulcer crater, the clot remains in contact with gastric contents. Acid-suppressive agents are used to stabilize the clot by raising the pH level of gastric contents. Several types of drugs are used. H_2-receptor antagonists prevent acid from being produced by parietal cells. Proton pump inhibitors prevent the transport of acid across the parietal cell membrane, whereas antacids buffer acid produced in the stomach.

Perforation is managed by immediately replacing fluid, blood, and electrolytes, administering antibiotics, and keeping the patient NPO. Maintain nasogastric suction to drain gastric secretions and thus prevent further peritoneal spillage. Carefully monitor intake and output and check vital signs at least hourly. Monitor the patient for clinical manifestations of septic shock, such as fever, pain, tachycardia, lethargy, or anxiety.

Pyloric obstruction is caused by edema, spasm, or scar tissue. Symptoms of obstruction related to difficulty in emptying the stomach include feelings of fullness, distention, or nausea after eating, as well as vomiting copious amounts of undigested food.

Treatment of obstruction is directed toward restoring fluid and electrolyte balance and decompressing the dilated stomach. Obstruction related to edema and spasm generally responds to medical therapy. First, the stomach must be decompressed with nasogastric suction. Next, interventions are directed at correcting metabolic alkalosis and dehydration. The NGT is clamped after about 72 hours. Check the patient for retention of gastric contents. If the amount retained is not more than 50 mL in 30 minutes, the health care provider may allow oral fluids. In some cases, surgical intervention may be required to treat PUD.

Surgical Management. Evidence-based guidelines for the treatment of PUD that include *H. pylori* treatment and the development of nonsurgical means of controlling bleeding have led to a decline in the need for surgical intervention. In PUD, surgical intervention may be used to:

- Treat patients who do not respond to medical therapy or other nonsurgical procedures
- Treat a surgical emergency that develops as a complication of PUD, such as perforation

Two general surgical approaches are available for PUD—minimally invasive surgery and conventional open surgery.

Minimally invasive surgery (MIS) via laparoscopy (a type of endoscope) may be used to remove a chronic gastric ulcer or treat hemorrhage from perforation. Several small incisions allow access to the stomach and duodenum. The patient may have partial stomach removal (subtotal gastrectomy), pyloroplasty (to open the pylorus), and/or a vagotomy (vagus nerve cutting) to control acid secretion. Acid-reduction surgery may not be necessary due to the increased use of PPIs and endoscopic procedures in the treatment of PUD. The advantages of MIS over traditional open surgical procedures include a shorter hospital stay, fewer complications, less pain, and better, quicker recovery.

CLINICAL JUDGMENT CHALLENGE

Prioritization, Delegation, and Supervision

A 67-year-old man drove himself to the emergency department (ED) after vomiting bright red blood twice within 6 hours. He is alert and oriented and admits to having a few drinks last weekend. He takes some medicine for his stomach, but he cannot recall the name of the drug. He reports intermittent dizziness and fatigue over the past 2 days. His skin is dry and pale, and his abdomen is slightly distended. He reports pain (4/10) in the mid-epigastric area. His BP is 140/90, heart rate is 110/min, respirations are 24/min, and temperature is 98.9° F.

1. What actions are appropriate in the care of this patient in the ED? As the nurse in the ER, what additional questions will you ask his wife?
2. What data will you document?
3. Which task is most appropriate to assign to the nursing assistant working with you?
4. You are performing additional assessment and history on the patient. Which finding should you immediately report to the health care provider?
5. What medication is the physician most likely to prescribe for emergency treatment of acute and severe bleeding of the patient's ulcer?

Community-Based Care

Patients may be discharged from the hospital as long as there is no evidence of ongoing bleeding, orthostatic changes, or cardiopulmonary distress or compromise. Those discharged after treatment for peptic ulcer disease (PUD) and/or complications secondary to the disease must face several challenges to manage the disease successfully. Long-term adherence to drug therapy may require the patient to take several drugs each day. Permanent lifestyle alterations in nutrition habits must also be made.

Home Care Management. Most patients are discharged to the home to continue their recovery. Those who have had major surgery or have had complications, such as hemorrhage, may require one or two visits from a home care nurse to assess

CHART 55-5 Home Care Assessment

The Patient with Ulcer Disease

Assess gastrointestinal and cardiovascular status, including:
- Vital signs, including orthostatic vital signs
- Skin color
- Presence of abdominal pain (location, severity, character, duration, precipitating factors, and relief measures)
- Character, color, and consistency of stools
- Changes in bowel elimination pattern
- Hemoglobin and hematocrit
- Bowel sounds; palpate for areas of tenderness

Assess nutritional status, including:
- Dietary patterns and habits
- Intake of coffee and alcohol
- Relationship of food to symptoms

Assess medication history:
- Use of steroids
- Use of NSAIDs
- Use of over-the-counter medications

Assess patient's coping style:
- Recent stressors
- Past coping style

Assess patient's understanding of illness and ability to adhere to the therapeutic regimen:
- Symptoms to report to health care provider
- Expected and side effects of medications
- Food and drug interactions
- Need for smoking cessation

clinical progress, especially if the patient is an older adult (Chart 55-5).

Self-Management Education. The primary focus of home care preparation is patient and family teaching regarding risk factors for the recurrence of PUD. Teach them how to recognize new complications and what to do if they occur, especially abdominal pain; nausea and vomiting; black, tarry stools; and weakness or dizziness.

Teach the patient and family about risk factors for recurring peptic ulcers. Help them plan ways to make needed lifestyle changes. For postsurgical patients, especially those who have undergone partial stomach removal, smaller meals may be required. Other postoperative nutrition changes are described on p. 1142 in the discussion of Self-Management Education in the Gastric Cancer section.

! NURSING SAFETY PRIORITY QSEN

Action Alert

Teach the patient who has had surgery for PUD to avoid any OTC product containing aspirin or other NSAID. Emphasize the importance of following the treatment regimen for *H. pylori* infection and healing the ulcer. Emphasize the importance of keeping all follow-up appointments. Help the patient identify situations that cause stress, describe feelings during stressful situations, and develop a plan for coping with stressors.

Health Care Resources. If needed, refer the patient and family to the National Digestive Diseases Information Clearinghouse (www.digestive.niddk.nih.gov/). This group provides information and support to patients who have digestive disorders.

◆ *Evaluation: Outcomes*

Evaluate the care of the patient with peptic ulcer disease (PUD) based on the identified priority patient problems. The expected outcomes are that the patient:
- Does not have active PUD or associated complications
- Verbalizes PAIN relief or control
- Adheres to the drug regimen and lifestyle changes to prevent recurrence and heal the ulcer
- Does not experience an upper GI bleed; if bleeding occurs, it will be promptly and effectively managed

GASTRIC CANCER

Most cancers of the stomach are adenocarcinomas. This type of cancer develops in the mucosal cells that form the innermost lining of any portion or all of the stomach. *Often there are no symptoms in the early stages and the disease is advanced when detected.*

❖ *PATHOPHYSIOLOGY*

Gastric cancer usually begins in the glands of the stomach mucosa. Atrophic gastritis and intestinal metaplasia (abnormal tissue development) are precancerous conditions. Inadequate acid secretion in patients with atrophic gastritis creates an alkaline environment that allows bacteria (especially *H. pylori*) to multiply. This INFECTION causes mucosa-associated lymphoid tissue (MALT) lymphoma, which starts in the stomach (McCance et al., 2014).

Gastric cancers spread by direct extension through the gastric wall and into regional lymphatics, which carry tumor deposits to lymph nodes. Direct invasion of and adherence to adjacent organs (e.g., the liver, pancreas, and transverse colon) may also result. Hematogenous spread via the portal vein to the liver and via the systemic circulation to the lungs and bones is the most common mode of metastasis. Peritoneal seeding of cancer cells from the tumor areas to the omentum, peritoneum, ovary, and pelvic cul-de-sac can also occur.

In people with *advanced* gastric cancer, there is invasion of the muscularis (stomach muscle) or beyond. These lesions are not cured by surgical resection. The overall 5-year survival rate of people with stomach cancer in the United States is poor because most patients have no symptoms until the disease advances.

Etiology and Genetic Risk

INFECTION with *H. pylori* is the largest risk factor for gastric cancer because it carries the cytotoxin-associated gene A *(CagA)* gene. Patients with pernicious anemia, gastric polyps, chronic atrophic gastritis, and **achlorhydria** (absence of secretion of hydrochloric acid) are 2 to 3 times more likely to develop gastric cancer.

The disease also seems to be positively correlated with eating pickled foods, nitrates from processed foods, and salt added to food. The ingestion of these foods over a long period can lead to atrophic gastritis, a precancerous condition. A low intake of fruits and vegetables is also a risk factor for cancer (McCance et al., 2014).

Gastric surgery seems to increase the risk for gastric cancer because of the eventual development of atrophic gastritis, which results in changes to the mucosa. Patients with Barrett's esophagus from prolonged or severe gastroesophageal reflux disease (GERD) have an increased risk for cancer in the cardia (at the point where the stomach connects to the esophagus).

Incidence and Prevalence

Generally, stomach cancer rates are about twice as high in males as in females. Over 70% of new cases and gastric cancer deaths occur in developing countries (Jemal et al., 2011). The highest incidence rates are in Eastern Asia, Eastern Europe, and South America, and the lowest rates are in North America and parts of Africa (Jemal et al., 2011). The average age for developing gastric cancer is 70 years (American Cancer Society, 2014).

Nurses are uniquely positioned to improve gastric cancer survival rates by ensuring that patients with high risk and suspicious symptoms are assessed and diagnosed early (Bailey, 2011). Maintaining functional status and quality of life during gastric cancer care is a priority for nursing care.

Health Promotion and Maintenance

Teach patients with gastritis and/or *H. pylori* INFECTION to follow the treatment regimen to ensure that gastritis heals and *H. pylori* infection is eliminated. *Stress the need for eating a well-balanced diet and limiting pickled foods, salted foods, and processed foods to help prevent gastric cancer.*

❖ PATIENT-CENTERED COLLABORATIVE CARE

◆ Assessment

Question the patient about known risk factors for the development of gastric cancer. Ask about preferred foods, especially pickled, salted, or smoked foods. Inquire whether the patient has ever been diagnosed with or treated for *H. pylori* INFECTION, gastritis, or pernicious anemia. Note whether he or she has a history of gastric surgery or polyps. Also ask whether any of the patient's immediate relatives have gastric cancer.

Although patients with *early* gastric cancer may be asymptomatic, indigestion (heartburn) and abdominal discomfort are the *most* common symptoms (Chart 55-6). These symptoms are often ignored, however, or a change in diet or use of antacids relieves them. As the tumor grows, these symptoms become more severe and do not respond to nutrition changes or antacids. Epigastric or back PAIN is also an early symptom that may go unrecognized.

In *advanced* gastric cancer, progressive weight loss, nausea, and vomiting can occur. Vomiting represents pronounced dilation, thickening of the stomach wall, or pyloric obstruction. Obstructive symptoms appear earlier with tumors located near the pylorus than with those in the fundus. Patients with advanced disease may have weakness, fatigue, and anemia. Physical assessment findings in advanced disease may be absent, or a palpable epigastric mass may suggest hepatomegaly (liver enlargement) from metastatic disease. Hard, enlarged lymph nodes in the left supraclavicular chain, left axilla, or umbilicus result from metastasis from gastric cancer. Masses on the right suggest metastasis in the perigastric lymph nodes or liver.

CHART 55-6 Key Features

Early Versus Advanced Gastric Cancer

Early Gastric Cancer*	Advanced Gastric Cancer
• Indigestion • Abdominal discomfort initially relieved with antacids • Feeling of fullness • Epigastric, back, or retrosternal pain	• Nausea and vomiting • Obstructive symptoms • Iron deficiency anemia • Palpable epigastric mass • Enlarged lymph nodes • Weakness and fatigue • Progressive weight loss

*NOTE: Many patients with early gastric cancer have no clinical manifestations.

In patients with advanced disease, anemia is evidenced by *low hematocrit* and hemoglobin values. Patients may have macrocytic or microcytic anemia associated with decreased iron or vitamin B_{12} absorption. *The stool may be positive for occult blood. Hypoalbuminemia* and *abnormal results of liver tests* (e.g., bilirubin and alkaline phosphatase) occur with advanced disease and with hepatic metastasis. The level of carcinoembryonic antigen (CEA) is elevated in advanced cancer of the stomach (Pagana & Pagana, 2014).

The health care provider uses esophagogastroduodenoscopy (EGD) with biopsy for definitive diagnosis of gastric cancer. (See Chapter 52 for a discussion of nursing care associated with this diagnostic test.) The lesion can be viewed directly, and biopsies of all visible lesions can be obtained to determine the presence of cancer cells. During the endoscopy, an endoscopic (endoluminal) ultrasound (EUS) of the gastric mucosa can also be performed. This technology allows the health care provider to evaluate the depth of the tumor and the presence of lymph node involvement, which permits more accurate staging of the disease. CT, positron emission tomography (PET), and MRI scans of the chest, abdomen, and pelvis are used in determining the extent of the disease and planning therapy.

◆ Interventions

Management of gastric cancer includes drug therapy, radiation, and/or surgery. Drug therapy and radiation may be used instead of surgery or as an adjunct before and/or after surgery.

Nonsurgical Management. The treatment of gastric cancer depends highly on the stage of the disease. Radiation and chemotherapy commonly prolong survival of patients with advanced gastric disease.

Combination *chemotherapy* with multiple cycles of drugs such as cisplatin (Platinol) and epirubicin (Elience) before and after surgery may be given. Bone marrow suppression, nausea, and vomiting are common adverse drug effects. Chapter 22 discusses the general nursing care of patients receiving chemotherapy.

Although gastric cancers are somewhat sensitive to the effects of radiation, the use of this treatment is limited because the disease is often widely spread to other abdominal organs on diagnosis. Organs such as the liver, kidneys, and spinal cord can endure only a limited amount of radiation. Intraoperative radiotherapy (IORT) is available in large tertiary care health care systems. Radiation may be used for palliative management when surgery is not an option.

The most common side effects of radiation include impaired skin integrity, fatigue, and anorexia. Nausea, vomiting, and diarrhea may occur about 1 week after treatment is initiated and diminish a month or more after treatment ends. (See Chapter 22 for more information on radiation therapy.)

Surgical Management. *Surgical resection by removing the tumor is the preferred method for treating gastric cancer.* The primary surgical procedures for the treatment of gastric cancer are total gastrectomy and subtotal (partial) gastrectomy. In early stages, laparoscopic surgery (minimally invasive surgery [MIS]) plus adjuvant chemotherapy or radiation may be curative. Patients having MIS have less PAIN, shorter hospital stays, rare postoperative complications, and quicker recovery. However, MIS is seldom performed because very few patients are diagnosed in the early stage of the disease.

Most patients with advanced disease are candidates for palliative surgical treatment. Metastasis in the supraclavicular lymph nodes, inguinal lymph nodes, liver, umbilicus, or perirectal wall indicates that the opportunity for cure by resection has been lost. Palliative resection may significantly improve the quality of life for a patient suffering from obstruction, hemorrhage, or PAIN.

Preoperative Care. Before conventional open-approach surgery, a nasogastric tube (NGT) is often inserted and connected to suction to remove secretions and empty the stomach. This allows surgery to take place without contamination of the peritoneal cavity by gastric secretions. The NGT remains in place for a few days *postoperatively* to prevent the accumulation of secretions, which may lead to vomiting or GI distention and pressure on the incision. Patients having laparoscopic surgery (minimally invasive surgery [MIS]) do not require an NGT.

Because weight loss is problematic for patients with gastric cancer, NUTRITION therapy is a vital aspect of preoperative and postoperative management. Preoperatively, compression by the tumor can prevent adequate nutritional intake. To correct malnutrition before surgery, the health care provider may prescribe enteral supplements to the diet and/or total parenteral nutrition (TPN). Vitamin, mineral, iron, and protein supplements are essential to correct nutritional deficits.

Other preoperative nursing measures for the patient undergoing open gastric surgery are the same as those for any patient undergoing abdominal surgery and general anesthesia (see Chapter 14).

Operative Procedures. The surgeon usually removes part or all of the stomach to take out the tumor. When the tumor is located in the mid-portion or distal (lower) portion of the stomach, a subtotal (partial) gastrectomy is typically performed. The omentum, spleen, and relevant nodes are also removed. The surgery may be performed as an MIS procedure or as an open conventional surgical technique, with or without robotic assistance.

For the patient with a removable growth in the proximal (upper) third of the stomach, a total gastrectomy is performed (Fig. 55-4). In this procedure the surgeon removes the entire stomach along with the lymph nodes and omentum. The surgeon sutures the esophagus to the duodenum or jejunum to reestablish continuity of the GI tract. More radical surgery involving removal of the spleen and distal pancreas is controversial, although the Whipple procedure may be used to prolong life. However, the complications of this drastic surgery are very serious and common. For patients with advanced disease, total gastrectomy is performed only when gastric bleeding or obstruction is present.

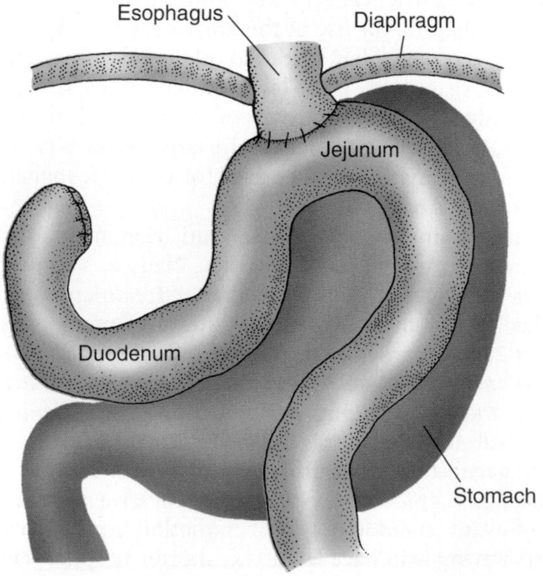

FIG. 55-4 Total gastrectomy with anastomosis of the esophagus to the jejunum (esophagojejunostomy) is the principal surgical intervention for extensive gastric cancer.

Patients with tumors at the gastric outlet who are not candidates for subtotal or total gastrectomy may undergo gastroenterostomy for palliation. The surgeon creates a passage between the body of the stomach and the small bowel, often the duodenum.

Postoperative Care. Provide the usual postoperative care for patients who have had general anesthesia to prevent atelectasis, paralytic ileus, wound infection, and peritonitis (see Chapter 16). Document and report any signs and symptoms of these complications immediately to the surgeon. Patients who have the laparoscopic surgery usually have less postoperative PAIN, fewer complications, and a shorter stay in the hospital.

Auscultate the lungs for adventitious sounds (crackles or reduced breath sounds), and monitor for the return of bowel sounds. Take vital signs as appropriate to detect signs of INFECTION or bleeding. Aggressive pulmonary exercises and early ambulation can help prevent respiratory complications and deep vein thrombosis. Also inspect the operative site every 8 to 12 hours for the presence of redness, swelling, or drainage, which indicates wound infection. Keep the head of the bed elevated to prevent aspiration from reflux.

Decreased patency caused by a clogged NGT can result in *acute gastric dilation* after surgery. This problem is manifested by epigastric PAIN and a feeling of fullness, hiccups, tachycardia, and hypotension. Irrigation or replacement of the NGT by request of the surgeon can relieve these symptoms.

Dumping syndrome is a term that refers to a group of vasomotor symptoms that occur after eating. This syndrome is believed to occur as a result of the rapid emptying of food contents into the small intestine, which shifts fluid into the gut, causing abdominal distention. Observe for *early* manifestations of this syndrome, which typically occur within 30 minutes of eating. Symptoms include vertigo, tachycardia, syncope, sweating, pallor, palpitations, and the desire to lie down. Report these manifestations to the surgeon, and encourage the patient to lie down. Monitor the patient for late symptoms.

Late dumping syndrome, which occurs 90 minutes to 3 hours after eating, is caused by a release of an excessive amount of insulin. The insulin release follows a rapid rise in the blood glucose level that results from the rapid entry of high-carbohydrate food into the jejunum. Observe for manifestations, including dizziness, light-headedness, palpitations, diaphoresis, and confusion.

Dumping syndrome is managed by nutrition changes that include decreasing the amount of food taken at one time and eliminating liquids ingested with meals. In collaboration with the dietitian, teach the patient to eat a high-protein, high-fat, low- to moderate-carbohydrate diet (Table 55-3). Acarbose may be used to decrease carbohydrate absorption. A somatostatin analog, octreotide (Sandostatin), 50 mcg subcutaneously 2 or 3 times daily 30 minutes before meals may be prescribed in severe cases. This drug decreases gastric and intestinal hormone secretion and slows stomach and intestinal transit time.

TABLE 55-3 **Diet for Dumping Syndrome**

FOOD GROUP	FOODS ALLOWED OR ENCOURAGED	FOODS TO USE WITH CAUTION	FOODS THAT MUST BE EXCLUDED
Soups		Fluids 1 hr before and after meals	Spicy soups
Meat and meat substitutes	8 oz or more per day: fish, poultry, beef, pork, veal, lamb, eggs, cheese, and peanut butter		Spicy meats or meat substitutes
Potatoes	Potato, rice, pasta, starchy vegetables (small amount)		Highly spiced potatoes or potato substitutes
Bread and cereal	White bread, rolls, muffins, crackers, and cereals (small amount)	Whole-grain bread, rolls, crackers, and cereals	Breads with frosting or jelly, sweet rolls, and coffee cake
Vegetables	Two or more cooked vegetables	Gas-producing vegetables, such as cabbage, onions, broccoli, or raw vegetables	
Fruits	Limit three per day: unsweetened cooked or canned fruits	Unsweetened juice or fruit drinks 30-45 min after meals; fresh fruit	Sweetened fruit or juice
Beverages	Dietetic drinks	Limit to 1 hr after meals; caffeine-containing beverages, such as coffee, tea, and cola; if tolerated, diet carbonated beverages	Milk shakes, malts, and other sweet drinks; regular carbonated beverages and alcohol
Fats	Margarine, oils, shortening, butter, bacon, and salad dressings	Mayonnaise	Any fats with milk products
Desserts	Fruit (see Fruits)	Sugar-free gelatin, pudding, and custard	All sweets, cakes, pies, cookies, candy, ice cream, and sherbet
Seasonings and miscellaneous	Diet jelly, diet syrups, sugar substitutes	Excessive amounts of salt	Excessive amounts of spices, sugar, jelly, honey, syrup, or molasses

General Principles

- Several small meals daily
- Relatively high fat and protein content
- Low roughage
- Relatively low carbohydrate content
- No milk, sweets, or sugars
- Liquid between meals *only*

Alkaline reflux gastropathy, also known as *bile reflux gastropathy,* is a complication of gastric surgery in which the pylorus is bypassed or removed. Endoscopic examination reveals regurgitated bile in the stomach and mucosal hyperemia. Symptoms include early satiety (satisfied quickly with little food), abdominal discomfort, and vomiting.

Delayed gastric emptying is often present after gastric surgery and usually resolves within 1 week. Edema at the anastomosis (surgical connection areas) or adhesions (scar tissue) obstructing the distal loop may cause mechanical blockage. Metabolic causes (e.g., hypokalemia, hypoproteinemia, or hyponatremia) should be considered. The edema is resolved with nasogastric suction, maintenance of fluid and electrolyte balance, and proper nutrition.

Several problems related to NUTRITION develop as a result of partial removal of the stomach, including deficiencies of vitamin B_{12}, folic acid, and iron; impaired calcium metabolism; and reduced absorption of calcium and vitamin D. These problems are caused by a reduction of intrinsic factor. The decrease results from the resection and from inadequate absorption because of rapid entry of food into the bowel. In the absence of intrinsic factor, clinical manifestations of pernicious anemia may occur. Assess for the development of atrophic glossitis secondary to vitamin B_{12} deficiency. In atrophic glossitis, the tongue takes on a shiny, smooth, and "beefy" appearance. The patient may also have signs of anemia secondary to folic acid and iron deficiency. Monitor the complete blood count (CBC) for signs of megaloblastic anemia (low red blood cell [RBC] level) and leukopenia (low white blood cell [WBC] level). These manifestations are corrected by the administration of vitamin B_{12}. The health care provider may also prescribe folic acid or iron preparations.

NCLEX EXAMINATION CHALLENGE

Physiological Integrity

A client has undergone a subtotal (partial) gastrectomy for gastric cancer and is scheduled to begin radiation therapy. What is the most important information for the nurse to include in the teaching plan for this client?

A. Management of alopecia
B. Medication management
C. Nutritional intake
D. Skin care

Community-Based Care

Patients who have undergone total gastrectomy and those who are debilitated with advanced gastric cancer are discharged to home with maximal assistance and support or to a transitional care unit or skilled nursing facility. Patients who have undergone subtotal gastrectomy and are not debilitated may be discharged to home with partial assistance for ADLs. Recurrence of cancer is common, and patients need regular follow-up examinations and imaging assessments. Collaborate with the case manager (CM) to ensure continuity of care and thorough follow-up with diagnostic testing.

Home Care Management. Gastric cancer is a life-threatening illness. Therefore the patient and family members require physical and emotional care. Assess their ability to cope with the disease and the possible need for end-of-life care. The adverse effects of gastric cancer treatment can be debilitating, and patients need to learn symptom management strategies. Hospice programs can help both the patient and the family cope with these physical and emotional needs.

Patients may fear returning home because of their inability for self-management. Enlisting family and health care resources for the patient may ease some of this anxiety. Provide the family with adequate information about community support systems to make the transition to home care easier. If the prognosis is poor, they need continued professional support from case managers, social workers, and/or nurses to cope with death and dying. (See Chapter 7 for a discussion of end-of-life care.)

Self-Management Education. Educate the patient and family about any continuing needs, drug therapy, and nutrition therapy. If patients are discharged to home with surgical dressings, teach the patient and family how to change them. Review the manifestations of incisional infection (e.g., fever, redness, and drainage) that they should report to their surgeon.

Patients who will be receiving radiation therapy or chemotherapy require instructions related to the side effects of these treatments. Nausea and vomiting are common side effects of chemotherapy, and instruction in the use of prescribed antiemetics may be needed. (See Chapter 22 for health teaching for patients receiving chemotherapy or radiation therapy.)

In collaboration with the dietitian, teach the patient and family about the type and quantity of foods that will provide optimal nutritional value. Interventions to minimize dumping syndrome and decrease gastric stimulants are also emphasized (see Table 55-3). Remind the patient to:

- Eat small, frequent meals
- Avoid drinking liquids with meals
- Avoid foods that cause discomfort
- Eliminate caffeine and alcohol consumption
- Begin a smoking-cessation program, if needed
- Receive B_{12} injections, as prescribed
- Lie flat after eating for a short time

Health Care Resources. A home care referral provides continued assessment, assistance, and encouragement to the patient and family. A home care nurse can help with care procedures and provide valuable psychological support. Additional referrals to a dietitian, professional counselor, or clergy/spiritual leader may be necessary. Referral to a hospice agency can be of great assistance for the patient with advanced disease. Hospice care may be delivered in the home or in an institutional setting. Appropriate support groups (e.g., I Can Cope, provided by the American Cancer Society [www.cancer.org/treatment/supportprogramsservices/i-can-cope]) can be a major resource.

NURSING CONCEPTS AND CLINICAL JUDGMENT REVIEW

What might you NOTICE if the patient is experiencing impaired digestion and NUTRITION as a result of a stomach disorder?

- Report of epigastric pain or indigestion before or after a meal
- Report of inability to tolerate certain foods
- Nausea and/or vomiting (with or without blood)
- Melena or frank blood in stools

What should you INTERPRET and how should you RESPOND to a patient experiencing impaired digestion and NUTRITION as a result of a stomach disorder?

Perform and interpret physical assessment, including:

- Taking vital signs
- Observing and documenting assessment findings
- Interpreting laboratory values and other diagnostic findings:
  - Presence of *H. pylori*
  - Decreased hemoglobin and hematocrit

Respond by:

- Maintaining airway, breathing, and circulation (ABCs)
- Placing the patient in a sitting position or on the left side to prevent aspiration if vomiting
- Preparing to assist with gastric lavage if hematemesis is present

On what should you REFLECT?

- Think about what else you could do to care for this patient.
- Consider with whom you should collaborate to improve or maintain digestion and nutrition for this patient.
- After patient interventions, monitor for changes in vital signs, hematocrit, and hemoglobin.

GET READY FOR THE NCLEX® EXAMINATION!

KEY POINTS

Review these Key Points for each NCLEX Examination Client Needs Category.

Safe and Effective Care Environment

- When caring for patients with gastric health problems, collaborate with the pharmacist, dietitian, health care provider, and/or case manager. **Teamwork and Collaboration** QSEN

Health Promotion and Maintenance

- Refer the patient to the American Cancer Society if gastric cancer is the diagnosis.
- Identify patients at risk for gastritis and PUD, especially older adults who take large amounts of NSAIDs and those with *H. pylori.* **Safety** QSEN
- Teach patients behaviors to prevent PUD, such as avoiding large consumption of caffeine, alcohol, coffee, aspirin, and other NSAIDs. Also teach them to avoid contaminated foods

and water and to avoid smoking (Chart 55-1). **Evidence-Based Practice** QSEN

- Teach patients the importance of adhering to *H. pylori* treatment to prevent the risk for gastric cancer.

Psychosocial Integrity

- Allow patients with gastric cancer to express feelings of grief, fear, and anxiety. **Patient-Centered Care** QSEN
- For patients with advanced gastric cancer, identify the need for end-of-life care, including referral to hospice care.

Physiological Integrity

- Recall that *acute* gastritis causes a rapid onset of epigastric PAIN and dyspepsia; *chronic* gastritis causes vague epigastric PAIN (usually relieved with food) and an intolerance to fatty and spicy foods (Chart 55-2).
- Be aware that assessment findings vary depending on whether the patient has a gastric or duodenal ulcer: patients with gastric ulcers may be malnourished and have PAIN that is worsened by ingestion of food; patients with duodenal ulcers are usually well nourished, have PAIN that is relieved by ingestion of food, and usually awaken with PAIN during the night (Table 55-2).
- For patients who have undergone a gastrectomy, collaborate with the dietitian and instruct the patient regarding diet changes to avoid abdominal distention and dumping syndrome. **Teamwork and Collaboration** QSEN
- Teach patients with abnormal symptoms (e.g., abdominal tenderness, abdominal PAIN that is relieved by food, or PAIN that becomes worse 3 hours after eating, dyspepsia, melena, and/or distention) to consult with their physician immediately for a prompt diagnosis and treatment.
- Teach patients that hematemesis is a medical emergency and that they should go to the emergency department for prompt treatment. **Safety** QSEN
- Teach the proper administration of antacids (one or two after meals). Tell patients that antacids can interfere with the effectiveness of certain drugs, such as phenytoin (Dilantin).
- Teach the proper administration of H_2 antagonists. Explain that they should be given at bedtime (Chart 55-3).
- Teach the proper administration of antisecretory agents, noting that most cannot be crushed because they are sustained-release or enteric-coated tablets.
- Monitor patients with ulcers for any of the signs and symptoms of upper GI bleeding that are listed in Chart 55-4. Report any of these symptoms if noted to a physician immediately.
- After an EGD, monitor the patient's vital signs, heart rhythm, and oxygen saturation frequently until they return to baseline. To prevent aspiration, assess the gag reflex and ensure that it is intact before giving the patient food or fluids. **Safety** QSEN
- Observe the patient for signs and symptoms of dumping syndrome after gastric surgery; teach the manifestations and management of this syndrome. Advise the patient to eat six small meals per day and to consume a diet high in protein and fat but low in carbohydrate-rich foods. Liquids should not be taken with meals. **Evidence-Based Practice** QSEN

56 CHAPTER

Care of Patients with Noninflammatory Intestinal Disorders

Donna D. Ignatavicius

http://evolve.elsevier.com/Iggy/

PRIORITY CONCEPTS

- Elimination
- Nutrition
- Pain
- Fluid and Electrolyte Balance

LEARNING OUTCOMES

Safe and Effective Care Environment

1. Prioritize nursing care for the patient with abdominal trauma.
2. Describe the importance of collaborating with health care team members to provide care for patients with colorectal cancer (CRC).

Health Promotion and Maintenance

3. Identify community-based resources for patients with CRC.
4. Teach people health promotion practices to prevent noninflammatory intestinal disorders.
5. Plan health teaching for patients to promote self-management when caring for a colostomy based on patient preferences and values.

Psychosocial Integrity

6. Assess patient and family response to a diagnosis of CRC.

Physiological Integrity

7. Develop a plan of care for a patient undergoing a minimally invasive inguinal hernia repair.
8. Interpret assessment findings for patients with CRC.
9. Explain the role of the nurse in managing the patient with CRC.
10. Develop an evidence-based perioperative plan of care for a patient undergoing a colon resection and colostomy.
11. Explain the differences between assessment findings associated with small-bowel and large-bowel obstructions.
12. Describe the postoperative care for a patient having a hemorrhoid surgical procedure.
13. Identify collaborative interventions for patients with malabsorption disorders.

Intestinal health problems may be inflammatory or noninflammatory. This chapter describes those disorders that are noninflammatory in origin. Noninflammatory intestinal problems often cause rectal bleeding, changing bowel patterns, and abdominal pain. If not diagnosed and managed early, some intestinal problems can lead to inadequate absorption of vital nutrients and therefore affect the need for NUTRITION and ELIMINATION. If these disorders become severe or progress, PAIN and problems with FLUID AND ELECTROLYTE BALANCE may occur.

IRRITABLE BOWEL SYNDROME

❖ PATHOPHYSIOLOGY

Irritable bowel syndrome (IBS) is a functional GI disorder that causes chronic or recurrent diarrhea, constipation, and/or abdominal pain and bloating. It is sometimes referred to as *spastic colon, mucous colon,* or *nervous colon* (Fig. 56-1). *IBS is the most common digestive disorder seen in clinical practice* and may affect as many as one in five people in the United States (McCance et al., 2014).

In patients with IBS, bowel motility changes and increased or decreased bowel transit times result in changes in the normal *bowel* ELIMINATION pattern to one of these classifications: diarrhea (IBS-D), constipation (IBS-C), alternating diarrhea and constipation (IBS-A), or a mix of diarrhea and constipation (IBS-M). Symptoms of the disease typically begin to appear in young adulthood and continue throughout the patient's life.

The etiology of IBS remains unclear. Research suggests that a combination of environmental, immunologic, genetic, hormonal, and stress factors play a role in the development and course of the disorder. Examples of environmental factors include foods and fluids like caffeinated or carbonated beverages and dairy products. Infectious agents have also been identified. Several studies have found that patients with IBS often have small-bowel bacterial overgrowth, which causes bloating and abdominal distention. Multiple normal flora and pathogenic agents have been identified, including *Pseudomonas*

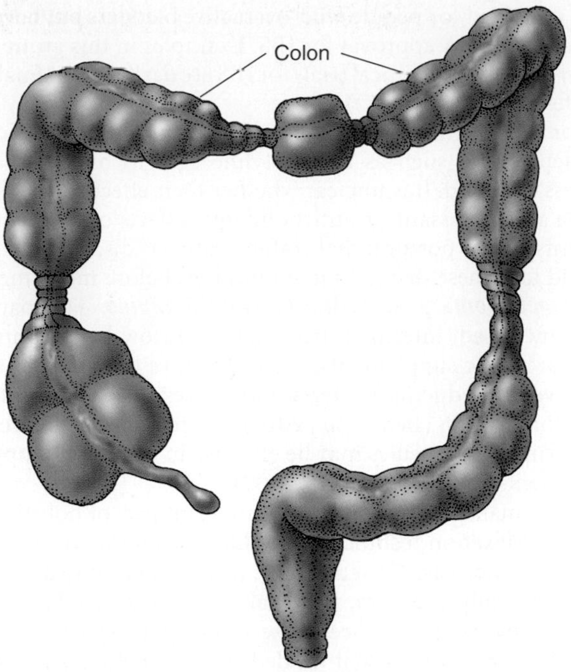

FIG. 56-1 Spastic contractions of the colon as they occur with irritable bowel syndrome.

aeruginosa (Kerckhoffs et al., 2011). Other researchers believe that these agents are less causative and serve as measurable biomarkers for the disease (Malinen et al., 2010).

Immunologic and genetic factors have also been associated with IBS, especially cytokine genes, including pro-inflammatory interleukins (IL), such as IL-6, and tumor necrosis factor (TNF)–alpha (Barkhordari et al., 2010). These findings may provide the basis of targeted drug therapy for the disease.

In the United States, women are 2 times more likely to have IBS than are men. This difference may be the result of hormonal differences. However, in other areas of the world, this distribution pattern may not occur. For example, researchers found that there is not a female predominance for the disease in Asian countries (Gwee et al., 2010).

Considerable evidence relates the role of stress and mental or behavioral illness, especially anxiety and depression, to IBS. Many patients diagnosed with IBS meet the criteria for at least one primary mental health disorder. Some researchers suggest that psychosocial problems may be a cause for IBS (Nicholl et al., 2008). However, the pain and other chronic symptoms of the disease may lead to secondary mental health disorders. For example, when diarrhea is predominant, patients fear that there will be no bathroom facilities available and can become very anxious. As a result, they may not want to leave their homes or travel on trips where bathrooms are not available at all times. The long-term nature of dealing with a chronic disease for which there is no cure can lead to secondary depression in some patients.

❖ PATIENT-CENTERED COLLABORATIVE CARE

◆ Assessment

Ask the patient about a history of weight change, fatigue, malaise, abdominal pain, changes in the bowel pattern (constipation, diarrhea, or an alternating pattern of both) or consistency of stools, and the passage of mucus. Patients with IBS do not usually lose weight. Ask whether the patient has had any GI infections. Collect information on all drugs the patient is taking, because some of them can cause symptoms similar to those of IBS. Ask about the NUTRITION history, including the use of caffeinated drinks or beverages sweetened with sorbitol or fructose, which can cause bloating or diarrhea.

The course of the illness is specific to each patient. Most patients can identify factors that cause exacerbations, such as diet, stress, or anxiety. Food intolerance may be associated with IBS. Dairy products (e.g., for those with lactose intolerance), raw fruits, and grains can contribute to bloating, **flatulence** (gas), and abdominal distention. Patients may keep a food diary to record possible triggers for IBS symptoms.

A flare-up of worsening cramps, abdominal pain, and diarrhea and/or constipation may bring the patient to the health care provider. One of the *most common concerns of patients with IBS is pain in the left lower quadrant of the abdomen.* Assess the location, intensity, and quality of the PAIN. Some patients have internal visceral (organ) hypersensitivity that can cause or contribute to the pain. Nausea may be associated with mealtime and defecation. The constipated stools are small and hard and are generally followed by several softer stools. The diarrheal stools are soft and watery, and mucus is often present in the stools. Patients with IBS often report belching, gas, anorexia, and bloating.

The patient generally appears well, with a stable weight, and nutritional and fluid status are within normal ranges. Inspect and auscultate the abdomen. Bowel sounds vary but are generally within normal range. With constipation, bowel sounds may be hypoactive; with severe diarrhea, they may be hyperactive.

Routine laboratory values (including a complete blood count [CBC], serum albumin, erythrocyte sedimentation rate [ESR], and stools for occult blood) are normal in IBS. Some health care providers request a *hydrogen breath test* (Lindberg, 2009). When small-intestinal bacterial overgrowth or malabsorption of nutrients is present, excess hydrogen is produced. Some of this hydrogen is absorbed into the bloodstream and travels to the lungs where it is exhaled. Patients with IBS often exhale an increased amount of hydrogen.

Teach the patient that he or she will need to be NPO (may have water) for at least 12 hours before the hydrogen breath test. At the beginning of the test, the patient blows into a hydrogen analyzer. Then, small amounts of test sugar are ingested, depending on the purpose of the test, and additional breath samples are taken every 15 minutes for 1 hour or longer (Pagana & Pagana, 2014).

◆ Interventions

The patient with IBS is usually managed on an ambulatory care basis and learns self-management strategies. Interventions include health teaching, drug therapy, and stress reduction. Some patients also use complementary and alternative therapies. A holistic approach to patient care is essential for positive outcomes (Bengtsson et al., 2010).

Dietary fiber and bulk help produce bulky, soft stools and establish regular bowel ELIMINATION habits. The patient should ingest about 30 to 40 g of fiber each day. Eating regular meals, drinking 8 to 10 cups of liquid each day, and chewing food slowly help promote normal bowel function.

Drug therapy depends on the main symptom of IBS. The health care provider may prescribe bulk-forming or antidiarrheal agents and/or newer drugs to control symptoms.

For the treatment of *constipation-predominant IBS (IBS-C)*, bulk-forming laxatives, such as *psyllium* hydrophilic mucilloid (Metamucil), are generally taken at mealtimes with a glass of water. The hydrophilic properties of these drugs help prevent dry, hard, or liquid stools. *Lubiprostone* (Amitiza) is an oral laxative approved for women with IBS-C, which increases fluid in the intestines to promote bowel ELIMINATION. Teach the patient to take the drug with food and water. Linaclotide (Linzess) is the newest drug for IBS-C, which works by simulating receptors in the intestines to increase fluid and promote bowel transit time. The drug also helps relieve PAIN and cramping that are associated with IBS. Teach patients to take this drug once a day about 30 minutes before breakfast.

Diarrhea-predominant IBS (IBS-D) may be treated with antidiarrheal agents, such as loperamide (Imodium), and psyllium (a bulk-forming agent). *Alosetron* (Lotronex), a selective serotonin (5-HT3) receptor antagonist, may be used with caution in women with IBS-D as a last resort when they have not responded to conventional therapy. Patients taking this drug must agree to report symptoms of colitis or constipation early because it is associated with potentially life-threatening bowel complications, including ischemic colitis (lack of blood flow to the colon).

! NURSING SAFETY PRIORITY QSEN

Drug Alert

Before the patient begins alosetron, take a thorough drug (including herbs) history, both prescribed and over the counter, because it interacts with many drugs in a variety of classes. Remind patients that they should not take psychoactive drugs and antihistamines while taking alosetron. Teach patients to report severe constipation, fever, increasing abdominal pain, increasing fatigue, darkened urine, bloody diarrhea, or rectal bleeding as soon as it occurs and stop the drug immediately (Lilley et al., 2014).

Many patients with IBS who have bloating and abdominal distention without constipation have success with *rifaximin* (Xifaxan), an antibiotic that works locally with little systemic absorption (Pimental et al., 2011). Although the drug has been approved for "traveler's diarrhea" and other illnesses, the U.S. Food and Drug Administration (FDA) has not yet approved its use for patients with IBS.

A newer group of drugs called *muscarinic-receptor antagonists* also inhibit intestinal motility. Some of these agents have been approved for people with overactive bladders but have not yet received FDA approval for IBS. Examples in this group currently undergoing clinical trials for IBS are darifenacin (Enablex) and fesoterodine (Toviaz).

For IBS in which PAIN is the predominant symptom, tricyclic antidepressants such as amitriptyline (Elavil) have also been successfully used. It is unclear whether their effectiveness is due to the antidepressant or anticholinergic effects of the drugs. If patients have postprandial (after eating) discomfort, they should take these drugs 30 to 45 minutes before mealtime.

Complementary and Alternative Therapies. For patients with increased intestinal bacterial overgrowth, recommend daily probiotic supplements. *Probiotics* have been shown to be effective for reducing bacteria and successfully alleviating GI symptoms of IBS (Lyra et al., 2010). There is also evidence that peppermint oil capsules may be effective in reducing symptoms for patients with IBS (Pirotta, 2009).

Stress management is also an important part of holistic care. Suggest relaxation techniques, meditation, and/or yoga to help the patient decrease GI symptoms. If the patient is in a stressful work or family situation, personal counseling may be helpful. Based on patient preference, make appropriate referrals or assist in making appointments if needed. The opportunity to discuss problems and attempt creative problem solving is often helpful. Teach the patient that regular exercise is important for managing stress and promoting regular bowel ELIMINATION.

HERNIATION

❖ *PATHOPHYSIOLOGY*

A **hernia** is a weakness in the abdominal muscle wall through which a segment of the bowel or other abdominal structure protrudes. Hernias can also penetrate through any other defect in the abdominal wall, through the diaphragm, or through other structures in the abdominal cavity.

The most important elements in the development of a hernia are congenital or acquired muscle weakness and increased intra-abdominal pressure. The most significant factors contributing to increased intra-abdominal pressure are obesity, pregnancy, and lifting heavy objects.

The most common types of abdominal hernias (Fig. 56-2) are indirect, direct, femoral, umbilical, and incisional (McCance et al., 2014).

- An **indirect inguinal hernia** is a sac formed from the peritoneum that contains a portion of the intestine or

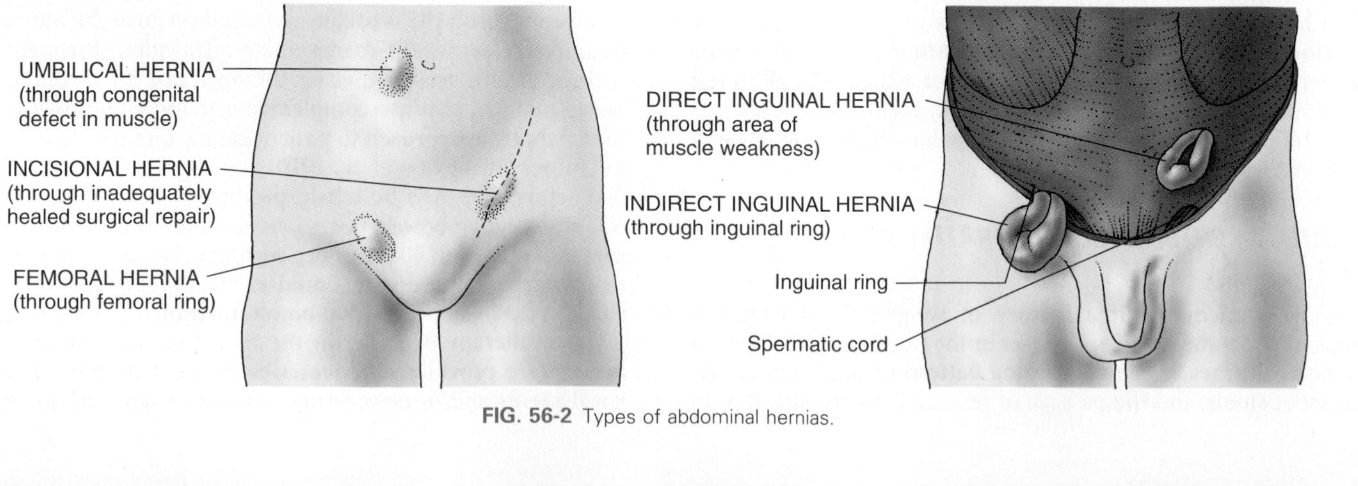

FIG. 56-2 Types of abdominal hernias.

omentum. The hernia pushes downward at an angle into the inguinal canal. In males, indirect inguinal hernias can become large and often descend into the scrotum.
- **Direct inguinal hernias**, in contrast, pass through a weak point in the abdominal wall.
- **Femoral hernias** protrude through the femoral ring. A plug of fat in the femoral canal enlarges and eventually pulls the peritoneum and often the urinary bladder into the sac.
- **Umbilical hernias** are congenital or acquired. Congenital umbilical hernias appear in infancy. Acquired umbilical hernias directly result from increased intra-abdominal pressure. They are most commonly seen in people who are obese.
- **Incisional**, or **ventral, hernias** occur at the site of a previous surgical incision. These hernias result from inadequate healing of the incision, which is usually caused by postoperative wound infections, inadequate nutrition, and obesity.

Hernias may also be classified as reducible, irreducible (incarcerated), or strangulated. A hernia is **reducible** when the contents of the hernial sac can be placed back into the abdominal cavity by gentle pressure. An **irreducible** (incarcerated) hernia cannot be reduced or placed back into the abdominal cavity. *Any hernia that is not reducible requires immediate surgical evaluation.*

A hernia is **strangulated** when the blood supply to the herniated segment of the bowel is cut off by pressure from the hernial ring (the band of muscle around the hernia). If a hernia is strangulated, there is ischemia and obstruction of the bowel loop. *This can lead to necrosis of the bowel and possibly bowel perforation. Signs of strangulation are abdominal distention, nausea, vomiting, pain, fever, and tachycardia.*

Indirect inguinal hernias, the most common type, occur mostly in men because they follow the tract that develops when the testes descend into the scrotum before birth. Direct hernias occur more often in older adults. Femoral and adult umbilical hernias are most common in obese or pregnant women. Incisional hernias can occur in people who have undergone abdominal surgery.

❖ PATIENT-CENTERED COLLABORATIVE CARE

◆ Assessment

The patient with a hernia typically comes to the health care provider's office, clinic, or the emergency department with a report of a "lump" or protrusion felt at the involved site. The development of the hernia may be associated with straining or lifting.

Perform an abdominal assessment inspecting the abdomen when the patient is lying and again when he or she is standing. If the hernia is reducible, it may disappear when the patient is lying flat. The advanced practice nurse or other health care provider asks the patient to strain or perform the Valsalva maneuver and observes for bulging. Auscultate for active bowel sounds. *Absent bowel sounds may indicate obstruction and strangulation, which is a medical emergency!*

To palpate an inguinal hernia, the health care provider gently examines the ring and its contents by inserting a finger in the ring and noting any changes when the patient coughs. *The hernia is never forcibly reduced; that maneuver could cause strangulated intestine to rupture.*

If a male patient suspects a hernia in his groin, the health care provider has him stand for the examination. Using the right hand for the patient's right side and the left hand for the patient's left side, the examiner pushes in the loose scrotal skin with the index finger, following the spermatic cord upward to the external inguinal cord. At this point, the patient is asked to cough and any palpable herniation is noted.

◆ Interventions

The type of treatment selected depends on patient factors such as age, as well as the type and severity of the hernia.

Nonsurgical Management. If the patient is not a surgical candidate (often an older man with multiple health problems), the health care provider may prescribe a truss for an inguinal hernia, usually for men. A **truss** is a pad made with firm material. It is held in place over the hernia with a belt to help keep the abdominal contents from protruding into the hernial sac. If a truss is used, it is applied only after the physician has reduced the hernia if it is not incarcerated. The patient usually applies the truss upon awakening. Teach him to assess the skin under the truss daily and to protect it with a light layer of powder.

Surgical Management. Most hernias are inguinal, and surgical repair is the treatment of choice. Surgery is usually performed on an ambulatory care basis for patients who have no pre-existing health conditions that would complicate the operative course. In same-day surgery centers, anesthesia may be regional or general and the procedure is typically laparoscopic. More extensive surgery, such as a bowel resection or temporary colostomy, may be necessary if strangulation results in a gangrenous section of bowel. Patients undergoing this extensive surgery are hospitalized for a longer period.

A **minimally invasive inguinal hernia repair** (MIIHR) through a laparoscope, also called **herniorrhaphy**, is the surgery of choice. A conventional open herniorrhaphy may be performed when laparoscopy is not appropriate. Patients having minimally invasive surgery (MIS) recover more quickly, have less PAIN, and develop fewer postoperative complications compared with those having the conventional surgery.

In addition to patient education about the procedure, the most important preoperative preparation is to teach the patient to remain NPO for the number of hours before surgery that the surgeon specifies. If same-day surgery is planned, remind the patient to arrange for someone to take him or her home and be available for the rest of the day at home. For patients having an open surgical approach, provide general preoperative care as described in Chapter 14.

During an MIIHR, the surgeon makes several small incisions, identifies the defect, and places the intestinal contents back into the abdomen. During a traditional herniorrhaphy, the surgeon makes an abdominal incision to perform this procedure. When a **hernioplasty** is also performed, the surgeon reinforces the weakened outside abdominal muscle wall with a mesh patch.

The patient who has had MIIHR is discharged from the surgical center in 3 to 5 hours, depending on recovery from anesthesia. Teach him or her to avoid strenuous activity for several days before returning to work and a normal routine. A stool softener may be needed to prevent constipation. Caution patients who are taking oral opioids for pain management to not drive or operate heavy machinery. Teach them to observe incisions for redness, swelling, heat, drainage, and increased pain and promptly report their occurrence to the surgeon. Remind patients that soreness and discomfort rather than severe, acute pain are common after MIS. Be sure to make a follow-up telephone call on the day after surgery to check on the patient's status.

General postoperative care of patients having a hernia repair is the same as that described in Chapter 16 *except that they should avoid coughing.* To promote lung expansion, encourage deep breathing and ambulation. With repair of an indirect inguinal hernia, the physician may suggest a scrotal support and ice bags applied to the scrotum to prevent swelling, which often contributes to pain. Elevation of the scrotum with a soft pillow helps prevent and control swelling.

In the immediate postoperative period, male patients who have had an inguinal hernia repair may experience difficulty voiding. Encourage them to stand to allow a more natural position for gravity to facilitate voiding and bladder emptying. Urine output of less than 30 mL per hour should be reported to the surgeon. Techniques to stimulate voiding such as allowing water to run may also be used. A fluid intake of at least 1500 to 2500 mL daily prevents dehydration, maintains urinary function, and minimizes constipation. A "straight" or intermittent ("in and out") catheterization is required if the patient cannot void. Chart 56-1 summarizes best nursing practices for postoperative care after an MIIHR.

Most patients have uneventful recoveries after a hernia repair. Surgeons generally allow them to return to their usual activities after surgery, with avoidance of straining and lifting for several weeks while subcutaneous tissues heal and strengthen.

Provide oral instructions and a written list of symptoms to be reported, including fever, chills, wound drainage, redness or separation of the incision, and increasing incisional pain. Teach the patient to keep the wound dry and clean with antibacterial soap and water. Showering is usually permitted in a few days (see Chart 56-1).

CHART 56-1 Best Practice for Patient Safety & Quality Care QSEN

Nursing Care of the Postoperative Patient Having a Minimally Invasive Inguinal Hernia Repair (MIIHR)

- Monitor vital signs, especially blood pressure, for indications of internal bleeding.
- Assess and manage incisional pain with oral analgesics; report and document severe pain that does not respond to drug therapy immediately.
- Encourage deep breathing after surgery; avoid excessive coughing.
- Encourage ambulation with assistance as soon as possible after surgery (within the first few hours).
- Apply ice packs as prescribed to the surgical area.
- Assist the patient to void by standing the first time after surgery.
- Teach patients at discharge to:
  - Rest for several days after surgery.
  - Observe the incision sites for redness or drainage, and report these findings to the surgeon.
  - Shower after 24 to 36 hours after removing any bandage (do not remove Steri-Strips); be aware that the Steri-Strips will fall off in about a week.
  - Monitor temperature for the first few days, and report the occurrence of a fever.
  - Do not lift more than 10 pounds until allowed by the surgeon.
  - Avoid constipation by eating high-fiber foods and drinking extra fluids.
  - Return to work when allowed by the surgeon, usually in 1 to 2 weeks, depending on the patient's work responsibilities.

NCLEX EXAMINATION CHALLENGE

Physiological Integrity

A nurse is caring for a client following a laparoscopic hernia repair surgery. Which assessment finding will the nurse report to the surgeon immediately?

A. Severe abdominal pain
B. Blood pressure of 140/86 mm Hg
C. Respiratory rate of 26 breaths per minute
D. Mild abdominal distention

COLORECTAL CANCER

PATHOPHYSIOLOGY

Colorectal refers to the colon and rectum, which together make up the large intestine, also known as the *large bowel.* Colorectal cancer (CRC) is cancer of the colon or rectum and is a major health problem worldwide. In the United States it is one of the most common malignancies. Patients often consider a diagnosis of cancer as a "death sentence," but colon cancer for many patients is highly curable.

Tumors occur in different areas of the colon, with about two thirds occurring within the rectosigmoid region as shown in Fig. 56-3. Most CRCs are **adenocarcinomas,** which are tumors that arise from the glandular epithelial tissue of the colon. They develop as a multi-step process affecting immunity, resulting in a number of molecular changes. These changes include loss of key tumor suppressor genes and activation of certain oncogenes that alter colonic mucosa cell division. The increased proliferation of the colonic mucosa forms polyps that can transform into malignant tumors. Most CRCs are believed to arise from adenomatous polyps that present as visible protrusions from the mucosal surface of the bowel (McCance et al., 2014).

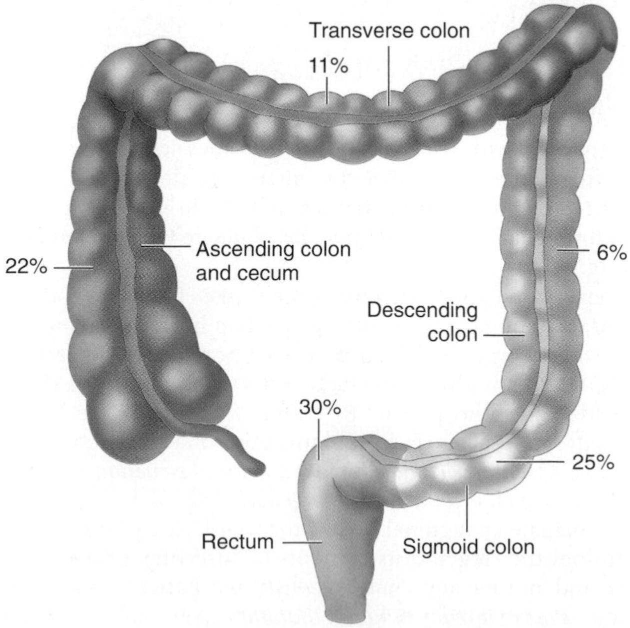

FIG. 56-3 The incidence of cancer in relation to colorectal anatomy.

CRC can metastasize by direct extension or by spreading through the blood or lymph. The tumor may spread locally into the four layers of the bowel wall and into neighboring organs. It may enlarge into the lumen of the bowel or spread through the lymphatics or the circulatory system. The circulatory system is entered directly from the primary tumor through blood vessels in the bowel or via the lymphatic system. The liver is the most common site of metastasis from circulatory spread. Metastasis to the lungs, brain, bones, and adrenal glands may also occur. Colon tumors can also spread by peritoneal seeding during surgical resection of the tumor. Seeding may occur when a tumor is excised and cancer cells break off from the tumor into the peritoneal cavity. For this reason, special techniques are used during surgery to decrease this possibility.

Complications related to the increasing growth of the tumor locally or through metastatic spread include bowel obstruction or perforation with resultant peritonitis, abscess formation, and fistula formation to the urinary bladder or the vagina. The tumor may invade neighboring blood vessels and cause frank bleeding. Tumors growing into the bowel lumen can gradually obstruct the intestine and eventually block it completely. Those extending beyond the bowel wall may place pressure on neighboring organs (uterus, urinary bladder, and ureters) and cause symptoms that mask those of the cancer. Chapter 21 discusses cancer pathophysiology in more detail.

Etiology and Genetic Risk

The major risk factors for the development of colorectal cancer (CRC) include being older than 50 years, genetic predisposition, personal or family history of cancer, and/or diseases that predispose the patient to cancer such as familial adenomatous polyposis (FAP), Crohn's disease, and ulcerative colitis (McCance et al., 2014). Only a small percentage of colorectal cancers are familial and transmitted genetically.

GENETIC/GENOMIC CONSIDERATIONS

Patient-Centered Care QSEN

People with a first-degree relative (parent, sibling, or child) diagnosed with colorectal cancer (CRC) have 3 to 4 times the risk for developing the disease. An autosomal dominant inherited genetic disorder known as *familial adenomatous polyposis (FAP)* accounts for 1% of CRCs. FAP is the result of one or more mutations in the adenomatous polyposis coli (APC) gene (McCance et al., 2014). In these very young patients, thousands of adenomatous polyps develop over the course of 10 to 15 years and have nearly a 100% chance of becoming malignant. By 20 years of age, most patients require surgical intervention, usually a colectomy with ileostomy or ileoanal pull-through, to prevent cancer. Chemotherapy may also be used for cancer prevention.

Hereditary nonpolyposis colorectal cancer (HNPCC) is another autosomal dominant disorder and accounts for a small percentage of all colorectal cancers. HNPCC is also caused by gene mutations, including *MLH1* and *MLH2*. People with these mutations have an 80% chance of developing CRC at an average of 45 years of age. They also tend to have a higher incidence of endometrial, ovarian, stomach, and ureteral cancers (Nussbaum et al., 2007). Genetic testing is available for both of these familial CRC syndromes. Refer patients for genetic counseling and possible testing if the patient prefers.

The role of infectious agents in the development of colorectal and anal cancer continues to be investigated. Some lower GI cancers are related to *Helicobacter pylori, Streptococcus bovis,* John Cunningham (JC) virus, and human papilloma virus (HPV) infections.

There is also strong evidence that long-term smoking, obesity, physical inactivity, and heavy alcohol consumption are risk factors for colorectal cancer (American Cancer Society [ACS], 2014). A high-fat diet, particularly animal fat from red meats, increases bile acid secretion and anaerobic bacteria, which are thought to be carcinogenic within the bowel. Diets with large amounts of refined carbohydrates that lack fiber decrease bowel transit time.

Incidence and Prevalence

Colorectal cancer (CRC) is the third most common cause of cancer death in the United States (ACS, 2014). It is not common before 40 years of age, but the incidence in younger adults is slowly increasing, most likely due to increases in HPV infections (Stubenrauch, 2010). The overall incidence of CRC has decreased over the past 20 years, probably as a result of increased cancer screenings (Wilkes, 2013). The disease is most common in African Americans, and their survival rate is lower than that of Euro-Americans (Caucasians). The possible reasons for this difference include less use of diagnostic testing (especially colonoscopy), decreased access to health care, lack of health insurance, cultural beliefs, and lack of education about the need for early cancer detection (Good et al., 2010; Oliver et al., 2012).

Health Promotion and Maintenance

People at risk can take action to decrease their chance of getting CRC and/or increase their chance of surviving it. For example, those whose family members have had hereditary CRC should be genetically tested for FAP and HNPCC. If gene mutations are present, the person at risk can collaborate with the health care team to decide what prevention or treatment plan to implement.

Teach people about the need for diagnostic screening. An integrative review by Rawl et al. (2012) found that most efforts to increase CRC screening interventions have focused on Euro-Americans. However, other groups are more at risk than Euro-Americans (see the Evidence-Based Practice box).

When an adult turns 40 years of age, he or she should discuss with the health care provider the need for colon cancer screening. The interval depends on level of risk. People of average risk who are 50 years of age and older and without a family history should undergo regular CRC screening. The screening includes fecal occult blood testing (FOBT) and colonoscopy every 10 years or double-contrast barium enema every 5 years. People who have a personal or family history of the disease should begin screening earlier and more frequently. Teach all patients to follow the American Cancer Society recommendations for CRC screening listed in Chart 56-2.

Teach people, regardless of risk, to modify their diets as needed to decrease fat, refined carbohydrates, and low-fiber foods. Encourage baked or broiled foods, especially those high in fiber and low in animal fat. Remind people to eat increased amounts of brassica vegetables, including broccoli, cabbage, cauliflower, and sprouts. These foods help protect the intestinal mucosa from colon cancer (ACS, 2014).

Teach people the hazards of smoking, excessive alcohol, and physical inactivity. Refer patients as needed for smoking- or alcohol-cessation programs, and recommend ways to increase regular physical exercise. These programs are discussed elsewhere in this text.

CHART 56-2 Best Practice for Patient Safety & Quality Care QSEN

Screening Recommendations for Men and Women Ages 50 Years and Older at Average Risk for Colorectal Cancer

PROCEDURE: CHOICE OF ONE OF THE FOLLOWING	INTERVAL AFTER SCREENING INITIATED AT AGE 50 YEARS	COMMENTS
FOBT and sigmoidoscopy	Every 5 years	FOBT procedure: two or three samples from three consecutive bowel movements obtained at home; tested by physician or nurse
OR		
Double-contrast barium enema	Every 5 years	
OR		
Colonoscopy	Every 10 years	

FOBT, Fecal occult blood testing.

EVIDENCE-BASED PRACTICE QSEN

How Effective are Interventions to Promote Colorectal Cancer Screening?

Rawl, S.M., Menon, U., Burness, A., & Breslau, E.S. (2012). Interventions to promote colorectal cancer screening: An integrative review. *Nursing Outlook, 60*(4), 172-181.

The researchers reviewed and evaluated 33 randomized trials of colorectal cancer screening (CRC) interventions that were published between 1997 and 2007 using a modified version of TREND criteria to draw conclusions. Significant effects of interventions were reported in 6 of the 10 trials that studied fecal occult blood testing, 4 of the 7 trials that focused on colonoscopy or sigmoidoscopy interventions, and 9 of the 16 trials that included any type of recommended CRC screening method. Most of these trials studied effectiveness of interventions in Euro-Americans (Caucasians). The authors concluded that further research is needed to examine factors that contribute to successful CRC screening. Other groups in addition to Euro-Americans should also be studied, especially given their risk for the disease.

Level of Evidence: 1

This study was an integrative review and evaluation of multiple randomized trials.

Commentary: Implications for Practice and Research

Nurses should continue to teach people about the need for and effectiveness of screening to detect CRC early for the best possible outcome. Further research is needed to explore the factors that enable many patients to have regular screening for CRC. This research should include diverse subjects for comparison and analysis.

❖ *PATIENT-CENTERED COLLABORATIVE CARE*

◆ *Assessment*

History. When taking a history, ask the patient about major risk factors, such as a personal history of breast, ovarian, or endometrial cancer (which can spread to the colon); ulcerative colitis; Crohn's disease; familial polyposis or adenomas; polyps; or a family history of CRC. Also assess the patient's participation in age-specific cancer screening guidelines. Ask about whether the patient uses tobacco and/or alcohol. Assess the patient's usual physical activity level.

Ask whether vomiting and changes in bowel ELIMINATION habits, such as constipation or change in shape of stool with or without blood, have been noted. The patient may also report fatigue (related to anemias), abdominal fullness, vague abdominal PAIN, or unintentional weight loss. These symptoms suggest advanced disease.

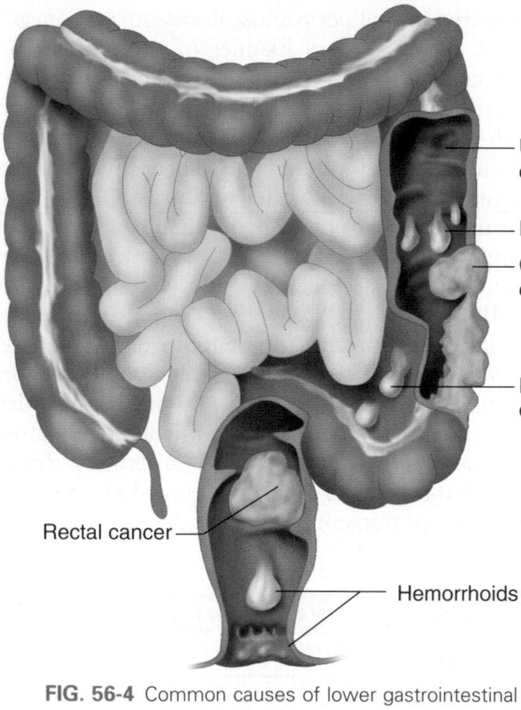

FIG. 56-4 Common causes of lower gastrointestinal bleeding.

Physical Assessment/Clinical Manifestations. The clinical manifestations of CRC depend on the location of the tumor. *However, the most common signs are rectal bleeding, anemia, and a change in stool consistency or shape.* Stools may contain microscopic amounts of blood that are not noticeably visible, or the patient may have mahogany (dark)-colored or bright red stools (Fig. 56-4). Gross blood is not usually detected with tumors of the right side of the colon but is common (but not massive) with tumors of the left side of the colon and the rectum.

Tumors in the transverse and descending colon result in symptoms of obstruction as growth of the tumor blocks the passage of stool. The patient may report "gas pains," cramping, or incomplete evacuation. Tumors in the rectosigmoid colon are associated with **hematochezia** (the passage of red blood via the rectum), straining to pass stools, and narrowing of stools. Patients may report dull pain. Right-sided tumors can grow quite large without disrupting bowel patterns or appearance because the stool consistency is more liquid in this part of the colon. These tumors ulcerate and bleed intermittently, so stools can contain mahogany (dark)-colored blood. A mass may be palpated in the lower right quadrant, and the patient often has anemia secondary to blood loss.

Examination of the abdomen begins with assessment for obvious distention or masses. Visible peristaltic waves accompanied by high-pitched or "tinkling" bowel sounds may indicate a partial bowel obstruction from the tumor. Total absence of bowel sounds indicates a complete bowel obstruction. Palpation and percussion are performed by the advanced practice nurse or other health care provider to determine whether the spleen or liver is enlarged or whether masses are present along the colon. The examiner may also perform a digital rectal examination to palpate the rectum and lower sigmoid colon for masses. Fecal occult blood screening should not be done with a specimen from a rectal examination because it is not reliable. A positive result could occur as a result of tissue trauma during the examination.

Psychosocial Assessment. The psychological consequences associated with a diagnosis of colorectal cancer (CRC) are many. Patients must cope with a diagnosis that instills fear and anxiety about treatment, feelings that life has been disrupted, a need to search for ways to deal with the diagnosis, and concern about family. They also have questions about why colon cancer affected them, as well as concerns about PAIN, possible body changes, and possible death. In addition, if the cancer is believed to have a genetic origin, there is anxiety concerning implications for immediate family members.

Laboratory Assessment. Hemoglobin and hematocrit values are often decreased as a result of the intermittent bleeding associated with the tumor. For some patients, that may be the first indication that a tumor is present. CRC that has metastasized to the liver causes liver enzymes to be elevated.

A positive test result for occult blood in the stool (**fecal occult blood test [FOBT]**) indicates bleeding in the GI tract. These tests can yield false-positive results if certain vitamins or drugs are taken before the test. Remind the patient to avoid aspirin, vitamin C, and red meat for 48 hours before giving a stool specimen. Also assess whether the patient is taking anti-inflammatory drugs (e.g., ibuprofen, corticosteroids, or salicylates). These drugs should be discontinued for a designated period before the test. Two or three separate stool samples should be tested on 3 consecutive days. Negative results do not completely rule out the possibility of CRC.

Carcinoembryonic antigen (CEA), an oncofetal antigen, is elevated in many people with CRC. The normal value is less than 5 ng/mL (Pagana & Pagana, 2014). This protein is not specifically associated with the colorectal cancer, and it may be elevated in the presence of other benign or malignant diseases and in smokers. CEA is often used to monitor the effectiveness of treatment and to identify disease recurrence.

Imaging Assessment. A *double-contrast barium enema* (air and barium are instilled into the colon) or colonoscopy provides better visualization of polyps and small lesions than does a barium enema alone. These tests may show an occlusion in the bowel where the tumor is decreasing the size of the lumen.

CT or *MRI* of the chest, abdomen, pelvis, lungs, or liver helps confirm the existence of a mass, the extent of disease, and the location of distant metastases. CT-guided virtual colonoscopy is growing in popularity and may be more thorough than traditional colonoscopy. However, treatments or surgeries cannot be performed when a virtual colonoscopy is used.

Other Diagnostic Assessment. A *sigmoidoscopy* provides visualization of the lower colon using a fiberoptic scope. Polyps can be visualized, and tissue samples can be taken for biopsy. Polyps are usually removed during the procedure. A *colonoscopy* provides views of the entire large bowel from the rectum to the ileocecal valve. As with sigmoidoscopy, polyps can be seen and removed and tissue samples can be taken for biopsy. *Colonoscopy is the definitive test for the diagnosis of colorectal cancer. These procedures and associated nursing care are discussed in Chapter 52.*

◆ Analysis

The priority NANDA-I nursing diagnoses and collaborative problems for patients with colorectal cancer (CRC) include:

1. Potential for colorectal cancer metastasis
2. Grieving related to cancer diagnosis (NANDA-I)

◆ Planning and Implementation

The primary approach to treating CRC is to remove the entire tumor or as much of the tumor as possible to prevent or slow metastatic spread of the disease. A patient-centered collaborative care approach is essential to meet the desired outcomes.

Preventing or Controlling Metastasis

Planning: Expected Outcomes. The patient with colorectal cancer (CRC) is expected to not have the cancer spread to vital organs. Thus the patient's life expectancy will be increased and the quality of life will be improved. However, if metastasis is present, the desired outcome is to ensure that the patient is as comfortable as possible and PAIN is well-managed.

Interventions. Although surgical resection is the primary method used to control the disease, several adjuvant (additional) therapies are used. Adjuvant therapies are administered before or after surgery to achieve a cure and prevent recurrence, if possible.

Nonsurgical Management. The type of therapy used is based on the pathologic staging of the disease. Several staging systems may be used.

The administration of preoperative *radiation therapy* has not improved overall survival rates for colon cancer, but it has been effective in providing local or regional control of the disease. Postoperative radiation has not demonstrated any consistent improvement in survival or recurrence. However, as a palliative measure, radiation therapy may be used to control PAIN, hemorrhage, bowel obstruction, or metastasis to the lung in advanced disease. For rectal cancer, unlike colon cancer, radiation therapy is almost always a part of the treatment plan. Reinforce information about the radiation therapy procedure to the patient and family, and monitor for possible side effects (e.g., diarrhea, fatigue). Chapter 22 describes the general nursing care of patients undergoing radiation therapy.

Adjuvant *chemotherapy* after primary surgery is recommended for patients with stage II or stage III disease to interrupt the DNA production of cells and destroy them. The drugs of choice are IV 5-fluorouracil (5-FU) with leucovorin (LV) (folinic acid) (5-FU/LV), capecitabine (Xeloda), or a combination of drugs referred to as *FOLFOX4.* The most frequently used FOLFOX4 combination for metastatic CRC is fluorouracil (5-FU), leucovorin (LV), and oxaliplatin (Eloxatin), a platinum analog. These drugs cannot discriminate between cancer and healthy cells. Therefore common side effects are diarrhea, mucositis, leukopenia, mouth ulcers, and peripheral neuropathy (Lilley et al., 2014).

Bevacizumab (Avastin) and panitumumab (Vectibix) are antiangiogenesis drugs, also known as *vascular endothelial growth factor (VEGF) inhibitors,* approved for advanced CRC. These drugs reduce blood flow to the growing tumor cells, thereby depriving them of necessary nutrients needed to grow (Wilkes, 2013). A VEGF inhibitor is usually given in combination with other chemotherapeutic agents.

Cetuximab (Erbitux), a monoclonal antibody known as an *epidermal growth factor receptor (EGFR) antagonist,* may also be given in combination with other drugs for advanced disease (Wilkes, 2013). This drug works by blocking factors that promote cancer cell growth.

Intrahepatic arterial chemotherapy, often with 5-FU, may be administered to patients with liver metastasis. Patients with CRC also receive drugs for relief of symptoms, such as opioid analgesics and antiemetics. Chapter 22 describes care of patients receiving chemotherapy in detail.

Surgical Management. Surgical removal of the tumor with margins free of disease is the best method of ensuring removal of CRC. The size of the tumor, its location, the extent of metastasis, the integrity of the bowel, and the condition of the patient determine which surgical procedure is performed for colorectal cancer (Table 56-1). Many regional lymph nodes are removed and examined for presence of cancer. The number of lymph nodes that contain cancer is a strong predictor of prognosis. The most common surgeries performed are **colon resection** (removal of the tumor and regional lymph nodes) with reanastomosis, **colectomy** (colon removal) with *colostomy (temporary or permanent) or ileostomy/ileoanal pull-through,* and **abdominoperineal (AP) resection**. A **colostomy** is the surgical creation of an opening of the colon onto the surface of the abdomen. An AP resection is performed when rectal tumors are present. The surgeon removes the sigmoid colon, rectum, and anus through combined abdominal and perineal incisions.

TABLE 56-1 Surgical Procedures for Colorectal Cancers in Various Locations

Right-Sided Colon Tumors
- Right hemicolectomy for smaller lesions
- Right ascending colostomy or ileostomy for large, widespread lesions
- Cecostomy (opening into the cecum with intubation to decompress the bowel)

Left-Sided Colon Tumors
- Left hemicolectomy for smaller lesions
- Left descending colostomy for larger lesions

Sigmoid Colon Tumors
- Sigmoid colectomy for smaller lesions
- Sigmoid colostomy for larger lesions
- Abdominoperineal resection for large, low sigmoid tumors (near the anus) with colostomy (the rectum and the anus are completely removed, leaving a perineal wound)

Rectal Tumors
- Resection with anastomosis or pull-through procedure (preserves anal sphincter and normal elimination pattern)
- Colon resection with permanent colostomy
- Abdominoperineal resection with colostomy

For patients having a colon resection, minimally invasive surgery (MIS) via laparoscopy is commonly performed today. This procedure results in shorter hospital stays, less pain, fewer complications, and quicker recovery compared with the conventional open surgical approach (Kapritsou et al., 2013).

Preoperative Care. Reinforce the physician's explanation of the planned surgical procedure. The patient is told as accurately as possible what anatomic and physiologic changes will occur with surgery. The location and number of incision sites and drains are also discussed.

Before evaluating the tumor and colon during surgery, the surgeon may not be able to determine whether a colostomy (or less commonly, an ileostomy) will be necessary. The patient is told that a colostomy is a possibility. If a colostomy is planned, the surgeon consults a certified wound, ostomy, continence nurse (CWOCN) to recommend optimal placement of the ostomy. The CWOCN teaches the patient about the rationale and general principles of ostomy care. In many settings, he or she marks the patient's abdomen to indicate a potential ostomy site that will decrease the risk for complications such as interference of the undergarments or a prosthesis with the ostomy appliance. Table 56-2 describes the role of the CWOCN.

The patient who requires low rectal surgery (e.g., AP resection) is faced with the risk for postoperative sexual dysfunction and urinary incontinence after surgery as a result of nerve damage during surgery. The surgeon discusses the risk for these problems with the patient before surgery and allows him or her to verbalize concerns and questions related to this risk. Reinforce teaching about abdominal surgery performed for the patient under general anesthesia, and review the routines for turning and deep breathing (see Chapter 14). Teach the patient about the method of PAIN management to be used after surgery such as IV patient-controlled analgesia (PCA), epidural analgesia, or other method.

If the bowel is not obstructed or perforated, elective surgery is planned. The patient may be instructed to thoroughly clean the bowel, or "bowel prep," to minimize bacterial growth and prevent complications. Mechanical cleaning is accomplished with laxatives and enemas or with "whole-gut lavage." The use of bowel preps is controversial, and some surgeons do not recommend it because of patient discomfort. Older adults may become dehydrated from this process.

TABLE 56-2 Preoperative Assessment by the CWOCN Prior to Ostomy Surgery

Key Points of Psychosocial Assessment
- Patient's and family's level of knowledge of disease and ostomy care
- Patient's educational level
- Patient's physical limitations (particularly sensory)
- Support available to patient
- Patient's type of employment
- Patient's involvement in activities such as hobbies
- Financial concerns regarding purchase of ostomy supplies

Key Points of Physical Assessment
- Before marking the placement for the ostomy, the nurse specialist considers:
  - Contour of the abdomen in lying, sitting, and standing positions
  - Presence of skinfolds, creases, bony prominences, and scars
  - Location of belt line
  - Location that is easily visible to the patient
  - Possible location in the rectus muscle

CWOCN, Certified wound, ostomy, continence nurse.

To reduce the risk for infection, the surgeon may prescribe one dose of oral or IV antibiotics to be given before the surgical incision is made. Teach patients that a nasogastric tube (NGT) may be placed for decompression of the stomach after surgery. A peripheral IV or central venous catheter is also placed for fluid and electrolyte replacement while the patient is NPO after surgery. Patients having minimally invasive surgeries do not need an NGT.

The patient with colorectal cancer faces a serious illness with long-term consequences of the disease and treatment. A case manager or social worker can be very helpful in identifying patient and family needs, as well as ensuring continuity of care and support.

Operative Procedures. For the conventional open surgical approach, the surgeon makes a large incision in the abdomen and explores the abdominal cavity to determine whether the tumor can be removed. For a colon resection, the portion of the colon with the tumor is excised and the two open ends of the bowel are irrigated before **anastomosis** (reattachment) of the colon. If an anastomosis is not feasible because of the location of the tumor or the bowel is inflamed, a colostomy is created.

A temporary or permanent colostomy may be created in the ascending, transverse, descending, or sigmoid colon (Fig. 56-5). One of several techniques is used to construct a colostomy. A loop **stoma** (surgical opening) is made by bringing a loop of colon to the skin surface, severing and everting the anterior wall, and suturing it to the abdominal wall. Loop colostomies are usually performed in the transverse colon and are usually temporary. An external rod may be used to support the loop until the intestinal tissue adheres to the abdominal wall. Care must be taken to avoid displacing the rod, especially during appliance changes.

An end stoma is often constructed, usually in the descending or sigmoid colon, when a colostomy is intended to be permanent. It may also be done when the surgeon oversews the distal stump of the colon and places it in the abdominal cavity, preserving it for future reattachment. An end stoma is constructed by severing the end of the proximal portion of the bowel and bringing it out through the abdominal wall.

The least common colostomy is the **double-barrel stoma**, which is created by dividing the bowel and bringing both the proximal and distal portions to the abdominal surface to create two stomas. The proximal stoma (closest to the patient's head) is the functioning stoma and eliminates stool. The distal stoma (farthest from the head) is considered nonfunctioning, although it may secrete some mucus. The distal stoma is sometimes referred to as a *mucous fistula.*

MIS colon resection or total colectomy allows complete tumor removal with an adequate surgical margin and removal of associated lymph nodes. Several small incisions are made, and a miniature video camera is placed within the abdomen to help see the area that is involved. This technique takes longer than the conventional procedure and requires specialized training. However, blood loss is less.

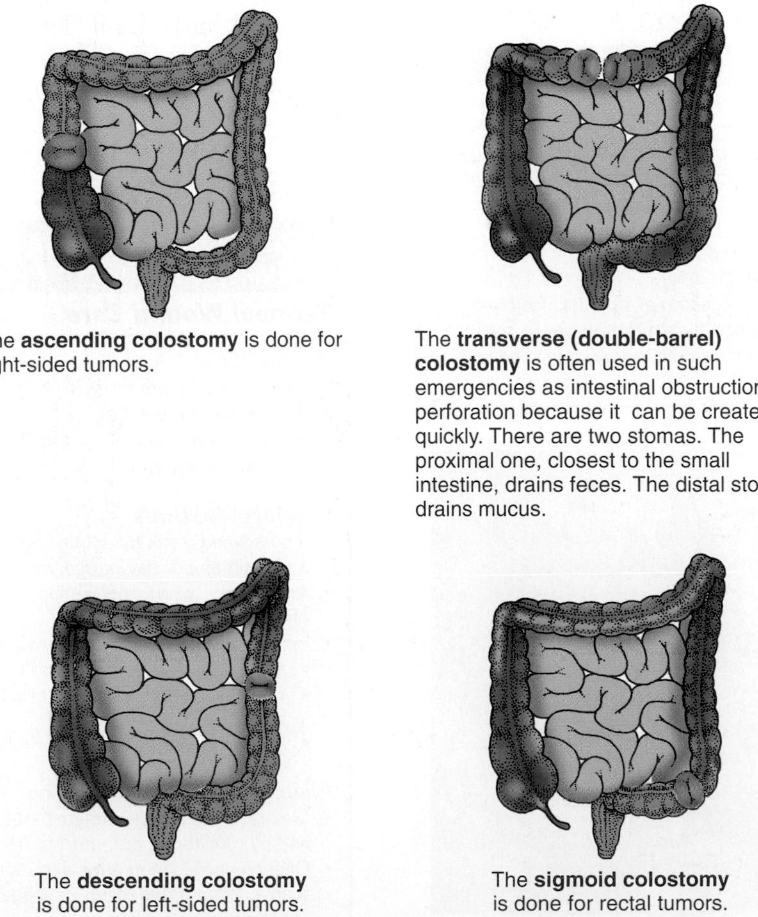

The **ascending colostomy** is done for right-sided tumors.

The **transverse (double-barrel) colostomy** is often used in such emergencies as intestinal obstruction or perforation because it can be created quickly. There are two stomas. The proximal one, closest to the small intestine, drains feces. The distal stoma drains mucus.

The **descending colostomy** is done for left-sided tumors.

The **sigmoid colostomy** is done for rectal tumors.

FIG. 56-5 Different locations of colostomies in the colon.

Postoperative Care. Patients who have an *open colon resection* without a colostomy receive care similar to that of those having any abdominal surgery (see Chapter 16). Other patients have surgeries that also require colostomy management. They typically have a nasogastric tube (NGT) after open surgery and receive IV PCA for the first 24 to 36 hours. After NGT removal, the diet is slowly progressed from liquids to solid foods as tolerated. The care of patients with an NGT is found on p. 1159 in the discussion of Interventions in the Intestinal Obstruction section.

By contrast, patients who have *laparoscopic (MIS) surgery* can eat solid foods very soon after the procedure. Because they usually have less PAIN, they are able to ambulate earlier than those who have the conventional approach. The hospital stay is usually shorter for the patient with MIS—less than 23 hours or 1 to 2 days, depending on the patient's age and general condition.

Colostomy Management. The patient who has a colostomy may return from surgery with a clear ostomy pouch system in place. A clear pouch allows the health care team to observe the stoma. If no pouch system is in place, a petrolatum gauze dressing is usually placed over the stoma to keep it moist. This is covered with a dry, sterile dressing. In collaboration with the CWOCN, place a pouch system as soon as possible. The colostomy pouch system, also called an *appliance,* allows more convenient and acceptable collection of stool than a dressing does.

Assess the color and integrity of the stoma frequently. A healthy stoma should be reddish pink and moist and protrude about ¾ inch (2 cm) from the abdominal wall (Fig. 56-6). During the initial postoperative period, the stoma may be slightly edematous. A small amount of bleeding at the stoma is common.

! NURSING SAFETY PRIORITY (QSEN)

Action Alert

Report any of these problems related to the colostomy to the surgeon:

- Signs of ischemia and necrosis (dark red, purplish, or black color; dry)
- Unusual bleeding
- Mucocutaneous separation (breakdown of the suture line securing the stoma to the abdominal wall)

Also assess the condition of the peristomal skin (skin around the stoma), and frequently check the pouch system for proper fit and signs of leakage. The skin should be intact, smooth, and without redness or excoriation.

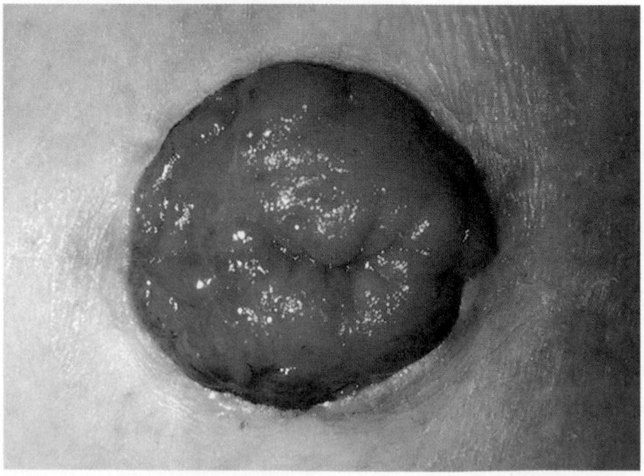

FIG. 56-6 A mature colostomy.

The colostomy should start functioning in 2 to 3 days postoperatively. When it begins to function, the pouch may need to be emptied frequently because of excess gas collection. It should be emptied when it is one-third to one-half full of stool. Stool is liquid immediately postoperatively but becomes more solid, depending on where in the colon the stoma was placed. For example, the stool from a colostomy in the ascending colon is liquid, the stool from a colostomy in the transverse colon is pasty, and the stool from a colostomy in the descending colon is more solid (similar to usual stool expelled from the rectum).

Wound Management. For an AP resection, the perineal wound is generally surgically closed and two bulb suction drains such as Jackson-Pratt drains are placed in the wound or through stab wounds near the wound. The drains help prevent drainage from collecting within the wound and are usually left in place for several days, depending on the character and amount of drainage. These drains are described in more detail in Chapter 16.

Monitoring drainage from the perineal wound and cavity is important because of the possibility of infection and abscess formation. Serosanguineous drainage from the perineal wound may be observed for 1 to 2 months after surgery. Complete healing of the perineal wound may take 6 to 8 months. This wound can be a greater source of discomfort than the abdominal incision and ostomy, and more care may be required. The patient may experience phantom rectal sensations because sympathetic innervation for rectal control has not been interrupted. Rectal PAIN and itching may occasionally occur after healing. Interventions may include use of antipruritic drugs, such as benzocaine, and warm compresses. Continually assess for signs of infection, abscess, or other complications, and implement methods for promoting wound drainage and comfort (Chart 56-3).

CHART 56-3 Best Practice for Patient Safety & Quality Care (QSEN)

Perineal Wound Care

Wound Care

- Place an absorbent dressing (e.g., abdominal pad) over the wound.
- Instruct the patient that he or she may:
  - Use a feminine napkin as a dressing
  - Wear jockey-type shorts rather than boxers

Comfort Measures

- If prescribed, soak the wound area in a sitz bath for 10 to 20 minutes 3 or 4 times per day or use warm/hot compresses or packs.
- Administer pain medication as prescribed, and assess its effectiveness.
- Instruct the patient about permissible activities. The patient should:
  - Assume a side-lying position in bed; avoid sitting for long periods
  - Use foam pads or a soft pillow to sit on whenever in a sitting position
  - Avoid the use of air rings or rubber donut devices

Prevention of Complications

- Maintain fluid and electrolyte balance by monitoring intake and output and by monitoring output from the perineal wound.
- Observe incision integrity, and monitor wound drains; watch for erythema, edema, bleeding, drainage, unusual odor, and excessive or constant pain.

NCLEX EXAMINATION CHALLENGE

Physiological Integrity

A nurse is assigned to care for a client who had an open partial colectomy and descending colostomy this morning. What assessment findings are expected for the client? **Select all that apply.**

A. The colostomy stoma is purple and dry.
B. The nasogastric tube is draining yellowish green fluid.
C. The client has pain that is controlled by analgesics.
D. The colostomy is not draining any stool.
E. The perineal incision is covered with a surgical dressing.

NURSING SAFETY PRIORITY (QSEN)

Action Alert

Refer patients who are at risk for or have familial CRC for genetic counseling. Specially trained nurses can discuss the purposes and goals of genetic testing. Ensure privacy and confidentiality. A review of the family history may provide important information concerning the pattern of colorectal cancer inheritance. To make an informed decision, the patient and family need information about the advantages, risks, and costs of appropriate genetic tests. Monitor the patient's response regarding genetic risk factors.

Assisting with the Grieving Process

Planning: Expected Outcomes. The expected outcomes are that the patient will verbalize feelings about the diagnosis and treatment and progress through the normal stages of grief.

Interventions. The patient and family are faced with a possible loss of or alteration in body functions. Medical and surgical interventions for the treatment of colorectal cancer may result in cure, disease control, or palliation. Interventions are designed to assist the patient and family in planning effective strategies for expressing feelings of grief and developing coping skills. Families and significant others may request that patients not be informed of the diagnosis of cancer, particularly if the patient is an older adult.

Observe and identify:

- The patient's and family's current methods of coping
- Effective sources of support used in past crises
- The patient's and family's present perceptions of the health problem
- Signs of anticipatory grief, such as denial, crying, anger, and withdrawal from usual relationships

Encourage the patient and family to verbalize feelings about the diagnosis, treatment, and anticipated alteration in body functions if a colostomy is planned. (See discussion of Operative Procedures on p. 1153 in the Surgical Management section.) Denial, sadness, anger, feelings of loss, and depression are normal responses to this change in body function. The patient will need to learn new methods for toileting and how to cope with these changes.

If a colostomy is planned, instruct the patient on what to expect about the appearance and care of the colostomy. Postoperatively, encourage him or her to look at and touch the stoma. When the patient is physically able, ask him or her to participate in colostomy care. Participation helps restore the patient's sense of control over his or her lifestyle and thus facilitates improved self-esteem. If culturally appropriate, encourage participation of family or other caregivers in colostomy care.

Assist the patient in identifying the nature of and reaction to the loss. Encourage the patient and family to verbalize feelings and identify fears to help move them through the appropriate phases of the grief process. Establish a trusting, ongoing relationship with the patient and family, and provide support through the personal grieving stages.

In collaboration with the social worker or chaplain, assist the patient in identifying personal coping strategies. Encourage him or her to implement cultural, religious, and social customs associated with the loss, and identify sources of community support. Modifications in lifestyle are needed for patients with CRC. Help the patient and family identify these changes and how best to make them. The chaplain, social worker, or case manager assists in discussions and decisions with them concerning treatment, the prognosis, and end-of-life decisions as appropriate.

Community-Based Care

Patients undergoing a colon resection by open approach are typically hospitalized for 2 to 3 days or longer, depending on the age of the patient and any complications or concurrent health problems. Collaborate with the case manager to assist patients and their families in coping with the immediate postoperative phase of recovery. After hospitalization for surgery, the patient is usually managed at home. Radiation therapy or chemotherapy is typically done on an ambulatory care basis. For the patient with advanced cancer, hospice care may be an option (see Chapter 7).

Home Care Management. Assess all patients for their ability for self-management within limitations. For those requiring assistance with care, home care visits by nurses or assistive nursing personnel can be provided.

For the patient who has undergone a colostomy, review the home situation to aid the patient in arranging for care. Ostomy products should be kept in an area (preferably the bathroom) where the temperature is neither hot nor cold (skin barriers may become stiff or melt in extreme temperatures) to ensure proper functioning. The home care nurse or CWOCN or enterostomal therapist (ET) may serve as a consultant after the patient is discharged home to ensure continuity of care (per The Joint Commission's National Patient Safety Goals).

No changes are needed in sleeping accommodations. A moisture-proof covering may initially be placed over the bed mattress if patients feel insecure about the pouch system. They may consume their usual diet on discharge.

Self-Management Education. Before discharge, teach the patient to avoid lifting heavy objects or straining on defecation to prevent tension on the anastomosis site. If he or she had the open surgical approach, the patient should avoid driving for 4 to 6 weeks while the incision heals. Patients who have had laparoscopy can usually return to all usual activities in 1 to 2 weeks.

NURSING SAFETY PRIORITY (QSEN)

Action Alert

A stool softener may be prescribed to keep stools at a soft consistency for ease of passage. Teach patients to note the frequency, amount, and character of the stools. In addition to this information, teach those with colon resections to watch for and report clinical manifestations of intestinal obstruction and perforation (e.g., cramping, abdominal pain, nausea, vomiting). Advise the patient to avoid gas-producing foods and carbonated beverages. Four to six weeks may be required to establish the effects of certain foods on bowel patterns.

Colostomy Care. Rehabilitation after surgery requires that patients and family members learn how to perform colostomy care. Provide adequate opportunity before discharge for patients to learn the psychomotor skills involved in this care. Plan sufficient practice time for learning how to handle, assemble, and apply all ostomy equipment. Teach patients and families or other caregivers about:

- The normal appearance of the stoma
- Signs and symptoms of complications
- Measurement of the stoma
- The choice, use, care, and application of the appropriate appliance to cover the stoma
- Measures to protect the skin adjacent to the stoma
- Nutrition changes to control gas and odor
- Resumption of normal activities, including work, travel, and sexual intercourse

The appropriate pouch system must be selected and fitted to the stoma. Patients with flat, firm abdomens may use either flexible (bordered with paper tape) or nonflexible (full skin barrier wafer) pouch systems. A firm abdomen with lateral creases or folds requires a flexible system. Patients with deep creases, flabby abdomens, a retracted stoma, or a stoma that is flush or concave to the abdominal surface benefit from a convex appliance with a stoma belt. This type of system presses into the skin around the stoma, causing the stoma to protrude. This protrusion helps tighten the skin and prevents leaks around the stoma opening onto the peristomal skin.

Measurement of the stoma is necessary to determine the correct size of the stomal opening on the appliance. The opening should be large enough not only to cover the peristomal skin but also to avoid stomal trauma. The stoma will shrink within 6 to 8 weeks after surgery. Therefore it needs to be measured at least once weekly during this time and as needed if the patient gains or loses weight. Teach the patient and family caregiver to trace the pattern of the stomal area on the wafer portion of the appliance and to cut an opening about $\frac{1}{8}$- to $\frac{1}{16}$-inch larger than the stomal pattern to ensure that stomal tissue will not be constricted.

Skin preparation may include clipping peristomal hair or shaving the area (moving from the stoma outward) to achieve a smooth surface, prevent unnecessary discomfort when the wafer is removed, and minimize the risk for infected hair follicles. Advise the patient to clean around the stoma with mild soap and water before putting on an appliance. He or she should avoid using moisturizing soaps to clean the area because the lubricants can interfere with adhesion of the appliance.

! NURSING SAFETY PRIORITY (QSEN)

Action Alert

Teach the patient and family to apply a skin sealant (preferably without alcohol) and allow it to dry before application of the appliance (colostomy bag) to facilitate less painful removal of the tape or adhesive. If peristomal skin becomes raw, stoma powder or paste or a combination may also be applied. The paste or other filler cream is also used to fill in crevices and creases to create a flat surface for the faceplate of the colostomy bag. If the patient develops a fungal rash, an antifungal cream or powder should be used.

Control of gas and odor from the colostomy is often an important outcome for patients with new ostomies. Although a leaking or inadequately closed pouch is the usual cause of odor, flatus can also contribute to the odor. Remind the patient that although generally no foods for ostomates are forbidden, certain foods and habits can cause flatus or contribute to odor when the pouch is open. Broccoli, beans, spicy foods, onions, Brussels sprouts, cabbage, cauliflower, cucumbers, mushrooms, and peas often cause flatus, as does chewing gum, smoking, drinking beer, and skipping meals. Crackers, toast, and yogurt can help prevent gas. Asparagus, broccoli, cabbage, turnips, eggs, fish, and garlic contribute to odor when the pouch is open. Buttermilk, cranberry juice, parsley, and yogurt help prevent odor. Charcoal filters, pouch deodorizers, or placement of a breath mint in the pouch helps eliminate odors. The patient should be cautioned to not put aspirin tablets in the pouch because they may cause ulceration of the stoma. Vents that allow release of gas from the ostomy bag through a deodorizing filter are available and may decrease the patient's level of self-consciousness about odor.

The patient with a sigmoid colostomy may benefit from colostomy irrigation to regulate elimination. However, most patients with a sigmoid colostomy can become regulated through diet. An irrigation is similar to an enema but is administered through the stoma rather than the rectum.

In addition to teaching the patient about the clinical manifestations of obstruction and perforation, ask the patient to report any fever or sudden onset of pain or swelling around the stoma. Other home care assessment is listed in Chart 56-4.

Psychosocial Concerns. The diagnosis of cancer can be emotionally immobilizing for the patient and family or significant others, but treatment may be welcomed because it may provide hope for control of the disease. Explore reactions to the illness and perceptions of planned interventions.

The patient's reaction to ostomy surgery may include:

- Fear of not being accepted by others
- Feelings of grief related to disturbance in body image
- Concerns about sexuality

Encourage the patient and family to verbalize their feelings. By teaching how to physically manage the ostomy, help them begin to restore self-esteem and improve body image. Inclusion of family and significant others in the rehabilitation process may help maintain relationships and raise self-esteem. Anticipatory

CHART 56-4 Home Care Assessment

The Patient with a Colostomy

Assess gastrointestinal status, including:
- Dietary and fluid intake and habits
- Presence or absence of nausea and vomiting
- Weight gain or loss
- Bowel elimination pattern and characteristics and amount of effluent (stool)
- Bowel sounds

Assess condition of stoma, including:
- Location, size, protrusion, color, and integrity
- Signs of ischemia, such as dull coloring or dark or purplish bruising

Assess peristomal skin for:
- Presence or absence of excoriated skin, leakage underneath drainage system
- Fit of appliance and effectiveness of skin barrier and appliance

Assess the patient's and family's coping skills, including:
- Self-care abilities in the home
- Acknowledgment of changes in body image and function
- Sense of loss

instruction includes information on leakage accidents, odor control measures, and adjustments to resuming sexual relationships.

Health Care Resources. Several resources are available to maintain continuity of care in the home environment and provide for patient needs that the nurse is not able to meet. Make referrals to community-based case managers or social workers, who can provide further emotional counseling, aid in managing financial concerns, or arrange for services in the home or long-term care facility as needed.

Provide information about the United Ostomy Associations of America, Inc. (www.uoaa.org), a self-help group of people who have ostomies. This group has literature such as the organization's publication *(Ostomy Quarterly)* and information about local chapters. The organization conducts a visitor program that sends specially trained visitors (who have an ostomy [ostomate]) to talk with patients. After obtaining consent, make a referral to the visitor program so that the volunteer ostomate can see the patient both preoperatively and postoperatively. A physician's consent for visitation may be necessary.

The local division or unit of the American Cancer Society (ACS) (www.cancer.org) can help provide necessary medical equipment and supplies, home care services, travel accommodations, and other resources for the patient who is having cancer treatment or surgery. Inform the patient and family of the programs available through the local division or unit. Other excellent web resources include Cancer Care (www.cancercare.org), Colon Cancer Alliance (www.ccalliance.org), and the National Cancer Institute (www.nci.gov).

Because of short hospital stays, patients with new ostomies receive much health teaching from nurses working for home health care agencies. This resource also helps provide physical care needs, medication management, and emotional support. If the patient has advanced colorectal cancer, a referral for hospice services in the home, nursing home, or other long-term care setting may be appropriate. The home health care nurse informs the patient and family about what ostomy supplies are needed and where they can be purchased. Price and location are considered before recommendations are made.

CLINICAL JUDGMENT CHALLENGE

Prioritization, Delegation, and Supervision

A 56-year-old woman returns from the postanesthesia care unit (PACU) after an open colon resection and colostomy for ascending colon cancer. She has IV fluids running at 100 mL/hr and is receiving morphine PCA. An NGT is in place connected to low suction, and she is NPO. Her abdominal dressing is dry and intact, and her oxygen saturation is 95% on 2 L/min of oxygen via nasal cannula. She is allowed out of bed to the bathroom or chair today. You are assigned to care for this patient for the rest of the day shift.

1. Upon the patient's admission to your unit at 11 AM, should you delegate taking the patient's vital signs to an experienced nursing technician? Why or why not?
2. At 5 PM, the patient states that she needs to go to the bathroom. Will you delegate this activity to the nursing technician? Why or why not?
3. While the patient was in the bathroom, her oxygen saturation level decreased to 88%. What is your best action at this time?
4. The patient's husband asks you about his wife's prognosis regarding her cancer survival. What is your best response at this time?

◆ *Evaluation: Outcomes*

Evaluate the care of the patient with colorectal cancer based on the identified priority patient problems. The expected outcomes are that the patient:

- Adjusts to actual or impending loss
- Is free of complications or metastasis associated with CRC
- States he or she has well-controlled pain and is as comfortable as possible (if metastasis is present)

INTESTINAL OBSTRUCTION

❖ *PATHOPHYSIOLOGY*

Intestinal obstructions can be partial or complete and are classified as mechanical or nonmechanical. In **mechanical obstruction,** the bowel is physically blocked by problems outside the intestine (e.g., adhesions), in the bowel wall (e.g., Crohn's disease), or in the intestinal lumen (e.g., tumors). **Nonmechanical obstruction** (also known as **paralytic ileus** or *adynamic ileus*) does not involve a physical obstruction in or outside the intestine. Instead, peristalsis is decreased or absent as a result of neuromuscular disturbance, resulting in a slowing of the movement or a backup of intestinal contents (McCance et al., 2014).

Intestinal contents are composed of ingested fluid, food, and saliva; gastric, pancreatic, and biliary secretions; and swallowed air. In both mechanical and nonmechanical obstructions, the intestinal contents accumulate at and above the area of obstruction. Distention results from the intestine's inability to absorb the contents and move them down the intestinal tract. To compensate for the lag, peristalsis increases in an effort to move the intestinal contents forward. This increase stimulates more secretions, which then leads to additional distention. The bowel then becomes edematous, and increased capillary permeability results. Plasma leaking into the peritoneal cavity and fluid trapped in the intestinal lumen decrease the absorption of fluid and electrolytes into the vascular space. Reduced circulatory blood volume (hypovolemia) and electrolyte imbalances typically occur. Hypovolemia ranges from mild to extreme (hypovolemic shock).

Specific problems related to FLUID AND ELECTROLYTE BALANCE and acid-base balance result, depending on the part of the intestine that is blocked. An obstruction high in the small intestine causes a loss of gastric hydrochloride, which can lead to *metabolic alkalosis.* Obstruction below the duodenum but above the large bowel results in loss of both acids and bases, so that acid-base balance is usually not compromised. Obstruction at the end of the small intestine and lower in the intestinal tract causes loss of alkaline fluids, which can lead to *metabolic acidosis* (McCance et al., 2014).

If hypovolemia is severe, renal insufficiency or even death can occur. Bacterial peritonitis with or without actual perforation can also result. Bacteria in the intestinal contents lie stagnant in the obstructed intestine. This is not a problem unless the blood flow to the intestine is compromised. However, with *closed-loop obstruction* (blockage in two different areas) or a **strangulated obstruction** (obstruction with compromised blood flow), the risk for peritonitis is greatly increased. Bacteria without blood supply can form and release an endotoxin into the peritoneal or systemic circulation and cause septic shock. With a strangulated obstruction, major blood loss into the intestine and the peritoneum can occur. Sepsis and bleeding can result in an increased intra-abdominal pressure (IAP) or acute

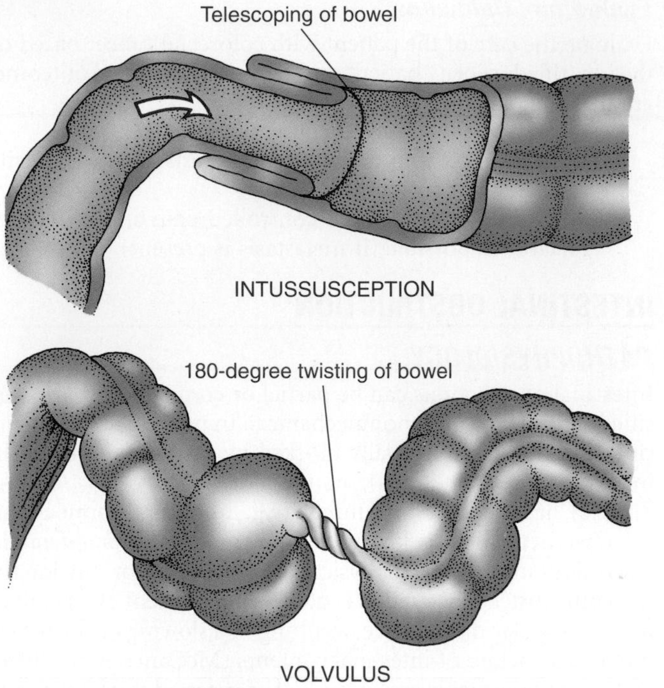

FIG. 56-7 Two major types of mechanical obstruction.

compartment syndrome (Lee, 2012). (See later discussion of IAP on p. 1163 of this chapter.)

Intestinal obstruction is a common and serious disorder caused by a variety of conditions and is associated with significant morbidity. It can occur anywhere in the intestinal tract, although the ileum in the small intestine (the narrowest part of the intestinal tract) is the most common site.

Mechanical obstruction can result from:

- Adhesions (scar tissue from surgeries or pathology)
- Benign or malignant tumor
- Complications of appendicitis
- Hernias
- Fecal impactions (especially in older adults)
- Strictures due to Crohn's disease or previous radiation therapy
- **Intussusception** (telescoping of a segment of the intestine within itself) (Fig. 56-7)
- **Volvulus** (twisting of the intestine) (see Fig. 56-7)
- Fibrosis due to disorders such as endometriosis
- Vascular disorders (e.g., emboli and arteriosclerotic narrowing of mesenteric vessels)

In people ages 65 years or older, diverticulitis, tumors, and fecal impaction are the most common causes of obstruction (McCance et al., 2014).

Postoperative ileus (POI) (paralytic ileus), or *nonmechanical* obstruction, is most commonly caused by handling of the intestines during abdominal surgery. In patients with POI, intestinal function is lost for a few hours to several days. Electrolyte disturbances, especially hypokalemia, predispose the patient to this problem. The ileus can also be a consequence of **peritonitis**, because leakage of colonic contents causes severe irritation and triggers an inflammatory response and infection (see discussion of peritonitis on p. 1170 in Chapter 57). Vascular insufficiency to the bowel, also referred to as *intestinal ischemia,* is another potential cause of an ileus. It results when arterial or venous thrombosis or an embolus decreases blood flow to the mesenteric blood vessels surrounding the intestines, as in heart failure or severe shock. Severe insufficiency of blood supply can result in infarction of surrounding organs (e.g., bowel infarction).

❖ PATIENT-CENTERED COLLABORATIVE CARE

◆ Assessment

History. Collect information about a history of gastrointestinal disorders, surgeries, and treatments. Question the patient about recent nausea and vomiting and the color of emesis. Perform a thorough PAIN assessment with particular attention to the onset, aggravating factors, alleviating factors, and patterns or rhythms of the pain. Severe pain that then stops and changes to tenderness on palpation may indicate perforation and should be reported promptly to the physician. Ask about the passage of flatus and the time, character, and consistency of the last bowel movement. Singultus (hiccups) is common with all types of intestinal obstruction. When an obstruction is suspected, keep the patient NPO and contact the physician promptly for further direction.

Assess for a family history of colorectal cancer (CRC), and ask about blood in the stool or a change in bowel pattern. Body temperature with uncomplicated obstruction is rarely higher than 100° F (37.8° C). A temperature higher than this, with or without guarding and tenderness, and a sustained elevation in pulse could indicate a strangulated obstruction or peritonitis. A fever, tachycardia, hypotension, increasing abdominal pain, abdominal rigidity, or change in color of skin overlying the abdomen should be reported to the attending physician immediately.

Physical Assessment/Clinical Manifestations. The patient with *mechanical* obstruction in the *small intestine* often has mid-abdominal PAIN or cramping. The pain can be sporadic, and the patient may feel comfortable between episodes. If strangulation is present, the pain becomes more localized and steady. Vomiting often accompanies obstruction and is more profuse with obstructions in the proximal small intestine. The vomitus may contain bile and mucus or be orange-brown and foul smelling as a result of bacterial overgrowth with low ileal obstruction. Prolonged vomiting can result in a disruption in FLUID AND ELECTROLYTE BALANCE. **Obstipation** (no passage of stool) and failure to pass flatus accompany complete obstruction. Diarrhea may be present in partial obstruction.

Mechanical colonic obstruction causes a milder, more intermittent colicky abdominal PAIN than is seen with small-bowel obstruction. Lower abdominal distention and obstipation may be present, or the patient may have ribbon-like stools if obstruction is partial. Alterations in bowel patterns and blood in the stools accompany the obstruction if colorectal cancer or diverticulitis is the cause.

On examination of the abdomen, observe for abdominal distention, which is common in all forms of intestinal obstruction. Peristaltic waves may also be visible. Auscultate for proximal high-pitched bowel sounds (**borborygmi**), which are associated with cramping early in the obstructive process as the intestine tries to push the mechanical obstruction forward. In later stages of mechanical obstruction, bowel sounds are absent, especially distal to the obstruction. Abdominal tenderness and rigidity are usually minimal. The presence of a tense, fluid-filled bowel loop mimicking a palpable abdominal mass may signal a closed-loop, strangulating small-bowel obstruction.

CHART 56-5 Key Features

Small-Bowel and Large-Bowel Obstructions

SMALL-BOWEL OBSTRUCTIONS	LARGE-BOWEL OBSTRUCTIONS
Abdominal discomfort or pain possibly accompanied by visible peristaltic waves in upper and middle abdomen	Intermittent lower abdominal cramping
Upper or epigastric abdominal distention	Lower abdominal distention
Nausea and early, profuse vomiting (may contain fecal material)	Minimal or no vomiting
Obstipation	Obstipation or ribbon-like stools
Severe fluid and electrolyte imbalances	No major fluid and electrolyte imbalances
Metabolic alkalosis	Metabolic acidosis (not always present)

In most types of *nonmechanical* obstruction, the PAIN is described as a constant, diffuse discomfort. Colicky cramping is not characteristic of this type of obstruction. Pain associated with obstruction caused by vascular insufficiency or infarction is usually severe and constant. On inspection, abdominal distention is typically present. On auscultation of the abdomen, note and document decreased bowel sounds in early obstruction and absent bowel sounds in later stages. Vomiting of gastric contents and bile is frequent, but the vomitus rarely has a foul odor and is rarely profuse. Obstipation may or may not be present. Chart 56-5 compares small-bowel and large-bowel obstructions.

Diagnostic Assessment. There is no definitive laboratory test to confirm a diagnosis of mechanical or nonmechanical obstruction. *White blood cell (WBC) counts* are normal unless there is a strangulated obstruction, in which case there may be leukocytosis (increased WBCs). *Hemoglobin, hematocrit, creatinine, and blood urea nitrogen (BUN)* values are often elevated, indicating dehydration. Serum sodium, chloride, and potassium are decreased. Elevations in serum amylase levels may be found with strangulating obstructions, which can damage the pancreas.

The health care provider obtains an *abdominal CT scan* as soon as an obstruction is suspected. Distention with fluid and gas in the small intestine with the absence of gas in the colon indicates an obstruction in the small intestine.

The diagnostic examination chosen depends on the suspected location of the obstruction. As an initial assessment, the health care provider may prescribe an *abdominal ultrasound* to evaluate the potential cause of the obstruction. The physician may perform endoscopy (sigmoidoscopy or colonoscopy) to determine the cause of the obstruction, except when perforation or complete obstruction is suspected.

◆ *Interventions*

Interventions are aimed at uncovering the cause and relieving the obstruction. Intestinal obstructions can be relieved by nonsurgical or surgical means. If the obstruction is partial and there is no evidence of strangulation, nonsurgical management may be the treatment of choice (Chart 56-6).

Nonsurgical Management. Paralytic ileus responds well to nonsurgical methods of relieving obstruction. Nonsurgical approaches are also preferred in the treatment of patients with terminal disease associated with bowel obstruction. In addition to being NPO, patients typically have a nasogastric tube (NGT) inserted to decompress the bowel by draining fluid and air. The tube is attached to suction.

CHART 56-6 Best Practice for Patient Safety & Quality Care QSEN

Nursing Care of Patients Who Have an Intestinal Obstruction

- Monitor vital signs, especially blood pressure, for indications of fluid balance.
- Assess the patient's abdomen at least twice a day for bowel sounds, distention, and passage of flatus.
- Monitor fluid and electrolyte status, including laboratory values.
- Manage the patient who has a nasogastric tube (NGT):
    - Monitor drainage.
    - Ensure tube patency.
    - Check tube placement.
    - Irrigate tube as prescribed.
    - Maintain the patient on NPO status.
    - Provide frequent mouth and nares care.
    - Maintain the patient in a semi-Fowler's position.
- Give analgesics for pain as prescribed.
- Give alvimopan (Entereg) as prescribed for patients with a postoperative ileus.
- Maintain parenteral nutrition if prescribed.

Nasogastric Tubes. Most patients with an obstruction have an NGT unless the obstruction is mild. A **Salem sump tube** is inserted through the nose and placed into the stomach. It is attached to low continuous suction. This tube has a vent ("pigtail") that prevents the stomach mucosa from being pulled away during suctioning. Levin tubes do not have a vent and therefore should be connected to low intermittent suction. They are used much less often than the Salem sump tubes.

! NURSING SAFETY PRIORITY QSEN

Action Alert

At least every 4 hours, assess the patient with an NGT for proper placement of the tube, tube patency, and output (quality and quantity). Monitor the nasal skin around the tube for irritation. Use a device that secures the tube to the nose to prevent accidental removal. Assess for peristalsis by auscultating for bowel sounds with the suction disconnected (suction masks peristaltic sounds).

Question the patient about the passage of flatus, and record flatus and the character of bowel movements daily. Flatus or stool means that peristalsis has returned. Assess for nausea, and ask the patient to report this manifestation.

Monitor any NGT for proper functioning. Occasionally NGTs move out of optimal drainage position or become plugged. In this case, note a decrease in gastric output or stasis of the tube's contents. Assess the patient for nausea, vomiting, increased abdominal distention, and placement of the tube. If the NGT is repositioned or replaced, confirmation of proper placement may be obtained by x-ray before use. After appropriate placement is established, aspirate the contents and irrigate the tube with 30 mL of normal saline every 4 hours or as requested by the health care provider.

Other Nonsurgical Interventions. Most types of nonmechanical obstruction respond to nasogastric decompression with medical treatment of the primary disorder. Incomplete mechanical obstruction can sometimes be successfully treated without surgery. Obstruction caused by lower fecal impaction usually resolves after disimpaction and enema administration. Intussusception may respond to hydrostatic pressure changes during a barium enema.

For patients with a postoperative ileus (POI), alvimopan (Entereg) may be given for short-term use. This drug is an oral, peripherally acting mu opioid receptor antagonist that increases GI motility (Russell et al., 2012).

IV fluid replacement and maintenance are indicated for all patients with intestinal obstruction because the patient is NPO and FLUID AND ELECTROLYTE BALANCE is lost (particularly potassium) through vomiting and nasogastric suction. On the basis of serum electrolytes and blood urea nitrogen (BUN) levels, the health care provider prescribes aggressive fluid replacement with 2 to 4 L of normal saline or lactated Ringer's solution with potassium added. Use care with patients who are susceptible to fluid overload (e.g., older adults with a history of heart or kidney failure). Monitor lung sounds, weight, and intake and output daily. Weight is the most reliable indicator of fluid balance. Blood replacement may be indicated in strangulated obstruction because of blood loss into the bowel or peritoneal cavity.

Monitor vital signs and other measures of fluid status (e.g., urine output, skin turgor, mucous membranes) every 2 to 4 hours, depending on the severity of the patient's symptoms. In collaboration with the dietitian, the physician may prescribe parenteral nutrition (PN), especially if the patient has had chronic nutritional problems and has been NPO for an extended period. Chapter 60 discusses the nursing care of patients receiving PN.

The patient with intestinal obstruction is usually thirsty, although some older adults have a decreased thirst response. Delegate frequent mouth care to unlicensed assistive personnel (UAP) to help maintain moist mucous membranes. Be sure to supervise this activity. A few ice chips may be allowed if the patient is not having surgery. Follow agency protocol or the physician's request regarding ice chips.

Abdominal distention can cause a great deal of discomfort, especially when it is severe. The colicky, crampy pain that comes and goes with mechanical obstruction and the nausea, vomiting, dry mucous membranes, and thirst contribute to the patient's discomfort. Continually assess the character and location of the pain, and immediately report any PAIN that significantly increases or changes from a colicky, intermittent type to a constant discomfort. These changes can indicate perforation of the intestine or peritonitis.

Opioid analgesics may be temporarily withheld in the diagnostic workup period so that clinical manifestations of perforation or peritonitis are not masked. Explain to the patient and family the rationale for not giving analgesics. In addition, if analgesics such as morphine are given, they may slow intestinal motility and can cause vomiting. Be alert to this side effect because nausea and vomiting are also signs of NG tube obstruction or worsening bowel obstruction.

Help the patient obtain a position of comfort with frequent position changes to promote increased peristalsis. A semi-Fowler's position helps alleviate the pressure of abdominal distention on the chest. This position is for comfort and promotion of thoracic excursion to facilitate breathing.

Discomfort is generally less with nonmechanical obstruction than with mechanical obstruction. With both types of obstruction, discomfort is aggravated by taking in food or fluids.

If strangulation is thought to be likely, the health care provider prescribes IV broad-spectrum antibiotics. In addition, in cases of partial obstruction or paralytic ileus, drugs that enhance gastric motility such as octreotide acetate (Sandostatin) may be used.

Surgical Management. In patients with complete mechanical obstruction and in some cases of incomplete mechanical obstruction, surgical intervention is necessary to relieve the obstruction. A strangulated obstruction is complete, and surgical intervention is always required. An **exploratory laparotomy** (a surgical opening of the abdominal cavity to investigate the cause of the obstruction) is initially performed for many patients with obstruction. More specific surgical procedures depend on the cause of the obstruction.

Preoperative Care. Provide general preoperative teaching for both the patient and family as discussed in Chapter 14. In cases of complete obstruction, the patient may feel too ill to want the information. Reinforce the information with the family or other caregiver. Depending on the cause and severity of the obstruction, as well as the expertise of the surgeon, patients have either minimally invasive surgery (MIS) via laparoscopy or a conventional open approach.

Operative Procedures. In the *conventional open surgical approach,* the surgeon makes a large incision, enters the abdominal cavity, and explores for obstruction and its cause, if possible (exploratory laparotomy). If adhesions are found, they are lysed (cut and released). Obstruction caused by a tumor or diverticulitis requires a colon resection with primary anastomosis or a temporary or permanent colostomy. If obstruction is caused by intestinal infarction, an embolectomy, thrombectomy, or resection of the gangrenous small or large bowel may be necessary. In severe cases a colectomy (removal of the entire colon) may be needed.

For the *MIS* approach, the specially trained surgeon makes several small incisions in the abdomen and places a video camera to view the abdominal contents to determine the extent of the obstruction. A laparoscope (type of endoscope) with a lighted end is inserted along with various surgical instruments to remove the problem. This procedure takes longer than the open approach, but blood loss is less and healing is faster. Robotic assistance may be used, depending on the experience of the surgeon and available equipment.

Postoperative Care. General postoperative care for the patient undergoing an *exploratory laparotomy* with lysis of adhesions, colon resection, thrombectomy, or embolectomy is similar to that described in Chapter 16. In addition, patients who had an open surgical approach have an NGT in place until peristalsis resumes. A clear liquid diet may be prescribed to encourage peristalsis return. As liquids are started, the NGT can be disconnected from suction and capped for 1 to 2 hours after the patient has taken clear liquids to determine if he or she is able to tolerate them. If the patient vomits after liquids, the suction is resumed. When the patient has return of peristalsis, the NGT suction is discontinued and the tube is clamped for a scheduled amount of time. If the patient does not experience nausea while the NGT is clamped, the tube is removed.

Most patients today have laparoscopic surgery (MIS) for mechanical intestinal obstructions. They usually do *not* have an NGT and can recover more quickly than those with the open surgical approach. The hospital stay for those having MIS to remove tumors, adhesions, and other obstructions may be as short as 1 to 2 days compared with 3 days or longer for the conventional surgical patients. Recovery is much quicker because there is less pain and there are fewer postoperative complications among those who had laparoscopic surgery.

CLINICAL JUDGMENT CHALLENGE

Patient-Centered Care; Teamwork and Collaboration; Informatics QSEN

An 82-year-old woman had open abdominal surgery 36 hours ago for removal of a large uterine tumor. As her nurse, you note that she continues to have no bowel sounds and has not passed flatus. Her abdomen is moderately distended and hard. She has reported several episodes of severe nausea and has no appetite but states that she has no pain. You suspect that the patient has a postoperative ileus but need more data before calling the surgeon.

1. What questions do you need to ask the patient and her family related to her current problem?
2. What other objective assessment data do you need before contacting the surgeon?
3. Using SBAR and data that you provide, how will you communicate the information about this patient to the surgeon?
4. What evidence-based collaborative interventions are appropriate for this patient immediately? Support your answer with Internet resources.
5. What information will you document in the electronic health record?
6. What electrolyte imbalances would you expect? How might her presentation be somewhat different from that of a younger adult and why?

Community-Based Care

All patients with intestinal obstruction are hospitalized for monitoring and treatment. The length of stay varies according to the type of obstruction, the treatment, and the presence of complications. Patients who have complicated obstruction, such as strangulation or incarceration, are at greater risk for peritonitis, sepsis, and shock.

Patients with nonmechanical (adynamic) intestinal obstruction are less likely to require a lengthy hospitalization because of the obstruction alone. Adynamic obstruction generally responds to NG suction and possible drug therapy within a few days. However, if the ileus occurs as a complication of an abdominal surgery, the hospital stay could be lengthy.

Home Care Management. For the patient who has had an intestinal obstruction, preparation for home care depends on the cause of the obstruction and the treatment required. Those who have resolution of obstruction without surgical intervention are assessed for their knowledge of strategies to avoid recurrent obstruction. For example, if fecal impaction was the cause of the obstruction, assess the patient's ability to carry out a bowel regimen independently (Chart 56-7). For those who have had surgery, evaluate their ability to function at home with the added tasks of incision care and possibly colostomy care.

CHART 56-7 Nursing Focus on the Older Adult

Preventing Fecal Impaction

- Teach the patient to eat high-fiber foods, including plenty of raw fruits and vegetables and whole-grain products.
- Encourage the patient to drink adequate amounts of fluids, especially water.
- Do not routinely administer a laxative; teach the patient that laxative abuse decreases abdominal muscle tone and contributes to an atonic colon.
- Encourage the patient to exercise regularly, if possible. Walking every day is an excellent exercise for promoting intestinal motility.
- Use natural foods to stimulate peristalsis, such as warm beverages and prune juice.
- Take bulk-forming products, such as Metamucil, to provide fiber.
- Check the patient's stool for amount and frequency; oozing of soft or diarrheal stool often indicates a fecal impaction.
- Have the patient sit on a toilet or bedside commode rather than on a bedpan for elimination.

Self-Management Education. Instruct the patient to report any abdominal pain or distention, nausea, or vomiting, with or without constipation, because these symptoms might indicate recurrent obstruction. The patient should be reassured, however, that recurrent paralytic ileus is not common.

Teach the patient who has had surgery about incision care, drug therapy, and activity limitations. Drug therapy consists of an oral opioid analgesic, such as oxycodone hydrochloride with acetaminophen (Tylox, Percocet, Endocet ♣), to be taken as needed for incisional discomfort. As with any opioid therapy, an over-the-counter laxative with a softener (e.g., Docusate with Senna) or polyethylene glycol (MiraLax) may be added to prevent constipation and possible recurrent obstruction.

The patient who had curative treatment of the underlying cause most likely requires less support than one who had treatment of obstruction related to a serious disease that will require further management. Encourage the patient to express fears and concerns about the future. Assess the patient's understanding and needs with regard to treatment plans.

Health Care Resources. The need for follow-up appointments depends on the cause of the obstruction and the treatment required. In collaboration with the case manager, make arrangements for a home care nurse if the patient needs help with incision or colostomy care.

ABDOMINAL TRAUMA

❖ PATHOPHYSIOLOGY

Abdominal trauma is defined as injury to the structures located between the diaphragm and the pelvis that occurs when the abdomen is subjected to blunt or penetrating forces. Organs injured may include the large or small bowel, liver, spleen, duodenum, pancreas, kidneys, and urinary bladder.

At least one half of all *blunt abdominal traumas* occur from motor vehicle crashes. Other causes of blunt trauma include falls, aggravated assaults, and contact sports. The spleen is the most commonly injured organ from *blunt* abdominal trauma. *Penetrating abdominal trauma* is caused by gunshot wounds (GSWs), stabbing, or impalement with an object. The liver is the most commonly injured organ from penetrating abdominal trauma. *Trauma is the leading cause of death in adults younger than 40 years in the United States.*

❖ PATIENT-CENTERED COLLABORATIVE CARE

◆ Assessment

*First, assess any patient experiencing trauma for **a**irway, **b**reathing, and **c**irculation (ABCs).*

! NURSING SAFETY PRIORITY (QSEN)

Critical Rescue

Once the patient with abdominal trauma has been assessed for airway, breathing, and circulation, focus on the risks for hemorrhage, shock, and peritonitis. Mental status, vital signs, and skin perfusion are *priority* nursing assessments, with skin perfusion being the most reliable clinical guide in assessing hypovolemic shock:

- In a person with mild shock, the skin is pale, cool, and moist.
- With moderate shock, diaphoresis is more marked and urine output ceases.
- With severe shock, changes in mental status are manifested by agitation, disorientation, and recent memory loss.

Assess for abdominal trauma by asking the patient about the presence, location, and quality of pain. Inspect the abdomen, flanks, back, genitalia, and rectum for contusions, abrasions, lacerations, ecchymosis, penetrating injuries, and asymmetry. All of the patient's clothes must be removed for this examination.

Inspection of the abdomen may reveal distention. To perform an adequate inspection, turn the patient while maintaining spinal immobilization. *Ecchymosis (bruising) may indicate internal bleeding. Ecchymosis present in the distribution of a lap seat belt should be reported to the health care provider immediately because the bowel or other major organ may be injured.*

Auscultate the abdomen for bowel sounds. Absent or diminished bowel sounds may be caused by the presence of blood, bacteria, or a chemical irritant in the abdominal cavity. Also auscultate for bruits in the abdomen, which could indicate renal artery injury.

Injury to the spleen is present in many people with left lower rib fractures. Liver injury may be present in those with right lower rib fractures. Dullness over hollow organs that normally contain gas, such as the stomach and the large and small intestines, may indicate the presence of blood or fluid. Light abdominal palpation identifies areas of tenderness, rebound tenderness, guarding, rigidity, and spasm. A palpated mass may be blood or a fluid collection.

The patient without obvious significant bleeding or definite signs of peritoneal irritation undergoes abdominal ultrasound, **diagnostic peritoneal lavage (DPL)**, and CT. For DPL, the physician inserts a large-bore catheter into the abdomen and allows fluid to enter the abdominal cavity. If the return drainage from the abdomen is pink or grossly bloody, the health care team prepares for surgery. Abdominal ultrasound or *focused abdominal sonography for trauma (FAST)* is used to diagnose blunt abdominal trauma and may replace CT and DPL for diagnosis. Patients with hemodynamic instability or peritonitis are candidates for immediate laparotomy.

◆ Interventions

Nonsurgical and surgical interventions are aimed at preserving or restoring hemodynamic stability, preventing or decreasing blood loss, and preventing complications. Patients with abdominal trauma from a vehicle crash often have other injuries such as multiple fractures. *The priority for care is to establish and maintain the ABCs.*

Emergency Care: Abdominal Trauma. Nursing interventions include placement of at least two large-bore IV catheters in the upper extremities. IV catheters are not used in the lower extremities; if the vasculature has been injured, fluid can pool in the abdomen. The health care provider may insert a central venous catheter to assist with rapid fluid volume infusion. IV fluids include saline, crystalloids, and possibly blood. Be sure that the patient is typed and crossmatched for as many as 4 to 8 units of packed red blood cells.

These laboratory values are monitored:

- Arterial blood gases
- Complete blood count (CBC)
- Serum electrolyte, glucose and amylase, and blood urea nitrogen (BUN) determinations
- Liver function tests
- Coagulation studies

Measuring arterial blood gases may help determine the severity of shock. Hemoglobin and hematocrit values do not initially reflect true blood loss; values can be skewed because of hemoconcentration from volume loss or the dilutional effects of IV fluids. Serial hemoglobin and hematocrit measurements may be more accurate in determining true blood loss. An elevated white blood cell (WBC) count may indicate a ruptured spleen or intestinal injury. Elevated levels of serum transaminases may indicate liver injury. Elevation of serum amylase activity may signal injury to the pancreas or the bowel. All laboratory work is compiled so that values can be compared and trended.

Continuous hemodynamic monitoring is begun in the emergency department. Insert an indwelling urinary (Foley) catheter unless there is blood at the urinary meatus. Initially and hourly thereafter, evaluate urine output for bleeding and specific gravity. Laboratory tests indicate the amount of blood and protein in the urine. If there is an open abdominal wound or evisceration, cover it with a sterile dry dressing unless the physician requests otherwise. Unless it is contraindicated, as in the case of a skull fracture, the physician or nurse inserts a nasogastric tube (NGT) to identify bleeding and minimize the risk for vomiting and aspiration. Antibiotics may be administered as prescribed to reduce the risk for peritonitis.

If the patient with known abdominal trauma has no definite clinical manifestations of active bleeding or organ injury, he or she is admitted to the hospital for observation. Many patients are admitted to the critical care unit. Blunt trauma can cause active, but often not obvious, damage.

! NURSING SAFETY PRIORITY (QSEN)

Critical Rescue

For the patient who has sustained abdominal trauma, assess for abdominal or referred pain and nausea. Every 15 to 30 minutes in the early postinjury period and then hourly, evaluate:

- Mental status
- Vital signs
- Clinical findings, such as vomiting, guarding, rigidity, or rebound tenderness
- Bowel sounds
- Urine output

Report any change immediately to the health care provider! It is more important to recognize the high risk for an active abdominal injury and assess for general signs of organ injury (e.g., hemorrhage and peritonitis) than to identify the exact nature of the abdominal injury. Opioid analgesics are given for pain after the physician's initial assessment is complete. Explain to the patient and family the rationale for delaying analgesics.

Intra-Abdominal Pressure Monitoring. Some patients are monitored for intra-abdominal pressure (IAP) using a continuous monitoring system. As the name implies, **intra-abdominal pressure** is pressure within the abdominal cavity. The normal IAP in healthy adults is 0 to 5 mm Hg, but obese patients often have a higher normal value (Lee, 2012). Increased IAP commonly occurs in patients with abdominal trauma. Other causes of IAP elevation include sepsis, burns, abdominal hemorrhage, and mechanical intestinal obstruction.

Nursing interventions to help *prevent* increased IAP in high-risk patients include (Lee, 2012):

- Record bowel movements.
- Check daily for fecal impaction.
- Provide measures to prevent constipation (e.g., increased fluids if tolerated, daily stool softener).
- Provide fluid replacement with hypertonic saline, crystalloids (e.g., 0.9% saline), or colloids (e.g., albumin, Dextran) as prescribed to expand plasma volume.
- Document intake and output.
- Monitor residuals for patients being tube-fed.
- Elevate the head of the bed to 20-30 degrees, depending on the patient's condition.
- Manage pain adequately.

When IAP becomes higher than the central venous pressure, the inferior vena cava and other abdominal vessels are compressed. This leads to impaired venous return, increased afterload, and decreased preload. The patient is then at risk for deep vein thrombosis and pulmonary embolism (PE). The patient has tachycardia and hypotension. As the IAP increases further, acidosis and ischemia occur. A sustained or repeated IAP of 12 mm Hg or higher is considered **intra-abdominal hypertension (IAH)**. **Abdominal acute compartment syndrome (AACS)** results when the IAP is sustained at greater than 20 mm Hg. Untreated AACS results in damage to the intestine and increases the risk for sepsis, multiple organ dysfunction syndrome (MODS), and death. Almost every body system can be affected (Lee, 2012).

For patients with abdominal trauma or other high-risk factors, the health care provider may request continuous or intermittent IAP monitoring in the critical care unit using a urinary manometer or transducer system. *Report any increase in IAP immediately to the health care provider.* AACS has a rapid onset after abdominal trauma (especially blunt trauma) and must be treated immediately using either a nonsurgical (vasopressor drugs and fluids) or surgical approach (fasciotomy). Surgery is risky because it increases the chance of embolic stroke and PE.

Surgical Management. For the patient with severe abdominal trauma, the surgeon performs an *exploratory laparotomy* and repairs abdominal injuries immediately if there are definite signs of peritoneal irritation. These signs include rebound tenderness, significant blood loss, evisceration, or a gunshot wound (GSW) with possible peritoneal involvement. After surgery, many of these patients are admitted to a critical care unit and mechanically ventilated.

Most stab wounds and GSWs require exploratory laparotomy. The surgeon explores and cleans superficial penetrating wounds. The patient does not require an exploratory laparotomy for superficial wounds.

Patients with multiple trauma stay in the hospital for a prolonged period. Before discharge from the hospital, teach the patient and family the signs and symptoms of abdominal bleeding whether or not surgery has been performed. Instruct them to report abdominal pain, nausea, vomiting, bloody or black stools, fever, weakness, and dizziness.

Hemorrhage can occasionally occur weeks after blunt abdominal trauma, despite medical evaluation or treatment. For the patient who has surgery or exploration of wounds, provide instructions on wound care before discharge from the hospital. Provide additional health teaching as the patient's overall condition requires.

NCLEX EXAMINATION CHALLENGE

Physiological Integrity

A client is admitted to the emergency department in severe pain with a gunshot wound to the right upper abdomen. Admitting vital signs are TPR 98-96-28; BP 118/70; oxygen saturation 94%. What is the nurse's priority when monitoring this client?

A. Open the airway to improve breathing.
B. Give oxygen via nasal cannula at 2 L/min.
C. Monitor vital signs frequently.
D. Determine how the client was shot and by whom.

POLYPS

❖ PATHOPHYSIOLOGY

Polyps in the intestinal tract are small growths covered with mucosa and attached to the surface of the intestine. Although most are benign, they are significant because some have the potential to become malignant.

Polyps are identified by their tissue type. Although only a very small number of adenomas progress to cancer, almost all colorectal cancers develop from an adenoma. Adenomas are further classified as villous or tubular. Of these, villous adenomas pose a greater cancer risk.

Familial adenomatous polyposis (FAP) and hereditary nonpolyposis colorectal cancer (HNPCC) are inherited syndromes characterized by progressive development of colorectal adenomas. Unless these syndromes are treated, colorectal cancer (CRC) inevitably occurs by the fourth to fifth decade of life. These conditions were discussed on p. 1149 in the Genetic/Genomic Considerations feature in the Colorectal Cancer section.

❖ PATIENT-CENTERED COLLABORATIVE CARE

Polyps are usually asymptomatic and are discovered during routine colonoscopy screening. However, they can cause gross rectal bleeding, intestinal obstruction, or intussusception (telescoping of the bowel). Biopsy specimens of polyps can be obtained and the entire polyp can be removed (polypectomy) with the use of a snare that fits through the sigmoidoscope or colonoscope. This often eliminates the need for abdominal surgery to remove a suspicious or definitely malignant polyp. The patient with FAP often requires a total colectomy (colon removal) to prevent the development of cancer.

Nursing care focuses on patient education. Instruct the patient about:

- The nature of the polyp
- Clinical manifestations to report to the health care provider
- The need for regular, routine monitoring or screening

If the patient has had a polypectomy, follow-up sigmoidoscopic or colonoscopic examinations are needed because there is an increased risk for developing multiple polyps.

Nursing care of the patient after a polypectomy of the colorectal area includes monitoring for abdominal distention and pain, rectal bleeding, mucopurulent drainage from the rectum, and fever. A small amount of blood might appear in the stool after a polypectomy, but this should be temporary.

HEMORRHOIDS

❖ PATHOPHYSIOLOGY

Hemorrhoids are unnaturally swollen or distended veins in the anorectal region. The veins involved in the development of hemorrhoids are part of the normal structure in the anal region. With limited distention, the veins function as a valve overlying the anal sphincter that assists in continence. Increased intra-abdominal pressure causes elevated systemic and portal venous pressure, which is transmitted to the anorectal veins. Arterioles in the anorectal region shunt blood directly to the distended anorectal veins, which increases the pressure. With repeated elevations in pressure from increased intra-abdominal pressure and engorgement from arteriolar shunting of blood, the distended veins eventually separate from the smooth muscle surrounding them. The result is prolapse of the hemorrhoidal vessels.

Hemorrhoids can be internal or external (Fig. 56-8). **Internal hemorrhoids**, which cannot be seen on inspection of the perineal area, lie above the anal sphincter. **External hemorrhoids** lie below the anal sphincter and can be seen on inspection of the anal region. Prolapsed hemorrhoids can become thrombosed or inflamed, or they can bleed (McCance et al., 2014).

Hemorrhoids are common and not significant unless they cause pain or bleeding. Caused by increased abdominal pressure, the condition worsens during pregnancy, constipation with straining, obesity, heart failure, prolonged sitting or standing, and strenuous exercise and weight lifting. Decreased fluid intake can also cause hemorrhoids because of the development of hard stool and subsequent constipation. Straining while evacuating stool causes them to enlarge.

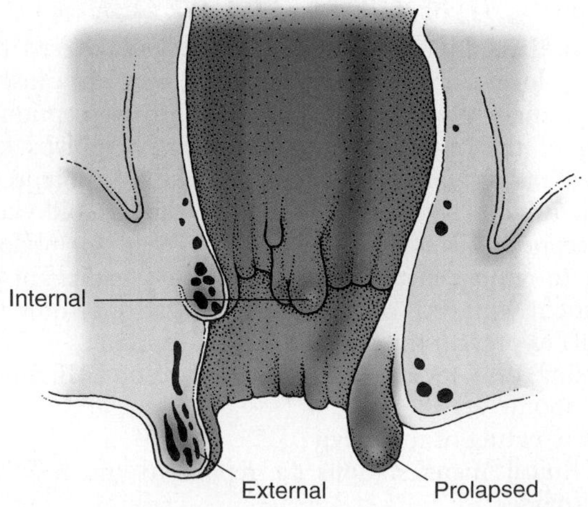

FIG. 56-8 Internal, external, and prolapsed hemorrhoids. *Internal hemorrhoids* lie above the anal sphincter and cannot be seen on inspection of the anal area. *External hemorrhoids* lie below the anal sphincter and can be seen on inspection of the anal region. Hemorrhoids that enlarge, fall down, and protrude through the anus are called *prolapsed hemorrhoids*.

Health Promotion and Maintenance

Prevention of constipation is the most important preventive measure. It can be prevented by increasing fiber in the diet, such as eating more whole grains and raw vegetables and fruits. Encourage patients to drink plenty of water unless otherwise contraindicated (e.g., kidney disease, heart disease). Remind the patient to avoid straining at stool. Remind him or her to exercise regularly with a gradual buildup in intensity. Maintaining a healthy weight also helps prevent hemorrhoids.

❖ PATIENT-CENTERED COLLABORATIVE CARE

◆ Assessment

The most common symptoms of hemorrhoids are bleeding, swelling, and prolapse (bulging). Blood is characteristically bright red and is present on toilet tissue or streaked in the stool. PAIN is a common symptom and is often associated with thrombosis, especially if thrombosis occurs suddenly. Other symptoms include itching and a mucous discharge. Diagnosis is usually made by inspection and digital examination.

◆ Interventions

Interventions are typically conservative and are aimed at reducing symptoms with a minimum of discomfort, cost, and time lost from usual activities. Local treatment and NUTRITION therapy are used when symptoms begin. Cold packs applied to the anorectal region for a few minutes at a time beginning with the onset of pain and tepid sitz baths 3 or 4 times per day are often enough to relieve discomfort, even if the hemorrhoids are thrombosed.

Topical anesthetics, such as lidocaine (Xylocaine), are useful for severe pain. Dibucaine (Nupercainal) ointment and similar products are available over the counter and may be applied for mild to moderate PAIN and itching. This ointment should be used only temporarily, however, because it can mask worsening symptoms and delay diagnosis of a severe disorder. If itching or inflammation is present, the health care provider prescribes a steroid preparation, such as hydrocortisone. Cleansing the anal area with moistened cleansing tissues rather than standard toilet tissue helps avoid irritation. The anal area should be cleansed gently by dabbing, rather than by wiping.

Diets high in fiber and fluids are recommended to promote regular bowel movements without straining. Stool softeners, such as docusate sodium (Colace), can be used temporarily. Irritating laxatives are avoided, as are foods and beverages that can make hemorrhoids worse. Spicy foods, nuts, coffee, and alcohol can be irritating. Remind patients to avoid sitting for long periods. The health care provider may prescribe mild oral analgesics for pain if the hemorrhoids are thrombosed.

Conservative treatment should alleviate symptoms in 3 to 5 days. If symptoms continue or recur frequently, the patient may require surgical intervention.

The surgeon can perform several procedures in an ambulatory care setting to remove symptomatic hemorrhoids (**hemorrhoidectomy**). The type of surgery (e.g., ultrasound or laser removal) depends on the degree of prolapse, whether there is thrombosis, and the overall condition of the patient. Complications of these procedures include PAIN, thrombosis of other hemorrhoids, infection, bleeding, and abscess formation. If the hemorrhoid is prolapsed, a circular stapling device may be used to excise a band of mucosa above the prolapse and restore the hemorrhoidal tissue back into the anal canal.

Teach patients with hemorrhoids about the need to eat high-fiber, high-fluid diets to promote regular bowel patterns before and after surgery. Advise them to avoid stimulant laxatives, which can be habit forming.

For patients who undergo any type of surgical intervention, monitor for bleeding and PAIN postoperatively and teach them to report these problems to their health care provider. Using moist heat (e.g., sitz baths or warm compresses) 3 or 4 times per day can help promote comfort.

! NURSING SAFETY PRIORITY (QSEN)

Action Alert

Tell the patient who has had surgical intervention for hemorrhoids that the first postoperative bowel movement may be very painful. Be sure that someone is with or near the patient when this happens. Some patients become light-headed and diaphoretic and may have syncope ("blackout").

The physician usually prescribes stool softeners such as docusate sodium (Colace) to begin preoperatively and continue after surgery. Analgesics and anti-inflammatory drugs are prescribed. A mild laxative should be administered if the patient has not had a bowel movement by the third postoperative day.

MALABSORPTION SYNDROME

❖ PATHOPHYSIOLOGY

Malabsorption is a syndrome associated with a variety of disorders and intestinal surgical procedures. It interferes with the ability to absorb nutrients and is a result of a generalized flattening of the mucosa of the small intestine. With various disorders, physiologic mechanisms limit absorption of nutrients because of one or more of these abnormalities:

- Bile salt deficiencies
- Enzyme deficiencies
- Presence of bacteria
- Disruption of the mucosal lining of the small intestine
- Altered lymphatic and vascular circulation
- Decrease in the gastric or intestinal surface area

The nutrient involved in malabsorption depends on the type and location of the abnormality in the intestinal tract.

Deficiencies of bile salts can lead to malabsorption of fats and fat-soluble vitamins. Bile salt deficiencies can result from decreased synthesis of bile in the liver, bile obstruction, or alteration of bile salt absorption in the small intestine.

Enzymes normally found in the intestine split disaccharides (complex sugars) to monosaccharides (simple sugars). Examples of these enzymes are lactase, sucrase, maltase, and isomaltase. Lactase deficiency is the most common disaccharide enzyme deficiency. Without sufficient amounts of this enzyme, the body is not able to break down lactose. Lactase deficiency can be due to genetic inheritance, injury to intestinal mucosa from viral hepatitis, or excessive bacteria in the intestine. Deficiencies of the other disaccharide enzymes are rare.

Pancreatic enzymes are also necessary for absorption of vitamin B_{12}. With destruction or obstruction of the pancreas or insufficient pancreatic stimulation, this nutrient is not well absorbed. Chronic pancreatitis, pancreatic carcinoma, resection of the pancreas, and cystic fibrosis can cause these malabsorption problems.

Loops of bowel can accumulate intestinal contents, resulting in bacterial overgrowth, when peristalsis is decreased. Bacteria at these sites break down bile salts, and fewer salts are available for fat absorption. They can also ingest vitamin B_{12}, which contributes to vitamin B_{12} deficiency. This process can occur after a gastrectomy.

Obstruction to lymphatic flow in the intestine can lead to loss of plasma proteins along with loss of minerals (e.g., iron, copper, calcium), vitamin B_{12}, folic acid, and lipids. Lymphatic obstruction can be caused by many conditions. Certain cancers such as lymphoma, inflammatory states, radiation enteritis, Crohn's disease, heart failure, and constrictive pericarditis are causes of lymphatic obstruction.

Interference with blood flow to the intestinal mucosa results in malabsorption. With intestinal surgery, there is loss of the surface area needed to facilitate absorption. Resection of the ileum results in vitamin B_{12}, bile salt, and other nutrient deficiencies. Gastric surgery is one of the most common causes of malabsorption and maldigestion. Other conditions associated with poor digestion and malabsorption include small-bowel ischemia and radiation enteritis.

❖ PATIENT-CENTERED COLLABORATIVE CARE

◆ Assessment

Chronic diarrhea is a classic symptom of malabsorption. It occurs as a result of unabsorbed nutrients, which add to the bulk of the stool, and unabsorbed fat. **Steatorrhea** (greater than normal amounts of fat in the feces) is a common sign. It is a result of bile salt deconjugation, nonabsorbed fats, or bacteria in the intestine. Not all patients with malabsorption have diarrhea. Instead, some have an increased stool mass. Other clinical manifestations include:

- Unintentional weight loss
- Bloating and flatus (carbohydrate malabsorption)
- Decreased libido
- Easy bruising (purpura)
- Anemia (with iron and folic acid or vitamin B_{12} deficiencies)
- Bone pain (with calcium and vitamin D deficiencies)
- Edema (caused by hypoproteinemia)

Serum laboratory studies reveal a decrease in mean corpuscular volume (MCV), mean corpuscular hemoglobin (MCH), and mean corpuscular hemoglobin concentration (MCHC). These decreases indicate hypochromic microcytic anemia resulting from iron deficiency. Increased MCV and variable MCH and MCHC values indicate macrocytic anemia resulting from vitamin B_{12} and folic acid deficiencies. Serum iron levels are low in protein malabsorption because of insufficient gastric acid for use of iron. Serum cholesterol levels may be low from decreased absorption and digestion of fat. Low serum calcium levels may indicate malabsorption of vitamin D and amino acids. Low levels of serum vitamin A (retinol) and carotene, its precursor, indicate a bile salt deficiency and malabsorption of fat. Serum albumin and total protein levels are low if protein is lost.

A quantitative *fecal fat analysis* is often elevated in either malabsorption or maldigestive disorders (Pagana & Pagana, 2014).

A *lactose tolerance test* is a type of disaccharidase analysis that may show an inability to digest foods and beverages that contain lactose. A hydrogen breath test can also be performed to detect this problem. The D-xylose absorption test can reveal low urine and serum D-xylose levels if malabsorption in the small intestine is present (Pagana & Pagana, 2014).

The *Schilling test* measures urinary excretion of vitamin B_{12} for diagnosis of pernicious anemia and a variety of other malabsorption syndromes. The *bile acid breath test* assesses the absorption of bile salt. If the patient has bacterial overgrowth, the bile salts will become deconjugated and the carbon dioxide level in the breath will peak earlier than expected.

Ultrasonography is used to diagnose pancreatic tumors and tumors in the small intestine that are causing malabsorption. X-rays of the GI tract reveal pancreatic calcifications, tumors, or other abnormalities that cause malabsorption. A CT scan may also be done.

◆ Interventions

Interventions for most malabsorption syndromes focus on (1) avoidance of substances that aggravate malabsorption and (2) supplementation of nutrients. Surgical management of the primary disease may be indicated. Drug therapy may also improve or resolve malabsorption.

NUTRITION management includes a low-fat diet for patients who have gallbladder disease, severe steatorrhea, or cystic fibrosis. A low-fat diet may or may not be indicated for pancreatic insufficiency because this disorder improves with enzyme replacement. Some clinicians believe that limitation of fat intake is not necessary with enzyme replacement. Dietary intake of fat is actually beneficial to the patient because it has a high number of calories. After a total gastrectomy, a high-protein, high-calorie diet and small, frequent meals are recommended. Lactose-free or lactose-restricted diets are available for patients with lactase deficiency, and gluten-free diets are available for those with celiac disease, discussed in Chapter 57.

The health care provider prescribes nutritional supplements according to the specific deficiency. Common supplements include:

- Water-soluble vitamins, such as folic acid and vitamin B complex
- Fat-soluble vitamins, such as vitamin A, vitamin D, and vitamin K
- Minerals, such as calcium, iron, and magnesium
- Pancreatic enzymes, such as pancrelipase (Pancrease, Viokase)

CHART 56-8 Best Practice for Patient Safety & Quality Care QSEN

Special Skin Care for Patients with Chronic Diarrhea

- Use medicated wipes or premoistened disposable wipes rather than toilet tissue to clean the perineal area.
- Clean the perineal area well with mild soap and warm water after each stool; rinse soap from the area well.
- If the physician allows, provide a sitz bath several times per day.
- Apply a thin coat of A+D Ointment or other medicated protective barrier, such as aloe products, after each stool.
- Keep the patient off the affected buttock area.
- For open areas, cover with thin DuoDerm or Tegaderm occlusive dressing to promote rapid healing.
- Observe for fungal or yeast infections, which appear as dark red rashes with "satellite" lesions. Obtain prescription for medication if this problem occurs.

Antibiotics are used to treat disorders involving bacterial overgrowth. Bacterial overgrowth can be caused by a variety of disorders but is often treated with tetracycline and metronidazole (Flagyl, Novonidazol 🍁).

Drug therapy is used to control the clinical manifestations of malabsorption. Antidiarrheal agents, such as diphenoxylate hydrochloride and atropine sulfate (Lomotil, N-Lomotil 🍁), are often used to control diarrhea and steatorrhea. Anticholinergics, such as dicyclomine hydrochloride (Bentyl, Bentylol 🍁), may be given before meals to inhibit gastric motility. IV fluids may be necessary to replenish fluid losses associated with diarrhea.

Provide special measures to protect the skin when chronic diarrhea occurs (Chart 56-8). Conduct an ongoing assessment for clinical manifestations of malabsorption, and relate these to activities and dietary intake. For example, patients with steatorrhea are monitored for FLUID AND ELECTROLYTE BALANCE and are encouraged to drink electrolyte-rich liquids liberally. Teach them the rationale for dietary, drug, and surgical management of nutritional deficiencies, and evaluate interventions on the basis of changes in or resolution of clinical manifestations.

NURSING CONCEPTS AND CLINICAL JUDGMENT REVIEW

What might you NOTICE if the patient has impaired absorption and inadequate NUTRITION as a result of noninflammatory intestinal disorders?

- Rectal bleeding
- Report of change in bowel habits
- Diarrhea or report of constipation
- Fatigue
- Vomiting
- Abdominal pain
- Change in bowel sounds (decreased or increased)
- Weight loss

What should you INTERPRET and how should you RESPOND to a patient with impaired absorption and inadequate NUTRITION as a result of noninflammatory intestinal disorders?

Perform and interpret focused physical assessment findings, including:

- Vital signs
- Complete pain assessment
- Abdominal assessment
- Current weight compared with previous weight

Respond by:

- Decreasing abdominal pain by placing patient in sitting position
- Starting IV (large-bore catheter) to replace fluids and electrolytes
- Giving blood transfusion as prescribed
- Providing rest
- Providing privacy and dignity

- Assisting with hygiene as needed
- Inserting nasogastric tube and connecting to low suction as needed
- Checking laboratory values of hemoglobin and hematocrit
- Checking stool for occult or frank blood
- Giving antidiarrheal drugs if prescribed
- Recording intake and output
- Assisting with ADLs and ambulation as needed

On what should you REFLECT?

- Continue to monitor for vomiting and diarrhea and for changes in pain.
- Think about what you need to document. Decide when you might need to call the health care provider or Rapid Response Team.
- Determine what health teaching and community resources may be needed for the patient and family.
- Think about what you can do to help prevent complications of the health problem.

GET READY FOR THE NCLEX® EXAMINATION!

KEY POINTS

Review these Key Points for each NCLEX Examination Client Needs Category.

Safe and Effective Care Environment

- Prioritize care for patients experiencing abdominal trauma: first assess airway, breathing, and circulation (ABCs), and then monitor vital signs, mental status, and skin perfusion to assess for hypovolemic shock. **Safety** QSEN
- Collaborate with the certified wound, ostomy, continence nurse (CWOCN) or enterostomal therapist (ET) when a patient is scheduled for or has a new colostomy. **Teamwork and Collaboration** QSEN
- Collaborate with the case manager/discharge planner, health care provider, and CWOCN to plan care for the patient with CRC. **Teamwork and Collaboration** QSEN

Health Promotion and Maintenance

- Refer patients with familial CRC syndromes for genetic counseling and testing. **Patient-Centered Care** QSEN
- Refer ostomy patients to the United Ostomy Associations of America, Inc. and the American Cancer Society for additional information and support groups. **Patient-Centered Care** QSEN
- Teach patients with irritable bowel syndrome (IBS) to avoid GI stimulants, such as caffeine, alcohol, and milk and milk products, and to manage stress. **Evidence-Based Practice** QSEN
- Instruct patients on dietary modifications to decrease the occurrence of colorectal cancer (CRC), such as eating a diet high in fiber and avoiding red meat. **Evidence-Based Practice** QSEN
- Teach adults 50 years and older to have routine screening for CRC as listed in Chart 56-2; people with genetic predispositions should have earlier and more frequent screening. **Evidence-Based Practice** QSEN
- Teach people to prevent or manage constipation to help avoid hemorrhoids; teach patients the importance of maintaining a healthy weight to decrease the risk for hemorrhoids. **Evidence-Based Practice** QSEN
- Teach patients and caregivers how to provide colostomy care, including dietary measures, skin care, and ostomy products. **Patient-Centered Care** QSEN

Psychosocial Integrity

- Assist the patient with CRC with the grieving process. **Patient-Centered Care** QSEN
- Be aware that having a colostomy is a life-altering event that can severely impact one's body image; issues related to sexuality and fear of acceptance should be discussed. **Patient-Centered Care** QSEN

Physiological Integrity

- Be aware that minimally invasive inguinal hernia repair is an ambulatory care procedure done via laparoscopy; postoperative management requires health teaching regarding rest for a few days and inspection of incisions for signs of infection (see Chart 56-1). **Evidence-Based Practice** QSEN
- Be aware that a strangulated hernia can cause ischemia and bowel obstruction, requiring immediate intervention. **Safety** QSEN
- Monitor patients who have conventional open herniorrhaphy for ability to void. **Safety** QSEN
- Recall that changes in bowel habits or stool characteristics and/or rectal bleeding are often associated with a diagnosis of CRC. **Safety** QSEN
- Keep the peristomal skin clean and dry; observe for leakage around the pouch seal. **Evidence-Based Practice** QSEN
- Provide meticulous perineal wound care for patients having an abdominoperineal (AP) resection, as described in Chart 56-3. **Safety** QSEN
- Document the characteristics of the colostomy stoma, which should be reddish pink and moist; report abnormalities such as ischemia and necrosis (purplish or black) or unusual bleeding to the surgeon. **Informatics** QSEN
- Recall that bowel sounds are altered in patients with obstruction; absent bowel sounds imply total obstruction. **Safety** QSEN
- Assess the patient's nasogastric tube for proper placement, patency, and output at least every 4 hours. **Safety** QSEN
- Monitor patients with bowel obstruction for signs and symptoms of fluid, electrolyte, and acid-base imbalances; patients with small bowel obstruction are at greater risk for problems with FLUID AND ELECTROLYTE BALANCE. **Safety** QSEN
- Teach patients having hemorrhoid surgery to take stool softeners before and after surgery to decrease discomfort during ELIMINATION. **Evidence-Based Practice** QSEN
- Provide comfort measures for the patient who has chronic diarrhea associated with malabsorption as described in Chart 56-8. **Patient-Centered Care** QSEN
- Reinforce teaching regarding supplements or dietary restrictions needed for malabsorption management. **Evidence-Based Practice** QSEN

57 CHAPTER

Care of Patients with Inflammatory Intestinal Disorders

Donna D. Ignatavicius

http://evolve.elsevier.com/Iggy/

PRIORITY CONCEPTS

- Elimination
- Inflammation
- Nutrition
- Pain
- Infection
- Fluid and Electrolyte Balance

LEARNING OUTCOMES

Safe and Effective Care Environment

1. Describe the importance of collaborating with health care team members to provide care for patients with inflammatory bowel disease (IBD).

Health Promotion and Maintenance

2. Develop a health teaching plan for patients to promote self-management when caring for ileostomy or other surgical diversion.
3. Identify community resources for patients and families regarding IBD.
4. Discuss ways that gastroenteritis can be prevented.

Psychosocial Integrity

5. Identify expected body image changes associated with having an ileostomy or other surgical diversion.

Physiological Integrity

6. Differentiate common types of acute inflammatory bowel disorders.
7. Develop an evidence-based collaborative plan of care for the patient who has appendicitis or peritonitis.
8. Compare and contrast the pathophysiology and clinical manifestations of ulcerative colitis and Crohn's disease.
9. Identify priority problems for patients with ulcerative colitis.
10. Explain the purpose of and nursing implications related to drug therapy for patients with IBD.
11. Plan evidence-based postoperative care for a patient undergoing surgery for IBD.
12. Develop a hospital discharge teaching plan for patients who have IBD.
13. Explain the role of NUTRITION therapy in managing the patient with diverticular disease.
14. Describe the comfort measures to relieve PAIN that the nurse can implement for the patient with anal disorders.

Inflammatory bowel health problems affect the small intestine, large intestine (colon), or both. Together, these organs are called the *intestinal tract*. Continued digestion of food and absorption of nutrients occur primarily in the small intestine (bowel) to meet the body's needs for energy. Water is reabsorbed in the large intestine to help maintain a fluid balance and promote the passage of waste products. When the intestinal tract and its nearby structures become inflamed, NUTRITION may be inadequate to meet a patient's needs. Bowel ELIMINATION changes, PAIN, INFECTION, and/or problems with FLUID AND ELECTROLYTE BALANCE can result from inflammatory bowel diseases that are chronic.

ACUTE INFLAMMATORY BOWEL DISORDERS

Appendicitis, gastroenteritis, and peritonitis are the most common acute inflammatory bowel problems. These disorders are potentially life threatening and can have major systemic complications if not treated promptly.

APPENDICITIS

❖ PATHOPHYSIOLOGY

Appendicitis is an acute INFLAMMATION of the vermiform appendix that occurs most often among young adults. It is the most common cause of right lower quadrant (RLQ) PAIN. The appendix usually extends off the proximal cecum of the colon just below the ileocecal valve. Inflammation occurs when the lumen (opening) of the appendix is obstructed (blocked), leading to infection as bacteria invade the wall of the appendix. The initial obstruction is usually a result of fecaliths (very hard pieces of feces) composed of calcium phosphate–rich mucus and inorganic salts. Less common causes are malignant tumors, helminthes (worms), or other INFECTIONS (McCance et al., 2014).

When the lumen is blocked, the mucosa secretes fluid, increasing the internal pressure and restricting blood flow, which results in PAIN. If the process occurs slowly, an abscess may develop, but a rapid process may result in peritonitis (INFLAMMATION and INFECTION of the peritoneum). *All complications of peritonitis are serious. Gangrene and sepsis can occur within 24 to 36 hours, are life threatening, and are some of the most common indications for emergency surgery. Perforation may develop within 24 hours, but the risk rises rapidly after 48 hours.* Perforation of the appendix also results in peritonitis with a temperature of greater than 101°F (38.3°C) and a rise in pulse rate.

CONSIDERATIONS FOR OLDER ADULTS

Patient-Centered Care QSEN

Appendicitis is relatively rare at extremes in age. However, perforation is more common in older people, causing a higher mortality rate. The diagnosis of appendicitis is difficult to establish in older adults because symptoms of pain and tenderness may not be as pronounced in this age-group. This difference results in treatment delay and an increased risk for perforation, peritonitis, and death.

PATIENT-CENTERED COLLABORATIVE CARE

Assessment

History taking and tracking the sequence of symptoms are important because nausea or vomiting before abdominal pain can indicate gastroenteritis. Abdominal PAIN followed by nausea and vomiting can indicate appendicitis. Ask about risk factors such as age, familial tendency, and intra-abdominal tumors. Classically, patients with appendicitis have cramplike pain in the epigastric or periumbilical area. Anorexia is a frequent symptom with nausea and vomiting occurring in many cases.

Perform a complete pain assessment. Initially, PAIN can present anywhere in the abdomen or flank area. As the INFLAMMATION and INFECTION progress, the pain becomes more severe and steady and shifts to the RLQ between the anterior iliac crest and the umbilicus. This area is referred to as *McBurney's point* (Fig. 57-1). *Abdominal pain that increases with cough or movement and is relieved by bending the right hip or the knees suggests perforation and peritonitis.* An advanced practice nurse or other health care provider assesses for muscle rigidity and guarding on palpation of the abdomen. The patient may report pain after release of pressure. This is referred to as "rebound" tenderness.

Laboratory findings do not establish the diagnosis, but often there is a moderate elevation of the *white blood cell (WBC) count* (leukocytosis) to 10,000 to 18,000/mm^3 with a "shift to the left" (an increased number of immature WBCs). A WBC elevation to greater than 20,000/mm^3 may indicate a perforated

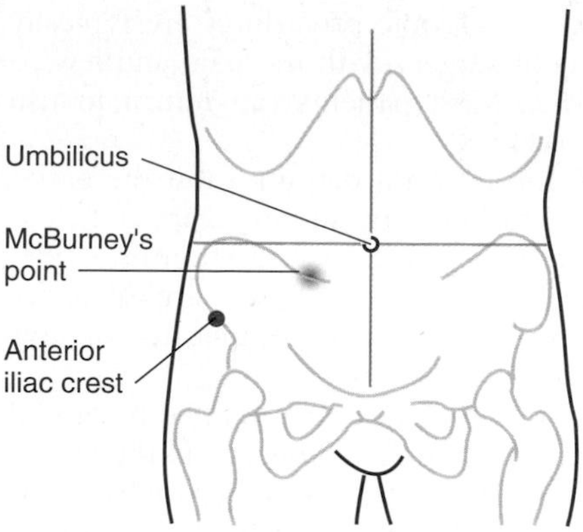

FIG. 57-1 McBurney's point is located midway between the anterior iliac crest and the umbilicus in the right lower quadrant. This is the classic area for localized tenderness during the later stages of appendicitis.

appendix. An *ultrasound* study may show the presence of an enlarged appendix. If symptoms are recurrent or prolonged, a CT scan can be used for diagnosis and may reveal the presence of a fecalith.

Interventions

All patients with suspected or confirmed appendicitis are hospitalized and most have surgery to remove the inflamed appendix.

Nonsurgical Management. Keep the patient with suspected or known appendicitis on NPO to prepare for the possibility of surgery and to avoid making the INFLAMMATION worse.

NURSING SAFETY PRIORITY QSEN

Action Alert

For the patient with suspected appendicitis, administer IV fluids as prescribed to maintain FLUID AND ELECTROLYTE BALANCE and to replace fluid volume. If tolerated, advise the patient to maintain a semi-Fowler's position so that abdominal drainage, if any, can be contained in the lower abdomen. Once the diagnosis of appendicitis is confirmed and surgery is scheduled, administer opioid analgesics and antibiotics as prescribed. *The patient with suspected or confirmed appendicitis should not receive laxatives or enemas, which can cause perforation of the appendix. Do not apply heat to the abdomen because this may increase circulation to the appendix and result in increased inflammation and perforation!*

Surgical Management. Surgery is required as soon as possible. An **appendectomy** is the removal of the inflamed appendix by one of several surgical approaches. Uncomplicated appendectomy procedures are done via laparoscopy. A **laparoscopy** is a minimally invasive surgical (MIS) procedure with one or more small incisions near the umbilicus through which a small endoscope is placed. Patients having this type of surgery for appendix removal have few postoperative complications (see Chapter 15). A newer procedure known as natural orifice transluminal endoscopic surgery (NOTES) (e.g., transvaginal endoscopic appendectomy) does not require an external skin incision. In this procedure the surgeon places the endoscope into the vagina or other orifice and makes a small incision to enter the peritoneal space. Patients having any type of laparoscopic procedures are typically discharged the same day of surgery with less pain and few complications after discharge. Most patients can return to usual activities in 1 to 2 weeks.

If the diagnosis is not definitive but the patient is at high risk for complications from suspected appendicitis, the surgeon may perform an exploratory laparotomy to rule out appendicitis. A **laparotomy** is an open surgical approach with a large abdominal incision for complicated or atypical appendicitis or peritonitis.

Preoperative teaching is often limited because the patient is in PAIN or may be transferred quickly to the operating suite for emergency surgery. The patient is prepared for general anesthesia and surgery as described in Chapter 14. After surgery, care of the patient who has undergone an appendectomy is the same as that required for anyone who has received general anesthesia (see Chapter 16).

If complications such as peritonitis or abscesses are found during *open* traditional surgery, wound drains are inserted and a nasogastric tube may be placed to decompress the stomach and prevent abdominal distention. Administer IV antibiotics and opioid analgesics as prescribed. Help the patient out of bed on the evening of surgery to help prevent respiratory complications, such as atelectasis. He or she may be hospitalized for as long as 3 to 5 days and return to normal activity in 4 to 6 weeks.

PERITONITIS

Peritonitis is a life-threatening, acute INFLAMMATION and INFECTION of the visceral/parietal peritoneum and endothelial lining of the abdominal cavity. Primary peritonitis is rare and indicates the peritoneum is infected via the bloodstream. This problem is not discussed here.

❖ PATHOPHYSIOLOGY

Normally the peritoneal cavity contains about 50 mL of sterile fluid (transudate), which prevents friction in the abdominal cavity during peristalsis. When the peritoneal cavity is contaminated by bacteria, the body first begins an inflammatory reaction walling off a localized area to fight the INFECTION. This local reaction involves vascular dilation and increased capillary permeability, allowing transport of leukocytes and subsequent phagocytosis of the offending organisms. If this walling-off process fails, the INFLAMMATION spreads and contamination becomes massive, resulting in diffuse (widespread) peritonitis.

Peritonitis is most often caused by contamination of the peritoneal cavity by bacteria or chemicals. Bacteria gain entry into the peritoneum by perforation (from appendicitis, diverticulitis, peptic ulcer disease) or from an external penetrating wound, a gangrenous gallbladder, bowel obstruction, or ascending infection through the genital tract. Less common causes include perforating tumors, leakage or contamination during surgery, and INFECTION by skin pathogens in patients undergoing continuous ambulatory peritoneal dialysis (CAPD). Common bacteria responsible for peritonitis include *Escherichia coli, Streptococcus, Staphylococcus, Pneumococcus,* and *Gonococcus.* Chemical peritonitis results from leakage of bile, pancreatic enzymes, and gastric acid (McCance et al., 2014).

When diagnosis and treatment of peritonitis are delayed, blood vessel dilation continues. The body responds to the continuing infectious process by shunting extra blood to the area of INFLAMMATION (hyperemia). Fluid is shifted from the extracellular fluid compartment into the peritoneal cavity, connective tissues, and GI tract (*"third spacing"*). This shift of fluid can result in a significant decrease in circulatory volume and *hypovolemic shock.* Severely decreased circulatory volume can result in insufficient perfusion of the kidneys, leading to acute kidney injury with impaired FLUID AND ELECTROLYTE BALANCE (McCance et al., 2014). Assess for clinical manifestations of these life-threatening problems.

Peristalsis slows or *stops* in response to severe peritoneal INFLAMMATION, and the lumen of the bowel becomes distended with gas and fluid. Fluid that normally flows to the small bowel and the colon for reabsorption accumulates in the intestine in volumes of 7 to 8 L daily. The toxins or bacteria responsible for the peritonitis can also enter the bloodstream from the peritoneal area and lead to bacteremia or **septicemia** (bacterial invasion of the blood).

Respiratory problems can occur as a result of increased abdominal pressure against the diaphragm from intestinal distention and fluid shifts to the peritoneal cavity. PAIN can interfere with respirations at a time when the patient has an increased oxygen demand because of the infectious process.

❖ PATIENT-CENTERED COLLABORATIVE CARE

◆ Assessment

Ask the patient about abdominal PAIN, and determine the character of the pain (e.g., cramping, sharp, aching), location of the pain, and whether the pain is localized or generalized. Ask about a history of a low-grade fever or recent spikes in temperature.

Physical findings of peritonitis (Chart 57-1) depend on several factors: the stage of the disease, the ability of the body to localize the process by walling off the infection, and whether the INFLAMMATION has progressed to generalized peritonitis. The patient most often appears acutely ill, lying still, possibly with the knees flexed. Movement is guarded, and he or she may report and show signs of pain (e.g., facial grimacing) with coughing or movement of any type. During inspection, observe for progressive abdominal distention, often seen when the inflammation markedly reduces intestinal motility. Auscultate for bowel sounds, which usually disappear with progression of the inflammation.

CHART 57-1 Key Features

Peritonitis

- Rigid, boardlike abdomen (classic)
- Abdominal pain (localized, poorly localized, or referred to the shoulder or chest)
- Distended abdomen
- Nausea, anorexia, vomiting
- Diminishing bowel sounds
- Inability to pass flatus or feces
- Rebound tenderness in the abdomen
- High fever
- Tachycardia
- Dehydration from high fever (poor skin turgor)
- Decreased urine output
- Hiccups
- Possible compromise in respiratory status

The cardinal signs of peritonitis are abdominal pain, tenderness, and distention. In the patient with *localized* peritonitis, the abdomen is tender on palpation in a well-defined area with rebound tenderness in this area. With *generalized* peritonitis, tenderness is widespread.

! NURSING SAFETY PRIORITY QSEN

Action Alert

For patients with peritonitis, assess for abdominal wall rigidity, which is a classic finding that is sometimes referred to as a "boardlike" abdomen. Monitor the patient for a high fever because of the infectious process. Assess for tachycardia occurring in response to the fever and decreased circulating blood volume. Observe whether he or she has dry mucous membranes and a low urine output seen with third spacing. Nausea and vomiting may also be present. Hiccups may occur as a result of diaphragmatic irritation. Be sure to document all assessment findings.

White blood cell (WBC) counts are often elevated to 20,000/mm^3 with a high neutrophil count. *Blood culture* studies may be done to determine whether septicemia has occurred and to identify the causative organism to enable appropriate therapy. The health care provider requests laboratory tests to assess FLUID AND ELECTROLYTE BALANCE and renal status, including blood urea nitrogen (BUN), creatinine, hemoglobin, and hematocrit. Oxygen saturation and end–carbon dioxide monitoring may be obtained to assess respiratory function and acid-base balance.

Abdominal x-rays can assess for free air or fluid in the abdominal cavity, indicating perforation. The x-rays may also show dilation, edema, and inflammation of the small and large intestines. An *abdominal ultrasound* may also be performed.

◆ Interventions

Patients with peritonitis are hospitalized because of the severe nature of the illness. If complications are extensive, the patients are often admitted to a critical care unit. Nursing interventions focus on the early identification of complications.

Nonsurgical Management. The health care provider prescribes hypertonic IV fluids and broad-spectrum antibiotics immediately after establishing the diagnosis of peritonitis. IV fluids are used to replace fluids collected in the peritoneum and bowel. Monitor daily weight and intake and output carefully. A nasogastric tube (NGT) decompresses the stomach and the intestine, and the patient is NPO. Apply oxygen as prescribed and according to the patient's respiratory status and oxygen saturation via pulse oximetry (e.g., Spo_2 less than 93%). Administer analgesics, and monitor for pain control. Document all PAIN assessments and interventions thoroughly.

Surgical Management. Abdominal surgery may be needed to identify and repair the cause of the peritonitis. If the patient is so critically ill that surgery would be life threatening, it may be delayed. Surgery focuses on controlling the contamination, removing foreign material from the peritoneal cavity, and draining collected fluid.

Exploratory laparotomy (surgical opening into the abdomen) or laparoscopy is used to remove or repair the inflamed or perforated organ (e.g., appendectomy for an inflamed appendix; a colon resection, with or without a colostomy, for a perforated diverticulum). Before the incision(s) is closed, the surgeon irrigates the peritoneum with antibiotic solutions. Several catheters may be inserted to drain the cavity and provide a route for irrigation after surgery.

The preoperative care is similar to that described in Chapter 14 for patients having general anesthesia. Chapter 16 describes general postoperative care for exploratory laparotomy. Multi-system complications can occur with peritonitis. Loss of fluids and electrolytes from the extracellular space to the peritoneal cavity, NGT suctioning, and NPO status require that the patient receives IV fluid replacement. Be sure that unlicensed assistive personnel (UAP) carefully measure intake and output. Fluid rates may be changed frequently based on laboratory values and patient condition.

! NURSING SAFETY PRIORITY QSEN

Action Alert

Monitor the patient's level of consciousness, vital signs, respiratory status (respiratory rate and breath sounds), and intake and output at least hourly immediately after abdominal surgery. Maintain the patient in a semi-Fowler's position to promote drainage of peritoneal contents into the lower region of the abdominal cavity. This position helps increase lung expansion.

If an open surgical procedure is needed, the INFECTION may slow healing of an incision or the incision may be partially open to heal by second or third intention. These wounds require special care involving manual irrigation or packing as prescribed by the surgeon. If the surgeon requests peritoneal irrigation through a drain, *maintain sterile technique during manual irrigation.* Assess whether the patient retains the fluid used for irrigation by comparing the amount of fluid returned with the amount of fluid instilled. Fluid retention could cause abdominal distention or pain.

Community-Based Care

The length of hospitalization depends on the extent and severity of the infectious process. Patients who have a localized abscess drained and who respond to antibiotics and IV fluids without multi-system complications are discharged in several days. Others may require mechanical ventilation or hemodialysis with longer hospital stays. Some patients may be transferred to a transitional care unit to complete their antibiotic therapy and recovery. Convalescence is often longer than for other surgeries because of multi-system involvement.

When discharged home, assess the patient's ability for self-management at home with the added task of incision care and a reduced activity tolerance. Provide the patient and family with written and oral instructions to report these problems to the health care provider immediately:

- Unusual or foul-smelling drainage
- Swelling, redness, or warmth or bleeding from the incision site
- A temperature higher than 101° F (38.3° C)
- Abdominal PAIN
- Signs of wound dehiscence or ileus

Patients with large incisions heal by second or third intention and may require dressings, solution, and catheter-tipped syringes to irrigate the wound. A home care nurse may be needed to assess, irrigate, or pack the wound and change the dressing as needed until the patient and family feel comfortable with the procedure. If the patient needs assistance with ADLs, a home care aide or temporary placement in a skilled care facility may be indicated. Collaborate with the case manager (CM) to determine the most appropriate setting for seamless continuing care in the community.

Review information about antibiotics and analgesics. For patients taking oral opioid analgesics such as oxycodone with acetaminophen (Tylox, Percocet, Endocet ♣) for any length of time, a stool softener such as docusate sodium (Colace, Regulex ♣) may be prescribed. Older adults are especially at risk for constipation from codeine-based drugs. Remind patients to avoid taking additional acetaminophen (Tylenol) to prevent liver toxicity.

Teach patients to refrain from any lifting for *at least* 6 weeks after an open surgical procedure. Other activity limitations are made on an individual basis with the physician's recommendation. Patients who have laparoscopic surgery can resume activities within a week or two and may not have any major restrictions.

NCLEX EXAMINATION CHALLENGE

Safe and Effective Care Environment

A client had a bowel resection yesterday for colorectal cancer. Which assessment finding does the nurse report immediately to the surgeon?

A. Abdominal discomfort
B. Mild abdominal distention
C. Distended, board-like abdomen
D. Minimal abdominal bowel sounds

GASTROENTERITIS

❖ PATHOPHYSIOLOGY

Gastroenteritis is a very common health problem worldwide that causes diarrhea and/or vomiting as a result of INFLAMMATION of the mucous membranes of the stomach and intestinal tract. It affects mainly the small bowel and can be caused by either viral or bacterial INFECTION. Viral gastroenteritis is the most common (Krenzer, 2012). Table 57-1 lists common types of gastroenteritis and their primary characteristics.

Norovirus (also known as Norwalk-like viruses) is the leading foodborne disease that causes gastroenteritis. It occurs most often between November and April because it is resistant to low temperatures and has a long viral shedding before and after the illness. Norovirus is transmitted (spread) through the fecal-oral route from person to person and from contaminated food and water. Infected people can also contaminate surfaces and objects in the environment. Vomiting causes the virus to become airborne. The incubation time is 1 to 2 days.

In most cases of gastroenteritis, the illness is self-limiting and lasts about 3 days. However, in people who are immunosuppressed or in older adults, dehydration and hypovolemia can occur as complications requiring medical attention and possibly hospitalization.

TABLE 57-1 Common Types of Gastroenteritis and Their Characteristics

TYPE	CHARACTERISTICS
Viral Gastroenteritis	
Epidemic viral	Caused by many parvovirus-type organisms Transmitted by the fecal-oral route in food and water Incubation period 10-51 hrs Communicable during acute illness
Norovirus (Norwalk viruses)	Transmitted by the fecal-oral route and possibly the respiratory route (vomitus) Incubation in 48 hrs Affects adults of all ages Older adults can become hypovolemic and experience electrolyte imbalances
Bacterial Gastroenteritis	
Campylobacter enteritis	Transmitted by the fecal-oral route or by contact with infected animals or infants Incubation period 1-10 days Communicable for 2-7 wks
Escherichia coli diarrhea	Transmitted by fecal contamination of food, water, or fomites
Shigellosis	Transmitted by direct and indirect fecal-oral routes Incubation period 1-7 days Communicable during the acute illness to 4 wk after the illness Humans possibly carriers for months

Health Promotion and Maintenance

Outbreaks of norovirus have occurred in prisons, cruise ships, nursing homes, college dormitories, and other places where large groups of people are in close proximity. Handwashing and sanitizing surfaces and other environmental items help prevent the spread of the illness. Hand sanitizers are often placed in public areas so that hands can be cleaned when washing with soap and water is inconvenient. Proper food and beverage preparation is also important to prevent contamination.

❖ PATIENT-CENTERED COLLABORATIVE CARE

◆ Assessment

The patient history can provide information related to the potential cause of the illness. Ask about recent travel, especially to tropical regions of Asia, Africa, or Central or South America. Some areas of Mexico may also be the source of gastroenteritis.

Also inquire if the patient has eaten at any restaurant in the past 24 to 36 hours. Some people have acquired gastroenteritis from eating in "fast food" restaurants or from food items purchased at a farmer's market or grocery store. Bacterial INFECTIONS have caused large outbreaks that resulted from contaminated spinach and lettuce in the United States.

The patient who has gastroenteritis usually looks ill. Nausea and vomiting typically occur first, followed by abdominal cramping and diarrhea.

For patients who are older or for those who have inadequate immune systems, weakness and cardiac dysrhythmias may occur from loss of potassium (hypokalemia) from diarrhea. Monitor for and document manifestations of hypokalemia and hypovolemia (dehydration).

! NURSING SAFETY PRIORITY (QSEN)

Action Alert

For patients with gastroenteritis, note any abdominal distention and listen for hyperactive bowel sounds. Depending on the amount of fluids and electrolytes lost through diarrhea and vomiting, patients may have varying degrees of dehydration manifested by:

- Poor skin turgor
- Fever (not common in older adults)
- Dry mucous membranes
- Orthostatic blood pressure changes (which can cause falls, especially for older adults)
- Hypotension
- Oliguria (scant urinary output)

In some cases, dehydration may be severe. Dehydration occurs rapidly in older adults. Monitor mental status changes, such as acute confusion, that result from hypoxia in the older adult. These changes may be the only clinical manifestation of dehydration in older adults.

◆ Interventions

For any type of gastroenteritis, encourage fluid replacement. The amount and route of fluid administration are determined by the patient's hydration status and overall health condition. Teach patients to drink extra fluids to replace fluid lost through vomiting and diarrhea. Oral rehydration therapy (ORT) may be needed for some patients to replace fluids and electrolytes. Examples of ORT solutions include Gatorade, Pedialyte, and Powerade. Depending on the patient's age and severity of dehydration, he or she may be admitted to the hospital for gastroenteritis or may stay in the emergency department or urgent care center until adequate hydration is restored.

Drugs that suppress intestinal motility may not be given for bacterial or viral gastroenteritis. *Use of these drugs can prevent the infecting organisms from being eliminated from the body.* If the health care provider determines that antiperistaltic agents are necessary, an initial dose of loperamide (Imodium) 4 mg can be administered orally, followed by 2 mg after each loose stool, up to 16 mg daily.

! NURSING SAFETY PRIORITY (QSEN)

Drug Alert

Diphenoxylate hydrochloride with atropine sulfate (Lomotil, Lomanate) reduces GI motility but is used sparingly because of its habit-forming ability. *The drug should not be used for older adults because it also causes drowsiness and could contribute to falls.*

Treatment with antibiotics may be needed if the gastroenteritis is due to bacterial infection with fever and severe diarrhea. Depending on the type and severity of the illness, examples of drugs that may be prescribed include ciprofloxacin (Cipro), levofloxacin (Levaquin), or azithromycin (Zithromax). If the gastroenteritis is due to shigellosis, anti-infective agents such as trimethoprim/sulfamethoxazole (Septra DS, Bactrim DS, Roubac 🍁) or ciprofloxacin (Cipro) are prescribed.

Frequent stools that are rich in electrolytes and enzymes, as well as frequent wiping and washing of the anal region, can irritate the skin. Teach the patient to avoid toilet paper and harsh soaps. Ideally, he or she can gently clean the area with warm water or an absorbent material, followed by thorough but gentle drying. Cream, oil, or gel can be applied to a damp, warm washcloth to remove stool that sticks to open skin. Special prepared skin wipes can also be used. Protective barrier cream can be applied to the skin between stools. Sitz baths for 10 minutes 2 or 3 times daily can also relieve discomfort.

If leakage of stool is a problem, the patient can use an absorbent cotton or panty liner and keep it in place with snug underwear. For patients who are incontinent, remind unlicensed assistive personnel (UAP) to keep the perineal and buttock areas clean and dry. The use of incontinent pads at night instead of briefs allows air to circulate to the skin and prevents irritation.

During the acute phase of the illness, teach the patient and family about the importance of fluid replacement. Teaching the patient and family about reducing the risk for transmission of gastroenteritis is also important (Chart 57-2).

CHRONIC INFLAMMATORY BOWEL DISEASE

Ulcerative colitis and Crohn's disease are the two most common inflammatory bowel diseases (IBDs) that affect adults. Comparisons and differences are listed in Table 57-2. Viral and bacterial gastroenteritis can cause symptoms similar to those of

CHART 57-2 Patient and Family Education: Preparing for Self-Management

Preventing Transmission of Gastroenteritis

Advise the patient to:

- Wash hands well for at least 30 seconds with an antibacterial soap, especially after a bowel movement, and maintain good personal hygiene.
- Restrict the use of glasses, dishes, eating utensils, and tubes of toothpaste for his or her own use. In severe cases, disposable utensils may be wise.
- Maintain clean bathroom facilities to avoid exposure to stool.
- Inform the health care provider if symptoms persist beyond 3 days.
- Do not prepare or handle food that will be consumed by others. If you (the patient) are employed as a food handler, the public health department should be consulted for recommendations about the return to work.

TABLE 57-2 Differential Features of Ulcerative Colitis and Crohn's Disease

FEATURE	ULCERATIVE COLITIS	CROHN'S DISEASE
Location	Begins in the rectum and proceeds in a continuous manner toward the cecum	Most often in the terminal ileum, with patchy involvement through all layers of the bowel
Etiology	Unknown	Unknown
Peak incidence at age	15-25 yr and 55-65 yr	15-40 yr
Number of stools	10-20 liquid, bloody stools per day	5-6 soft, loose stools per day, non-bloody
Complications	Hemorrhage Nutritional deficiencies	Fistulas (common) Nutritional deficiencies
Need for surgery	Infrequent	Frequent

IBD, and other problems must be ruled out before a definitive diagnosis is made.

The approach to each patient is individualized. Encourage patients to self-manage their disease by learning about the illness, treatment, drugs, and complications.

ULCERATIVE COLITIS

❖ PATHOPHYSIOLOGY

Ulcerative colitis (UC) creates widespread INFLAMMATION of mainly the rectum and rectosigmoid colon but can extend to the entire colon when the disease is extensive. Distribution of the disease can remain constant for years. UC is a disease that is associated with periodic remissions and exacerbations (flare-ups) (McCance et al., 2014). Many factors can cause exacerbations, including intestinal INFECTIONS. Older adults with UC are at high risk for impaired FLUID AND ELECTROLYTE BALANCE as a result of diarrhea, including dehydration and hypokalemia.

The intestinal mucosa becomes hyperemic (has increased blood flow), edematous, and reddened. In more severe INFLAMMATION, the lining can bleed and small erosions, or ulcers, occur. Abscesses can form in these ulcerative areas and result in tissue necrosis (cell death). Continued edema and mucosal thickening can lead to a narrowed colon and possibly a partial bowel obstruction. Table 57-3 lists the categories of the severity of UC.

The patient's stool typically contains blood and mucus. Patients report **tenesmus** (an unpleasant and urgent sensation to defecate) and lower abdominal colicky PAIN relieved with defecation. Malaise, anorexia, anemia, dehydration, fever, and weight loss are common. Extraintestinal manifestations such as migratory polyarthritis, ankylosing spondylitis, and erythema nodosum are present in a large number of patients. The common complications of UC, including extraintestinal manifestations, are listed in Table 57-4.

Etiology and Genetic Risk

The exact cause of UC is unknown, but a combination of genetic, immunologic, and environmental factors likely contributes to disease development. A genetic basis of the disease has been supported because it is often found in families and twins. Immunologic causes, including autoimmune dysfunction, are likely the etiology of extraintestinal manifestations of the disease. Epithelial antibodies in the immunoglobulin G (IgG) class have been identified in the blood of some patients with UC (McCance et al., 2014).

With long-term disease, cellular changes can occur that increase the risk for colon cancer. Damage from pro-inflammatory cytokines, such as specific interleukins (ILs) (e.g., IL-1, IL-6, IL-8) and tumor necrosis factor (TNF)–alpha, have cytotoxic effects on the colonic mucosa (McCance et al., 2014).

Incidence and Prevalence

Chronic inflammatory bowel disease (IBD) affects about 1.4 million people in the United States and is split about equally between ulcerative colitis (UC) and Crohn's disease (discussed later). Peak age for being diagnosed with UC is between 30 and

TABLE 57-3 American College of Gastroenterologists Classification of UC Severity

SEVERITY	STOOL FREQUENCY	SIGNS/SYMPTOMS
Mild	<4 stools/day with/without blood	Asymptomatic Laboratory values usually normal
Moderate	>4 stools/day with/without blood	Minimal symptoms Mild abdominal pain Mild intermittent nausea Possible increased C-reactive protein* or ESR†
Severe	>6 bloody stools/day	Fever Tachycardia Anemia Abdominal pain Elevated C-reactive protein* and/or ESR†
Fulminant	>10 bloody stools/day	Increasing symptoms Anemia may require transfusion Colonic distention on x-ray

UC, Ulcerative colitis.
*C-reactive protein is a sensitive acute-phase serum marker that is evident in the first 6 hours of an inflammatory process.
†ESR (erythrocyte sedimentation rate) may be helpful but is less sensitive than C-reactive protein.

TABLE 57-4 Complications of Ulcerative Colitis and Crohn's Disease

COMPLICATION	DESCRIPTION
Hemorrhage/perforation	Lower gastrointestinal bleeding results from erosion of the bowel wall.
Abscess formation	Localized pockets of infection develop in the ulcerated bowel lining.
Toxic megacolon	Paralysis of the colon causes dilation and subsequent colonic ileus, possibly perforation.
Malabsorption	Essential nutrients cannot be absorbed through the diseased intestinal wall, causing anemia and malnutrition (most common in Crohn's disease).
Nonmechanical bowel obstruction	Obstruction results from toxic megacolon or cancer.
Fistulas	In Crohn's disease in which the inflammation is transmural, fistulas can occur anywhere but usually track between the bowel and bladder resulting in pyuria and fecaluria.
Colorectal cancer	Patients with ulcerative colitis with a history longer than 10 years have a high risk for colorectal cancer. This complication accounts for about one third of all deaths related to ulcerative colitis.
Extraintestinal complications	Complications include arthritis, hepatic and biliary disease (especially cholelithiasis), oral and skin lesions, and ocular disorders, such as iritis. The cause is unknown.
Osteoporosis	Osteoporosis occurs especially in patients with Crohn's disease.

40 years and again at 55 to 65 years. Women are more often affected than men in their younger years, but men have the disease more often as middle-aged and older adults (McCance et al., 2014).

CULTURAL CONSIDERATIONS

Patient-Centered Care QSEN

Ulcerative colitis is more common among Jewish persons than among those who are not Jewish and among whites more than non-whites (McCance et al., 2014). The reasons for these cultural differences are not known.

❖ PATIENT-CENTERED COLLABORATIVE CARE

◆ Assessment

History. Collect data on family history of IBD, previous and current therapy for the illness, and dates and types of surgery. Obtain a NUTRITION history, including intolerance of milk and milk products and fried, spicy, or hot foods. Ask about usual bowel ELIMINATION pattern (color, number, consistency, and character of stools), abdominal pain, tenesmus, anorexia, and fatigue. Note any relationship between diarrhea, timing of meals, emotional distress, and activity. Inquire about recent (past 2 to 3 month) exposure to antibiotics suggesting *Clostridium difficile* infection. Has the patient traveled to or emigrated from tropical areas? Ask about recent use of NSAIDs that can cause a flare-up of the disease. Ask about any extraintestinal symptoms such as arthritis, mouth sores, vision problems, and skin disorders.

Physical Assessment/Clinical Manifestations. Symptoms vary with an acuteness of onset. Vital signs are usually within normal limits in mild disease. In more severe cases, the patient may have a low-grade fever (99° to 100° F [37.2° to 37.8° C]). The physical assessment findings are usually nonspecific, and in milder cases the physical examination may be normal. Viral and bacterial infections cause symptoms similar to those of UC.

Note any abdominal distention along the colon. Fever associated with tachycardia may indicate peritonitis, dehydration, and bowel perforation. Assess for clinical manifestations associated with extraintestinal complications, such as inflamed joints and lesions inside the mouth.

Psychosocial Assessment. Many patients are very concerned about the frequency of stools and the presence of blood. *The inability to control the disease symptoms, particularly diarrhea, can be disruptive and stress producing.* Severe illness may limit the patient's activities outside the home with fear of fecal incontinence resulting in feeling "tied to the toilet." Severe anxiety and depression may result. Eating may be associated with pain and cramping and an increased frequency of stools. Mealtimes may become unpleasant experiences. Frequent visits to health care providers and close monitoring of the colon mucosa for abnormal cell changes can be anxiety provoking.

Assess the patient's understanding of the illness and its impact on his or her lifestyle. Encourage and support the patient while exploring:

- The relationship of life events to disease exacerbations
- Stress factors that produce symptoms
- Family and social support systems
- Concerns regarding the possible genetic basis and associated cancer risks of the disease
- Internet access for reliable education information

Laboratory Assessment. As a result of chronic blood loss, hematocrit and hemoglobin levels may be low, which indicates anemia and a chronic disease state. *An increased WBC count, C-reactive protein, or erythrocyte sedimentation rate (ESR) is consistent with inflammatory disease.* Blood levels of sodium, potassium, and chloride may be *low* as a result of frequent diarrheal stools and malabsorption through the diseased bowel (Pagana & Pagana, 2014). Hypoalbuminemia (decreased serum albumin) is found in patients with extensive disease from losing protein in the stool.

Other Diagnostic Assessment. *Magnetic resonance enterography (MRE)* is the major examination used to study the bowel in patients who have IBD. Teach the patient that he or she will need to fast for 4 to 6 hours prior to the test. To have the test, the patient drinks a contrast medium, which can cause diarrhea. The patient has the opportunity to go to the restroom before positioning on the MRI table. The patient then lies prone while the first of two doses of glucagon are given subcutaneously. This substance helps to slow the bowel's activity and motility (Grossman, 2011).

A *colonoscopy* may be done to aid in diagnosis, but the bowel prep can be especially uncomfortable for patients with inflammatory bowel disease (IBD). Frequent colonoscopies are recommended when patients have longer than a 10-year history of UC involving the entire colon because they are at high risk for colorectal cancer. In some cases, a *CT scan* may be done to confirm the disease or its complications. *Barium enemas* with air contrast can show differences between UC and Crohn's disease and identify complications, mucosal patterns, and the distribution and depth of disease involvement. In early disease, the barium enema may show incomplete filling as a result of inflammation and fine ulcerations along the bowel contour, which appear deeper in more advanced disease.

◆ Analysis

The priority NANDA-I nursing diagnoses and collaborative problems for patients with ulcerative colitis include:

1. Diarrhea related to inflammation of the bowel mucosa (NANDA-I)
2. Acute Pain and Chronic Pain related to inflammation and ulceration of the bowel mucosa and skin irritation (NANDA-I)
3. Potential for lower GI bleeding and resulting anemia

◆ Planning and Implementation

Decreasing Diarrhea

Planning: Expected Outcomes. The major concern for a patient with ulcerative colitis is the occurrence of frequent, bloody diarrhea and fecal incontinence from tenesmus. Therefore, with treatment, the patient is expected to have decreased diarrhea, formed stools, and control of bowel movements.

Interventions. Many measures are used to relieve symptoms and to reduce intestinal motility, decrease INFLAMMATION, and promote intestinal healing. Nonsurgical and/or surgical management may be needed.

Nonsurgical Management. Nonsurgical management includes drug and NUTRITION therapy. The use of physical and emotional rest is also an important consideration. Teach the patient to record color, volume, frequency, and consistency of stools to determine severity of the problem.

Monitor the skin in the perianal area for irritation and ulceration resulting from loose, frequent stools. Stool cultures may be sent for analysis if diarrhea continues. Have the patient weigh himself or herself 1 or 2 times per week. If the patient is hospitalized, remind unlicensed assistive personnel to weigh him or her on admission and daily in the morning before breakfast and document all weights.

NCLEX EXAMINATION CHALLENGE

Physiological Integrity

The nurse is caring for an older client who experiences an exacerbation of ulcerative colitis with severe diarrhea. What is the nurse's priority for care?

A. Monitor skin for breakdown.
B. Monitor heart rate and rhythm.
C. Maintain intake and output records.
D. Auscultate bowel sounds frequently.

Drug Therapy. Common drug therapy for UC includes aminosalicylates, glucocorticoids, antidiarrheal drugs, and immunomodulators. Teach patients about side effects and adverse drug events (ADEs) and when to call their health care provider.

The *aminosalicylates* are drugs commonly used to treat mild to moderate UC and/or maintain remission. Several aminosalicylic acid compounds are available. These drugs, also called *5-ASAs,* are thought to have an anti-inflammatory effect by inhibiting prostaglandins and are usually effective in 2 to 4 weeks.

Sulfasalazine (Azulfidine, Azulfidine EN-tabs), the first aminosalicylate approved for UC, is metabolized by the intestinal bacteria into 5-ASA, which delivers the beneficial effects of the drug, and sulfapyridine, which is responsible for unwanted side effects.

Glucocorticoids, such as prednisone and prednisolone, are corticosteroid therapies prescribed during exacerbations of the disease. Prednisone (Deltasone, Winpred) 40 to 65 mg daily is typically prescribed, but the dose may be increased as acute flare-ups occur. Once clinical improvement occurs, the corticosteroids are tapered because of the adverse effects that commonly occur with long-term steroid therapy (e.g., hyperglycemia, osteoporosis, peptic ulcer disease, increased risk for infection). For patients with rectal INFLAMMATION, topical steroids in the form of small retention enemas may be prescribed.

! NURSING SAFETY PRIORITY (QSEN)

Drug Alert

Teach patients taking sulfasalazine to report nausea, vomiting, anorexia, rash, and headache to the health care provider. With higher doses, hemolytic anemia, hepatitis, male infertility, or agranulocytosis can occur. This drug is in the same family as sulfonamide antibiotics. Therefore assess the patient for an allergy to sulfonamide or other drugs that contain sulfa *before* the patient takes the drug. The use of a thiazide diuretic is also a contraindication for sulfasalazine (Lilley et al., 2014).

Mesalamine (Asacol, Pentasa, Rowasa, Apriso, Canasa) is better tolerated than sulfasalazine because none of its preparations contain sulfapyridine. Asacol is an enteric-coated drug and is released in the terminal ileum and right side of the colon. Pentasa and Apriso are delayed- and extended-release drugs that work throughout the colon and rectum. Rowasa can be given as an enema, and Canasa can be given as a suppository. These preparations have minimal systemic absorption and therefore have fewer side effects. Table 57-5 lists commonly used 5-ASA drugs.

To provide symptomatic management of diarrhea, *antidiarrheal drugs* may be prescribed. These drugs are given very cautiously, however, because they can cause colon dilation and toxic megacolon. Common antidiarrheal drugs include diphenoxylate hydrochloride and atropine sulfate (Lomotil) and loperamide (Imodium).

Immunomodulators are drugs that alter a person's immune response. Alone, they are often not effective in the treatment of ulcerative colitis. However, in combination with steroids, they may offer a synergistic effect to a quicker response, thereby decreasing the amount of steroids needed. Biologic response modifiers (BRMs) used for UC (and Crohn's disease, discussed later in this chapter) include infliximab (Remicade) and adalimumab (Humira). Although not approved as a first-line therapy for ulcerative colitis, *infliximab* (Remicade) may be used for refractory disease or for severe complications, such as **toxic megacolon** (massive dilation of the colon that can lead to gangrene and peritonitis) and extraintestinal manifestations. Remicade is an immunoglobulin G (IgG) monoclonal antibody that reduces the activity of tumor necrosis factor (TNF) to decrease INFLAMMATION. Adalimumab (Humira) is another monoclonal antibody approved for refractory (not responsive to other therapies) cases. BRMs are used more commonly in management

TABLE 57-5 Recommended Doses for 5-ASA Medications

GENERIC NAME	TRADE NAME	DOSAGE AVAILABLE	RECOMMENDED DOSE
Sulfasalazine	Azulfidine Azulfidine En-tabs Azulfidine oral suspension (50 mg/mL)	500 mg tablets 250 mg/5 mL liquid	3-4 g daily in divided doses Children >2 yr: 30 mg/kg/day not to exceed 2 g/day
Mesalamine	Asacol Pentasa Rowasa enemas Rowasa suppository	400 mg tablets 500 mg tablets 4 g/60 mL 1000 mg/supp	800 mg three times daily 1 g four times daily At bedtime Twice daily or at bedtime
Olsalazine (rarely used)	Dipentum	250 mg tablets	1 g daily in two divided doses
Balsalazide	Colazal	750 mg tablets	3 tablets three times daily

5-ASA, 5-aminosalicylic acid.

of Crohn's disease. These drugs cause immunosuppression and should be used with caution. *Teach the patient to report any signs of a beginning* INFECTION, *including a cold, and to avoid large crowds or others who are sick!*

Several newer monoclonal antibodies are awaiting FDA approval for use in patients with IBD. One of these drugs, vedolizumab, is an intestinal-specific leukocyte traffic inhibitor in that it prevents white blood cells from migrating to inflamed bowel tissue.

Nutrition Therapy and Rest. Patients with severe symptoms who are hospitalized are kept NPO to ensure bowel rest. The physician may prescribe total parenteral NUTRITION (TPN) for severely ill and malnourished patients during severe exacerbations. Chapter 60 describes this therapy in detail. Patients with less severe symptoms may drink elemental formulas such as Vivonex PLUS or Vivonex T.E.N, which are absorbed in the small bowel and reduce bowel stimulation.

Diet is not a major factor in the inflammatory process, but some patients with ulcerative colitis (UC) find that caffeine and alcohol increase diarrhea and cramping. For some patients, raw vegetables and other high-fiber foods can cause GI symptoms. Lactose-containing foods may be poorly tolerated and should be reduced or eliminated. Teach patients that carbonated beverages, pepper, nuts and corn, dried fruits, and smoking are common GI stimulants that could cause discomfort. Each patient differs in his or her food and fluid tolerances.

During an exacerbation of the disease, patient activity is generally restricted because rest can reduce intestinal activity, provide comfort, and promote healing. Ensure that the patient has easy access to a bedpan, bedside commode, or bathroom in case of urgency or tenesmus.

Complementary and Alternative Therapies. In addition to dietary changes, complementary and alternative therapies may be used to supplement traditional management of ulcerative colitis. Examples include herbs (e.g., flaxseed), selenium, and vitamin C. Biofeedback, hypnosis, yoga, acupuncture, and ayurveda (a combination of diet, yoga, herbs, and breathing exercises) may also be helpful. These therapies need further study to validate their effectiveness, but some patients find them helpful.

Surgical Management. Some patients with ulcerative colitis require surgery to help manage their disease when medical therapies alone are not effective. In some cases, surgery is performed for complications of UC such as toxic megacolon, hemorrhage, dysplastic biopsy results, and colon cancer.

Preoperative Care. General preoperative teaching related to abdominal surgery is described in Chapter 14. If a temporary or permanent ileostomy is planned, provide an in-depth explanation to the patient and family. An **ileostomy** is a procedure in which a loop of the ileum is placed through an opening in the abdominal wall (**stoma**) for drainage of fecal material into a pouching system worn on the abdomen. The external pouching system consists of a solid skin barrier (wafer) to protect the skin and a fecal collection device (pouch), similar to the system used for patients with colostomies (discussed in Chapter 56).

If an ileostomy is planned, the surgeon consults with a certified wound, ostomy, continence nurse (CWOCN) before surgery for recommendations on the best location of the stoma. A visit from an **ostomate** (a patient with an ostomy) may be helpful before surgery. Parenteral antibiotics are given within 1 hour of surgical opening based on current best evidence and per The Joint Commission's National Patient Safety Goals.

Operative Procedures. Any one of several surgical approaches may be used for the patient with UC. Minimally invasive procedures, such as laparoscopic, laparoscopic-assisted, hand-assisted, and robotic-assisted surgery, are common for patients with ulcerative colitis in large tertiary care centers (Kessler et al., 2011). Laparoscopic surgery usually involves one or several small incisions but often takes longer to perform than the open surgical approach. A newer procedure, natural orifice transluminal endoscopic surgery (NOTES), can be performed via the anus or vagina for selected patients if the surgeon has been trained in the procedure. Patients may have moderate sedation or general anesthesia for minimally invasive surgical procedures and are not typically admitted to critical care units for continuing postoperative care.

Patients who are obese, have had previous abdominal surgeries, or have dense scar tissue (adhesions) may not be candidates for laparoscopic procedures. The conventional open surgical approach involves an abdominal incision and is done under general anesthesia. Patients with open procedures are typically admitted to critical care units for short-term stabilization.

Restorative Proctocolectomy with Ileo Pouch–Anal Anastomosis (RPC-IPAA). This procedure has become the gold standard for patients with UC. In some centers, the surgery is performed via laparoscopy (laparoscopic RPC-IPAA). It is usually a two-stage procedure that includes the removal of the colon and most of the rectum (Fig. 57-2). The anus and anal sphincter remain intact. The surgeon then surgically creates an internal pouch (reservoir) using the last 1½ feet of the small intestine. The pouch, sometimes called a *J-pouch, S-pouch,* or *pelvic pouch,* is then connected to the anus. A temporary ileostomy through the abdominal skin is created to allow healing of the internal pouch and all anastomosis sites. It also allows for an increase in the capacity of the internal pouch. In the *second* surgical stage, the loop ileostomy is closed. The time interval between the first and second stages varies, but many patients have the second surgical stage to close the ileostomy within 1 to 2 months of the first surgery.

Usually bowel continence is excellent after this procedure, but some patients have leakage of stool during sleep. They may take antidiarrheal drugs to help control this problem.

Total Proctocolectomy with a Permanent Ileostomy. Total proctocolectomy with a permanent ileostomy is done for patients who are not candidates for or do not want the ileo-anal pouch. The procedure involves the removal of the colon, rectum, and anus with surgical closure of the anus (Fig. 57-3, *A*). The surgeon brings the end of the ileum out through the abdominal wall and forms a stoma, or **ostomy.**

! NURSING SAFETY PRIORITY (QSEN)

Critical Rescue

The ileostomy stoma (Fig. 57-3, *B*) is usually placed in the right lower quadrant of the abdomen below the belt line. It should not be prolapsed or retract into the abdominal wall. *Assess the stoma frequently. It should be pinkish to cherry red to ensure an adequate blood supply. If the stoma looks pale, bluish, or dark, report these findings to the health care provider immediately!*

With an ileostomy, initially after surgery the output is a loose, dark green liquid that may contain some blood. Over time, a process called "ileostomy adaptation" occurs. The small intestine begins to perform some of the functions that had

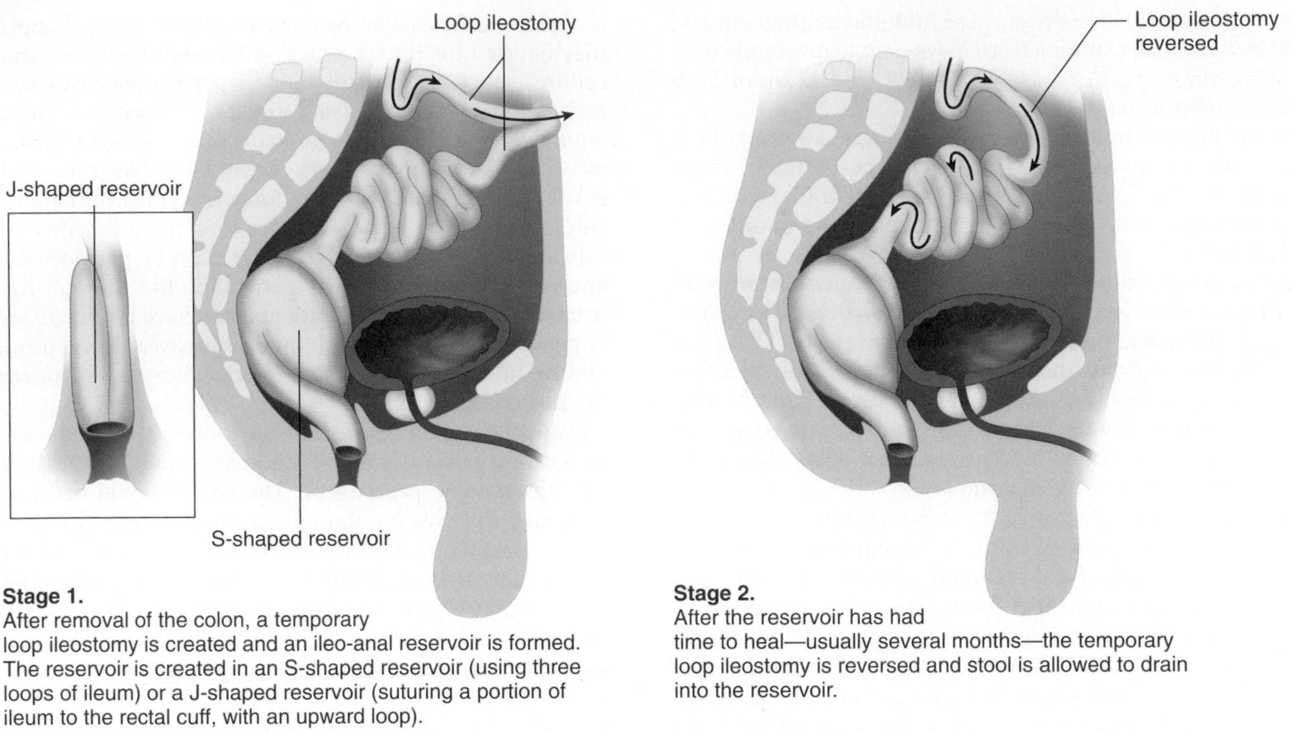

FIG. 57-2 The creation of an ileo-anal reservoir.

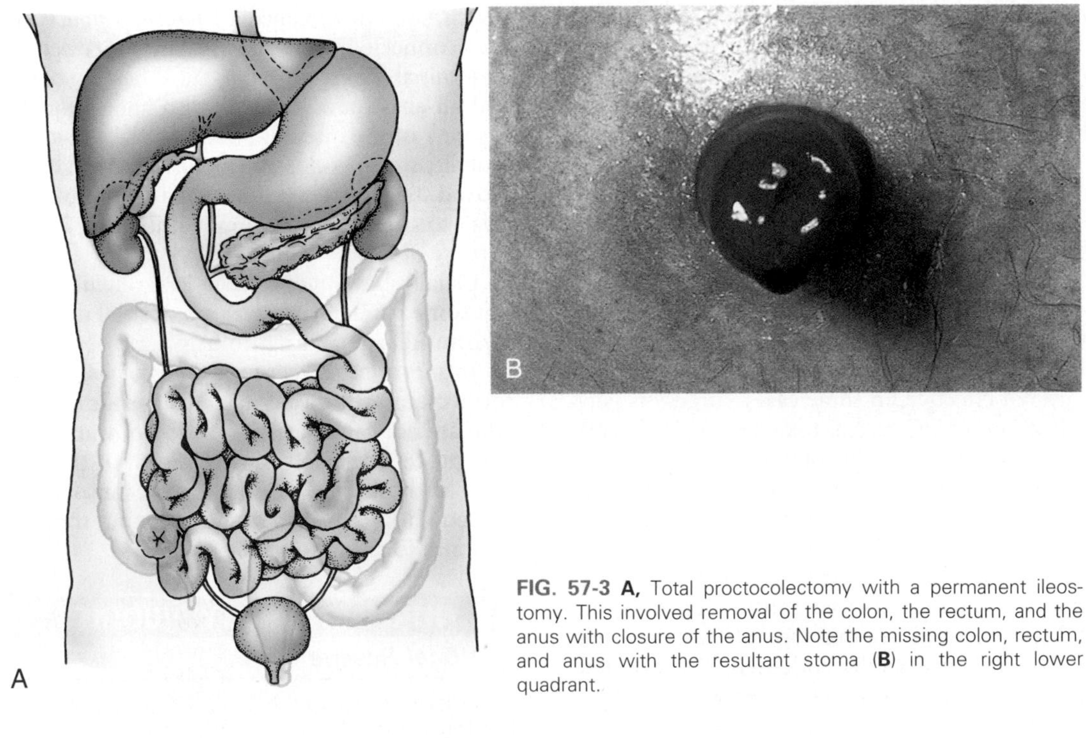

FIG. 57-3 A, Total proctocolectomy with a permanent ileostomy. This involved removal of the colon, the rectum, and the anus with closure of the anus. Note the missing colon, rectum, and anus with the resultant stoma (**B**) in the right lower quadrant.

previously been done by the colon, including the absorption of increased amounts of sodium and water. Stool volume decreases, becomes thicker (pastelike), and turns yellow-green or yellow-brown. The effluent (fluid material) usually has little odor or a sweet odor. Any foul or unpleasant odor may be a symptom of a problem such as blockage or infection.

The ostomy drains frequently, and the stool is irritating. *The patient must wear a pouch system at all times.* The stool from the small intestine contains many enzymes and bile salts, which can quickly irritate and excoriate the skin. *Skin care around the stoma is a priority!* A pouch system with a skin barrier (gelatin or pectin) provides sufficient protection for most patients. Other products are also available.

Postoperative Care. Provide general postoperative care after surgery, as described in Chapter 16. The few patients requiring open-approach surgery for ulcerative colitis have a large abdominal incision. At first they are NPO and a nasogastric tube (NGT) is used for suction. The tube is removed in 1 to 2 days as the drainage decreases, and fluids and food are slowly introduced. The patient having minimally invasive surgery (MIS) usually does not have an NGT.

In collaboration with the CWOCN, help the patient adjust and learn the required care. The ileostomy usually begins to drain within 24 hours after surgery at more than 1 L per day. Be sure that fluids are replaced by adding an additional 500 mL or more each day to prevent dehydration. After about a week of high-volume output, the drainage slows and becomes thicker. During this period, some patients need antidiarrheal drugs.

The hospital stay is usually from 1 to 4 days, depending on whether the patient has laparoscopic or conventional open surgery. Patients having MIS have less pain from surgery and faster restoration of bowel function when compared with other surgical patients, but the incidence of complications is about the same (Fajardo et al., 2010).

For those who have the RPC-IPAA procedure, remind them that the internal pouch can become inflamed. This problem is usually effectively treated with metronidazole (Flagyl) for 7 to 10 days. Teach patients that after the second stage of surgery, they might have burning during bowel ELIMINATION because gastric acid cannot be well absorbed by the ileum. Also instruct them to omit foods that can cause odors or gas, such as cabbage, asparagus, Brussels sprouts, and beans. Teach patients to eliminate foods that cannot be well digested, such as nuts and corn. Each patient differs in which foods he or she can tolerate.

Surgery for UC may result in altered body image. However, it may be viewed as positive because the patient will have fewer symptoms and feel more comfortable than before the procedure. Patients have to adjust to having an ostomy before they can resume their presurgery activities.

NCLEX EXAMINATION CHALLENGE

Physiological Integrity

The health care provider prescribes prednisone (Deltasone) for a client with ulcerative colitis. What health teaching is most important before the client begins the medication?

A. Determine if the client's insurance pays for the drug.
B. Teach the client to take the drug at night.
C. Ask the client if he has any allergies to sulfa-type drugs.
D. Teach the client the importance of avoiding crowds.

Minimizing Pain

Planning: Expected Outcomes. The desired outcome for the patient is that he or she will verbalize decreased PAIN as a result of collaborative, evidence-based pain management interventions.

Interventions. Pain control requires pharmacologic and nonpharmacologic measures. Physical discomfort can contribute to emotional distress. A variety of symptom-reducing interventions and supportive measures are used. Surgery also reduces pain for many patients.

The purpose of pain management is alleviation of pain or a reduction in pain to a level of comfort that is acceptable to the patient. Increases in PAIN may indicate the development of complications such as peritonitis (see earlier discussion in this chapter). Assist the patient in reducing or eliminating factors that can cause or increase the pain experience. For example, he or she may benefit from NUTRITION changes to decrease abdominal discomfort such as cramping and bloating.

Antidiarrheal drugs may be needed to control diarrhea, thus reducing the discomfort. However, they must be used with caution and for a short time because toxic megacolon can develop.

Perineal skin can be irritated by contact with loose stools and frequent cleaning. Explain special measures for skin care. Use of medicated wipes is soothing if the rectal area is tender or sensitive from the use of toilet tissue (Chart 57-3). A number of ostomy manufacturers (e.g., Hollister, ConvaTec) produce a system for skin care that may help prevent and heal perineal skin irritation. These systems usually include a skin-cleaning solution, a moisturizing and healing cream, and a petroleum jelly–like barrier that prevents contact of moisture and stool with the skin.

Monitoring for Lower GI Bleeding

Planning: Expected Outcomes. For patients who experience GI bleeding, the patient with UC is expected to have a reduction in or cessation of bleeding with prompt collaborative care. If possible, patients are expected to remain free of complications of the disease that can cause bleeding, such as perforation.

Interventions. The primary nursing priority is to monitor the patient closely for signs and symptoms of GI bleeding resulting from the disease or its complications.

CHART 57-3 Best Practice for Patient Safety & Quality Care QSEN

Pain Control and Skin Care for Patients with Inflammatory Bowel Disease

PATIENT PROBLEM	INTERVENTIONS
Abdominal pain (particularly with exacerbations of the disease)	Administer analgesics. Assist with frequent positioning. Identify foods that increase pain. Perform a comprehensive pain assessment. Observe for signs and symptoms of peritonitis. Evaluate effectiveness of pain management. Teach music therapy, guided imagery.
Skin excoriation and/or irritation from frequent bowel movements	Encourage good skin care with a mild soap and water after each bowel movement. Gently pat the area dry. Identify foods that increase diarrhea. Sitz baths may be of benefit. Apply a thin coat of A+D Ointment or aloe cream. Use medicated wipes instead of tissue. Ensure appropriate ostomy supplies that fit well. Antidiarrheal medications may help, but use with caution. Observe for symptoms related to megacolon (fever, leukocytosis, tachycardia, distended abdomen with 3-view abdominal x-ray noting an enlarged colon).

! NURSING SAFETY PRIORITY (QSEN)

Critical Rescue

For the patient with ulcerative colitis, monitor stools for blood loss. The blood may be bright red (frank bleeding) or black and tarry (melena). Monitor hematocrit, hemoglobin, and electrolyte values, and assess vital signs. Prolonged slow bleeding can lead to anemia. Observe for fever, tachycardia, and signs of fluid volume depletion. Changes in mental status may occur, especially among older adults, and may be the first indication of dehydration or anemia.

If symptoms of GI bleeding begin, notify the health care provider immediately. Blood products are often prescribed for patients with severe anemia. Prepare for the blood transfusion by inserting a large-bore IV catheter if it is not already in place. Chapter 40 outlines nursing actions during blood transfusion.

If the patient has lower GI bleeding of more than 0.5 mL per minute, a *GI bleeding scan* may be useful to localize the site of the bleeding (Pagana & Pagana, 2014). This test cannot indicate the cause of the bleeding, however, and may take several hours to administer. Patients in the critical care unit are not candidates for the test because they must leave the unit for the test.

Community-Based Care

Home Care Management. The patient with ulcerative colitis provides self-management at home but may require hospitalization during severe exacerbations or surgery. In addition, those who have extraintestinal problems often need ongoing collaborative care for joint and/or skin problems.

Home care management focuses on controlling clinical manifestations and monitoring for complications. For patients returning home or transferring to nursing home or transitional care after surgery, ongoing respiratory care, incision care (if applicable), ostomy care, and PAIN management should be continued.

Self-Management Education. Teach the patient about the nature of ulcerative colitis, including its acute episodes, remissions, and symptom management. Also stress that even though the cause is unknown, relapses can be prevented with proper health care. Teach patients taking immunosuppressive drugs, such as corticosteroids and biologic response modifiers (monoclonal antibodies), to report signs of possible infection, such as sore throat, to the health care provider. Remind them to avoid crowds and anyone who has an INFECTION. Review the purpose of drug therapy, when drugs should be taken, side effects, and adverse drug events.

Instruct the patient about measures to reduce or control abdominal PAIN, cramping, and diarrhea. Also teach the patient and family about symptoms associated with disease exacerbation that should be reported to the health care provider, such as fever higher than 101° F (38.3° C), tachycardia, palpitations, and an increase in diarrhea, abdominal pain, or nausea/vomiting. Provide written information and contact numbers for the health care provider.

There is no special diet for a patient with an ileostomy. However, teach the patient to avoid any foods that cause gas. Examples include high-fiber foods like nuts, raw cabbage, corn, celery, apples with peels, and popcorn. The patient needs to learn what foods he or she tolerates best and adjust the diet accordingly.

If the patient has undergone a temporary or permanent surgical diversion, collaborate with the CWOCN to explain and demonstrate required care so that the patient can self-manage or the family/caregiver can assist. Also teach the importance of including adequate amounts of salt and water in the diet because the ileostomy increases the loss of these substances. Urge the patient to be cautious in situations that lead to heavy sweating or fluid loss, such as strenuous physical activity, high environmental heat, and episodes of diarrhea and vomiting.

Finding the best ostomy pouching system is a major issue for many patients. An effective system is one that:

- Protects the skin
- Contains the effluent (drainage) and reduces odor, if any
- Remains securely attached to the skin for a dependable period of time

Most patients desire an adhesive barrier that will last for 3 to 7 days. The barrier must create a solid seal to prevent the enzymes in the drainage from irritating the skin. Solid barriers are classified as "regular wear" or "extended wear." A person with a high output may want an extended-wear barrier. A special cream can be used to help fill any uneven skin surfaces and provide a consistent seal. Pouches are also individualized by the patient. Large pouches can hold more but are heavy when full. Patients also have to consider the costs of the various systems and if or how much their insurance will pay for them. Chart 57-4 describes the main aspects of ileostomy care, including skin care.

A patient with an ileostomy may have many concerns about management at home and about sexual and social adjustments. Considering possible sexual issues helps the patient identify and discuss these concerns with the sex partner. For example, a change in positioning during intercourse may alleviate apprehension. Social situations may cause anxiety related to decreased self-esteem and a disturbance in body image. Encourage the patient to discuss possible concerns in addressing and resolving these potentially stressful events. Clinical depression is common among patients with ulcerative colitis. Refer patients to appropriate mental health resources if depression is suspected.

Some hospitals provide community support groups for their patients with inflammatory bowel disease (IBD). These groups help patients and their families cope with the psychological impact of IBD and educate them about NUTRITION and complementary and alternative therapies (see the Evidence-Based Practice box).

Health Care Resources. If the patient needs assistance with self-management at home, collaborate with the case manager or social worker to arrange the services of a home care aide or nurse. A home care nurse can provide assessment and guidance in integrating ostomy care into the patient's lifestyle. The nurse may also teach about wound care, including the monitoring of wound healing, if needed (Chart 57-5). The patient and family need to know where to purchase ostomy supplies, along with the name, size, and manufacturer's order number.

For patients with a permanent ileostomy, locate a community ostomy support group by contacting the United Ostomy Associations of America (www.uoaa.org). The United Ostomy Association of Canada serves the needs of Canadian patients (www.ostomycanada.ca). A local support group or the Crohn's and Colitis Foundation of America (www.ccfa.org) may be helpful in obtaining supplies and providing education for ostomates. Inform the patient and family of available ostomy ambulatory care clinics and ostomy specialists. If the patient agrees,

CHART 57-4 Patient and Family Education: Preparing for Self-Management

Ileostomy Care

Skin Protection

- Use a skin barrier to protect your skin from contact with contents from the ostomy.
- Use skin care products, such as skin sealants and ostomy skin creams. If your skin continues to come into contact with ostomy contents, select a product to fill in problem areas and provide an even skin surface.
- Watch your skin for any irritation or redness.

Pouch Care

- Empty your pouch when it is one-third to one-half full.
- Change the pouch during inactive times, such as before meals, before retiring at night, on waking in the morning, and 2 to 4 hours after eating.
- Change the entire pouch system every 3 to 7 days.

Nutrition

- Chew food thoroughly.
- Be cautious of high-fiber and high-cellulose foods. You may need to eliminate these from the diet if they cause severe problems (diarrhea, constipation, or blockage). Examples include corn, peanuts, coconut, Chinese vegetables, string beans, tough-fiber meats, shrimp and lobster, rice, bran, and vegetables with skins (tomatoes, corn, and peas).

Drug Therapy

- Avoid taking enteric-coated and capsule medications.
- Inform any health care provider who is prescribing medications for you that you have an ostomy. Before having prescriptions filled, inform your pharmacist that you have an ostomy.
- Do not take any laxative or enemas. You should usually have loose stool and should contact a physician if no stool has passed in 6 to 12 hours.

Symptoms to Watch for

- Report any drastic increase or decrease in drainage to your health care provider.
- If stomal swelling, abdominal cramping, or distention occurs or if ileostomy contents stop draining:
  - Remove the pouch with faceplate.
  - Lie down, assuming a knee-chest position.
  - Begin abdominal massage.
  - Apply moist towels to the abdomen.
  - Drink hot tea.
  - If none of these maneuvers is effective in resuming ileostomy flow or if abdominal pain is severe, call your health care provider right away.

a visit from an ostomate can be continued after discharge to home.

◆ *Evaluation: Outcomes*

Evaluate the care of the patient with ulcerative colitis based on the identified priority patient problems. Expected outcomes may include that the patient will:

- Verbalize decreased PAIN
- Gain control over bowel elimination
- Not experience lower GI bleeding
- Self-manage the ileostomy (temporary or permanent)
- Maintain peristomal skin integrity
- Demonstrate behaviors that integrate ostomy care into his or her lifestyle if a permanent ileostomy is performed

CHART 57-5 Home Care Assessment

The Patient with Inflammatory Bowel Disease

Assess gastrointestinal function and nutritional status, including:
- Abdominal cramping or pain
- Bowel elimination pattern, specifically frequency, characteristics, and amount of stools and presence or absence of blood in stools
- Food and fluid intake (include relationship of specific foods to cramping and stools)
- Weight gain or loss
- Signs and symptoms of dehydration
- Presence or absence of fever, rectal tenesmus, or urgency
- Bowel sounds
- Condition of perianal skin, including presence or absence of perianal fistula or abscess

Assess patient's and family's coping skills, including:
- Current and ongoing stress level and coping style
- Availability of support system

Assess home environment, including:
- Adequacy and availability of bathroom facilities
- Opportunity for rest and relaxation

Assess ability to self-manage therapeutic regimen, including:
- Drug therapy
- Signs and symptoms to report
- Nutrition therapy
- Availability of community resources
- Importance of follow-up care

EVIDENCE-BASED PRACTICE QSEN

Is a Support Group for Patients with Inflammatory Bowel Disease Helpful?

McMaster, K., Aguinaldo, L., & Parekh, N.K. (2012). Evaluation of an ongoing psychoeducational inflammatory bowel disease support group in an adult outpatient setting. *Gastroenterology Nursing, 35*(6), 383-390.

In this study, researchers evaluated the use of an ongoing open psychoeducational support group for adult patients with inflammatory bowel disease (IBD) in an outpatient tertiary care setting. The sample was 18 adults who attended more than two meetings of the support group. The support group focused on diet and nutrition, psychological impact of IBD, and complementary and alternative medicine. Subjects completed several tools, including the Client Satisfaction Questionnaire, Multidimensional Support Scale, demographic data tool, and a brief open-ended qualitative questionnaire developed by the researchers.

The results showed that the participants in the support group were very satisfied with the support group and the peer support they received. The study demonstrated that the support group for IBD clients was effective.

Level of Evidence: 5

This study was a very small descriptive study that collected both quantitative and qualitative data.

Commentary: Implications for Practice and Research

Patients who have IBD need ongoing support and education in the community to cope with their disease. Nurses are in a prime position to facilitate these groups and help patients gain knowledge as well as emotional support as they learn to cope with their disease. This research was a small pilot study that needs a larger sample in a multi-setting research design.

CROHN'S DISEASE

❖ *PATHOPHYSIOLOGY*

Crohn's disease (CD) is a chronic inflammatory disease of the small intestine (most often), the colon, or both. It can affect the

GI tract from the mouth to the anus but most commonly affects the terminal ileum. CD is a slowly progressive and unpredictable disease with involvement of multiple regions of the intestine with normal sections in between (called "skip lesions" on x-rays). Like ulcerative colitis (UC), this disease is recurrent with remissions and exacerbations.

Crohn's disease presents as INFLAMMATION that causes a thickened bowel wall. Strictures and deep ulcerations (cobblestone appearance) also occur, which put the patient at risk for developing bowel **fistulas** (abnormal openings between two organs or structures). The result is severe diarrhea and malabsorption of vital nutrients. Anemia is common, usually from iron deficiency or malabsorption issues (McCance et al., 2014).

The complications associated with Crohn's disease are similar to those of ulcerative colitis (see Table 57-4). Hemorrhage is more common in ulcerative colitis, but it can occur in CD as well. Severe malabsorption by the small intestine is more common in patients with CD because UC may not involve the small bowel to any significant extent. *Therefore patients with CD can become very malnourished and debilitated.*

Rarely, cancer of the small bowel and colon develop but can occur after the disease has been present for 15 to 20 years. Fistula formation is a common complication of CD but is rare in UC. Fistulas can occur between segments of the intestine or manifest as cutaneous fistulas (opening to the skin) or perirectal abscesses. They can also extend from the bowel to other organs and body cavities, such as the bladder or vagina (Fig. 57-4). Some patients develop intestinal obstruction, which at first is secondary to INFLAMMATION and edema. Over time, fibrosis and scar tissue develop and obstruction results from a narrowing of the bowel. Most patients with CD require surgery at some time.

Almost a million people in the United States have Crohn's disease. Most have symptoms and are diagnosed as adolescents or young adults.

GENETIC/GENOMIC CONSIDERATIONS

Patient-Centered Care QSEN

The exact cause of CD is unknown. A combination of genetic, immune, and environmental factors may contribute to its development. About 10% to 20% of patients have a positive family history for the disease (Nussbaum et al., 2007). The discovery of a mutation in the *NOD2/CARD15* gene on chromosome 16 seems to be associated with some patients who have CD. This gene is found in monocytes that normally recognize and destroy bacteria.

Pro-inflammatory cytokines, such as tumor necrosis factor–alpha (TNF-alpha) and interleukins (ILs) (e.g., IL-6 and IL-8), are immunologic factors that contribute to the etiology of CD (McCance et al., 2014). Many of the drugs used for the disease inhibit or block one or more of these factors.

Other risk factors include tobacco use, Jewish ethnicity, and living in urban areas (McCance et al., 2014). CD is more common in people of Ashkenazi Jewish background than in any other group (Nussbaum et al., 2007). The reasons for these factors have not been established. It was once thought that stress and nutrition play a role in the *development* of CD, but these factors have not been proven. However, inadequate NUTRITION can worsen the patient's symptoms.

❖ PATIENT-CENTERED COLLABORATIVE CARE

◆ Assessment

Crohn's disease is made worse by bacterial INFECTION. A detailed history is needed to identify manifestations specific to the disease. Ask about recent unintentional weight loss, the frequency and consistency of stools, the presence of blood in the stool, fever, and abdominal pain.

Perform a thorough abdominal assessment. Assess for manifestations of the disease, and evaluate the patient's NUTRITION and hydration status.

When inspecting the abdomen, assess for distention, masses, or visible peristalsis. Inspection of the perianal area may reveal ulcerations, fissures, or fistulas. During auscultation, bowel sounds may be decreased or absent with severe inflammation or obstruction. An increase in high-pitched or rushing sounds may be present over areas of narrowed bowel loops. Muscle guarding, masses, rigidity, or tenderness may be noted on palpation by the advanced practice nurse or other health care provider.

The clinical presentation of Crohn's disease varies greatly from person to person. Most patients report diarrhea, abdominal pain, and low-grade fever. Fever is common with fistulas, abscesses, and severe INFLAMMATION. If the disease occurs in only the ileum, diarrhea occurs 5 or 6 times per day, often with a soft, loose stool. **Steatorrhea** (fatty diarrheal stools) is common. Rarely, stools may contain bright red blood.

Abdominal pain from the inflammatory process is usually constant and often located in the right lower quadrant. The patient also may have PAIN around the umbilicus before and

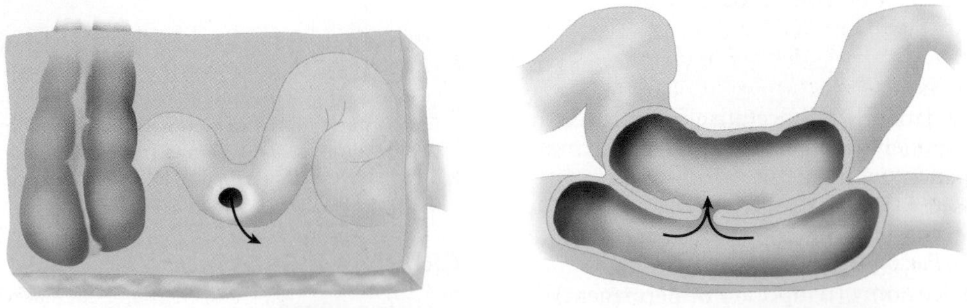

FIG. 57-4 The types of fistulas that are complications of Crohn's disease.

after bowel movements. If the lower colon is diseased, pain is common in both lower abdominal quadrants.

Most patients with Crohn's disease have *weight loss.* Nutritional problems are the result of increased catabolism from chronic INFLAMMATION, anorexia, malabsorption, or self-imposed dietary restrictions. These problems result in impaired FLUID AND ELECTROLYTE BALANCE and vital nutrient deficiencies.

The inflammatory bowel changes decrease the small bowel's ability to absorb nutrients, which may be made worse by surgery and fistulas.

! NURSING SAFETY PRIORITY (QSEN)

Action Alert

For the patient with Crohn's disease, be especially alert for manifestations of peritonitis (discussed earlier in this chapter), small-bowel obstruction, and nutritional and fluid imbalances. Early detection of a change in the patient's status helps reduce these life-threatening complications.

The patient who has Crohn's disease (CD) needs a complete psychosocial assessment. The chronic nature of the problem and the associated complications can greatly affect patients and their families. Lifestyle changes are necessary to cope with such a disruptive and painful chronic illness. Assess the patient's coping skill, and help identify support systems. Similar to problems associated with other chronic diseases, clinical depression and severe anxiety disorders are common among patients with CD.

The health care provider requests many laboratory studies for patients with Crohn's disease. The results of laboratory tests often indicate the extent and severity of INFLAMMATION or complications that occur with the disease.

Anemia is common as a result of slow bleeding and poor nutrition. Serum levels of folic acid and vitamin B_{12} are generally low because of malabsorption, further contributing to anemia. Amino acid malabsorption and protein-losing enteropathy may result in *decreased albumin* levels. C-reactive protein and ESR may be elevated to indicate INFLAMMATION. White blood cells (WBCs) in the urine may show INFECTION (pyuria), which is caused by ureteral obstruction or an enterovesical (bowel to bladder) fistula. If severe diarrhea or fistula is present, the patient may have fluid and electrolyte losses, particularly potassium and magnesium. Assess the patient for clinical manifestations that can occur as a result of electrolyte losses (see Chapter 11).

X-rays show the narrowing, ulcerations, strictures, and fistulas common with Crohn's disease. *Magnetic resonance enterography (MRE)* is performed to determine bowel activity and motility as discussed on p. 1175 in this chapter. An *abdominal ultrasound or CT* scan may also be performed. In acute illness, these tests may be deferred until the risk for perforation lessens. If the patient has lower GI bleeding of more than 0.5 mL per minute, a *GI bleeding scan* may be useful to localize the site of the bleeding (Pagana & Pagana, 2014).

◆ Interventions

Collaborative care for patients with Crohn's disease is similar to that described on p. 1175 in the Nonsurgical Management discussion in the Ulcerative Colitis section. Specific interventions vary with the severity of disease and the complications that are present.

Drug Therapy. Drugs used to manage Crohn's disease (CD) are similar to those used in the treatment of ulcerative colitis (UC). For mild to moderate disease, 5-ASA drugs may be very effective (see p. 1183 in the Drug Therapy discussion in the Ulcerative Colitis section).

Most patients have moderate to severe disease and need stronger drug therapy to control their symptoms. Two agents that may be prescribed for CD are azathioprine (Imuran) and mercaptopurine (Purinethol). These drugs suppress the immune system and can lead to serious INFECTIONS. Methotrexate (MTX) may also be given to suppress immune activity of the disease.

A group of biologic response modifiers (BRMs), also known as *monoclonal antibody drugs,* have been approved for use in Crohn's disease when other drugs have been ineffective. These drugs inhibit tumor necrosis factor (TNF)–alpha, which decreases the inflammatory response. Examples of commonly used drugs for patients with CD include infliximab (Remicade), adalimumab (Humira), natalizumab (Tysabri), and certolizumab pegol (Cimzia). These agents are not given to patients with a history of cancer, heart disease, or multiple sclerosis.

! NURSING SAFETY PRIORITY (QSEN)

Drug Alert

Both infliximab and certolizumab pegol must be given in a health care setting, such as a physician's office, via parenteral routes. Adalimumab (Humira) is self-administered by subcutaneous injection every other week. If needed, instruct patients on how to give themselves a subcutaneous injection. Teach patients to report injection site reactions, including redness and swelling. Remind them that headache, abdominal pain, and nausea and vomiting are common side effects. Teach them to avoid crowds, such as malls and large shopping centers, and people with infection. Reinforce the need to report any INFECTION, including a cold or sore throat, to the health care provider immediately.

Natalizumab is given IV under medical supervision every 4 weeks for moderate to severe CD and is given when other drugs are not effective. Although the use of this drug has decreased the length of hospital stays (Dudley-Brown et al., 2009), natalizumab can cause **progressive multifocal leukoencephalopathy** (PML), a deadly infection that affects the brain. Before giving the drug, be sure that the patient is free of all INFECTIONS. Teach patients the importance of reporting any cognitive, motor, or sensory changes immediately to the health care provider.

Although glucocorticoids can be effective for patients with Crohn's disease, sepsis can result from abscesses or fistulas that may be present. These drugs mask the symptoms of infection. Therefore they must be used with caution. Monitor the patient closely for signs of infection. Metronidazole (Flagyl, Novonidazol 🍁) has been helpful in patients with fistulas.

Nutrition Therapy. Long-standing nutritional deficits can have severe consequences for the patient with Crohn's disease. Poor NUTRITION can lead to inadequate fistula and wound healing, loss of lean muscle mass, decreased immune responses, and increased morbidity and mortality. During severe exacerbations of the disease, the patient may be hospitalized to provide bowel rest and nutritional support with total parenteral nutrition (TPN). For less severe exacerbations, an elemental or semi-elemental product such as Vivonex PLUS may be prescribed to induce remission. These products are absorbed in the jejunum and therefore permit the distal small intestine and colon to rest. Nutritional supplements such as Ensure or Sustacal can be added then to provide nutrients and more calories. Teach the patient to avoid GI stimulants, such as caffeinated beverages and alcohol.

Fistula Management. Fistulas (abnormal tracts between two or more body areas) are common with acute exacerbations of Crohn's disease. They can be between the bowel and bladder (enterovesical), between two segments of bowel (enteroenteric), between the skin and bowel (enterocutaneous), or between the bowel and vagina (enterovaginal) (see Fig. 57-4). The patient with one or more fistulas often has complications such as systemic infections, skin problems, malnutrition, and impaired FLUID AND ELECTROLYTE BALANCE. Treatment of the patient with a fistula is complicated and includes nutrition and electrolyte therapy, skin care, and prevention of infection.

! NURSING SAFETY PRIORITY QSEN

Action Alert

Adequate NUTRITION and FLUID AND ELECTROLYTE BALANCE are priorities in the care of the patient with a fistula. GI secretions are high in volume and rich in electrolytes and enzymes. The patient is at high risk for malnutrition, dehydration, and hypokalemia (decreased serum potassium). Assess for these complications, and collaborate with the health care team to manage them. Monitor urinary output and daily weights. A decrease indicates possible dehydration, which should be treated immediately by providing additional fluids.

The patient requires at least 3000 calories daily to promote healing of the fistula. If he or she cannot take adequate oral fluids and nutrients, total enteral nutrition (TEN) or TPN may be prescribed. For patients who do not require TEN or TPN, collaborate with the dietitian to:

- Carefully monitor the patient's tolerance to the prescribed diet.
- Assist the patient in selecting high-calorie, high-protein, high-vitamin, low-fiber meals.
- Offer enteral supplements, such as Ensure and Vivonex PLUS.
- Record food intake for accurate calorie counts.

Providing enteral supplements, recording intake and output, and taking daily weights may be delegated to unlicensed assistive personnel (UAP) under the supervision of the RN.

Collaborate with the certified wound, ostomy, and continence nurse (CWOCN) to select the most appropriate wound management for each patient.

! NURSING SAFETY PRIORITY QSEN

Action Alert

For patients with fistulas, preserving and protecting the skin is the nursing priority. Be sure that wound drainage is not in direct contact with skin because intestinal fluid enzymes are caustic! Clean the skin promptly to prevent skin breakdown or fungal infection, which can cause major discomfort for the patient.

Enzymes and bile in the stool contribute to the problem of skin irritation and excoriation. Skin irritation needs to be prevented. This may be accomplished through the use of skin barriers, pouching systems, and insertion of drains (Fig. 57-5). Skin barriers or dressings are used when the fistula drainage is less than 100 mL in 24 hours. A pouch is used for heavily draining fistulas to reduce the risk for skin breakdown and measure the **effluent** (drainage). However, they are very challenging because of location and drainage amount. Treatment with an antifungal powder applied to the skin around the fistula is often very helpful to prevent or treat *Candida* infection.

For some fistulas, pouching may not be possible because of their location. Drainage may need to be managed using regulated wall suction or a negative-pressure wound therapy device. Continuous low wall suction is attached to a suction catheter in the wound bed of the fistula, not into the fistula tract. These systems are not meant for long-term management.

Negative-pressure wound therapy (e.g., VAC therapy) promotes wound healing by secondary intention as it prepares the wound bed for closure, reduces edema, promotes granulation and perfusion, and removes exudate and infectious material. It should not be used for patients who are at risk for bleeding or only for the purpose of drainage containment. Chapter 25 describes this therapy in detail.

Patients with fistulas are also at high risk for intra-abdominal abscesses and sepsis. Antibiotic therapy is commonly prescribed. Observe for signs of sepsis (systemic INFECTION), such as fever, abdominal pain, or a change in mental status. Monitor for increased WBC levels that could indicate a systemic infection.

Other helpful interventions for the patient with CD are those that relax the patient and soothe the GI tract. Such therapies may include naturopathy, herbs (e.g., ginger), acupuncture, hypnotherapy, and ayurveda (a combination of diet, herbs, yoga, breathing exercises). The evidence supporting the use of these substances for CD is lacking, but many patients find them helpful for overall physical and emotional health. Teach patients about the availability of these therapies, and recommend that they include them in their collaborative plan of care.

? CLINICAL JUDGMENT CHALLENGE

Patient-Centered Care; Teamwork and Collaboration; Informatics QSEN

A young woman has an exacerbation of Crohn's disease with multiple diarrheal stools each day. She has been taking adalimumab (Humira) for the past 2 years to control the disease. However, she has been especially stressed in her doctoral program because she is applying for an internship for clinical psychology. The process is very competitive, and she is concerned that she may not be successful in finding a suitable internship site. She is worried that her flare-up will put her behind in her program.

1. What is your best response to the patient at this time?
2. What patient assessments will you perform on admission and why?
3. Based on the patient data provided, what priority problems do you identify?
4. Using best current evidence, how will you plan care with other members of the health care team? What members of the health care team will be involved in this patient's care and why?

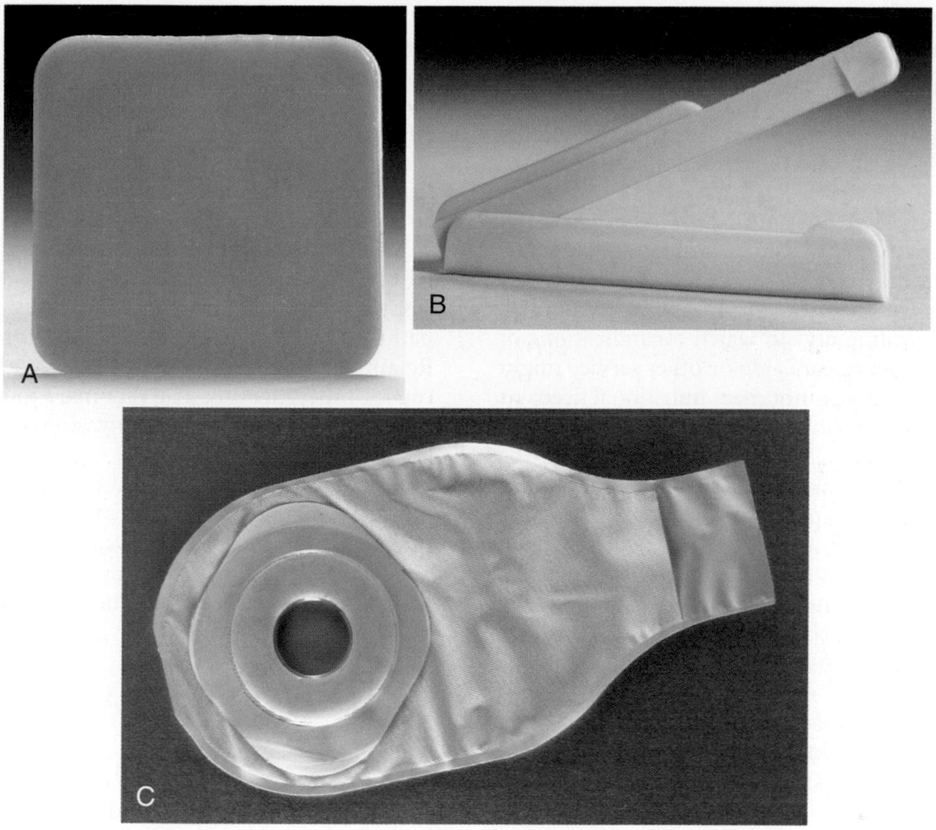

FIG. 57-5 Skin barriers, such as wafers **(A)** are cut to fit $\frac{1}{8}$ inch around the fistula. A drainable pouch **(B)** is applied over the wafer and clamped **(C)** until the pouch is to be emptied. Effluent should drain into the bag and not contact the skin.

Surgical Management. Surgery for Crohn's disease may be performed for those patients who have not improved with medical management or for those who have complications from the disease. Surgery to manage CD is not as successful as that for ulcerative colitis because of the extent of the disease. The patient with a fistula may undergo resection of the diseased area. Other indications for surgical treatment include perforation, massive hemorrhage, intestinal obstruction or strictures, abscesses, or cancer.

In some cases, a resection (removal of part of the small bowel) can be performed as minimally invasive surgery (MIS) via laparoscopy. This surgery involves one or more small incisions, less pain, and a quicker surgical recovery when compared with traditional open surgery. Both small-bowel resection (usually the ileum) and ileocecal resection can be done using this procedure. For other patients, an open surgical approach is used to allow for better visual access to the bowel.

Stricturoplasty may be performed for bowel strictures related to Crohn's disease. This procedure increases the bowel diameter. Care before and after each of these surgical procedures is similar to care for patients undergoing other types of abdominal surgery (see Chapters 14 and 16).

Community-Based Care

The discharge care plan for the patient with Crohn's disease is similar to that for the patient with ulcerative colitis (see p. 1180 in the discussion of Community-Based Care in the Ulcerative Colitis section). Collaborate with the case manager and CWOCN or wound nurse to help the patient plan self-management.

The interventions that were started to manage the disease are continued. Reinforce measures to control the disease and related symptoms and manage nutrition. Teach the patient and family to make arrangements for the patient to have easy access to the bathroom, as well as privacy to perform fistula care, if needed.

The health teaching plan for Crohn's disease is similar to that for the patient with ulcerative colitis. Teach the patient about the usual course of the disease, symptoms of complications, and when to notify the health care provider. Provide health teaching for drug therapy, including purpose, dose, and side effects. In addition to other drugs, vitamin supplements, including monthly vitamin B_{12} injections, may be needed because of the inability of the ileum to absorb these nutrients. In collaboration with the dietitian, instruct the patient to follow a low-residue, high-calorie diet and to avoid foods that cause discomfort, such as milk, gluten (wheat products), and other GI stimulants like caffeine.

Remind the patient to take rest periods, especially during exacerbations of the disease. If stress appears to increase symptoms of the disease, recommend stress management techniques, counseling, and/or physical activity to improve quality of life (Crumbock et al., 2009). For long-term follow-up, teach the patient about the increased risk for bowel cancer and the importance of having frequent colonoscopies.

If a patient has a fistula, explain and demonstrate wound care. Provide the opportunity for the patient to practice this care in the hospital. Ideally, he or she should be independent in fistula care before leaving the hospital. However, because of location of the fistula (perirectal or vaginal) or a large abdomen, assistance may be needed. If this is the case, teach a family member or other caregiver how to manage the wound. Patients may be transferred to a transitional or skilled nursing unit for collaborative care.

Patients who are discharged to home after undergoing resection and anastomosis may require visits from a home care nurse to assess the surgical wound and monitor for complications (see Chart 57-5). Assess the patient's and family's ability to monitor the progress of fistula healing and to watch for indications of INFECTION and sepsis. A home care aide or other service might be helpful for the patient who cannot meet nutritional needs or who needs help with grocery shopping and meal preparation.

In collaboration with the CM, assist with obtaining the equipment and supplies for fistula care, such as skin barriers and wound drainage bags. A support group sponsored by the United Ostomy Associations of America (www.uoaa.org) or a local hospital in the community may also be available to help with meeting physical and psychosocial needs.

DIVERTICULAR DISEASE

Diverticula are pouchlike herniations of the mucosa through the muscular wall of any portion of the gut but most commonly the colon. **Diverticulosis** is the presence of many abnormal pouchlike herniations (diverticula) in the wall of the intestine. Acute **diverticulitis** is the INFLAMMATION of diverticula.

❖ PATHOPHYSIOLOGY

Diverticula can occur in any part of the small or large intestine but usually occur in the sigmoid colon (Fig. 57-6). The muscle of the colon hypertrophies, thickens, and becomes rigid, and herniation of the mucosa and submucosa through the colon wall is seen. Diverticula seem to occur at points of weakness in the intestinal wall, often at areas where blood vessels interrupt the muscle layer. Muscle weakness develops as part of the aging process or as a result of a lack of fiber in the diet.

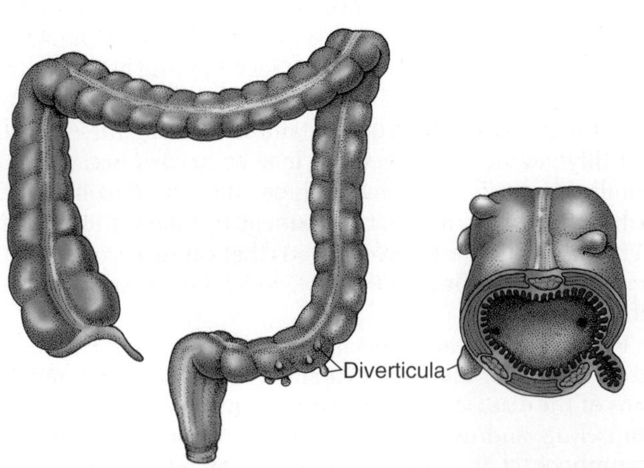

FIG. 57-6 Several abnormal outpouchings, or herniations, in the wall of the intestine, which are diverticula. These can occur anywhere in the small or large intestine but are found most often in the colon. Diverticulitis is the inflammation of a diverticulum that occurs when undigested food or bacteria become trapped in the diverticulum.

Without INFLAMMATION, diverticula cause few problems. If undigested food or bacteria become trapped in a diverticulum, however, blood supply to that area is reduced. Bacteria invade the diverticulum, resulting in diverticulitis, which then can perforate and develop a local abscess. A perforated diverticulum can progress to an intra-abdominal perforation with peritonitis (inflammation of the peritoneum). Lower GI bleeding may also occur.

High intraluminal pressure forces the formation of a pouch in the weakened area of the mucosa, frequently near blood vessels. Diets low in fiber that cause less bulky stool and constipation have been implicated in the formation of diverticula. Retained undigested food in diverticula is suggested to be one cause of diverticulitis. The retained food reduces blood flow to that area and makes bacterial invasion of the sac easier (McCance et al., 2014).

The exact incidence of diverticulosis is unknown, but millions of people are affected by the problem. It is found in two thirds of adults older than 80 years, with more men than women affected. African Americans have more diverticular disease than do Caucasians (Hall, 2011). The causes for these differences are not known.

❖ PATIENT-CENTERED COLLABORATIVE CARE

◆ Assessment

The patient with *diverticulosis* usually has no symptoms. Unless pain or bleeding develops, the condition may go undiagnosed. Diverticula are most often diagnosed during routine colonoscopy. Occasionally, diverticulosis will cause symptoms. For the patient with uncomplicated diverticulosis, ask about intermittent pain in the left lower quadrant and a history of constipation. If diverticulitis is suspected, ask about a history of low-grade fever, nausea, and abdominal PAIN. Inquire about recent bowel ELIMINATION patterns because constipation may develop as a result of intestinal INFLAMMATION. Also ask about any bleeding from the rectum.

The patient with *diverticulitis* may have abdominal PAIN, most often localized to the left lower quadrant. It is intermittent at first but becomes progressively steady. Occasionally, pain may be just above the pubic bone or may occur on one side. Abdominal pain is generalized if peritonitis has occurred. Nausea and vomiting are common. The patient's temperature is elevated, ranging from a low-grade fever to 101°F (38.3°C). Chills may be present. Often an increased heart rate (tachycardia) occurs with fever.

CONSIDERATIONS FOR OLDER ADULTS

Patient-Centered Care QSEN

The first sign of peritonitis in older adults may be a sudden change in mental status (e.g., acute confusion). For those who have dementia, the confusion worsens. Fever and chills may not be present due to normal physiologic changes associated with aging.

On examination of the abdomen, observe for distention. The patient may report tenderness over the involved area. Localized muscle spasm, guarded movement, and rebound tenderness may be present with peritoneal irritation. If generalized peritonitis is present, profound guarding occurs; rebound tenderness is more widespread; and sepsis, hypotension, or hypovolemic shock can occur. If the perforated diverticulum is close to the rectum, the health care provider may palpate a tender mass during the rectal examination. Blood pressure checks may show orthostatic changes. *If bleeding is massive, the patient may have hypotension and dehydration that result in shock.*

For the patient with uncomplicated diverticulosis, laboratory studies are not indicated. The patient with diverticulitis, however, has an *elevated white blood cell (WBC) count. Decreased hematocrit and hemoglobin* values are common if chronic or severe bleeding occurs. Stool tests for occult blood, if requested, are sometimes positive. Abdominal x-rays may be done to evaluate for free air and fluid indicating perforation. A CT scan may be performed to diagnose an abscess or thickening of the bowel related to diverticulitis.

Abdominal ultrasonography, a noninvasive test, may also reveal bowel thickening or an abscess. The health care provider may recommend a colonoscopy 4 to 8 weeks *after the acute phase* of the illness to rule out a tumor in the large intestine, particularly if the patient has rectal bleeding.

◆ Interventions

Patients are managed on an ambulatory care basis if the symptoms are mild. Monitor the patient for any prolonged or increased fever, abdominal PAIN, or blood in the stool. The patient with moderate to severe diverticulitis may be hospitalized, especially if the patient is older or has complications. Manifestations suggesting the need for admission are a temperature higher than 101° F (38.3° C), persistent and severe abdominal PAIN for more than 3 days, and/or lower GI bleeding.

Nonsurgical Management. A combination of drug and nutrition therapy with rest is used to decrease the INFLAMMATION associated with diverticular disease. Broad-spectrum antimicrobial drugs, such as metronidazole (Flagyl) plus trimethoprim/sulfamethoxazole (TMZ) (Bactrim or Bactrim DS, Septra) or ciprofloxacin (Cipro), are often prescribed. A mild analgesic may be given for PAIN. Chart 57-6 lists nursing interventions needed for care of older adults with diverticulitis.

The patient with more severe PAIN may be admitted to the hospital for IV fluids to correct dehydration and IV drug therapy. For patients with moderate to severe diverticulitis, an opioid analgesic may alleviate pain.

Laxatives and enemas are avoided because they increase intestinal motility. Assess the patient on an ongoing basis for manifestations of impaired FLUID AND ELECTROLYTE BALANCE.

Teach the patient to rest during the acute phase of illness. Remind him or her to refrain from lifting, straining, coughing, or bending to avoid an increase in intra-abdominal pressure, which can result in perforation of the diverticulum. NUTRITION therapy should be restricted to low fiber or clear liquids based on symptoms. The patient with more severe symptoms is NPO. A nasogastric tube (NGT) is inserted if nausea, vomiting, or abdominal distention is severe. Infuse IV fluids as prescribed for hydration. In collaboration with the dietitian, the patient increases dietary intake slowly as symptoms subside. When INFLAMMATION has resolved and bowel function returns to normal, a fiber-containing diet is introduced gradually.

Surgical Management. Diverticulitis can result in rupture of the diverticulum with peritonitis, pelvic abscess, bowel obstruction, fistula, persistent fever or PAIN, or uncontrolled bleeding. The surgeon performs emergency surgery if peritonitis, bowel obstruction, or pelvic abscess is present. Colon resection, with or without a colostomy, is the most common surgical procedure for patients with diverticular disease. Chapter 56 discusses the nursing care for patients with this procedure.

CHART 57-6 Nursing Focus on the Older Adult

Diverticulitis

- Provide antibiotics, analgesics, and anticholinergics as prescribed. Observe older patients carefully for side effects of these drugs, especially confusion (or increased confusion), urinary retention or failure, and orthostatic hypotension.
- Do not give laxatives or enemas. Teach the patient and the family about the importance of avoiding these measures.
- Encourage the patient to rest and to avoid activities that may increase intra-abdominal pressure, such as straining and bending.
- While diverticulitis is active, provide a *low*-fiber diet. When the inflammation resolves, provide a *high*-fiber diet. Teach the patient and family about these diets and when they are appropriate.
- Because older patients do not always experience the typical pain or fever expected, observe carefully for other signs of active disease, such as a sudden change in mental status.
- Perform frequent abdominal assessments to determine distention and tenderness on palpation.
- Check stools for occult or frank bleeding.

Community-Based Care

The length of stay for patients hospitalized for diverticulitis ranges from 1 to 4 days, depending on the response to treatment and if surgery is performed. Discharge plans vary according to the treatment. The patient who has surgical intervention has the added responsibilities of incision care and possibly colostomy care with temporary limitations placed on activities.

Patients with diverticular disease need education regarding a high-fiber diet. Encourage the patient with *diverticulosis* to eat a diet high in cellulose and hemicellulose types of fiber. These substances can be found in wheat bran, whole-grain breads, and cereals. Teach the patient to eat at least 25 to 35 g of fiber per day. Fresh fruits and vegetables with high fiber content are added to provide bulk to stools.

If not accustomed to eating high-fiber foods, teach the patient to add them to the diet gradually to avoid flatulence and abdominal cramping. If he or she cannot tolerate the recommended fiber requirement, a bulk-forming laxative, such as psyllium hydrophilic mucilloid (Metamucil), can be taken to increase fecal size and consistency. Teach the patient to drink plenty of fluids to help prevent bloating that may occur with a high-fiber diet. Alcohol should be avoided because it irritates the bowel. Foods containing seeds or indigestible material that may block a diverticulum, such as nuts, corn, popcorn, cucumbers, tomatoes, figs, and strawberries, may be eliminated. Teach the patient that dietary fat intake should not exceed 30% of the total daily caloric intake.

Teach the patient to avoid all fiber when symptoms of *diverticulitis* are present, because high-fiber foods are then irritating. As INFLAMMATION resolves, fiber can gradually be added until progression to a high-fiber diet is established. The patient who has undergone surgery is usually taking solid food by the time of discharge from the hospital.

Provide oral and written instructions on incision care and the signs and symptoms to report to the health care provider for the patient who had abdominal surgery. If a colostomy was created, reinforce ostomy care as needed. Encourage the patient to express concerns about body image. Allow time and address sexual concerns regarding the changed body image.

Instruct the patient with any type of diverticular disease, orally and in writing, about the manifestations of acute diverticulitis, including fever, abdominal PAIN, and bloody, mahogany, or tarry stools. Advise patients to avoid the use of laxatives (other than bulk-forming types) and enemas. Reassure them that this disorder should not cause problems if a proper diet is followed.

In collaboration with the case manager, arrange for a home care nurse, if needed, to assess wound healing and proper functioning of the ostomy and the appliance. If the patient is interested, arrange for a visit from an ostomy volunteer (ostomate) or an ostomy nurse. For information about other community resources, remind the patient to contact the United Ostomy Associations of America (www.uoaa.org).

NCLEX EXAMINATION CHALLENGE

Physiological Integrity

The nurse is teaching a client about nutrition and diverticulitis. Which statement by the client indicates a need for further teaching?

A. "I should eat more foods low in fiber."
B. "I will not drink any alcohol."
C. "I can have any fruits that I want."
D. "I need to avoid nuts and corn."

CELIAC DISEASE

Celiac disease (CD) was once thought to be a rare disease, but many cases in adults between 30 and 50 years old have been diagnosed in the past 10 years. CD is a multi-system autoimmune disease with an estimated incidence of about 3 million Americans; most are not diagnosed (Strauch & Cotter, 2011). Patients who have other autoimmune diseases, such as rheumatoid arthritis and diabetes mellitus type 1, are at the highest risk for the disease.

CD is a chronic INFLAMMATION of the small intestinal mucosa that can cause bowel wall atrophy and malabsorption. Like many inflammatory disorders, it is thought to be caused by a combination of genetic, immunologic, and environmental factors. The primary complication of CD is cancer, specifically non-Hodgkin's lymphoma or GI cancers.

Patients with CD have varying clinical manifestations with cycles of remission and exacerbation (flare-up). Classic symptoms include anorexia, diarrhea and/or constipation, steatorrhea (fatty stools), abdominal PAIN, abdominal bloating and distention, and weight loss. Some patients have no symptoms. Still others have atypical symptoms that affect every body system (Chart 57-7).

Dietary management is the only available treatment for achieving disease remission. In most cases, a gluten-free diet (GFD) results in healing the intestinal mucosa after about 2 years (Strauch & Cotter, 2011). Gluten is the primary substance in wheat and wheat-based products. Teach patients to carefully check for hidden sources of gluten that are in foods, food additives, drugs, and cosmetics. Patients often take vitamin and mineral supplements to replace those lost in avoiding gluten foods.

CHART 57-7 Key Features

Celiac Disease

Classic Symptoms	Atypical Symptoms
• Weight loss	• Osteoporosis
• Anorexia	• Joint pain and inflammation
• Diarrhea and/or constipation	• Lactose intolerance
• Steatorrhea	• Iron deficiency anemia
• Abdominal pain and distention	• Depression
• Vomiting	• Migraines
	• Epilepsy
	• Autoimmune disorders
	• Stomatitis
	• Early menopause
	• Protein-calorie malnutrition

ANAL DISORDERS

ANORECTAL ABSCESS

Anorectal abscess is a localized area of induration and pus caused by INFLAMMATION of the soft tissue near the rectum or anus. It is most often the result of obstruction of the ducts of glands in the anorectal region. Feces, foreign bodies, or trauma can be the cause of the obstruction and stasis, leading to INFECTION that spreads into nearby tissue.

Rectal PAIN is often the first symptom. There may be no other manifestations at first, but local swelling, redness, and tenderness are present within a few days after the onset of pain. If the abscess becomes chronic, discharge, bleeding, and pruritus (itching) may exist. Fever occurs if larger abscesses are present.

Anorectal abscesses are managed by surgical incision and drainage (I&D). The physician can often excise (surgically remove) simple perianal and ischiorectal abscesses using a local anesthetic. For patients with more extensive abscesses, a regional or general anesthetic may be needed. Systemic antibiotics are given only for patients who are immunocompromised, are diabetic, have valvular disease or a prosthetic valve, or are obese.

NURSING SAFETY PRIORITY QSEN

Action Alert

For patients with an anorectal abscess, nursing interventions are focused on comfort and helping the patient maintain optimal perineal hygiene. Encourage the use of warm sitz baths, analgesics, bulk-producing agents, and stool softeners after the surgery until healing occurs. *Stress the importance of good perineal hygiene after all bowel movements and the maintenance of a regular bowel pattern with a high-fiber diet.*

Patients are often embarrassed about having anal problems. Provide privacy and maintain the patient's dignity during the examination and treatment.

ANAL FISSURE

An **anal fissure** is a tear in the anal lining, which can be very painful. Smaller fissures occur with straining to have a stool, such as with diarrhea or constipation. Larger, deeper fissures may occur as a result of another disorder (e.g., Crohn's disease, tuberculosis, leukemia, neoplasm) or from trauma (e.g., from a foreign body, anal intercourse, perirectal surgery).

An *acute* anal fissure is superficial and usually resolves on its own or heals quickly with conservative treatment. *Chronic* fissures recur, and surgical treatment may be needed. Pain during and after defecation and bright red blood in the stool are the most common symptoms. Other manifestations include pruritus, urinary frequency or retention, dysuria, and **dyspareunia** (painful intercourse).

The diagnosis is made by stretching and inspecting the perianal skin. If the patient is having pain at the time of the examination, diagnostic testing is usually limited to inspection. If he or she is not in severe PAIN, a digital examination and possibly a sigmoidoscopy are performed. When painless or multiple fissures are present, a colonoscopy may be performed to rule out any inflammatory bowel disorder.

Management of an acute fissure is usually aimed at local PAIN relief and softening of stools to reduce trauma to the area. Teach the patient to use warm sitz baths, analgesics, and bulk-producing agents (e.g., psyllium hydrophilic mucilloid [Metamucil]) to help minimize the pain from defecation. Topical anti-inflammatory agents (hydrocortisone creams and suppositories) may be helpful for some patients.

Explain PAIN control measures to the patient. Remind him or her to notify the health care provider if pain is not relieved within a few days. If fissures do not respond to management within several days to weeks, surgical repair under a local anesthetic may be needed. Teach the patient to report any drainage or bleeding from the rectum to the health care provider.

ANAL FISTULA

An anal fistula, or *fistula in ano,* is an abnormal tract leading from the anal canal to the perianal skin. Most anal fistulas result from anorectal abscesses, which are caused by obstruction of anal glands (see Anorectal Abscess, p. 1188). Fistulas can also occur with tuberculosis, Crohn's disease, or cancer. Intermittent discharge is usually noted over the perianal area.

The patient with an anal fistula has pruritus (itching), purulent discharge, and tenderness or PAIN that is worsened by bowel movements. A proctoscope may be used to identify the source of symptoms and to locate the fistula. Because fistulas do not heal spontaneously, surgery is necessary. To perform a fistulotomy, the surgeon opens the tissue over the tract and scrapes the base. The incision site then heals by secondary intention. For a fistula higher in the anus, a special surgical technique is used to preserve important sphincters. After surgery, instruct the patient about sitz baths, analgesics, and the use of bulk-producing agents or stool softeners to reduce pain.

PARASITIC INFECTION

❖ PATHOPHYSIOLOGY

Parasites can enter and invade the GI tract and cause INFECTION. They commonly enter through the mouth (oral-fecal transmission) from contaminated food or water, oral-anal sexual practices, or contact with feces from a contaminated person. Common parasites that cause infection in humans are *Giardia lamblia,* which causes giardiasis; *Entamoeba histolytica,* which causes amebiasis (amebic dysentery); and *Cryptosporidium. Handwashing is the best way to prevent the spread of parasitic infections.*

G. lamblia is a protozoal parasite that causes superficial invasion, destruction, and INFLAMMATION of the mucosa in the small intestine. This organism occurs in cysts and trophozoites (sporozoan parasites). Trophozoites die rapidly after they leave the body in stool. Cysts, however, can remain alive in the right type of environment for weeks or months. Humans who eliminate cysts are infectious. Flies can spread the cysts, and the problem is more common in areas that use human excrement for fertilizer. Humans are hosts to this organism, but beavers and dogs may be reservoirs for infection.

Giardiasis is a well-recognized problem in international travelers, campers, and immunosuppressed patients. In the United States, giardiasis is prevalent and is the most common parasitic INFECTION. This disorder affects only the intestinal system, causing acute diarrhea, chronic diarrhea, or malabsorption syndrome. The acute phase usually is self-limiting, lasting days or weeks. The chronic phase can last for years. Diarrhea is usually mild in both forms, but it can be severe. As stools increase in frequency, they become more watery, greasy, frothy, and malodorous with mucus. Weight loss and weakness are also common. Malabsorption can occur with diarrhea that continues for longer than 3 weeks. Manifestations result from malabsorption of fat, protein, and vitamin B_{12} and lactase deficiency.

Humans are the only known hosts for *E. histolytica* (also known as *amebiasis*). This organism also occurs in cysts and trophozoites. Amebiasis occurs worldwide, but it is most common in tropical areas. Prevalence rates are high in areas with poor sanitation, crowding, and poor nutrition. Amebiasis causes tens of thousands of deaths annually worldwide. The disease causes less severe symptoms and often goes undiagnosed in temperate climates.

E. histolytica either feeds on bacteria in the intestine or invades and ulcerates the mucosa of the large intestine. The parasite can be limited to the GI tract (intestinal amebiasis), or it can extend outside the intestines (extraintestinal amebiasis). People can have intestinal amebiasis without having any symptoms, or symptoms can range from mild to severe.

Cryptosporidium is manifested by diarrhea. This INFECTION occurs most commonly in immunosuppressed patients, particularly those with human immune deficiency virus (HIV). It can also occur in children and older adults from contaminated swimming pools. (See Chapter 19 for a discussion of HIV infection.)

Chagas disease is caused by the *Trypanosoma cruzi* parasite, which is most commonly transmitted to people in poverty areas of Latin America by the triatomine (kissing) bug. Patients first develop an acute infection, followed by an intermediate asymptomatic period and a chronic infection. Patients with chronic Chagas disease often develop cardiac dysrhythmias or heart failure, as well as colon or esophagus dilation causing impaired digestion and bowel elimination. An estimated 300,000 people in the United States have the disease (most in the southern areas of the United States), which can be transmitted through blood transfusions and organ transplantations. The CDC has targeted Chagas disease as one of five neglected parasitic infections that require public health action as the number of cases is expected to increase (CDC, 2014).

❖ PATIENT-CENTERED COLLABORATIVE CARE

◆ Assessment

A thorough history can help determine potential sources of exposure to parasitic INFECTION. A history of travel to parts of the world where such infections are prevalent increases suspicion for infection with parasites. GI symptoms related to travel may be delayed as long as 1 to 2 weeks after the return home. Immigrants (newcomers) may have the infection upon entering a new country. A NUTRITION history is especially helpful if several people in a group become ill. Common water supplies or bodies of water may be infected with *Giardia* or *Cryptosporidium*. Trichinosis should be considered if the patient has eaten pork products.

Mild to moderate *E. histolytica* infestation causes the daily passage of several strongly foul-smelling stools, possibly with mucus but without blood, accompanied by abdominal cramping, flatulence (gas), fatigue, and weight loss.

The infected patient usually experiences remissions and recurrences. Severe amebic dysentery is manifested by frequent, more liquid, and foul-smelling stools with mucus *and* blood. Fever up to 104° F (40° C), **tenesmus** (feeling the urge to defecate), generalized abdominal tenderness, and vomiting can also occur. The ulcerations of invading amebiasis that occur in the colon can cause pain, bleeding, and obstruction. Ulcerations can also occur in the rectum, resulting in formed stool with blood. Complications are rare but include appendicitis and bowel perforation.

Extraintestinal amebiasis can occur without symptoms of intestinal INFECTION. The most common form is amebic liver abscess, which causes symptoms of fever, PAIN, and an enlarged liver. The abscess can rupture, and death can result if the infection and complications are not treated.

The diagnosis of *amebiasis* is made by examining the stool for parasites. Because *E. histolytica* is difficult to detect, serial stool examinations are needed if the disease is suspected. The use of sigmoidoscopy may detect ulcerations in the rectum or colon. Exudate obtained during sigmoidoscopic examination is studied for the parasite. The white blood cell (WBC) count can be very high when severe dysentery is present.

The diagnosis of *giardiasis* is also confirmed by the presence of parasites in the stool. Because organisms may not be detected for at least 1 week after symptoms appear, multiple stool samples should be examined.

◆ *Interventions*

Treatment for all types of *amebiasis* involves the use of amebicide drugs. Metronidazole (Flagyl, Novonidazol 🍁) and diloxanide furoate (Entamide) or diloxanide furoate and tetracycline hydrochloride (Sumycin) followed by chloroquine are commonly prescribed. The patient with severe dysentery requires IV fluid replacement and possibly opiates, such as diphenoxylate hydrochloride and atropine sulfate (Lomotil), to control bowel motility. The patient with extraintestinal amebiasis or severe dehydration is hospitalized, especially the older adult. The patient with asymptomatic, mild, or moderate disease is treated with drug therapy on an ambulatory care basis. Therapy effectiveness is based on the examination of at least three stools at 2- to 3-day intervals, starting 2 to 4 weeks after drug therapy has been completed. *Teach patients the importance of keeping their follow-up appointments and taking all drugs as prescribed.*

Treatment for *giardiasis* is drug therapy. Metronidazole is the drug of choice, 250 mg orally 3 times daily for 5 days. Tinidazole (Fasigyn) can be used as an alternative. Stools are examined 2 weeks after treatment to assess for drug effectiveness.

! NURSING SAFETY PRIORITY (QSEN)

Action Alert

Explain modes of transmission of parasitic infections and means to avoid the spread of INFECTION and recurrent contact with parasitic organisms. *Inform the patient that the infection can be transmitted to others until amebicides effectively kill the parasites. Teach the patient to:*

- Avoid contact with stool.
- Keep toilet areas clean.
- Wash hands meticulously with an antimicrobial soap after bowel movements.
- Maintain good personal hygiene by bathing or showering daily.
- Avoid stool from dogs and beavers.

Advise the patient to avoid sexual practices that allow rectal contact until drug therapy is completed. *All household and sexual partners should have stool examinations for parasites.* If the water supply is suspected as the source, a sample is obtained and sent for analysis. Multiple infections are common in households, often as a result of contaminated water supplies. Well water and water from areas with inadequate or no filtration equipment can be sources of contamination.

Infection with *Cryptosporidium* is usually self-limiting in people who have normal immune function. Drug therapy for patients who are immunosuppressed may include paromomycin (Paromycin), an aminoglycoside antibiotic. Teach patients that this drug can cause dizziness.

NURSING CONCEPTS AND CLINICAL JUDGMENT REVIEW

What might you NOTICE if the patient has impaired digestion and inadequate NUTRITION as a result of inflammatory intestinal problems?

- Report of nausea
- Vomiting
- Report of epigastric or abdominal pain
- Diarrhea (sometimes bloody)
- Elevated temperature
- Weakness

Perform and interpret focused physical assessment findings, including:

- Vital signs
- Complete pain assessment
- Skin turgor and mucous membrane dryness
- Abdominal assessment
- Current and previous weight
- History of recent food intake
- History of recent travel

What should you INTERPRET and how should you RESPOND to a patient with impaired digestion and inadequate NUTRITION as a result of inflammatory intestinal problems?

Respond by:

- Preventing pain and aspiration by placing the patient in a sitting position

- Placing an IV catheter (large-bore) to replace fluids
- Providing privacy, and assisting with hygiene
- Providing rest
- Checking laboratory values for hemoglobin and hematocrit (anemia)
- Checking serum electrolytes (dehydration, hypokalemia)
- Giving antidiarrheal drugs if prescribed
- Recording intake and output
- Assisting with ADLs and ambulation as needed

On what should you REFLECT?

- Continue to monitor for vomiting and diarrhea and changes in pain level.
- Think about what you need to document.
- Decide when you might need to call the health care provider or Rapid Response Team (for hospitalized patients).
- Determine what health teaching and community resources may be needed for this patient and family.
- Think about what you can do to help prevent complications of the health problem.

GET READY FOR THE NCLEX® EXAMINATION!

KEY POINTS

Review these Key Points for each NCLEX Examination Client Needs Category.

Safe and Effective Care Environment

- Collaborate with a CWOCN, health care provider, and case manager to plan care for patients with IBD. **Teamwork and Collaboration** QSEN

Health Promotion and Maintenance

- Teach patients to use INFECTION control measures to prevent transmission of gastroenteritis as stated in Chart 57-2.
- Teach patients how to self-manage an ileostomy or other surgical diversion, including skin care, pouch management, and stoma assessment (see Chart 57-4).
- Remind patients and families about community resources for IBD, including the United Ostomy Associations of America and the Crohn's and Colitis Foundation of America.

Psychosocial Integrity

- Be aware that all inflammatory bowel diseases (acute and chronic) are very disruptive to one's daily routine; living with IBD requires a lifetime of modifications.
- Recognize that having a chronic bowel disease or an ileostomy impacts the patient's body image and self-esteem; assess for coping strategies that the patient has previously used, and identify personal support systems, such as family members, to assist in coping.

Physiological Integrity

- Assess for the classic clinical manifestations of appendicitis, which include abdominal pain, nausea and vomiting, and abdominal tenderness upon palpation (McBurney's point); some patients also have leukocytosis.
- Recognize that perforation (rupture) of the appendix requires prompt intervention and can result in peritonitis.
- Assess for the key features of peritonitis as listed in Chart 57-1.
- Assess for signs and symptoms of dehydration in patients who have acute and chronic inflammatory bowel disorders.
- Administer antidiarrheal medications as prescribed to decrease stools and therefore prevent dehydration in patients with acute and chronic inflammatory bowel disorders.
- Be aware that there are two major types of chronic inflammatory bowel disease (IBD): ulcerative colitis (UC) and Crohn's disease; both have similarities but also have differences (see Table 57-2).
- Be alert for GI bleeding in the patient with chronic inflammatory bowel disease (IBD).
- Be aware that patients with Crohn's disease are at high risk for malnutrition as a result of an inability to absorb nutrients via the small intestine.
- Priority problems for patients with ulcerative colitis include diarrhea, pain, and potential for lower GI bleeding.
- Monitor for complications of UC as listed in Table 57-4.
- Provide nursing interventions for patients with IBD as listed in Chart 57-3.
- Teach patients with IBD to avoid GI stimulants, such as alcohol and caffeine; each patient's response to foods differs.
- Administer 5-aminosalicylic acid (5-ASA) drugs as prescribed (e.g., Pentasa) to decrease inflammation in patients with UC; most of these same drugs are also used for Crohn's disease management.
- Administer infliximab (Remicade) or other monoclonal antibody agent as prescribed for patients with Crohn's disease; these drugs may also be useful for those with UC in selected cases.
- Observe for manifestations of lower GI bleeding in patients with chronic inflammatory and diverticular disease.
- Teach patients with diverticulosis to eat a high-fiber diet; diverticulitis requires a low-fiber diet.
- Teach older patients how to self-manage diverticulitis as outlined in Chart 57-6.
- Instruct patients with diverticulosis about NUTRITION modifications, such as avoiding nuts, foods with seeds, and GI stimulants.
- Be aware that patients with celiac disease (CD) vary in their clinical manifestations; some have no symptoms, some have classic symptoms, and some have atypical symptoms (see Chart 57-7).
- Teach patients with CD about the need to consume a strict gluten-free diet, which avoids wheat and wheat-based products.
- Be aware that GI problems, including diarrhea, may also be caused by parasites and food poisoning.
- Instruct patients with anorectal disorders to use sitz baths, bulk-forming agents (e.g., Metamucil), and stool softeners to decrease pain.

58 CHAPTER

Care of Patients with Liver Problems

Jennifer Powers and Lara Carver

http://evolve.elsevier.com/Iggy/

PRIORITY CONCEPTS

- INFLAMMATION
- INFECTION
- PAIN
- FLUID AND ELECTROLYTE BALANCE

LEARNING OUTCOMES

Safe and Effective Care Environment

1. Describe the need to collaborate with health care team members to provide care for patients with liver INFLAMMATION and necrosis.
2. Identify community resources for patients with chronic liver disease.

Health Promotion and Maintenance

3. Develop a health teaching plan for patients and families to prevent hepatitis and its spread to others.
4. Develop a health teaching plan for patients and families to prevent or slow the progress of alcohol-induced cirrhosis.

Psychosocial Integrity

5. Explain the psychosocial needs of patients with liver problems.

Physiological Integrity

6. Identify risk factors for developing hepatic cirrhosis.
7. Interpret laboratory test findings commonly seen in patients with cirrhosis.
8. Analyze assessment data from patients with cirrhosis to determine priority patient problems.
9. Develop an evidence-based collaborative plan of care for the patient with late-stage cirrhosis.
10. Describe the role of the nurse in monitoring for and managing potentially life-threatening complications of cirrhosis.
11. Identify emergency interventions for the patient with bleeding esophageal varices.
12. Explain the role of the nurse when assisting with a paracentesis procedure.
13. Describe treatment options for patients with cancer of the liver.
14. Describe the interventions to prevent complications that result from liver transplantation, including INFECTION.

The liver is the largest and one of the most vital internal organs, performing more than 400 functions and affecting every system in the body. When the liver is diseased or damaged, it cannot accomplish these functions. As a result, *digestion, nutrition, and metabolism* can be severely affected. Liver diseases range in severity from mild hepatic INFLAMMATION to chronic end-stage cirrhosis.

CIRRHOSIS

Cirrhosis is extensive, irreversible scarring of the liver, usually caused by a chronic reaction to hepatic INFLAMMATION and necrosis. The disease typically develops slowly and has a progressive, prolonged, destructive course resulting in end-stage liver disease. The most common causes for cirrhosis in the United States are chronic alcoholism, chronic viral hepatitis, nonalcoholic steatohepatitis (NASH), bile duct disease, and genetic diseases (Table 58-1).

❖ *PATHOPHYSIOLOGY*

Cirrhosis is characterized by widespread fibrotic (scarred) bands of connective tissue that change the liver's normal makeup. INFLAMMATION caused by either toxins or disease results in extensive degeneration and destruction of **hepatocytes** (liver cells). As cirrhosis develops, the tissue becomes nodular. These nodules can block bile ducts and normal blood flow throughout the liver. Impairments in blood and lymph flow result from compression caused by excessive fibrous tissue. In early disease, the liver is usually enlarged, firm, and hard. As the pathologic process continues, the liver shrinks in size, resulting in decreased liver function, which can occur in weeks to years. Some patients with cirrhosis have no symptoms until serious complications occur. The impaired liver function results in elevated serum liver enzymes (Pagana & Pagana, 2014).

Cirrhosis of the liver can be divided into several common types, depending on the cause of the disease (McCance et al., 2014):

TABLE 58-1 Common Causes of Cirrhosis

• Alcoholic liver disease	• Drugs and chemical toxins
• Viral hepatitis	• Gallbladder disease
• Autoimmune hepatitis	• Metabolic/genetic causes
• Steatohepatitis (from fatty liver)	• Cardiovascular disease

- Postnecrotic cirrhosis (caused by viral hepatitis [especially hepatitis C] and certain drugs or other toxins)
- Laennec's or alcoholic cirrhosis (caused by chronic alcoholism)
- Biliary cirrhosis (also called *cholestatic;* caused by chronic biliary obstruction or autoimmune disease)

Complications of Cirrhosis

Common problems and complications associated with hepatic cirrhosis depend on the amount of damage sustained by the liver. In **compensated cirrhosis**, the liver is scarred but can still perform essential functions without causing major symptoms. In **decompensated cirrhosis**, liver function is impaired with obvious manifestations of liver failure.

The loss of hepatic function contributes to the development of metabolic abnormalities. Hepatic cell damage may lead to these common complications:

- Portal hypertension
- Ascites and esophageal varices
- Coagulation defects
- Jaundice
- Portal-systemic encephalopathy (PSE) with hepatic coma
- Hepatorenal syndrome
- Spontaneous bacterial peritonitis

Portal Hypertension. **Portal hypertension**, a persistent increase in pressure within the portal vein greater than 5 mm Hg, is a major complication of cirrhosis (Minano & Garcia-Tsao, 2010). It results from increased resistance to or obstruction (blockage) of the flow of blood through the portal vein and its branches. The blood meets resistance to flow and seeks collateral (alternative) venous channels around the high-pressure area.

Blood flow backs into the spleen, causing **splenomegaly** (spleen enlargement). Veins in the esophagus, stomach, intestines, abdomen, and rectum become dilated. Portal hypertension can result in ascites (excessive abdominal [peritoneal] fluid), esophageal varices (distended veins), prominent abdominal veins (caput medusae), and hemorrhoids.

Ascites and Gastroesophageal Varices. **Ascites** is the collection of free fluid within the peritoneal cavity caused by increased hydrostatic pressure from portal hypertension (McCance et al., 2014). The collection of plasma protein in the peritoneal fluid reduces the amount of circulating plasma protein in the blood. When this decrease is combined with the inability of the liver to produce albumin because of impaired liver cell functioning, the serum colloid osmotic pressure is decreased in the circulatory system. The result is a fluid shift from the vascular system into the abdomen, a form of "third spacing." As a result, the patient may have hypovolemia and edema at the same time.

Massive ascites may cause renal vasoconstriction, triggering the renin-angiotensin system. This results in sodium and water retention, which increases hydrostatic pressure and the vascular volume and leads to more ascites.

As a result of portal hypertension, the blood backs up from the liver and enters the esophageal and gastric veins. **Esophageal varices** occur when fragile, thin-walled esophageal veins become distended and tortuous from increased pressure. The potential for varices to bleed depends on their size; size is determined by direct endoscopic observation. Varices occur most often in the distal esophagus but can be present also in the stomach and rectum.

Bleeding esophageal varices is a life-threatening medical emergency. Severe blood loss may occur, resulting in shock from hypovolemia. The bleeding may be either **hematemesis** (vomiting blood) or **melena** (black, tarry stools). Loss of consciousness may occur before any observed bleeding. Variceal bleeding can occur spontaneously with no precipitating factors. However, any activity that increases abdominal pressure may increase the likelihood of a variceal bleed, including heavy lifting or vigorous physical exercise. In addition, chest trauma or dry, hard food in the esophagus can cause bleeding.

Patients with portal hypertension may also have **portal hypertensive gastropathy.** This complication can occur with or without esophageal varices. Slow gastric mucosal bleeding occurs, which may result in chronic slow blood loss, occult-positive stools, and anemia.

Splenomegaly (enlarged spleen) results from the backup of blood into the spleen. The enlarged spleen destroys platelets, causing thrombocytopenia (low serum platelet count) and increased risk for bleeding. Thrombocytopenia is often the first clinical sign that a patient has liver dysfunction.

Biliary Obstruction. In patients with cirrhosis, the production of bile in the liver is decreased. This prevents the absorption of fat-soluble vitamins (e.g., vitamin K). Without vitamin K, clotting factors II, VII, IX, and X are not produced in sufficient quantities and the patient is susceptible to bleeding and easy bruising. These abnormalities are confirmed by coagulation studies. Some patients have a genetic predisposition to obstruction of the bile duct that leads to biliary cirrhosis—usually from gallbladder disease or an autoimmune form of the disease called *primary biliary cirrhosis (PBC).*

Jaundice (yellowish coloration of the skin) in patients with cirrhosis is caused by one of two mechanisms: hepatocellular disease or intrahepatic obstruction (Fig. 58-1). *Hepatocellular* jaundice develops because the liver cells cannot effectively excrete bilirubin. This decreased excretion results in excessive circulating bilirubin levels. *Intrahepatic obstructive* jaundice results from edema, fibrosis, or scarring of the hepatic bile channels and bile ducts, which interferes with normal bile and bilirubin excretion. Patients with jaundice often report pruritus (itching).

Hepatic Encephalopathy. **Hepatic encephalopathy** (also called **portal-systemic encephalopathy [PSE]**) is a complex cognitive syndrome that results from liver failure and cirrhosis. Patients report sleep disturbance, mood disturbance, mental status changes, and speech problems early as this complication begins. Hepatic encephalopathy may be reversible with early intervention. Later neurologic symptoms include an altered level of consciousness, impaired thinking processes, and neuromuscular problems.

Hepatic encephalopathy may develop slowly in patients with chronic liver disease and go undetected until the late stages. Symptoms develop rapidly in acute liver dysfunction. Four stages of development have been identified (Table 58-2). The patient's symptoms may gradually progress to coma or fluctuate among the four stages.

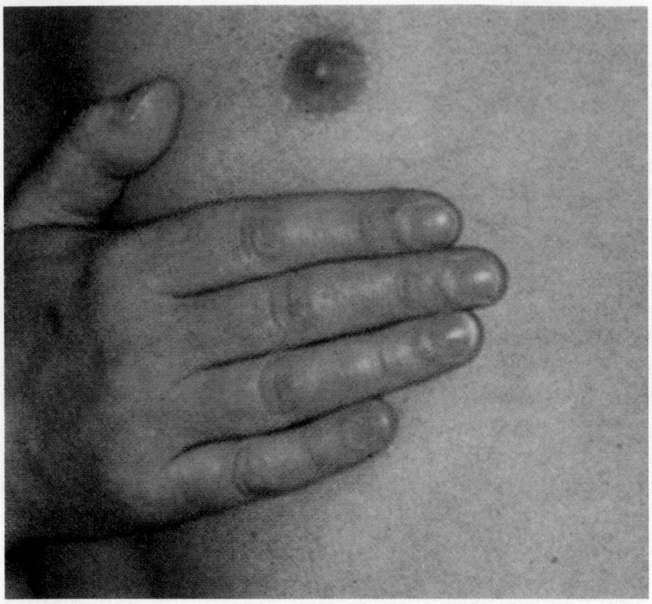

FIG. 58-1 Jaundice as a result of liver dysfunction such as cirrhosis and hepatitis.

TABLE 58-2 Stages of Hepatic Encephalopathy

Stage I
- Subtle manifestations that may not be recognized immediately
- Personality changes
- Behavior changes (agitation, belligerence)
- Emotional lability (euphoria, depression)
- Impaired thinking
- Inability to concentrate
- Fatigue, drowsiness
- Slurred or slowed speech
- Sleep pattern disturbances

Stage II
- Continuing mental changes
- Mental confusion
- Disorientation to time, place, or person
- Asterixis (hand flapping)

Stage III
- Progressive deterioration
- Marked mental confusion
- Stuporous, drowsy but arousable
- Abnormal electroencephalogram tracing
- Muscle twitching
- Hyperreflexia
- Asterixis (hand flapping)

Stage IV
- Unresponsiveness, leading to death in most patients progressing to this stage
- Unarousable, obtunded
- Usually no response to painful stimulus
- No asterixis
- Positive Babinski's sign
- Muscle rigidity
- Fetor hepaticus (characteristic liver breath—musty, sweet odor)
- Seizures

The exact mechanisms causing hepatic encephalopathy are not clearly understood but probably are the result of the shunting of portal venous blood into the central circulation so that the liver is bypassed. As a result, substances absorbed by the intestine are not broken down or detoxified and may lead to metabolic abnormalities, such as elevated serum ammonia and gamma-aminobutyric acid (GABA). Elevated serum ammonia results from the inability of the liver to detoxify protein by-products and is common in patients with hepatic encephalopathy. However, it is not a clear indicator of the presence of encephalopathy. Some patients may have major impairment without high elevations of serum ammonia, and elevations of ammonia can occur without evidence of encephalopathy.

Factors that may lead to hepatic encephalopathy in patients with cirrhosis include:
- High-protein diet
- INFECTION
- Hypovolemia (decreased fluid volume)
- Hypokalemia (decreased serum potassium)
- Constipation
- GI bleeding (causes a large protein load in the intestines)
- Drugs (e.g., hypnotics, opioids, sedatives, analgesics, diuretics, illicit drugs)

The prognosis depends on the severity of the underlying cause, the precipitating factors, and the degree of liver dysfunction.

Other Complications. The development of **hepatorenal syndrome (HRS)** indicates a poor prognosis for the patient with liver failure. It is often the cause of death in these patients. This syndrome is manifested by:
- A sudden decrease in urinary flow (<500 mL/24 hr) (oliguria)
- Elevated blood urea nitrogen (BUN) and creatinine levels with abnormally decreased urine sodium excretion
- Increased urine osmolarity

HRS often occurs after clinical deterioration from GI bleeding or the onset of hepatic encephalopathy. It may also complicate other liver diseases, including acute hepatitis and fulminant liver failure.

Patients with cirrhosis and ascites may develop acute *spontaneous bacterial peritonitis (SBP)*. Those who are particularly susceptible are patients with very advanced liver disease. This may be the result of low concentrations of proteins; proteins normally provide some protection against bacteria.

The bacteria responsible for SBP are typically from the bowel and reach the ascitic fluid after migrating through the bowel wall and transversing the lymphatics. Clinical manifestations vary but may include fever, chills, and abdominal PAIN and tenderness. However, manifestations can also be minimal with only mild symptoms in the absence of fever. Worsening encephalopathy and increased jaundice may also be present without abdominal symptoms.

The diagnosis of SBP is made when a sample of ascitic fluid is obtained by paracentesis for cell counts and culture. An ascitic fluid leukocyte count of more than 250 polymorphonuclear (PMN) leukocytes may indicate the need for treatment.

Etiology and Genetic Risk

Hepatitis C is the second leading cause of cirrhosis and liver failure in the United States. It is an infectious bloodborne illness that usually causes chronic disease. INFLAMMATION caused by INFECTION over time leads to progressive scarring of the liver. It usually takes decades for cirrhosis to develop, although alcohol use in combination with hepatitis C may speed the process.

Hepatitis B and hepatitis D are the most common causes of cirrhosis worldwide. Hepatitis B also causes INFLAMMATION and low-grade damage over decades that can ultimately lead to cirrhosis. Hepatitis D virus can infect the liver but only in people who already have hepatitis B (see discussion of hepatitis on p. 1203).

Cirrhosis may also occur as a result of nonalcoholic fatty liver disease (NAFLD), a rapidly growing health care concern. NAFLD is associated with obesity, diabetes mellitus type 2, and metabolic syndrome. It is the most common cause of liver disease in the world (World Gastroenterology Organisation, 2012). This disease can progress to liver cancer, cirrhosis, or failure, causing a premature death. Up to 25% of Americans may have NAFLD (American Liver Foundation, 2010) (see p. 1208). The Patatin-like phospholipase domain-containing 3 gene (PNPLA3) has been identified as a risk gene for the disease. Hispanics have this gene more often than other ethnic groups and are therefore at the highest risk for NAFLD (Houghton-Rahrig et al., 2014).

Another common cause of cirrhosis is excessive and prolonged alcohol use. Alcohol has a direct toxic effect on the hepatocytes and causes liver inflammation (**alcoholic hepatitis**). The liver becomes enlarged, with cellular degeneration and infiltration by fat, leukocytes, and lymphocytes. Over time, the inflammatory process decreases and the destructive phase increases. Early scar formation is caused by fibroblast infiltration and collagen formation. Damage to the liver tissue progresses as malnutrition and repeated exposure to the alcohol continue. If alcohol is withheld, the fatty infiltration and INFLAMMATION are reversible. If alcohol use continues, widespread scar tissue formation and fibrosis infiltrate the liver as a result of cellular necrosis. The long-term use of illicit drugs, such as cocaine, has similar effects on the liver.

GENDER HEALTH CONSIDERATIONS

Patient-Centered Care QSEN

The amount of alcohol necessary to cause cirrhosis varies widely from person to person, and there are gender differences. In women, it may take as few as two or three drinks per day over a minimum of 10 years. In men, perhaps six drinks per day over the same time period may be needed to cause disease. However, a smaller amount of alcohol over a long period of time can increase memory loss from alcohol toxicity of the cerebral cortex. Binge drinking can increase risk for hepatitis and fatty liver.

Incidence and Prevalence

The American Liver Foundation (2011) released the following statistics on the prevalence of liver disease in the United States:

- More than 30 million people in the United States have liver disease—or 1 in 10 Americans.
- Four million Americans have hepatitis C, and more than 1 million Americans have hepatitis B.

Combined, the incidence of chronic liver disease and cirrhosis are the twelfth most common cause of death in the United States, and about 28,000 adults die from them each year.

❖ *PATIENT-CENTERED COLLABORATIVE CARE*

◆ *Assessment*

History. Obtain data from patients with suspected cirrhosis, including age, gender, and employment history, especially history of exposure to alcohol, drugs (prescribed and illicit), and chemical toxins. Keep in mind that all exposures are important regardless of how long ago they occurred. Determine whether there has ever been a needle stick injury. Sexual history and orientation may be important in determining an infectious cause for liver disease, because men having sex with men (MSM) are at high risk for hepatitis A, hepatitis B, and hepatitis C. People with hepatitis can develop cirrhosis (American Liver Foundation, 2011).

Inquire about whether there is a family history of alcoholism and/or liver disease. Ask the patient to describe his or her alcohol intake, including the amount consumed during a given period. Is there a history of illicit drug use, including oral, IV, and intranasal forms? Is there a history of tattoos? If so, when and where were they done? Has the patient been in the military or in prison? Is the patient a health care worker, firefighter, or police officer? For patients previously or currently in an alcohol or drug recovery program, how long have they been sober? This information is sensitive and often difficult for the patient to answer. Be sure to establish why you are asking these questions, and accept answers in a nonjudgmental manner. Provide privacy during the interview. For many people, the behaviors causing the liver disease occurred years before the onset of their current illness and they are regretful and often embarrassed.

Ask the patient about previous medical conditions, such as an episode of jaundice or acute viral hepatitis, biliary tract disorders (such as cholecystitis), viral INFECTIONS, surgery, blood transfusions, autoimmune disorders, obesity, altered lipid profile, heart failure, respiratory disorders, or liver injury.

Physical Assessment/Clinical Manifestations. Because cirrhosis has a slow onset, many of the *early* manifestations are vague and nonspecific. Assess for:

- Fatigue
- Significant change in weight
- GI symptoms, such as anorexia and vomiting
- Abdominal PAIN and liver tenderness (both of which may be ignored by the patient)

Liver function problems are often found during a routine physical examination or when laboratory tests are completed for an unrelated illness or problem. The patient with *compensated cirrhosis* may be completely unaware that there is a liver problem. The first sign may present before the onset of symptoms when routine laboratory tests, presurgical evaluations, or life and health insurance assessments show abnormalities. These tests could indicate abnormal liver function or thrombocytopenia, requiring a more thorough diagnostic workup.

The development of late signs of *advanced cirrhosis* (also called "end-stage liver failure") usually cause the patient to seek medical treatment. GI bleeding, jaundice, ascites, and spontaneous bruising indicate poor liver function and complications of cirrhosis.

Thoroughly assess the patient with liver dysfunction or failure because it affects every body system. The clinical picture and course vary from patient to patient depending on the severity of the disease. Assess for:

- Obvious yellowing of the skin (jaundice) and sclerae (icterus)
- Dry skin
- Rashes
- Purpuric lesions, such as **petechiae** (round, pinpoint, red-purple lesions) or **ecchymoses** (large purple, blue, or yellow bruises)
- Warm and bright red palms of the hands (palmar erythema)
- Vascular lesions with a red center and radiating branches, known as "**spider angiomas**" (telangiectases, spider nevi, or vascular spiders), on the nose, cheeks, upper thorax, and shoulders
- Ascites (abdominal fluid)
- Peripheral dependent edema of the extremities and sacrum

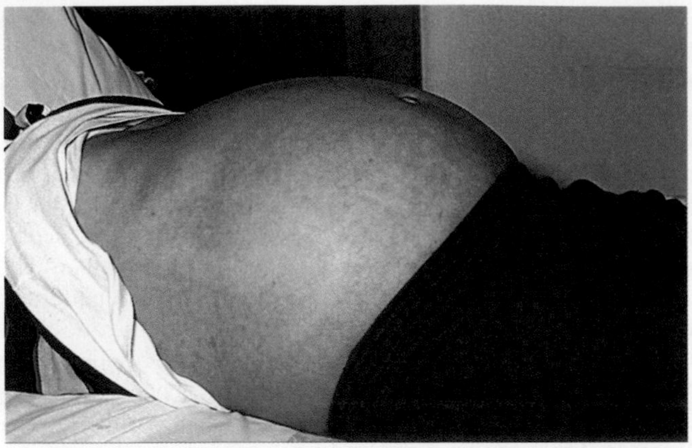

FIG. 58-2 Patient with abdominal ascites in late-stage cirrhosis.

- Vitamin deficiency (especially fat-soluble vitamins A, D, E, and K)

Abdominal Assessment. *Massive* ascites can be detected as a distended abdomen with bulging flanks (Fig. 58-2). The umbilicus may protrude, and dilated abdominal veins (caput medusae) may radiate from the umbilicus. Ascites can cause physical problems. For example, orthopnea and dyspnea from increased abdominal distention can interfere with lung expansion. The patient may have difficulty maintaining an erect body posture, and problems with balance may affect walking. Inspect and palpate for the presence of inguinal or umbilical hernias, which are likely to develop because of increased intra-abdominal pressure. *Minimal* ascites is often more difficult to detect, especially in the obese patient.

When performing an assessment of the abdomen, keep in mind that **hepatomegaly** (liver enlargement) occurs in many cases of early cirrhosis. Splenomegaly is common in nonalcoholic causes of cirrhosis. As the liver deteriorates, it may become hard and small.

Measure the patient's abdominal girth to evaluate the progression of ascites (see Fig. 58-2). To measure abdominal girth, the patient lies flat while the nurse or other examiner pulls a tape measure around the largest diameter (usually over the umbilicus) of the abdomen. The girth is measured at the end of exhalation. Mark the abdominal skin and flanks to ensure the same tape measure placement on subsequent readings. *Taking daily weights, however, is the most reliable indicator of fluid retention.*

Other Physical Assessment. Observe vomitus and stool for blood. This may be indicated by frank blood in the excrement or by a positive fecal occult blood test (FOBT) (Hema-Check, Hematest). Gastritis, stomach ulceration, or oozing esophageal varices may be responsible for the blood in the stool. Note the presence of **fetor hepaticus**, which is the distinctive breath odor of chronic liver disease and hepatic encephalopathy and is characterized by a fruity or musty odor.

Amenorrhea (no menstrual period) may occur in women, and men may exhibit testicular atrophy, **gynecomastia** (enlarged breasts), and impotence as a result of inactive hormones. Patients with problems of the hematologic system caused by hepatic failure may have bruising and petechiae (small, purplish hemorrhagic spots on the skin).

Continually assess the patient's neurologic function. Subtle changes in mental status and personality often progress to coma—a late complication of encephalopathy. Monitor for **asterixis**—a coarse tremor characterized by rapid, nonrhythmic extensions and flexions in the wrists and fingers (hand-flapping).

Psychosocial Assessment. The patient with hepatic cirrhosis may undergo subtle or obvious personality, cognitive, and behavior changes, such as agitation. He or she may experience sleep pattern disturbances or may exhibit signs of emotional lability (fluctuations in emotions), euphoria (a very elevated mood), or depression. A psychosocial assessment identifies needs and helps guide care.

Repeated hospitalizations are common for patients with cirrhosis. It is a life-altering chronic disease, impacting not only the patient but also the immediate and extended family members and significant others. There are significant emotional, physical, and financial changes. Substance use may continue even as health worsens. It is important, whenever possible, to use resources available to these patients and their families. Collaborate with social workers, substance use counselors, and mental health/behavioral health care professionals as needed for patient assessment and management.

Part of the psychosocial assessment is determining if the patient is alcohol-dependent. If this is the case, observe and prepare for alcohol withdrawal (Donnelly et al., 2012). Care of the patient experiencing withdrawal can be a medical emergency. Consult mental health textbooks or references for this chapter for more information about caring for the alcohol-dependent patient.

NCLEX EXAMINATION CHALLENGE

Physiological Integrity

A client previously diagnosed with liver cirrhosis visits the medical clinic. What assessment findings does the nurse expect in this client? **Select all that apply.**

A. Ecchymosis
B. Soft abdomen
C. Moist, clammy skin
D. Jaundice
E. Ankle edema
F. Fever

Laboratory Assessment. Laboratory study abnormalities are common in patients with liver disease (Table 58-3). Serum levels of *aspartate aminotransferase* (AST), *alanine aminotransferase* (ALT), and *lactate dehydrogenase* (LDH) are typically elevated because these enzymes are released into the blood during hepatic INFLAMMATION. However, as the liver deteriorates, the hepatocytes may be unable to create an inflammatory response and the AST and ALT may be normal. ALT levels are more specific to the liver, whereas AST can be found in muscle, kidney, brain, and heart. An AST/ALT ratio greater than 2 is usually found in alcoholic liver disease (Pagana & Pagana, 2014).

Increased *alkaline phosphatase* and gamma-glutamyl transpeptidase (GGT) levels are caused by biliary obstruction and therefore may increase in patients with cirrhosis. Alkaline phosphatase is a nonspecific bone, intestinal, and liver enzyme. However, alkaline phosphatase also increases when bone disease, such as osteoporosis, is present. Total serum *bilirubin* levels also rise. Indirect bilirubin levels increase in patients with cirrhosis because of the inability of the failing liver to excrete bilirubin. Therefore bilirubin is present in the urine (urobilinogen) in

TABLE 58-3 Assessment of Abnormal Laboratory Findings in Liver Disease

ABNORMAL FINDING	SIGNIFICANCE
Serum Enzymes	
Elevated serum aspartate aminotransferase (AST)	Hepatic cell destruction, hepatitis
Elevated serum alanine aminotransferase (ALT)	Hepatic cell destruction, hepatitis (most specific indicator)
Elevated lactate dehydrogenase (LDH)	Hepatic cell destruction
Elevated serum alkaline phosphatase	Obstructive jaundice, hepatic metastasis
Elevated gamma-glutamyl transpeptidase (GGT)	Biliary obstruction, cirrhosis
Bilirubin	
Elevated serum total bilirubin	Hepatic cell disease
Elevated serum direct conjugated bilirubin	Hepatitis, liver metastasis
Elevated serum indirect unconjugated bilirubin	Cirrhosis
Elevated urine bilirubin	Hepatocellular obstruction, viral or toxic liver disease
Elevated urine urobilinogen	Hepatic dysfunction
Decreased fecal urobilinogen	Obstructive liver disease
Serum Proteins	
Increased serum total protein	Acute liver disease
Decreased serum total protein	Chronic liver disease
Decreased serum albumin	Severe liver disease
Elevated serum globulin	Immune response to liver disease
Other Tests	
Elevated serum ammonia	Advanced liver disease or portal-systemic encephalopathy (PSE)
Prolonged prothrombin time (PT) or international normalized ratio (INR)	Hepatic cell damage and decreased synthesis of prothrombin

increased amounts. Fecal urobilinogen concentration is decreased in patients with biliary tract obstruction. These patients have light- or clay-colored stools.

Total serum *protein* and *albumin* levels are decreased in patients with severe or chronic liver disease as a result of decreased synthesis by the liver (Pagana & Pagana, 2014). Loss of osmotic "pull" proteins like albumin promotes the movement of intravascular fluid into the interstitial tissues (e.g., ascites). Prothrombin time/*international normalized ratio* (PT/INR) is prolonged because the liver decreases the production of prothrombin. The platelet count is low, resulting in a characteristic thrombocytopenia of cirrhosis. Anemia may be reflected by decreased red blood cell (RBC), hemoglobin, and hematocrit values. The white blood cell (WBC) count may also be decreased. *Ammonia* levels are usually elevated in patients with advanced liver disease. Serum creatinine may be elevated in patients with deteriorating kidney function. Dilutional hyponatremia (low serum sodium) may occur in patients with ascites.

Imaging Assessment. Plain x-rays of the abdomen may show hepatomegaly, splenomegaly, or massive ascites. A CT scan may be requested.

MRI is another test used to diagnose the patient with liver disease. It can reveal mass lesions, giving additional specific information. This information is helpful in determining whether the condition is malignant or benign.

Other Diagnostic Assessment. *Ultrasound (US) of the liver is often the first assessment for a person with suspected liver disease to detect ascites, hepatomegaly, and splenomegaly.* It can also determine the presence of biliary stones or biliary duct obstruction. Liver US is useful in detecting portal vein thrombosis and evaluating whether the direction of portal blood flow is normal.

Some patients being assessed for liver disease require biopsies to determine the exact pathology and the extent of disease progression. This procedure can be problematic because a large number of patients are at risk for bleeding. Even a **percutaneous** (through the skin) biopsy can pose a significant risk to the patient. To minimize this risk, an interventional radiologist can perform a liver biopsy using a long sheath through a jugular vein that then is threaded into the hepatic vein and liver. A tissue sample is obtained for microscopic evaluation. If a biopsy procedure is not possible, a radioisotope liver scan may be used to identify cirrhosis or other diffuse disease.

The physician may request *arteriography* if US is not conclusive in finding portal vein thrombosis. To evaluate the portal vein and its branches, a portal venogram may be performed instead, by passing a catheter into the liver and into the portal vein. This procedure is described on p. 1200 in the Transjugular Intrahepatic Portal-Systemic Shunt section.

The physician may perform an **esophagogastroduodenoscopy (EGD)** to directly visualize the upper GI tract to detect complications of liver failure. These complications may include bleeding or oozing esophageal varices, stomach irritation and ulceration, or duodenal ulceration and bleeding. EGD is performed by introducing a flexible fiberoptic endoscope into the mouth, esophagus, and stomach while the patient is under moderate sedation. A camera attached to the scope permits direct visualization of the mucosal lining of the upper GI tract. An **endoscopic retrograde cholangiopancreatography (ERCP)** uses the endoscope to inject contrast material via the sphincter of Oddi to view the biliary tract and allow for stone removals, sphincterotomies, biopsies, and stent placements if required. These procedures are described in more detail in Chapter 52.

◆ Analysis

The priority NANDA-I nursing diagnoses and collaborative problems for patients with cirrhosis include:

1. Excess Fluid Volume related to third spacing of abdominal and peripheral fluid (NANDA-I)
2. Potential for hemorrhage due to portal hypertension
3. Potential for hepatic encephalopathy due to shunting of portal venous blood and/or increased serum ammonia levels

◆ Planning and Implementation

Managing Fluid Volume

Planning: Expected Outcomes. The patient with cirrhosis is expected to have less excess fluid volume as evidenced by decreased ascites and peripheral edema and adequate circulatory volume. If ascites continues, the patient will not have respiratory distress and will manage ascites by adhering to the collaborative plan of care (see the Concept Map for liver failure due to cirrhosis on p. 1198).

CONCEPT MAP

CIRRHOSIS

PAIN

F/E BALANCE

INFECTION

INFLAMMATION

HISTORY

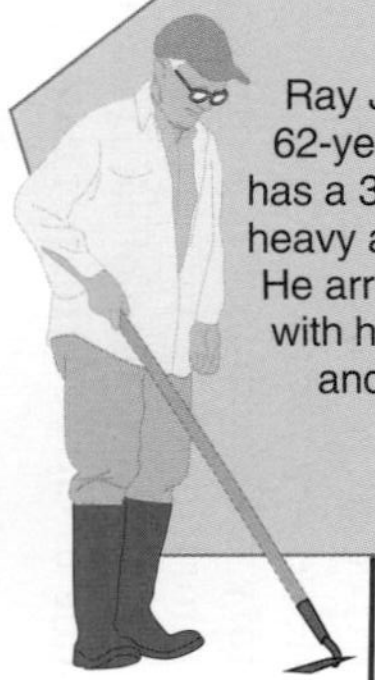

Ray Jones, a 62-year-old farmer, has a 30-year history of heavy alcoholic intake. He arrives in the ED with hematemesis and melena.

Objective Data

- Patient states he feels lightheaded and dizzy when he stands up.
- VS on admission: BP – 100/60; HR – 116, T – 100.8° F; RR – 24
- Pulse ox – 92%; HGB – 11 g/dL; HCT – 33%
- Platelets 100,000
- Ascites, caput medusa, and hemorrhoids present

Pathophysiology of Cirrhosis

- A slow, progressive, irreversible destruction of hepatocytes; scarring of the liver and reduced blood flow through the liver
- Digestion, nutrition, and metabolism severely affected
- Eventually end-stage liver failure occurs

Data Synthesis

PATIENT PROBLEMS

- Excess Fluid Volume related to third spacing of abdominal and peripheral fluid
- Potential for hemorrhage due to portal hypertension
- Potential for hepatic encephalopathy due to shunting of portal venous blood and/or increased serum ammonia levels

Planning

EXPECTED OUTCOMES

- Have less excess fluid volume as evidenced by decreased ascites and peripheral edema and adequate circulatory volume
- If ascites continues, no respiratory distress will develop
- Manage ascites by adhering to the collaborative plan of care
- Free of bleeding episodes or managed immediately if bleeding occurs
- Lab values within normal limits
- No development of encephalopathy or decrease in LOC; immediate management if it occurs
- Highest quality of life possible
- Abstain from alcohol or drugs

INTERVENTIONS

1 Physical Assessment/Clinical Manifestations

Assess for jaundice and icterus; dry skin; rashes; petechiae; ecchymosis; palmar erythema; spider angiomas on the nose, cheeks, upper thorax, and shoulders; ascites; peripheral dependent edema of the extremities and sacrum. Listen to bowel sounds; assess for abdominal wall rigidity. *Evaluates the effects of chronic inflammation and necrosis resulting from cirrhosis.*

2 Nursing Safety Priority: Action Alert!

Monitor for and manage potentially life-threatening complications of cirrhosis with ascites, esophageal varices, coagulation defects, jaundice, encephalopathy, hepatic coma, hepatorenal syndrome, spontaneous bacterial peritonitis. *Prevents hemorrhage and death.*

3 Preventing INFECTION

Monitor for signs of acute spontaneous bacterial peritonitis (SBP) (low grade fever, loss of appetite, abdominal pain, change in mental state) that can result from low concentrations of proteins. *Proteins provide some protection against bacteria.*

4 Interpretation of Lab Values

Monitor blood urea nitrogen (BUN), serum protein, hemoglobin, hematocrit, platelets, and electrolytes. *Helps determine fluid and electrolyte status. Elevated BUN, decreased serum proteins, and increased hematocrit may indicate hypovolemia. Indicates destroyed platelets caused by splenomegaly (which causes thrombocytopenia and increased risk for bleeding).*

5 Drug Therapy

Administer antibiotics, propranolol (Inderal), and vasoconstrictive drugs as prescribed. *Prevents or controls bleeding and infection in patients with esophageal varices.*

6 Fluid Status

Monitor the effect of diuretic therapy by daily weights, measuring daily intake and output, measuring abdominal girth, documenting peripheral edema, and assessing electrolyte levels. *Identifies serious problems with FLUID AND ELECTROLYTE BALANCE such as dehydration, hypokalemia, and hypernatremia.*

7 Sodium Restriction

Teach the patient about decreased sodium in the diet (1 to 2 g). Review how to read nutritional labels. Avoid table salt; use lemon, vinegar, parsley, oregano, and pepper instead. *Helps to manage electrolyte imbalance of hypernatremia with low-sodium diet controlling fluid accumulation in the abdominal cavity.*

8 Regulating Activity

Decrease activity that increases abdominal pressure, such as heavy lifting or vigorous physical exercise, chest trauma, or dry, hard food in the esophagus. *Such increased activity can cause bleeding and increases the likelihood of a variceal bleed.*

9 Nursing Priority: Preventing INFECTION

Teach the patient to use cool to warm water on skin and not too much soap. Teach UAP to use lotion to soothe the skin. Protect skin integrity and assess for open areas from scratching. *Maintains skin integrity and prevents INFECTION.*

10 Level of Consciousness (LOC)

Monitor for changes in LOC in the patient with an acute bleed or with hepatic encephalopathy. *Signifies decreased perfusion to the brain.*

Concept Map by Deanne A. Blach, MSN, RN

Interventions. Fluid accumulations are minimal during the early stages of ascites. Therefore interventions are aimed at preventing the accumulation of additional fluid and moving the existing fluid collection. Nonsurgical treatment measures are used to treat ascites in most cases.

Supportive measures to control abdominal ascites include nutrition therapy, drug therapy, paracentesis, and respiratory support. The patient's FLUID AND ELECTROLYTE BALANCE is also carefully monitored. If the patient is jaundiced, he or she will likely scratch the skin because the excess bilirubin products cause irritation and pruritus (itching).

! NURSING SAFETY PRIORITY (QSEN)

Action Alert

For skin irritation and pruritus associated with jaundice, teach the patient to use cool rather than warm water on the skin and to not use an excessive amount of soap. Teach unlicensed assistive personnel to use lotion to soothe the skin. Assess for open skin areas from scratching, which could become infected.

Nutrition Therapy. The health care provider usually places the patient with abdominal ascites on a low-sodium diet as an initial means of controlling fluid accumulation in the abdominal cavity. The amount of daily sodium (Na^+) intake restriction varies, but a 1- to 2-gram (2000 mg) Na^+ restriction may be tried first. In collaboration with the dietitian, explain the purpose of the restriction and advise the patient and family to read the sodium content labels on all food and beverages. Table salt should be completely excluded. Low-sodium diets may be distasteful, so suggest alternative flavoring additives such as lemon, vinegar, parsley, oregano, and pepper. Remind the patient that seasoned and salty food is an acquired taste; in time, he or she will become used to the decrease in dietary sodium.

In general, patients with late-stage cirrhosis are malnourished and have multiple dietary deficiencies. Vitamin supplements such as thiamine (due to alcohol withdrawal), folate, and multivitamin preparations are typically added to the IV fluids because the liver cannot store vitamins. For patients with biliary cirrhosis, bile may not be available for fat-soluble vitamin transport and absorption. Oral vitamins are prescribed when IV fluid administration is discontinued.

Drug Therapy. The health care provider usually prescribes a *diuretic* to reduce fluid accumulation and to prevent cardiac and respiratory problems. Monitor the effect of diuretic therapy by weighing the patient daily, measuring daily intake and output, measuring abdominal girth, documenting peripheral edema, and assessing electrolyte levels. Serious FLUID AND ELECTROLYTE imbalances, such as dehydration, hypokalemia (decreased potassium), and hyponatremia (decreased sodium), may occur with loop diuretic therapy. Depending on the diuretic selected, the provider may prescribe an oral or IV potassium supplement. Some clinicians prescribe furosemide (Lasix) and spironolactone (Aldactone) as a combination diuretic therapy for the treatment of ascites. Because these drugs work differently, they are used for maintenance of sodium and potassium balance. For example, furosemide causes potassium loss, whereas spironolactone conserves it in the body.

All patients with ascites have the potential to develop **spontaneous bacterial peritonitis (SBP)** from bacteria in the collected ascitic fluid. In some patients, mild symptoms such as low-grade fever and loss of appetite occur. In others, there may be abdominal PAIN, fever, and change in mental status. When performing an abdominal assessment, listen for bowel sounds and assess for abdominal wall rigidity. Quinolones such as norfloxacin (Noroxin) are the drugs of choice for SBP. If the patient is allergic to this class of *antibiotics,* combination antibiotics like trimethoprim-sulfamethoxazole (Bactrim) are given.

CHART 58-1 Best Practice for Patient Safety & Quality Care (QSEN)

The Patient with Paracentesis

- Explain the procedure, and answer patient questions.
- Obtain vital signs, including weight.
- *Ask the patient to void before the procedure to prevent injury to the bladder!*
- Position the patient in bed with the head of the bed elevated.
- Monitor vital signs per protocol or physician's request.
- Measure the drainage, and record accurately.
- Describe the collected fluid.
- Label and send the fluid for laboratory analysis; document in the patient record that specimens were sent.
- After the physician removes the catheter, apply a dressing to the site; assess for leakage.
- Maintain bedrest per protocol.
- Weigh the patient after the paracentesis; document in the patient record weight both before and after paracentesis.

Paracentesis. For some patients, abdominal **paracentesis** may be needed. Nursing implications associated with this procedure are described in Chart 58-1. The procedure is performed at the bedside, in an interventional radiology department, or in an ambulatory care setting. The physician inserts a trocar catheter or drain into the abdomen to remove the ascitic fluid from the peritoneal cavity. This procedure is done using ultrasound for added safety. In some situations, a short-term ascites drain catheter may be placed while the patient is awaiting surgical intervention, or tunneled ascites drains (e.g., PleurX drains) can allow a patient or family caregiver to drain ascitic fluid at home.

If SBP is suspected, a sample of fluid is withdrawn and sent for cell count and culture. If the patient has symptoms of infection, the physician may prescribe antibiotics while awaiting the culture results.

Respiratory Support. Excessive ascitic fluid volume may cause the patient to have respiratory problems. He or she may develop *hepatopulmonary syndrome.* Dyspnea develops as a result of increased intra-abdominal pressure, which limits thoracic expansion and diaphragmatic excursion. Auscultate lungs every 4 to 8 hours for crackles that could indicate pulmonary complications, depending on the patient's overall condition.

! NURSING SAFETY PRIORITY (QSEN)

Action Alert

For the patient with hepatopulmonary syndrome, monitor his or her oxygen saturation with pulse oximetry. If needed, apply oxygen therapy to ease breathing. Elevate the head of the bed to at least 30 degrees or as high as the patient wants to improve breathing. This position, with his or her feet elevated to decrease dependent ankle edema, often relieves dyspnea. Weigh the patient daily, or delegate and supervise this activity.

FLUID AND ELECTROLYTE BALANCE problems are common as a result of the disease or treatment. Laboratory tests, such as blood urea nitrogen (BUN), serum protein, hematocrit, and electrolytes, help determine fluid and electrolyte status. An elevated BUN, decreased serum proteins, and increased hematocrit may indicate hypovolemia.

If medical management fails to control ascites, the physician may choose to divert ascites into the venous system by creating a shunt. Patients with ascites are poor surgical risks. The transjugular intrahepatic portal-systemic shunt (TIPS) is a nonsurgical procedure that is used to control long-term ascites and to reduce variceal bleeding. This procedure is described in the discussion of Interventions in the Preventing or Managing Hemorrhage section that follows.

NCLEX EXAMINATION CHALLENGE

Psychosocial Integrity

The nurse is providing teaching for a client scheduled for a paracentesis. Which statement by the client indicates the teaching has been successful?

A. "I must not use the bathroom prior to the procedure."
B. "I will lie on my stomach while the procedure is performed."
C. "I will not be allowed to eat or drink anything the night before surgery."
D. "The physician will likely remove 2 to 3 liters of fluid from my abdomen."

Preventing or Managing Hemorrhage

Planning: Expected Outcomes. The patient is expected to be free of bleeding episodes. However, if he or she has a hemorrhage, it is expected to be controlled by prompt, evidence-based interdisciplinary interventions. Esophageal variceal bleeds are the most common type of upper GI bleeding.

Interventions. All patients with cirrhosis should be screened for esophageal varices by endoscopy to detect them early *before they bleed.* If patients have varices, they are placed on preventive therapy. If acute bleeding occurs, early interventions are used to manage it. *Because massive esophageal bleeding can cause rapid blood loss, emergency interventions are needed.*

Drug Therapy. The role of early drug therapy is to *prevent* bleeding and INFECTION in patients who have varices. A nonselective *beta-blocking agent* such as propranolol (Inderal) is usually prescribed to prevent bleeding. By decreasing heart rate and the hepatic venous pressure gradient, the chance of bleeding may be reduced (Felicilda-Reynaldo, 2012b).

Up to 20% of cirrhotic patients who are admitted to the hospital due to upper GI bleeding have bacterial infections, and even more patients develop health care–associated infections, usually urinary tract infections or pneumonia (McCance et al., 2014). INFECTION is one of the most common indicators that patients will have an acute variceal bleed (AVB). Therefore cirrhotic patients with GI bleeding should receive *antibiotics* when admitted to the hospital.

If bleeding occurs, the health care team intervenes quickly to control it by combining vasoactive drugs with endoscopic therapies. *Vasoactive* drugs, such as vasopressin and octreotide acetate (Sandostatin), reduce blood flow through vasoconstriction to decrease portal pressure. Octreotide also suppresses secretion of gastrin, serotonin, and intestinal peptides, which decreases GI blood flow to help with pressure reduction within the varices (Felicilda-Reynaldo, 2012b).

Endoscopic Therapies. Endoscopic therapies include ligation of the bleeding veins or sclerotherapy. Both procedures have been very effective in controlling bleeding and improving patient survival rates. Esophageal varices may be managed with **endoscopic variceal ligation (EVL) (banding)**. This procedure involves the application of small "O" bands around the base of the varices to decrease the blood supply to the varices. The patient is unaware of the bands, and they cause no discomfort.

Endoscopic sclerotherapy (EST), also called **injection sclerotherapy**, may be done to stop bleeding. The varices are injected with a sclerosing agent via a catheter. This procedure is associated with complications such as mucosal ulceration, which could result in further bleeding.

Rescue Therapies. If rebleeding occurs, rescue therapies are used. These procedures include a second endoscopic procedure, balloon tamponade and esophageal stents, and shunting procedures. Short-term esophagogastric balloon tamponade using a Minnesota or **Sengstaken-Blakemore tube** with esophageal stents is a very effective way to control bleeding. However, the procedure can cause potentially life-threatening complications, such as aspiration, asphyxia, and esophageal perforation (Augustin et al., 2010). Similar to a nasogastric tube, the tube is placed through the nose and into the stomach. An attached balloon is inflated to apply pressure to the bleeding variceal area. Before this tamponade, the patient is usually intubated and placed on a mechanical ventilator to protect the airway. This therapy is used if the patient is not able to have a second endoscopy or TIPS procedure.

Transjugular Intrahepatic Portal-Systemic Shunt. The transjugular intrahepatic portal-systemic shunt (TIPS) is a nonsurgical procedure performed in interventional radiology departments. This procedure is used for patients who have not responded to other modalities for hemorrhage or long-term ascites. If time permits, patients have a Doppler ultrasound to assess jugular vein anatomy and patency. The patient receives heavy IV sedation or general anesthesia for this procedure. The radiologist places a large sheath through the jugular vein. A needle is guided through the sheath and pushed through the liver into the portal vein. A balloon enlarges this tract, and a stent keeps it open. Most patients also have a Doppler ultrasound study of the liver after the TIPS procedure to record the blood flow through the shunt.

Serious complications of TIPS are not common. Patients are usually discharged in 1 or 2 days and are followed up with ultrasounds for the first year after the shunt is placed. Some shunts require re-opening at least once during the first year as an ambulatory care procedure.

Other Interventions. Depending on the procedure done to control esophageal bleeding, patients usually have a nasogastric tube (NGT) inserted to detect any new bleeding episodes. Patients often receive packed red blood cells, fresh frozen plasma, dextran, albumin, and platelets through large-bore IV catheters.

Monitor vital signs every hour, and check coagulation studies, including prothrombin time (PT), partial thromboplastin time (PTT), platelet count, and international normalized ratio (INR). Additional interventions for upper GI bleeding are discussed in Chapter 55.

Preventing or Managing Hepatic Encephalopathy

Planning: Expected Outcomes. The patient is expected to be free of encephalopathy. However, if it occurs, it is expected that the interdisciplinary team will intervene early to prevent further health problems or death.

Interventions. The poorly functioning liver cannot convert ammonia and other by-products of protein metabolism to a less toxic form. They are carried by the circulatory system to the brain, where they affect cerebral function. Interventions are planned around the management of slowing or stopping the accumulation of ammonia in the body.

Because ammonia is formed in the GI tract by the action of bacteria on protein, nonsurgical treatment measures to decrease ammonia production include dietary limitations and drug therapy to reduce bacterial breakdown.

Nutrition Therapy. Patients with cirrhosis have increased nutritional requirements—high-carbohydrate, moderate-fat, and high-protein foods. However, the diet may be changed for those who have elevated serum ammonia levels with signs of encephalopathy. Patients should have a moderate amount of protein and fat foods and simple carbohydrates. Strict protein restrictions are not required because patients need protein for healing. In collaboration with the dietitian, be sure to include family members or significant others in nutrition counseling. The patient is often weak and unable to remember complicated guidelines. Brief, simple directions regarding dietary dos and don'ts are recommended. Keep in mind any financial, cultural, or personal preferences when discussing food choices, as well as the patient's food allergies.

Drug Therapy. Drugs are used sparingly because they are difficult for the failing liver to metabolize. In particular, opioid analgesics, sedatives, and barbiturates should be restricted, especially for the patient with a history of encephalopathy.

Several types of drugs, however, may eliminate or reduce ammonia levels in the body. These include lactulose (e.g., Evalose, Heptalac) or lactitol and nonabsorbable antibiotics (Felicilda-Reynaldo, 2012a). The health care provider may prescribe *lactulose* (or lactitol) to promote the excretion of ammonia in the stool. This drug is a viscous, sticky, sweet-tasting liquid that is given either orally or by NG tube. The purpose is to obtain a laxative effect. Cleansing the bowels may rid the intestinal tract of the toxins that contribute to encephalopathy. It works by increasing osmotic pressure to draw fluid into the colon and prevents absorption of ammonia in the colon. The drug may be prescribed to the patient who has manifested signs of encephalopathy, regardless of the stage. The desired effect of the drug is production of two or three soft stools per day and a decrease in patient confusion caused by this complication.

Observe for response to lactulose. The patient may report intestinal bloating and cramping. Serum ammonia levels may be monitored but do not always correlate with symptoms. Hypokalemia and dehydration may result from excessive stools. Remind unlicensed nursing personnel to help the patient with skin care if needed to prevent breakdown caused by excessive stools.

Several *nonabsorbable antibiotics* may be given if lactulose does not help the patient meet the desired outcome or if he or she cannot tolerate the drug. These drugs should not be given together. Older adults can become weak and dehydrated from having multiple stools. Neomycin sulfate (Mycifradin) or rifaximin (Xifaxan), both broad-spectrum antibiotics, may be given to act as an intestinal antiseptic (Felicilda-Reynaldo, 2012a). These drugs destroy the normal flora in the bowel, diminishing protein breakdown and decreasing the rate of ammonia production. Maintenance doses of neomycin are given orally but may also be administered as a retention enema. Long-term use has the potential for kidney toxicity and therefore is not commonly used. It cannot be used for patients with existing kidney disease.

Metronidazole (Flagyl, Novonidazol 🍁) is another broad-spectrum antibiotic with similar action to neomycin, but it can cause peripheral neuropathy. Vancomycin (Vancocin) may also be given, but its long-term use can lead to resistance (Felicilda-Reynaldo, 2012a).

Frequently assess for changes in level of consciousness and orientation. Check for asterixis (liver flap) and fetor hepaticus (liver breath). These signs suggest worsening encephalopathy. Thiamine supplements and benzodiazepines may be needed if the patient is at risk for alcohol withdrawal.

CLINICAL JUDGMENT CHALLENGE

Safety; Evidence-Based Practice QSEN

A 60-year-old man is admitted to the emergency department (ED) with a report of vomiting bright red blood. He has had liver cirrhosis for the past 10 years and states that he has been drinking heavily since his wife died last year. His blood pressure is 106/68, and his pulse rate is 94. His abdomen is distended, and he is having some difficulty breathing; his respirations are 34 per minute. You are assigned to care for this patient.

1. For what complications is this patient at risk and why? What causes these complications?
2. In what position will you place the patient and why? What evidence supports your answer? Why do you think he has tachypnea?
3. The physician suspects that he has bleeding gastroesophageal varices. What laboratory tests will he likely request and why?
4. Vasopressin is prescribed for the patient, and several large-bore IV lines are inserted. What is the purpose of this drug for this patient?
5. How will you know if the drug was effective?
6. If the drug is not effective in treating the patient, what other options are available for his management?

Community-Based Care

If the patient with late-stage cirrhosis survives life-threatening complications, he or she is usually discharged to the home or to a long-term care facility after treatment measures have managed the acute medical problems. A home care referral may be needed if the patient is discharged to the home. These chronically ill patients are often readmitted multiple times, and community-based care is aimed at optimizing comfort, promoting independence, supporting caregivers, and preventing rehospitalization. Patients with end-stage disease may benefit from hospice care. Collaborate with the case manager (CM) or other discharge planner to coordinate interdisciplinary continuing care.

Home Care Management. In collaboration with the patient, family, and case manager, assess physical adaptations needed to prepare the patient's home for recovery. Referrals for physical therapy, nutrition therapy, and transportation for physician and laboratory follow-up may be needed. The patient's rest area needs to be close to a bathroom because diuretic and/or lactulose therapy increases the frequency of urination and stools. If the patient has difficulty reaching the toilet, additional equipment (e.g., bedside commode) is necessary. Special adult-size incontinence pads or briefs may be helpful if the patient has an

CHART 58-2 Patient and Family Education: Preparing for Self-Management

Cirrhosis

Nutrition Therapy
- Consume a diet that adheres to the guidelines set by your physician, nurse, or dietitian.
- If you have excessive fluid in your abdomen, follow the low-sodium diet prescribed for you.
- Eat small, frequent meals that are nutritionally well balanced.
- Include in your diet daily supplemental liquids (e.g., Ensure or Ensure Plus) and a multivitamin.

Drug Therapy
- Take the diuretic or preventive beta blocker prescribed for you. If you experience muscle weakness, irregular heartbeat, or light-headedness, contact your health care provider right away.
- Take the medication prescribed for you that helps prevent gastrointestinal bleeding.
- Take the lactulose syrup as prescribed to maintain two or three bowel movements every day.
- Do *not* take any other medication (prescribed or over the counter) unless specifically prescribed by your health care provider.

Alcohol Abstinence
- Do not consume any alcohol.
- Seek support services for help if needed.

altered mental status and has incontinence. If the patient has shortness of breath from massive ascites, elevating the head of the bed and maintaining the patient in a semi-Fowler's to high-Fowler's position may help alleviate respiratory distress. Alternatively, a reclining chair with an elevated foot rest may be used.

Self-Management Education. The patient is discharged to the home setting with an individualized teaching plan (Chart 58-2) that includes nutrition therapy, drug therapy, and alcohol abstinence, if needed. The patient who has a tunneled ascites drain (e.g., PleurX drain) will need to be taught how to access the drain and remove excess fluid. *Review the home care instructions that are provided with the drainage system with both the patient and family/caregiver. Remind them to not remove more than 2000 mL from the abdomen at one time to prevent hypovolemic shock.*

The patient with encephalopathy often finds that small, frequent meals are best tolerated. If the patient's nutritional intake or albumin/pre-albumin is decreased after discharge, multivitamin supplements and supplemental liquid feedings (e.g., Ensure, Boost) are usually needed. Teach patients to avoid excessive vitamins and minerals that can be toxic to the liver, such as fat-soluble vitamins, excessive iron supplements, and niacin. Remind patients to check with their health care provider before taking any vitamin supplement.

The patient is often discharged while receiving diuretics. Provide instructions regarding the health care provider's prescription for the diuretic. Teach about side effects of therapy, such as hypokalemia. The patient may need to take a potassium supplement if he or she is taking a diuretic that is not potassium-sparing.

If the patient has had problems with bleeding from gastric ulcers, the primary care provider may prescribe an H_2-receptor antagonist agent or proton pump inhibitor to reduce acid reflux (see Chapter 55). Patients who have had episodes of spontaneous bacterial peritonitis (SBP) may be on a daily maintenance antibiotic.

Teach family members how to recognize signs of encephalopathy and to contact the health care provider if these signs develop. Reinforce that constipation, bleeding, and infections can increase the risk for encephalopathy.

Advise the patient to avoid all over-the-counter drugs, especially NSAIDs and hepatic toxic herbs, vitamins, and minerals. Reinforce the need to keep appointments for follow-up medical care. Remind the patient and family to notify the health care provider immediately if any GI bleeding (overt bleeding or melena) is noted so that re-evaluation can begin quickly.

! NURSING SAFETY PRIORITY QSEN

Action Alert

One of the most important aspects of ongoing care for the patient with cirrhosis is to stress the need to avoid acetaminophen (Tylenol), alcohol, and illicit drugs. By avoiding these substances, the patient may:
- Prevent further fibrosis of the liver from scarring
- Allow the liver to heal and regenerate
- Prevent gastric and esophageal irritation
- Reduce the incidence of bleeding
- Prevent other life-threatening complications

Health Care Resources. The patient with chronic cirrhosis may require a home care nurse for several visits after hospital discharge. The home care nurse can monitor the effectiveness of treatment in controlling ascites. The encephalopathic patient may need to be monitored for adherence to drug therapy and alcohol abstinence, if appropriate. Individual and group therapy sessions may be arranged to assist patients in dealing with alcohol abstinence if they are too ill to attend a formal treatment program. Because some patients may have alienated relatives over the years because of substance use, it may be necessary to help them identify a friend, neighbor, or person in their recovery group for support. If needed, refer the patient and family to self-help groups, such as Alcoholics Anonymous and Al-Anon.

The patient with cirrhosis may also desire spiritual or other psychosocial support. Finances are frequently a problem for the chronically ill patient and family; social support and community services need to be identified. The American Liver Foundation (www.liverfoundation.org) and American Gastroenterological Association (www.gastro.org) are excellent sources for more information about liver disease.

For patients who are not candidates for liver transplantation, address end-of-life issues. Discuss options such as hospice care with patients and their families (see Chapter 7). Be aware that they will go through a grieving process and will perhaps be in denial or very angry.

Evaluation: Outcomes

Evaluate the care of the patient with cirrhosis based on the identified priority patient problems. The expected outcomes include that the patient will:
- Have a decrease in or have no ascites
- Have electrolytes within normal limits (WNL)
- Not have hemorrhage or will be managed immediately if bleeding occurs
- Not develop encephalopathy or will be managed immediately if it occurs
- Have the highest quality of life possible
- Successfully abstain from alcohol or drugs (if disease is caused by these substances)

NCLEX EXAMINATION CHALLENGE

Physiological Integrity

Which intervention will the nurse include in the plan of care for a client with severe liver disease?

A. Encourage the client to eat a low-protein, high-carbohydrate diet.
B. Administer Kayexalate enemas.
C. Instruct the client to eat a high-protein, low-carbohydrate diet.
D. Teach the client to participate in frequent, vigorous physical activities.

HEPATITIS

❖ PATHOPHYSIOLOGY

Hepatitis is the widespread INFLAMMATION of liver cells. *Viral* hepatitis is the most common type and can be either acute or chronic. Less common types of hepatitis are caused by chemicals, drugs, and some herbs. This section discusses hepatitis caused by a virus. **Viral hepatitis** results from an infection caused by one of five major categories of viruses:

- Hepatitis A virus (HAV)
- Hepatitis B virus (HBV)
- Hepatitis C virus (HCV)
- Hepatitis D virus (HDV)
- Hepatitis E virus (HEV)

Some cases of viral hepatitis are not caused by any of these viruses. These patients have non–A-E hepatitis.

Liver injury with INFLAMMATION can develop after exposure to a number of drugs and chemicals by inhalation, ingestion, or parenteral (IV) administration. **Toxic and drug-induced hepatitis** can result from exposure to hepatotoxins (e.g., industrial toxins, alcohol, and drugs). Hepatitis may also occur as a secondary INFECTION during the course of infections with other viruses, such as Epstein-Barr, herpes simplex, varicella-zoster, and cytomegalovirus.

After the liver has been exposed to any causative agent (e.g., a virus), it becomes enlarged and congested with inflammatory cells, lymphocytes, and fluid, resulting in right upper quadrant pain and discomfort. As the disease progresses, the liver's normal lobular pattern becomes distorted as a result of widespread inflammation, necrosis, and hepatocellular regeneration. This distortion increases pressure within the portal circulation, interfering with the blood flow into the hepatic lobules. Edema of the liver's bile channels results in obstructive **jaundice** (yellowing of the skin).

Classification of Hepatitis and Etiologies

The five major types of acute viral hepatitis vary by mode of transmission, manner of onset, and incubation periods. Hepatitis cases must be reported to the local public health department, which then notifies the Centers for Disease Control and Prevention (CDC).

Hepatitis A. The causative agent of **hepatitis A**, hepatitis A virus (HAV), is a ribonucleic acid (RNA) virus of the enterovirus family. *It is a hardy virus and survives on human hands.* The virus is resistant to detergents and acids but is destroyed by chlorine (bleach) and extremely high temperatures.

Hepatitis A usually has a mild course similar to that of a typical flu-like INFECTION and often goes unrecognized. It is spread most often by the fecal-oral route by fecal contamination either from person-to-person contact (e.g., oral-anal sexual activity) or by consuming contaminated food or water. Common sources of infection include shellfish caught in contaminated water and food contaminated by food handlers infected with HAV. The incubation period of hepatitis A is usually 15 to 50 days, with a peak of 25 to 30 days. The disease is usually not life threatening, but its course may be more severe in people older than 40 years and those with pre-existing liver disease such as hepatitis C (McCance et al., 2014).

In a small percentage of hepatitis A cases, severe illness with extrahepatic manifestations can occur. Advanced age and conditions such as chronic liver disease may cause widespread damage that requires a liver transplant. In some cases, death may occur. The incidence of hepatitis A is particularly high in non-affluent countries in which sanitation is poor. However, over 35,000 cases are diagnosed each year in the United States (American Liver Foundation, 2010). Some adults have hepatitis A and do not know it. The course is similar to that of a GI illness, and the disease and recovery are usually uneventful.

Hepatitis B. The **hepatitis B** virus (HBV) is not transmitted like HAV. It is a double-shelled particle containing DNA composed of a core antigen (HBcAg), a surface antigen (HBsAg), and another antigen found within the core (HBeAg) that circulates in the blood. HBV may be spread through these common modes of transmission (Lok & McMahon, 2009):

- Unprotected sexual intercourse with an infected partner
- Sharing needles
- Accidental needle sticks or injuries from sharp instruments primarily in health care workers (low incidence)
- Blood transfusions (that have not been screened for the virus, before 1992)
- Hemodialysis
- Close person-to-person contact by open cuts and sores

In addition, patients who are immunosuppressed either by disease or drug therapy are more likely to develop hepatitis B.

The clinical course of hepatitis B may be varied. Symptoms usually occur within 25 to 180 days of exposure and include (McCance et al., 2014):

- Anorexia, nausea, and vomiting
- Fever
- Fatigue
- Right upper quadrant pain
- Dark urine with light stool
- Joint PAIN
- Jaundice

Blood tests confirm the disease, although many people with hepatitis B have no symptoms.

Most adults who get hepatitis B recover, clear the virus from their body, and develop immunity. However, a small percentage of people do not develop immunity and become carriers. **Hepatitis carriers** can infect others even though they are not sick and have no obvious signs of hepatitis B. Chronic carriers are at high risk for cirrhosis and liver cancer. Because of the high number of newcomers from endemic areas, the incidence of hepatitis B has increased in the United States.

Hepatitis C. The causative virus of **hepatitis C** (HCV) is an enveloped, single-stranded RNA virus. Transmission is blood to blood. The rate of sexual transmission is very low in a single-couple relationship but increases with multiple sex partners.

HCV is spread most commonly by:

- Illicit IV drug needle sharing (highest incidence)
- Blood, blood products, or organ transplants received before 1992

- Needle stick injury with HCV-contaminated blood (health care workers at high risk)
- Unsanitary tattoo equipment
- Sharing of intranasal cocaine paraphernalia

The disease is **not** transmitted by casual contact or by intimate household contact. However, those infected are advised not to share razors, toothbrushes, or pierced earrings because microscopic blood may be on these items.

The average incubation period is 7 weeks. Acute infection and illness are not common. Most people are completely unaware that they have been infected. They are asymptomatic and not diagnosed until many months or years after the initial exposure when an abnormality is detected during a routine laboratory evaluation or when liver problems occur. Unlike with hepatitis B, most people infected with hepatitis C do not clear the virus and a chronic infection develops.

HCV usually does its damage over decades by causing a chronic inflammation in the liver that eventually causes the liver cells to scar. This scarring may progress to cirrhosis (McCance et al., 2014).

Hepatitis D. **Hepatitis D** (delta hepatitis) is caused by a defective RNA virus that needs the helper function of HBV. It occurs only with HBV to cause viral replication. This usually develops into chronic disease. The incubation period is about 14 to 56 days. As with hepatitis B, the disease is transmitted primarily by parenteral routes, especially in patients who are IV drug users. Having sexual contact with a person with HDV is also a high risk factor (McCance et al., 2014).

Hepatitis E. The **hepatitis E** virus (HEV) causes a waterborne infection associated with epidemics in the Indian subcontinent, Asia, Africa, the Middle East, Mexico, and Central and South America. Many large outbreaks have occurred after heavy rains and flooding. Like hepatitis A, hepatitis E is caused by fecal contamination of food and water.

In the United States, hepatitis E has been found only in international travelers. It is transmitted via the fecal-oral route, and the clinical course resembles that of hepatitis A. Hepatitis E has an incubation period of 15 to 64 days. There is no evidence at this time of a chronic form of the disease. The disease tends to be self-limiting and resolves on its own (McCance et al., 2014).

Complications of Hepatitis

Failure of the liver cells to regenerate, with progression of the necrotic process, results in a severe acute and often fatal form of hepatitis known as **fulminant hepatitis**. Hepatitis is considered to be chronic when liver inflammation lasts longer than 6 months. **Chronic hepatitis** usually occurs as a result of hepatitis B or hepatitis C. Superimposed infection with hepatitis D virus (HDV) in patients with chronic hepatitis B may also result in chronic hepatitis. Chronic hepatitis can lead to cirrhosis and liver cancer. Many patients have multiple infections, especially the combination of HBV with either HCV, HDV, or HIV infections (McCance et al., 2014).

Incidence and Prevalence

The incidence of hepatitis A and hepatitis B is declining as a result of CDC recommendations for vaccination. However, hepatitis B and hepatitis C are a concern because of their association with cirrhosis and liver cancer. Although exact numbers are not known, it is estimated that about 200 million people worldwide have the hepatitis C virus (HCV), making this type of hepatitis the most common type. Currently there is no vaccine for HCV. Therefore it is expected that the cases of HCV will rise over the next several decades as a result of increasing illicit drug use. This increase will require a major increase in transplantations and lead to many more deaths (Lok & McMahon, 2009).

Health Promotion and Maintenance

Hepatitis vaccines for infants, children, and adolescents have helped decrease the incidence of hepatitis A and hepatitis B. Some adults also are advised to receive these immunizations.

Measures for preventing hepatitis A in adults include:

- Proper handwashing, especially after handling shellfish
- Avoiding contaminated food or water (including tap water in countries with high incidence)
- Receiving immunoglobulin within 14 days if exposed to the virus
- Receiving the HAV vaccine before traveling to areas where the disease is common (e.g., Mexico, Caribbean)
- Receiving the vaccine if living or working in enclosed areas with others, such as college dormitories, correctional institutions, day-care centers, and long-term care facilities

Several HAV vaccines are available (e.g., Havrix and Vaqta). Both of these vaccines are made of inactivated hepatitis A virus and are given in the deltoid muscle.

Several vaccines can also provide protection against hepatitis B (HBV) infection (e.g., Engerix-B and Recombivax-HB). Twinrix is a combination HAV and HBV vaccine that is also available for adults. Examples of groups for whom immunization against HBV should be used include (Lok & McMahon, 2009):

- People who have sexual intercourse with more than one partner
- People with sexually transmitted disease (STD) or a history of STD
- Men having sex with men (MSM)
- People with any chronic liver disease (such as hepatitis C or cirrhosis)
- Patients with human immune deficiency virus (HIV) infection
- People who are exposed to blood or body fluids in the workplace, including health care workers, firefighters, and police
- People in correctional facilities
- Patients needing immunosuppressant drugs
- Family members, household members, and sexual contacts of people with HBV infection

Additional measures to prevent viral hepatitis for health care workers and others in contact with infected patients are listed in Charts 58-3 and 58-4.

❖ PATIENT-CENTERED COLLABORATIVE CARE

◆ Assessment

History. Begin by asking the patient whether he or she has had known exposure to a person with hepatitis. For the patient who presents with few or no symptoms of liver disease but has abnormal laboratory tests (e.g., elevated alanine aminotransferase [ALT] or aspartate aminotransferase [AST] level), the history may need to include additional questions regarding risk factors such as:

- Exposure to either inhaled or ingested chemical
- Use of herbal supplements

CHART 58-3 Best Practice for Patient Safety & Quality Care QSEN

Prevention of Viral Hepatitis in Health Care Workers

- Use Standard Precautions to prevent the transmission of disease between patients or between patients and health care staff (see Chapter 23).
- Eliminate needles and other sharp instruments by substituting needleless systems. (Needle sticks are the major source of hepatitis B transmission in health care workers.)
- Take the hepatitis B vaccine (e.g., Recombivax HB), which is given in a series of three injections. This vaccine also prevents hepatitis D by preventing hepatitis B.
- For postexposure prevention of hepatitis A, seek medical attention immediately for immunoglobulin (Ig) administration.
- Report all cases of hepatitis to the local health department.

CHART 58-4 Patient and Family Education: Preparing for Self-Management

Health Practices to Prevent Viral Hepatitis

- Maintain adequate sanitation and personal hygiene. Wash your hands before eating and after using the toilet.
- Drink water treated by a water purification system.
- If traveling in underdeveloped or non-industrialized countries, drink only bottled water. Avoid food washed or prepared with tap water, such as raw vegetables, fruits, and soups. Avoid ice.
- Use adequate sanitation practices to prevent the spread of the disease among family members.
- Do not share bed linens, towels, eating utensils, or drinking glasses.
- Do not share needles for injection, body piercing, or tattooing.
- Do not share razors, nail clippers, toothbrushes, or Waterpiks.
- Use a condom during sexual intercourse, or abstain from this activity.
- Cover cuts or sores with bandages.
- If ever infected with hepatitis, never donate blood, body organs, or other body tissue.

- Use of any new prescribed drug or over-the-counter (OTC) medication
- Recent ingestion of shellfish
- Exposure to a possibly contaminated water source
- Travel to another country
- Sexual activities with men, women, or both and whether it was protected or unprotected
- Illicit drug use, IV or intranasal
- For health care workers, recent needle stick exposure
- Body piercing or tattooing
- Close living accommodations (e.g., military barracks, correctional institutions, overcrowded dormitories, long-term care facilities, day-care centers) or employment in any such setting
- Blood or blood products or organ transplants received before 1992
- Military service
- Place of birth (United States or other country) and parents' place of birth
- History of alcohol use (how many drinks each day or week)
- Human immune deficiency virus (HIV)

Physical Assessment/Clinical Manifestations. Assess whether the patient has:

- Abdominal PAIN
- Changes in skin or sclera (icterus)
- **Arthralgia** (joint pain) or **myalgia** (muscle pain)
- Diarrhea/constipation
- Changes in color of urine or stool
- Fever
- Lethargy
- Malaise
- Nausea/vomiting
- Pruritus (itching)

Lightly palpate the right upper abdominal quadrant to assess for liver tenderness. The patient may report right upper quadrant pain with jarring movements. Inspect the skin, sclerae, and mucous membranes for jaundice. He or she may present for medical treatment only after jaundice appears, believing that other vague symptoms are related to a flu-like syndrome.

Jaundice in hepatitis results from intrahepatic obstruction and is caused by edema of the liver's bile channels. Dark urine and clay-colored stools are often reported by the patient. If possible, obtain a urine and stool specimen for visual inspection and laboratory analysis. The patient may also have skin abrasions from scratching because of pruritus (itching).

Psychosocial Assessment. Viral hepatitis has various presentations, but for most infected people the initial course is mild with few or no symptoms. The long-term complications of fibrosis and cirrhosis cause the more serious problem. This is especially true for patients who have chronic HBV and HCV INFECTION.

Emotional problems for affected patients may center on their feeling sick and fatigued. General malaise, inactivity, and vague symptoms contribute to depression. Some patients often feel guilty and are remorseful about decisions made that caused the disease. These feelings are most likely to occur when the source of infection is from drug use. Family members may be angry that the patient caused the disease.

Infectious diseases such as hepatitis continue to have a social stigma. The patient may feel embarrassed by the precautions that are imposed in the hospital and continue to be necessary at home. This embarrassment may cause the patient to limit social interactions. Patients may be afraid that they will spread the virus to family and friends.

Family members are sometimes afraid of getting the disease and may distance themselves from the patient. Allow them to verbalize these feelings, and explore the reasons for these fears. Educate the patient and family members about modes of transmission, and clarify information as needed.

Patients may be unable to return to work for several weeks during the acute phases of illness. The loss of wages and the cost of hospitalization for a patient without insurance coverage may produce great anxiety and financial burden. This situation may last for months or years if hepatitis becomes chronic.

Laboratory Assessment. Hepatitis A, hepatitis B, and hepatitis C are usually confirmed by acute elevations in levels of liver enzymes, indicating liver cellular damage, and by specific serologic markers.

Levels of ALT and AST may possibly rise into the thousands in acute or fulminant cases of hepatitis. Alkaline phosphatase levels may be normal or elevated. Serum total bilirubin levels are elevated and are consistent with the clinical appearance of jaundice. Elevated levels of bilirubin are also present in the urine (Pagana & Pagana, 2014).

The presence of *hepatitis A* is established when hepatitis A virus (HAV) antibodies (anti-HAV) are found in the blood. Ongoing INFLAMMATION of the liver by HAV is indicated by the presence of immunoglobulin M (IgM) antibodies, which persist in the blood for 4 to 6 weeks. Previous infection is identified by the presence of immunoglobulin G (IgG) antibodies. These antibodies persist in the serum and provide permanent immunity to HAV.

The presence of the *hepatitis B* virus (HBV) is established when serologic testing confirms the presence of hepatitis B antigen-antibody systems in the blood and a detectable viral count (HBV polymerase chain reaction [PCR] DNA). Antigens located on the surface (shell) of the virus (HBsAg) and IgM antibodies to hepatitis B core antigen (anti-HBcAg IgM) are the most significant serologic markers. The presence of these markers establishes the diagnosis of hepatitis B. *The patient is infectious as long as hepatitis B surface antigen (HBsAg) is present in the blood.* Persistence of this serologic marker after 6 months or longer indicates a carrier state or chronic hepatitis. HBsAg levels normally decline and disappear after the acute hepatitis B episode. The presence of antibodies to HBsAb in the blood indicates recovery and immunity to hepatitis B. *People who have been vaccinated against HBV have a positive HBsAg because they also have immunity to the disease* (Pagana & Pagana, 2014).

Enzyme-linked immunosorbent assay (ELISA) is the initial screening test for patients suspected of being infected with *hepatitis C* virus (HCV). It is also the most commonly used enzyme test for HCV antibodies (anti-HCV). The antibodies can be detected within 4 weeks of the infection (Pagana & Pagana, 2014). A more specific assay called the *recombinant immunoblot assay (RIBA)* can be used as a confirmatory test. These tests show that the patient has been exposed to HCV and has developed the antibody. To identify the actual circulating virus, the HCV PCR RNA test is used. This confirms active virus and can measure the viral load. A newer diagnostic tool called the *OraQuick HCV Rapid Antibody Test* was approved by the Food and Drug Administration in the United States in 2010. It has the advantage of providing a quick diagnosis of the disease as a point-of-care test.

The presence of *hepatitis D* virus (HDV) can be confirmed by the identification of intrahepatic delta antigen or, more often, by a rise in the hepatitis D virus antibodies (anti-HDV) titer. This increase can be seen within a few days of INFECTION (Pagana & Pagana, 2014).

Hepatitis E virus (HEV) testing is usually reserved for travelers in whom hepatitis is present but the virus cannot be detected. Hepatitis E antibodies (anti-HEV) are found in people infected with the virus.

Other Diagnostic Assessment. *Liver biopsy* may be used to confirm the diagnosis of hepatitis and to establish the stage and grade of liver damage. Characteristic changes help the pathologist distinguish among a virus, drug, toxin, fatty liver, iron, and other disease. It is usually performed in an ambulatory care setting as a percutaneous procedure (through the skin) after a local anesthetic is given. If coagulation is abnormal, however, it may be done using either a CT-guided or transjugular route to reduce the risk for pneumothorax or hemothorax. *Ultrasound* also may be used.

◆ Interventions

The patient with viral hepatitis can be mildly or acutely ill depending on the severity of the inflammation. Most patients are not hospitalized, although older adults and those with dehydration may be admitted for a short-term stay. The plan of care for all patients with viral hepatitis is based on measures to rest the liver, promote cellular regeneration, and prevent complications, if possible.

During the acute stage of viral hepatitis, interventions are aimed at resting the inflamed liver to promote hepatic cell regeneration. *Rest* is an essential intervention to reduce the liver's metabolic demands and increase its blood supply. Collaborative care is generally supportive. The patient is usually tired and expresses feelings of general malaise. Complete bedrest is usually not required, but rest periods alternating with periods of activity are indicated and are often enough to promote hepatic healing. Individualize the patient's plan of care and change it as needed to reflect the severity of symptoms, fatigue, and the results of liver function tests and enzyme determinations. Activities such as self-care and ambulating are gradually added to the activity schedule as tolerated.

The diet should be high in carbohydrates and calories with moderate amounts of fat and protein after nausea and anorexia subside. Small, frequent meals are often preferable to three standard meals. Ask the patient about food preferences because favorite foods are tolerated better than randomly selected foods. Encourage the patient to eat foods that are appealing. High-calorie snacks may be needed. Supplemental vitamins are often prescribed.

Drugs of any kind are used sparingly for patients with hepatitis to allow the liver to rest. An antiemetic to relieve nausea

EVIDENCE BASED PRACTICE QSEN

Do Patients with Chronic Hepatitis C Use Complementary and Alternative Therapies?

Richmond, J.A., Bailey, D.E. Jr., McHutchinson, J.G., & Muir, A.J. (2010). The use of mind-body medicine and prayer among adult patients with hepatitis C. *Gastroenterology Nursing, 33*(3), 201-216.

The researchers studied the use of mind-body therapies and prayer as part of a larger, exploratory, descriptive study on the use of complementary and alternative medicine by patients with hepatitis C who were treated at one tertiary care center. According to a self-administered survey of 105 participants and semi-structured interviews of 28 participants in the study, most had used mind-body medicine in the past 12 months. The most commonly used therapies were prayer, deep breathing, and meditation to promote general well-being and relieve tension and anxiety.

Level of Evidence: 4

This study did not use an experimental design.

Commentary: Implications for Practice and Research

This exploratory descriptive study showed that patients with chronic hepatitis C use complementary and alternative medicine (CAM) in their everyday lives to promote their health and increase their quality of life. Nurses need to ensure that they ask patients about the use of CAM and which therapies are most helpful so that they can be continued as part of the patient's plan of care.

This research was the first to explore the use of CAM with this population of patients and serves as a pilot study for further research using larger sample sizes of diverse patients in multiple health care settings.

TABLE 58-4 Drug Therapy for Chronic Hepatitis B and Hepatitis C

MEDICATION	NURSING IMPLICATIONS	COMMENTS
Chronic Hepatitis B		
Tenofovir (Viread)	Monitor kidney function. Can cause bone de-mineralization. Teach risk for falls to prevent fractures.	Purpose of treatment is to achieve sustained suppression of hepatitis B virus (HBV) replication and remission of liver disease.
Adefovir (Hepsera)	Monitor kidney function.	
Lamivudine (Epivir-HBV)	Monitor kidney function. Dose is altered if co-infection with human immune deficiency virus (HIV) present.	
Entecavir (Baraclude)	Monitor kidney function.	
Chronic Hepatitis C		
Telaprevir (Incivek) Boceprevir (Victrelis) in combination with HIV medications if co-infection present PegIFN/RBV (interferon/ribavirin)	Monitor complete blood count (CBC) for anemia. Monitor chemistry panel for impaired kidney and liver function, along with electrolytes abnormalities. Peg/IFN administered subcutaneously. Instruct patients that they cannot miss a dose.	As a result of shared routes of transmission, co-infection with HIV is common.

CLINICAL JUDGMENT CHALLENGE

Patient-Centered Care; Safety QSEN

You are a nurse working in the emergency department (ED) of the local community hospital. You receive report from the night nurse regarding a 50-year-old man who has just returned to the United States from a month-long trip to the southern parts of Africa. For the past 2 weeks, he has been experiencing fevers on and off, malaise, anorexia, and mild abdominal discomfort. He has been taking acetaminophen (Tylenol) for fevers and abdominal discomfort. His past medical history is significant for elevated cholesterol for which he takes only atorvastatin (Lipitor) every day. While reviewing his social history, you note that the patient reported that he is a nonsmoker, drinks 6 or 7 alcoholic drinks daily, is married, and has three children. He had his gallbladder removed when he was 43 years old.

His current vital signs are: blood pressure 126/82 mm Hg; heart rate 100 beats/min; respirations 22 breaths/min; temperature 101°F orally; pulse oximetry reading 98% on room air. The ED physician orders the following:

Diet: nothing by mouth

Laboratory studies: complete blood count and chemistry panel, urinalysis, blood cultures

STAT electrocardiogram (ECG) and chest x-ray

Start: 0.9% normal saline intravenously to run at 100 mL/hr

The results of his recent laboratory work are:

	LABORATORY RESULT	NORMAL RANGE
White blood cells	13,000/mm³	(4,000-12,000/mm³)
Red blood cells	7.0 million/mm³	(3.5-5.5 million/mm³)
Hemoglobin	18 g/dL	(12-16 g/dL)
Hematocrit	52%	(36-46%)
Sodium	135 mEq/L	(135-145 mEq/L)
Potassium	3.5 mEq/L	(3.5-4.5 mEq/L)
Magnesium	1.5 mEq/L	(1.5-2.5 mEq/L)
Serum aspartate aminotransferase (AST)	780 IU/L	(10-34 IU/L)
Serum alanine aminotransferase (ALT)	922 IU/L	(10-40 IU/L)
Blood urea nitrogen (BUN)	30 mg/dL	(8-24 mg/dL)
Creatinine	2.0 mg/dL	0.6-1.1 mg/dL
Urinalysis	Negative for blood, protein, glucose	
Blood culture	Negative for any bacterial growth	
ECG	Sinus tachycardia	
Chest x-ray	Lung fields without any noted infiltrates or masses	

1. In reviewing Mr. Goldman's laboratory values, which findings indicate abnormal liver function?
2. While reviewing Mr. Goldman's medical history, what information most likely increases his risk for abnormal liver function?
3. With further medical workup in the ED, the physician determines that Mr. Goldman is suffering from acute hepatitis A. The patient asks you how he contracted the virus. What is your best response?
4. You are educating the patient's family about receiving vaccinations against hepatitis. What information will you provide to promote their safety?

may be prescribed. However, due to the life-threatening nature of chronic hepatitis B and hepatitis C, a number of drugs are given, including antiviral and immunomodulating drugs (Table 58-4). Similar to patients with other chronic diseases, patients with hepatitis often use complementary and alternative therapies to promote general well-being and improve quality of life (see the Evidence-Based Practice box). Be sure to ask patients about their use of these therapies and incorporate them into the collaborative plan of care.

Community-Based Care. Home care management varies according to the type of hepatitis and whether the disease is acute or chronic. A primary focus in any case is preventing the spread of the infection. For hepatitis transmitted by the fecal-oral route, careful handwashing and sanitary disposal of feces are important. Education is therefore very important. Collaborate with the certified infection control practitioner and infectious disease specialist if needed in caring for these patients. These experts can also suggest resources for the patient and family.

CHART 58-5 Patient and Family Education: Preparing for Self-Management

Viral Hepatitis

- Avoid all medications, including over-the-counter drugs such as acetaminophen (Tylenol, Exdol ♣), unless prescribed by your physician.
- Avoid all alcohol.
- Rest frequently throughout the day, and get adequate sleep at night.
- Eat small, frequent meals with a high-carbohydrate, moderate-fat, and moderate-protein content.
- Avoid sexual intercourse until antibody testing results are negative.
- Follow the guidelines for preventing transmission of the disease (see Chart 58-4).

! NURSING SAFETY PRIORITY (QSEN)

Action Alert

Teach the patient with viral hepatitis and the family to use measures to prevent infection transmission (see Chart 58-4). *In addition, instruct the patient to avoid alcohol and to check with the health care provider before taking any medication or vitamin, supplement, or herbal preparation.*

Encourage the patient to increase activity gradually to prevent fatigue. Suggest that he or she eat small, frequent meals of high-carbohydrate foods (Chart 58-5).

FATTY LIVER (STEATOSIS)

Fatty liver is caused by the accumulation of fats in and around the hepatic cells. It may be caused by alcohol use or other factors. Nonalcoholic fatty liver disease (NAFLD) and nonalcoholic steatohepatitis (NASH) are types of fatty liver disease. Causes include:

- Diabetes mellitus
- Obesity
- Elevated lipid profile

Fatty infiltration of the liver may result from faulty fat metabolism in the liver and the movement of fatty acids from adipose tissue (fat). Many patients are asymptomatic. The most common and typical finding is an elevated ALT and AST or normal ALT and elevated AST (part of a group of liver function tests [LFTs]).

MRI, ultrasound, and nuclear medicine examinations can be used to confirm excessive fat in the liver. A percutaneous biopsy can also confirm the diagnosis. Interventions are aimed at removing the underlying cause of the infiltration. Weight loss, glucose control, and aggressive treatment using lipid-lowering agents are recommended. Monitoring liver function tests is essential in disease management.

LIVER TRAUMA

The liver is one of the most common organs to be injured in patients with abdominal trauma. Damage or injury should be suspected whenever any upper abdominal or lower chest trauma is sustained. The liver is often injured by steering wheels in vehicular crashes. Common injuries include simple lacerations, multiple lacerations, avulsions (tears), and crush injuries.

The liver is a highly vascular organ and receives almost a third of the body's cardiac output. When hepatic trauma occurs, blood loss can be massive. *Observe for early signs of hypovolemic shock* (Chart 58-6).

CHART 58-6 Key Features

Liver Trauma

- Right upper quadrant pain with abdominal tenderness
- Abdominal distention and rigidity
- Guarding of the abdomen
- Increased abdominal pain exaggerated by deep breathing and referred to the right shoulder (Kehr's sign)
- Indicators of hemorrhage and hypovolemic shock:
  - Hypotension
  - Tachycardia
  - Tachypnea
  - Pallor
  - Diaphoresis
  - Cool, clammy skin
  - Confusion or other change in mental state

An ultrasound or CT scan of the abdomen is often done to determine the presence of a hematoma (blood clot). A decreased hematocrit may confirm suspected blood loss. Clinical manifestations include right upper quadrant PAIN with abdominal tenderness, distention, guarding, and rigidity. Abdominal pain exaggerated by deep breathing and referred to the right shoulder may indicate diaphragmatic irritation.

Liver trauma is managed in a conservative manner through new diagnostic and therapeutic modalities such as enhanced critical care monitoring and damage control surgery (Ahmed & Vernick, 2011). Patients with hepatic trauma may require multiple blood products such as packed red blood cells and fresh frozen plasma, as well as massive volume infusion to maintain adequate hydration. After surgery, the patient is admitted to a critical care unit. Monitor the patient for persistent or new bleeding. Closely monitor complete blood count and coagulation studies for trends in changes.

CANCER OF THE LIVER

❖ PATHOPHYSIOLOGY

Cancers may be *primary* tumors (hepatocellular carcinoma) starting in the liver, or they may be *metastatic* cancers that spread from another organ to the liver. They are most often seen in regions of Asia and the Mediterranean area. Worldwide, the disease kills about 1 million people each year and affects Vietnamese men more than any other group. Black and Hispanic populations have twice the rate of the disease as Euro-Americans, and older adults are affected more than other age-groups (Rossi et al., 2010). In the United States and worldwide, the incidence of liver cancer is increasing because there is an increase in cases of hepatitis C.

Chronic INFECTION with HBV and HCV frequently lead to cirrhosis, which is a risk factor for developing liver cancer. It is important to remember that cirrhosis from any cause, including alcoholic liver disease, increases the risk for cancer.

❖ PATIENT-CENTERED COLLABORATIVE CARE

◆ Assessment

In the early stage of cancer, most patients are without symptoms. Later in the disease, they report weight loss, anorexia, and weakness. Ask the patient if he or she has or has had recent abdominal PAIN, the most common concern. It is most often felt in the right upper quadrant before jaundice, bleeding, ascites, and edema develop. Palpation may reveal an enlarged, nodular liver.

Elevated serum *alpha-fetoprotein* (AFP) (a tumor marker for cancers of the liver, testis, and ovary) and increased *alkaline phosphatase* are also common (Pagana & Pagana, 2014). Ultrasound (US) and contrast-enhanced CT are both useful in detecting metastasis. If the primary tumor site is not known, a CT- or ultrasound-guided liver biopsy can confirm the diagnosis, although this procedure is risky because of possible bleeding and spread of the cancer cells.

◆ Interventions

Surgical resection and liver transplantation offer the only treatments for long-term survival from liver cancer. Unfortunately, most patients are not candidates for surgical removal because their tumors are unresectable. Tunneled abdominal drains, such as the PleurX drainage system, may be used at home by the patient and family to remove excess ascitic fluid. *Teach them how to empty the drain and maintain the system. Remind them not to remove more than 2000 mL of fluid at one time to prevent hypovolemic shock.*

Selective internal radiation therapy (SIRT) has been successful for some patients. Other palliative approaches include hepatic artery embolization, ablation techniques, and drug therapy. *Hepatic artery embolization* causes cell death by blocking blood supply to the tumor in the liver. It is performed under moderate sedation by an interventional radiologist who threads a catheter through the femoral artery to inject small beads into the hepatic artery to block blood flow. The patient usually stays overnight in the hospital for observation in case of bleeding. This procedure may be followed by infusing a chemotherapy agent directly into the hepatic artery (chemoembolization).

Common *ablation* procedures include radiofrequency ablation (RFA), percutaneous ethanol injection, and cryotherapy. RFA uses energy waves to heat cancer cells and kill them. It is most often performed as an ambulatory care procedure using a percutaneous laparoscopic approach. Ethanol may also be injected directly into the tumor to destroy tumor cells, although this procedure is not as commonly done as RFA (Rossi et al., 2010). Cryotherapy uses liquid nitrogen to freeze and destroy liver tumors. The general nursing care for patients having these procedures is described in Chapter 22.

Chemotherapy may be administered orally or IV. However, it is not effective in many cases. Examples of drugs used are doxorubicin (Adriamycin), 5-fluorouracil (5-FU), and cisplatin. Sorafenib (Nexavar) is a kinase inhibitor that is approved for inoperable liver cancer. Other drugs are targeted therapies that are being investigated and used with some success.

Another drug route is a catheter-directed method directly into the hepatic artery, a procedure called *hepatic arterial infusion (HAI)*. The interventional radiologist places a catheter into the artery that supplies the tumor and injects a mixture of chemotherapy and contrast agent into the tumor. This procedure has the unique effect of depositing chemotherapeutic drugs directly into the tumor without causing major systemic effects. Chapter 22 describes the general nursing care for patients receiving chemotherapy.

Patients with advanced liver cancer usually need end-of-life care and hospice services. Collaborate with the case manager to help patients and their families find the best community resources that meet their needs. Chapter 7 describes end-of-life care and hospice services in detail.

LIVER TRANSPLANTATION

❖ PATHOPHYSIOLOGY

Liver transplantation has become a common procedure worldwide. The patient with end-stage liver disease or acute liver failure who has not responded to conventional medical or surgical intervention is a potential candidate for liver transplantation. Many diseases can cause liver failure. Cirrhosis (scarring of the liver) is the most common reason for liver transplants. Other common reasons for liver transplants are chronic hepatitis B and hepatitis C, bile duct diseases, autoimmune liver disease, primary liver cancer, alcoholic liver disease, and fatty liver disease (American Liver Foundation, 2012).

Transplantation Considerations

The patient for potential transplantation has extensive physiologic and psychological assessment and evaluation by physicians and transplant coordinators. Alternative treatment should be extensively explored before committing a patient for a liver transplant. Patients who are *not* considered candidates for transplantation are those with:

- Severe cardiovascular instability with advanced cardiac disease
- Severe respiratory disease
- Metastatic tumors
- Inability to follow instructions regarding drug therapy and self-management

Liver transplantation has become the most effective treatment for an increasing number of patients with acute and chronic liver diseases. Inclusion and exclusion criteria vary among transplantation centers and are continually revised as treatment options change and surgical techniques improve.

Donor livers are obtained primarily from trauma victims who have not had liver damage. They are distributed through a nationwide program—the United Network of Organ Sharing (UNOS). This system distributes donor livers based on regional considerations and patient acuity. Candidates with the highest level of acuity receive highest priority.

The donor liver is transported to the surgery center in a solution that preserves the organ for up to 8 hours. The diseased liver is removed through an incision made in the upper abdomen. The new liver is carefully put in its place and is attached to the patient's blood vessels and bile ducts. The procedure can take many hours to complete and requires a highly specialized team and large volumes of fluid and blood replacement.

Living donors have also been used and are usually close family members or spouse. This is done on a voluntary basis after careful psychological and physiologic preparation and testing. The donor's liver is resected (usually removal of one lobe) and implanted into the recipient after removal of the diseased liver. In both the donor and the recipient, the liver regenerates and grows in size to meet the demands of the body.

Transplantation Complications

Although liver transplantations are commonly done, complications can occur. Some problems can be medically managed, whereas others require removal of the transplant. The two most common complications are acute graft rejection and infection.

The success rate for transplantations has greatly improved since the introduction many years ago of cyclosporine (cyclosporin A), an immunosuppressant drug. Today, many other anti-rejection drugs are used. (See Chapter 20 for a complete discussion of rejection and preventive drug therapy.)

! NURSING SAFETY PRIORITY QSEN

Action Alert

For the patient who has undergone liver transplantation, monitor for clinical manifestations of rejection, which may include tachycardia, fever, right upper quadrant or flank pain, decreased bile pigment and volume, and increasing jaundice. Laboratory findings include elevated serum bilirubin, rising ALT and AST levels, elevated alkaline phosphatase levels, and increased prothrombin time/international normalized ratio (PT/INR).

Transplant rejection is treated aggressively with immunosuppressive drugs. As with all rejection treatments, the patient is at a greater risk for infection. If therapy is not effective, liver function rapidly deteriorates. Multi-system organ failure, including respiratory and renal involvement, develops along with diffuse coagulopathies and portal-systemic encephalopathy (PSE). The only alternative for treatment is emergency retransplantation.

INFECTION is another potential threat to the transplanted graft and the patient's survival. Vaccinations and prophylactic antibiotics are helpful in prevention. Immunosuppressant therapy, which must be used to prevent and treat organ rejection, significantly increases the patient's risk for infection. Other risk factors include the presence of multiple tubes and intravascular lines, immobility, and prolonged anesthesia.

In the early post-transplantation period, common INFECTIONS include pneumonia, wound infections, and urinary tract infections. Opportunistic infections usually develop after the first postoperative month and include cytomegalovirus, mycobacterial infections, and parasitic infections. Latent infections such as tuberculosis and herpes simplex may be reactivated.

The physician prescribes broad-spectrum antibiotics for prophylaxis during and after surgery. Obtain culture specimens from all lines and tubes and collect specimens for culture at predetermined time intervals as dictated by the agency's policy. If an INFECTION is detected, the physician prescribes organism-specific anti-infective agents.

The biliary anastomosis is susceptible to breakdown, obstruction, and infection. If leakage occurs or if the site becomes necrotic or obstructed, an abscess can form or peritonitis, bacteremia, and cirrhosis may develop. Observe for potential complications, which are listed in Table 58-5.

❖ PATIENT-CENTERED COLLABORATIVE CARE

Care of the patient undergoing liver transplantation requires an interdisciplinary team approach. Receiving a transplant has a major psychosocial impact. Transplant complications cause patients to be very anxious. In collaboration with the members of the health care team, assure them and their families that these problems are common and usually successfully treated.

After the patient is identified as a candidate and a donor organ is procured, the actual liver transplantation surgical procedure usually takes many hours. The length of the procedure can vary greatly.

In the immediate postoperative period, the patient is managed in the critical care unit and requires aggressive

TABLE 58-5 Assessment and Prevention of Common Postoperative Complications Associated with Liver Transplantation

ASSESSMENT	PREVENTION
Acute Graft Rejection	
Occurs from the 4th to 10th postoperative day Manifested by tachycardia, fever, right upper quadrant (RUQ) or flank pain, diminished bile drainage or change in bile color, or increased jaundice Laboratory changes: (1) increased levels of serum bilirubin, transaminases, and alkaline phosphatase; (2) prolonged prothrombin time	Prophylaxis with immunosuppressant agents, such as cyclosporine Early diagnosis to treat with more potent anti-rejection drugs
Infection	
Can occur at any time during recovery Manifested by fever or excessive, foul-smelling drainage (urine, wound, or bile); other indicators depend on location and type of infection	Antibiotic prophylaxis; vaccinations Frequent cultures of tubes, lines, and drainage Early removal of invasive lines Good handwashing Early diagnosis and treatment with organism-specific anti-infective agents
Hepatic Complications (Bile Leakage, Abscess Formation, Hepatic Thrombosis)	
Manifested by decreased bile drainage, increased RUQ abdominal pain with distention and guarding, nausea or vomiting, increased jaundice, and clay-colored stools Laboratory changes: increased levels of serum bilirubin and transaminases	If present, keep T-tube in dependent position and secure to patient; empty frequently, recording quality and quantity of drainage Report manifestations to physician immediately May necessitate surgical intervention
Acute Renal Failure	
Caused by hypotension, antibiotics, cyclosporine, acute liver failure, or hypothermia Indicators of hypothermia: shivering, hyperventilation, increased cardiac output, vasoconstriction, and alkalemia Early indicators of renal failure: changes in urine output, increased blood urea nitrogen (BUN) and creatinine levels, and electrolyte imbalance	Monitor all drug levels with nephrotoxic side effects Prevent hypotension Observe for early signs of renal failure, and report them immediately to the physician

! NURSING SAFETY PRIORITY QSEN

Action Alert

For the patient who has had a liver transplantation, monitor the temperature frequently per hospital protocol, and report elevations, increased abdominal pain, distention, and rigidity, which are indicators of peritonitis. Nursing assessment also includes monitoring for a change in neurologic status that could indicate encephalopathy from a nonfunctioning liver. Report signs of clotting problems (e.g., bloody oozing from a catheter, petechiae, ecchymosis) to the surgeon immediately because they may indicate impaired function of the transplanted liver.

monitoring and care. Assess for signs and symptoms of complications of surgery, and immediately report them to the surgeon (see Table 58-5).

Post–liver transplant patients are living longer today than ever. Teach patients to be aware of side effects of immunosuppressive drugs, such as hypertension, nephrotoxicity, and gastrointestinal disturbances. Remind them that long-term management of care includes surveillance for malignancy, metabolic syndrome, and diabetes. Teaching the patient self-examination for skin, breast, and testicular malignancies is important as well as reminders for annual Papanicolaou (Pap) smears and other cancer screening tests. Post-transplant patients need to maintain lifestyle changes to increase their longevity after surgery (Clayton, 2011; Lucey et al., 2013).

NURSING CONCEPTS AND CLINICAL JUDGMENT REVIEW

What might you NOTICE if the patient is experiencing inadequate digestion, nutrition, and metabolism as a result of impaired liver function?

- Jaundice
- Icterus
- Report of nausea and anorexia
- Vomiting
- Weight loss
- Bruising or bleeding
- Ascites

What should you INTERPRET and how should you RESPOND to a patient experiencing inadequate digestion, nutrition, and metabolism as a result of impaired liver function?

Perform and interpret physical assessment findings, including:

- Assessing respiratory status to check for dyspnea or shallow breathing
- Checking level of consciousness and cognition
- Taking vital signs (looking for fever or decreased BP) and oxygen saturation
- Checking for blood in the vomitus
- Performing an abdominal assessment, including measuring girth
- Checking urine for dark color and stool for clay-colored appearance
- Taking current weight, and comparing with previous weight
- Assessing skin for open areas
- Checking most recent laboratory values for coagulation studies and LFTs

Respond by:

- Applying oxygen to assist in ease of breathing
- Keeping head of bed elevated to at least 30 degrees
- Maintaining rest
- Collaborating with dietitian and pharmacist as needed
- Prioritizing and pacing activities to prevent fatigue
- Monitoring patient closely for complications, such as bleeding; calling the Rapid Response Team if bleeding occurs

On what should you REFLECT?

- Monitor the patient for restored digestion and nutrition, such as increased appetite.
- Think about what may have caused the liver problem.
- Consider for what complications the patient is at risk.
- Think about what members of the health care team need to provide care for this patient.

GET READY FOR THE NCLEX® EXAMINATION!

KEY POINTS

Review these Key Points for each NCLEX Examination Client Needs Category.

Safe and Effective Care Environment

- When caring for patients with cirrhosis, collaborate with the dietitian, physician, and pharmacist. **Teamwork and Collaboration** QSEN
- Refer patients with liver disorders to the American Liver Foundation; refer dying patients to hospice and other community resources as needed. **Patient-Centered Care** QSEN

Health Promotion and Maintenance

- Follow the guidelines listed in Chart 58-3 to prevent viral hepatitis in the workplace. **Evidence-Based Practice** QSEN
- Teach patients to take precautions to prevent viral hepatitis in the community as described in Chart 58-4. **Evidence-Based Practice** QSEN
- For patients with viral hepatitis, instruct them to follow the guidelines listed in Chart 58-5. **Safety** QSEN
- Teach patients to avoid alcohol and illicit drugs to prevent or slow the progression of alcohol-induced cirrhosis; remind them not to take any medication (including over-the-counter drugs) without checking with their health care provider. **Safety** QSEN

Psychosocial Integrity

- Recognize that patients with cirrhosis have mental and emotional changes due to hepatic encephalopathy. **Patient-Centered Care** QSEN
- Be aware that patients with cirrhosis and/or chronic hepatitis may feel guilty about their disease because of past habits such as drug and alcohol use. **Patient-Centered Care** QSEN
- Be aware that family members and friends may fear getting hepatitis from the patient. **Patient-Centered Care** QSEN
- Be aware that patients having liver transplantation have major concerns about the possibility of complications, such as organ rejection. **Patient-Centered Care** QSEN

Physiological Integrity

- Be aware that cirrhosis has many causes other than alcohol use (see Table 58-1). **Patient-Centered Care** QSEN

- Observe for clinical manifestations of hepatic encephalopathy (PSE) as listed in Table 58-2. **Safety** QSEN
- Monitor laboratory values of patients suspected of or diagnosed with cirrhosis of the liver as listed in Table 58-3. **Informatics** QSEN
- Monitor the patient with cirrhosis for bleeding and neurologic changes. **Safety** QSEN
- Provide care for the patient having a paracentesis as described in Chart 58-1. **Safety** QSEN
- Administer drug therapy to decrease ammonia levels (which cause PSE) in patients with cirrhosis, such as lactulose and nonabsorbable antibiotics. **Safety** QSEN
- Differentiate the five major types of hepatitis: A, B, C, D, and E. Hepatitis D occurs only with Hepatitis B and is transmitted most commonly by blood and body fluid exposure. Hepatitis A is transmitted via the fecal-oral route. Hepatitis C is the most common type and is also transmitted via blood and body fluids. **Evidence-Based Practice** QSEN
- Be aware that patients with chronic viral hepatitis often develop cirrhosis and cancer of the liver. **Evidence-Based Practice** QSEN
- Recognize that potent immunomodulators and antivirals are given to treat hepatitis B and hepatitis C; teach patients on immunomodulators to avoid large crowds and people who have INFECTIONS. **Safety** QSEN
- Monitor for bleeding in the patient with liver trauma; assume that any abdominal trauma has damaged the liver. **Safety** QSEN
- Monitor the patient having a liver transplantation for complications, such as those described in Table 58-5. **Safety** QSEN
- Report and document elevated temperature, increased abdominal PAIN and rigidity, bleeding, and/or neurologic status changes as possible indicators of liver transplantation complications. **Evidence-Based Practice** QSEN

Care of Patients with Problems of the Biliary System and Pancreas

Lara Carver and Jennifer Powers

http://evolve.elsevier.com/Iggy/

PRIORITY CONCEPTS

- PAIN
- NUTRITION
- INFLAMMATION

LEARNING OUTCOMES

Safe and Effective Care Environment

1. Collaborate with health care team members to provide care for patients with pancreatic disorders.
2. Identify community-based resources for patients with pancreatic disorders.

Health Promotion and Maintenance

3. Teach people about health promotion practices to prevent gallbladder disease.
4. Teach people about evidence-based health promotion practices to prevent pancreatitis.

Psychosocial Integrity

5. Describe the psychosocial needs of patients with pancreatic cancer and their families.

Physiological Integrity

6. Identify risk factors for gallbladder disease.
7. Interpret diagnostic test results associated with gallbladder disease.
8. Compare postoperative care of patients undergoing a traditional cholecystectomy with that of patients having laparoscopic cholecystectomy.
9. Compare and contrast the pathophysiology of acute and chronic pancreatitis.
10. Interpret laboratory test results associated with acute pancreatitis.
11. Interpret common assessment findings associated with acute and chronic pancreatitis.
12. Prioritize nursing care for patients with acute pancreatitis and patients with chronic pancreatitis.
13. Explain the use and precautions associated with enzyme replacement for chronic pancreatitis.
14. Develop a postoperative plan of care for patients having a Whipple procedure.

The biliary system (liver and gallbladder) and pancreas secrete enzymes and other substances that promote food digestion in the stomach and small intestine. When these organs do not work properly, the person has impaired *digestion,* which may result in inadequate NUTRITION. Collaborative care for patients with problems of the biliary system and pancreas includes the need to promote nutrition for healthy cellular function. This chapter focuses on problems of the gallbladder and pancreas. Liver disorders are described in Chapter 58.

Because of the close anatomic location of these organs, disorders of the gallbladder and pancreas may extend to other organs if the primary health problem is not treated early. INFLAMMATION is caused by **obstruction** (blockage) in the biliary system from gallstones, edema, stricture, or tumors. For example, gallstones in the cystic duct cause cholecystitis. Gallstones lodged in the ampulla of Vater block the flow of bile and pancreatic secretions, which can result in pancreatitis. These problems frequently cause the patient to have moderate to severe abdominal PAIN.

CHOLECYSTITIS

❖ *PATHOPHYSIOLOGY*

Cholecystitis is an INFLAMMATION of the gallbladder that affects many people, most commonly in affluent countries. It may be either acute or chronic, although most patients have the acute type.

Acute Cholecystitis

Two types of acute cholecystitis can occur: calculous and acalculous cholecystitis. The most common type is **calculous cholecystitis,** in which chemical irritation and INFLAMMATION result from gallstones (**cholelithiasis**) that obstruct the cystic duct (most often), gallbladder neck, or common bile duct (choledocholithiasis) (Fig. 59-1). When the gallbladder is inflamed, trapped bile is reabsorbed and acts as a chemical irritant to the gallbladder wall. Reabsorbed bile, in combination with impaired circulation, edema, and distention of the gallbladder, causes ischemia and infection. The result is tissue sloughing with

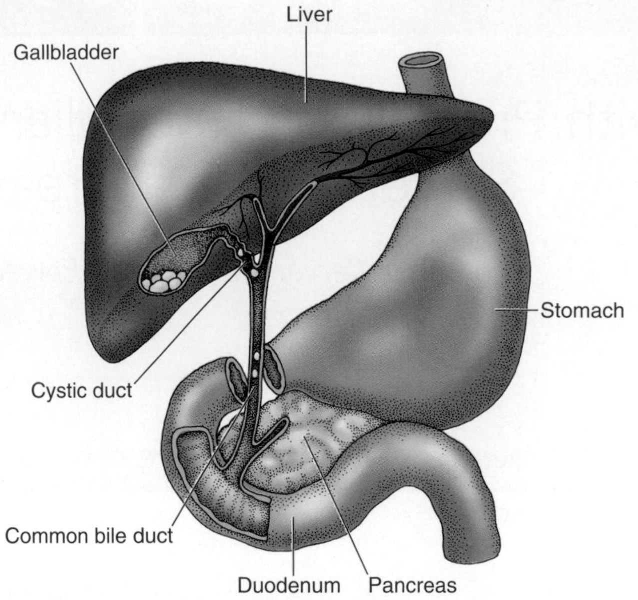

FIG. 59-1 Gallstones within the gallbladder and obstructing the common bile and cystic ducts.

necrosis and gangrene within the gallbladder itself. The gallbladder wall may eventually perforate (rupture). If the perforation is small and localized, an abscess may form. **Peritonitis**, infection of the peritoneum, may result if the perforation is large.

The exact pathophysiology of gallstone formation is not clearly understood, but abnormal metabolism of cholesterol and bile salts plays an important role in their formation. The gallbladder provides an excellent environment for the production of stones because it only occasionally mixes its normally abundant mucus with its highly viscous, concentrated bile. Impaired gallbladder motility can lead to stone formation by delaying bile emptying and causing biliary stasis.

Gallstones are composed of substances normally found in bile, such as cholesterol, bilirubin, bile salts, calcium, and various proteins. They are classified as either cholesterol stones or pigment stones. Cholesterol calculi form as a result of metabolic imbalances of cholesterol and bile salts. They are the most common type found in people in the United States (McCance et al., 2014).

Bacteria can collect around the stones in the biliary system. Severe bacterial invasion can lead to life-threatening *suppurative* cholangitis when symptoms are not recognized quickly and pus accumulates in the ductal system.

Acalculous cholecystitis (INFLAMMATION occurring without gallstones) is typically associated with biliary stasis caused by any condition that affects the regular filling or emptying of the gallbladder. For example, a decrease in blood flow to the gallbladder or anatomic problems such as twisting or kinking of the gallbladder neck or cystic duct can result in pancreatic enzyme reflux into the gallbladder, causing inflammation. Sphincter of Oddi dysfunction (SOD) can also occur to cause reflux and inflammation (Pfadt & Carlson, 2011). Most cases of this type of cholecystitis occur in patients with:

- Sepsis
- Severe trauma or burns
- Long-term total parenteral nutrition
- Multi-system organ failure
- Major surgery
- Hypovolemia

Chronic Cholecystitis

Chronic cholecystitis results when repeated episodes of cystic duct obstruction cause chronic INFLAMMATION. Calculi are almost always present. In chronic cholecystitis, the gallbladder becomes fibrotic and contracted, which results in decreased motility and deficient absorption.

Pancreatitis and cholangitis (bile duct INFLAMMATION) can occur as chronic complications of cholecystitis. These problems result from the backup of bile throughout the biliary tract. Bile obstruction leads to jaundice.

Jaundice (yellow discoloration of the skin and mucous membranes) and **icterus** (yellow discoloration of the sclera) can occur in patients with acute cholecystitis but are most commonly seen in those with the *chronic* form of the disease. Obstructed bile flow caused by edema of the ducts or gallstones contributes to *extrahepatic* **obstructive jaundice**. Jaundice in cholecystitis may also be caused by direct liver involvement. Inflammation of the liver's bile channels or bile ducts may cause *intrahepatic* obstructive jaundice, resulting in an increase in circulating levels of bilirubin, the major pigment of bile.

In a person with obstructive jaundice, the normal flow of bile into the duodenum is blocked, allowing excessive bile salts to accumulate in the skin. This accumulation of bile salts leads to **pruritus** (itching) or a burning sensation. The bile flow blockage also prevents bilirubin from reaching the large intestine, where it is converted to urobilinogen. Because urobilinogen accounts for the normal brown color of feces, clay-colored stools result. Water-soluble bilirubin is normally excreted by the kidneys in the urine. When an excess of circulating bilirubin occurs, the urine becomes dark and foamy because of the kidneys' effort to clear the bilirubin.

Etiology and Genetic Risk

A familial or genetic tendency appears to play a role in the development of cholelithiasis, but this may be partially related to familial nutrition habits (excessive dietary cholesterol intake) and sedentary lifestyles. Genetic-environment interactions may contribute to gallstone production. For example, current studies are investigating DNA expression sequences that program some people to make and secrete more cholesterol into bile, leading to the increase in cholesterol-containing gallstones. The main risk factors for developing gallstones are obesity, type 2 diabetes, dyslipidemia, and insulin resistance. Independent risk factors for developing gallstones are increase in age, female gender, and family history (Agostino et al., 2013). Also, people who experience rapid weight loss and certain intestinal diseases affecting the normal absorption of nutrients, such as Crohn's disease, are at risk for gallstones. The highest frequency of gallstone production lies among the American-Indian and Mexican-American populations (McCance, et al., 2014). Risk factors for cholecystitis are listed in Table 59-1.

The incidence of chronic cholecystitis is increased in young, thin women, especially those who are athletic (e.g., ballerinas and gymnasts). These women have chronic pain that is often misdiagnosed as gastritis.

TABLE 59-1 Risk Factors for Cholecystitis

- Women
- Aging
- American Indian, Mexican American, or Caucasian
- Obesity
- Rapid weight loss or prolonged fasting
- Increased serum cholesterol
- Women on hormone replacement therapy (HRT)
- Cholesterol-lowering drugs
- Family history of gallstones
- Prolonged total parenteral nutrition
- Crohn's disease
- Gastric bypass surgery
- Sickle cell disease
- Glucose intolerance/diabetes mellitus
- Pregnancy
- Genetic factors

GENDER HEALTH CONSIDERATIONS

Patient-Centered Care QSEN

Women who are between 20 and 60 years of age are twice as likely to develop gallstones as are men. Obesity is a major risk factor for gallstone formation, especially in women. Pregnancy and drugs such as hormone replacements and birth control pills alter hormone levels and delay muscular contraction of the gallbladder, decreasing the rate of bile emptying. The incidence of gallstones is higher in women who have had multiple pregnancies. Combinations of causative factors increase the incidence of stone formation, especially in women. Therefore some clinicians refer to the patient most at risk for acute cholecystitis and gallstones by the four Fs:

- Female
- Forty
- Fat
- Fertile

❖ PATIENT-CENTERED COLLABORATIVE CARE

◆ Assessment

Physical Assessment/Clinical Manifestations. Obtain the patient's height, weight, and vital signs, or delegate these activities to unlicensed assistive personnel (UAP). Ask about food preferences, and determine whether excessive fat and cholesterol are part of the diet. Typically, diets high in fat, high in calories, low in fiber, and high in refined white carbohydrates place patients at higher risk for developing gallstones. Inquire if any foods cause pain. Question whether any GI symptoms occur when fatty food is eaten: **flatulence** (gas), **dyspepsia** (indigestion), **eructation** (belching), anorexia, nausea, vomiting, and abdominal PAIN or discomfort.

Patients with cholecystitis present with abdominal PAIN, although clinical manifestations vary in intensity and frequency (Chart 59-1). Ask the patient to describe the PAIN, including its intensity and duration, precipitating factors, and any measures that relieve it. Pain may be described as indigestion of varying intensity, ranging from a mild, persistent ache to a steady, constant pain in the right upper abdominal quadrant. It may radiate to the right shoulder or scapula. In some cases the abdominal pain of chronic cholecystitis may be vague and nonspecific. The usual pattern is episodic. Patients often refer to acute pain episodes as "gallbladder attacks."

The severe PAIN of **biliary colic** is produced by obstruction of the cystic duct of the gallbladder or movement of one or more stones. When a stone is moving through or is lodged within the duct, tissue spasm occurs in an effort to get the stone through the small duct.

CHART 59-1 Key Features

Cholecystitis

- Episodic or vague upper abdominal pain or discomfort that can radiate to the right shoulder
- Pain triggered by a high-fat or high-volume meal
- Anorexia
- Nausea and/or vomiting
- Dyspepsia (indigestion)
- Eructation (belching)
- Flatulence (gas)
- Feeling of abdominal fullness
- Rebound tenderness (Blumberg's sign)
- Fever
- Jaundice, clay-colored stools, dark urine, steatorrhea (most common with chronic cholecystitis)

CONSIDERATIONS FOR OLDER ADULTS

Patient-Centered Care QSEN

Older adults and patients with diabetes mellitus may have atypical manifestations of cholecystitis, including the absence of pain and fever. Localized tenderness may be the only presenting sign. The older patient may become acutely confused (delirium) as the first manifestation of gallbladder disease.

! NURSING SAFETY PRIORITY QSEN

Critical Rescue

Biliary colic may be so severe that it occurs with tachycardia, pallor, diaphoresis, and prostration (extreme exhaustion). Assess the patient for possible shock caused by biliary colic. Notify the health care provider or Rapid Response Team if these manifestations occur. Stay with the patient, and keep the head of the bed flat.

Ask patients to describe their daily activity or exercise routines to determine whether they are sedentary. Sedentary lifestyle, rapid weight loss, prolonged fasting, and pregnancy are risk factors for developing gallstones. Question whether there is a family history of gallbladder disease. Ask the patient about taking current or previous hormone replacement therapy (HRT). If the patient is female, ask if she is taking or has recently been on oral contraceptives (birth control pills).

Assessment for rebound tenderness (**Blumberg's sign**) and deep palpation are performed only by physicians and advanced practice nurses. To elicit rebound tenderness, the health care provider pushes his or her fingers deeply and steadily into the patient's abdomen and then quickly releases the pressure. PAIN that results from the rebound of the palpated tissue may indicate peritoneal inflammation. Deep palpation below the liver border in the right upper quadrant may reveal a sausage-shaped mass, representing the distended, inflamed gallbladder. Percussion over the posterior rib cage worsens localized abdominal pain.

In *chronic* cholecystitis, patients may have slowly developing symptoms and may not seek medical treatment until late symptoms such as jaundice (yellowing of the skin), clay-colored stools, and dark urine occur from biliary obstruction. Yellowing of the sclera (icterus) and oral mucous membranes may also be present. **Steatorrhea** (fatty stools) occurs because fat absorption is decreased because of the lack of bile. Bile is needed for the absorption of fats and fat-soluble vitamins in the intestine. As with any inflammatory process, the patient may have an elevated temperature of 99° to 102° F (37.2° to 38.9° C), tachycardia, and dehydration from fever and vomiting.

CONSIDERATIONS FOR OLDER ADULTS

Patient-Centered Care QSEN

> Older adults become dehydrated much quicker than other age-groups, and they may not present with a fever. Monitor for a new onset of disorientation or acute confusion due to decreased blood volume available to oxygenate the cells of the brain (hypoxia).

Diagnostic Assessment. A differential diagnosis rules out other diseases that may cause similar symptoms, such as peptic ulcer disease, hepatitis, and pancreatitis. An increased *white blood cell* (WBC) count indicates INFLAMMATION. Serum levels of *alkaline phosphatase, aspartate aminotransferase (AST),* and *lactate dehydrogenase (LDH)* may be elevated, indicating abnormalities in liver function in patients with severe biliary obstruction. The direct (conjugated) and indirect (unconjugated) *serum bilirubin levels* are also elevated. If the pancreas is involved, serum amylase and lipase levels are elevated.

Calcified gallstones are easily viewed on abdominal x-ray. Stones that are not calcified cannot be seen. *Ultrasonography (US) of the right upper quadrant is the best initial diagnostic test for cholecystitis.* It is safe, accurate, and painless. Acute cholecystitis is seen as edema of the gallbladder wall and pericholecystic fluid.

A hepatobiliary scan (sometimes called a HIDA scan) can be performed to visualize the gallbladder and determine patency of the biliary system. In this nuclear medicine test, a radioactive tracer or chemical is injected intravenously. About 20 minutes after the injection, a gamma camera tracks the flow of the tracer from the gallbladder to determine the ejection rate of bile into the biliary duct. A decreased bile flow indicates gallbladder disease with obstruction. Teach patients having this test to have nothing by mouth before the procedure. Remind the patient that the camera is large and close to the body for most of the procedure.

When the cause of cholecystitis or cholelithiasis is not known or the patient has manifestations of biliary obstruction (e.g., jaundice), an *endoscopic retrograde cholangiopancreatography* (ERCP) may be performed. Some patients have the less invasive and safer *magnetic resonance cholangiopancreatography* (MRCP), which can be performed by an interventional radiologist. For this procedure, the patient is given oral or IV contrast material (gadolinium) before having an MRI scan (Griffin et al., 2011). Before the test, ask the patient about any history of urticaria (hives) or other allergy. MRI is also contraindicated in patients with pacemaker or other incompatible devices. Gadolinium does not contain iodine, which decreases the risk for an allergic response. Chapter 52 discusses these tests in more detail.

◆ *Interventions*

Acute cholecystitis is diagnosed on the basis of clinical findings, laboratory tests, and abdominal imaging. If acute infection of the gallbladder is diagnosed, emergency cholecystectomy is usually performed the same or the following day. Laparoscopic cholecystectomy is the treatment of choice for patients with acute and long-term chronic cholecystitis. This minimally invasive procedure achieves the desired outcomes of shorter recovery time, decreased expense, less postoperative pain, and minimal scarring after surgery.

Nonsurgical Management. Many people with gallstones have no symptoms. Acute PAIN is present when gallstones partially or totally obstruct the cystic or common bile duct. Most patients find that they need to avoid fatty foods to prevent further episodes of biliary colic. Withhold food and fluids if nausea and vomiting occur. IV therapy is used for hydration.

Drug Therapy. *Acute biliary pain requires opioid analgesia, such as morphine or hydromorphone (Dilaudid). All opioids may cause some degree of sphincter of Oddi spasm.*

Ketorolac (Toradol, Acular), an NSAID, may be used for mild to moderate pain. Be sure to monitor the patient for signs and symptoms of GI distress and pain because the drug can cause GI bleeding. The health care provider prescribes antiemetics to control nausea and vomiting. IV antibiotic therapy may also be given, depending on the cause of cholecystitis or as a one-time dose for surgery.

An option for a small number of patients with cholelithiasis (gallstones) is the use of oral bile acid dissolution or gallstone stabilizing agents. Drugs such as ursodiol (Actigall) and chenodiol (Chenodal) may be given for up to 2 years to dissolve or stabilize gallstones. A gallbladder ultrasound is required every 6 months for the first year of therapy to determine the effectiveness of the drug. Teach patients on this type of drug therapy to report diarrhea, vomiting, or severe abdominal PAIN, especially if it radiates to the shoulders, to their health care provider immediately. Remind them to take the medication with food and milk (Felicilda-Reynaldo, 2012).

Other Nonsurgical Interventions. For some patients with small stones or for those who are not good surgical candidates, a treatment that is commonly used for kidney stones can be used to break up gallstones—*extracorporeal shock wave lithotripsy (ESWL).* This procedure can be used only for patients who have a normal weight, cholesterol-based stones, and good gallbladder function. The patient lies on a water-filled pad, and shock waves break up the large stones into smaller ones that can be passed through the digestive system. During the procedure, he or she may have PAIN from the movement of the stones or duct or gallbladder spasms. A therapeutic bile acid, such as ursodeoxycholic acid (UDCA), may be used after the procedure to help dissolve the remaining stone fragments.

Another treatment option in people who cannot have surgery is the insertion of a percutaneous transhepatic biliary catheter (drain) using CT or ultrasound guidance to open the blocked duct(s) so that bile can flow (cholecystostomy). Catheters can be placed several ways, depending on the condition of the biliary ducts, in an internal, external, or internal/external drain. Biliary catheters usually divert bile from the liver into the duodenum to bypass a stricture. When all of the bile enters the duodenum, it is called an *internal* drain. However, in some cases a patient has an *internal/external* drain in which part of the bile empties into a drainage bag. Patients who need this drain for an extended period may have the external drain capped. If jaundice or leakage around the catheter site occurs, teach the patient to reconnect the catheter to a drainage bag and have a follow-up cholangiogram injection done by an interventional radiologist. An *external* only catheter is connected either temporarily or permanently to a drainage bag. A reduction in bile drainage indicates that the drain is no longer working.

Surgical Management. Cholecystectomy is a surgical removal of the gallbladder. One of two procedures is performed: the laparoscopic cholecystectomy and, far less often, the traditional open approach cholecystectomy.

Laparoscopic Cholecystectomy. Laparoscopic cholecystectomy, a minimally invasive surgery (MIS), is the "gold standard" and is performed far more often than the traditional open approach. The advantages of MIS when compared with the open approach include:

- Complications are not common.
- The death rate is very low.
- Bile duct injuries are rare.
- Patient recovery is quicker.
- Postoperative PAIN is less severe.

The laparoscopic procedure (often called a "lap chole") is commonly done on an ambulatory care basis in a same-day surgery suite. The surgeon explains the procedure, and the nurse answers questions and reinforces the instructions. Reinforce what to expect after surgery, and review pain management, deep-breathing exercises, incisional care, and leg exercises to prevent deep vein thrombosis. There is no special preoperative preparation other than the routine preparation for surgery under general anesthesia described in Chapter 14. An IV antibiotic is usually given immediately before or during surgery (Society of American Gastrointestinal and Endoscopic Surgeons [SAGES], 2013).

During the surgery the surgeon makes a very small midline puncture at the umbilicus. Additional small incisions may be needed, although single-incision laparoscopic cholecystectomy (SILC) using a flexible endoscope is often done (Salam, 2010). The abdominal cavity is insufflated with 3 to 4 liters of carbon dioxide. Gasless laparoscopic cholecystectomy using abdominal wall lifting devices is a more recent innovation in some centers. This technique results in improved pulmonary and cardiac function. A trocar catheter is inserted, through which a laparoscope is introduced. The laparoscope is attached to a video camera, and the abdominal organs are viewed on a monitor. The gallbladder is dissected from the liver bed, and the cystic artery and duct are closed. The surgeon aspirates the bile and crushes any large stones, if present, and then extracts the gallbladder through the umbilical port.

Removing the gallbladder with the laparoscopic technique reduces the risk for wound complications. Some patients have mild to severe discomfort from carbon dioxide retention in the abdomen, which may be felt throughout the thorax and shoulders.

! NURSING SAFETY PRIORITY QSEN

Action Alert

After a laparoscopic cholecystectomy, assess the patient's oxygen saturation level frequently until the effects of the anesthesia have passed. Remind the patient to perform deep-breathing exercises every hour.

Other postoperative care for the patient after a laparoscopic procedure is similar to that for any patient having minimally invasive endoscopic surgery (see Chapter 16). Offer the patient food and water when fully awake, and monitor for the nausea and/or vomiting that often results from anesthesia. If needed, administer an antiemetic drug, such as ondansetron hydrochloride (Zofran), either IV push or as a disintegrating tablet. Several drug doses may be needed. Maintain an IV line to administer fluids until nausea and/or vomiting subside. Be sure to have the head of the bed elevated in the same-day surgery unit to prevent aspiration from vomiting. After nausea subsides, assist the patient to the bathroom to void. Early ambulation also promotes absorption of the carbon dioxide, which can decrease postoperative discomfort.

Administer an oral or IV push opioid as needed immediately after surgery. Continuous IV pain control is usually not required because there is only one or a few small incisions, which are covered with Steri-Strips and small adhesive bandages (e.g., Band-Aids) or are surgically glued. The glue or Steri-Strips lose their adhesiveness in about a week to 10 days and can be removed or fall off as the incision heals.

The patient is usually discharged from the hospital or surgery center the same day, although older and obese patients may stay overnight. Provide postoperative teaching regarding pain management, incision care, and follow-up appointments. Teach the patient to use ice and oral opioids for incisional pain, if needed, for a few days. For abdominal or thoracic discomfort from carbon dioxide retention, many patients report that heat application is helpful. The patient is typically allowed to bathe or shower the day after surgery.

After laparoscopic surgery, the patient can return to usual activities much sooner than those having an open cholecystectomy. Instruct the patient to rest for the first 24 hours and then begin to resume usual activities Most patients are able to resume usual activities within a week.

Some patients are able to return to their usual diet after surgery, while others must carefully monitor their diet to avoid high-fat foods. A large intake of fatty foods may result in abdominal pain and diarrhea, which could result in a mild post-cholecystectomy syndrome (PCS) (see later discussion of PCS on p. 1218). Teach patients to introduce foods high in fat one at a time to determine which foods are best tolerated.

A new minimally invasive surgical procedure is *natural orifice transluminal endoscopic surgery* (NOTES) for removal of or repair of organs. Surgery can be performed on many body organs through the mouth, vagina, and rectum. For removal of the gallbladder, the vagina is used most often in women because it can be easily decontaminated with Betadine or other antiseptic and allows easy access into the peritoneal cavity. The surgeon makes a small internal incision through the cul-de-sac of Douglas between the rectum and uterine wall to access the gallbladder. The main advantages of this procedure are the lack of visible incisions and minimal, if any, postoperative complications (Navarra et al., 2010).

Traditional Cholecystectomy. Use of the open surgical approach (abdominal laparotomy) has greatly declined during the past 25 years. Patients who have this type of surgery usually have severe biliary obstruction and the ducts are explored to ensure patency.

The surgical nurse provides the usual preoperative care and teaching in the operating suite on the day of surgery (see Chapter 14). The surgeon removes the gallbladder through an incision and explores the biliary ducts for the presence of stones or other cause of obstruction. The surgeon usually inserts a drainage tube such as a Jackson-Pratt (JP) drain. This tube is placed in the gallbladder bed to prevent fluid accumulation. The drainage is usually serosanguineous (serous fluid mixed with blood) and is stained with bile in the first 24 hours after surgery. Antibiotic therapy is given to prevent infection.

Patient care for a patient who has had a traditional open cholecystectomy is similar to the care for any patient who has had abdominal surgery under general anesthesia as described in Chapter 16. Postoperative incisional PAIN after a traditional cholecystectomy is controlled with opioids using a patient-controlled analgesia (PCA) pump. Encourage the patient to use coughing and deep-breathing exercises when pain is controlled and the incision is splinted.

Antiemetics may be necessary for episodes of postoperative nausea and vomiting. Administer the antiemetic early, as prescribed, to prevent retching associated with vomiting and thus to decrease pain related to muscle straining.

Provide care for the incision and the surgical drain. The surgeon typically removes the surgical dressing and drain within 24 hours after surgery.

The patient is NPO until fully awake postoperatively. Document the patient's level of consciousness, vital signs, and pain level. Assess the surgical incision for signs of infection, such as excessive redness or purulent drainage. Report changes to the surgeon immediately. Begin ambulation as soon as possible to prevent deep vein thrombosis and promote peristalsis.

Advance the diet from clear liquids to solid foods as peristalsis returns. The patient usually resumes solid foods and is discharged to home 1 to 2 days after surgery, depending on any complications and the patient's general condition. In the early postoperative period, if bile flow is reduced, a low-fat diet may reduce discomfort and prevent nausea. For most patients, a special diet is not required. Advise them to eat nutritious meals and avoid excessive intake of fatty foods, especially fried food, butter, and "fast food." If the patient is obese, recommend a weight-reduction program.

Teach the patient to keep the incision clean and report any changes that may indicate infection. Remind him or her to report repeated abdominal or epigastric pain with vomiting and/or diarrhea that may occur several weeks to months after surgery. These symptoms indicate possible **postcholecystectomy syndrome (PCS)**. There are multiple causes of PCS, some of which are related to the biliary system and others are not. Common causes of PCS are listed in Table 59-2. Not all patients experience PCS. Often the PAIN returns because of one of the underlying conditions listed in Table 59-2, not as a result of the cholecystectomy itself (Girometti et al., 2010).

Management depends on the exact cause but usually involves the use of endoscopic retrograde cholangiopancreatography (ERCP) to find the cause of the problem and repair it. This procedure and related nursing care are described in Chapter 52. Collaborative care includes pain management, antibiotics, nutrition and hydration therapy (possibly short-term parenteral nutrition), and control of nausea and vomiting.

TABLE 59-2 Common Causes of Postcholecystectomy Syndrome

Biliary	Non-Biliary
• Pseudocyst	• Coronary artery disease
• Common bile duct (CBD) leak	• Intercostal neuritis
• CBD or pancreatic duct stricture or obstruction	• Unexplained pain syndrome
• Sphincter of Oddi dysfunction	• Psychiatric or neurologic disorder
• Retained or new CBD gallstone	
• Pancreatic or liver mass	
• Primary sclerosing cholangitis	
• Diverticular compression	

NCLEX EXAMINATION CHALLENGE

Physiological Integrity

The nurse is providing discharge instructions for a client who has undergone a laparoscopic cholecystectomy. Which instruction will the nurse include in the discharge teaching?

A. Keep dressings in place for 4 weeks.
B. Report bile-colored drainage from any of the incisions.
C. Expect dark, tarry stools after surgery.
D. Be aware that no dietary changes will be necessary.

ACUTE PANCREATITIS

❖ PATHOPHYSIOLOGY

Acute pancreatitis is a serious and, at times, life-threatening INFLAMMATION of the pancreas. This process is caused by a premature activation of excessive pancreatic enzymes that destroy ductal tissue and pancreatic cells, resulting in autodigestion and fibrosis of the pancreas. The pathologic changes occur in different degrees. The severity of pancreatitis depends on the extent of inflammation and tissue damage. Pancreatitis can range from mild involvement evidenced by edema and inflammation to **necrotizing hemorrhagic pancreatitis (NHP)**. NHP is diffusely bleeding pancreatic tissue with fibrosis and tissue death.

The pancreas is unusual in that it functions as both an exocrine gland and an endocrine gland. The primary *endocrine* disorder is diabetes mellitus and is discussed in Chapter 64. The *exocrine* function of the pancreas is responsible for secreting enzymes that assist in the breakdown of starches, proteins, and fats. These enzymes are normally secreted in the inactive form and become activated once they enter the small intestine. Early activation (i.e., activation within the pancreas rather than the intestinal lumen) results in the inflammatory process of pancreatitis. Direct toxic injury to the pancreatic cells and the production and release of pancreatic enzymes (e.g., trypsin, lipase, elastase) result from the obstructive damage. After pancreatic duct obstruction, increased pressure may contribute to ductal rupture allowing spillage of trypsin and other enzymes into the pancreatic parenchymal tissue. Autodigestion of the pancreas occurs as a result (Fig. 59-2). In *acute* pancreatitis, four major pathophysiologic processes occur: lipolysis, proteolysis, necrosis of blood vessels, and INFLAMMATION.

The hallmark of pancreatic necrosis is enzymatic fat necrosis of the endocrine and exocrine cells of the pancreas caused by the enzyme *lipase.* Fatty acids are released during this *lipolytic process* and combine with ionized calcium to form a soap-like product. The initial rapid lowering of serum calcium levels is not readily compensated for by the parathyroid gland. Because the body needs ionized calcium and cannot use bound calcium, hypocalcemia occurs (McCance et al., 2014).

Proteolysis involves the splitting of proteins by hydrolysis of the peptide bonds, resulting in the formation of smaller polypeptides. Proteolytic activity may lead to thrombosis and

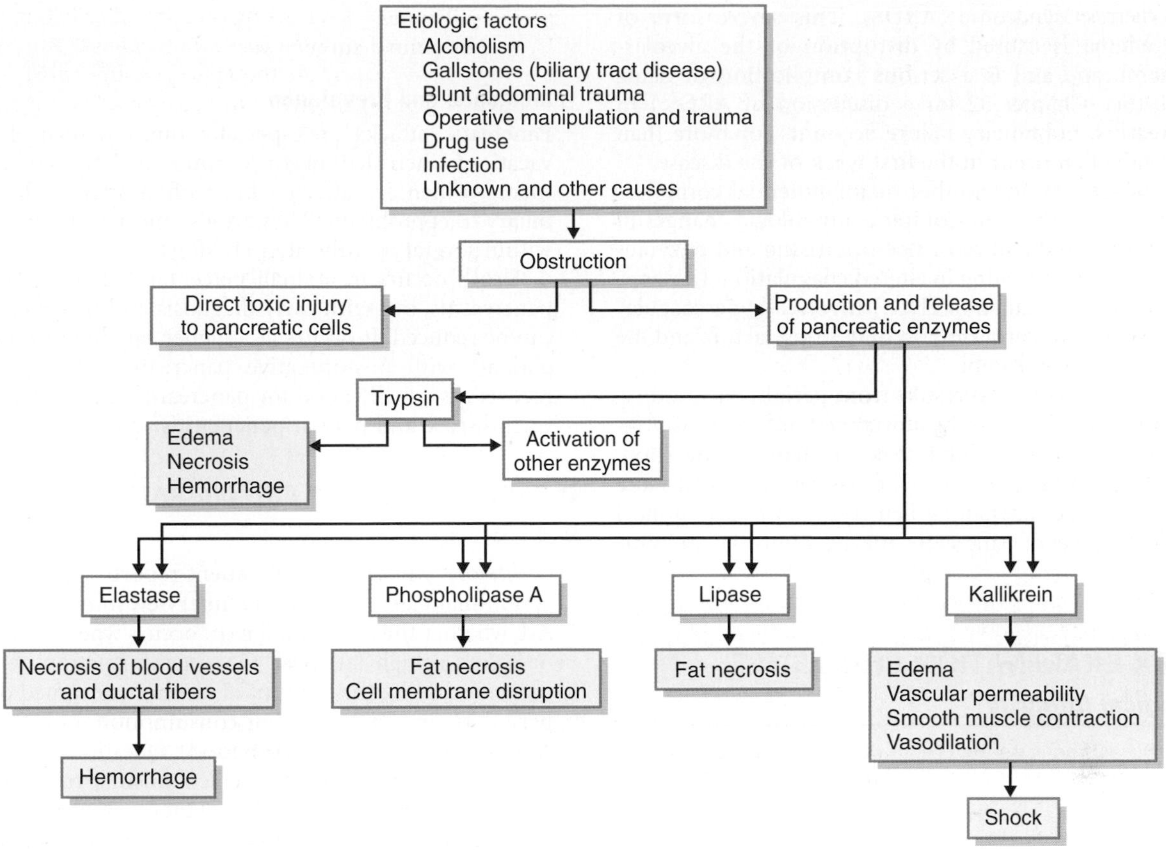

FIG. 59-2 The process of autodigestion in acute pancreatitis.

gangrene of the pancreas. Pancreatic destruction may be localized and confined to one area or may involve the entire organ.

Elastase is activated by trypsin and causes elastic fibers of the blood vessels and ducts to dissolve. The *necrosis of blood vessels* results in bleeding, ranging from minor bleeding to massive hemorrhage of pancreatic tissue. Another pancreatic enzyme, kallikrein, causes the release of vasoactive peptides, bradykinin, and a plasma kinin known as *kallidin.* These substances contribute to vasodilation and increased vascular permeability, further compounding the hemorrhagic process. This massive destruction of blood vessels by necrosis may lead to generalized hemorrhage with blood escaping into the retroperitoneal tissues. *The patient with hemorrhagic pancreatitis is critically ill, and extensive pancreatic destruction and shock may lead to death. The majority of deaths in patients with acute pancreatitis result from irreversible shock.*

The *inflammatory stage* occurs when leukocytes cluster around the hemorrhagic and necrotic areas of the pancreas. A secondary bacterial process may lead to suppuration (pus formation) of the pancreatic parenchyma or the formation of an abscess. (See discussion of Pancreatic Abscess on p. 1226.) Mild infected lesions may be absorbed. When infected lesions are severe, calcification and fibrosis occur. If the infected fluid becomes walled off by fibrous tissue, a pancreatic pseudocyst is formed. (See discussion of Pancreatic Pseudocyst on p. 1226.)

Complications of Acute Pancreatitis

Acute pancreatitis may result in severe, life-threatening complications (Table 59-3). Jaundice occurs from swelling of the head of the pancreas, which slows bile flow through the common bile duct. The bile duct may also be compressed by calculi (stones) or a pancreatic pseudocyst. The resulting total bile flow obstruction causes severe jaundice. Intermittent hyperglycemia occurs from the release of glucagon, as well as the decreased release of insulin due to damage to the pancreatic islet cells. Total destruction of the pancreas may occur, leading to type 1 diabetes mellitus (McCance et al., 2014).

TABLE 59-3 Potential Complications of Acute Pancreatitis

- Pancreatic infection (causes septic shock)
- Hemorrhage (necrotizing hemorrhagic pancreatitis [NHP])
- Acute kidney failure
- Paralytic ileus
- Hypovolemic shock
- Pleural effusion
- Acute respiratory distress syndrome (ARDS)
- Atelectasis
- Pneumonia
- Multi-organ system failure
- Disseminated intravascular coagulation (DIC)
- Type 2 diabetes mellitus

Left lung pleural effusions frequently develop in the patient with acute pancreatitis. *Atelectasis and pneumonia may occur also, especially in older patients.*

Multi-system organ failure is caused by necrotizing hemorrhagic pancreatitis (NHP). The patient is at risk for acute respiratory distress syndrome (ARDS). This severe form of pulmonary edema is caused by disruption of the alveolar-capillary membrane and is a serious complication of acute pancreatitis. (See Chapter 32 for a discussion of ARDS.) In acute pancreatitis, pulmonary failure accounts for more than half of all deaths that occur in the first week of the disease.

Coagulation defects are another major potential complication and may result in death. Complex physiologic changes in the pancreas cause the release of necrotic tissue and enzymes into the bloodstream, resulting in altered coagulation. Disseminated intravascular coagulation (DIC) involves hypercoagulation of the blood, with consumption of clotting factors and the development of microthrombi.

Shock in acute pancreatitis results from peripheral vasodilation from the released vasoactive substances and the retroperitoneal loss of protein-rich fluid from proteolytic digestion. Hypovolemia may result in decreased renal perfusion and acute renal failure. Paralytic (adynamic) ileus results from peritoneal irritation and seepage of pancreatic enzymes into the abdominal cavity.

NCLEX EXAMINATION CHALLENGE

Physiological Integrity

The nurse closely monitors the client with acute pancreatitis for which complication?

A. Duodenal ulcer
B. Infection
C. Pneumonia
D. Heart failure

Etiology and Genetic Risk

In many cases the cause of pancreatitis is not known, but many factors can injure the pancreas. The most common cause is biliary tract disease, with gallstones accounting for almost half of the cases of obstructive pancreatitis (McCance et al., 2014). Acute pancreatitis may occur as a result of trauma from surgical manipulation after biliary tract, pancreatic, gastric, and duodenal procedures, such as cholecystectomy, the Whipple procedure, and partial gastrectomy. The trauma may also occur as a complication of the diagnostic procedure *endoscopic retrograde cholangiopancreatography (ERCP)*, although this rarely occurs.

Other causative factors include:

- Trauma: external (blunt trauma, stab wounds, gunshot wounds [GSWs])
- Pancreatic obstruction: tumors, cysts, or abscesses; abnormal organ structure
- Metabolic disturbances: hyperlipidemia, hyperparathyroidism, or hypercalcemia
- Renal disturbances: failure or transplantation
- Familial, inherited pancreatitis
- Penetrating gastric or duodenal ulcers, resulting in peritonitis
- Viral infections, such as coxsackievirus B and human immune deficiency virus [HIV] infection
- Alcoholism
- Toxicities of drugs, including opiates, sulfonamides, thiazides, steroids, and oral contraceptives (less common)
- Cigarette smoking
- Cystic fibrosis
- Gallstones
- Abdominal surgery

Incidence and Prevalence

Pancreatic "attacks" are especially common during holidays and vacations when alcohol consumption may be high, especially in men. Women are affected most often after cholelithiasis and biliary tract problems. They are also most at risk for pancreatitis within several months after childbirth.

Death occurs in a small percentage of patients with acute pancreatitis, but with early diagnosis and treatment, mortality can be reduced. It occurs at a higher rate in *older adults* and in patients with postoperative pancreatitis. The prognosis for recovery is usually good for pancreatitis associated with biliary tract disease and poor if pancreatitis accompanies alcoholism.

❖ PATIENT-CENTERED COLLABORATIVE CARE

◆ Assessment

History. Most often the patient reports severe and constant abdominal pain. Conduct the interview *after pain is controlled.* Ask whether the abdominal PAIN occurs when drinking alcohol or eating a high-fat meal. Obtain information about alcohol usage, including the amount of alcohol consumed during what period of time (i.e., years of consumption, how much usually consumed over a particular period). Question the patient about a family or personal history of alcoholism, pancreatitis, trauma, or biliary tract disease. Ask whether any abdominal surgical interventions, such as cholecystectomy, or diagnostic procedures, such as ERCP, have been performed recently.

Ask about other medical problems known to cause pancreatitis, including peptic ulcer disease, renal failure, vascular disorders, hyperparathyroidism, and hyperlipidemia. Inquire about recent viral infections. Ask the patient or family member to list all prescription and over-the-counter (OTC) drugs taken recently, including nutritional and herbal supplements.

Physical Assessment/Clinical Manifestations. The diagnosis of pancreatitis is made based on the clinical presentation combined with the results of diagnostic studies—both laboratory and imaging assessments. Clinical manifestations of acute pancreatitis vary widely and depend on the severity of the inflammation. Typically, a patient is diagnosed after presenting with severe abdominal PAIN in the mid-epigastric area or left upper quadrant. Assess the intensity and quality of pain. The patient often states that the pain had a sudden onset and radiates to the back, left flank, or left shoulder. The pain is described as intense, **boring** (feeling that it is going through the body), and continuous and is worsened by lying in the supine position. Often the patient finds relief by assuming the fetal position (with the knees drawn up to the chest and the spine flexed) or by sitting upright and bending forward. He or she may report weight loss resulting from nausea and vomiting. Obtain the patient's weight.

When performing an abdominal assessment, inspect for:

- Generalized jaundice
- Gray-blue discoloration of the abdomen and periumbilical area
- Gray-blue discoloration of the flanks, caused by pancreatic enzyme leakage to cutaneous tissue from the peritoneal cavity

Listen for bowel sounds; absent or decreased bowel sounds usually indicate paralytic (adynamic) ileus. On light palpation, note abdominal tenderness, rigidity, and guarding as a result of peritonitis. A palpable mass may be found if a pancreatic pseudocyst is present. Pancreatic ascites creates a dull sound on percussion.

Monitor and record vital signs frequently to assess for elevated temperature, tachycardia, and decreased blood pressure, or delegate and supervise this activity. Respiratory problems, such as left lung pleural effusions, atelectasis, and pneumonia, are common in patients with acute pancreatitis. Auscultate the lung fields for adventitious sounds or diminished breath sounds, and observe for dyspnea or orthopnea.

! NURSING SAFETY PRIORITY (QSEN)

Critical Rescue

For the patient with acute pancreatitis, monitor for significant changes in vital signs that may indicate the life-threatening complication of shock. Hypotension and tachycardia may result from pancreatic hemorrhage, excessive fluid volume shifting, or the toxic effects of abdominal sepsis from enzyme damage. Observe the patient for changes in behavior and level of consciousness (LOC) that may be related to alcohol withdrawal, hypoxia, or impending sepsis with shock.

Psychosocial Assessment. If excessive alcohol is a causative factor, tactfully explore the patient's alcohol intake history. Provide patient privacy, and establish a trusting relationship. Discuss the intake of alcohol and the reasons for overindulging. Using the CAGE questionnaire to assist with determining alcohol use may be beneficial. Ask him or her when increased drinking episodes occur and, in particular, whether binges occur during holidays, vacations, or weekends or revolve around particular activities, such as television viewing. Question the patient about any recent traumatic or stressful event that may have contributed to increased alcohol consumption, such as the death of a family member or a job loss.

Laboratory Assessment. Diagnostic laboratory abnormalities are typical in patients with acute pancreatitis (Table 59-4).

TABLE 59-4 Causes of Diagnostic Laboratory Abnormalities in Acute Pancreatitis

ABNORMAL FINDING	CAUSE
Cardinal Diagnostic Tests	
Increased *serum* amylase	Pancreatic cell injury
Elevated *serum* lipase	Pancreatic cell injury
Elevated *serum* trypsin	Pancreatic cell injury
Elevated *serum* elastase	Pancreatic cell injury
Other Diagnostic Tests	
Elevated serum glucose	Pancreatic cell injury, resulting in impaired carbohydrate metabolism; decreased insulin release
Decreased serum calcium and magnesium	Fatty acids combined with calcium; seen in fat necrosis
Elevated bilirubin	Hepatobiliary obstructive process
Elevated alanine aminotransferase (ALT)	Hepatobiliary involvement
Elevated aspartate aminotransferase (AST)	Hepatobiliary involvement
Elevated leukocyte count	Inflammatory response

A variety of pancreatic and non-pancreatic disorders can cause increased serum amylase levels. In patients with pancreatitis, *amylase* levels usually increase within 12 to 24 hours and remain elevated for 2 to 3 days. Persistent elevations may be an indicator of pancreatic abscess or pseudocyst (Pagana & Pagana, 2014).

Lipase also helps determine the presence of acute pancreatitis. Serum levels may rise later than amylase and remain elevated for up to 2 weeks. Because these levels stay elevated for such a long time, the health care provider may find this test useful in diagnosing patients who are not examined until several days after the initial onset of symptoms. An increase in lipase and amylase in the urine is also expected (Pagana & Pagana, 2014).

If pancreatitis is accompanied by biliary dysfunction (biliary pancreatitis), serum *bilirubin* and *alkaline phosphatase* levels are usually elevated. A sensitive indicator of biliary obstruction in acute pancreatitis is serum *alanine aminotransferase (ALT)*. A threefold or greater rise in concentration indicates that the diagnosis of acute biliary pancreatitis is valid. Elevated *white blood cell (WBC) count and differential, erythrocyte sedimentation rate (ESR),* and serum *glucose* levels are also common in acute pancreatitis. The levels often correlate with disease severity.

Decreased serum *calcium* and *magnesium* levels are seen with fat necrosis. Calcium levels may fall and remain decreased for 7 to 10 days. Those that consistently remain below 8 mg/dL are associated with a poor prognosis. Other tests include the basic metabolic panel (BMP), complete blood count (CBC), triglycerides, serum total protein, and albumin. The blood urea nitrogen (BUN), serum glucose, and triglycerides are usually elevated. Hemoconcentration is common as a result of third-space fluid loss. Leukocytosis (elevated WBCs) and thrombocytopenia (decreased platelets) are common (Pagana & Pagana, 2014). Albumin levels are decreased because cytokines (e.g., tumor necrosis factor [TNF]) released as part of the inflammatory response allow it to move from the bloodstream into the extravascular space. The presence of C-reactive protein suggests possible pancreatic INFLAMMATION and necrosis.

Imaging Assessment. Abdominal ultrasound is the most sensitive test to diagnose causes of pancreatitis, such as gallstones, and can be performed at the bedside. However, it is not helpful in viewing the pancreas because of overlying bowel gas. Therefore *contrast-enhanced computed tomography (CT)* provides a more reliable image and diagnosis of acute pancreatitis. This noninvasive technique may also be used to rule out pancreatic pseudocyst or ductal calculi.

An abdominal x-ray may also reveal gallstones. A chest x-ray may show elevation of the left side of the diaphragm or pleural effusion. Pancreatic stones are best diagnosed through ERCP.

◆ *Analysis*

The priority NANDA-I nursing diagnoses and collaborative problems for patients with acute pancreatitis include:

1. Acute Pain related to pancreatic inflammation and enzyme leakage (NANDA-I)
2. Inadequate nutrition related to the inability to ingest food and absorb nutrients

◆ *Planning and Implementation*

Managing Acute Pain

Planning: Expected Outcomes. The patient with acute pancreatitis is expected to state that he or she has a decrease in or absence of abdominal PAIN, as evidenced by a pain intensity scale measurement.

Interventions. The priorities for patient care are to provide supportive care by relieving symptoms, to decrease INFLAMMATION, and to anticipate or treat complications. *As for any patient, continually assess for and support the ABCs (airway, breathing, and circulation).* In collaboration with the respiratory therapist, if available, provide oxygen and other respiratory support as needed. The collaborative plan of care depends on the severity of the illness.

Abdominal pain is the most common symptom of pancreatitis. The main focus of nursing care is aimed at controlling PAIN by interventions that decrease GI tract activity, thus decreasing pancreatic stimulation. Pain assessment to measure the effectiveness of these interventions is an essential part of nursing care.

Nonsurgical Management. *Mild* pancreatitis requires hydration with IV fluids, pain control, and drug therapy. The health care team initially attempts to relieve pain with nonsurgical interventions, which include fasting and rest, drug therapy, and comfort measures. If the patient has a life-threatening complication or requires frequent assessment, he or she is admitted to a critical care unit for invasive hemodynamic monitoring.

To rest the pancreas and reduce pancreatic enzyme secretion, withhold food and fluids (NPO) during the acute period. The health care provider prescribes IV isotonic fluid administration to maintain hydration. IV replacement of calcium and magnesium may also be needed. Measure and document intake and output. Some patients have an indwelling urinary catheter to obtain accurate measurements.

Nasogastric drainage and suction are reserved for more *severely ill* patients who have continuous vomiting or biliary obstruction. Gastric decompression using a nasogastric tube (NGT) prevents gastric juices from flowing into the duodenum.

! NURSING SAFETY PRIORITY QSEN

Action Alert

Because paralytic (adynamic) ileus is a common complication of acute pancreatitis, prolonged nasogastric intubation may be necessary. Assess frequently for the return of peristalsis by asking the patient if he or she has passed flatus or had a stool. The return of bowel sounds is not reliable as an indicator of peristalsis return; passage of flatus or a bowel movement is the most reliable indicator. See the discussion of intestinal obstructions in Chapter 57 on p. 1157.

To decrease PAIN, the primary drug class used is opioid. Other drugs may also be prescribed. Pain management for acute pancreatitis typically begins with the administration of opioids by patient-controlled analgesia (PCA). Drugs such as morphine or hydromorphone (Dilaudid) are typically used because meperidine (Demerol) can cause seizures, especially in older adults. Other options that have been used successfully to manage acute pain include IV or transdermal fentanyl and epidural analgesia.

In *mild* pancreatitis, the pain usually subsides in 2 to 3 days. However, with *severe* acute pancreatitis, the abdominal pain and tenderness may persist for up to 2 weeks. The dosages and intervals of drug administration are individualized according to the severity of the disease and the symptoms.

Histamine receptor antagonists (e.g., ranitidine [Zantac]) and proton pump inhibitors (e.g., omeprazole [Prilosec]) help decrease gastric acid secretion. Antibiotics may be used, but they are indicated primarily for patients with acute necrotizing pancreatitis. The health care provider will prescribe appropriate antibiotics, if needed.

Helping the patient assume a side-lying position (with the legs drawn up to the chest) may decrease the abdominal PAIN of pancreatitis ("fetal position"). Sitting with the knees flexed toward the chest is also helpful.

If the patient is NPO or has an NGT, remind assistive nursing personnel to implement frequent oral and nares hygiene measures to keep mucous membranes moist and free of INFLAMMATION or crusting. Because of the drying effect of drugs and the absence of oral fluids, the mouth and oral cavity may be extremely dry, resulting in considerable discomfort and possibly parotitis (inflammation of the parotid [salivary] glands).

! NURSING SAFETY PRIORITY QSEN

Action Alert

For the patient with acute pancreatitis, monitor his or her respiratory status every 4 to 8 hours or more often as needed, and provide oxygen to promote comfort in breathing. Respiratory complications such as pleural effusions increase patient discomfort. Fluid overload can be detected by assessing for weight gain, listening for crackles, and observing for dyspnea. Carefully monitor for signs of respiratory failure.

Observe for signs and symptoms of hypocalcemia by assessing for Chvostek's and Trousseau's signs. These tests cause muscle spasms after stimulating the associated nerves. Chapter 11 discusses assessment and interventions for patients with hypocalcemia in more detail.

Lowering the patient's anxiety level may also substantially reduce pain. Explain all procedures and other aspects of patient care thoroughly. Provide reassurance, offer diversional activities such as music and reading material, and encourage visitors to direct attention away from the pain.

If pancreatitis was caused by gallstones, an ERCP with a **sphincterotomy** (opening of the sphincter of Oddi) may be performed on an urgent or emergent basis. If this procedure is not successful, surgery is required. ERCP is described in detail in Chapter 52.

Surgical Management. Surgical intervention for acute pancreatitis is usually not indicated. However, if an ERCP is not successful in removing gallstones, a laparoscopic cholecystectomy may be performed as described on p. 1217 in the discussion of Surgical Management in the Cholecystitis section.

Complications of pancreatitis, such as pancreatic pseudocyst and abscess, may also require surgical intervention. Laparoscopy (minimally invasive surgery [MIS]) may be done to drain an abscess or pseudocyst. For patients who are high surgical risks, pseudocysts or abscesses can be treated by percutaneous drainage under CT guidance.

Promoting Nutrition

Planning: Expected Outcomes. The patient with acute pancreatitis is expected to have adequate NUTRITION to meet his or her metabolic needs.

Interventions. The patient is maintained on NPO status in the early stages of pancreatitis. Antiemetics for nausea and vomiting are prescribed as needed. Patients who have severe pancreatitis and are unable to eat for 24 to 48 hours after illness onset may begin jejunal tube feeding unless paralytic ileus is present. *Early* NUTRITIONAL intervention enhances immune system functioning and may prevent complications and worsening inflammation. Enteral feeding is preferred over total parenteral nutrition (TPN) because it causes fewer episodes of glucose elevation and other complications associated with TPN. Be sure that the patient is weighed every day. Collaborate with the health care provider, dietitian, and pharmacist to plan and implement the most appropriate nutritional intervention. Chapter 60 describes collaborative care of patients receiving enteral feeding and TPN.

When food is tolerated during the healing phase, the health care provider prescribes small, frequent, moderate- to high-carbohydrate, high-protein, low-fat meals. Foods should be bland with little spice. GI stimulants such as caffeine-containing foods (tea, coffee, cola, and chocolate), as well as alcohol, should be avoided. Monitor the patient beginning to resume oral food intake for nausea, vomiting, and diarrhea. *If any of these symptoms occur, notify the health care provider immediately.*

To boost caloric intake, commercial liquid nutritional preparations supplement the diet. The health care provider may also prescribe fat-soluble and other vitamin and mineral replacement supplements. Glutamine, omega-3 fatty acids, fiber, antioxidants, and/or nucleotides may be added to the patient's nutrition plan.

Community-Based Care

Home care preparation is individualized for each patient's circumstances. Some patients may be severely weakened from their acute illness and need to confine activity to one floor, limiting stair climbing and other strenuous activities until they regain their strength. Collaborate with the case manager to plan the best place for the patient to recover and resources that may be needed.

Education needs to be started early in the hospitalization period—as soon as the acute episodes of pain have subsided. Assess the patient's and family's knowledge of the disease.

The desired outcomes for discharge planning and education are to avoid further episodes of pancreatitis and prevent progression to a chronic disease. If the patient uses alcohol, instruct him or her to abstain from drinking to prevent further pain attacks and extension of inflammation and pancreatic insufficiency. Tell the patient that if alcohol is consumed, acute PAIN will return and further autodigestion of the pancreas may lead to chronic pancreatitis.

Teach the patient to notify the health care provider after discharge to home if acute abdominal PAIN or biliary tract disease (as evidenced by jaundice, clay-colored stools, or darkened urine) occurs. These signs and symptoms are possible indicators of complications or disease progression.

Patients with acute pancreatitis may require several visits by a home care nurse if the hospital course was complicated. In these cases, home care may be needed for wound care and assistance with ADLs. The patient requires medical follow-up with the primary care physician or nurse practitioner to monitor the disease process. For those with alcoholism, provide information about groups such as Alcoholics Anonymous (AA). Family members may attend support groups such as Al-Anon and Alateen.

◆ *Evaluation: Outcomes*

Evaluate the care of the patient with acute pancreatitis based on the identified priority patient problems. The expected outcomes include that the patient will:

- Have control of abdominal PAIN, as indicated by self-report
- Have adequate NUTRITION available to meet metabolic needs

CLINICAL JUDGMENT CHALLENGE

Patient-Centered Care; Evidence-Based Practice; Teamwork and Collaboration; Informatics QSEN

A 78-year-old man is admitted from home to the medical unit with acute pancreatitis secondary to a history of gallstones, hypertension, osteoarthritis, and type 2 diabetes mellitus. He has lost 20 pounds (9 kg) in the past 2 months and reports severe boring-like abdominal pain, fatigue, and weakness. On physical assessment, he has decreased bowel sounds in all quadrants, crackles in the bases of his lungs, and signs of dehydration. Vital signs are: T, 100° F; P, 110; R, 36; and BP, 102/58.

What is the priority for this patient's care at this time? What current evidence supports your answer? Where would you look for current evidence that would help you answer this question? (Be specific in your answer.)

1. What laboratory findings would you expect him to have? Why?
2. With whom should you collaborate to meet the desired outcomes for his care?
3. What community support and health teaching is he going to require when he is discharged?

CHRONIC PANCREATITIS

❖ PATHOPHYSIOLOGY

Chronic pancreatitis is a progressive, destructive disease of the pancreas that has remissions and exacerbations ("flare-ups"). INFLAMMATION and fibrosis of the tissue contribute to pancreatic insufficiency and diminished function of the organ.

Chronic pancreatitis can be classified into several categories. *Alcoholism* is the primary risk factor for **chronic calcifying pancreatitis (CCP)**, the most common type. In the early stages of the disease, pancreatic secretions precipitate as insoluble proteins that plug the pancreatic ducts and flow of pancreatic juices. As the protein plugs become more widespread, the cellular lining of the ducts changes and ulcerates. This inflammatory process causes fibrosis of the pancreatic tissue. Intraductal calcification and marked pancreatic tissue destruction (necrosis) develop in the late stages. The organ becomes hard and firm as a result of cell atrophy and pancreatic insufficiency.

Chronic calcifying pancreatitis is found predominantly in men, but the incidence in women is increasing. In women, chronic pancreatitis occurs more commonly among those with biliary tract disease (cholecystitis and cholelithiasis).

Chronic obstructive pancreatitis develops from INFLAMMATION, spasm, and obstruction of the sphincter of Oddi, often from cholelithiasis (gallstones). Inflammatory and sclerotic lesions occur in the head of the pancreas and around the ducts, causing an obstruction and backflow of pancreatic secretions. (See Complications of Acute Pancreatitis, p. 1219.)

Autoimmune pancreatitis is a chronic inflammatory process in which immunoglobulins invade the pancreas. Other organs may also be infiltrated, including the lungs and liver. Whereas other types of chronic pancreatitis may predispose the patient to pancreatic cancer, there is no evidence that autoimmune pancreatitis is a risk factor (Novotny et al., 2010).

Idiopathic and **hereditary chronic pancreatitis** may be associated with *SPINK1* and *CFTR* gene mutations (Midha et al., 2010). The protein encoded by the *SPINK1* gene is a trypsin inhibitor. The *CFTR* gene is associated with cystic fibrosis. Research on these gene mutations can help develop targeted drug therapy for treatment of these diseases.

Pancreatic insufficiency in any type of chronic pancreatitis causes loss of *exocrine* function. Most patients with chronic pancreatitis have decreased pancreatic secretions and bicarbonate. Pancreatic enzyme secretion must be greatly reduced to produce steatorrhea resulting from severe malabsorption of fats. These characteristic stools are pale, bulky, and frothy and have an offensive odor. The action of colonic bacteria on unabsorbed lipids and proteins is responsible for the extremely foul odor. On inspection of the stools, the fat content is visible. In severe chronic pancreatitis, stool fat output may be more than 40 g/day.

Fat malabsorption also contributes to weight loss and muscle wasting (a decrease in muscle mass) and leads to general debilitation. Protein malabsorption results in a "starvation" edema of the feet, legs, and hands caused by decreased levels of circulating albumin.

The loss of pancreatic *endocrine* function is responsible for the development of diabetes mellitus in patients with chronic pancreatic insufficiency. (See Chapter 64 for a complete discussion of diabetes mellitus.)

The patient with chronic pancreatitis may have pulmonary complications, such as pleuritic pain, pleural effusions, and pulmonary infiltrates. Pancreatic ascites may decrease diaphragmatic excursion and lung expansion, resulting in impaired ventilation. In the ill patient with chronic pancreatitis, acute respiratory distress syndrome (ARDS) may develop.

❖ PATIENT-CENTERED COLLABORATIVE CARE

◆ Assessment

Many of the clinical manifestations of chronic pancreatitis differ from those of an acute INFLAMMATION. Abdominal PAIN is the major clinical manifestation for most types of pancreatitis (Chart 59-2). For those with chronic pancreatitis, pain is typically described as a continuous burning or gnawing dullness with periods of acute exacerbation (flare-ups). The pain is very intense and relentless. The frequency of acute exacerbations may increase as the pancreatic fibrosis develops.

CHART 59-2 Key Features

Chronic Pancreatitis

- Intense abdominal pain (major clinical manifestation) that is continuous and burning or gnawing
- Abdominal tenderness
- Ascites
- Possible left upper quadrant mass (if pseudocyst or abscess is present)
- Respiratory compromise manifested by adventitious or diminished breath sounds, dyspnea, or orthopnea
- Steatorrhea; clay-colored stools
- Weight loss
- Jaundice
- Dark urine
- Polyuria, polydipsia, polyphagia (diabetes mellitus)

Perform an abdominal assessment. Abdominal tenderness is less intense in patients with chronic pancreatitis than in those with acute pancreatitis. A mass may be palpated in the left upper quadrant, which may suggest a pancreatic pseudocyst or abscess. Massive pancreatic ascites may be present, producing dullness on abdominal percussion. Because respiratory complications can occur, auscultate the lung fields for adventitious sounds or decreased aeration and observe for dyspnea or orthopnea.

Ask the patient to collect a random stool specimen if able, or ask him or her to describe the stools. The specimen may show **steatorrhea** (foul-smelling fatty stools that may increase in volume as pancreatic insufficiency progresses and lipase production decreases). Assess for unintentional weight loss, muscle wasting, jaundice, dark urine, and the manifestations of diabetes mellitus, such as polyuria (increased urinary output), polydipsia (excessive thirst), and polyphagia (increased appetite).

Diagnosis is based on the patient's clinical manifestations and laboratory and imaging assessment. *Endoscopic retrograde cholangiopancreatography* (ERCP) is done to visualize the pancreatic and common bile ducts. *Imaging studies* such as CT scanning, contrast-enhanced MRI, abdominal ultrasound (US), and endoscopic ultrasound (EUS) are also useful in making the diagnosis. In chronic pancreatitis, laboratory findings include normal or moderately elevated serum *amylase* and *lipase* levels. Obstruction of the intrahepatic bile duct can cause elevated serum *bilirubin* and *alkaline phosphatase* levels. Intermittent elevations in serum *glucose* levels are common and can be detected by blood glucose monitoring, both fasting and non-fasting.

◆ Interventions

The focus of caring for the patient with chronic pancreatitis is to manage PAIN, assist in maintaining sufficient NUTRITION, and prevent recurrence.

Nonsurgical Management. Nonsurgical interventions include primarily drug and NUTRITION therapy. The major intervention for the PAIN of chronic pancreatitis is drug therapy. Medicate the patient as prescribed according to the assessment of the intensity of pain. Evaluate the effectiveness of the drug intervention. Opioid analgesia is most frequently used initially, but dependency may occur. Non-opioid analgesics may be tried to relieve pain. (See Chapter 3 for other interventions for chronic pain.)

Pancreatic-enzyme replacement therapy (PERT) is the standard of care to prevent malnutrition, malabsorption, and excessive weight loss (Chart 59-3). Pancrelipase is usually prescribed in capsule or tablet form and contains varying amounts of amylase, lipase, and protease. Teach patients not to chew or crush pancrelipase delayed-release capsules (Creon) or enteric tablets, and teach them to take the medications with all meals and snacks.

The dosage of pancreatic enzymes depends on the severity of the malabsorption. Record the number and consistency of stools per day to monitor the effectiveness of enzyme therapy. If pancreatic enzyme treatment is effective, the stools should become less frequent and less fatty.

CHART 59-3 Patient and Family Education: Preparing for Self-Management

Enzyme Replacement for the Patient with Chronic Pancreatitis

- Take pancreatic enzymes with meals and snacks and follow with a glass of water.
- Administer enzymes after antacid or H_2 blockers. (Decreased pH inactivates drug.)
- Swallow the tablets or capsules without chewing to minimize oral irritation and to allow the drug to be released slowly.
- If you cannot swallow the capsule, pierce the gelatin casing and place contents in applesauce.
- Do not mix enzyme preparations in protein-containing foods.
- Wipe your lips after taking enzymes to avoid skin irritation.
- Do not crush enteric-coated preparations.
- Follow up on all scheduled laboratory testing. (Pancrelipase can cause an increase in uric acid levels.)

! NURSING SAFETY PRIORITY QSEN

Action Alert

If the patient has diabetes, the health care provider prescribes insulin or oral hypoglycemic agents for glucose control. Patients maintained on total parenteral nutrition (TPN) are particularly susceptible to elevated glucose levels and usually require regular insulin additives to the solution. Closely monitor blood glucose so that hyperglycemia is controlled. Check finger-stick blood glucose (FSBG) or sugar (FSBS) levels every 2 to 4 hours. Chapter 60 describes in detail the care associated with TPN.

The health care provider may also prescribe drug therapy to decrease gastric acid. Gastric acid destroys the lipase needed to break down fats. Controlling the acidity of the stomach with H_2 blockers or proton pump inhibitors or neutralizing stomach acid with oral sodium bicarbonate may enhance the effectiveness of PERT.

Protein and fat malabsorption result in significant weight loss and decreased muscle mass in the patient with chronic pancreatitis. Therefore the nutritional interventions for acute pancreatitis are also used for chronic pancreatitis. The patient often limits food intake to avoid increased pain. For this reason, nutrition maintenance is often difficult to achieve. Patients receive either total parenteral nutrition (TPN) or total enteral nutrition (TEN), including vitamin and mineral replacement.

Collaborate with the dietitian to teach the patient about long-term dietary management. He or she needs an increased number of calories, up to 4000 to 6000 calories/day, to maintain weight. Those foods high in carbohydrates and protein also assist in the healing process. Foods high in fat are avoided because they cause or increase diarrhea. Teach all patients to avoid alcohol. Alcohol-cessation programs may be recommended.

Surgical Management. Surgery is not a primary intervention for the treatment of chronic pancreatitis. However, it may be indicated for ongoing abdominal PAIN, incapacitating relapses of pain, or complications such as abscesses and pseudocysts.

The underlying pathologic changes determine the procedure indicated. Using laparoscopy, the surgeon incises and drains an abscess or pseudocyst. Laparoscopic cholecystectomy or choledochotomy (incision of the common bile duct) may be indicated if biliary tract disease is an underlying cause of pancreatitis. If the pancreatic duct sphincter is fibrotic, the surgeon performs a sphincterotomy (incision of the sphincter) to enlarge it. Endoscopic sphincterotomy may be used for patients who are poor surgical candidates.

In some cases laparoscopic distal pancreatectomy may be appropriate for resection of the distal pancreas or pancreas head. Endoscopic pancreatic necrosectomy and natural orifice transluminal endoscopic surgery (NOTES) are becoming more common for removing necrosed pancreatic tissue. Both procedures are performed through the GI wall without a visible skin incision. The NOTES procedure is discussed in Surgical Management on p. 1217 in the Cholecystitis section.

In a few cases, pancreas transplantation may be done. However, this procedure is performed most often for patients with severe, uncontrolled diabetes. Chapter 64 discusses pancreas transplantation.

CHART 59-4 Patient and Family Education: Preparing for Self-Management

Prevention of Exacerbations of Chronic Pancreatitis

- Avoid things that make your symptoms worse, such as drinking caffeinated beverages.
- Avoid alcohol ingestion; refer to self-help group for assistance.
- Avoid nicotine.
- Eat bland, low-fat, high-protein, and moderate-carbohydrate meals; avoid gastric stimulants, such as spices.
- Eat small meals and snacks high in calories.
- Take the pancreatic enzymes that have been prescribed for you with meals.
- Rest frequently; restrict your activity to one floor until you regain your strength.

Community-Based Care

Collaborate with the hospital-based case manager (CM) or discharge planner about home care or follow-up in another setting. A community-based CM may continue to follow the patient after hospital discharge. If the patient is discharged to home, the living area should be limited to one floor until he or she regains strength and can increase activity. Teach patients and families that toilet facilities must be easily accessible because of chronic steatorrhea and frequent defecation. If they are not easily accessible, a bedside commode is obtained for the home.

Because there is no known cure for chronic pancreatitis, patient and family education is aimed at preventing acute episodes of the disease, providing long-term care, and promoting health maintenance (Chart 59-4). Teach the patient to avoid known irritating substances, such as caffeinated beverages (stimulates the GI system) and alcohol. Collaborate with the dietitian in diet teaching, which focuses on eating bland, low-fat, frequent meals and avoiding rich, fatty foods. Stress the importance of adhering to the nutritional recommendations. Written instructions are essential, with consideration of personal and cultural food preferences.

Remind the patient and family members or significant others of the importance of adhering to pancreatic enzyme replacement. The patient must take the prescribed enzymes with meals and snacks to aid in the digestion of food and promote the absorption of fats and proteins. Teach the patient to take the enzymes before or at the beginning of the meal. Instruct him or her to report any increase in abdominal distention, cramping, and foul-smelling, frothy, fatty stools to the health care provider so that these supplements may be increased as needed. Remind the patient to report any skin breakdown so that therapeutic interventions to promote skin integrity can be started. Abdominal fistulas are common and present a difficult challenge because pancreatic secretions irritate the skin.

The frequency of defecation (whether continent or incontinent) poses challenging skin care problems. Instruct the patient to keep the skin dry and free of the abrasive fatty stools, which damage the skin. The skin should be cleaned thoroughly after each stool and a moisture barrier applied to prevent breakdown and maintain skin integrity. Many products on the market actively repel stool from the skin.

If the patient develops diabetes mellitus as a result of chronic pancreatitis, management of elevated glucose levels after discharge from the hospital may require oral antidiabetic agents or insulin injections. If this is the case, collaborate with the certified diabetic educator (CDE) to provide in-depth teaching concerning diabetes, its signs and symptoms, medical management, drug therapy, nutrition therapy, blood glucose monitoring, and general care.

Chronic illnesses are devastating for families. The high costs of medical insurance, medical treatment, and drug therapy cause serious financial problems. Often the patient with chronic pancreatitis is unable to work. Collaborate with the CM about ways to assist the patient with resources for financial help.

The patient may require several home visits by nurses, depending on the severity of the chronic health problems and home maintenance and support needs. The nurse assesses the patient for PAIN, enzyme therapy, and psychosocial adaptation to a chronic illness. Refer him or her and the family to a counselor or a self-help group, such as Alcoholics Anonymous (www.aa.org) and Al-Anon (www.al-anon.org), if appropriate.

NCLEX EXAMINATION CHALLENGE

Physiological Integrity

Which foods will the nurse teach the client with chronic pancreatitis to avoid? **Select all that apply.**

A. Blueberries
B. Green beans
C. Bacon
D. Baked fish
E. Fried potatoes

PANCREATIC ABSCESS

Pancreatic abscesses are the most serious complication of acute necrotizing pancreatitis. If untreated, they are always fatal. After surgery, the recurrence rate is high. The abscesses form from collections of purulent liquefaction of the necrotic pancreas.

Patients with pancreatic abscesses often appear more seriously ill than those with pseudocysts. Clinical manifestations are similar. However, the temperature in patients with abscesses may spike to as high as 104° F (40° C). Drainage via the percutaneous method or laparoscopy should be performed as soon as possible to prevent sepsis. Antibiotic treatment alone does not resolve the abscess. Death rates remain high even after surgical drainage. Many patients require multiple drainage procedures for repeated abscesses.

PANCREATIC PSEUDOCYST

❖ PATHOPHYSIOLOGY

Pancreatic pseudocysts, or false cysts, are so named because, unlike true cysts, they do not have an epithelial lining. They are encapsulated, saclike structures that form on or surround the pancreas. The pseudocyst wall is inflamed, vascular, and fibrotic. It may contain up to several liters of straw-colored or dark brown viscous fluid, the enzymatic exudate of the pancreas (McCance et al., 2014). Risk factors for pseudocysts are acute pancreatitis, abdominal trauma, and chronic pancreatitis.

❖ PATIENT-CENTERED COLLABORATIVE CARE

◆ Assessment

A pseudocyst can be palpated as an epigastric mass in about half of all cases. The primary presenting symptom is epigastric pain radiating to the back. Other common clinical manifestations include abdominal fullness, nausea, vomiting, and jaundice. Pseudocysts are diagnosed and their growth and resolution monitored by serial pancreatic diagnostic testing. Complications of pseudocyst formation include:

- Hemorrhage
- Infection
- Obstruction of the bowel, biliary tract, or splenic vein
- Abscess
- Fistula formation
- Pancreatic ascites

◆ Interventions

Pseudocysts may spontaneously resolve, or they may rupture and produce hemorrhage. Surgical intervention is necessary if the pseudocyst does not resolve within 6 to 8 weeks or if complications develop. To provide external drainage, the surgeon inserts a sump drainage tube to remove pancreatic secretions and exudate. Pancreatic fistulas are common after surgery, and skin breakdown from corrosive pancreatic enzymes in patients who have external drainage presents a major nursing care challenge.

PANCREATIC CANCER

❖ PATHOPHYSIOLOGY

Cancer of the pancreas is a leading cause of cancer deaths each year in the United States. It is difficult to diagnose early because the pancreas is hidden and surrounded by other organs. Treatment has limited results, and 5-year survival rates are low (American Cancer Society [ACS], 2013).

Pancreatic tumors usually originate from epithelial cells of the pancreatic ductal system. If the tumor is discovered in the early stages, the tumor cells may be localized within the glandular organ. However, this is highly unlikely. Most often, the tumor is discovered in the late stages of development and may be a well-defined mass or is diffusely spread throughout the pancreas.

The tumor may be a primary cancer, or it may result from metastasis from cancers of the lung, breast, thyroid, kidney, or skin. Primary tumors are generally adenocarcinomas and grow in well-differentiated glandular patterns. They grow rapidly and spread to surrounding organs (stomach, duodenum, gallbladder, and intestine) by direct extension and invasion of lymphatic and vascular systems. This highly metastatic lesion may eventually invade the lung, peritoneum, liver, spleen, and lymph nodes.

Clinical manifestations depend on the site of origin or metastasis. The head of the pancreas is the most common site. The tumors are usually small lesions with poorly defined margins. Jaundice results from tumor compression and obstruction of the common bile duct and from gallbladder dilation, causing the organ to enlarge.

Cancers of the body and tail of the pancreas are usually large and invade the entire tail and body. These tumors may be palpable abdominal masses, especially in the thin patient. Through metastatic spread via the splenic vein, metastasis to the liver may cause **hepatomegaly** (enlargement of the liver up to 2 to 3 times its normal size). Cancers of the body and tail spread more extensively than do pancreatic head carcinomas, with invasion of the retroperitoneum, vertebral column, spleen, adrenal glands, colon, or stomach. Regardless of where it originates, it spreads rapidly through the lymphatic and venous systems to other organs.

Venous thromboembolism is a common complication of pancreatic cancer. Necrotic products of the pancreatic tumor are believed to have thromboplastic properties resulting in the blood's hypercoagulable state. In addition, the patient is at high risk because of decreased mobility and extensive surgical manipulation.

The exact cause of pancreatic cancer is unknown. High-risk populations are those in their sixth to eighth decades of life and those with a personal history of smoking.

GENETIC/GENOMIC CONSIDERATIONS

Patient-Centered Care QSEN

A small number of those with pancreatic cancer have an inherited risk. Mutations in certain oncogenes have been identified. Mutations have also been revealed in tumor suppressor genes, such as *p16* and *BRCA2*—the same mutation that makes some women susceptible to breast and ovarian cancer. Genes responsible for hereditary nonpolyposis colorectal cancer can also increase a person's risk for pancreatic cancer (ACS, 2013).

Other risk factors associated with the disease include:

- Diabetes mellitus
- Chronic pancreatitis
- Cirrhosis
- High intake of red meat, especially processed meat like steak
- Long-term exposure to chemicals such as gasoline and pesticides
- Obesity
- Older age
- Male gender
- Cigarette smoking
- Family history
- Genetic syndromes

CHART 59-5 Key Features

Pancreatic Cancer

- Jaundice
- Clay-colored (light) stools
- Dark urine
- Abdominal pain: usually vague, dull, or nonspecific that radiates into the back
- Weight loss
- Anorexia
- Nausea or vomiting
- Glucose intolerance
- Splenomegaly (enlarged spleen)
- Flatulence
- Gastrointestinal bleeding
- Ascites (abdominal fluid)
- Leg or calf pain (from thrombophlebitis)
- Weakness and fatigue

❖ PATIENT-CENTERED COLLABORATIVE CARE

◆ Assessment

Pancreatic cancer often presents in a slow and vague manner. The presenting symptoms depend somewhat on the location of the tumor. The first sign may be jaundice, which suggests late, advanced disease (Chart 59-5). Jaundice occurs because the gallbladder and liver are commonly involved. As the tumor spreads, the yellow skin color associated with obstructive jaundice progressively worsens. Ask the patient whether the color of the stool and urine has changed. As a result of the obstructive process, the stool is clay colored and the urine is dark and frothy. Inspect the skin for dryness and scratch marks, indicating pruritus from jaundice caused by bile salt collection. Assess the sclera for icterus (yellowing) and the mucous membranes for signs of jaundice.

The enlarged gallbladder and liver may be palpable. In advanced cases of pancreatic carcinoma, the tumor may be felt as a firm, fixed mass in the left upper abdominal quadrant or epigastric region.

The most common concern is fatigue, which is described as a diminished energy level and an increased need for rest relative to the level of activity. The patient notices an inability to perform usual physical or intellectual activities.

Question the patient about abdominal PAIN, which is usually described as a vague, constant dullness in the upper abdomen and nonspecific in nature. Pain also indicates advanced stages of the disease and may be related to eating or activity. Ask whether the patient has pain in other areas of the body. Referred back pain may be caused by pressure on the nerve plexus. Some patients have leg or calf pain with swelling and redness as a result of deep vein thrombosis or thrombophlebitis.

Weigh the patient to determine the extent of weight loss and whether it has occurred rapidly. Ask about food intake and intolerances. Anorexia accompanied by early satiety, nausea, flatulence (gas), and vomiting is common. GI bleeding may develop from esophageal or gastric varices caused by the tumor pressing on the portal vein. A new diagnosis of diabetes is found in some patients.

In addition to the focused history, perform a general abdominal assessment. In particular, observe for distention and swelling, which may be **ascites** (abdominal fluid). Percussion over the ascitic abdomen elicits dullness, seen in the advanced stages of the disease process.

No specific blood tests diagnose pancreatic cancer. Serum *amylase* and *lipase* levels, as well as *alkaline phosphatase* and *bilirubin* levels, are increased. The degree of elevation depends on the acuteness or chronicity of the pancreatic and biliary damage. Elevated *carcinoembryonic antigen* (CEA) levels occur in most patients with pancreatic cancer. This test may provide early information about the presence of tumor cells. Other tumor markers such as CA 19-9 and CA 242 have been found to be useful serologic tests for monitoring a proven diagnosis and for continuing surveillance for potential spread or recurrence (Pagana & Pagana, 2014).

Abdominal *ultrasound* and *contrast-enhanced CT* are the most commonly used imaging techniques for confirming a tumor and can differentiate the tumor from a cyst. Endoscopic ultrasonography can also be performed to sample tissue for diagnosis and provide information on tumor type and size (Tonolini et al., 2012). Contrast harmonic echo-endoscopic ultrasound increases the accuracy of diagnosing solid pancreatic masses (Fusaroli et al., 2010).

Endoscopic retrograde cholangiopancreatography (ERCP) also provides visual diagnostic data. An alternative to ERCP is a percutaneous transhepatic biliary cholangiogram with placement of a percutaneous transhepatic biliary drain (PTBD). This drain decompresses the blocked biliary system by draining bile, either internally, externally, or both. Aspiration of pancreatic ascitic fluid by abdominal paracentesis may reveal cancer cells and elevated amylase levels.

◆ Interventions

Management of the patient with pancreatic cancer is geared toward preventing tumor spread and decreasing pain. These measures are not curative, only palliative. The cancers are often metastatic and recur despite treatment.

Nonsurgical Management. As in other types of cancer, chemotherapy or radiation is used to relieve pain by shrinking the tumor. It may be used before, after, or instead of surgery. *Chemotherapy* has had limited success in increasing survival time. In most cases, combining agents has been more successful than single-agent chemotherapy. 5-Fluorouracil (5-FU), a commonly used drug, may be given alone or with gemcitabine (Gemzar) for locally advanced, or unresectable, pancreatic cancers. Gemcitabine may also be given with capecitabine (Xeloda), docetaxel (Taxotere), and/or erlotinib (Tarceva), a targeted agent for unresectable or metastatic tumors. Some patients receive three or four drugs and have had more tumor shrinkage as a result. Observe for adverse drug effects, such as fatigue, rash, anorexia, and diarrhea. Chapter 22 discusses nursing implications of chemotherapy in more detail.

Other targeted therapies being investigated include growth factor inhibitors, anti-angiogenesis factors, and kinase inhibitors (also known as *tyrosine kinase inhibitors*). Kinase inhibitors are a newer group of drugs that focus on cancer cells with little or no effect on healthy cells. Chapter 22 describes general nursing interventions associated with chemotherapy.

To control pain, the patient takes high doses of opioid analgesics (usually morphine) as prescribed and uses other comfort measures before the pain escalates and peaks. Because of the poor prognosis, drug dependency is not a consideration. Chapter 3 describes in detail the care of the patient with chronic cancer PAIN.

Intensive external beam *radiation* therapy to the pancreas may offer pain relief by shrinking tumor cells, alleviating obstruction, and improving food absorption. It does not improve survival rates. Implantation of radioactive iodine (^{125}I) seeds, in combination with systemic or intra-arterial administration of floxuridine (FUDR), has also been used. The patient may experience discomfort during and after the radiation treatments. Chapter 22 describes radiation therapy in more detail.

For patients experiencing biliary obstruction who are high surgical risks, **biliary stents** placed percutaneously (through the skin) can ensure patency to relieve pain. These stents are devices made of plastic materials that keep the ducts of the biliary system open. Using another approach, self-expandable stents may be inserted endoscopically to relieve obstruction.

Surgical Management. Complete surgical resection of the pancreatic tumor offers the patient with pancreatic cancer the only effective treatment, but it is done only in patients with small tumors. *Partial pancreatectomy* is the preferred surgery for tumors smaller than 3 centimeters in diameter (Grützmann et al., 2011). Recent technologic advances have expanded the role of **minimally invasive surgery (MIS)** via laparoscopy in the staging, palliation, and removal of pancreatic cancers. The procedure selected depends on the purpose of the surgery and stage of the disease. For example, if the patient has a biliary obstruction, a laparoscopic procedure to relieve the obstruction is performed. This procedure diverts bile drainage into the jejunum.

For larger tumors, the surgeon may perform either a *radical pancreatectomy* or the *Whipple procedure (pancreaticoduodenectomy)*. These procedures have traditionally been done using an open surgical approach. Because of new advances in laparoscopic technology using a hand-assist device, this method is beginning to replace the conventional method. Some surgeons are not yet trained in how to perform this technique. Therefore the traditional open surgical approach remains the most common method of performing these surgeries.

Preoperative Care. The patient with pancreatic cancer may be a poor surgical risk because of malnutrition and debilitation. Specific care depends on the type of surgical approach being used.

Often, in the late stages of pancreatic cancer or before the Whipple procedure, the physician inserts a small catheter into the jejunum (**jejunostomy**) so that enteral feedings may be given. This feeding method is preferred to prevent reflux and to facilitate absorption. Feedings are started in low concentrations and volumes and are gradually increased as tolerated. Provide feedings using a pump to maintain a constant volume, and assess for diarrhea frequency to determine tolerance. Chapter 60 provides additional information about enteral feeding.

For optimal NUTRITION, TPN may be necessary in addition to tube feedings or as a single measure to provide nutrition. When central venous access is required, a peripherally inserted central catheter (PICC) or other type of IV catheter may be necessary. Meticulous IV line care is an important nursing measure to prevent catheter sepsis. Sterile dressing changes and site observation are extremely important. Additional nursing care measures for the patient receiving TPN are given in Chapter 60. Monitor nutrition indicators such as serum prealbumin and albumin.

For the laparoscopic procedure, no bowel preparation is needed. However, either approach requires that the patient have nothing by mouth (NPO) for at least 6 to 8 hours before surgery.

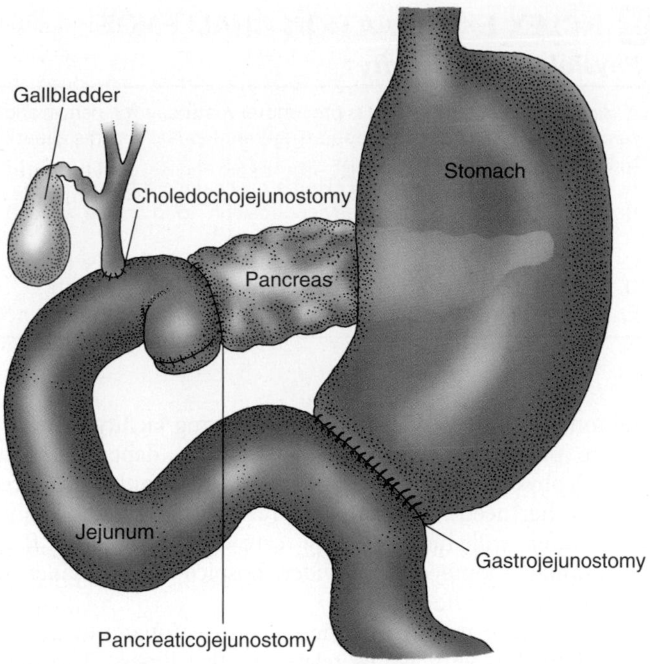

FIG. 59-3 The three anastomoses that constitute the Whipple procedure: choledochojejunostomy, pancreaticojejunostomy, and gastrojejunostomy.

Surgeon preference and agency policy determine the preferred protocol for preoperative preparation.

Operative Procedures. The **Whipple procedure (radical pancreaticoduodenectomy)** involves extensive surgical manipulation and is used most often to treat cancer of the head of the pancreas. The procedure entails removal of the proximal head of the pancreas, the duodenum, a portion of the jejunum, the stomach (partial or total **gastrectomy**), and the gallbladder, with anastomosis of the pancreatic duct (**pancreaticojejunostomy**), the common bile duct (**choledochojejunostomy**), and the stomach (**gastrojejunostomy**) to the jejunum (Fig. 59-3). In addition, the surgeon may remove the spleen (**splenectomy**).

Postoperative Care. In addition to routine postoperative care measures, the patient who has undergone an open radical pancreaticoduodenectomy requires intensive nursing care and is usually admitted to a surgical critical care unit. Observe for multiple potential complications of the open Whipple procedure as listed in Table 59-5.

The patient's primary benefits of MIS are a shorter postoperative recovery and less pain than with traditional open procedures. The patient having the laparoscopic Whipple surgery or radical pancreatectomy is also less at risk for severe complications. For patients having one of these procedures, observe for and implement preventive measures for these surgical complications:

- Diabetes (Check blood glucose often.)
- Hemorrhage (Monitor pulse, blood pressure, skin color, and mental status [e.g., LOC].)
- Wound infection (Monitor temperature, and assess wounds for redness and induration [hardness].)
- Bowel obstruction (Check bowel sounds and stools.)
- Intra-abdominal abscess (Monitor temperature and patient's report of severe pain.)

Immediately after surgery the patient is NPO and usually has a nasogastric tube (NGT) to decompress the stomach. Monitor GI drainage and tube patency. In open surgical approaches, biliary drainage tubes are placed during surgery to remove drainage and secretions from the area and to prevent stress on the anastomosis sites. Assess the tubes and drainage devices for tension or kinking, and maintain them in a dependent position.

TABLE 59-5 Potential Complications of the Whipple Procedure

Cardiovascular Complications • Hemorrhage at anastomosis sites with hypovolemia • Myocardial infarction • Heart failure • Thrombophlebitis **Pulmonary Complications** • Atelectasis • Pneumonia • Pulmonary embolism • Acute respiratory distress syndrome • Pulmonary edema **Metabolic Complications** • Unstable diabetes mellitus • Renal failure	**Gastrointestinal Complications** • Adynamic (paralytic) ileus • Gastric retention • Gastric ulceration • Bowel obstruction from peritonitis • Acute pancreatitis • Hepatic failure • Thrombosis to mesentery **Wound Complications** • Infection • Dehiscence • Fistulas: pancreatic, gastric, and biliary

Monitor the drainage for color, consistency, and amount. The drainage should be serosanguineous. The appearance of clear, colorless, bile-tinged drainage or frank blood with an increase in output may indicate disruption or leakage of an anastomosis site. Most of the disruptions of the site occur within 7 to 10 days after surgery. Hemorrhage can occur as an early or late complication.

Place the patient in the semi-Fowler's position to reduce tension on the suture line and anastomosis site as well as to optimize lung expansion. Stress can be decreased by maintaining NGT drainage at a low or high intermittent suction level to keep the remaining stomach (if a partial gastrectomy is done) or the jejunum (if a total gastrectomy is done) free of excessive fluid buildup and pressure. The NGT also reduces stimulation of the remaining pancreatic tissue.

The development of a fistula (an abnormal passageway) is the most common and most serious postoperative complication. Biliary, pancreatic, or gastric fistulas result from partial or total breakdown of an anastomosis site. The secretions that drain from the fistula contain bile, pancreatic enzymes, or gastric secretions, depending on which site is ruptured. *These secretions, particularly pancreatic fluid, are corrosive and irritating to the skin, and internal leakage causes chemical peritonitis.* **Peritonitis** (inflammation and infection of the peritoneum causing boardlike abdominal rigidity) requires treatment with multiple antibiotics. *If you suspect any postoperative complications resulting from MIS or open surgical approaches, call the surgeon immediately and provide assessment findings that support your concerns.*

Because the *open* Whipple procedure is extensive and can take many hours to complete, maintaining fluid and electrolyte balance can be difficult. Patients often have significant intraoperative blood loss and postoperative bleeding. The intestine is exposed to air for long periods, and fluid evaporates. Significant losses of fluid and electrolytes occur from the NGT and other drainage tubes. In addition, these patients may be malnourished and have low serum levels of protein and albumin, which maintain colloid osmotic pressure within the circulating system. Reduction in the serum osmotic pressure makes the patient likely to develop third spacing of body fluids, with fluid moving from the vascular to the interstitial space, resulting in shock. These problems are less likely to occur when MIS is used. Therefore, when possible, the trained surgeon prefers to perform laparoscopic Whipple procedures to shorten operating time and prevent the many complications that can occur.

NURSING SAFETY PRIORITY QSEN

Action Alert

To detect early signs of hypovolemia and prevent shock, closely monitor vital signs for decreased blood pressure and increased heart rate, decreased vascular pressures with a pulmonary artery catheter (Swan-Ganz catheter) (in ICU setting), and decreased urine output. Be alert for pitting edema of the extremities, dependent edema in the sacrum and back, and an intake that far exceeds output. Maintain sequential compression devices to prevent deep vein thrombosis.

Maintenance of prescribed IV isotonic fluid replacement with colloid replacements is important. Monitor hemoglobin and hematocrit values to assess for blood loss and the need for blood transfusions. Review electrolyte values for decreased serum levels of sodium, potassium, chloride, and calcium. IV fluid concentrations must be altered to correct these electrolyte imbalances. The physician prescribes replacement of electrolytes as needed.

Immediately after the Whipple procedure, the patient may have hyperglycemia or hypoglycemia as a result of stress and surgical manipulation of the pancreas. Most of the endocrine cells (responsible for insulin and glucagon secretion) are located in the body and tail of the pancreas. In some patients, up to half of the gland remains and diabetes does not develop. However, a large number of patients are diabetic before surgery. For patients having a radical pancreatectomy, administer insulin as prescribed because the entire pancreas is removed. Monitor glucose levels frequently during the early postoperative period, and administer insulin injections as prescribed.

Community-Based Care

The patient with pancreatic cancer is usually followed by a case manager (CM), both in the hospital and in the home or other community-based setting. Collaborate with the CM to ensure that the patient receives cost-effective treatment and that his or her needs are met.

Home Care Management. The stage of progression of pancreatic cancer and available home care resources determine whether the patient can be discharged to home or whether additional care is needed in a skilled nursing facility or with a hospice provider. Home care preparations depend on the patient's physical and activity limitations and should be tailored to his or her needs. Coordinate care with the patient, family, or whoever will be providing care after discharge from the hospital—home care provider, hospice care provider, or extended-care provider.

NCLEX EXAMINATION CHALLENGE

Physiological Integrity

A client had an open Whipple procedure yesterday for pancreatic cancer. Which nursing interventions are appropriate for this client? **Select all that apply.**

A. Monitor and document the client's nasogastric tube drainage.
B. Place the client in a side-lying position to promote wound drainage.
C. Assess the abdomen for signs of peritonitis.
D. Monitor the client's hemoglobin and hematocrit.
E. Check the client's blood glucose frequently.

The patient and family need compassionate emotional support to deal with issues related to this illness. The diagnosis of pancreatic cancer can frighten and overwhelm the patient and family. Assist family members in looking realistically and objectively at the amount of physical care required. Tell family members that their own physical and emotional health are at risk during this stressful period and that supportive counseling may be needed. If the family does not have a religious affiliation or a spiritual leader (e.g., a minister or a rabbi) to provide support, suggest alternative counseling options. Refer patients and families to the certified hospital chaplain if desired. It is appropriate for the nurse to make the initial contact or appointment according to the patient's or family's wishes.

Self-Management Education. When the patient is discharged to home, many interventions are palliative and aimed at managing symptoms such as pain. In many cases the diagnosis of pancreatic cancer is made a few months before death occurs. The patient needs time to adjust to the diagnosis, which is usually made too late for cure or prolonged survival. Help the patient identify what needs to be done to prepare for death, including end-of-life care. For example, he or she may want to write a will or see family members and friends whom he or she has not seen recently. The patient needs to make known to family members or others his or her specific requests for the funeral or memorial service. These actions help prepare for death in a dignified manner. Chapter 7 discusses in detail anticipatory grieving and preparation for death, as well as symptom management during the end of life.

Health Care Resources. Regular home care nursing and assistive nursing personnel visits may be scheduled to assist the patient and family by providing physical, psychological, and supportive care. Supply information about local palliative and hospice care (see Chapter 7) and cancer support groups.

NURSING CONCEPTS AND CLINICAL JUDGMENT REVIEW

What might you NOTICE if the patient is experiencing inadequate digestion and NUTRITION as a result of gallbladder and pancreatic disorders?

- Report of intense abdominal pain
- Report of nausea, especially after food
- Report of anorexia
- Vomiting
- Jaundice
- Report of weight loss
- Dark urine
- Clay-colored stools

What should you INTERPRET and how should you RESPOND to a patient experiencing inadequate digestion and NUTRITION as a result of gallbladder and pancreatic disorders?

Perform and interpret physical assessment, including:

- Taking vital signs to assess for hypovolemia and fever
- Assessing respiratory status, including breath sounds
- Conducting a complete pain assessment if possible
- Weighing the patient
- Checking laboratory values, especially enzyme levels like amylase and lipase, liver function studies, and CBC
- Assessing vomitus for quality and amount

Respond by:

- Keeping the patient's head of the bed elevated and knees flexed
- Providing pain management by comfort measures and analgesia
- Providing oxygen if the patient is having dyspnea or adventitious breath sounds
- Reassuring the patient who may be concerned about possible cancer

On what should you REFLECT?

- Observe the patient for improvement in signs and symptoms, including pain control.
- Think about what could have caused the health problem.
- Think about what else you could do to help the patient meet desired outcomes.
- Plan health teaching for patient discharge.

GET READY FOR THE NCLEX® EXAMINATION!

KEY POINTS

Review these Key Points for each NCLEX Examination Client Needs Category.

Safe and Effective Care Environment

- Collaborate with the dietitian, pharmacist, health care provider, and case manager when planning care for patients with pancreatic cancer. **Teamwork and Collaboration** QSEN
- Refer patients with end-stage pancreatic cancer for palliative and hospice care.
- Refer patients with pancreatitis who use excessive alcohol to community resources such as Alcoholics Anonymous. **Patient-Centered Care** QSEN

Health Promotion and Maintenance

- Recognize that obese, middle-aged women are most likely to have gallbladder disease. **Patient-Centered Care** QSEN
- Teach patients to avoid losing weight too quickly and to keep weight under control to help prevent gallbladder disease. **Evidence-Based Practice** QSEN
- Teach patients to avoid excessive alcohol consumption to help prevent alcohol-induced acute pancreatitis.
- Instruct patients about ways to prevent exacerbations of chronic pancreatitis as outlined in Chart 59-4.

Psychosocial Integrity

- Refer patients with pancreatic cancer for support services such as spiritual leaders and counselors for coping strategies and facilitation of the grieving process.
- Help prepare the pancreatic cancer patient and family for the death and dying process.

Physiological Integrity

- Be aware that autodigestion of the pancreas causes severe PAIN in patients with acute pancreatitis (see Fig. 59-2).
- Monitor serum laboratory values, especially amylase and lipase (both elevated), in patients with pancreatitis (see Table 59-4).
- Assess for common clinical manifestations of cholecystitis as listed in Chart 59-1.
- For patients with acute pancreatitis, provide PAIN management including opioid analgesia. **Patient-Centered Care** QSEN
- Recognize that acute PAIN relief is the first priority for patients with acute pancreatitis. **Evidence-Based Practice** QSEN
- Be aware that patients with biliary and pancreatic disorders are at high risk for biliary obstruction, a serious and painful complication.
- Assess for common clinical manifestations of chronic pancreatitis as listed in Chart 59-2.
- Document health teaching about enzyme replacement therapy as described in Chart 59-3. **Informatics** QSEN
- Assess patients with presenting clinical manifestations of pancreatic cancer as described in Chart 59-5.
- Observe for and implement interventions to prevent life-threatening complications of the Whipple procedure as outlined in Table 59-5. **Safety** QSEN

60 CHAPTER

Care of Patients with Malnutrition: Undernutrition and Obesity

Cherie R. Rebar, Nicole Heimgartner, Laura Willis

http://evolve.elsevier.com/Iggy/

PRIORITY CONCEPTS

- NUTRITION
- FLUID AND ELECTROLYTE BALANCE

LEARNING OUTCOMES

Safe and Effective Care Environment

1. Collaborate with the health care team members when providing care for patients with malnutrition or obesity.
2. Protect bariatric patients from injury.
3. Select appropriate activities to delegate to unlicensed assistive personnel to promote a patient's NUTRITION.

Health Promotion and Maintenance

4. Provide care that meets the special nutrition needs of older adults.
5. Recall the *2010 Dietary Guidelines for Americans* recommendations.
6. Teach overweight and obese patients the importance of lifestyle changes to promote health.
7. Perform a nutrition screening for all patients to determine if they are at high risk for NUTRITION health problems.

Psychosocial Integrity

8. Assess patient responses to being obese.
9. Explain how to reduce the psychological impact for the patient who is having bariatric surgery.

Physiological Integrity

10. Interpret findings of a nutrition screening and assessment.
11. Calculate body mass index (BMI), and interpret findings.
12. Describe the risk factors for malnutrition, especially for older adults.
13. Explain why serum visceral protein levels indicate change in NUTRITION status.
14. Identify the role of supplements in restoring or maintaining nutrition.
15. Explain how to prevent complications of total parenteral nutrition (TPN).
16. Explain how to maintain enteral tube patency.
17. Describe evidence-based practices to prevent aspiration for patients with nasoenteric tubes.
18. Explain the medical complications associated with obesity.
19. Identify the role of drug therapy in the management of obesity.
20. Prioritize nursing care for patients having bariatric surgery.
21. Develop a discharge teaching plan for patients having bariatric surgery.

Carbohydrates, protein, and fat are nutrients in food that supply the body with energy. In healthy people, most of this energy undergoes digestion and is absorbed from the GI tract. Food energy is used to maintain body temperature, respiration, cardiac output, muscle function, protein synthesis, and the storage and metabolism of food sources. Therefore proper NUTRITION plays a major role in promoting and maintaining health.

Energy balance refers to the relationship between energy used and energy stored. Weight loss occurs when energy used is more than intake. If food intake is more than energy used, weight is gained. Body proteins are used for energy when calorie intake is insufficient. The body attempts to meet its calorie requirements even if it is at the expense of protein needs.

NUTRITION STANDARDS FOR HEALTH PROMOTION AND MAINTENANCE

The role of NUTRITION in disease has been a subject of interest for many years. The current focus is on health promotion and the prevention of disease by healthy eating and exercise. The Institute of Medicine of The National Academies (2014) has developed the **Dietary Reference Intakes (DRIs)** to serve as a nutrition guide that provides a scientific basis for food guidelines in the United States and Canada. Age, gender, and life stage influence the nutrient reference values of more than 40 nutrient substances (The Institute of Medicine of The National Academies, 2014). In the United States, the **Dietary Guidelines for Americans** are revised by the U.S. Department of Agriculture

(USDA) and the U.S. Department of Health and Human Services (DHHS) every 5 years. The 2010 guidelines emphasize the need to include preferences of specific racial/ethnic groups, vegetarians, and other populations when selecting foods to maintain a healthful diet that is balanced with moderation and variety. If alcohol is consumed, it should be limited to one drink per day for women and two drinks for men (U.S. Department of Agriculture [USDA], 2010). Examples of other guidelines are listed in Table 60-1.

To remind people about healthy eating habits, the USDA designed "MyPlate," a picture to demonstrate that half of each meal should consist of fruits and vegetables (Fig. 60-1). When grains are consumed, half of them should be whole grains rather than refined grain products.

Some people follow vegetarian diet patterns for health, environmental, or moral reasons. In general, vegetarians are leaner than those who consume meat. The **lacto-vegetarian** eats milk, cheese, and dairy foods but avoids meat, fish, poultry, and eggs. The **lacto-ovo-vegetarian** includes eggs in his or her diet. The **vegan** eats only foods of plant origin. Some people among these groups eat fish as well. Vegans can develop anemia as a result of vitamin B_{12} deficiency. Therefore they should include a daily source of vitamin B_{12} in their diets, such as a fortified breakfast cereal, fortified soy beverage, or meat substitute. All vegetarians should ensure that they get adequate amounts of calcium, iron, zinc, and vitamins D and B_{12}. Well-planned vegetarian diets can provide adequate NUTRITION. The Academy of Nutrition and Dietetics (2013) publishes a number of credible resources regarding vegetarian health at www.eatright.org.

TABLE 60-1 Examples of *2010 Dietary Guidelines for Americans*

- Control total calorie intake to manage body weight.
- Consume less than 300 mg per day of dietary cholesterol.
- Increase intake of fat-free or low-fat milk and milk products, such as milk, yogurt, cheese, or fortified soy products.
- Choose a variety of protein foods, which include seafood, lean meat and poultry, eggs, beans and peas, soy products, and unsalted nuts and seeds.
- Reduce the intake of calories from solid fats and added sugars.
- Reduce daily sodium intake to less than 2300 mg and further reduce intake to 1500 mg among persons who are 51 years of age or older and those of any age who are African American or have hypertension, diabetes, or chronic kidney disease.
- Limit the consumption of foods that contain refined grains, especially refined grains that contain solid fats, added sugars, and sodium.
- Increase vegetable and fruit intake.

Source: *Dietary Guidelines for Americans Council.* (2014). Retrieved September 2014, from http://www.fns.usda.gov/dietary-guidelines-americans-2010

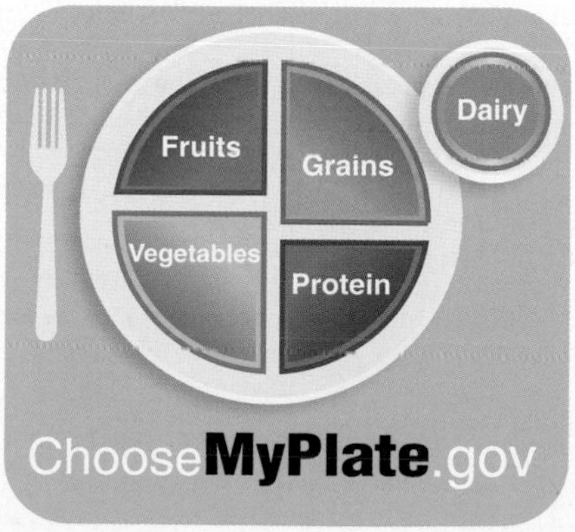

FIG. 60-1 The U.S. Department of Agriculture MyPlate.

CULTURAL CONSIDERATIONS

***Patient-Centered Care* QSEN**

Many people have specific food preferences based on their ethnicity or race. For example, for people of Hispanic descent, tortillas, beans, and rice *may* be desired over pasta, risotto, and potatoes. *Never assume that a person's racial or ethnic background means that he or she eats only foods associated with his or her primary ethnicity.* Health teaching about nutrition should incorporate any cultural preferences.

Some people have food allergies or intolerances. For instance, lactose intolerance (lactose is found in milk and milk products) is a common problem that occurs in a number of ethnic groups. It is found more often in Mexican Americans and black people as well as in some American Indian groups, Asian Americans, and Ashkenazi Jews. A small percentage of white people, particularly those of Mediterranean descent (e.g., Greek, Italian), are also lactose intolerant. The cause of **lactose intolerance** is an inadequate amount of the lactase enzyme, which converts lactose into absorbable glucose. Patients may benefit from learning more about the management of lactose intolerance from resources provided by organizations such as the American Dietetic Association or the Dieticians of Canada.

CONSIDERATIONS FOR OLDER ADULTS

***Patient-Centered Care* QSEN**

The USDA recommends that older adults drink eight glasses of water a day and eat plenty of fiber to prevent or manage constipation. It also suggests daily calcium and vitamins D and B_{12} supplements and a reduction in sodium and cholesterol-containing foods.

One of the most recent publications from Health Canada on Nutrition is the Canada Food Guide. Compared with previous documents, it includes more culturally diverse foods, information on *trans* fats, customized individual recommendations, and exercise guidelines. Several booklets can be purchased to help people select the best foods and nutrients from the new guide, such as *Eating Well with Canada's Food Guide* (Minister of Health Canada, 2011). In addition, Canada has published a separate booklet to address the special needs of some of its indigenous people. The *Eating Well with Canada's Food Guide—First Nations, Inuit, and Métis* includes berries, wild plants, and wild game to reflect the values and traditions for aboriginal people living in Canada (Health Canada, 2011).

NUTRITION ASSESSMENT

Nutrition status reflects the balance between nutrient requirements and intake. Common factors that affect these requirements include age, gender, disease, infection, and psychological stress. Eating behavior, economic implications, emotional stability, disease, drug therapy, and cultural factors influence nutrient intake. Malnutrition (also called *undernutrition*) and obesity, discussed later in this chapter, are common nutrition health problems that may lead to many comorbidities and complications, including death.

Evaluation of nutrition status is an important part of total patient assessment and includes:

- Review of the nutrition history
- Food and fluid intake record
- Laboratory data
- Food-drug interactions
- Health history and physical assessment
- Anthropometric measurements
- Psychosocial assessment

Monitor the NUTRITION status of a patient during hospitalization as an important part of your initial assessment. Collaborate with the interdisciplinary health care team to identify patients at risk for nutrition problems.

Initial Nutrition Screening

An initial screening provides an inexpensive, quick way of determining which patients need more extensive nutrition assessment by the health care team. The Joint Commission Patient Care Standards require that a nutrition screening occur within 24 hours of the patient's hospital admission. If indicated, an in-depth nutrition assessment should be performed. When patients are in the hospital for more than a week, nutrition assessment should be part of the daily plan of care.

The initial **nutrition screening** includes inspection, measured height and weight, weight history, usual eating habits, ability to chew and swallow, and any recent changes in appetite or food intake. Examples of questions that help identify patients at risk for nutrition problems are part of the history and physical assessment (Chart 60-1).

The Mini Nutritional Assessment (MNA), a two-part tool that has been tested worldwide, provides a reliable, rapid assessment for patients in the community and in any health care setting. The *first* part (A-F) is a screening section that takes 3 minutes to complete and asks about food intake, mobility, and body mass index (BMI) (described on p. 1235). It also screens for weight loss, acute illness, and psychological health problems. If the patient scores 11 points or less, the *second* part (G-R) of the MNA is completed, for an additional 12 questions. The entire assessment takes only minutes to complete (Fig. 60-2). The MNA Short Form can be used as a stand-alone tool to evaluate whether the older patient is well nourished, at risk for malnutrition, or malnourished. The alternative is to take the patient's calf circumference, which can be a reliable alternative if BMI is unavailable.

Anthropometric Measurements

Anthropometric measurements are noninvasive methods of evaluating NUTRITION status. These measurements include height and weight and assessment of body mass index (BMI).

Obtain a current *height and weight* to provide a baseline. Be sure to obtain accurate measurements because patients tend to overestimate height and underestimate weight. Measurements taken days or weeks later may indicate an early change in nutrition status. *You may delegate this activity to unlicensed assistive personnel (UAP) under your supervision.*

Patients should be measured and weighed while wearing minimal clothing and no shoes. Determine the height in inches or centimeters using the measuring stick of a weight scale if the

CHART 60-1 Best Practice for Patient Safety & Quality Care QSEN

Nutrition Screening Assessment

General

- Does the patient have any conditions that cause nutrient loss, such as malabsorption syndromes, draining abscesses, wounds, fistulas, or prolonged diarrhea?
- Does the patient have any conditions that increase the need for nutrients, such as fever, burns, injury, sepsis, or antineoplastic therapies?
- Has the patient been NPO for 3 days or more?
- Is the patient receiving a modified diet or a diet restricted in one or more nutrients?
- Is the patient being enterally or parenterally fed?
- Does the patient describe food allergies, lactose intolerance, or limited food preferences?
- Has the patient experienced a recent unexplained weight loss?
- Is the patient on drug therapy—either prescription, over-the-counter, or herbal/natural products?

Gastrointestinal

- Does the patient report nausea, indigestion, vomiting, diarrhea, or constipation?
- Does the patient exhibit glossitis (tongue inflammation), stomatitis (oral inflammation), or esophagitis?
- Does the patient have difficulty chewing or swallowing?
- Does the patient have a partial or total GI obstruction?
- What is the patient's state of dentition?

Cardiovascular

- Does the patient have ascites or edema?
- Is the patient able to perform ADLs?
- Does the patient have heart failure?

Genitourinary

- Is fluid intake about equal to fluid output?
- Does the patient have an ostomy?
- Is the patient hemodialyzed or peritoneally dialyzed?

Respiratory

- Is the patient receiving mechanical ventilatory support?
- Is the patient receiving oxygen via nasal prongs?
- Does the patient have chronic obstructive pulmonary disease (COPD) or asthma?

Integumentary

- Does the patient have abnormal nail or hair changes?
- Does the patient have rashes or dermatitis?
- Does the patient have dry or pale mucous membranes or decreased skin turgor?
- Does the patient have pressure areas on the sacrum, hips, heels, or ankles?

Extremities

- Does the patient have pedal edema?
- Does the patient have cachexia?

Modified with courtesy of Ross Products Division, Abbott Laboratories, Columbus, OH.

Nestlé NutritionInstitute

Mini Nutritional Assessment MNA®

Last name: First name:

Sex: Age: Weight, kg: Height, cm: Date:

Complete the screen by filling in the boxes with the appropriate numbers. Add the numbers for the screen. If score is 11 or less, continue with the assessment to gain a Malnutrition Indicator Score.

Screening

A Has food intake declined over the past 3 months due to loss of appetite, digestive problems, chewing or swallowing difficulties?
0 = severe decrease in food intake
1 = moderate decrease in food intake
2 = no decrease in food intake ☐

B Weight loss during the last 3 months
0 = weight loss greater than 3 kg (6.6lbs)
1 = does not know
2 = weight loss between 1 and 3kg (2.2 and 6.6lbs)
3 = no weight loss ☐

C Mobility
0 = bed or chair bound
1 = able to get out of bed/chair but does not go out
2 = goes out ☐

D Has suffered psychological stress or acute disease in the past 3 months
0 = yes 2 = no ☐

E Neuropsychological problems
0 = severe dementia or depression
1 = mild dementia
2 = no psychological problems ☐

F Body Mass Index (BMI) (weight in kg) / height in m^2)
0 = BMI less than 19
1 = BMI 19 to less than 21
2 = BMI 21 to less than 23
3 = BMI 23 or greater ☐

Screening score
(subtotal max. 14 points) ☐☐

12-14 points:	Normal nutritional status
8-11 points:	At risk of malnutrition
0-7 points:	Malnourished

For a more in-depth assessment, continue with questions G-R

Assessment

G Lives independently (not in nursing home or hospital)
1 = yes 0 = no ☐

H Takes more than 3 prescription drugs per day
0 = yes 1 = no ☐

I Pressure sores or skin ulcers
0 = yes 1 = no ☐

Ref. 1. Vellas B, Villars H, Abellan G, *et al.* Overview of MNA® - Its History and Challenges. *J Nut Health Aging.* 2006; **10**:**456**-465.
2. Rubenstein LZ, Harker JO, Salva A, Guigoz Y, Vellas B. Screening for Undernutrition in Geriatric Practice: Developing the Short-Form Mini Nutritional Assessment (MNA-SF). *J. Geront.* 2001; **56A**: M366-377
3. Guigoz Y. The Mini-Nutritional Assessment (MNA®) Review of the Literature – What does it tell us? *J Nutr Health Aging.* 2006; **10**: 466-487.

J How many full meals does the patient eat daily?
0 = 1 meal
1 = 2 meals
2 = 3 meals ☐

K Selected consumption markers for protein intake
- At least one serving of dairy products (milk, cheese, yoghurt) per day yes ☐ no ☐
- Two or more servings of legumes or eggs per week yes ☐ no ☐
- Meat, fish or poultry every day yes ☐ no ☐

0.0 = if 0 or 1 yes
0.5 = if 2 yes
1.0 = if 3 yes ☐.☐

L Consumes two or more servings of fruit or vegetables per day?
0 = no 1 = yes ☐

M How much fluid (water, juice, coffee, tea, milk...) is consumed per day?
0.0 = less than 3 cups
0.5 = 3 to 5 cups
1.0 = more than 5 cups ☐.☐

N Mode of feeding
0 = unable to eat without assistance
1 = self-fed with some difficulty
3 = self-fed without any problem ☐

O Self view of nutritional status
0 = views self as being malnourished
1 = is uncertain of nutritional state
2 = views self as having no nutritional problem ☐

P In comparison with other people of the same age, how does the patient consider his/her health status?
0.0 = not as good
0.5 = does not know
1.0 = as good
2.0 = better ☐.☐

Q Mid-arm circumference (MAC) in cm
0.0 = MAC less than 21
0.5 = MAC 21 to 22
1.0 = MAC 22 or greater ☐.☐

R Calf circumference (CC) in cm
0 = CC less than 31
1 = CC 31 or greater ☐

Assessment (max. 16 points) ☐☐.☐

Screening score ☐☐.☐

Total Assessment (max. 30 points) ☐☐.☐

Malnutrition Indicator Score

24 to 30 points	☐	Normal nutritional status
17 to 23.5 points	☐	At risk of malnutrition

FIG. 60-2 The Mini Nutritional Assessment (MNA).

patient can stand. He or she should stand erect and look straight ahead, with the heels together and the arms at the sides. For patients who cannot stand or those who cannot stand erect (e.g., some older adults), use a sliding-blade **knee height caliper**, if available. This device uses the distance between the patient's patella and heel to estimate height. It is especially useful for patients who have knee or hip contractures.

Remind UAP to weigh ambulatory patients with an upright balance-beam or digital scale. Non-ambulatory patients can be weighed with a digital wheelchair or bed scale.

! NURSING SAFETY PRIORITY QSEN

Action Alert

For daily or sequential weights, obtain the weight at the same time each day, if possible, preferably before breakfast. Conditions such as congestive heart failure and renal disease cause weight gain; dehydration and conditions such as cancer cause weight loss. *Weight is the most reliable indicator of fluid gain or loss, so accurate weights are essential!*

Normal weights for adult men and women are available from several reference standards, such as the Metropolitan Life tables. Some health care professionals prefer these tables because they consider body-build differences by gender and body frame size.

Changes in body weight can be expressed by three different formulas:

Weight as a percentage of ideal body weight (IBW):

$$\%IBW = \frac{\text{Current weight}}{\text{Ideal body weight}} \times 100$$

Current weight as a percentage of usual body weight (UBW):

$$\%UBW = \frac{\text{Current weight}}{\text{Usual body weight}} \times 100$$

Change in weight:

$$\text{Weight change} = \frac{\text{Usual weight} - \text{Current weight}}{\text{Usual weight}} \times 100$$

An unintentional weight loss of 10% over a 6-month period at any time significantly affects nutrition status and should be evaluated. Depending on the patient's needs, weights may need to be taken daily, several times a week, or weekly for monitoring status and the effectiveness of nutrition support.

In the health care setting, *assessment of body fat* is usually calculated by the dietitian. For people who participate in a structured exercise program in the community, this assessment is typically performed by a fitness trainer or physical therapist.

The **body mass index (BMI)** is a measure of nutrition status that does not depend on frame size (Centers for Disease Control and Prevention [CDC], 2012). It indirectly estimates total fat stores within the body by the relationship of weight to height. *Therefore an accurate height is as important as an accurate weight.*

A simple calculation for estimating BMI can be programmed into handheld computers or calculators using one of these two formulas:

$$BMI = \frac{\text{Weight (lb)}}{\text{Height (in inches)}^2} \times 703$$

$$BMI = \frac{\text{Weight (kg)}}{\text{Height (in meters)}^2}$$

BMI can also be determined using a table that is linked with height and weight. The least risk for malnutrition is associated with scores between 18.5 and 25. BMIs above and below these values are associated with increased health risks (CDC, 2012a).

CONSIDERATIONS FOR OLDER ADULTS

Patient-Centered Care QSEN

Body weight and BMI usually increase throughout adulthood until about 60 years of age. As people get older, they often become less hungry and eat less, even if they are healthy. Ideally, older adults should have a BMI between 23 and 27.

The average daily energy intake expended by this group tends to be more than the average energy intake. This physiologic change has been called the "anorexia of aging" (Champion, 2011). Many older adults are underweight, leading to undernutrition and increased risk for illness.

NCLEX EXAMINATION CHALLENGE

Health Promotion and Maintenance

An older adult is admitted to the hospital with pressure ulcers and septicemia. His height is 5 feet, 8 inches (1.72 meters), and he weighs 302 pounds (137 kg). His current body mass index (BMI) is _______. (Round your answer to the nearest tenth.)

Skinfold measurements estimate body fat and can be measured by either the nurse or the dietitian. The *triceps and subscapular* skinfolds are most commonly measured using a special caliper. Both are compared with standard measurements and recorded as percentiles.

The *midarm circumference (MAC) and calf circumference (CC)* can be obtained to measure muscle mass and subcutaneous fat. These measurements are needed if the Mini Nutritional Assessment tool is used. To measure MAC, place a flexible tape around the upper arm at the midpoint, taking care to hold the tape firmly but gently to avoid compressing the tissue. This measurement is usually recorded in centimeters. The midarm muscle mass (MAMM) measures the amount of muscle in the body and is a sensitive indicator of protein reserves. It can be computed from the MAC and the triceps skinfold measure. The CC is obtained using a similar procedure on the calf.

MALNUTRITION

❖ PATHOPHYSIOLOGY

Protein-energy malnutrition (PEM), also known as **protein-calorie malnutrition (PCM)**, may present in three forms: marasmus, kwashiorkor, and marasmic-kwashiorkor. **Marasmus** is generally a calorie malnutrition in which body fat and protein are wasted. Serum proteins are often preserved. **Kwashiorkor** is a lack of protein quantity and quality in the presence of adequate calories. Body weight is more normal, and serum proteins are low. **Marasmic-kwashiorkor** is a combined protein and energy malnutrition. This problem often presents clinically when metabolic stress is imposed on a chronically starved patient. The outcome of unrecognized or untreated PEM is often dysfunction or disability and increased morbidity and mortality.

Malnutrition (also called *undernutrition)* is a multinutrient problem because foods that are good sources of calories and protein are also good sources of other nutrients. In the malnourished patient, protein catabolism exceeds protein intake and synthesis, resulting in negative nitrogen balance, weight loss, decreased muscle mass, and weakness.

The functions of the liver, heart, lungs, GI tract, and immune system decrease in the patient with malnutrition. A decrease in serum proteins (**hypoproteinemia**) occurs as protein synthesis in the liver decreases. Vital capacity is also reduced as a result of respiratory muscle atrophy. Cardiac output diminishes. Malabsorption occurs because of atrophy of GI mucosa and the loss of intestinal villi.

Common complications of *severe* malnutrition in adults include:

- Leanness and **cachexia** (muscle wasting with prolonged malnutrition)
- Decreased activity tolerance
- Lethargy
- Intolerance to cold
- Edema
- Dry, flaking skin and various types of dermatitis
- Poor wound healing
- Infection, particularly postoperative infection and sepsis
- Possible death

Malnutrition results from inadequate nutrient intake, increased nutrient losses, and increased nutrient requirements. Inadequate nutrient intake can be linked to poverty, lack of education, substance abuse, decreased appetite, and a decline in functional ability to eat independently, particularly in older adults. Infectious diseases, such as tuberculosis and human immune deficiency virus (HIV) infection, can also cause PEM. Diseases that produce diarrhea and infections leading to anorexia result in negative calorie and protein balance. Anorexia then leads to poor food intake. Vomiting causes decreased intestinal absorption with increased nutrient losses. Medical treatments such as chemotherapy can also cause malnutrition. In addition, catabolic processes, such as that caused by prolonged immobility, increase nutrient requirements and metabolic losses.

Inadequate nutrient intake can result also when a person is admitted to the hospital or long-term care facility. For example, decreased staffing may not allow time for patients who need to be fed, especially older adults, who may eat slowly. Many diagnostic tests, surgery, trauma, and unexpected medical complications require a period of NPO or cause **anorexia** (loss of appetite). In a systematic integrative review, Tappenden et al. (2013) reviewed strategies needed to address the needs of hospitalized patients to prevent or treat malnutrition (see the Evidence-Based Practice box).

CULTURAL CONSIDERATIONS

Patient-Centered Care QSEN

In some cases, malnutrition results when the provided meals are different from what the patient usually eats. Be sure to identify specific food preferences that the patient can eat and enjoy that are in keeping with his or her cultural practices.

CONSIDERATIONS FOR OLDER ADULTS

Patient-Centered Care QSEN

Older adults in the community or in any health care setting are most at risk for poor nutrition, especially PEM. Risk factors include physiologic changes of aging, environmental factors, and health problems. Chart 60-2 lists some of these major factors. Chapter 2 discusses nutrition for older adults in more detail.

EVIDENCE-BASED PRACTICE QSEN

The Critical Role of Nutrition in Improving Quality of Care

Tappenden, K.A., Quatrara, B., Parkhurst, M.L., Malone, A.M., Fanjiang, G., & Ziegler, T.R. (2013). Critical role of nutrition in improving quality of care: An interdisciplinary call to action to address adult hospital malnutrition. *MEDSURG Nursing, 22*(3), 147-165.

Health care costs have increased tremendously in the United States over the past decades. With substantial changes coming in health care policy that affect the way that health care is delivered, health care facilities will need to continue searching for ways to deliver the best care at the most reasonable cost. At least one third of patients come to the hospital in a state of malnourishment, and others become malnourished after admission. Therefore ways for addressing adult hospital malnutrition are very important for both quality of care and cost containment.

The Alliance to Advance Patient Nutrition (Alliance) reflects combined efforts of the Academy of Medical-Surgical Nurses (AMSN), the Academy of Nutrition and Dietetics (AND), the American Society for Parenteral and Enteral Nutrition (ASPEN), the Society of Hospital Medicine (SHM), and Abbott Nutrition to help achieve positive patient outcomes and support improving patient nutrition. The Alliance recommends a number of strategies for meeting these outcomes, such as:

- Include nutrition as a component of all health care team member conversations and in conversation with patients and family members.
- Provide thorough explanations about the patient's nutrition status, nutrition recommendations, nutrition interventions, and post-discharge nutrition care; document these interventions in the electronic health record.
- Ensure that the patient and/or family member is given comprehensive follow-up nutrition assessment, education, and follow-up appointment recommendations at the time of discharge.
- Provide comprehensive, clear, standardized written instructions for nutrition care at home.
- Prioritize nutrition as part of self-management education, taking into consideration dietary intake, weight change, access to food, and other concerns that may affect nutrition status.

Level of Evidence: 1

The clinical evidence presented was collected and presented as a result of a systematic integrative review conducted by numerous professional health care organizations.

Commentary: Implications for Practice and Research

Quality of care, cost implications, and recovery are of primary concern for all patients who are malnourished. Collaborative efforts among the health care team members can (1) provide a more consistent and reliable approach to addressing nutrition needs for hospitalized patients, (2) avoid overlapping charges that may arise from a lack of communication, and (3) create a best practice approach for teaching the patient and family about meeting nutrition needs at the time of discharge. Nurses who work directly with patients are in a key position to provide consistent, comprehensive nutrition education; this can result in better meeting the nutrition needs of patients who are hospitalized, as well as prepare them better for self-management upon discharge.

CHART 60-2 Nursing Focus on the Older Adult

Risk Assessment for Malnutrition

Assess for:
- Decreased appetite
- Weight loss
- Poor-fitting or no dentures/poor dental health
- Poor eyesight
- Dry mouth
- Limited income
- Lack of transportation
- Inability to prepare meals because of functional decline or fatigue
- Loneliness and/or depression
- Chronic constipation (e.g., in patients with Alzheimer's disease)
- Decreased meal enjoyment
- Chronic physical illness
- "Failure to thrive" (a combination of three of five symptoms, including weakness, slow walking speed, low physical activity, unintentional weight loss, exhaustion)
- Prescription and over-the-counter (OTC) drugs (including herbs, vitamins, and minerals)
- Acute or chronic pain

Acute PEM may develop in patients who were adequately nourished before hospitalization but experience starvation while in a catabolic state from infection, stress, or injury. *Chronic* PEM can occur in those who have cancer, end-stage kidney or liver disease, or chronic neurologic disease.

Eating disorders such as anorexia nervosa and bulimia nervosa, which are seen most often in teens and young adults, also lead to malnutrition. **Anorexia nervosa** is a self-induced starvation resulting from a fear of fatness, even though the patient is underweight. **Bulimia nervosa** is characterized by episodes of binge eating in which the patient ingests a large amount of food in a short time. The binge eating is followed by some form of purging behavior, such as self-induced vomiting or excessive use of laxatives and diuretics. If not treated, death can result from starvation, infection, or suicide. Information about eating disorders can be found in textbooks on mental/behavioral health nursing.

❖ PATIENT-CENTERED COLLABORATIVE CARE

◆ Assessment

History. Review the medical history to determine the possibility of increased metabolic needs or NUTRITION losses, chronic disease, trauma, recent surgery of the GI tract, drug and alcohol use, and recent significant weight loss. Each of these conditions can contribute to malnutrition. For older adults, explore mental status changes and note poor eyesight, diseases affecting major organs, constipation or incontinence, and slowed reactions. Review prescription and over-the-counter (OTC) drugs, including vitamin, mineral, herbal, and other nutrition supplements.

For patients who live independently in the community, the nurse may assess their performance of instrumental activities of daily living (IADLs). Functional status can best be evaluated for institutionalized patients by assessing their ADL performance. Poor NUTRITION is a major contributing factor to decreased functional ability.

In collaboration with the dietitian, obtain information about the patient's usual daily food intake, eating behaviors, change in appetite, and recent weight changes. If the patient is able to communicate, ask him or her to describe the usual foods eaten daily, cultural food preferences, and the times of meals and snacks. If available, ask the family these questions if the patient cannot communicate. If the patient cannot understand the questions due to language differences, locate an interpreter to assist with communication. The dietitian can more thoroughly analyze the diet, if necessary, based on your initial nutrition screening.

Ask about changes in eating habits as a result of illness, and document any change in appetite, taste, and weight loss. *A weight loss of 5% or more in 30 days, a weight loss of 10% in 6 months, or a weight that is below ideal may indicate malnutrition.*

! NURSING SAFETY PRIORITY (QSEN)

Action Alert

When assessing for malnutrition, assess for difficulty or pain in chewing or swallowing. *Unrecognized dysphagia is a common problem among nursing home residents and can cause malnutrition, dehydration, and aspiration pneumonia.* Ask the patient whether any foods are avoided and why. Ask UAP to report any choking while the patient eats. Record the occurrence of nausea, vomiting, heartburn, or any other symptoms of discomfort with eating.

Ask the patient about dental health problems, including the presence of dentures. Dentures or partial plates that do not fit well interfere with food intake. Dental caries (decay) or missing teeth may also cause discomfort while eating.

Physical Assessment/Clinical Manifestations. Assess for manifestations of various nutrient deficiencies (Table 60-2). Inspect the patient's hair, eyes, oral cavity, nails, and musculoskeletal and neurologic systems. Examine the condition of the skin, including any reddened or open areas. Anthropometric measurements may also be obtained as described on p. 1234. The nurse or UAP monitors all food and fluid intake and notes any mouth pain or difficulty in chewing or swallowing. A 3-day caloric intake may be collected and then calculated by the dietitian.

Psychosocial Assessment. The psychosocial history provides information about the patient's economic status, occupation, educational level, gender orientation, ethnicity/race, living and cooking arrangements, and mental status. Determine whether financial resources are adequate for providing the necessary food. If resources are inadequate, the social worker or case manager may refer the patient and family to available community services. Chapter 2 discusses NUTRITION in older adults in more detail.

Laboratory Assessment. Laboratory tests supply objective data that can support subjective data and identify deficiencies. Interpret laboratory data carefully with regard to the total patient; focusing on an isolated value may yield an inaccurate conclusion.

A low *hemoglobin* level may indicate anemia, recent hemorrhage, or hemodilution caused by FLUID retention. Hemoglobin may also be decreased secondary to conditions such as low serum albumin, infection, catabolism, or chronic disease. High levels may indicate hemoconcentration or dehydration or may be found secondary to liver disease.

TABLE 60-2 Manifestations of Nutrient Deficiencies

SIGN/SYMPTOM	POTENTIAL NUTRIENT DEFICIENCY
Hair	
Alopecia	Zinc
Easy to remove	Protein
Lackluster hair	Protein
"Corkscrew" hair	Vitamin C
Decreased pigmentation	Protein
Eyes	
Xerosis of conjunctiva	Vitamin A
Corneal vascularization	Riboflavin
Keratomalacia	Vitamin A
Bitot's spots	Vitamin A
Gastrointestinal Tract	
Nausea, vomiting	Pyridoxine
Diarrhea	Zinc, niacin
Stomatitis	Pyridoxine, riboflavin, iron
Cheilosis	Pyridoxine, iron
Glossitis	Pyridoxine, zinc, niacin, folic acid, vitamin B_{12}
Magenta tongue	Vitamin A, riboflavin
Swollen, bleeding gums	Vitamin C
Fissured tongue	Niacin
Hepatomegaly	Protein
Skin	
Dry and scaling	Vitamin A
Petechiae/ecchymoses	Vitamin C
Follicular hyperkeratosis	Vitamin A
Nasolabial seborrhea	Niacin
Bilateral dermatitis	Niacin
Extremities	
Subcutaneous fat loss	Calories
Muscle wastage	Calories, protein
Edema	Protein
Osteomalacia, bone pain, rickets	Vitamin D
Hematologic	
Anemia	Vitamin B_{12}, iron, folic acid, copper, vitamin E
Leukopenia, neutropenia	Copper
Low prothrombin time, prolonged clotting time	Vitamin K, manganese
Neurologic	
Disorientation	Niacin, thiamine
Confabulation	Thiamine
Neuropathy	Thiamine, pyridoxine, chromium
Paresthesia	Thiamine, pyridoxine, vitamin B_{12}
Cardiovascular	
Congestive heart failure, cardiomegaly, tachycardia	Thiamine
Cardiomyopathy	Selenium
Cardiac dysrhythmias	Magnesium

Courtesy of Ross Products Division, Abbott Laboratories, Columbus, OH.

Low *hematocrit* levels may reflect anemia, hemorrhage, excessive FLUID, renal disease, or cirrhosis. High hematocrit levels may indicate dehydration or hemoconcentration.

Serum albumin, thyroxine-binding prealbumin, and transferrin are measures of **visceral proteins**. Serum *albumin* is a plasma protein that reflects the nutrition status of the patient a few weeks before testing; therefore it is not considered to be a sensitive test. Patients who are dehydrated often have high levels of albumin, and those with fluid excess have a lowered value. The normal serum albumin level for men and women is 3.5 to 5.0 g/dL or 35 to 50 g/L (SI units) (Pagana & Pagana, 2014).

Thyroxine-binding **prealbumin (PAB)** is a plasma protein that provides a more sensitive indicator of nutrition deficiency because of its short half-life of 2 days. Depending on the laboratory test used, the normal PAB range is 15 to 36 mg/dL or 150 to 360 mg/L (SI units) (Pagana & Pagana, 2014). Although not used as commonly, serum **transferrin**, an iron-transport protein, can be measured directly or calculated as an indirect measurement of total iron-binding capacity (TIBC). It has a short half-life of 8 to 10 days and therefore is also a more sensitive indicator of protein status than albumin.

Cholesterol levels normally range between 160 and 200 mg/dL in adult men and women. Values are typically low with malabsorption, liver disease, pernicious anemia, end-stage cancer, or sepsis. A cholesterol level below 160 mg/dL has been identified as a possible indicator of malnutrition. Cholesterol testing is discussed in more detail in Chapter 36.

Total lymphocyte count (TLC) can be used to assess immune function. Malnutrition suppresses the immune system and leaves the patient more likely to get an infection. When a patient is malnourished, the TLC is usually decreased to below $1500/mm^3$.

◆ Analysis

The priority problem for the patient with malnutrition is Imbalanced Nutrition: Less Than Body Requirements related to inability to ingest or digest food or absorb nutrients (NANDA-I).

◆ Planning and Implementation

Improving Nutrition

Planning: Expected Outcomes. The patient with malnutrition is expected to have nutrients available to meet his or her metabolic needs as evidenced by normal serum proteins and adequate hydration.

Interventions. The preferred route for food intake is through the GI tract because it enhances the immune system and is safer, easier, less expensive, and more enjoyable.

Meal Management. The dietitian calculates the nutrients required daily and plans the patient's diet. In collaboration with the health care provider and dietitian, provide high-calorie, nutrient-rich foods (e.g., milkshakes, cheese, supplement drinks like Boost or Ensure). Assess the patient's food likes and dislikes. A feeding schedule of six small meals may be tolerated better than three large ones. A pureed or dental soft diet may be easier for those who have problems chewing or are **edentulous** (toothless).

! NURSING SAFETY PRIORITY QSEN

Action Alert

Malnourished ill patients often need to be encouraged to eat. Instruct UAP who are feeding patients to keep food at the appropriate temperature and to provide mouth care before feeding. Assess for other needs, such as pain management, and provide interventions to make the patient comfortable. Pain can prevent patients from enjoying their meals. Remove bedpans, urinals, and emesis basins from sight. Provide a quiet environment, which is conducive to eating. Soft music may calm those with advanced dementia or delirium. Appropriate time should be taken so that the patient does not feel rushed through a meal.

CONSIDERATIONS FOR OLDER ADULTS

Patient-Centered Care QSEN

Some patients, especially older adults, may take a long time to eat even small quantities of food because they tend to be less hungry than younger adults. If available, suggest that family members bring in favorite or ethnic foods that the patient might be more likely to eat. Teach them about ways to encourage the patient to increase food intake. Chart 60-3 describes additional interventions to promote food intake in older adults.

Restorative feeding programs help nursing home residents who need special assistance. These residents often eat in a separate dining area so that time and attention can be given to them. Some nursing homes have designated food and nutrition nursing assistants and/or trained volunteers who are primarily responsible for promoting and maintaining nutrition and hydration. Delegate appropriate feeding tasks, and supervise these UAPs during resident mealtime.

Nutrition Supplements. If the patient cannot take in enough nutrients in food, fortified **medical nutrition supplements (MNSs)** (e.g., Ensure, Sustacal, Carnation Instant Breakfast [also available as lactose-free supplement]) may be given, especially to older adults. Many commercial enteral products are available. For patients with medical diagnoses such as liver and renal disease or diabetes, special products that meet those needs are available (e.g., Glucerna for diabetic patients). Nutrition supplements used in acute care, long-term care, and home care can be costly. In addition, patients may refuse them and the supplements are then wasted. In a classic study, Bender et al. (2000) found that a more successful alternative to having the MNS given by nursing assistant staff in the nursing home was to have the supplements delivered by nurses during their usual medication passes. In this study, the nurses gave 60 mL or more of the MNS at least 4 times a day with the residents' medications. As a result, the patients gained weight and had fewer pressure ulcers, thus making the program very cost-effective and providing positive clinical outcomes.

Nutrition supplements are supplied as liquid formulas, powders, soups, coffee, and puddings in a variety of flavors. They come in different degrees of sweetness and are also available as modular supplements that provide single nutrients. Examples of modular supplements are Polycose glucose polymers for carbohydrates and Resource Beneprotein for protein, both available in liquid and powder form. Carbohydrate modulars are useful only if additional calories are needed. Protein modulars are indicated when metabolic stress causes a need for higher protein intake.

The dietitian may ask the nursing staff to keep a food and fluid intake record for at least 3 consecutive days to help assess the patient's nutrition status. Delegate this activity to UAP under your supervision. UAP also weigh the patient daily, every 3 days, or once a week, depending on the health care setting and severity of malnutrition.

Drug Therapy. Multivitamins, zinc, and an iron preparation are often prescribed to treat or prevent anemia. Monitor the patient's hemoglobin and hematocrit levels. Drug therapy can affect nutrition and elimination. For example, iron can cause constipation and zinc can cause nausea and vomiting.

If the patient still does not receive enough nutrition by mouth using the interventions just mentioned, request nutrition therapy in the form of **specialized nutrition support (SNS)**. SNS consists of either total enteral nutrition (TEN) or total parenteral nutrition (TPN).

Total Enteral Nutrition. Patients often cannot meet the desired outcomes of adequate nutrition via their usual oral intake because of increased metabolic demands or a decreased

CHART 60-3 Nursing Focus on the Older Adult

Promoting Nutrition Intake

- Be sure that patient is toileted and receives mouth care before mealtime.
- Be sure that patient has glasses and hearing aids in place, if appropriate, during meals.
- Be sure that bedpans, urinals, and emesis basins are removed from sight.
- Give analgesics to control pain and/or antiemetics for nausea at least 1 hour before mealtime.
- Remind unlicensed assistive personnel (UAP) to have patient sit in chair, if possible, at mealtime.
- If needed, open cartons and packages and cut up food at the patient's and/or family's request.
- Observe the patient during meals for food intake.
- Ask the patient about food likes and dislikes and ethnic food preferences.
- Encourage self-feeding, or feed the patient slowly; *delegate* this activity to UAP if desired.
- If feeding patient, sit at eye-level if culturally appropriate.
- Create an environment that is conducive to eating and socialization and relaxation, if possible.
- Decrease distractions, such as environmental noise from television, music, or other people.
- Provide adequate, nonglaring lighting.
- Keep patient away from offensive or medicinal odors.
- Keep eye contact with the patient during the meal if culturally appropriate.
- Serve snacks with activities, especially in long-term care settings; *delegate* this activity to UAP if desired.
- Document the percentage of food eaten at each meal and snack; *delegate* this activity to UAP if appropriate.
- Ensure that meals are visually appealing, appetizing, appropriately warm or cold, and properly prepared.
- Do not interrupt patients during mealtimes for nonurgent procedures or rounds.
- Assess for need for supplements between meals and at bedtime.
- Review the patient's drug profile, and discuss with the health care provider the use of drugs that might be suppressing appetite.
- If the patient is depressed, be sure that the depression is treated by the health care provider.

ability to eat. Therefore TEN using enteral tube feeding may be necessary to supplement oral intake or to provide total nutrition.

Patients likely to receive TEN can be divided into three groups:

- Those who can eat but cannot maintain adequate NUTRITION by oral intake of food alone
- Those who have permanent neuromuscular impairment and cannot swallow
- Those who do not have permanent neuromuscular impairment but cannot eat because of their condition

Patients in the first group are often older adults or patients receiving cancer treatment who cannot meet their calorie and protein needs. In some cases, this artificial nutrition and hydration may not be desired. For example, some patients have advance directives stating that they do not want to be kept alive by artificial nutrition and hydration if certain conditions exist. *However, legal and ethical questions arise when patients are not able to make their wishes known!*

For many years it was believed that withholding food and fluids would cause discomfort. Terminally or chronically ill patients who do not eat and drink may not suffer. In fact, they may be more comfortable if food and fluids are withheld. *The decision to feed is complex, and there is no clear right or wrong answer. To compound this legal and ethical dilemma, medical complications (e.g., aspiration, pressure ulcers) are common in older adults who are tube-fed.*

Decisions about these dilemmas are aided by the advice of interdisciplinary ethics committees in health care facilities. When clinicians are making decisions about the desirability of tube feedings in these cases, the focus should be on achieving consensus by:

- Reviewing what is known about tube feedings, especially their risks and benefits
- Reviewing the medical facts about the patient
- Investigating any available evidence that would help understand the patient's wishes
- Obtaining the opinions of all stakeholders in the situation
- Delaying any action until consensus is achieved

Those in the second group of patients likely to receive TEN usually have permanent swallowing problems and require some type of feeding tube for delivery of the enteral product on a long-term basis. Examples of conditions that can cause permanent swallowing problems are strokes, severe head trauma, and advanced multiple sclerosis. Patients in the third group receive enteral NUTRITION for as long as their illness lasts. The feeding is discontinued when the patient's condition improves and he or she can eat again. TEN is contraindicated for patients in states of significant hemodynamic compromise, such as those with diffuse peritonitis, severe acute or chronic pancreatitis, intestinal obstruction, intractable vomiting or diarrhea, and paralytic ileus (Bankhead et al., 2009).

Many commercially prepared enteral products are available. A therapeutic combination of carbohydrates, fat, vitamins, minerals, and trace elements is available in liquid form. Differences among products allow the dietitian to select the right formula for each patient. A prescription from the health care provider is required for enteral nutrition, but the dietitian usually makes the recommendation and computes the amount and type of product needed for each patient.

NCLEX EXAMINATION CHALLENGE

Health Promotion and Maintenance

An older client tells the nurse that he does not have an appetite. His wife states that he refuses to eat the food she cooks. What instructions will the nurse provide for the client and wife? **Select all that apply.**

A. "Place the fork in his hand and leave the room."
B. "As long as you drink fluids, you do not need food."
C. "Let him choose what foods he might desire."
D. "Eat meals together, to make mealtime feel special."
E. "Take your time eating, and do not rush through meals."
F. "Use nutrition supplements such as Ensure throughout the day."

Methods of Administering Total Enteral Nutrition. TEN is administered as "tube feedings" through one of the available GI tubes, either through a nasoenteric or enterostomal tube. It can be used in the patient's home or any health care setting.

A **nasoenteric tube (NET)** is any feeding tube inserted nasally and then advanced into the GI tract, such as a Keofeed, Entriflex, or Dobbhoff tube. Commonly used NETs include the **nasogastric (NG) tube** and the smaller (small-bore) **nasoduodenal tube (NDT)** (Fig. 60-3, *A*). A nasojejunal tube (NJT) is also available but is used less often than the other NETs.

The NDTs are used for delivering *short-term* enteral feedings (usually less than 4 weeks) because they are easy to use and are safer for the patient at risk for aspiration *if the tip of the tube is placed below the pyloric sphincter of the stomach and into the duodenum.* Small-bore polyurethane or silicone tubes from 8 to 12 Fr external diameter are preferred. The smaller tubes are more comfortable and are less likely to cause complications such as nasal irritation, sinusitis, tissue erosion, and pulmonary compromise.

Enterostomal feeding tubes are used for patients who need *long-term* enteral feeding. The most common types are gastrostomies and jejunostomies. The surgeon directly accesses the GI tract using various surgical, endoscopic, and laparoscopic techniques.

A **gastrostomy** is a stoma created from the abdominal wall into the stomach, through which a short feeding tube is inserted by the surgeon. It may require a small abdominal incision or may be placed endoscopically. This tube is called a **percutaneous endoscopic gastrostomy (PEG)** or dual-access gastrostomy-jejunostomy (PEG/J) tube. The PEG requires monitored conscious sedation for placement and is secure and durable. An alternative to either device is the **low-profile gastrostomy device (LPGD)** (Fig. 60-3, *B* and *C*). The LPGD is available with a firm or balloon-style internal bumper or retention disk. An anti-reflux valve keeps GI contents from leaking onto the skin. This device is less irritating to the skin, longer lasting, and more cosmetically pleasing. It also allows greater patient independence. However, skin-level devices do not allow easy access for checking **residuals** (the amount of feeding that remains in the stomach).

Jejunostomies are used less often than gastrostomies. A **jejunostomy** is used for long-term feedings when it is desirable to bypass the stomach, such as with gastric disease, upper GI obstruction, and abnormal gastric or duodenal emptying.

Tube feedings are administered by bolus feeding, continuous feeding, and cyclic feeding. **Bolus feeding** is an intermittent feeding of a specified amount of enteral product at set intervals

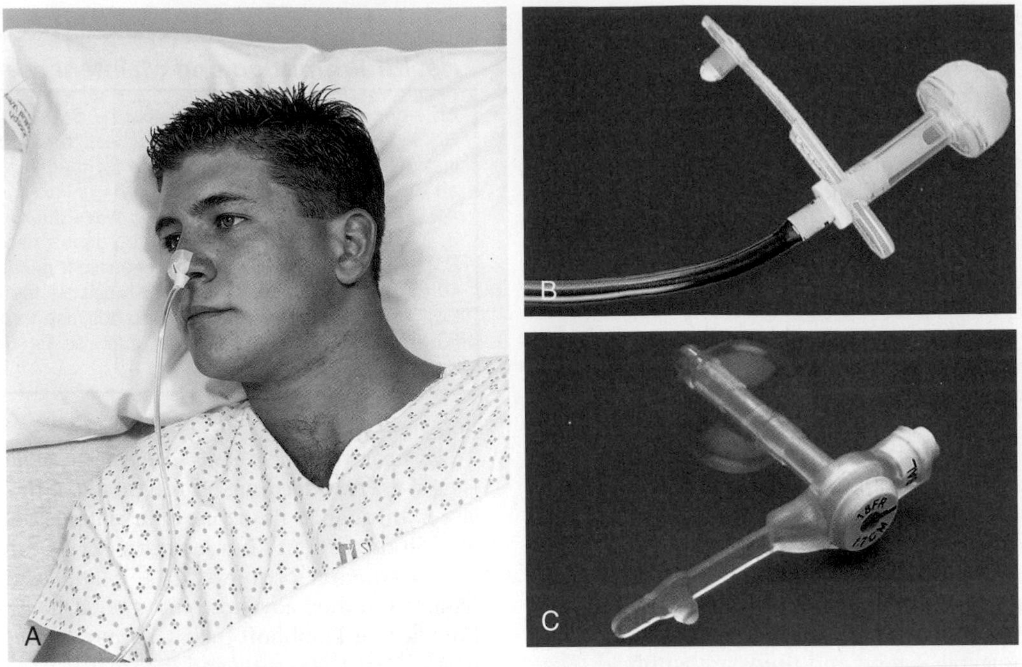

FIG. 60-3 Feeding tubes used for total enteral nutrition. **A,** Nasoduodenal tube. **B** and **C,** Gastrostomy tubes.

during a 24-hour period, typically every 4 hours. This method can be accomplished manually or by infusion through a mechanical pump or controller device. Another method of tube feeding is continuous enteral feeding. **Continuous feeding** is similar to IV therapy in that small amounts are continuously infused (by gravity drip or by a pump or controller device) over a specified time. The most commonly seen method, **cyclic feeding**, is the same as continuous feeding except the infusion is stopped for a specified time in each 24-hour period, usually 6 hours or longer ("down time"). Down time typically occurs in the morning to allow bathing, treatments, and other activities.

Infusion rates for cyclic feedings (and to some extent for intermittent bolus feeding) vary with the total amount of solution to be infused, the specific composition of the product, and the response of the patient to the feeding. The health care provider and dietitian usually decide the type, rate, and method of tube feeding, as well as the amount of additional water ("free water") needed. If the patient can swallow small amounts of food, he or she may also eat orally while the tube is in place.

The nurse is responsible for the care and maintenance of the feeding tube and the enteral feeding. Chart 60-4 lists best practices for the patient receiving TEN.

Complications of Total Enteral Nutrition. The nursing priority for care is patient safety, including preventing, assessing, and managing complications associated with tube feeding. Some complications of therapy result from the type of tube used to administer the feeding, and others result from the enteral product itself. The most common problem is the development of an obstructed ("clogged") tube. Use the tips in Chart 60-5 to maintain tube patency.

Patients receiving TEN are at risk for several other complications, including refeeding syndrome, tube misplacement and dislodgement, abdominal distention and nausea/vomiting, and FLUID AND ELECTROLYTE imbalance, often associated with diarrhea. These problems can be prevented if the patient is carefully monitored and complications are detected early.

Refeeding Syndrome. **Refeeding syndrome** is a potentially life-threatening metabolic complication that can occur when nutrition is restarted for a patient who is in a *starvation* state. When a patient is starved for nutrition, the body breaks down fat and protein, rather than carbohydrates, for energy. Protein catabolism leads to muscle and cell loss, often in major organs like the heart, liver, and lungs. The body's cells lose valuable electrolytes, including potassium and phosphate, into the plasma. Insulin secretion decreases in response to these changes. When *refeeding* begins, insulin production resumes and the cells take up glucose and electrolytes from the bloodstream, thus depleting serum levels.

! NURSING SAFETY PRIORITY QSEN

Critical Rescue

The electrolyte shift of refeeding syndrome can cause cardiovascular, respiratory, and neurologic problems, primarily as a result of hypophosphatemia, according to a classic study by Mehanna et al. (2008). Observe for clinical manifestations of this electrolyte imbalance, including shallow respirations, weakness, acute confusion, seizures, and increased bleeding tendency. Report and document your findings immediately. More information on fluid and electrolyte imbalance can be found in Chapter 11.

Refeeding syndrome can be prevented if patients are carefully assessed and managed for nutrition needs. Interventions to supplement or replace NUTRITION should be implemented early before the patient is in a starvation state. Patients receiving parenteral nutrition (described on pp. 1244-1245 later in this chapter) also may experience refeeding syndrome.

Tube Misplacement and Dislodgement. A serious complication is misplacement or dislodgement of the tube, *which can cause aspiration and possible death. Immediately remove any tube that you suspect is dislodged!* The Joint Commission's National Patient Safety Goals and the Centers for Medicare and Medicaid Services require all health care facilities to establish and

CHART 60-4 **Best Practice for Patient Safety & Quality Care** QSEN

Tube Feeding Care and Maintenance

- If nasogastric or nasoduodenal feeding is prescribed, use a soft, flexible, small-bore feeding tube (smaller than 12 Fr). *The initial placement of the tube should be confirmed by x-ray study.* Secure the tube with tape or a commercial attachment device after applying a skin protectant; change the tape regularly.
- Check tube placement by x-ray study when the correct position of the tube is in question; *an x-ray study is the most reliable method.*
- Per The Joint Commission's National Patient Safety Goals, if a gastrostomy or jejunostomy tube is used, assess the insertion site for signs of infection or excoriation (e.g., excessive redness, drainage). Rotate the tube 360 degrees each day, and check for in-and-out play of about ¼ inch (0.6 cm). If the tube cannot be moved, notify the health care provider immediately because the retention disk may be embedded in the tissue. Cover the site with a dry, sterile dressing, and change the dressing at least once a day.
- Check and record the residual volume every 4 to 6 hours or per facility policy by aspirating stomach contents into a syringe. If residual feeding is obtained, check with the health care provider for the appropriate intervention (usually to slow or stop the feeding for a time) or use the American Society of Parenteral and Enteral Nutrition (ASPEN) best practice recommendations.
- Check the feeding pump to ensure proper mechanical operation.
- Ensure that the enteral product is infused at the prescribed rate (mL/hr).
- Change the feeding bag and tubing every 24 to 48 hours; label the bag with the date and time of the change with your initials. Use an irrigation set for no more than 24 hours.
- For continuous or cyclic feeding, add only 4 hours of product to the bag at a time to prevent bacterial growth. *A closed system is preferred, and each set should be used no longer than 24 hours.*
- Wear clean gloves when changing or opening the feeding system or adding product; wipe the lid of the formula can with clean gauze; wear sterile gloves for critically ill or immunocompromised patients.
- Label open cans with date and time opened; cover, and keep refrigerated. Discard any unused open cans after 24 hours.
- *Do not use blue (or any color) food dye in formula because it does not assess aspiration and can cause serious complications.*
- To prevent aspiration, keep the head of the bed elevated at least 30 degrees during the feeding and for at least 1 hour after the feeding for bolus feeding; continuously maintain semi-Fowler's position for patients receiving cyclic or continuous feeding.
- Monitor laboratory values, especially blood urea nitrogen (BUN), serum electrolytes, hematocrit, prealbumin, and glucose.
- Monitor for complications of tube feeding, especially diarrhea.
- Monitor and carefully record the patient's weight and intake and output as requested by the physician or dietitian.

implement procedures and systems to prevent patient harm from medical complications.

Several techniques should be used to confirm proper placement to prevent harm and to keep the patient safe. *An x-ray is the most accurate confirmation method and should always be done upon initial tube insertion.* After the initial placement is confirmed, check the placement before each intermittent feeding or at least every 4 to 8 hours during feeding. Also check placement before each drug administration.

The traditional auscultatory method for checking tube placement may not be reliable, especially for patients with small-bore tubes. In this method, the nurse instills 20 to 30 mL of air into the tube ("insufflation") while listening over the epigastric area (stomach) with a stethoscope. *The resulting "whooshing" sound does not guarantee correct tube placement!*

Although some patients have respiratory distress if the tube is misplaced into the lungs, others do not. Therefore better methods for ensuring patient safety are being researched. Several safer procedures have been recommended for checking tube placement *after the initial placement has been confirmed by x-ray.* These methods include:

- Testing aspirated contents for pH, bilirubin, trypsin, or pepsin
- Assessing for carbon dioxide using capnometry

Some hospitals and nursing homes support testing the *pH of GI contents* at the bedside. To perform this procedure, aspirate a sample of the GI content, observe its color, and test its pH. When aspirating fluid, wait at least 1 hour after drug administration and then flush the tube with 20 mL of air to clear it. Collect the aspirate, and test it with pH paper. The pH of gastric fluid ranges from 0 to 4.0. If the tube has moved down into the intestines, the pH will be between 7.0 and 8.0. If the tube is in the lungs, the pH will be greater than 6.0. The pH may also be as high as 6 if the patient takes certain drugs, such as H_2 blockers (e.g., ranitidine [Zantac] and famotidine [Pepcid]). Because these drugs affect pH, bilirubin testing or capnometry may be more reliable and valid methods for predicting tube location.

Capnometry can determine if carbon dioxide is emitted from the tube (Grmec et al., 2011). A device to measure the presence of the gas is attached to the end of the tube after placement. The test is positive for carbon dioxide if the tube is placed into the lungs, rather than the stomach. *The tube should be immediately removed if the gas is detected.*

CHART 60-5 **Best Practice for Patient Safety & Quality Care** QSEN

Maintaining a Patent Feeding Tube

- Flush the tube with 20 to 30 mL of water (or the amount prescribed by the health care provider or dietitian):
  - At least every 4 hours during a continuous tube feeding
  - Before and after each intermittent tube feeding
  - Before and after drug administration (use warm water)
  - After checking residual volume
- If the tube becomes clogged, use 30 mL of water for flushing, applying gentle pressure with a 50-mL piston syringe.
- Avoid the use of carbonated beverage, except for existing clogs *when water is not effective.* Do not use cranberry juice.
- Whenever possible, use liquid medications instead of crushed tablets unless liquid forms cause diarrhea; make sure that the drug is compatible with the feeding solution.
- Do not mix drugs with the feeding product before giving. Crush tablets as finely as possible, and dissolve in warm water. *(Check to see which tablets are safe to crush. For example, do not crush slow-acting [SA] or slow-release [SR] drugs.)*
- Consider use of automatic flush feeding pump such as Flexiflo or Kangaroo.

! NURSING SAFETY PRIORITY QSEN

Action Alert

If enteral tubes are misplaced or become dislodged, the patient is likely to aspirate. Aspiration pneumonia is a life-threatening complication associated with TEN, especially for older adults. Observe for increasing temperature and pulse, as well as for other signs of dehydration such as dry mucous membranes and decreased urinary output. Auscultate lungs every 4 to 8 hours to check for diminishing breath sounds, especially in lower lobes. Patients may become short of breath and report chest discomfort. A chest x-ray confirms this diagnosis, and treatment with antibiotics is started.

Abdominal Distention and Nausea/Vomiting. Abdominal distention, nausea, and vomiting during tube feeding are often caused by overfeeding. To *prevent* overfeeding, check gastric residual volumes every 4 to 6 hours, depending on facility policy and the needs of the patient. The American Society of Parenteral and Enteral Nutrition (ASPEN) (2011) recommends holding a feeding if the gastric residual volumes are more than 200 mL on two consecutive assessments. In some facilities, feedings are temporarily held if the gastric residual is 100 mL or more, depending on the patient. After a period of rest, the feeding can be restarted at a lower flow rate.

A problem with frequent residual assessments is that the formula may clog the tube during aspiration, even if flushed with water. If the patient's residual volumes have been low or zero and he or she has no abdominal distention, nausea, or vomiting, consider discontinuing these assessments, depending on facility policy.

FLUID AND ELECTROLYTE Imbalances. Patients receiving enteral nutrition therapy are at an increased risk for FLUID *imbalances.* They are often older or debilitated and may also have cardiac or renal problems. Fluid imbalances associated with enteral nutrition are usually related to the body's response to increased serum osmolarity, but *fluid overload* from too much tube feeding can also occur.

Osmolarity is the amount or concentration of particles dissolved in solution. This concentration exerts a specific osmotic pressure within the solution. Normal osmolarity of extracellular fluid (ECF) ranges between 270 and 300 mOsm. Enteral feeding products range in osmolarity from isotonic (about 300 mOsm) to extremely hypertonic (600 mOsm). Electrolytes (including sodium) contribute to this hypertonicity, but more of the osmolarity is determined by the concentration of proteins and sugar molecules in the enteral product. Even when the product is isotonic, the ECF can become hyperosmolar unless some hypotonic FLUIDS are also administered to the patient. This situation is most likely to develop in patients who are unconscious, unable to respond to the thirst reflex, on fluid restrictions, or receiving hyperosmotic enteral preparations.

Because increased plasma osmolarity is largely a result of extra glucose and proteins (which tend to remain in the plasma rather than move to interstitial spaces), the plasma osmotic pressure (water-pulling pressure) is increased. In this situation, intracellular and interstitial water move into and expand the plasma volume. This volume expansion results in an increased renal excretion of water (in patients with normal renal function) and leads to osmotic *dehydration.*

CONSIDERATIONS FOR OLDER ADULTS

Patient-Centered Care QSEN

If patients do *not* have normal renal and cardiac function, expansion of the plasma volume can lead to circulatory overload and pulmonary edema, especially in older adults. Therefore early identification of patients at risk for impairment of renal and/or cardiac function is important. Assess for signs and symptoms of circulatory overload, such as peripheral edema, sudden weight gain, crackles, dyspnea, increased blood pressure, and bounding pulse. Collaborate with the dietitian and health care provider to plan the correct amount of fluid to be provided.

Excessive *diarrhea* may develop when hyperosmolar enteral preparations are delivered quickly. This situation can also lead to *dehydration* through excessive water loss. Collaborate with the health care provider and dietitian for recommendations to prevent diarrhea. The dietitian usually changes the feeding to a more iso-osmolar formula. Most of these formulas can be started full strength but slowly at 15 to 20 mL/hr. The rate is gradually increased as the patient tolerates and as the expected nutrition outcome is achieved.

If diarrhea continues, especially if it has a very foul odor, evaluate the patient for *Clostridium difficile* or other infectious organisms. Contamination can occur because of repeated and often faulty handling of the feeding solution and system. *Per The Joint Commission's National Patient Safety Goals, wear clean gloves when changing systems and adding product. Sterile gloves may help prevent infection in critically ill or immunocompromised patients. A closed feeding system is preferred over an open one because the chance of contamination is lessened* (see Chart 60-4). Tubes with ports also minimize contamination by eliminating the need to open the feeding system to administer drugs.

In some cases, diarrhea may be the result of multiple liquid medications, such as elixirs and suspensions that have a very high osmolarity. Examples include acetaminophen (Tylenol), furosemide (Lasix), and phenytoin (Dilantin). Patients receiving multiple liquid drugs should be evaluated by the health care provider to determine whether their drug regimen can be changed to prevent diarrhea. Diluting these liquids may also be an option.

Depending on the patient's state of health, some electrolyte imbalances can be avoided. This is achieved by the use of enteral preparations containing lower concentrations of the electrolytes that the patient cannot handle well. For example, renal patients with high potassium levels receive a special formula that is used for this imbalance.

The two most common electrolyte imbalances associated with enteral nutrition therapy are hyperkalemia and hyponatremia. Both of these conditions may be related to hyperglycemia-induced hyperosmolarity of the plasma and the resultant osmotic diuresis. Risk for disturbances in FLUID AND ELECTROLYTE BALANCE are discussed in detail in Chapter 11.

Parenteral Nutrition. When a patient cannot effectively use the GI tract for NUTRITION, either partial or total parenteral nutrition therapy may be needed. This form of IV therapy differs from standard IV therapy in that any or all nutrients (carbohydrates, proteins, fats, vitamins, minerals, and trace elements) can be given. One liter of IV fluid containing 5% dextrose, which is often used as standard therapy, provides only 170 kcal. A hospitalized patient typically receives 3 to 4 L a day, for a total number of calories ranging between 500 and 700 a day. This calorie intake is not sufficient when the patient requires IV therapy for a prolonged period and cannot eat an adequate diet or has increased calorie needs for tissue repair and building.

Partial Parenteral Nutrition. Partial, or peripheral, parenteral nutrition (PPN) is usually given through a cannula or catheter in a large distal vein of the arm or through a peripherally inserted central catheter (PICC line). (See Chapter 13 for care of patients with PICC lines.) The alternative is used for some patients who can eat but are not able to take in enough nutrients to meet their needs. The patient must have adequate peripheral vein access and be able to tolerate large volumes of fluid to have PPN. Two types of solutions are commonly used in various combinations for PPN: IV fat (lipid) emulsions (IVFEs) and amino acid–dextrose solutions. IVFEs are usually given using a piggyback method.

NURSING SAFETY PRIORITY QSEN

Critical Rescue

For patients receiving fat emulsions, monitor for manifestations of fat overload syndrome, especially in those who are critically ill. These manifestations include fever, increased triglycerides, clotting problems, and multi-system organ failure. Discontinue the IVFE infusion and report any of these changes to the health care provider immediately if this complication is suspected.

Most IVFEs (20% fat emulsion) are isotonic, but the tonicity of commercially prepared amino acid–dextrose solutions ranges from 300 mOsm to nearly 900 mOsm for PPN. Amino acid–dextrose solutions are considered more stable than IVFEs, and therefore additives (e.g., vitamins, minerals, electrolytes, trace elements) tend to be mixed with them. These solutions must be delivered through an in-line filter and are administered by an infusion pump for an accurate and constant delivery rate.

Some PPN products are a *mixture* of lipids (10% or 20% fat emulsion) and an amino acid–dextrose (usually 10%) solution. This mixture of three types of nutrients is referred to as a *3:1, total nutrient admixture (TNA),* or *triple-mix solution.*

Total Parenteral Nutrition. When the patient requires intensive NUTRITION support for an extended time, the health care provider prescribes centrally administered **total parenteral nutrition (TPN).** TPN is delivered through access to central veins, usually through a PICC line or the subclavian or internal jugular veins. Central venous catheters and associated nursing care are described in detail in Chapter 13.

Total parenteral nutrition solutions contain higher concentrations of dextrose and proteins, usually in the form of synthetic amino acids or protein hydrolysates (3% to 5%). These solutions are hyperosmotic (3 to 6 times the osmolarity of normal blood). The base solutions are available as commercially prepared solutions. The hospital or community pharmacist adds components (specific electrolytes, minerals, trace elements, and insulin) according to the patient's nutrition needs. This therapy provides needed calories and spares body proteins from catabolism for energy requirements.

The TPN solutions are administered with an infusion pump. The osmolarity of the fluid and the concentrations of the specific components make controlled delivery essential.

Patients receiving parenteral nutrition fluids are at risk for a wide variety of serious and potentially life-threatening complications. Complications may result from the solutions or from the peripheral or central venous catheter. The following discussion is limited to the complications that involve FLUID AND ELECTROLYTE BALANCE. Complications of IV cannulas and central venous catheters are discussed in Chapter 13, including infection and sepsis.

Patients receiving parenteral nutrition therapy are at high risk for fluid imbalance. Not only is fluid delivered directly into the venous system but also the extreme hyperosmolarity of the solutions stimulates fluid shifts between body fluid compartments. The hyperosmolarity is caused by their amino acid and dextrose concentrations. Increased dextrose causes hyperglycemia (increased blood glucose). As a result, some of the dextrose moves into the interstitial and intracellular spaces, where it is metabolized. However, dextrose remains in the plasma volume when the solutions are administered too rapidly, without enough insulin coverage, or in the presence of hyponatremia and hypokalemia. The result is a shift of water from the interstitial and intracellular spaces into the plasma. Expansion of the plasma volume together with hyperglycemia can cause osmotic diuresis and lead to serious dehydration and hypovolemic shock. If the patient also has cardiac or renal dysfunction, he or she may develop fluid overload, congestive heart failure, and pulmonary edema. Monitor the infusion rate of the parenteral fluid, and give insulin as prescribed.

Monitor for these complications by taking daily weights and by documenting accurate intake and output while the patient is receiving parenteral nutrition. Serum glucose and electrolyte values are also monitored (Chart 60-6). Report any major changes or abnormalities to the health care provider, and document all assessments and interventions.

CHART 60-6 Best Practice for Patient Safety & Quality Care QSEN

Care and Maintenance of Total Parenteral Nutrition

- Check each bag of total parenteral nutrition (TPN) solution for accuracy by comparing it with the physician's or pharmacist's prescription.
- Monitor the IV pump for accuracy in delivering the prescribed hourly rate.
- If the TPN solution is temporarily unavailable, give 10% dextrose/water ($D_{10}W$) or 20% dextrose/water ($D_{20}W$) until the TPN solution can be obtained.
- If the TPN administration is not on time ("behind"), do not attempt to "catch up" by increasing the rate.
- Monitor the patient's weight daily or according to facility protocol.
- Monitor serum electrolytes and glucose daily or per facility protocol. (Many facilities require finger-stick blood sugars [FSBSs] every 4 hours, especially if the patient is receiving insulin. Urine testing for ketones may also be requested.)
- Monitor for, report, and document complications, including fluid and electrolyte imbalances.
- Monitor and carefully record the patient's intake and output.
- Assess the patient's IV site for signs of infection or infiltration (see Chapter 13).
- Change the IV tubing every 24 hours or per facility protocol.
- Change the dressing around the IV site every 48 to 72 hours or per facility protocol.
- Before administering TPN, have a second nurse check the prescription and solution to prevent patient harm.

Patients receiving TPN are at an increased risk for many different disturbances of FLUID AND ELECTROLYTE BALANCE, depending on the composition of the solution and whether a fluid imbalance occurs. The health care provider usually requests frequent determinations of serum electrolyte levels to detect these imbalances. The risk for metabolic and electrolyte complications is reduced when the rate of administration is carefully controlled and patients are closely monitored for response to treatment. Potassium and sodium imbalances are common, especially when insulin is also administered as part of the therapy. Calcium imbalances, particularly hypercalcemia, are associated with TPN, although immobility may play more of a role than the actual therapy in developing this imbalance (National Institutes of Health [NIH], 2013a).

Community-Based Care

Malnourished patients can be cared for in a variety of settings, including the acute care hospital, transitional care unit, nursing home, or their own home. Malnutrition is often diagnosed when the patient is admitted to the acute care hospital or shortly after hospitalization if complications such as poor wound healing or sepsis occur. If the patient is severely compromised, he or she may require admission to a traditional nursing home for either transitional or long-term care. If adequate home support is available, he or she may be discharged to home in the care of a family member or other caregiver. Home care nurses may be needed to monitor and direct the care.

Home Care Management. The malnourished patient needs a variety of resources at home to continue aggressive NUTRITION support. If he or she can consume food by the oral route, the case manager or other discharge planner determines whether financial resources are available for the necessary nutrition supplements. If the hospital provides ambulatory nutrition counseling services, the patient is scheduled for follow-up after discharge for assessment of weight gain.

Self-Management Education. The dietitian teaches the malnourished patient and family about high-calorie, high-protein diet and NUTRITION supplements. In collaboration with the pharmacist, review specific parenteral solutions with the patient and family or significant others.

Reinforce the importance of adhering to the prescribed diet, and review any drugs the patient may be taking. If using an iron preparation, teach the importance of taking the drug immediately before or during meals. Caution the patient that iron tends to cause constipation. For the older adult already susceptible to constipation, emphasize the importance of measures for prevention, including adequate fiber intake, adequate fluids, and exercise.

Some patients are discharged to home with enteral or parenteral nutrition. Teach the family or other caregiver how to continue these therapies. Remind caregivers to consider the psychosocial aspects of these alternative methods for nutrition. For example, the caregiver can bring the enteral product and napkin to the patient on a decorative tray to make the feeding experience more elegant and "normal." Moving the feeding equipment out of view of the patient when it is not in use is also helpful.

Health Care Resources. The malnourished patient discharged to home on enteral or parenteral nutrition support needs the specialized services of a home nutrition therapy team. This team generally consists of the physician, nurse, dietitian, pharmacist, and case manager or social worker. Several commercial companies supply these services to patients at home in addition to the feeding supplies and formulas and health teaching.

◆ Evaluation: Outcomes

Evaluate the care of the malnourished patient based on the identified priority patient problem. The primary expected outcome is that he or she has available nutrients to meet the metabolic demands for maintaining weight and total protein and has adequate hydration.

OBESITY

❖ PATHOPHYSIOLOGY

Obesity is not just one disease; it includes many conditions with varying causes. The terms *obesity* and *overweight* are often used interchangeably, but they refer to different health problems. For both problems, the patient often does not consume enough healthy nutrients and may not receive adequate nutrition. **Overweight** is an increase in body weight for height compared with a reference standard, or up to 10% greater than ideal body weight (IBW) and a body mass index (BMI) of 25 to 29. This weight may not reflect excess body fat. For example, well-developed athletes may appear overweight because of increased muscle (lean) mass, in which the proportion of muscle to fat is greater than average (NIH, 2013b).

Obesity refers to an excess amount of body fat when compared with lean body mass. The normal amount of body fat in *men* is between 15% and 20% of body weight. For *women,* the normal amount is 18% to 32%. An obese person weighs at least 20% above the upper limit of the normal range for ideal body weight and has a BMI of 30 or more. **Morbid obesity,** also called *extreme obesity,* refers to a weight that has a severely negative effect on health—usually more than 100% above IBW and a BMI over 40.

More than one third of Americans are obese (CDC, 2012b). About 10% or more of adults are morbidly obese. *This problem is the second leading cause of preventable deaths in the United States, second only to smoking, and has become a national crisis.* Obesity across the life span is considered an epidemic in the United States and Canada. Worldwide, it is recognized as a major global health problem, costing billions of dollars for health care and lost productivity.

The pathophysiology of obesity is very complex. A number of chemicals in the body, including hormones known as *adipokines,* work together to affect appetite and fat metabolism:

- **Leptin:** a hormone released by fat cells and possibly by gastric cells; it also acts on the hypothalamus to control appetite
- **Adiponectin:** an anti-inflammatory and insulin-sensitizing hormone
- **Resistin:** a hormone produced by fat cells that creates resistance to insulin activity
- **Inflammatory cytokines:** such as inflammatory interleukins and tumor necrosis factor–alpha
- **Apolipoprotein E:** one of several regulators of lipoprotein metabolism
- **Cholecystokinin:** a hormone that stimulates digestive juices and may work with leptin to increase or decrease appetite
- **Ghrelin:** the "hunger hormone" that is secreted in the stomach; increases in a fasting state and decreases after a meal

Some adipokines are neuropeptides, including orexins and anorexins, which play a role in body weight. **Orexins** are appetite stimulants; examples are ghrelin secreted by the stomach and peptide YY from the intestines. **Anorexins** decrease appetite and include leptin and insulin (McCance et al., 2014). Increased circulating plasma levels of orexins are associated with the development of obesity. However, in some people, high levels of leptin may not be effective in suppressing appetite—a condition known as *leptin resistance.* In this case, overeating and excessive weight gain can result. Hyperleptinemia also stimulates the autonomic nervous system and contributes to blood vessel inflammation and ventricular hypertrophy. These actions may help explain why obese patients are most at risk for hypertension, atherosclerosis, and heart disease (Kulie et al., 2011). Obesity is also associated with insulin resistance, which predisposes obese patients to type 2 diabetes mellitus (see Chapter 64) (NIH, 2013b).

The distribution of excess body fat rather than the degree of obesity has been used to predict increased health risks. For example, the waist circumference (WC) is a stronger predictor of coronary artery disease (CAD) than is the BMI. A WC greater than 35 inches (89 cm) in women and a WC greater than 40 inches (102 cm) in men indicate central obesity (National Institute of Diabetes and Digestive and Kidney Diseases, 2012). Central obesity is a major risk factor for CAD, stroke, type 2 diabetes, some cancers (e.g., colon, breast), sleep apnea, and early death (NIH, 2013b).

The waist-to-hip ratio (WHR) is also a predictor of CAD. This measure differentiates peripheral lower body obesity from central obesity. A WHR of 0.95 or greater in men (0.8 or greater in women) indicates android obesity with excess fat at the waist and abdomen.

Complications of Obesity

The major complications of obesity affect primarily the cardiovascular and respiratory systems. However, excess weight can also cause degeneration of the musculoskeletal system, especially the weight-bearing joints like hips and knees (osteoarthritis). Obese people are also more susceptible to infections and infectious diseases than are thinner people and tend to heal more slowly. Table 60-3 lists some of the most common complications of obesity.

Etiology and Genetic Risk

The causes of obesity involve complex interrelationships of many environmental, genetic, and behavioral factors. One of the most common causes of being overweight or obese is eating *high-fat and high-cholesterol diets.* Obesity is associated with diet when it contains a significant amount of *saturated* fat, which increases low-density lipoproteins (LDL, or LDL-C for low-density lipoproteins cholesterol). *Trans* fatty acids (TFAs), saturated fats, and cholesterol are linked to obesity and CAD (American Heart Association, 2013). By contrast, monounsaturated and polyunsaturated fats are healthy fats.

Physical inactivity has been identified as another cause of overweight and obesity. The major barriers to increasing physical activity include a lack of time, learned behaviors regarding a sedentary lifestyle, or decreased mobility associated with prolonged illness. Regular exercise is associated with lower death rates for adults of any age. It also increases lean muscle, decreases body fat, aids in weight control, and enhances psychological well-being. Although some people think that regular exercise has to include joining a fitness program or exercising for long periods, simple forms of exercise like walking 20 minutes provide the same type of benefit. Older adults can engage in this type of exercise. It does not cost money (like joining a program) and provides health benefits such as strengthening joints and improving cardiovascular health.

TABLE 60-3 Common Complications of Obesity

• Type 2 diabetes mellitus	• Obesity hypoventilation syndrome
• Hypertension	• Depression and other mental health/behavioral health problems
• **Hyperlipidemia** (increased serum lipids)	• Urinary incontinence
• Coronary artery disease (CAD)	• **Cholelithiasis** (gallstones)
• Stroke	• Gout
• Peripheral artery disease (PAD)	• Chronic back pain
• Metabolic syndrome	• Early osteoarthritis
• Obstructive sleep apnea	• Decreased wound healing

Another cause of obesity is *drug therapy.* Some prescribed drugs contribute to weight gain when they are taken on a long-term basis. Examples include:

- Corticosteroids
- Estrogens and certain progestins
- Nonsteroidal anti-inflammatory drugs (NSAIDs)
- Antihypertensives
- Antidepressants and other psychoactive drugs
- Antiepileptic drugs
- Certain oral antidiabetic agents

GENETIC/GENOMIC CONSIDERATIONS

Patient-Centered Care QSEN

Familial and genetic factors seem to play a very important role in obesity. When both parents are overweight, about 80% of their children will be overweight. If neither parent is overweight, fewer than 10% of the children will be overweight. In studies of identical twins, nonidentical twins, and parent-sibling relationships, about 50% of the difference in body fatness is transmitted to children and about 50% of this amount is genetically controlled (McCance et al., 2014).

Genetic composition may predispose some people but not others to obesity. Leptin, the hormone encoded by the *ob* gene, appears to send a message to the brain that the body has stored enough fat. This message serves as a signal to stop eating. In some obese people, other gene mutations have been identified, including an abnormality of the melanocortin-4 receptor that inhibits appetite in families with a history of obesity.

People who have **Prader-Willi syndrome (PWS)**, a complex neurodevelopmental genetic disorder, are typically morbidly obese. This disorder results from a hypothalamic-pituitary dysfunction that prevents appetite control (Yearwood et al., 2011).

Health Promotion and Maintenance

Obesity is a major public health problem and is associated with many complications, including death. As a result of this increasing problem, the *Healthy People 2020* agenda addresses the need to reduce the proportion of children, adolescents, and adults who are obese. *Healthy People 2020 objectives for Nutrition and Weight Status* include specific population targets related to obesity and healthy nutrition habits (Table 60-4). In

TABLE 60-4 Meeting *Healthy People 2020* Sample Objectives and Targets: Nutrition and Weight Status

- Reduce the proportion of adults who are obese (by 10%).
- Increase the proportion of adults who are at a healthy weight (by 10%).
- Increase the proportion of physician visits made by adult patients that include counseling about nutrition or diet (by 15.2%).
- Increase the proportion of primary care physicians who regularly assess body mass index (BMI) in their adult patients (by 10%).
- Increase the contribution of total vegetables to the diets of the population aged 2 years and older (to 1.1 cups per 1000 calories).
- Increase the contribution of fruits to the diets of the population aged 2 years and older (to 0.9 cups per 1000 calories).
- Reduce consumption of saturated fat in the population aged 2 years and older (by 9.5%).

collaboration with the dietitian, teach the importance of weight management and exercise to improve health. Even a 5% weight loss can drastically decrease the risk for coronary artery disease (CAD) and diabetes mellitus (NIH, 2013b). Nurses who practice healthful behaviors and value a healthy lifestyle are more likely to be seen by patients as credible teachers of this information (Marchiondo, 2014).

❖ PATIENT-CENTERED COLLABORATIVE CARE

◆ Assessment

History. In addition to taking a complete history regarding present and past health problems, collect this information about the patient in collaboration with the dietitian:

- Economic status
- Usual food intake
- Eating behavior
- Cultural background
- Attitude toward food
- Appetite
- Chronic diseases
- Drugs (prescribed and OTC, including herbal preparations)
- Physical activity/functional ability
- Family history of obesity
- Developmental level

A nutrition history usually includes a 24-hour recall of food intake and the frequency with which foods are consumed. The adequacy of the diet can be evaluated by comparing the amount and types of foods consumed daily with the established standards. The dietitian then provides a more detailed analysis of nutrition intake.

Physical Assessment/Clinical Manifestations. Obtain an accurate height and weight. The dietitian calculates the percentage of ideal body weight (% IBW) and the body mass index (BMI). He or she may also:

- Measure the waist circumference
- Calculate the waist-to-hip ratio
- Determine arm and calf circumferences

Examine the skin of the obese patient for reddened or open areas. Lift skinfold areas, such as pendulous breasts and abdominal aprons (**panniculus**), to observe for *Candida* (yeast) (a condition called *intertrigo*) or other infections or lesions. Infection of the panniculus is referred to as **panniculitis.**

Psychosocial Assessment. Obtain a psychosocial history to determine the patient's circumstances and emotional factors that might prevent successful therapy or that might be worsened by therapy. Interview the patient to determine his or her perception of current weight and weight reduction. Some patients do not view weight as a problem, which affects planning, treatment, and outcome. Ask the patient questions about his or her health beliefs related to being overweight, such as:

- What does food mean to you?
- Do you want to lose weight?
- What prevents you from losing weight?
- What do you think will motivate you to lose weight?
- How do you think you might benefit from losing weight?

Many patients report that they have tried multiple diets to lose weight but either the diets have not worked or they regained the weight they had initially lost. People who attempt restrictive diets become easy targets for the billion-dollar weight-loss industry, yet most dieters regain lost weight. This problem can be even more concerning for the older adult who loses weight and then regains it. Studies have shown that this cycle may contribute to loss of lean muscle mass, especially in older men (Lee et al., 2010).

The results of dieting and other efforts can lead to a sense of failure and lowered self-esteem, which often stimulates more overeating. Many overweight and obese people eat in response to environmental and emotional stressors rather than because they are hungry. Ask patients to identify their perceived stressors and what triggers their need for food.

Lifestyle changes are difficult without adequate family and community support. Assess useful coping strategies and support systems that the patient can employ during treatment for obesity.

Explore the patient's history to assess:

- Attempts at weight-reduction diets and outcomes
- Effects of obesity on lifestyle
- Effects of obesity on social interactions
- Mental health/behavioral health problems, such as depression
- Effects of obesity on intimate relationships, especially sexuality

Obese men often experience erectile dysfunction (ED), which can cause or worsen depression. Women often experience changes in their menstrual cycles and may have problems getting pregnant.

◆ Interventions

Weight is lost when energy used is greater than intake. Weight loss may be accomplished by nutrition modification with or without the aid of drugs and in combination with a regular exercise program. Patients who may be candidates for surgical treatment include those who have:

- Repeated failure of nonsurgical interventions
- A BMI equal to or greater than 40
- Weight more than 100% above IBW (i.e., morbidly obese)

Nonsurgical Management. Various nutrition approaches and drug therapy have been attempted to help obese patients achieve permanent weight loss.

Diet Programs. Diets for helping people lose weight include fasting, very-low-calorie diets, balanced and unbalanced low-energy diets, and novelty diets.

Short-term fasting programs have not been successful in treating morbidly obese patients, and prolonged fasting does not produce permanent benefits. Most patients regain the weight that was lost by this method. In addition, the risks associated with fasting (e.g., severe ketosis) require close medical supervision.

Very-low-calorie diets generally provide 200 to 800 calories/day. Two types of these diets are the *protein-sparing modified fast* and the *liquid formula diet.* The protein-sparing modified fast provides protein of high biologic value (1.5 g/kg of desirable body weight daily) within a limited number of calories. The diet produces rapid weight loss while preserving lean body mass. The liquid formula diet provides between 33 and 70 g of protein daily.

Both diets require an initial cardiac evaluation, supervision by an interdisciplinary health care team with monitoring by a physician, nutrition counseling by a dietitian, and supplementation with vitamins and minerals. These diets are only one part of a weight-reduction program. Patients who are on these diets should receive nutrition education, psychological counseling, exercise, and behavior therapy. Comparable weight losses have been achieved with both diets, but again, most patients regain the weight they lost.

Nutritionally balanced diets generally provide about 1200 calories/day with a conventional distribution of carbohydrate, protein, and fat. Vitamin and mineral supplements may be necessary if energy intakes fall below 1200 calories for women and 1800 calories for men. This diet provides conventional foods that are economical and easy to obtain. Thus the outcome of weight loss is facilitated, and it is hoped that loss is maintained. For example, Weight Watchers is an organization that provides education about nutritionally balanced diets based on a point system. They offer on-site weekly group support meetings or the option of an online community.

Unbalanced low-energy diets, such as the low-carbohydrate diet (e.g., Atkins or South Beach diet), restrict one or more nutrients. Protein and vegetables are encouraged, but certain carbohydrates and high-fat foods are not. Although they remain controversial in the medical community, these diets are extremely popular. Scientific outcome data have been conflicting.

Novelty diets, such as the grapefruit diet, the Cookie diet, and the Hollywood diet, are often nutritionally *inadequate.* This type of diet implies that a certain food or liquid increases metabolic rate or accelerates the oxidation of body fat. Weight loss is achieved because energy is restricted by food choice, but patients do not sustain weight loss after stopping the diet.

Nutrition Therapy. Nutrition recommendations for each patient are developed through close interaction among the patient, family, physician, nurse, and dietitian. The diet must meet the patient's needs, habits, and lifestyle and should be realistic.

The dietitian develops a diet plan and instructs the patient. At a minimum, the diet should:

- Have a scientific rationale
- Be nutritionally adequate for all nutrients
- Have a low risk-benefit ratio
- Be practical and conducive to long-term success

Calorie estimates are easily calculated. Resting metabolic rate is determined using a gender-specific formula that incorporates the appropriate activity factor. This figure reflects the total calories needed daily for maintaining current weight. To encourage a weight loss of 1 pound (0.45 kg) a week, the dietitian subtracts 500 calories each day. To encourage a weight loss of 2 pounds (0.9 kg) a week, 1000 calories each day are subtracted. The amount of weight lost varies with the patient's food intake, level of physical activity, and water losses. A reasonable expected outcome of 5% to 10% loss of body weight has been shown to improve glycemic control and reduce cholesterol and blood pressure. These benefits continue if the weight loss is sustained.

Exercise Program. Along with change in eating habits, a major intervention to manage obesity is to increase the type and amount of daily exercise to burn calories. For most people, adding exercise to a nutrition intervention produces more weight loss than just dieting alone. More of the weight lost is fat, which preserves lean body mass. An increase in exercise can reduce the waist circumference and the waist-to-hip ratio.

Teach patients that increasing and maintaining physical activity levels are important in maintaining weight loss. Many overweight or obese patients are so unfit that it may take several months of conditioning before they can exercise sufficiently to lose weight.

A minimum-level workout should be developed so that consistency can be achieved. The expected outcome is to maintain a lifetime of increased physical activity. The patient is likely to be less fatigued and discouraged with a low-intensity, short-duration program. Encourage sedentary (physically inactive) patients to increase their activity by walking 30 to 40 minutes at least 5 days each week. The activity may be performed all at once or divided over the course of the day. Remind the patient to exercise only under the supervision of the physician. All members of the interdisciplinary team should encourage and support any increase in physical activity. Structured national programs with support staff may be helpful for some patients. The staff typically offers diet counseling as well as cardiovascular and muscle-toning activities.

Drug Therapy. A BMI of 30 or a BMI of 27 with comorbidities is one indicator for the use of drug therapy. **Anorectic drugs** suppress appetite, which reduces food intake and, over time, may result in weight loss. The Food and Drug Administration (FDA) in the United States has pulled several drugs off the market and not approved other drugs due to concerns about cardiovascular complications associated with long-term use. Prescription drugs still available for the *long-term* treatment of obesity include orlistat (Xenical), lorcaserin (Belviq), and phentermine-topiramate (Qsymia).

Orlistat inhibits lipase and leads to partial hydrolysis of triglycerides. Because fats are only partially digested and absorbed, caloric intake is decreased. Most patients taking this drug have GI symptoms that include loose stools, abdominal cramps, and nausea unless they reduce their fat intake to less than 30% of their food intake each day. Therefore the drug should be used with caution and limited to adults between 18 and 75 years of age. Treatment is usually not extended beyond 12 months. A lower-dose 60-mg orlistat tablet (Alli) is the only *over-the-counter* weight-loss aid product that has received FDA approval for long-term use.

Lorcaserin (Belviq) works by activating the serotonin 2C receptor in the brain to help decrease appetite and create a sense of feeling full after eating small amounts of food (Mayo Clinic, 2014). Side effects may include headaches, dizziness, dry mouth, and constipation. Teach patients to report the signs of the rare but serious side effect of serotonin syndrome, including suicidal thoughts, psychiatric concerns, and problems with memory or comprehension (Mayo Clinic, 2014).

Phentermine-topiramate (Qsymia) combines a short-term weight-loss drug (phentermine) with a drug that is used to control seizures (topiramate) (Mayo Clinic, 2014). Side effects may include an increased heart rate, hand and feet tingling, insomnia, dizziness, dry mouth, and constipation. Teach patients that a rare but serious side effect that is associated with this drug is suicidal thoughts, which should immediately be reported to the prescribing health care provider (Mayo Clinic, 2014).

Other sympathomimetic drugs suppress appetite for *short-term* use along with a structured weight-management and exercise program. These drugs act on the central nervous system, including suppressing the appetite center in the hypothalamus. Examples include phentermine (Adipex-P), diethylpropion (Tenuate, Tenuate Dospan), and phendimetrazine (Bontril).

! NURSING SAFETY PRIORITY (QSEN)

Drug Alert

Patients with hypertension, heart disease, and hyperthyroidism should not take anorectic drugs because they may worsen their symptoms. These drugs are not prescribed for any patient taking psychoactive agents because they cause similar side effects. Teach patients who are candidates for sympathomimetic drugs about side effects, which include:

- Palpitations
- Diarrhea or constipation
- Restlessness
- Insomnia
- Dry mouth
- Blurred vision (especially with Bontril)
- Change in sex drive or activity
- Anxiety

Behavioral Management. Behavioral management of obesity helps the patient change daily eating habits to lose weight. Self-monitoring techniques include keeping a record of foods eaten (food diary), exercise patterns, and emotional and situational factors. Stimulus control involves controlling the external cues that promote overeating. Reinforcement techniques are used to self-reward the behavior change. Cognitive restructuring involves modifying negative beliefs by learning positive coping self-statements. Counseling by health care professionals must continue before, during, and after treatment. The 12-step program offered by Overeaters Anonymous (www.oa.org) has helped many people lose weight, especially those who are compulsive eaters.

Complementary and Alternative Therapies. Many complementary and alternative therapies have been tested and used for obesity. These modalities aim to suppress appetite and therefore limit food intake to lose weight:

- Acupuncture
- Acupressure
- Ayurveda (a combination of holistic approaches)
- Hypnosis

Surgical Management. At any weight, some patients seek to improve their appearance by having a variety of cosmetic procedures to reduce the amount of adipose tissue in selected areas of the body. A typical example of this type of surgery is **liposuction**, which can be done in a physician's office or ambulatory surgery center. Although the patient's appearance improves, if weight gain continues, the fatty tissue will return. This procedure is not a solution for people who are morbidly obese.

Morbidly obese people who do not respond to traditional interventions may be considered for a major surgical procedure aimed at producing permanent weight loss. Patients with a body mass index (BMI) of 40 or greater or a BMI of 35 or greater along with additional risk factors are considered for surgery. Surgery has been perceived as a last resort to address weight issues, but it *is the only method that has a long-term impact on morbid obesity.*

Bariatrics. **Bariatrics** is a branch of medicine that manages patients with obesity and its related diseases. Surgical procedures include these three types: gastric restrictive, malabsorption, or both. *Restrictive* surgeries decrease the volume capacity of the stomach to limit the amount of food that can be eaten at one time. As the name implies, *malabsorption* procedures interfere with the absorption of food and nutrients from the GI tract.

Every year more than 200,000 people in the United States have bariatric surgical procedures (American Society for Bariatric Surgery, 2013), and that number continues to increase. The surgeon may use a conventional open approach or minimally invasive surgery (MIS). Most patients have MIS by having either the laparoscopic adjustable gastric band (LAGB) procedure or the laparoscopic sleeve gastrectomy (LSG). Both procedures are classified as restrictive surgeries (Virji, 2011). The decision of whether the patient is a candidate for the MIS is based on weight, body build, history of abdominal surgery, and co-existing medical complications. With any surgical approach, patients must agree to modify their lifestyle and follow stringent protocols to lose weight and keep the weight off. After bariatric surgery, many patients no longer have complications of obesity, such as diabetes mellitus, hypertension, depression, or sleep apnea.

Preoperative Care. Preoperative care is similar to that for any patient undergoing abdominal surgery or laparoscopy (see Chapter 14). However, obese patients are at increased surgical risks of pulmonary and thromboembolitic complications, as well as death. Some surgeons require limited weight loss before bariatric surgery to decrease these complications. Patients also have a thorough psychological assessment and testing to detect depression, substance abuse, or other mental health/behavioral health problem that could interfere with their success after surgery. Cognitive ability, coping skills, development, motivation, expectations, and support systems are also assessed. Patients who are not alert and oriented or do not have sufficient strength and mobility are not considered for bariatric surgery. *The primary role of the nurse is to reinforce health teaching in preparation for surgery.* Most bariatric surgical centers provide education sessions for groups of patients who plan to have the procedure.

Operative Procedures. *Gastric restriction* surgeries allow for normal digestion without the risk for nutrition deficiencies. In the LAGB procedure, the surgeon places an adjustable band to create a small proximal stomach pouch through a laparoscope (Fig. 60-4, *A*). The band may or may not be inflatable. For example, the REALIZE band requires that saline be injected into a balloon to control the tightness of the band. This type of procedure is considered to be restrictive; malabsorption complications usually do not occur (Virji, 2011). For the LSG, the surgeon removes the portion of the stomach where ghrelin, the "hunger hormone," is secreted. Restrictive surgeries are the easiest to perform. However, weight lost is often regained after a period of time. By contrast, patients having the malabsorption procedures maintain 60% to 70% of their weight loss even after 20 years.

The most common *malabsorption surgery* performed in the United States is the *Roux-en-*Y *gastric bypass (RNYGB),* which is often done as a robotic-assistive surgical procedure. This procedure results in quick weight loss, but it is more invasive with a higher risk for postoperative complications. In RNYGB, most commonly just called a **gastric bypass**, gastric resection is combined with malabsorption surgery (Virji, 2011). The patient's stomach, duodenum, and part of the jejunum are bypassed so that fewer calories can be absorbed (see Fig. 60-4, *B*).

Postoperative Care. Postoperative care depends on the type of surgery—the conventional open approach or the minimally invasive technique. Although many patients have MIS, they are

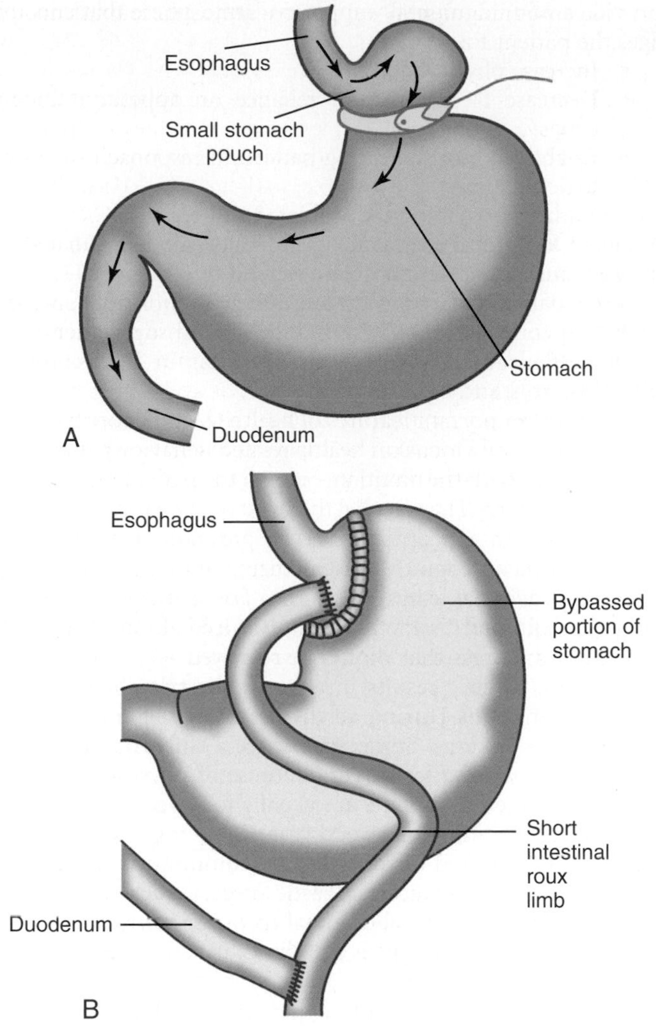

FIG. 60-4 Bariatric surgical procedures. **A,** Adjustable banded gastroplasty. **B,** Roux-en-Y gastric bypass (RNYGB).

considered as having major abdominal surgery along with all its risks and are cared for accordingly. These patients may require less than 24 hours in the hospital; some may need 1 to 2 days. Patients with open procedures may need several days to recover.

Patients having one of the MIS procedures have less pain, scarring, and blood loss. They typically have a faster recovery time and a faster return to daily activities.

The priority for immediate care of postoperative bariatric surgery patients is airway management. Patients with short and thick necks often have compromised airways and need aggressive respiratory support—possibly mechanical ventilation in the critical care unit.

All patients experience some degree of pain, but it is usually less severe when MIS is done. Patients may use patient-controlled analgesia (PCA) with morphine for up to the first 24 hours. All patients receive oral opioid analgesic agents as prescribed after the PCA is discontinued. Liquid forms of drug therapy are preferred. Acute pain management is discussed in detail in Chapter 3.

Care of the bariatric surgical patient is similar to that of any patient having abdominal or laparoscopic surgery. *A major focus is patient and staff safety.* Special bariatric equipment and accommodations, including an extra-wide bed and additional personnel for moving the patient, are needed for both the surgical suite and postoperative care units. Weight-rated beds must be wide enough to allow the patient to turn. Bed rails should not be touching the body because they can cause pressure areas. Pressure between skinfolds, as well as tubes and catheters, can also cause skin breakdown. Monitor the skin in these areas, and keep it clean and dry.

! NURSING SAFETY PRIORITY QSEN

Action Alert

Some patients who have bariatric surgery have a nasogastric (NG) tube put in place, especially after open surgical procedures. In gastroplasty procedures, the NG tube drains both the proximal pouch and the distal stomach. Closely monitor the tube for patency. *Never reposition the tube because its movement can disrupt the suture line!* The NG tube is removed on the second day if the patient is passing flatus.

Clear liquids are introduced slowly if the patient can tolerate water, and 1-ounce cups are used for each serving. Pureed foods, juice, and soups thinned with broth, water, or milk are added to the diet 24 to 48 hours after clear liquids are tolerated. Typically, the patient can increase the volume to 1 ounce over 5 minutes or until satisfied, but the diet is limited to liquids or pureed foods for 6 weeks. The patient then progresses to regular food, with an emphasis on nutrient-dense foods. Nausea, vomiting, or discomfort occurs if too much liquid is ingested.

! NURSING SAFETY PRIORITY QSEN

Critical Rescue

Anastomotic leaks are the most common serious complication and cause of death after gastric bypass surgery. Monitor for manifestations of this life-threatening problem, including increasing back, shoulder, or abdominal pain; restlessness, and unexplained tachycardia and oliguria (scant urine). Report any of these findings to the surgeon immediately!

In addition to the postoperative complications typically associated with abdominal and laparoscopic surgeries, bariatric patients have special needs and risks, such as the risk for anastomotic leaks (a leak of digestive juices and partially digested food through an anastomosis).

Implement these measures to prevent complications:

- Apply an abdominal binder to prevent wound dehiscence for open surgical procedures.
- Place the patient in semi-Fowler's position or use bi-level or continuous positive airway pressure (BiPAP or CPAP) ventilation at night to improve breathing and decrease risk for sleep apnea or other pulmonary complications, such as pneumonia and atelectasis.
- Monitor oxygen saturation; provide oxygen at 2 L/min as prescribed.
- Apply sequential compression stockings and administer prophylactic anticoagulant (usually heparin) therapy as prescribed to help prevent thromboembolitic complications, including pulmonary embolism (PE), a Joint Commission Core Measure intervention to prevent venous thromboembolism (VTE).

- Observe skin areas and folds for redness, excoriation, or breakdown to treat these problems early.
- Use absorbent padding between folds to prevent pressure areas and skin breakdown; make sure that tubes and catheters are not causing pressure as well.
- Remove urinary catheter within 24 hours after surgery to prevent urinary tract infection per the National Patient Safety Goals.
- Assist the patient out of bed on the day of surgery; encourage and assist with turning every 2 hours using an appropriate weight-bearing overhead trapeze. Collaborate with the physical or occupational therapist if needed for transfers or ambulation assistive devices, such as walkers.
- Ambulate patient as soon as possible to prevent postoperative complications, such as deep vein thrombosis and pulmonary embolus.
- Measure and record abdominal girth daily, as requested.
- In collaboration with the dietitian, provide six small feedings and plenty of fluids to prevent dehydration.
- Observe for signs and symptoms of **dumping syndrome** (caused by food entering the small intestine instead of the stomach) after *gastric bypass,* such as tachycardia, nausea, diarrhea, and abdominal cramping.

CLINICAL JUDGMENT CHALLENGE

Patient-Centered Care; Evidence-Based Practice; Teamwork and Collaboration; Informatics QSEN

A 32-year-old morbidly obese woman had a laparoscopic sleeve gastrectomy procedure yesterday afternoon as part of a long-term plan for weight loss. She tells you that despite having had surgery, she is afraid she will not live long enough to see her children grow up. She is diaphoretic, with respirations of 32 per minute. You notice that she is wringing her hands as she talks.

1. What patient problems do you think she is having at this time? What data support your answer?
2. What priority health assessments will you perform at this time, and why?
3. How will you respond to her problems at this time, and why?
4. With which members of the health care team will you collaborate to address the patient's immediate concerns?
5. When she is ready for discharge, what health teaching will you provide related to the *Healthy People 2020 and 2010 Dietary Guidelines for Americans?* Find the complete evidence-based documents online, and develop a teaching plan for this patient.
6. To which community resources would you refer this patient, and why?

Community-Based Care

Obese patients are cared for in a variety of settings, including the acute care hospital and transitional care unit (particularly after surgery) or in their own home. Obesity is a chronic, lifelong problem. Diets, drug therapy, exercise, and behavior modification can produce short-term weight losses with reasonable safety. However, most patients who do lose weight often regain the weight. Treatment of obesity should focus on the long-term reduction of health risks and medical problems associated with obesity, improving quality of life, and promoting a health-oriented lifestyle. Interdisciplinary team members need to provide a nonjudgmental, supportive atmosphere that encourages the patient to:

- Increase physical activity
- Decrease fat intake and reliance on appetite-reducing drugs
- Establish a normal eating pattern in response to physiologic hunger
- Address psychological problems and concerns

Frequent long-term ambulatory care follow-up coordinated by a case manager is essential for successful treatment.

Teach patients that bowel changes are common after surgery, including constipation. Vitamin and mineral supplements are often needed after surgery, especially vitamin D, B-complex vitamins, iron, and calcium.

The most important features of health teaching for any obese patient and family focus on health-related behavior patterns. In collaboration with the dietitian, counsel the patient on a healthful eating pattern. The physical therapist or exercise physiologist recommends an appropriate exercise program. A psychologist may recommend cognitive restructuring approaches that help alter dysfunctional eating patterns. For patients who have surgery, additional discharge teaching is needed. Chart 60-7 lists the important areas that should be reviewed.

Bariatric surgery results in a major lifestyle change and a variety of emotions. During weight loss, the patient may become depressed or anxious. Some experience a "hibernation phase" for about a month after surgery because of physical and emotional adjustments. Patients are usually followed closely by the surgeon and dietitian for several years. Encourage them to keep all appointments and to adhere to the community-based treatment plan to ensure success. Plastic surgery, such as **panniculectomy** (removal of the abdominal apron, or **panniculus**), may be performed after weight is stabilized, usually in about 18 to 24 months.

Provide the patient with a list of available community resources, such as Overeaters Anonymous (www.oa.org) and the American Obesity Association (www.obesity.org). For surgical patients, the American Society for Metabolic and Bariatric Surgery (www.asmbs.org) may be helpful.

CHART 60-7 Patient and Family Education: Preparing for Self-Management

Discharge Teaching for the Patient After Bariatric Surgery

Nutrition: Diet progression, nutrient (including vitamin and mineral) supplements, hydration guidelines

Drug therapy: Analgesics and antiemetic drugs, if needed; drugs for other health problems

Wound care: Clean procedure for open or laparoscopic wounds; cover during shower or bath

Activity level: Restrictions, such as avoiding lifting; activity progression; return to driving and work

Signs and symptoms to report: Fever; excessive nausea or vomiting; epigastric, back, or shoulder pain; red, hot, and/or draining wound(s); pain, redness, or swelling in legs; chest pain; difficulty breathing

Follow-up care: Health care provider office or clinic visits, support groups and other community resources, counseling for patient and family

Continuing education: Nutrition and exercise classes; follow-up visits with dietitian

NURSING CONCEPTS AND CLINICAL JUDGMENT REVIEW

What might you NOTICE if the patient is experiencing inadequate NUTRITION as a result of malnutrition or obesity?

Malnutrition:
- Weight below ideal body weight or report of unexplained weight loss of 10 lbs (4.5 kg) in 6 months
- Dry, flaky skin
- Brittle nails and hair
- Leanness
- Activity intolerance
- Report of lethargy or fatigue
- Weakness
- Complications, such as infections, pressure ulcers, poor healing

Obesity:
- Weight at least 20% above ideal
- Excessive fat
- Shortness of breath during activity or at rest
- Slowed movement
- Change in gait or limping
- Complications, such as type 2 diabetes mellitus, hypertension, depression

What should you INTERPRET and how should you RESPOND to a patient experiencing inadequate NUTRITION as a result of malnutrition or obesity?

Perform and interpret assessments, including:
- Taking and recording height and weight
- Calculating BMI based on height and weight
- Checking laboratory values for hematocrit and hemoglobin and visceral proteins
- Taking complete medical history to determine associated complications and cause of nutrition problem
- Assessing impact of nutrition status on daily life, including ADLs
- Assessing coping mechanisms, especially for patients who are morbidly obese

Respond by:
- Teaching patients about their need for a healthy nutrition state
- Teaching patients how to either lose or gain weight, depending on their specific problem (e.g., nutrition supplements for malnutrition; restrictive diet and exercise for obesity)
- Teaching patients to weigh frequently
- Monitoring changes in serum visceral proteins (especially prealbumin) as an indicator of improved nutrition for malnourished patients
- Initiating total enteral or total parenteral nutrition as prescribed for malnutrition
- Informing morbidly obese patients about bariatric surgery options

On what should you REFLECT?
- Monitor patient for indicators of improved nutrition (e.g., increased prealbumin and weight for malnutrition; weight loss and decreased fat for obesity).
- Think about what may have caused these nutrition problems and how they can be prevented.
- Think about what else you can do to improve nutritional health of patients you care for.

GET READY FOR THE NCLEX® EXAMINATION!

KEY POINTS

Review these Key Points for each NCLEX Examination Client Needs Category.

Safe and Effective Care Environment
- Collaborate with the interdisciplinary health care team, especially the dietitian, health care provider, and case manager, when caring for patients with malnutrition or obesity. **Teamwork and Collaboration** QSEN
- Be sure that bariatric furniture and equipment are available for the obese patient in the hospital or other health care setting; avoid pressure on skinfold areas. **Safety** QSEN

Health Promotion and Maintenance
- Perform nutrition screening for all patients to determine if they are at risk (see Charts 60-1 and 60-2).
- Recall the recommendations included in the *2010 Dietary Guidelines for Americans* as listed in Table 60-1.
- Older patients are at increased risk for malnutrition (see Chart 60-2).
- Implement interventions to promote nutrition intake in older adults as specified in Chart 60-3. **Patient-Centered Care** QSEN

Psychosocial Integrity
- Be aware that some obese patients may not view their weight as a problem and are therefore unlikely to be part of a weight-reduction plan.
- Recognize that obesity can cause depression or anxiety, low self-esteem, and a disturbed body image.
- Be aware of legal and ethical issues related to tube-feeding older adults with chronic or terminal illness.

Physiological Integrity
- Review serum prealbumin, hemoglobin, and hematocrit levels to identify patients at nutrition risk.
- Assess patients with severe malnutrition for common complications, such as edema, lethargy, and dry, flaking skin.

- Provide evidence-based nursing interventions for managing total enteral nutrition as listed in Chart 60-4. **Evidence-Based Practice** QSEN
- Maintain feeding tube patency for patients receiving total enteral nutrition as described in Chart 60-5. **Safety** QSEN
- Ensure that feeding tube placement is verified by x-ray; check placement every 4 to 8 hours by aspirating gastric contents and assessing pH for nasogastric tubes. **Safety** QSEN
- Place patients receiving tube feeding in a semi-Fowler's position at all times to prevent aspiration; check residual contents every 4 hours or as designated per facility policy. **Safety** QSEN
- Use gloves when changing feeding system tubing or adding product; use sterile gloves when working with critically ill or immunocompromised patients.
- Use a feeding pump when the patient receives continuous or cyclic tube feeding.
- For patients receiving enteral or parenteral nutrition at home, teach family members or other caregivers how to provide NUTRITION while avoiding complications.
- Teach patients who are undernourished to eat high-protein, high-calorie foods and nutrition supplements.
- Provide care for patients receiving total parenteral nutrition as specified in Chart 60-6. **Evidence-Based Practice** QSEN
- Recall that normal body mass index (BMI) for adults should be between 18.5 and 25; older adults should have a BMI between 23 and 27. A BMI of 27 to 30 indicates overweight, over 30 indicates obesity, and 40 and greater indicates morbid obesity.
- Recall that obesity causes early onset of many chronic illnesses, such as osteoarthritis, diabetes mellitus, hypertension, and coronary artery disease. Pulmonary problems (e.g., obstructive sleep apnea), delayed wound healing, and infections are also common.
- Instruct obese patients about the importance of health care provider–approved exercise for weight reduction.
- Recognize that many people are following low-carbohydrate rather than low-fat diets to lose weight.
- Remember that bariatric surgery includes gastric restriction procedures or gastric bypass; a panniculectomy may be performed to remove skinfolds once weight is stabilized.
- Be alert for signs and symptoms of anastomotic leak after bariatric surgery, including severe pain, restlessness, anxiety, and unexplained tachycardia. **Safety** QSEN
- Provide postoperative care for patients having bariatric surgery to prevent complications such as wound dehiscence, respiratory distress, skin breakdown, and thromboembolitic complications, such as pulmonary embolism. Establishing and maintaining an airway is the priority for patients having bariatric surgery! **Safety** QSEN
- Observe for complications, such as dumping syndrome in patients who have a gastric bypass. Tachycardia, nausea, diarrhea, and abdominal cramping are common manifestations of dumping syndrome.
- Provide discharge teaching for patients having bariatric surgery as described in Chart 60-7.

CHAPTER 61

Assessment of the Endocrine System

M. Linda Workman

http://evolve.elsevier.com/Iggy/

PRIORITY CONCEPTS

- NUTRITION
- ELIMINATION

LEARNING OUTCOMES

Health Promotion and Maintenance

1. Teach all people measures to take to protect the endocrine system.

Psychosocial Integrity

2. Reduce the psychological impact for the patient and family regarding the assessment and testing of the endocrine system.

Physiological Integrity

3. Apply the principles of anatomy, physiology, and the aging process to assess the endocrine system and homeostasis.
4. Perform a focused assessment of endocrine function, incorporating information about genetic risk, age-related changes, and NUTRITION affecting endocrine function.
5. Coordinate appropriate care for patients and proper handling of specimens during testing of NUTRITION, ELIMINATION, and the endocrine system.

The tissues and organs of the endocrine system are located in many body areas (Fig. 61-1). Endocrine glands secrete **hormones**, which are natural chemicals that exert their effects on specific tissues known as **target tissues**. Target tissues are usually located some distance from the endocrine gland, with no connecting duct between the endocrine gland and its target tissue. For this reason, endocrine glands are called "ductless" glands and use the blood to transport secreted hormones to the target tissues (McCance et al., 2014). Endocrine glands include:

- Hypothalamus (a neuroendocrine gland)
- Pituitary gland
- Adrenal glands
- Thyroid gland
- Islet cells of the pancreas
- Parathyroid glands
- Gonads

The endocrine system working with the nervous system controls overall body function and regulation, including metabolism, NUTRITION, ELIMINATION, temperature, fluid and electrolyte balance, growth, and reproduction. Many interactions must occur between the endocrine system and all other body systems to ensure that each system maintains a constant normal balance (**homeostasis**) in response to environmental changes. For example, this regulation keeps the internal body temperature at or near 98.6° F (37° C), even when environmental temperatures vary. Other actions keep the serum sodium level between 136 and 145 mEq/L (mmol/L), regardless of whether a healthy person eats 2 g or 12 g of sodium per day.

Table 61-1 lists hormones secreted by various endocrine glands. Hormones travel through the blood to all body areas but exert their actions only on target tissues. They recognize their target tissues and exert their actions by binding to receptors on or within the target tissue cells. In general, each receptor site type is specific for only one hormone. Hormone-receptor actions work in a "lock and key" manner in that only the correct hormone (key) can bind to and activate the receptor site (lock) (Fig. 61-2). Binding a hormone to its receptor causes the target tissue to change its activity, producing specific responses.

Disorders of the endocrine system usually are related to:

- An excess of a specific hormone
- A deficiency of a specific hormone
- A receptor defect

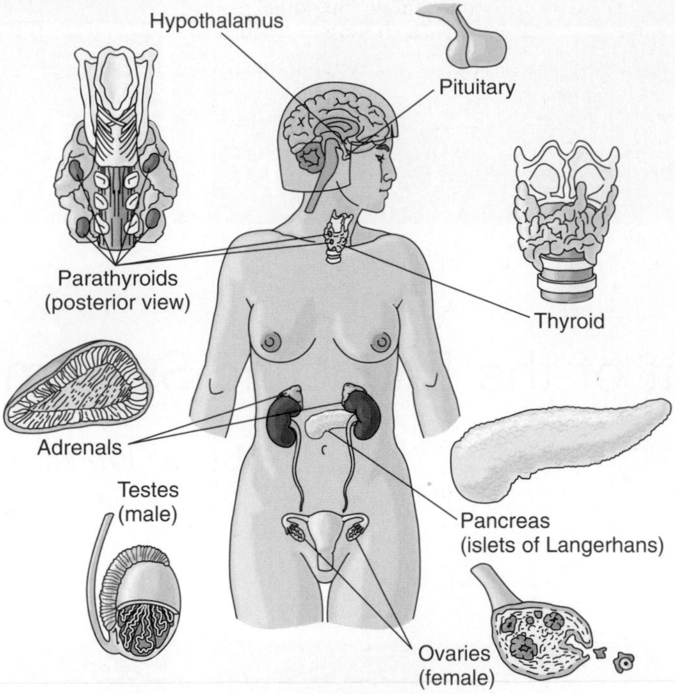

FIG. 61-1 The locations of various glands within the endocrine system.

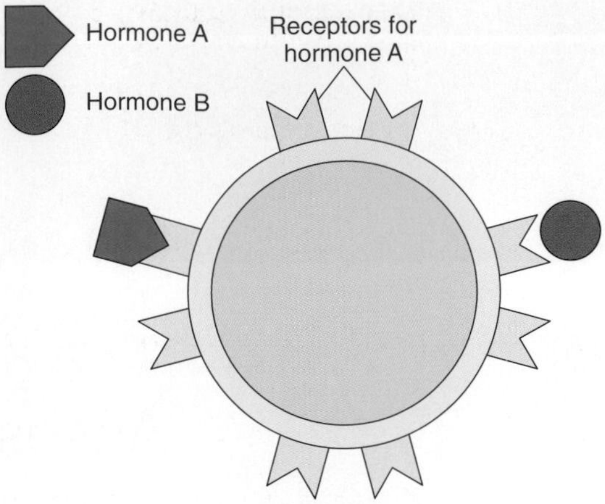

FIG. 61-2 "Lock and Key" hormone-receptor binding. *Hormone A* fits and binds to its receptors, causing a change in cell action. *Hormone B* does not fit or bind to receptors; no change in cell action results.

TABLE 61-1 Principal Hormones of the Endocrine Glands

GLAND	HORMONES
Hypothalamus	Corticotropin-releasing hormone (CRH) Thyrotropin-releasing hormone (TRH) Gonadotropin-releasing hormone (GnRH) Growth hormone–releasing hormone (GHRH) Growth hormone–inhibiting hormone (somatostatin GHIH) Prolactin-inhibiting hormone (PIH) Melanocyte-inhibiting hormone (MIH)
Anterior pituitary	Thyroid-stimulating hormone (TSH), also known as *thyrotropin* Adrenocorticotropic hormone (ACTH, corticotropin) Luteinizing hormone (LH), also known as *Leydig cell–stimulating hormone (LCSH)* Follicle-stimulating hormone (FSH) Prolactin (PRL) Growth hormone (GH) Melanocyte-stimulating hormone (MSH)
Posterior pituitary	Vasopressin (antidiuretic hormone [ADH]) Oxytocin
Thyroid	Triiodothyronine (T_3) Thyroxine (T_4) Calcitonin
Parathyroid	Parathyroid hormone (PTH)
Adrenal cortex	Glucocorticoids (cortisol) Mineralocorticoids (aldosterone)
Ovary	Estrogen Progesterone
Testes	Testosterone
Pancreas	Insulin Glucagon Somatostatin

ANATOMY AND PHYSIOLOGY REVIEW

The control of cellular function by any hormone depends on a series of reactions working through negative feedback control mechanisms. Hormone secretion usually depends on the body's need for the final action of that hormone. When a body condition starts to move away from the normal range and a specific response is needed to correct this change, secretion of the hormone capable of starting the correcting action or response is stimulated until the need (demand) is met, and the body condition returns to the normal range. As the correction occurs, hormone secretion decreases (and may halt). This control of hormone synthesis is "**negative feedback**" because the hormone causes the *opposite* action of the initial condition change.

An example of a simple negative feedback hormone response is the control of insulin secretion. When blood glucose levels start to rise above normal, the hormone *insulin* is secreted. Insulin increases glucose uptake by the cells, causing a *decrease* in blood glucose levels. Thus the action of insulin (decreasing blood glucose levels) is the opposite of or negative to the condition that stimulated insulin secretion (elevated blood glucose levels).

Some hormones have more complex interactions for negative feedback. These interactions involve a series of reactions in which more than one endocrine gland, as well as the final target tissues, is stimulated. In this situation, the first hormone in the series may have another endocrine gland or glands as its target tissue. The final result of complex negative feedback for endocrine function is still opposite of the initiating condition.

An example of complex control is the interaction of the hypothalamus and the anterior pituitary with the adrenal cortex (Fig. 61-3). Low blood levels of cortisol from the adrenal cortex stimulate the secretion of corticotropin-releasing hormone (CRH) in the hypothalamus. CRH stimulates the anterior pituitary gland to secrete adrenocorticotropic hormone (ACTH). ACTH then triggers the release of cortisol from the adrenal cortex, the final endocrine gland in this series. The rising blood levels of cortisol inhibit CRH release from the hypothalamus. Without CRH, the anterior pituitary gland stops secretion of ACTH. In response, normal blood cortisol levels are maintained.

The normal blood level range of each hormone is well defined. Excesses or deficiencies of hormone secretion can lead to pathologic conditions.

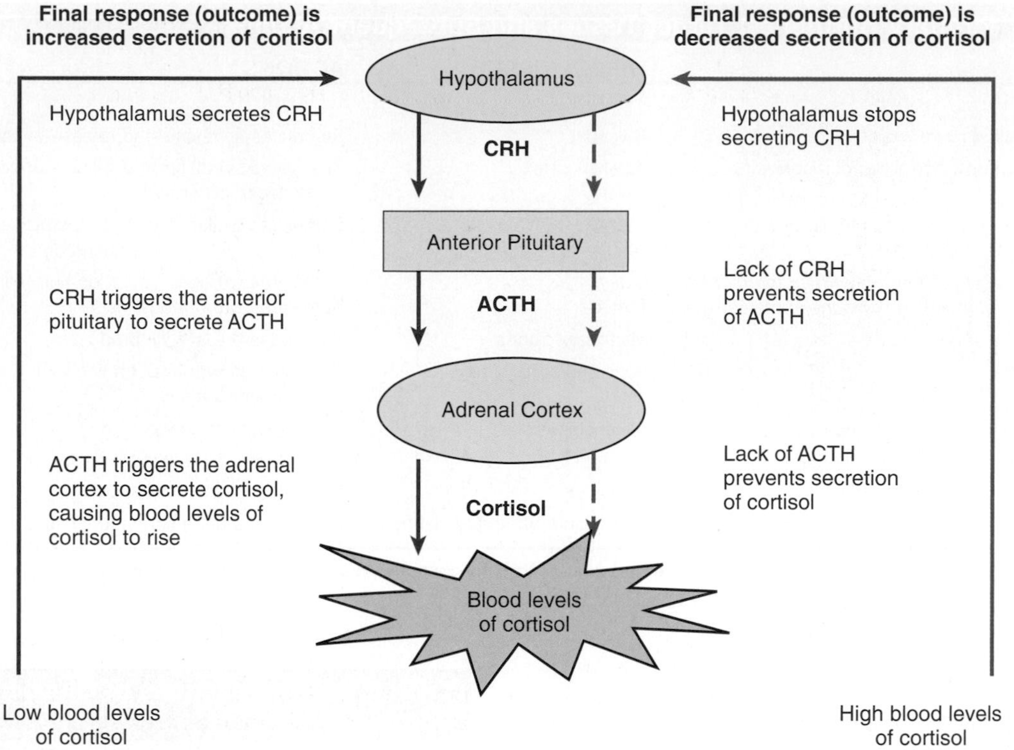

FIG. 61-3 Examples of positive and negative feedback control of hormone secretion. *ACTH,* Adrenocorticotropic hormone; *CRH,* corticotropin-releasing hormone.

Hypothalamus and Pituitary Glands

The hypothalamus is a small area of nerve and endocrine tissue located beneath the thalamus in the brain. Nerve fibers connect the hypothalamus to the rest of the central nervous system. The hypothalamus shares a small, closed circulatory system with the anterior pituitary gland, known as the *hypothalamic-hypophysial portal system.* This system allows hormones produced in the hypothalamus to travel directly to the anterior pituitary gland so that only very small amounts are wasted in systemic circulation.

The function of the hypothalamus is to produce regulatory hormones (see Table 61-1). Some of these hormones are released into the blood and travel to the anterior pituitary, where they either stimulate or inhibit the release of anterior pituitary hormones.

The pituitary gland is located at the base of the brain in a protective pocket of the sphenoid bone (see Fig. 61-1). It is divided into the anterior lobe (*adenohypophysis*) and the posterior lobe (*neurohypophysis*). Nerve fibers in the hypophysial stalk connect the hypothalamus to the posterior pituitary (Fig. 61-4).

In response to the releasing hormones of the hypothalamus, the anterior pituitary secretes some tropic hormones that stimulate other endocrine glands. Other pituitary hormones, such as prolactin, produce their effect directly on final target tissues (Table 61-2).

The hormones of the posterior pituitary—vasopressin (antidiuretic hormone [ADH]) and oxytocin—are produced in the hypothalamus and delivered to the posterior pituitary where they are stored. These hormones are released into the blood when needed.

Other factors can affect the release of hormones from the pituitary gland. Drugs, diet, lifestyle, and pathologic conditions can increase or decrease pituitary hormone secretion.

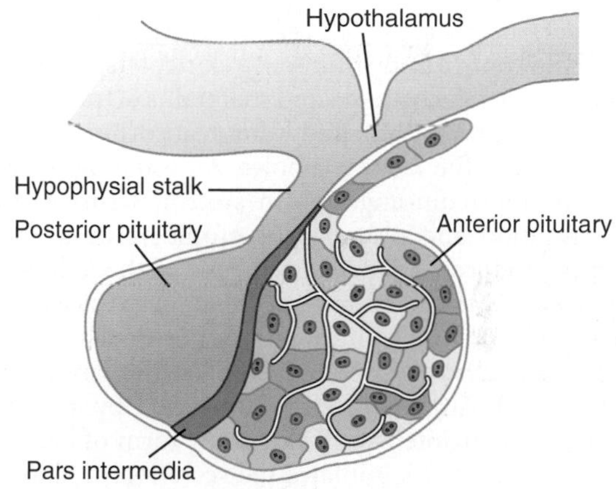

FIG. 61-4 The hypothalamus, hypophysial stalk, anterior pituitary gland, and posterior pituitary gland.

Gonads

The **gonads** are the male and female reproductive endocrine glands. Male gonads are the testes, and female gonads are the ovaries. Function of these glands begins at puberty when, under the influence of gonadotropic hormones secreted by the anterior pituitary, maturation of the glands and the external genitalia occurs. The testes are stimulated to produce testosterone, and the ovaries are stimulated to produce estrogen. The function of the gonads is detailed in Chapter 69.

Adrenal Glands

The adrenal glands are vascular, tent-shaped organs on the top of each kidney that have an outer cortex and an inner medulla (see Fig. 61-1). The adrenal hormones have effects throughout the body.

TABLE 61-2 Pituitary Hormones: Target Tissues and Subsequent Actions

HORMONE	TARGET TISSUE	ACTIONS
Anterior Pituitary		
TSH (thyroid-stimulating hormone or thyrotropin)	Thyroid	Stimulates synthesis and release of thyroid hormone
ACTH (adrenocorticotropic hormone, corticotropin)	Adrenal cortex	Stimulates synthesis and release of corticosteroids and adrenocortical growth
LH (luteinizing hormone [known as *Leydig cell–stimulating hormone* in males])	Ovary Testis	Stimulates ovulation and progesterone secretion Stimulates testosterone secretion
FSH (follicle-stimulating hormone [known as *interstitial cell–* or *Sertoli cell–stimulating hormone* in males])	Ovary Testis	Stimulates estrogen secretion and follicle maturation Stimulates spermatogenesis
PRL (prolactin)	Mammary glands	Stimulates breast milk production
GH (growth hormone)	Bone and soft tissue	Promotes growth through lipolysis, protein anabolism, and insulin antagonism
MSH (melanocyte-stimulating hormone)	Melanocytes	Promotes pigmentation
Posterior Pituitary*		
Vasopressin (antidiuretic hormone [ADH])	Kidney	Promotes water reabsorption
Oxytocin	Uterus and mammary glands	Stimulates uterine contractions and ejection of breast milk

*These hormones are synthesized in the hypothalamus and are stored in the posterior pituitary gland. They are transported from the hypothalamus down the hypothalamic stalk to the posterior pituitary while bound to proteins known as *neurophysins*.

Adrenal Cortex

The adrenal cortex makes up about 90% of the adrenal gland and has cells divided into three layers. The main hormone types secreted by the cortex are the mineralocorticoids and the glucocorticoids. In addition, the cortex also secretes small amounts of sex hormones.

Mineralocorticoids are produced and secreted by the adrenal cortex to help control body fluids and electrolytes. **Aldosterone** is the major mineralocorticoid and maintains extracellular fluid volume. It promotes sodium and water reabsorption and potassium excretion in the kidney tubules. Aldosterone secretion is regulated by the renin-angiotensin system, serum potassium ion concentration, and adrenocorticotropic hormone (ACTH).

Renin is produced by specialized cells of the kidney arterioles. Its release is triggered by a decrease in extracellular fluid volume from blood loss, sodium loss, or posture changes. Renin converts renin substrate (angiotensinogen), a plasma protein, to angiotensin I. Angiotensin I is converted by a converting enzyme to form angiotensin II, the active form of angiotensin. In turn, angiotensin II stimulates the secretion of aldosterone. Chapter 11 (Fig. 11-6) further explains the renin-angiotensin system. Aldosterone causes the kidney to reabsorb sodium and water to bring the plasma volume and osmolarity back to normal.

Serum potassium level also controls aldosterone secretion. It is secreted whenever the serum potassium level increases above normal by as little as 0.1 mEq/L. Aldosterone then enhances kidney excretion of potassium to reduce the blood potassium level back to normal.

Glucocorticoids are produced by the adrenal cortex and are essential for life. The main glucocorticoid produced by the adrenal cortex is **cortisol**. Cortisol affects:

- The body's response to stress
- Carbohydrate, protein, and fat metabolism
- Emotional stability
- Immune function
- Sodium and water balance

Cortisol also influences other important body processes. For example, it must be present for catecholamine action and maintaining the normal excitability of the heart muscle cells. Glucocorticoid functions are listed in Table 61-3.

TABLE 61-3 Functions of Glucocorticoid Hormones

- Prevent hypoglycemia by increasing liver gluconeogenesis and inhibiting peripheral glucose use
- Maintain excitability and responsiveness of cardiac muscle
- Increase lipolysis, releasing glycerol and free fatty acids
- Increase protein catabolism
- Degrade collagen and connective tissue
- Increase the number of mature neutrophils released from bone marrow
- Exert anti-inflammatory effects that decrease the migration of inflammatory cells to sites of injury
- Maintain behavior and cognitive functions

Glucocorticoid release is regulated directly by the anterior pituitary hormone *ACTH* and indirectly by the hypothalamic corticotropin-releasing hormone *(CRH)*. The release of CRH and ACTH is affected by the serum level of free cortisol, the normal sleep-wake cycle, and stress.

As described earlier and shown in Fig. 61-3, when blood cortisol levels are low, the hypothalamus secretes CRH, which triggers the pituitary to release ACTH. Then ACTH triggers the adrenal cortex to secrete cortisol. Adequate or elevated blood levels of cortisol *inhibit* the release of CRH and ACTH. This inhibitory effect is an example of a negative feedback system.

Glucocorticoid release peaks in the morning and reaches its lowest level 12 hours after each peak. Emotional, chemical, or physical stress increases the release of glucocorticoids.

Sex hormones (androgens and estrogens) are secreted in low levels by the adrenal cortex in both genders. Adrenal secretion of these hormones is usually not significant because the gonads (ovaries and testes) secrete much larger amounts of estrogens and androgens. In women, however, the adrenal gland is the major source of androgens.

NCLEX EXAMINATION CHALLENGE

Physiological Integrity

What effect on circulating levels of sodium and glucose does the nurse expect in a client who has been taking an oral cortisol preparation for 2 years because of a respiratory problem?

A. Decreased sodium; decreased glucose
B. Decreased sodium; increased glucose
C. Increased sodium; decreased glucose
D. Increased sodium; increased glucose

Adrenal Medulla

The adrenal medulla is a sympathetic nerve ganglion that has secretory cells. Stimulation of the sympathetic nervous system causes the release of adrenal medullary hormones, the **catecholamines** (which include epinephrine and norepinephrine). These hormones travel to all areas of the body through the blood and exert their effects on target cells. The adrenal medullary hormones are not essential for life because they also are secreted by other body tissues, but they do play a role in the stress response.

The adrenal medulla secretes about 15% norepinephrine (NE) and 85% epinephrine. Hormone effects vary with the specific receptor in the cell membranes of the target tissue.

These receptors are of two types: alpha adrenergic and beta adrenergic, which are further classified as $alpha_1$ and $alpha_2$ receptors and $beta_1$, $beta_2$, and $beta_3$ receptors. NE acts mainly on alpha-adrenergic receptors, and epinephrine acts mainly on beta-adrenergic receptors.

Catecholamines exert their actions on many target organs (Table 61-4). Activation of the sympathetic nervous system, which then releases adrenal medullary catecholamines, is an important part of the stress response. Catecholamines are secreted in small amounts at all times to maintain homeostasis. Stress triggers increased secretion of these hormones, resulting in the "fight-or-flight" response, a state of heightened physical and emotional awareness.

Thyroid Gland

The thyroid gland is in the anterior neck, directly below the cricoid cartilage (Fig. 61-5). It has two lobes joined by a thin strip of tissue *(isthmus)* in front of the trachea.

The thyroid gland is composed of follicular and parafollicular cells. Follicular cells produce the thyroid hormones **thyroxine (T_4)** and **triiodothyronine (T_3)**. Parafollicular cells produce **thyrocalcitonin** (TCT or calcitonin), which helps regulate serum calcium levels.

Control of metabolism occurs through T_3 and T_4. Both hormones increase metabolism, which causes an increase in oxygen use and heat production in all tissues. Most circulating T_4 and T_3 is bound to plasma proteins. The free hormone moves into the cell, where it binds to its receptor in the cell nucleus. Once in the cell, T_4 is converted to T_3, the most active thyroid hormone. The conversion of T_4 to T_3 is impaired by stress, starvation, dyes, and some drugs. Cold temperatures increase the conversion. Table 61-5 lists thyroid hormone functions.

Secretion of T_3 and T_4 is controlled by the hypothalamic-pituitary-thyroid gland axis negative feedback mechanism. The hypothalamus secretes thyrotropin-releasing hormone (TRH). TRH triggers the anterior pituitary gland to secrete thyroid-stimulating hormone (TSH), which then stimulates the thyroid

TABLE 61-4 Catecholamine Receptors and Effects of Adrenal Medullary Hormone Stimulation on Selected Organs and Tissues

ORGAN OR TISSUE	RECEPTORS	EFFECTS
Heart	$Beta_1$	Increased heart rate Increased contractility
Blood vessels	Alpha $Beta_2$	Vasoconstriction Vasodilation
Gastrointestinal tract	Alpha Beta	Increased sphincter tone Decreased motility
Kidneys	$Beta_2$	Increased renin release
Bronchioles	$Beta_2$	Relaxation; dilation
Bladder	Alpha $Beta_2$	Sphincter contractions Relaxation of detrusor muscle
Skin	Alpha	Increased sweating
Fat cells	Beta	Increased lipolysis
Liver	Alpha	Increased gluconeogenesis and glycogenolysis
Pancreas	Alpha	Decreased glucagon and insulin release
	Beta	Increased glucagon and insulin release
Eyes	Alpha	Dilation of pupils

TABLE 61-5 Functions of Thyroid Hormones in Adults

- Control metabolic rate of all cells
- Promote sufficient pituitary secretion of growth hormone and gonadotropins
- Regulate protein, carbohydrate, and fat metabolism
- Exert effects on heart rate and contractility
- Increase red blood cell production
- Affect respiratory rate and drive
- Increase bone formation and decrease bone resorption of calcium
- Act as insulin antagonists

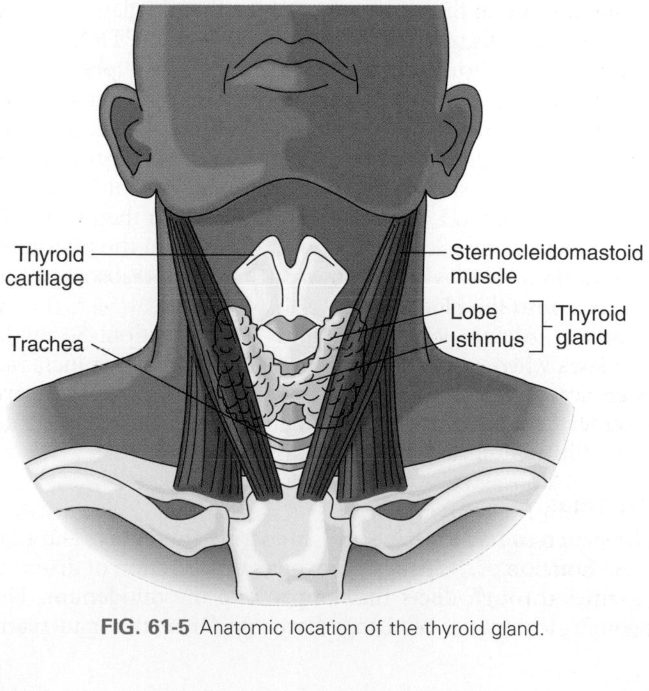

FIG. 61-5 Anatomic location of the thyroid gland.

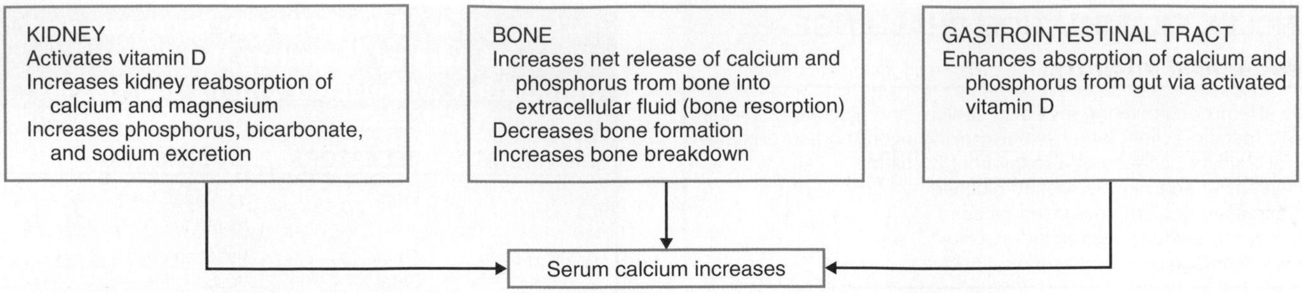

FIG. 61-6 Effects of parathyroid hormone on target tissues to maintain calcium balance.

gland to make and release thyroid hormones. If thyroid hormone levels are high, TRH and TSH release is inhibited. If thyroid hormone levels are low, release of TRH and TSH is increased. Cold and stress are two factors that cause the hypothalamus to secrete TRH, which then stimulates the anterior pituitary to secrete TSH.

Dietary intake of protein and iodine is needed to produce thyroid hormones. Iodine is absorbed from the intestinal tract as iodide. The thyroid gland withdraws iodide from the blood and concentrates it. After iodide is in the thyroid, it combines with the amino acid *tyrosine* to form T_4 and T_3. These hormones bind to thyroglobulin and are stored in the follicular cells of the thyroid gland. With stimulation, T_4 and T_3 are released into the blood. They enter many cells, where they bind to DNA receptors and turn on genes important in metabolism to regulate basal metabolic rate (BMR).

Calcium and phosphorus balance occurs partly through the actions of calcitonin (thyrocalcitonin [TCT]), which also is produced in the thyroid gland. Calcitonin lowers serum calcium and serum phosphorus levels by reducing bone resorption (breakdown). Its actions are opposite of parathyroid hormone.

The serum calcium level determines calcitonin secretion. Low serum calcium levels suppress the release of calcitonin. Elevated serum calcium levels increase its secretion.

Parathyroid Glands

The parathyroid glands consist of four small glands located close to or within the back surface of the thyroid gland (see Fig. 61-1). These cells secrete parathyroid hormone (PTH).

Parathyroid hormone regulates calcium and phosphorus metabolism by acting on bones, the kidneys, and the GI tract (Fig. 61-6). Bone is the main storage site of calcium. PTH increases **bone resorption** (bone release of calcium into the blood from bone storage sites), thus increasing serum calcium. In the kidneys, PTH activates vitamin D, which then increases the absorption of calcium and phosphorus from the intestines. In the kidney tubules, PTH allows calcium to be reabsorbed and put back into the blood.

Serum calcium levels determine PTH secretion. Secretion decreases when serum calcium levels are high, and it increases when serum calcium levels are low. PTH and calcitonin work together to maintain normal calcium levels in the blood and extracellular fluid.

Pancreas

The pancreas has exocrine and endocrine functions. The exocrine function of the pancreas involves the secretion of digestive enzymes through ducts that empty into the duodenum. The cells in the islets of Langerhans perform the pancreatic endocrine functions (Fig. 61-7). About one million islet cells are found throughout the pancreas.

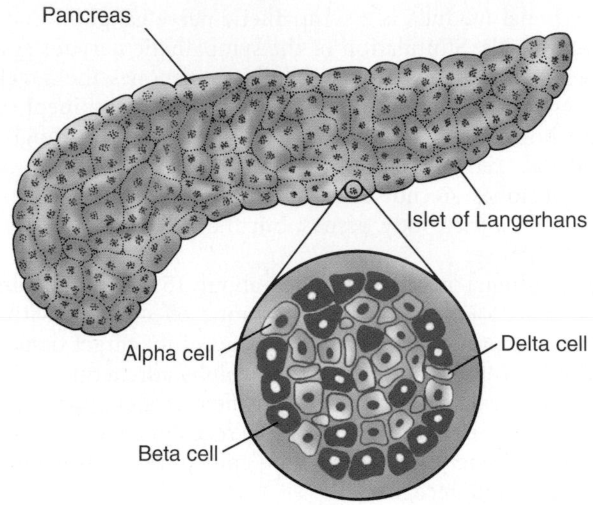

FIG. 61-7 The cells of the islets of Langerhans of the pancreas.

The islets have three distinct cell types: alpha cells, which secrete glucagon; beta cells, which secrete insulin; and delta cells, which secrete somatostatin. Glucagon and insulin affect carbohydrate, protein, and fat metabolism. Somatostatin, which is secreted not only in the pancreas but also in the intestinal tract and the brain, inhibits the release of glucagon and insulin from the pancreas. It also inhibits the release of gastrin, secretin, and other GI peptides.

Glucagon is a hormone that increases blood glucose levels. It is triggered by decreased blood glucose levels and increased blood amino acid levels. This hormone helps prevent hypoglycemia. Chapter 64 discusses glucagon function in more detail.

Insulin promotes the movement and storage of carbohydrate (CHO), protein, and fat. It lowers blood glucose levels by enhancing glucose movement across cell membranes and into the cells of many tissues. Basal levels of insulin are secreted continuously to control metabolism. Insulin secretion rises in response to an increase in blood glucose levels. More information on insulin is presented in Chapter 64.

Endocrine Changes Associated with Aging

The effects of aging on the endocrine system vary. The three endocrine tissues that usually have reduced function with aging are the gonads, the thyroid gland, and the endocrine pancreas (Touhy & Jett, 2014). It is difficult to distinguish normal from abnormal endocrine activity in older adults because of chronic illness, changes in diet and activity, sleep disturbances, decreased

CHART 61-1 Nursing Focus on the Older Adult

Changes in the Endocrine System Related to Aging

CHANGES	CLINICAL FINDINGS	NURSING ACTIONS/ADAPTATIONS
Decreased antidiuretic hormone (ADH) production	Urine is more dilute and may not concentrate when fluid intake is low.	The patient is at greater risk for dehydration. Assess the older patient more frequently for dehydration. If fluids are not restricted because of another health problem, teach unlicensed assistive personnel (UAP) to offer fluids at least every 2 hours while awake.
Decreased ovarian production of estrogen	Bone density decreases.	Teach the patient to engage in regular exercise and weight-bearing activity to maintain bone density. Handle the patient carefully to avoid injury from pathologic fractures.
	Skin is thinner, drier, and at greater risk for injury.	Avoid pulling or dragging the patient. Use minimal tape on the skin. Assist patients confined to bed or chairs to change positions at least every 2 hours. Teach patients to use skin moisturizers.
	Perineal and vaginal tissues become drier, and the risk for cystitis increases.	Perform or assist the patient to perform perineal care at least twice daily. Unless another health problem requires fluid restriction, encourage all women to drink at least 2 liters of fluids daily. Teach sexually active women to urinate immediately after sexual intercourse. Teach sexually active women that using vaginal lubricants with sexual activity can reduce discomfort and the risk for tissue damage.
Decreased glucose tolerance	Weight becomes greater than ideal along with: ▪ Elevated fasting blood glucose level ▪ Elevated random blood glucose level ▪ Slow wound healing ▪ Frequent yeast infections ▪ Polydipsia ▪ Polyuria	Obtain a family history of obesity and type 2 diabetes. Encourage the patient to engage in regular exercise and to keep body weight within 10 lbs of ideal. Teach patients the clinical manifestations of diabetes, and instruct them to report any of these manifestations to the health care provider. Suggest diabetes testing for any patient with: ▪ Persistent vaginal candidiasis ▪ Failure of a foot or leg skin wound to heal in 2 weeks or less ▪ Increased hunger and thirst ▪ Noticeable decrease in energy level
Decreased general metabolism	Less tolerant of cold. Decreased appetite. Decreased heart rate and blood pressure (BP).	Can be difficult to distinguish from hypothyroidism. Check for additional manifestations of: ▪ Lethargy ▪ Constipation (as a change from usual bowel habits) ▪ Decreased cognition ▪ Slowed speech ▪ Body temperature consistently below 97° F (36° C) ▪ Heart rate below 60 beats/min Teach patients to dress warmly in cool or cold weather.

metabolism, and the use of drugs that may affect hormone function. Consider these factors when assessing the older adult with endocrine dysfunction.

Encourage the older adult to participate in regular screening examinations, including fasting and random blood glucose checks, calcium level determinations, and thyroid function testing. Chart 61-1 lists the endocrine changes that occur in the older adult.

ASSESSMENT METHODS

Patient History

Use a systems approach to obtain the history of patients with a possible endocrine problem. This approach can be difficult because of the variety and combination of clinical manifestations. Physical, psychosocial, and laboratory findings are needed for a complete assessment of endocrine function.

The age and gender of the patient provide baseline assessment data. Certain disorders are more common in older than in younger patients, such as diabetes mellitus, loss of ovarian function, and decreased thyroid function.

Manifestations of endocrine disorders can be gender related, such as the sexual effects of hyperpituitarism and hypopituitarism (see Chapter 62). Thyroid problems are more common in women (McCance et al., 2014). Assess for a history of endocrine dysfunction, manifestations that could indicate an endocrine disorder, and hospitalizations. Ask about past and current drugs, such as hydrocortisone, levothyroxine, oral contraceptives, and antihypertensive agents. The use of exogenous hormone drugs, when not needed for hormone replacement, can cause serious dysfunction in many endocrine glands. Use the opportunity to warn patients about the dangers of misusing hormone-based drugs such as androgens and thyroid hormones.

Nutrition History

NUTRITION changes or GI tract disturbances may reflect many different endocrine problems. Ask about a history of nausea, vomiting, and abdominal pain. An increase or decrease in food or fluid intake may also indicate specific disorders. For example, diabetes insipidus triggers excessive thirst and adrenal hypofunction triggers salt craving. Hunger and thirst also are associated with diabetes mellitus. Rapid changes in weight without diet changes are often associated with several endocrine disorders, including diabetes mellitus and thyroid problems.

NUTRITION deficiencies from an inadequate diet, especially of protein and iodide-containing foods (salt-water fish and seafood, iodized table salt), may be a cause of an endocrine disorder. Teach the patient about a well-balanced diet that includes at least 60 g of protein daily, less animal fat, and fewer concentrated simple sugars. Teach patients who do not eat saltwater fish on a regular basis to use iodized salt in food preparation.

Family History and Genetic Risk

Ask the patient about any family history of obesity, growth or development difficulties, diabetes mellitus, infertility, or thyroid disorders. These problems may have an autosomal dominant, recessive, or cluster pattern of inheritance.

Current Health Problems

Focus on the patient's reason for seeking health care, asking questions such as:

- Did manifestations occur gradually, or was the onset sudden?
- Have you been treated for this problem in the past?
- How have the current problems affected your activities of daily living?

These questions can provide clues to specific endocrine disorders. Also explore changes in energy levels, ELIMINATION patterns, sexual and reproductive functions, and physical features.

Energy level changes occur with many endocrine problems, especially thyroid problems (see Chapter 63) and adrenal problems (see Chapter 62). Ask the patient about any change in ability to perform ADLs, and assess his or her current energy level. For instance, has he or she been sleeping longer or are fatigue and generalized weakness present?

ELIMINATION is affected by the endocrine system. Identify the patient's past pattern of elimination to determine deviations from the normal routine. Ask about the amount and frequency of urination. Does he or she urinate frequently in large amounts? Does the patient wake during the night to urinate (**nocturia**), or is pain present with urination (**dysuria**)? Information about the frequency of bowel movements and their consistency and color may provide clues to problems in fluid balance or metabolic rate (i.e., thyroid function).

Sexual and reproductive functions are greatly affected by endocrine disturbances. Ask women about any changes in the menstrual cycle, such as increased flow, duration, and frequency of menses; pain or excessive cramping; or a change in the regularity of menses. Ask men whether they have experienced impotence. Ask men and women about a change in libido (sexual desire) or any fertility problems.

Physical appearance changes can reflect an endocrine problem. Discuss any changes that the patient perceives in physical features. Ask about changes in:

- Hair texture and distribution
- Facial contours and eye protrusion
- Voice quality
- Body proportions
- Secondary sexual characteristics

For example, ask a man whether he is shaving less often or a woman if she has noticed an increase in facial hair. These changes may be associated with pituitary, thyroid, parathyroid, or adrenal dysfunction.

Physical Assessment

Inspection

An endocrine problem can change physical features because of its effect on growth and development, sex hormone levels, fluid and electrolyte balance, and metabolism. Different clinical findings can occur with many endocrine disorders or with nonendocrine problems.

Use a head-to-toe approach for inspection. Observe the patient's general appearance, and assess height, weight, fat distribution, and muscle mass in relation to age. Heredity and age rather than a health problem may be responsible for some physical features (e.g., short stature).

When examining the head, focus on abnormalities of facial structure, features, and expression, such as:

- Prominent forehead or jaw
- Round or puffy face
- Dull or flat expression
- Exophthalmos (protruding eyeballs and retracted upper lids)

Check the lower neck for a visible enlargement of the thyroid gland. Normally the thyroid tissue cannot be observed. The isthmus may be noticeable when the patient swallows. Jugular vein distention may be seen on inspection of the neck and can indicate fluid overload.

Observe skin color, and look for areas of pigment loss (hypopigmentation) or excess (hyperpigmentation). Fungal skin infections, slow wound healing, bruising, and petechiae are often seen in patients with adrenal hyperfunction. Skin infections, foot ulcers, and slow wound healing often occur with diabetes mellitus. With some types of adrenal gland dysfunction, the skin over joints, as well as any scar tissue, may show increased pigmentation due to increased levels of adrenocorticotropic hormone (ACTH) and melanocyte-stimulating hormone.

Vitiligo (patchy areas of pigment loss) is seen with primary hypofunction of the adrenal glands and is caused by autoimmune destruction of melanocytes in the skin. This is seen most often on the face, neck, arms, and legs. Mucous membranes may have large areas of uneven pigmentation. Document the location, color, distribution, and size of skin color changes.

Inspect the fingernails for malformation, thickness, or brittleness, all of which may suggest thyroid gland problems. Examine the extremities and the base of the spine for edema, which suggests a fluid and electrolyte imbalance.

Check the trunk for any abnormalities in chest size and symmetry. Truncal obesity and the presence of a "buffalo hump" between the shoulders on the back may indicate adrenocortical excess. Hormonal imbalance may also change secondary sexual characteristics. Inspect the breasts of both men and women for size, symmetry, pigmentation, and discharge. **Striae** (reddish purple "stretch marks") on the breasts or abdomen are often seen with adrenocortical excess.

Assess the patient's hair distribution for indications of endocrine gland dysfunction. Changes can include **hirsutism** (excessive growth of body hair, especially on the face, chest, and the center abdominal line of women), excessive scalp hair loss, or changes in hair texture.

Examination of the genitalia may reveal a dysfunction in hormone secretion. Observe the size of the scrotum and penis or of the labia and clitoris in relation to standards for the patient's age. The distribution and quantity of pubic hair are often affected in hypogonadism.

Palpation

The thyroid gland and the testes can be examined by palpation. Chapters 69 and 72 discuss examination of the testes. The thyroid gland is palpated for size, symmetry, general shape, and the presence of nodules or other irregularities.

Palpate the thyroid gland by standing either behind or in front of the patient. The posterior approach may be easier (Jarvis, 2016). Having the patient swallow sips of water during the examination helps you palpate the thyroid gland, which is not easily felt when normal.

Ask the patient to sit and to lower the chin. Using the posterior approach, place both your thumbs on the back of the patient's neck, with the fingers curved around to the front of the neck on either side of the trachea. Ask the patient to swallow, and locate the thyroid as you feel it rising. To examine the right lobe, turn the patient's head to the right and gently displace the trachea to the right with your left fingers. Placing your fingers between the trachea and the neck muscles, palpate the right lobe with your right hand. Reverse this procedure to examine the left lobe.

! NURSING SAFETY PRIORITY QSEN

Action Alert

Always palpate the thyroid gently because vigorous palpation can stimulate a thyroid storm in a person who has or is suspected to have hyperthyroidism.

Auscultation

Auscultate the chest to assess cardiac rate and rhythm to use later as a means of assessing treatment effectiveness. Some endocrine problems induce dysrhythmias. Many endocrine problems can cause dehydration and volume depletion. Document any difference in the patient's blood pressure and pulse in the lying, standing, or sitting positions (orthostatic vital signs).

If an enlarged thyroid gland is palpated, auscultate the area of enlargement for bruits. Hypertrophy of the thyroid gland causes an increase in vascular flow, which may result in bruits.

Psychosocial Assessment

Assess the patient's coping skills, support systems, and health-related beliefs. Many endocrine problems can change a patient's behaviors, personality, and psychological responses. Ask whether the patient has noticed a change in how stress is handled, frequency of crying, or degree of patience and anger expression. The patient may not recognize these changes in himself or herself. When possible, ask the family about changes in the patient's behaviors or personality.

A number of endocrine disorders affect the patient's perception of self. For example, body features can change significantly in disorders of the pituitary, adrenal, and thyroid glands. Infertility, impotence, and other changes in sexual function may result from endocrine dysfunction. Encourage the patient to express his or her feelings and concerns about a change in appearance or in sexual function. Ask about any difficulty in coping with such changes.

Patients with endocrine problems may require lifelong drugs and follow-up care. Assess their readiness to learn and ability to carry out specific self-management skills. Patients may also face financial difficulties resulting from a prolonged medical regimen or loss of employment. A referral to social service agencies may be needed.

CHART 61-2 Best Practice for Patient Safety & Quality Care QSEN

Endocrine Testing

For Blood Tests:

- Check your laboratory's method of handling hormone test samples for tube type, timing, drugs to be administered as part of the test, etc. For example, blood samples drawn for catecholamines must be placed on ice and taken to the laboratory immediately.
- Explain the procedure and any restrictions to the patient.
- If you are drawing blood samples from an IV line, clear the line thoroughly. Do not use a double- or triple-lumen line to obtain samples; contamination or dilution from another port is possible.
- Emphasize the importance of taking a drug prescribed for the test on *time*. Tell the patient to set an alarm if the drug is to be taken during the night.

For Urine Tests:

- Instruct the patient to begin the urine collection (whether for 2, 4, 8, 12, or 24 hours) by first emptying his or her bladder.
- Remind the patient to *not* save the urine specimen that begins the collection. The timing for the urine collection begins *after* this specimen.
- Tell the patient to note the time of the discarded specimen and to plan to collect all urine from this time until the end of the urine collection period.
- To end the collection, instruct the patient to empty his or her bladder at the end of the timed period and *add* that urine to the collection.
- Check with the laboratory to determine any special handling of the urine specimen (e.g., Is a preservative needed? Does the container need to be kept cold?).
- If needed, make sure that the preservative has been added to the collection container at the *beginning* of the collection.
- Tell the patient about any preservative and the need to avoid splashing urine from the container, because some preservatives make the urine caustic.
- If the specimen must be kept cool or cold, instruct the patient to place the container in an inexpensive cooler with ice. The specimen container should not be kept with food or drinks.

Diagnostic Assessment

Laboratory Assessment

Laboratory tests are an essential part of the diagnostic process for possible endocrine problems. Fluids commonly used for these tests include blood, urine, and saliva (Klee, 2011). Always check with the agency's laboratory for proper collection and handling of the specimen. The specialized testing for specific disorders is described in Chapters 62 to 64. Best practices for the collection of specimens for general endocrine testing are listed in Chart 61-2.

Assays. An assay measures the level of a specific hormone in blood or other body fluid. The most common assays for endocrine testing are antibody-based immunologic assays and chromatographic assays, which include mass spectrometry. These assays are very sensitive and can detect even minute quantities of a given hormone. Many different hormone concentrations can be analyzed at the same time by the mass spectrometry method.

Stimulation/Suppression Tests. Measurement of specific hormone blood levels does not always distinguish between the normal and the abnormal. The wide normal range for some hormones makes it necessary to trigger responses by stimulation or suppression tests.

For the patient who might have an underactive endocrine gland, a stimulus may be used to determine whether the gland is capable of normal hormone production. This method is called *stimulation testing.* Measured amounts of selected hormones are given to stimulate the target gland to maximum production. Hormone levels are then measured and compared with expected normal values. Failure of the hormone level to rise with stimulation indicates hypofunction.

Suppression tests are used when hormone levels are high or in the upper range of normal. Drugs or other substances known to normally suppress hormone production are administered. Failure of suppression of hormone production during testing indicates hyperfunction.

Venous Sampling. Blood samples are taken directly from veins that drain a specific endocrine gland, and hormone levels are measured. Unexpected blood hormone levels may indicate the location of a mass, a dysfunctional gland, or a dysfunctional part of a gland.

Urine Tests. Hormone levels and their metabolites in the urine can be measured to determine endocrine function. Because many of the endocrine hormones are secreted in a pulsatile fashion, measurement of a specific hormone in a 24-hour urine collection, rather than as a single blood or urine sample, better reflects specific gland function, such as the adrenal gland. Teach the patient how to collect a 24-hour urine sample (see also Chart 61-2).

Certain hormones require additives in the container at the beginning of the collection. Instruct the patient not to discard the preservative from the container and to use caution when handling it because some are caustic. Remind him or her that this collection is timed for *exactly* 24 hours. Instruct the patient to avoid taking any unnecessary drugs during endocrine testing because some drugs can interfere with the assay.

Tests for Glucose. Tests for functions of the islet cells of the pancreas measure the *result* of pancreatic islet cell function.

NCLEX EXAMINATION CHALLENGE

Health Promotion and Maintenance

Which precaution or action is most important for the nurse to teach the client who is to collect a 24-hour urine specimen for endocrine testing?

A. Eat a normal diet during the collection period.
B. Wear gloves when you urinate to prevent contamination of the specimen.
C. Urinate at the end of 24 hours and add that sample to the collection container.
D. Avoid walking, running, dancing, or any vigorous exercise during the collection period.

Blood glucose values and the oral glucose tolerance test help diagnose diabetes mellitus. The glycosylated hemoglobin (A1C) value reveals the *average* blood glucose level over a period of 2 to 3 months. (See Chapter 64 for diabetes mellitus testing.)

Imaging Assessment

Anterior, posterior, and lateral skull x-rays may be used to view the sella turcica, the bony pocket in the skull where the pituitary gland rests. Erosion of the sella turcica indicates invasion of the wall from an abnormal growth.

MRI with contrast is the most sensitive method of imaging the pituitary gland, although CT scans can also be used to evaluate it. The thyroid, parathyroid glands, ovaries, and testes are evaluated by ultrasound. CT scans are used to evaluate the adrenal glands, ovaries, and pancreas.

Other Diagnostic Assessment

Needle biopsy is a relatively safe and quick ambulatory surgery procedure used to indicate the composition of thyroid nodules. It is used to determine whether surgical intervention is needed.

NURSING CONCEPTS AND CLINICAL JUDGMENT REVIEW

What might you NOTICE in a patient with adequate NUTRITION related to endocrine function?

Vital signs:
- Heart rate and rhythm within normal range
- Oxygen saturation of 95% or higher
- Body temperature within normal range

Physical assessment:
- Weight proportionate to height; does not appear underweight or overweight
- Muscle development even with no muscle loss or excess
- Skin color and texture normal (no jaundice, striae, waxiness, edema, excessive dryness, or severe acne)
- Body hair distribution appropriate for gender
- Scalp hair thickness similar to family members with no recent changes
- Menstrual periods regular

Psychological assessment:
- Oriented and appropriate affect
- Not confused and does not have rapid changes of emotions that are out of proportion to existing situation
- Energy level good; can engage in desired work, recreational, and personal activities
- Sleep average 6 to 8 hours, feeling rested on awakening

Laboratory assessment:
- Hormone levels and production within normal limits for age and gender
- Serum electrolyte levels within normal limits
- Blood glucose levels within normal limits

GET READY FOR THE NCLEX® EXAMINATION!

KEY POINTS

Review these Key Points for each NCLEX Examination Client Needs Category.

Health Promotion and Maintenance

- Teach all patients that misusing hormones or steroids can have an adverse effect on endocrine function. **Patient-Centered Care** QSEN

Psychosocial Integrity

- Encourage the patient to express concerns about a change in appearance, sexual function, or fertility as a result of a possible endocrine problem. **Patient-Centered Care** QSEN
- Explain all diagnostic procedures, restrictions, and follow-up care to the patient scheduled for endocrine tests. **Patient-Centered Care** QSEN
- Ask family members about changes in the patient's personality or behavior. **Patient-Centered Care** QSEN

Physiological Integrity

- Be aware that the onset of endocrine problems can be slow and insidious or abrupt and life threatening.
- Ask the patient about other family members with endocrine disorders, because some problems have a genetic component. **Evidence-Based Practice** QSEN
- Ask the patient what prescribed and over-the-counter drugs are taken on a regular basis, because some drugs can alter endocrine function. **Patient-Centered Care** QSEN
- Follow the laboratory's procedures for collecting and handling specimens for endocrine function studies. **Evidence-Based Practice** QSEN
- Differentiate normal from abnormal laboratory test findings and clinical manifestations for patients with possible endocrine problems. **Patient-Centered Care** QSEN

62 CHAPTER

Care of Patients with Pituitary and Adrenal Gland Problems

M. Linda Workman

http://evolve.elsevier.com/Iggy/

PRIORITY CONCEPTS

- Fluid and Electrolyte Balance
- Glucose Regulation

LEARNING OUTCOMES

Safe and Effective Care Environment

1. Protect the patient with pituitary or adrenal gland problems from injury and from problems associated with changes in FLUID AND ELECTROLYTE BALANCE.

Health Promotion and Maintenance

2. Identify the teaching priorities for the patient taking hormone replacement therapy for pituitary or adrenal hypofunction.

Psychosocial Integrity

3. Reduce the psychological impact for the patient and family experiencing pituitary or adrenal gland problems.

Physiological Integrity

4. Interpret clinical changes and laboratory data to determine the effectiveness of therapy for diabetes insipidus and for syndrome of inappropriate antidiuretic hormone (SIADH).
5. Prioritize nursing care for the patient with acute adrenal insufficiency and poor GLUCOSE REGULATION.
6. Coordinate nursing care for the patient with Cushing's disease or syndrome.
7. Coordinate care for the patient with hyperaldosteronism or pheochromocytoma.

Pituitary and adrenal gland problems alter hormone levels and change the function of many tissues and organs. When too much or too little of one or more hormones is secreted, the effects may induce physical and psychological changes. The anterior pituitary gland regulates growth, metabolism, and sexual development. The posterior pituitary gland secretes **vasopressin** (antidiuretic hormone [ADH]). Problems in this gland result in changes in FLUID AND ELECTROLYTE BALANCE. The adrenal gland secretes hormones that influence homeostasis and are life sustaining. Nursing care for the patient with pituitary or adrenal gland disorders includes assessment, patient education, evaluation of patient response to therapy, and providing support.

A complete assessment is performed to detect specific clinical findings. The patient also often undergoes many diagnostic tests and relies on the nurse for explanations. Surgical intervention may be indicated. The patient often needs lifelong hormone replacement therapy, and physical and emotional support are critical.

DISORDERS OF THE ANTERIOR PITUITARY GLAND

The anterior pituitary gland (adenohypophysis) controls growth, metabolic activity, and sexual development through the actions of these hormones:

- Growth hormone (GH; somatotropin)
- Thyrotropin (thyroid-stimulating hormone [TSH])
- Corticotropin (adrenocorticotropic hormone [ACTH])
- Follicle-stimulating hormone (FSH)
- Luteinizing hormone (LH)
- Melanocyte-stimulating hormone (MSH)
- Prolactin (PRL)

Disorders of the anterior pituitary gland can result from problems within the anterior pituitary gland itself *(primary pituitary dysfunction),* from problems in the hypothalamus that change pituitary function *(secondary pituitary dysfunction),* or from the influence of exogenous drugs. Regardless of the problem, one or more hormones may be undersecreted *(pituitary hypofunction)* or oversecreted *(pituitary hyperfunction).*

HYPOPITUITARISM

❖ PATHOPHYSIOLOGY

A person with hypopituitarism has a deficiency of one or more anterior pituitary hormones. If only one hormone is affected, the condition is known as *selective hypopituitarism.* Decreased production of *all* of the anterior pituitary hormones *(panhypopituitarism)* is rare.

More often, one hormone has greatly decreased secretion and the secretion of other hormones is reduced to a lesser degree. Deficiencies of *adrenocorticotropic hormone (ACTH)* and *thyroid-stimulating hormone (TSH)* are the *most* life threatening because they cause a decrease in the secretion of vital hormones from the adrenal and thyroid glands. Adrenal gland hypofunction is discussed on pp. 1273-1276; hypothyroidism is discussed in Chapter 63.

Deficiency of the **gonadotropins** (luteinizing hormone [LH] and follicle-stimulating hormone [FSH]—hormones that stimulate the gonads to produce sex hormones) changes sexual function in both men and women. In men, gonadotropin deficiency results in testicular failure with decreased testosterone production that may cause sterility. In women, gonadotropin deficiency results in ovarian failure, amenorrhea, and infertility.

Growth hormone (GH) deficiency changes tissue growth patterns indirectly as a result of reduced liver production of somatomedins. These substances, especially somatomedin C, trigger growth and maintenance activities in bone, cartilage, and other tissues throughout life.

GH deficiency results from decreased GH production, failure of the liver to produce somatomedins, or a failure of tissues to respond to the somatomedins. Deficiency in children leads to short stature and general growth retardation. Deficiency in adults does not affect height but increases the rate of bone destructive activity, leading to thinner bones (**osteoporosis**) and an increased risk for fractures.

The cause of hypopituitarism varies. Benign or malignant pituitary tumors can compress and destroy pituitary tissue. Pituitary function can be impaired by malnutrition or rapid loss of body fat. Shock or severe hypotension reduces blood flow to the pituitary gland, leading to hypoxia and infarction. Other causes of hypopituitarism include head trauma, brain tumors or infection, radiation or surgery of the head and brain, and acquired immune deficiency syndrome (AIDS). *Idiopathic hypopituitarism* has an unknown cause.

Postpartum hemorrhage is the most common cause of pituitary infarction, which results in decreased hormone secretion. This clinical problem is known as *Sheehan's syndrome*. The pituitary gland normally enlarges during pregnancy, and when hypotension results from hemorrhage, ischemia and necrosis of the gland occur. Usually this condition develops immediately after delivery, although some cases have occurred up to several years later.

❖ PATIENT-CENTERED COLLABORATIVE CARE

◆ Assessment

Changes in physical appearance and target organ function occur with deficiencies of specific pituitary hormones (Chart 62-1). Gonadotropin (LH and FSH) deficiency results in the loss of or change in secondary sex characteristics in men and women. In male patients, look for facial and body hair loss. Ask about impotence and decreased *libido* (sex drive). Women may report **amenorrhea** (absence of menstrual periods), **dyspareunia** (painful intercourse), infertility, and decreased libido. In female patients, check for dry skin, breast atrophy, and a decrease or absence of axillary and pubic hair.

Neurologic manifestations of hypopituitarism as a result of tumor growth often first occur as changes in vision. Assess the patient's visual acuity, especially peripheral vision, for changes or loss. Headaches, **diplopia** (double vision), and limited eye movement are common.

CHART 62-1 Key Features

Pituitary Hypofunction

DEFICIENT HORMONE	CLINICAL MANIFESTATIONS
Anterior Pituitary Hormones	
Growth hormone (GH)	Decreased bone density Pathologic fractures Decreased muscle strength Increased serum cholesterol levels
Gonadotropins (luteinizing hormone [LH], follicle-stimulating hormone [FSH])	Women: ▪ Amenorrhea ▪ Anovulation ▪ Low estrogen levels ▪ Breast atrophy ▪ Loss of bone density ▪ Decreased axillary and pubic hair ▪ Decreased libido Men: ▪ Decreased facial hair ▪ Decreased ejaculate volume ▪ Reduced muscle mass ▪ Loss of bone density ▪ Decreased body hair ▪ Decreased libido ▪ Impotence
Thyroid-stimulating hormone (thyrotropin) (TSH)	Decreased thyroid hormone levels Weight gain Intolerance to cold Scalp alopecia Hirsutism Menstrual abnormalities Decreased libido Slowed cognition Lethargy
Adrenocorticotropic hormone (ACTH)	Decreased serum cortisol levels Pale, sallow complexion Malaise and lethargy Anorexia Postural hypotension Headache Hypoglycemia Hyponatremia Decreased axillary and pubic hair (women)
Posterior Pituitary Hormones	
Vasopressin (antidiuretic hormone [ADH])	Diabetes insipidus: ▪ Greatly increased urine output ▪ Low urine specific gravity (<1.005) ▪ Hypotension ▪ Dehydration ▪ Increased plasma osmolarity ▪ Increased thirst ▪ Output does not decrease when fluid intake decreases

Laboratory findings vary widely. Some pituitary hormone levels may be measured directly. As described in Chapter 61, laboratory assessment of some pituitary hormones involves measuring the *effects* of the hormones rather than measuring the actual hormone levels. For example, blood levels of triiodothyronine (T_3) and thyroxine (T_4) from the thyroid, as well as testosterone and estradiol from the gonads, are measured easily. If levels of one or all of these hormones are low or in the low-normal range, further pituitary evaluation is necessary.

Pituitary problems may cause changes in the sella turcica (the bony nest where the pituitary gland rests) that can be seen with skull x-rays (McCance et al., 2014). Changes may include enlargement, erosion, and calcifications as a result of pituitary tumors. CT and MRI can more distinctly define bone or soft-tissue lesions. An angiogram may be used to rule out the presence of an aneurysm or other vascular problems in the area before surgery.

◆ *Interventions*

Management of the adult with hypopituitarism focuses on replacement of deficient hormones. Men who have gonadotropin deficiency receive sex steroid replacement therapy with androgens (testosterone). The most effective routes of androgen replacement are parenteral and transdermal. Therapy begins with high-dose testosterone and is continued until **virilization** (presence of male secondary sex characteristics) is achieved, with responses that include increases in penis size, libido, muscle mass, bone size, and bone strength. Chest, facial, pubic, and axillary hair growth also increase. Patients usually report improved self-esteem and body image after therapy is initiated. The dose may then be decreased, but therapy continues throughout life. Therapy to increase fertility requires gonadotropin-releasing hormone (GnRH) injections in addition to testosterone therapy (Melmed et al., 2011).

Androgen therapy is avoided in men with prostate cancer. Side effects of therapy include **gynecomastia** (male breast tissue development), acne, baldness, and prostate enlargement.

Women who have gonadotropin deficiency receive hormone replacement with a combination of estrogen and progesterone. The risk for hypertension or *thrombosis* (formation of blood clots in deep veins) is increased with estrogen therapy, especially among smokers. Emphasize measures to reduce risk and the need for regular health visits. For inducing pregnancy, clomiphene (Clomid) may be given to trigger ovulation. Gonadotropin-releasing hormone (GnRH) and human chorionic gonadotropin (hCG) can be used to stimulate ovulation if therapy with clomiphene fails.

Adult patients with GH deficiency may be treated with subcutaneous injections of human GH (hGH). Injections are given at night to mimic normal GH release.

NCLEX EXAMINATION CHALLENGE

Safe and Effective Care Environment

For which client does the nurse question the prescription for androgen replacement therapy?

A. 35-year-old man who has had a vasectomy
B. 48-year-old man who takes prednisone for severe asthma
C. 62-year-old man with a history of prostate cancer
D. 70-year-old man who has hypertension and type 2 diabetes

HYPERPITUITARISM

❖ *PATHOPHYSIOLOGY*

Hyperpituitarism is hormone oversecretion that occurs with pituitary tumors or tissue hyperplasia (tissue overgrowth). Tumors occur most often in the anterior pituitary cells that produce growth hormone (GH), prolactin (PRL), and adrenocorticotropic hormone (ACTH). Overproduction of PRL also may occur in response to tumors that overproduce GH and ACTH. Excess ACTH may occur with increased secretion of melanocyte-stimulating hormone (MSH).

GENETIC/GENOMIC CONSIDERATIONS

Patient-Centered Care QSEN

One cause of hyperpituitarism is multiple endocrine neoplasia, type 1 (*MEN1*), in which there is inactivation of the suppressor gene *MEN1* (Manchester, 2013). This problem has an autosomal dominant inheritance pattern and is usually expressed as a benign tumor that affects the pituitary, parathyroid glands, and pancreas. In the pituitary, this problem causes excessive production of growth hormone and acromegaly. Ask a patient with acromegaly whether either parent also has this problem or has had a tumor of the pancreas or parathyroid glands.

The most common cause of hyperpituitarism is a pituitary adenoma—a benign tumor of one or more tissues within the anterior pituitary. Adenomas are classified by size, invasiveness, and the hormone secreted. As an adenoma gets larger and compresses brain tissue, neurologic changes, as well as endocrine problems, may occur. Such manifestations may include visual disturbances, headache, and increased intracranial pressure.

Prolactin (PRL)-secreting tumors are the most common type of pituitary adenoma. Excessive PRL inhibits the secretion of gonadotropins and sex hormones in men and women, resulting in *galactorrhea* (breast milk production), amenorrhea, and infertility.

Overproduction of GH in adults results in *acromegaly* (Fig. 62-1). The onset may be gradual with slow progression, and changes may remain unnoticed for years before diagnosis of the disorder. Early detection and treatment are essential to prevent irreversible changes in the soft tissues, such as those of the face, hands, feet, and skin. Other changes include increased skeletal thickness, hypertrophy of the skin, and enlargement of many organs, such as the liver and heart. Some changes may be reversible after treatment, but skeletal changes are permanent.

Bone thinning and bone cell overgrowth occur slowly. Breakdown of joint cartilage and hypertrophy of ligaments, vocal cords, and eustachian tubes are common. Nerve entrapment and poor GLUCOSE REGULATION with hyperglycemia (elevated blood glucose levels) are common.

Excess ACTH overstimulates the adrenal cortex. The result is excessive production of glucocorticoids, mineralocorticoids, and androgens, which leads to the development of Cushing's disease and problems with FLUID AND ELECTROLYTE BALANCE (see Hypercortisolism [Cushing's Disease], pp. 1276-1281).

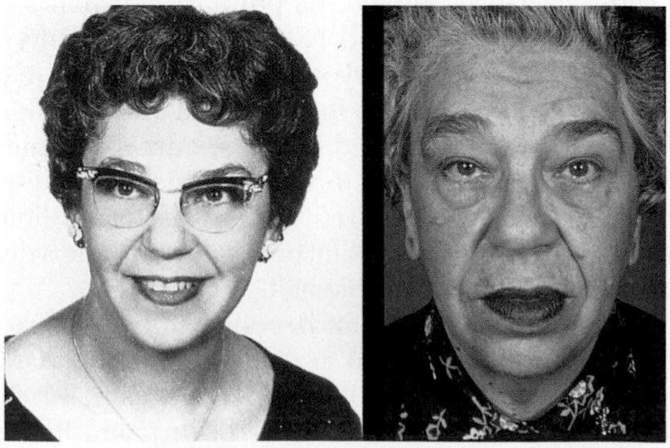

FIG. 62-1 The progression of acromegaly.

Usually, hyperpituitarism is caused by hormone-secreting benign tumors (*adenomas*) arising from one pituitary cell type. It can also be caused by hypothalamic problems that lead to excessive production of releasing hormones, which overstimulate the normal pituitary gland.

❖ PATIENT-CENTERED COLLABORATIVE CARE

◆ Assessment

The manifestations of hyperpituitarism vary with the hormone produced in excess. Obtain the patient's age, gender, and family history. Ask about any change in hat, glove, ring, or shoe size and the presence of fatigue. The patient with high GH levels may have backache and joint pain from bone changes. Ask specifically about headaches and changes in vision.

The patient with hypersecretion of PRL often reports sexual function difficulty. Ask women about menstrual changes, decreased libido, painful intercourse, and any difficulty in becoming pregnant. Ask men whether they have experienced decreased libido and impotence.

Changes in appearance and target organ function occur with excesses of specific anterior pituitary hormones (Chart 62-2). Manifestations of GH excess are increases in lip and nose sizes, a prominent brow ridge, and increases in head, hand, and foot sizes. The patient with hyperpituitarism often seeks health care because of these dramatic changes in appearance.

In a person with hyperpituitarism, usually only one hormone is produced in excess because the cell types within the pituitary gland are so individually organized. The most common hormones produced in excess with hyperpituitarism are PRL, ACTH, and GH.

Imaging assessment for hyperpituitarism is the same as for hypopituitarism. Skull x-rays are used to identify abnormalities of the sella turcica. CT scans and MRI can define soft-tissue lesions, and angiography can rule out an aneurysm or vascular malformations.

Suppression testing can help diagnose hyperpituitarism. For example, high blood glucose levels suppress the release of GH. Giving 100 g of oral glucose or 0.5 g/kg of body weight is followed by serial GH level measurements. GH levels that do not fall below 5 ng/mL indicate a positive (abnormal) result.

◆ Interventions

The expected outcomes of management for the patient who has hyperpituitarism are to return hormone levels to normal or near normal, reduce or eliminate headache and visual disturbances, prevent complications, and reverse as many of the body changes as possible.

Nonsurgical Management. Encourage the patient to express concerns about his or her altered physical appearance. Help him or her identify personal strengths and positive characteristics. Galactorrhea, gynecomastia, and reduced sexual functioning can disturb self-image and personal identity. Reassure the patient that treatment may reverse some of these problems.

Drug therapy may be used alone or in combination with surgery and radiation. The most common drugs used are the dopamine agonists *bromocriptine mesylate* (Parlodel) and *cabergoline* (Dostinex). These drugs stimulate dopamine receptors in the brain and inhibit the release of GH and PRL. In most cases, small tumors decrease until the pituitary gland is of normal size. Large pituitary tumors usually decrease to some extent.

CHART 62-2 **Key Features**

Anterior Pituitary Hyperfunction

Prolactin (PRL)

- Hypogonadism (loss of secondary sexual characteristics)
- Decreased gonadotropin levels
- Galactorrhea
- Increased body fat
- Increased serum prolactin levels

Growth Hormone (GH)

Acromegaly

- Thickened lips
- Coarse facial features
- Increasing head size
- Lower jaw protrusion
- Enlarged hands and feet
- Joint pain
- Barrel-shaped chest
- Hyperglycemia
- Sleep apnea
- Enlarged heart, lungs, and liver

Adrenocorticotropic Hormone (ACTH)

Cushing's Disease (Pituitary)

- Elevated plasma cortisol levels
- Weight gain
- Truncal obesity
- "Moon face"
- Extremity muscle wasting
- Loss of bone density
- Hypertension
- Hyperglycemia
- Striae and acne

Thyrotropin (Thyroid-Stimulating Hormone [TSH])

- Elevated plasma TSH and thyroid hormone levels
- Weight loss
- Tachycardia and dysrhythmias
- Heat intolerance
- Increased GI motility
- Fine tremors

Gonadotropins (Luteinizing Hormone [LH], Follicle-Stimulating Hormone [FSH])

Men:

- Elevated LH and FSH levels
- Hypogonadism or hypergonadism

Women:

- Normal LH and FSH levels

Side effects of bromocriptine include **orthostatic hypotension** (postural hypotension), gastric irritation, nausea, headaches, abdominal cramps, and constipation. Give and teach patients to take bromocriptine with a meal or a snack to reduce some of these side effects. Treatment starts with a low dose and is gradually increased until the desired level (usually 7.5 mg/day) is reached. *If pregnancy occurs, the drug is stopped immediately.*

! NURSING SAFETY PRIORITY QSEN

Drug Alert

Teach patients taking bromocriptine to seek medical care immediately if chest pain, dizziness, or watery nasal discharge occurs because of the possibility of serious side effects, including cardiac dysrhythmias, coronary artery spasms, and cerebrospinal fluid leakage.

Other agents used for acromegaly are the somatostatin analogs, especially octreotide (Sandostatin) and lanreotide (Somatuline), and a growth hormone receptor blocker, pegvisomant (Somavert). Octreotide inhibits GH release through negative feedback. Pegvisomant blocks growth hormone (GH) receptor activity and blocks production of insulin-like growth factor (IGF). Combination therapy with monthly injections of a somatostatin analog and weekly injections of pegvisomant have provided good control of the disease for some patients.

Radiation therapy does not have immediate effects in reducing pituitary hormone excesses, and several years may pass before a therapeutic effect can be seen. The use of the gamma knife and other more precise methods of delivering radiation to pituitary tumors has reduced the long-term side effects of this therapy. These side effects include hypopituitarism, optic nerve damage, and other eye and vision problems.

Surgical Management. Surgical removal of the pituitary gland and tumor (**hypophysectomy**) is the most common treatment for hyperpituitarism. Successful surgery decreases hormone levels, relieves headaches, and may reverse changes in sexual functioning.

Preoperative Care. Explain that because nasal packing is present for 2 to 3 days after surgery, it will be necessary to breathe through the mouth, and a "mustache" dressing ("drip pad") will be placed under the nose. Instruct the patient not to brush teeth, blow the nose, or bend forward after surgery. These activities can increase intracranial pressure (ICP) and delay healing, as can coughing and sneezing.

Operative Procedures. Usually a minimally invasive endoscopic transnasal approach is used instead of the more traditional transsphenoidal approach. The endoscopic approach uses smaller-diameter instruments and results in less damage to nasal structures. The procedure is performed with the patient under general anesthesia. After the gland is removed, a muscle graft is taken, often from the thigh, to support the area and prevent leakage of cerebrospinal fluid (CSF). Nasal packing is inserted after the incision is closed, and a mustache dressing is applied. If the tumor cannot be reached by either the endoscopic transnasal approach or the transsphenoidal approach, a craniotomy may be indicated (see Chapter 45).

Postoperative Care. Monitor the patient's neurologic responses, and document any changes in vision or mental status, altered level of consciousness, or decreased strength of the extremities. Observe the patient for complications such as transient diabetes insipidus (discussed on p. 1271), CSF leakage, infection, and increased ICP.

Teach the patient to report any postnasal drip or increased swallowing, which might indicate leakage of CSF. Keep the head of the bed elevated after surgery. Assess nasal drainage for quantity, quality, and the presence of glucose (which indicates that the fluid is CSF). A light yellow color at the edge of the clear drainage on the dressing is called the "halo sign" and indicates CSF. If the patient has persistent, severe headaches, CSF fluid may have leaked into the sinus area. Most CSF leaks resolve with bedrest, and surgical intervention is rarely needed.

Teach the patient to avoid coughing early after surgery because it increases pressure in the incision area and may lead to a CSF leak. Remind the patient to perform deep-breathing exercises hourly while awake to prevent pulmonary problems. Patients may have mouth dryness from mouth breathing. Instruct the patient to rinse the mouth frequently and to apply a lubricating jelly to dry lips.

CHART 62-3 Best Practice for Patient Safety & Quality Care QSEN

The Patient After Hypophysectomy

- Monitor the patient's neurologic status hourly for the first 24 hours and then every 4 hours.
- Monitor fluid balance, especially for output greater than intake.
- Encourage the patient to perform deep-breathing exercises.
- Instruct the patient to not cough, blow the nose, or sneeze.
- Instruct the patient to use dental floss and oral mouth rinses rather than tooth brushing until the surgeon gives permission.
- Instruct the patient to avoid bending at the waist to prevent increasing intracranial pressure.
- Monitor the nasal drip pad for the type and amount of drainage.
- Teach the patient to avoid constipation and subsequent "straining."
- Teach the patient self-administration of the prescribed hormones.

CHART 62-4 Focused Assessment

The Patient Who Has Undergone Nasal Hypophysectomy for Hyperpituitarism

Assess cardiovascular status:
- Vital signs, including apical pulse, pulse pressure, presence or absence of orthostatic hypotension, and the quality/rhythm of peripheral pulses

Assess cognition and mental status

Assess condition of operative site:
- Observe nasal area for drainage:
  If present, note color, clarity, and odor
  Test clear drainage for the presence of glucose

Assess neuromuscular status:
- Reactivity of patellar and biceps reflexes
- Oral temperature
- Handgrip strength
- Steadiness of gait
- Distant and near visual acuity
- Pupillary responses to light

Assess kidney function:
- Observe urine specimen for color, odor, cloudiness, and amount

Ask about:
- Headaches or visual disturbances
- Ease of bowel movements
- 24-hour fluid intake and output
- Over-the-counter and prescribed drugs taken

Assess patient's understanding of illness and adherence with treatment:
- Manifestations to report to health care provider
- Drug plan (correct timing and dose)

Assess for manifestations of infection, especially meningitis, such as headache, fever, and nuchal (neck) rigidity. The surgeon may prescribe antibiotics, analgesics, and antipyretics.

If the entire pituitary gland has been removed, replacement of thyroid hormones and glucocorticoids is lifelong. Best practices for care after surgery are listed in Chart 62-3.

After surgery the patient needs daily self-management regimens and frequent checkups. Chart 62-4 lists areas for focused assessment for the patient at home after a hypophysectomy. Review drug regimens and manifestations of infection and cerebral edema with the family.

After a hypophysectomy, advise the patient to avoid activities that might interfere with healing. Teach him or her to avoid bending over from the waist to pick up objects or tie shoes because this position increases ICP. Teach the patient to bend the knees and then lower the body to pick up fallen objects. ICP also increases when the patient strains to have a bowel movement. Suggest techniques to prevent constipation, such as eating high-fiber foods, drinking plenty of fluids, and using stool softeners or laxatives.

Teach the patient to avoid toothbrushing, which can disturb the operative site, for about 2 weeks after surgery. Frequent mouth care with mouthwash and daily flossing provide adequate oral hygiene. A decreased sense of smell is expected after surgery and usually lasts 3 to 4 months.

Hormone replacement with vasopressin may be needed to maintain fluid balance (see discussion of Interventions starting below in the Diabetes Insipidus section). If the anterior portion of the pituitary gland is removed, instruct the patient in cortisol, thyroid, and gonadal hormone replacement. Teach the patient to report the return of any manifestations of hyperpituitarism immediately to the primary health care provider.

DISORDERS OF THE POSTERIOR PITUITARY GLAND

Disorders of the posterior pituitary gland (**neurohypophysis**) occur with deficiency or excess of the hormone *vasopressin* (antidiuretic hormone [ADH]). ADH deficiency causes diabetes insipidus, and ADH excess causes the syndrome of inappropriate antidiuretic hormone (SIADH). Both types of problems disturb FLUID AND ELECTROLYTE BALANCE.

DIABETES INSIPIDUS

❖ PATHOPHYSIOLOGY

Diabetes insipidus (DI) is a water loss problem caused by either an ADH deficiency or an inability of the kidneys to respond to ADH. The result of DI is the excretion of large volumes of dilute urine because the distal kidney tubules and collecting ducts do not reabsorb water; this leads to **polyuria** (excessive water loss through urination), dehydration, and disturbed FLUID AND ELECTROLYTE BALANCE. Electrolyte imbalances most commonly include increased serum sodium levels.

Dehydration from this massive water loss increases plasma osmolarity, which stimulates the sensation of thirst. Thirst promotes increased fluid intake and aids in maintaining water homeostasis. *If the thirst mechanism is poor or absent or if the person is unable to obtain water, dehydration becomes more severe and can lead to death.*

! NURSING SAFETY PRIORITY QSEN

Critical Rescue

Ensure that no patient suspected of having DI is deprived of fluids for more than 4 hours, because he or she cannot reduce urine output. Continued urine output without adequate fluid intake leads to severe dehydration.

ADH deficiency is classified as nephrogenic, drug-related, primary, or secondary, depending on whether the problem is caused by insufficient production of ADH or an inability of the kidney to respond to the presence of ADH (John & Day, 2012).

Primary diabetes insipidus is caused by a defect in the hypothalamus or posterior pituitary gland, resulting in a lack of ADH production or release. *Secondary diabetes insipidus* most often results from tumors in or near the hypothalamus or pituitary gland, head trauma, infectious processes, brain surgery, or metastatic tumors.

Drug-related diabetes insipidus is usually caused by lithium carbonate (Eskalith, Lithobid, Carbolith ♣) and demeclocycline (Declomycin). These drugs can interfere with the response of the kidneys to ADH.

CHART 62-5 Key Features

Diabetes Insipidus

Cardiovascular Manifestations
- Hypotension
- Tachycardia
- Weak peripheral pulses
- Hemoconcentration

Kidney/Urinary Manifestations
- Increased urine output
- Dilute, low specific gravity

Skin Manifestations
- Poor turgor
- Dry mucous membranes

Neurologic Manifestations
- Decreased cognition*
- Ataxia*
- Increased thirst
- Irritability*

*Occurs when access to water is limited and rapid dehydration results.

GENETIC/GENOMIC CONSIDERATIONS

***Patient-Centered Care* QSEN**

Nephrogenic diabetes insipidus is a genetic disorder in which the kidney tubules do not respond to the actions of ADH. The result is poor water reabsorption by the kidney although the actual amount of hormone produced is not deficient. This problem is most commonly inherited as an X-linked recessive disorder in which the *AVPR2* gene coding for the ADH receptor is mutated and only males are affected (Online Mendelian Inheritance in Man [OMIM], 2011). There is also an autosomal form of the disorder in which the *AQP2* gene is mutated and both males and females are affected (OMIM, 2012). When assessing a patient with DI, always ask whether anyone else in the family has ever had this disorder.

❖ PATIENT-CENTERED COLLABORATIVE CARE

◆ Assessment

Most manifestations of DI are related to dehydration (Chart 62-5). Key manifestations are an increase in urination and excessive thirst. Ask about a history of recent surgery, head trauma, or drug use (e.g., lithium). Although increased fluid intake prevents serious volume depletion, the patient who is deprived of fluids or who cannot increase oral fluid intake may develop shock from fluid loss. Manifestations of dehydration (e.g., poor skin turgor, dry or cracked mucous membranes) may be present. (See Chapter 11 for discussion of dehydration.)

Water loss produces changes in blood and urine tests. The first step in diagnosis is to measure a 24-hour fluid intake and output without restricting food or fluid intake. DI is considered if urine output is more than 4 L during this period and is greater than the volume ingested. The amount of urine excreted in 24 hours may vary from 4 to 30 L/day. Urine is dilute with a low specific gravity (less than 1.005) and low osmolarity (50 to 200 mOsm/kg).

◆ Interventions

Management focuses on controlling manifestations with drug therapy. The most preferred drug is desmopressin acetate (DDAVP), a synthetic form of vasopressin given orally or intranasally in a metered spray. The frequency of dosing varies with patient responses. Teach patients that each metered spray delivers 10 mcg and those with mild DI may need only one or two doses in 24 hours. For more severe DI, one or two metered doses 2 or 3 times daily may be needed. During severe dehydration, ADH may be given IV or IM. Ulceration of the mucous membranes, allergy, a sensation of chest tightness, and lung inhalation of the spray may occur with use of the intranasal preparations. If side effects occur or if the patient has an upper respiratory infection, oral or subcutaneous vasopressin is used rather than the intranasal form.

! NURSING SAFETY PRIORITY QSEN

Drug Alert

The parenteral form of desmopressin is 10 times stronger than the oral and intranasal forms, and the dosage must be reduced.

For the hospitalized patient with DI, nursing management focuses on early detection of dehydration and maintaining adequate hydration. Interventions include accurately measuring fluid intake and output, checking urine specific gravity, and recording the patient's weight daily.

Urge the patient to drink fluids in an amount equal to urine output. If fluids are given IV, ensure the patency of the access catheter and accurately monitor the amount infused hourly.

The patient with permanent DI requires lifelong drug therapy. Assess his or her ability to follow instructions and adjust dosages. Teach that polyuria and polydipsia are indications of the need for another dose.

Drugs for DI induce water retention and can cause fluid overload (see Chapter 11). *Teach all patients taking these drugs to weigh themselves daily to identify weight gain.* Stress the importance of using the same scale and weighing at the same time of day while wearing a similar amount of clothing. If a weight gain of more than 2.2 lbs (1 kg) or other signs of water toxicity occur (e.g., persistent headache, acute confusion), instruct the patient or family that the patient must go to the emergency department or call 911. Instruct him or her to wear a medical alert bracelet identifying the disorder and drugs.

SYNDROME OF INAPPROPRIATE ANTIDIURETIC HORMONE

❖ PATHOPHYSIOLOGY

The **syndrome of inappropriate antidiuretic hormone (SIADH)** or *Schwartz-Bartter syndrome* is a problem in which vasopressin (antidiuretic hormone [ADH]) is secreted even when plasma osmolarity is low or normal. A decrease in plasma osmolarity normally inhibits ADH production and secretion. SIADH occurs with many conditions (e.g., cancer therapy) and with specific drugs, including selective serotonin reuptake inhibitors and fluoroquinolone antibiotics (Yam & Eraly, 2012). Table 62-1 lists common causes of SIADH.

In SIADH, ADH continues to be released even when plasma is hypo-osmolar, leading to disturbances of FLUID AND ELECTROLYTE BALANCE. Water is *retained,* which results in dilutional **hyponatremia** (a decreased serum sodium level) and fluid overload. The increase in blood volume increases the kidney filtration and inhibits the release of renin and aldosterone, which increase urine sodium loss and leads to greater hyponatremia.

TABLE 62-1 Conditions Causing the Syndrome of Inappropriate Antidiuretic Hormone

Malignancies	CNS Disorders
• Small cell lung cancer • Pancreatic, duodenal, and GU carcinomas • Thymoma • Hodgkin's lymphoma • Non-Hodgkin's lymphoma	• Trauma • Infection • Tumors (primary or metastatic) • Strokes • Porphyria • Systemic lupus erythematosus
Pulmonary Disorders	**Drugs**
• Viral and bacterial pneumonia • Lung abscesses • Active tuberculosis • Pneumothorax • Chronic lung diseases • Mycoses • Positive-pressure ventilation	• Exogenous ADH • Chlorpropamide • Vincristine • Cyclophosphamide • Carbamazepine • Opioids • Tricyclic antidepressants • General anesthetics • Fluoroquinolone antibiotics

ADH, Antidiuretic hormone; *CNS,* central nervous system; *GU,* genitourinary.

❖ PATIENT-CENTERED COLLABORATIVE CARE

◆ Assessment

Ask the patient about his or her medical history, which may reveal conditions that can cause SIADH. Information about these conditions should be obtained:

- Recent head trauma
- Cerebrovascular disease
- Tuberculosis or other pulmonary disease
- Cancer
- All past and current drug use

The early manifestations of SIADH are related to water retention. GI disturbances, such as loss of appetite, nausea, and vomiting, may occur first. Weigh the patient, and document any recent weight gain. Use this information to monitor responses to therapy. In SIADH, free water (not salt) is retained and dependent edema is not usually present, even though water is retained.

Water retention, hyponatremia, and fluid shifts affect central nervous system function, especially when the serum sodium level is below 115 mEq/L. The patient may have lethargy, headaches, hostility, disorientation, and a change in level of consciousness. Lethargy and headaches can progress to decreased responsiveness, seizures, and coma. Assess deep tendon reflexes, which are usually decreased.

Vital sign changes include full and bounding pulse (caused by the increased fluid volume) and hypothermia (caused by central nervous system disturbance). Chapter 11 presents other findings that occur with hyponatremia.

Water retention causes urine volume to decrease and urine osmolarity to increase. At the same time, plasma volume increases and plasma osmolarity decreases. Elevated urine sodium levels and specific gravity reflect increased urine concentration. Serum sodium levels are decreased, often as low as 110 mEq/L, because of fluid retention and sodium loss.

Radioimmunoassay of ADH along with clinical manifestations can help diagnose SIADH, but this test is usually not used for a definitive diagnosis.

◆ Interventions

Medical interventions for SIADH focus on restricting fluid intake, promoting the excretion of water, replacing lost sodium, and interfering with the action of ADH. Nursing interventions focus on monitoring response to therapy, preventing complications, teaching the patient and family about fluid restrictions and drug therapy, and preventing injury.

Fluid restriction is essential because fluid intake further dilutes plasma sodium levels. In some cases, fluid intake may be kept as low as 500 to 1000 mL/24 hr (John & Day, 2012). Dilute tube feedings with saline rather than water, and use saline to irrigate GI tubes. Mix drugs to be given by GI tube with saline.

Measure intake, output, and daily weights to assess the degree of fluid restriction needed. A weight gain of 2.2 lbs (1 kg) or more per day or a gradual increase over several days is cause for concern. A 2.2-lb (1kg) weight increase is equal to a 1000-mL fluid retention (1 kg = 1 L). Keep the mouth moist by offering frequent oral rinsing (remind the patient not to swallow the rinses).

Drug therapy with tolvaptan (Samsca) or conivaptan (Vaprisol) is used to treat SIADH when hyponatremia is present in hospitalized patients. These drugs are vasopressin antagonists that promote water excretion without causing sodium loss. Tolvaptan is an oral drug, and conivaptan is given IV. Tolvaptan has a black box warning that rapid increases in serum sodium levels (those greater than a 12 mEq/L increase in 24 hours) have been associated with central nervous system demyelination that can lead to serious complications and death. In addition, when this drug is used at higher dosages or for longer than 30 days, there is a significant risk for liver failure and death (Food and Drug Administration [FDA], 2013).

> **! NURSING SAFETY PRIORITY (QSEN)**
>
> ***Drug Alert***
>
> Administer tolvaptan or conivaptan only in the hospital setting so that serum sodium levels can be monitored closely for the development of hypernatremia.

Diuretics may be used to manage SIADH when sodium levels are near normal and heart failure is present. Be aware of the diuretic effects on sodium loss. Sodium loss can be potentiated, further contributing to the problems caused by SIADH. For milder SIADH, demeclocycline (Declomycin), an oral antibiotic, may help correct the disturbed FLUID AND ELECTROLYTE BALANCE, although it is not approved for this problem (Crawford & Harris, 2012).

Hypertonic saline (i.e., 3% sodium chloride [3% NaCl]) may be used to treat SIADH when the serum sodium level is very low (John & Day, 2012; Robinson & Verbalis, 2011). Give IV saline cautiously because it may add to existing fluid overload and promote heart failure. If the patient needs routine IV fluids, a saline solution rather than a water solution is prescribed.

Monitor the patient's response to therapy to prevent the fluid overload of SIADH from becoming worse, leading to pulmonary edema and heart failure. Any patient with SIADH, regardless of age, is at risk for these complications. The older adult or one who also has cardiac problems, kidney problems, pulmonary problems, or liver problems is at greater risk.

Monitor for increased fluid overload (bounding pulse, increasing neck vein distention, crackles in lungs, increasing peripheral edema, reduced urine output) at least every 2 hours. *Pulmonary edema can occur very quickly and can lead to death.* Notify the health care provider of any change that indicates the fluid overload is not responding to therapy or is worse.

Providing a safe environment is critical when the serum sodium level falls below 120 mEq/L. Possible neurologic changes and the risk for seizures increase as a result of osmotic fluid shifts into brain tissue. Observe for and document changes in the patient's neurologic status. Assess for subtle changes, such as muscle twitching, before they progress to seizures or coma. Check orientation to time, place, and person every 2 hours because disorientation or confusion may be present. Reduce environmental noise and lighting to prevent overstimulation.

Flow sheets with continuing information about the level of consciousness, neurologic assessments, and laboratory data are helpful in detecting neurologic trends. The frequency of neurologic checks depends on the patient's status. For the patient with SIADH who is hyponatremic but alert, awake, and oriented, checks every 4 hours are sufficient. For the patient who has had a change in level of consciousness, perform neurologic checks at least every hour. Inspect the environment every shift, making sure that basic safety measures, such as siderails being securely in place, are observed.

> **? NCLEX EXAMINATION CHALLENGE**
>
> ***Physiological Integrity***
>
> Which urine properties indicate to the nurse that the client with syndrome of inappropriate antidiuretic hormone (SIADH) is responding to interventions?
>
> A. Urine output volume increased; urine specific gravity increased
> B. Urine output volume increased; urine specific gravity decreased
> C. Urine output volume decreased; urine specific gravity increased
> D. Urine output volume decreased; urine specific gravity decreased

DISORDERS OF THE ADRENAL GLAND

ADRENAL GLAND HYPOFUNCTION

❖ PATHOPHYSIOLOGY

Adrenocortical steroid production may decrease as a result of inadequate secretion of adrenocorticotropic hormone (ACTH), dysfunction of the hypothalamic-pituitary control mechanism, or direct dysfunction of adrenal gland tissue. Manifestations may develop gradually or occur quickly with stress. In acute adrenocortical insufficiency (**adrenal crisis**), life-threatening manifestations may appear without warning.

Insufficiency of adrenocortical steroids causes problems through the loss of aldosterone and cortisol action. Decreased cortisol levels result in poor GLUCOSE REGULATION with **hypoglycemia** (low blood glucose levels). Glomerular filtration and gastric acid production decrease, leading to reduced urea nitrogen excretion, which causes anorexia and weight loss.

Reduced aldosterone secretion causes disturbances of FLUID AND ELECTROLYTE BALANCE, especially of potassium, sodium, and water. Potassium excretion is decreased, causing

CHART 62-6 Best Practice for Patient Safety & Quality Care QSEN

Emergency Care of the Patient with Acute Adrenal Insufficiency

Hormone Replacement
- Start rapid infusion of normal saline or dextrose 5% in normal saline.
- Initial dose of hydrocortisone sodium (Solu-Cortef) is 100 to 300 mg or dexamethasone 4 to 12 mg as an IV bolus.
- Administer additional 100 mg of hydrocortisone sodium by continuous IV infusion over the next 8 hours.
- Give hydrocortisone 50 mg IM concomitantly every 12 hours.
- Initiate an H_2 histamine blocker (e.g., ranitidine) IV for ulcer prevention.

Hyperkalemia Management
- Administer insulin (20 to 50 units) with dextrose (20 to 50 mg) in normal saline to shift potassium into cells.
- Administer potassium binding and excreting resin (e.g., Kayexalate).
- Give loop or thiazide diuretics.
- Avoid potassium-sparing diuretics, as prescribed.
- Initiate potassium restriction.
- Monitor intake and output.
- Monitor heart rate, rhythm, and ECG for manifestations of hyperkalemia (slow heart rate; heart block; tall, peaked T waves; fibrillation; asystole).

Hypoglycemia Management
- Administer IV glucose, as prescribed.
- Administer glucagon, as needed and prescribed.
- Maintain IV access.
- Monitor blood glucose level hourly.

ECG, Electrocardiogram.

TABLE 62-2 Causes of Primary and Secondary Adrenal Insufficiency

Primary Causes	Secondary Causes
• Autoimmune disease*	• Pituitary tumors
• Tuberculosis	• Postpartum pituitary necrosis
• Metastatic cancer	• Hypophysectomy
• AIDS	• High-dose pituitary or whole-brain radiation
• Hemorrhage	
• Gram-negative sepsis	
• Adrenalectomy	
• Abdominal radiation therapy	
• Drugs (mitotane) and toxins	

AIDS, Acquired immune deficiency syndrome.
*Most common cause.

CHART 62-7 Key Features

Adrenal Insufficiency

Neuromuscular Manifestations
- Muscle weakness
- Fatigue
- Joint/muscle pain

Gastrointestinal Manifestations
- Anorexia
- Nausea, vomiting
- Abdominal pain
- Constipation or diarrhea
- Weight loss
- Salt craving

Skin Manifestations
- Vitiligo
- Hyperpigmentation

Cardiovascular Manifestations
- Anemia
- Hypotension
- Hyponatremia
- Hyperkalemia
- Hypercalcemia

hyperkalemia. Sodium and water excretion are increased, causing hyponatremia and hypovolemia. Potassium retention also promotes reabsorption of hydrogen ions, which can lead to acidosis.

Low adrenal androgen levels decrease the body, axillary, and pubic hair, especially in women, because the adrenals produce most of the androgens in females. The severity of manifestations is related to the degree of hormone deficiency.

Acute adrenal insufficiency, or **Addisonian crisis**, is a life-threatening event in which the need for cortisol and aldosterone is greater than the available supply. It often occurs in response to a stressful event (e.g., surgery, trauma, severe infection), especially when the adrenal hormone output is already reduced. The problems are the same as those of chronic insufficiency but are more severe. *Unless intervention is initiated promptly, however, sodium levels fall and potassium levels rise rapidly. Severe hypotension results from the blood volume depletion that occurs with the loss of aldosterone.* Best practices for emergency care of patients with acute adrenal insufficiency are listed in Chart 62-6.

Adrenal insufficiency (Addison's disease) is classified as primary or secondary. Causes of primary and secondary adrenal insufficiency are listed in Table 62-2. A common cause of secondary adrenal insufficiency is the sudden cessation of long-term glucocorticoid therapy. This therapy suppresses production of glucocorticoids through negative feedback by causing atrophy of the adrenal cortex. Glucocorticoid drugs must be withdrawn gradually to allow for increasing pituitary production of ACTH and activation of adrenal cells to produce cortisol.

❖ PATIENT-CENTERED COLLABORATIVE CARE

◆ Assessment

History. Ask about manifestations and factors that cause adrenal hypofunction. Ask about any change in activity level, because lethargy, fatigue, and muscle weakness are often present. Include questions about salt intake, because salt craving often occurs with hypofunction.

GI problems, such as anorexia, nausea, vomiting, diarrhea, and abdominal pain, often occur. Ask about weight loss during the past months. Women may have menstrual changes related to weight loss, and men may report impotence.

Ask whether the patient has had radiation to the abdomen or head. Document medical problems (e.g., tuberculosis or previous intracranial surgery) and all past and current drugs, especially steroids, anticoagulants, opioids, and cancer drugs.

Physical Assessment/Clinical Manifestations. The manifestations of adrenal insufficiency vary, and the severity is related to the degree of hormone deficiency (Chart 62-7). In patients with primary insufficiency, plasma ACTH and melanocyte-stimulating hormone (MSH) levels are elevated in response to the adrenal-hypothalamic-pituitary feedback system. Elevated MSH levels result in areas of increased pigmentation (Fig. 62-2). In primary autoimmune disease, patchy areas of decreased pigmentation may occur because of destruction of skin melanocytes. Body hair may also be decreased. In secondary disease, skin pigmentation is not changed.

Assess for abnormal GLUCOSE REGULATION with hypoglycemia (e.g., sweating, headaches, tachycardia, and tremors) and fluid depletion (postural hypotension and dehydration).

Hyperkalemia (elevated blood potassium levels) can cause dysrhythmias with an irregular heart rate and can result in cardiac arrest.

Psychosocial Assessment. Depending on the degree of imbalance, patients may appear lethargic, depressed, confused, and even psychotic. Assess the patient's orientation to person, place, and time. Families may report that the patient has wide mood swings and is forgetful.

Diagnostic Assessment. Laboratory findings include low serum cortisol, low fasting blood glucose, low sodium, elevated potassium, and increased blood urea nitrogen (BUN) levels (Chart 62-8). In primary disease, the eosinophil count and ACTH level are elevated. Plasma cortisol levels do not rise during provocation tests.

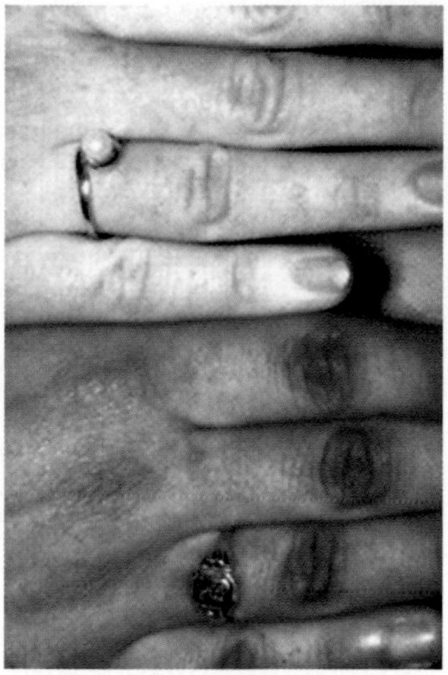

FIG. 62-2 The increased pigmentation seen in primary adrenocortical insufficiency.

Urinary 17-hydroxycorticosteroids are the glucocorticoid metabolites, and 17-ketosteroid levels reflect the adrenal androgen metabolites. Both levels are in the low or low-normal range in adrenal hypofunction.

An ACTH stimulation (provocation) test is the most definitive test for adrenal insufficiency. ACTH 0.25 to 1 mg is given IV, and plasma cortisol levels are obtained at 30-minute and 1-hour intervals. In primary insufficiency, the cortisol response is absent or very decreased. In secondary insufficiency, it is increased. When acute adrenal insufficiency is suspected, treatment is started without stimulation testing (Stewart & Krone, 2011).

Imaging Assessment. Skull x-rays, CT, MRI, and arteriography may help determine the cause of pituitary problems leading to adrenal insufficiency. CT scans may show adrenal gland atrophy.

◆ Interventions

Nursing interventions focus on promoting fluid balance, monitoring for fluid deficit, and preventing poor GLUCOSE REGULATION with hypoglycemia. *Because hyperkalemia can cause dysrhythmias with an irregular heart rate and result in cardiac arrest, assessing cardiac function is a nursing priority.* Assess vital signs every 1 to 4 hours, depending on the patient's condition and the presence of dysrhythmias or postural hypotension. Weigh the patient daily, and record intake and output. Monitor laboratory values to identify hemoconcentration (e.g., increased hematocrit or BUN). Chapter 11 discusses fluid volume deficit in detail.

Cortisol and aldosterone deficiencies are corrected by replacement therapy. Hydrocortisone corrects glucocorticoid deficiency (Chart 62-9). Oral cortisol replacement regimens vary. The most common drug used for this purpose is prednisone. Generally, divided doses are given, with two-thirds given in the morning and one-third in the late afternoon to mimic the normal release of this hormone. Although most patients do

CHART 62-8 Laboratory Profile

Adrenal Gland Assessment

TEST	NORMAL RANGE FOR ADULTS	SIGNIFICANCE OF ABNORMAL FINDINGS: HYPOFUNCTION OF THE ADRENAL GLAND	SIGNIFICANCE OF ABNORMAL FINDINGS: HYPERFUNCTION OF THE ADRENAL GLAND
Sodium	136-145 mEq/L	Decreased	Increased
Potassium	3.5-5.0 mEq/L	Increased	Decreased
Glucose	70-110 mg/dL (fasting) *Older adults:* slightly increased	Normal to decreased	Normal to increased
Calcium	9-10.5 mg/dL (total) 4.5-5.6 mg/dL (ionized) *Older adults:* slightly decreased	Increased	Decreased
Bicarbonate	23-30 mEq/L	Increased	Decreased
BUN	10-20 mg/dL *Older adults:* may be slightly higher	Increased	Normal
Cortisol (serum)	6 AM to 8 AM: 5-23 mcg/dL or 138-635 SI units (nmol/L) 4 PM to 6 PM: 3-13 mcg/dL or 83-359 SI units (nmol/L)	Decreased	Increased
Cortisol (salivary)	7 AM to 9 AM: 180-750 ng/dL 3 PM to 5 PM: <401 ng/dL 11 PM to midnight: <100 ng/dL		

Pagana, K., & Pagana, T. (2014). *Mosby's manual of diagnostic and laboratory tests* (5th ed.). St. Louis: Mosby.
BUN, Blood urea nitrogen; *SI,* International System of Units.

CHART 62-9 Common Examples of Drug Therapy

Hypofunction of the Adrenal Gland

DRUG AND USUAL DOSAGE	NURSING INTERVENTIONS	RATIONALES
Cortisone 25-50 mg orally daily	Instruct the patient to take the drug with meals or a snack.	GI irritation can occur.
Hydrocortisone (Cortef, Hycort 🍁) 20-50 mg orally	Instruct the patient to report these signs or symptoms of excessive drug therapy: ▪ Rapid weight gain ▪ Round face ▪ Fluid retention	Cushing's syndrome, which indicates a need for dosage adjustment, can occur.
Prednisone (Winpred 🍁) 5-10 mg orally daily	Instruct the patient to report illness, such as: ▪ Severe diarrhea ▪ Vomiting ▪ Fever	Other conditions may indicate a need for dosage change. The usual daily dosage may not be adequate during periods of illness or severe stress.
Fludrocortisone (Florinef) 0.05-0.2 mg orally daily	Monitor the patient's blood pressure. Instruct the patient to report weight gain or edema.	Hypertension is a potential side effect. Sodium-related fluid retention is possible.

NURSING SAFETY PRIORITY QSEN

Drug Alert

Prednisone and prednisolone are sound-alike drugs, and care is needed not to confuse them. Although they are both corticosteroids, they are not interchangeable because prednisolone is several times more potent than prednisone and dosages are not the same.

well on this regimen, some may not tolerate the dosage or may need more.

An additional mineralocorticoid hormone, such as fludrocortisone (Florinef), may be needed to maintain or restore FLUID AND ELECTROLYTE BALANCE (especially sodium and potassium). Dosage adjustment may be needed, especially in hot weather when more sodium is lost because of excessive perspiration. *Salt restriction or diuretic therapy should not be started without considering whether it might lead to an adrenal crisis.*

ADRENAL GLAND HYPERFUNCTION

The adrenal gland may oversecrete just one hormone or all adrenal hormones. Hypersecretion by the adrenal cortex results in hypercortisolism (e.g., **Cushing's disease** or **Cushing's syndrome**), **hyperaldosteronism** (excessive mineralocorticoid production), or excessive androgen production. Hyperstimulation of the adrenal medulla caused by a tumor (**pheochromocytoma**) results in excessive secretion of catecholamines (epinephrine and norepinephrine).

CLINICAL JUDGMENT CHALLENGE

Patient-Centered Care; Quality Improvement; Safety QSEN

The patient is a 32-year-old woman admitted to your unit after surgery for fractures of the left arm and leg resulting from a car crash. She is awake and able to verify her medical history of rheumatoid arthritis and her usual daily oral medications. These are 10 mg of prednisone, naproxen 800 mg twice daily, oral contraceptives, calcium 600 mg, and one multiple vitamin tablet. All of these are prescribed for her to receive during her hospitalization. She is concerned about pain management and how long the recovery will be for the fractures. She is friendly, somewhat anxious, asks many questions, and wants to do "her part" to ensure good recovery. Over the next 4 days, she has become quieter, mumbles that her head and stomach hurt, and now does not recognize the assistant who has been providing her daily care. When she receives her medications, she has difficulty picking them up. The nursing assistant remarks that taking her pulse is difficult because it is so slow and irregular. When you assess the patient, she is so weak that she is unable to lift her arm for a blood pressure check. Her blood pressure is 92/50, which is down from the 128/84 reading on admission. You also verify that her heart beat is slow and irregular.

1. What other assessment data should you obtain immediately and why?
2. What is the most likely cause of the changes in this patient's physical and mental status?
3. How could this problem have been avoided?
4. What specifically would be the nurse's role in preventing this problem?
5. What could be done to prevent this problem from happening again?

HYPERCORTISOLISM (CUSHING'S DISEASE)

❖ *PATHOPHYSIOLOGY*

Cushing's disease is the excess secretion of cortisol from the adrenal cortex, causing many problems. It is caused by either a problem in the adrenal cortex itself, a problem in the anterior pituitary gland, or a problem in the hypothalamus. In addition, glucocorticoid therapy can also lead to problems of hypercortisolism.

The presence of excess glucocorticoids, regardless of the cause, affects metabolism and all body systems. An increase in total body fat results from slow turnover of plasma fatty acids. This fat is redistributed, producing truncal obesity, "buffalo hump," and "moon face" (Fig. 62-3). Increases in the breakdown of tissue protein result in decreased muscle mass and muscle strength, thin skin, and fragile capillaries. The effects on minerals lead to bone density loss.

High levels of corticosteroids kill lymphocytes and shrink organs containing lymphocytes, such as the spleen and the lymph nodes. White blood cell cytokine production is decreased. These changes reduce the protection of the inflammatory and immune responses.

In most cases, increased androgen production also occurs and causes acne, **hirsutism** (increased body hair growth), and occasionally clitoral hypertrophy in women. Increased androgens disrupt the normal ovarian hormone feedback mechanism, decreasing the ovary's production of estrogens and progesterone. **Oligomenorrhea** (scant or infrequent menses) results.

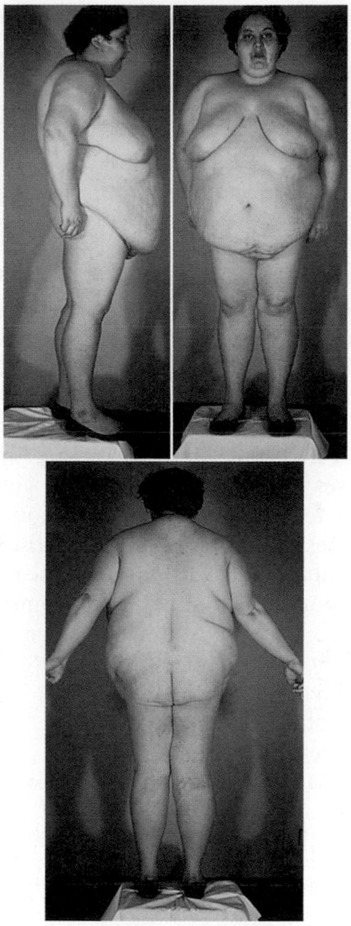

FIG. 62-3 The typical appearance of a patient with Cushing's disease or syndrome. Note truncal obesity, moon face, buffalo hump, thinner arms and legs, and abdominal striae.

Etiology

Cushing's disease or syndrome is a group of clinical problems caused by an excess of cortisol. Table 62-3 lists causes of cortisol excess. When the anterior pituitary gland oversecretes adrenocorticotropic hormone (ACTH), this hormone causes hyperplasia of the adrenal cortex in both adrenal glands and an excess of most hormones secreted by the adrenal cortex. (See Fig. 61-3 in Chapter 61.) This problem is known as **pituitary Cushing's disease** because the tissue causing the problem is the pituitary. When the excess glucocorticoids are caused by a problem in the actual adrenal cortex, usually a benign tumor (adrenal adenoma), the problem is called **adrenal Cushing's disease** and usually occurs in only one adrenal gland. When glucocorticoid excess results from drug therapy for another health problem, it is known as **Cushing's syndrome**.

Incidence and Prevalence

The most common cause of Cushing's disease is a pituitary adenoma. Women are more likely than men to develop Cushing's disease. The actual incidence of Cushing's syndrome from chronic use of exogenous corticosteroids is not known. However, because these drugs are commonly used to control serious chronic inflammatory conditions such as asthma, other respiratory problems, and rheumatoid arthritis, Cushing's syndrome is more common than Cushing's disease and affects both genders equally.

TABLE 62-3 Conditions Causing Increased Cortisol Secretion

Endogenous Secretion (Cushing's Disease)
- Bilateral adrenal hyperplasia*
- Pituitary adenoma increasing the production of ACTH (pituitary Cushing's disease)
- Malignancies: carcinomas of the lung, GI tract, pancreas
- Adrenal adenomas or carcinomas

Exogenous Administration (Cushing's Syndrome)
- Therapeutic use of ACTH or glucocorticoids—most commonly for treatment of:
  - Asthma
  - Autoimmune disorders
  - Organ transplantation
  - Cancer chemotherapy
  - Allergic responses
  - Chronic fibrosis

ACTH, Adrenocorticotropic hormone.
*Most common cause.

❖ PATIENT-CENTERED COLLABORATIVE CARE

◆ Assessment

History. Ask about the patient's other health problems and drug therapies, because glucocorticoid therapy is a common cause of hypercortisolism. Regardless of cause, the patient has many changes because of the widespread effect of excessive cortisol. The patient may report weight gain and an increased appetite. Ask about changes in activity or sleep patterns, fatigue, and muscle weakness. Ask about bone pain or a history of fractures, because osteoporosis is common in hypercortisolism. Ask about a history of frequent infections and easy bruising. Women often stop menstruating. GI problems include ulcer formation from increased hydrochloric acid secretion and decreased production of protective gastric mucus.

Physical Assessment/Clinical Manifestations. The patient with hypercortisolism has specific physical changes, although all body systems are affected (see Fig. 62-3 and Chart 62-10). Changes in fat distribution may result in fat pads on the neck, back, and shoulders ("buffalo hump"); an enlarged trunk with thin arms and legs; and a round face ("moon face"). Other changes include muscle wasting and weakness. Assess and document changes, and use these findings to prioritize patient problems.

Skin changes result from increased blood vessel fragility and include bruises, thin or translucent skin, and wounds that have not healed. Reddish purple **striae** ("stretch marks") occur on the abdomen, thighs, and upper arms because of the destructive effect of cortisol on collagen.

Acne and a fine coating of hair may occur over the face and body. In women, look for the presence of hirsutism, clitoral hypertrophy, and male pattern balding related to androgen excess.

Cardiac changes occur as a result of disturbed FLUID AND ELECTROLYTE BALANCE, especially water and mineral metabolism. Both sodium and water are reabsorbed and retained, leading to hypervolemia and edema formation. Blood pressure is elevated, and pulses are full and bounding.

Musculoskeletal changes occur as a result of nitrogen depletion and mineral loss. Muscle mass decreases, especially in arms and legs (see Fig. 62-3). Muscle weakness increases the risk for

CHART 62-10 Key Features

Hypercortisolism (Cushing's Disease/Syndrome)

General Appearance
- Moon face
- Buffalo hump
- Truncal obesity
- Weight gain

Cardiovascular Manifestations
- Hypertension
- Frequent dependent edema
- Bruising
- Petechiae

Musculoskeletal Manifestations
- Muscle atrophy (most apparent in extremities)
- Osteoporosis (bone density loss)
  - Pathologic fractures
  - Decreased height with vertebral collapse
  - Aseptic necrosis of the femur head
  - Slow or poor healing of bone fractures

Skin Manifestations
- Thinning skin
- Striae and increased pigmentation

Immune System Manifestations
- Increased risk for infection
- Decreased immune function
- Decreased inflammatory responses
- Manifestations of infection/inflammation may be masked

ACTH, Adrenocorticotropic hormone.

falls. Bone is thinner as a result of mineral loss, and osteoporosis is common, increasing the risk for pathologic fractures.

GLUCOSE REGULATION is affected by hypercortisolism. Fasting blood glucose levels are high because the liver releases glucose and the insulin receptors are less sensitive, so blood glucose does not move as easily into the tissues. Muscle mass loss also reduces glucose uptake.

Immune changes caused by excess cortisol result in immunosuppression and an increased risk for infection. Excess cortisol reduces the number of circulating lymphocytes, inhibits macrophage activity, reduces antibody synthesis, and inhibits production of cytokines and inflammatory chemicals (e.g., histamine) (McCance et al., 2014). The risk for infection is higher, and the patient may not have the expected manifestations (fever, purulent exudate, redness in the affected area) when an infection is present.

Psychosocial Assessment. Hypercortisolism can result in emotional instability, and patients often say that they do not feel like themselves. Ask about mood swings, irritability, confusion, or depression. Ask the patient whether he or she has been crying or laughing inappropriately or has had difficulty concentrating. Family members often report changes in the patient's mental or emotional status. The excess hormones stimulate the central nervous system, heightening the awareness of and responses to sensory stimulation. The patient often reports sleep difficulties and fatigue.

Laboratory Assessment. Laboratory tests include blood, salivary, and urine cortisol levels. These are high in patients with any type of hypercortisolism. Plasma ACTH levels vary, depending on the cause of the problem. In pituitary Cushing's disease, ACTH levels are elevated. In adrenal Cushing's disease or when Cushing's syndrome results from chronic steroid use, ACTH levels are low.

Salivary cortisol levels may be used to detect hypercortisolism. Saliva is easily and painlessly collected with the use of a salivary specimen cushion placed in the cheek next to the salivary gland. A normal salivary cortisol level is lower than 2.0 ng/mL. Higher levels indicate hypercortisolism.

Urine is tested to measure levels of free cortisol and the metabolites of cortisol and androgens (17-hydroxycorticosteroids and 17-ketosteroids). In Cushing's disease, levels of urine cortisol and androgens are all elevated in a 24-hour specimen, as are urine calcium, potassium, and glucose levels.

Dexamethasone suppression testing can screen for hypercortisolism and may take place overnight or over a 3-day period. Set doses of dexamethasone are given. A 24-hour urine collection follows drug administration. When urinary 17-hydroxycorticosteroid excretion and cortisol levels are suppressed by dexamethasone, Cushing's disease is not present.

Additional laboratory findings that accompany hypercortisolism include:
- Increased blood glucose level
- Decreased lymphocyte count
- Increased sodium level
- Decreased serum calcium level

Imaging Assessment. Imaging for hypercortisolism includes x-rays, CT scans, MRI, and arteriography. These images can identify lesions of the adrenal or pituitary glands, lung, GI tract, or pancreas.

◆ Analysis

The priority NANDA-I nursing diagnoses and collaborative problems for patients with Cushing's disease or Cushing's syndrome include:
1. Fluid overload
2. Risk for Injury related to skin thinning, poor wound healing, and bone density loss (NANDA-I)
3. Risk for Infection (NANDA-I)
4. Potential for acute adrenal insufficiency

◆ Planning and Implementation

Expected outcomes of hypercortisolism management are the reduction of plasma cortisol levels, removal of tumors, and restoration of normal or acceptable body appearance. When the disorder is caused by pituitary or adrenal problems, cure is possible. When caused by drug therapy for another health problem, the focus is to prevent complications from hypercortisolism.

Restoring Fluid Volume Balance

Planning: Expected Outcomes. The patient with hypercortisolism is expected to achieve and maintain an acceptable FLUID AND ELECTROLYTE BALANCE. Indicators include that these parameters are within or close to the normal range:
- Blood pressure
- Stable body weight
- Serum electrolytes

Interventions. Interventions for patients with fluid overload from hypercortisolism focus on ensuring patient safety, restoring FLUID AND ELECTROLYTE BALANCE, and providing supportive care. Depending on the cause, surgical management may be used to reduce cortisol production.

Nonsurgical Management. Patient safety, drug therapy, nutrition therapy, and monitoring are the basis of nonsurgical interventions for hypercortisolism and fluid overload.

Patient safety includes preventing fluid overload from becoming worse, leading to pulmonary edema and heart failure. Any patient with fluid overload, regardless of age, is at risk for these complications. The older adult or one who has coexisting cardiac problems, kidney problems, pulmonary problems, or liver problems is at greater risk.

Monitor for indicators of fluid overload (bounding pulse, increasing neck vein distention, lung crackles, increasing peripheral edema, reduced urine output) at least every 2 hours. *Pulmonary edema can occur very quickly and can lead to death.* Notify the health care provider of any change that indicates fluid overload either is not responding to therapy or is worse.

The patient with fluid overload and dependent edema is at risk for skin breakdown. Use a pressure-reducing or pressure-relieving overlay on the mattress. Assess skin pressure areas, especially the coccyx, elbows, hips, and heels, daily for redness or open areas. For patients receiving oxygen by mask or nasal cannula, check the skin around the mask, nares, and ears and under the elastic band. Assist the patient to change positions every 2 hours, or ensure that others delegated to perform this intervention are diligent in this action.

Drug therapy involves the use of drugs that interfere with adrenocorticotropic hormone (ACTH) production or adrenal hormone synthesis for temporary relief. Metyrapone (Metopirone), aminoglutethimide (Elipten, Cytadren), and ketoconazole use different pathways to decrease cortisol production (Hunt, 2012). For patients with hypercortisolism resulting from increased ACTH production, cyproheptadine (Periactin) may be used because it interferes with ACTH production. Mitotane (Lysodren) is an adrenal cytotoxic agent used for inoperable tumors causing hypercortisolism. For people with increased ACTH production who have type 2 diabetes and who do not respond to other drug therapies, another drug is mifepristone (Korlym), which is a synthetic steroid that blocks glucocorticoid receptors (Aschenbrenner, 2012).

! NURSING SAFETY PRIORITY (QSEN)

Drug Alert

Mifepristone (Korlym) cannot be used during pregnancy because it also blocks progesterone receptors and would cause termination of the pregnancy.

A new drug to manage hypercortisolism resulting from a pituitary adenoma is pasireotide (Signifor). This drug binds to somatostatin receptors on the adenoma and inhibits tumor production of corticotropin. Lower levels of corticotropin lead to lower levels of cortisol production in the adrenal glands (McKeage, 2013). This subcutaneous drug does not work for people whose tumors do not have somatostatin receptors. In addition, many patients taking this drug have problems with hyperglycemia.

Monitor the patient for response to drug therapy, especially weight loss and increased urine output. Observe for manifestations of problems with FLUID AND ELECTROLYTE BALANCE, especially changes in electrocardiogram (ECG) patterns. Assess laboratory findings, especially sodium and potassium values, whenever they are drawn.

Nutrition therapy for the patient with hypercortisolism may involve restrictions of both fluid and sodium intake to control fluid volume. Review the patient's serum sodium levels whenever fluid overload is present. Often sodium restriction involves only "no added salt" to ordinary table foods when fluid overload is mild. For more pronounced fluid overload, the patient may be restricted to anywhere from 2 g/day to 4 g/day of sodium. When sodium restriction is ongoing, teach the patient and family how to check food labels for sodium content and how to keep a daily record of sodium ingested. Explain to the patient and family the reason for any fluid restriction and the importance of adhering to the prescribed restriction.

Monitoring intake and output and weight can indicate therapy effectiveness. Ensure that unlicensed assistive personnel (UAP) understand that these measurements need to be accurate, not just estimated, because treatment decisions are based on these findings. Schedule fluid offerings throughout the 24 hours. Teach UAP to check urine for color and character and to report these findings. Check the urine specific gravity (a specific gravity below 1.005 may indicate fluid overload). If IV therapy is used, infuse only the amount prescribed.

Fluid retention may not be visible. Remember that rapid weight gain is the best indicator of fluid retention and overload. Each 1 lb (about 500 g) of weight gained equates to 500 mL of retained water. Weigh the patient at the same time daily (before breakfast), using the same scale. Have the patient wear the same type of clothing for each weigh-in.

Radiation therapy is rarely used to treat hypercortisolism caused by pituitary adenomas because it is not always effective and often destroys normal tissue. Chapter 45 discusses radiation therapy to the head.

Surgical Management. The surgical treatment of adrenocortical hypersecretion depends on the cause of the disease. When adrenal hyperfunction is due to increased pituitary secretion of ACTH, removal of a pituitary adenoma using minimally invasive techniques may be attempted. Sometimes a total *hypophysectomy* (surgical removal of the pituitary gland) is needed. (See earlier discussion of hypophysectomy on pp. 1270-1271.) If hypercortisolism is caused by an adrenal tumor, an *adrenalectomy* (removal of the adrenal gland) may be needed.

Preoperative Care. Disturbances of FLUID AND ELECTROLYTE BALANCE are corrected before surgery. Continue to monitor blood potassium, sodium, and chloride levels. Dysrhythmias from potassium imbalance may occur, and cardiac monitoring is needed. Problems with GLUCOSE REGULATION and hyperglycemia are controlled before surgery.

The patient with hypercortisolism is at risk for complications of infections and fractures. Prevent infection with handwashing and aseptic technique. Decrease the risk for falls by raising top siderails and encouraging the patient to ask for assistance when getting out of bed. A high-calorie, high-protein diet is prescribed before surgery.

Glucocorticoid preparations are given before surgery. The patient continues to receive glucocorticoids during surgery to prevent adrenal crisis because the removal of the tumor results in a sudden drop in cortisol levels. Before surgery, discuss the need for long-term drug therapy.

Operative Procedures. A unilateral adrenalectomy is performed when one gland is involved. A bilateral adrenalectomy is needed when ACTH-producing tumors cannot be treated by other means or when both adrenal glands are diseased. Surgery is most often performed by laparoscopic adrenalectomy, a minimally invasive surgical approach. If necessary, an open surgery through the abdomen or the lateral flank can be performed.

Postoperative Care. After an adrenalectomy, the patient is usually sent to a critical care unit. Immediately after surgery, assess the patient every 15 minutes for shock (e.g., hypotension; a rapid, weak pulse; and a decreasing urine output) resulting from insufficient glucocorticoid replacement. Monitor vital signs, central venous pressure, pulmonary wedge pressure, intake and output, daily weights, and serum electrolyte levels.

After a bilateral adrenalectomy, patients require lifelong glucocorticoid and mineralocorticoid replacement, starting immediately after surgery. In unilateral adrenalectomy, hormone replacement continues until the remaining adrenal gland increases hormone production. This therapy may be needed for up to 2 years after surgery.

NCLEX EXAMINATION CHALLENGE

Health Promotion and Maintenance

The client who is about to have a unilateral adrenalectomy for an adenoma that is causing hypercortisolism asks the nurse if she will have to continue the severe sodium restriction after surgery. What is the nurse's best response?

A. "No, once the tumor has been removed and your cortisol levels have normalized, you will not retain excess sodium anymore."
B. "No, after surgery you will have to take oral cortisol, which can be easily controlled so that your sodium levels do not rise."
C. "Yes, the fact that you are retaining sodium and have high blood pressure is related to your age and lifestyle, not the tumor."
D. "Yes, sodium is very bad for people and everyone needs to eliminate sodium completely from their diets for the rest of their lives."

Preventing Injury. The patient who has hypercortisolism is at risk for injury from skin breakdown, bone fractures, and GI bleeding. Prevention of these injuries is a major nursing care focus.

Planning: Expected Outcomes. The patient with hypercortisolism is expected to avoid injury. Indicators include:

- Skin is intact.
- Minimal or no bruising is present.
- Bones are intact.
- Stools, vomitus, and other GI secretions contain no gross or occult blood.

Interventions. Priority nursing interventions for prevention of injury focus on skin assessment and protection, coordinating care to ensure gentle handling, and patient teaching regarding drug therapy for prevention of GI ulcers.

Skin injury is a continuing risk even after surgery has corrected the cortisol excess because the changes induced in the skin and blood vessels remain for weeks to months. Assess the skin for reddened areas, excoriation, breakdown, and edema. If mobility is decreased, turn the patient every 2 hours and pad bony prominences.

Instruct the patient to avoid activities that can result in skin trauma. Teach him or her to use a soft toothbrush and an electric shaver. Instruct patients to keep the skin clean and to dry it thoroughly after washing. Excessive dryness can be prevented by using a moisturizing lotion.

Adhesive tape often causes skin breakdown. Use tape sparingly, and remove it carefully. After venipuncture, the patient may have increased bleeding because of blood vessel fragility. Exert pressure over the site for longer than normal to prevent bleeding and bruising.

Pathologic fractures from bone density loss and osteoporosis are possible for months to years after cortisol levels return to normal. Teach the patient about safety issues and dietary needs. When helping the patient move in bed, use a lift sheet instead of grasping him or her. Remind the patient to call for help when ambulating. Review the use of walkers or canes, if needed. Teach UAP to use a gait belt when walking with a patient who has bone density loss.

Coordinate with a dietitian to teach the patient about nutrition therapy. A high-calorie diet is prescribed that includes increased amounts of calcium and vitamin D. Generous amounts of milk, cheese, yogurt, and green leafy and root vegetables add calcium to promote bone density. Advise the patient to avoid caffeine and alcohol, which increase the risk for GI ulcers and may promote bone density loss.

GI bleeding is common with hypercortisolism. Cortisol (1) inhibits production of the thick, gel-like mucus that protects the stomach lining, (2) decreases blood flow to the area, and (3) triggers the release of excess hydrochloric acid. Although surgery reduces the hypercortisolism, the normal mucus and increased blood flow may take weeks to return. Interventions focus on drug therapy to reduce irritation, protect the GI mucosa, and decrease the secretion of hydrochloric acid.

Antacids buffer stomach acids and protect the GI mucosa. Teach the patient that these drugs should be taken on a regular schedule rather than on an as-needed basis.

When histamine binds to the H_2 receptors in the gastric mucosa, a series of actions release hydrochloric acid. Drugs that block the H_2-receptor site and reduce hydrochloric acid production include cimetidine (Tagamet, Peptol 🍁, Novo-Cimetine 🍁), ranitidine (Zantac, Apo-Ranitidine 🍁), famotidine (Pepcid), and nizatidine (Axid). Omeprazole (Losec 🍁, Prilosec) and esomeprazole (Nexium) inhibit the gastric proton pump and prevent the formation of hydrochloric acid.

Instruct the patient to reduce alcohol and caffeine consumption, smoking, and fasting, because these conditions cause gastric irritation. NSAIDs and drugs that contain aspirin or other salicylates can cause gastritis and intensify GI bleeding. These should be avoided or limited.

Preventing Infection. Glucocorticoids reduce both inflammation and the immune responses, increasing the risk for infection. For the patient who is taking glucocorticoid replacement therapy, the risk is ongoing. For the patient who is recovering from surgery to prevent hypercortisolism, the infection risk continues for weeks after surgery.

Planning: Expected Outcomes. The patient with hypercortisolism is expected to remain free from infection and avoid situations that increase the risk for infection. Indicators include these manifestations and behaviors:

- Does not have fever and foul-smelling or purulent drainage
- Does not have cough, chest pain, and dyspnea
- Does not have urinary frequency, urgency, or pain and burning
- Avoids crowds and large gatherings
- Obtains appropriate vaccinations
- Washes hands frequently

Interventions. Protect the patient with hypercortisolism from infection. All personnel must use extreme care during all nursing procedures. Thorough handwashing is important. Anyone with an upper respiratory tract infection who enters the patient's room must wear a mask. Observe strict aseptic technique when performing dressing changes or any invasive procedure.

Continually assess the patient for possible infection. Manifestations may not be obvious because hypercortisolism suppresses infection manifestations. Fever and the formation of pus depend on the presence of white blood cells (WBCs). The patient who is immunosuppressed may have a severe infection without pus and with only a low-grade fever.

Monitor the patient's daily complete blood count (CBC) with differential WBC count, especially neutrophils. Inspect the mouth during every shift for lesions and mucosa breakdown. Assess the lungs every 8 hours for crackles, wheezes, or reduced breath sounds. Assess all urine for odor and cloudiness. Ask about any urgency, burning, or pain on urination.

Take vital signs at least every 4 hours to assess for fever. A temperature elevation of even 1° F (or 0.5° C) above baseline is significant for a patient who is immunosuppressed and indicates infection until it has been proven otherwise.

Skin care is important for preventing infection because the skin may be the patient's only intact defense. Teach him or her about hygiene, and urge daily bathing. If the patient is immobile, turn him or her every 1 to 2 hours and apply skin lubricants.

Perform pulmonary hygiene every 2 to 4 hours. Listen to the lungs for crackles, wheezes, or reduced breath sounds. Urge the patient to deep breathe or to use an incentive spirometer every hour while awake.

Preventing Acute Adrenal Insufficiency. The patient most at risk for acute adrenal insufficiency is the one who has Cushing's syndrome as a result of glucocorticoid drug therapy. The exogenous drug inhibits the feedback control pathway (see Fig. 61-3 in Chapter 61), preventing the hypothalamus from secreting corticotropin-releasing hormone (CRH). The lack of CRH inhibits secretion of ACTH from the anterior pituitary gland. Without normal levels of ACTH, the adrenal glands atrophy and completely stop production of the corticosteroids. As a result, the patient completely depends on the exogenous drug. If the drug is stopped, even for a day or two, the atrophied adrenal glands cannot produce the glucocorticoids and the patient develops acute adrenal insufficiency, a life-threatening condition. Management of this problem is described on p. 1274.

! NURSING SAFETY PRIORITY QSEN

Drug Alert

Teach patients who are taking a corticosteroid for more than a week to not stop the drug suddenly. Gradual drug tapering should be done under the care of the health care provider.

Community-Based Care

Home Care Management. The patient with hypercortisolism usually has muscle weakness and fatigue for some weeks after surgery and remains at risk for falls and other injury. These problems may necessitate one-floor living for a short time, and a home health aide may be needed to assist with hygiene, meal preparation, and maintenance.

CHART 62-11 Patient and Family Education: Preparing for Self-Management

Cortisol Replacement Therapy

- Take your medication in divided doses—the first dose in the morning and the second dose between 4 PM and 6 PM.
- Take your medication with meals or snacks.
- Weigh yourself daily, and keep a record to show your health care provider.
- Increase your dosage as directed by your health care provider for increased physical stress or severe emotional stress.
- Never skip a dose of medication. If you have persistent vomiting or severe diarrhea and cannot take your medication by mouth for 24 to 36 hours, call your physician. If you cannot reach your physician, go to the nearest emergency department. You may need an injection to take the place of your usual oral medication.
- Always wear your medical alert bracelet or necklace.
- Make regular visits for health care follow-up.
- Learn how to give yourself an intramuscular injection of hydrocortisone.

Self-Management Education. The patient taking exogenous glucocorticoids who is discharged to home remains at continuing risk for problems with FLUID AND ELECTROLYTE BALANCE, especially fluid volume excess. Teach him or her and the family to monitor the patient's weight. Suggest that a record of these daily weights be kept to show the health care provider at any checkups. Also, instruct the patient to call the health care provider if more than 3 lbs are gained in a week or more than 1 to 2 lbs are gained in a 24-hour period.

Lifelong hormone replacement is needed after bilateral adrenalectomy. Teach the patient and family about adherence to the drug regimen and its side effects (Chart 62-11).

Protecting the patient from infection at home is important. Urge him or her to use proper hygiene and to avoid crowds or others with infections. Encourage the patient and all people living in the same home with him or her to have yearly influenza vaccinations. Stress that the patient should immediately notify the physician if he or she has a fever or any other indication of infection. Chart 40-10 in Chapter 40 lists guidelines for patients for infection prevention.

Health Care Resources. Immediately after returning home, the patient may need a support person to stay and provide more attention than could be given by a visiting nurse or home care aide. Contact with the health care team is needed for follow-up and identification of potential problems. The patient taking corticosteroid therapy may have manifestations of adrenal insufficiency if the dosage is inadequate. Suggest that the patient obtain and wear a medical alert bracelet listing the condition and the drug replacement therapy.

◆ Evaluation: Outcomes

Evaluate the care of the patient with hypercortisolism based on the identified priority patient problems. The expected outcomes are that the patient should:

- Maintain FLUID AND ELECTROLYTE BALANCE
- Remain free from injury
- Remain free from infection
- Not experience acute adrenal insufficiency

Specific indicators for these outcomes are listed for each priority patient problem under the Planning and Implementation section (see earlier).

HYPERALDOSTERONISM

❖ PATHOPHYSIOLOGY

Hyperaldosteronism is an increased secretion of aldosterone with mineralocorticoid excess. Primary hyperaldosteronism *(Conn's syndrome)* in adults results from excessive secretion of aldosterone from one or both adrenal glands, usually caused by an adrenal adenoma. In secondary hyperaldosteronism, excessive secretion of aldosterone is caused by the high levels of angiotensin II that are stimulated by high plasma renin levels. Some causes include kidney hypoxia, diabetic nephropathy, and excessive use of some diuretics. Some forms of hyperaldosterone secretion have a genetic basis and are diagnosed in childhood.

Increased aldosterone levels cause disturbances of FLUID AND ELECTROLYTE BALANCE, which then trigger the kidney tubules to retain sodium and excrete potassium and hydrogen ions. Hypernatremia, hypokalemia, and metabolic alkalosis result. Sodium retention increases blood volume, which raises blood pressure, increasing the risk for strokes, heart attacks, and kidney damage. (See Chapter 11 for discussion of electrolyte imbalances.)

❖ PATIENT-CENTERED COLLABORATIVE CARE

◆ Assessment

Hypokalemia and elevated blood pressure are the most common problems of the patient with hyperaldosteronism. He or she may have headache, fatigue, muscle weakness, dehydration, and loss of stamina. **Polydipsia** (excessive fluid intake) and **polyuria** (excessive urine output) occur less frequently. **Paresthesias** (sensations of numbness and tingling) may occur if potassium depletion is severe (Crawford, & Harris, 2011).

Hyperaldosteronism is diagnosed on the basis of laboratory studies, x-rays, and imaging with CT or MRI. Serum potassium levels are decreased, and sodium levels are elevated. Plasma renin levels are low, and aldosterone levels are high. Hydrogen ion loss leads to metabolic alkalemia (elevated blood pH). Urine has a low specific gravity and high aldosterone levels.

◆ Interventions

Surgery is the most common treatment for hyperaldosteronism. One or both adrenal glands may be removed. Surgery is not performed, however, until the patient's potassium levels are normal. Drugs used to increase potassium levels include spironolactone (Aldactone, Spirono, Sincomen 🍁), a potassium-sparing diuretic and aldosterone antagonist. Potassium supplements may be prescribed to increase potassium levels before surgery. The patient may also benefit from a low-sodium diet before surgery.

The patient who has undergone a unilateral adrenalectomy may need temporary glucocorticoid replacement. Replacement is lifelong if both adrenal glands are removed. Glucocorticoids are given before surgery to prevent adrenal crisis. The patient receiving long-term replacement therapy should wear a medical alert bracelet. (See the discussion of adrenalectomy on pp. 1279-1280 in the Hypercortisolism [Cushing's Disease] section for more discussion of care after surgery and patient education.)

When surgery cannot be performed, spironolactone therapy is continued to control hypokalemia and hypertension. Because spironolactone is a potassium-sparing diuretic, hyperkalemia can occur in patients who have impaired kidney function or excessive potassium intake. Advise the patient to avoid potassium supplements and foods rich in potassium. Hyponatremia can occur with spironolactone therapy, and the patient may need increased dietary sodium. Instruct the patient to report manifestations of hyponatremia, such as dryness of the mouth, thirst, lethargy, or drowsiness. Teach patients to report any additional side effects of spironolactone therapy, including gynecomastia, diarrhea, drowsiness, headache, rash, **urticaria** (hives), confusion, erectile dysfunction, hirsutism, and amenorrhea. Additional drug therapy to control hypertension is often needed.

PHEOCHROMOCYTOMA

❖ PATHOPHYSIOLOGY

Pheochromocytoma is a catecholamine-producing tumor that arises in the adrenal medulla. These tumors usually occur as a single lesion in one adrenal gland, although they can be bilateral or in the abdomen. Pheochromocytomas are usually benign, but at least 10% are malignant.

The tumors produce, store, and release epinephrine and norepinephrine (NE). Excessive epinephrine and NE stimulate adrenergic receptors and can have wide-ranging adverse effects mimicking the action of the sympathetic division of the autonomic nervous system.

The cause is unknown, but some pheochromocytomas occur with inherited disorders such as neurofibromatosis (type 1), multiple endocrine neoplasia (MEN-2), Von Hippel-Lindau disease, and pheochromocytoma-paraganglioma syndrome (OMIM, 2014). These tumors are rare; they occur at any age but appear most commonly in patients between 30 and 50 years of age (Young, 2011).

❖ PATIENT-CENTERED COLLABORATIVE CARE

◆ Assessment

The patient often has intermittent episodes of hypertension or attacks that range from a few minutes to several hours. During these episodes, the patient has severe headaches, palpitations, profuse diaphoresis, flushing, apprehension, or a sense of impending doom. Pain in the chest or abdomen, with nausea and vomiting, can also occur. Increased abdominal pressure, defecation, and vigorous abdominal palpation can provoke a hypertensive crisis. Drugs such as tricyclic antidepressants, droperidol, glucagon, metoclopramide, phenothiazines, and naloxone can induce a hypertensive crisis in the patient with pheochromocytoma. Foods or beverages high in tyramine (e.g., aged cheese, red wine) also induce hypertension. The patient may also report heat intolerance, weight loss, and tremors.

The most common diagnostic test is blood and 24-hour urine collection for fractionated metanephrine and catecholamine levels, all of which are elevated in the presence of a pheochromocytoma. Another test that may be conducted when catecholamine levels are not consistent is the clonidine suppression test (Young, 2011). MRI or CT scans can precisely locate tumors in the adrenal gland, as well as in the chest or abdomen.

◆ Interventions

Surgery is the main treatment for a pheochromocytoma. One or both adrenal glands are removed (depending on whether the tumor is bilateral). After surgery, nursing interventions focus on promoting adequate tissue perfusion, nutritional needs, and comfort measures.

Hypertension is the hallmark of the disease and the most common serious complication after surgery. Monitor the blood pressure regularly, and place the cuff consistently on the same arm, with the patient in lying and standing positions. Identify stressors that may lead to a hypertensive crisis, and attempt to reduce them. Teach the patient to not smoke, drink caffeine-containing beverages, or change position suddenly. Provide a diet rich in calories, vitamins, and minerals.

! NURSING SAFETY PRIORITY (QSEN)

Action Alert

Do not palpate the abdomen of a patient with a pheochromocytoma, because this action could stimulate a sudden release of catecholamines and trigger severe hypertension.

The patient often benefits from hydration before surgery because decreased blood volume increases the risk for hypotension during and after surgery. Assess the patient's hydration status, and report manifestations of dehydration or fluid overload.

The patient's blood pressure is stabilized with adrenergic blocking agents such as phenoxybenzamine (Dibenzyline) starting 7 to 10 days before surgery because of the increased risk for severe hypertension during surgery. The drug dosages are adjusted until blood pressure is controlled and hypertensive attacks do not occur. The blood volume expands, and blood pressure in the supine position returns to normal.

Anesthetic agents and touching of the tumor during surgery can cause a catecholamine release. Short-acting alpha-adrenergic blockers are given by IV bolus or continuous infusion for a hypertensive crisis.

Nursing care after surgery is similar to that for the patient who has undergone an adrenalectomy (see Hypercortisolism [Cushing's Disease], pp. 1279-1280). Monitor the patient for hypertension and for hypotension (from the sudden decrease in catecholamine levels) and for hypovolemia. Hemorrhage and shock are possible, and plasma expanders or fluids may be needed. Monitor vital signs, as well as fluid intake and output. If opioids are given, check for their effect on blood pressure.

When tumors are inoperable, management is medical, with alpha-adrenergic and beta-adrenergic blocking agents. For these patients, self-measurement of blood pressure with home monitoring equipment is essential. (See Chapter 36 for teaching priorities and community-based care of the patient with chronic hypertension.)

NURSING CONCEPTS AND CLINICAL JUDGMENT REVIEW

What might you NOTICE if the patient is experiencing disturbances of FLUID AND ELECTROLYTE BALANCE and GLUCOSE REGULATION as a result of adrenal gland hypofunction?

Assessment:
- Postural hypotension
- Irregular heart rate
- Sweating
- Headaches
- Tachycardia
- Tremors
- Muscle weakness
- Forgetfulness
- Lethargy and confusion
- Salt craving

What should you INTERPRET and how should you RESPOND to a patient experiencing disturbances of FLUID AND ELECTROLYTE IMBALANCE and GLUCOSE REGULATION as a result of adrenal gland hypofunction?

Interpret by:
- Taking vital signs
- Assessing cognition
- Assessing blood pressure in the sitting and standing positions
- Assessing muscle strength and function

Interpret laboratory values, including:
- Blood glucose levels
- Serum potassium levels
- Serum sodium levels
- Serum cortisol levels
- Blood urea nitrogen levels

Respond by:
- Ensuring fluid intake
- Providing adequate calorie and carbohydrate intake
- Monitoring for fluid deficit
- Obtaining daily weights
- Measuring intake and output
- Administering prescribed hormone replacements
- Assisting the patient with ambulation
- Monitoring electrocardiograph changes

On what should you REFLECT?
- Observe the patient for evidence of improved fluid and electrolyte balance and glucose regulation.
- Think about what patient education focus could help reduce the intensity of disturbances of fluid and electrolyte balance and glucose regulation in the future.

GET READY FOR THE NCLEX® EXAMINATION!

KEY POINTS

Review these Key Points for each NCLEX Examination Client Needs Category.

Safe and Effective Care Environment

- Handle all patients with bone density loss carefully, using lift sheets whenever possible. **Safety** QSEN
- Use good handwashing techniques before providing any care to a patient who is immunosuppressed. **Safety** QSEN
- Ensure that hormone replacement drugs are given as close to the prescribed times as possible. **Safety** QSEN

Health Promotion and Maintenance

- Instruct the patient with adrenal insufficiency to wear a medical alert bracelet and to carry simple carbohydrates with him or her at all times. **Patient-Centered Care** QSEN
- Teach the patient and family about the clinical manifestations of infection and when to seek medical advice. **Patient-Centered Care** QSEN
- Teach patients who have permanent endocrine hypofunction the proper techniques and timing of hormone replacement therapy. **Patient-Centered Care** QSEN
- Teach patients taking bromocriptine to seek medical care immediately if chest pain, dizziness, or watery nasal discharge occurs. **Safety** QSEN
- Teach patients with diabetes insipidus the proper way to self-administer desmopressin orally or by nasal spray. **Patient-Centered Care** QSEN
- Teach patients who are taking a corticosteroid for more than a week to not stop the drug suddenly. **Safety** QSEN

Psychosocial Integrity

- Encourage the patient and family to express concerns about a change in health status. **Patient-Centered Care** QSEN
- Explain all treatment procedures, restrictions, and follow-up care to the patient. **Patient-Centered Care** QSEN
- Allow patients who experience a change in physical appearance to mourn this change. **Patient-Centered Care** QSEN

Physiological Integrity

- During the immediate period after a hypophysectomy, teach the patient to avoid activities that increase intracranial pressure (e.g., bending at the waist, straining to have a bowel movement, coughing). **Patient-Centered Care** QSEN
- Measure intake and output accurately on patients who have either diabetes insipidus or syndrome of inappropriate antidiuretic hormone (SIADH). **Evidence-Based Practice** QSEN
- Teach the patient with diabetes insipidus the manifestations of dehydration. **Evidence-Based Practice** QSEN
- Ensure that no patient suspected of having DI is deprived of fluids for more than 4 hours. **Safety** QSEN
- Administer tolvaptan or conivaptan only in the hospital setting. **Safety** QSEN
- Do not confuse prednisone with prednisolone. **Safety** QSEN
- Do not palpate the abdomen of a patient who has a pheochromocytoma. **Safety** QSEN
- Work with physicians, dietitians, and pharmacists to help the patient experiencing problems of the pituitary or adrenal gland to achieve and maintain FLUID AND ELECTROLYTE BALANCE and GLUCOSE REGULATION. **Teamwork and Collaboration** QSEN

CHAPTER 63

Care of Patients with Problems of the Thyroid and Parathyroid Glands

M. Linda Workman

http://evolve.elsevier.com/Iggy/

PRIORITY CONCEPTS

- NUTRITION
- THERMOREGULATION

LEARNING OUTCOMES

Safe and Effective Care Environment

1. Protect the patient with thyroid or adrenal parathyroid gland problems from injury and complications.

Health Promotion and Maintenance

2. Identify the teaching priorities and NUTRITION needs for the patient taking hormone replacement therapy for thyroid or parathyroid problems.

Psychosocial Integrity

3. Reduce the psychological impact for the patient and family experiencing thyroid or parathyroid gland problems.

Physiological Integrity

4. Interpret clinical changes and laboratory data to determine the effectiveness of interventions for thyroid problems.
5. Prioritize nursing care for the patient experiencing severe thyrotoxicosis (thyroid storm) and impaired THERMOREGULATION.
6. Coordinate nursing care for the patient during the first 24 hours after thyroid or parathyroid surgery.
7. Coordinate care for the patient who has hyperparathyroidism.
8. Coordinate care for the patient who has hypoparathyroidism.

The hormones secreted from the thyroid and parathyroid glands affect metabolism, THERMOREGULATION, NUTRITION, electrolyte balance, and excitable membrane activity. Problems of either gland often have many effects and manifestations. Mild disturbances produce subtle problems. More severe disturbances may produce life-threatening problems.

THYROID DISORDERS

HYPERTHYROIDISM

❖ PATHOPHYSIOLOGY

Hyperthyroidism is excessive thyroid hormone secretion from the thyroid gland. The manifestations of hyperthyroidism are called **thyrotoxicosis**, regardless of the origin of the thyroid hormones. This term is correct even when a person takes a large amount of synthetic thyroid hormones that manifests as thyrotoxicosis although he or she does not have hyperthyroidism. Thyroid hormones increase metabolism in all body organs, producing many different manifestations. Hyperthyroidism can be temporary or permanent, depending on the cause.

The excessive thyroid hormones stimulate most body systems, causing hypermetabolism and increased sympathetic nervous system activity. Manifestations are listed in Chart 63-1.

Thyroid hormones stimulate the heart, increasing both heart rate and stroke volume. These responses increase cardiac output, systolic blood pressure, and blood flow (McCance et al., 2014).

Elevated thyroid hormone levels affect protein, fat, and glucose metabolism. Protein buildup and breakdown are increased, but breakdown exceeds buildup, causing a net loss of body protein known as a **negative nitrogen balance**. Glucose tolerance is decreased, and the patient has **hyperglycemia** (elevated blood glucose levels). Fat metabolism is increased, and body fat decreases. Although the patient has an increased appetite, the increased metabolism causes weight loss and NUTRITION deficits.

Thyroid hormones are produced in response to the stimulation hormones secreted by the hypothalamus and anterior pituitary glands. Thus oversecretion of thyroid hormones changes the secretion of hormones from the hypothalamus and the anterior pituitary gland through negative feedback (see Chapter 61). Thyroid hormones also have some influence over sex hormone production. Women have menstrual problems and decreased fertility. Both men and women with hyperthyroidism have an increased **libido** (sexual interest).

Etiology and Genetic Risk

Hyperthyroidism has many causes. The most common form of the disease is Graves' disease, also called *toxic diffuse goiter.*

CHART 63-1 **Key Features**

Hyperthyroidism

Skin Manifestations
- Diaphoresis (excessive sweating)
- Fine, soft, silky body hair
- Smooth, warm, moist skin
- Thinning of scalp hair

Cardiopulmonary Manifestations
- Palpitations
- Chest pain
- Increased systolic blood pressure
- Tachycardia
- Dysrhythmias
- Rapid, shallow respirations

Gastrointestinal Manifestations
- Weight loss
- Increased appetite
- Increased stools

Neurologic Manifestations
- Blurred or double vision
- Eye fatigue
- Increased tears
- Injected (red) conjunctiva
- Photophobia
- Exophthalmos*
- Eyelid retraction, eyelid lag
- Globe lag
- Hyperactive deep tendon reflexes
- Tremors
- Insomnia

Metabolic Manifestations
- Increased basal metabolic rate
- Heat intolerance
- Low-grade fever
- Fatigue

Psychological/Emotional Manifestations
- Decreased attention span
- Restlessness and irritability
- Emotional lability
- Manic behavior

Reproductive Manifestations
- Amenorrhea
- Increased libido

Other Manifestations
- Goiter
- Wide-eyed or startled appearance (exophthalmos)*
- Enlarged spleen
- Muscle weakness and wasting

*Present in Graves' disease only.

Graves' disease is an autoimmune disorder resulting from Hashimoto's thyroiditis (HT) (Mandel et al., 2011). HT results in the production of autoantibodies to different substances and structures within the thyroid gland. In Graves' disease, these antibodies (thyroid-stimulating immunoglobulins [TSIs]) attach to the thyroid-stimulating hormone (TSH) receptors on the thyroid tissue. The thyroid gland responds by increasing the glandular cells, which enlarges the gland, forming a **goiter**, and overproduces thyroid hormones (**thyrotoxicosis**). When HT causes production of antibodies to other structures within the thyroid gland, hypothyroidism results. (See the discussion of Etiology on pp. 1291-1292) in the Hypothyroidism section.)

In Graves' disease, all the general manifestations of hyperthyroidism are present. In addition, other manifestations specific to Graves' disease may occur, including **exophthalmos** (abnormal protrusion of the eyes) and **pretibial myxedema** (dry, waxy swelling of the front surfaces of the lower legs that resembles benign tumors or keloids). *Not all patients with a goiter have hyperthyroidism.*

Hyperthyroidism caused by multiple thyroid nodules is termed **toxic multinodular goiter**. The nodules may be enlarged thyroid tissues or benign tumors (adenomas). These patients usually have had a goiter for years. The manifestations are milder than those seen in Graves' disease, and the patient does not have exophthalmos or pretibial myxedema.

Hyperthyroidism also can be caused by excessive use of thyroid replacement hormones. This type of problem is called **exogenous hyperthyroidism**.

GENETIC/GENOMIC CONSIDERATIONS

Patient-Centered Care QSEN

Susceptibility to Graves' disease is associated with mutations in several genes, including *GRD1*, *GRD2*, *GRDX1*, and *GRDX2*. The pattern of inheritance appears to be autosomal recessive with sex limitation to females and reduced penetrance. Graves' disease also has a strong association with other autoimmune disorders, such as diabetes mellitus, vitiligo, and rheumatoid arthritis. It often occurs in both members of identical twins (Online Mendelian Inheritance in Man [OMIM], 2014). Be sure to ask the patient with Graves' disease whether any other family members have the problem.

Incidence and Prevalence

Hyperthyroidism is a common endocrine disorder. Graves' disease can occur at any age but is diagnosed most often in women between 20 and 40 years of age (Mandel et al., 2011). Toxic multinodular goiter usually occurs after the age of 50 years and affects women 4 times more often than men (McCance et al., 2014).

❖ PATIENT-CENTERED COLLABORATIVE CARE

◆ Assessment

History. Many changes and problems occur because hyperthyroidism affects all body systems, although changes may occur over such a long period that not all patients are aware of them. Record age, gender, and usual weight. The increased metabolic rate affects NUTRITION. The patient may report a recent unplanned weight loss, an increased appetite, and an increase in the number of bowel movements per day.

A hallmark of hyperthyroidism is poor THERMOREGULATION with heat intolerance. The patient may have increased sweating even when environmental temperatures are comfortable for others. He or she often wears lighter clothing in cold weather. The patient may also report palpitations or chest pain as a result of the cardiovascular effects. Ask about changes in breathing patterns, because dyspnea (with or without exertion) is common.

Visual changes may be the earliest problem the patient or family notices, especially exophthalmos with Graves' disease (Fig. 63-1). Ask about changes in vision, such as blurring or double vision, and tiring of the eyes.

Ask whether there has been a change in energy level or in the ability to perform ADLs. Fatigue and insomnia are common. Family and friends may report that the patient has become irritable or depressed.

Ask women about changes in menses, because amenorrhea or a decreased menstrual flow is common. Initially, both men and women may have an increase in libido, but this changes as the patient becomes more fatigued.

Ask about previous thyroid surgery or radiation therapy to the neck, because some people remain hyperthyroid after surgery or are resistant to radiation therapy. Ask about past and current drugs, especially the use of thyroid hormone replacement or antithyroid drugs.

Physical Assessment/Clinical Manifestations. Exophthalmos is common in patients with Graves' disease. The wide-eyed or "startled" look is due to edema in the extraocular muscles and increased fatty tissue behind the eye, which pushes the eyeball forward and may cause problems with focusing.

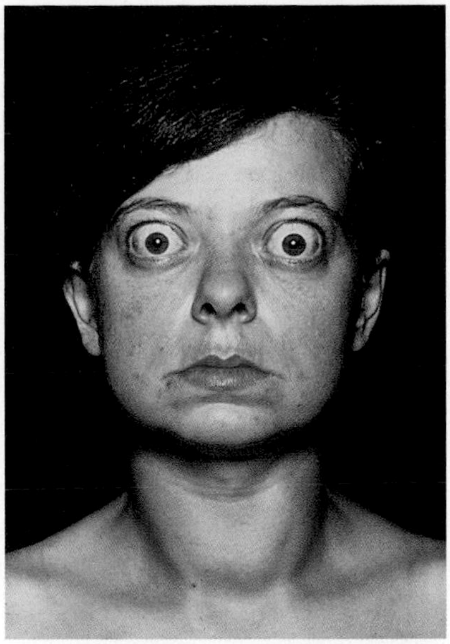

FIG. 63-1 Exophthalmos.

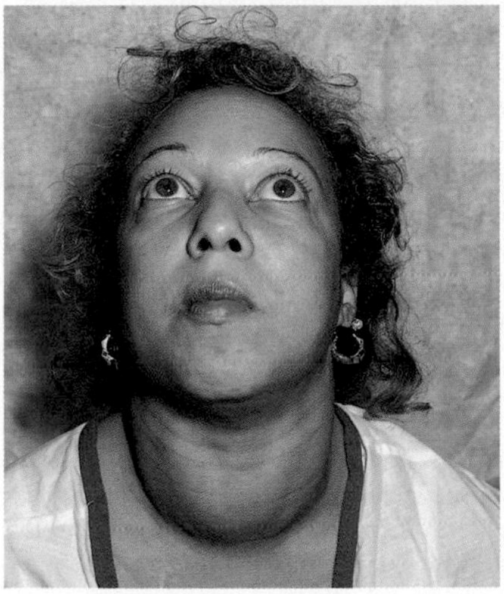

FIG. 63-2 Goiter.

Pressure on the optic nerve may impair vision. If the eyelids fail to close completely and the eyes are unprotected, they may become dry and corneal ulcers may develop. Observe the eyes for excessive tearing and a bloodshot appearance. Ask about sensitivity to light (**photophobia**).

Two other eye problems are common in all types of hyperthyroidism: eyelid retraction (eyelid lag) and globe (eyeball) lag. In eyelid lag, the upper eyelid fails to descend when the patient gazes slowly downward. In globe lag, the upper eyelid pulls back faster than the eyeball when the patient gazes upward. During assessment, ask the patient to look down and then up, and document the response.

Observe the size and symmetry of the thyroid gland. Palpate the thyroid gland to assess its size and consistency. In goiter, a generalized thyroid enlargement, the thyroid gland may increase to 4 times its normal size (Fig. 63-2). Goiters are common in Graves' disease and are classified by size (Table 63-1). Bruits (turbulence from increased blood flow) may be heard in the neck with a stethoscope. (See Chapter 61 for thyroid palpation and auscultation.)

TABLE 63-1 Goiter Classification

GOITER GRADE	DESCRIPTION
0	No palpable or visible goiter.
1	Mass is not visible with neck in the normal position. Goiter can be palpated and moves up when the patient swallows.
2	Mass is visible as swelling when the neck is in the normal position. Goiter is easily palpated and is usually asymmetric.

The cardiovascular problems of hyperthyroidism include increased systolic blood pressure, tachycardia, and dysrhythmias. Usually the diastolic pressure is decreased, causing a widened pulse pressure.

Inspect the hair and skin. Fine, soft, silky hair and smooth, warm, moist skin are common. Many patients notice thinning of scalp hair. Muscle weakness and hyperactive deep tendon reflexes are common. Observe motor movements of the hands for tremors. The patient may appear restless, irritable, and fatigued.

Psychosocial Assessment. The patient often has wide mood swings, irritability, decreased attention span, and manic behavior. Hyperactivity often leads to fatigue because of the inability to sleep well. Some patients describe their activity as having two modes—either "full speed ahead" or "completely stopped." Ask whether he or she cries or laughs without cause or has difficulty concentrating. Family members often report a change in the patient's mental or emotional status.

Laboratory Assessment. Testing for hyperthyroidism involves measurement of blood values for triiodothyronine (T_3), thyroxine (T_4), and thyroid-stimulating hormone (TSH). Antibodies to the TSH receptor (thyrotropin receptor [TRAbs]) are measured to diagnose Graves' disease. The most common changes in laboratory tests for hyperthyroidism are listed in Chart 63-2.

Other Diagnostic Assessment. *Thyroid scan* evaluates the position, size, and functioning of the thyroid gland. Radioactive iodine (RAI [^{123}I]) is given by mouth, and the uptake of iodine by the thyroid gland (radioactive iodine uptake [RAIU]) is measured. The half-life of ^{123}I is short, and radiation precautions are not needed. Pregnancy should be ruled out before the scan is performed. The normal thyroid gland has an uptake of 5% to 35% of the given dose at 24 hours. RAIU is increased in hyperthyroidism and can be used to identify active thyroid nodules. It is no longer the most common test for thyroid function (Mandel et al., 2011).

Ultrasonography of the thyroid gland can determine its size and the general composition of any masses or nodules. This procedure takes about 30 minutes to perform and is painless.

Electrocardiography (ECG) usually shows tachycardia. Other ECG changes with hyperthyroidism include atrial fibrillation, dysrhythmias, and changes in P and T waveforms.

◆ Interventions

Because Graves' disease is the most common form of hyperthyroidism, the interventions discussed in the following sections include those specific for the problems that occur with Graves' disease. The purposes of medical management are to decrease the effect of thyroid hormone on cardiac function and to reduce

CHART 63-2 **Laboratory Profile**

Thyroid Function

TEST	NORMAL RANGE FOR ADULTS	SIGNIFICANCE OF ABNORMAL FINDINGS	
		HYPERTHYROIDISM	HYPOTHYROIDISM
Serum T_3	70-205 ng/dL, or 1.2-3.4 SI units	Increased	Decreased
Serum T_4 (total)	4-12 mcg/dL, or 51-154 SI units	Increased	Decreased
Free T_4 index	0.8-2.8 ng/dL, or 10-36 SI units	Increased	Decreased
TSH stimulation test (thyroid stimulation test)	>10% in RAIU or >1.5 mcg/dL	N/A (test differentiates primary from secondary hypothyroidism)	No response in primary hypothyroidism Normal response in secondary hypothyroidism
Thyroid-stimulating immunoglobulins (TSI)	<130% of basal activity	Elevated in Graves' disease Normal in other types of hyperthyroidism	No change
Thyrotropin receptor antibodies (TRAb)	Titer: 0%	80%-95% indicates Graves' disease	No response
TSH	0.3-5.0 μU/mL or 0.3-5.0 SI units	Low in Graves' disease High in secondary or tertiary hyperthyroidism	High in primary disease Low in secondary or tertiary disease

Data from Pagana, K., & Pagana, T. (2014). *Mosby's manual of diagnostic and laboratory tests* (5th ed.). St. Louis: Mosby.
N/A, Nonapplicable; *SI,* International System of Units; *T_3,* triiodothyronine; *T_4,* thyroxine; *TSH,* thyroid-stimulating hormone.

NCLEX EXAMINATION CHALLENGE

Physiological Integrity

Which manifestations are most often seen in general hyperthyroidism? **Select all that apply.**

A. Increased appetite
B. Cold intolerance
C. Constipation
D. Eyelid retraction
E. Insomnia
F. Palpitations
G. Tremors
H. Weight gain

thyroid hormone secretion. The priorities for nursing care focus on monitoring for complications, reducing stimulation, promoting comfort, and teaching the patient and family about therapeutic drugs and procedures.

Nonsurgical Management. *Monitoring* includes measuring the patient's apical pulse, blood pressure (BP), and temperature at least every 4 hours. Instruct the patient to report immediately any palpitations, dyspnea, vertigo, or chest pain. Increases in temperature may indicate a rapid worsening of the patient's condition and the onset of *thyroid storm,* a life-threatening event that occurs with uncontrolled hyperthyroidism and is characterized by high fever and severe hypertension. *Immediately report a temperature increase of even one degree Fahrenheit.* If this task is delegated to unlicensed assistive personnel (UAP), instruct them to report the patient's temperature to you as soon as it has been obtained. If temperature is elevated, immediately assess the patient's cardiac status. If the patient has a cardiac monitor, check for dysrhythmias.

Reducing stimulation helps prevent increasing the manifestations of hyperthyroidism and the risk for cardiac complications. Encourage the patient to rest. Keep the environment as quiet as possible by closing the door to his or her room, limiting visitors, and eliminating or postponing nonessential care or treatments.

Promoting comfort includes reducing the room temperature to decrease discomfort caused by heat intolerance. Instruct UAP to ensure the patient always has a fresh pitcher of ice water and to change the bed linen whenever it becomes damp from diaphoresis. Suggest that the patient take a cool shower or sponge bath several times each day. For patients with exophthalmos, prevent eye dryness by encouraging the use of artificial tears.

Drug therapy with antithyroid drugs is the initial treatment for hyperthyroidism. Chart 63-3 lists teaching priorities for the patient receiving drug therapy for hyperthyroidism. The preferred drugs are the thionamides, especially methimazole (Tapazole). Propylthiouracil (PTU) is used less often because of its liver toxic effects (Mandel et al., 2011). These drugs block thyroid hormone production by preventing iodide binding in the thyroid gland. The response to these drugs is delayed because the patient may have large amounts of stored thyroid hormones that continue to be released.

NURSING SAFETY PRIORITY (QSEN)

Drug Alert

Although similar in action, methimazole and propylthiouracil are not interchangeable. The dosages for propylthiouracil are much higher than those for methimazole.

NURSING SAFETY PRIORITY (QSEN)

Drug Alert

Methimazole can cause birth defects and should not be used during pregnancy, especially during the first trimester. Instruct women to notify their health care provider if pregnancy occurs.

Iodine preparations may be used for short-term therapy before surgery. They decrease blood flow through the thyroid gland, reducing the production and release of thyroid hormones. Improvement usually occurs within 2 weeks, but it may be weeks before metabolism returns to normal. This treatment

CHART 63-3 Common Examples of Drug Therapy

Hyperthyroidism

DRUG/USUAL DOSAGE	NURSING INTERVENTION	RATIONALE
Thionamides Reduce manifestations of hyperthyroidism by preventing the new formation of thyroid hormones by inhibiting thyroid binding of iodide.		
Propylthiouracil (PTU, Propyl-Thyracil ♣) Initial dose 100-150 mg orally every 8 hr Maintenance dose 50-150 mg orally every 8 hr	Teach patient to avoid crowds and people who are ill.	Drug reduces blood cell counts and the immune response, increasing the risk for infection.
	Teach patient to report darkening of the urine, a yellow appearance to the skin or whites of the eyes.	These manifestations may indicate liver toxicity or failure, a possible side effect of the drug.
	Teach patient to check for weight gain, slow heart rate, and cold intolerance.	These indicate hypothyroidism and may require a lower drug dose.
Methimazole (Northyx, Tapazole) Initial dose 5-20 mg orally every 8 hr Maintenance dose 1-4 mg orally every 8 hr	Remind women to notify their health care providers if they become pregnant.	This drug causes birth defects and should not be used during pregnancy.
	Teach patient to avoid crowds and people who are ill.	Drug reduces blood cell counts and the immune response, increasing the risk for infection.
	Teach patient to check for weight gain, slow heart rate, and cold intolerance.	These indicate hypothyroidism and may require a lower drug dose.
Iodine and Iodine-Containing Agents The sudden excess of iodine rapidly inhibits thyroid hormone release and dramatically (but temporarily) resolves the cardiac and other manifestations of hyperthyroidism. For initial treatment of severe hyperthyroidism or thyroid storm.		
Lugol's solution Saturated solution of potassium iodide (SSKI) Dosages vary depending on the agent, how the drug is administered, and the severity of the manifestations	Administer these drugs orally 1 hour *after* a thionamide has been given.	Initially, the iodine agents can cause an increase in the production of thyroid hormones. Giving a thionamide first prevents this initial increase in thyroid hormone production.
	Check patient for a fever or rash, and ask about a metallic taste, mouth sores, sore throat, or GI distress.	These are manifestations of *iodism*, a toxic effect of the drugs, and may require that the drug be discontinued.

can result in hypothyroidism, and the patient is monitored closely for the need to adjust the drug regimen.

Beta-adrenergic blocking drugs such as propranolol (Inderal, Detensol ♣) may be used as supportive therapy. These drugs relieve diaphoresis, anxiety, tachycardia, and palpitations but do not inhibit thyroid hormone production. See Chapters 34 and 36 for a discussion of the actions and nursing implications of these agents.

Radioactive iodine (RAI) therapy is not used in pregnant women because ^{131}I crosses the placenta and can damage the fetal thyroid gland. The patient with hyperthyroidism may receive RAI in the form of oral ^{131}I. The dosage depends on the thyroid gland's size and sensitivity to radiation. The thyroid gland picks up the RAI, and some of the cells that produce thyroid hormone are destroyed by the local radiation. Because the thyroid gland stores thyroid hormones to some degree, the patient may not have complete symptom relief until 6 to 8 weeks after RAI therapy. Additional drug therapy for hyperthyroidism is still needed during the first few weeks after RAI treatment.

RAI therapy is performed on an outpatient basis. One dose may be sufficient, although some patients need a second or third dose. The radiation dose is low and is usually completely eliminated within a month; however, the source is unsealed and some radioactivity is present in the patient's body fluids and stool for a few weeks after therapy. Radiation precautions are needed to prevent exposure to family members and other people. Chart 63-4 lists precautions to teach the patient during the first few weeks after receiving ^{131}I.

The degree of thyroid destruction varies. Some patients become hypothyroid as a result of treatment. The patient then needs lifelong thyroid hormone replacement. All patients who have undergone RAI therapy should be monitored regularly for changes in thyroid function.

Surgical Management. Surgery to remove all or part of the thyroid gland is the preferred management for Graves' disease. It is also used when a large goiter causes tracheal or esophageal compression or when hyperthyroidism does not respond to drug therapy. Removal of all (**total thyroidectomy**) or part (**subtotal thyroidectomy**) of the thyroid tissue decreases the production of thyroid hormones. After a total thyroidectomy, patients must take lifelong thyroid hormone replacement.

Preoperative Care. The patient is treated with thionamide drug therapy first to have near-normal thyroid function (**euthyroid**) before thyroid surgery. Iodine preparations also are used to decrease thyroid size and vascularity, thereby reducing the risk for hemorrhage and the potential for thyroid storm during surgery.

Hypertension, dysrhythmias, and tachycardia must be controlled before surgery. The patient with hyperthyroidism may need to follow a high-protein, high-carbohydrate diet for days or weeks before surgery.

Teach the patient to perform deep-breathing exercises. Stress the importance of supporting the neck when coughing or moving by placing both hands behind the neck to reduce strain on the incision. Explain that hoarseness may be present for a few days as a result of endotracheal tube placement during surgery.

Reassure the patient by calmly explaining the surgery and the care after surgery. Remind him or her that a drain as well as a dressing may be in place after surgery. Answer any questions the patient and family have.

Operative Procedures. Many thyroidectomies are now performed as minimally invasive surgeries or mini-incision surgeries. With these surgeries, as with the traditional open approach, the parathyroid glands and recurrent laryngeal nerves are avoided to reduce the risk for complications and injury. Usually, general anesthesia is used even for the minimally invasive techniques.

CHART 63-4 Patient and Family Education: Preparing for Self-Management

Safety Precautions for the Patient Receiving an Unsealed Radioactive Isotope

- Use a toilet that is not used by others for at least 2 weeks after receiving the radioactive iodine.
- Sit to urinate (males and females) to avoid splashing the seat, walls, and floor.
- Flush the toilet 3 times after each use.
- If urine is spilled on the toilet seat or floor, use paper tissues or towels to clean it up, bag them in sealable plastic bags, and take them to the hospital's radiation therapy department.
- Men with urinary incontinence should use condom catheters and a drainage bag rather than absorbent gel-filled briefs or pads.
- Women with urinary incontinence should use facial tissue layers in their clothing to catch the urine rather than absorbent gel-filled briefs or pads. These tissues should then be flushed down the toilet exclusively used by the patient.
- Using a laxative on the second and third days after receiving the radioactive drug helps you excrete the contaminated stool faster (this also decreases the exposure of your abdominal organs to radiation).
- Wear only machine-washable clothing, and wash these items separately from others in your household.
- After washing your clothing, run the washing machine for a full cycle on empty before it is used to wash the clothing of others.
- Avoid close contact with pregnant women, infants, and young children for the first week after therapy. Remain at least 3 feet (about 1 meter) away from these people, and limit your exposure to them to no more than 1 hour daily.
- Some radioactivity will be in your saliva during the first week after therapy. Precautions to avoid exposing others to this contamination (both household members and trash collectors) include:
  - Not sharing toothbrushes or toothpaste tubes
  - Using disposable tissues rather than cloth handkerchiefs, and either flushing used ones down the toilet or keeping them in a plastic bag and turning them in to the radiation department of the hospital for disposal
  - Using disposable utensils, plates, and cups
  - Selecting foods that can be eaten completely and do not result in a saliva-coated remnant (Foods to avoid are fruit with a core that can be contaminated, meat with a bone [e.g., chicken wings or legs, ribs])

Data from Al-Shakhrah, I. (2008). Radioprotection using iodine-131 for thyroid cancer and hyperthyroidism: A review. *Clinical Journal of Oncology Nursing, 12*(6), 905-912.

With a subtotal thyroidectomy, the remaining thyroid tissues are sutured to the trachea. With a total thyroidectomy, the entire thyroid gland is removed but the parathyroid glands are left with an intact blood supply to prevent causing hypoparathyroidism.

Postoperative Care. *Monitoring the patient for complications is the most important nursing action after thyroid surgery.* Monitor vital signs every 15 minutes until the patient is stable and then every 30 minutes. Increase or decrease the monitoring of vital signs based on changes in the patient's condition.

Assess the patient's level of discomfort. Use pillows to support the head and neck. Place the patient, while he or she is awake, in a semi-Fowler's position. Avoid positions that cause neck extension. Give prescribed drugs for pain control as needed.

Assist the patient to deep-breathe every 30 minutes to 1 hour. Suction oral and tracheal secretions when necessary.

Thyroid surgery can cause hemorrhage, respiratory distress, parathyroid gland injury (resulting in **hypocalcemia** [low serum calcium levels] and **tetany** [hyperexcitability of nerves and muscles]), damage to the laryngeal nerves, and thyroid storm. Remain alert to the potential for complications, and identify manifestations early.

Hemorrhage is most likely to occur during the first 24 hours after surgery. Inspect the neck dressing and behind the patient's neck for blood. A drain may be present, and a moderate amount of serosanguineous drainage is normal. Hemorrhage may be seen as bleeding at the incision site or as respiratory distress caused by tracheal compression with swelling of the site.

Respiratory distress can result from swelling, tetany, or damage to the laryngeal nerve resulting in spasms. Laryngeal **stridor** (harsh, high-pitched respiratory sounds) is heard in acute respiratory obstruction. Keep emergency tracheostomy equipment in the patient's room. Check that oxygen and suctioning equipment are nearby and in working order.

! NURSING SAFETY PRIORITY QSEN

Critical Rescue

When stridor, dyspnea, or other symptoms of obstruction appear after thyroid surgery, notify the Rapid Response Team.

Hypocalcemia and tetany may occur if the parathyroid glands are removed or damaged or their blood supply is impaired during thyroid surgery, resulting in decreased parathyroid hormone (PTH) levels. Ask the patient hourly about tingling around the mouth or of the toes and fingers. Assess for muscle twitching as a sign of calcium deficiency. Calcium gluconate or calcium chloride for IV use should be available in an emergency situation. (For information on the later signs of hypocalcemia, see the discussion of postoperative care on p. 1297 in the Hyperparathyroidism section and p. 1298 in the Assessment discussion in the Hypoparathyroidism section. Hypocalcemia is also discussed in Chapter 11.)

Laryngeal nerve damage may occur during surgery. This problem results in hoarseness and a weak voice. Assess the patient's voice at 2-hour intervals, and document any changes. Reassure the patient that hoarseness is usually temporary.

Thyroid storm or **thyroid crisis** is a life-threatening event that occurs in patients with uncontrolled hyperthyroidism and occurs most often with Graves' disease. Manifestations develop quickly. It is often triggered by stressors such as trauma, infection, diabetic ketoacidosis, and pregnancy. Other conditions that can lead to thyroid storm include vigorous palpation of the goiter, exposure to iodine, and radioactive iodine (RAI) therapy. Although thyroid storm after surgery is less common because of drug therapy before thyroid surgery, it can still occur.

The manifestations of thyroid storm are caused by excessive thyroid hormone release, which dramatically increases metabolic rate. *Key manifestations include fever, tachycardia, and systolic hypertension.* The patient may have abdominal pain, nausea, vomiting, and diarrhea. Often he or she is very anxious and has tremors. As the crisis progresses, the patient may become restless, confused, or psychotic and may have seizures, leading to coma. *Even with treatment, thyroid storm may lead to death.*

! NURSING SAFETY PRIORITY QSEN

Critical Rescue

When caring for a patient with hyperthyroidism, even after a thyroidectomy, immediately report a temperature increase of even 1°F because it may indicate an impending thyroid crisis.

CHART 63-5 **Best Practice for Patient Safety & Quality Care** QSEN

Emergency Care of the Patient During Thyroid Storm

- Maintain a patent airway and adequate ventilation.
- Give oral antithyroid drugs as prescribed: methimazole (Tapazole), up to 60 mg daily; propylthiouracil (PTU, Propyl-Thyracil 🍁), 300 to 900 mg daily.
- Administer sodium iodide solution, 2 g IV daily as prescribed.
- Give propranolol (Inderal, Detensol 🍁), 1 to 3 mg IV as prescribed. Give slowly over 3 minutes. The patient should be connected to a cardiac monitor, and a central venous pressure catheter should be in place.
- Give glucocorticoids as prescribed: hydrocortisone, 100 to 500 mg IV daily; prednisone, 4 to 60 mg IV daily; or dexamethasone, 2 mg IM every 6 hours.
- Monitor continually for cardiac dysrhythmias.
- Monitor vital signs every 30 minutes.
- Provide comfort measures, including a cooling blanket.
- Give non-salicylate antipyretics as prescribed.
- Correct dehydration with normal saline infusions.
- Apply cooling blanket or ice packs to reduce fever.

Emergency measures to prevent death vary with the intensity and type of manifestations. Interventions focus on maintaining airway patency, providing adequate ventilation, reducing fever, and stabilizing the hemodynamic status. Chart 63-5 outlines the best practices for emergency management of thyroid storm.

Eye and vision problems of Graves' disease are not corrected by treatment for hyperthyroidism, and management is symptomatic. Teach the patient with mild problems to elevate the head of the bed at night and to use artificial tears. If **photophobia** (sensitivity to light) is present, dark glasses may be helpful. For those who cannot close the eyelids completely, recommend gently taping the lids closed with nonallergenic tape at bedtime. These actions prevent eye irritation and injury. If pressure behind the eye continues and forces the eye forward, the blood supply to the eye can be compromised, leading to ischemia and blindness.

In severe cases, short-term steroid therapy is prescribed to reduce swelling and halt the infiltrative process. Prednisone (Deltasone, Winpred 🍁) is given in high doses (often 120 mg daily) at first and then is tapered down according to the patient's response. Explain the need to reduce the prednisone gradually, and review its side effects with the patient.

Other management strategies include external radiation combined with lower-dose steroid therapy. Surgical intervention (orbital decompression) may be needed if loss of sight or damage to the eyeball is possible. Rituximab injections are an experimental approach for this problem (Mandel et al., 2011).

Health teaching includes reviewing with the patient and family the manifestations of hyperthyroidism and instructing the patient to report any increase or recurrence of these. Also teach about the manifestations of hypothyroidism (discussed in the next section) and the need for thyroid hormone replacement. Reinforce the need for regular follow-up because hypothyroidism can occur several years after radioactive iodine therapy.

The discharged patient may continue to have mood changes as a result of hyperthyroidism. Explain the reason for mood swings to the patient and family, and reassure them that these will decrease with continued treatment.

NCLEX EXAMINATION CHALLENGE

Safe and Effective Care Environment

For which assessment finding in a client who has severe hyperthyroidism does the nurse notify the Rapid Response Team?

A. An increase in premature ventricular heart contractions from 4 per minute to 5 per minute
B. An increase in or widening of pulse pressure from 40 mm Hg to 46 mm Hg
C. An increase in temperature from 99.5° F (37.5° C) to 101.3° F (38.5° C)
D. An increase of 20 mL of urine output per hour

HYPOTHYROIDISM

PATHOPHYSIOLOGY

The manifestations of hypothyroidism (Chart 63-6) are the result of decreased metabolism from low levels of thyroid hormones. Thyroid cells may fail to produce sufficient levels of thyroid hormones (THs) for several reasons. Sometimes the cells themselves are damaged and no longer function normally. At other times the thyroid cells are functional but the person does not ingest enough of the substances needed to make thyroid hormones, especially iodide and tyrosine. When the production of thyroid hormones is too low or absent, the blood levels of TH are very low and the patient has a decreased metabolic rate. This lowered metabolism causes the hypothalamus and anterior pituitary gland to make stimulatory hormones, especially thyroid-stimulating hormone (TSH), in an attempt to trigger hormone release from the poorly responsive thyroid gland. The TSH binds to thyroid cells and causes the thyroid gland to enlarge, forming a goiter, although thyroid hormone production does not increase.

Most tissues and organs are affected by the low metabolic rate caused by hypothyroidism. Cellular energy is decreased, and metabolites that are compounds of proteins and sugars called *glycosaminoglycans (GAGs)* build up inside cells. This GAG buildup increases the mucus and water, forms cellular edema, and changes organ texture. The edema is mucinous and called **myxedema**, rather than edema caused by water alone. This edema changes the patient's appearance (Fig. 63-3). Nonpitting edema forms everywhere, especially around the eyes, in the hands and feet, and between the shoulder blades. The tongue thickens, and edema forms in the larynx, making the voice husky. All general physiologic function is decreased.

Myxedema coma is a rare, serious complication of untreated or poorly treated hypothyroidism. The decreased metabolism causes the heart muscle to become flabby and the chamber size to increase. The result is decreased cardiac output and decreased perfusion to the brain and other vital organs, which makes the already slowed cellular metabolism worse, resulting in tissue and organ failure. *The mortality rate for myxedema coma is extremely high, and this condition is a life-threatening emergency.* Myxedema coma can be caused by a variety of events, drugs, or conditions.

Etiology

Most cases of hypothyroidism in the United States occur as a result of thyroid surgery and radioactive iodine (RAI) treatment of hyperthyroidism. Worldwide, hypothyroidism is common in areas where the soil and water have little natural

CHART 63-6 Key Features

Hypothyroidism

Skin Manifestations
- Cool, pale or yellowish, dry, coarse, scaly skin
- Thick, brittle nails
- Dry, coarse, brittle hair
- Decreased hair growth, with loss of eyebrow hair
- Poor wound healing

Pulmonary Manifestations
- Hypoventilation
- Pleural effusion
- Dyspnea

Cardiovascular Manifestations
- Bradycardia
- Dysrhythmias
- Enlarged heart
- Decreased activity tolerance
- Hypotension

Metabolic Manifestations
- Decreased basal metabolic rate
- Decreased body temperature
- Cold intolerance

Psychological/Emotional Manifestations
- Apathy
- Depression
- Paranoia

Gastrointestinal Manifestations
- Anorexia
- Weight gain
- Constipation
- Abdominal distention

Neuromuscular Manifestations
- Slowing of intellectual functions:
  - Slowness or slurring of speech
  - Impaired memory
  - Inattentiveness
- Lethargy or somnolence
- Confusion
- Hearing loss
- Paresthesia (numbness and tingling) of the extremities
- Decreased tendon reflexes
- Muscle aches and pain

Reproductive Manifestations

Women
- Changes in menses (amenorrhea or prolonged menstrual periods)
- Anovulation
- Decreased libido

Men
- Decreased libido
- Impotence

Other Manifestations
- Periorbital edema
- Facial puffiness
- Nonpitting edema of the hands and feet
- Hoarseness
- Goiter (enlarged thyroid gland)
- Thick tongue
- Increased sensitivity to opioids and tranquilizers
- Weakness, fatigue
- Decreased urine output
- Easy bruising
- Iron deficiency anemia
- Vitamin deficiencies

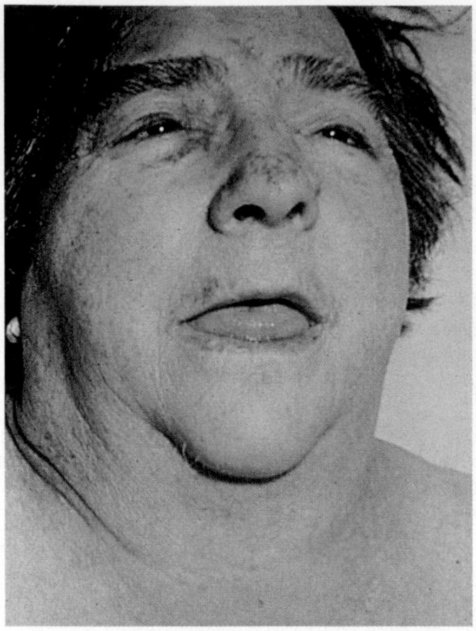

FIG. 63-3 Myxedema.

TABLE 63-2 Causes of Hypothyroidism

Primary Causes

Decreased Thyroid Tissue
- Surgical or radiation-induced thyroid destruction
- Autoimmune thyroid destruction
- Congenital poor thyroid development
- Cancer (thyroidal or metastatic)

Decreased Synthesis of Thyroid Hormone
- Endemic iodine deficiency
- Drugs:
  - Lithium
  - Propylthiouracil
  - Sodium or potassium perchlorate
  - Aminoglutethimide

Secondary Causes

Inadequate Production of Thyroid-Stimulating Hormone
- Pituitary tumors, trauma, infections, or infarcts
- Congenital pituitary defects
- Hypothalamic tumors, trauma, infections, or infarcts

iodide, causing endemic goiter. Hypothyroidism is also caused by a variety of other conditions (Table 63-2).

Incidence and Prevalence

Hypothyroidism occurs most often in women between 30 and 60 years of age. Women are affected 7 to 10 times more often than men (McCance et al., 2014).

❖ *PATIENT-CENTERED COLLABORATIVE CARE*

◆ *Assessment*

History. A decrease in thyroid hormones produces many manifestations related to decreased metabolism. However, changes may have occurred slowly and the patient may not have noticed them. Ask him or her to compare activity now with that of a year ago. The patient often reports an increase in time spent sleeping, sometimes up to 14 to 16 hours daily. Generalized weakness, anorexia, muscle aches, and paresthesias may also be present. Constipation and cold intolerance are common. Ask whether more blankets at night or extra clothing, even in warm weather, has been needed. Some changes may be subtle and are often missed, especially in older adults.

Both men and women may report a decreased libido. Women may have had difficulty becoming pregnant or have changes in menses (heavy, prolonged bleeding or amenorrhea). Men may have problems with impotence and infertility.

Ask about current or previous use of drugs, such as lithium, thiocyanates, aminoglutethimide, sodium or potassium perchlorate, or cobalt. All these drugs can impair thyroid hormone production. In particular, the cardiac drug *amiodarone* (Cordarone) often has damaging effects on the thyroid gland (Mosher, 2011). Also ask whether the patient has ever been treated for hyperthyroidism and what specific treatment was used.

Physical Assessment/Clinical Manifestations. Observe the patient's overall appearance. Fig. 63-3 shows the typical appearance of an adult with hypothyroidism. Common changes include coarse features, edema around the eyes and face, a blank expression, and a thick tongue. The patient's overall muscle movement is slow. He or she may not speak clearly and may take a longer time to respond to questions.

Cardiac and respiratory functions are decreased. Heart rate may be below 60 beats per minute, and respiratory rate may be slow. Body temperature is often lower than 97° F.

Weight gain is very common, even when the person is not overeating. Weigh the patient, and ask whether the result is the same or different from his or her weight a year ago.

Depending on the cause of hypothyroidism, the patient may have a goiter. However, some types of hypothyroidism do not induce a goiter and some types of hyperthyroidism do. The presence of a goiter suggests a thyroid problem but does not indicate whether the problem is excessive hormone secretion or too little hormone secretion.

Psychosocial Assessment. Hypothyroidism causes many problems in psychosocial functioning. Depression is the most common reason for seeking medical attention. Family members often bring the patient for the initial evaluation. The patient may be too lethargic, apathetic, or drowsy to recognize changes in his or her condition. Families may report that the patient is withdrawn and has reduced mental function. Assess his or her attention span and memory, both of which can be impaired by hypothyroidism. The mental slowness can contribute to social isolation.

Laboratory Assessment. Laboratory findings for hypothyroidism are the opposite of those for hyperthyroidism. Triiodothyronine (T_3) and thyroxine (T_4) serum levels are decreased. TSH levels are high in primary hypothyroidism but can be decreased or near normal in patients with secondary hypothyroidism (see Chart 63-2). Patients older than 80 years may have lower-than-normal levels of thyroid hormones without manifestations of hypothyroidism, and hormone replacement is not used until other manifestations are present (Touhy & Jett, 2014).

◆ Analysis

The priority NANDA-I nursing diagnoses and collaborative problems for patients with hypothyroidism include:

1. Impaired Gas Exchange related to decreased energy, obesity, muscle weakness, and fatigue (NANDA-I)
2. Hypotension related to altered heart rate and rhythm as a result of decreased myocardial metabolism
3. Altered cognitive functioning related to impaired brain metabolism and edema
4. Potential for myxedema coma

◆ Planning and Implementation

Both cardiac and respiratory problems are serious, and their management is a priority. The most common cause of death among patients with myxedema coma is respiratory failure.

Improving Gas Exchange

Planning: Expected Outcomes. The patient with hypothyroidism is expected to have improved gas exchange. Indicators include:

- Maintenance of Spo_2 of at least 90%
- Absence of cyanosis
- Maintenance of cognitive orientation

Interventions. Observe and record the rate and depth of respirations. Measure oxygen saturation by pulse oximetry, and apply oxygen if the patient has hypoxemia. Auscultate the lungs for a decrease in breath sounds. If hypothyroidism is severe, the patient may require ventilatory support. Severe respiratory distress often occurs with myxedema coma.

Sedating a patient with hypothyroidism can make gas exchange worse and is avoided if possible. When sedation is needed, the dosage is reduced because hypothyroidism increases sensitivity to these drugs. For the patient receiving sedation, assess for adequate gas exchange.

Preventing Hypotension

Planning: Expected Outcomes. The patient with hypothyroidism is expected to have adequate cardiovascular function and tissue perfusion. Indicators include that the patient:

- Maintains heart rate above 60 beats/min
- Maintains blood pressure within normal limits for his or her age and general health
- Has no dysrhythmias, peripheral edema, or neck vein distention

Interventions. The patient with hypothyroidism can have decreased blood pressure, bradycardia, and dysrhythmias. Nursing priorities are monitoring for condition changes and preventing complications. Monitor blood pressure and heart rate and rhythm, and observe for manifestations of shock (e.g., hypotension, decreased urine output, changes in mental status).

If hypothyroidism is chronic, the patient may have cardiovascular disease. *Instruct the patient to report episodes of chest pain or chest discomfort immediately.*

The patient with hypothyroidism requires lifelong thyroid hormone replacement. Synthetic hormone preparations are usually prescribed. The most common is levothyroxine sodium (Synthroid, T_4, Eltroxin 🍁). Therapy is started with low doses and gradually increased over a period of weeks. *The patient with more severe symptoms of hypothyroidism is started on the lowest dose of thyroid hormone replacement.* This precaution is very important when the patient has known cardiac problems. Starting at too high a dose or increasing the dose too rapidly can cause severe hypertension, heart failure, and myocardial infarction (Brent & Davies, 2011). *Teach patients, as well as their families, who are beginning thyroid replacement hormone therapy to take the drug exactly as prescribed and not to change the dose or schedule without consulting the prescriber. Also teach them not to switch brands because the response to different drug brands can vary.*

Assess the patient for chest pain and dyspnea during initiation of therapy. The final dosage is determined by blood levels of TSH and the patient's physical responses. The dosage and time required for symptom relief vary with each patient. Monitor for and teach the patient and family about the manifestations of hyperthyroidism (see Chart 63-1), which can occur with replacement therapy.

Supporting Cognition

Planning: Expected Outcomes. The patient with hypothyroidism is expected to have cognitive function at the same level as before the thyroid problem started. Indicators include that the patient consistently:

- Demonstrates immediate memory
- Communicates clearly and appropriately for age and ability
- Is attentive during conversations

CHART 63-7 Best Practice for Patient Safety & Quality Care QSEN

Emergency Care of the Patient During Myxedema Coma

- Maintain a patent airway.
- Replace fluids with IV normal or hypertonic saline as prescribed.
- Give levothyroxine sodium IV as prescribed.
- Give glucose IV as prescribed.
- Give corticosteroids as prescribed.
- Check the patient's temperature hourly.
- Monitor blood pressure hourly.
- Cover the patient with warm blankets.
- Monitor for changes in mental status.
- Turn every 2 hours.
- Institute Aspiration Precautions.

Interventions. Observe for and record the presence and severity of lethargy, drowsiness, memory deficit, poor attention span, and difficulty communicating. These problems should decrease with thyroid hormone treatment, and mental awareness usually returns to the patient's normal level within 2 weeks. Orient the patient to person, place, and time, and explain all procedures slowly and carefully. Provide a safe environment.

Family members may have difficulty coping with the patient's behavior. Encourage them to accept the mood changes and mental slowness as manifestations of the disease. Remind the family that these problems should improve with therapy.

Preventing Myxedema Coma. Any patient with hypothyroidism who has any other health problem or who is newly diagnosed is at risk for myxedema coma. Factors leading to myxedema coma include acute illness, surgery, chemotherapy, discontinuing thyroid replacement therapy, and the use of sedatives or opioids. Problems that often occur with this condition include:

- Coma
- Respiratory failure
- Hypotension
- Hyponatremia
- Hypothermia
- Hypoglycemia

! NURSING SAFETY PRIORITY QSEN

Action Alert

Myxedema coma can lead to shock, organ damage, and death. Assess the patient with hypothyroidism at least every 8 hours for changes that indicate increasing severity, especially changes in mental status, and report these promptly to the health care provider.

Treatment is instituted quickly according to the patient's manifestations and without waiting for laboratory confirmation. Best practices for emergency care of the patient with myxedema coma are listed in Chart 63-7.

Community-Based Care

Hypothyroidism is usually chronic. Patients usually live in the community and are managed on an outpatient basis. Patients in acute care settings, subacute care settings, and rehabilitation centers may have long-standing hypothyroidism in addition to other health problems. Ensure that whoever is responsible for overseeing the patient's daily care is aware of the condition and understands its management.

CHART 63-8 Nursing Focus on the Older Adult

Thyroid Problems

Teach the patient these facts about changes in the thyroid gland related to aging:

- Thyroid hormone secretion decreases with age, but the hormone level remains stable because storage site clearance of the hormone also decreases with age.
- The basal metabolic rate decreases with age, which changes body composition from predominantly muscular to predominantly fatty.
- Older patients require lower doses of replacement thyroid hormone. Too large a dose may adversely affect the heart muscle.

Home Care Management. The patient with hypothyroidism does not usually require changes in the home unless cognition has decreased to the point that he or she poses a danger to himself or herself. Activity intolerance and fatigue may necessitate one-floor living for a short time. If manifestations have not improved before discharge, discuss the need for extra heat or clothing because of cold intolerance. The patient may need help with the drug regimen. Discuss this issue with the family and patient, and develop a plan for drug therapy. One person should be clearly designated as responsible for drug preparation and delivery so that doses are neither missed nor duplicated.

Self-Management Education. *The most important educational need for the patient with hypothyroidism is about hormone replacement therapy and its side effects.* Emphasize the need for lifelong drugs, and review the manifestations of both hyperthyroidism and hypothyroidism. Teach the patient to wear a medical alert bracelet. Teach the patient and family when to seek medical interventions for dosage adjustment and the need for periodic blood tests of hormone levels. Instruct the patient to not take any over-the-counter (OTC) drugs without consulting his or her health care provider because thyroid hormone preparations interact with many other drugs. Older patients may need additional information about the effects of aging on the thyroid gland (Chart 63-8).

Advise the patient to maintain NUTRITION by eating a well-balanced diet with adequate fiber and fluid intake to prevent constipation. Caution him or her that use of fiber supplements may interfere with the absorption of thyroid hormone. Thyroid hormones should be taken on an empty stomach. Remind the patient about the importance of adequate rest.

Assist the family in understanding that the time required for resolution of hypothyroidism varies. During this time the patient may continue to have mental slowness. Teach the family to orient the patient often and to explain everything clearly, simply, and as often as needed.

Teach the patient to monitor himself or herself for therapy effectiveness. The two easiest parameters to check are need for sleep and bowel elimination. When the patient requires more sleep and is constipated, the dose of replacement hormone may need to be increased. When the patient has difficulty getting to sleep and has more bowel movements than normal for him or her, the dose may need to be decreased.

Health Care Resources. Immediately after returning home, the patient may need a support person to stay and provide day and night attention. Contact with the health care team is needed for follow-up and identification of potential problems. The patient taking thyroid drugs may have manifestations

CHART 63-9 Focused Assessment

The Patient with Thyroid Dysfunction

Assess cardiovascular status:
- Vital signs, including apical pulse, pulse pressure, presence or absence of orthostatic hypotension, and the quality and rhythm of peripheral pulses
- Presence or absence of peripheral edema
- Weight gain or loss

Assess cognition and mental status:
- Level of consciousness
- Orientation to time, place, and person
- Ability to accurately read a seven-word sentence containing no words greater than three syllables
- Ability to count backward from 100 by 3s

Assess condition of skin and mucous membranes:
- Moistness of skin, most reliable on chest and back
- Skin temperature and color

Assess neuromuscular status:
- Reactivity of patellar and biceps reflexes
- Oral temperature
- Handgrip strength
- Steadiness of gait
- Presence or absence of fine tremors in the hand

Ask about:
- Sleep in the past 24 hours
- Patient warm enough or too warm indoors
- 24-hour diet recall
- 24-hour activity recall
- Over-the-counter and prescribed drugs taken
- Last bowel movement

Assess patient's understanding of illness and adherence with therapy:
- Manifestations to report to health care provider
- Drug therapy plan (correct timing and dose)

of hypothyroidism if the dosage is inadequate or may have manifestations of hyperthyroidism if the dosage is too high. A home care nurse performs a focused assessment at every home visit to the patient with thyroid dysfunction (Chart 63-9).

◆ Evaluation: Outcomes

Evaluate the care of the patient with hypothyroidism based on the identified priority patient problems. The expected outcomes are that with proper management the patient should:

- Maintain normal cardiovascular function
- Maintain adequate respiratory function
- Experience improvement in thought processes

Specific indicators for these outcomes are listed for each patient problem in the Planning and Implementation section (see earlier).

THYROIDITIS

❖ PATHOPHYSIOLOGY

Thyroiditis is an inflammation of the thyroid gland. There are three types: acute, subacute, and chronic. Chronic thyroiditis (Hashimoto's disease) is the most common type.

Acute thyroiditis is caused by bacterial invasion of the thyroid gland. Manifestations include pain, neck tenderness, malaise, fever, and dysphagia (difficulty swallowing). It usually resolves with antibiotic therapy.

Subacute or granulomatous thyroiditis results from a viral infection of the thyroid gland after a cold or other upper respiratory infection. Manifestations include fever, chills, dysphagia, and muscle and joint pain. Pain can radiate to the ears and the jaw. The thyroid gland feels hard and enlarged on palpation. Thyroid function can remain normal, although hyperthyroidism or hypothyroidism may develop.

Chronic thyroiditis (Hashimoto's disease) is a common type of hypothyroidism that affects women more often than men, usually when patients are in their 30s to 50s (Brent & Davies, 2011). Hashimoto's disease is an autoimmune disorder that is usually triggered by a bacterial or viral infection. The thyroid is invaded by antithyroid antibodies and lymphocytes, causing selective thyroid tissue destruction. When large amounts of the gland are destroyed, serum thyroid hormone levels are low and secretion of thyroid-stimulating hormone (TSH) is increased.

CLINICAL JUDGMENT CHALLENGE

Patient-Centered Care; Safety QSEN

The patient, a 45-year-old former school teacher, is residing in a skilled nursing facility to recover from a tibia-fibula fracture that is being managed with an external fixation system. On admission 2 weeks ago, she told you that she felt she was "getting old too fast." She explained that she had gained 54 pounds in the previous 6 months, had no energy, was often constipated, and was always cold. She teared up and said that her ability to concentrate was so bad that not only could she no longer help her high school children with their homework but also that she didn't recognize the step hazard that caused her to fall and break her ankle. Today the nursing assistant assigned to her care reports that the patient's pulse is only 42 beats per minute and that her temperature was 96° F even with two blankets. When you enter her room, she is sleeping and an untouched breakfast tray is on her table.

1. What are the priority assessment data you should obtain? Provide a rationale for your choices.
2. Should oxygen be applied? Why or why not?
3. What indications do you have that the changes in her health status are not related to complications of her fractured ankle?
4. What manifestations of hypothyroidism are in her history and present during this assessment?

❖ PATIENT-CENTERED COLLABORATIVE CARE

The manifestations of Hashimoto's disease are dysphagia and painless enlargement of the gland. Diagnosis is based on circulating antithyroid antibodies and needle biopsy of the thyroid gland. Serum thyroid hormone levels and TSH levels vary with disease stage.

The patient is given thyroid hormone to prevent hypothyroidism and to suppress TSH secretion, which decreases the size of the thyroid gland. Surgery (subtotal thyroidectomy) is needed if the goiter does not respond to thyroid hormone, is disfiguring, or compresses other structures. Nursing interventions focus on promoting comfort and teaching the patient about hypothyroidism, drugs, and surgery.

THYROID CANCER

❖ PATHOPHYSIOLOGY

The four distinct types of thyroid cancer are papillary, follicular, medullary, and anaplastic (American Cancer Society, 2014). The initial manifestation of thyroid cancer is a single, painless lump or nodule in the thyroid gland. Additional manifestations depend on the presence and location of **metastasis** (spread of cancer cells).

Papillary carcinoma, the most common type of thyroid cancer, occurs most often in younger women. It is a slow-growing tumor that can be present for years before spreading to nearby lymph nodes. When the tumor is confined to the thyroid gland, the chance for cure is good with a partial or total thyroidectomy.

Follicular carcinoma occurs most often in older patients. The cancer invades blood vessels and spreads to bone and lung tissue. It can adhere to the trachea, neck muscles, great vessels, and skin, resulting in **dyspnea** (difficulty breathing) and **dysphagia** (difficulty swallowing). When the tumor involves the recurrent laryngeal nerves, the patient may have a hoarse voice.

Medullary carcinoma is most common in patients older than 50 years. This tumor often occurs as part of multiple endocrine neoplasia (MEN) type II, a familial endocrine disorder. The tumor usually secretes calcitonin, adrenocorticotropic hormone (ACTH), prostaglandins, and serotonin.

Anaplastic carcinoma is a rapid-growing, aggressive tumor that directly invades nearby structures. Manifestations include stridor (harsh, high-pitched respiratory sounds), hoarseness, and dysphagia.

A hallmark of thyroid cancer is an elevated serum thyroglobulin (Tg) level. The normal range of Tg for men is 0.5 to 53.0 ng/mL and for women is 0.5 to 43.0 ng/mL (Pagana & Pagana, 2014).

❖ PATIENT-CENTERED COLLABORATIVE CARE

Radiation therapy is used most often for anaplastic carcinoma because this cancer has usually metastasized at diagnosis. The patient is treated with **ablative** (enough to destroy the tissue) amounts of RAI. (See Chart 63-4 for precautions to teach the patient receiving unsealed RAI therapy.) If spread has occurred to the neck or mediastinum, external radiation is also applied. If thyroid cancer does not respond to RAI, chemotherapy is initiated.

Surgery is the treatment of choice for other types of thyroid cancer. A total thyroidectomy is usually performed with dissection of lymph nodes in the neck if regional lymph nodes are involved. (See the postoperative care discussion in the Surgical Management section for Hyperthyroidism on p. 1290.) Suppressive doses of thyroid hormone are usually taken for 3 months after surgery. Thyroglobulin levels are monitored after surgery. A rising level indicates the probable presence of cancer cells.

The patient is hypothyroid after treatment for thyroid cancer. Nursing interventions then focus on teaching the patient about the management of hypothyroidism. (See discussion of Patient-Centered Collaborative Care on pp. 1293-1294 in the Hypothyroidism section.)

PARATHYROID DISORDERS

HYPERPARATHYROIDISM

❖ PATHOPHYSIOLOGY

The parathyroid glands maintain calcium and phosphate balance (see Fig. 61-6 in Chapter 61). Serum calcium level is normally maintained within a narrow range. Increased levels of parathyroid hormone (PTH) act directly on the kidney, causing increased kidney reabsorption of calcium and increased phosphorus excretion. In hyperparathyroidism, these processes cause **hypercalcemia** (excessive calcium) and **hypophosphatemia** (inadequate blood phosphorus level).

TABLE 63-3 Causes of Parathyroid Dysfunction

Causes of Hyperparathyroidism
- Parathyroid tumor or cancer
- Congenital hyperplasia
- Neck trauma or radiation
- Vitamin D deficiency
- Chronic kidney disease with hypocalcemia
- Parathyroid hormone–secreting carcinomas of the lung, kidney, or GI tract

Causes of Hypoparathyroidism
- Surgical or radiation-induced thyroid ablation
- Parathyroidectomy
- Congenital dysgenesis
- Idiopathic (autoimmune) hypoparathyroidism
- Hypomagnesemia

In bone, excessive PTH levels increase bone *resorption* (bone loss of calcium) by decreasing *osteoblastic* (bone production) activity and increasing *osteoclastic* (bone destruction) activity. This process releases calcium and phosphorus into the blood and reduces bone density. With chronic calcium excess and hypercalcemia, calcium is deposited in soft tissues.

Although the exact triggering mechanisms are unknown, primary hyperparathyroidism results when one or more parathyroid glands do not respond to the normal feedback of serum calcium levels. The most common cause is a benign tumor in one parathyroid gland. Table 63-3 lists other causes of hyperparathyroidism.

❖ PATIENT-CENTERED COLLABORATIVE CARE

◆ Assessment

Manifestations of hyperparathyroidism may be related either to the effects of excessive PTH or to the effects of the accompanying hypercalcemia.

Ask about any bone fractures, recent weight loss, arthritis, or psychological stress. Ask whether the patient has received radiation treatment to the head or neck. The patient with chronic disease may have a waxy pallor of the skin and bone deformities in the extremities and back.

High levels of PTH cause kidney stones and deposits of calcium in the soft tissue of the kidney. Bone lesions are due to an increased rate of bone destruction and may result in pathologic fractures, bone cysts, and osteoporosis.

GI problems (e.g., anorexia, nausea, vomiting, epigastric pain, constipation, weight loss) are common when serum calcium levels are high. Elevated serum gastrin levels are caused by hypercalcemia and lead to peptic ulcer disease. Fatigue and lethargy may be present and worsen as the serum calcium levels increase. When serum calcium levels are greater than 12 mg/dL, the patient may have psychosis with mental confusion, which leads to coma and death if left untreated. (See Chapter 11 for more information about hypercalcemia.)

Serum PTH, calcium, and phosphorus levels and urine cyclic adenosine monophosphate (cAMP) levels are the laboratory tests used to detect hyperparathyroidism (Chart 63-10). X-rays may show kidney stones, calcium deposits, and bone lesions. Loss of bone density occurs in the patient with chronic hyperparathyroidism. Other diagnostic tests include arteriography, CT scans, venous sampling of the thyroid for blood PTH levels,

CHART 63-10 Laboratory Profile

Parathyroid Function

		SIGNIFICANCE OF ABNORMAL FINDINGS	
TEST	NORMAL RANGE FOR ADULTS	HYPERPARATHYROIDISM	HYPOPARATHYROIDISM
Serum calcium	Total: 9.0-10.5 mg/dL or 2.25-2.75 SI units Ionized (active): 4.64-5.28 mg/dL or 1.16-1.32 SI units	Increased in primary hyperparathyroidism	Decreased
Serum phosphorus	3.0-4.5 mg/dL or 0.97-1.45 SI units *Older adults:* May be slightly lower	Decreased	Increased
Serum magnesium	1.3-2.1 mEq/L	Increased	Decreased
Serum parathyroid hormone	C-terminal 50-330 pg/mL N-terminal 8-25 pg/mL Whole 10-65 pg/mL	Increased	Decreased
Vitamin D (calciferol)	25-80 ng/mL	Variable	Decreased
Urine cAMP	18.3-45.4 nmol/L in a 24-hour urine collection specimen	Increased	Decreased

Data from Pagana, K., & Pagana, T. (2014). *Mosby's manual of diagnostic and laboratory tests* (5th ed.). St. Louis: Mosby.
cAMP, Cyclic adenosine monophosphate; *SI,* International System of Units.

and ultrasonography. Explain the procedures and care for the patient undergoing diagnostic tests.

◆ *Interventions*

Surgical management is the treatment of choice for patients with hyperparathyroidism. For those who are not candidates for surgery, medication can help control the problems. Priority nursing interventions focus on monitoring and preventing injury.

Nonsurgical Management. *Diuretic and hydration therapies* are used for reducing serum calcium levels in patients who have milder disease. Usually furosemide (Lasix, Uritol 🍁), a diuretic that increases kidney excretion of calcium, is used together with IV saline in large volumes to promote calcium excretion.

Drug therapy for patients who have more severe manifestations of primary or secondary hyperparathyroidism or who have hypercalcemia related to parathyroid cancer involves the use of cinacalcet (Sensipar). This drug is the first in a new class of drugs known as *calcimimetics.* When taken orally, the drug binds to calcium-sensitive receptors on parathyroid tissue. This binding reduces PTH production and release. The result is decreased serum calcium levels, stabilization of other minerals, and decreased progression of PTH-induced bone complications. The initial dose is low (30 mg orally twice daily) and is gradually increased to the maximum maintenance dose of 90 mg three times daily. The patient's serum calcium must be monitored for hypocalcemia on a regular basis for the duration of therapy.

For patients who do not respond to cinacalcet, oral phosphates are used to inhibit bone resorption and interfere with calcium absorption. IV phosphates are used only when serum calcium levels must be lowered rapidly. Calcitonin decreases the release of skeletal calcium and increases the kidney excretion of calcium. It is not effective when used alone because of its short duration of action. The therapeutic effects are greatly enhanced if calcitonin is given along with glucocorticoids.

Monitor cardiac function and intake and output every 2 hours during hydration therapy. Continuous cardiac monitoring may be needed. Compare recent ECG tracings with the patient's baseline tracings. Especially look for changes in the T waves and the QT interval, as well as changes in rate and rhythm. Monitor serum calcium levels, and immediately report any sudden drop to the health care provider. Sudden drops in calcium levels may cause tingling and numbness in the muscles.

Preventing injury is important because the patient with chronic hyperparathyroidism often has significant bone density loss and is at risk for pathologic fractures. Teach unlicensed assistive personnel (UAP) to handle the patient carefully. Use a lift sheet to reposition the patient rather than pulling him or her.

Surgical Management. Surgical management of hyperparathyroidism is a parathyroidectomy. Before surgery the patient is stabilized and calcium levels are decreased to near normal.

The operative procedure can be performed as minimally invasive surgery, mini-incision surgery, or with a traditional transverse incision in the lower neck. All four parathyroid glands are examined for enlargement. If a tumor is present on one side but the other side is normal, the surgeon removes the glands containing tumor and leaves the remaining glands on the opposite side intact. If all four glands are diseased, they are all removed.

Nursing care before and after surgical removal of the parathyroid glands is the same as that for thyroidectomy. See the Preoperative Care section on p. 1289 and the Postoperative Care section on p. 1290 for specific nursing interventions.

The remaining glands, which may have atrophied as a result of PTH overproduction, require several days to several weeks to return to normal function. A hypocalcemic crisis can occur during this critical period, and the serum calcium level is assessed frequently after surgery. Check serum calcium levels whenever they are drawn until calcium levels stabilize. Monitor for manifestations of hypocalcemia, such as tingling and twitching in the extremities and face. Check for Trousseau's and Chvostek's signs, either of which indicates potential tetany (see Chapter 11).

The recurrent laryngeal nerve can be damaged. Assess the patient for changes in voice patterns and hoarseness.

When hyperparathyroidism is due to **hyperplasia** (tissue overgrowth), three glands plus half of the fourth gland are usually removed. If all four glands are removed, a small portion and may be implanted in the forearm, where it produces PTH and maintains calcium homeostasis. If all these maneuvers fail, the patient will need lifelong treatment with calcium and vitamin D because the resulting hypoparathyroidism is permanent (see next section).

HYPOPARATHYROIDISM

❖ PATHOPHYSIOLOGY

Hypoparathyroidism is a rare endocrine disorder in which parathyroid function is decreased. Problems are directly related to a lack of parathyroid hormone (PTH) secretion or to decreased effectiveness of PTH on target tissue. Whether the problem is a lack of PTH secretion or an ineffectiveness of PTH on tissues, the result is the same: *hypocalcemia.*

Iatrogenic hypoparathyroidism, the most common form, is caused by the removal of all parathyroid tissue during total thyroidectomy or by surgical removal of the parathyroid glands.

Idiopathic hypoparathyroidism can occur spontaneously. The exact cause is unknown, but an autoimmune basis is suspected. It may occur with other autoimmune disorders such as adrenal insufficiency, hypothyroidism, diabetes mellitus, pernicious anemia, and vitiligo.

Hypomagnesemia (decreased serum magnesium levels) may also cause hypoparathyroidism. Hypomagnesemia is seen in patients with malabsorption syndromes, chronic kidney disease, and malnutrition. It causes impairment of PTH secretion and may interfere with the effects of PTH on the bones, kidneys, and calcium regulation.

❖ PATIENT-CENTERED COLLABORATIVE CARE

◆ Assessment

Ask about any head or neck surgery or radiation therapy because these treatments may damage the parathyroid glands and cause hypoparathyroidism. Also ask whether the neck has ever sustained a serious injury in a car crash or by strangulation. Assess whether the patient has any manifestations of hypoparathyroidism, which may range from mild tingling and numbness to muscle tetany. Tingling and numbness around the mouth or in the hands and feet reflect mild to moderate hypocalcemia. Severe muscle cramps, spasms of the hands and feet, and seizures (with no loss of consciousness or incontinence) reflect a more severe hypocalcemia. The patient or family may notice mental changes ranging from irritability to psychosis.

The physical assessment may show excessive or inappropriate muscle contractions that cause finger, hand, and elbow flexion. This can signal an impending attack of tetany. Check for Chvostek's sign and Trousseau's sign; positive responses indicate potential tetany (see Chapter 11). Bands or pits may encircle the crowns of the teeth, which indicate a loss of calcium from the teeth with enamel loss.

Diagnostic tests for hypoparathyroidism include electroencephalography (EEG), blood tests, and CT scans. EEG changes revert to normal with correction of hypocalcemia. Serum calcium, phosphorus, magnesium, vitamin D, and urine cyclic adenosine monophosphate (cAMP) levels may be used in the diagnostic workup for hypoparathyroidism (see Chart 63-10). The CT scan can show brain calcifications, which indicate chronic hypocalcemia.

◆ Interventions

Nonsurgical management of hypoparathyroidism focuses on correcting hypocalcemia, vitamin D deficiency, and hypomagnesemia. For patients with acute and severe hypocalcemia, IV calcium is given as a 10% solution of calcium chloride or calcium gluconate over 10 to 15 minutes. Acute vitamin D deficiency is treated with oral calcitriol (Rocaltrol), 0.5 to 2 mg daily. Acute hypomagnesemia is corrected with 50% magnesium sulfate in 2-mL doses (up to 4 g daily) IV. Long-term oral therapy for hypocalcemia involves the intake of calcium, 0.5 to 2 g daily, in divided doses.

Long-term therapy for vitamin D deficiency is 50,000 to 400,000 units of oral ergocalciferol daily. The dosage is adjusted to keep the patient's calcium level in the low-normal range (slightly hypocalcemic), enough to prevent symptoms of hypocalcemia. It must also be low enough to prevent increased urine calcium levels, which can lead to stone formation.

Nursing management includes teaching about the drug regimen and interventions to reduce anxiety. Teach the patient to eat foods high in calcium but low in phosphorus. Milk, yogurt, and processed cheeses are avoided because of their high phosphorus content. *Stress that therapy for hypocalcemia is lifelong.* Advise the patient to wear a medical alert bracelet. With adherence to the prescribed drug and diet regimen, the calcium level usually remains high enough to prevent a hypocalcemic crisis.

NCLEX EXAMINATION CHALLENGE

Safe and Effective Care Environment

When taking the blood pressure of a client receiving treatment for hyperparathyroidism, the nurse observes the client's hand to undergo flexion contractions. What is the nurse's interpretation of this observation?

A. Hyperphosphatemia
B. Hypophosphatemia
C. Hypercalcemia
D. Hypocalcemia

NURSING CONCEPTS AND CLINICAL JUDGMENT REVIEW

What might you NOTICE in a patient with hyperthyroidism who demonstrates inadequate THERMOREGULATION?

Vital signs:

- Blood pressure elevated with a widened pulse pressure
- Heart rate rapid and irregular
- Temperature above 100° F

Physical assessment:

- Excessive sweating
- Smooth, warm, moist skin
- Underweight for height
- Fine hand tremors

Psychosocial assessment:

- Decreased attention span

- Restlessness and irritability
- Emotional lability

Laboratory assessment:
- Elevated T_3 and T_4 levels
- Abnormal TSH levels

What should you INTERPRET and how should you RESPOND to a patient experiencing inadequate THERMOREGULATION as a result of hyperthyroidism?

Perform and interpret physical assessment, including:
- Assessing body temperature
- Assessing cardiac effectiveness
- Checking deep tendon reflexes

Respond by:
- Maintaining a calm approach
- Cooling the environment
- Offering a sponge bath or shower
- Avoiding palpation of the neck or thyroid gland
- Maintaining a patent airway
- Administering prescribed drugs appropriately
- Notifying the health care provider of changes in cardiac or neurologic status

On what should you REFLECT?
- Think about how the environment could be made more calming.
- Think about what emergency equipment might be needed.

GET READY FOR THE NCLEX® EXAMINATION!

KEY POINTS

Review these Key Points for each NCLEX Examination Client Needs Category.

Safe and Effective Care Environment
- Keep the environment of a patient at risk for thyroid storm cool, dark, and quiet. **Safety** QSEN
- Keep emergency suctioning and tracheotomy equipment in the room of a patient who has had thyroid or parathyroid surgery. **Safety** QSEN
- Use a lift sheet to move or reposition a patient with hypocalcemia. **Safety** QSEN

Health Promotion and Maintenance
- Teach all patients to take antithyroid drugs or thyroid hormone replacement therapy as prescribed. **Patient-Centered Care** QSEN
- Teach patients to use clinical manifestations (e.g., the number of bowel movements per day, the ability to sleep) as indicators of therapy effectiveness and when the dose of thyroid hormone replacement may need to be adjusted. **Patient-Centered Care** QSEN
- Include the person who prepares the patient's meals when teaching about dietary electrolyte restrictions. **Patient-Centered Care** QSEN
- Collaborate with the registered dietitian to teach patients about diets that are restricted in calcium or phosphorus. **Teamwork and Collaboration** QSEN

Psychosocial Integrity
- Be accepting of patient behavior. **Patient-Centered Care** QSEN
- Remind patients and family members that changes in cognition and behavior related to thyroid problems are usually temporary. **Patient-Centered Care** QSEN
- Encourage the patient who has a permanent change in appearance (e.g., exophthalmia) to mourn the change. **Patient-Centered Care** QSEN

Physiological Integrity
- Be aware that:
  - The presence of a goiter indicates a problem with the thyroid gland but can accompany either hyperthyroidism or hypothyroidism.
  - Although similar in action, methimazole and propylthiouracil are not interchangeable.
  - Methimazole can cause birth defects and should not be used during pregnancy, especially during the first trimester.
- When stridor, dyspnea, or other symptoms of obstruction appear after thyroid surgery, notify the Rapid Response Team. **Safety** QSEN
- When caring for a patient with hyperthyroidism, even after a thyroidectomy, immediately report a temperature increase of even 1°F because it may indicate an impending thyroid crisis. **Evidence-Based Practice** QSEN
- Assess the cardiopulmonary status of any patient with hypothyroidism for decreased perfusion or decreased gas exchange at least every 8 hours. **Patient-Centered Care** QSEN
- Use sedating drugs or opioids sparingly with patients who have hypothyroidism. **Patient-Centered Care** QSEN
- Monitor the hydration status of patients who have hypercalcemia. **Patient-Centered Care** QSEN
- Assess the patient with hypoparathyroidism for manifestations of hypocalcemia, especially numbness or tingling around the mouth and a positive Chvostek's sign or Trousseau's sign. **Patient-Centered Care** QSEN

64 CHAPTER

Care of Patients with Diabetes Mellitus

Margaret Elaine McLeod

http://evolve.elsevier.com/Iggy/

PRIORITY CONCEPTS

- Glucose Regulation
- Tissue Integrity
- Sensory Perception
- Perfusion
- Infection
- Pain
- Nutrition

LEARNING OUTCOMES

Safe and Effective Care Environment

1. Protect the patient who has diabetes mellitus from injury.
2. Protect the patient who has diabetes mellitus from infection.

Health Promotion and Maintenance

3. Teach all people how to prevent or delay development of type 2 diabetes.
4. Teach people who have diabetes to prevent or delay long-term complications of the disorder.
5. Teach all patients with diabetes and their family members how to self-manage their disease.
6. Teach the patient with diabetes and the family the importance of foot care and good nutrition.
7. Work with other health care professionals to help the patient and family experiencing diabetes mellitus achieve health goals.

Psychosocial Integrity

8. Reduce the psychological impact of diabetes mellitus for the patient and family.
9. Work with other members of the health care team to ensure that patient values, preferences, and expressed needs related to diabetes mellitus are respected.

Physiological Integrity

10. Compare the risk factors, age of onset, manifestations, and pathologic mechanisms of type 1 and type 2 diabetes mellitus.
11. Apply knowledge of anatomy, physiology, and pathophysiology to assess the adequacy of glucose regulation for the patient with diabetes.
12. Ensure that pain is appropriately managed for the patient with diabetes.
13. Evaluate laboratory data and clinical manifestations to determine effectiveness of the prescribed dietary, drug, and exercise therapies for diabetes.
14. Prioritize care for the patient with diabetes experiencing hypoglycemia, ketoacidosis, or hyperglycemic-hyperosmolar state (HHS).
15. Coordinate care for the patient with diabetes in the community.

Diabetes mellitus (DM) resulting in poor glucose regulation is a major public health problem, and its complications, especially hypertension and **hyperlipidemia** (high blood lipid levels), cause many serious health problems. In the United States, DM is a leading cause of blindness, end-stage kidney disease, and foot or leg amputations. Many people have undiagnosed diabetes, and among those who are diagnosed, many continue to have high blood glucose levels. The complications of DM can be greatly reduced with **glycemic** (blood glucose) control along with management of hypertension and hyperlipidemia. Thus nursing priorities focus on helping the patient with diabetes achieve and maintain lifestyle changes that prevent long-term complications by keeping blood glucose levels and cholesterol levels as close to normal as possible.

Because DM is a chronic metabolic disease affecting glucose regulation, it requires lifelong behavioral and lifestyle changes for best management. A collaborative approach helps the patient be successful in achieving desired outcomes. As part of the team, you will plan, organize, and coordinate care with other health care team members to provide care and promote the patient's health and well-being.

❖ PATHOPHYSIOLOGY

Classification of Diabetes

For all types of diabetes mellitus (DM), the main feature is chronic **hyperglycemia** (high blood glucose level) resulting from problems with glucose regulation that include reduced

TABLE 64-1 Classification of Diabetes Mellitus

Type 1 Diabetes
- Beta-cell destruction leading to absolute insulin deficiency
- Autoimmune
- Idiopathic

Type 2 Diabetes
- Ranges from insulin resistance with relative insulin deficiency to secretory deficit with insulin resistance

Other Conditions Resulting in Hyperglycemia
- Genetic defects of beta-cell function
- Genetic defects in insulin action
- Pancreatic diseases (pancreatitis, trauma, cancer, cystic fibrosis, hemochromatosis)
- Endocrinopathies: acromegaly, Cushing's disease, glucagonoma, pheochromocytoma, hyperthyroidism, aldosteronism
- Drug- or chemical-induced hyperglycemia
- Infections: congenital rubella, cytomegalovirus, human immune deficiency virus
- Genetic syndromes associated with diabetes: Down syndrome, Klinefelter syndrome, Turner's syndrome, Huntington disease, and others

Gestational Diabetes Mellitus (GDM)
- Glucose intolerance with onset or first recognition during pregnancy

Data from American Diabetes Association (ADA). (2014d). Position statement: Diagnosis and classification of diabetes mellitus. *Diabetes Care, 37*(Suppl. 1), S81-S90.

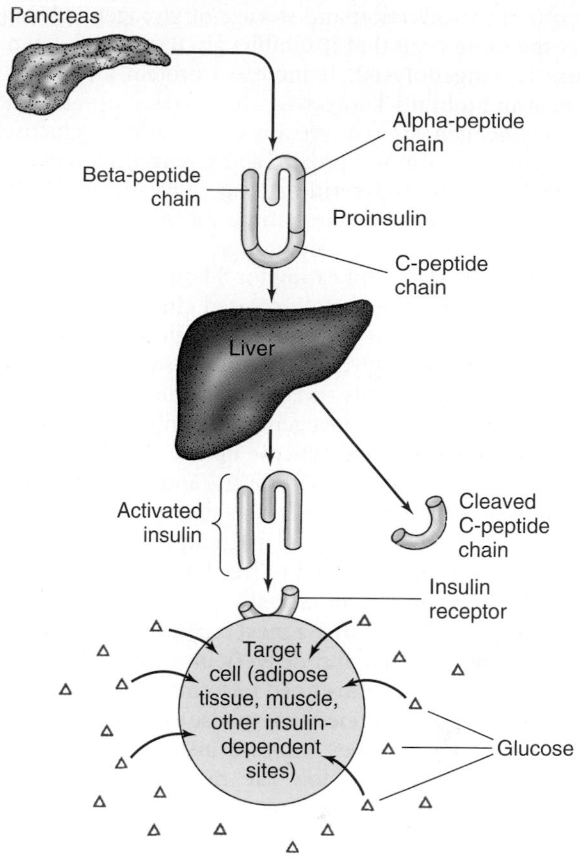

FIG. 64-1 Proinsulin, secreted by and stored in the beta cells of the islets of Langerhans in the pancreas, is transformed by the liver into active insulin. Insulin attaches to receptors on target cells, where it promotes glucose transport into the cells through the cell membranes.

insulin secretion or reduced insulin action (McCance et al., 2014). The disease is classified by the underlying problem causing a lack of insulin or its action and the severity of the insulin deficiency. Table 64-1 outlines the types of DM.

The Endocrine Pancreas

The pancreas has exocrine functions that are related to digestion and endocrine functions for blood GLUCOSE REGULATION. The endocrine portion of the pancreas has about 1 million small glands, the islets of Langerhans, scattered through the organ. The islet cells are only a small portion of the gland. The two types of islet cells important to glucose regulation are the *alpha* cells, which secrete glucagon, and the *beta* cells, which produce insulin and amylin. **Glucagon** is a "counterregulatory" hormone that has actions opposite those of insulin. It prevents *hypoglycemia* (low blood glucose levels) by triggering the release of glucose from cell storage sites. Insulin prevents hyperglycemia by allowing body cells to take up, use, and store carbohydrate, fat, and protein.

Active insulin is a protein made up of 51 amino acids. It is initially produced as inactive *proinsulin,* a prohormone that contains an additional amino acid chain (the C-peptide chain). Proinsulin is converted into active insulin by removal of the C-peptide (Fig. 64-1).

Insulin is secreted daily directly into liver circulation in a two-step manner. It is secreted at low levels during fasting (basal insulin secretion) and at increased levels after eating (**prandial**). An early burst of insulin secretion occurs within 10 minutes of eating. This is followed by an increasing release that lasts until the blood glucose level is normal.

Glucose Regulation and Homeostasis

Glucose is the main fuel for central nervous system (CNS) cells. Because the brain cannot produce or store much glucose, it needs a continuous supply from circulation to prevent neuron dysfunction and cell death. Other organs can use both glucose and fatty acids to generate energy. Glucose is stored inside cells as glycogen in the liver and muscles, and free fatty acids are stored as triglyceride in fat cells. Fat is the most efficient means of storing energy, with 9 calories of stored energy per gram. Protein and carbohydrate have only 4 calories per gram. During a prolonged fast or after illness, proteins are broken down and some of the amino acids are converted into glucose.

Several organs and hormones play a role in maintaining GLUCOSE REGULATION. During fasting, when the stomach is empty, blood glucose is maintained between 60 and 150 mg/dL (3.3 and 8.3 mmol/L) by a balance between glucose uptake by cells and glucose production by the liver. Insulin plays a pivotal role in this process.

Movement of glucose into some cells requires the presence of specific carrier proteins, known as glucose transport (GLUT) proteins, along with insulin. Insulin is like a "key" that opens "locked" membranes to glucose, allowing blood glucose to move into cells to generate energy. Insulin starts this action by binding to insulin receptors on the cell membranes, which changes membrane permeability to glucose.

Insulin exerts many effects on metabolism and cellular processes in all tissues and organs. The main metabolic effects of insulin are to stimulate glucose uptake in skeletal muscle and heart muscle and to suppress liver production of glucose and very-low-density lipoprotein (VLDL). In the liver, insulin promotes the production and storage of glycogen (**glycogenesis**) at the same time that it inhibits glycogen breakdown into glucose (**glycogenolysis**). It increases protein and lipid (fat) synthesis and inhibits **ketogenesis** (conversion of fats to acids) and **gluconeogenesis** (conversion of proteins to glucose). In muscle, insulin promotes protein and glycogen synthesis. In fat cells, it promotes triglyceride storage. Overall, insulin keeps blood glucose levels from becoming too high and helps keep blood lipid levels in the normal range.

In the *fasting state* (not eating for 8 hours), insulin secretion is suppressed, which leads to increased gluconeogenesis in the liver and kidneys, along with increased glucose generation by the breakdown of liver glycogen. In the fed state, insulin released from pancreatic beta cells reverses this process. Instead, glycogen breakdown and gluconeogenesis are inhibited. At the same time, insulin also enhances glucose uptake and use by cells and reduces both fat breakdown (**lipolysis**) and protein breakdown (**proteolysis**). When more glucose is present in liver cells than can be used for energy or stored as glycogen, insulin causes the excess glucose to be converted to free fatty acids (FFAs). These extra FFAs are deposited in fat cells.

Glucose in the blood after a meal is controlled by the emptying rate of the stomach and delivery of nutrients to the small intestine where they are absorbed into circulation. Incretin hormones (e.g., GLP-1), secreted in response to food in the stomach, have several actions. They increase insulin secretion, inhibit glucagon secretion, and slow the rate of gastric emptying, thereby preventing hyperglycemia after meals.

Counterregulatory hormones increase blood glucose by actions opposite those of insulin when more energy is needed. Glucagon is the main counterregulatory hormone. Other hormones that increase blood glucose levels are epinephrine, norepinephrine, growth hormone, and cortisol. The combined actions of insulin and counterregulatory hormones (discussed in the next section) participate in GLUCOSE REGULATION and keep blood glucose levels in the range of 60 to 100 mg/dL (3.3 to 5.6 mmol/L) to support brain function. When blood glucose levels fall, insulin secretion stops and glucagon is released. Glucagon causes glucose release from the liver. Liver glucose is made through breakdown of glycogen to glucose (glycogenolysis) and conversion of amino acids into glucose. When liver glucose is unavailable, the breakdown of fat (lipolysis) and the breakdown of proteins (proteolysis) provide fuel for energy.

NCLEX EXAMINATION CHALLENGE

Physiological Integrity

How is hypoglycemia prevented in the healthy person who does not have diabetes even after fasting for 8 hours?

A. Metabolism is so slow when a person sleeps without eating for 8 hours that blood glucose does not enter cells to be used for energy. As a result, hypoglycemia does not occur.
B. Fasting for 8 hours triggers conversion of proteins into glycogen (glycogenesis) so that hyperglycemia develops rather than hypoglycemia.
C. Lipolysis (fat breakdown) in fat stores occurs, converting fatty acids into glucose to maintain blood glucose levels.
D. The secretion of glucagon prevents hypoglycemia by promoting glucose release from liver storage sites.

TABLE 64-2 Physiologic Response to Insufficient Insulin

- Decreased glycogenesis (conversion of glucose to glycogen)
- Increased glycogenolysis (conversion of glycogen to glucose)
- Increased gluconeogenesis (formation of glucose from noncarbohydrate sources such as amino acids and lactate)
- Increased lipolysis (breakdown of triglycerides to glycerol and free fatty acids)
- Increased ketogenesis (formation of ketones from free fatty acids)
- Proteolysis (breakdown of protein with amino acid release in muscles)

Absence of Insulin

Insulin for GLUCOSE REGULATION is needed to move glucose into many body tissues. The lack of insulin in diabetes, from either a lack of production or a problem with insulin use at its cell receptor, prevents some cells from using glucose for energy. The body then breaks down fat and protein in an attempt to provide energy and increases levels of counterregulatory hormones to make glucose from other sources. Table 64-2 outlines responses to insufficient insulin.

Without insulin, glucose builds up in the blood, causing high blood glucose levels (**hyperglycemia**). Hyperglycemia causes fluid and electrolyte imbalances, leading to the classic manifestations of diabetes: polyuria, polydipsia, and polyphagia.

Polyuria is frequent and excessive urination and results from an osmotic diuresis caused by excess glucose in the blood and urine. With diuresis, electrolytes are excreted in the urine and water loss is severe. Dehydration results, and **polydipsia** (excessive thirst) occurs. Because the cells receive no glucose, cell starvation triggers **polyphagia** (excessive eating). Despite eating, the person remains in cellular starvation until insulin is available to move glucose into the cells.

With insulin deficiency, fats break down, releasing free fatty acids. Conversion of fatty acids to **ketone bodies** (small acids) provides a backup energy source. Ketone bodies or "ketones" are abnormal breakdown products that collect in the blood when insulin is not available, leading to a type of metabolic acidosis known as ketoacidosis.

Dehydration with diabetes leads to hemoconcentration (increased blood concentration); hypovolemia (decreased blood volume); thick, concentrated blood; poor tissue PERFUSION; and hypoxia (poor tissue oxygenation), especially to the brain. Hypoxic cells do not metabolize glucose efficiently, the Krebs' cycle is blocked, and lactic acid increases, causing more acidosis.

The excess acids caused by absence of insulin increase hydrogen ion (H^+) and carbon dioxide (CO_2) levels in the blood, causing anion-gap metabolic acidosis. These products trigger the brain to increase the rate and depth of respiration in an attempt to "blow off" carbon dioxide and acid. This type of breathing is known as **Kussmaul respiration**. Acetone is exhaled, giving the breath a "rotting fruit" odor. When the lungs can no longer offset acidosis, the blood pH drops. Arterial blood gas studies show a metabolic acidosis (decreased pH with decreased arterial bicarbonate [HCO_3^-] levels) and compensatory respiratory alkalosis (decreased partial pressure of arterial carbon dioxide [$Paco_2$]).

Insulin lack initially causes potassium depletion. With the increased fluid loss from hyperglycemia, excessive potassium is excreted in the urine, leading to low serum potassium levels.

High serum potassium levels may occur in acidosis because of the shift of potassium from inside the cells to the blood. Serum potassium levels in DM, then, may be low (**hypokalemia**), high (**hyperkalemia**), or normal, depending on hydration, the severity of acidosis, and the patient's response to treatment. Chapter 12 discusses acid-base balance and acidosis in more detail.

Acute Complications of Diabetes

Three glucose-related emergencies can occur in patients with diabetes:

- Diabetic ketoacidosis (DKA) caused by lack of insulin and ketosis
- Hyperglycemic-hyperosmolar state (HHS) caused by insulin deficiency and profound dehydration
- Hypoglycemia from too much insulin or too little glucose

All three problems require emergency treatment and can be fatal if treatment is delayed or incorrect. These problems and their interventions are described later, starting on p. 1330.

Chronic Complications of Diabetes

Diabetes mellitus (DM) can lead to health problems and early death because of changes in large blood vessels (**macrovascular**) and small blood vessels (**microvascular**) in tissues and organs (McCance et al., 2014). Complications result from poor tissue PERFUSION and cell death. Macrovascular complications, including coronary heart disease, cerebrovascular disease, and peripheral vascular disease, lead to increased early death. Microvascular complications of blood vessel structure and function lead to **nephropathy** (kidney dysfunction), **neuropathy** (nerve dysfunction), and **retinopathy** (vision problems). Causes of these diabetic vascular complications include:

- Chronic hyperglycemia thickens basement membranes, which causes organ damage.
- Glucose toxicity directly or indirectly affects functional cell integrity.
- Chronic ischemia in small blood vessels causes connective tissue hypoxia and microischemia.

Chronic high blood glucose levels are the main cause of microvascular complications and allow premature development of macrovascular complications. Other risk factors contributing to poor health outcomes for people with DM include smoking, physical inactivity, obesity, hypertension, and high blood fat and cholesterol levels. Many of these factors can be modified to reduce complications related to DM.

Hyperglycemia from poor GLUCOSE REGULATION is a critical factor for long-term complications in patients with type 1 DM. Intensive therapy to maintain blood glucose levels as close to normal as possible delays the onset and progression of retinopathy, nephropathy, neuropathy, and macrovascular disease for patients with type 1 and type 2 DM. For every percentage point decrease in A1C (glycosylated hemoglobin A1C), a risk reduction of at least 25% to 30% for kidney and eye complications has been shown (American Diabetes Association [ADA], 2014b).

Macrovascular Complications

Cardiovascular Disease. Diabetes mellitus (DM) is associated with a reduced life span, largely as a result of cardiovascular disease (CVD). Most patients with DM die as a result of a thrombotic event, usually myocardial infarction (MI). Systolic and diastolic heart failure are associated with DM. Patients with DM are more likely to develop left ventricular dysfunction with heart failure and fatal cardiac dysrhythmias after MI.

Patients with diabetes, those with prediabetes, and those with metabolic syndrome are at increased risk for CVD (ADA, 2014f). This risk affects women to a greater degree than men and is influenced by the patient's ethnic group. Diabetes is now considered a "coronary heart disease risk equivalent" and a target for aggressive reduction of risk factors.

Patients with diabetes often have the traditional CVD risk factors of obesity, high blood lipid levels, hypertension, and sedentary lifestyle. Cigarette smoking and a positive family history also increase risk for CVD. Kidney disease, indicated by **albuminuria** (presence of albumin in the urine), increases the risk for coronary heart disease and mortality from MI. Patients with DM often have higher levels of C-reactive protein (CRP), an inflammatory marker associated with increased risk for cardiovascular problems and death. In addition, the presence of diabetic retinopathy is associated with an increased risk for mortality and cardiovascular events in both type 1 and type 2 DM.

Cardiovascular complication rates can be reduced through aggressive management of hyperglycemia, hypertension, and hyperlipidemia. The American Diabetes Association (ADA) recommends that blood pressure be maintained below 140/80 mm Hg and that low-density lipoprotein (LDL) cholesterol remains below 100 mg/dL (2.60 mmol/L) for patients without manifestations of CVD and below 70 mg/dL (1.8 mmol/L) for patients with manifestations of CVD (ADA, 2014f). Lifestyle modifications that focus on reducing saturated fat, *trans* fat, and cholesterol intake; increasing intake of omega-3 fatty acids, fiber, and plant sterols; weight loss (if indicated); and increasing physical activity are recommended to improve the lipid profile for patients with DM (ADA, 2013).

Priority nursing actions focus on interventions to reduce modifiable risk factors associated with CVD, such as smoking cessation, diet, exercise, blood pressure control, maintaining prescribed aspirin use, and maintaining prescribed lipid-lowering drug therapy. Many patients with DM do not have the traditional and more obvious manifestations of myocardial infarction (i.e., crushing chest pain radiating down the left arm or up the jaw). Instead the manifestations are more subtle. These include dyspnea with or without cough, extreme fatigue, and sudden onset of nausea and vomiting. Teach patients to report any of these subtle manifestations of MI to their health care provider for evaluation.

Cerebrovascular Disease. The risk for stroke is 2 to 4 times higher in people with DM compared with those who do not have the disease. Diabetes also increases the likelihood of severe carotid atherosclerosis. Hypertension, hyperlipidemia, nephropathy, peripheral vascular disease, and alcohol and tobacco use further increase the risk for stroke in people with DM.

DM also affects stroke outcomes. Patients with DM are likely to suffer irreversible brain damage with carotid emboli that produce only transient ischemic attacks in people without DM. Elevated blood glucose levels at the time of the stroke may lead to greater brain injury and higher mortality.

Microvascular Complications

Eye and Vision Complications. Legal blindness (a corrected visual acuity of 20/200 or less) is 25 times more common in patients with DM. Diabetic retinopathy (DR) is strongly related to the duration of diabetes. After 20 years of DM, nearly all patients with type 1 disease and most with type 2 disease have some degree of retinopathy. Unfortunately, DR has few manifestations until vision loss occurs.

The cause and progression of DR are related to problems that block retinal blood vessels and cause them to leak, leading to retinal hypoxia. Nonproliferative diabetic retinopathy causes structural problems in retinal vessels, including areas of poor retinal circulation, edema, hard fatty deposits in the eye, and retinal hemorrhages. Fluid and blood leak from the retinal vessels and cause retinal edema and hard exudates.

Other retinal problems include optic nerve atrophy from hypoxia and venous beading. **Venous beading** is the abnormal appearance of retinal veins in which areas of swelling and constriction along a segment of vein resemble links of sausage. It occurs in areas of retinal ischemia. Nonproliferative diabetic retinopathies develop slowly and rarely reduce vision to the point of blindness.

Proliferative diabetic retinopathy is the growth of new retinal blood vessels, also known as "neovascularization." When retinal blood flow is poor and hypoxia develops, retinal cells secrete growth factors that stimulate formation of new blood vessels in the eye. These new vessels are thin, fragile, and bleed easily, leading to eye hemorrhage and vision loss.

Visual SENSORY PERCEPTION loss from DR has several mechanisms. Central vision may be impaired by macular edema, characterized by increased blood vessel permeability and deposits of hard exudates at the center of the retina. This problem is the main cause of vision loss in the person with DM. Monthly injections of ranibizumab (Lucentis) into the vitreous can improve vision for some people with macular edema (Aschenbrenner, 2012). Vision loss also occurs from macular degeneration, corneal scarring, and changes in lens shape or clarity.

Hyperglycemia may cause blurred vision, even with eyeglasses. Hypoglycemia may cause double vision. Cataracts occur at a younger age and progress faster among patients with DM. Open-angle glaucoma also is more common in patients with DM. The management of cataracts and glaucoma is the same as for patients who do not have diabetes (see Chapter 47).

Control of blood glucose, blood pressure, and blood lipid levels is important in preventing DR. Thus patients with DM should have routine ophthalmic evaluations to detect vision problems early before vision loss occurs. The ADA recommends eye care examinations with an ophthalmologist every year after a person has been diagnosed with type 2 diabetes and yearly for a person who has had type 1 diabetes for more than 5 years (Chou et al., 2014). Not all people with DM understand the importance of these annual eye screenings (see the Evidence-Based Practice box).

EVIDENCE-BASED PRACTICE QSEN

Why Do Adults with Diabetes Forego Annual Eye Care?

Chou, C., Sherrod, C., Zhang, Z., Barker, L., Bullard, K., Crews, J., et al. (2014). Barriers to eye care among people aged 40 years and older with diagnosed diabetes, 2006-2010. *Diabetes Care, 37*(1), 180-188.

Both type 1 and type 2 diabetes mellitus (DM) are associated with major eye problems and blindness. Extensive research has shown that maintaining tight glucose control and having at least annual ophthalmologic evaluations can reduce or delay eye complications. Previous studies have indicated that vision impairment related to DM has increased by 20% in less than 10 years. The purposes of this large retrospective and descriptive study were to determine (1) about what percentage of people with diabetes mellitus were following the recommended guidelines of annual eye examinations from the time of diagnosis of type 2 DM and starting at 5 years after initial diagnosis of type 1 DM, and (2) what were the barriers to eye care for those who were not following the recommended guidelines. The researchers re-analyzed the existing data previously collected through the Behavior Risk Factor Surveillance System (BRFSS), an annual state-based random-digit-dialed telephone survey, from 22 states between the years 2006 and 2010. The defined categories of barriers to eye care were (1) cost, lack of insurance; (2) no need, have not thought of it, no reason to; (3) no eye doctor, transportation issues, couldn't get an appointment; and (4) other (everything else). More than 27,000 people who were diagnosed with DM responded to the survey.

Of the subjects with DM, 23.5% (more than 6500) reported not having had an eye examination in the previous 12 months. The barrier categories cited among these subjects were: 39.7% category **1,** 32.3% category **2,** 6.4% category **3,** and 20.5% category **4**. The majority of subjects citing barrier category **1** issues were women between the ages of 40 years and 64 years, those who have lower annual incomes, those of Hispanic or African-American ethnicity, and those who had less formal education. The majority of subjects citing barrier category **2** issues were white men, those with higher incomes, those with more formal education, and those with diagnosed visual problems. The researchers indicated that the cost issue was not surprising because Medicare does cover an annual eye examination for people older than 65 years, and the younger subjects may not have had sufficient funds or insurance to cover this cost. The surprising results were the people, especially those who already had some degree of visual problem, who said they believed there was essentially "no need" for an annual eye examination.

Level of Evidence: 4

Although very large, the study was retrospective and descriptive in nature without randomization of subject selection or assignment. The data collected relied on subject self-report and was subject to social desirability bias in that more subjects may have reported receiving annual eye examinations than actually participated in the health-seeking behavior. Also, subjects did not include people without telephones, those who had only cell phone access, those residing in institutions, and those with undiagnosed diabetes. In addition to the study size and the fact that many ethnic groups were represented, a major strength was the detailed questions asked about the barriers to eye care behaviors. The methods of statistical analysis were appropriate for the research questions posed.

Commentary: Implications for Practice and Research

The results of this study indicate that cost is a significant barrier to annual eye care for people with diabetes. Perhaps this barrier will change with the implementation of the Affordable Care Act. Nurses can help people with diabetes check their insurance policies to determine what types of eye care are covered and encourage them to make use of this benefit. Of equal concern is the subjects' beliefs that there is no compelling need for annual eye care. It is possible that some patients think that all vision issues over age 65 years are related to old age and are unavoidable. Nurses can help patients with DM understand that annual eye care can slow the progression of existing vision problems and may help prevent blindness. Other strategies for increasing adherence to annual eye care include reminders from the health care provider and nurses' asking patient's with DM during any encounter when the last eye care appointment was and reinforcing the importance of this health care behavior. More research is needed to determine specifically why patients with DM believe that annual eye care is not necessary so that more targeted interventions could be developed.

CONSIDERATIONS FOR OLDER ADULTS

Patient-Centered Care QSEN

The older patient with diabetic retinopathy also has visual changes from aging, and his or her ability to perform self-care may be seriously affected. The patient with retinopathy may have blurred vision, distorted central vision, fluctuating vision, loss of color perception, and mobility problems resulting from loss of depth perception. It is especially important to assess the patient's ability to measure and inject insulin and to monitor blood glucose levels to determine if adaptive devices are needed to assist in self-management activities.

Diabetic Peripheral Neuropathy. **Diabetic peripheral neuropathy** (DPN) is a progressive deterioration of nerve function that results in loss of SENSORY PERCEPTION. It is a common complication of DM and often involves all parts of the body. Damage to sensory nerve fibers results in either pain or loss of sensation. Damage to motor nerve fibers results in muscle weakness. Damage to nerve fibers in the autonomic nervous system can cause dysfunction in every part of the body. The combination of interacting factors leading to the nerve damage in DPN are:

- Hyperglycemia, long duration of DM, hyperlipidemia, low insulin levels
- Damaged blood vessels leading to reduced neuronal oxygen and other nutrients
- Autoimmune neuronal inflammation
- Increased genetic susceptibility to nerve damage
- Smoking and alcohol use

Hyperglycemia leads to DPN through blood vessel changes and reduced tissue PERFUSION that cause nerve hypoxia. Both the axon and its myelin sheath are damaged by reduced blood flow, resulting in blocked nerve impulse transmission. Excessive glucose is converted to sorbitol, which collects in nerves and impairs motor nerve conduction. Common diabetic neuropathies are listed in Table 64-3. Autonomic nervous system neuropathy leads to problems in cardiovascular, GI, and urinary function. Keeping blood glucose levels in the normal range can slow the development and progression of diabetic neuropathies.

Diabetic neuropathy can be focal or diffuse, each with different causes and rates of progression. *Diffuse neuropathies* are the most common neuropathies in DM and involve widespread nerve function loss and SENSORY PERCEPTION loss. The onset is slow, affects both sides of the body, involves motor and sensory nerves, progresses slowly, is permanent, and includes autonomic nerve dysfunction. Late complications include foot ulcers and deformities.

Focal neuropathies in DM affect a single nerve or nerve group and usually are caused by an acute ischemic event that leads to nerve damage or nerve death. Ischemic neuropathies occur when the blood supply to a nerve or nerve group is disrupted. Manifestations begin suddenly, affect only one side of the body area, and are self-limiting. The most common neuropathies affect the nerves that control the eye muscles. Manifestations begin with pain on one side of the face near the affected eye. The eye muscles become paralyzed, resulting in double vision. The problem usually resolves in 2 to 3 months.

Cardiovascular autonomic neuropathy (CAN) affects sympathetic and parasympathetic nerves to the heart and blood vessels. This problem contributes to left ventricular dysfunction, painless myocardial infarction, and exercise intolerance. Most often, CAN leads to **orthostatic hypotension** (postural hypotension) and **syncope** (brief loss of consciousness on standing). These problems result from failure of the heart and arteries to adjust to position changes by increasing heart rate and vascular tone. As a result, blood flow to the brain is interrupted briefly. Orthostatic hypotension and syncope increase the risk for falls, especially among older adults.

Autonomic neuropathy can affect the entire GI system. Common GI problems from diabetic neuropathy include gastroesophageal reflex, delayed gastric emptying and gastric retention, early satiety, heartburn, nausea, vomiting, and anorexia. Sluggish movement of the small intestine can lead to bacterial overgrowth, which causes bloating, gas, and diarrhea. Diarrhea caused by diabetes is chronic, may be severe, and often occurs at night. Constipation, the most common GI problem with DM, is intermittent and may alternate with bouts of diarrhea. **Gastroparesis** (delay in gastric emptying) is a cause of hypoglycemia.

TABLE 64-3 Features of Diabetic Neuropathy

	COMPLICATION	MANIFESTATION
Diffuse Neuropathies		
Distal symmetric polyneuropathy	Sensory alterations	Paresthesias: burning/tingling sensations, starting in toes and moving up legs Dysesthesias: burning, stinging, or stabbing pain Anesthesia: loss of sensation
	Motor alterations in intrinsic muscles of foot	Foot deformities: high arch, claw toes, hammertoes; shift of weight-bearing to metatarsal heads and tips of toes
Autonomic neuropathy	Anhidrosis	Drying, cracking of skin
	Gastrointestinal	Delayed gastric emptying, gastric retention, early satiety, bloating, nausea, vomiting, anorexia, constipation, diarrhea
	Neurogenic bladder	Atonic bladder, urinary retention
	Impotence	Erectile dysfunction
	Cardiovascular autonomic neuropathy	Early fatigue, weakness with exercise, orthostatic hypotension
	Defective counterregulation	Loss of warning signs of hypoglycemia
Focal Neuropathies		
Focal ischemia	Thoracolumbar radiculopathy with sensory and reflex loss	Pain radiating across back, side, and front of chest or abdomen
	Cranial nerve palsies, third and sixth nerves	Sudden diplopia or ptosis; eye pain
	Amyotrophy	Pain; asymmetric weakness; wasting of iliopsoas, quadriceps, and adductor muscles

Urinary problems from neuropathy result in incomplete bladder emptying and urine retention, which lead to urinary INFECTION and kidney problems. Manifestations include frequency, urgency, and incontinence.

Diabetic Nephropathy. **Nephropathy** is a pathologic change in the kidney that reduces kidney function and leads to kidney failure. Diabetes is the leading cause of chronic kidney disease (CKD) and end-stage kidney disease (ESKD) in the United States. Risk factors include a 10- to 15-year history of DM, poor blood glucose control, uncontrolled hypertension, and genetic predisposition. Patients who have a genetic predisposition appear to have higher serum uric acid levels and higher levels of tumor necrosis factor receptors. When a person has these genetic differences, the risk for progression of kidney problems to ESKD is greater even when blood glucose levels are controlled (Krolewski et al., 2014). The onset of diabetic kidney disease may be prevented and the progression to ESKD can be delayed by maintaining optimum blood GLUCOSE REGULATION, keeping blood pressure within the normal ranges, and using drug therapy to protect the kidneys (ADA, 2014b; Krolewski et al., 2014; Zitkus, 2012). Drugs that protect the kidneys are the angiotensin-converting enzyme (ACE) inhibitors and the angiotensin receptor blockers (ABRs).

Kidney disease causes progressive albumin excretion and declining glomerular filtration rate (GFR). Early manifestations of nephropathy are **microalbuminuria** (small amounts of albumin in the urine) and elevated serum uric acid levels. Annual testing for microalbuminuria is recommended for patients who have had type 1 DM for at least 5 years and in everyone with type 2 DM (ADA, 2014b).

Chronic high blood glucose levels cause hypertension in kidney blood vessels and excess kidney tissue PERFUSION. The increased pressure damages the kidney in many ways. The blood vessels become leakier, especially in the glomerulus. This leakiness allows filtration of albumin and other proteins, which then form deposits in the kidney tissue and blood vessels. Blood vessels narrow, decreasing kidney oxygenation and leading to kidney cell hypoxia and cell death. These processes worsen over time, with scarring of glomerular blood vessels and loss of urine filtration ability, leading to kidney failure.

Kidney damage is also related to hypertension for patients with DM and cardiovascular disease. Both systolic and diastolic hypertension speed the progression of diabetic nephropathy.

Male Erectile Dysfunction. Erectile dysfunction (ED) is the inability to achieve or maintain a sufficient penile erection for satisfactory sexual performance. ED occurs at a higher rate and 10 to 15 years earlier among men with DM as compared with the general population. It is related to poor blood GLUCOSE REGULATION, obesity, hypertension, heavy cigarette smoking, and the presence of other chronic vascular complications. Chapter 72 discusses erectile function problems in depth.

Cognitive Dysfunction. People age 65 years or older with diabetes are at a significantly higher risk for developing all types of dementia as compared with people who do not have the disease. Chronic hyperglycemia with microvascular disease contributes to neuron damage, brain atrophy, and cognitive impairment (Acee, 2012). These problems occur more frequently and are more severe in patients with longer-duration DM and increase the complications of neuropathy and retinopathy. Depression is highly prevalent in people with diabetes and is associated with worse outcomes.

TABLE 64-4 Differentiation of Type 1 and Type 2 Diabetes

FEATURES	TYPE 1	TYPE 2
Former names	Juvenile-onset diabetes Ketosis-prone diabetes Insulin-dependent diabetes mellitus (IDDM)	Adult-onset diabetes Ketosis-resistant diabetes Non–insulin-dependent diabetes mellitus (NIDDM)
Age at onset	Usually younger than 30 yr, occurs at any age	Peaks in 50s; may occur earlier
Symptoms	Abrupt onset, thirst, hunger, increased urine output, weight loss	Frequently none; thirst, fatigue, blurred vision, vascular or neural complications
Etiology	Viral infection	Not known
Pathology	Pancreatic beta-cell destruction	Insulin resistance Dysfunctional pancreatic beta cell
Antigen patterns	*HLA-DR, HLA-DQ*	None
Antibodies	ICAs present at diagnosis	None
Endogenous insulin and C-peptide	None	Low, normal, or high
Inheritance	Complex	Dominant, multifactorial
Nutritional status	Usually nonobese	60% to 80% obese
Insulin	All dependent on insulin	Required for 20% to 30%
Medical nutrition therapy	Mandatory	Mandatory

ICAs, Islet cell antibodies.

NCLEX EXAMINATION CHALLENGE

Physiological Integrity

Which health problems are considered results of microvascular complications from long-term or poorly controlled diabetes mellitus?

A. Obesity and hyperglycemia
B. Systolic hypertension and heart failure
C. Retinal hemorrhage and male erectile dysfunction
D. Diabetic ketoacidosis and hyperglycemic-hyperosmolar state

Etiology and Genetic Risk

Type 1 Diabetes. Type 1 diabetes mellitus (DM) is an autoimmune disorder in which beta cells are destroyed in a genetically susceptible person (Table 64-4). The immune system fails to recognize normal body cells as "self," and immune system cells and antibodies take destructive actions against the insulin-secreting cells in the islets. People with certain tissue types are more likely to develop autoimmune diseases, including type 1 DM. Viral infections, such as mumps and coxsackievirus infection, may trigger autoimmune destructive actions (McCance et al., 2014).

Type 2 Diabetes and Metabolic Syndrome. Type 2 DM is a progressive disorder in which the person has a combination of insulin resistance and decreased beta-cell secretion of insulin. Insulin resistance (a reduced cell response to insulin) develops

GENETIC/GENOMIC CONSIDERATIONS

Patient-Centered Care QSEN

Risk for type 1 diabetes is determined by inheritance of genes coding for the *HLA-DR* and *HLA-DQA* and *DQB* tissues types (ADA, 2014d). However, inheritance of these genes only increases the risk and most people with these genes do not develop type 1 DM. Development of DM is an interactive effect of genetic predisposition and exposure to certain environmental factors. It is unclear why some genetically susceptible people develop diabetes and others do not. Ask patients newly diagnosed with type 1 diabetes whether any other relatives have diabetes or other autoimmune disease.

from obesity and physical inactivity in a genetically susceptible person. It occurs before the onset of type 2 DM and often is accompanied by the cardiovascular risk factors of hyperlipidemia, hypertension, and increased clot formation. Most patients with type 2 DM are obese (ADA, 2014d). The specific causes of type 2 DM are not known, although insulin resistance and beta-cell failure have many genetic and nongenetic causes. Heredity plays a major role in the development of type 2 DM, although not all gene variations that increase the risk for type 2 DM are known.

Metabolic syndrome is the simultaneous presence of metabolic factors known to increase risk for developing type 2 DM and cardiovascular disease. Features of the syndrome include:

- Abdominal obesity: waist circumference of 40 inches (100 cm) or more for men and 35 inches (88 cm) or more for women
- Hyperglycemia: fasting blood glucose level of 100 mg/dL or more or on drug treatment for elevated glucose
- Abnormal A1C: between 5.5% and 6.0%
- Hypertension: systolic BP of 130 mm Hg or more or diastolic BP of 85 mm Hg or more or on drug treatment for hypertension
- Hyperlipidemia: triglyceride level of 150 mg/dL or more or on drug treatment for elevated triglycerides; high-density lipoprotein (HDL) cholesterol less than 40 mg/dL for men or less than 50 mg/dL for women

Any one of these health problems increases the rate of atherosclerosis and the risk for stroke, coronary heart disease, and early death. Teach patients about the lifestyle changes that can improve health (Bosak, 2012a). (See the Health Promotion and Maintenance section below.)

Incidence and Prevalence

More than 57 million American adults have prediabetes, defined as impaired fasting glucose (IFG) or impaired glucose tolerance (IGT) or an A1C level between 5.5% and 6.0%. IFG (fasting blood glucose levels of 100 mg/dL [5.6 mmol/L] to 125 mg/dL [6.9 mmol/L] and IGT (2-hr oral glucose tolerance values of 140 mg/dL [7.8 mmol/L] to 199 mg/dL [11.0 mmol/L]) are considered risk factors for diabetes and for cardiovascular disease. Over a 3- to 5-year period, people with prediabetes have a fivefold to fifteenfold higher risk for developing type 2 DM than do those with normal blood glucose levels. IFG and IGT are associated with obesity (especially abdominal or central obesity), dyslipidemia with high triglycerides and/or low HDL cholesterol, and hypertension (ADA, 2014d).

In the United States, nearly 26 million people are living with DM and another 79 million have prediabetes. This means

TABLE 64-5 Indications for Testing People for Type 2 Diabetes

- Testing for diabetes should be considered in people 45 years of age and older, particularly in those with a BMI greater than 25 kg/m^2. If normal, it should be repeated at 3-year intervals.
- Testing should be considered at a younger age or be carried out more frequently in people who are overweight (BMI >25 kg/m^2) and have these additional associated factors:
  - Have a first-degree relative with diabetes
  - Are physically inactive
  - Are members of a high-risk ethnic population (e.g., African American, Hispanic American, American Indian, Asian American, or Pacific Islander)
  - Deliver a baby weighing more than 9 pounds or have been diagnosed with GDM
  - Are hypertensive (>140/90 mm Hg)
  - Have a high-density lipoprotein (HDL) cholesterol level less than 35 mg/dL (0.90 mmol/L) and/or a triglyceride level greater than 250 mg/dL (2.82 mmol/L)
  - Have polycystic ovary syndrome
  - Have IFG or IGT on previous testing
  - Have a history of vascular disease

BMI, Body mass index; *GDM,* gestational diabetes mellitus; *IFG,* impaired fasting glucose, *IGT,* impaired glucose tolerance.
Data from American Diabetes Association (ADA). (2014d). Position statement: Diagnosis and classification of diabetes mellitus. *Diabetes Care, 37*(Suppl. 1), S81-S90.

almost one third of the total U.S. population are affected by diabetes (CDC, 2011).

About 90% of people with diabetes have type 2 DM (ADA, 2014d). It is diagnosed most often among middle-aged and older adults, affecting about 9.6% of patients ages 20 to 59 years and 20.9% of patients ages 60 years and older. It is more common among men than women (National Institute of Diabetes and Digestive and Kidney Diseases [NIDDK], 2011). With the prevalence of obesity rising in North America, diabetes will become even more common.

CULTURAL CONSIDERATIONS

Patient-Centered Care QSEN

Racial and ethnic minorities have a higher prevalence and greater burden of diabetes compared with whites, and some minority groups also have higher rates of complications. The risk for diabetes is 77% higher among African Americans than non-Hispanic white Americans. At nearly 16.1%, American Indians and Alaska Indians have the highest age-adjusted prevalence of diabetes among U.S. racial and ethnic groups (Chow et al., 2012). The increase in obesity and sedentary lifestyles in the U. S. population intensifies this growing problem. The ADA has identified patients who should be tested for diabetes in Table 64-5.

The overall clinical outcomes for minority patients with diabetes are worse than for non-Hispanic whites with DM. Possible factors for these outcome differences include lack of access to health care, lifestyle issues, mistrust of the health care system, reduced financial resources, and lack of knowledge about the relationship between glucose control and complications. Be alert to the risk for diabetes whenever you are interviewing or assessing people who belong to these higher risk racial or ethnic groups.

Health Promotion and Maintenance

Diabetes causes many preventable but devastating complications and is a major public health problem. Control of diabetes and its complications is a major focus for health promotion

CHART 64-1 Laboratory Profile

Blood Glucose Values

TEST	NORMAL RANGE FOR ADULTS	SIGNIFICANCE OF ABNORMAL RESULTS
Fasting blood glucose test	<100 mg/dL (5.6 mmol/L) Older adults: Levels rise 1 mg/dL per decade of age	Levels >100 mg/dL (5.6 mmol/L) but <126 mg/dL (7.0 mmol/L) indicate impaired fasting glucose (IFG). Levels >126 mg/dL (7.0 mmol/L) obtained on at least two occasions are diagnostic of diabetes, even in older adults.
Glucose tolerance test (2-hr post-load result)	<140 mg/dL (7.8 mmol/L)	Levels >140 mg/dL (7.8 mmol/L) and <200 mg/dL (11.1 mmol/L) indicate impaired glucose tolerance (IGT). Levels >200 mg/dL (11.1 mmol/L) indicate provisional diagnosis of diabetes.
Glycosylated hemoglobin (A1C) test	4%-6%	Levels of 5.7 to 6.4% indicate increased risk for development of diabetes. Levels >8% indicate poor diabetes control and need for adherence to regimen or changes in therapy.

Data from American Diabetes Association (ADA). (2014d). Position statement: Diagnosis and classification of diabetes mellitus. *Diabetes Care, 37*(Suppl. 1), S81-S90.

activities. No interventions are successful in preventing type 1 DM, but health promotion activities focus on controlling hyperglycemia to reduce its long-term complications.

Adopting a low calorie diet that results in weight loss and increasing physical activity improve metabolic and cardiac risk factors. These improvements include reducing hypertension, increasing heart rate variability between resting rate and exercise rate, lowering triglyceride levels, increasing high-density lipoprotein cholesterol (the "good" cholesterol) levels, and reducing low-density lipoprotein cholesterol (the "bad" cholesterol) levels.

Teach all patients with DM that tight control of blood glucose levels can prevent many complications. Urge all patients with DM to regularly follow up with their health care provider or endocrinologist, to have their eyes and vision tested yearly by an ophthalmologist, and to have urine microalbumin levels assessed yearly. Early detection of changes in the eye or kidney permits adjustments in treatment regimens that can slow or halt progression of retinopathy and nephropathy. Encourage all people to maintain weight within an appropriate range for height and body build and to engage in physical activity at least 3 times per week (Bosak, 2012b).

❖ PATIENT-CENTERED COLLABORATIVE CARE

◆ Assessment

History. Ask about risk factors and manifestations related to diabetes. Age is important because type 2 diabetes mellitus (DM) is more common in older patients, especially among African Americans and Mexican Americans. Ask women how large their children were at birth, because many women who develop type 2 DM had gestational diabetes mellitus (GDM) or glucose intolerance during pregnancy (ADA, 2014d). These women often have given birth to infants weighing 9 pounds or more.

Assessing weight and weight change is important, because excess weight and obesity are risk factors for type 2 DM. The patient with type 1 DM often has weight loss with increased appetite during the weeks before diagnosis. For both types of DM, patients usually have fatigue, polyuria, and polydipsia. Ask about recent major or minor infections. In particular, ask women about frequent vaginal yeast infections. Ask all patients whether they have noticed that small skin injuries become infected more easily or take longer to heal. Also ask whether they have noticed any changes in vision or in the sense of touch.

TABLE 64-6 Criteria for the Diagnosis of Diabetes

A1C >6.5%. The test should be performed in a laboratory using a method that is NGSP certified and standardized to the DCCT assay.

Or

Fasting blood glucose greater than 126 mg/dL (7.0 mmol/L). *Fasting* is defined as no caloric intake for at least 8 hours.

Or

Two-hour blood glucose equal to or greater than 200 mg/dL (11.1 mmol/L) during oral glucose tolerance test. The test should be performed using a glucose load containing the equivalent of 75 g anhydrous glucose dissolved in water.

Or

In a patient with classic manifestations of hyperglycemia or hyperglycemic crisis, a random blood glucose concentration greater than 200 mg/dL (11.1 mmol/L). *Casual* is defined as any time of the day without regard to time since last meal. The classic symptoms of diabetes include polyuria, polydipsia, and unexplained weight loss.

Note: In the absence of unequivocal hyperglycemia, the first three criteria should be confirmed by repeat testing.

Data from American Diabetes Association (ADA). (2014d). Position statement: Diagnosis and classification of diabetes mellitus. *Diabetes Care, 37*(Suppl. 1), S81-S90.

DCCT, Diabetes Control and Complications Trial; *NGSP,* National Glycohemoglobin Standardization Program.

Laboratory Assessment

Diagnosis of Diabetes. Diabetes can be diagnosed by assessing blood glucose levels. The ADA defines normal blood glucose values in Chart 64-1. A test result indicating DM should be repeated to rule out laboratory error unless manifestations of hyperglycemia or hyperglycemic crisis are also present. Table 64-6 lists criteria for the diagnosis of diabetes.

The diagnosis of diabetes mellitus includes elevated glycosylated hemoglobin levels. **Glycosylated hemoglobin (A1C)** is a standardized test that measures how much glucose permanently attaches to the hemoglobin molecule. Because glucose binds to many proteins, including hemoglobin, through a process called *glycosylation,* the higher the blood glucose level is over time, the more glycosylated hemoglobin becomes. The ADA defines A1C levels greater than 6.5% as diagnostic of DM (ADA, 2014d; Funnell, 2014).

Fasting plasma glucose (FPG) (fasting blood glucose [FBG]) is used to diagnose diabetes in nonpregnant adults. The patient should have no caloric intake for at least 8 hours (water is permitted). The blood sample needs to be obtained before insulin or oral antidiabetic agents have been taken. A diagnosis of diabetes is made with two separate test results greater than 126 mg/dL (7 mmol/L) (ADA, 2014d). *Random* or *casual* plasma (blood) glucose greater than 200 mg/dL (7.0 mmol/L) is used to diagnose diabetes in patients with severe classic hyperglycemia or hyperglycemic crisis.

Oral glucose tolerance testing (OGTT) is the most sensitive test for the diagnosis of DM. It is often used to diagnose gestational diabetes mellitus (GDM) during pregnancy and is not routinely used for general diagnosis.

Other blood tests for diabetes can help determine whether a patient has type 1 or type 2 DM. Type 1 DM results from autoimmune destruction of the beta cells of the pancreas. Markers of this destruction include islet cell autoantibodies (ICAs), autoantibodies to insulin, and autoantibodies to glutamic acid decarboxylase (GAD65). ICAs are present in 85% to 90% of people with new-onset type 1 DM.

Measurement of C-peptide levels indicates beta secretory function of the pancreas. Low to absent C-peptide levels diagnose type 1 DM, as well as late-stage type 2 DM when the ability of the pancreas to secrete insulin is severely impaired.

Screening for Diabetes. Measurement of islet cell antibodies may identify people who are at risk for developing type 1 DM. Testing to detect prediabetes and type 2 DM should be considered in patients older than 45 years and those defined as overweight (body mass index [BMI] greater than 25 kg/m^2). Testing is considered for patients who are younger than 45 years and are overweight if they have additional risk factors for diabetes or have other health problems associated with diabetes. Screening for diabetes usually is done with either hemoglobin A1C levels or fasting plasma glucose levels (ADA, 2014d). The use of portable glucose meters for the diagnosis of diabetes is not recommended because of imprecise results and variance in results among the different glucose monitors (Sacks, 2011).

Ongoing Assessment. *Glycosylated hemoglobin assays* are useful because blood glucose permanently attaches to hemoglobin. The higher the blood glucose level is over time, the more glycosylated hemoglobin becomes. Thus glycosylated hemoglobin A1C (A1C) is a good indicator of the average blood glucose levels because it shows the average blood glucose level during the previous 120 days—the life span of red blood cells. A1C testing can help assess long-term glycemic control and predict the risk for complications. *Unlike the fasting blood glucose test, A1C test results are not altered by eating habits the day before the test.* This testing is performed at diagnosis and at specific intervals to evaluate the treatment plan. A1C testing is recommended at least twice yearly in patients who are meeting expected treatment outcomes and have stable blood glucose control. Quarterly assessment is recommended for patients whose therapy has changed or who are not meeting prescribed glycemic levels (ADA, 2014d). Table 64-7 shows the correlation between A1C and mean blood glucose levels.

When glucose binds to amino groups on serum proteins, especially albumin, the glycosylated protein product is called *fructosamine.* This product increases with elevated blood glucose levels in the same way as hemoglobin does but can indicate blood glucose control over a shorter period. These measures are useful for short-term follow-up of treatment changes or in patients with hemoglobin abnormalities in which A1C is not an accurate reflection of glucose control. Available tests are called

TABLE 64-7 Correlation Between A1C Level and Mean Blood Glucose Levels

A1C (%)	MEAN BLOOD GLUCOSE Mg/dL	MEAN BLOOD GLUCOSE mmol/L
6	126	7.0
7	154	8.6
8	183	10.2
9	212	11.8
10	240	13.4
11	269	14.9
12	298	16.5

Data from American Diabetes Association (ADA). (2013). Standards of medical care in diabetes—2013. *Diabetes Care, 36*(Suppl. 1), S19.

glycosylated serum albumin (GSA), glycosylated serum protein (GSP), and *fructosamine.*

Urine Tests. *Ketone bodies* are a product of fat metabolism, and the presence of moderate to high urine ketones (hyperketonuria) indicates a severe lack of insulin. Hyperketonuria in the presence of hyperglycemia is a medical emergency that, when detected early, can be managed with insulin and careful monitoring. Urine testing for ketones should be performed during acute illness or stress, when blood glucose levels consistently exceed 300 mg/dL (16.7 mmol/L), during pregnancy, or when any manifestations of ketoacidosis are present. Ketone testing is recommended for patients with diabetes participating in a weight-loss program. Hyperketonuria without hyperglycemia suggests that weight loss is occurring without disrupting blood glucose control.

Ketone bodies appear in urine in the same proportion as they do in blood but are affected by urine volume and concentration. Thus urine ketone bodies are not used to evaluate the effectiveness of treatment for ketoacidosis.

Tests for kidney function are important in detecting kidney disease in diabetes. Persistent albuminuria in the range of 30 to 299 mg/24 hr is an indicator of early-stage diabetic nephropathy in type 1 diabetes and a marker for development of nephropathy in type 2 diabetes. Persistent albuminuria is also a marker for increased cardiovascular risk (ADA, 2014f). Screening for increased urinary albumin excretion can be performed by measurement of albumin-to-creatinine ratio in a random spot collection.

Serum creatinine is used to estimate kidney function (e.g., glomerular filtration rate) and to stage the level of chronic kidney disease. In patients with nephropathy, a rise in serum creatinine level is related to both poor blood glucose control and hypertension.

Urine glucose testing is an indirect measurement of blood glucose and is not accurate. This test is not used for monitoring DM management.

◆ Analysis

The priority NANDA-I nursing diagnoses and collaborative problems for patients with diabetes include:

1. Risk for Injury related to hyperglycemia (NANDA-I)
2. Potential for impaired wound healing related to endocrine and vascular effects of diabetes
3. Risk for Injury related to diabetic neuropathy (NANDA-I)

4. Acute Pain and Chronic Pain related to diabetic neuropathy (NANDA-I)
5. Risk for Injury related to diabetic retinopathy–induced reduced vision (NANDA-I)
6. Potential for kidney disease related to impaired kidney circulation
7. Potential for hypoglycemia
8. Potential for diabetic ketoacidosis
9. Potential for hyperglycemic-hyperosmolar state and coma

◆ Planning and Implementation

The management of diabetes mellitus (DM) is complex and involves extensive patient education. The Concept Map on p. 1311 highlights care issues for the patient with type 2 DM.

Preventing Injury from Hyperglycemia

Planning: Expected Outcomes. The patient with diabetes is expected to manage DM and prevent disease progression by maintaining blood glucose levels in his or her target range. Indicators are that the patient consistently demonstrates these behaviors:

- Performs treatment regimen as prescribed
- Follows recommended diet
- Monitors blood glucose using correct testing procedures
- Seeks health care if blood glucose levels fluctuate outside of recommended parameters
- Meets recommended activity levels
- Uses drugs as prescribed
- Maintains optimum weight
- Problem solves about barriers to self-management

Interventions

Nonsurgical Management. Nonsurgical management of diabetes mellitus (DM) involves nutrition interventions, blood glucose monitoring, a planned exercise program, and often, drugs to lower blood glucose levels. The nurse, together with the patient, physician, dietitian, pharmacist, case manager, and other health care professionals, plans, coordinates, and delivers care.

The American Diabetes Association (ADA) has proposed these treatment outcomes for glycosylated hemoglobin (A1C) and blood glucose levels (ADA, 2014d):

- A1C levels are maintained at 6.5% or below.
- The majority of premeal blood glucose levels are 70 to 130 mg/dL (3.9 to 7.2 mmol/L).
- Peak after-meal blood glucose levels are less than 180 mg/dL (<10.0 mmol/L).

Drug Therapy. Drug therapy is indicated when a patient with type 2 DM does not achieve blood glucose control with diet changes, regular exercise, and stress management. Several categories of drugs are available to lower blood glucose levels. Patients with type 1 DM require insulin therapy for blood glucose control.

Drugs are started at the lowest effective dose and increased every 1 to 2 weeks until the patient reaches desired blood glucose control or the maximum dosage. If the maximum dosage of one agent does not control blood glucose levels, a second agent with a different mechanism of action may be added. Insulin therapy is indicated for the patient with type 2 DM when blood glucose cannot be controlled with the use of two or three different antidiabetic agents.

Antidiabetic drugs are not a substitute for dietary modification and exercise. Teach the patient about the need for continuing dietary restrictions and regular exercise while taking antidiabetic drugs.

! NURSING SAFETY PRIORITY (QSEN)

Drug Alert

To avoid adverse drug interactions, teach the patient who is taking an antidiabetic drug to consult with his or her primary care provider or pharmacist before using *any* over-the-counter drugs.

Drug Selection. The choice of antidiabetic drug is based on cost, the patient's ability to manage multiple drug dosages, age, and response to the drugs. Shorter-acting agents (e.g., glipizide) are preferable in older patients, those with irregular eating schedules, or those with liver, kidney, or cardiac dysfunction. Longer-acting agents (e.g., glyburide, glimepiride) with once-a-day dosing are better for adherence. Beta-cell function in type 2 DM often declines over time, reducing the effectiveness of some drugs. The treatment regimen for a patient with type 2 DM may eventually require insulin therapy either alone or with other antidiabetic drugs.

Antidiabetic Drugs. Some antidiabetic drugs are oral agents, and others require subcutaneous injection. Chart 64-2 lists common antidiabetic drugs in each category.

Insulin Secretogogues. Insulin secretagogues stimulate insulin release from pancreatic beta cells and are used for patients who are still able to produce insulin.

Sulfonylurea Agents. Sulfonylurea agents lower fasting blood glucose levels by triggering the release of insulin from beta cells. Many drugs interact with sulfonylureas. Be sure to consult a drug reference book or pharmacologist when instructing patients who are prescribed a drug from this class.

Meglitinide Analogs. Meglitinide analogs are classified as insulin secretagogues and have actions and adverse effects similar to those of sulfonylureas. They tend to increase meal-related insulin secretion.

Biguanides. Metformin (Glucophage) does not increase insulin secretion. It decreases liver glucose production and decreases intestinal absorption of glucose. It also improves insulin sensitivity by increasing peripheral glucose uptake and utilization.

! NURSING SAFETY PRIORITY (QSEN)

Drug Alert

Metformin can cause lactic acidosis in patients with renal insufficiency and should not be used by anyone with kidney disease. To prevent kidney damage, the drug should be withheld after using contrast material or any surgical procedure requiring anesthesia until adequate kidney function is established.

Insulin Sensitizers. Thiazolidinediones (TZDs) increase cellular utilization of glucose, which lowers blood glucose levels. Both of the TZDs—rosiglitazone (Avandia) and pioglitazone (Actos)—are associated with an increased risk for heart-related deaths, bone fracture, and macular edema. The Food and Drug Administration (FDA) has issued a black box warning indicating that these drugs are not to be used by patients who have symptomatic heart failure or other specific types of cardiovascular disease (Sisson et al., 2012). (A **Black Box Warning** is a government designation indicating that a drug has at least one serious side effect and must be used with caution.)

CONCEPT MAP

DIABETES MELLITUS TYPE 2

PERFUSION · NUTRITION · PAIN · INFECTION · SENSORY PERCEPTION · GLUCOSE REGULATION · TISSUE INTEGRITY

HISTORY

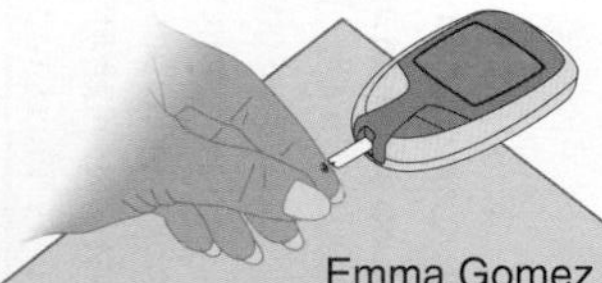

Emma Gomez is an Hispanic woman with a 20-year history of diabetes type 2. She has peripheral vascular disease and vision changes. She is admitted for gastroenteritis and a blood glucose (BG) level of 330 mg/dL.

↓ Subjective Data

SUBJECTIVE DATA

"My vision is blurred and I have trouble with my central vision. Sometimes my vision gets a little better. I'm scared I'm going to fall when I come down the stairs because I can't tell how deep the steps are."

→ Objective Data

LAB VALUES

- Hyperglycemia
  - BG 330 mg/dL
- Central obesity
  - waist 39 inches
- Drug treatment for ↑ BG
- Hypertension: 160/90 mm Hg
- Triglycerides ↑ level 250 mg/dL
- HDL cholesterol 40 mg/dL

↑ Data Synthesis (from Subjective Data and Lab Values)

PATIENT PROBLEMS

- Risk for Injury due to hyperglycemia; diabetic neuropathy; diabetic retinopathy
- Potential for impaired wound healing due to endocrine and vascular effects
- PAIN due to diabetic neuropathy
- Potential for kidney disease due to impaired kidney circulation, hypoglycemia, diabetic ketoacidosis, hyperglycemic-hyperosmolar state, and coma

↑ Planning

EXPECTED OUTCOMES

- Manage DM and prevent progression by maintaining BG levels in expected range
- Seek care if BG levels fluctuate outside normal parameters
- Meet recommended activity level
- Use drugs as prescribed
- Maintain optimum weight
- Problem solve about barriers to self-management

INTERVENTIONS

1 Nursing Safety Priority: Critical Rescue!

Assess vital signs, provide fluids for hydration, intervene to manage BP of 160/90 mm Hg, and treat high BG level. *Treats gastroenteritis and reduces the risk of a CVA and continued vascular damage. Drug therapy may be required to achieve desired outcomes.*

2 Early Detection

Teach about tight control of BG, regular eye checkups, and urine assessment for microalbumin and ketones. *Checks for early detection of* SENSORY PERCEPTION *(retinopathy) and* PERFUSION *issues (hypertensive kidney disease, nephropathy) which permits adjustments in treatment.*

3 Interpretation of Lab Values

- Monitor K^+ levels closely (it can be decreased, increased, or normal). *Potassium levels vary depending on hydration, the severity of any acidosis, and the patient's response to treatment.*
- Teach the patient to keep BG in the range of 60-100 mg/dL and maintain A_{1c} levels below 7%. *Monitors history of glucose regulation. Maintaining near normal levels delays problems with visual* SENSORY PERCEPTION, INFECTION, PERFUSION, *and* TISSUE INTEGRITY *(retinopathy, nephropathy, neuropathy, macrovascular disease).*

4 GLUCOSE REGULATION

Review with the patient the treatment regimen including nutrition, monitoring BG, when to seek medical care, recommended activity levels, using drug therapy correctly, optimum weight, and problem solving about barriers to self-management. *Prevents injury from hyperclycemia.*

5 Nursing Safety Priority: Drug Alert!

Teach the patient who is taking an antidiabetic drug to consult with the health care provider or pharmacist before using any over-the-counter drugs. *Prevents adverse drug interactions.*

6 Maintaining Nutrition

Evaluate an individualized nutritional plan in collaboration with dietitian: food intake during illness; activity level; amount of carbohydrates, fat, and fiber; consumption of alcohol, weight, and financial constraints. *Determines whether present habits are effective, need reinforcement, or require change.*

7 Preventing Complications

Teach the patient to recognize symptoms of hypoglycemia or hyperglycemia (and treatments), and when to call the health care provider. *Prevents development of diabetic ketoacidosis, prevents frequent episodes of hypoglycemia. Establishes what dietary changes are needed during illness.*

8 Health Promotion Activities – Risk Factors

Teach the patient to report decreased TISSUE PERFUSION: dyspnea, cough, extreme fatigue, and sudden onset of nausea and vomiting. *Improves CVD risk factors if the patient addresses smoking cessation, nutrition, exercise, blood pressure control, aspirin use, and adhering to prescribed lipid-lowering drug therapy.*

9 Racial and Ethnic Considerations

Explore issues related to lack of access to health care, lifestyle, mistrust of the health care system, limited financial resources, and lack of knowledge. *Racial and ethnic differences affect clinical outcomes for patients with diabetes.*

Concept Map by Deanne A. Blach, MSN, RN

CHART 64-2 Common Examples of Drug Therapy

Diabetes Mellitus

DRUG/CLASS	ROUTE OF ADMINISTRATION	SIDE EFFECTS
Secretagogues—Lower fasting plasma (blood) glucose levels by triggering the release of insulin from beta cells.		
Second-Generation Sulfonylurea Agents		
Glipizide (Glucotrol)	Oral	Hypoglycemia Weight gain Interacts with many drugs
Glimepiride (Amaryl)	Oral	Hypoglycemia
Meglitinide Analogs**—**Lower fasting plasma (blood) glucose levels by triggering the release of insulin from beta cells.		
Repaglinide (Prandin)	Oral	Hypoglycemia
Nateglinide (Starlix)	Oral	Hypoglycemia
Biguanides		
Metformin (Glucophage)	Oral	Abdominal discomfort (diarrhea, nausea, vomiting, flatulence, indigestion) Lactic acidosis Interacts with contrast material and can induce acute kidney injury
Insulin Sensitizers—Do not increase insulin secretion. Decrease liver glucose production, reducing fasting plasma (blood) glucose release, and improve insulin receptor sensitivity. TDZs also increase cellular utilization of glucose.		
Thiazolidinediones (TZDs)		
Pioglitazone (Actos)	Oral	Increased risk for heart-related deaths; not to be used by patients with symptomatic heart failure Increased risk for bone fracture and macular edema Increased risk for liver impairment Increased risk for bladder cancer
Rosiglitazone (Avandia)	Oral	Increased risk for heart-related deaths; not to be used by patients with symptomatic heart failure Increased risk for bone fracture and macular edema Increased risk for liver impairment
Alpha-Glucosidase Inhibitors—Prevent after-meal hyperglycemia by inhibiting enzymes in the intestinal tract, reducing the rate of digestion of starches, and delaying absorption of carbohydrate from the small intestine.		
Acarbose (Precose)	Oral	Abdominal discomfort (diarrhea, nausea, vomiting, flatulence, bloating, indigestion) Elevates serum transaminase levels and reduces liver function Drug accumulates in patients with kidney impairment
Miglitol (Glyset)	Oral	Abdominal discomfort (diarrhea, nausea, vomiting, flatulence, bloating, indigestion) Elevates serum transaminase levels and reduces liver function Drug accumulates in patients with kidney impairment
Incretin Mimetics (GLP-1 agonists)—Act like natural "gut" hormones that work with insulin to lower plasma (blood) glucose levels. They lower glucagon secretion from the pancreas, leading to reduced liver glucose production. Also reduce blood glucose levels by delaying gastric emptying, slowing the rate of nutrient absorption into the blood, and reducing food intake.		
Albiglutide (Tanzeum)	Subcutaneous injection (once weekly)	Increased risk for pancreatitis Increased risk for thyroid cancer
Exenatide (Byetta)	Subcutaneous injection	Increased risk for pancreatitis Increased risk for hypersensitivity reactions, including Stevens-Johnson syndrome
Exenatide extended release (Bydureon)	Subcutaneous injection	Increased risk for pancreatitis Increased risk for thyroid cancer
Liraglutide (Victoza)	Subcutaneous injection	Increased risk for pancreatitis Increased risk for thyroid cancer
DPP-4 Inhibitors—DPP-4 is an enzyme that breaks down the natural gut hormones (GLP-1 and GIP). DPP-4 inhibitors increase the amount of natural substances that work with insulin to lower glucagon secretion from the pancreas, leading to reduced liver glucose production. Also reduce blood glucose levels by delaying gastric emptying, slowing the rate of nutrient absorption into the blood, and reducing food intake.		
Sitagliptin (Januvia)	Oral	Increased risk for acute pancreatitis
Saxagliptin (Onglyza)	Oral	Increased risk for acute pancreatitis
Linagliptin (Tradjenta)	Oral	Increased risk for acute pancreatitis
Alogliptin (Nesina)	Oral	Increased risk for acute pancreatitis Kazano (alogliptin/metformin combination) carries black box warning for lactic acidosis
Amylin Analogs—Similar to amylin, a naturally occurring hormone produced by beta cells in the pancreas that is co-secreted with insulin and lowers blood glucose levels by delaying gastric emptying and triggering satiety.		
Pramlintide (Symlin)	Subcutaneous injection	Severe hypoglycemia Nausea and vomiting
Fixed Combinations—There are many fixed combinations of oral drugs available. The side effects of these combination drugs are the same as for each component of the combination. When a drug that has the side effect of hypoglycemia is combined with a drug that does not alone produce hypoglycemia, the development of hypoglycemia is still very much a risk for the combination agent.		

Alpha-Glucosidase Inhibitors. Alpha-glucosidase inhibitors prevent after-meal hyperglycemia by delaying absorption of carbohydrate from the small intestine. These drugs inhibit enzymes in the intestinal tract, reducing the rate of digestion of starches and the absorption of glucose. This action prevents a sudden blood glucose surge after meals. These drugs do not cause hypoglycemia unless given with sulfonylureas or insulin.

Incretin Mimetics. Incretin mimetics work like the natural "gut" hormones—glucagon-like peptide-1 (GLP-1) and glucose-dependent insulinotropic polypeptide (GIP)—that are released by the intestine in response to food intake and act with insulin to perform GLUCOSE REGULATION. Drugs in this class include the GLP-1 agonists *exenatide* (Byetta), *exenatide extended-release* (Bydureon), and the glucagon-like peptide-1 (GLP-1) agonists *liraglutide* (Victoza) and *albiglutide* (Tanzeum). These drugs are used in addition to diet and exercise to improve glycemic control in adults with type 2 DM. Liraglutide carries a black box warning for thyroid tumors and is not to be used by patients with a history of medullary thyroid carcinoma.

! NURSING SAFETY PRIORITY QSEN

Drug Alert

Albiglutide (Tanzeum) is only administered once per week, not daily like other incretin mimetics.

DPP-4 Inhibitors. The natural incretins *GLP* and *GIP* are rapidly metabolized and inactivated by the enzyme *DPP-4 (dipeptidyl peptidase 4)*. DPP-4 inhibitors work by reducing the inactivation of the incretin hormones so that they remain available for blood GLUCOSE REGULATION. The four DPP-4 inhibitors approved for use in patients with type 2 DM are sitagliptin (Januvia), saxagliptin (Onglyza), linagliptin (Tradjenta), and alogliptin (Nesina) (Sisson et al., 2012).

! NURSING SAFETY PRIORITY QSEN

Drug Alert

All four DPP-4 inhibitors and the incretin mimetic *liraglutide* are associated with an increased risk for pancreatitis. Warn patients taking these drugs to immediately report these manifestations to the health care provider: jaundice; sudden onset of intense abdominal pain that radiates to the back, left flank, or left shoulder; or gray-blue discoloration of the abdomen or periumbilical area.

Amylin Analogs. Amylin analogs are drugs similar to amylin, a naturally occurring hormone produced by pancreatic beta cells that works with and is co-secreted with insulin in response to blood glucose elevation. Amylin levels are deficient in patients with type 1 DM who are also deficient in insulin. Pramlintide (Symlin), an analog of amylin, is approved for patients with either type 1 or type 2 DM treated with insulin. It works by three mechanisms: delaying gastric emptying; reducing after-meal blood glucose levels; and triggering satiety (in the brain). (Satiety leads to decreased caloric intake and eventual weight loss.)

! NURSING SAFETY PRIORITY QSEN

Drug Alert

Do not mix pramlintide and insulin in the same syringe because the pH of the two drugs is not compatible.

Sodium-Glucose Co-transport Inhibitors. Sodium-glucose co-transport inhibitors are the newest class of antidiabetic drugs. They lower blood glucose levels by preventing kidney reabsorption of the glucose that was filtered from the blood into the urine. Thus the filtered glucose is excreted in the urine rather than moved back into the blood. These oral drugs include *canagliflozin* (Invokana) and *dapagliflozin* (Farxiga).

Combination Agents. Combination agents combine drugs with different mechanisms of action. Glucovance, for example, combines glyburide with metformin. Combining drugs with different mechanisms of action may be highly effective in maintaining desired blood glucose control. Some patients may need a combination of oral agents and insulin to control blood glucose levels.

Insulin Therapy. Insulin therapy is needed for type 1 DM and also may be used for type 2 DM. The safety of insulin therapy in older patients may be affected by reduced vision, mobility and coordination problems, and decreased memory. There are many types of insulin and regimens to achieve normal blood glucose levels. Because insulin is a small protein that is quickly digested and inactivated in the GI tract, it must be administered as an injection.

Types of Insulin. Insulin is manufactured using DNA technology to produce pure human insulin. Insulin analogs are synthetic human insulins in which the structure of the insulin molecule is altered to change the rate of absorption and duration of action within the body (Dokken, 2013). An example is Lispro insulin, a rapid-acting insulin analog that is created by switching the positions of lysine and proline in one area of the insulin molecule.

Rapid-, short-, intermediate-, and long-acting forms of insulin can be injected separately, and some can be mixed in the same syringe. Insulin is available in concentrations of 100 units/mL (U-100) or 500 units/mL (U-500). U-500 is indicated only for patients with severe insulin resistance whose total daily insulin dose exceeds 200 units.

Teach the patient that the insulin types, the injection technique, the site of injection, and the patient response can all affect the absorption, onset, degree, and duration of insulin activity. Reinforce that changing insulins may affect blood glucose control and should be done only under supervision of the health care provider. Table 64-8 outlines the time activity of human insulin.

Insulin Regimens. Insulin regimens try to duplicate the normal insulin release pattern from the pancreas. The pancreas produces a constant *(basal)* amount of insulin that balances liver glucose production with glucose use and maintains normal blood glucose levels between meals. The pancreas also produces additional *(prandial)* insulin to prevent blood glucose elevation after meals. The insulin dose required for blood glucose control varies among patients. A usual starting dose is between 0.5 and 1 unit/kg of body weight per day. For multiple-dose regimens or continuous subcutaneous insulin infusion (CSII), basal insulin makes up about 40% to 50% of the total daily dosage, with the remainder divided into premeal doses of rapid-acting insulin analogs or regular insulin. Basal insulin coverage is provided by intermediate-acting insulin such as NPH insulin or by

TABLE 64-8 Time Activity of Pharmaceutical Insulin

PREPARATION	BRAND	ONSET (Hr)	PEAK (Hr)	DURATION (Hr)
Rapid-Acting Insulin				
Insulin aspart	NovoLog	0.25	1-3	3-5
Insulin glulisine	Apidra	0.3	0.5-1.5	3-4
Human lispro injection	Humalog	0.25	0.5-1.5	5
Short-Acting Insulin				
Regular human insulin injection	Humulin R Novolin R ReliOn R	0.5 0.5 0.5	2-4 2.5-5 2.5-5	5-7 8 8-12
Humulin R (Concentrated U-500)	Humulin R (U-500)	1.5	4-12	24
Intermediate-Acting Insulin				
Isophane Insulin NPH injection	Humulin N Novolin N ReliOn N	1.5 1-4 1-4	4-12 4-14 4-14	16-24+ 10-24+ 10-24+
70% human insulin isophane suspension/30% human insulin injection	Humulin 70/30 Novolin 70/30 ReliOn 70/30	0.5	2-12	24
50% human insulin isophane suspension/50% human insulin injection	Humulin 50/50	0.5	3-5	24
70% insulin aspart protamine suspension/30% insulin aspart injection	NovoLog Mix 70/30	0.25	1-4	24
75% insulin lispro protamine suspension/25% insulin lispro injection	Humalog Mix 75/25	0.25	1-2	24
Long-Acting Insulin				
Insulin glargine injection	Lantus	2-4	None	24
Insulin detemir injection	Levemir	1	6-8	5.7-24

long-acting insulin analogs, such as insulin glargine (Lantus) or insulin detemir (Levemir). Dosages are adjusted based on the results of blood glucose monitoring.

Single daily injection protocols require insulin injection only once daily. This protocol may include one injection of intermediate- or long-acting insulin or a combination of short- and intermediate-acting insulin. Many patients with type 2 diabetes combine once-daily insulin injection with oral agent therapy.

Multiple-component insulin therapy combines short- and intermediate-acting insulin injected twice daily. Two thirds of the daily dose is given before breakfast and one third before the evening meal. Ratios of intermediate-acting and regular insulin are based on results of blood glucose monitoring.

Intensified regimens include a basal dose of intermediate- or long-acting insulin and a bolus dose of short- or rapid-acting insulin designed to bring the *next* blood glucose value into the target range. Blood glucose elevations above the target range are treated with "correction" doses of short- or rapid-acting insulin. The patient's blood glucose patterns determine insulin dosage. Frequency of blood glucose monitoring is based on the timed action of insulin and may occur as often as 8 times daily. Blood glucose testing 1 to 2 hours after meals and within 10 minutes before the next meal helps determine the adequacy of the bolus dose. The patient determines the effects of basal insulin by monitoring blood glucose levels before breakfast (fasting) and before the evening meal.

Patients on intensified insulin regimens need extensive education to achieve target blood glucose values. They need to know how to adjust insulin doses and understand NUTRITION therapy for dietary flexibility and target blood glucose values. Patients must also be able to accurately monitor blood glucose levels so that therapy decisions can be based on accurate data.

Regardless of the specific insulin regimen, adherence to insulin injection schedules is critical in achieving glycemic control and maintaining A1C levels below the 6.5% needed to reduce long-term complications. At times, skipping an occasional insulin dose may be related to an unusual meal pattern for a day or a change in exercise.

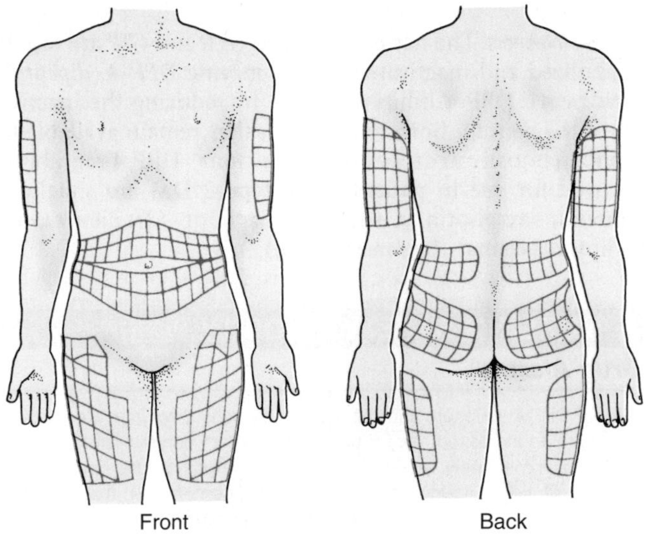

FIG. 64-2 Common insulin injection areas and sites.

Factors Influencing Insulin Absorption. Many factors affect insulin absorption and availability, including injection site; timing, type, or dose of insulin used; and physical activity.

Injection site area affects the speed of insulin absorption. Fig. 64-2 shows common insulin injection areas. Absorption is fastest in the abdomen, and except for a 2-inch radius around the navel, it is the preferred injection site area. Rotating injection site areas prevents lipohypertrophy (increased fat deposits in the skin) and lipoatrophy (loss of fatty tissue, leaving an uneven appearance). Rotation *within* one anatomic site is preferred to rotation from one area to another to prevent day-to-day changes in absorption.

Absorption rate is determined by insulin properties. The longer the duration of action, the more unpredictable is absorption. Larger doses of insulin also prolong the absorption. Factors that increase blood flow from the injection site, such as local application of heat, massage of the area, and exercise of the injected area, increase insulin absorption. Scarred sites often become favorite injection sites because they are less sensitive to pain, but these areas usually slow the rate of insulin absorption.

Injection depth changes insulin absorption. Usually, injections are made into the subcutaneous tissue. IM injection has a faster absorption and is not used for routine insulin use. Most patients lightly grasp a fold of skin and inject at a 90-degree angle; however, a 45-degree angle is advised for frail older adults and those who are cachexic. Aspiration for blood is not needed. Patients with high body mass index (BMI) levels can use 4 mm or 5 mm needles to inject insulin at a 90-degree angle without pinching a skinfold before injection. Assess the older patient's ability to inject insulin, and arrange for assistance when self-care is no longer possible.

Timing of injection affects blood glucose levels. The interval between premeal injections and eating, known as "lag time," affects blood glucose levels after meals. Insulin lispro, insulin aspart, and insulin glulisine have rapid onsets of action and should be given within 10 minutes before mealtime when blood glucose is in the target range. If hyperglycemia or hypoglycemia is not present, these insulins can be given at any time from 10 minutes before mealtime to just before eating or even immediately after eating. Regular insulin should be given at least 20 to 30 minutes before eating when glucose levels are within the target range. When blood glucose levels are above the target range, the lag time should be increased to permit insulin to begin to have an effect sooner. Rapid-acting insulin analogs can be given 15 minutes before and regular insulin 30 to 60 minutes before eating a meal. When blood glucose levels are below the target range, injection of regular insulin should be delayed until immediately before eating and injection of rapid-acting insulin should be delayed until sometime after eating the meal.

Mixing insulins can change the time of peak action. Mixtures of short- and intermediate-acting insulins produce a more normal blood glucose response in some patients than does a single dose. The patient's response to mixed insulin may differ from the response to the same insulins given separately.

! NURSING SAFETY PRIORITY QSEN

Drug Alert

Do not mix any other insulin type with insulin glargine, with insulin detemir, or with any of the premixed insulin formulations, such as Humalog Mix 75/25.

Complications of Insulin Therapy. Hypoglycemia from insulin excess has many causes. Its effects and treatment are discussed on p. 1330 in the Preventing Hypoglycemia section.

Lipoatrophy is a loss of fat tissue in areas of repeated injection that results from an immune reaction to impurities in insulin. Treatment consists of injection of insulin at the edge of the atrophied area. *Lipohypertrophy* is an increased swelling of fat that occurs at the site of repeated insulin injections. The overlying skin has decreased sensitivity, and the area can become large and unsightly. Treatment consists of rotating the injection site among different body areas.

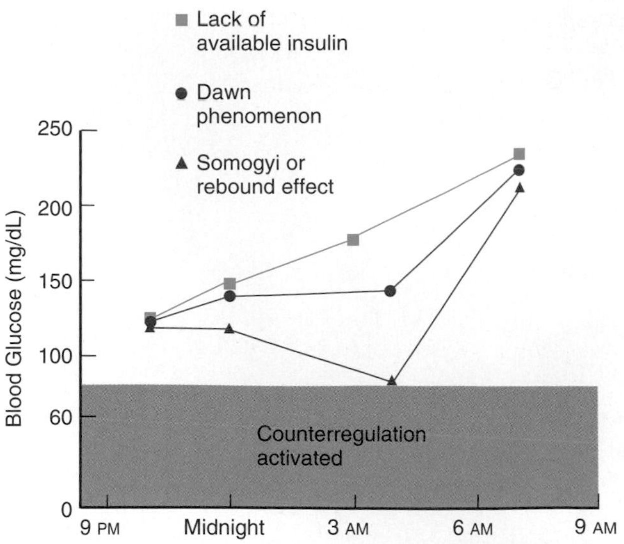

FIG. 64-3 Three blood glucose phenomena in patients with diabetes.

Two conditions of fasting hyperglycemia can occur (Fig. 64-3). *Dawn phenomenon* results from a nighttime release of growth hormone that causes release of liver glucose resulting in blood glucose elevations at about 5 to 6 AM. It is managed by providing more insulin for the overnight period (e.g., giving the evening dose of intermediate-acting insulin at 10 PM). *Somogyi phenomenon* is morning hyperglycemia from the counterregulatory response to nighttime hypoglycemia resulting in release of liver glucose. It is managed by ensuring adequate dietary intake at bedtime and evaluating the insulin dose and exercise programs to prevent conditions that lead to hypoglycemia. Both problems are diagnosed by blood glucose monitoring during the night. Help identify these problems, and teach the patient and family about management.

Alternative Methods of Insulin Administration. Many methods of insulin delivery are available in addition to traditional subcutaneous injections.

Continuous subcutaneous infusion of a basal dose of insulin (CSII) with increases in insulin at mealtimes is more effective in controlling blood glucose levels than other schedules. It allows flexibility in meal timing, because if a meal is skipped, the additional mealtime dose of insulin is not given. CSII is given by an externally worn pump containing a syringe and reservoir with rapid-acting insulin and is connected to the patient by an infusion set. Teach him or her to adjust the amount of insulin based on data from blood glucose monitoring. Rapid-acting insulin analogs are used with insulin infusion pumps (Hughes, 2012a) (Fig. 64-4).

Problems with CSII include skin infections that can occur when the infusion site is not cleaned or the needle is not changed every 2 to 3 days. CSII may lead to more episodes of ketoacidosis than other methods of insulin delivery because of inexperience in pump use, INFECTION, accidental cessation or obstruction of the infusion, or mechanical pump problems (Hughes, 2012a). Stress the importance of testing for ketones when blood glucose levels are greater than 300 mg/dL (16.7 mmol/L).

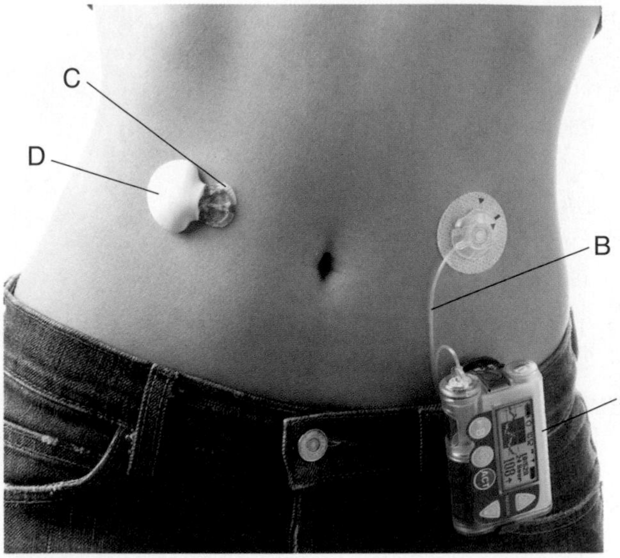

FIG. 64-4 The MiniMed Paradigm REAL-Time Insulin Pump and Continuous Glucose Monitoring System. **A,** Pump. **B,** Injection cannula. **C,** Glucose sensor. **D,** Data transmitter.

Patients using CSII need intensive education. Because of the risk for hypoglycemia or hyperglycemia, he or she must be able to operate the pump, adjust the settings, and respond appropriately to alarms. Removing the pump for any length of time can result in hyperglycemia. Provide supplemental insulin schedules for times when the pump is not operational. CSII is more costly than traditional insulin injections, and not all costs are covered by insurance.

Injection devices include a needleless system and a pen-type injector in addition to traditional insulin syringes. With a needleless device, the needle is replaced by an ultrathin liquid stream of insulin forced through the skin under high pressure known as "jet injection." Insulin given by jet injection is absorbed at a faster rate and has a shorter duration of action. Cost is a drawback to this system.

Patient Education: Drugs. Provide specific instructions about insulin therapy, new drug therapies, and self-monitoring of blood glucose levels.

Insulin storage varies by use. Teach patients to refrigerate insulin that is not in use to maintain potency, prevent exposure to sunlight, and inhibit bacterial growth. Insulin in use may be kept at room temperature for up to 28 days to reduce irritation at the injection site caused by cold insulin.

To prevent loss of drug potency, teach the patient to avoid exposing insulin to temperatures below 36° F (2.2° C) or above 86° F (30° C), to avoid excessive shaking, and to protect insulin from direct heat and light. Insulin should not be allowed to freeze. Insulin glargine (Lantus) should be stored in a refrigerator (36° to 46° F [2.2° to 7.8° C]) even when in use. Teach patients to discard any unused insulin after 28 days.

Teach patients to always have a spare bottle of each type of insulin used. A slight loss in potency may occur for bottles in use for more than 30 days, even when the expiration date has not passed. Prefilled syringes are stable up to 30 days when refrigerated. Store prefilled syringes in the upright position, with the needle pointing upward, so that insulin particles do not clog it. Teach patients to roll, not shake, prefilled syringes between the hands before using.

CHART 64-3 Patient and Family Education: Preparing for Self-Management

Subcutaneous Insulin Administration

- Wash your hands.
- Inspect the bottle for the type of insulin and the expiration date.
- Gently roll the bottle of intermediate-acting insulin in the palms of your hands to mix the insulin.
- Clean the rubber stopper with an alcohol swab.
- Remove the needle cover, and pull back the plunger to draw air into the syringe. The amount of air should be equal to the insulin dose. Push the needle through the rubber stopper, and inject the air into the insulin bottle.
- Turn the bottle upside down, and draw the insulin dose into the syringe.
- Remove air bubbles in the syringe by tapping on the syringe or injecting air back into the bottle. Redraw the correct amount.
- Make certain the tip of the plunger is on the line for your dose of insulin. Magnifiers are available to assist in measuring accurate doses of insulin.
- Remove the needle from the bottle. Recap the needle if the insulin is not to be given immediately.
- Select a site within your injection area that has not been used in the past month.
- Clean your skin with an alcohol swab. Lightly grasp an area of skin, and insert the needle at a 90-degree angle.
- Push the plunger all the way down. This will push the insulin into your body. Release the pinched skin.
- Pull the needle straight out quickly. Do not rub the place where you gave the shot.
- Dispose of the syringe and needle without recapping in a puncture-proof container.

Dose preparation is critical for insulin effectiveness and patient safety. Teach patients that the person giving the insulin needs to inspect the insulin before each use for changes (e.g., clumping, frosting, precipitation, or change in clarity or color) that may indicate loss in potency. Rapid-acting, short-acting, and glargine insulins should be clear. Preparations containing NPH insulin should be uniformly cloudy after gently rolling the vial between the hands. If potency is questionable, another vial of the same type of insulin should be used.

Syringes are the most commonly used method to administer insulin. The standard insulin syringes are marked in insulin units. They are available in 1-mL (100-U), ½-mL (50-U), and $\frac{3}{10}$-mL (30-U) sizes. The unit scale on the barrel of the syringe differs with the syringe size and manufacturer. Insulin syringe needles are measured in 28-, 29-, 30-, and 31-gauge and in lengths of 6 mm, 8 mm, and 12.7 mm. To ensure accurate insulin measurement, instruct the patient to always buy the same type of syringe. Chart 64-3 reviews instructions for drawing up a single insulin injection.

Disposable needles should be used only once. Reuse of an insulin syringe and needle can compromise insulin sterility. A reason not to reuse smaller (30- and 31-gauge) needles is that even with one injection, the needle tip can become bent to form a hook, which can lacerate tissue or break off to leave needle fragments in the skin (Fig. 64-5). Teach the patient to discard the syringe and needle after one use. Information on needle disposal can be obtained at www.safeneedledisposal.org.

Pen-type injectors hold small, lightweight, prefilled insulin cartridges. The injectors are easy to carry and make intensive therapy with multiple injections easier. These devices allow greater accuracy than traditional insulin syringes, especially

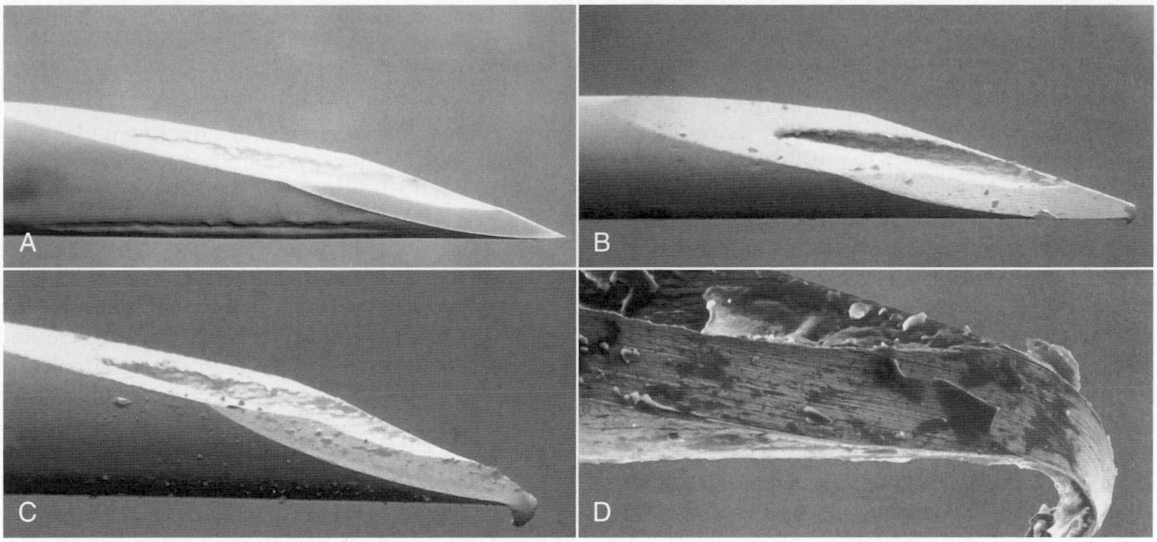

FIG. 64-5 Reuse of an insulin needle. **A,** A new needle. **B,** A needle that has been used once. **C,** A needle that has been used twice. **D,** A needle that has been used 6 times.

when measuring small doses. Discuss proper storage for prefilled insulin pens or cartridges. Ensure that the product is appropriate to the patient's unique needs. *Pen-type injectors are not designed for independent use by visually impaired patients or by those with cognitive impairment.* Ensure that the patient has received education on its use. Each syringe or cartridge has specific requirements. Patients using the FlexPen (Novo Nordisk) must be able to attach a needle and to perform an air shot of 2 units to ensure that a dose of insulin is administered. The Institute for Safe Medication Practices (ISMP) and The Joint Commission's National Patient Safety Goals identify insulin as a *High-Alert* drug. (**High-Alert drugs** are those that have an increased risk for causing patient harm if given in error.) The ISMP cautions that digital displays on some of the newer insulin pens can be misread. If the pen is held upside down, as a left-handed person might do, a dose of 52 units actually appears to be a dose of 25 units and a dose of 12 units looks like a dose of 21 units.

NCLEX EXAMINATION CHALLENGE

Health Promotion and Maintenance

Which statement made by a client who is learning about self-injection of insulin indicates to the nurse that clarification is needed about injection site selection and rotation?

A. "The abdominal site is best because it is closest to the pancreas."
B. "I can reach my thigh best, so I will use different areas of the same thigh."
C. "By rotating sites within one area, my chance of having skin changes is less."
D. "If I change my injection site from the thigh to an arm, the insulin absorption may be different."

Patient Education: Blood Glucose Monitoring. Self-monitoring of blood glucose (SMBG) levels provides information to assess effectiveness of the management plan. SMBG allows patients and providers to evaluate patient response to therapy and assess whether glycemic targets are being reached. Results of SMBG are useful in preventing hypoglycemia and adjusting drug therapy, diet therapy, and physical activity. Assessment of blood glucose levels is very important for these situations:

- Manifestations of hypoglycemia/hyperglycemia
- Hypoglycemic unawareness
- Periods of illness
- Before and after exercise
- Gastroparesis
- Adjustment of diabetes drugs
- Evaluation of other drug therapies (e.g., steroids)
- Preconception planning
- Pregnancy

Technique for SMBG follows principles that are the same for most self-monitoring systems. The finger is pricked, a drop of blood flows over or is drawn into a testing strip or disc impregnated with chemicals, and the glucose value is displayed in mg/dL or mmol/L. Most meters display blood glucose results on a screen. For vision-impaired patients, "talking-meters" are available to allow independence in blood glucose monitoring.

Data obtained from SMBG are evaluated along with other measures of blood glucose (e.g., A1C values) or periodic laboratory blood glucose tests. Even when SMBG is performed correctly, the results are affected by hematocrit values (anemia falsely elevates glucose values; polycythemia falsely depresses them) and may be unreliable in the hypoglycemic or severe hyperglycemic ranges.

The performance of SMBG systems depends on accuracy of the specific blood glucose meter, operator proficiency, and test strip quality. Results are influenced by the size and quality of the blood sample; the meter's calibration to the strip in use; and environmental conditions of altitude, temperature, and moisture. Patient-specific conditions influencing results include hematocrit level, triglyceride level, high levels of substances such as ascorbic acid in blood, and the presence of hypotension or hypoxia.

Accuracy of the blood glucose monitor is ensured when the manufacturer's directions are followed. The most common source of error is related to the skill of the user rather than to errors of the instrument. Common errors involve failure to obtain a sufficient blood drop, poor storage of test strips, using expired strips, and not changing the code number on the meter to match the strip bottle code. Help the patient select a meter based on cost, ease of use, and availability of repair and servicing. Provide training, explain and demonstrate procedures, assess visual acuity, and check the patient's ability to perform the procedure using "teach-back" strategies. Glucose meters are designed to reduce user error as much as possible. Newer meters have fewer steps, include error signals for inadequate sample size, "lock out" if control solutions are not tested, and store hundreds of SMBG results. (See the *Consumer Guide* published yearly in the January edition of *Diabetes Forecast* [forecast.diabetes.org] for information to help patients determine which blood glucose meter best meets their needs.)

Accuracy and precision vary widely among capillary blood glucose monitoring devices. Teach patients to properly calibrate ("code") the machine. Instruct them to re-check the calibration and re-test if they obtain a test result that is unusual for them and whenever they are in doubt about test accuracy. Continued retraining of patients performing SMBG helps ensure accurate results because performance accuracy deteriorates over time. Laboratory glucose determinations are more accurate than SMBG.

Frequency of testing varies with the drug schedules and the patient's prescribed therapy target outcomes. The ADA recommends that patients taking multiple insulin injections or using insulin pump therapy monitor glucose levels 3 or more times daily. For patients taking less-frequent injections of insulin, non-insulin therapy, or diet therapy alone, SMBG is useful for evaluation of therapy.

Blood glucose therapy target goals are set individually for each patient. The health care team works with him or her to reach target blood glucose levels. The ADA recommends that patients with type 1 diabetes aim for A1C values less than 6.5%, premeal glucose levels of 70 to 130 mg/dL (3.9 to 7.2 mmol/L), and postmeal glucose levels less than 180 mg/dL (10.0 mmol/L) (ADA, 2013).

Infection control measures are needed for SMBG. The chance of becoming infected from blood glucose monitoring processes is reduced by handwashing before monitoring and by not reusing lancets. *Instruct patients to not share their blood glucose monitoring equipment.* Hepatitis B virus can survive in a dried state for at least 1 week. INFECTION can be spread by the lancet holder even when the lancet itself has been changed. Small particles of blood can stick to the device and infect multiple users. Regular cleaning of the meter is critical for infection control. Remind health care staff who perform blood glucose testing and family members who help with testing to wear gloves.

Many meters allow data to be downloaded by a cable or by infrared technology to a computer that has diabetes management software (Hunt et al., 2014). Some meters allow entry of additional data such as insulin dose, amounts of carbohydrate eaten, or exercise. A radio link to an insulin pump allows automatic transfer of glucose readings to a calculator that assists the patient in deciding on an appropriate insulin dose. Some patients use smart phone applications to record and trend or graph serial blood glucose levels, insulin dosages, food intake, and other data. This information can be sent to the health care provider electronically or downloaded and printed.

Once the patient learns the technical aspects of meter use, help him or her use the results of SMBG to achieve glycemic control. Post-meal glucose monitoring provides information about the effects of the size and content of their meals. SMBG allows the patient to assess effects of exercise on glucose control and provides critical information to help patients who take insulin to exercise safely. Teach patients how to use SMBG results to adjust the treatment plan. Patients should make agreed upon adjustments in the treatment plan when results are consistently out of range for a 3-day period when no change in meal plan, medications, or activity has occurred.

The U.S. Food and Drug Administration issued an Important Safety Information Notice about blood glucose measurement following use of parenteral maltose, parenteral galactose, oral xylose-containing products, and the peritoneal dialysis solution *icodextrin* (EXTRANEAL). Galactose and xylose are found in some foods, herbs, and dietary supplements; they are also used in diagnostic tests. Some meters and test strips read these substances as glucose and falsely report the blood glucose as elevated. There have been insulin overdoses with severe hypoglycemia, coma, and death when patients have used this falsely elevated glucose reading in calculating an insulin dose. The Core Measures of The Joint Commission and other agencies recommend meters and test strips that use a technology in which *only glucose* in the blood is recognized for accurate blood glucose monitoring.

! NURSING SAFETY PRIORITY (QSEN)

Action Alert

Prevent hypoglycemia by ensuring that appropriate blood glucose testing products are used for patients receiving parenteral maltose, parenteral galactose, and oral xylose products.

It is important that staff understand the potential for hypoglycemia when patients are admitted to the hospital. In that instance, it is safest to monitor blood glucose patterns by laboratory methods. Blood glucose monitoring needs to be performed with a system in which the test strips use a different enzyme technology. The best resource for guidance in selecting a glucose monitoring system that is not reactive to maltose interference is the manufacturer of the test strip. Some manufacturers produce test strips that use more than one type of enzyme technology.

Alternate site testing allows patients to obtain blood from sites other than the fingertip and is available on many meters. However, use caution when interpreting results obtained from alternate sites. Comparison studies have shown wide variation between fingertip and alternate sites and the variation is most evident during times when blood glucose levels are rapidly changing. Teach patients that there is a lag time for blood glucose levels between the fingertip and other sites when blood glucose levels are changing rapidly and that the fingertip reading is the only safe choice at those times.

! NURSING SAFETY PRIORITY (QSEN)

Critical Rescue

Teach patients with a history of hypoglycemic unawareness ***not*** to test at alternative sites.

Continuous glucose monitoring (CGM) systems monitor glucose levels in interstitial fluid to provide real-time glucose information to the user. The system consists of three parts: a disposable sensor that measures glucose levels, a transmitter that is attached to the sensor, and a receiver that displays and stores glucose information. After an initiation or warm-up period, the sensor gives glucose values every 1 to 5 minutes. Sensors may be used for 3 to 7 days, depending on the manufacturer. CGM provides information about the current blood glucose level, provides short-term feedback about results of treatment, and provides warnings when glucose readings become dangerously high or low. Most available sensors require at least two capillary glucose readings per day for calibration of the sensor. Sensor accuracy depends on these calibrations. There may be a lag time between the capillary glucose measurement and the glucose sensor value. If the blood glucose value is changing rapidly, the time between capillary and interstitial glucose values may be as long as 30 minutes. For this reason, capillary glucose readings need to be checked on all extreme values and before any corrective treatment is given.

The costs for CGM systems are substantial, starting with the cost of the device. There are additional monthly charges for disposable sensors and for the glucose test strips used to calibrate the sensors and perform FDA-required capillary glucose testing before treatment decisions are made. *Continuous glucose monitoring is meant to supplement, not replace, finger stick tests. Insulin should be given only after confirming the results of any of the continuous glucose monitoring systems.*

Nutrition Therapy. Effective self-management of diabetes requires that NUTRITION, including the meal plan, education, and counseling programs be "patientized" for each patient. A registered dietitian (RD) should be a member of the treatment team. The nurse, RD, patient, and family work together on all aspects of the meal plan, which must be realistic and as flexible as possible. Plans that consider the patient's cultural background, financial status, and lifestyle are more likely to be successful. The desired outcomes of NUTRITION and diet therapy are listed in Table 64-9.

Principles of Nutrition in Diabetes. No one meal plan is right for all patients with diabetes. Each patient's NUTRITION recommendations are based on blood glucose monitoring results, total blood lipid levels, and A1C levels. These tests help determine whether current meal and exercise patterns need adjustment or whether present habits need reinforcement. The RD individually develops a meal plan based on the patient's usual food intake, weight-management expectations, and lipid and blood glucose patterns (ADA, 2014e). Day-to-day consistency in the timing and amount of food eaten helps control blood glucose. Patients receiving insulin therapy need to eat at times that are coordinated with the timed action of insulin. Teach patients using intense insulin therapy to adjust premeal insulin to allow for timing and quantity changes in their meal plan.

TABLE 64-9 Desired Outcomes of Nutrition Therapy for the Patient With Diabetes

- Achieving and maintaining blood glucose levels in the normal range or as close to normal as is safely possible
- Achieving and maintaining a blood lipid profile that reduces the risk for vascular disease
- Achieving blood pressure levels in the normal range or as close to normal as is safely possible
- Preventing or slowing the rate of development of the chronic complications of diabetes by modifying nutrient intake and lifestyle
- Addressing patient nutrition needs taking into account personal and cultural preferences and willingness to change
- Maintaining the pleasure of eating by limiting food choices only when indicated by scientific evidence
- Meeting the nutrition needs of unique times of the life cycle, particularly for pregnant and lactating women and for older adults with diabetes
- Providing self-management training for patients treated with insulin or insulin secretagogues for exercising safely, including the prevention and treatment of hypoglycemia, and managing diabetes during acute illness

Carbohydrate intake and available insulin are responsible for postmeal glucose levels, and managing carbohydrate intake is the main strategy for achieving GLUCOSE REGULATION and glycemic control. The recommendation for the patient with diabetes is a diet containing 45% of calories from carbohydrate, with a minimum intake of 130 g carbohydrate/day. However, the upper limit on daily carbohydrate intake is now considered somewhat flexible so that individual patient NUTRITION needs can be met with some variation in the carbohydrate-protein mix distribution (ADA, 2014e). The diet should include carbohydrate from fruit, vegetables, whole grains, legumes, and low-fat milk products.

The percentage of calories from carbohydrates is determined for each patient. Various starches have different blood glucose responses. The *total amount* of carbohydrate consumed each day rather than the source of the carbohydrate is still important.

Dietary fat and cholesterol intake for people with diabetes is the same as the Institute of Medicine's (IOM) recommendations for the general population to reduce the risk for cardiovascular disease. These recommendations are based on the issue that fat *quality* is more important in lipid control than is fat *quantity* (ADA, 2014e). Current recommendations are:

- Limiting total fat intake to 20% to 35% of daily calorie intake
- Choosing monounsaturated and polyunsaturated fats over saturated fats and *trans* fats
- Limiting dietary cholesterol to less than 200 mg/day
- Having two or more servings of fatty fish per week (with the exception of commercially fried fish) to provide n-3 polyunsaturated fatty acids

Trans fatty acids increase the risk for cardiovascular disease and are found in hard margarine and in foods prepared with or fried in hydrogenated and partly hydrogenated oils. Teach the patient to limit the amount of commercially fried foods and bakery goods eaten.

Further dietary fat restrictions for diabetes are determined by the RD based on specific lipid levels. Adults with diabetes should be tested annually for abnormalities of fasting serum cholesterol, triglyceride, HDL cholesterol, and calculated LDL cholesterol levels.

Protein intake of 15% to 20% of total daily calories is appropriate for patients with diabetes and normal kidney function. Some patients may need a higher percentage of calories from protein, substituted from carbohydrates, to maintain satiety and control blood glucose levels. Diets higher in protein have demonstrated improvement in insulin response but do not prevent hypoglycemia (ADA, 2014e). In patients with progressive kidney disease, reducing protein intake is needed and the level of protein reduction must be individualized.

Fiber improves carbohydrate metabolism and lowers cholesterol levels. Recommendations for the person with diabetes are the same as for the general population, which include foods containing a minimum of 25 g of fiber daily for women and 38 g daily for men (ADA, 2014e). Teach the patient to select a variety of fiber-containing foods such as legumes, fiber-rich cereals (more than 5 g fiber/serving), fruits, vegetables, and whole-grain products because they provide vitamins, minerals, and other substances important for good health.

Teach the patient that adding high-fiber foods to the diet gradually can reduce abdominal cramping, loose stools, and flatulence. An increase in fluid intake should accompany increased fiber intake. Teach the patient to pay careful attention to blood glucose levels because hypoglycemia can result when dietary fiber intake increases significantly.

Sucrose, fructose, and nonnutritive sweeteners (NNSs) are present in a variety of foods. Dietary sucrose does not increase blood glucose more than equal amounts of other starches. Intake of sucrose and sucrose-containing foods by patients with diabetes does not need to be restricted out of a concern for causing hyperglycemia. Sucrose can be included in the meal plan as long as it is adequately covered with insulin or other glucose-lowering agents; however, all people with diabetes are encouraged to avoid sugar sweetened beverages (SSBs) (ADA, 2014e). The use of nonnutritive sweeteners to enhance the taste of food while not disturbing blood glucose control is desirable. Foods sweetened with high-fructose corn syrup should be avoided by people with diabetes because this substance has been found to increase the levels of triglycerides and other lipids. Free fructose, such as that found in fruit, does not appear to alter lipid metabolism in the way that foods containing high-fructose corn syrup do (ADA, 2014e).

Alcohol consumption can affect blood glucose levels. Levels are not affected by *moderate* use of alcohol when diabetes is well controlled. Teach patients with diabetes that two alcoholic beverages for men and one for women daily can be ingested with, and in addition to, the usual meal plan. (One alcoholic beverage equals 12 ounces of beer, 5 ounces of wine, or 1.5 ounces of distilled spirits.) Because alcohol raises blood triglycerides, reducing or abstaining from alcohol is important for patients with high blood lipid levels.

! NURSING SAFETY PRIORITY QSEN

Action Alert

Because of the potential for alcohol-induced hypoglycemia, instruct the patient with diabetes to ingest alcohol only with or shortly after meals.

Patient Education: Prescribed Nutrition Plan. Reinforce NUTRITION information provided by the RD. The patient with DM must understand how to adjust food intake during illness, planned exercise, and social occasions (e.g., restaurant meals) when the usual time of eating may be delayed. He or she may be unable to follow the prescribed plan because of an inability to read or understand printed materials. Share dietary information with the person who prepares the meals. The RD sees each patient at least yearly to identify changes in lifestyle and make appropriate diet therapy changes. Some patients, such as those with weight-control problems or low incomes, may need more frequent evaluation and counseling.

Meal Planning Strategies. Many meal planning approaches for good NUTRITION are available. Each approach emphasizes different aspects of nutrition.

Carbohydrate (CHO) counting is a simple approach to NUTRITION and meal planning that uses label information of the nutrition content of packaged food items. Because fat and protein have little effect on after-meal blood glucose levels, CHO counting focuses on the nutrient that has the greatest impact on these levels. It uses total grams of carbohydrate, regardless of the food source. The RD determines the number of grams of carbohydrate to be eaten at each meal and snack and helps the patient make appropriate food choices. This method is effective in achieving overall blood glucose control when carbohydrate intake is consistent from day to day.

Patients using intensive insulin or pump therapies can use CHO counting to determine insulin coverage. After the amount of insulin needed to cover the usual meal is determined, insulin may be added or subtracted for changes in carbohydrate intake. An initial formula of 1 unit of rapid-acting insulin for each 15 g of carbohydrate provides flexibility to meal plans. The patient determines the grams of carbohydrate in a specific meal or snack by reading labels or weighing and measuring each item. The total grams of carbohydrate are used to calculate the bolus dose of insulin based on his or her prescribed insulin-to-carbohydrate ratio.

People at high risk for type 2 diabetes are encouraged to achieve moderate weight loss (7% total body weight), participate in regular physical activity (150 minutes per week), and reduce caloric and dietary fat intake. These at-risk people are also encouraged to increase fiber intake to at least 14 g per 1000 calories consumed and to eat foods containing whole grains.

Special considerations for type 1 diabetes include developing insulin regimens that conform to the patient's preferred meal routines, food preferences, and exercise patterns. Patients using rapid-acting insulin by injection or an insulin pump should adjust insulin doses based on the carbohydrate content of the meals and snacks. Insulin-to-carbohydrate ratios are developed and are used to provide mealtime insulin doses. Blood glucose monitoring before and 2 hours after meals determines whether the insulin-to-carbohydrate ratio is correct. For patients who are on fixed insulin regimens and do not adjust premeal insulin dosages, consistency of timing of meals and the amount of CHO eaten at each meal is important to prevent hypoglycemia.

Exercise can cause hypoglycemia if insulin is not decreased before activity. For planned exercise, reduction in insulin dosage is used for hypoglycemia prevention. For unplanned exercise, intake of additional CHO is usually needed. Moderate exercise increases glucose utilization by 2 to 3 mg/kg/min. A 70-kg (154-lb) person would need about 10 to 15 g additional CHO per hour of moderate-intensity activity. More CHO is needed for intense activity.

It is important for patients with type 1 diabetes to avoid gaining weight. Chronic high insulin levels (**hyperinsulinemia**) can occur with intensive management schedules and may result in weight gain. These patients may need to manage hyperglycemia by restricting calories rather than increasing insulin. Weight gain can be minimized by following the prescribed meal plan, getting regular exercise, and avoiding overtreatment of hypoglycemia.

Special considerations for type 2 diabetes focus on lifestyle changes. Many patients with type 2 diabetes are overweight and insulin resistant. NUTRITION therapy stresses lifestyle changes that reduce calories eaten and increase calories expended through physical activity. Many patients also have abnormal blood fat levels and hypertension (metabolic syndrome), making reductions of saturated fat, cholesterol, and sodium desirable. A moderate caloric restriction (250 to 500 calories less than average daily intake) and an increase in physical activity improve diabetes control and weight control. Decreases of more than 10% of body weight can result in significant improvement in A1C. Decreasing intake of cholesterol-raising fatty acids helps reduce the risk for cardiovascular disease.

When patients with type 2 diabetes need insulin, consistency in timing and carbohydrate content of meals is important. Division of the total daily calories into three meals or into smaller meals and snacks is based on patient preference.

CONSIDERATIONS FOR OLDER ADULTS

Patient-Centered Care QSEN

Older patients are at increased risk for poor nutrition, hypoglycemia, and especially dehydration, a factor in the development of hyperglycemic-hyperosmolar state (HHS). Many factors contribute to malnutrition. Nutrition needs of the older adult change as the person's taste, smell, and appetite diminish and his or her ability to obtain and prepare food decreases. Older patients who prepare their own food or have tooth loss or poorly fitting dentures may not eat enough food. Neuropathy with gastric retention or diarrhea compounds poor food intake. Impaired cognition and depression may disrupt self-care. Older patients may have a marginal food supply because of inadequate income, may have poor understanding of meal-planning needs, or may live alone and have reduced incentive to prepare or eat proper meals. They may eat in restaurants or live in situations in which they have little control over meal preparation. Regular visits by home health nurses can assist older patients in following a diabetic meal plan.

A realistic approach to nutrition therapy is essential for the older patient with diabetes. Changing the eating habits of 60 to 70 years is very difficult. The nurse, dietitian, and patient assess the patient's usual eating patterns. Teach the older patient taking antidiabetic drugs about the importance of eating meals and snacks at the same time every day, eating the same amount of food from day to day, and eating all food allowed on the diet.

Exercise Therapy. Regular exercise is an essential part of diabetic management. It has beneficial effects on carbohydrate metabolism and insulin sensitivity. Programs of increased physical activity and weight loss reduce the incidence of type 2 diabetes in patients with impaired glucose tolerance (American Association of Diabetes Educators [AADE], 2011).

Blood glucose levels remain stable in physically active patients without diabetes because of the balance between glucose use by exercising muscles and glucose production by the liver. The patient with type 1 DM cannot make the hormonal changes needed to maintain stable blood glucose levels during exercise. Without an adequate insulin supply, cells cannot use glucose. Low insulin levels trigger release of glucagon and epinephrine (counterregulatory hormones) to increase liver glucose production, further raising blood glucose levels. In the absence of insulin, free fatty acids become the source of energy. Exercise in the patient with uncontrolled diabetes results in further hyperglycemia and the formation of ketone bodies. He or she may have prolonged elevated blood glucose levels after vigorous exercise.

Exercise in the person with diabetes also can cause hypoglycemia because of increased muscle glucose uptake and inhibited glucose release from the liver. It can occur during exercise and for up to 24 hours after exercise. Replacement of muscle and liver glycogen stores, along with increased insulin sensitivity after exercise, causes insulin requirements to drop.

Benefits of Exercise. Appropriate exercise results in better blood GLUCOSE REGULATION and reduced insulin requirements for patients with type 1 DM. Exercise also increases insulin sensitivity, which enhances cell uptake of glucose and promotes weight loss.

Regular exercise decreases risk for cardiovascular disease. It decreases most blood lipid levels and increases high-density lipoproteins (HDLs). Exercise decreases blood pressure and improves cardiovascular function. Regular vigorous physical activity prevents or delays type 2 DM by reducing body weight, insulin resistance, and glucose intolerance.

Adjustments for Diabetes Complications. Exercise in the presence of long-term complications of diabetes often requires some adjustment. Vigorous aerobic or resistance exercise should be avoided in the presence of proliferative diabetic retinopathy or severe nonproliferative diabetic retinopathy. Teach the patient with retinopathy to avoid the *Valsalva maneuver* (breath holding while bearing down) and activities that increase blood pressure. Heavy lifting, rapid head motion, or jarring activities can cause vitreous hemorrhage or retinal detachment. Decreased pain sensation in the extremities increases the risk for skin breakdown and infection and for joint destruction. Teach patients with diabetic peripheral neuropathy (DPN) to wear proper footwear and to examine their feet daily for lesions. Teach anyone with a foot injury or open sore to engage in non-weight-bearing activities such as swimming, bicycling, seated yoga, or arm exercises. Those with autonomic neuropathy are at increased risk for exercise-induced injury from impaired temperature control, postural hypotension, and impaired thirst with risk for dehydration. Physical activity also can increase urine protein excretion. Encourage high-risk patients to start with short periods of low-intensity exercise and to increase the intensity and duration slowly (ADA, 2013).

Safety Assessment. Assessment before initiating an exercise program is necessary to ensure patient safety. Although current ADA guidelines do not recommend routine screening for patients with diabetes who have no manifestations of cardiovascular disease, be alert to conditions that might predispose the patient to injury or that contraindicate certain types of exercise. Regular physical activity increases the risk for both musculoskeletal injury and life-threatening cardiovascular events. Patients with diabetes often take drugs to reduce blood pressure, to normalize blood lipid concentrations, and to inhibit platelet activity. These drugs may increase fall risk, change physiologic response to exercise and physical activity, alter muscle performance, and increase bleeding risk (Sisson et al., 2012). The ADA recommends screening when any of these conditions exist:

- Chest pain or discomfort
- Abnormal electrocardiogram (ECG) suggestive of ischemia or infarction
- Peripheral or carotid occlusive disease
- Age older than 35 years with sedentary lifestyle in a patient who plans a vigorous exercise program
- Two or more risk factors in addition to diabetes, such as dyslipidemia, hypertension, tobacco use
- Family history for premature coronary artery disease, or microalbuminuria or macroalbuminuria of more than 10 years' duration
- Age older than 25 years and type 1 diabetes of more than 15 years' duration
- Severe autonomic neuropathy, severe diabetic peripheral neuropathy, history of foot lesions, and unstable proliferative retinopathy

Screening for coronary artery disease before an exercise program is started is recommended for patients with cardiovascular risk factors. Exercise treadmill testing (ETT) is used to determine if a person can exercise to 85% of his or her predicted heart rate without having ischemic changes. It also provides information about exercise capacity and functional status. Failure to achieve 85% of the predicted heart rate is associated with increased incidence of death.

Other studies to determine the risk for exercise-induced problems include medical stress tests with vasodilator therapy and stress echocardiography. Additional tests may be performed to determine the presence of obstructive lesions in coronary arteries.

Advise people with DM to perform at least 150 min/wk of moderate-intensive aerobic physical activity or 75 min/wk of vigorous aerobic physical activity or an equivalent combination of the two. In the absence of contraindications, patients with type 2 diabetes are urged to perform resistance exercise 3 times a week, targeting all major muscle groups (ADA 2013). The ADA recommends that there be no more than 2 consecutive days without aerobic physical activity.

A 5- to 10-minute warm-up period with stretching and low-intensity exercise before exercise prepares the skeletal muscles, heart, and lungs for a progressive increase in exercise intensity. After the activity session, a cool-down should be performed similarly to the warm-up. The cool-down should last 5 to 10 minutes and gradually bring the heart rate down to pre-exercise level.

Guidelines for exercise are based on blood glucose levels and urine ketone levels. Recommend that the patient test blood glucose before exercise, at intervals during exercise, and after exercise to determine if it is safe to exercise and to evaluate the effects of exercise. The absence of urine ketones indicates that enough insulin is available for glucose transport and that exercise should be effective in lowering blood glucose levels. *When urine ketones are present, the patient should **NOT** exercise.* Ketones indicate that current insulin levels are not adequate and

! NURSING SAFETY PRIORITY QSEN

Critical Rescue

Teach patients with type 1 diabetes to perform vigorous exercise only when blood glucose levels are 100 to 250 mg/dL (5.6 to 13.8 mmol/L) and no ketones are present in the urine.

CONSIDERATIONS FOR OLDER ADULTS

Patient-Centered Care QSEN

With age, the ability of the heart and lungs to deliver oxygen to tissues and organs declines. Muscle strength and power decline gradually. Connective tissue becomes less elastic, affecting range of motion and flexibility. Limited range of motion can alter gait, increasing risk for falls. Older adults who remain active can limit losses in muscle mass and function.

The emphasis for any activity program is on changing sedentary behavior to active behavior at any level. Encourage sedentary older adults to begin with low-intensity physical activity. Start low-intensity activities in short sessions (less than 10 minutes); include warm-up and cool-down components with active stretching. Changes in activity levels should be gradual. Formal evaluation by a physical therapist or occupational therapist may be needed. Examples of specific exercise can be found at www.geri.com.

CHART 64-4 Patient and Family Education: Preparing for Self-Management

Exercise

- Teach the patient about the relationship between regularly scheduled exercise and blood glucose levels, blood lipid levels, and complications of diabetes.
- Reinforce the level of exercise recommended for the patient based on his or her physical health.
- Instruct the patient to wear appropriate footwear designed for exercise.
- Remind the patient to examine his or her feet daily and after exercising.
- Remind the patient to stay hydrated and not to exercise in extreme heat or cold.
- Warn the patient not to exercise within 1 hour of insulin injection or near the time of peak insulin action.
- Teach patients how to prevent hypoglycemia during exercise:
  - Do not exercise unless blood glucose level is at least 80 and less than 250 mg/dL.
  - Have a carbohydrate snack before exercising if 1 hour has passed since the last meal or if the planned exercise is high intensity.
  - Carry a simple sugar to eat during exercise if symptoms of hypoglycemia occur.
  - Ensure that identification information about diabetes is carried during exercise.
- Remind the patient to check blood glucose levels more frequently on days in which exercise is performed and that extra carbohydrate and less insulin may be needed during the 24-hour period after extensive exercise.

that exercise would elevate blood glucose levels. Carbohydrate foods should be ingested to raise blood glucose levels above 100 mg/dL (5.6 mmol/L) before engaging in exercise. Chart 64-4 lists tips to teach the patient and family about self-management and exercise.

Blood Glucose Control in Hospitalized Patients. Hyperglycemia in hospitalized patients occurs for many reasons and is associated with poor outcomes (Kubacka, 2014). In patients without a previous diagnosis of diabetes, elevated blood glucose is often "stress hyperglycemia." Hyperglycemia may result from decline in basic level of GLUCOSE REGULATION caused by illness, decreased physical activity, withholding of antidiabetic drugs, use of drugs that cause hyperglycemia such as corticosteroids, and initiation of tube feedings or parenteral nutrition (Freeland & Funnell, 2012).

Hyperglycemia among medical-surgical patients is linked with higher infection rates, longer hospital stays, increased need for intensive care, and greater mortality. Admission glucose levels greater than 198 mg/dL (10.9 mmol/L) are associated with greater risk for mortality and complications. Hypoglycemia, defined as blood glucose values lower than 40 mg/dL (2.2 mmol/L), is an independent risk factor for mortality.

Current American Association of Clinical Endocrinologists (AACE) and ADA Core Measures recommend treatment protocols that maintain blood glucose levels between 140 and 180 mg/dL (7.8 and 10.0 mmol/L) for critically ill patients. For the majority of non–critically ill patients, premeal glucose targets should be lower than 140 mg/dL (7.8 mmol/L) with random blood glucose values less than 180 mg/dL (10.0 mmol/L). To prevent hypoglycemia, insulin regimens should be reviewed if blood glucose levels fall below 100 mg/dL (5.6 mmol/L) and should be modified when blood glucose levels are less than 70 mg/dL (3.9 mmol/L) (ADA, 2013).

Continuous IV insulin solutions are the most effective method for achieving glycemic targets in the intensive care setting. Scheduled subcutaneous injection with basal, meal, and correction elements is the preferred method for achieving and maintaining glucose control in non–critically ill patients. Using correction dose or "supplemental insulin" to correct premeal hyperglycemia in addition to scheduled prandial and basal insulin is recommended. The correction dose is determined by the patient's insulin sensitivity and current blood glucose level.

Prevention of hypoglycemia is also part of managing blood glucose levels. Causes of inpatient hypoglycemia include an inappropriate insulin type, mismatch between insulin type and/or timing of food intake, and altered eating plan without insulin dosage adjustment. The Joint Commission (TJC), together with the ADA, has established Core Measures for preventing hypoglycemia in the inpatient care of people with diabetes (The Joint Commission [TJC], 2014). These involve protocols for hypoglycemia treatment that direct staff to provide carbohydrate replacement if the patient is alert and able to swallow or to administer 50% dextrose intravenously or glucagon by subcutaneous injection if the patient cannot swallow.

There is confusion about whether to give or to hold insulin from a patient who is NPO. Administration of rapid-acting or short-acting insulin, as well as amylin and incretin mimetics, will cause hypoglycemia if a patient is not eating. Basal insulin should be administered when the patient is NPO because it controls baseline glucose levels. Insulin mixtures are not administered because they contain some short-acting or rapid-acting insulin and will cause hypoglycemia.

Surgical Management. Surgical interventions for diabetes include a pancreas transplantation. When successful, this procedure eliminates the need for insulin injections, blood glucose monitoring, and many dietary restrictions. It can eliminate the acute complications related to blood glucose control but is only partially successful in reversing long-term diabetes complications. Pancreatic transplant is successful when the patient no longer needs insulin therapy and all blood measures of glucose are normal.

Transplantation requires lifelong drug therapy to prevent graft rejection. These drug regimens have toxic side effects that restrict their use to patients who have serious progressive complications of diabetes. In addition, some anti-rejection drugs have the effect of increasing blood glucose levels. Pancreas-alone transplants are most often considered for patients with severe metabolic complications and for those with consistent failure of insulin-based therapy to prevent acute complications.

Pancreas transplantation is considered in patients with diabetes and end-stage kidney disease who have had or plan to have a kidney transplant. Normal blood glucose levels after pancreas transplantation improve kidney graft survival. Pancreas graft survival is better when performed at the time of the kidney transplant.

Whole-Pancreas Transplantation. Improved surgical techniques and newer anti-rejection drugs have improved transplantation outcomes. The 1-year survival rate for patients is above 95%, with more than 83% of patients remaining free of insulin injection and diet restrictions after 1 year. The degree of tissue-type matching affects the results.

Pancreatic transplantation is performed in one of three ways: pancreas transplant alone (PTA), pancreas after kidney (PAK) transplant, and simultaneous pancreas and kidney (SPK) transplant. SPK transplant is the ideal procedure for patients with DM and uremia.

Operative Procedure. Most pancreatic transplants are from cadaver donors using a total pancreas still attached to the exit of the pancreatic duct. The recipient's pancreas is left in place, and the donated pancreas is placed in the pelvis. The insulin released by the pancreas graft is secreted into the bloodstream. The new pancreas also produces about 800 to 1000 mL of fluid daily, which is diverted to either the bladder or the bowel.

Excretion of pancreatic fluids can cause dehydration and electrolyte imbalance, and drainage of these fluids into the urinary bladder causes irritation. When the pancreas is attached to the bladder, the loss of fluid rich in bicarbonate may cause acidosis.

Rejection Management. A combination of drugs and antibodies is used to reverse rejection. (See Chapter 17 for a listing of agents used to prevent or manage transplant rejection.) Patients undergoing anti-rejection therapy first receive drugs to prevent viral, bacterial, and fungal infection because of the risk for opportunistic INFECTIONS. Most patients receiving high-dose steroids, as well as those on chronic long-term steroid therapy, will require dosage adjustments in insulin to achieve desired levels of glucose control.

In most episodes of rejections, kidney problems occur before pancreatic problems. An increase in serum creatinine indicates rejection of both the transplanted kidney and the pancreas. In patients with bladder drainage of pancreatic hormones, a decrease in the urine amylase level by 25% is an indication to treat rejection. High blood glucose levels are a later marker of rejection and usually indicate irreversible graft failure.

Long-Term Effects. Long-term anti-rejection therapy increases the risk for INFECTION, cancer, and atherosclerosis. When insulin drains into systemic rather than portal (liver) circulation, blood insulin levels rise (hyperinsulinemia) and increase the risk for hypertension and macrovascular disease.

Complications. Complications are common in patients taking long-term anti-rejection therapy. Monitor laboratory values, fluid and electrolyte status, physical changes, and changes in vital signs to identify possible complications. Early removal of IV and intra-arterial lines, use of sterile technique with dressing changes and catheter irrigations, strict handwashing by all health care personnel, and good pulmonary hygiene help prevent INFECTION.

Complications immediately after surgery include thrombosis, pancreatitis, anastomosis leak with INFECTION, and rejection of the transplanted pancreas. Pancreatic blood vessel thrombosis occurs in about 30% of patients after transplantation. Observe for and report any sudden drop in urine amylase levels, rapid increases in blood glucose, gross **hematuria** (bloody urine), and tenderness or pain in the graft area (iliac fossa). Pancreatitis in the transplanted organ occurs to some degree in all patients after surgery. Report elevations in serum amylase that persist after 48 to 96 hours.

The most serious complication of enteric-drained pancreas transplantation is leaking and INFECTION with intra-abdominal abscess formation. Observe for and report elevation in temperature, abdominal discomfort, and elevation in white blood cell (WBC) count. Bladder-drained pancreas transplantation has a lower rate of intra-abdominal abscess formation. However, drainage of bicarbonate-rich fluid with pancreatic enzymes into the urinary bladder can cause urinary tract infections, cystitis, urethritis, and balanitis. Metabolic acidosis occurs from the loss of large amounts of alkaline pancreatic secretions.

Assess for and document manifestations of rejection. In acute rejection, decreased kidney function is indicated by increased serum creatinine, decreased urine output, hypertension, increased weight, graft tenderness, and fever. Proteinuria is often the first indicator of chronic graft rejection. Check for increased blood amylase, lipase, or glucose; decreased urine amylase; graft tenderness; hyperglycemia; and fever. *It is especially important to assess for* INFECTION *and start appropriate therapy. Fever can indicate both infection and rejection.*

Monitor for side effects of the anti-rejection drugs. Cyclosporine (Neoral) is toxic to the kidney. Indications of toxicity are elevated creatinine and decreased urine output. Monitor WBC counts daily, because azathioprine (Imuran) can suppress bone marrow function. Common side effects of tacrolimus (Prograf) are hypertension, kidney toxicity, neurotoxicity, GI toxicity, and glucose intolerance. Prednisone has many side effects, including elevated blood glucose levels.

Islet Cell Transplantation. Islet cell transplantation eliminates the need for insulin and protects against the complications of diabetes. Wider use of this procedure is hindered by the limited supply of beta cells available for transplantation and by issues related to rejection. Islet cells from tissue-typed (HLA-matched) cadaver pancreas glands are injected into the portal vein. The new cells lodge in the liver and begin to function, secreting insulin and maintaining near-perfect blood glucose control.

Islet cell transplantation may successfully restore long-term endogenous insulin production and glycemic control in patients with type 1 diabetes and unstable baseline control. Most patients undergoing this procedure eventually have a progressive loss of islet cell function. Very few islet cell transplant recipients have remained insulin-free for more than 4 years. The reasons for this gradual loss of function are not known and make this procedure a long-term but temporary intervention. It is considered an experimental procedure.

Enhancing Surgical Recovery

Planning: Expected Outcomes. The patient with diabetes undergoing a surgical procedure is expected to recover completely without complications. Indicators include:

- Wound healing
- Absence of infection
- Maintenance of blood glucose levels within expected range

Interventions. Surgery is a physical and emotional stressor, and the patient with diabetes has a higher risk for complications. Anesthesia and surgery cause a stress response with release of counterregulatory hormones that elevate blood glucose. Stress hormones suppress insulin action, increasing the risk for ketoacidosis. Hyperglycemic-hyperosmolar state (HHS) is a common complication after major surgery and is associated with increased mortality. Diuresis from hyperglycemia can cause dehydration and increases the risk for kidney failure.

Complications of diabetes increase the risk for surgical complications. Patients with DM are at higher risk for hypertension, ischemic heart disease, cerebrovascular disease, MI, and cardiomyopathy. Heart failure is a serious risk factor and must be improved before surgery. Autonomic neuropathy may result in sudden tachycardia, bradycardia, or postural hypotension. The patient with DM is at risk for acute kidney injury and urinary retention after surgery, especially if he or she has albumin in the urine (indicator of kidney damage). Nerves to the intestinal wall and sphincters can be impaired, leading to delayed gastric emptying and reflux of gastric acid, which increases the risk for aspiration with anesthesia. Autonomic neuropathy may cause paralytic ileus after surgery.

Preoperative Care. Patients undergoing major surgery are admitted to the hospital 2 to 3 days before surgery to optimize blood glucose control. Sulfonylureas are discontinued 1 day before surgery. Metformin (Glucophage) is stopped at least 24 hours before surgery and restarted only after kidney function is normal. All other oral drugs are stopped the day of surgery. Patients taking long-acting insulin may need to be switched to intermediate-acting insulin forms 1 to 2 days before surgery.

Preoperative blood glucose levels should be less than 200 mg/dL (11.1 mmol/L). Higher levels are associated with increased INFECTION rates and impaired wound healing.

Plan ahead for pain control after surgery. PAIN, a stressor, triggers the release of counterregulatory hormones, increasing blood glucose levels and insulin needs. Opioid analgesics slow GI motility and alter blood glucose levels. The older patient who receives opioids is more at risk for confusion, paralytic ileus, hypoventilation, hypotension, and urinary retention. Patient-controlled analgesia (PCA) systems reduce respiratory complications and confusion. (See Chapter 3 for pain interventions and Chapter 14 for general preoperative care.)

Intraoperative Care. IV infusion of insulin, glucose, and potassium is standard therapy for perioperative management of diabetes. In accordance with The Joint Commission's NPSGs, the objective is to keep the blood glucose level between 140 and 180 mg/dL (7.8 and 10.0 mmol/L) during surgery to prevent hypoglycemia and reduce risks from hyperglycemia (TJC, 2014). Insulin/glucose infusion rates are based on hourly capillary glucose tests. Higher insulin doses may be needed because stress releases glucagon and epinephrine. Patients with DM usually receive about 5 g of glucose per hour during surgery to prevent hypoglycemia, ketosis, and protein breakdown.

Monitor the patient's temperature—it may be lowered deliberately in some surgical procedures and inadvertently in others. Low operating room temperatures and large incisions also lower body temperature. Hypothermia decreases metabolic needs, depresses heart rate and contractility, causes vasoconstriction, and impairs insulin release, resulting in high blood glucose levels. Monitor arterial blood gas values for acidosis.

Postoperative Care. Hyperglycemia is associated with increased mortality after surgical procedures. Current AACE and ADA Core Measures recommend insulin protocols that maintain blood glucose between 140 and 180 mg/dL (7.8 and 10.0 mmol/L) for critically ill patients (ADA, 2013).

Protocols and computer-based programs can be used to determine the insulin infusion rate required to maintain blood glucose levels within a defined target range. Many insulin infusion algorithms are implemented by nursing staff. Continue glucose and insulin infusions as prescribed until the patient is stable and can tolerate oral feedings. Short-term insulin therapy may be needed after surgery for the patient who usually uses oral agents. For those receiving insulin therapy, dosage adjustments may be required until the stress of surgery subsides.

Monitoring. Patients with autonomic neuropathy or vascular disease need close monitoring to avoid hypotension or respiratory arrest. Those who take beta blockers for hypertension need close monitoring for hypoglycemia because these drugs mask manifestations of hypoglycemia. Patients with increased protein or nitrogen waste products in the blood may have problems with fluid management. Check central venous pressure or pulmonary artery pressure as needed.

Glucose levels are a sensitive marker of counterregulatory hormones, which are often activated before patients become febrile. Hyperglycemia often occurs before a fever.

! NURSING SAFETY PRIORITY QSEN

Critical Rescue

When a patient who has had reasonably controlled blood glucose levels in the hospital develops an unexpected rise in blood glucose values, check for wound infection.

Hyperkalemia (high blood potassium level) is common in patients with mild to moderate kidney failure and can lead to cardiac dysrhythmia. In other patients, **hypokalemia** (low blood potassium level) may occur and be made worse by insulin and glucose given during surgery. Monitor the cardiac rhythm and serum potassium values.

Cardiovascular monitoring by continuous electrocardiograms (ECGs) is recommended for older patients with diabetes, those with long-standing type 1 DM, and those with heart disease. Patients with diabetes are at higher risk for MI after surgery with a higher mortality rate. Changes in ECG or in potassium level may indicate a silent MI.

Kidney monitoring, especially observing fluid balance, helps detect acute kidney injury (AKI). Diagnosis of kidney impairment may require the use of x-ray studies using dyes, which may be nephrotoxic. Management of INFECTION may require the use of nephrotoxic antibiotics. Ensure adequate hydration when these drugs are used. Check for impending kidney failure by assessing fluid and electrolyte status.

Nutrition. Patients requiring clear or full liquid diets should receive about 200 g of carbohydrate daily in equally divided amounts at meals and snack times. Initial liquids should not be sugar-free. Most patients require 25 to 35 calories per kg of body weight every 24 hours. After surgery, food intake is initiated as quickly as possible with progression from clear liquids to solid foods occurring as rapidly as tolerated. Returning to a normal meal plan as soon as possible after surgery promotes healing and metabolic balance. When oral foods are tolerated, make sure the patient takes at least 150 to 200 g of carbohydrate daily to prevent hypoglycemia.

If total parenteral nutrition (TPN) is used after surgery, severe hyperglycemia may occur. Monitor blood glucose often to determine the need for supplemental insulin.

Preventing Injury from Peripheral Neuropathy

Planning: Expected Outcomes. The patient with diabetes is expected to identify factors that increase the risk for injury, practice proper foot care, and maintain skin TISSUE INTEGRITY on the feet. Indicators include that the patient consistently demonstrates these behaviors:

- Cleanses and inspects the feet daily
- Wears properly fitting shoes
- Avoids walking in bare feet
- Trims toenails properly
- Reports nonhealing breaks in the skin of the feet to the health care provider

Interventions. Patients with DM need intensive teaching about foot care. *Foot injury is the most common complication of diabetes leading to hospitalization.* Once a failure of TISSUE INTEGRITY has occurred and an ulcer has developed, there is an increased risk for wound progression that will eventually lead to amputation. Almost all lower extremity amputations are preceded by foot ulcers. The 5-year mortality rate after leg or foot amputation ranges from 39% to 67% (National Institute of Diabetes and Digestive and Kidney Diseases [NIDDK], 2011). Neuropathy is the main factor for development of a diabetic ulcer, and an inadequate vascular supply is the main cause of poor healing (Thomas, 2013).

Motor neuropathy damages the nerves of foot muscles, resulting in foot deformities. These deformities create pressure points that gradually cause reduced TISSUE INTEGRITY with skin breakdown and ulceration. Thinning or shifting of the fat pad under the metatarsal heads decreases cushioning and increases areas of pressure. In claw toe deformity, toes are hyperextended and increase pressure on the metatarsal heads ("ball" of the foot). These changes predispose the patient to callus formation, ulceration, and INFECTION. The Charcot foot is a type of diabetic foot deformity with many abnormalities, often including a hallux valgus (turning inward of the great toe) (Fig. 64-6). The foot is warm, swollen, and painful. Walking collapses the arch, shortens the foot, and gives the sole of the foot a "rocker bottom" shape.

Autonomic neuropathy causes loss of normal sweating and skin temperature regulation, resulting in dry, thinning skin. Skin cracks and fissures increase the risk for INFECTION. Sensory neuropathy may cause PAIN, tingling, or burning (Funnell, 2014). More often it produces numbness and reduced SENSORY PERCEPTION. Without sensation, the patient does not notice injuries and loss of TISSUE INTEGRITY in the foot and does not treat them. Peripheral arterial disease reduces the blood supply to the foot, increasing the risk for ulcer formation and reducing the rate of ulcer healing (McCance et al., 2014).

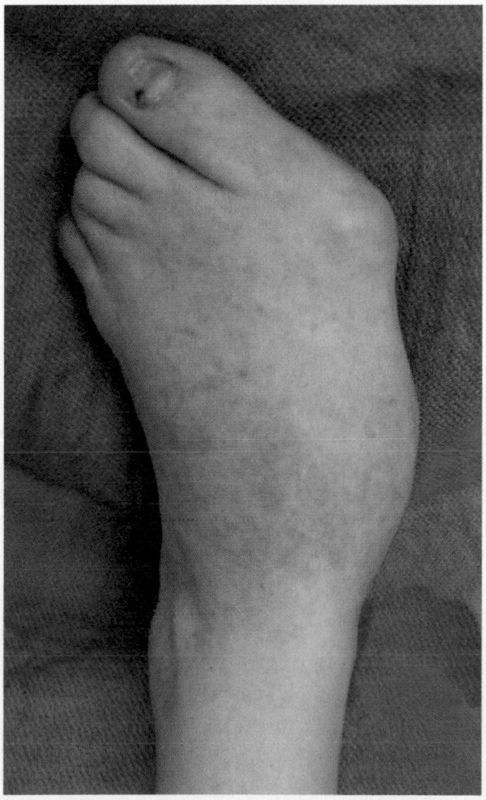

FIG. 64-6 A "Charcot foot" type of diabetic foot deformity.

Foot injuries can be caused by walking barefoot, wearing ill-fitting shoes, sustaining thermal injuries from heat (e.g., hot water bottles, heating pads, baths), or chemical burns from over-the-counter corn treatments. These injuries can lead to loss of TISSUE INTEGRITY and to amputation.

Ulcers result from continued pressure. Plantar ulcers (on the sole, usually the ball) are from standing or walking. Those on the top or sides of the foot usually are from shoes. The increased pressure causes calluses. Ulcers usually form over or around the great toe, under the metatarsal heads, and on the tops of claw toes.

Loss of TISSUE INTEGRITY with broken skin increases the risk for INFECTION. Skin tends to break in areas of pressure. Infection is common in diabetic foot ulcers and, once present, is difficult to treat. Infection also impairs GLUCOSE REGULATION, leading to higher blood glucose levels and reduced immune defenses, which further increases the risk for infection.

Prevention of High-Risk Conditions. Neuropathy of the feet and legs can be delayed by keeping blood glucose levels as near to normal as possible. Poor blood glucose control increases the risk for neuropathy and amputation. Urge smoking cessation to reduce the risk for vascular complications.

The risk for ulcers or amputation increases with duration of diabetes. Other associated factors are male gender; poor glucose control; and cardiovascular, retinal, or kidney complications. Foot-related risks include poor gait and stepping mechanics, peripheral neuropathy, increased pressure (callus, erythema, hemorrhage under a callus, limited joint mobility, foot deformities, or severe nail pathology), peripheral vascular disease, and a history of ulcers or amputation.

Peripheral Neuropathy Management. The feet should be evaluated closely at least annually. Chart 22-9 in Chapter 22 lists self-management activities for prevention of injury from peripheral neuropathy, and Table 64-10 lists foot risk categories.

Complete a full foot assessment as outlined in Chart 64-5. Sensory examination with Semmes-Weinstein monofilaments is a practical measure of the risk for foot ulcers. The nylon monofilament is mounted on a holder standardized to exert a 10-g force. A person who cannot feel the 10-g pressure at any point is at increased risk for ulcers. To perform the examination:

- Provide a quiet and relaxed setting. Ask the patient to close his or her eyes during the test.
- Test the monofilament on the patient's cheek so he or she knows what to expect.
- Test the sites noted in Fig. 64-7.
- Apply the monofilament at a right angle to the skin surface.
- Apply enough force to bend the filament using a smooth, not jabbing, motion (Fig. 64-8).

TABLE 64-10 Foot Risk Categories

RISK CATEGORIES	MANAGEMENT CATEGORIES
Risk Category 0	***Management Category 0***
• Has protective sensation • No evidence of peripheral vascular disease • No evidence of foot deformity	• Comprehensive foot examination once a year • Patient education to include advice on appropriate footwear
Risk Category 1	***Management Category 1***
• Does not have protective sensation • May have evidence of foot deformity	• Evaluation every 3-6 months • Consider referral to a specialist to assess need for specialized treatment and follow-up • Patient education
Risk Category 2	***Management Categories 2 & 3***
• Does not have protective sensation • Evidence of peripheral vascular disease	• Evaluation every 1-3 months • Referral to a specialist • Prescription footwear • Consider vascular consultation for combined follow-up • Patient education
Risk Category 3	
• History of ulcer or amputation	

CHART 64-5 Focused Assessment

The Diabetic Foot

Assess the patient for risk for diabetic foot problems:
- History of previous ulcer
- History of previous amputation
- Assess the foot for abnormal skin and nail conditions:
- Dry, cracked, fissured skin
- Ulcers
- Toenails: thickened, long nails; ingrown nails
- Tinea pedis; onychomycosis (mycotic nails)

Assess the foot for status of circulation:
- Manifestations of claudication
- Presence or absence of dorsalis pedis or posterior tibial pulse
- Prolonged capillary filling time (greater than 25 seconds)
- Presence or absence of hair growth on the top of the foot

Assess the foot for evidence of deformity:
- Calluses, corns
- Prominent metatarsal heads (metatarsal head is easily felt under the skin)
- Toe contractures: clawed toes, hammertoes
- Hallux valgus or bunions
- Charcot foot ("rocker bottom")

Assess the foot for loss of strength:
- Limited ankle joint range of motion
- Limited motion of great toe

Assess the foot for loss of protective sensation:
- Numbness, burning, tingling
- Semmes-Weinstein monofilament testing at 10 points on each foot

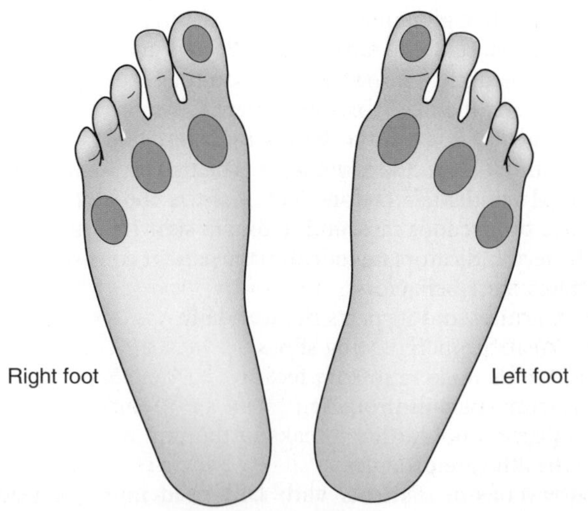

FIG. 64-7 Placement sites of monofilaments for testing of protective sensation.

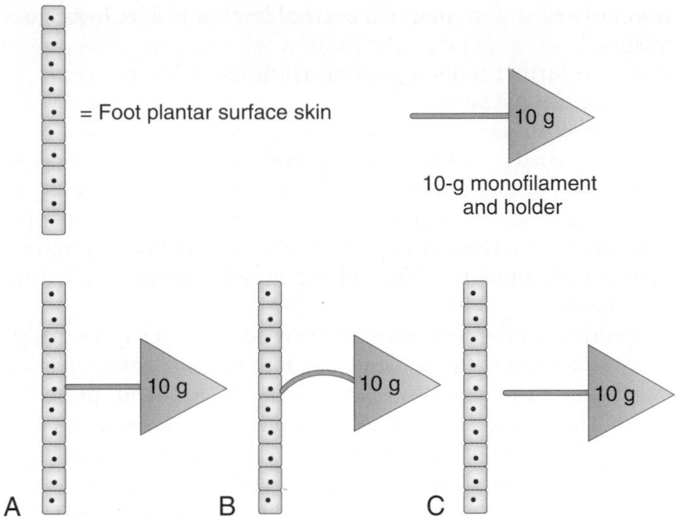

FIG. 64-8 Correct technique for sensation testing with 10-g monofilament. **A,** Apply monofilament to designated areas of the foot sole (intact skin only; see Fig. 64-7). **B,** Apply pressure to the filament either until the patient states he or she can feel the pressure or until the filament bends (see pp. 1326-1327). **C,** Quickly remove the filament without sliding it or touching other areas of the foot. *BUN,* Blood urea nitrogen; Ca^{2+}, calcium; HCO_3^-, bicarbonate; K^+, potassium; Mg^{2+}, magnesium; Na^+, sodium; PO_4, phosphate.

- The approach, contact, and removal of the filament at each site should take 1 to 2 seconds.
- Apply the filament along the perimeter and **not** on an ulcer site, callus, scar, or necrotic tissue. Do not slide the filament across the skin or make repeated contact at the test site.

Randomize the sequence of applying the filament throughout the examination. Have the patient identify where the filament touched rather than asking "Do you feel this?"

Footwear. All patients with any degree of peripheral neuropathy are at risk for loss of TISSUE INTEGRITY and need to wear protective shoes. It is best to be fitted by an experienced shoe fitter, such as a certified podiatrist. The shoe should be ½ to ⅝ inch longer than the longest toe. Heels should be less than 2 inches high. Shoes that are too tight damage tissue. Instruct the patient to change shoes by midday and again in the evening. Socks or stockings need to fit properly and be appropriate for the planned activity. Socks should feel soft and have no thick seams, creases, or holes. They should pad the foot and absorb excess moisture. Teach patients to avoid tight stockings or those that have constricting bands. Patients with toe deformities should buy custom shoes with high, wide toe boxes and extra depth. Those with severely deformed feet, such as Charcot feet, need specially molded shoes. All new shoes need a long break-in period with frequent inspection for irritation or blistering.

Foot Care. Teach patients about preventive foot care and the need for examination of the feet and legs at each visit to a health care provider. Identify patients with high-risk foot conditions. Explain problems caused by loss of protective SENSORY PERCEPTION, the importance of monitoring the feet daily, proper care of the feet (including nail and skin care), and how to select appropriate footwear.

Assess the patient's ability to inspect all areas of the foot and to perform foot care. Teach family members how to inspect and care for the patient's feet if the patient cannot. Chart 64-6 lists foot care instructions for self-management.

CHART 64-6 Patient and Family Education: Preparing for Self-Management

Foot Care Instructions

- Inspect your feet daily, especially the area between the toes.
- Wash your feet daily with lukewarm water and soap. Dry thoroughly.
- Apply moisturizing cream to your feet after bathing. Do not apply to the area between your toes.
- Change into clean cotton socks every day.
- Do not wear the same pair of shoes 2 days in a row, and wear only shoes made of breathable materials, such as leather or cloth.
- Check your shoes for foreign objects (nails, pebbles) before putting them on. Check inside the shoes for cracks or tears in the lining.
- Purchase shoes that have plenty of room for your toes. Buy shoes later in the day, when feet are normally larger. Break in new shoes gradually.
- Wear socks to keep your feet warm.
- Trim your nails straight across with a nail clipper. Smooth the nails with an emery board.
- See your physician or nurse immediately if you have blisters, sores, or infections. Protect the area with a dry, sterile dressing. Do not use adhesive tape to secure dressing to the skin.
- Do not treat blisters, sores, or infections with home remedies.
- Do not smoke.
- Do not step into the bathtub without checking the temperature of the water with your wrist or thermometer. Optimal temperature is 95° F (35° C). Maximum temperature is 110° F (43° C).
- Do not use very hot or cold water. Never use hot water bottles, heating pads, or portable heaters to warm your feet.
- Do not treat corns, blisters, bunions, calluses, or ingrown toenails yourself.
- Do not go barefooted.
- Do not wear sandals with open toes or straps between the toes.
- Do not cross your legs or wear garters or tight stockings that constrict blood flow.
- Do not soak your feet.

Wound Care. The standards of care for diabetic ulcers are a moist wound environment, débridement of necrotic tissue, and elimination of pressure (offloading). Proper wound care and débridement are presented in Chapter 25.

Eliminating pressure on an infected area is essential to wound healing. Teach patients with foot ulcers to not wear a shoe on the affected foot while the ulcer is healing. Those with poor SENSORY PERCEPTION may keep walking on an ulcer because it does not hurt. This results in pressure necrosis that delays healing and increases ulcer size. Pressure is reduced by specialized orthotic devices, custom-molded shoe inserts, or shoe adjustments that redistribute weight.

Offloading redistributes force away from ulcer sites and pressure points to wider areas of the foot. Available products include total-contact casting, half shoes, removable cast walkers, wheelchairs, and crutches. Total-contact casts redistribute pressure over the bottom of the foot. Casting material is molded to the foot and leg to spread pressure along the entire surface of contact, reducing vertical force. The almost complete elimination of motion of the total-contact cast reduces plantar shear forces. The cast is removed 24 to 48 hours after application to inspect the foot and cast fit. The cast is replaced and then removed and reapplied weekly until the ulcer is healed. *Teach the patient that foot ulcers will recur unless weight is permanently redistributed.*

NCLEX EXAMINATION CHALLENGE
Health Promotion and Maintenance

While assessing the client who has had diabetes for 15 years, the nurse finds that he has decreased sensory perception in both feet. What is the nurse's best first action?
A. Document the finding as the only action.
B. Examine the feet for manifestations of injury.
C. Test the sensory perception of the client's hands.
D. Tell the client that he now has peripheral neuropathy.

Managing Pain

Planning: Expected Outcomes. The patient with neuropathic pain is expected to experience relief of PAIN. Indicators include these consistent behaviors:
- Uses preventive measures
- Uses available resources to increase comfort
- Reports that pain is controlled

Interventions. Neuropathic PAIN results from damage anywhere along the nerve. Many patients with diabetes suffer from the painful neuropathy. Manifestations of diabetic neuropathy include:
- Burning
- Muscle cramps
- Piercing, stabbing, or darting pain
- Metatarsalgia (feeling as if you are walking on marbles)
- Hyperalgesia (exaggerated pain response)
- Allodynia (pain in response to normally nonpainful stimuli)
- Tingling, numbness, and loss of proprioception in lower extremities

Maintaining normal blood glucose levels and avoiding extreme fluctuations prevent neuropathy and relieve manifestations. Rapid improvement in blood glucose control may actually trigger acute peripheral neuropathy.

Several pharmacologic agents are used to manage neuropathic PAIN. The anticonvulsants *gabapentin* (Neurontin) and *pregabalin* (Lyrica) and the serotonin-norepinephrine reuptake inhibitor (SNRI) *duloxetine* (Cymbalta) are used in management of neuropathic pain. Tricyclic antidepressants such as amitriptyline hydrochloride (Elavil, Levate 🍁) and nortriptyline (Pamelor) are widely used for pain but are not approved for this purpose and have some significant side effects. Their use is contraindicated for older adults and those with cardiovascular disease.

The burning of neuropathy may respond to capsaicin cream 0.075% (Axsain 🍁, Zostrix-HP). Teach the patient to apply it 4 times daily for several weeks. The pain may worsen for several days after therapy is started before improving.

Unpleasant symptoms are noted with abrupt discontinuation of many of these drugs. A gradual reduction in the dose is recommended to prevent side effects.

Provide support and information on measures to reduce pain. Even having a bed cradle to lift bed clothes off hypersensitive skin can be beneficial. Assist the patient to maintain stable glucose control. *All patients with neuropathy are at increased risk for foot ulcers and require more frequent assessment and education in routine foot management.*

Preventing Injury from Reduced Vision

Planning: Expected Outcomes. The patient with diabetes is expected to be free of injury related to reduced visual SENSORY PERCEPTION and to maintain current level of vision. Indicators include:
- No further reduction of visual fields
- No double vision

Interventions

Blood Glucose Control. Poor blood GLUCOSE REGULATION (control), proteinuria, diastolic hypertension, and long duration of diabetes are risk factors for vision loss among people with diabetes (ADA, 2014a). Surgical intervention for retinal hemorrhage or new retinal blood vessel growth can reduce vision loss.

Besides regular eye examinations to evaluate retinopathy, urge the patient with impaired vision to have an optometrist or ophthalmologist assess the remaining vision and prescribe appropriate vision support. A functional vision assessment, performed by a low-vision technician, rehabilitation teacher, or diabetes educator, determines the patient's use of lighting, contrast, non-optical and low-vision devices, large-print options, and use of central or peripheral vision. Many low-vision reading aids are available as described in Chapter 47. The American Foundation for the Blind maintains a list of services for visually impaired people that is organized by type of service and geographic area. More information is available at (800) 232-5463 and www.afb.org.

Environmental Management. Not all visually impaired patients need special devices. Adjustments in lighting, contrast, color, distance, type size of printed materials, and eye movement often improve visual abilities. Chapter 47 describes general methods of enhancing vision. For the patient with diabetes and low vision, coding objects such as vials of insulin with bright colors or with felt-tipped markers helps identify the correct bottle. Bringing the blood glucose lancet or insulin syringe close to the eye makes it easier to see.

Prefilled insulin pens are not approved for use by people with severe visual impairment unless they are assisted by a person with good vision who is trained to use the pen correctly. Adaptive devices can help the patient self-administer insulin independently. Some syringes may have a magnifier attached to the syringe. Other devices include preset dose gauges (which measure the space between the end of the syringe barrel and the plunger) to help the patient draw up the correct amount of insulin by feeling this distance. The blind patient can accurately measure insulin by using products such as the Count-A-Dose Insulin Measuring Device. This device is designed to be used with the BD Lo-Dose syringe. It holds two insulin vials and has a slot to direct the syringe needle into the vials' rubber stoppers. The patient draws insulin into the syringe by turning a thumbwheel, which clicks for each unit (clicks can be both heard and felt). (See the *Consumer Guide* published yearly in the January edition of *Diabetes Forecast* [forecast.diabetes.org] for information to help patients determine which adaptive devices best meet their needs.) When teaching the patient to use an adaptive device, stress:
- Differentiating between bottles of fast-acting and slower-acting insulin by wrapping a rubber band around the fast-acting insulin bottle
- Ensuring proper placement of the device on the syringe
- Holding the insulin bottle upright when measuring insulin
- Avoiding air bubbles in the syringe by pulling a small amount of insulin into the syringe, moving the plunger in and out 3 times, and measuring insulin on the fourth draw

Design a system to determine how many doses can be drawn from a bottle so the patient does not inject air from an empty bottle instead of insulin.

Specialized adaptive equipment also is available to assist with blood glucose monitoring techniques. Assist the patient to select a blood glucose monitoring device best suited to his or her level of visual impairment. Some monitors have large display screens and easy-to-use features. Fully audio systems are available for patients who are visually impaired. The monitor uses no coding, has automatic turn-on with test strip insertion, and has a button for repeating the last message. Assess the ability of the patient to obtain an adequate blood sample and to apply it to the test strip. Commercially made blood drop guides can assist with this task.

CLINICAL JUDGMENT CHALLENGE

Patient-Centered Care QSEN

During a clinic visit, you are reviewing the records of a 39-year-old patient who was diagnosed 5 years ago with type 2 diabetes. You discover that, although he has always been extremely near-sighted, he has not seen an ophthalmologist for 4 years. He has gained 12 lbs since his last visit a year ago. His laboratory values show a fasting blood glucose level of 96 mg/dL, an A1C of 8.2%, a total cholesterol of 322 mg/dL, and an LDL of 190 mg/dL. When you ask him about ophthalmology follow-up and point out his laboratory values, he replies that because he is taking prescribed antidiabetic medication, he believes that he won't have all the diabetes complications that his father had. He further tells you that he did have his eyes checked by an optometrist to make sure his prescription was accurate but that because he is younger than 40 years, he does not need intraocular pressure measurements.

1. How should you interpret his laboratory values in terms of his personal glucose regulation?
2. Should you address his weight gain? Why or why not?
3. Is he correct in thinking that an ophthalmologist visit is not necessary at this time? Explain your response.
4. Is he correct in believing that taking antidiabetic medication will prevent complications of diabetes? Explain your response.
5. How do you propose to assist this patient in managing his diabetes?

Reducing the Risk for Kidney Disease

Planning: Expected Outcomes. The patient with diabetes is expected to maintain a normal urine elimination pattern. Indicators include:

- Urine protein levels within normal limits
- 24-hour intake and output balance
- Blood urea nitrogen (BUN) and serum creatinine within the normal ranges
- Serum electrolytes within the normal ranges

Interventions

Prevention. Diabetic kidney disease is more likely to develop in patients with poor blood glucose control. Progression to end-stage kidney disease (ESKD) can be delayed or prevented by normalizing blood pressure, correcting hyperlipidemia, and restricting dietary protein. Control of hypertension is essential for the reduction of diabetic nephropathy (ADA, 2014b). Both systolic and diastolic hypertension greatly accelerate the progression of diabetic kidney disease.

Stress the need for evaluation of kidney function according to the ADA Standards of Care. Serum creatinine should be measured at least annually for an estimation of GFR in all patients with diabetes (ADA, 2013). An annual test for microalbuminuria is performed for patients who have had type 1 DM for over 5 years and in all those with type 2 DM starting at diagnosis and during pregnancy.

Persistent albuminuria in the range of 30 to 299 mg/24 hr (formerly called *microalbuminuria*) is the earliest stage of nephropathy in type 1 DM and a marker for the development of nephropathy in type 2 DM. Patients with albumin levels greater than 300 mg/24 hr (formerly called *macroalbuminuria*) are likely to progress to end-stage kidney disease (ESKD) (ADA, 2014b). Screening for increased urinary albumin excretion is performed by measurement of the albumin-creatinine ratio in a spot collection.

Aggressive control of blood glucose and hypertension in patients without microalbuminuria can avoid nephropathy. Once microalbuminuria develops, management focuses on controlling blood pressure and blood glucose, restricting dietary protein, avoiding nephrotoxic agents, promptly treating urinary tract infections, and preventing dehydration.

Control of blood pressure and blood glucose levels requires the patient's participation and effort. Prescribed drugs must be taken according to schedules, and dietary restrictions must be maintained. Teach patients about the roles of blood pressure and blood glucose levels in kidney disease. Help them maintain normal blood glucose levels and blood pressure levels below 140/80 mm Hg. Stress the need for yearly screening for microalbuminuria.

Smoking cessation is important in halting the progression of diabetic kidney disease for patients with type 1 and type 2 diabetes. Teach the patient about the risks of smoking, and refer him or her to appropriate resources for assistance in smoking cessation.

Any urinary tract INFECTION (UTI) can lead to kidney infection and further reduce kidney function. Explain the manifestations of UTI. Urge the patient to take antibiotics exactly as prescribed, completing the entire course of treatment. Reinforce the need for follow-up urine cultures to reduce the risk for kidney damage. Avoid indwelling urinary catheters when possible.

Drugs can affect kidney function either through toxic effects on the kidney or by an acute but reversible reduction in function. The most common nephrotoxic drugs are antifungal agents and aminoglycoside antibiotics. Outside the hospital, the leading nephrotoxic agents are NSAIDs such as ibuprofen (Advil) or naproxen (Aleve), when used long-term. To prevent accidental ingestion of nephrotoxic drugs, teach the patient to check with a health care provider before taking over-the-counter drugs or herbal remedies.

Radiocontrast dyes can also affect kidney function, especially in patients with preexisting kidney problems. Monitor IV hydration before and after contrast is used to prevent contrast-induced nephropathy in patients with diabetes.

Drug Therapy. Use of angiotensin-converting enzyme (ACE) inhibitors (ACEIs) or angiotensin receptor blockers (ARBs) is recommended for all patients with microalbuminuria or advanced stages of nephropathy (ADA, 2013). ACE inhibitors reduce the level of albuminuria and the rate of progression of kidney disease, although they do not appear to prevent microalbuminuria. Monitor serum potassium levels for development of hyperkalemia.

Nutrition Therapy. Patients with nephropathy should restrict protein intake to 0.8 g/kg of body weight per day. Once the glomerular filtration rate (GFR) starts falling, further reducing protein may slow the decline in kidney function. Because lifelong dietary restrictions are difficult, provide ongoing teaching to encourage adherence.

Fluid and Electrolyte Management. Fluid and electrolyte management can prevent more loss of kidney function. Avoiding dehydration is important for kidney PERFUSION and function. The most common cause of dehydration in patients with diabetes is overuse of diuretics. Teach patients to report edema or symptoms of orthostatic hypotension, and provide ongoing education to promote nutrition therapy.

Dialysis for patients with DM and kidney failure is the same as for patients without diabetes (see Chapter 68). The dosage of insulin needs to be adjusted when dialysis starts.

Preventing Hypoglycemia. Hypoglycemia (low blood glucose level) induces specific manifestations and resolves when blood glucose concentration is raised. Once blood glucose levels fall below 70 mg/dL (3.88 mmol/L), a sequence of events begins with release of counterregulatory hormones, stimulation of the autonomic nervous system, and production of *neurogenic* and *neuroglycopenic* manifestations. Peripheral autonomic manifestations, including sweating, irritability, tremors, anxiety, tachycardia, and hunger, serve as an early warning system and occur before the manifestations of confusion, paralysis, seizure, and coma occur from brain glucose deprivation. *Neuroglycopenic symptoms* occur when brain glucose *gradually declines* to a low level. *Neurogenic symptoms* result from autonomic nervous activity triggered by a *rapid decline* in blood glucose (Table 64-11).

Central nervous system (CNS) function depends on a continuous supply of glucose in the blood. The brain cannot make glucose and stores only a few minutes' supply as glycogen. This needed supply is not maintained when the blood glucose level falls below critical levels.

The first defense against falling blood glucose levels in the nondiabetic person is decreased insulin secretion, decreased glucose use, and increased glucose production. Normally, insulin secretion decreases when blood glucose levels drop to about 83 mg/dL (4.5 mmol/L). Counterregulatory hormones are activated at about 67 mg/dL (3.7 mmol/L), a level well above the threshold for manifestations of hypoglycemia. The main counterregulatory hormone is glucagon. Epinephrine also becomes important in patients with DM who are deficient in glucagon. Both glucagon and epinephrine raise blood glucose levels by stimulating liver glycogen breakdown and conversion of protein to glucose. Epinephrine also limits insulin secretion.

Type 1 DM disrupts the body's response to hypoglycemia, usually within 1 to 5 years of diagnosis. Regulation of circulating insulin levels is lost because insulin comes from an injection rather than from the pancreas. As blood glucose levels fall, insulin levels do not decrease. Over time, the pancreas loses its ability to secrete glucagon in response to hypoglycemia. After a few more years of type 1 DM, the response of epinephrine to falling blood glucose levels does not occur until the blood glucose level is very low. These problems greatly increase the risk for severe hypoglycemia.

A second problem with long-standing type 1 DM is *hypoglycemic unawareness,* in which patients no longer have the warning manifestations of impending hypoglycemia that should prompt them to take preventive action (Mompoint-Williams et al., 2012). This problem occurs most often in patients who have had type 1 DM for 30 years or longer.

The blood glucose level at which manifestations of hypoglycemia occur varies among patients. Thus clinical criteria used to categorize hypoglycemia are based on manifestation severity rather than blood glucose levels. In mild hypoglycemia, the patient remains alert and able to self-manage symptoms. In severe hypoglycemia, neurologic function is so impaired that he or she needs another person's help to increase blood glucose levels.

Planning: Expected Outcomes. The patient with DM is expected to have decreased episodes of hypoglycemia and remain oriented to person, place, and time, as indicated by a Glasgow Coma Scale score above 7.

Interventions. A blood glucose level below 70 mg/dL (3.9 mmol/L) alerts you to assess for manifestations of hypoglycemia (Table 64-11; see also Table 64-12).

Blood Glucose Management. Monitor blood glucose levels before giving antidiabetic drugs, before meals, before bedtime, and when the patient is symptomatic. All patients who take insulin, those taking long-acting insulin secretagogues (glyburide [glibenclamide]), and those taking metformin in combination with glyburide (Glucovance) are at risk for hypoglycemia.

TABLE 64-11 Manifestations of Hypoglycemia

Neuroglycopenic Manifestations	Neurogenic Manifestations
• Weakness	• Adrenergic:
• Fatigue	• Shaky/tremulous
• Difficulty thinking	• Heart pounding
• Confusion	• Nervous/anxious
• Behavior changes	• Cholinergic:
• Emotional instability	• Sweaty
• Seizures	• Hungry
• Loss of consciousness	• Tingling
• Brain damage	
• Death	

TABLE 64-12 Differentiation of Hypoglycemia and Hyperglycemia

FEATURE	HYPOGLYCEMIA	HYPERGLYCEMIA
Skin	Cool, clammy	Warm, moist
Dehydration	Absent	Present
Respirations	No particular or consistent change	Rapid, deep*; Kussmaul type; acetone odor ("fruity" odor) to breath
Mental status	Anxious, nervous,* irritable, mental confusion,* seizures, coma	Varies from alert to stuporous, obtunded, or frank coma
Manifestations	Weakness,* double vision, blurred vision, hunger, tachycardia, palpitations	None specific for DKA Acidosis; hypercapnia; abdominal cramps, nausea and vomiting Dehydration: decreased neck vein filling, orthostatic hypotension, tachycardia, poor skin turgor
Glucose	<70 mg/dL (3.9 mmol/L)	>250 mg/dL (13.8 mmol/L)
Ketones	Negative	Positive

DKA, Diabetic ketoacidosis.
*Classic symptoms.

This risk is increased if they are older, have liver or kidney impairment, or are taking drugs that enhance the effects of antidiabetic drugs. Proper patient selection, drug dosage, and instructions are important factors in avoiding severe hypoglycemia. Hypoglycemia may be difficult to recognize in those who take beta-blocking drugs. Manifestations are less intense and less obvious. Manifestations of hypoglycemia in older patients may be mistaken for other conditions.

The most common causes of hypoglycemia are:

- Too much insulin compared with food intake and physical activity
- Insulin injected at the wrong time relative to food intake and physical activity
- The wrong type of insulin injected at the wrong time
- Decreased food intake resulting from missed or delayed meals
- Delayed gastric emptying from gastroparesis
- Decrease liver glucose production after alcohol ingestion
- Increased insulin sensitivity as a result of regular exercise and weight loss
- Decreased insulin clearance from progressive kidney failure

Nutrition Therapy. When the patient is hypoglycemic, start carbohydrate replacement per physician prescription or standing protocols—usually ingestion of 15 to 20 g of glucose. If the patient can swallow, give a liquid form of carbohydrate, although any carbohydrate source can be used. Ingestion of 15 to 20 g of glucose is the preferred management for blood glucose levels less than 70 mg/dL (3.9 mmol/L), repeated in about 15 minutes if manifestations have not improved or if blood glucose levels are still less than 70. The amount of carbohydrate should be increased to 30 g for glucose levels less than 50 mg/dL (2.8 mmol/L).

Ten grams (g) of oral glucose raises blood glucose levels by about 40 mg/dL over 30 minutes, and 20 g of oral glucose raises blood glucose levels by about 60 mg/dL over 45 minutes. Specific recommendations are listed in Chart 64-7.

The blood glucose level determines the form and amount of glucose used. The response should be apparent in 10 to 20 minutes; however, test blood glucose again in about 60 minutes because additional management may be needed. Fluid is absorbed much more quickly from the GI tract than are solids. Concentrated sweet fluids, such as juice with sugar added or a soft drink, may slow absorption.

Management of hypoglycemia requires ingestion of glucose or glucose-containing foods. The blood glucose response correlates better with the glucose content rather than the carbohydrate content of the food. Adding protein to carbohydrate does NOT improve blood glucose response and does NOT prevent subsequent hypoglycemia. Adding fat may retard and then prolong the blood glucose response, resulting in post-treatment hyperglycemia. Commercially available products provide predictable glucose absorption.

Drug Therapy. Glucagon given subcutaneously or IM and 50% dextrose given IV are used for patients who cannot swallow. Glucagon is the main counterregulatory hormone to insulin and is used as first-line therapy for severe hypoglycemia in DM. It converts liver glycogen to glucose but is not effective in severely starved patients. Take care to prevent aspiration in patients receiving glucagon, because it often causes vomiting. Give 50% dextrose carefully to avoid extravasation because it is hyperosmolar and can damage tissue. The effects of glucagon and dextrose are temporary. After the patient responds and is no longer nauseated, give a simple sugar followed by a small snack or meal. IV glucose is used to maintain mild hyperglycemia. Diazoxide (Proglycem) or octreotide (Sandostatin) may be required to treat sulfonylurea-induced hypoglycemia. Evaluate response by monitoring blood glucose levels for several hours because manifestations may persist. A target blood glucose level is 70 to 110 mg/dL (3.9 to 6.2 mmol/L).

CHART 64-7 Patient and Family Education: Preparing for Self-Management

Management of Hypoglycemia at Home

For *mild* hypoglycemia (hungry, irritable, shaky, weak, headache, fully conscious; blood glucose usually less than 60 mg/dL [3.4 mmol/L]):

- Treat the symptoms of hypoglycemia with 10 to 15 g of carbohydrate. You may use one of these:
  - Glucose tablets or glucose gel (dosage is printed on the package)
  - ½ cup of fruit juice
  - ½ cup of regular (nondiet) soft drink
  - 8 ounces of skim milk
  - 6 to 10 hard candies
  - 4 cubes of sugar
  - 4 teaspoons of sugar
  - 6 saltines
  - 3 graham crackers
  - 1 tablespoon of honey or syrup
- Re-test blood glucose in 15 minutes.
- Repeat this treatment if symptoms do not resolve.
- Eat a small snack of carbohydrate and protein if your next meal is more than an hour away.

For *moderate* hypoglycemia (cold, clammy skin; pale; rapid pulse; rapid, shallow respirations; marked change in mood; drowsiness; blood glucose usually less than 40 mg/dL [2.2 mmol/L]):

- Treat the symptoms of hypoglycemia with 15 to 30 g of rapidly absorbed carbohydrate.
- Take additional food, such as low-fat milk or cheese, after 10 to 15 minutes.

For *severe* hypoglycemia (unable to swallow; unconsciousness or convulsions; blood glucose usually less than 20 mg/dL [1.0 mmol/L]):

- Treatment administered by family members:
  - Administer 1 mg of glucagon as intramuscular or subcutaneous injection.
  - Administer a second dose in 10 minutes if the person remains unconscious.
  - Notify a primary care provider immediately, and follow instructions.
  - If still unconscious, transport the person to the emergency department.
  - Give a small meal when the person wakes up and is no longer nauseated.

! NURSING SAFETY PRIORITY QSEN

Critical Rescue

For the patient with *severe* hypoglycemia (unable to swallow, unconscious or convulsing, blood glucose usually less than 20 mg/dL [1.0 mmol/L]), treat by:

1. Giving glucagon 1 mg subcutaneously or IM
2. Repeating the dose in 10 minutes if the patient remains unconscious
3. Notifying the primary health care provider immediately, and following instructions

Prevention Strategies. Teach the patient how to prevent hypoglycemia by avoiding its four common causes: (1) excess insulin, (2) deficient intake or absorption of food, (3) exercise, and (4) alcohol intake.

Insulin excess from variable absorption of insulin can cause hypoglycemia even when insulin is injected correctly. Increased insulin sensitivity can occur with weight loss, exercise programs, and resolution of an INFECTION. Differences in insulin formulation can result in hypoglycemia. Teach the patient to not change insulin brands without medical supervision.

Deficient food intake from inadequate or incorrectly timed meals can result in hypoglycemia. Changes in gastric absorption may cause hypoglycemia in patients with delayed gastric emptying, which is more severe with solid meals, and is made worse by illness or poor glucose control. Teach the patient the importance of regularity in timing and quantity of food eaten.

Exercise often causes blood glucose levels to fall in a patient with type 1 DM. Prolonged exercise increases cellular glucose uptake for several hours after exercise. Teach the patient about blood glucose monitoring and carbohydrate consumption before and during exercise.

Alcohol inhibits liver glucose production and leads to hypoglycemia. It interferes with the counterregulatory response to hypoglycemia and impairs glycogen breakdown, making exercise-induced hypoglycemia more severe. Teach the patient to ingest alcohol only with or shortly *after* eating a meal with enough carbohydrate to prevent hypoglycemia. Warn patients to avoid excess alcohol at bedtime to prevent nighttime hypoglycemia.

Patient and Family Education. The cause of hypoglycemia may be subtle. At the onset of menses, a fall in hormone levels decreases insulin needs and contributes to hypoglycemia. When patients switch to a new bottle of insulin, hypoglycemia may occur because the fresh insulin has greater potency. Some patients have hypoglycemia when they change injection sites. Beta-blocking drugs mask manifestations that are warning signs and thus predispose patients to severe hypoglycemia. Some episodes of hypoglycemia occur without an obvious cause.

Many patients who have been treated in the emergency department for hypoglycemia do not receive adequate prevention instructions and are at continuing risk. Help each patient develop a personal treatment plan for hypoglycemia. The exact glucose rise from a set amount of carbohydrate varies; however, using the estimate that each 5 g of carbohydrate raises blood glucose about 20 mg/dL is a good starting plan. For example, the patient may be directed to take:

- 20 to 30 g of carbohydrate if the blood glucose level is 50 mg/dL (2.8 mmol/L) or less
- 10 to 15 g of carbohydrate if the blood glucose level is 51 to 70 mg/dL (2.9 to 3.9 mmol/L)

Use blood glucose monitoring results to revise or reinforce this plan.

Encourage the patient to wear a medical alert bracelet, and help him or her obtain one. This bracelet is helpful if the patient becomes hypoglycemic and is unable to provide self-care.

Teach the patient and family about the manifestations of hypoglycemia. Emphasize that delaying a meal for more than 30 minutes raises the risk for hypoglycemia when using some insulin regimens. Instruct him or her to keep a carbohydrate source nearby at all times. Teach the patient and family how to administer glucagon.

Hypoglycemia is a major risk for patients receiving intensive insulin protocols who engage in exercise programs. Explain that nightmares or headaches on days after prolonged or severe exercise may indicate hypoglycemia.

Establishing Treatment Plans. Blood glucose monitoring directs hypoglycemia management. Treatment continues until blood glucose levels reach and stay in the target range. Once blood glucose control is regained, the patient should identify the specific cause of the episode and take specific measures to prevent recurrence.

CONSIDERATIONS FOR OLDER ADULTS

Patient-Centered Care QSEN

Patients in the older age-groups are especially vulnerable to hypoglycemia. Age-related declines in kidney function and liver enzyme activity may interfere with the metabolism of sulfonylureas and insulin, thereby potentiating their hypoglycemic effects. Older patients with diabetes have impaired epinephrine release and a diminished glucagon response to falling blood glucose levels. They often have a reduced awareness of hypoglycemic manifestations. Confusion and any impairment in psychomotor performance when blood sugars are low prevent the older adult from taking appropriate steps to return the blood sugar to normal.

Instruct the older patient and family to check blood glucose values when symptoms such as unsteadiness, light-headedness, poor concentration, trembling, or sweating occur. Assess eating patterns to make sure sufficient foods are eaten at appropriate times. Encourage a patient with a poor appetite to eat a small snack at bedtime to prevent hypoglycemia during the night.

The highest rates of severe and fatal episodes of hypoglycemia are associated with the use of glyburide in patients older than 70 years. Drug regimens that require that meals be eaten on time increase the potential for hypoglycemic reactions. Complex regimens that require multiple decision points should be simplified, especially for patients with decreased functional status (Seaquist et al., 2013).

CLINICAL JUDGMENT CHALLENGE

Safety; Quality Improvement; Teamwork and Collaboration QSEN

The patient is a 60-year-old-woman who is 1 day postoperative after a total knee replacement. She has type 2 diabetes and just recently was switched from oral antidiabetic drugs to an insulin regimen. She let her nurse know that her on-demand lunch has been ordered. The nurse tests her blood and gives her the prescribed short-acting insulin dose. An hour later the physical therapist finds her pale, confused, and clammy. Her lunch tray is on her table and appears untouched.

1. Is her condition consistent with hyperglycemia or hypoglycemia? Explain your choice.
2. What is your first action? Provide a rationale.
3. What is the most likely cause leading to this problem?
4. What could be done on this nursing care unit to prevent such an incident from happening again?

Preventing Diabetic Ketoacidosis. Diabetic ketoacidosis (DKA) is characterized by uncontrolled hyperglycemia, metabolic acidosis, and increased production of ketones. This condition results from the combination of insulin deficiency and an increase in hormone release that leads to increased liver and kidney glucose production and decreased glucose use in peripheral tissues (Fig. 64-9). Laboratory diagnosis of DKA is shown in Table 64-13. All of these changes increase ketoacid production with resultant ketonemia and metabolic acidosis.

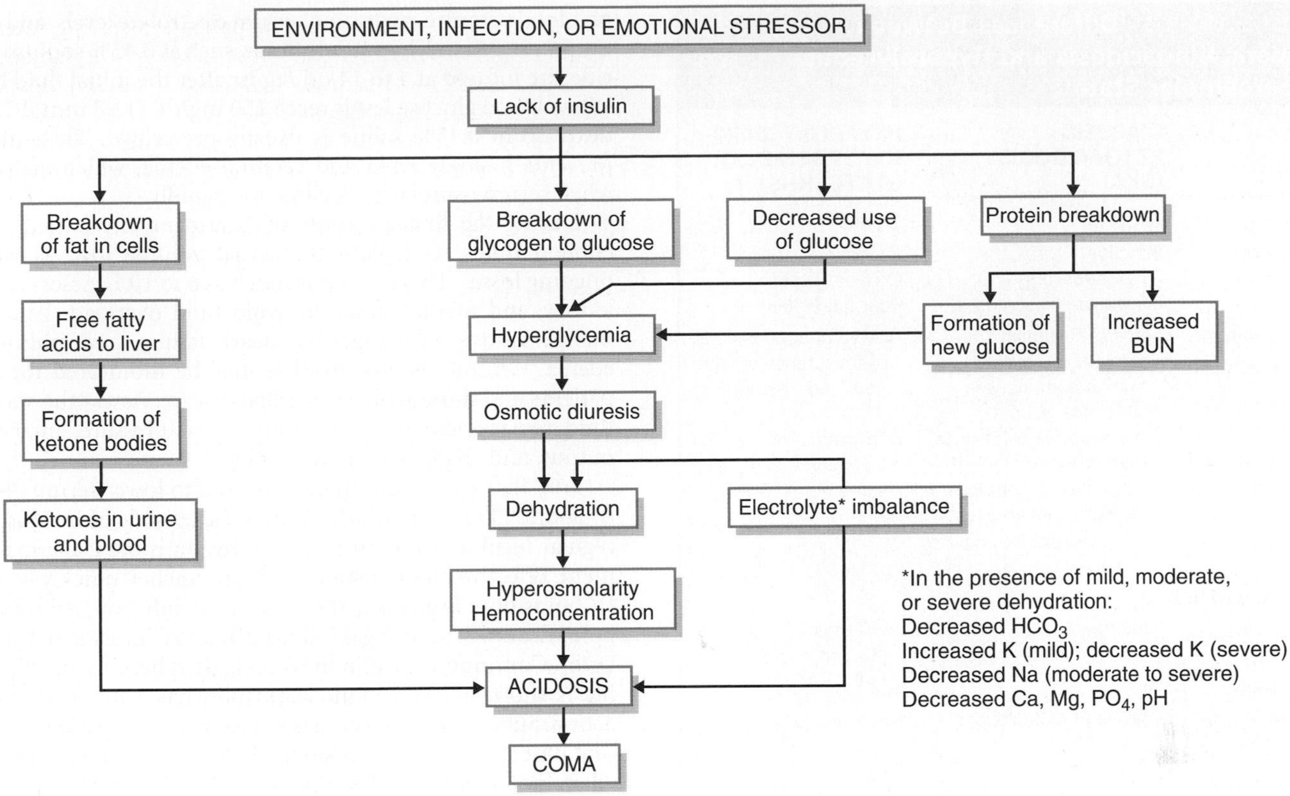

FIG. 64-9 The pathophysiologic mechanism of diabetic ketoacidosis (DKA).

DKA occurs most often in patients with type 1 DM but also can occur in those with type 2 DM who are under severe stress (e.g., trauma, surgery, infection). Some people with type 2 diabetes have a syndrome known as *ketosis-prone diabetes* or *KPD* (Palmer & Jessup, 2012). This problem is not yet fully characterized, and it is important to remember that regardless of whether the patient with DKA has type 1 or type 2 diabetes, management of the acute episode is the same. The most common precipitating factor for DKA is INFECTION. *Death occurs in up to 10% of these cases even with appropriate treatment.*

Hyperglycemia leads to osmotic diuresis with dehydration and electrolyte loss. Classic manifestations of DKA include polyuria, polydipsia, polyphagia, vomiting, abdominal pain, dehydration, weakness, confusion, shock, and coma. Mental status can vary from total alertness to profound coma. As ketone levels rise, the pH of the blood decreases and acidosis occurs. **Kussmaul respirations** (very deep and rapid respirations) cause respiratory alkalosis in an attempt to correct metabolic acidosis by exhaling carbon dioxide. Initial serum sodium levels may be low or normal. Initial potassium levels depend on how long DKA existed before treatment. After therapy starts, serum potassium levels drop quickly.

Planning: Expected Outcomes. The patient is expected to have few episodes of hyperglycemia and avoid diabetic ketoacidosis. Indicators include that the patient consistently demonstrates these behaviors:

- Maintains blood glucose levels within the prescribed target range
- Adjusts insulin doses to match eating patterns and blood glucose levels during illness
- Maintains easily digestible liquid diet containing carbohydrate and salt when nauseated
- Describes correct procedure for urine ketone testing
- Describes when to seek help from health care professional

Interventions

Blood Glucose Management. Monitor for manifestations of DKA (see Table 64-13 and Fig. 64-9). Document and use these findings to determine therapy effectiveness. *First assess the airway, level of consciousness, hydration status, electrolytes, and blood glucose level.* Check the patient's blood pressure, pulse, and respirations every 15 minutes until stable. Record urine output, temperature, and mental status every hour. When a central venous catheter is present, assess central venous pressure every 30 minutes or as prescribed. After treatment starts and these values are stable, monitor and record vital signs every 4 hours. Use blood glucose values to assess therapy and determine when to switch from saline to dextrose-containing solutions.

Fluid and Electrolyte Management. *Closely assess the patient's fluid status.* Assess for acute weight loss, thirst, decreased skin turgor, dry mucous membranes, and oliguria with a high specific gravity. Also assess for weak and rapid pulse, flattened neck veins, increased temperature, decreased central venous pressure, muscle weakness, postural hypotension, and cool, clammy, and pale skin to determine if the patient is at risk for dehydration and shock.

Manifestations of fluid volume excess include acute weight gain, full and bounding pulses, distended neck veins, pulmonary crackles, peripheral edema, and elevated central venous pressure. Acute pulmonary edema can develop quickly. Hypertension is common, especially in patients with kidney failure.

Expected manifestations of fluid balance are altered by age-related changes, by other medical conditions, and by drugs. Age-related skin changes, such as loss of elasticity and dryness, make

TABLE 64-13 Differences Between Diabetic Ketoacidosis and Hyperglycemic-Hyperosmolar State

	DIABETIC KETOACIDOSIS (DKA)	HYPERGLYCEMIC-HYPEROSMOLAR STATE (HHS)
Onset	Sudden	Gradual
Precipitating factors	Infection Other stressors Inadequate insulin dose	Infection Other stressors Poor fluid intake
Manifestations	Ketosis: Kussmaul respiration, "rotting fruit" breath, nausea, abdominal pain Dehydration or electrolyte loss: polyuria, polydipsia, weight loss, dry skin, sunken eyes, soft eyeballs, lethargy, coma	Altered central nervous system function with neurologic symptoms Dehydration or electrolyte loss: same as for DKA
Laboratory Findings		
Serum glucose	>300 mg/dL (16.7 mmol/L)	>600 mg/dL (33.3 mmol/L)
Osmolarity	Variable	>320 mOsm/L
Serum ketones	Positive at 1:2 dilutions	Negative
Serum pH	<7.35	>7.4
Serum HCO_3^-	<15 mEq/L	>20 mEq/L
Serum Na^+	Low, normal, or high	Normal or low
BUN	>30 mg/dL; elevated because of dehydration	Elevated
Creatinine	>1.5 mg/dL; elevated because of dehydration	Elevated
Urine ketones	Positive	Negative

BUN, Blood urea nitrogen; *HCO_3^-*, bicarbonate; *Na^+*, sodium.

skin turgor an unreliable indicator of dehydration. With severe hyperglycemia, the kidneys are less able to respond to changes in pH or fluid and electrolyte balance, to concentrate urine, or to regulate blood osmolarity. The risk for kidney failure rises with age, and acidosis occurs more quickly. Cardiovascular disease can cause fluid retention. In patients with poor kidney function and excess fluid volume, assess for edema around the eyes and in the limbs, increasing blood pressure, jugular venous distention, and orthostatic hypotension. Edema occurs with excess interstitial fluid and often is not apparent until interstitial volume increases by 2 to 3 L. Jugular venous pressure increases with volume overload. In severe volume depletion, the jugular venous pulsation may not be visible even with the patient lying flat.

Tachycardia is a compensatory mechanism to increase cardiac output. Older adults may not exhibit tachycardia if they are taking beta blockers or calcium channel blockers. Dry mucous membranes may be caused by anticholinergic drugs, and postural hypotension may occur with antihypertensive therapy.

The first outcome of fluid therapy is to restore volume and maintain PERFUSION to the brain, heart, and kidneys. Typically, initial infusion rates of 0.9% sodium chloride are 15 to 20 mL/kg/hr during the first hour.

The second outcome of replacing total body fluid losses is achieved more slowly. The choice for fluid replacement depends on blood pressure, hydration, serum electrolyte levels, and urine output. In general, hypotonic fluids, such as 0.45% sodium chloride, are infused at 4 to 14 mL/kg/hr after the initial fluid bolus. When blood glucose levels reach 250 mg/dL (13.8 mmol/L), 5% dextrose in 0.45% saline is usually prescribed. This solution prevents hypoglycemia and cerebral edema, which can occur when serum osmolarity declines too rapidly.

During the first 24 hours of treatment, the patient needs enough fluids to replace the actual volume lost, as well as ongoing losses. This may be as much as 6 to 10 L. Assess cardiac, kidney, and mental status to avoid fluid overload. Watch for manifestations of congestive heart failure and pulmonary edema. Central venous pressure may be monitored for older patients and those with myocardial disease. Assess the status of fluid replacement by monitoring blood pressure, intake and output, and changes in daily weight.

Drug Therapy. Insulin therapy is used to lower serum glucose by about 50 to 75 mg/dL/hr. Unless the episode of DKA is mild, regular insulin by continuous IV infusion is the usual management. Effective blood insulin levels are reached quickly when an IV bolus dose is given at the start of the infusion. An initial IV bolus dose of 0.1 unit/kg is followed by an IV infusion of 0.1 unit/kg/hr. Continuous insulin infusion is used because insulin half-life is short and subcutaneous insulin has a delayed onset of action. Subcutaneous insulin is started when the patient can take oral fluids and ketosis has stopped. DKA is considered resolved when blood glucose is less than 200 mg/mL along with a serum bicarbonate level higher than 18 mEq/L, venous pH higher than 7.3, and a calculated ion gap less than 12 mEq/L. Assess therapy effectiveness by hourly blood glucose measurements.

Acidosis Management. The key feature of DKA is elevation in blood ketone concentration (measured as serum β-hydroxybutyrate). Accumulation of ketoacids results in an increased anion gap metabolic acidosis. A normal anion gap is between 7 and 9 mEq/L; an anion gap greater than 10 to12 mEq/L indicates metabolic acidosis.

Mild to moderate hyperkalemia is common in patients with hyperglycemia. Insulin therapy, correction of acidosis, and volume expansion decrease serum potassium concentration. To prevent hypokalemia, potassium replacement is initiated after serum levels fall below the upper limit of normal (5.0 mEq/L). *Assess for manifestations of hypokalemia, including fatigue, malaise, confusion, muscle weakness, shallow respirations, abdominal distention or paralytic ileus, hypotension, and weak pulse.* An ECG shows conduction changes related to potassium. Hypokalemia is a common cause of death in the treatment of DKA.

! NURSING SAFETY PRIORITY QSEN

Critical Rescue

Before giving IV potassium-containing solutions, make sure the urine output is at least 30 mL/hr.

Bicarbonate is used only for severe acidosis. Sodium bicarbonate, given by slow IV infusion over several hours, is indicated when the arterial pH is 7.0 or less or the serum bicarbonate level is less than 5 mEq/L (5 mmol/L).

Patient and Family Education. Exploring the factors leading to DKA helps in planning specific educational efforts. Teach the patient and family to check blood glucose levels every 4 to 6 hours as long as manifestations such as anorexia, nausea, and vomiting are present and as long as glucose levels exceed 250 mg/dL (13.8 mmol/L). Teach them to check urine ketone levels when blood glucose levels exceed 300 mg/dL (16.7 mmol/L).

Teach the patient to prevent dehydration by maintaining food and fluid intake. Unless another health problem is present that requires fluid restriction, suggest that he or she drink at least 2 L of fluid daily and increase this amount when INFECTION is present. When nausea is present, instruct the patient to take liquids containing both glucose and electrolytes (e.g., soda pop, diluted fruit juice, and sports drinks [Gatorade]). Small amounts of fluid may be tolerated even when vomiting is present. When the blood glucose level is normal or elevated, the patient should take 8 to 12 ounces (240 to 360 mL) of calorie-free and caffeine-free liquids every hour while awake to prevent dehydration.

Liquids containing carbohydrate can be taken if the diabetic patient cannot eat solid food. Ingesting at least 150 g of carbohydrate daily reduces the risk for starvation ketosis. After consulting a primary care provider, urge the patient to take additional rapid-acting (lispro) or short-acting (regular) insulin based on blood glucose levels.

Instruct the patient and family to consult the health care provider when these problems occur:

- Blood glucose exceeds 250 mg/dL (13.8 mmol/L).
- Ketonuria lasts for more than 24 hours.
- The patient cannot take food or fluids.
- Illness lasts more than 1 to 2 days.

Also instruct them to detect hyperglycemia by monitoring blood glucose whenever the patient is ill. Illness can result in dehydration with DKA, hyperglycemic-hyperosmolar state, or both. The sooner the patient seeks treatment, the less severe the metabolic alteration. He or she should not omit insulin therapy during illness. Chart 64-8 lists guidelines for the ill patient.

CLINICAL JUDGMENT CHALLENGE

Prioritization, Delegation, and Supervision

The patient, a 21-year-old college student, was brought to the emergency department (ED) by his roommate. He reports abdominal pain, polyuria for the past 2 days, vomiting several times prior to arrival, and extreme thirst. He appears flushed, and his lips and mucous membranes are dry and cracked. His skin turgor is poor. He demonstrates deep, rapid respirations; there is a rotting fruit odor to his breath. He has type 1 diabetes and "may have skipped a few doses of insulin because of cramming for final exams." He is alert and talking but is having trouble focusing on questions.

Vital signs: Blood pressure, 110/60; Pulse, 110/min; Respirations, 32/min; Temperature, 100.8° F; Fingerstick glucose, 485 mg/dL; Oxygen saturation, 99%.

1. You have completed triage assessment and history. Should you now notify his parents for permission to treat him? Why or why not?
2. Should you apply oxygen at this time? Why or why not?
3. Should you call his primary care provider? Why or why not?
4. Your work plan includes checking hourly vital signs, assessing blood glucose levels, updating the roommate about the patient's condition, and measuring the patient's emesis. Which task(s) is (are) appropriate to assign to the new nursing assistant? Provide a rationale for your choices.
5. In caring for this patient, what immediate intervention do you anticipate the ED physician will order to be performed first? Provide a rationale for your choice.
6. What IV solution do you anticipate the ED physician will order for initial fluid replacement?

CHART 64-8 Patient and Family Education: Preparing for Self-Management

Sick-Day Rules

- Notify your health care provider that you are ill.
- Monitor your blood glucose at least every 4 hours.
- Test your urine for ketones when your blood glucose level is greater than 240 mg/dL (13.8 mmol/L).
- Continue to take insulin or oral antidiabetic agents.
- To prevent dehydration, drink 8 to 12 ounces of sugar-free liquids every hour that you are awake. If your blood glucose level is below your target range, drink fluids that contain sugar.
- Continue to eat meals at regular times.
- If unable to tolerate solid food because of nausea, consume more easily tolerated foods or liquids equal to the carbohydrate content of your usual meal.
- Call your primary care provider for any of these danger signals:
  - Persistent nausea and vomiting
  - Moderate or large ketones
  - Blood glucose elevation after two supplemental doses of insulin
  - High (101.5° F [38.6° C]) temperature or increasing fever; fever for more than 24 hours
- Treat symptoms (e.g., diarrhea, nausea, vomiting, fever) as directed by your primary care provider.
- Get plenty of rest.

Preventing Hyperglycemic-Hyperosmolar State. Hyperglycemic-hyperosmolar state (HHS) is a hyperosmolar (increased blood osmolarity) state caused by hyperglycemia. The processes of HHS are outlined in Fig. 64-10. Both HHS and diabetic ketoacidosis (DKA) are caused by hyperglycemia and dehydration. HHS differs from DKA in that ketone levels are absent or low and blood glucose levels are much higher. Blood glucose levels may exceed 600 mg/dL (33.3 mmol/L), and blood osmolarity may exceed 320 mOsm/L. Table 64-13 lists the differences between DKA and HHS.

HHS results from a sustained osmotic diuresis. Kidney impairment in HHS allows for extremely high blood glucose levels. As blood concentrations of glucose exceed the renal threshold, the kidney's capacity to reabsorb glucose is exceeded.

Decreased blood volume, caused by osmotic diuresis, or underlying kidney disease, common in many older patients with diabetes, results in further deterioration of kidney function. The decreased volume further reduces glomerular filtration rate, causing the glucose level to increase. Decreased kidney PERFUSION from hypovolemia further impairs kidney function.

CONSIDERATIONS FOR OLDER ADULTS

Patient-Centered Care QSEN

HHS occurs most often in older patients with type 2 diabetes mellitus, many of whom did not know that they had diabetes. Mortality rates in older patients are as high as 40% to 70%. The onset of HHS is slow and may not be recognized. The older patient often seeks medical attention later and is sicker than the younger patient. HHS does not occur in adequately hydrated patients. Older patients are at greater risk for dehydration and HHS because of age-related changes in thirst perception, poor urine-concentrating abilities, and use of diuretics. Stress to all older adults, especially those who have diabetes, the importance of maintaining hydration.

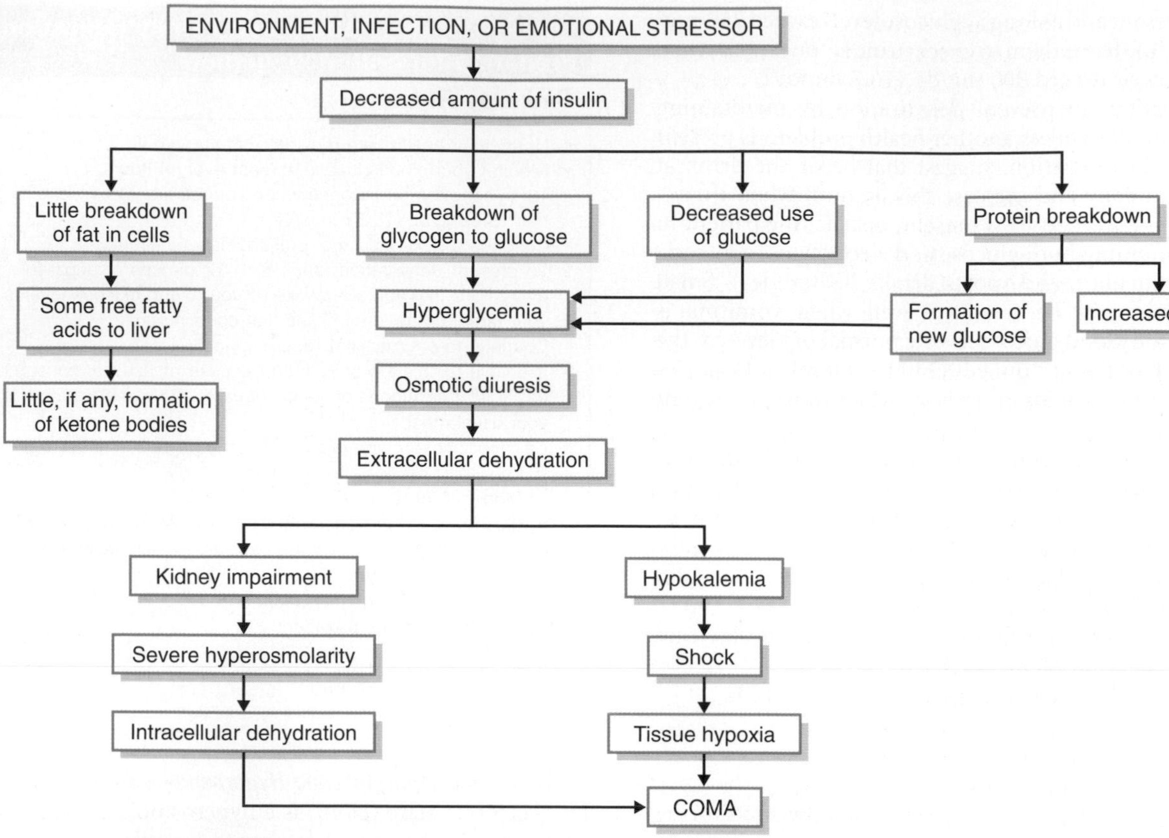

FIG. 64-10 The pathophysiologic mechanism of hyperglycemic-hyperosmolar state (HHS). *BUN,* Blood urea nitrogen.

Myocardial infarction, sepsis, pancreatitis, stroke, and some drugs (glucocorticoids, diuretics, phenytoin [Dilantin], beta blockers, and calcium channel blockers) also may cause HHS. Central nervous system (CNS) changes range from confusion to complete coma. Unlike DKA, patients with HHS may have seizures and reversible paralysis. The degree of neurologic impairment is related to serum osmolarity, with coma occurring once serum osmolarity is greater than 350 mOsm/L (350 mmol/L).

The development of HHS rather than DKA is related to residual insulin secretion. In HHS, the patient secretes just enough insulin to prevent ketosis but not enough to prevent hyperglycemia. The hyperglycemia of HHS is more severe than that of DKA, greatly increasing blood osmolarity, leading to extreme diuresis with severe dehydration and electrolyte loss.

Planning: Expected Outcomes. The patient with DM is expected to have few episodes of hyperglycemia and avoid HHS. Indicators include that the patient consistently demonstrates these behaviors:

- Maintains blood glucose levels within the target range
- Uses antidiabetic drugs appropriately
- Remains well hydrated
- Describes when to seek help from health care professionals

Interventions

Monitoring. Assess for manifestations of HHS. (See Tables 64-12 and 64-13 for manifestations of hyperglycemia.) Continually assess fluid status.

Fluid Therapy. The expected outcome of therapy is to rehydrate the patient and restore normal blood glucose levels within 36 to 72 hours. The choice of fluid replacement and the rate of infusion are critical in managing HHS. The severity of the CNS problems is related to the level of blood hyperosmolarity and cellular dehydration. Re-establishing fluid balance in brain cells is a difficult and slow process, and many patients do not recover baseline CNS function until hours after blood glucose levels have returned to normal.

The *first* priority for fluid replacement in HHS is to increase blood volume. In shock or severe hypotension, normal saline is used. Otherwise, half-normal saline (0.45% sodium chloride) is used. Infuse fluids at 1 L/hr until central venous pressure or pulmonary capillary wedge pressure begins to rise or until blood pressure and urine output are adequate. The rate is then reduced to 100 to 200 mL/hr. Half of the estimated fluid deficit is replaced in the first 12 hours, and the rest is given over the next 36 hours. Body weight, urine output, kidney function, and the presence or absence of pulmonary congestion and jugular venous distention determine the rate of fluid infusion. In patients with congestive heart failure, kidney disease, or acute kidney injury, monitor central venous pressure. *Assess the patient hourly for signs of cerebral edema—abrupt changes in mental status, abnormal neurologic signs, and coma.* Lack of

! NURSING SAFETY PRIORITY QSEN

Critical Rescue

For patients being managed for hyperglycemic-hyperosmolar state, immediately report changes in the level of consciousness; changes in pupil size, shape, or reaction; or seizures.

improvement in level of consciousness may indicate inadequate rates of fluid replacement or reduction in plasma (blood) osmolarity. Regression after initial improvement may indicate a too-rapid reduction in blood osmolarity. A slow but steady improvement in CNS function is the best evidence that fluid management is satisfactory.

Continuing Therapy. IV insulin is administered after adequate fluids have been replaced. The typical intervention is an initial bolus dose of 0.15 unit per kg IV followed by an infusion of 0.1 unit per kg per hour until blood glucose levels fall to 250 mg/dL (13.9 mmol/L). A reduction of blood glucose of 50 to 70 mg/dL per hour is the expected outcome. Monitor the patient closely for hypokalemia. Total body potassium depletion is often unrecognized because the blood potassium level may be normal or high as a result of dehydration. The potassium level may drop quickly when insulin therapy is started. Potassium replacement is initiated once urine output is adequate. Serum electrolytes are checked every 1 to 2 hours until stable, and the cardiac rhythm is monitored continuously for signs of hypokalemia or hyperkalemia. Patient education and interventions to minimize dehydration are similar to those for ketoacidosis.

Community-Based Care

Self-Management Education. Diabetes is a self-managed chronic disease requiring those affected to be actively involved in their own care. The concept of diabetes self-management refers to the patient's daily responsibility for almost all tasks involved in diabetes care. Education about blood glucose control for those with or at risk for diabetes occurs in a variety of health care settings. Physicians, nurses, registered dietitians, pharmacists, social workers, and psychologists all participate in the education. People with diabetes are best able to learn through educational efforts that are tailored to their individual needs.

Assessing Learning Needs and Readiness to Learn. First assess the patient's learning needs and readiness to learn. This assessment establishes what the patient already knows and what he or she needs to know. It also helps you determine the patient's ability and desire to learn. Assess the needs of both patient and family before teaching (Hughes, 2012b). Table 64-14 lists areas to include in this assessment.

Patients want information that applies directly to them. Find out what concerns the patient most about having diabetes, and ask what he or she wants to learn. Start with what the patient already knows, and build on that base. Make sure that the patient's knowledge is current and applies to his or her type of diabetes.

Your assessment may indicate that the patient is not ready to learn needed self-management behaviors. With the patient's permission, you would then teach a family member or someone close to the patient about diabetes management. You would also provide written materials on diabetes management as well as telephone numbers for the patient to call when he or she is ready to learn.

Assessing Physical, Cognitive, and Emotional Limitations. Assessing the patient's literacy is essential in developing a plan of care and providing self-management education. It is important to measure the patient's ability to read and understand written materials and conduct math calculations. Assess the patient's education and reading level to determine what level of information to present. It is important to match the literacy level of materials to the literacy level of the patient. Simplify the information you present by replacing technical terms with plain language (words people use in everyday conversation).

TABLE 64-14 Assessment of Learning Needs for the Patient with Diabetes

- Health and medical history
- Nutrition history and practices
- Physical activity and exercise behaviors
- Prescription and over-the-counter medications and complementary and alternative therapies and practices
- Factors that influence learning such as education and literacy levels, perceived learning needs, motivation to learn, and health beliefs
- Diabetes self-management behaviors, including experience with self-adjusting the treatment plan
- Previous diabetes self-management training, actual knowledge, and skills
- Physical factors including age, mobility, visual acuity, hearing, manual dexterity, alertness, attention span, and ability to concentrate or special needs or limitations requiring adaptive support and use of alternative skills
- Psychosocial concerns, factors, or issues including family and social support
- Current mental health status
- History of substance use including alcohol, tobacco, and recreational drugs
- Occupation, vocation, education level, financial status, and social, cultural, and religious practices
- Access to and use of health care resources

Assess the patient's ability to read printed information, insulin labels, and markings on syringes and equipment. Many with type 2 diabetes have age-related visual problems made worse by blurred vision caused by fluctuating blood glucose levels. Assess the patient's ability to reason with numbers. Determine whether the patient has the math skills needed to interpret a food label or to make adjustments in insulin doses based on glucose readings.

Assess manual dexterity for any physical limitations that may alter the teaching plan. A hand injury, tremors, or severe arthritis often leads to dosing errors with a standard syringe and may require a change in insulin preparation.

Individual learning styles vary. Visual learners think in terms of pictures and remember things best by seeing something written or by seeing visual aids. Auditory learners learn best through hearing. Kinesthetic or tactile learners learn best through touching, feeling, and experiencing what they are trying to learn. Tactile learners remember best by writing or physically manipulating the equipment. Successful diabetes self-management education uses all three learning styles by providing written handouts, discussing steps involved in a procedure such as insulin administration or self-monitoring of blood glucose, and encouraging the learner to touch and manipulate equipment. Confirm that the patient understands your instructions by having him or her "teach back" the information to you.

Tailor educational sessions to the time available and to the condition of the patient. Hospitalized people require only basic education when they are acutely ill. In these situations, it is appropriate to teach basic survival skills or focused problem-solving skills while reserving more detailed education for follow-up sessions.

Survival Skills Information. The initial phase of diabetes education involves teaching information necessary for the survival of anyone diagnosed with diabetes. Survival information includes:

- Simple information on pathophysiology of diabetes
- Learning how to prepare and administer insulin or how to take oral drugs for diabetes
- Recognition, treatment, and prevention of hypoglycemia and hyperglycemia
- Basic diet information
- Monitoring of blood glucose and ketones
- Sick-day management
- Where to buy diabetes supplies and how to store them
- When and how to notify the health care provider

In-Depth Education. In-depth education and counseling involve teaching more detailed information about survival skills and about actions for avoiding long-term complications. Educational sessions with patient and family are needed to "patientize" the diabetes regimen for *their* needs and abilities.

The person with diabetes needs to understand the pathology of diabetes. He or she should be able to discuss the action of insulin in the body and the effects of insulin deficiency. He or she should also be able to explain the effects of diet, drugs, and activity on blood glucose. The patient should be able to relate maintaining normal blood glucose levels to preventing complications. This includes relating changes in glucose level to the possible need for a change in insulin dosage.

Provide education about the manifestations of hypoglycemia along with the prescribed treatment options if the patient takes any drugs that will lower blood glucose levels. Educate patients and their families about common causes of hypoglycemia such as changes in drug regimen, increase in physical activity, and delayed or missed meals. Review manifestations of hypoglycemia at each visit. Advise patients to check their blood glucose levels before driving and make sure they have easy-to-reach snacks or fast-acting sugars with them at all times. Encourage them to always wear a medical ID tag or bracelet and to contact their health care provider if they experience low blood glucose levels more than twice a week.

Many patients require combination drug therapy to achieve GLUCOSE REGULATION in addition to aspirin and drugs to lower lipids and blood pressure. If the patient takes an oral antidiabetic drug, ask him or her to identify the drugs and describe the prescribed schedule. Determine if the patient is able to administer insulin accurately by having him or her "teach back" injection techniques. Ask the patient to discuss the onset, peak, and duration of the insulin used. The patient must be able to state when insulin is to be injected, where insulin is injected, and how insulin is stored. Review formulas for self-adjustment in insulin (when permitted by the health care provider), and explain blood glucose monitoring requirements needed to evaluate the effects of additional insulin. Stress the dangers of skipping doses. Review drug interactions, especially with older patients taking oral antidiabetic drugs.

Teach patients receiving diet therapy alone, glucose-lowering drugs, or fixed insulin doses to eat consistent amounts of carbohydrate at meals and snacks. Patients who adjust mealtime doses of insulin or those on insulin pump therapy can be taught to match their insulin dose to the carbohydrate content of their diet. The patient needs to understand what to eat, how much to eat, and when to eat. Stress the importance of eating on time, the dangers of skipping meals, and how to maintain food intake during illness. Ask the patient to describe the meal plan and explain the adjustments needed to meet diabetic diet requirements. Include the family member usually responsible for buying groceries and preparing meals in this teaching.

Regular physical activity is important for physical fitness, weight management, and blood glucose control. Assist all patients to identify activities they can do to achieve the goal of moderate-intensity activity 3 or more days a week. For patients taking insulin and/or insulin secretagogues, physical activity can cause hypoglycemia if drug dosage or carbohydrate intake is not increased. Review how to perform physical activities safely. Instruct the patient on blood glucose levels that are safe for exercise, the frequency of glucose monitoring during exercise, drug adjustments before exercise, food required before exercise, and what food to have available during exercise. He or she should be aware of the risk for injury during exercise and be able to explain the importance of protective footwear.

Self-monitoring of blood glucose provides immediate information on a person's blood glucose level and provides feedback on the effects of recent activity, drugs, and meals. The nurse's role includes teaching skills of performing the test, educating how to interpret results, and problem solving to adjust behaviors and therapy based on the information. Teach patients how to recognize when blood glucose levels are out of range, how to adjust therapy and behaviors based on self-monitoring of blood glucose (SMBG) results, and how to verify the effects of these adjustments by performing subsequent glucose testing. Also, show patients who use insulin how to use SMBG to adjust dosages to achieve glucose control while avoiding episodes of hypoglycemia.

Teach patients sick-day procedures when initially diagnosed with diabetes. Hyperglycemia often develops before INFECTION manifestations and can serve as a warning that infection is developing. Provide guidelines for the frequency of glucose testing, for ketone testing, and for insulin adjustment for those patients able to self-adjust insulin doses.

Psychosocial Preparation. The diagnosis of diabetes may represent a loss of control and flexibility. Life becomes ordered, and routines must be followed. Certain events surrounding diabetes are predictable. Taking an insulin injection and not eating for several hours causes hypoglycemia. Poorly controlled diabetes leads to complications and premature death. Tight control of blood glucose levels prevents complications.

The stress of diabetes is in addition to the demands of normal daily life. The patient must be able to integrate the demands of diabetes into daily and recreational schedules while keeping blood glucose stable.

Patients are more likely to adhere to disease management activities when the strategies make sense and seem effective. Other factors promoting adherence include the patient's belief that the activity is important, having confidence in himself or herself, and having support. Assist in healthy psychological adaptation to diabetes by providing successful educational experiences. Mastery of blood glucose monitoring helps the patient feel that he or she has control over the disease. Knowing the effects of extra activities, extra food, or extra insulin is helpful in learning to adjust the regimen.

Feeling a sense of control over the condition promotes a positive attitude about diabetes. Success in injecting insulin provides concrete evidence that he or she can master the disease. Teach by breaking a task into small, achievable units to ensure mastery. For example, a patient may begin learning how to inject insulin by first obtaining an accurate dose.

Devote as much teaching time as possible to insulin injection and blood glucose monitoring. Patients with newly diagnosed diabetes are often fearful of giving themselves injections. After

CHART 64-9 Focused Assessment

The Insulin-Dependent Patient with Diabetes During a Home or Clinic Visit

- Assess overall mental status, wakefulness, ability to converse.
- Take vital signs and weight:
  - Fever could indicate infection.
  - Are blood pressure and weight within target range? If not, why?
- Question patient regarding any change in visual acuity; check current visual acuity.
- Inspect oral mucous membranes, gums, and teeth.
- Question patient about injection areas used; inspect areas being used; assess whether patient is using areas and sites appropriately.
- Inspect skin for intactness, wounds that have not healed, new sores, ulcers, bruises, or burns; assess any previously known wounds for infection, progression of healing.
- Question patient regarding foot care.
- Assess lower extremities and feet for peripheral pulses, lack of or decreased sensation, abnormal sensations, breaks in skin integrity, condition of toes and nails.
- Question patient regarding color and consistency of stools and frequency of bowel movements; assess abdomen for bowel sounds.
- Review patient's home health diary:
  - Is blood glucose within targeted range? If not, why?
  - Is glucose monitoring being recorded often enough?
  - Is the patient's food intake adequate and appropriate? If not, why?
  - Is exercise occurring regularly? If not, why?
- Assess patient's ability to perform self-monitoring of blood glucose.
- Assess patient's procedures for obtaining and storing insulin and syringes, cleaning equipment, disposing of syringes and needles.
- Assess patient's insulin preparation and injection technique.

this technique has been mastered, they become less anxious and are able to attend to other tasks.

Recognize that not everyone will adapt to diabetes. Some patients are unable to progress beyond the survival level. Major depression affects many patients with diabetes, having an impact on quality of life and all aspects of functioning, including self-management behaviors. Refer those who have significant problems coping with the day-to-day demands of diabetes to mental health counseling for appropriate treatment.

Home Care Management. Patients with diabetes self-manage their disease. Each day they decide what to eat, whether to exercise, and whether to take prescribed drugs. Maintaining blood glucose control depends on the accuracy of self-management skills. The nurse provides support and education to empower the patient to make informed decisions. Self-management education allows patients to identify their problems and provides techniques to help them make decisions, take appropriate actions, and alter these actions as needed.

Provide information about resources. The patient must know whom to contact in case of emergency. Older adults who live alone need to have daily telephone contact with a friend or neighbor. The patient may also need help shopping and preparing meals. He or she may have limited access to transportation and may not have sufficient supplies of food, particularly in bad weather. Because of the likelihood of visual problems in older patients, they may need assistance in preparing insulin syringes for injection or in monitoring blood glucose. Make referrals to home care or public health agencies as needed. Chart 64-9 identifies areas for assessment during a home or clinic visit.

TABLE 64-15 Outcome Criteria for Diabetes Teaching

Before being discharged to home, the patient with diabetes or the significant other should be able to:

- Tell why insulin or an oral hypoglycemic agent is being prescribed
- Name which insulin or oral hypoglycemic agent is being prescribed, and name the dosage and frequency of administration
- Discuss the relationship between mealtime and the action of insulin or the oral hypoglycemic agent
- Discuss plans to follow diabetic diet instructions
- Prepare and administer insulin accurately
- Test blood for glucose, or state plans for having blood glucose levels monitored
- Test urine for ketones, and state when this test should be done
- Verbalize how to store insulin
- List manifestations that indicate a hypoglycemic reaction
- Tell what carbohydrate sources are used to treat hypoglycemic reactions
- Tell what manifestations indicate hyperglycemia
- Tell what dietary changes are needed during illness
- Verbalize when to call the physician or the nurse (frequent episodes of hypoglycemia, manifestations of hyperglycemia)
- Verbalize the procedures for proper foot care

◆ *Evaluation: Outcomes*

Evaluate the care of the patient with diabetes based on the identified priority patient problems. Outcome success for diabetes education is the ability of the patient to maintain blood glucose levels within their established target range. General outcome criteria are listed below and in Table 64-15. More specific outcomes are listed with each priority patient problem. The expected outcomes include that the patient should:

- Achieve blood glucose control
- Avoid acute and chronic complications of diabetes
- Avoid injury
- Experience relief of pain
- Maintain optimal visual SENSORY PERCEPTION
- Maintain a urine output in the expected range
- Have an optimal level of mental status functioning
- Have decreased episodes of hypoglycemia
- Have decreased episodes of hyperglycemia

Specific indicators for these outcomes are listed for each priority patient problem under the Planning and Implementation section (see earlier).

NURSING CONCEPTS AND CLINICAL JUDGMENT REVIEW

What might you NOTICE in a patient with diabetes mellitus who demonstrates adequate GLUCOSE REGULATION?

Vital signs:

- Blood pressure less than 140/80
- Heart rate and rhythm within the normal range
- Temperature within the normal range

Physical assessment:

- Skin intact, especially on the feet, no open wounds or sores that have failed to heal
- Weight proportionate to height; does not appear overweight or underweight
- Vision adequate for safety and participation in ADLs
- No report of pain, tingling, numbness, or burning in extremities

Psychological assessment:

- Oriented and not confused
- Willing to learn and participate in self-care
- Energy level good; can engage in desired work, recreational, and personal activities

Laboratory assessment:

- A1C levels are maintained at 6.5% or below.
- The majority of premeal blood glucose levels are 70 to 130 mg/dL (3.9 to 7.2 mmol/L).
- Peak after-meal blood glucose levels are less than 180 mg/dL (<10.0 mmol/L).
- Urine is free from ketone bodies and albumin.
- 24-hour intake and output balance.
- Blood urea nitrogen (BUN) and serum creatinine are within the normal ranges.
- Serum electrolytes are within the normal ranges.

GET READY FOR THE NCLEX® EXAMINATION!

KEY POINTS

Review these Key Points for each NCLEX Examination Client Needs Category.

Safe and Effective Care Environment

- Use aseptic technique during any invasive procedure when caring for a patient with diabetes. **Safety** QSEN
- Administer antidiabetic drugs and insulin in a safe manner. **Safety** QSEN
- Ensure that meals are available immediately after the patient receives an antidiabetic drug or insulin. **Safety** QSEN
- Use good handwashing techniques before providing any care to a patient who has diabetes. **Safety** QSEN

Health Promotion and Maintenance

- Encourage all patients to maintain weight within an appropriate range. **Evidence-Based Practice** QSEN
- Encourage all patients, including patients with diabetes, to participate regularly in exercise or physical activity appropriate to their health status. **Patient-Centered Care** QSEN
- Teach the patient and family about the manifestations of INFECTION and when to seek medical advice.
- Instruct patients with diabetes to wear a medical alert bracelet. **Safety** QSEN
- Instruct patients to not share blood glucose monitoring equipment. **Evidence-Based Practice** QSEN
- Reinforce to all patients with diabetes that tight control over blood glucose levels reduces the risk for the vascular complications of diabetes. **Patient-Centered Care** QSEN
- Remind patients with diabetes to have yearly eye examinations by an ophthalmologist. **Evidence-Based Practice** QSEN
- Teach patients with peripheral neuropathy to use a bath thermometer to test water for bathing, to avoid walking barefoot, and to inspect their feet daily. **Safety** QSEN
- Assess patients' visual acuity and peripheral tactile sensation to determine needed adjustments in teaching self-medication and self-monitoring of blood glucose levels.
- Instruct all patients with diabetes to avoid becoming dehydrated and to drink at least 2 L of water each day unless another medical condition requires fluid restriction. **Patient-Centered Care** QSEN
- Instruct patients who are taking sulfonylurea drugs about an increased risk for hypoglycemic reactions. **Patient-Centered Care** QSEN
- Teach patients who are taking metformin the clinical manifestations of lactic acidosis (fatigue, dizziness, difficulty breathing, stomach discomfort, irregular heartbeat). **Safety** QSEN
- Warn patients to not take over-the-counter drugs with their oral antidiabetic drugs without consulting their primary care provider.
- Teach patients to rotate insulin injection sites within one area rather than to other areas, to prevent changes in absorption. **Evidence-Based Practice** QSEN
- Use return demonstration and "teach-back" strategies when teaching the patient about drug regimen, insulin injection, blood glucose monitoring, and foot assessment. **Patient-Centered Care** QSEN
- Teach patients to administer an accurate dose of insulin using a prefilled or disposable insulin pen.
- Teach patients who experience Somogyi phenomenon (early morning hyperglycemia) to ensure an adequate dietary intake at bedtime.
- Instruct patients to always carry a glucose source.
- Teach patients who exercise to test urine for ketone bodies if blood glucose levels are greater than 250 mg/dL before engaging in strenuous exercise.
- Instruct patients in foot care as outlined in Chart 64-6.

Psychosocial Integrity

- Explore with the patient what the diagnosis of diabetes means to him or her. **Patient-Centered Care** QSEN
- Allow the patient the opportunity to express concerns about the diagnosis of diabetes or the treatment regimen.

- Explain all procedures, restrictions, drugs, and follow-up care to the patient and family.
- Instruct the patient and family on the manifestations of complications and when to seek assistance. **Safety** QSEN
- Pace your education sessions to match the learning needs and style of the patient. **Patient-Centered Care** QSEN

Physiological Integrity

- Never dilute or mix insulin glargine with any other insulin or solution. **Safety** QSEN
- Avoid injecting insulin within a 2-inch radius of the umbilicus.
- Avoid IM insulin injection.
- Assist patients who have PAIN from peripheral neuropathy to determine what pain-relieving drugs and techniques work best for them.
- Assess the patient's A1C level for indications of adherence to prescribed regimens and their effectiveness.
- Start carbohydrate replacement per physician prescription or standing protocols immediately on identifying a patient with hypoglycemia. **Safety** QSEN
- Give glucagon subcutaneously or IM and 50% dextrose IV to patients identified with hypoglycemia who cannot swallow. **Evidence-Based Practice** QSEN
- First assess the airway, level of consciousness, hydration status, electrolytes, and blood glucose level of any patient with diabetic ketoacidosis.
- Use blood glucose values to assess therapy effectiveness and determine when to switch from saline to dextrose-containing solutions in a patient with diabetic ketoacidosis.
- Continually assess fluid status and level of consciousness in a patient with hyperglycemic-hyperosmolar state (HHS) during the resuscitation period.
- Immediately report manifestations of cerebral edema (abrupt changes in mental status; changes in level of consciousness; changes in pupil size, shape, or reaction; seizures) in a patient with HHS to the health care provider. **Safety** QSEN
- Collaborate with the health care provider, diabetes nurse educator, registered dietitian, pharmacist, social worker, and case manager to individualize patient care for the person with diabetes in any care setting. **Teamwork and Collaboration** QSEN
- Refer patients newly diagnosed with diabetes to local resources and support groups.

CONCEPT OVERVIEW

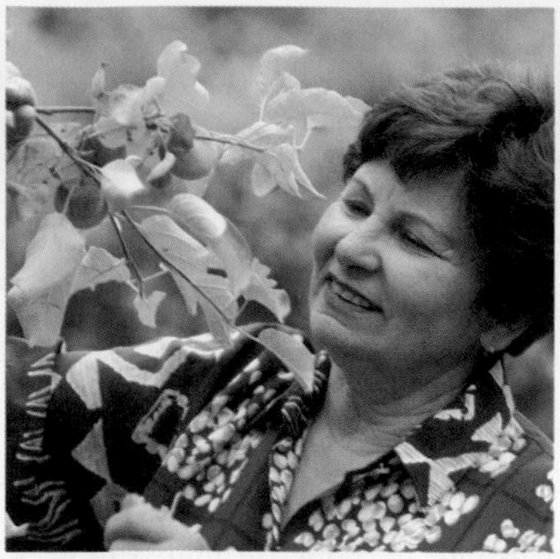

Urinary Elimination

Adequate urinary elimination is essential for body fluid homeostasis—the ability of the body to maintain its internal environment at a "steady state" and within very narrow ranges of normal, regardless of external changes. Urinary ELIMINATION alone is defined as the passage of urine through the urinary tract by means of the urinary sphincter and urethra (Giddens, 2013). However, urine cannot be eliminated unless it is first formed in the kidneys from the blood. The kidneys perform the actual work of determining which substances in body fluid will be eliminated and which will be retained. So kidney function is critical for urinary ELIMINATION to be able to maintain homeostasis of all body fluids.

The body works best when blood and other extracellular fluids maintain volumes within the normal ranges and maintain the proper ranges of electrolytes. Serious health problems and death occur when these electrolytes are much higher or lower than normal ranges. When blood volume is too high, hypertension develops and damages vital organs. When blood volume is too low, hypotension can be so severe that vital organs are not perfused with oxygen and become hypoxic. In addition, protein waste products containing nitrogen, such as urea, act as a poison and must be prevented from getting too high. Humans ingest many foods and liquids that contain water, electrolytes, and substances that will be converted to waste products. Without control mechanisms to balance the intake of these substances with their ELIMINATION, we would rapidly accumulate too much of everything and die.

As part of the renal/urinary system, the kidneys are responsible for maintaining this balance of what is taken into the body, what is allowed to remain in the body, and what is eliminated from the body. Although some products are eliminated in the stool, there is no discrimination or adjustment in bowel ELIMINATION. Urinary ELIMINATION, however, allows a person to eat and drink almost anything (except poisons and infectious organisms) in almost any amount without upsetting the homeostatic balance for body water, electrolytes, waste products, and blood pressure. For example, on one day a person may drink 2 L of fluids and eat food that contains 2 g of sodium and 5 g of potassium. The next day this same person may drink 3 L of fluids and eat food that contains 12 g of sodium and 10 g of potassium. Yet because the kidneys selectively adjust to change the amount of each substance that gets eliminated, the blood pressure, serum sodium, and serum potassium levels remain the same and within the normal ranges on both days. A "steady-state" or homeostatic balance of these substances is maintained because the kidneys adjust the output to match the intake (Fig. 1).

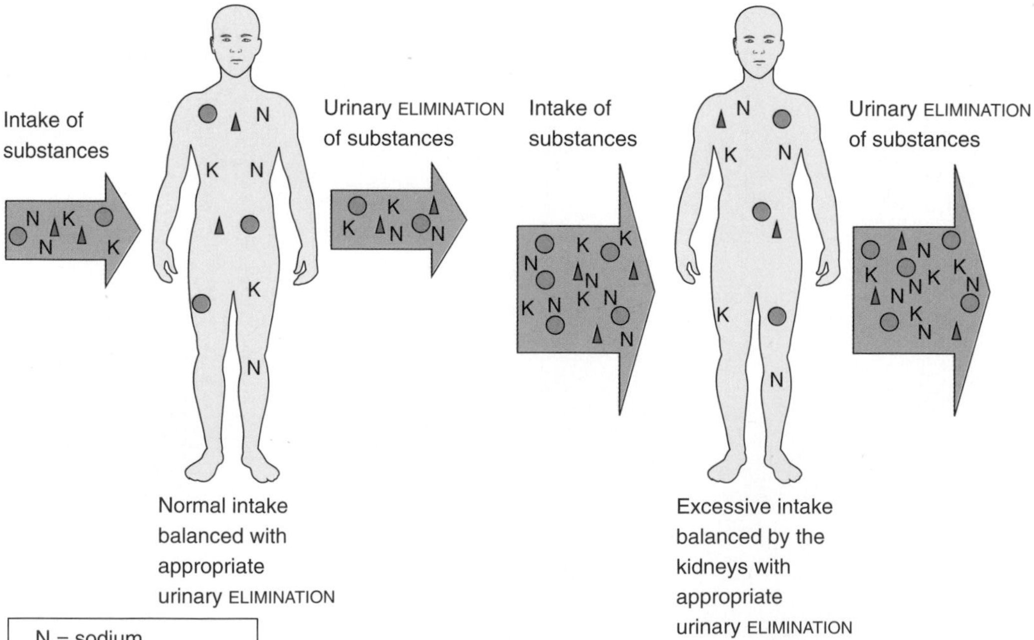

FIG. 1

When kidney function is impaired to any degree as a result of renal/urinary problems, urinary ELIMINATION is not adequate and the steady-state homeostasis of water, electrolyte, and waste products is disrupted (Fig. 2). Without intervention, this lack of steady state leads to excesses of body water, electrolytes, and nitrogenous waste products that interfere with normal organ function and can cause death.

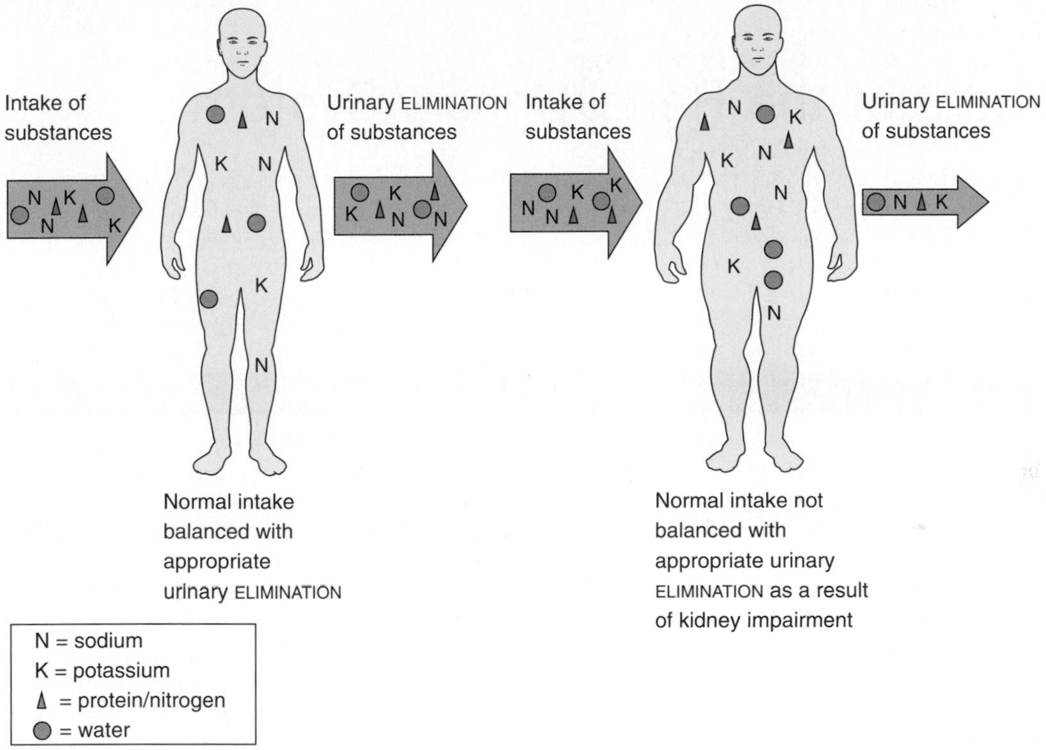

FIG. 2

65 CHAPTER

Assessment of the Renal/Urinary System

Chris Winkelman

http://evolve.elsevier.com/Iggy/

PRIORITY CONCEPTS

- ELIMINATION
- FLUID AND ELECTROLYTE BALANCE
- ACID-BASE BALANCE

LEARNING OUTCOMES

Safe and Effective Care Environment

1. Use principles of infection control when assessing a patient's kidney and urinary ELIMINATION for adequate FLUID AND ELECTROLYTE BALANCE and ACID-BASE BALANCE.

Health Promotion and Maintenance

2. Teach all people about the importance of maintaining an adequate oral fluid intake for FLUID AND ELECTROLYTE BALANCE.
3. Teach about or assist with cleansing of the perineum or urinary meatus after using the toilet and during daily bathing or showering.
4. Teach all people how to protect the kidneys and urinary system from toxic substances.

Psychosocial Integrity

5. Reduce the psychological impact for the patient and family regarding the assessment and testing of the renal/urinary system.

Physiological Integrity

6. Perform a focused assessment of kidney and urinary function, incorporating information from anatomy and physiology, including genetic risk and age-related changes affecting kidney and urinary function.
7. Coordinate appropriate care for patients after invasive and noninvasive testing of kidney and urinary function.
8. Use correct technique to assess the kidneys and urinary system.
9. Prioritize nursing care for the patient during the first 24 hours after invasive procedures, especially those requiring contrast material.

The renal system includes the kidneys and the entire urinary tract. The ureters, bladder, and urethra are the drainage route for the excretion of urine. Structural or functional problems in the kidneys or urinary tract may alter FLUID AND ELECTROLYTE BALANCE and ACID-BASE BALANCE.

The kidneys help maintain health in many ways. *Most important, they maintain body fluid volume and composition and filter waste products for ELIMINATION.* The kidneys also help regulate blood pressure and ACID-BASE BALANCE, produce erythropoietin for red blood cell (RBC) synthesis, and convert vitamin D to an active form.

Assessment of the patient at risk for or with actual problems of the kidneys or urinary system begins with a history and physical assessment. Understanding the anatomy, physiology, and diagnostic tests of the renal system helps you in problem solving about kidney and urinary tract function in the clinical setting. It also assists you in teaching the patient about the purpose of procedures and in physically and emotionally preparing the patient for assessment.

ANATOMY AND PHYSIOLOGY REVIEW

Kidneys

Structure

Gross Anatomy. The two kidneys are located behind the peritoneum, not in the abdominal cavity, one on either side of the spine (Fig. 65-1). The adult kidney is 4 to 5 inches (10 to 13 cm) long, 2 to 3 inches (5 to 7 cm) wide, and about 1 inch (2.5 to 3 cm) thick. The left kidney is slightly longer and narrower than the right kidney. Larger-than-usual kidneys may indicate obstruction or polycystic disease. Smaller-than-usual kidneys may indicate chronic kidney disease (CKD).

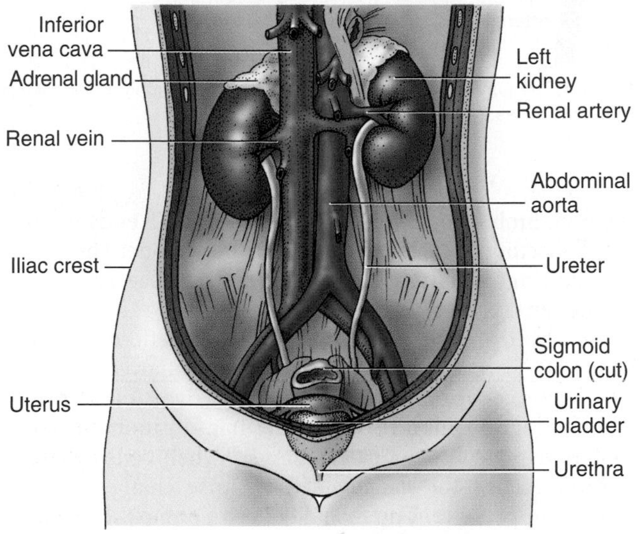

FIG. 65-1 Anatomic location of the kidneys and structures of the urinary system.

Variation in kidney shape and number is not uncommon and does not always indicate a problem in kidney function. Some people have more than two kidneys or may have only one large, horseshoe-shaped kidney. As long as tests of kidney function are normal, these variations are of no significance.

Several layers of tissue surround the kidney, providing protection and support. The outer surface of the kidney is a layer of fibrous tissue called the **capsule** (Fig. 65-2). It covers most of the kidney except the **hilum**, which is the area where the kidney blood vessels and nerves enter and exit. It is also where the ureter exits. The capsule is surrounded by layers of fat and connective tissue.

Lying beneath the capsule are the two layers of functional kidney tissue—the cortex and the medulla. The **renal cortex** is the outer tissue layer. The **medulla** is the medullary tissue lying below the cortex in the shape of many fans. Each "fan" is called a *pyramid.* The **renal columns** are cortical tissue that dips down into the interior of the kidney and separates the pyramids.

The tip of each pyramid is called a **papilla**. The papillae drain urine into the collecting system. A cuplike structure called a **calyx** collects the urine at the end of each papilla. The calices join together to form the **renal pelvis**, which narrows to become the ureter.

The kidneys have a rich blood supply and receive a blood flow from 600 to 1300 mL/min. The blood supply to each kidney comes from the renal artery, which branches from the abdominal aorta. The renal artery divides into progressively smaller arteries, supplying all blood to areas of the kidney tissue and the nephrons. The smallest arteries (**afferent arterioles**) feed the nephrons directly to form urine.

Venous blood from the kidneys starts with the capillaries surrounding each nephron. These capillaries drain into progressively larger veins, with blood eventually returned to the inferior vena cava through the renal vein.

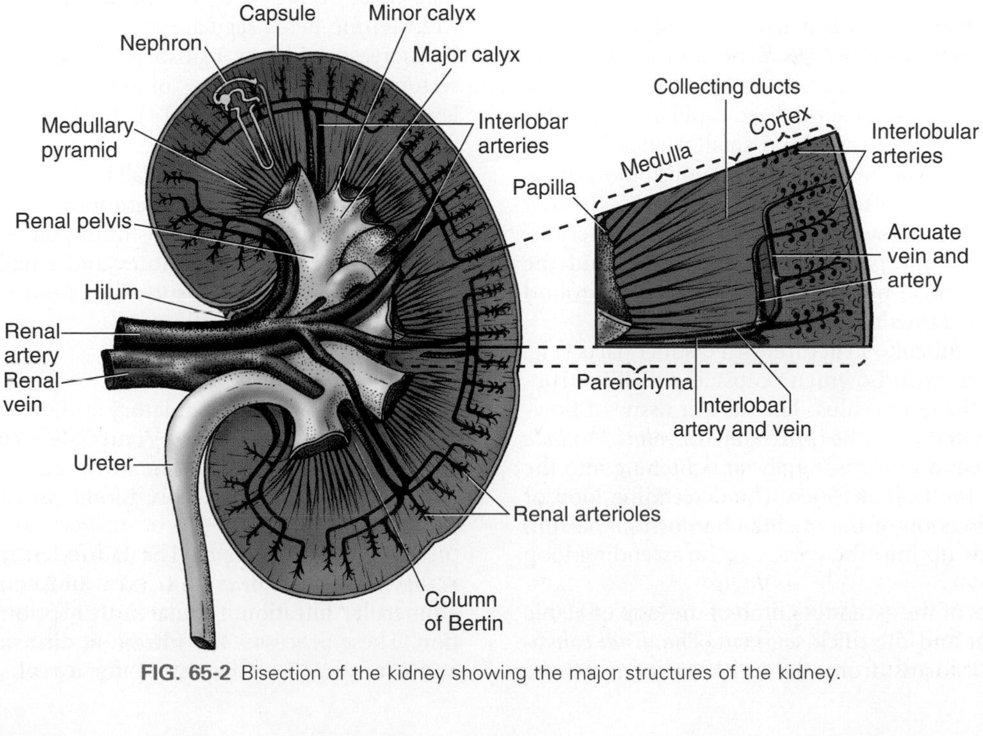

FIG. 65-2 Bisection of the kidney showing the major structures of the kidney.

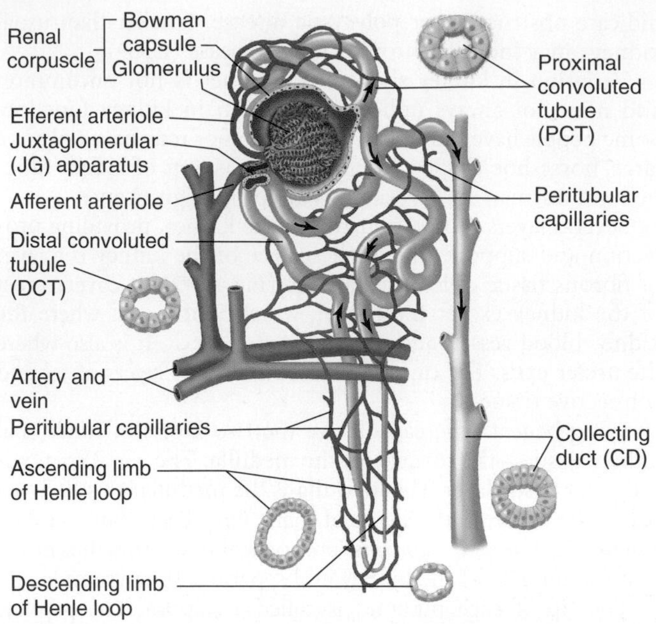

FIG. 65-3 Anatomy of the nephron—the functional unit of the kidney. The differences in appearance in tubular cells seen in a cross section reflect the differing functions of each nephron segment. Note that the particular nephron labeled here is a juxtamedullary nephron.

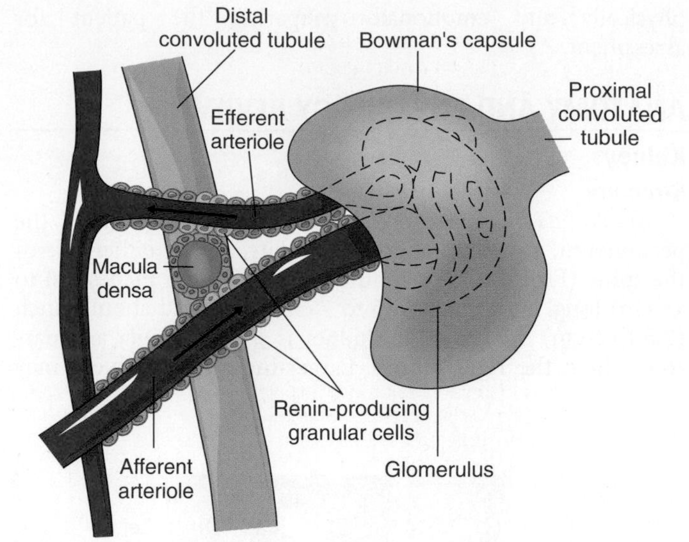

FIG. 65-4 The juxtaglomerular complex showing juxtaglomerular cells and the macula densa.

Microscopic Anatomy. The **nephron** is the functional unit of the kidney, which forms urine from blood. There are about 1 million nephrons per kidney, and each nephron separately makes urine from blood.

There are two types of nephrons: *cortical nephrons* and *juxtamedullary nephrons.* The cortical nephrons are short and lie totally within the renal cortex. The juxtamedullary nephrons (about 20% of all nephrons) are longer, and their tubes and blood vessels dip deeply into the medulla. The purpose of these longer nephrons is to concentrate urine during times of low fluid intake to allow continued excretion of body wastes with less fluid loss.

Blood supply to the nephron is delivered through the afferent arteriole—the smallest, most distal portion of the renal arterial system. From the afferent arteriole, blood flows into the **glomerulus**, which is a series of specialized capillary loops. It is through these capillaries that water and small particles are filtered from the blood to make urine. The remaining blood leaves the glomerulus through the **efferent arteriole**, which is the first vessel in the kidney's venous system. From the efferent arteriole, blood exits into either the *peritubular capillaries* around the tubular part of the cortical nephrons or the *vasa recta* around the tubular part of juxtamedullary nephrons.

Each nephron is a tubelike structure with distinct parts (Fig. 65-3). The tube begins with Bowman's capsule, a saclike structure that surrounds the glomerulus. The tubular tissue of Bowman's capsule narrows into the *proximal convoluted tubule (PCT).* The PCT twists and turns, finally straightening into the descending limb of the *loop of Henle.* The descending loop of Henle dips in the direction of the medulla but forms a hairpin loop and comes back up into the cortex as the ascending loop of Henle.

The two segments of the ascending limb of the loop of Henle are the thin segment and the thick segment. The *distal convoluted tubule (DCT)* forms from the thick segment of the ascending limb of the loop of Henle. The DCT ends in one of many collecting ducts located in the kidney tissue. The urine in the collecting ducts passes through the papillae and empties into the renal pelvis.

Special cells in the afferent arteriole, the efferent arteriole, and the DCT are known as the **juxtaglomerular complex** (Fig. 65-4). These cells produce and store **renin**, which is a hormone that helps regulate blood flow, glomerular filtration rate (GFR), and blood pressure. Renin is secreted when sensing cells in the DCT (called the *macula densa*) sense changes in blood volume and pressure. The macula densa lies next to the renin-producing cells. Renin is produced when the macula densa cells sense that blood volume, blood pressure, or blood sodium level is low. Renin then converts renin substrate (angiotensinogen) into angiotensin I. This leads to a series of reactions that cause secretion of the hormone *aldosterone* (Fig. 65-5). Aldosterone helps regulate FLUID AND ELECTROLYTE BALANCE by increasing kidney reabsorption of sodium and water and restoring blood pressure, blood volume, and blood sodium levels (McCance et al., 2014). It also promotes excretion of potassium (see Chapter 11).

The glomerular capillary wall has three layers (Fig. 65-6): the endothelium, the basement membrane, and the epithelium. The endothelial and epithelial cells lining these capillaries are separated by pores that filter water and small particles from the blood into Bowman's capsule. This fluid is called the "filtrate" or "early urine."

Function

The kidneys have both regulatory and hormonal functions. The regulatory functions control FLUID AND ELECTROLYTE BALANCE and ACID-BASE BALANCE. The hormonal functions control red blood cell (RBC) formation, blood pressure, and vitamin D activation.

Regulatory Functions. The kidney processes that maintain FLUID AND ELECTROLYTE BALANCE and ACID-BASE BALANCE are glomerular filtration, tubular reabsorption, and tubular secretion. These processes use filtration, diffusion, active transport, and osmosis. (See Chapter 11 for a review of these actions.)

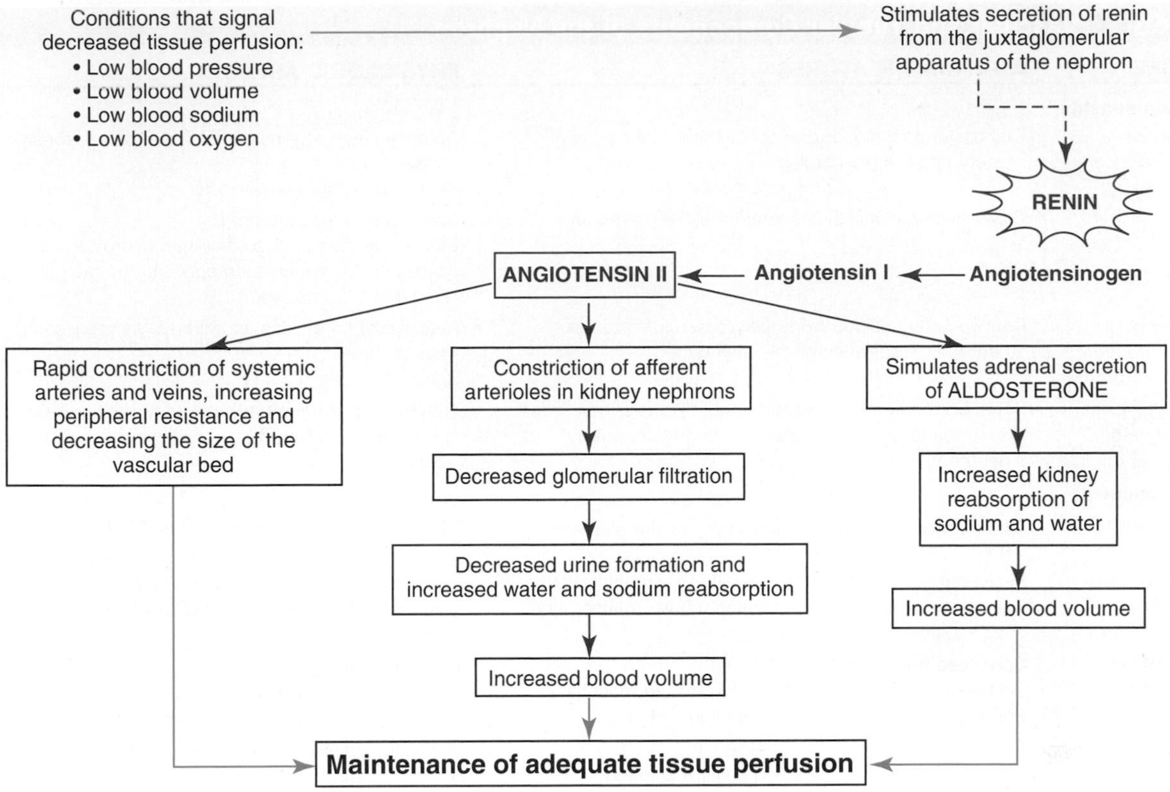

FIG. 65-5 The role of aldosterone, renin substrate (angiotensinogen), angiotensin I, and angiotensin II in the renal regulation of water and sodium.

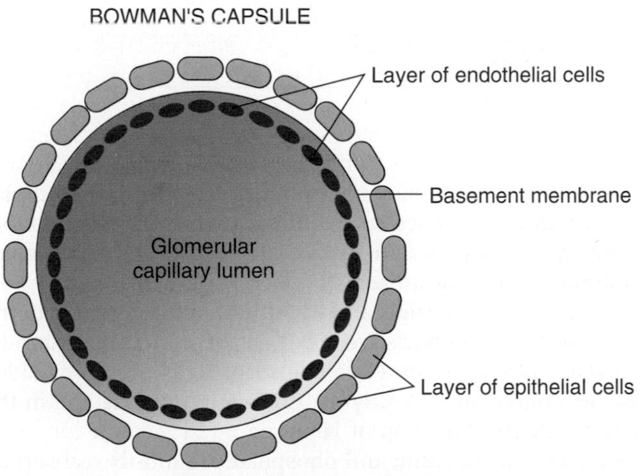

FIG. 65-6 Glomerular capillary wall.

Table 65-1 lists the functions of nephron tubules and blood vessels.

Glomerular filtration is the first process in urine formation. As blood passes from the afferent arteriole into the glomerulus, water, electrolytes, and other small particles (e.g., creatinine, urea nitrogen, glucose) are filtered across the glomerular membrane into the Bowman's capsule to form *glomerular* filtrate. As the filtrate enters the proximal convoluted tubule (PCT), it is called *tubular filtrate.*

Large particles, such as blood cells, albumin, and other proteins, are too large to filter through the glomerular capillary walls. *Therefore these substances are not normally present in the final urine.*

About 180 L of glomerular filtrate is formed from the blood each day. The rate of filtration is expressed in milliliters per minute. Normal glomerular filtration rate (GFR) averages 125 mL/min. If the entire amount of filtrate were excreted as urine, death would occur quickly from dehydration. Actually, only about 1 to 3 L is excreted each day as urine. The rest is reabsorbed back into the circulatory system (McCance et al., 2014).

GFR is controlled by blood pressure and blood flow. The kidneys self-regulate their own blood pressure and blood flow, which keeps GFR constant. GFR is controlled by selectively constricting and dilating the afferent and efferent arterioles. When the afferent arteriole is constricted or the efferent arteriole is dilated, pressure in the glomerular capillaries falls and filtration decreases. When the afferent arteriole is dilated or the efferent arteriole is constricted, pressure in the glomerular capillaries rises and filtration increases. This way the kidney maintains a constant GFR, even when systemic blood pressure changes. When systolic pressure drops below 65 to 70 mm Hg, these self-regulation processes are not effective at maintaining GFR.

Tubular reabsorption is the second process in urine formation. This reabsorption of most of the filtrate keeps normal urine output at 1 to 3 L/day and prevents dehydration. As the filtrate passes through the tubular parts of the nephron, most of the water and electrolytes is reabsorbed from the tubular lumen of the nephron and into the peritubular capillaries. This process returns most water, electrolytes, and other particles to the blood.

TABLE 65-1 Vascular and Tubular Components of the Nephron

STRUCTURE	ANATOMIC FEATURES	PHYSIOLOGIC ASPECTS
Vascular Components		
Afferent arteriole	Delivers arterial blood from the branches of the renal artery into the glomerulus	Autoregulation of renal blood flow via vasoconstriction or vasodilation Renin-producing granular cells
Glomerulus	Capillary loops with thin, semipermeable membrane	Site of glomerular filtration Glomerular filtration occurs when hydrostatic pressure (blood pressure) is greater than opposing forces (tubular filtrate and oncotic pressure)
Efferent arteriole	Delivers arterial blood from the glomerulus into the peritubular capillaries or the vasa recta	Autoregulation of renal blood flow via vasoconstriction or vasodilation Renin-producing granular cells
Peritubular capillaries (PTCs) and vasa recta (VR)	PTCs: surround tubular components of cortical nephrons VR: surround tubular components of juxtamedullary nephrons	Tubular reabsorption and tubular secretion allow movement of water and solutes to or from the tubules, interstitium, and blood
Tubular Components		
Bowman's capsule (BC)	Thin membranous sac surrounding ⅞ of the glomerulus	Collects glomerular filtrate (GF) and funnels it into the tubule
Proximal convoluted tubule (PCT)	Evolves from and is continuous with Bowman's capsule Specialized cellular lining facilitates tubular reabsorption	Site for reabsorption of sodium, chloride, water, glucose, amino acids, potassium, calcium, bicarbonate, phosphate, and urea
Loop of Henle	Continues from PCT Juxtamedullary nephrons dip deep into the medulla Permeable to water, urea, and sodium chloride	Regulation of water balance
Descending limb (DL)	Continues from the loop of Henle Permeable to water, urea, and sodium chloride	Regulation of water balance
Ascending limb (AL)	Emerges from DL as it turns and is redirected up toward the renal cortex	Potassium and magnesium reabsorption in the thick segment Thin segment is impermeable to water
Distal convoluted tubule (DCT)	Evolves from AL and twists so the macula densa cells lie adjacent to the juxtaglomerular cells of afferent arteriole	Site of additional water and electrolyte reabsorption, including bicarbonate Potassium and hydrogen secretion
Collecting ducts	Collect formed urine from several tubules and deliver it into the renal pelvis	Receptor sites for antidiuretic hormone regulation of water balance

The tubules return about 99% of all filtered water back into the body (Fig. 65-7). Most water reabsorption occurs in the PCT. Water reabsorption continues as the filtrate flows down the descending loop of Henle. The thin and thick segments of the ascending loop of Henle are *not* permeable to water, and water reabsorption does not occur here.

The distal convoluted tubule (DCT) can be permeable to water, and some water reabsorption occurs as the filtrate continues to flow through the tubule. The membrane of the DCT may be made more permeable to water when *vasopressin,* also known as *antidiuretic hormone* (ADH), and aldosterone are present. Vasopressin increases tubular permeability to water, allowing water to leave the tube and be reabsorbed back into the capillaries. Vasopressin also increases arteriole constriction. Arteriole constriction alters blood pressure, which then affects the amounts of fluid and particles that exit glomerular capillaries. Aldosterone promotes the reabsorption of sodium in the DCT. Water reabsorption occurs as a result of the movement of sodium (where sodium goes, water follows).

The ability of the kidneys to vary the volume or concentration of urine helps regulate water balance regardless of fluid intake. In this way, the healthy kidney can prevent dehydration when fluid intake is low and can prevent circulatory overload when fluid intake is high.

In addition to water, some types of particles in the tubular filtrate also are returned to the blood by *tubular reabsorption.* About 50% of all urea in the filtrate is reabsorbed, although creatinine is not reabsorbed.

Most sodium, chloride, and water reabsorption occurs in the PCT. The collecting ducts are the other site of sodium, chloride, and water reabsorption. Here reabsorption is caused by aldosterone. Potassium is mostly reabsorbed in the PCT and in the thick segment of the loop of Henle.

Bicarbonate, calcium, and phosphate are mostly reabsorbed in the PCT. Bicarbonate reabsorption helps ACID-BASE BALANCE and maintains a normal blood pH. Blood levels of calcitonin and parathyroid hormone (PTH) (see Chapters 11 and 63) control calcium balance.

The kidney reabsorbs some of the glucose filtered from the blood. However, there is a limit to how much glucose the kidney can reabsorb. This limit is called the **renal threshold** or **transport maximum (tm)** for glucose reabsorption. The usual renal threshold for glucose is about 220 mg/dL. This means that at a blood glucose level of 220 mg/dL or less, all glucose is reabsorbed and returned to the blood, with no glucose present in final urine. When blood glucose levels are greater than 220 mg/dL, some glucose stays in the filtrate and is present in the urine. Normally, almost all glucose and most proteins are reabsorbed and are not present in the urine.

TABLE 65-2 Kidney Hormones and Hormones Influencing Kidney Function

	SITE	ACTION
Kidney Hormones		
Renin	Renin-producing granular cells	Raises blood pressure as result of angiotensin (local vasoconstriction) and aldosterone (volume expansion) secretion
Prostaglandins	Kidney tissues	Regulate intrarenal blood flow by vasodilation or vasoconstriction
Bradykinins	Juxtaglomerular cells of the arterioles	Increase blood flow (vasodilation) and vascular permeability
Erythropoietin	Kidney parenchyma	Stimulates bone marrow to make red blood cells
Activated vitamin D	Kidney parenchyma	Promotes absorption of calcium in the GI tract
Hormones Influencing Kidney Function		
Vasopressin (Antidiuretic hormone [ADH])	Released from posterior pituitary	Makes DCT and CD permeable to water to maximize reabsorption and produce a concentrated urine
Aldosterone	Released from adrenal cortex	Promotes sodium reabsorption and potassium secretion in DCT and CD; water and chloride follow sodium movement
Natriuretic hormones	Cardiac atria, cardiac ventricles, brain	Cause tubular secretion of sodium

CD, Collecting duct; *DCT,* distal convoluted tubule.

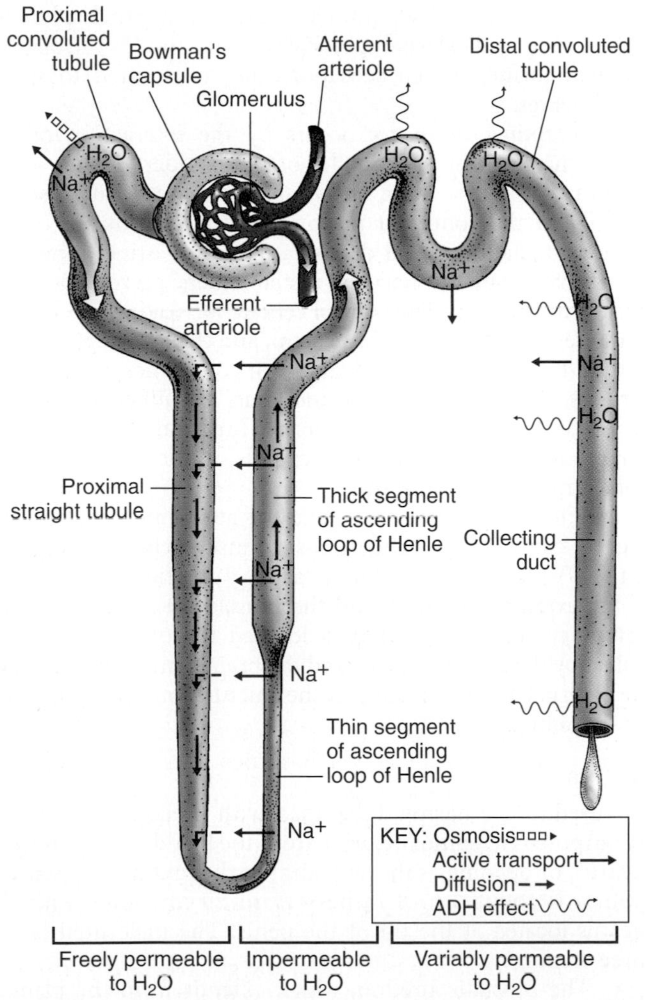

FIG. 65-7 Sodium and water reabsorption by the tubules of a cortical nephron. *ADH,* Antidiuretic hormone; *Na⁺,* sodium.

! NURSING SAFETY PRIORITY QSEN

Action Alert

Report the presence of glucose or proteins in the urine of a patient undergoing a screening examination to the health care provider because this is an abnormal finding and requires further assessment.

Tubular secretion is the third process of urine formation. It allows substances to move from the blood into the early urine. During tubular secretion, substances move from the peritubular capillaries in reverse, across capillary membranes, and into the cells that line the tubules. From the cells, these substances are moved into the urine and are excreted from the body. Potassium (K^+) and hydrogen (H^+) ions are some of the substances moved in this way to maintain FLUID AND ELECTROLYTE BALANCE and ACID-BASE BALANCE (pH).

Hormonal Functions. The kidneys produce renin, prostaglandins, erythropoietin, and activated vitamin D (Table 65-2). Other kidney products, such as the kinins, change kidney blood flow and capillary permeability. The kidneys also help break down and excrete insulin.

Renin, as discussed on p. 1346 in the Microscopic Anatomy section, assists in blood pressure control. It is formed and released when there is a decrease in blood flow, blood volume, or blood pressure through the renal arterioles or when too little sodium is present in kidney blood. These conditions are detected through the receptors of the juxtaglomerular complex.

Renin release causes the production of *angiotensin II* through a series of steps (see Fig. 65-5). Angiotensin II increases systemic blood pressure through powerful blood vessel constricting effects and triggers the release of aldosterone from the adrenal glands. Aldosterone increases the reabsorption of sodium in the distal tubule of the nephron. Therefore more water is reabsorbed, which increases blood volume and blood pressure. When blood flow to the kidney is reduced, this system also prevents fluid loss and maintains circulating blood volume (see Chapter 11).

Prostaglandins are produced in the kidney and many other tissues. Those produced specifically in the kidney help regulate glomerular filtration, kidney vascular resistance, and renin production. They also increase sodium and water excretion.

Erythropoietin is produced and released in response to decreased oxygen tension in the kidney's blood supply. It triggers red blood cell (RBC) production in the bone marrow. When kidney function is poor, erythropoietin production decreases and the person develops anemia.

Vitamin D activation occurs through a series of steps. Some of these steps take place in the skin when it is exposed to sunlight, and then more processing occurs in the liver. From there, vitamin D is converted to its active form in the kidney. Activated vitamin D is needed to absorb calcium in the intestinal tract and to regulate calcium balance (McCance et al., 2014).

Ureters

Each kidney has a single ureter—a hollow tube that connects the renal pelvis with the urinary bladder. The ureter is about ½ inch (1.25 cm) in diameter and about 12 to 18 inches (30 to 45 cm) in length. The diameter of the ureter narrows in three areas:

- In the upper third of the ureter, at the point in which the renal pelvis becomes the ureter, is a narrowing known as the **ureteropelvic junction (UPJ)**.
- The ureter also narrows as it bends toward the abdominal wall (aortoiliac bend).
- Each ureter narrows at the point it enters the bladder; this point is called the **ureterovesical junction (UVJ)**.

The ureter tunnels through bladder tissue for a short distance and then opens into the bladder at the trigone (Fig. 65-8).

The ureter has three layers: an inner lining of mucous membrane *(urothelium)*, a middle layer of smooth muscle fibers, and an outer layer of fibrous tissue. The middle layer of muscle fibers is controlled by several nerve pathways from the lower spinal cord.

Contractions of the smooth muscle in the ureter move urine from the kidney pelvis to the bladder. Stretch receptors in the kidney pelvis regulate this movement. For example, a large volume of urine in the kidney pelvis triggers the stretch receptors, which respond by increasing ureteral contractions and ureter peristalsis.

Urinary Bladder

Structure

The urinary bladder is a muscular sac (see Fig. 65-8) that lies directly behind the pubic bone. In men, the bladder is in front of the rectum. In women, it is in front of the vagina.

The bladder is composed of the *body* (the rounded sac portion) and the *bladder neck* (posterior urethra), which connects to the bladder body. The bladder has three linings—an inner lining of epithelial cells *(urothelium)*, middle layers of smooth muscle *(detrusor muscle)*, and an outer lining. The *trigone* is an area on the posterior wall between the points of ureteral entry (ureterovesical junctions [UVJs]) and the urethra.

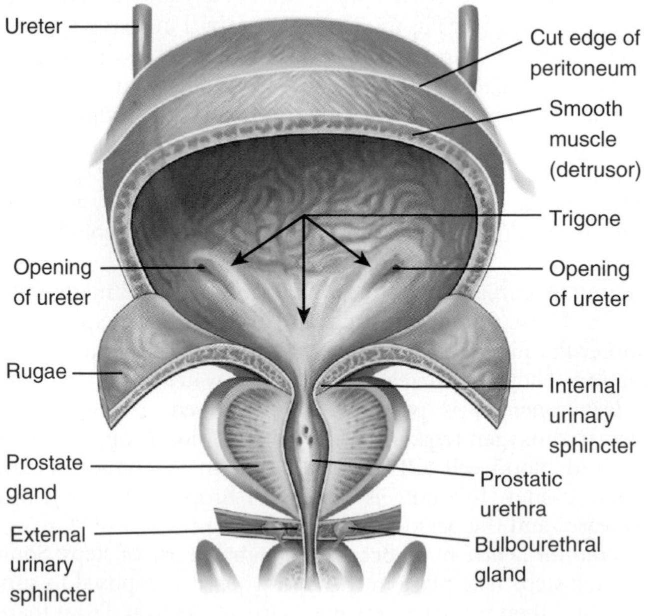

FIG. 65-8 Gross anatomy of the urinary bladder.

The **internal urethral sphincter** is the smooth detrusor muscle of the bladder neck and elastic tissue. The **external urethral sphincter** is skeletal muscle that surrounds the urethra. In men, the external sphincter surrounds the urethra at the base of the prostate gland. In women, the external sphincter is at the base of the bladder. The pudendal nerve from the spinal cord controls the external sphincter.

Function

The bladder stores urine, provides continence, and enables voiding. The secretions of the urothelium lining the bladder resist bacteria.

Continence is the ability to voluntarily control bladder emptying. Continence occurs during bladder filling through the combination of detrusor muscle relaxation, internal sphincter muscle tone, and external sphincter contraction. As the bladder fills with urine, stretch sensations are transmitted to spinal sacral nerves.

Maintaining continence occurs by the interaction of the nerves that control the muscles of the bladder, bladder neck, urethra, and pelvic floor, as well as by factors that close the urethra. In the continent person, the smooth muscle of the detrusor remains relaxed during a period of urine filling and storage. Sympathetic nervous system fibers prevent detrusor muscle contraction. The control centers for voiding are located in the cerebral cortex, the brainstem, and the lower spinal cord. For urethral closure to be adequate for continence, the mucosal surfaces must be in contact and must be adhesive. Contact depends on the presence and proper function of the involved nerves and muscles. Adhesion depends on the adequate secretion of mucus-like substances.

Micturition (voiding) is a reflex of autonomic control that triggers contraction of the detrusor muscle (closing the ureter at the UVJ to prevent backflow) at the same time as relaxation of the external sphincter and the muscles of the pelvic floor. Voluntary voiding occurs as a learned response and is controlled by the cerebral cortex and the brainstem. Contraction of the external sphincter inhibits the micturition reflex and prevents voiding.

Urethra

The urethra is a narrow tube lined with mucous membranes. Its purpose is to eliminate urine from the bladder. The **urethral meatus**, or opening, is the end point of the urethra. In men, the urethra is about 6 to 8 inches (15 to 20 cm) long, with the meatus located at the tip of the penis. The male urethra has three sections:

- The prostatic urethra, which extends from the bladder through the prostate gland
- The membranous urethra, which extends from the prostate to the wall of the pelvic floor
- The cavernous urethra, which is external and extends through the length of the penis

In women, the urethra is about 1 to 1½ inches (2.5 to 3.75 cm) long and exits the bladder through the pelvic floor. The meatus lies slightly below the clitoris and directly in front of the vagina and rectum.

Kidney and Urinary System Changes Associated with Aging

Kidney Changes

Changes occur in the kidney as a result of the aging process and can affect health (Chart 65-1) (Touhy & Jett, 2014). The kidney loses cortical tissue and gets smaller with age. This cortical loss is caused by reduced blood flow to the kidney. The medulla is not affected by aging, and the juxtamedullary nephron functions are preserved. The glomerular and tubular linings thicken. Both the number of glomeruli and their surface areas decrease with aging. Tubule length decreases. These changes reduce the ability of the older adult to filter blood and excrete waste products.

Blood flow to the kidney declines by about 10% per decade as blood vessels thicken. This means that blood flow to the kidney is not as adaptive in older adults, leaving nephrons more vulnerable to damage during episodes of either hypotension or hypertension.

Glomerular filtration rate (GFR) decreases with age. By age 65 years, the GFR is about 65 mL/min (half the rate of a young adult) and increases the risk for fluid overload. This decline is more rapid in patients with diabetes, hypertension, or heart failure. The combination of reduced kidney mass, reduced blood flow, and decreased GFR contributes to reduced drug clearance and a greater risk for drug reactions and kidney damage from drugs and contrast dyes in older adults.

Tubular changes with aging decrease the ability to concentrate urine, resulting in **urgency** (a sense of a nearly uncontrollable need to urinate) and **nocturnal polyuria** (increased urination at night). The regulation of sodium, acids, and bicarbonate is less efficient. Along with an age-related impairment in the thirst mechanism, these changes increase the risk for disturbances of FLUID AND ELECTROLYTE BALANCE, such as dehydration and **hypernatremia** (increased blood sodium levels) in the older adult. Hormonal changes include a decrease in renin secretion, aldosterone levels, and activation of vitamin D.

Urinary Changes

Changes in detrusor muscle elasticity lead to decreased bladder capacity and reduced ability to retain urine. The urge to void may cause immediate bladder emptying because the urinary sphincters lose tone and often become weaker with age. In women, weakened muscles in the pelvic floor shorten the urethra and promote incontinence. In men, an enlarged prostate gland makes starting the urine stream difficult and may cause urinary retention.

CULTURAL CONSIDERATIONS

Patient-Centered Care QSEN

African Americans have more rapid age-related decreases in GFR than do white people. Kidney excretion of sodium is less effective in hypertensive African Americans who have high sodium intake, and the kidneys have about 20% less blood flow as a result of anatomic changes in small blood vessels and intrarenal responses to renin. Thus African-American patients are at greater risk for kidney failure than are white patients (Jarvis, 2016). Remind African Americans that yearly health examinations should include urinalysis, checking for the presence of microalbuminuria, and evaluating serum creatinine.

CHART 65-1 Nursing Focus on the Older Adult

Changes in the Renal System Related to Aging

PHYSIOLOGIC CHANGE	NURSING INTERVENTIONS	RATIONALES
Decreased glomerular filtration rate (GFR)	Monitor hydration status.	The ability of the kidneys to regulate water balance decreases with age.
	Ensure adequate fluid intake.	The kidneys are less able to conserve water when necessary.
	Administer potentially nephrotoxic agents or drugs carefully.	Dehydration reduces kidney blood flow and increases the nephrotoxic potential of many agents. Acute or chronic kidney failure may result.
Nocturia	Ensure adequate nighttime lighting and a hazard-free environment.	Falls and injuries are common among older patients seeking bathroom facilities.
	Ensure the availability of a bedside toilet, bedpan, or urinal.	Using these items instead of getting up to the bathroom can help prevent falls.
	Discourage excessive fluid intake for 2-4 hr before the patient goes to bed.	Excessive fluid intake at night may increase nocturia.
	Evaluate drugs and timing.	Some drugs increase urine output.
Decreased bladder capacity	Encourage the patient to use the toilet, bedpan, or urinal at least every 2 hr.	Emptying the bladder on a regular basis may avoid overflow urinary incontinence.
	Respond as soon as possible to the patient's indication of the need to void.	A quick response may alleviate episodes of urinary stress incontinence.
Weakened urinary sphincters and shortened urethra in women	Provide thorough perineal care after each voiding.	The shortened urethra increases the potential for bladder infections.
		Good perineal hygiene may prevent skin irritations and urinary tract infection (UTI).
Tendency to retain urine	Observe the patient for urinary retention (e.g., bladder distention) or urinary tract infection (e.g., dysuria, foul odor, confusion).	Urinary stasis may result in a UTI, which may lead to bloodstream infections, urosepsis, or septic shock.
	Provide privacy, assistance, and voiding stimulants such as warm water over the perineum as needed.	Nursing interventions can help initiate voiding.
	Evaluate drugs for possible contribution to retention.	Anticholinergic drugs promote urinary retention.

ASSESSMENT METHODS

Patient History

Demographic information, such as age, gender, race, and ethnicity, is important to consider as nonmodifiable risk factors in the patient with any kidney or urinary problem. A sudden onset of hypertension in patients older than 50 years suggests possible kidney disease. Clinical changes with adult polycystic kidney disease typically occur in patients in their 40s or 50s. In men older than 50 years, altered urine patterns accompany prostate disease.

Anatomic gender differences make some disorders worse or more common. For example, men rarely have ascending urinary tract infections. Women have a shorter urethra and more commonly develop cystitis (bladder inflammation, most often with infection) because bacteria pass more readily into the bladder.

Ask the patient about any previous kidney or urologic problems, including tumors, infections, stones, or urologic surgery. A history of any chronic health problems, especially diabetes mellitus or hypertension, increases the risk for development of kidney disease because these disorders damage kidney blood vessels.

Exposure to certain dyes during imaging can harm the kidneys. Iodinated contrast used for CT scans is associated with both acute and chronic kidney damage. High osmolarity contrast agents can also contribute to kidney function impairment. Exposure to gadolinium-enhanced MRI can result in nephrogenic systemic fibrosis.

Ask the patient about chemical exposures at the workplace or with hobbies. Exposure to hydrocarbons (e.g., gasoline, oil), heavy metals (especially mercury and lead), and some gases (e.g., chlorine, toluene) can impair kidney function. Use this opportunity to teach patients who come into contact with chemicals at work or during leisure-time activities to avoid direct skin or mucous membrane contact with these chemicals. Use of heroin, cocaine, methamphetamine, ecstasy, and volatile solvents (inhalants) has also been associated with kidney damage.

Specifically ask the patient whether he or she has ever been told about the presence of protein or albumin in the urine. The question "Have you ever been told that your blood pressure is high?" may prompt a response different from the one to the question "Do you have high blood pressure?" Ask women about health problems during pregnancy (e.g., proteinuria, high blood pressure, gestational diabetes, urinary tract infections). Obtain information about:

- Chemical or environmental toxin exposure in occupational, diagnostic, or other settings
- Recent travel to geographic regions that pose infectious disease risks
- Recent trauma or injury, particularly to the abdomen or pelvic or genital areas
- A history of altered patterns of urinary ELIMINATION

Socioeconomic status may influence health care practices. Prevention, early detection, and treatment of kidney or urinary problems may be limited by lack of insurance or access to health care, lack of transportation, and reduced income. Low income may also result in difficulty following medical advice, having prescriptions filled, adhering to dietary instructions, and keeping follow-up appointments.

Education level may affect health-seeking practices and the patient's understanding of a disease or its manifestations. Recurring urinary tract infections can result from not completing a course of antibiotic therapy or from not following up to ensure the infection is cleared and risks are well-managed.

The patient's health beliefs affect the approach to health and illness. Cultural background or religious affiliation may influence the belief system.

The language used by patients may be different from that used by the health care professional. When obtaining a history, listen to and explore the terms used by the patient. By using the patient's own terms, you may help him or her provide a more complete description of the problem and may decrease the patient's discomfort when discussing bodily functions.

Nutrition History

Ask the patient with known or suspected kidney or urologic disorders about his or her usual diet and any recent changes in the diet. Note any excessive intake or omission of certain food categories. Ask about food and fluid intake. Assess how much and what types of fluids the patient drinks daily, especially fluids with a high calorie or caffeine content. Use this opportunity to teach the patient the importance of drinking sufficient fluid to cause urine to be dilute (clear or very light yellow). If another medical problem does not require fluid restriction, health care providers recommend about 2 liters of fluid daily to prevent dehydration and cystitis. If the patient has followed a diet for weight reduction, the details of the diet plan are important and collaboration with a dietitian may be needed. A high-protein intake can result in temporary kidney problems. For example, a patient at risk for calculi (stone) formation who ingests large amounts of protein or has a poor fluid intake may form new stones.

Ask about any change in appetite or taste. These manifestations can occur with the buildup of nitrogenous waste products from kidney impairment. Changes in thirst or fluid intake may also cause changes in urine output. Endocrine disorders may also cause changes in thirst, fluid intake, and urine output. (See Chapter 61 for a discussion of endocrine influences on fluid balance.)

Medication History

Identify all of the patient's prescription drugs because many can impair kidney function. Ask about the duration of drug use and whether there have been any recent changes in prescribed drugs. Drugs for diabetes mellitus, hypertension, cardiac disorders, hormonal disorders, cancer, arthritis, and psychiatric disorders are potential causes of kidney problems. Antibiotics, such as gentamicin (Garamycin, Cidomycin 🍁), may also cause acute kidney injury. Drug-drug interactions and drug–contrast dye interactions also may lead to kidney dysfunction.

Explore the past and current use of over-the-counter (OTC) drugs or agents, including dietary supplements, vitamins and minerals, herbal agents, laxatives, analgesics, acetaminophen, and NSAIDs. Many of these agents affect kidney function. For example, dietary supplementation with synthetic creatine, used to increase muscle mass, has been associated with compromised kidney function. High-dose or long-term use of NSAIDs or acetaminophen can seriously reduce kidney function. Some agents are associated with hypertension, hematuria, or proteinuria, which may occur before kidney dysfunction.

Family History and Genetic Risk

The family history of the patient with a suspected kidney or urologic problem is important because some disorders have a familial inheritance pattern. Ask whether his or her siblings, parents, or grandparents have had kidney problems. Past terms used for kidney disease include *Bright's disease, nephritis,* and *nephrosis.* Although nephritis is a current term describing an inflammatory process in the kidney and nephrosis is a current term describing a degenerative process in the kidney, these terms have been used by lay people for years to describe any kidney problem. Adult polycystic kidney disease, which is a genetic disorder, can occur in either gender.

Current Health Problem

The effects of severe kidney impairment are evident in all body systems. Therefore document all of the patient's current health problems. Ask him or her to describe all health concerns, because some kidney disorders cause systemic problems or problems in other body systems. Recent upper respiratory problems, achy muscles or joints, or GI problems may be related to problems of kidney function.

Assess the kidney and urologic system by asking about any changes in the appearance (color, odor, clarity) of the urine, pattern of urination, ability to initiate or control voiding, and other unusual manifestations. For example, urine that is reddish, dark brown or black, greenish, or different from the usual yellowish color usually prompts the patient to seek health care assistance. Urine typically has a mild but distinct odor of ammonia. An increase in the intensity of color, a change in odor quality, or a decrease in urine clarity may suggest infection.

Ask about changes in urination patterns, such as **incontinence** (involuntary bladder emptying), **nocturia** (urination at night), frequency, or an increase or decrease in the amount of urine. The normal urine output for adults is about 1500 to 2000 mL/day or within 500 mL of the volume of fluid ingested daily. Ask about how close the urine output is to the volume of fluid ingested. The patient usually does not know the exact amount of urine produced. A bladder diary may provide useful data. Also ask whether:

- Initiating urine flow is difficult
- A burning sensation or other discomfort occurs with urination
- The force of the urine stream is decreased (in men)
- Persistent dribbling of urine is present

The onset of pain in the flank, in the lower abdomen or pelvic region, or in the perineal area usually triggers concern and may prompt the patient to seek assistance. Ask about the onset, intensity, and duration of the pain, its location, and its association with any activity or event.

Pain associated with kidney or ureteral irritation is often severe and spasmodic. Pain that radiates into the perineal area, groin, scrotum, or labia is described as *renal colic.* This pain occurs with distention or spasm of the ureter, such as in an obstruction or the passing of a stone. Renal colic pain may be intermittent or continuous and may occur with pallor, diaphoresis, and hypotension. These general manifestations occur because of the location of the nerve tracts near or in the kidneys and ureters.

Because the kidneys are close to the GI organs and the nerve pathways are similar, GI manifestations may occur with kidney problems. These renointestinal reflexes often complicate the description of the kidney problem.

Uremia is the buildup of nitrogenous waste products in the blood as a result of some degree of kidney impairment. Manifestations include anorexia, nausea and vomiting, muscle cramps, **pruritus** (itching), fatigue, and lethargy.

Physical Assessment

The physical assessment of the patient with a known or suspected kidney or urologic disorder includes general appearance, a review of body systems, and specific structure and functions of the kidney and urinary system.

Assess the patient's general appearance, and check the skin for the presence of any rashes, bruising, or yellowish discoloration. The skin and tissues may show edema, especially in the **pedal** (foot), **pretibial** (shin), and sacral tissues and around the eyes. Use a stethoscope to listen to the lungs to determine whether fluid is present. Weigh the patient and measure blood pressure as a baseline for later comparisons.

Assess the level of consciousness and level of alertness. Record any deficits in memory, concentration, or thought processes. Family members may report subtle changes. Cognitive changes may be the result of the buildup of waste products when kidney disease is present.

Assessment of the Kidneys, Ureters, and Bladder

Assess the kidneys, ureters, and bladder during an abdominal assessment (Jarvis, 2016). Auscultate before percussion and palpation because these activities can enhance bowel sounds and obscure abdominal vascular sounds.

Inspect the abdomen and the flank regions with the patient in both the supine and the sitting positions. Observe the patient for asymmetry (e.g., swelling) or discoloration (e.g., bruising or redness) in the flank region, especially in the area of the costovertebral angle (CVA). The CVA is located between the lower portion of the twelfth rib and the vertebral column.

Listen for a bruit by placing a stethoscope over each renal artery on the midclavicular line. A **bruit** is an audible swishing sound produced when the volume of blood or the diameter of the blood vessel changes. It often occurs with blood flow through a narrowed vessel, as in renal artery stenosis.

Kidney palpation is usually performed by a physician or advanced practice nurse. It can help locate masses and areas of tenderness in or around the kidney. Lightly palpate the abdomen in all quadrants. Ask about areas of tenderness or pain, and examine nontender areas first. The outline of the bladder may be seen as high as the umbilicus in patients with severe bladder distention. *If tumor or aneurysm is suspected, palpation may harm the patient.*

Because the kidneys are located deep and posterior, palpation is easier in thin patients who have little abdominal musculature. For palpation of the right kidney, the patient is in a supine position while the examiner places one hand under the right flank and the other hand over the abdomen below the lower right part of the rib cage. The lower hand is used to raise the flank, and the upper hand depresses the abdomen as the patient takes a deep breath (Fig. 65-9) (Jarvis, 2016). The left kidney is deeper and often cannot be palpated. A transplanted kidney is readily palpated in either the lower right or left abdominal quadrant. The normal kidney is smooth, firm, and nontender.

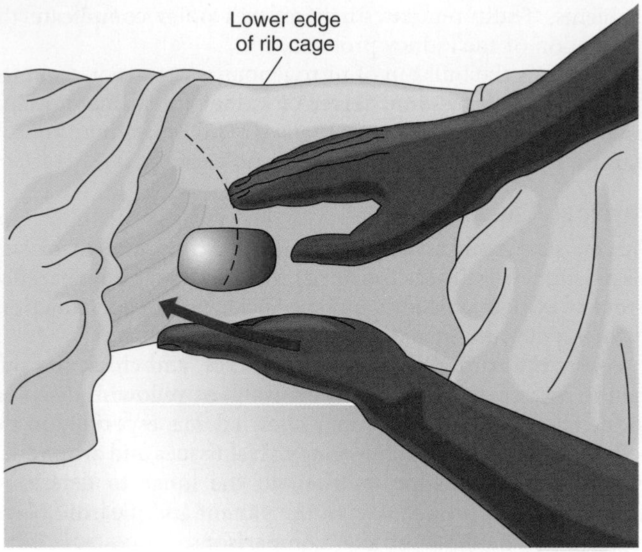

FIG. 65-9 Advanced technique for palpation of the kidney.

A distended bladder sounds dull when percussed. After gently palpating to determine the outline of the distended bladder, begin percussion on the lower abdomen and continue in the direction of the umbilicus until dull sounds are no longer produced. If you suspect bladder distention, use a portable bladder scanner to determine the amount of retained urine.

If the patient reports flank pain or tenderness, percuss the nontender flank first. Have the patient assume a sitting, side-lying, or supine position, and then form one of your hands into a clenched fist. Place your other hand flat over the CVA of the patient. Then quickly deliver a firm thump to your hand over the CVA area (Jarvis, 2016). Costovertebral tenderness often occurs with kidney infection or inflammation. Patients with inflammation or infection in the kidney or nearby structures may describe their pain as severe or as a constant, dull ache.

Assessment of the Urethra

Using a good light source and wearing gloves, inspect the urethra by examining the meatus and the tissues around it. Record any unusual discharge such as blood, mucus, or pus. Inspect the skin and mucous membranes of surrounding tissues. Record the presence of lesions, rashes, or other abnormalities of the penis or scrotum or of the labia or vaginal opening. Urethral irritation is suspected when the patient reports discomfort with urination. Use this opportunity to remind women to clean the perineum by wiping from front to back, never from back to front. Teach them that the front-to-back technique keeps organisms in stool from coming close to the urethra and decreases the risk for infection.

GENDER HEALTH CONSIDERATIONS

Patient-Centered Care QSEN

Women from other cultures may have undergone female circumcision. This procedure alters the anatomic appearance of the vulvar-perineal area and increases the risk for urinary tract infections. It also makes urethral inspection or catheterization difficult. Document any noted anatomic changes, and ask the patient to describe her hygiene practices for this area.

Psychosocial Assessment

Concerns about the urologic system may evoke fear, anger, embarrassment, anxiety, guilt, or sadness in the patient. Childhood learning often includes privacy with regard to toilet habits. Urologic disorders may bring up forgotten memories of difficult toilet training and bedwetting or of childhood experiences of exploring one's body. The patient may ignore manifestations or delay seeking health care because of emotional responses or cultural taboos about the urogenital area.

NCLEX EXAMINATION CHALLENGE

Health Promotion and Maintenance

The client arrives at the primary health care clinic with a problem of new abdominal pain and blood in her urine. She is afebrile. Which information is most important for the nurse to obtain from this client's history?

A. Kidney cancer in the client's family
B. Injury or trauma to the abdomen or pelvis
C. Treatment for a urinary tract infection in the past 12 months
D. Recent exposure to heavy metals, drugs, or other nephrotoxins

Diagnostic Assessment

Laboratory Assessment

Blood Tests. *Serum creatinine* is produced when muscle and other proteins are broken down. Because protein breakdown is usually constant, the serum creatinine level is a good indicator of kidney function. Serum creatinine levels are slightly higher in men than in women because men tend to have a larger muscle mass than do women. Similarly, people with greater muscle mass or muscle mass turnover (e.g., athletes) may have a slightly-higher-than-average serum creatinine level. Muscle mass and the amount of creatinine produced decrease with age. Because of decreased rates of creatinine clearance, however, the serum creatinine level remains relatively constant in older adults unless kidney disease is present.

No common pathologic condition other than kidney disease increases the serum creatinine level. The serum creatinine level does not increase until at least 50% of the kidney function is lost, and therefore *any* elevation of serum creatinine values is important and should be assessed further. Creatinine is excreted by the kidneys.

NURSING SAFETY PRIORITY QSEN

Action Alert

A serum creatinine of 1.5 mg/dL or greater places a patient at risk for acute kidney injury (AKI) from iodinated contrast dyes and some drugs. Monitor both baseline and trend values to determine risk for and actual kidney damage, especially among patients exposed to agents that can cause kidney dysfunction. Promptly inform the health care provider of increases in serum creatinine greater than 1.5 times the baseline and urine output values of less than 0.5 mL/kg/hr for 6 or more hours.

Blood urea nitrogen (BUN) measures the effectiveness of kidney excretion of urea nitrogen, a by-product of protein breakdown in the liver. Urea nitrogen is produced mostly from liver metabolism of food sources of protein. The kidneys filter urea nitrogen from the blood and excrete the waste in urine.

CHART 65-2 Laboratory Profile

Kidney Function Blood Studies

TEST	NORMAL RANGE FOR ADULTS	SIGNIFICANCE OF ABNORMAL FINDINGS
Serum creatinine	*Males:* 0.6-1.2 mg/dL (0.053-0.106 mmol/L; 53-106 μmol/L) *Females:* 0.5-1.1 mg/dL (0.044-0.097 mmol/L; 44-97μmol/L) *Older adults:* may be decreased	An *increased level* indicates kidney impairment. A *decreased level* may be caused by a decreased muscle mass.
Blood urea nitrogen (BUN)	10-20 mg/dL (3.6-7.1 mmol/L) *Older adults:* 60-90 yr: 8-23 mg/dL (2.9-8.2 mmol/L) Older than 90 yr: 10-31 mg/dL (3.6-11.1 mmol/L)	An *increased level* may indicate liver or kidney disease, dehydration or decreased kidney perfusion, a high-protein diet, infection, stress, steroid use, GI bleeding, or other situations in which blood is in body tissues. A *decreased level* may indicate malnutrition, fluid volume excess, or severe hepatic damage.
BUN/creatinine ratio	6-25 (BUN divided by creatinine)	An *increased ratio* may indicate fluid volume deficit, obstructive uropathy, catabolic state, or a high-protein diet. A *decreased ratio* may indicate fluid volume excess.

Data from Pagana, K., & Pagana, T. (2014). *Mosby's manual of diagnostic and laboratory tests* (5th ed.). St. Louis: Mosby.

Other factors influence the BUN level, and an elevation does not always mean kidney disease is present (Chart 65-2). For example, rapid cell destruction from infection, cancer treatment, or steroid therapy may elevate BUN level. In addition, blood is a protein. Blood in the tissues rather than in the blood vessels is reabsorbed as if it were a general protein. Thus reabsorbed blood protein is processed by the liver and increases BUN levels. This means that injured tissues can result in increased BUN levels even when kidney function is normal. Also, BUN is increased by protein turnover in exercising muscle and is elevated as a result of concentration during dehydration.

The liver must function properly to produce urea nitrogen. When liver and kidney dysfunction are present, urea nitrogen levels are actually *decreased* because the liver failure limits urea production. The BUN level is not always elevated with kidney disease and is not the best indicator of kidney function. However, an elevated BUN level suggests kidney dysfunction.

Blood urea nitrogen to serum creatinine ratio can help determine whether non–kidney-related factors, such as low cardiac output or red blood cell destruction, are causing the elevated BUN level. When blood volume is deficient (e.g., dehydration) or cardiac output is low, the BUN level rises more rapidly than the serum creatinine level. As a result, the ratio of BUN to creatinine is *increased.*

When both the BUN and serum creatinine levels increase at the same rate, the BUN/creatinine ratio remains normal. However, elevations of ***both*** serum creatinine and BUN levels suggest kidney dysfunction that is not related to dehydration or poor perfusion.

Blood osmolarity is a measure of the overall concentration of particles in the blood and is a good indicator of hydration status. The kidneys excrete or reabsorb water to keep blood osmolarity in the range of 285 to 295 mOsm/L. Osmolarity is slightly higher in older adults (285 to 301 mOsm/L). When blood osmolarity is decreased, the release of vasopressin (antidiuretic hormone [ADH]) is inhibited. Without vasopressin, the distal tubule and collecting ducts are *not* permeable to water. As a result, water is *excreted,* not reabsorbed, and blood osmolarity increases. When blood osmolarity increases, vasopressin is released. Vasopressin increases the permeability of the distal tubule to water. Then water is reabsorbed and blood osmolarity decreases.

Urine Tests

Urinalysis. Urinalysis is a part of any complete physical examination and is especially useful for patients with suspected kidney or urologic disorders (Chart 65-3). Ideally, the urine specimen is collected at the morning's first voiding. Specimens obtained at other times may be too dilute. The specimen may be collected by several techniques (Table 65-3).

Urine color comes from urochrome pigment. Color variations may result from increased levels of urochrome or other pigments, changes in the concentration or dilution of the urine, and the presence of drug metabolites in the urine. Urine smells faintly like ammonia and is normally clear without *turbidity* (cloudiness) or haziness.

Specific gravity is the concentration of particles, including electrolytes and wastes, in urine. A high specific gravity indicates concentrated urine, such as might occur from dehydration, decreased kidney blood flow, or excess vasopressin associated with stress, surgery, anesthetic agents, and certain drugs (e.g., morphine, some oral antidiabetic drugs) or syndrome of inappropriate antidiuretic hormone (SIADH) (see Chapter 62). A low specific gravity indicates dilute urine that may occur from high fluid intake, diuretic drugs, or diabetes insipidus (DI) (see Chapter 62).

Specific gravity refers to the density of urine compared with distilled water, which has a specific gravity of 1.000. The normal specific gravity of urine ranges from 1.005 to about 1.030. Kidney disease diminishes the concentrating ability of the kidney, and chronic kidney disease (CKD) may be associated with a low (dilute) specific gravity.

pH is a measure of urine acidity or alkalinity. A pH value less than 7 is acidic, and a value greater than 7 is alkaline. Urine pH is affected by diet, drugs, systemic disturbances of ACID-BASE BALANCE, and kidney tubular function. For example, a high-protein diet produces acidic urine, whereas a high intake of citrus fruit produces alkaline urine.

Urine specimens become more alkaline when left standing unrefrigerated for more than 1 hour, when bacteria are present, or when a specimen is left uncovered. Alkaline urine increases cell breakdown; thus the presence of red blood cells may be missed on analysis. In addition, alkalinity promotes bacterial overgrowth. Ensure that urine specimens are covered and delivered to the laboratory promptly or

CHART 65-3 **Laboratory Profile**

Urinalysis

TEST	NORMAL RANGE FOR ADULTS	SIGNIFICANCE OF ABNORMAL FINDINGS
Color	Yellow	*Dark amber* indicates concentrated urine. *Very pale yellow* indicates dilute urine. *Dark red* or *brown* indicates blood in the urine. Brown may indicate increased bilirubin level. Red also may indicate the presence of myoglobin. *Other color* changes may result from diet or drugs.
Odor	Specific aroma, similar to ammonia	*Foul smell* indicates possible infection, dehydration, or ingestion of certain foods or drugs.
Turbidity	Clear	*Cloudy urine* indicates infection, sediment, or high levels of urine protein.
Specific gravity	Usually 1.005-1.030; possible range 1.000-1.040 *Older adult:* Decreased	*Increased* in decreased kidney perfusion, inappropriate ADH secretion, or heart failure. *Decreased* in chronic kidney disease, diabetes insipidus, malignant hypertension, diuretic administration, and lithium toxicity.
pH	Average: 6; possible range: 4.6-8	*Changes* are caused by diet, drugs, infection, age of specimen, acid-base imbalance, and kidney disease.
Glucose	Fresh specimen, negative 50-300 mg/day in a 24-hour specimen	*Presence* reflects hyperglycemia or a decrease in the kidney threshold for glucose.
Ketones	None	*Presence* occurs with diabetic ketoacidosis, prolonged fasting, anorexia nervosa.
Protein	0-0.8 mg/dL 50-80 mg in a 24-hour specimen at rest <250 mg in a 24-hour specimen with exercise	*Increased* amounts may indicate stress, infection, recent strenuous exercise, or glomerular disorders.
Bilirubin (urobilinogen)	None	*Presence* suggests liver or biliary disease or obstruction.
Red blood cells (RBCs)	0-2 per high-power field	*Increased* is normal with catheterization or menses but may reflect tumor, stones, trauma, glomerular disorders, cystitis, or bleeding disorders.
White blood cells (WBCs)	0-4 per low-power field	*Increased* may indicate an infection or inflammation in the kidney and urinary tract, kidney transplant rejection, or exercise.
Casts	None	*Increased* indicates bacteria, protein, or urinary calculi.
Crystals	None	*Presence* may indicate that the specimen has been allowed to stand.
Bacteria	<1000 colonies/mL	*Increased* indicates the need for urine culture to determine the presence of urinary tract infection.
Parasites	None	*Presence* of *Trichomonas vaginalis* indicates infection, usually of the urethra, prostate, or vagina.
Leukoesterase	None	*Presence* suggests urinary tract infection.
Nitrites	None	*Presence* suggests urinary *Escherichia coli.*

Data from Pagana, K., & Pagana, T. (2014). *Mosby's manual of diagnostic and laboratory tests* (5th ed.). St. Louis: Mosby.
ADH, Antidiuretic hormone.

refrigerated. During systemic acidosis or alkalosis, the kidneys, along with blood buffers and the lungs, normally respond to keep serum pH normal. Chapter 12 discusses ACID-BASE BALANCE and imbalance.

Protein is not normally present in the urine. Levels greater than 30 mg/hr, or 200 mcg/min, are abnormal. Protein molecules are too large to pass through intact glomerular membranes. When glomerular membranes are not intact, protein molecules pass through and are excreted in the urine. Increased membrane permeability is caused by infection, inflammation, or immunologic problems. Some systemic problems cause production of abnormal proteins, such as globulin. Detection of abnormal protein types requires electrophoresis.

A random finding of **proteinuria** (usually albumin in the urine) followed by a series of negative (normal) findings does not imply kidney disease. If infection is the cause of the proteinuria, urinalyses after resolution of the infection should be negative for protein. Persistent proteinuria needs further investigation.

Microalbuminuria is the presence of albumin in the urine that is not measurable by a urine dipstick or usual urinalysis procedures. Specialized assays are used to quickly analyze a freshly voided urine specimen for microscopic levels of albumin. The normal microalbumin levels in a freshly voided specimen should range between 2.0 and 20 mg/mmol for men and between 2.8 and 28 mg/mmol for women. Higher levels indicate microalbuminuria and could mean mild or early kidney disease, especially in patients with diabetes mellitus. In 24-hour urine specimens, levels of 30 to 300 mg/24 hr, or 20 to 200 mcg/min, indicate microalbuminuria.

Glucose is filtered by the glomerulus and is reabsorbed in the proximal tubule of the nephron. When the blood glucose level rises above 220 mg/dL, the renal threshold for reabsorption is exceeded and glucose "spills over" into urine. Changes in the renal threshold for glucose occur in many patients, such as those with infection or severe stress.

Ketone bodies are formed from the incomplete metabolism of fatty acids. Three types of ketone bodies are acetone,

TABLE 65-3 Collection of Urine Specimens

NURSING INTERVENTIONS	RATIONALES
Voided Urine	
Collect the first specimen voided in the morning.	Urine is more concentrated in the early morning.
Send the specimen to the laboratory as soon as possible.	After urine is collected, cellular breakdown results in more alkaline urine.
Refrigerate the specimen if a delay is unavoidable.	Refrigeration delays the alkalinization of urine. Bacteria are more likely to multiply in an alkaline environment.
Clean-Catch Specimen	
Explain the purpose of the procedure to the patient.	Correct technique is needed to obtain a valid specimen.
Instruct the patient to self-clean before voiding: Instruct the female patient to separate the labia and use the sponges and solution provided to wipe with three strokes over the urethra. The first two wiping strokes are over each side of the urethra; the third wiping stroke is centered over the urethra (from front to back). Instruct the male patient to retract the foreskin of the penis and to similarly clean the urethra, using three wiping strokes with the sponge and solution provided (from the head of the penis downward).	Surface cleaning is necessary to remove secretions or bacteria from the urethral meatus.
Instruct the patient to initiate voiding after cleaning. The patient then stops and resumes voiding into the container. Only 1 ounce (30 mL) is needed; the remainder of the urine may be discarded into the commode.	A midstream collection further removes secretions and bacteria because urine flushes the distal portion of the internal urethra.
Ensure that the patient understands the procedure.	An improperly collected specimen may result in inappropriate or incomplete treatment.
Assist the patient as needed.	The patient's understanding and the nurse's assistance ensure proper collection.
Catheterized Specimen	
For non-indwelling (straight) catheters: Avoid routine use.	The one-time passage of a urinary catheter may be necessary to obtain an uncontaminated specimen for analysis or to measure the volume of residual urine.
Follow the facility's procedures for catheterization technique.	These procedures minimize bacterial entry.
For indwelling catheters:	Urine is collected from an indwelling catheter or tubing when patients have catheters for continence or long-term urinary drainage.
Apply a clamp to the drainage tubing, distal to the injection port.	Clamping allows urine to collect in the tubing at the location where the specimen is obtained.
Clean the injection port cap of the catheter drainage tubing with an appropriate antiseptic. Povidone-iodine solution or alcohol is acceptable.	Surface contamination is prevented by following the cleaning procedures.
Attach a sterile 5-mL syringe into the port, and aspirate the quantity of urine required.	A minimum of 5 mL is needed for culture and sensitivity (C&S) testing.
Inject the urine sample into a sterile specimen container. Remove the clamp to resume drainage. Properly dispose of the syringe.	A sterile container is used for C&S specimens.
24-Hour Urine Collection	
Instruct the patient thoroughly.	A 24-hr collection of urine is necessary to quantify or calculate the rate of clearance of a particular substance.
Provide written materials to assist in instruction. Place signs appropriately. Inform all personnel or family caregivers of test in progress.	Instructional materials for patients, signs, etc. remind patients and staff to ensure that the total collection is completed.
Check laboratory or procedure manual on proper technique for maintaining the collection (e.g., on ice, in a refrigerator, or with a preservative).	Proper technique prevents breakdown of elements to be measured.
On initiation of the collection, ask the patient to void, discard the urine, and note the time. If a Foley catheter is in use, empty the tubing and drainage bag at the start time and discard the urine. Collect all urine of the next 24 hr. Twenty-four hours after initiation, ask the patient to empty the bladder and add that urine to the container.	Proper techniques ensure that *all* urine formed within the 24-hr period is collected.
Do not remove urine from the collection container for other specimens.	Urine in the container is not considered a "fresh" specimen and may be mixed with preservative.

acetoacetic acid, and beta-hydroxybutyric acid. *Normally there are no ketones in urine.* Ketone bodies are produced when fat is used instead of glucose for cellular energy. Ketones present in the blood are partially excreted in the urine.

Leukoesterase is an enzyme found in some white blood cells, especially neutrophils. When the number of these cells increases in the urine or they are broken (lysed), the urine then contains leukoesterase. The presence of leukoesterase and nitrites in the urine is a sensitive screen for assessing urinary tract infections. A normal reading is no leukoesterase in the urine. A positive test (+ sign) is an indication of a urinary tract infection.

Nitrites are not usually present in urine. Many types of bacteria, when present in the urine, convert nitrates (normally found in urine) into nitrites. A positive test enhances the sensitivity of the leukoesterase test to detect urinary tract infection.

Sediment is precipitated particles in the urine. These particles include cells, casts, crystals, and bacteria. Normally, urine contains few, if any, cells. Types of cells abnormally present in the urine include tubular cells (from the tubule of the nephron), epithelial cells (from the lining of the urinary tract), red blood cells (RBCs), and white blood cells (WBCs). WBCs may indicate a urinary tract or kidney infection. RBCs may indicate *glomerulonephritis, acute tubular necrosis, pyelonephritis,* kidney trauma, or kidney cancer.

Casts are clumps of materials or cells. When cells, bacteria, or proteins are present in the urine, minerals and sticky materials clump around them and form a cast of the distal renal tubule and collecting duct. Casts are described by the type of particle they have surrounded (e.g., hyaline [protein-based] or cellular [from RBCs, WBCs, or epithelial cells]) or the stage of cast breakdown (whole cell or granular from cell breakdown). Although an isolated urinalysis with sediment from casts may be the result of strenuous exercise, repeated findings with sediment are more likely to be associated with disease.

Urine crystals come from mineral salts as a result of diet, drugs, or disease. Common salt crystals are formed from calcium, oxalate, urea, phosphate, magnesium, or other substances. Some drugs, such as the sulfates, can also form crystals.

Bacteria multiply quickly, so the urine specimen must be analyzed promptly to avoid falsely elevated counts of bacterial colonization. Normally urine is sterile, but it is easily contaminated by perineal bacteria during collection.

Recent advances in technology and molecular biology are leading to new diagnostic tests using urine, including identification of biomarkers of disease and profiling for specific proteins. Markers are being used in investigation to identify early-onset kidney dysfunction, target therapy, and predict responsiveness to intervention. Markers for angiogenesis and kidney cell adhesion, regulation, and apoptosis will likely contribute to clinical diagnostics in the future.

Urine for Culture and Sensitivity. Urine is analyzed for the number and types of organisms present. Manifestations of infection and unexplained bacteria in a urine specimen are indications for urine culture and sensitivity testing. Bacteria from urine are placed in a medium with different antibiotics. In this way we can know which antibiotics are effective in killing or stopping the growth of the organisms (organisms are "sensitive") and which are not effective (organisms are "resistant"). A clean-catch or catheter-derived specimen is best for culture and sensitivity testing.

Composite Urine Collections. Some urine collections are made for a specified number of hours (e.g., 24 hours) for more precise analysis of one or more substances. These collections are often used to measure urine levels of creatinine or urea nitrogen, sodium, chloride, calcium, catecholamines, or other components (Chart 65-4). For a composite urine specimen, *all* urine within the designated time frame must be collected (see Table 65-3). If other urine must be obtained while the collection is in progress, measure and record the amount collected but not added to the timed collection.

The urine collection may need to be refrigerated or stored on ice to prevent changes in the urine during the collection time. Follow the procedure from the laboratory for urine storage, including whether a preservative is to be added. The urine collection must be free from fecal contamination. Menstrual blood and toilet tissue also contaminate the specimen and can invalidate the results.

The collection of urine for a 24-hour period is often more difficult than it seems. With hospitalized patients, the cooperation of staff personnel, the patient, family members, and visitors is essential. Placing signs in the bathroom, instructing the patient and family, and emphasizing the need to save the urine are helpful.

Creatinine Clearance. Creatinine clearance is a calculated measure of glomerular filtration rate (GFR) and kidney function. The patient's age, gender, height, weight, diet, and activity level influence the expected amount of excreted creatinine. Thus these factors are considered when interpreting creatinine clearance test results. Decreases in the creatinine clearance rate may require reducing drug doses and often signifies the need to further explore the cause of kidney deterioration.

Commonly, creatinine clearance is calculated from serum creatinine, age, weight, urine creatinine, gender, and race. Current guidelines suggest clinical laboratories report an estimate of GFR whenever a serum creatinine is ordered, based on the modified diet in renal disease (MDRD) study equation (National Kidney Disease Education Program, 2012). The MDRD equation does not require urine to estimate GFR. The estimated GFR (eGFR) for the MDRD equation is >60 mL/min/1.73 m^2 (Pagana & Pagana, 2014). An alternate approach for calculation is the Cockcroft-Gault equation, and this equation has traditionally been used to determine the need for drug dose adjustment (Dong & Quan, 2010).

While expensive and time consuming, creatinine clearance to estimate GFR can be based on a 24-hour urine collection, although urine can be collected for shorter periods (e.g., 8 or 12 hours). The analysis compares the urine creatinine level with the blood creatinine level, and therefore a blood specimen for creatinine must also be collected. The range for normal creatinine clearance is 107 to 239 mL/min for men and 87 to 107 mL/min for women tested with a 24-hour urine collection. Values decrease 6.5 mL/min per decade of life for adults older than 40 years because of age-related decline in GFR.

Urine Electrolytes. Urine samples can be analyzed for electrolyte levels (e.g., sodium, chloride). Normally the amount of sodium excreted in the urine is nearly equal to that consumed. Urine sodium levels of less than 10 mEq/L indicate that the tubules are able to conserve (reabsorb) sodium.

Urine Osmolarity. Osmolarity measures the concentration of particles in solution. The particles in urine contributing to osmolarity include electrolytes, glucose, urea, and creatinine. Urine osmolarity can vary from 50 to 1400 mOsm/L, depending on the patient's hydration status and kidney function. With average fluid intake, the range for urine osmolarity is 300 to 900 mOsm/L. Electrolytes, acids, and other wastes of normal metabolism are continually produced. These particles are the solute load that must be excreted in the urine on a regular basis. This is referred to as *obligatory solute excretion.* If the patient loses excessive fluids, the kidney response is to save water while ridding the body of wastes by excreting small amounts of highly

CHART 65-4 **Laboratory Profile**

24-Hour Urine Collections

COMPONENT	NORMAL RANGE FOR ADULTS	SIGNIFICANCE OF ABNORMAL FINDINGS
Creatinine	*Males:* 1-2 g/24 hr or 14-26 mg/kg/24 hr (124-230 μmol/kg/24 hr or 7.1-17.7 mmol/24 hr) *Females:* 0.6-1.8 g/24 hr or 11-20 mg/kg/24 hr (97-177 μmol/kg/24 hr or 5.3-15.9 mmol/24 hr) *Older adults:* 10 mg/kg/24 hr (88.4 μmol/kg/24 hr) at 90 yr	*Decreased amounts* indicate a deterioration in function caused by kidney disease. *Increased amounts* occur with infections, exercise, diabetes mellitus, and meat meals.
Urea nitrogen	12-20 g/24 hr (0.43-0.71 mmol/24 hr)	*Decreased amounts* occur when kidney damage or liver disease is present. *Increased amounts* commonly result from a high-protein diet, dehydration, trauma, or sepsis.
Sodium	40-220 mEq/24 hr (40-220 mmol/24 hr)	*Decreased* in hemorrhage, shock, hyperaldosteronism, and prerenal acute kidney injury. *Increased* with diuretic therapy, excessive salt intake, hypokalemia, and acute tubular necrosis.
Chloride	110-250 mEq/24 hr (110-250 mmol/24 hr) *Older adults:* 95-195 mEq/24 hr (95-195 mmol/24 hr)	*Decreased* in certain kidney diseases, malnutrition, pyloric obstruction, prolonged nasogastric tube drainage, diarrhea, diaphoresis, heart failure, and emphysema. *Increased* with hypokalemia, adrenal insufficiency, and massive diuresis.
Calcium	100-400 mg/24 hr (2.50-7.50 mmol/kg/24 hr)	*Decreased* with hypocalcemia, hypoparathyroidism, nephrosis, and nephritis. *Increased* with calcium kidney stones, hyperparathyroidism, sarcoidosis, certain cancers, immobilization, and hypercalcemia.
*Total catecholamines	<100 mcg/24 hr (<591 mmol/24 hr)	*Increased* with pheochromocytoma, neuroblastomas, stress, or heavy exercise.
Protein	1-14 mg/dL (10-140 mg/L) or 50-80 mg/24 hr at rest	*Increased* in glomerular disease, nephrotic syndrome, diabetic nephropathy, urinary tract malignancies, and irritations.

Data from Pagana, K., & Pagana, T. (2014). *Mosby's manual of diagnostic and laboratory tests* (5th ed.). St. Louis: Mosby.
*Epinephrine and norepinephrine only; dopamine is not measured.

concentrated urine. Diet, drugs, and activity can change urine osmolarity. Thus urine with an increased osmolarity is concentrated urine with less water and more solutes. Urine with a decreased osmolarity is dilute urine with more water and fewer solutes.

NCLEX EXAMINATION CHALLENGE

Physiological Integrity

The client's urinalysis shows all of these abnormal results. Which result does the nurse report to the health care provider immediately?

A. pH 7.8
B. Protein 31 mg
C. Sodium 15 mEq/L
D. Leukoesterase and nitrate positive

Bedside Sonography/Bladder Scanners. The use of portable ultrasound scanners in the hospital and rehabilitation setting by nurses is a noninvasive method of estimating bladder volume (Fig. 65-10). Bladder scanners are used to screen for post-void residual volumes and to determine the need for intermittent catheterization based on the amount of urine in the bladder

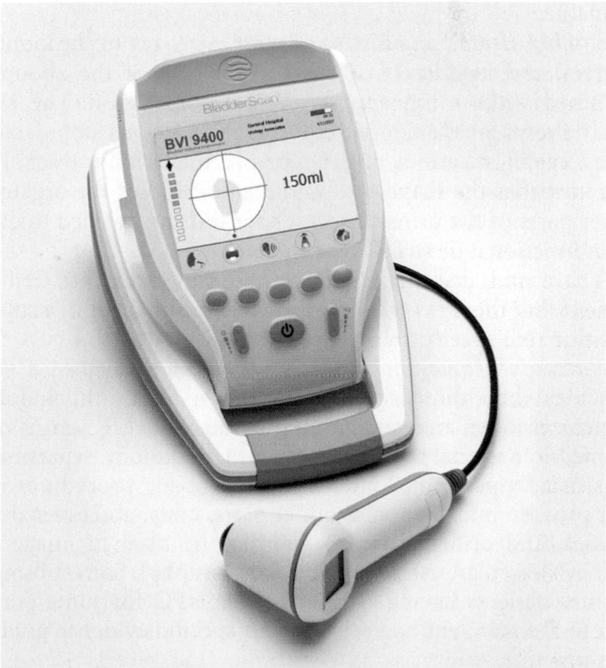

FIG. 65-10 The "BladderScan" BVI 9400, a handheld portable bladder scanner.

rather than the time between catheterizations. There is no discomfort with the scan, and no patient preparation beyond an explanation of what to expect is required.

Explain why the procedure is being done and what sensations the patient might experience during the procedure. For example, "This test will measure the amount of urine in your bladder. I will place a gel pad just above your pubic area and then place the probe, which is a little bigger and heavier than a stethoscope, on the gel."

Before scanning, select the male or female icon on the bladder scanner. Using the female icon allows the scanner software to subtract the volume of the uterus from any measurement. Use the male icon on all men and on women who have undergone a hysterectomy.

Place an ultrasound gel pad right above the symphysis pubis (pubic bone), or moisten the round dome of the scan head area with 5 mL of conducting gel to improve ultrasound conduction. Use gel on the scanner head for obese patients and those with heavy body hair in the area to be scanned. Place the probe midline over the abdomen about 1½ inches (4 cm) above the pubic bone. Aim the scan head so the ultrasound is projected toward the expected location of the bladder, typically toward the patient's coccyx. Press and release the scan button. The scan is complete with the sound of a beep, and a volume is displayed. Two readings are recommended for best accuracy. An aiming icon on the portable bladder scanner indicates whether the bladder image is centered on the crosshairs of the scan head. If the crosshairs on the aiming icon are not centered on the bladder, the measured volume may not be accurate.

TABLE 65-4 Radiologic and Special Diagnostic Tests for Patients with Disorders of the Kidney and Urinary System

TEST	PURPOSE
Radiography of kidneys, ureters, and bladder (KUB) (plain film of abdomen)	To screen for the presence of two kidneys To measure kidney size To detect gross obstruction in kidneys or urinary tract
Computed tomography (CT)	To measure kidney size To evaluate contour to assess for masses or obstruction in kidneys or the urinary tract To assess renal blood flow
Magnetic resonance imaging (MRI)	Similar to CT Useful for staging of cancers
Ultrasonography (US) Can be used with a dye	To identify the size of the kidneys or obstruction (e.g., tumors, stones) in the kidneys or the lower urinary tract
(Nuclear) Renal scan	To evaluate renal perfusion To estimate glomerular filtration rate To provide functional information without exposing the patient to iodinated contrast dye
Cystoscopy	To identify abnormalities of the bladder wall and urethral and ureteral occlusions To treat small obstructions or lesions via fulguration, lithotripsy, or removal with a stone basket
Cystography and cystourethrography	To outline bladder's contour when full and examine structure during voiding To examine the structure of the urethra To detect backward urine flow
Metabolic imaging with positron emission tomography (PET)	To evaluate cysts, tumors, and other lesions, eliminating the need for biopsy in some patients

Imaging Assessment

Many imaging procedures are used to diagnose abnormalities within the urinary system (Table 65-4). Explain the procedures thoroughly to the patient, prepare him or her, and provide follow-up care. Patient education materials for many urologic tests have been developed by professional organizations such as the Society for Urologic Nurses and Associates and are freely available.

Kidney, Ureter, and Bladder X-rays. An x-ray of the kidneys, ureters, and bladder (KUB) is a plain film of the abdomen obtained without any specific patient preparation. The KUB study shows gross anatomic features and obvious stones, strictures, calcifications, or obstructions in the urinary tract. This test identifies the shape, size, and relationship of the organs to other parts of the urinary tract. Other tests are needed to diagnose functional or structural problems.

There is no discomfort or risk from this procedure. Tell the patient that the x-ray will be taken while he or she is in a supine position. No specific follow-up care is needed.

Computed Tomography. Inform the patient that a CT scan provides three-dimensional information about the kidneys, ureters, bladder, and surrounding tissues. The CT scan is performed in a special room, usually in the radiology department. It is usually performed after other diagnostic procedures and can provide information about tumors, cysts, abscesses, other masses, and obstruction. CT can also be used to image the kidney's vascular system (i.e., CT angiography). Some hospitals require patients having CT scans to be NPO for some period before the scan, although there is no specific evidence guiding this practice.

Determine whether the scan requires administration of a dye. Oral or injected contrast dye is usually given before starting the imaging procedure. Dye use may be omitted in patients at risk for contrast-induced acute kidney injury, but the images produced are less distinct.

When a dye is used, ensure that there is sufficient oral or intravenous intake to dilute and excrete the dye. Typically, the radiologist will specify a total fluid intake of 1 liter or a variable rate to maintain urine output at 1 to 2 mL/kg/hr for up to 6 hours. When no contrast or dye is used, there is no special postprocedure care.

The contrast dye is potentially kidney-damaging (nephrotoxic). *Contrast-induced nephropathy* is the onset of *acute kidney failure* within 24 to 72 hours after the administration of iodinated contrast medium (Wood, 2012). The risk for *contrast-induced nephropathy* is greatest in patients who are older, dehydrated, have pre-existing renal insufficiency (e.g., serum creatinine levels greater than 1.5 mg/dL or estimated GFR <45 mL/min), or are also taking other nephrotoxic drugs (Davenport et al., 2014). Chart 65-5 lists assessment questions to ask before a patient undergoes testing that uses contrast material.

In addition, patients taking metformin are at risk for lactic acidosis when they receive iodinated contrast media. Metformin should be discontinued at least 24 hours before the time

CHART 65-5 **Best Practice for Patient Safety & Quality Care** QSEN

Assessing the Patient About to Undergo a Kidney Test or Procedure Using Contrast Medium

Before the procedure:

- Ask the patient if he or she has ever had a reaction to contrast media. (Such a patient has the highest risk for having another reaction.)
- Ask the patient about a history of asthma. (Patients with asthma have been shown to be at greater risk for contrast reactions than the general public. When reactions do occur, they are more likely to be severe.)
- Ask the patient about known hay fever or food or drug allergies, especially to seafood, eggs, milk, or chocolate. (Contrast reactions have been reported to be as high as 15% in these patients.)
- Ask the patient to describe any specific allergic reactions (e.g., hives, facial edema, difficulty breathing, bronchospasm).
- Assess for a history of renal impairment and for conditions that have been implicated in increasing the chance of developing kidney failure after contrast media (e.g., diabetic nephropathy, class IV heart failure, dehydration, concomitant use of potentially nephrotoxic drugs such as the aminoglycosides or NSAIDs, and cirrhosis).
- Ask the patient if he or she is taking metformin (Glucophage). (Metformin must be discontinued at least 24 hours before any study using contrast media because the life-threatening complication of lactic acidosis, although rare, could occur.)
- Assess hydration status by checking blood pressure, heart and respiratory rates, mucous membranes, skin turgor, and urine concentration.
- Ask the patient when he or she last ate or drank anything.

of a procedure and for at least 48 hours after the procedure. Kidney function should be re-evaluated before the patient resumes metformin therapy.

! NURSING SAFETY PRIORITY QSEN

Drug Alert

Ensure that the patient who is prescribed metformin does not receive the drug after a procedure requiring IV contrast material until adequate kidney function has been determined.

All patients at risk for contrast-induced nephrotoxicity need regular assessment and collaboration with the health care provider to maintain hydration and decrease the risk for kidney damage following a dye-enhanced CT scan. Sodium bicarbonate in a liter of intravenous fluid or oral acetylcysteine (an antioxidant) may be used preprocedure to prevent contrast-induced nephrotoxic effects in radiologic procedures; however, protection provided to the kidneys is not consistent in clinical trials (Lameire & Kellum, 2013). Diuretics may be given immediately after the dye is injected to enhance dye excretion in patients who are well hydrated.

Magnetic Resonance Imaging of the Kidney. MRI provides improved contrast between normal and abnormal tissue in the renal system compared with a CT scan. As with all MRIs, the patient with metal implants (pins, pacemaker, joint replacement, aneurysmal clips, or other cosmetic or medical devices) is not eligible for this test because the magnet can move the metal implant. Gadolinium-based contrast agents have been linked with nephrogenic systemic fibrosis (Pagana & Pagana, 2014) and should not be used in patients with renal impairment, usually defined as a serum creatinine above 1.5 mg/dL or an estimated GFR less than 45 mL/min. Adults older than 60 years should be carefully evaluated for renal impairment (see the Kidney and Urinary System Changes Associated with Aging section on p. 1351).

Kidney Ultrasonography. Inform the patient that ultrasonography does not cause discomfort and is without risk. This test usually requires a full bladder. Ask the patient to drink water, if needed, to help fill the bladder. This test applies sound waves to structures of different densities to produce images of the kidneys, ureters, and bladder and surrounding tissues. Ultrasonography allows assessment of kidney size, cortical thickness, and status of the calices. The test can identify obstruction in the urinary tract, tumors, cysts, and other masses without the use of contrast dye.

The patient undergoing kidney ultrasound is usually placed in the prone position. Sonographic gel is applied to the skin over the back and flank areas to enhance sound-wave conduction. A transducer in contact with and moving across the skin delivers sound waves and measures the echoes. Images of the internal structures are produced. Skin care to remove the gel is all that is needed after ultrasonography.

Renal Scan. This imaging test is used to examine the perfusion, function, and structure of the kidneys, using the IV administration of a radioisotope. It does not use an iodinated dye and so may be used in preference to a CT scan when the patient is allergic to iodine or has impaired kidney function that places him or her at risk for kidney injury from contrast dyes.

Patient Preparation and Procedural Care. No fasting or sedation is used. A peripheral IV catheter is inserted to give the radioisotope. While the patient lies in a prone or sitting position, a camera is passed over the kidney area and records the isotope uptake on film, minutes after it is given. After initial images, the patient may be given furosemide or captopril to better visualize kidney function and blood flow. The isotope is eliminated 6 to 24 hours after the procedure. Encourage the patient to drink fluids to aid in excretion of the isotope. Because only tracer doses of radioisotopes are used, no precautions are needed related to radioactive exposure.

Renal Arteriography (Angiography). Renal arteriography allows dye to enter the renal blood vessels and generates images to determine blood vessel size and abnormalities. This test has largely been replaced by other imaging techniques (e.g., nuclear renal scans, ultrasonography, computed tomography) and is seldom used as a stand-alone diagnostic procedure. The most common use of renal arteriography is at the time of a renal angioplasty or other intervention.

Cystoscopy and Cystourethroscopy

Patient Preparation. Cystoscopy and cystourethroscopy are endoscopic procedures and require completion of a preoperative checklist and a signed informed consent statement. The urologist provides a complete description of and reasons for the procedure, and the nurse reinforces this information. Cystoscopy may be performed for diagnosis or treatment. This test is used to examine for bladder trauma (cystoscopy) or urethral trauma (cystourethroscopy) and to identify causes of urinary tract obstruction. Cystoscopy also may be used to remove bladder tumors or to plant radium seeds into a tumor, dilate the urethra and ureters with or without stent placement, stop areas of bleeding, or resect an enlarged prostate gland.

Cystoscopy may be performed under general anesthesia or under local anesthesia with sedation. The patient's age and general health and the expected duration of the procedure are considered in the decision about anesthesia. A light evening meal may be eaten. Usually the patient is NPO after midnight on the night before the cystoscopy. A bowel preparation with laxatives or enemas is performed the evening before the procedure.

Procedure. The cystoscopy is performed in a designated cystoscopic examination room. If the procedure is performed in a surgical suite under general anesthesia, the usual surgical support personnel are present (see Chapter 15). This procedure is often performed in clinics, ambulatory surgery or short-procedure units, or a urologist's office.

Assist the patient onto a table, and after sedation, place him or her in the lithotomy position. After the anesthesia is given and the area cleansed and draped, the urologist inserts a cystoscope through the urethra into the urinary bladder. This examination commonly includes the use of both the cystoscope and the urethroscope.

Follow-up Care. After this procedure with general anesthesia, the patient is returned to a postanesthesia care unit (PACU) or area. If local anesthesia and sedation were used, he or she may be returned directly to the hospital room. Ambulatory care patients undergoing cystoscopic examinations are transferred to an area for monitoring before discharge to home. Monitor for airway patency and breathing, changes in vital signs (including temperature), and changes in urine output. Also observe for the complications of bleeding and infection.

A catheter may or may not be present after cystoscopy. The patient without a catheter has urinary frequency as a result of irritation from the procedure. The urine may be pink tinged, but gross bleeding is not expected. Bleeding or the presence of clots may obstruct the catheter and decrease urine output. Monitor urine output, and notify the urologist of obvious blood clots or a decreased or absent urine output. Irrigate the Foley catheter with sterile saline, if prescribed. Notify the urologist if the patient has a fever (with or without chills) or an elevated white blood cell (WBC) count, which suggests infection. Urge the patient to take oral FLUIDS to increase urine output (which helps prevent clotting) and to reduce the burning sensation on urination.

Cystography and Cystourethrography. These tests are a series of x-rays or a continuous radiographic visualization by fluoroscopy. During the imaging, a dye fills the bladder and the bladder is emptied. Images show structure and function of the bladder and urethra. Tumors, rupture or perforation of the bladder and urethra, abnormal backflow of urine, and distortion from trauma or other pelvic masses can be seen.

Patient Preparation and Procedural Care. Explain the procedure to the patient. A urinary catheter is temporarily needed to instill contrast dye directly into the bladder for both procedures. The dye is needed to enhance x-ray visibility of the lower urinary tract and is not absorbed into the bloodstream, which reduces the risk for contrast-induced kidney injury.

After bladder filling, x-rays are taken from the front, back, and side positions. For the voiding cystourethrogram (VCUG), the patient is requested to void and x-rays are taken during the voiding. A VCUG is obtained to determine whether urine refluxes (flows backward) into the ureter. The cystogram is used in cases of trauma when urethral or bladder injury is suspected or for patients with recurrent *pyelonephritis* (kidney infection).

Monitor for infection as a result of catheter placement. In this test, the dye is not nephrotoxic because it does not enter the bloodstream and does not reach the kidney. Encourage fluid intake to dilute the urine and reduce the burning sensation from catheter irritation after removal. Monitor for changes in urine output because pelvic or urethral trauma may be present.

Retrograde Procedures. **Retrograde** means going against the normal flow of urine. A retrograde examination of the ureters and the pelvis of both kidneys *(pyelogram)*, the bladder *(cystogram)*, and the urethra *(urethrogram)* involves instilling dye into the lower urinary tract. Because the dye is instilled directly to obtain an outline of the structures of interest, the dye does not enter the bloodstream. Therefore the patient is not at risk for dye-induced acute kidney injury (AKI) or a systemic allergic response.

The patient is prepared for retrograde procedures (retrograde pyelography, retrograde cystography, and retrograde urethrography) in the same way as for cystoscopy. Retrograde x-rays are obtained during the cystoscopy. After placement of the cystoscope by the urologist, catheters are placed into each ureter and contrast dye is instilled into each ureter and kidney pelvis. The catheters are removed by the urologist, and x-rays are taken to outline these structures as the dye is excreted. The procedure identifies obstruction or structural abnormalities.

For patients undergoing retrograde cystoscopy or urethrography, contrast dye is instilled similarly into the bladder or urethra. Cystography and urethrography identify structural problems, such as fistulas, diverticula, and tumors.

After retrograde procedures, monitor the patient for infection caused by placing instruments in the urinary tract. Because these procedures are performed during cystoscopic examination, follow-up care is the same as that for cystoscopy.

Other Diagnostic Assessments

Urodynamic Studies. Urodynamic studies examine the processes of voiding and include:

- Tests of bladder capacity, pressure, and tone
- Studies of urethral pressure and urine flow
- Tests of perineal voluntary muscle function

These tests are often used along with voiding urographic or cystoscopic procedures to evaluate problems with urine flow and disorders of the lower urinary tract (Gray, 2011; Gray, 2012a; Gray, 2012b).

Cystometrography (CMG) can determine how well the bladder wall (detrusor) muscle functions and how sensitive it is to stretching as the bladder fills. This test provides information about bladder capacity, bladder pressure, and voiding reflexes.

Explain the procedure, and inform the patient that a urinary catheter will be needed temporarily during the procedure. Ask the patient to void normally. Record the amount and time of voiding. Insert a urinary catheter to measure the residual urine volume. The cystometer is attached to the catheter, and fluid is instilled via the catheter into the bladder. The point at which the patient first notes a feeling of the urge to void and the point at which he or she notes a strong urge to void are recorded. Bladder capacity and bladder pressure readings are recorded graphically. The patient is asked to void when the bladder instillation is complete (about 500 mL). The residual urine after voiding is recorded, and the catheter is removed.

Electromyography of the perineal muscles may be performed during this examination.

For any procedure that involves inserting instruments into the urinary tract, monitor for infection. Record the patient's temperature, the character of the urine, and urine output volume.

Urethral pressure profile (also called a *urethral pressure profilometry [UPP]*) can provide information about the nature of urinary incontinence or urinary retention.

Explain the procedure, and inform the patient that a urinary catheter will be needed temporarily during the procedure. A special catheter with pressure-sensing capabilities is inserted into the bladder. Variations in the pressure of the smooth muscle of the urethra are recorded as the catheter is slowly withdrawn.

As with any study involving inserting instruments into the urinary tract, monitor the patient for manifestations of infection.

Urine stream testing is used to evaluate pelvic muscle strength and the effectiveness of pelvic muscles in stopping the flow of urine. It is useful in assessing urinary incontinence.

Explain the procedure, and reassure the patient that efforts will be made to ensure privacy. The patient is asked to begin urinating. Three to five seconds after urination begins, the examiner gives the patient a signal to stop urine flow. The length of time required to stop the flow of urine is recorded.

Cleaning the perineal area, as after any voiding, is all that is necessary after the urine stream test.

Electromyography (EMG) of the perineal muscles tests the strength of the muscles used in voiding. This information may help identify methods of improving continence. Inform the patient that some mild, temporary discomfort may accompany placement of the electrodes. In EMG of the perineal muscles, electrodes are placed in either the rectum or the urethra to measure muscle contraction and relaxation. After the completion of EMG, administer analgesics as prescribed to promote the patient's comfort.

NCLEX EXAMINATION CHALLENGE

Safe and Effective Care Environment

Which assessments are most important for the nurse to perform when monitoring a client who returns to the medical-surgical unit after a dye-enhanced CT scan?

A. Body temperature and urine odor
B. Kidney tenderness and flank pain
C. Urine volume and color
D. Specific gravity and pH

Kidney Biopsy

Patient Preparation. Explain that a kidney biopsy can help determine a cause of unexplained kidney problems and can help direct or change therapy. Most kidney biopsies are performed **percutaneously** (through skin and other tissues) using ultrasound or CT guidance. The patient signs an informed consent and is NPO for 4 to 6 hours before the procedure.

Because of the risk for bleeding after the biopsy, coagulation studies such as platelet count, activated partial thromboplastin time (aPTT), prothrombin time (PT), and bleeding time are performed before surgery. Hypertension is aggressively managed before and after the procedure because high blood pressure can make stopping the bleeding after the biopsy more difficult. Uremia also increases the risk for bleeding, and dialysis may be prescribed before a biopsy. A blood transfusion may be needed to correct anemia before biopsy.

Procedure. In a percutaneous biopsy, the nephrologist or radiologist obtains tissue samples without an incision. Patients receive sedation and are monitored throughout the procedure. The patient is placed in the prone position on the procedure table. The entry site is selected after taking preliminary images. The area is prepped and sterilely draped. A local anesthetic is injected, and the physician then inserts the biopsy device into the tissues toward the kidney. Needle depth and placement are confirmed by ultrasound or CT. While the patient holds his or her breath, the needle is advanced into the renal cortex. Samples are then taken with a spring-loaded coring biopsy needle and sent for pathologic study.

Follow-up Care. After a percutaneous biopsy, the major risk is bleeding from the biopsy site. For 24 hours after the biopsy, monitor the dressing site, vital signs (especially fluctuations in blood pressure), urine output, hemoglobin level, and hematocrit. Even if the dressing is dry and there is no hematoma, the patient could be bleeding from the site. An internal bleed is not readily visible but is suspected with flank pain, decreasing blood pressure, decreasing urine output, or other signs of hypovolemia or shock.

The patient follows a plan of strict bedrest, lying in a supine position with a back roll for additional support for 2 to 6 hours after the biopsy. The head of the bed may be elevated, and the patient may resume oral intake of food and fluids. After bedrest, the patient may have limited bathroom privileges if there is no evidence of bleeding.

Monitor for hematuria, the most common complication of kidney biopsy. Hematuria occurs microscopically in most patients, but 5% to 9% have gross hematuria. This problem usually resolves without treatment in 48 to 72 hours after the biopsy but can persist for 2 to 3 weeks. In rare cases, transfusions and surgery are required. There should be no obvious blood clots in the urine.

The patient may have some local pain after the biopsy. If aching originates at the biopsy site and begins to radiate to the flank and around the front of the abdomen, bleeding may have started or a hematoma is forming around the kidney. This pattern of discomfort with bleeding occurs because blood in the tissues around the kidney increases pressure on local nerve tracts.

If bleeding occurs, IV fluid, packed red blood cells, or both may be needed to prevent shock. In general, a small amount of bleeding creates enough pressure to compress bleeding sites. This is called a "tamponade effect." If tamponade does not occur and bleeding is extensive, surgery for hemostasis or even nephrectomy may be needed. A hematoma in, on, or around the kidney may become infected, requiring treatment with antibiotics and surgical drainage.

If no bleeding occurs, the patient can resume general activities after 24 hours. Instruct him or her to avoid lifting heavy objects, exercising, or performing other strenuous activities for 1 to 2 weeks after the biopsy procedure. Driving may also be restricted. Refer to Chapter 16 for general postoperative care for the patient who has undergone an open kidney biopsy.

CLINICAL JUDGMENT CHALLENGE

Safety; Patient-Centered Care QSEN

At the start of the shift, you are assessing an 86-year-old patient who is awaiting surgery for a hip repair after a fall 12 hours ago at home. You are collecting a clean-catch urine specimen, using a bedpan, as part of the preoperative preparation. You observe that when she voids, the urine odor is foul and the urine is cloudy and full of sediment. She reports some urgency but notes that she had urgency before her fall.

1. What assessment information will you document in the chart?
2. What additional information should you ask the patient and what else should you consider?
3. Organize your thoughts into a SBAR communication (Chapter 1)
4. Who should you notify and why?

NURSING CONCEPTS AND CLINICAL JUDGMENT REVIEW

In addition to normal ranges indicating FLUID AND ELECTROLYTE BALANCE and ACID-BASE BALANCE, what might you NOTICE in a patient with adequate urinary ELIMINATION?

Vital signs:
- Body temperature is within normal range.
- Blood Pressure is within normal range.

Physical assessment:
- Daily urine output is within 500 mL of daily fluid intake.
- Skin texture is normal (no edema or superficial crystals present).
- Skin color is appropriate for ethnicity with no excessive yellowing, bruising, or petechiae.
- Urine is clear and some variation of yellow in color.
- Patient voids 300 to 500 mL per voiding.
- Patient does not report pain or burning on urination.
- Patient has no difficulty starting or stopping the stream of urine.
- Patient is continent of urine and can maintain continence without sensation of urgency.
- Patient is alert and oriented.

Psychological assessment:
- Patient is able to communicate concerns about the urinary tract system.
- Patient is aware and informed about kidney function and diagnostic tests.

Laboratory assessment:
- Hematocrit and hemoglobin are within normal limits (no anemia).
- BUN and creatinine are within normal limits.
- Serum electrolytes are within normal ranges.
- Urinalysis shows no bacteria, blood, sediment, or protein.

GET READY FOR THE NCLEX® EXAMINATION!

KEY POINTS

Review these Key Points for each NCLEX Examination Client Needs Category.

Safe and Effective Care Environment
- Use sterile technique when inserting a catheter or any other instrument into the urinary system. **Safety** QSEN
- Use Contact Precautions with any patient who has drainage from the genitourinary tract. **Safety** QSEN
- Wear gloves when testing or handling urine. **Safety** QSEN
- Evaluate risk for kidney injury from diagnostic testing by asking about allergy to contrast dye or iodine and adverse reactions following the use of diagnostic agents such as gadolinium in MRI.
- Ask the patient about the use of prescribed and over-the-counter drugs that increase risk for kidney dysfunction.
- Verify that informed consent has been obtained and that the patient has a clear understanding of the potential risks before he or she undergoes invasive procedures to assess the kidneys and urinary function. **Safety** QSEN

Health Promotion and Maintenance
- Teach patients to clean the perineal area after voiding, after having a bowel movement, and after sexual intercourse. **Evidence-Based Practice** QSEN
- Urge all patients to maintain an adequate fluid intake (sufficient to dilute urine to a light yellow color). A minimum of 2 L/day may be recommended unless another health problem requires fluid restriction.
- Teach patients who come into contact with chemicals in their workplaces or for leisure-time activities to avoid direct skin or mucous membrane contact with these chemicals. **Safety** QSEN

Psychosocial Integrity
- Allow the patient the opportunity to express fear or anxiety about tests of the kidneys and urinary tract or about a potential change in kidney function. **Patient-Centered Care** QSEN
- Assess the patient's level of comfort in discussing issues related to elimination and the urogenital area.

- Explain all diagnostic procedures, restrictions, and follow-up care to the patient scheduled for tests.
- Provide as much privacy as possible for patients undergoing examination or testing of the kidney/urinary tract. **Patient-Centered Care** QSEN
- Use language and terminology that the patient can understand during discussions of kidney/urinary assessment. **Patient-Centered Care** QSEN

Physiological Integrity

- Ask the patient about kidney problems in any other members of the family, because some problems have a genetic component.
- Ask the patient about current and past drug use (prescribed, over-the-counter, and illicit), and evaluate drug use for potential nephrotoxicity.
- Use laboratory data to distinguish between dehydration and kidney impairment. **Evidence-Based Practice** QSEN
- Describe how to obtain a sterile urine specimen from a urinary catheter.
- Assess urine output closely after any procedure in which contrast dye is used IV. **Evidence-Based Practice** QSEN
- Assess the patient for bleeding or manifestations of infection after any invasive test of kidney/urinary function.
- Inform health care providers about any manifestations of complications following invasive or noninvasive tests of urinary and kidney structure or function.

66 CHAPTER

Care of Patients with Urinary Problems

Chris Winkelman

http://evolve.elsevier.com/Iggy/

PRIORITY CONCEPTS

- ELIMINATION
- PAIN
- INFECTION
- INFLAMMATION

LEARNING OUTCOMES

Safe and Effective Care Environment

1. Assess the appropriateness for continuing therapy with indwelling urinary catheters.
2. Prevent INFECTION when caring for a patient with a urinary problem.

Health Promotion and Maintenance

3. Encourage everyone to have adequate fluid intake daily.
4. Teach people how to reduce or prevent urinary tract INFECTION and injury and urinary incontinence.

Psychosocial Integrity

5. Reduce the psychological impact of urinary problems for the patient and family.

Physiological Integrity

6. Coordinate care to prevent urinary tract INFECTION among hospitalized patients.
7. Compare the pathophysiology and manifestations of stress incontinence, urge incontinence, overflow incontinence, mixed incontinence, and functional incontinence.
8. Coordinate nursing care for the patient who has invasive bladder cancer.

The ureters, bladder, and urethra make up the urinary system. Their functions are to store the urine made by the kidney and eliminate it from the body. Problems in the urinary system can interfere with urinary ELIMINATION when the mechanics of moving urine out of the body are disrupted. Such problems can reduce control of fluids, electrolytes, nitrogenous wastes, and blood pressure.

Urinary problems affect the storage or ELIMINATION of urine. Both acute and chronic urinary problems are common and costly. More than 20 million people in the United States are treated annually for urinary tract infections, cystitis, kidney and ureter stones, or urinary incontinence (U.S. Renal Data Systems, 2012). Although life-threatening complications are rare with urinary problems, patients may have functional, physical, and psychosocial changes that reduce quality of life. Nursing interventions are directed toward prevention, detection, and management of urologic disorders.

INFECTIOUS DISORDERS

Infections of the urinary tract and kidneys are common, especially among women. Manifestations of urinary tract INFECTION (UTI) account for more than 7 million health care visits and 1 million hospital admissions annually in the United States (U.S. Renal Data Systems, 2012). Total direct and indirect costs for adult urinary tract infections are estimated at $1.6 billion each year. UTIs are the most common health care–associated INFECTION (Dudeck et al., 2013).

Urinary tract infections are described by their location in the tract. Acute infections in the lower urinary tract include *urethritis* (urethra), *cystitis* (bladder), and *prostatitis* (prostate gland). Acute *pyelonephritis* is an upper urinary tract (kidney) infection. Although the vocabulary for these infected sites reflects an inflammatory condition *(-itis)*, the most common cause of INFLAMMATION in the urinary tract is INFECTION. Thus these terms are often used interchangeably to refer to either an infectious process or a noninfectious inflammatory process. Several risk factors are associated with occurrence of UTIs (Table 66-1).

The presence of bacteria in the urine is **bacteriuria** and can occur with any urologic infection. When bacteriuria is without manifestations of infection, it is called *colonization,* or *asymptomatic bacterial urinary tract infection or ABUTI,* and is more common in older adults. This problem may progress to acute infection or renal insufficiency when the patient has other conditions, and only then does it require treatment.

Urinary tract INFECTIONS are typically categorized as *uncomplicated* or *complicated.* An acute, uncomplicated UTI is usually cystitis or pyelonephritis in premenopausal, nonpregnant, otherwise healthy women. With an uncomplicated UTI, there

TABLE 66-1 Factors Contributing to Urinary Tract Infections

FACTOR	MECHANISM
Obstruction	Incomplete bladder emptying creates a continuous pool of urine in which bacteria can grow, prevents flushing out of bacteria, and allows bacteria to ascend more easily to higher structures. Bacteria have a greater chance of multiplying the longer they remain in residual urine. Overdistention of the bladder damages the mucosa and allows bacteria to invade the bladder wall.
Stones (calculi)	Large stones can obstruct urine flow. The rough surface of a stone irritates mucosal surfaces and creates a spot where bacteria can establish and grow. Bacteria can live within stones and cause re-infection.
Vesicoureteral reflux	Bacteria-laden urine is forced backward from the bladder up into the ureters and kidneys, where pyelonephritis can develop. Reflux of sterile urine can cause kidney scarring, which may promote kidney dysfunction.
Diabetes mellitus	Excess glucose in urine provides a rich medium for bacterial growth. Peripheral neuropathy affects bladder innervation and leads to a flaccid bladder and incomplete bladder emptying.
Characteristics of urine	Alkaline urine promotes bacterial growth. Concentrated urine promotes bacterial growth.
Gender	**Women** Susceptibility to periurethral colonization with coliform bacteria is increased, especially as estrogen levels fall during menopause. Use of douches, perfumed pads or toilet tissue, diaphragms, or spermicide (including spermicide-coated condoms) in women can inflame periurethral tissue and contribute to colonization. Bladder displacement during pregnancy predisposes women to cystitis and the development of pyelonephritis. A diaphragm or pessary that is too large can obstruct urine flow or traumatize the urethra. **Men** With increased age, the prostate enlarges and may obstruct the normal flow of urine, producing stasis. With increased age, prostatic secretions lose their antibacterial characteristics and predispose to bacterial proliferation in the urine. Sexually transmitted diseases may cause urethral strictures that obstruct the flow of urine and predispose to urinary stasis.
Age	Urinary stasis may be caused by incomplete bladder emptying as a result of an enlarged prostate in men and cystocele and vaginal prolapse in women. Neuromuscular conditions that cause incomplete bladder emptying, such as Parkinson disease and stroke, affect older adults more frequently. The use of drugs with intentional or unintentional anticholinergic properties in older adults contributes to delayed bladder emptying. Fecal incontinence contributes to periurethral contamination. Low estrogen in menopausal women adversely affects the cells of the vagina and urethra, making them more susceptible to infections.
Sexual activity	Sexual intercourse is the strongest risk factor for uncomplicated cystitis, particularly in young women. Irritation of the perineum and urethra during intercourse can promote migration of bacteria from the perineal area to the urinary tract in some women. Inadequate vaginal lubrication may exacerbate potential urethral irritation. Bacteria may be introduced into the man's urethra during anal intercourse or during vaginal intercourse with a woman who has a bacterial vaginitis.
Recent use of antibiotics	Antibiotics change normal protective flora, providing opportunity for pathogenic bacterial overgrowth and colonization.

is no anatomic or functional abnormality of the urinary tract. Complicated UTIs are associated with conditions that increase the risk for treatment failure or serious outcomes. These conditions or factors include obstruction, pregnancy, male gender, diabetes, neurogenic bladder, renal insufficiency, and immunosuppression (Hooton, 2012). Complicated UTIs require greater vigilance to avoid or to detect adverse events from the infection and a longer course of antimicrobial treatment. They also may require additional diagnostics to identify and manage other related health problems (comorbidities).

CYSTITIS

❖ PATHOPHYSIOLOGY

Cystitis is an inflammatory condition of the bladder. Commonly, it refers to INFLAMMATION from an INFECTION of the bladder. However, cystitis can be caused by inflammation without infection. Drugs, chemicals, or radiation, for example, cause bladder inflammation without an infecting organism. Irritants, such as feminine hygiene spray, spermicidal jellies, or long-term use of a catheter can cause cystitis without infection. Cystitis may sometimes occur as a complication of other disorders, such as gynecologic cancers, pelvic inflammatory disorders, endometriosis, Crohn's disease, diverticulitis, lupus, or tuberculosis. **Interstitial cystitis** is an inflammatory disease that has no known cause.

Microbes, most commonly bacteria, move up the urinary tract from the external urethra to the bladder to cause infectious cystitis. Less commonly, spread of INFECTION through the blood and lymph fluid can occur. Mucin produced by cells lining the bladder helps maintain mucosal integrity and prevents cellular damage. Mucin may also prevent bacteria from adhering to urothelial cells. Bladder irritating factors, like concentrated urine, may interfere with the production and effectiveness of mucin.

Etiology and Genetic Risk

UTIs, like other INFECTIONS, are the result of interactions between a pathogen and the host. Usually, a high bacterial *virulence* (ability to invade and infect) is needed to overcome normal host resistance. However, a compromised host is more likely to become infected even with bacteria that have low virulence. Invading bacteria with special adhesions are more likely to cause ascending UTIs that start in the urethra or bladder and move up into the ureter and kidney. Patient-specific genetic factors such as innate inflammatory response may influence the risk for UTI.

Infectious cystitis is most commonly caused by pathogens from the bowel or, in some cases, the vagina (Hooton, 2012). About 90% of UTIs are caused by *Escherichia coli.* Less common organisms include *Staphylococcus saprophyticus, Klebsiella pneumoniae,* and organisms from the *Proteus* and *Enterobacter* species (Brusch, 2013). Other infecting microbes causing infectious cystitis are viruses, mycobacteria, parasites, and yeast (fungus), especially *Candida* species.

In most cases, organisms adhere to the perineal area and move into the urethra as a result of irritation, trauma, or instrumentation of the urinary tract. Infecting organisms then migrate to the bladder. Small urine volume or infrequent voiding, sexual intercourse, urinary tract obstruction, instrumentation, use of catheters not drained to gravity, and *vesicoureteral reflux* (backward flow of urine at the ureteral-bladder junction) are all associated with the ascending migration of infecting organisms.

Catheters are the most common factor placing patients at risk for UTIs in the hospital and long-term care settings (Mori, 2014). Within 48 hours of catheter insertion, bacterial colonization along the urethra and the catheter itself begins. About 50% of patients with indwelling catheters become infected within 1 week of catheter insertion.

How a catheter-related INFECTION occurs varies between genders. Bacteria from a woman's perineal area are more likely to ascend to the bladder by moving along the urethra. The shorter urethra in women aids in the ascending organism migration. In men, bacteria tend to gain access to the bladder from the catheter itself. Any break in the closed urinary drainage system allows bacteria to move through the lumen of the catheter. The external catheter surface also provides route for migration. Best practices to reduce the risk for catheter contamination and catheter-related UTIs are listed in Chart 66-1.

Organisms other than bacteria cause cystitis. Fungal INFECTIONS, such as those caused by *Candida,* can occur during long-term antibiotic therapy, because antibiotics change normal protective flora that reduce the adherence and virulence of pathogenic bacteria. Patients who are severely immunosuppressed, are receiving corticosteroids or other immunosuppressive agents, or have diabetes mellitus or acquired immune deficiency syndrome (AIDS) are at higher risk for fungal UTIs.

Viral and parasitic infections are rare and usually are transferred to the urinary tract from an INFECTION at another body site. For example, *Trichomonas,* a parasite found in the vagina, can also be found in the urine. Treatment of the vaginal infection also resolves the UTI.

Noninfectious cystitis may result from chemical exposure, such as to drugs (e.g., cyclophosphamide [Cytoxan, Procytox♣]); from radiation therapy; and from immunologic responses, as with systemic lupus erythematosus (SLE).

Interstitial cystitis is a rare, chronic INFLAMMATION of the entire lower urinary tract (bladder, urethra, and adjacent pelvic muscles) that is not a result of INFECTION. The condition affects women 10 times more often than men, and the diagnosis is difficult to make. Manifestations are PAIN associated with bladder filling or voiding, usually accompanied by frequency, urgency, and nocturia (McCance et al., 2014). Pain occurs in suprapubic or pelvic areas, sometimes radiating to the groin, vulva, or rectum. Results from urinalysis and urine culture are negative for infection (Quillin & Erickson, 2012).

Although cystitis is not life threatening, infectious cystitis can lead to life-threatening complications, including pyelonephritis and sepsis. Severe kidney damage from an ascending INFECTION that began as cystitis is a rare complication unless the patient also has other predisposing factors, such as anatomic abnormalities, pregnancy, obstruction, reflux, calculi, or diabetes.

The urinary tract is the INFECTION source of severe sepsis or septic shock in about 10% to 30% of cases (Wagenlehner et al., 2013). The spread of the infection from the urinary tract to the bloodstream is termed **urosepsis**. Urosepsis is associated with complicated urinary tract infections and is more common among older adults. Sepsis is a systemic reaction to infection that can lead to overwhelming organ failure, shock, and death.

CHART 66-1 Best Practice for Patient Safety & Quality Care (QSEN)

Minimizing Catheter-Related Infection

- Maintain good hand hygiene.
- Insert urinary catheters for appropriate use only, including:
  - Acute urinary retention or bladder obstruction
  - Accurate measurement of urine volume in critically ill patients
  - Perioperative situations that involve urologic surgery
  - Monitor urine output when large-volume infusions or diuretics are used
  - Patient requires immobilization from unstable spine or pelvic fractures
- Assess patients daily to determine the need for an indwelling catheter; the strongest predictor of a catheter-associated urinary tract infection (CAUTI) is the length of time the catheter dwells in a patient.
- Consider appropriate alternatives to an indwelling catheter such as an external device in men.
- Use sterile technique when inserting the urinary catheter.
- When emptying the urine bag, do not allow the tip of the outflow tube to touch the urine collection container. Use a dedicated container for each patient or resident.
- Select a small-size catheter, and do not overfill the balloon.
- Maintain a closed system by ensuring that catheter tubing connections are sealed securely; disconnections can introduce pathogens into the urinary tract.
- Maintain unobstructed urine flow by keeping the tubing patent and urine collection bags below the level of the bladder at all times; elevating the collection bag above the bladder causes reflux from the bag into the urinary tract.
- Monitor and report CAUTI rates, and promote ongoing best practices.
- Secure the catheter to the patient's thigh (women) or lower abdomen (men); catheter movement can cause urethral friction and irritation.
- Perform daily catheter care by washing the perineum and proximal portion of the catheter with soap and water and drying gently (removes pathogens and reduces pathogenic population).
- Consider the use of coated catheters for patients requiring indwelling catheters for more than 3 to 5 days. This coating reduces bacterial colonization along the catheter.

Application of antiseptic solutions or antibiotic ointments to the perineal area of catheterized patients has not been demonstrated to have any beneficial effect.

Adapted from Dumont, C., & Wakeman, J. (2010). Preventing catheter-associated UTIs: Survey report. *Nursing2010, 40*(12), 24-30.

Sepsis has a high mortality and prolongs hospitalization (see Chapter 37).

Incidence and Prevalence

The incidence of UTI is second only to that of upper respiratory infections in primary care. Patients who have **frequency** (an urge to urinate frequently in small amounts), **dysuria** (PAIN or burning with urination), and **urgency** (the feeling that urination will occur immediately) account for more than 8 million health care visits annually (Foxman, 2010). About 60% of these patients will have a confirmed UTI (Lowe & Ryan-Wenger, 2012).

CONSIDERATIONS FOR OLDER ADULTS

Patient-Centered Care QSEN

The prevalence of UTIs varies with age and gender. Women of any age are more commonly affected with UTIs than are men. In men, the incidence of UTI greatly increases after 73 years of age. In women, the prevalence of UTIs increases from 20% among all women to 50% among those older than 80 years (U.S. Renal Data Systems, 2012). Skin and mucous membrane changes from a lack of estrogen appear to account for much of the increased risk in older women. Prostate disease increases risk for UTIs in men. Ask about manifestations of UTI whenever you are assessing an older adult.

Health Promotion and Maintenance

Although cystitis is common, in many cases it is preventable. In the health care setting, reducing the use and duration of indwelling urinary catheters is a major prevention strategy. When catheters must be used in institutional settings, strict attention to sterile technique during insertion is essential to reduce the risk for UTIs (see Chart 66-1). Long-term placement of urinary catheters requires aseptic technique for insertion. When *intermittent catheterization* is used in the home setting, a clean technique may be used (Newman & Willson, 2011).

! NURSING SAFETY PRIORITY QSEN

Action Alert

Ensuring that urinary catheters are used appropriately and discontinued as early as possible is everyone's responsibility. Do not allow catheters to remain in place for staff convenience.

Certain changes in fluid intake patterns, urinary ELIMINATION patterns, and hygiene patterns can help prevent or reduce cystitis in the general population. For example, a liberal water intake of 2.2 L for women and 3 L for men can promote general health. Another strategy to promote health is to have sufficient fluid intake to cause 1.5 L of clear or light yellow urine daily. Other strategies to prevent cystitis and other UTIs are listed in Chart 66-2. Although these strategies do not have consistent or high-quality evidence to support a reduced risk for UTI when followed, they are low risk and reasonable (Hooton, 2012).

CHART 66-2 Patient and Family Education: Preparing for Self-Management

Preventing a Urinary Tract Infection

- Drink fluid liberally, as much as 2 to 3 liters daily if not contraindicated by health conditions.
- Be sure to get enough sleep, rest, and nutrition daily to maintain immunologic health.
- If spermicides are used, consider changing to another method of contraception.
- *[For women]* Clean your perineum (the area between your legs) from front to back.
- *[For women]* Avoid using or wearing irritating substances such as douches, scented lubricants for intercourse, bubble bath, tight-fitting underwear, and scented toilet tissue. Wear loose-fitting cotton underwear.
- *[For women]* Empty your bladder before and after intercourse.
- *[For both women and men]* Gently wash the perineal area before intercourse.
- Do not routinely delay urination because the flow of urine can help remove bacteria that may be colonizing the urethra or bladder.
- If you experience burning when you urinate, if you have to urinate frequently, or if you find it difficult to begin urinating, notify your physician or other health care provider right away, especially if you have a chronic medical condition (e.g., diabetes) or are pregnant.
- Consider using one or more of these therapies to reduce the risk for developing a urinary tract infection:
  - Taking cranberry substances (juice, capsules, or tablets) daily. Avoid high fructose cranberry juice to minimize calories and high glucose urine favorable to bacterial reproduction.
  - Ingesting apple cider vinegar, 2 tablespoons 3 times daily in juice.
  - Applying topical estrogen to the perineal area, if postmenopausal. Topical estrogen normalizes vaginal flora. Oral estrogens are not effective.
  - Ingesting D-mannose 500 mg tablet or 0.5-1 teaspoon of powder; D-mannose is thought to block adhesion of *E. coli* to the epithelium in the urinary tract.

Adapted from Hooton, T.M. (2012). Clinical practice: Uncomplicated urinary tract infection. *New England Journal of Medicine, 366*(11), 1028-1037.

❖ PATIENT-CENTERED COLLABORATIVE CARE

◆ Assessment

Physical Assessment/Clinical Manifestations. Frequency, urgency, and dysuria are the common manifestations of a urinary tract INFECTION (UTI), but other manifestations may be present (Chart 66-3). Urine may be cloudy, foul smelling, or blood tinged. Ask the patient about risk factors for UTI during the assessment (see Table 66-1). For noninfectious cystitis, the Pelvic Pain and Urgency/Frequency (PUF) patient symptom scale can identify patients with interstitial cystitis (Richmond, 2010).

Before performing the physical assessment, ask the patient to void so that the urine can be examined and the bladder emptied before palpation. Assess vital signs to help identify the presence of INFECTION (e.g., fever, tachycardia, and tachypnea). Inspect the lower abdomen, and palpate the bladder. Distention after voiding indicates incomplete bladder emptying.

Using Standard Precautions, record any lesions around the urethral meatus and vaginal opening. To help differentiate between a vaginal and a urinary tract INFECTION, note whether there is any vaginal discharge. Vaginal discharge and irritation are more indicative of vaginal infection. Women often report burning with urination when normal acidic urine touches labial tissues that are inflamed or ulcerated by vaginal infections or sexually transmitted diseases (STDs). Maintain privacy with drapes during the examination.

The prostate is palpated by digital rectal examination (DRE) for size, change in shape or consistency, and tenderness. The physician or advanced practice nurse performs the DRE.

Laboratory Assessment. Laboratory assessment for a UTI is a urinalysis with testing for leukocyte esterase and nitrate. The

CHART 66-3 Key Features

Urinary Tract Infection

Common Clinical Manifestations
- Frequency
- Urgency
- Dysuria
- Hesitancy or difficulty in initiating urine stream
- Low back pain
- Nocturia
- Incontinence
- Hematuria
- Pyuria
- Bacteriuria
- Retention
- Suprapubic tenderness or fullness
- Feeling of incomplete bladder emptying

Rare Clinical Manifestations
- Fever
- Chills
- Nausea or vomiting
- Malaise
- Flank pain

Clinical Manifestations that May Occur in the Older Adult
- The only manifestation may be something as vague as increasing mental confusion or frequent, unexplained falls.
- A sudden onset of incontinence or a worsening of incontinence may be the only manifestation of an early urinary tract infection (UTI).
- Fever, tachycardia, tachypnea, and hypotension, even without any urinary manifestations, may be signs of urosepsis.
- Loss of appetite, nocturia, and dysuria are common manifestations.

combination of a positive leukocyte esterase and nitrate is 68% to 88% sensitive in the diagnosis of a UTI (Lowe & Ryan-Wenger, 2012). However, when a urinalysis includes a microscopic count of bacteria, white blood cells (WBCs), and red blood cells (RBCs), the additional testing is more expensive and may not improve diagnostic accuracy. The presence of more than 20 epithelial cells/high-power field (hpf) suggests contamination. The presence of 100,000 colonies/mL or the presence of three or more WBCs (**pyuria**) with RBCs (**hematuria**) indicates INFECTION.

A urinalysis is performed on a clean-catch midstream specimen. If the patient cannot produce a clean-catch specimen, you may need to obtain the specimen with a small-diameter (6 Fr) catheter. For a routine urinalysis, 10 mL of urine is needed; smaller quantities are sufficient for culture.

A urine culture confirms the type of organism and the number of colonies. Urine culture is expensive, and initial results take at least 48 hours. It is indicated when the UTI is complicated, when it does not respond to usual therapy, or when the diagnosis is uncertain. A UTI is confirmed when more than 10^5 colony-forming units are in the urine from any patient. In patients who also have manifestations of UTI, as few as 10^3 colony-forming units may be used to confirm the infection. The presence of many different types of organisms in low colony counts usually indicates that the specimen is contaminated. Sensitivity testing follows culture results when complicating factors are present (e.g., stones or recurrent infection), when the patient is older, or to ensure the appropriate antibiotics are prescribed.

Occasionally the serum WBC count may be elevated, with the differential WBC count showing a "left shift" (see Chapter 17). This shift indicates that the number of immature WBCs is increasing in response to the INFECTION. As a result, the number of bands, or immature WBCs, is elevated. Left shift most often occurs with urosepsis and rarely occurs with uncomplicated cystitis, which is a local rather than a systemic infection.

Other Diagnostic Assessment. The diagnosis of cystitis is based on the history, physical examination, and laboratory data. If urinary retention and obstruction of urine outflow are suspected, pelvic ultrasound or CT may be needed to locate the site of obstruction or the presence of calculi. Voiding cystourethrography (see Chapter 65) is needed when urine reflux is suspected.

Cystoscopy (see Chapter 65) may be performed when the patient has recurrent UTIs (more than three or four a year). A urine culture is performed first to ensure that no infection is present. If INFECTION is present, the urine is sterilized with antibiotic therapy before the procedure to reduce the risk for sepsis. Cystoscopy identifies abnormalities that increase the risk for cystitis. Such abnormalities include bladder calculi, bladder diverticula, urethral strictures, foreign bodies (e.g., sutures from previous surgery), and **trabeculation** (an abnormal thickening of the bladder wall caused by urinary retention and obstruction). Retrograde pyelography, along with the cystoscopic examination, shows outlines and images of the drainage tract.

Cystoscopy is needed to accurately diagnose interstitial cystitis. A urinalysis usually shows WBCs and RBCs but no bacteria. Common findings in interstitial cystitis are a small-capacity bladder, the presence of Hunner's ulcers (a type of bladder lesion), and small hemorrhages after bladder distention.

◆ *Interventions*

Nonsurgical Management. The expected outcome is to maintain an optimal urine ELIMINATION pattern. Nursing interventions for the management of cystitis focus on comfort and teaching about drug therapy, fluid intake, and prevention measures.

Drug Therapy. Drugs used to treat bacteriuria and promote patient comfort include urinary antiseptics or antibiotics, analgesics, and antispasmodics. Cure of a UTI depends on the antimicrobial levels achieved in the urine. Fluconazole is the drug of choice for treatment of *Candida* (fungal) infections. Antispasmodic drugs decrease bladder spasm and promote complete bladder emptying.

Antibiotic therapy is used for bacterial UTIs (Chart 66-4). Guidelines for uncomplicated cystitis recommend nitrofurantoin, trimethoprim/sulfamethoxazole, or fosfomycin as first-line therapy (Brusch, 2013; Hooton, 2012; Hopkins et al., 2014). Longer antibiotic treatment (7 to 21 days) and sometimes different agents are required for hospitalized patients and those with complicated UTIs (e.g., pregnant women and patients with anatomic, functional or metabolic derangements that affect the urinary tract).

! NURSING SAFETY PRIORITY QSEN

Drug Alert

Two of the fluoroquinolone antibiotics, Tequin and Noroxin, are designated as sound-alike, look-alike agents with other drugs and could easily be administered in error. Take care to not confuse Tequin with Tegretol, an oral anticonvulsant, or with Ticlid, a platelet inhibitor. Take care to not confuse Noroxin with Neurontin, an oral anticonvulsant.

CHART 66-4 Common Examples of Drug Therapy

Urinary Tract Infections

DRUG/DOSAGE	NURSING INTERVENTIONS	RATIONALES
Antimicrobials		
Sulfonamides—Reduce Bacteria in the Urinary Tract By Direct Killing (Trimethoprim) and By Inhibiting Bacterial Reproduction (Sulfamethoxazole).		
Trimethoprim*/ sulfamethoxazole (Bactrim, Bacter-Aid, Septra, Sulfatrim, Sultrex, Roubac 🍁) 160 mg trimethoprim/800 mg sulfamethoxazole orally every 12 hr	Ask patients about drug allergies, especially to sulfa drugs, before beginning drug therapy.	Allergies to sulfa drugs are common and require changing the drug therapy.
	Teach patients to drink a full glass of water with each dose and to have an overall fluid intake of 3 L daily.	Sulfamethoxazole can form crystals that precipitate in the kidney tubules. Fluid intake prevents this complication.
	Teach patients to keep out of the sun or to wear protective clothing outdoors and use a sunscreen.	This drug increases skin sensitivity to the sun and can lead to severe sunburns, even in darker-skinned patients.
	Caution patients to complete the drug regimen even if the symptoms improve or disappear sooner.	Not completing the drug regimen can lead to an infection recurrence and to bacterial drug resistance.
Fluoroquinolones—Reduce Bacteria in the Urinary Tract By Direct Killing (Bactericidal Actions) and By Inhibiting Bacterial Reproduction (Bacteriostatic Actions).		
Ciprofloxacin (Cipro, ProQuin) 250 mg orally twice daily Levofloxacin (Levaquin) 400 mg orally daily	Teach patients taking the extended-release drugs to swallow them whole, not to crush or chew the tablets.	Crushing or chewing the tablet releases all the drug at once, ruining the extended effect.
	Warn patients to not take the drug within 2 hours of taking an antacid.	Many antacids (especially those containing magnesium or aluminum) interfere with drug absorption.
	Teach patients how to take their pulse, to monitor it twice daily while on this drug, and to notify the prescriber if new-onset irregular heartbeats occur.	This class of drugs can induce serious cardiac dysrhythmias.
	Teach patients to keep out of the sun or to wear protective clothing outdoors and use a sunscreen.	Most quinolones increase skin sensitivity to the sun and can lead to severe sunburns even in darker-skinned patients.
	Caution patients to complete the drug regimen even if the symptoms improve or disappear sooner.	Not completing the drug regimen can lead to an infection recurrence and to bacterial drug resistance.
Penicillins—Reduce Bacteria in the Urinary Tract By Direct Killing (Bactericidal Actions) As a Result of Interrupting Bacterial Cell Wall Synthesis.		
Amoxicillin (Amoxil) 500 mg orally every 12 hr Amoxicillin/ clavulanate (Augmentin, Clavulin 🍁) 500 mg/125 mg orally every 12 hr	Ask patients about drug allergies to penicillin before beginning drug therapy.	Allergies to penicillin are common and require changing the drug therapy.
	Teach patients to take the drug with food.	Taking it with food reduces the risk for GI upset.
	Instruct patients to call the prescriber if severe or watery diarrhea develops.	A complication of penicillin therapy is pseudomembranous colitis, which may require discontinuing the drug.
	Suggest that women who take oral contraceptives use an additional method of birth control while taking this drug.	Penicillin appears to reduce the effectiveness of estrogen-containing oral contraceptives.
	Caution patients to complete the drug regimen even if the symptoms improve or disappear sooner.	Not completing the drug regimen can lead to an infection recurrence and to bacterial drug resistance.
Cephalosporins—Reduce Bacteria in the Urinary Tract By Direct Killing (Bactericidal Actions) As a Result of Interrupting Bacterial Cell Wall Synthesis.		
Cefdinir, cefaclor, or cefpodoxime 250-500 mg orally daily	Ask about drug allergies to penicillin or cephalosporins before beginning drug therapy.	Drugs in this class are structurally similar to penicillin. Anyone with allergies to penicillin is likely to be allergic to the cephalosporins.
	Instruct patients to call the prescriber if severe or watery diarrhea develops.	A complication of penicillin therapy is pseudomembranous colitis, which may require discontinuing the drug.
	Caution patients to complete the drug regimen even if the symptoms improve or disappear sooner.	Not completing the drug regimen can lead to an infection recurrence and to bacterial drug resistance.
Other		
Fosfomycin (Monurol)—Reduces bacteria in the urinary tract by direct killing (bactericidal actions) as a result of interrupting bacterial cell wall synthesis.		
3 g orally as a one-time dose	Instruct patients to mix the contents of a package in about ½ cup of cold water, stir well, and drink all the liquid.	This oral drug is available as granules that must be dissolved before taking.
	Avoid taking this drug when also taking metoclopramide or any other drug that increases GI motility.	Drugs that increase GI motility reduce the absorption of fosfomycin.

Continued

CHART 66-4 Common Examples of Drug Therapy—cont'd

Urinary Tract Infections

DRUG/DOSAGE	NURSING INTERVENTIONS	RATIONALES
Nitrofurantoin (Furadantin, Macrobid, Macrodantin, Nephronex 🍁, Urotoin)—*Usually reduce bacteria in the urinary tract by inhibiting bacterial reproduction (bacteriostatic actions).*		
100 mg orally every 12 hr	Teach patients to shake the bottle well before measuring the drug.	Drug is a suspension and requires shaking to ensure homogeneity.
	Suggest that patients obtain a calibrated spoon for liquid drugs and to not use household spoons.	Household spoons are not accurate for measuring drugs.
	Teach patients to drink a full glass of water with each dose and to have an overall fluid intake of at least 3 L daily.	Drug precipitates in the kidney tubules and damages the kidney. Fluid intake prevents this complication.
	Caution patients to complete the drug regimen even if the symptoms improve or disappear sooner.	Not completing the drug regimen can lead to an infection recurrence and to bacterial drug resistance.
Bladder Analgesics—*Reduce Bladder Pain and Burning on Urination by Exerting a Topical Analgesic or Local Anesthetic Effect on the Mucosa of the Urinary Tract.*		
Phenazopyridine (Azo-Dine, Prodium, Pyridiate, Pyridium, Uristat, Phenazo 🍁) 200 mg orally 3 times daily, after meals	Remind patients that this drug will not treat an infection, only the symptoms.	Drug does not have any antibacterial actions.
	Teach patients to take the drug with or immediately after a meal.	Food reduces the risk for GI disturbances.
	Warn patients that urine will turn red or orange.	This expected response to the drug may stain clothing or toilets.
Antispasmodics—*Relieve Bladder Spasms by Inhibiting Nerve Stimulation to the Bladder Muscle.*		
Hyoscyamine (Anaspaz, Cystospaz, many others) 0.125-0.25 mg orally 3 to 4 times daily	Teach patients to notify the prescriber if blurred vision or other eye problems, confusion, dizziness or fainting spells, fast heartbeat, fever, or difficulty passing urine occurs.	These are manifestations of drug toxicity.
	Teach patients to wear dark glasses in sunlight or other bright-light areas.	Drug dilates the pupil and increases eye sensitivity to light.

*Trimethoprim can be given alone to patients with a sulfa allergy.

NCLEX EXAMINATION CHALLENGE

Safe and Effective Care Environment

A client in the community health clinic is prescribed trimethoprim/sulfamethoxazole for cystitis. The client reports developing hives to "something called Septra." What is the nurse's best action?

A. Reassure the client that Septra is not trimethoprim/sulfamethoxazole.
B. Highlight this important information in the client's medical record.
C. Place an allergy alert band on the client's wrist.
D. Notify the prescriber immediately.

Long-term, low-dose antibiotic therapy is sometimes used for chronic, recurring INFECTION caused by structural abnormalities or stones. Trimethoprim 100 mg daily may be used for long-term management of the older patient with frequent UTIs. For women who have recurrent UTIs after intercourse, antibiotics may be prescribed to be taken after intercourse. The three most common drug treatment regimens are (1) one low-dose tablet of trimethoprim (TMP) (Proloprim, Trimpex),(2) TMP/sulfamethoxazole (half or single-strength Bactrim, Cotrim, Septra), or (3) nitrofurantoin (Macrodantin, Nephronex 🍁, Novo Furantoin 🍁).

GENDER HEALTH CONSIDERATIONS

Patient-Centered Care QSEN

Pregnant women with a bacterial UTI require prompt and aggressive treatment because cystitis can lead to acute pyelonephritis during pregnancy. Pyelonephritis in pregnancy can cause preterm labor and adversely affect the fetus. Remind pregnant patients to contact their health care provider whenever manifestations of UTI are present.

Fluid Intake. Urge patients to drink enough fluid to maintain a diluted urine throughout the day and night unless fluid restriction is needed for another health problem. Some urologists recommend sufficient fluid intake to result in at least 1.5 L of urine output or 7 to 12 voidings daily. Food can provide 20% or more of fluid intake, particularly the intake of fruits and vegetables.

Drinking 50 mL of concentrated cranberry juice daily appears to decrease the ability of bacteria to adhere to the epithelial cells lining the urinary tract, decreasing the incidence of recurrent symptomatic UTIs in some patients. Cranberry juice, tablets, or capsules must be consumed for more than 4 weeks to affect the ability of *E. coli* to adhere to the urinary tract (Stapleton et al., 2012). Cranberry products have not consistently demonstrated effectiveness but are a low-cost and low-risk intervention (Hooton, 2012). It is important to note that cranberry juice is an irritant to the bladder with interstitial cystitis and should be avoided by patients with this condition. Avoiding caffeine, carbonated beverages, and tomato products may decrease bladder irritation during cystitis.

Comfort Measures. A warm sitz bath 2 or 3 times a day for 20 minutes may provide comfort and some relief of local symptoms. If burning with urination is severe or urinary retention occurs, teach the patient to sit in the sitz bath and urinate into the warm water. Urinary tract analgesics or antispasmodics may also provide comfort (see Chart 66-4).

Surgical Management. Surgery for cystitis treats the conditions that increase the risk for recurrent UTIs (e.g., removal of obstructions and repair of vesicoureteral reflux). Procedures may include cystoscopy (see Chapter 65) to identify and remove calculi or obstructions.

Community-Based Care

Assess the patient's level of understanding of the problem. His or her knowledge about factors that promote the development of cystitis determines the teaching interventions planned.

Teach the patient how to take prescribed drugs. Stress the need for correct spacing of doses throughout the day and the need to complete all of the prescribed antibiotics. If the drug will change the color of the urine, as it does with phenazopyridine (Pyridium, Urogesic, Phenazo ♣), inform the patient to expect this change.

Patients may associate discomfort with sexual activities and have feelings of guilt and embarrassment. Open and sensitive discussions with a woman who has recurrences of UTI after sexual intercourse can help her find techniques to handle the problem (see Chart 66-2). Explore with her the factors that contribute to her INFECTIONS, such as sexual penetration when the bladder is full, diaphragm use, and her general resistance to infection. Some positions during intercourse may reduce urethral irritation and subsequent cystitis. Remind the patient that vigorous cleaning of the perineum with harsh soaps and vaginal douching may irritate the perineal tissues and *increase* the risk for UTI. At the patient's request, discuss the problem with her and her partner to help them find ways of maintaining their intimate relationship.

URETHRITIS

❖ PATHOPHYSIOLOGY

Urethritis is an INFLAMMATION of the urethra. In men, manifestations include burning or difficulty urinating and a discharge from the urethral meatus. The most common cause of urethritis in men is sexually transmitted diseases (STDs). These include gonorrhea or nonspecific urethritis caused by *Ureaplasma* (a gram-negative bacterium), *Chlamydia* (a sexually transmitted gram-negative bacterium), or *Trichomonas vaginalis* (a protozoan found in both the male and female genital tract).

In women, urethritis causes manifestations similar to those of cystitis. Urethritis is known by several other terms: *pyuria-dysuria syndrome, frequency-dysuria syndrome, trigonitis syndrome,* and *urethral syndrome.* Urethritis is most common in postmenopausal women and is probably caused by tissue changes related to low estrogen levels.

❖ PATIENT-CENTERED COLLABORATIVE CARE

Ask the patient about a history of STD, painful or difficult urination, discharge from the penis or vagina, and discomfort in the lower abdomen. Urinalysis may show **pyuria** (white blood cells [WBCs] in the urine) without a large number of bacteria. However, results of urethral culture may indicate an STD. In women, the diagnosis may be made when urinalysis and urethral culture are negative for bacteria and there is no evidence of interstitial cystitis but manifestations persist. In such cases, pelvic examination may reveal tissue changes from low estrogen levels in the vagina. Urethroscopy may show low estrogen changes with INFLAMMATION of urethral tissues.

STDs and INFECTION are treated with antibiotic therapy. More information on STDs can be found in Chapter 74.

Postmenopausal women often have improvement in their urethral symptoms with the use of estrogen vaginal cream. Estrogen cream applied locally to the vagina increases the amount of estrogen in the urethra as well, and irritating manifestations are reduced.

NONINFECTIOUS DISORDERS

URETHRAL STRICTURES

Urethral strictures are narrowed areas of the urethra. These problems may be caused by complications of an STD (usually gonorrhea) and by trauma during catheterization, urologic procedures, or childbirth. About one third of urethral strictures have no obvious cause. Strictures occur more often in men than in women. They may be a factor in other urologic problems, such as recurrent UTIs, urinary incontinence, and urinary retention.

The most common manifestation of urethral stricture is obstruction of urine flow. Strictures rarely cause pain. Because urine stasis can result when flow is obstructed, the patient is at risk for developing a UTI and may have overflow incontinence. **Overflow incontinence** is the involuntary loss of urine when the bladder is overdistended. Assess the patient for these two problems.

A urethral stricture is treated surgically. Dilation of the urethra (using a local anesthetic) is only a temporary measure, not a curative one. Stent placement can be used in some patients. The best chance of long-term cure is with **urethroplasty**, which is the surgical removal of the affected area with or without grafting to create a larger opening. The recurrence rate after surgery is still high, and most patients need repeated procedures. The urethral stricture location and length are the most important factors affecting choice of interventions and recovery.

URINARY INCONTINENCE

❖ PATHOPHYSIOLOGY

Continence is the control over the time and place of urination and is unique to humans and some domestic animals. It is a learned behavior in which a person can suppress the urge to urinate until a socially appropriate location is available (e.g., a toilet). Efficient bladder emptying (i.e., coordination between bladder contraction and urethral relaxation) is needed for continence.

Incontinence is an involuntary loss of urine severe enough to cause social or hygienic problems. It is *not* a normal consequence of aging or childbirth and often is a stigmatizing and an underreported health problem. Many people suffer in silence, are socially isolated, and may be unaware that treatment is available. In addition, the cost of incontinence can be enormous.

Continence occurs when pressure in the urethra is greater than pressure in the bladder. For normal voiding to occur, the urethra must relax and the bladder must contract with enough pressure and duration to empty completely. Voiding should occur in a smooth and coordinated manner under a person's conscious control. Incontinence has several possible causes and can be either temporary or chronic (Table 66-2). Temporary causes usually do not involve a disorder of the urinary tract. The most common types of adult urinary incontinence are stress incontinence, urge incontinence, overflow incontinence, functional incontinence, and a mixed form.

TABLE 66-2 **Types of Urinary Incontinence**

TYPE	DEFINITION/DESCRIPTION	CAUSE	CLINICAL MANIFESTATIONS
Stress incontinence	The involuntary loss of urine during activities that increase abdominal and detrusor pressure. Patients cannot tighten the urethra sufficiently to overcome the increased detrusor pressure; leakage of urine results.	Weakening of bladder neck supports; associated with childbirth. Intrinsic sphincter deficiency caused by such congenital conditions as epispadias (abnormal location of the urethra on the dorsum of the penis) or myelomeningocele. Acquired anatomic damage to the urethral sphincter (from repeated incontinence surgeries, prostatectomy, radiation therapy, and trauma).	Urine loss with physical exertion, cough, sneeze, or exercise. Usually only small amounts of urine are lost with each exertion. Normal voiding habits (≤8 times per day, ≤2 times per night). Post-void residual usually ≤50 mL. Pelvic examination shows hypermobility of the urethra or bladder neck with Valsalva maneuvers.
Urge incontinence	The involuntary loss of urine associated with a strong desire to urinate. Patients cannot suppress the signal from the bladder muscle to the brain that it is time to urinate.	Unknown.	An abrupt and strong urge to void. May have loss of large amounts of urine with each occurrence.
Detrusor hyperreflexia (reflex incontinence)	The abnormal detrusor contractions result from neurologic abnormalities.	Central nervous system (CNS) lesions from stroke, multiple sclerosis, and parasacral spinal cord lesions. Local irritating factors such as caffeine, medications, or bladder tumor.	Post-void residual ≤50 mL.
Overflow incontinence	The involuntary loss of urine associated with overdistention of the bladder when the bladder's capacity has reached its maximum. The urethra is obstructed, so it fails to relax sufficiently to allow urine to flow, resulting in incomplete bladder emptying or complete urinary retention, causing overflow incontinence.	Diabetic neuropathy; side effects of medication; after radical pelvic surgery or spinal cord damage; outlet obstruction. Causes external to the mechanism of the urethra: an enlarged prostate (male patients) and large genital prolapse (female patients). When the cause is intrinsic to the urethra, abnormal contraction of the skeletal muscle occurs, causing obstruction. This condition, called *detrusor dyssynergia,* is seen in patients with spinal cord injuries and multiple sclerosis.	Bladder distention, often up to the level of the umbilicus. Constant dribbling of urine.
Mixed incontinence	A combination of stress, urge, and overflow incontinence.	As with each separate disorder.	As with each separate disorder.
Functional incontinence	Leakage of urine caused by factors other than disease of the lower urinary tract.		Quantity and timing of urine leakage vary; patterns are difficult to discern.
Transient causes	Transient causes improve with treatment of the underlying condition.	Loss of cognitive functioning. Loss of awareness that urination is to occur in a socially acceptable place.	Altered mental state, as in delirium, confusion, depression, dementia, sepsis, mental illness, or severe psychological stress.
		Abnormal openings in the urinary tract, such as a fistula or diverticulum.	Urinary drainage noted from areas other than the urinary meatus.
		Drugs, such as sedatives, hypnotics, diuretics, anticholinergics, decongestants, antihypertensives, and calcium channel blockers.	Some drugs cause altered mental state; others cause increased urine production.
		Diabetes insipidus or psychogenic polydipsia.	Increased urine output.
		Inability to get to toileting facilities.	Restraints, restricted mobility.
		Direct bladder pressure or urethral obstruction.	Constipation or fecal impaction.
Permanent causes	Permanent causes are organic but may be improved with treatment.	Cognitive impairment. Traumatic or surgical effects. Those factors contributing to stress incontinence, urge incontinence, and overflow incontinence. Structural or functional defects of the bladder or the sphincters. Injuries or diseases of the spinal cord, brainstem, or cerebral cortex (neurogenic bladder). Congenital defects, including exstrophy of the bladder (bladder turned "inside out") and spina bifida.	Clinical manifestations depend on the cause.

Stress incontinence is the most common type. Its main feature is the loss of small amounts of urine during coughing, sneezing, jogging, or lifting. In the continent person, the urethra can be relaxed and tightened under conscious control because skeletal muscles of the pelvic floor surround it. When a person feels the urge to urinate, the conscious contraction of the urethra can override a bladder contraction if the urethral contraction is strong enough.

Patients with *stress incontinence* cannot tighten the urethra enough to overcome the increased bladder pressure caused by contraction of the detrusor muscle. This is common after childbirth, when the pelvic muscles are stretched and weakened. The weakened pelvic floor allows the urethra to move during exertion. If the pelvic muscles are not strengthened, this condition continues. Low estrogen levels after menopause also contribute to stress incontinence. Vaginal, urethral, and pelvic floor muscles become thin and weak without estrogen.

Urge incontinence is the perception of an urgent need to urinate as a result of bladder contractions regardless of the urine volume in the bladder. Normally when the bladder is full, contraction of the smooth muscle fibers of the bladder detrusor muscle signals the brain that it is time to urinate. Continent people override that signal and relax the detrusor muscle for the time it takes to locate a toilet. Those who suffer from urge incontinence cannot suppress the signal and have a sudden strong urge to void and often leak large amounts of urine at this time. Urge incontinence is also known as an *overactive bladder* (OAB). Overactivity may have no known cause or may be the result of abnormal detrusor contractions related to other problems. Such problems include stroke and other neurologic problems, other urinary tract problems, and irritation from concentrated urine, artificial sweeteners, caffeine, alcohol, and citric intake. Drugs, such as diuretics, and nicotine can also irritate the bladder.

Mixed incontinence is the presence of more than one type of incontinence. Often urine loss is related to both stress and urge incontinence. The manifestations mimic more than one subtype. This category is more common in older women.

Overflow incontinence occurs when the detrusor muscle fails to contract and the bladder becomes overdistended. This type of incontinence (also known as *reflex incontinence* or *underactive bladder*) occurs when the bladder has reached its maximum capacity and some urine must leak out to prevent bladder rupture. Causes for the underactive (acontractile) bladder may or may not be determined.

The urethra can be obstructed and fail to relax enough to allow urine flow. Incomplete bladder emptying or urinary retention from urethral obstruction results in overflow incontinence.

Functional incontinence is incontinence occurring as a result of factors other than the abnormal function of the bladder and urethra. A common factor is the loss of cognitive function in patients affected by dementia. To maintain continence, a person must be aware that urination needs to occur in a socially acceptable place. Patients with dementia may not have that awareness.

Etiology

Incontinence may have temporary or permanent causes. Evaluation of the incontinent patient means considering all possible causes, beginning with those that are temporary and correctable. Surgical and traumatic causes of urinary incontinence are related to procedures or surgery in the lower pelvic structures, which are areas that contain complex nerve pathways. Radical urologic, prostatic, and gynecologic procedures for treatment of pelvic cancers may result in urinary incontinence. Injury to segments S2 to S4 of the spinal cord may cause incontinence from impairment of normal nerve pathways.

Inappropriate bladder contraction may result from disorders of the brain and nervous system or from bladder irritation due to chronic INFECTION, stones, chemotherapy, or radiation therapy. Other causes of bladder contraction failure include the neuropathies associated with diabetes mellitus and syphilis. Constipation can lead to temporary urinary incontinence. Some drugs, such as anticholinergics, calcium channel blockers, diuretics, and sedatives, can cause or worsen urinary incontinence.

CONSIDERATIONS FOR OLDER ADULTS

Patient-Centered Care QSEN

Many factors contribute to urinary incontinence in older adults (Chart 66-5). An older person may have decreased mobility from many causes. In inpatient settings, mobility is limited when the older patient is placed on bedrest. Vision and hearing impairments may also prevent the patient from locating a call light to notify the nurse or assistive personnel of the need to void. Assess for these factors, and minimize them to prevent urinary incontinence. Getting out of bed to urinate is a common cause of falls among older adults.

CHART 66-5 Nursing Focus on the Older Adult

*Factors Contributing to Urinary Incontinence**

Drugs

- Central nervous system depressants, such as opioid analgesics, decrease the patient's level of consciousness and the urge to void, and they contribute to constipation.
- Diuretics cause frequent voiding, often of large amounts of urine.
- Multiple drugs can contribute to changes in mental status or mobility, and they can irritate the bladder.
- Anticholinergic drugs or drugs with anticholinergic side effects are especially challenging because they affect both cognition and the ability to void. Monitor patient responses to these drugs early in treatment.

Disease

- Cerebrovascular accidents and other neurologic disorders decrease mobility, sensation, or cognition.
- Arthritis decreases mobility and causes pain.
- Parkinson disease causes muscle rigidity and an inability to initiate movement.

Depression

- Depression decreases the energy necessary to maintain continence.
- Decreased self-esteem and feelings of self-worth decrease the importance to the patient of maintaining continence.

Inadequate Resources

- Patients who need assistive devices (e.g., eyeglasses, cane, walker) may be afraid to ambulate without them or without personal assistance.
- Products that help patients manage incontinence are often costly.
- No one may be available to assist the patient to the bathroom or help with incontinence products.

*These factors are in addition to the physiologic changes of aging given in Chapter 2.

Incidence and Prevalence

Incontinence is a major health problem. As many as 25% to 45% of woman report some degree of urinary incontinence with roughly half as many men reporting this condition (Buckley et al., 2010). It is most common in older adults and in at least one half of all nursing home residents.

Increased risk for urinary incontinence occurs with pregnancy, childbirth, diabetes mellitus, and increased body mass (Buckley et al., 2010). Urinary incontinence can occur as an isolated condition or with other chronic health problems. In addition, impairments from central nervous system diseases (i.e., dementia, stroke, multiple sclerosis, Parkinson disease) and musculoskeletal disorders (i.e., osteoporosis, osteoarthritis, low back pain) contribute to reduced leg strength and mobility limitations resulting in the onset and severity of urinary incontinence (McCance et al., 2014). More than 35% of adults admitted to the hospital develop urinary incontinence (Dowling-Castronovo & Bradway, 2012). Because the problem is so common among older adults, it is recommended that all people older than 65 years be screened for urinary incontinence (DuBeau, 2013).

❖ PATIENT-CENTERED COLLABORATIVE CARE

◆ Assessment

History. Effective screening includes asking patients to respond "always," "sometimes," or "never" to these questions:

- Do you ever leak urine or water when you don't want to?
- Do you ever leak urine or water when you cough, laugh, or exercise?
- Do you ever leak urine or water on the way to the bathroom?
- Do you ever use pads, tissue, or cloth in your underwear to catch urine?

If any answer is "always" or "sometimes," proceed with a focused assessment (Chart 66-6). Incontinence may be underreported because health care professionals do not ask patients about urine loss. *Do not assume that patients will volunteer the information without specifically being asked.*

Physical Assessment/Clinical Manifestations. Assess the abdomen to estimate bladder fullness, to rule out palpable hard stool, and to evaluate bowel sounds. Urinary incontinence is confirmed by evaluating the force and character of the urine stream during voiding. Asking the patient to cough while wearing a perineal pad is useful in evaluating stress incontinence; a wet pad on forceful coughing may indicate stress incontinence.

For women, inspect the external genitalia to determine whether there is apparent urethral or uterine prolapse, cystocele (herniation of the bladder into the vagina), or rectocele. These conditions occur with pelvic floor muscle weakness. A health care provider puts on an examination glove and inserts two fingers into the vagina to assess the strength of these muscles. Strength is described as *weak, adequate,* or *strong* based on the amount of pressure felt by the health care provider as the patient tightens her vaginal muscles. Describe and document the color, consistency, and odor of any secretions from the genitourinary orifices. The urine stream interruption test (i.e., asking a patient to voluntarily start and stop urine flow during a void at least twice) is another method of determining pelvic muscle strength. For men, inspect the urethral meatus for any discharge.

CHART 66-6 Focused Assessment

The Patient with Urinary Incontinence

Note the presence of risk factors for urinary incontinence:
- Age
- If female, menopausal status
- Neurologic disease:
  - Parkinson disease
  - Dementia
  - Multiple sclerosis
  - Stroke
  - Spinal injury
- Diabetes mellitus
- Childbirth
- Urologic procedures
- Prescribed and over-the-counter drugs
- Bowel patterns
- Stress/anxiety level

Detail the symptoms of urinary incontinence:
- Leakage
- Frequency
- Urgency
- Nocturia
- Sensation of full bladder before leakage

Obtain a 24-hour intake-and-output record or a voiding diary:
- Time and amount of oral intake and continent voiding
- Time and estimated amount of incontinent leakages
- Activity around the time of leakage

Assess the patient's:
- Mobility
- Self-care ability
- Cognitive ability
- Communication patterns

Assess the environment for barriers to toileting:
- Privacy
- Restrictive clothing
- Access to toilet

A digital rectal examination (DRE) is performed by the health care provider on both male and female patients. It provides information about the nerve integrity to the bladder. The examiner determines whether there is tactile sensation in the anal area by observing whether the rectal sphincter is relaxed or contracted on digital insertion. Because nerve supply to the bladder is similar to nerve supply to the rectum, the presence of tactile sensation and a rectal sphincter that contracts suggest that the nerve supply to the bladder is intact. Impaction of stool is a cause of transient urinary incontinence and can be detected during a rectal examination. The health care provider assesses for prostate enlargement in men as a possible cause of incontinence.

Laboratory Assessment. A urinalysis is useful to rule out INFECTION. This test is the first step in the assessment of incontinent patients of any age. The presence of red blood cells (RBCs), white blood cells (WBCs), leukocyte esterase, or nitrites is an indication for culturing the urine. Any infection is treated before further assessment of incontinence.

Imaging Assessment. Determine the amount of post-void residual urine (urine remaining in the bladder immediately after voiding) by portable ultrasound. With a health care provider's order, catheterizing the patient immediately after voiding can also be used to assess residual volume. Additional imaging is rarely needed unless surgery is being considered. CT is most useful for locating abnormalities in kidneys and ureters. A voiding cystourethrogram (VCUG) or urodynamic testing may be performed to assess the size, shape, support, and function of the urinary tract system. Urodynamic testing (see Chapter 65) may take several hours and more than one visit. Electromyography (EMG) of the pelvic muscles may be a part of the urodynamic studies.

◆ Analysis

The priority NANDA-I nursing diagnoses and collaborative problems for patients with urinary incontinence include:

1. Stress Urinary Incontinence related to weak pelvic muscles and structural supports (NANDA-I)
2. Urge Urinary Incontinence related to decreased bladder capacity, bladder spasms, diet, and neurologic impairment (NANDA-I)
3. Reflex Urinary Incontinence related to neurologic impairment (NANDA-I)
4. Functional Urinary Incontinence related to impaired cognition or neuromuscular limitations (NANDA-I)
5. Total urinary incontinence (mixed) related to many causes

◆ Planning and Implementation

Several interventions are useful for each type of incontinence in addition to drugs, surgical repair, and nutrition therapy.

Reducing Stress Urinary Incontinence

Planning: Expected Outcomes. With appropriate therapy, the patient with stress urinary incontinence is expected to develop urinary continence. Indicators include that the patient rarely or never demonstrates these problems:

- Urine leakage between voidings
- Urine leakage with increased abdominal pressure (e.g., sneezing, laughing, lifting)

Interventions. Initial interventions for patients with stress incontinence include keeping a diary, behavioral interventions, and drugs. Surgery also may be an option if other interventions are not effective. Explain the purpose of a detailed diary in which the patient records times of urine leakage, activities, and foods eaten. The diary is then used by the health care provider to plan and evaluate interventions. Collection devices, absorbent pads, and undergarments may be used during the sometimes lengthy process of assessment and treatment and by those patients who elect not to pursue further interventions.

Nonsurgical Management. Drug therapy and behavioral interventions (primarily diet and exercise) for stress incontinence require the patient's active participation for success. Nursing interventions focus on teaching patients about the drugs and behavioral strategies and on providing ongoing encouragement, clarification, and support to maximize intervention effects.

Pelvic floor (Kegel) exercise therapy for women with stress incontinence strengthens the muscles of the pelvic floor (circumvaginal muscles). These muscles become strengthened, as any other skeletal muscle does, by frequent, systematic, and repeated contractions. Pelvic floor muscle training improves not only continence but also quality of life in women with urinary incontinence (Fan et al., 2013).

The most important step in teaching pelvic muscle exercises is to help the patient learn which muscle to exercise. During the pelvic examination in women and the rectal examination in men or women, instruct the patient to tighten the pelvic muscles around your fingers. Then provide feedback about the strength of the contraction. Starting and stopping the urine stream or stopping the passage of flatus indicates that the patient has correctly identified the pelvic muscles. Biofeedback devices, such as electromyography or perineometers, measure the strength of contraction. A perineometer is a tampon-shaped instrument inserted into the vagina to measure the strength of pelvic muscle contractions. The graph shows the amplitude of muscle contraction to the patient as a method of biofeedback. Alternatively, retention of a vaginal weight also shows that the patient has identified the proper muscle (see discussion on vaginal cone therapy below).

Instructions for pelvic muscle exercises are given in Chart 66-7. Although improvement may take several months, most patients notice a positive change after 6 weeks. Teach patients to continue the exercises 10 times daily to improve and maintain pelvic muscle strength.

Nutrition therapy in the form of weight reduction is helpful for obese patients because stress incontinence is made worse by increased abdominal pressure from obesity (Wilde et al., 2014). Teach the patient to avoid bladder irritants in the diet that can contribute to urgency and frequency. For example, caffeine is a bladder irritant (Jura et al., 2011). Stress the importance of maintaining an adequate fluid intake, especially water. Refer the patient to a registered dietitian as needed.

Drug therapy can be useful for some people with stress incontinence. Because bladder pressure is greater than urethral resistance in patients with stress incontinence, drugs may be used to improve urethral resistance (Chart 66-8).

Topical estrogen to the perineal and vaginal orifice is used to treat postmenopausal women with stress incontinence, although it is not known exactly how this drug helps improve continence. Estrogen may increase the blood flow and tone of the muscles around the vagina and urethra, thus improving the patient's ability to contract those muscles during times of increased intra-abdominal stress.

Vaginal cone therapy involves using a set of five small, cone-shaped weights. They are of equal size but of varying weights and are used together with pelvic muscle exercise. The woman inserts the lightest cone, labeled *1,* into her vagina (Fig. 66-1),

CHART 66-7 Patient and Family Education: Preparing for Self-Management

Pelvic Muscle Exercises

- The pelvic muscles are composed of a sling of muscles that support your bladder, urethra, and vagina. Like any other muscles in your body, you can make your pelvic muscles stronger by alternately contracting (tightening) and relaxing them in regular exercise periods. By strengthening these muscles, you will be able to stop your urine flow more effectively.
- To identify your pelvic muscles, sit on the toilet with your feet flat on the floor about 12 inches apart. Begin to urinate, and then try to stop the urine flow. Do not strain down, lift your bottom off the seat, or squeeze your legs together. When you start and stop your urine stream, you are using your pelvic muscles.
- To perform pelvic muscle exercises, tighten your pelvic muscles for a slow count of 10 and then relax for a slow count of 10. Do this exercise 15 times while you are lying down, sitting up, and standing (a total of 45 exercises). Repeat—and this time rapidly contract and relax the pelvic muscles 10 times. This should take no more than 10 to 12 minutes for all three positions, or 3 to 4 minutes for each set of 15 exercises.
- Begin with 45 exercises a day in three sets of 15 exercises each. You will notice faster improvement if you can do this twice a day, or a total of 20 minutes each day. Remember to exercise in all three positions so your muscles learn to squeeze effectively despite your position. At first, it is helpful to have a designated time and place to do these exercises because you will have to concentrate to do them correctly. After you have been doing them for several weeks, you will notice improvement in your control of urine. However, many people report that improvement may take as long as 3 months.

CHART 66-8 Common Examples of Drug Therapy

Urinary Incontinence

DRUG/DOSAGE	NURSING INTERVENTIONS	RATIONALES
Hormones—Thought to Enhance Nerve Conduction to the Urinary Tract, Improve Blood Flow, and Reduce Tissue Deterioration of the Urinary Tract.		
*Estrogen vaginal cream daily or an estrogen-containing ring inserted monthly	Teach patients that a thin application of the cream is all that is needed.	Topical use minimizes the amount of estrogen absorbed and distributed in the body. A thick application increases risk for systemic distribution.
	Teach patients that it takes 4-6 wks to achieve continence benefits and that benefits disappear after about 4 weeks after discontinuing regular use.	Topical administration via a cream or ring avoids systemic adverse drug effects from this hormone but also takes longer for effects.
Antispasmodics—Reduce Incontinence By Causing Bladder Muscle Relaxation.		
Oxybutynin (Ditropan) 5 mg orally 3-4 times daily; (Ditropan XL) 5-10 mg orally daily	Ask whether the patient has glaucoma before starting the drug.	Anticholinergics can increase intraocular pressure and make glaucoma worse.
	Suggest that patients increase fluid intake and use hard candy to moisten the mouth.	Dry mouth is a common side effect of drugs in this category.
	Teach patients to increase fluid intake and the amount of dietary fiber.	Constipation is a common side effect of drugs in this category.
	Teach patients to monitor urine output and to report an output significantly lower than intake to the health care provider.	Drugs in this category can cause urinary retention.
	Instruct patients taking the extended-release forms of these drugs not to chew or crush the tablet/capsule.	Crushing or chewing the tablet/capsule releases all the drug at once, ruining the extended effect and increasing the possibility of side effects.
Anticholinergics—Suppress Involuntary Bladder Contraction, Increase Urine Volume and May Increase the Bladder Capacity.		
Tolterodine (Detrol) 2 mg orally twice daily; (Detrol LA) 4 mg orally daily	Ask whether the patient has glaucoma before starting the drug.	These drugs can increase intraocular fluid and pressure.
Propantheline (Pro-Banthine, Propanthel) 7.5-30 mg orally 3-4 times daily	Do not use these drugs if prostate hypertrophy co-exists.	These drugs can worsen urinary retention from prostate hypertrophy.
Dicyclomine (Barmine, Bentyl) 10-40 mg orally 3-4 times daily	Teach patients to avoid dehydration and increase the amount of dietary fiber to avoid constipation.	These drugs can cause significant constipation.
Trospium (Sanctura) 20 mg orally every 12 hr Darifenacin (Enablex) 7.5-15 mg orally daily Solifenacin (Vesicare) 5-10 mg orally daily Fesoterodine (Toviaz) 4-8 mg orally daily	Evaluate kidney function before starting and at least annually.	These drugs may have decreased renal clearance and should either be avoided or administered in a reduced dose in patients with renal insufficiency.
	Instruct the patient to avoid crushing or chewing tablets.	Most of the once-daily drugs are a long-acting formulation and should not be crushed or chewed.
Alpha Adrenergic Agonists—Increase Contractile Force of the Urethral Sphincter, Increasing Resistance to Urine Outflow.		
*Midorine (ProAmatine, Orvaten) 2.5-5 mg orally every 8-12 hr *Pseudoephedrine (Sudafed, SudoGest) 30 mg orally; also comes in an extended-release formulation	Teach the patient to monitor his or her blood pressure periodically when starting the drug.	These drugs can cause a supine hypertension; do not use with severe cardiac disease.
$Beta_3$ Blockers—Relax the Detrusor Smooth Muscle to Increase Bladder Capacity and Urine Storage.		
Mirabegron (Myrbetriq) 25 mg orally daily	Teach the patient to periodically obtain a blood pressure and to inform the health care provider if the systolic or diastolic values increase more than 10 mm Hg or above 180/110.	Because it is a selective beta blocker, there is some potential to increase blood pressure.
	If the patient is taking warfarin, avoid this drug or schedule additional blood testing for potential increased risk for bleeding.	This drug may interact with warfarin due to similar metabolic pathways, resulting in prolonged international normalized ratio (INR), the test to evaluate warfarin effects.
Antidepressants: Tricyclics and Serotonin-Norepinephrine Reuptake Inhibitors (SNRIs)—Increase Norepinephrine and Serotonin Levels, Which Are Thought to Strengthen the Urinary Sphincters. They Also Have Anticholinergic Actions.		
Tricyclics Imipramine (Tofranil, Novo-Pramine) 25-100 mg orally 4 times daily Amitriptyline (Elavil, Levate) 10-25 mg orally daily	Warn patients not to combine these drugs with other antidepressant drugs. Instruct patients to inform their provider if they take drugs to manage hypertension.	These drugs have significant drug-drug interactions with other antidepressants and with some antihypertensive drugs, leading to hypertensive crisis.
	Teach patients to change positions slowly, especially in the morning.	These drugs cause dizziness and orthostatic hypotension and can increase the risk for falls.
SNRI *Duloxetine (Cymbalta) 20-60 mg orally daily	Teach patients the same interventions as for anticholinergic agents.	These drugs have anticholinergic activity and produce the same side effects.

*These drugs are used off-label and do not have United States Food and Drug Administration (FDA) approval for use. However, they are commonly used to manage incontinence syndromes.

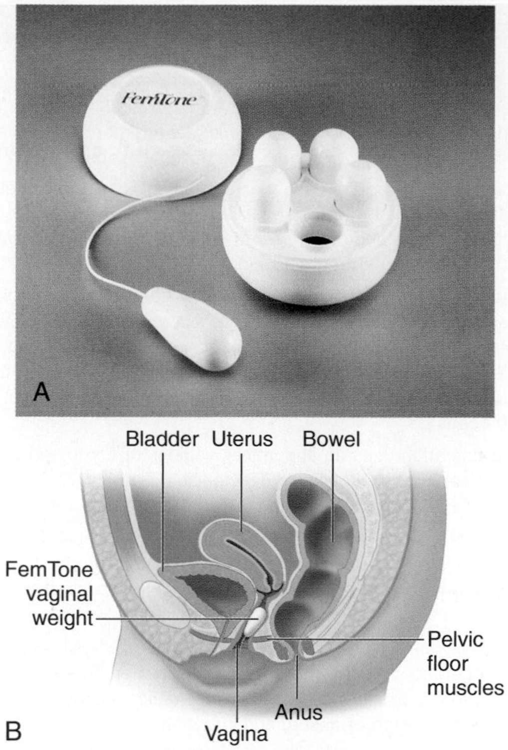

FIG. 66-1 A, FemTone vaginal weights, or cones. The number on the top of each cone represents increasing weight up to the heaviest cone, a *5*. **B,** Diagram showing the correct positioning of a vaginal weight, or cone, in place.

with the string to the outside, for a 1-minute test period. If she can hold the first cone in place without its slipping out while she walks around, she proceeds to the second cone, labeled *2*, and repeats the procedure. The patient begins her treatment with the heaviest cone she can comfortably hold in her vagina for the 1-minute test period. Treatment periods are 15 minutes twice a day. When the patient can comfortably hold the cone in her vagina for the 15-minute period, she progresses to the next heaviest weight. Treatment is completed with the cone labeled *5*.

Weighted vaginal cones can help strengthen the pelvic muscles and decrease stress incontinence but may not help pelvic prolapse. Vaginal cones do not require a prescription.

Other interventions for stress incontinence include behavior modification, psychotherapy, and electrical stimulation devices to strengthen urethral contractions. Many intravaginal and intrarectal electrical stimulation devices have been used with varying degrees of success.

A ring-shaped *pessary* inserted into the vagina may help with a prolapsed uterus or bladder when this condition is contributing to urinary incontinence. A prolapse occurs when the supportive tissue in the vagina weakens and stretches, allowing pelvic organs to protrude into the vaginal lumen. The pessary presses against the wall of the vagina to reposition pelvic organs. Generally, a pessary is removed and cleaned with soap and water on a monthly basis by the patient but can be done by the nurse for adults with cognitive or musculoskeletal impairment.

Urethral occlusion devices can be particularly helpful for activity-induced incontinence. One device, the Reliance insert, is like a tiny tampon that the patient inserts into the urethra. After insertion, the patient inflates a tiny balloon, which rests at the bladder neck and prevents the flow of urine. To void, the patient pulls a string to deflate the balloon and removes the device. The applicator is reusable, although the tampon part is disposed of after each void.

Electrical stimulation with either an intravaginal or intrarectal electrical stimulation device is available to treat both urge and stress incontinence. Treatment consists of stimulating sensory nerves to decrease the sensation of urgency. It is done as an office-based procedure 1 to 3 times weekly for 6 to 8 weeks.

Magnetic resonance therapy involves targeted urinary tract nerves and muscles for depolarization. The patient sits on a chair containing a magnetic device, which induces depolarization and helps reduce stress-induced incontinence similar to drug-induced relaxation of muscle and nerves.

Surgical Management. Stress incontinence may be treated by a surgical sling or bladder suspension procedure (Table 66-3). A sling procedure creates a sling around the bladder neck and urethra using strips of body tissue or synthetic material (mesh). Bladder suspension procedures are more extensive, and the surgeon sutures tissue near the bladder neck to a pubic bone ligament to provide support and prevent sagging. A third surgical procedure is the injection of bulking agents into the urethral wall to provide resistance to urine outflow. Bulking agents include collagen, carbon-coated zirconium beads, and silicone implants (Shultz, 2012).

Preoperative Care. Teach the patient about the procedure, and clarify the surgeon's explanation of events surrounding the surgery. Extensive urodynamic testing (see Chapter 65) is often performed before surgery, and you must explain the need for such thorough assessment to the patient and family.

Postoperative Care. After surgery, assess for and intervene to prevent or detect complications. For prevention of movement or traction on the bladder neck, secure the urethral catheter with tape or a tube holder. If a suprapubic catheter is used instead of a urethral catheter, monitor the dressing for urine leakage and other drainage. Catheters are usually in place until the patient can urinate easily and has residual urine volume after voiding of less than 50 mL. (See Chapters 14 and 16 for a discussion of general care before and after surgery.)

Reducing Urge Urinary Incontinence

Planning: Expected Outcomes. The patient with urinary incontinence is expected to use techniques to prevent or manage urge incontinence. Indicators include that the patient often or consistently demonstrates these behaviors:

- Responds to urge in a timely manner
- Gets to toilet between urge and passage of urine
- Avoids substances that stimulate the bladder (e.g., caffeine, alcohol)

Interventions. Interventions for patients with urge incontinence or overactive bladder (OAB) include neuromodulation, drugs, and behavioral interventions. *Neuromodulation* therapy, which involves stimulation of the nerves to the bladder, can be used to manage urge incontinence. The device requires minor surgery to place the device. Other types of surgery are not the recommended treatment of this condition.

Drug Therapy. Because the hypertonic bladder contracts involuntarily in patients with urge incontinence, drugs that relax the smooth muscle and increase the bladder's capacity are prescribed (see Chart 66-8). The most effective drugs are anticholinergics, such as propantheline (Pro-Banthine, Propanthel

TABLE 66-3 **Surgical Procedures for Stress Incontinence**

PROCEDURE	PURPOSE	NURSING CONSIDERATIONS
Anterior vaginal repair (colporrhaphy)	Elevates the urethral position and repairs any cystocele.	Because the operation is performed by vaginal incision, it is often done in conjunction with a vaginal hysterectomy. Recovery is usually rapid, and a urethral catheter is in place for 24-48 hr.
Retropubic suspension (Marshall-Marchetti-Krantz or Burch colposuspension)	Elevates the urethral position and provides longer-lasting results.	The operation requires a low abdominal incision and a urethral or suprapubic catheter for several days postoperatively. Recovery takes longer, and urinary retention and detrusor instability are the most frequent complications.
Needle bladder neck suspension (Pereyra or Stamey procedure)	Elevates the urethral position and provides longer-lasting results without a long operative time.	The combined vaginal approach with a needle and a small suprapubic skin incision does not allow direct vision of the operative site; however, the high complication rates may be due to the selection of patients who, because of their medical condition, are not good candidates for longer retropubic procedures.
Pubovaginal sling procedures	A sling made of synthetic or fascial material is placed under the urethrovesical junction to elevate the bladder neck.	The operation uses an abdominal, vaginal, or combined approach to treat intrinsic sphincter deficiencies. Temporary or permanent urinary retention is common postoperatively.
Midurethral sling procedures	A tensionless vaginal sling is made from polypropylene mesh (or other materials) and placed near the urethrovesical junction to increase the angle, which inhibits movement of urine into the urethra with lower intravesicular pressures.	This ambulatory surgery procedure uses a vaginal approach to improve symptoms of stress incontinence. Temporary or permanent urinary retention is common postoperatively.
Artificial sphincters	A mechanical device to open and close the urethra is placed around the anatomic urethra.	The operation is done more frequently in men. The most common complications include mechanical failure of the device, erosion of tissue, and infection.
Periurethral injection of collagen or Siloxane	Implantation of small amounts of an inert substance through several small injections provides support around the bladder neck.	The procedure can be done in an ambulatory care setting and can be repeated as often as necessary. Certain compounds may migrate after injection; an allergy test to bovine collagen must be performed before implantation.

🍁), and anticholinergics with smooth muscle relaxant properties, such as oxybutynin (Ditropan and Ditropan XL), tolterodine (Detrol and Detrol LA), and dicyclomine hydrochloride (Baramine, Bentyl, Spasmoban 🍁). This class of drugs has serious side effects and is used along with behavioral interventions. These drugs inhibit the nerve fibers that stimulate bladder contraction. Tricyclic antidepressants with anticholinergic and alpha-adrenergic agonist activity, such as imipramine (Tofranil, Novopramine 🍁), have been used successfully. The effectiveness of other drugs, such as flavoxate (Urispas) and the antihistamines, NSAIDs, beta-adrenergic agonists, and calcium channel blockers, has yet to be determined.

Another drug therapy for urge incontinence is onabotulinumtoxinA (Botox), which received approval in 2013 from the U.S. Food and Drug Administration (FDA) for this use. The drug is injected during cystoscopy into multiple areas of the detrusor muscle of the bladder. Usually, 10 to 30 different sites are injected during one treatment session. This treatment relaxes the detrusor muscle and relieves the urge to urinate. Some patients have had relief of incontinence for as long as 6 to 9 months after injection. Side effects may include urinary retention, painful urination, and an increased incidence of urinary tract infections. For most patients who experience urinary retention, the condition is temporary but does require intermittent self-catheterization.

! NURSING SAFETY PRIORITY QSEN

Drug Alert

Teach patients taking the extended-release forms of anticholinergic drugs to swallow the tablet or capsule whole without chewing it or crushing it. Chewing or crushing the tablet/capsule ruins the extended-release feature, allowing the entire dose to be absorbed quickly, which increases drug side effects.

Nutrition Therapy. Teach the patient to avoid foods that irritate the bladder such as caffeine and alcohol. Spacing fluids at regular intervals throughout the day (e.g., 120 mL every hour or 240 mL every 2 hours) and limiting fluids after the dinner hour (e.g., only 120 mL at bedtime) help avoid fluid overload on the bladder and allow urine to collect at a steady pace.

Behavioral Interventions. Behavioral interventions for urge incontinence include bladder training, habit training, exercise therapy, and electrical stimulation. Interventions for urinary bladder training and urinary habit training are listed in Chart 66-9. Behavioral interventions involve a great deal of patient participation. Provide ongoing encouragement, clarification, and support to increase the effects of all interventions. Behavioral interventions are often combined with drug therapy for greatest effect.

Bladder training is an education program for the patient that begins with a thorough explanation of the problem of urge incontinence. Instead of the bladder being in control of the patient, the patient learns to control the bladder. For the program to succeed, he or she must be alert, aware, and able to resist the urge to urinate (Wilde et al., 2014).

Start a schedule for voiding, beginning with the longest interval that is comfortable for the patient, even if the interval is only 30 minutes. Instruct the patient to void every 30 minutes and to ignore any urge to urinate between the set intervals. Once he or she is comfortable with the starting schedule, increase the interval by 15 to 30 minutes. Instruct the patient

CHART 66-9 **Best Practice for Patient Safety & Quality Care** QSEN

Bladder Training and Habit Training to Reduce Urinary Incontinence

Bladder Training

- Assess patient's awareness of bladder fullness and ability to cooperate with training regimen.
- Assess the patient's 24-hour voiding pattern for 2 to 3 consecutive days.
- Base the initial interval of toileting on the voiding pattern (e.g., 45 minutes).
- Teach the patient to void every 45 minutes on the first day and to ignore or suppress the urge to urinate between the 45-minute intervals.
- Take the patient to the toilet or remind him or her to urinate at the 45-minute intervals.
- Provide privacy for toileting and run water in the sink to promote the urge to urinate at this time.
- If the patient is not consistently able to resist the urge to urinate between the intervals, reduce the intervals by 15 minutes.
- Continue this regimen for at least 24 hours or for as many days as it takes for the patient to be comfortable with this schedule and not urinate between the intervals.
- When the patient remains continent between the intervals, increase the intervals by 15 minutes daily until a 3- to 4-hour interval is comfortable for the patient.
- Praise successes. If incontinence occurs, work with the patient to re-establish an acceptable toileting interval.

Habit Training

- Assess the patient's 24-hour voiding pattern for 2 to 3 days.
- Base the initial interval of toileting on the voiding pattern (e.g., 2 hours).
- Assist the patient to the toilet or provide a bedpan/urinal every 2 hours (or whatever has been determined to be an appropriate toileting interval for the individual patient).
- During the toileting, remind the patient to void and provide cues such as running water.
- If the patient is incontinent between scheduled toileting, reduce the time interval by 30 minutes until the patient is continent between voidings.
- Assist the patient to toilet and prompt to void at prescribed intervals.
- Do not leave the patient on the toilet or bedpan for longer than 5 minutes.
- Ensure that all nursing staff members comply with the established toileting schedule and do not apply briefs or encourage the patient to "just wet the bed."
- Reduce toileting interval by 30 minutes if there are more than two incontinence episodes in 24 hours.
- If the patient remains continent at the toileting interval, attempt to increase the interval by 30 minutes until a 3- to 4-hour continence interval is reached.
- Praise the patient for successes, and spend extra time socializing with the patient.
- When incontinence occurs, ensure that the patient and bed are cleaned appropriately but do not spend extra time socializing with the patient.
- Discuss daily record of continence with staff to provide reinforcement and encourage compliance with toileting schedule.
- Include unlicensed assistive personnel in all aspects of the habit training.

to follow the new schedule until he or she achieves success again. As the interval increases, the bladder gradually tolerates more volume. Teach him or her relaxation and distraction techniques to maximize success in the retraining. Provide positive reinforcement for maintaining the prescribed schedule.

Habit training (scheduled toileting) is a type of bladder training that is successful in reducing incontinence in cognitively impaired patients. To use habit training, caregivers assist the patient in voiding at specific times (e.g., every 2 hours on the even hours). The goal is to get the patient to the toilet before incontinence occurs. The focus is on reducing incontinence. When that has been achieved, the focus may change to increase bladder capacity by gradually lengthening the voiding intervals, but this is only secondary.

! NURSING SAFETY PRIORITY QSEN

Action Alert

Habit training is undermined when absorbent briefs are used in place of timed toileting. Do not tell patients to "just wet the bed." A common cause of falls in health care facilities is related to patient efforts to get out of bed unassisted to use the toilet. Work with all staff members, including unlicensed assistive personnel (UAP), to implement consistently the toileting schedule for habit training.

Prompted voiding, a supplement to habit training, attempts to increase the patient's awareness of the need to void and to prompt him or her to ask for toileting assistance. Habit training otherwise relies completely on a time schedule.

Exercise therapy with pelvic muscle exercises for urge incontinence is helpful and is taught in the same way as for stress incontinence (see Chart 66-7). Improved urethral resistance helps the patient overcome abnormal detrusor contractions long enough to get to the toilet.

Reducing Reflex Urinary Incontinence

Planning: Expected Outcomes. With appropriate intervention, the patient with reflex incontinence is expected to achieve continence. Indicators include that the patient often or consistently demonstrates these behaviors:

- Recognizes the urge to void
- Maintains a predictable pattern of voiding
- Responds to urge in a timely manner
- Empties bladder completely
- Keeps urine volume in the bladder under 300 mL

Interventions. Interventions for the patient with reflex (overflow) incontinence caused by obstruction of the bladder outlet may include surgery to relieve the obstruction. The most common procedures are prostate removal (see Chapter 72) and repair of uterine prolapse (see Chapter 71).

Drug Therapy. Drugs are prescribed for short-term management of urinary retention, often after surgery. They are not used in long-term management of overflow incontinence caused by a hypotonic bladder. The most commonly used drug is bethanechol chloride (Urecholine), an agent that increases bladder pressure.

Behavioral Interventions. The most effective common behavioral interventions are bladder compression and intermittent self-catheterization.

Bladder compression uses techniques that promote bladder emptying and include the Credé method, the Valsalva maneuver, double-voiding, and splinting.

For the Credé method, teach the patient how to press over the bladder area, increasing its pressure, or to trigger nerve stimulation by tugging at pubic hair or massaging the genital area. These techniques manually assist the bladder in emptying. In the Valsalva maneuver, breathing techniques increase chest and abdominal pressure. This increased pressure is then directed toward the bladder during exhalation. With the technique of double-voiding, the patient empties the bladder and then, within a few minutes, attempts a second bladder emptying.

For women who have a large *cystocele* (prolapse of the bladder into the vagina), a technique called *splinting* both compresses the bladder and moves it into a better position. The woman inserts her fingers into her vagina, gently lifts the cystocele, and begins to urinate. A *pessary,* described earlier, can also provide relief from cystocele-related incontinence.

Intermittent self-catheterization is often used to help patients with long-term problems of incomplete bladder emptying. It is effective, can be learned fairly easily, and remains the preferred method of bladder emptying in patients who have incontinence as a result of a neurogenic bladder (Newman & Willson, 2011). These points are important in teaching the technique:

- Proper handwashing and cleaning of the catheter reduce the risk for INFECTION.
- A small lumen and good lubrication of the catheter prevent urethral trauma.
- A regular schedule for bladder emptying prevents distention and mucosal trauma.

Patients must be able to understand instructions and have the manual dexterity to manipulate the catheter. Caregivers or family members in the home can also be taught to perform straight catheterization using clean (rather than sterile) technique with good outcomes (Kannankeril et al., 2011).

Reducing Functional Urinary Incontinence

Planning: Expected Outcomes. The patient with functional urinary incontinence is expected to remain dry. Indicators include that the patient often or consistently demonstrates these behaviors:

- Uses urine containment or collection measures to ensure dryness
- Manages clothing independently

Interventions. Causes of functional (or chronic intractable) incontinence vary greatly. Some are reversible, and others are not. The focus of intervention is treatment of reversible causes. When incontinence is not reversible, urinary habit training (see Chart 66-9) is used to establish a predictable pattern of bladder emptying to prevent incontinence. A final strategy focuses on containment of the urine and protection of the patient's skin. Nonsurgical interventions include applied devices, containment, and catheterization.

Applied devices include intravaginal pessaries for women and penile clamps for men. The intravaginal pessary supports the uterus and vagina and helps maintain the correct position of the bladder. (See Chapter 71 for further discussion of pessaries.) The penile clamp is applied around the outside of the penis to compress the urethra and prevent urine leakage.

Adverse outcomes from pessaries and penile clamps include damage to the tissues from pressure and INFECTION from colonization of damaged tissues. Both devices require that the patient have either manual dexterity or a caregiver to apply and remove the device. Instruct the patient or caregivers in the use of these devices. Male patients may use an external collecting device, such as a condom catheter. Design of an effective external collecting device for women has not been as successful.

Containment is achieved with absorbent pads and briefs designed to collect urine and keep the patient's skin and clothing dry. Many types and sizes of pads are available:

- Shields or liners inserted inside a panty
- Undergarments that are full-size pads with waist straps
- Plastic-lined protective underpants
- Combination pad and pant systems
- Absorbent bed pads

A major concern with the use of protective pads is the risk for skin breakdown. Materials and costs vary. Some are reusable; others are disposable. The disposal of these products raises ecologic concerns. Avoid use of the word "diaper" when discussing these adult protective pants, however, because of the association of diapers with a baby.

Catheterization for control of incontinence may be intermittent or involve an indwelling catheter. Intermittent catheterization is preferred to an indwelling catheter because of the reduced risk for INFECTION. An indwelling urinary catheter is appropriate for patients with skin breakdown who need a dry environment for healing, for those who are terminally ill and need comfort, and for those who are critically ill and require precise measurement of urine output.

Reducing Total or Mixed Urinary Incontinence. Mixed or total urinary incontinence is a combination of two or more types of involuntary urine loss syndromes. For example, stress incontinence and urge incontinence often occur together in women during and after menopause. For the patient with mixed or total incontinence, combinations of assessment techniques (as discussed under each syndrome) are used. Interventions are also combined to promote continence. The problems and interventions for mixed incontinence are the same as for each specific type of incontinence separately. After identifying the specific types of incontinence an individual patient has, apply the appropriate priority patient problems, interventions, and expected outcomes discussed earlier with each incontinence type.

CULTURAL CONSIDERATIONS

Patient-Centered Care QSEN

Compared with white women, Asian and black women are less likely to report urinary incontinence. In addition, black women are more likely to report remission or cessation of urinary incontinence and Asian women are more likely to report improvement or a decrease of manifestations over a 2-year period when compared with white women. These cultural differences in urinary incontinence and recovery may be a result of differences in pelvic floor anatomy and function, including smaller pelvic floor area and higher urethral closure pressure in black women (Townsend et al., 2011).

CLINICAL JUDGMENT CHALLENGE

Patient-Centered Care; Evidence-Based Practice QSEN

The patient is a 52-year-old perimenopausal woman who reports a small loss of urine with coughing, laughing, and occasionally bending over. Recently she has started to leak urine just as she arrives in the bathroom but before she sits on the toilet. She states her mother has had a continuing problem with incontinence for years and seldom leaves her home. The patient wants to continue to lead an active lifestyle and wants to discuss options for preventing progression of this embarrassing condition.

1. What other information should you obtain from this patient?
2. What type or types of incontinence is she most likely to have from the information she has provided thus far?
3. Is this problem likely to be genetic? Why or why not?
4. What will you tell her regarding options for care?
5. She asks if there is anything she can do now to help reduce her urine leakage. How do you respond?

Community-Based Care

Community-based care for the patient with urinary incontinence considers his or her personal, physical, emotional, and social resources. Important personal resources for self-care include mobility, vision, and manual dexterity. When planning care, consider who will be the primary caregiver and what factors may influence the effectiveness of the plan. A recent comparative effectiveness review from the Agency for Healthcare Research and Quality (AHRQ) (2012) reports that some drugs for urinary incontinence can provide benefit but that adverse drug events, overall, lead to poor adherence. This report also provides information that nonpharmacologic and nonsurgical treatments provide significant clinical benefit with low risk for adverse effects but that these interventions are also associated with poor adherence. Ongoing relationships with health care providers may improve adherence.

Home Care Management. Assess the home environment for barriers that limit access to the bathroom. Eliminate hazards that might slow walking or lead to a fall. Such hazards include throw rugs, furniture with legs that extend into the walking area, slippery waxed or polished floors, and poor lighting.

If the patient must climb stairs to reach a bathroom, handrails should be installed and stairs kept free of obstacles. Toilet seat extenders may help provide the right level and height of seating so that maximal abdominal pressure may be applied for voiding. Portable commodes may be obtained when ambulatory access to toilets is impractical. Physical and occupational therapists are valuable resources for assisting with home care management.

Self-Management Education. Teach the patient and family about the cause of the specific type of incontinence, and discuss available treatment options for its management. The teaching plan addresses the prescribed drugs (purpose, dosage, method and route of administration, and expected and potential side effects). Instruct the patient and family about the importance of weight reduction and dietary modification to help control incontinence. Remind the patient who smokes that nicotine can contribute to bladder irritation and that coughing can cause urine leakage.

When external devices or protective pads are needed, describe the possible options and help the patient make a selection best for his or her lifestyle and resources. For patients who will use intermittent catheterization or those with artificial urinary sphincters, demonstrate the correct technique to the patient or caregiver. Evaluate return demonstrations for correct technique. Chart 66-10 also addresses teaching.

Psychosocial Preparation. The embarrassment of incontinence can be devastating to self-esteem, body image, and relationships. Sexual intimacy is often adversely affected by incontinence. The unpredictable nature of incontinence creates anxiety. Patients may be embarrassed to seek help, and even when resources are identified, they may need help to feel comfortable in using the resources. Buying supplies at a local store may threaten privacy.

Accept and acknowledge the personal concerns of the patient and caregiver. Never make their concerns seem trivial. As he or she learns the specifics of the plan that will allow control of urinary incontinence, the confidence to resume social interactions should return. Many continence supplies can be purchased online and delivered directly to the home to maintain privacy.

CHART 66-10 Patient and Family Education: Preparing for Self-Management

Urinary Incontinence

- Maintain a normal body weight to reduce the pressure on your bladder.
- Do not try to control your incontinence by limiting your fluid intake. Adequate fluid intake is necessary for kidney function and health maintenance.
- If you have a catheter in your bladder, follow the instructions given to you about maintaining the sterile drainage system.
- If you are discharged with a suprapubic catheter in your bladder, inspect the entry site for the tube daily, clean the skin around the opening gently with warm soap and water, and place a sterile gauze dressing on the skin around the tube. Report any redness, swelling, drainage, or fever to your physician.
- Do not put anything into your vagina, such as tampons, drugs, hygiene products, or exercise weights, until you check with your physician at your 6-week checkup after surgery.
- Do not have sexual intercourse until after your 6-week postoperative checkup.
- Do not lift or carry anything heavier than 5 pounds or participate in any strenuous exercise until your physician gives you postoperative clearance. In some cases, this could be as long as 3 months.
- Avoid exercises, such as running, jogging, step or dance aerobic classes, rowing, cross-country ski or stair-climber machines, and mountain biking. Brisk walking without any additional hand, leg, or body weights is allowed. Swimming is allowed after all drains and catheters have been removed and your incision is completely healed.
- If Kegel exercises are recommended, ask your nurse for specific instructions.

Health Care Resources. Referral to home care agencies for help with personal care and to continence clinics that specialize in evaluation and treatment may be helpful. In many continence clinics, nurses collaborate with physicians and other health care professionals to evaluate and manage patients. The treatment plan is specific for each patient; supplies and products are custom selected.

Patients may benefit from education and from the support of others who experience similar concerns. The National Association for Continence (NAFC) (www.nafc.org), Access to Continence Care and Treatment (www.wellweb.com/INCONT/acct/contents.htm), and the Wound, Ostomy, and Continence Nurses (www.wocn.org) publish newsletters and educational materials written with easy-to-understand explanations. The American Foundation for Urologic Disease (www.afud.com) provides information on many areas of bladder dysfunction. Local hospitals often have local NAFC-approved support groups.

NCLEX EXAMINATION CHALLENGE

Safe and Effective Care Environment

For which hospitalized client does the nurse recommend the ongoing use of a urinary catheter?

A. 36-year-old woman who is blind and is receiving diuretics
B. 46-year-old man who has paraplegia and is admitted for asthma management
C. 56-year-old woman who is admitted with a vaginal-rectal fistula and has diabetes
D. 66-year-old man who has severe osteoarthritis and is a high risk for falling

◆ *Evaluation: Outcomes*

Evaluate the care of the patient with urinary incontinence based on the identified priority patient problems. The expected outcomes are that the patient will:

- Describe the type of urinary incontinence experienced
- Demonstrate knowledge of proper use of drugs and correct procedures for self-catheterization, use of the artificial sphincter, or care of an indwelling urinary catheter
- Demonstrate effective use of the selected exercise or bladder-training program
- Select and use incontinence interventions, devices, and products
- Have a reduction in the number of incontinence episodes

Specific indicators for these outcomes are listed for each priority patient problem under the Planning and Implementation section (see earlier).

UROLITHIASIS

❖ *PATHOPHYSIOLOGY*

Urolithiasis is the presence of *calculi* (stones) in the urinary tract. Stones often do not cause manifestations until they pass into the lower urinary tract, where they can cause excruciating PAIN. **Nephrolithiasis** is the formation of stones in the kidney. Formation of stones in the ureter is **ureterolithiasis**.

Urologic stones are caused by many disorders. However, the exact mechanism of stone formation is not entirely understood. Everyone excretes crystals in the urine at some time, but fewer than 10% of people form stones. Most stones contain calcium as one part of the stone complex. Struvite (15%), uric acid (8%), and cystine (3%) are more rare compositions of stones. Formation of stones involves three conditions:

- Slow urine flow, resulting in supersaturation of the urine with the particular element (e.g., calcium) that first becomes crystallized and later becomes the stone
- Damage to the lining of the urinary tract (e.g., abrasion from crystals)
- Decreased amounts of inhibitor substances in the urine that would otherwise prevent supersaturation and crystal aggregation

High urine acidity (as with uric acid and cystine stones) or alkalinity (as with calcium phosphate and struvite stones), as well as drugs (e.g., triamterene, indinavir, acetazolamide), contributes to stone formation.

One example of a metabolic problem causing stone formation begins when excessive amounts of calcium are absorbed through the intestinal tract leading to hypercalciuria. As blood circulates through the kidneys, the excess calcium is filtered into the urine, causing supersaturation of calcium in the urine. If fluid intake is poor, such as when a patient is dehydrated, supersaturation is more likely to occur and the risk for calcium combining with another compound to form a larger molecule increases. Calcium complexes often serve as a center for other deposits, and eventually a stone forms.

Stones that form in the kidney and then pass into the ureter often lodge in areas where the ureter bends or slightly changes shape. When the stone occludes the ureter and blocks the flow of urine, the ureter dilates. Enlargement of the ureter is called **hydroureter**.

The PAIN associated with ureteral spasm is excruciating and may cause the patient to go into shock from stimulation of nearby nerves. **Hematuria** (bloody urine) may result from damage to the urothelial lining. If the obstruction is not removed, urinary stasis can cause INFECTION and impair kidney function on the side of the blockage. As the blockage persists, **hydronephrosis** (enlargement of the kidney caused by blockage of urine lower in the tract and filling of the kidney with urine) and permanent kidney damage may develop.

TABLE 66-4 Metabolic Defects That Commonly Cause Kidney Stones

METABOLIC DEFICIT	ETIOLOGY
Hypercalcemia	
Primary	Absorptive: increased intestinal calcium absorption Renal: decreased kidney tubular excretion of calcium
Secondary	Resorptive: hyperparathyroidism, vitamin D intoxication, kidney tubular acidosis, prolonged immobilization
Hyperoxaluria	
Primary	Genetic: autosomal recessive trait resulting in high oxalate production
Secondary	Dietary: excess oxalate from foods such as spinach, rhubarb, Swiss chard, cocoa, beets, wheat germ, pecans, peanuts, okra, chocolate, and lime peel
Hyperuricemia	
Primary	Gout is an inherited disorder of purine metabolism (20% of patients with gout have uric acid calculi)
Secondary	Increased production or decreased clearance of purine from myeloproliferative disorders, thiazide diuretics, carcinoma
Struvite	Made of magnesium ammonium phosphate and carbonate apatite; formed by urea splitting by bacteria, most commonly, *Proteus mirabilis;* needs an alkaline urine to form
Cystinuria	Autosomal recessive defect of amino acid metabolism that precipitates insoluble cystine crystals in the urine

Etiology and Genetic Risk

The cause of urolithiasis is unknown. At least 90% of patients who form stones have a metabolic risk factor. Table 66-4 lists some metabolic problems that cause stone formation. Patients who are white, older, obese, or have diabetes or gout (hyperuricemia) have increased risk for stone formation (Rodgers, 2013). Other conditions associated with stone formation and recurrence are hyperparathyroidism, urinary tract obstruction, inflammatory bowel diseases, and a history of GI problems (Fink et al., 2013).

Diet is not considered a risk for stone formation. However, calcium and vitamin D supplementation as well as high-dose

GENETIC/GENOMIC CONSIDERATIONS

Patient-Centered Care QSEN

Family history has a strong association with stone formation and recurrence. More than 30 genetic variations are associated with the formation of kidney stones. Single gene disorders are rare. More commonly, nephrolithiasis is a complex disease, with genetic variation in intestinal calcium absorption, kidney calcium transport, or kidney phosphate transport all associated with stone formation. Always ask a patient with a renal stone whether other family members have also had this problem.

ascorbic acid (vitamin C) intake have been implicated in stone formation (Fletcher, 2013; Rosa et al., 2013). Conversely, high intake of fluids, fruits, and vegetables, low consumption of protein, and a balanced intake of calcium, fats, and carbohydrates are prescribed to prevent and treat recurrent urolithiasis (Fink et al., 2013).

Incidence and Prevalence

The incidence of stone disease is high and varies with geographic location, race, and family history. About 12% of adults will have at least one episode of renal stone disease. The incidence is higher in men; however, struvite stones are twice as common in women. Recurrence rates vary depending on the type of treatment. The recurrence rate of untreated calcium oxalate stones is 35% to 50% in 5 to 10 years. A higher recurrence of stones occurs in patients with a family history of stone disease and in those who had their first occurrence by age 25 years.

CULTURAL CONSIDERATIONS

Patient-Centered Care QSEN

The incidence of stone disease is most common in the southeastern United States, Japan, and western Europe. Calcium stone disease is more common in men than in women and tends to occur in young adults or during early middle adulthood. Kidney stone disease occurs more often in younger adults than older adults and more commonly among white people (Rodgers, 2013). For patients in these higher-risk groups, nursing care includes teaching family members, as well as patients, about the manifestations of a stone and interventions to reduce stone formation.

❖ PATIENT-CENTERED COLLABORATIVE CARE

◆ Assessment

Ask the patient about a personal or family history of urologic stones. Obtain a diet history, focusing on fluid intake patterns and supplemental vitamin or mineral intake. If he or she has a history of stone formation, ask about past treatment, whether chemical analysis of the stone was performed, and what preventive measures are followed.

The major manifestation of stones is severe PAIN, commonly called **renal colic**. Flank pain suggests that the stone is in the kidney or upper ureter. Flank pain that extends toward the abdomen or to the scrotum and testes or the vulva suggests that stones are in the ureters or bladder. Pain is most intense when the stone is moving or when the ureter is obstructed.

Renal colic begins suddenly and is often described as "unbearable." Nausea, vomiting, pallor, and diaphoresis often accompany the PAIN. A large stationary stone in the kidney (staghorn calculus), however, rarely causes much pain because it is not moving. Frequency and dysuria occur when a stone reaches the bladder. **Oliguria** (scant urine output) or **anuria** (absence of urine output) suggests obstruction, possibly at the bladder neck or urethra. *Urinary tract obstruction is an emergency and must be treated immediately to preserve kidney function.*

Assess the patient for bladder distention. He or she may appear pale, ashen, and diaphoretic and may suffer from excruciating PAIN. Vital signs may be moderately elevated with pain; body temperature and pulse are elevated with INFECTION. Blood pressure may decrease if the severe pain causes shock.

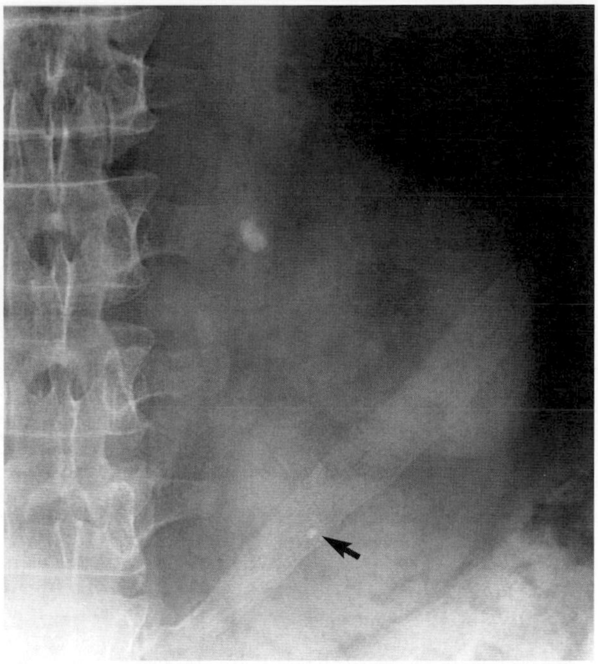

FIG. 66-2 Urinary stones on x-ray of the kidneys, ureters, and bladder (KUB).

Urinalysis is performed in patients with suspected stones. Hematuria is common, and blood may make the urine appear smoky or rusty. RBCs are usually caused by stone-induced trauma on the lining of the ureter, bladder, or urethra. WBCs and bacteria may be present as a result of urinary stasis. Increased *turbidity* (cloudiness) and odor indicate that INFECTION may also be present. Microscopic examination of the urine may identify crystals from which stones could form. Urinary pH is measured to determine acidity or alkalinity.

The serum WBC count is elevated with INFECTION. Increases in the serum calcium, serum phosphate, or serum uric acid levels indicate excess minerals are present and may contribute to stone formation.

Stones are easily seen on x-rays of the kidneys, ureters, and bladder (KUB) (Fig. 66-2), CT, and ultrasound, with ultrasound being used most commonly for screening. Noncontrast CT is the most sensitive procedure to identify urinary tract stones and can confirm the presence, shape, and location of the stones.

◆ Interventions

Nursing interventions focus on PAIN management and prevention of INFECTION and urinary obstruction. Most patients can expel the stone without invasive procedures. The most important factors regarding whether a stone will pass on its own are its composition, size, and location. The larger the stone and the higher up in the urinary tract it is, the less likely it is to be passed. When the stone is passed, it should be captured and sent to the laboratory for analysis. Other interventions are needed when the patient does not pass the stone spontaneously (Fig. 66-3).

Managing Pain. Nonsurgical and surgical approaches are used to assist the patient with a kidney stone achieve an acceptable degree of PAIN relief.

Nonsurgical Management. Nonsurgical measures to relieve pain include strategies to enhance stone passing, as well as direct pain management.

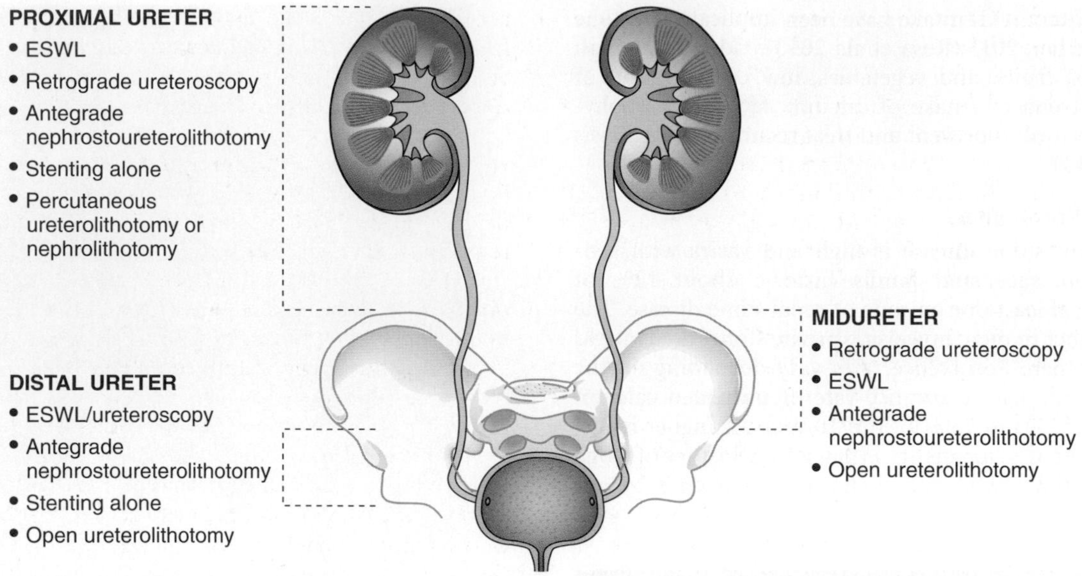

FIG. 66-3 Treatment options for ureteral stones. *ESWL,* Extracorporeal shock wave lithotripsy.

Drug therapy is needed in the first 24 to 36 hours when PAIN is most severe. Opioid analgesics are used to control the severe pain caused by stones in the urinary tract and may be given IV for rapid pain relief. NSAIDs such as ketorolac (Toradol) or ketoprofen (Nexcede) in the acute phase may be quite effective. When NSAIDs are used, the risk for bleeding is increased and the use of extracorporeal shock wave lithotripsy is delayed.

Control of PAIN is more effective when drugs are given at regularly scheduled intervals or by a constant delivery system (e.g., skin patch) instead of PRN. Spasmolytic drugs, such as oxybutynin chloride (Ditropan) and propantheline bromide (Pro-Banthine, Propanthel 🍁), are important for control of pain (see Chart 66-8). Give the drugs, and assess the response by asking the patient to rate the discomfort on a pain-rating scale.

Other management techniques include avoiding overhydration and underhydration in the acute phase to help make the passage of a stone less painful. Strain the urine and teach the patient to strain it to monitor for stone passage. Send any stone passed to the laboratory for analysis because preventive therapy is based on stone composition.

Two drugs may be used to aid in stone expulsion: a thiazide diuretic and allopurinol. These drugs, combined with a high fluid intake, increase urine volume or decrease urine pH and help increase the excretion of stones or stone fragments (Rosa et al., 2013). Citrate may be used to alter urine pH and interrupt intrarenal conditions that promote stone production.

Lithotripsy, also known as *shock wave lithotripsy (SWL),* is the use of sound, laser, or dry shock waves to break the stone into small fragments. The patient receives moderate sedation and lies on a flat table with the lithotriptor aimed at the stone, which is located by fluoroscopy. A local anesthetic cream is applied to the skin site over the stone 45 minutes before the procedure. During the procedure, cardiac rhythm is monitored by electrocardiography (ECG) and the shock waves are delivered in synchrony with the R wave. Shock waves at the rate of 60 to 120/min are applied over 30 to 45 minutes (Li et al., 2013). Continuous ECG monitoring for dysrhythmia and fluoroscopic observation for stone destruction are maintained.

After lithotripsy, strain the urine to monitor the passage of stone fragments. Bruising may occur on the flank of the affected side. Occasionally a stent is placed in the ureter before SWL to ease passage of the stone fragments.

Surgical Management. Minimally invasive surgical and open surgical procedures are used if urinary obstruction occurs or if the stone is too large to be passed.

Minimally Invasive Surgical Procedures. Minimally invasive surgical (MIS) procedures include stenting, ureteroscopy, percutaneous ureterolithotomy, and percutaneous nephrolithotomy.

Stenting is performed with a **stent**—a small tube that is placed in the ureter by ureteroscopy. The stent dilates the ureter and enlarges the passageway for the stone or stone fragments. This totally internal procedure prevents the passing stone from coming in contact with the ureteral mucosa, thereby reducing PAIN, bleeding, and INFECTION risk, all of which could block the ureter. A Foley catheter may be placed to facilitate passage of the stone through the urethra.

Ureteroscopy is an endoscopic procedure. The ureteroscope is passed through the urethra and bladder into the ureter. Once the stone is seen, it is removed using grasping baskets, forceps, or loops. Lithotripsy also can be performed through the ureteroscope. A Foley catheter may be placed to facilitate passage of the stone fragments through the urethra.

Percutaneous ureterolithotomy or nephrolithotomy is the removal of a stone in the ureter or kidney through the skin. The patient lies prone or on the side and receives local or general anesthesia. The physician identifies the ideal entry point with fluoroscopy and then passes a needle into the collecting system of the kidney. Once a tract has been made in the kidney, other equipment, such as an **intracorporeal** (inside the body) ultrasonic or laser lithotriptor, can be used to break up and remove the stone. An endoscope with a special attachment to grasp and extract the stone can be used. Often a nephrostomy tube is left in place at first to prevent the stone fragments from passing through the urinary tract.

Monitor the patient for complications after the procedure. Complications include bleeding at the site or through the tube, pneumothorax, and INFECTION. Monitor nephrostomy tube drainage for volume and the presence of blood in the urine, which is normal for the first 24 to 48 hours after tube placement. Provide routine nephrostomy tube care, with sterile dressing changes and tube flushing (if ordered).

Open Surgical Procedures. When other stone removal attempts have failed or when risk for a lasting injury to the ureter or kidney is possible, an *open ureterolithotomy* (into the ureter), *pyelolithotomy* (into the kidney pelvis), or *nephrolithotomy* (into the kidney) procedure may be performed. These procedures are used for a large or impacted stone.

Preoperative Care. Explain to the patient how, when, and where the procedure will be performed. Describe what he or she can expect to see, hear, and feel before and after the procedure. The patient is given nothing by mouth and also receives a bowel preparation before the procedure. (See Chapter 14 for routine care before surgery.)

Operative Procedures. The retroperitoneal area is entered through a large flank incision, as for nephrectomy (see Chapter 67), pyelolithotomy, or nephrolithotomy and through a lower abdominal incision for ureterolithotomy. The urinary tract is entered surgically, and the stone is removed. Before closure, tubes and drains may be placed (e.g., nephrostomy tube, ureteral stent, Penrose or other wound drainage device, and Foley catheter).

Postoperative Care. Follow routine procedures for assessment of the patient who has received anesthesia. (See Chapter 16 for routine care after surgery.) Monitor the amount of bleeding from incisions and in the urine. Maintain adequate fluid intake. Strain the urine to monitor the passage of stone fragments. Teach the patient how to prevent future stones through dietary changes, including consistent daily fluid intake to avoid dehydration and supersaturation.

Preventing Infection. Control of INFECTION before invasive procedures is critical for the prevention of urosepsis. Interventions include giving appropriate antibiotics, either to eliminate an existing infection or to prevent new infections, and maintaining adequate nutrition and fluid intake. Because infection always occurs with struvite stone formation, the health care team plans for long-term infection prevention.

Drug therapy involves the use of broad-spectrum antibiotics, such as the aminoglycosides (e.g., gentamicin [Garamycin]) and cephalosporins (e.g., cephalexin [Keflex, Novo-Lexin 🍁]). The broad coverage is effective against gram-negative organisms. After the results of the culture and sensitivity (C&S) studies are obtained, more specific antibiotics may be prescribed. C&S studies are often done 48 hours after the start of antibiotic therapy and again 48 hours after completion of the prescribed course of therapy.

Blood levels of antibiotics may be measured to ensure that adequate levels have been reached. If the blood level of the antibiotic is not adequate, organisms may not be completely eliminated. Evidence of a new infection (e.g., chills, fever, and altered mental status) warrants the collection of a urine sample for repeat C&S tests.

For the patient with struvite stones, periodic and long-term monitoring of the urine for infection is needed. Urine cultures are checked monthly for 3 months and then quarterly for 1 year. Drugs that prevent bacteria from splitting urea, such as acetohydroxamic acid (Lithostat) and hydroxyurea (Hydrea), are often prescribed long-term for patients with struvite stones. Serum creatinine levels are monitored in patients receiving acetohydroxamic acid, and the drug is stopped if creatinine levels are above 2 mg/dL. Review interventions aimed at preventing urinary tract infection (UTI). (See Health Promotion discussion on p. 1369 in the Cystitis section.)

Nutrition therapy ideally includes adequate calorie intake with a balance of all food groups. Encourage a fluid intake sufficient to dilute urine to a light color throughout the 24-hour day (typically 2 to 3 L/day) unless another health problem requires fluid restriction.

Preventing Obstruction. Measures to prevent urinary obstruction by stones include a high intake of fluids (3 L/day or more) and accurate measures of intake and output. Fluid intake sufficient to provide diluted urine helps prevent dehydration, promotes urine flow, and decreases the chance of crystals forming a stone. Interventions also depend on the type of stone the patient has formed. Drugs, diet modification, and fluid intake are the major strategies used to prevent future stones.

Drug therapy to prevent obstruction depends on what is causing stone formation and the type of stone formed. Teach the patient the reason for the drug, and assess for side effects or adverse drug reactions. Some drugs may need to be avoided because they may contribute to stone formation.

Drugs to treat *hypercalciuria* (high levels of calcium in the urine) include thiazide diuretics (e.g., chlorothiazide [Diuril] or hydrochlorothiazide [HydroDIURIL, Urozide 🍁]). These drugs promote calcium reabsorbtion from the renal tubules back into the body, thereby reducing urine calcium loads. For patients with *hyperoxaluria* (high levels of oxalic acid in the urine), allopurinol (Zyloprim) or febuxostat (Uloric) is used.

For patients with hyperuricemia or chronic gout, both allopurinol and febuxostat help prevent the formation of urate (uric acid) stones. To alkalinize the urine, drugs such as potassium citrate, 50% sodium citrate, and sodium bicarbonate are used. Lemon or orange juice may also be ingested as a daily source of citrate. The desired urine pH is 6 to 6.5. Because the normal urine pH averages 5 to 6, the desired values are termed *alkaline.*

For patients with *cystinuria* (high levels of cystine in the urine), both alpha-mercaptopropionylglycine (AMPG) and captopril (Capoten) lower urine cystine levels. They are used when hydration and urine alkalinization have not been successful.

Statins, drugs used to manage hypercholesterolemia, have also been found to reduce the incidence of stone recurrence (Sur et al., 2013). In general, with one stone, patients are advised to increase fluid intake. With two or more stones, drug therapy is advised based on the type of stone as described above (Fink et al., 2013).

Nutrition therapy depends on the type of stone formed (Table 66-5). Collaborate with the dietitian to plan for and teach the appropriate diet to the patient (Türk et al., 2011).

Other measures can help the stone pass more quickly. Urge the patient to walk as often as possible. Walking promotes passage of stones and reduces bone calcium resorption. Check the urine pH daily, and strain all urine with filter paper or a special urine sieve/strainer to collect passed stones and fragments.

Self-management education includes the key points listed in Chart 66-11. Follow-up care to evaluate effects of intervention includes a 24-hour urine collection and serum chemical analysis. The patient often has great anxiety and fear that a stone and its PAIN may recur. In addition to anxiety about the pain, the risk for repeated surgical interventions or permanent and

TABLE 66-5 Dietary Treatment for Kidney and Urinary Stones

STONE TYPE	DIETARY INTERVENTIONS	RATIONALES
Calcium oxalate	Avoid oxalate sources, such as spinach, black tea, and rhubarb. Decrease sodium intake.	Reduction of urinary oxalate content may help prevent these stones from forming. Urinary pH is not a factor. High sodium intake reduces kidney tubular calcium reabsorption.
Calcium phosphate	Limit intake of foods high in animal protein to 5-7 servings per week and never more than 2 per day. Some patients may benefit from a reduced calcium intake (milk, other dairy products). Decrease sodium intake.	Reduction of protein intake reduces acidic urine and prevents calcium precipitation. Reduction of urine calcium concentration may prevent calcium precipitation and crystallization. High sodium intake reduces kidney tubular calcium reabsorption.
Struvite (magnesium ammonium phosphate)	Limit high-phosphate foods, such as dairy products, organ meats, and whole grains.	Reduction of urinary phosphate content may help prevent these stones from forming.
Uric acid (urate)	Decrease intake of purine sources, such as organ meats, poultry, fish, gravies, red wines, and sardines.	Reduction of urinary purine content may help prevent these stones from forming.
Cystine	Limit animal protein intake (as above). Encourage oral fluid intake (500 mL every 4 hours while awake and 750 mL at night).	Reduces urinary uric acid. Increased fluid helps dilute the urine and prevents the cystine crystals from forming.

CHART 66-11 Patient and Family Education: Preparing for Self-Management

Urinary Calculi

- Finish your entire prescription of antibiotics to ensure that you will not get a urinary tract infection.
- You may resume your usual daily activities.
- Remember to balance regular exercise with sleep and rest.
- You may return to work 2 days to 6 weeks after surgery, depending on the type of intervention, your personal tolerance, and your physician's directives.
- Depending on the type of stone you had, your diet may be restricted to prevent further stone formation.
- Remember to drink at least 3 L of fluid a day to dilute potential stone-forming crystals, prevent dehydration, and promote urine flow.
- Monitor urine pH as directed (possibly up to 3 times per day).
- Expect bruising after lithotripsy. The bruising may be quite extensive and may take several weeks to resolve.
- Your urine may be bloody for several days after surgery.
- Pain in the region of the kidneys or bladder may signal the beginning of an infection or the formation of another stone. Report any pain, fever, chills, or difficulty with urination immediately to your physician or nurse.
- Keep follow-up appointments to check on infection, and have repeat cultures done.

NCLEX EXAMINATION CHALLENGE

Health Promotion and Maintenance

The client passes a urinary stone that laboratory analysis indicates is composed of calcium oxalate. Based on this analysis, which instruction does the nurse specifically include for dietary prevention of the problem?

A. "Increase your intake of meat, fish, and cranberry juice."
B. "Avoid citrus fruits and citrus juices such as oranges."
C. "Avoid dark green leafy vegetables such as spinach."
D. "Decrease your intake of dairy products, especially milk."

serious kidney damage is of major concern. Psychosocial preparation is enhanced when patients know what to expect and what actions to take if problems develop. Reassure the patient that preventive and health promotion activities help prevent recurrence.

UROTHELIAL CANCER

❖ PATHOPHYSIOLOGY

Urothelial cancers are malignant tumors of the *urothelium*—the lining of transitional cells in the kidney, renal pelvis, ureters, urinary bladder, and urethra. Most urothelial cancers occur in the bladder, and the term *bladder cancer* describes this condition.

In North America, most urinary tract cancers are transitional cell carcinomas of the bladder (ACS, 2014; Canadian Cancer Society, 2014). The second most common site of urinary tract cancer is the kidney and renal pelvis. Urothelial cancers are usually low grade, have multiple points of origin *(multifocal)*, and are recurrent. Once the cancer spreads beyond the transitional cell layer, it is highly invasive and can spread beyond the bladder. Because of the nature of this cancer, patients may have recurrence up to 10 years after being cancer free (ACS, 2014).

Tumors confined to the bladder mucosa are treated by simple excision, whereas those that are deeper but not into the muscle layer are treated with excision plus **intravesical** (inside the bladder) chemotherapy. Cancer that has spread deeper into the bladder muscle layer is treated with more extensive surgery, often a **radical cystectomy** (removal of the bladder and surrounding tissue) with urinary diversion. Chemotherapy and radiation therapy are used in addition to surgery. If untreated, the tumor invades surrounding tissues, spreads to distant sites (liver, lung, and bone), and ultimately leads to death.

Exposure to toxins, especially chemicals used in hair dyes and the rubber, paint, electric cable, and textile industries, increases the risk for bladder cancer. The greatest risk factor for bladder cancer is tobacco use. Other risks include *Schistosoma haematobium* (a parasite) INFECTION, excessive use of drugs containing phenacetin, and long-term use of cyclophosphamide (Cytoxan, Procytox 🍁).

In the United States and Canada, about 82,690 new cases of bladder cancer are diagnosed each year, and about 17,780 deaths occur each year from the disease (ACS, 2014; Canadian Cancer Society, 2014). This cancer is rare in adults younger than 40 years and is most common after 60 years of age.

Health Promotion and Maintenance

Many people believe that tobacco use is associated with cancers only of organs that come into direct contact with it, such as the lungs. However, many compounds in tobacco enter the bloodstream and affect other organs, such as the bladder. Therefore encourage everyone who smokes to quit and nonsmokers not to start (see the Health Promotion and Maintenance section of Chapter 27 on pp. 494-496). Just as important, encourage anyone who comes into contact with dry, liquid, or gaseous chemicals to take precautions. Some people work with chemicals, and others may come into contact with them while engaging in hobbies. Many chemicals and fumes can enter the body through contact with skin and with mucous membranes in the respiratory tract. Use of personal protective equipment, such as gloves and masks, can reduce this contact. Also encourage anyone who works with chemicals to shower or bathe and change clothing as soon as contact is completed.

NCLEX EXAMINATION CHALLENGE

Physiological Integrity

A 65-year-old client is seeing his primary care provider for an annual examination. Which assessment finding alerts the nurse to an increased risk for bladder cancer?

A. Smoking
B. Urine with a high specific gravity
C. Recurrent urinary tract infections
D. History of cancer in another organ or tissue

PATIENT-CENTERED COLLABORATIVE CARE

Assessment

Physical Assessment/Clinical Manifestations. Ask about the patient's perception of his or her general health. Document the gender and age of the patient. Ask about active and passive exposure to cigarette smoke. To detect exposure to harmful environmental agents, ask the patient to describe his or her occupation and hobbies in detail. Also ask the patient to describe any change in the color, frequency, or amount of urine and any abdominal discomfort.

Observe the patient's overall appearance, especially skin color and nutrition status. Inspect, percuss, and palpate the abdomen for asymmetry, tenderness, and bladder distention.

Examine the urine for color and clarity. Blood in the urine is often the first manifestation of bladder cancer. It may be gross or microscopic and is usually painless and intermittent. Dysuria, frequency, and urgency occur when INFECTION or obstruction is also present.

Psychosocial Assessment. Assess the patient's emotions, including his or her response to a tentative diagnosis of bladder cancer, and note anxiety, fear, sadness, anger, or guilt. Early manifestations are painless, and many patients ignore the blood in the urine because it is intermittent. They also may be reluctant to seek treatment because they suspect a sexually transmitted disease (STD). As a result, they may have guilt or anger about their own delays in seeking medical attention.

Assess the patient's coping methods and available support from family members. Social support may provide motivation and improve coping during recovery from treatment.

Diagnostic Assessment. The only significant finding on a routine urinalysis is gross or microscopic hematuria. Cytologic testing on voided urine specimens usually is not helpful. Bladder-wash specimens and bladder biopsies are the most specific tests for cancer.

Cystoscopy is usually performed to evaluate painless hematuria. A biopsy of a visible bladder tumor can be performed during cystoscopy. This is essential for staging and is usually performed in an ambulatory care surgery center. Cystoureterography may be used to identify obstructions, especially where the ureter joins the bladder. CT scans show tumor invasion of surrounding tissues. Ultrasonography shows masses but is less valuable for tumor staging. MRI may help assess deep, invasive tumors.

Interventions

Therapy for the patient with bladder cancer usually begins with surgical removal of the tumor for diagnosis and staging of disease. For tumors extending beyond the mucosa, surgery is followed by intravesical chemotherapy or immunotherapy. High-grade or recurrent tumors are treated with more radical surgery plus intravesical chemotherapy, radiotherapy, or both. Systemic chemotherapy is reserved for patients with distant metastases. (See Chapter 22 for general care of the patient receiving chemotherapy or radiation therapy.)

Nonsurgical Management. Prophylactic immunotherapy with intravesical instillation of bacille Calmette-Guérin (BCG), a live virus compound, is used to prevent tumor recurrence of superficial cancers. This procedure is more effective than single-agent chemotherapy. Usually the agent is instilled in an outpatient cancer clinic and allowed to dwell in the bladder for a specified length of time, usually 2 hours. When the patient urinates, live virus is excreted with the urine.

Teach patients receiving this treatment to prevent contact of the live virus with other members of the household by not sharing a toilet with others for at least 24 hours after instillation. Instruct men to urinate while sitting down to avoid splashing the urine. After 24 hours, the toilet should be completely cleaned using a solution of 10% liquid bleach. If only one toilet is available in the household, teach the patient to flush the toilet after use and follow this by adding one cup of undiluted bleach to the bowl water. The bowl is then flushed after 15 minutes and the seat and flat surfaces of the toilet wiped with a cloth containing a solution of 10% liquid bleach. Instruct the patient to wear gloves during the cleaning and to dispose of the cloth after sealing it in a plastic bag.

Underwear or other clothing that has come into contact with the urine during the immediate 24 hours after instillation should be washed separately from other clothing in a solution of 10% liquid bleach. Sexual intercourse is avoided for 24 hours after the instillation.

Multiagent chemotherapy is successful in prolonging life after distant metastasis has occurred but rarely results in a cure. Radiation therapy is also useful in prolonging life.

Surgical Management. The type of surgery for bladder cancer depends on the type and stage of the cancer and the patient's general health. Complete bladder removal *(cystectomy)* with additional removal of surrounding muscle and tissue offers the best chance of a cure for large, invasive bladder cancers. Four alternatives for urine ELIMINATION are used after cystectomy: ileal conduit; continent pouch; bladder reconstruction, also known as *neobladder;* and ureterosigmoidostomy.

Preoperative Care. Specific patient education depends on the type and extent of the planned surgical procedure.

Coordinate education before surgery with the patient, surgeon, and enterostomal therapist (ET) or wound, ostomy, and continence nurse. Discuss the type of planned urinary diversion and the selection of a site for the stoma. Including the patient in this planning improves the chances for the patient to have a positive attitude about body image and a positive self-image. Use educational counseling to ensure understanding about self-care practices, methods of pouching, control of urine drainage, and management of odor.

The site selected for the stoma should be visible to the patient and avoid folds of skin, bones, and scar tissue. When possible, the waistline or belt area is avoided. Prepare the patient for the number and type of drains that will be present after surgery. General care before surgery is discussed in Chapter 14.

Operative Procedures. Transurethral resection of the bladder tumor (TURBT) or partial cystectomy is performed for small, early, superficial tumors. In a partial (segmental) cystectomy, a portion of the bladder is removed when there is only a single isolated bladder tumor.

When the entire bladder must be removed (complete cystectomy), the ureters are diverted into a collecting reservoir. Techniques for urinary diversion are shown in Fig. 66-4. With an ileal conduit, the ureters are surgically placed in the ileum and urine is collected in a pouch on the skin around the stoma. More often, continent reservoirs or "neobladders" are created from an intestinal graft. With cutaneous ureterostomy or ureteroureterostomy, the ureter opening is brought out onto the skin. The cutaneous ureterostomies may be located on either side of the abdomen or side by side.

Postoperative Care. After cutaneous ureterostomy, an external pouch covers the ostomy to collect urine. Work with the ET to focus care on the wound, the skin, and urinary drainage. (See Chapter 56 for ostomy care.)

The patient with a Kock's pouch, a continent reservoir, may have a Penrose drain and a plastic Medena catheter in the stoma. The drain removes lymphatic fluid or other secretions; the catheter ensures urine drainage so that incisions can heal. The patient with a neobladder usually requires 2 to 4 days in the intensive care unit (ICU) and will have a drain at first in the event the neobladder requires irrigation. Later, irrigation can be performed with intermittent catheterization. Irrigation is performed to ensure patency. There is no sensation of bladder fullness with a neobladder because sensory nerves are not attached. As a result, the patient will need to learn new cues to void, such as prescribed times or noticing a feeling of neobladder pressure. General care after surgery is discussed in Chapter 16.

Different types of drains and nephrostomy catheters are used, sometimes on a temporary basis, to drain urine from the kidney. Some are totally internal, with no drainage to the outside. Others may drain exclusively to the outside and urine is collected in a pouch or bag. For this type of drainage system, urine output remains constant. Decreased or no drainage is cause for concern and must be reported to the surgeon or nephrologist, as is leakage around the catheter. Some nephrostomy tubes are connected both to the new bladder (internal drainage) and to an external drainage system. With this type of system, urine output from the external portion of the catheter is variable. With any drainage system, intervention is needed if the external catheter is partially or completely pulled out accidentally. Immediately notify the surgeon or nephrologist. If the catheter remains partially in place, secure it from further movement. This action may result in a re-insertion process rather than a total replacement.

Community-Based Care

Self-Management Education. Teach the patient and family about drugs, diet and fluid therapy, the use of external pouching systems, and the technique for catheterizing a continent reservoir.

With some procedures, the patient may need electrolyte replacement to prevent long-term deficits. Teach him or her to avoid foods that are known to produce gas if the urinary diversion uses the intestinal tract. When intestinal production of gas is excessive, flatus can induce incontinence.

Patients who have a neobladder created often have extreme weight loss during the first few weeks after surgery. Collaborate with a dietitian to develop a diet plan specific to the patient to meet his or her caloric needs.

! NURSING SAFETY PRIORITY QSEN

Action Alert

INFECTION is common in patients who have a neobladder. Teach patients and family members the manifestations of infection and the importance of reporting them immediately to the surgeon.

Instruct the patient and family about any changes in self-care activities related to the urinary diversion. In collaboration with the enterostomal therapist, demonstrate external pouch application, local skin care, pouch care, methods of adhesion, and drainage mechanisms. If a Kock's pouch has been created, teach the patient how to use a catheter to drain the pouch. For all instruction, observe at least one return demonstration or "teach-back" session by the patient or the caregiver. Ideally, the patient assumes responsibility for self-care before discharge.

Assist the patient to prepare for the impact of urinary diversion on self-image, body image, sexual functioning, and self-esteem. Counseling provides information and support to reduce feelings of powerlessness.

Through discussions with the patient about common social situations, help him or her gain control over new toileting practices. Men with a urinary diversion into the sigmoid colon need to learn the habit of sitting to urinate. For patients of either gender, promote confidence in social situations by encouraging frequent emptying of urinary collection devices before traveling or attending social functions. Resumption of sexual activity is a major concern for many, regardless of age. Address this topic openly and with sensitivity. Cystectomy causes impotence in men, but treatment is available (see Chapter 72).

Health Care Resources. The United Ostomy Association and the American Cancer Society have educational materials that may be useful to patients. Refer patients and family members to local chapters or units of these organizations. In some areas, local support groups have meetings to assist others and to send visitors to provide peer counseling and support. Home care personnel may assist with follow-up, easing the transition from hospital to home. The Wound, Ostomy, and Continence Nurses Society has educational programs and a journal for the care of patients with ostomies.

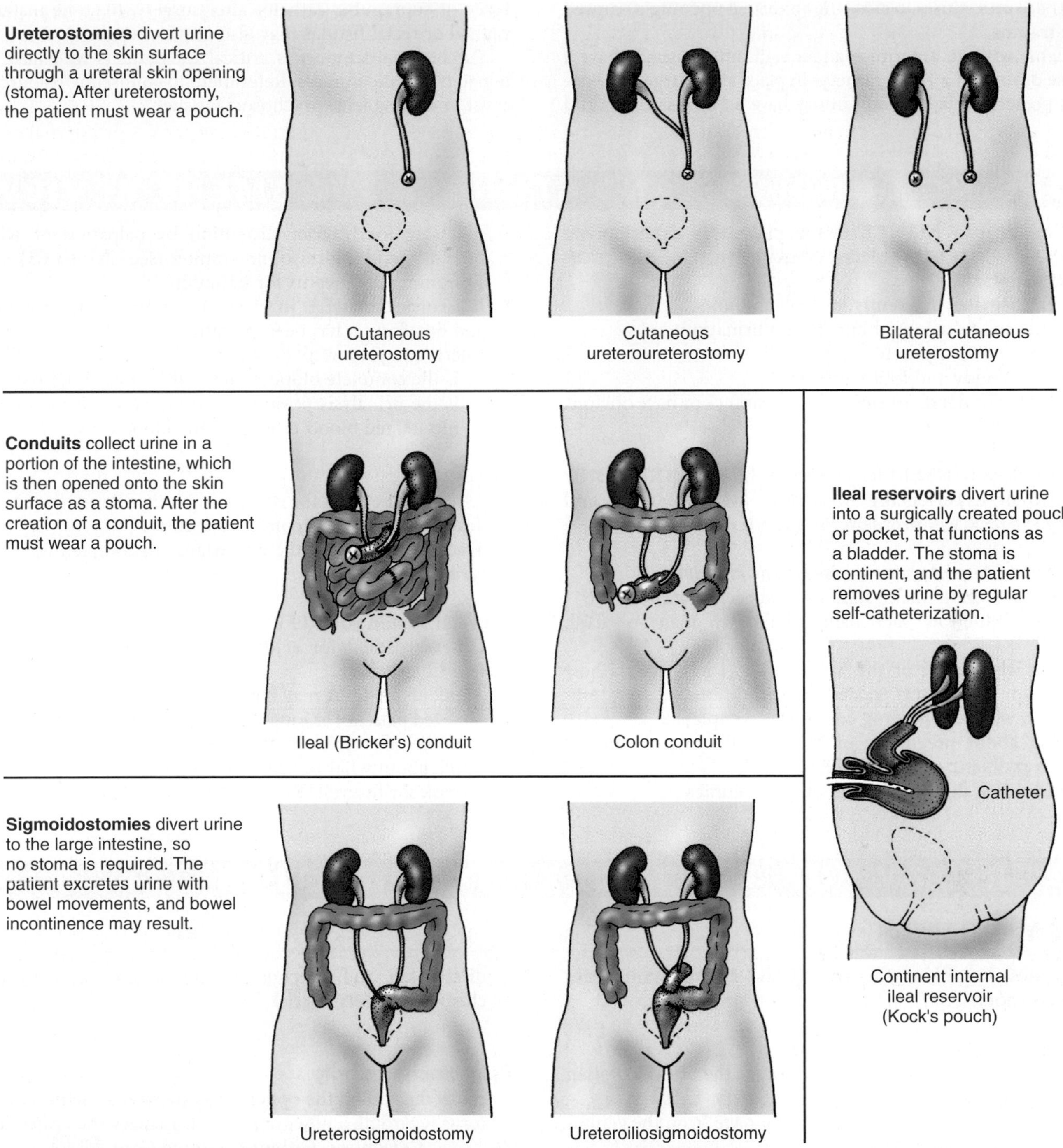

FIG. 66-4 Urinary diversion procedures used in the treatment of bladder cancer.

BLADDER TRAUMA

❖ PATHOPHYSIOLOGY

Bladder trauma can be caused by penetrating or blunt injury to the lower abdomen. Penetrating injury may occur by stabbing, gunshot wound, or other trauma in which objects pierce the abdominal wall. A fractured pelvis with puncture of the bladder by bone fragments is the most common cause of bladder trauma. Bladder trauma may also be a result of sexual assault.

Blunt trauma compresses the abdominal wall and the bladder. A seat belt may compress the bladder hard enough to cause injury, especially when the bladder is full or distended.

❖ PATIENT-CENTERED COLLABORATIVE CARE

Patients with a penetrating bladder wound often have anuria or hematuria. In the emergency department, initial assessment includes inspection of the urinary meatus for blood.

Bladder trauma, other than a simple contusion, requires surgical intervention. When bone fractures are present, they are stabilized before bladder repair to prevent further bladder damage. Surgical interventions include repairing the bladder wall and peritoneal membrane. Usually, repairs of the bladder are procedures to close the abnormal opening(s) caused by the trauma.

Patients with an anterior bladder wall injury usually have a Penrose drain and a Foley catheter in place after surgery. Those with a posterior bladder wall injury have a Penrose drain and Foley or suprapubic catheter after surgery. In some instances, vaginal or rectal fistulas may also require repair.

Psychosocial support is critical for patients who have sustained traumatic injuries. Refer them to counseling resources to assist in dealing with psychosocial issues.

NURSING CONCEPTS AND CLINICAL JUDGMENT REVIEW

What might you NOTICE if the patient is experiencing urinary ELIMINATION problems, INFLAMMATION, or INFECTION from cystitis?

- Patient urinates frequently in small amounts.
- Patient reports pain and burning on urination.
- Patient reports suprapubic pain.
- Urine is cloudy and foul-smelling.
- Urine may be darker or smoky in appearance or have obvious blood in it.

What should you INTERPRET and how should you RESPOND to a patient experiencing INFECTION, INFLAMMATION, and urinary ELIMINATION problems as a result of a UTI?

Perform and interpret physical assessment, including:

- Asking how long manifestations have been present
- Asking about low back pain (midline in men) or flank pain
- Asking whether he or she has had a UTI in the past; how long ago; how it was treated; and if antibiotics were prescribed, whether the drug course was completed
- Asking about pregnancy or the presence of any chronic health problem, especially diabetes
- Determining fluid intake and output volumes
- Assessing for bladder distention by palpation or with a bedside bladder ultrasound scanner (see Chapter 65)
- Examining the meatus for irritation
- If a Foley catheter is in place, determining why it is in use and how long it has been present
- Interpreting laboratory values:
  - Is the complete blood count within normal limits?
  - Is the urinalysis positive for bacteria, leukocyte esterase, nitrate, red blood cells, or white blood cells?

Respond by:

- Assessing the need for continuing indwelling catheter
- Teaching the patient comfort measures
- Teaching the patient the importance of completing the prescribed drug regimen

On what should you REFLECT?

- Observe patient for evidence of improved urinary output (see Chapter 65).
- Think about what may have caused this infection in a hospitalized patient (or long-term care resident) and what steps could be taken to prevent a similar episode.
- Think about what patient-teaching focus could help reduce the risk for future UTI.

GET READY FOR THE NCLEX® EXAMINATION!

KEY POINTS

Review these Key Points for each NCLEX Examination Client Needs Category.

Safe and Effective Care Environment

- Use sterile technique when inserting a catheter or any other instrument into the urinary system. **Safety** QSEN
- Use Contact Precautions with any drainage from the genitourinary tract. **Safety** QSEN
- Determine whether there is an ongoing need for an indwelling catheter. **Evidence-Based Practice** QSEN

Health Promotion and Maintenance

- Teach patients to clean the perineal area daily, after voiding, after having a bowel movement, and after sexual intercourse. **Patient-Centered Care** QSEN
- Encourage all patients to maintain an adequate fluid intake.
- Instruct women who have stress incontinence the proper way to perform pelvic floor strengthening exercises. **Patient-Centered Care** QSEN
- Urge anyone who smokes to stop smoking.
- Teach patients who come into contact with chemicals in their workplaces or with leisure-time activities to avoid direct skin and mucous membrane contact with these chemicals. **Safety** QSEN

Psychosocial Integrity

- Allow the patient the opportunity to express feelings or concerns regarding a potential chronic urinary tract disorder or a cancer diagnosis. **Patient-Centered Care** QSEN
- Use a nonjudgmental approach in caring for patients with urinary incontinence.
- Avoid referring to protective pads or pants as "diapers."
- Recognize the need for the patient undergoing cystectomy and urinary diversion to grieve about the body image change. **Patient-Centered Care** QSEN
- Assess the patient's level of comfort in discussing issues related to ELIMINATION and the urogenital area. **Patient-Centered Care** QSEN
- Use language and terminology during kidney/urinary assessment that the patient is comfortable using. **Patient-Centered Care** QSEN
- Refer patients to community resources and support groups.

Physiological Integrity

- Identify hospitalized patients at risk for bacteriuria and urosepsis.
- Report immediately any condition that obstructs urine flow.
- Instruct patients with UTI to complete all prescribed antibiotic therapy even when manifestations of INFECTION are absent.
- Evaluate daily the indications for maintaining indwelling catheters and discontinue their use as soon as possible. **Evidence-Based Practice** QSEN
- Teach patients the expected side effects and any adverse reactions to prescribed drugs.
- Assess the patient's manual dexterity and cognitive awareness before teaching a regimen of intermittent self-catheterization. **Patient-Centered Care** QSEN

67 CHAPTER

Care of Patients with Kidney Disorders

Chris Winkelman

http://evolve.elsevier.com/Iggy/

PRIORITY CONCEPTS

- Elimination
- Pain
- Fluid and Electrolyte Balance
- Acid-Base Balance
- Inflammation
- Infection

LEARNING OUTCOMES

Safe and Effective Care Environment

1. Collaborate with members of the health care team when providing care to patients with various types of kidney disorders.
2. Prioritize collaborative interventions for patients with kidney disorders and after nephrectomy.
3. Assess presence and extent of pain and suffering for patients with kidney disease.

Health Promotion and Maintenance

4. Teach patients who have other health problems that affect kidney function and elimination to manage these problems and maintain kidney health.
5. Instruct patients who are at risk for or who have kidney changes involving infection or inflammation to manage kidney health appropriately.

Psychosocial Integrity

6. Reduce the psychological impact of kidney disorders for the patient and family.

Physiological Integrity

7. Identify adults at highest risk for development of an acute or chronic kidney disorder that affects fluid and electrolyte balance.
8. Perform focused kidney/urinary assessment and re-assessment.

The role of the kidneys in urinary elimination is to filter wastes and maintain fluid and electrolyte balance, as well as acid-base balance. Any problem that disrupts kidney function limits the ability to meet these roles and has the potential to impair general homeostasis (Fig. 67-1). The kidneys work together with many other organ systems. Thus kidney disorders affect systemic health and can lead to life-threatening outcomes. Kidney disorders are classified as congenital, obstructive, infectious, glomerular, and degenerative. Kidney tumors and kidney trauma are also described in this chapter. Acute kidney injury (AKI) and chronic kidney disease (CKD) are discussed in Chapter 68.

CONGENITAL DISORDERS

POLYCYSTIC KIDNEY DISEASE

PATHOPHYSIOLOGY

Polycystic kidney disease (PKD) is an inherited disorder in which fluid-filled cysts develop in the nephrons (Fig. 67-2). In the dominant form, only a few nephrons have cysts until the person reaches his or her 30s. In the recessive form of the disease, nearly all nephrons have cysts from birth. Cysts develop throughout the nephron as a result of abnormal cell division.

Over time, small cysts become much larger (up to centimeters in diameter) and more widely distributed. The growing cysts damage the glomerular and tubular membranes. As the cysts fill with fluid and enlarge, the nephron and kidney function become less effective.

The kidney tissue is eventually replaced by nonfunctioning cysts, which look like clusters of grapes (see Fig. 67-2). The kidneys become very large. Each cystic kidney may enlarge to 2 or 3 times its normal size, becoming as large as a football, and may weigh 10 pounds or more each. Other abdominal organs are displaced, and the patient has pain. The fluid-filled cysts are also at increased risk for infection, rupture, and bleeding, which increase pain.

Most patients with PKD have high blood pressure. The cause of hypertension is related to kidney ischemia from the enlarging cysts. As the vessels are compressed and blood flow to the kidneys decreases, the renin-angiotensin system is activated, raising blood pressure. Control of hypertension is a top priority because proper treatment can disrupt the process that leads to further kidney damage.

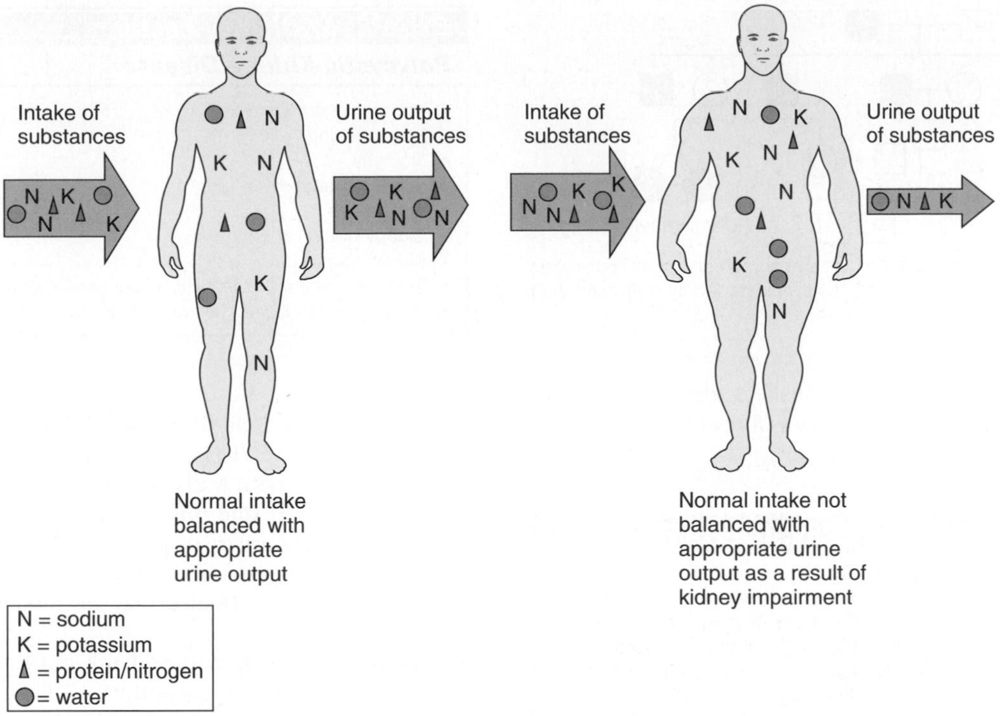

FIG. 67-1 Unbalanced body water, electrolytes, and waste products as a result of kidney problems that prevent adjustments in urinary elimination.

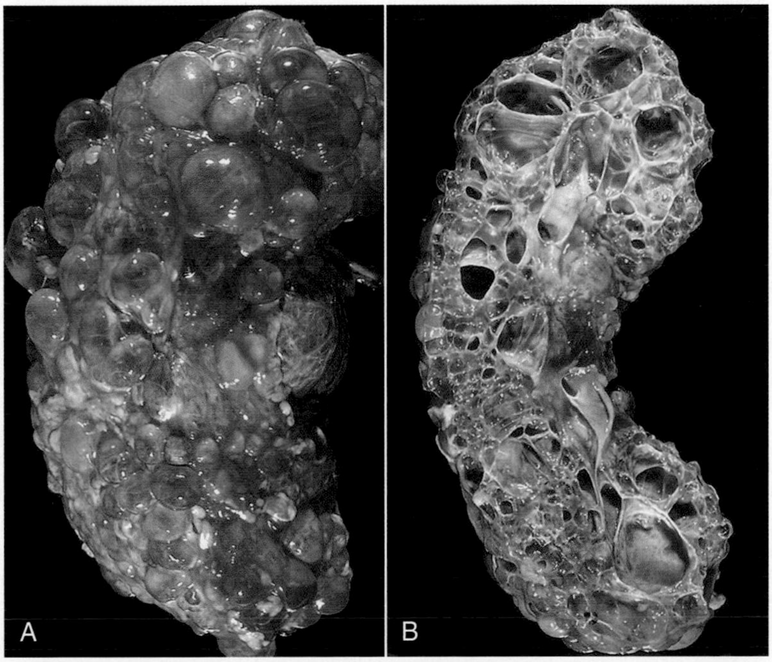

FIG. 67-2 External surface **(A)** and internal surface **(B)** of a polycystic kidney.

Cysts may occur also in other tissues, such as the liver and blood vessels. They may reduce liver function. In addition, the incidence of cerebral *aneurysms* (outpouching and thinning of an artery wall) is higher in patients with PKD. These aneurysms may rupture, causing bleeding and sudden death. For reasons as yet unknown, kidney stones occur in many patients with PKD. Heart valve problems (e.g., mitral valve prolapse), left ventricular hypertrophy, and colonic diverticula also are common in patients with PKD (McCance et al., 2014).

Etiology and Genetic Risk

PKD has several forms and can be inherited as either an autosomal dominant trait or, less commonly, as an autosomal recessive trait. People who inherit the recessive form of PKD usually

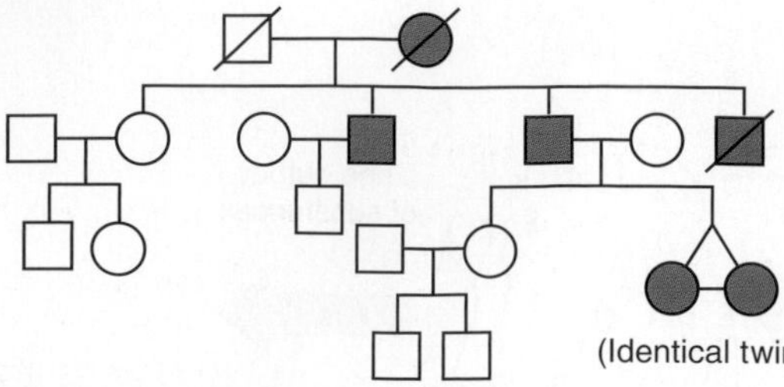

FIG. 67-3 Four-generation pedigree for autosomal dominant polycystic kidney disease (ADPKD). *Colored-in symbols* indicate family members with ADPKD. *Slashes* indicate the person has died.

die in early childhood. The 5% to 10% incidence of PKD in patients with no family history occurs as a result of a new gene mutation.

GENETIC/GENOMIC CONSIDERATIONS

Patient-Centered Care QSEN

The autosomal dominant form of PKD (ADPKD) is the most common form of polycystic disease. Children of parents who have the autosomal dominant form of PKD have a 50% chance of inheriting the gene mutation that causes the disease (*PKD1*). Fig. 67-3 shows a typical pedigree for a family with ADPKD. Presentation of ADPKD can vary for age of onset, manifestations, and illness severity, even within one family. However, it is fully penetrant, meaning that nearly 100% of people who inherit a PKD gene mutation will develop kidney cysts by age 30 (Online Mendelian Inheritance in Man [OMIM], 2014). Half of these people develop chronic kidney disease (CKD) by age 50 years. ADPKD-1 is the most common and most severe form of the autosomal dominant disease. ADPKD-2 has a slower rate of cyst formation, so manifestations occur later in life and progression to end-stage kidney disease (ESKD) and other complications is delayed.

There is no way to prevent PKD among people who have the genetic mutation, although early detection and management of hypertension may slow the progression of kidney damage. Genetic counseling may be useful for adults who have a parent with PKD. Family history analysis is a simple assessment that can be used to help identify people at risk for PKD (see Fig. 67-3).

Incidence and Prevalence

PKD is a common disorder, affecting about 600,000 people in the United States (National Kidney Foundation, 2013). It is more common in white people than in people of other races. Men and women have an equal chance of inheriting the disease because the gene responsible for PKD is not located on the sex chromosomes.

❖ *PATIENT-CENTERED COLLABORATIVE CARE*

◆ *Assessment*

History. Explore the family history of a patient with suspected or actual PKD, and ask whether either parent was known to have PKD or whether there is any family history of kidney disease. Important information to obtain is the age at which the problem was diagnosed in the parent and any related complications. Ask about constipation, abdominal discomfort, a change in urine color or frequency, high blood pressure, headaches, and a family history of sudden death from a stroke.

CHART 67-1 Key Features

Polycystic Kidney Disease

- Abdominal or flank pain
- Hypertension
- Nocturia
- Increased abdominal girth
- Constipation
- Bloody or cloudy urine
- Kidney stones
- Sodium wasting and inability to concentrate urine in early stage
- Progression to kidney failure with anuria

Physical Assessment/Clinical Manifestations. Chart 67-1 lists key features of PKD. PAIN is often the first manifestation. Inspect the abdomen. A distended abdomen is common as the cystic kidneys swell and push the abdominal contents forward. Polycystic kidneys are easily palpated because of their increased size. Proceed with *gentle* abdominal palpation because the cystic kidneys and nearby tissues may be tender and palpation is uncomfortable.

The patient also may have flank PAIN as a dull ache or as sharp and intermittent discomfort. Dull, aching pain is caused by increased kidney size with distention or by INFECTION within the cyst. Sharp, intermittent pain occurs when a cyst ruptures or a stone is present. When a cyst ruptures, the patient may have bright red or cola-colored urine. Infection is suspected if the urine is cloudy or foul smelling or if there is **dysuria** (pain on urination).

Nocturia (the need to urinate excessively at night) is an early manifestation and occurs because of decreased urine concentrating ability. Patients with early PKD waste sodium and water. As kidney function further declines, the patient has increasing hypertension, edema, and uremic manifestations such as anorexia, nausea, vomiting, pruritus, and fatigue (see Chapter 68). Because berry aneurysms often occur in patients with PKD, a severe headache with or without neurologic or vision changes requires attention.

Psychosocial Assessment. As an inherited disorder, PKD may cause psychosocial responses. The patient often has seen the effects and problems of the disease in close family members. He or she may have had a parent who died or close relatives who required dialysis or transplantation. While obtaining the family history, listen carefully for spoken and unspoken feelings of anger, resentment, futility, sadness, or anxiety. Such feelings may need further exploration. The focus of the feelings may be one or both parents or the process of diagnosis and treatment. Feelings of guilt and concern for the patient's children may also complicate the issue.

Diagnostic Assessment. Urinalysis shows **proteinuria** (protein in the urine) once the glomeruli are involved. **Hematuria** (blood in the urine) may be gross or microscopic. Bacteria in the urine indicate INFECTION, usually in the cysts. Obtain a urine sample for culture and sensitivity testing when there is evidence of infection. As kidney function declines, serum creatinine and blood urea nitrogen (BUN) levels rise. With decreasing kidney function, creatinine clearance decreases. Changes in kidney handling of sodium may cause either sodium losses or sodium retention.

Diagnostic studies to detect cysts include renal ultrasound, CT, and MRI.

◆ *Interventions*

Interventions for the patient with PKD include PAIN management and prevention of INFECTION, constipation, hypertension, and chronic kidney disease. Newer drug therapies are being evaluated to interrupt the pathways that promote malignant cyst formation such as molecular signaling for cell division or endothelial growth (Aguiari et al., 2013). When the disease progresses and the kidneys no longer function to clear wastes, care becomes similar to that needed for the patient with end-stage kidney disease (ESKD) (see Chapter 68).

Managing Pain. PAIN management strategies include drug therapy and complementary approaches. A combination may be most effective. NSAIDs are used cautiously because they can reduce kidney blood flow. Aspirin-containing compounds are avoided to reduce the risk for bleeding.

If cyst INFECTION causes discomfort, antibiotics such as trimethoprim/sulfamethoxazole (Bactrim, Septra, Trimpex) or ciprofloxacin (Cipro) are prescribed. (See Chart 66-4 in Chapter 66.) These drugs enter the cyst wall. Monitor the serum creatinine levels because antibiotic therapy can be nephrotoxic. Apply dry heat to the abdomen or flank to promote comfort when kidney cysts are infected. When PAIN is severe, cysts can be reduced by needle aspiration and drainage; however, they usually refill.

Teach the patient methods of relaxation and comfort using deep breathing, guided imagery, or other strategies. The expected outcome is patient self-management. (See Chapter 3 for pain management.)

Preventing Constipation. Teach the patient who has adequate urine output how to prevent constipation by maintaining adequate fluid intake, increasing dietary fiber when fluid intake is more than 2500 mL/24 hr, and exercising regularly. Explain that pressure on the large intestine may occur as the polycystic kidneys increase in size. The patient should know that these recommendations for bowel management might change, particularly if ESDK also develops. Advise him or her about the use of stool softeners and bulk agents, including the careful use of laxatives, to prevent chronic constipation.

Controlling Hypertension and Preventing End-Stage Kidney Disease. Blood pressure control is necessary to reduce cardiovascular complications and slow the progression of kidney dysfunction. Nursing interventions include education to promote self-management and understanding. When kidney impairment results in decreased urine concentration with nocturia and low urine specific gravity, urge the patient to drink at least 2 L of fluid per day to prevent dehydration, which can further reduce kidney function. Restricting sodium intake may help control blood pressure. See Chapter 36 for a detailed discussion about the causes and management of hypertension.

Drug therapy for blood pressure control includes antihypertensive agents and diuretics. Antihypertensive agents include angiotensin-converting enzyme (ACE) inhibitors, calcium channel blockers, beta blockers, and vasodilators (see Chapter 36). ACE inhibitors may help control the cell growth aspects of PKD and reduce microalbuminuria.

Teach the patient and family how to measure and record blood pressure. Help the patient establish a schedule for self-administering drugs, monitoring daily weights, and keeping blood pressure records (Chart 67-2). Explain the potential side effects of the drugs. Make available written materials, such as drug teaching cards and booklets.

CHART 67-2 Patient and Family Education: Preparing for Self-Management

Polycystic Kidney Disease

- Measure and record your blood pressure daily, and notify your health care provider for consistent changes in blood pressure.
- Take your temperature if you suspect you have a fever. If a fever is present, notify your physician or nurse.
- Weigh yourself every day at the same time of day and with the same amount of clothing; notify your physician or nurse if you have a sudden weight gain.
- Limit your intake of salt to help control your blood pressure.
- Notify your physician or nurse if your urine smells foul or has blood in it.
- Notify your physician or nurse if you have a headache that does not go away or if you have visual disturbances.
- Monitor bowel movements to prevent constipation.

Many patients may have salt wasting and should not follow a sodium-restricted diet. As the disease progresses, the protein intake may be limited to slow the development of ESKD. Assist the patient and family in understanding the diet plan and why it was prescribed. Work closely with the dietitian to foster the patient's understanding. Also refer the patient for nutrition counseling.

Health Care Resources

The Polycystic Kidney Research Foundation (www.pkdcure.org) and the National Kidney & Urologic Diseases Clearinghouse (NKUDIC) of the National Institute of Diabetes and Digestive and Kidney Diseases (www2.niddk.nih.gov) conduct research and provide education about PKD. Many pamphlets are available; there is a fee for some materials. Chapters of the National Kidney Foundation (NKF) and the American Association of Kidney Patients (AAKP) also have resources for information and support.

NCLEX EXAMINATION CHALLENGE

Health Promotion and Maintenance

Which statement made by the client who is newly diagnosed with polycystic kidney disease (PKD) indicates to the nurse that additional teaching for self-management is needed?

A. "I will need to increase my daily water intake."
B. "I will restrict my sodium to less than 2 g daily."
C. "Now I will need to take a blood pressure drug daily."
D. "If I become sexually active or plan to have a family, I will seek genetic counseling."

OBSTRUCTIVE DISORDERS

HYDRONEPHROSIS, HYDROURETER, AND URETHRAL STRICTURE

❖ *PATHOPHYSIOLOGY*

Hydronephrosis and hydroureter are problems of urine outflow obstruction. Urethral strictures also obstruct urine outflow. Prompt recognition and treatment are crucial to prevent permanent kidney damage.

In **hydronephrosis**, the kidney enlarges as urine collects in the renal pelvis and kidney tissue. Because the capacity of the renal pelvis is normally 5 to 8 mL, obstruction in the renal

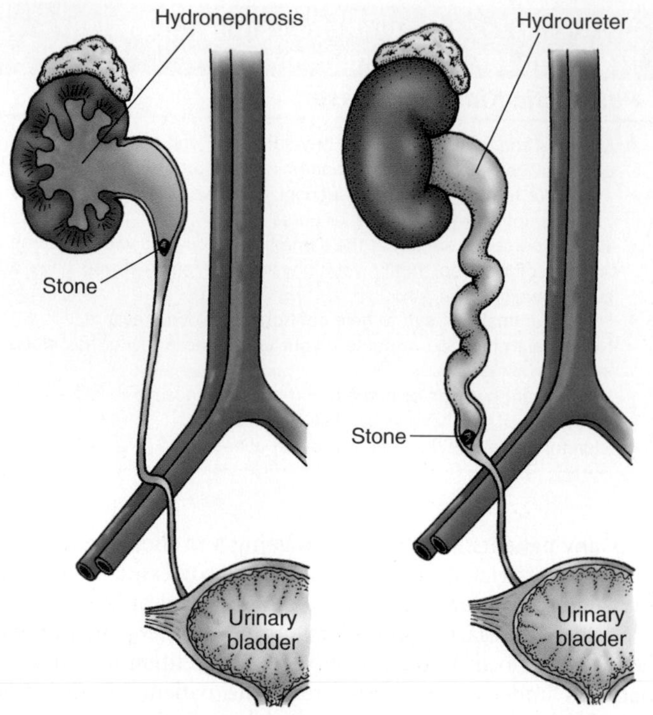

FIG. 67-4 Hydronephrosis is caused by obstruction in the upper part of the ureter. Hydroureter is caused by obstruction in the lower part of the ureter.

pelvis or at the point where the ureter joins the renal pelvis quickly distends the renal pelvis. Kidney pressure increases as the volume of urine increases. Over time, sometimes in only a matter of hours, the blood vessels and kidney tubules can be damaged extensively (Fig. 67-4).

In patients with **hydroureter** (enlargement of the ureter), the effects are similar but the obstruction is in the ureter rather than in the kidney. The ureter is most easily obstructed where the iliac vessels cross or where the ureters enter the bladder. Ureter dilation occurs above the obstruction and enlarges as urine collects (see Fig. 67-4).

In patients with a **urethral stricture**, the obstruction is very low in the urinary tract, causing bladder distention before hydroureter and hydronephrosis. The problems and kidney damage are similar without prompt treatment.

Urinary obstruction causes damage when pressure builds up directly on kidney tissue. Tubular filtrate pressure also increases in the nephron as drainage through the collecting system is impaired. With this added pressure, glomerular filtration decreases or ceases. Necrosis of the affected kidney can occur. Nitrogen waste products (urea, creatinine, and uric acid) and *electrolytes* (sodium, potassium, chloride, and phosphorus) are retained, and ACID-BASE BALANCE is impaired.

Causes of hydronephrosis or hydroureter include tumors, stones, trauma, structural defects, and fibrosis (Pengo et al., 2013). In patients with cancer, obstructed ureters may result from the tumors themselves, pelvic radiation, or surgical treatment. Early treatment of the causes can prevent hydronephrosis and hydroureter and prevent permanent kidney damage. The time needed to prevent permanent damage depends on the patient's kidney health. Permanent damage can occur in less than 48 hours in some patients and after several weeks in other patients.

❖ PATIENT-CENTERED COLLABORATIVE CARE

◆ Assessment

Obtain a history from the patient, focusing on known kidney or urologic disorders. A history of childhood urinary tract problems may indicate previously undiagnosed structural defects. Ask about his or her usual pattern of urine ELIMINATION, especially amount, frequency, color, clarity, and odor. Ask about recent flank or abdominal PAIN. Chills, fever, and malaise may be present with a urinary tract infection (UTI).

Inspect each flank to identify asymmetry, which may occur with a kidney mass, and *gently* palpate the abdomen to locate areas of tenderness. Palpate and percuss the bladder to detect distention, or use a bedside bladder scanner. Gentle pressure on the abdomen may cause urine leakage, which reflects a full bladder and possible obstruction.

Urinalysis may show bacteria or white blood cells if INFECTION is present. When urinary tract obstruction is prolonged, microscopic examination may show tubular epithelial cells. Blood chemistries are normal unless glomerular filtration has decreased. Blood creatinine and blood urea nitrogen (BUN) levels increase with a reduced glomerular filtration rate (GFR). Serum electrolyte levels may be altered with elevated blood levels of potassium, phosphorus, and calcium along with a metabolic acidosis (bicarbonate deficit).

Urinary outflow obstruction can be seen with ultrasound (US) or CT.

◆ Interventions

Urinary retention and potential for INFECTION are the primary problems. Failure to treat the cause of obstruction leads to infection and ESKD.

Urologic Interventions. If the stricture is caused by a stone, it can be located and removed using cystoscopic or retrograde urogram procedures. The urologist uses a cystoscope to guide a stone basket over the stone and removes it through the bladder. After stone removal, a plastic stent is usually left in the ureter for a few weeks to improve urine flow in the area irritated by the stone. The stent is later removed by another cystoscopic procedure.

Radiologic Interventions. When a stricture is causing hydronephrosis and cannot be corrected with urologic procedures, a **nephrostomy** is performed. Most nephrostomy drains provide only external drainage (diversion). Other styles of nephrostomy drains enter the kidney but extend to the bladder. These tubes can drain urine out to a bag or past a ureteral stricture and into the bladder, so there is both an internal and external component to the nephrostomy tubing. Externally, a fully external or an internal/external diversion drain appears the same. The urine output will fluctuate more if all urine goes to the bladder before external drainage.

Patient Preparation. If possible, the patient is kept NPO for 4 to 6 hours before the procedure. Clotting studies (e.g., international normalized ratio [INR], prothrombin time [PT], and partial thromboplastic time [PTT]) should be normal or corrected. Drugs are used to reduce hypertension. The patient receives moderate sedation for the procedure.

Procedure. The patient is placed in the prone position. The kidney is located under ultrasound or fluoroscopic guidance, and a local anesthetic is given. A needle is placed into the kidney, a soft-tipped guidewire is placed through the needle, and then a catheter is placed over the wire. The catheter tip remains in the renal pelvis, and the external end is connected to a drainage bag. The procedure immediately relieves the pressure and prevents further damage. The nephrostomy tube remains in place until the obstruction is resolved (with or without further intervention).

Follow-up Care. Assess the amount of drainage in the collection bag. The amount of drainage depends on whether a ureteral catheter is also being used (with a separate drainage bag). Patients with ureteral tubes may have all urine pass through to the bladder or may have urine drain into the collection bags. The type of urine drainage expected should be clearly communicated in the chart. If urine is expected to drain into the collection bag, assess the amount of drainage hourly for the first 24 hours. When urine drains only into the collection bag and not into the bladder, the minimum expected drainage is 30 mL/hr. If the amount of drainage decreases and the patient has back PAIN, the tube may be clogged or dislodged.

Monitor the nephrostomy site for leaking urine or blood. Urine drainage may be red-tinged for the first 12 to 24 hours after the procedure and should gradually clear. Assess the patient for manifestations of INFECTION, including fever or a change in urine character.

! NURSING SAFETY PRIORITY (QSEN)

Critical Rescue

After nephrostomy, notify the physician immediately when the drainage decreases or stops, drainage becomes cloudy or foul-smelling, the nephrostomy site leaks blood or urine, or the patient has back PAIN.

NCLEX EXAMINATION CHALLENGE

Physiological Integrity

When providing care to a client who has undergone a nephrostomy for hydronephrosis, which observation alerts the nurse to a possible complication?

A. Urine output of 15 mL/hr
B. Tenderness at the surgical site
C. Blood urea nitrogen (BUN) of 23 mg/dL
D. Pink-tinged urine draining from the nephrostomy

INFECTIOUS DISORDERS: PYELONEPHRITIS

In the healthy person, urine is normally sterile and remains sterile if there is no obstruction to urine passage in the kidney and urinary tract. When any structural abnormality is present, the risk for damage as a result of INFECTION is greatly increased. **Urinary tract infection (UTI)** is an infection in this normally sterile system. **Pyelonephritis** is a bacterial infection in the kidney and renal pelvis.

PATHOPHYSIOLOGY

Pyelonephritis is either the presence of active organisms in the kidney or the effects of kidney INFECTION. **Acute pyelonephritis** is the active bacterial infection, whereas **chronic pyelonephritis** results from repeated or continued upper urinary tract infections or the effects of such infections. Chronic pyelonephritis often occurs with a urinary tract defect, with obstruction, or, most commonly, when urine refluxes from the bladder back into the ureters. **Reflux** is the reverse or upward flow of urine toward the renal pelvis and kidney.

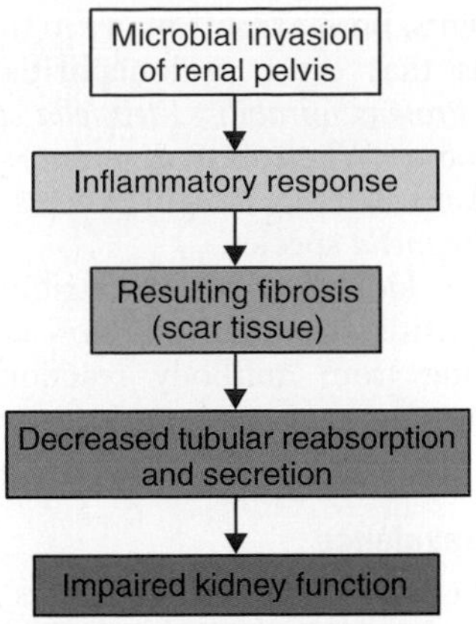

FIG. 67-5 Pathophysiology of pyelonephritis.

In pyelonephritis, organisms move up from the urinary tract into the kidney tissue. Descending infection transmitted by organisms in the blood may occur, but not often. Bacteria trigger the inflammatory response, and local edema results.

Acute pyelonephritis involves acute tissue INFLAMMATION, tubular cell necrosis, and possible abscess formation. **Abscesses**, which are pockets of INFECTION, can occur anywhere in the kidney. The infection is scattered within the kidney; healthy tissues can lie next to infected areas. Fibrosis and scar tissue develop from the inflammation. The calices thicken, and scars develop in the interstitial tissue.

Reflux of infected urine from the bladder into the ureters and kidney is responsible for most cases of chronic pyelonephritis. Reflux within the kidney can occur when some papillae in the kidney do not close properly. INFLAMMATION and fibrosis lead to deformity of the renal pelvis and calices. Repeated or continuous INFECTION creates additional scar tissue, changing blood vessel, glomerular, and tubular structure. As a result, filtration, reabsorption, and secretion are impaired and kidney function is reduced (Fig. 67-5).

Etiology and Genetic Risk

Single episodes of *acute pyelonephritis* result from bacterial INFECTION, with or without obstruction or reflux. *Chronic pyelonephritis* usually occurs with structural deformities, urinary stasis, obstruction, or reflux. Conditions that lead to urinary stasis include prolonged bedrest and paralysis. Obstruction can be caused by stones, kidney cancer, scarring from pelvic radiotherapy or surgery, recurrent infection, or injury. Reflux may occur from scarring or as a result of anatomic anomalies. Reflux also results from bladder tumor, prostate enlargement, or urinary tract stones. Reduced bladder tone from diabetic neuropathy, spinal cord injury, and neurodegenerative diseases (e.g., spina bifida, multiple sclerosis) contributes to reflux and increases the risk for pyelonephritis.

Pyelonephritis from an ascending INFECTION may follow manipulation of the urinary tract (e.g., placement of a urinary catheter), particularly in patients who are immunosuppressed or who have diabetes mellitus. In patients with chronic kidney stone disease, stones may retain organisms, resulting in ongoing infection and kidney scarring. Drug use can also contribute to pyelonephritis. In particular, high-dose or prolonged use of NSAIDs can lead to papillary necrosis and reflux.

The most common pyelonephritis-causing infecting organism is *Escherichia coli*. *Enterococcus faecalis* is common in hospitalized patients. Both organisms are in the intestinal tract. Other organisms that cause pyelonephritis in hospitalized patients include *Proteus mirabilis, Klebsiella* species, and *Pseudomonas aeruginosa*. When the INFECTION is bloodborne, common organisms include *Staphylococcus aureus* and the *Candida* and *Salmonella* species.

Other causes of kidney scarring contributing to increased risk for pyelonephritis are INFLAMMATION and inflammatory responses resulting from antibody reactions, cell-mediated immunity against the bacterial antigens, or autoimmune reactions.

Incidence and Prevalence

About 250,000 cases of acute pyelonephritis occur each year, resulting in more than 100,000 hospitalizations in the United States (U.S. Renal Data Systems, 2012). Chronic pyelonephritis is more common in women, although the exact incidence and prevalence are not known. After 65 years of age, rates of pyelonephritis for men increase greatly because of the increased incidence of prostatitis.

CHART 67-3 Key Features

Acute Pyelonephritis

- Fever
- Chills
- Tachycardia and tachypnea
- Flank, back, or loin pain
- Tender costovertebral angle (CVA)
- Abdominal, often colicky, discomfort
- Nausea and vomiting
- General malaise or fatigue
- Burning, urgency, or frequency of urination
- Nocturia
- Recent cystitis or treatment for urinary tract infection (UTI)

CHART 67-4 Key Features

Chronic Pyelonephritis

- Hypertension
- Inability to conserve sodium
- Decreased urine-concentrating ability, resulting in nocturia
- Tendency to develop hyperkalemia and acidosis

❖ PATIENT-CENTERED COLLABORATIVE CARE

◆ Assessment

History. Ask about a history of urinary tract INFECTIONS (UTIs), diabetes mellitus, stone disease, and defects of the genitourinary tract. Determine whether the UTIs occurred with pregnancy, and ask the patient about any previous episodes of pyelonephritis or similar problems. Ask about disease or treatment that causes immunosuppression, because they can also increase risk for pyelonephritis. Recurrences are common and may lead to a decline of kidney function. Ensure that a woman is not pregnant before radiographic imaging.

Physical Assessment/Clinical Manifestations. Ask about specific manifestations of acute pyelonephritis (Chart 67-3). Chronic pyelonephritis has a less dramatic presentation, with manifestations related to the INFECTION or reduced kidney function. Ask the patient to describe any vague urinary manifestations or abdominal discomfort. Inquire about any history of repeated low-grade fevers. Changes in urine color or odor may accompany bacteriuria. Chart 67-4 lists the kidney effects of chronic pyelonephritis.

Inspect the flanks, and gently palpate the costovertebral angle (CVA). Inspect both CVAs for enlargement, asymmetry, edema, or redness, all of which can indicate inflammation. If there is no tenderness to light palpation in either CVA, an advanced practice nurse firmly percusses each area. Tenderness or discomfort may indicate INFECTION or INFLAMMATION.

Psychosocial Assessment. The patient with any problem in the genitourinary area may have feelings of anxiety, embarrassment, or guilt. Listen carefully for signs of anxiety or specific fears, and prevent embarrassment during assessment. Feelings of guilt, often associated with sexual habits or practices, may be masked through delay in seeking treatment or through vague, nonspecific responses to specific or direct questions. Encourage patients to tell their own story in familiar, comfortable language.

Laboratory Assessment. Urinalysis shows a positive leukocyte esterase and nitrite dipstick test and the presence of white blood cells and bacteria. Occasional red blood cells, white blood cell casts, and protein may be present. The urine is cultured to determine whether gram-positive or gram-negative organisms are causing the INFECTION. The urine sample for culture and sensitivity testing, obtained by the clean-catch method, shows the bacterial species and susceptibility or resistance of the specific organism to various antibiotics. In patients with recurrent episodes of pyelonephritis or upper UTIs, more specific testing of bacterial antigens and antibodies may help determine whether the same organism is responsible for the recurrent infections.

Blood cultures are obtained for specific organisms. Other blood tests include the C-reactive protein and erythrocyte sedimentation rate to determine the presence of INFLAMMATION.

Imaging Assessment. An x-ray of the kidneys, ureters, and bladder (KUB) or CT is performed to visualize anatomy, INFLAMMATION, fluid accumulation, abscess formation, and defects in kidneys and the urinary tract. These tests also identify stones, tumors, or prostate enlargement. Urine reflux caused by incompetent bladder-ureter valve closure can be seen with a cystourethrogram. (See Chapter 65 for more information on imaging assessment.)

Other Diagnostic Assessment. Other diagnostic tests include examining antibody-coated bacteria in urine, testing for certain enzymes (e.g., lactate dehydrogenase isoenzyme 5), and radionuclide renal scan. Examining urine for antibody-coated bacteria helps identify patients who may need long-term antibiotic therapy. High-molecular-weight enzymes in urine, such as lactate dehydrogenase isoenzyme 5, are present with any kidney tissue deterioration problem and give trend data. The renal scan can identify active pyelonephritis or abscesses in or around the kidney.

◆ Analysis

The priority NANDA-I nursing diagnoses and collaborative problems for patients with pyelonephritis include:

1. Acute Pain (flank and abdominal) related to inflammation and infection (NANDA-I)
2. Potential for chronic kidney disease and end-stage kidney disease related to infectious tissue destruction

◆ Planning and Implementation

Managing Pain

Planning: Expected Outcomes. With proper intervention, the patient with pyelonephritis is expected to achieve an acceptable state of comfort. Indicators include that he or she often or consistently demonstrates these behaviors:

- Uses pharmacologic relief measures
- Uses NSAIDs appropriately
- Reports PAIN controlled

Interventions. Interventions may be nonsurgical or surgical. The use of several techniques that crush stones, such as lithotripsy and percutaneous ultrasonic pyelolithotomy (see Chapter 66), has decreased the need for surgery.

Nonsurgical Management. Interventions include the use of drug therapy, nutrition and fluid therapy, and teaching to ensure the patient's understanding of the treatment.

Drug therapy with antibiotics is prescribed to treat the INFECTION. At first, the antibiotics are broad spectrum. After urine and blood culture and sensitivity results are known, more specific antibiotics may be prescribed. Urinary antiseptic drugs (e.g., nitrofurantoin [Macrodantin]) may also be prescribed to provide comfort.

Nutrition therapy involves ensuring that the patient's nutrition intake has adequate calories from all food groups for healing to occur. Fluid intake is recommended at 2 L/day, sufficient to result in dilute (pale yellow) urine, unless another health problem requires fluid restriction.

Surgical Management. Surgical interventions can correct structural problems causing urine reflux or obstruction of urine outflow or can remove the source of infection.

Antibiotics are given, usually IV, to achieve adequate blood levels or sterile blood culture results. Teach the patient the nature and purpose of the proposed surgery, the expected outcome, and how he or she can participate.

The surgical procedures may be one of these: **pyelolithotomy** (stone removal from the kidney), **nephrectomy** (removal of the kidney), ureteral diversion, or reimplantation of ureter to restore proper bladder drainage.

A pyelolithotomy is needed for removal of a large stone in the kidney pelvis that blocks urine flow and causes INFECTION. Nephrectomy is a last resort when all other measures to clear the infection have failed. For patients with poor ureter valve closure or dilated ureters, **ureteroplasty** (ureter repair or revision) or ureteral reimplantation (through another site in the bladder wall) preserves kidney function and eliminates infections.

Preventing End-Stage Kidney Disease

Planning: Expected Outcomes. The patient is expected to conserve existing kidney function for as long as possible and have a slow progression to end-stage kidney disease (ESKD) once the damage has occurred. Indicators include that he or she consistently demonstrates these behaviors:

- Describes the role of antibiotics and self-administration of drugs
- Explains and offers techniques to ensure adequate nutrition and hydration
- Describes the plan for post-treatment follow-up, including knowledge of recurrent manifestations
- Modifies prescribed regimen as directed by a health care professional

Interventions. Specific antibiotics are prescribed to treat the INFECTION. Stress the importance of completing the drug therapy as directed. Discuss with the patient and family the importance of regular follow-up examinations and completing the recommended diagnostic tests.

Blood pressure control is needed to slow the progression of kidney dysfunction. When kidney impairment decreases concentrating ability, encourage the patient to drink sufficient fluid during waking hours to prevent dehydration because dehydration could further reduce kidney function. When dietary protein is restricted, refer the patient to the dietitian as needed. Other interventions related to the progression of chronic kidney disease are covered in Chapter 68.

Community-Based Care

Pyelonephritis causes fear and anxiety in the patient and family. The severity of the acute process and its potential to develop into a chronic process are frightening. The patient and the family need reassurance that treatment and preventive measures can be successful.

Home Care Management. If no surgery is performed, the patient may need help with self-care, nutrition, and drug management at home. If surgery is performed, he or she may need help with incision care, self-care, and transportation for follow-up appointments.

Self-Management Education. After assessing the patient's and family's understanding of pyelonephritis and its therapy, explain:

- Drug regimen (purpose, timing, frequency, duration, and possible side effects)
- The role of nutrition and adequate fluid intake
- The need for a balance between rest and activity, including any limitations after surgery
- The manifestations of disease recurrence
- The use of previously successful coping mechanisms

Advise the patient to complete all prescribed antibiotic regimens and to report any side effects or unusual manifestations to the health care provider rather than stopping the drugs. Refer the patient and family for nutrition counseling as needed, because many patients have special nutrition needs, such as those for diabetes or pregnancy.

Health Care Resources. The patient may also briefly need a home health care nurse to help with drug or nutrition therapy at home. Housekeeping services may be helpful while he or she is regaining strength.

◆ Evaluation: Outcomes

Evaluate the care of the patient with pyelonephritis based on the identified priority patient problems. Expected outcomes may include that the patient will:

- Report that PAIN is controlled
- Be knowledgeable about the disease, its treatment, and interventions to prevent or reduce disease progression

Specific indicators for these outcomes are listed for each priority patient problem in the Planning and Implementation section (see earlier).

IMMUNOLOGIC KIDNEY DISORDERS

Glomerulonephritis (GN) is the third leading cause of end-stage kidney disease (ESKD) (U.S. Renal Data Systems, 2012). Whether the disease starts in the kidney or occurs as the result of other health problems, the glomeruli are usually injured (Table 67-1). For disease that starts in the kidney, a genetic basis

TABLE 67-1 Primary Glomerular Diseases and Syndromes

- Acute glomerulonephritis
- Rapidly progressive glomerulonephritis (RPGN)
- Chronic glomerulonephritis
- Nephrotic syndrome
- Persistent, vague urinary abnormalities with few or no symptoms

TABLE 67-2 Secondary Glomerular Diseases and Syndromes

• Systemic lupus erythematosus (SLE)	• Multiple myeloma
• Schönlein-Henoch purpura	• Viral hepatitis B
• Goodpasture's syndrome	• Viral hepatitis C
• Systemic necrotizing vasculitis	• Cirrhosis
• Wegener's granulomatosis	• Sickle cell disease
• Periarteritis nodosa (also called *polyarteritis nodosa*)	• Nonstreptococcal postinfectious acute glomerulonephritis
• Amyloidosis	• Infective endocarditis
• Diabetic glomerulopathy	• Hemolytic-uremic syndrome
• HIV-associated nephropathy	• Thrombotic thrombocytopenic purpura
• Alport's syndrome	

HIV, Human immune deficiency virus.

and immune-inducing INFLAMMATION problems are common. In addition, systemic diseases and INFECTIONS can have kidney effects and cause glomerular injury (Table 67-2). Conditions that lead to glomerular disease include systemic lupus erythematous and diabetic nephropathy.

Each type of disease or syndrome has a specific pathophysiology and clinical manifestations. Their *glomerular* effects are caused by injury to the glomeruli and result in proteinuria, hematuria, decreased glomerular filtration rate (GFR), edema, and hypertension. The extent and duration of kidney injury, prognosis, and specific cause vary among these syndromes.

Immunologic changes injure the glomeruli, interstitium, or tubules, and the effects may be acute or chronic. Both antibody and cellular immune responses leading to INFLAMMATION are involved. The resultant kidney disorder can be systemic or confined to the kidneys.

Most forms of INFLAMMATION-induced glomerulonephritis (GN) occur with a collection of immune complexes in the glomeruli (Fig. 20-4 in Chapter 20). An immune complex is made up of antigens (foreign substances within the body) and antibodies. The antigen can be part of any normal kidney tissue, or it can be dissolved in a body fluid (e.g., blood). Bacteria and viruses are also antigens. Exposure to bacteria, viruses, drugs, or other toxins is believed to be the trigger for glomerular injury.

Antibody reaction with antigens can cause immune complexes to form and become deposited in glomerular tissue, leading to INFLAMMATION. These complexes trigger many inflammatory mediators, such as complement, white blood cells, and blood clotting proteins, which also damage the kidney tissue. Actions that cause tissue injury include damage to cell membranes, local edema, movement of white blood cells to the site of inflammation, and platelet activation.

TABLE 67-3 Infectious Causes of Acute Glomerulonephritis

- Group A beta-hemolytic *Streptococcus*
- Staphylococcal or gram-negative bacteremia or sepsis
- Pneumococcal, *Mycoplasma,* or *Klebsiella* pneumonia
- Syphilis
- Visceral abscesses
- Infective endocarditis
- Hepatitis B
- Infectious mononucleosis
- Measles
- Mumps
- Rocky Mountain spotted fever
- Cytomegalovirus infection
- Histoplasmosis
- Toxoplasmosis
- Varicella
- *Chlamydia psittaci* infection
- Coxsackievirus infection
- Any bacterial, parasitic, fungal, or viral infection (potentially)

ACUTE GLOMERULONEPHRITIS

❖ PATHOPHYSIOLOGY

An INFECTION often occurs before the kidney manifestations of acute glomerulonephritis (GN). The onset of manifestations is about 10 days from the time of infection. Usually patients recover quickly and completely from acute GN. The term *acute nephritic syndrome* also describes this disorder.

Most causes of acute GN are infectious (Table 67-3) or are related to other systemic diseases (see Table 67-2). The incidence of acute GN is unknown. GN after a systemic streptococcal infection is more common in men.

❖ PATIENT-CENTERED COLLABORATIVE CARE

◆ Assessment

History. Ask about recent INFECTION, particularly of the skin or upper respiratory tract, and about recent travel or other possible exposures to viruses, bacteria, fungi, or parasites. Recent illnesses, surgery, or other invasive procedures may suggest infections. Ask about any known systemic diseases, such as systemic lupus erythematosus (SLE), which could cause acute GN.

Physical Assessment/Clinical Manifestations. Inspect the patient's skin for lesions or recent incisions, including body piercings. Assess the face, eyelids, hands, and other areas for edema because edema is present in most patients with acute GN. Assess for fluid overload and circulatory congestion that may accompany the fluid and sodium retention occurring with acute GN. Ask about any difficulty in breathing or shortness of breath. Assess for crackles in the lung fields, an S_3 heart sound (gallop rhythm), and neck vein distention.

Ask about changes in voiding patterns and any change in urine color, volume, clarity, or odor. Microscopic blood in the urine occurs, and patients often describe their urine as smoky, reddish brown, rusty, or cola colored. Ask about dysuria or oliguria. Weigh him or her to assess for fluid retention.

Take the patient's blood pressure, and compare it with the baseline blood pressure. Mild to moderate hypertension occurs with acute GN as a result of fluid and sodium retention. The patient may have fatigue, a lack of energy, anorexia, nausea, and vomiting if uremia from severe kidney impairment is present.

CONSIDERATIONS FOR OLDER ADULTS

Patient-Centered Care QSEN

The less common manifestations of acute GN are more likely to occur in older adults. Circulatory congestion often is present, causing acute GN to be easily confused with congestive heart failure (CHF). Ask any older adult with CHF about voiding patterns to determine whether the problem may be related to acute GN.

Laboratory Assessment. Urinalysis shows red blood cells *(hematuria)* and protein *(proteinuria)*. An early morning specimen of urine is preferred for urinalysis because the urine is most acidic and formed elements are more intact at that time. Microscopic examination often shows red blood cell casts, as well as casts from other substances.

The glomerular filtration rate (GFR), either estimated from a single serum and urine creatinine value or measured by the 24-hour urine test for creatinine clearance, may be decreased to 50 mL/min. The older patient may have a greater decline in GFR.

A 24-hour urine collection for total protein assay is obtained. The protein excretion rate for patients with acute GN may be increased from 500 mg/24 hr to 3 g/24 hr. Serum albumin levels are decreased because of the protein lost in the urine and because of fluid retention causing dilution.

Specimens from the blood, skin, or throat are obtained for culture, if indicated. Serum creatinine and blood urea nitrogen provide information about kidney function and may be elevated, indicating impairment. Other serum tests include antistreptolysin O titers, C3 complement levels, cryoglobulins (immunoglobulin G [IgG]), antinuclear antibodies (ANAs), and circulating immune complexes.

Antistreptolysin-O titers are increased after group A beta-hemolytic *Streptococcus* INFECTION. Complement levels are decreased when the complement system is activated. Type III cryoglobulins may be found during acute illness. ANAs suggest an autoimmune response with INFLAMMATION, and systemic lupus erythematosus (SLE) is just one possibility. Immune complexes containing IgG and C3 are often detected.

Other Diagnostic Assessment. A kidney biopsy provides a precise diagnosis of the condition, assists in determining the prognosis, and helps outline treatment (see Chapter 65). The specific tissue features are determined by light microscopy, immunofluorescent stains, and electron microscopy to identify cell type, the presence of immunoglobulins, or the type of tissue deposits.

◆ Interventions

Interventions focus on managing INFECTION, preventing complications, and providing appropriate patient education.

Managing infection as a cause of acute GN begins with appropriate antibiotic therapy. Penicillin, erythromycin, or azithromycin is prescribed for GN caused by streptococcal INFECTION. Check the patient's known allergies before giving any drug. To prevent infection spread, antibiotics for people in immediate close contact with the patient also may be prescribed. Stress personal hygiene and basic infection control principles (e.g., handwashing) to prevent spread of the organism. Teach patients the importance of completing the entire course of the prescribed antibiotic.

Preventing complications is an important nursing intervention. For patients with fluid overload, hypertension, and edema, diuretics and sodium and water restrictions are prescribed. The usual fluid allowance is equal to the 24-hour urine output plus 500 to 600 mL. Patients with oliguria usually have increased serum levels of potassium and blood urea nitrogen (BUN). Potassium and protein intake may be restricted to prevent hyperkalemia and uremia. Antihypertensive drugs may be needed to control hypertension (see Chapter 36).

Nausea, vomiting, or anorexia indicates that uremia is present. Dialysis is necessary if uremic manifestations or fluid volume excess cannot be controlled (see Chapter 68). **Plasmapheresis** (removal and filtering of the plasma to eliminate antibodies) also may be used (see Chapter 40).

Coordinate care to conserve patient energy. Balance activity with rest to maintain function. Relaxation techniques and participation in diversional activities can reduce emotional stress.

Preparing for self-management includes teaching the patient and family members about the purpose of prescribed drugs, the dosage and schedule, and potential adverse side effects. Ensure that they understand diet and fluid restrictions. Advise the patient to measure weight and blood pressure daily at the same time each day. Instruct him or her to notify the health care provider of any sudden increase in weight or blood pressure.

If short-term dialysis is required to control FLUID AND ELECTROLYTE BALANCE or uremic manifestations, explain peritoneal or vascular access care and dialysis schedules and routines (also see Chapter 68).

RAPIDLY PROGRESSIVE GLOMERULONEPHRITIS

Rapidly progressive glomerulonephritis (RPGN), a type of acute nephritis, is also called *crescentic glomerulonephritis* because of the presence of crescent-shaped cells in the Bowman's capsule. RPGN develops over several weeks or months and causes loss of kidney function. Patients become quite ill quickly and have manifestations of kidney impairment (hypertension, oliguria, disturbed FLUID AND ELECTROLYTE BALANCE, and uremic symptoms).

The patient may have had previous INFECTION or systemic disease, such as systemic lupus erythematosus (SLE). When associated with SLE, steroid therapy is recommended (Hahn et al., 2012). Regardless of treatment, RPGN often progresses to end-stage kidney disease (ESKD).

CHRONIC GLOMERULONEPHRITIS

❖ PATHOPHYSIOLOGY

Chronic glomerulonephritis, or *chronic nephritic syndrome*, develops over 20 to 30 years or even longer. The exact onset of the disorder is rarely identified. Often the cause of the disease is not known. Mild proteinuria and hematuria, hypertension, fatigue, and occasional edema are often the only manifestations.

Although the exact cause is not known, changes in the kidney tissue result from hypertension, INFECTION and INFLAMMATION, or poor blood flow to the kidneys. Kidney tissue atrophies, and the number of functional nephrons is greatly reduced. Biopsy in the late stages of atrophy may show glomerular changes, cell loss, protein and collagen deposits, and fibrosis of the kidney tissue. Microscopic examination shows deposits of immune complexes and inflammation.

The loss of nephrons reduces glomerular filtration. Hypertension and renal arteriolar sclerosis are often present. The glomerular damage allows proteins to enter the urine. Chronic glomerulonephritis always leads to ESKD (see Chapter 68).

❖ PATIENT-CENTERED COLLABORATIVE CARE

◆ Assessment

History. Ask about other health problems, including systemic diseases, kidney or urologic disorders, infectious diseases (e.g., streptococcal infections), and recent exposures to INFECTION. Ask about overall health status and whether increasing fatigue and lethargy have occurred.

Identify the patient's voiding pattern. Ask whether the frequency of urine ELIMINATION has increased or the quantity of urine has decreased. Ask about changes in urine color, odor, or clarity and whether dysuria or incontinence has occurred. Nocturia is a common manifestation.

Assess the patient's general comfort, and ask whether new-onset dyspnea has occurred, because fluid overload can occur with decreased urine output. Ask about and observe for changes in mental functioning (e.g., irritability, an inability to read, or incapacity during job-related functions) or disturbed concentration. Changes in memory and the ability to concentrate occur as waste products collect in the blood.

Physical Assessment/Clinical Manifestations. Assess for systemic circulatory overload. Auscultate lung fields for crackles, observe the respiratory rate and depth, and measure blood pressure and weight. Auscultate the heart for rate, rhythm, and the presence of an S_3 heart sound. Inspect the neck veins for venous engorgement, and check for edema of the feet and ankles, on the shins, and over the sacrum.

Assess for uremic manifestations, such as slurred speech, ataxia, tremors, or asterixis (flapping tremor of the fingers or the inability to maintain a fixed posture with the arms extended and wrists hyperextended). Inspect skin for a yellowish color, texture changes, bruises, rashes, or eruptions. Ask about itching, and document areas of dryness or any excoriation from scratching.

Diagnostic Assessment. Urine output decreases, and urinalysis shows protein, usually less than 2 g in a 24-hour collection. The specific gravity is fixed at a constant level of dilution (around 1.010) despite variable fluid intake. Red blood cells and casts may be in the urine.

The glomerular filtration rate (GFR), measured by creatinine clearance, is low. The serum creatinine level is elevated, usually greater than 6 mg/dL but may be as high as 30 mg/dL or more. The BUN is increased, often as high as 100 to 200 mg/dL.

Decreased kidney function causes disturbed FLUID AND ELECTROLYTE BALANCE. Sodium retention is common, but dilution of the plasma from excess fluid can result in a falsely normal serum sodium level (135 to 145 mEq/L) or a low sodium level (less than 135 mEq/L). When oliguria develops, potassium is not excreted and hyperkalemia occurs when levels exceed 5.4 mEq/L.

Hyperphosphatemia develops with serum levels greater than 4.7 mg/dL. Serum calcium levels are usually at the lower end of the normal range (9.0 to 10.5 mg/mL) or are slightly below normal.

Disturbances of ACID-BASE BALANCE with acidosis develop from hydrogen ion retention and loss of bicarbonate. However, there may be a decrease in serum carbon dioxide (CO_2) levels as patients breathe more rapidly to compensate for the acidosis. If respiratory compensation is present, the pH of arterial blood is between 7.35 and 7.45. A pH of less than 7.35 means that the patient's respiratory system is not completely compensating for the acidosis (see Chapter 12).

The kidneys are abnormally small on x-ray or CT. A kidney biopsy is important in the early stages of glomerulonephritis, when protein or blood is first present in the urine. Tissue changes include INFLAMMATION with a variety of cells infiltrating the glomerular tissue, deposits of immune complexes, and blood vessel sclerosis. In advanced disease, when the kidneys are small, biopsy is not usually performed.

◆ Interventions

Interventions focus on slowing the progression of the disease and preventing complications. Management consists of diet changes, fluid intake sufficient to prevent reduced blood flow to the kidneys, and drug therapy to control the problems from uremia. Eventually the patient requires dialysis or transplantation to prevent death. (Care for the patient requiring dialysis or transplantation is discussed in Chapter 68.)

NEPHROTIC SYNDROME

❖ PATHOPHYSIOLOGY

Nephrotic syndrome (NS) is a condition of increased glomerular permeability that allows larger molecules to pass through the membrane into the urine and then be excreted. This process causes massive loss of protein into the urine, edema formation, and decreased plasma albumin levels. Many agents and disorders are possible causes of NS.

The most common cause of glomerular membrane changes is an immune or inflammatory process. Defects in glomerular filtration can also occur as a result of genetic defects of the glomerular filtering system, such as Fabry disease. Altered liver activity may occur with nephrotic syndrome, resulting in increased lipid production and hyperlipidemia.

❖ PATIENT-CENTERED COLLABORATIVE CARE

The main feature of nephrotic syndrome (NS) is severe proteinuria (with more than 3.5 g of protein in a 24-hour urine sample). Patients also have low serum albumin levels of less than 3 g/dL, high serum lipid levels, fats in the urine, edema, and hypertension (Chart 67-5). Renal vein thrombosis often occurs at the same time as NS, either as a cause of the problem or as an effect. NS may progress to end-stage kidney disease (ESKD), but treatment can prevent progression in most patients.

Management varies depending on what process is causing the disorder (identified by kidney biopsy). Immunologic processes may improve with suppressive therapy using steroids and

CHART 67-5 Key Features

Nephrotic Syndrome

Sudden onset of these manifestations:
- Massive proteinuria
- Hypoalbuminemia
- Edema (especially facial and periorbital)
- Lipiduria
- Hyperlipidemia
- Increased coagulation
- Reduced kidney function

cytotoxic or immunosuppressive agents. Angiotensin-converting enzyme (ACE) inhibitors can decrease protein loss in the urine, and cholesterol-lowering drugs can improve blood lipid levels. Heparin may reduce vascular defects and improve kidney function. Diet changes are often prescribed. If the glomerular filtration rate (GFR) is normal, dietary intake of complete proteins is needed. If the GFR is decreased, dietary protein intake must be decreased. Mild diuretics and sodium restriction may be needed to control edema and hypertension. Assess the patient's hydration status, because vascular dehydration is common. If the plasma volume is depleted, kidney problems worsen. Acute kidney injury (AKI) may be avoided if good blood flow to the kidney is maintained.

IMMUNOLOGIC INTERSTITIAL AND TUBULOINTERSTITIAL DISORDERS

Problems can arise in the kidney tissues around the nephrons, as well as in the nephrons. These interstitial and tubulointerstitial disorders in the kidney are usually caused by immune problems and INFLAMMATION. The kidney changes may be acute or chronic. The acute effects often occur with drugs such as penicillins, cephalosporins, sulfonamides, or NSAIDs. Chronic interstitial nephritis has many causes, including NSAID use, complement activation, cyclosporin use, polycystic kidney disease, autoimmune disorders, inflammation, multiple myeloma, sickle cell disease, obstructive disorders, and radiation nephritis. Drug-induced problems often occur with a rash or an elevated eosinophil count. Fever is common in interstitial nephritis of unknown cause. Progression to ESKD occurs unless the cause is identified and removed.

DEGENERATIVE DISORDERS

Degenerative disorders that change kidney function often occur with a multisystem disorder. Many of these degenerative disorders result from changes in kidney blood vessels.

NEPHROSCLEROSIS

❖ *PATHOPHYSIOLOGY*

Nephrosclerosis is a problem of thickening in the nephron blood vessels, resulting in narrowing of the vessel lumens. This change decreases kidney blood flow, and the tissue is chronically hypoxic. Ischemia and fibrosis develop over time.

Nephrosclerosis occurs with hypertension, atherosclerosis, and diabetes mellitus. The more severe the hypertension, the greater the risk for severe kidney damage. Nephrosclerosis is rarely seen when blood pressure is consistently below 160/110 mm Hg. The changes caused by hypertension may be reversible or may progress to end-stage kidney disease (ESKD) within months or years. (Hypertension is the second leading cause of ESKD.)

> **CULTURAL CONSIDERATIONS**
>
> ***Patient-Centered Care*** QSEN
>
> Hypertension is more common in African Americans and American Indians, and the risks for ESKD from hypertension are also greater for these ethnic groups (U.S. Renal Data Systems, 2012). Between 25 and 45 years of age, the ratio of African Americans to Caucasians at risk for ESKD from hypertension is nearly 20:1. At any health care encounter with an African-American patient or an American-Indian patient, blood pressure should always be assessed. If hypertension is present, treatment and patient education can help reduce the risk for development of ESKD.

❖ *PATIENT-CENTERED COLLABORATIVE CARE*

Management focuses on controlling blood pressure and reducing albuminuria to preserve kidney function. Although many antihypertensive drugs may lower blood pressure, the patient's response is important in ensuring long-term adherence to the prescribed therapy. Factors that promote adherence include once-a-day dosing, low cost, and minimal side effects.

Lack of knowledge or misinformation about hypertension poses many challenges to health care providers working with patients who have hypertension. When kidney disease occurs, adherence to therapy is even more important for preserving health.

Many drugs can control high blood pressure (see Chapter 36), and more than one agent may be needed for best control. Angiotensin-converting enzyme (ACE) inhibitors are very useful in reducing hypertension and preserving kidney function. Diuretics can maintain fluid and electrolyte balance in the presence of kidney function insufficiency. Hyperkalemia needs to be prevented when potassium-sparing diuretics, alone or in combination with other diuretics, are used to treat hypertensive patients with known kidney disease.

RENOVASCULAR DISEASE

❖ *PATHOPHYSIOLOGY*

Processes affecting the renal arteries may severely narrow the lumen and greatly reduce blood flow to the kidney tissues. Uncorrected renovascular disease, such as renal artery stenosis, atherosclerosis, or thrombosis, causes ischemia and atrophy of kidney tissue.

Patients with renovascular disease often have a sudden onset of hypertension, particularly in those older than 50 years. Patients with high blood pressure but with no family history of hypertension also may potentially have renal artery stenosis (RAS). RAS from atherosclerosis or blood vessel hyperplasia is the main cause of renovascular disease. Other causes include thrombosis and renal vessel aneurysms.

Atherosclerotic changes in the renal artery often occur along with sclerosis in the aorta and other vessels. Changes in the renal artery are often located where the renal artery and aorta meet. Fibrotic changes of the blood vessel wall occur throughout the length of the renal artery.

❖ *PATIENT-CENTERED COLLABORATIVE CARE*

◆ *Assessment*

Key features of renovascular disease are listed in Chart 67-6. Hypertension usually first occurs after 40 to 50 years of age, and

> **CHART 67-6 Key Features**
>
> ***Renovascular Disease***
>
> - Significant, difficult-to-control high blood pressure
> - Poorly controlled diabetes or sustained hyperglycemia
> - Elevated serum creatinine
> - Decreased creatinine clearance

often the patient does not have a family history of hypertension. Diagnosis is made by magnetic resonance angiography (MRA), renal ultrasound, radionuclide imaging, or renal arteriography. MRA provides an excellent image of the renal vasculature and kidney anatomy. Radionuclide imaging is a noninvasive way of evaluating kidney blood flow and excretory function. Combining radionuclide imaging with ingestion of an angiotensin-converting enzyme (ACE) inhibitor, such as captopril, improves the accuracy of the test. A renal arteriogram makes the features of the renal blood vessels visible.

◆ *Interventions*

Identifying the type of defect, extent of narrowing, and condition of the surrounding blood vessels is critical for treatment choice. The patient's overall health and the size of the atrophied kidney also affect management decisions. Many patients with renovascular disease also have cardiovascular disease, and both conditions require treatment.

RAS may be managed by drugs to control blood pressure and by procedures to restore the blood supply to the kidney. Drugs may control high blood pressure but may not lead to long-term preservation of kidney function. In young and middle-aged adults, a lifetime of treatment with many drugs for high blood pressure makes treatment difficult and the outcomes uncertain.

Endovascular techniques are nonsurgical approaches to repair RAS. Stent placement with or without balloon angioplasty is an example of an endovascular intervention (see Chapter 36). After the procedure, the patient usually remains under close observation for 24 hours to monitor for sudden blood pressure fluctuations as the kidneys adjust to increased blood flow. Endovascular techniques are less risky and require less time for recovery than does renal artery bypass surgery (Escobar & Campbell, 2012).

Renal artery bypass surgery is a major procedure and requires 2 or more months for recovery. A bypass may be performed for either one or both renal arteries. A synthetic blood vessel graft is inserted to redirect blood flow from the abdominal aorta into the renal artery, beyond the area of narrowing. A splenorenal bypass can also restore blood flow to the kidney. The process is similar to other arterial bypass procedures (see Chapter 38).

DIABETIC NEPHROPATHY

❖ *PATHOPHYSIOLOGY*

Diabetes mellitus (DM) is the leading cause of end-stage kidney disease (ESKD) in North America (U.S. Renal Data Systems, 2012). About 36% of patients requiring dialysis or kidney transplantation have DM (U.S. Renal Data Systems, 2012). Diabetic nephropathy occurs with either type 1 or type 2 DM. Severity of diabetic kidney disease is related to the degree of hyperglycemia the patient generally experiences. With poor control of hyperglycemia, the complicating problems of atherosclerosis, hypertension, and neuropathy (which promotes loss of bladder tone, urinary stasis, and urinary tract infection) are more severe and more likely to cause kidney damage.

❖ *PATIENT-CENTERED COLLABORATIVE CARE*

Diabetic nephropathy is a vascular complication of diabetes. Its first manifestation is microalbuminuria, and screening for small amounts of protein in the urine should begin 5 years after the diagnosis of type 1 DM and annually after type 2 DM is diagnosed. Diabetic kidney disease is progressive.

Structural and functional changes occur in the kidneys of patients with diabetes. Initially, kidney size is slightly increased and glomerular filtration rates (GFRs) are higher than normal. Any proteinuria (albuminuria) indicates the need for aggressive treatment and a thorough diagnostic workup for comorbidities. See Chapter 64 for a detailed discussion of kidney issues in patients with diabetes.

Patients with diabetes are always considered to be at risk for ESKD. If possible, nephrotoxic agents (e.g., iodinated contrast media, aminoglycosides) and dehydration are avoided. Patients with worsening kidney function may begin to have frequent hypoglycemic episodes and a reduced need for insulin or antidiabetic agents. Explain that the kidneys metabolize and excrete insulin. When kidney function is reduced, the insulin is available for a longer time and thus less of it is needed. Some patients may believe this means their diabetes is improving with reduced insulin needs, but that is not accurate. Instead, it is an indication of worsening complications.

Desired outcomes of care to prevent the development of microalbuminuria and delay the progression to ESKD in patients with DM include:

- Achieving glycemic control (e.g., A1C <6.5%)
- Normalizing blood pressure (goal of 130/80 mm Hg or 125/75 mm Hg if proteinuria is greater than 1.0 g/24 hr and serum creatinine is greater than 1.5 mg/dL)
- Using drugs that block renin-angiotensin-aldosterone system (e.g. aldosterone)
- Treating dyslipidemia (so that the low-density lipoprotein [LDL] cholesterol is less than 100 mg/dL)

(See Chapter 64 for specific information on diabetic nephropathy.)

NCLEX EXAMINATION CHALLENGE

Health Promotion and Maintenance

When assessing a client with diabetic nephropathy, which question about self-management should the nurse ask to determine whether the client is currently following best practices to slow the progression of this condition?

A. "Have you increased your protein intake to promote healing of the damaged nephrons?"
B. "Do you avoid contact sports to reduce the risk for causing trauma to your kidneys?"
C. "How do you manage your diet to keep your blood glucose levels in the target range?"
D. "Have you increased your fluid intake based on urine output?"

RENAL CELL CARCINOMA

❖ *PATHOPHYSIOLOGY*

Renal cell carcinoma (RCC) is the most common type of kidney cancer and is also known as *adenocarcinoma of the kidney.* As with other cancers, the healthy tissue of the kidney is damaged and replaced by cancer cells.

Systemic effects occurring with this cancer type are called *paraneoplastic syndromes* and include anemia, erythrocytosis, hypercalcemia, liver dysfunction with elevated liver enzymes, hormonal effects, increased sedimentation rate, and hypertension.

Anemia and erythrocytosis may seem confusing; however, most patients with this cancer have *either* anemia *or* erythrocytosis, not both at the same time. There is some blood loss from

TABLE 67-4 Staging Kidney Tumors

Stage I. Tumors up to 2.5 cm are situated within the capsule of the kidney. The renal vein, perinephric fat, and adjacent lymph nodes have no tumor.
Stage II. Tumors are larger than 2.5 cm and extend beyond the capsule but are within Gerota's fascia. The renal vein and lymph nodes are not involved.
Stage III. Tumors extend into the renal vein, lymph nodes, or both.
Stage IV. Tumors include invasion of adjacent organs beyond Gerota's fascia or metastasize to distant tissues.

Data from American Cancer Society. (2014). *Cancer facts and figures 2014.* Report No. 00-300M–No. 500814. Atlanta: Author.

hematuria, but the small amount lost does not cause anemia. The cause of the anemia and the erythrocytosis is related to kidney cell production of erythropoietin. At times, the tumor cells produce large amounts of erythropoietin, causing erythrocytosis. At other times, the tumor cells destroy the erythropoietin-producing kidney cells and anemia results.

Parathyroid hormone produced by tumor cells can cause hypercalcemia. Other hormone changes include increased renin levels (causing hypertension) and increased human chorionic gonadotropin (hCG) levels, which decrease libido and change secondary sex features.

RCC has five distinct carcinoma cell types: clear cell, papillary cell, chromophobe cell, collecting duct carcinoma, and unclassified type (Patel et al., 2012). A few RCCs are hereditary. The most well-known genetic syndrome that includes kidney cancer is von Hippel-Lindau syndrome. These cancers are highly vascular and may occur with cancers of the pancreas, central nervous system, and adrenal glands.

Kidney tumors are classified into four stages (Table 67-4). Complications include metastasis and urinary tract obstruction. The cancer usually spreads to the adrenal gland, liver, lungs, long bones, or the other kidney. When the cancer surrounds a ureter, hydroureter and obstruction may result.

The causes of nonhereditary RCC are unknown, but the risk is slightly higher for people who use tobacco or are exposed to cadmium and other heavy metals, asbestos, benzene, and trichloroethylene. Men are slightly more likely to acquire RCC, as are obese, African-American, or hypertensive people.

Kidney cancers account for about 64,000 new cases and 13,860 deaths annually in the United States (American Cancer Society [ACS], 2014). In Canada, 6000 new cases and 1750 deaths from kidney cancers occur each year (Canadian Cancer Society, 2014). The 5-year survival rate is 60% in the United States. Renal cell carcinoma occurs most often in patients between 55 and 60 years of age (Patel et al., 2012).

CLINICAL JUDGMENT CHALLENGE

Safety; Patient-Centered Care QSEN

The 56-year-old African-American woman is admitted for treatment of newly diagnosed renal cell carcinoma. You find her daughter in the hallway crying. She has heard that her mother has undergone genetic testing related to her cancer diagnosis and wonders if she is at increased risk for the same condition. She was with her mother during the renal scan before admission and is also worried that this exposure to a radioactive isotope will cause cancer in her.

1. Is renal cell carcinoma commonly inherited, and why is genetic testing done?
2. Do renal scan radioisotopes require radiation precautions? Why or why not?
3. What risk factors are associated with renal cell carcinoma?
4. How can you evaluate whether your information was understood by the daughter and if follow-up is needed?

❖ PATIENT-CENTERED COLLABORATIVE CARE

◆ Assessment

History. Ask the patient about age, known risk factors (e.g., smoking or chemical exposures), weight loss, changes in urine color, abdominal or flank discomfort, and fever. Also ask whether any other family member has ever been diagnosed with cancer of the kidney, bladder, ureter, prostate gland, uterus, ovary, or appendix.

Physical Assessment/Clinical Manifestations. Few patients with renal cell cancer have flank PAIN, obvious blood in the urine, and a kidney mass that can be palpated. Ask about the nature of the flank or abdominal discomfort. Patients often describe the pain as dull and aching. The pain may be more intense if bleeding into the tumor or kidney occurs. Inspect the flank area, checking for asymmetry or an obvious bulge. An abdominal mass may be felt through *gentle* palpation. A renal bruit may be heard on auscultation.

Bloody urine is a *late* common manifestation. Blood may be visible as bright red flecks or clots, or the urine may appear smoky or cola colored. Without gross hematuria, microscopic examination may or may not reveal red blood cells.

Inspect the skin for pallor, darkening of the nipples, and, in men, breast enlargement *(gynecomastia)* caused by changing hormone levels. Other findings may include muscle wasting, weakness, poor nutrition status, and weight loss. All tend to occur late in the disease.

Diagnostic Assessment. Urinalysis may show red blood cells. Hematologic studies show decreased hemoglobin and hematocrit values, hypercalcemia, increased erythrocyte sedimentation rate, and increased levels of adrenocorticotropic hormone (ACTH), human chorionic gonadotropin (hCG), cortisol, renin, and parathyroid hormone. Elevated serum creatinine and blood urea nitrogen (BUN) levels indicate impaired kidney function.

Kidney masses may be detected by CT scan or MRI. Ultrasound is also used to detect masses or for initial screening. Kidney biopsy may be considered to help target therapy.

◆ Interventions

Interventions focus on controlling the cancer and preventing metastasis (ACS, 2014).

Nonsurgical Management. Radiofrequency or cryo-ablation can slow tumor growth. It is a minimally invasive procedure carried out after MRI has precisely located the tumor. The procedure is used most commonly for patients who have only one kidney or who are not surgical candidates.

Chemotherapy has limited effectiveness against this cancer type. Use of biological response modifiers (BRMs) such as interleukin-2 (IL-2), interferon (INF), and tumor necrosis factor (TNF) has lengthened survival time (see Chapters 17 and 22). Newer targeted therapy agents, sorafenib (Nexavar) and temsirolimus (Torisel), were approved as treatment for patients with advanced renal cell carcinoma. Sorafenib, an oral drug taken daily, is a multikinase inhibitor that slows cancer cell division and inhibits blood vessel growth in the tumor. Temsirolimus is a weekly IV infusion that blocks a protein that is needed for cell division, inhibiting cell cycle progression. Other targeted drugs used to treat RCC are sunitinib (Sutent), everolimus (Afinitor), and pazopanib (Votrient) (Patel et al., 2012). These drugs have increased survival time of patients with advanced RCC.

Surgical Management. Renal cell carcinoma is usually treated surgically by *nephrectomy* (kidney removal). Renal cell tumors are highly vascular, and blood loss during surgery is a major concern. Before surgery, the arteries supplying the kidney may be occluded (embolized) by the interventional radiologist to reduce bleeding during nephrectomy.

Preoperative Care. Instruct the patient about surgical routines (see Chapters 14, 15, and 16). Explain the probable site of incision and the presence of dressings, drains, or other equipment after surgery. Reassure the patient about PAIN relief. Care before surgery may include giving blood and fluids IV to prevent shock.

Operative Procedures. The patient is placed on his or her side with the kidney to be removed uppermost. The trunk area is flexed to increase exposure of the kidney area. Removal of the eleventh or twelfth rib may be needed to provide better access to the kidney. The surgeon removes either part or all of the kidney and all visible tumor. The renal artery, renal vein, and fascia also may be removed after tying off the ureter. A drain may be placed in the wound before closure. The adrenal gland may be removed when the tumor is near this organ.

When a *radical* nephrectomy is performed, local and regional lymph nodes are also removed. The surgical approach may be transthoracic (as discussed in the previous paragraph), lumbar, or through the abdomen, depending on the size and location of the tumor. Radiation therapy may follow a radical nephrectomy.

Postoperative Care. Refer to Chapter 16 for care of the patient after surgery. Nursing priorities are focused on assessing kidney function to determine effectiveness of the remaining kidney, PAIN management, and preventing complications.

Monitoring includes assessing for hemorrhage and adrenal insufficiency. Inspect the patient's abdomen for distention from bleeding. Check the bed linens under the patient, because blood may pool there. Hemorrhage or adrenal insufficiency causes hypotension, decreased urine output, and an altered level of consciousness.

A decrease in blood pressure is an early indication of both hemorrhage and adrenal insufficiency. With hypotension, urine output also decreases immediately. Large water and sodium losses in the urine occur in patients with adrenal insufficiency. As a result, a large urine output is followed by hypotension and oliguria (less than 400 mL/24 hr or less than 25 mL/hr). IV replacement of fluids and packed red blood cells may be needed.

The second kidney is expected to provide adequate function, but this may take days or weeks. Assess urine output hourly for the first 24 hours after surgery (urine output of 0.5 mL/kg/hr or about 30 to 50 mL/hr is acceptable). A low urine output of less than 25 to 30 mL/hr suggests decreased blood flow to the remaining kidney and potential for acute kidney injury (AKI). The hemoglobin level, hematocrit values, and white blood cell count may be measured every 6 to 12 hours for the first day or two after surgery.

Monitor the patient's temperature, pulse rate, and respiratory rate at least every 4 hours. Accurately measure and record fluid intake and output. Weigh the patient daily.

The patient may be in a special care unit for 24 to 48 hours after surgery for monitoring of bleeding and adrenal insufficiency. A drain placed near the site of incision removes residual fluid. Because of the discomfort of deep breathing, the patient is at risk for atelectasis. Fever, chills, thick sputum, or decreased breath sounds suggest pneumonia.

Managing PAIN after surgery usually requires opioid analgesics (e.g., hydromorphone [Dilaudid] and morphine [Statex ♣]) given intravenously. The incision was made through major muscle groups used with breathing and movement. Liberal use of analgesics is needed for 3 to 5 days after surgery to manage pain. Oral agents may be tried when the patient can eat and drink.

Preventing complications focuses on INFECTION and management of adrenal insufficiency. Antibiotics may be prescribed during and after surgery to prevent infection. The need for additional antibiotics is based on evidence of infection. Assess the patient at least every 8 hours for manifestations of systemic infection or local wound infection.

Adrenal insufficiency is possible as a complication of kidney and adrenal gland removal. Although only one adrenal gland may be affected, the remaining gland may not be able to secrete sufficient glucocorticoids immediately after surgery. Steroid replacements may be needed in some patients. Chapter 62 discusses the manifestations of acute adrenal insufficiency in detail along with specific nursing interventions.

KIDNEY TRAUMA

❖ PATHOPHYSIOLOGY

Trauma to one or both kidneys is a concern in penetrating wounds or blunt injuries to the back, flank, or abdomen. Another cause of kidney trauma is iatrogenic from urologic procedures, extracorporeal shock wave lithotripsy, kidney biopsy, or percutaneous renal procedures. Blunt trauma accounts for most kidney injuries. Kidney injury has been classified into five grades based on the severity of the injury. Grade one consists of low-grade injury in the form of kidney bruising, and grade five represents the most severe trauma associated with shattering of the kidney and tearing its blood supply. Anyone can suffer kidney trauma. Strategies to prevent trauma are reviewed in Chart 67-7.

❖ PATIENT-CENTERED COLLABORATIVE CARE

◆ Assessment

Obtain a history of the patient's usual health and the events involved in the trauma from the patient, a witness, or

CHART 67-7 Patient and Family Education: Preparing for Self-Management

Preventing Kidney and Genitourinary Trauma

- Wear a seat belt.
- Practice safe walking habits.
- Use caution when riding bicycles and motorcycles.
- Wear appropriate protective clothing when participating in contact sports.
- Avoid all contact sports and high-risk activities if you have only one kidney.

emergency personnel. Documenting the mechanism of injury can help the provider determine the severity of the injury. For example, most blunt trauma from car crashes has low severity. Critical information to acquire is a history of kidney or urologic disease, surgical intervention, or health problems such as diabetes mellitus or hypertension.

Ureteral or renal pelvic injury often causes diffuse abdominal PAIN. Urine outside of the urinary tract may be visible. Ask the patient about pain in the flank or abdomen. Is the pain dull? Sharp? Constant? Intermittent? Made worse by coughing?

Patients with kidney injuries should be assessed with initial attention to the basic ABCDEs outlined in Advanced Trauma Life Support protocols. Take the patient's blood pressure, apical and peripheral pulses, respiratory rate, and temperature. Inspect both flanks for bruising, asymmetry or penetrating injuries. Also inspect the abdomen, chest, and lower back for bruising or penetrating wounds. Percuss the abdomen for distention. Inspect the urethra for blood.

Urinalysis shows hemoglobin or red blood cells from tissue damage or kidney blood vessel rupture. Microscopic examination may also show red blood cell casts, which suggest tubular damage. Hemoglobin and hematocrit values decrease with blood loss (see discussion of shock in Chapter 37).

Diagnostic procedures include ultrasound and CT. CT scan shows greater detail about blood vessel and tissue integrity. Hematomas within or through the kidney capsule can be seen, along with the integrity and patency of the urinary tract. If the patient is being taken to the operating room emergently, a one-shot high dose of ionic or nonionic IV contrast dye can be given, followed by an abdominal x-ray (KUB) to visualize the traumatic injury and any organ damage.

◆ *Interventions*

Nonsurgical Management. *Drug therapy* is used for bleeding prevention or control. The need for clotting factors, vitamin K, and platelets is assessed, and they are given as needed.

Fluid therapy is given to restore circulating blood volume and ensure adequate blood flow to the kidneys. Crystalloid solutions replace water and some electrolytes and include 0.9% sodium chloride (normal saline solution [NSS]), 5% dextrose in 0.45% sodium chloride, and lactated Ringer's solution. When bleeding is extensive, packed red blood cell replacement restores hemoglobin and promotes oxygenation. Fresh frozen plasma or clotting factors may help with uncontrolled bleeding. Plasma volume expanders, such as dextran or albumin, help restore plasma oncotic pressure and reduce the onset or severity of shock or fluid displacement to interstitial tissues.

During fluid restoration, give fluids at the prescribed rate and monitor the patient for indications of shock. Take vital signs as often as every 5 to 15 minutes. Measure and record urine output hourly. Output should be greater than 0.5 mL/kg/hr.

The interventional radiologist may use percutaneous or other instrumentation to drain collections of fluid or to embolize (clot) an artery or artery segment or place a stent to repair the urethra or ureters.

! NURSING SAFETY PRIORITY QSEN

Action Alert

If the urethral opening is bleeding, consult with the physician before attempting urinary catheterization.

Surgical Management. Most kidney injuries are managed without surgery. Many serious injuries can be treated with minimally invasive techniques such as angiographic embolization, which accesses the arteries of the kidneys through large blood vessels in the groin, similar to a cardiac catheterization. Surgery to explore the injured kidney occurs when the patient is hemodynamically unstable and appears to be losing a lot of blood from the kidney. Patients with other significant abdominal injuries, such as injuries to the bowel, spleen, or liver, who require a laparotomy may also undergo inspection and repair of the injured kidney at the same time. The aim of surgical management is to repair the injured kidney. However, if the kidney is severely injured (usually Grade 5 injury), the surgeon performs a nephrectomy.

Community-Based Care

Teach the patient and family how to assess for INFECTION and other complications following kidney trauma. The most common complications are urine leakage and delayed bleeding. Instruct the patient to check the pattern and frequency of urine ELIMINATION and to note whether the color, clarity, and amount appear normal. The development of an abscess surrounding the kidney also can occur. Instruct the patient to seek medical attention for worsening hematuria, a worrisome change, or PAIN with voiding. Chills, fever, lethargy, and cloudy, foul-smelling urine indicate a urinary tract INFECTION or abscess formation. Traumatic kidney injury can also cause hypertension from changes in perfusion and activation of the renin-angiotensin-aldosterone system (see Chapter 65 and Fig. 65-5). Advise the patient to seek medical care promptly for all new and concerning manifestations.

NURSING CONCEPTS AND CLINICAL JUDGMENT REVIEW

What might you NOTICE if the patient is experiencing problems with urinary ELIMINATION as a result of acute pyelonephritis?

- Patient urinates frequently in small amounts.
- Patient reports pain and burning on urination.
- Patient reports back or flank pain.
- Urine is cloudy and foul-smelling
- Urine may be darker or smoky or have obvious blood in it.

What should you INTERPRET and how should you RESPOND to a patient experiencing problems with urinary ELIMINATION as a result of acute pyelonephritis?

Perform and interpret physical assessment, including:

- Asking how long manifestations have been present
- Asking about low back (midline in men) or flank pain

- Asking whether he or she has had a UTI in the past; how long ago; how it was treated; and if, antibiotics were prescribed, whether the drug course was completed
- Asking about the presence of pregnancy or any chronic health problem, especially diabetes
- Asking about any nausea or vomiting and its duration
- Determining fluid intake and output volumes
- Assessing for pain over the right and left kidneys
- Weighing the patient, and asking whether this weight is more or less than his or her usual weight
- Assessing for fever and chills
- Assessing for tachycardia
- Interpreting laboratory values:
  - Is the complete blood count with differential elevated?
  - Are the BUN and serum creatinine levels elevated?
  - Is the urinalysis positive for bacteria, leukocyte esterase, nitrate, red blood cells, white blood cells, or casts?

Respond by:
- Providing for pain control
- Teaching the patient the importance of completing the prescribed antibiotic drug regimen

On what should you REFLECT?
- Observe patient for evidence of improved urinary output (see Chapter 65).
- Think about what may have caused this infection and what steps could be taken to prevent a similar episode.
- Think about what patient teaching focus could help reduce the risk for future pyelonephritis and its complications.

GET READY FOR THE NCLEX® EXAMINATION!

KEY POINTS

Review these Key Points for each NCLEX Examination Client Needs Category.

Safe and Effective Care Environment
- Report immediately any condition that obstructs urine flow. **Safety** QSEN
- Check the blood pressure and urine output frequently in patients who have any type of kidney problem.
- Report immediately to the health care provider any sudden decrease of urine output in a patient with kidney disease or kidney trauma. In general, adult urine output expectations are 0.5-1 mL/kg/hr. **Safety** QSEN

Health Promotion and Maintenance
- Encourage patients with diabetes to achieve tight glycemic control.
- Encourage patients with hypertension to follow their treatment regimens to maintain blood pressure within the target range.
- Teach patients at risk for urinary tract INFECTION (UTI) to maintain a daily fluid intake of 2 L unless another health problem requires fluid restriction.
- Teach patients on antibiotic therapy for a UTI to complete the drug regimen. **Evidence-Based Practice** QSEN
- Teach all people strategies to prevent kidney trauma.

Psychosocial Integrity
- Allow the patient the opportunity to express fear or anxiety regarding the potential for chronic kidney disease and end-stage kidney disease. **Patient-Centered Care** QSEN
- Assess the patient's level of comfort in discussing issues related to ELIMINATION and the genitourinary area.
- Use language the patient is comfortable with during assessment of the kidney and urinary system. **Patient-Centered Care** QSEN
- Explain treatment procedures to patients and families.
- Refer patients with polycystic kidney disease to a geneticist or a genetic counselor.
- Refer patients to community resources, support groups, and information organizations such as the National Kidney Foundation, the Polycystic Kidney Disease Foundation, and the American Association of Kidney Patients.

Physiological Integrity
- Instruct patients with any type of kidney problem to weigh daily and to notify their health care provider if there is a sudden weight gain. **Patient-Centered Care** QSEN
- Teach patients the expected side effects and any adverse reactions to prescribed drugs, especially as they relate to kidney function.
- Teach patients the manifestations of disease recurrence and when to seek medical help.
- Explain the genetics of autosomal dominant polycystic kidney disease.
- Use laboratory data and clinical manifestations to determine the effectiveness of therapy for pyelonephritis.
- Be aware of the clinical manifestations of hydronephrosis.
- Be aware of the relationship between hypertension and kidney disease.

CHAPTER 68

Care of Patients with Acute Kidney Injury and Chronic Kidney Disease

Chris Winkelman

http://evolve.elsevier.com/Iggy/

PRIORITY CONCEPTS

- ELIMINATION
- ACID-BASE BALANCE
- FLUID AND ELECTROLYTE BALANCE
- INFECTION
- INFLAMMATION
- PERFUSION

LEARNING OUTCOMES

Safe and Effective Care Environment

1. Collaborate with members of the health care team to reduce patient risk for kidney INFLAMMATION, kidney INFECTION, and acute kidney injury (AKI).
2. Implement interventions to protect patients with chronic kidney disease (CKD) from related systemic complications that affect ELIMINATION, FLUID AND ELECTROLYTE BALANCE, and ACID-BASE BALANCE.
3. Implement interventions to maintain patency of hemodialysis or peritoneal access when this renal replacement therapy occurs.

Health Promotion and Maintenance

4. Assess risk for AKI in patients with hemodynamic instability.
5. Collaborate with the patient and health care team to promote adequate nutrition and FLUID AND ELECTROLYTE BALANCE when AKI or CKD is diagnosed.
6. Teach transplant recipients and their families about the importance of adhering to anti-rejection therapy.

Psychosocial Integrity

7. Promote communication about patient preferences and values to plan care related to treatment for kidney failure.
8. Teach patients to use *high-quality* community resources for self-management.

Physiological Integrity

9. Compare the pathophysiology and causes of AKI with those of CKD.
10. Establish priorities in the care of patients with AKI and CKD.
11. Discuss interventions to prevent AKI.
12. Discuss the mechanisms of peritoneal dialysis (PD) and hemodialysis (HD) as renal replacement therapies.
13. Coordinate nursing care for the patient with CKD or end-stage kidney disease (ESKD).
14. Prioritize nursing care for the patient who receives a kidney transplant.

The loss of kidney function affects the ability to maintain normal processes of urinary ELIMINATION, FLUID AND ELECTROLYTE BALANCE, and ACID-BASE BALANCE. Kidney function loss also interrupts the activity of every organ system, particularly the immune, endocrine, skeletal, and cardiovascular systems. Acute kidney injury (AKI) is most common in the acute care setting, whereas chronic kidney disease (CKD) is more likely to be seen in community settings or as a co-existing condition in acute care settings. The characteristics of AKI and CKD are described in Table 68-1.

Both types of kidney dysfunction can result in end-stage kidney disease (ESKD), requiring renal replacement therapy (e.g., dialysis) or kidney transplant. ESKD reduces independence, shortens life, and decreases quality of life. Many diseases and conditions are associated with the onset and severity of kidney function loss.

As described in Chapter 65, kidney functions include excretion of waste, FLUID AND ELECTROLYTE BALANCE, regulation of ACID-BASE BALANCE, and hormone secretion. When kidney function declines gradually, it is diagnosed as CKD, also known as *chronic renal failure (CRF)*. The patient may have many years of abnormal serum blood urea nitrogen and creatinine values, sometimes called *renal insufficiency,* before the uremia of ESKD develops. During this time of decreased kidney function, the patient may also experience acute kidney injury (AKI). The combination of AKI and CKD, called *acute-on-chronic kidney injury,* can accelerate loss of kidney function. Low nephron numbers from CKD contribute to the progression of kidney disease (Taal et al., 2012).

When kidney decline is sudden, the functioning nephrons are overworked and kidney failure may develop with the loss of only 50% of functioning nephrons. Acute kidney injury affects

TABLE 68-1 Characteristics of Acute Kidney Injury and Chronic Kidney Disease

CHARACTERISTIC	ACUTE KIDNEY INJURY	CHRONIC KIDNEY DISEASE
Onset	Sudden (hours to days)	Gradual (months to years)
% of nephron involvement	50%-95%	Varies by stage; generally symptomatic with 75% loss and dialysis with 90%-95% loss
Duration	May not progress; full recovery (return to baseline) possible ESKD occurs in 10%-20% with lifetime reliance on dialysis or kidney transplant	Progressive and permanent Treatment and lifestyle can slow progression and delay onset of ESKD
Prognosis	Good when kidney function is maintained or returns High mortality associated with renal replacement therapy requirements of prolonged illness	Fatal without a renal replacement therapy (dialysis or transplantation) Reduced life span and potential for complex medical regimen even with optimal treatment

ESKD, End-stage kidney disease.

many body systems. Chronic kidney disease affects *every* body system. The problems that occur with kidney function loss are related to disturbances of FLUID AND ELECTROLYTE BALANCE, disturbances of ACID-BASE BALANCE, buildup of nitrogen-based wastes, and loss of kidney hormone function.

When kidney function declines to the point that the kidneys can no longer maintain homeostasis by urine ELIMINATION, renal replacement therapy is needed to prevent death from life-threatening consequences.

ACUTE KIDNEY INJURY

Pathophysiology

Acute kidney injury (AKI) has now replaced the older terminology of *acute renal failure.* AKI is a rapid reduction in kidney function resulting in a failure to maintain FLUID AND ELECTROLYTE BALANCE and ACID-BASE BALANCE. AKI occurs over a few hours or days. Most experts described AKI as one of three classes (risk, injury, and failure or Stages 1, 2, and 3 [Table 68-2]). One expert group also describes two outcomes (loss of function and end-stage kidney disease [ESKD]) following AKI. Severity of AKI is based on increases in serum creatinine and decreased urine output. Although glomerular filtration rate (GFR) is accepted as the best overall indicator of kidney function, it is not measured during acute and critical illness (Puzantian & Townsend, 2013). GFR represents the sum filtration rate of all functional nephrons. Estimations of GFR from serum creatinine are not considered accurate during critical illness. Values from direct measurements can be altered during acute and critical illness when diuretics or IV fluids are used (Moore et al., 2012; Puzantian & Townsend, 2013). Direct

TABLE 68-2 The RIFLE and KDIGO Classification Systems for Severity and Outcomes of Acute Kidney Injury

	GLOMERULAR FILTRATION RATE (GFR)* CRITERIA	URINE OUTPUT CRITERIA
RIFLE Classification		
Risk stage	Serum creatinine increased × 1.5 or GFR decrease >25%	<0.5 mL/kg/hr for ≥6 hr
Injury stage	Serum creatinine increased × 2 or GFR decrease >50%	<0.5 mL/kg/hr for ≥12 hr
Failure stage	Serum creatinine increased × 3 or GFR decrease ≥75% or an absolute serum creatinine ≥354 μmol/L with an acute rise ≥4 μmol/L	<0.3 mL/kg/hr for ≥24 hr or anuria for ≥12 hr
Outcome: **L**oss	Persistent acute kidney injury (AKI), requiring renal replacement therapy for >4 wk	
Outcome: **E**nd-stage kidney disease	Requiring dialysis >3 mo	
KDIGO Classification		
Stage 1	Serum creatinine increased × 1.5-1.9 baseline or by ≥26.2 μmol/L	<0.5 mL/kg/hr for 6-12 hr
Stage 2	Serum creatinine increased × 2-2.9 baseline	<0.5 mL/kg/hr for ≥12 hr
Stage 3	Serum creatinine increased × 3 baseline or serum creatinine ≥354 μmol/L with an acute rise ≥44 μmol/L or initiation of renal replacement therapy	<0.3 mL/kg/hr for ≥24 hr or anuria for ≥12 hr

RIFLE, **R**isk, **I**njury, **F**ailure, **L**oss, **E**nd-Stage Kidney Failure; *KDIGO*, **K**idney **D**isease: **I**mproving **G**lobal **O**utcomes

*GFR must be directly measured, not estimated (Chapter 65 describes serum and urine measurement of GFR).

measurement of GFR uses a 24-hour urinary creatinine analysis or the clearance of IV-administered markers like inulin, nonradioactive contrast agents or radioisotope compounds.

AKI not only affects kidney function but also causes systemic effects and complications described in Table 68-3. These complications increase discomfort and risk for death in the patient with new AKI. Duration of oliguria or anuria is closely correlated with lack of recovery of kidney function; the longer the duration of oliguria or anuria, the less likely the patient will return to full or baseline kidney function (Davies & Leslie, 2012).

Etiology

The causes of AKI are reduced PERFUSION to the kidneys, damage to kidney tissue, and obstruction. Diseases and conditions associated with reduced kidney PERFUSION, kidney damage, and urinary obstruction are listed in Table 68-4. (The diseases in Table 68-3 are described elsewhere in this text.) Notice that several conditions resulting in AKI are listed more than once in Table 68-4. For example, coagulopathy (disorders of bleeding and clotting; see Chapter 40) reduces perfusion, causes INFLAMMATION and direct tissue damage, and creates obstruction of urinary flow. Coagulopathy causes prerenal, intrarenal, and postrenal AKI.

TABLE 68-3 Complications from Acute Kidney Injury

Metabolic
- Metabolic acidosis
- Hyperkalemia
- Hyponatremia
- Hypocalcemia
- Hypophosphatemia

Cardiopulmonary
- Peripheral and pulmonary edema
- Heart failure
- Pulmonary embolism
- Pericarditis
- Pericardial effusion
- Hypertension
- Myocardial infarction

Neurologic
- Neuromuscular irritability or weakness
- Asterixis
- Seizures
- Mental status changes

Immune/Infectious
- Pneumonia
- Sepsis

Gastrointestinal
- Nausea
- Vomiting
- Decreased peristalsis
- Enteral nutrition intolerance
- Malnutrition
- Ulcer formation
- Bleeding

Hematologic
- Bleeding
- Thrombosis
- Anemia

Renal
- Permanent kidney damage
- Chronic kidney disease (CKD)
- End-stage kidney disease (ESKD)

Other
- Hiccups
- Elevated parathyroid hormone
- Low thyroid hormone

AKI is more likely to occur in hospitalized adults who are older or who have pre-existing hypertension, diabetes, peripheral vascular disease, liver disease, or chronic kidney disease (CKD). Prolonged mechanical ventilation (see Chapter 32) also is an independent risk factor for the development of AKI (Akker et al., 2013).

Traditionally, AKI caused by reduced PERFUSION is classed as **prerenal failure**. It is the most common cause of AKI in acute care. Damage to kidney tissue is classed as **intrarenal** or **intrinsic renal failure** and reflects injury to the glomeruli, nephrons, or tubules. Obstruction of urine flow is also called **postrenal failure**. Although the usefulness of this classification system is a source of controversy, it does provide a framework to guide care for both prevention and treatment of AKI (Fournir, 2013). When AKI occurs in patients who already have CKD, it is called **acute-on-chronic kidney disease**. Any of these conditions can occur together such as acute prerenal and intrarenal failure occurring in someone who already has CKD. Multiple pathologies are more likely to result in end-stage kidney disease (ESKD).

With prerenal or postrenal pathology, the kidney compensates by the three responses of constricting kidney blood vessels, activating the renin-angiotensin-aldosterone pathway, and releasing antidiuretic hormone (ADH). These responses increase blood volume and improve kidney PERFUSION. However, these same responses reduce urine volume, resulting in **oliguria** (urine output less than 400 mL/day) and **azotemia** (the retention and buildup of nitrogenous wastes in the blood). Toxins can also cause blood vessel constriction in the kidney, leading to reduced kidney blood flow, oliguria, and azotemia.

INFLAMMATION, INFECTION, and damage from toxins (Table 68-5) cause intracellular changes of the tubular system in kidney tissue. Immune-mediated complexes can also damage nephrons. With extensive tubular damage, tubular cells slough and nephrons lose the ability to repair themselves. The presence of tubular debris and sediment in urine from kidney tissue damage (intrarenal failure) is sometimes termed *acute tubular necrosis.* This term is no longer favored because supportive evidence is limited for the pathologic processes and clinical diagnosis (Moore et al., 2012).

Even with severe AKI, categorized as loss of function ("L" in *RIFLE* or stage 2 in *KDIGO* in Table 68-2), some people have return of kidney function. It is the responsibility of all health care professionals to be alert to the possibility of AKI and implement prevention strategies when risk factors are present. *Timely implementation of interventions to remove the cause of AKI may*

TABLE 68-4 Diseases and Conditions that Contribute to Acute Kidney Injury

Perfusion Reduction (Prerenal Causes)
- Blood or fluid loss (e.g., surgery or trauma; hemorrhagic or hypovolemic shock)
- Blood pressure drugs resulting in hypotension
- Heart attack or heart failure resulting in low ejection fraction and low cardiac output
- Infection (e.g., sepsis, septic shock)
- Liver failure
- Use of aspirin, ibuprofen (e.g., Advil, Motrin IB), naproxen (e.g., Aleve), or NSAIDs
- Severe allergic reaction (anaphylaxis)
- Severe burns
- Severe dehydration
- Renal artery stenosis
- Bleeding or clotting in the kidney blood vessels (coagulopathy)
- Atherosclerosis or cholesterol deposits that block blood flow in the kidneys

Kidney Damage (Intrinsic or Intrarenal Causes)
- Glomerulonephritis or inflammation of the glomeruli
- Bleeding in the kidney
- Thrombi or emboli in the kidney blood vessels
- Hemolytic uremic syndrome, a condition of premature destruction of red blood cells caused by infection
- Systemic infection (sepsis)
- Local infection (pyelonephritis)
- Lupus, an immune system disorder causing glomerulonephritis
- Drugs, such as certain chemotherapy agents, antibiotics, dyes used during imaging tests (contrast-induced nephropathy), many antibiotics, and zoledronic acid (Reclast, Zometa), used to treat osteoporosis and high blood calcium levels (hypercalcemia)
- Multiple myeloma, a cancer of the plasma cells
- Scleroderma, a group of rare diseases affecting the skin and connective tissues
- Thrombotic thrombocytopenic purpura (TTP), a rare platelet disorder that increases clotting
- Ingested toxins, such as alcohol, heavy metals, and cocaine
- Vasculitis, an inflammation of blood vessels
- Ischemia in kidney tissue, including hypoxemia from respiratory and cardiac arrest

Urine Flow Obstruction (Postrenal Causes)
- Bladder cancer
- Cervical cancer
- Colon cancer
- Prostate cancer
- Enlarged prostate (prostate hypertrophy)
- Kidney stones (nephrolithiasis and ureterolithiasis)
- Nerve damage involving the nerves that control the bladder (neurogenic bladder)
- Blood clots in the urinary tract

TABLE 68-5 Examples of Potentially Nephrotoxic Substances

Drugs	Other Drugs
Antibiotics/Antimicrobials	• Acetaminophen
• Amphotericin B	• Captopril
• Colistimethate	• Cyclosporine
• Methicillin	• Fluorinate anesthetics
• Polymyxin B	• Metformin
• Rifampin	• *D*-Penicillamine
• Sulfonamides	• Phenazopyridine hydrochloride
• Tetracycline hydrochloride	• Quinine
• Vancomycin	
	Other Substances
Aminoglycoside Antibiotics	***Organic Solvents***
• Gentamicin	• Carbon tetrachloride
• Kanamycin	• Ethylene glycol
• Neomycin	
• Netilmicin sulfate	***Non-drug Chemical Agents***
• Tobramycin	• Radiographic contrast dye (e.g., iodinated dyes, high-osmolar dyes, and gadolinium)
Chemotherapy agents	
• Cisplatin	
• Cyclophosphamide	• Pesticides
• Methotrexate	• Fungicides
	• Myoglobin (from breakdown of skeletal muscle)
Nonsteroidal Anti-inflammatory Drugs (NSAIDs)	
• Celecoxib	***Heavy Metals and Ions***
• Flurbiprofen	• Arsenic
• Ibuprofen	• Bismuth
• Indomethacin	• Copper sulfate
• Ketorolac	• Gold salts
• Meclofenamate	• Lead
• Meloxicam	• Mercuric chloride
• Nabumetone	
• Naproxen	
• Oxaprozin	
• Rofecoxib	
• Tolmetin	

prevent ESKD and need for lifelong renal replacement therapy or a renal transplant.

Incidence and Prevalence

The reported prevalence of AKI from United States data ranges from 1% (community-acquired) up to 7.1% (hospital-acquired) of all hospital admissions. As many as 30% of patients admitted to an ICU experience an episode of AKI (Fournir, 2013). Transient azotemia and oliguria occur in as many as 40% of all inpatients (Uchino et al., 2010). AKI is associated with an in-hospital and 1-year mortality rate of up to 60% (Ralib et al., 2013).

Health Promotion and Maintenance

Keep in mind that severe blood volume depletion can lead to kidney injury even in people who have no known kidney problems. Urge all healthy people to avoid dehydration by drinking 2 to 3 L of water daily. This is especially important for athletes or any person who performs strenuous exercise or work and sweats heavily.

Nurses have an essential role in the prevention of AKI in hospitalized patients. Always be on the lookout for signs of impending kidney dysfunction through physical assessment and close monitoring of laboratory values. Early recognition and correction of problems causing reduced kidney blood flow often restore function before tissue damage can occur. Evaluate the patient's fluid status. Accurately measure intake and output and check body weight to identify changes in fluid balance. Note the characteristics of the urine, and report new sediment, hematuria (smoky or red color), foul odor, or other worrisome changes. It is important to immediately report to the health care provider a urine output of less than 0.5 mL/kg/hr that persists for more than 2 hours. Some experts suggest that 0.3 mL/kg/hr for more than 2 hours should be reported (Ralib et al., 2013). Waiting for 6 hours of oliguria to meet RIFLE criteria may promote kidney damage—act early!

! NURSING SAFETY PRIORITY QSEN

Critical Rescue

In any acute care setting, preventing volume depletion and providing intervention early when volume depletion occurs are nursing priorities. Reduced PERFUSION from volume depletion is a common cause of AKI. Recognize the manifestations of volume depletion (low urine output, decreased systolic blood pressure, decreased pulse pressure, orthostatic hypotension, thirst, rising blood osmolarity). Intervene early with oral fluids, or in the patient who is unable to take or tolerate oral fluid, request an increase in IV fluid rate from the health care provider to prevent permanent kidney damage.

Monitor laboratory values for any changes that reflect poor kidney function. A clinically significant increase in creatinine, especially when the increase occurs over hours or a few days, is a concern and should be reported urgently to the health care providers. Other laboratory values that help monitor kidney function include serum blood urea nitrogen (BUN); serum potassium, sodium, and osmolarity; and urine specific gravity and electrolytes.

Be aware of nephrotoxic substances that the patient may ingest or be exposed to (see Table 68-5). Question any prescription for potentially nephrotoxic drugs, and validate the dose before the patient receives the drug. Many antibiotics have nephrotoxic side effects. NSAIDs can cause or increase the risk for AKI. Combining two or more nephrotoxic drugs dramatically increases the risk for AKI. If a patient must receive a known nephrotoxic drug, closely monitor laboratory values, including BUN, creatinine, and drug peak and trough levels, for indications of reduced kidney function. When nephrotoxic agents are used, nephrons may be protected by administering a pretreatment oral or IV bolus of fluid volume.

❖ PATIENT-CENTERED COLLABORATIVE CARE

◆ Assessment

History. The accurate diagnosis of AKI, including its cause, depends on a detailed history. Ask the patient about recent surgery or trauma, transfusions, or other factors that might lead to reduced kidney blood flow. Obtain a drug history, especially treatment with antibiotics and NSAIDs. Ask about recent imaging procedures requiring injection of a contrast dye. Coexisting conditions of advanced age, diabetes mellitus, long-term hypertension, systemic lupus erythematosus, major or systemic INFECTION (sepsis), systemic INFLAMMATION from any cause, and coagulopathy or treatment for bleeding or clotting disorders increase the risk for AKI.

CHART 68-1 Laboratory Profile

Kidney Disease

TEST	NORMAL RANGE FOR ADULTS	VALUES IN KIDNEY DISEASE
Serum creatinine	*Male:* 0.6-1.2 mg/dL *Female:* 0.5-1.1 mg/dL *Older adults:* Decreased	**In Chronic Kidney Disease** May increase by 0.5-1.0 mg/dL every 1-2 yr May be as high as 15-30 mg/dL *before* manifestations of severe CKD are present **In Acute Kidney Injury** Increase of 1-2 mg/dL every 24-48 hr May increase 1-6 mg/dL in 1 wk or less
Blood urea nitrogen	10-20 mg/dL *Older adults:* May be slightly increased	**In Chronic Kidney Disease** May reach 180-200 mg/dL *before* manifestations develop **In Acute Kidney Injury** Often increases by 10-20 mg/dL at same pace as serum creatinine level May reach 80-100 mg/dL within 1 wk
Serum sodium	136-145 mEq/L; 136-145 mmol/L (SI units)	Normal, increased, or decreased
Serum potassium	3.5-5.0 mEq/L; 3.5-5.0 mmol/L (SI units)	Increased
Serum phosphorus (phosphate)	3.0-4.5 mg/dL; 0.97-1.45 mmol/L (SI units) *Older adults:* May be slightly decreased	Increased
Serum calcium	Total calcium: 9.0-10.5 mg/dL; 2.25-2.75 mmol/L (SI units) Ionized calcium: 4.5-5.6 mg/dL; 1.05-1.3 mmol/L (SI units) *Older adults:* Slightly decreased	Decreased
Serum magnesium	1.3-2.1 mEq/L; 0.65-1.05 mmol/L	Increased
Serum carbon dioxide combining power (bicarbonate)	23-30 mEq/L (venous); 23-30 mmol/L (SI units)	Decreased
Arterial blood pH	7.35-7.45	Decreased (in metabolic acidosis) or normal
Arterial blood bicarbonate (HCO_3^-)	21-28 mEq/L	Decreased
Arterial blood $PaCO_2$	35-45 mm Hg	Decreased
Hemoglobin	*Female:* 12-16 g/dL; 7.4-9.9 mmol/L (SI units) *Male:* 14-18 g/dL; 8.7-11.2 mmol/L (SI units) *Older adults:* Slightly decreased	Decreased
Hematocrit	*Female:* 37%-47% *Male:* 42%-52% *Older adults:* May be slightly decreased	Decreased to 20%
Blood osmolarity	285-295 mOsm/kg or mmol/kg (SI)	Elevated in volume-depleted states, increasing the risk for acute kidney injury

Data from Pagana, K., & Pagana, T. (2014). *Mosby's manual of diagnostic and laboratory tests* (5th ed.). St. Louis: Mosby.
CKD, Chronic kidney disease; *SI,* International System of Units.

To identify immune-mediated acute glomerulonephritis, ask about acute illnesses such as influenza, colds, gastroenteritis, and sore throats. Ask whether urine color is darker or appears smoky.

Anticipate AKI following any episode of hypotension, shock, burns, or heart failure exacerbation. Any problem in which the blood volume is depleted can contribute to AKI such as extensive bowel preparations, being NPO before surgery, or dehydration from exercise.

Consider whether there is a history of urinary obstructive problems. Ask the patient about any difficulty in starting the urine stream, changes in the amount or appearance of the urine, narrowing of the urine stream, nocturia, urgency, or manifestations of kidney stones. Also ask about any cancer history that may cause urinary obstruction.

Physical Assessment/Clinical Manifestations. The manifestations of AKI are related to the buildup of nitrogenous wastes (**azotemia**), decreased urine output (**oliguria**), as well as to the underlying cause. As AKI progresses in severity, the patient may have manifestations of fluid overload (because in AKI, fluid is not eliminated) including pulmonary crackles, dependent and generalized edema, decreased oxygenation (low peripheral oxygenation or SpO_2), increased respiratory rate, and dyspnea. See Chapter 11 for further assessment related to fluid overload.

Laboratory Assessment. The many changes in laboratory values in the patient with AKI are similar to those occurring in chronic kidney disease (CKD) (Chart 68-1). A rising serum creatinine is more likely to indicate prolonged or permanent kidney damage. Expect to see rising BUN levels and abnormal blood electrolytes values. Patients with AKI, however, usually do *not* have the anemia associated with CKD unless there is blood loss from another condition (e.g., surgery, trauma) or when BUN levels are high enough to break (lyse) red blood cells.

In early AKI, urine tests provide important information. Urine sodium levels may reflect an inability to concentrate urine. Urine may be dilute with a specific gravity near 1.000 or concentrated with a specific gravity greater than 1.030. The presence of urine sediment (e.g., red blood cells [RBCs], RBC casts, and tubular cells), myoglobin, or hemoglobin may contribute to nephron damage.

Imaging Assessment. Ultrasonography is useful in the diagnosis of kidney and urinary tract obstruction. Dilation of the renal calyces and collecting ducts, as well as stones, can be detected. Ultrasonography can show kidney size and patency of the ureters.

CT scans without contrast dye can determine adequacy of kidney blood flow and identify obstruction or tumors. Contrast dyes are usually avoided to prevent further kidney damage. An MRI may be used in place of CT scan at some medical centers.

X-rays of the pelvis or kidneys, ureters, and bladder (KUB) may be used to provide an initial screening view of kidneys and the urinary tract to determine the cause of AKI. Enlarged kidneys with obstruction may show hydronephrosis. X-rays can show stones obstructing the renal pelvis, ureters, or bladder. More commonly, ultrasound is used to screen for hydronephrosis.

A nuclear medicine study called *MAG3* may be used to determine the nature of the kidney failure and measure GFR. A renal scan can determine whether blood flow to the kidneys is sufficient. Cystoscopy or retrograde pyelography may be needed to identify obstructions of the lower urinary tract.

Other Diagnostic Assessments. Kidney biopsy is performed if the cause of AKI is uncertain and manifestations persist or an immunologic disease is suspected. Prepare the patient before the test, particularly managing both hypotension and hypertension. Hypertension can contribute to intrarenal hemorrhage following needle biopsy. Provide follow-up care. Be aware of all test results, and understand how they might affect the treatment regimen. (See Chapter 65 for a detailed discussion of diagnostic tests related to the kidney.)

NCLEX EXAMINATION CHALLENGE

Safe and Effective Care Environment

An 84-year-old male client is being admitted after surgery to remove a section of his bowel (colectomy) following a diagnosis of colon cancer. His urine output from an indwelling urinary catheter after 3 hours in the postanesthesia care unit plus the amount in the bag on admission to the medical-surgical unit totals 100 mL. The urine is cloudy and dark yellow. He also has a history of hypertension. After evaluating the patency of the collection device, what is the most appropriate action for the nurse to perform?

A. Notify the health care provider of the low urine output.
B. Increase the rate of IV fluids until urine output is 0.5mL/kg/hr.
C. Continue to assess the client and re-evaluate urine output in 4 hours.
D. Ask about his typical voiding patterns and about any previous episodes of urinary problems.

◆ *Interventions*

A reduction in blood flow to the kidneys may initially not be recognized when there is no associated drop in systemic blood pressure (Davies & Leslie, 2012). Autoregulation and the renin-angiotensin-aldosterone system effectively maintain normal kidney blood flow and glomerular filtration rate. However, these mechanisms may not be working well in the critically ill patient. Thus current guidelines suggest that a mean arterial pressure (MAP) of 65 mm Hg be maintained to promote kidney PERFUSION. The calculation of MAP is illustrated in Table 68-6.

TABLE 68-6 Calculation of Mean Arterial Pressure (MAP)

MAP = (SBP + [2 × DBP]) ÷ 3

Example:

Blood pressure 130/80; SBP = 130; DBP = 80
(130 + [2 × 80]) ÷ 3 =
(130 + 160) ÷ 3 =
290 ÷ 3 =
96.666 = 97 mm Hg. **NOTE:** this value of 97 mm Hg is safe in relation to kidney perfusion and reduces risk for acute kidney injury (AKI) and progression of chronic kidney disease (CKD). A normal range for MAP is 70-110 mm Hg for healthy adults.

Abbreviations: SBP = systolic blood pressure; DBP = diastolic blood pressure

MAP is often displayed as a component of automated blood pressure measurement devices and during intra-arterial blood pressure measurement at the ICU bedside. Observations about peripheral edema, increased daily weight, and reduced urine output can identify patients with a positive fluid balance from AKI. Blood sampling of patients at risk for AKI allows monitoring of kidney function and early recognition of elevated serum creatinine. Communicate these observations early and often to the provider so that interventions can promote kidney health and interrupt the progression of AKI when it occurs. Surviving kidney tubule cells possess a remarkable ability to regenerate and proliferate, and early identification can both stop progression of AKI and aid in recovery of kidney function.

Not all patients with AKI experience oliguria. Inflammatory causes of AKI may allow proteins to enter the glomerulus, and these proteins can hold fluid in the filtrate, causing a *polyuria* (excess urine output). During AKI with high-volume urine output, hypovolemia and electrolyte *loss* are the main problems. The patient in the diuretic phase of AKI needs a plan of care that focuses on fluid and electrolyte *replacement* and monitoring. Onset of polyuria can be the start of recovery from AKI.

Base the desired outcomes of care on collaboration and communication with health care team members. Update the plan of care for either restriction or liberal administration of fluid based on timely and accurate health care team communication.

Frequent serum monitoring, close surveillance of intake and output, drug therapy, nutrition, careful administration of fluids and minerals, and renal replacement therapy are commonly used to manage AKI.

Drug Therapy. The health care team should consult the inpatient pharmacist for drug adjustment based on kidney function. As kidney function changes, drug dosages are changed. It is important to be knowledgeable about the site of drug metabolism and especially careful when giving drugs. Continuously monitor the patient with AKI for adverse drug events and interactions of the drugs that he or she is receiving. Diuretics may be used to increase urine output in AKI. Diuretic-induced urine output does not preserve kidney function or stop AKI, but diuretics do rid the body of retained fluid and electrolytes in the patient with AKI that has not progressed to ESKD.

Fluid challenges are often used to promote kidney PERFUSION. In patients without fluid overload, 500 to 1000 mL of normal saline may be infused over 1 hour. Patients with AKI often require central venous pressure (CVP) monitoring. When cardiac disease is also present and worsening, measurement of pulmonary arterial pressure by means of a pulmonary artery catheter for accurate evaluation of hemodynamic status may be needed. During fluid challenges, closely assess the response to fluid and slow the infusion if indications of fluid overload, particularly respiratory distress, occur.

Calcium channel blockers may be used to treat AKI resulting from nephrotoxins. These drugs prevent the movement of calcium into the kidney cells, maintain kidney cell integrity, and improve kidney blood flow. If they do not improve GFR as estimated by serum creatinine (described in Chapter 65), calcium channel blockers are stopped.

Investigation is ongoing to identify biomarkers that can indicate kidney injury early. Neutrophil gelatinase-associated lipocalin (NGAL) and kidney injury molecule-1 (KIM-1) are promising new biomarkers to identify AKI and guide treatment (Obermüller et al., 2014; Vanmassenhove et al., 2013).

Nutrition Therapy. Patients who have AKI often have a high rate of *catabolism* (protein breakdown). Increases in metabolism and protein breakdown may be related to the stress of illness and the increase in blood levels of catecholamines, cortisol, and glucagon. The rate of protein breakdown correlates with the severity of uremia and azotemia. Catabolism causes the breakdown of muscle for protein and increases azotemia.

A registered dietitian will calculate the patient's protein and caloric needs. Whereas this occurs for all patients admitted to an ICU, a consult may need to be requested for inpatients outside of the ICU or for those in the community settings. Work with the dietitian to establish a diet with specified amounts of protein, sodium, and fluids. For the patient who does not require dialysis, 0.6 g/kg of body weight or 40 g/day of protein is usually prescribed. For patients who do require dialysis, the protein level needed will range from 1 to 1.5 g/kg. The amount of dietary sodium ranges from 60 to 90 mEq/kg. If high blood potassium levels are present, dietary potassium is restricted to 60 to 70 mEq/kg. The daily amount of fluid permitted is calculated to be equal to the urine volume plus 500 mL. Assess food intake every shift to ensure that caloric intake is adequate.

Many patients with AKI are too ill or their appetite is too poor to meet caloric goals. For these patients, nutrition support is needed. Nutrition support can include oral supplements, enteral nutrition, or parenteral nutrition (hyperalimentation). The purposes of nutrition support in AKI are to provide sufficient nutrients to maintain or improve nutrition status, to preserve lean body mass, to restore or maintain fluid balance, and to preserve kidney function.

There are several kidney-specific formulations of oral supplements and enteral solutions (e.g., Nepro, Suplena Renalcal, and NovaSource Renal). As a rule, specialty tube feedings for kidney patients are lower in sodium, potassium, and phosphorus and higher in calories than are standard feedings. Enteral nutrition, delivered with a nasogastric or nasojejunal tube (these tubes can also be placed orally), is an effective route to deliver nutrition support. If TPN is used, the IV solutions are mixed to meet the patient's specific needs. Because kidney function is unstable in AKI, continuously monitor fluid balance (intake and output) and serum electrolyte levels to indicate how the supplementation affects FLUID AND ELECTROLYTE BALANCE. IV fat emulsion (Intralipid) infusions can provide a nonprotein source of calories. In uremic patients, fat emulsions are used in place of glucose to avoid the problems of excessive sugars.

Renal Replacement Therapy. Renal replacement therapy (RRT), also called *dialysis,* is used for patients with loss of kidney function. Indications for dialysis use include symptomatic uremia (pericarditis, neuropathy, or unexplained decline in cognition), persistent or rapidly rising high potassium levels (i.e., greater than 6.5 mEq/L), severe metabolic acidosis (pH less than 7.1), or fluid overload that compromises tissue PERFUSION. When AKI is associated with drug or alcohol intoxication, RRT also can remove toxins.

Immediate vascular access for RRT in patients with AKI is made by placement of a catheter specific for dialysis (Fig. 68-1). The catheter is placed in a central vein using best practices to avoid catheter-associated bloodstream infections (see Chapter 13, pp. 193-196). Placement of a dialysis catheter requires informed consent and a "time-out" similar to other surgical procedures (see Chapter 14, Care of Preoperative Patients). The catheter is not used to acquire blood samples, give drugs or fluid, or monitor central venous pressure. Provide site care in accordance with institutional policy and best practices to avoid catheter-related bloodstream INFECTION (CR-BSI).

A long-term dialysis catheter may be placed in the radiology department using a tunneling technique. The patient receives moderate sedation. Under ultrasound or fluoroscopic guidance, the physician makes a small incision where the internal jugular vein passes behind the clavicle. A 6- to 8-cm tunnel is created away from the site of the incision. A long-term hemodialysis catheter is inserted through the tunnel and into the jugular vein. Keeping a segment of the catheter within the subcutaneous tissues before entering the jugular vein reduces the risk for INFECTION. These centrally placed catheters are dedicated to dialysis alone and require aseptic dressing changes as for all central venous catheters.

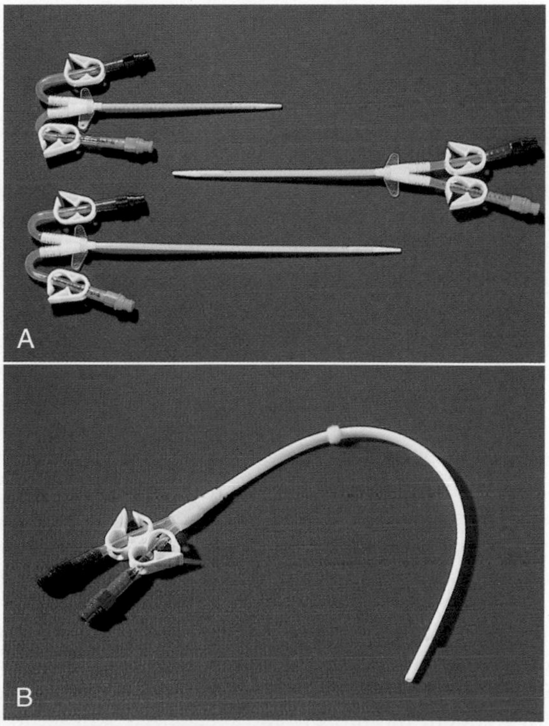

FIG. 68-1 Subclavian dialysis catheters. These catheters are radiopaque tubes that can be used for hemodialysis access. The Y-shaped tubing allows arterial outflow and venous return through a single catheter. **A,** Mahurkar catheters, made of polyurethane and used for short-term access. **B,** A PermCath catheter, made of silicone and used for long-term access.

Dialysis catheters have two lumens—one for outflow and one for inflow. This allows the patient's blood to flow out and, once dialyzed, to be returned through the inflow lumen. Some catheters have a third lumen for the dialysis nurse to sample venous blood or give drugs and fluid during dialysis.

Intermittent Versus Continuous Renal Replacement Therapy. Renal replacement therapy (RRT) is a supportive strategy to purify blood, substituting for the normal function of the kidney. Particles are separated from blood based on the different ability of particles to pass through (diffuse) a membrane. RRT can be delivered intermittently, continuously, or as a hybrid of these treatment approaches to hospitalized patients. There is no difference in the number of patients who go on to recover kidney function based on the type of RRT administered during AKI. Mortality is significant, regardless of modality, among patients with AKI who require RRT, and this mortality is around 50% while in the hospital (Elseviers et al., 2010).

Intermittent RRT, sometimes called *hemodialysis,* is delivered over 3 to 6 hours. Generally a technician or nurse with specialized training brings the dialysis machine to the bedside of a critically ill patient. Patients who do not need intensive care may be transported to an inpatient dialysis unit for the duration of the RRT treatment.

Intermittent RRT uses a dialysis machine to mix and monitor the dialysate. Dialysate is the fluid that helps remove the unwanted particles and waste products from blood. Dialysate is prescribed by the health care provider as an admixture to restore electrolytes and minerals to normal levels in the blood. The machine also monitors the flow of blood while it is outside of the body. Alarms are set and monitored by the dialysis technician or nurse to ensure safe and effective flow. This type of RRT has a long history of safety and effectiveness in ESKD. It is usually delivered 3 or 4 times weekly and may require anticoagulation in the dialysis circuit. However, this high-intensity treatment creates shifts of fluid and electrolytes that may not be tolerated in acutely and critically ill patients.

Continuous renal replacement therapies (RRTs), also known as *hemofiltration,* are alternative methods for removing wastes and restoring FLUID AND ELECTROLYTE BALANCE in hospitalized adults with AKI who are too unstable to tolerate the changes in blood pressure that occur with intermittent conventional hemodialysis. In all hemodialysis, blood is passed through a filter to remove waste and undesired particles. Unlike intermittent hemodialysis, continuous RRT removes and returns blood over 12 to 24 hours each day. Another difference between continuous RRT and intermittent hemodialysis is the approach used to remove particles from blood. Hemofiltration uses ultrafiltration, whereas diffusion is used in intermittent dialysis to remove toxins and other particles. *Ultrafiltration* is the separation of particles from a suspension by passage through a filter with very fine pores. In ultrafiltration, the separation is performed by convective transport. During intermittent hemodialysis, separation depends on differential diffusion. Some approaches to continuous RRT combine ultrafiltration with diffusion (combined hemofiltration and hemodialysis).

Continuous RRT occurs only in the ICU because of (1) the need for frequent monitoring and specialized skill set to maintain safety during *extracorporeal circulation* (blood flow outside the body) and (2) the need for ongoing replacement of fluid and electrolytes. Many agencies require nurses who deliver continuous RRT to attend classes and demonstrate competency in care annually. The American Nephrology Nurses Association provides resources for RRT policies and procedures.

There are several strategies to provide hemofiltration to critically ill patients. Continuous venovenous hemofiltration (CVVH) is more commonly used. CVVH is powered by a pump that drives blood from the patient catheter into the dialyzer (filter). The ultrafiltrate fluid is then collected into a bag for disposal. There may be a second pump that acts on the ultrafiltrate tubing to create negative pressure and increase fluid removal. Replacement fluid is infused via the inflow circuit in some systems. The pump increases the risk for an air embolus, but RRT systems should have alarms that detect air. These systems may also use anticoagulants but at lower doses than needed for systems using arterial access. CVVH can also be combined with dialysis (continuous venovenous hemofiltration and dialysis [CVVHD]). CVVHD is similar to intermittent RRT except that the rates of blood circulation and waste formation are much slower with CVVHD, thus the need for continuous therapy (Golestaneh et al., 2012).

Another modality for RRT is a hybrid of continuous and intermittent approaches. Slow continuous ultrafiltration (SCUF) provides slow removal of fluid over 12 to 24 hours. It can be useful when azotemia or uremia is not a concern (Streets & Vickers, 2012). Sustained low-efficiency dialysis (SLED) uses the dialysis machine to deliver prolonged dialysis for 12 to 24 hours. Lower blood flow and dialysate flow rates remove both particles and water and may be better tolerated by the unstable or critically ill patient, with fewer episodes of hypotension.

Continuous RRT is expensive and resource intensive (Allegretti et al., 2013; Golestaneh et al., 2012). It requires consultation and collaboration with the nephrologist and, often, with nurses specialized in dialysis delivery. Clear evidence about when to start or stop RRT when AKI occurs does not yet exist. Conservative management of FLUID AND ELECTROLYTE BALANCE, ACID-BASE BALANCE, and drug therapy is an acceptable and reasonable approach to manage AKI. This approach may be associated with less mortality up to 2 years following RRT for AKI.

Posthospital Care. The care for a patient with AKI after discharge from the hospital varies, depending on the status of the kidney function when the patient is discharged. The course of AKI varies, with recovery lasting up to several months. If the kidney injury is resolving, follow-up care may be provided by a nephrologist or by the family physician in consultation with the

NCLEX EXAMINATION CHALLENGE

Physiological Integrity

The nurse is completing documentation for a client with acute kidney injury who is being discharged today. The nurse notices that the client has a serum potassium level of 5.8 mEq/L. Which is the priority nursing action?

A. Asking the client to drink an extra 500 mL of water to dilute the electrolyte concentration and then re-checking the serum potassium level.
B. Encouraging the client to eat potassium-binding foods and to contact his or her primary care provider within 24 hours.
C. Checking the remaining values on the electrolyte panel and informing the primary care provider of all results before the client is discharged.
D. Applying a cardiac monitor and evaluating the client's muscle strength and muscle irritability.

nephrologist. Frequent medical visits are necessary, as are scheduled laboratory blood and urine tests to monitor kidney function. A dietitian can plan modifications to the patient's diet according to the degree of kidney function and ongoing nutrition needs. Fluid restrictions and daily weights may be advised to avoid fluid overload while kidneys are recovering.

About 10% of patients who receive RRT for AKI in the hospital experience ESKD and require chronic intermittent dialysis or renal transplantation (Allegretti et al., 2013). In patients who require dialysis at discharge following AKI, follow-up care is similar to that needed for patients with ESKD from CKD (see Community-Based Care, pp. 1444-1446). Depending on their level of independence and family support, patients may also need home care nursing or social work assistance.

CHRONIC KIDNEY DISEASE

❖ PATHOPHYSIOLOGY

Unlike acute kidney injury (AKI), chronic kidney disease (CKD) is a progressive, irreversible disorder and kidney function does *not* recover (Taal et al., 2012). When kidney function is too poor to sustain life, CKD becomes end-stage kidney disease (ESKD). Terms used with CKD include azotemia (buildup of nitrogen-based wastes in the blood), uremia (azotemia with clinical manifestations [Chart 68-2]), and uremic syndrome. See Table 68-1 for a comparison of AKI and CKD.

Stages of Chronic Kidney Disease

The kidneys fail in an organized fashion involving five stages based on estimated glomerular filtration rate (GFR). Direct measurement (described in Chapter 65, using a 3-hour or 24-hour urine collection) is advised for the most accurate estimation of GFR. The five stages of CKD are described in Table 68-7. CKD starts with a normal GFR but increased risk for kidney damage. In the first stage, the person may have a normal GFR (greater than 90 mL/min) but urine findings or structural abnormalities or genetic trait point to kidney disease. The patient is at increased risk for kidney damage from INFECTION, INFLAMMATION, pregnancy, dehydration, and hypotension or hypertension. Careful management of conditions like diabetes, hypertension, and heart failure can slow the progression of CKD even before GFR changes and manifestations of CKD occur (Wynne et al., 2012).

In the next stage, *mild CKD*, GFR is reduced, ranging between 60 and 89 mL/min. Kidney nephron damage has occurred, and there may be slight elevations of metabolic wastes in the blood because of nephron loss. Levels of blood urea nitrogen (BUN), serum creatinine, uric acid, and phosphorus are not sensitive enough to define this stage. Increased output of dilute urine may occur at this stage of CKD and contribute to severe dehydration.

CHART 68-2 Key Features

Uremia

- Metallic taste in the mouth
- Anorexia
- Nausea
- Vomiting
- Muscle cramps
- Uremic "frost" on skin
- Itching
- Fatigue and lethargy
- Hiccups
- Edema
- Dyspnea
- Paresthesias

! NURSING SAFETY PRIORITY (QSEN)

Action Alert

Teach patients with mild CKD that carefully managing fluid volume, blood pressure, electrolytes, and other kidney-damaging diseases by following prescribed drug and nutrition therapies can prevent damage and slow the progression to ESKD.

In *moderate CKD*, GRF reduction continues and ranges between 30 and 59 mL/min. Nephron damage is greater, and azotemia is present. Ongoing management of the underlying conditions that cause nephron damage is essential, especially glycemic and blood pressure control. Restriction of fluids, proteins, and electrolytes is needed.

Over time, patients progress to *severe CKD* (the fourth stage) and *end-stage kidney disease* (ESKD) (the fifth stage). Excessive amounts of urea and creatinine build up in the blood, and the kidneys cannot maintain homeostasis. Severe impairments of FLUID AND ELECTROLYTE BALANCE and ACID-BASE BALANCE occur. Without renal replacement therapy, death results from ESKD.

TABLE 68-7 Stages of Chronic Kidney Disease

STAGE	ESTIMATED GLOMERULAR FILTRATION RATE	INTERVENTION
Stage 1 At risk; normal kidney function but urine findings or structural abnormalities or genetic trait point to kidney disease	>90 mL/min	Screen for risk factors and manage care to reduce risk: • Uncontrolled hypertension • Diabetes mellitus • Chronic kidney or urinary tract infection • Family history of genetic kidney diseases • Exposure to nephrotoxic substances
Stage 2 Mild chronic kidney disease (CKD); reduced kidney function; laboratory values and other findings (e.g. structural changes) point to kidney disease	60-89 mL/min	Focus on reduction of risk factors
Stage 3 Moderate CKD	30-59 mL/min	Implement strategies to slow disease progression
Stage 4 Severe CKD	15-29 mL/min	Manage complications Discuss patient preferences and values Educate about options and prepare for renal replacement therapy
Stage 5 End-stage kidney disease (ESKD)	<15 mL/min	Implement renal replacement therapy or kidney transplantation

Kidney Changes

CKD with greatly reduced GFR causes many problems, including abnormal urine production, severe disruption of FLUID AND ELECTROLYTE BALANCE, and metabolic abnormalities. Because healthy nephrons become larger and work harder, urine production and water ELIMINATION are sufficient to maintain essential homeostasis until about three fourths of kidney function is lost. As the disease progresses, the ability to produce diluted urine is reduced, resulting in urine with a fixed osmolarity *(isosthenuria)*. As kidney function continues to decline, the BUN increases and urine output decreases. At this point, the patient is at risk for fluid overload.

Metabolic Changes

Urea and creatinine excretion are disrupted by CKD. Creatinine comes from proteins present in skeletal muscle. The rate of creatinine excretion depends on muscle mass, physical activity, and diet. Without major changes in diet or physical activity, the serum creatinine level is constant. Creatinine is partially excreted by the kidney tubules, and a decrease in kidney function leads to a buildup of serum creatinine. Urea is made from protein metabolism and is excreted by the kidneys. The BUN level normally varies directly with protein intake.

Sodium excretion changes are common. Early in CKD, the patient is at risk for *hyponatremia* (sodium depletion) because there are fewer healthy nephrons to reabsorb sodium. Thus sodium is lost in the urine. Polyuria of mild to moderate CKD also causes sodium loss.

In the later stages of CKD, kidney excretion of sodium is reduced as urine production decreases. Then sodium retention and high serum sodium levels *(hypernatremia)* can occur with only modest increases in dietary sodium intake. This problem leads to severe disruption of FLUID AND ELECTROLYTE BALANCE (see Chapter 11). Sodium retention causes hypertension and edema.

Even with sodium retention, the serum sodium level may appear normal because plasma water is retained at the same time. If fluid retention occurs at a greater rate than sodium retention, the serum sodium level is falsely low because of dilution (see Chart 68-1).

Potassium excretion occurs mainly through the kidney. Any increase in potassium load during the later stages of CKD can lead to **hyperkalemia** (high serum potassium levels). Normal serum potassium levels of 3.5 to 5 mEq/L are maintained until the 24-hour urine output falls below 500 mL. High potassium levels then develop quickly, reaching 7 to 8 mEq/L or greater. Life-threatening changes in cardiac rate and rhythm result from this elevation due to abnormal depolarization and repolarization. Other factors contribute to high potassium levels in CKD, including the ingestion of potassium in drugs, failure to restrict dietary potassium, tissue breakdown, blood transfusions, and bleeding or hemorrhage. (See Chapter 11 for discussion of potassium problems.)

ACID-BASE BALANCE is affected by CKD. In the early stages, blood pH changes little because the remaining healthy nephrons increase their rate of acid excretion. As more nephrons are lost, acid excretion is reduced and metabolic acidosis results (see Chapter 12).

Many factors lead to acidosis in CKD. First, the kidneys cannot excrete excessive hydrogen ions (acids). Normally, tubular cells move hydrogen ions into the urine for excretion, but ammonium and bicarbonate are needed for this movement to occur. In patients with CKD, ammonium production is decreased and reabsorption of bicarbonate does not occur. This process leads to a buildup of hydrogen ions and reduced levels of bicarbonate *(base deficit)*. High potassium levels further reduce kidney ammonium production and excretion.

As CKD worsens and acid retention increases, increased respiratory action is needed to keep blood pH normal. The respiratory system adjusts or compensates for the increased blood hydrogen ion levels (acidosis or decreased pH) by increasing the rate and depth of breathing to excrete carbon dioxide through the lungs. This breathing pattern, called **Kussmaul respiration**, increases with worsening kidney disease. Serum bicarbonate measures the extent of metabolic acidosis (bicarbonate deficit). Patients with CKD usually need alkali replacement to counteract acidosis.

Calcium and phosphorus balance is disrupted by CKD. A complex, balanced normal reciprocal relationship exists between calcium and phosphorus (used interchangeably with phosphate) and is influenced by vitamin D (see Chapter 11). The kidney produces a hormone needed to activate vitamin D, which then enhances intestinal absorption of calcium.

Normally, excess dietary phosphorus is excreted by the kidneys in the urine. In CKD, phosphorus overload leads to secretion of a phosphaturic hormone from bone (Fukagawa et al., 2013). This hormone, fibroblast growth factor 3 (GG3), contributes to mineral imbalance.

Parathyroid hormone (PTH) controls the amount of phosphorus in the blood by causing tubular excretion of phosphorus when there is an excess. An early effect of CKD is reduced phosphorus excretion (Fig. 68-2). As plasma phosphorus levels increase *(hyperphosphatemia)*, calcium levels decrease *(hypocalcemia)*. Chronic low blood calcium levels stimulate the parathyroid glands to release more PTH. Under the influence of additional PTH, calcium is released from storage areas in bones

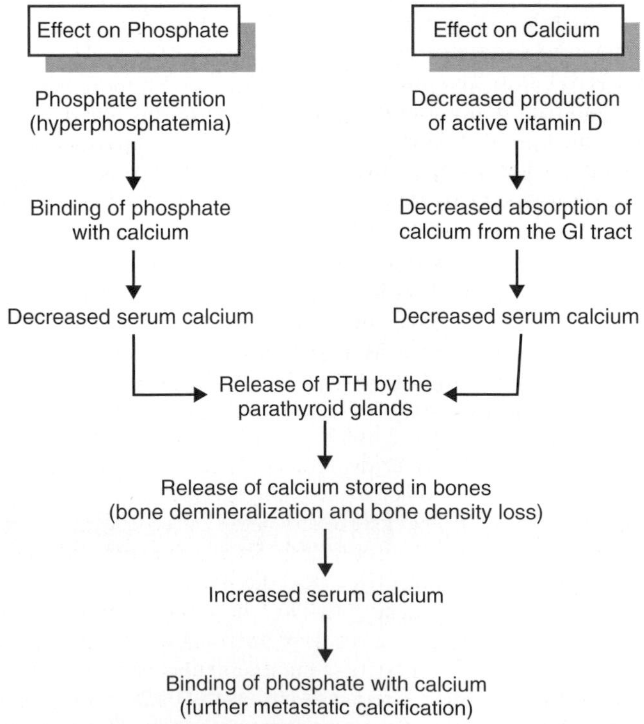

FIG. 68-2 The effects of kidney dysfunction on phosphorus and calcium balance. *PTH,* Parathyroid hormone.

(bone resorption), which results in bone density loss. The extra calcium from the bone is needed to balance the excess plasma phosphorus level. The problem of low blood calcium levels is made worse with severe CKD because kidney cell damage also reduces production of active vitamin D. Thus less calcium is absorbed through the intestinal tract in the absence of sufficient vitamin D.

The problems in bone metabolism and structure caused by CKD-induced low calcium levels and high phosphorus levels are called **renal osteodystrophy**. Bone mineral loss causes bone pain, spinal sclerosis, fractures, bone density loss, osteomalacia, and tooth calcium loss.

Crystals formed from excessive calcium phosphorus are called *metastatic calcifications* and may precipitate in many body areas. When the plasma level of the calcium-phosphorus product (serum calcium level multiplied by the serum phosphorus level) exceeds 70 mg/dL, the crystals may lodge in the kidneys, heart, lungs, major blood vessels, joints, eyes (causing conjunctivitis), and brain. Skin itching increases with calcium-phosphorus imbalances.

Calcium is also deposited in atherosclerotic plaques and in the intima of blood vessels. Vascular calcium deposits are a marker of significant risk for cardiovascular disease.

Cardiac Changes

Hypertension is common in most patients with CKD. This problem may be either the cause or the result of CKD. In patients who have other causes of hypertension such as atherosclerosis, the increased blood pressure damages the glomerular capillaries and eventually ESKD results.

CKD itself elevates blood pressure by causing fluid and sodium overload and dysfunction of the renin-angiotensin-aldosterone system. Hypertension alone can damage kidney arterioles, reducing PERFUSION. A decrease in kidney blood flow results in the production and release of a number of signaling chemicals, including renin, to improve blood flow to the kidney. The release of renin triggers the production of angiotensin and aldosterone. Angiotensin causes blood vessel constriction and increases blood pressure. Aldosterone, a hormone released by the adrenal glands, stimulates kidney tubules to reabsorb sodium and water. These actions increase plasma volume and raise blood pressure. However, in the presence of CKD, an increase in blood pressure may not result in increased blood flow, and the production of renin continues, which creates a cycle of vasoconstriction in kidney arterioles and peripheral arterioles. The result is severe hypertension that worsens kidney function. Hypertension with CKD is difficult to manage. Many patients with CKD have heart damage and heart enlargement from the long-term hypertension that results in coronary artery damage and poor coronary artery perfusion.

Hyperlipidemia occurs in CKD from changes in fat metabolism that increase triglyceride, total cholesterol, and low-density lipoprotein (LDL) levels. These changes increase the patient's risk for coronary artery disease and acute cardiac events. Problems with lipids and atherosclerosis are significantly increased for the patient with both CKD and diabetes.

Heart failure may occur in CKD because it increases the workload on the heart as a result of anemia, hypertension, and fluid overload. Left ventricular enlargement and heart failure are common in ESKD. Uremia may cause *uremic cardiomyopathy*, the uremic toxin effect on the myocardium. Heart failure also may occur in these patients because of hypertension and coronary artery disease. Cardiac disease is a leading cause of death in patients with ESKD.

Pericarditis also occurs in patients with CKD. The pericardial sac becomes inflamed by uremic toxins or INFECTION. If it is not treated, this problem leads to pericardial effusion, cardiac tamponade, and death. Manifestations include shortness of breath from low cardiac output, severe chest pain, tachycardia, narrow *pulse pressure* (close values for systolic and diastolic blood pressure), low-grade fever, and a pericardial friction rub that can be heard with a stethoscope placed over the left sternal border. Dysrhythmias may occur with uremia and uremic pericarditis. Treatment of tamponade requires removal of pericardial fluid by placement of a needle, catheter, or drainage tube into the pericardium.

Hematologic Changes

Anemia is a common problem in patients in the later stages of CKD, and it worsens the CKD manifestations. The causes of anemia include a decreased erythropoietin level that decreases red blood cell (RBC) production, decreased RBC survival time resulting from uremia, iron and folic acid deficiencies, and increased bleeding as a result of impaired platelet function.

Gastrointestinal Changes

Uremia affects the entire GI system. The flora of the mouth change with uremia. The mouth contains the enzyme *urease*, which breaks down urea into ammonia. The ammonia generated then causes *halitosis* (bad breath) and *stomatitis* (mouth INFLAMMATION).

Anorexia, nausea, vomiting, and hiccups are common in patients with uremia. The specific cause of these problems is unknown but may be related to high BUN and creatinine levels as well as acidosis.

Peptic ulcer disease is common in patients with uremia, but the exact cause is unclear. Uremic colitis with watery diarrhea or constipation may also be present with uremia. Ulcers may occur in the stomach or intestine, causing erosion of blood vessels. The blood loss caused by these erosions may lead to hemorrhagic shock from severe GI bleeding.

Etiology and Genetic Risk

The causes of CKD are complex (Table 68-8). More than 100 different disease processes can result in progressive loss of kidney function (see also Chapter 67). Two main causes of CKD leading to dialysis are hypertension and diabetes mellitus. African-American patients are much more likely to develop ESKD and to have hypertensive ESKD.

Incidence and Prevalence

The number of patients being treated for CKD is increasing, particularly among people older than 65 years. Over 871,000 people in the United States are being treated for ESKD (U.S. Renal Data Systems [USRDS], 2014). As many as 25% of patients receiving treatment for ESKD die in the first year of dialysis. Chart 68-3 addresses the prevention of kidney and urinary problems.

Health Promotion and Maintenance

The health-promotion activities to prevent or delay the onset of CKD focus on controlling the diseases that lead to its development, such as diabetes mellitus and hypertension. Educating and encouraging the patient to accept lifestyle modifications

TABLE 68-8 Selected Causes of Chronic Kidney Disease

Glomerular Disease
- Glomerulonephritis
- Basement membrane disease
- Goodpasture's syndrome
- Intercapillary glomerulosclerosis

Tubular Disease
- Chronic hypercalcemia
- Chronic potassium depletion
- Fanconi's syndrome
- Heavy metal (lead) poisoning

Vascular Disease of the Kidney
- Ischemic disease of the kidney
- Bilateral renal artery stenosis
- Nephrosclerosis
- Hyperparathyroidism

Inherited or Genetic Conditions
- Hypoplastic kidneys
- Medullary cystic disease
- Polycystic kidney disease

Infection
- Pyelonephritis
- Tuberculosis

Systemic Vascular Disease
- Intrarenal renovascular hypertension
- Extrarenal renovascular hypertension

Metabolic Kidney Disease
- Diabetes
- Amyloidosis
- Gout (hyperuricemic nephropathy)
- Milk-alkali syndrome
- Sarcoidosis

Connective Tissue Disease
- Progressive systemic sclerosis
- Systemic lupus erythematosus
- Polyarteritis

Urinary Tract Disease
- Obstructive uropathy

NOTE: List is not all-inclusive.

and how to implement them are incorporated into the plan of care in an ongoing manner. Diet adjustments (e.g., sodium, protein, and cholesterol restriction), weight maintenance (i.e., achieve body mass index of 22-25 kg/m^2), cessation of smoking, participation in 30 to 60 minutes of moderate-intensity exercise daily, and limitation of alcohol to 1 or 2 drinks daily are examples of lifestyle recommendations for the patient with CKD (Saccomano & DeLuca, 2012). Identifying patients who have diabetes or hypertension at an early stage is critical to CKD prevention. Teach patients to adhere to drug and diet regimens and to engage in regular physical activity to prevent the blood vessel changes and cascade of kidney cell damage that lead to CKD. Instruct patients with diabetes to keep their blood glucose levels within the prescribed range. Teach patients with hypertension that drug therapy reduces vessel damage. Lifestyle changes in diet and activity promote health and healthy kidneys. Urge patients with diabetes or hypertension to have yearly testing for microalbuminuria along with serum creatinine and BUN.

Teach everyone treated for an INFECTION anywhere in the kidney/urinary system to take all antibiotics as prescribed. Urge everyone to drink at least 2 L of water daily unless a health problem requires fluid restriction. Caution people who use NSAIDs to use the lowest dose for the briefest time period because these drugs interfere with blood flow to the kidney. High-dose and long-term NSAID use reduces kidney function.

❖ PATIENT-CENTERED COLLABORATIVE CARE

◆ Assessment

History. When taking a history from a patient with risk for or actual chronic kidney disease (CKD), document the patient's age and gender. Accurately measure weight and height, and ask about usual weight and recent weight gain or loss. Weight gain may indicate fluid retention from poor kidney function. Weight loss may be the result of anorexia from high blood urea levels.

Obtain a complete history of kidney and urologic disorders, long-term health problems, and drug use. Long-term health problems such as hypertension, diabetes, systemic lupus erythematosus, arthritis, cancer, and tuberculosis can cause decreased kidney function. Ask the patient about family members' kidney disease that might indicate a genetic problem.

Document the use of current and past prescription and over-the-counter drugs because many drugs are nephrotoxic and can cause kidney damage (see Table 68-5). Inquire about contrast-induced nephropathy by asking if the patient has had x-rays or CT scan with dye.

Examine the patient's dietary habits, and discuss any present GI problems. A change in the taste of foods often occurs with CKD. Patients may report that sweet foods are not as appealing or that meats have a metallic taste. Ask about the presence of nausea, vomiting, anorexia, hiccups, diarrhea, or constipation. These manifestations may be the result of excess wastes that the body cannot excrete because of kidney disease.

Ask about the patient's energy level and any recent injuries or bleeding. Explore changes in his or her daily routine as a possible *result* of fatigue. Fatigue is a common and often profound problem among patients with CKD, particularly among patients receiving dialysis (Horigan et al., 2012). Weakness, drowsiness, and shortness of breath suggest impending pulmonary edema or neurologic degeneration. Ask about bruising or bleeding, which can be caused by hematologic changes from uremia.

CHART 68-3 Patient and Family Education: Preparing for Self-Management

Prevention of Kidney and Urinary Problems

- Be alert to the general appearance of your urine. Note any changes in its color, clarity, or odor.
- Changes in the frequency or volume of urine passage occur with changes in fluid intake. More frequent or infrequent voiding not associated with changes in fluid intake may signal health problems.
- Any discomfort or distress with the passage of urine is not normal. Pain, burning, urgency, aching, or difficulty with initiating urine flow or complete bladder emptying is of some concern.
- The kidneys need 1 to 2 liters of fluid a day to flush out your body wastes. Water is the ideal flushing agent.
- Avoid sugary, high-calorie drinks; they provide low-quality calories that contribute to weight gain and hyperglycemia-induced diuresis.
- Changes in kidney function are often silent for many years. Periodically ask your health care provider to measure your kidney function with a blood test (serum creatinine) and a urinalysis.
- If you have a history of kidney disease, diabetes mellitus, hypertension (high blood pressure), or a family history of kidney disease, you should know your serum creatinine level and your glomerular filtration rate (either estimated from serum creatinine or measured with a 24-hour creatinine urine collection). At least one checkup per year that includes laboratory blood and urine testing of kidney function is recommended.
- If you are identified as having decreased kidney function, ask about whether any prescribed drug, diagnostic test, or therapeutic procedure will present a risk to your current kidney function. Evaluate the contribution of diet to risk for kidney disease with your health care provider or a dietitian. Check out all nonprescription drugs with your physician or pharmacist before using them.

Discuss urine ELIMINATION in detail, including frequency of urination, appearance of the urine, and any difficulty starting or controlling urination. These data can help identify urologic problems that may influence existing kidney function.

NCLEX EXAMINATION CHALLENGE

Health Promotion and Maintenance

A 60-year-old African-American client is newly diagnosed with mild chronic kidney disease (stage 2 CKD). She has a history of diabetes, and her current A1C is 8.0%. She asks the nurse whether any of the following factors could have caused this problem. Which factor should the nurse indicate may have influenced the development of CKD?

A. She heavily salted her food as a child and teenager but added no extra salt to her food as an adult.
B. Her chronic hyperglycemia causes blood vessel changes in the kidney that can damage kidney tissue.
C. Her paternal grandparents had type 2 diabetes and hypertension.
D. She drinks 2 cups of coffee with cream daily.

Physical Assessment/Clinical Manifestations. CKD causes changes in all body systems (Chart 68-4). Most manifestations are related to changes in FLUID AND ELECTROLYTE BALANCE, ACID-BASE BALANCE, and buildup of nitrogenous wastes.

Neurologic manifestations of CKD and uremic syndrome vary (see Chart 68-4). Observe for problems ranging from lethargy to seizures or coma, which may indicate uremic encephalopathy. Assess for sensory changes that appear in a glove-and-stocking pattern over the hands and feet (peripheral neuropathy). Check for weakness in the upper and lower extremities (e.g., uremic neuropathy).

If untreated, encephalopathy can lead to seizures and coma. Dialysis is used for CKD when neurologic problems result. The manifestations of encephalopathy may resolve with dialysis. However, improvement in neuropathy is limited if it is severe and motor function is impaired.

Cardiovascular manifestations of CKD and uremia result from fluid overload, hypertension, heart failure (HF), pericarditis, potassium-induced dysrhythmias, and cholesterol/calcium (plaque) deposits in blood vessels. Assess for manifestations of reduced sodium and water excretion. Circulatory overload, if untreated, leads to hypertension, pulmonary edema, peripheral edema, and HF.

Assess heart rate and rhythm, listening for extra sounds (particularly an S_3), irregular patterns, or a pericardial friction rub. Unless a dialysis vascular access has been created, measure blood pressure in each arm. Assess the jugular veins for distention, and assess for edema of the feet, shins, and sacrum and around the eyes. Crackles during lung auscultation and shortness of breath with exertion and at night suggest fluid overload.

Respiratory manifestations of CKD also vary (e.g., breath that smells like urine [*uremic fetor* or uremic halitosis], deep sighing, yawning, shortness of breath). Observe the rhythm, rate, and depth of breathing. Tachypnea and **hyperpnea** (increased depth of breathing) occur with metabolic acidosis.

With severe metabolic acidosis, extreme increases in rate and depth of ventilation (Kussmaul respirations) occur. A few patients have pneumonitis, or *uremic lung*. In these patients, assess for thick sputum, reduced coughing, tachypnea, and fever. A pleural friction rub may be heard with a stethoscope. Patients often have pleuritic pain with breathing. Auscultate the lungs for crackles, which indicate fluid overload.

Hematologic manifestations of CKD include anemia and abnormal bleeding. Check for indicators of anemia (e.g., fatigue, pallor, lethargy, weakness, shortness of breath, dizziness). Check for abnormal bleeding by observing for bruising, petechiae, purpura, mucous membrane bleeding in the nose or gums, or intestinal bleeding (black, tarry stools [**melena**]).

GI manifestations of CKD include foul breath and mouth INFLAMMATION or ulceration. Document any abdominal pain, cramping, or vomiting. Test all stools for occult blood.

Skeletal manifestations of CKD are related to osteodystrophy from poor absorption of calcium and continuous bone calcium

CHART 68-4 Key Features

Severe Chronic and End-Stage Kidney Disease

Neurologic Manifestations
- Lethargy and daytime drowsiness
- Inability to concentrate or decreased attention span
- Seizures
- Coma
- Slurred speech
- Asterixis (jerky movements or "flapping" of the hands)
- Tremors, twitching, or jerky movements
- Myoclonus
- Ataxia (alteration in gait)
- Paresthesias

Cardiovascular Manifestations
- Cardiomyopathy
- Hypertension
- Peripheral edema
- Heart failure
- Uremic pericarditis
- Pericardial effusion
- Pericardial friction rub
- Cardiac tamponade
- Cardiorenal syndrome

Respiratory Manifestations
- Uremic halitosis
- Tachypnea
- Deep sighing, yawning
- Kussmaul respirations
- Uremic pneumonitis
- Shortness of breath
- Pulmonary edema
- Pleural effusion
- Depressed cough reflex
- Crackles

Hematologic Manifestations
- Anemia
- Abnormal bleeding and bruising

Gastrointestinal Manifestations
- Anorexia
- Nausea
- Vomiting
- Metallic taste in the mouth
- Changes in taste acuity and sensation
- Uremic colitis (diarrhea)
- Constipation
- Uremic gastritis (possible GI bleeding)
- Uremic fetor (breath odor)
- Stomatitis

Urinary Manifestations
- Polyuria, nocturia (early)
- Oliguria, anuria (later)
- Proteinuria
- Hematuria
- Diluted, straw-colored urine appearance (early)
- Concentrated and cloudy urine appearance (later)

Integumentary Manifestations
- Decreased skin turgor
- Yellow-gray pallor
- Dry skin
- Pruritus
- Ecchymosis
- Purpura
- Soft-tissue calcifications
- Uremic frost (late, premorbid)

Musculoskeletal Manifestations
- Muscle weakness and cramping
- Bone pain
- Fractures
- Renal osteodystrophy

Reproductive Manifestations
- Decreased fertility
- Infrequent or absent menses
- Decreased libido
- Impotence
- Sexual dysfunction

loss. Adults with osteodystrophy have thin, fragile bones that are at risk for pathologic fractures with even slight trauma. Vertebrae become more compact and may bend forward, leading to an overall loss of height. Ask about changes in height and any unexplained bone pain. Observe for spinal curvatures and any unusual bumps or protrusions in bone areas that may indicate fractures. Handle the patient carefully during examination and care.

Urine manifestations in CKD reflect the kidneys' decreasing function. At first, urine amount, frequency, and appearance change. Protein, sediment, or blood may be in the urine.

The amount and composition of the urine change as kidney function decreases. With the onset of mild to moderate CKD, the urine may be more dilute and clearer because tubular reabsorption of water is reduced. The actual urine output in a patient with CKD varies with the amount of remaining kidney function. The patient with severe CKD or ESKD usually has oliguria, but some patients continue to produce 1 L or more daily. Daily urine volume usually changes again after dialysis is started. A long duration of oliguria is an indication that recovery of kidney function is not to be expected.

Skin manifestations of CKD occur as a result of uremia. Pigment is deposited in the skin, causing a yellowish coloration, or darkening when skin is brown or bronze. The anemia of CKD causes a sallowness, appearing as a faded suntan on lighter-skinned patients.

Skin oils and turgor are decreased in patients with uremia. A distressing problem of uremia is severe *pruritus* (itching). **Uremic frost**, a layer of urea crystals from evaporated sweat, may appear on the face, eyebrows, axillae, and groin in patients with advanced uremic syndrome. Assess for bruises *(ecchymosis)*, purple patches *(purpura)*, and rashes.

Psychosocial Assessment. Chronic kidney disease (CKD) and its treatment disrupt many aspects of a patient's life. Psychosocial assessment and support are part of the nurse's role from the time that CKD is first diagnosed. Ask about the patient's understanding of the diagnosis and what the treatment regimen means to him or her (e.g., diet, drugs, dialysis). Assess for anxiety and for the coping styles used by the patient or family members. Issues affected by CKD include family relations, social activity, work patterns, body image, and sexual activity. The long-term nature of severe CKD and ESKD, the many treatment options, and the uncertainties about the course of the disease and its treatment require ongoing psychosocial assessment.

Laboratory Assessment. CKD causes extreme changes in many laboratory values (see Chart 68-1). Monitor these blood values: creatinine, blood urea nitrogen (BUN), sodium, potassium, calcium, phosphorus, bicarbonate, hemoglobin, and hematocrit. Also monitor GFR for trends.

A urinalysis is performed. In the early stages of CKD, urinalysis may show excessive protein, glucose, red blood cells (RBCs) and white blood cells (WBCs), and decreased or fixed specific gravity. Urine osmolarity is usually decreased. As CKD progresses, urine output decreases dramatically and osmolarity increases.

Glomerular filtration rate (GFR) can be estimated from serum creatinine levels, age, gender, race, and body size. But this type of estimation is generally considered for screening rather than for staging of CKD. Estimation of GFR based on serum creatinine is also useful to calculate drug dose or drug frequency when reduced renal function is a concern. However, to determine stage of CKD, a urine collection of 3 hours to 24 hours is usually done.

In severe CKD, measurements of the serum creatinine and BUN levels may be used to determine the presence and degree of uremia. Serum creatinine levels may increase gradually over a period of years, reaching levels of 15 to 30 mg/dL or more, depending on the patient's muscle mass. BUN levels are directly related to dietary protein intake. Without protein restriction, BUN levels may rise to 10 to 20 times the value of the serum creatinine level. With dietary protein restriction, BUN levels are elevated but less than those of non–protein-restricted patients. Fluid balance also affects BUN.

Imaging Assessment. Few x-ray findings are abnormal with CKD. Bone x-rays of the hand can show renal osteodystrophy. With long-term ESKD, the kidneys shrink (except for ESKD caused by polycystic kidney disease) and may be 8 to 9 cm or smaller. This small size results from atrophy and fibrosis. If CKD progresses suddenly, a kidney ultrasound or CT scan without contrast medium may be used to rule out an obstruction. (See Chapter 65 for a complete description of diagnostic tests for kidney function.)

◆ Analysis

The patient with CKD usually has had a progressive reduction of kidney function and is often hospitalized for adjustment of the treatment plan. The focus of care is to manage problems and prevent complications. The priority NANDA-I nursing diagnoses and collaborative problems for patients with CKD include:

1. Excess Fluid Volume related to the inability of diseased kidneys to maintain body fluid balance (NANDA-I)
2. Potential for pulmonary edema related to fluid overload
3. Decreased Cardiac Output related to reduced stroke volume, dysrhythmias, fluid overload, and increased peripheral vascular resistance (NANDA-I)
4. Inadequate nutrition related to inability to ingest, digest, or absorb food and nutrients as a result of physiologic factors
5. Risk for Infection related to skin breakdown, immune-related kidney dysfunction, or malnutrition (NANDA-I)
6. Risk for Injury related to effects of kidney disease on bone density, blood clotting, and drug elimination (NANDA-I)
7. Fatigue related to kidney disease, anemia, and reduced energy production (NANDA-I)
8. Anxiety related to threat to or change in health status, economic status, relationships, role function, systems, or self-concept; situational crisis; threat of death; lack of knowledge about diagnostic tests, disease process, treatment; loss of control; or disrupted family life (NANDA-I)

◆ Planning and Implementation

The Concept Map on p. 1425 discusses nursing care issues related to patients who have end-stage kidney disease (ESKD).

Managing Fluid Volume

Planning: Expected Outcomes. The patient with CKD is expected to achieve and maintain an acceptable FLUID AND ELECTROLYTE BALANCE. Indicators include that blood pressure, central venous pressure, and electrolytes are normal or nearly normal. Body weight is stable (±2 lbs overnight and 5 lbs weekly) and does not increase more than 3 pounds between dialysis sessions.

CONCEPT MAP

END-STAGE KIDNEY DISEASE

- PERFUSION
- ACID-BASE BALANCE
- INFECTION
- FLUID AND ELECTROLYTE BALANCE
- INFLAMMATION
- ELIMINATION

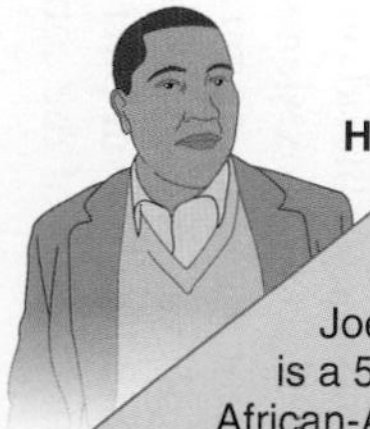

History

Joe Brown is a 55-year-old African-American man who has a lengthy history of type 2 diabetes, coronary artery disease, and hyperlipidemia. He has had complete loss of kidney function for 4 months. His vital signs are T – 100° F; P – 104 and irregular; R – 32; BP – 160/100 mm Hg.

- Age 55, male, height 5'9", 225 lbs, recent weight gain of 8 lbs.
- History of kidney stones, uncontrolled DM type 2, drug use, hypertension, and hyperlipidemia. Family history of polycystic kidney disease.
- Chronic use of NSAIDs for arthritis pain.
- Reports that desserts "don't taste sweet like before" and meat leaves a metallic taste. Some nausea and anorexia.
- Reports feeling weak and tired and is often short of breath. He has several bruises on his arms and legs at different stages.
- States he urinates dark-colored urine in small amounts a few times a day.

Data Synthesis →

PATIENT PROBLEMS

- Excess Fluid Volume due to inability of kidneys to maintain body fluid balance
- Potential for pulmonary edema due to fluid overload
- Decreased Cardiac Output due to reduced stroke volume, dysrhythmias, fluid overload, and increased peripheral vascular resistance
- Inadequate nutrition due to inability to ingest, digest, or absorb food and nutrients as a result of physiologic factors
- Risk for Infection related to skin breakdown, immune-related kidney dysfunction, or malnutrition
- Risk for Injury due to effects of kidney disease on bone density, blood clotting, and drug elimination
- Fatigue related to kidney disease, anemia, and reduced energy production
- Anxiety due to threat to or change in health status, economic status, relationships, role function, systems, or self-concept; situational crisis; threat of death; lack of knowledge about diagnostic tests, disease process, treatment; loss of control; or disrupted family life

Planning ↑

EXPECTED OUTCOMES

- Achieve an acceptable fluid balance
- Maintain a stable body weight
- No exhibiting signs of pulmonary edema
- Maintain adequate cardiac output
- Maintain adequate nutrition
- Remain free of infection
- Remain free of injury
- Decreased fatigue

INTERVENTIONS

1 Physical Assessment

Assess for presence of S_3 or pericardial friction rub, chest pain, jugular vein distention, edema, fatigue, dyspnea, crackles, weight change, skin integrity, pruritus, skin discoloration, mental status, seizure activity, sensory changes, LE weakness, anorexia, nausea, vomiting, stomatitis, melena, urine amount/frequency/appearance, bone pain, presence of hyperglycemia secondary to diabetes, signs of bleeding disorders (petechiae, purpura, ecchymosis). *Guides patient care; assesses for signs of kidney failure.*

2 Fluid Management

Monitor vital signs, intake and output, weight, hydration status, treat hypertension with drug therapy. *Monitors for fluid overload; sodium retention causes hypertension and edema.*

3 Monitoring for Pulmonary Edema

- Assess for restlessness, anxiety, tachycardia, shortness of breath, crackles, decreased breath sounds, frothy, blood-tinged sputum, and diaphoresis. *Indicates pulmonary edema, uremic injury to lung blood vessels causes inflammation.*
- Position the patient in high Fowler's; give oxygen, loop diuretics, and measure urine output every 15-30 minutes. *Decreases fluid volume; improves gas exchange and* PERFUSION.
- Monitor vital signs and assess breath sounds at least every 2 hours. *Evaluates the patient's response to treatment.*

4 Maintaining Acid-Base Balance

Ensure participation in renal replacement therapies, either peritoneal dialysis (PD) or hemodialysis (HD). *Improves fluid, electrolyte, and acid-base balance; removes nitrogenous wastes.*

5 Interpretation of Lab Values

Monitor lab values – Blood urea nitrogen (BUN), serum creatinine, creatinine clearance, complete blood count, electrolytes. *Determines the effectiveness of therapy for kidney failure.*

6 Monitoring Cardiac Output

Assess for signs of heart failure. Administer calcium channel blockers, ACE inhibitors, alpha-adrenergic and beta-adrenergic blockers, and vasodilators. *Controls blood pressure, which is essential to preserve kidney function.*

7 Enhancing Nutrition

Collaborate with the dietitian to determine calories; protein, fluid, potassium, sodium, and phosphorus restrictions; vitamin and mineral supplements. *Provides a balance of food and fluids to prevent malnutrition and avoid complications.*

8 Preventing Infection

Provide meticulous skin care; inspect vascular access site or peritoneal dialysis catheter site for redness, swelling, pain, and drainage. Monitor vital signs for fever and tachycardia. *Prevents and detects early signs of infection.*

9 Health Promotion and Maintenance

Teach the patient and family the importance of adhering to prescribed fluid and dietary restrictions, medications, and dialysis as scheduled. *Promotes health and reduces complications.*

10 Psychosocial Integrity

Encourage the expression of concerns about risks for death and lifestyle disruption; determine the presence of anxiety or maladaptive behavior. Refer to community health or support groups. *Minimizes the impact that depression, anxiety, and nonacceptance have on mental well-being.*

Concept Map by Deanne A. Blach, MSN, RN

CHART 68-5 Best Practice for Patient Safety & Quality Care (QSEN)

Managing Fluid Volume

- Weigh the patient daily at the same time each day, using the same scale, with the patient wearing the same amount and type of clothing, and graph the results.
- Observe the weight graph for trends (1 L of water weighs 1 kg).
- Accurately measure all fluid intake and output.
- Teach the patient and family about the need to keep fluid intake within prescribed restricted amounts and to ensure that the prescribed daily amount is evenly distributed throughout the 24 hours.
- Monitor for these manifestations of fluid overload at least every 4 hours:
  - Decreased urine output
  - Rapid, bounding pulse
  - Rapid, shallow respirations
  - Presence of dependent edema
  - Auscultation of crackles or wheezes
  - Presence of distended neck veins in a sitting position
  - Decreased oxygen saturation
  - Elevated blood pressure
  - Narrowed pulse pressure
- Assess level of consciousness and degree of cognition.
- Ask about the presence of headache or blurred vision.

Interventions. Management of the patient with CKD includes drug therapy, nutrition therapy, fluid restriction, and dialysis. Dialysis using extracorporeal blood circulation (hemodialysis) is done intermittently for 3 to 4 hours, typically 3 days per week. Alternatively, some patients with ESKD receive peritoneal dialysis. PD uses the peritoneum as the dialyzing membrane. The dialysate is infused through a catheter implanted in the peritoneum. Dialysis for ESKD is described on pp. 1431-1437 in this chapter.

The purpose of fluid management is to attain fluid balance and prevent complications of fluid overload (Chart 68-5). Monitor the patient's intake and output and hydration status. Assess for manifestations of fluid overload (e.g., lung crackles, edema, distended neck veins).

Drug therapy with diuretics is prescribed for patients with mild to severe CKD to increase urinary ELIMINATION of fluid. The increased urine output produced from these drugs helps reduce fluid overload and hypertension in patients who still have some urine output. Diuretics are seldom used in ESKD after dialysis is started because, as kidney function is reduced, these drugs can have harmful side effects on the remaining kidney cells and on a patient's hearing.

Assess fluid status by obtaining daily weights and reviewing intake and output. Daily weight gain in these patients indicates fluid retention rather than true body weight gain. Estimate the amount of fluid retained: 1 kg of weight equals about 1 L of fluid retained. Weigh the patient daily at the same time each day, on the same scale, wearing the same amount of clothing, and after voiding (if the patient is not anuric). Monitor weight for changes before and after dialysis.

Fluid restriction is often needed. Consider all forms of fluid intake, including oral, IV, and enteral sources, when calculating fluid intake. Assist the patient in spreading oral fluid intake over a 24-hour period. Monitor his or her response to fluid restriction, and notify the health care provider if manifestations of fluid overload persist or worsen.

Preventing Pulmonary Edema

Planning: Expected Outcomes. The patient with CKD is expected to remain free of pulmonary edema by maintaining optimal fluid balance. Indicators include that the patient has no breathing difficulty and no adventitious lung sounds (e.g., crackles, wheezes) with auscultation and that oxygen saturation remains greater than 92%.

Interventions. In the patient with CKD, pulmonary edema can result from left-sided heart failure related to fluid overload or from blood vessel injury. In left-sided heart failure, the heart is unable to eject blood adequately from the left ventricle, leading to an increased pressure in the left atrium and in the pulmonary blood vessels. The increased pressure causes fluid to cross the capillaries into the pulmonary tissue, forming edema (McCance et al., 2014). Pulmonary edema can also occur from injury to the lung blood vessels as a result of uremia. This condition causes INFLAMMATION and capillary leak. Fluid then leaks from pulmonary circulation into the lung tissue and the alveoli. It may also leak into the pleural space, causing a *pleural effusion*.

Assess the patient for early indicators of pulmonary edema, such as restlessness, anxiety, rapid heart rate, shortness of breath, and crackles that begin at the base of the lungs. As pulmonary edema worsens, the level of fluid in the lungs rises. Auscultation reveals increased crackles and decreased breath sounds. The patient may have frothy, blood-tinged sputum. As cardiac and pulmonary function decrease further, the patient becomes diaphoretic and cyanotic.

The patient with pulmonary edema usually is admitted to the hospital for aggressive treatment and continuous cardiac monitoring. Place the patient in a high-Fowler's position and give oxygen to improve gas exchange. Drug therapy with kidney failure and pulmonary edema is difficult because of potential adverse drug effects on the kidneys. Loop diuretics such as IV furosemide (Lasix) are used to manage pulmonary edema. Kidney impairment increases the risk for *ototoxicity* (ear damage with hearing loss) with furosemide; thus IV doses are given cautiously. Diuresis usually begins within 5 minutes of giving IV furosemide. Measure urine output every 15 to 30 minutes during the acute episode and every hour thereafter until the patient is stabilized. Monitor vital signs and assess breath sounds at least every 2 hours to evaluate the patient's response to this treatment.

IV morphine sulfate (1 to 2 mg) can be prescribed to reduce myocardial oxygen demand by triggering blood vessel dilation and to provide sedation. Dosage adjustments are needed to achieve the desired response and avoid respiratory depression. Monitor the patient's respiratory rate, oxygen saturation, and blood pressure hourly during this therapy. Other drugs that dilate blood vessels, such as nitroglycerin, may be given as a continuous infusion to reduce pulmonary pressure from left heart failure. Monitor vital signs at least hourly because this drug combination may cause severe hypotension.

Monitor serum electrolyte levels daily, and report abnormalities to the health care provider so that imbalances can be corrected quickly. If using electrocardiogram (ECG) monitoring, identify dysrhythmias as they occur and report changes in rhythm that affect consciousness or blood pressure immediately to the health care provider. Monitor oxygen saturation levels by pulse oximetry, and consult with the respiratory therapist for the optimal method to deliver oxygen (e.g., facemask, nasal cannula, or noninvasive mechanical support [see Chapter 28]). Monitor the patient for worsening of the condition, manifested as increasing hypoxemia. He or she may require temporary intubation and mechanical ventilation if respiratory failure occurs.

Patients with CKD who have existing cardiac problems, high blood pressure, or chronic fluid retention are at increased risk for developing pulmonary edema. They are less likely to respond quickly to treatment and are more likely to develop problems related to drug therapy. Ultrafiltration may be used with these patients to reduce fluid volume.

Increasing Cardiac Output

Planning: Expected Outcomes. The patient with CKD is expected to attain and maintain adequate cardiac output. Indicators include that systolic and diastolic blood pressures, ejection fraction, peripheral pulses, and cognitive status are either normal or nearly normal.

Interventions. Many patients with long-standing hypertension are at risk for CKD and accelerated progression of kidney failure once CKD occurs. *Therefore blood pressure control is essential in preserving kidney function.* To control blood pressure, calcium channel blockers, angiotensin-converting enzyme (ACE) inhibitors, alpha-adrenergic and beta-adrenergic blockers, and vasodilators may be prescribed. ACE inhibitors are the most effective drugs to slow the progression of CKD in patients with hypertension. Calcium channel blockers can improve the GFR and blood flow within the kidney.

More information on the specific drugs for blood pressure control can be found in Chapter 36. Indications vary depending on the patient, and these drugs are used carefully to avoid complications. Different dosages and combinations may be tried until blood pressure control is adequate and side effects are minimized.

Teach the patient and family to measure blood pressure daily. Evaluate their ability to measure and record blood pressure accurately using their own equipment. Re-check measurement accuracy on a regular basis. Teach the patient and family about the relationship of blood pressure control to diet and drug therapy. Instruct the patient to weigh daily and to bring records of blood pressure measurements, drug administration times, and weights for discussion with the physician, nurse, or registered dietitian.

Assess the patient on an ongoing basis for manifestations of reduced cardiac output, heart failure, and dysrhythmias. These topics are discussed in Chapters 35 through 38.

Enhancing Nutrition

Planning: Expected Outcomes. The patient with CKD is expected to maintain adequate nutrition. The patient should have a protein-caloric intake appropriate for his or her weight-to-height ratio, muscle tone, and laboratory values (serum albumin, hematocrit, hemoglobin).

Interventions. The nutrition needs and diet restrictions for the patient with CKD vary according to the degree of kidney function and the type of renal replacement therapy used (Table 68-9). The purpose of nutrition therapy is to provide the food and fluids needed to prevent malnutrition and avoid complications from CKD.

The patient is referred to a dietitian for dietary teaching and planning. Work with the dietitian to teach the patient about diet changes that are needed as a result of CKD. Common changes include control of protein intake; fluid intake limitation; restriction of potassium, sodium, and phosphorus intake; taking vitamin and mineral supplements; and eating enough calories to meet metabolic need.

Protein restriction early in the course of the disease prevents some of the problems of CKD and may preserve kidney function. Protein is restricted on the basis of the degree of kidney impairment (reduced GFR) and the severity of the manifestations. Buildup of waste products from protein breakdown is the main cause of uremia.

The glomerular filtration rate (GFR) and treatment of CKD is used to guide safe levels of protein intake. A patient with a severely reduced GFR who is *not* undergoing dialysis is usually permitted 0.55 to 0.60 g of protein per kilogram of body weight (e.g., 40 g of protein daily for a 150-lb [70-kg] adult). If protein is lost in the urine, protein is added to the diet in amounts equal to that lost in the urine. Protein requirements are calculated based on actual body weight (corrected for edema), not ideal body weight.

The patient with ESKD receiving dialysis needs more protein because some protein is lost through dialysis. Protein requirements are tailored according to the patient's post-dialysis, or "dry," weight. Generally, patients receiving dialysis are allowed about 1 to 1.5 g of protein/kg/day. Peritoneal dialysis (PD) patients are allowed 1.2 to 1.5 g of protein/kg/day because protein is lost with each exchange. Suggested protein-containing foods are milk, meat, or eggs. If protein intake is not adequate, significant muscle wasting can occur. BUN and serum prealbumin and albumin levels are used to monitor the adequacy of protein intake. Decreased serum prealbumin or albumin levels indicate poor protein intake.

Sodium restriction is needed in patients with little or no urine output. Both fluid and sodium retention cause edema, hypertension, and heart failure (HF). Most patients with CKD retain sodium; a few cannot conserve sodium.

Estimate fluid and sodium retention status by monitoring the patient's body weight and blood pressure. In uremic patients not receiving dialysis, sodium is limited to 1 to 3 g daily and fluid intake depends on urine output. In patients receiving dialysis, the sodium restriction is 2 to 4 g daily and fluid intake

TABLE 68-9 Dietary Restrictions Needed for Severe Kidney Disease

DIETARY COMPONENT	WITH CHRONIC UREMIA	WITH HEMODIALYSIS	WITH PERITONEAL DIALYSIS
Protein	0.55-0.60 g/kg/day	1.0-1.5 g/kg/day	1.2-1.5 g/kg/day
Fluid	Depends on urine output but may be as high as 1500-3000 mL/day	500-700 mL/day plus amount of urine output	Restriction based on fluid weight gain and blood pressure
Potassium	60-70 mEq/day	70 mEq/day	Usually no restriction
Sodium	1-3 g/day	2-4 g/day	Restriction based on fluid weight gain and blood pressure
Phosphorus	700 mg/day	700 mg/day	800 mg/day

is limited to 500 to 700 mL plus the amount of any urine output. Instruct the patient not to add salt at the table or during cooking. Many foods are significant sources of sodium (e.g., processed foods, fast foods, potato chips, pretzels, pickles, ham, bacon, sausage) and difficult to moderate or remove from one's diet. Inattention to sodium intake can increase the duration or number of dialysis treatments and contribute to *disequilibrium syndrome* (feeling "zonked") following dialysis.

Potassium restriction may be needed because high blood potassium levels can cause dangerous cardiac dysrhythmias. Monitor the ECG for tall, peaked T waves caused by hyperkalemia. Document serum potassium levels. Instruct the patient with ESKD to limit potassium intake to 60 to 70 mEq/day. Teach him or her to read labels of seasoning agents carefully for sodium and potassium content. Chart 11-6 in Chapter 11 lists common foods that are low in potassium and are permitted, along with foods that are high in potassium and should be avoided. Instruct patients to avoid salt substitutes composed of potassium chloride. Those receiving peritoneal dialysis or who are producing urine may not need potassium restriction.

Phosphorus restriction for control of phosphorus levels is started early in CKD to avoid renal osteodystrophy (bone defects). Monitor serum phosphorus levels. Dietary phosphorus restrictions and drugs to assist with phosphorus control may be prescribed. Phosphate binders must be taken at mealtimes. Most patients with CKD already restrict their protein intake, and because high-protein foods are also high in phosphorus, this reduces phosphorus intake. Chapter 11 lists foods high in potassium, sodium, and phosphorus. Cinacalcet (Sensipar), a drug to control parathyroid hormone excess, is also used to manage hyperphosphatemia and hypocalcemia.

Vitamin and mineral supplementation is needed daily for most patients with CKD. Low-protein diets are also low in vitamins, and water-soluble vitamins are removed from the blood during dialysis. Anemia also is a problem in patients with CKD because of the limited iron content of low-protein diets and decreased kidney production of erythropoietin. Thus supplemental iron is needed. Calcium and vitamin D supplements may be needed, depending on the patient's serum calcium levels and bone status.

Nutrition needs for patients undergoing peritoneal dialysis (PD) are slightly different from those for patients undergoing dialysis. Because protein is lost with the dialysate in PD, replacing lost protein is needed. Often 1.2 to 1.5 g of protein per kilogram of body weight per day is recommended. Patients may have anorexia and have difficulty eating enough protein. High-calorie oral supplements may also be needed (e.g., Magnacal Renal, Ensure Plus). Sodium restriction varies with fluid weight gain and blood pressure. Usually dietary potassium does not need to be restricted because the dialysate is potassium-free. Any potassium restriction is determined by serum potassium levels.

Collaborate with the dietitian to assess each patient's nutrition needs. Teach the patient the dietary regimen, and evaluate his or her understanding of and adherence to it. Give the patient and family written examples of the diet to promote adherence. Help patients adapt diet restrictions to their budget, ethnic background, and food preferences.

Preventing Infection

Planning: Expected Outcomes. The patient with CKD is expected to remain free of INFECTION. Indicators include that the patient will have only mild or no fever, no lymph node enlargement, negative urine culture, negative dialysis access site culture, and white blood cell count either within the normal range or only slightly elevated.

Interventions. Provide meticulous care to any areas where skin is not intact (e.g., incisions, site of drains, puncture sites, cracked or excoriated skin, pressure ulcers), and provide preventive skin care to intact areas. For patients with ESKD undergoing dialysis, inspect the vascular access site or peritoneal dialysis catheter insertion site every shift for redness, swelling, pain, and drainage. Monitor vital signs for manifestations of INFECTION (e.g., fever, tachycardia).

Preventing Injury

Planning: Expected Outcomes. The patient with CKD is expected to remain free of injury. Indicators include that the patient should not have any of these problems:

- Pathologic fractures
- Toxic side effects from drug therapy
- Bleeding

Interventions. *Injury prevention strategies* are needed because the patient with long-standing CKD may have brittle, fragile bones that fracture easily and cause little pain. When lifting or moving a patient with fragile bones, use a lift sheet rather than pulling the patient. Teach unlicensed assistive personnel (UAP) the correct use of lift sheets. Observe for normal range of joint motion and for any unusual surface bumps or depressions over bony areas.

Managing drug therapy in patients with CKD is a complex clinical problem. Many over-the-counter drugs contain agents that alter kidney function. Therefore it is important to obtain a detailed drug history. Know the use of each drug, its side effects, and its site of metabolism.

Certain drugs must be avoided, and the dosages of others must be adjusted according to the degree of remaining kidney function. As the patient's kidney function decreases, repeated dosage adjustments are necessary. Assess for side effects and indications of drug toxicity, and notify the prescriber as appropriate.

! NURSING SAFETY PRIORITY (QSEN)

Drug Alert

Monitor the patient with severe CKD or ESKD closely for drug-related complications, and ensure that dosages are adjusted as needed. Consult with the pharmacist to determine safe effective doses.

Many drugs are routinely given to patients with CKD, and some of the common drugs are detailed in Chart 68-6. Know the rationale for these drugs and the indicated nursing interventions. Many patients also have cardiac disease and may require cardiac drugs such as digoxin. Patients with severe CKD and ESKD are particularly at risk for digoxin toxicity because the drug is excreted by the kidneys. When caring for patients with CKD who are receiving digoxin, monitor for indications of

! NURSING SAFETY PRIORITY (QSEN)

Drug Alert

Doses of digoxin are much lower than for most drugs. When digoxin is administered to older adults with kidney disease, the prescribed daily dose may be even lower (0.0625 mg). Check and recheck the dosage before administering digoxin to a patient with kidney disease.

toxicity, such as nausea, vomiting, anorexia, visual changes, restlessness, headache, fatigue, confusion, bradycardia, and tachycardia. Monitor the serum drug levels to be certain they are in the therapeutic range (0.8-2 ng/mL). Also closely monitor the serum potassium levels of any patient receiving digoxin.

Drugs to control an excessively high phosphorus level include phosphate-binding agents. Non-calcium binders may be preferred to reduce the risk for extraskeletal deposition of calcium and subsequent vessel disease or stone formation (Lewis, 2012). These drugs help prevent renal osteodystrophy and related

CHART 68-6 Common Examples of Drug Therapy

Chronic Kidney Disease

DRUG/DOSAGE	ACTION/PURPOSE	NURSING INTERVENTIONS	RATIONALES
Loop Diuretics			
Furosemide (Lasix) Bumetanide (Bumex, Burinex) Dose varies with severity of kidney damage; not effective in ESKD	Manage volume overload when urinary elimination is still present.	Monitor intake and output.	Generally the expected outcome is for output to be greater than intake by 500-1000 mL per 24 hr.
		Monitor electrolytes.	Loop diuretics result in loss of potassium; this can be a desired effect in patients with hyperkalemia
Vitamins and Minerals			
Phosphate Binders: Calcium acetate (PhosLo) 2-4 capsules with each meal Calcium carbonate (Caltrate, Oystercal, others) 2-4 capsules with each meal Lanthanum carbonate (Fosrenol) 500-1000 mg tablets Sevelamer (Renagel, Renvela) 400-800 mg Taken just before or with meals	High blood phosphorus levels cause hypocalcemia and osteodystrophy. These drugs bind to dietary phosphorous and phosphate, typically by using calcium to form an insoluble calcium phosphate such that neither mineral is absorbed from the gastrointestinal tract. These are non-calcium, non-aluminum phosphate binders.	Teach patients to take drugs with meals. Teach patients not to take these drugs within 2 hours of other schedule drugs. Teach patients to separate administration of phosphate binders from other scheduled drugs by 2 or more hours. Monitor both serum phosphorus and calcium levels. Monitor for constipation.	Oral phosphate binders reduce hyperphosphatemia common in severe CKD and ESKD. Many of these drugs can bind with other oral drugs—notably cardiovascular drugs and antibiotics. Drugs that use calcium to bind phosphorus can cause hypercalcemia. Bound phosphorus is excreted in feces. These drugs can cause significant constipation leading to fecal impaction or ileus. Manage constipation with stool softeners like docusate or bowel stimulants such as senna.
		Teach patients to report muscle weakness, slow or irregular pulse, or confusion to the prescriber.	These are manifestations of hypophosphatemia, which require dosage adjustment.
Multivitamins and vitamin B supplements: Folic acid (vitamin B_9, Folvite, Novo-Folacid 🍁) 1 mg orally daily	When the patient is receiving dialysis, many essential vitamins and minerals are removed from the blood. Replacement is needed to prevent severe deficiencies.	Teach patients to take the drugs after dialysis. Teach patients to take iron supplements (ferrous sulfate) with meals.	Dialysis removes the drug from the blood. Food reduces nausea and abdominal discomfort.
Iron Salts: Ferrous sulfate (Feosol, Novoferrosulfa 🍁) 325 mg orally three or four times daily Iron sucrose (Venofer) 20 mg/mL; 100 mg per dialysis session		Teach patients to take stool softeners daily while taking iron supplements.	Oral iron preparations cause constipation, and most patients with kidney disease must reduce their fluid intake, further increasing the risk for constipation.
		Remind patients that iron supplements change the color of the stool.	Knowing the expected side effects decreases anxiety when they appear.
Vitamin D: Calcitriol (Rocaltrol, Calcijex, Vectical) 0.25-0.5 mcg capsules or 1 mcg/mL solution Paricalcitol (Zemplar) 1-4 mcg capsules or injectable solution	This is the active form of vitamin D. It is used to suppress parathyroid production and secretion and to treat hypocalcemia.	Monitor serum levels of vitamin D and calcium.	Monitor for hypocalcemia or evidence of vitamin D toxicity.
Doxercalciferol (Hectorol) 0.25-2.5 mg, given 3 times/weekly at dialysis	This is a vitamin D analog that does not require activation by the kidneys.		

Continued

CHART 68-6 **Common Examples of Drug Therapy—cont'd**

Chronic Kidney Disease

DRUG/DOSAGE	ACTION/PURPOSE	NURSING INTERVENTIONS	RATIONALES
Erythropoietin-Stimulating Agents (ESAs)			
Epoetin alfa (Epogen, Procrit, generic) 50-100 units/kg subcutaneously or IV three times a week for patients on dialysis Darbepoetin alfa (Aranesp) 0.45 mcg/kg subcutaneously or IV once weekly for patients on dialysis	Drug prevents anemia by stimulating red blood cell growth and maturation in the bone marrow.	Monitor hemoglobin values. Start when hemoglobin is less than 10 g/dL and the rate of decline indicates the likelihood of requiring a red blood cell transfusion. Once the hemoglobin level is greater than 11 g/dL, reduce or interrupt dose. Teach patients to report any of these side effects to the prescriber as soon as possible: chest pain, difficulty breathing, high blood pressure, rapid weight gain, seizures, skin rash or hives, swelling of feet or ankles.	Drug can induce serious cardiovascular problems, such as myocardial infarction (MI).
Parathyroid Hormone Modulator			
Cinacalcet (Sensipar) 30-180 mg daily	Reduce parathyroid hormone levels. This drug increases the sensitivity to calcium on the chief cell receptors in the parathyroid gland.	Monitor levels of serum calcium. Teach the patient to monitor for diarrhea and muscle pain (myalgia).	This drug should not be used in severe hypocalcemia (levels less than 8.4 mg/dL).

CKD, Chronic kidney disease; *ESKD,* end-stage kidney disease.

injuries. Stress the importance of taking these agents and all prescribed drugs.

Hypophosphatemia (low serum phosphorus levels) is a complication of phosphate binding, especially in patients who are not eating adequately but who are continuing to take phosphate-binding drugs. *Hypercalcemia* (high serum calcium levels) also is a possible complication for patients taking calcium-containing compounds to control phosphorus excess. In patients taking aluminum-based phosphate binders for prolonged periods, aluminum deposits may cause bone disease or permanent neurologic problems. Monitor the patient for muscle weakness, anorexia, malaise, tremors, and bone pain.

Teach patients with kidney disease to avoid antacids containing magnesium. These patients cannot excrete magnesium and thus should avoid additional intake.

Some drugs, in addition to those used to treat kidney failure, require special attention. These drugs include antibiotics, opioids, antihypertensives, diuretics, insulin, and heparin.

Many antibiotics are safe for patients with CKD, but those excreted by the kidney require dose adjustment. To prevent complications of bloodstream INFECTION from mouth bacteria, prophylactic antibiotic treatment is given to patients with CKD before any dental procedures. The antibiotic used varies with the patient's needs and the health care provider's preference.

Give opioid analgesics cautiously in patients with severe CKD or ESKD because the effects often last longer. Patients with uremia are sensitive to the respiratory depressant effects of these drugs. Because opioids are broken down by the liver and not the kidneys, the dosages are often the same regardless of the level of kidney function. Monitor the patient's reactions closely after opioids are given to determine whether adjustments are needed.

As CKD progresses, the patient with diabetes often requires reduced doses of insulin or antidiabetic drugs because the failing kidneys do not excrete or metabolize these drugs well. Thus the drugs are effective longer, increasing the risk for hypoglycemia. Monitor blood glucose levels at least 4 times daily to assess whether a dosage change is needed.

Poor platelet function and capillary fragility in CKD make anticoagulant therapy risky. Monitor patients receiving heparin, warfarin, or any anticoagulant every shift for bleeding. See Chapter 40 for more information on caring for patients at increased risk for bleeding.

Minimizing Fatigue

Planning: Expected Outcomes. The patient with chronic kidney disease (CKD) is expected to conserve energy by balancing activity and rest. Indicators include that the patient will be able to participate in self-care activities, have interest in surroundings, and demonstrate mental concentration.

Interventions. Some causes of fatigue in the patient with CKD include vitamin deficiency, anemia, and buildup of urea. All patients are given vitamin and mineral supplements because of diet restrictions and vitamin losses from dialysis. Avoid giving these supplements before hemodialysis (HD) treatment because they will be dialyzed out of the body and the patient will receive no benefit.

The anemic patient with CKD is treated with agents to stimulate red blood cell production (Dutka, 2012). The outcome of this therapy is to maintain a hemoglobin level around 10 g/dL. This therapy is effective in triggering bone marrow production of red blood cells if the patient has adequate iron stores. Iron supplements may be needed if patients are iron deficient. Many who receive these drugs report improved appetite and sexual function along with decreased fatigue. The increased production of all blood cells from this therapy may increase blood pressure. The improved appetite challenges patients in their attempts to maintain protein, potassium, and fluid restrictions and requires additional education.

Reducing Anxiety

Planning: Expected Outcomes. The patient with CKD is expected to have reduced tension and apprehension. Indicators include that the patient consistently demonstrates these behaviors:

- Seeks information to reduce anxiety
- Uses effective coping strategies
- Reports an absence of anxiety manifestations

Interventions. The nurse coordinates a team of health care professionals to support and counsel the patient and family, often over many years of treatment. The nurse has the most contact with the patient when he or she is hospitalized or undergoing in-center dialysis treatments. Perform an ongoing assessment of the patient's anxiety level. Observe behavior for cues indicating anxiety (e.g., anxious facial expressions, clenching of hands, tapping of feet, withdrawn posture, absence of eye contact, an increased pulse rate). Evaluate the support systems, such as the involvement of family and friends with the patient's care.

Unfamiliar settings and lack of knowledge about treatments and tests can increase the patient's anxiety level. Explain all procedures, tests, and treatments. Identify the patient's knowledge needs about kidney disease. Provide instruction at a level he or she can understand using a variety of written and visual materials.

Provide continuity of care, whenever possible, by using a consistent nurse-patient relationship to decrease anxiety and promote discussions of concerns. As you develop the nurse-patient relationship, encourage the patient to discuss current problems or concerns.

Encourage the patient to ask questions and discuss fears about the diagnosis. An open atmosphere that allows for discussion can decrease anxiety. Facilitate discussions with family members about the prognosis and the impact on lifestyle.

Renal Replacement Therapies

Renal replacement therapy (RRT) is needed when the pathologic changes of stage 4 and stage 5 CKD are life threatening or pose continuing discomfort. When the patient can no longer be managed with conservative therapies, such as diet, drugs, and fluid restriction, dialysis is indicated. Transplantation may be discussed at any time.

Hemodialysis

Intermittent hemodialysis (HD) is the most common RRT used with ESKD (Table 68-10). Dialysis removes excess fluids and waste products and restores chemical and electrolyte balance. HD involves passing the patient's blood through an artificial semipermeable membrane to perform the filtering and excretion functions of the kidney. This therapy usually requires technicians to provide meticulous care to the machines delivering HD and nurses to implement and supervise direct care. Such measures are essential to safe HD. Technical or human error can lead to avoidable complications (e.g., hemolysis, air embolism, dialysate error, contamination).

Patient Selection. Any patient may be considered for intermittent HD therapy. Starting HD depends on manifestations from disruptions of FLUID AND ELECTROLYTE BALANCE and waste and toxin accumulation, not the GFR alone (Yeun et al., 2012). Dialysis is started immediately for patients who have:

- Fluid overload that does not respond to diuretics (including fluid overload with pericarditis)
- Symptomatic hyperkalemia
- Calciphylaxis (a condition of thrombosis and skin necrosis that can occur in stage 5 CKD)
- Symptomatic toxin ingestion such as drug overdose or poisoning that is dialyzable (see Table 68-13)

Most commonly, hemodialysis for CKD is started when uremic manifestations (e.g., nausea and vomiting, decreased attention span, decreased cognition, and pruritus) are present.

Many patients survive for years with HD therapy, and others may live only a few months. How long the patient survives using HD therapy depends on his or her age, the cause of CKD, and the presence of other diseases, such as cardiovascular disease or diabetes. General patient selection criteria are:

- Irreversible kidney failure when other therapies are unacceptable or ineffective
- No disorders that would seriously complicate HD
- Patient values and preferences
- Expected ability to continue or resume roles at home, work, or school

TABLE 68-10 Comparison of Hemodialysis and Peritoneal Dialysis

HEMODIALYSIS	PERITONEAL DIALYSIS
Advantages	
More efficient clearance of wastes	Flexible schedule for exchanges
Short time needed for treatment	Few hemodynamic changes during and following exchanges
	Less dietary and fluid restrictions
Complications	
Disequilibrium syndrome	Protein loss
Muscle cramps and back pain	Peritonitis
Headache	Hyperglycemia from dialysate
Itching	Respiratory distress
Hemodynamic and cardiac adverse events (hypotension, cell lysis contributing to anemia, cardiac dysrhythmias)	Bowel perforation
	Infection
	Weight gain; discomfort from "carrying" 1-2 liters in abdomen during dwell time; potential for back pain or development of hernia
Infection	
Increased risk for subdural and intracranial hemorrhage from anticoagulation and changes in blood pressure during dialysis	
Contraindications	
Hemodynamic instability or severe cardiac disease	Extensive peritoneal adhesions, fibrosis, or active inflammatory gastrointestinal disease (e.g., diverticulitis, inflammatory bowel conditions)
Severe vascular disease that prevents vascular access	Ascites or massive central obesity
Serious bleeding disorders	Recent abdominal surgery
Uncontrolled diabetes	
Access	
Vascular access route	Intra-abdominal catheter
Procedure	
Complex; requires a second person trained in the technique whether completed at home or at a dialysis unit/center	Simple, easier to complete at home compared with at-home hemodialysis
Special training for center personnel and in-home use; requires at least two people to manage process	Less complex training; typically managed by patient; can be managed by one person

Dialysis Settings. Patients with CKD may receive HD treatments in many settings, depending on specific needs. Regardless of the setting for therapy, they need ongoing nursing support to maintain this complex and lifesaving treatment.

Patients may be dialyzed in a hospital-based center if they have recently started treatment or have complicated conditions that require close supervision. Stable patients not requiring intense supervision may be dialyzed in a community or free-standing dialysis center. Selected patients may participate in complete or partial self-care in an ambulatory care center or with in-home HD.

In-home HD is the least disruptive and allows the patient to adapt the regimen to his or her lifestyle. Many cannot participate in in-home dialysis because they lack a skilled partner to assist with the therapy and manage the dialysis machine. Some patients and partners find the use of in-home dialysis to be too stressful. In addition, a water treatment system must be installed in the home to provide a safe, clean water supply for the dialysis process. More compact and more easily managed systems have contributed to the growth of in-home HD (Yeun et al., 2012).

Procedure. Dialysis works using the passive transfer of toxins by diffusion. **Diffusion** is the movement of molecules from an area of higher concentration to an area of lower concentration. The rate of diffusion during dialysis is most dependent on the difference in the solute concentrations between the patient's blood and the dialysate. Large molecules, such as RBCs and most plasma proteins, cannot pass through the membrane.

When HD is started, blood and **dialysate** (dialyzing solution) flow in opposite directions across an enclosed semipermeable membrane. The dialysate contains a balanced mix of electrolytes and water that closely resembles human plasma. On the other side of the membrane is the patient's blood, which contains nitrogen waste products, excess water, and excess electrolytes. During HD, the waste products move from the blood into the dialysate because of the difference in their concentrations (diffusion). Some water is also removed from the blood into the dialysate by *osmosis*. Electrolytes can move in either direction, as needed, and take some fluid with them. Potassium and sodium typically move out of the plasma into the dialysate. Bicarbonate and calcium generally move from the dialysate into the plasma. This circulating process continues for a preset length of time, removing nitrogenous wastes and reestablishing FLUID AND ELECTROLYTE BALANCE, as well as restoring ACID-BASE BALANCE. Water volume may be removed from the plasma by applying positive or negative pressure to the system.

The HD system includes a dialyzer, dialysate, vascular access routes, and an HD machine. The artificial kidney, or **dialyzer** (Fig. 68-3), has four parts: a blood compartment, a dialysate compartment, a semipermeable membrane, and an enclosed support structure.

Dialysate is made from water and chemicals and is free of any waste products or drugs. Often dialysate is made in the pharmacy in an acute care setting. It may be made by technicians in dialysis centers. Because bacteria and other organisms are too large to pass through the membrane, dialysate is not sterile. The water used in dialysate must meet specific standards and usually requires special treatment before mixing the dialysate. The dialysate composition may be altered according to the patient's needs for management of electrolyte imbalances. During HD, the dialysate is warmed to 100° F (37.8° C) to increase the diffusion rate and to prevent hypothermia.

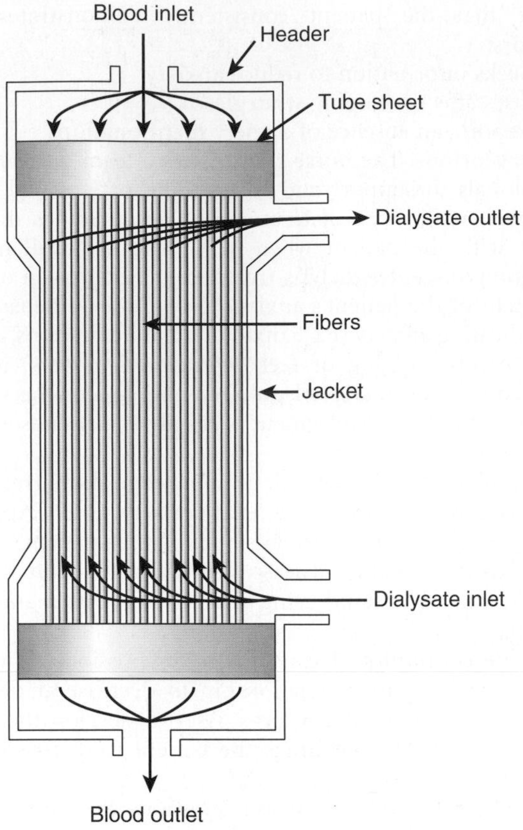

FIG. 68-3 Hollow fiber dialyzer (artificial kidney) used in hemodialysis.

The HD machine has built-in safety features such as the ability to record patient vital signs, blood and dialysate flows, arterial and venous pressures, delivered dialysis dose, plasma volume changes and thermal changes. If any of these problems are detected, an alarm sounds to protect the patient from life-threatening complications.

All dialyzers function in a similar manner. Fig. 68-4 shows a comparison of fluid and particle movement across the dialyzer membranes, comparing intermittent HD with continuous renal replacement circuits. For intermittent HD, the number and length of treatments depend on the amount of wastes and fluid to be removed, the clearance capacity of the dialyzer, and the blood flow rate to and from the machine. Fig. 68-5 shows a typical intermittent dialysis machine. Most patients receive three 4-hour treatments over the course of a week. For those with some ongoing urine production, two 5- to 6-hour treatments a week may be adequate. If the patient gains large amounts of fluid, a longer HD treatment time may be needed to remove the fluid without hypotension or severe side effects.

Anticoagulation. Blood clotting can occur during dialysis. Anticoagulation, usually with heparin, is most often delivered into the blood circuit via a pump. In patients with high risk for bleeding, a reduced dose, regional anticoagulation (using citrate rather than heparin for anticoagulation or reversing heparin actions by administering protamine before returning blood to the patient), or no anticoagulation may be used. Patient response to heparin varies, and the dose is adjusted on the basis of each patient's need.

Heparin remains active in the body for 4 to 6 hours after dialysis, increasing the patient's risk for hemorrhage during and immediately after HD treatments. Invasive procedures must be

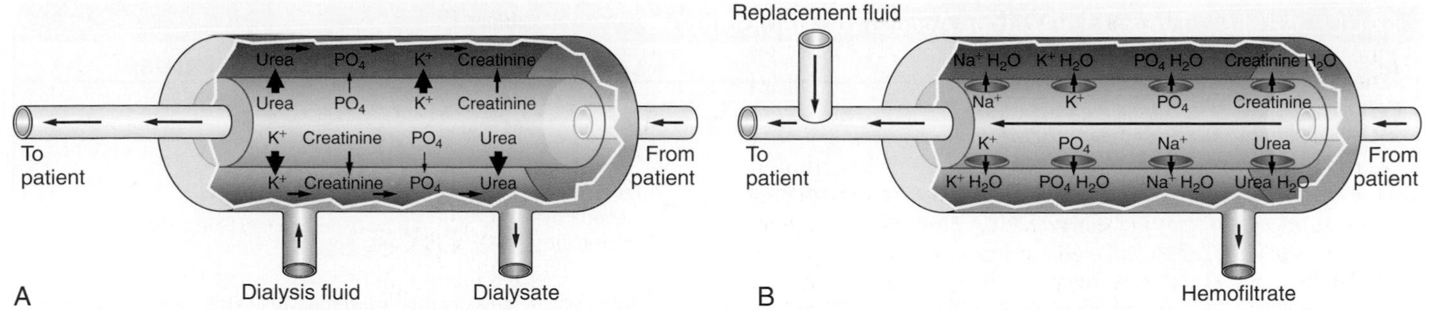

FIG. 68-4 Comparison of hemodialysis and hemofiltration fluid and solute movements across the membrane. Demonstrates this movement in hemodialysis **(A)** and in hemofiltration **(B)**. The *arrows* that cross the membrane indicate the predominant direction of movement of each solute through the membrane; the relative size of the *arrows* indicates the net amounts of the solute transferred. Other *arrows* indicate the direction of flow.

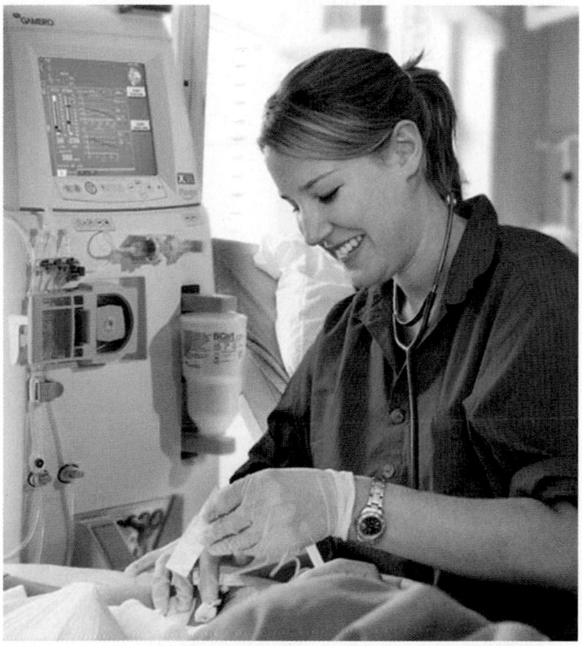

FIG. 68-5 Renal replacement therapy with an intermittent hemodialysis machine.

avoided during that time. Monitor him or her closely for any manifestations of bleeding or hemorrhage. Protamine sulfate is an antidote to heparin and always should be available in the dialysis setting.

Vascular Access. Vascular access is required for hemodialysis (Table 68-11 and Fig. 68-6). The procedure requires the easy availability of a large amount of blood flow: at least 250 to 300 mL/min, usually for a period of 3 to 4 hours. Normal venous cannulation does not provide this high rate of blood flow.

Long-term vascular access is internal for most patients having long-term HD (see Table 68-11). The two common choices are an internal arteriovenous (AV) fistula or an AV graft (see Fig. 68-6 *A*, *B*, and *C*). *AV fistulas* are formed by surgically connecting an artery to a vein. The vessels used most often are the radial or brachial artery and the cephalic vein of the nondominant arm. Fistulas increase venous blood flow to 250 to 400 mL/min, the amount needed for effective dialysis.

Time is needed after anastomosis for the AV fistula to develop. As the AV fistula "matures," the increased pressure of the arterial blood flow into the vein causes the vessel walls to thicken. This thickening increases their strength and durability for repeated cannulation. Patients differ in the amount of time needed for the fistula to mature. Some fistulas may not be ready for use for as long as 4 months after the surgery, and a temporary vascular access (AV shunt or HD catheter) is used during this time. Fig. 68-7 shows a mature fistula.

To access a fistula, cannulate it by inserting two needles—one toward the venous blood flow and one toward the arterial blood flow. This procedure allows the HD machine to draw the blood out through the arterial needle and return it through the venous needle.

Arteriovenous grafts are used when the AV fistula does not develop or when complications limit its use. The polytetrafluoroethylene (PTFE) graft is a synthetic material (GORE-TEX). This type of graft is commonly used for older patients using HD. Figs. 68-6, *A*, and 68-7 show a patient's fistula.

Precautions. Some precautions are needed to ensure the functioning of an internal AV fistula or AV graft. First assess for adequate circulation in the fistula or graft as well as in the lower portion of the arm. Check distal pulses and capillary refill in the arm with the fistula or graft. Then check for a bruit or a thrill by auscultation or palpation over the access site. Chart 68-7 lists best practices for care of the patient with an HD access.

! NURSING SAFETY PRIORITY QSEN

Action Alert

Because repeated compression can result in the loss of the vascular access, avoid taking the blood pressure or performing venipunctures in the arm with the vascular access. Do not use an AV fistula or graft for delivery of IV fluids.

Complications. Complications can occur with any type of access. The most common problems are thrombosis or stenosis, INFECTION, aneurysm formation, ischemia, and heart failure. Table 68-12 lists strategies to prevent access complications.

Thrombosis, or clotting of the AV access, is the most frequent complication. Most grafts fail because of high-pressure arterial flow entering the venous system. The muscle layers of the veins react to this increased pressure by thickening. The venous thickening reduces or occludes blood flow. An interventional radiologist can re-open failing grafts with the injection of a thrombolytic drug (e.g., tPA) to dissolve the clot. The clot usually dissolves within minutes, and often a stricture is revealed

TABLE 68-11 Types of Vascular Access for Hemodialysis

ACCESS TYPE	DESCRIPTION	LOCATION	TIME TO INITIAL USE
Permanent			
AV fistula	An internal anastomosis of an artery to a vein	Forearm Upper arm	2-4 mo or longer
AV graft	Synthetic vessel tubing tunneled beneath the skin, connecting an artery and a vein	Forearm Upper arm Inner thigh	1-2 wk
Temporary			
Dialysis catheter	A specially designed catheter with separate lumens for blood outflow and inflow	Subclavian, internal jugular, or femoral vein	Immediately after insertion and x-ray confirmation of placement
Subcutaneous device	An internal device with two metallic access ports and two catheters inserted into large central veins	Subclavian	

AV, Arteriovenous.

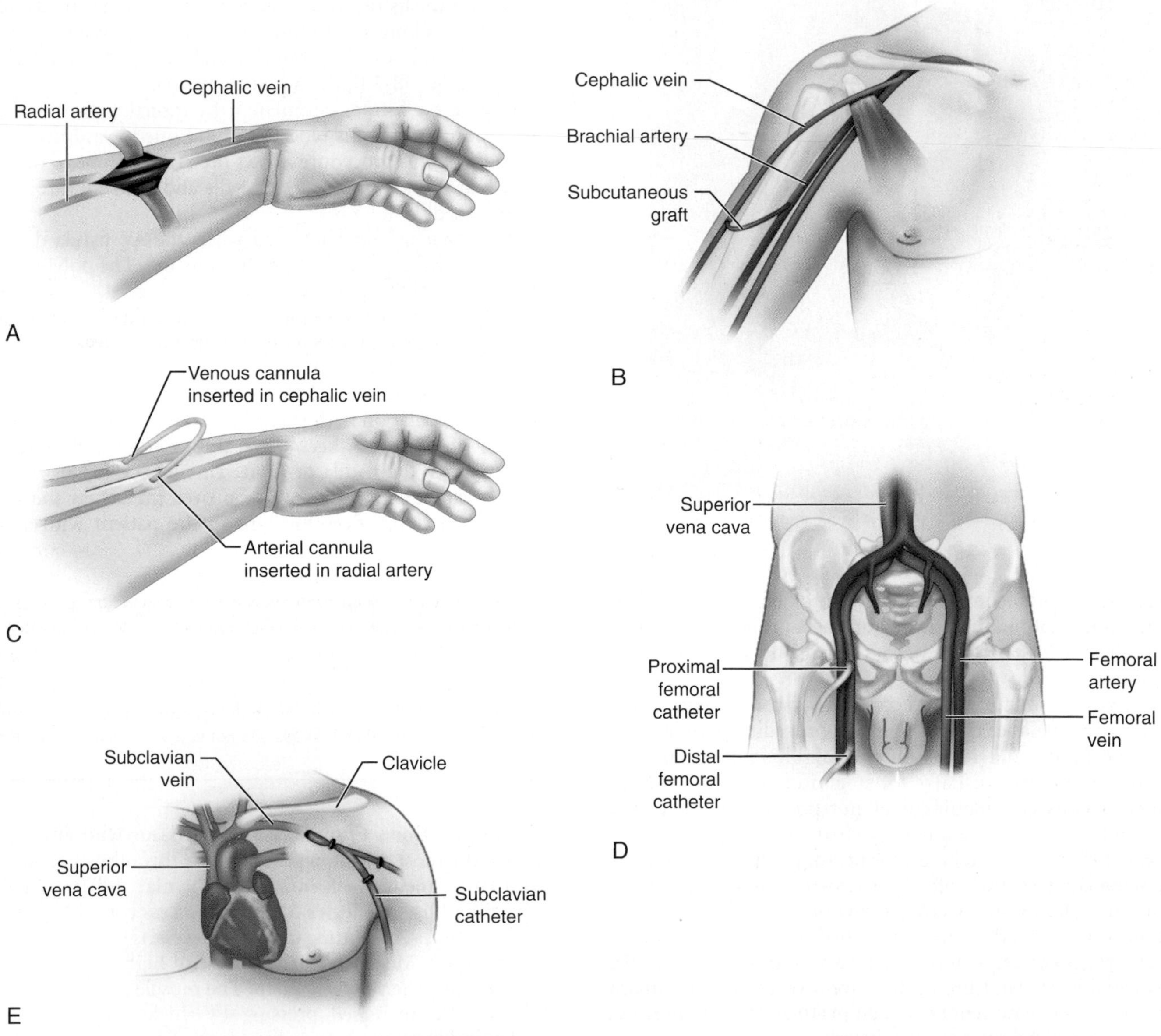

FIG. 68-6 Frequently used means for gaining vascular access for hemodialysis include arteriovenous fistula **(A),** arteriovenous graft **(B),** external arteriovenous shunt **(C),** femoral vein catheterization **(D),** and subclavian vein catheterization **(E)**. **A** and **B** are options for long-term vascular access for hemodialysis. **C, D,** and **E** are used for short-term access for intermittent hemodialysis or for continuous renal replacement therapy in acute care.

TABLE 68-12 Interventions for Preventing Complications in Hemodialysis Vascular Access

ACCESS TYPE	BLEEDING	INFECTION	CLOTTING
AV fistula or AV graft	Apply pressure to the needle puncture sites.	Prepare skin using best practices before cannulation. Typically 2% chlorhexidine is used, similar to central line skin preparation. Between hemodialysis sessions, the patient should wash the area with antibacterial soap and rinse with water.	Avoid constrictive devices. Rotate needle insertion sites with each hemodialysis treatment. Assess for thrill and bruit.
Hemodialysis catheters (temporary and permanent)	Monitor the access site.	Use aseptic technique to dress site and access catheter.	Place a heparin or heparin/saline dwell solution after hemodialysis treatment. Do not use access except for dialysis treatments.

AV, Arteriovenous.

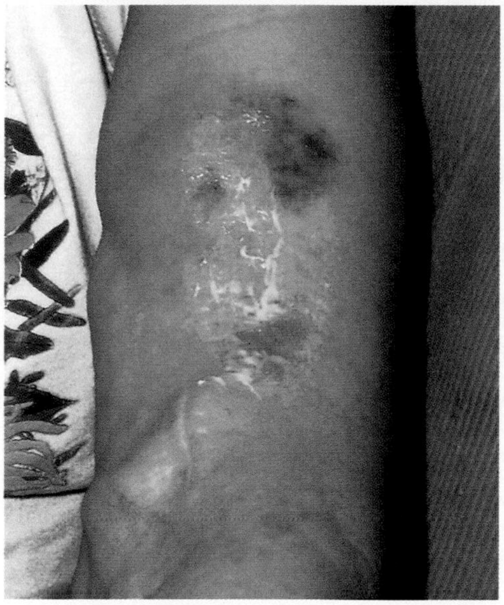

FIG. 68-7 A mature fistula for hemodialysis access. The increased pressure from the anastomosed artery forced blood into the vein. This process caused the vein to dilate enough for fistula needles to be placed for hemodialysis. When the vein is sufficiently dilated, a process that takes 8 to 12 weeks, the fistula is said to be "developed" or "mature."

at the point where the graft and the vein connect. The stricture can be corrected by balloon angioplasty.

Most infections of the vascular access are caused by *Staphylococcus aureus* introduced during cannulation. Prepare the skin with an antibacterial agent according to agency policy before cannulation to prevent INFECTION.

Aneurysms can form in the fistula and are caused by repeated needle punctures at the same site. Large aneurysms may cause loss of the fistula's function and require surgical repair.

Ischemia occurs in a few patients with vascular access when the fistula decreases arterial blood flow to areas below the fistula *(steal syndrome)*. Manifestations vary from cold or numb fingers to gangrene. If the collateral circulation is poor, the fistula may need to be surgically tied off and a new one created in another area to preserve extremity circulation.

Shunting of blood directly from the arterial system to the venous system, through the fistula, can cause heart failure in patients with limited cardiac function. This complication is rare, but if it does occur, the fistula may need to be revised to reduce arterial blood flow.

Temporary Vascular Access. Temporary access with special catheters can be used for patients requiring immediate HD. A catheter designed for HD may be inserted into the subclavian, internal jugular, or femoral vein. The lumens of these devices are much smaller than the permanent accesses, and more time (4 to 8 hours) is required to complete a dialysis session.

Subcutaneous devices may also be surgically inserted to provide temporary access for HD. Implanted beneath the skin, these devices are composed of two small metallic ports with attached catheters that are inserted into large central veins. The ports of subcutaneous devices have internal mechanisms that open when needles are inserted and close when needles are removed. Blood from one port flows from the body to the HD machine and returns to the body via the other port. These devices may be ideal for patients waiting for permanent access placement or a kidney transplant.

CHART 68-7 Best Practice for Patient Safety & Quality Care QSEN

Caring for the Patient with an Arteriovenous Fistula or Arteriovenous Graft

- Do not take blood pressure readings using the extremity in which the vascular access is placed.
- Do not perform venipunctures or start an IV line in the extremity in which the vascular access is placed.
- Palpate for thrills and auscultate for bruits over the vascular access site every 4 hours while the patient is awake.
- Assess the patient's distal pulses and circulation in the arm with the access.
- Elevate the affected extremity postoperatively.
- Encourage routine range-of-motion exercises.
- Check for bleeding at needle insertion sites.
- Assess for manifestations of infection at needle sites.
- Instruct the patient not to carry heavy objects or anything that compresses the extremity in which the vascular access is placed.
- Instruct the patient not to sleep with his or her body weight on top of the extremity in which the vascular access is placed.

AV, Arteriovenous.

CLINICAL JUDGMENT CHALLENGE

Evidence-Based Practice; Patient-Centered Care **QSEN**

The patient just completed a vascular "mapping" procedure with an angiogram to plan the site of an AV fistula for hemodialysis. You are considering the care priorities for the patient's return when the AV fistula is formed.

1. What are important teaching points for the period immediately following AV fistula formation?
2. The patient asks if there is anything she can do to make this AV fistula last a long time. How should you respond to promote best practices in AV fistula self-management?
3. What else should this patient know about AV fistula care?

TABLE 68-13 Examples of Dialyzable Drugs

Consult the pharmacist, nephrologist, or dialysis nurse to plan the best time to administer a drug based on the dialysis schedule.

Aminoglycosides
- Amikacin
- Gentamicin
- Tobramycin

Antituberculosis Agents
- Ethambutol
- Isoniazid

Antiviral and Antifungal Agents
- Acyclovir
- Ganciclovir
- Fluconazole

Cephalosporins
- Cefaclor
- Cefazolin
- Cefoxitin
- Ceftizoxime
- Ceftriaxone
- Cefuroxime
- Cefepime

Anticonvulsants
- Ethosuximide
- Gabapentin
- Phenobarbital

Penicillins
- Amoxicillin
- Ampicillin
- Cloxacillin
- Dicloxacillin
- Mezlocillin
- Penicillin G
- Ticarcillin

Miscellaneous
- Aztreonam
- Cimetidine
- Vitamins
- Clavulanic acid
- Allopurinol
- Enalapril
- Aspirin

Hemodialysis Nursing Care. Many drugs are dialyzable (i.e., can be partially removed from the blood during dialysis). Coordinate with the health care provider to assess the patient's drug regimen and determine which drugs should be held until after HD treatment. Table 68-13 lists common dialyzable drugs that should be given *after* rather than before HD. Consult the dialysis nurse or nephrologists to determine if antihypertensive drugs should be given before a scheduled dialysis treatment; some short-acting antihypertensives can contribute to hypotension during dialysis (Ryan, 2012).

The time required to complete an HD treatment usually is at least 4 hours. During this time patients may use various distraction techniques to prevent boredom. This time can be used also for brief health teaching opportunities (see the Quality Improvement box).

Post-Dialysis Care. Closely monitor the patient immediately and for several hours after dialysis for any side effects from the treatment. Common problems include hypotension, headache, nausea, vomiting, dizziness, and muscle cramps.

Obtain vital signs and weight for comparison with pre-dialysis measurements. Blood pressure and weight are expected to be reduced as a result of fluid removal. Hypotension may require rehydration with IV fluids, such as normal saline. The patient's temperature may also be elevated because the dialysis machine warms the blood slightly. If he or she has a fever, sepsis may be present and a blood sample is needed for culture and sensitivity.

The heparin required during HD increases the risk for excessive bleeding. All invasive procedures must be avoided for 4 to 6 hours after dialysis. Continually monitor the patient for hemorrhage during and for at least 1 hour after dialysis (Chart 68-8).

Complications of Hemodialysis. Few adverse events occur during a 3- to 4-hour HD treatment under current practice protocols. Improved water treatment, more physiologic solutions, and improvements in HD equipment and procedures

CHART 68-8 Best Practice for Patient Safety & Quality Care QSEN

Caring for the Patient Undergoing Hemodialysis

- Weigh the patient before and after dialysis.
- Know the patient's dry weight.
- Discuss with the health care provider whether any of the patient's drugs should be withheld until after dialysis.
- Be aware of events that occurred during previous dialysis treatments.
- Measure blood pressure, pulse, respirations, and temperature.
- Assess for manifestations of orthostatic hypotension.
- Assess the vascular access site.
- Observe for bleeding.
- Assess the patient's level of consciousness.
- Assess for headache, nausea, and vomiting.

QUALITY IMPROVEMENT QSEN

Using Hemodialysis Time as a Teachable Moment

Wilson, B., & Lawrence, J. (2013). Implementation of a foot assessment program in a regional satellite hemodialysis setting. *Canadian Association of Nephrology Nurses and Technologists Journal, 23*(2), 41-47.

Because many patients receiving hemodialysis (HD) also have diabetes, the authors designed a quality improvement project to implement guidelines for foot care among their patients in an ambulatory care HD setting. The program included a one-time full assessment of risk for all patients followed by a monthly foot check for all patients with diabetes. Results included early identification of patients with a foot problem, timelier referral for treatment of foot problems, and a high degree of staff and patient satisfaction with the program.

Commentary: Implications for Practice and Research

This is an example of translating guidelines into practice and using guidelines in an uncommon setting to provide consistent assessment for diabetic patients at high risk for impaired self-management. Although the guidelines were Canadian and the implementation occurred in a single site, the steps to translating a guideline into practice and evaluating adherence to practice can be followed by other sites interested in delivering high-quality care to high-risk patients who receive hemodialysis.

! NURSING SAFETY PRIORITY QSEN

Critical Rescue

Hypotension can occur in up to 50% of HD treatments (Yeun et al., 2012). Heat transfer from warmed solutions can result in vasodilation and a drop in blood pressure. When this occurs, consider reducing the temperature of the dialysate to 35° C (95° F). A shift of fluid from the intravascular to extravascular space related to the difference in electrolytes concentrations between HD solutions and blood also contributes to low blood pressure. Whereas modest declines in blood pressure can be addressed by adjusting the rate of extracorporeal blood flow and placing the patient in a legs-up (Trendelenburg) position, sustained or symptomatic hypotension is treated with a fluid bolus of 100 to 250 mL of normal saline or sometimes albumin or mannitol. A second bolus may be needed. If hypotension persists, consider that new-onset myocardial injury or pericardial disease may be a contributing factor and administer oxygen, reduce the blood flow, and notify the health care provider urgently. Discontinue HD when hypotension continues despite cooling dialysate or providing up to two bolus infusions.

have significantly improved safe care for patients receiving this treatment. Complications during HD include hypotension, dialysis disequilibrium syndrome, cardiac events, and reactions to dialyzers.

Dialysis disequilibrium syndrome may develop during HD or after HD has been completed. It is characterized by mental status changes and can include seizures or coma; it is uncommon to observe this severity of disequilibrium syndrome with today's HD practice. A mild form of disequilibrium syndrome includes manifestations of nausea, vomiting, headaches, fatigue, and restlessness. It is thought to be the result of a rapid reduction in electrolytes and other particles (**solutes**) in a short time frame. Maintaining a low blood flow or reducing blood flow with the onset of manifestations can prevent this syndrome.

Cardiac events during HD are associated with underlying cardiovascular disease, especially left ventricular hypertrophy, coronary vascular disease, and a history of cardiac dysrhythmias. These conditions are described in Chapters 35, 36, and 38. Cardiac events leading to a full cardiac arrest are most concerning in an ambulatory care or in-home HD setting. Although cardiac arrest is a rare event, the setting should be equipped with an automatic defibrillator and staff or family trained in cardiopulmonary resuscitation. Often cardiac arrest is related to new-onset cardiac ischemia. The patient then needs to be managed in an acute care setting in which the presence of myocardial disease can be evaluated and cardiac treatment optimized.

Pericardial disease is a complication of patients with ESKD. Assess the patient's heart sounds for the presence of a pericardial rub prior to dialysis. Intensification of dialysis may be used to treat this complication. Other treatment might include NSAID use or surgery as described on p. 1421.

Reactions to dialyzers still occur, although more biocompatible membranes and careful attention to rinsing the dialyzer before use (to eliminate sterilizing agents) have reduced this type of adverse event during HD. Reactions occur during a "first-time" use of the filter and resemble an anaphylactic episode early during HD, with profound hypotension (Chapter 20 describes anaphylactic reactions). With suspected dialyzer reactions, the nurse does not return the blood to the patient and discontinues HD. Corticosteroids may be used to treat the immune reaction.

Other potential complications of recurrent HD require the nurse to monitor the level of consciousness and vital signs frequently during treatment and to slow or stop HD when manifestations occur. Hypoglycemia is a rare adverse HD event and more likely to occur when the patient has diabetes. Hypoglycemia is managed by providing glucose and increasing dialysis glucose concentration in subsequent treatments. Hemorrhage can occur when needle dislodgement or circuit connections become loose and is amplified by the anticoagulation treatment to maintain circuit patency. Some hemolysis will occur because of mechanical trauma to red blood cells, contributing to the anemia of CKD and, perhaps, sensations of dyspnea or chest tightness.

Infectious diseases transmitted by blood transfusion are a serious complication of long-term HD. Two of the most serious blood-transmitted infections are hepatitis and human immune deficiency virus (HIV) infection. *Hepatitis B infection* and *hepatitis C infection* in patients with CKD have decreased because the use of erythropoietin-stimulating agents (ESAs) has reduced the need for blood transfusions to maintain red blood cell counts. Hepatitis is a problem because of the blood access and the risk for contamination during HD. The viruses can be transmitted through the use of contaminated needles or instruments, by entry of contaminated blood through open wounds in the skin or mucous membranes, or through transfusions with contaminated blood. Monitor all patients receiving HD for manifestations of hepatitis (see Chapter 58).

HIV is a bloodborne virus that poses some risk for patients undergoing HD. Fortunately, the risks for HIV transmission are reduced by the consistent practice of Standard Precautions, routine screening of donated blood for HIV, and decreased need for blood transfusions with CKD and ESKD. Patients who have been undergoing HD or who received frequent transfusions during the early to middle 1980s are at risk for acquired immune deficiency syndrome (AIDS) (see Chapter 19).

CONSIDERATIONS FOR OLDER ADULTS

Patient-Centered Care QSEN

Between the years 2000 and 2010, a threefold increase in the number of older adults diagnosed with CKD occurred (Elliott, 2012). In 2010, the number of patients ages 60 years and older increased to more than 25% of patients beginning ESKD therapy (USRDS, 2014). The overall mean age for new patients requiring dialysis is 64.6. Patients older than 65 years who are receiving HD are more at risk for dialysis-induced hypotension. These patients require more frequent monitoring during and after dialysis.

Peritoneal Dialysis

Peritoneal dialysis (PD) allows exchanges of wastes, fluid, and electrolytes to occur in the peritoneal cavity. PD is slower than hemodialysis (HD), however, and more time is needed to achieve the same effect. Other disadvantages of PD are the protein loss in outflow fluid, risk for peritoneal injury, and potential discomfort from indwelling fluid. Advantages and complications are listed in Table 68-10. The use of PD has deceased and currently accounts for less than 10% of dialysis (USRDS, 2014).

Patient Selection. Most patients with CKD can select either HD or PD. For those who are unstable and those who cannot tolerate anticoagulation, PD is less hazardous than HD. For some patients, vascular access problems may eliminate HD as an option. At times a patient may use PD until a new arteriovenous (AV) fistula matures. PD is often the treatment of choice for older adults because it offers more flexibility if his or her status changes frequently.

Peritoneal dialysis *cannot* be performed if peritoneal adhesions are present or if extensive intra-abdominal surgery has been performed. In these cases, the surface area of the peritoneal membrane is not sufficient for adequate dialysis exchange. Peritoneal membrane fibrosis may occur after repeated INFECTION, which decreases membrane permeability.

Procedure. A siliconized rubber (Silastic) catheter is surgically placed into the abdominal cavity for infusion of dialysate (Fig. 68-8). Usually 1 to 2 L of dialysate is infused by gravity *(fill)* into the peritoneal space over a 10- to 20-minute period, according to the patient's tolerance. The fluid stays *(dwells)* in the cavity for a specified time prescribed by the physician. The fluid then flows out of the body *(drains)* by gravity into a drainage bag. The peritoneal outflow contains the dialysate and the excess water, electrolytes, and nitrogen-based waste products. The dialyzing fluid is called peritoneal *effluent* on outflow. The three phases of the process (infusion, or "fill"; dwell; and outflow, or drain) make up one PD exchange. The number and frequency of PD exchanges are prescribed by the physician, depending on manifestations and laboratory data.

Process. Peritoneal dialysis occurs through diffusion and osmosis across the semipermeable peritoneal membrane and capillaries. The peritoneal membrane is large and porous. It allows solutes (particles) and water to move from an area of higher concentration in the blood to an area of lower concentration in the dialyzing fluid (diffusion).

The peritoneal cavity is rich in capillaries and is a ready access to the blood supply. The fluid and waste products dialyzed from the patient move through the blood vessel walls, the interstitial tissues, and the peritoneal membrane and are removed when the dialyzing fluid is drained from the body.

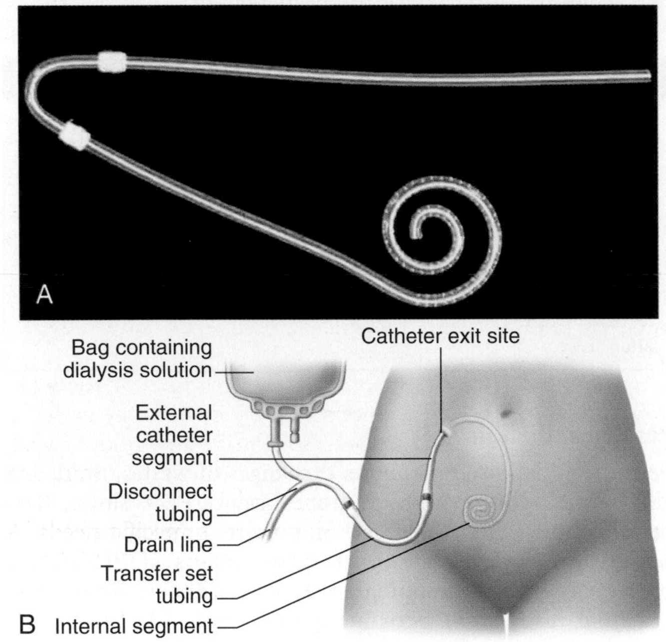

FIG. 68-8 Peritoneal dialysis catheter. **A,** The actual Silastic peritoneal dialysis catheter. **B,** Positioning of the Silastic catheter within the abdominal cavity.

PD efficiency is affected by many factors. INFECTION can cause scarring and reduce capillary blood flow. Vascular disease and decreased PERFUSION of the peritoneum reduce PD diffusion. For PD, water removal depends on the concentration of the dialysate. PD efficiency can be altered by the *tonicity* (i.e., number of particles per liter of fluid) of the dialysate. Increasing the dialysate glucose concentration makes the solution more hypertonic. The more hypertonic the solution, the greater the osmotic pressure for water filtration and fluid removal from the patient during an exchange. The dialysate concentration is prescribed on the basis of the patient's fluid status.

Dialysate Additives. Heparin may be added to the dialysate to prevent clotting of the catheter or tubing. Usually intraperitoneal (IP) heparin is needed only after new catheter placement or if peritonitis occurs. IP heparin is not absorbed systemically and does not affect blood clotting.

Other agents that may be given in the dialysate include potassium and antibiotics. Commercially prepared dialysate does not contain potassium. Some patients need potassium added to the dialysate to prevent hypokalemia. Antibiotics may be given by the IP route when peritonitis is present or suspected. Potassium and antibiotics are not mixed in the same dialysate bag because interactions may reduce the antibiotic effect.

Types of Peritoneal Dialysis. Many types of PD are available, including continuous ambulatory PD, multiple-bag continuous ambulatory PD, automated PD, intermittent PD, and continuous-cycle PD. The type selected depends on the patient's ability and lifestyle. The two most commonly used types of PD are continuous ambulatory peritoneal dialysis and continuous cycling peritoneal dialysis.

Continuous ambulatory peritoneal dialysis (CAPD) is performed by the patient with the infusion of four 2-L exchanges of dialysate into the peritoneal cavity. Each time, the dialysate remains for 4 to 8 hours, and these exchanges occur 7 days a week (Figs. 68-9 through 68-11). During the dwell period, the patient can use a continuous connect system or disconnect and

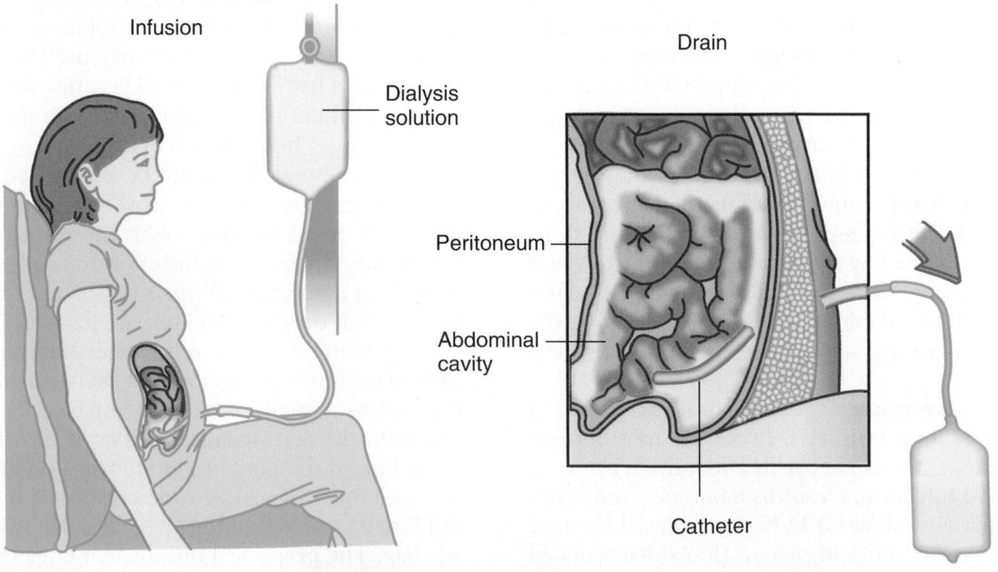

FIG. 68-9 Peritoneal dialysis exchange for control of fluids, electrolytes, nitrogenous wastes, blood pressure, and acid-base balance. The peritoneal membrane acts as the dialyzing membrane.

reconnect at a later time. Most long-term patients with PD prefer to complete exchanges overnight with an automated cycler (automatic peritoneal dialysis [APD], described below).

With the continuous *connect* system (straight transfer set), the dialysate bag is attached to the catheter by 48-inch tubing. The empty bag and tubing are folded and worn beneath the clothing until they are used for outflow. After draining, the patient removes the bag and connects a new bag to repeat the process.

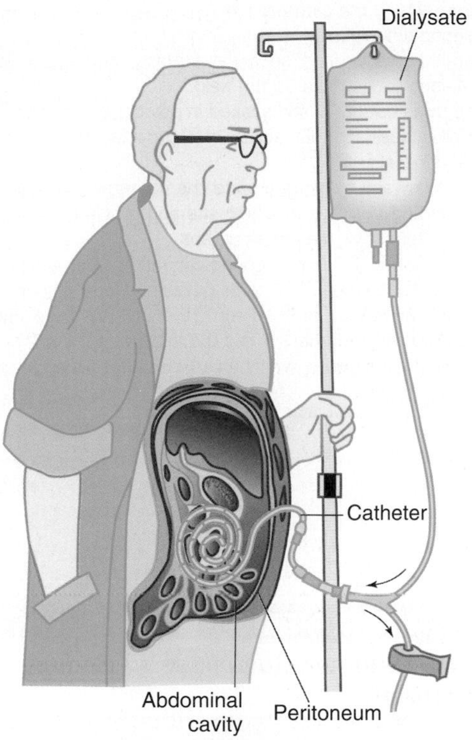

FIG. 68-10 A patient performing continuous ambulatory peritoneal dialysis (CAPD). Note that the patient can walk with this setup.

With the *disconnect system* (Y–transfer set), the patient removes the connecting tubing and empties the dialysate bag after inflow and attaches a cap to the PD catheter. The disconnect system eliminates the need to wear the tubing and bag but requires opening the system 2 extra times with each exchange. The extra opening of the system increases the risk for INFECTION.

With CAPD, no machine is necessary and no partner is required. However, it is best for a partner also trained in CAPD to be available as a support for the patient if illness occurs. Devices to assist in the safe, sterile connection of the tubing spike into the dialysate bag are available. These are useful for patients with poor vision, limited manual dexterity, or reduced hand and arm strength. CAPD allows constant removal of fluid and wastes and more closely resembles kidney action than HD. Some patients even perform their own exchanges while hospitalized.

Continuous-cycle peritoneal dialysis (CCPD) is a form of automated dialysis that uses an automated cycling machine. Exchanges occur at night while the patient sleeps. The final exchange of the night is left to dwell through the day and is drained the next evening as the process is repeated. CCPD offers the advantage of 24-hour dialysis, as in CAPD, but the sterile catheter system is opened less often.

Automated peritoneal dialysis (APD) may be used in the acute care setting, the ambulatory care dialysis center, or the patient's home. APD uses a cycling machine for dialysate inflow, dwell, and outflow according to preset times and volumes. A warming chamber for dialysate is part of the machine (Fig. 68-12). The functions are programmed for the patient's specific needs. A typical prescription calls for 30-minute exchanges (10/10/10 for inflow, dwell, and outflow) for a period of 8 to 10 hours. The machines have many safety monitors and alarms and are relatively simple to learn to use.

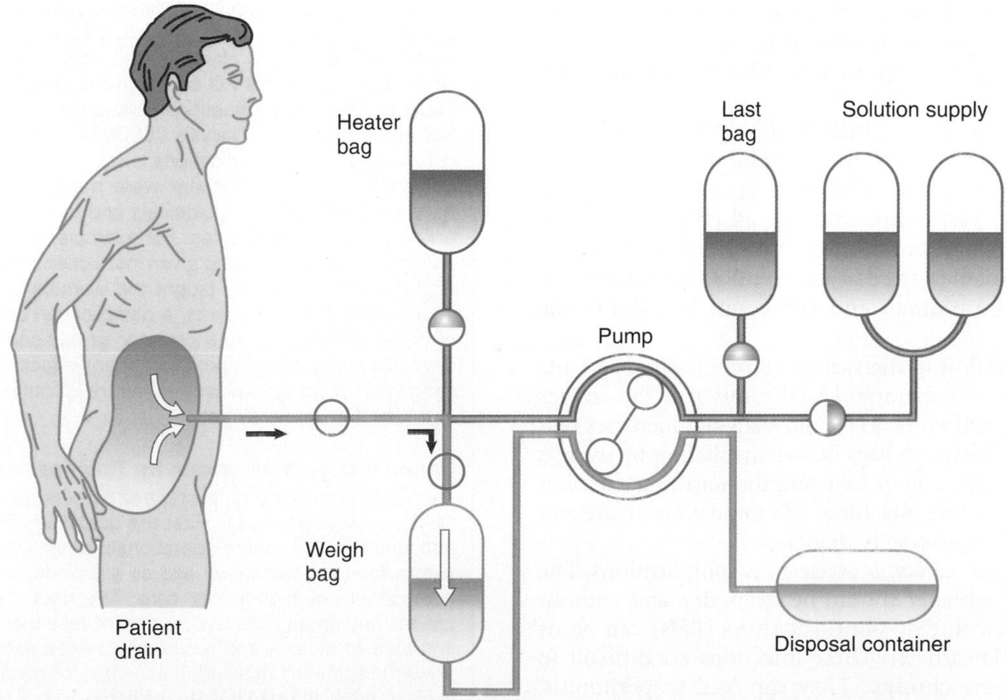

FIG. 68-11 Peritoneal dialysis machine circuit in automated peritoneal dialysis (APD).

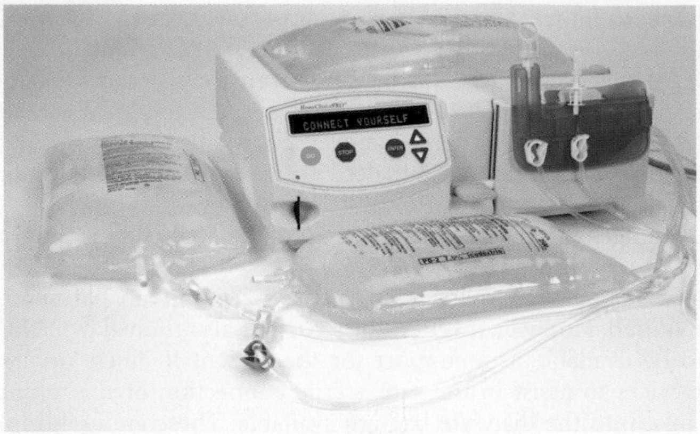

FIG. 68-12 A cycler machine for automated peritoneal dialysis at home.

Automated peritoneal dialysis has several advantages. It permits in-home dialysis while the patient sleeps, allowing him or her to be dialysis-free during waking hours. The incidence of peritonitis is reduced with APD because fewer connections and disconnections are needed. Also, APD can be used to deliver larger volumes of dialysis solution for patients who need higher clearances.

Intermittent peritoneal dialysis (IPD) combines osmotic pressure gradients with true dialysis. The patient usually requires exchanges of 2 L of dialysate at 30- to 60-minute intervals, allowing 15 to 20 minutes of drain time. For most patients, 30 to 40 exchanges of 2 L three times weekly are needed. IPD treatments can be automated or manual.

Complications. Complications are possible with PD, but many can be prevented with meticulous care and appropriate patient education for self-management. Problems and complications are more common when evidence-based guidelines for catheter care are not followed (see the Quality Improvement box regarding PD catheters).

Peritonitis is the major complication of PD, most commonly caused by connection site contamination. To prevent peritonitis, use meticulous sterile technique when caring for the PD catheter and when hooking up or clamping off dialysate bags (Chart 68-9).

Manifestations of peritonitis include cloudy dialysate outflow (effluent), fever, abdominal tenderness, abdominal pain, general malaise, nausea, and vomiting. *Cloudy or opaque effluent is the earliest indication of peritonitis.* Examine all effluent for color and clarity to detect peritonitis early. When peritonitis is suspected, send a specimen of the dialysate outflow for culture and sensitivity study, Gram stain, and cell count to identify the infecting organism.

Pain during the inflow of dialysate is common when patients are first started on PD therapy. Usually this pain no longer occurs after a week or two of PD. Cold dialysate increases discomfort. Warm the dialysate bags before instillation by using a heating pad to wrap the bag or by using the warming chamber of the automated cycling machine. *Microwave ovens are* ***not*** *recommended for the warming of dialysate.*

Exit site and tunnel infections are serious complications. The exit site from a PD catheter should be clean, dry, and without pain or INFLAMMATION. Exit-site INFECTIONS (ESIs) can occur with any type of PD catheter. These infections are difficult to treat and can become chronic. They can lead to peritonitis, catheter failure, and hospitalization. Dialysate leakage and

CHART 68-9 Best Practice for Patient Safety & Quality Care (QSEN)

Caring for the Patient with a Peritoneal Dialysis Catheter

- Mask yourself and your patient. Wash your hands.
- Put on sterile gloves. Remove the old dressing. Remove the contaminated gloves.
- Assess the area for signs of infection, such as swelling, redness, or discharge around the catheter site.
- Use aseptic technique:
  - Open the sterile field on a flat surface, and place two precut 4 × 4–inch gauze pads on the field.
  - Place three cotton swabs soaked in povidone-iodine or other solution prescribed by your health care provider on the field. Put on sterile gloves.
- Use cotton swabs to clean around the catheter site. Use a circular motion starting from the insertion site and moving away toward the abdomen. Repeat with all three swabs.
- As an alternative (if recommended by your health care provider or clinic), cleanse the area with sterile gauze pads using soap and water. Use a circular motion starting from the insertion site and moving away toward the abdomen. Rinse thoroughly.
- Apply precut gauze pads over the catheter site. Tape only the edges of the gauze pads.

QUALITY IMPROVEMENT (QSEN)

Follow PD Catheter Guidelines to Reduce Complications

Wong, L.P., Yamamoto, K.T., Reddy, V., Cobb, D., Chamberlin, A., Pham, H., et al. (2014). Patient education and care for peritoneal dialysis catheter placement: A quality improvement study. *Peritoneal Dialysis International, 34*(1), 12-23.

Although there are practice guidelines for placement of a peritoneal dialysis (PD) catheter, it is unknown if these recommendations are followed. The authors observed the care of 46 new patients at a single site—a regional PD center in the United States Northwest. Patients completed a questionnaire derived from the International Society for Peritoneal Dialysis (ISPD) catheter guidelines and were followed for early complications.

Results indicated that there were many and serious deviations from the ISPD catheter guidelines and that these deviations were linked to adverse outcomes. For example, after insertion, 20% of patients reported not being given instructions for follow-up care and 46% reported not being taught the warning signs of PD catheter infection. In 41% of patients, a complication developed, with 30% of patients experiencing a catheter or exit-site problem and 11% developing infection. Improving patient education and care coordination for PD catheter placement were identified as the next steps in the quality improvement (QI) cycle.

Commentary: Implications for Practice and Research

This study shows the initial steps of gathering information in a Plan-Do-Study-Act cycle of QI. First the guidelines for care were identified, and then they were operationalized as a patient questionnaire with a focus on education and as a provider checklist to observe components of high-quality care. The data were then linked to patient outcomes. The association of less-than-optimal education and care to serious and recurrent adverse patient outcomes is a powerful approach to develop essential interventions with the next cycle in order to provide safe, effective care.

pulling or twisting of the catheter increase the risk for ESIs. A Gram stain and culture should be performed when exit sites have purulent drainage.

Tunnel infections occur in the path of the catheter from the skin to the cuff. Manifestations include redness, tenderness, and pain. ESIs are treated with antimicrobials. Deep cuff infections may require catheter removal.

Poor dialysate flow is usually related to constipation. To prevent constipation, a bowel preparation is prescribed before placement of the PD. An enema before starting PD may also prevent flow problems. Teach patients to eat a high-fiber diet and to use stool softeners to prevent constipation. Other causes of flow difficulty include kinked or clamped connection tubing, the patient's position, fibrin clot formation, and catheter displacement.

Ensure that the drainage bag is lower than the patient's abdomen to enhance gravity drainage. Inspect the connection tubing and PD system for kinking or twisting. Ensure that clamps are open. If inflow or outflow drainage is still inadequate, reposition the patient to stimulate inflow or outflow. Turning the patient to the other side or ensuring that he or she is in good body alignment may help. Having the patient in a supine low-Fowler's position reduces abdominal pressure. Increased abdominal pressure from sitting or standing or from coughing contributes to leakage at the PD catheter site.

Fibrin clot formation may occur after PD catheter placement or with peritonitis. Milking the tubing may dislodge the fibrin clot and improve flow. An x-ray is needed to identify PD catheter placement. If displacement has occurred, the physician repositions the PD catheter.

Dialysate leakage is seen as clear fluid coming from the catheter exit site. When dialysis is first started, small volumes of dialysate are used. It may take patients 1 to 2 weeks to tolerate a full 2-L exchange without leakage around the catheter site. Leakage occurs more often in obese patients, those with diabetes, older adults, and those on long-term steroid therapy. During periods of catheter leak, patients may require hemodialysis (HD) support.

Other complications of PD include bleeding, which is expected when the catheter is first placed, and bowel perforation, which is serious. When PD is first started, the outflow may be bloody or blood tinged. This condition normally clears within a week or two. After PD is well-established, the effluent should be clear and light yellow. Observe for and document any change in the color of the outflow. Brown-colored effluent occurs with a bowel perforation. If the outflow is the same color as urine and has the same glucose level, a bladder perforation is probable. Cloudy or opaque effluent indicates INFECTION.

Nursing Care During Peritoneal Dialysis. In the hospital setting, PD is routinely started and monitored by the nurse. Before the treatment, assess baseline vital signs, including blood pressure, apical and radial pulse rates, temperature, quality of respirations, and breath sounds. Weigh the patient, always on the same scale, before the procedure and at least every 24 hours while receiving treatment. Weight should be checked after a drain and before the next fill to monitor the patient's "dry weight." Baseline laboratory tests, such as electrolyte and glucose levels, are obtained before starting PD and are repeated at least daily during the PD treatment.

Continually monitor the patient during PD. Take and record vital signs every 15 to 30 minutes. Assess for respiratory distress, pain, or discomfort. Check the dressing around the catheter exit site every 30 minutes for wetness during the procedure. Monitor the prescribed dwell time, and initiate outflow. Assess blood glucose levels in patients who absorb glucose.

Observe the outflow pattern (outflow should be a continuous stream after the clamp is completely open). Measure and record the total amount of outflow after each exchange. Maintain accurate inflow and outflow records when hourly PD exchanges are performed. When outflow is less than inflow, the difference is retained by the patient during dialysis and is counted as fluid intake. Weigh the patient daily to monitor fluid status.

Kidney Transplantation

Dialysis and kidney transplant are life-sustaining *treatments* for end-stage kidney disease (ESKD). Kidney transplant is not considered a "cure." Each patient, in consultation with a nephrologist, determines which type of therapy is best suited to his or her physical condition and lifestyle. About 17,000 to 18,000 kidney transplants are performed yearly in the United States. Currently about 159,000 people are awaiting kidney transplant in North America. The median time on the waiting list is 678 days (USRDS, 2014).

Candidate Selection Criteria. Candidates for transplantation must be free of medical problems that might increase the risks from the procedure. The usual age-range for kidney transplant is 2 to 70 years. Patients older than 70 years are considered for transplant on an individual basis because complications are more common in the older adult.

The patient is thoroughly assessed before he or she is considered for a kidney transplant. Patients who have advanced, uncorrectable cardiac disease are excluded from the procedure because these problems are made worse by transplantation. Other conditions that preclude kidney transplant include metastatic cancer, chronic INFECTION, and severe psychosocial problems such as alcoholism or chemical dependency. Long-standing pulmonary disease increases the risk for complications and death from respiratory infection. Patients with diseases of the GI system, such as peptic ulcers and diverticulosis, require treatment before consideration for transplantation because some diseases are made worse by the large doses of steroids used after surgery.

The urinary system is completely evaluated to ensure normal urine flow. Many patients with ESKD have not used their lower urinary tract for years, and ureteral or bladder problems may require surgical correction before a kidney is transplanted.

Patients with a recent history of cancer are treated with dialysis because of the shortage of donor organs and the uncertain life expectancy of these patients. In addition, the drugs used after the procedure increase the risk for cancer recurrence. If more than 2 to 5 years have passed since cancer eradication, the patient can be considered for a transplant.

Diabetes mellitus and other endocrine problems cause great risks. Patients with these problems can have a kidney transplant but require intense observation and management to limit complications. Other pre-existing conditions are considered on an individual basis, depending on the patient's health status. Kidney transplantation is considered for most patients with ESKD and is the optimal therapy for many people.

Donors. Kidney donors may be living donors (related or unrelated to the patient), non-heart-beating donors (NHBDs), and cadaveric donors. The available kidneys are matched on the basis of tissue type similarity between the donor and the recipient. NHBDs are persons declared dead by cardiopulmonary criteria. Kidneys from NHBDs are removed (harvested) immediately after death in cases in which patients have previously given consent for organ donation. If immediate removal must be delayed, the organ is preserved by infusing a cool preservation solution into the abdominal aorta after death is declared and until surgery can be performed. Cadaveric donors are usually people who suffered irreversible brain injury, most often as a result of trauma. These donors are maintained with mechanical ventilation and must have sufficient PERFUSION for the kidneys to remain viable.

The size of the kidney is seldom a problem in adults. Kidneys transplanted from children become larger to meet adult needs within a few months.

Organs from living *related* donors (LRDs) have the highest rates of kidney graft survival (90%). A living donor is one who is medically compatible with the recipient (Ficorelli et al., 2013). LRDs are usually at least 18 years old and are seldom older than 65 years, although there are reports of donors age 70 years with good outcomes for both the donor and recipient (Berger et al., 2011). Physical criteria for donors include:

- Absence of systemic disease and INFECTION
- No history of cancer
- No hypertension or kidney disease
- Adequate kidney function as determined by diagnostic studies

LRDs must express a clear understanding of the surgery and a willingness to give up a kidney. Some transplant centers require a psychiatric evaluation to assess the donor's motivation.

A paired or chain exchange donation can be done when two kidney donor/recipient pairs have blood types that are not compatible (Gentry et al., 2011). The recipients trade donors so that each recipient can receive a kidney with a compatible blood type and tissue type (Fig. 68-13). Once the evaluations of all

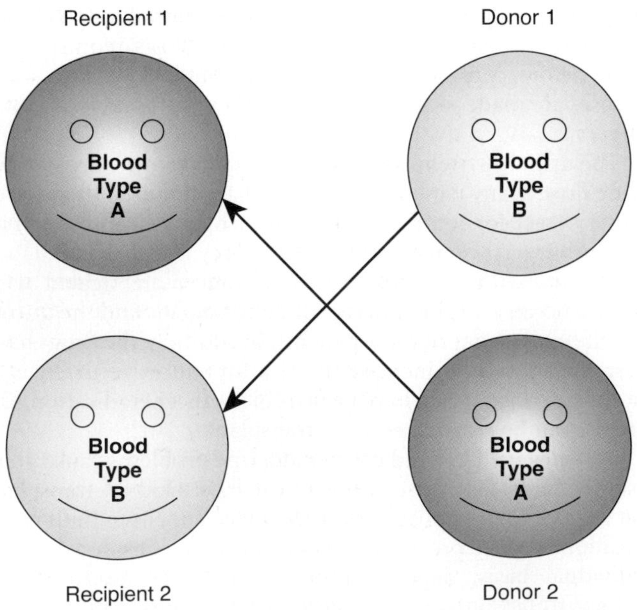

FIG. 68-13 An example of a paired exchange kidney donation. *Donor 1* is related to or acquainted with *recipient 1* and has agreed to donate a kidney but is not a blood type or tissue type match with *recipient 1. Donor 1* is compatible with *recipient 2* and agrees to donate a kidney to *recipient 2* if *donor 2* agrees to donate a kidney to *recipient 1 with confirmed compatibility to recipient 1.*

donors and recipients are completed, the series of kidney transplant operations are scheduled to occur consecutively (www.paireddonaton.org).

Because of advances in immunosuppressant therapy and medical management, the United Network for Organ Sharing (UNOS) reported 1-year kidney transplant graft survival to be almost 95% for all centers in the United States during 2012 (UNOS, 2014).

Preoperative Care. Many issues related to patient health and the actual transplant procedure must be addressed before surgery. The *Clinical Pathway* on the *Evolve* website highlights care needs for the patient undergoing kidney transplantation.

Immunologic studies are needed because the major barrier to transplant success after a suitable donor kidney is available is the body's ability to reject "foreign" tissue. This immunologic process can attack the transplanted kidney and destroy it. For immunologic problems to be overcome, tissue typing is performed on all candidates. These studies include simple blood typing and human leukocyte antigen (HLA) studies, as well as other tests. A donated kidney *must* come from a donor who is the same blood type as the recipient. The HLAs are the main immunologic feature used to match transplant recipients with compatible donors. The more similar the antigens of the donor are to those of the recipient, the more likely the transplant will be successful and rejection will be avoided (see Chapter 17).

Nursing actions before surgery include teaching about the procedure and care after surgery, in-depth patient assessment, coordination of diagnostic tests, and development of treatment plans. See Chapter 14 for more discussion of standard preoperative nursing care.

The patient usually requires dialysis within 24 hours of the surgery and often receives a blood transfusion before surgery. Usually blood from the kidney donor is transfused into the recipient. This procedure increases graft survival of organs from living related donors (LRDs).

Operative Procedures. The donor nephrectomy procedure varies depending on whether the donor is a non-heart-beating donor (NHBD), cadaveric donor, or living donor (Beach et al., 2011). The NHBD or cadaveric donor nephrectomy is a sterile autopsy procedure performed in the operating room. All arterial and venous vessels and a long piece of ureter are preserved. After removal, the kidneys are preserved until time for implantation into the recipient. The technique for kidney removal from living donors is a laparoscopic procedure. Donors need postoperative nursing care and support for the psychological adjustment to loss of a body part.

Transplantation surgery usually takes several hours. The new kidney is usually placed in the right or left anterior iliac fossa (Fig. 68-14) instead of the usual kidney position. This placement allows easier connection of the ureter and the renal artery and vein. It also allows for easier kidney palpation. The recipient's own failed kidneys are not removed unless chronic kidney INFECTION is present or, as in the case of polycystic kidney disease, the nonfunctioning, enlarged kidneys cause pain. After surgery, the patient is taken to the postanesthesia care unit and then, when stable, to a designated unit in the transplant center or to a critical care unit.

Postoperative Care. Care of the recipient after surgery requires that nurses be knowledgeable about the expected clinical findings and potential complications. Nursing care includes ongoing physical assessment, especially evaluation of kidney function. The most common complications occurring in

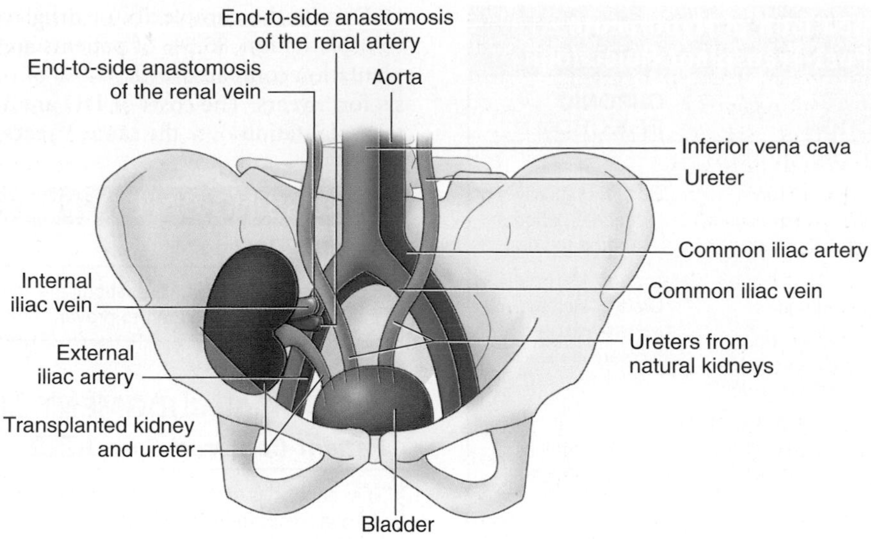

FIG. 68-14 Placement of a transplanted kidney in the right iliac fossa.

patients after renal transplant are rejection and INFECTION. Immunosuppressive drug therapy used to prevent tissue rejection impairs healing and increases the risk for INFECTION.

Urologic management is essential to graft success. A urinary catheter is placed for accurate measurements of urine output and decompression of the bladder. Decompression prevents stretch on sutures and ureter attachment sites on the bladder.

Assess urine output at least hourly during the first 48 hours. An abrupt decrease in urine output may indicate complications such as rejection, acute kidney injury (AKI), thrombosis, or obstruction. Examine the urine color. The urine is pink and bloody right after surgery and gradually returns to normal over several days to several weeks, depending on kidney function. Obtain daily urine specimens for urinalysis, glucose measurement, the presence of acetone, specific gravity measurement, and culture (if needed).

Occasionally, continuous bladder irrigation is prescribed to decrease blood clot formation, which could increase pressure in the bladder and endanger the graft. Perform routine catheter care, according to agency policy, to reduce catheter-associated urinary tract infection (CAUTI). The catheter is removed as soon as possible to avoid INFECTION—usually 3 to 5 days after surgery. After surgery, the function of the transplanted kidney (graft) can result in either oliguria or diuresis. Oliguria may occur as a result of ischemia and AKI, rejection, or other complications. To increase urine output, the health care provider may prescribe diuretics and osmotic agents. Closely monitor the patient's fluid status because fluid overload can cause hypertension, heart failure, and pulmonary edema. Evaluate his or her fluid status by weighing daily, measuring blood pressure every 2 to 4 hours, and measuring intake and output.

Instead of oliguria, the patient may have diuresis, especially with a kidney from a living related donor (LRD). Monitor intake and output, and observe for disruptions of FLUID AND ELECTROLYTE BALANCE, such as low potassium and sodium levels. Excessive diuresis may cause hypotension.

Complications. Many complications are possible after kidney transplantation. Early detection and intervention improve the chances for graft survival.

! NURSING SAFETY PRIORITY QSEN

Critical Rescue

Notify the physician immediately about hypotension or excessive diuresis (e.g., unanticipated urine output 500-1000 mL greater than intake over 12-24 hours or other goal for intake and output [I&O]) because hypotension reduces blood flow and oxygen to the new kidney, threatening graft survival.

Rejection is the most serious complication of transplantation and is the leading cause of graft loss. A reaction occurs between the tissues of the transplanted kidney and the antibodies and cytotoxic T-cells in the recipient's blood. These substances treat the new kidney as a foreign invader and cause tissue destruction, thrombosis, and eventual kidney necrosis.

The three types of rejection are hyperacute, acute, and chronic. Acute rejection is the most common type with kidney transplants. It is treated with increased immunosuppressive therapy and often can be reversed. Rejection is diagnosed by manifestations, a CT or renal scan, and kidney biopsy. Table 68-14 lists the features of the three types of rejection. Chapter 17 discusses their causes and treatment.

Ischemia from delayed transplantation following harvesting can contribute to AKI. Newly transplanted patients with AKI may need dialysis until adequate urine output returns and the blood urea nitrogen (BUN) and creatinine levels normalize. Biopsy can be used to determine if oliguria is the result of AKI or rejection.

Thrombosis of the major renal blood vessels may occur during the first 2 to 3 days after the transplant. A sudden decrease in urine output may signal impaired PERFUSION resulting from thrombosis. Ultrasound of the kidney may show decreased or absent blood supply. Emergency surgery is required to prevent ischemic damage or graft loss.

Renal artery stenosis may result in hypertension. Other manifestations include a bruit over the artery anastomosis site and decreased kidney function. A CT or renal scan can quantify the blood flow to the kidney. The involved artery may be repaired surgically or by balloon angioplasty in the radiology

TABLE 68-14 Comparison of Hyperacute, Acute, and Chronic Post-Transplant Rejection

HYPERACUTE REJECTION	ACUTE REJECTION	CHRONIC REJECTION
Onset		
Within 48 hours after surgery	1 week to any time postoperatively; occurs over days to weeks	Occurs gradually during a period of months to years
Clinical Manifestations		
Increased temperature	Oliguria or anuria	Gradual increase in BUN and serum creatinine levels
Increased blood pressure	Temperature over 100° F (37.8° C)	
Pain at transplant site	Increased blood pressure Enlarged, tender kidney Lethargy Elevated serum creatinine, BUN, potassium levels Fluid retention	Fluid retention Changes in serum electrolyte levels Fatigue
Treatment		
Immediate removal of the transplanted kidney	Increased doses of immunosuppressive drugs	Conservative management until dialysis is required

BUN, Blood urea nitrogen.

department. The decision to perform a balloon repair is determined by the amount of healing time after the surgery.

Other vascular problems include vascular leakage or thrombosis, both of which require an emergency transplant nephrectomy.

Other complications may involve the surgical wound or urinary tract. Wound problems, such as hematomas, abscesses, and lymphoceles (cysts containing lymph fluid), increase the risk for infection and exert pressure on the new kidney. INFECTION is a major cause of death in the transplant recipient. Prevention of infection is essential. Strict aseptic technique and handwashing must be rigorously enforced. Transplant recipients may not have the usual manifestations of infection because of the immunosuppressive therapy. Low-grade fevers, mental status changes, and vague reports of discomfort may be the only manifestations before sepsis. Always consider the possibility of infection with any patient after a kidney transplant. Urinary tract complications include ureteral leakage, fistula, or obstruction; stone formation; bladder neck contracture; and graft rupture. Surgical intervention may be required.

Immunosuppressive Drug Therapy. The success of kidney transplantation depends on changing the patient's immunologic response so that the new kidney is not rejected as a foreign organ. Immunosuppressive drugs protect the transplanted organ. These drugs include corticosteroids, inhibitors of T-cell proliferation and activity (azathioprine, mycophenolic acid, cyclosporine, and tacrolimus), mTOR inhibitors (to disrupt stimulatory T-cell signals), and monoclonal antibodies. Chapter 17 discusses the mechanisms of action for these agents and the associated patient responses. Patients taking these drugs are at an increased risk for death from INFECTION.

Some patients do not follow the regimen correctly and are at high risk for losing the transplanted kidney. Work with the patient to ensure adherence to the drug regimen.

Despite the complexity of drug regimens following kidney transplantation, 85.5% of patients are living 5 years after transplantation compared with 35.8% of patients who receive dialysis for 5 years. The costs of HD are 3 times the cost of kidney transplantation over the same 5 years (USRDS, 2014).

! NURSING SAFETY PRIORITY QSEN

Action Alert

Teach patients and families about the importance of adhering to the anti-rejection drug regimen to prevent transplant rejection.

? CLINICAL JUDGMENT CHALLENGE

Patient-Centered Care QSEN

The patient is a 64-year-old man with ESKD who has been on hemodialysis for 3 years while waiting for a kidney transplant. He expresses frustration with the wait from time to time and has told you that he fears that he will be considered too old to receive a kidney if much more time goes by. He states that he feels "chained" to the dialysis center.

1. How should you respond to his concern about age possibly affecting his ability to be a transplant recipient?
2. How do you respond to his feeling about being chained to the dialysis center?
3. What other resources can you offer to help him be informed and deal with the emotional aspects of dialysis?

Community-Based Care

Home Care Management. Because of the complex nature of CKD, its progressive course, and many treatment options, a case manager is helpful in planning, coordinating, and evaluating care. As kidney disease progresses, the patient is seen by a physician or nurse practitioner regularly. Together with the dietitian and social worker, evaluate the home environment and determine equipment needs before discharge. Once the patient is discharged, home care nurses direct care and monitor progress.

Provide health teaching about the diet in kidney disease and the progression of disease. As CKD approaches end-stage kidney disease (ESKD), one of these treatment methods is chosen: hemodialysis (HD), peritoneal dialysis (PD), or transplantation. For each form of treatment, the patient and partner must learn about the procedures and consider his or her personal lifestyle, support systems, and methods of coping. Decision making about treatment type or even whether to pursue treatment is difficult for patients and families. Provide information and emotional support to assist patients with these decisions.

Teach patients who select hemodialysis (HD) about the machine and vascular access care. If in-home HD is selected, preparations are needed for the appropriate equipment, including a water treatment system. Referral to a home health care agency is essential for a successful transition to at-home HD. A home care visit occurs before discharge to coordinate equipment setup. Family members or agency staff must be available to respond to alarms during treatment. Because nocturnal HD is a growing modality, additional safety considerations must be addressed, including a plan for treatment discontinuation or generator backup during power outages. Regardless of whether the treatment occurs at home or in a center, promote independence through teaching and best practices in self-management.

The patient receiving PD needs extensive training in the procedure. He or she also needs help in obtaining equipment and the many supplies needed. Home care nurses assess patients, monitor vital signs, assess adherence with drug and diet regimens, and monitor for manifestations of peritonitis.

The nurse plays a vital role in the long-term care of the patient with a kidney transplant. Facilitate acceptance and understanding of the anti-rejection drug regimen as a part of daily life. Carefully monitor for indications of graft rejection and for complications, such as INFECTION. Chart 68-10 describes the focused assessment for the patient following kidney transplant.

Self-Management Education. Instruct patients and family members in all aspects of nutrition therapy, drug therapy, and complications. Teach them to report complications, such as fluid overload and INFECTION. When a patient has a specific form of therapy, such as dialysis or transplantation, focus teaching on the chosen type of intervention. Assess the need for immunizations, and request a prescription to administer needed ones before transplantation.

CHART 68-10 Focused Assessment

The Patient Following Kidney Transplant

Assess cardiovascular and respiratory status, including:
- Vital signs, with special attention to blood pressure
- Presence of S_3 or pericardial friction rub
- Presence of chest pain
- Presence of edema (periorbital, pretibial, sacral)
- Jugular vein distention
- Presence of dyspnea
- Presence of crackles, beginning at the lung bases and extending upward

Assess nutritional status, including:
- Weight gain or loss
- Presence of anorexia, nausea, or vomiting

Assess kidney status, including:
- Amount, frequency, and appearance of urine (in non-anuric patients)
- Presence of bone pain
- Presence of hyperglycemia secondary to diabetes

Assess hematologic status, including:
- Presence of petechiae, purpura, ecchymoses
- Presence of fatigue or shortness of breath

Assess gastrointestinal status, including:
- Presence of stomatitis
- Presence of melena

Assess integumentary status, including:
- Skin integrity
- Presence of pruritus
- Presence of skin discoloration

Assess neurologic status, including:
- Changes in mental status
- Presence of seizure activity
- Presence of sensory changes
- Presence of lower extremity weakness

Assess laboratory data, including:
- BUN
- Serum creatinine
- Creatinine clearance
- CBC
- Electrolytes

Assess psychosocial status, including:
- Presence of anxiety
- Presence of maladaptive behavior

BUN, Blood urea nitrogen; *CBC*, complete blood count.

Hemodialysis (HD) is the most complex form of therapy for the patient and family to understand. Even if patients receive HD in a dialysis center instead of at home, they are expected to have some knowledge of the process. Teach the patient or a family member to care for the vascular access and to report signs of INFECTION and stenosis. Those who plan to have in-home HD will need a partner. Both the patient and the partner must be taught the entire process of HD and must be able to perform it independently before the patient is discharged.

Peritoneal dialysis (PD) involves extensive health teaching for the patient and family. Emphasize sterile technique because peritonitis is the most common complication of PD. Instruct patients to report any manifestation of peritonitis, especially cloudy effluent and abdominal pain. If peritonitis develops, teach patients how to give themselves antibiotics by the intraperitoneal (IP) route. Stress the importance of completing the antibiotic regimen. Remind patients that repeated episodes of peritonitis can reduce the effectiveness of PD, which may require the transfer to HD.

The patient receiving a kidney transplant also needs extensive health teaching. Provide instruction about drug regimens, home monitoring, immunosuppression, manifestations of rejection, INFECTION, and prescribed changes in the diet and activity level.

Psychosocial Preparation. Provide psychological support for the patient and family. Help the patient adjust to the diagnosis of kidney failure and eventually accept the treatment regimens.

Many patients view dialysis as a cure instead of lifelong management. For many patients, reduction of uremic manifestations in the first weeks after starting dialysis treatment creates a sense of well-being (the "honeymoon" period). They feel better physically, and their mood may be happy and hopeful. At this time they tend to overlook the discomfort and inconvenience of dialysis. Use this time to begin health teaching. Stress that although manifestations are reduced, not to expect a complete return to the previous state of well-being before ESKD.

Many patients become discouraged during the first year of treatment. This mood state may last a few months to a year or longer. The difficulties of incorporating dialysis into daily life are staggering, and patients may become depressed as problems occur. They may struggle with the idea of having to be permanently dependent on a disruptive therapy. Patients may feel helpless and dependent. Some people may deny the need for dialysis or may not adhere to drug therapy and diet restrictions. Monitor any behaviors that may contribute to nonadherence, and suggest psychiatric referrals. Help the patient and family focus on the positive aspects of the treatments. Continue health education with patients as active participants and decision makers.

Most patients with CKD eventually enter a phase of acceptance or resignation. Each person reacts differently. To make this long-term adaptation, the patient must adjust to continuous change. Concerns depend on the patient's health and specific treatment method.

After patients have accepted or become resigned to the chronic aspect of their disease, they usually attempt to return to their previous activities. Resuming the previous level of activity, however, may not be possible. Help patients develop realistic expectations that allow them to lead active, productive lives.

Health Care Resources. Professionals from many disciplines are resources for the patient with ESKD. Home care nurses monitor the patient's status and evaluate maintenance of the prescribed treatment regimen (HD or PD). Social services are often involved because of the complex process of applying for financial aid to pay for the required medical care. A physical therapist may be beneficial in helping to improve the patient's functional health. A dietitian can assist the patient and family members in understanding special dietary needs. A psychiatric evaluation may be needed if depressive symptoms are present. Pharmacists provide invaluable insight and teaching about drug therapy and adjustments to meet outcomes. Clergy and pastoral care specialists offer spiritual support.

Patients with CKD are routinely followed by a physician, usually a nephrologist. Organizations such as the National Kidney Foundation (NKF), the American Kidney Fund, and the National Association of Patients on Hemodialysis and Transplantation (NAPHT) may be helpful to patients and families.

◆ Evaluation: Outcomes

Evaluate the care of the patient with CKD based on the identified priority problems. The expected outcomes are that with appropriate management the patient should:

- Achieve and maintain appropriate FLUID AND ELECTROLYTE BALANCE
- Maintain an adequate nutrition status
- Avoid INFECTION at the vascular access site
- Use effective coping strategies
- Report an absence of physical manifestations of anxiety
- Prevent or slow systemic complications of CKD, including osteodystrophy

Specific indicators for these outcomes are listed for each priority problem under the Planning and Implementation section (see earlier).

NURSING CONCEPTS AND CLINICAL JUDGMENT REVIEW

What might you NOTICE if the patient is experiencing reduced PERFUSION and altered urinary ELIMINATION related to acute kidney injury?

- Hemodynamic instability, especially hypotension and tachycardia that persist or recur
- Urine output (elimination) of less than 0.5 mL/kg/hr for more than 2 hours; some experts suggest reporting urine output of less than 0.3 mL/kg/hr for more than 2 hours.
- Serum creatinine increased above baseline or admission values
- Patient reports of back or flank pain
- Urine that has sediment or is dark or smoky or has obvious blood in it
- Signs of abnormalities in fluid and electrolytes including dehydration and abnormal serum and urine potassium and sodium values

How should you INTERPRET and how should you RESPOND to a patient experiencing complications from INFECTION, INFLAMMATION, disturbances in FLUID AND ELECTROLYTE BALANCE, and altered ACID-BASE BALANCE as a result of chronic kidney disease?

Perform and interpret physical assessment, including:

- Asking how long manifestations have been present
- Determining fluid intake and output volumes
- Weighing the patient, and asking whether this weight is more or less than the usual weight
- Assessing for tachycardia, hypertension, and hypotension
- Assessing for pulmonary congestion
- Assessing for skin tissue integrity related to risk for injury from uremia and edema
- Interpreting laboratory values:
  - BUN and serum creatinine levels elevated with altered cognition
  - Serum potassium level elevated with potential for cardiac dysrhythmias
  - Low serum calcium indicating risk for renal osteodystrophy
  - Arterial pH or venous base deficit

Respond by:

- Ensuring hemodynamic stability
- Monitoring urine output
- Monitoring for fluid overload and, after dialysis, dehydration
- Evaluating laboratory results regularly with physical assessment
- Evaluating patient risk for falls or other unsafe situations
- Promoting best practices related to care of the patient with vascular access for hemodialysis
- Providing education about drugs used to manage CKD and kidney transplant

On what should you REFLECT?

- Observe patient for evidence of improved urine output after implementing the plan of care for AKI.
- Plan care to avoid periods of inadequate kidney perfusion from hypotension and dehydration.
- Identify and evaluate the effect of interventions to minimize the risk for infection, including appropriate administration of immunizations, particularly in patients with CKD and altered immunity from kidney transplant.
- Think about topics for patient teaching that could help prevent complications from AKI or progressive CKD.
- Explore how patient preferences and values affect patient decisions about self-management in CKD.
- Explain how immunosuppression in kidney transplant patients and patients with ESKD alters immune responses, including inflammation.
- Consider how timeliness (routine versus urgent versus immediate) and accuracy (e.g., isolated versus trend, and complete versus focused data) of communication to the health care provider or other health care team members can avoid or reduce complications, worsening CKD, transplant rejection, and severity of AKI.
- Inform health care providers about signs of local or systemic infection, vital signs that are not within normal ranges or ranges that are not acceptable for the patient, abnormal laboratory results, or other changes in patient status that require urgent assessment and intervention.

GET READY FOR THE NCLEX® EXAMINATION!

KEY POINTS

Review these Key Points for each NCLEX Examination Client Needs Category.

Safe and Effective Care Environment

- Use sterile technique when initiating and providing renal replacement therapy. **Safety** QSEN
- Implement fall precautions and consider physical therapy referral for patients with CKD osteodystrophy to prevent fractures. **Safety** QSEN
- Use skin protective measures to reduce injury and pressure ulcer formation in patients with CKD. **Safety** QSEN
- Communicate to health care providers patient assessments that indicate dehydration or hypovolemia to avoid inadequate kidney PERFUSION. **Teamwork and Collaboration** QSEN
- Avoid taking blood pressure measurements or drawing blood from an arm with a vascular access (AV fistula or graft). **Safety** QSEN
- Do not use a renal replacement vascular access device (the AV fistula or graft site) to give IV fluids. **Safety** QSEN

Health Promotion and Maintenance

- Encourage patients with AKI, CKD, or end-stage kidney disease (ESKD) to follow fluid and dietary restrictions regarding sodium, potassium, and protein.
- Teach patients the expected side effects, any adverse reactions to prescribed drugs, and when to contact the prescriber. **Safety** QSEN
- Teach patients using peritoneal dialysis the manifestations of peritonitis. **Patient-Centered Care** QSEN
- Teach patients receiving immunosuppressive therapy for kidney transplantation to assess themselves daily for fever, general malaise, and nausea or vomiting, as well as weight gain, indicating new fluid retention. **Patient-Centered Care** QSEN

Psychosocial Integrity

- Allow patients the opportunity to express concerns about the disruption of lifestyle and considerations for end-of-life care as a result of kidney failure. **Patient-Centered Care** QSEN
- Use language and terminology that are comfortable for the patient. **Patient-Centered Care** QSEN
- Assess the patient for depression and nonacceptance of the diagnosis or treatment plan. **Patient-Centered Care** QSEN
- Refer patients to community resources and support groups. **Informatics** QSEN

Physiological Integrity

- Report immediately any condition that obstructs urine flow. **Safety** QSEN
- Collaborate with the dietitian to teach patients about needed fluid, sodium, potassium, or dietary protein restriction. **Teamwork and Collaboration** QSEN
- Inform the health care provider urgently or immediately about hemodynamic instability, change in cognition, manifestations of INFECTION, newly abnormal serum electrolytes, and urine output less than 0.5mL/kg/hr for more than 2-4 hours (unless the patient is oliguric or anuric from ESKD). **Teamwork and Collaboration** QSEN
- Teach patients in the early stages of CKD the manifestations of dehydration. **Patient-Centered Care** QSEN
- Teach patients in the later stages of CKD the manifestations of fluid overload and hyperkalemia. **Patient-Centered Care** QSEN
- Avoid all invasive procedures in the 4 to 6 hours following hemodialysis. **Evidence-Based Practice** QSEN

CONCEPT OVERVIEW

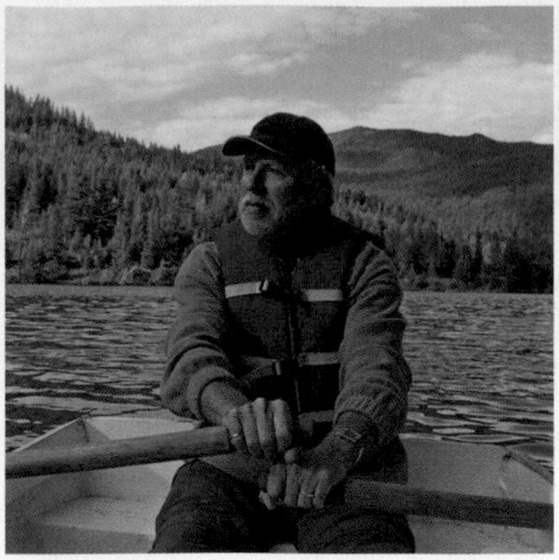

Sexuality

Unlike the physiologic human needs introduced in other section openers of this text, *sexuality* is a complex integration of many physiologic, emotional, social, and cultural aspects of well-being. It is closely associated with self-concept, self-esteem, role relationships, sexual response, gender identity, and reproduction. Sexuality comprises other related human needs, such as belonging, intimacy (e.g., touching, kissing), sharing, and caring. When these needs are met, a person is sexually healthy (Fig. 1).

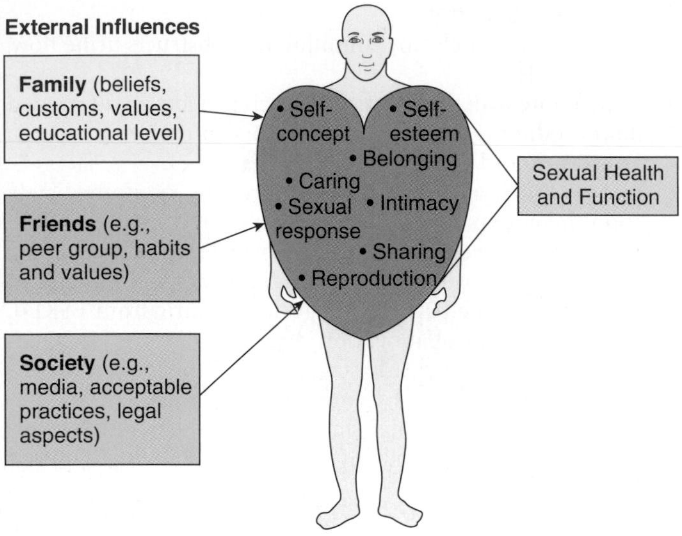

FIG. 1

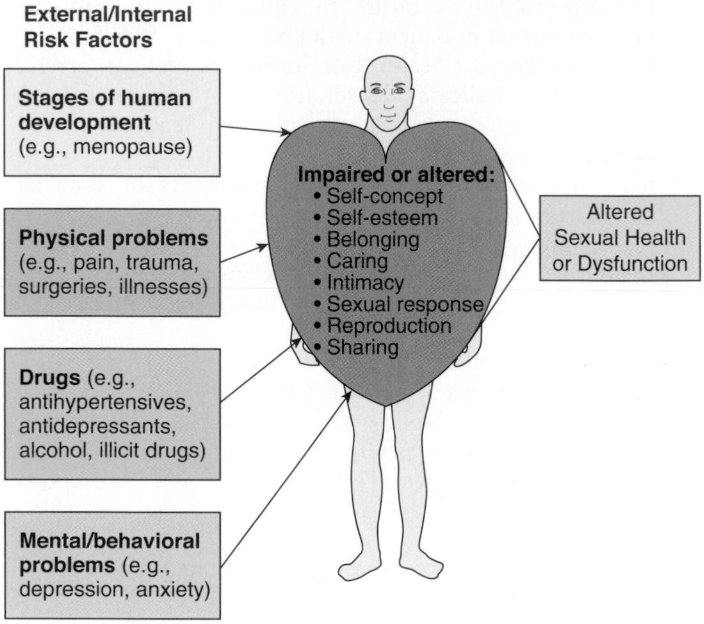

FIG. 2

Sexuality, therefore, is a vital part of one's holistic being from birth to death. During the stages of human development, a person's attitudes, beliefs, and values related to sexuality are influenced and shaped by the environment, including family, friends, and society. For example, cultural beliefs affect the nature of physical sexual pleasure. The media also play a large role in developing one's views on sexuality. Some societies, such as the United States, tend to value youth and beauty more than aging and wisdom. As a result, people in these societies may feel less physically attractive and desirable for intimacy and belonging as they age.

Various external and internal risk factors can alter or impair sexual health. In many cases, they cause physical sexual dysfunction, which then affects emotional needs such as self-esteem (Fig. 2). These factors include:

- Stages of human development
- Physical health problems
- Drugs
- Mental/behavioral health problems

The *stages of human development* typically influence human sexuality, especially when menopause occurs in middle adulthood. Although each woman's response is different, menopause may result in a decreased libido (desire for sexual contact or intercourse). Relationships with her sexual partner(s) are altered, and interpersonal conflict can occur.

Physical health problems also can negatively affect sexual health. For example, chronic pain may cause decreased physical contact and a lowered self-concept along with chronic fatigue and decreased energy. Sexual dysfunction commonly occurs in people with chronic diseases such as diabetes and hypertension. Reproductive diseases (e.g., sexually transmitted diseases, testicular cancer) and their treatments (e.g., radiation therapy, surgery) can also affect sexuality, both physically and emotionally. Physical trauma such as spinal cord injury may prevent a person from having sexual intercourse.

Certain prescription or recreational *drugs* can cause impotence (inability to have an erection) or infertility. Alcohol and many antihypertensive agents, antidepressants, and illicit drugs interfere with sexual function in men.

Mental/behavioral health problems can also result in altered sexual health. Common examples include depression and severe anxiety states. In some cases, concern about physical performance can lead to sexual dysfunction.

CHAPTER 69

Assessment of the Reproductive System

Donna D. Ignatavicius

http://evolve.elsevier.com/Iggy/

PRIORITY CONCEPTS

- PAIN
- SEXUALITY
- INFECTION

LEARNING OUTCOMES

Health Promotion and Maintenance

1. Teach patients about recommended guidelines for selected reproductive screening tests.

Psychosocial Integrity

2. Identify general psychological responses to reproductive health problems that affect SEXUALITY.

Physiological Integrity

3. Review the anatomy and physiology of the male and the female reproductive systems.
4. Identify reproductive changes associated with aging and their implications for nursing care.
5. Perform a focused physical assessment of the patient with male or female reproductive system problems.
6. Explain the use of laboratory testing for patients with suspected or actual reproductive health problems.
7. Develop an evidence-based teaching plan for a patient undergoing endoscopic studies for reproductive health problems.

The first health care professional to assess the patient with a reproductive system health problem or hear a patient's concern about a reproductive problem is often the nurse. These problems typically affect the need for SEXUALITY, both its physical and psychosocial aspects, and are difficult for many people to discuss. Assessment of the male and the female reproductive systems should be part of every complete physical assessment. *Be aware of and sensitive to differences in sexual orientation and practices.*

This chapter reviews the focused reproductive system assessment that a nurse generalist performs. An advanced practice nurse or other health care provider performs the comprehensive reproductive examination. A more detailed discussion of human SEXUALITY is found in a fundamentals or basic nursing text.

ANATOMY AND PHYSIOLOGY REVIEW

Structure and Function of the Female Reproductive System

The female reproductive system is located both outside (external) and inside (internal) the body.

External Genitalia

The external female genitalia, or **vulva**, extend from the mons pubis to the anal opening. The mons pubis is a fat pad that covers the symphysis pubis and protects it during coitus (sexual intercourse).

The labia majora are two vertical folds of adipose tissue that extend posteriorly from the mons pubis to the perineum. The size of the labia majora varies depending on the amount of fatty tissue present. The skin over the labia majora is usually darker than the surrounding skin and is highly vascular. It protects inner vulval structures and enhances sexual arousal.

The labia majora surround two thinner, vertical folds of reddish epithelium called the *labia minora.* The labia minora are highly vascular and have a rich nerve supply. Emotional or physical stimulation produces marked swelling and sensitivity. Numerous sebaceous glands in the labia minora lubricate the entrance to the vagina. The clitoris is a small, cylindric organ that is composed of erectile tissue with a high concentration of sensory nerve endings. During sexual arousal, the clitoris becomes larger and increases sexual sensation.

The vestibule is a longitudinal area between the labia minora, the clitoris, and the vagina that contains Bartholin glands and the openings of the urethra, Skene's glands (paraurethral glands), and vagina. The two Bartholin glands, located deeply toward the back on both sides of the vaginal opening, secrete lubrication fluid during sexual excitement. Their ductal openings are usually not visible.

The area between the vaginal opening and the anus is the perineum. The skin of the perineum covers the muscles, fascia, and ligaments that support the pelvic structures.

Internal Genitalia

The internal female genitalia are shown in Fig. 69-1. The vagina is a hollow tube that extends from the vestibule to the uterus. Ovarian hormones (primarily *estrogen*) influence the amounts of glycogen and lubricating fluid secreted by the vaginal cells. The normal vaginal bacteria (flora) interact with the secretions to produce lactic acid and maintain an acidic pH (3.5 to 5) in the vagina. This acidity helps prevent infection in the vagina.

At the upper end of the vagina, the uterine cervix projects into a cup-shaped vault of thin vaginal tissue. The recessed pockets around the cervix permit palpation of the internal pelvic organs. The posterior area provides access into the peritoneal cavity for diagnostic or surgical purposes.

The uterus (or "womb") is a thick-walled, muscular organ attached to the upper end of the vagina. This inverted pear–shaped organ is located within the true pelvis, between the bladder and the rectum. The uterus is made up of the body and the cervix.

The cervix is a short (1 inch [2.5 cm]), narrowed portion of the uterus and extends into the vagina. The surfaces of the cervix and the canal are the sites for Papanicolaou (Pap) testing. (See discussion on p. 1454.)

The fallopian tubes (uterine tubes) insert into the fundus of the uterus and extend laterally close to the ovaries. They provide a duct between the ovaries and the uterus for the passage of ova and sperm. In most cases, the ovum is fertilized in these tubes.

The ovaries are a pair of almond-shaped organs located near the lateral walls of the upper pelvic cavity. After menopause, they become smaller. These small organs develop and release ova and produce the sex steroid hormones (estrogen, progesterone, androgen, and relaxin). Adequate amounts of these hormones are needed for normal female growth and development and to maintain a pregnancy.

Breasts

The female breasts are a pair of mammary glands that develop in response to secretions from the hypothalamus, pituitary gland, and ovaries. The breasts are an accessory of the reproductive system that nourish the infant after birth.

Breast tissue is composed of a network of glandular and ductal tissue, fibrous tissue, and fat. The proportion of each component of breast tissue depends on genetic factors, nutrition, age, and obstetric history. The breasts are supported by

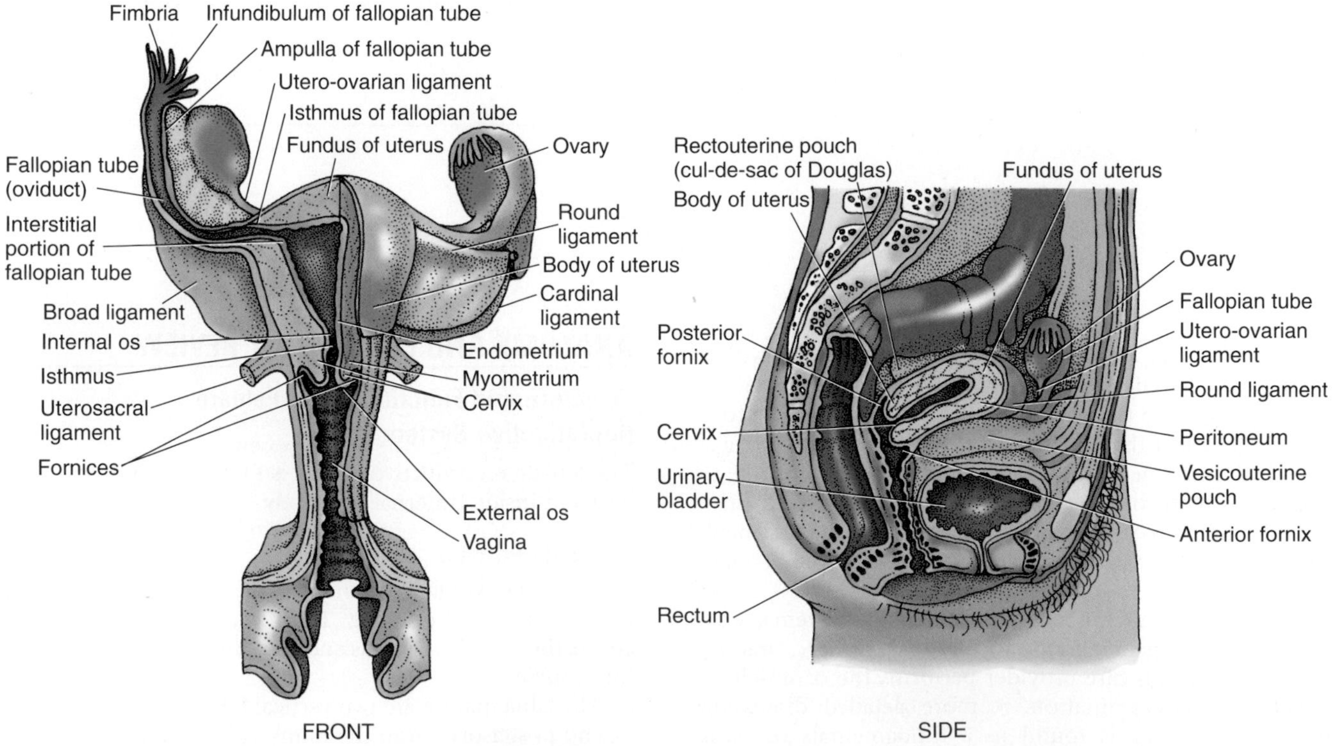

FIG. 69-1 Internal female genitalia.

ligaments that are attached to underlying muscles. They have abundant blood supply and lymph flow that drain from an extensive network toward the axillae (Fig. 69-2).

Structure and Function of the Male Reproductive System

The male reproductive system also consists of external and internal genitalia. The primary male hormone for sexual development and function is *testosterone.* Testosterone production is fairly constant in the adult male. Only a slight and gradual reduction of testosterone production occurs in the older adult male until he is in his 80s. Low testosterone levels decrease muscle mass, reduce skin elasticity, and lead to changes in sexual performance.

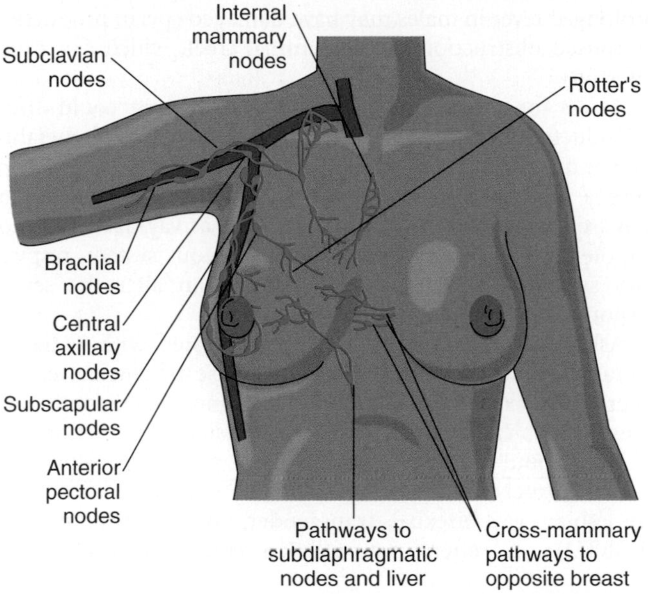

FIG. 69-2 Lymphatic drainage of the female breast.

The penis is an organ for urination and intercourse consisting of the body or shaft and the glans penis (the distal end of the penis). The glans is the smooth end of the penis and contains the opening of the urethral meatus. The urethra is the pathway for the exit of both urine and semen. A continuation of skin covers the glans and folds to form the prepuce (foreskin). Surgical removal of the foreskin (**circumcision**) for religious or cultural reasons is a common procedure in the United States and other Western countries.

The scrotum is a thin-walled, fibromuscular pouch that is behind the penis and suspended below the pubic bone. This pouch protects the testes, epididymis, and vas deferens in a space that is slightly cooler than inside the abdominal cavity. The scrotal skin is darkly pigmented and contains sweat glands, sebaceous glands, and few hair follicles. It contracts with cold, exercise, tactile stimulation, and sexual excitement.

The internal male genitalia are shown in Fig. 69-3. The major organs are the testes and prostate gland. The testes are a pair of oval organs in the scrotum that produce sperm and testosterone. Each testis is suspended in the scrotum by the spermatic cord, which provides blood, lymphatic, and nerve supply to the testis. Sympathetic nerve fibers are located on the arteries in the cord, and sympathetic and parasympathetic fibers are on the vas deferens. When the testes are damaged, these autonomic nerve fibers transmit excruciating PAIN and a sensation of nausea.

The epididymis is the first portion of a ductal system that transports sperm from the testes to the urethra and is a site of sperm maturation. The vas deferens, or ductus deferens, is a firm, muscular tube that continues from the tail of each epididymis. The end of each vas deferens is a reservoir for sperm and tubular fluids. They merge with ducts from the seminal vesicle to form the ejaculatory ducts at the base of the prostate

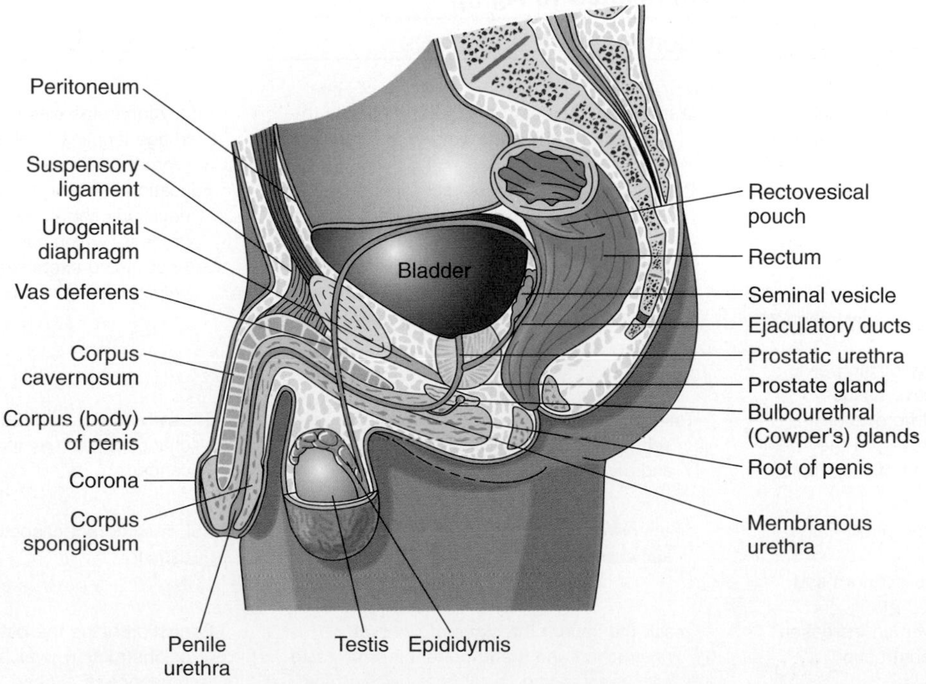

FIG. 69-3 Internal male genitalia.

gland. Sperm from the vas deferens and secretions from the seminal vesicles move through the ejaculatory duct to mix with prostatic fluids in the prostatic urethra.

The prostate gland is a large accessory gland of the male reproductive system that can be palpated via the rectum. The gland secretes a milky alkaline fluid that adds bulk to the semen, enhances sperm movement, and neutralizes acidic vaginal secretions. Men older than 50 years commonly have an enlarged prostate (benign prostatic hyperplasia [BPH]), which can cause problems such as overflow incontinence and nocturia (nighttime urination). Prostate function depends on adequate levels of testosterone.

REPRODUCTIVE CHANGES ASSOCIATED WITH AGING

Age affects the function of both the male and the female reproductive systems. Many changes in the reproductive system occur as people age (Chart 69-1).

ASSESSMENT METHODS

Patient History

Establish a trusting relationship with the patient. Many patients are hesitant to share their reproductive history or concerns about SEXUALITY. Respect their choice to refuse to answer questions about their reproductive problems or sexual practices. Assess the patient's health habits, such as diet, sleep, and exercise patterns. Low levels of body fat may be related to ovarian dysfunction. Assess for alcohol, tobacco, and drug use (prescribed, over-the-counter [OTC], and illicit drugs), because **libido** (sex drive), sperm production, and the ability to have or sustain an erection can be affected by these substances.

Ask female patients about the date and result of their most recent Pap test, breast self-examination, and vulvar self-examination. Determine when male patients older than 50 years had their last prostate examination and prostate-specific antigen test.

Ask about childhood illnesses that could have an effect on the reproductive system. For example, mumps in men may cause **orchitis** (painful inflammation and swelling of the testes) and can lead to testicular atrophy and sterility. Also ask whether the patient has had any infections. Pelvic inflammatory disease or a ruptured appendix followed by peritonitis can cause pelvic scarring and strictures or adhesions in the fallopian tubes. **Salpingitis** (uterine tube INFECTION) is often caused by chlamydia and can result in female infertility. A history of infections or prolonged fever in males may have damaged sperm production or caused obstruction of the seminal tract, which can cause infertility.

Assess for chronic illnesses or surgeries that could affect reproductive function. Disorders that affect a woman's metabolism or nutrition can depress ovarian function and cause **amenorrhea** (absence of menses). Patients with diabetes mellitus may experience physiologic changes such as vaginal dryness or impotence. Chronic disorders of the nervous system, respiratory system, or cardiovascular system can alter the sexual response.

Ask whether the patient has been treated with radiation therapy. Inquire about the prolonged use of corticosteroids, internal or external estrogen, testosterone, or chemotherapy drugs, which can lead to reproductive system dysfunction.

Data about sexual activity are vital parts of the patient's history. Sexual orientation should not be assumed. Patients who are lesbian, gay, bisexual, transgender, and queer/questioning (LGBTQ) are often not fully assessed by health care

CHART 69-1 Nursing Focus on the Older Adult

Changes in the Reproductive System Related to Aging

PHYSIOLOGIC CHANGE	NURSING INTERVENTIONS	RATIONALES
Women		
Graying and thinning of the pubic hair Decreased size of the labia majora and clitoris	Discuss changes with the patient (applies to all structures for both women and men).	Education helps prevent problems with body image (applies to all structures for both women and men).
Drying, smoothing, and thinning of the vaginal walls	Provide information about vaginal estrogen therapy and water-soluble lubricants.	Education enables the patient to make informed decisions about the treatment of vaginal dryness, which can cause painful intercourse.
Decreased size of the uterus Atrophy of the endometrium Decreased size and marked convolution of the ovaries Loss of tone and elasticity of the pelvic ligaments and connective tissue	Provide information about Kegel exercises to strengthen pelvic muscles. Urinary incontinence can be a major problem.	Strengthening exercises may prevent or reduce pelvic relaxation and urinary incontinence.
Increased flabbiness and fibrosis of the breasts, which hang lower on the chest wall; decreased erection of the nipples	Teach or reinforce the importance of breast self-awareness, clinical breast examinations, and mammography.	These methods can detect masses or other changes that may indicate the presence of cancer.
Men		
Graying and thinning of the pubic hair	Teach or reinforce the importance of testicular self-examination (TSE).	TSE may detect changes that may indicate cancer.
Increased drooping of the scrotum and loss of rugae		
Prostate enlargement, with an increased likelihood of urethral obstruction	Teach the patient the signs of urethral obstruction and the importance of prostate cancer screening.	Education helps the patient detect enlargement or obstruction, which may indicate the presence of cancer.

professionals. These patients feel more comfortable sharing this information about their reproductive health and sexual activity when approached in a caring, nonjudgmental way. Chapter 1 describes sensitive interviewing techniques that are appropriate for LGBTQ patients. Chapter 73 in this unit discusses assessment and care of transgender patients in detail.

CULTURAL CONSIDERATIONS

Patient-Centered Care QSEN

Other cultural beliefs and practices influence lifestyle and sexual activity. A person's religious beliefs often influence specific sexual practices, the acceptable number of sexual partners, and contraceptive use. Be sensitive to these differences by being nonjudgmental and showing acceptance.

Nutrition History

A nutrition history is important when assessing the reproductive system. Fatigue and low libido may occur as a result of poor diet and anemia. The World Cancer Research Fund estimates that about one quarter to one third of the new *preventable* cancer cases expected to occur in the United States in 2014 will be related to overweight or obesity, physical inactivity, and poor nutrition (American Cancer Society [ACS], 2014a). Ask the patient to recall his or her dietary intake for a recent 24-hour period to assess nutritional quality.

Assess the patient's height, weight, and body mass index. The patient may be hesitant to discuss practices such as bingeing, purging, anorexic behaviors, or excessive exercise. A certain level of body fat and weight is necessary for the onset of menses and the maintenance of regular menstrual cycles. Decreased body fat results in insufficient estrogen levels.

GENDER HEALTH CONSIDERATIONS

Patient-Centered Care QSEN

Women have special nutrition needs. Heavy menstrual bleeding, particularly in women who have intrauterine devices, may require iron supplements. Teach all women about their body's need for calcium. Although adequate calcium intake throughout life is needed, it is especially important during and after menopause to help prevent osteoporosis due to decreased estrogen production (see Chapter 50).

Family History and Genetic Risk

The family history helps determine the patient's risk for conditions that affect reproductive functioning. A delayed or early development of secondary sex characteristics may be a familial pattern.

The current age and health status of family members are important. Evidence of medical diseases or reproductive problems in family members (e.g., diabetes, endometriosis, reproductive cancer) provides a fuller understanding of the patient's current symptoms. For example, daughters of women who were given diethylstilbestrol (DES) to control bleeding during pregnancy are at increased risk for infertility and reproductive tract cancer.

Specific *BRCA1* and *BRCA2* gene mutations increase the overall risk for breast or ovarian cancer (ACS, 2014c). Men with first-degree relatives (e.g., father, brother) with prostate cancer

CHART 69-2 Best Practice for Patient Safety & Quality Care QSEN

Assessing the Patient with Reproductive Health Problems

PATIENT CONCERN	NURSING ASSESSMENT
Pain	Type and intensity of pain Location and duration of pain Factors that relieve or worsen pain Relationship to menstrual, sexual, urinary, or GI function Medications
Bleeding	Presence or absence of bleeding Character and amount of bleeding Relationship of bleeding to events or other factors (e.g., menstrual cycle) Onset and duration of bleeding Presence of associated symptoms, such as pain
Discharge	Amount and character of discharge Presence of genital lesions, bleeding, itching, or pain Presence of symptoms or discharge in sexual partner
Masses	Location and characteristics of mass Presence of associated symptoms, such as pain Relationship to menstrual cycle

are at greater risk for the disease than are men in the general population.

Current Health Problems

Patients often seek medical attention as a result of PAIN, bleeding, discharge, and masses (Chart 69-2). Pain related to reproductive system disorders may be confused with symptoms usually associated with GI or urinary health problems (e.g., urinary frequency). Ask the patient to describe the nature of the pain, including its type, intensity, timing and location, duration, and relationship to menstrual, sexual, urinary, or GI function. Assess the factors that exacerbate (worsen) or relieve the pain. Ask about sleeping patterns and if pain or other symptoms affect the ability to get adequate rest (Ruhl, 2010).

Heavy *bleeding* or a lack of bleeding may concern the patient. The possibility of pregnancy in any sexually active woman with amenorrhea must be considered. Postmenopausal bleeding needs to be evaluated. Ask the patient to describe the amount and characteristics of abnormal vaginal bleeding. Assess whether the bleeding occurs in relation to the menstrual cycle or menopause, intercourse, trauma, or strenuous exercise. For male patients, ask about the presence of penile bleeding. Ask any patient who has abnormal bleeding about associated symptoms, such as PAIN, cramping or abdominal fullness, a change in bowel habits, urinary difficulties, and weight changes.

Discharge from the male or female reproductive tract can cause irritation of the surrounding tissues, itching, PAIN, embarrassment, and anxiety. Ask about the amount, color, consistency, odor, and chronicity of discharge that may be present from orifices used during sexual activity. Drugs (e.g., antibiotics) and clothing (e.g., tight jeans, synthetic underwear fabric) may cause or worsen genital discharge. Many types of discharge are caused by sexually transmitted diseases (STDs) or other INFECTION (see Chapter 74).

Masses in the breasts, testes, or inguinal area must be evaluated. Patients can sometimes relate changes in character or size of masses to menstrual cycles, heavy lifting, straining, or trauma. Ask about associated symptoms such as tenderness, heaviness, PAIN, dimpling, and tender lymph nodes.

Physical Assessment

Assessment of the Female Reproductive System

The nurse generalist does not perform a comprehensive female or male reproductive examination. However, you should perform a focused assessment related to specific concerns of the patient. The primary care provider conducts a more detailed gynecologic assessment as described below; the generalist nurse often assists with the examination.

Immediately before the pelvic and breast examinations, ask the patient to empty her bladder and undress completely. Drape the patient adequately to provide modesty throughout the examination. Remove drapes only over the region being examined, and replace them after that area has been assessed. Mirrors can be used to facilitate teaching if the patient so desires. The examination should be performed in a room that has adequate lighting for body inspection, that has comfortable temperature, and that ensures privacy.

The physical examination of the female reproductive system includes the breasts (see Chapter 70), cardiovascular system, and abdomen. The patient's arms should be at her sides or over her chest to allow better relaxation of the abdominal muscles. During the gynecologic examination, the primary care provider palpates for symptomatic and asymptomatic abdominopelvic masses, which can be of reproductive, intestinal, or urinary tract origin. Gynecologic masses, such as ovarian masses, may be further differentiated from lesions on the body of the uterus during the bimanual portion of the pelvic examination.

Inspection of the female genitalia and the pelvic examination are usually performed at the end of a head-to-toe physical assessment. The patient is often more apprehensive about these portions of the examination than about any other part. PAIN or lack of privacy during previous pelvic or breast examinations may prevent the patient from relaxing.

Other than determining pregnancy or infertility, a pelvic examination is indicated to assess for:

- Menstrual irregularities
- Unexplained abdominal or vaginal PAIN
- Vaginal discharge, itching, sores, or INFECTION
- Rape trauma or other pelvic injury
- Physical changes in the vagina, cervix, and uterus

Assessment of the Male Reproductive System

Unless a male patient seeks health care for a specific problem, the health care provider may not perform a reproductive assessment, depending on the setting and the age of the patient. Men are often embarrassed and anxious when the reproductive system is assessed. The patient may be concerned about discomfort, the developmental stage of his genitalia, or the possibility of an erection during the examination. If he does have an erection, the examiner should assure him that this is a normal response to a tactile stimulus (touch) and should continue the examination.

Explain each step of the assessment procedure before it is performed. The patient needs to be reassured that the health care provider will stop and change the assessment plan or technique if the patient experiences pain during the examination. Teach relaxation techniques and provide nonjudgmental support during the examination to increase comfort.

Psychosocial Assessment

The psychosocial assessment may provide information about factors that affect the patient's health status. During the social history, ask about sources of support, strengths, and coping reactions to illness or dysfunction.

A patient's personal experiences, culture, and/or spiritual beliefs may influence his or her ability to enjoy a satisfactory sexual life. These factors may include:

- Sexual trauma or abuse inflicted during childhood or adulthood
- Punishment for masturbation
- Psychological trauma
- Cultural influences, such as the idea of female passivity during intercourse
- Concerns about sexual partners or sexual lifestyle
- Use of alcohol or street drugs

Fears may affect the patient's satisfaction with SEXUALITY or body image. He or she may also be concerned about the potential or actual reaction of family members to reproductive health problems (see Chart 69-2). Use nonjudgmental listening to continue development of trust between yourself and the patient, allowing the patient to openly express feelings or concerns.

Diagnostic Assessment

Laboratory Assessment

Chart 69-3 summarizes important laboratory tests associated with reproductive function. The **Papanicolaou test (Pap test)**, or **Pap smear**, is a cytologic study that is effective in detecting precancerous and cancerous cells within the female patient's cervix. It is done immediately before the pelvic examination. A speculum is inserted into the vagina, and several samples of cells from the cervix are obtained with a small brush or spatula. The specimens are placed on a glass slide and sent to the laboratory for examination.

The Pap test should be scheduled between the patient's menstrual periods so that the menstrual flow does not interfere with laboratory analysis. Teach women not to douche, use vaginal medications or deodorants, or have sexual intercourse for at least 24 hours before the test, because these may interfere with test interpretation.

The American Cancer Society (ACS) advises all women to begin having an annual Pap test at 21 years of age. Women younger than 21 years should not be tested (ACS, 2014a). Between ages 21 and 29 years, women should have a Pap test every 3 years; women between ages 30 and 65 years should have a Pap test plus a human papilloma virus (HPV) test ("co-testing") every 5 years. More information on the HPV test is found later in this chapter. In the absence of co-testing, this population should still have a Pap test every 3 years. According to the ACS, women older than 65 years who have had regular cervical cancer testing with normal results should not receive Pap tests (ACS, 2014a). Recommended guidelines from other health care organizations suggest a Pap test every 3 years for women older than 60 years. Those who have had a history of a serious cervical precancerous lesion should be tested annually for at least 20 years after that diagnosis, regardless of age (ACS, 2014a).

Other types of laboratory testing include cytologic vaginal *cultures,* which can detect bacterial, viral, fungal, and parasitic disorders. Examination of cells from the vaginal walls can evaluate estrogen balance.

The **human papilloma virus (HPV) test** can identify many high-risk types of HPV INFECTION associated with the

CHART 69-3 **Laboratory Profile**

Reproductive Assessment

TEST	NORMAL RANGE FOR ADULTS	SIGNIFICANCE OF ABNORMAL FINDINGS
Serum Studies		
Follicle-stimulating hormone (FSH) (Follitropin)	*Men:* 1.42-15.4 IU/L *Women:* follicular phase, 1.37-9.9 IU/L; midcycle, 6.17-17.2 IU/L; luteal phase, 1.09-9.2 IU/L; postmenopause, 19.3-100.6 IU/L	Decreased levels indicate possible infertility, anorexia nervosa, neoplasm. Elevations indicate possible Turner's syndrome.
Luteinizing hormone (LH) (Lutropin)	*Men:* 1.24-7.8 IU/L *Women:* follicular phase, 1.68-15 IU/L; midcycle, 21.9-56.6 IU/L; luteal phase, 0.61-16.3 IU/L; postmenopause, 14.2-52.3 IU/L	Decreased levels indicate possible infertility, anovulation. Elevations indicate possible ovarian failure, Turner's syndrome.
Prolactin	*Men:* 3-13 ng/mL *Women:* 3-27 ng/mL Pregnant women: 20-400 ng/mL	Elevations indicate possible galactorrhea (breast discharge), pituitary tumor, disease of hypothalamus or pituitary gland, hypothyroidism.
Estradiol	*Men:* 10-50 pg/mL *Women:* follicular phase, 20-350 pg/mL; midcycle, 150-750 pg/mL; luteal phase, 30-450 pg/mL; postmenopause, ≤20 pg/mL	Elevations of estradiol, total estrogens, and estriol in men indicate possible gynecomastia, decreased body hair, increased fat deposits, feminization, testicular tumor; in women, ovarian tumor.
Estriol	Men and nonpregnant women: N/A	Decreased levels of estradiol, total estrogens, and estriol in women indicate possible amenorrhea, climacteric, impending miscarriage, hypothalamic disorders.
Progesterone	*Men:* 10-50 ng/dL *Women:* follicular phase, <50 ng/dL; luteal phase, 300-2500 ng/dL; postmenopausal, <40 ng/dL	Decreased levels in women indicate possible inadequate luteal phase, amenorrhea. Elevations in women indicate possible ovarian luteal cysts. Decreased levels may indicate ovarian neoplasm, ovarian dysfunction.
Testosterone	*Men:* 280-1080 ng/dL *Women:* <70 ng/dL	Increased levels in men indicate possible testicular tumor, hyperthyroidism. Decreased levels in men indicate possible hypogonadism. Elevations in women indicate possible adrenal neoplasm, ovarian neoplasm, polycystic ovary syndrome.
Prostate-specific antigen	*Men:* 0-2.5 ng/mL	Increased levels may indicate prostatitis, benign prostatic hyperplasia, prostate cancer.
Urine Studies		
Total estrogens	*Men:* 4-25 mcg/24 hr *Women:* 4-60 mcg/24 hr	Elevations indicate possible testicular tumors. Decreased levels indicate possible ovarian dysfunction.
Pregnanediol	*Men:* 0-1.9 mg/24 hr *Women:* follicular phase, <2.6 mg/24 hr; luteal phase, 2.6-10.6 mg/24 hr	Elevations indicate possible luteal ovarian cysts, ovarian neoplasms, adrenal disorders. Decreased levels indicate possible amenorrhea.
17-Ketosteroids	Men (20-50 yr): 6-20 mg/24 hr Women (20-50 yr): 6-17 mg/24 hr Values decrease with age	Elevations indicate possible Cushing's syndrome, increased androgen or cortisol production, severe stress. Decreased levels indicate possible Addison's disease, hypopituitarism.

Data from Pagana, K.D., & Pagana, T.J. (2014). *Mosby's manual of diagnostic and laboratory tests* (12th ed.). St. Louis: Mosby.
1 mcg, 1 microgram or 1 millionth of a gram; *1 ng,* 1 nanogram or 1 billionth of a gram; *1 pg,* 1 picogram or 1 trillionth of a gram.

development of cervical cancer. This test can be done at the same time as the Pap test for women older than 30 years and for women of any age who have had an abnormal Pap test result (ACS, 2014a). It does not take the place of the Pap test because it tests for viruses that can cause cell changes in the cervix that, if not treated, could lead to cancer. Cells are collected from the cervix and sent to a laboratory for analysis. Women who have normal Pap test results and no HPV infection are at very low risk for developing cervical cancer. Conversely, women with an abnormal Pap test result and a positive HPV test are at higher risk if not treated.

Serum levels of follicle-stimulating hormone (FSH), luteinizing hormone (LH), and prolactin are helpful in the diagnosis of male and female reproductive tract disorders. No nutrition restrictions are necessary before the test. Serum testing can also detect estrogen, progesterone, and testosterone levels in men and women. See Chart 69-3 for normal values and the significance of abnormal findings.

Serologic studies detect antigen-antibody reactions that occur in response to foreign organisms. This form of diagnostic testing is helpful only after an infection has become well established. Serologic testing can be used in the evaluation of exposure to organisms causing syphilis, rubella, and herpes simplex virus type 2 (HSV2). Results may be read as *nonreactive, weakly reactive,* or *reactive.* A single titer is not as revealing as serial titers, which can detect the rise in antibody reactions as the body continues to fight the infection (see Chapter 74).

The *prostate-specific antigen (PSA)* test is used to screen for prostate cancer and to monitor the disease after treatment. PSA levels less than 2.5 ng/mL may be considered normal, although there is no agreement on that value and how it is affected by age. Elevated PSA levels may be associated with prostate cancer. Older men, particularly African-American men, often have a higher normal PSA, especially as they age (Pagana & Pagana, 2014). Chapter 72 discusses this test in more detail.

NCLEX EXAMINATION CHALLENGE

Health Promotion and Maintenance

A 27-year-old client asks the nurse if she needs a Pap smear. Her last Pap test was 2 years ago, and the results were normal. What is the appropriate nursing response?

A. "Yes, you need a Pap test this year."
B. "You are not due for another Pap test until next year."
C. "A Pap smear is not needed unless you are sexually active."
D. "You do not need a Pap smear, but you should have an HPV test."

Imaging Assessment

Computed Tomography. CT scans for reproductive system disorders involve the abdomen and the pelvis. Health care providers can detect and evaluate masses and identify lymphatic enlargement from metastasis. This scan can differentiate solid tissue masses from cystic or hemorrhagic structures.

Hysterosalpingography. A **hysterosalpingogram** is an x-ray that uses an injection of a contrast medium to visualize the cervix, uterus, and fallopian tubes (American Congress of Obstetricians and Gynecologists [ACOG], 2011). This test is used to evaluate tubal anatomy and patency and uterine problems such as fibroids, tumors, and fistulas. The study should not be attempted for at least 6 weeks after abortion, delivery, or dilation and curettage. Other contraindications include reproductive tract infection and uterine bleeding.

The examination is best performed in the first half (days 1-14) of the patient's menstrual cycle, which reduces the chance that the patient may be pregnant (ACOG, 2011). Patients preparing to have a hysterosalpingogram should be instructed to follow the recommendations of their health care provider, which may include taking an over-the-counter pain reliever before the procedure (ACOG, 2011).

On the day of the examination, confirm the date of the patient's last menstrual period. Ask about allergies to iodine dye or shellfish. The health care provider will share benefits and risks of the procedure with the patient. You, as the nurse, may witness the signed informed consent. Be aware that the patient may experience some nausea and vomiting, abdominal cramping, or faintness during the procedure. Provide support and assistance with relaxation techniques as needed.

After the patient is placed in lithotomy position, the health care provider will insert a speculum to view the cervix. Dye is injected through the cervix to fill and highlight the interior of the cervix, uterus, and fallopian tubes. If the fallopian tubes are patent, the contrast material spills into the peritoneal cavity. Usually, only two or three views are obtained to show the path and distribution of the contrast medium.

The patient may experience pelvic PAIN after the study and should receive analgesic medications as ordered. Inform her that she may also have referred PAIN to the shoulder because of irritation of the phrenic nerve. Provide a perineal pad after the test to prevent soiling of clothes as the dye drains from the cervix. Instruct the patient to contact her health care provider if bloody discharge continues for 4 days or longer and to immediately report any signs of infection, such as lower quadrant PAIN, fever, malodorous discharge, or tachycardia.

Mammography. **Mammography** is an x-ray of the soft tissue of the breast. Mammograms assess differences in the density of breast tissue. They are especially helpful in evaluating poorly defined masses, multiple masses or nodules, nipple changes or discharge, skin changes, and PAIN. Mammography can detect about 78% of cancers that are not palpable by physical examination in women younger than 50 years and 83% in women older than 50 years (Susan G. Komen, 2013). However, some actual cancers may not appear on mammography or may appear as benign (ACS, 2014b).

In young women's breasts, there is little difference in the density between normal glandular tissue and malignant tumors, which makes the mammogram less useful for evaluation of breast masses in these women. For this reason, annual screening mammograms are not recommended for women younger than 40 years (ACS, 2014b). In older women, the amount of fatty tissue is higher and the fatty tissue appears lighter than cancers. Cancer and cysts may have the same density. Cysts usually have smooth borders, and cancers often have starburst-shaped margins.

No dietary restrictions are necessary before the mammogram. Remind the patient not to use creams, lotions, powders, or deodorant on the breasts or underarms before the study because these products may be visible on the mammogram and lead to misdiagnosis. If there is any possibility that the patient is pregnant, the test should be rescheduled. Explain the purpose of the study and its anticipated discomforts. Provide a gown and privacy to undress above the waist. Allow the patient to express concerns about the mammogram and the presence of any lumps.

When performing a standard mammogram, a technician positions the patient next to the x-ray machine with one breast exposed. A film plate and the platform of the machine are placed on opposite sides of the breast to be examined. The technician includes as much breast tissue as possible between the plates. The woman may experience some temporary discomfort when the breast is compressed (for about a minute for each of four positions). The entire test takes about 15 minutes. The patient usually is asked to wait until the films are reviewed in case a view needs to be repeated. If a digital mammogram is performed, the images are recorded and saved as computer files (ACS, 2014b).

Inform the patient when to expect the report of the results. Because this is a time when the patient is anxious about the health of her breasts, teach or reinforce the importance of breast self-awareness and provide instructions as needed.

Other Diagnostic Assessment

Ultrasonography. Ultrasonography (US) is a technique that is used to assess fibroids, cysts, and masses. It can be used to monitor the progress of tumor regression after medical treatment. US is also helpful in differentiating solid tumors from cysts in breast examinations. In men, ultrasound can test for varicoceles, scrotal abnormalities, and problems of the ejaculatory ducts and seminal vesicles and the vas deferens (Pagana & Pagana, 2014).

For an abdominal, breast, or scrotal scan, the technician exposes the area and applies gel to the area to be scanned, which provides better transmission of sound waves from the transducer through the patient's skin. The transducer is moved in a linear pattern across the area being tested to outline and define soft-tissue masses and to differentiate tumor type, ascites, and encapsulated fluid.

For a *transvaginal* or *transrectal* scan, the transducer is covered with a condom onto which transmission gel has been placed. The transducer is then inserted into the vagina or rectum as indicated. Women should have an empty or only partially filled bladder if they are having a transvaginal ultrasound. Patients having an internal ultrasound should be informed that they might feel some mild discomfort associated with pressure of the probe (Levin, 2012).

Magnetic Resonance Imaging. MRI uses a magnetic field and radiofrequency energy to scan for pelvic tumors. This scan distinguishes between normal and malignant tissues. MRIs are used in addition to mammograms to assess for breast cancer in women who have a genetic risk (ACS, 2014c). The use of MRI in evaluating patients with dense breast tissue may reduce the need for biopsy.

Endoscopic Studies

Colposcopy. A colposcope allows three-dimensional magnification and intense illumination of epithelium with suspected disease. Colposcopy is suited for inspection of a female patient's cervical epithelium, vagina, and vulvar epithelium. Because it provides accurate site selection, this procedure can locate the exact site of precancerous and malignant lesions for biopsy.

Inform the patient that she should not douche or use vaginal preparations for 24 to 48 hours before the test. This nearly painless procedure is better tolerated if it is explained in advance and if the actual colposcope instrument is shown to the patient. Explain that the health care provider may take a biopsy while performing colposcopy.

Provide the patient with a gown and privacy, and instruct her to undress from the waist down. Assist the patient to the lithotomy position. The health care provider locates the cervix or vaginal site through a speculum examination. Lubricants other than water should not be used. Cells in the area may be stained or left unstained to enhance visibility. The cervix will be cleaned and moistened with normal saline to increase the visibility of vascular patterns and the junction between the columnar epithelium and the squamous epithelium. Acetic acid is applied to the cervix to draw moisture from the tissue and to accentuate important features. The health care provider then uses a colposcope or colpomicroscope to inspect the area in question, and a biopsy specimen can be taken if abnormal cells are seen. (See Cervical Biopsy section on p. 1458.)

After the procedure, allow the patient to rest for a few minutes, especially if she had a biopsy performed. Provide privacy and supplies to clean the perineum and a perineal pad to absorb any dye or discharge. Inform the patient that she may wish to wear a sanitary pad, as mild cramping, spotting, or dark or black-colored discharge (from medication applied to the cervix to reduce bleeding) may occur for several days (Johns Hopkins Medicine, 2014). Remind the patient to take pain relievers as recommended by her health care provider but to avoid aspirin to decrease the chance of bleeding. The patient should be instructed to refrain from douching, using tampons, and having sexual intercourse for 1 week (or as instructed by the health care provider) (Johns Hopkins Medicine, 2014).

Laparoscopy. Laparoscopy is a direct examination of the pelvic cavity through an endoscope. This procedure can rule out an ectopic pregnancy, evaluate ovarian disorders and pelvic masses, and aid in the diagnosis of infertility and unexplained pelvic PAIN. Laparoscopy is also used during surgical procedures such as:

- Tubal sterilization
- Ovarian biopsy
- Cyst aspiration
- Removal of endometriosis tissue
- Lysis of adhesions around the fallopian tubes
- Retrieval of "lost" intrauterine devices

A laparoscopy may be used instead of a laparotomy for minor surgical procedures because it uses small incisions, involves less discomfort, and does not require overnight hospitalization.

The surgeon describes benefits and risks of the procedure to the patient. Risks include complications associated with the use of general anesthesia, postoperative shoulder pain from irritation of the phrenic nerve, effects of carbon dioxide gas and/or peritoneal stretching (Taş et al., 2013), irritation at the incision site, and the rare occurrence of infection or electrical burns. As the nurse, you may witness the patient signing the informed consent. A laparoscopy can be performed with a regional or general anesthetic.

After the patient is anesthetized and placed in the lithotomy position, a urinary catheter is inserted to drain the bladder. The operating table is placed in slight Trendelenburg position to allow the intestines to fall away from the pelvis. The cervix is held with a cannula to allow movement of the uterus during laparoscopy (Fig. 69-4). The surgeon inserts a needle below the umbilicus to infuse carbon dioxide (CO_2) into the pelvic cavity, which distends the abdomen and permits better visualization of the organs. After the trocar and cannula are in place in the abdominal cavity, the surgeon removes the trocar and inserts the laparoscope. The surgeon can then visualize the pelvic cavity and reproductive organs. Further instrumentation is possible through one or more small incisions. The laparoscope is removed at the end of the procedure, and the abdomen is deflated. The small incision is closed with absorbable sutures and dressed with an adhesive bandage.

The patient is usually discharged on the day of the procedure. Discomfort from the incision is managed by oral analgesics. The greatest discomfort is due to referred shoulder PAIN. Most of these sensations disappear within 48 hours. Instruct the patient to change the small adhesive bandage as needed and to observe the incision for signs of infection or hematoma. Remind

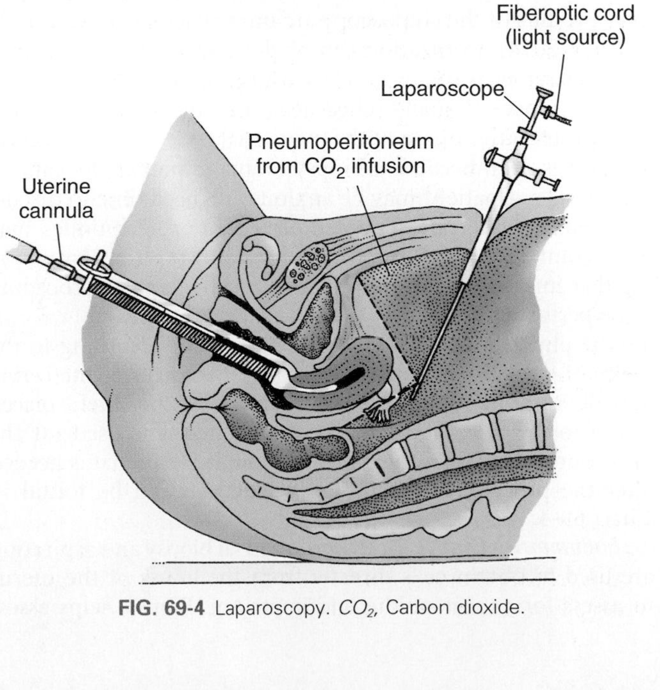

FIG. 69-4 Laparoscopy. *CO_2,* Carbon dioxide.

her also to avoid strenuous activity for the first week after the procedure.

Hysteroscopy. Hysteroscopy is a procedure that uses a fiberoptic camera to visualize the uterus to diagnose and treat causes of abnormal bleeding (Cleveland Clinic, 2013). The hysteroscope includes a fiberoptic camera that is inserted into the vagina to examine the cervix and uterus. Diagnostic hysteroscopy is used to diagnose new problems with the uterus or to confirm results from other tests (Cleveland Clinic, 2013). Hysteroscopy can also be used before or during other procedures (e.g., laparoscopy) for infertility and unexplained bleeding. The procedure is best performed 5 days after menses has ceased to reduce the possibility of pregnancy.

The physician informs the patient of benefits and risks associated with the procedure and obtains consent. You may witness the patient signing the informed consent. The preparation is the same as for a pelvic examination. After the patient is placed in lithotomy position, she is usually anesthetized with a paracervical or other regional block before the cervix is dilated. The physician inserts the hysteroscope through the cervix. Because this distends the uterus, cells can be pushed through the fallopian tubes and into the pelvic cavity. Therefore hysteroscopy is contraindicated in patients with suspected cervical or endometrial cancer, in those with infection of the reproductive tract, and in pregnant patients.

Care is the same as that after a pelvic examination. Analgesics may be prescribed if the patient has cramping or shoulder PAIN.

Biopsy Studies

Cervical Biopsy. In a cervical biopsy, cervical tissue is removed for cytologic study. A biopsy is indicated for an identifiable cervical lesion, regardless of the cytologic findings. The health care provider usually performs a biopsy in conjunction with colposcopy as a follow-up to a suspicious Pap test finding. The procedure may be performed in a clinic or office setting.

Several techniques can be used for a cervical biopsy. If a lesion is clearly visible, an endocervical curettage can be performed as an ambulatory care procedure and with little or no anesthetic. **Conization** (removal of a cone-shaped sample of tissue) and loop electrosurgical excision procedures (LEEPs) are usually not done unless the cervical biopsy findings are positive or the results of the colposcopy are unsatisfactory (Lowdermilk & Perry, 2014). Conization can be done as a cold-knife procedure, a laser excision, or an electrosurgical incision.

The biopsy is usually scheduled when the woman is in the early proliferative phase of the menstrual cycle, when the cervix is least vascular. Because a biopsy evaluates potentially cancerous cells, your patient may be anxious and need time to discuss her feelings and fears. The use of relaxation techniques may assist comfort. Assist her into the lithotomy position, recognizing that further preparation depends on the type of procedure to be performed.

The physician may anesthetize the patient according to the needs of the chosen procedure. He or she visualizes the cervix and obtains the tissue sample, which is immediately placed into a formalin solution. The type of anesthetic used for the procedure determines the type of immediate care that is needed after the procedure. Discharge instructions can be found in Chart 69-4.

CHART 69-4 Patient and Family Education: Preparing for Self-Management

The Patient Recovering from Cervical Biopsy

- Do not lift any heavy objects until the site is healed (about 2 weeks).
- Rest for 24 hours after the procedure.
- Report any excessive bleeding (more than that of a normal menstrual period) to your health care provider.
- Report signs of infection (fever, increased pain, foul-smelling drainage) to your health care provider.
- Do not douche, use tampons, or have vaginal intercourse until the site is healed (about 2 weeks).
- Keep the perineum clean and dry by using antiseptic solution rinses (as directed by your health care provider) and changing pads frequently.

Endometrial Biopsy. Both endometrial biopsy and aspiration are used to obtain cells directly from the lining of the uterus to assess for cancer of the endometrium. Biopsy helps assess menstrual disturbances (especially heavy bleeding) and infertility (corpus luteum dysfunction).

When menstrual disturbances are being evaluated, the biopsy is generally done in the immediate premenstrual period to provide an index of progesterone influence and ovulation. A biopsy performed in the second half of the menstrual cycle (about days 21 and 22) evaluates corpus luteum function and the presence or absence of a persistent secretory endometrium. Postmenopausal women may undergo biopsies at any time.

Menstrual data should be obtained from the patient and are included on the specimen request for the pathologist. Prepare the patient in the same way as you would for a pelvic examination. Advise her that she may experience some cramping when the cervix is dilated. Analgesia before the procedure and relaxation and breathing techniques during the procedure may be helpful to make her more comfortable.

An endometrial biopsy is usually done as an office procedure with or without anesthesia. After the uterus is measured and the cervix dilated, the physician inserts the curette or intrauterine cannula into the uterus. A portion of the endometrium is withdrawn using either the cuplike end of the curette or suction equipment and is placed into a formalin solution to be sent for histologic examination. The patient will likely have moderate cramping. Allow her to rest on the examining table until the cramping has subsided. Provide a perineal pad and a wipe to clean the perineum. Teach her that spotting may be present for 1 to 2 days but any signs of infection or excessive bleeding should be reported to the physician. Instruct the patient to avoid intercourse or douching until all discharge has ceased.

Breast Biopsy. All breast masses should be evaluated for the possibility of cancer. It is important to recognize that breast cancer can occur in men as well as women (National Cancer Institute, 2014). Fibrocystic lesions, fibroadenomas, and intraductal papillomas can be differentiated by biopsy. Any discharge from the breasts is examined histologically.

Provide instructions to the patient depending on the type of biopsy performed and the type of anesthesia used. The patient usually receives a local anesthetic, and the tissue either is aspirated through a large-bore needle (core-needle biopsy) or is removed using a small incision to extract multiple samples of tissue.

Aspirated fluid from benign cysts may appear clear to dark green–brown. Bloody fluid suggests cancer. These specimens undergo histologic evaluation. If cancer is found, the tissue is evaluated for estrogen receptor analysis. Chapter 70 discusses types of breast cancer and their relationship to estrogen receptors.

Teach that discomfort after the procedure is usually mild and can be controlled with analgesics or the use of ice or heat, depending on the type and extent of the biopsy. Educate the patient about how to assess the area or incision for bleeding and edema. Tell women to wear a properly supportive bra continuously for 1 week after surgery or as recommended by their surgeon. Remind the patient that numbness around the biopsy site may last several weeks. If cancer is identified, provide emotional support and reinforce information about follow-up treatment options.

Prostate Biopsy. When prostate cancer is suspected, a biopsy must be performed. This can be done by transurethral biopsy, by inserting a needle through the area of skin between the anus and scrotum, or, most commonly, by transrectal biopsy (Mayo Clinic, 2013). Preparation for the procedure depends on the technique used to puncture the gland.

Explain to the patient that he may experience some discomfort. Teach him about breathing and relaxation techniques that may be helpful to use during the procedure. Because the purpose of this procedure is to evaluate prostate cells for cancer, allow him time to discuss his anxieties and fears.

Assist the patient who is undergoing transrectal biopsy into the side-lying position with his knees pulled up toward his chest (Mayo Clinic, 2013). The physician will cleanse the area, apply gel, and then insert a thin ultrasound probe into the patient's rectum to anesthetize (if needed) and guide the biopsy needle into place. The biopsy is collected over a 5- to 10-minute period. The patient may experience a brief, uncomfortable feeling each time the needle collects a sample.

After prostate biopsy, educate the patient to take the entire prescribed antibiotic. Remind him that he may experience slight soreness, light rectal bleeding, and blood in the urine or stools for a few days. Semen may be red or rust-colored for several weeks. Teach the patient to contact his health care provider if he has prolonged or heavy bleeding, worsening pain, swelling in the area of biopsy, and/or difficulty urinating (Mayo Clinic, 2013). Rarely, sepsis can develop after a prostate biopsy. Teach the patient to contact his health care provider immediately if he experiences fever, pain when urinating, or penile discharge.

NCLEX EXAMINATION CHALLENGE

Physiological Integrity

A client has undergone a transrectal biopsy for suspected prostate cancer. The nurse teaches which postoperative condition should immediately be reported to the health care provider?

A. Fever the next morning
B. Blood in urine 1 day postprocedure
C. Scant rectal bleeding for 2 days
D. Reddish-tinted semen 3 weeks after biopsy

NURSING CONCEPTS AND CLINICAL JUDGMENT REVIEW

What might you EXPECT to see in a patient without reproductive health problems that affect SEXUALITY?

Physical assessment:

- No vaginal bleeding other than normal menstruation
- No unusual vaginal discharge
- No penile bleeding or discharge
- No masses or lesions on internal or external genitalia
- Reports ability to have intercourse without pain

Psychosocial assessment:

- Reports satisfaction with sexual activity
- Reports satisfaction with body image

Laboratory assessment:

- Sex hormones within normal limits for age and gender
- Prostate-specific antigen within normal limits for age

GET READY FOR THE NCLEX® EXAMINATION!

KEY POINTS

Review these Key Points for each NCLEX Examination Client Needs Category.

Health Promotion and Maintenance

- Encourage women to follow recommended Pap screening guidelines for early detection of precancerous and cancerous cells from the cervix. **Evidence-Based Practice** QSEN
- Assess and respect cultural preferences when identifying risks for certain reproductive problems and when evaluating health promotion practices. **Patient-Centered Care** QSEN

Psychosocial Integrity

- Allow the patient to express fear or anxiety regarding potential changes in sexual or reproductive function.
- Assess the patient's level of comfort in discussing issues related to reproductive health and SEXUALITY. **Patient-Centered Care** QSEN
- Encourage patients to express feelings of anxiety or discomfort related to genital examinations and testing of the reproductive system.

Physiological Integrity

- Urge patients with PAIN, bleeding, discharge, masses, or changes in reproductive function to see their health care provider. **Safety** QSEN
- Provide privacy for patients undergoing examination or testing of the reproductive system.

- Recognize that reproductive changes occur with aging, as described in Chart 69-1.
- Recall the selected laboratory tests used for diagnosing reproductive health problems as outlined in Chart 69-3.
- Explain all diagnostic procedures, restrictions, and follow-up care to the patient scheduled for tests.
- Teach women to report symptoms of infection to their health care provider after endoscopic procedures and biopsies of the breast, cervix, and endometrium. **Safety** QSEN
- Instruct men to report symptoms of infection to their health care provider after a transrectal biopsy of the prostate. **Safety** QSEN

CHAPTER 70

Care of Patients with Breast Disorders

Mary Justice

http://evolve.elsevier.com/Iggy/

PRIORITY CONCEPTS

- INFECTION
- PAIN
- SEXUALITY

LEARNING OUTCOMES

Safe and Effective Care Environment

1. Collaborate with health care team members to identify community resources for patients with breast cancer.

Health Promotion and Maintenance

2. Describe the three-pronged approach to early detection of breast masses: mammography, clinical breast examination (CBE), and breast self-awareness.
3. Teach patients who choose breast self-examination (BSE) as an option to use correct technique.
4. Explain the options available to a person at high genetic risk for breast cancer.
5. Evaluate patient risk factors for breast cancer.

Psychosocial Integrity

6. Reduce the psychosocial impact for the patient and family who have received a diagnosis of breast cancer.
7. Discuss SEXUALITY issues with the patient having breast surgery.
8. Describe body image changes that can result from breast cancer surgery.

Physiological Integrity

9. Compare assessment findings associated with benign breast lesions with those of malignant breast lesions.
10. Explain implications of breast reduction and breast augmentation.
11. Discuss treatment options for breast cancer.
12. Develop a personalized postoperative collaborative plan of care for a patient with breast cancer, including PAIN management.
13. Describe the role of radiation and drug therapy in the care of patients with breast cancer.
14. Identify the role of complementary and alternative therapies in breast cancer management.
15. Explain evidence-based options that are available to a woman considering breast reconstruction.

Breast disorders may be benign or cancerous. Changes in the breast can cause a great deal of anxiety for women. An ever-increasing amount of health information is communicated through various types of media that often leads to anxiety and confusion about one's risk for breast cancer (Justice et al., 2012). As a result, many women seek advice for breast changes that they perceive to be abnormal. Nurses are often in the position of assisting patients by providing accurate information about benign breast disorders and breast cancer.

BENIGN BREAST DISORDERS

Benign breast conditions are very common. Noncancerous changes to breast tissue can present as breast lumps, discomfort or PAIN, and nipple changes (Amin et al., 2013). Most breast lumps are benign. Because the incidence of breast disease is related to age, breast disorders are described below in an age-related order (Table 70-1).

FIBROADENOMA

Fibroadenomas are the most common benign tumor in women during the reproductive years. However, they also may occur in a few postmenopausal women. A **fibroadenoma** is a mass of connective tissue that is unattached to the surrounding breast tissue and is usually discovered by the woman herself or during mammography. Although the immediate fear is that of breast cancer, the risk for cancer occurring within a fibroadenoma is very small. On clinical examination, the tumors are oval, freely mobile, and rubbery. Their size varies from smaller than 0.4 inch (1 cm) in diameter to as large as 6 inches (15 cm) in diameter.

Fibroadenomas may occur anywhere in the breast. The health care provider may request a breast ultrasound examination or may perform a needle aspiration to establish whether the lump is cystic (fluid-filled) or solid. If the lesion is solid, excision in an ambulatory care setting using local anesthesia is sometimes the treatment of choice.

TABLE 70-1 Typical Presentation of Benign Breast Disorders

BREAST DISORDER	DESCRIPTION	INCIDENCE
Fibroadenoma	Most common benign lesion; solid mass of connective tissue that is unattached to the surrounding tissue	During teenage years into the 30s (most commonly)
Fibrocystic breast condition	Breast PAIN and tender lumps; the lumps are rubbery, ill defined, and commonly found in the upper outer quadrant of the breast	Onset late teens and 20s; usually subsides after menopause
Ductal ectasia	Hard, irregular mass or masses with nipple discharge, enlarged axillary nodes, redness, and edema; difficult to distinguish from cancer	Women approaching menopause
Intraductal papilloma	Mass in duct that results in nipple discharge; mass is usually not palpable	Women 40 to 55 yr of age

FIBROCYSTIC BREAST CONDITION

❖ *PATHOPHYSIOLOGY*

Fibrocystic changes of the breast include a range of changes involving the lobules, ducts, and stromal tissues of the breast. Because these changes affect at least half of women over the life span, they are referred to as **fibrocystic breast condition (FBC)** rather than *fibrocystic disease.* This condition most often occurs in premenopausal women between 20 and 50 years of age and is thought to be caused by an imbalance in the normal estrogen-to-progesterone ratio. Typical symptoms include breast PAIN and tender lumps or swelling in the breasts. The symptoms are more noticeable before a woman's menstrual period (American Cancer Society [ACS], 2013a).

The two main features of FBC are fibrosis and cysts. Areas of fibrosis are made up of fibrous connective tissue and are firm or hard. Cysts are spaces filled with fluid lined by breast glandular cells. Microcysts are small, nonpalpable cysts inside the breast glands. Macrocysts occur when fluid continues to build up. They often enlarge in response to monthly hormonal changes, stretching the surrounding breast tissue, and become PAINful. Symptoms usually resolve after menstruation and then recur before the next menstrual period in a cyclic fashion. Breast ultrasound is used to confirm the presence of a cyst.

Postmenopausal women taking hormone replacement therapy (HRT) may develop FBC or experience worsening of symptoms. Having cysts or fibrosis does not increase a woman's chance of developing breast cancer. However, if a lump is very firm or has other features raising the concern about cancer, mammography is indicated. A needle biopsy or a surgical biopsy may be needed to make sure cancer is not present. Biopsy may be indicated in these situations:

- No fluid is aspirated.
- The mammogram shows suspicious findings.
- A mass remains palpable after aspiration.
- The aspirated fluid reveals cancer cells.

Symptoms often resolve after menopause when estrogen decreases.

❖ *PATIENT-CENTERED COLLABORATIVE CARE*

Management of FBC focuses on the symptoms of the condition. Suggest supportive measures for women with mild discomfort. The use of analgesics or limiting salt intake before menses to help decrease swelling may be helpful. Teach patients that wearing a supportive bra, even to bed, can reduce PAIN by decreasing tension on the ligaments. Local application of ice or heat may provide temporary relief of pain. For a small number of women, draining the cysts by needle aspiration can help relieve painful symptoms. Many women find relief with the reduction of dietary caffeine and other stimulants, although research has not found stimulants to have a significant impact on FBC (ACS, 2013a).

In women with severe symptoms of FBC, hormonal drugs such as oral contraceptives or selective estrogen receptor modulators (SERMs) may be prescribed to suppress oversecretion of estrogen and correct luteal insufficiency. Vitamin supplements have also been suggested to relieve symptoms, but research has not consistently shown these to be effective; some may have dangerous side effects if taken in large doses. Diuretics may be prescribed to decrease premenstrual breast engorgement.

! NURSING SAFETY PRIORITY (QSEN)

Drug Alert

Explain to women the benefits and risks associated with hormonal drug therapy for FBC, such as stroke, liver disease, and increased intracranial pressure. Teach them to seek medical attention immediately if any signs or symptoms of these complications occur.

Encourage the patient to continue prescribed drug therapy, and monitor the effectiveness of these interventions. Teach the patient to become familiar with the normal feel and texture of her breasts so she is aware of any changes.

DUCTAL ECTASIA

Ductal ectasia is a benign breast problem that is usually seen in women approaching menopause. It occurs when a breast duct dilates and its walls thicken, causing the duct to become blocked. The ducts in the subareolar area are most often affected. These ducts become distended and filled with cellular debris, which activates an inflammatory response. Two manifestations result from these changes:

- A mass develops that feels hard, has irregular borders, and may be tender.
- A greenish brown nipple discharge, enlarged axillary nodes, and redness and edema over the site of the mass are noted.

Ductal ectasia does not affect a woman's breast cancer risk. However, if a mass is present, it may be difficult to distinguish it from breast cancer. Because the risk for breast cancer is increased among women in the menopause age-group, accurate diagnosis is vital. A microscopic examination of the nipple discharge is performed to detect any atypical or malignant cells, and the affected area is excised. Nursing care is directed at reducing the anxiety associated with the threat of breast cancer and at supporting the woman through the diagnostic and treatment procedures. Ductal ectasia may improve without treatment. Warm compresses and antibiotics may be helpful. If symptoms do not improve, the abnormal duct may be surgically removed.

INTRADUCTAL PAPILLOMA

Intraductal papilloma occurs most often in women 40 to 55 years of age. A benign process in the epithelial lining of the duct forms a **papilloma** (pedunculated outgrowth of tissue). As it grows, trauma and erosion within the duct result in a bloody or serous nipple discharge. A mass is rarely palpable.

Diagnosis is aimed first at ruling out breast cancer. Microscopic examination of the nipple discharge and surgical excision of the mass and ductal area are usually indicated.

ISSUES OF LARGE-BREASTED WOMEN

Although Western society emphasizes large breasts as a positive attribute, women with excessive breast tissue often have health problems and discomfort. For instance, a woman with large breasts may have difficulty finding clothes that fit well and in which she feels attractive. The breast size may be out of proportion to the rest of the body, which adds to the problem of finding clothes that fit. Larger bras are expensive and may need to be specially ordered. The woman may have large dents in the shoulders from bra straps. In addition, many large-breasted women develop fungal INFECTIONS under the breasts, especially in hot weather, because it is difficult to keep this area dry and exposed to air.

Backaches from the added weight are also common. If well-fitting bras do not help and obesity is not part of the problem, the only alternative for this condition may be breast reduction surgery. The surgeon removes excess breast tissue and then repositions the nipple and remaining skin flaps to produce the best cosmetic effect. This operation is a major surgical procedure and is called a **reduction mammoplasty**.

The decision to have the procedure is usually made after years of living with the discomfort of excessive breast size. Listen to the woman verbalize her feelings, and reinforce information as appropriate. The nursing care after surgery is similar to that for the woman having reconstructive surgery. (See discussion of Breast Reconstruction, p. 1476, in the Surgical Management section.)

ISSUES OF SMALL-BREASTED WOMEN

Some women choose to have **breast augmentation** surgery to increase or improve the size, shape, or symmetry of their breasts. Most health insurers do not pay for this procedure. Most surgeries involve the implantation of saline-filled or silicon prostheses. Some are constructed from the women's own tissue in much the same way as for reconstruction after mastectomy. *Saline* implants are filled with sterile saline and can be filled with the amount needed to get the shape and firmness the woman wants. If the implant shell leaks, the saline will be safely absorbed by the body. *Silicone* implants are filled with an elastic gel, which can leak into the breast and will not be absorbed. The plastic surgeon reviews the advantages and disadvantages of each implant or natural procedure.

After surgery, the patient can be discharged to home the same day or the day after. Remind the family or significant other that someone should stay with her for at least 24 hours after surgery. The incisions may or may not have dressings depending on the surgeon and type of surgery.

! NURSING SAFETY PRIORITY (QSEN)

Action Alert

Before breast augmentation surgery, teach the patient to stop smoking (to promote healing), avoid aspirin and other NSAIDs, and avoid herbs that can cause bleeding during the procedure, such as garlic, *Ginkgo biloba,* and ginseng. Tell her that the incisions will be hidden as much as possible, either under the pectoral muscle or directly behind the breast tissue as a submammary placement. One or more wound drains will be inserted during surgery, and she will need to know how to care for those drains at home. Review possible postoperative complications, including INFECTION and implant leakage, which can cause severe PAIN and possible fever.

! NURSING SAFETY PRIORITY (QSEN)

Action Alert

Remind the patient after breast augmentation that for the first few days she should expect soreness in her chest and arms. Her breasts will feel tight and sensitive, and the skin over her breasts may feel warm or may itch. Teach the patient that she will have difficulty raising her arms over her head and should not lift, push, or pull anything until the surgeon permits. Teach her to also avoid strenuous activity or twisting above her waist. Remind the patient to walk every few hours to prevent deep vein thrombi. Tell her to expect some swelling of the breasts for 3 to 4 weeks after surgery.

An important issue for patients who have breast augmentation surgery is breast cancer surveillance. Breast self-examination (BSE) and clinical breast examination (CBE) can still be performed because the prosthesis is placed behind the woman's normal breast tissue, actually pushing it forward. However, screening mammography may not be as sensitive because the amount of visualized breast tissue is decreased. Additional x-rays, called *implant displacement views,* may be used to examine the breast tissue more completely (ACS, 2013a). Although there is no conclusive evidence that breast augmentation increases breast cancer risk, further research is needed regarding diagnosis and prognosis of breast cancer among women with cosmetic breast implants (Lavigne et al., 2013). Teach women desiring cosmetic breast augmentation about the differences in breast cancer screening.

GYNECOMASTIA

Gynecomastia literally means "female breasts" and is a symptom rather than a disease. It is usually a benign condition of breast enlargement in *men* (Fig. 70-1). However, gynecomastia can be a result of a primary cancer such as lung or testicular cancer. The enlargement is usually bilateral but may be asymmetric in a few cases. The condition is caused by abnormal growth of the glandular tissue, including the mammary ducts and ductal tissue. In many instances it is difficult to determine gynecomastia from breast enlargement related to excess adipose tissue. Other causes of gynecomastia include:

- Drugs, such as anti-androgen agents and corticosteroids
- Aging
- Obesity
- Underlying disease causing estrogen excess, such as malnutrition, liver disease, or hyperthyroidism
- Androgen-deficiency states, such as age, chronic kidney disease, or alcoholism

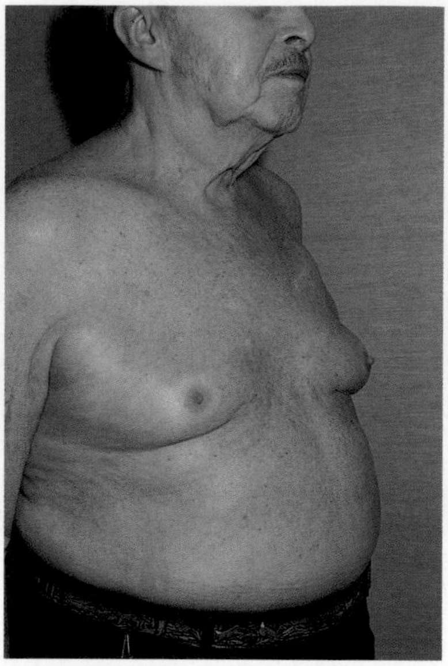

FIG. 70-1 Gynecomastia.

Although gynecomastia is not common, men with abnormal breast findings, especially a breast mass, should be carefully evaluated for breast cancer.

BREAST CANCER

PATHOPHYSIOLOGY

Excluding skin cancers, breast cancer is the most commonly diagnosed cancer in women and is second only to lung cancer as a cause of female cancer deaths (ACS, 2013b). Therefore most references in this section are to women with breast cancer. Because of the high incidence of the disease, almost every woman knows of someone with the disease. Thus most women have strong reactions to the threat of breast cancer. These reactions greatly influence health habits, including breast self-examination (BSE) and the patient's readiness to seek care when a suspicious area is discovered. Nurses play a key role in early detection by educating women about screening guidelines, risk factors for breast cancer, and BSE. Men should also be taught about this disease.

Early detection is the key to effective treatment and survival. The 5-year relative survival rate is lower for women who are diagnosed with an advanced stage of breast cancer. The 5-year survival rate for localized breast cancer is 98.6%, whereas the rate drops to 83.8% when the cancer has spread to the regional lymph nodes (ACS, 2013b). Survival drops dramatically when breast cancer is metastatic (spread to distant sites).

Cancer of the breast begins as a single transformed cell that grows and multiplies in the epithelial cells lining one or more of the mammary ducts or lobules. It is a heterogeneous disease, having many forms with different clinical presentations and responses to therapy (Weigelt et al., 2010). Some breast cancers will present as a palpable lump in the breast, whereas others show up only on a mammogram.

There are two broad categories of breast cancer: noninvasive and invasive. About 20% are *noninvasive;* the remaining 80% are invasive. As long as the cancer remains within the duct, it is noninvasive. The cancer is classified as *invasive* when it penetrates the tissue surrounding the duct. Most of these cancers arise from the intermediate ducts. Metastasis occurs when cancer cells leave the breast via the blood and lymph systems, which permits spread of these cells to distant sites. The most common sites of metastasis are bone, lung, brain, and liver. The course of metastatic breast cancer is related to the site affected and to the function impaired. The processes involved in cancer development are described in Chapter 21.

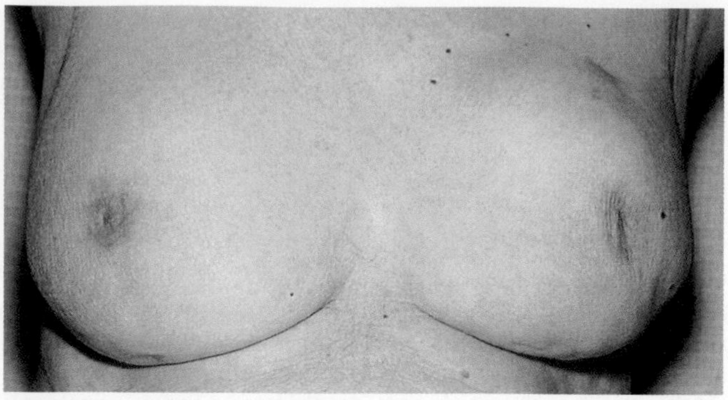

FIG. 70-2 Skin dimpling on a breast as a result of fibrosis or breast cancer.

Noninvasive Breast Cancers

Ductal carcinoma in situ (DCIS) is an early *noninvasive* form of breast cancer. In DCIS, cancer cells are located within the duct and have not invaded the surrounding fatty breast tissue. Because of mammography screening and earlier detection, the number of women diagnosed with DCIS has increased. If left untreated, it is estimated that 14% to 53% of DCIS would become invasive and spread into the breast tissue surrounding the ducts over a period of 10 years (Morgan et al., 2011). Currently there is no way to determine which DCIS lesions will progress to invasive cancer and which ones will remain unchanged. This uncertainty causes anxiety and decisional conflict in many women diagnosed with DCIS. It is important to convey to patients the ways in which DCIS differs from invasive cancer and that DCIS cells lack the biologic capacity to metastasize.

Another type of noninvasive cancer is **lobular carcinoma in situ (LCIS)**. This cancer is rare and occurs as an abnormal cell growth in the lobules (milk-producing glands) of the breast. It is not a true cancer, but having LCIS increases one's risk for developing a separate breast cancer later. It is usually diagnosed before menopause in women 40 to 50 years of age. Traditionally, LCIS is treated with close observation only. Women with LCIS and other breast cancer risk factors may want to consider prophylactic treatment options such as tamoxifen, raloxifene, or prophylactic mastectomy (ACS, 2013a).

Invasive Breast Cancers

The most common type of invasive breast cancer is **infiltrating ductal carcinoma**. As the name implies, the disease originates in the mammary ducts and grows in the epithelial cells lining these ducts. Once invasive, the cancer grows into the tissue around it in an irregular pattern. If a lump is present, it is felt as an irregular, poorly defined mass. As the tumor continues to grow, **fibrosis** (replacement of normal cells with connective tissue and collagen) develops around the cancer. This fibrosis may cause shortening of Cooper's ligaments and the resulting typical skin dimpling that is seen with more advanced disease (Fig. 70-2). Another sign, sometimes indicating late-stage breast

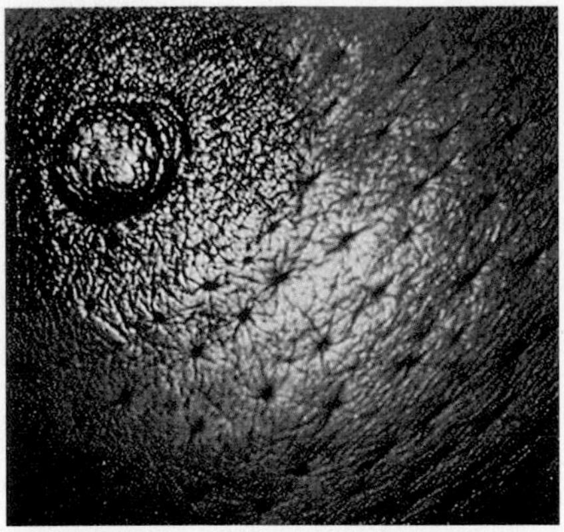

FIG. 70-3 Breast edema giving the skin an "orange peel" *(peau d'orange)* appearance.

cancer, is an edematous thickening and pitting of breast skin called *peau d'orange* (orange peel skin) (Fig. 70-3).

A rare but highly aggressive form of invasive breast cancer is **inflammatory breast cancer** (IBC). Symptoms include swelling, skin redness, and PAIN in the breasts. IBC seldom presents as a palpable lump and may not show up on a mammogram. Because it is usually diagnosed at a later stage than other types of breast cancer, it is often harder to treat successfully (ACS, 2013a).

Breast Cancer in Men

Male breast cancer is rare, occurring in fewer than 1% of all cases. The average age of onset is 68 years (Mattarella, 2010). Causes are not completely understood, but there is a strong association between male breast cancer, family history, and genetic factors. (See discussion of genetic risk below.)

Men usually present with a hard, painless, subareolar mass; gynecomastia may be present. Occasionally the man may have nipple discharge, retraction, erosion, or ulceration. Because *men* usually do not suspect breast cancer when they feel a lump, diagnosis frequently is delayed (Mattarella, 2010). Thus men have a slightly lower overall survival than do women. However, there are more similarities than differences between male and female breast cancer (Greif et al., 2012). Treatment of breast cancer in men is the same as in women at a similar stage of disease.

Breast Cancer in Young Women

Media coverage and accounts of women with breast cancer often portray women younger than 60 years, misleading many to overestimate the incidence of breast cancer in younger women (National Breast Cancer Coalition [NBCC], 2012). Nevertheless, about 4.6% of breast cancer cases occur in women younger than 40 years (ACS, 2013b). Genetic predisposition is a stronger risk factor for younger women than older women (Pollán, 2010). Younger women frequently present with more aggressive forms of the disease, and the number of cases of advanced breast cancer in younger women is increasing (Johnson et al., 2013). Screening tools can be less effective for this group because the breasts are denser; therefore regular screening mammograms before the age of 40 years are not recommended for average-risk women (ACS, 2013a). Nurses should encourage women who have symptoms to seek evaluation and not watch and wait. Younger women with breast cancer face unique issues associated with treatment. These include surgical menopause, infertility after treatment, and sexual dysfunction (Kedde et al., 2013).

Etiology and Genetic Risk

There is no single known cause for breast cancer. *Being an older woman or man is the primary risk factor, although some people are at higher risk than others.* Several breast cancer risk factors have been identified; some are modifiable, whereas others are not (ACS, 2013b). Risk factors have varying degrees of influence on breast cancer development. Having several risk factors increases one's risk more than having a single risk factor. Table 70-2 lists major breast cancer risk factors according to the varying degree of risk. Assist women to clarify that not all risk factors are the same.

GENETIC/GENOMIC CONSIDERATIONS

Patient-Centered Care QSEN

Mutations in several genes, such as *BRCA1* and *BRCA2*, are related to hereditary breast cancer. People who have specific mutations in either one of these genes are at a high risk for developing breast cancer as well as ovarian cancer. However, only 5% to 10% of all breast cancers are hereditary. Only women with a strong family history and a reasonable suspicion that a mutation is present have genetic testing for *BRCA* mutations (ACS, 2013a). Encourage women to talk with a genetics counselor to carefully consider the benefits and potential harmful consequences of genetic testing before these tests are done.

Knowledge of modifiable risk factors can help women develop strategies for prevention of breast cancer. These include avoiding weight gain and obesity, engaging in regular physical activity, and minimizing alcohol intake. Breast-feeding for a year or more has been shown to have a protective influence on breast cancer as does avoidance of hormone replacement therapy (HRT) for menopausal symptoms. Encourage women seeking help for menopausal symptoms to discuss the benefits and risks of hormonal therapy with their health care provider. Environmental causes of breast cancer are the subject of increasing research and concern for many women. Environmental estrogens found to influence breast cancer development in animals include DDT found in pesticides, perfluorooctanoic acid (PFOA) found in nonstick cookware, and bisphenol A (BPA) found in plastic food containers. More research is needed to discover the effect of these chemicals on human breast cancer (Schmidt, 2012), but many women are choosing to avoid them as a precaution. (See the Evidence-Based Practice box.)

Incidence and Prevalence

The American Cancer Society estimated the incidence of breast cancer in the United States to be 232,340 in 2013. Breast cancer is the second leading cause of cancer death in women, exceeded only by lung cancer, and 39,629 are likely to die of the disease (ACS, 2013b).

Health Promotion and Maintenance

The American Cancer Society (ACS) establishes evidence-based guidelines for breast cancer screening in women. Guidelines have not been recommended for screening men in the general population because breast cancer in men is so uncommon (ACS, 2013a). Encourage men with a strong family history or known genetic mutations to discuss screening with their health care provider.

TABLE 70-2 Risk Factors for Breast Cancer

FACTORS	COMMENTS
High Increased Risk (Relative Risk >4.0)	
Female gender	Ninety-nine percent of all breast cancers occur in women.
Age >65 years	Risk increases across all ages until age 80 years.
Genetic factors	Inherited mutations of *BRCA1* and/or *BRCA2* increase risk.
History of a previous breast cancer	The risk for developing a cancer in the opposite breast is 5 times greater than for the average population at risk.
Breast density	Dense breasts contain more glandular and connective tissue, which increases the risk for developing breast cancer.
Atypical hyperplasia	Biopsy-confirmed atypical hyperplasia is a high relative risk.
Moderate Increased Risk (Relative Risk 2.1–4.0)	
Family history	Two first-degree relatives with breast cancer increases risk.
Ionizing radiation	Women who received frequent low-level radiation exposure to the thorax had an increased risk, especially if the exposure occurred during periods of rapid breast formation.
High postmenopausal bone density	High estrogen levels over time both strengthen bone and increase breast cancer risk.
Low Increased Risk (Relative Risk 1.1–2.0)	
Reproductive history Nulliparity OR First child born after age 30 years	Childless women have an increased risk, as do women who bear their first child near or after age 30.
Menstrual history Early menstruation OR Late menopause OR Both	The risk for breast cancer rises as the interval between menarche and menopause increases. Women who undergo bilateral oophorectomy before age 35 years have less risk for breast cancer than women who undergo natural menopause.
Recent oral contraceptive use	There is a slight increase in breast cancer risk in women taking oral contraceptives. The risk returns to normal after 10 years of stopping the pill.
Recent hormone replacement therapy (HRT)	Use of HRT containing both estrogen and progestin increases risk; risk diminishes after 5 years of discontinuation.
Obesity	Postmenopausal obesity (especially increased abdominal fat), increased body mass, insulin resistance, and hyperglycemia have been reported to be associated with an increased risk for breast cancer.
Other Risk Factors	
Alcohol	Risk is dose-dependent; consumption of 3 to 14 drinks per week is associated with a slight increase in risk; risk increases with increased consumption.
High socioeconomic status	Breast cancer incidence is greater in women of higher education and socioeconomic background. This relationship is possibly related to lifestyle differences, such as later age at first birth.
Jewish heritage	Women of Ashkenazi Jewish heritage have higher incidences of *BRCA1* and *BRCA2* genetic mutations.

Modified from American Cancer Society. (2013). *Breast cancer facts & figures 2011-2012*. Atlanta: Author.

EVIDENCE-BASED PRACTICE QSEN

Does Night-Shift Work Increase the Risk for Breast Cancer?

Kamdar, B., Tergas, A., Mateen, F., Bhayani, N., & Oh, J. (2013). Night-shift work and risk of breast cancer: A systematic review and meta-analysis. *Breast Cancer Research and Treatment, 138*(1), 291-301.

Researchers conducted a systematic review and meta-analysis of studies examining night-shift work and its relationship with breast cancer. Previous studies have suggested that night-shift workers, such as flight attendants and nurses, may lack adequate melatonin, which may contribute to an increase in breast cancer risk. Fifteen studies were included in the analysis. The researchers determined that the findings of these studies were limited due to unmeasured confounding and substantial heterogeneity observed among the studies. They concluded there is weak evidence to support previous findings that night-shift work is associated with an increased breast cancer risk.

Level of Evidence: 1

The study utilized a systematic review of the literature and meta-analysis of multiple studies to make conclusions.

Commentary: Implications for Practice and Research

Nurses should be aware of the validity of publicized studies as well as ongoing research in this area. This meta-analysis found lack of consistencies among studies about shift work and breast cancer risk. Future studies involving large sample sizes and diverse occupational and geographic populations are necessary. The increasing number of around-the-clock workers raises important public health and policy issues.

CULTURAL CONSIDERATIONS

Patient-Centered Care QSEN

One of every 8 women in the United States will develop breast cancer by age 70 years. Euro-American women older than 40 years are at a greater risk than other racial/ethnic groups, but the rate of breast cancer in African-American women *younger than 40 years* is higher than for others in that age-group. African-American women have a higher death rate at any age when compared with other women with the disease (ACS, 2013b). Cultural disparities with regard to breast cancer stage and mortality are persistent. Ooi et al. (2011) found that non-Hispanic white women are more likely to present with an earlier-stage breast cancer than American-Indian/Alaska-Native, Asian-Indian/Pakistani, Black, Filipino, Hawaiian, Mexican, Puerto Rican, and Samoan women. These groups are also more likely to present with more aggressive breast cancer that is harder to treat, such as *triple negative breast cancer*. In this type of breast cancer, cells lack receptors for estrogen, progesterone, and the protein *HER2*. African-American and Puerto Rican women have the highest risk for triple negative breast cancer. Breast cancer death rates are highest in African-American, Hawaiian, Puerto Rican, and Samoan women. Cultural disparities should be addressed with targeted interventions that are appropriate for specific cultural and ethnic groups. Nurses need to be culturally competent to assist women to overcome barriers to care.

NCLEX EXAMINATION CHALLENGE

Health Promotion and Maintenance

The nurse is caring for four clients. Which client does the nurse recognize as having the highest risk for development of breast cancer?

A. 45-year-old male with gynecomastia
B. 40-year-old female whose father had colon cancer
C. 50-year-old male whose mother had ovarian cancer
D. 65-year-old female with history of a prior episode of breast cancer

The ACS recommendation for early detection by screening for breast masses is a screening mammogram for women ages 40 years and older and a clinical breast examination (CBE) by a health care professional at least every 3 years for women 20 to 40 years old. Monthly breast self-examination (BSE) is less emphasized today than in the past several decades. It is recommended as an option to women to increase breast self-awareness beginning at age 20.

NURSING SAFETY PRIORITY (QSEN)

Action Alert

Teach women that no single method for early detection of breast cancer is effective when used alone. The best approach for average-risk women is screening mammogram, clinical breast examination, and breast self-awareness.

Mammography

The use of mammography (x-ray of the breasts) screening for healthy, average-risk women continues to be studied for its effectiveness. In 2009, the U.S. Preventive Services Task Force (USPSTF) recommended raising the screening age for average-risk women from 40 to 50 years (USPSTF, 2009). Scientific evidence shows there are benefits as well as risks associated with mammography, and disagreement exists about the emphasis that should be placed on each one. However, the ACS and The American College of Obstetricians and Gynecologists (ACOG) continue to recommend that all women ages 40 years and older have a screening mammogram annually (ACOG, 2011). Educate women on the advantages and disadvantages of breast screening techniques so that they can make informed decisions about the screening methods best suited to their individual situations (Association of Women's Health, Obstetric, and Neonatal Nursing [AWHONN], 2010).

According to guidelines of the American Society of Clinical Oncology, women who are asymptomatic following breast cancer treatment should be screened with annual mammograms, without additional tests (Khatcheressian et al., 2013). A small number of women who have known genetic mutations and/or other high risk factors for breast cancer should have screening with MRI in addition to annual mammography (ACS, 2013a). Encourage women with moderate risk factors to discuss with their health care provider the benefits and limitations of adding MRI screening to their annual mammograms. MRI screening is not recommended for women with low breast cancer risk factors.

Breast ultrasound is sometimes used in addition to mammography when problems are found during routine screening and for some women with dense breast tissue. Although the use of ultrasound has added benefits over mammography alone, it is not recommended as part of routine breast cancer screening for women who are average risk for breast cancer (ACS, 2013a).

Breast Self-Awareness/Self-Examination

Nurses working with women should teach them the importance of becoming familiar with the appearance and feel of their breasts. Any changes detected by the woman should be reported to her health care provider. Teach a woman that lumps are not necessarily abnormal. For premenopausal women, lumps can come and go with the menstrual cycle. Most lumps that are detected and tested are not cancerous.

Some women may want to practice regular breast self-examination (BSE) as a method for breast self-awareness. Evidence shows that monthly BSE is no more beneficial than women simply being aware of what is normal for their own breasts and women are just as likely to find a lump by chance (ACS, 2013a). However, BSE should be presented as an option to women beginning in their early 20s. In addition to breast self-awareness, emphasis should be placed on mammography and clinical breast examination for early detection of breast cancer. The combined approach is better than any single test (ACS, 2013a). A woman who chooses to perform BSE should be taught the correct technique and have it reviewed by a health care professional during her clinical breast examination.

The BSE technique is similar for women and men. Use teaching models of normal and abnormal breasts when teaching BSE. Discuss the proper timing for BSE. Instruct premenopausal women to examine their breasts 1 week after the menstrual period. At this time, hormonal influence on breast tissue is decreased, so fluid retention and tenderness are reduced. Teach women whose breast tissue is no longer influenced by hormonal fluctuations, such as after a total hysterectomy or menopause, to pick a day each month to do BSE, such as the first day of the month. Chart 70-1 describes the procedure for breast self-examination and may be used as a patient resource.

Clinical Breast Examination

Clinical breast examination (CBE) is typically performed by advanced practice nurses and other health care providers. Clinicians who perform CBE ideally go through simulation training and exposure to patients to become proficient at the technique

CONSIDERATIONS FOR OLDER ADULTS

Patient-Centered Care (QSEN)

As women age, the breast tissue becomes flattened and elongated and is suspended loosely from the chest wall. On palpation, the breast tissue of the older woman has a finer, more granular feel than the lobular feel in a younger woman. The inframammary ridge may be more prominent as a result of atrophy of the breast tissue. Breast examination in older adults may be easier because of tissue atrophy and relaxation of the suspensory ligaments.

Women in nursing homes and other long-term care facilities often do not have clinical breast examinations and may not be deliberately aware of the normal appearance and feel of their breasts. Teach the importance of breast self-awareness and reporting any breast changes the woman may notice. Teach BSE as an option for older women who are comfortable with and able to perform this method. Collaborate with the health care provider to ensure that residents have clinical breast examinations.

CHART 70-1 Best Practice for Patient Safety & Quality Care QSEN

Performing Breast Self-Examination

1. Lie down on your back, and place your right arm behind your head. Lying down spreads the breast tissue evenly over the chest wall, making it easier to feel all the breast tissue.
2. Use the finger pads of the three middle fingers on your left hand to feel for lumps in the right breast. Use overlapping dime-size circular motions of the finger pads to feel the breast tissue.
3. Use three different levels of pressure to feel all the breast tissue. Light pressure is needed to feel the tissue closest to the skin; medium pressure to feel a little deeper; and firm pressure to feel the tissue closest to the chest and ribs. It is normal to feel a firm ridge in the lower curve of each breast.
4. Move around the breast in an up-and-down pattern starting at an imaginary line drawn straight down your side from the underarm and moving across the breast to the middle of the chest bone (sternum or breastbone). Be sure to check the entire breast area going down until you feel only ribs, and up to the neck.
5. Repeat the exam on your left breast, putting your left arm behind your head and using the finger pads of your right hand to do the exam.
6. While standing in front of a mirror with your hands pressing firmly down on your hips, look at your breasts for any changes of size, shape, contour, or dimpling and look at your nipples and breast skin for redness or scaling. (The pressing-down-on-the-hips position contracts the chest wall muscles and enhances any breast changes.)
7. Examine each underarm while sitting up or standing and with your arm only slightly raised so you can easily feel in this area. Raising your arm straight up tightens the tissue in this area and makes it harder to examine.

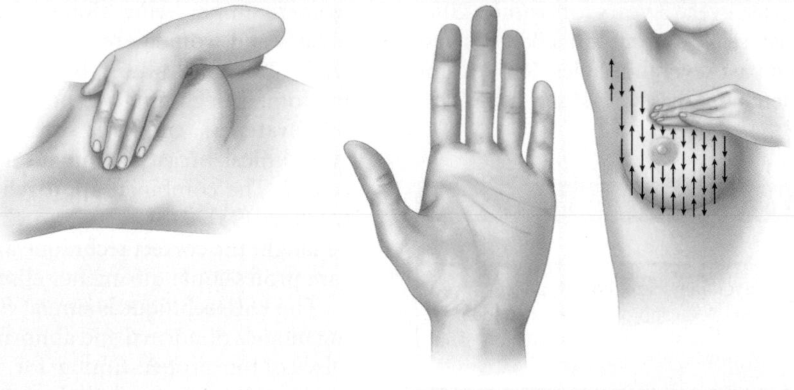

Adapted from the American Cancer Society. (2013). *Detailed guide: How to examine your breasts.* Atlanta: Author. Available from www.cancer.org.

(Bryan & Snyder, 2013). It is recommended that the CBE be part of a periodic health assessment, at least every 3 years for women in their 20s and 30s, and every year for asymptomatic women at least 40 years of age (ACS, 2013a). Teach patients what to expect during this examination. First, they will be asked to undress from the waist up. The examiner inspects the breasts for abnormalities in size and shape and for skin and nipple changes. Then, using the pads of the fingers, the examiner palpates the breasts for any lumps and, if present, whether such lumps are attached to the skin or deeper tissues. The area under both arms is also examined.

Options for High-Risk Women

Women with a personal history of breast cancer are at risk for developing a recurrence or a new breast cancer. Those with known *BRCA1* and *BRCA2* genetic mutations, strong family history, or other high-risk factors are also considered high-risk. Women in this category usually practice *close surveillance* as a prevention option. It is referred to as "secondary prevention" and is used to detect cancer early in the initial stages. In addition to annual mammography and clinical breast examination, high-risk women are recommended to have an annual breast MRI screening (ACS, 2013a). Close surveillance may begin as early as age 30 years, but evidence is limited regarding the best age at which to start screening. Encourage high-risk women to discuss their personal preferences for close surveillance with their health care providers.

Options currently available for reducing a woman's breast cancer risk are **prophylactic mastectomy** (preventive surgical removal of one or both breasts), prophylactic **oophorectomy** (removal of the ovaries), and anti-estrogen chemopreventive drugs. Although each option significantly reduces the risk for breast cancer, no option completely eliminates it. Each option has its own risks and potentially serious complications.

Even though a woman may decide to have a *prophylactic mastectomy,* there is a small risk that breast cancer will develop in residual breast glandular tissue because no mastectomy reliably removes all mammary tissue. Women must also understand that breast reconstruction after a prophylactic mastectomy is very different from breast augmentation. It is a more complex surgical procedure with a greater potential for complications. The decision to have this type of surgery can be a very difficult one to make. Women may find it helpful to reach out to a breast cancer support organization and talk to someone who has been through a prophylactic mastectomy. The majority of patients express long-term satisfaction with this surgical procedure (Soran et al., 2013).

Women undergoing *oophorectomy* will likely experience menopausal symptoms, although some estrogen remains in body fat tissue. *Anti-estrogen drugs* reduce breast cancer recurrence but carry other risks such as blood clots and endometrial cancer. Encourage women to carefully consider the benefits and risks of breast cancer–risk-reducing options and to discuss them with their health care provider.

❖ PATIENT-CENTERED COLLABORATIVE CARE

◆ Assessment

History. Often the history is taken after a mass has been discovered but before a diagnosis has been made for a woman or man with breast cancer. For some patients, the history may be obtained at the time they are seen for treatment of an identified cancer. The interview should focus on three major areas: risk factors, the breast mass, and health maintenance practices.

Record age, gender, marital status, weight, and height. Marital status and identifying the patient's primary support person provide information about who should be included in the patient's care, teaching, and support.

CULTURAL CONSIDERATIONS

Patient-Centered Care QSEN

Remember that some cultures do not allow the man to be part of a woman's care or only women are allowed to care for her (e.g., Arab Muslim women). Other cultures are male-predominant and all decisions about female care are made by the man (e.g., Nigerian women).

Ask specific information on personal and family histories of breast cancer. In addition to increasing the woman's own risk, these factors also affect any sisters' or daughters' risk and should be part of later counseling.

Ask about the woman's gynecologic and obstetric history, including:

- Age at menarche
- Age at menopause
- Symptoms of menopause
- Age at first child's birth
- Number of children/pregnancies

Prolonged hormonal stimulation (e.g., early menses, late menopause) increases a woman's risk, as do birth of the first child after 30 years of age and nulliparity (having no children).

A history of the breast mass or lump reveals not only the course of the disease but also information related to health care–seeking practices and health-promoting behaviors. Ask the patient about how, when, and by whom the mass was discovered and the time between discovery and seeking care. If the patient found the mass, ask how it was discovered. The answer to this question reveals the need for discussion and teaching about health promotion practices, regardless of whether the mass proves to be cancerous. If there was a delay between discovery and seeing the health care provider, ask what caused the delay. These questions are linked to the psychosocial assessment but also reveal the length of time that the tumor has been present. Ask what procedures have been performed to diagnose the problem. Also, ask patients if they have noticed any other changes in their body within the past year. This information can help determine whether there has been obvious cancer spread. Ask especially about the presence of joint or bone PAIN.

Ask about the use of alcohol intake, because this is a factor that may increase breast cancer risk. Ask what prescribed and over-the-counter (OTC) drugs are used—specifically, hormonal supplements such as estrogen and natural or herbal substances that stimulate hormones. Estrogen can be taken orally, intravaginally, or via a transdermal patch. Document the type and form of hormones (birth control pills or patches, supplements) and length of use.

CHART 70-2 Best Practice for Patient Safety & Quality Care QSEN

Assessing a Breast Mass

- Identify the location of the mass by using the "face of the clock" method.
- Describe the shape, size, and consistency of the mass.
- Assess whether the mass is fixed or movable.
- Note any skin changes around the mass, such as dimpling *(peau d'orange)*, increased vascularity, nipple retraction, and ulceration.
- Assess the adjacent lymph nodes—both axillary and supraclavicular nodes.
- Ask patients if they experience pain or soreness in the area around the mass.

Physical Assessment/Clinical Manifestations. Document in the electronic medical record any abnormal findings from the clinical breast examination. Describe specific information about a breast mass (Chart 70-2) such as location, using the "face of the clock" method; shape; size; consistency; and whether the mass is mobile or fixed to the surrounding tissue. Note any skin change, such as *peau d'orange* (dimpling, orange peel appearance), redness and warmth, nipple retraction, or ulceration, which can indicate advanced disease. Document the location of any enlargements of axillary and supraclavicular lymph nodes. Evaluate the presence of PAIN or soreness in the affected breast.

Psychosocial Assessment. A breast cancer diagnosis is usually an unanticipated event in the life of a woman who feels physically well. It initiates a sudden and distressing transition into a potentially life-threatening illness. Feelings of fear, shock, and disbelief are predominant as a woman learns about her disease and faces numerous treatment decisions. Psychological distress is common at cancer diagnosis and at the end of treatment. A previous history of mental illness, age, and life circumstances can contribute to increased psychological distress (Williams, 2012). Encourage expression of feelings, and determine if a referral to a breast cancer support group would be helpful. Talking with someone who has been through the experience is particularly helpful in dealing with the emotional aspects of the disease.

Assess the patient's need for information. Some people may not be ready for a lot of information at first. Most want to know how advanced the disease is, the likelihood of cure, treatment options and side effects, how treatment will affect their life and self-image, how family or partners will be affected, and what is required for home self-management. A previous experience with cancer, especially with other people who had breast cancer, influences the reactions to the disease. Ask patients and family members whether they have known anyone with breast cancer, and explore their feelings about the disease. The Internet is a primary source of information through which breast cancer information is sought and shared. Increasingly, the information on the Internet is provided by patients themselves (Quinn et al., 2013). Clarify health information the patient has received on the Internet, and provide current information about the stage of the disease and treatment options.

Assess the patient for problems related to SEXUALITY. Sexual dysfunction affects most breast cancer survivors in some way.

Sometimes the sexual dysfunction is related to the loss of a breast and the threat to one's femininity, but many women also equate a breast cancer diagnosis and treatment effects with the aging process (Klaeson et al., 2011). Lack of libido (sexual desire) related to hormonal changes, psychological distress, and severe anxiety is commonly experienced by women with breast cancer. If the patient does not discuss sexual concerns voluntarily, ask about the frequency of and satisfaction with sexual relations with her partner. Use resources that provide education about alternative expressions of intimacy and a focus on pleasure rather than performance. Refer the patient and her partner to counseling if appropriate.

GENDER HEALTH CONSIDERATIONS

Patient-Centered Care QSEN

Research is limited about breast cancer and women who identify as lesbian, but it is thought that breast cancer is more common in this group (Beredjick, 2012). A possible explanation is that risk factors for breast cancer, such as smoking, alcohol use, obesity, and infrequent pregnancy, are more common in this group (ACS, 2013a). Lesbian and bisexual women are less likely to have health insurance and get regular cancer screenings (see Chapter 73). Factors include fear and distrust of culturally incompetent health care providers. They may also be less focused on their breasts and breast cancer risk. Nurses' awareness and sensitivity to these issues help establish trust. Emphasize the importance of screening and early detection. Assess the need for referrals to support organizations such as the National LGBT Cancer Network (2013).

Laboratory Assessment. The diagnosis of breast cancer relies on pathologic examination of tissue from the breast mass. After the diagnosis of cancer is established, laboratory tests, including pathologic study of the lymph nodes, help detect possible metastases. Elevated liver enzyme levels indicate possible liver metastases, and increased serum calcium and alkaline phosphatase levels suggest bone metastases.

Imaging Assessment. Mammography is a sensitive screening tool for breast cancer. The uniqueness of this test results from its ability to reveal preclinical lesions (masses too small to be palpated manually). Most breast centers now use *digital mammography*—a system that is able to read, file, and transmit mammograms electronically. Women should be screened with mammography annually beginning at age 40 years (ACS, 2013a). Patient preparation and the procedure for mammography are discussed in Chapter 69. Some women may voice concern about radiation exposure with mammograms. Reassure them the dose is very small and the risk for harm from radiation is minimal (ACS, 2013b). Breast *tomosynthesis* is an emerging technology that is similar to mammography but uses three-dimensional images. It has the potential to improve detection of breast cancer by better differentiating suspicious from normal tissue (Alakhras et al., 2013). Although tomosynthesis has been approved by the Food and Drug Administration (FDA), its role in breast cancer screening and diagnosis has not yet been established (ACS, 2013a).

Ultrasonography of the breast is an additional diagnostic tool used to clarify findings on mammography. If the mammogram reveals a lesion, ultrasonography is helpful in differentiating a fluid-filled cyst from a solid mass. Mammography screening combined with ultrasound may be effective for detecting cancers in women with dense breasts, but currently it is not recommended for routine breast cancer screening (ACS, 2013a).

MRI is used for screening high-risk women and better examination of suspicious areas found by a mammogram (ACS, 2013b). MRI is more expensive than mammography. Most insurance companies will cover a portion of the cost if the woman is shown to be high risk. Although higher-quality images are produced, there is concern about high costs and access to quality breast MRI services for high-risk women (ACS, 2013b).

If the patient has an invasive breast cancer, other imaging tests may be done to rule out metastases. A chest x-ray is done to screen for lung metastases. Bone, liver, and brain scans and CT scans of the chest and abdomen can reveal distant metastases.

Other Diagnostic Assessment. Whereas imaging techniques serve as tools for screening and more precise visualization of potential breast cancers, *breast biopsy (pathologic examination of the breast tissue) is the only definitive way to diagnose breast cancer.* Breast tissue is obtained by one of several types of biopsies (see Chapter 69). Tissue samples are analyzed by a pathologist to determine the presence of breast cancer. If breast cancer is identified, it is classified according to the size and type of breast cancer, the histologic grade, and the type of receptors on the cells. These characteristics are used to guide treatment. For example, a small, noninvasive breast cancer may be treated only with lumpectomy and radiation, whereas a larger, aggressive tumor (one with a high histologic grade) may be treated with a mastectomy and chemotherapy, followed by radiation. Cancer cells that contain estrogen receptors (*ER positive*) or progesterone receptors (*PR positive)* have a better prognosis and usually respond to hormonal therapy. If the type of breast cancer is *HER2,* or one in which the *neu* gene product is overexpressed, it may be treated successfully with trastuzumab (Herceptin), which is a breast cancer *targeted therapy* for this specific type.

Most women, even those with very small tumors, receive some sort of treatment in addition to surgery for breast cancer. Research has focused on ways to predict clinical outcomes so that low-risk women may avoid unnecessary treatments. Gene expression profiling systems, such as Oncotype DX and MammaPrint, have been developed to help predict clinical outcomes by analyzing genes in breast cancer tissue. Some clinicians use this information in addition to the pathologic analysis for guiding treatment decisions. These multi-gene tests have been shown to be accurate predictors of patient prognosis and response to therapy in breast cancer (Jankowitz & Lee, 2013). Their role in clinical practice continues to evolve.

◆ *Analysis*

The priority NANDA-I nursing diagnoses and collaborative problems for patients with breast cancer include:

1. Ineffective Coping related to unanticipated breast cancer diagnosis (NANDA-I)
2. Potential for metastasis of cancer to other parts of the body

◆ *Planning and Implementation*

Developing Coping Strategies

Planning: Expected Outcomes. The patient with breast cancer is expected to report the use of methods to help increase coping ability and reduce anxiety. The patient will maintain relationships and participate as an active partner in management of her disease.

Interventions. The anxiety and uncertainty for the patient with breast cancer begin the moment a lump is discovered or when a mammogram reveals an abnormality. These feelings may be related to past experiences and personal associations with the disease. Assess the patient's perceptions of his or her own situation. Allow the patient to ventilate these feelings even if a diagnosis has not been established.

If the mass has been diagnosed as cancer, many people feel a partial sense of relief to be dealing with a known entity. A feeling of shock or disbelief usually occurs. It is difficult to accept a diagnosis of cancer when one feels basically well. Patients and their families or significant others deal in individual ways with the mix of feelings. Flexibility is the key to nursing care. Adjust your approach to care as the patient's emotional state changes. Those who have an interval between the diagnosis and treatment during which they actively participate in the choice of treatment cope more effectively after surgery, no matter which treatment is chosen.

An integral part of the plan to meet these emotional needs is the use of outside resources. Health care providers working with breast cancer may know other patients willing to make a preoperative visit. For example, the patient who is worried in particular about the side effects of radiation therapy may benefit more from talking to someone who has undergone radiation than from talking to the nurse or health care provider. Be sure to assess his or her preference.

Assess the patient's need for knowledge. Some may want to read and discuss any available information. Provide accurate information, and clarify any misinformation the patient may have received by the media, on the Internet, or from family and friends. The American Cancer Society (www.cancer.org) and Breastcancer.org (www.breastcancer.org) are two Internet sources that provide evidence-based information in language a lay person can understand.

! NURSING SAFETY PRIORITY QSEN

Action Alert

Women are exposed to many misconceptions and much misinformation about breast cancer through various media. Clarify misconceptions and provide current information regarding risk factors, screening recommendations, and treatment for breast cancer.

Decreasing the Risk for Metastasis

Planning: Expected Outcomes. The patient with breast cancer is expected to remain free of metastases or recurrence of disease, if possible. If cancer recurs, the patient will experience optimal health outcomes, including potential palliation and end-of-life care.

Interventions. There are many surgical and nonsurgical options for breast cancer treatment. Because of the various options, the patient with breast cancer often faces difficult decisions. Although patients are living longer with metastatic disease, the 5-year survival rate remains low. Once cancer is diagnosed, the extent and location of metastases determine the overall therapeutic strategy. The emphasis of breast cancer treatment is on preventing or stopping the spread of tumor cells that leads to distant metastasis. Treatment is tailored specifically to each patient, taking into account other health problems and the patient's ability to tolerate a particular therapy.

Nonsurgical Management. For patients with breast cancer at a stage for which surgery is the main treatment, follow-up with adjuvant (in addition to surgery) radiation, chemotherapy, hormone therapy, or targeted therapy is commonly prescribed. For those who cannot have surgery or whose cancer is too advanced, these therapies are used to promote comfort (palliation). These options are discussed in the Adjuvant Therapy section on p. 1476.

Complementary and Alternative Therapies. Women with breast cancer often cope with distressing symptoms related to the disease itself or the side effects of chemotherapy, radiation, and hormonal therapy. Common symptoms associated with these therapies include PAIN, nausea, hot flashes, anxiety, depression, and fatigue. Physical and emotional symptoms associated with breast cancer may be eased with the use of complementary and alternative medicine (CAM). Up to 80% of women use some form of CAM during breast cancer treatment (Wyatt et al., 2010). The most frequently used types of CAM are biologically based therapies such as vitamins, special cancer diets, and herbal therapy. Prayer is also widely used. Other types of CAM are mind-body or body-based such as guided imagery and massage. Encourage women to seek a practitioner with a certification or license for the specific type of CAM therapy. In some states, a certification or license is required for acupuncture, chiropractic therapy, massage, and shiatsu. Some types of CAM can be self-taught or done alone after a few sessions of instruction. Table 70-3 lists complementary therapies for specific symptoms associated with breast cancer and its treatments.

Although the use of CAM can improve quality of life, its use does not alter the outcome of breast cancer and should not be used in place of standard treatment (Saquib et al., 2012). Encourage patients who are interested in trying CAM therapies to check with their health care provider before using them. Refer patients to reliable resources for information about CAM. The website *breastcancer.org* provides accurate information about complementary therapies and the extent to which they have been researched in breast cancer patients. Cost may be a factor in decision making since not all insurances provide

TABLE 70-3 Complementary and Alternative Medicine (CAM) for Breast Cancer

SYMPTOM	CAM
Physical	
Pain	Acupuncture, chiropractic therapy, hypnosis, massage, music, reiki, shiatsu
Nausea/vomiting	Acupuncture, aromatherapy, ginger, hypnosis, progressive muscle relaxation, shiatsu
Fatigue	Acupuncture, massage, meditation, reiki, tai chi, yoga
Hot flashes	Acupuncture, black cohosh, flaxseed
Muscle tension	Aromatherapy, massage, shiatsu
Emotional	
Anxiety/stress/fear	Aromatherapy, guided imagery, hypnosis, journaling, massage, meditation, music therapy, progressive muscle relaxation, prayer, support groups, tai chi, yoga
Depression	Aromatherapy, yoga, journaling, progressive muscle relaxation

NURSING SAFETY PRIORITY (QSEN)

Action Alert

Teach women that some complementary and alternative therapies can have risks and side effects for women with breast cancer. Acupuncture should be avoided in women experiencing lymphedema, bleeding disorders, or a low white blood cell count from chemotherapy. There is concern that soy and soy products also may not be safe for women with breast cancer.

coverage for CAMs. Teach the patient that all ingested CAM agents potentially risk interaction with conventional drugs.

Surgical Management. The most common types of breast surgeries are shown in Fig. 70-4. Although controversy exists concerning the best treatment for breast cancer, experts agree that the mass itself should be removed to reduce the risk for local recurrence. A large tumor is sometimes treated with chemotherapy, called **neoadjuvant therapy**, to shrink the tumor before it is surgically removed. An advantage of this therapy is that cancers can be removed by lumpectomy rather than mastectomy.

Axillary lymph nodes are analyzed for the presence of cancer and staging purposes. Axillary lymph node dissection (ALND) is usually done when there are palpable axillary lymph nodes or when cancer is suspected to be at a later stage. Sentinel lymph node biopsy (SLNB) is a much less invasive approach now preferred by most surgeons for analyzing lymph nodes in early-stage breast cancers with low to moderate risk for lymph node involvement. SLNB is shown in Fig. 70-5. In this method, the sentinel lymph node is identified during breast surgery by injecting the breast with radioisotope and/or dye that travels via lymphatic pathways to the sentinel lymph node. The nodes that take up the dye (or give off a certain level of radiation picked up by a handheld counter) are removed and examined for the presence of cancer cells. It is believed that if cancer cells have traveled through the lymph channels, the cells will lodge in the sentinel nodes. Travel beyond these nodes to higher-level nodes may occur as a secondary event. Therefore the absence of cancer cells in the sentinel nodes is an indicator that no other nodes in the regional area are involved.

Preoperative Care. Care of the patient facing surgery for breast cancer focuses on psychological preparation and preoperative teaching. Priority nursing interventions are directed toward relieving anxiety and providing information to increase patient knowledge. *Include the spouse or partner, who may be experiencing similar stress and confusion, in the health teaching unless the patient's culture does not permit this approach.*

Review the type of procedure planned. Use open-ended questions (e.g., "What type of surgery are you having? Can you explain what will happen?") to assess the current level of knowledge. Provide postoperative information, including:

- The need for a drainage tube
- The location of the incision
- Mobility restrictions
- The length of the hospital stay (if any)
- The possibility of adjuvant therapy
- General preoperative and postoperative information needed by any surgical patient (see Chapters 14 and 16)

Supplement teaching with written or electronic materials for the patient and family to take home as references. This information should include whom to call in case there are any

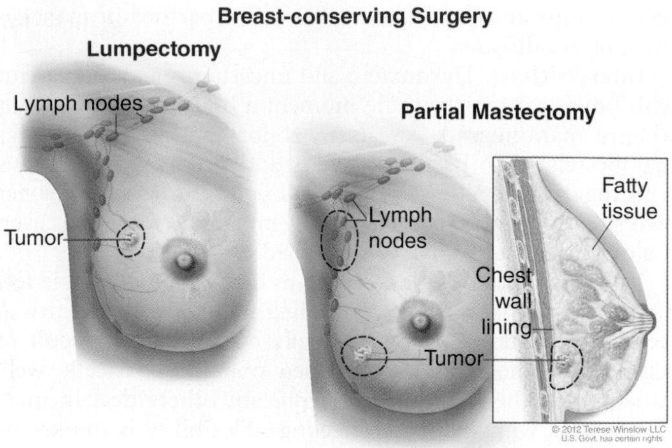

Breast-conserving surgery. Dotted lines show the area containing the tumor that is removed and some of the lymph nodes that may be removed.

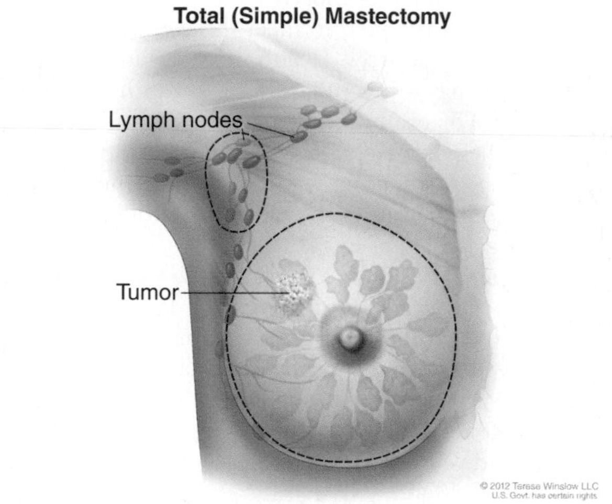

Total (simple) mastectomy. The dotted line shows where the entire breast is removed. Some lymph nodes under the arm may also be removed.

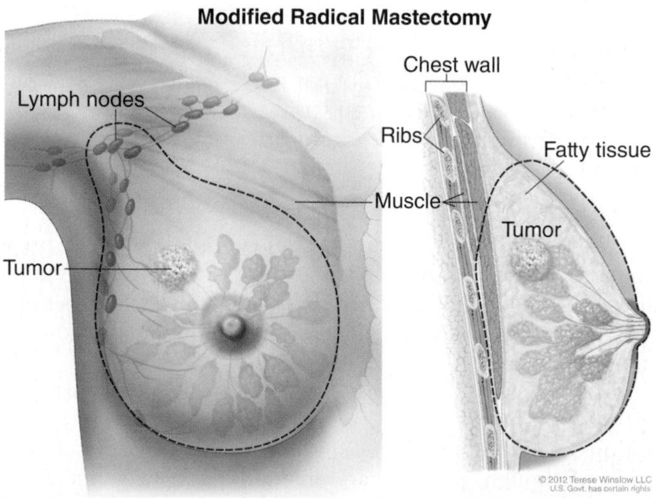

Modified radical mastectomy. The dotted line shows where the entire breast and some lymph nodes are removed. Part of the chest wall muscle may also be removed.

FIG. 70-4 Surgical treatment for breast cancer.

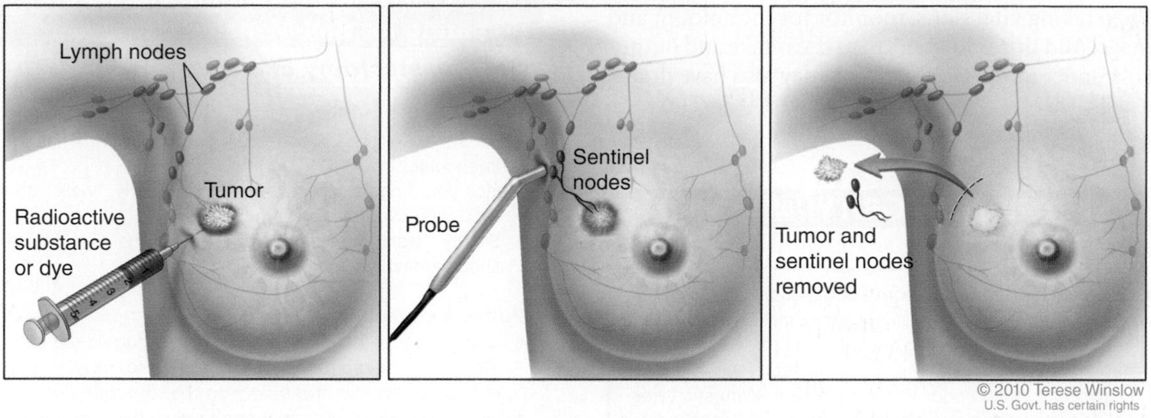

FIG. 70-5 Sentinel lymph node biopsy of the breast.

complications. Address body image issues before surgery to correct misconceptions about appearance after surgery. If available, suggest that patients and their caregivers attend classes before surgery in an ambulatory care setting, such as a breast cancer center, to promote successful early discharge from the hospital. Programs that provide emotional support, information, and opportunities for discussion related to SEXUALITY, body image, and preoperative and postoperative care enhance the recovery of the short-stay mastectomy patient.

Operative Procedures. Types of breast surgeries are shown in Fig. 70-5. During **breast-conserving surgery**, such as a *lumpectomy,* the surgeon removes the tumor and a small amount of tissue rather than the entire breast. A partial mastectomy is surgery to remove part of the breast that contains cancer and some normal tissue around it. *Margins* refer to the distance between the tumor and the edge of the surrounding tissue. The desired outcome of breast-conserving surgery is to obtain negative *margins* in which no cancer cells extend to the edge of the tissue. Typically, radiation therapy follows to kill any residual tumor cells.

Breast-conserving procedures are usually performed in same-day surgical settings. The cosmetic results of these surgeries are good to excellent, and the psychological benefits of avoiding breast removal are significant for patients who choose this option.

Despite advances in breast-conserving surgery, mastectomy remains a popular option for breast cancer treatment and women are increasingly choosing it for prophylactic treatment (McLaughlin, 2013). Typically, indications for a mastectomy include multi-centric disease (tumor is present in different quadrants of the breast), inability to have radiation therapy, presence of a large tumor in a small breast, and patient preference. Mastectomy does not conserve the breast; the affected breast is completely removed. A total (simple) mastectomy is surgery to remove the whole breast that has cancer. A modified radical mastectomy removes the breast tissue, lymph nodes, and sometimes, part of the underlying chest wall muscle. If reconstruction is to be performed at the same time as the mastectomy, less-invasive techniques, such as incising a ½-inch flap of skin around the nipple (excising the same amount of breast tissue as with conventional mastectomy), may be performed. Skin flaps or expanders may be used to create a breast mound at the time of the original procedure.

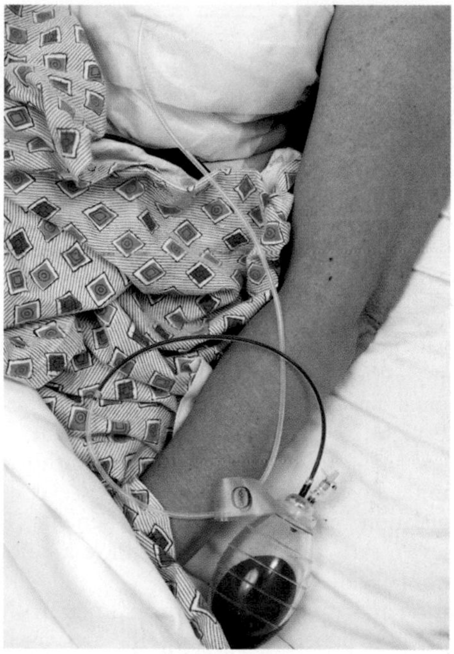

FIG. 70-6 Jackson-Pratt drain in place after a mastectomy.

Postoperative Care. Before the patient returns from surgery, inform the staff to avoid using the affected arm for measuring blood pressure, giving injections, or drawing blood. He or she returns from the postanesthesia care unit (PACU) as soon as vital signs return to baseline levels and if no complications have occurred. Assess vital signs on a schedule of decreasing frequency, such as every 30 minutes for 2 times, every hour for 2 times, and then every 4 hours. During these checks, assess the dressing for bleeding.

During a *modified radical mastectomy,* the surgeon places one or two drainage tubes, usually Jackson-Pratt drains, under the skin flaps and attaches the tubes to a small collection chamber (Fig. 70-6). Gentle suction is exerted, and fluid that would accumulate under the flaps and delay healing is collected. Various drains are available, but all allow the drainage to be seen and measured. When taking vital signs, monitor for the amount and color of drainage. Add this information to the intake and output record. Patients undergoing a *lumpectomy* may also have drainage tubes (usually Jackson-Pratt drains) placed if the lump is large or if axillary node dissection is performed.

! NURSING SAFETY PRIORITY (QSEN)

Action Alert

Per TJC National Patient Safety Goal recommendations, to decrease the chance of surgical site infection, carefully observe the surgical wound after breast surgery for signs of swelling and infection throughout recovery. Assess the incision and flap of the post-mastectomy patient for signs of bleeding, infection, and poor tissue perfusion. With short hospital stays, drainage tubes are usually removed about 1 to 3 weeks after hospital discharge when the patient returns for an office visit. The drainage amount should be less than 25 mL in a 24-hour period. Inform the patient that tube removal may be uncomfortable although these tubes lie just under the skin. Provide or suggest analgesia before they are removed. Document all findings, and report any abnormalities to the surgeon immediately.

Assess the patient's position to ensure that the drainage tubes or collection device is not pulled or kinked. The patient should have the head of the bed up at least 30 degrees with the affected arm (the arm on the same side as the axillary dissection) elevated on a pillow while awake. Keeping the affected arm elevated promotes lymphatic fluid return after removal of lymph nodes and channels. Provide other basic comfort measures, such as repositioning and analgesics as prescribed on a regular basis until PAIN ceases. Patient-controlled analgesia may be used for some patients for a short time depending on the type of surgery that was performed.

The hospital stay after breast surgery is short, often same-day or just overnight, and recovery is usually not complicated. Because some managed care plans will not authorize an overnight stay in the hospital after a mastectomy, several states have enacted legislation mandating inpatient benefits. The patient who chooses an early discharge should have a home care visit within 24 hours of the discharge.

Ambulation and a regular diet are resumed by the day after surgery. While the patient is walking, the arm on the affected side may need to be supported at first. Gradually, the arm should be allowed to hang straight by the side. Instruct the patient to avoid the hunched-back position with the arm flexed because of the risk for elbow contracture. Beginning exercises that do not stress the incision can usually be started on the first day after surgery. These exercises include squeezing the affected hand around a soft, round object (a ball or rolled washcloth) and flexion/extension of the elbow. The progression to more strenuous exercises depends on the subsequent procedures planned (e.g., reconstruction) and the surgeon's prescription.

As soon as the patient is ambulatory and surgical PAIN is under control, he or she is discharged to home. Common instructions for exercises after mastectomy are listed in Chart 70-3.

Breast Reconstruction. Breast reconstruction after or during mastectomy for women is common with few complications. Patients consult with the plastic surgeon to discuss the type of reconstruction, timing of the procedure, and technique desired. Many women prefer reconstruction immediately after mastectomy using their own tissue (autogenous reconstruction). Breast reconstruction at the time of mastectomy, both autogenous and prosthetic, may lessen the psychological strain associated with undergoing a mastectomy.

The surgeon should offer the option of breast reconstruction before surgery is performed. If the woman does not choose immediate reconstructive surgery, a temporary prosthesis can be used. Refer the patient to the American Cancer Society's *Reach to Recovery* program (www.cancer.org). In this program, a volunteer who has had breast cancer surgery visits the woman at home, offering information on breast forms, clothing, coping with breast cancer, and possible reconstructive options. For this intervention to be as helpful as possible, the volunteer should be about the same age as the patient and have experienced the same surgical procedure.

Evaluate the woman's level of satisfaction with her prosthesis several weeks after surgery. Assess her attitude by asking about future plans for restoring appearance. Although reconstruction is not appropriate for some women and others may not be

CHART 70-3 Patient and Family Education: Preparing for Self-Management

Post-mastectomy Exercises

Hand Wall Climbing
- Face the wall, and put the palms of your hands flat against the wall at shoulder level.
- Flex your fingers so that your hands slowly "walk" up the wall.
- Stop when your arms are fully extended.
- Slowly "walk" your hands back down the wall until they return to shoulder level.

Pulley Exercise
- Drape a 6-foot-long rope over a shower curtain rod or over the top of a door. If you use a door for this exercise, have someone put a nail or hook at the top of the door so that the rope does not slip off.
- Grab the ends of the rope, one in each hand, and extend your arms out to your sides until they are straight.
- Keeping your arms straight, pull down with your left arm to raise your right arm as high as you can.
- Pull down with your right arm to raise your left arm as high as you can.

Rope Turning
- Tie a rope to the knob of a closed door.
- Hold the other end of the rope and step back from the door until your arm is almost straight out in front of you.
- Swing the rope in a circle. Start with small circles, and gradually increase to larger circles as you become more flexible.

? NCLEX EXAMINATION CHALLENGE

Physiological Integrity

The nurse is assigned to care for a client who has undergone a modified radical left mastectomy for breast cancer. When delegating care, which statement by the nursing assistant would require further teaching by the nurse?

A. "I will report urine intake and output to you."
B. "If the client appears to be in pain, I will tell you right away."
C. "It is important for me to take blood pressure on the client's left arm."
D. "When ambulating, I will assist the client to stand straight with arms hanging at the side."

TABLE 70-4 Examples of Breast Reconstruction Procedures

PROCEDURE	DESCRIPTION
Implantation	An implant matching the size of the other breast is placed under the muscle on the operative side to create a breast mound. 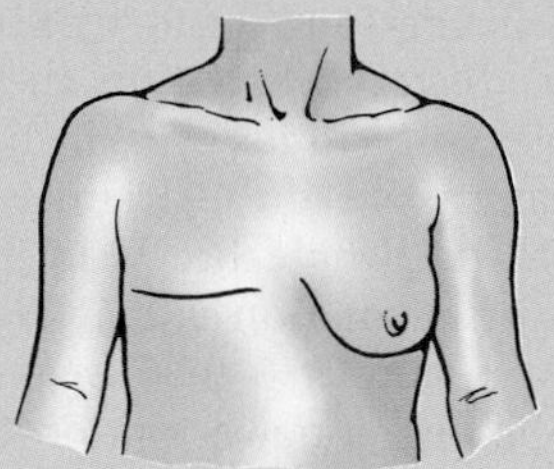 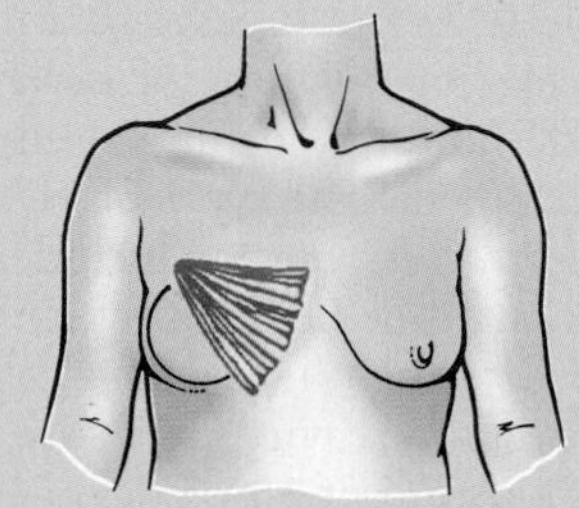
Tissue expansion	A tissue expander is placed under the muscle and gradually expanded with saline to stretch the overlying skin and create a pocket. After several weeks, the tissue expander is exchanged for an implant. 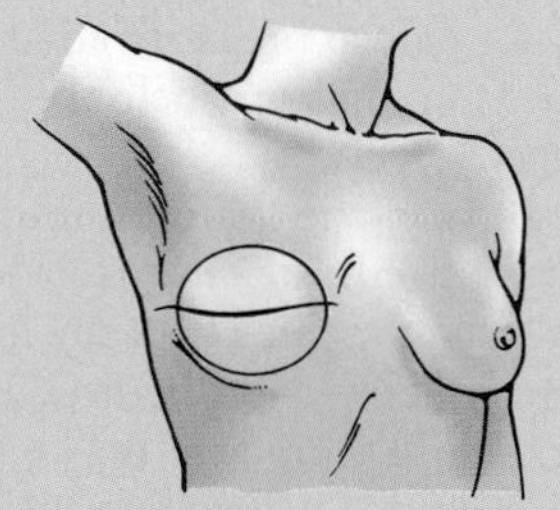
Myocutaneous flaps	A flap of skin, fat, and muscle is transferred from the donor site to the operative area. The flap contains an appropriate amount of fat to match the other breast and is similar in appearance to breast tissue. A blood supply is established by reanastomosis of vessels from the operative area to those with the flap when possible. A new nipple may be created with tissue from areas such as the labia or upper, inner thigh. Nipples can also be created by tattooing. Latissimus dorsi musculocutaneous flap 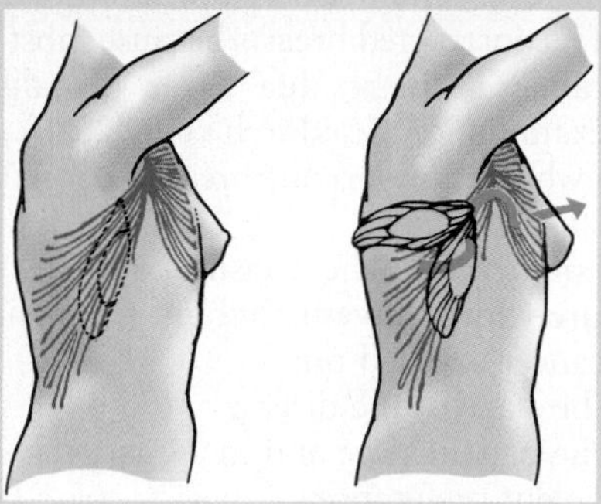 Abdominal myocutaneous flap 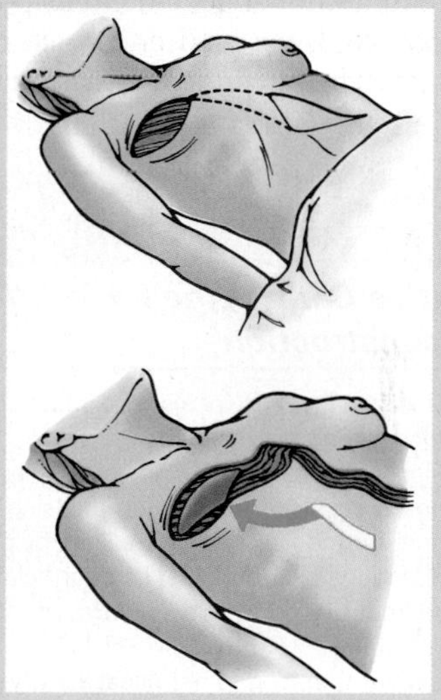

interested in it, the surgeon should discuss the indications and contraindications, advantages and disadvantages, and typical recovery. If immediate reconstruction is chosen, the surgeon should be aware of this before surgery so that plans can be coordinated with those of the plastic surgeon.

Several procedures are available for restoring the appearance of the breast (Table 70-4). Reconstruction may begin during the original operative procedure or later in one to several stages. Common types of breast reconstruction are:

- Breast expanders (saline or gel)
- Autologous reconstruction using the patient's own skin, fat, and muscle

Breast expanders are the most common method of breast reconstruction used today in the United States. A tissue expander is a balloon-like device with a resealable metal port that is placed under the pectoralis muscle. A small amount of normal saline is injected intraoperatively into the expander to partially inflate it. The patient then receives additional weekly saline injections for about 6 to 8 weeks until the expander is fully inflated. When full expansion is achieved, the tissue expander is then exchanged for a permanent implant during surgery in an ambulatory care center. The permanent implant is filled with either saline or silicone gel. Despite earlier claims that silicone gel caused autoimmune diseases like lupus and arthritis, silicone implants have been safely used in the majority of women who choose this type of breast implant.

Autologous reconstruction using the patient's own skin, fat, and muscle is advantageous because the donor site tissue is similar in consistency to the natural breast. Therefore the results more closely resemble a real breast as compared with implant reconstruction. Flap donor sites include the latissimus dorsi flap (back muscle); transverse rectus abdominis myocutaneous flap, known as the *TRAM flap* (abdominal muscle); and the gluteal flap (buttock muscle). Reconstruction of the nipple-areola complex is the last stage in the reconstruction of the breast. If necessary, a new nipple may be created with other body tissue, such as from the labia, abdomen, or inner thigh.

Women who have had a mastectomy and breast reconstruction in one breast should have close surveillance breast cancer screening in the contralateral (opposite) breast, including imaging with mammography or mammography and MRI. Mammography and MRI are not recommended to be routinely done in reconstructed breasts because most local recurrences of breast cancer in the residual tissue are palpable during clinical breast examination (Zakhireh et al., 2010). Nursing care of the woman who has undergone breast reconstruction is outlined in Chart 70-4.

Adjuvant Therapy. The decision to follow the original surgical procedure with **adjuvant therapy** (in addition to surgery) for breast cancer is based on:

- The stage of the disease
- The patient's age and menopausal status
- Patient preferences
- Pathologic examination
- Hormone receptor status
- Presence of a known genetic predisposition

Adjuvant therapy for breast cancer consists of radiation therapy and drug therapy. The purpose of radiation therapy is to reduce the risk for local recurrence of breast cancer. Drug therapy includes chemotherapy, targeted therapy, and/or hormonal therapy. These drugs destroy breast cancer cells that may be present anywhere in the body. They are typically delivered after surgery for breast cancer, although **neoadjuvant** chemotherapy may be given to reduce the size of a tumor before surgery. Hormonal therapy is a chemoprevention option for high-risk women with a personal history of breast cancer.

Radiation Therapy. Radiation therapy is administered after breast-conserving surgery to kill breast cancer cells that may remain near the site of the original tumor. This therapy can be delivered to the whole breast or to only part of the breast. Whole-breast irradiation is delivered by external beam radiation over a period of 5 to 6 weeks. Partial breast irradiation (PBI) has become a newer option for women with early-stage breast cancer. PBI is a convenient alternative to whole breast radiation. Less time is needed for completion, and outcomes are comparable to whole breast radiation (Edwards et al., 2013). The advantage of this type of radiation is that it is delivered over a much shorter time interval, eliminating the need for daily trips for treatment. The types of methods available for delivering *partial-breast irradiation* include:

- Interstitial brachytherapy, in which several catheters loaded with a radioactive source are inserted at the lumpectomy cavity and surrounding margin, is given over a period of 4 to 5 days.
- Balloon brachytherapy, also known as *MammoSite,* involves the use of a single balloon-tipped catheter that is surgically placed near the tumor bed. The catheter is loaded with a radiation source and inflated to conform to the total cavity. Ten total treatments are given, with at least 6 hours between each treatment.
- Intraoperative radiation therapy is the most accelerated form of partial breast irradiation. It utilizes a high single dose of radiation delivered during the lumpectomy surgery.

Nursing care for the patient undergoing radiation therapy includes patient education and side effect management. Skin changes are a major side effect during this therapy (see Chapter 22). If brachytherapy is planned, instruct patients about the procedure. Assure them that they will be radioactive only while the radiation source is dwelling inside the breast tissue.

CHART 70-4 Best Practice for Patient Safety & Quality Care QSEN

Postoperative Care of the Patient After Breast Reconstruction

- Assess the incision and flap for signs of infection (excessive redness, drainage, odor) during dressing changes.
- Assess the incision and flap for signs of poor tissue perfusion (duskiness, decreased capillary refill) during dressing changes.
- Avoid pressure on the flap and suture lines by positioning the patient on her nonoperative side and avoiding tight clothing.
- Monitor and measure drainage in collection devices, such as for Jackson-Pratt drains.
- Teach the patient to return to her usual activity level gradually and to avoid heavy lifting.
- Remind the patient to avoid sleeping in the prone position.
- Teach the patient to avoid participation in contact sports or other activities that could cause trauma to the chest.
- Teach the patient to minimize pressure on the breast during sexual activity.
- Remind the patient to refrain from driving until advised by the physician.
- Remind the patient to ask at the 6-week postoperative visit when full activity can be resumed.
- Reassure the patient that optimal appearance may not occur for 3 to 6 months postoperatively.
- If implants have been inserted, teach the proper method of breast massage to enhance expansion and prevent capsule formation (consult with the physician).
- Emphasize breast self-awareness; if the patient performs breast self-examination (BSE), review her technique.
- Remind the patient of the importance of clinical breast examination and follow-up surveillance by her physician.

! NURSING SAFETY PRIORITY QSEN

Action Alert

Teach women undergoing brachytherapy for breast cancer that radiation is contained in the temporary implant. The risk for others to be exposed to radiation is very small. Body fluids and items contacted by patients with brachytherapy are not radioactive. However, during the time the radiation is delivered, it is recommended they limit visitors, including pregnant women and children.

Chemotherapy. Chemotherapy for breast cancer is delivered systemically via the central IV route, such as an implantable venous access device (Port-a-Cath). Its purpose is to kill undetected breast cancer cells that may have left the original tumor and moved to more distant sites. Chemotherapy is recommended for treatment of invasive breast cancer after surgery (adjuvant chemotherapy). It may also be given before surgery to reduce the size of the tumor (neoadjuvant chemotherapy). Chemotherapy is most effective when combinations of more than one drug are used. Table 70-5 lists common chemotherapy agents used in breast cancer and their mechanism of action. Chemotherapy drugs are usually delivered in four to six cycles, with each period of treatment followed by a rest period to give the body time to recover from the effects of the drugs. Each cycle is 2 to 3 weeks long. The total treatment time is 3 to 6 months, although treatment may be longer for advanced breast cancer. Many combinations of drugs are used, and no one combination has been proven to be superior over others (ACS, 2013a). A common chemotherapy regimen for breast cancer treatment is Cytoxan, Adriamycin, and fluorouracil, which is also known as 5-FU (CAF). In early-stage breast cancer, chemotherapy regimens lower the risk for breast cancer recurrence. In advanced breast cancer, chemotherapy regimens reduce cancer size in many patients.

Nurses must be very proficient in the preparation and administration of chemotherapy drugs and knowledgeable about various venous access devices. They must also be able to manage the distressing symptoms associated with side effects of chemotherapy. Chapter 22 discusses general nursing management of alopecia, nausea and vomiting, mucositis, and bone marrow suppression. Fatigue and sleep disturbance are often major concerns as side effects of chemotherapy.

! NURSING SAFETY PRIORITY QSEN

Action Alert

Teach patients undergoing chemotherapy with anthracyclines such as doxorubicin (Adriamycin) to be aware of cardiotoxic effects. Instruct them to report excessive fatigue, shortness of breath, chronic cough, and edema to the health care provider.

Chemotherapy is unpleasant and expensive and can have life-threatening short-term and long-term side effects. Because more women are living longer with breast cancer, long-term effects are increasingly emerging. Although targeted therapy is effective with fewer side effects, some side effects are nevertheless life threatening. For example, cardiac toxicity is a risk associated with the use of Herceptin, particularly when it is combined with other chemotherapy. Chemotherapy and ovarian suppression can result in infertility, a devastating effect for women of childbearing age. Hormonal therapy can result in long-term ill effects from bone loss. Discuss patient concerns, provide accurate information, and assist him or her in decision making.

Targeted Therapy. Targeted cancer therapies are drugs that target specific characteristics of cancer cells, such as a protein, an enzyme, or the formation of new blood vessels. The advantage of targeted therapy over traditional chemotherapy is that targeted therapy is less likely to harm normal, healthy cells and therefore it has fewer side effects. Table 70-5 lists targeted chemotherapy drugs used in breast cancer. One of the first targeted therapies developed for breast cancer is the monoclonal antibody *trastuzumab* (Herceptin). This drug targets the *HER2/neu* gene product in breast cancer cells. Several other targeted therapies have been developed since Herceptin.

Hormonal Therapy. Table 70-5 lists hormonal therapy drugs used in breast cancer prevention and treatment. The purpose of hormonal therapy is to reduce the estrogen available to breast tumors to stop or prevent their growth. *Premenopausal* women whose main estrogen source is the ovaries may benefit from

TABLE 70-5 Drug Therapy for Breast Cancer

CATEGORY	MECHANISM OF ACTION	AGENTS
Chemotherapy		
Anthracyclines	Inhibit DNA synthesis in susceptible cells	doxorubicin (Adriamycin) (A) epirubicin (Ellence) (E) daunorubicin (Cerubidine) mitoxantrone (Novantrone)
Taxanes	Inhibit microtubule network in rapidly dividing cells	docetaxel (Taxotere) (D) paclitaxel (Taxol) (P) paclitaxel, protein-bound (Abraxane)
Alkylating agents	Interfere with the replication of susceptible cells	cyclophosphamide (Cytoxan) (C) thiotepa (Thioplex)
Antimetabolites	Inhibit DNA synthesis and cellular replication in rapidly dividing cells	methotrexate (Mexate) (M) fluorouracil (5-FU) (F) capecitabine (Xeloda) gemcitabine (Gemzar)
Additional Chemotherapy Drugs Used in Advanced Breast Cancer		
Vinca alkaloids	Interfere with genes, stopping cells from reproducing	vinorelbine (Navelbine) vincristine (Oncovin)
Platinum-based	Weakens or destroys breast cancer cells by damaging genetic material	carboplatin (Paraplatin)
Microtubule inhibitor	Disrupts cells division by interfering with microtubulin	eribulin (Halaven)
Epothilone	Interferes with cancer cell division	ixabepilone (Ixempra)
Antitumor antibiotic	Damages genes, interfering with reproduction	mitomycin (Mutamycin)
Targeted Therapy	Selectively targets critical steps in the processes required for tumor growth, viability, or invasion	trastuzumab (Herceptin) lapatinib (Tykerb) pertuzumab (Perjeta) everolimus (Afinitor) T-DM1 (Kadcyla)
Hormonal Therapy		
LH-RH agonists	Block release of LH and FSH, thereby preventing ovarian production of estrogen	goserelin (Zoladex) leuprolide (Lupron)
Selective estrogen receptor modulators (SERMs)	Bind to estrogen receptors; have both agonist and antagonist properties (selectively block action of estrogen in the breast but not in other organs)	tamoxifen (Nolvadex) raloxifene (Evista) toremifene (Fareston)
Aromatase inhibitors	Prevent conversion of adrenal and ovarian androgens to estrogens by inhibiting the aromatase enzyme	anastrozole (Arimidex) letrozole (Femara) exemestane (Aromasin)
Estrogen receptor down-regulators	Induce degradation of estrogen receptor	fulvestrant (Faslodex)

FSH, Follicle-stimulating hormone; *LH,* luteinizing hormone; *LH-RH,* luteinizing hormone–releasing hormone.

LH-RH agonists that inhibit estrogen synthesis. These drugs include leuprolide (Lupron) and goserelin (Zoladex), which suppress the hypothalamus from making luteinizing hormone–releasing hormone (LH-RH). When LH-RH is inhibited, the ovaries do not produce estrogen. Although the suppression of ovarian function decreases breast cancer risk, the drastic drop in estrogen causes significant menopausal symptoms. Therefore the decision to use these drugs is not made lightly.

Selective estrogen receptor modulators (SERMs), on the other hand, do not affect ovarian function. Rather, they block the effect of estrogen in women who have estrogen receptor (ER)–positive breast cancer. SERMs are also used as chemoprevention in women at high risk for breast cancer and in women with advanced breast cancer. For women with hormone receptor–positive breast cancer, tamoxifen reduces the chances of the cancer coming back by about half (ACS, 2013a). A recent study demonstrated that taking tamoxifen for 10 years, rather than 5 years, achieves the best benefit for risk reduction (Davies et al., 2013). Common side effects of SERMs include hot flashes and weight gain. Rare but serious side effects of these drugs include endometrial cancer and thromboembolic events.

Aromatase inhibitors (AIs) are used in *postmenopausal* women whose main source of estrogen is not the ovaries but, rather, body fat. AIs reduce estrogen levels by inhibiting the conversion of androgen to estrogen through the action of the enzyme *aromatase.* AIs are beneficial when given to postmenopausal women for up to 5 years. Treatment with AIs usually follows treatment with tamoxifen. Studies are underway to determine whether it is beneficial to take AIs longer than 5 years (ACS, 2013a). A side effect of AIs, not seen with tamoxifen, is loss of bone density. Women taking AIs are candidates for bone-strengthening drugs and must be closely monitored for osteoporosis. Fulvestrant (Faslodex), a second-line hormonal therapy for postmenopausal women with advanced breast cancer, is used after other hormonal treatments have stopped working.

Stem Cell Transplantation. Autologous or allogeneic stem cell transplantation is an option for patients with a high risk for recurrence or who have advanced disease. **Autologous bone marrow transplantation** (taken from the patient's bone marrow), peripheral blood stem cell transplantation (taken from circulating blood), or **allogeneic bone marrow transplantation** (taken from a healthy donor's bone marrow or peripheral blood) is performed as a means of rescue therapy after very high doses of chemotherapy. The general care of the patient undergoing bone marrow or stem cell transplantation is discussed in Chapter 22.

Community-Based Care

Home Care Management. In collaboration with the case manager and members of the interdisciplinary health care team, make the appropriate referrals for care after discharge. Preoperative teaching and arrangements for home care management and referrals (*Reach to Recovery,* social services, home care) can be started before surgery or other treatment.

The patient who has undergone breast surgery can be discharged to the home setting unless other physical disabilities exist. Some are discharged the day after surgery with Jackson-Pratt or other types of drains in place. Many patients are discharged to home on the day of surgery. Older adults should not be sent home without a family member or friend who can stay with them for 1 to 2 days. These patients may need some assistance at home with drain care, dressings, and ADLs because of PAIN and impaired range of motion of the affected arm. Summaries of continuing care instructions are given in Charts 70-5 and 70-6.

CHART 70-5 Patient and Family Education: Preparing for Self-Management

Recovery from Breast Cancer Surgery

- There may be a dry gauze dressing over the incision when you leave the hospital. You may change this dressing if it becomes soiled.
- A small, dry dressing will be around the site where a drain is placed. Often there is some leakage of fluid around the drain. Check the gauze dressing for drainage, and change it if it becomes soiled. Some leakage is normal, but if the dressing becomes soaked more than once a day, call your health care provider.
- You have been taught how to empty the reservoir from your drain and how to measure the volume of drainage. You should empty the reservoir twice a day and record the measurements.
- Drains are generally removed when drainage is less than 25 mL in 24 hours.
- Drains are often removed at the same time as the stitches or staples, generally 7 to 10 days (could be as long as 3 weeks if needed) after surgery.
- You may take sponge baths or tub baths, making certain that the area of the drain and incision stays dry. You may shower after the stitches, staples, and drains are removed.
- You can begin using your arm for normal activities, such as eating or combing your hair. Exercises involving the wrist, hand, and elbow, such as flexing your fingers, circular wrist motions, and touching your hand to your shoulder, are very good. You can usually resume more strenuous exercises after the drains have been removed.
- You can expect some discomfort or mild pain after surgery, but within 4 to 5 days, most women have no need for pain medication or require medication only at bedtime.
- Numbness in the area of the surgery and along the inner side of the arm from the armpit to the elbow occurs in almost all women. It is the injury to the nerves that causes sensation to the skin in those areas. Women have described sensations of heaviness, pain, tingling, burning, and "pins and needles." Neuropathic pain is sometimes relieved by gabapentin (Neurontin). These sensations change over the months and usually resolve by 1 year.
- Pamphlets on exercises, hand and arm care, and general facts about breast cancer are available from us or from a volunteer visitor. The American Cancer Society has volunteers who have had surgery similar to yours and are available to visit you.

Teach patients that activities involving stretching or reaching for heavy objects should be avoided temporarily. This restriction can be discussed with a family member or significant other who can perform these tasks or place the objects within easy reach.

Self-Management Education. The teaching plan for the patient after surgery includes:

- Measures to improve body image
- Information about interpersonal relationships and roles
- Exercises to regain full range of motion
- Measures to prevent INFECTION of the incision (per The Joint Commission's National Patient Safety Goals)
- Measures to avoid lymphedema
- Measures to avoid injury, INFECTION, and swelling of the affected arm (per The Joint Commission's National Patient Safety Goals)
- Care of the incision and drainage device

Teach incisional care to the patient, family, and/or other caregiver. The patient may wear a light dressing to prevent irritation. Explain that no lotions or ointments should be used on the area

CHART 70-6 Home Care Assessment

Patients Recovering from Breast Cancer Surgery

Assess cardiovascular, respiratory, and urinary status:
- Vital signs
- Lung sounds
- Urine output patterns

Assess for pain and effectiveness of analgesics.
Assess dressing and incision site:
- Excess drainage
- Manifestations of infection
- Wound healing
- Intact staples

Assess drain and site:
- Drainage around drain site and in drain reservoir
- Color and amount of drainage
- Manifestations of infection

Review patient's recordings of drainage.
Evaluate patient's ability to care for and empty drain reservoir.
Assess status of affected extremity:
- Range of motion
- Ability to perform exercise regimen
- Lymphedema

Assess nutritional status:
- Food and fluid intake
- Presence of nausea and vomiting
- Bowel sounds

Assess functional ability:
- Activities of daily living
- Mobility and ambulation

Assess home environment:
- Safety
- Structural barriers

Assess patient's compliance and knowledge of illness and treatment plan:
- Follow-up appointment with surgeon
- Manifestations to report to health care provider
- Hand and arm care guidelines
- Referral to *Reach to Recovery*

Assess patient and caregiver coping skills:
- Whether patient and/or caregiver has looked at incision site
- Patient's and/or caregiver's reaction to incision site

and that the use of deodorant under the affected arm should be avoided until healing is complete. Although swelling and redness of the scar itself are normal for the first few weeks, swelling, redness, increased heat, and tenderness of the surrounding area indicate INFECTION and should be reported to the surgeon immediately. If a lymph node dissection was performed, instruct the patient to elevate the affected arm on a pillow for at least 30 minutes a day for the first 6 months. Ask the patient to have someone bring a loose-fitting, non-wire bra or camisole for her to try before discharge with a soft, cotton-filled or polyester fiber–filled form supplied by the hospital or by *Reach to Recovery*. The patient wears this form until the incision is completely healed and the health care provider approves the fitting of a more sophisticated prosthesis, usually 6 to 8 weeks after discharge. Encourage the patient to dress in loose-fitting street clothes at home, not pajamas, to further enhance a positive self-image.

Teach the patient to continue performing the exercises that began in the hospital. Active range-of-motion exercises should begin 1 week after surgery or when sutures and drains are removed. Emphasize that reaching and stretching exercises should continue only to the point of PAIN or pulling, never beyond that. Some YWCA locations have a free program called *ENCORE*, which supports women and men following breast cancer surgery. The program includes exercise to music, exercise in water, and peer psychological support. Patients may participate as early as 3 weeks after surgery. Before discharge, the surgeon may prescribe precautions or limitations specific to plans for future procedures, such as reconstruction.

Lymphedema, an abnormal accumulation of protein fluid in the subcutaneous tissue of the affected limb after a mastectomy, is a commonly overlooked topic in health teaching. Risk factors include injury or INFECTION of the extremity, obesity, presence of extensive axillary disease, and radiation treatment. Once it develops, it can be very difficult to manage, and *lifelong measures must be taken to prevent it.* Nurses play a vital role in educating patients about this complication. Teach your patient to immediately report symptoms of lymphedema such as sensations of heaviness, aching, fatigue, numbness, tingling, and/or swelling in the affected arm, as well as swelling in the upper chest (Mohler & Mondry, 2013).

! NURSING SAFETY PRIORITY (QSEN)

Action Alert

Provide information needed to help the patient avoid INFECTION and subsequent lymphedema of the affected arm after the mastectomy. Teach the importance of avoiding having blood pressure measurements taken on, having injections in, or having blood drawn from the arm on the side of the mastectomy. Instruct the patient to wear a mitt when using the oven, wear gloves when gardening, and treat cuts and scrapes appropriately. If lymphedema occurs, early intervention provides the best chance for control. Nurses should not assume that women with lymphedema are disabled; they are able to live full lives within this limitation (Ridner et al., 2012). A referral to a lymphedema specialist may be necessary for the patient to be fitted for a compression sleeve and/or glove, to be taught exercises and manual lymph drainage, and to discuss ways to modify daily activities to avoid worsening the problem. Management is directed toward measures that promote drainage of the affected arm. Teach patients, especially those who have had axillary lymph nodes removed, that measures to prevent lymphedema are lifelong and include avoiding trauma to the arm on the side of the mastectomy.

Psychosocial Preparation. Concerns about appearance after surgery are common and are often a threat to the patient's self-concept as a woman. Before breast surgery, the woman and her partner can benefit from an explanation of the expected postoperative appearance. After a modified radical mastectomy, the chest wall is fairly smooth and has a horizontal incision from the axilla to the midchest area. After breast-conserving surgery, scars vary according to the amount of breast tissue removed. Women are sometimes shown pictures of post-mastectomy reconstruction but are disappointed with their own results. Emphasize that scars will fade and edema will lessen with time. Scars may be red and raised at first, but these features lessen in the first few months. After surgery, encourage the woman to look at her incision when she is ready. Do not push her to accept this body image change immediately.

Much of one's body image is a reflection of how others respond. Therefore the response of the patient's family or partner to the surgery is crucial in determining the effect on self-concept. These people may also need the support of the nurse. They may have concerns about their ability to accept the changes and need to discuss these feelings with an objective listener. They may also need help with communicating their feelings, both negative and positive, with their loved one. Involving them in teaching may also help reinforce learning and increase retention.

Discuss sexual concerns before discharge. Most surgeons recommend avoiding sexual intercourse for 4 to 6 weeks. Patients may prefer to lay a pillow over the surgical site or to wear a bra, camisole, or T-shirt to prevent contact with the surgical site during intercourse. He or she may be embarrassed to discuss the topic of *SEXUALITY*. Be sensitive to possible concerns, and approach the subject first.

For young women, issues related to childbearing may be a concern. Chemotherapy and radiation are considered serious teratogenic (birth defect–causing) agents. Advise sexually active patients receiving chemotherapy or radiotherapy to use birth control during therapy. The method and length of birth control should be discussed with the health care provider.

Health Care Resources. Resources available to the patient after discharge include personal support and community programs. After discharge, the spouse or partner may need help in planning support for home responsibilities. For example, a partner who may be assuming additional duties at home and work may feel stressed. Discussing the need for ongoing emotional support is also beneficial to both the patient and partner. Leaving the hospital and appearing normal do not end the anxiety and fear. Identifying a support person with whom the patient or couple can explore these feelings and discussing the need to ventilate feelings enhance personal and family recovery.

Numerous support and educational resources are available to those diagnosed with breast cancer. Nurses must provide accurate and current information to patients who may have obtained inaccurate information from various media. There are over 2 million breast cancer survivors in the United States, and many men and women are active in breast cancer support and advocacy organizations. National breast cancer organizations are accessible online, and many of them have local affiliates. Examples of such organizations are Susan G. Komen for the Cure, the National Breast Cancer Coalition, Y-Me, Sisters Network, Young Survival Coalition, and Pink Ribbon Girls. Local support organizations can be accessed through the health care provider, the local hospital, wellness centers, home care agencies, or by word of mouth. The American Cancer Society (ACS) (www.cancer.org) is a comprehensive resource for information and support.

CLINICAL JUDGMENT CHALLENGE

Patient-Centered Care; Safety; Evidence-Based Practice QSEN

A 46-year-old Caucasian lesbian woman is diagnosed with breast cancer and scheduled for a radical right mastectomy and chemotherapy. She tells you that she often feared developing cancer because her mother and aunt were both diagnosed with breast cancer in their 40s. She says she is fearful because her employer does not offer insurance and she is not eligible to be covered under her partner's insurance plan. She also shares that she feels sad because she has been attempting to get pregnant for the first time and she now realizes that this will not be possible for the foreseeable future.

1. What evidence-based risk factors does this patient have?
2. What discharge instructions will you provide for her and why?
3. What will you teach the patient about chemotherapy to maintain her safety?
4. How might you help address the patient's emotional concerns?

NURSING CONCEPTS AND CLINICAL JUDGMENT REVIEW

What might you NOTICE if a patient is experiencing impaired SEXUALITY as a result of breast cancer or other disorder?

- Breast swelling or lump (with or without pain)
- Discharge from nipple(s)
- Skin dimpling or orange peel appearance
- Asymmetric breast tissue
- Very large or very small breasts
- Skin redness and warmth

What should you INTERPRET and how should you RESPOND to a patient having impaired SEXUALITY as a result of breast cancer or other disorder?

Perform and interpret physical assessment, including:

- Taking a thorough patient and family history
- Examining each breast, comparing sides, and documenting
- Assessing pain and documenting
- Assessing psychosocial reaction to the breast changes

Respond by:

- Checking recent mammogram test or other imaging assessment results
- Acknowledging patient's concerns about body image and sexuality changes
- Asking the patient about resources for support that have been used in the past for coping with crisis
- Preparing the patient for testing and possible biopsy
- Listening to the patient's concerns in a nonjudgmental manner

On what should you REFLECT?

- Consider what health care resources (team members) the patient and family will need throughout disease management.
- Think about what other community resources the patient and family will need.
- Observe the patient's progress in adapting to body image changes.

GET READY FOR THE NCLEX® EXAMINATION!

KEY POINTS

Review these Key Points for each NCLEX Examination Client Needs Category.

Safe and Effective Care Environment

- In collaboration with the health care team, identify community resources for patients with breast cancer, including *Reach to Recovery* of the American Cancer Society. **Teamwork and Collaboration** QSEN

Health Promotion and Maintenance

- Identify patients at high risk for breast cancer, especially women with family history of breast cancer at a young age; those who have had early menarche, late menopause, or first pregnancy after 30 years of age; or those who are nullipara.
- Discuss benefits and risks of options available to women who are high risk for breast cancer, including close surveillance and prophylactic surgery.
- Teach women to become self-aware of breasts and any breast changes; teach breast self-examination (BSE) to women who choose this method of breast self-awareness. **Patient-Centered Care** QSEN
- Encourage women to have screening mammography according to recommended guidelines. Baseline screening should begin at 40 years of age and continue yearly. In high-risk women, screening should be started earlier. **Evidence-Based Practice** QSEN
- Encourage women to have a clinical breast examination (CBE) according to recommended guidelines. **Evidence-Based Practice** QSEN

Psychosocial Integrity

- Assess patients' reactions to the diagnosis of breast cancer and the effect of breast cancer treatment on their body image and SEXUALITY. **Patient-Centered Care** QSEN
- Identify resources that facilitate patients' grief work and coping skills.
- Allow patients opportunities to express feelings of grief, fear, and anxiety.
- Teach women ways to minimize surgical area deformity and enhance body image, such as use of a breast implant (prosthesis) or the option of breast reconstruction.
- Address the reactions of family and significant others to the diagnosis of breast cancer; provide support and education.

Physiological Integrity

- Assess benign lumps as mobile and round or oval; assess possible malignant lumps as fixed and irregularly shaped, often in the upper outer breast quadrant.
- A breast reduction is an option to promote comfort for women with very large, heavy breasts.
- A breast augmentation is an elective procedure for women with small breasts or for women who desire reconstruction after breast removal.
- After breast cancer surgery, assess vital signs, dressings, drainage tubes, and amount of drainage.
- Notify the health care team that the arm of the surgical mastectomy side should not be used for blood pressures, blood drawing, or injections. **Safety** QSEN
- Assess the return of arm and shoulder mobility after breast surgery and axillary dissection.
- Assess for the presence of lymphedema, and assist the patient to perform therapeutic measures to reduce lymphedema in the affected arm. **Safety** QSEN
- Teach the patient measures to prevent lymphedema after axillary node dissection.
- Observe for and report other complications of breast cancer surgery or breast reconstruction, especially infection and inadequate vascular perfusion. **Safety** QSEN
- After an axillary lymph node dissection, elevate the affected arm on a pillow.
- Radiation and drug therapy are used most often as adjuvant therapy after breast surgery but may be used before surgery to shrink the tumor.

71 CHAPTER

Care of Patients with Gynecologic Problems

Donna D. Ignatavicius

http://evolve.elsevier.com/Iggy/

PRIORITY CONCEPTS

- Infection
- Pain
- Sexuality
- Elimination

LEARNING OUTCOMES

Safe and Effective Care Environment

1. Collaborate with members of the health care team when providing care for patients with gynecologic cancers.
2. Teach patients about community-based resources for patients with gynecologic health problems.
3. Develop a community-based plan of care for patients with gynecologic cancers.

Health Promotion and Maintenance

4. Identify risk factors for gynecologic cancers.
5. Describe evidence-based health promotion and maintenance measures to help prevent or early-detect gynecologic cancers.

Psychosocial Integrity

6. Reduce the psychological impact for the patient who has received a diagnosis of a gynecologic health problem.
7. Discuss ways to help patients adapt to physical changes, including impaired SEXUALITY, caused by gynecologic problems and their treatment.

Physiological Integrity

8. Describe the mechanisms of action, side effects, and nursing implications of drug therapy for endometriosis.
9. Develop a teaching plan for a patient with a vaginal inflammation or INFECTION.
10. Prioritize care after surgery for the woman undergoing an anterior and/or posterior repair.
11. Develop a plan of care for a patient undergoing a hysterectomy.
12. Explain the purpose and side effects of radiation and chemotherapy for patients with gynecologic cancers.
13. Teach patients about complementary and alternative therapies that they may wish to explore.

Common gynecologic symptoms that women experience are PAIN, vaginal discharge, and bleeding. Some patients also have urinary ELIMINATION symptoms associated with their gynecologic problem. Women are often hesitant to seek medical attention for these problems because of fear of a life-threatening disease diagnosis or concern about privacy and dignity. Be sensitive to the woman's concerns and encourage discussion about menstrual or other reproductive problems. Teach women about their bodies, and help them recognize when professional help should be sought. Teach them how to make informed decisions about treatments. Assess the effects of gynecologic disorders on SEXUALITY in any setting. These health problems often impair sexual function and therefore can affect the woman's relationship with her partner. Remember that SEXUALITY affects a woman's sense of being, self-esteem, and body image.

ENDOMETRIOSIS

❖ *PATHOPHYSIOLOGY*

Endometriosis is endometrial (inner uterine) tissue implantation *outside* the uterine cavity. The tissue typically appears on the ovaries and the cul-de-sac (posterior rectovaginal wall) and less commonly on other pelvic organs and structures (Fig. 71-1). A "chocolate" cyst, also called an *endometrioma,* is an area of endometriosis on an ovary. The disease affects millions of women in their 30s and 40s. Endometriosis responds to cyclic hormonal stimulation just as if it were in the uterus. Monthly cyclic bleeding occurs at the **ectopic** (out of place) site of implantation, which irritates and scars the surrounding tissue. Scarring can lead to adhesions, causing infertility (inability to become pregnant). Endometriosis progresses slowly and regresses during pregnancy and at menopause. The most common site for endometriosis is the ovaries (Saul, 2013). Although cancer of the endometrium is possible, simply having endometriosis does not mean that a patient is at high risk. Estrogen, tamoxifen, hereditary conditions, and amount of body fat are more strongly linked to development of endometrial cancer (National Cancer Institute [NCI], 2013a).

The cause of endometriosis is unknown. Retrograde menstruation, a condition in which the menstrual blood (which contains endometrial cells) may flow back through the fallopian tube, emptying into the pelvic cavity (instead of outside the

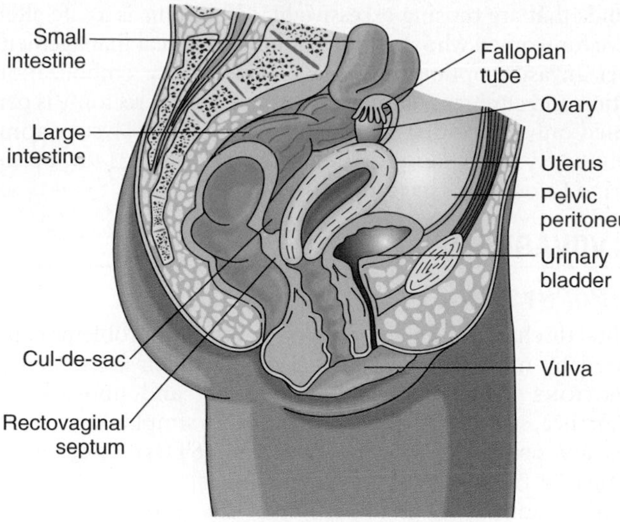

FIG. 71-1 Common sites of endometriosis.

body), is thought to be a cause. The displaced cells stick to surfaces within the pelvic cavity and grow, thicken, and bleed during each menstrual cycle. Embryonic cell growth, surgical scar implantation, endometrial cell transport (via the lymphatic system), and immune system disorders are also thought to be possible causes for endometriosis (Mayo Clinic, 2013).

❖ PATIENT-CENTERED COLLABORATIVE CARE

◆ Assessment

Take a detailed history, including the woman's menstrual history, sexual history (including any patient concerns regarding history of abuse), and bleeding characteristics. A thorough menstrual history includes onset, duration, flow type and characteristics, and regularity. *PAIN is the most common symptom of endometriosis.* The pain usually peaks just before the menstrual flow. It is usually located in the lower abdomen, causing many women to feel a sense of rectal pressure. The degree of pain is not related to the extent of the endometriosis but, instead, to the site. Often, women with minimal disease have more severe pain than do women with extensive disease. Other manifestations include **dyspareunia** (painful sexual intercourse), painful defecation, low backache, and infertility. GI disturbances such as nausea and diarrhea are also common.

A pelvic examination performed by the health care provider may reveal pelvic tenderness, tender nodules in the posterior vagina, and limited movement of the uterus. A psychosocial assessment may reveal anxiety because of uncertainty about the diagnosis or frustration because of PAIN. The woman may also have concerns about her self-concept if she is infertile but wants to become pregnant.

Diagnostic tests may rule out pelvic inflammatory disease caused by chlamydia or gonorrhea. Serum cancer antigen *CA-125* may be positive in women with endometriosis (Mayo Clinic, 2011). Transvaginal ultrasound is used to determine whether pelvic masses are endometriosis or malignant.

◆ Interventions

Hormonal and surgical management may be used, depending on the symptoms, the extent of disease, the woman's desire for childbearing, and her treatment option preferences. Collaborative care consists of interventions that:

- Reduce PAIN
- Restore sexual function
- Alleviate anxiety related to the disease and the uncertainty of the diagnosis
- Educate the patient about the disease and its treatment
- Alleviate fear related to the possibility of laparoscopy or surgery
- Prevent self-concept disturbance related to infertility

Nonsurgical Management. Several resources, such as the Endometriosis Association (www.endometriosisassn.org) and RESOLVE (an organization for infertile couples) (www.resolve.org), offer information on endometriosis that is helpful for patients and caregivers.

Menstrual cycle control using oral contraceptives or progestins, such as oral medroxyprogesterone acetate (Provera, Alti-MPA🍁 Novo-Medrone🍁) and norethindrone acetate (Aygestin, Norlutate🍁), may be prescribed. Injectable forms of progestins, such as medroxyprogesterone acetate (Depo-Provera), may be more convenient because these drugs are given less frequently.

Continuous low-level heat using wearable heat packs may provide temporary PAIN relief. Relaxation techniques, yoga, massage, and biofeedback may decrease muscle tissue hypoxia and hypertonicity and relieve ischemia by increasing blood flow to the affected areas. Calcium and magnesium may also relieve muscle cramping for some patients.

Surgical Management. Surgical management of endometriosis for a woman who wants to remain fertile involves ablation, a laparoscopic removal of endometrial implants and adhesions, in a same-day surgical setting. Chapter 16 describes the general postoperative care for patients having surgery. The surgeon may use a laser to treat endometriosis by vaporizing adhesions and endometrial implants. Teach patients that temporary postoperative PAIN from carbon dioxide, used during laparoscopy to better visualize internal organs, can occur in the shoulders and chest.

DYSFUNCTIONAL UTERINE BLEEDING

❖ PATHOPHYSIOLOGY

Dysfunctional uterine bleeding (DUB) is excessive and frequent bleeding (more than every 21 days). It is a diagnosis of exclusion, made after ruling out anatomic or systemic conditions such as drug therapy or disease. DUB occurs most often at the beginning or end of a woman's reproductive years—when ovulation is becoming established or when it is becoming irregular at or after menopause.

Normally the menstrual cycle is a series of delicately timed hormonal events regulated by hypothalamic, pituitary, ovarian, and uterine functions. **Menses**, the sloughing of the endometrial lining, is an expected result. DUB occurs when there is a hormonal imbalance, generally when the ovaries fail to ovulate. This decreases progesterone production, which is needed to mature the uterine lining and prevent overgrowth. Without progesterone, prolonged estrogen stimulation causes the endometrium to grow past its hormonal support, causing disordered shedding of uterine lining. Most cases of DUB are classified into two types: anovulatory DUB (most common) and ovulatory DUB. Common risk factors for DUB during the reproductive years are listed in Table 71-1.

TABLE 71-1 Risk Factors for Dysfunctional Uterine Bleeding

- Obesity
- Extreme weight loss or gain
- Age older than 40 years
- High stress levels
- Polycystic ovary disease
- Long-term drug use (e.g., oral contraceptives)
- Excessive exercise

❖ PATIENT-CENTERED COLLABORATIVE CARE

◆ Assessment

Take a complete menstrual history. Ask about illnesses, changes in weight or nutritional intake, exercise, drug ingestion, and whether the woman experiences PAIN.

Assess for symptoms of anemia or systemic disease, such as:

- Renal or hepatic disease
- Abnormal weight
- Signs of hormonal dysfunction, such as thyroid enlargement or male hair pattern
- Evidence of abdominal PAIN or masses

The health care provider inspects the external genitalia, does a bimanual pelvic examination, performs a Papanicolaou (Pap) test to assess for the presence of cervical cancer, and does a rectal examination to identify INFECTIONS, lesions, or tenderness. Vaginal specimens are also tested for sexually transmitted diseases (STDs) such as chlamydia. Women at high risk for endometrial cancer should also have an endometrial biopsy. Risk factors are described later in this chapter.

A complete blood count may be taken to determine whether the patient is anemic. Thyroid-stimulating hormone and reproductive hormone levels may also be evaluated.

Transvaginal ultrasound may reveal **leiomyomas** (fibroids) and measure an excessively thick endometrium. *Sonohysterography* uses vaginal ultrasound to visualize the uterus after sterile saline is infused through the cervix, thus outlining the inner uterine cavity (American Congress of Obstetricians and Gynecologists [ACOG], 2011).

◆ Interventions

Nonsurgical Management. As with endometriosis, hormone manipulation is usually the treatment of choice for women with anovulatory DUB. The drugs used depend on the severity of bleeding and age of the patient. Progestin or combination hormone therapy (estrogen and progestin) may be given when bleeding is heavy and acute. For nonemergent bleeding, contraceptives (oral or patch) provide the progestin (artificial progesterone) needed to stabilize the endometrial lining. Progestin-only pills (e.g., norethindrone [Aygestin, Norlutate🍁]) or long-acting progestins (e.g., injectable medroxyprogesterone acetate [Depo-Provera]) are preferable for women older than 35 years who smoke or are at risk for thrombophlebitis.

Explain the desired outcomes and the side effects of these drugs, and evaluate the woman's knowledge of the effects, dosage, and schedule. Remind her to take the drug exactly as prescribed and not to skip a dose or run out of it. If bleeding worsens, teach her to call her health care provider immediately.

Surgical Management. Removal of the built-up uterine lining, called **endometrial ablation**, stops the blood flow to fibroids that are causing excessive bleeding. This is a safe alternative for women who do not respond to medical management. Other invasive options include uterine artery embolization, dilation and curettage, and hysterectomy. A hysterectomy is performed only after other treatments have failed. (Hysterectomy is discussed under Surgical Management on p. 1489 of the Uterine Leiomyoma section.)

VULVOVAGINITIS

❖ PATHOPHYSIOLOGY

Vaginal discharge and itching are two common problems experienced by most women at some time in their lives. Vaginal INFECTIONS may be transmitted sexually and non-sexually. Gonorrhea, syphilis, chlamydia, and herpes simplex virus infections are sexually transmitted diseases (STDs) discussed in Chapter 74.

Vulvovaginitis is inflammation of the lower genital tract resulting from a disturbance of the balance of hormones and flora in the vagina and vulva. It may be characterized by itching, change in vaginal discharge, odor, or lesions. The most common causes include:

- Fungal (yeast) INFECTIONS *(Candida albicans)*
- Bacterial vaginosis
- STDs *(Trichomonas vaginalis)*
- Postmenopausal vaginal atrophy
- Changes in the normal flora or pH (from douching)
- Chemical irritant or allergens (vaginal spray, fabric dyes, detergent) or foreign body (tampon)
- Drugs, especially antibiotics
- Immunosuppression from diabetes or human immune deficiency virus (HIV)

Primary INFECTIONS that affect the vulva include *herpes genitalis* and *condylomata acuminata* (human papilloma virus, venereal warts) (see Chapter 74). Secondary infections of the vulva are caused by organisms responsible for the many types of vaginitis, including *candidiasis.* Pediculosis pubis (crab lice, or "crabs") and scabies (itch mite) are common parasitic infestations of the skin of the vulva. Other causes of vulvitis include:

- Atrophic vaginitis
- Lichen planus (thickened, leathery skin from scratching)
- Vulvar leukoplakia (postmenopausal atrophy and thickening of vulvar tissues)
- Vulvar cancer
- Urinary incontinence

Some women may have an *itch-scratch-itch cycle,* in which the itching leads to scratching, which causes excoriation that then must heal. As healing takes place, itching occurs again. If the cycle is not interrupted, the chronic scratching may lead to the white, thickened skin of lichen planus. This dry, leathery skin cracks easily, increasing the risk for infection.

❖ PATIENT-CENTERED COLLABORATIVE CARE

Assess for vulvovaginitis by asking questions about the symptoms, assisting with a pelvic examination, and obtaining vaginal smears for laboratory testing. Ask if the patient is experiencing an itching or burning sensation, **erythema** (redness), edema, and/or superficial skin ulcers. Use a nonjudgmental approach and provide reassurance during the assessment because the patient may be embarrassed or afraid to discuss her symptoms.

CHART 71-1 Patient and Family Education: Preparing for Self-Management

Vaginal Infections

- Your risk for getting vaginal infections increases if you have sex with more than one person.
- When you have a vaginal infection, do not have sexual intercourse, if possible, or at least make sure that your partner wears a condom.
- All sexual partners may need to be treated for infection.
- The only way to identify what infection you have is to be examined by a health care provider and to follow up to get the results of laboratory tests.
- Take all of your medicine as prescribed, not just until your symptoms go away.

Encourage her to talk about her problem and its effect on her sexual health.

Interventions for vulvovaginitis depend on the specific vaginal INFECTION. Proper health habits can benefit treatment. Instruct the patient to get enough rest and sleep, observe good dietary habits, exercise regularly, and use good personal hygiene. Teach her about how to manage her infection (Chart 71-1) and how to prevent further infections (Chart 71-2).

Wet compresses, warm or tepid sitz baths for 30 minutes several times a day, and topical drugs such as estrogens and lidocaine can help relieve itching. Encourage the patient to wear breathable fabrics such as cotton and to avoid irritants or allergens in products such as laundry detergents or bath products.

Treatment of pediculosis and scabies is used if needed and includes:

- Applying lindane (Kwell, Kwellada ♣) lotion, shampoo, or cream to the affected area as directed
- Cleaning affected clothes, bedding, and towels
- Disinfecting the home environment (lice cannot live for more than 24 hours away from the body)

NCLEX EXAMINATION CHALLENGE

Health Promotion and Maintenance

A client tells the nurse that she has vaginal itching. Which client statement would cause the nurse to further assess for symptoms of vaginitis? **Select all that apply.**

A. "I always use the same detergent when washing clothes."
B. "All of my immunizations, including Gardasil, are up to date."
C. "I've scratched so hard that it gets raw, but then it feels better for awhile."
D. "My boyfriend and I broke up last month, but we are together again now."
E. "My health care provider prescribed antibiotics for my sinus infection last week."

TOXIC SHOCK SYNDROME

❖ PATHOPHYSIOLOGY

Toxic shock syndrome (TSS) can result from menstruation and tampon use. Other conditions associated with TSS include surgical wound INFECTION, nonsurgical infections, gynecologic surgeries, and use of internal contraceptives.

In INFECTION related to menstruation, menstrual blood provides a growth medium for *Staphylococcus aureus* (or, less frequently, Group A *Streptococcus* [GAS], also known as *Streptococcus pyogenes*). Exotoxins produced from the bacteria cross the vaginal mucosa to the bloodstream via microabrasions from tampon insertion or prolonged use. TSS can be fatal. Extensive public education has led to a decreased number of women developing the infection.

CHART 71-2 Patient and Family Education: Preparing for Self-Management

Prevention of Vulvovaginitis

- Wear cotton underwear.
- Avoid wearing tight clothing, such as pantyhose or tight jeans, because they can cause chafing. You can also get hot and sweaty, which can increase the risk for infection.
- Always wipe front to back after having a bowel movement or urinating.
- During bath or shower, cleanse inner labial mucosa with water, not soap.
- Do not douche or use feminine hygiene sprays.
- If your sexual partner has an infection of the sex organs, do not have intercourse with him or her until he or she has been treated.
- You are more likely to get an infection if you are pregnant, have diabetes, take oral contraceptive drugs, or are menopausal.
- Practice vulvar self-examination monthly.

CHART 71-3 Patient and Family Education: Preparing for Self-Management

Prevention of Toxic Shock Syndrome

- Wash your hands before inserting a tampon.
- Do not use a tampon if it is dirty.
- Insert the tampon carefully to avoid injuring the delicate tissue in your vagina.
- Change your tampon every 3 to 6 hours.
- Do not use superabsorbent tampons.
- Use sanitary napkins (instead of tampons) at night.
- Call your health care provider if you suddenly experience a high temperature, vomiting, or diarrhea.
- Do not use tampons at all if you have had toxic shock syndrome.
- Not using tampons almost guarantees that you will not get toxic shock syndrome.

❖ PATIENT-CENTERED COLLABORATIVE CARE

TSS usually develops within 5 days after the onset of menstruation. Most common symptoms include fever, rash, myalgias, sore throat, edema, and hypotension (Low, 2013). The rash associated with TSS often looks like a sunburn, and patients often develop broken capillaries in the eyes and skin. Educate all women on prevention of TSS (Chart 71-3).

Treatment includes removal of the INFECTION source, such as a tampon; restoring fluid and electrolyte balance; administering drugs to manage hypotension; and IV antibiotics. Other measures may include transfusions to reverse low platelet counts and corticosteroids to treat skin changes.

PELVIC ORGAN PROLAPSE

❖ PATHOPHYSIOLOGY

The pelvic organs are supported by a sling of muscles and tendons, which sometimes become weak and no longer able to hold an organ in place. Uterine prolapse, the most common type of pelvic organ prolapse (POP), can be caused by neuromuscular damage of childbirth; increased intra-abdominal

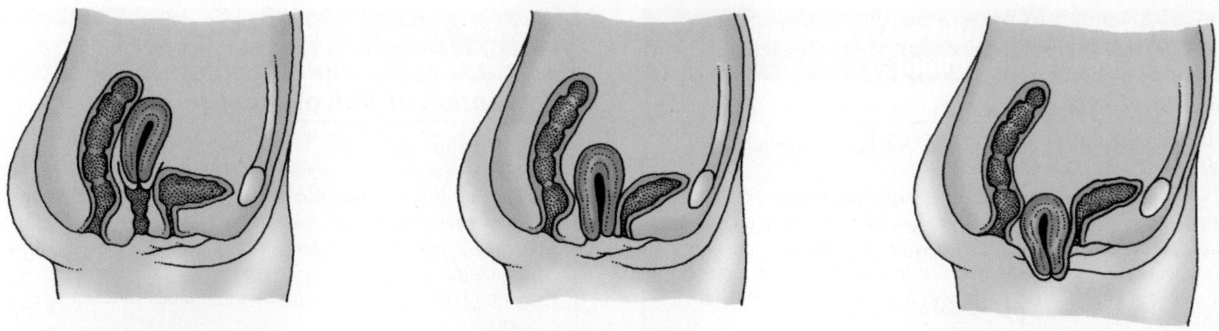

In **grade I uterine prolapse**, the uterus bulges into the vagina, but the cervix does not protrude through the entrance to the vagina.

In **grade II uterine prolapse**, the uterus bulges farther into the vagina, and the cervix protrudes through the entrance to the vagina.

In **grade III uterine prolapse**, the body of the uterus and the cervix protrude through the entrance to the vagina. The vagina is turned inside out.

FIG. 71-2 Types of uterine prolapse.

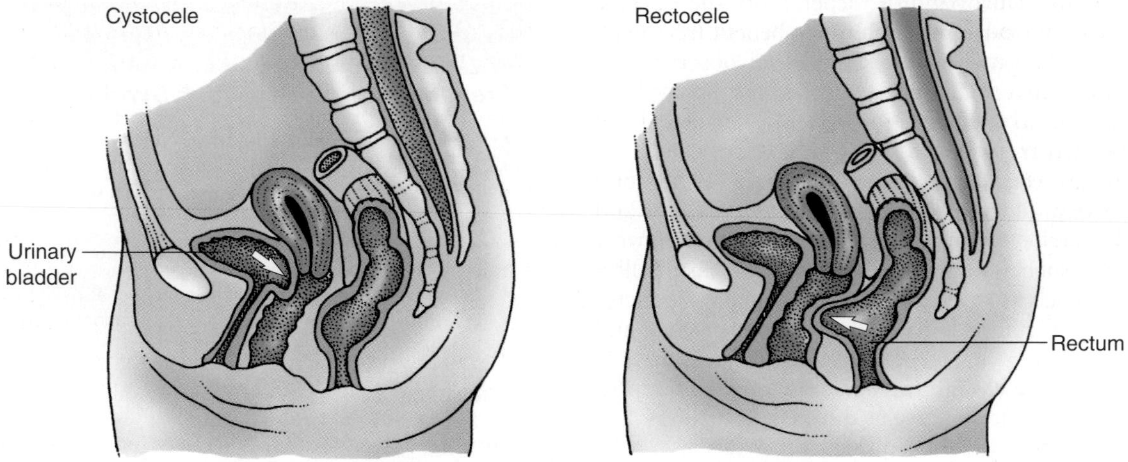

FIG. 71-3 In cystocele, the urinary bladder is displaced downward, causing bulging of the anterior vaginal wall. In rectocele, the rectum is displaced, causing bulging of the posterior vaginal wall.

pressure related to pregnancy, obesity, or physical exertion; or weakening of pelvic support due to decreased estrogen. The stages of uterine prolapse are described by the degree of descent of the uterus (Fig. 71-2) through the pelvic floor.

Whenever the uterus is displaced, other structures such as the bladder, rectum, and small intestine can protrude through the vaginal walls (Fig. 71-3). A **cystocele** is a protrusion of the bladder through the vaginal wall (urinary bladder prolapse), which can lead to stress urinary incontinence (SUI) and urinary tract infections (UTIs). A **rectocele** is a protrusion of the rectum through a weakened vaginal wall (rectal prolapse).

❖ PATIENT-CENTERED COLLABORATIVE CARE

◆ Assessment

Patients with suspected uterine prolapse may report a feeling of "something falling out," dyspareunia (painful intercourse), backache, and heaviness or pressure in the pelvis. A pelvic examination may reveal a protrusion of the cervix or anterior vaginal wall when the woman is asked to bear down. Listen to her concerns, and note signs of anxiety or depression from having long-term symptoms.

Ask the patient whether she has urinary ELIMINATION problems, such as difficulty emptying her bladder, urinary frequency and urgency, a urinary tract infection, or **stress urinary incontinence (SUI)** (loss of urine during activities that increase intra-abdominal pressure, such as laughing, coughing, sneezing, or lifting heavy objects). These symptoms may be associated with a *cystocele* (bladder prolapse).

Diagnostic tests include cystography (to show the presence of bladder herniation), measurement of residual urine by bladder ultrasound, and urine culture and sensitivity testing. Radiographic imaging of urinary anatomy and voiding function is useful in determining the degree of *cystocele* (prolapse).

Rectocele assessment usually includes symptoms of constipation, hemorrhoids, fecal impaction, and feelings of rectal or vaginal fullness. A vaginal and rectal examination may show a bulge of the posterior vaginal wall when the woman is asked to bear down.

◆ Interventions

Interventions are based on the degree of the POP. Conservative treatment is preferred over surgical treatment when possible.

Nonsurgical Management. Teach women to improve pelvic support and tone by doing pelvic floor muscle exercises (PFMEs, or Kegel exercises). Space-filling devices such as pessaries or spheres can be worn in the vagina to elevate the uterine prolapse. Intravaginal estrogen therapy may be prescribed for the postmenopausal woman to prevent atrophy and weakening of vaginal walls. Women with bladder symptoms may benefit from bladder training and attention to complete emptying. Management of a rectocele focuses on promoting bowel elimination. The health care provider usually prescribes a high-fiber diet, stool softeners, and laxatives.

Surgical Management. Surgery may be recommended for severe symptoms of POP, with preference given to the least invasive approach. Address the fears and concerns of the patient and her family.

Transvaginal repair for pelvic organ prolapse (POP) using surgical vaginal mesh or tape is a commonly performed minimally invasive technique. It is particularly useful for women who are very obese. Depending on the procedure that is planned, the patient has either local or general anesthesia. The surgeon creates a sling with the mesh or tape, and the woman is discharged the same day. Procedures done under local anesthesia can be done in the surgeon's office. Since 2008, patient report of complications associated with the use of transvaginal mesh has required the U.S. Food and Drug Administration (2011) to release an initial report and update advising about the safety and effectiveness of the use of this product for POP. Complications associated with the use of transvaginal mesh for POP include vaginal mesh erosion, painful sexual intercourse, infection, urinary ELIMINATION problems, bleeding, and organ perforation (U.S. Food and Drug Administration [USFDA], 2011). Three deaths associated with this procedure (two bowel perforations and one hemorrhage) were also reported between 2008 and 2010 (USFDA, 2011).

! NURSING SAFETY PRIORITY QSEN

Action Alert

To help the patient decide if she should have any surgical procedure using mesh or tape, be sure that she is provided with information regarding informed consent prior to surgery. Reinforce information about possible adverse events, the signs and symptoms of infection, and when she should contact her surgeon. Provide the patient with the manufacturer's labeling and written information.

Teach patients who have had the mesh or tape procedure to avoid strenuous exercise, heavy lifting, and sexual intercourse for 6 weeks. After 6 weeks, the patient may gradually begin to return to regular activities but must be educated about prevention of increasing intra-abdominal pressure (e.g., constipation, weight-lifting, cigarette smoking) for a minimum of 3 months to allow proper healing and prevent POP recurrence (Lazarou, 2012).

Alternatives to minimally invasive surgery are open surgical techniques. An **anterior colporrhaphy** (anterior repair) tightens the pelvic muscles for better *bladder* support. A vaginal surgical approach is used and may be done as a laparoscopic-assisted procedure. Nursing care for a woman undergoing an anterior repair is similar to that for a woman undergoing a vaginal hysterectomy.

After surgery, instruct the patient how to splint her abdomen to protect sutures and to limit her activities. Teach her to *avoid lifting anything heavier than 5 pounds, strenuous exercises, and sexual intercourse for 6 weeks.* For discomfort, she may use heat either as a moist heating pad or warm compresses applied to the abdomen. A hot bath may also be helpful. Sutures do not need to be removed because some are absorbable and others will fall out as healing occurs. Tell the woman to notify her health care provider if she has signs of INFECTION, such as fever, persistent PAIN, or purulent, foul-smelling discharge. Encourage her to keep her follow-up appointment after surgery.

Posterior colporrhaphy (posterior repair) reduces *rectal* bulging. If both a cystocele and a rectocele are present, an *anterior and posterior colporrhaphy (A&P repair)* is performed.

The nursing care after a posterior repair is similar to that after any rectal surgery. After surgery, a low-residue (low-fiber) diet is usually prescribed to decrease bowel movements and allow time for the incision to heal. Instruct the patient to avoid straining when she does have a bowel movement so that she does not put pressure on the suture line. Bowel movements are often painful, and she may need pain medication before having a stool. Provide sitz baths or delegate this activity to unlicensed nursing personnel to relieve the woman's discomfort. Health teaching for the patient undergoing a posterior repair is similar to that for the patient undergoing an anterior repair. Vaginal hysterectomy may accompany any uterine prolapse repair surgery unless the woman wants to become pregnant. This procedure is described on p. 1489.

BENIGN NEOPLASMS

OVARIAN CYST

Functional ovarian cysts can occur in a woman of any age but are rare after menopause. Other cysts and tumors of the ovaries are not related to the menstrual cycle but arise from ovarian tissue. Primary assessment involves pelvic examination and transvaginal ultrasound. Further testing with CT, MRI, or laparoscopic biopsy to rule out cancer may be needed. Some ovarian cysts disappear over time, and others cause discomfort for a prolonged period. Laparoscopic surgery to remove the cyst or ovary may be needed.

UTERINE LEIOMYOMA

❖ *PATHOPHYSIOLOGY*

Leiomyomas, also called **fibroids** or **myomas,** are benign, slow-growing solid tumors of the uterine myometrium (muscle layer). They are classified according to their position in the layers of the uterus: intramural, submucosal, and subserosal (Fig. 71-4).

Intramural leiomyomas are contained in the uterine wall within the myometrium. *Submucosal* leiomyomas protrude into the cavity of the uterus and can cause bleeding and disrupt pregnancy. *Subserosal* leiomyomas protrude through the outer surface of the uterine wall and may extend to the broad ligament, pressing other organs (McCance et al., 2014).

Although most fibroids develop within the uterine wall, a few may appear in the cervix. Pedunculated leiomyomas are attached by a pedicle (stalk) to the outside of the uterus and occasionally break off and attach to other tissues (parasitic fibroids).

Although the cause is not known, leiomyomas develop from excessive local growth of smooth muscle cells. This may be a genetic error causing a lack of ability to halt growth. The growth of leiomyomas may be related to stimulation by estrogen, progesterone, and growth hormone. This explains why fibroids sometimes enlarge during pregnancy and diminish in size after menopause.

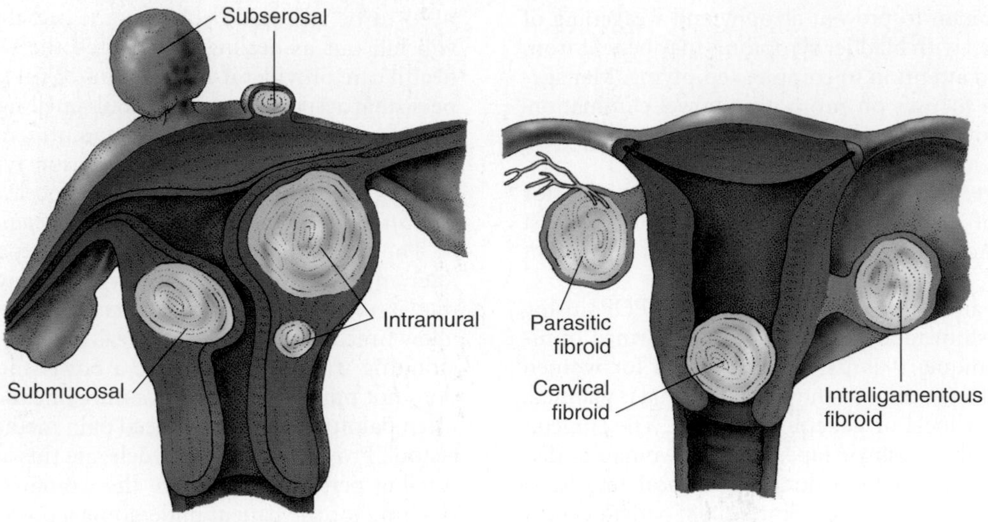

FIG. 71-4 Classification of uterine leiomyomas.

The incidence of leiomyomas increases as women get older. Women who have never been pregnant also are at a high risk. Many women have asymptomatic fibroids, whereas others have severe symptoms.

❖ PATIENT-CENTERED COLLABORATIVE CARE

◆ Assessment

Women with fibroids usually do not have pain, although acute PAIN may occur with twisting of the fibroid on its stalk. *The patient often seeks medical attention because of heavy vaginal bleeding.* Ask about how many tampons or menstrual pads she uses a day. She may report a feeling of pelvic pressure, constipation, or urinary frequency or retention. These symptoms result when an enlarged fibroid presses on other organs. The patient may notice that her abdomen has increased in size. Assess the woman's abdomen for distention or enlargement. Ask if she has dyspareunia (painful intercourse) and/or infertility (inability to become pregnant).

Abdominal, vaginal, and rectal examinations usually reveal the presence of a uterine enlargement. Further diagnostic procedures are needed to differentiate benign tumors from cancerous ones.

Symptoms such as dyspareunia may significantly lower the patient's quality of life. A woman who is symptomatic may fear that she has cancer or may have anxiety about abnormal bleeding or her failure to conceive. She may also be concerned if surgery is recommended if she desires pregnancy. Assess the woman's feelings and concerns about her symptoms and fears of the unknown. If hysterectomy is recommended, explore the significance of the loss of the uterus for the woman and her partner. Discuss SEXUALITY issues with the patient based on your assessment.

A complete blood count may identify iron deficiency anemia (related to bleeding). A pregnancy test is done to determine whether pregnancy is the cause of the uterine enlargement. An endometrial biopsy may be performed to evaluate for endometrial cancer.

Transvaginal ultrasound alone or with saline infusion (saline sonogram) provides a picture of a submucosal fibroid that may protrude into the uterine cavity. The health care provider may then choose to directly view a tumor and perform a biopsy using *laparoscopy* (for tumors on the outside of the uterus) or *hysteroscopy* (for tumors accessible inside the uterus). *MRI* can differentiate between benign and malignant lesions.

◆ Interventions

Asymptomatic fibroids do not need treatment. Management depends on the size and location of the tumor and the woman's desire for future pregnancy. Women who still desire pregnancy can take drug therapy or have magnetic resonance–guided focused ultrasound surgery or laparoscopic myomectomy to remove the tumor. Uterine artery embolization and hysterectomy are choices for women who no longer desire pregnancy.

Nonsurgical Management. If the woman is menopausal, the fibroids usually shrink and surgery may not be necessary. *Teach the patient who is receiving hormone replacement therapy for menopausal symptoms that the fibroids may continue to grow because of estrogen stimulation.*

If the woman has few symptoms or desires childbearing, the health care provider may recommend intermittent observation and examination. As with dysfunctional uterine bleeding, mild leiomyoma symptoms can be managed with oral contraception.

Magnetic resonance–guided focused ultrasound is a noninvasive, painless technique for women with few smaller fibroids who wish to preserve their fertility. The woman lies prone on an MRI scanner, which provides a three-dimensional image of the pelvis. The radiologic clinician then guides a focused pulse of ultrasound to heat the tumor to destroy it.

An alternative to surgery for the woman who does not desire pregnancy is **uterine artery embolization** (also called *uterine fibroid embolization [UFE]*) under conscious sedation. The interventional radiologist uses a percutaneous catheter inserted through the femoral artery to inject polyvinyl alcohol pellets into the uterine artery. The resulting blockage starves the tumor of circulation, allowing it (or them) to shrink.

Before discharge, tell the patient to observe for postembolectomy syndrome—a flu-like illness that some women develop that lasts about 5 to 7 days (Northwest Radiology

NURSING SAFETY PRIORITY (QSEN)

Action Alert

After uterine artery embolization, the woman may have severe cramping within the first 24 hours caused by decreased blood flow to the uterus. Cramping can last from a few days to 2 weeks. Assess her pain level, and provide analgesics as needed. If a vascular closure device is used at the arterial insertion site (most commonly), raise the head of the bed. Help the patient ambulate in about 2 hours after the procedure. If a closure device was not used, keep her on bedrest with the legs immobilized for 4 hours before ambulating to prevent bleeding. Patients generally recover quickly, returning to normal activities within 7 to 10 days after the procedure (Storck, 2012.)

Associates, 2014). Teach her to resume usual activities slowly. Most patients can return to work or daily routine within a week. She should avoid strenuous activity until the physician recommends it.

Surgical Management. When possible, minimally invasive surgical (MIS) techniques are performed, such as a myomectomy. If not, a hysterectomy is the procedure of choice.

Uterus-Sparing Surgeries. If the woman desires children, the surgeon may perform a laparoscopic or hysteroscopic **myomectomy** (the removal of leiomyomas from the uterus) (Bradley, 2013). During this procedure, a laser may be used to remove the tumors. This minimally invasive procedure is usually performed in the early phase of the menstrual cycle to minimize blood loss and to avoid the possibility of interrupting an unsuspected pregnancy. A small percentage of leiomyomas recur after surgery. Scarring makes the uterus more likely to rupture during labor, so future deliveries will be planned cesarean deliveries. Nursing care is similar to that for a woman undergoing a hysterectomy (see below).

In selected cases (e.g., submucous fibroids, menorrhagia), a *transcervical endometrial resection (TCER)* is performed via hysteroscopy. A hysteroscope (endoscope) is inserted into the uterus, and the endometrium is destroyed using diathermy (heat) or radioablation.

NURSING SAFETY PRIORITY (QSEN)

Critical Rescue

Monitor for rare but potential complications of hysteroscopic surgery, which include:

- Fluid overload (fluid used to distend the uterine cavity can be absorbed)
- Embolism
- Hemorrhage
- Perforation of the uterus, bowel, or bladder and ureter injury
- Persistent increased menstrual bleeding
- Incomplete suppression of menstruation

Monitor for any indications of these problems, and report signs and symptoms, such as severe pain and heavy bleeding, to the surgeon immediately. Scarring may cause a small risk for complications in future pregnancies.

Hysterectomy. Leiomyomas are the most common reason for hysterectomies. Hysterectomies may be performed abdominally, vaginally, or with laparoscopic or robotic assistance based on the patient's clinical reason for hysterectomy and the surgeon's area of technical expertise (Falcone, 2014).

A *total abdominal hysterectomy (TAH)* is usually performed for leiomyomas larger than the size of a 16-week pregnancy. The uterus and cervix are most often removed by laparoscopic-assisted minimally invasive surgery (MIS), which requires one or more very small umbilical incisions. The traditional open surgery is performed through a horizontal bikini incision. A *total vaginal hysterectomy (TVH)* requires no skin incision because the uterus is removed through the vagina.

TABLE 71-2 Common Gynecologic Surgeries

Total Hysterectomy	All of the uterus, including the cervix, is removed. The procedure may be vaginal or abdominal, with laparoscopic or robotic assistance.
Bilateral Salpingo-Oophorectomy (BSO)	Fallopian tubes and ovaries are removed.
Panhysterectomy	Total abdominal hysterectomy and BSO: The uterus, ovaries, and fallopian tubes are removed.
Radical Hysterectomy	The uterus, cervix, adjacent lymph nodes, the upper third of the vagina, and the surrounding tissues (parametrium) are removed.

Some surgeons use robotic technology to assist in performing a TAH, although it is much more expensive than a traditional vaginal or laparoscopic approach (ACOG, 2013). Robotic surgery is helpful when performing hysterectomies on patients who are extremely obese (Gallo et al., 2012). In both vaginal and abdominal hysterectomies, the surgeon removes the uterus from the five supporting ligaments, which are then attached to the vaginal cuff so that normal depth of the vagina is maintained (Table 71-2).

Preoperative teaching by the health care team begins in the surgeon's office. Explain procedures that routinely take place before surgery, including laboratory tests and expected drugs such as a prophylactic antibiotic. Depending on the type of surgical technique planned, teach about the need for turning, coughing, and deep-breathing exercises; incentive spirometry; early ambulation; and PAIN relief. (See Chapter 14 for a discussion of general patient care before surgery.)

Psychological assessment is essential. Assess the significance of the surgery for the woman and her partner related to SEXUALITY. If it involves loss of the uterus, she may feel a great loss if she wishes to become pregnant. Many women relate their uterus to self-image and femininity or believe that their sexual function is related to their uterus. Although surgical menopause by hysterectomy can create loss of libido and vaginal changes if the ovaries are also removed, teach the patient that vaginal estrogen cream and gentle dilation can help correct that. Reassure her regarding any misperceptions about the effects of hysterectomy, such as association with masculinization and weight gain. Assess the patient's support system. She may fear rejection by her sexual partner. Include the partner in all teaching sessions (if the patient prefers) unless this practice is not culturally acceptable.

Patients who have *uterus-sparing surgeries* usually go home the same day of surgery. They often experience less postoperative PAIN and fewer complications when compared with patients who have their uterus and cervix removed. Teach patients that they usually return to usual daily activities in 2 weeks but sexual intercourse should be avoided for at least 6 weeks.

Postoperative care of the woman who has undergone a *TAH* is similar to that of any patient who has had laparoscopic or

CHART 71-4 Focused Assessment

Postoperative Nursing Care of the Patient after Total Abdominal Hysterectomy

- Assess cardiovascular, respiratory, renal, and gastrointestinal status, including:
  - Vital signs
  - Heart, lung, and bowel sounds
  - Urine output
  - Temperature and color of the skin
  - Red blood cell, hemoglobin, and hematocrit levels
  - Activity tolerance
  - Dressing and drains for color and amount of drainage
  - Perineal pads for vaginal bleeding and clots
  - Fluid intake (IVs until peristalsis returns and patient is tolerating oral intake)
- Teach the patient to use these interventions to prevent postoperative complications:
  - Cough and deep-breathing exercises
  - Incentive spirometry
  - Sequential compression devices
  - Ambulation
  - Avoidance of heavy lifting or strenuous activity
  - Adequate hydration
- Assess the home care teaching needs of the patient related to the illness and surgery, including:
  - Physiologic effects of the surgery
  - Signs or symptoms to report
  - Side or toxic effects of medications
  - Activity limitations related to driving and use of stairs
  - Follow-up care
  - Postoperative restrictions related to sexual activity, use of tampons, and bathing
  - Care of wound and/or drains
- Assess the patient's coping skills and reaction to the diagnosis and surgical procedure.

traditional open abdominal surgery (see Chapter 16). Assess (Chart 71-4):

- Vaginal bleeding (there should be less than one saturated perineal pad in 4 hours)
- Abdominal bleeding at the incision site(s) (a small amount is normal)
- Intactness of the incision(s)
- Urine output per urinary catheter for 24 hours or less (for open surgery only)
- PAIN

Specific postoperative interventions for a *vaginal hysterectomy* include:

- Assessment of vaginal bleeding (there should be less than one saturated pad in 4 hours)
- Urinary catheter care
- Perineal care

NCLEX EXAMINATION CHALLENGE

Physiological Integrity

A client returns from surgery after a total vaginal hysterectomy. Upon initial assessment, which finding by the nurse requires immediate intervention?

A. Clean, intact dressing
B. Excessive vaginal bleeding
C. Temperature of 99° F
D. Client statement that pain is "4" on scale of 0-10

CHART 71-5 Patient and Family Education: Preparing for Self-Management

Care after a Total Vaginal or Abdominal Hysterectomy

Expected Physical Changes

- You will no longer have a period, although you may have some vaginal discharge for a few days after you go home.
- It will not be possible for you to become pregnant, and birth control methods are no longer needed. (Condoms should still be used to decrease the chance of getting a sexually transmitted disease [STD].)
- If your ovaries were removed, you may have some menopause symptoms such as hot flushes, night sweats, and vaginal dryness.
- It is normal to tire more easily and require more sleep and rest during the first few weeks after surgery.

Activity

- Limit stair climbing to fewer than 5 times per day.
- Do not lift anything heavier than 5 to 10 lbs.
- Gradually increase walking as exercise, but stop before you become fatigued.
- Avoid the sitting position for any extended period. When you sit, do not cross your legs at the knees.
- Avoid jogging, aerobic exercise, participating in sports, and any strenuous activity for 2 to 6 weeks, depending on what type of surgical procedure was performed.
- Do not drive until your surgeon has told you it is alright.

Sexual Activity

- Do not engage in sexual intercourse for 4 to 6 weeks or as prescribed by your surgeon.
- If you had a vaginal "repair" as part of your surgery, the first time you have intercourse you may have some tenderness or pain because the vaginal walls are tighter. Careful intercourse and the use of water-based lubricants can help reduce this discomfort. This discomfort usually goes away with time and stretching of the vagina.

Complications

- Take your temperature twice each day for the first 3 days after surgery. Report fevers of over 100° F (38° C).
- Check your incision, if you have any, daily for signs of infection (increasing redness, open areas, drainage that is thick or foul-smelling, incision pain).

Symptoms to Report to Your Surgeon

- Increased vaginal drainage or change in drainage (bloodier, thicker, foul-smelling)
- Temperature over 100° F (38° C)
- Pain, tenderness, redness, or swelling in your calves
- Pain or burning on urination

Community-Based Care

If the patient had a hysterectomy, teach her to limit stair climbing for several weeks. If she lives alone and is not permitted to drive for several weeks, she may need to arrange for transportation for follow-up surgical visits.

Teach the woman who has undergone an abdominal hysterectomy about the expected physical changes, any activity restrictions, diet, sexual activity, wound care, complications, and the need for follow-up care. Chart 71-5 lists areas to include for health teaching.

Generally, women are more accepting of surgery if they have completed childbearing, have interests outside the home, work, have no misconceptions about the effects of hysterectomy, and have support from the family, especially their sexual partner. Psychological reactions can occur months to years after surgery, particularly if sexual functioning and libido are diminished. Women identified as being at high risk for psychological problems may need long-term follow-up care or referral. They may need to be counseled about signs of depression. Intermittent sadness is normal, but continued feelings of low self-esteem or loss of interest or pleasure in usual activities and pastimes is not expected and should be evaluated. Provide written materials, and focus on the positive aspects of the woman's life to help decrease adverse psychological reactions.

BARTHOLIN CYST

Bartholin cyst is a common disorder of the vulva. It results from obstruction of the duct of the Bartholin gland. The secretory function of the gland continues, and the fluid fills the obstructed duct. The main causes of the obstruction are INFECTION, thickened mucus near the ductal opening, or trauma, such as lacerations.

The patient may be asymptomatic if the cyst is small. Ask if she has dyspareunia (painful intercourse) or inadequate genital lubrication. Assess for swelling in the perineal area. A large cyst usually causes constant local pain and may cause difficulty walking or sitting. Assessment of the vulva reveals a unilateral swelling immediately beneath the skin in the posterior portion of the vulva. The cyst may appear brown or bloody, depending on its contents. Vaginal discharge may be present with a Bartholin *abscess* if an infection, such as one caused by a sexually transmitted organism, is present (Braun, 2014).

If the cyst is draining, a fluid sample is sent to the laboratory to culture for gonorrhea and/or other organisms. If the woman is older than 40 years, a biopsy of the cyst may be done to identify possible cancer.

If the woman is asymptomatic, no intervention is needed. An abscess usually ruptures spontaneously within 72 hours of forming. Teach the patient to take over-the-counter or prescribed analgesics and apply moist heat (sitz baths or hot wet packs) to the vulva. Cultures most often reveal *Escherichia coli* or *S. aureus,* for which antibiotics are prescribed.

Simple incision and drainage (I&D) may provide temporary relief. However, cysts tend to recur when the opening of the duct re-obstructs. Usually the surgeon establishes a permanent opening for drainage. **Marsupialization** (formation of a pouch that is a new duct opening) is performed using local, regional, or general anesthesia. Discomfort after surgery may be relieved with analgesics and sitz baths. Prophylactic antibiotics may be prescribed.

The Bartholin glands may be totally removed in older women when cancer is suspected or if infections with abscess formation recur. Care after surgery includes:

- Application of ice packs or sitz baths several times a day for comfort and promotion of healing
- Analgesics for PAIN
- Prophylactic antibiotics
- Assessment of the incision for signs of healing or INFECTION

CERVICAL POLYP

Cervical polyps are *pedunculated* (on stalks) tumors that arise from the mucosa and extend through the opening of the cervical os. Although the cause is not completely understood, they may result from a hyperplasia (overgrowth) of the endocervical epithelium in response to estrogen, chronic inflammation, and/or clogged blood vessels in the cervix (Storck, 2014). Polyps may also be due to inflammation or to localized vascular congestion of the cervical blood vessels. They are the most common benign growth of the cervix and occur most often in women older than 40 years who have had several children.

Some patients are asymptomatic; others may have premenstrual or postmenstrual bleeding, experience bleeding after douching or intercourse, and/or have leukorrhea (white or yellow mucus) (Storck, 2014). A speculum examination may reveal a small single polyp or multiple polyps. They are bright red, are soft and fragile, and may bleed when touched.

Polyp removal is usually accomplished as a simple office procedure. The base of the polyp is grasped with a clamp, and the polyp is gently twisted off and sent to the pathology laboratory for evaluation. Cautery usually stops any bleeding at the site of removal and is also effective when removing larger polyps (Storck, 2014). The woman does not feel any pain during the procedure. Instruct her to avoid tampon use, douches, and sexual intercourse for a week or until healing has taken place.

GYNECOLOGIC CANCERS

ENDOMETRIAL (UTERINE) CANCER

❖ *PATHOPHYSIOLOGY*

Endometrial cancer (cancer of the inner uterine lining) is the most common gynecologic malignancy (Nguyen et al., 2013). This chapter includes two other common gynecologic cancers, but the disease can affect any organ in the reproductive tract.

Endometrial cancer grows slowly in most cases, and early symptoms of vaginal bleeding generally lead to prompt evaluation and treatment. As a result, this type of cancer has a good prognosis. *Adenocarcinoma* is the most common type of tumor. It arises from the glandular part of the endometrium and usually follows endometrial hyperplasia (overgrowth).

The initial growth of the cancer is within the uterine cavity, followed by extension into the myometrium and the cervix. Stage I endometrial cancer is confined to the endometrium. Stage II cancer also involves the cervix, and stage III reaches the vagina or lymph nodes. Stage IV endometrial cancer has spread to the bowel or bladder mucosa and/or beyond the pelvis (McCance et al., 2014).

Metastasis outside the uterus occurs in these ways:

- Through lymphatic spread to the ovaries and parametrial, pelvic, inguinal, and para-aortic lymph nodes
- By blood to the lungs, liver, or bones
- By transtubal or intra-abdominal spread to the peritoneal cavity

Etiology and Genetic Risk

Endometrial cancer is strongly associated with conditions causing prolonged exposure to estrogen without the protective effects of progesterone. Risk factors for endometrial cancer are listed in Table 71-3. Although most cases of endometrial cancer do not have a genetic predisposition, it is more common in families who have gene mutations for hereditary nonpolyposis colon cancer (HNPCC) (National Cancer Institute [NCI], 2013b).

Incidence and Prevalence

In 2013, it was estimated that there will be 49,560 new cases of endometrial cancer in the United States, with 8,910 deaths associated with this condition. White women get the disease more

TABLE 71-3 Risk Factors for Endometrial (Uterine) Cancer and Cervical Cancer

ENDOMETRIAL (UTERINE) CANCER	CERVICAL CANCER
• Women in reproductive years • Family history of endometrial cancer or HNPCC • Diabetes mellitus • Hypertension • Obesity • Uterine polyps • Late menopause • Nulliparity (no childbirths) • Smoking • Tamoxifen (Nolvadex) given for breast cancer	• Girls and young women • Infection with HPV • Multiparity (multiple births) • Smoking • Younger than 18 years at first intercourse • Multiple sex partners • African American • Oral contraceptive use • History of STDs • Obesity or poor diet • Family history of cervical cancer • HIV/AIDS • Lower socioeconomic status • Sexual partner had a previous partner who developed cervical cancer • Intrauterine exposure to DES

AIDS, Acquired immune deficiency syndrome; *DES,* diethylstilbestrol; *HIV,* human immune deficiency virus; *HNPCC,* hereditary nonpolyposis colon cancer; *HPV,* human papilloma virus; *STDs,* sexually transmitted diseases.

often than African-American women, but African-American women die more often from the disease (American Cancer Society [ACS], 2013a). The causes for these differences are not known.

❖ PATIENT-CENTERED COLLABORATIVE CARE

◆ Assessment

Physical Assessment/Clinical Manifestations. *The main symptom of endometrial cancer is postmenopausal bleeding. Ask the patient how many tampons or menstrual pads she uses each day.* Some women also have a watery, bloody vaginal discharge, low back or abdominal PAIN, and low pelvic PAIN (caused by pressure of the enlarged uterus). Ask the patient to describe the exact location and intensity of her discomfort. A pelvic examination may reveal the presence of a palpable uterine mass or uterine polyp. The uterus is enlarged if the cancer is advanced.

Laboratory Assessment. Several laboratory tests are used to determine the overall condition of the woman with possible or confirmed endometrial cancer. For example, the complete blood count typically shows anemia because the patient has heavy bleeding. Serum tumor markers to assess for metastasis include CA-125 (cancer antigen–125) and alpha-fetoprotein (AFP), both of which may be elevated when ovarian cancer is present (Pagana & Pagana, 2013). A human chorionic gonadotropin (hCG) level may be taken to rule out pregnancy before treatment for cancer begins. Genetic testing may be done for the mutation causing hereditary nonpolyposis colorectal cancer (HNPCC) if there is a family history of this disease.

Other Diagnostic Assessment. *Transvaginal ultrasound* and *endometrial biopsy* are the gold standard tests to determine the presence of endometrial thickening and cancer. Saline may be infused during the ultrasound to improve the image of the uterine cavity. The clinician then collects an endometrial biopsy from inside the uterus via a thin, flexible suction curette through the cervix (Pagana & Pagana, 2013).

Other diagnostic tests to determine the patient's overall health status and the presence of metastasis (cancer spread) include:

- Chest x-ray
- Intravenous pyelography (IVP) or excretory urography to assess renal function and to assess for renal metastasis
- Abdominal ultrasound
- CT of the pelvis
- MRI of the abdomen and pelvis
- Liver and bone scans to assess for distant metastasis

Some women also have a hysteroscopic examination of the uterus and proctosigmoidoscopy depending on the stage of their cancer.

Psychosocial Assessment. Before a diagnosis is made, the woman may deny that the symptoms are related to cancer. During the diagnostic phase, the woman may express fears and concerns about having the disease. After the diagnosis is confirmed, she may express disbelief, anger, depression, anxiety, or withdrawal behaviors. Assess these emotional reactions, and encourage the patient to discuss her feelings. Ask her about how she copes with other stressful events, and assess her support systems.

◆ Analysis

The priority NANDA-I nursing diagnoses and collaborative problems for patients with endometrial cancer include:

1. Potential for disease metastasis
2. Ineffective Coping related to the diagnosis of cancer and fear of dying (NANDA-I)

◆ Planning and Implementation

Reducing the Risk for Metastasis

Planning: Expected Outcomes. The patient is expected to be free of metastatic disease if she has been diagnosed without obvious metastasis. For patients whose cancer has already spread, the expected outcomes are to have the highest quality life for as long as possible. In some cases, palliation and end-of-life care are needed.

Interventions. Surgical removal and cancer staging of the tumor with adjacent lymph nodes are the most important interventions for endometrial cancer. Cancer staging is often done using minimally invasive techniques, such as laparoscopic or robotic-assisted procedures.

Surgical Management. For stage I disease, the gynecology oncologist usually removes the uterus, fallopian tubes, and ovaries (**total hysterectomy** and **bilateral salpingo-oophorectomy [BSO]**), as well as peritoneum fluid or washings for cytologic examination. Laparoscopic surgery has fewer complications, shorter hospital stay, and less cost. A radical hysterectomy with bilateral pelvic lymph node dissection and removal of the upper third of the vagina is performed for stage II cancer. Nursing care for a radical hysterectomy is the same as that for a simple hysterectomy except that the woman's hospitalization is usually longer and her convalescence may be extended. (See p. 1489 for discussion of hysterectomy in this chapter.) Radical surgery and node dissection can also be done as a minimally invasive procedure using laparoscopic or robotic-assisted technology.

Nonsurgical Management. Nonsurgical interventions (radiation therapy and chemotherapy) are typically used postoperatively and depend on the surgical staging.

Radiation Therapy. The oncologist may prescribe radiation therapy to be delivered by external beam and/or brachytherapy for stage II and stage III cancers. Women with stage II disease may use brachytherapy (internal) radiation to prevent recurrence of vaginal cancer and improve survival.

The purpose of *brachytherapy* is to prevent disease recurrence. The radiologist places an applicator within the woman's uterus through the vagina. After the correct position of the applicator is confirmed by x-ray, the radioactive isotope is placed in the applicator and remains for several minutes. This procedure may be repeated between 2 and 5 times once or twice a week. Some patients also have external beam radiation while having brachytherapy treatment sessions. There are no restrictions for the woman to stay away from her family or the public between treatments.

While the radioactive implant is in place, radiation is emitted that can affect other people. The amount of time needed for the therapy depends on the amount of radiation emitted from the source. The radiologist calculates the time needed for a specific dose of radiation.

Inform the patient that she is restricted to bedrest during the treatment session. Excessive movement in bed is restricted to prevent dislodgment of the radioactive source. Chart 71-6 lists the health teaching for the patient having brachytherapy for gynecologic cancer. Teach patients about when to call the health care provider after each treatment session.

External beam radiation therapy (EBRT or XRT) may be used to treat any stage of endometrial cancer in combination with surgery, brachytherapy, and/or chemotherapy. Depending on the extent of the tumor, the treatment is given on an ambulatory care basis for 4 to 6 weeks. Tissue around the tumor and pelvic wall nodes also are treated. *Teach the patient to monitor for signs of skin breakdown, especially in the perineal area; to avoid sunbathing; and to avoid washing the markings outlining the treatment site.* Chapter 22 discusses nursing care of patients receiving radiation therapy in more detail.

Drug Therapy. *Chemotherapy* is used as palliative treatment in advanced and recurrent disease when it has spread to distant parts of the body, but it is not always effective. Although the combination can vary, three of the most common agents used for endometrial cancer are doxorubicin (Adriamycin), cisplatin (Platinol), and paclitaxel (Taxol). Chapter 22 describes chemotherapy and general nursing care during treatment.

Every woman experiences cancer differently. Many complementary therapies have evidence of benefit in decreasing the side effects of drug therapy and boosting the immune system. Provide your patient with information that will help her make informed, evidence-based decisions. Encourage her to check with her oncologist and/or pharmacist because some alternative therapies can be harmful or interfere with cancer treatment. Current evidence-based information is available at the American Cancer Society website (www.cancer.org) about mind-body therapies, healing touch, herbs, vitamins, nutrition, and biologic therapies.

CHART 71-6 Best Practice for Patient Safety & Quality Care (QSEN)

Health Teaching for the Patient Having Brachytherapy for Gynecologic Cancer

- Teach the patient to report any of these signs and symptoms to the health care provider immediately:
  - Heavy vaginal bleeding
  - Urethral burning for more than 24 hours
  - Blood in the urine
  - Extreme fatigue
  - Severe diarrhea
  - Fever over 100° F (38° C)
  - Abdominal pain
- Teach the patient that she is not radioactive between treatments and there are no restrictions on her interactions with others.

Helping the Patient Develop Coping Strategies

Planning: Expected Outcomes. The patient is expected to develop coping strategies that will help her deal with the diagnosis and collaborative care for endometrial cancer.

Interventions. Women need to discuss their concerns about the presence of cancer and the potential for recurrence. Provide emotional support, and create an atmosphere that encourages them to ask questions or express their fears and concerns. Include family members or significant others in discussions when the patient desires and when this is possible.

Reactions to radiation therapy vary. Some women feel "radioactive" or "unclean" after treatments and may exhibit withdrawal behaviors. Reassure them by correcting any misconceptions. Patients who have chemotherapy may be upset if **alopecia** (hair loss) occurs. Warn them of this possibility before treatment starts. Wigs, scarves, or turbans can be worn until the hair grows back. Many women select these replacements before they lose their hair. Others shave their heads and begin wearing them immediately as the treatment begins. Tell women about these options so that they can make decisions with which they are personally comfortable.

Often patients experience emotional crises because of the physical effects of cancer treatments. Radical hysterectomy may be seen as mutilating. Both radiation and chemotherapy have side effects that change physical appearance and body image. Women may have a grief reaction to these changes. The feelings of loss depend on the visibility of the loss and the loss of function. Help the patient adapt to the body changes. Using a calm and accepting approach, encourage self-management as soon as her physical condition is stable.

Death can occur with or without treatment. The patient and family want the woman to pass the 5-year survival mark without a recurrence of disease. If there is a recurrence, they may be hostile and have manifestations of a grief reaction. Encourage patients and their families to discuss their feelings. Refer to support services such as certified hospital chaplain or other spiritual leader, social worker, or counselor. Response to loss and grieving is discussed in Chapter 7.

Community-Based Care

Home Care Management. The woman with endometrial cancer is managed at home unless surgery is indicated. After surgery, she is usually discharged to her home. Home care after surgery for endometrial cancer is the same as that after a hysterectomy. (See discussion off Hysterectomy on p. 1489 in the Uterine Leiomyoma section.) Patients who are receiving chemotherapy or radiation therapy are treated on an ambulatory care basis. Most women are surprised by the fatigue caused by radiation and chemotherapy. Help the patient and her family plan daily activities around trips to the clinic or the health care provider's office. If the tumor recurs and cure is not likely, the woman and her family need to think about hospice care and whether she can be cared for in the home.

Self-Management Education. Teach the patient to report vaginal or rectal bleeding, foul-smelling discharge, abdominal PAIN or distention, and hematuria to the health care provider. These symptoms may be the result of the disease or its treatment.

The high dose of radiation causes sterility, and vaginal shrinkage can occur. Vaginal dilators can be used with water-soluble lubricants for 10 minutes each day until sexual activity resumes, generally within 4 weeks (ACS, 2013b). Reassure the woman that she is not radioactive and that her partner will not "catch" cancer by engaging in sexual intercourse.

Review all prescribed drugs, including the dosage and schedule, effects, and side effects. Emphasize the importance of keeping appointments for follow-up care.

Health Care Resources. In the United States, local American Cancer Society chapters provide written materials about endometrial cancer and information about local support groups. Each province in Canada also has a division of the Canadian Cancer Society (www.cancer.ca). If the patient is in the terminal stages of cancer, hospice care may be appropriate (see Chapter 7). If nursing care is needed at home, the hospital nurse or case manager makes referrals to a home health care agency. A referral to a social services agency may be needed if the patient cannot meet the financial demands of treatment and long-term follow-up.

CERVICAL CANCER

❖ *PATHOPHYSIOLOGY*

The uterine cervix is covered with squamous cells on the outer cervix and columnar (glandular) cells that line the endocervical canal. Papanicolaou (Pap) tests sample cells from both areas as a screening test for cervical cancer. The squamo-columnar junction is the *transformation zone* where most cell abnormalities occur. The adolescent has more columnar cells exposed on the outer cervix, which may be one reason she is more vulnerable to sexually transmitted diseases (STDs) and human immune deficiency virus (HIV). In contrast, in the menopausal woman, the squamo-columnar junction may be higher up in the endocervical canal, making it difficult to sample for a Pap test.

Premalignant changes are described on a continuum from *atypia* (suspicious) to *cervical intraepithelial neoplasia (CIN)* to *carcinoma in situ (CIS),* which is the most advanced premalignant change. It generally takes years for the cervical cells to transform from normal to premalignant to invasive cancer. CIN, sometimes called *dysplasia,* is graded on a scale of 1 to 3 depending on the appearance of the cervical tissue under a microscope (ACS, 2014b). Not much tissue appears abnormal in CIN1 (mild dysplasia), which is thought to be the least serious cervical pre-cancer; more tissue appears abnormal in CIN2 (moderate dysplasia). Most tissue looks abnormal in CIN3 (severe dysplasia as well as carcinoma *in situ*), which is the most serious pre-cancer (ACS, 2014b).

Most cervical cancers arise from the squamous cells on the outside of the cervix. The other cancers arise from the mucus-secreting glandular cells (adenocarcinoma) in the endocervical canal. The disease spreads by direct extension to the vaginal mucosa, lower uterine segment, parametrium, pelvic wall, bladder, and bowel. Metastasis is usually confined to the pelvis, but distant spread can occur through lymphatic spread and the circulation to the liver, lungs, or bones.

Etiology

Human papilloma virus infection (HPV) is the most common type of STD in the United States (Centers for Disease Control and Prevention [CDC], 2014b). Almost all women will have HPV sometime in their life, but not all types lead to cancer. Most cases of cervical cancer are caused by certain types of HPV. The high-risk HPV types, especially strains 16 and 18, impair the tumor-suppressor gene and cause most of the cervical cancers. The unrestricted tissue growth can spread, becoming invasive and metastatic. Strains 6 and 11 are associated with genital warts (McCance et al., 2014). Risk factors for cervical cancer are listed in Table 71-3.

Incidence and Prevalence

Invasive cancer of the cervix is the third most common cancer of the female genital system, after ovarian and uterine cancer. The number of cases of cervical cancer (and deaths from cervical cancer) has decreased significantly over the past 40 years because more women regularly get Pap tests (CDC, 2014a).

Health Promotion and Maintenance

Girls and young women (ages 9 through 26 years) should receive one of the two currently used HPV vaccines, *Gardasil* and *Cervarix,* ideally before their first sexual contact to receive protection against the highest-risk HPV types that are responsible for most cervical cancers. It is also given for boys and young men (ages 9 through 26 years) to prevent genital warts because it protects against the 6 and 11 HPV strains and to prevent anal cancer, which is caused by HPV strains 16 and 18 (Merck Sharpe & Dohme Corporation, 2014). Cervarix protects girls and women ages 9 through 25 years against INFECTION for HPV strains 16 and 18 to prevent cervical cancer (GlaxoSmithKline, 2012).

Teach all young adults and parents of minors about the importance of receiving the vaccine and the need to have the entire series (3 injections over 6 months). Tell them that the most frequent side effects are related to local irritation from the injections (e.g., PAIN, redness). Other common side effects include nausea, vomiting, dizziness, headache, and diarrhea.

The American Cancer Society (ACS) recommends that women have periodic pelvic examinations and Pap tests to screen for cervical cancer early. Teach women that they should begin these screening precautions at the age of 21 years. Between ages 21 and 29 years, women should have a Pap test every 3 years; women between ages 30 and 65 years should have a Pap test plus a human papilloma virus (HPV) test ("co-testing") every 5 years. More information on the HPV test is found later in this chapter. In the absence of co-testing, this population should still have a Pap test every 3 years. According to the ACS, women older than 65 years who have had regular cervical cancer testing with normal results should not receive Pap tests (ACS, 2014a). Recommended guidelines from other health care organizations suggest a Pap test every 3 years for women older than 60 years. Those who have had a history of a serious cervical pre-cancerous lesion should be tested annually for at least 20 years after that diagnosis, regardless of age (ACS, 2014a).

❖ *PATIENT-CENTERED COLLABORATIVE CARE*

◆ *Assessment*

Physical Assessment/Clinical Manifestations. The patient who has preinvasive cancer is often asymptomatic. *The classic symptom of invasive cancer is painless vaginal bleeding.* Ask the patient if she has had or now has bleeding. It may start as spotting between menstrual periods or after sexual intercourse or douching. As the cancer grows, bleeding increases in frequency, duration, and amount and may become continuous.

Ask the woman if she has a watery, blood-tinged vaginal discharge that becomes dark and foul-smelling (occurs as the disease progresses). Leg pain (along the sciatic nerve) or swelling of one leg may be a late symptom or may indicate recurrent disease. Flank pain may be a late symptom of hydronephrosis, indicating advanced cancer pressing on the ureters, backing up the urine into the kidney. Ask the patient if she has had other signs of recurrence or metastasis such as:

- Unexplained weight loss
- Dysuria (painful urination)
- Pelvic PAIN (caused by pressure of the tumor on the bladder or the bowel)
- Hematuria (bloody urine)
- Rectal bleeding
- Chest PAIN
- Coughing

A physical examination may not reveal any abnormalities in early preinvasive cervical cancer. The internal pelvic examination may identify late-stage disease.

Diagnostic Assessment. If Pap results are abnormal, an *HPV-typing DNA test* of the cervical sample can determine the presence of one or more high-risk types. The health care provider may perform a colposcopic examination to view the transformation zone. Colposcopy is a procedure in which application of an acetic acid solution is applied to the cervix. The cervix is then examined under magnification with a bright filter light that enhances the visualization of the characteristics of dysplasia or cancer. If abnormal tissue is recognized, multiple biopsies of the cervical tissue are performed.

If atypical glandular cells are suspected, the health care provider may perform an *endocervical curettage* (scraping of the endocervix wall) as well. Inform her that a small amount of bleeding is expected for up to 2 weeks after the biopsies.

◆ *Interventions*

Interventions for the woman with cervical cancer are similar to those for endometrial cancer: surgery, which is possibly followed by radiation and chemotherapy for later-stage disease.

Surgical Management. Early stage I management techniques include local cervical ablation therapies of electrosurgical excision, laser therapy, or cryosurgery. Small tumors that are only microinvasive are managed with excisional conization or hysterectomy. Early-stage *invasive* cancers are managed with radical surgery and radiation. Advanced inoperable cancers are treated with radiation. Factors that influence the choice of localized treatment versus surgical intervention include patient overall health, desire for future childbearing, tumor size, stage, cancer cell type, degree of lymph node involvement, and patient preference.

Early Surgical Procedures. The loop electrosurgical excision procedure (LEEP) is short (10 to 30 minutes) and is performed in a physician's office or in an ambulatory care setting with a local anesthetic injected into the cervix. A thin loop-wire electrode that transmits a painless electrical current is used to cut away affected tissue. LEEP is both a diagnostic procedure and a treatment, because it provides a specimen that can be examined by a pathologist to ensure the lesion was completely removed. Little discomfort is associated with this procedure.

CHART 71-7 Patient and Family Education: Preparing for Self-Management

Care after Local Cervical Ablation Therapies

- Refrain from sexual intercourse.
- Do not use tampons.
- Do not douche.
- Take showers rather than tub baths.
- Avoid lifting heavy objects.
- Report any heavy vaginal bleeding, foul-smelling drainage, or fever.

The usual time period for these restrictions is 3 weeks. Your health care provider may prescribe a different (longer or shorter) time frame for you.

Spotting after the procedure is common. Teach patients to adhere for 3 weeks to the restrictions listed in Chart 71-7.

Laser therapy is also an office procedure used for early cancers. A laser beam is directed to the abnormal tissues, where energy from the beam is absorbed by the fluid in the tissues, causing them to vaporize. A small amount of bleeding occurs with the procedure, and the woman may have a slight vaginal discharge. Healing occurs in 6 to 12 weeks. A disadvantage of this procedure is that no specimen is available for study.

Cryotherapy involves freezing of the cancer, causing subsequent necrosis. The procedure is often painless, although some women have slight cramping after the procedure. The patient has a heavy watery discharge for several weeks after the procedure. Instruct her to follow the restrictions in Chart 71-7.

In cases of microinvasive cancer, a *conization* can remove the affected tissue while still preserving fertility. This procedure is done when the lesion cannot be visualized by colposcopic examination. A cone-shaped area of cervix is removed surgically and sent to the laboratory to determine the extent of the cancer. Potential complications from this procedure include hemorrhage and uterine perforation Long-term follow-up care is needed because new cancers can develop.

Hysterectomy. A total hysterectomy may be performed as treatment of microinvasive cancer if the woman does not want children or more children. A laparoscopic approach is commonly used. A radical hysterectomy and bilateral pelvic lymph node dissection may be as effective as radiation is for treating cancer that has extended beyond the cervix but not to the pelvic wall. Care for patients undergoing hysterectomy is found in the Uterine Leiomyoma section on pp. 1489-1491.

Nonsurgical Management. *Radiation therapy* is reserved for invasive cervical cancer. Brachytherapy and external beam radiation therapy are used in combination, depending on the extent and location of the lesion. The procedure is similar to that described on pp. 1492-1493 for endometrial cancer.

A combination of chemotherapy with cisplatin (Platinol) and radiation may also be used. This treatment modality shows increased survival times but increased toxicity for many patients. Examples of other drugs used alone or in combination include paclitaxel (Taxol), carboplatin, fluorouracil (5-FU), and mitomycin. See Chapter 22 for more information about the general nursing care for the patient on chemotherapy and radiation.

OVARIAN CANCER

❖ *PATHOPHYSIOLOGY*

Most ovarian cancers are epithelial tumors that grow on the surface of the ovaries. These tumors grow rapidly, spread

TABLE 71-4 Risk Factors for Ovarian Cancer

• Older than 40 years	• Colorectal cancer
• Family history of ovarian or breast cancer or HNPCC	• Infertility
• Diabetes mellitus	• *BRCA1* or *BRCA2* gene mutations
• Nulliparity	• Early menarche/late menopause
• Older than 30 years at first pregnancy	• Endometriosis
• Breast cancer	• Obesity/high-fat diet

HNPCC, Hereditary nonpolyposis colon cancer.

quickly, and are often bilateral. Tumor cells spread by direct extension into nearby organs and through blood and lymph circulation to distant sites (McCance et al., 2014). Free-floating cancer cells also spread through the abdomen to seed new sites, usually accompanied by ascites (abdominal fluid).

Ovarian cancer seems to be disordered growth in response to excessive exposure to estrogen. This would explain the protective effects of pregnancies and oral contraceptive use, both of which interrupt the monthly estrogen exposure. Table 71-4 lists known and suspected risk factors for ovarian cancer.

Ovarian cancer is the leading cause of death from female reproductive cancers, but it is not the most common type of cancer (ACS, 2013a). The incidence increases in women older than 50 years, and most are diagnosed after menopause. Family history accounts for a small percentage of cases. These women carry *BCRA1* or *BCRA2* genetic mutations. Of these, some choose to have an elective **bilateral salpingo-oophorectomy (BSO)** (removal of both ovaries and fallopian tubes) to prevent ovarian cancer.

Survival rates are low because ovarian cancer is often not detected until its late stages. It is important for nurses to teach women to *"think ovarian"* if they have vague abdominal and GI symptoms.

Health Promotion and Maintenance

Health promotion measures to help prevent ovarian cancer include maintaining a normal weight and eating a well-balanced diet. Women who have had tubal ligation, used oral contraception, and breast-fed their children also have less risk for having the disease (ACS, 2014a).

❖ PATIENT-CENTERED COLLABORATIVE CARE

◆ Assessment

Most women with ovarian cancer have had mild symptoms for several months but may have thought they were due to normal perimenopausal changes or stress. They may report abdominal pain or swelling or have vague GI disturbances such as dyspepsia (indigestion) and gas. Ask the patient if she has had urinary frequency or incontinence, unexpected weight loss, and/or vaginal bleeding.

Complications of advanced metastatic cancer include:

- Pleural effusion
- Ascites
- Lymphedema
- Intestinal obstruction
- Malnutrition

On pelvic examination, an abdominal mass may not be palpable until it reaches a size of 4 to 6 inches (10 to 15 cm). Any enlarged ovary found after menopause should be evaluated as though it were malignant. A Pap smear is of limited value for detecting ovarian cancer.

A cancer antigen test, *CA-125*, measures the presence of damaged endometrial and uterine tissue in the blood. It may be elevated if ovarian cancer is present, but it can also be elevated in patients with endometriosis, fibroids, pelvic inflammatory disease, pregnancy, and even menses (Pagana & Pagana, 2013). It is also useful for monitoring a patient's progress during and after treatment. Transvaginal ultrasonography, chest radiography, and CT are part of a complete workup to evaluate for metastasis. Complete blood work includes a liver profile if there is ascites.

The woman with ovarian cancer has concerns similar to those described for the patient with endometrial cancer (see p. 1493 of this chapter). Because the cancer is often diagnosed in an advanced stage, thoughts of death and dying, menopause, and loss of fertility come as a shock.

CLINICAL JUDGMENT CHALLENGE

Patient-Centered Care; Evidence-Based Practice; Informatics; Teamwork and Collaboration QSEN

A 34-year-old woman is diagnosed with ovarian cancer today. She tells you that she "can't believe this," and that "this must be the wrong diagnosis." She states that she and her husband had planned to get pregnant later this year and that she "cannot lose" her ovaries. However, she is scheduled to have a bilateral salpingo-oophorectomy and hysterectomy in 2 days. Her oncologist told her that after she recovers from surgery, she may need to have adjuvant chemotherapy to destroy any remaining cancer cells.

1. What preoperative teaching will you provide for this patient and why?
2. How will you address this patient's statements about disbelief of the diagnosis?
3. How will you approach the patient's feelings about getting pregnant later this year?
4. Do you believe that this patient understands the implications of a bilateral salpingo-oophorectomy? If not, what would be your next nursing action?
5. What will you tell her about chemotherapy that may be necessary after surgery?
6. Where would you search for evidence about her expected quality of life and prognosis?
7. To what community resources would you refer this patient after discharge?

◆ Interventions

Nursing care of the patient with ovarian cancer is similar to that for endometrial or cervical cancer. The options for treatment depend on the extent of the cancer and usually include surgery first, followed by chemotherapy. Radiation is used for more widespread cancers.

Surgical Management. Diagnosis depends on surgical exploration. Exploratory laparotomy (abdominal surgery) is performed to diagnose, treat, and stage ovarian tumors. A total abdominal hysterectomy, bilateral salpingo-oophorectomy (removal of the ovaries and fallopian tubes), and pelvic and para-aortic lymph node dissection are usually performed. Very large tumors that cannot be removed are debulked (cytoreduction). These procedures can be performed via laparoscopic technique to decrease recovery time, minimize PAIN, and reduce postoperative complications. (See p. 1489 for discussion of laparoscopic hysterectomy in this chapter.) Ovarian cancer is staged during surgery.

Nursing care of the patient is similar to that for any patient having abdominal surgery (see Chapter 16). As for any patient after abdominal surgery, assess vital signs and PAIN and maintain catheters and drains. Teach her the importance of antiembolism stockings, incentive spirometry, and early ambulation. Infections after ovarian cancer surgery commonly affect the respiratory and urinary tracts. Assess vital signs, and monitor the quantity and quality of urine output.

Nonsurgical Management. After cytoreduction and staging of ovarian cancer, chemotherapy is the treatment that is used most often. For all stages of ovarian cancer, cisplatin (Platinol), carboplatin, and taxanes of all types are the most common postoperative *drugs* used for treating ovarian cancer. They may be given IV and/or intraperitoneally. Intraperitoneal (IP) therapy is described in Chapter 13. New drugs continue to be tested that use monoclonal antibodies, hormones, and agents that target cell growth and tumor blood supply.

Community-Based Care

Patients having surgery usually return to their home. Teach them to avoid tampons, douches, and sexual intercourse for at least 6 weeks or as instructed by the health care provider. Remind them to keep their follow-up surgical appointment and talk with the health care provider about resuming usual activities. Refer patients and their families to Gilda's Club (www.gildasclub.org) and the National Ovarian Cancer Coalition (NOCC) (www.ovarian.org) for more information and support groups. In Canada, the National Ovarian Cancer Association (www.ovariancanada.org) is available for the same purpose.

For patients with advanced metastatic disease, collaborate with the case manager, patient, and family for possible referral to hospice. Chapter 7 discusses end-of-life care and hospice in detail. The woman who is faced with the diagnosis of advanced ovarian cancer is usually very anxious about dying. Encourage her to discuss her feelings. Provide realistic assurance, as well as accurate information about treatments. Patients report their most distressing moments in the hospital were when they thought they were not getting adequate information. Encourage them to use their support systems of family members, friends, and clergy, including the hospital chaplain. Grief counseling is very appropriate. A visit from another woman who has survived a similar disease or referral to a support group may decrease fears. Refer the patient who fears passing the *BRCA1* or *BRCA2* gene to her daughter for genetic counseling and testing.

Ovarian cancer has a high recurrence rate. After recurrence, the cancer is treatable but no longer curable. If this occurs, the patient may deny symptoms at first or express feelings of anger and grief. The family is often fearful of the outcome. Provide encouragement and support during this difficult time, and help the patient and her family work through their grief and prepare for death.

NURSING CONCEPTS AND CLINICAL JUDGMENT REVIEW

What might you NOTICE if the patient is experiencing impaired SEXUALITY as a result of gynecologic problems?

- Irregular or abnormal vaginal bleeding
- Vaginal discharge
- Report of perineal itching or burning
- Report of painful intercourse
- Abdominal distention and discomfort
- Report of irritability, anxiety, or depression
- Report of decreased libido

What should you INTERPRET and how should you RESPOND to the patient experiencing impaired SEXUALITY as a result of gynecologic problems?

Perform and interpret physical assessment, including:

- Conducting an abdominal assessment
- Conducting a thorough pain assessment
- Checking for bleeding and amount (number of pads or tampons)
- Listening to patient's concerns about her sexuality

Respond by:

- Helping the patient into a sitting position
- Providing pain-relief measures, such as heat and analgesia
- Referring the patient to a sexual or intimacy counselor (including the patient's partner if desired)

On what should you REFLECT?

- Think about what else you can do to help provide psychosocial support.
- Prepare for complications, such as hemorrhage, if the patient is bleeding.
- Evaluate pain level after interventions.

GET READY FOR THE NCLEX® EXAMINATION!

KEY POINTS

Review these Key Points for each NCLEX Examination Client Needs Category.

Safe and Effective Care Environment

- Refer patients with gynecologic problems to appropriate community resources such as the American Cancer Society and the Endometriosis Association. **Teamwork and Collaboration** QSEN
- Collaborate with the case manager when planning care for patients with gynecologic cancers. **Teamwork and Collaboration** QSEN

Health Promotion and Maintenance

- Teach women to follow the American Cancer Society's screening guidelines to prevent and early-detect for gynecologic cancers.

- Teach all women to have regular Pap tests based on their risk factors.
- Teach women to practice safe sex to prevent INFECTION of the reproductive organs.
- Teach women about risk factors for gynecologic cancers as described in Tables 71-3 and 71-4.
- Teach women how to prevent toxic shock syndrome (TSS) as listed in Chart 71-3. **Safety** QSEN

Psychosocial Integrity

- Explain all tests, procedures, and treatments, especially if they cause PAIN during or after the procedures.
- Assess the patient's anxiety before any gynecologic surgery, and encourage the patient to discuss her feelings. **Patient-Centered Care** QSEN
- Encourage women who are having procedures that may interfere with fertility and/or SEXUALITY to express feelings of fear or grief. **Patient-Centered Care** QSEN
- Encourage women with chronic or serious health problems to consider using support groups or counseling.

Physiological Integrity

- Urge any woman who experiences postmenopausal vaginal bleeding to consult with her gynecologic health care provider as soon as possible. **Safety** QSEN
- Assess for symptoms of problems associated with urinary ELIMINATION.
- Assess for symptoms associated with toxic shock syndrome.
- Teach patients about specific restrictions after local cervical ablation therapy (see Chart 71-7).
- When caring for a patient who has a radioactive implant, use best practices as described in Chart 71-6. **Teamwork and Collaboration** QSEN
- Teach the patient who is going home after a hysterectomy how to monitor for INFECTION and other complications. **Safety** QSEN
- Instruct patients receiving external beam radiation to the abdomen to gently wash the area; to not apply creams or lotions (unless prescribed by the radiologist); to not wash off marking; to avoid exposing the area to sunlight or temperature extremes; and to wear soft, nonirritating clothing.

CHAPTER 72

Care of Patients with Male Reproductive Problems

Donna D. Ignatavicius

http://evolve.elsevier.com/Iggy/

PRIORITY CONCEPTS

- Pain
- Elimination
- Infection
- Reproduction

LEARNING OUTCOMES

Safe and Effective Care Environment

1. Collaborate with health care team members to provide care for patients with male reproductive health problems.

Health Promotion and Maintenance

2. Teach men and their partners about community resources for reproductive cancers.
3. Develop a health teaching plan for men to prevent or detect early male reproductive cancers.

Psychosocial Integrity

4. Explain the psychosocial needs of men who have male reproductive problems.

Physiological Integrity

5. Identify the clinical manifestations of benign prostatic hyperplasia (BPH) as they affect urinary ELIMINATION.
6. Describe the nursing implications for pharmacologic management of BPH.
7. Develop an evidence-based postoperative plan of care for a patient undergoing surgery for benign prostatic hyperplasia.
8. Evaluate patient risk factors for male reproductive cancers.
9. Identify complementary and alternative therapies to incorporate into the patient's plan of care.
10. Discuss treatment options for prostate cancer with patients, partners, and/or families.
11. Provide preoperative teaching for patients having a radical prostatectomy.
12. Identify adverse effects of radiation therapy for male reproductive cancers.
13. Develop a community-based plan of care for a man with prostate cancer.
14. Describe the options for treating erectile dysfunction.
15. Identify cultural considerations related to male reproductive problems.
16. Develop a plan of care for a patient with testicular cancer, including fertility issues.
17. Compare the assessment and treatment for hydrocele, spermatocele, and varicocele.

Male reproductive problems can range from short-term INFECTIONS to long-term health care problems that require end-of-life care. Any health issue that affects the male reproductive system can affect the human needs for SEXUALITY and urinary ELIMINATION. For example, some patients have surgeries that damage essential nerves that are needed to have an erection. Others have disorders that psychologically prevent the patient from engaging in his usual sexual activity.

The role of the nurse and other health care team members is to be open, supportive, and nonjudgmental when caring for men with reproductive problems. Respect the man's privacy at all times.

BENIGN PROSTATIC HYPERPLASIA

PATHOPHYSIOLOGY

Benign prostatic hyperplasia (BPH) is a very common health problem, but the exact cause is unclear. It is likely the result of a combination of aging and the influence of androgens that are present in prostate tissue, such as dihydrotestosterone (DHT) (McCance et al., 2014). With aging and increased DHT levels, the glandular units in the prostate undergo nodular tissue **hyperplasia** (an increase in the number of cells). This altered tissue promotes local inflammation by attracting cytokines and other substances (McCance et al., 2014).

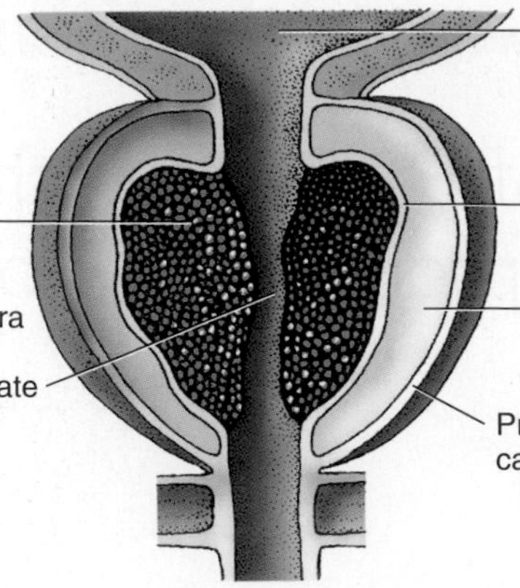

FIG. 72-1 Benign prostatic hyperplasia (BPH) grows inward, causing narrowing of the urethra.

As the prostate gland enlarges, it extends upward into the bladder and inward, causing *bladder outlet obstruction* (Fig. 72-1). In response, the urinary system is affected in several ways. First, the detrusor (bladder) muscle thickens to help urine push past the enlarged prostate gland (McCance et al., 2014). In spite of the bladder muscle change, the patient has increased residual urine (stasis) and chronic urinary retention. The increased volume of residual urine often causes **overflow urinary incontinence**, in which the urine "leaks" around the enlarged prostate causing dribbling. Urinary stasis can also result in urinary tract INFECTIONS and bladder calculi (stones).

In a few patients, the prostate becomes very large and the man cannot void (acute urinary retention [AUR]). The patient with this problem requires emergent care. In other patients, chronic urinary retention may result in a backup of urine and cause a gradual dilation of the ureters (**hydroureter**) and kidneys (**hydronephrosis**) if BPH is not treated. These urinary ELIMINATION problems can lead to chronic kidney disease as described in Chapter 68.

❖ PATIENT-CENTERED COLLABORATIVE CARE

◆ Assessment

History. When taking a history, several standardized assessment tools are used to help the health care provider determine the severity of lower urinary tract symptoms (LUTS) associated with prostatic enlargement. One of the most commonly used assessments is the International Prostate Symptom Score (I-PSS), which incorporates the American Urological Association Symptom Index (AUA-SI) (Fig. 72-2) as questions 1 through 7. The additional question included on the I-PSS is the effect of the patient's urinary symptoms on quality of life. Most patients complete the questions as a self-administered tool because it is available in many languages. If the patient is illiterate (does not read) or does not feel like reading the questions, the nurse or health care provider can ask them. Be sure that older men wear their glasses or contact lenses if needed.

Physical Assessment/Clinical Manifestations. Ask about the patient's current urinary ELIMINATION pattern. Assess for urinary frequency and urgency. Determine the number of times the patient awakens during the night to void (**nocturia**). Other symptoms of LUTS include:

- Difficulty in starting (hesitancy) and continuing urination
- Reduced force and size of the urinary stream ("weak" stream)
- Sensation of incomplete bladder emptying
- Straining to begin urination
- Post-void (after voiding) dribbling or leaking

If frequency and nocturia do not occur with restricted urinary flow, the patient may have an INFECTION or other bladder problem. Ask whether the patient has had **hematuria** (blood in the urine) when starting the urine stream or at the end of voiding. BPH is a common cause of hematuria in older men.

The health care provider examines the patient for physical changes of the prostate gland. Remind the patient to void before the physical examination. Inspect and palpate the abdomen for a distended bladder. The health care provider may percuss the bladder. If the patient has a sense of urgency when gentle pressure is applied, the bladder may be distended. Obese patients are best assessed by percussion or bedside ultrasound bladder scanner rather than by inspection or palpation.

Prepare the patient for the prostate gland examination. Tell him that he may feel the urge to urinate as the prostate is palpated. Because the prostate is close to the rectal wall, it is easily examined by digital rectal examination (DRE). If needed, help the patient bend over the examination table or assume a side-lying fetal position, whichever is the easiest position for him. The health care provider examines the prostate for size and consistency. BPH presents as a uniform, elastic, nontender enlargement, whereas cancer of the prostate gland feels like a stony-hard nodule. Advise the patient that after the prostate gland is palpated, it may be massaged to obtain a fluid sample for examination to rule out **prostatitis** (inflammation and possible INFECTION of the prostate), a common problem that can occur with BPH. If the patient has bacterial prostatitis, he is treated with broad-spectrum antibiotic therapy to prevent the spread of infection (McCance et al., 2014).

Psychosocial Assessment. Patients who have nocturia and other LUTS may be irritable or depressed as a result of interrupted sleep and annoying visits to the bathroom. Assess the effect of sleep interruptions on the patient's mood and mental status.

Post-void dribbling and overflow incontinence may cause embarrassment and prevent the patient from socializing or leaving his home. For some patients, this social isolation can affect quality of life and lead to clinical depression and/or severe anxiety. Johnson et al. (2010) found a strong correlation between depression and BPH in older men. Depressed patients were 3 times more likely to have severe symptoms.

Laboratory Assessment. A *urinalysis* and urine *culture* are typically obtained to diagnose urinary tract infection and microscopic hematuria. If INFECTION is present, the urinalysis measures the number of white blood cells (WBCs).

Other laboratory studies that may be performed include:

- A *complete blood count* (CBC) to evaluate any evidence of systemic infection (elevated WBCs) or anemia (decreased red blood cells [RBCs]) from hematuria
- *Blood urea nitrogen* (BUN) and serum creatinine levels to evaluate renal function (both are usually elevated with kidney disease)
- A *prostate-specific antigen* (PSA) and a serum acid phosphatase level if prostate cancer is suspected (both are typically elevated in patients who have prostate cancer)
- *Culture and sensitivity* of prostatic fluid (if expressed during the examination)

International Prostate Symptom Score (I-PSS)

Patient Name:________________________ **Date of Birth:**________________ **Date Completed**________________

In the past month:	Not at All	Less Than 1 in 5 Times	Less Than Half the Time	About Half the Time	More Than Half the Time	Almost Always	Your Score
1. Incomplete Emptying How often have you had the sensation of not emptying your bladder?	0	1	2	3	4	5	
2. Frequency How often have you had to urinate less than every 2 hours?	0	1	2	3	4	5	
3. Intermittency How often have you found you stopped and started again several times when you urinated?	0	1	2	3	4	5	
4. Urgency How often have you found it difficult to postpone urination?	0	1	2	3	4	5	
5. Weak Stream How often have you had a weak urinary stream?	0	1	2	3	4	5	
6. Straining How often have you had to strain to start urination?	0	1	2	3	4	5	
	None	**1 Time**	**2 Times**	**3 Times**	**4 Times**	**5 Times**	
7. Nocturia How many times do you typically get up at night to urinate?	0	1	2	3	4	5	
Total I-PSS Score							

Score: 1-7: Mild 8-19: Moderate 20-35: Severe

Quality of Life Due to Urinary Symptoms	Delighted	Pleased	Mostly Satisfied	Mixed	Mostly Dissatisfied	Unhappy	Terrible
If you were to spend the rest of your life with your urinary condition just the way it is now, how would you feel about that?	**0**	**1**	**2**	**3**	**4**	**5**	**6**

FIG. 72-2 The International Prostate Symptom Score (I-PSS).

Continued

About the I-PSS

The International Prostate Symptom Score (I-PSS) is based on the answers to seven questions concerning urinary symptoms and one question concerning quality of life. Each question concerning urinary symptoms allows the patient to choose one out of six answers indicating increasing severity of the particular symptom. The answers are assigned points from 0 to 5. The total score can therefore range from 0 to 35 (asymptomatic to very symptomatic).

The questions refer to the following urinary symptoms:

Questions	Symptom
1	Incomplete emptying
2	Frequency
3	Intermittency
4	Urgency
5	Weak Stream
6	Straining
7	Nocturia

Question 8 refers to the patient's perceived quality of life.

The first seven questions of the I-PSS are identical to the questions appearing on the American Urological Association (AUA) Symptom Index, which currently categorizes symptoms as follows:

Mild (symptom score less than or equal to 7)
Moderate (symptom score range 8 to 19)
Severe (symptom score range 20 to 35)

The International Scientific Committee (SCI), under the patronage of the World Health Organization (WHO) and the International Union Against Cancer (UICC), recommends the use of only a single question to assess the quality of life. The answers to this question range from "delighted" to "terrible," or 0 to 6. Although this single question may or may not capture the global impact of benign prostatic hyperplasia (BPH) symptoms or quality of life, it may serve as a valuable starting point for a doctor-patient conversation.

The SCI has agreed to use the symptom index for BPH, which has been developed by the AUA Measurement Committee, as the official worldwide symptoms assessment tool for patients suffering from prostatism.

The SCI recommends that physicians consider the following components for a basic diagnostic workup: history; physical examination; appropriate labs such as U/A, creatinine, etc.; and DRE or other evaluation to rule out prostate cancer.

FIG. 72-2, cont'd

Other Diagnostic Assessment. Imaging studies that are typically performed are *transabdominal ultrasound* and/or *transrectal ultrasound (TRUS)*. The patient having a TRUS lies on his side while the transducer is inserted into the rectum for viewing the prostate and surrounding structures. A tissue biopsy may also be done if the health care provider is uncertain whether the prostatic problem is benign or malignant.

In some cases the physician uses a cystoscope to view the interior of the bladder, the bladder neck, and the urethra. This examination is used to study the presence and effect of bladder neck obstruction and is usually done in an ambulatory care setting. See Chapter 66 for a detailed description of *cystoscopy* and the nursing care needed for patients having this procedure.

Residual urine may be determined by *bladder ultrasound* immediately after the patient voids. As an alternative, because the patient voids before cystoscopy, residual urine may be measured when the cystoscope is inserted. *Urodynamic pressure-flow studies* may help diagnose and grade bladder outlet obstruction and detrusor muscle function.

◆ Analysis

The priority NANDA-I nursing diagnosis for the patient with benign prostatic hyperplasia (BPH) is Impaired

Urinary Elimination related to bladder outlet obstruction (NANDA-I).

◆ Planning and Implementation

Improving Urinary Elimination

Planning: Expected Outcomes. The patient with BPH is expected to have a normal urinary ELIMINATION pattern without urinary hesitancy, urgency, or infection.

Interventions. Patients with symptomatic BPH are first treated with nonsurgical interventions, such as drug therapy. The Concept Map on p. 1504 shows nursing assessment and collaborative interventions for the patient with BPH.

Nonsurgical Management. Drug therapy is a popular option for treating BPH. For patients with acute urinary retention (AUR) or for those who do not respond to or cannot tolerate drug therapy, noninvasive procedures or surgery is the treatment of choice.

Drug Therapy. Drugs from two major categories may be used alone, but most commonly they are given in combination. The health care provider usually prescribes a *5-alpha reductase inhibitor (5-ARI) as first-line drug therapy.* Examples of these drugs are finasteride (Proscar) and dutasteride (Avodart). Normally, testosterone is converted to DHT in the prostate gland by the enzyme *5-alpha reductase.* By taking an enzyme-inhibiting agent, the patient's DHT levels decrease, which results in reducing the enlarged prostate.

! NURSING SAFETY PRIORITY QSEN

Drug Alert

Remind patients who are being treated with a 5-ARI for BPH that they may need to take it for as long as 6 months before improvement is noticed. Teach them about possible side effects, which include erectile dysfunction (ED), decreased libido (sexual desire), and dizziness due to orthostatic hypotension. *Remind them to change positions carefully and slowly!*

The alpha-adrenergic receptors in prostatic smooth muscle enable the prostate gland to respond to *alpha-1 selective blocking agents,* such as tamsulosin (Flomax), alfuzosin (Uroxatral), doxazosin (Cardura, Cardura-1♣), and silodosin (Rapaflo). Tamsulosin is also available as an over-the-counter (OTC) drug. These drugs relax smooth muscles in the prostate gland, creating less urinary resistance and improved urinary flow. They also cause peripheral vasodilation and reduced peripheral vascular resistance.

! NURSING SAFETY PRIORITY QSEN

Drug Alert

If giving alpha blockers in an inpatient setting, assess for orthostatic (postural) hypotension, tachycardia, and syncope ("blackout"), especially after the first dose is given to older men. If the patient is taking the drug at home, teach him to be careful when changing position and to report any weakness, lightheadedness, or dizziness to the health care provider immediately. Bedtime dosing may decrease the risk for problems related to hypotension. Teach patients taking a 5-ARI or alpha-blocking drug to keep all appointments for follow-up laboratory testing because both drug classes can cause liver dysfunction.

The most effective drug therapy approach for many patients is a combination of a 5-ARI drug and an alpha-1 selective blocking agent. A commonly prescribed drug regimen is finasteride and doxazosin. Newer drugs, such as Jalyn, provide a combination of dutasteride and tamsulosin in a once-a-day capsule.

Other drugs may be helpful in managing specific urinary symptoms. For example, low-dose oral desmopressin, a synthetic antidiuretic analog, has been used successfully for nocturia (Wang et al., 2011). Tadalafil (Cialis), a drug usually given to treat erectile dysfunction, has also been approved for some men with BPH because it can improve lower urinary tract symptoms.

Complementary and Alternative Therapies. Although many men use *Serenoa repens* (saw palmetto extract), a plant extract, to help manage the urinary symptoms associated with BPH, studies on the effectiveness of this herb have not shown that it is effective (Barry et al., 2011). Teach patients who want to try these herbs and other natural substances that scientific evidence to prove they are useful is lacking. However, if they choose to take them, remind them to check with their health care provider before taking any OTC natural substance. Some herbs interfere with prescription drugs the patient may be taking for other health problems.

Other Nonsurgical Interventions. Other interventions that may reduce obstructive symptoms include those that cause the release of prostatic fluid such as frequent sexual intercourse. This approach is helpful for the man whose obstructive symptoms result from an enlarged prostate with a large amount of retained prostatic fluid.

Teach patients with BPH to avoid drinking large amounts of fluid in a short time; to avoid alcohol, diuretics, and caffeine; and to void as soon as they feel the urge. These measures are aimed at preventing overdistention of the bladder, which may result in loss of detrusor muscle tone. Teach patients to avoid any drugs that can cause urinary retention, especially anticholinergics, antihistamines, and decongestants. *Emphasize the importance of telling any health care provider about the diagnosis of BPH so that these drugs are not prescribed.*

If drug therapy or other measures are not helpful in relieving urinary symptoms, several noninvasive techniques are available to destroy excess prostate tissue using a variety of heat methods (**thermotherapy**). These procedures are often done in a physician's office or another ambulatory care setting. Examples include:

- **Transurethral needle ablation (TUNA)** (low radiofrequency energy shrinks the prostate)
- **Transurethral microwave therapy (TUMT)** (high temperatures heat and destroy excess tissue)
- **Interstitial laser coagulation (ILC)**, also called **contact laser prostatectomy (CLP)** (laser energy coagulates excess tissue)
- **Electrovaporization of the prostate (EVAP)** (high-frequency electrical current cuts and vaporizes excess tissue)

Prostatic stents may be placed into the urethra to maintain permanent patency after a procedure for destroying or removing prostatic tissue. All of these highly technical treatments use local or regional anesthesia and do not require an indwelling urinary catheter. They are also associated with less risk for complications such as intraoperative bleeding and erectile dysfunction when compared with traditional surgical approaches. Patients can return to their usual activities in a day or two.

CONCEPT MAP

PAIN — ELIMINATION — SEXUALITY

BENIGN PROSTATIC HYPERPLASIA (BPH)

HISTORY

Davey Smitt, a 64-year-old with BPH, is admitted with a urinary tract infection (UTI), hematuria, and hydronephrosis. His wife says their sexual relationship has been nonexistent due to her husband's BPH. He has used saw palmetto extract for his urinary symptoms with some relief.

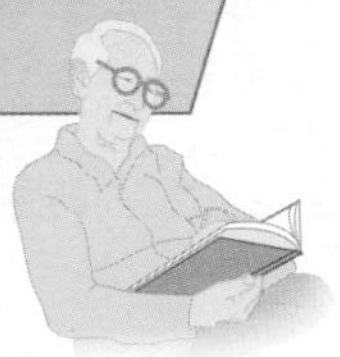

Pathophysiology

As the prostate gland enlarges, bladder outlet obstruction occurs and the patient develops urinary stasis and retention.

- Increased volume of residual → overflow incontinence → urine "leaks" around enlarged prostate → dribbling
- Urinary stasis → UTI and bladder calculi
- Chronic retention → backup of urine causes gradual dilation of ureters, hydronephrosis if not treated

Data Synthesis

PRIORITY PATIENT PROBLEMS

Impaired Urinary Elimination related to bladder outlet obstruction

Planning

EXPECTED OUTCOMES

Normal urinary elimination pattern without urinary hesitancy, urgency, or infection

INTERVENTIONS

1 Nonjudgment

Respect privacy at all times. *Being open, supportive, and nonjudgmental when caring for the patient with SEXUALITY issues facilitates trust.*

2 Physical Assessment of Elimination

Perform focused assessment of urinary pattern: frequency, hesitancy, urgency, presence of weak stream, nocturia, sensation of incomplete emptying, straining, hematuria, and post-void dribbling. *Evaluates whether BPH is causing hematuria. If frequency and nocturia do not occur with this elimination problem of restricted urinary flow, it may be infection or other bladder problem.*

3 Drug Therapy

Explain the mechanisms of action, side effects, and implications for drug therapy for BPH. *Minimizes side effects and the potential for injury.*

4 Nursing Safety Priority: Drug Alert!

- Assess for orthostatic hypotension, tachycardia, and syncope from alpha blockers. *Minimizes potential for injury from falls from orthostatic hypotension.*
- Instruct the patient to report weakness, lightheadedness, or dizziness; monitor liver function, and side effects, including erectile dysfunction, and decreased libido. *Providing accurate discharge information prevents serious complications.*

5 Interpretation of Lab Values

- Obtain urinalysis (U/A) and culture, and complete blood count. *U/A and culture detects UTI and hematuria; ↑ WBC is sign of infection, ↓ RBC indicates anemia from hematuria.*
- Obtain blood urea nitrogen (BUN) and serum creatinine, prostate-specific antigen (PSA), and serum acid phosphatase level. *BUN and serum creatinine increase detects renal dysfunction; increased PSA and serum phosphatase detects prostate cancer.*
- Obtain culture and sensitivity of prostatic fluid if expressed during the exam. *Rules out prostatitis.*

6 Reducing Obstructive Symptoms

- Instruct the patient to avoid large amounts of fluid, alcohol, diuretics, caffeine; void as soon as the urge is felt. *Promotes ELIMINATION and prevents bladder overdistention.*
- Inform the patient that frequent sexual intercourse can reduce obstructive symptoms. *Relieves symptoms in the patient who has a large amount of retained prostatic fluid.*
- Teach to avoid anticholinergics, antihistamines, and decongestants. *These medications cause urinary retention.*

7 Psychosocial Integrity and Sexuality

Assess the patient's acceptance of body image related to BPH and its impact on sleep and sexual function that affects mood and mental status. *Evaluates irritability or depression that may occur with nocturia. Evaluates embarrassment of postvoid incontinence that can prevent socialization. Evaluates effect on SEXUALITY.*

8 Herbal Remedies

Remind the patient to check with the provider before taking complementary therapies. *Teaches patients that scientific evidence is lacking. Some herbs such as saw palmetto used for urinary symptoms can interfere with prescription drugs.*

9 Treatment Options – TURP

If surgery is a chosen treatment option, consider the patient's general physical condition, size of prostate, patient preferences, anxiety, and misconceptions. *Assists with options for treatment of BPH and prevents postoperative complications.*

Concept Map by Deanne A. Blach, MSN, RN

Surgical Management. For patients who are not candidates for nonsurgical management or do not want to take drugs or have other treatment options, surgery may be performed. The gold standard continues to be a **transurethral resection of the prostate (TURP)** in which the enlarged portion of the prostate is removed through an endoscopic instrument. The newer holmium laser enucleation of the prostate (HoLEP) procedure is a minimally invasive surgical technique that is gaining popularity. For a few men, an open prostatectomy (entire prostate removal) may be performed. (See discussion of Surgical Management on p. 1509 in the Prostate Cancer section.) Some or all of these criteria indicate the need for surgery:

- Acute urinary retention (AUR)
- Chronic urinary tract infections secondary to residual urine in the bladder
- Hematuria
- Hydronephrosis

Preoperative Care. When planning surgical interventions, the patient's general physical condition, the size of the prostate gland, and the man's preferences are considered. The patient may have many fears and misconceptions about prostate surgery, such as believing that automatic loss of sexual functioning or permanent incontinence will occur. Assess the patient's anxiety, correct any misconceptions about the surgery, and provide accurate information to him and his family. Regardless of the type of surgery to be performed, reinforce information about anesthesia (see Chapter 15). Remind patients taking anticoagulants that the drugs will be discontinued prior to a TURP or open prostate surgery to prevent postoperative bleeding. Other general preoperative care is described in Chapter 14.

The patient may have other medical problems that increase the risk for complications of general anesthesia and may be advised to have regional anesthesia. Epidural and spinal anesthesia are the most common types of anesthesia used for a TURP. Because the patient is awake, it is easier to assess for hyponatremia (low serum sodium), fluid overload, and water intoxication, which can result from large-volume bladder irrigations.

After a TURP, all patients have an indwelling urethral catheter. *Be sure that they know that they will feel the urge to void while the catheter is in place.* Tell the patient that he will likely have traction on the catheter that may cause discomfort. However, reassure him that analgesics will be prescribed to relieve his pain. Explain that it is normal for the urine to be blood-tinged after surgery. Small blood clots and tissue debris may pass while the catheter is in place and immediately after it is removed. Some patients also have a continuous bladder irrigation (CBI) depending on the procedure performed.

Operative Procedures. The traditional TURP is a "closed" surgery. To perform the procedure, the surgeon inserts a resectoscope (an instrument similar to a cystoscope, but with a cutting and cauterizing loop) through the urethra. The enlarged portion of the prostate gland is then removed in small pieces (prostate chips). A similar procedure is the transurethral incision of the prostate (TUIP) in which small cuts are made into the prostate to relieve pressure on the urethra. This alternate technique is used for smaller prostates. To prevent bleeding and excess clotting, a fibrinolytic inhibitor like tranexamic acid (Cyklokapron) may be used during surgery.

The disadvantage of a TURP is that, because only small pieces of the gland are removed, remaining prostate tissue may continue to grow and cause urinary obstruction, requiring additional TURPs. Also, urethral trauma from the resectoscope with resulting urethral strictures is possible.

In many large medical centers around the world, specialists can perform newer surgical treatments, such as the *holmium laser enucleation of the prostate (HoLEP)* (Eltabey et al., 2010). For this procedure, the surgeon uses the laser to remove the obstructive prostatic tissue and then pushes the tissue into the bladder for removal. Very little blood is lost during the short procedure and is therefore safe for patients taking anticoagulants.

Postoperative Care. After both the TURP and HoLEP procedures, a urinary catheter is placed into the bladder. Traction is often applied on the catheter for the patient having a TURP by pulling it taut and taping it to the patient's abdomen or thigh. If the catheter is taped to the patient's thigh, instruct him to keep his leg straight. The patient having the HoLEP procedure has a urinary catheter overnight, but the patient with a TURP may have a catheter and continuous bladder irrigation (CBI) in place for several days. In some cases the patient is discharged with the catheter in place.

For patients with a CBI, a 3-way urinary catheter is used to allow drainage of urine and inflow of a bladder irrigating solution. Be sure to maintain the flow of the irrigant to keep the urine clear. When measuring the fluid in the urinary drainage bag, be sure to subtract the amount of irrigating solution that was used to determine actual urinary output.

NCLEX EXAMINATION CHALLENGE

Physiological Integrity

A client has a urinary catheter and continuous bladder irrigation after a transurethral resection of the prostate this morning. The amount of bladder irrigating solution that has infused over the past 12 hours is 1000 mL. The amount of fluid in the urinary drainage bag is 1725 mL. The nurse records that the client had ____ mL urinary output in the past 12 hours.

CONSIDERATIONS FOR OLDER ADULTS

Patient-Centered Care QSEN

When caring for older men who may become confused after surgery, reorient them frequently and remind them not to pull on the catheter. If the patient is restless or "picks" at tubes, provide a familiar object such as a family picture for him to hold for distraction and a feeling of security. Do not restrain the patient unless all other alternatives have failed.

Remind the patient that because of the urinary catheter's large diameter and the pressure of the retention balloon on the internal sphincter of the bladder, he will feel the urge to void continuously. This is a normal sensation, not a surgical complication. Advise the patient not to try to void around the catheter, which causes the bladder muscles to contract and may result in painful spasms. Chart 72-1 summarizes the nursing care for patients having a TURP.

If the bleeding is *venous,* the urine output is burgundy, with or without any change in vital signs. *Inform the surgeon of any bleeding.* Closely monitor the patient's hemoglobin (Hgb) and hematocrit (Hct) levels for anemia as a result of blood loss.

When the urinary catheter is removed, the patient may experience burning on urination and some urinary frequency,

CHART 72-1 Best Practice for Patient Safety & Quality Care (QSEN)

Care of the Patient After Transurethral Resection of the Prostate

- Monitor the patient closely for signs of infection. Older men undergoing prostate surgery often also have underlying chronic diseases (e.g., cardiovascular disease, chronic lung disease, diabetes).
- Help the patient out of the bed to the chair as soon as permitted to prevent complications of immobility. Older men may need assistance because of underlying changes in the musculoskeletal system (e.g., decreased range of motion, stiffness in joints). These patients are at *high risk* for falls.
- Assess the patient's pain every 2 to 4 hours, and intervene as needed to control pain.
- Provide a safe environment for the patient. Anticipate a temporary change in mental status for the older patient in the immediate postoperative period as a result of anesthetics and unfamiliar surroundings. Reorient the patient frequently. Keep catheter tubes secure.
- Maintain the rate of the continuous bladder irrigation to ensure clear urine without clots and bleeding.
- Use normal saline solution for the intermittent bladder irrigant unless otherwise prescribed. Normal saline solution is isotonic.
- Monitor the color, consistency, and amount of urine output.
- Check the drainage tubing frequently for external obstructions (e.g., kinks) and internal obstructions (e.g., blood clots, decreased output).
- Assess the patient for reports of severe bladder spasms with decreased urinary output, which may indicate obstruction.
- If the urinary catheter is obstructed, irrigate the catheter per agency or surgeon protocol.
- Notify the physician immediately if the obstruction does not resolve by hand irrigation or if the urinary return becomes ketchup-like.

! NURSING SAFETY PRIORITY (QSEN)

Critical Rescue

After a TURP, monitor the patient's urine output every 2 hours and vital signs, including pain assessment, every 4 hours for the first postoperative day. Assess for postoperative bleeding. *Patients who undergo a TURP or open prostatectomy are at risk for severe bleeding or hemorrhage after surgery. Although rare, bleeding is most likely within the first 24 hours.* Blood transfusions may be given after a TURP surgery but are not needed after the HoLEP procedure. Bladder spasms or movement may trigger fresh bleeding from previously controlled vessels. This bleeding may be arterial or venous, but venous bleeding is more common.

If arterial bleeding occurs, the urinary drainage is bright red or ketchup-like with numerous clots. Notify the surgeon immediately, and irrigate the catheter with normal saline solution per physician or hospital protocol. In rare instances the surgeon may prescribe aminocaproic acid (Amicar) to control bleeding. If this drug does not work, surgical intervention may be needed to clear the bladder of clots and to stop bleeding.

dribbling, and leakage. Reassure him that these symptoms are normal and will decrease. The patient may also pass small clots and tissue debris for several days after the TURP. *Instruct him to increase fluid intake to at least 2000 to 2500 mL daily, which helps decrease dysuria and keep the urine clear.* An older patient who has renal disease or who is at risk for heart failure may not be able to tolerate this much fluid. By the time of discharge (usually 2 to 3 days after surgery depending on age and progress), he should be voiding 150 to 200 mL of clear yellow urine every 3 to 4 hours. By discharge, pain is minimal and analgesics may not be required.

Observe for other possible but uncommon complications of TURP, such as INFECTION and incontinence. Teach the patient that sexual function should not be affected after surgery but that retrograde ejaculation is possible. In this case, most of the semen flows backwards into the bladder so only a small amount will be ejaculated from the penis.

Community-Based Care

The patient with benign prostatic hyperplasia (BPH) is typically managed at home. Patients who have surgery are also discharged to their home or other setting from where they were admitted. Some patients, especially those who have had a TURP, may have temporary loss of control of urination or a dribbling of the urine. Reassure the patient that these symptoms are almost always temporary and will resolve. Also remind him that REPRODUCTION ability should not be affected by surgery.

Assist the patient and his family in finding ways to keep his clothing dry until sphincter control returns. Instruct him to contract and relax his sphincter frequently to re-establish urinary ELIMINATION control (Kegel exercises). External urinary (condom) catheters are not used except in extreme cases because they may give the patient a false sense of security and delay urinary control.

Patients having the HoLEP procedure typically stay in the hospital overnight and usually have no urinary symptoms after surgery. This procedure may soon replace the TURP as the gold standard for surgical management of the patient with BPH.

NCLEX EXAMINATION CHALLENGE

Physiological Integrity

A client had a transurethral resection of the prostate (TURP) with continuous bladder irrigation yesterday. The staff nurse notes that the urinary drainage is bright red and thick. What is the nurse's best action?

A. Notify the charge nurse as soon as possible.
B. Increase the rate of the bladder irrigation.
C. Document the assessment in the medical record.
D. Prepare the patient for a blood transfusion.

PROSTATE CANCER

❖ *PATHOPHYSIOLOGY*

Prostate cancer is the second most common type of cancer in men in the world and if found early has a nearly 100% cure rate. Men older than 65 years have the greatest risk for the disease. In the United States, it affects African-American men more commonly than Euro-American men and at an earlier age. The exact cause for this difference is not known (Hegarty & Bailey, 2011).

Testosterone and dihydrotestosterone (DHT) are the major androgens (male hormones) in the adult male. Testosterone is produced by the testis and circulates in the blood. DHT is a testosterone derivative in the prostate gland. In some patients the prostate grows very rapidly, leading to noncancerous high-grade prostatic intraepithelial neoplasia (PIN). Patients with PIN are at a higher risk for developing prostate cancer than are men who do not have that growth pattern.

Many prostate tumors are androgen-sensitive (McCance et al., 2014). Most are adenocarcinomas and arise from

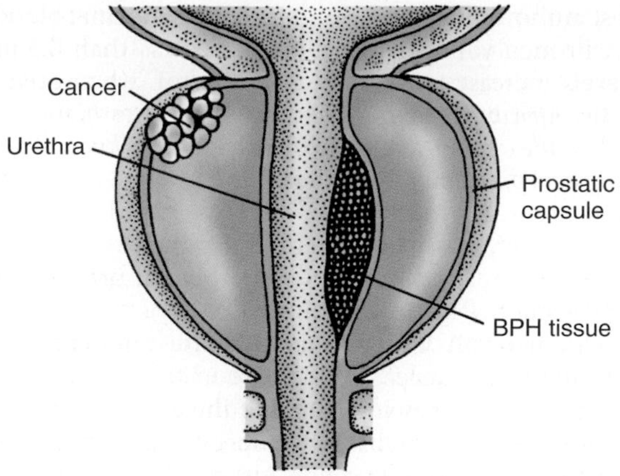

FIG. 72-3 The prostate gland with cancer and benign prostatic hyperplasia (BPH). Note that cancer normally arises in the periphery of the gland, whereas BPH occurs in the center of the gland.

epithelial cells located in the posterior lobe or outer portion of the gland (Fig. 72-3).

Of all malignancies, prostate cancer is one of the slowest growing, and it metastasizes (spreads) in a predictable pattern. Common sites of metastasis are the nearby lymph nodes, bones, lungs, and liver (McCance et al., 2014). The bones of the pelvis, sacrum, and lumbar spine are most often affected. Chapter 21 describes staging categories of localized and advanced cancers.

Prostate cancer is caused by a number of factors. Advanced age is the leading risk factor. Race is the second most common risk factor, and family history of prostate cancer is the third most common risk factor for this malignancy. The risk increases twofold for men who have a first-degree relative (brother, father) with the disease.

CULTURAL CONSIDERATIONS

Patient-Centered Care QSEN

Race is the second most common risk factor for prostate cancer because the disease affects African Americans more often than other ethnic/racial groups, followed by Caucasians (Euro-Americans) and Hispanic-American men. The reasons for these differences are not known but may be related to socioeconomic factors, health care access, health insurance, education, and diet (Dunn & Kazer, 2011).

Other risk factors that may play a role are eating a diet high in animal fat (e.g., red meat) and complex carbohydrates or having a low-fiber intake. Men who have had a vasectomy or those who were exposed to environmental toxins, such as arsenic, may also be at increased risk for the disease (McCance et al., 2014). Although controversial, some researchers believe that excessive intake of vitamin E and omega-3 fish oil supplements may increase the risk for prostate cancer (American Cancer Society [ACS], 2014a).

GENETIC/GENOMIC CONSIDERATIONS

Patient-Centered Care QSEN

Many gene mutations play a role in various types of prostate cancer. Some men with the most aggressive prostate cancers have *BRCA2* mutations similar to those women who have *BRCA2*-associated breast and ovarian cancers. The most common genetic factor that increases the risk for prostate cancer is a mutation in the glutathione S-transferase *(GST P1)* gene. This gene is normally part of the pathway that helps prevent cancer (McCance et al., 2014).

EVIDENCE-BASED PRACTICE QSEN

What Are the Evidence-Based Recommendations for Prostate-Specific Antigen Screening for Prostate Cancer?

O'Rourke, M.E. (2011). The prostate-specific antigen screening conundrum: Examining the evidence. *Seminars in Oncology Nursing, 27*(4), 251-259.

The researchers reviewed the current guidelines and recommendations for prostate-specific antigen (PSA) screening from a variety of nursing and medical literature. They found multiple recommendations from randomized controlled trials (RCTs) and various national and international organizations, including the National Comprehensive Cancer Network, The American College of Preventive Medicine, and the Advisory Committee on Cancer Prevention of the European Union. However, there was no consensus regarding the normal values of PSA for age-groups or when PSA screening is needed. Most guidelines made adjustments for age and race because the PSA normal value is likely to increase as a man ages and African-American men tend to have higher normal PSA values than other groups.

Level of Evidence: 1

The researchers used a systematic literature review of RCTs and guidelines from various professional international and national organizations.

Commentary: Implications for Practice and Research

Nurses need to explain to men that there is no consensus regarding PSA screening. Instead, men should talk with their primary health care provider and identify risk factors that may influence the decision for PSA screening. More RCTs are needed to establish guidelines for prostate screening to assist health care providers as they counsel their patients.

Health Promotion and Maintenance

Teach men about the most recent American Cancer Society (ACS) guidelines for prostate cancer screening and early detection (ACS, 2014a). The current recommendations are that men should make an informed decision about whether to have prostate cancer screening. Although not agreed upon by all authoritative sources, starting at the age of 50 years, men should discuss the options of having prostate-specific antigen testing with their health care provider (see the Evidence-Based Practice box). Men at a higher risk for prostate cancer, including African Americans or men who have a first-degree relative with prostate cancer before the age of 65 years, should have this discussion at age 45 years. Men who have multiple first-degree relatives with prostate cancer at an early age should discuss screening at age 40 years (O'Rourke, 2011).

Although a family history of prostate cancer cannot be changed, certain nutritional habits can be altered to possibly decrease the risk for the disease. First, teach men to eat a healthy, balanced diet, including decreasing animal fat (e.g., red meat). Instead of red meat, remind them to eat more fish and other foods high in *omega-3 fatty acids* because they are thought to be helpful in preventing cancer. Also reinforce the need to increase fruits, vegetables, and high-fiber foods (Carmody et al., 2012).

❖ PATIENT-CENTERED COLLABORATIVE CARE

◆ Assessment

History. Assess the patient's age, race/ethnicity, and family history of prostate cancer. Ask about his nutritional habits, especially focusing on the intake of red meat, fish, and fruits and vegetables. Assess whether the patient has any problems with urinary ELIMINATION. Take a drug history to determine if he is taking any medication that could affect voiding. The first symptoms that the man may report are related to bladder outlet obstruction, such as difficulty in starting urination, frequent bladder INFECTIONS, and urinary retention. Ask about urinary frequency, **hematuria** (blood in the urine), and **nocturia** (voiding during the night). Ask if he has had any PAIN during intercourse, especially when ejaculating. Inquire if the patient has had or currently has any other pain (particularly bone pain), a symptom associated with advanced prostate cancer. Ask him if he has had any recent unexpected weight loss.

Take a sexual history for recent changes in desire or function. Ask about current or previous sexually transmitted diseases, penile discharge, or scrotal pain or swelling.

Physical Assessment/Clinical Manifestations. Most *early* cancers are diagnosed while the patient is having a routine physical examination or is being treated for benign prostatic hyperplasia (BPH). Gross blood in the urine (hematuria) is a common clinical manifestation of *late* prostate cancer. Assess for PAIN in the pelvis, spine, hips, or ribs. Complete a thorough pain assessment. Palpate for swollen lymph nodes, especially in the groin areas. Pain and swollen nodes also indicate advanced disease that has spread. Take and record the patient's weight because unexpected weight loss is also common when the disease is advanced.

Prepare the patient for a digital rectal examination (DRE). On rectal examination, a prostate that is found to be stony hard and with palpable irregularities or indurations is suspected to be malignant.

Psychosocial Assessment. A diagnosis of any type of cancer causes fear and anxiety for most people. Some men, particularly African Americans, develop the disease in their 40s and 50s when they are perhaps planning their retirements, putting their children through college, and/or enjoying their middle years. Assess the reaction of the patient to the diagnosis, and observe how his family reacts to the illness. Men may describe their feelings as shock, fear, anger, and "roller coaster." Expect that patients usually go through the grieving process and may be in denial or depressed. Determine what support systems they have, such as spiritual leaders or community group support, to help them through diagnosis, treatment, and recovery.

One of the biggest concerns for the man may be his ability for sexual function after cancer treatment. Tell him that function will depend on the type of treatment he has. Common surgical techniques used today do not involve cutting the perineal nerves that are needed for an erection. A dry climax may occur if the prostate is removed because it produces most of the fluid in the ejaculate. Refer the patient to his surgeon (urologist), sex therapist, or intimacy counselor if available.

Laboratory Assessment. **Prostate-specific antigen (PSA)** is a glycoprotein produced by the prostate. *PSA analysis is used as a screening test for prostate cancer.* If the test is performed, it should be drawn before the DRE because the examination can cause an increase in PSA due to prostate irritation.

Most authoritative sources agree that the normal blood level of PSA in men younger than 50 years is less than 2.5 ng/mL. PSA levels increase to as high as 6.5 ng/mL when men reach their 70s. *African-American men have a slighter higher normal value, but the reason for this difference is not known. Because other prostate problems also increase the PSA level, it is not specifically diagnostic for cancer.* The level associated with prostate cancer, however, is usually much higher than those occurring with problems such as prostatitis and benign prostatic hyperplasia (Pagana & Pagana, 2014).

An elevated PSA level should decrease a few days after a prostatectomy for cancer. An increase in the PSA level several weeks after surgery may indicate that the disease has recurred.

Because PSA is not absolutely specific to prostate cancer, another test, *early prostate cancer antigen (EPCA-2),* may be a serum marker for prostate cancer. It can detect changes in the prostate gland early and is a very sensitive test. EPCA-2 may also eliminate the need to perform a biopsy of prostate tissue (Pagana & Pagana, 2014).

Other Diagnostic Assessment. After assessments by DRE and PSA, most patients have a *transrectal ultrasound (TRUS)* of the prostate in an ambulatory care or imaging setting. The technician inserts a small probe into the rectum and obtains a view of the prostate using sound waves. If prostate cancer is suspected, a *biopsy* is usually performed in the physician's office to obtain an accurate diagnosis. Prior to the procedure, the physician uses lidocaine jelly on the ultrasound probe and/or injects lidocaine into the prostate gland to promote patient comfort (Dunn & Kazer, 2011).

! NURSING SAFETY PRIORITY QSEN

Action Alert

After a *transrectal ultrasound with biopsy,* instruct the patient about possible complications, although rare, including hematuria with clots, signs of infection, and perineal pain. Teach him to report fever, chills, bloody urine, and any difficulty voiding. Advise him to avoid strenuous physical activity and to drink plenty of fluids, especially in the first 24 hours after the procedure. Teach him that a small amount of bleeding turning the urine pink is expected during this time. However, bright red bleeding should be reported to the health care provider immediately.

After prostate cancer is diagnosed, the patient has additional imaging and blood studies to determine the extent of the disease. Common tests include lymph node biopsy, CT of the pelvis and abdomen, and MRI to assess the status of the pelvic and para-aortic lymph nodes. A radionuclide bone scan may be performed to detect metastatic bone disease. An enlarged liver or abnormal liver function study results indicate possible liver metastasis.

Patients with advanced prostate cancer often have *elevated* levels of *serum acid phosphatase.* Most men with bone metastasis have *elevated serum alkaline phosphatase* levels and severe PAIN.

◆ Interventions

As with any cancer, accurate staging and grading of prostate tumors guide treatment planning and monitoring during the course of the disease. Patients are faced with several treatment options. A urologist and oncologist are needed to help patients make the best decision. Because prostate cancer is slow growing with late metastasis, older men who are asymptomatic and have other illnesses may choose observation without immediate active treatment, especially if the cancer is early stage. This option is known as **active surveillance (AS)**. This form of treatment involves initial surveillance with active treatment only if the symptoms become bothersome. The average time from diagnosis to start of treatment is up to 10 years. During the AS period, men are monitored at regular intervals through DRE and PSA testing. Factors that are considered in choosing AS include potential side effects of treatment (e.g., urinary incontinence, erectile dysfunction), estimated life expectancy, and the risk for increased morbidity and mortality from not seeking active treatment (Hegarty & Bailey, 2011).

Patients who have very early–stage cancer of the prostate who choose AS require close follow-up by their health care provider. If obstruction occurs, a transurethral resection of the prostate (TURP) may be done. The care of patients having this procedure is described in the discussion of Surgical Management on p. 1505 in the Benign Prostatic Hyperplasia section.

Specific management is based on the extent of the disease and the patient's physical condition. The patient may undergo surgery for a biopsy, staging and removal of the tumor, or palliation to control the spread of disease or relieve distressing symptoms. As with AS, the health care provider and patient must weigh the benefits of treatment against potential adverse effects such as incontinence and erectile dysfunction (ED).

Surgical Management. *Surgery is the most common intervention for a cure.* Minimally invasive surgery (MIS) or, less commonly, an open surgical technique for radical prostatectomy (prostate removal) is usually performed. A **bilateral orchiectomy** (removal of both testicles) is another palliative surgery that slows the spread of cancer by removing the main source of testosterone.

Preoperative Care. Preoperative care depends on the type of surgery that will be done. Minimally invasive surgery (MIS) is most appropriate for localized prostate cancer and is used as a curative intervention. The most common procedure is the *laparoscopic radical prostatectomy (LRP),* most often with robotic assistance (Chitlik, 2011). Other newer procedures include transrectal high-intensity focused ultrasound (HIFU) and cryosurgery. Patients who qualify for LRP must have a PSA less than 10 ng/mL and have no previous hormone therapy or abdominal surgeries. Remind the patient that the advantages of this procedure over open surgery are (Dunn & Kazer, 2011):

- Decreased hospital stay (1 to 2 days)
- Minimal bleeding
- Smaller or no incisions and less scarring
- Less postoperative discomfort
- Decreased time for urinary catheter placement
- Fewer complications
- Faster recovery and return to usual activities
- Nerve-sparing advantages

For the patient undergoing an *open* radical prostatectomy, provide preoperative care as for any patient having surgery (see Chapter 14).

Operative Procedures. For the *LRP procedure,* the patient is placed in lithotomy positioning with steep Trendelenburg. Nurses in the OR ensure that the patient maintains a balanced body temperature and positions the patient to prevent injury (Chitlik, 2011). The urologist makes one or more small punctures or incisions into the abdomen. A laparoscope with a camera on the end is inserted through one of the incisions while other instruments are inserted into the other incisions. The robotic system may be used to control the movement of the instruments by a remote device. The prostate is removed along with nearby lymph nodes, but perineal nerves are not affected.

The *open* radical prostatectomy can be performed via several surgical approaches, depending on the patient's desired outcomes and the staging of the disease. The transperineal and retropubic (nerve-sparing) approaches are most commonly used. The surgeon removes the entire prostate gland along with the prostatic capsule, the cuff at the bladder neck, the seminal vesicles, and the regional lymph nodes. The remaining urethra is connected to the bladder neck. The removal of tissue at the bladder neck allows the seminal fluid to travel upward into the bladder rather than down the urethral tract, resulting in retrograde ejaculations.

Postoperative Care. Provide postoperative care of the patient after *open* radical prostatectomy as summarized in Chart 72-2. Nursing interventions include all the typical care for a patient undergoing major surgery. Maintaining hydration, caring for wound drains (open procedure), managing PAIN, and preventing pulmonary complications are important aspects of nursing care. (See general postoperative care in Chapter 16.)

Assess the patient's pain level, and monitor the effectiveness of PAIN management with opioids given as patient-controlled analgesia (PCA), a common method of delivery during the first 24 hours after surgery. Administer a stool softener if needed to prevent possible constipation from the drugs. Patients having the minimally invasive surgery have much less pain and fewer complications.

The patient has an indwelling urinary catheter to straight drainage to promote urinary ELIMINATION. Monitor intake and output every shift and record, or delegate this activity to and supervise unlicensed assistive personnel (UAP). An antispasmodic may be prescribed to decrease bladder spasm induced by the indwelling urinary catheter. The time for catheter removal depends on the type of procedure that is performed and overall patient condition. Those with open surgical procedures use the catheter for 7 to 10 days or longer.

CHART 72-2 Best Practice for Patient Safety & Quality Care (QSEN)

Care of the Patient After an Open Radical Prostatectomy

- Encourage the patient to use patient-controlled analgesia (PCA) as needed.
- Help the patient get out of bed into a chair on the night of surgery and ambulate by the next day.
- Maintain the sequential compression device until the patient begins to ambulate.
- Monitor the patient for deep vein thrombosis and pulmonary embolus.
- Keep an accurate record of intake and output, including Jackson-Pratt or other drainage device drainage.
- Keep the urinary meatus clean using soap and water.
- Avoid rectal procedures or treatments.
- Teach the patient how to care for the urinary catheter because he may be discharged with the catheter in place.
- Teach the patient how to use a leg bag.
- Emphasize the importance of not straining during bowel movement. Advise the patient to avoid suppositories or enemas.
- Remind the patient about the importance of follow-up appointments with the physician to monitor progress.

Ambulation should begin no later than the day after surgery. Provide assistance in walking the patient when he first gets out of bed. Assess for scrotal or penile swelling from the disrupted pelvic lymph flow. If this occurs, elevate the scrotum and penis and apply ice to the area intermittently for the first 24 to 48 hours.

Many patients who have the minimally invasive techniques are discharged in 1 to 3 days after surgery and can resume usual activities in about a week or two. Those who have open procedures are discharged in 2 to 3 days or longer, depending on their progress.

Remind patients that common potential long-term complications of open radical prostatectomy are erectile dysfunction (ED) and urinary incontinence. For ED, drugs such as sildenafil (Viagra) may be effective. *Urge incontinence* may occur because the internal and external sphincters of the bladder lie close to the prostate gland and are often damaged during the surgery. Kegel perineal exercises may reduce the severity of urinary incontinence after radical prostatectomy. Teach the patient to contract and relax the perineal and gluteal muscles in several ways. For one of the exercises, teach him to:

1. Tighten the perineal muscles for 3 to 5 seconds as if to prevent voiding, and then relax.
2. Bear down as if having a bowel movement.
3. Relax and repeat the exercise.

Show him how to inhale through pursed lips while tightening the perineal muscles and how to exhale when he relaxes. To regain urinary control, teach the patient to practice holding an object, such as a pencil, in the fold between the buttock and the thigh. He may also sit on the toilet with the knees apart while voiding and start and stop the stream several times.

Nonsurgical Management. Nonsurgical management may be an adjunct to surgery or alternative intervention if the cancer is widespread or the patient's condition or age prevents surgery. Available modalities include radiation therapy, hormone therapy, and chemotherapy (less often).

Radiation Therapy. External or internal radiation therapy may be used in the treatment of prostate cancer or as "salvage" treatments when cancer recurs. It may also be done for palliation of the patient's symptoms.

External beam radiation therapy (EBRT or XRT) comes from a source outside the body. Patients are usually treated 5 days a week for 4 to 6 weeks (Dunn & Kazer, 2011). Three-dimensional conformal radiation therapy (3D-CRT) can more accurately target prostate tissue and can reduce side effects such as damage to the rectum. An advanced type of this radiation called *intensity-modulated radiation therapy* provides very high doses to the prostate. EBRT can also be used to relieve pain from bone metastasis or given following radical prostatectomy. Teach patients that external beam radiation causes ED in many men well after the treatment is completed.

Teach patients that other complications from EBRT include urinary frequency, diarrhea, and *acute radiation cystitis,* which causes persistent pain and hematuria. Symptoms are usually mild to moderate and subside in 6 weeks after treatment. Drugs to prevent urinary urgency such as tolterodine (Detrol LA) may be prescribed. Teach the patient to avoid caffeine and continue drinking plenty of water and other fluids.

Radiation proctitis (rectal mucosa inflammation) may also develop but is less likely with 3D-CRT. The man reports rectal urgency and cramping and passes mucus and blood. Teach him to report these symptoms to the health care provider. Like cystitis, this problem usually resolves in 4 to 6 weeks after the treatment stops. If proctitis occurs, teach patients to limit spicy or fatty foods, caffeine, and dairy products.

Low-dose brachytherapy (internal radiation) can be delivered by implanting low-dose radiation seeds, needles, or wires directly into and around the prostate gland. This treatment includes ultrasonically guided interstitial or radioactive implantation. These procedures are done on an ambulatory care basis and are the most cost-effective treatment for early-stage prostate cancer. Reassure the patient that the dose of radiation is low and that the radiation will not pose a hazard to him or others. Teach him that ED, urinary incontinence, and rectal problems do occur in a small percentage of cases. Fatigue is also common and may last for several months after the treatment stops. Chapter 22 describes general nursing care for patients having radiation therapy.

Drug Therapy. Drug therapy may consist of either hormone therapy (androgen deprivation therapy [ADT]) or chemotherapy.

Hormone Therapy. Because most prostate tumors are hormone dependent, patients with extensive tumors or those with metastatic disease may be managed by androgen deprivation. Luteinizing hormone–releasing hormone (LH-RH) agonists or anti-androgens can be used.

Examples of *LH-RH agonists* are leuprolide (Lupron), goserelin (Zoladex), and triptorelin (Trelstar). These drugs first stimulate the pituitary gland to release the luteinizing hormone (LH). After about 3 weeks, the pituitary gland "runs out" of LH, which reduces testosterone production by the testes.

! NURSING SAFETY PRIORITY QSEN

Drug Alert

Teach patients taking LH-RH agonists that side effects include "hot flashes," erectile dysfunction, and decreased **libido** (desire to have sex). Some men also have **gynecomastia** (breast tenderness and growth). These drugs can also cause osteoporosis. Bisphosphonates like pamidronate (Aredia) are prescribed to prevent bone fractures. They can also be used to slow the damage caused by bone metastasis.

Anti-androgen drugs, also known as *androgen deprivation therapy (ADT),* work differently in that they block the body's ability to use the available androgens (Dunn & Kazer, 2011). These drugs are the major treatment for metastatic disease. Examples include flutamide (Eulexin, Euflex ♣), bicalutamide (Casodex), and nilutamide (Nilandron). These drugs inhibit tumor progression by blocking the uptake of testicular and adrenal androgens at the prostate tumor site.

Anti-androgens may be used alone or in combination with LH-RH agonists for a total or maximal androgen blockade (hormone ablation). Patients who have this drug combination often have "hot flashes" similar to those experienced by menopausal women, and they can decrease the patient's perceived quality of life. Ask the patient if he has been experiencing this problem. Megestrol acetate may be prescribed for this uncomfortable condition.

Chemotherapy. Systemic chemotherapy may be an option for patients whose cancer has spread and for whom other therapies have not worked. For example, small cell prostate cancer is rare and is more responsive to chemotherapy than to hormone therapy. Docetaxel (Taxotere) plus prednisone given every 3 weeks is the preferred treatment. A combination of cisplatin (Platinol) and etoposide (VP-16, VePesid) may also be effective for this type of cancer. Chapter 22 describes general nursing care for patients receiving chemotherapy.

Community-Based Care

Patient-centered collaborative care of the man with prostate cancer should include his partner, if any, and family. The diagnosis and treatment of cancer greatly affect couples who survive the disease. Recognize that the patient and partner have specific physical and psychosocial needs that should be addressed before hospital discharge and management should continue in the community setting.

Patients with prostate cancer may require care in a wide variety of settings: at the hospital, the radiation therapy department, the oncologist's office, or home at any stage of the disease process. Specific interventions depend on which treatment the patient had or if he had a combination of treatments. This section focuses on the needs of those who had a radical prostatectomy.

Home Care Management. Discharge planning and health teaching start early, even before surgery. A patient can better plan home care management when he knows what to expect. Collaborate with the case manager to coordinate the efforts of various health care providers, surgical unit nursing staff, and possibly a home care nurse. As specified by The Joint Commission and other accrediting agencies, continuity of care is essential when caring for this patient because he may need weeks or months of therapies.

Self-Management Education. An important area of teaching for the patient going home after an *open* radical prostatectomy may be urinary catheter care. An indwelling urinary catheter may be in place for up to several weeks, depending on the surgical technique that was used. Teach him and his family how to care for the catheter, use a leg bag, and identify manifestations of INFECTION and other complications. See Chart 72-3 for patient and family education.

Encourage the patient to walk short distances. Lifting may be restricted to no more than 15 pounds for up to 6 weeks if an open procedure was done. Remind him to maintain an upright position and not walk bent or flexed. Vigorous exercise such as running or jumping should be avoided for at least 12 weeks and then gradually introduced. By contrast, patients having the minimally invasive laparoscopic surgery can usually return to work or usual activities in about a week.

Teach the patient to not strain to defecate. A stool softener may be prescribed to reduce the need for straining. If an opioid is prescribed for PAIN management, encourage the patient to drink adequate water to prevent constipation.

If the patient had an *open* radical prostatectomy, teach him to shower for the first 2 to 3 weeks rather than soak in a bathtub. Patients who had a laparoscopic procedure can usually shower in 1 to 2 days. Teach them to remove the small bandage but leave the Steri-Strips in place (they should fall off in about a week). Show patients how to inspect the incision or puncture site(s) daily for signs of INFECTION. Remind them to keep all follow-up appointments. PSA blood tests are taken 6 weeks after surgery and then every 4 to 6 months to monitor progress.

Health Care Resources. Refer the patient and partner to agencies or support groups such as the American Cancer Society's *Man to Man* program to help cope with prostate cancer. This program provides one-on-one education, personal visits, educational presentations, and the opportunity to engage in open and candid discussions. Another prostate cancer support group is *Us TOO International* (www.ustoo.com) sponsored by the Prostate Cancer Education and Support Network. This group provides education and support with national and international chapters. Information can also be obtained from the Prostate Cancer Foundation (www.prostatecancerfoundation.org) or the National Prostate Cancer Coalition (www.fightprostatecancer.org). Other personal and community support services such as spiritual leaders or churches and synagogues are also important to many patients.

For same-sex couples surviving prostate cancer, *Malecare* (http://malecare.org) is an excellent resource. This nonprofit organization provides support groups for gay and bisexual men and their partners (Galbraith et al., 2011). Another resource is *A Gay Man's Guide to Prostate Cancer,* which was updated in 2011.

Some men have erectile dysfunction (ED) for the first 3 to 18 months after a prostatectomy. Refer them to a specialist who can help with this problem. (ED is discussed briefly in the Erectile Dysfunction section, p. 1512.) Refer patients with urinary incontinence to a urologist who specializes in this area. Drug therapy and other strategies may be used. Chapter 66 discusses incontinence management in detail.

CHART 72-3 **Patient and Family Education: Preparing for Self-Management**

Urinary Catheter Care at Home

- Once a day, gently wash the first few inches of the catheter starting at the penis and washing outward with mild soap and water.
- Rinse and dry the catheter well.
- If you have not been circumcised, push the foreskin back to clean the catheter site; when finished, push the foreskin forward.
- Change the drainage bag at least once a week as needed:
  - Hold the catheter with one hand and the tubing with the other hand, and twist in opposite directions to disconnect.
  - Place the end of the catheter in a clean container to catch leakage of urine.
  - Remove the rubber cap from the tubing of the leg bag or clean drainage bag.
  - Clean the end of the new tubing with alcohol swabs.
  - Insert the end of the new tubing into the catheter, and twist to connect securely.
- Clean the drainage bag just removed by pouring a solution of one part vinegar to two parts water through the tubing and bag. Rinse well with water, and allow the bag to dry.

CLINICAL JUDGMENT CHALLENGE

Patient-Centered Care QSEN

A urologist tells a 70-year-old man that his biopsy revealed stage 2 prostate cancer. The patient has lived with his male life partner for 20 years; they are both very upset about his diagnosis and prognosis. The urologist states that the patient is a candidate for laparoscopic prostatectomy.

1. As the office nurse, what is your best response to the patient and his partner at this time?
2. How would you describe his likely prognosis?
3. What health teaching will the patient and partner need?
4. What community resources will you recommend and why?

PROSTATITIS

❖ PATHOPHYSIOLOGY

Prostatitis is an inflammation of the prostate gland. Duration of symptoms, presence or absence of WBCs in the urine, and urinary culture results determine the classification.

Bacterial prostatitis often occurs with urethritis or an INFECTION of the lower urinary tract. Organisms may reach the prostate via the bloodstream or the urethra. The most common organisms are *Escherichia coli, Enterobacter, Proteus,* and group D streptococci. Acute bacterial prostatitis may be manifested by fever, chills, **dysuria** (painful urination), urethral discharge, and a boggy, tender prostate. Gentle palpation of the prostate usually results in a urethral discharge, which has WBCs in the prostatic secretions.

Chronic bacterial prostatitis generally occurs in older men and has a less dramatic presentation than acute bacterial prostatitis and without the systemic manifestations. The patient reports experiencing hesitancy, urgency, dysuria, difficulty initiating and terminating the flow of urine, and decreased strength and volume of urine. Also, there may be discomfort in the perineum, scrotum, and penis.

❖ PATIENT-CENTERED COLLABORATIVE CARE

The patient with chronic prostatitis usually reports backache, perineal PAIN, mild dysuria, and urinary frequency. Hematuria may be present. The prostate may feel irregularly enlarged, firm, and slightly tender when palpated. The patient often has an elevated serum WBC count and prostate-specific antigen (PSA) level.

Complications of prostatitis are **epididymitis** (inflammation of the epididymis) and **cystitis** (inflammation of the bladder). The patient with either acute or chronic bacterial prostatitis is likely to develop urinary tract INFECTIONS. Sexual functioning may be impaired because of discomfort.

Early diagnosis and treatment of prostatitis with antimicrobials are important. Treatment may last from weeks to many months because there is poor penetration of antibiotics into prostatic tissue. Acute bacterial prostatitis may require hospitalization with aggressive IV antibiotics.

Emphasize the importance of comfort measures, such as sitz baths, muscle relaxants, and NSAIDs. Stool softeners are prescribed to prevent straining and rectal irritation of the prostate during a bowel movement. Alpha blockers such as tamsulosin (Flomax) may be given to promote voiding. Teach patients to avoid alcohol, coffee, tea, and spicy foods that irritate symptoms. Instruct them to avoid over-the-counter cold preparations containing decongestants or antihistamines that may cause urinary retention.

Teach the patient with chronic prostatitis about the long-term nature of the problem. Because prostatitis can cause other urinary tract INFECTIONS, explain the importance of long-term antibiotic therapy and increasing fluid intake. Remind him to take the prescribed antibiotics on schedule. Because sulfamethoxazole-trimethoprim (Bactrim, Septra) diffuses into the prostatic fluid, it is often the antibiotic of choice. *Before drug administration, be sure that the patient does not have any allergy to sulfa drugs.*

Teach the patient about activities that drain the prostate (sexual intercourse, masturbation), which may help in the management of chronic prostatitis. Inform him that prostatitis is not infectious or contagious.

ERECTILE DYSFUNCTION

❖ PATHOPHYSIOLOGY

Erectile dysfunction (ED), also known as *impotence,* is the inability to achieve or maintain an erection for sexual intercourse. It affects millions of men in the United States. There are two major types of ED: organic and functional.

Organic ED is a gradual deterioration of function. The man first notices diminishing firmness and a decrease in frequency of erections. Causes include (McCance, et al., 2014):

- Inflammation of the prostate, urethra, or seminal vesicles
- Surgical procedures such as prostatectomy
- Pelvic fractures
- Lumbosacral injuries
- Vascular disease, including hypertension
- Chronic neurologic conditions, such as Parkinson disease or multiple sclerosis
- Endocrine disorders, such as diabetes mellitus (a major cause) or thyroid disorders
- Smoking and alcohol consumption
- Drugs, such as antihypertensives
- Poor overall health that prevents sexual intercourse

If the patient has episodes of ED, it usually has a *functional* (psychological) cause. Men with functional ED usually have normal nocturnal (nighttime) and morning erections. Onset is usually sudden and follows a period of high stress.

❖ PATIENT-CENTERED COLLABORATIVE CARE

If possible, the physician determines the cause of the ED through a variety of diagnostic testing, including measuring serum hormone levels and using Doppler ultrasonography to determine blood flow to the penis. The most common intervention for ED is drug therapy. Other interventions include vacuum devices, intracorporal injections, intraurethral applications, and prostheses (implants).

First-line oral drugs used to manage ED, phosphodiesterace-5 (PDE-5) inhibitors, work by relaxing the smooth muscles in the corpora cavernosa so blood flow to the penis is increased. The veins exiting the corpora are compressed, limiting outward blood flow and resulting in penile **tumescence** (swelling). Teach patients to take the pill 1 hour before sexual intercourse. For some drugs, such as sildenafil (Viagra) and vardenafil (Levitra), sexual stimulation is needed within ½ to 1 hour to promote the erection. With other drugs, such as tadalafil (Cialis), erection can be stimulated over a longer period. Because the erection occurs more naturally compared with other treatment options, most men and their partners prefer this option.

! NURSING SAFETY PRIORITY (QSEN)

Drug Alert

Instruct patients taking PDE-5 inhibitors to abstain from alcohol before sexual intercourse because it may impair the ability to have an erection. Common side effects of these drugs include dyspepsia (heartburn), headaches, facial flushing, and stuffy nose. If more than one pill a day is being taken, leg and back cramps, nausea, and vomiting also may occur. *Teach men who take nitrates to avoid PDE-5 inhibitors because the vasodilation effects can cause a profound hypotension and reduce blood flow to vital organs.* For patients who cannot take these drugs or do not respond to them, other methods are available to achieve an erection.

The basic design of a *vacuum constriction device (VCD)* is a cylinder that fits over the penis and sits firmly against the body. Using a pump, a vacuum is created to draw blood into the penis to maintain an erection. A rubber ring (tension band) is placed around the base of the penis to maintain the erection, and the cylinder is removed.

Injecting the penis with vasodilating drugs can make the penis erect by engorging it with blood. The most common agents used for this purpose include (Lilley et al., 2014):

- Alprostadil (Caverject), a synthetic vasodilator identical to prostaglandin E_1 produced in the body
- Paverine, also a vasodilator
- Phentolamine (Regitine), an alpha-1, alpha-2 selective adrenergic receptor antagonist
- A combination of any or all of these drugs

Adverse drug effects include priapism (prolonged erection), penile scarring, fibrosis, bleeding, bruising at the injection site, pain, infection, and vasovagal responses.

Penile implants (prostheses) are used when other modalities fail. Devices include semirigid, flexible, or hydraulic inflatable and multi-component or one-piece instruments. The three-piece inflatable device is the most commonly implanted prosthesis. A reservoir is placed in the scrotum. Tubes carry the fluid into the inflatable pieces that are placed in the penis. To inflate the prosthesis, the man squeezes the pump located in the scrotum. To deflate the prosthesis, a release button is activated. Advantages include the man's ability to control his erections. The major disadvantages include device failure and infection. The device is implanted as an ambulatory care surgical procedure. *Teach the patient to observe the surgical site for bleeding and* INFECTION.

NCLEX EXAMINATION CHALLENGE

Health Promotion and Maintenance

The nurse is teaching a client about taking sildenafil (Viagra) for erectile dysfunction. Which statement by the client indicates a need for further teaching?

A. "I should have sex within an hour after taking the drug."
B. "I should avoid alcohol when on the drug or it might not work well."
C. "I can expect to maybe get a stuffy nose or headache when I take the drug."
D. "If I have chest pain during sex, I should take a nitroglycerin tablet."

TESTICULAR CANCER

PATHOPHYSIOLOGY

Testicular cancer is a rare cancer that most often affects men between 20 and 35 years of age but can affect men of any age (American Cancer Society [ACS], 2014b). It usually strikes men at a productive time of life and thus has significant economic, social, and psychological impact on the patient and his family and/or partner. With early detection by testicular self-examination (TSE) (Chart 72-4) and treatment, testicular cancer has a 95% cure rate (Viatori, 2012). It can occur in one testicle or both.

Primary testicular cancers fall into two major groups:

- Germ cell tumors arising from the sperm-producing cells (account for most testicular cancers)
- Non–germ cell tumors arising from the stromal, interstitial, or Leydig cells that produce testosterone (account for a very small percentage of testicular cancers)

Testicular germ cell tumors are classified into two broad categories: seminomas and nonseminomas (Table 72-1). The most common type of testicular tumor is *seminoma.* Patients with seminomas have the most favorable prognoses because the tumors are usually localized, metastasize late, and respond to treatment (Viatori, 2012). They often are diagnosed when they are still confined to the testicles and retroperitoneal lymph nodes.

Non–germ cell tumors are classified as either *interstitial cell tumors* or *androblastomas* (testicular adenomas). Most of these tumors do not metastasize. Interstitial cell tumors arise from the Leydig cells, which secrete testosterone into the bloodstream. Androblastomas sometimes secrete estrogen, which accounts for the feminization and **gynecomastia** (breast enlargement) occasionally seen in these men.

The risk for testicular tumors is higher in males who have an undescended testis (**cryptorchidism**) or have human immune deficiency virus (HIV) infection (McCance, et al., 2014).

CHART 72-4 Patient and Family Education: Preparing for Self-Management

Testicular Self-Examination

- Examine your testicles monthly immediately after a bath or a shower, when your scrotal skin is relaxed.
- Examine each testicle by gently rolling it between your thumbs and fingers. Testicular tumors tend to appear deep in the center of the testicle.
- Look and feel for any lumps; smooth, rounded masses; or any change in the size, shape, or consistency of the testes.
- Report any lump or swelling to your doctor as soon as possible.

TABLE 72-1 Classification of Testicular Tumors

GERM CELL (GERMINAL) TUMORS	NON–GERM CELL (NONGERMINAL) TUMORS
• Seminoma	• Interstitial cell tumor
• Nonseminoma:	• Androblastoma
• Embryonal carcinoma	
• Teratoma	
• Choriocarcinoma	

GENETIC/GENOMIC CONSIDERATIONS

Patient-Centered Care QSEN

Men are at a higher risk for testicular cancer if they have a family history of the disease (Viatori, 2012). The incidence is higher among identical twins, brothers, and other close male relatives. Euro-American men are at a higher risk for testicular cancer than men of other races or ethnicities (Viatori, 2012). The reason for these differences is not known.

Primary testicular cancer is rarely bilateral. Other cancers such as leukemia, lymphoma, and metastatic carcinomas may invade the testes. A man with bilateral testicular tumors is more likely to have metastatic disease to the testes than primary cancer.

❖ PATIENT-CENTERED COLLABORATIVE CARE

◆ Assessment

Physical Assessment/Clinical Manifestations. When taking a history from a patient with a suspected testicular tumor, consider the risk factors. Assess for other risk factors, including a history or presence of an undescended testis and a family history of testicular cancer.

The most common manifestation is a painless, hard swelling or enlargement of the testicle. Patients with discomfort such as heaviness or aching in the lower abdomen or the scrotum may have metastatic disease. Determine how long any manifestations have been present.

Assess the patient's family situation. Is the patient sexually active? If so, what is his sexual preference? Does he have children? Does he want children in the future? Depending on the treatment plan chosen, would he be interested in sperm storage in a sperm bank?

If the man has one healthy testis, he can function sexually and may not have any problem with REPRODUCTION. If he has a retroperitoneal lymph node dissection or chemotherapy, he may become sterile because of treatment effects on the sperm-producing cells or surgical trauma to the sympathetic nervous system resulting in retrograde ejaculations.

The testes, lymph nodes, and abdomen should be thoroughly examined. Patients may feel embarrassed about having this examination. Provide privacy, and explain the procedure to the patient. Inspect the testicles for swelling or a lump that the patient reports is painless. An advanced practice nurse or other health care provider palpates the testes for lumps and swelling that are not visible (Chart 72-5). The presence of any testicular PAIN, lymph node swelling, bone pain, abdominal masses, sudden hydrocele (fluid in the scrotum), or gynecomastia often indicates metastatic disease.

Psychosocial Assessment. Because testicular cancer and its treatment often lead to sexual dysfunction, pay close attention to the psychosocial aspects of the disease. Sexuality is an issue for men of any age, but it may be even more of an issue for younger men. Even if the cancer is detected at an early stage and the patient is cured after surgery, he may be afraid that he will be sexually deficient. He may also think of himself as "less than a whole person." These fears can disrupt the psychosocial and sexual development of young males and can threaten their identity. The patient may be afraid that he will be unable to perform sexually, will no longer be sexually attractive or desirable, and will face rejection. Feelings of sexual inadequacy may be denied, repressed, or displaced, causing increased stress on the man's personal and work relationships.

Assess the man's support systems, including his partner, family members, and friends. Ask him where he feels that he can be supported, such as a religious or spiritual group, community club, or social group. Friends are often very helpful during this difficult time.

Laboratory Assessment. Common serum tumor markers that confirm a diagnosis of testicular cancer are:

- Alpha-fetoprotein (AFP)
- Beta human chorionic gonadotropin (hCG)
- Lactate dehydrogenase (LDH)

Serum testosterone levels are increased when the tumor affects the Leydig cells, which produce this hormone. Drugs such as alcohol and antiepileptic drugs can also cause an increase in testosterone (Pagana & Pagana, 2014).

Other Diagnostic Assessment. When a patient has a change in testis size, shape, or texture, *ultrasonography* can determine whether the mass is solid or fluid filled. It also can help differentiate benign masses from malignant ones.

After the diagnosis of testicular cancer, the patient should have a *CT* scan of the abdomen and the chest to identify small metastatic lesions. *Lymphangiography* shows a view of the body's lymph system to look for spread to other areas.

MRI is used to detect enlarged lymph nodes and abnormal nodules in certain organs that may indicate metastasis from the testicles. Chest x-rays and bone scans may also be performed if metastasis is suspected.

◆ Interventions

At diagnosis, the incidence of **oligospermia** (low sperm count) and **azoospermia** (absence of living sperm) is common in patients with testicular cancer. This problem is thought to be related to higher testicular temperatures created by cancer cell metabolism. The man may not discover that he has reduced sperm count until he has a sperm count performed before surgery.

Health teaching about REPRODUCTION, fertility, and sexuality is started in the pretreatment phase. Review the normal reproductive function, as well as the possible effects of cancer and its treatment on reproductive function. Explore with the patient various reproductive options if desired (Chart 72-6). A sperm bank facility provides comprehensive information on

CHART 72-5 Focused Assessment

The Patient with a Testicular Lump

- Obtain a medical history from the patient:
  - When was the lump discovered?
  - Are there any other symptoms (sensation of heaviness, dragging in testicle, pain, discharge from penis)?
  - Is there a history of cryptorchidism?
- An advanced practice nurse or other health care provider will assess the genital system. They will:
  - Inspect and palpate the scrotal contents, have the patient perform a Valsalva maneuver, and palpate for a varicocele.
  - Any lump or enlargement that does not transilluminate should be suspected as malignant.
- Palpate for any enlarged lymph nodes. Always wear gloves during the examination of the male genitalia. The most common areas for lymphadenopathy are in the inguinal or supraclavicular regions.
- Assess the abdomen for a possible mass or hepatomegaly.

CHART 72-6 Patient and Family Education: Preparing for Self-Management

Sperm Banking

- You may want to investigate sperm storage in a sperm bank as a way to preserve your sperm for future use.
- No one knows how long sperm can be stored successfully, but pregnancies have resulted from sperm stored for longer than 10 years.
- Check with the sperm bank to see how much it charges to process and store your sperm and to see whether you must pay when the service is provided.
- Investigate whether your health insurance company will reimburse you for sperm collection and storage.

semen collection, storage of semen, the storage contract, costs, and the insemination process.

When preparing the patient for the collection and storage of sperm, assume the role of patient advocate and keep in mind the effect of the cancer diagnosis. The psychological benefit of having stored sperm may be important for the man and may influence his response to treatment. For some men, knowing that the potential for being a father still exists may help them cope with other fears, such as alopecia or erectile dysfunction (ED).

Suggest that the patient arrange for semen storage, if desired, as soon as possible after diagnosis. Sperm collection should be completed before he begins radiation therapy or chemotherapy or undergoes a radical lymph node dissection. After radiation therapy or chemotherapy has been started, the patient is at increased risk for producing mutagenic sperm, which may not be viable or may result in fetal abnormalities.

The patient's diagnosis and his physical condition may not allow treatment to be postponed, thus making sperm storage impossible. Also, some men may have personal or religious beliefs that do not allow sperm storage. For those who are not candidates for sperm storage in a sperm bank and for those who choose not to bank, discuss other options for REPRODUCTION such as donor insemination or adoption.

Surgical Management. Surgery is the main treatment for testicular cancer. For stage 0 or 1 (localized disease), the surgeon performs a unilateral **orchiectomy** to remove the affected testicle. Every effort is made to remove the cancerous testis as an intact organ to prevent releasing cancer cells into the surgical site. Depending on the type and stage of the cancer, radical retroperitoneal lymph node dissection (RPLND) may also be done.

Preoperative Care. Like most patients with cancer, the man with testicular cancer is very apprehensive. Offer support, and reinforce the teaching provided by the surgeon. Teach the patient and his family or partner about what to expect after surgery. For patients with very early disease, minimally invasive surgery (MIS) using a laparoscope is performed rather than using an open incision. For patients having MIS, teach them that carbon dioxide may be used as part of the surgery. Carbon dioxide can cause chest or shoulder pain from diaphragmatic irritation after the procedure.

Operative Procedures. Most patients with seminoma have only one surgery to remove the diseased testicle through the groin (inguinal) for a cure. A frozen section of the tumor is examined to confirm the type and stage of the cancer. A gel-filled silicone prosthesis may be surgically implanted into the scrotum at the time of the orchiectomy or later if the patient desires. Reassure the patient that this procedure does not impair fertility or sexual function. He cosmetically appears to have two testes (reconstructive surgery).

Some men have more advanced disease or tumor types that are more aggressive. Two options are available for the lymph node dissection: a traditional open approach and minimally invasive surgery (MIS) using a laparoscope. To perform the *open* approach, the surgeon removes the retroperitoneal nodes in the iliac and lumbar regions. Because the blood supply and the lymphatic vessels of the testes and kidneys are directly related, an extensive midline incision from the xiphoid process to the pubis is necessary. Removal of the sympathetic ganglia eliminates peristalsis in the vas deferens and contractions of the seminal vesicles. This disruption results in sterility because the man's ejaculate no longer contains sperm. However, having a normal erection and experiencing orgasm usually are not affected.

The MIS procedure involves using a laparoscope through several small "keyhole" incisions through which the nodes are dissected for examination. This technique shortens the time the patient is in the operating suite, minimizes bleeding, and causes less pain after surgery. The patient has fewer postoperative complications and a shorter hospital stay.

Postoperative Care. Nursing care for the patient after surgery depends on the type of surgical procedure that was performed and the extent of the disease process.

! NURSING SAFETY PRIORITY QSEN

Action Alert

Because of the length of the *open* orchiectomy and lymph node dissection approach, manipulation of the abdominal and retroperitoneal viscera, and the loss of lymphatic fluid, observe, assess, and report any complications of this major abdominal surgery (e.g., paralytic ileus) (see Chapter 16). Monitor vital signs (including pain), hydration, and pulmonary function carefully for the first 24 to 48 hours. Ambulate the patient as soon as possible, and teach him how to use the incentive spirometer. Assess the patency of the urinary catheter. Be sure the patient wears antiembolism stockings or devices, and provide care for surgical incisions and wound drains.

The patient having the *laparoscopic* procedure may have a urinary catheter in place for 1 to 2 days. The other advantages of the MIS procedure are that patients have less pain and fewer complications than those who had the open surgery. Chapter 15 describes laparoscopic surgery in detail.

? NCLEX EXAMINATION CHALLENGE

Physiological Integrity

A client had an orchiectomy and laparoscopic radical retroperitoneal lymph node dissection this morning. What is the nurse's priority for care?

A. Assess the client's pain level and provide pain management.
B. Ensure that the client's urinary catheter is draining clear yellow urine.
C. Observe the client's incision for redness, swelling, and drainage.
D. Apply oxygen therapy via nasal cannula at 2 L/min.

Nonsurgical Management. Combination *chemotherapy* may be used as adjuvant therapy for nonseminomatous testicular tumors or as primary treatment when there is evidence of metastatic disease. Many drug regimens are used, including varying combinations of bleomycin, etoposide, and cisplatin (BEP). The specific combination of drugs and the frequency, cycling, and duration of treatment vary from patient to patient, depending on the extent of the disease and the protocol being followed. Chapter 22 discusses the general nursing care for the patient receiving chemotherapy.

Patients having chemotherapy are at risk for certain health problems that are associated with these drugs. Examples of these problems include hypertension, hyperlipidemia, lung toxicity, anemia, and leukemia (Viatori, 2012). Teach patients taking these drugs about the long-term effects for which they should be continually and carefully monitored by their health care providers.

After orchiectomy for localized disease, *external beam radiation therapy* (EBRT) may be used. The remaining testis is shielded with a lead cup to preserve reproductive function. Even with these precautions, the patient may have a temporary decreased sperm count as a result of radiation scatter. Normally the sperm count returns to the pretreatment level within 24 to 30 months after the radiation treatment is completed. If metastases develop outside the lymphatic system, the man may still be cured with radiation therapy if the area of involvement is limited. If lymphatic involvement is extensive or if the visceral organs are involved, combination chemotherapy is used.

Community-Based Care

The patient is usually hospitalized for multiple days after an *open* radical retroperitoneal lymph node dissection but for just 1 to 2 days for the *MIS* laparoscopic procedure.

After an open *orchiectomy,* unless the patient has a wound complication, he is discharged without a dressing on the inguinal incision. A scrotal support may be needed for several days. He may want to wear a dry dressing to prevent clothing from rubbing on the sutures and causing irritation. Tell him that the sutures will be removed in the physician's office 7 to 10 days after surgery.

! NURSING SAFETY PRIORITY QSEN

Action Alert

For the patient who has undergone testicular surgery, emphasize the importance of scheduling a follow-up visit with the surgeon to examine the incision for healing and complications. Instruct him to notify the surgeon if chills, fever, increasing tenderness or pain around the incision, drainage, or dehiscence of the incision occurs. These manifestations may indicate INFECTION for which antibiotics are needed. Instruct the patient who had a laparoscopic orchiectomy that he will be able to resume most of his usual activities within 1 week after discharge. He can take a shower in 1 or 2 days after surgery, but be sure he does not remove the Steri-Strips. These strips will loosen and fall off in about a week after surgery.

Patients who also had an *open retroperitoneal lymph node dissection* recover more slowly. They should not lift anything over 15 pounds, should avoid stair climbing, and should not drive a car for several weeks. Be sure that bathroom facilities are on the first floor of the house where he can easily access them.

Explain the importance of performing monthly testicular self-examination (TSE) on the remaining testis and scheduling follow-up examinations with the physician. The patient who has had testicular cancer should schedule tests for urinary and serum levels of tumor markers and CT or MRI studies as part of his routine follow-up for at least 3 years.

Depending on the pathologic findings and the stage of the cancer, the patient may need further treatment. This information may not be known at the time of discharge. If it is known that the patient needs further surgery, he and his family need information about the future surgery. If it is known that he must undergo radiation therapy or chemotherapy, he needs education about these treatments as soon as possible.

The man who has testicular cancer needs emotional support. If permanent sterility occurs and sperm storage has not been feasible, he may desire counseling about other reproductive options. Refer the patient to agencies or support groups, such as the American Fertility Society (www.theafa.org) or RESOLVE: The National Infertility Association (www.resolve.org) (organizations for infertile couples).

OTHER PROBLEMS AFFECTING THE TESTES AND ADJACENT STRUCTURES

Problems that develop inside the scrotum usually occur as a mass or as scrotal edema. Some problems produce pain, but others do not. Fig. 72-4 shows some of the most common conditions found in adult men, including hydrocele, spermatocele, and varicocele. In addition to local comfort measures, these masses are either drained or removed surgically. Scrotal support, heat, and analgesics are needed after surgery. Teach patients to follow up with their health care provider.

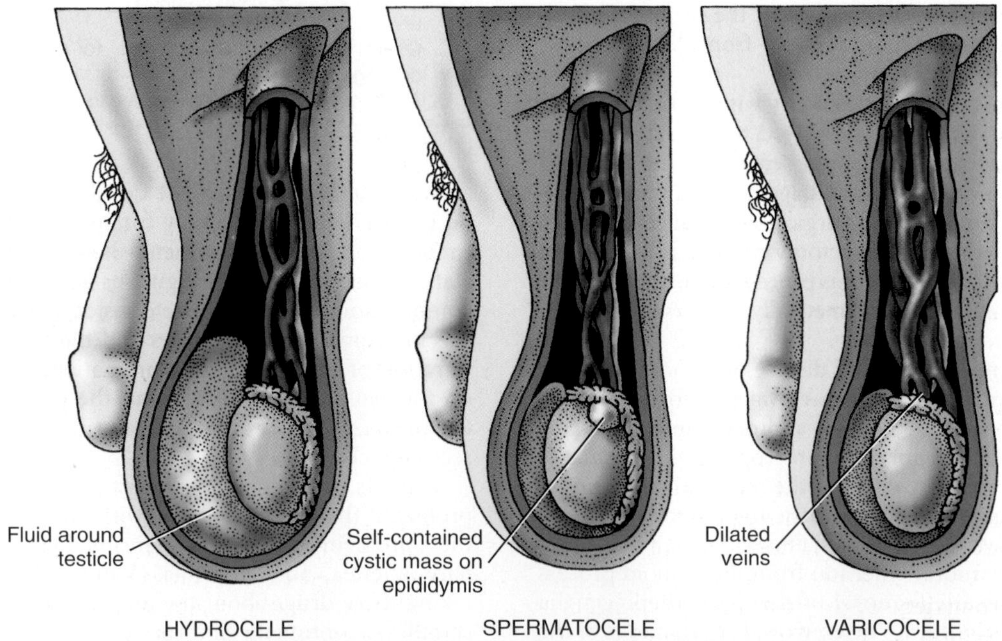

FIG. 72-4 Common problems affecting the testes and adjacent structures.

NURSING CONCEPTS AND CLINICAL JUDGMENT REVIEW

What might you NOTICE if the patient is experiencing impaired SEXUALITY as a result of male reproductive problems?

- Lump or swelling in prostate or scrotum
- Report of pain in scrotum or during ejaculation
- Report of difficulty voiding (e.g., starting urine stream)
- Hematuria
- Report of dribbling of urine (incontinence)
- Report of inability to have a penile erection
- Report of decreased libido

What should you INTERPRET and how should you RESPOND to a patient experiencing impaired SEXUALITY as a result of male reproductive problems?

Perform and interpret physical assessment, including:

- Conducting a complete pain assessment
- Inspecting and palpating bladder for distention
- Inspecting and palpating scrotum for swelling or masses
- Palpating lymph nodes for swelling, especially in the inguinal areas
- Sending urine sample for urinalysis and culture
- Checking most recent laboratory values for PSA, CBC, and serum tumor markers

Respond by:

- Catheterizing patient if retaining urine
- Providing pain-relief measures, such as ice or medication as prescribed
- Elevating scrotum if swollen
- Arranging for consultation with sex or intimacy therapist if patient desires

On what should you REFLECT?

- Evaluate patient for need for indwelling urinary catheter.
- Evaluate effectiveness of actions to control pain and swelling.
- Think about what additional resources the patient will need to cope with his problem.

GET READY FOR THE NCLEX® EXAMINATION!

KEY POINTS

Review these Key Points for each NCLEX Examination Client Needs Category.

Safe and Effective Care Environment

- Teach patients with prostate cancer about American Cancer Society's *Man to Man* program and the American Foundation for Urologic Disease's *Us TOO International* program to help men and their partners cope with prostate cancer.
- Teach patients to report signs of INFECTION when caring for a urinary catheter in the home. **Safety** QSEN

Health Promotion and Maintenance

- Teach men at risk for prostate cancer to follow the current American Cancer Society's screening and early detection guidelines. **Evidence-Based Practice** QSEN
- Teach men how to perform testicular self-examination as described in Chart 72-4.
- Teach uncircumcised men the importance of keeping the penis clean to prevent penile cancer.

Psychosocial Integrity

- Because most patients with testicular cancer are young and middle-aged adults, assess their reaction to the possible loss of REPRODUCTION ability.
- Because of the high incidence of erectile dysfunction after radical prostatectomy, assess the patient's adjustment to these changes in body function. **Patient-Centered Care** QSEN
- Assess the patient's anxiety before prostate surgery, and allow him to express feelings of fear or grief. **Patient-Centered Care** QSEN

Physiological Integrity

- Perform a focused physical assessment for patients reporting lumps or swelling in their genital area; inspect and palpate bladder and scrotum.
- Observe for and report complications after radical prostatectomy, including infection, severe PAIN, urinary infection, urinary ELIMINATION problems, and erectile dysfunction. **Safety** QSEN
- Observe for and report bloody urine with clots after TURP; increase continuous bladder irrigation or irrigate the bladder per agency or surgeon protocol. **Safety** QSEN
- Maintain traction on the urinary catheter and continuous bladder irrigation after a TURP. **Safety**
- Teach patients about drug therapies (5-ARIs and alpha blocking agents) used to treat BPH, including side effects such as orthostatic hypotension, erectile dysfunction, decreased libido, dizziness, and liver dysfunction. **Safety** QSEN
- Teach patients to avoid any drugs that can cause urinary retention, especially anticholinergics, antihistamines, and decongestants if BPH is present. **Evidence-Based Practice** QSEN
- Remind patients wanting to use complementary and alternative therapies to check with their health care providers before using them.
- Eating a well-balanced diet with plenty of fish and fruits and vegetables may help prevent prostate cancer.
- Reinforce the man's option for managing prostate cancer; some procedures and drugs cause erectile dysfunction and incontinence either temporarily or permanently.
- Use the information listed in Chart 72-3 to teach patients urinary catheter care after prostate cancer surgery.

- Teach patients about not lifting more than 15 lb (6.8 kg) after open prostate surgery. **Safety** QSEN
- Options for erectile dysfunction (ED) include drug therapy (most common), vacuum assist devices, penile injections, transurethral suppositories, or penile implants.
- Be aware that African-American middle-aged men are the most at risk for prostate cancer; Euro-American young men are the most at risk for testicular cancer.
- Teach patients to report symptoms of radiation cystitis or proctitis to their health care provider as soon as possible; these complications resolve in 4 to 6 weeks after the end of radiation therapy.
- Teach patients and their partners about hormone therapy used to manage prostate cancer: LH-RH agonists and anti-androgen drugs.
- Be aware that sexually transmitted diseases (STDs) are a major cause of male reproductive system INFECTIONS.

CHAPTER 73

Care of Transgender Patients

Donna D. Ignatavicius and Stephanie M. Ignatavicius

http://evolve.elsevier.com/Iggy/

PRIORITY CONCEPTS

- SEXUALITY
- REPRODUCTION

LEARNING OUTCOMES

Safe and Effective Care Environment

1. Describe the need to collaborate with members of the health care team to provide high-quality care for transgender patients.
2. Explain the role of the nurse as a leader to promote advocacy for transgender people.

Health Promotion and Maintenance

3. Develop a health teaching plan for transgender patients who take hormone therapy and/or have gender reassignment surgery.
4. Identify appropriate resources for accurate trans-health information and ongoing preventive health care.

Psychosocial Integrity

5. Discuss how to use culturally sensitive terminology when providing care for transgender patients.
6. Identify the major sources of stress that contribute to transgender health issues.
7. Explain the major challenges for transgender patients in obtaining health care.

Physiological Integrity

8. Describe the side effects and adverse effects of feminizing and masculinizing hormone therapy, including effects of SEXUALITY and REPRODUCTION.
9. Identify laboratory test values that require monitoring for patients taking hormone therapy.
10. Describe the preoperative care needed for male-to-female or female-to-male patients having genital surgery.
11. Prioritize postoperative nursing care for patients having feminizing or masculinizing genital surgery.

The American Nurses Association (ANA) *Code of Ethics* states that the nurse practices with compassion and respect for the dignity and worth of every patient (ANA, 2001). The Institute of Medicine and the Quality and Safety Education for Nurses (QSEN) Institute further identified the need for nurses to be competent in patient-centered care (see Chapter 1). This competency ensures that nurses provide care with sensitivity and respect for diverse patients, even if those patients have values and preferences different from their own (ANA, 2001). Diversity is often discussed as ethnicity and race, but other cultural aspects such as sexual orientation and gender identity are part of the diverse human experience. An estimated 9 million people in the United States identify themselves as sexual and gender minorities (Gates, 2011).

People of minority sexual and gender identities are often grouped under one population category described by the acronym LGBTQ—lesbian, gay, bisexual, transgender, and queer/questioning (people who do not feel they belong in any other subgroup) (Table 73-1) (Eliason et al., 2013; Pettinato, 2012). Some literature includes only "LGBT." These evolving labels are misleading regarding people who identify as transgender. The grouping of SEXUALITY (sexual attraction and behavior) and gender identity (sense of maleness or femaleness) suggests that these two concepts are related or dependent upon one another, but they are different. *LGB* refers to specific sexual orientation. However, transgender people may identify as heterosexual, homosexual, both, or neither. Nurses and other health care professionals should not assume that transgender patients have the same experiences or health care needs as those who identify as lesbian, gay, or bisexual.

PATIENT-CENTERED TERMINOLOGY

Commonly, gender is categorized as one of two terms: *male* and *female.* For the majority of people, these descriptors are accurate. However, some people do not clearly fit into either category and may define themselves as *transgender.* Identifying oneself as transgender is not a choice or lifestyle but, rather, an inner sense of being born in the wrong body. When transgender people pursue ways of affirming their physical body and

TABLE 73-1 Appropriate Terminology Associated with Transgender Health

TERM	DEFINITION
Coming out	A lesbian, gay, bisexual, transgender, and queer/questioning (LGBTQ) person's public disclosure regarding sexual orientation or gender identity
Female-to-male	An adjective to describe people who were female at birth and are changing (or have changed) to a more masculine body or male
Gender dysphoria	Emotional or psychological distress caused by an incongruence between one's natal (birth) sex and gender identity
Gender identity	A person's inner sense of being a male, a female, or an alternative gender (e.g., genderqueer)
Genderqueer	An identity label used by some people whose gender identity does not conform to one of the two categories of male or female
Male-to-female	An adjective to describe people who were male at birth and are changing (or have changed) to a more feminine body or female
Sex (also called *natal sex*)	The gender assigned at one's birth
Sex reassignment surgery (SRS) (also called *gender reassignment surgery* or *gender affirmation surgery*)	A group of surgical procedures that change primary and/or secondary sex characteristics to affirm a person's gender identity
Transgender	An adjective to describe a person who crosses or transcends culturally defined categories of gender
Transition	The period of time when transgender people change from the gender role associated with their sex to a different gender role
Transsexual	Term often used by health care professionals to describe people who want to change or have changed their primary and/or secondary sex characteristics

appearance with their gender identity, their interaction with the health care system requires knowledge, respect, compassion, and specialized nursing care.

Using appropriate terminology is essential to demonstrating respect (see Table 73-1). Of utmost importance is the distinction between gender and sex. Gender, also known as **gender identity**, describes a person's inner sense of maleness or femaleness and is not related to reproductive anatomy. Gender identity describes one's social role as a man or a woman (American Psychiatric Association [APA], 2013). Sex, also known as *biological* or **natal sex**, refers to a person's genital anatomy present at birth (Edwards-Leeper & Spack, 2013).

When babies are born, the gender of the child is determined by the genitalia present, but there is no way of knowing the child's true sense of gender. The sense of gender and feelings toward maleness or femaleness can develop in children as early as age 2 years and is usually present in most children during the early elementary years. Transgender people feel a mismatch between their gender identity and natal sex, often extending back into early childhood. When this incongruence occurs, they can experience **gender dysphoria**, or discomfort with one's natal sex (APA, 2013; Edwards-Leeper & Spack, 2013). Some people who have gender dysphoria may seek interventions for sex reassignment to transition to the preferred gender.

The term "transgender" is often used as an umbrella description for all people whose gender identity and presentation do not conform to social expectations (Aramburu Alegria, 2011). In this text, **transgender** describes patients who self-identify as the opposite gender or a gender that does not match their natal sex (APA, 2013; Jenner, 2010). For proper usage, transgender should be used only in adjective form. For example, a patient "is transgender," "identifies as transgender," or "is a transgender patient." Note that "transgender" never ends in "-ed." The term "transgender" should not be used as a noun, and a patient should never be described as "*a* transgender."

According to *The Diagnostic and Statistical Manual of Mental Disorders* (APA, 2013), prevalence of gender dysphoria ranges from 5 to 14 in 1000 natal males and from 2 to 3 in 1000 natal females. However, these data describe the number of people who experience discontent with the gender they were assigned at birth and do not give an accurate estimate of the number of people who identify as transgender. Other studies have shown that the prevalence of transgender people is between 1 in 11,900 and 1 in 200,000 people (Coleman et al., 2011). Most scholars suggest that the prevalence is much higher, and more research is needed to collect more accurate demographic data for this population.

Another common term is **transsexual**, which generally describes a person who has modified his or her natal body to match the appropriate gender identity, either through cosmetic, hormonal, or surgical means (APA, 2013; Jenner, 2010). "Transsexual" can be used as both an adjective and a noun, such that a patient can be described "as transsexual" or "as a transsexual." People who were born with anatomically male parts but identify as and/or live as female are known as "male-to-female" or "MtF." Male-to-female people are also known as "transwomen," with the gender descriptor indicating the current-lived gender identity. Conversely, "transmen" are natal females who identify as and/or live as men. They are described as "female-to-male" or "FtM."

Transgender people are sometimes described as "transvestites" or "cross-dressers," often in a judgmental or negative manner. These terms should not be used unless the patient identifies as such. Other terms, such as "tranny," "he-she," or "shemale," are offensive and hurtful. These terms and other negative comments should never be used.

A patient may self-identify with any of the above terms or choose not to be defined at all. Become familiar with appropriate terms and concepts, but do not force definitions on your patients. Instead, if you are unsure how to address patients, during your nursing assessment ask them how they define their gender identity.

TRANSGENDER HEALTH ISSUES

Transgender people (also referred to as *trans-people*) encounter frequent discrimination and are faced with numerous stressful situations related to their identity. Sources of stress such as job discrimination and bias-related harassment can have an impact on patients' physical and psychological health. In a 2011 national survey on discrimination, the majority of transgender people had experienced mistreatment in the workplace. Also, almost half of transgender respondents reported loss of job or denial of promotion due to their transgender identity (Grant et al., 2011). As a result, they may be homeless, use alcohol or drugs as coping mechanisms, and ignore their health needs (Grant et al., 2011). In some cases they may turn to sex work (prostitution) as a mechanism for survival (Chestnut et al., 2013; Grant et al., 2011). Only a small subset of primarily MtF transgender people engage in sex work, which can expose them to human immune deficiency virus (HIV) and sexually transmitted disease (STD).

Transgender people are also vulnerable to bias-related violence and verbal harassment, including threats and intimidation (Chestnut et al., 2013; Shipherd et al., 2011). MtF people are more than 2 times more likely to experience physical violence and discrimination than non-transwomen; the likelihood of harassment is even greater for transwomen of color (Chestnut et al., 2013). A recent report indicated that half of LGBTQ-related hate crime homicides in the United States were committed against transwomen (Chestnut et al., 2013). Factors that increase this risk for violence include poverty, homelessness, and sex work.

Having an identity that puts a person at risk for violence and mistreatment can lead to emotional distress, particularly if the person has been directly victimized. Transgender people who have experienced traumatic situations may demonstrate manifestations of posttraumatic stress disorder (PTSD) and/or depression (Shipherd et al., 2011). They may turn to a variety of coping strategies to deal with distress, some of which can negatively impact physical health. In a 2010 national survey, 26% of transgender people reported current or previous alcohol or drug use to cope with discrimination and mistreatment; however, the number of people who use substances recreationally may be higher (Grant et al., 2010). Rates of smoking in the transgender community are higher than the rates in the LGB community and general population of U.S. adults. Most important, major life stressors, emotional distress, and lack of resources can lead to suicidal ideation or suicide attempt when all other methods of coping have failed. In a sample of over 7000 transgender adults, 41% reported at least one suicide attempt in their lifetime (Grant et al., 2010).

STRESS AND TRANSGENDER HEALTH

Transgender people have additional sources of stress when attempting to access health care, such as lack of health insurance due to unemployment. This barrier to health care causes them to postpone both acute and preventive medical care. For those people who are insured, coverage for health care related to gender transition (gender reassignment), such as hormone use and surgery, is often denied (Grant et al., 2010; Lombardi, 2010).

When transgender people gain access to health care, they are often fearful and anxious about the providers and setting. In particular, they may be hesitant to disclose their transgender status due to fear of discrimination or ridicule (Aramburu Alegria, 2011; Lombardi, 2010). They may also fear that this information will be documented in health records and shared with family members. This reluctance is increased if they have had previous negative experiences with health care providers. One national survey found that 19% of transgender adults were refused health care services due to their gender identity, while 28% reported receiving verbal harassment in a health care setting. Male-to-female transgender people were more likely to encounter discrimination and avoid health care due to these experiences (Grant et al., 2010). Even with providers who seem tolerant and caring with transgender patients, there is still a risk for patients overhearing jokes in the hallway and defamatory comments (Rounds et al., 2013).

Another source of stress faced by many transgender people is lack of health care–professional knowledge regarding health care needs (Aramburu Alegria, 2011; Jenner, 2010). When this situation occurs, transgender patients are put in a position of acting as health care experts, which can limit the quality of their care. While most transgender patients generally expect their providers to have some level of knowledge or know where to seek answers (Rounds et al., 2013), at least half of them find they have to teach their providers. When they encounter providers who are unfamiliar with the specific health care needs of their population, patient confidence is likely to diminish drastically and affect desire for future health care.

Whereas transgender patients may encounter providers who do not understand or who overlook their gender identity, some may encounter health care professionals who over-focus on it. Although it is important to be generally knowledgeable about a patient's gender status and understand how it may affect health care needs, this factor is not always relevant for every health problem. For example, transgender patients with fractures or influenza do not need to be extensively questioned about their gender identity. Whereas there are instances in which the presenting manifestations require transgender-specific care, there are also many other instances that require the same health care that all patients receive. At these times, most transgender patients prefer to be treated as any other patient (Rounds et al., 2013). Therefore use sound clinical judgment to decide if one's gender identity impacts patient assessment and care.

NEED TO IMPROVE TRANSGENDER HEALTH CARE

During the past few years, several national documents were published by the U.S. Department of Health and Human Services and private health care organizations that call for improvement in LGBTQ health care. These important publications include:

- *Healthy People 2020*
- The Institute of Medicine's (IOM) report on LGBT health
- The Joint Commission field guide for care of LGBT patients
- World Professional Association for Transgender Health standards of care

The U.S. Department of Health and Human Services' *Healthy People 2010* publication did *not* include the need to improve health care for LGBT people. As a result of this omission, a companion document was developed by the Gay and Lesbian Medical Association (GLMA) to address special health care needs of this population across the life span. Ten common health problems affecting the LGBT group were identified, including cancer, nutrition and weight, and sexually transmitted disease.

The *Healthy People 2020* agenda added objectives for improving the health of LGBT people, including the need to recognize and address the special health needs of transgender patients of all ages.

One major objective is to develop a system to identify patients who identify as LGBTQ. This objective is similar to the recommendation in the Institute of Medicine's (IOM) publication entitled *The Health of LGBT People: Building a Foundation for Better Understanding* (IOM, 2011).

The IOM LGBT health report calls for the need for more research to identify the special health care concerns of LGBT people of all ages. To help meet this outcome, the document outlined the need to collect more demographic data to better identify this population. LGBTQ people need to feel safe when disclosing this very personal information.

In 2011, The Joint Commission (TJC) published a similar document that recommends ways for health care agencies to create a welcoming and safe environment for LGBT patients. In response to growing attention to the need for cultural competence for all health care professionals and to provide quality health care for sexual and gender minority patients, TJC published a field guide for health care agencies to improve LGBT patient care (TJC, 2011). Chart 73-1 lists the recommendations for health care agencies in designing a safe environment for LGBT patient care. Fig. 73-1 shows an example of a "safe zone" image that should be used to reassure these patients that they are in a safe place where they can receive respectful and knowledgeable quality care.

Also in 2011, the World Professional Association for Transgender Health (WPATH) updated its standards of care (Coleman et al., 2011). This document outlines core principles that nurses and other health care professionals should follow when caring for transgender patients (Table 73-2).

CHART 73-1 Best Practice for Patient Safety & Quality Care (QSEN)

The Joint Commission Recommendations for Creating a Safe, Welcoming Environment for LGBTQ Patients

- Post the *Patients' Bill of Rights* and nondiscrimination policies in a visible place.
- Make waiting rooms inclusive of LGBTQ patients and families, such as posting *Safe Zone,* rainbow, or pink triangle signs.
- Designate unisex or single-stall restrooms.
- Ensure that visitation policies are equitable for families of LGBTQ patients.
- Avoid assumptions about any patient's sexual orientation and gender identity.
- Include gender-neutral language on all medical forms and documents; e.g., "partnered" in addition to married, single, or divorced categories.
- Reflect the patient's choice of terminology in communication and documentation.
- Provide information on special health concerns for LGBTQ patients.
- Become knowledgeable about LGBTQ health needs and care.
- Refer LGBTQ patients to qualified health care professionals as needed.
- Provide community resources for LGBTQ information and support as needed.

Adapted from The Joint Commission (TJC). (2011). *Advancing effective communication, cultural competence, and patient- and family-centered care for the lesbian, gay, bisexual, and transgender community.* Retrieved September 2013, from www.jointcommission.org/lgbt.

❖ PATIENT-CENTERED COLLABORATIVE CARE

◆ Assessment

As with any patient, it is best to ask during the nursing history and physical assessment how he or she prefers to be addressed. For example, for non-transgender patients, some people may go by a nickname or by their middle name and prefer to be addressed as such. For transgender patients, it is not uncommon for driver's licenses, insurance cards, and other forms of identification to retain their birth names (and by extension, birth sex) because it can be difficult to change this information,

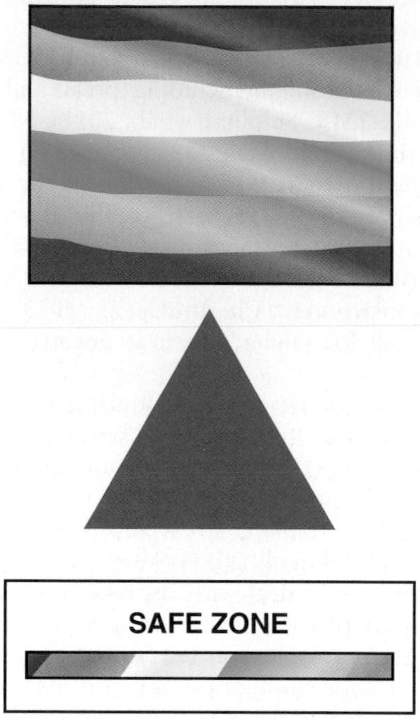

FIG. 73-1 The Safe Zone—rainbow or pink triangle signs welcome LGBTQ patients in a health care agency.

TABLE 73-2 Core Principles for Health Care Professionals Who Care for Transgender Patients

- Become knowledgeable about the health care needs of transgender and other gender-nonconforming people.
- Become knowledgeable about the treatment options for transgender patients and required follow-up care.
- Do not assume that all transgender patients are the same; treat each one as an individual and develop an individualized plan of care.
- Demonstrate respect for patients with nonconforming gender identities.
- Provide culturally sensitive care and use appropriate terminology that affirms the patient's gender identity.
- Facilitate patient access to appropriate and knowledgeable health care providers.
- Seek informed consent before providing treatment.
- Offer continuity of care or refer patients for ongoing quality health care.
- Advocate for patients within their families and communities.

Adapted from Coleman, E., Bockting, W., Botzer, M., Cohen-Kettenis, P., DeCuypere, G., Fladman, J., et al., (2011). Standards of care for the health of transsexual, transgender, and gender-nonconforming people (Version 7). *International Journal of Transgenderism, 13,* 165-232; Rounds, K.E., McGrath, B.B., & Walsh, E. (2013). Perspectives on provider behaviors: A qualitative study of sexual and gender minorities regarding quality of care. *Contemporary Nurse, 44*(1), 99-110.

particularly if a person is in the process of transitioning. Therefore nurses may receive patient documentation with misleading patient data. For example, a nurse may receive a health care record listing a male name and birth sex yet encounter a patient presenting as female in appearance. It can be offensive and embarrassing for the patient who clearly identifies as female to be called "Mister," "sir," or the male birth name. Not only does it communicate disrespect, it also signals to the patient that she may receive inadequate care or that the environment is unsafe.

In addition to preferred names, correct pronoun usage is also important. Each patient has his or her own preference. For example, an MtF patient may visit a clinic during lunch hour at work. Because the patient has not disclosed the transgender identity at work, this patient maintains male dress and demeanor at the office. Though the patient may identify as female and live as female at home, the patient may request the nurse to use male pronouns (he, him, his) to match the patient's current presentation and may not disclose the transgender identity to the nurse. Conversely, even though the patient presents at the time as male, the patient may request the nurse to use female pronouns (she, her, hers) because the patient identifies with a female gender identity.

In general, use pronouns that match the patient's physical presentation and dress. Even though the biological sex may not match, patients presenting as female should be addressed as female and patients presenting as male should be addressed as male. With changing styles and trends, it can sometimes be difficult to assess by clothing alone. However, with a patient whose birth sex is listed as female yet presents in traditionally male attire, facial hair, and a men's hairstyle, it is most appropriate to address this patient as male. Understandably, the clinical setting can be fast-paced and nurses may encounter multiple patients at a time; however, taking time to use clinical judgment is important. Appropriately interacting with a transgender patient can sometimes mean the difference between the patient continuing to seek health care or not.

In a few cases, patients may not identify as male or female and prefer to not use male or female pronouns. These patients often feel that the binary gender system in which a person must fit clearly into one category or the other is too limiting. Though this is a small subset of the transgender population, it is important to be aware of this subculture in case you encounter a patient who refuses to identify with a specific gender or instead identifies as genderqueer (the Q in LGBTQ). Genderqueer patients may request the use of gender neutral pronouns, or they may use these pronouns in the nurse's presence. For many genderqueer people, the pronoun "they" is preferred instead of "he" or "she."

Getting used to using the correct name or pronoun can take some time. Occasionally, nurses will know their patient's preferred name or pronoun but accidentally say the wrong one. Transgender patients encounter this situation often and typically anticipate an error at times. When this error occurs, it is best to self-correct and continue with care rather than make a prolonged apology. Focusing too much on the error may make the patient more uncomfortable because more attention has been drawn to the situation. Most transgender patients, particularly those who live full time in their gender-affirming role, wish to be treated like any other patient.

History. Interventions for transgender people who experience gender dysphoria (discomfort with one's natal sex) include one or more of these options (Coleman et al., 2011):

- Changes in gender expression that may involve living part time or full time in another gender role
- Psychotherapy to explore gender identity and expression, improve body image, or strengthen coping mechanisms
- Hormone therapy to feminize or masculinize the body
- Surgery to change primary and/or secondary sex characteristics (e.g., the breasts/chest, facial features, internal and/or external genitalia)

During the health history, inquire about which interventions the patient has had, if any, or if there are plans to have them in the future. Ask about current use of *drug therapy,* including hormones and other feminizing or masculinizing agents, including silicone injections. These medications are usually prescribed by endocrinologists or other specialists in transgender health care, but some patients may obtain them from nonmedical sources, including the Internet.

Exogenous hormone therapy can cause adverse health problems and requires careful patient monitoring, including laboratory testing. For example, estrogen therapy can cause increased health risks such as increased blood clotting causing venous thromboembolism (VTE), elevated blood glucose, hypertension, estrogen-dependent cancers, and fluid retention (Brennan et al., 2012). Smoking and obesity increase these risks. The risks also increase with higher doses of the medication. Ask the patient about a history of these problems.

Inquire about the patient's *surgical history.* For the MtF patient, ask about breast surgery and any surgical changes to the genitalia, such as a penectomy (removal of the penis) and vaginoplasty (creation of a vagina). The MtF patient still has the prostate gland. For older patients, ask about any problems with prostate health problems, such as urinary dribbling and retention. For the FtM patient, ask whether a hysterectomy, bilateral salpingo-oophorectomy (BSO), mastectomy, phalloplasty (creation of a penis), and/or scrotoplasty (creation of a scrotum) was performed.

Keep in mind that health insurance usually does not cover the cost of the transition process and patients may seek alternative care. For example, hormones may be obtained illegally or from countries that do not have quality controls for medication. MtF patients may seek silicone for creating breasts from nonmedical people, causing a high risk for hepatitis C and silicone complications (Brennan et al., 2012). Ask patients about the use of these alternatives as a part of their transition process.

Physical Assessment. Be sure to review the transgender patient's health record carefully before performing a physical assessment. Be culturally sensitive, nonjudgmental, and respectful during the assessment. Be aware that transgender patients may be young, middle-aged, or older adults.

CONSIDERATIONS FOR OLDER ADULTS

Patient-Centered Care QSEN

Transgender patients who are older than 65 years lived in an era when most of them concealed their sexual orientation and true gender identity due to social stigma. These people have not been well studied as a group, but research indicates that those who lived with a partner have fewer mental health problems and better self-esteem compared with those who lived alone (Brennan et al., 2012).

When assessing transgender patients, be aware that they will be in varying stages of transition. Some patients present with no obvious physical signs that they are in the process of transitioning. Others have had gender reassignment surgery such that their new appearance matches their gender identity. Realize a transgender patient's genitalia may not match his or her physical appearance.

Psychosocial Assessment. If gender and SEXUALITY are relevant to the patient's presenting health problem, ask specific questions to determine how these factors may impact care. Reassure patients that their responses are confidential and will not be shared with any family, friends, or significant others without the patient's permission. However, evidence of abuse must be reported as mandated by law. Appropriate screening questions about gender and sexuality include (Coleman et al., 2011):

- Are you experiencing any challenges, concerns, or anxiety related to your sexuality?
- Related to your gender, how do you identify?
- Are you experiencing any sadness, depression, or thoughts of hurting yourself?
- Have you experienced any violence or discrimination in your personal or work life?
- Are you currently being seen by a counselor or psychologist related to your sexuality and gender identity? If so, why?

If the responses to these questions indicate that the patient has potential or actual mental health problems, consult with the health care provider for further evaluation by a qualified mental health care professional, such as a clinical psychologist.

◆ Interventions

Nurses care for transgender patients who are transitioning or have completed gender reassignment. They may care for them for health problems related to their transition process or for problems that are unrelated to the patient's SEXUALITY or gender identity. In general, care for transgender patients with most health problems is the same as for any other patient. However, some interventions such as hormone therapy may affect nursing assessment and care. As a leader in health care, advocate for transgender patients and provide health teaching to promote their health. Encourage them to include their sexual partner, if any, in discussions about the transition process.

Nonsurgical Management. The primary nonsurgical interventions for transgender patients include drug (hormone) therapy, counseling about REPRODUCTION and reproductive health, and vocal therapy. The type of intervention depends on whether the patient is transitioning from MtF or FtM.

Drug Therapy. Drug therapy may be started after a psychosocial assessment by a qualified mental health care professional and informed consent has been obtained. According to WPATH's most recent standards of care, the criteria for hormone therapy include:

- Continuing and well-documented gender dysphoria
- Patient ability to make a fully informed decision and give consent to treatment
- Patient older than 18 years
- Well-controlled existing medical or mental health problems, if any

Drugs for MtF Patients. Patients transitioning from male to female (MtF) typically take a combination of estrogen therapy and androgen-reducing medications to achieve feminizing effects. Expected physical changes from *estrogen therapy* are breast enlargement, thinning hair, decreased testicular size, decreased erectile function, and increased body fat compared with muscle mass (Table 73-3). Because oral estrogen (ethinyl estradiol) can increase the risk for venous thromboembolism, transdermal estrogen (Climara) or injectable estradiol is preferred for use in transgender patients. The typical dosing is two 0.1-mg patches changed twice weekly (Aramburu Alegria, 2011). Injectable estradiol is usually prescribed in a dose between 5 and 20 mg IM every 2 weeks. Progesterone may also be prescribed for 10 days each month.

Before the first dose of transdermal estrogen, teach the patient to apply the patch to an area that is hairless to ensure good contact with the skin. When changing to a new patch, wash any excess drug from the skin where the previous patch was applied.

Teach patients taking any form of estrogen about side effects such as headache, breast tenderness, nausea/vomiting, and weight gain (often due to fluid retention) or loss. Tell them to report increased feelings of anxiety or depression to their health care provider. Estrogens can also cause estrogen-dependent cancers, hypertension (due to fluid retention), venous thromboembolism (VTE) such as deep vein thrombosis (DVT), and gallbladder disease (Brennan et al., 2012). Teach patients to follow up with their health care provider to monitor for these potential adverse drug effects. Diagnostic testing is part of follow-up and monitoring, as listed in Table 73-3.

TABLE 73-3 Feminizing Drug Therapy for MtF Patients: Expected Changes and Monitoring

Expected Physical Changes
- Enlargement of breast tissue (gynecomastia)
- Decreased testicular size
- Decreased erectile function
- Decreased libido (sex drive)
- Decreased body hair growth
- Decreased male pattern baldness
- Increased fat compared with muscle
- Softening of skin

Laboratory/Imaging Studies
- Chemistry panel (including glucose and electrolytes)
- Liver function tests
- Lipid profile
- Complete blood count
- Prostate-specific antigen (PSA) if recommended for age-group
- Mammogram (when breast tissue develops)
- Papanicolaou (Pap) smear (if vagina present)

NCLEX EXAMINATION CHALLENGE

Physiological Integrity

The nurse provides health teaching for a client receiving estrogen therapy. Which statement by the client indicates a need for further teaching?

A. "I need to check my blood pressure frequently when taking this drug."
B. "I will call my doctor if I have any redness or swelling in my legs."
C. "I will drink extra fluids because this drug will cause me to urinate a lot."
D. "I will eat more oranges and bananas to replace the potassium I lose."

In addition to estrogen therapy, androgen-reducing agents (anti-androgens) are often given to block the effects of testosterone, including (Coleman et al., 2011):

- Spironolactone (Aldactone), a low-cost diuretic that also inhibits testosterone secretion and androgen binding to androgen receptors.
- 5-alpha reductase inhibitors (e.g., finasteride [Proscar]), drugs typically used to treat benign prostatic hyperplasia (BPH). These drugs block the conversion of testosterone to a more active ingredient to decrease the hair loss associated with estrogen therapy and shrink prostate tissue.
- GnRH agonists (e.g., goserelin [Zoladex]), neurohormones that block the gonadotropin-releasing hormone receptor, thus inhibiting the release of the follicle-stimulating hormone (FSH) and luteinizing hormone (LH). These drugs are more expensive and are available only as implants and parenteral preparations.

! NURSING SAFETY PRIORITY (QSEN)

Drug Alert

Teach patients taking *spironolactone* to monitor their blood pressure and have periodic laboratory tests to assess for hyperkalemia if the health care provider determines them to be at risk for these drug effects. Remind them that increased serum potassium can cause cardiac dysrhythmias and skeletal muscle spasticity.

Common side effects of finasteride and other *5-alpha reductase inhibitors* include dizziness, cold sweats, and chills. These manifestations typically decrease over time. If patients continue to have these side effects, instruct them to contact their health care provider.

Teach patients receiving *GnRH agonists* how to self-administer subcutaneous injections. Major side effects of these drugs are tachycardia and other cardiac dysrhythmias. Remind patients to follow up with their health care provider to monitor heart rate and rhythm. Teach them to call 911 if they experience chest pain.

Drugs for FtM Patients. Testosterone is the major drug used for achieving masculinizing effects in transgender people transitioning from female to male; however, much of the available drug converts to estrogen in the body (Coleman et al., 2011). This drug can be taken orally, transdermally, or parenterally (IM). Buccal and implantable forms of testosterone are also available. Oral testosterone (Andriol) is the least effective form of the drug. Depo-Testosterone, the most common IM preparation, is usually started in a low dose and increased to 100 to 200 mg every 1 to 2 weeks (Lilley et al., 2014). Teach patients the importance of not sharing needles to prevent bloodborne diseases such as hepatitis C.

AndroGel and Androderm are topical forms that are more expensive than other testosterone preparations but may provide more consistent (though slower) results. A new topical form of the drug, Axiron, can be applied to the armpits to increase serum testosterone levels. For all topical testosterone preparations, be sure that the patient washes his hands between applications and covers the area with clothing.

Expected effects of testosterone therapy include deepening of the voice, increased libido (sex drive), increased body hair growth, breast and ovarian atrophy, clitoral enlargement, and cessation of menses (Aramburu Alegria, 2011; Jenner, 2010) (Table 73-4). Teach the patient taking testosterone that some of these changes take up to a year to appear. If menses does not stop in the first few months of drug therapy, the patient is placed on Depo-Provera (progesterone) every 3 months until the testosterone becomes effective.

TABLE 73-4 Masculinizing Drug Therapy for FtM Patients: Expected Changes and Monitoring

Expected Changes	Laboratory/Imaging Studies
• Voice deepening • Body hair growth (hirsutism) • Breast atrophy • Increased libido • Increased aggression • Clitoral growth • Redistribution of fat • Laryngeal prominence	• Lipid profile • Liver function tests • Complete blood count • Papanicolaou (Pap) smear (if vagina present) • Mammogram (if breast tissue present)

Common side effects of testosterone therapy include edema, acne, seborrhea (oily skin), headaches, weight gain, and possible psychotic symptoms. Before taking this medication, the patient is screened for a history of liver and heart disease. Testosterone therapy can cause increased liver enzymes, increased low-density lipoproteins (LDLs, or "bad" cholesterol), and decreased high-density lipoproteins (HDLs, or "good" cholesterol). Increased blood glucose and decreased clotting factors can also occur when taking the drug (Aramburu Alegria, 2011). Teach patients that these changes can lead to diabetes, heart disease, and stroke. Therefore remind patients that they need to follow up with their health care providers for careful monitoring for these complications, including having extensive diagnostic and laboratory testing (see Table 73-4).

Reproductive Health Options. Using feminizing or masculinizing hormone therapy affects reproductive health, especially fertility. Therefore be sure that patients know their options for REPRODUCTION, if desired, *before* transition begins (Coleman et al., 2011). MtF patients may want to consider sperm banking prior to drug therapy or gender reassignment surgery if they desire to have a biologic child. FtM patients may want to consider oocyte (egg) or embryo freezing. These frozen gametes or embryo could be implanted in a surrogate woman to become pregnant and carry to birth. Inform patients that these options are expensive, but be sure all patients are informed. Be sure to include the patient's sexual partner, if any, in discussions related to reproductive options.

Voice and Communication Therapy. Communication is an essential aspect of human behavior and gender expression. Voice deepening for transgender people who are transitioning from female to male is accomplished by taking masculinizing hormones, such as testosterone. However, feminizing hormones have no effect on the adult MtF voice.

MtF patients may seek assistance from a voice and communication specialist to help them develop certain vocal characteristics, such as pitch and intonation. Vocal therapy can assist in management of gender dysphoria and be a positive step in the transition process. Specialists include speech-language pathologists and speech-voice clinicians. Remind patients to seek a specialist who is licensed, knowledgeable in transgender health, and has specialized training in assessment and development of communication skills for transgender patients (Coleman et al., 2011).

The purpose of vocal therapy is to help patients adapt their voice and communication such that it is authentic and reflects their gender identity. The voice therapist should take the patient's communication preferences and style into consideration as part of the assessment process to develop an individualized treatment plan. Some patients choose follow-up sessions for vocal therapy following voice feminization surgery, also called *feminization laryngoplasty.* This surgery is described in the next section.

Surgical Management. Many transgender people are satisfied with their gender identity, role, and self-expression without surgery. Surgery, particularly procedures that affect the external or internal genitalia, is usually the last and most carefully considered option for transitioning from one's natal sex to one's inner gender identity. These procedures are often referred to as **gender** or **sex reassignment surgery (SRS)**. The patient has a number of surgical options to achieve either feminizing or masculinizing effects. Regardless of the procedure performed, the nurse collaborates with the patient, family, and health care team to promote positive outcomes for the transition process.

Gender reassignment surgeries are procedures that alter anatomically normal structures. Not all surgeons feel comfortable in performing procedures that could "harm" transgender patients. However, these procedures help treat gender dysphoria (discomfort with one's natal sex) (Coleman et al., 2011). Some patients elect to undergo the full range of surgeries, whereas others choose to have only some or none of them. Most health insurance plans do not cover their cost (Aramburu Alegria, 2011).

Genital surgeries "below the waist" are the most invasive procedures. The criteria for genital surgery depend on the type of surgery being requested. For example, most surgeons (usually urologists or plastic surgeons) require 12 months of hormone therapy plus one or two referrals from qualified psychotherapists for MtF patients who desire an orchiectomy (removal of testes). The same requirements are needed for FtM patients who desire a hysterectomy (uterus removal) and bilateral salpingo-oophorectomy (BSO, or removal of both fallopian tubes and ovaries) (Reed, 2011).

The psychotherapist assesses the patient's readiness for genital surgery and hormone therapy, including a discussion of risks and out-of-pocket costs. The patient's support system is assessed to ensure that the patient makes the best possible decision and achieves the desired outcomes.

For MtF patients requesting a vaginoplasty (creation of a vagina) or FtM patients desiring a phalloplasty (creation of a penis), the required criteria include 12 continuous months of living in a gender role that is congruent with the patient's gender identity. It is also recommended that these patients have regular visits with a mental health care professional (Coleman et al., 2011).

Feminizing Surgeries for MtF Patients. Feminizing surgeries are performed for MtF patients to create a functional and/or aesthetic (cosmetic) female anatomy, including (Brennan et al., 2012; Coleman et al., 2011):

- Breast/chest surgeries, such as breast augmentation (mammoplasty to increase breast tissue).
- Genital surgeries, such as partial penectomy (removal of the penis), orchiectomy (removal of the testes), vaginoplasty and labiaplasty vulvoplasty (creation of a vagina and labia/vulva), clitoroplasty (creation of a clitoris).
- Other surgeries, such as facial feminizing surgery (to achieve feminine facial contour), liposuction (fatty tissue removal), often from the waist or abdominal area, vocal feminizing surgery, gluteal augmentation (to enlarge buttocks), and other body-contouring procedures.

Breast augmentation creates breast tissue for the MtF patient through the use of silicone or saline implants. Although not a prerequisite, it is recommended that MtF patients take feminizing hormones for 12 months prior to surgery for the best results (Coleman et al., 2011). Perioperative care of any patient having this procedure is discussed in Chapter 70 on p. 1463.

Voice surgery, such as reduction thyroid chondroplasty, is performed to decrease the size of the "Adam's apple." The procedure is done through a bronchoscope for cosmetic purposes. Nursing care of the patient having a bronchoscopy is discussed in Chapter 27.

The most common "below the waist" genital surgeries for MtF patients are bilateral *orchiectomy* to remove the testes and vaginoplasty with partial penectomy. Orchiectomy procedures and associated nursing care are the same for the transgender patient as they are for other natal males (see Chapter 72 for a detailed discussion).

A **vaginoplasty** is the construction of a neovagina (new vagina) usually with inverted penile tissue (obtained during a partial penectomy) or a colon graft. The procedure also includes creating a clitoris and labia using scrotal or penile tissue and skin grafts. Using penile tissue creates a less appealing appearance and low patient satisfaction (Reed, 2011).

Preoperative Care. In addition to the required criteria to qualify for a vaginoplasty (also called *transvaginal surgery*), the transgender patient is medically evaluated like any other presurgical patient. Patients who have poorly controlled diabetes with vascular complications, coronary artery disease, or other systemic disease that limits functional ability are not candidates for gender reassignment surgery. Chapter 14 describes general preoperative care for any patient.

The surgeon explains the options for selected procedures, postoperative care expectations, and potential for complications after surgery. Postoperative recovery for transvaginal surgery takes a long time and has a high complication rate (Reed, 2011). Overweight patients have a higher incidence of wound infection and may have problems with adequate ventilation (breathing) and ambulation after surgery. Refer these patients for nutritional counseling as needed.

Written and verbal preoperative instructions are provided by the surgeon, including optional methods of body hair removal. A bowel preparation may be started 24 hours before surgery and includes a clear liquid diet, laxatives, and Fleet's enemas. Increased fluids are recommended until the patient goes to bed the night before surgery because the bowel "prep" can be very dehydrating. Antimicrobials such as neomycin sulfate and metronidazole (Flagyl) are typically given on the day of surgery to minimize the risk for infection.

Some surgeons require that the patient take supplements to prevent bruising and promote tissue healing, such as vitamin C. Patients who are very thin are encouraged to eat a high-protein diet. A powdered protein supplement with arginine (an amino acid) may also be prescribed to promote wound healing.

Patients have a number of laboratory tests to ensure they are healthy before surgery. Adequate hemoglobin and hematocrit (H&H) levels are especially important because some blood is lost during surgery. For patients who have low H&H levels, an erythropoietin such as epoetin alfa (Procrit) or IM testosterone with iron is given. Most patients choose testosterone because it is a lower-cost drug.

Operative Procedures. Because surgery requires multiple procedures to create a female anatomy, the patient is on the operating table for about 5 hours. The surgery may be performed in a hospital or specialized center for transgender surgeries. After general or epidural anesthesia is administered, the patient is placed in a lithotomy position (feet in stirrups) for the procedure. Epidural anesthesia is preferred for patients who are asthmatic or obese. The patient is transferred to the postanesthesia care unit (PACU) with a perineal dressing and packing, Jackson-Pratt drain, and indwelling urinary catheter.

Postoperative Care. Provide general postoperative care as described in Chapter 16. In addition, immediately after surgery, apply an ice pack to the perineum to decrease pain and bruising. Monitor the patient's pain level carefully, and offer analgesia as needed. Genital surgery is painful because there is a high concentration of nerve endings in the perineum.

Although not a common postoperative complication, monitor the patient for bleeding. Observe the surgical dressing and surrounding area for oozing or bright red blood. Report and document any indication of bleeding immediately to the surgeon, and keep the patient in bed.

Encourage the patient to drink liquids after surgery; discontinue the patient's IV line once oral fluids are tolerated. Evaluate the patient's intake and output every 8 to 12 hours.

! NURSING SAFETY PRIORITY QSEN

Action Alert

Patients are in a lithotomy position for an extended period during surgery. Therefore, after surgery, monitor lower extremity neurovascular status and encourage the patient to move the legs often during the first 24 hours after surgery. Report and document any unexpected findings, such as continued numbness or inability to move the lower legs or feet. Patients who had epidural anesthesia are not able to move their legs for several hours after surgery until the effect of the drug diminishes.

All patients stay in the hospital for at least one night after surgery, but some patients may stay longer depending on the number and complexity of the surgical procedures. Some agencies transfer the patient the day after surgery to a local hotel for continued follow-up and monitoring by a health care professional (usually a nurse) (Reed, 2011). Collaborate with the case manager for discharge planning and follow-up care.

The Jackson Pratt drain is removed typically in 3 to 5 days after surgery when drainage is less than 15 to 20 mL in a 24-hour period. In about a week after surgery, the surgical pressure dressing, packing, and external sutures are removed.

At this time, patients are taught how to douche and insert vaginal stents to dilate the vagina. Sexual intercourse also helps keep the vagina dilated. Remind patients that routine douching and douching after intercourse are needed to prevent infection in the new vagina. A solution of vinegar and water or a commercial product such as Massengill can be used. Vaginal stents (also called *dilators*) must be inserted several times a day for months after surgery. The stent should remain in the vagina for 30 to 45 minutes or as instructed by the surgeon. Teach patients the importance of using the stents with water-based lubrication. Collaborate with the surgeon to determine patient-specific instructions.

The urinary catheter is removed between postoperative day 7 and 12. Early removal can cause urinary retention (Reed, 2011).

TABLE 73-5 Postoperative Complications of Vaginoplasty Surgery

Most Serious Complications
- Vaginal-rectal fistula
- Rectal perforation
- Bleeding

Other Complications
- Surgical wound infection
- Urinary leakage/incontinence
- Chronic urinary tract infections
- Urinary meatus stenosis
- Vaginal stenosis
- Vaginal collapse
- Labial hematoma
- Inadequate vaginal length or width
- Lack of sensation
- Lack of sexual pleasure

Patients should continue follow-up visits with their health care provider for manifestations of complications. One of the worst complications is a vaginal-rectal fistula, which is caused by rectal perforation during surgery (Reed, 2011). Teach patients to report any leakage of stool into the vagina immediately to their surgeon. The treatment for this complication is a temporary colostomy and fistula wound management for many months. Other surgical complications of vaginoplasty are listed in Table 73-5.

In addition to physical complications after surgery, some MtF patients are not satisfied with the quality of the results. For example, the neovagina may not be functional for sexual intercourse. Some patients request another surgery to achieve more satisfying results.

? NCLEX EXAMINATION CHALLENGE

Physiological Integrity

A client is admitted to the postanesthesia care unit (PACU) following a vaginoplasty. Which nursing interventions are appropriate for this client? **Select all that apply.**

A. Irrigate the nasogastric tube every 4 hours.
B. Keep the client in a sitting position to facilitate breathing.
C. Apply an ice pack to the perineal area.
D. Monitor drainage from the Jackson-Pratt tube.
E. Perform frequent neurovascular assessments of the legs.

Masculinizing Surgeries for FtM Patients. Masculinizing surgeries are performed for FtM patients to create a functional and/or aesthetic male anatomy, including (Brennan et al., 2012; Coleman et al., 2011):

- Breast/chest surgeries, usually a bilateral mastectomy (removal of both breasts) and chest reconstruction.
- Genital surgeries, such as a hysterectomy and bilateral BSO, vaginectomy (removal of the vagina), phalloplasty (creation of an average-size male penis) with ureteroplasty (creation of a urethra) or metoidioplasty (creation of a small penis using hormone-enhanced clitoral tissue), and scrotoplasty (creation of a scrotum) with insertion of testicular prostheses.
- Other surgeries, such as liposuction, pectoral muscle implants, and other body-contouring procedures.

Care of transgender patients having a mastectomy, hysterectomy, and bilateral salpingo-oophorectomy (BSO) is similar to care for any patient having these procedures as described elsewhere in this text. If the transgender patient has not had previous abdominal surgery, a laparoscopic procedure is preferred for the hysterectomy and BSO surgery.

Surgery to create a penis has not been as successful as other gender reassignment procedures. Procedures to create a male anatomy are not performed as often as MtF surgeries. Phalloplasties are the most difficult reconstructive genital surgeries to perform and usually require several stages. Skin flaps from the radial forearm, anterior lateral thigh, or back are used to create the penis. Fat grafts may be needed to increase penile girth, and buccal mucosal tissue may be used to create the urethra. A penile prosthesis or implant is not inserted until months after surgery until the initial surgical healing has occurred.

Complications from phalloplasty include urinary tract stenosis, donor graft site scarring, and occasionally necrosis of the neopenis (new penis). In addition to these physical problems, the patient may not be satisfied with the results of the surgery, such as an inadequate length of the penis. For this reason, most FtM patients do not have this procedure and prefer to have only a laparoscopic hysterectomy and BSO (Coleman et al., 2011).

CLINICAL JUDGMENT CHALLENGE

Patient-Centered Care; Teamwork and Collaboration QSEN

A 58-year-old male-appearing patient visits the gender identity clinic to discuss the desire to have sex reassignment surgery (SRS). As the clinical nurse, you take the patient's history and find that the patient was married to a woman for 30 years and had three children. The couple divorced 3 months ago when the patient's wife discovered that her husband identified as a woman. The couple's children have no contact with the patient since they found out that their father has been dressing as a woman for the past few weeks. The patient is employed as the vice-president of a large commercial construction company and has health insurance. The patient is interested in learning about his options for male-to-female transitioning.

1. How would you address this patient?
2. What other data do you need to collect for the patient's history and why?
3. What options for transitioning to a female does this patient have?
4. Is SRS the best first step for MtF patients? Why or why not?
5. After a physical examination, the clinic physician prescribed estrogen and spironolactone for the patient. What instructions will you provide for the patient before beginning drug therapy?
6. What health teaching does the patient need regarding ongoing follow-up and monitoring while taking these feminizing drugs?
7. With whom might you need to collaborate to manage the patient's care now and in the future?

Community-Based Care

Transgender patients often take hormone therapy for many years. Teach them that ongoing follow-up with a qualified health care professional is needed to maintain health and detect any complications, such as diabetes or cardiovascular problems, as early as possible.

Long-term follow-up with the surgeon after gender reassignment is essential to detect and treat the frequent complications that occur. Assess the patient's support systems and coping strategies, including financial status and health insurance benefits. Collaborate with the case manager to ensure a smooth transition into the community, including the need for any ongoing mental health counseling or therapy.

Urogenital care is also needed for patients who have gender reassignment surgery. FtM patients usually do not have a vaginectomy and therefore may experience vaginal atrophy causing itching and burning. Recommend that they seek gynecologic care to treat this problem, although the examination can be physically and emotionally painful.

MtF patients need counseling about sexuality, genital hygiene, and prevention of sexually transmitted diseases. They are also at a high risk for frequent urinary tract infections as a result of a shortened urethra and urinary incontinence as a result of genital surgery (Coleman et al., 2011). Teach patients the importance of having follow-up care for these problems.

Preventive health care screenings for transgender patients are also important. For example, the MtF patient requires prostate health care screenings like natal males. Mammograms are also recommended to monitor for early signs of breast cancer.

A number of community resources and organizations are available for transgender support and information, such as:

- National Coalition for LGBT Health (http://lgbthealth.webolutionary.com/content/resources)
- National Resource Center for LGBT Aging (www.lgbtagingcenter.org)
- Services and Advocacy for Gay, Lesbian, Bisexual, and Transgender Elders (www.sageusa.org)
- University of San Francisco Center for Transgender Health (www.transhealth.ucsf.edu)
- World Professional Association for Transgender Health (www.wpath.org)

GET READY FOR THE NCLEX® EXAMINATION!

KEY POINTS

Review these Key Points for each NCLEX Examination Client Needs Category.

Safe and Effective Care Environment

- Depending on identified health care needs, collaborate with the primary health care provider, mental health professional, surgeon, pharmacist, and/or vocal/speech specialist when caring for the transgender patient. **Teamwork and Collaboration** QSEN
- Advocate for the transgender patient who is often distrustful of health care professionals and fearful when seeking health care. **Patient-Centered Care** QSEN

Health Promotion and Maintenance

- Teach patients taking hormone therapy about the need for ongoing health care monitoring for adverse drug events and health complications. **Safety** QSEN

- Refer the transgender patient and significant others, as appropriate, to community resources for information and support, such as the University of San Francisco Center for Transgender Health and the Services and Advocacy for Gay, Lesbian, Bisexual, and Transgender Elders (SAGE) organization.

Psychosocial Integrity
- Use culturally sensitive and accurate language when communicating with transgender patients; use pronouns that match the patient's physical appearance and dress unless the patient requests a specific term (see Table 73-1). **Patient-Centered Care** QSEN
- Provide transgender care with dignity and respect for all patients.
- Be aware that transgender people often have gender dysphoria, which presents an inner conflict between the person's natal (birth) sex and perceived gender identity.
- Assess transgender patients for sources of stress in the community that can lead to health issues, such as depression, anxiety, and substance abuse.
- Be aware that transgender patients may avoid health care settings because they are often unemployed, have no health insurance, and/or fear lack of respect and understanding based on previous experiences. **Patient-Centered Care** QSEN

Physiological Integrity
- Monitor for expected, side, and adverse effects of hormone therapy as described in Tables 73-3 and 73-4.
- Recognize that patients receiving hormone therapy need to have periodic laboratory testing to monitor for complications as listed in Tables 73-3 and Table 73-4. **Evidence-Based Practice** QSEN
- Provide preoperative care for a patient having a vaginoplasty, including teaching about bowel preparation, food and fluid intake, hair removal methods, and the need for informed consent.
- Monitor for potentially life-threatening complications of sex reassignment surgery, such as fistula development, bleeding, and wound infection.

74 CHAPTER

Care of Patients with Sexually Transmitted Disease

Shirley E. Van Zandt

http://evolve.elsevier.com/Iggy/

PRIORITY CONCEPTS

- Infection
- Pain
- Sexuality

LEARNING OUTCOMES

Safe and Effective Care Environment

1. Maintain patient confidentiality and privacy related to sexually transmitted diseases (STDs).

Health Promotion and Maintenance

2. Educate patients with STDs and their partners on self-care measures.
3. Describe the role of expedited partner therapy in reducing STD recurrence.
4. Develop a teaching plan for young adults and other at-risk people about risk factors, prevention, and treatment for STDs.
5. Explain the importance of respect for patients' personal values and beliefs regarding practices associated with SEXUALITY.

Psychosocial Integrity

6. Assess patients' and their partners' responses to a diagnosis of STD.
7. Reduce the psychological impact for the patient who has been diagnosed with STD.

Physiological Integrity

8. Compare the stages of syphilis.
9. Identify the role of drug therapy in managing patients with STDs.
10. Develop a health teaching plan for patients on how to self-manage their STD, including antibiotic therapy.
11. Describe the assessment findings, including PAIN, that are typical in patients with STDs.
12. Develop a collaborative plan of care for a patient with pelvic inflammatory disease (PID).
13. Identify three sexually transmitted vaginal INFECTIONS.

OVERVIEW

Sexually transmitted diseases (STDs) are caused by infectious organisms that have been passed from one person to another through intimate contact—usually oral, vaginal, or anal intercourse. Some organisms that cause these diseases are transmitted only through sexual contact. Other organisms are transmitted also by parenteral exposure to infected blood, fecal-oral transmission, intrauterine transmission to the fetus, and perinatal transmission from mother to neonate (Table 74-1). The term **sexually transmitted infections (STIs)** is used to describe the same group of health problems. This terminology is intended to focus on the management of acute INFECTIONS and to decrease the social stigma of labeling them as diseases. If the STI continues to recur and become chronic, the term *STD* is used. *STD continues to be the most acceptable term used by the Centers for Disease Control and Prevention (CDC) and is therefore used in this chapter.*

Improved diagnostic techniques, increased knowledge about organisms that can be sexually transmitted, and changes in sexual attitudes and practices have led to an increasing number of reported cases of STDs. *Sexual issues are often sensitive, personal, and controversial, and nurses must respect the patients' lifestyle. Providing confidentiality is essential for patients to receive correct information, make informed decisions, and obtain appropriate care.*

The prevalence of STDs is a major public health concern worldwide. Populations at greatest risk for acquiring STDs and suffering from their complications are pregnant women, adolescents, and men who have sex with men (MSM). External factors such as an increasing population, cultural factors (e.g., earlier first intercourse), political and economic policies, incidences of sexual abuse and sexual trafficking, and international travel and migration affect the prevalence of STDs.

TABLE 74-1 Sexually Transmitted Diseases

- Human immune deficiency virus infection
- Chancroid
- Syphilis
- Lymphogranuloma venereum
- Genital herpes simplex virus infection
- Genital warts
- Gonococcal infection
- Chlamydia infection
- Nongonococcal urethritis
- Mucopurulent cervicitis
- Epididymitis
- Pelvic inflammatory disease
- Sexually transmitted enteritis
- Sexually transmitted proctitis
- Trichomoniasis
- Candidal infection
- Bacterial vaginosis
- Viral hepatitis
- Cytomegalovirus infection
- Ectoparasitic infection:
  - Pediculosis pubis
  - Scabies

From Centers for Disease Control and Prevention (CDC). (2010). Sexually transmitted diseases treatment guidelines, 2010. *Morbidity and Mortality Weekly Report, 59*(RR-12), 1-110.

CONSIDERATIONS FOR OLDER ADULTS

Patient-Centered Care QSEN

Another factor contributing to STD prevalence is the increasing number of older adults that will continue as the baby boomers age. People older than 50 years may not realize their risk for STDs or feel comfortable discussing their sexuality with health care providers. Providers may also lack awareness of the sexual activity of older adults. Be sure to teach older adults who are sexually active about their risk for developing STDs (Jeffers & DiBartolo, 2011).

In the United States, one of the greatest factors associated with STD prevalence is the secrecy that surrounds SEXUALITY, sexual behavior, and intimacy in the American culture. The stigma of STDs in the United States has been associated with higher rates of STDs as compared with rates in other developed countries. The prevalence of STDs is also affected by changing human physiology patterns such as earlier onset of menarche, comorbidities associated with human immune deficiency virus (HIV) and diabetes, treatments given for cancer or organ transplantation, and disparities in access to health care. Substance abuse has also been identified as a significant risk factor because of the effects illicit drugs have on sexual risk-taking behavior.

STDs cause complications that can contribute to severe physical and emotional suffering, including infertility, ectopic pregnancy, cancer, and death. Some of the most common complications caused by sexually transmitted organisms are listed in Table 74-2.

Chlamydia infection, gonorrhea, syphilis, chancroid, human immune deficiency virus (HIV) INFECTION, and acquired immune deficiency syndrome (AIDS) are reportable to local health authorities in every state (Centers for Disease Control and Prevention [CDC], 2013f). Other STDs such as genital herpes (GH) may or may not be reported, depending on local legal requirements. Positive results can be reported by clinicians and laboratories. Reports are kept strictly confidential.

Nurses in a variety of settings are responsible for identifying people at risk for STDs, caring for patients with diagnosed STDs, and preventing further cases through education and case finding. Nurses in primary care community settings and acute care settings have a responsibility to recognize patients who are at risk for or who have STDs, possibly while being treated for another unrelated health problem.

The CDC provides regularly updated guidelines for treatment of STDs. These best practice guidelines provide information, treatment standards, and counseling advice to help decrease the spread of these diseases and their complications (CDC, 2010b).

Evidence from the U.S. Preventive Services Task Force (USPSTF) has shown that education and counseling about STDs needs to be of high intensity and on multiple occasions for it to change behavior (USPSTF, 2014b). Health education messages that are short, nonspecific, and not related to the person's sexual behaviors have little effect in lowering the risk for acquiring STDs.

GENDER HEALTH CONSIDERATIONS

Patient-Centered Care QSEN

Because of the very vascular and large surface area of the mucous membranes of the vagina, women are more easily infected with STDs and are at greater risk for STD-related health problems than are men. Young women who are sexually active with men have the greatest risk for contracting an STD. Younger adults have greater rates of sexual activity, including more partners and more unprotected sex than older adults. Women are more vulnerable to infections because of the exposure of cervical basal epithelium cells. Lesbian women have a decreased risk for STDs because of fewer partners, although many have or have had sex with men.

Some young women may also be at high risk because they:

- Lack knowledge about the risk for disease
- Believe that they are not vulnerable to disease
- Mistakenly believe that contraceptives also protect them from STDs
- Drink alcohol in binges, which promotes risky sexual behavior

Postmenopausal women also may be at risk for STDs because many perceive that pregnancy is no longer likely and thus do not use barrier protection. Changing social relationships (e.g., divorce and widowhood in the middle years) has changed risk for exposure to STDs. Physiologic changes during menopause such as mucosal tears from vaginal atrophy may also place them at risk.

Women have more asymptomatic infections that may delay diagnosis and treatment. Many STDs reside in the cervical os and cause little change in vaginal discharge or vulvar tissue so women are not aware that they are infected. This delay increases the likelihood of complications from STDs, including ascending infections that may cause reproductive organ damage and illness. Embarrassment, denial, or fear about STDs may further delay treatment, increasing the potential for serious complications.

INFECTIONS ASSOCIATED WITH ULCERS

SYPHILIS

❖ *PATHOPHYSIOLOGY*

Syphilis is a complex sexually transmitted disease (STD) that can become systemic and cause serious complications, including death. The causative organism is a spirochete called *Treponema pallidum*. Although the organism can be seen only with a darkfield microscope, several serologic tests are used to screen for the presence of syphilis antibody. *T. pallidum* is damaged by dry air or any known disinfectant. The organisms die within

TABLE 74-2 Complications Caused by Sexually Transmitted Organisms

COMPLICATION	CAUSATIVE ORGANISMS
Salpingitis, infertility, and ectopic pregnancy	*Neisseria gonorrhoeae* *Chlamydia trachomatis* *Mycoplasma hominis* *Ureaplasma urealyticum*
Reproductive loss (abortion/miscarriage)	*N. gonorrhoeae* *C. trachomatis* Herpes simplex virus *M. hominis* *U. urealyticum* *Treponema pallidum*
Puerperal infection	*N. gonorrhoeae* *C. trachomatis*
Perinatal infection	Hepatitis B virus Human immune deficiency virus Human papilloma virus *N. gonorrhoeae* *C. trachomatis* Herpes simplex virus *T. pallidum* Cytomegalovirus Group B streptococcus
Cancer of genital area	Human papilloma virus
Male urethritis	*M. hominis* Herpes simplex virus *N. gonorrhoeae* *C. trachomatis* *U. urealyticum*
Vulvovaginitis	Herpes simplex virus *Trichomonas vaginalis* Bacterial vaginosis *Candida albicans*
Cervicitis	*N. gonorrhoeae* *C. trachomatis* Herpes simplex virus
Proctitis	*N. gonorrhoeae* *C. trachomatis* Herpes simplex virus *Campylobacter jejuni* *Shigella* species *Entamoeba histolytica*
Hepatitis	*T. pallidum* Hepatitis A, hepatitis B, and hepatitis C viruses
Dermatitis	*Sarcoptes scabiei* *Phthirus pubis*
Genital ulceration or warts	*C. trachomatis* Herpes simplex virus Human papilloma virus *T. pallidum* *Haemophilus ducreyi* *Calymmatobacterium granulomatis*

hours at temperatures of 105.8° to 107.6°F (41° to 42°C) and are not airborne. *The* INFECTION *is usually transmitted by sexual contact and blood exposure, but transmission can occur through close body contact such as kissing.*

Syphilis progresses through four stages: primary, secondary, latent, and tertiary. The appearance of an ulcer called a **chancre** is the first sign of *primary* syphilis. It develops at the site of entry (inoculation) of the organism from 10 to 90 days after exposure (3 weeks is average). Chancres may be found on any area of the skin or mucous membranes but occur most often on the genitalia, lips, nipples, and hands and in the mouth, anus, and rectum.

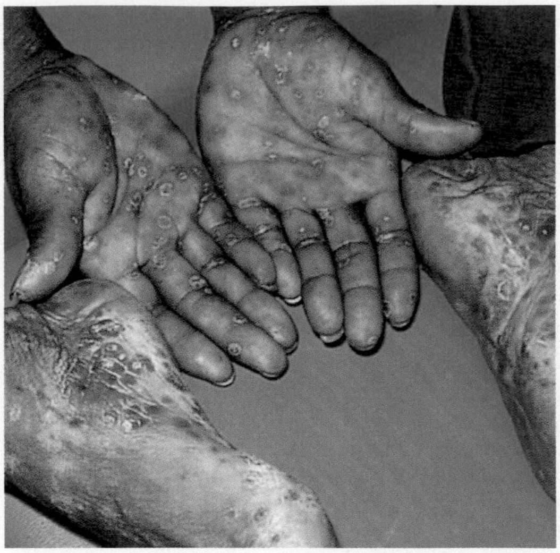

FIG. 74-1 Palmar and plantar secondary syphilis.

During this highly infectious stage, the chancre begins as a small papule. Within 3 to 7 days, it breaks down into its typical appearance: a painless, indurated, smooth, weeping lesion. Regional lymph nodes enlarge, feel firm, and are not painful. Without treatment, the chancre usually disappears within 6 weeks. However, the organism spreads throughout the body and the patient is still infectious.

Secondary syphilis develops 6 weeks to 6 months after the onset of primary syphilis. During this stage, syphilis is a systemic disease because the spirochetes circulate throughout the bloodstream. Commonly mistaken for influenza, manifestations include flu-like symptoms (malaise, low-grade fever, headache, muscular aches, sore throat) and a generalized rash. There is no typical appearance of this rash except for its presence on the palms and soles of the feet and on mucous membranes. It can appear as diffuse macules (reddish brown), papules (usually less than 5 mm) or pustules, scaly psoriasis-like lesions (Fig. 74-1), or gray-white wart-like lesions (condylomata lata). *All of these lesions are highly contagious and should not be touched without gloves.* Patchy alopecia on the scalp or facial hair (missing part of the eyebrow, "moth-eaten" appearance) is another symptom. The rash subsides without treatment in 4 to 12 weeks.

After the second stage of syphilis, there is a period of latency. *Early latent* syphilis occurs during the first year after INFECTION, and infectious lesions can recur. *Late latent* syphilis is a disease of more than 1 year's duration after INFECTION. This stage is not infectious except to the fetus of a pregnant woman. Patients with latent syphilis may or may not have reactive serologic test (e.g., Venereal Disease Research Laboratory [VDRL]) findings.

Tertiary, or late, syphilis occurs after a highly variable period, from 4 to 20 years. This stage develops in untreated cases and can mimic other conditions because any organ system can be affected. Manifestations of late syphilis include:

- Benign lesions (gummas) of the skin, mucous membranes, and bones
- Cardiovascular syphilis, usually in the form of aortic valvular disease and aortic aneurysms
- Neurosyphilis, causing central nervous system symptoms (e.g., meningitis, hearing loss, generalized paresis [weakness])

CULTURAL CONSIDERATIONS

Patient-Centered Care QSEN

Disparity exists between racial and ethnic groups in the incidence of primary and secondary syphilis. In the most recent reports from 2011, the rates increased among Hispanics, American Indians/Alaska Natives (from 2.5 to 2.7 cases per 100,000 population), Euro-Americans (from 2.1 to 2.3 cases per 100,000 population), and most dramatically (33%) among Asian/Pacific Islanders but impressively have decreased among African Americans. Nevertheless, African Americans have a 7 times greater rate of acquiring syphilis than whites. Compared with Euro-Americans, the 2011 rate for Hispanics was 2 times higher (CDC, 2013a). The reason for these differences is unclear, but status of health literacy and lack of access to health care may be factors.

GENDER HEALTH CONSIDERATIONS

Patient-Centered Care QSEN

Unique needs regarding sexual health and prevention and treatment of sexually related infections of lesbian, gay, bisexual, transgender, and questioning (LGBTQ) patients should be identified and addressed by the nurse. Because of discrimination, health care inequities, and health care provider lack of understanding, the overall health status of people in these populations may be poor. LGBTQ people may have difficulty finding health care that identifies and addresses their particular risks and concerns. Taking a health history that provides opportunity for the patient to identify his or her sexual orientation, sexual identity, and sexual activity is crucial. Especially among transgender people, opportunities for physical examination are avoided or missed by both the patient and care provider because of fears of being misunderstood or inadequately prepared to give or receive appropriate care (Williamson, 2010).

The CDC does not currently collect or report the incidence or prevalence of STDs among transgender people. There have been estimates from self-report that 11% to 28% of the transgender community are infected with HIV (Cobos & Jones, 2009).

Men who have sex with men (MSM) are at greatest risk for contracting primary and secondary syphilis and made up 75% of cases of these diseases in 2012 (CDC, 2014a). These men are 17 times more likely to have anal cancer than heterosexual men, and those infected with HIV are at even greater risk. Infection with high-risk human papilloma virus (HPV) has been associated with greater risk for anal cancers among this population (CDC, 2012a).

A common perception that women who have sex with women (WSW) are at very low or no risk for getting STDs has not been supported in research because of the lack of data. Bacterial, viral, and protozoal infections have all been reported among WSW (CDC, 2014c). Identifying risk in this population may depend more on asking about sexual practices such as use of sex objects or oral-anal, digital-anal, or digital-vaginal sex. Being aware of these practices can increase the nurse's ability to identify risk factors for patients.

Assuming that lesbian women or gay men have sex only with same-gender partners or similarly assuming that heterosexual patients never have sexual encounters with partners of their same sex may limit the accuracy of the nurse's risk assessment. Nurses must be aware that patients may not reveal that they are bisexual. Establish a trusting relationship and be culturally sensitive and nonjudgmental when working with LGBTQ patients. Chapter 1 describes recommendations for communicating with this population. Chapter 73 discusses the special health care needs of transgender patients.

Health Promotion and Maintenance

One of the *Healthy People 2020* objectives is to completely eliminate syphilis in the United States (U.S. Department of Health and Human Services [USDHHS], 2014) (Table 74-3). One of the primary tools for prevention of sexually transmitted diseases (STDs), including syphilis, is education. All people, regardless of age, gender, ethnicity, socioeconomic status, education level, or sexual orientation, are susceptible to these diseases. Health literacy, motivation, and perceived risk can affect the health status of any patient. STDs are largely preventable through safer sex practices. *Do not assume that a person is not sexually active because of his or her age, education, marital status, profession, or religion.* Discuss prevention methods, including safer sex, with all patients who are or may become sexually active.

TABLE 74-3 Meeting *Healthy People 2020* Objectives and Targets for Improvement: Sexually Transmitted Diseases

- Reduce the proportion of adolescents and young adults with *Chlamydia trachomatis* infections (by 10%).
- Reduce the proportion of females ages 15 to 44 years who have ever required treatment for pelvic inflammatory disease (by 10%).
- Reduce gonorrhea rates (by 10%).
- Reduce sustained domestic transmission of primary and secondary syphilis (by 10%).
- Reduce the proportion of females with human papilloma virus (HPV) infection (no specific target).
- Reduce the proportion of young adults with genital herpes due to herpes simplex type 2 (by 10%).

Safer sex practices are those that reduce the risk for nonintact skin or mucous membranes coming in contact with infected body fluids and blood. These practices include:

- Using a latex or polyurethane condom for genital and anal intercourse
- Using a condom or latex barrier (dental dam) over the genitals or anus during oral-genital or oral-anal sexual contact
- Wearing gloves for finger or hand contact with the vagina or rectum
- Abstinence
- Mutual monogamy
- Decreasing the number of sexual partners

❖ PATIENT-CENTERED COLLABORATIVE CARE

◆ Assessment

Assessment of the patient who has manifestations of syphilis begins with a history to gather information about any ulcers or rash. Take a sexual history and conduct a risk assessment to include whether previous testing or treatment for syphilis or other STDs has ever been done (Chart 74-1). Ask about allergic reactions to drugs, especially penicillin. A woman may report inguinal lymph node enlargement resulting from a chancre in the vagina or cervix that is not easily visible to her. She may state a history of sexual contact with a male partner who had an ulcer that she noticed during the encounter. Men usually discover the chancre on the penis or scrotum.

Conduct a physical examination, including inspection and palpation, to identify manifestations of syphilis. *Wear gloves while palpating any lesions because of the highly contagious treponemes that are present.* Observe for and document rashes of any type because of the variable presentation of secondary syphilis.

After the physical examination, the health care provider obtains a *specimen of the chancre* for examination under a

CHART 74-1 Focused Assessment

The Patient with a Sexually Transmitted Disease

Assess history of present illness:
- Chief concern
- Onset
- Symptoms by quality and quantity, precipitating and palliative factors
- Any treatments taken (self-prescribed or over-the-counter products)

Assess past medical history:
- Major health problems—including any history of STDs/PID or immunosuppression
- Surgeries—obstetric and gynecologic, circumcision

Assess current health status:
- Menstrual history for irregularities
- Sexual history:
  - Type and frequency of sexual activity
  - Number of lifetime and past 6 months sexual contacts/partners; monogamous
  - Sexual orientation
- Contraception history
- Medications
- Allergies
- Lifestyle risks—drugs, alcohol, tobacco

Assess preventive health care practices:
- Papanicolaou (Pap) tests
- Regular STD screening
- Use of barrier contraceptives to prevent STDs and pregnancy

Assess physical examination findings:
- Vital signs
- Oropharyngeal findings
- Abdominal findings
- Genital or pelvic findings
- Anorectal findings

Assess laboratory data:
- Urinalysis
- Hematology
- ESR or CRP if PID is being considered
- Cervical, urethral, oral, rectal specimens
- Lesion samples for microbiology and virology
- Pregnancy testing

CRP, C-reactive protein; *ESR*, erythrocyte sedimentation rate; *PID*, pelvic inflammatory disease; *STDs*, sexually transmitted diseases.

darkfield microscope. Diagnosis of primary or secondary syphilis is confirmed if *T. pallidum* is present.

Blood tests are also used to diagnose syphilis. The usual screening and/or diagnostic nontreponemal tests are the *Venereal Disease Research Laboratory (VDRL)* serum test and the more sensitive *rapid plasma reagin (RPR)*. These tests are based on an antibody-antigen reaction that determines the presence and amount of antibodies produced by the body in response to an INFECTION by *T. pallidum*. They become reactive 2 to 6 weeks after infection. VDRL titers are also used to monitor treatment effectiveness. The antibodies are not specific to *T. pallidum*, and false-positive reactions often occur from such conditions as viral INFECTIONS, hepatitis, and systemic lupus erythematosus (SLE) (Pagana & Pagana, 2014).

If a VDRL result is positive, the health care provider requests or the laboratory may automatically perform a more specific treponemal test, such as the *fluorescent treponemal antibody absorption (FTA-ABS)* test or the *microhemagglutination assay for T. palladum (MHA-TP)*, to confirm the infection. These tests are more sensitive for all stages of syphilis, although false-positive results may still occur. Patients who have a reactive test will have this positive result for their entire life, even after sufficient treatment. This poses a challenge when receiving a positive result for a patient who denies a history of or does not know he or she had syphilis.

◆ *Interventions*

Patient-centered collaborative care includes drug therapy and health teaching to resolve the INFECTION and prevent infection transmission to others.

Drug Therapy. Benzathine penicillin G given IM as a single 2.4 million-unit dose is the evidence-based treatment for primary, secondary, and early latent syphilis (CDC, 2010b). Patients in the late latent stage receive the same dose every week for 3 weeks (CDC, 2010b). A different regimen, found in the CDC's *STD Treatment Guidelines,* is recommended for patients who are HIV-infected or pregnant.

! NURSING SAFETY PRIORITY QSEN

Drug Alert

Allergic reactions to benzathine penicillin G can occur. Monitor for allergic manifestations (e.g., rash, edema, shortness of breath, chest tightness, anxiety). Penicillin desensitization is recommended for penicillin-allergic patients. *Keep all patients at the health care agency for at least 30 minutes after they have received the antibiotic so that manifestations of an allergic reaction can be detected and treated. The most severe reaction is anaphylaxis. Treatment should be available and implemented immediately if symptoms occur.* Chapter 17 describes the management of drug allergies in detail.

After treatment, the CDC recommends follow-up evaluation including blood tests at 6, 12, and 24 months. Repeat treatment may be needed if the patient does not respond to the initial antibiotic.

The *Jarisch-Herxheimer reaction* may also follow antibiotic therapy for syphilis. This reaction is caused by the rapid release of products from the disruption of the cells of the organism. Symptoms include generalized aches, pain at the injection site, vasodilation, hypotension, and fever. They are usually benign and begin within 2 hours after therapy with a peak at 4 to 8 hours. This reaction may be treated symptomatically with analgesics and antipyretics.

Self-Management Education. Teach about the cause of INFECTION (sexual transmission); treatment, including side effects; possible complications of untreated or incompletely treated disease; and the need for follow-up care.

! NURSING SAFETY PRIORITY QSEN

Drug Alert

Discuss with the patient with syphilis the importance of partner notification and treatment, including the risk for re-infection if the partner goes untreated. All sexual partners must be prophylactically treated as soon as possible, preferably within 90 days of the syphilis diagnosis.

Inform the patient that the disease will be reported to the local health authority and that all information will be held in strict confidence. Encourage the patient to provide accurate information for this follow-up to ensure that all at-risk partners are treated appropriately. Provide a setting that offers privacy and encourages open discussion. Urge the patient to keep follow-up appointments. For primary and secondary syphilis, medication treatment will be completed at the first visit, which may suggest to the patient that no further visits are indicated or important. Remind the patient that follow-up for partners and assessment that symptoms have resolved are imperative and part of continuing care. Recommend sexual abstinence until the treatment of both the patient and partner(s) is completed.

The emotional responses to syphilis vary and may include feelings of fear, depression, guilt, and anxiety. Patients may experience guilt if they have infected others or anger if a partner has infected them. If further psychosocial interventions are needed, encourage the patient to discuss these feelings or refer him or her to other resources such as psychotherapy, self-help support groups, or STD clinics.

NCLEX EXAMINATION CHALLENGE

Physiological Integrity

The nurse gives a client an IM dose of penicillin G for primary syphilis. Which client statement indicates a need for further teaching?

A. "I will wait in the clinic for 30 minutes to be sure I do not have a reaction."
B. "When I get home, I will call my partner to tell them about my diagnosis."
C. "If I have sex with someone, I do not have to worry about spreading the disease."
D. "I plan to return to see my primary care provider for follow-up in 6, 12, and 24 months."

GENITAL HERPES

PATHOPHYSIOLOGY

Genital herpes (GH) is an acute, recurring, incurable viral disease. It is the most common STD in the United States, with 17.0% of Americans currently infected with herpes simplex virus type 2 (HSV-2) and 57.7% with type 1 (HSV-1) (Warren et al., 2011).

The prevalence among African Americans is 39.2%, disproportionately affecting African-American women (48.0%) (CDC, 2010a). These rates are based on the presence of HSV-2 antibodies in the blood of those tested, the majority of whom have had no symptoms and most have never received a diagnosis of GH INFECTION (CDC, 2010a).

Two serotypes of herpes simplex virus (HSV) affect the genitalia: type 1 (HSV-1) and type 2 (HSV-2). Most *nongenital* lesions such as cold sores are caused by HSV-1, transmitted via oral-oral contact. Historically, HSV-2 caused most of the genital lesions. However, this distinction is academic because the transmission, symptoms, diagnosis, and treatment are nearly identical for the two types. Either type can produce oral or genital lesions through oral-genital or genital-genital contact with an infected person. HSV-2 recurs and sheds asymptomatically more often than HSV-1. Most people with GH have not been diagnosed because they have mild symptoms and shed virus intermittently, with possibly only 10% to 25% of those with HSV-2 realizing they have GH (Patel & Rompalo, 2012).

The incubation period of genital herpes is 2 to 20 days, with the average period being 1 week. Many people do not have symptoms during the primary outbreak. When subsequent outbreaks of genital herpes occur, they are usually more severe and occasionally require hospitalization.

Recurrences are not caused by re-infection. Additional episodes are usually less severe and of shorter duration than the primary INFECTION episode. Some patients have no symptoms at all during recurrence or viral reactivation. *However, there is viral shedding and the patient is infectious.* Long-term complications of GH include the risk for neonatal transmission and an increased risk for acquiring HIV infection.

PATIENT-CENTERED COLLABORATIVE CARE

Assessment

The diagnosis of GH is based on the patient's history and physical examination (see Chart 74-1). Ask the patient if he or she felt itching or a tingling sensation in the skin 1 to 2 days before the outbreak, known as the *prodrome.* These sensations are usually followed by the appearance of **vesicles** (blisters) in a typical cluster on the penis, scrotum, vulva, vagina, cervix, or perianal region at the site of inoculation. The blisters rupture spontaneously in a day or two and leave painful ulcerations that can become extensive. Assess for other symptoms such as headaches, fever, general malaise, and swelling of inguinal lymph nodes. Ask if urination is painful. External dysuria is a painful symptom when urine passes over the eroded areas. Patients with urinary retention may need to be catheterized. Lesions resolve within 2 to 6 weeks.

After the lesions heal, the virus remains in a dormant state in the sacral nerve ganglia. Periodically, the virus may activate and symptoms recur. These recurrences may be triggered by many factors, including stress, fever, sunburn, poor nutrition, menses, and sexual activity. Assess the patient for these risk factors to provide anticipatory guidance for prevention of outbreaks.

GH is confirmed through a viral cell culture or polymerase chain reaction (PCR) assays of the lesions. PCR is the more sensitive test and is currently the gold standard; however, it is very expensive and usually not available. Fluid from inside the blister obtained within 48 hours of the first outbreak will yield the most reliable results because accuracy decreases as the blisters begin to heal (Patel & Rompalo, 2012). Serology testing, which is glycoprotein G antibody-based, can identify the HSV type, either 1 or 2. Serologic tests are used to identify INFECTION in high-risk groups such as HIV-positive patients, patients who have partners with HSV, or men who have sex with men (MSM) (CDC, 2010b). Antibodies may take up to 12 weeks to develop, so false-negative results can occur if tested too soon after the initial infection. Because 80% to 90% of the population will become positive over their lifetime, using the antibody serology test to screen for infection in the general population is not effective or appropriate (Patel & Rompalo, 2012).

Interventions

The desired outcomes of treatment for HSV-infected patients are to decrease the discomfort from painful ulcerations, promote healing without secondary infection, decrease viral shedding, and prevent INFECTION transmission (Chart 74-2).

Drug Therapy. Antiviral drugs are used to treat GH. *The drugs decrease the severity, promote healing, and decrease the frequency of recurrent outbreaks but do not cure the infection.*

Drug therapy should be offered to anyone with an initial outbreak of GH regardless of the severity of the symptoms. Topical therapy is not recommended. Acyclovir (Zovirax, Avirax 🍁), famciclovir (Famvir), or valacyclovir (Valtrex) may be prescribed. The main differences in these drugs are cost and

CHART 74-2 Best Practice for Patient Safety & Quality Care QSEN

Care of or Self-Management for the Patient with Genital Herpes

- Administer oral analgesics as prescribed.
- Apply local anesthetic sprays or ointments as prescribed.
- Apply ice packs or warm compresses to the patient's lesions.
- Administer sitz baths 3 or 4 times a day.
- Urge an increase in fluid intake to replace fluid lost through open lesions.
- Encourage frequent urination.
- Pour water over the patient's genitalia while voiding, or encourage voiding while the patient is sitting in a tub of water or standing in a shower.
- Catheterize the patient as necessary.
- Encourage genital hygiene, and encourage keeping the skin clean and dry.
- Wash hands thoroughly after contact with lesions, and launder towels that have had direct contact with lesions.
- Wear gloves when applying ointments or making any direct contact with lesions.
- Advise the patient to avoid sexual activity when lesions are present.
- Advise the patient to use latex or polyurethane condoms during all sexual exposures.
- Instruct the patient in the use, side effects, and risks versus benefits of antiviral agents.
- Advise the patient to discuss the diagnosis of genital herpes (GH) with current and new partners.

frequency of use. Dosage and length of treatment differ for primary outbreaks (7 to 10 days) and recurrent outbreaks (1 to 5 days). Therapy for recurrent outbreaks is most beneficial if it is started within 1 day of the appearance of lesions or during the period of itching or tingling before lesions appear. Intermittent or continuous (daily) suppressive antiviral therapy is offered to patients to lessen the severity and frequency of or prevent outbreaks, even for those with infrequent recurrent episodes.

Suppression reduces recurrences in most patients, but it does not prevent viral shedding, even when symptoms are absent (CDC, 2010b). Patients receiving continuous therapy should periodically (possibly once a year) be reassessed for recurrences, usually by stopping the antiviral drug temporarily.

IV acyclovir and hospitalization may be indicated for patients with severe HSV infections, such as disseminated disease or encephalitis. These are severe complications of genital herpes and may be fatal.

Self-Management Education. Nursing interventions focus on patient education about the INFECTION, sexual transmission, the potential for recurrent episodes, and the correct use and possible side effects of antiviral therapy. Frank discussion about sexual activity, including whether the patient has new or multiple partners, is an essential component of the nurse's intervention.

! NURSING SAFETY PRIORITY QSEN

Action Alert

Remind patients to abstain from sexual activity while GH lesions are present. Sexual activity can be painful, and likelihood of viral transmission is higher. Urge condom use during all sexual exposures because of the increased risk for HSV transmission from viral shedding, which can occur even when lesions are not present. Teach the patient about how to use condoms (Chart 74-3).

CHART 74-3 Patient and Family Education: Preparing for Self-Management

Use of Condoms

- Use latex or polyurethane condoms rather than natural membrane condoms.
- Use a condom with every sexual encounter (including oral, vaginal, and anal).
- Female condoms (Reality)—polyurethane or nitrile sheaths in the vagina—are effective in preventing transmission of viruses, including HIV.
- Condoms infrequently (2 per 100) break during sexual intercourse.
- Keep condoms (especially latex) in a cool, dry place, out of direct sunlight.
- Do not use condoms that are in damaged packages or that are brittle or discolored.
- Always handle a condom with care to avoid damaging it with fingernails, teeth, or other sharp objects.
- Put condoms on before any genital contact. Hold the condom by the tip and unroll it on the penis. Leave a space at the tip to collect semen.
- If you use a lubricant with condoms, make sure that the lubricant is water based and washes away with water. Oil-based products damage latex condoms.
- Use of spermicide (nonoxynol-9) with condoms, either lubricated condoms or vaginal application, has *not* been proven to be more or less effective against STDs than use without spermicide. Spermicide-coated condoms have been associated with *Escherichia coli* urinary tract infections in women. *Nonoxynol-9 may increase risk for transmission of HIV during vaginal intercourse and anal intercourse. Its use is discouraged.*
- If a condom breaks, replace it immediately.
- After ejaculation, withdraw the erect penis carefully, holding the condom at the base of the penis to prevent the condom from slipping off.
- Never use a condom more than once.

Modified from Centers for Disease Control and Prevention (CDC). (2010). Sexually transmitted diseases treatment guidelines, 2010. *Morbidity and Mortality Weekly Report, 59*(RR-12), 4-5.
HIV, Human immune deficiency virus; *STDs,* sexually transmitted diseases.

Assess the patient's and partner's emotional responses to the diagnosis of genital herpes. Many people are initially shocked and need reassurance that they can manage the disease. Infected patients may have feelings of disbelief, uncleanness, isolation, and loneliness. They may also be angry at their partner(s) for transmitting the INFECTION or fear rejection because they have the infection. Help patients cope with the diagnosis by being sensitive and supportive during assessments and interventions. Encourage social support, and refer patients to support groups (e.g., local support groups of the National Herpes Resource Center [www.ashasexualhealth.org/std-sti/Herpes.html]) and therapists. Symptomatic care may include oral analgesics, topical anesthetics, sitz baths, and increased oral fluid intake (Bavis et al., 2009).

Emphasize the risk for neonatal INFECTION to all patients, both male and female. Men and women who have genital herpes need to inform their pregnancy care provider of their history. Uninfected women will be advised to avoid unprotected intercourse with infected partners during pregnancy to avoid the risk for a new primary infection and outbreak during pregnancy. People who have tested serology positive to HSV-1 or HSV-2 but have never had GH symptoms should be counseled with the same information as for those who have symptoms (CDC, 2010b).

INFECTIONS OF THE EPITHELIAL STRUCTURES

CONDYLOMATA ACUMINATA (GENITAL WARTS)

❖ PATHOPHYSIOLOGY

Condylomata acuminata (also known as *genital warts*) are caused by certain types of *human papilloma virus (HPV)*, 90% of which are types 6 and 11 or low-risk HPV (Datta et al., 2012; Mark et al., 2012). These types *rarely* result in invasive cancer of the genital tract such as cervical cancer. *However, HPV types 16, 18, 31, 33, and 35, considered high-risk HPV, can be found on the skin of the genitalia and increase the risk for genital cancers, especially cervical cancer.* INFECTION with several HPV types can occur at the same time. The presence of one strain increases the risk for acquiring a higher-risk strain. Genital warts are the most common viral disease that is sexually transmitted and are often seen with other infections. Among American women ages 14 to 59 years, 26.8% are infected with either high- or low-risk HPV (Datta et al., 2012).

HPV INFECTION has been established as the primary risk factor for development of cervical cancer (Datta et al., 2012). Sites commonly affected by INFECTION include the urinary meatus, labia, vagina, cervix, penis, scrotum, anus, and perineal area. The incubation period is usually 2 to 3 months. There is growing evidence that HPV infection through oral and anal sex, especially in men who have sex with men (MSM), may be a risk factor for developing oral and anal cancers (Kim, 2010).

❖ PATIENT-CENTERED COLLABORATIVE CARE

◆ Assessment

The diagnosis of condylomata acuminata is made by examination of the lesions. They are initially small, white or flesh-colored papillary growths that may grow into large cauliflower-like masses (Fig. 74-2). Multiple warts usually occur in the same area. Bleeding may occur if the wart is disturbed. Warts may disappear or resolve on their own without treatment. They may occur once or recur at the original site. Warts can occur on the external or internal surfaces of the genitalia, including the mucosal surfaces of the vagina and urethra.

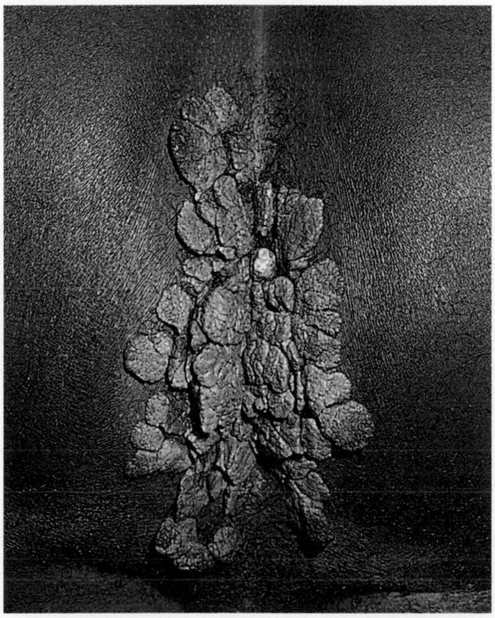

FIG. 74-2 Perianal condylomata acuminata.

Screening for HPV and dysplasia of the cervix is done by obtaining cervical specimens for Papanicolaou (Pap) and HPV DNA testing. The frequency of screening has changed significantly as new understanding about the course of HPV infection has evolved. Identifying high-risk strains of HPV and correlating with abnormal Pap smear findings is now the standard of care (Schiffman et al., 2011). High-risk HPV may coexist with low-risk HPV, the likely cause of the warts. The diagnosis should include consideration of condyloma lata or secondary syphilis since STDs frequently coexist. A VDRL test, HIV test, and cultures for chlamydia and gonorrhea infections are done. Condylomata lata (secondary syphilis) can resemble condylomata acuminata (genital warts). If a wartlike lesion bleeds easily, appears infected, is atypical, or persists, a biopsy of the lesion is performed to rule out other pathologic problems such as cancer. A biopsy of warts that are seen on the cervix should be performed prior to any treatment to eradicate them.

◆ Interventions

The outcome of treatment is to remove the warts. No current therapy eliminates the HPV infection, and recurrences after treatment are likely. It is not known whether removal of visible warts decreases the risk for disease transmission.

Drug Therapy. Patients may apply podofilox (Condylox) 0.5% cream or gel twice daily for 3 days with no treatment for the next 4 days. This regimen should be repeated for four cycles. Other options are imiquimod (Aldara) 5% cream applied topically at bedtime 3 times a week and sinecatechins 15% ointment (made from green tea extract) applied 3 times a day, both until the warts disappear or for up to 16 weeks. Imiquimod boosts the immune system rather than simply destroying the warts. These self-treatments are less expensive than those performed in the health care provider's office, but they take longer for healing. *Teach patients that over-the-counter (OTC) wart treatments should not be used on genital tissue (CDC, 2010b).*

Cryotherapy, trichloroacetic acid (TCA) or bichloroacetic acid (BCA), and podophyllin (Pododerm) are provider-applied treatments. **Cryotherapy** (freezing), usually with liquid nitrogen, can be used every 1 to 2 weeks until lesions are resolved. TCA/BCA (80% to 90%) can be applied weekly. Podophyllin resin can be applied weekly but needs to be washed off 1 to 4 hours after application. Extensive warts have been treated with the carbon dioxide laser, intra-lesion interferon injections, and surgical removal (CDC, 2010b).

Self-Management Education. *The priority nursing intervention is patient and sexual partner education about the mode of transmission, incubation period, treatment, and complications, especially the association with cervical cancer.* Reinforce instructions about local care of the lesions or patient-applied treatment for self-management.

! NURSING SAFETY PRIORITY (QSEN)

Drug Alert

Teach patients that after treatment with cryotherapy, podophyllin, or TCA, they may experience discomfort, bleeding, or discharge from the site or sloughing of parts of warts. Instruct patients to keep the area clean (shower or bath) and dry. Teach them to be alert for any signs or symptoms of infection or side effects of the treatment.

Inform patients that recurrence is likely, especially in the first 3 months, and that repeated treatments may be needed. Urge all patients to have complete STD testing, since exposure to one STD may increase risk for contracting another. Sexual partners should also be evaluated and offered treatment if warts are present. Teach patients to avoid intimate sexual contact until external lesions are healed. Recommend condoms to help reduce transmission even after warts have been treated (see Chart 74-3). Encourage women to have a Pap test annually, starting at age 21 years; after they have had three normal smears, they should have a Pap test every 3 years if no new risk factors are present (e.g., new partner, other STDs) (Murphy & Mark, 2012). The presence of warts should increase suspicion that the patient may have had exposure to other STDs, which warrants additional testing.

Gardasil (Merck Sharpe & Dohme Corporation, 2014) is used to provide immunity for HPV types 6 and 11 (predominantly types causing warts, low risk for cervical cancer) and 16 and 18 (high risk for cervical cancer). Initially approved for females, the vaccine is now also recommended for males ages 9 to 26 years. Cervarix (GlaxoSmithKline, 2012) may be given to 9- to 25-year-old females and protects only against HPV types 16 and 18. Both vaccines are recommended before onset of sexual activity (and before age 26 years) and possible exposure to HPV. Because exposure to HPV is likely for most sexually active young adults, vaccination protects them against the strains to which they have not yet been exposed. Vaccination is also especially encouraged for MSM and immunocompromised young adults up to the age of 26 years (CDC, 2012a).

CHLAMYDIA INFECTION

❖ PATHOPHYSIOLOGY

Chlamydia trachomatis is an intracellular bacterium and the causative agent of genital chlamydia infections. It invades the epithelial tissues in the reproductive tract. The incubation period ranges from 1 to 3 weeks, but the pathogen may be present in the genital tract for months without producing symptoms.

C. trachomatis is reportable to local health departments in all states. Diagnosed cases continue to increase yearly, which reflects more sensitive screening tests and increased public health efforts to screen high-risk people. Each year there are an estimated 2.9 million new cases in the United States (CDC, 2013a), with 1.4 million reported to the CDC in 2011 (CDC, 2012c). Because it is frequently asymptomatic, the estimated incidence is about double of what is reported. African-American women between 15 and 24 years of age are at the highest risk for the disease (CDC, 2012c).

In women, 20% to 40% of those infected will develop pelvic inflammatory disease (PID) if not treated, discussed later in this chapter on p. 1541.

❖ PATIENT-CENTERED COLLABORATIVE CARE

◆ Assessment

Obtain a complete history including a genitourinary review of systems and psychosocial history. This will include a sexual history (see Chart 74-1). In particular, ask about:

- Presence of symptoms, including vaginal or urethral discharge, **dysuria** (painful urination), pelvic pain, irregular bleeding
- Any history of sexually transmitted diseases (STDs)
- Whether sexual partners have had symptoms or a history of STDs
- Whether patient has had a new or multiple sexual partner(s)
- Whether patient or partner has had unprotected intercourse

About 70% of chlamydia infections are asymptomatic in women. For men and women, their history may reveal only risk factors associated with *C. trachomatis,* such as new or multiple sexual partners, age younger than 26 years and female, or a male having sex with a male (MSM). As with all interviews concerning sexual behavior, use a nonjudgmental approach and provide privacy and confidentiality.

GENDER HEALTH CONSIDERATIONS

Patient-Centered Care QSEN

For men, ask about dysuria, frequent urination, and a mucoid discharge that is more watery and less copious than a gonorrheal discharge. *These manifestations indicate urethritis, the main symptom of chlamydia infection in men.* Some men have the discharge only in the morning on arising. Complications include epididymitis, prostatitis, infertility, and Reiter's syndrome, a type of connective tissue disease discussed in Chapter 18.

In contrast, many women have no symptoms. Those with symptoms have mucopurulent vaginal discharge (typically yellow and more opaque), urinary frequency, and abdominal discomfort or pain. Cervical bleeding, from infected and therefore fragile tissue, may present as spotting or bleeding between menses and frequently after intercourse. Complications of infection with *C. trachomatis* include salpingitis (inflammation of the fallopian tubes), PID, ectopic pregnancy, and infertility. These health problems are discussed in detail in maternal-child textbooks.

Diagnosis is made by sampling cells from the endocervix, urethra, or both, easily obtained with a swab. Because chlamydiae can reproduce only inside cells, cervical (or host) cells that harbor the organism (or parts of it) are required in the sample. Tissue culture (the gold standard) obtained from the cervical os during the female pelvic examination or male urethral examination obtained by swabbing has been replaced by genetic tests. As with gonorrhea, the nucleic acid amplification tests (NAATs) and gene amplification tests (ligand chain reaction [LCR] and polymerase chain reaction [PCR] transcription-mediated amplification) are the newest methods of detecting *Chlamydia* in endocervical samples, urethral swabs, and urine. They are more sensitive tests than the tissue culture. Samples can be obtained by swab by the examining clinician or by a patient-collected urine specimen. This urine self-collection method has been found to be more acceptable and highly sensitive and specific. The acceptability of urine testing has resulted in increased identification of asymptomatic people.

All sexually active women 24 years old or younger, and all women older than 25 years with new or multiple partners, should be screened annually for *Chlamydia* (CDC, 2010b; USPSTF, 2014a). There is no recommendation for or against screening asymptomatic men, regardless of age or other risk, and low-risk asymptomatic women.

◆ Interventions

The treatment of choice for chlamydia infections is azithromycin (Zithromax) 1 g orally in a single dose or doxycycline (Monodox, Doxy-Caps, Doxycin) 100 mg orally twice daily for 7 days. The one-dose course, although more expensive, is preferred because of the ease in completing the treatment. Directly observing the patient taking the medication in the health care setting assures the nurse of compliance. Drugs that are prescribed for patients with allergies to these drugs include erythromycin, ofloxacin, and levofloxacin, all for 7 days (CDC, 2010b).

Sexual partners should be treated and tested for other STDs. Expedited partner therapy, or patient-delivered partner therapy, shows signs of reducing chlamydia INFECTION rates (CDC, 2010b). **Expedited partner therapy (EPT)** is the practice of treating sexual partners of patients diagnosed with chlamydia infection or gonorrhea by providing prescriptions or medication to the patient, which they can take to their partner(s), without the health care provider examining the partner(s) (CDC, 2013c). Legal questions have arisen about whether a drug can be prescribed without a relationship between the health care provider and the patient, but many states have now ruled that this is appropriate and legal (CDC, 2013d). When patients have been given the drug to give to their partner, rates of infection have decreased and more partners have reported receiving treatment (CDC, 2013c; Trelle et al., 2007).

Patient and partner education is a crucial nursing intervention. Explain:

- The sexual mode of transmission
- The incubation period
- The high possibility of asymptomatic infections and the usual symptoms if present
- Treatment of infection with antibiotics and need for completion of course of treatment
- The need for abstinence from sexual intercourse until the patient and partner(s) have all completed treatment (7 days from the start of treatment, including a single-dose regimen)
- That women should be re-screened for re-infection 3 to 12 months after treatment because of the high risk for PID; also, that there is less evidence of the need for re-screening of treated men, but it should be considered
- The need to return for evaluation if symptoms recur or new symptoms develop (most recurrences are re-infections from a new or untreated partner)
- Complications of untreated or inadequately treated infection, which may include PID, ectopic pregnancy, or infertility

GONORRHEA

PATHOPHYSIOLOGY

Gonorrhea is a sexually transmitted bacterial INFECTION that occurs in both men and women. The causative organism is *Neisseria gonorrhoeae,* a gram-negative intracellular diplococcus. It is transmitted by direct sexual contact with mucosal surfaces (vaginal intercourse, orogenital contact, or anogenital contact).

The first symptoms of gonorrhea may appear 3 to 10 days after sexual contact with an infected person. The disease can be present without symptoms and can be transmitted or progress without warning. In women, ascending spread of the organism can cause pelvic INFECTION (**pelvic inflammatory disease [PID]**), **endometritis** (endometrial infection), **salpingitis** (fallopian tube infection), and pelvic peritonitis. Rare complications of gonorrhea in adults include arthritis, meningitis, hepatitis, and disseminated infection (Bleich et al., 2012).

CULTURAL CONSIDERATIONS

Patient-Centered Care QSEN

Significant disparity exists between age and racial groups. In 2011, young (ages 15-24 years) African-American women had the highest gonorrhea rate, followed by young African-American men (CDC, 2012c). The reasons for these differences are not known, although lack of access to health care may be a factor.

In 2011, 321,849 new gonococcal infections were diagnosed and reported, but the CDC estimates that this represents only about half of the cases that occurred (CDC, 2012c). Over the years, gonorrhea has become resistant to penicillin, tetracycline, and ciprofloxacin and recently to cefixime. Cefixime is no longer the drug of choice because of the development of oral cephalosporin-resistant *N. gonorrhoeae.* Intramuscular injection of Rocephin (ceftriaxone) 250 mg in a single dose is now the drug of choice (CDC, 2012d).

PATIENT-CENTERED COLLABORATIVE CARE

Assessment

A complete history includes reviewing the genitourinary systems, including taking a sexual history that includes sexual orientation and sites of sexual exposure or intercourse. Assess for allergies to antibiotics (see Chart 74-1). Establish a trusting relationship and use a nonjudgmental approach to gather more complete information. This approach may decrease the patient's anxiety and fear about having an STD.

The infection can be asymptomatic in both men and women, but women have asymptomatic, or "silent," infections more often than do men. If symptoms are present, men usually notice dysuria and a penile discharge that can be either profuse, yellowish green fluid or scant, clear fluid. The urethra is most commonly affected, but infection can extend to the prostate, the seminal vesicles, and the epididymis. Men seek curative treatment sooner, usually because they have symptoms, and thereby avoid some of the serious complications.

Women may report a change in vaginal discharge (yellow, green, profuse, odorous), urinary frequency, or dysuria. The cervix and urethra are the most common sites of infection.

Anal manifestations may include itching and irritation, rectal bleeding or diarrhea, and painful defecation. Assess the mouth for a reddened throat, ulcerated lips, tender gingivae, and lesions in the throat. Fig. 74-3 shows common sites of gonococcal infections.

If fever occurs, this may be a sign of an ascending (PID or epididymitis) or systemic infection (disseminated gonococcal infection). Symptoms could include joint or tendon pain, either in a single joint or as migratory arthralgias, especially of the knees, elbows, fingers or toes, and a rash usually on the palms and soles. The rash can be pustular or maculopapular (Bleich et al., 2012).

Clinical symptoms of gonorrhea can resemble those of chlamydia INFECTION and need to be differentiated. *Molecular testing for* N. gonorrhoeae *is currently the most widely used standard and preferred over cultures or microscopic examinations.* These nucleic acid amplification tests (NAATs) are highly sensitive and specific. During examination, providers can swab the male urethra or female cervix to obtain specimens. These specimens can be placed in medium for molecular testing, cultured

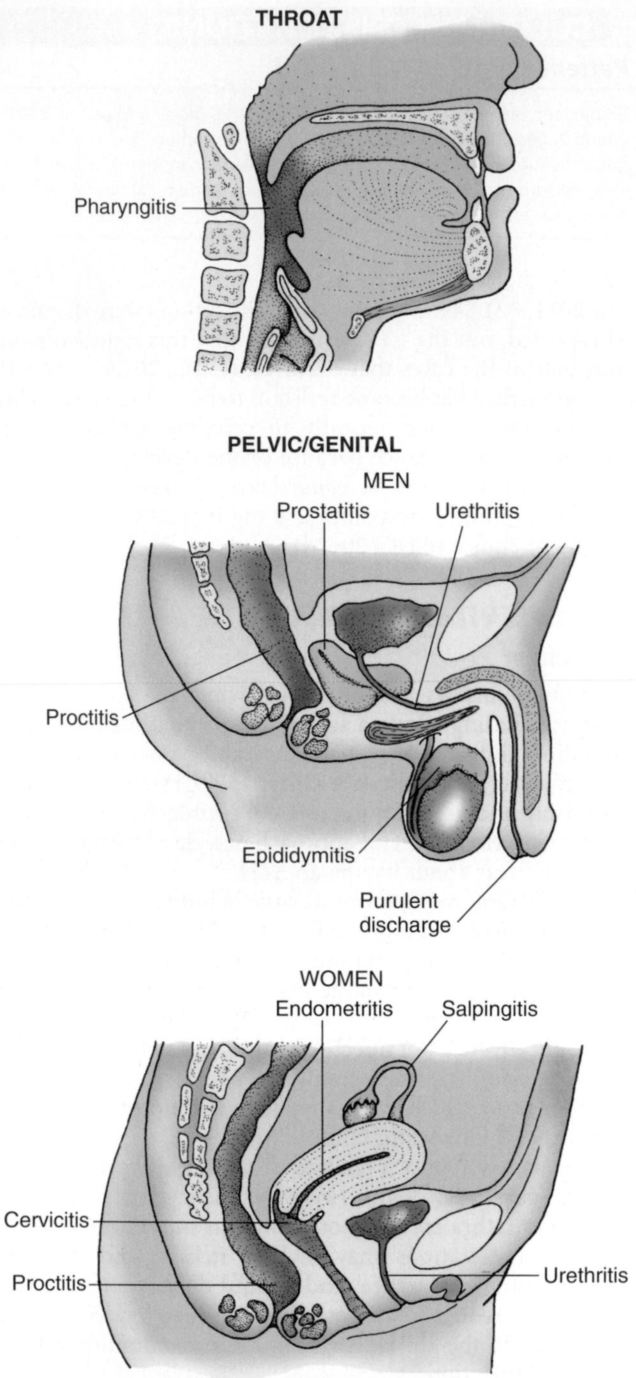

FIG. 74-3 Areas of involvement of gonorrhea in men and women.

on chocolate agar (gold standard), or viewed microscopically after Gram staining (male urethral specimens only). Patient-collected urine or vaginal swabs can also be used to diagnose both gonorrhea and chlamydia infections, allowing for testing without a full examination.

In men, gonorrhea can be diagnosed by Gram staining smears of urethral discharge that has been swabbed onto a glass slide, dried, and stained. The presence of gram-negative diplococci is diagnostic for gonococcal urethritis in men. If the man has symptoms, Gram stains are very sensitive and specific for gonorrhea and allow for immediate diagnosis and treatment in the clinical setting. Without symptoms, Gram stains are less reliable. Smears do not confirm the diagnosis in women because the female genital tract normally harbors other *Neisseria* organisms that resemble *N. gonorrhoeae.*

All patients with gonorrhea should be tested for syphilis, chlamydia, hepatitis B and hepatitis C, and HIV infection and, if possible, examined for HSV and HPV, because they may have been exposed to these STDs as well. Sexual partners who have been exposed in the past 30 days should be examined, and specimens should be obtained.

◆ Interventions

Uncomplicated gonorrhea is treated with antibiotics. Chlamydia infection, which is 4 times more common, is frequently found in patients with gonorrhea. Because of this, patients treated for gonorrhea should also be managed with drugs that treat chlamydia infection.

Drug Therapy. Drug therapy recommended by the CDC is ceftriaxone (Rocephin) 250 mg IM *plus* azithromycin (Zithromax) 1 g orally in a single dose *or* doxycycline (Monodox, Doxy-Caps, Doxycin 🍁) 100 mg orally twice daily for 1 week to treat a presumed co-infection with *Chlamydia* (up to 40%), unless a negative *Chlamydia* result has been obtained. These combinations seem to be effective for all mucosal gonorrheal infections; treatment failure is rare (CDC, 2012d). A test of cure is not required for treatment with ceftriaxone. Advise the patient to return for a follow-up examination if symptoms persist after treatment. Re-infection is usually the cause of these symptoms.

Sexual partners must be treated, not only evaluated, to prevent re-infection. Sexual partners also need to receive education about the INFECTION.

Because the best treatment for gonorrhea is injected Rocephin (ceftriaxone), expedited partner therapy (EPT) is not ideal for treating gonorrhea. If there is concern that the partner may not come to a health care facility for treatment, providing oral cefixime as an alternative has been recommended by the CDC. Because of the potential for resistance of gonorrhea to cefixime, a test of cure is recommended after treatment is completed.

Gonorrhea infection can become disseminated (disseminated gonococcal infection [DGI]), requiring hospitalization and IV or IM ceftriaxone 1 g every 24 hours. If symptoms resolve within 24 to 48 hours, the patient may be discharged to home to continue oral antibiotic therapy (cefixime 400 mg twice a day) for at least a week (CDC, 2010b).

Meningitis and endocarditis occur rarely. Hospitalization of patients with these problems is recommended for the initial treatment. Treatment includes IV antibiotic therapy, usually ceftriaxone 1 to 2 g every 12 hours. If meningitis or endocarditis is present, therapy is continued for 10 to 14 days for meningitis and at least 4 weeks for endocarditis. Collaborate with the infectious disease specialist for management of these INFECTIONS.

Self-Management Education. Teach the patient about transmission and treatment of gonorrhea. The use of medication to treat chlamydia infection at the same time as treating gonorrhea should be explained to the patient since the likelihood of co-infection is high. Discuss the possibility of re-infection, including the risk for pelvic inflammatory disease (PID), and resultant problems such as ectopic pregnancy, infertility, and chronic pelvic pain. Instruct patients to cease sexual activity until the antibiotic therapy is completed and they no longer have symptoms; but if abstinence is not possible, urge men and women to use condoms. Explain that gonorrhea is a *reportable disease.*

When a diagnosis of gonorrhea is made, patients may have feelings of fear or guilt. They may be concerned that they have contracted other STDs or see the disease as a punishment for promiscuity or "unnatural" sex acts. They may believe that acquiring gonorrhea (or any STD) is a risk that they must take to pursue their desired lifestyle. Such feelings can impair relationships with sexual partners. Encourage patients to express their feelings, and offer other information and professional resources to assist them in having a correct understanding of their diagnosis and treatment. Ensuring privacy during your discussion with them and maintaining confidentiality of personal health information are essential in meeting psychosocial needs.

CLINICAL JUDGMENT CHALLENGE

Patient-Centered Care; Teamwork and Collaboration QSEN

A 39-year-old gay man has been diagnosed with a chlamydial infection and provided with treatment for the infection. After learning how the infection is transmitted, he states that he and his partner "broke up" briefly 3 months ago and he wonders if his partner became involved with someone who transmitted the infection to him. One week later, the patient and his partner return to the health care center. The partner states that he "slept with another man" during the break-up. As the nurse, you explain that medication treatment is available with expedited partner therapy (EPT) for the person the partner became involved with during the break-up. The patient becomes angry and tells his partner, "I don't want you ever speaking to him again!"

1. What is the best therapeutic approach for working with this patient and his partner?
2. How will you further explain to this couple the need for EPT for the other person?
3. In your presence, the patient tells his partner that he cannot imagine ever talking with "that jerk you slept with." What emotional feelings is this patient experiencing? How will you respond to the patient's statement?
4. Develop a collaborative plan of care for this patient to ensure that the needs of all involved parties will be met.

OTHER GYNECOLOGIC CONDITIONS

PELVIC INFLAMMATORY DISEASE

PATHOPHYSIOLOGY

Pelvic inflammatory disease (PID) is a complex infectious process in which organisms from the lower genital tract migrate from the endocervix upward through the uterine cavity into the fallopian tubes. The spread of INFECTION to other organs and tissues of the upper genital tract occurs from direct contact with mucosal surfaces or through the fimbriated ends of the tubes to the ovaries, parametrium, and peritoneal cavity (Fig. 74-4). This may involve one or more pelvic structures, including the uterus, fallopian tubes, and adjacent pelvic structures. The most common site is the fallopian tube. Resulting infections include:

- Endometritis (infection of the endometrial cavity)
- Salpingitis (inflammation of the fallopian tubes)
- Oophoritis (ovarian infection)
- Parametritis (infection of the parametrium)

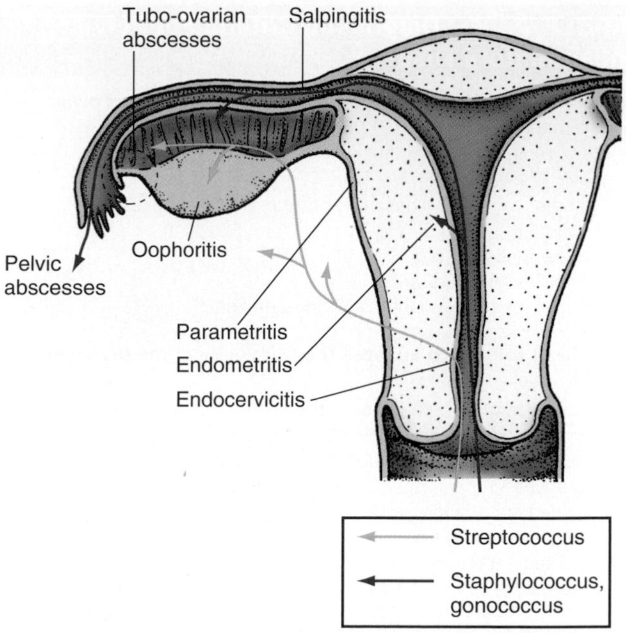

FIG. 74-4 The spread of pelvic inflammatory disease.

- Peritonitis (infection of the peritoneal cavity)
- Tubal or tubo-ovarian abscess

Usually multiple pathogens are involved in the development of PID. Sexually transmitted organisms are most often responsible, especially *C. trachomatis* and *N. gonorrhoeae.* Organisms that are part of the vaginal flora can also cause PID including *Gardnerella vaginalis, Haemophilus influenzae, Staphylococcus, Streptococcus, Mycoplasma, Escherichia coli,* and other aerobic and anaerobic organisms. There is increasing evidence that the anaerobes involved in bacterial vaginosis may have a role in the development of PID and increase the risk for INFECTION with HIV, *N. gonorrhoeae, C. trachomatis,* and HSV (CDC, 2010b; Sweet, 2012).

The organisms invade the pelvis from an infection ascending from the vagina or cervix. Infections are spread during sexual intercourse, during childbirth (including the postpartum period), and after abortion. *Sepsis and death can occur, especially if treatment is delayed or inadequate.*

PID is one of the leading causes of infertility and is related to the increase in the number of ectopic pregnancies reported in the United States. It is an acute syndrome resulting in tenderness in the tubes and ovaries (adnexa) and, typically, dull pelvic pain. However, many women experience only mild discomfort or menstrual irregularity, whereas others have acute pain, which can affect their gait. Others experience no symptoms at all—so-called "silent" or "subclinical" PID. The diagnosis and treatment of this disease are challenging. Irreversible scarring or stricture, causing sterility, may occur before it is diagnosed (Sweet, 2012).

Because of variations in patient manifestations, the diagnosis is difficult because women may have subtle symptoms not typical of the disease. Delay in diagnosis and treatment may add to complications of PID in the upper genital tract. The disease is usually diagnosed on the basis of clinical signs and symptoms. The Centers for Disease Control and Prevention (CDC) (2013e) has set minimum criteria for diagnosis, but no laboratory or physical examination techniques alone are both sensitive and specific (Table 74-4).

TABLE 74-4 Diagnostic Criteria For Pelvic Inflammatory Disease

Minimum Criteria for Initiating Empiric Treatment for Pelvic Inflammatory Disease

- Sexually active woman and at risk for STDs
- Pelvic or lower abdominal pain
- No other cause for illness can be found (e.g., appendicitis)

and

- Uterine tenderness *or*
- Adnexal tenderness *or*
- Cervical motion tenderness (chandelier sign)

Additional Criteria to Increase the Specificity of the Diagnosis of PID

- Oral temperature >101° F (>38.3° C)
- Abnormal cervical or vaginal mucopurulent discharge
- Presence of white blood cells on saline microscopy of vaginal secretions
- Elevated erythrocyte sedimentation rate
- Elevated C-reactive protein
- Laboratory documentation of cervical infection with *Neisseria gonorrhoeae* or *Chlamydia trachomatis*

Definitive Criteria for Diagnosing PID, Warranted in Selected Cases

- Histopathologic evidence of endometritis on endometrial biopsy
- Transvaginal sonography or MRI techniques showing thickened, fluid-filled tubes with or without free pelvic fluid or tubo-ovarian complex, or Doppler studies suggesting pelvic infection
- Laparoscopic abnormalities consistent with PID

Modified from Centers for Disease Control and Prevention (CDC). (2014). *Sexually transmitted diseases treatment guidelines, 2010: Pelvic inflammatory diseases.* Retrieved November 2014, from www.cdc.gov/std/treatment/2010/pid.htm
PID, Pelvic inflammatory disease; *STDs,* sexually transmitted diseases.

❖ PATIENT-CENTERED COLLABORATIVE CARE

◆ Assessment

History. Obtain a complete history of the symptoms with menstrual, obstetric, sexual, and family history and a history of previous episodes of pelvic inflammatory disease (PID) or other sexually transmitted diseases (see Chart 74-1). Assess for contraceptive use, a history of reproductive surgery, and other risk factors previously discussed. Ask the patient if sexual abuse has occurred. If so, encourage her to discuss what happened and whether she was seen by a health care provider.

Many of the same factors that place women at risk for STDs also place them at risk for PID. Risk factors for sexually active women include:

- Age younger than 26 years
- Multiple sexual partners
- Intrauterine device (IUD) placed within the previous 3 weeks
- Smoking
- A history of PID
- Chlamydial or gonococcal infection; bacterial vaginosis
- A history of sexually transmitted diseases (STDs)

Physical Assessment/Clinical Manifestations. *One of the most frequent symptoms of PID is lower abdominal or pelvic pain.* Conduct a complete pain assessment. Other symptoms include irregular vaginal bleeding (spotting or bleeding between periods), dysuria (painful urination), an increase or change in vaginal discharge, dyspareunia (painful sexual intercourse), malaise, fever, and chills.

Observe whether the patient has discomfort with movement. Often the patient has a hunched-over gait to protect her abdomen. She may find it difficult to independently get on the examination table or stretcher. Assess for lower abdominal tenderness, possibly with rigidity or rebound tenderness. A pelvic examination by the health care provider may reveal yellow or green cervical discharge and a reddened or **friable** cervix (a cervix that bleeds easily). Criteria for accurate diagnosis of PID are listed in Table 74-4. The diagnosis of PID is usually based on health history, physical examination, and laboratory tests. Imaging studies and laparoscopy are not generally used to make the diagnosis.

Psychosocial Assessment. The woman who has symptoms of PID is usually anxious and fearful of the examination and unknown diagnosis. She may need much reassurance and support during the physical examination because her abdomen may be very tender or painful. Explain what is taking place to help promote comfort during the examination.

Because PID is often associated with an STD, the woman may feel embarrassed or uncomfortable discussing her symptoms or history. Use a nonjudgmental approach, and encourage the patient to express her feelings and concerns. Determining the patient's ability to follow through with the treatment plan is essential in deciding whether hospitalization should be considered.

Laboratory Assessment. The health care provider obtains specimens from the cervix, urethra, and rectum to determine the presence of *N. gonorrhoeae* or *C. trachomatis.* The white blood cell (WBC) count, erythrocyte sedimentation rate (ESR), and C-reactive protein may be elevated but are not specific for PID. A sensitive test that detects human chorionic gonadotropin (hCG) in urine or blood should be performed to determine whether the patient is pregnant. Microscopic examination of vaginal discharge should be done to evaluate for the presence of more than 10 WBCs per high-power field, which correlates with infection. Bacterial vaginosis can be found by observing the diagnostic "clue" cells with microscopic examination of vaginal discharge.

Other Diagnostic Assessment. Abdominal *ultrasonography* may be used to determine the presence of appendicitis and tubo-ovarian abscesses that need to be ruled out when the diagnosis of PID is made. Transvaginal ultrasound and *MRI* are used in some cases to detect tubal wall thickening, fluid-filled tubes, and free pelvic fluid or a tubo-ovarian abscess, all associated with PID. *Endometrial biopsy* also has been used to increase the accuracy of the diagnosis.

◆ Analysis

The priority collaborative problem for patients with pelvic inflammatory disease (PID) is infection related to invasion of pelvic organs by pathogens.

◆ Planning and Implementation

Managing Infection

Planning: Expected Outcomes. The patient with PID is expected to have her infection resolved, be free of abdominal pain, and prevent re-infection.

Interventions. *Patient-centered collaborative care includes* antibiotic therapy and self-management measures.

Uncomplicated PID is usually treated on an ambulatory care basis. The CDC (2010b) recommends hospitalization for PID if the patient:

- Has appendicitis, ectopic pregnancy, or other surgical emergency that has not been excluded
- Is pregnant
- Does not respond to oral antibiotic therapy
- Is unable to follow or tolerate treatment on an ambulatory care basis
- Has severe illness, nausea and vomiting, or high fever
- Has a tubo-ovarian abscess

There are no recommendations about whether HIV-infected women should be hospitalized. Assess the ability of high-risk women for self-management at home. The patient's health status and availability of support systems are important considerations for home care. If the infection has not responded to treatment, the patient may need to be hospitalized for IV antibiotic therapy and further evaluation.

The CDC recommends oral and/or parenteral antibiotics for PID (CDC, 2010b). Drug therapy is required for 14 days. If the woman has not responded to oral antibiotics, she is hospitalized for IV antibiotic therapy and further evaluation. Inpatient therapy involves a combination of several IV antibiotics until the woman shows signs of improvement (e.g., decreased pelvic tenderness for at least 24 hours). Then oral antibiotics are continued at home until the course of treatment has lasted 14 days.

Antibiotic therapy relieves pain by destroying the pathogens and decreasing the inflammation caused by infection. Other pain-relief measures include taking mild analgesics and applying heat to the lower abdomen or back. As with any INFECTION, encourage the patient to increase her intake of fluids and to eat nutritious foods that can promote healing. *Teach the patient to rest in a semi-Fowler's position and encourage limited ambulation to promote gravity drainage of the infection that may help relieve pain.*

! NURSING SAFETY PRIORITY QSEN

Action Alert

Instruct women who are being treated for PID on an ambulatory care basis to avoid sexual intercourse for the full course of treatment and until their symptoms have resolved. Ask them to check their temperature twice a day. Teach them to report an increase in temperature to their health care provider. Remind them to be seen by the health care provider within 72 hours from starting antibiotic treatment and then 1 and 2 weeks from the time of the initial diagnosis.

In a small number of patients, the pain and tenderness may not be relieved by antibiotic therapy. The surgeon may perform a laparoscopy to remove an abscess through one or more subumbilical incisions to provide better access to the fallopian tubes. Before surgery, provide information about hospital routines and procedures. After surgery, the care of the woman with PID is similar to that of any patient after laparoscopic abdominal surgery. One difference is that she may have a wound drain for drainage of abscess fluid that may not have been completely removed during surgery. Observe, measure, and record wound drainage every 4 to 8 hours as requested.

Community-Based Care. If the woman is hospitalized, collaborate with the case manager or discharge planner before the woman is discharged to home. Teach the patient with PID to see her health care provider for follow-up to assess for complications and assess that the infection has resolved. The ongoing role of the nurse is to assess for any continued risk for contracting PID again, signs of persistent or recurrent infection, and education to prevent exposure to and infection with all STDs (e.g., decrease the number of partners, consistently use condoms). Establish an atmosphere of trust that encourages the woman to return frequently, if needed, for education or reassurance.

CHART 74-4 Patient and Family Education: Preparing for Self-Management

Oral Antibiotic Therapy for Sexually Transmitted Diseases

- Take your medicine for the number of times a day it is prescribed and until it is completed.
- Your sexual partner must be treated if you have a sexually transmitted disease (STD). Expedited partner therapy is one way to ensure partners are treated.
- Be sure to return for your follow-up appointment after completing your antibiotic treatment.
- Call if you have any questions or concerns.
- Do not have sex until after you and your partner complete your antibiotic therapy. This should be at least 7 days, even if treatment is one dose.
- Drink at least 8 to 10 glasses of fluid a day to help heal your infection, while taking your antibiotics.
- Do not take antacids containing calcium, magnesium, or aluminum, such as Tums, Maalox, or Mylanta, with your antibiotics. They may decrease the effectiveness of the antibiotic.
- Take your antibiotics on an empty stomach unless your health care provider instructs you to take them with food.

Home Care Management. Parenteral antibiotic therapy may be given at home, but usually the health care provider changes the treatment regimen to oral antibiotics before hospital discharge.

Self-Management Education. Patient teaching focuses on providing information about PID, identifying symptoms that suggest persistent or recurrent infection (persistent pelvic pain, dysmenorrhea, low backache, fever), and urging completion of antibiotic treatment, rest, and healthy nutrition to resolve the infection and prevent complications. Review information for oral antibiotic therapy (Chart 74-4).

Counsel the patient to contact her sexual partner(s) for examination and treatment. All sexual partners should be treated for gonorrhea and chlamydia infection regardless of whether they have symptoms. Remind the patient about follow-up care, and counsel her about the complications that can occur after an episode of PID. These problems include increased risk for recurrence, ectopic pregnancy, and infertility. Chronic pelvic pain may also develop.

Discuss contraception and the patient's need or desire for it. This discussion includes the use of condoms that can decrease the risk for future episodes of PID. Consider the likelihood that the patient had unprotected (from pregnancy and STDs) intercourse, which resulted in PID. Contraception that includes the use of condoms is an important health message to be communicated. Help the patient understand that having sexual intercourse with multiple partners increases the risk for recurrent episodes. Douching has also been suggested as a risky behavior for development of PID and/or infection with *Chlamydia* or *N. gonorrhoeae.*

Psychosocial concerns may require counseling. A patient who has PID may exhibit a variety of feelings (guilt, disgust, anger) about having a condition that may have been transmitted to her sexually. These feelings may affect her relationship with significant others and future sexual partners. She may also have concerns about future fertility if PID has damaged or scarred the fallopian tubes and other reproductive organs. Provide nonjudgmental emotional support, and allow time for her to discuss her feelings. The primary provider of care may refer the patient to a mental health care provider as another appropriate option.

NCLEX EXAMINATION CHALLENGE

Physiological Integrity

A client with pelvic inflammatory disease returns to her primary care provider's office 3 days after starting treatment with oral antibiotics. Which symptom does the nurse recognize that requires immediate intervention?

A. Mild nausea
B. Temperature of 101°F
C. Report of two diarrheal stools daily after starting antibiotic
D. Expression of anxiety that her partner will "catch" the infection

Health Care Resources. The cost of antibiotics for patients with PID and other STDs may be a concern for those who are uninsured, underinsured, or impoverished. In collaboration with the case manager or social worker, help locate community resources for free or discounted drugs for women who cannot afford them. Ask the patient directly if she has the ability to pay for the drug and her follow-up visits, regardless of her apparent financial status.

If infertility is a result of PID, the patient may need referral to a clinic specializing in infertility treatment and counseling. She can also contact support groups for infertile couples, which exist in many local communities.

◆ *Evaluation: Outcomes*

Evaluate the care of the patient with PID based on the identified priority patient problem. The expected outcomes include that the patient should:

- Show evidence that the infection has resolved
- Report or demonstrate that pain is relieved or reduced and that she feels more comfortable
- Demonstrate a plan for ensuring treatment of her partner, obtaining antibiotics, and returning for follow-up care

VAGINAL INFECTIONS

Vaginal INFECTION associated with sexual activity may produce vaginal discharge or vulvar irritation. The common causes of vaginal infection that can be but are not always sexually transmitted include:

- *Trichomonas vaginalis*
- *Candida,* primarily *Candida albicans*
- Bacteria that produce bacterial vaginosis, including *Gardnerella vaginalis, Mycoplasma hominis,* and anaerobes including *Prevotella* and *Mobiluncus* species

Men can also get these infections but are not always symptomatic.

Trichomoniasis and candida infections are limited to the vagina. They can be very irritating and bothersome but do not cause any long-term problems. The partner must also be treated for *trichomoniasis* for the infection to be resolved. *Candidiasis* does not usually require partner treatment. However, if the male partner is symptomatic (irritation of the genital skin), treatment is indicated. It is important to remember that *Candida* is a normal flora on the skin and vagina. Although it can be transmitted sexually, candidiasis occurs in women regardless of their sexual activity. Also, antibiotics that change the normal flora of the vagina contribute to infection.

Bacterial vaginosis (BV) has been implicated in upper genital tract infections. Women undergoing surgery of the upper genital tract should be evaluated and treated if BV is found. Chapter 71 describes the management of each of these infections.

OTHER SEXUALLY TRANSMITTED DISEASES

Less common diseases in the United States that are transmitted by sexual contact are lymphogranuloma venereum, chancroid, and granuloma inguinale. Like syphilis, all of these diseases are associated with ulcers but they are seen most often in less developed countries. As newcomers migrate into the United States and international travel increases, these STDs may become more common. Ask patients suspected of these infections whether they have traveled out of the United States and whether they had sexual contact with people who live in other countries.

NURSING CONCEPTS AND CLINICAL JUDGMENT REVIEW

What might you OBSERVE if the patient has altered SEXUALITY as a result of a sexually transmitted disease (STD)?

- Report of heavy and abnormal vaginal discharge
- Report of urinary frequency or dysuria
- Ulcers, blisters, or warts in the genital area
- Low-grade fever
- Report of malaise
- Report of vaginal, penile, or anal itching or irritation
- Report of abdominal pain (pelvic inflammatory disease [PID])
- Anxious behavior
- Depressive symptoms
- Report of disinterest in sexual activity
- Changes in relationships (e.g., ending a long-term relationship)

What should you INTERPRET and how should you RESPOND to a patient with altered SEXUALITY as a result of STD?

Perform and interpret focused physical assessment, including:

- Vital signs
- Pain intensity and quality
- Posture and mobility
- Skin inspection (genital area)

Respond by:
- Reporting and documenting all findings
- Helping patient with abdominal pain into a semi-Fowler's position
- Providing pain-control measures
- Teaching patient about prescribed antibiotic or antiviral therapy
- Teaching patient to avoid sexual intercourse while being treated
- Teaching patient the importance of treating all sexual partners
- Teaching patient and partner(s) about safer sex practices
- Providing support and listening to the patient and partner(s) without judgment

On what should you REFLECT?
- Examine your feelings about patients who make sexual choices different from your own.
- Think about what else you could do to help patients meet their physical and emotional needs during this time.
- Determine what other health teaching may be needed for this patient.
- Monitor the patient's response to pain-control interventions.

GET READY FOR THE NCLEX® EXAMINATION!

KEY POINTS

Review these Key Points for each NCLEX Examination Client Needs Category.

Safe and Effective Care Environment
- Maintain patient and partner confidentiality and privacy at all times. **Patient-Centered Care** QSEN
- Use gloves when examining the patient's genitalia or skin lesions. **Safety** QSEN

Health Promotion and Maintenance
- Teach patients to not have sexual intercourse during their treatment for sexually transmitted disease (STD). **Safety** QSEN
- Assume that all adult patients may be sexually active, regardless of age or stage of life. Sexually transmitted diseases are still spread within the older adult population because perception of risk is lower.
- Educate young women about increased vulnerability to STDs; women's vaginal mucous membranes place them at higher risk for contracting an STD, and young women statistically have more partners and more unprotected sex, which further increases their risk. **Safety** QSEN
- Teach the patient about the availability of expedited partner therapy; be sure that both the patient and the partner take all doses of the drug.
- Encourage all patients who are sexually active to use condoms during sexual intimacy (see Chart 74-3).
- Urge sexually active people, especially those younger than 26 years (or those older than 26 years if at high risk), to have STD screenings at least annually.
- Treat all patients, regardless of diagnosis, gender identity, or sexual orientation, with respect.
- Respect the sexual choices of all patients. **Patient-Centered Care** QSEN

Psychosocial Integrity
- Provide privacy for patients undergoing examination or testing for STDs.
- Allow the patient to express fears and/or anxiety regarding a diagnosis of STD. **Patient-Centered Care** QSEN
- Refer patients newly diagnosed with an STD to local resources and support groups as needed based on their response. **Teamwork and Collaboration** QSEN
- Encourage all patients who have an STD to inform their sexual partner(s) of their health status.

Physiological Integrity
- Assess patients with STD using the guidelines in Chart 74-1. **Evidence-Based Practice** QSEN
- Recognize that each stage of syphilis has unique symptoms and it is important to not overlook symptoms that resolve.
- Understand that patients without symptoms may still be infected with an STD.
- Encourage patients to adhere to their entire anti-infective drug regimen (see Chart 74-4), even after they begin to feel better.
- Teach patients the expected side effects and possible adverse reactions to prescribed drugs.
- Teach patients about the short-term and long-term complications of STD using the information in Table 74-2.
- Be aware that PID is diagnosed based on the criteria in Table 74-4. **Evidence-Based Practice** QSEN

BIBLIOGRAPHY

Asterisk indicates a classic or definitive work on this subject.

General References

This list represents references that are cited in the majority of chapters in this text.

Giddens, J. F. (2013). *Concepts for nursing practice.* St. Louis: Elsevier.

Jarvis, C. (2016). *Physical examination & health assessment* (7th ed.). St. Louis: Elsevier Saunders.

Lilley, L. L., Collins, S. R., & Snyder, J. S. (2014). *Pharmacology and the nursing process* (7th ed.). St. Louis: Mosby.

McCance, K., Huether, S., Brashers, V., & Rote, N. (2014). *Pathophysiology: The biologic basis for disease in adults and children* (7th ed.). St. Louis: Mosby.

Pagana, K. D., & Pagana, T. J. (2014). *Mosby's manual of diagnostic and laboratory tests* (5th ed.). St. Louis: Mosby.

Quality and Safety Education for Nurses (QSEN) (2014). *Pre-licensure KSAs (knowledge, skill, and attitudes).* Retrieved July 2014, from <http://qsen.org/competencies/pre-licensure-ksas/>.

Touhy, T., & Jett, K. (2014). *Ebersole and Hess' gerontological nursing healthy aging* (4th ed.). St. Louis: Mosby.

Chapter 1

Academy of Medical-Surgical Nurses (AMSN) (2012). *Scope and standards of medical-surgical nursing practice* (5th ed.). Pitman, NJ: Author.

Alfaro-LeFevre, R. (2012). *Critical thinking, clinical reasoning, and clinical judgment: A practical approach to outcome-focused thinking* (5th ed.). Philadelphia: Saunders.

American Nurses Association (ANA) (2010). *Code of ethics for nurses with interpretive statements.* Retrieved March 30, 2014, from <www.nursingworld.org/MainMenuCategories/EthicsStandards/CodeofEthicsforNurses>.

Benner, P. E., Malloch, K., & Sheets, V. (2010). *Nursing pathways for patient safety.* St. Louis: Mosby.

Bogert, S., Ferrell, C., & Rutledge, D. N. (2010). Experience with family activation of rapid response teams. *Medsurg Nursing, 19,* 215–222.

Burns, K. (2011). Nurse-physician rounds: A collaborative approach to improving communication, efficiencies, and perception of care. *Medsurg Nursing, 20,* 194–199.

*Donaldson, N., Shapiro, S., Scott, M., Foley, M., & Spetz, J. (2009). Leading successful rapid response teams: A multi-site implementation evaluation. *Journal of Nursing Administration, 39,* 176–181.

Evans, D., Grunawalt, J., McClish, D., Wood, W., & Friese, C. R. (2012). Bedside shift-to-shift nursing report: Implementation and outcomes. *Medsurg Nursing, 21*(5), 281–284, 292.

Flicek, C. L. (2012). Communication: A dynamic between nurses and physicians. *Medsurg Nursing, 21,* 385–386.

Furst, C. M., Finto, D., Malouf-Todaro, N., Moore, C., Orr, D., Santos, J., et al. (2013). Changing times: Enhancing clinical practice through evolving technology. *Medsurg Nursing, 22*(2), 131–134.

Gasarian, P. K., Henneman, E. A., & Chandler, G. E. (2010). Nurse decision making in the pre-arrest period. *Clinical Nursing Research, 19,* 21–37.

Hicks, D. (2012). Cultural competence and the Hispanic population. *Medsurg Nursing, 21,* 314–315.

*Institute for Healthcare Improvement (IHI) (2005). *Protecting 5 million lives from harm.* Accessed March 30, 2014, from <www.ihi.org>.

*Institute of Medicine (IOM) (2000). *To err is human: Building a safer health care system.* Washington, DC: National Academies Press.

*Institute of Medicine (IOM) (2003). *Health professions education: A bridge to quality.* Washington, DC: National Academies Press.

Institute of Medicine (IOM) (2011). *The health of lesbian, gay, bisexual, and transgender people: Building a foundation for better understanding.* Washington, DC: National Academies Press.

Joint Commission Center for Transforming Healthcare (2010). *Joint Commission Center for Transforming Healthcare tackles miscommunication among caregivers.* Accessed March 30, 2014, from <www.centerfortransforminghealthcare.org>.

Maklebust, J. (2011). Engaging the patient and family as partners in practice. *Nursing, 41*(6), 23–24.

Maxson, P. M., Derby, K. M., Wrobleski, D. M., & Foss, D. M. (2012). Bedside nurse-to-nurse handoff promotes patient safety. *Medsurg Nursing, 21,* 140–144.

Melnyk, B. M., & Fineout-Overholt, E. (2011). *Evidence-based practice in nursing and healthcare* (2nd ed.). Philadelphia: Lippincott Williams & Wilkins.

Morrison, D., & Sanders, C. (2011). Huddling for optimal care outcomes. *Nursing, 41*(12), 22–24.

Pettinato, M. (2012). Providing care for LGBTQ patients. *Nursing, 42*(12), 22–27.

Quality and Safety Education for Nurses (QSEN) (2011). *Competency KSAs (pre-licensure).* Accessed November 1, 2012, from <www.qsen.org>.

Robert, R. R., & Petersen, S. (2013). Critical thinking at the bedside. *Medsurg Nursing, 22*(2), 85–93.

Schneider, M. A. (2012). Nurse-physician collaboration: Its time has come. *Nursing, 42*(7), 50–53.

Shafer, L., & Aziz, M. G. (2013). Shaping a unit's culture through effective nurse-led quality improvement. *Medsurg Nursing, 22*(4), 229–236.

Sherwood, G., & Barnsteiner, J. (2012). *Quality and safety in nursing: A competency approach to improving outcomes.* Hoboken, NJ: Wiley-Blackwell.

The Joint Commission (TJC) (2011). *Speak Up initiatives: The Joint Commission's award-winning patient safety program.* Accessed March 30, 2014, from <www.jointcommission.org/speakup.aspx>.

Yoder-Wise, P. S. (2011). *Leading and managing in nursing* (5th ed.). St. Louis: Mosby.

Chapter 2

Berryman, S. N., Jennings, J., Ragsdale, S., Lofton, T., Huff, D. C., & Rooker, J. S. (2012). Beers criteria for potentially inappropriate medication use in older adults. *Medsurg Nursing, 21*(3), 129–133.

Brown-O'Hara, R. (2013). Geriatric syndromes and their implications for nursing. *Nursing, 43*(1), 1–3.

Dossa, A., Bokhour, B., & Hoenig, H. (2012). Care transitions from the hospital to home for patients with mobility impairments: Patient and family caregiver experiences. *Rehabilitation Nursing, 37,* 277–285.

Eldelman, M., & Ficorelli, C. T. (2012). Keeping older adults safe at home. *Nursing, 42,* 65–66.

Fink, A., Morton, S. C., Beck, J. C., Hays, R. D., Spritzer, K., Oishi, S., et al. (2002). The alcohol-related problems survey: Identifying hazardous and harmful drinking in older primary care patients. *Journal of the American Geriatrics Society, 50*(10), 1717–1722.

Fredriksen-Goldsen, K. I. (2011). Resilience and disparities among lesbian, gay, bisexual, and transgender older adults. *Public Policy and Aging Report, 21*(3), 3–7.

*Fulmer, T. (2007). How to try this: Fulmer SPICES. *American Journal of Nursing, 107*(10), 40–48.

Gerber, L. (2013). Bringing home effective nursing care for the homeless. *Nursing, 43*(3), 32–38.

Graham, B. C. (2012). Examining evidence-based interventions to prevent inpatient falls. *Medsurg Nursing, 21,* 267–270.

*Greenberg, S. A. (2007). How to try this: The Geriatric Depression Scale—Short Form. *The American Journal of Nursing, 107*(10), 60–69.

Lee, L. Y., Lee, D. T., & Woo, J. (2010). The psychosocial effect of Tai Chi on nursing home residents. *Journal of Clinical Nursing, 19*(7–8), 927–938.

McCaffrey, R., Hanson, C., & McCaffrey, W. (2010). Garden walking for depression: A research report. *Holistic Nursing Practice, 24*(5), 252–259.

Messina, B. A., & Escallier, L. A. (2011). Taking the "hyper" out of pharmacotherapy. *Nursing, 41*(7), 51–53.

National Institute on Alcohol Abuse and Alcoholism (NIAAA) (2011). *Older adults and alcohol problems*. Retrieved October 17, 2013, from <www.pubs.niaaa.nih.gov/publications/socialworkeducationmodule>.

National Institute of Mental Health (NIMH) (2011). *Older adults and depression*. Retrieved March 30, 2014, from <www.nimh.nih.gov/health/topics/depression>.

Phillips, L. A. (2013). Delirium in geriatric patients: Identification and prevention. *Medsurg Nursing*, *22*, 9–12.

Planton, J., & Edlund, B. J. (2010). Strategies for reducing polypharmacy in older adults. *Journal of Gerontological Nursing*, *36*(1), 8–12.

*Rocchiccioli, J. T., & Sanford, J. T. (2009). Revisiting geriatric failure to thrive. *Journal of Gerontological Nursing*, *35*(1), 18–24.

Rogers, C., Keller, C., & Larkey, L. K. (2010). Perceived benefits of meditative movement in older adults. *Geriatric Nursing*, *31*(1), 37–51.

*Sendelbach, S., & Guthrie, P. F. (2009). Evidence-based guideline—Acute confusion/delirium: Identification, assessment, treatment, and prevention. *Journal of Gerontological Nursing*, *35*(11), 11–17.

Stark, S. (2012). Elder abuse: Screening, intervention, and prevention. *Nursing*, *42*(10), 24–29.

Strunk, J., Townsend-Rocchiccioli, J., & Sanford, J. T. (2013). The aging Hispanic in America: Challenges for nurses in a stressed health care environment. *Medsurg Nursing*, *22*, 45–50.

Swan, B. A., Becker, J., Brawer, R., & Sciamanna, C. N. (2011). Factors influencing the implementation of a point-of-care screening tool for delirium. *Medsurg Nursing*, *20*, 318–322.

Swartzell, K. L., Fulton, J. S., & Friesth, B. M. (2013). Relationship between occurrence of falls and fall-risk scores in an acute care setting using the Hendrich II Fall Risk Model. *Medsurg Nursing*, *22*(3), 180–187.

Toner, F., & Claros, E. (2012). Preventing, assessing, and managing constipation in older adults. *Nursing*, *42*(12), 32–38.

Tzeng, H.-M., & Yin, C.-Y. (2010). Nurses response time to call lights and fall occurrences. *Medsurg Nursing*, *19*(5), 266–272.

Tzeng, H.-M., & Yin, C.-Y. (2012). Toileting-related inpatient falls in adult acute care settings. *Medsurg Nursing*, *21*, 372–377.

U.S. Census Bureau (2013). *Projections of the population by selected age groups and sex for the United States 2010 to 2050*. Retrieved March 30, 2014, from <http://www.census.gov/population/projections/data/national/2008/summarytables.html>.

Vitale, S. A. (2012). What your patient needs to know about CAM. *Nursing*, *42*(8), 59–61.

Volkert, D., Saegitz, C., Gueldenzoph, H., Sieber, C. C., & Stehle, P. (2010). Underdiagnosed malnutrition and nutrition-related problems in geriatric patients. *Journal of Nutrition, Health & Aging*, *14*(5), 387–392.

Williams, K. N., & Kemper, S. (2010). Interventions to reduce cognitive decline in aging. *Journal of Psychosocial Nursing and Mental Health Services*, *48*(5), 42–51.

Wooten, A. C. (2010). An integrative review of Tai Chi research: An alternative form of physical activity to improve balance and prevent falls in older adults. *Orthopedic Nursing*, *29*(2), 108–118.

Chapter 3

Allred, K. D., Byers, J., & Sole, M. L. (2010). The effect of music on postoperative pain and anxiety. *Pain Management Nursing*, *11*, 15–25.

*American Geriatrics Society (AGS). (2009). The pharmacological management of persistent pain in older persons. *Journal of the American Geriatrics Society*, *57*(8), 1331–1346.

American Society of Anesthesiologists (ASA) Task Force on Acute Pain Management. (2012). Practice guidelines for acute pain management in the perioperative setting: An updated report by the American Society of Anesthesiologists Task Force on Acute Pain Management. *Anesthesiology*, *116*(2), 248–273.

Arnstein, P., Broglio, K., Wuhrman, E., & Kean, M. B. (2010). *American Society for Pain Management Nursing (ASPMN) position statement: Use of placebos in pain management* (revised). Retrieved November 15, 2013, from <http://aspmn.org/Organization/documents/Placebo_Position_FINAL.pdf>.

Bruckenthal, P. (2010). Integrating nonpharmacologic and alternative strategies into a comprehensive management approach for older adults with pain. *Pain Management Nursing*, *11*(2), S23–S31.

Catterall, W. A., & Mackie, K. (2011). Local anesthetics. In L. L. Brunton, B. A. Chabner, & B. C. Knoolmann (Eds.), *Goodman & Gilman's pharmacologic basis of therapeutics* (12th ed., pp. 565–582). New York: McGraw-Hill.

Curtis, K., Osadchuk, A., & Katz, J. (2011). An eight-week yoga intervention is associated with improvements in pain, psychological functioning and mindfulness, and changes in cortisol levels in women with fibromyalgia. *Journal of Pain Research*, *2011*(4), 189–201.

Dworkin, R. H., O'Connor, A. B., Audette, J., Baron, R., Gourlay, G. K., Haanpää, M. L., et al. (2010). Recommendations for pharmacological management of neuropathic pain. *Mayo Clinical Proceedings*, *85*, S3–S14.

Fillingim, R. B., King, C. D., Ribeiro-Dasilva, M. C., Rahim-Williams, B., & Riley, J. L. (2009). Sex, gender, and pain: A review of recent clinical and experimental findings. *Journal of Pain*, *10*(5), 447–485.

Fouladbakhsh, J. M., Szczesny, S., Jenuwine, E. S., & Vallerand, A. H. (2011). Nondrug therapies for pain management among rural older adults. *Pain Management Nursing*, *12*(2), 70–81.

*Gordon, D. B., Dahl, J., Phillips, P., Frandsen, J., Cowley, C., Foster, R. L., et al. (2004). The use of "as needed" range orders for opioid analgesics in the management of acute pain: A consensus statement of the ASPMN and the APS. *Pain Management Nursing*, *5*(2), 53–58.

Herr, K. (2010). Pain in the older adult: An imperative across all health care settings. *Pain Management Nursing*, *11*(2), S1–S10.

Herr, K., Coyne, P. J., McCaffery, M., Manworren, R., & Merkel, S. (2011). *American Society for Pain Management Nursing position statement with clinical practice recommendations: Pain assessment in the patient unable to self report* (revised). Retrieved January 1, 2014, from <http://aspmn.org/Organization/documents/UPDATED_NonverbalRevisionFinalWEB.pdf>.

Ho, K. T., & Gan, T. J. (2009). Opioid-related adverse effects and treatment options. In R. S. Sinatra, O. A. de Leon-Casasola, B. Ginsberg, & E. R. Viscusi (Eds.), *Acute pain management* (pp. 406–415). New York: Cambridge University Press.

Institute of Medicine (IOM) (June 2011). *Relieving pain in America: A blueprint for transforming prevention, care, education, and research*. Retrieved November 15, 2013, from <www.iom.edu/~/media/Files/Report%20Files/2011/Relieving-Pain-in-America-A-Blueprint-for-Transforming-Prevention-Care-Education-Research/Pain%20Research%202011%20Report%20Brief.pdf>.

Jarzyna, D., Junquist, C., Pasero, C., Willens, J., Nisbet, A., Oakes, L., et al. (2011). American Society for Pain Management evidence-based guideline on monitoring for opioid-induced sedation and respiratory depression. *Pain Management Nursing*, *12*(3), 118–145.

Kwekkeboom, K. L., Cherwin, C. H., Lee, J. W., & Wanta, B. (2010). Mind-body treatments for the pain-fatigue-sleep disturbance symptom cluster in persons with cancer. *Journal of Pain and Symptom Management*, *39*, 126–138.

Liberto, L. A., & Fornili, K. S. (2013). Managing pain in opioid-dependent patients in general hospital settings. *Medsurg Nursing*, *22*(1), 33–37.

*McCaffery, M. (1968). *Nursing practice and theories related to cognition, bodily pain, and man-environment interactions*. Los Angeles: University of California at Los Angeles Students' Store.

National Center for Complementary and Alternative Medicine (NCCAM) (2010). *What is CAM?* Retrieved November 15, 2013, from <http://nccam.nih.gov/health/whatiscam/>.

Nicolas, M. K., Asghari, A., Corbett, M., Smeets, R. J., Wood, B. M., Overton, S., et al. (2012). Is adherence to pain self-management strategies associated with improved pain, depression and disability in those with disabling chronic pain? *European Journal of Pain*, *16*(1), 93–104.

Oliver, J., Coggins, C., Compton, P., Haggan, S., Matteliano, D., Stanton, M., et al. (2012). American Society for Pain Management Nursing position statement: Pain management in patients with substance use disorders. *Pain Management Nursing*, *13*(3), 169–183. Retrieved November 15, 2013, from <http://aspmn.org/Organization/documents/PainManagementinPatientswithSubstanceAbuseDisorders.pdf>.

Pasero, C. (2011). Persistent post-surgical and post-trauma pain. *Journal of Perianesthesia Nursing*, *26*(1), 38–41.

Pasero, C., & McCaffery, M. (2011). *Pain assessment and pharmacologic management.* St. Louis: Mosby.

Pasero, C., & Stannard, D. (2012). Role of IV acetaminophen in acute pain management: A case-illustrated review. *Pain Management Nursing, 13*(2), 107–124. Retrieved November 15, 2013, from <www.medscape.com/viewarticle/764841_5>.

Portenoy, R. K. (2011). Treatment of cancer pain. *The Lancet, 377*(9784), 2236–2247.

Quality and Safety Education for Nurses (QSEN) (2011). *Competency KSAs (pre-licensure).* Retrieved November 15, 2013, from <www.qsen.org>.

*Snidvongs, S. (2008). Gender differences in responses to medications and side effects of medications. *Pain Clinical Updates, 16*(5), 1–6.

Tate, J. A., Seaman, J. B., & Happ, M. B. (2012). Overcoming barriers to pain assessment: Communicating pain information with intubated older adults. *Geriatric Nursing, 33*(4), 310–313.

Turk, D. C., Wilson, H. D., & Cahana, A. (2011). Treatment of chronic non-cancer pain. *The Lancet, 377*(9784), 2226–2235.

Wu, C. L., & Raja, S. N. (2011). Treatment of acute postoperative pain. *The Lancet, 377*(9784), 2215–2225.

*Wuhrman, E., Cooney, M. F., Dunwoody, C. J., Eksterowicz, N., Merkel, S., Oakes, L. L., et al. (2007). Authorized and unauthorized ("PCA by Proxy") dosing of analgesic infusion pumps: Position statement with clinical practice recommendations. *Pain Management Nursing, 8*(1), 4–11.

Yaksh, T. L., & Wallace, M. S. (2011). Opioids, analgesia, and pain management. In L. L. Brunton, B. A. Chabner, & B. C. Knoolmann (Eds.), *Goodman & Gilman's pharmacologic basis of therapeutics* (12th ed., pp. 481–526). New York: McGraw-Hill.

Chapter 4

Badzek, L., Henaghan, M., Turner, M., & Monsen, R. (2013). Ethical, legal, and social issues in the translation of genomics into health care. *Journal of Nursing Scholarship, 45*(1), 15–24.

Beery, T., & Workman, M. L. (2012). *Genetics and genomics in nursing and health care.* Philadelphia: F.A. Davis.

Berkman, B., & Hull, S. (2014). The right not to know in the genomic era: Time to break from tradition? *American Journal of Bioethics, 14*(3), 28–31.

Bielinski, S., Olson, J., Pathak, J., Weinshilboum, R.M., Wang, L., Lyke, K.J., et al. (2014). Preemptive genotyping for personalized medicine: Design of the right drug, right dose, right time—using genomic data to individualize treatment protocol. *Mayo Clinic Proceedings, 89*(1), 25–33.

Calzone, K. A., Jenkins, J., Nicol, N., Skirton, H., Feero, W. G., & Green, E. D. (2013). Relevance of genomics to healthcare and nursing practice. *Journal of Nursing Scholarship, 45*(1), 1–2.

Cheek, D. (2013). What you need to know about pharmacogenomics. *Nursing, 43*(3), 44–48.

Conley, Y. P., Biesecker, L. G., Gonsalves, S., Merkle, C. J., Kirk, M., & Aouizerat, B. E. (2013). Current and emerging technology approaches in genomics. *Journal of Nursing Scholarship, 45*(1), 5–14.

Crockett-Maillet, G. (2010). Know the red flags of hereditary cancers. *The Nurse Practitioner Journal, 35*(7), 39–43.

Giarelli, E., & Reiff, M. (2012). Genomic literacy and competent practice: Call for research on genomics in nursing education. *Nursing Clinics of North America, 47*(4), 529–545.

Greco, K., & Mahon, S. (2012). Genomic health care has arrived, but are nurses competent to deliver it? *American Nurse Today, 7*(11), 37–38.

Kirk, M., Calzone, K., Arimori, N., & Tonkin, E. (2011). Genetic-genomics competencies and nursing regulation. *Journal of Nursing Scholarship, 43*(2), 107–116.

Manuck, S., & McCaffery, J. (2014). Gene environment interaction. *Annual Review of Psychology, 65*(1), 41–70.

Chapter 5

American Nurses Association (2010). *Nursing: Scope and standards of practice* (2nd ed.). Silver Spring, MD: Author.

Burnett, M., Lewis, M., Joy, T., & Jarrett, K. (2012). Participating in clinical nursing research: Challenges and solutions of the bedside nurse champion. *Medsurg Nursing, 21*(5), 309–311.

*Carlson, C. (2009). Use of three evidence-based postoperative pain assessment practices by registered nurses. *Pain Management Nursing, 10*(4), 174–187.

*Cronenwett, L., Sherwood, G., Barnsteiner, J., Disch, J., Johnson, J., Mitchell, P., et al. (2007). Quality and safety education for nurses. *Nursing Outlook, 55*(3), 122–131.

Fleming, K. (2008). Asking answerable questions. In N. Cullum, D. Ciliska, R. B. Haynes, & S. Marks (Eds.), *Evidence-based nursing.* Oxford, UK: Blackwell.

*DiCenso, A., Guyatt, G., & Ciliska, D. (2005). *Evidence-based nursing: A guide to clinical practice.* St. Louis: Mosby.

*Ervin, N. E. (2002). Evidence-based nursing practice: Are we there yet? *Journal of the New York State Nurses' Association, 33*(2), 11–16.

Fineout-Overholt, E., Melnyk, B. M., Stillwell, S. B., & Williamson, K. M. (2010). Critical appraisal of the evidence: Part 1—An introduction to gathering, evaluating, and recording the evidence. *The American Journal of Nursing, 110*(10), 47–52.

Fineout-Overholt, E., & Stillwell, S. B. (2011). Asking compelling clinical questions. In B. M. Melnyk & E. Fineout-Overholt (Eds.), *Evidence-based practice in nursing and healthcare: A guide to best practice* (2nd ed.). Philadelphia: Lippincott Williams & Wilkins.

Gélinas, C. (2010). Nurses' evaluation of the feasibility and the clinical utility of the critical-care pain observation tool. *Pain Management Nursing, 11*(2), 115–125.

*Hall, D. (2007). Evaluation of 3 pain assessment tools for use with critically ill adult patients. *American Journal of Critical Care, 16*(3), 309–310.

Institute of Medicine (IOM); Board on Health Care Services (2011). *Standards for developing trustworthy clinical practice guidelines: Clinical practice guidelines we can trust* (Report Brief). Washington, DC: National Academies Press. Available online at <www.nap.edu>.

*Institute of Medicine (IOM); Committee on the Health Professions Education Summit (2003). *Health professions education: A bridge to quality.* Washington, DC: National Academies Press.

*Institute of Medicine (IOM); Committee on Quality of Health Care in America (2001). *Crossing the quality chasm: A new health care system for the 21st century.* Washington, DC: National Academies Press.

Institute of Medicine (IOM); Committee on the Robert Wood Johnson Foundation Initiative on the Future of Nursing (2010). *The future of nursing: Leading change, advancing health* (Report Brief). Washington, DC: National Academies Press. Available online at <www.nap.edu>.

Keane, K. M. (2012). Validity and reliability of the critical care pain observation tool: A replication study. *Pain Management Nursing, 14*(4), e216–e225.

*Langley, G. J., Moen, R. G., Nolan, K. M., Nolan, T. W., Norman, C. L., & Provost, L. P. (2009). *The improvement guide: A practical approach to enhancing organizational performance* (2nd ed.). San Francisco: Jossey-Bass.

*Levin, R. F. (2008). Translating research evidence for WOCN practice—Evidence levels and quality ratings: What do they mean? *World Council of Enterostomal Therapists Journal, 28*(1), 30–31.

*Levin, R. F. (2009). Evidence-based practice—Implementing practice changes: Walk before you run. *Research and Theory in Nursing Practice, 23*(2), 85–87.

Levin, R. F. (2013). Formulating clinical questions: Follow my lips. In R. F. Levin & H. R. Feldman (Eds.), *Teaching evidence-based practice in nursing: A guide for academic and clinical settings* (pp. 75–83). New York: Springer.

Levin, R. F., Burke, R. E., & Kealey, S. B. (2013). Searching the sea of evidence: It takes a library. In R. F. Levin & H. R. Feldman (Eds.), *Teaching evidence-based practice in nursing: A guide for academic and clinical settings* (pp. 103–118). New York: Springer.

Levin, R. F., & Jacobs, S. K. (2012). Developing and evaluating clinical practice guidelines: A systematic approach. In M. Boltz, E. Capezuti, T. Fulmer, & D. Zwicker (Eds.), *Evidence-based geriatric nursing protocols* (4th ed.). New York: Springer.

Levin, R. F., Keefer, J. M., Marren, J., Vetter, M., Lauder, B., & Sobolewski, S. (2010). Evidence-based practice improvement: Merging 2 paradigms. *Journal of Nursing Care Quality, 25*(2), 117–126.

Levin, R. F., Melnyk, B. M., Fineout-Overholt, E., Barnes, M., & Vetter, M. (2011). Fostering evidence-based practice to improve nurse and cost outcomes in a community health setting: A pilot test of the ARCC model. *Nursing Administration Quarterly, 35*(1), 1–13.

Melnyk, B. M., & Fineout-Overholt, E. (2010). ARCC (Advancing Research and Clinical Practice through Close Collaboration): A model for system-wide implementation and sustainability of evidence-based practice. In J. Rycroft-Malone & T. Bucknall (Eds.), *Models and frameworks for implementing evidence-based practice: Linking evidence to action*. Oxford: Wiley-Blackwell.

Melnyk, B. M., & Fineout-Overholt, E. (2011). *Evidence-based practice in nursing and healthcare: A guide to best practice* (2nd ed.). Philadelphia: Lippincott Williams & Wilkins.

*Pravikoff, D. S., Tanner, A. B., & Pierce, S. T. (2005). Readiness of U.S. nurses for evidence-based practice: Many don't understand or value research and have had little or no training to help them find evidence on which to base their practice. *American Journal of Nursing, 105*(9), 40–52.

*Reavy, K., & Tavernier, S. (2008). Nurses reclaiming ownership of their practice: Implementation of an evidence-based practice model and process. *Journal of Continuing Education in Nursing, 39*(4), 166–172.

Rycroft-Malone, J., & Bucknall, T. (2010). Using theory and frameworks to facilitate the implementation of evidence into practice. *Worldviews on Evidence-Based Nursing, 7*(2), 57.

*Sackett, D. L., Straus, S. E., Richardson, W. S., Rosenberg, W., & Haynes, R. B. (2000). *Evidence-based medicine: How to practice and teach EBM* (2nd ed.). Edinburgh: Churchill Livingston.

Stetler, C. B. (2010). Stetler model. In J. Rycroft-Malone & T. Bucknall (Eds.), *Models and frameworks for implementing evidence-based practice: Linking evidence to action*. Oxford: Wiley-Blackwell.

Stillwell, S. B., Fineout-Overholt, E., Melnyk, B. M., & Williamson, K. M. (2010). Evidence-based practice, step by step: Asking the clinical question—A key step in evidence-based practice. *American Journal of Nursing, 110*(3), 58–61.

The Joint Commission (TJC) (2010). *Approaches to pain management* (2nd ed.). Oakbrook Terrace, IL: Author.

Titler, M. (2010). Iowa model of evidence-based practice. In J. Rycroft-Malone & T. Bucknall (Eds.), *Models and frameworks for implementing evidence-based practice: Linking evidence to action*. Oxford: Wiley-Blackwell.

*Wilding, J., Manias, E., & McCoy, D. (2009). Pain assessment and management in patients after abdominal surgery from PACU to the postoperative unit. *Journal of Perianesthesia Nursing, 24*(4), 233–240.

*Wolosin, R. (2008). Safety and satisfaction: Where are the connections? *Patient Safety & Quality Healthcare, May/June*, Available online at <www.psqh.com>.

*Worral, P. S., Levin, R. F., & Arsenault, D. C. (2009-2010). Documenting an EBP project: Guidelines for what to include and why. *Journal of the New York State Nurses Association, 40*(2), 12–19.

Chapter 6

American Nurses' Association (2012). *Safe patient handling practices*. Retrieved April 2014, from <www.anasafepatienthandling.org>.

*Association of Rehabilitation Nurses (ARN) (2002). *Practice guidelines for the management of constipation in adults*. Glenview, IL: Author.

*Association of Rehabilitation Nurses (ARN) (2008a). *Standards and scope of rehabilitation nursing practice*. Glenview, IL: Author.

*Association of Rehabilitation Nurses (ARN) (2008b). *The specialty practice of rehabilitation nursing: A core curriculum* (5th ed.). Skokie, IL: Author.

Coggrave, M. J., & Norton, C. (2010). The need for manual evacuation and oral laxatives in the management of neurogenic bowel dysfunction after spinal cord injury: A randomized controlled trial of a stepwise protocol. *Spinal Cord, 48*(6), 504–510.

Cournan, M. (2012). Bladder management in female stroke survivors: Translating research into practice. *Rehabilitation Nursing, 37*, 220–230.

Frisina, P. G., Guellnitz, R., & Alverzo, J. (2010). A time series of falls and injury in the inpatient rehabilitation setting. *Rehabilitation Nursing, 35*(4), 141–146, 166.

*Granger, C. V., & Gresham, G. E. (1984). *Functional assessment in rehabilitation medicine*. Baltimore: Williams & Wilkins.

Krebs, H. I. (2012). Robotic therapy: The tipping point. *American Journal of Physical Medicine and Rehabilitation, 91*(11 Suppl. 3), 290–297.

Pardee, C., Bricker, D., Rundquist, J., MacRae, C., & Tebben, C. (2012). Characteristics of neurogenic bowel in spinal cord injury and perceived quality of life. *Rehabilitation Nursing, 37*, 128–135.

Poslawsky, I. E., Schuurmans, M. J., Lindeman, E., & Hafsteinsdottir, T. B. (2010). A systematic review of nursing rehabilitation of stroke patients with aphasia. *Journal of Clinical Nursing, 19*(1–2), 17–32.

Pryor, J. (2010). Nurses create a rehabilitation milieu. *Rehabilitation Nursing, 35*(3), 123–128.

*Pullen, R. L. (2008). Transferring a patient from bed to wheelchair. *Nursing, 38*(2), 46–48.

*Rieg, L. S., Mason, C. H., & Preston, K. (2006). Spiritual care: Practical guidelines for rehabilitation nurses. *Rehabilitation Nursing, 31*(6), 249–256.

Sievert, K. D., Amend, B., Gakis, G., Toomey, P., Badke, A., Kaps, H. P., et al. (2010). Early sacral neuromodulation prevents urinary incontinence after complete spinal cord injury. *Annals of Neurology, 67*(1), 74–84.

Stein, J. (2012). Robotics in rehabilitation: Technology as destiny. *American Journal of Physical Medicine and Rehabilitation, 91*(11 Suppl. 3), S199–S203.

U.S. National Library of Medicine (NIH) (2011). *Cranberry*. Retrieved February 2013, from <www.nlm.nih.gov/medlineplus/druginfo/natural/958.html>.

Waters, T. R., & Rockefeller, K. (2010). Safe patient handling for rehabilitation professionals. *Rehabilitation Nursing, 35*(5), 216–222.

*Whipple, K. (2007). Therapeutic use of assistive technology: A clinical perspective. *Rehabilitation Nursing, 32*(2), 48–50.

Chapter 7

Abrahm, J. L. (2011). Advances in palliative medicine and end-of-life care. *Annual Review of Medicine, 62*, 187–199.

*American Association of Colleges of Nursing (2002). *Peaceful death competencies: Recommended competencies and curricular guidelines for end-of-life nursing care*. Washington, DC: Author.

Arnstein, P. R., & Robinson, E. M. (2011). Is palliative sedation right for your patient? *Nursing, 41*(8), 50–54.

Buck, H. G. (2012). Refusing artificial nutrition and hydration in advanced illness. *Nursing, 42*(9), 12–13.

Byock, I. (2012). *The best care possible*. New York: Avery.

Clabots, S. (2012). Strategies to help initiate and maintain the end-of-life discussion with patients and family members. *Medsurg Nursing, 21*(4), 197–204.

Clarke, V., & Holtslander, L. (2010). Incorporating the medicine wheel teaching in the care of Aboriginal people. *Journal of Palliative Care, 26*(1), 34–36.

Doka, K. J., & Tucci, A. S. (Eds.), (2011). *Spirituality and end-of-life care*. Washington, DC: Hospice Foundation of America.

Ferrell, B. (2010). Palliative care research: Nursing response to emergent society needs. *Nursing Science Quarterly, 23*(3), 221–225.

Ferrell, B., & Coyle, N. (Eds.), (2010). *Oxford textbook of palliative nursing* (3rd ed.). New York: Oxford University Press.

Giger, J. N. (2013). *Transcultural nursing: Assessment and intervention* (6th ed.). St. Louis: Mosby.

Gillick, M. R. (2010). Reversing the code status of advance directives? *New England Journal of Medicine, 362*, 1239–1240.

Goldstein, N. E., & Morrison, R. S. (2013). *Evidence-based practice of palliative medicine*. Philadelphia: Saunders.

Hoyert, D. L., & Xu, J. (2011). Deaths: Preliminary data for 2011. *National Vital Statistics Reports, 61*(6), 1–52. National Center for Health Statistics. Retrieved December 2013, from <www.cdc.gov/nchs/data/nvsr/nvsr61/nvsr61_06.pdf>.

Kazanowski, M. (2012). Suffering and palliative care at the end of life. In K. Perrin, C. Sheehan, M. Potter, & M. Kazanowski (Eds.), *Palliative care nursing: Caring for suffering patients* (pp. 119–159). New York: Springer.

Kelley, A. S., Deb, P., Du, Q., Aldridge Carlson, M. D., & Morrison, R. S. (2013). Hospice enrollment saves money for Medicare and improves care quality across a number of different lengths-of-stay. *Health Affairs*, *32*(3), 552–561.
Kirk, T., Coyle, N., Poppito, S., & Bigoney, R. (2010). *Palliative sedation and existential suffering: A dialogue between medicine, nursing, philosophy, and psychology*. Boston: American Academy of Hospice and Palliative Medicine.
Lachman, V. (2010). Do-not-resuscitate orders: Nurse's role requires moral courage. *Medsurg Nursing*, *19*(4), 249–251.
Lachman, V. D. (2011). Nurse's role in increasing patient access to hospice care. *Medsurg Nursing*, *20*(4), 200–203.
Matzo, M. L., & Sherman, D. W. (Eds.), (2010). *Palliative care nursing: Quality care to the end of life* (3rd ed.). New York: Springer.
*National Consensus Project for Quality Palliative Care Task Force (2009). *Clinical practice guidelines for quality palliative care* (2nd ed.). Pittsburgh: Author.
*National Hospice and Palliative Care Organization. (2007). *Caring connections*. Retrieved February 2013, from <www.caringinfo.org>.
National Hospice and Palliative Care Organization (2012). *NHPCO facts and figures: Hospice care in America*. Author.
Peberdy, M. A., Ornato, J. P., Larkin, G. L., Braithwaite, R. S., Kashner, T. M., Carey, S. M., National Registry of Cardiopulmonary Resuscitation Investigators, et al. (2008). Survival from in-hospital cardiac arrest during nights and weekends. *Journal of the American Medical Association*, *299*(7), 785–792.
Perrin, K. (2010). Communicating with seriously ill and dying patients, their families, and their healthcare providers. In M. Matzo & D. W. Sherman (Eds.), *Palliative care nursing* (3rd ed.). New York: Springer.
Perrin, K. (2012). Ethical responsibilities and issues in palliative care. In K. Perrin, C. Sheehan, M. Potter, & M. Kazanowski (Eds.), *Palliative care nursing: Caring for suffering patients* (pp. 77–117). New York: Springer.
Perrin, K. (2013). Caring for the ICU patient at the end of life. In K. Perrin & C. E. MacLeod (Eds.), *Understanding the essentials of critical care nursing* (pp. 510–530). Boston: Pearson.
Quill, T., Holloway, R., Shah, M. S., Caprio, T. V., Olden, A. M., & Storey, C. P. (2010). *Primer of palliative care* (5th ed.). Glenview, IL: American Academy of Hospice and Palliative Medicine.
Sessanna, L. (2010). End-of-life care needs and preferences among independent community dwelling older adults 65 years or older. *Journal of Hospice and Palliative Nursing*, *12*(6), 360–369.
Silveira, M. J., Kim, S. Y. H., & Langa, K. M. (2010). Advance directives and outcomes of surrogate decision-making before death. *New England Journal of Medicine*, *362*, 1211–1218.
Steed, M. (2012). Palliative care: Are you asking the right questions? *Nursing*, *42*(10), 59–61.
*Support Study Principal Investigators. (1995). A controlled trial to improve care for seriously ill hospitalized patients: The Study to Understand Prognoses and Preferences for Outcomes and Risks of Treatments (SUPPORT). *Journal of the American Medical Association*, *274*, 1591–1598.
Teno, J. M., Gozalo, P. L., Bynum, J. P., Leland, N. E., Miller, S., Morden, N. E., et al. (2013). Change in end-of-life care for Medicare beneficiaries' site of death, place of care, and health care transitions in 2000, 2005, and 2009. *Journal of the American Medical Association*, *309*(5), 470–477.
Tian, J., Kaufman, D., Zarich, S., Ong, P., Amoateng-Adjepong, Y., & Manthous, C. (2010). Outcomes of critically ill patients who received cardiopulmonary resuscitation. *American Journal of Respiratory and Critical Care Medicine*, *182*(4), 501–506.

Chapter 8

Aachargya, R. P., Gastmans, C., & Denier, Y. (2011). Emergency department triage: An ethical analysis. *BMC Emergency Medicine*, *11*(16).
Alberts, M. J., Latchaw, R. E., Jagoda, A., Wechsler, L. R., Crocco, T., George, M. G., et al. (2011). Revised and updated recommendations for the establishment of primary stroke centers: A summary statement from the brain attack coalition. *Stroke*, *42*(9), 2651–2665.
Alexander, D., Kinsley, T. L., & Waszinski, C. (2013). Journey to a safe environment: Fall prevention in an emergency department at a level I trauma center. *JEN: Journal of Emergency Nursing*, *39*(4), 346–352.
American College of Surgeons Committee on Trauma (2006). *Resources for optimal care of the injured patient 2006*. Chicago: Author.
*American College of Surgeons Committee on Trauma (2008). *Advanced trauma life support course for doctors student manual* (8th ed.). Chicago: Author.
Blouin, A. S. (2011). Improving hand-off communication: New solutions for nurses. *Journal of Nursing Care Quality*, *26*(2), 97–100.
Centers for Disease Control and Prevention (CDC) (2010). *FastStats: Emergency department visits*. Retrieved April 2014, from <www.cdc.gov/nchs/fastats/ervisits.htm>.
Centers for Medicare and Medicaid Services (2013). *Critical access hospitals*. Retrieved April 2014, from <www.cms.gov/Medicare/Provider-Enrollment-and-Certification/CertificationandComplianc/CAHs.html>.
*Cooper, G., & Laskowski-Jones, L. (2006). Development of trauma care systems. *Prehospital Emergency Care*, *10*(3), 328–331.
Dateo, J. (2013). What factors increase the accuracy and inter-rater reliability of the emergency severity index among emergency nurses in triaging adult patients? *Journal of Emergency Nursing*, *39*(2), 203–207.
Davis, D. T., Johannigman, J. A., & Pritts, T. A. (2012). New strategies for massive transfusion in the bleeding trauma patient. *Journal of Trauma Nursing*, *19*(2), 69–75.
Desy, P., Howard, P. K., Perhats, C., & Li, S. (2010). Alcohol screening, brief intervention, and referral to treatment conducted by emergency nurses: An impact evaluation. *Journal of Emergency Nursing*, *36*(6), 538–545.
Feagan, L. M., & Fisher, N. J. (2011). Impact of education on provider attitudes toward family witnessed resuscitation. *Journal of Emergency Nursing*, *37*(3), 231–239.
Gerber, L. (2013). Bringing home effective nursing care for the homeless. *Nursing*, *43*(3), 32–38.
Gurney, D., & Westergard, A. M. (2014). Chapter 5: Initial assessment. In D. Gurney (Ed.), *TNCC: Trauma nursing core course provider manual* (7th ed.). Des Plaines, IL: Emergency Nurses Association.
Harding, A. D. (2011). Education and culture: Mitigation for workplace violence. *Journal of Emergency Nursing*, *37*(3), 256–257.
Hewitt, L. N., Bhavsar, P., & Phelan, H. (2011). The secrets women keep: Intimate partner violence screening in the female trauma patient. *The Journal of Trauma: Injury, Infection and Critical Care*, *70*(2), 320–323.
*Howard, P. K. (2009). Crowding: A report of the ENA ED crowding work team. *Journal of Emergency Nursing*, *35*(1), 55–56.
Institute of Medicine (IOM) Board on Health Care Services (2010). *Regionalizing emergency care workshop summary*. Washington, DC: National Academies Press. Retrieved April 2014, from <www.nap.edu/catalog.php?record_id=12872>.
*Johnson, D., & Parker, D. (2009). Managers Forum—Cutting-edge discussion of management, policy, and program issues in emergency care: Canine security (Solheim, J., & Papa, A. [Eds.]). *Journal of Emergency Nursing*, *35*(5), 469–470.
Kisner, T., & Johnson-Anderson, H. (2010). Simulation on a shoestring budget. *Nursing*, *40*(8), 32–35.
*Laskowski-Jones, L. (2008). Change management at the hospital front door: Integrating automatic patient tracking in a high volume emergency department and Level I trauma center. *Nurse Leader*, *6*(2), 52–57.
Laskowski-Jones, L. (2009). Responding to trauma: Your priorities in the first hour. *Nursing*, *39*, 7–12.
Moore, K. M. (2011). The four horsemen of the apocalypse of trauma. *Journal of Emergency Nursing*, *37*(3), 294–295.
Mower-Wade, D., & Pirrung, J. M. (2010). Advanced practice nurses making a difference: Implementation of a formal rounding process. *Journal of Trauma Nursing*, *17*(2), 69–71.
National Alliance to End Homelessness (2012). *The state of homelessness in America 2012*. Retrieved April 2014, from <www.endhomelessness.org/content/article/detail/4361>.
National Center for Injury Prevention and Control (NCIPC) (2012). *Injury prevention and control: Data & statistics* (WISQARS). Retrieved April 2014, from <www.cdc.gov/injury/wisqars/index.html>.

Nikki, L., Lepisto, S., & Paavilainen, E. (2013). Experiences of family members of elderly patients in the emergency department: A qualitative study. *International Emergency Nursing, 20*(4), 193–200.

Nolan, M. R. (2009). Older patients in the emergency department: What are the risks? *Journal of Gerontological Nursing, 35*(12), 14–18.

Popovich, M. A., Boyd, C., Dachenhaus, T., & Kusler, D. (2012). Improving stable patient flow through the emergency department by utilizing evidence-based practice: One hospital's journey. *Journal of Emergency Nursing, 38*(5), 474–478.

Richardson, K. (2014). Front-gate triage. *JEN: Journal of Emergency Nursing, 40*(2), 198–200.

Robertson, D. J. (2013). An integrative review: Triage protocols and the effect on ED length of stay. *JEN: Journal of Emergency Nursing, 39*(4), 398–408.

Sadowski, L. S., Kee, R. A., VanderWeele, T. J., & Buchanan, D. (2009). Effect of a housing and case management program on emergency department visits and hospitalizations among chronically ill homeless adults. *The Journal of the American Medical Association, 301*(17), 1771–1778.

Shelton, R. (2010). ESI: A better triage system? *Nursing Critical Care, 5*(6), 34–37.

Strickler, J. (2010). Traumatic hypovolemic shock: Halt the downward spiral. *Nursing, 40*(10), 34–39.

The Joint Commission (TJC) (2013). *National Patient Safety Goals.* Retrieved April 2014, from <http://www.jointcommission.org/standards_information/npsgs.aspx>.

Touhy, T. A., & Jett, K. (2012). *Ebersole & Hess' toward healthy aging: human needs and nursing response* (8th ed.). St. Louis: Mosby.

U.S. Department of Health and Human Services (2013). *Read the law.* Retrieved April 2014, from <www.hhs.gov/healthcare/rights/law/index.html>.

Watkins, L. M., & Patrician, P. A. (2014). Handoff communication for the emergency department to primary care. *Advanced Emergency Nursing Journal, 36*(1), 44–51.

Chapter 9

*American Heart Association (2011). *Advanced cardiovascular life support provider manual.* Dallas: Author.

Arnold, T. C. (Last updated July 30, 2012). *Brown recluse spider envenomation treatment and management.* Retrieved April 2014, from *Medscape reference: drugs, diseases & procedures* <http://emedicine.medscape.com/article/772295-overview>.

*Auerbach, P. S. (2009). *Medicine for the outdoors: The essential guide to first aid and medical emergencies* (5th ed.). St. Louis: Mosby.

*Auerbach, P. S. (2012). *Wilderness medicine* (6th ed.). Philadelphia: Mosby.

Auerbach, P. S., Della-Giustina, D., & Ingebretsen, R. (2010). *Advanced wilderness life support* (4th ed.). Utah: AdventureMed.

*Auerbach, P. S., Donner, H. J., & Weiss, E. A. (2013). *Field guide to wilderness medicine* (4th ed.). St. Louis: Mosby.

*Bledsoe, G. H., Manyak, M. J., & Townes, D. A. (2009). *Expedition & wilderness medicine.* New York: Cambridge University Press.

Boyer, L. V., Binford, G. J., & Degan, J. A. (2012). Spider bites. In P. S. Auerbach (Ed.), *Wilderness medicine* (6th ed., pp. 975–996). Philadelphia: Mosby.

Bush, S. P. (2012). *Rattlesnake envenomation (updated November 14, 2012).* Available on *Medscape website.* Retrieved April 2014, from <http://emedicine.medscape.com/article/771455-overview>.

Cardwell, M. D. (2011). Recognizing dangerous snakes in the United States and Canada: A novel 3-step identification method. *Wilderness & Environmental Medicine, 22*(4), 304–308.

Choo, K. J., Simons, F. E., & Sheikh, A. (2013). Glucocorticoids for the treatment of anaphylaxis. *Evidence-Based Child Health, 8*(4), 1279–1294.

Cusack, L., de Crespigny, C., & Athanasos, P. (2011). Heatwaves and their impact on people with alcohol, drug and mental health conditions: A discussion paper on clinical practice considerations. *Journal of Advanced Nursing, 67*(4), 915–922.

Davis, C., Engeln, A., Johnson, E., McIntosh, S. E., Zafren, K., Islas, A. A., et al. (2012). Wilderness Medical Society practice guidelines for the prevention and treatment of lightning injuries. *Wilderness & Environmental Medicine, 23*, 260–269.

Fougera Pharmaceuticals, Inc. (2008). *CroFab—Crotalidae Polyvalent Immune Fab (Ovine).* Retrieved April 2014, from <www.savagelabs.com/Products/CroFab/Home/crofab_frame.htm>.

*Guoen, J., Shenghua, L., Rili, G., Mitchell, A., & Yanping, S. (2009). High altitude disease: Consequences of genetic and environmental interactions. *North American Journal of Medicine and Science, 2*(3), 74–80.

Hackett, P. H., & Roach, R. C. (2012). High altitude medicine and physiology. In P. S. Auerbach (Ed.), *Wilderness medicine* (6th ed., pp. 2–33). Philadelphia: Mosby.

Hausfater, P., Doumenc, B., Chopin, S., Le Manach, Y., Dautheville, S., Hericord, P., et al. (2010a). Elevation of cardiac troponin I during non-exertional heat-related illnesses in the context of a heat wave. *Critical Care, 14*(3), R99.

Hausfater, P., Megarbane, B., Dautheville, S., Patzak, A., Andronikof, M., Andre, S., et al. (2010b). Prognostic factors in non-exertional heatstroke. *Intensive Care Medicine, 36*, 272–280.

*Johnson, C., Anderson, S. R., Dallimore, J., Winser, S., & Warrell, D. A. (2008). *Oxford handbook of expedition and wilderness medicine.* New York: Oxford University Press.

Jones, P., Moran, K., & Webber, J. (2013). Drowning terminology: Not what it used to be. *New Zealand Medical Journal, 126*(1386), 114–116.

Krau, S. D. (2013). Bites and stings: Epidemiology and treatment. *Critical Care Nursing Clinics of North America, 25*(2), 143–150.

Krau, S. D. (2013). Heat-related illness: A hot topic in critical care. *Critical Care Nursing Clinics of North America, 25*(2), 251–262.

Krau, S. D. (2013). The impact of heat on morbidity and mortality. *Critical Care Nursing Clinics of North America, 25*(2), 243–250.

Laskowski-Jones, L. (2009). Winter emergencies: Managing ski and snowboard injuries. *Nursing, 39*(11), 24–30.

Laskowski-Jones, L. (2010). Summer emergencies: Can you take the heat? *Nursing, 40*(6), 24–32.

Leikin, S. M., Korley, F. K., Wang, E. E., & Leikin, J. B. (2012). The spectrum of hypothermia: From environmental exposure to therapeutic uses and medical simulation. *Disease-A-Month, 58*(1), 6–32.

Lin, C. J., Wu, C. J., Chen, H. H., & Lin, H. C. (2011). Multiorgan failure following mass wasp stings. *Southern Medical Journal, 104*(5), 378–379.

Mattis, J. G., & Yates, A. M. (2011). Heatstroke: Helping patients keep their cool. *Nurse Practitioner, 36*(5), 48–52.

*Mitchell, A. (2006). Africanized killer bees: A case study. *Critical Care Nurse, 26*(3), 23–32.

Norris, R. (2011). *Coral snake envenomation.* Retrieved April 2014 from *Medscape Reference: Drugs, Diseases & Procedures* <http://emedicine.medscape.com/article/771701-overview>.

Norris, R. L., Bush, S. P., & Smith, J. C. (2012). Bites by venomous reptiles in Canada, the United States, and Mexico. In P. S. Auerbach (Ed.), *Wilderness medicine* (6th ed., pp. 1011–1039). Philadelphia: Mosby.

O'Brien, K. K., Leon, L. R., & Kenefick, R. W. (2012). Clinical management of heat-related illnesses. In P. S. Auerbach (Ed.), *Wilderness medicine* (6th ed., pp. 232–238). Philadelphia: Mosby.

Paden, M., Franjic, L., & Halcomb, S. (2013). Hyperthermia caused by drug interactions and adverse reactions. *Emergency Medicine Clinics of North America, 31*(4), 1035–1044.

Simon, R. B., & Simon, D. A. (2014). Illness at high altitudes. *Nursing, 44*(7), 36–41.

Smallheer, B. A. (2013). Bee and wasp stings: Reactions and anaphylaxis. *Critical Care Nursing Clinics of North America, 25*(2), 151–164.

Suchard, J. R. (2011). "Spider bite" lesions are usually diagnosed as skin and soft tissue infections. *Journal of Emergency Medicine, 41*(5), 473–481.

*Suchard, J. R. (2012). Scorpion envenomation. In P. S. Auerbach (Ed.), *Wilderness medicine* (6th ed., pp. 996–1011). Philadelphia: Mosby.

Szpilman, D., Bierens, J. J., Handley, A. J., & Orlowski, J. P. (2012). Drowning. *New England Journal of Medicine, 366*, 2102–2110.

Vetter, R. S. (2013). Spider envenomation in North America. *Critical Care Nursing Clinics of North America, 25*(2), 205–223.

Weimer, S., Staubil, L., & Makic, M. B. F. (2013). Fending off disaster for a frostbite victim. *American Nurse Today, 8*(1), 20.

Wilbeck, J., & Gresham, C. (2013). North American snake and scorpion envenomations. *Critical Care Nursing Clinics of North America*, *25*(2), 173–190.

Chapter 10

Adler, E., & Bauer, L. (2011). Condition gray: Inside the hospital as the Joplin tornado hit. *The Kansas City Star*. Retrieved April 2014, from <www.kansascity.com/2011/06/18/2959600/condition-gray-inside-the-hospital.html>.

*American Nurses Association (ANA) (2001). *Code of ethics for nurses with interpretive statements*. Washington, DC: Author.

Bulson, J. A., & Bulson, T. (2011). Nursing process and critical thinking linked to disaster preparedness. *Journal of Emergency Nursing*, *37*(5), 477–483.

Busby, S., & Witucki-Brown, J. (2011). Theory development for situational awareness in multi-casualty incidents. *Journal of Emergency Nursing*, *37*(5), 444–452.

Caramenico, A. (2013). In emergencies, hospital preparedness goes beyond planning. *FierceHealthcare.com*. Retrieved April 2014, from <www.fiercehealthcare.com/story/emergencies-hospital-preparedness-goes-beyond-planning/2013-04-18>.

Centers for Medicare and Medicaid Services (CMS) (2012). *Life safety code requirements*. Retrieved April 2014, from <www.cms.gov/Medicare/Provider-Enrollment-and-Certification/CertificationandComplianc/LSC.html>.

Chaffee, M. (2006). Making the decision to report to work in a disaster. *American Journal of Nursing*, *106*(9), 54–57.

*Claudius, I., Behar, S., Ballow, S., Wood, R., Stevenson, K., Blake, N., et al. (2008). Disaster drill exercise documentation and management: Are we drilling to standard? *Journal of Emergency Nursing*, *34*(6), 504–508.

Evans, M. (2012). Recovery mode. *Modern Healthcare*, *42*(50), 6–7.

Federal Emergency Management Agency (FEMA) (2013). *Resources*. Retrieved April 2014, from <www.fema.gov/resources>.

Hyer, K., & Brown, L. M. (2008). The Impact of Event Scale—Revised. *American Journal of Nursing*, *108*(11), 60–68.

International Critical Incident Stress Foundation, Inc. (2013). *Mission statement*. Retrieved April 2014, from <www.icisf.org/who-we-are>.

Kallman, M., & Feury, K. J. (2011). Preparing for patient surge in an emergency department during a disaster. *Journal of Emergency Nursing*, *37*(2), 184–185.

*Laskowski-Jones, L. (2008). Change management at the hospital front door: Integrating automatic patient tracking in a high volume emergency department and Level I trauma center. *Nurse Leader*, *6*(2), 52–57.

Laskowski-Jones, L. (2010). When disaster strikes: Ready, or not? (Editorial). *Nursing*, *40*(4), 6.

Letner, J. (2011). A fist coming out of the sky: Six miles of terror. *The Joplin Globe*. Retrieved April 2014, from <www.joplinglobe.com/local/x564433625/A-fist-coming-out-of-the-sky-Six-miles-of-terror>.

Merchant, R. M., Leigh, J. E., & Lurie, N. (2010). Health care volunteers and disaster response: first, be prepared. *New England Journal of Medicine*, *362*(10), 872–873.

National Fire Protection Association (2013). *Codes and standards*. Retrieved April 2014, from <www.nfpa.org/codes and standards.aspx>.

Olchin, L., & Krutz, A. (2012). Nurses as first responders to a mass casualty: Are you prepared? *Journal of Trauma Nursing*, *19*(2), 122–129.

Smith, J. S. (2010). Mass casualty events: Are you prepared? *Nursing*, *40*(4), 40–45.

Somes, J., & Donatelli, N. S. (2012). Disaster planning considerations involving the geriatric patient, Part I. *Journal of Emergency Nursing*, *38*(5), 479–481.

The Joint Commission (2008). *Standards FAQs: Emergency management*. Retrieved April 2014, from <www.jointcommission.org/standards_information/jcfaqdetails.aspx?StandardsFaqId=392&ProgramId=47>.

U.S. Department of Health & Human Services (2013). *National Disaster Medical System*. Retrieved April 2014, from <www.phe.gov/Preparedness/responders/ndms/Pages/default.aspx>.

Wielawski, I. M. (2006). The health legacy of September 11: Five years later illness and memories haunt many. *American Journal of Nursing*, *106*(9), 27–28.

Yin, H., He, H., Arbon, P., Zhu, J., Tan, J., & Zhang, L. (2012). Optimal qualifications, staffing and scope of practice for first responder nurses in disaster. *Journal of Clinical Nursing*, *21*(1–2), 264–271.

Chapter 11

Collins, M., & Claros, E. (2011). Recognizing the face of dehydration. *Nursing*, *41*(8), 26–31.

Cottrell, D. (2012). Managing acute hyperkalemia. *Nursing*, *42*(10), 68.

Crawford, A., & Harris, H. (2011a). Balancing act: Hypomagnesemia and hypermagnesemia. *Nursing*, *41*(10), 52–55.

Crawford, A., & Harris, H. (2011b). Balancing act: Na+ and K+. *Nursing*, *41*(7), 44–50.

Crawford, A., & Harris, H. (2011c). IV fluids: What nurses need to know. *Nursing*, *41*(5), 30–38.

Crawford, A., & Harris, H. (2012). Balancing act: Calcium and phosphorus. *Nursing*, *42*(1), 36–42.

McGraw, M. (2012). Beer potomania: Drink in this atypical cause of hyponatremia. *Nursing*, *42*(7), 24–30.

Nguyen, T., & Wang, A. (2012). Hyperphosphatemia: Consequences and management strategies. *The Journal for Nurse Practitioners*, *8*(1), 56–60.

Schreiber, M. (2013a). Understanding hypernatremia. *Nursing Critical Care*, *8*(3), 8–10.

Schreiber, M. (2013b). Understanding hyponatremia. *Nursing Critical Care*, *8*(2), 8–10.

Scotto, C., Fridline, M., Menhart, C., & Klions, H. (2014). Preventing hypokalemia in critically ill patients. *American Journal of Critical Care*, *23*(2), 145–149.

Stannard, D. (2012). Hypertonic saline for perioperative fluid management. *Journal of Perianesthesia Nursing*, *27*(2), 115–117.

Thomsen, G., Berdjian, L., Rodriguez, L., & Hopkins, R. (2012). Clinical outcomes of a furosemide infusion protocol in edematous patients in the intensive care unit. *Critical Care Nurse*, *32*(6), 25–33.

Trissel, L. (2013). *Handbook on injectable drugs* (17th ed.). Bethesda, MD: American Society of Hospital-System Pharmacists.

Chapter 12

Barnette, L., & Kautz, D. (2013). Creative ways to teach arterial blood gas interpretation. *Dimensions of Critical Care Nursing*, *32*(2), 84–87.

Blevins, S. (2014). Making ABGs simple. *Medsurg Nursing*, *23*(3), 185–186.

*Jones, M. (2010). Basic interpretation of metabolic acidosis. *Critical Care Nurse*, *30*(5), 63–69.

Chapter 13

Aguiar, T. (2010). *Intraosseous access: Not just for emergencies anymore*. Presentation at the Infusion Nurses Society annual meeting: Las Vegas, NV.

Alekseyev, S., Byrne, M., Carpenter, A., Franker, C., Kidd, C., & Hulton, L. (2012). Prolonging the life of a patient's IV: An integrative review of intravenous securement devices. *Medsurg Nursing*, *21*(5), 285–292.

Alexandrou, E., Ramjan, L. M., Spencer, T., Frost, S. A., Salamonson, Y., Davidson, P., et al. (2011). The use of midline catheters in the adult acute care setting: Clinical implications and recommendations for practice. *Journal for the Association of Vascular Access*, *16*(1), 35–41.

*Almadrones, L. (2007). Evidence-based research for intraperitoneal chemotherapy in epithelial ovarian cancer. *Clinical Journal of Oncology Nursing*, *11*(2), 211–216.

Bard Access Systems (2011). *PowerPICC Solo2 Catheter: Overview*. Retrieved December 2013, from <www.bardaccess.com/nurse-powerpiccsolo.php>.

Bard, C. R. (2013). *PowerGlide midline catheter*. Bard Access Systems. Retrieved December 2013, from <www.bardaccess.com/midline-powerglide.php>.

Breland, B. D. (2010). Continuous quality improvement using intelligent infusion pump data analysis. *American Journal of Health-System Pharmacy*, *67*, 1446–1455.

Candon, H. L., Amirov, C., & Toen, J. V. (2010). A multifaceted intervention to address a case cluster of cellulitis associated with hypodermoclysis in a geriatric complex continuing care unit. *Canadian Journal of Infection Control*, *25*(2), 101–106.

Centers for Disease Control and Prevention (CDC) (2011). *2011 guidelines for prevention of intravascular catheter-related infections.* Retrieved September 2013, from <www.cdc.gov/hicpac/bsi/07-bsi-background-info-2011.htmles-2011.html>.

Clemence, B. J., & Maneval, R. E. (2014). Risk factors associated with catheter-related upper extremity deep vein thrombosis in peripherally inserted central venous catheter: Literature review—Part 1. *Journal of Infusion Therapy, 37*(3), 187–196.

Connolly, S., Korzemba, H., Harb, G., Lebel, F., & Syltevik, C. (2011). Techniques for hyaluronidase-facilitated subcutaneous fluid administration with recombinant human hyaluronidase: The increased flow utilizing subcutaneously enabled administration technique (INFUSE AT) study. *Journal of Infusion Nursing, 43*(5), 300–307.

Crawford, A., & Harris, H. (2011). IV fluids: What nurses need to know. *Nursing, 41*(5), 30–39.

Davenport, D. E., & Utterback, V. A. (2011). Physics and flushes: The science supporting why we do what we do. *Nursing, 41*(8), 65–66.

Dumont, C., Getz, O., & Miller, S. (2014). Evaluation of midline vascular access: A descriptive study. *Nursing, 44*(10), 60–66.

*Earhart, A., & Kaminski, D. (2007). Evidence-based practice in infusion nursing: 2007 NACNS national conference abstracts. *Clinical Nurse Specialist, 21*(2), 107.

*Fowler, R., Gallagher, J. V., Isaacs, S. M., Ossman, E., Pepe, P., & Wayne, M. (2007). The role of intraosseous vascular access in the out-of-hospital environment. *Prehospital Emergency Care, 11*(1), 63–66.

Garcia, L. S., & Isenberg, H. D. (2010). *Clinical microbiology procedures handbook* (3rd ed.). Washington, DC: ASM Press.

Genentech USA, Inc. (2011). *Cathflo(r) Activase (r) (Alteplase).* Retrieved December 2013, from <www.cathflo.com>.

*Griswold-Theodorson, S., Hanna, H., Handly, N., Pugh, B., Fojtik, J., Saks, M., et al. (2009). Improving patient safety with ultrasonography guidance during internal jugular central venous catheter placement by novice practitioners. *Simulation in Healthcare, 4*(4), 212–216.

*Hadaway, L. C. (2009). Managing vascular access device occlusions, Part 1. *Nursing, 39*(1), 10.

Hadaway, L. C. (2010a). Infusion therapy equipment. In M. Alexander, A. Corrigan, L. Gorski, J. Hankins, & R. Perucca (Eds.), *Infusion nursing; An evidence-based approach* (3rd ed.). St. Louis: Saunders.

Hadaway, L. C. (2010b). Preventing and managing peripheral extravasation. *Nursing, 39*(10), 26–27.

Hayek, S. M., Deer, T. R., Pope, J. E., Panchal, S. J., & Patel, V. B. (2011). Intrathecal therapy for cancer and non-cancer pain. *Pain Physician, 14*(3), 219–248.

Infusion Nurses Society (INS). (2011). Infusion nursing standards of practice. *Journal of Infusion Nursing, 34*(1S), S8.

*Jarvis, W. R., Murphy, C., Hall, K. K., Fogle, P. J., Karchmer, T. B., Harrington, G., et al. (2009). Health care-associated bloodstream infections associated with negative- or positive-pressure or displacement mechanical valve needleless connectors. *Clinical Infectious Diseases, 49*(12), 1821–1827.

*Khalidi, N., Kovacevich, D. S., Papke-O'Donnell, L. F., & Btaiche, I. (2009). Impact of the positive pressure valve on vascular access device occlusions and bloodstream infections. *Journal of the Association for Vascular Access, 14*(2), 84–91.

*Macha, D. B., Nelson, R. C., Howle, L. E., Hollingsworth, J. W., & Schindera, S. T. (2009). Central venous catheter integrity during mechanical power injection of iodinated contrast medium. *Radiology, 253*(3), 870–878.

*Madigan, K. (2008). Now, intraosseous infusions for adults. *American Nurse Today, 3*(1), 11–12.

McGoldrick, M. (2010). Infection prevention and control. In M. Alexander, L. Gorski, J. Hankins, & R. Perucca (Eds.), *Infusion nursing: An evidence-based approach* (3rd ed.). St. Louis: Saunders.

McHugh, M. E., Miller-Saultz, D., Wuhrman, E., & Kosharskyy, B. (2012). Interventional pain management in the palliative care patient. *International Journal of Palliative Nursing, 18*(9), 426–433.

Mitchell, M. D., Anderson, B. J., Williams, K., & Umscheid, C. A. (2009). Heparin flushing and other interventions to maintain patency of central venous catheters: A systematic review. *Journal of Advanced Nursing, 65*(10), 2007–2021.

*Moran, J. E., Ash, S. R., & ASDIN Clinical Practice Committee. (2008). Locking solutions for hemodialysis catheters: Heparin and citrate—a position paper by ASDIN. *Seminars in Dialysis, 21*(5), 490–492.

Ness, K. K., Hudson, M. M., Pui, C. H., Green, D. M., Krull, K. R., Huang, T. T., et al. (2012). Neuromuscular impairments in adult survivors of childhood acute lymphoblastic leukemia: Associations with physical performance and chemotherapy doses. *Cancer, 118*(3), 828–838.

O'Grady, N. P., Alexander, M., Burns, L. A., Dellinger, E. P., Garland, J., Heard, S. O., et al. (2011). *Guidelines for the prevention of intravascular catheter-related infections.* Atlanta: Centers for Disease Control and Prevention.

Perucca, R. (2010). Peripheral venous access devices. In M. Alexander, A. Corrigan, L. Gorski, J. Hankins, & R. Perucca (Eds.), *Infusion nursing: An evidence-based approach* (3rd ed.). St. Louis: Saunders.

Phillips, L., Brown, L., Campbell, T., Miller, J., Proehl, J., & Youngberg, B. (2010). Recommendations for the use of intraosseous vascular access for emergent and nonemergent situations in various health care settings: A consensus paper. *Critical Care Nurse, 30*(6), e1–e7.

Santolim, T. Q., Santos, L. A., Giovani, A. M., & Dias, V. C. (2012). The strategic role of the nurse in the selection of IV devices. *British Journal of Nursing, 21*(21), S28–S32.

Scales, K. (2011). Use of hypodermoclysis to manage dehydration. *Nursing Older People, 23*(5), 16–22.

The Joint Commission (2014). *National Patient Safety Goals: NPSG.01.03.01 eliminate transfusion errors related to patient misidentification.* Retrieved April 2014, from <www.jointcommission.org/hap_2014_npsg/>.

Thompson, C. D., Vital-Carona, J., & Faustino, E. V. (2012). The effect of tubing dwell time on insulin absorption during intravenous insulin infusions. *Diabetes Technology & Therapeutics, 14*(10), 912–916.

Watts, D., & Kremer, M. J. (2011). Complex regional pain syndrome: A review of diagnostics, pathophysiologic mechanisms, and treatment implications for certified registered nurse anesthetists. *AANA Journal, 79*(6), 505–510.

Weeks, K. A. (2012). Intermittent IV infusions in acute care: Special considerations. *Nursing, 42*(11), 66–68.

White, A., Lopez, F., & Stone, P. (2010). Developing and sustaining an ultrasound-guided peripheral intravenous access program for emergency nurses. *Advanced Emergency Nursing Journal, 32*(2), 173–188.

Chapter 14

AmbulatorySurgeryCenter Association (2013). *Advancing surgical care.* Retrieved April 2014, <www.ascassociation.org/AdvancingSurgicalCare/AboutASCs/History>.

American Society of PeriAnesthesia Nurses (ASPAN) (2012). *2012-2014 Perianesthesia nursing standards, practice recommendations and interpretive statements.* Cherry Hill, NJ: Author.

Association of periOperative Registered Nurses (AORN) (2014a). Perioperative explications for the ANA code of ethics for nurses. In *Perioperative standards and recommended practices* (pp. 21–42). Denver: Author.

Association of periOperative Registered Nurses (AORN) (2014b). *Position statement on perioperative care of patients with do-not-resuscitate (DNR) orders.* Retrieved August 2014, from <http://www.aorn.org/Clinical_Practice/Position_Statements/Position_Statements.aspx>.

Association of periOperative Registered Nurses (AORN) (2014c). Position statement on verification of correct site, correct procedure, and correct patient. In *Perioperative standards and recommended practices* (pp. 640–643). Denver: Author.

Association of periOperative Registered Nurses (AORN) (2014d). Recommended practices for perioperative patient skin antisepsis. In *Perioperative standards and recommended practices* (pp. 73–85). Denver: Author.

Bradley, S. (2014). Infection prevention practices in ambulatory surgery centers. *The American Journal of Nursing, 114*(7), 64–67.

Crenshaw, J. (2011). Preoperative fasting: Will the evidence ever be put into practice? *American Journal of Nursing, 111*(10), 38–43.

*Doerflinger, D. (2009). Older adult surgical patients: Presentation and challenges. *AORN Journal, 90*(2), 223–240.

Elpern, E., Killeen, K., Patel, G., & Senecal, G. (2013). The application of intermittent pneumatic compression devices for thromboprophylaxis. *The American Journal of Nursing, 113*(4), 30–36.

Graham, D., Faggionato, E., & Timberlake, A. (2011). Preventing perioperative complications in the patient with a high body mass index. *AORN Journal, 94*(4), 334–344.

Johnson, J. (2011). Preoperative assessment of high-risk orthopedic surgery patients. *Nurse Practitioner, 36*(7), 40–47.

Larkin, B., Mitchell, K., & Petrie, K. (2012). Translating evidence to practice for mechanical venous thromboembolism prophylaxis. *AORN Journal, 96*(5), 513–527.

McEwen, D. (2011). Ambulatory surgery. In J. C. Rothrock (Ed.), *Alexander's care of the patient in surgery* (14th ed.). St. Louis: Mosby.

MDConsult (2012). *Propofol monograph.* Retrieved April 2014, from <www.mdconsult.com/das/pharm/body/407435066-4/0/full/519?infotype=2>.

Rock, M., & Hoebeke, R. (2014). Informed consent: Whose duty to inform? *Medsurg Nursing, 23*(3), 189–191, 194.

Rothrock, J. C. (2011). *Alexander's care of the patient in surgery* (14th ed.). St. Louis: Mosby.

*Sendelbach, S. (2010). Preoperative fasting doesn't mean nothing after midnight. *The American Journal of Nursing, 110*(9), 64–65.

Spruce, L., & Braswell, M. L. (2012). Implementing AORN recommended practices for electrosurgery. *AORN Journal, 95*(3), 373–387.

Tanner, J., Norrie, P., & Melen, K. (2011). Preoperative hair removal to reduce surgical site infection. *The Cochrane Library, 11*, 1–50.

The Joint Commission (2014). *National Patient Safety Goals.* Retrieved April 2014, from <www.jointcommission.org/patientsafety/nationalpatientsafetygoals/>.

Chapter 15

Adams, D., & Dervay, K. (2012). Pharmacology of procedural sedation. *AACN Advanced Critical Care, 23*(4), 349–354.

AmbulatorySurgeryCenter Association (2013). *Advancing surgical care.* Retrieved April 2014, <www.ascassociation.org/AdvancingSurgicalCare/AboutASCs/History>.

Association of periOperative Registered Nurses (AORN) (2014a). *Perioperative standards and recommended practices: For inpatient and ambulatory settings.* (2014 Ed.), Denver: Author.

Association of periOperative Registered Nurses (AORN) (2014b). *Position statement: AORN position statement on RN first assistants.* Retrieved August 2014, from <http://www.aorn.org/Clinical_Practice/Position_Statements/Position_Statements.aspx>.

Association of periOperative Registered Nurses (AORN) (2010c). *Position statement: Perioperative care of patients with do not resuscitate (DNR) orders.* Retrieved Augustl 2014, from <http://www.aorn.org/Clinical_Practice/Position_Statements/Position_Statements.aspx>.

Association of periOperative Registered Nurses (AORN) (2014d). Recommended practices for cleaning and care of surgical instruments and powered equipment. In *Perioperative standards and recommended practices* (pp. 541–560). Denver: Author.

Association of periOperative Registered Nurses (AORN) (2014e). Recommended practices for Disinfection, high-level. In *Perioperative standards and recommended practices* (pp. 515–528). Denver: Author.

Association of periOperative Registered Nurses (AORN) (2014f). Recommended practices for information management. In *Perioperative standards and recommended practices* (pp. 443–464). Denver: Author.

Association of periOperative Registered Nurses (AORN) (2014g). Recommended practices for environmental cleaning in the perioperative setting. In *Perioperative standards and recommended practices* (pp. 255–276). Denver: Author.

Association of periOperative Registered Nurses (AORN) (2014h). Recommended practices for laser safety in the practice settings. In *Perioperative standards and recommended practices* (pp. 141–154). Denver: Author.

Association of periOperative Registered Nurses (AORN) (2014i). Recommended practices for managing the patient receiving moderate sedation/analgesia. In *Perioperative standards and recommended practices* (pp. 471–480). Denver: Author.

Association of periOperative Registered Nurses (AORN) (2014j). Recommended practices for positioning the patient in the perioperative practice setting. In *Perioperative standards and recommended practices* (pp. 481–500). Denver: Author.

Association of periOperative Registered Nurses (AORN) (2014k). Recommended practices for preoperative patient skin antisepsis. In *Perioperative standards and recommended practices* (pp. 73–88). Denver: Author.

Association of periOperative Registered Nurses (AORN) (2014l). Recommended practices for sharps safety. In *Perioperative standards and recommended practices* (pp. 351–374). Denver: Author.

Association of periOperative Registered Nurses (AORN) (2014m). Recommended practices for sterile technique. In *Perioperative standards and recommended practices* (pp. 89–118). Denver: Author.

Association of periOperative Registered Nurses (AORN) (2014n). Recommended practices for sterilization. In *Perioperative standards and recommended practices* (pp. 575–602). Denver: Author.

Association of periOperative Registered Nurses (AORN) (2014o). Recommended practices for surgical attire. In *Perioperative standards and recommended practices* (pp. 49–60). Denver: Author.

Association of periOperative Registered Nurses (AORN) (2014p). Recommended practices for hand hygiene in the perioperative setting. In *Perioperative standards and recommended practices* (pp. 61–72). Denver: Author.

Association of periOperative Registered Nurses (AORN) (2014q). Recommended practices for traffic patterns in the perioperative practice setting. In *Perioperative standards and recommended practices* (pp. 110–122). Denver: Author.

Association of periOperative Registered Nurses (AORN) (2014r). Position statement on verification of correct site, correct procedure, and correct patient. In *Perioperative standards and recommended practices* (pp. 640–643). Denver: Author.

Centers for Disease Control and Prevention (2014). *National health statistics report: Surgical site infection (SSI) event.* Retrieved August 2014, from <www.cdc.gov/nhsn/pdfs/pscmanual/9pscssicurrent.pdf>.

*Dawson, R., von Fintel, N., & Naim, S. (2010). Sedation assessment using the Ramsay scale. *Emergency Nurse, 18*(3), 18–20.

DeLamar, L. (2011). Anesthesia. In J. C. Rothrock (Ed.), *Alexander's care of the patient in surgery* (14th ed.). St. Louis: Mosby.

Johnson, J. (2011). Preoperative assessment of high-risk orthopedic surgery patients. *Nurse Practitioner, 36*(7), 40–47.

Malignant Hyperthermia Association of the United States (2014). *Emergency therapy for MH acute phase treatment.* Retrieved August 2014, from <www.mhaus.org/healthcare-professionals/#.UPGIEGeN58F>.

Mitchell-Brown, F. (2012). Malignant hyperthermia: Turn down the heat. *Nursing, 42*(5), 38–44.

Norred, C. (2012). Anesthesia-induced anaphylaxis. *American Association of Nurse Anesthetists Journal, 80*(2), 129–140.

Online Mendelian Inheritance in Man (OMIM) (2013). *Malignant Hyperthermia, Susceptibility to, 1;MHS1.* Retrieved August 2014, from <www.omim.org/entry/145600>.

Rothrock, J. C. (2011). *Alexander's care of the patient in surgery* (14th ed.). St. Louis: Mosby.

The Joint Commission (TJC) (2014). *National Patient Safety Goals.* Retrieved August 2014, from <www.jointcommission.org/patientsafety/nationalpatientsafetygoals/>.

Tschannen, D., Bates, O., Talsma, A., & Guo, Y. (2012). Patient-specific and surgical characteristics in the documentation of pressure ulcers. *American Journal of Critical Care, 21*(2), 116–125.

*Ulmer, B. (2010). Best practices for minimally invasive procedures. *AORN Journal, 91*(5), 558–575.

World Health Organization (2014). *WHO: Good hand hygiene by health workers protects patients from drug resistant infections*. Retrieved August 2014, from <www.who.int/mediacentre/news/releases/2014/hand-hygiene/en/>.

Chapter 16

American Society of PeriAnesthesia Nurses (ASPAN) (2012). *2012-2014 Perianesthesia nursing standards, practice recommendations and interpretive statements*. Cherry Hill, NJ: Author.

Association of periOperative Registered Nurses (AORN) (2014f). Recommended practices for information management. In *Perioperative standards and recommended practices* (pp. 443–464). Denver: Author.

Brooks, P. (2012). Postoperative delirium in elderly patients. *American Journal of Nursing, 112*(9), 38–49.

Collins, A. (2011). Postoperative nausea and vomiting in adults: Implications for critical care. *Critical Care Nurse, 31*(6), 36–45.

Eby, A. (2012). Best practices in postoperative feeding. *Nursing, 42*(6), 20–22.

Kibler, V. A., Hayes, R. M., Johnson, D. E., Anderson, L. W., Just, S. L., & Wells, N. L. (2012). Early postoperative ambulation: Back to basics. *American Journal of Nursing, 112*(4), 63–69.

Massey, R. (2012). Return of bowel sounds indicating an end of postoperative ileus: Is it time to cease this long-standing nursing tradition? *Medsurg Nursing, 21*(3), 146–150.

Myles, M. (2012). Preventing postoperative complications: Surgical Care Improvement Project guidelines. *Medsurg Nursing, 21*(6), 383–384.

Rothrock, J. C. (2011). *Alexander's care of the patient in surgery* (14th ed.). St. Louis: Mosby.

Sullivan, J. M. (2011). Caring for older adults after surgery. *Nursing, 41*(4), 48–51.

The Joint Commission (2014). *National Patient Safety Goals*. Retrieved January 2013, from <www.jointcommission.org/patientsafety/nationalpatientsafetygoals/>.

Ward, C. (2012). Fast track program to prevent postoperative ileus. *Medsurg Nursing, 21*(4), 214–220.

Ward, C. (2014). Procedure-specific postoperative pain management. *Medsurg Nursing, 23*(2), 107–110.

Wronski, S. (2014). Chew on this: Reducing postoperative ileus with chewing gum. *Nursing, 44*(8), 19–23.

Chapter 17

Abbas, A., Lichtman, A., & Pillai, S. (2012). *Cellular and molecular immunology* (7th ed.). Philadelphia: Saunders.

Alexander, E., & Susla, G. (2013). Postoperative transplant immunosuppression in the critical care unit. *AACN Advanced Critical Care, 24*(4), 345–350.

Kaufman, C. (2011). The secret life of lymphocytes. *Nursing, 41*(6), 50–54.

Chapter 18

*Almada, P., & Archer, R. (2009). Planning ahead for better outcomes: Preparation for joint replacement surgery begins at home! *Orthopaedic Nursing, 28*(1), 3–8.

Antonelli, M. C., & Starz, T. W. (2012). Assessing for risk and progression of osteoarthritis: The nurse's role. *Orthopaedic Nursing, 31*(2), 98–102.

Arthritis Foundation (2013a). *Gout*. Retrieved December 2013, from <www.arthritis.org/conditions-treatments/disease-center/gout/>.

Arthritis Foundation (2013b). *Osteoarthritis*. Retrieved December 2013, from <www.arthritis.org/conditions-treatments/disease-center/osteoarthritis/>.

Arthritis Foundation (2013c). *Who gets rheumatoid arthritis?* Retrieved December 2013, from <www.arthritis.org/who-gets-rheumatoid-arthritis.php>.

*Barbay, K. (2009). Research evidence for the use of preoperative exercise in patients preparing for total hip or total knee arthroplasty. *Orthopaedic Nursing, 28*(3), 127–133.

Cranwell-Bruce, L. A. (2011). Biological disease modifying anti-rheumatic drugs. *Medsurg Nursing, 20*(3), 147–151.

Davies, P. S. (2011). New developments in the treatment of osteoarthritis. *Pain Management Nursing, 12*(1), 817–822.

Firestein, G. S., Budd, R. C., Gabriel, S. E., McInnes, I. B., & O'Dell, J. R. (2013). *Kelley's textbook of rheumatology* (9th ed.). Philadelphia: Saunders.

Fouladbakhsh, J. (2012). Complementary and alternative modalities to relieve osteoarthritis symptoms. *Orthopaedic Nursing, 31*(2), 115–121.

*Galimba, J. (2009). Promoting the use of periarticular modal drug injection for total knee arthroplasty. *Orthopaedic Nursing, 28*(5), 250–254.

Gillaspie, M. (2010). Better pain management after total joint arthroplasty: A quality improvement approach. *Orthopaedic Nursing, 29*(1), 20–24.

Horse, J. S. (2010). Improving clinical outcomes with continuous passive motion: An interactive educational approach. *Orthopaedic Nursing, 29*(1), 27–33.

Kim, I.-S., Chung, S.-H., Park, Y.-J., & Kang, H. Y. (2012). The effectiveness of an aquarobic exercise program for patients with osteoarthritis. *Applied Nursing Research, 25*(3), 181–189.

Lupus Foundation of America (2014). *What is lupus?* Retrieved June 2014, from <http://www.lupus.org/answers/entry/what-is-lupus>.

Marchese, N. M., & Primer, S. R. (2013). Targeting Lyme disease. *Nursing, 43*(5), 28–33.

Mazaleski, A. (2011). Postoperative total joint replacement class for support persons: Enhancing patient and family centered care using a quality improvement model. *Orthopaedic Nursing, 30*(6), 361–364.

McFadden, B. (2013). Is there a safe coital position after a total hip arthroplasty? *Orthopaedic Nursing, 32*(4), 223–228.

Nelson, D. E. (2011). Perioperative care of the patient with rheumatoid arthritis. *AORN Journal, 94*(3), 290–300.

*Nussbaum, R. L., McInnes, R., & Willard, H. (2007). *Thompson & Thompson genetics in medicine* (7th ed.). Philadelphia: Saunders.

Parker, R. J. (2011). Evidence-based practice: Caring for a patient undergoing total knee arthroplasty. *Orthopaedic Nursing, 30*(1), 4–8.

Pellatino, M. (2012). Providing care for GLBTQ patients. *Nursing, 42*(12), 22–28.

*Pullen, R. L., Jr., Brewer, S., & Ballard, A. (2009). Putting a face on systemic lupus erythematosus. *Nursing, 39*(8), 22–28.

Regan, E. R., Phillips, F., & Magri, T. (2013). Get a leg (or two) up on total knee arthroplasty. *Nursing, 43*(7), 32–37.

*Remadevi, R., & Szallisi, A. (2008). Adlea (ALGRX-4975), an injectable capsaicin (TRPV1 receptor agonist) formulation for long-lasting pain relief. *Drugs, 11*(2), 120–132.

*Rutledge, D. N., Mouttapa, M., & Wood, P. B. (2009). Symptom clusters in fibromyalgia: Potential utility in patient assessment and treatment evaluation. *Nursing Research, 58*, 359–366.

Scleroderma Foundation (2013). *What is scleroderma?* Retrieved December 2013, from <www.scleroderma.org/site/PageServer?pagename=patients_whatis#.Ur0aYbSJI5M>.

Simmons, S. (2011). Recognizing and managing rheumatoid arthritis. *Nursing, 41*(7), 34–40.

Thomas, K. M., & Sethares, K. A. (2010). Is guided imagery effective in reducing pain and anxiety in the postoperative total joint arthroplasty patient? *Orthopaedic Nursing, 29*(6), 393–399.

Valdes, A. M., & Spector, T. D. (2011). The genetic epidemiology of osteoarthritis. *Current Opinions in Rheumatology, 22*(2), 139–143.

Shin, S. Y., & Kolanowski, A. M. (2010). Best evidence of psychosocially focused nonpharmacologic therapies for symptom management in older adults with osteoarthritis. *Pain Management Nursing, 11*(4), 234–244.

Zhang, W. W., Nuki, G., Moskowitz, R., Abramson, S., Altman, R. D., Arden, N. K., et al. (2010). OARSI recommendations for the management of hip and knee osteoarthritis, Part III: Changes in evidence following systematic cumulative update of research published through January 2009. *Osteoarthritis and Cartilage, 18*(4), 476–499.

Chapter 19

AmericanAcademy of HIV Medicine (2012). *AAHIVM fundamentals of HIV medicine for the HIV specialist* (12th ed.). Washington, DC: Author.

Anastasi, J., Capili, B., & Chang, M. (2013). HIV peripheral neuropathy and foot care management: A review of assessment and relevant guidelines. *The American Journal of Nursing, 113*(12), 34–40.

Aschenbrenner, D. (2012). Truvada: The first drug approved to prevent HIV infection. *The American Journal of Nursing, 112*(11), 20–21.

Blanc, F., Sok, T., Laureillard, D., Borand, L., Rekacewicz, C., Nerrienet, E., et al. (2011). Earlier versus later start of antiretroviral therapy in HIV-infected adults with tuberculosis. *New England Journal of Medicine, 365*(16), 1471–1481.

Carr, R., & Traufler, R. (2011). Immune reconstitution inflammatory syndrome in HIV-infected patients: What a critical-care nurse needs to know. *Dimensions of Critical Care Nursing, 30*(3), 139–143.

*Centers for Disease Control and Prevention (CDC). (1987). Public Health Service guidelines for counseling and antibody testing to prevent HIV infection and AIDS. *Morbidity and Mortality Weekly Report, 36*(31), 509–515.

*Centers for Disease Control and Prevention (CDC). (1991). Recommendations for preventing transmission of human immunodeficiency virus and hepatitis B virus to patients during exposure-prone invasive procedures. *Morbidity and Mortality Weekly Report, 40*(RR–8), 1–9.

*Centers for Disease Control and Prevention (CDC). (2005). Updated Public Health Service guidelines for the management of health-care worker exposure to HIV and recommendations for postexposure prophylaxis. *Morbidity and Mortality Weekly Report, 54*(RR–9), 1–22.

*Centers for Disease Control and Prevention (CDC). (2008). Recommendations and reports: Appendix A—AIDS-defining conditions. *Morbidity and Mortality Weekly Report, 57*(RR–10), 9.

*Centers for Disease Control and Prevention (CDC). (2009). Guidelines for prevention and treatment of opportunistic infections in HIV infected adults and adolescents. *Morbidity and Mortality Weekly Report, 58*(RR–4), 1–207.

Centers for Disease Control and Prevention (CDC) (2013a). *HIV in the United States: At a glance.* Retrieved December 2013, from <www.cdc.gov/hiv/resources/factsheets/PDF/stats_basics_factsheet.pdf>.

Centers for Disease Control and Prevention (CDC) (2013b). *HIV surveillance report, 2011* (Vol. 23). Retrieved April 2014, from <www.cdc.gov/hiv/topics/surveillance/resources/reports/>.

Cohen, M., Chen, Y., McCauley, M., Gamble, T., Hosseinipour, M., Kumarasamy, N., et al. (2011). Prevention of HIV-1 infection with early antiretroviral therapy. *New England Journal of Medicine, 365*(6), 493–505.

Foster, V., Clark, P., Holstad, M., & Burgess, E. (2012). Factors associated with risky sexual behaviors in older adults. *Journal of the Association of Nurses in AIDS Care, 23*(6), 487–499.

Hoogbruin, A. (2011). Complementary and alternative therapy (CAT) use and highly active antiretroviral therapy (HAART): Current evidence in the literature, 2000-2009. *Journal of Clinical Nursing, 20*(7–8), 925–939.

Kaufman, C. (2011). The secret life of lymphocytes. *Nursing, 41*(6), 50–54.

Keithley, J., & Swanson, B. (2013). HIV-associated wasting. *Journal of the Association of Nurses in AIDS Care, 24*(1S), S103–S111.

Kirton, C. (2011). The changing HIV epidemic. *Nursing, 41*(1), 36–43.

Kuznar, W., & Kayyali, A. (2011). Tuberculosis prevention in HIV-positive adults with latent disease. *The American Journal of Nursing, 111*(11), 59.

Lanier, Y., & Sutton, M. (2013). Reframing the context of preventive health care services and prevention of HIV and other sexually transmitted infections for young men: New opportunities to reduce racial/ethnic sexual health disparities. *American Journal of Public Health, 103*(2), 262–269.

New York State Department of Health AIDS Institute (2014). *Free compilation of current guidelines for clinical practice.* Retrieved April 2014, from <www.hivguidelines.org>.

Nokes, K., Johnson, M. O., Webel, A., Rose, C. D., Phillips, J. C., Sullivan, K., et al. (2012). Focus on increasing treatment self-efficacy to improve human immunodeficiency virus treatment adherence. *Journal of Nursing Scholarship, 44*(4), 403–410.

Pettinato, M. (2012). Providing care for GLBTQ patients. *Nursing, 42*(12), 22–27.

Starr, M., & Bradley-Springer, L. (2014). Nursing in the fourth decade of the HIV epidemic. *The American Journal of Nursing, 114*(3), 38–47.

World Health Organization (WHO) (2013). *Global epidemic: HIV/AIDS online questions and answers.* Retrieved April 2014, from <www.who.int/features/qa/71/en/index.html>.

Chapter 20

Abbas, A., Lichtman, A., & Pillai, S. (2012). *Cellular and molecular immunology* (7th ed.). Philadelphia: Saunders.

Arnold, J., & Williams, P. (2011). Anaphylaxis: Recognition and management. *American Family Physician, 84*(10), 1111–1118.

Bostock-Cox, B. (2013). Dealing with emergencies in general practice: Anaphylaxis. *Practice Nurse, 43*(4), 24–26.

Catanzaro, J., & Dinkel, S. (2014). Sjogren's syndrome: The hidden disease. *Medsurg Nursing, 23*(4), 219–221.

Caton, E., & Flynn, M. (2013). Management of anaphylaxis in the ED: A clinical audit. *International Emergency Nursing, 21*(1), 64–70.

Holmes, S., & Scullion, J. (2012). Allergic rhinitis: Assessment and treatment. *Nurse Prescribing, 10*(5), 222–228.

Norred, C. (2012). Anesthesia-induced anaphylaxis. *AANA Journal, 80*(2), 129–150.

Poetzsch, B. (2012). Sjögren syndrome. *Journal of the American Academy of Physician Assistants, 25*(1), 67–68.

Ruiz, C. (2012). Act immediately against anaphylaxis. *American Nurse Today, 7*(7), 18.

Simons, E., Ardusso, L., Bilo, M. B., El-Gamal, Y., Ledford, D., Ring, J., et al. (2011). World Allergy Organization guidelines for the assessment and management of anaphylaxis. *The World Allergy Organization Journal, 4*(2), 13–37.

Vacca, V., & McMahon-Bowen, E. (2013). Anaphylaxis. *Nursing, 43*(11), 16–17.

Wade, J. (2012). Care of the type 1 latex allergy patient. *Australian Nursing Journal, 19*(9), 30–33.

Chapter 21

American Cancer Society (ACS) (2010). *Cancer prevention and early detection: Facts & figures—2010.* Report No. 8600.10. Atlanta: Author.

American Cancer Society (ACS) (2012). *Cancer facts and figures for Hispanics/Latinos—2012-2014.* Report No. 862313. Atlanta: Author.

American Cancer Society (ACS) (2013). *Cancer facts and figures for African Americans—2013-2014.* Report No. 861413. Atlanta: Author.

American Cancer Society (ACS) (2014). *Cancer facts and figures—2014.* Report No. 00-300M–No. 500814. Atlanta: Author.

Beery, T. A., & Workman, M. L. (2012). *Genetics and genomics in nursing and health care.* Philadelphia: F.A. Davis.

Calzone, K., Masny, A., &Jenkins, J. (Eds.). (2010). *Genetics and genomics in oncology nursing practice.* Pittsburgh: Oncology Nursing Society.

Canadian Cancer Society, Statistics Canada (2014). *Canadian Cancer Statistics, 2014.* Toronto: Canadian Cancer Society.

Feero, G., Guttmacher, E., & Collins, F. (2010). Genomic medicine: An updated primer. *New England Journal of Medicine, 362*, 2001–2011.

Santos, E. M., Edwards, Q. T., Floria-Santos, M., Rogatto, S. R., Achatz, M. I., & MacDonald, D. J. (2013). Integration of genomics in cancer care. *Journal of Nursing Scholarship, 45*(1), 43–51.

U.S. Department of Health and Human Services (USDHHS), Public Health Service, National Toxicology Program (2011). *Report on carcinogens* (12th ed.). Retrieved August 2014, from <http://ntp.niehs.nih.gov/go/roc12>.

Chapter 22

Abbas, A., Lichtman, A., & Pillai, S. (2012). *Cellular and molecular immunology* (7th ed.). Philadelphia: Saunders.

Agostinis, P., Berg, K., Cengel, K. A., Foster, T. H., Girotti, A. W., Gollnick, S. O., et al. (2011). Photodynamic therapy of cancer: An update. *CA: A Cancer Journal for Clinicians, 61*(4), 250–281.

American Cancer Society (2014). *Cancer facts and figures—2014.* Report No. 00-300M–No. 500814. Atlanta: Author.

Barak, F., Amoyal, M., & Kalichman, L. (2013). Using a simple diary for management of nausea and vomiting during chemotherapy. *Clinical Journal of Oncology Nursing, 17*(5), 479–481.

Beatty, K., Winkelman, C., Bokar, J., & Mazanec, P. (2011). Targeted therapies. *AACN Advanced Critical Care, 22*(4), 323–334.

Bergstrom, K. (2011). Development of a radiation skin care protocol and algorithm using the Iowa Model of Evidence-Based Practice.

Clinical Journal of Oncology Nursing, 15(5), 593–595.
Binner, M., Ross, D., & Browner, I. (2011). Chemotherapy-induced peripheral neuropathy: Assessment of oncology nurses' knowledge and practice. *Oncology Nursing Forum, 38*(4), 448–454.
Borsellino, M., & Young, M. (2011). Anticipatory coping: Taking control of hair loss. *Clinical Journal of Oncology Nursing, 15*(3), 311–315.
Boucher, J., Habin, K., & Underhill, M. (2014). Cancer genetics and genomics: Essentials for oncology nurses. *Clinical Journal of Oncology Nursing, 18*(3), 355–359.
Buck, H. (2012). Real-world symptom management. *Nursing, 42*(3), 18–19.
Byar, K., & Workman, M. (2012). Targeted therapies to treat cancer. In J. Kee, E. Hayes, & L. McCuistion (Eds.), *Pharmacology: A nursing process approach* (7th ed., pp. 543–567). St. Louis: Saunders.
Canadian Cancer Society, Statistics Canada (2014). *Canadian cancer statistics, 2014*. Toronto: Canadian Cancer Society.
Cherwin, C. (2012). Gastrointestinal symptom representation in cancer symptom clusters: A synthesis of the literature. *Oncology Nursing Forum, 39*(2), 157–165.
Dalby, C., Nesbitt, M., Frechette, C., Kennerley, K., Lacoursiere, L., & Buswell, L. (2013). Standardization of initial chemotherapy teaching to improve care. *Clinical Journal of Oncology Nursing, 17*(5), 472–475.
Davey, M. (2013). Improving adherence to oral anticancer therapy. *Nursing, 43*(9), 31–36.
Davidson, W., Teleni, L., Muller, J., Ferguson, M., McCarthy, A. L., Vick, J., et al. (2012). Malnutrition and chemotherapy-induced nausea and vomiting: Implications for practice. *Oncology Nursing Forum, 39*(4), E340–E345.
Denshar, R., Vanek, R., & Mazanec, P. (2011). Oncologic emergencies: New decade, new perspectives. *AACN Advanced Critical Care, 22*(4), 337–348.
Given, B. A., Given, C. W., & Sherwood, P. R. (2012). Family and caregiver needs over the course of the cancer trajectory. *Journal of Supportive Oncology, 10*(2), 57–64.
Gonzales, T. (2013). Chemotherapy extravasations: Prevention, identification, management, and documentation. *Clinical Journal of Oncology Nursing, 17*(1), 61–66.
Held-Warmkessel, J. (2011). Taming three high-risk chemotherapy complications. *Nursing, 41*(11), 30–37.
Kanaskie, M. (2012). Chemotherapy-related cognitive changes: A principle-based concept analysis. *Oncology Nursing Forum, 39*(3), E241–E248.
Limburg, C., Maxwell, C., & Mautner, B. (2014). Prevention and treatment of bone loss in patients with nonmetastatic breast or prostate cancer who receive hormone ablation therapy. *Clinical Journal of Oncology Nursing, 18*(2), 223–230.
Mackiewicz, T. (2012). Prevention of tumor lysis syndrome in an outpatient setting. *Clinical Journal of Oncology Nursing, 16*(2), 189–193.
Maloney, K., & Denno, M. (2011). Tumor lysis syndrome: Prevention and detection to enhance patient safety. *Clinical Journal of Oncology Nursing, 15*(6), 601–603.
Myers, J. (2012). Chemotherapy-related cognitive impairment: The breast cancer experience. *Oncology Nursing Forum, 39*(1), E31–E40.
Neuss, M., Polovich, M., McNiff, K., Esper, P., Gilmore, T., LeFebvre, K., et al. (2013). 2013 updated American Society of Clinical Oncology/Oncology Nursing Society chemotherapy safety standards including standards for the safe administration and management of oral chemotherapy. *Oncology Nursing Forum, 40*(3), 225–233.
Northouse, L. L. (2012). Helping patients and their family caregivers cope with cancer. *Oncology Nursing Forum, 39*(5), 500–506.
Poirier, P. (2011). The impact of fatigue on role functioning during radiation therapy. *Oncology Nursing Forum, 38*(4), 457–465.
Polovich, M., & Martin, S. (2011). Nurses' use of hazardous drug-handling precautions and awareness of national safety guidelines. *Oncology Nursing Forum, 38*(6), 718–726.
Proud, C. (2014). Radiogenomics: The promise of personalized treatment in radiation oncology? *Clinical Journal of Oncology Nursing, 18*(2), 185–189.
Running, A., & Turnbeaugh, E. (2011). Oncology pain and complementary therapy: A review of the literature. *Clinical Journal of Oncology Nursing, 15*(4), 374–379.
Ruppert, R. (2011). Radiation therapy 101: What you need to know to help cancer patients understand their treatment and cope with side effects. *American Nurse Today, 6*(1), 24–29.
Santos, E. M. M., Edwards, Q. T., Floria-Santos, M., Rogatto, S. R., Achatz, M. I. W., & MacDonald, D. J. (2013). Integration of genomics in cancer care. *Journal of Nursing Scholarship, 45*(1), 43–51.
Schulmeister, L. (2014). Safe management of chemotherapy: Infusion-related complications. *Clinical Journal of Oncology Nursing, 18*(3), 283–287.
Serra, D., Parris, C. R., Carper, E., Homel, P., Fleishman, S. B., Harrison, L. B., et al. (2012). Outcomes of guided imagery in patients receiving radiation therapy for breast cancer. *Clinical Journal of Oncology Nursing, 16*(6), 617–622.
Shaw, C., & Taylor, L. (2012). Treatment-related diarrhea in patients with cancer. *Clinical Journal of Oncology Nursing, 16*(4), 413–417.
Sheldon, L. K., Harris, D., & Arcieri, D. (2012). Psychosocial concerns in cancer care: The role of the oncology nurse. *Clinical Journal of Oncology Nursing, 16*(3), 316–319.
Tofthagen, C., McAllister, D., & McMillan, S. (2011). Peripheral neuropathy in patients with colorectal cancer receiving oxaliplatin. *Clinical Journal of Oncology Nursing, 15*(2), 182–188.
Vachani, C., Di Lullo, G., Hampshire, M. K., Hill-Kayser, C. E., & Metz, J. M. (2011). Nursing resources: Preparing patients for life after cancer treatment. *American Journal of Nursing, 111*(4), 51–55.
Walton, A. M., Mason, S., Busshart, M., Spruill, A. D., Cheek, S., Lane, A., et al. (2012). Safe handling: Implementing hazardous drug precautions. *Clinical Journal of Oncology Nursing, 16*(3), 251–254.
Wanchai, A., Armer, J., & Stewart, B. (2011). Nonpharmacologic supportive strategies to promote quality of life in patients experiencing cancer-related fatigue: A systematic review. *Clinical Journal of Oncology Nursing, 15*(2), 203–214.
Wiencek, C., Ferrell, B., & Jackson, M. (2011). The meaning of our work: Caring for the critically ill patient with cancer. *AACN Advanced Critical Care, 22*(4), 397–407.
Yagasaki, K., & Kumatsu, H. (2013). The need for a nursing presence in oral chemotherapy. *Clinical Journal of Oncology Nursing, 17*(5), 512–516.
Yu, H., Friedlander, D. R., Patel, S., & Hu, J. C. (2013). The current status of robotic oncologic surgery. *CA: A Cancer Journal for Clinicians, 63*(1), 45–56.

Chapter 23

Alspach, J. G. (2014). About that health care icon dangling around your neck: Do we have some cleaning up to do? *Critical Care Nurse, 34*(4), 11–14.
*Backman, C., Zoutman, D. E., & Marck, P. B. (2008). An integrative review of the current evidence on the relationship between hand hygiene interventions and the incidence of health care–associated infections. *American Journal of Infection Control, 36*(5), 333–348.
Barnes, B. E., & Sampson, D. A. (2011). A literature review on community-acquired methicillin-resistant *Staphylococcus aureus* in the United States: Clinical information for primary care nurse practitioners. *Journal of the Academy of Nurse Practitioners, 23*(1), 23–32.
*Centers for Disease Control and Prevention (CDC). (2002). Guideline for hand hygiene in health-care settings: Recommendations of the Healthcare Infection Control Practices Advisory Committee and the HICPAC/SHEA/APIC/IDSA Hand Hygiene Task Force. *Morbidity and Mortality Weekly Report, 51*(RR–16), 1–44.
Centers for Disease Control and Prevention (CDC) (2013). *2012 CRE toolkit: Guidance for control of carbapenem-resistant Enterobacteriaceae, Part 1: Facility-level CRE prevention*. Retrieved January 2014, from <www.cdc.gov/hai/organisms/cre/cre-toolkit/f-level-prevention-supmeasures.html>.
Centers for Disease Control and Prevention (CDC) (2014). *Ebola (Ebola virus disease)*. Retrieved October 2014, from <www.cdc.gov/vhf/ebola>.
*Childs, S. G. (2008). Biofilm: The pathogenesis of slime glycocalyx. *Orthopedic Nursing, 27*(6), 361–368.

Foulk, K. C., Tocydlowski, P., Snow, T. M., McCloud, K., Cuevas, M., Bishop, D., et al. (2012). Infusing fun into quality and safety initiatives. *Nursing, 41*(11), 14–16.

Grossman, S., & Mager, D. (2010). *Clostridium difficile:* Implications for nursing. *Medsurg Nursing, 19*(3), 155–158.

Kassakian, S. Z., Mermel, L. A., Jefferson, J. A., Parenteau, S. L., & Machan, J. T. (2011). Impact of chlorhexidine bathing on hospital-acquired infections among general medical patients. *Infection Control and Hospital Epidemiology, 32*(3), 238–243.

*Lo, S. F., Hayter, M., Change, C. J., Wu, W. Y., & Lee, L. L. (2008). A systematic review of silver-releasing dressings in the management of infected chronic wounds. *Journal of Clinical Nursing, 17*(15), 1973–1985.

Lopez-Bushnell, K., Demaroy, W. S., & Jaco, C. (2014). Reducing sepsis mortality. *Medsurg Nursing, 23*(1), 9–14.

Ly, E. (2013). A closer look at hantavirus. *Nursing, 43*(9), 65–66.

Mori, C. (2014). A-voiding catastrophe: Implementing a nurse-driven protocol. *Medsurg Nursing, 23*(1), 15–21, 28.

Myers, F. (2011). Beyond mainstream: Making the case for fecal bacteriotherapy. *Nursing, 41*(12), 50–53.

Palese, A., Buchini, S., Deroma, L., & Bartone, F. (2010). The effectiveness of the ultrasound bladder scanner in reducing urinary tract infections: A meta-analysis. *Journal of Clinical Nursing, 19*(21–22), 2970–2979.

*Parker, D., Callan, L., Harwood, J., Thompson, D. L., Wilde, M., & Gray, M. (2009). Nursing interventions to reduce the risk of catheter-associated urinary tract infection, Part 1: Catheter selection. *Journal of Wound, Ostomy, Continence Nursing, 36*(1), 23–34.

Powers, J., Peed, J., Burns, L., & Ziemba-Davis, M. (2012). Chlorhexidine bathing and microbial contamination in patients' bath basins. *American Journal of Critical Care, 21*(5), 338–342.

Powers, J., & Fortney, S. (2014). Bed baths: Much more than a basic nursing task. *Nursing, 44*(10), 67–68.

Ramage, G., Culshaw, S., Jones, B., & Williams, C. (2010). Are we any closer to beating the biofilm: Novel methods of biofilm control. *Current Opinion in Infectious Disease, 23*(6), 560–566.

Rosini, J. M., & Srivastava, N. (2013). Understanding vancomycin levels. *Nursing, 43*(11), 66–67.

*Siegel, J. D., Rhinehart, E., Jackson, M., Chiarello, L., & Healthcare Infection Control Practices Advisory Committee (2007). *Guidelines for isolation precautions: Preventing transmission of infectious agents in healthcare settings 2007.* Atlanta: CDC.

Simko, L. (2012). Breaking sterility: Dealing with procedural violations in health care. *Nursing, 42*(8), 22–26.

Snow, M. (2011). *Clostridium difficile:* Trouble for adults and children. *Nursing, 41*(8), 67–68.

Stickler, D. J., & Feneley, R. C. (2010). The encrustation and blockage of long-term indwelling catheters: A way forward in prevention and control. *Spinal Cord, 48*(11), 784–790.

Upshaw-Owens, M., & Bailey, C. A. (2012). Preventing hospital-associated infection: MRSA. *Medsurg Nursing, 21*(2), 77–80.

Chapter 24

American Cancer Society (2014). *Cancer facts and figures—2014.* Report No. 00-300M–No. 500814. Atlanta: Author.

Cross, H. H. (2014). Obtaining a wound swab culture specimen. *Nursing, 44*(7), 68–69.

*Gaskin, F. C. (1986). Detection of cyanosis in the person with dark skin. *Journal of National Black Nurses' Association, 1*(1), 52–60.

LeBlanc, K., & Baranowski, S. (2011). Skin tears: State of the science: Consensus statements for the prevention, prediction, assessment, and treatment of skin tears. *Advances in Skin & Wound Care, 24*(9), 2–15.

Marks, J., & Miller, J. (2013). *Lookingbill and Marks' principles of dermatology* (5th ed.). Philadelphia: Saunders.

McEnroe-Petitte, D. (2011). Melanoma. *Nursing, 41*(5), 45.

Siegel, V. (2012). Adding patient education of skin cancer and sun-protective behaviors to the skin assessment screening on admission to hospitals. *Medsurg Nursing, 21*(3), 183–184.

The Skin Cancer Foundation (2014). *Understanding melanoma—Warning signs: The ABCDEs of melanoma.* Retrieved September 2014, from <www.skincancer.org/skin-cancer-information/melanoma>.

Chapter 25

Ackerman, C. (2011). "Not on my watch": Treating and preventing pressure ulcers. *Medsurg Nursing, 20*(2), 86–93.

Adams, S., Sabesan, V., & Easley, M. (2012). Wound healing agents. *Critical Care Nursing Clinics of North America, 24*(2), 255–260.

Alderden, J., Whitney, J., Taylor, S., & Zaratkiewicz, S. (2011). Risk profile characteristics associated with outcomes of hospital-acquired pressure ulcers: A retrospective review. *Critical Care Nurse, 31*(4), 30–42.

Ambutas, S., Staffileno, B., & Fogg, L. (2014). Reducing nasal pressure ulcers with an alternative taping device. *Medsurg Nursing, 23*(2), 96–100.

American Cancer Society (ACS) (2014). *Cancer facts and figures 2014.* Report No. 00-300M–No. 500814. Atlanta: Author.

Armour-Burton, T., Fields, W., Outlaw, L., & Deleon, E. (2013). The healthy skin project: Changing nursing practice to prevent and treat hospital-acquired pressure ulcers. *Critical Care Nurse, 33*(3), 32–39.

Ayello, E., & Baranoski, S. (2014). Wound care and prevention. *Nursing, 44*(4), 32–40.

Barnes, E., & Murray, B. (2013). Bedbugs: What nurses need to know. *The American Journal of Nursing, 113*(10), 58–62.

Beitz, J. (2012). Wound debridement: Therapeutic options and care considerations. *Critical Care Nursing Clinics of North America, 24*(2), 239–253.

Bolton, L., Girolami, S., & Hurlow, J. (2013). The AAWC pressure ulcer guidelines. *The American Journal of Nursing, 113*(9), 58–63.

Bryce, J., & Passoni, C. (2013). Nursing management of patients with metastatic melanoma receiving ipilimumab. *Oncology Nursing Forum, 40*(3), 215–218.

Cooper, K. (2012). Drug reaction, skin care, skin loss. *Critical Care Nurse, 32*(4), 52–58.

Cowdell, F. (2011). Older people, personal hygiene, and skin care. *Medsurg Nursing, 20*(5), 235–240.

Cross, H. H. (2014). Obtaining a wound swab culture specimen. *Nursing, 44*(7), 68–69.

Demidova-Rice, T., Hamblin, M., & Herman, I. (2012a). Acute and impaired wound healing: Pathophysiology and current methods for drug delivery,Part 1: Normal and chronic wounds: Biology, causes, and approaches to care. *Advances in Skin & Wound Care, 25*(7), 304–314.

Demidova-Rice, T., Hamblin, M., & Herman, I. (2012b). Acute and impaired wound healing: Pathophysiology and current methods for drug delivery, Part 2: Role of growth factors in normal and pathological wound healing: Therapeutic potential and methods of delivery. *Advances in Skin & Wound Care, 25*(8), 349–370.

Estilo, M., Angeles, A., Perez, T., Hernandez, M., & Valdez, M. (2012). Pressure ulcers in the intensive care unit: New perspectives on an old problem. *Critical Care Nurse, 32*(3), 65–70.

Goldberg, S., & Diegelmann, R. (2012). Wound healing primer. *Critical Care Nursing Clinics of North America, 24*(2), 165–178.

LeBlanc, K., & Christensen, D. (2011). Demystifying skin tears, Part 2. *Nursing, 41*(7), 16–17.

LeBlanc, K., & Baranoski, S. (2014). Skin tears: Best practices for care and prevention. *Nursing, 44*(5), 36–46.

Li, D., & Korniewicz, D. (2013). Determination of the effectiveness of electronic health records to document pressure ulcers. *Medsurg Nursing, 22*(1), 17–25.

Lyder, C. H., Wang, Y., Metersky, M., Curry, M., Kliman, R., Verzier, N. R., et al. (2012). Hospital-acquired pressure ulcers: Results from the national Medicare Patient Safety Monitoring System study. *Journal of the American Geriatrics Society, 60*(9), 1603–1608.

Marks, J. G., Jr., & Miller, J. (2013). *Lookingbill & Mark's principles of dermatology* (5th ed.). Philadelphia: Saunders.

Mayo, T., & Cantrell, W. (2014). Putting onchomycosis under the microscope. *The Nurse Practitioner, 39*(5), 8–11.

Moreira, M., & Markovchick, M. (2012). Wound management. *Critical Care Nursing Clinics of North America, 24*(2), 215–237.

Napierkowski, D. (2013). Uncovering common bacterial skin infections. *The Nurse Practitioner, 38*(3), 30–37.

National Pressure Ulcer Advisory Panel, European Pressure Ulcer Advisory Panel, & Pan Pacific Pressure Injury Alliance (2014). *Prevention and treatment of pressure ulcers: Quick reference guide.* Perth, Australia: Cambridge Media. Retrieved Septermber 2014, from <www.npuap.org/wp-content/uploads/2014/08/Quick-Reference-Guide-DIGITAL-NPUAP-EPUAP-PPPIA.pdf>.

Nelson, M., & Harris, R. (2013). Pressure ulcer alert! *Nursing, 43*(11), 64–67.

Online Mendelian Inheritance in Man (OMIM) (2014a). *Melanoma, cutaneous malignant, Susceptibility to, 1; CMM1.* Retrieved September 2014, from <www.omim.org/entry/155600>.

Online Mendelian Inheritance in Man (OMIM) (2014b). Psoriasis, Susceptibility1; *PSORS1.* Retrieved September 2014, from <www.omim.org/entry/177900>.

Passalacqua, S., DiRocco, Z., DiPietro, C., Mozzetta, A., Tabolli, S., Scoppola, A., et al. (2012). Information needs of patients with melanoma: A nursing challenge. *Clinical Journal of Oncology Nursing, 16*(6), 625–632.

Posthauer, M. E. (2012). The role of nutrition in wound care. *Advances in Skin & Wound Care, 25*(2), 62–63.

Rock, R. (2011). Get positive results with negative-pressure wound therapy. *American Nurse Today, 6*(1), 49–51.

Rubin, K. (2012). Managing immune-related adverse events to ipilimumab: A nurse's guide. *Clinical Journal of Oncology Nursing, 16*(2), E69–E75.

Sardina, D. (2013). Is your wound-cleansing practice up to date? *American Nurse Today, 8*(7), 37–38.

Schaefer, P. (2011). Urticaria: Evaluation and treatment. *American Family Physician, 83*(9), 1078–1084.

The Skin Cancer Foundation (2014). *Understanding melanoma—Warning signs: The ABCDEs of melanoma.* Retrieved September 2014, from <www.skincancer.org/skin-cancer-information/melanoma>.

van Rijswijk, L. (2013). Measuring wounds to improve outcomes. *The American Journal of Nursing, 113*(8), 60–61.

Williams, J., & Barbul, A. (2012). Nutrition and wound healing. *Critical Care Nursing Clinics of North America, 24*(2), 179–200.

Wong, J., & Woo, J. Y. (2012). The safety of systemic treatments that can be used for geriatric psoriasis patients: A review. *Dermatology Research and Practice, 2012,* 1–4.

Woo, K., Coutts, P., & Sibbald, R. G. (2012). Continuous topical oxygen for the treatment of chronic wounds: A pilot study. *Advances in Skin & Wound Care, 25*(12), 543–547.

Yu, N., Long, X., Lujan-Hernandez, J., Hassan, K., Bai, M., Wang, Y., et al. (2013). Marjolin's ulcer: A preventable malignancy arising from scars. *World Journal of Surgical Oncology,* doi:10.1186/1477-7819-11-313; Retreived September 2014, from <http://www.wjso.com/content/11/1/313>.

Chapter 26

Alharbi, Z., Piatkowski, A., Dembinski, R., Reckort, S., Grieb, G., Kauczok, J., et al. (2012). Treatment of burns in the first 24 hours: Simple and practical guide by answering 10 questions in a step-by-step form. *World Journal of Emergency Surgery, 7*(1), 13–22.

American Burn Association (ABA) (2012). *National Burn Repository: Summary of the findings 2002-2011.* Website <www.ameriburn.org>.

Aziz, Z., Abu, S. F., & Chong, N. J. (2012). A systematic review of silver-containing dressings and topical silver agents (used with dressings) for burn wounds. *Burns, 38*(3), 307–318.

Badger, K., & Royse, D. (2012). Describing compassionate care: The burn survivor's perspective. *Journal of Burn Care & Research, 33*(6), 772–780.

Bidwell, K., Miller, S., Coffey, R., Calvitti, K., Porter, K., & Murphy, C. (2013). Evaluation of the safety and efficacy of a nursing-driven midazolam protocol for management of procedural pain associated with burn injuries. *Journal of Burn Care & Research, 34*(1), 176–182.

Bishop, S., Walker, M., & Spivak, I. (2013). Family presence in the adult burn intensive care unit during dressing changes. *Critical Care Nurse, 33*(1), 14–23.

Brown-Guttovz, H. (2011). Burn injury. *Nursing, 41*(5), 72.

Butcher, M., & Swales, B. (2012). Assessment and management of patients with burns. *Nursing Standard, 27*(2), 50–56.

Carrougher, G., Martinez, E., McMullen, K., Fauerbach, J., Holavanahalli, R., Herndon, D., et al. (2012). Pruritus in adult burn survivors: Prevalence and risk factors associated with increased intensity. *Journal of Burn Care & Research, 34*(1), 94–101.

Coffey, R., & Murphy, C. (2012). Effects of alcohol use and abuse on critically ill burn patients. *Critical Care Nursing Clinics of North America, 24*(1), 1–7.

Culleiton, A., & Simko, L. (2013a). Caring for patients with burn injuries. *Nursing, 43*(8), 26–34.

Culleiton, A., & Simko, L. (2013b). Caring for patients with burn injuries. *Nursing Critical Care, 8*(1), 14–22.

Culleiton, A., & Simko, L. (2013c). Managing burn injuries in the ICU. *Nursing Critical Care, 8*(2), 22–30.

Dahl, O., Wickman, M., & Wengstrom, Y. (2012). Adapting to life after burn injury: Reflections on care. *Journal of Burn Care & Research, 33*(5), 595–605.

Fahlstrom, K., Boyle, C., & Makic, M. B. (2013). Implementation of a nurse-driven burn resuscitation protocol: A quality improvement project. *Critical Care Nurse, 33*(1), 25–35.

Hardwicke, J., Thomsom, R., Bamford, A., & Moiemen, N. (2013). A pilot evaluation study of high resolution digital thermal imaging in the assessment of burn depth. *Burns, 39*(1), 76–81.

Herndon, D. (2013). *Total burn care* (4th ed.). Philadelphia: Saunders.

Laing, C. (2013). Acute carbon monoxide toxicity: Be alert for this easy-to-miss illness. *Nursing Critical Care, 8*(1), 30–34.

Lewis, C. (2013). Stem cell application in acute burn care and reconstruction. *Journal of Wound Care, 11*(1), 7–16.

Murabit, A., & Tredget, E. (2012). Review of burn injuries secondary to home oxygen. *Journal of Burn Care & Research, 33*(2), 212–217.

Park, Y., Choi, Y., Lee, H., Moon, D., Kim, S., Lee, J., et al. (2013). The impact of laser Doppler imaging on the early decision-making process for surgical intervention in adults with indeterminate burns. *Burns, 39*(4), 655–661.

Silverstein, P., Heimbach, D., Meites, H., Latenser, B., Mozingo, D., Mullins, F., et al. (2011). An open, parallel, randomized, comparative, multicenter study to evaluate the cost-effectiveness, performance, tolerance, and safety of a silver-containing soft silicone foam dressing (intervention) vs sulfadiazine cream. *Journal of Burn Care & Research, 32*(6), 617–626.

Weimer, S., Staubli, L., & Makic, M. B. (2013). Fending off disaster for a frostbite victim. *American Nurse Today, 8*(1), 20.

Williams, F., Ludwik, K., Jeschke, M., & Herndon, D. (2011). What, how, and how much should burn patients be fed? *Surgical Clinics of North America, 91*(3), 609–629.

Chapter 27

American Lung Association (2012). *The LBGT community: A priority population for tobacco control.* Retrieved May 2014, from <www.lung.org/stop-smoking/tobacco-control-advocacy/reports-resources/tobacco-policy-trend>.

Baker, K., Barsamian, J., Leone, D., Donovan, B., Williams, D., Carnevale, K., et al. (2013). Routine dyspnea assessment on unit admission. *The American Journal of Nursing, 113*(11), 42–49.

Barnette, L., & Kautz, D. (2013). Creative ways to teach arterial blood gas interpretation. *Dimensions of Critical Care Nursing, 32*(2), 84–87.

Bauman, M., & Cosgrove, C. (2012). Understanding end-tidal CO2 monitoring. *American Nurse Today, 7*(11), 12–17.

Butler, K., Fallin, A., & Ridner, L. (2012). Evidence-based smoking cessation for college students. *Nursing Clinics of North America, 47*(1), 21–30.

Carlisle, H. (2014). The case for capnography in patients receiving opioids. *American Nurse Today, 9*(9), 22–26.

Fiala, S., Morris, D., & Pawlak, R. (2012). Measuring indoor air quality of hookah lounges. *American Journal of Public Health, 102*(11), 2043–2045.

Grief, S. (2011). Nicotine dependence: Health consequences, smoking cessation therapies, and pharmacotherapy. *Primary Care Clinics in Office Practice, 38*(1), 23–39.

Johnson, C., Anderson, M. A., & Hill, P. (2012). Comparison of pulse oximetry measures in a healthy population. *Medsurg Nursing, 21*(2), 70–75.

King, B. A., Dube, S. R., & Tynan, M. A. (2012). Current tobacco use among adults in the United States: Findings from the National Adult Tobacco Survey. *American Journal of Public Health, 102*, 93–100.

Lee, J., Blosnich, J., & Melvin, C. (2012). Up in smoke: Vanishing evidence of tobacco disparities in the Institute of Medicine's report on sexual and gender minority health. *American Journal of Public Health, 102*(11), 2041–2043.

MacIntyre, N. (2012). The future of pulmonary function testing. *Respiratory Care, 57*(1), 154–161.

Meridith, T., & Massey, D. (2011). Respiratory assessment 1: More key skills to improve care. *Journal of Cardiovascular Nursing, 6*(2), 63–68.

Murgu, S., Pecson, J., & Colt, H. (2011). Flexible bronchoscopy assisted by noninvasive positive pressure ventilation. *Critical Care Nurse, 31*(3), 70–76.

Passion, C., Matsumoto, K., & Day, D. (2011). Benzocaine puts a patient in a bind. *American Nurse Today, 6*(11), 25.

Riker, C., Lee, K., Darville, E., & Hahn, E. (2012). E-cigarettes: Promise or peril? *Nursing Clinics of North America, 47*(1), 159–171.

Ruppel, G., & Enright, P. (2012). Pulmonary function testing. *Respiratory Care, 57*(1), 165–175.

Wesley, C. (2014). Understanding acquired methemoglobinemia. *Nursing, 44*(2), 67.

Chapter 28

Abdo, W., & Heunks, L. (2012). Oxygen-induced hypercapnia in COPD: Myths and facts. *Critical Care, 16*(5), 323–326.

Ambutas, S., Staffileno, B., & Fogg, L. (2014). Reducing nasal pressure ulcers with an alternative taping device. *Medsurg Nursing, 23*(2), 96–100.

Bullard, D., Brothers, K., Davis, C., Kingsley, E., & Waters, J., III. (2012). Contraindications to nasopharyngeal airway insertion. *Nursing, 42*(10), 66–67.

Carlisle, H. (2014). The case for capnography in patients receiving opioids. *American Nurse Today, 9*(9), 22–26.

Dailey, C., Tola, D., & Kesten, K. (2012). Providing safe passage: Rapid sequence intubation for advanced practice nursing. *AACN Advanced Critical Care, 23*(3), 270–283.

Lamar, J. (2012). Relationship of respiratory care bundle with incentive spirometry to reduced pulmonary complications in a medical general practice unit. *Medsurg Nursing, 21*(1), 33–36.

Mac Sweeney, R., McAuley, D. F., & Matthay, M. A. (2011). Acute lung failure. *Seminars in Respiratory and Critical Care Medicine, 32*(5), 607–625.

Makic, M. B., Martin, S., Burns, S., Philbrick, D., & Rauen, C. (2013). Putting evidence into nursing practice: Four traditional practices not supported by the evidence. *Critical Care Nurse, 33*(2), 28–42.

Morris, L., McIntosh, E., & Whitmer, A. (2014). The importance of tracheostomy progression in the intensive care unit. *Critical Care Nurse, 34*(1), 40–48.

Morris, L., Whitmer, A., & McIntosh, E. (2013). Tracheostomy care and complications in the intensive care unit. *Critical Care Nurse, 33*(5), 18–30.

Murabit, A., & Tredget, E. (2012). Review of burn injuries secondary to home oxygen. *Journal of Burn Care & Research, 33*(2), 212–217.

Overdyk, F., & Guerra, J. (2011). Improving outcomes in med-surg patients with opioid-induced respiratory depression. *American Nurse Today, 6*(11), 26–30.

Rahu, M., Grap, M., Cohn, J., Munro, C., Lyon, D., & Sessler, C. (2013). Facial expression as an indicator of pain in critically ill intubated adults during endotracheal suctioning. *American Journal of Critical Care, 22*(5), 412–422.

Reed, C., Reineck, C., & Fonseca, I. (2011). Communicating with intubated patients: A new approach. *American Nurse Today, 6*(7), 34–35.

Simons, S., & Abdallah, L. (2012). Bedside assessment of enteral tube placement: Aligning practice with evidence. *American Journal of Nursing, 112*(2), 40–47.

Sole, M. L., Su, X., Talbert, S., Penover, D., Kalita, S., Jimenez, E., et al. (2011). Evaluation of an intervention to maintain endotracheal tube cuff pressure within therapeutic range. *American Journal of Critical Care, 20*(2), 109–118.

Stepter, C. (2012). Maintaining placement of temporary enteral feeding tubes in adults: A critical appraisal of the evidence. *Medsurg Nursing, 21*(2), 61–68.

Chapter 29

American Cancer Society (ACS) (2014). *Cancer facts and figures, 2014*. 01-300M–No. 500814. Atlanta: Author.

Ardilio, S. (2011). Calculating nutrition needs for a patient with head and neck cancer. *Clinical Journal of Oncology Nursing, 15*(5), 457–459.

Boucher, J., Olson, L., & Piperdi, B. (2011). Preemptive management of dermatologic toxicities associated with epidermal growth factor receptor inhibitors. *Clinical Journal of Oncology Nursing, 15*(5), 501–508.

Callaway, C. (2011). Rethinking the head and neck cancer population: The human papillomavirus association. *Clinical Journal of Oncology Nursing, 15*(2), 165–170.

Canadian Cancer Society, Statistics Canada (2014). *Canadian cancer statistics, 2014*. Toronto: Canadian Cancer Society.

Carlucci, M., Smith, M., & Corbridge, S. (2013). Poor sleep, hazardous breathing. *The Nurse Practitioner, 38*(3), 20–28.

Fletcher, B., Cohen, M., Schumacher, K., & Lydiatt, W. (2012). A blessing and a curse: Head and neck cancer survivors' experiences. *Cancer Nursing, 35*(2), 126–132.

Haisfield-Wolfe, M. E., McGuire, D., & Krumm, S. (2012). Perspectives on coping among patients with head and neck cancer receiving radiation. *Oncology Nursing Forum, 39*(3), E249–E257.

Happ, M. B., Garrett, K., Thomas, D., Tate, J., George, E., Houze, M., et al. (2011). Nurse-patient communication interactions in the intensive care unit. *American Journal of Critical Care, 20*(2), e28–e40.

Mannix, C., Bartholomay, M., Doherty, C., Lewis, M., & Bilodeau, M. L. (2012). A feasibility study of low-cost, self-administered skin care interventions in patients with head and neck cancer receiving chemoradiation. *Clinical Journal of Oncology Nursing, 16*(3), 278–285.

Mason, H., DeRubeis, M., Foster, J., Tayloe, J., & Worden, F. (2013). Outcomes evaluation of a weekly nurse practitioner-managed symptom management clinic for patients with head and neck cancer treated with chemotherapy. *Oncology Nursing Forum, 40*(6), 581–586.

McLaughlin, L. (2013). Taste dysfunction in head and neck cancer survivors. *Oncology Nursing Forum, 40*(1), E4–E13.

Nance-Floyd, B. (2011). Tracheostomy care: An evidence-based guide to suctioning and dressing changes. *American Nurse Today, 6*(7), 14–17.

National Comprehensive Cancer Network (2013). *Practice guidelines in oncology: Head and neck cancers*. (version 2.2013). Fort Washington, PA: Author.

Poetker, D. (2013). Adults with epistaxis. *Patient Management Perspectives in Otolaryngology, 42*(6), 1–26.

Reed, C., Reineck, C., & Fonseca, I. (2011). Communicating with intubated patients: A new approach. *American Nurse Today, 6*(7), 34–35.

Simmons, S., & Pruitt, B. (2012). Sounding the alarm for patients with obstructive sleep apnea. *Nursing, 42*(4), 35–41.

Suzuki, M. (2012). Quality of life, uncertainty, and perceived involvement in decision making in patients with head and neck cancer. *Oncology Nursing Forum, 39*(6), 541–548.

Vacca, V., & Poirier, W. (2013). Action STAT: Posterior epistaxis. *Nursing, 43*(1), 72.

Woidtke, R. (2013). Adult obstructive sleep apnea: Taking a patient-centered approach. *American Nurse Today, 8*(7), 12–15.

Zeien, J. (2011). Create your own tracheostomy and laryngectomy teaching aids. *Nursing, 41*(2), 17–18.

Chapter 30

Abdo, W., & Heunks, L. (2012). Oxygen-induced hypercapnia in COPD: Myths and facts. *Critical Care, 16*(5), 323–326.

American Cancer Society (ACS) (2014). *Cancer facts and figures—2014*. No. 01-300M–No. 500814. Atlanta: Author.

Bauman, M., & Handley, C. (2011). Chest-tube care: The more you know, the easier it gets. *American Nurse Today, 6*(9), 27–31.

Beery, T. A., & Workman, M. L. (2012). *Genetics and genomics in nursing and health care.* Philadelphia: F.A. Davis.

Burt, L., & Corbridge, S. (2013). COPD exacerbations: Evidence-based guidelines for identification, assessment, and management. *American Journal of Nursing, 113*(2), 34–43.

Cagle, P., & Chirieac, L. (2012). Advances in treatment of lung cancer with targeted therapy. *Archives of Pathology & Laboratory Medicine, 136*(5), 504–509.

Centers for Disease Control and Prevention (CDC). (2012). Summary of health statistics for U.S. adults: National Health Interview Survey, 2011. *Vital and Health Statistics, Series 10*, (256). Retrieved June 2014, from <www.cdc.gov/nchs/data/series/sr_10/sr10_256.pdf>.

Centers for Disease Control and Prevention (CDC) (2014a). *FastStats—Asthma.* Retrieved June 2014, from <www.cdc.gov/nchs/fastats/asthma.htm>.

Centers for Disease Control and Prevention (CDC) (2014b). *FastStats—Chronic obstructive pulmonary disease (COPD).* Retrieved June 2014, from <www.cdc.gov/nchs/fastats/copd.htm>.

Cystic Fibrosis Foundation (2014). *About cystic fibrosis.* Retrieved June 2014, from <www.cff.org/AboutCF/>.

Demerouti, E., Manginas, A., Athanassopoulis, G., Karatasakis, G., Leontiadis, E., & Pavlides, G. (2013). Successful epoprostenol withdrawal in pulmonary arterial hypertension: Case report and literature review. *Respiratory Care, 58*(2), e1–e5.

Esguerra-Gonzalez, A., Ilagan-Honorio, M., Fraschilla, S., Kehoe, P., Lee, A., Marcarian, T., et al. (2013). Pain after lung transplant: High frequency chest wall oscillation vs chest physiotherapy. *American Journal of Critical Care, 22*(2), 115–125.

Fuentes, A., Coralic, A., & Dawson, K. (2012). A new epoprostenol formulation for the treatment of pulmonary artery hypertension. *American Journal of Health-System Pharmacists, 69*, 1389–1393.

Global Initiative for Asthma (GINA) (2014). *Pocket guide for asthma management and prevention.* Retrieved June 2014, from <www.ginasthma.org/Guidelines/guidelines-resources.html>.

Global Initiative for Chronic Obstructive Lung Disease (GOLD) (2014). *Global strategy for the diagnosis, management, and prevention of chronic obstructive pulmonary disease.* Retrieved June 2014, from <www.goldcopd.org/>.

Grant, M., Sun, M., Fujinami, R., Sidhu, R., Otis-Green, S., Juarez, G., et al. (2013). Family caregiver burden, skills, preparedness, and quality of life in non–small cell lung cancer. *Oncology Nursing Forum, 40*(4), 337–346.

Held-Warmkessel, J., & Schiech, L. (2014). Non-small cell lung cancer: Recent advances. *Nursing, 44*(2), 32–42.

Kessenich, C., & Bacher, K. (2014). Alpha-1 antitrypsin deficiency. *The Nurse Practitioner, 39*(7), 12–14.

Kingman, M., & Chin, K. (2013). Safety recommendations for administering intravenous prostacyclins in the hospital. *Critical Care Nurse, 33*(5), 32–34, 36–41.

Lareau, S., & Hodder, R. (2012). Teaching inhaler use in chronic obstructive pulmonary disease patients. *Journal of the American Academy of Nurse Practitioners, 24*(2), 113–120.

Lehto, R. H. (2014). Lung cancer screening guidelines: The nurse's role in patient education and advocacy. *Clinical Journal of Oncology Nursing, 18*(3), 338–342.

Lewis, D., & Scullion, J. (2012). Palliative and end-of-life care for patients with idiopathic pulmonary fibrosis: Challenges and dilemmas. *International Journal of Palliative Nursing, 18*(7), 331–337.

Makic, M. B., Martin, S., Burns, S., Philbrick, D., & Rauen, C. (2013). Putting evidence into practice: Four traditional practices not supported by the evidence. *Critical Care Nurse, 33*(2), 28–42.

Nakano, S., & Tluczek, A. (2014). Genomic breakthroughs in the diagnosis and treatment of cystic fibrosis. *The American Journal of Nursing, 114*(6), 36–43.

Neufeld, K., & Keith, L. (2012). Care of patients with cystic fibrosis. *AORN Journal, 96*(5), 529–536.

O'Laughlen, M., & Rance, K. (2012). Update on asthma management in primary care. *The Nurse Practitioner, 37*(11), 32–40.

Online Mendelian Inheritance in Man (OMIM) (2013a). *Adenocarcinoma of the lung.* Retrieved June 2014, from <www.omim.org/entry/211980>.

Online Mendelian Inheritance in Man (OMIM) (2013b). *Asthma, susceptibility to.* Retrieved June 2014, from <www.omim.org/entry/600807>.

Online Mendelian Inheritance in Man (OMIM) (2013c). *Cystic fibrosis; CF.* Retrieved June 2014, from <www.omim.org/entry/219700>.

Online Mendelian Inheritance in Man (OMIM) (2013d). *Pulmonary hypertension, primary.* Retrieved June 2014, from <www.omim.org/entry/178600>.

Pruitt, B. (2011). Assessing and managing asthma: A global initiative for asthma update. *Nursing, 41*(5), 46–52.

Roberts-Collins, C., Tagney, J., Tulloh, R., & Garratt, V. (2013). Being mindful of pulmonary arterial hypertension. *British Journal of Cardiac Nursing, 8*(3), 127–133.

Smith, B., & Tasota, F. (2011). Smoking out the dangers of COPD. *Nursing, 41*(4), 32–39.

Weber, C., Silver, M., Cromer, D., Kaminski, S., Wirick, T., & Vallejo, J. (2011). Under pressure: Pulmonary arterial hypertension. *Critical Care Nurse, 31*(4), 87–94.

World Health Organization (WHO). (2011). Dasatinib: Pulmonary artery hypertension. *WHO Drug Information, 25*(4), 360.

World Health Organization (WHO). (2012). Ambrisentan: Idiopathic pulmonary fibrosis. *WHO Drug Information, 28*(3), 270.

Chapter 31

Acerra, J. (2014). Pharyngitis. *Medscape Reference.* Retrieved June 2014, from <http://emedicine.medscape.com/article/764304-overview>.

American Lung Association (ALA) (2010a). *Trends in pneumonia and influenza morbidity and mortality.* Retrieved June 2014, from <www.lungusa.org/finding-cures/our-research/trend-reports/pi-trend-report.pdf>.

American Lung Association (ALA) (2010b). *Trends in tuberculosis morbidity and mortality.* Retrieved June 2014, from <www.lungusa.org/finding-cures/our-research/trend-reports/TB-Trend-Report.pdf>.

Aung, K. (2013). Viral pharyngitis. *Medscape Reference.* Retrieved June 2014, from <http://emedicine.medscape.com/article/225362-overview#a0199>.

2012 Beers Criteria Update Expert Panel. (2012). American Geriatrics Society updated Beers criteria for potentially inappropriate medication use in older adults. *Journal of the American Geriatrics Society.* Retrieved June 2014, from <www.americangeriatrics.org/files/documents/beers/2012BeersCriteria_JAGS.pdf>.

Barclay, L. (2013). MERS-CoV: Different from SARS, comorbidities may be key. *Medscape Reference.* Retrieved June, 2014, from <http://www.medscape.com/viewarticle/808465>.

Bocka, J. J. (2014). Pertussis. *Medscape Reference.* Retrieved June 2014, from <http://emedicine.medscape.com/article/967268-overview>.

Brook, I. (2013). Acute sinusitis. *Medscape Reference.* Retrieved June 2014, from <http://emedicine.medscape.com/article/232670-overview>.

Buhrow, S. (2013). Coccidioidomycosis: A differential diagnosis for visitors to the southwest. *The American Journal of Nursing, 113*(11), 52–55.

CDC urges better flu, pertussis vaccination (2012). *Hospital Employee Health*, 3–4.

Centers for Disease Control and Prevention (CDC) (2010a). *Cover your cough.* Retrieved June 2014, from <www.cdc.gov/flu/protect/covercough.htm>.

Centers for Disease Control and Prevention (CDC) (2010b). *2009 H1N1: Overview of a pandemic.* Retrieved June 2014, from <www.cdc.gov/h1n1flu/yearinreveiw.htm>.

Centers for Disease Control and Prevention (CDC). (2010c). Prevention & control of influenza with vaccines: Recommendations of the Advisory Committee on Immunization Practices (ACIP). *Morbidity and Mortality Weekly Report, 59*, 1–62.

Centers for Disease Control and Prevention (CDC) (2012). *CDC fast facts: Pertussis.* Retrieved June 2014, from <www.cdc.gov/pertussis/fast-facts.html>.

Centers for Disease Control and Prevention (CDC) (2013). *HIV and tuberculosis.* Retrieved June 2014, from <www.cdc.gov/hiv/resources/factsheets/PDF/hivtb.htm>.

Centers for Disease Control and Prevention (CDC) (2014a). *Information on avian influenza.* Retrieved June 2014, from <www.cdc.gov/flu/avianflu/>.

Centers for Disease Control and Prevention (CDC) (2014b). *Key facts about seasonal flu vaccine.* Retrieved June 2014, from <www.cdc.gov/flu/protect/keyfacts.htm>.

Centers for Disease Control and Prevention (CDC) (2014c). *Global Tuberculosis.* Retrieved June, 2014, from <http://www.cdc.gov/tb/topic/globaltb/>.

Centers for Disease Control and Prevention (CDC) (2014d). Middle East Respiratory Syndrome (MERS). *Medscape Reference.* Retrieved June, 2014, from <http://www.cdc.gov/CORONAVIRUS/MERS/INDEX.HTML>.

Cunha, B. (2014). Anthrax. *Medscape Reference.* Retrieved June 2014, from <http://emedicine.medscape.com/article/212127-overview>.

Dambaugh, L. A. (2012). A review of influenza: Implications for the geriatric population. *Critical Care Nursing Clinics of North America, 24*, 573–580.

Echevarria, I., & Schwoebel, A. (2012). Development of an intervention model for the prevention of aspiration pneumonia in high-risk patients on a medical-surgical unit. *Medsurg Nursing, 21*(5), 303–308.

Gler, M., Skripconoka, V., Sanchez-Garavito, E., Xiao, H., Cabrera-Rivero, J., Vargas-Vasquez, D., et al. (2012). Delamanid for multidrug-resistant pulmonary tuberculosis. *The New England Journal of Medicine, 366*(23), 2151–2160.

Gould, D. (2011). The challenges of caring for patients with influenza. *Nursing Older People, 23*(10), 28–34.

Heavey, E. (2013). Does the BCG vaccine protect against TB? *Nursing, 43*(10), 62.

Kamangar, N. (2013). Lung abscess. *Medscape Reference.* Retrieved June 2014, from <http://emedicine.medscape.com/article/299425-overview>.

Krouse, H. J., & Krouse, J. (2014). Allergic rhinitis: Diagnosis through management. *The Nurse Practitioner, 39*(4), 20–29.

Medication Update. (2014). FDA approves first adjuvanted vaccine to prevent H5N1 avian flu. *The Nurse Practitioner, 39*(2), 56.

Plosker, G. L. (2012). A/H5N1 prepandemic influenza vaccine (whole virion, vero cell-derived, inactivated) [Vepacel®]. *Drugs, 72*(11), 1543–1557.

Roark, D. C. (2012). Working toward perfection on the pneumonia core measure. *Journal of Emergency Nursing, 38*, 127–129.

Schweon, S. J. (2011). Pertussis: Not just for kids anymore. *Nursing, 41*(10), 61–62.

Scott, S., & Kardos, C. (2012). Community-acquired, health care-associated, and ventilator-associated pneumonia: Three variations of a serious disease. *Critical Care Nursing Clinics of North America, 24*(3), 431–441.

Shah, U. K. (2014a). Tonsillitis and peritonsillar abscess. *Medscape Reference.* Retrieved June 2014, from <http://emedicine.medscape.com/article/871977-overview>.

Shah, U. K. (2014b). Tonsillitis and peritonsillar abscess treatment and management. *Medscape Reference.* Retrieved June 2014, from <http://emedicine.medscape.com/article/871977-treatment>.

Sheikh, J. (2014). Allergic rhinitis. *Medscape Reference.* Retrieved June 2014, from <http://emedicine.medscape.com/article/134825-overview>.

Thornton, K., Alston, M., Dye, H., & Williamson, S. (2011). Are saline irrigations effective in relieving chronic rhinosinusitis symptoms? A review of the evidence. *The Journal for Nurse Practitioners, 7*(8), 680–686.

Todd, B. (2014). Middle east respiratory syndrome (MERS-CoV). *The American Journal of Nursing, 114*(1), 56–59.

World Health Organization (WHO) (2014a). *Global tuberculosis report 2013: Executive summary.* Retrieved June 2014, from <www.who.int/tb/data>.

World Health Organization (WHO) (2014b). *Global tuberculosis report 2013: Factsheet.* Retrieved June 2014, from <www.who.int/tb/publications/factsheets/en/index.html>.

World Health Organization (WHO) (2013). *What is multi-drug resistant tuberculosis and how do we treat it.* Retrieved June 2014, from <www.who.int/features/qu/79/en/>.

Zwanger, M. (2013). Empyema and abscess pneumonia. *Medscape Reference.* Retrieved June 2014, from <http://emedicine.medscape.com/article/807499-overview>.

Chapter 32

Amidei, C., & Sole, M. (2013). Physiological responses to passive exercise in adults receiving mechanical ventilation. *American Journal of Critical Care, 22*(4), 337–348.

ARDS Foundation (2013). *Facts about ARDS.* Retrieved June 2014, from <http://ardsfoundation.com>.

Aust, M. (2014). Compact clinical guide to mechanical ventilation: Foundations of practice for critical care nurses. *Critical Care Nurse, 34*(2), 80.

Bekken, N. (2011). Strategies for nursing care of adult patients with acute respiratory failure. *Mosby's Nursing Consult Clinical Updates.* Retrieved June 2014, from <www.nursingconsult.com/nursing/clinical-updates/full-text?clinical_update_id=203829&specId=0&sortBy=title-a&parentpage=search&sort_order=Relevance&contact_hours>.

Benson, A. B. (2012). Pulmonary complications of transfused blood components. *Critical Care Nursing Clinics of North America, 24*, 403–418.

Bjerke, H. S. (2012). Flail chest. *Medscape Reference.* Retrieved June 2014, from <http://emedicine.medscape.com/article/433779-overview>.

Booker, S., Murff, S., Kitko, L., & Jablonski, R. (2013). Mouth care to reduce ventilator-associated pneumonia. *The American Journal of Nursing, 113*(10), 24–30.

Bortolotto, S. J., & Makic, M. B. (2012). Understanding advanced modes of mechanical ventilation. *Critical Care Nursing Clinics of North America, 24*(4), 443–456.

Bull, A. (2014). Primary care of chronic dyspnea in adults. *The Nurse Practitioner, 39*(8), 34–40.

Carlisle, H. (2014). The case for capnography in patients receiving opioids. *American Nurse Today, 9*(9), 22–26.

Carroll, P., Shirato, S., & Beach, P. R. (2013). Acute respiratory distress syndrome/acute lung injury. *Mosby's Nursing Consult Evidence-Based Nursing Monographs.* Retrieved June 2014, from <www.nursingconsult.com/nursing/evidence-based-nursing/monograph?monograph_id=216675>.

Daley, B. (2014). Pneumothorax. *Medscape Reference.* Retrieved April 2013, from <http://emedicine.medscape.com/article/424547-overview>.

Day, M. (2011). On alert for iatrogenic pneumothorax. *Nursing, 41*(6), 66–67.

Dechert, R. E., Haas, C. F., & Ostwani, W. (2012). Current knowledge of acute lung injury and acute respiratory distress syndrome. *Critical Care Nursing Clinics of North America, 24*, 377–401.

Dennison, R. D., Johnson, J. M., & Blair, M. (2011). *Pass CEN!* Philadelphia: Elsevier.

Drumright, K., Jukenbeck, S., & Judd, C. (2013). The ABCs of acute PE. *Nursing Made Incredibly Easy, 11*(2), 45–49.

Duff, J., Walker, K., Omari, A., & Stratton, C. (2013). Prevention of venous thromboembolism in hospitalized patients: Analysis of reduced cost and improved clinical outcomes. *Journal of Vascular Nursing, 31*, 9–14.

Ferri, F. (2013). Acute respiratory distress syndrome. *Ferri's clinical advisor 2013.* St. Louis: Mosby.

Garg, K. (2013). Acute pulmonary embolism (Helical CT). *Medscape Reference.* Retrieved June 2014, from <http://emedicine.medscape.com/article/361131-overview>.

Golembiewski, J. A. (2011). Dabigatran: A new oral anticoagulant. *Journal of Perianesthesia Nursing, 26*(6), 420–423.

Grossbach, I., Chlan, L., & Tracy, M. (2011). Overview of mechanical ventilatory support and management of patient- and ventilator-related responses. *Critical Care Nurse, 31*(3), 30–44.

Grossbach, I., Stranberg, S., & Chlan, L. (2011). Promoting effective communication for patients receiving mechanical ventilation. *Critical Care Nurse, 31*(3), 46–60.

Hiller, B., Wilson, C., Chamberlain, D., & King, L. (2013). Preventing ventilator-associated pneumonia through oral care, product selection, and application method. *AACN Advanced Critical Care, 24*(1), 38–58.

Hussey, L. (2013). Reducing mortality in pulmonary embolism through prevention and careful management. *Mosby's Nursing Consult.* Retrieved June 2014, from <www.nursingconsult.com/nursing/clinical-updates/full-text?clinical_update_id=197598&specId=0&sortBy=title-a&parentpage=search&sort_order=Relevance&contact_hours>.

Kessenich, C., & Erigo-Backman, R. (2012). Computed tomography angiography and pulmonary embolism. *The Nurse Practitioner, 37*(10), 10–11.

Kiypshi-Teo, H., Cabana, M. O., Froelicher, E. S., & Blegen, M. A. (2014). Adherence to institution-specific ventilator-associated pneumonia prevention guidelines. *American Journal of Critical Care, 23*(3), 201–215.

Kydonaki, K., Huby, G., & Tocher, J. (2014). Difficult to wean patients: Cultural factors and their impact on weaning decision-making. *Journal of Clinical Nursing, 23*(5/6), 683–693.

Landeen, C., & Smith, H. L. (2014). Examination of pneumonia risks and risk levels in trauma patients with pulmonary contusion. *Journal of Trauma Nursing, 21*(2), 41–49.

Lee, A. (2014). Factor V Leiden. *Nursing, 44*(6), 10–12.

Lian, J. (2013). Using ABGs to optimize mechanical ventilation. *Nursing, 43*(6), 46–52.

Mancini, M. C. (2012a). Blunt chest trauma. *Medscape Reference*. Retrieved June 2014, from <http://emedicine.medscape.com/article/428723-overview>.

Mancini, M. C. (2012b). Hemothorax. *Medscape Reference*. Retrieved June 2014, from <http://emedicine.medscape.com/article/2047916-overview>.

Mathay, M. A., & Zemans, R. L. (2011). The acute respiratory distress syndrome: Pathogenesis and treatment. *Annual Review of Pathology, 6*, 147–163.

McLean, B. A. (2012). Acute respiratory failure and intensive measures. *Critical Care Nursing Clinics of North America, 24*, 361–375.

McLenon, M. (2012). Acute pulmonary embolism. *Critical Care Nursing Quarterly, 35*(2), 173–182.

Mellott, K. G., Grap, M., Munro, C. L., Sessler, C. N., Wetzel, P. A., Nilsestuen, J. O., et al. (2014). Patient ventilator asynchrony in critically ill adults: Frequency and types. *Heart and Lung, 43*(3), 231–243.

Mendez, M., Lazar, M., DiGiovine, B., Schuldt, S., Behrendt, R., Peters, M., et al. (2013). Dedicated multidisciplinary ventilator bundle team and compliance with sedation vacation. *American Journal of Critical Care, 22*(1), 54–60.

Messing, J. A., Gail, V., & Sarani, B. (2014). Successful management of severe flail chest via early operative intervention. *Journal of Trauma Nursing, 21*(2), 83–85.

Morris, P. E., Griffin, L., Berry, M., Thompson, C., Hite, R. D., Winkelman, C., et al. (2011). Receiving early mobility during an ICU admission is a predictor of improved outcomes in acute respiratory failure. *American Journal of Medical Sciences, 341*, 373–377.

Morton, P. G., & Fontaine, D. K. (2013). *Essentials of critical care nursing: A holistic approach*. Philadelphia: Lippincott Williams & Wilkins.

Munro, N., & Ruggiero, M. (2014). Ventilator-associated pneumonia bundle. *AACN Advanced Critical Care, 25*(2), 163–178.

Online Mendelian Inheritance in Man (OMIM) (2013). *Coagulation factor V; F5*. Retrieved July 2014, from <www.omim.org/entry/612309>.

Ouellette, D. R. (2014). Pulmonary embolism treatment and management. *Medscape Reference*. Retrieved June 2014, from <http://emedicine.medscape.com/article/300901-treatment>.

Poirier, W., & Vacca, V. (2013). Flail chest. *Nursing, 43*(12), 10–11.

Powers, K., & Talbot, L. (2011). Fat embolism syndrome after femur fracture with intramedullary nailing: Case report. *American Journal of Critical Care, 20*(3), 264–265, 267.

Riley, P. (2013). Measuring, monitoring heparin: A discussion of anti factorXa versus aPTT. *Advance for Medical Laboratory Professionals, 25*(2), 10–11.

Ruiz, C. (2011). Thwarting a pneumothorax. *American Nurse Today, 6*(5), 32.

Smithburger, P. L., Campbell, S., & Kane-Gill, S. L. (2013). Alteplase treatment of acute pulmonary embolism in the intensive care unit. *Critical Care Nurse, 33*(2), 17–26.

Urden, L. D., Stacy, K. M., & Lough, M. E. (2012). *Priorities in critical care nursing* (6th ed.). St. Louis: Mosby.

Warren, E. (2013). A practice guide to anticoagulation. *Prescribing Nurse, 43*(2), 29–33.

Williams, K. (2013). Extracorporeal membrane oxygenation for acute respiratory distress syndrome in adults. *AACN Advanced Critical Care, 24*(2), 149–158.

Wright, A. D., & Flynn, M. (2011). Using the prone position for ventilated patients with respiratory failure: A review. *Nursing in Critical Care, 16*(1), 19–27.

Chapter 33

American Heart Association (AHA) (2013). *Diet and lifestyle recommendations* (updated: March 19, 2013). Retrieved July 2014, from <www.heart.org/HEARTORG/GettingHealthy/Diet-and-Lifestyle-Recommendations_UCM_305855_Article.jsp>.

*Cheek, D., & Tester, J. (2008). Women and heart disease: What's new? *Nursing, 38*(1), 37–42.

Go, A. S., Mozaffarian, D., Roger, V. L., Benjamin, E. J., Berry, J. D., Borden, W. B., et al. (2013). Heart disease and stroke statistics—2014 update: A report from the American Heart Association. *Circulation*. Retrieved July 2014, from <http://circ.ahajournals.org/content/early/2013/12/18/01.Circ0000441139.102102.80.citation>.

*Howie-Esquivel, J., & White, M. (2008). Biomarkers in acute cardiovascular disease. *Journal of Cardiovascular Nursing, 23*(2), 124–131.

James, P. A., Oparil, S., Carter, B. L., Cushman, W. C., Dennison-Himmelfarb, C., Handler, J., et al. (2014). 2014 evidence-based guidelines for the management of high blood pressure in adults: report from the panel members appointed to the Eighth Joint National Committee (JNC 8). *The Journal of the American Medical Association, 311*(5), 507–520.

Johnson, C. J., Anderson, M. A., & Hill, P. D. (2012). Comparison of pulse oximetry in a health population. *Medsurg Nursing, 21*(2), 70–73.

Landgraf, J., Wishner, S. H., & Kloner, R. A. (2010). Comparison of automatic oscillometric versus auscultatory blood pressure measurement. *American Journal of Cardiology, 106*(3), 386–388.

Pearson, T. L. (2010). Ankle brachial index as a prognostic tool for women with coronary artery disease. *Journal of Cardiovascular Nursing, 25*(1), 20–24.

Sanborn, T. A., Ebrahimi, R., Manoukian, S. V., McLaurin, B. T., Cox, D. A., Feit, F., et al. (2010). Impact of femoral vascular closure devices and antithrombotic therapy on access site bleeding in acute coronary syndromes. *Circulation: Cardiovascular Interventions, 3*(1), 57–62.

Sulzbach-Hoke, L. M., Ratcliffe, S. J., Kimmel, S. E., Kolansky, D. M., & Polomano, R. (2010). Predictors of complications following sheath removal with percutaneous coronary intervention. *Journal of Cardiovascular Nursing, 25*(3), e1–e8.

*The New York Heart Association (1964). *Diseases of the heart and blood vessels: Nomenclature and criteria for diagnosis* (6th ed.). Boston: Little, Brown.

*Wright, J. D., Hirsch, R., & Wang, C. Y. (2009). One-third of U.S. adults embraced most heart healthy behaviors in 1999-2002. *National Center for Health Statistics Data Brief, (17)*. Hyattsville, MD: National Center for Health Statistics. Retrieved July 2014, from <www.cdc.gov/nchs/data/databriefs/db17.htm>.

Chapter 34

American Heart Association (AHA) (2010). *Highlights of the 2010 American Heart Association Guidelines for CPR and ECC*. Retrieved June 2013, from <www.heart.org/idc/groups/heart-public/@wcm/@ecc/documents/downloadable/ucm_317350.pdf>.

Anderson, J., Halperin, J., Albert, N., Bozkurt, B., Brindis, R., Curtis, L., et al. (2013). Management of patients with atrial fibrillation (compilation of 2006 ACCF/AHA/ESC and 2011 ACCF/AHA/HRS recommendations). *Journal of the American College of Cardiology, 61*(18), 1935–1944.

Barekatain, A., & Razavi, M. (2012). Antiarrhythmic therapy in atrial fibrillation: Indications, guidelines and safety. *Texas Heart Institute, 39*(4), 532–534.

Batista, L., Lima, F., Januzzi, J., Donahue, V., Snydeman, C., & Greer, D. (2010). Feasibility and safety of combined percutaneous coronary intervention and therapeutic hypothermia following cardiac arrest. *Resuscitation, 81*(4), 398–403.

Berdowski, J., Blom, M., Bardai, A., Tan, H., Tijessen, J., & Koster, R. (2011). Impact of onsite or dispatched automated external defibrillator use on survival after out of hospital cardiac arrest. *Circulation, 124*, 2225–2232.

Berry, E., & Padgett, H. (2012). Management of patients with atrial fibrillation: Diagnosis and treatment. *Nursing Standard, 26*(22), 47–56.

Bosen, D. (2011). Pacing therapies for atrial fibrillation. *Nursing*, 11–12. doi:10.1097/01.NURSE.0000394518.21592.1a.

Buck, H. G. (2012). CPR in older adults: What's the evidence? *Nursing, 42*(5), 14–15.

Calkins, H., Kuck, K., Cappato, R., Brugada, J., Camm, A., Chen, S., et al. (2012). 2012 HRS/EHRA/ECAS expert consensus statement on catheter and surgical ablation of atrial fibrillation: Recommendations for patient selection, procedural techniques, patient management and follow-up, definitions, endpoints and research trial design. *Heart Rhythm, 9*(4), 632–696.

Chalupka, A. N. (2010). Radiofrequency catheter ablation for atrial fibrillation. *American Association of Occupational Health Nurses, 58*(5), 220.

Cheng, J. M. (2010). New and emerging antiarrhythmic and anticoagulant agents for atrial fibrillation. *American Journal of Health-System Pharmacy, 67*(9), S26–S34.

Chilukuri, K., Dalal, D., Gadrey, S., Marine, J. E., MacPherson, E., Henrikson, C. A., et al. (2010). A prospective study evaluating the role of obesity and obstructive sleep apnea for outcomes after catheter ablation of atrial fibrillation. *Journal of Cardiovascular Electrophysiology, 21*(5), 521–525.

Chinitz, J., Halperin, J., Reddy, V., & Fuster, V. (2012). Rate or rhythm control for atrial fibrillation: Update and controversies. *The American Journal of Medicine, 125*, 1049–1056.

Craig, K. J., & Day, M. P. (2011). Are you up to date on the latest BLS and ACLS guidelines? *Nursing, 41*(5), 40–44.

Cronin, E., & Varma, N. (2012). Remote monitoring of cardiovascular implanted electronic devices: A paradigm shift for the 21st century. *Expert Reviews, 9*(4), 367–376.

Dagres, N., & Anastasiou-Nana, M. (2010). Atrial fibrillation and obesity: An association of increasing importance. *Journal of the American College of Cardiology, 55*(21), 2328–2329.

DeVon, H. A., Hogan, N., Ochs, A. L., & Shapiro, M. (2010). Time to treatment for acute coronary syndromes: The cost of indecision. *Journal of Cardiovascular Nursing, 25*(2), 106–114.

Dobromir, D., & Nattel, S. (2010). New antiarrhythmic drugs for treatment of atrial fibrillation. *The Lancet, 375*(9721), 1212–1223.

Franks, M., & Lawson, L. (2012). Body surface mapping improves diagnosis of acute myocardial infarction in the emergency department. *Advanced Emergency Nursing Journal, 34*(1), 32–40.

Garlitski, A. C., & Estes, N. A. I. I. I. (2010). Emerging therapies for atrial fibrillation: Is the paradigm shifting? *Journal of Interventional Cardiac Electrophysiology, 28*(1), 1–4.

Go, A., Mozaffarian, D., Roger, V., Benjamin, E., Berry, J., Borden, W., et al. (2013). Heart disease and stroke statistics—2013 update: A report from the American Heart Association. *Circulation, 127*, e6–e245.

Green, J. M., & Chiaramida, A. J. (2010). *12-lead EKG confidence: A step-by-step guide*. New York: Springer.

Hallas, C., Burke, J., White, D., & Connelly, D. (2010). A prospective 1-year study of changes in neuropsychological functioning after implantable cardioverter-defibrillator surgery. *Circulation: Arrhythmia and Electrophysiology, 3*, 170–177.

Harden, J. (2011). Taking a cool look at therapeutic hypothermia. *Nursing, 41*(9), 46–52.

*Hardin, S. R., & Steele, J. R. (2008). Atrial fibrillation among older adults: Pathophysiology, symptoms, and treatment. *Journal of Gerontological Nursing, 34*(7), 26–32.

Johnson, T., Jadick, E., & Knippers, L. (2011). Atrial fibrillation ablation. *American Journal of Nursing, 111*(2), 58–61.

Jost, D., Degrange, H., Verret, C., Hersan, O., Banville, I. L., Chapman, F. W., et al. (2010). A randomized controlled trial of the effect of automated external defibrillator cardiopulmonary resuscitation protocol on outcome from out-of-hospital cardiac arrest. *Circulation, 121*, 1614–1622.

Keseg, D. P. (2010). Reducing interruptions: Continuous compression CPR & minimally interrupted CPR result in improved survival. *A Journal of Emergency Medical Services, 35*(1), 14–17.

Kireyev, D., Fernandez, S., Gupta, V., Arkhipow, M., & Paris, J. (2012). Targeting tachycardia: Diagnostic tips and tools. *Journal of Family Practice, 61*(5), 258–263.

Lee, G., Sanders, P., & Kalman, J. (2012). Catheter ablation of atrial arrhythmias: State of the art. *Lancet, 380*, 1509–1519.

Link, M. (2012). Evaluation and initial treatment of supraventricular tachycardia. *New England Journal of Medicine, 367*, 1438–1448. doi:10.1056/NEJMcp1111259.

Marcus, G. M., Olgin, J. E., Whooley, M., Vittinghoff, E., Stone, K. L., Mehra, R., et al. (2010). Racial differences in atrial fibrillation prevalence and left atrial size. *American Journal of Medicine, 123*(4), 375.e1–375.e7.

Michaels, A. D., Spinler, S. A., Leeper, B., Ohman, E. M., Alexander, K. P., Newby, L. K., et al. (2010). Medication errors in acute cardiovascular and stroke patients: A scientific statement from the American Heart Association. *Circulation, 121*, 1664–1682.

Mooney, T. (2013). Use of dabigatran to prevent stroke in patients with atrial fibrillation. *Nursing Standard, 27*(27), 35–41.

Palmer, B. (2011). Systematic cardiac rhythm strip analysis. *Medsurg Nursing, 20*(2), 96–97.

Patel, M. R., Mahaffey, K. W., Garg, J., Pan, G., Singer, D. E., Hacke, W., ROCKET AF Steering Committee for the ROCKET AF Investigators, et al. (2011). Rivaroxaban versus warfarin in nonvalvular atrial fibrillation. *New England Journal of Medicine, 365*(10), 883–891.

Pelter, M. (2010). Time to treatment for acute coronary syndromes: The cost of indecision. *Journal of Cardiovascular Nursing, 25*(2), 115–116.

Richards, G. (2012). An overview of atrial fibrillation. *Nursing Standard, 26*(52), 47–56.

Rose, E., Chinitz, L. A., Holmes, D. S., & Aizer, A. (2010). A novel mechanism of failure to detect atrial arrhythmias by pacemakers and implantable cardioverter defibrillators. *Journal of Cardiovascular Electrophysiology, 21*(3), 325–328.

Ruiter, J. H., Mulder, E., Schuchert, A., Burri, H., Stuhlinger, M. C., Hartikainen, J., et al. (2010). The feasibility of fully automated pacemaker advice in treating atrial tachyarrhythmias. *Pacing & Clinical Electrophysiology, 33*(5), 605–614.

Sellers, M. B., & Newby, L. K. (2011). Atrial fibrillation, anticoagulants, fall risk, and outcomes in elderly patients. *American Heart Journal, 161*(2), 241–246.

Tedrow, U. B., Conen, D., Ridker, P. M., Cook, N. R., Koplan, B. A., Manson, J. E., et al. (2010). The long- and short-term impact of elevated body mass index on the risk of new atrial fibrillation: The WHS (Women's Health Study). *Journal of the American College of Cardiology, 55*(21), 2319–2327.

Tracy, C., Epstein, A., Darbar, D., DiMarco, J., Dunbar, S., Estes, M., et al. (2012). 2012 ACCF/AHA/HRS focused update of the 2008 guidelines for device based therapy of cardiac rhythm abnormalities. *Journal of the American College of Cardiology, 60*(14), 1247–1313. doi:10.1016/j.jacc2012.08.009.

Wann, L. S., Curtis, A. B., Ellenbogen, K. A., Estes, N. A., III, Ezekowitz, M. D., Jackman, W. M., et al. (2011). 2011 ACCF/AHA/HRS focused update on the management of patients with atrial fibrillation (update on dabigatran): A report of the American College of Cardiology Foundation/American Heart Association Task Force on Practice Guidelines. *Journal of the American College of Cardiology, 57*(11), 1330–1337.

Whinnett, Z., Sohaib, S., & Davies, D. (2012). Diagnosis and management of supraventricular tachycardia. *British Medical Journal, 345*(e7769), 1–9. doi:10.1136/bmj.e7769.

Wilber, D. J., Pappone, C., Neuzil, P., De Paola, A., Marchlinski, F., Natale, A., et al. (2010). Comparison of antiarrhythmic drug therapy and radiofrequency catheter ablation in patients with paroxysmal atrial fibrillation. *Journal of the American Medical Association, 303*(4), 333–340.

Wokhlu, A., Monahan, K. H., Hodge, D. O., Asirvatham, S. J., Friedman, P. A., Munger, T. M., et al. (2010). Long-term quality of life after ablation of atrial fibrillation: The impact of recurrence, symptom relief, and placebo effect. *Journal of the American College of Cardiology, 55*(21), 2308–2316.

Yeung, J., & Perkins, G. D. (2010). Timing of drug administration during CPR and the role of simulation. *Resuscitation, 81*(3), 265–266.

Zak, J. (2010). Ablation to treat atrial fibrillation: Beyond rhythm control. *Critical Care Nurse, 30*, 68–78. doi:10.4037/ccn2010335.

Zarraga, I., & Kron, I. (2013). Oral anticoagulation in elderly adults with atrial fibrillation: Integrating new options with old concepts. *Journal of the American Geriatrics Society, 61*, 143–150. doi:10.1111/jgs.12042.

Zishiri, E., Cronin, E., Williams, S., Blackstone, S., Ellis, S., Smedira, N., et al. (2011). Abstract 9816: Use of the wearable cardioverter defibrillator and survival after coronary artery revascularization in patients with left ventricular dysfunction. *Circulation, 124*, A9816.

Chapter 35

Albert, N. M. (2012). Fluid management strategies in heart failure. *Critical Care Nurse, 32*(2), 20–32.

Boyde, M., Turner, C., Thompson, D., & Stewart, S. (2011). Educational interventions for patients with heart failure: A systematic review of randomized controlled trials. *Journal of Cardiovascular Nursing, 26*(4), E27–E35.

Cary, T., & Pearce, J. (2013). Aortic stenosis: Pathophysiology, diagnosis, and medical management of nonsurgical patients. *Critical Care Nurse, 33*(2), 58–72.

Chen, W., Tran, K., & Maisel, A. (2010). Biomarkers in heart failure. *Heart, 96*, 314–320.

Christensen, D. (2012). Physiology of continuous-flow pumps. *Advanced Critical Care, 23*(1), 46–54.

Clerico, A., Giannoni, A., Vittorini, S., & Emdin, M. (2012). The paradox of low BNP levels in obesity. *Heart Failure Reviews, 17*(1), 81–96.

Cooper, K. L. (2011). Care of the lower extremities in patients with acute decompensated heart failure. *Critical Care Nurse, 31*(4), 21–29.

DeBeradinis, B., & Januzzi, J. L., Jr. (2012). Use of biomarkers to guide outpatient therapy of heart failure. *Current Opinion in Cardiology, 27*(6), 661–668.

DiSalvo, T., Acker, M., Dec, W., & Byrne, J. (2010). Mitral valve surgery in advanced heart failure. *Journal of the American College of Cardiology, 55*(4), 271–282.

Dudzinski, D., Mak, G., & Hung, J. (2012). Pericardial diseases. *Current Problems in Cardiology, 37*(3), 75–118.

Dworakowski, R., Prendergast, B., Wendler, O., & MacCarthy, P. (2010). Treatment of acquired valvular heart disease: Percutaneous alternatives. *Clinical Medicine, 10*(2), 181–187.

Eisen, H. J. (2014). *Prevention and treatment of cardiac allograft vasculopathy*. Retrieved December 8, 2014, from: <http://www.uptodate.com/content/prevention-and-1.com>.

Fard, A., Taub, P., Iqbal, N., & Maisel, A. (2012). Natriuretic peptides in the hospital: Risk stratification and treatment titration. In A. Maisel (Ed.), *Cardiac biomarkers: Expert advice for clinicians* (pp. 128–139). London: JP Medical Publishers.

Go, A. S., Mozaffarian, D., Roger, V. L., Benjamin, E. J., Berry, J. D., Borden, W. B., et al. (2013). Heart disease and stroke statistics—2013 update: A report from the American Heart Association. *Circulation, 127*(1), 2–245.

Hannibal, G. (2012). ECG characteristics of acute pericarditis. *Advanced Critical Care, 23*(3), 341–344.

Hoen, B., & Duval, X. (2013). Clinical practice. Infective endocarditis. *The New England Journal of Medicine, 368*(15), 1425–1433.

*Hoercher, K. J., Vacha, C. J., & McCarthy, P. M. (2002). Left ventricular splints and wraps for end-stage heart failure: A new approach in the new millennium. *Journal of Cardiovascular Nursing, 16*(3), 82–86.

Hull, C. (2012). Treating calcific aortic stenosis: An evolving science. *Medsurg Nursing, 21*(2), 82–87.

Imazio, M., Brucato, A., Cemin, R., Ferrua, S., Belli, R., Maestroni, S., et al. (2011). Colchicine for recurrent pericarditis (CORP): A randomized trial. *Annals of Internal Medicine, 155*(7), 409–414.

Jacoby, D. L., DePasquale, E. C., & McKenna, W. J. (2013). Hypertrophic cardiomyopathy: Diagnosis, risk stratification and treatment. *Canadian Medical Association Journal, 185*(2), 127–134.

*Jessup, M., Abraham, W. T., Casey, D. E., Feldman, A. M., Francis, G. S., Ganiats, T. G., et al. writing on behalf of the 2005 guideline update for the diagnosis and management of chronic heart failure in the adult writing committee. (2009). 2009 Focused update: ACCF/AHA guidelines for the diagnosis and management of heart failure in adults: A report of the American College of Cardiology Foundation/American Heart Association Task Force on Practice Guidelines. *Circulation, 119*(14), 1977–2016.

Litton, K. (2011). Demystifying ventricular assist devices. *Critical Care Nursing Quarterly, 34*(3), 200–207.

Manning, S. (2011). Bridging the gap between hospital and home: A new model of care for reducing readmission rates in chronic heart failure. *Journal of Cardiovascular Nursing, 26*(5), 368–376.

McConaghy, J., & Oza, R. (2013). Outpatient diagnosis of acute chest pain in adults. *American Family Physician, 87*(3), 177–182.

*Nishimura, R., Carabello, B., Faxon, D., Freed, M., Lytle, B., O'Gara, P., et al. (2008). ACC/AHA 2008 guideline update on valvular heart disease: Focused update on infective endocarditis: A report of the American College of Cardiology/American Heart Association Task Force on Practice Guidelines: Endorsed by the Society of Cardiovascular Anesthesiologists, Society for Cardiovascular Angiography and Interventions, and Society of Thoracic Surgeons. *Circulation, 118*(8), 887–896.

Ramani, G., Uber, P., & Mehra, M. (2010). Chronic heart failure: Contemporary diagnosis and management. *Mayo Clinic Proceedings, 85*(2), 180–195.

Ray, S. (2010). Changing epidemiology and natural history of valvular heart disease. *Clinical Medicine, 10*(2), 168–171.

Rogers, J., Aaronson, K., Boyle, A., Russell, S., Milano, C., Pagani, F., et al. (2010). Continuous flow left ventricular assist device improves functional capacity and quality of life of advanced heart failure patients. *Journal of the American College of Cardiology, 55*(17), 1826–1834.

Rowland, C. (2012). Pump it up with an LVAD left ventricular assist device. *Nursing, 42*(4), 47–50.

Saunders, M. (2010). A comparison of employed and unemployed caregivers of older heart failure patients. *Holistic Nursing Practice, 24*(1), 16–22.

Seward, J., & Casaclang-Verzosa, G. (2010). Infiltrative cardiovascular diseases. *Journal of the American College of Cardiology, 55*(17), 1769–1779.

Sherrid, M., & Arabadjian, M. (2012). A primer of disopyramide treatment of obstructive hypertrophic cardiomyopathy. *Progress in Cardiovascular Diseases, 54*(6), 483–492.

Streets, K., & Vickers, S. (2012). Is this patient with heart failure a candidate for ultrafiltration? *Nursing, 42*(6), 30–36.

Suter, P., Gorski, L., Hennessey, B., & Suter, W. (2012). Best practices for heart failure: A focused review. *Home Healthcare Nurse, 30*(7), 394–405.

Yancy, C., Jessup, M., Bozkurt, B., Butler, J., Casey, D., Drazner, M., et al. (2013). 2013 ACCF/AHA Guideline for the management of heart failure: Executive Summary: A report of the American College of Cardiology Foundation/American Heart Association Task Force on Practice Guidelines. *Journal of the American College of Cardiology, 62*(16), 1495–1539.

Chapter 36

*ALLHAT Officers and Coordinators for the ALLHAT Collaborative Research Group. (2002a). Major outcomes in high-risk hypertensive patients randomized to angiotensin-converting enzyme inhibitor or calcium channel blocker vs diuretic. The Antihypertensive and Lipid-Lowering Treatment to Prevent Heart Attack Trial (ALLHAT). *Journal of the American Medical Association, 288*(23), 2981–2997.

*ALLHAT Officers and Coordinators for the ALLHAT Collaborative Research Group. (2002b). Major outcomes in moderately hypercholesterolemic, hypertensive patients randomized to pravastatin vs usual care. The Antihypertensive and Lipid-Lowering Treatment to Prevent Heart Attack Trial (ALLHAT-LLT). *Journal of the American Medical Association, 288*(23), 2998–3007.

Anderson, D. J., Anderson, M. A., & Hill, P. D. (2010). Location of blood pressure measurement. *Medsurg Nursing, 19*(5), 287–294.

Anthony, M. (2013). Nursing assessment of deep vein thrombosis. *Medsurg Nursing, 22*(2), 95–98.

Armstrong, K. E. (2013). Stop the reflux: An update on treatment for symptomatic varicose veins. *Nursing, 43*(2), 27–34.

Bailey, D. G., Dresser, D., & Arnold, J. M. O. (2013). Grapefruit-medication interactions: Forbidden fruit or avoidable consequences. *CMAJ: Canadian Medical Association Journal, 185*, 309–316.

Baldwin, S. (2011). Helping patients manage hypertension. *Nursing, 41*(8), 60–63.

Braverman, A. C. (2010). Acute aortic dissection. *Circulation, 122*(2), 184.

Carlson, D. S. (2012). Action Stat: Acute aortic dissection. *Nursing, 42*(7), 72.

Coke, L. A. (2011). Vascular risk assessment of the older CV patient: The Ankle-Brachial Index (ABI). *Medsurg Nursing, 20*(1), 47–48.

Day, M. W. (2011). Action Stat: Hypertensive emergency. *Nursing, 41*(8), 11.

Eckel, R. H., Jakicic, J. M., Ard, J. D., Hubbard, V. S., de Jesus, J. M., Lee, I. M., et al. (2014). 2013 AHA/ACC guideline on lifestyle management to reduce cardiovascular risk: A report of the American College of Cardiology/American Heart Association Task Force on Practice Guidelines. *Circulation, 129*(25 Suppl. 2), S76–S99.

*Gay, V., Hamilton, R., Heiskell, S., & Sparks, A. M. (2009). Influence of bedrest or ambulation in the clinical treatment of acute deep vein thrombosis on patient outcomes: A review and synthesis of the literature. *Medsurg Nursing, 18*(5), 293–299.

Go, A. S., Mozaffarian, D., Roger, V. L., Benjamin, E. J., Berry, J. D., Borden, W. B., et al. (2013). Heart disease and stroke statistics—2013 update: A report from the American Heart Association. *Circulation, 127*(1), e6–e245.

Hiratzka, L. F., Bakris, G. L., Beckman, J. A., Bersin, R. M., Carr, V. F., Casey, D. E., et al. (2010). *Guidelines for the diagnosis and management of patients with thoracic aortic disease.* Philadelphia: Lippincott Williams & Wilkins.

James, P. A., Oparil, S., Carter, B. L., Cushman, W. C., Dennison-Himmelfarb, C., Handler, J., et al. (2014). 2014 evidence-based guidelines for the management of high blood pressure in adults: Report from the panel members appointed to the Eighth National Committee (JNC 8). *Journal of the American Medical Association, 311*(5), 507–520. Retrieved December 2013, from <http://jama.jamanetwork.com/article.aspx?articleid=1791497>.

Michaels, K., & Regan, N. (2013). Teaching patients INR self-management. *Nursing, 43*(5), 67–69.

National Center for Complementary and Alternative Medicine (2013). *Herbs at a glance: Garlic.* Retrieved June 2013, from <http://nccam.nih.gov/health/garlic/ataglance.htm>.

*National Cholesterol Education Program (2002). *Third Report of the Expert Panel on Detection, Evaluation, and Treatment of High Blood Cholesterol in Adults (Adult Treatment Panel III). NIH Publication No. 02-5215.* Bethesda, MD: National Heart, Lung, and Blood Institute.

National Heart, Lung, and Blood Institute (2012). *What is the DASH eating plan?* Retrieved December 2013, from <www.nhlbi.nih.gov/health/health-topics/topics/dash/>.

Pezzotti, W., & Freuler, M. (2012). Using anticoagulants to steer clear of clots. *Nursing, 42*(2), 26–34.

Stone, N. J., Robinson, J., Lichtenstein, A. H., Merz, N. B., Blum, C. B., Eckel, R. H., et al. (2014). 2013 ACC/AHA guidelines on the treatment of blood cholesterol to reduce atherosclerotic cardiovascular risk in adults: A report of the American College of Cardiology/American Heart Association Task Force on Practice Guidelines. *Circulation, 129*(25 Suppl. 2), S1–S45.

Van Tongeren, R., Bastiaansen, A., Van Wissen, R., Le Cessie, S., Hamming, J., & Van Bockel, J. (2010). A comparison of the Doppler-derived maximal systolic acceleration versus the ankle-brachial pressure index or detecting and quantifying peripheral arterial occlusive disease in diabetic patients. *Journal of Cardiovascular Surgery, 51*(3), 391–398.

*Verdecchia, P., Angeli, F., Mazzotta, G., Gentile, G., & Reboldi, G. (2009). Home blood pressure measurements will not replace 24-hour ambulatory blood pressure monitoring. *Hypertension, 54*, 188–195.

Woo, K. Y., & Gowie, B. G. (2013). Understanding compression for venous leg ulcers. *Nursing, 43*(1), 66–68.

Chapter 37

Abbas, A., Lichtman, A., & Pillai, S. (2012). *Cellular and molecular immunology* (7th ed.). Philadelphia: Saunders.

Bernstein, M., & Lynn, S. (2013). Helping patients survive sepsis. *American Nurse Today, 8*(1), 24–28.

Day, D., Matsumoto, K., & Passion, C. (2013). Acute traumatic coagulopathy: The latest intervention strategies. *American Nurse Today, 8*(11), 8–11.

Dellinger, R. P., Levy, M., Rhodes, A., Annane, D., Gerlach, H., Opal, S. M., et al. (2013). Surviving sepsis campaign: International guidelines for management of severe sepsis and septic shock: 2012. *Critical Care Medicine, 41*(2), 580–637.

Dumont, C., & Nesselrodt, D. (2012). Preventing CLABSI: Central line-associated bloodstream infections. *Nursing, 42*(6), 41–46.

Earhart, A. (2013). Recognizing, preventing, and troubleshooting central line complications. *American Nurse Today, 8*(11), 18–22.

Kilburn, F., Baily, P., & Price, D. (2013). Sepsis: Recognizing the next event. *Nursing, 43*(10), 14–16.

Kleinpell, R., Aitken, L., & Schorr, C. (2013). Implications of the new international sepsis guidelines for nursing care. *American Journal of Critical Care, 22*(3), 212–222.

Kleinpell, R., & Schorr, C. (2014). Targeting sepsis as a performance improvement metric: Role of the nurse. *AACN Advanced Critical Care, 25*(2), 179–180.

Lopez-Bushnell, K., Demaray, W., & Jaco, C. (2014). Reducing sepsis mortality. *Medsurg Nursing, 23*(1), 9–14.

Mann-Salinas, E., Engebretson, J., & Batchinsky, A. (2012). A complex systems review of sepsis: Implications for nursing. *Dimensions of Critical Care Nursing, 32*(1), 12–17.

Schell-Chaple, H., & Lee, M. (2014). Reducing sepsis deaths: A systems approach to early detection and management. *American Nurse Today, 9*(7), 26–30.

Walkey, A., Wiener, R., & Lindenauer, P. (2013). Utilization patterns and outcomes associated with central venous catheter in septic shock: A population-based study. *Critical Care Medicine, 41*(6), 1450–1457.

Chapter 38

Allen, J., & Dennison, C. (2010). Randomized trials of nursing interventions for secondary prevention in patients with coronary artery disease and heart failure. *Journal of Cardiovascular Nursing, 25*(3), 207–220.

American Heart Association (AHA) (2013). *Diet and lifestyle recommendations* (updated: March 19, 2013). Retrieved May 2013, from <www.heart.org/HEARTORG/GettingHealthy/Diet-and-Lifestyle-Recommendations_UCM_305855_Article.jsp>.

Berra, K., Fletcher, B., & Handberg, E. (2011). Antiplatelet therapy in acute coronary syndromes. *Journal of Cardiovascular Nursing, 26*(3), 239–249.

Cayla, G., Silvain, J., O'Connor, S., Collet, J., & Montalescot, G. (2012). Current antiplatelet options for NSTE-ACS patients. *QJM: Monthly Journal of the Association of Physicians, 105*, 935–948.

Cossette, S., Frasure-Smith, N., Dupuis, J., Juneau, M., & Guertin, M. (2012). Randomized control trial of tailored nursing interventions to improve cardiac rehabilitation enrollment. *Nursing Research, 61*(2), 111–120.

Crea, F., & Liuzzo, G. (2013). Pathogenesis of acute coronary syndromes. *Journal of the American College of Cardiology, 61*(1), 1–11.

Dechant, L. (2012). UA/NSTEMI: Are you following the latest guidelines? *Nursing, 42*(9), 26–33.

Dolansky, M. A., Xu, F., Zullio, M., Shishehbor, B., Moore, S. M., & Rimm, A. A. (2010). Post-acute care services received by older adults following a cardiac event: A population-based analysis. *Journal of Cardiovascular Nursing, 25*(4), 342–349.

Flicker, L. (2010). Cardiovascular risk factors, cerebrovascular disease burden and healthy brain aging. *Clinics in Geriatric Medicine, 26*(1), 17–27.

Gara, P., Kushner, F., Ascheim, D., Casey, D., Chung, M., de Lemos, J., et al. (2013). 2013 ACCF/AHA guideline for the management of ST-elevation myocardial infarction. *Circulation, 127*, e362–e425.

Go, A., Mozaffarian, D., Roger, V., Benjamin, E., Berry, J., Borden, W., et al. (2013). Heart disease and stroke statistics—2013 update: A report from the American Heart Association. *Circulation, 127*, e6–e245.

*Grundy, S. M., Cleeman, J. I., Daniels, S. R., Donato, K. A., Eckel, R. H., Franklin, B. A., et al. (2005). Diagnosis and management of the metabolic syndrome: An American Heart Association/National Heart, Lung, and Blood Institute scientific statement. *Circulation, 112*(17), 2735–2752.

*Harris, W. S., Mozaffarian, D., Rimm, E., Kris-Etherton, P., Rudel, L. L., Appel, L. J., et al. (2009). Omega-6 fatty acids and risk for cardiovascular disease: A science advisory from the American Heart Association Nutrition Subcommittee of the Council on Nutrition, Physical Activity and Metabolism; Council on Cardiovascular Nursing; and Council on Epidemiology and Prevention. *Circulation, 119*(6), 902–907.

Hillis, D., Smith, P., Anderson, J., Bittl, J., Bridges, C., Byrne, J., et al. (2011). 2011 ACCF/AHA guideline for coronary artery bypass graft surgery: Executive summary: A report of the American College of Cardiology Foundation/ American Heart Association Task Force on Practice Guidelines. *Circulation, 124*, 2610–2642.

Housholder-Hughes, S. (2011). Non-ST-segment elevation acute coronary syndrome. *AACN Advanced Critical Care, 22*(2), 113–124.

Jneid, H., Anderson, J., Wright, R., Adams, C., Bridges, C., Casey, D., et al. (2012). 2012 ACCF/AHA focused update of the guideline for the management of patients with unstable angina/non-ST-elevation myocardial infarction (Updating the 2007 guideline and replacing the 2011 focused update). *Circulation, 126*, 875–910.

Leeper, B., Cyr, A., & Martin, K. (2011). Acute coronary syndrome. *Critical Care Nursing Clinics of North America, 23*, 547–557.

Lindholm, D., Varenhorst, C., Cannon, C., Harrington, R., Himmelmann, A., Maya, J., et al. (2013). Ticagrelor vs. clopidogrel in patients with non-ST-elevation acute coronary syndrome: Results from the PLATO trial. *Journal of the American College of Cardiology, 61*(10_Suppl).

McConaghy, J., & Oza, R. (2013). Outpatient diagnosis of acute chest pain in adults. *American Family Physician, 87*(3), 177–182.

McSweeney, J. C., O'Sullivan, P., Cleves, M. A., Lefler, L. L., Cody, M., Moser, D. K., et al. (2010). Racial differences in women's prodromal and acute symptoms of myocardial infarction. *American Journal of Critical Care, 19*(1), 63–73.

*NHLBI. (2004). *Third report of the national cholesterol education program expert panel on detection, evaluation and treatment of high blood cholesterol in adults (adult treatment panel III)*. <www.nhlbi.nih.gov>.

Pettinato, M. (2012). Providing care for GLBTQ patients. *Nursing, 42*(12), 22–27.

Rowland, C. A. (2012). Pump it up with an LVAD. *Nursing, 42*(4), 47–50.

Sanz, J., Moreno, P. R., & Fuster, V. (2010). The year in atherothrombosis. *Journal of the American College of Cardiology, 55*(14), 1487–1498.

Scirica, B. (2010). Acute coronary syndrome: Emerging tools for diagnosis and risk assessment. *Journal of the American College of Cardiology, 55*(14), 1403–1415.

Sherrod, M. M., Sherrod, N. M., Spitzer, M. T., & Cheek, D. J. (2013). AHA recommendations for preventing heart disease in women. *Nursing, 43*(5), 61–66.

Shin, J., Martin, R., & Suls, J. (2010). Meta-analytic evaluation of gender differences and symptom measurement strategies in acute coronary syndromes. *Heart and Lung: The Journal of Critical Care, 39*, 283–295.

Summers, K., Martin, K., & Watson, K. (2010). Impact and clinical management of depression in patients with coronary artery disease. *Pharmacotherapy, 30*(3), 304–322.

Thygesen, K., Alpert, J., Jaffe, A., Simoons, M., Chaitman, B., White, H., et al. (2012). Third universal definition of myocardial infarction. *Circulation, 126*, 2020–2035.

Weustink, A. C., Mollet, N. R., Neefjes, L. A., Meijboom, W. B., Galema, T. W., van Mieghem, C. A., et al. (2010). Diagnostic accuracy and clinical utility of noninvasive testing for coronary artery disease. *Annals of Internal Medicine, 152*(10), 630–639.

Chapter 39

Karch, A. (2012). Pharmacology review: Drugs that alter blood coagulation. *American Nurse Today, 7*(11), 26–30.

Pezzotti, W., & Freuler, M. (2012). Using anticoagulants to steer clear of clots. *Nursing, 42*(2), 26–34.

Rauen, C. (2012). Beyond the bloody mess: Hematologic assessment. *Critical Care Nurse, 32*(5), 42–46.

Straznitskas, A., & Giarratano, M. (2014). Emergent reversal of oral anticoagulation: Review of current treatment strategies. *AACN Advanced Clinical Care, 25*(1), 5–12.

Chapter 40

AABB (2013). *Circular information for the use of human blood and blood components*. Retrieved July 2014, from <www.aabb.org/tm/coi/Documents/coi1113.pdf>.

Albrecht, T. (2014). Physiologic and psychological symptoms experienced by adults with acute leukemia: An integrative literature review. *Oncology Nursing Forum, 41*(3), 286–295.

American Cancer Society (ACS) (2014). *Cancer facts and figures 2014*. Report No. 01-300M–No. 500814. Atlanta: Author.

Baker, M., & McKiernan, P. (2011). Management of chronic graft-versus-host disease. *Clinical Journal of Oncology Nursing, 15*(4), 429–432.

Beery, T., & Workman, M. L. (2012). *Genetics and genomics in nursing and health care*. Philadelphia: F.A. Davis.

Byar, K., & Workman, M. (2012). Targeted therapies to treat cancer. In J. Kee, E. Hayes, & L. McCuistion (Eds.), *Pharmacology: A nursing process approach* (7th ed.). St. Louis: Saunders.

Card, E., Nelson, D., Jeskey, M., Miller, A., Michaels, D., Hardeman, W., et al. (2012). Early detection of a blood transfusion reaction utilizing a wireless remote monitoring device. *Medsurg Nursing, 21*(5), 299–302.

Chiffelle, R., & Kenny, K. (2013). Exercise for fatigue management in hematopoietic stem cell transplantation recipients. *Clinical Journal of Oncology Nursing, 17*(3), 241–242.

Elgin, K., Cozzi, K., Fowler, M., Perry, S., Davis, M., Conaway, M., et al. (2011). Maintaining patency with packed red blood cell infusions: Comparison of IV normal saline infusions vs. normal saline syringe method. *Medsurg Nursing, 20*(3), 134–138.

Hardwick, J., Osswald, M., & Walker, D. (2013). Acute pain transfusion reaction. *Oncology Nursing Forum, 40*(6), 543–545.

Hitch, D. (2013). What every nurse should know about hemophilia. *American Nurse Today, 8*(3), 22–26.

Jenerette, C., & Leak, A. (2012). The role of oncology nurses in the care of adults with sickle cell disease. *Clinical Journal of Oncology Nursing, 16*(6), 633–635.

Johnson, N. (2013). Ocular graft-versus-host disease after allogeneic transplantation. *Clinical Journal of Oncology Nursing, 17*(6), 621–626.

Kasberg, H., Brister, L., & Barnard, B. (2011). Aggressive disease, aggressive treatment: The adult hematopoietic stem cell transplant patient in the intensive care unit. *AACN Advanced Critical Care, 22*(4), 349–364.

Kessler, C. (2013). Priming blood transfusion tubing: A critical review of the blood transfusion process. *Critical Care Nurse, 33*(3), 80–83.

Kessler, D., Shaz, B., & Grima, K. (2012). Advances in blood transfusion. *American Nurse Today, 7*(3), 8–11.

Kurtin, S. (2012). Myelodysplastic syndromes: The challenge of developing clinical guidelines and supportive care strategies for a rare disease. *Clinical Journal of Oncology Nursing, S16*(3), S5–S7.

Kurtin, S., & Faiman, B. (2013). The changing landscape of multiple myeloma: Implications for oncology nurses. *Clinical Journal of Oncology Nursing, S17*(6), S2, S7–S11.

Ladizinski, B., Bazakas, A., Mistry, N., Alavi, A., Sibbald, R., & Salcido, R. (2012). Sickle cell disease and leg ulcers. *Advances in Skin & Wound Care, 25*(9), 420–428.

Leak, A., Smith, S., Crandell, J., Jenerette, C., Bailey, D., Zimmerman, S., et al. (2013). Demographic and disease characteristics associated with non-Hodgkin lymphoma survivors' quality of life: Does age matter? *Oncology Nursing Forum, 40*(2), 157–162.

Mangan, P., Gleason, C., & Miceli, T. (2013). Autologous hematopoietic stem cell transplantation for multiple myeloma. *Clinical Journal of Oncology Nursing, 17*(6), 43–47.

MD Consult. <www.mdconsult.com>.

Myers, F., & Reyes, C. (2011). Blood cultures: 5 steps to doing it right. *Nursing, 41*(3), 62–63.

Myers, M., & Eckes, E. (2012). A novel approach to pain management in persons with sickle cell disease. *Medsurg Nursing, 21*(5), 293–298.

National Hemophilia Foundation (2014). *MASAC recommendation regarding the use of recombinant clotting factor products with respect to pathogen transmission.* Retrieved July 2014, <www.hemophilia.org/Researchers-Healthcare-Providers/Medical-and-Scientific-Advisory-Council-MASC/All-MASAC-Recommendations/Rexommendation-Regarding-the-Use-of-recombinant-Clotting-Factor-Products-with-Respect-toPathogen-Transmission>.

Orton, C. (2012). Vitamin B12 (cobalamin) deficiency in the older adult. *The Journal for Nurse Practitioners, 8*(7), 547–553.

Parsh, B., & Kumar, D. (2012). Understanding sickle cell disease. *Nursing, 42*(8), 64.

Radovich, P. (2011). The multiple causes and myriad presentations of thrombocytopenia. *American Nurse Today, 6*(1), 9–12.

Simmons, S. (2012). To B or not to B? The inside scoop on vitamin B12. *Nursing, 42*(12), 55–59.

Simoneau, A. (2013). Treating chronic myeloid leukemia: Improving management through understanding of the patient experience. *Clinical Journal of Oncology Nursing, 14*(3), 67–72.

Slater, S. (2012). Plerixafor. *Journal of the Advanced Practitioner in Oncology, 3*(1), 49–54.

The Joint Commission (TJC) (2014). *Implementation guide for The Joint Commission patient blood management performance measures.* Retrieved July 2014, from <www.jointcommission.org/patient_blood_management_performance_measures_project/>.

Thoele, K. (2014). Engraftment syndrome in hematopoietic stem cell transplantations. *Clinical Journal of Oncology Nursing, 18*(3), 349–354.

Tolich, D., Blackmur, S., Stahorsky, K., & Wabeke, D. (2013). Blood management: Best practice transfusion strategies. *Nursing, 43*(1), 40–47.

United States National Library of Medicine (2014). *Genetics home reference: Sickle cell disease.* Retrieved October 2014, from <http://ghr.nlm.nih.gov/condition/sickle-cell-disease>.

Chapter 41

Adamis, D., Sharma, N., Whelan, P. J., & Macdonald, A. J. (2010). Delirium scales: A review of current evidence. *Aging & Mental Health, 14*(5), 543–555.

Barr, J., Fraser, G. L., Puntillo, K., Ely, E. W., Gélinas, C., Dasta, J. F., et al. (2013). Clinical practice guidelines for the management of pain, agitation, and delirium in adult patients in the intensive care unit. *Critical Care Medicine, 41*(1), 263–306.

Centers for Medicare & Medicaid (2014). *Recommend Core Measures.* Retrieved July 2014, from <http://www.cms.gov/Regulations-and-Guidance/Legislation/EHRIncentivePrograms/Recommended_Core_Set.html>.

Emmett, M., Fenves, A. Z., & Schwartz, J. C. (2012). Approach to the patient with kidney disease. In M. W. Taal, G. M. Chertow, P. A. Marsden, K. Skorecki, A. S. L. Yu, & B. M. Benner (Eds.), *Brenner and Rector's the kidney* (9th ed.). Philadelphia: Saunders.

Faraklas, I., Holt, B., Tran, S., Lin, H., Saffle, J., & Cochran, A. (2013). Impact of a nursing-driven sleep hygiene protocol on sleep quality. *Journal of Burn Care and Research, 34*(2), 249–254.

Hickey, J. V. (2013). *The clinical practice of neurological and neuosurgical nursing* (7th ed.). Philadelphia: Lippincott Williams & Wilkins.

Holsinger, T., Plassman, B. L., Stechuchak, K. M., Burke, J. R., Coffman, C. J., & Williams, J. W. (2012). Screening for cognitive impairment: Comparing the performance of four instruments in primary care. *Journal of the American Geriatrics Society, 60*(6), 1027–1036.

Iacono, L. A., Wells, C., & Mann-Finnerty, K. (2014). Standardizing neurological assessments. *The Journal of Neuroscience Nursing, 46*(2), 125–132.

Iverson, D. J., Gronseth, G. S., Reger, M. A., Classen, S., Dubinsky, R. M., & Rizzo, M. (2010). Practice parameter update: Evaluation and management of driving risk in dementia: Report of the Quality Standards Subcommittee of the American Academy of Neurology. *Neurology, 74*(16), 1316–1324.

Institute for magnetic resonance safety, education, and research (2014). *MRI Safety.* Retrieved July 2014. from, <http://www.mrisafety.com/>.

Rank, W. (2013). Performing a focused neurologic assessment. *Nursing, 43*(12), 37–40.

Rattray, J. E., Lauder, W., Ludwick, R., Johnstone, C., Zeller, R., Winchell, J., et al. (2011). Indicators of acute deterioration in adult patients nursed in acute wards: A factorial survey. *Journal of Clinical Nursing, 20*(5–6), 723–732.

Saliba, D., Buchanan, J., Edelen, M. O., Streim, J., Ouslander, J., Berlowitz, D., et al. (2012). Brief interview for mental status. *Journal of the American Medical Directors Association, 13*(7), 611–617.

Schmidt, C. W. (2012). CT scans: Balancing health risks and medical benefits. *Environmental Health Perspectives, 120*(3), A118–A121.

Wijdicks, E. F. M., Varelas, P. N., Gronseth, G. S., & Greer, D. M. (2010). Evidence-based guideline update: Determining brain death in adults. *Neurology, 74*(23), 1911–1918.

Chapter 42

A.D.A.M. Medical Encyclopedia (2014). *Huntington's disease.* Retrieved July 2014, from <www.ncbi.nlm.nih.gov/pubmedhealth/PMH0001775/>.

Babtain, F. A. (2012). Management of women with epilepsy: Practical issues faced when dealing with women with epilepsy. *Neurosciences (Riyadh), 17*(2), 115–120.

Bettens, K., Sleegers, K., & Van Broeckhoven, C. (2013). Genetic insights in Alzheimer's disease. *Lancet Neurology, 12*(1), 92–104.

Carod-Artel, F. J. (2014). Tackling chronic migraine: Current perspectives. *Journal of Pain Research, 7*(online), 185–194.

Corbett, A., Stevens, J., Aarsland, D., Day, S., Moniz-Cook, E., Woods, R., et al. (2012). Systematic review of services providing information and/or advice to people with dementia and/or their caregivers. *International Journal of Geriatriatric Psychiatry, 27*(6), 628–636.

Coskun, P., Wyrembak, J., Schriner, S. E., Chen, H. W., Marciniack, C., Laferla, F., et al. (2012). A mitochondrial etiology of Alzheimer and Parkinson disease. *Biochimica et Biophysica Acta, 1820*(5), 553–564.

Cranwell-Bruce, L. A. (2010). Drugs for Parkinson's disease. *Medsurg Nursing, 19*(6), 347–350.

D'Arcy, Y. (2014). Preventing migraine headaches in adults. *Nursing, 44*(1), 58–61.

Diener, H. C., Dodick, D. W., Turkel, C. C., Demos, G., Degryse, R. E., Earl, N. L., et al. (2014). *European Jounal of Neurology, 21*(6), 651–659.

Eggenberger, E., Heimerl, K., & Bennett, M. I. (2013). Communication skills training in dementia care: A systematic review of effectiveness, training content, and didactic methods in different care settings. *International Psychogeriatrics, 25*(3), 345–358.

Ellison, D., Williams, M. L., Moodt, G., & Farrar, F. C. (2010). Electrodiagnostic studies. *Critical Care Nursing Clinics of North America, 22*(1), 7–18.

Epilepsy Foundation. (2014). Retrieved July 2014 from <www.epilepsyfoundation.org/>.

Haahr, A., Kirkevold, M., Hall, E. O., & Ostergaard, K. (2011). Living with advanced Parkinson's disease: A constant struggle with unpredictability. *Journal of Advanced Nursing, 67*(2), 408–417.

Hauser, L. (2012). Migraines and perimenopause: Helping women in midlife manage and treat migraine. *Nursing for Women's Health, 16*(3), 247–250.

Heavey, E. (2010). An update on meningococcal meningitis. *Nursing, 40*(10), 61–62.

Huntington's Disease Society of America (HDSA) (2014). *About Huntington disease.* Retrieved July 2014, from <www.hdsa.org/>.

Kropelin, T. F., Neyens, J. C., Halfens, R. J., Kempen, G. I., & Hamers, J. P. (2013). Fall determinants in older long-term care residents with dementia: A systematic review. *International Psychogeriatrics, 25*(4), 549–563.

Johnson, D. K., Niedens, M., Wilson, J. R., Swartzendruber, L., Yeager, A., & Jones, K. (2013). Treatment outcomes of a crisis intervention program for dementia with severe psychiatric complications: The Kansas bridge project. *Gerontologist, 53*(1), 102–112.

Kumar, K. R., Lohmann, K., & Klein, C. (2012). Genetics of Parkinson disease and other movement disorders. *Current Opinion in Neurology, 25*(4), 466–474.

Kwok, T., Bai, X., Chui, M. Y., Lai, C. K., Ho, D. W., Ho, F. K., et al. (2012). Effect of physical restraint reduction on older patients' hospital length of stay. *Journal of the American Medical Directors Association, 13*(7), 645–650.

Leuzy, A., & Gauthier, S. (2012). Ethical issues in Alzheimer's disease: An overview. *Expert Review of Neurotherapeutics, 12*(5), 557–567.

Lin, J. J., Mula, M., & Hermann, B. P. (2012). Uncovering the neurobehavioural comorbidities of epilepsy over the lifespan. *Lancet, 380*(9848), 1180–1192.

Marcus, D. A. (2014). *Tools for sufferers.* Retrieved July 2014, from <www.headaches.org/education/Tools_for_Sufferers>.

Mauskop, A. (2012). Nonmedication, alternative, and complementary treatments for migraine. *Continuum (Minneap Minn), 18*(4), 796–806.

Mayeux, R., & Stern, Y. (2012). Epidemiology of Alzheimer disease. *Cold Spring Harbor Perspectives in Medicine, 2*(8), 1–26.

Modgill, G., Jette, N., Wang, J. L., Becker, W. J., & Patten, S. B. (2012). A population-based longitudinal community study of major depression and migraine. *Headache, 52*(3), 422–432.

Mohler, R., Richter, T., Kopke, S., & Meyer, G. (2012). Interventions for preventing and reducing the use of physical restraints in long-term geriatric care: A Cochrane review. *Journal of Clinical Nursing, 21*(21–22), 3070–3081.

Moloney, M. F., & Cranwell-Bruce, L. A. (2010). Pharmacologic management of migraine headaches. *Nurse Practitioner, 35*(9), 16–22.

Moyle, W., Borbasi, S., Wallis, M., Olorenshaw, R., & Gracia, N. (2011). Acute care management of older people with dementia: A qualitative perspective. *Journal of Clinical Nursing, 20*(3–4), 420–428.

National Institute of Neurological Disorders and Stroke (NINDS) (2014). *Parkinson's disease.* Retrieved July 2014, from <www.ninds.nih.gov/disorders/parkinsons_disease/parkinsons_disease.htm>.

Niemeijer, A., Frederiks, B., Depla, M., Eefsting, J., & Hertogh, C. (2013). The place of surveillance technology in residential care for people with intellectual disabilities: Is there an ideal model of application. *Journal of Intellectual Disability Research, 57*(3), 201–215.

Overstreet, M. (2011). West Nile virus. *Nursing, 42*(6), 43.

Park, N. H. (2012). Parkinson disease. *JAAPA: Official Journal of the American Academy of Physician Assistants, 25*(5), 73–74.

Parkinson's Disease Foundation (2014). *About Parkinson's disease.* Retrieved July 2014, from <www.pdf.org/>.

Plesh, O., Adams, S. H., & Gansky, S. A. (2012). Self-reported comorbid pains in severe headaches or migraines in a U.S. national sample. *Headache, 52*(6), 946–956.

Rausa, M., Cevoli, S., Sancisi, E., Grimaldi, D., Pollutri, G., Casoria, M., et al. (2013). Personality traits in chronic daily headache patients with and without psychiatric comorbidity: An observational study in a tertiary care headache center. *Journal of Headache and Pain, 14*, 22.

Richter, T., Meyer, G., Mohler, R., & Kopke, S. (2012). Psychosocial interventions for reducing antipsychotic medication in care home residents. *Cochrane Database of Systematic Reviews*, (12), CD008634.

Roberts, B. R. (2010). Caring for patients with Parkinson's disease. *Nursing, 40*(7), 58–64.

Saliba, D., Buchanan, J., Edelen, M. O., Streim, J., Ouslander, J., Berlowitz, D., et al. (2012). MDS 3.0: Brief interview for mental status. *Journal of the American Medical Directors Association, 13*(7), 611–617.

Seitz, D. P., Brisbin, S., Herrmann, N., Rapoport, M. J., Wilson, K., Gill, S. S., et al. (2012). Efficacy and feasibility of nonpharmacological interventions for neuropsychiatric symptoms of dementia in long term care: A systematic review. *Journal of the American Medical Directors Association, 13*(6), 503–506.

Subramaniam, P., & Woods, B. (2012). The impact of individual reminiscence therapy for people with dementia: Systematic review. *Expert Review of Neurotherapeutics, 12*(5), 545–555.

Te Boekhorst, S., Depla, M. F., Francke, A. L., Twisk, J. W., Zwijsen, S. A., & Hertogh, C. M. (2012). Quality of life of nursing-home residents with dementia subject to surveillance technology versus physical restraints: An explorative study. *International Journal of Geriatric Psychiatry, 28*(4), 356–363.

The Joint Commission (2013). *2014 National Patient Safety Goals.* Retrieved July 2014, from <www.jointcommission.org/assets/1/18/NPSG_Chapter_Jan2014_OME.pdf>.

Tolson, D., & Morley, J. E. (2012). Physical restraints: Abusive and harmful. *Journal of the American Medical Directors Association, 13*(4), 311–313.

Van Mierlo, L. D., Meiland, F. J., Van der Roest, H. G., & Droes, R. M. (2012). Personalised caregiver support: Effectiveness of psychosocial interventions in subgroups of caregivers of people with dementia. *International Journal of Geriatric Psychiatry, 27*(1), 1–14.

Vasilevskis, E. E., Pandharipande, P. P., Girard, T. D., & Ely, E. W. (2010). A screening, prevention, and restoration model for saving the injured brain in intensive care unit survivors. *Critical Care Medicine, 38*(Suppl. 10), S683–S691.

Vervloet, M., Linn, A. J., van Weert, J. C. M., de Bakker, D. H., Bouvy, M. L., & van Dijk, L. (2012). The effectiveness of interventions using electronic reminders to improve adherence to chronic medication: a systematic review of the literature. *Journal of the American Medical Informatics Association, 19*(online), 696–704.

Weitzel, T., Robinson, S., Barnes, M. R., Berry, T. A., Holmes, J. M., Mercer, S., et al. (2011). The special needs of the hospitalized patient with dementia. *Medsurg Nursing, 20*(1), 13–18.

Yang, M. H., Wang, P. H., Wang, S. J., Sun, W. Z., Oyang, Y. J., & Fuh, J. L. (2012). Women with endometriosis are more likely to suffer from migraines: A population-based study. *PLoS ONE, 7*(3), e33941.

Zwijsen, S. A., Depla, M. F., Niemeijer, A. R., Francke, A. L., & Hertogh, C. M. (2012). Surveillance technology: An alternative to physical restraints? A qualitative study among professionals working in nursing homes for people with dementia. *International Journal of Nursing Studies, 49*(2), 212–219.

Chapter 43

Ahmad, F., Wang, M. Y., & Levi, A. D. (2013). Hypothermia for acute spinal cord injury: A review. *World Neurosurgery, S1878–8750*(13).

American Nurses Association (ANA) (2013). *Safe patient handling and mobility: interprofessional national standards across the care continuum.* Silver Spring, MD: ANA.

Andersen, P. M., Abrahams, S., Borasio, G. D., de Carvalho, M., Chio, A., Van Damme, P., et al. (2012). EFNS guidelines on the clinical management of amyotrophic lateral sclerosis (MALS): Revised report of an EFNS task force. *European Journal of Neurology, 19*(3), 360–375.

Bailey, J., Dijkers, M. P., Gassaway, J., Thomas, J., Lingefelt, P., Kreider, S. E., et al. (2012). Relationship of nursing education and care management inpatient rehabilitation interventions and patient characteristics to outcomes following spinal cord injury: The SCIRehab project. *Journal of Spinal Cord Medicine, 35*(6), 593–610.

Bergman, D., & Peterson, D. (2011). *Chiropractic technique* (3rd ed.). St. Louis: Mosby.

Costa-Black, K. M., Loisel, P., Anema, J. R., & Pransky, G. (2010). Back pain and work. *Best Practice & Research: Clinical Rheumatology, 24*(2), 227–240.

Courtois, F., Rodrigue, X., Cote, I., Boulet, M., Vezina, J. G., Charvier, K., et al. (2012). Sexual function and autonomic dysreflexia in men with spinal cord injuries: How should we treat? *Spinal Cord, 50*(12), 869–877.

de Carvalho, M., & Swash, M. (2011). Amyotrophic lateral sclerosis: An update. *Current Opinion in Neurology, 24*(5), 497–503.

Duddy, M., Haghikia, A., Cocco, E., Eggers, C., Drulovic, J., Carmona, O., et al. (2011). Managing MS in a changing treatment landscape. *Journal of Neurology, 258*(5), 728–739.

Forrest, G., Huss, S., Patel, V., Jeffries, J., Myers, D., Barber, C., et al. (2012). Falls on an inpatient rehabilitation unit: Risk assessment and prevention. *Rehabilitation Nursing, 37*(2), 56–61.

Frankel, D., & James, H. (2011). *Living with multiple sclerosis.* New York: National Multiple Sclerosis Society.

Furlan, J. C., Noonan, V., Singh, A., & Fehlings, M. G. (2011a). Assessment of disability in patients with acute traumatic spinal cord injury: A systematic review of the literature. *Journal of Neurotrauma, 28*(8), 1413–1430.

Furlan, J. C., Noonan, V., Singh, A., & Fehlings, M. G. (2011b). Assessment of impairment in patients with acute traumatic spinal cord injury: A systematic review of the literature. *Journal of Neurotrauma, 28*(8), 1445–1477.

Gunduz, H., & Binak, D. F. (2012). Autonomic dysreflexia: An important cardiovascular complication in spinal cord injury patients. *Cardiology Journal, 19*(2), 215–219.

Hart, E. S., & Puttaswamy, M. K. (2013). Epidural abscess with spinal cord compression. *Orthopaedic Nursing, 32*(4), 229–230.

Juknis, N., Cooper, J. M., & Volshteyn, O. (2012). The changing landscape of spinal cord injury. *Handbook of Clinical Neurology, 109*, 149–166.

Krassioukov, A. (2012). Autonomic dysreflexia: Current evidence related to unstable arterial blood pressure control among athletes with spinal cord injury. *Clinical Journal of Sport Medicine, 22*(1), 39–45.

Kuijpers, T., van Middelkoop, M., Rubinstein, S. M., Ostelo, R., Verhagen, A., Koes, B. W., et al. (2011). A systematic review on the effectiveness of pharmacological interventions for chronic non-specific low-back pain. *European Spine Journal, 20*(1), 40–50.

Lucas, S. M. (2012). Malignant spinal cord compression. *Nursing, 42*(2), 72.

Ludolph, A. C., Brettschneider, J., & Weishaupt, J. H. (2012). Amyotrophic lateral sclerosis. *Current Opinion in Neurology, 25*(5), 530–535.

*Miller, R. G., Jackson, C. E., Kasarskis, E. J., England, J. D., Forshew, D., Johnston, W., Quality Standards Subcommittee of the American Academy of Neurology, et al. (2009). Practice parameter update: The care of the patient with amyotrophic lateral sclerosis—Multidisciplinary care, symptom management, and cognitive/behavioral impairment (an evidence-based review): Report of the Quality Standards Subcommittee of the American Academy of Neurology. *Neurology, 73*(15), 1227–1233.

Miller, R. G., Mitchell, J. D., & Moore, D. H. (2012). Riluzole for amyotrophic lateral sclerosis (ALS)/motor neuron disease (MND). *Cochrane Database of Systematic Reviews*, (3), CD001447.

Mior, S., Gamble, B., Barnsley, J., Cote, P., & Cote, E. (2013). Changes in primary care physician's management of low back pain in a model of interprofessional collaborative care: An uncontrolled before-after study. *Chiropractic and Manual Therapies, 21*(1), 6.

National Multiple Sclerosis Society (2014a). *What we know about MS*. Retrieved July 20142013, from <www.nationalmssociety.org/about-multiple-sclerosis/what-we-know-about-ms/treatments/medications/tecfidera/index.aspx>.

National Multiple Sclerosis Society (2014b). *Who gets MS*. Retrieved July 2014, from <www.nationalmssociety.org/about-multiple-sclerosis/what-we-know-about-ms/who-gets-ms/index.aspx>.

National Spinal Cord Injury Statistical Center (2014). *Spinal cord injury facts and figures at a glance*. Retrieved July 2014, from <www.nscisc.uab.edu/PublicDocuments/fact_figures_docs/Facts2014.pdf>.

Nayduch, D. A. (2010). Back to basics: Identifying and managing acute spinal cord injury. *Nursing, 40*(9), 24–30.

*Nelson, A., Harwood, K. J., Tracey, C. A., & Dunn, K. L. (2008). Myths and facts about safe patient handling in rehabilitation. *Rehabilitation Nursing, 33*(1), 10–17.

Newland, P. K., Riley, M. A., Fearing, A. D., Neath, A. A., & Gibson, D. (2010). Pain in women with relapsing-remitting multiple sclerosis and healthy women: Relationship to demographic variables. *Medsurg Nursing, 19*(3), 177–182.

Newman, S. D. (2010). Evidence-based advocacy: using Photovoice to identify barriers and facilitators to community participation after spinal cord injury. *Rebailatation Nursing, 35*(2), 47–49.

Norton, C., & Chelvanayagam, S. (2010). Bowel problems and coping strategies in people with multiple sclerosis. *British Journal of Nursing, 19*(4), 220, 221–226.

Parkinson, L., Sibbritt, D., Bolton, P., van Rotterdam, J., & Villadsen, I. (2013). Well-being outcomes of chiropractic intervention for lower back pain: A systematic review. *Clinical Rheumatology, 32*(2), 167–180.

Patton, K. T., & Thibodeau, G. A. (2014). *The human body in health and disease* (6th ed.). St. Louis: Mosby.

Rubinstein, S. M., van Middelkoop, M., Kuijpers, T., Ostelo, R., Verhagen, A. P., de Boer, M. R., et al. (2010). A systematic review on the effectiveness of complementary and alternative medicine for chronic non-specific low-back pain. *European Spine Journal, 19*(8), 1213–1228.

Scherer, K., & Bedlack, R. S. (2012). Diaphragm pacing in amyotrophic lateral sclerosis: A literature review. *Muscle and Nerve, 46*(1), 1–8.

Stahel, P. F., VanderHeiden, T., & Finn, M. A. (2012). Management strategies for acute spinal cord injury: Current options and future perspectives. *Current Opinion in Critical Care, 18*(6), 651–660.

van Middelkoop, M., Rubinstein, S. M., Kuijpers, T., Verhagen, A. P., Ostelo, R., Koes, B. W., et al. (2011). A systematic review on the effectiveness of physical and rehabilitation interventions for chronic non-specific low back pain. *European Spine Journal, 20*(1), 19–39.

van Middelkoop, M., Rubinstein, S. M., Verhagen, A. P., Ostelo, R. W., Koes, B. W., & van Tulder, M. W. (2010). Exercise therapy for chronic nonspecific low-back pain. *Best Practice & Research: Clinical Rheumatology, 24*(2), 193–204.

Wegner, I., Widyahening, I. S., van Tulder, M. W., Blomberg, S. E., de Vet, H. C., Brønfort, G., et al. (2013). Traction of low-back pain with or without sciatica. *Cochrane Database of Systematic Reviews*, online doi:10.1002/14651858.CD003010.pub5.

Zychowicz, M. E. (2013). Pathophysiology of heterotopic ossification. *Orthopaedic Nursing, 32*(3), 173–177.

Chapter 44

Abbott, S. A. (2010). Diagnostic challenge: Myasthenia gravis in the emergency department. *Journal of the American Academy of Nurse Practitioners, 22*(9), 468–473.

Arcila-Londono, X., & Lewis, R. A. (2012). Guillain-Barré syndrome. *Seminars in Neurology, 32*(3), 179–186.

Centers for Disease Control and Prevention (CDC) (2014). *Guillain-Barré syndrome*. Retrieved July 2014, from <www.cdc.gov/flu/protect/vaccine/guillainbarre.htm>.

Cranwell-Bruce, L. A. (2011). Drug treatment for peripheral neuropathy. *Medsurg Nursing, 20*(5), 269–272.

Diaz-Manera, J., Rojas Garcia, R., & Illa, I. (2012). Treatment strategies for myasthenia gravis: An update. *Expert Opinion on Pharmacotherapy, 13*(13), 1873–1883.

Forrest, G., Huss, S., Patel, V., Jeffries, J., Myers, D., Barber, C., et al. (2012). Falls on an inpatient rehabilitation unit: Risk assessment and prevention. *Rehabilitation Nursing, 37*(2), 56–61.

Ibrahim, S. (2012). Trigeminal neuralgia: Diagnostic criteria, clinical aspects and treatment outcomes: A retrospective study. *Gerodontology, 31*(2), 89–94.

Kaplan, A. (2012). Complications of apheresis. *Seminars in Dialysis, 25*(2), 152–158.

Khan, F., & Amatya, B. (2012). Rehabilitation interventions in patients with acute demyelinating inflammatory polyneuropathy: A systematic review. *European Journal of Physical and Rehabilitation Medicine, 48*(3), 507–522.

Liang, C. L., & Han, S. (2013). Neuromuscular junction disorders. *Physical Medicine and Rehabilitation, 5*(Suppl. 5), S81–S88.

Lui, H., Li, H., Xu, M., Chung, K. F., & Zhang, B. P. (2010). A systematic review on acupuncture for trigeminal neuralgia. *Alternative Therapies in Health and Medicine, 16*(3), 30–35.

National Institute of Neurological Disease and Stroke (2014a). *Restless leg syndrome*. Retrieved July 2014, from <www.ninds.nih.gov/disorders/restless_legs/restless_legs.htm>.

National Institute of Neurological Disease and Stroke (2014b). *Trigeminal neuralgia information page*. Retrieved July 2014, from <www.ninds.nih.gov/disorders/trigeminal_neuralgia/trigeminal_neuralgia.htm>.

Novak, C. (2012). Peripheral nerve injuries. *MedScape Reference*. Retrieved April 2013, from <http://emedicine.medscape.com/article/1270360>.

Patwa, H. S., Chaudhry, V., Katzerg, H., Rae-Grant, A. D., & So, Y. T. (2012). Evidence-based guideline: Intravenous immunoglobulin in the treatment of nueromuscular disorders. *Neurology, 78*(13), 1009–1015.

Rajabally, Y. A. (2012). Treatment of Guillain-Barré syndrome: A review. *Inflammation and Allergy Drug Targets, 11*(4), 330–334.

Sejvar, J. J., Baughman, A. L., Wise, M., & Morgan, O. W. (2011). Population incidence of Guillain-Barré syndrome: A systematic review and meta-analysis. *Neuroepidemiology, 36*(2), 123–133.

Silber, M. H. (2013). Sleep-related movement disorders. *Continuum (Minneap Minn), 19*(1 Sleep Disorders), 170–184.

Simmons, S. (2010). Guillain-Barré syndrome. *Nursing, 40*(1), 24–29.

Walsh, M. T. (2012). Interventions in the disturbances in the motor and sensory environment. *Journal of Hand Therapy, 25*(2), 202–218.

Chapter 45

American Heart Association (2014). *Get with the guidelines® educational materials.* Retrieved August 2014, from <http://www.heart.org/HEARTORG/HealthcareResearch/GetWithTheGuidelines/Get-With-The-Guidelines-Educational-Materials_UCM_310980_Article.jsp>.

Aw, D., & Sharma, J. C. (2012). Antiplatelets in secondary stroke prevention: Should clopidogrel be the first choice? *Postgraduate Medical Journal, 88*(1035), 34–37.

Beal, C. C. (2010). Gender and stroke symptoms: A review of the current literature. *Journal of Neuroscience Nursing, 42*(2), 80–87.

Bousser, M. G. (2012). Stroke prevention: An update. *Frontiers of Medicine, 6*(1), 22–34.

Cahill, J. E., & Armstrong, T. S. (2011). Caring for an adult with a malignant primary brain tumor. *Nursing, 41*(6), 28–33.

Cameron, V. (2013). Best practices for stroke patient and family education in the acute care setting: A literature review. *Medsurg Nursing, 22*(3), 51–55.

Centers for Disease Control and Prevention (CDC) (2013a). *Injury prevention & control: Traumatic brain injury.* Retrieved Ocotber, 2014, from <www.cdc.gov/TraumaticBrainInjury>.

Centers for Disease Control and Prevention (CDC) (2013b). *Stroke.* Retrieved October, 2014, from <www.cdc.gov/stroke/>.

Courman, M. (2012). Bladder management in female stroke survivors: Translating research into practice. *Rehabilitation Nursing, 37*(5), 220–230.

Defazio, M. V., Rammo, R. A., Robles, J. R., Bramlett, H. M., Dietrich, W. D., & Bullock, M. R. (2013). The potential utility of blood-derived biochemical markers as indicators of early clinical trends following severe traumatic brain injury. *World Neurosurgery, 81*(1), 151–158.

Howard, G., Cushman, M., Kissela, B. M., Kleindorfer, D. O., McClure, L. A., Safford, M. M., Racial Differences in Stroke Investigators, et al. (2011). Traditional risk factors as the underlying cause of racial disparities in stroke: Lessons from the half-full (empty?) glass. *Stroke, 42*(12), 3369–3375.

Hughes, P. (2011). Comprehensive care of adults with acute ischemic stroke. *Critical Care Nursing Clinics of North America, 23*(4), 661–675.

Knauft, W., Chhabra, J., & McCullough, L. D. (2010). Emergency department arrival times, treatment, and functional recovery in women with acute ischemic stroke. *Journal of Woman's Health, 19*(4), 681–688.

Lakoski, S. G., Le, A. H., Muntner, P., Judd, S. E., Safford, M. M., Levine, D. A., et al. (2011). Adiposity, inflammation, and risk for death in black and white men and women in the United States: The Reasons for Geographic and Racial Differences in Stroke (REGARDS) study. *Journal of Clinical Endocrinology and Metabolism, 96*(6), 1805–1814.

Lee, L. K., Bateman, B. T., Wang, S., Schumacher, H. C., Pile-Spellman, J., & Saposnik, G. (2012). Trends in the hospitalization of ischemic stroke in the United States, 1998-2007. *International Journal of Stroke, 7*(3), 195–201.

Mink, J., & Miller, J. (2011a). Opening the window of opportunity for treating acute ischemic stroke. *Nursing, 41*(1), 24–32.

Mink, J., & Miller, J. (2011b). Stroke, Part 2: Respond aggressively to hemorrhagic stroke. *Nursing, 41*(3), 36–42.

Müller, B., Evangelopoulos, D. S., Bias, K., Wildisen, A., Zimmermann, H., & Exadaktylos, A. K. (2011). Can S-100B serum protein help to save cranial CT resources in a peripheral trauma centre? A study and consensus paper. *Emergency Medicine Journal, 28*(11), 938–940.

Muttikkal, T. J., & Wintermark, M. (2013). MRI patterns of global hypoxic-ischemic injury in adults. *Journal of Neuroradiology, 40*(3), 164–171.

Norton, C., Feltz, S. J., Brocker, A., & Granitto, M. (2013). Tackling long-term consequences of concussion. *Nursing, 43*(1), 50–55.

Oran, N. T., & Oran, I. (2010). Carotid angioplasty and stenting in carotid artery stenosis: Neuroscience nursing implications. *The Journal of Neuroscience Nursing, 42*(1), 3–11.

Perry, L., Hamilton, S., Williams, J., & Jones, S. (2013). Nursing interventions for improving nutritional status and outcomes of stroke patients: Descriptive reviews of processes and outcomes. *Worldviews on Evidence-based Nursing, 10*(1), 17–40.

Rank, W. (2012). Making repairs with endovascular surgical neuroradiology. *Nursing, 42*(12), 41–45.

Rank, W. (2013). Aneurysmal subarachnoic hemorrhage. *Nursing, 43*(5), 43–50.

Schnieder, M., & Schneider, M. D. E. (2012). Recognizing post stroke depression. *Nursing, 42,* 60–63.

Simmons, S. (2012). Recognizing stroke in women. *Nursing, 42*(3), 30–36.

Simpson, J. R., Zahuranec, D. B., Lisabeth, L. D., Sanchez, B. N., Skolarus, L. E., Mendizabal, J. E., et al. (2010). Mexican Americans with atrial fibrillation have more recurrent strokes than do non-Hispanic whites. *Stroke, 41*(10), 2132–2136.

Smania, N., Avesani, R., Roncari, L., Ianes, P., Girardi, P., Varalta, V., et al. (2013). Factors predicting functional and cognitive recovery following severe traumatic, anoxic, and cerebrovascular brain damage. *Journal of Head Trauma Rehabilitation, 28*(2), 131–140.

The Joint Commission (2014). *Stroke.* Retrieved October 2014, from <http://www.jointcommission.org/stroke/>.

Thompson, H. J., & Mauk, K. (2011). *Care of the patient with mild traumatic brain injury.* Retrieved October 2014, from <www.rehabnurse.org/uploads/files/cpgmtbi.pdf>.

Wijdicks, E. F., Varelas, P. N., Gronseth, G. S., Greer, D. M., & American Academy of Neurology. (2010). Evidence-based guideline update: Determining brain death in adults: Report of the Quality Standards Subcommittee of the American Academy of Neurology. *Neurology, 74*(23), 1911–1918.

Chapter 46

See General References.

Chapter 47

American Cancer Society (2014). *Cancer facts and figures 2014.* Report No. 00-300M–No. 500814. Atlanta: Author.

Corneal abrasion. (2013). Corneal abrasion. *Nursing, 43*(2), 49.

Foundation Fighting Blindness. (2012). Retrieved October 2014, from <www.blindness.org>.

Huber, M., Hofmann, W., & Drager, D. (2013). Ophthalmic drugs as part of polypharmacy in nursing home residents with glaucoma. *Drugs and Aging, 30*(1), 31–38.

Kerr, E. (2013). Back to basics: Age-related macular degeneration. *Nursing and Residential Care, 15*(7), 484–487.

National Eye Institute of the National Institutes of Health (2012). *Prevalence of adult vision impairment and age-related eye diseases in America.* Retrieved July 2014, from <www.nei.nih.gov/eyedata/adultvision_usa.asp>.

Newton, M., & Sanderson, A. (2013). The effect of visual impairment on patients' falls risk. *Nursing Older People, 25*(8), 16–21.

Online Mendelian Inheritance in Man (OMIM) (2014). *Retinitis pigmentosa.* Retrieved October 2014, from <www.omim.org/entry/268000>.

Russo, A., & Bowden, D. (2013). Visual impairment: Setting sights on an independent life. *Nursing & Residential Care, 15*(1), 38–40.

Warren, M. (2013). Promoting health literacy in older adults with low vision. *Topics in Geriatric Rehabilitation, 29*(2), 107–115.

Watkinson, S. (2013). Assessment and management of patients with acute red eye. *Nursing Older People, 25*(5), 27–34.

Chapter 48

Alm, M. (2012). Hope to cope. *Hearing Health, 28*(4), 14–15.

Barbara, M., Biagini, M., & Monini, S. (2011). The totally implantable middle ear device "Esteem" for rehabilitation of severe sensorineural hearing loss. *Acta Oto-Laryngologica, 131*(4), 399–404.

Bridges, J., Lataille, A., Buttorff, C., White, S., & Niparko, J. K. (2012). Consumer preferences for hearing aid attributes: A comparison of rating and conjoint analysis methods. *Trends in Amplification, 16*(1), 40–48.

Haynes, D. (2014). Defining Ménière's disease. *Hearing Health, Winter*, 34–37.

Holmes, A., Shrivastav, R., Krause, L., Siburt, H., & Schwartz, E. (2012). Speech based optimization of cochlear implants. *International Journal of Audiology, 51*(6), 806–816.

*National Institute on Deafness and other Communication Disorders (NIDCD) (2010). *Ménière's disease*. Retrieved October 2014, from <www.nidcd.nih.gov/health/balance/pages/meniere.aspx>.

National Institute on Deafness and other Communication Disorders (NIDCD) (2014). *Statistics about hearing, balance, ear infections and deafness*. Retrieved October 2014, from <www.nidcd.nih.gov/health/statistics/pages/hearing.aspx>.

National Institute on Deafness and other Communication Disorders (NIDCD) (2012). *Noise-induced hearing loss*. Retrieved October 2014, from <www.nidcd.nih.gov/health/statistics/pages/noise.aspx>.

Online Mendelian Inheritance in Man (OMIM) (2014). *Gap junction proteins, beta-2; GJB2*. Retrieved October 2014, from <www.omim.org/entry/121011>.

Oyler, A. (2012). The American hearing loss epidemic. *The American Speech-Language Hearing Association LEADER, 17*(2), 5–7.

Richardson, K. J. (2014). Deaf culture: Competencies and best practices. *The Nurse Practitioner, 39*(5), 20–28.

Ruppert, S., & Fay, V. (2012). Tinnitus evaluation in primary care. *The Nurse Practitioner, 37*(10), 20–26.

Shuler, G., Mistler, L., Torrey, K., & Depukat, R. (2013). Bridging communication gaps with the deaf. *Nursing, 43*(11), 24–30.

Spyridakou, C. (2012). Hearing loss: A health problem for all ages. *Primary Health Care, 22*(4), 16–20.

Chapter 49

Chou, R., Deyo, R. A., & Jarvik, J. G. (2012). Appropriate use of lumbar imaging for evaluation of low back pain. *Radiology Clinics of North America, 50*(4), entire issue.

*Collyott, C. L., & Brooke, M. V. (2008). Evaluation and management of joint pain. *Orthopaedic Nursing, 27*(4), 246–250.

Doheny, M. O., Sedlak, C. A., Estok, P. J., & Zeller, R. A. (2011). Bone density, health beliefs, and osteoporosis preventing behaviors in men. *Orthopaedic Nursing, 30*(4), 266–272.

Esoga, P. I., & Seidl, K. L. (2012). Best practices in orthopedic inpatient care. *Orthopaedic Nursing, 31*(4), 236–240.

Kamienski, M., Tate, D., & Vega, M. (2011). The silent thief: Diagnosis and management of osteoporosis. *Orthopaedic Nursing, 30*(3), 162–171.

*Kress, T., Krueger, D., & Ziccardi, S. (2008). Creatine kinase: An assay with muscle. *Nursing, 38*(10), 62.

Mosher, C. M. (2010). *An introduction to orthopaedic nursing* (4th ed.). Chicago: National Association of Orthopaedic Nurses.

*Nussbaum, R. L., McInnes, R. R., & Willard, H. F. (2007). *Thompson & Thompson genetics in medicine* (7th ed.). Philadelphia: Saunders.

Schoen, D. C. H. (2010). *Adult orthopaedic nursing*. Philadelphia: Lippincott-Williams-Wilkins.

Smith, M. A., & Smith, W. T. (2010). Rotator cuff tears: An overview. *Orthopaedic Nursing, 29*(5), 319–322.

Chapter 50

Chang, S. F., Yang, R. S., Chung, U. L., Chen, C. M., & Cheng, M. H. (2010). Perception of risk factors and DXA T-score among at-risk females of osteoporosis. *Journal of Clinical Nursing, 19*(13–14), 1795–1802.

Cohen, H. V. (2010). Bisphosphonate-associated osteonecrosis of the jaw—Patient care considerations: Overview for the orthopaedic nursing healthcare professional. *Orthopaedic Nursing, 29*(3), 176–180.

Crawford, A., & Harris, H. (2012). Balancing act: Calcium and phosphorus. *Nursing, 42*(1), 36–42.

Doheny, M. O., Sedlak, C. A., Estok, P. J., & Zeller, R. A. (2011). Bone density, health beliefs, and osteoporosis preventing behaviors in men. *Orthopaedic Nursing, 30*(4), 266–272.

Doheny, M. O., Sedlak, C. A., Zeller, R., & Estok, P. J. (2010). Validation of the Osteoporosis Smoking Health Belief instrument. *Orthopaedic Nursing, 29*(1), 11–16.

*Gloth, F. M., III, & Simonson, W. (2008). Osteoporosis is underdiagnosed in skilled nursing facilities: A large-scale heel BMD screening study. *Journal of the American Medical Directors Association, 9*(3), 190–193.

Greene, D., & Dell, R. M. (2010). Outcomes of an osteoporosis disease-management program managed by nurse practitioners. *Journal of the American Academy of Nurse Practitioners, 22*(6), 326–329.

Institute for Safe Medication Practices (2013). *ISMPs list of high-alert medications*. Retrieved June 2013, from <www.ismp.org/Tools/highalertmedications.pdf>.

*Johnson, M. A., Davery, A., Park, S., Hausman, D. B., & Poon, L. W. (2008). Age, race and season predict vitamin D status in African American and white octogenarians and centenarians. *Journal of Nutrition and Health Aging, 12*(10), 690–695.

Kamienski, M., Tate, D., & Vega, M. (2011). The silent thief: Diagnosis and management of osteoporosis. *Orthopaedic Nursing, 30*(3), 162–171.

*Lee, J. (2009). Complication related to bisphosphonate therapy: Osteonecrosis of the jaw. *Journal of Infusion Nursing, 32*(6), 330–335.

*Najat, D., Garner, T., Hagen, T., Shaw, B., Sheppard, P. W., Falchetti, A., et al. (2009). Characterization of a non-UBA domain missense mutation of sequestosome (SQSTM1) in Paget's disease of bone. *Journal of Bone and Mineral Research, 24*(4), 632–642.

National Institute of Arthritis and Musculoskeletal and Skin Diseases (2013). *Information for patients about Paget's disease of bone*. Retrieved June 2013, from <www.niams.nih.gov/Health_Info/Bone/pagets/patient_info.asp>.

National Osteoporosis Foundation (NOF) (2010). *Clinician's guide to prevention and treatment of osteoporosis*. Washington, DC: Author.

*Nussbaum, R., McInnes, R., & Willard, H. (2007). *Thompson & Thompson: Genetics in medicine* (7th ed.). Philadelphia: Saunders.

*Parikh, S., Avorn, J., & Solomon, D. H. (2009). Pharmacological management of osteoporosis in nursing home populations: A systematic review. *Journal of the American Geriatrics Society, 57*(2), 327–334.

*Sadler, C., & Huff, M. (2007). African-American women: Health beliefs, lifestyle, and osteoporosis. *Orthopaedic Nursing, 26*(2), 96–101.

Sambrook, P. N., Cameron, I. D., Chen, J. S., March, L. M., Simpson, J. M., Cumming, R. G., et al. (2010). Oral bisphosphonates are associated with reduced mortality in frail older people: A prospective five-year study. *Osteoporosis International, 21*(10), [Epub ahead of print].

Seton, M., Moses, A. M., Bode, R. K., & Schwartz, C. (2011). Paget's disease of bone: The skeletal distribution, complications, and quality of life as perceived by patients. *Bone, 48*(2), 281–285.

Sutcliffe, A. (2010). Paget's: The neglected bone disease. *International Journal of Orthopaedic and Trauma Nursing, 14*, 142–149.

Swislocki, A., Green, J. A., Heinrich, G., Barnett, C. A., Meadows, I. D., Harmon, E. B., et al. (2010). Prevalence of osteoporosis in men in a VA rehabilitation center. *American Journal of Managed Care, 16*(6), 427–433.

*Voda, S. C. (2009a). Dangerous curves: Treating adult idiopathic scoliosis. *Nursing, 39*(12), 42–46.

*Voda, S. C. (2009b). Help older men bone up on osteoporosis. *Nursing, 39*(12), 66–67.

Chapter 51

Al-Shaer, D., Hill, P. D., & Anderson, M. A. (2011). Nurses' knowledge and attitudes regarding pain assessment and intervention. *Medsurg Nursing, 20*(1), 7–12.

*Altizer, L. L. (2008). Colles' fracture. *Orthopaedic Nursing, 27*(2), 140–145.

Barry, M. (2010). Bringing Achilles tendinopathy to heel. *Nursing, 40*(10), 30–33.

Chang, H. J., Burke, A. E., & Glass, R. M. (2010). Achilles tendinopathy. *Journal of the American Medical Association, 303*(2), 188.

Friedrich, J. B., & Shin, A. Y. (2012). Management of forearm compartment syndrome. *Critical Care Nursing Clinics of North America, 24*(2), 261–274.

Guarin, P. L. B. (2013). How effective are nerve blocks after orthopedic surgery: A quality improvement study. *Nursing, 43*(6), 63–66.

*Herr, K., & Titler, M. (2009). Acute pain assessment and pharmacological management practices for the older adult with a hip fracture: Review of ED trends. *Journal of Emergency Nursing, 35*(4), 312–320.

Hershey, K. (2013). Fracture complications. *Critical Care Nursing Clinics of North America, 25*(2), 321–331.

*Hsu, E. (2009). Practical management of complex regional pain syndrome. *American Journal of Therapeutics, 16*(2), 147–154.

Huisstede, B. M., Randsdorp, M. S., Coert, J. H., Glerum, S., van Middlekoop, M., & Koes, B. W. (2010). Carpal tunnel syndrome, Part II—Effectiveness of surgical treatments: A systematic review. *Archives of Physical Medicine and Rehabilitation, 91*(7), 1005–1024.

*Ketz, A. K. (2008). Pain management in the traumatic amputee. *Critical Care Nursing Clinics of North America, 20*(1), 51–57.

*Lowe, J., & Tariman, J. D. (2008). Lower extremity amputations: Black men with diabetes overburdened. *Advance for Nurse Practitioners, 16*(11), 28.

Montana, C., & Kautz, D. D. (2011). Turning the nightmare of complex regional pain syndrome into a time of healing, renewal, and hope. *Medsurg Nursing, 20*(3), 139–142.

Nahm, E.-S., Resnick, B., Orwig, D., Magaziner, J., & Degrezia, M. (2010). Exploration of informal caregiving following hip fractures. *Geriatric Nursing, 31*(4), 254–262.

Nahm, E.-S., Resnick, B., Plummer, L., & Park, B. K. (2013). Use of discussion boards in an online hip fracture resource center for caregivers. *Orthopaedic Nursing, 32*(2), 89–96.

National Institute of Neurological Disorders and Stroke (2011). *Complex regional pain syndrome fact sheet.* Retrieved March 2011, from <www.ninds.nih.gov/disorders/reflex_sympathetic_dystrophy/detail.htm>.

Pirrung, J., & Mower-Wade, D. (2014). Early recognition and treatment of pelvic fractures. *Nursing, 44*(9), 38–46.

Pullen, R. L. (2010). Caring for a patient after amputation. *Nursing, 40*(1), 15.

Satryb, S. A., Wilson, T. J., & Patterson, M. M. (2011). Casting: All wrapped up. *Orthopedic Nursing, 30*(1), 37–41.

Smith, M. A., & Smith, W. T. (2010). Rotator cuff tears: An overview. *Orthopaedic Nursing, 29*(5), 319–322.

Sweitzer, V., Rondeau, D., Guido, V., & Rasmor, M. (2013). Interventions to improve outcomes in the elderly after hip fracture. *Journal for Nurse Practitioners, 9*(4), 238–242.

Uchiyama, S., Itsubo, T., Nakamura, K., Kato, H., Yasutomi, T., & Momose, T. (2010). Current concepts of carpal tunnel syndrome: Pathophysiology, treatment, and evaluation. *Journal of Orthopaedic Science, 15*(1), 1–13.

Voda, S. C. (2011). Bad breaks: A nurse's guide to distal radius fractures. *Nursing, 41*(8), 34–40.

Walsh, C. R. (2013). Wrist fractures in adults: Getting a grip. *Nursing, 43*(4), 38–44.

Chapter 52

American Cancer Society (2014). *American Cancer Society guidelines for the early detection of cancer.* Retrieved January 2014, from <www.cancer.org/healthy/findcancerearly/cancerscreeningguidelines/american-cancer-society-guidelines-for-the-early-detection-of-cancer>.

Bittler, R. D. (2011). Splenic injury due to colonoscopy: Nursing considerations. *Gastroenterology Nursing, 34*(5), 357–364.

Bjorkman, I., Karlsson, F., Lundberg, A., & Frisman, G. H. (2013). Gender differences when using sedative music during colonoscopy. *Gastroenterology Nursing, 36*(1), 14–20.

Bourque, A. L., Sullivan, M. E., & Winter, M. R. (2012). Reiki as a pain management adjunct in screening colonoscopy. *Gastroenterology Nursing, 35*(5), 308–312.

Bruesehoff, M. P. (2010). ERCP—Much ado about blockages: Update your knowledge about the diagnostic and therapeutic uses for endoscopic retrograde cholangiopancreatography. *Nursing, 40*(9), 46–50.

Devitt, J., Shellman, L., Gardner, K., & Nichols, L. W. (2011). Using positioning after a colonoscopy for patient comfort management. *Gastroenterology Nursing, 34*(2), 93–100.

Dudley-Brown, S. (2012). The importance of the physical examination. *Gastroenterology Nursing, 35*(5), 350–352.

Ellett, M. L. (2010). A literature review of the safety and efficacy of using propofol for sedation in endoscopy. *Gastroenterology Nursing, 33*(2), 113–117.

Hulse, R. S., Stuart-Shor, E. M., & Russo, J. (2010). Endoscopic procedure with a modified Reiki intervention: A pilot study. *Gastroenterology Nursing, 33*(1), 20–26.

Keske, L. A., & Letizia, M. (2010). *Clostridium difficile* infection: Essential information for nurses. *Medsurg Nursing, 19*(6), 329–333.

Mikocka-Walus, A. A., Moulds, L. G., Rollbusch, N., & Andrews, J. M. (2012). "It's a tube up your bottom: It makes people nervous": The experience of anxiety in initial colonoscopy patients. *Gastroenterology Nursing, 35*(6), 392–401.

Munson, G. W., Van Norstrand, M. D., O'Donnell, J. J., Hammes, N. L., & Francis, D. L. (2011). Intraprocedural evaluation of comfort for sedated outpatient upper endoscopy and colonoscopy: The La Crosse (WI) Intra-Endoscopy Sedation Comfort Score. *Gastroenterology Nursing, 34*(4), 296–301.

Muscarella, L. F. (2010). Evaluation of the risk of transmission of bacterial biofilms and *Clostridium difficile* during gastrointestinal endoscopy. *Gastroenterology Nursing, 33*(1), 28–35.

Tas, A. (2013). Periorbital ecchymosis following an upper gastrointestinal endoscopy. *Gastroenterology Nursing, 36*(1), 72.

Van Dongen, M. (2012). Enhancing bowel preparation for colonoscopy: An integrative review. *Gastroenterology Nursing, 35*(1), 36–44.

Welliver, M. (2012). Why capnography for procedural sedation? *Gastroenterology Nursing, 35*(6), 423–425.

Chapter 53

Agency for Toxic Substances and Disease Registry (2014). *ToxFAQs for polycyclic aromatic hydrocarbons (PAHs.* Retrieved July 2014, from <www.atsdr.cdc.gov/>.

AHFS® Consumer Medication Information (2013). *Thalidomide.* Retrieved July 2014, from <www.nlm.nih.gov/medlineplus/druginfo/meds/a699032.html>.

Alterburg, A., & Zouboulis, C. (2014). *Current concepts in the treatment of recurrent aphthous stomatitis.* Retrieved July 2014, from <www.skintherapyletter.com/2008/13.7/1.html>.

American Dietetic Association (2014). *Position of the American Dietetic Association: Oral health and nutrition.* Retrieved July 2014, from <www.eatright.org>.

Baldwin, C., Spiro, A., Ahern, R., & Emery, P. W. (2012). Oral nutritional interventions in malnourished patients with cancer: A systematic review and meta-analysis. *Journal of the National Cancer Institute, 104*(5), 371–385.

Broutian, T., Pickard, R., Tong, Z., Xiao, W., Kahle, L., Graubard, B., et al. (2012). Prevalence of oral HPV infection in the United States, 2009-2010. *Journal of the American Medical Association, 307*(7), 693–703.

Cancer Research UK (2014). *Types of mouth and oropharyngeal cancer.* Retrieved July 2014, from <www.cancerhelp.org.uk>.

Livestrong.com (2014). *Cautions for family members of persons receiving radiation treatment for cancer.* Retrieved July 2014, from <www.livestrong.com>.

Moriya, S., Tei, K., Murata, A., Muramatsu, M., Inoue, N., & Miura, H. (2012). Relationships between Geriatric Oral Health Assessment Index scores and general physical status in community-dwelling older adults. *Gerodontology, 29*(2), e998–e1004.

National Institutes of Health (2014). *Genetics home reference: TP53.* Retrieved July 2014, from <www.ghr.nlm.nih.gov/gene/TP53>.

North Carolina State Health Plan (2012). *Thalidomide.* Retrieved July 2014, from <www.shpnc.org/library/pdf/pharmacy/thalomid.pdf>.

Oral Cancer Foundation (OCF) (2014). *Oral cancer facts.* Retrieved July 2014, from <www.oralcancerfoundation.org>.

OralCDx (2013). *The OralCDx brush test.* Retrieved July 2014, from <www.sopreventable.com>.

Prendergast, V., Jakobsson, U., Renvert, S., & Hallberg, I. (2012). Effects of a standard versus comprehensive oral care protocol among intubated neuroscience ICU patients: Results of a randomized controlled trial. *Journal of Neuroscience Nursing, 44*(3), 134–146.

van der Meulen, I. C., de Leeuw, J. R. J., Gamel, C. J., & Hafsteinsdóttir, T. B. (2012). Educational intervention for patients with head and neck cancer in the discharge phase. *European Journal of Oncology Nursing, 17*(2), 220–227.

World Health Organization (2014). *Oral health.* Retrieved July 2014, from <www.who.int/mediacentre/factsheets/fs318/en/>.

Chapter 54

American Cancer Society (ACS) (2012). *Cancer facts and figures 2012.* Retrieved August 2014, from <www.cancer.org/acs/groups/content/@epidemiologysurveilance/documents/document/acspc-031941.pdf>.

American Cancer Society (ACS) (2014a). *Chemotherapy for cancer of the esophagus.* Retrieved August 2014, from <www.cancer.org/cancer/esophaguscancer/detailedguide/esophagus-cancer-treating-chemotherapy>.

American Cancer Society (ACS) (2014b). *Targeted therapy for cancer of the esophagus.* Retrieved June 2013, from <www.cancer.org/cancer/esophaguscancer/detailedguide/esophagus-cancer-treating-targeted-therapy>.

Buckley, F., & Roberts, K. (2014). *Laparoscopic Nissen fundoplication.* Retrieved August 2014, from <http://emedicine.medscape.com/article/1892517-overview>.

*Chait, M. M. (2010). Gastroesophageal reflux disease: Important considerations for older patients. *World Journal of Gastrointestinal Endoscopy, 2*(12), 388–396.

Harvard Health Publications (2011). *Proton-pump inhibitors.* Retrieved August 2014, from <www.health.harvard.edu/newsletters/Harvard_Health_Letter/2011/April/proton-pump-inhibitors>.

National Cancer Institute at the National Institutes of Health (2013). *A snapshot of esophageal cancer.* Retrieved August 2014, from <www.cancer.gov/researchandfunding/snapshots/esophageal>.

National Guideline Clearinghouse (NGC) (2013). *Guideline synthesis: Diagnosis and management of gastroesophageal reflux disease (GERD).* Retrieved August 2014, from <http://www.guideline.gov/content.aspx?id=43847&search=gerd>.

National Institutes of Health (2013). *Esophageal monometry.* Retrieved August 2014, from <www.nlm.nih.gov/medlineplus/ency/article/003884.htm>.

*Nussbaum, R. L., McInnes, R. R., & Willard, H. F. (2007). *Thompson and Thompson's genetics in medicine.* Philadelphia: Saunders.

Patel, D., & Siddiqui, R. (2013). Fully covered esophageal stents: Role in benign disease. *Practical Gastroenterology,* 39–46. Retrieved August 2014, from <www.practicalgastro.com/pdf/May13/D-Patel.pdf>.

Solomon, M., & Reynolds, J. C. (2012). Esophageal reflux disease and its complications. In *Geriatric gastroenterology.* New York: Springer.

The Ohio State University Wexner Medical Center (OSUWMC) (2014). *Diagnosing GERD.* Retrieved August 2014, from <http://medicalcenter.osu.edu/patientcare/healthcare_services/digestive_disorders/gerd_heartburn/diagnosing_treating_gerd/diagnosing_gerd/Pages/index.aspx>.

University of Michigan Health System (2012). *Gastroesophageal reflux disease (GERD).* Retrieved August 2014, from <www.guideline.gov/content.aspx?id=37564>.

Chapter 55

Abe, N., Takeuchi, H., Yanagida, O., Sugiyama, M., & Atomi, Y. (2010). Surgical indications and procedures for bleeding peptic ulcer. *Digestive Endoscopy, 22*(Suppl. 1), S35–S37.

American Cancer Society (2014). *Stomach cancer.* Retrieved January 2014, from <www.cancer.org/acs/groups/cid/documents/webcontent/003141-pdf.pdf>.

Bailey, K. (2011). An overview of gastric cancer and its management. *Cancer Nursing Practice, 10*(6), 31–37.

Bosaeus, I., & Bergbom, I. (2010). Patients' experiences of the recovery period 12 months after upper gastrointestinal surgery. *Gastroenterology Nursing, 33*(6), 422–431.

DeRanieri, J. T. (2013). *Peptic ulcer disease.* Retrieved July 2013, from <www.nursingconsult.com/nursing/evidence-based-nursing/monograph?monograph_id=219951>.

Howlader, N., Noone, A. M., Krapcho, M., Neyman, N., Aminou, R., Altekruse, S. F., et al. (Eds.), (2012). *SEER cancer statistics review, 1975-2009 (Vintage 2009 Populations).* Bethesda, MD: National Cancer Institute. Retrieved July 2013, from <http://seer.cancer.gov/csr/1975_2009_pops09/>.

Jemal, A., Bray, F., Center, M. M., Ferlay, J., Ward, E., & Forman, D. (2011). Global cancer statistics. *CA: A Cancer Journal for Clinicians, 61,* 69–90.

Kwok, C. S., Yeong, J. K., & Loke, Y. K. (2010). Meta-analysis: Risk of fractures with acid-suppressing medication. *Bone, 48*(4), 768–776.

Mayhew, M. S. (2011). Long-term safety of proton pump inhibitors. *Journal for Nurse Practitioners, 7*(4), 323–324.

National Cancer Institute (2012). *Surveillance, epidemiology and end results (SEER) stat fact sheet: Cancer of the stomach.* Retrieved April 2013, from <http://seer.cancer.gov/statfacts/html/stomach.html#content>.

National Cancer Institute (2013). *Fact sheet: Helicobacter pylori and cancer.* Retrieved April 2013, from <www.cancer.gov/cancertopics/factsheet/Risk/h-pylori-cancer>.

National Digestive Diseases Information Clearinghouse (2012). *H. pylori and peptic ulcers. National Institute of Diabetes and Digestive and Kidney Diseases home page.* Retrieved April 2013, from <www.digestive.niddk.nih.gov/ddiseases/pubs/hpylori/index.aspx>.

Saif, W. W., Makrilia, N., Zalonis, A., Merikas, M., & Syrigos, K. (2010). Gastric cancer in the elderly: An overview. *European Journal of Surgical Oncology, 36*(8), 709–717.

Yang, D., Hendifar, A., Lenz, C., Togawa, K., Lurje, G., Pohl, A., et al. (2011). Survival of metastatic gastric cancer: Significance of age, sex and race/ethnicity. *Journal of Gastrointestinal Oncology, 2*(2), 77–84.

Zarowitz, B. J. (2011). The challenge of discontinuing proton pump inhibitors. *Geriatric Nursing, 32*(4), 276–278.

Chapter 56

American Cancer Society (ACS) (2014). *Cancer facts and figures 2014.* Atlanta: Author.

Barkhordari, E., Rezaei, N., Ansaripour, B., Larki, P., Alighardashi, M., Ahmad-Ashtiani, H. R., et al. (2010). Proinflammatory cytokine gene polymorphisms in irritable bowel syndrome. *Journal of Clinical Immunology, 30*(1), 74–79.

Bengtsson, M., Ulander, K., Borgdal, E. B., & Ohlsson, B. (2010). A holistic approach for planning care of patients with irritable bowel syndrome. *Gastroenterology Nursing, 33*(2), 98–108.

Berger, A. M., Grem, J. L., Visovsky, C., Marunda, H. A., & Yurkovich, J. M. (2010). Fatigue and other variables during adjuvant chemotherapy for colon and rectal cancer. *Oncology Nursing Forum, 37*(1), 59–69.

Carlsson, E., Berndtsson, I., Hallen, A. M., Lindholm, E., & Persson, E. (2010). Concerns and quality of life before surgery and during the recovery period in patients with rectal cancer and an ostomy. *Journal of Wound, Ostomy, and Continence Nursing, 37*(6), 654–661.

Good, K., Niziolek, J., Yoshida, C., & Rowlands, A. (2010). Insights into barriers that prevent African Americans from seeking colorectal screenings: A qualitative study. *Gastroenterology Nursing, 33*(3), 204–208.

Gwee, K. A., Bak, Y. T., Ghoshal, U. C., Gonlachanvit, S., Lee, O. Y., Fock, K. M., et al. (2010). Asian consensus on irritable bowel syndrome. *Journal of Gastroenterology and Hepatology, 25*(7), 1189–1205.

*Hamlyn, S. (2008). Reducing the incidence of colorectal cancer in African Americans. *Gastroenterology Nursing, 31*(1), 39–42.

Herman, J., Pokkunuri, V., Braham, L., & Pimentel, M. (2010). Gender distribution in irritable bowel syndrome is proportional to the severity of constipation relative to diarrhea. *Gender Medicine: The Journal for the Study of Sex & Gender Differences, 7*(3), 240–246.

Kapritsou, M., Korkolis, D. P., & Knostantinou, E. A. (2013). Open or laparoscopic surgery for colorectal cancer: A retrospective comparative study. *Gastroenterology Nursing, 36*(1), 37–41.

Kerckhoffs, A. P., Ben-Amor, K., Samsom, M., van der Rest, M. E., de Vogel, J., Knol, J., et al. (2011). Molecular analysis of faecal and duodenal samples reveals significantly higher prevalence and numbers of *Pseudomonas aeruginosa* in irritable bowel syndrome. *Journal of Medical Microbiology, 60,* 236–245.

Lee, R. K. (2012). Intra-abdominal hypertension and acute compartment syndrome: A comprehensive overview. *Critical Care Nurse, 22*(1), 19–32.

*Lindberg, D. A. (2009). Hydrogen breath testing in adults: What is it and why is it performed? *Gastroenterology Nursing, 32*(1), 19–24.

Lyra, A., Krogius-Kurikka, L., Nikkila, J., Malinen, E., Kajander, K., Kurikka, K., et al. (2010).

Effect of a multispecies probiotic supplement on quantity of irritable bowel syndrome-related intestinal microbial phylotypes. *BMC Gastroenterology, 10*, 110.

Malinen, E., Krogius-Kurikka, L., Lyra, A., Nikkila, J., Jaaskelainen, A., Rinttila, T., et al. (2010). Association of symptoms with gastrointestinal microbiota in irritable bowel syndrome. *World Journal of Gastroenterology, 16*(36), 4532–4540.

*Nicholl, B. I., Halder, S. L., Macfarlane, G. L., Thompson, D. G., O'Brien, S., Musleh, M., et al. (2008). Psychosocial risk markers for new onset irritable bowel syndrome: Results of a large prospective population-based study. *Pain, 137*(1), 147–155.

*Nussbaum, R. L., McInnes, R. R., & Willard, H. F. (2007). *Thompson and Thompson's genetics in medicine*. Philadelphia: Saunders.

Oliver, J. S., Worley, C. B., DeCoster, J., Palardy, L., Kim, G., Reddy, A., et al. (2012). Disparities in colorectal cancer screening behaviors: Implications for African American men. *Gastroenterology Nursing, 35*(2), 93–98.

Pimental, M., Lembo, A., Chey, W. D., Zakko, S., Ringel, Y., Yu, J., et al. (2011). Rifaximin therapy for patients with irritable bowel syndrome without constipation. *New England Journal of Medicine, 364*(1), 22–32.

*Pirotta, M. (2009). Irritable bowel syndrome: The role of complementary medicines in treatment. *Australian Family Physician, 389*(12), 966–968.

Rawl, S. N., Memon, U., Burness, A., & Breslau, E. S. (2012). Interventions to promote colorectal cancer screening: An integrative review. *Nursing Outlook, 60*(4), 172–181.

Russell, S., Champange, B., & Techner, L. (2012). Alvimopan for acceleration of GI recovery after bowel resection. *Medsurg Nursing, 21*(3), 151–157.

Stubenrauch, J. M. (2010). Rectal cancer rates rising in patients under 40. *The American Journal of Nursing, 110*(11), 15.

Walker, C. A., & Lochman, V. D. (2013). Gaps in the discharge process for patients with an ostomy: An ethical perspective. *Medsurg Nursing, 22*(1), 61–64.

Wilkes, G. (2013). *What's new in colon cancer: Update for the practicing nurse*. Retrieved July 2013, from <www.nursingconsult.com/nursing/clinical-updates/full-text?clinical_update_id=198216>.

Wilkes, G., & Hartshorn, K. (2012). Clinical update: Colon, rectal, and anal cancers. *Seminars in Oncology Nursing, 28*(4), 1–22.

Chapter 57

Centers for Disease Control and Prevention. (2014). *Parasites-American trypanosomiasis*. Retrieved from: <http://www.cdc.gov/parasites/chagas>; December 2014.

Cooper, J. M., Collier, J., James, V., & Hawkey, C. J. (2010). Beliefs about personal control and self-management in 30-40 year olds living with inflammatory bowel disease: A qualitative study. *International Journal of Nursing Studies, 47*(12), 1500–1509.

Cronin, E. (2010). Prednisolone in the management of patients with Crohn's disease. *British Journal of Nursing, 19*(21), 1333–1336.

*Crumbock, S. C., Loeb, S. J., & Fick, D. M. (2009). Physical activity, stress, disease activity, and quality of life in adults with Crohn disease. *Gastroenterology Nursing, 32*(3), 188–195.

Dolejs, S., Kennedy, G., & Heise, C. P. (2011). Small bowel obstruction following restorative proctocolectomy: Affected by a laparoscopic approach? *Journal of Surgical Research*, [Epub ahead of print].

*Dudley-Brown, S., Nag, A., Cullinan, C., Ayers, M., Hass, S., & Panjabi, S. (2009). Health-related quality-of-life evaluation of Crohn disease patients after receiving natalizumab therapy. *Gastroenterology Nursing, 32*(5), 327–339.

Fajardo, A. D., Dharmarajan, S., George, V., Hunt, S. R., Birnbaum, E. H., Fleshman, J. W., et al. (2010). Laparoscopic versus open 2-stage ileal pouch: Laparoscopic approach allows for faster restoration of intestinal continuity. *Journal of the American College of Surgeons, 211*(3), 377–383.

Grossman, V. A. (2011). Inflammatory bowel disease and MR enterography. *Journal of Radiology Nursing, 30*(1), 4–5.

Hall, M. A. (2011). Diagnosing diverticular disease. *Journal for Nurse Practitioners, 7*(7), 606–607.

Harris, H., & Jelemensky, L. (2014). Managing the ups and downs of ulcerative colitis. *Nursing, 44*(8), 36–43.

Kessler, H., Mudter, J., & Hohenberger, W. (2011). Recent results of laparoscopic surgery in inflammatory bowel disease. *World Journal of Gastroenterology, 17*(9), 1116–1125.

Krenzer, M. E. (2012). Viral gastroenteritis in the adult population. *Critical Care Nursing Clinics of North America, 24*(4), 541–553.

McMaster, K., Aguinaldo, L., & Parekh, N. K. (2012). Evaluation of an ongoing psychoeducational inflammatory bowel disease support group in an adult outpatient setting. *Gastroenterology Nursing, 35*(6), 383–390.

*Nussbaum, R. L., McInnes, R. R., & Willard, H. F. (2007). *Thompson & Thompson genetics in medicine* (7th ed.). Philadelphia: Saunders.

Pihl-Lesnovska, K., Hjortswang, H., Ek, A. C., & Frisman, G. H. (2010). Patients' perspective of factors influencing quality of life while living with Crohn disease. *Gastroenterology Nursing, 33*(1), 37–44.

Ryan, M., & Grossman, S. (2011). Celiac disease: Implications for patient management. *Gastroenterology Nursing, 34*(3), 225–228.

Smith, M. M., & Goodfellow, L. (2011). The relationship between quality of life and coping strategies of adults with celiac disease adhering to a gluten-free diet. *Gastroenterology Nursing, 34*(6), 460–468.

Spencer, C. (2010). Ulcerative colitis. *Nursing Standard, 24*(52), 59.

Strauch, K. A., & Cotter, V. T. (2011). Celiac disease: An overview and management for primary care nurse practitioners. *Journal for Nurse Practitioners, 7*(7), 588–594.

Chapter 58

Ahmed, N., & Vernick, J. (2011). Management of liver trauma in adults. *Journal of Emergencies, Trauma/Shock, 4*, 114–119.

American Liver Foundation (2010). *Hepatitis B*. New York: Author.

American Liver Foundation (2011). *Position statement on hepatitis A and vaccination*. New York: Author.

American Liver Foundation (2012). *Liver transplant*. Retrieved August 2014, from <www.liverfoundation.org/abouttheliver/info/transplant/>.

Augustin, S., Gonzalez, A., & Genesca, J. (2010). Acute esophageal variceal bleeding: Current strategies and new perspectives. *World Journal of Hepatology, 2*(7), 261–274.

Clayton, M. (2011). Assessing patients before and after a liver transplant. *Practice Nursing, 22*(5), 236–241.

Donnelly, G., Kent-Wilkinson, A., & Rush, A. (2012). The alcohol-dependent patient in the hospital: Challenges for nursing. *Medsurg Nursing, 21*(1), 9–14.

Elliott, D. T., Geyer, C., & Doty, L. (2012). Managing alcohol withdrawal in hospitalized patients. *Nursing, 42*(4), 22–30.

Felicilda-Reynaldo, R. F. D. (2012a). Ammonia abolishers: Antibiotics for hepatic encephalopathy. *Medsurg Nursing, 21*(3), 173–176.

Felicilda-Reynaldo, R. F. D. (2012b). Block the bleed: Pharmacologic therapies for gastroesophageal variceal bleeding. *Medsurg Nursing, 21*(2), 107–110.

Houghton-Rahrig, L., Schutte, D., Fenton, J. I., & Awad, J. (2014). Nonalcoholic fatty liver disease and the *PNPLA3* gene. *Medsurg Nursing, 23*(2), 101–106.

Lee, H., Park, W., Yang, J. H., & You, K. S. (2010). Management of hepatitis B virus infection. *Gastroenterology Nursing, 33*(2), 120–126.

*Lok, A. S. F., & McMahon, B. J. (2009). AASLD: Chronic hepatitis B: Update 2009. *Hepatology, 50*(3), 661–662.

Lucey, M. R., Terrault, N., Ojo, L., Hay, J. E., Neuberger, J., Blumberg, E., et al. (2013). Long-term management of the successful adult liver transplant: 2012 Practice Guideline by the American Association for the Study of Liver Diseases and the American Society of Liver Transplantation. *Liver Transplantation, 19*, 3–26.

Minano, C., & Garcia-Tsao, G. (2010). Clinical pharmacology of portal hypertension. *Gastroenterology Clinics of North America, 39*(3), 681–695.

Morrison, D., Sgrillo, J., & Daniels, L. H. (2014). Managing alcoholic liver disease. *Nursing, 44*(11), 30–40.

Richmond, J. A., Bailey, D. E., Jr., McHutchinson, J. G., & Muir, A. J. (2010). The use of mind-body medicine and prayer among adult patients with hepatitis C. *Gastroenterology Nursing, 33*(3), 201–216.

Rossi, L., Zoratto, F., Papa, A., Iodice, F., Minozzi, M., Frati, L., et al. (2010). Current approach in the treatment of hepatocellular carcinoma.

World Journal of Gastroenterology Oncology, 2(9), 348–359.

Rugari, S. M. (2010). Longitudinal quality of life in liver transplant recipients. *Gastroenterology Nursing, 33*(2), 219–230.

Sulkowski, M. S. (2013). Current management of hepatitis C virus infection in patients with HIV co-infection. *The Journal of Infectious Diseases, 207*(Suppl. 1), S26–S32.

Yee, H. S., Change, M. F., Pocha, C., Lim, J., Ross, D., Morgan, T. R., et al. (2012). Update on the management and treatment of hepatitis C virus infection: Recommendations from the Department of Veterans Affairs Hepatitis C Resource Center Program and the National Hepatitis C Program Office. *American Journal of Gastroenterology, 104*, 1–21.

World Gastroenterology Organisation (WGO) (2012). *World Gastroenterology Organisation global guidelines: Nonalcoholic fatty liver disease and nonalcoholic steatohepatitis.* Milwaukee, WI: Author.

Chapter 59

Agostino, D. I., Wang, D. Q., Bonfrate, L., & Portincasa, P. (2013). Current views on genetics and epigenetics of cholesterol gallstone disease. *Cholesterol*, [Epub ahead of print].

American Cancer Society (ACS) (2013). *Cancer facts and figures—2013.* Atlanta: Author.

Bharwani, N., Patel, S., Prabhusesal, S., Fortheringham, T., & Power, N. (2011). Acute pancreatitis: The role of imaging in diagnosis and management. *Clinical Radiology, 66*(2), 164–175.

Conwell, D. L., & Wu, B. U. (2012). Chronic pancreatitis: Making the diagnosis. *Clinical Gastroenterology and Hepatology, 10*, 1088–1095.

Culp, B. L., Cedillo, V. E., & Arnold, D. (2012). Single-incision laparoscopic cholecystectomy versus traditional four-port cholecystectomy. *Baylor University Medical Center Proceedings, 25*(4), 319–323.

Felicilda-Reynaldo, R. F. D. (2012). Oral gallstone dissolution therapies. *Medsurg Nursing, 21*(1), 41–44.

Fusaroli, P., Spada, A., Mancino, M. G., & Caletti, G. (2010). Contrast harmonic echo-endoscopic ultrasound improves accuracy in diagnosis of solid pancreatic masses. *Journal of Gastroenterology and Hepatology, 8*(7), 629–634.

Gee, C. (2011). Pancreatic cancer: A whistle-stop tour. *Gastrointestinal Nursing, 9*(7), 41–45.

Girometti, R., Brondani, G., Cereser, L., Como, G., Del Pin, M., Bazzocchi, M., et al. (2010). Post-cholecystectomy syndrome: Spectrum of biliary findings at magnetic resonance cholangiopancreatography. *The British Journal of Radiology, 83*, 351–361.

Griffin, N., Charles-Edwards, G., & Grant, L. (2011). Magnetic resonance cholangiopancreatography: The ABC of MRCP. *Insights Imaging, 3*, 11–21.

Grützmann, R., Post, S., Saeger, H. D., & Niedergethmann, M. (2011). Intraductal papillary mucinous neoplasia (IPMN) of the pancreas: Its diagnosis, treatment, and prognosis. *Deutsches Ärzteblatt International, 108*(46), 788–794.

Huang, L., Ma, B., He, F., & Yang, S. (2012). Electrocardiographic, cardiac enzymes, and magnesium in patients with severe acute pancreatitis. *Gastroenterology Nursing, 35*(4), 256–260.

Hubb, H. A., & Saunders, M. (2011). The yellow bird of jaundice: Recognizing biliary obstruction. *Nursing, 41*(10), 28–36.

Huffman, J. L., & Schenker, S. (2010). Acute acalculous cholecystitis: A review. *Clinical Gastroenterology and Hepatology, 8*, 15–22.

Midha, S., Khajuria, R., Shastri, S., Kabra, M., & Garg, P. K. (2010). Idiopathic chronic pancreatitis in India: Phenotypic characterization and strong genetic susceptibility due to SPINK1 and CFTR gene mutations. *Gut, 59*(6), 800–807.

Navarra, G., La Malfa, G., Lazzara, S., Ullo, G., & Curro, G. (2010). SILS and NOTES cholecystectomy: A tailored approach. *Journal of Laparoendoscopic and Advanced Surgical Techniques, 20*(6), 511–514.

Novotny, I., Dite, P., Lata, J., Nechutova, H., & Klanicka, B. (2010). Autoimmune pancreatitis: Recent advances. *Digestive diseases, 28*(2), 334–338.

Pfadt, E., & Carlson, D. S. (2011). Sphincter of Oddi dysfunction. *Nursing, 41*(8), 42–45.

Salam, M. A. (2010). Single incision laparoscopic surgery. *Journal of Urology, 13*, 2.

Simmons, S. (2010). Gallstones. *Nursing, 37*(11), 37.

Society of American Gastrointestinal and Endoscopic Surgeons (SAGES) (2010). *Guidelines for the clinical application of laparoscopic biliary tract surgery.* Retrieved December 2013, from <www.sages.org/publications/guidelines/guidelines-for-the-clinical-application-of-laparoscopic-biliary-tract-surgery/>.

Targarona, E. M., Maldonado, M., Marzol, J. A., & Marinello, F. (2010). Natural orifice transluminal endoscopic surgery: The transvaginal route moving forward from cholecystectomy. *World Journal of Gastroenterology Surgery, 2*(6), 179–186.

Tonolini, M., Ravelli, A., Villa, C., & Bianco, R. (2012). Urgent MRI with MR cholangiopancreatography (MRCP) of acute cholecystitis and related complications: Diagnostic role and spectrum of imaging findings. *Emergency Radiology, 19*, 341–348.

Chapter 60

Academy of Nutrition and Dietetics (2013). *It's about eating right.* Retrieved September 2014, from <www.eatright.org/Public/content.aspx?id=6372>.

American Heart Association (2014). *Know your fats.* Retrieved September 2014, from <www.heart.org/HEARTORG/Conditions/Cholesterol/PreventionTreatmentofHighCholesterol/Know-Your-Fats_UCM_305628_Article.jsp>.

American Society for Bariatric Surgery (2011). *Longitudinal assessment of bariatric surgery.* Retrieved September 2014, from <http://win.niddk.nih.gov/publications/labs.htm#howmany>.

American Society of Parenteral and Enteral Nutrition (ASPEN). (2011). Retrieved September 2014, from:< https://www.nutritioncare.org/Guidelines_and_Clinical_Practice/Clinical_Guidelines/>.

*Bankhead, R., Boullata, J., Brantley, S., Corkins, M., Guenter, P., Krenitsky, J., et al. (2009). Enteral nutrition administration. In A.S.P.E.N. enteral nutrition practice recommendations. *Journal of Parenteral Enteral Nutrition, 33*(2), 149–158.

*Bender, S., Pusateri, M., Cook, A., Ferguson, M., & Hall, J. C. (2000). Malnutrition: Role of the TwoCal® HN Med Pass Program. *Medsurg Nursing, 9*(6), 284–296.

Centers for Disease Control and Prevention (CDC) (2012). *About BMI for adults.* Retrieved January 2014, from <www.cdc.gov/healthyweight/assessing/bmi/adult_bmi/>.

Champion, A. (2011). Anorexia of aging. *Annals of Long Term Care, 19*(10), 18–24.

Grmec, Š., Lah, K., & Mally, Š. (2011). Capnometry/capnography in prehospital cardiopulmonary resuscitation. In A. Gullo (Ed.), *Anaesthesia, pharmacology, intensive care and emergency medicine APICE* (pp. 47–56). Milan: Springer.

Health Canada (2011). *Eating well with Canada's Food Guide: First Nations, Inuit, and Métis.* Retrieved September 2014, from <www.hc-sc.gc.ca/fn-an/food-guide-aliment/index_e.html>.

Kulie, T., Slattengren, A., Redmer, J., Counts, H., Eglash, A., & Schranger, S. (2011). Obesity and women's health: An evidence-based review. *Journal of the American Board of Family Medicine, 24*(1), 75–78.

*Lee, J., Visser, M., Tylavsky, F., Kritchevsky, S., Schwartz, A., Sahyoun, N., et al. (2010). Weight loss and regain and effects on body composition: The health, aging, and body composition study. *The Journals of Gerontology, Series A, 65*(1), 78–83.

Marchiondo, K. (2014). Stemming the obesity epidemic: Are nurses credible coaches? *Medsurg Nursing, 23*(3), 155–158.

Mayo Clinic (2014). *Obesity: Treatment and drugs.* Retrieved September 2014, from <www.mayoclinic.com/health/obesity/DS00314/DSECTION=treatments-and-drugs>.

*Mehanna, H. M., Moledina, J., & Travis, J. (2008). Refeeding syndrome: What it is, and how to prevent and treat it. *BMJ, 336*, 1495–1498.

Minister of Health Canada (2011). *Eating well with Canada's food guide.* Retrieved January 2014, from <www.hc-sc.gc.ca/fn-an/alt_formats/hpfb-dgpsa/pdf/food-guide-aliment/view_eatwell_vue_bienmang-eng.pdf>.

National Institute of Diabetes and Digestive and Kidney Diseases (2012). *Weight and waist measurement: Tools for adults.* Retrieved September 2014, from <https://fhs.umr.com/print/UM0868.pdf>.

National Institutes of Health (NIH) (2013a). *General information about parathyroid cancer.*

National Cancer Institute. Retrieved September 2014, from <http://www.cancer.gov/cancertopics/pdq/treatment/parathyroid/Patient/page1>.

National Institutes of Health (NIH) (2013b). *What are overweight and obesity*. National Heart, Lung, and Blood Institute. Retrieved September 2014, from <www.nhlbi.nih.gov/health/health-topics/topics/obe/>.

Tappenden, K. A., Quatrara, B., Parkhurst, M. L., Malone, A. M., Fanjiang, G., & Ziegler, T. R. (2013). Critical role of nutrition in improving quality of care: An interdisciplinary call to action to address adult hospital malnutrition. *Medsurg Nursing, 22*(3), 147–165.

The Institute of Medicine of the National Academies (2014). *Dietary references intakes and application tables*. Retrieved September 2014, from <www.iom.edu/Activities/Nutrition/SummaryDRIs/DRI-Tables.aspx>.

U.S. Department of Agriculture (USDA) (2010). *Dietary guidelines for Americans, 2010*. Retrieved September 2014, from <http://www.fns.usda.gov/dietary-guidelines-americans-2010>.

Virji, A. (2011). *Obesity and weight loss (bariatric surgery)*. Retrieved September 2014, from <www.essentialevidenceplus.com.ezproxy.midwives.org/content/eee/155>.

Yearwood, E., McCulloch, M., Tucker, M., & Riley, J. (2011). Care of the patient with Prader-Willi syndrome. *Medsurg Nursing, 20*(3), 113–122.

Chapter 61

Klee, G. (2011). Laboratory techniques for recognition of endocrine disorders. In S. Melmed, K. Polonsky, P. R. Larsen, & H. Kronenberg (Eds.), *Williams' textbook of endocrinology* (12th ed.). Philadelphia: Saunders.

Lamberts, S. (2011). Endocrinology and aging. In S. Melmed, K. Polonsky, P. R. Larsen, & H. Kronenberg (Eds.), *Williams' textbook of endocrinology* (12th ed.). Philadelphia: Saunders.

Melmed, S., Polonsky, K., Larsen, P. R., & Kronenberg, H. (Eds.), (2011). *Williams' textbook of endocrinology* (12th ed.). Philadelphia: Saunders.

Spiegel, A., Carter-Su, C., Taylor, S., & Kulkarni, R. (2011). Mechanism of action of hormones that act at the cell surface. In S. Melmed, K. Polonsky, P. R. Larsen, & H. Kronenberg (Eds.), *Williams' textbook of endocrinology* (12th ed.). Philadelphia: Saunders.

Chapter 62

Aschenbrenner, D. (2012). Drug watch: FDA approves first drug for endogenous Cushing's syndrome. *The American Journal of Nursing, 112*(6), 26–27.

Collins, M., & Claros, E. (2011). Recognizing the face of dehydration. *Nursing, 41*(8), 26–31.

Crawford, A., & Harris, H. (2011). Balancing act: Na+ and K+. *Nursing, 41*(7), 44–50.

Crawford, A., & Harris, H. (2012). SIADH: Fluid out of balance. *Nursing, 42*(9), 50–58.

Hunt, D. (2012). Is it Addison's disease or Cushing syndrome? *American Nurse Today, 7*(1), 8–11.

John, C., & Day, M. (2012). Central neurogenic diabetes insipidus, syndrome of inappropriate secretion of antidiuretic hormone, and cerebral salt-wasting syndrome in traumatic brain injury. *Critical Care Nurse, 32*(2), e1–e7.

Manchester, C. (2013). Multiple endocrine neoplasia: The enigma of MEN. *AACN Advanced Critical Care, 24*(3), 304–313.

McKeage, K. (2013). Pasireotide: A review of its use in Cushing's disease. *Drugs, 73*(6), 563–574.

Melmed, S., Kleinberg, D., & Ho, K. (2011). Pituitary physiology and diagnostic evaluation. In S. Melmed, K. Polonsky, P. R. Larsen, & H. Kronenberg (Eds.), *Williams' textbook of endocrinology* (12th ed.). Philadelphia: Saunders.

Melmed, S., Polonsky, K., Larsen, P. R., & Kronenberg, H. (Eds.), (2011). *Williams' textbook of endocrinology* (12th ed.). Philadelphia: Saunders.

Online Mendelian Inheritance in Man (OMIM) (2012). *Diabetes insipidus, nephrogenic, Autosomal*. Retrieved August 2014, from <www.omim.org/entry/125800>.

Online Mendelian Inheritance in Man (OMIM) (2011). *Diabetes insipidus, nephrogenic, X-linked*. Retrieved January 2014, from <www.omim.org/entry/304800>.

Online Mendelian Inheritance in Man (OMIM) (2014). *Pheochromocytoma, Susceptibility to*. Retrieved August 2014, from <www.omim.org/entry/171300>.

*Radovich, P. (2010). Primary adrenal insufficiency: Elusive and potentially life-threatening. *American Nurse Today, 5*(3), 37–39.

Robinson, A., & Verbalis, J. (2011). Posterior pituitary. In S. Melmed, K. Polonsky, P. R. Larsen, & H. Kronenberg (Eds.), *Williams' textbook of endocrinology* (12th ed.). Philadelphia: Saunders.

Stewart, P., & Krone, N. (2011). The adrenal cortex. In S. Melmed, K. Polonsky, P. R. Larsen, & H. Kronenberg (Eds.), *Williams' textbook of endocrinology* (12th ed.). Philadelphia: Saunders.

United States Food and Drug Administrations (USFDA) (2013). *Samsca (Tolvaptan): Drug Safety Communication-FDA limits duration and usage due to possible liver injury leading to organ transplant or death*. Retrieved August 2014, from <www.fda.gov/Safety/MedWatch/SafetyInformation/SafetyAlertsforHumanMedicalProducts/ucm350185>.

Yam, F., & Eraly, S. (2012). Syndrome of inappropriate antidiuretic hormone associated with moxifloxacin. *American Journal of Health-System Pharmacists, 69*(3), 217–220.

Young, W. (2011). Endocrine hypertension. In S. Melmed, K. Polonsky, P. R. Larsen, & H. Kronenberg (Eds.), *Williams' textbook of endocrinology* (12th ed.). Philadelphia: Saunders.

Chapter 63

American Cancer Society (2014). *Cancer facts and figures 2014*. Report No. 00-300M–No. 500814. Atlanta: Author.

Brent, G., & Davies, T. (2011). Hypothyroidism and thyroiditis. In S. Melmed, K. Polonsky, P. R. Larsen, & H. Kronenberg (Eds.), *Williams' textbook of endocrinology* (12th ed.). Philadelphia: Saunders.

Bringhurst, F. R., Demay, M., & Kronenberg, H. (2011). Hormones and disorders of mineral metabolism. In S. Melmed, K. Polonsky, P. R. Larsen, & H. Kronenberg (Eds.), *Williams' textbook of endocrinology* (12th ed.). Philadelphia: Saunders.

Burton, J. (2011). Hyperthyroidism. *Medsurg Nursing, 20*(3), 152–153.

Burton, J. (2012). Primary hypothyroidism. *Medsurg Nursing, 21*(3), 169–170.

Crawford, A., & Harris, H. (2011). Balancing act: Hypomagnesemia and hypermagnesemia. *Nursing, 41*(10), 52–55.

Crawford, A., & Harris, H. (2012). Thyroid imbalances: Dealing with disorderly conduct. *Nursing, 42*(11), 45–50.

Hampton, J. (2013). Thyroid gland emergencies: Thyroid storm and myxedema coma. *AACN Advanced Critical Care, 24*(3), 325–332.

Kapustin, J., & Schofield, D. (2012). Hyperparathyroidism: An incidental finding. *The Nurse Practitioner, 37*(11), 9–14.

Mandel, S., Larsen, P. R., & Davies, T. (2011). Thyrotoxicosis. In S. Melmed, K. Polonsky, P. R. Larsen, & H. Kronenberg (Eds.), *Williams' textbook of endocrinology* (12th ed.). Philadelphia: Saunders.

Melmed, S., Polonsky, K., Larsen, P. R., & Kronenberg, H. (Eds.), (2011). *Williams' textbook of endocrinology* (12th ed.). Philadelphia: Saunders.

Mosher, M. (2011). Amiodarone-induced hypothyroidism and other adverse effects. *Dimensions of Critical Care Nursing, 30*(2), 87–93.

Online Mendelian Inheritance in Man (OMIM) (2014). *Graves disease, susceptibility to, 1*. Retrieved November 2014, from <www.omim.org/entry/275000>.

Salvatore, D., Davies, T., Schlumberger, M., Hay, I., & Larsen, P. R. (2011). Thyroid physiology and diagnostic evaluation of patients with thyroid disorders. In S. Melmed, K. Polonsky, P. R. Larsen, & H. Kronenberg (Eds.), *Williams' textbook of endocrinology* (12th ed.). Philadelphia: Saunders.

Woodhouse, K. (2012). Thyrotoxicosis: Evaluation and treatment of a multinodular goiter. *The Nurse Practitioner, 37*(7), 6–10.

Chapter 64

Acee, A. (2012). Type 2 diabetes and vascular dementia: Assessment and clinical strategies of care. *Medsurg Nursing, 21*(6), 349–353.

American Association of Diabetes Educators (AADE) (2011). *AADE position statement:*

Diabetes and physical activity. <Diabeteseducator.org/>.

American Diabetes Association (ADA). (2013). Position statement: Standard of medical care in diabetes—2013. *Diabetes Care, 36*(Suppl. 1), S11–S66.

American Diabetes Association (ADA). (2014a). Diabetic retinopathy and other ocular findings in the Diabetes Control and Complications Trial/Epidemiology of Diabetes Interventions and Complications Study. *Diabetes Care, 37*(1), 17–23.

American Diabetes Association (ADA). (2014b). Kidney disease and related findings in the Diabetes Control and Complications Trial/ Epidemiology of Diabetes Interventions and Complications Study. *Diabetes Care, 37*(1), 24–30.

American Diabetes Association (ADA). (2014c). National standards: National standards for diabetes self-management education and support. *Diabetes Care, 37*(Suppl. 1), S144–S153.

American Diabetes Association (ADA). (2014d). Position statement: Diagnosis and classification of diabetes mellitus. *Diabetes Care, 37*(Suppl. 1), S81–S90.

American Diabetes Association (ADA). (2014e). Position statement: Nutritional recommendations and interventions for diabetes. *Diabetes Care, 37*(Suppl. 1), S120–S143.

American Diabetes Association (ADA). (2014f). Update on cardiovascular outcomes at 30 years of the Diabetes Control and Complications Trial/Epidemiology of Diabetes Interventions and Complications Study. *Diabetes Care, 37*(Suppl. 1), S39–S43.

Aschenbrenner, D. (2012). First drug approved for treating diabetic macular edema. *The American Journal of Nursing, 112*(12), 20.

Bosak, K. (2012a). Managing metabolic syndrome in women. *The Nurse Practitioner, 37*(8), 14–20.

Bosak, K. (2012b). Managing metabolic syndrome: Focus on physical activity. *The Journal for Nurse Practitioners, 8*(3), 206–211.

Brady, V. (2013). Management of hyperglycemia in the intensive care unit: When glucose reaches critical levels. *Critical Care Nursing Clinics of North America, 25*(1), 7–13.

Carter, B., Barba, B., & Kautz, D. (2013). Culturally tailored education for African Americans with type 2 diabetes. *Medsurg Nursing, 22*, 105–109, 123.

Centers for Disease Control and Prevention (2011). *National diabetes fact sheet: National estimates and general information on diabetes and prediabetes in the United States.* Atlanta: U.S. Department of Health and Human Services.

Chou, C., Sherrod, C., Zhang, Z., Barker, L., Bullard, K., Crews, J., et al. (2014). Barriers to eye care among people aged 40 years and older with diagnosed diabetes, 2006-2010. *Diabetes Care, 37*(1), 180–188.

Chow, E., Foster, H., Gonzales, V., & McIver, L. (2012). The disparate impact of diabetes on racial/ethnic minority populations. *Clinical Diabetes, 30*(3), 130–133.

Crawford, K. (2013). Guidelines for care of the hospitalized patient with hyperglycemia and diabetes. *Critical Care Nursing Clinics of North America, 25*(1), 1–6.

Dokken, B. (2013). How insulin analogues can benefit patients. *The Nurse Practitioner, 38*(2), 44–48.

Freeland, B., & Funnell, M. (2012). Corticosteroid-induced hyperglycemia. *Nursing, 42*(11), 68–69.

Funnell, M. (2014). Managing the pain of diabetic peripheral neuropathy. *Nursing, 44*(7), 64–65.

Glover, T., & Galvan, E. (2013). Diabetes and heart failure. *Critical Care Nursing Clinics of North America, 25*(1), 93–99.

Hughes, L. (2012a). Assessing a patient with an insulin pump. *Nursing, 42*(9), 62–64.

Hughes, L. (2012b). Think "SAFE": Four crucial elements for diabetes education. *Nursing, 42*(1), 58–61.

Hunt, C., Sanderson, B., & Ellison, K. J. (2014). Support for diabetes using technology: A pilot study to improve self-management. *Medsurg Nursing, 23*(8), 231–237.

Kopecky, C. (2013). Use of noninsulin antidiabetic medications in hospitalized patients. *Critical Care Nursing Clinics of North America, 25*(1), 39–53.

Krolewski, A., Niewczas, M., Skupien, J., Gohda, T., Smiles, A., Eckfeldt, J., et al. (2014). Early progressive renal decline precedes the onset of microalbuminuria and its progression to macroalbuminuria. *Diabetes Care, 37*(Suppl. 1), S226–S234.

Kubacka, B. (2014). A balancing act: Achieving glycemic control in hospitalized patients. *Nursing, 44*(1), 30–37.

Levesque, C. (2013a). Management of hypertension in patients with diabetes. *Critical Care Nursing Clinics of North America, 25*(1), 71–91.

Levesque, C. (2013b). Perioperative care of patients with diabetes. *Critical Care Nursing Clinics of North America, 25*(1), 21–29.

Link, D. (2013). New paradigms in managing chronic kidney disease. *The Clinical Advisor, 16*(1), 18–23.

Martin, A. (2013). Intravenous insulin infusions: What nurses need to know. *Critical Care Nursing Clinics of North America, 25*(1), 15–20.

McCrea, D. (2013). Management of the hospitalized diabetes patient with an insulin pump. *Critical Care Nursing Clinics of North America, 25*(1), 111–121.

Mompoint-Williams, D., Watts, P., & Appel, S. (2012). Detecting and treating hypoglycemia in patients with diabetes. *Nursing, 42*(8), 50–52.

National Institute of Diabetes and Digestive and Kidney Diseases (NIDDK) of the National Institutes of Health (2011). *National Diabetes Information Clearing House: National diabetes statistics, 2011.* Retrieved September 2014, from <www.diabetes.niddk.nih.gov/statistics/>.

National Kidney Foundation. (2012). KDOQI clinical practice guidelines for diabetes and CKD: 2012 update. *American Journal of Kidney Diseases, 60*(5), 850–886.

Palmer, C., & Jessup, A. (2012). Ketoacidosis in patients with type 2 diabetes. *The Nurse Practitioner, 37*(5), 13–17.

Sacks, D., Arnold, M., Bakris, G., Bruns, D., Horvath, A., Kirkman, M., et al. (2011). Guidelines and recommendations for laboratory analysis in the diagnosis and management of diabetes mellitus. *Diabetes Care, 34*(6), 61–99.

Seaquist, E., Anderson, J., Childs, B., Cryer, P., Dagogo-Jack, S., Fish, L., et al. (2013). Hypoglycemia and diabetes: A report of a workgroup of the American Diabetes Association and the Endocrine Society. *Journal of Clinical Endocrinology and Metabolism, 98*(5), 1845–1859.

Sibbald, R., Ayello, E., Alavi, A., Ostrow, B., Lowe, J., Botros, M., et al. (2012). Screening for the high-risk diabetic foot: A 60-second tool. *Advances in Skin & Wound Management, 25*(10), 465–476.

Sisson, E., Mills, J., & Chin, L. (2012). Recent safety updates on type 2 diabetes medications. *The American Journal of Nursing, 112*(12), 49–53.

Smith, J., & Clinard, V. (2013). Diabetes and sudden cardiac death. *US Pharmacist, 38*(2), 38–42.

The Joint Commission (TJC) (2014). *Advanced certification in inpatient diabetes.* Retrieved September 2014, from <www.jointcommision.org/certification/inpatient_diabetes.aspx>.

Thomas, D. (2013). Clinical management of diabetic ulcers. *Clinics in Geriatric Medicine, 29*(2), 433–441.

Trotter, B., Conaway, M., & Burns, S. (2013). Relationship of glucose values to sliding scale insulin (correctional insulin) dose delivery and meal time in acute care patients with diabetes mellitus. *Medsurg Nursing, 22*(2), 99–104, 135.

Young, J. (2011). Educating staff nurses on diabetes: Knowledge enhancement. *Medsurg Nursing, 20*(3), 143–146, 150.

Zitkus, B. (2012). Type 2 diabetes mellitus: An evidence-based update. *The Nurse Practitioner, 37*(7), 28–37.

Chapter 65

Brenner, B. M. (Ed.), (2012). *Brenner & Rector's the kidney* (9th ed.). Philadelphia: Saunders.

Davenport, M., Khalatbari, S., & Ellis, J. (2014). The challenges in assessing contrast-induced nephropathy: Where are we now? *American Journal of Roentgenology, 202*(4), 784–789.

*Dong, K., & Quan, D. (2010). Appropriately assessing renal function for drug dosing. *Nephrology Nursing Journal, 37*(3), 304–308.

Gray, M. (2011). Traces: Making sense of urodynamics testing—part 3: Electromyography of the pelvic floor muscles. *Urologic Nursing, 31*(1), 31–38.

Gray, M. (2012a). Traces: Making sense of urodynamics testing—part 9: Evaluation of detrusor response to bladder filling. *Urologic Nursing, 32*(1), 21–28.

Gray, M. (2012b). Traces: Making sense of urodynamics testing—part 12: Videourodynamics testing. *Urologic Nursing, 32*(4), 193–202.

Lameire, N., & Kellum, J. (2013). Contrast-induced acute kidney injury and renal support for acute kidney injury: A KDIGO summary (Part 2). *Critical Care, 17*(1), 205.

National Kidney Disease Education Program (NKDEP) (2012). *GFR MDRD Calculator for adults (conventional units).* Retrieved October 2014, from <nkdep.nih.gov/lab-evaluation/gfr-calculators/adults-conventional-unit.asp>.

Puzantian, H. V., & Townsend, R. R. (2013). Understanding kidney function assessment: The basics and advances. *Journal of the American Association of Nurse Practitioners, 25*(7), 334–341.

Society of Urologic Nurses and Associates (2014). *Patient Education.* Retrieved October 2014, from <https://www.suna.org/resource/patient-education>.

U.S. Renal Data Systems (2013). *USRDS 2013 annual data report: Atlas of chronic kidney disease and end-stage renal disease in the United States.* Bethesda, MD: The National Kidney and Urologic Diseases Information Clearinghouse (NKUDIC). National Institutes of Health.

Wood, S. (2012). Contrast-induced nephropathy in critical care. *Critical Care Nurse, 32*(6), 15–24.

Chapter 66

Agency for Healthcare Research and Quality (AHRQ) (2012). *Non-surgical treatments for urinary incontinence in adult women: Diagnosis and comparative effectiveness. AHRQ Comparative Effectiveness Reviews.* Rockville, MD: Author. Retrieved October 2014, from <http://effectivehealthcare.ahrq.gov/index.cfm/search-for-guides-reviews-and-reports/?productid=1021&pageaction=displayproduct>.

American Cancer Society (ACS) (2014). *Cancer facts and figures 2014.* Report No. 01-300M–No. 500814. Atlanta: Author.

Bagga, H. S., Tasian, G. E., Fisher, P. B., McCulloch, C. E., McAninch, J. W., & Breyer, B. N. (2013). Product related adult genitourinary injuries treated at emergency departments in the United States from 2002 to 2010. *Journal of Urology, 189*(4), 1362–1368.

Bernard, M. S., Hunter, K. F., & Moore, K. N. (2012). A review of strategies to decrease the duration of indwelling urethral catheters and potentially reduce the incidence of catheter-associated urinary tract infections. *Urologic Nursing, 32*(1), 29–37.

Brenner, B. (2012). *Brenner & Rector's the kidney* (9th ed.). Philadelphia: Saunders.

Brusch, J. L. (2013). *Cystitis in females.* emedicine, 5. Accessed October 2014, from <http://emedicine.medscape.com/article/233101-overview#showall>.

*Buckley, B. S., Lapitan, M. C., & Epidemiology Committee of the Fourth International Consultation on Incontinence, Paris. (2010). Prevalence of urinary incontinence in men, women, and children—current evidence: Findings of the Fourth International Consultation on Incontinence. *Urology, 76*(2), 265–270.

Canadian Cancer Society, Statistics Canada (2014). *Canadian Cancer Statistics, 2014.* Toronto: Canadian Cancer Society.

Centers for Disease Control and Prevention (CDC) (2013). *Guideline for prevention of catheter-associated urinary tract infections, 2013.* Retrieved February2014, from <www.cdc.gov/>.

Christian, R. (2014). Do prophylactic antibiotics reduce UTI risk after urodynamic studies? *The American Journal of Nursing, 114*(2), 20.

Dowling-Castronovo, A., & Bradway, C. (2012). *Urinary incontinence. Nursing Standard of Practice Protocol: Urinary incontinence in older adults admitted to acute care. Evidence Based Geriatric Topics.* Retrieved October 2014, from <http://consultgerirn.org/topics/urinary_incontinence/want_to_know_more>.

DuBeau, C. B. (2013). *Approach to women with urinary incontinence. UpToDate.* Retrieved October 2014, from <www.uptodate.com/contents/clinical-presentation-and-diagnosis-of-urinary-incontinence>.

Dudeck, M. A., Horan, T. C., Peterson, K. D., Allen-Bridson, K., Morrell, G., Anttila, A., et al. (2013). National Healthcare Safety Network report, data summary for 2011, device-associated module. *American Journal of Infection Control, 41*(4), 286–300.

Fan, H. L., Chan, S. S., Law, T. S., Cheung, R. Y., & Chung, T. K. (2013). Pelvic floor muscle training improves quality of life of women with urinary incontinence: A prospective study. *The Australian and New Zealand Journal of Obstetrics & Gynaecology, 53*(3), 298–304.

Fink, H. A., Wilt, T. J., Eidman, K. E., Garimella, P. S., MacDonald, R., Rutks, I. R., et al. (2013). Medical management to prevent recurrent nephrolithiasis in adults: A systematic review for an American College of Physicians Clinical Guideline. *Annals of Internal Medicine, 158*(7), 535–543.

Fletcher, R. H. (2013). The risk of taking ascorbic acid. *JAMA Internal Medicine, 173*(5), 375–394.

*Foxman, B. (2010). The epidemiology of urinary tract infection. *Nature Reviews: Urology, 7*(12), 653–660.

Hooton, T. M. (2012). Clinical practice: Uncomplicated urinary tract infection. *New England Journal of Medicine, 366*(11), 1028–1037.

Hopkins, L., McCroskey, D., Reeves, G., & Tanabe, P. (2014). Implementing a urinary tract infection clinical practice guideline in an ambulatory urgent care practice. *The Nurse Practitioner, 39*(4), 50–54.

Jura, Y. H., Townsend, M. K., Curhan, G. C., Resnick, N. M., & Grodstein, F. (2011). Caffeine intake, and the risk of stress, urgency and mixed urinary incontinence. *Journal of Urology, 185*(5), 1775–1780.

Kannankeril, A., Lam, H., Reyes, E., & McCartney, J. (2011). Urinary tract infection rates associated with re-use of catheters in clean intermittent catheterization of male veterans. *Urologic Nursing, 31*(1), 41–48.

Li, K., Lin, T., Zhang, C., Fan, X., Xu, K., Bi, L., et al. (2013). Optimal frequency of shock wave lithotripsy in urolithiasis treatment: A systematic review and meta-analysis of randomized controlled trials. *Journal of Urology, 190*(4), 1260–1267.

Lowe, N. K., & Ryan-Wenger, N. A. (2012). Uncomplicated UTIs in women. *Nurse Practitioner, 37*(5), 41–48.

Mori, C. (2014). A-voiding catastrophe: Implementing a nurse-driven protocol. *Medsurg Nursing, 23*(1), 15–21, 28.

Myles, M. L. (2011). Urinary diversions. *Medsurg Nursing, 20*(2), 94–95.

Newman, D. K., & Willson, M. M. (2011). Review of intermittent catheterization and current best practices. *Urologic Nursing, 31*(1), 12–28, 48.

Pelvic Pain and Urgency Frequency symptom scale: PUF questionnaire. (2005). Retrieved October 2014, from <www.orthoelmiron.com/orthoelmiron/hcptools_puf.html?host>.

Quillin, R. B., & Erickson, D. R. (2012). Practical use of the new American Urological Association interstitial cystitis guidelines. *Current Urology Reports, 13*(5), 394–401.

Ragnarsdóttir, B., Lutay, N., Grönberg-Hernandez, J., Köves, B., & Svanborg, C. (2011). Genetics of innate immunity and UTI susceptibility. *Nature Reviews: Urology, 8*(8), 449–468.

*Richmond, C. F. (2010). Interstitial cystitis—chronic, common, and sometimes complicated to treat. *American Nurse Today, 5*(11), 19–24.

Rodgers, A. L. (2013). Race, ethnicity and urolithiasis: A critical review. *Urolithiasis, 41*(2), 99–103.

Rosa, M., Usai, P., Miano, R., Kim, F. J., Finazzi Agro, E., Bove, P., et al. (2013). Recent finding and new technologies in nephrolithiasis: A review of the recent literature. *BMC Urology, 13*, 10.

Scemons, D. (2013). Urinary incontinence in adults. *Nursing, 43*(11), 52–60.

Shultz, J. M. (2012). Rethink urinary incontinence in older women. *Nursing, 42*(11), 32–40.

Stapleton, A. E., Dziura, J., Hooton, T. M., Cox, M. E., Yarova-Yarovaya, Y., Chen, S., et al. (2012). Recurrent urinary tract infection and urinary *Escherichia coli* in women ingesting cranberry juice daily: A randomized controlled trial. *Mayo Clinic Proceedings, 87*(2), 143–150.

Sur, R. L., Masterson, J. H., Palazzi, K. L., L'Esperance, J. O., Auge, B. K., Chang, D. C., et al. (2013). Impact of statins on nephrolithiasis in hyperlipidemic patients: A 10-year review of an equal access health care system. *Clinical Nephrology, 79*(5), 351–355.

Townsend, M. K., Curhan, G. C., Resnick, N. M., & Grodstein, F. (2011). Original research: Rates of remission, improvement, and progression of urinary incontinence in Asian, Black, and White women. *American Journal of Nursing, 111*(4), 26–33.

Türk, C., Knoll, T., Petrik, A., Sarica, K., Straub, M., Seitz, C., et al. (2011). *Guidelines for urolithiasis*. Retrieved October 2014, from <www.uroweb.org/gls/pdf/18_Urolithiasis.pdf>.

U.S. Renal Data Systems (2012). *USRDS 2011 annual data report*. Bethesda, MD: The National Kidney and Urologic Diseases Information Clearinghouse (NKUDIC). National Institutes of Health.

Wagenlehner, F. M., Lichtenstern, C., Rolfes, C., Mayer, K., Uhle, F., Weidner, W., et al. (2013). Diagnosis and management for urosepsis. *International Journal of Urology, 20*(10), 963–970.

Wilde, M. L., Bliss, D., Booth, J., Cheater, F., & Tannenbaum, C. (2014). Self-management of urinary and fecal incontinence. *The American Journal of Nursing, 114*(1), 38–45.

Chapter 67

Aguiari, G., Catizone, L., & Del Senno, L. (2013). Multidrug therapy for polycystic kidney disease: A review and perspective. *American Journal of Nephrology, 37*(2), 175–182.

American Cancer Society (2014). *Cancer facts and figures 2014*. Report No. 00-300M–No. 500814. Atlanta: Author.

Aragona, F., Pepe, P., Patane, D., Malfa, P., D'Arrigo, L., & Pennisi, M. (2012). Management of severe blunt renal trauma in adult patients: A 10-year retrospective review from an emergency hospital. *BJU International, 110*(5), 744–748.

Aschenbrenner, D. (2012). New drug approved for advanced renal cell cancer. *American Journal of Nursing, 112*(5), 22–23.

Brenner, B. (Ed.), (2012). *Brenner & Rector's the kidney* (9th ed.). Philadelphia: Saunders.

Byar, K., & Workman, M. (2012). Targeted therapies to treat cancer. In J. Kee, E. Hayes, & L. McCuistion (Eds.), *Pharmacology: A nursing process approach* (7th ed.). St. Louis: Saunders.

Canadian Cancer Society, Statistics Canada (2014). *Canadian Cancer Statistics, 2014*. Toronto: Canadian Cancer Society.

Davies, H., & Leslie, G. (2012). Acute kidney injury and the critically ill patient. *Dimensions of Critical Care Nursing, 31*(3), 135–152.

Escobar, G. A., & Campbell, D. N. (2012). Randomized trials in angioplasty and stenting of the renal artery: Tabular review of the literature and critical analysis of their results. *Annals of Vascular Surgery, 26*(3), 434–442.

Fournier, M. (2013). Stemming the rising tide of acute kidney injury. *American Nurse Today, 8*(1), 12–16.

Hahn, B. H., McMahon, M. A., Wilkinson, A., Wallace, W. D., Daikh, D. I., Fitzgerald, J. D., et al. (2012). American College of Rheumatology guidelines for screening, treatment, and management of lupus nephritis. *Arthritis Care & Research (Hoboken), 64*(6), 797–808.

Isaac, S. (2012). Contrast-induced nephropathy: Nursing implications. *Critical Care Nurse, 32*(3), 41–47.

Kidney stones. (2012). Kidney stones. *Nursing, 42*(12), 29.

National Kidney Foundation (2013). *Polycystic kidney disease*. Retrieved October 2014, from <www.kidney.org/atoz/content/polycystic.cfm>.

Online Mendelian Inheritance in Man (OMIM) (2014). *Polycystic kidney disease 1; PKD1*. Retrieved October 2014, from <www.omim.org/entry/173900>.

Patel, C., Ahmed, A., & Ellsworth, P. (2012). Renal cell carcinoma: A reappraisal. *Urologic Nursing, 32*(4), 182–190.

Pengo, M. F., Soloni, P., Cecchin, D., Maiolino, G., Rossi, G. P., & Caló, L. A. (2013). Pelvic-ureteric junction obstruction and hypertension with target organ damage: A case report and review of the literature. *Blood Pressure, 22*(5), 336–339.

U.S. Renal Data Systems (2012). *USRDS 2011 annual data report*. Bethesda, MD: The National Kidney and Urologic Diseases Information Clearinghouse (NKUDIC). National Institutes of Health.

Wood, S. (2012). Contrast-induced nephropathy in critical care. *Critical Care Nurse, 32*(6), 15–23.

Chapter 68

Akker, J. P., Egal, M., & Groeneveld, A. B. (2013). Invasive mechanical ventilation as a risk factor for acute kidney injury in the critically ill: A systematic review and meta-analysis. *Critical Care, 17*(3), R98.

Allegretti, A. S., Steele, D. J., David-Kasdan, J. A., Bajwa, E., Niles, J. L., & Bhan, I. (2013). Continuous renal replacement therapy outcomes in acute kidney injury and end stage renal disease: A cohort study. *Critical Care, 17*(3), R109.

American Nephrology Nurses Association (ANNA) (2011). *Nephrology Nursing Process of Care: Apheresis and Therapeutic Plasma Exchange and Continuous Renal Replacement Therapy*. Pitman, NJ: Author.

Beach, P. R., Hallett, A. M., & Zaruca, K. (2011). Organ donation after circulatory death: Vital partnerships. *The American Journal of Nursing, 111*(5), 32–38.

Beal-Lloyd, D., & Groh, C. J. (2012). Dialysis and sexuality. *Nephrology Nursing Journal, 39*(4), 281–283.

Berger, J. C., Muzaale, A. D., James, N., Hoque, M., Wang, J. M., Montgomery, R. A., et al. (2011). Living kidney donors ages 70 and older: Recipient and donor outcomes. *Clinical Journal of the American Society of Nephrology, 6*(12), 2887–2893.

Davies, H., & Leslie, G. (2012). Acute kidney injury and the critically ill patient. *Dimensions of Critical Care Nursing, 31*(3), 135–152.

Dutka, P. (2012). Erythropoiesis-stimulating agents for the management of anemia of chronic kidney disease: Past advancements and current innovations. *Nephrology Nursing Journal, 39*(6), 447–457.

Elliott, R. W. (2012). Demographics of the older adult and chronic kidney disease: A literature review. *Nephrology Nursing Journal, 39*(6), 491–496.

Elseviers, M. M., Lins, R. L., Van der Niepen, P., Hoste, E., Malbrain, M. L., Damas, P., et al. (2010). Renal replacement therapy is an independent risk factor for mortality in critically ill patients with acute kidney injury. *Critical Care, 14*(6), R221.

Ficorelli, C. T., Edelman, M., & Weeks, B. H. (2013). Living donor renal transplant: A gift of life. *Nursing, 43*(1), 58–62.

Fournir, M. (2013). Stemming the rising tide of acute kidney injury. *American Nurse Today, 8*(1), 12–16.

Fukagawa, M., Komaba, H., & Kakuta, T. (2013). Hyperparathyroidism in chronic kidney disease patients: An update on current pharmacotherapy. *Expert Opinion on Pharmacotherapy, 14*(7), 863–871.

Gentry, S. E., Montgomery, R. A., & Segev, D. L. (2011). Kidney paired donation: Fundamentals, limitations, and expansions. *American Journal of Kidney Diseases, 57*(1), 144–151.

Golestaneh, L., Richter, B., & Amato-Hayes, M. (2012). Logistics of renal replacement therapy: Relevant issues for critical care nurses. *American Journal of Critical Care, 21*(2), 126–130.

Horigan, A., Rocchiccioli, J., & Trimm, D. (2012). Dialysis and fatigue: Implications for nurses—A case study analysis. *Medsurg Nursing, 21*(3), 158–163, 175.

Lewis, R. (2012). Mineral and bone disorders in chronic kidney disease: New insights into mechanism and management. *Annals of Clinical Biochemistry, 49*(Pt. 5), 432–440.

Moore, E. M., Bellomo, R., & Nichol, A. D. (2012). The meaning of acute kidney injury and its relevance to intensive care and anaesthesia. *Anaesthesia and Intensive Care, 40*(6), 929–948.

Obermüller, N., Geiger, H., Weipert, C., & Urbschat, A. (2014). Current developments in early diagnosis of acute kidney injury. *International Urology and Nephrology, 46*(1), 1–7.

Prescott, A. M., Lewington, A., & O'Donoghue, D. (2012). Acute kidney injury: Top ten tips. *Clinical Medicine, 12*(4), 328–332.

Puzantian, H. V., & Townsend, R. R. (2013). Understanding kidney function assessment: The basics and advances. *Journal of the American Association of Nurse Practitioners, 25*(7), 334–341.

Ralib, A. M., Pickering, J. W., Shaw, G. M., & Endre, Z. H. (2013). The urine output definition of acute kidney injury is too liberal. *Critical Care, 17*(3), R112.

Ricci, Z., Cruz, D. N., & Ronco, C. (2011). Classification and staging of acute kidney injury: Beyond the RIFLE and AKIN criteria. *Nature Reviews. Nephrology*, *7*(4), 201–208.

Ryan, E. J. (2012). When do (or don't) you administer drugs to patients on hemodialysis? *Nursing*, *42*(8), 47–49.

Saccomano, S. J., & DeLuca, D. A. (2012). Living with chronic kidney disease: Related issues and treatment. *Nurse Practitioner*, *37*(8), 32–38.

Streets, K. W., & Vickers, S. M. (2012). Is this patient with heart failure a candidate for ultrafiltration? *Nursing*, *42*(6), 30–36.

Taal, M. W. (2012). Risk factors and chronic kidney disease. In M. W. Taal, G. M. Chertow, K. Skorecki, A. S. L. Yu, & B. M. Brenner (Eds.), *Brenner and Rector's the kidney* (9th ed.). Philadelphia: Saunders.

Taal, M. W., Chertow, G. M., Skorecki, K., Yu, A. S. L., & Brenner, B. M. (2012). *Brenner and Rector's the kidney* (9th ed.). Philadelphia: Saunders.

Uchino, S., Bellomo, R., Bagshaw, S. M., & Goldsmith, D. (2010). Transient azotaemia is associated with a high risk of death in hospitalized patients. *Nephrology, Dialysis, Transplantation*, *25*(6), 1833–1839.

United Network for Organ Sharing online (UNOS). (2014). Retrieved October 2014, from <www.unos.org>.

U.S. Renal Data Systems (USRDS) (2014). *USRDS 2013 annual data report*. Bethesda, MD: The National Kidney and Urologic Diseases Information Clearinghouse (NKUDIC). National Institutes of Health. Retrieved October 2014, from <http://kidney.niddk.nih.gov/statistics/index.aspx>.

Vanmassenhove, J., Vanholder, R., Nagler, E., & Van Biesen, W. (2013). Urinary and serum biomarkers for the diagnosis of acute kidney injury: An in-depth review of the literature. *Nephrology, Dialysis, Transplantation*, *28*(2), 254–273.

Wilson, B., & Lawrence, J. (2013). Implementation of a foot assessment program in a regional satellite hemodialysis setting. *Canadian Association of Nephrology Nurses and Technologists Journal*, *23*(2), 41–47.

Wong, L. P., Yamamoto, K. T., Reddy, V., Cobb, D., Chamberlin, A., Pham, H., et al. (2014). Patient education and care for peritoneal dialysis catheter placement: A quality improvement study. *Peritoneal Dialysis International*, *34*(1), 12–23.

Wynne, J., Narveson, S. Y., & Littmann, L. (2012). Cardiorenal syndrome. *Heart and Lung: The Journal of Critical Care*, *41*(2), 157–160.

Yeun, J. Y., Ornt, D., & Depner, T. A. (2012). Hemodialysis. In M. W. Taal, G. M. Chertow, K. Skorecki, A. S. L. Yu, & B. M. Brenner (Eds.), *Brenner and Rector's the kidney* (9th ed.). Philadelphia: Saunders.

Chapter 69

American Cancer Society (ACS) (2014a). *Cancer facts and figures 2013-2014*. Retrieved October 2014, from <www.cancer.org/acs/groups/content/@epidemiologysurveilance/documents/document/acspc-036845.pdf>.

American Cancer Society (ACS) (2014b). *Mammograms*. Retrieved October 2014, from <www.cancer.org/cancer/breastcancer/moreinformation/breastcancerearlydetection/breast-cancer-early-detection-acs-recs-mammograms>.

American Cancer Society (ACS) (2014c). *American Cancer Society recommendations for early breast cancer detection in women without breast symptoms*. Retrieved October 2014, from <www.cancer.org/cancer/breastcancer/moreinformation/breastcancerearlydetection/breast-cancer-early-detection-acs-recs>.

American Congress of Obstetricians and Gynecologists (ACOG) (2011). *Hysterosalpingography*. Retrieved October 2014, from <www.acog.org/~/media/For%20Patients/faq143.pdf?dmc=1&ts=20130827T1635426695>.

Cleveland Clinic (2013). *What is hysteroscopy?* Retrieved October 2014, from <http://my.clevelandclinic.org/services/hysteroscopy/hic_what_is_hysteroscopy.aspx>.

Johns Hopkins Medicine (2014). *Cervical biopsy*. Retrieved October 2014, from <www.hopkinsmedicine.org/healthlibrary/test_procedures/gynecology/cervical_biopsy_92,P07767/>.

Levin, K. (2012). *Transvaginal ultrasound*. Retrieved October 2014, from <www.nlm.nih.gov/medlineplus/ency/article/003779.htm>.

Lowdermilk, D. L., & Perry, S. E. (2014). *Maternity and women's health care* (11th ed.). St. Louis: Mosby.

Mayo Clinic (2013). *Prostate biopsy*. Retrieved October 2014, from <www.mayoclinic.com/health/prostate-biopsy/MY00182/DSECTION=what-you-can-expect>.

National Cancer Institute at the National Institutes of Health (2014). *General information about male breast cancer*. Retrieved October 2014, from <www.cancer.gov/cancertopics/pdq/treatment/malebreast/Patient/page1#Keypoint3>.

*Ruhl, C. (2010). Sleep is a vital sign: Why assessing sleep is an important part of women's health. *Nursing for Women's Health*, *14*(3), 243–247.

Susan G. Komen (2013). *Accuracy of mammograms*. Retrieved October 2014, from <http://ww5.komen.org/BreastCancer/AccuracyofMammograms.html>.

Taş, B., Donatsky, A. M., & Gögenur, I. (2013). Techniques to reduce shoulder pain after laparoscopic surgery for benign gynaecological disease: A systematic review. *Gynecological Surgery*, *10*(3), 169–175.

U.S. Preventive Services Task Force (2013). *Screening for HIV*. Retrieved October 2014, from <www.uspreventiveservicestaskforce.org/uspstf/uspshivi.htm>.

Chapter 70

Alakhras, M. M., Bourne, R. R., Rickard, M. M., Ng, K. H., Pietrzyk, M. M., & Brennan, P. C. (2013). Digital tomosynthesis: A new future for breast imaging? *Clinical Radiology*, *68*(5), e225–e236.

American Cancer Society (ACS) (2013a). *Breast cancer detailed guide*. Atlanta: Author.

American Cancer Society (ACS) (2013b). *Breast cancer facts & figures 2011-2012*. Atlanta: Author.

American College of Obstetricians and Gynecologists (ACOG). (2011). Annual mammogram should start at age 40 years. *Contemporary OB/GYN*, *56*(9), 20.

Amin, A. L., Purdy, A. C., Mattingly, J. D., Kong, A. L., & Termuhlen, P. M. (2013). Multidisciplinary breast management benign breast disease. *Surgical Clinics of North America*, *93*(2), 299–308.

Association of Women's Health, Obstetric, and Neonatal Nursing (AWHONN). (2010). Breast cancer screening: A AWHONN position statement. *Journal of Obstetric, Gynecologic, & Neonatal Nursing*, *39*(5), 608–610.

Beredjick, C. (2012). The lesbian breast cancer link. *Advocate*, *1062*, 16.

Bryan, T., & Snyder, E. (2013). The clinical breast exam: A skill that should not be abandoned. *JGIM: Journal of General Internal Medicine*, *28*(5), 719–722.

Davies, C., Hongchao, P., Godwin, J., Gray, R., Arriagada, R., Raina, V., et al. (2013). Long-term effects of continuing adjuvant tamoxifen to 10 years versus stopping at 5 years after diagnosis of oestrogen receptor-positive breast cancer: ATLAS, a randomised trial. *Lancet*, *381*(9869), 805–816.

Edwards, J., Herzberg, S., Shook, J., Beirne, T., & Schomas, D. (2013). Breast conservation therapy utilizing partial breast brachytherapy for early-stage cancer of the breast: A retrospective review from the Saint Luke's Cancer Institute. *American Journal of Clinical Oncology*, [epub ahead of print].

Greif, J. M., Pezzi, C. M., Klimberg, S., Bailey, L., & Zurack, M. (2012). Gender differences in breast cancer: Analysis of 13,000 breast cancers in men from the National Cancer Data Base. *Annals of Surgical Oncology*, *19*, 3199–3204.

Jankowitz, R. C., & Lee, A. V. (2013). The evolving role of multi-gene tests in breast cancer management. *Oncology*, *27*(3), 210–214.

Johnson, R. H., Chien, F. L., & Bleyer, A. (2013). Incidence of breast cancer with distant involvement among women in the United States, 1976-2009. *Journal of the American Medical Association*, *309*(8), 800–805.

Justice, M., Greenburg, G., Hernick, A. D., & Monroe, P. (2012). Disseminating research findings to the community: Breast cancer advocates conduct education forums. *Environmental Justice*, *5*(3), 128–132.

Kamdar, B., Tergas, A., Mateen, F., Bhayani, N., & Oh, J. (2013). Night-shift work and risk of breast cancer: A systematic review and meta-analysis. *Breast Cancer Research and Treatment*, *138*(1), 291–301.

Kedde, H., Wiel, H. B., Weijmar Schultz, W. C., & Wijsen, C. (2013). Sexual dysfunction in young women with breast cancer. *Supportive Care in Cancer*, *21*(1), 271–280.

Khatcheressian, J., Hurley, P., Bantug, E., Esserman, L., Grunfeld, E., Halberg, F., et al.

(2013). Breast cancer follow-up and management after primary treatment: American Society of Clinical Oncology clinical practice guideline update. *Journal of Clinical Oncology, 31*(7), 961–965.

Klaeson, K. K., Sandell, K. K., & Bertero, C. M. (2011). To feel like an outsider: Focus group discussions regarding the influence on sexuality caused by breast cancer treatment. *European Journal of Cancer Care, 20*(6), 728–737.

Lavigne, E., Holowaty, E. J., Pan, S. Y., Villeneuve, P. J., Johnson, K. C., Furgusson, D. A., et al. (2013). Breast cancer detection and survival among women with cosmetic breast implants: Systematic review and meta-analysis of observational studies. *British Medical Journal, 346*(f2399), 1–12.

Mattarella, A. (2010). Breast cancer in men. *Radiologic Technology, 81*(4), 361M–378M.

McLaughlin, S. (2013). Surgical management of the breast: Breast conservation therapy and mastectomy. *The Surgical Clinics of North America, 93*(2), 411–428.

Mohler, E., & Mondry, T. (2013). *Patient education: Lymphedema after breast cancer surgery (Beyond the basics)*. Retrieved January 2014, from <www.uptodate.com>.

Morgan, S. D., Redman, S., D'Este, C., & Rogers, K. (2011). Knowledge, satisfaction with information, decisional conflict and psychological morbidity amongst women diagnosed with ductal carcinoma in situ (DCIS). *Patient Education and Counseling, 84*, 62–68.

National Breast Cancer Coalition (NBCC) (2012). *Breast cancer deadline 2020: 2nd annual progress report*. Washington, DC: Author.

National LGBT Cancer Network (2013). *About us*. New York: Author.

Ooi, S., Martinez, M., & Li, C. (2011). Disparities in breast cancer characteristics and outcomes by race/ethnicity. *Breast Cancer Research and Treatment, 127*(3), 729–738.

Pollán, M. (2010). Epidemiology of breast cancer in young women. *Breast Cancer Research and Treatment, 123*(Suppl.), 3–6. doi:10.1007/s10549-010-1098-2.

Quinn, E., Corrigan, M., McHugh, S., Murphy, D., O'Mullane, J., Hill, A., et al. (2013). Who's talking about breast cancer? Analysis of daily breast cancer posts on the internet. *Breast, 22*(1), 24–27.

Ridner, S. H., Sinclair, V., Deng, J., Bonner, C. M., Kidd, N., & Dietrich, M. S. (2012). Breast cancer survivors with lymphedema. *Clinical Journal of Oncology Nursing, 16*(6), 609–614.

Saquib, J., Parker, B., Natarajan, L., Madlensky, L., Saquib, N., Patterson, R., et al. (2012). Prognosis following the use of complementary and alternative medicine in women diagnosed with breast cancer. *Complementary Therapies in Medicine, 20*(5), 283–290.

Schmidt, C. (2012). IOM issues report on breast cancer and the environment. *Environmental Health Perspectives, 120*(2), a60–a61.

Soran, A., Ibrahim, A., Kanbour, M., McGuire, K., Balci, F., Polat, A., et al. (2013). Decision making and factors influencing long-term satisfaction with prophylactic mastectomy in women with breast cancer. *American Journal of Clinical Oncology*, [epub ahead of print].

*U.S. Preventive Services Task Force (USPSTF). (2009). Screening for breast cancer: U.S. Preventive Services Task Force recommendations statement. *Annals of Internal Medicine, 151*, 716–726.

Wanchai, A., Armer, J. M., & Stewart, B. R. (2010). Complementary and alternative medicine use among women with breast cancer: A systematic review. *Clinical Journal of Oncology Nursing, 14*(4), 45–55.

Weigelt, B., Geyer, F., & Reis-Filho, J. (2010). Histological types of breast cancer: How special are they? *Molecular Oncology, 4*(3), 192–208.

Williams, A. F. (2012). Living with and beyond breast cancer. *Journal of Community Nursing, 26*(1), 6.

Wyatt, G., Sikorskii, A., Wills, C., & Su, H. (2010). Complementary and alternative medicine use, spending, and quality of life in early stage breast cancer. *Nursing Research, 59*(1), 58–66.

Zakhireh, J., Fowble, B., & Esserman, L. (2010). Application of screening principles to the reconstructed breast. *Journal of Clinical Oncology, 28*(1), 173–180.

Chapter 71

American Cancer Society (ACS) (2014a). *Cancer facts and figures 2013-2014*. Retrieved November 2014, from <www.cancer.org/acs/groups/content/@epidemiologysurveilance/documents/document/acspc-036845.pdf>.

American Cancer Society (ACS) (2014b). *Cervical cancer prevention and early detection*. Retreived November 2014, from <http://www.cancer.org/acs/groups/cid/documents/webcontent/003167-pdf.pdf>.

American Cancer Society (ACS) (2012). *New screening guidelines for cervical cancer*. Retrieved January 2014, from <www.cancer.org/cancer/news/new-screening-guidelines-for-cervical-cancer>.

American Cancer Society (ACS) (2013a). *Cancer facts and figures 2013*. Retrieved November 2014, from <www.cancer.org/acs/groups/content/@epidemiologysurveilance/documents/document/acspc-036845.pdf>.

American Cancer Society (ACS) (2013b). *Sex and pelvic radiation therapy*. Retrieved November 2014, from <www.cancer.org/treatment/treatmentsandsideeffects/physicalsideeffects/sexualsideeffectsinwomen/sexualityforthewoman/sexuality-for-women-with-cancer-pelvic-rad>.

American Cancer Society (ACS) (2014). *Ovarian cancer prevention*. Retrieved November 2014, from <www.cancer.gov/cancertopics/pdq/prevention/ovarian/Patient/page3>.

American Congress of Obstetricians and Gynecologists (ACOG) (2011). *Sonohysterography FAQ*. Retrieved November 2014, from <www.acog.org/~/media/For%20Patients/faq175.pdf?dmc=1&ts=20130830T2133066904>.

American Congress of Obstetricians and Gynecologists (ACOG) (2013). *Statement on robotic surgery by ACOG*. Retrieved November 2014, from <www.acog.org/About_ACOG/News_Room/News_Releases/2013/Statement_on_Robotic_Surgery>.

Bradley, L. (2013). *Hysteroscopic myomectomy*. Retrieved November 2014, from <www.uptodate.com/contents/hysteroscopic-myomectomy>.

Braun, R. (2014). *Bartholin cyst*. Retrieved November 2014, from <www.emedicinehealth.com/bartholin_cyst/page3_em.htm#bartholins_cyst_symptoms>.

Centers for Disease Control and Prevention (CDC) (2014a). *Cervical cancer statistics*. Retrieved November 2014, from <www.cdc.gov/cancer/cervical/statistics/>.

Centers for Disease Control and Prevention (CDC) (2014b). *Genital HPV infection: Fact sheet*. Retrieved November 2014, from <www.cdc.gov/std/hpv/stdfact-hpv.htm>.

Falcone, T. (2014). *Overview of hysterectomy*. Retrieved November 2014, from <www.uptodate.com/contents/overview-of-hysterectomy?detectedLanguage=en&source=search_result&search=hysterectomy+robotic&selectedTitle=3~7&provider=noProvider>.

Gallo, T., Kashani, S., Patel, D. A., Elsahwi, K., Silasi, D. A., & Azodi, M. (2012). Robotic-assisted laparoscopic hysterectomy: Outcomes in obese and morbidly obese patients. *Journal of the Society of Laparoendoscopic Surgeons, 16*(3), 421.

GlaxoSmithKline (2012). *Cervarix*. Retrieved November 2014, from <http://www.cervarix.ca/>.

Lazarou, G. (2012). *Pelvic organ prolapse treatment and management*. Retrieved November 2014, from <http://emedicine.medscape.com/article/276259-treatment#a1134>.

Low, D. (2013). Toxic shock syndrome: Major advances in pathogenesis, but not treatment. *Critical Care Clinics, 29*, 651–675.

Mayo Clinic (2011). *Endometriosis: Definition*. Retrieved January 2014, from <www.mayoclinic.com/health/ca-125-test/MY00590>.

Mayo Clinic (2013). *Endometriosis: Causes*. Retrieved January 2014, from <www.mayoclinic.com/health/endometriosis/DS00289/DSECTION=causes>.

Merck Sharpe & Dohme Corporation (2014). *Gardasil*. Retrieved November 2014, from <http://www.gardasil.com/>.

National Cancer Institute (NCI) (2013a). *Endometrial cancer treatment: Endometrial cancer prevention*. Retrieved November 2014, from <www.cancer.gov/cancertopics/pdq/prevention/endometrial/Patient/page3>.

National Cancer Institute (NCI) (2013b). *A snapshot of endometrial cancer: Incidence and mortality*. Retrieved November 2014, from <http://www.cancer.gov/researchandfunding/snapshots/endometrial>.

Nguyen, M., LaFargue, C., Pua, T., & Tedjarati, S. (2013). Grade 1 endometrioid endometrial carcinoma presenting with pelvic bone metastasis: A case report and review of the literature. *Case Reports in Obstetrics and Gynecology, 2013*, doi:10.1155/2013/807205.

Northwest Radiology Associates (2014). *Uterine fibroid embolization: FAQ*. Retrieved November 2014, from <www.fibroiddoc.com/faq/>.

Saul, T. (2013). *Emergent treatment of endometriosis*. Retrieved November 2014, from <http://emedicine.medscape.com/article/795771-overview>.

Storck, S. (2012). *Uterine artery embolization*. Retrieved November 2014, from <www.nlm.nih.gov/medlineplus/ency/article/007384.htm>.

Storck, S. (2014). *Cervical polyps*. Retrieved November 2014, from <www.nlm.nih.gov/medlineplus/ency/article/001494.htm>.

Turandot, S. (2013). *Emergent treatment of endometriosis*. Retrieved November 2014, from <http://emedicine.medscape.com/article/795771-overview>.

U.S. Food and Drug Administration (USFDA) (2011). *Urogynecologic surgical mesh: Update on the safety and effectiveness of transvaginal placement for pelvic organ prolapse*. Retrieved November 2014, from <www.fda.gov/downloads/MedicalDevices/Safety/AlertsandNotices/UCM262760.pdf>.

Chapter 72

American Cancer Society (ACS) (2014a). *Prostate cancer*. Retrieved November 2014, from <www.cancer.org/cancer/prostatecancer/detailedguide/prostate-cancer-key-statistics>.

American Cancer Society (ACS) (2014b). *Testicular cancer*. Retrieved November 2014, from <www.cancer.org/cancer/testicularcancer/detailedguide/testicular-cancer-key-statistics>.

Barry, M. J., Meleth, S., Lee, J. Y., Kreder, K. J., Avins, A. A., Nickel, J. C., et al. (2011). Effect of increasing doses of saw palmetto extract on lower urinary tract symptoms: A randomized trial. *Journal of the American Medical Association, 306*, 1344–1351.

*Bohenkamp, S., & Yoder, L. H. (2009). The medical-surgical nurse's guide to testicular cancer. *Medsurg Nursing, 18*(2), 116–124.

Carmody, J. F., Olendzki, B. C., Merriam, P. A., Liu, Q., Qiao, Y., & Ma, Y. (2012). A novel measure of dietary change in a prostate cancer dietary program incorporating mindfulness training. *Journal of the Academy of Nutrition and Dietetics, 112*(11), 1822–1827.

Chitlik, A. (2011). Safe positioning for robotic-assisted laparoscopic prostatectomy. *AORN Journal: Association of periOperative Registered Nurses, 94*(1), 37–48.

Cranwell-Bruce, L. A. (2010). Drugs for erectile dysfunction. *Medsurg Nursing, 19*(3), 185–187.

Dunn, M. W., & Kazer, M. W. (2011). Prostate cancer overview. *Seminars in Oncology Nursing, 27*(4), 244–250.

Eltabey, M. A., Sherif, H., & Hussein, A. A. (2010). Holmium laser enucleation versus transurethral resection of the prostate. *Canadian Journal of Urology, 17*(6), 5447–5452.

Galbraith, M. E., Fink, R., & Wilkins, G. G. (2011). Couples surviving prostate cancer: Challenges in their lives and relationships. *Seminars in Oncology Nursing, 27*(4), 300–308.

Hegarty, J., & Bailey, D. E. (2011). Active surveillance as a treatment option for prostate cancer. *Seminars in Oncology Nursing, 27*(4), 260–266.

Johnson, T. V., Abbasi, A., Ehrlich, S. S., Kleris, R. S., Chirumamilla, S. L., Schoenberg, E. D., et al. (2010). Major depression drives severity of American Urological Association Symptom Index. *Urology, 76*(6), 1317–1320.

King, D. (2012). Benign prostatic hyperplasia. *Nursing, 42*(5), 37.

*Leman, E. S., Cannon, G. W., Trock, B. J., Sokoll, L. J., Chan, D. W., Mangold, R., et al. (2007). EPCA-2: A highly specific serum marker for prostate cancer. *Urology, 69*(4), 714–720.

Maliski, S. L., Connor, S. E., Oduro, C., & Litwin, M. S. (2011). Access to health care and quality of life for underserved men with prostate cancer. *Seminars in Oncology Nursing, 27*(4), 267–277.

O'Rourke, M. E. (2011). The prostate-specific antigen screening conundrum: Examining the evidence. *Seminars in Oncology Nursing, 27*(4), 251–259.

Perlman, G., & Drescher, J. (2011). *A gay man's guide to prostate cancer*. Binghamton, NY: Haworth Medical Press.

Roehrborn, C. G. (2011). Male lower urinary tract symptoms (LUTS) and benign prostatic hyperplasia (BPH). *Medical Clinics of North America, 95*(1), 87–100.

*Tackland, J., MacDonald, R., Rutks, I., & Wilt, T. J. (2009). *Serenoa repens* for benign prostatic hyperplasia. *Cochrane Database of Systematic Reviews*, (2), CD001423. Retrieved August 24, 2013, from <www.ncbi.nlm.nih.gov/pubmed/19370565>.

Viatori, M. (2012). Testicular cancer. *Seminars in Oncology Nursing, 28*(3), 180–189.

Wang, C. J., Lin, Y. N., Huang, S. W., & Chang, C. H. (2011). Low dose oral desmopressin for nocturnal polyuria in patients with benign prostatic hyperplasia: A double-blind, placebo controlled, randomized study. *Journal of Urology, 185*(1), 219–223.

Zarowitz, B. J. (2010). Opportunity to optimize management of benign prostatic hyperplasia. *Geriatric Nursing, 31*(6), 441–445.

Chapter 73

*American Nurses Association (ANA) (2001). *Code of ethics for nurses*. Washington, DC: Author.

American Psychiatric Association (APA) (2013). *Diagnostic and statistical manual of mental disorders* (5th ed.). Washington, DC: Author.

Aramburu Alegria, C. (2011). Transgender identity and health care: Implications for psychosocial and physical evaluation. *Journal of the American Academy of Nurse Practitioners, 23*, 175–182.

Brennan, A. M., Barnsteiner, J., Siantz, M. L., Cotter, V. T., & Everett, J. (2012). Lesbian, gay, bisexual, transgendered, or intersexed content for nursing curricula. *Journal of Professional Nursing, 28*(2), 96–104.

Chestnut, S., Dixon, E., & Jindasurat, C. (2013). *Lesbian, gay, bisexual, transgender, queer, and HIV-affected hate violence in 2012*. National Coalition of Anti-Violence Programs. Retrieved September 2014, from <www.avp.org/storage/documents/ncavp_2012_hvreport_final.pdf>.

Coleman, E., Bockting, W., Botzer, M., Cohen-Kettenis, P., DeCuypere, G., Fladman, J., et al. (2011). Standards of care for the health of transsexual, transgender, and gender-nonconforming people (Version 7). *International Journal of Transgenderism, 13*, 165–232.

Conron, K. J., Mimiago, M. J., & Landers, S. J. (2010). A population-based study of sexual orientation identity and gender differences in African Americans. *American Journal of Public Health, 100*, 1953–1960.

Edwards-Leeper, L., & Spack, N. P. (2013). Psychological evaluation and medical treatment of transgender youth in an interdisciplinary "Gender Management Services" (GeMS) in a major pediatric center. In J. Drescher & W. Byne (Eds.), *Treating transgender children and adolescents: An interdisciplinary discussion*. New York: Routledge.

Eliason, M. J., Chinn, P., Dibble, S. L., & DeJoseph, J. (2013). Open the door for LGBTQ patients. *Nursing, 43*(8), 44–50.

Gates, G. (2011). *How many people are gay, lesbian, bisexual, or transgender?* Williams Institute on Sexual Orientation and Gender Identify Law and Public Policy at UCLA School of Law. Retrieved September 2014, from <http://wiwp.law.ucla.edu/wp-content/uploads/Gates-How-Many-People-LGBT-Apr-2011.pdf>.

Grant, J. M., Mottet, L. A., & Tanis, J. (2010). *National transgender discrimination survey report on health and health care*. National Center for Transgender Equality and National Gay and Lesbian Task Force. Retrieved September 2014, from <http://transequality.org/PDFs/NTDSReportonHealth_final.pdf>.

Grant, J. M., Mottet, L. A., & Tanis, J. (2011). *Injustice at every turn: A report of the national transgender discrimination survey*. National Center for Transgender Equality and National Gay and Lesbian Task Force. Retrieved September 2014, from <http://transequality.org/PDFs/Executive_Summary.pdf>.

Institute of Medicine (IOM) (2011). *The health of LGBT people: Building a foundation for better understanding*. Washington, DC: National Academies Press.

Jenner, C. O. (2010). Transsexual primary care. *Journal of the American Academy of Nurse Practitioners, 22*, 403–408.

Lombardi, E. (2010). Transhealth: A review and guidance for future research—Proceedings from The Summer Institute at the Center for Research on Health and Sexual Orientation, University of Pittsburgh. *Journal of Transgenderism, 12*, 211–229.

Pettinato, M. (2012). Providing care for GLBTQ patients. *Nursing, 42*(12), 22–27.

Reed, H. M. (2011). Aesthetic and functional male to female genital and perineal surgery: Feminizing vaginoplasty. *Seminars in Plastic Surgery, 25*(2), 163–174.

Rounds, K. E., McGrath, B. B., & Walsh, E. (2013). Perspectives on provider behaviors: A qualitative study of sexual and gender minorities regarding quality of care. *Contemporary Nurse, 44*(1), 99–110.

Shipherd, J. C., Maguen, S., Skidmore, W. C., & Abramovitz, S. M. (2011). Potentially traumatic events in a transgender sample: Frequency and associated symptoms. *Traumatology, 17*, 56–67.

Spack, N. P. (2013). Management of transgenderism. *Journal of the American Medical Association, 309*, 478–484.

The Joint Commission (TJC) (2011). *Advancing effective communication, cultural competence, and patient- and family-centered care for the lesbian, gay, bisexual, and transgender community*. Retrieved September 2014, from <www.jointcommission.org/lgbt>.

Chapter 74

Augenbraum, M. (2012). Genital ulcer disease. In M. J. Zenilman & M. Shahmanesh (Eds.), *Sexually transmitted infections: Diagnosis, management and treatment* (pp. 155–163). Sudbury, MA: Jones & Bartlett Learning.

*Bavis, M. P., Smith, D. Y., & Siomos, M. Z. (2009). Genital herpes: Diagnosis, treatment, and counseling in the adolescent patient. *Journal for Nurse Practitioners, 5*(6), 415–420.

Bleich, A. T., Sheffield, J. S., Wendel, G. D., Sigman, A., & Cunningham, G. (2012). Disseminated gonococcal infection in women. *Obstetrics and Gynecology, 119*(3), 597–602.

Centers for Disease Control and Prevention (CDC). (2010a). Seroprevalence of herpes simplex virus type 2 among persons aged 14-49 years—United States, 2005-2008. *Morbidity and Mortality Weekly Report, 59*(15), 456–459.

Centers for Disease Control and Prevention (CDC). (2010b). Sexually transmitted diseases treatment guidelines, 2010. *Morbidity and Mortality Weekly Report, 59*(RR–12), 1–110.

Centers for Disease Control and Prevention (CDC) (2012a). *HPV vaccine information for clinicians—Fact sheet*. Retrieved November 2014, from <www.cdc.gov/std/hpv/stdfact-hpv-vaccine-hcp.htm>.

Centers for Disease Control and Prevention (CDC). (2012b). National and state vaccination coverage among adolescents aged 13-17 years—United States, 2011. *Morbidity and Mortality Weekly Report, 61*(34), 671–677. Retrieved November 2014, from <www.cdc.gov/mmwr/preview/mmwrhtml/mm6134a3.htm>.

Centers for Disease Control and Prevention (CDC) (2012c). *Sexually transmitted disease surveillance 2011*. Atlanta: U.S. Department of Health and Human Services. Retrieved November 2014, from <www.cdc.gov/std/stats11/Surv2011.pdf>.

Centers for Disease Control and Prevention (CDC). (2012d). Update to CDC's sexually transmitted diseases treatment guidelines, 2010: Oral cephalosporins no longer a recommended treatment for gonococcal infections. *Morbidity and Mortality Weekly Report, 61*(31), 590–594.

Centers for Disease Control and Prevention (CDC) (2013a). *CDC fact sheet: Incidence, prevalence, and cost of sexually transmitted infections in the United States*. Retrieved November 2014, from <www.cdc.gov/std/stats/STI-Estimates-Fact-Sheet-Feb-2013.pdf>.

Centers for Disease Control and Prevention (CDC) (2013c). *Guidance on the use of expedited partner therapy in the treatment of gonorrhea*. Retrieved November 2014, from <www.cdc.gov/std/ept/GC-Guidance.htm>.

Centers for Disease Control and Prevention (CDC) (2013d). *Legal status of expedited partner therapy (EPT)*. Retrieved November 2014, from <www.cdc.gov/std/ept/legal/default.htm>.

Centers for Disease Control and Prevention (CDC) (2013e). *Pelvic inflammatory disease treatment: Guidelines, research, & updates*. Retrieved November 2014, from <www.cdc.gov/std/PID/treatment.htm>.

Centers for Disease Control and Prevention (CDC). (2013f). Summary of notifiable diseases, United States, 2011. *Morbidity and Mortality Weekly Report, 60*(53), 1–118. Retrieved November 2014, from <www.cdc.gov/mmwr/PDF/wk/mm6053.pdf>.

Centers for Disease Control and Prevention (CDC) (2014a). *Expedited partner therapy*. Atlanta: U.S. Department of Health and Human Services. Retrieved November 2014, from <www.cdc.gov/std/ept/>.

Centers for Disease Control and Prevention (CDC) (2014b). *Gay and bisexual men's health: Sexually transmitted diseases*. Retrieved November 2014, from <www.cdc.gov/msmhealth/STD.htm>.

Centers for Disease Control and Prevention (CDC) (2014c). *Sexually transmitted diseases: Treatment Guidelines 2010, Special populations*. Retrieved November 2014, from <www.cdc.gov/std/treatment/2010/specialpops.htm#wsw>.

Centers for Disease Control and Prevention (CDC). (2014d). *Syphilis: CDC Fact Sheet*. Retrieved November 2014, from <www.cdc.gov/std/syphilis/stdfact-syphilis-detailed.htm>.

*Cobos, D. G., & Jones, J. (2009). Moving forward: Transgender persons as change agents in health care access and human rights. *Journal of the Association of Nurses in AIDS Care, 20*(5), 341–347.

Datta, D., Dunne, E. F., Saraiya, M., & Markowitz, L. (2012). Human papillomaviruses. In M. J. Zenilman & M. Shahmanesh (Eds.), *Sexually transmitted infections: Diagnosis, management and treatment*. Sudbury, MA: Jones & Bartlett Learning.

Fenton, K. A., & French, P. (2012). Infectious syphilis. In M. J. Zenilman & M. Shahmanesh (Eds.), *Sexually transmitted infections: Diagnosis, management and treatment* (pp. 80–82). Sudbury, MA: Jones & Bartlett Learning.

GlaxoSmithKline. (2012). *Cervarix*. Retrieved November 2014, from <http://www.cervarix.ca/>.

Holmes, K. K., Sparling, P. F., Stamm, W. E., Wasserheit, J. N., Corey, L., et al. (Eds.), (2008). *Sexually transmitted diseases* (4th ed.). New York: McGraw-Hill.

Jeffers, L. A., & DiBartolo, M. C. (2011). Raising health care provider awareness of sexually transmitted disease in patients over 50. *Medsurg Nursing, 20*(6), 285–290.

Johns Hopkins Point of Care-IT Center (2014). *Antibiotic guide*. Retrieved November 2014, from <www.hopkinsguides.com/hopkins/ub>.

Kim, J. J. (2010). Targeted human papillomavirus vaccination of men who have sex with men in the USA: A cost-effectiveness modeling analysis. *The Lancet Infectious Diseases, 10*(12), 845–852.

Koester, K. A., Collins, S. P., Fuller, S. M., Galindo, G. R., Gibson, S., & Steward, W. T. (2013). Sexual healthcare preferences among gay and bisexual men: A qualitative study in San Francisco, California. *PLoS ONE, 8*(8), e71546.

Mark, H., Jordan, E. T., Cruz, J., & Warren, N. (2012). What's new in sexually transmitted infection management: Changes in the 2010 guidelines from the Centers for Disease Control and Prevention. *Journal of Midwifery & Women's Health, 57*(3), 276–284.

Markowitz, L. E., Hariri, S., Lin, C., Dunne, E. F., Steinau, M., McQuillan, G., et al. (2013). Reduction in human papillomavirus (HPV) prevalence among young women following HPV vaccine introduction in the United States, National Health and Nutrition Examination Surveys, 2003-2010. *Journal of Infectious Diseases, 208*(3), 385–393.

Merck Sharpe & Dohme Corporation (2014). *Gardasil*. Retrieved November 2014, from <http://www.gardasil.com/>.

Murphy, J., & Mark, H. (2012). Cervical cancer screening in the era of human papillomavirus testing and vaccination. *Journal of Midwifery & Women's Health, 57*(6), 569–576.

Owusu-Edusei, K., Chesson, H. W., Gift, T. L., Tao, G., Mahajan, R., Ocfemia, M. C., et al. (2013). The estimated direct medical cost of selected sexually transmitted infections in the United States, 2008. *Sexually Transmitted Diseases, 40*(3), 197–201.

Patel, R., & Rompalo, A. (2012). Genital herpes infections. In M. J. Zenilman & M.

Shahmanesh (Eds.), *Sexually transmitted infections: Diagnosis, management and treatment* (pp. 165–176). Sudbury, MA: Jones & Bartlett Learning.

Satterwhite, C. L., Torrone, E., Meites, E., Dunne, E. F., Mahajan, R., Banez Ocfemia, M. C., et al. (2013). Sexually transmitted infections among U.S. women and men: Prevalence and incidence estimates, 2008. *Sexually Transmitted Diseases, 40*(3), 187–193.

Schiffman, M., Wentzensen, N., Wacholder, S., Kinney, W., Gage, J. C., & Castle, P. E. (2011). Human papillomavirus testing in the prevention of cervical cancer. *Journal of the National Cancer Institute, 103*, 368–383.

*Spinola, S. M. (2008). Chancroid and *Haemophilus ducreyi*. In K. K. Holmes, P. F. Sparling, W. E. Stamm, P. Piot, J. N. Wasserheit, L. Corey, et al. (Eds.), *Sexually transmitted diseases* (4th ed., pp. 689–699). New York: McGraw-Hill.

Sweet, R. L. (2012). Pelvic inflammatory disease: Current concepts of diagnosis and management. *Current Infectious Diseases Reports*, [epub ahead of print].

*Trelle, S., Shang, A., Nartey, L., Cassell, J. A., & Low, N. (2007). Improved effectiveness of partner notification for patients with sexually transmitted infections: Systematic review. *BMJ, 334*(7589), 354.

U.S. Department of Health and Human Services (USDHHS), Office of Disease Prevention and Health Promotion (2014). *Healthy People 2020*. Retrieved November 2014, from <www.healthypeople.gov/hp2020/>.

U.S. Preventive Services Task Force (USPSTF) (2014a). *Guide to clinical preventive services, 2014: Recommendations of the U.S. Preventive Services Task Force*. Rockville, MD: Agency for Healthcare Research and Quality. Retrieved November 2014, from <http://www.ahrq.gov/professionals/clinicians-providers/guidelines-recommendations/guide/index.html>.

U.S. Preventive Services Task Force (USPSTF) (2014b). *Sexually transmitted infections: Behavioral Counseling. U.S. Preventive Services Task Force recommendation statement*. AHRQ Publication. 08-05123-EF-2. Retrieved November 2014, from <www.uspreventiveservicestaskforce.org/uspstf08/sti/stirs.htm>.

Warren, T., Gilbert, L., & Mark, H. (2011). Availability of serologic and virologic testing for herpes simplex virus in the largest sexually transmitted disease clinics in the United States. *Sexually Transmitted Diseases, 38*(4), 267–269.

Williamson, C. (2010). Providing care to transgender persons: A clinical approach to primary care, hormones, and HIV management. *Journal of the Association of Nurses in AIDS Care, 21*(3), 221–229.

Zenilman, M. J., & Shahmanesh, M. (2012). *Sexually transmitted infections: Diagnosis, management and treatment*. Sudbury, MA: Jones & Bartlett Learning.

GLOSSARY

A

abdominal acute compartment syndrome (AACS) A complication after abdominal trauma that occurs when the intraabdominal pressure is sustained at greater than 200 mm Hg.

abdominoperineal (AP) resection The surgical removal of the sigmoid colon, rectum, and anus through combined abdominal and perineal incisions. This resection is performed when rectal tumors are present.

ablative The process or act of removing.

abscess A localized collection of pus caused by an inflammatory response to bacteria in tissues or organs.

absolute neutrophil count (ANC) The percentage and actual number of mature circulating neutrophils; used to measure a patient's risk for infection. The higher the numbers, the greater the resistance to infection.

absorption The uptake from the intestinal lumen of nutrients produced by digestion.

acalculia Difficulty with math calculations; caused by brain injury or disease.

acalculous cholecystitis Inflammation of the gallbladder occurring in the absence of gallstones; typically associated with biliary stasis caused by any condition that affects the regular filling or emptying of the gallbladder.

acclimatization The process of adapting to a high altitude; involves physiologic changes that help the body compensate for less available oxygen in the atmosphere.

accommodation The process of maintaining a clear visual image when the gaze is shifted from a distant object to a near object. The eye adjusts its focus by changing the curvature of the lens.

achlorhydria The absence of hydrochloric acid from gastric secretions.

acid A substance that releases hydrogen ions when dissolved in water. The strength of an acid is measured by how easily it releases hydrogen ions in solution.

acidosis An acid-base imbalance in which blood pH is below normal.

acinus The structural unit of the lower respiratory tract consisting of a respiratory bronchiole, an alveolar duct, and an alveolar sac.

Acorn cardiac support device A polyester mesh jacket that is placed over the ventricles to provide support and avoid overstretching the myocardial muscle in the patient with heart failure; reduces heart muscle hypertrophy and assists with improvement of ejection fraction.

acoustic neuroma A benign tumor of cranial nerve VIII; symptoms include damage to hearing, facial movements, and sensation. The tumor can enlarge into the brain, damaging structures in the cerebellum.

active euthanasia Purposeful action that directly causes death; not supported by most professional organizations, including the American Nurses Association.

active immunity Resistance to infection that occurs when the body responds to an invading antigen by making specific antibodies against the antigen. Immunity lasts for years and is natural by infection or artificial by stimulation (e.g., vaccine) of the body's immune defenses.

active surveillance (AS) Observation for cancer, without immediate active treatment.

activities of daily living (ADLs) The activities performed in the course of a normal day, such as bathing, dressing, feeding, and ambulating.

activity therapist See *recreational therapist.*

acute Having relatively greater intensity; marked by a sudden onset and short duration.

acute adrenal insufficiency A life-threatening event in which the need for cortisol and aldosterone is greater than the available supply. Also called "addisonian crisis."

acute arterial occlusion The sudden blockage of an artery, typically in the lower extremity, in the patient with chronic peripheral arterial disease.

acute compartment syndrome (ACS) A complication of a fracture characterized by increased pressure within one or more compartments and causing massive compromise of circulation to the area. Compartments are sheaths of inelastic fascia that support and partition muscles, blood vessels, and nerves in the body.

acute coronary syndrome (ACS) A disorder, including unstable angina and myocardial infarction, that results from obstruction of the coronary artery by ruptured atherosclerotic plaque and leads to platelet aggregation, thrombus formation, and vasoconstriction.

acute gastritis Inflammation of the gastric mucosa or submucosa after exposure to local irritants. Various degrees of mucosal necrosis and inflammatory reaction occur in acute disease. Complete regeneration and healing usually occur within a few days.

acute hematogenous infection An infection resulting from bacteremia, disease, or nonpenetrating trauma that is disseminated by the blood through the circulation.

acute kidney injury (AKI) A rapid decrease in kidney function, leading to the collection of metabolic wastes in the body; formerly called "acute renal failure (ARF)."

acute-on-chronic kidney disease A condition in which acute kidney injury occurs in addition to chronic kidney disease.

acute pain The unpleasant sensory and emotional experience associated with tissue damage that results from acute injury, disease, or surgery.

acute pancreatitis A serious inflammation of the pancreas characterized by a sudden onset of abdominal pain, nausea, and vomiting. It is caused by premature activation of pancreatic enzymes that destroy ductal tissue and pancreatic cells and results in autodigestion and fibrosis of the pancreas.

acute paronychia Inflammation of the skin around the nail, which usually occurs with a torn cuticle or an ingrown toenail.

acute pericarditis An inflammation or alteration of the pericardium, the membranous sac that encloses the heart; may be fibrous, serous, hemorrhagic, purulent, or neoplastic.

acute pyelonephritis Active bacterial infection in the kidney.

acute respiratory distress syndrome (ARDS) Respiratory failure marked by hypoxemia that persists even when 100% oxygen is given, as well as decreased pulmonary compliance, dyspnea, noncardiac-associated bilateral pulmonary edema, and dense pulmonary infiltrates on x-ray.

acute sialadenitis Inflammation of a salivary gland; can be caused by infectious agents, irradiation, or immunologic disorders.

adaptive immunity The immunity that a person's body makes (or can receive) as an adaptive response to invasion by organisms or foreign proteins; occurs either naturally or artificially through lymphocyte responses and can be either active or passive.

addisonian crisis Acute adrenal insufficiency; a life-threatening event in which the need for cortisol and aldosterone is greater than the available supply.

adenocarcinoma Tumor that arises from the glandular epithelial tissue.

adenohypophysis The anterior lobe of the pituitary gland, which makes up about 70% of the gland.

adiponectin An anti-inflammatory and insulin sensitizing hormone.

adipose Fatty.

adjuvant A substance that aids another substance, such as a cancer treatment that uses chemotherapy in addition to surgery.

adjuvant therapy Chemotherapy that is used along with surgery or radiation.

adrenal crisis Acute adrenocortical insufficiency, which can be life threatening.

adrenal Cushing's disease An excess of glucocorticoids caused by a problem in the adrenal cortex, usually a benign tumor (adrenal adenoma). This usually occurs in only one adrenal gland.

advance directive (AD) A written document prepared by a competent person to specify what, if any, extraordinary actions he or she would want when no longer able to make decisions about personal health care.

adverse drug event (ADE) An unintended harmful reaction to an administered drug.

aerosolization Transmission via fine airborne droplets.

aesthetic plastic surgery Plastic surgery that is cosmetic and aims to alter a person's physical appearance.

afferent arteriole The smallest, most distal portion of the renal arterial system that supplies blood to the nephron. From the afferent arteriole, blood flows into the glomerulus, a series of specialized capillary loops.

after-drop A continued decrease in core body temperature after a victim is removed from a cold environment; results from equilibration of core and peripheral blood temperature and counter-current cooling of the blood perfusing cold tissue.

afterload The pressure or resistance that the ventricles must overcome to eject blood through the semilunar valves and into the peripheral blood vessels; the amount of resistance is directly related to arterial blood pressure and blood vessel diameter.

agglutination A clumping action that results during the antibody-binding process when antibodies link antigens together to form large and small immune complexes.

agnosia A general term for a loss of sensory comprehension; may include an inability to write, comprehend reading material, or use an object correctly.

agraphia Loss of the ability to write; caused by brain injury or disease.

Airborne Precautions Infection control guidelines from the Centers for Disease Control and Prevention; used for patients with infections spread by the airborne transmission route, such as tuberculosis. Negative airflow rooms are required to prevent the airborne spread of microbes.

akinesia Slow or no movement, as seen in a patient with Parkinson disease. Also called "bradykinesia."

albuminuria The presence of albumin in the urine.

alcoholic hepatitis Liver inflammation caused by the toxic effect of alcohol on hepatocytes. The liver becomes enlarged, with cellular degeneration and infiltration by fat, leukocytes, and lymphocytes.

aldosterone The chief mineralocorticoid produced by the adrenal cortex. Aldosterone increases kidney reabsorption of sodium and water, thus restoring blood pressure, blood volume, and blood sodium levels. Aldosterone secretion is regulated by the renin-angiotensin system, serum potassium ion concentration, and adrenocorticotropic hormone.

alexia Complete inability to understand written language; caused by brain injury or disease.

alkaline reflux gastropathy A complication of gastric surgery in which the pylorus is bypassed or removed. Endoscopic examination reveals regurgitated bile in the stomach and mucosal hyperemia. Symptoms include early satiety, abdominal discomfort, and vomiting. Also called "bile reflux gastropathy."

alkalosis An acid-base imbalance in which blood pH is above normal.

allele An alternate form (or variation) of a gene.

allergen A foreign protein that is capable of causing a hypersensitivity response, or allergy, that ranges from uncomfortable (itchy, watery eyes or sneezing) to life threatening (allergic asthma, anaphylaxis, bronchoconstriction, or circulatory collapse); causes a release of natural chemicals, such as histamine, in the body.

allergy An increased or excessive response to the presence of a foreign protein or allergen (antigen) to which the patient has been previously exposed.

allogeneic bone marrow transplantation The transplantation of bone marrow from a sibling.

allograft A graft of tissue or bone between individuals of the same species but a different genotype; the donor may be a cadaver or a living person, either related or unrelated. Also called "homograft."

alopecia Hair loss.

alveolitis Inflammation of the alveoli.

amaurosis fugax A transient, brief episode of blindness in one eye.

ambulatory A term that refers to a patient who goes to the hospital or physician's office for treatment and returns home on the same day.

ambulatory aid Assistive device such as a cane or a walker.

ambulatory pump Infusion therapy pump generally used with a home care patient to allow a return to his or her usual activities while receiving infusion therapy.

amenorrhea The absence of menstrual periods in women.

amnesia Loss of memory.

amputation The removal of a limb or other appendage of the body.

amyotrophic lateral sclerosis (ALS) A progressive and degenerative disease of the motor system that is characterized by atrophy of the hands, forearms, and legs and results in paralysis and death. There is no known cause, no cure, no specific treatment, no standard pattern of progression, and no method of prevention. Also called "Lou Gehrig's disease."

anaerobic Lacking adequate oxygen.

anaerobic cellular metabolism Metabolism without oxygen.

anal fissure A painful ulcer at the margin of the anus.

analgesia Pain relief or pain suppression.

anaphylaxis The widespread reaction that occurs in response to contact with a substance to which the person has a severe allergy (antigen); characterized by blood vessel and bronchiolar smooth muscle involvement causing widespread blood vessel dilation, decreased cardiac output, and bronchoconstriction; results in cell damage and the release of large amounts of histamine, severe hypovolemia, vascular collapse, decreased cardiac contraction, and dysrhythmias and causes extreme whole-body hypoxia.

anasarca Generalized edema.

anastomosis Surgical reattachment. Also a general term meaning "a connection."

anatomic dead space Places in which air flows but the structures are too thick for gas exchange.

anemia A clinical sign of some abnormal condition related to a reduction in one of the following: number of red blood cells, amount of hemoglobin, or hematocrit (percentage of packed red blood cells per deciliter of blood).

anergy The inability to mount an immune response to an antigen.

anesthesia An induced state of partial or total loss of sensation with or without loss of consciousness.

aneuploid (aneuploidy) An abnormal karyotype with more or fewer than 23 pairs of chromosomes.

aneurysm A permanent localized dilation of an artery (to at least 2 times its normal diameter) that forms when the middle layer (media) of the artery is weakened, stretching the inner (intima) and outer (adventitia) layers. As the artery widens, tension in the wall increases and further widening occurs, thus enlarging the aneurysm.

aneurysmectomy A surgical procedure performed to excise an aneurysm.

angina pectoris Literally, "strangling of the chest"; a temporary imbalance between the ability of the coronary arteries to supply oxygen and the demand for oxygen by the cardiac muscle. As a result, the patient experiences chest discomfort.

angioedema Diffuse swelling resulting from a vascular reaction in the deep tissues; can occur in a patient having an anaphylactic reaction.

anion Ion that has a negative charge.

anisocoria A difference in the size of the pupils.

ankle-brachial index (ABI) A ratio derived by dividing the ankle blood pressure by the brachial blood pressure; this calculation is used to assess the vascular status of the lower extremities. To obtain the ABI, a blood pressure cuff is applied to the lower extremities just above the malleoli. The systolic pressure is measured by Doppler ultrasound at both the dorsalis pedis and posterior tibial pulses. The higher of these two pressures is then divided by the higher of the two brachial pulses.

anomia Inability to find words.

anorectal abscess A localized induration and fluctuance that is caused by inflammation of the soft tissue near the rectum or anus and is most often the result of obstruction of the ducts of glands in the anorectal region by feces, foreign bodies, or trauma.

anorectic drugs Drugs that suppress appetite, which reduces food intake and, over time, may result in weight loss; may be prescribed for obese patients in a comprehensive weight reduction program.

anorexia The loss of appetite for food.

anorexia nervosa An eating disorder of self-induced starvation resulting from a fear of fatness, even though the patient is underweight.

anorexin Neuropeptide that decreases appetite.

anoxic Completely lacking oxygen.

antalgic (gait) A term that refers to an abnormality in the stance phase of gait. When part of one leg is painful, the person shortens the stance phase on the affected side.

anterior colporrhaphy Surgery for severe symptoms of cystocele in which the pelvic muscles are tightened for better bladder support.

anterior nares The nostrils or external openings into the nasal cavities.

antibody-mediated immunity (AMI) or antibody-mediated immune system The defense response that produces antibodies directed against certain pathogens. The antibodies inactivate the pathogens and protect against future infection from that microorganism.

antidepressants A group of drugs that help manage clinical depression.

antiepileptic drugs (AEDs) A class of drugs used to control seizures. Also called "anticonvulsants."

antigen A foreign protein or allergen that is capable of causing an immune response; protein on the surface of a cell.

anuria Complete lack of urine output; usually defined as less than 100 mL/24 hr.

aortic regurgitation The flow of blood from the aorta back into the left ventricle during diastole; occurs when the aortic valve leaflets do not close properly during diastole and the annulus (the valve ring that attaches to the leaflets) is dilated or deformed.

aortic stenosis Narrowing of the aortic valve orifice and obstruction of left ventricular outflow during systole.

aphasia Inability to use or comprehend spoken or written language due to brain injury or disease.

apheresis A procedure in which whole blood is withdrawn from the patient, a blood component (e.g., stem cells) is filtered out, and the plasma is returned to the patient.

aphonia Inability to produce sound; complete but temporary loss of the voice.

aphthous stomatitis Noninfectious stomatitis.

apical impulse The pulse located at the left fifth intercostal space in the midclavicular line in the mitral area (the apex of the heart). Also called the "point of maximal impulse."

apolipoprotein E One of several regulators of lipoprotein metabolism.

appendectomy Surgical removal of the inflamed appendix.

appendicitis Acute inflammation of the vermiform appendix, which is the blind pouch attached to the cecum of the colon, usually located in the right iliac region just below the ileocecal valve.

approximated In a clean laceration or a surgical incision to be closed with sutures or staples, the act of bringing together the wound edges with the skin layers lined up in correct anatomic position so they can be held in place until healing is complete.

apraxia The loss of the ability to carry out a purposeful motor activity.

aqueous humor The clear, watery fluid that is continually produced by the ciliary processes and fills the anterior and posterior chambers of the eye. This fluid drains through the canal of Schlemm into the blood to maintain balanced intraocular pressure (pressure within the eye).

arcus senilis An opaque ring within the outer edge of the cornea caused by fat deposits. Its presence does not affect vision.

areflexic bladder Urinary retention and overflow (dribbling) caused by injuries to the lower motor neuron at the spinal cord level of S2 to S4 (e.g., multiple sclerosis and spinal cord injury below T12). Bladder emptying may be achieved by performing a Valsalva maneuver or tightening the abdominal muscles. The effectiveness of these maneuvers should be ascertained by catheterizing the patient for residual urine after voiding. Also called "flaccid bladder."

arrhythmogenic right ventricular cardiomyopathy (dysplasia) A form of cardiomyopathy that results from the replacement of myocardial tissue with fibrous and fatty tissue.

arterial revascularization The surgical procedure most commonly used to increase arterial blood flow in the affected limb of a patient with peripheral arterial disease.

arterial ulcers A painful complication in the patient with peripheral arterial disease. Typically, the ulcer is small and round, with a "punched out" appearance and well-defined borders. Ulcers develop on the toes (often the great toe), between the toes, or on the upper aspect of the foot. With prolonged occlusion, the toes can become gangrenous.

arteriography Angiography of the arterial vessels; this invasive diagnostic procedure involves fluoroscopy and the use of a contrast medium and is performed when an arterial obstruction, narrowing, or aneurysm is suspected.

arteriosclerosis A thickening, or hardening, of the arterial wall.

arteriotomy A surgical opening into an artery.

arteriovenous malformation (AVM) An abnormality that occurs during embryonic development, resulting in a tangled mass of malformed, thin-walled, dilated vessels. The congenital absence of a capillary network in these vessels forms an abnormal communication between the arterial and venous systems and increases the risk that the vessels may rupture, causing bleeding, such as into the subarachnoid space or into the intracerebral tissue with brain AVMs. In the absence of the capillary network, the thin-walled veins are subjected to arterial pressure.

arthralgia Pain in a joint.

arthritis Inflammation of one or more joints.

arthrodesis The surgical fusion of a joint.

arthrogram An x-ray study of a joint after contrast medium (air or solution) has been injected to enhance its visualization.

arthroscopy Procedure in which a fiberoptic tube is inserted into a joint for direct visualization of the ligaments, menisci, and articular surfaces of the joint.

articulations Joint surfaces.

artifact In the electrocardiogram, interference that is seen on the monitor or rhythm strip and may look like a wandering or fuzzy baseline; can be caused by patient movement, loose or defective electrodes, improper grounding, or faulty equipment.

ascending tracts Groups of nerves that originate in the spinal cord and end in the brain.

ascites The accumulation of free fluid within the peritoneal cavity. Increased hydrostatic pressure from portal hypertension causes this fluid to leak into the peritoneal cavity.

assistive/adaptive device Any item that enables the patient to perform all or part of an activity independently.

assistive technology Electronic equipment that increases the ability of disabled patients to care for themselves.

asterixis A coarse tremor characterized by rapid, nonrhythmic extensions and flexions in the wrists and fingers; a motor disturbance seen in portal-systemic encephalopathy. Also called a "liver flap" or "flapping tremor."

asthma A chronic respiratory condition in which reversible airflow obstruction in the airways occurs intermittently.

astigmatism A refractive error caused by unevenly curved surfaces on or in the eye (especially of the cornea) that distort vision.

ataxia Gait disturbance or loss of balance.

atelectasis Collapse of alveoli.

atelectrauma Shear injury to alveoli from opening and closing.

atherectomy An invasive nonsurgical technique in which a high-speed, rotating metal burr uses fine abrasive bits to scrape plaque from inside an artery while minimizing damage to the vessel surface.

atherosclerosis A type of arteriosclerosis that involves the formation of plaque within the arterial wall; the leading contributor to coronary artery and cerebrovascular disease.

atrial fibrillation (AF) A cardiac dysrhythmia in which multiple rapid impulses from many atrial foci, at a rate of 350 to 600 times per minute, depolarize the atria in a totally disorganized manner, with no P waves, no atrial contractions, a loss of the atrial kick, and an irregular ventricular response.

atrial gallop An abnormal fourth heart sound that occurs as blood enters the ventricles during the active filling phase at the end of ventricular diastole; may be heard in patients with hypertension, anemia, ventricular hypertrophy, myocardial infarction, aortic or pulmonic stenosis, and pulmonary emboli.

atrioventricular (AV) junction In the cardiac conduction system, the area consisting of a transitional cell zone, the atrioventricular (AV) node itself, and the bundle of His. The AV node lies just beneath the right atrial endocardium, between the tricuspid valve and the ostium of the coronary sinus.

attenuated The quality of making a substance weaker; for example, antigens that are used to make vaccines are specially processed to make them less likely to grow in the body.

atypical angina Angina that manifests itself as indigestion, pain between the shoulders, an aching jaw, or a choking sensation that occurs with exertion. Many women experience atypical angina.

atypical migraine The least common of the three types of migraine headaches, after migraines with aura and migraines without aura; the atypical category includes menstrual and cluster migraines.

aura A sensation that signals the onset of a headache or seizure; the patient may experience visual changes, flashing lights, or double vision.

autoamputation of the distal digits A condition in which the tips of the digits fall off spontaneously; can occur in severe cases of Raynaud's phenomenon.

autoantibodies Antibodies directed against self tissues of cells.

autocontamination The occurrence of infection in which the patient's own normal flora overgrows and penetrates the internal environment.

autodigestion Self-digestion. Specifically, the process of the stomach digesting itself if there is a break in its protective mucosal barrier.

autogenous Belonging to the person, such as a person's vein being moved from one part of the body to another.

autoimmune pancreatitis A chronic inflammatory form of pancreatitis that can also affect the bile ducts, kidneys, and other major connective tissues.

autologous blood transfusion Reinfusing the patient's own blood during surgery.

autologous bone marrow transplantation A type of bone marrow transplant in which patients receive their own stem cells, which were collected before high-dose chemotherapy.

autologous donation The donation of a patient's own blood before scheduled surgery for use, if needed, during the surgery to eliminate transfusion reactions and reduce the risk of bloodborne disease.

autolysis The spontaneous disintegration of tissue by the action of the patient's own cellular enzymes.

automaticity The ability of a cell to initiate an impulse spontaneously and repetitively; in cardiac electrophysiology, the ability of primary pacemaker cells (SA node, AV junction) to generate an electrical impulse.

autonomic dysreflexia (AD) A syndrome that affects the patient with an upper spinal cord injury; characterized by severe hypertension and headache, bradycardia, nasal stuffiness, and flushing; caused by a noxious stimulus, usually a distended bladder or constipation. This is a neurologic emergency and must be promptly treated to prevent a hypertensive brain attack.

autonomic nervous system (ANS) The part of the nervous system that is not under conscious control; consists of the sympathetic nervous system and the parasympathetic nervous system.

autonomy Ethical principle that implies a person's self-determination and self-management.

autosome Any of the 22 pairs of human chromosomes containing genes that code for all the structures and regulatory proteins needed for normal function but do not code for the sexual differentiation of a person.

axial loading A mechanism of injury that involves vertical compression. An example is a diving accident, in which the blow to the top of the head causes the vertebrae to shatter and pieces of bone enter the spinal canal and damage the cord.

azoospermia The absence of living sperm in the semen.

azotemia An excess of nitrogenous wastes (urea) in the blood.

B

B-type natriuretic peptide (BNP) A peptide produced and released by the ventricles when the patient has fluid overload as a result of heart failure (HF).

Babinski's sign Dorsiflexion of the great toe and fanning of the other toes, which is an abnormal reflex in response to testing the plantar reflex with a pointed (but not sharp) object; indicates the presence of central nervous system disease. The normal response is plantar flexion of all toes.

bacteremia The presence of bacteria in the bloodstream.

bacteriuria Bacteria in the urine.

bad death A death embodied by pain, not having one's wishes followed at the end of one's life, isolation, abandonment, and constant agonizing about losses associated with death.

Baker's cyst Enlarged popliteal bursa.

banding See *endoscopic variceal ligation.*

barbiturate coma The use of drugs such as pentobarbital sodium or sodium thiopental at dosages to maintain complete unresponsiveness; used for patients whose increased intracranial pressure cannot be controlled by other means. These drugs decrease the metabolic demands of the brain and cerebral blood flow, stabilize cell membranes, decrease the formation of vasogenic edema, and produce a more uniform blood supply. The patient in a barbiturate coma requires mechanical ventilation, sophisticated hemodynamic monitoring, and intracranial pressure monitoring.

bariatrics Branch of medicine that manages obesity and its related diseases.

baroreceptors Sensory receptors in the arch of the aorta and at the origin of the internal carotid arteries that are stimulated when the arterial walls are stretched by an increased blood pressure.

Barrett's epithelium Columnar epithelium (instead of the normal squamous cell epithelium) that develops in the lower esophagus during the process of healing from gastroesophageal reflux disease. It is considered premalignant and is associated with an increased risk of cancer in patients with prolonged disease.

Barrett's esophagus Ulceration of the lower esophagus caused by exposure to acid and pepsin, leading to the replacement of normal distal squamous mucosa with columnar epithelium as a response to tissue injury.

base A substance that binds (reduces) free hydrogen ions in solution. Strong bases bind hydrogen ions easily; weak bases bind less readily.

Basic Cardiac Life Support (BCLS) Procedure that involves ventilating the patient who has stopped breathing, as well as giving chest compressions in the absence of a carotid pulse. Also known as "cardiopulmonary resuscitation (CPR)."

Bell's palsy Acute paralysis of cranial nerve VII; characterized by a drawing sensation and paralysis of all facial muscles on the affected side. The patient cannot close the eye, wrinkle the forehead, smile, whistle, or grimace. The face appears masklike and sags. Also called "facial paralysis."

beneficence The ethical principle of preventing harm and ensuring the patient's well-being.

benign Altered cell growth that is harmless and does not require intervention.

benign tumor cells Normal cells growing in the wrong place or at the wrong time.

bereavement Grief and mourning experienced by the survivor before and after a death.

bicaval technique Surgical technique in heart transplantation in which the intact right atrium of the donor heart is preserved by anastomoses at the recipient's superior and inferior vena cavae.

bifurcation The point of division of a single structure into two branches.

bigeminy A type of premature complex that exists when normal complexes and premature complexes occur alternately in a repetitive two-beat pattern, with a pause occurring after each premature complex so that complexes occur in pairs.

bilateral orchiectomy The surgical removal of both testes, typically performed as palliative surgery in patients with prostate cancer. It is not intended to cure the prostate cancer but to arrest its spread by removing testosterone.

bilateral salpingo-oophorectomy (BSO) Surgical removal of both fallopian tubes and both ovaries.

biliary colic Intense pain due to obstruction of the cystic duct of the gallbladder from a stone moving through or lodged within the duct. Tissue spasm occurs in an effort to mobilize the stone through the small duct.

biliary stent A plastic or metal device that is placed percutaneously to keep a duct of the biliary system open in patients experiencing biliary obstruction.

biofilm A complex group of microorganisms that functions within a "slimy" gel coating on medical devices.

biological response modifiers (BRMs) A class of immunomodulating drugs that attempt to modify the course of disease. Also called "biologics."

biologics See *biological response modifiers.*

biomedical technician Member of the health care team who maintains the safety of adaptive and electronic devices by monitoring their function and making repairs as needed.

biotrauma Inflammatory response–mediated damage to alveoli.

bivalve To cut a cast lengthwise into two equal pieces.

black box warning A governmental designation indicating that a drug has at least one serious side effect and must be used with caution.

bladder ultrasound Less invasive test to determine postvoiding residual urine volumes for the patient with a reflex (upper motor neuron) or uninhibited bladder; often used to measure residual urine in the bladder of patients with spinal cord injury.

blanch To whiten or lighten.

blast phase cell Immature cell that divides.

bloodborne metastasis The release of tumor cells into the blood; the most common cause of cancer spread.

blood pressure (BP) The force of blood exerted against the vessel walls.

blood stem cells Immature, unspecialized (undifferentiated) cells that are capable of becoming any type of blood cell, depending on the body's needs.

Blumberg's sign Pain felt on abrupt release of steady pressure (rebound tenderness) over the site of abdominal pain.

body mass index (BMI) A measure of nutritional status that does not depend on frame size;

indirectly estimates total fat stores within the body by the relationship of weight to height.

bolus feeding A method of tube feeding that involves intermittent feeding of a specified amount of enteral product at specified times during a 24-hour period, typically every 4 hours.

bone biopsy Procedure in which the physician extracts a specimen of bone tissue for microscopic examination to confirm the presence of infection or neoplasm; not commonly done today.

bone mineral density (BMD) The quality of bone that determines bone strength. It peaks between 30 and 35 years of age, when both bone resorption activity and bone-building activity occur at a constant rate. When bone resorption activity exceeds bone-building activity, bone density decreases.

bone reduction Realignment of fractured bone ends for proper healing.

bone resorption Loss of bone density due to demineralization resulting from the release of calcium from storage areas in bones.

bone scan A radionuclide test in which radioactive material is injected for visualization of the entire skeleton; used to detect tumors, arthritis, osteomyelitis, osteoporosis, vertebral compression fractures, and unexplained bone pain.

borborygmus (borborygmi) Bowel sounds, especially loud gurgling sounds, resulting from hypermotility of the bowel.

boring In pain, the type of intense pain that feels like it is going through the body.

Bouchard's nodes Swelling at the proximal interphalangeal joints in osteoarthritis involving the hands.

bowel retraining A program for patients with neurologic problems that is designed to include a combination of suppository use and a consistent toileting schedule.

bradycardia Slowness of the heart rate; characterized as a pulse rate less than 50 to 60 beats/min.

bradydysrhythmia An abnormal heart rhythm characterized by a heart rate less than 60 beats/min.

bradykinesia Slow or no movement, as seen in a patient with Parkinson disease. Also called "akinesia."

brain abscess A collection of pus that forms in the extradural, subdural, or intracerebral area of the brain as a result of a purulent infection, usually due to bacteria invading the brain directly or indirectly.

brain attack Stroke; disruption in the normal blood supply to the brain, either as an interruption in blood flow (ischemic stroke) or as bleeding within or around the brain (hemorrhagic stroke). A medical emergency that occurs suddenly, a stroke should be treated immediately to prevent neurologic deficit and permanent disability. Formerly called "cerebrovascular accident," the National Stroke Association now uses the term "brain attack" to describe stroke.

brain herniation syndrome In the patient with untreated increased intracranial pressure, protrusion (herniation) of the brain downward toward the brainstem or laterally from a unilateral lesion within one cerebral hemisphere, causing irreversible brain damage and possibly death.

breakthrough pain Additional pain that "breaks through" the pain that is being managed by mainstay analgesic drugs.

breast augmentation Cosmetic surgical procedure to enhance the size, shape, or symmetry of the breasts.

breast-conserving surgery Surgical method for breast cancer that removes the bulk of the tumor rather than the entire breast.

Broca's aphasia See *expressive aphasia.*

Broca's area An important speech area of the cerebrum. It is located in the frontal lobe and is composed of neurons responsible for the formation of words, or speech.

bronchoscopy Insertion of a tube in the airway, usually as far as the secondary bronchi, for the purpose of visualizing airway structures and obtaining tissue samples for biopsy or culture.

bruit Swishing sound in the larger arteries (carotid, aortic, femoral, and popliteal) that can be heard with a stethoscope or Doppler probe; may indicate narrowing of the artery and is usually associated with atherosclerotic disease.

bulbar Pertaining to the muscles involved in facial expression, chewing, and speech.

bulimia nervosa An eating disorder that is characterized by episodes of binge eating in which the patient ingests a large amount of food in a short time, followed by purging behavior such as self-induced vomiting or excessive use of laxatives and diuretics.

bunion Hallux valgus deformity of the foot in which lateral deviation of the great toe causes the first metatarsal head to become enlarged.

bunionectomy Surgical removal of the hallux valgus deformity (bunion) of the foot.

butterfly rash A dry, scaly, raised rash on the face; the major skin manifestation of systemic lupus erythematosus.

C

cachexia Extreme body wasting and malnutrition that develop from an imbalance between food intake and energy use.

calciphylaxis A condition of thrombosis and skin necrosis that can occur in stage 5 chronic kidney disease.

calculi Abnormal formations of a mass of mineral salts that can occur in the body; forms in the kidney when excess calcium precipitates out of solution. Also called "stones."

calculous cholecystitis Inflammation of the gallbladder usually following and created by obstruction of the cystic duct by a stone (calculus).

callus The loose, fibrous, vascular tissue that forms at the site of a fracture as the first phase of healing and is normally replaced by hard bone as healing continues.

calyx The anatomic term for a cuplike structure.

Canadian Triage Acuity Scale (CTAS) A standardized model for triage in which lists of descriptors are used to establish the triage level.

cancellous The softer tissue inside bones that contains large spaces, or trabeculae, that are filled with red and yellow marrow.

candidiasis An infection caused by the fungus *Candida albicans.*

canthus The place where the upper and lower eyelids meet at the corner of either side of the eye.

capillary closing pressure The amount of pressure needed to occlude skin capillary blood flow.

capillary leak syndrome The response of capillaries to the presence of biologic chemicals (mediators) that change blood vessel integrity and allow fluid to shift from the blood in the vascular space into the interstitial tissues.

Caplan's syndrome The presence of pneumoconiosis and rheumatoid nodules in the lungs; noted primarily in coal miners and asbestos workers.

capsule The layer of fibrous tissue on the outer surface of the kidney, which provides protection and support. The renal capsule itself is surrounded by layers of fat and connective tissue.

carboxyhemoglobin Carbon monoxide on oxygen-binding sites of the hemoglobin molecule.

carcinoembryonic antigen (CEA) An oncofetal antigen that may be elevated in 70% of people with colorectal cancer. CEA is not specifically associated with the colorectal cancer and may be elevated in the presence of other benign or malignant diseases and in smokers. CEA is often used to monitor the effectiveness of treatment and to identify disease recurrence.

carcinogen Any substance that changes the activity of the genes in a cell so that the cell becomes a cancer cell.

carcinogenesis Cancer development.

cardiac axis In electrocardiography (ECG), the direction of electrical current flow in the heart. The relationship between the cardiac axis and the lead axis is responsible for the deflections seen on the ECG pattern.

cardiac catheterization The most definitive but most invasive test in the diagnosis of heart disease; involves passing a small catheter into the heart and injecting contrast medium.

cardiac index A calculation of cardiac output requirements to account for differences in body size; determined by dividing the cardiac output by the body surface area.

cardiac markers Serum studies that include troponin, creatine kinase–MB, and myoglobin.

cardiac output (CO) The volume of blood ejected by the heart each minute; normal range in adults is 4 to 7 L/min.

cardiac rehabilitation The process of actively assisting the patient with cardiac disease to achieve and maintain a productive life while remaining within the limits of the heart's ability to respond to increases in activity and stress. *Phase 1* begins with the acute illness and ends with discharge from the hospital. *Phase 2* begins after discharge and continues through convalescence at home. *Phase 3* refers to long-term conditioning.

cardiac resynchronization therapy (CRT) In patients with some types of heart failure, the use of a permanent pacemaker alone or in combination with an implantable cardioverter-defibrillator to provide biventricular pacing.

cardiac tamponade Compression of the myocardium by fluid that has accumulated around the heart; this compresses the atria and ventricles, prevents them from filling adequately, and reduces cardiac output.

cardiogenic shock Post–myocardial infarction heart failure in which necrosis of more than 40% of the left ventricle has occurred. Also called "class IV heart failure."

cardiomegaly Enlarged heart.

cardiomyopathy A subacute or chronic disease of cardiac muscle; classified into four categories based on abnormalities in structure and function: dilated, hypertrophic, restrictive, and arrhythmogenic.

cardiopulmonary bypass (CPB) Diversion of the blood from the heart to a bypass machine, where it is heparinized, oxygenated, and returned to the circulation through a cannula placed in the ascending aortic arch or femoral artery to provide oxygenation, circulation, and hypothermia during induced cardiac arrest for coronary artery bypass surgery. This process ensures a motionless operative field and prevents myocardial ischemia.

cardioversion A synchronized countershock that may be performed in emergencies for hemodynamically unstable ventricular or supraventricular tachydysrhythmias or electively for stable tachydysrhythmias that are resistant to medical therapies. The shock depolarizes a critical mass of myocardium simultaneously during intrinsic depolarization and is intended to stop the re-entry circuit and allow the sinus node to regain control of the heart.

carina The point at which the trachea branches into the right and left mainstem bronchi.

carpal tunnel syndrome (CTS) A common condition in which the median nerve in the wrist becomes compressed, causing pain and numbness.

carrier (1) A person who harbors an infectious agent without symptoms of active disease; (2) in genetics, a person who has one mutated allele for a recessive genetic disorder. A carrier does not usually have any manifestations of the disorder but can pass the mutated allele to his or her children.

case management The process of assessment, planning, implementation, evaluation, and interaction for patients who have complex health problems and incur a high cost to the health care system. Goals include promoting quality of life, decreasing fragmentation and duplication of care across health care settings, and maintaining cost-effectiveness.

caseation necrosis A type of necrosis in which tissue is turned into a granular mass.

cast A rigid device that immobilizes the affected body part while allowing other body parts to move. It is most commonly used for fractures but may also be applied to correct deformities (e.g., clubfoot) or to prevent deformities (e.g., those seen in some patients with rheumatoid arthritis).

cataract A lens opacity that distorts the image projected onto the retina.

catechol O-methyltransferases (COMTs) Enzymes that inactivate dopamine.

catecholamines Hormones (dopamine, epinephrine, and norepinephrine) released by the adrenal medulla in response to stimulation of the sympathetic nervous system.

cation Ion that has a positive charge.

cell-mediated immunity Microbial resistance that is mediated by the action of specifically sensitized T-lymphocytes.

cellulitis An acute, spreading, edematous inflammation of the deep subcutaneous tissues; usually caused by infection of a wound or burn.

central IV therapy IV therapy in which a vascular access device (VAD) is placed in a central blood vessel, such as the superior vena cava.

cerebral angiography (arteriography) Visualization of the cerebral circulation (carotid and vertebral arteries) after injecting a contrast medium into an artery (usually the femoral).

cerebral blood flow (CBF) Useful in evaluating cerebral vasospasm; can be measured in many areas of the brain with the use of radioactive substances.

cerebral perfusion pressure (CPP) The pressure gradient over which the brain is perfused. It is influenced by oxygenation, cerebral blood volume, blood pressure, cerebral edema, and intracranial pressure (ICP) and is determined by subtracting the mean ICP from the mean arterial pressure. A cerebral perfusion pressure above 70 mm Hg is generally accepted as an appropriate goal of therapy.

cerebral salt wasting (CSW) The primary cause of hyponatremia in the neurosurgical population; characterized by hyponatremia, decreased serum osmolality, and decreased blood volume. It is thought to result from the extrarenal influence of atrial natriuretic factor.

cerumen The wax produced by glands within the external ear canal; helps protect and lubricate the ear canal.

cervical polyp Tumor that arises from the mucosa and extends to the opening of the cervical os. Polyps result from hyperplasia of the endocervical epithelium, inflammation, or an abnormal local response to hormonal stimulation or localized vascular congestion of the cervical blood vessels. Polyps are the most common benign growth of the cervix.

$CHADS_2$ scoring system Acronymn for Congestive heart failure, Hypertension, Age ≥ 75 years, Diabetes mellitus, Stroke. Determines if a patient with atrial fibrillation needs preventive anticoagulant therapy.

chalazion An inflammation of a sebaceous gland in the eyelid.

chancre The ulcer that is the first sign of syphilis. It develops at the site of entry (inoculation) of the organism, usually 3 weeks after exposure. The lesion may be found on any area of the skin or mucous membranes but occurs most often on the genitalia, lips, nipples, and hands and in the oral cavity, anus, and rectum.

chemotherapy The treatment of cancer with chemical agents that have systemic effects; used to cure and to increase survival time.

chemotherapy-induced peripheral neuropathy (CIPN) The loss of sensory or motor function of peripheral nerves associated with exposure to certain anticancer drugs.

chest tube A drain placed in the pleural space to allow closed–chest drainage, which restores intrapleural pressure and allows re-expansion of the lung after surgery in patients who have undergone thoracotomy (incision of the chest wall).

Cheyne-Stokes respirations Common sign of nearing death in which apnea alternates with periods of rapid breathing.

choked disc See *papilledema.*

cholecystectomy The surgical removal of the gallbladder.

cholecystitis Inflammation of the gallbladder.

cholecystokinin A hormone that stimulates digestive juices and may work with leptin to increase or decrease appetite.

choledochojejunostomy Surgical anastomosis of the common bile duct with the jejunum.

cholelithiasis The presence of gallstones.

cholesteatoma A benign overgrowth of squamous cell epithelium.

cholesterol Serum lipid that includes high-density lipoproteins and low-density lipoproteins.

cholinergic crisis Overmedication with cholinesterase inhibitors.

cholinesterase inhibitors Drugs that improve cholinergic neurotransmission in the central nervous system by delaying the destruction of acetylcholine by acetylcholinesterase, thus delaying the onset of cognitive decline. These are approved for symptomatic treatment of Alzheimer's disease but do not affect the course of the disease.

chondroitin A supplement that may play a role in strengthening cartilage.

choreiform movement Rapid, jerky movement.

chronic Having a slow onset and symptoms that persist for an extended period.

chronic calcifying pancreatitis (CCP) Alcohol-induced chronic pancreatitis that is characterized by protein precipitates that plug the ducts and lead to ductal obstruction, atrophy, and dilation. The epithelium of the ducts undergoes histologic changes, resulting in metaplasia (cell replacement) and ulceration. This inflammatory process causes fibrosis of the pancreatic tissue.

chronic constrictive pericarditis A fibrous thickening of the pericardium that prevents adequate filling of the ventricles and eventually results in cardiac failure; caused by chronic pericardial inflammation due to tuberculosis, radiation therapy, trauma, kidney failure, or metastatic cancer.

chronic fatigue syndrome (CFS) A chronic illness characterized by severe fatigue for 6 months or longer, usually following flu-like symptoms. At least four of the following criteria are required for diagnosis: sore throat; substantial impairment in short-term memory or concentration; tender lymph nodes; muscle pain;

multiple joint pain with redness or swelling; headaches of a new type, pattern, or severity; unrefreshing sleep; and postexertional malaise lasting more than 24 hours.

chronic gastritis A patchy, diffuse inflammation of the mucosal lining of the stomach. Chronic gastritis usually heals without scarring but can progress to hemorrhage and ulcer formation.

chronic health problem A condition that has existed for at least 3 months.

chronic hepatitis Chronic liver inflammation that usually occurs as a result of hepatitis B or C. Superimposed infection with hepatitis D virus (HDV) in patients with chronic hepatitis B may also result in chronic hepatitis. Can lead to cirrhosis and liver cancer.

chronic kidney disease (CKD) A condition characterized by loss of kidney function over time.

chronic obstructive pancreatitis Pancreatitis that develops from inflammation, spasm, and obstruction of the sphincter of Oddi. Inflammatory and sclerotic lesions occur in the head of the pancreas and around the ducts, causing obstruction and backflow of pancreatic secretions.

chronic osteomyelitis Bone infection that persists over a long time due to misdiagnosis or inadequate treatment. Also called "subchronic osteomyelitis."

chronic pain Pain that persists or recurs for indefinite periods (usually more than 3 months), often involves deep body structures, is poorly localized, and is difficult to describe. Also called "persistent pain."

chronic pancreatitis A progressive, destructive disease of the pancreas characterized by remissions and exacerbations. Inflammation and fibrosis of the tissue contribute to pancreatic insufficiency and diminished function of the organ.

chronic paronychia Inflammation of the skin around the nail that persists for months. People at risk for chronic paronychia are those with frequent exposure to water, such as homemakers, bartenders, and laundry workers.

chronic pyelonephritis A kidney disorder that results from repeated or continued upper urinary tract infections or the effects of such infections.

chronic stable angina (CSA) Type of angina characterized by chest discomfort that occurs with moderate to prolonged exertion and in a pattern that is familiar to the patient.

chyme The liquid formed when food is transformed during the digestion process in the gastrointestinal tract.

circle of Willis At the base of the brain, the ring formed by the anterior, middle, and posterior cerebral arteries where they are joined together by small communicating arteries.

circumcision The surgical removal of the prepuce or foreskin of the penis.

circumferential Referring to something that completely surrounds an extremity or the thorax.

cirrhosis Liver disease that is characterized by extensive scarring of the liver and is usually caused by a chronic irreversible reaction to hepatic inflammation and necrosis; disease typically develops insidiously and has a prolonged, destructive course.

classic heat stroke A form of heat stroke in which the body's ability to dissipate heat is significantly impaired; occurs over time as a result of long-term exposure to a hot, humid environment such as a home without air-conditioning in the high heat of the summer.

clinical practice guideline An "official recommendation" based on evidence to diagnose and/or manage a health problem (e.g., pain management).

clinical psychologist Member of the health care team who counsels patients and families on their psychological problems and on strategies to cope with disability.

clinically competent The condition of being legally competent and having decisional capacity.

clonic (rhythmic) Pertaining to a state of alternating muscle stiffness followed by rhythmic jerking motions, as in a tonic-clonic seizure.

clonus The sudden, brief, jerking contraction of a muscle or muscle group often seen in seizures. Also called "myoclonus."

closed fracture A fracture that does not extend through the skin and therefore has no visible wound. Also called "simple fracture."

closed reduction A nonsurgical method for managing a simple fracture. While applying a manual pull, or traction, on the bone, the health care provider manipulates the bone ends so they realign.

closed traumatic brain injury A type of traumatic primary brain injury that occurs as the result of blunt trauma; the integrity of the skull is not violated, and damage to brain tissue depends on the degree and mechanisms of injury.

***C. difficile*–associated disease (CDAD)** Clinical manifestations that are caused by *Clostridium difficile* as a potential result of antibiotic therapy use, especially in older adults.

clubbing Changes in the tissue beds of the fingers and toes, with the base of the nail becoming spongy; results from chronic oxygen deprivation in the tissue beds.

cluster headache A type of oculotemporal or oculofrontal headache marked by unilateral, excruciating, nonthrobbing pain that is felt deep in and around the eye and may radiate to the forehead, temple, cheek, ear, occiput, or neck. Average duration is 10 to 45 minutes. Headaches occur every 8 to 12 hours and up to 24 hours daily at the same time for about 6 to 8 weeks (hence the term "cluster"), followed by remission for 9 months to a year. Cause and mechanism are unknown but have been attributed to vasoreactivity and oxyhemoglobin desaturation.

clysis See *hypodermoclysis.*

coagulopathy Clotting abnormalities.

cognition The ability of the brain to process, store, retrieve, and manipulate information.

cognitive therapist A member of the rehabilitative health care team, usually a neuropsychologist, who works primarily with patients who have experienced head injuries and have cognitive impairments.

cohorting The practice of grouping patients who are colonized or infected with the same pathogen.

cold antibody anemia A form of immunohemolytic anemia (in which the immune system attacks a person's own red blood cells for unknown reasons) that occurs with complement protein fixation on immunoglobulin M (IgM). In this condition, the arteries in the hands and feet constrict profoundly in response to cold temperatures or stress.

cold phase A phase after peripheral nerve trauma resulting in complete denervation in which the skin appears cyanotic, mottled, or reddish blue and feels cool compared with the contralateral unaffected extremity. The cold phase follows the warm phase, which lasts 2 to 3 weeks after injury.

colectomy Surgical removal of part or all of the colon.

collaboration The planning, implementing, and evaluation of patient care using an interdisciplinary (ID) plan of care.

collateral circulation Circulation that provides blood to an area with altered tissue perfusion through smaller vessels that develop and compensate for the occluded vessels.

colon interposition A surgical procedure that may be performed in patients with an esophageal tumor when the tumor involves the stomach or the stomach is otherwise unsuitable for anastomosis. In colon interposition, a section of right or left colon is removed and brought up into the thorax to substitute for the esophagus.

colon resection Surgery performed for colorectal cancer in which the tumor and regional lymph nodes are removed.

colonoscopy The endoscopic examination of the entire large bowel.

colostomy The surgical creation of an opening between the colon and the surface of the abdomen.

colposcopy Examination of the cervix and vagina using a colposcope, which allows three-dimensional magnification and intense illumination of epithelium with suspected disease. This procedure can locate the exact site of precancerous and malignant lesions for biopsy.

command center See *emergency operations center.*

commando procedure Mnemonic for combined neck dissection, mandibulectomy, and oropharyngeal resection—a procedure in which the surgeon removes a segment of the mandible with the oral lesion and performs a radical neck dissection.

communicable The ability of an infection, such as influenza, to be transmitted from person to person.

communicating hydrocephalus Form of hydrocephalus that occurs when the flow of cerebrospinal fluid (CSF) is blocked after it exits the ventricles; this form is "communicating" because CSF can still flow between the ventricles, which remain open.

compartment syndrome A condition in which increased tissue pressure in a confined anatomic space causes decreased blood flow to the area, leading to hypoxia and pain.

compensated cirrhosis A form of cirrhosis in which the liver has significant scarring but is still able to perform essential functions without causing significant symptoms.

compensatory mechanism The means of producing compensation. Also called "adaptive mechanism."

complement activation and fixation Actions triggered by some classes of antibodies that can remove or destroy antigen.

complete spinal cord injury An injury in which the spinal cord has been severed or damaged in a way that eliminates all innervation below the level of the injury.

complex regional pain syndrome (CRPS) A complex disorder that includes debilitating pain, atrophy, autonomic dysfunction (excessive sweating, vascular changes), and motor impairment (most notably muscle paresis), probably caused by an abnormally hyperactive sympathetic nervous system. This syndrome most often results from traumatic injury and commonly occurs in the feet and hands; formerly called "reflex sympathetic dystrophy (RSD)."

compliance In respiratory physiology, a measure of elasticity within the lung. Also, a patient's fulfillment of a caregiver's prescribed course of treatment.

compound fracture See *open fracture.*

compression fracture A fracture that is produced by a loading force applied to the long axis of cancellous bone. These fractures commonly occur in the vertebrae of patients with osteoporosis.

computed tomography coronary angiography (CTCA) 64-slice diagnostic scan used to diagnose coronary artery disease in symptomatic patients.

conductive hearing loss Hearing loss that results from any physical obstruction of sound wave transmission (e.g., a foreign body in the external canal, a retracted or bulging tympanic membrane, or fused bony ossicles).

conductivity The ability of a cell to transmit an electrical stimulus from cell membrane to cell membrane.

congestive heart failure (CHF) Former term for "left-sided heart failure." Categorized as either systolic heart failure or diastolic heart failure, which may be acute or chronic and mild to severe.

conization The removal of a cone-shaped sample of tissue from the cervix for cytologic study.

conjunctivae The mucous membranes of the eye that line the undersurface of the eyelids (palpebral conjunctiva) and cover the sclera (bulbar conjunctiva).

connective tissue disease (CTD) A group of diseases that are the major focus of rheumatology (the study of rheumatic diseases); most are musculoskeletal disorders.

consensual response In assessing pupillary reaction to light, a slight constriction of the pupil of the eye not being tested when a penlight is brought in from the side of the patient's head and shined into the eye being tested as soon as the patient opens his or her eyes.

consolidation Solidification; lack of air spaces in the lung, such as occurs in pneumonia.

constipation The passage of hard, dry stool fewer than 3 times a week (as defined by the Association of Rehabilitation Nurses).

contact laser prostatectomy (CLP) Procedure for treating benign prostatic hyperplasia that uses laser energy to coagulate excess tissue. Also called "interstitial laser coagulation (ILC)."

Contact Precautions Infection control guidelines from the Centers for Disease Control and Prevention; used for patients with infections spread by direct contact or contact with items in the patient's environment, such as pediculosis.

contiguous Something in direct contact with, or adjacent to, another area or structure.

continence The ability to voluntarily control emptying the bladder and colon. Continence is a learned behavior whereby a person can suppress the urge to urinate until a socially appropriate location is available.

continuous feeding A method of tube feeding in which small amounts of enteral product are continuously infused (by gravity drip or by a pump or controller device) over a specified time.

continuous positive airway pressure (CPAP) A respiratory treatment that improves obstructive sleep apnea in patients with heart failure.

contractility The ability of a cell to contract in response to an impulse. In cardiac electrophysiology, the ability of atrial and ventricular muscle cells to shorten their fiber length in response to electrical stimulation, generating sufficient pressure to propel blood forward. Contractility is the mechanical activity of the heart.

contraction The closure of a wound as new collagen replaces damaged tissue, pulling the wound edges inward along the path of least resistance.

contralateral Pertaining to the opposite side.

contrecoup injury Bruising of the brain tissue, with damage occurring on the side opposite the site of impact.

control therapy drugs Drugs used every day, regardless of symptoms, to reduce airway responsiveness to prevent asthma attacks from occurring.

contusion A bruise; when referring to closed head injury, a bruising of brain tissue usually found at the site of impact (coup injury). Compare with *contrecoup injury.*

cor pulmonale Right-sided heart failure caused by pulmonary disease.

cordectomy Excision of a vocal cord in surgery for laryngeal cancer.

cornea The clear layer that forms the external coat on the front of the eye.

corneal abrasion Scrape or scratch of the cornea that disrupts its integrity.

corneal ulceration Deep disruption of the corneal epithelium that extends into the stromal layer and is caused by bacteria, protozoa, or fungi.

coronary artery bypass graft (CABG) A surgical procedure in which occluded coronary arteries are bypassed with the patient's own venous or arterial blood vessels or synthetic grafts.

coronary artery disease (CAD) Disease affecting the arteries that provide blood, oxygen, and nutrients to the myocardium; partial or complete blockage of the blood flow through the coronary arteries, causing ischemia and infarction of the myocardium, angina pectoris, and acute coronary syndromes. Also known as "coronary heart disease" or simply "heart disease."

coronary artery vasculopathy (CAV) A form of coronary artery disease that presents as diffuse plaque in the arteries of the donor heart in patients who have received a heart transplant.

cortisol The main glucocorticoid produced by the adrenal cortex.

coryza The common cold, or acute viral rhinitis.

cough assist A technique for assisting the tetraplegic patient to cough. Place his or her hands on either side of the rib cage or upper abdomen below the diaphragm; then, as the patient inhales, push upward to help expand the lungs and cough.

craniotomy Surgical incision into the cranium.

creatine kinase (CK) An enzyme specific to cells of the brain, myocardium, and skeletal muscle. Its appearance in the blood indicates tissue necrosis or injury, with levels following a predictable rise and fall during a specified period.

Credé maneuver A technique used to assist in urination in which a patient places his or her hand in a cupped position directly over the bladder area and pushes inward and downward gently as if massaging the bladder to empty.

crepitus A continuous grating sensation caused when irregular cartilage or bone fragments rub together and which may be felt or heard as a joint is put through passive range of motion; also, a crackling sensation that can be felt on a patient's chest, indicating that air is trapped within the tissues.

CREST syndrome In patients with systemic sclerosis, the combination of calcinosis (calcium deposits), Raynaud's phenomenon, esophageal dysmotility, sclerodactyly (scleroderma of the digits), and telangiectasia (spider-like hemangiomas).

cricothyroidotomy Surgical procedure in which an opening is made between the thyroid cartilage and cricoid cartilage ring and results in a tracheostomy. Also called "cricothyrotomy." The procedure is used in an emergency for access to the lower airways.

crises In the patient with sickle cell disease, periodic episodes of extensive cellular sickling that have a sudden onset and can occur as often as weekly or as seldom as once a year.

critical access hospital A small rural facility of 15 or fewer inpatient beds that provides around-the-clock emergency care services 7 days per week. Considered a necessary provider of health care to community residents who are not close to other hospitals in a given region.

cross-contamination A type of contamination in which organisms from another person or from the environment are transmitted to the patient.

cryotherapy (1) A way of decreasing muscle pain by "cooling down" the area with a local, short-acting gel or cream, such as after physical therapy; (2) in ophthalmologic surgery, use of a freezing probe to repair retinal detachment.

cryptorchidism Failure of the testes to descend into the scrotum.
culture A procedure for identifying a microorganism by cultivating and isolating it in tissue cultures or artificial media.
Curling's ulcer Acute ulcerative gastroduodenal disease, which may develop within 24 hours of a severe burn injury because of reduced gastrointestinal blood flow and mucosal damage.
Cushing's disease (Cushing's syndrome) Hypercortisolism caused by oversecretion of hormones by the adrenal cortex.
Cushing's triad A classic yet late sign of increased intracranial pressure (ICP) manifested by severe hypertension with a widened pulse pressure and bradycardia. As ICP increases, the pulse becomes thready, irregular, and rapid. Cerebral blood flow increases in response to hypertension.
Cushing's ulcer Acute ulcerative gastroduodenal disease that may develop as a result of increased intracranial pressure.
cutaneous (superficial) reflexes Superficial reflexes. Usually the plantar and abdominal reflexes are tested.
cyanosis Bluish or darkened discoloration of the skin and mucous membranes; results from an increased amount of deoxygenated hemoglobin.
cyclic feeding A method of tube feeding similar to continuous feeding (see definition of *continuous feeding*) except the infusion is stopped for a specified time in each 24-hour period ("down time"); the down time typically occurs in the morning to allow bathing, treatments, and other activities.
cystitis Inflammation of the bladder.
cystocele Herniation of the bladder into the vagina.
cytokines Small protein hormones produced by white blood cells.
cytotoxic Having cell-damaging effects.

D

dandruff An accumulation of patchy or diffuse white or gray scales on the surface of the scalp.
death When illness or trauma overwhelms the compensatory mechanisms of the body and the lungs and heart cease to function.
death rattle Loud, wet respirations caused by secretions in the respiratory tract and oral cavity of a patient who is near death.
débridement The removal of infected tissue from a healing wound.
debriefing After a mass casualty incident or disaster, (1) the provision of sessions for small groups of staff in which teams are brought in to discuss effective coping strategies (critical incident stress debriefing), and (2) the administrative review of staff and system performance during the event to determine opportunities for improvement in the emergency management plan.
debris Dead cells and tissues in a wound.
decerebrate posturing Abnormal posturing and rigidity characterized by extension of the arms and legs, pronation of the arms, plantar flexion, and opisthotonos; usually associated with dysfunction in the brainstem area. Also called "decerebration."
decerebration See *decerebrate posturing.*
decompensated cirrhosis A form of cirrhosis in which liver function is significantly impaired with obvious manifestations of liver failure.
decompressive craniectomy Removal of a section of the skull in the patient with uncontrolled intracranial pressure (ICP); allows for additional space for edema without increasing ICP.
decorticate posturing Abnormal posturing seen in the patient with lesions that interrupt the corticospinal pathways. The arms, wrists, and fingers are flexed with internal rotation and plantar flexion of the legs. Also called "decortication."
decortication See *decorticate posturing.*
deep tendon reflexes Tested as part of the neurologic assessment. An intact reflex arc is indicated when the muscle contracts in response to the tendon being struck with a reflex hammer.
deep vein thrombophlebitis Presence of a thrombus associated with inflammation in the deep veins, usually in the legs. Compared with superficial thrombophlebitis, it presents a greater risk for pulmonary embolism. Also called "deep vein thrombosis."
deep vein thrombosis (DVT) Common term for "deep vein thrombophlebitis."
defibrillation An asynchronous countershock that depolarizes a critical mass of myocardium simultaneously to stop the re-entry circuit, allowing the sinus node to regain control of the heart.
dehiscence A partial or complete separation of the outer layers of a wound, sometimes described as a "splitting open" of the wound.
dehydration Fluid intake less than what is needed to meet the body's fluid needs.
delayed union Term describing a fracture that has not healed within 6 months of injury.
delegation The process of transferring to a competent person the authority to perform a selected nursing task or activity in a selected patient care situation.
delirium An acute state of confusion, usually short-term and reversible within 3 weeks. Often seen among older adults in a hospital or other unfamiliar setting.
dementia A syndrome of slowly progressive cognitive decline with global impairment of intellectual function. The most common type is Alzheimer's disease.
demyelination Destruction of myelin between the nodes of Ranvier; a major pathologic finding in multiple sclerosis or Guillain-Barré syndrome.
depolarization The ability of a cell to respond to a stimulus by initiating an impulse. Also called "excitability."
depression A response to multiple life stresses, a single situation, a primary disorder, or a problem associated with dementia; this response can range from mild, transient feelings of sadness to a severe sense of helplessness and hopelessness.
dermal papillae Fingerlike projections of dermal tissue that anchor the epidermis to the dermis.
dermatomes Specific areas of the skin that receive sensory input from spinal nerves.
descending tracts Groups of nerves that begin in the brain and end in the spinal cord.
desquamation The shedding or peeling of skin.
diabetic peripheral neuropathy (DPN) A progressive deterioration of nerves that results in loss of nerve function (sensory perception). A common complication of diabetes, it often involves all parts of the body.
diagnostic peritoneal lavage (DPL) Test that determines the presence of internal bleeding following abdominal trauma.
dialysate The solution used in dialysis. It is composed of water, glucose, sodium chloride, potassium, magnesium, calcium, and bicarbonate; dialysate composition may be altered according to the patient's needs for treatment of electrolyte imbalances.
dialyzer The apparatus used to perform hemodialysis. Also known as the "artificial kidney," it has four parts: a blood compartment, a dialysate compartment, a semipermeable membrane, and an enclosed structure to support the membrane.
diaphragmatic pacing A pacemaker for the phrenic nerve to cause the diaphragm to contract (leading to inhalation). Also known as "phrenic nerve pacing."
diastole The phase of the cardiac cycle that consists of relaxation and filling of the atria and ventricles; normally about two thirds of the cardiac cycle.
diastolic blood pressure The amount of pressure/force against the arterial walls during the relaxation phase of the heart.
diastolic heart failure Heart failure that occurs when the left ventricle is unable to relax adequately during diastole, which prevents the ventricle from filling with sufficient blood to ensure adequate cardiac output.
Dietary Guidelines for Americans Recommendations made by the USDA and U.S. Department of Health and Human Services to help people maintain nutritional health; updated every 5 years.
Dietary Reference Intakes (DRIs) Nutrition guide developed by the Institute of Medicine of the National Academies that provides a scientific basis for food guidelines in the United States and Canada.
diffuse axonal injury (DAI) A type of closed head injury that is usually related to high-speed acceleration/deceleration, as with motor vehicle crashes. There is significant damage to axons in the white matter, and there are lesions in the corpus callosum, midbrain, cerebellum, and upper brainstem. Patients with severe injury may present with immediate coma, and most survivors require long-term care.
diffuse cutaneous systemic sclerosis Skin thickening on the trunk, face, and proximal and distal extremities in patients with systemic sclerosis.
diffuse light reflex A description of a light reflex that is spotty or multiple because of a changed eardrum shape from either retraction or bulging.
diffusion The spontaneous, free movement of particles (solute) across a permeable membrane down a concentration gradient; that is, from an

area of higher concentration to an area of lower concentration.

digestion The mechanical and chemical process in which complex foodstuffs are broken down into simpler forms that can be used by the body.

digoxin toxicity A reaction to therapy with digitalis derivatives (digoxin) that is identified by monitoring serum digoxin and potassium levels (hypokalemia potentiates digitalis toxicity). Signs of toxicity are nonspecific (anorexia, fatigue, changes in mental status). Toxicity may cause dysrhythmia, most commonly premature ventricular contractions.

dilated cardiomyopathy (DCM) A type of cardiomyopathy that involves extensive damage to the myofibrils and interference with myocardial metabolism. There is normal ventricular wall thickness but dilation of both ventricles and impairment of systolic function.

dilation Increase in the diameter of blood vessels.

diplopia Double vision.

direct current stimulation (DCS) The placement of an implantable device to promote bone fusion; used as an adjunct for patients for whom spinal fusion may be difficult.

direct inguinal hernia A sac formed from the peritoneum that contains a portion of the intestine and passes through a weak point in the abdominal wall.

direct response Pupil constriction in response to bringing a penlight in from the side of the patient's head and shining the light in the eye being tested as soon as the patient opens his or her eyes.

directly observed therapy (DOT) A technique in which a health care professional watches the patient swallow prescribed drugs.

disabling health problem Any physical or mental health problem that can cause disability.

disaster A mass casualty incident in which the number of casualties exceeds the resource capabilities of a particular community or hospital facility.

disaster triage tag system A system that categorizes triage priority by colored and numbered tags.

discoid lesion Round lesion in patients who have discoid lupus erythematosus; evident when exposed to sunlight or ultraviolet light.

disease-modifying antirheumatic drugs (DMARDs) Drugs prescribed to slow the progression of mild rheumatoid disease before it worsens, such as hydroxychloroquine, sulfasalazine, or minocycline.

disequilibrium A condition in which the hydrostatic pressure is not the same in the two fluid spaces on either side of a permeable membrane.

disinfection A method of infection control in which the level of disease-causing organisms is reduced but the organisms are not killed; adequate when an item is entering a body area that has resident bacteria or normal flora, such as the respiratory tract.

diskitis Disk inflammation.

dislocation of a joint Occurrence of the articulating surfaces of two or more bones moving away from each other.

dissociate The act of separating and releasing ions.

diverticula Sacs resulting from the herniation of the mucosa and submucosa of a tubular organ into surrounding tissue.

diverticulitis The inflammation of one or more diverticula.

diverticulosis The presence of many abnormal pouchlike herniations (diverticula) in the wall of the intestine.

dizziness A disturbed sense of a person's relationship to space.

DNR Do not resuscitate; order from a physician or other authorized health care provider who instructs that CPR not be attempted in the event of cardiac or respiratory arrest.

dopamine agonist A class of drugs that mimic dopamine. Dopamine agonists stimulate dopamine receptors and are typically the most effective during the first 3 to 5 years of use. Prescribed for the patient with Parkinson disease to reduce dyskinesias (problems with movement).

dose-dense chemotherapy Chemotherapy that uses higher doses more often for aggressive cancer treatment, especially breast cancer.

double-barrel stoma The least common type of colostomy, which is created by dividing the bowel and bringing both the proximal and distal portions to the abdominal surface to create two stomas.

doubling time The amount of time it takes for a tumor to double in size.

Droplet Precautions Infection control guidelines from the Centers for Disease Control and Prevention; used for patients with infections spread by the droplet transmission route, such as influenza.

drug holiday Period of time lasting up to 10 days in which the patient with Parkinson disease receives no drug therapy.

dual x-ray absorptiometry (DXA or DEXA) A type of radiographic scan that measures bone mineral density in the hip, wrist, or vertebral column; used as a screening and diagnostic tool for diagnosis and for follow-up evaluation of treatment of osteoporosis.

ductal carcinoma in situ (DCIS) An early, noninvasive form of breast cancer in which cancer cells are located within the duct and have not invaded the surrounding fatty breast tissue.

ductal ectasia A benign breast disease caused by dilation and thickening of the collecting ducts in the subareolar area. The ducts become distended and filled with cellular debris, which activates an inflammatory response. It is usually seen in women approaching menopause.

dumping syndrome A constellation of vasomotor symptoms that typically occur within 30 minutes after eating; believed to occur as a result of the rapid emptying of gastric contents into the small intestine, which shifts fluid into the gut and causes abdominal distention. Early manifestations include vertigo, tachycardia, syncope, sweating, pallor, and palpitations.

Dupuytren's contracture A slowly progressive contracture of the palmar fascia that results in flexion of the fourth or fifth digit of the hand and occasionally affects the third digit. Although a fairly common problem, the cause is unknown. It usually occurs in older men, tends to occur in families, and can be bilateral.

durable power of attorney for health care (DPOAHC) A legal document in which a person appoints someone else to make health care decisions in the event he or she becomes incapable of making decisions.

dysarthria Slurred speech.

dysfunctional uterine bleeding (DUB) A nonspecific term to describe bleeding that is excessive or abnormal in amount or frequency without predisposing anatomic or systemic conditions. Such bleeding occurs most often at either end of the span of a woman's reproductive years, when ovulation is becoming established or when it is becoming irregular at menopause.

dyskinesia Difficulty with movement.

dyslexia Problems understanding written language; caused by brain injury or disease.

dysmetria The inability to direct or limit movement.

dyspareunia Painful sexual intercourse.

dyspepsia Indigestion or heartburn following meals.

dysphagia Difficulty in swallowing.

dysphasia Slurred speech.

dyspnea Difficulty in breathing or breathlessness.

dyspnea on exertion (DOE) Dyspnea that is associated with activity, such as climbing stairs.

dysrhythmia A disorder of the heartbeat involving a disturbance in cardiac rhythm; irregular heartbeat.

dystrophic Pertaining to or characterized by dystrophy; abnormal.

dystrophin A muscle protein that maintains muscle integrity by sending signals to coordinate smooth, synchronous muscle fiber contraction. Faulty action of this protein causes muscular dystrophy.

dysuria Painful urination.

E

Eaton-Lambert syndrome A form of myasthenia gravis that affects the muscles of the trunk and the pelvic and shoulder girdles; often observed in combination with small cell carcinoma of the lung. Although weakness increases after exertion, there may be a temporary increase in muscle strength during the first few contractions, followed by a rapid decline.

ecchymoses Large purple, blue, or yellow bruises of the skin resulting from small hemorrhages; these bruises are larger than petechiae.

ecchymotic Pertaining to a bruise.

ECG caliper A measurement tool used in analysis of an electrocardiographic (ECG) rhythm strip.

echocardiography In cardiovascular assessment, the use of ultrasound waves to assess cardiac structure and mobility, particularly of the valves; a noninvasive, risk-free test that is easily performed at the bedside or on an ambulatory care basis.

echolalia Automatic repetition of what another person says.

ectopic Out of place.

ectropion A turning outward and sagging of the eyelid, which is caused by relaxation of the orbicular muscle.
edema Tissue swelling as a result of the accumulation of excessive fluid in the interstitial spaces.
edentulous Without teeth.
efferent arterioles The extremely small blood vessels that carry the remaining blood out of the glomerulus (once the glomerulus has filtered the blood to make urine) and into one of two additional capillary systems (the peritubular capillaries or the vasa recta).
effluent Drainage.
effusion An accumulation of fluid, such as in a joint (where it may limit movement).
ejection fraction The percentage of blood ejected from the heart during systole.
electrical bone stimulation The use of an electronic device (e.g., magnetic coils applied on the skin or over a cast to deliver a pulsed magnetic field) to promote bone union after a fracture. The exact mechanism of action is unknown, but this procedure is based on research showing that bone has inherent electrical properties that are used in healing.
electrocardiogram (ECG) A graphic recording of the electrical current generated by the heart. The ECG provides information about cardiac dysrhythmias, myocardial ischemia, site and extent of myocardial infarction, cardiac hypertrophy, electrolyte imbalances, and effectiveness of cardiac drugs. It is a routine part of cardiovascular evaluation and is a valuable diagnostic test.
electroencephalography (EEG) A recording of the electrical activity of the cerebral hemispheres; it represents the voltage changes in various areas of the brain as determined by recording the difference between two electrodes.
electrolyte A substance in body fluids that carries an electrical charge. Also called an "ion."
electromyography (EMG) A recording of the electrical activity of peripheral nerves by testing muscle activity.
electrophysiologic study (EPS) In cardiovascular assessment, an invasive procedure performed in a catheterization laboratory during which programmed electrical stimulation of the heart is used to induce and evaluate lethal dysrhythmias and conduction abnormalities to permit accurate diagnosis and effective treatment. The study is used in patients who have survived cardiac arrest, have recurrent tachydysrhythmias, or experience unexplained syncopal episodes.
electrovaporization of the prostate (EVAP) Procedure for treating benign prostatic hyperplasia with high-frequency electrical current to cut and vaporize excess tissue.
embolectomy Removal of a blood clot.
embolic stroke Damage to the brain when a blood clot forms somewhere in the body (usually the heart) and travels through the bloodstream to block one or more of the arteries supplying the brain.
embolus The occurrence of inflammation and thickening of the vein wall around a clot (thrombus).
emergence Recovery from anesthesia.
emergency medical technician (EMT) Prehospital care provider who supplies basic life-support interventions such as oxygen, basic wound care, splinting, spinal immobilization, and monitoring of vital signs.
emergency medicine physician A member of the emergency health care team with education and training in the specialty of emergency patient management.
emergency operations center (EOC) A designated location in the Hospital Incident Command System (HICS) with accessible communication technology. Also called the "command center."
emergency preparedness A goal or plan to meet the extraordinary need for hospital beds, staff, drugs, personal protective equipment, supplies, and medical devices such as mechanical ventilators.
Emergency Severity Index (ESI) A standardized model for triage that categorizes both patient acuity and resource utilization into five levels, from most urgent to least urgent.
emergent triage In a three-tiered triage scheme, the category that includes any condition or injury that poses an immediate threat to life or limb, such as crushing chest pain or active hemorrhage.
emetogenic A substance that induces nausea and vomiting.
emmetropia The state of perfect refraction of the eye; with the lens at rest, light rays from a distant source are focused into a sharp image on the retina.
emotional abuse The intentional use of threats, humiliation, intimidation, and isolation to another person.
emotional lability Having uncontrollable emotions; for example, the patient laughs and then cries unexpectedly for no apparent reason.
empyema A collection of pus in the pleural space.
encephalitis An inflammation of the brain parenchyma (brain tissue) and meninges that affects the cerebrum, brainstem, and cerebellum; usually caused by a virus.
endometrial ablation Procedure for dysfunctional uterine bleeding that removes a built-up uterine lining using a laser, roller ball, or balloon.
endometrial cancer Cancer of the inner uterine lining.
endometriosis The abnormal occurrence of endometrial tissue outside the uterine cavity.
endometritis An infection of the endometrium.
endoscope A tube that allows viewing and manipulation of internal body areas.
endoscopic retrograde cholangiopancreatography (ERCP) The visual and radiographic examination of the liver, gallbladder, bile ducts, and pancreas by means of an endoscope and the injection of radiopaque dye to identify the cause and location of obstruction.
endoscopic variceal ligation (EVL) The application of small "O" bands around the base of the esophageal varices to cut off their blood supply. Also called "banding."
endoscopy The direct visualization of the gastrointestinal tract by means of a flexible fiberoptic endoscope.
endothelin A secretion produced by the endothelial cells when they are stretched.
endovascular stent graft The repair of an abdominal aortic aneurysm using a stent made of flexible material; the stent is inserted through a skin incision into the femoral artery by way of a catheter-based system.
end-stage kidney disease (ESKD) Acute renal failure combined with chronic renal insufficiency, resulting in the inability of the kidney to excrete waste products normally. The patient may need hemodialysis or a kidney transplant.
energy conservation Strategies to reduce the fatigue associated with chronic and disabling conditions, such as allowing rest periods and setting priorities.
engraftment The successful transplantation of cells in the patient's bone marrow.
enophthalmos Backward displacement of the eyeball into the orbit so that the eye appears sunken.
enteroscopy Visualization of the small intestine.
enterostomal feeding tube A tube used for patients who need long-term enteral feeding; the physician directly accesses the gastrointestinal tract using surgical, endoscopic, or laparoscopic techniques.
entropion The turning inward of the eyelid, causing the eyelashes to rub against the eye.
enucleation The surgical removal of the entire eyeball.
envenomation Venom injection from a snakebite.
epididymitis Inflammation of the epididymis.
epidural Term for the space between the dura mater and vertebrae; it consists of fat, connective tissue, and blood vessels.
epidural hematoma An accumulation of clotted blood resulting from arterial bleeding into the space between the dura and the skull; a neurosurgical emergency.
epiglottis A leaf-shaped, elastic structure that is attached along one edge to the top of the larynx; it closes over the glottis during swallowing to prevent food from entering the trachea and opens during breathing and coughing.
epiglottitis Infection or inflammation of the epiglottis and supraglottic structures that results in swelling. If swelling is great enough, the airway can be obstructed.
epilepsy A chronic disorder characterized by recurrent, unprovoked seizure activity; may be caused by an abnormality in electrical neuronal activity, an imbalance of neurotransmitters, or a combination of both.
epistaxis Nosebleed.
erectile dysfunction (ED) The inability to achieve or maintain a penile erection sufficient for sexual intercourse.
ergonomics An applied science in which the workplace is designed to increase worker comfort (thus reducing injury) while increasing efficiency and productivity.
erosion Ulceration.
eructation The act of belching.
erythema Redness of the skin.
erythema migrans A round or oval flat or slightly raised rash.

erythrocyte A red blood cell (RBC). Red blood cells are the major cells in the blood and are responsible for tissue oxygenation.

erythroplakia A velvety red mucosal lesion, most often occurring in the oral cavity.

erythropoiesis The selective maturation of stem cells into mature erythrocytes.

eschar The crust of dead tissue that forms from coagulated particles of destroyed dermis in a patient with a full-thickness burn injury.

escharotomy Incision made through tight eschar to relieve pressure and allow normal blood flow and breathing.

esophageal stricture Narrowing of the esophageal opening.

esophageal varices The distention of fragile, thin-walled esophageal veins due to increased pressure; the increased pressure is a result of portal hypertension, in which the blood backs up from the liver and enters the esophageal and gastric vessels that carry it into the systemic circulation.

esophagectomy The surgical removal of all or part of the esophagus.

esophagitis Inflammation of the esophagus.

esophagogastroduodenoscopy (EGD) The visual examination of the esophagus, stomach, and duodenum by means of a fiberoptic endoscope.

esophagogastrostomy The surgical creation of a communication between the stomach and the esophagus; it involves the removal of part of the esophagus and proximal stomach.

essential hypertension Elevated blood pressure that is not caused by a specific disease. The major risk factor is a family history of hypertension. Also called "primary hypertension."

euploid Having the correct number of chromosome pairs for the species.

euploidy The normal diploid number for a cell.

eustachian tube Tube that connects the nasopharynx with the middle ear and opens during swallowing to equalize pressure within the middle ear.

euthyroid Having normal thyroid function.

euvolemia A state of balanced fluid intake and output.

evidence-based practice (EBP) A QSEN competency in which the nurse integrates best current evidence with clinical expertise and patient/family preferences and values for delivery of optimal health care.

evisceration The total separation of all layers of a wound and the protrusion of internal organs through the open wound.

evoked potentials Tests to measure the electrical signals to the brain generated by hearing, touch, or sight. Also called "evoked response."

exacerbation An increase in severity of a disease. Also called "flare-up."

excitability The ability of a cell to respond to a stimulus by initiating an impulse. Also called "depolarization." In cardiac electrophysiology, it is the ability of non-pacemaker myocardial cells to respond to an electrical impulse generated from pacemaker cells and to depolarize.

exercise electrocardiography In cardiovascular assessment, a test that assesses cardiovascular response to an increased workload. Also called "exercise tolerance" or a "stress test." Exercise electrocardiography helps determine the functional capacity of the heart, screens for coronary artery disease, and identifies dysrhythmias that develop during exercise. It also aids in evaluating the effectiveness of antidysrhythmic drugs.

exercise tolerance See *exercise electrocardiography.*

exertional dyspnea Breathlessness or difficulty breathing that develops during activity or exertion.

exertional heat stroke A form of heat stroke with a sudden onset, typically due to strenuous physical activity in hot, humid conditions. Lack of acclimatization to hot weather and wearing clothing too heavy for the environment are common contributing factors.

exogenous Originating outside the body.

exogenous hyperthyroidism Hyperthyroidism caused by excessive use of thyroid replacement hormones.

exophthalmos Abnormal protrusion of the eyeball (proptosis).

expedited partner therapy (EPT) Therapy used to treat chlamydia in which patients are given a drug or prescription with specific instructions for administration to their partners without direct evaluation by a health care provider. Also called "patient-delivered partner therapy."

exploratory laparotomy A surgical opening of the abdominal cavity to investigate the cause of an obstruction or peritonitis.

exposure (1) The final component of the primary survey that allows for thorough assessment of the trauma patient; (2) in radiation therapy, the amount of radiation that is delivered to a tissue.

expressed gene When a particular gene has been "turned on."

expressive aphasia A type of aphasia resulting from damage in Broca's area of the frontal lobe of the brain. A motor speech problem in which the patient understands what is said but is unable to communicate verbally and has difficulty writing; rote speech and automatic speech, such as responses to a greeting, are often intact. The patient is aware of the deficit and may become frustrated and angry. Also called "Broca's aphasia" or "motor aphasia."

expressivity In genetics, the degree of expression a person has when a specific autosomal dominant gene is present. The gene is always expressed, but some people have more severe results.

external fixation A system in which pins or wires are passed through skin and bone and connected to a rigid external frame to immobilize a fracture during healing.

external fixator See *external fixation.*

external hemorrhoid A hemorrhoid that lies below the anal sphincter and can be seen on inspection of the anal region.

external otitis A painful irritation or infection of the skin of the external ear, with resulting allergic response or inflammation. When it occurs in patients who participate in water sports, external otitis is called "swimmer's ear."

external urethral sphincter The sphincter composed of the skeletal muscle that surrounds the urethra.

extracapsular Located outside the joint capsule.

extracellular fluid (ECF) The portion of total body water (about one third) that is in the space outside the cells. This space also includes interstitial fluid, blood, lymph, bone, and connective tissue water, and the transcellular fluids.

extracranial-intracranial bypass A surgical procedure in which the surgeon performs a craniotomy and bypasses the blocked artery by making a graft (bypass) from the first artery to the second artery to establish blood flow around the blocked artery and re-establish blood flow to the involved areas.

extramedullary tumor A tumor found within the spinal dura but outside the cord.

extrapulmonary Involving nonpulmonary tissues.

extravasation Escape of fluids or drugs into the subcutaneous tissue; a complication of intravenous infusion.

extrinsic factor In hematology, an event (e.g., trauma) that occurs outside the blood to cause platelet plugs to form.

extubation The removal of an endotracheal tube.

F

facial paralysis See *Bell's palsy.*

facilitated diffusion Diffusion across a cell membrane that requires the assistance of a transport system or membrane-altering system. Also called "facilitated transport."

facilitated transport See *facilitated diffusion.*

failed back surgery syndrome (FBSS) A combination of organic, psychological, and socioeconomic factors in patients for whom back surgery is not successful. Discouraged by repeated surgical procedures, these patients must continue long-term nonsurgical management of pain, including nerve blocks.

fall An unintentional change in body position that results in the patient's body coming to rest on the floor or ground.

fallophobia In some older adults, the fear of falling and sustaining a serious injury.

far point (of vision) The farthest point at which the eye can see an object.

fascia An inelastic tissue that surrounds groups of muscles, blood vessels, and nerves in the body.

fasciculation Abnormal, involuntary twitching of a muscle.

fasciotomy A surgical procedure in which an incision is made through the skin and subcutaneous tissues into the fascia of the affected compartment to relieve the pressure in and restore circulation to the affected area in the patient with acute compartment syndrome.

fat embolism syndrome (FES) A serious complication, usually resulting from a fracture, in which fat globules are released from the yellow bone marrow into the bloodstream. This syndrome usually occurs within 48 hours of the fracture and can result in respiratory failure or death, often from pulmonary edema.

fatigue (stress) fracture A fracture that results from excessive or repeated strain and stress on a bone.

fatty liver Caused by the accumulation of fats in and around the hepatic cells. It may be caused by alcohol abuse or other factors. Also known as "steatosis."

fecal occult blood test (FOBT) A diagnostic test that measures the presence of blood in the stool from gastrointestinal bleeding; this is a common finding associated with colorectal cancer.

Felty's syndrome The combination of rheumatoid arthritis, hepatosplenomegaly (enlarged liver and spleen), and leukopenia.

femoral hernia A hernia that protrudes through the femoral ring.

fetor hepaticus The distinctive fruity or musty breath odor of chronic liver disease and portal-systemic encephalopathy.

fibrinolysis The breakdown of a clot.

fibrinolytic Drug that targets the fibrin component of the coronary thrombosis; used to dissolve thrombi in the coronary arteries and restore myocardial blood flow; examples include tissue plasminogen activator, anisoylated plasminogen-streptokinase activator complex, and reteplase.

fibroadenoma A solid, slowly enlarging, benign mass of connective tissue that is unattached to the surrounding breast tissue and is typically discovered by the patient herself. The mass is usually round, firm, easily movable, nontender, and clearly delineated from the surrounding tissue.

fibrocystic breast condition (FBC) Physiologic nodularity of the breast that is thought to be caused by an imbalance in the normal estrogen-to-progesterone ratio. It is the most common breast problem of women between 20 and 30 years of age.

fibroids See *leiomyomas.*

fibromyalgia syndrome (FMS) A chronic pain syndrome characterized by pain and tenderness at specific sites in the back of the neck, upper chest, trunk, low back, and extremities along with fatigue, sleep disturbances, and headache.

fibrosis Replacement of normal cells with connective tissue and collagen (scar tissue).

fidelity Ethical principle that refers to the agreement that nurses will keep their obligations or promises to patients to follow through with care.

filter The movement of fluid from the space with higher hydrostatic pressure through the membrane into the space with lower hydrostatic pressure.

filtration The movement of fluid through a cell or blood vessel membrane because of hydrostatic pressure differences on both sides of the membrane.

financial abuse Mismanagement or misuse of the patient's property or resources.

first heart sound (S_1) Sound created by the closure of the mitral and tricuspid valves (atrioventricular valves).

first intention Healing in which the wound can be easily closed and dead space eliminated without granulation, which thus shortens the phases of tissue repair. Inflammation resolves quickly, and connective tissue repair is minimal, resulting in a thin scar.

fistula An abnormal opening between two adjacent organs or structures.

five cardinal manifestations of inflammation Warmth, redness, swelling, pain, and decreased function.

fixed occlusion Wiring the jaws together in the mouth closed position.

flaccid bladder See *areflexic bladder.*

flaccid paralysis Paralysis of a part of the body that is characterized by loss of muscle tone due to hypotonia; may be seen in the patient who has experienced a brain attack.

flail chest Inward movement of the thorax during inspiration, with outward movement during expiration; results from multiple rib fractures caused by blunt chest trauma that leaves a segment of the chest wall loose.

flatulence The presence of an excessive amount of gas in the stomach or intestines.

fluid overload An excess of body fluid. Also called "overhydration."

folliculitis A superficial bacterial infection involving only the upper portion of the hair follicle.

forensic nurse examiner (RN-FNE) Emergency department specialist who is trained to recognize evidence of abuse and to intervene on the patient's behalf and who obtains patient histories, collects forensic evidence, and offers counseling and follow-up care for victims of rape, child abuse, and domestic violence.

fracture A break or disruption in the continuity of a bone.

fremitus Vibration.

frequency (1) The highness or lowness of tones (expressed in hertz). The greater the number of vibrations per second, the higher the frequency (pitch) of the sound; the fewer the number of vibrations per second, the lower the pitch; (2) an urge to urinate frequently in small amounts.

fresh frozen plasma (FFP) Plasma that is frozen immediately after donation so that the clotting factors are preserved.

friable Easily crumbled or damaged.

frostbite A cold injury characterized by the degree of tissue freezing and the resultant damage it produces. Frostbite injuries can be superficial, partial, or full thickness.

frostnip A form of superficial frostbite (typically on the face, fingers, or toes) that produces pain, numbness, and pallor but is easily remedied with the application of warmth and does not induce tissue injury.

Fulmer SPICES A framework that identifies six serious "marker conditions" that can lead to longer hospital stays for patients, higher medical costs, and deaths.

fulminant hepatitis A severe acute and often fatal form of hepatitis caused by failure of the liver cells to regenerate, with progression to necrosis.

furuncle A localized inflammation of the skin caused by bacterial infection, usually *Staphylococcus,* of a hair follicle. Also called "a boil."

G

gallium scan A test that is similar to the bone scan but uses the radioisotope *gallium citrate* and is more specific and sensitive in detecting bone problems. This substance also migrates to brain, liver, and breast tissue and therefore is used to examine these structures when disease is suspected.

gamma globulin See *immunoglobulin.*

ganglion A round, cystlike lesion, often overlying a wrist joint or tendon.

gastrectomy The surgical removal of part or all of the stomach.

gastric bypass A type of gastric restriction surgery in which gastric resection is combined with malabsorption surgery. The patient's stomach, duodenum, and part of the jejunum are bypassed so that fewer calories can be absorbed. Also known as a "Roux-en-Y gastric bypass," or "RNYGB."

gastric lavage Procedure of irrigating the stomach in which a large-bore nasogastric tube is inserted into the stomach and room-temperature solution is instilled in volumes of 200 to 300 mL. The solution and blood are repeatedly withdrawn manually until returns are clear or light pink and without clots.

gastritis An inflammation of the gastric mucosa (stomach lining).

gastroenteritis An increase in the frequency and water content of stools or vomiting as a result of inflammation of the mucous membranes of the stomach and intestinal tract. It affects primarily the small bowel and can be of either viral or bacterial origin.

gastroesophageal reflux (GER) Condition that occurs as a result of backward flow of stomach contents into the esophagus.

gastroesophageal reflux disease (GERD) An upper gastrointestinal disease caused by the backward flow (reflux) of gastrointestinal contents into the esophagus.

gastrojejunostomy Surgical anastomosis of the stomach to the jejunum.

gastroparesis Delay in gastric emptying.

gastrostomy A stoma created from the abdominal wall into the stomach.

gel phenomenon In patients with rheumatoid arthritis, morning stiffness that lasts between 45 minutes and several hours after awakening.

gender dysphoria Discomfort with one's natal sex.

gender identity A person's inner sense of maleness or femaleness not related to reproductive anatomy.

gender reassignment surgery See *sex reassignment surgery.*

gene The deoxyribonucleic acid (DNA) in the form of chromosomes within the nucleus of each cell that contains the instructions for making all the different proteins any organism makes. Every human cell with a nucleus contains the entire set of human genes.

general anesthesia A reversible loss of consciousness induced by inhibiting neuronal impulses in the central nervous system.

generalized seizure One of the three broad categories of seizure disorders along with partial seizures and unclassified seizures. There are six types: tonic-clonic, tonic, clonic, absence, myoclonic, and atonic (akinetic).

genetics The science concerned with the general mechanisms of heredity and the variation of inherited traits.

genital herpes (GH) An acute, recurring, incurable viral disease of the genitalia caused by the herpes simplex virus and transmitted through contact with an infected person. An outbreak typically is preceded by a tingling sensation of the skin followed by the appearance of vesicles (blisters) on the penis, scrotum, vulva, perineum, vagina, cervix, or perianal region. The blisters rupture spontaneously, leaving painful erosions. After the lesions heal, the virus remains dormant, periodically reactivating with a recurrence of symptoms.

genome The complete set of human genes. Each human cell with a nucleus contains the entire set of human genes. The human genome contains about 35,000 individual genes.

genomic health care The application of known genetic variation to enhance health care to individuals and their families.

genomics The science focusing on the function of all of the human DNA, including genes and noncoding DNA regions.

genotype The actual alleles for a genetic trait, not just what can be observed.

genu valgum A deformity in which the knees are abnormally close together and the space between the ankles is increased. Also called "knock-knee."

genu varum A deformity in which the knees are abnormally separated and the lower extremities are bowed inward. Also called "bowleg."

Geriatric Depression Scale—Short Form (GDS-SF) A valid and reliable screening tool to help determine if an older patient has clinical depression.

geriatric failure to thrive (GFTT) A complex syndrome including under-nutrition, impaired physical functioning, depression, and cognitive impairment.

geriatric syndromes Major health issues that are associated with late adulthood in community and inpatient settings.

ghrelin The "hunger hormone" that is secreted in the stomach; increases in a fasting state and decreases after a meal.

Glasgow Coma Scale (GCS) An objective and widely accepted tool for neurologic assessment and documentation of level of consciousness. It establishes baseline data for eye opening, motor response, and verbal response. The patient is assessed and assigned a numeric score for each of these areas. A score of 15 represents normal neurologic functioning, and a score of 3 represents a deep coma state.

glaucoma A group of ocular diseases resulting in increased intraocular pressure, causing reduced blood flow to the optic nerve and retina and followed by tissue damage.

glomerulus A series of specialized capillary loops that receive blood from the afferent arteriole and then filter water and small particles from the blood to make urine. The remaining blood leaves the glomerulus via the efferent arteriole.

glossectomy The partial or total surgical removal of the tongue.

glossitis A smooth, beefy red tongue.

glottis The opening between the true vocal cords inside the larynx.

glucagon A hormone secreted by the pancreas that increases blood glucose levels. It is a "counterregulatory" hormone that has actions opposite those of insulin. It causes the release of glucose from cell storage sites whenever blood glucose levels are low.

gluconeogenesis The conversion of proteins and amino acids to glucose in the body.

glucosamine A supplement that may decrease inflammation.

glycemic A term referring to blood glucose.

glycogenesis The production of glycogen in the body.

glycogenolysis The breakdown of glycogen into glucose.

glycoprotein (GP) IIb/IIIa inhibitors Drugs that target the platelet component of the thrombus. They are administered intravenously to prevent fibrinogen from attaching to activated platelets at the site of a thrombus and are given to patients with acute coronary syndromes (especially unstable angina and non–Q-wave myocardial infarction). Examples include abciximab, eptifibatide, and tirofiban.

glycosylated hemoglobin (A1C) A standardized test that measures how much glucose permanently attaches to the hemoglobin molecule. A1C levels greater than 6.5% are diagnostic of diabetes mellitus.

"go bag" See *personal readiness supplies.*

goiter Enlargement of the thyroid gland.

gonadotropins Hormones that stimulate the ovaries and testes to produce sex hormones.

gonads The male and female reproductive endocrine glands. Male gonads are the testes, and female gonads are the ovaries.

goniometer An instrument for measuring angles; also refers to a tool used to measure joint range of motion.

good death A death that is free from avoidable distress and suffering for patients, families, and caregivers; in agreement with patients' and families' wishes; and consistent with clinical practice standards.

gout A systemic disease in which urate crystals deposit in the joints and other body tissues, causing inflammation.

grading System of classifying cellular aspects of a cancer tumor.

granulation The formation of scar tissue for wound healing to occur.

granuloma Growth that develops in the lungs of patients with sarcoidosis and contains lymphocytes, macrophages, epithelioid cells, and giant cells; scar tissue.

Graves' disease Toxic diffuse goiter characterized by hyperthyroidism, enlargement of the thyroid gland, abnormal protrusion of the eyes, and dry, waxy swelling of the front surfaces of the lower legs.

gray (gy) Unit of measurement for an absorbed radiation dose.

gray matter In the spinal cord, neuron cell bodies.

grief The emotional feeling related to the perception of loss.

grommet A polyethylene tube that is surgically placed through the tympanic membrane to allow continuous drainage of middle-ear fluids in the patient with otitis media.

ground substance A lubricant composed of protein and sugar groups that surrounds the dermal cells and fibers and contributes to the skin's normal suppleness and turgor.

guardian A person appointed to make health care decisions for a patient who is determined to not be legally competent.

Guillain-Barré syndrome (GBS) An acute autoimmune disorder characterized by varying degrees of motor weakness and paralysis. It may be referred to by a variety of other names, such as "acute idiopathic polyneuritis" and "polyradiculoneuropathy."

gynecomastia Abnormal enlargement of the breasts in men.

H

H_2-receptor antagonists A group of drugs that inhibit gastric acid secretion by blocking the effects of histamine on parietal cell receptors in the stomach.

half-life Time it takes for the amount of drug in the body to be reduced by 50%.

halitosis A foul odor of the mouth.

hallux valgus A common deformity of the foot that occurs when the great toe deviates laterally at the metatarsophalangeal joint; sometimes referred to as a "bunion."

halo fixator A static traction device used for immobilization of the cervical spine. Four pins or screws are inserted into the skull, and a metal halo ring is attached to a plastic vest or cast when the spine is stable, allowing increased patient mobility.

hammertoe The dorsiflexion of any metatarsophalangeal joint with plantar flexion of the adjacent proximal interphalangeal joint. The second toe is most often affected.

hand hygiene Infection control protocol that refers to both handwashing and alcohol-based hand rubs.

health care–associated infection (HAI) Infections associated with the provision of health care; for example, microorganisms can enter the body through the genitourinary tract in patients with indwelling urinary catheters.

heart failure A general term for the inadequacy of the heart to pump blood throughout the body, causing insufficient perfusion of body tissues with vital nutrients and oxygen. Also called "pump failure."

heart rate (HR) Term referring to the number of times the ventricles contract each minute.

heart transplantation A surgical procedure in which a heart from a donor with a comparable body weight and ABO compatibility is transplanted into a recipient less than 6 hours after procurement. It is the treatment of choice for patients with severe dilated cardiomyopathy and may be considered for patients with restrictive cardiomyopathy.

heat exhaustion A syndrome primarily caused by dehydration from heavy perspiration and inadequate fluid and electrolyte consumption during heat exposure over hours to days; if left untreated, can be a precursor to heat stroke.

heat stroke A true medical emergency in which the victim's heat regulatory mechanisms fail and are unable to compensate for a critical elevation in body temperature; if uncorrected, organ dysfunction and death will ensue.

Heberden's nodes Swelling at the distal interphalangeal joints in osteoarthritis that involves the hands.

hematemesis The vomiting of blood.

hematochezia The passage of red blood via the rectum.

hematocrit The percentage of packed red blood cells per deciliter of blood.

hematogenous tuberculosis A form of tuberculosis that spreads throughout the body when a large number of organisms enter the blood. Also called "miliary tuberculosis."

hematopoiesis The production of blood cells, which occurs in the red marrow of bones.

hematuria Blood in the urine.

hemianopsia Blindness in half of the visual field of one or both eyes. Also called "hemianopia."

hemiarthroplasty Surgical replacement of part of the shoulder joint, typically the humeral component, as an alternative to total shoulder arthroplasty.

hemiparesis Weakness on one side of the body.

hemiplegia Paralysis on one side of the body.

hemoconcentration Elevated plasma levels of hemoglobin, hematocrit, serum osmolarity, glucose, protein, blood urea nitrogen, and electrolytes that occur when only the water is lost and other substances remain.

hemodilution Excessive water in the vascular space.

hemoglobin A (HbA) Normal adult hemoglobin. The molecule has two alpha chains and two beta chains of amino acids.

hemoglobin S (HbS) An abnormal beta chain of hemoglobin associated with sickle cell disease that is sensitive to low oxygen content of red blood cells.

hemolytic The characteristic of destroying red blood cells.

hemolytic anemia Anemia caused by the destruction of red blood cells.

hemoptysis Coughing up blood or blood-stained sputum.

hemorrhoid Unnaturally swollen or distended vein in the anorectal region.

hemorrhoidectomy The excision of a hemorrhoid.

hemostasis The multi-step process of controlled blood clotting.

heparin-induced thrombocytopenia (HIT) The aggregation of platelets into "white clots" that can cause thrombosis, usually in the form of an acute arterial occlusion; occurs with heparin administration. Also called "white clot syndrome."

hepatic encephalopathy See *portal-systemic encephalopathy.*

hepatitis The widespread inflammation of liver cells.

hepatitis A Hepatitis that is caused by the hepatitis A virus (HAV) and is characterized by a mild course similar to that of a typical viral syndrome and often goes unrecognized. It is spread via the fecal-oral route by oral ingestion of fecal contaminants. Sources of infection include contaminated water, shellfish caught in contaminated water, and food contaminated by infected food handlers. The virus may also be spread by oral-anal sexual activity. The incubation period is usually 15 to 50 days. The disease is usually not life threatening but may be more severe in people older than 40 years. It can also complicate preexisting liver disease.

hepatitis B A form of hepatitis that is caused by the hepatitis B virus (HBV), which is shed in the body fluids of infected people and asymptomatic carriers. It is spread through unprotected sexual intercourse with an infected partner, needle sharing, blood transfusions, and other modes. Symptoms usually occur within 25 to 180 days of exposure and include nausea, fever, fatigue, joint pain, and jaundice. Most adults who get hepatitis B recover, clear the virus from their body, and develop immunity; however, up to 10% of patients with the disease do not develop immunity and become carriers.

hepatitis C Hepatitis that is caused by the hepatitis C virus (HCV). Transmission is blood to blood, most commonly by needle sharing or needle stick injury with contaminated blood. The rate of sexual transmission is very low; it is not spread by casual contact and is rarely transmitted from mother to fetus. The average incubation period is 7 weeks. Most people are asymptomatic and are not diagnosed until long after the initial exposure when an abnormality is detected during a routine laboratory evaluation or when symptoms of liver impairment appear. Hepatitis C causes chronic inflammation in the liver that eventually causes the hepatocytes to scar and may progress to cirrhosis.

hepatitis carrier Person who has had hepatitis B but has not developed immunity. Hepatitis carriers can infect others even though they are not sick and demonstrate no obvious signs of disease. Chronic carriers are at high risk for cirrhosis and liver cancer.

hepatitis D The hepatitis D virus (HDV) co-infects with hepatitis B virus (HBV) and needs the presence of HBV for viral replication. HDV can co-infect a patient with HBV or can occur as a superinfection in a patient with chronic HBV. Superinfection usually develops into chronic HDV infection. The incubation period is 14 to 56 days. As with HBV, the disease is transmitted primarily by parenteral routes.

hepatitis E Hepatitis E virus (HEV) was originally identified by its association with water-borne epidemics of hepatitis in the Indian subcontinent. Since then, it has occurred in epidemics in Asia, Africa, the Middle East, Mexico, and Central and South America, typically after heavy rains and flooding. In the United States, hepatitis E has been found only in travelers returning from endemic areas. The virus is transmitted via the fecal-oral route, and the clinical course resembles that of hepatitis A. HEV has an incubation period of 15 to 64 days. There is no evidence at this time of a chronic form of hepatitis E.

hepatocyte Liver cell.

hepatomegaly Enlargement of the liver.

hepatorenal syndrome (HRS) A state of progressive oliguric renal failure associated with hepatic failure, resulting in functional impairment of kidneys with normal anatomic and morphologic features. It indicates a poor prognosis for the patient with hepatic failure and is often the cause of death in patients with cirrhosis.

hereditary chronic pancreatitis Pancreatitis that may be associated with *SPINK1* and *CFTR* gene mutations.

heritability The risk that a disorder can be transmitted to one's children in a recognizable pattern.

hernia A weakness in the abdominal muscle wall through which a segment of the bowel or other abdominal structure protrudes.

herniated nucleus pulposus (HNP) The protrusion (herniation) of the pulpy material from the center of a vertebral disk; herniated disks occur most often between the fourth and fifth lumbar vertebrae (L4-5) but may occur at other levels. A herniation in the lumbosacral area can press on the adjacent spinal nerve (usually the sciatic nerve), causing severe burning or stabbing pain into the leg or foot, or it may press on the spinal cord itself, causing leg weakness and bowel and bladder dysfunction. The specific area of pain depends on the level of herniation.

hernioplasty Surgical repair of a hernia in which the surgeon reinforces the weakened outside muscle wall with a mesh patch.

herniorrhaphy The surgical repair of a hernia.

heterotopic ossification Abnormal bony overgrowth, often into muscle; seen as a complication of prolonged immobility in patients with spinal cord injury.

hiatal hernia Protrusion of the stomach through the esophageal hiatus of the diaphragm and into the thorax. Also called "diaphragmatic hernia."

high-alert drug A drug that has an increased risk for causing patient harm if given in error.

high altitude disease (HAD) See *high altitude illnesses.*

high altitude illnesses Pathophysiologic responses in the body caused by exposure to low partial pressure of oxygen at high elevations.

high altitude pulmonary edema (HAPE) A form of acute mountain sickness often seen with high altitude cerebral edema. Clinical indicators include persistent dry cough, cyanosis of the lips and nail beds, tachycardia and tachypnea at rest, and rales auscultated in one or both lungs. Pink, frothy sputum is a late sign.

high-density lipoproteins (HDLs) Part of the total cholesterol value that should be more than 45 mg/dL for men and more than 55 mg/dL for women; "good" cholesterol.

highly sensitive C-reactive protein (hsCRP) A serum marker of inflammation and a common and critical component to the development of atherothrombosis.

high-output heart failure Heart failure that occurs when cardiac output remains normal or above normal. It is usually caused by increased metabolic needs or hyperkinetic conditions such as septicemia (fever), anemia, and hyperthyroidism. This type of heart failure is different from left- and right-sided heart failure, which are typically low-output states, and is not as common as other types.

hilum The area of the kidney in which the renal artery and nerve plexus enter and the renal vein and ureter exit. This area is not covered by the renal capsule.

hirsutism Abnormal growth of body hair, especially on the face, chest, and the linea alba of the abdomen of women.

homeostasis The narrow range of normal conditions (e.g., body temperature, blood electrolyte values, blood pH, blood volume) in the human body; the tendency to maintain a constant balance in normal body states.

homeostatic mechanism A safeguard or control mechanism within the human body that prevents dangerous changes.

homocysteine An essential sulfur-containing amino acid that is produced when dietary protein breaks down; elevated values (greater than 15 mmol/L) may be a risk factor for the development of cardiovascular disease.

homonymous hemianopsia Condition in which there is blindness in the same side of both eyes.

hordeolum An infection of the sweat glands in the eyelid.

hormone Chemical produced in the body that exerts its effects on specific tissues known as "target tissues."

hospice An interdisciplinary approach to facilitate quality of life and a "good" death for patients near the end of their lives, with care provided in a variety of settings.

Hospital Incident Command System (HICS) An organizational model for disaster management in which roles are formally structured under the hospital or long-term care facility incident commander, with clear lines of authority and accountability for specific resources.

hospital incident commander As defined in a hospital's emergency response plan, the person (either an emergency physician or administrator) who assumes overall leadership for implementing the institutional plan at the onset of a mass casualty incident. The hospital incident commander has a global view of the entire situation, facilitates patient movement through the system, and brings in resources to meet patient needs.

hospitalist Family practitioner or internist employed by a hospital.

human leukocyte antigen (HLA) Antigen that is present on the surfaces of nearly all body cells as a normal part of the person and acts as an antigen only if it enters another person's body.

human papilloma virus (HPV) test A test that can identify many high-risk types of HPV associated with the development of cervical cancer.

humoral immunity A type of immunity provided by antibodies circulating in body fluids.

Huntington disease (HD) A hereditary disorder transmitted as an autosomal dominant trait at the time of conception (formerly called "Huntington chorea"). Men and women between 35 and 50 years of age are affected; clinical onset is gradual. The two main symptoms are progressive mental status changes (leading to dementia) and choreiform movements (rapid, jerky movements) in the limbs, trunk, and facial muscles.

hydrocephalus The abnormal accumulation of cerebrospinal fluid within the skull.

hydronephrosis Abnormal enlargement of the kidney caused by a blockage of urine lower in the tract and filling of the kidney with urine.

hydrophilic Tending to absorb water readily.

hydrophobic Not readily absorbing water; waterproof.

hydrostatic pressure The force of the weight of water molecules pressing against the confining walls of a space.

hydrotherapy The application of water for treatment of injury or disease.

hydroureter Abnormal distention of the ureter.

hyperacusis An intolerance for sound levels that do not bother other people.

hyperaldosteronism Excessive mineralocorticoid production.

hypercalcemia A total serum calcium level above 10.5 mg/dL or 2.75 mmol/L, which can cause fatigue, anorexia, nausea and vomiting, constipation, polyuria, and serious damage to the urinary system.

hypercapnia Increased arterial carbon dioxide levels.

hypercarbia Increased partial pressure of arterial carbon dioxide ($PaCO_2$) levels.

hypercellularity An abnormal number of cells.

hyperemia Increased blood flow to an area.

hyperesthesia Abnormally increased sensation.

hyperextension A mechanism of injury that occurs when a part of the body is suddenly accelerated and then decelerated, causing extreme extension.

hyperflexion A mechanism of injury that occurs when a part of the body is suddenly and force fully accelerated forward, causing extreme flexion.

hyperglycemia Abnormally high levels of blood glucose.

hyperinsulinemia Chronic high blood insulin levels.

hyperkalemia An elevated level of potassium in the blood.

hyperlipidemia An elevation of serum lipid (fat) levels in the blood.

hypermagnesemia A serum magnesium level above 2.1 mEq/L.

hypernatremia An excessive amount of sodium in the blood.

hyperopia An error of refraction that occurs when the eye does not refract light enough, causing images to fall (converge) behind the retina and resulting in poor near vision. Also called "farsightedness."

hyperosmotic Describes fluids with osmolarities (solute concentrations) greater than 300 mOsm/L; hyperosmotic fluids have a greater osmotic pressure than do isosmotic fluids and tend to pull water from the isosmotic fluid space into the hyperosmotic fluid space until an osmotic balance occurs. Also called "hypertonic."

hyperpharmacy See *polypharmacy.*

hyperphosphatemia A serum phosphorus level above 4.5 mg/dL.

hyperpituitarism Hormone oversecretion that occurs with pituitary tumors or hyperplasia.

hyperplasia Growth that causes tissue to increase in size by increasing the number of cells; abnormal overgrowth of tissue.

hyperpnea An abnormal increase in the depth of respiratory movements.

hypersensitivity An overreaction to a foreign substance.

hypertension A cardiovascular condition pertaining to people who have a systolic blood pressure of 140 mm Hg or higher or a diastolic blood pressure of 90 mm Hg or higher or who take medication to control blood pressure; approximately 1 of every 5 Americans has hypertension.

hypertensive crisis A severe elevation in blood pressure (greater than 180/120 mm Hg) that can cause damage to organs such as the kidneys or heart.

hyperthermia Elevated body temperature; fever.

hyperthyroidism A condition caused by excessive production of thyroid hormone.

hypertonia A condition of excessive muscle tone, which tends to cause fixed positions or contractures of the involved extremities and restricted range of motion of the joints.

hypertonic See *hyperosmotic.*

hypertriglyceridemia Elevated levels (150 mg/dL or above) of triglyceride in the blood.

hypertrophic cardiomyopathy (HCM) A type of cardiomyopathy that involves disarray of the myocardial fibers and asymmetric ventricular hypertrophy; leads to a stiff left ventricle that results in diastolic filling abnormalities.

hypertrophy The enlargement or overgrowth of an organ; tissue increases in size by the enlargement of each cell.

hyperuricemia An excess of uric acid in the blood.

hyperventilation A state of increased rate and depth of breathing.

hyperviscous The quality of being thicker than normal.

hypervolemia Increased plasma volume; or fluid excess.

hypocalcemia A total serum calcium level below 9.0 mg/dL or 2.25 mmol/L.

hypocapnia Decreased arterial carbon dioxide levels.

hypodermoclysis The slow infusion of isotonic fluids into subcutaneous tissue.

hypoesthesia Abnormally decreased sensation.

hypoglycemia Abnormally low levels of glucose in the blood.

hypokalemia A decreased serum potassium level; a common electrolyte imbalance.

hyponatremia A serum sodium level below 136 mEq/L (mmol/L).

hypo-osmotic Describes fluids with osmolarities of less than 270 mOsm/L. Hypo-osmolar fluids have a lower osmotic pressure than isosmotic fluids, and water tends to be pulled from the hypo-osmotic fluid space into the isosmotic fluid space until an osmotic balance occurs. Also called "hypotonic."

hypophonia Soft voice.

hypophosphatemia Inadequate levels of phosphate in the blood (below 3.0 mg/dL).
hypophysectomy Surgical removal of the pituitary gland.
hypoproteinemia A decrease in serum proteins.
hypothalamic-hypophysial portal system The small, closed circulatory system that the hypothalamus shares with the anterior pituitary gland, which allows hormones produced in the hypothalamus to travel directly to the anterior pituitary gland.
hypothalamus A structure within the brain; an integral part of autonomic nervous system control (controlling temperature and other functions) that is essential in intellectual function.
hypothermia A core body temperature less than 95° F (35° C).
hypotonia An abnormal condition of inadequate muscle tone, with an inability to maintain balance.
hypotonic See *hypo-osmotic.*
hypoventilation A state in which gas exchange at the alveolar-capillary membrane is inadequate so that too little oxygen reaches the blood and carbon dioxide is retained.
hypovolemia Abnormally decreased volume of circulating fluid in the body; fluid deficit.
hypoxemia (hypoxemic) Decreased blood oxygen levels; hypoxia.
hypoxia A reduction of oxygen supply to the tissues.
hysterosalpingogram An x-ray of the cervix, uterus, and fallopian tubes that is performed after injection of a contrast medium. This test is used in infertility workups to evaluate tubal anatomy and patency and uterine problems such as fibroids, tumors, and fistulas.
hysteroscopy Examination of the interior of the uterus and cervical canal using an endoscope.

I

icterus Yellow discoloration of the sclerae.
idiopathic chronic pancreatitis Pancreatitis that may be associated with *SPINK1* and *CFTR* gene mutations.
idiopathic seizure See *unclassified seizure.*
ileostomy The surgical creation of an opening into the ileum, usually by bringing the end of the terminal ileum through the abdominal wall and forming a stoma, or ostomy.
immediate memory Short-term or new memory. Test by asking the patient to repeat two or three unrelated words to make sure they were heard; after about 5 minutes, while continuing the examination, ask the patient to repeat the words.
immunity Resistance to infection; usually associated with the presence of antibodies or cells that act on specific microorganisms.
immunocompetent Having proper functioning of the body's ability to maintain itself and defend against disease.
immunoglobulin Antibody. Also called "gamma globulin."
impermeable Not porous.
implanted port A device used for long-term or frequent infusion therapy; consists of a portal body, a dense septum over a reservoir, and a catheter that is surgically implanted on the upper chest or upper extremity.
inactivation The process of binding an antibody to an antigen to cover the antigen's active site and to make the antigen harmless without destroying it. Also called "neutralization."
incisional hernia Protrusion of the intestine at the site of a previous surgical incision resulting from inadequate healing. Most often caused by postoperative wound infections, inadequate nutrition, and obesity. Also called "ventral hernia."
incomplete spinal cord injury An injury in which the spinal cord has been damaged in a way that allows some function or movement below the level of the injury.
incontinence Involuntary loss of urine or stool severe enough to cause social or hygienic problems.
independent living skills See *instrumental activities of daily living (IADLs).*
indirect inguinal hernia A sac formed from the peritoneum that contains a portion of the intestine or omentum. The hernia pushes downward at an angle into the inguinal canal. In males, indirect inguinal hernias can become large and often descend into the scrotum.
indolent Slow-growing.
induration Hardening.
infarction Necrosis, or cell death.
infective endocarditis A microbial infection (e.g., viruses, bacteria, fungi) involving the endocardium; previously called "bacterial endocarditis."
inferior vena cava filtration Surgical procedure in which the surgeon inserts a filter device percutaneously into the inferior vena cava of a patient with recurrent deep vein thrombosis (to prevent pulmonary emboli) or pulmonary emboli that do not respond to medical treatment. The device is meant to trap emboli in the inferior vena cava before they progress to the lungs. Holes in the device allow blood to pass through, thus not significantly interfering with the return of blood to the heart.
inferior wall myocardial infarction A type of myocardial infarction that occurs in patients with obstruction of the right coronary artery, causing significant damage to the right ventricle.
infiltrating ductal carcinoma The most common type of breast cancer; it originates in the mammary ducts and grows in the epithelial cells lining these ducts.
infiltration The leakage of IV solution into the tissues around the vein.
inflammatory breast cancer A rare but highly aggressive form of invasive breast cancer. Symptoms include swelling, skin redness, and pain in the breasts.
inflammatory cytokines Proteins produced primarily by white blood cells that assist in the inflammatory and immune responses of the body (e.g., tumor necrosis factor, interleukins).
inflow disease Chronic peripheral arterial disease with obstruction at or above the common iliac artery, abdominal aorta, or profunda femoris artery. The patient experiences discomfort in the lower back, buttocks, or thighs after walking a certain distance. The pain usually subsides with rest.
informatics A QSEN competency in which the nurse uses information and technology to communicate, manage knowledge, mitigate error, and support decision making.
infratentorial Located below the tentorium of the cerebellum.
infusate A solution that is infused into the body.
infusion therapy The delivery of parenteral medications and fluids through a variety of catheter types and locations using multiple techniques and procedures, such as intravenous and intra-arterial therapy to deliver solutions into the vascular system.
inpatient A patient who is admitted to a hospital.
inpatient rehabilitation facilities (IRFs) Freestanding rehabilitation hospitals, rehabilitation or skilled units within hospitals (e.g., transitional care units), and skilled nursing facilities to which the patient is typically admitted for 1 to 3 weeks or longer.
insensible water loss Water loss from the skin, lungs, and stool that cannot be controlled.
instrumental activities of daily living (IADLs) Special activities performed in the course of a day such as using the telephone, shopping, preparing food, and housekeeping. Also called "independent living skills."
insufflation The practice of injecting gas or air into a cavity before surgery to separate organs and improve visualization.
intensity A quality of sound that is expressed in decibels; generally, having a high degree of energy or activity.
intensivist A physician who specializes in critical care.
intention tremor A tremor that occurs when performing an activity.
interbody cage fusion Cagelike spinal device that is implanted into the space where a disk was removed. Bone graft tissue grows into and around the cage and creates a stable spine at that level.
intercostally Located between the ribs.
intermittent claudication A characteristic leg pain experienced by patients with chronic peripheral arterial disease. Typically, patients can walk only a certain distance before a cramping muscle pain forces them to stop. As the disease progresses, the patient can walk only shorter and shorter distances before pain recurs. Ultimately, pain may occur even at rest.
internal derangement A broad term for disturbances of an injured knee joint.
internal fixation The use of metal pins, screws, rods, plates, or prostheses to immobilize a fracture during healing. The surgeon makes an incision (open reduction) to gain access to the broken bone and implants one or more devices.
internal hemorrhoid A hemorrhoid that is located above the anal sphincter and cannot be seen on inspection of the perineal area.
internal urethral sphincter The smooth detrusor muscle that lines the interior of the bladder neck.

interstitial cystitis A bladder inflammation of unknown etiology that occurs predominantly in women and is characterized by urinary frequency and pain on bladder filling.

interstitial fluid A portion of the extracellular fluid that is between cells, sometimes called the "third space."

interstitial laser coagulation (ILC) Procedure for treating benign prostatic hyperplasia that uses laser energy to coagulate excess tissue. Also called "contact laser prostatectomy (CLP)."

intra-abdominal hypertension (IAH) Condition of sustained or repeated intra-abdominal pressure of 12 mm Hg or higher.

intra-abdominal pressure Pressure contained within the abdominal cavity.

intra-aortic balloon pump (IABP) An intra-aortic counterpulsation device. It may be used as an invasive intervention to improve myocardial perfusion during an acute myocardial infarction, reduce preload and afterload, and facilitate left ventricular ejection. It is also used when patients do not respond to drug therapy with improved tissue perfusion, decreased workload of the heart, and increased cardiac contractility.

intra-arterial infusion therapy The use of catheters placed into arteries to obtain repeated arterial blood samples, to monitor various hemodynamic pressures continuously, and to infuse chemotherapy agents or fibrinolytics.

intracapsular Located within the joint capsule.

intracellular fluid (ICF) The portion of total body water (about two thirds) that is found inside the cells.

intracerebral hemorrhage Bleeding within the brain tissue caused by the tearing of small arteries and veins in the subcortical white matter.

intracorporeal Situated or occurring inside the body.

intramedullary tumor Tumor originating within the spinal cord in the central gray matter and anterior commissure. It is often malignant.

intraocular pressure (IOP) Pressure of the fluid within the eye; may be measured by methods that involve direct contact with the eye or by noncontact techniques.

intraoperative During surgery.

intraosseous (IO) therapy Infusion therapy that is delivered to the vascular network in the long bones.

intraperitoneal (IP) infusion therapy The administration of antineoplastic agents into the peritoneal cavity.

intrapulmonary Within the respiratory tract.

intrarenal/intrinsic renal failure Decreased renal function resulting from damage to the glomeruli, interstitial tissue, or tubules. It can contribute to acute renal failure.

intrathecal Referring to the spine.

intravascular ultrasonography (IVUS) In cardiac catheterization, the use of a flexible catheter with a miniature transducer that emits sound waves. Sound waves are reflected off the plaque and the arterial wall, creating an image of the blood vessel; used as an alternative to injecting a contrast medium into the coronary arteries.

intravenous (systemic) fibrinolytic therapy The intravenous administration of thrombolytic agents to dissolve a thrombus.

intravesical Situated inside the bladder.

intrinsic factor A substance normally secreted by the gastric mucosa and needed for intestinal absorption of vitamin B_{12}. A deficiency of intrinsic factor and the resulting failure to absorb vitamin B_{12} lead to pernicious anemia.

intussusception The telescoping of a segment of the intestine within itself.

invasive hemodynamic monitoring System used in critical care areas to provide quantitative information about vascular capacity, blood volume, pump effectiveness, and tissue perfusion. It directly measures pressures in the heart and great vessels.

ion A substance found in body fluids that carries an electrical charge. Also called "electrolyte."

iontophoresis A treatment for lower back pain in which a small electrical current and dexamethasone are typically used.

ipsilateral Occurring on the same side.

iris The colored portion of the external eye; its center opening is the pupil. Muscles of the iris contract and relax to control pupil size and the amount of light entering the eye.

irreducible hernia A hernia that cannot be reduced or placed back into the abdominal cavity; requires immediate surgical evaluation.

irritability An overresponse to stimuli.

irritable bowel syndrome (IBS) A chronic gastrointestinal disorder characterized by chronic or recurrent diarrhea, constipation, and/or abdominal pain and bloating. Also called "spastic colon," "mucous colon," or "nervous colon."

ischemia Blockage of blood flow through a blood vessel resulting in a lack of oxygen. Prolonged severe ischemia can cause irreversible damage to tissue.

ischemic Cell dysfunction or death from a lack of oxygen resulting from decreased blood flow in a body part.

ischemic stroke A type of brain attack caused by occlusion of a cerebral artery by either a thrombus or an embolus. About 80% of all brain attacks are ischemic.

isoelectric Having equal electric potentials, such as in the heart.

isosmotic Having the same osmotic pressures. Also called "isotonic" or "normotonic."

isotonic See *isosmotic.*

J

jaundice A syndrome characterized by excessive circulating bilirubin levels. Liver cells cannot effectively excrete bilirubin, and skin and mucous membranes become characterized by a yellow coloration.

jejunostomy The surgical creation of an opening between the jejunum and the surface of the abdominal wall.

joint The place at which two or more bones come together. Also referred to as "articulation" of the joint. The primary function is to provide movement and flexibility in the body.

jugular venous distention (JVD) Enlargement of the jugular vein of the neck; caused by an increase in jugular venous pressure.

juxtaglomerular complex Specialized cells that produce and store renin in the afferent arteriole, efferent arteriole, and distal collecting tubule; taken together, the juxtaglomerular cells and the macula densa.

K

karyotype Technique used to make an organized arrangement of all the chromosomes within one cell during the metaphase section of mitosis.

keratin The protein produced by keratinocytes; makes the outermost skin layer waterproof.

keratinocytes Basal skin cells attached to the basement membrane of the epidermis that undergo cell division and differentiation to continuously renew skin tissue integrity and maintain optimal barrier function. As basal cells divide, keratinocytes are pushed upward and flattened to form the stratified layers of the epithelium (malpighian layers).

keratoconjunctivitis sicca A condition of the eyes that results from changes in tear composition, lacrimal gland malfunction, or altered tear distribution. Also called "dry eye syndrome."

keratoconus The degeneration of the corneal tissue resulting in abnormal corneal shape.

keratoplasty Corneal transplant. The surgical removal of diseased corneal tissue and replacement with tissue from a human donor cornea.

ketogenesis The conversion of fats to acids in the body.

ketone bodies Substances, including acetone, that are produced as by-products of the incomplete metabolism of fatty acids. When insulin is not available (as in uncontrolled diabetes mellitus), they accumulate in the blood and cause metabolic acidosis. Also called "ketones."

knee height caliper Device that uses the distance between the patella and heel to estimate height.

Kupffer cells Phagocytic cells that are part of the body's reticuloendothelial system and are involved in the protective function of the liver. Kupffer cells engulf harmful bacteria and anemic red blood cells.

Kussmaul respiration A type of breathing that occurs when excess acids caused by the absence of insulin increase hydrogen ion and carbon dioxide levels in the blood. This state triggers an increase in the rate and depth of respiration in an attempt to excrete more carbon dioxide and acid.

kwashiorkor Lack of protein quantity and quality in the presence of adequate calories. Body weight is somewhat normal, and serum proteins are low.

kyphoplasty A minimally invasive surgery for managing vertebral fractures in patients with osteoporosis. Bone cement is injected into the fracture site to provide pain relief, and an inflated balloon is used to restore height to the vertebra.

L

labyrinthectomy Surgical removal of the labyrinth; used as a radical treatment of Ménière's disease when medical therapy is ineffective and the patient already has significant hearing loss.

labyrinthitis An infection of the labyrinth of the ear; may occur as a complication of acute or chronic otitis media.

laceration A type of wound characterized by tearing or mangling and usually caused by sharp objects and projectiles.

lacrimal gland A small gland that produces tears; located in the upper outer part of each ocular orbit.

lacto-ovo-vegetarian A vegetarian diet pattern in which milk, cheese, eggs, and dairy foods are eaten but meat, fish, and poultry are avoided.

lactose intolerance The inability to convert lactose (found in milk and dairy products) to glucose and galactose in the body.

lacto-vegetarian A vegetarian diet pattern in which milk, cheese, and dairy foods are eaten but meat, fish, poultry, and eggs are avoided.

laparoscopy A minimally invasive procedure in which the surgeon makes several small incisions near the umbilicus through which a small endoscope is placed to examine the abdomen; direct examination of the pelvic cavity through an endoscope.

laparotomy An open surgical approach in which a large abdominal incision is made.

laryngectomee A person who has had a laryngectomy.

laryngopharynx The area behind the larynx that extends from the base of the tongue to the esophagus. It is the critical dividing point at which solid foods and fluids are separated from air.

larynx The "voice box"; it is composed of several cartilages and is located above the trachea and just below the throat at the base of the tongue; part of the upper respiratory tract.

laser An acronym for light amplification by stimulated emission of radiation. As a surgical tool, a laser emits a high-powered beam of light that cuts tissue more cleanly than do scalpel blades. A laser creates intense heat, rapidly clots blood vessels or tissue, and turns target tissue (e.g., a tumor) into vapor.

latency period The time between the initiation of a cell and the development of an overt tumor.

latex allergy Reactions to exposure to latex in gloves and other medical products; reactions include rashes, nasal or eye symptoms, and asthma.

latrodectism A syndrome caused by the venom of a black widow spider bite in which neurotransmitter releases from nerve terminals to cause severe abdominal pain, muscle rigidity and spasm, hypertension, and nausea and vomiting.

lead In an ECG, the provider of one view of the heart's electrical activity.

lead axis In electrocardiography, the imaginary line that joins the positive and negative poles of the lead systems.

left shift An increase in the band cells (immature neutrophils) in the white blood cell differential count; an early indication of infection.

left-sided heart (ventricular) failure Inadequacy of the left ventricle of the heart to pump adequately; results in decreased tissue perfusion from poor cardiac output and pulmonary congestion from increased pressure in the pulmonary vessels; typical causes include hypertensive, coronary artery, or valvular disease involving the mitral or aortic valve. Most heart failure begins with failure of the left ventricle and progresses to failure of both ventricles.

legally competent A person 18 years of age or older, a pregnant or a married minor, a legally emancipated (free) minor who is self-supporting, or a person not declared incompetent by a court of law.

leiomyomas Benign, slow-growing solid tumors of the uterine myometrium (muscle layer). These are the most commonly occurring pelvic tumors. Also called "myomas" and "fibroids."

lens The circular, convex structure of the eye that lies behind the iris and in front of the vitreous body. Normally transparent, the lens bends the rays of light entering through the pupil so they focus on the retina. The curve of the lens changes to focus on near or distant objects.

leptin A hormone that is released by fat cells and possibly by gastric cells; it also acts on the hypothalamus to control appetite.

leukemia A type of cancer with uncontrolled production of immature white blood cells in the bone marrow; the bone marrow becomes overcrowded with immature, nonfunctional cells, and the production of normal blood cells is greatly decreased.

leukocyte White blood cell (WBC); this immune system cell protects the body from the effects of invasion by organisms.

leukopenia A reduction in the number of white blood cells.

leukoplakia White, patchy lesions on a mucous membrane.

levels of evidence Term used to refer to the status, rank, or strength of evidence.

LGBTQ Acronym for "lesbian, gay, bisexual, transgender, and queer/questioning" culture.

libido Sexual desire.

lichenified An abnormal thickening of the skin to a leathery appearance; can occur in patients with chronic dermatitis because of their continual rubbing of the area to relieve itching.

Lichtenberg figures Branching or ferning marks that appear on the skin as a result of a lightning strike. Also called "keraunographic markings" or "erythematous arborization."

life review A structured process of reflecting on one's life that is often facilitated by an interviewer.

light reflex The reflection of the otoscope's light off the eardrum in the form of a clearly demarcated triangle of light in the normal ear.

limited cutaneous systemic sclerosis Thick skin that is usually limited to sites distal to the elbow and knee but also involves the face and neck.

lipid Fat, including cholesterol and triglycerides, that can be measured in the blood.

lipolysis The decomposition or splitting up of fat to provide fuel for energy when liver glucose is unavailable.

liposuction A cosmetic procedure to reduce the amount of adipose tissue in selected areas of the body.

lithotripsy The use of sound, laser, or dry shock wave energy to break a kidney stone into small fragments. Also called "extracorporeal shock wave lithotripsy."

living will A legal document that instructs physicians and family members about what life-sustaining treatment is wanted (or not wanted) if the patient becomes unable to make decisions.

lobectomy Surgical removal of an entire lung lobe.

lobular carcinoma in situ (LCIS) A noninvasive form of breast cancer that does not show up as a calcified cluster on a mammogram and is therefore most often diagnosed incidentally during a biopsy for another problem.

local anesthesia Anesthesia that is delivered by applying it to the skin or mucous membranes of the area to be anesthetized or by injecting it directly into the tissue around an incision, wound, or lesion.

locus The specific chromosome location for a gene.

log rolling Turning technique in which the patient turns all at once while his or her back is kept as straight as possible.

loop electrosurgical excision procedure (LEEP) Diagnostic procedure/treatment in which a thin loop-wire electrode that transmits a painless electrical current is used to cut away affected cervical cancer tissue.

lordosis The anterior concavity in the curvature of the lumbar and cervical spine when viewed from the side; a common finding in pregnancy and abdominal obesity.

Lou Gehrig's disease See *amyotrophic lateral sclerosis (ALS)*.

low back pain (LBP) Pain in the lumbosacral region of the back caused by muscle strain or spasm, ligament sprain, disk degeneration, or herniation of the nucleus pulposus from the center of the disk. Herniated disks occur most often between the fourth and fifth lumbar vertebrae (L4-5) but may occur at other levels.

low-density lipoproteins (LDLs) Part of the total cholesterol value that should be less than 130 mg/dL; "bad" cholesterol.

lower esophageal sphincter (LES) The portion of the esophagus proximal to the gastroesophageal junction; when at rest, the sphincter is closed to prevent reflux of gastric contents into the esophagus.

low-intensity pulsed ultrasound A method using ultrasonic waves to promote bone union in slow-healing fractures or for new fractures as an alternative to surgery.

low-profile gastrostomy device (LPGD) A gastrostomy device that uses a firm or balloon-style internal bumper or retention disk; an antireflux valve keeps gastric contents from leaking onto the skin.

loxoscelism Systemic effects from the injected toxin of a spider bite.

lumbar puncture (spinal tap) The insertion of a spinal needle into the subarachnoid space between the third and fourth (sometimes the fourth and fifth) lumbar vertebrae to withdraw spinal fluid for analysis.

lumen The inside cavity of a tube or tubular organ, such as a blood vessel or airway.

lung compliance The quality of elasticity of the lungs.

lunula The white crescent-shaped portion of the nail at the lower end of the nail plate.

lurch An abnormality in the swing phase of gait; occurs when the muscles in the buttocks or legs are too weak to allow the person to change weight from one foot to the other.

Lyme disease A systemic infectious disease that is caused by the spirochete *Borrelia burgdorferi* and results from the bite of an infected deer tick. Signs and symptoms include a large "bull's-eye" circular rash, malaise, fever, headache, and muscle or joint aches.

lymphadenopathy Persistently enlarged lymph nodes.

lymphedema Abnormal accumulation of protein fluid in the subcutaneous tissue of the affected limb after a mastectomy.

lymphoblastic Pertaining to abnormal leukemic cells that come from the lymphoid pathways and develop into lymphocytes.

lymphocytic Pertaining to abnormal leukemic cells that come from the lymphoid pathways.

lymphokine Cytokine produced by T-cells.

lysis Breakage, for example, of a cell membrane.

M

macrocytic anemia A form of vitamin B_{12} deficiency anemia characterized by abnormally large precursor cells.

macrovascular Referring to large blood vessels.

macular Referring to a macula, a discolored spot on the skin that is not raised above the surface.

macular degeneration The deterioration of the macula, the area of central vision.

magnesium (Mg^{2+}) A mineral that forms a cation when dissolved in water.

magnetoencephalography (MEG) A noninvasive imaging technique that measures the magnetic fields produced by electrical activity in the brain via extremely sensitive devices such as superconducting quantum interference devices (SQUIDs).

malabsorption A syndrome associated with a variety of disorders and intestinal surgical procedures and characterized by impaired intestinal absorption of nutrients.

malignant Referring to cancer.

malignant cell growth Altered cell growth that is serious and, without intervention, leads to death; cancer.

malignant hypertension A severe type of elevated blood pressure that rapidly progresses, with systolic blood pressure greater than 200 mm Hg and diastolic blood pressure greater than 150 mm Hg (greater than 130 mm Hg when there are pre-existing complications).

malignant transformation The process of changing a normal cell into a cancer cell.

mammography An x-ray of the soft tissue of the breast.

mandibulectomy Surgical removal of the jaw.

marasmic-kwashiorkor A combined protein and energy malnutrition that often presents clinically when metabolic stress is imposed on a chronically starved patient.

marasmus A calorie malnutrition in which body fat and protein are wasted but serum proteins are often preserved.

marsupialization Surgical formation of a pouch that is a new duct opening.

mass casualty event A situation affecting the public health that is defined based on the resource availability of a particular community or hospital facility. When the number of casualties exceeds the resource capabilities, a disaster situation is recognized to exist.

mastication The process of chewing.

mastoiditis An acute or chronic infection of the mastoid air cells caused by untreated or inadequately treated otitis media.

maze procedure An open chest surgical technique often performed with coronary artery bypass grafting for patients in atrial fibrillation with decompensation.

mean arterial pressure (MAP) The arterial blood pressure (between 60 and 70 mm Hg) necessary to maintain perfusion of major body organs, such as the kidneys and brain.

mechanical débridement Method of débriding a wound by mechanical entrapment and detachment of dead tissue.

mechanical obstruction The physical obstruction of the bowel by disorders outside the intestine (e.g., adhesions or hernias) or by blockages in the lumen of the intestine (e.g., tumors, inflammation, strictures, or fecal impactions).

mediastinal shift A shift of central thoracic structures toward one side; seen on chest x-ray.

mediastinitis Infection of the mediastinum.

medical command physician As defined in a hospital's emergency response plan, the person responsible for determining the number, acuity, and medical resource needs of victims arriving from the incident scene and for organizing the emergency health care team response to injured or ill patients.

medical harm Physician incidents and all errors caused by members of the health care team or system that lead to patient injury or death.

medical nutrition supplements (MNSs) Enteral products taken by patients who cannot consume enough nutrients in their usual diet (e.g., Ensure, Boost).

medication overuse headache See *rebound headache.*

medulla A general term for the most interior portion of an organ or structure.

melena Blood in the stool, with the appearance of black tarry stools.

memory cell A type of B-lymphocyte that remains sensitized but does not start to produce antibodies until the next exposure to the same antigen.

Ménière's disease Tinnitus, one-sided sensorineural hearing loss, and vertigo that is related to overproduction or decreased reabsorption of endolymphatic fluid and causes a distortion of the entire inner canal system.

meninges The immediate protective covering of the brain and the spinal cord.

meningioma A type of benign brain tumor that arises from the coverings of the brain (the meninges) and causes compression and displacement of adjacent brain tissue.

meningitis Inflammation, usually bacterial or viral, of the arachnoid and pia mater of the brain and spinal cord and the cerebrospinal fluid. May be caused by bacteria or viruses; symptoms are the same regardless of the causative organism.

meniscectomy Surgical excision of a meniscus, as in a knee joint.

menses The monthly flow of blood from the genital tract of women.

metabolic syndrome A collection of related health problems with insulin resistance as a main feature. Other features include obesity, low levels of physical activity, hypertension, high blood levels of cholesterol, and elevated triglyceride levels. Metabolic syndrome increases the risk for coronary heart disease. Also called "syndrome X."

metastasis The growth and spread of cancer.

metastasize To spread cancer from the main tumor site to many other body sites.

metastatic Referring to disease, such as cancer, that transfers from one organ to another organ or part not directly connected; pertains to additional tumors that form after cancer cells move from the primary location by breaking off from the original group and establishing remote colonies.

methemoglobinemia The conversion of normal hemoglobin to methemoglobin.

microalbuminuria The presence of very small amounts of albumin in the urine that are not measurable by a urine dipstick or usual urinalysis procedures. Specialized assays are used to analyze a freshly voided urine specimen for microscopic levels of albumin.

microcytic Abnormally small in size, such as an abnormally small red blood cell.

microvascular Referring to small blood vessels.

microvascular decompression A surgical procedure to relieve the pain of trigeminal neuralgia by relocating a small artery that compresses the trigeminal nerve as it enters the pons. The surgeon carefully lifts the loop of the artery off the nerve and places a small silicone sponge between the vessel and the nerve.

midline catheter A type of catheter that is 6 to 8 inches long and inserted through the veins of the antecubital fossa; used in therapies lasting from 1 to 4 weeks.

migraine headache An episodic familial disorder manifested by a unilateral, frontotemporal, throbbing pain that is often worse behind one eye or ear. It is often accompanied by a sensitive scalp, anorexia, photophobia, and nausea with or without vomiting. Three categories of migraine headache are migraines with aura, migraines without aura, and atypical migraines.

migratory arthritis In the early stage of rheumatoid arthritis, symptoms that are migrating or involve more joints.

miliary tuberculosis See *hematogenous tuberculosis.*

minimally invasive direct coronary artery bypass (MIDCAB) Surgical procedure that does not require cardiopulmonary bypass and may be used for patients with a lesion of the left anterior descending artery. Also known as "keyhole" surgery.

minimally invasive esophagectomy (MIE) A laparoscopic surgical procedure to remove part of the esophagus; may be performed in patients with early-stage cancer.

minimally invasive inguinal hernia repair (MIIHR) Surgical repair of an inguinal hernia through a laparoscope, which is the treatment of choice.

minimally invasive surgery (MIS) A general term for any surgery performed using laparoscopic technique.

Minimum Data Set (MDS) 3.0 Interdisciplinary tool required by the U.S. Centers for Medicare and Medicaid Services (CMS) to assess patients (residents) in nursing homes.

miosis Constriction of the pupil of the eye.

mitosis Cell division.

mitotic index The percentage of actively dividing cells within a tumor.

mitral regurgitation Inability of the mitral valve to close completely during systole, which allows the backflow of blood into the left atrium when the left ventricle contracts; usually due to fibrosis and calcification caused by rheumatic disease. Also called "mitral insufficiency."

mitral stenosis Thickening of the mitral valve due to fibrosis and calcification and usually caused by rheumatic fever. The valve leaflets fuse and become stiff, the chordae tendineae contract, and the valve opening narrows, preventing normal blood flow from the left atrium to the left ventricle. As a result, left atrial pressure rises, the left atrium dilates, pulmonary artery pressures increase, and the right ventricle hypertrophies.

mitral valve prolapse (MVP) Dysfunction of the mitral valve that occurs because the valvular leaflets enlarge and prolapse into the left atrium during systole; usually benign but may progress to pronounced mitral regurgitation.

mixed conductive-sensorineural hearing loss A profound hearing loss that results from a combination of both conductive and sensorineural types of hearing loss.

modifiable risk factor A factor in disease development that can be altered or controlled by the patient. Examples include elevated serum cholesterol levels, cigarette smoking, hypertension, impaired glucose tolerance, obesity, physical inactivity, and stress.

monokine Cytokine made by macrophages, neutrophils, eosinophils, and monocytes.

morbid obesity A weight that has a severely negative effect on health; usually more than 100% above ideal body weight or a body mass index greater than 40.

morbidity An illness or an abnormal condition or quality.

mortality Death.

Morton's neuroma Plantar digital neuritis, a condition in which a small tumor grows in a digital nerve of the foot. The patient usually describes the pain as an acute, burning sensation in the web space that involves the entire surface of the third and fourth toes.

motor Facilitating movement.

motor aphasia See *expressive aphasia.*

motor cortex Area in the frontal lobe of the brain that controls voluntary movement.

mourning The outward social expression of loss.

mucositis Open sores on mucous membranes.

multi-casualty event A disaster event in which a limited number of victims or casualties are involved and can be managed by a hospital using local resources.

multigated blood pool scanning In nuclear cardiology, cardiac blood pool imaging is a noninvasive test to evaluate cardiac motion and calculate ejection fraction by using a computer to synchronize the patient's electrocardiogram with pictures obtained by a gamma-scintillation camera. In multigated blood pool scanning, the computer breaks the time between R waves into fractions of a second, called "gates." The camera records blood flow through the heart during each gate. By analyzing information from multiple gates, the computer can evaluate ventricular wall motion and calculate ejection fraction (percentage of the left ventricular volume that is ejected with each contraction) and ejection velocity.

multiple organ dysfunction syndrome (MODS) The sequence of inadequate blood flow to body tissues, which deprives cells of oxygen and leads to anaerobic metabolism with acidosis, hyperkalemia, and tissue ischemia; this is followed by dramatic changes in vital organs and leads to the release of toxic metabolites and destructive enzymes.

multiple sclerosis (MS) A chronic autoimmune disease that affects the myelin sheath and conduction pathway of the central nervous system. It is one of the leading causes of neurologic disability in persons 20 to 40 years of age.

murmur Abnormal heart sound that reflects turbulent blood flow through normal or abnormal valves; murmurs are classified according to their timing in the cardiac cycle (systolic or diastolic) and their intensity depending on their level of loudness.

muscle biopsy The extraction of a muscle specimen for the diagnosis of atrophy (as in muscular dystrophy) and inflammation (as in polymyositis).

muscular dystrophy (MD) A group of degenerative myopathies characterized by weakness and atrophy of muscle without nervous system involvement. At least nine types have been clinically identified and can be broadly categorized as slowly progressive or rapidly progressive.

mutation A change in deoxyribonucleic acid (DNA) that is passed from one generation to another.

myalgia Muscle aches/muscle pain.

myasthenia gravis (MG) A chronic autoimmune disease of the neuromuscular junction. It is characterized by remissions and exacerbations, with fatigue and weakness primarily in the muscles innervated by the cranial nerves and in the skeletal and respiratory muscles. It ranges from mild disturbances of the ocular muscles to a rapidly developing, generalized weakness that may lead to death from respiratory failure.

myasthenic crisis Undermedication with cholinesterase inhibitors.

mydriasis Dilation of the pupil of the eye.

myelin sheath A white, lipid covering of the axon.

myelocytic Pertaining to leukemias in which the abnormal cells come from the myeloid pathways.

myelogenous Pertaining to leukemias in which the abnormal cells come from the myeloid pathways.

myelography Radiography of the spine after injection of contrast medium into the subarachnoid space of the spine; used to visualize the vertebral column, intervertebral disks, spinal nerve roots, and blood vessels.

myocardial hypertrophy Enlargement of the myocardium.

myocardial infarction (MI) Injury and necrosis of myocardial tissue that occurs when the tissue is abruptly and severely deprived of oxygen; usually caused by atherosclerosis of a coronary artery, rupture of the plaque, subsequent thrombosis, and occlusion of blood flow.

myocardial nuclear perfusion imaging (MNPI) The use of radionuclide techniques in which radioactive tracer substances are used to view, record, and evaluate cardiovascular abnormalities; useful for detecting myocardial infarction and decreased myocardial blood flow and for evaluating left ventricular ejection.

myocardium The heart muscle.

myoglobin A low–molecular-weight heme protein found in cardiac and skeletal muscle; an early marker of myocardial infarction.

myoglobinuria The release of muscle myoglobulin into the urine.

myomas See *leiomyomas.*

myomectomy The surgical removal of leiomyomas with preservation of the uterus.

myopathy A problem in muscle tissue.

myopia An error of refraction that occurs when the eye over-refracts or over-bends the light and focuses images in front of the retina; this results in normal near vision but poor distance vision. Also called "nearsightedness."

myositis Inflammation of a muscle.

myosplint Electrical stimulation of tension splints in the heart to help the ventricle change to a more normal shape in the patient with heart failure; under investigation in Europe and the United States.

myringoplasty Surgical reconstruction of the eardrum.

myringotomy The surgical creation of a hole in the eardrum; performed to drain middle-ear fluids and relieve pain in the patient with otitis media (middle-ear infection).

myxedema Dry, waxy swelling of the skin that is accompanied by nonpitting edema (especially around the eyes, in the hands and feet, and between the shoulder blades) and is associated with primary hypothyroidism.

myxedema coma A rare, serious complication of untreated or poorly treated hypothyroidism in which decreased metabolism causes the heart muscle to become flabby and the chamber size to increase, resulting in decreased cardiac output and decreased perfusion to the brain and other vital organs.

N

nadir In cancer treatment therapy, the period of greatest bone marrow suppression, when the patient's platelet count may be very low.

nasoduodenal tube (NDT) A tube that is inserted through a nostril and into the small intestine.

nasoenteric tube (NET) Any feeding tube that is inserted nasally and then advanced into the gastrointestinal tract.

nasogastric (NG) tube A tube that is inserted through a nostril and into the stomach for liquid feeding or for withdrawing gastric contents.

nasotracheal The route for inserting a tube into the trachea via the nose.

natal sex A person's genital anatomy present at birth. Also known as "biological sex."

National Patient Safety Goals (NPSGs) Goals published by The Joint Commission that require health care organizations to focus on specific priority safety practices.

natural chemical débridement Method of débriding a wound by creating an environment that promotes self-digestion of dead tissues by bacterial enzymes.

near point of vision The closest distance at which the eye can see an object clearly.

near-drowning Recovery after submersion in a liquid medium (usually water); this term is no longer used because language that describes drowning incidents has been standardized.

near-syncope Dizziness with an inability to remain in an upright position.

necrotizing hemorrhagic pancreatitis (NHP) Inflammation of the pancreas that is characterized by diffusely bleeding pancreatic tissue with fibrosis and tissue death. This form affects about 20% of patients with pancreatitis.

needle thoracostomy A quick, temporary method of chest decompression in which a large-bore needle is used to vent trapped air pending chest tube insertion.

negative deflection In electrocardiography, the flow of electrical current in the heart (cardiac axis) away from the positive pole and toward the negative pole.

negative feedback control mechanism The condition of maintaining a constant output of a system by exerting an inhibitory control on a key step by a product of that system. Used in a series of reactions that control hormone secretion and cellular activity based on responses to correct any movement away from normal function. An example of a simple negative feedback hormone response is the control of insulin secretion in which the action of insulin (decreasing blood glucose levels) is the opposite of the condition that stimulated insulin secretion (elevated blood glucose levels).

negative nitrogen balance A net loss of protein that occurs when the breakdown (degradation) of protein exceeds buildup (synthesis).

neglect In nursing, failure to provide for a patient's basic needs.

neoadjuvant therapy Treatment of a cancerous tumor with chemotherapy to shrink the tumor before it is surgically removed.

neoplasia Any new or continued cell growth not needed for normal development or replacement of dead and damaged tissues.

nephrectomy The surgical removal of the kidney.

nephrolithiasis The formation of stones in the kidney.

nephron The "working" unit of the kidney where urine is formed from blood. Each kidney consists of about 1 million nephrons, and each nephron separately makes urine. There are two types of nephrons: cortical and juxtamedullary.

nephropathy Pathologic change in the kidney that reduces kidney function and leads to renal failure.

nephrosclerosis Thickening in the nephron blood vessels that results in narrowing of the vessel lumen, with decreased renal blood flow and chronically hypoxic kidney tissue.

nephrostomy The surgical creation of an opening directly into the kidney; performed to divert urine externally and prevent further damage to the kidney when a stricture is causing hydronephrosis and cannot be corrected with urologic procedures.

nephrotic syndrome (NS) A condition of increased glomerular permeability that allows larger molecules to pass through the membrane into the urine and be removed from the blood. This process causes massive loss of protein into the urine, edema formation, and decreased plasma albumin levels.

neuraxial Referring to the epidural or spinal area.

neuritic plaques Degenerating nerve terminals found particularly in the hippocampus, an important part of the limbic system, and marked by increased amounts of an abnormal protein called "beta amyloid"; a characteristic change of the brain found in patients with Alzheimer's disease.

neurofibrillary tangles Tangled masses of fibrous elements throughout the neurons; a classic finding at autopsy in the brains of patients with Alzheimer's disease.

neurogenic shock Hypotension and bradycardia associated with cervical spinal injuries and caused by a loss of autonomic function. The patient is at greatest risk in the first 24 hours after injury.

neuroglia cells Cells of varying size and shape that provide protection, structure, and nutrition for the neurons.

neurohypophysis The posterior lobe of the pituitary gland that stores hormones produced in the hypothalamus.

neuroma A sensitive tumor consisting of nerve cells and nerve fibers.

neuron Excitable nerve cell that processes and transmits information through electrical and chemical signals.

neuropathic pain A type of chronic non-cancer pain that results from a nerve injury. Examples of causes include diabetic neuropathy, postherpetic neuralgia, radiculopathy (spinal nerve damage), and trigeminal neuralgia. Neuropathic pain is described as burning, shooting, stabbing, and the sensation of "pins and needles."

neurotransmitter Regulatory chemical that exerts inhibitory (slowing down) or excitatory (speeding up) activity at postsynaptic nerve cell membranes. Acetylcholine, norepinephrine, epinephrine, dopamine, and serotonin are neurotransmitters.

neurovascular assessment Assessment of the neuromuscular system that includes inspection of skin color, temperature, and capillary refill distal to an injury, surgical procedure, or cast. Palpation of pulses in the extremities below level of injury and assessment of sensation, movement, and pain in the injured part give a complete assessment.

neutralization See *inactivation.*

neutropenia Decreased numbers of leukocytes, especially neutrophils, which causes immunosuppression.

neutrophilia Increased number of circulating neutrophils.

nevus A mole; a benign skin growth of the pigment-forming cells.

new-onset angina Cardiac chest pain that occurs for the first time.

nitroglycerin (NTG) A drug prescribed for patients with angina. It increases collateral blood flow, redistributes blood flow toward the subendocardium, and causes dilation of the coronary arteries.

nits Lice eggs.

***N*-methyl-D-aspartate (NMDA) receptor antagonist** A group of drugs that block excess amounts of glutamate, which damages nerve cells in the brain; used to treat Alzheimer's disease.

nociception Term used to describe how pain becomes a conscious experience.

nociceptive pain Pain related to the skin, musculoskeletal structures, or body organs.

nociceptors Sensory neurons that respond to pain or other noxious stimuli.

nocturia The need to urinate excessively at night. Also called "nocturnal polyuria."

nocturnal polyuria See *nocturia.*

nonadherence In health care, accidental failure by a patient to take medication.

noncompliance In health care, deliberate failure by a patient to take medication.

nonmaleficence Ethical principle that emphasizes the importance of preventing harm and ensuring the patient's well-being.

nonmechanical obstruction Intestinal obstruction that does not involve a physical obstruction in or outside the intestine. Instead, decreased or absent peristalsis results in a slowing of the movement or a backup of intestinal contents. This is also known as "paralytic ileus" or "adynamic ileus" because it is a result of neuromuscular disturbance.

nonmodifiable risk factor Factor in disease development that cannot be altered or controlled by the patient. Examples include age, gender, family history, and ethnic background.

non–ST-segment elevation myocardial infarction (NSTEMI) Myocardial infarction in which the patient typically has ST and T-wave changes on a 12-lead ECG; this indicates myocardial ischemia.

nonsustained ventricular tachycardia (NSVT) Occurrence of three or more successive premature ventricular complexes.

nontunneled percutaneous central venous catheter (CVC) A type of catheter, usually 15 to 20 cm long and with dual or triple lumens, that is inserted through the subclavian vein in the upper chest or through the jugular veins in the neck using sterile technique.

nonurgent In a three-tiered triage scheme, the category that includes patients who can generally tolerate waiting several hours for health care services without a significant risk of clinical deterioration, such as those with sprains, strains, or simple fractures.

normal flora The microorganisms living in or on the human host without causing disease; the bacteria that are characteristic of each body location. Normal flora often compete with and prevent infection from unfamiliar microorganisms attempting to invade a body site.

normal sinus rhythm (NSR) The rhythm originating from the sinoatrial node (dominant pacemaker), with atrial and ventricular rates of 60 to 100 beats/min and regular atrial and ventricular rhythms.

normotonic See *isosmotic.*

North American pit vipers The Crotalidae, one of two families of indigenous poisonous snakes in North America; named for the characteristic depression between each eye and nostril. They include rattlesnakes, copperheads, and water moccasins and account for most poisonous snakebites in the United States.

nosocomial (infection) Acquired in an inpatient health care setting; for example, infections that were not present at hospital admission. Also called "hospital-acquired infections" and "health care–associated infections."

nothing by mouth (NPO) No eating, drinking (including water), or smoking.

nuchal rigidity Stiff neck, which can be a sign of cerebrospinal fluid leak; nuchal rigidity is not checked until a spinal cord injury has been ruled out.

nucleotide The final form of a base that actually gets put into the strand of deoxyribonucleic acid. A nucleoside becomes a complete nucleotide by the attachment of phosphate groups.

nursing assistant A member of the rehabilitative health care team who assists the registered nurse in the care of patients.

nursing technician See *nursing assistant.*

nutritional screening A screening by the health care provider that includes visual inspection, measured height and weight, weight history, usual eating habits, ability to chew and swallow, and any recent changes in appetite or food intake. The screening is a way to determine which patients need more extensive nutritional assessment.

nutritional status Reflects the balance between nutrient requirements and intake.

nystagmus Involuntary, rapid eye movements.

O

obesity An increase in body weight at least 20% above the upper limit of the normal range for ideal body weight, with an excess amount of body fat; in an adult, a body mass index greater than 30.

obligatory urine output The minimum amount of urine per day needed to dissolve and excrete toxic waste products.

obstipation The inability to pass stool; intractable constipation.

obstruction Blockage.

obstructive jaundice Jaundice caused by an impediment to the flow of bile from the liver to the duodenum; may be caused by edema of the ducts or gallstones.

obstructive sleep apnea A breathing disruption during sleep that lasts at least 10 seconds and occurs a minimum of 5 times in an hour.

Occupational Safety and Health Administration (OSHA) A federal agency that protects workers from injury or illness at their place of employment.

occupational therapist (OT, OTR) A member of the rehabilitation health care team who works to develop the patient's fine motor skills used for activities of daily living and the skills related to coordination and cognitive retraining.

odynophagia Pain on swallowing.

oligomenorrhea Scant or infrequent menses.

oligospermia Low sperm count.

oliguria Decreased excretion of urine in relation to amount of fluid intake; usually defined as urine output less than 400 mL/day.

oncogene Proto-oncogene that has been "turned on" and can cause cells to change from normal cells to cancer cells.

oncogenesis Cancer development.

oncovirus Virus that causes cancer.

oophorectomy Surgical removal of the ovary.

open fracture A fracture in which the skin surface over the broken bone is disrupted, causing an external wound. Also called "compound fracture."

open reduction The reduction of a fracture after surgical incision into the site to allow direct visualization of the fracture. See *internal fixation.*

open traumatic brain injury A type of traumatic primary brain injury that occurs with a skull fracture or when the skull is pierced by a penetrating object. The integrity of the brain and the dura is violated and there is exposure to outside contaminants, with damage to the underlying vessels, dural sinus, brain, and cranial nerves.

opportunistic infection Infection caused by organisms that are present as part of the normal environment and would be kept in check by normal immune function.

optic disc The point at the inside back of the eye where the optic nerve enters the eyeball. It appears as a creamy pink to white depressed area in the retina and contains only nerve fibers and no photoreceptor cells.

optic fundus The area at the inside back of the eye that can be seen with an ophthalmoscope.

optic nerve The nerve of sight; connects the optic disc to the brain.

orbit The bony socket of the skull that surrounds and protects the eye along with the attached muscles, nerves, vessels, and tear-producing glands.

orchiectomy The surgical removal of one or both testes.

orchitis An acute testicular inflammation resulting from trauma or infection.

orexin Neuropeptide that is an appetite stimulant.

orotracheal The route for inserting a tube into the trachea via the mouth.

orthopnea Shortness of breath that occurs when lying down but is relieved by sitting up.

orthostatic Pertaining to or caused by standing erect.

orthostatic hypotension A decrease in blood pressure (20 mm Hg systolic and/or 10 mm Hg diastolic) that occurs during the first few seconds to minutes after changing from a sitting or lying position to a standing position. Also called "postural hypotension."

orthotopic The most common type of transplantation procedure in which a diseased organ is removed and a donor organ is grafted in its place. For example, during heart transplantation, the surgeon removes the diseased heart and leaves the posterior walls of the patient's atria, which serve as the anchor for the donor heart; anastomoses are made between the recipient and donor atria, aorta, and pulmonary arteries.

osmolality The number of milliosmoles in a kilogram of solution.

osmolarity The number of milliosmoles in a liter of solution.

osmosis The movement of a solvent across a semipermeable membrane (a membrane that allows the solvent but not the solute to pass through) from a lesser to a greater concentration.

ossiculoplasty Replacement of the ossicles within the middle ear.

osteitis deformans See *Paget's disease.*

osteoarthritis Noninflammatory form of arthritis characterized by the progressive deterioration and loss of cartilage in one or more joints; most common form of arthritis.

osteoblast Cell associated with formation of bone.

osteoclast Cell associated with destruction or resorption of bone.

osteocyte Bone cell.

osteomalacia Abnormal softening of the bone tissue characterized by inadequate mineralization of osteoid. It is the adult equivalent of rickets (vitamin D deficiency) in children.

osteomyelitis An inflammation of bone tissue caused by pathogenic microorganisms; produces an increased vascularity and edema often involving the surrounding soft tissues.

osteonecrosis The death of bone tissue, usually because the blood supply to the bone is disrupted. Usually a complication of a hip fracture or any fracture in which there is displacement of bone.

osteopenia A condition of low bone mass that occurs when there is a disruption in the bone remodeling process.

osteophyte Bone spur.

osteoporosis A metabolic disease in which bone demineralization results in decreased density and subsequent fractures.

osteotomy Surgical resection of bone.

ostomate A patient with an ostomy.
ostomy The surgical creation of an opening, usually referring to an opening in the abdominal wall; stoma.
otorrhea Ear discharge.
otosclerosis Irregular bone growth around the ossicles.
otoscope An instrument used to examine the ear; consists of a light, a handle, a magnifying lens, and a pneumatic bulb for injecting air into the external canal to test mobility of the eardrum.
ototoxic Having a toxic effect on the inner ear structures.
outflow disease Chronic peripheral arterial disease with obstruction at or below the superficial femoral or popliteal artery. The patient experiences burning or cramping in the calves, ankles, feet, and toes after walking a certain distance; the pain usually subsides with rest.
outpatient A patient who goes to the hospital for treatment and returns home on the same day.
overflow urinary incontinence The involuntary loss of urine when the bladder is overdistended.
overweight An increase in body weight for height compared with a reference standard (e.g., the Metropolitan Life height and weight tables) or 10% greater than ideal body weight. However, this weight may not reflect excess body fat, which in an adult is a body mass index of 25 to 30.
ovoid pupil In evaluating pupils for size and reaction to light, the midstage between a normal-size pupil and a dilated pupil; indicates the development of increased intracranial pressure.
oxygen concentrator A machine that removes nitrogen, water vapor, and hydrocarbons from room air. Also known as "oxygen extractor."
oxygen dissociation The transfer of oxygen from hemoglobin to tissues.

P

P wave In the electrocardiogram, the deflection representing atrial depolarization.
pack-years The number of packs of cigarettes per day multiplied by the number of years the patient has smoked; used in recording the patient's smoking history.
Paget's disease A metabolic disorder of bone remodeling, or turnover, in which increased resorption or loss results in bone deposits that are weak, enlarged, and disorganized. Also known as "osteitis deformans."
pain An unpleasant sensory and emotional experience associated with actual or potential tissue damage; the most reliable indication of pain is the patient's self-report.
palliation Relieving symptoms.
palliative care A compassionate and supportive approach to patients and families who are living with life-threatening illnesses; involves a holistic approach that provides relief of symptoms experienced by the dying patient.
palpitations A feeling of fluttering in the chest, an unpleasant awareness of the heartbeat, and an irregular heartbeat; may result from a change in heart rate or rhythm or from an increase in the force of heart contractions.
pancreatic abscess A collection of purulent material that results from extensive inflammatory necrosis of the pancreas after infection by organisms such as *Escherichia coli;* the most serious complication of pancreatitis. It is fatal if left untreated.
pancreatic pseudocyst A false cyst, so named because, unlike a true cyst, it does not have an epithelial lining. It is an encapsulated saclike structure that forms on or surrounds the pancreas and develops as a complication of acute or chronic pancreatitis. It may contain up to several liters of straw-colored or dark-brown viscous fluid, the enzymatic exudate of the pancreas.
pancreaticojejunostomy Surgical anastomosis of the pancreatic duct with the jejunum.
pancytopenia A deficiency of all three cell types (red blood cells, white blood cells, and platelets) of the blood.
pandemic A general epidemic spread over a wide geographic area and affecting a large proportion of the population.
panniculectomy The surgical removal of any panniculus, most often the abdominal apron; usually done as a follow-up to bariatric surgery in an obese patient.
panniculitis Infection of the panniculus.
panniculus A layer of membrane; also used to refer to skinfold areas in the obese patient.
pannus Vascular granulation tissue composed of inflammatory cells that forms in a joint space; erodes articular cartilage and eventually destroys bone.
Papanicolaou test (Pap smear) A cytologic study that is effective in detecting precancerous and cancerous cells obtained from the cervix.
papilla The anatomic term for a small, nipple-shaped projection or structure.
papilledema Edema and hyperemia of the optic disc; a sign of increased intracranial pressure found on ophthalmoscopic examination. Also called a "choked disc."
papilloma A pedunculated outgrowth of tissue.
papillotomy An incision of a papilla, a small nipple-shaped projection or structure.
papular Referring to a papule, a small, solid elevation of the skin.
paracentesis A procedure in which the physician inserts a trocar catheter into the abdomen to remove and drain ascitic fluid from the peritoneal cavity.
paradoxical blood pressure An exaggerated decrease in systolic pressure by more than 10 mm Hg during the inspiratory phase of the respiratory cycle (normal is 3 to 10 mm Hg); clinical conditions that may produce a paradoxical blood pressure include pericardial tamponade, constrictive pericarditis, and pulmonary hypertension. Also known as "paradoxical pulse" and "pulsus paradoxus."
paradoxical chest wall movement The "sucking inward" of the loose chest area during inspiration and a "puffing out" of the same area during expiration in a patient with a flail chest.
paradoxical pulse See *paradoxical blood pressure.*
paradoxical splitting Abnormal splitting of the S_2 heart sound heard in patients with severe myocardial depression; causes early closure of the pulmonic valve or a delay in aortic valve closure.
paralysis Absence of movement.
paralytic ileus Absence of peristalsis.
paramedic Prehospital care provider for patients who require care that exceeds basic life support resources. Advanced life support (ALS) may include cardiac monitoring, advanced airway management and intubation, establishing IV access, and administering drugs en route to the emergency department.
paranasal sinuses The air-filled cavities within the bones that surround the nasal passages. Lined with ciliated membrane, the sinuses provide resonance during speech and decrease the weight of the skull.
paraparesis Weakness that involves only the lower extremities, as seen in lower thoracic and lumbosacral injuries or lesions.
paraplegia Paralysis that involves only the lower extremities, as seen in lower thoracic and lumbosacral injuries or lesions.
paresis Weakness.
paresthesia Abnormal or unusual nerve sensations of touch, such as tingling and burning.
parietal cells Cells lining the wall of the stomach that secrete hydrochloric acid and produce intrinsic factor.
Parkinson disease (PD) A debilitating neurologic disease that affects motor ability and is characterized by four cardinal symptoms: tremor, rigidity, akinesia (slow movement), and postural instability. It is the third most common neurologic disorder of older adults. Also called "paralysis agitans."
parotidectomy The surgical removal of the parotid glands.
paroxysmal nocturnal dyspnea (PND) In the patient with heart disease, difficulty breathing that develops after lying down for several hours and causes the patient to awaken abruptly with a feeling of suffocation and panic. Occurs because the heart is unable to compensate for the increased volume when blood from the lower extremities is redistributed to the venous system, which increases venous return to the heart. A diseased heart is ineffective in pumping the additional fluid into the circulatory system, and pulmonary congestion results.
paroxysmal supraventricular tachycardia (PSVT) A form of supraventricular tachycardia that occurs when the rhythm is intermittent, initiated suddenly by a premature complex such as a premature atrial complex, and terminated suddenly with or without intervention.
partial left ventriculectomy (PLV) A ventricular reconstructive procedure that involves removing a triangle-shaped section of the weakened heart in the left lateral ventricle to reduce the ventricle's diameter and decrease wall tension. Also known as "heart reduction surgery" and "Batista procedure."
partial seizure One of the three broad categories of seizure disorders along with generalized seizure and unclassified seizure. Partial seizures are of two types: complex and simple. Partial seizures begin in a part of one cerebral

hemisphere; some can evolve into generalized tonic-clonic, tonic, or clonic seizures. They are most often seen in adults and in general are less responsive to medical treatment. Also called "focal seizures" or "local seizures."

passive euthanasia See *withdrawing or withholding life-sustaining therapy.*

passive immunity Resistance to infection that is of short duration (days or months) and either natural by transplacental transfer from the mother or artificial by injection of antibodies (e.g., immunoglobulin).

patellofemoral pain syndrome (PFPS) A health problem that occurs most often in people who are runners or who overuse their knee joints. For that reason, it is sometimes referred to as "runner's knee." These patients describe pain as being behind or around their patella (knee cap) in one or both knees.

pathogen Any microorganism capable of producing disease.

pathogenicity The ability to cause disease.

pathologic (spontaneous) fracture A fracture that occurs after minimal trauma to a bone that has been weakened by a disease such as bone cancer or osteoporosis.

patient-centered care A QSEN competency in which the nurse recognizes the patient or designee as the source of control and full partner in providing compassionate and coordinated care based on respect for the patient's preferences, values, and needs.

patient-controlled analgesia A method that allows the patient to control the dosage of opioid analgesic received by using an infusion pump to deliver the desired amount of medication through a conventional IV route.

PDSA Acronym for plan, do, study, act, which is one of the steps of the evidence-based practice improvement (EBPI) model.

pedal Pertaining to the feet.

pediculosis An infestation by human lice.

pedigree A graph of a family history for a specific trait or health problem over several generations.

pelvic inflammatory disease (PID) Any infection of the pelvis involving the upper genital tract beyond the cervix in women. It occurs when organisms from the lower genital tract migrate from the endocervix upward through the uterine cavity into the fallopian tubes.

pelvic organ prolapse (POP) Condition in which the sling of muscles and tendons that support the pelvic organs becomes weak and is no longer able to hold them in place.

penetrance In genetics, how often or how well a gene is expressed when it is present within a population.

penetrating trauma Injuries caused by piercing; classified by the velocity of the vehicle (e.g., knife or bullet) causing the injury. Low-velocity injuries from knife wounds cause damage directly at the site; high-velocity injuries from gunshot wounds cause both direct and indirect damage. Also called "penetrating injury."

peptic ulcer A mucosal lesion of the stomach or duodenum.

peptic ulcer disease (PUD) The impairment of gastric mucosal defenses so they no longer protect the epithelium from the effects of acid and pepsin.

percutaneous Performed through the skin and other tissues.

percutaneous alcohol septal ablation Surgical procedure for hypertrophic cardiomyopathy (HCM) in which alcohol is injected into a target septal branch of the left anterior descending coronary artery to produce a small septal infarction. This procedure also widens the left ventricular outflow tract.

percutaneous coronary intervention (PCI) See *percutaneous transluminal coronary angioplasty (PTCA).*

percutaneous endoscopic gastrostomy (PEG) A stoma created from the abdominal wall into the stomach for insertion of a short feeding tube.

percutaneous stereotactic rhizotomy (PSR) Procedure performed under general anesthesia to treat trigeminal neuralgia; a hollow needle is passed through the inside of the patient's cheek into the trigeminal nerve fibers, and a heating current (radiofrequency thermocoagulation) goes through the needle to destroy some of the fibers.

percutaneous transhepatic cholangiography (PTC) The radiographic study of the biliary duct system using an iodinated dye instilled via a percutaneous needle inserted through the liver into the intrahepatic ducts. It may be performed when a patient has jaundice or persistent upper abdominal pain, even after cholecystectomy, but it is rarely performed as a diagnostic procedure.

percutaneous transluminal coronary angioplasty (PTCA) A nonsurgical method of improving arterial flow by opening the vessel lumen and creating a smooth inner vessel surface. One or more arteries are dilated with a balloon catheter advanced through a cannula, which is inserted into or above an occluded or stenosed artery. Also called "percutaneous vascular intervention" and "percutaneous coronary intervention (PCI)."

percutaneous vascular intervention See *percutaneous transluminal coronary angioplasty.*

pericardial effusion Complication of pericarditis that occurs when the space between the parietal and visceral layers of the pericardium fills with fluid.

pericardial friction rub An abnormal sound that originates from the pericardial sac and occurs with the movements of the heart during the cardiac cycle; usually transient and a sign of inflammation, infection, or infiltration; may be heard in patients with pericarditis resulting from myocardial infarction, cardiac tamponade, or post-thoracotomy.

pericardiectomy Surgical excision of the pericardium (the sac around the heart).

pericardiocentesis Withdrawal of pericardial fluid through a catheter inserted into the pericardial space to relieve the pressure on the heart.

pericarditis An inflammation of the tissue (pericardium) surrounding the heart.

perichondrium A tough, fibrous tissue layer that surrounds the ear cartilage and gives shape to the pinna.

periodontal disease Gum disease in which mandibular bone loss has occurred.

perioperative The operative experience consisting of the preoperative, intraoperative, and postoperative time periods.

peripheral blood stem cells (PBSCs) Stem cells that are collected from peripheral blood for transplantation into the patient.

peripheral chemoreceptors Several 1- to 2-mm collections of tissue identified in the carotid arteries and along the aortic arch.

peripheral IV therapy IV therapy in which a vascular access device (VAD) is placed in a peripheral vein, usually in the arm.

peripheral vascular disease (PVD) Any disorder that alters the natural flow of blood through the arteries and veins of the peripheral circulation.

peripherally inserted central catheter (PICC) A long catheter inserted through a vein of the antecubital fossa (inner aspect of the bend of the arm) or the middle of the upper arm.

peritonitis Acute inflammation of the visceral/parietal peritoneum and endothelial lining of the abdominal cavity, or peritoneum.

peritonsillar abscess (PTA) A complication of acute tonsillitis. The infection spreads from the tonsil to the surrounding tissue, which forms an abscess.

periungual lesion Skin lesion around the nail bed.

permeable The quality of being porous.

pernicious anemia A form of megaloblastic anemia caused by failure to absorb vitamin B_{12} because of a deficiency of intrinsic factor (normally secreted by the gastric mucosa) needed for intestinal absorption of vitamin B_{12}.

PERRLA An acronym that stands for the phrase "Pupils should be equal in size, round and regular in shape, and react to light and accommodation."

personal emergency preparedness plan An individual plan that outlines specific arrangements in the event of disaster, such as childcare, pet care, and older adult care.

personal protective equipment (PPE) Infection control protocol that refers to the use of gloves, isolation gowns, face protection, and respirators with N95 or higher filtration.

personal readiness supplies A preassembled disaster supply kit for the home and/or automobile that contains clothing and basic survival supplies. Also called a "go bag."

petechiae Pinpoint red spots on the mucous membranes, palate, conjunctivae, or skin.

pH A measure of the free hydrogen ion level in body fluid.

pH monitoring examination The most accurate testing method of diagnosing GERD, accomplished by placing a small catheter into the distal esophagus or esophageal wall (depending on the specific technique). The patient then records a diary of activities and symptoms over a 24- to 48-hour period while pH is continuously monitored.

phagocytosis The process of engulfing, ingesting, killing, and disposing of an invading organism by neutrophils and macrophages; a key process of inflammation.

Phalen's maneuver Test to determine the presence of carpal tunnel syndrome (CTS); a positive test for CTS causes paresthesia in the medial nerve distribution of the palm of the hand in 60 seconds.

phantom limb pain (PLP) A frequent complication of amputation in which the patient perceives sensation in the absent (amputated) foot or hand. This sensation usually diminishes over time.

pharmacist Member of the health care team who oversees the prescription and preparation of medications and provides the team with essential information regarding drug safety.

pharmacologic stress echocardiogram A form of echocardiography in which either dobutamine (increases heart's contractility) or adenosine (dilates coronary arteries) is given to the patient; usually used when patients cannot tolerate exercise.

phenotype Any genetic characteristic that can actually be observed or, in some cases, determined by laboratory test.

pheochromocytoma A tumor of the adrenal medulla, which can cause excessive secretion of catecholamines.

phlebitis Inflammation of a vein, which can predispose patients to thrombosis.

phlebothrombosis Presence of a thrombus in a vein without inflammation.

phonophobia Abnormal sensitivity to sound.

phonophoresis Treatment for back pain in which a topical drug (e.g., lidocaine, hydrocortisone) is applied followed by continuous ultrasound for 10 minutes.

photophobia Abnormal sensitivity to light.

photopsia The appearance of bright flashes of light due to the onset of retinal detachment.

physiatrist A physician who specializes in rehabilitative medicine.

physical abuse The use of a physical force, such as hitting, burning, pushing, and molesting the patient, that results in bodily injury.

physical therapist (PT, RPT) A member of the rehabilitation health care team who helps the patient achieve mobility and who teaches techniques for performing certain activities of daily living.

piggyback set See *secondary administration set.*

pitting Indentation of the skin; often occurs with edema.

pituitary Cushing's disease Oversecretion of ACTH by the anterior pituitary gland, which causes hyperplasia of the adrenal cortex in both adrenal glands and an excess of most hormones secreted by the adrenal cortex.

plantar fasciitis An inflammation of the plantar fascia, which is located in the area of the arch of the foot. It is often seen in athletes, especially runners.

plasma cell A short-lived B-lymphocyte that begins functioning immediately to produce antibodies against sensitizing antigens.

plasmapheresis The separation of plasma from whole blood, after which the blood cells are returned to the patient without the plasma to eliminate antibodies.

plethoric A flushed appearance of the skin.

pleura The continuous smooth membrane composed of two surfaces that totally enclose the lungs.

pleural effusion Fluid in the pleural space.

pleuritic chest pain A stabbing pain on taking a deep breath.

plexus Cluster of nerves.

ploidy The number and appearance of chromosomes; used to describe cancer cells.

pluripotent stem cell The precursor cell involved in the production of red blood cells.

pneumonectomy Removal of an entire lung, including all blood vessels.

pneumonia Excess fluid in the lungs resulting from an inflammatory process that can include infection.

pneumothorax Air in the pleural (chest) cavity.

podagra Inflammation of the metatarsophalangeal joint of the great toe.

point of maximal impulse (PMI) See *apical impulse.*

polycystic kidney disease (PKD) An inherited disorder in which fluid-filled cysts develop in the kidneys.

polycythemia vera (PV) A disease that involves massive production of red blood cells, leukocytes, and platelets.

polydipsia Excessive intake of water.

polymorphism A variation in form.

polyp An abnormal outgrowth from a mucous membrane.

polyphagia Excessive eating.

polypharmacy The use of many drugs to treat multiple health problems for older adults. Also known as "hyperpharmacy."

polyuria Frequent and excessive urination.

pores Openings or spaces.

portal hypertension An abnormal persistent increase in pressure within the portal vein; a major complication of cirrhosis.

portal hypertensive gastropathy A complication that can occur in patients with portal hypertension, with or without esophageal varices. Slow gastric mucosal bleeding may result in chronic slow blood loss, occult positive stools, and anemia.

portal-systemic encephalopathy (PSE) A clinical disorder seen in hepatic failure and cirrhosis; it is manifested by neurologic symptoms and is characterized by an altered level of consciousness, impaired thinking processes, and neuromuscular disturbances. Also called "hepatic encephalopathy" and "hepatic coma."

positive deflection In electrocardiography, the flow of electrical current in the heart (cardiac axis) toward the positive pole.

positive inotropic agents Drugs that increase myocardial contractility and are prescribed to improve cardiac output.

postanesthesia care unit (PACU) Recovery room.

postcholecystectomy syndrome (PCS) The occurrence of the clinical manifestations of biliary tract disease following cholecystectomy; caused by residual or recurring calculi, inflammation, or stricture of the common bile duct.

post-concussion syndrome A group of clinical manifestations following a concussion that consist of personality changes, irritability, headaches, dizziness, restlessness, nervousness, insomnia, memory loss, and depression. The prolonged pattern is classified as post-trauma syndrome.

posterior colporrhaphy The surgical procedure to repair a rectocele by strengthening pelvic supports and reducing the bulging.

posteroanterior Back to front; position for standard chest x-rays.

postherpetic neuralgia Pain that persists after herpes zoster lesions have resolved.

postictal stage Referring to the time immediately after a seizure.

postoperative period After surgery.

postpericardiotomy syndrome Symptoms, including pericardial and pleural pain, pericarditis, friction rub, elevated temperature and white blood cell count, and dysrhythmias, that occur in patients after cardiac surgery; may occur days to weeks after surgery and seems to be associated with blood that remains in the pericardial sac.

postrenal failure Decrease in renal function related to an obstruction in the flow of urine. It can progress to acute renal failure.

postural hypotension See *orthostatic hypotension.*

posture A person's body build and alignment when standing and walking.

post-void residual (PVR) The amount of urine remaining in the bladder within 20 minutes after voiding.

power air purifying respirator (PAPR) Device with a high efficiency particulate air (HEPA) filter and battery to promote positive pressure air flow; more effective than an N95 respirator.

PQRST A mnemonic (memory device) that may help in the current problem assessment of patients with gastrointestinal tract disorders. The letters represent these areas: P, precipitating or palliative (What brings it on? What makes it better or worse?); Q, quality or quantity (How does it look, feel, or sound?); R, region or radiation (Where is it? Does it spread anywhere?); S, severity scale (How bad is it [on a scale of 0 to 10]? Is it getting better, worse, or staying the same?); T, timing (Onset, duration, and frequency?).

PR interval In the electrocardiogram, the interval measured from the beginning of the P wave to the end of the PR segment; represents the time required for atrial depolarization as well as impulse delay in the atrioventricular node and travel time to the Purkinje fibers.

PR segment In the electrocardiogram, the isoelectric line from the end of the P wave to the beginning of the QRS complex, when the electrical impulse is traveling through the atrioventricular node, where it is delayed.

Prader-Willi syndrome (PWS) A complex neurodevelopmental genetic disorder that results from a hypothalamic-pituitary dysfunction that prevents appetite control. Patients with this syndrome are typically morbidly obese.

prandial (insulin secretion) The increased levels of insulin that are secreted after eating. Within 10 minutes of eating, an early burst of insulin secretion occurs, which is followed by an increasing insulin release that lasts as long as hyperglycemia is present.

prealbumin (PAB) A protein secreted by the liver that binds thyroxine.

precipitation The formation of large, insoluble antigen-antibody complexes during the antibody-binding process.

prediabetes An impaired fasting glucose (IFG) or impaired glucose tolerance (IGT).

prehospital care provider Typically, any of the first caregivers encountered by the patient if he or she is transported to the emergency department by an ambulance or helicopter.

preictal phase Referring to events that a patient experiences before a seizure, such as the presence of an aura.

pre-infarction angina Chest pain that occurs in the days or weeks before a myocardial infarction.

preload The degree of myocardial fiber stretch at the end of diastole and just before contraction; determined by the amount of blood returning to the heart from both the venous system (right heart) and the pulmonary system (left heart).

premature atrial complex (contraction) (PAC) In the electrocardiogram, an early complex that occurs when atrial tissue becomes irritable. This ectopic focus fires an impulse before the next sinus impulse is due, thus usurping the sinus pacemaker. The premature P wave from the atrial focus is early and has a shape different from that of the P wave generated from the sinus node.

premature complex In the electrocardiogram, an early complex that occurs when a cardiac cell or cell group other than the sinoatrial node becomes irritable and fires an impulse before the next sinus impulse is generated. After the premature complex, there is a pause before the next normal complex, which creates an irregularity in the rhythm.

premature ventricular complex (PVC) In the electrocardiogram, an early ventricular complex is followed by a pause that results from increased irritability of ventricular cells. The QRS complexes may be unifocal or uniform (of the same shape), or multifocal or multiform (of different shapes).

preoperative Before surgery.

prerenal failure Condition that causes inadequate kidney perfusion; can progress to acute renal failure.

presbycusis The loss of hearing, especially for high-pitched sounds; occurs as a result of aging.

presbyopia An age-related impairment of vision characterized by a loss of lens elasticity and the ability of the eye to accommodate. The near point of vision increases, and near objects must be placed farther from the eye to be seen clearly.

presence A type of communication that consists of listening and acknowledging the legitimacy of the patient's and/or family's pain.

pressure ulcer Tissue damage caused when the skin and underlying soft tissue are compressed between a bony prominence and an external surface for an extended period; commonly occurs over the sacrum, hips, and ankles.

pretibial Pertaining to the front of the leg below the knee.

pretibial myxedema Dry, waxy swelling of the front surfaces of the lower legs.

primary angle-closure glaucoma A form of glaucoma characterized by a narrowed angle and forward displacement of the iris so that movement of the iris against the cornea narrows or closes the chamber angle, obstructing the outflow of aqueous humor. It can have a sudden onset and is an emergency. Also called "closed-angle glaucoma," "narrow-angle glaucoma," or "acute glaucoma."

primary arthroplasty A total joint arthroplasty procedure that has been performed for the first time.

primary gout The most common type of gout; results from one of several inborn errors of purine metabolism.

primary lesions In describing skin disease, the initial reaction to a problem that alters one of the structural components of the skin.

primary open-angle glaucoma (POAG) The most common form of primary glaucoma; characterized by reduced outflow of aqueous humor through the chamber angle. Because the fluid cannot leave the eye at the same rate it is produced, intraocular pressure gradually increases.

primary prevention Strategies used to avoid or delay the actual occurrence of a specific disease.

primary progressive multiple sclerosis (PPMS) A type of multiple sclerosis (MS) that involves a steady and gradual neurologic deterioration without remission of symptoms. Patients with this type of MS are usually between 40 and 60 years of age at onset of the disease and experience progressive disability with no acute attacks.

primary survey Priorities of care addressed in order of immediate threats to life as part of the initial assessment in the emergency department. Survey is based on an "ABC" mnemonic with "D" and "E" added for trauma patients: airway/cervical spine (A), breathing (B), circulation (C), disability (D), and exposure (E).

primary tumor The original tumor, usually identified by the tissue from which it arose (parent tissue), such as in breast cancer or lung cancer.

progressive multifocal leukoencephalopathy (PML) Rare disease affecting the white matter of the brain caused by a virus that attacks the cells that make myelin; occurs most often in patients who are immunosuppressed.

progressive-relapsing multiple sclerosis (PRMS) A type of multiple sclerosis (MS) that occurs in only 5% of patients with MS. It is characterized by the absence of periods of remission, and the patient's condition does not return to baseline. Progressive cumulative symptoms and deterioration occur over several years.

proliferative diabetic retinopathy A form of retinopathy associated with diabetes mellitus in which a network of fragile new blood vessels develops, leaking blood and protein into surrounding tissue. The new blood vessels are stimulated by retinal hypoxia that results from poor capillary perfusion of the retinal tissues. New blood vessels grow in the retina, onto the iris, and into the back of the vitreous. The vitreous contracts and pulls away from the retina, causing blood vessels to break and bleed into the vitreous.

promoter In oncology, a substance that promotes or enhances growth of the initiated cancer cell; may be a hormone, drug, or chemical.

pronator drift Occurs in a patient with muscle weakness due to cerebral or brainstem reasons. The arm on the weak side tends to fall, or "drift," with the palm pronating (turning inward) after the patient has closed his or her eyes and held the arms perpendicular to the body with the palms up for 15 to 30 seconds; part of the neurologic assessment.

prophylactic mastectomy Highly controversial practice of surgically removing the breast in order to reduce the risk of breast cancer.

proportionate palliative sedation A care management approach involving the administration of drugs such as benzodiazepines for the purpose of lowering patient consciousness.

proprioception (proprioceptive) Awareness of body position and movement.

prosopagnosia The inability to recognize oneself and other familiar faces; occurs in patients in the later stages of Alzheimer's disease.

prostaglandins Chemicals that are produced in the cells and cause inflammation and swelling.

prostate-specific antigen (PSA) A glycoprotein produced solely by the prostate. The normal blood level of PSA is less than 4 ng/mL; levels are higher in patients with increased prostatic tissue as a result of benign prostatic hyperplasia, prostatic infarction, prostatitis, and prostate cancer. Levels associated with prostate cancer are usually much higher than those occurring with other prostate tissue enlargement.

prostatitis Inflammation of the prostate.

protein-calorie malnutrition (PCM) A disorder of nutrition that may present in three forms: marasmus, kwashiorkor, and marasmic-kwashiorkor. Also called "protein-energy malnutrition."

protein-energy malnutrition (PEM) See *protein-calorie malnutrition.*

protein synthesis The process by which genes are used to make the proteins needed for physiologic function.

proteinuria The presence of protein in the urine.

proteolysis The breakdown of proteins to provide fuel for energy when liver glucose is unavailable.

proton pump inhibitor (PPI) A group of drugs that inhibit the proton pump in the stomach to decrease gastric acid production.

pruritus An unpleasant itching sensation.

psoriasis A chronic, autoimmune disorder of the skin with exacerbations and remissions. It results from overstimulation of the immune system (Langerhans' cells) in the skin that activates T-lymphocytes. The features include increased skin cell division in patchy areas forming scaly plaques.

psoriatic arthritis (PsA) A syndrome of inflammatory arthritis associated with psoriasis, the skin condition characterized by a scaly, itchy rash.

psychiatric crisis nurse team An emergency department specialty team whose nurses interact with patients and families in crisis.

psychotropic drugs Antipsychotic and neuroleptic drugs. These are appropriately given to patients with emotional and behavioral health problems (e.g., hallucinations and delusions) that accompany dementia but are sometimes inappropriately used for agitation, combativeness, or restlessness. They are considered chemical restraints because they decrease mobility and patients' ability to care for themselves.

ptosis Drooping of the eyelid.

pulmonary artery occlusive pressure (PAOP) See *pulmonary artery wedge pressure.*

pulmonary artery wedge pressure (PAWP) Measurement of pressure in the left atrium using a balloon-tipped catheter introduced into the pulmonary artery. When the balloon at the catheter tip is inflated, the catheter advances and wedges in a branch of the pulmonary artery. The tip of the catheter is able to sense pressures transmitted from the left atrium, which reflect left ventricular end-diastolic pressure. Also called "pulmonary artery occlusive pressure."

pulmonary autograph The relocation of the patient's own pulmonary valve to the aortic position for aortic valve replacement (Ross procedure).

pulmonary embolism (PE) A collection of particulate matter, most commonly a blood clot, that enters venous circulation and lodges in the pulmonary vessels, obstructing pulmonary blood flow and leading to decreased systemic oxygenation, pulmonary tissue hypoxia, and potential death.

pulmonary empyema A collection of pus in the pleural space most commonly caused by a pulmonary infection.

pulse deficit The difference between the apical and peripheral pulses.

pulse pressure The difference between the systolic and diastolic pressures.

pulse therapy Any therapy given at a high dose for a short duration.

pulsus alternans A type of pulse in which a weak pulse alternates with a strong pulse despite a regular heart rhythm; seen in patients with severely depressed cardiac function.

punctum The opening through which tears drain; located at the nasal side of the eyelid edges.

pupil The opening through which light enters the eye; located in the center of the iris of the eye.

Purkinje cells In the cardiac conduction system, the cells that make up the bundle of His, bundle branches, and terminal Purkinje fibers. These cells are responsible for the rapid conduction of electrical impulses throughout the ventricles, leading to ventricular depolarization and subsequent ventricular muscle contraction.

purpura Purple patches on the skin that may be caused by blood disorders, vascular abnormalities, or trauma.

pyelolithotomy The surgical removal of a stone from the kidney.

pyelonephritis A bacterial infection in the kidney and renal pelvis (the upper urinary tract).

pyloromyotomy An incision through the serosa and muscularis of the pylorus, down to the mucosa; created to prevent gastric motility disturbances in patients who have undergone esophagectomy.

pyuria The presence of white blood cells (pus) in the urine.

Q

QRS complex In the electrocardiogram, the portion consisting of the Q, R, and S waves, representing ventricular depolarization.

QRS duration In the electrocardiogram, the time required for depolarization of both ventricles; measured from the beginning of the QRS complex to the J point (the junction where the QRS complex ends and the ST segment begins).

QT interval In the electrocardiogram, the time from the beginning of the QRS complex to the end of the T wave. It represents the total time required for ventricular depolarization and repolarization.

quadriceps-setting exercise Postoperative leg exercise performed by straightening the legs and pushing the back of the knees into the bed.

quadrigeminy A type of premature complex consisting of a repetitive four-beat pattern; usually occurs as three sequential normal complexes followed by a premature complex and a pause, with the same pattern repeating itself in a four-beat pattern.

quadriparesis Weakness that involves all four extremities; seen with cervical spinal cord injury.

qualitative question A clinical question that focuses on the meanings and interpretations of human phenomena or experience of people and usually analyzes the content of what a person says during an interview or what a researcher observes.

quality improvement A QSEN competency in which the nurse uses data to monitor the outcomes of care processes and uses improvement methods to design and test changes to continuously improve the quality and safety of health care systems.

quantitative question A clinical question that asks about the relationship between or among defined, measurable phenomena and includes statistical analysis of information that is collected to answer a question.

R

radiation dose The amount of radiation absorbed by the tissue.

radiation proctitis Rectal mucosa inflammation that results from external beam radiation therapy.

radical cystectomy Removal of the bladder and surrounding tissue with urinary diversion.

radicular Referring to a nerve root.

radiculopathy Referring to radicular pain; spinal nerve root involvement.

radiofrequency catheter ablation An invasive procedure that uses radiofrequency waves to abolish an irritable focus that is causing a supraventricular or ventricular tachydysrhythmia.

Rapid Response Team Team of critical care experts who save lives and decrease the risk for harm by providing care to patients before a respiratory or cardiac arrest occurs. Also called "Medical Emergency Team."

RBC Red blood cell.

rebound headache Headache that occurs as a side effect of a drug that has relieved an initial migraine headache. Also called "medication overuse headache."

recall memory Recent memory, which can be tested during the history taking by asking about items such as the dates of clinic or physician appointments.

receptive aphasia A type of aphasia caused by injury to Wernicke's area in the temporoparietal area of the brain and characterized by an inability to understand the spoken and written word; both reading and writing ability are equally affected. Although the patient can talk, the language is often meaningless and neologisms (made-up words) are common parts of speech. Also called "Wernicke's aphasia" or "sensory aphasia."

reconstructive plastic surgery Type of plastic surgery that corrects or improves functional defects that have occurred as a result of congenital problems, trauma and scarring, or other types of therapy.

recreational therapist A member of the health care team who works to help patients continue or develop hobbies or interests. Also called "activity therapist."

rectocele A protrusion of the rectum through a weakened vaginal wall.

red reflex A reflection of light on the retina seen as a red glare during ophthalmoscopic examination. An absent red reflex may indicate a lens opacity or cloudiness of the vitreous.

redirection An intervention to help with communication problems in patients with dementia; consists of attracting the patient's attention before conversing, keeping the environment as free of distractions as possible, and speaking directly to the patient in a distinct manner using clear and short sentences.

reducible hernia A hernia that can be placed back into the abdominal cavity by gentle pressure.

reduction mammoplasty Breast reduction surgery in which the surgeon removes excess breast tissue and then repositions the nipple and remaining skin flaps to produce an optimal cosmetic effect.

Reed-Sternberg cell A specific cancer cell type, found in lymph nodes, that is a marker for Hodgkin's lymphoma.

re-epithelialization In partial-thickness (superficial) wounds involving damage to the epidermis and upper layers of the dermis, a form of healing by means of the production of new skin cells by undamaged epidermal cells in the basal layer of the dermis.

refeeding syndrome Life-threatening metabolic complication that can occur when nutrition is restarted for a patient who is in a starvation state.

reflex arc A closed circuit of spinal and peripheral nerves that requires no control by the brain.

reflex sympathetic dystrophy (RSD) See *complex regional pain syndrome.*

reflux Reverse or backward flow.

reflux esophagitis Damage to the esophageal mucosa, often with erosion and ulceration, in patients with gastroesophageal reflux disease.

refraction The bending of light rays.
refractory hypoxemia Low blood oxygen levels that persist even when 100% oxygen is given.
regional anesthesia A type of local anesthesia that blocks multiple peripheral nerves in a specific body region.
registered dietitian (RD) Member of the health care team who ensures patients meet their nutritional needs. Also called "nutritionist."
regurgitation Flowing in the opposite direction from normal, as the occurrence of warm fluid traveling up the throat, unaccompanied by nausea, in the patient with gastroesophageal reflux disease.
rehabilitation The process of learning to live with chronic and disabling conditions by returning the patient to the fullest possible physical, mental, social, vocational, and economic capacity.
rehabilitation case manager Nurse or other health care professional who coordinates health care for patients undergoing rehabilitation in home or acute care settings.
rehabilitation nurse Nurse who coordinates the efforts of health care team members for patients undergoing rehabilitation in the inpatient setting; may be designated as the patient's case manager.
relapsing-remitting multiple sclerosis (RRMS) A type of multiple sclerosis that occurs in 85% of cases and is characterized by a mild or moderate course, depending on the degree of disability. Relapses develop over 1 to 2 weeks and resolve over 4 to 8 months, after which the patient returns to baseline.
reliever drugs Drugs used in asthma therapy to stop an asthma attack once it has started.
religions Formal belief systems that provide a framework for making sense of life, death, and suffering and responding to universal spiritual questions; a formal expression of spirituality.
relocation stress syndrome Physiologic or psychosocial distress following transfer from one environment to another, such as after admission to a hospital or nursing home. Also called "relocation trauma."
reminiscence The process of randomly reflecting on memories of events in one's life.
remote memory Long-term memory of events; can be tested by asking patients about their birth date, schools attended, city of birth, or anything from the past that can be verified.
renal colic Severe pain associated with distention or spasm of the ureter, such as with an obstruction or the passing of a stone; the pain radiates into the perineal area, groin, scrotum, or labia. Pain may be intermittent or continuous and may be accompanied by pallor, diaphoresis, and hypotension.
renal columns Cortical tissue that dips into the interior of the kidney and separates the pyramids in the medulla. Also called "columns of Bertin."
renal cortex The outermost layer of functional kidney tissue lying beneath the renal capsule.
renal osteodystrophy The problems in bone metabolism and structure caused by renal failure–induced hypocalcemia and hyperphosphatemia.
renal pelvis The expansion from the upper end of the ureter into which the calices of the kidney open.
renal threshold The limit to the amount of glucose that the kidney can reabsorb as glucose is filtered from the blood. Also called the "transport maximum."
renin A hormone that is produced in the juxtaglomerular complex of the kidney and helps regulate blood flow, glomerular filtration rate, and blood pressure. Renin is secreted when sensing cells (macula densa) in the distal convoluted tubule sense changes in blood volume and pressure.
repetitive stress injury (RSI) Injury caused by repeated movements of the same part of the body (e.g., carpal tunnel syndrome).
replicate The reproduction of DNA that occurs each time a cell divides.
resident An individual who lives in an inpatient facility and has all the rights of anyone living in his or her home.
residuals Amount of feeding that remains in the stomach after enteral nutrition.
resistin A hormone produced by fat cells that creates resistance to insulin activity.
resorption In referring to bone, the loss of bone minerals and density; the release of free calcium from bone storage sites directly into the extracellular fluid.
restorative aide A member of the health care team, often with the nursing department, who assists the therapists, especially in the long-term care setting.
restraint Any device (physical restraint) or drug (chemical restraint) that prevents the patient from moving freely.
restrictive cardiomyopathy A form of cardiomyopathy that restricts the filling of the ventricles; a type of lung disease that prevents good expansion and recoil of the gas exchange unit.
restrictive (lung disorder) Any lung disorder that prevents good expansion and recoil of the gas exchange unit.
resurfacing Regrowth of new skin cells across the open area of a wound as it heals.
resuscitation phase The first phase of a burn injury, beginning at the onset of injury and continuing to about 48 hours.
rete pegs The fingers of epidermal tissue that project into the dermis.
reticular activating system (RAS) Special cells throughout the brainstem that constitute the system that controls awareness and alertness.
retina The innermost layer of the eye, made up of sensory receptors that transmit impulses to the optic nerve. It contains blood vessels and two types of photoreceptors called "rods" and "cones." Rods work at low light levels and provide peripheral vision; cones are active at bright light levels and provide color and central vision.
retinal detachment Separation of the retina from the epithelium.
retinal hole A break in the retina; can be caused by trauma or can occur with aging.
retinal tear Jagged and irregularly shaped break in the retina resulting from traction on the retina.
retinopathy Inflammation of the retina. Also used as a general term for vision problems.
retrograde Going against the normal direction of flow.
retroviruses The family of viruses that includes the human immune deficiency virus.
revision arthroplasty Surgical replacement of a prosthesis that has loosened and is causing pain.
rhabdomyolysis The breakdown or disintegration of muscle tissue; associated with excretion of myoglobin in the urine.
rheumatic carditis Inflammatory lesions in the heart due to a sensitivity response that develops after an upper respiratory tract infection with group A beta-hemolytic streptococci, which occurs in about 40% of patients with rheumatic fever. Inflammation results in impaired contractile function of the myocardium, thickening of the pericardium, and valvular damage. Also called "rheumatic endocarditis."
rheumatic disease Any disease or condition involving the musculoskeletal system.
rheumatoid arthritis (RA) A chronic, progressive, systemic, inflammatory autoimmune disease process that primarily affects the synovial joints; one of the most common connective tissue diseases and the most destructive to the joints.
rhinitis An inflammation of the nasal mucosa.
rhinoplasty A surgical reconstruction of the nose done for cosmetic purposes and improvement of airflow.
rhinorrhea Watery drainage from the nose; a "runny" nose.
rickets Vitamin D deficiency in children.
right-sided heart (ventricular) failure The inability of the right ventricle to empty completely, resulting in increased volume and pressure in the systemic veins and systemic venous congestion with peripheral edema.
robotic technology Technology that provides mechanical parts for extremities when they are not functional or have been amputated.
Romberg sign Swaying or falling when the patient is standing with arms at the sides, feet and knees close together, and eyes closed; a test of equilibrium in neurologic assessment.
rotation A mechanism of injury in which the head is turned excessively beyond the normal range.
rubor Dusky red discoloration of the skin.
rugae Folds, as of a mucous membrane.

S

S_3 gallop The third heart sound; an early diastolic filling sound that indicates an increase in left ventricular pressure and may be heard on auscultation in patients with heart failure.
safety A QSEN competency in which the nurse minimizes risk of harm to patients and providers through both system effectiveness and individual performance.
Salem sump tube Tube inserted through the nose and placed into the stomach that is attached to low continuous suction. It has a vent ("pigtail") that prevents the stomach mucosa from being pulled away during suctioning.
salpingitis Infection of the fallopian tube.

sanguineous Having a bloody appearance.

sarcoidosis A granulomatous disorder of unknown cause that can affect any organ but most often involves the lung.

SBAR Acronym for a formal method of communication between two or more members of the health care team. It is used most often when there is an unmet patient need or problem but can also be used to communicate continuing care issues when a patient is discharged from one agency to another. It consists of four steps: Situation, Background, Assessment, Recommendation.

scabies A contagious skin disease caused by mite infestations.

sclera The external white layer of the eye.

scleroderma See *systemic sclerosis.*

sclerotherapy The injection of a sclerosing agent via a catheter, usually in an endoscopic procedure, to stop variceal bleeding.

sclerotic Hard, or hardening.

scoliosis An abnormal lateral curve in the spine, which normally should be a straight vertical line.

scotomas Changes in peripheral vision.

sebum A mildly bacteriostatic, fat-containing substance produced by the sebaceous glands. Sebum lubricates the skin and reduces water loss from the skin surface.

second intention Healing of deep tissue injuries or wounds with tissue loss in which a cavity-like defect requires gradual filling of the dead space with connective tissue, which prolongs the repair process.

secondary administration set A short conduit that is attached to the primary administration set at a Y-injection site and is used to deliver intermittent medications. Also called a "piggyback set."

secondary gout Gout involving hyperuricemia.

secondary hypertension Elevated blood pressure that is related to a specific disease (e.g., kidney disease) or medication (e.g., estrogen).

secondary lesion Describing skin disease in terms of changes in the appearance of the primary lesion. These changes occur with progression of an underlying disease or in response to a topical or systemic therapeutic intervention.

secondary prevention Early detection of a disease or condition, sometimes before signs and symptoms are evident, to prevent or limit permanent disability or death.

secondary progressive multiple sclerosis (SPMS) A type of multiple sclerosis that begins with a relapsing-remitting course and later becomes steadily progressive. Attacks and partial recoveries may continue to occur.

secondary survey In the emergency department, a more comprehensive head-to-toe assessment performed to identify other injuries or medical issues that need to be managed or that might impact the course of treatment.

secondary tumor Additional tumor that is established when cancer cells move from the primary location to another area in the body. Also called "metastatic tumor."

seizure An abnormal, sudden, excessive, uncontrolled electrical discharge of neurons within the brain that may result in an alteration in consciousness, motor or sensory ability, and/or behavior. A single seizure may occur for no known reason; however, seizures may be due to a pathologic condition of the brain, such as a tumor.

self-tolerance In immunology, the ability to recognize self cells versus non-self cells, which is necessary to prevent healthy body cells from being destroyed along with invading cells.

Sengstaken-Blakemore tube Tube similar to a nasogastric tube that is placed through the nose and into the stomach in which an attached balloon is inflated to apply pressure to bleeding variceal areas of the esophagus.

sensitivity The likelihood that infecting bacterial organisms will be killed or stopped by a particular antibiotic drug. Sensitivity is determined by testing different antibiotics against the organisms. Organisms are "sensitive" if the antibiotic is effective in stopping their growth; organisms are "resistant" if the antibiotic is not effective.

sensorineural hearing loss Hearing loss that results from a defect in the cochlea, the eighth cranial nerve, or the brain itself. Exposure to loud noises and music may cause this type of hearing loss as a result of damage to the cochlear hair cells.

sensory Facilitating sensation.

sensory aphasia See *receptive aphasia.*

sentinel event As defined by The Joint Commission, an unexpected occurrence involving serious physical or psychological injury or the risk thereof and requiring an intense analysis of the contributing factors and corrective action.

sepsis Systemic infection.

septic shock The type of shock that occurs when large amounts of toxins and endotoxins produced by bacteria are released into the blood, causing a whole-body inflammatory reaction.

septicemia Systemic disease associated with sepsis; the presence of pathogens in the blood.

sequestrum A piece of necrotic bone that has separated from surrounding bone tissue; a common complication of osteomyelitis.

serologic testing Laboratory testing that is performed to identify pathogens by detecting antibodies to the organism.

serositis Inflammation of a serous membrane, such as the pleura or peritoneum.

serous Having a serum-like appearance, or yellow color.

serum sickness A type III hypersensitivity reaction that develops first as a skin rash and occurs within 3 to 21 days of the administration of antivenin (Crotalidae) polyvalent. This allergic response is often accompanied by other manifestations such as fever, arthralgias (joint pains), and pruritus (itching).

severe acute respiratory syndrome (SARS) An easily spread respiratory infection first identified in China in November 2002. At first appearing as an atypical pneumonia, it is caused by a new, more virulent form of coronavirus, and there is no known effective treatment.

severe sepsis The progression of sepsis with an amplified inflammatory response.

sex chromosomes The pair of chromosomes containing the genes for sexual differentiation in humans. In males, the sex chromosomes are an X and a Y; in females, the sex chromosomes are two Xs.

sex reassignment surgery (SRS) Surgery, particularly procedures that affect the external or internal genitalia, that transitions an individual from one's natal sex to one's inner gender identity. Also known as "gender reassignment surgery."

sexually transmitted infections (STIs) Any of a group of diseases caused by infectious organisms that have been passed from one person to another through intimate contact. Some organisms that cause these diseases are transmitted only through sexual contact. Other organisms are transmitted by parenteral exposure to infected blood, fecal-oral transmission, intrauterine transmission to the fetus, and perinatal transmission from mother to neonate. Also known as "sexually transmitted diseases (STDs)."

SHARE Acronym standing for Standardize critical content, Hardwire within your system, Allow opportunity to ask questions, Reinforce quality and measurement, Educate and coach.

shift to the left An increased number of immature neutrophils found on a differential count in patients with infections; can be characterized by changes in percentages of different types of leukocytes. Also known as "left shift."

shock The whole-body response to poor tissue oxygenation. Any problem that impairs oxygen delivery to tissues and organs can start the syndrome of shock and lead to a life-threatening emergency.

short peripheral catheter A catheter that consists of a plastic cannula built around a sharp stylet for venipuncture, which extends slightly beyond the cannula and is advanced into the vein.

sialagogue An agent that stimulates the flow of saliva.

simple fracture See *closed fracture.*

single-photon emission computed tomography (SPECT) A diagnostic tool using a radiopharmaceutical (agent that enables radioisotopes to cross the blood-brain barrier) that is administered by IV injection, after which the patient is scanned.

sinoatrial (SA) node In the cardiac conduction system, the primary pacemaker of the heart; located close to the epicardial surface of the right atrium near its junction with the superior vena cava. It can spontaneously and rhythmically generate electrical impulses at a rate of 60 to 100 beats/min. Also called the "sinus node."

sinus arrhythmia A variant of normal sinus rhythm that results from changes in intrathoracic pressure during breathing; heart rate increases slightly during inspiration and decreases slightly during exhalation. Atrial and ventricular rates are between 60 and 100 beats/min, and atrial and ventricular rhythms are irregular.

sinus bradycardia A cardiac dysrhythmia caused by a decreased rate of sinus node discharge, with a heart rate that is less than 60 beats/min.

sinus tachycardia A cardiac dysrhythmia caused by an increased rate of sinus node discharge, with a heart rate that is more than 100 beats/min.

sinusitis An inflammation of the mucous membranes of the sinuses.

SIRS Acronym for systemic inflammatory response syndrome, an inflammatory state affecting the whole body.

Sjögren's syndrome In patients with advanced rheumatoid arthritis, the triad of dry eyes, dry mouth, and dry vagina caused by the obstruction of secretory ducts and glands by inflammatory cells and immune complexes.

skilled nursing facility (SNF) Part of either a hospital or long-term care (nursing home) setting in which care is reimbursed through Medicare Part A for the first 21 days after admission.

skinfold measurement Measurement that estimates body fat.

smart pump An infusion pump with dosage calculation software.

social justice Ethical principle that refers to equality and fairness—that all patients should be treated equally and fairly, regardless of age, gender, religion, race, ethnicity, or education.

social worker Member of the health care team who helps patients identify support services and resources and who coordinates transfers to or discharges from the rehabilitation setting.

sodium (Na^+) A mineral that is the major cation in the extracellular fluid and maintains extracellular fluid (ECF) osmolarity.

solute A particle dissolved or suspended in the water portion (solvent) of body fluids; a solution consists of a solute and a solvent.

solvent The water portion of fluids.

spastic bladder Incontinence characterized by sudden, gushing voids, usually without completely emptying the bladder; caused by neurologic problems affecting the upper motor neuron, such as with spinal cord injuries above the twelfth thoracic vertebra.

spastic paralysis Paralysis of a part of the body that is characterized by spasticity of muscles due to hypertonia; may be seen in the patient who has experienced a brain attack.

specialized nutrition support (SNS) Total nutritional intake orally or intravenously with commercially prepared products (either total enteral nutrition or total parenteral nutrition).

speech-language pathologist (SLP) A member of the rehabilitation health care team who evaluates and retrains patients with speech, language, or swallowing problems.

sphincter of Oddi The sheath of muscle fibers surrounding the papillary opening of the duodenum.

sphincterotomy A procedure for opening a sphincter.

spider angiomas See *telangiectasias.*

spinal fusion (arthrodesis) A surgical procedure to stabilize the spine after repeated laminectomies have been unsuccessful. Chips of bone are removed (typically from the iliac crest) or are obtained from donor bone; the chips are grafted between the vertebrae for support and to strengthen the back.

spinal shock See *spinal shock syndrome.*

spinal shock syndrome Loss of reflex activity below the level of a spinal lesion; occurs immediately after injury as a result of disruption in the communication pathways between the upper motor neurons and the lower motor neurons. Also called "spinal shock."

spinal stenosis Narrowing of the spinal canal; typically seen in people older than 60 years.

spirituality The connection to self, others, the environment, and a "higher power."

spiritual counselor Counselor who specializes in spiritual assessments and care, usually a member of the clergy.

splenectomy Surgical removal of the spleen.

splenomegaly Enlargement of the spleen.

splint Any object or device that extends to the joints above and below a fracture to immobilize it.

splinter hemorrhage Black longitudinal line or small red streak on the distal third of the nail bed; seen in patients with infective endocarditis.

spondee Two-syllable words in which there is generally equal stress on each syllable, such as *airplane, railroad,* and *cowboy;* used in testing speech reception threshold.

spondylolisthesis Condition in which one vertebra slips forward on the one below it, often as a result of spondylolysis. This problem causes pressure on the nerve roots, leading to pain in the lower back and into the buttocks.

spondylolysis A defect in one of the vertebrae; usually found in the lumbar spine.

spontaneous bacterial peritonitis (SBP) Bacterial infection of the abdominal peritoneum caused by ascites; often seen in patients with cirrhosis of the liver.

spore An encapsulated, inactive organism.

sprain Excessive stretching of a ligament.

ST segment In the electrocardiogram, the line (normally isoelectric) representing early ventricular repolarization. It occurs from the J point to the beginning of the T wave.

ST-elevation myocardial infarction (STEMI) Myocardial infarction in which the patient typically has ST elevation in two contiguous leads on a 12-lead ECG; this indicates myocardial infarction/necrosis.

staging System of classifying clinical aspects of a cancer tumor.

Standard Precautions Infection control guidelines from the Centers for Disease Control and Prevention stating that all body excretions, secretions, and moist membranes and tissues are potentially infectious; combines protective measures from Universal Precautions and Body Substance Isolation.

stasis dermatitis In patients with venous insufficiency, discoloration of the skin along the ankles, which extends up to the calf.

stasis ulcer In patients with long-term venous insufficiency, ulcer formed as a result of edema or minor injury to the limb; typically occurs over the malleolus.

status epilepticus Prolonged seizures lasting more than 5 minutes or repeated seizures over the course of 30 minutes; a potential complication of all types of seizures.

steatorrhea An excessive amount of fat in the stool.

stem cell An immature, undifferentiated cell produced by the bone marrow.

stent A small tube that is placed in a tubular structure to dilate it; a wirelike device that may be used along with percutaneous transluminal angioplasty to help keep the vessel open.

stereotactic pallidotomy A surgical treatment for the patient with Parkinson disease when drugs are ineffective in symptom management. An electrode is used to create a lesion in a targeted area within the pallidum, with the goal of reducing tremor and rigidity.

sterilization A method of infection control in which all living organisms and bacterial spores are destroyed; used on items that invade human tissue where bacteria are not commonly found.

stoma The surgical creation of an opening; usually refers to an opening in the abdominal wall.

stomatitis Inflammation of the oral mucosa; characterized by painful single or multiple ulcerations that impair the protective lining of the mouth. The ulcerations are commonly referred to as "canker sores."

strain Excessive stretching of a muscle or tendon when it is weak or unstable; sometimes referred to as "muscle pulls."

strangulated hernia A tightly constricted hernia that compromises the blood supply to the herniated segment of the bowel as a result of pressure from the hernial ring (the band of muscle around the hernia); leads to ischemia and obstruction of the bowel loop, with necrosis of the bowel and possibly bowel perforation.

strangulated obstruction Intestinal obstruction with compromised blood flow.

stratum corneum The outermost layer of the skin.

stress test See *exercise electrocardiography.*

stress ulcers Multiple shallow erosions of the proximal stomach and occasionally the duodenum.

stress urinary incontinence (SUI) Loss of urine during activities that increase intra-abdominal pressure, such as laughing, coughing, sneezing, or lifting heavy objects.

striae Reddish purple streaks on the skin. Also called "stretch marks."

stricture Narrowing.

stridor A high-pitched crowing sound caused by laryngospasm or edema above or below the glottis; heard during respiration.

stroke See *brain attack.*

stroke volume (SV) The amount of blood ejected by the left ventricle during each heartbeat.

subarachnoid space Term for the space between the arachnoid mater and pia mater of the spinal cord. Also called "subarachnoid."

subcutaneous emphysema The presence of bubbles under the skin because of air trapping; an uncommon late complication of fracture.

subcutaneous infusion therapy Infusion therapy that is delivered under the skin when patients cannot tolerate oral medications, when intramuscular injections are too painful, or when vascular access is not available.

subcutaneous nodule Characteristic round, movable, nontender swelling under the skin of the arm or fingers in patients with severe rheumatoid arthritis.

subdural hematoma (SDH) The collection of clotted blood that typically results from venous bleeding into the space beneath the dura and above the arachnoid.

subdural space Term for the space between the dura mater and the middle layer (arachnoid).

subluxation Partial joint dislocation.

submucous resection (SMR) Surgical procedure to straighten a deviated septum when chronic symptoms or discomfort occur. Also called "nasoseptoplasty."

substernally Located below the ribs.

subtotal thyroidectomy The surgical removal of part of the thyroid tissue.

sundowning In patients with Alzheimer's disease, increased confusion at night or when excessively fatigued.

superinfection Reinfection or a second infection of the same type.

supervision Guidance or direction, evaluation, and follow-up by the nurse to ensure that the task or activity is performed appropriately.

supratentorial Located within the cerebral hemispheres, in the area above the tentorium of the cerebellum; the tentlike fold of dura that surrounds the cerebellar hemisphere and supports the occipital lobe.

supraventricular tachycardia (SVT) A form of tachycardia that involves the rapid stimulation of atrial tissue at a rate of 100 to 280 beats/min. It is most often due to a re-entry mechanism in which one impulse circulates repeatedly throughout the atrial pathway, re-stimulating the atrial tissue at a rapid rate.

surfactant A fatty protein secreted by type II pneumocytes to reduce surface tension in the alveoli.

surveillance Term used to describe the tracking of infections by health care agencies.

susceptibility The risk of the host to infection; may be increased by the breakdown of host defenses against pathogens.

swimmer's ear See *external otitis.*

sympathectomy Surgical cutting of the sympathetic nerve branches via endoscopy through a small axillary incision.

sympathetic tone A state of partial blood vessel constriction caused when nerves from the sympathetic division of the autonomic nervous system continuously stimulate vascular smooth muscle.

synapse The area through which impulses are transmitted to their eventual destination.

syncope Transient loss of consciousness (blackouts), most commonly caused by decreased perfusion to the brain.

syndrome of inappropriate antidiuretic hormone (SIADH) Persistent hyponatremia, hypovolemia, and inappropriately elevated urine osmolality that occurs when vasopressin (antidiuretic hormone) is secreted even when plasma osmolarity is low or normal.

synovectomy The surgical removal of synovium.

synovial joint Type of joint lined with synovium, a membrane that secretes synovial fluid for lubrication and shock absorption.

synovitis Inflammation of synovial membrane.

syphilis A complex sexually transmitted disease that can become systemic and cause serious complications and even death. It is caused by the spirochete *Treponema pallidum,* which is found in the mouth, intestinal tract, and genital areas of people and animals. The infection is usually transmitted by sexual contact, but transmission can occur through close body contact and kissing.

syringe pump Pump for infusion therapy that uses a battery-powered piston to push the plunger continuously at a selected mL/hr rate; limited to small-volume continuous or intermittent infusions.

systemic Affecting the body system as a whole.

systemic lupus erythematosus (SLE) A chronic, progressive, inflammatory connective tissue disorder that can cause major body organs and systems to fail; characterized by spontaneous remissions and exacerbations.

systemic sclerosis (SSc) A chronic connective tissue disease characterized by inflammation, fibrosis, and sclerosis of the skin and vital organs. Also called "scleroderma" and formerly called "progressive systemic sclerosis."

systole The phase of the cardiac cycle that consists of the contraction and emptying of the atria and ventricles.

systolic blood pressure The amount of pressure/force generated by the left ventricle to distribute blood into the aorta with each contraction of the heart.

systolic heart failure (systolic ventricular dysfunction) Heart failure that results when the heart is unable to contract forcefully enough during systole to eject adequate amounts of blood into the circulation.

T

T wave In the electrocardiogram, the deflection that follows the ST segment and represents ventricular repolarization.

tachycardia An excessively fast heart rate; characterized as a pulse rate greater than 100 beats/min.

tachydysrhythmia An abnormal heart rhythm with a rate greater than 100 beats/min.

tactile (vocal) fremitus A vibration of the chest wall produced when the patient speaks; can be palpated on the chest wall.

target tissues The tissues that respond specifically to a given hormone.

taut Tightly stretched.

teamwork and collaboration A QSEN competency in which the nurse functions effectively within nursing and interprofessional teams, fostering open communication, mutual respect, and shared decision making to achieve quality patient care.

telangiectasias Vascular lesions with a red center and radiating branches. Also called "spider angiomas," "spider nevi," or "vascular spiders."

telemetry In electrocardiography (ECG), the use of a battery-powered transmitter system for monitoring an ambulatory patient; allows freedom of movement within a certain radius without losing transmission of the ECG.

temporal field blindness A decrease in lateral peripheral vision.

temporary pacing A nonsurgical intervention for cardiac dysrhythmia that provides a timed electrical stimulus to the heart when either the impulse initiation or the intrinsic conduction system of the heart is defective.

tendon Any one of many bands of tough, fibrous tissue that attach muscles to bones.

tendon transplant Removal of a tendon from one part of the body and transplantation into the affected area to replace a ruptured tendon that cannot be repaired surgically.

tenesmus Straining, especially painful straining to defecate.

teratogenic Tending to produce birth defects.

tetany Continuous contractions of muscle groups; hyperexcitability of nerves and muscles.

tetraplegia Another term for *quadriplegia* (paralysis that involves all four extremities).

thalamotomy An alternative to stereotactic pallidotomy as a surgical treatment for the patient with Parkinson disease; uses thermocoagulation of brain cells to reduce tremor. Usually only unilateral surgery is performed to benefit the side of the body most affected by the disease.

thalamus A structure within the brain; functions as the "central switchboard" for the central nervous system.

thallium scan A test that is similar to the bone scan but uses the radioisotope *thallium* and is more sensitive in diagnosing the extent of disease in patients with osteosarcoma.

The Joint Commission An organization that offers peer evaluation for accreditation every 3 years for all types of health care agencies that meet their standards. Formerly known as the *Joint Commission for Accreditation of Healthcare Organizations (JCAHO).*

therapeutic hypothermia Treatment that lowers the body core temperature to reduce the risk of cell, tissue, and organ damage from a low or absent blood flow. Usually follows cardiac arrest.

thermotherapy Technique for treating benign prostatic hyperplasia that uses a variety of heat methods to destroy excess prostate tissue.

third intention Delayed primary closure of a wound with a high risk for infection. The wound is intentionally left open for several days until inflammation has subsided and is then closed by first intention.

thoracentesis The aspiration of pleural fluid or air from the pleural space.

threshold In evaluating hearing, the lowest level of intensity at which pure tones and speech are heard by a patient; in general, the lowest level at which a stimulus is perceived.

thrombectomy Removal of a clot (thrombus) from a blood vessel.

thrombocytopenia A reduction in the number of blood platelets below the level needed for normal coagulation, resulting in an increased tendency to bleed.

thrombophlebitis The presence of a thrombus associated with inflammation; usually occurs in the deep veins of the lower extremities.

thrombosis The formation of a blood clot (thrombus) within a blood vessel.

thrombotic stroke Damage to the brain when blood flow is impaired from a clot, resulting in blockage to one or more of the arteries supplying blood to the brain.

thrombus A blood clot believed to result from an endothelial injury, venous stasis, or hypercoagulability.

thymectomy Removal of the thymus gland.

thymoma An encapsulated tumor of the thymus gland.

thyrocalcitonin (TCT) A hormone produced and secreted by the parafollicular cells of the thyroid gland to help regulate serum calcium levels; secreted in response to excess plasma calcium.

thyroiditis Inflammation of the thyroid gland.

thyroid storm (thyroid crisis) A life-threatening event that occurs in patients with uncontrolled hyperthyroidism and is usually caused by Graves' disease. Key manifestations include fever, tachycardia, and systolic hypertension.

thyrotoxicosis The condition caused by excessive amounts of thyroid hormones.

thyroxine (T_4) A hormone that is produced by the follicular cells of the thyroid gland and increases metabolism.

Tinel's sign Test that confirms a diagnosis of carpal tunnel syndrome; a positive test causes palmar paresthesias when the area of the median nerve is tapped lightly.

tinnitus A continuous ringing or noise perception in the ears.

titration Adjustment of IV fluid rate on the basis of the patient's urine output plus serum electrolyte values.

TNM (tumor, node, metastasis) System developed by the American Joint Committee on Cancer to describe the anatomic extent of cancers.

toe brachial pressure index (TBPI) Toe systolic pressure divided by brachial (arm) systolic pressure; may be performed instead of or in addition to ankle-brachial index to determine arterial perfusion in the feet and toes.

tonic phase Pertaining to a state of stiffening or rigidity of the muscles, particularly of the arms and legs, and immediate loss of consciousness of a tonic-clonic seizure.

tonsillitis An inflammation and infection of the tonsils and lymphatic tissues located on each side of the throat.

tophi A collection of uric acid crystals that form hard, irregular, painless nodules on the ears, arms, and fingers of patients with gout.

topical chemical débridement Method of débriding a wound by applying topical enzyme preparations to loosen necrotic tissue.

torn meniscus Tear of the knee meniscus (medial or lateral) in which the patient typically has pain, swelling, and tenderness in the knee.

torsades de pointes A type of ventricular tachycardia that is related to a prolonged QT interval.

total hysterectomy Removal of the uterus and cervix; the procedure may be vaginal or abdominal.

total joint arthroplasty (TJA) Surgical creation of a joint, or total joint replacement; commonly performed in patients with osteoarthritis. Also called "total joint replacement (TJR)."

total joint replacement (TJR) See *total joint arthroplasty.*

total parenteral nutrition (TPN) Provision of intensive nutritional support for an extended time; delivered to the patient through access to central veins, usually the subclavian or internal jugular veins.

total thyroidectomy The surgical removal of all of the thyroid tissue.

touch discrimination Part of the neurologic examination. The patient closes his or her eyes while the practitioner touches the patient with a finger and asks that the patient point to the area touched.

toxic and drug-induced hepatitis Liver inflammation resulting from exposure to hepatotoxins (e.g., industrial toxins, alcohol, and medications).

toxic epidermal necrolysis (TEN) A rare acute drug reaction of the skin that results in diffuse erythema and blister formation, with mucous membrane involvement and systemic toxicity.

toxic megacolon Acute enlargement of the colon along with fever, leukocytosis, and tachycardia; usually associated with ulcerative colitis.

toxic multinodular goiter Hyperthyroidism caused by multiple thyroid nodules, which may be enlarged thyroid tissues or adenomas, and a goiter that has been present for several years.

toxic shock syndrome (TSS) A severe illness caused by a toxin produced by certain strains of *Staphylococcus aureus*. It was first recognized in 1980 as related to menstruation and tampon use. It is characterized by abrupt onset of a high fever and headache, sore throat, vomiting, diarrhea, generalized rash, and hypotension. The most common manifestations are skin changes (initially a rash that resembles a severe sunburn and changes to a macular erythema similar to a drug-related rash).

toxidrome A syndrome related to drug toxicity.

toxin Protein molecule released by bacteria that affects host cell at a distant site. Continued multiplication of a pathogen is sometimes accompanied by toxin production.

trabeculation An abnormal thickening of the bladder wall caused by urinary retention and obstruction.

tracheostomy The (tracheal) stoma, or opening, that results from a tracheotomy.

tracheotomy The surgical incision into the trachea for the purpose of establishing an airway.

trachoma A chronic conjunctivitis caused by *Chlamydia trachomatis.*

traction The application of a pulling force to a part of the body to provide reduction, alignment, and rest.

transcellular fluid Any of the fluids in special body spaces, including cerebrospinal fluid, synovial fluid, peritoneal fluid, and pleural fluid.

transcutaneous pacing Temporary pacing that is accomplished through the application of two large external electrodes.

transesophageal echocardiography (TEE) A form of echocardiography performed transesophageally (through the esophagus); an ultrasound transducer is placed immediately behind the heart in the esophagus or stomach to examine cardiac structure and function.

transferrin An iron-transport protein that can be measured directly or calculated as an indirect measurement of total iron-binding capacity.

transgender Patients who self-identify as the opposite gender or a gender that does not match their natal sex.

transient ischemic attack (TIA) A brief attack (lasting a few minutes to less than 24 hours) of focal neurologic dysfunction caused by a brief interruption in cerebral blood flow, possibly resulting from cerebral vasospasm or transient systemic arterial hypertension. Repeated attacks may damage brain tissue; multiple attacks indicate significant increased risk for brain attack.

transmyocardial laser revascularization A new surgical procedure for patients with unstable angina and inoperable coronary artery disease with areas of reversible myocardial ischemia. After a single-lung intubation, a left anterior thoracotomy is performed and the heart is visualized. A laser is used to create 20 to 24 long, narrow channels through the left ventricular muscle to the left ventricle. The channels eventually allow oxygenated blood to flow from the left ventricle during diastole to nourish the muscle.

transport maximum See *renal threshold.*

transsexual A person who has modified his or her natal body to match the appropriate gender identity, either through cosmetic, hormonal, or surgical means.

transurethral microwave therapy (TUMT) Procedure for treating benign prostatic hyperplasia using high temperatures to heat and destroy excess tissue.

transurethral needle ablation (TUNA) Procedure for treating benign prostatic hyperplasia using low radiofrequency energy to shrink the prostate.

transurethral resection of the prostate (TURP) The traditional "closed" surgical procedure for removal of the prostate. In this procedure, the surgeon inserts a resectoscope (an instrument similar to a cystoscope, but with a cutting and cauterizing loop) through the urethra. The enlarged portion of the prostate gland is then resected in small pieces.

trauma Bodily injury.

trauma center Specialty care facility that provides competent and timely trauma services to patients depending on its designated level of capability.

trauma system An organized and integrated approach to trauma care designed to ensure that all critical elements of trauma care delivery are aligned to meet the injured patient's needs.

triage In the emergency department, sorting or classifying patients into priority levels depending on illness or injury severity, with the highest acuity needs receiving the quickest evaluation and treatment.

triage officer In a hospital's emergency response plan, the person who rapidly evaluates each patient who arrives at the hospital. In a large hospital, this person is generally a physician who is assisted by triage nurses; however, a nurse may assume this role when physician resources are limited.

trigeminy A type of premature complex consisting of a repetitive three-beat pattern; usually occurs as two sequential normal complexes followed by a premature complex and a pause, with the same pattern repeating itself in triplets.

trigger points In patients with fibromyalgia syndrome, tender areas that can typically be palpated to elicit pain in a predictable, reproducible pattern.

triglycerides Serum lipid profile that includes the measurement of cholesterol and lipoproteins.

triiodothyronine (T_3) A hormone produced by the follicular cells of the thyroid gland.

troponin A myocardial muscle protein released into the bloodstream after injury to myocardial muscle. Because it is not found in healthy patients, any rise in values indicates cardiac necrosis or acute myocardial infarction.

truss A device, usually a pad made with firm material, that is held in place over the hernia with a belt to keep the abdominal contents from protruding into the hernial sac.

tuberculosis (TB) A highly communicable disease caused by *Mycobacterium tuberculosis.* It is the most common bacterial infection worldwide.

tumescence The condition of being swollen.

tunneled central venous catheter A type of catheter used for long-term infusion therapy in which a portion of the catheter lies in a subcutaneous tunnel, separating the points where the catheter enters the vein from where it exits the skin.

turbidity Cloudiness of a solution.

turbinates Three bony projections that protrude into the nasal cavities from the walls of the internal portion of the nose.

turgor The condition of being swollen and congested; indicates the amount of skin elasticity; the normal resiliency of a pinched fold of skin.

tyrosine kinase inhibitors (TKIs) Drugs with the main action of inhibiting activation of tyrosine kinases. There are many different TKIs. Some are unique to the cell type; others may be present only in cancer cells that express a specific gene mutation. As a result, the different TKI drugs are effective in disrupting the growth of some cancer cell types and not others.

U

U wave In the electrocardiogram, the deflection that follows the T wave and may result from slow repolarization of ventricular Purkinje fibers. When present, it is of the same polarity as the T wave, although generally smaller. Abnormal prominence of the U wave suggests an electrolyte abnormality or other disturbance.

ulcerative colitis (UC) A chronic inflammatory process that affects the mucosal lining of the colon or rectum; one of a group of bowel diseases of unknown etiology characterized by remissions and exacerbations. It can result in loose stools containing blood and mucus, poor absorption of vital nutrients, and thickening of the colon wall.

umbilical hernia Protrusion of the intestine at the umbilicus; can be congenital or acquired. Congenital umbilical hernias appear in infancy. Acquired umbilical hernias directly result from increased intra-abdominal pressure and are most commonly seen in obese people.

unclassified seizure One of the three broad categories of seizure disorders along with partial seizure and generalized seizure. They occur for no known reason, do not fit into the generalized or partial classifications, and account for about half of all seizure activity. Also called "idiopathic seizures."

uncus The inner part of the temporal lobe of the brain that can move downward and cause pressure on the brainstem; the vital sign center.

undermining Separation of the skin layers at the wound margins from the underlying granulation tissue.

unilateral body neglect syndrome In the patient who has had a brain attack, an unawareness of the existence of the paralyzed side. For example, the patient may believe he or she is sitting up straight when actually he or she is leaning to one side. Another typical example is the patient who washes or dresses only one side of the body.

Unna boot A wound dressing constructed of gauze moistened with zinc oxide; used to promote venous return in the ambulatory patient with a stasis ulcer and to form a sterile environment for the ulcer. The boot is applied to the affected limb, from the toes to the knee, after the ulcer has been cleaned with normal saline solution and covered with an elastic wrap. The dressing hardens like a cast.

upper endoscopy See *esophagogastroduodenoscopy.*

upper esophageal sphincter (UES) The ring-like band of muscle fibers at the upper end of the esophagus. When at rest, the sphincter is closed to prevent air from entering into the esophagus during respiration.

upper GI (gastrointestinal) radiographic series The radiographic visualization of the gastrointestinal tract from the oral part of the pharynx to the duodenojejunal junction; used to detect disorders of structure or function of the esophagus (barium swallow), stomach, or duodenum.

uremia The accumulation of nitrogenous wastes in the blood (azotemia); a result of renal failure, with clinical symptoms including nausea and vomiting.

uremic frost A layer of urea crystals from evaporated sweat; may appear on the face, eyebrows, axilla, and groin in patients with advanced uremic syndrome.

uremic syndrome The systemic clinical and laboratory manifestations of end-stage kidney disease.

ureterolithiasis Formation of stones in the ureter.

ureteropelvic junction (UPJ) The narrow area in the upper third of the ureter at the point at which the renal pelvis becomes the ureter.

ureteroplasty Surgical repair of the ureter.

ureterovesical junction (UVJ) The point at which each ureter becomes narrow as it enters the bladder.

urethral meatus The opening at the endpoint of the urethra.

urethral stricture An obstruction that occurs low in the urinary tract due to decreased diameter of the urethra, causing bladder distention before hydroureter and hydronephrosis.

urethritis An inflammation of the urethra that causes symptoms similar to urinary tract infection.

urethroplasty Surgical treatment of the urethral stricture to remove the affected area with or without grafting to create a larger opening.

urgency The feeling that urination will occur immediately.

urgent triage In a three-tiered triage scheme, the category that includes patients who should be treated quickly but in whom an immediate threat to life does not currently exist, such as those with abdominal pain or displaced fractures or dislocations.

urinary tract infection (UTI) An infection in the normally sterile urinary system. The unobstructed and complete passage of urine from the renal and urinary systems is critical in maintaining a sterile urinary tract. When any structural abnormality is present, the risk for damage as a result of infection is greatly increased.

urolithiasis The presence of calculi (stones) in the urinary tract.

urosepsis The spread of an infection from the urinary tract to the bloodstream, resulting in systemic infection accompanied by fever, chills, hypotension, and altered mental status.

urticaria A transient vascular reaction of the skin marked by the development of wheals (hives).

uterine artery embolization Treatment for leiomyomas in which a radiologist uses a percutaneous catheter inserted through the femoral artery to inject polyvinyl alcohol pellets into the uterine artery. The resulting blockage starves the tumor of circulation, allowing it (or them) to shrink.

uterine prolapse Downward displacement of the uterus into the vagina.

uvea The middle layer of the eye, which consists of the choroid, ciliary body, and iris. The choroid has many blood vessels that supply nutrients to the retina.

V

vagal maneuver Nonsurgical management of cardiac dysrhythmias that is intended to induce vagal stimulation of the cardiac conduction system, specifically the sinoatrial and atrioventricular nodes. Vagal maneuvers may be attempted to terminate supraventricular tachydysrhythmia.

vaginoplasty The construction of a new vagina in a male-to-female patient, usually with inverted penile tissue or a colon graft, and the creation of a clitoris and labia using scrotal or penile tissue and skin grafts.

validation therapy For the patient with moderate or severe Alzheimer's disease, the process of recognizing and acknowledging the patient's feelings and concerns without reinforcing an erroneous belief (e.g., if the patient is looking for his or her deceased mother).

Valsalva maneuver A form of vagal stimulation of the cardiac conduction system in which the health care provider instructs the patient to bear down as if straining to have a bowel movement.

valvular regurgitation Regurgitation of any heart valve. See also *mitral regurgitation*.

variant (Prinzmetal's) angina A type of angina caused by coronary vasospasm (vessel spasm); usually associated with elevation of the ST segment on an electrocardiogram obtained during anginal attacks.

varicose veins Distended, protruding veins that appear darkened and tortuous; common in patients older than 30 years whose occupations require prolonged standing. As the vein wall weakens and dilates, venous pressure increases and the valves become incompetent (defective). The incompetent valves enhance the vessel dilation, and the veins become tortuous and distended.

vascular access device (VAD) A catheter; a plastic tube placed in a blood vessel to deliver fluids and medications.

vasculitis Blood vessel inflammation.

vasoconstriction Decrease in diameter of blood vessels.

vasopressin Secretion of the posterior pituitary gland. Also known as "antidiuretic hormone" or "ADH."

vasospasm A sudden and transient constriction of a blood vessel.

Vaughn-Williams classification System used to categorize antidysrhythmic agents according to their effects on the action potential of cardiac cells.

vegan A vegetarian diet pattern in which only foods of plant origin are eaten.

venous beading A complication of diabetes; the abnormal appearance of retinal veins in which areas of swelling and constriction along a segment of vein resemble links of sausage. Such bleeding occurs in areas of retinal ischemia and is a predictor of proliferative diabetic retinopathy.

venous insufficiency Alteration of venous efficiency by thrombosis or defective valves; caused by prolonged venous hypertension, which stretches the veins and damages the valves, resulting in further venous hypertension, edema, and, eventually, venous stasis ulcers, swelling, and cellulitis.

venous thromboembolism (VTE) A term that refers to both deep vein thrombosis and pulmonary embolism; obstruction by a thrombus.

ventilator-associated lung injury (VALI) Damage from prolonged ventilation causing loss of surfactant, increased inflammation, fluid leakage, and noncardiac pulmonary edema. Also known as "ventilator-induced lung injury."

ventilator-induced lung injury (VILI) See *ventilator-associated lung injury.*

ventral hernia See *incisional hernia.*

ventricular asystole The complete absence of any ventricular rhythm. There are no electrical impulses in the ventricles and therefore no ventricular depolarization, no QRS complex, no contraction, no cardiac output, and no pulse, respirations, or blood pressure. The patient is in full cardiac arrest.

ventricular fibrillation (VF) A cardiac dysrhythmia that results from electrical chaos in the ventricles; impulses from many irritable foci fire in a totally disorganized manner so that ventricular contraction cannot occur; there is no cardiac output or pulse and therefore no cerebral, myocardial, or systemic perfusion. This rhythm is rapidly fatal if not successfully terminated within 3 to 5 minutes.

ventricular gallop An abnormal third heart sound that arises from vibrations of the valves and supporting structures and is produced during the rapid passive filling phase of ventricular diastole when blood flows from the atrium to a noncompliant ventricle. In patients older than 35 years, it is an early sign of heart failure or ventricular septal defect.

ventricular remodeling (1) Progressive myocyte (myocardial cell) contractile dysfunction over time; results from activation of the renin-angiotensin system caused by reduced blood flow to the kidneys, a common occurrence in low-output states; (2) after a myocardial infarction, permanent changes in the size and shape of the left ventricle due to scar tissue; such remodeling may decrease left ventricular function, cause heart failure, and increase morbidity and mortality.

ventricular tachycardia (VT) An abnormal heart rhythm that occurs with repetitive firing of an irritable ventricular ectopic focus, usually at a rate of 140 to 180 beats/min or more.

ventriculomyomectomy The surgical excision of a portion of the hypertrophied ventricular septum to create a widened outflow tract in patients with obstructive hypertrophic cardiomyopathy. Also called "ventricular septal myectomy."

veracity Ethical principle that requires that the nurse is obligated to tell the truth to the best of his or her knowledge.

vertebroplasty A minimally invasive surgery for managing vertebral fractures in patients with osteoporosis. Bone cement is injected directly into the fracture site to provide immediate pain relief.

vertigo A sense of spinning movement that may result from diseases of the inner ear.

vesicants Chemicals or drugs that cause tissue damage on direct contact or extravasation.

vesicle In health care, a small bladder or blister.

vestibule A longitudinal area between the labia minora, the clitoris, and the vagina that contains Bartholin glands and the openings of the urethra, Skene's glands (paraurethral glands), and vagina.

viral hepatitis Inflammation of the liver that results from an infection caused by one of five major categories of viruses (hepatitis A, B, C, D, or E). Viral hepatitis is the most common type and can be either acute or chronic.

viral load testing Test that measures the presence of human immune deficiency virus genetic material (ribonucleic acid) or other viral proteins in the patient's blood.

Virchow's triad The occurrence of stasis of blood flow, endothelial injury, or hypercoagulability; often associated with thrombus formation.

viremia The presence of viruses in the blood.

virilization The presence of male secondary sex characteristics.

virtual colonoscopy A noninvasive alternative to the colonoscopy procedure. A scanner is used to view the colon.

virulence A term used to describe the frequency with which a pathogen causes disease (degree of communicability) and its ability to invade and damage a host. Virulence can also indicate the severity of the disease; often used as a synonym for *pathogenicity.*

visceral proteins Proteins such as albumin that circulate in the bloodstream and may be produced by the liver.

vitiligo An abnormality of the skin characterized by patchy areas of pigment loss with increased pigmentation at the edges. It is seen with primary hypofunction of the adrenal glands and is due to autoimmune destruction of melanocytes in the skin.

vitreous body The clear, thick gel that fills the vitreous chamber of the eye (the space between the lens and the retina). This gel transmits light and shapes the eye.

vocational counselor A member of the rehabilitative health care team who assists the patient with job placement, training, or further education.

volutrauma Damage to the lung by excess volume delivered to one lung over the other.

volvulus Obstruction of the bowel caused by twisting of the bowel.

vulvovaginitis Inflammation of the lower genital tract resulting from a disturbance of the balance of hormones and flora in the vagina and vulva.

W

warm antibody anemia A form of immunohemolytic anemia (in which the immune system attacks a person's own red blood cells for unknown reasons) that occurs with immunoglobulin G antibody excess and may be triggered by drugs, chemicals, or other autoimmune problems.

warm phase A phase lasting 2 to 3 weeks after peripheral nerve trauma resulting in complete denervation; the extremity is warm, and the skin appears flushed or rosy. The warm phase is gradually superseded by a cold phase.

water brash Reflex salivary hypersecretion that occurs in response to reflux in the patient with gastroesophageal reflux disease.

WBC White blood cell.

weaning The process of going from ventilatory dependence to spontaneous breathing.

wedge resection Removal of small, localized areas of disease.

Wernicke's aphasia See *receptive aphasia.*

Wernicke's area An important speech area of the cerebrum. It is located in the temporal lobe and plays a significant role in higher-level brain function. It enables the processing of words into coherent thought and recognition of the idea behind written or printed words (language).

Whipple procedure (radical pancreaticoduodenectomy) A surgical treatment for cancer of the head of the pancreas. The procedure entails removal of the proximal head of the pancreas, the duodenum, a portion of the jejunum, the stomach (partial or total gastrectomy), and the gallbladder, with anastomosis of the pancreatic duct (pancreaticojejunostomy), the common bile duct (choledochojejunostomy), and the stomach (gastrojejunostomy) to the jejunum.

white matter In the spinal cord, myelinated axons that surround the gray matter (neuron cell bodies).

Williams position A position in which the patient lies in the semi-Fowler's position and flexes the knees to relax the muscles of the lower back and relieve pressure on the spinal nerve root. This is typically more comfortable and therapeutic for the patient with low back pain.

withdrawing or withholding life-sustaining therapy The withdrawal or withholding of one or more therapies that might prolong the life of a person who cannot be cured by the therapy; the withdrawal of therapy does not directly cause death. Formerly called "passive euthanasia."

work-related musculoskeletal disorders (MSDs) Disorders caused by heavy lifting and dependent transfers by staff members.

X

xenograft Tissue transplanted (grafted) from another species; for example, a heart valve transplanted from a pig to a human.

xerostomia Abnormal dryness of the mouth caused by a severe reduction in the flow of saliva.

x-ray Radiation that is generated by machine.

NCLEX® EXAMINATION CHALLENGES—ANSWER KEY

Chapter 2
p. 12 C
p. 15 C
p. 21 D

Chapter 3
p. 33 A, B, E
p. 34 B
p. 37 C
p. 41 0.4 mL
p. 44 B

Chapter 4
p. 62 D

Chapter 6
p. 79 D
p. 88 A

Chapter 7
p. 97 A, B, D, E
p. 99 A, B, C, E

Chapter 8
p. 112 A
p. 118 C

Chapter 9
p. 122 B
p. 132 A, B, C, D, E
p. 135 C

Chapter 10
p. 141 D
p. 144 A, B, E

Chapter 11
p. 158 D
p. 163 D
p. 165 B
p. 170 D

Chapter 12
p. 183 C

Chapter 13
p. 190 D, A, C, B
p. 193 100

Chapter 14
p. 216 C
p. 222 A
p. 225 C

Chapter 15
p. 244 D
p. 248 C

Chapter 16
p. 261 C
p. 263 D
p. 271 A

Chapter 17
p. 281 B

Chapter 18
p. 294 B, C, E
p. 300 B, D, E
p. 302 A
p. 308 B, C, E, F
p. 317 A, B, C, E
p. 320 C

Chapter 19
p. 332 B
p. 332 C
p. 340 D
p. 342 A

Chapter 20
p. 354 B
p. 355 D

Chapter 21
p. 365 C
p. 369 D

Chapter 22
p. 377 A
p. 383 C
p. 387 B
p. 394 C

Chapter 23
p. 405 C
p. 406 B, E

Chapter 24
p. 424 C
p. 430 B

Chapter 25
p. 453 B
p. 458 D
p. 461 C

Chapter 26
p. 475 D
p. 479 B
p. 485 A

Chapter 27
p. 500 C
p. 503 A
p. 506 C

Chapter 28
p. 516 D
p. 522 C
p. 527 A

Chapter 29
p. 533 C
p. 537 C
p. 539 D

Chapter 30
p. 557 B
p. 564 D
p. 569 D
p. 579 C

Chapter 31
p. 587 B
p. 593 A
p. 598 A, B, D

Chapter 32
p. 608 A, E
p. 616 A
p. 619 D

Chapter 33
p. 634 D
p. 645 C

Chapter 34
p. 663 C
p. 668 A, D
p. 669 C
p. 673 D

Chapter 35
p. 683 B, C, E
p. 686 D
p. 687 B
p. 697 B

Chapter 36
p. 709 A
p. 717 C
p. 722 B
p. 733 D
p. 735 A

Chapter 37
p. 746 C
p. 749 B
p. 753 D

Chapter 38
p. 761 B, D, F
p. 768 79
p. 778 C

Chapter 39
p. 792 B
p. 795 C

Chapter 40
p. 801 D
p. 806 A
p. 809 B
p. 814 C
p. 826 B

Chapter 41
p. 839 B
p. 848 A

Chapter 42
p. 857 C
p. 862 A, B, D
p. 876 C
p. 879 D

Chapter 43
p. 891 D
p. 897 A

Chapter 44
p. 916 A, C, D
p. 928 C

Chapter 45
p. 933 A, B, E
p. 938 B, A, D, C
p. 942 D
p. 953 D
p. 961 C

Chapter 46
p. 971 C

Chapter 47
p. 985 D
p. 989 C
p. 989 A
p. 994 C

Chapter 48
p. 1002 D
p. 1008 A
p. 1009 A

Chapter 49
p. 1023 B, E
p. 1027 D

Chapter 50
p. 1034 B
p. 1039 C

Chapter 51
p. 1061 A, C, D
p. 1066 A
p. 1073 C
p. 1075 A, B, E

Chapter 52
p. 1091 C
p. 1093 A, D, E

Chapter 53
p. 1102 A
p. 1105 C
p. 1107 A, E, F

Chapter 54
p. 1114 A
p. 1118 A, B, C, E

Chapter 55
p. 1132 C, B, A, D
p. 1134 A, C, E
p. 1141 D

Chapter 56
p. 1148 A
p. 1155 B, C, D
p. 1163 C

Chapter 57
p. 1172 C
p. 1176 A
p. 1179 D
p. 1188 C

Chapter 58
p. 1196 A, D, E
p. 1200 D
p. 1203 A

Chapter 59
p. 1218 B
p. 1220 C
p. 1226 C, E
p. 1230 A, C, D, E

Chapter 60
p. 1236 45.9
p. 1241 C, D, E, F

Chapter 61
p. 1259 D
p. 1264 C

Chapter 62
p. 1268 C
p. 1273 B
p. 1280 A

Chapter 63
p. 1288 A, D, E, F, G
p. 1291 C
p. 1298 D

Chapter 64
p. 1302 D
p. 1306 C
p. 1317 A
p. 1328 B

Chapter 65
p. 1354 B
p. 1359 D
p. 1363 C

Chapter 66
p. 1372 D
p. 1383 C
p. 1388 C
p. 1389 A

Chapter 67
p. 1397 B
p. 1399 A
p. 1406 C

Chapter 68
p. 1416 A
p. 1418 C
p. 1423 B

Chapter 69
p. 1456 B
p. 1459 A

Chapter 70
p. 1467 D
p. 1474 C

Chapter 71
p. 1485 C, D, E
p. 1490 B

Chapter 72
p. 1506 725
p. 1507 B
p. 1514 D
p. 1516 B

Chapter 73
p. 1525 C
p. 1528 C, D, E

Chapter 74
p. 1536 C
p. 1545 B

ILLUSTRATION CREDITS

Chapter 1

1-1, From Potter, P., Perry, A., Stocker, P., & Hall, A. (2011). *Basic nursing* (7th ed.). St. Louis: Mosby; **1-2,** from Sorrentino, S. (2011). *Mosby's textbook for long-term care nursing assistants* (6th ed.). St. Louis: Mosby.

Chapter 2

2-3, From the Aging Clinical Research Center (ACRC), a joint project of Stanford University and the VA Palo Alto Health Care System, Palo Alto, CA, funded by the National Institute of Aging and the Department of Veterans Affairs.

Chapter 3

3-1, Modified from Pasero, C., & McCaffery, M. (2011). *Pain assessment and pharmacologic management.* St. Louis: Mosby; **3-2,** from Melzack, R. (1975). The McGill Pain Questionnaire: Major properties and scoring methods. *Pain, 1,* 272-281; **3-3,** Copyright 1983 Wong-Baker FACES Foundation.

Chapter 4

4-2, Modified from Nussbaum, R., McInnes, R., & Willard, H. (2007). *Thompson & Thompson: Genetics in medicine* (7th ed.). Philadelphia: Saunders; **4-5,** modified from Jorde, L., Carey, J., Bamshad, M., & White, R. (2000). *Medical genetics* (2nd ed.). St. Louis: Mosby; **4-8,** modified from Jorde, L., Carey, J., & Bamshad, M. (2010). *Medical genetics* (4th ed.). St. Louis: Mosby.

Chapter 5

5-1, © 2010. Rona F. Levin & Jeffrey M. Keefer; **5-2,** © 2010. R.E. Burke & R.F. Levin; **5-3,** © 2007. Visiting Nurse Service of New York and Rona F. Levin.

Chapter 6

6-1, From Scott, K., Webb, M., & Sorrentino, S. (2011). *Long-term caring* (2nd ed.). Sydney: Mosby Australia; **6-5,** from Potter, P., Perry, A., Stockert, P., & Hall, A. (2013). *Fundamentals of nursing* (8th ed.). St. Louis: Mosby.

Chapter 7

7-1, © 2005. National Hospice and Palliative Care Organization, 2007 Revised. All rights reserved. Reproduction and distribution by an organization or organized group without the written permission of the National Hospice and Palliative Care Organization is expressly forbidden. Visit caringinfo.org for more information.

Chapter 9

9-1, From Auerbach, P. S. (2012). *Wilderness medicine* (6th ed.). Philadelphia: Mosby; courtesy Michael Cardwell & Carl Barden Venom Laboratory; **9-2,** from Auerbach, P. S. (2012). *Wilderness medicine* (6th ed.). Philadelphia: Mosby; courtesy Sherman Minton, MD; **9-3,** from Auerbach, P. S. (2012). *Wilderness medicine* (6th ed.). Philadelphia: Mosby; courtesy Michael Cardwell & Jude McNally; **9-4,** from Auerbach, P. S. (2012). *Wilderness medicine* (6th ed.). Philadelphia: Mosby; courtesy Indiana University Medical Center; **9-5,** from Auerbach, P. S. (2012). *Wilderness medicine* (6th ed.). Philadelphia: Mosby; courtesy Paul S. Auerbach, MD; **9-6,** from Auerbach, P. S. (2012). *Wilderness medicine* (6th ed.) Philadelphia: Mosby; **9-7,** from Auerbach, P. S. (2008). *Wilderness medicine* (5th ed.). Philadelphia: Mosby; courtesy Cameron Bangs, MD.

Chapter 10

10-2, Courtesy Meg Blair, PhD, RN; **10-3,** courtesy Jeanne McConnell, MSN, RN.

Chapter 11

11-2, 11-7, 11-9, ©1992 by M. Linda Workman. All rights reserved.

Chapter 12

12-3, 12-12, ©1992 by M. Linda Workman. All rights reserved.

Chapter 13

13-1, From Perry, A., Potter, P., & Ostendorf, W. (2014). *Clinical nursing skills & techniques* (8th ed.). St. Louis: Mosby; **13-2, 13-16,** courtesy and © Becton, Dickinson and Company; **13-3,** courtesy AccuVein, LLC; **13-7,** courtesy Edwards Lifesciences, Irvine, CA; **13-11,** courtesy NowMedical, Chadds Ford, PA; **13-12,** from Lilley, L., Collins, S., & Snyder, J. (2014). *Pharmacology and the nursing process* (7th ed.). St. Louis: Mosby; **13-14,** courtesy Kimberly-Clark Corporation; **13-15,** courtesy Venetec International, San Diego, CA; **13-17,** courtesy I.V. House, Hazelwood, MO; **13-18,** from Lopez, J. H., & Reyes-Ortiz, A. (2010). Subcutaneous hydration by hypodermoclysis. *Reviews in Clinical Gerontology, 20,* 105-113.

Chapter 14

14-1, From World Health Organization: Surgical safety checklist, ed 1. Available at www.who.int/patientsafety/safesurgery/en/. © World Health Organization, 2009. **14-2,** courtesy Christiana Care Health Services, Newark, DE; **14-4,** from Perry, A. G., & Potter, P. A. (2010). *Clinical nursing skills and techniques* (7th ed.). St. Louis: Mosby; **14-5,** from Angelo, R., Ryu, R., & Esch, J. (2010). *AANA advanced arthroscopy: the shoulder.* Philadelphia: Saunders.

Chapter 15

15-1, Courtesy Christiana Care Health Services, Newark, DE; **15-3, A,** from Patell, A., Whang, P., & Vaccaro, A. (2008). Overview of computer-assisted image-guided surgery of the spine. *Seminars in Spine Surgery, 20*(3), 186-194; **15-3, B,** from Miller, R., & Pardo, M. (2011). *Basics of anesthesia* (6th ed.). Philadelphia: Saunders; **15-5,** redrawn with permission by Intuitive Surgical, Inc., 2007.

Chapter 16

16-1, Courtesy Forrest General Hospital, Hattiesburg, MS; **16-2, 16-4,** from Harkreader, H., Hogan, M. A., & Thobaben, M. (2007). *Fundamentals of nursing: Caring and clinical judgment* (3rd ed.). Philadelphia: Saunders; **16-3, A,** from Sirois, M. (2011). *Principles and practice of veterinary technology* (3rd ed.). St. Louis: Mosby; **16-3, B,** courtesy 2014 C. R. Bard, Inc. Covington, GA. Used with permission; **16-3 C, D,** courtesy C.R. Bard, Inc., Covington, GA.

Chapter 17

17-3, Modified from Goldman, L., & Schafer, A. (Eds.). (2012). *Goldman's Cecil medicine* (24th ed.). Philadelphia: Saunders.

Chapter 18

18-2, From Sainani, G. S. (2010). *Manual of clinical and practical medicine.* New Delhi: Elsevier India; **18-3, A,** from Jebson, L.R., & Coons, D.D. (1998). Total hip arthroplasty. *Surgical Technologist, 30*(10), 12-21; **B,** from Mercier, L.R. (2000). *Practical orthopaedics* (5th ed.). St. Louis: Mosby; **18-6,** from Damjanov, I. (2006). *Pathophysiology for the health professions* (3rd ed.). Philadelphia: Saunders; **18-9,** from Goldman L., & Ausiello, D. (2007). *Cecil medicine* (23rd ed.). Philadelphia: Saunders; **18-10,** from Currie, G., & Douglas, G. (2011). *Flesh and bones of medicine.* Edinburgh: Mosby Ltd.

Chapter 19

19-1, From Kumar, V., Abbas, A., & Fausto, N. (2010). *Robbins & Cotran pathologic basis of disease* (8th ed.). Philadelphia: Saunders; **19-3,** from McCance, K.L., & Huether, S.E. (2002). *Pathophysiology: The biologic basis for disease in adults and children* (4th ed.). St. Louis: Mosby; **19-4A,** adapted from New York State Department of Health AIDS Institute. Clinical Guidelines Development Program. (2013). Recommendations for non-occupational post-exposure prophylaxis for HIV infection. New York: Author. www.hivguidelines.org.; **19-4B,** adapted from New York State Department of Health AIDS Institute. Clinical Guidelines Development Program. (2012). Recommendations for occupational post-exposure prophylaxis for HIV infection. New York: Author. www.hivguidelines.org.; **19-5,** from Marks, J., & Miller, J. (2006). *Lookingbill & Marks' principles of dermatology* (4th ed.). Philadelphia: Saunders; **19-6,** from Leonard, P. C. (2012). *Building a medical vocabulary* (8th ed.). St. Louis: Saunders.

Chapter 20

20-2, Courtesy Dey, Napa, CA; **20-3,** from Auerbach, P. (2008). *Wilderness medicine* (5th ed.). Philadelphia: Mosby; courtesy Sheryl Olson.

Chapter 22

22-2, From Weinzweig, J., & Weinzweig, N. (2005). *The mutilated hand,* St. Louis: Mosby; **22-3,** from Workman, M.L., & LaCharity, L. (2011). *Understanding pharmacology: Essentials for medication safety.* St. Louis: Saunders; **22-4,** from Kee, J., Hayes, E., & McCuistion, L. (2012). *Pharmacology: A nursing process approach,* St. Louis: Saunders; **22-6,** from Forbes, C.D., & Jackson, W.F. (2003). *Colour atlas and text of clinical medicine* (3rd ed.). London: Mosby.

Chapter 23

23-1, A, From deWit, S.C. (2014). *Fundamental concepts and skills for nursing* (4th ed.). Philadelphia: Saunders; **B,** from Currance, P. (2006). *Medical response to weapons of mass destruction.* Philadelphia: Mosby/JEMS.

Chapter 24

24-10, Modified from Marks, J., & Miller, J. (2013). *Lookingbill and Marks' principles of dermatology* (5th ed.). Philadelphia: Saunders.

Chapter 25

25-3, Modified from Swaim, S.F. (1980). *Surgery of traumatized skin.* Philadelphia: Saunders; **25-5,** from Barbara Braden & Nancy Bergstrom. © 1988. Reprinted with permission; **25-6,** illustrations from the National Pressure Ulcer Advisory Panel and European Pressure Ulcer Advisory Panel. (2009). *Pressure ulcer prevention and treatment: Clinical practice guideline.* Washington, DC: NPUAP. Used with permission; **25-9,** from The Centers for Disease Control and Prevention, Atlanta, GA (www.bt.cdc.gov/agent/anthrax/anthrax-images/); **25-15,** courtesy Stevens Johnson Syndrome Foundation, Littleton, CO.

Chapter 26

26-15, from Herndon, D. N. (2012). *Total burn care* (4th ed.). Philadelphia: Saunders.

Chapter 27

27-12, From Young, A.P., & Proctor, D. (2008). *Kinn's the medical assistant: An applied learning approach* (10th ed.). St. Louis: Saunders; **27-13,** from Harkreader, H., Hogan, M.A., & Thobaben, M. (2007). *Fundamentals of nursing: Caring and clinical judgment* (3rd ed.). Philadelphia: Saunders.

Chapter 28

28-3, 28-9, 28-10, From Perry, A. G., Potter, P. A., & Ostendorf, W. R. (2014). *Clinical nursing skills and techniques* (8th ed.). St. Louis: Mosby; **28-11,** courtesy Chad Therapeutics, Chatsworth, CA; **28-13,** courtesy Mallinckrodt, Inc., Shiley Tracheostomy Products, St. Louis, MO; **28-14,** courtesy J.T. Posey Company, Arcadia, CA; **28-15,** courtesy Dale Medical Products, Inc., Plainville, MA.

Chapter 29

29-1, From Tardy, M.E. (1997). *Rhinoplasty: The art and science.* Philadelphia: Saunders. Used with permission; **29-2, A,** courtesy Invotec International, Jacksonville, FL.

Chapter 30

30-3, From Jarvis, C. (2012). *Physical examination and health assessment* (6th ed.). Philadelphia: Saunders; **30-4,** from Aehlert, B. (2011). *Paramedic practice today: Above and beyond.* St. Louis: Mosby; **30-9,** modified from Gift, A. (1989). A dyspnea assessment guide. *Critical Care Nurse, 9*(8), 79. Used with permission; **30-10,** from Swartz, M.H. (2009). *Textbook of physical diagnosis: History and examination* (6th ed.). Philadelphia: Saunders; **30-11,** courtesy Axcan Pharma, Mont-Saint-Hilaire, Quebec, Canada; **30-12,** modified © 2015 Hill-Rom Services, Inc. Reprinted With Permission—All Rights Reserved; **30-16,** courtesy Atrium Medical Corporation, Hudson, NH.

Chapter 31

31-1, Courtesy Covidien, AG, Switzerland; **31-2,** illustration from Workman, M.L., & LaCharity, L. (2011). *Understanding pharmacology.* St. Louis: Saunders; photo from Kumar, V., Abbas, A., Fausto, N., & Aster, J. (2009). *Robbins and Cotran pathologic basis for disease* (8th ed.). Philadelphia: Saunders; **31-3,** from Zitelli, B.J., McIntire, S. C., & Nowalk, A. J. (2012). *Zitelli and Davis' atlas of pediatric physical diagnosis* (6th ed.). Philadelphia: Saunders; courtesy Kenneth Schuitt, MD.

Chapter 32

32-2, A, courtesy Sims Porter, Inc.; **32-3,** © Dräger Medical AG & Co. KG, Lübeck, Germany. All rights reserved. No portion hereof may be reproduced, saved or stored in a data processing system, electronically or mechanically copied or otherwise recorded by any other means without express prior written permission; **32-4,** from McCance, K.L. Huether S.E., Brashers, V.L., & Rote, N.S. (2010). *Pathophysiology: The biologic basis for disease in adults and children* (6th ed.). St. Louis: Mosby.

Chapter 33

33-5, From Sahrmann, S. (2011). *Movement system impairment syndromes of the extremities, cervical and thoracic spines.* St. Louis: Mosby; **33-9,** From Baker, T., Nikolic, G., & O'Connor, S. (2008). *Practical cardiology,* ed 2, Sydney: Churchill Livingstone Australia.

Chapter 34

34-10, Reproduced with permission of Medtronic, Inc., Minneapolis, MN; **34-15,** courtesy Philips Medical Systems, Andover, MA.

Chapter 35

35-1, From McCance, K.L., & Huether, S.E. (2002). *Pathophysiology: The biologic basis for disease in adults and children* (4th ed.). St. Louis: Mosby; **35-2,** courtesy Abiomed, Inc., Danvers, MA; **35-4, A, B,** courtesy Medtronic, Inc., Minneapolis, MN; **C** courtesy Baxter Healthcare Corporation, Edwards CVS Division, Santa Ana, CA.

Chapter 36

36-4, From Brooks, M., & Jenkins, M.P. (2008). Acute and chronic ischaemia of the limb. *Surgery 26*(1), 17-20; **36-8,** from Forbes, C.D., & Jackson, W.F. (2003). *Colour atlas and text of clinical medicine* (3rd ed.). London: Mosby.

Chapter 38

38-1, From Huether S.E., McCance, K.L., Brashers, V.L., & Rote, N.S. (2012). *Understanding pathophysiology* (5th ed.). St. Louis: Mosby.

Chapter 40

40-3, From Feldman, M., Friedman, L., & Brandt, L. (2010). *Sleisenger and Fordtran's gastrointestinal and liver disease* (9th ed.). Philadelphia: Saunders; **40-4,** from Leonard, P.C. (2012). *Building a medical vocabulary: With Spanish translations* (8th ed.). St. Louis: Saunders; **40-7,** from deWit, S.C., & O'Neill, P. (2014). *Fundamental concepts and skills for nursing* (4th ed.). St. Louis: Saunders.

Chapter 41

41-3, Modified from Thibodeau, G.A., & Patton, K.T. (2007). *Anatomy and physiology* (6th ed.). St. Louis: Mosby.

Chapter 42

42-1, From Salvo, S.G. (2014). *Mosby's pathology for massage therapists* (3rd ed.). St. Louis: Mosby; **42-2, A,** from Mini-Mental State Examination © 1975, 1998, 2001 by MiniMental, LLC. All rights reserved. Published 2001 by Psychological Assessment Resources, Inc. May not be reproduced in whole or in part in any form or by any means without written permission of Psychological Assessment Resources, Inc., 16204 N. Florida Ave., Lutz, FL 33549; (800) 331-8378, www4.parinc.com/. **B,** from Seidel, H.M., Ball, J.W., Dains, J.E., Benedict, G.W. (2003). *Mosby's guide to physical examination* (5th ed.). St. Louis: Mosby.

Chapter 43

43-1, From Patton, K.T., & Thibodeau, G.A. (2014). *The human body in health & disease* (6th ed.). St. Louis: Mosby; **43-5,** from Harkreader, H. (2007). *Fundamentals of nursing: Caring and clinical judgment* (3rd ed.). Philadelphia: Saunders.

Chapter 45

45-3, From Seidel, H.M., Ball, J.W., Dains, J.E., Flynn, J.A., Solomon, B.S., & Stewart, R.W. (2011). *Mosby's guide to physical examination* (7th ed.). St. Louis: Mosby; **B,** modified from Stein, H.A., Slatt, B.J., & Stein, R.M. (1994). *The ophthalmic assistant* (6th ed.). St. Louis: Mosby. **45-10,** from Flint, P.W., Haughey, B.H., Lund, V.J., Niparko, J.K., Richardson, M.A.,

Robbins, K.T., et al. (2010). *Cummings otolaryngology: Head & neck surgery* (5th ed.). Philadelphia: Mosby; courtesy Elekta, Inc.

Chapter 46

46-11, Courtesy Medtronic Ophthalmics, Minneapolis, MN.

Chapter 47

47-5, from Patton, K.T., & Thibodeau, G.A. (2010). *Anatomy and physiology* (7th ed.). St. Louis: Mosby; **47-8,** from Workman, M.L., LaCharity, L., & Kruchko, S.C. (2011). *Understanding pharmacology.* St. Louis: Saunders.

Chapter 50

50-3, From Johal, S., Sawalha, S., & Pasapula, C. (2010). Post-traumatic acute hallux valgus: A case report. *The Foot, 29*(2), 87-89; **50-4,** from Hochberg, M., Silman, A., Smolen, J., Weinblatt, M., & Weisman, M. (2011). *Rheumatology* (5th ed). Philadelphia: Mosby.

Chapter 51

51-3, 51-5, 51-10, Courtesy Smith & Nephew, Inc., Orthopaedics Divisions, Memphis, TN; **51-4,** from Perry, A.G., Potter, P.A., & Elkin, M.K. (2012). *Nursing interventions & clinical skills* (5th ed.). St. Louis: Mosby; **51-6,** from McCance, K.L., Huether, S.E., Brashers, V.L., & Rote, N.S. (2010). *Pathophysiology: The biologic basis for disease in adults and children* (6th ed.). St. Louis: Mosby; **51-8,** from Douglas, G., Robertson, C., & Nicol, F. (2011). *Macleod exploración clínica* (12th ed.). Barcelona: Elsevier; **51-14,** courtesy Zimmer, Inc., Warsaw, IN; **51-15,** from Darby, M., & Walsh, M. (2010). *Dental hygiene: theory and practice* (3rd ed.). St. Louis: Saunders.

Chapter 53

53-1, From Friedman-Kien, A.E., & Cockerell, C.J. (1996). *Color atlas of AIDS* (2nd ed.). Philadelphia: Saunders.

Chapter 56

56-6, From Evans, S. (2009). *Surgical pitfalls.* Philadelphia: Saunders.

Chapter 57

57-3, B, From Perry, A.G., & Potter, P.A. (2006). *Clinical nursing skills & techniques* (6th ed.). St. Louis: Mosby; courtesy ConvaTec, Princeton, NJ; **57-5,** courtesy ConvaTec, a Bristol-Myers Squibb Company, Princeton, NJ.

Chapter 58

58-1, From Leonard, P. (2011). *Quick & easy medical terminology* (6th ed.). St. Louis: Saunders; **58-2,** from Talley, N., & O'Connor, S. (2010). *Clinical examination: a systematic guide to physical diagnosis* (6th ed.). Sydney: Churchill Livingstone Australia.

Chapter 60

60-1, From U.S. Department of Agriculture, 2011, www.ChooseMyPlate.gov; **60-2,** ® Société des Produits Nestlé S.A., Vevey, Switzerland, Trademark Owners; **60-3, A,** from Lilley, L., Rainforth Collins, S., Harrington, S., & Snyder, J. (2011). *Pharmacology and the nursing process* (6th ed.). St. Louis: Mosby; **B,** from Harkreader, H. (2007). *Fundamentals of nursing* (3rd ed.). St. Louis: Saunders; courtesy C.R. Bard, Inc., Billerica, MA; **C,** from Harkreader, H. (2007). *Fundamentals of nursing* (3rd ed.). St. Louis: Saunders; courtesy Ballard Medical Products, Draper, UT.

Chapter 61

61-4, From Guyton, A., & Hall, J. (2006). *Textbook of medical physiology* (11th ed.). Philadelphia: Saunders.

Chapter 62

62-1, Courtesy of the Group for Research in Pathology Educations (GRIPE), Oklahoma City, OK; **62-2,** from Wilson J.D., Foster, D., Kronenberg, H., & Larsen, P.R. (1998). *Williams textbook of endocrinology* (9th ed.). Philadelphia: Saunders; courtesy Dr. H. Patrick Higgins; **62-3,** from Wenig B.M., Heffess, C.S., & Adair, C.F. (1997). *Atlas of endocrine pathology.* Philadelphia: Saunders.

Chapter 64

64-4, Courtesy Medtronic Diabetes, Northridge, CA; **64-5,** courtesy Becton, Dickinson and Company, Franklin Lakes, NJ; **64-6,** from Frykberg, R.G., Zgonis, T., Armstrong, D.G., Driver, V.R., Giurini, J.M., Kravitz, S.R., et al. (2006). Diabetic foot disorders: A clinical practice guideline—2006 revision. *The Journal of Foot and Ankle Surgery, 45*(5), S1-S66.

Chapter 65

65-3, From Patton, K.T., & Thibodeau, G.A. (2014). *The human body in health & disease* (6th ed.). St. Louis: Mosby; **65-8,** modified from Patton, K.T., & Thibodeau, G.A. (2013). *Anatomy & physiology* (8th ed.). St. Louis: Mosby; **65-10,** Courtesy Verathon Corporation, Bothell, WA.

Chapter 66

66-1, A, Courtesy ConvaTec, A Bristol-Meyers Squibb Company, a Division of E.R. Squibb & Sons, Inc., Princeton, NJ; **66-2,** from Pollack, H.M. (2000). *Clinical urography* (2nd ed.). Philadelphia: Saunders; **66-3,** modified from Singal, R.K., & Denstedt, J.D. (1997). Contemporary management of ureteral stones. *The Urologic Clinics of North America, 24*(1), 59-70.

Chapter 67

67-2, From Kumar, V., Abbas, A., Fausto, N., & Aster, J. (2010). *Robbins and Cotran pathologic basis of disease* (8th ed.). Philadelphia: Saunders.

Chapter 68

68-1, Courtesy Kendall Company, Bothell, WA; **68-3, 68-4,** from Feehally, J., Floege, J., & Johnson, R. (2007). *Comprehensive clinical nephrology* (3rd ed.). Philadelphia: Mosby; **68-5,** courtesy Gambro Lundia AB, Lund, Sweden; **68-8, A,** from Geary, D.F., & Schaefer, F. (2008). *Comprehensive pediatric nephrology.* Philadelphia: Mosby; **68-12,** courtesy Baxter International, Inc., Deerfield, IL.

Chapter 70

70-1, From Swartz, M.H. (2009). *Textbook of physical diagnosis: History and examination* (6th ed.). Philadelphia: Saunders; **70-2,** from Mansel, R., & Bundred, N. (1995). *Color atlas of breast disease.* St. Louis: Mosby; **70-3,** from Gallager, H.S., Leis, H.P. Jr., Snyderman, R.K., & Urban, J.A. (1978). *The breast.* St. Louis: Mosby; **70-4, 70-5,** © 2010 Terese Winslow. U.S. Govt. has certain rights.

Chapter 72

72-2, Adapted from the American Urological Association Practice Guidelines Committee. (2003). Guideline on the management of benign prostatic hyperplasia (BPH). *Journal of Urology, 170*(2 Pt 1), 530-547.

Chapter 74

74-1, 74-2, From Morse, S., Ballard, R., Holmes, K., & Moreland, A. (2003). *Atlas of sexually transmitted diseases and AIDS* (3rd ed.). Edinburgh: Mosby.

INDEX

Page numbers followed by "f" indicate figures, "t" indicate tables, and "b" indicate boxes.

B

D

H